Drug Information Handbook

For Perioperative Nursing

Including

Drug and Herbal Interaction References, Geriatric and Pediatric Dosing, and Abbreviations and Measurements

Adapted from Lexi-Comp's
Anesthesiology & Critical Care Drug Handbook, 6th Edition
and the
Drug Information Handbook for the Advance Practice Nursing, 6th Edition

Developed in collaboration with AORN

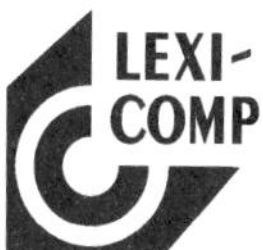

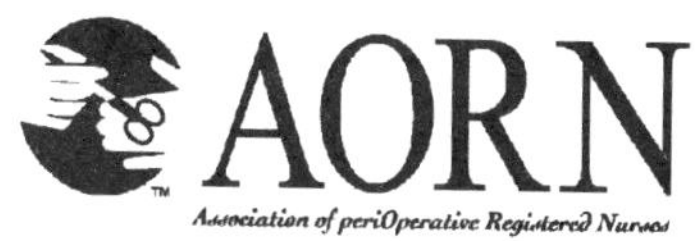

LEXI-COMP'S

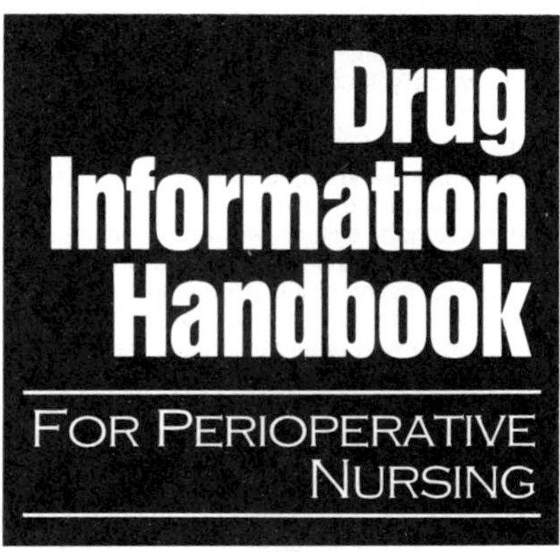

Including

Drug and Herbal Interaction References, Geriatric and Pediatric Dosing, and Abbreviations and Measurements

Adapted from

Anesthesiology and Critical Care Drug Handbook, 6th Edition

Andrew J. Donnelly, PharmD, MBA; Verna L. Baughman, MD;
Jeffrey P. Gonzales, PharmD, BCPS; Elizabeth A. Tomsik, PharmD, BCPS

Drug Information Handbook for Advanced Practice Nursing, 6th Edition

Beatrice B. Turkoski, RN, PhD; Brenda R. Lance, RN, MSN;
Mark F. Bonfiglio BS, PharmD, RPh

AORN Advisory Panel

Rodney Hicks, MSN, MPA
Linda J. Wanzer, MSN
Cheryl A. Reilly, MSN
Stella Harrington, BSN
Sharon Giarrizzo-Wilson, RN, BSN/MS

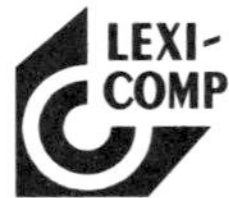

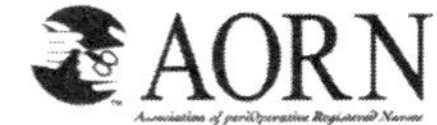

This data is intended to serve the user as a handy reference and not as a complete drug information resource. It does not include information on every therapeutic agent available. The publication covers 677 commonly used drugs and is specifically designed to present important aspects of drug data in a more concise format than is typically found in medical literature or product material supplied by manufacturers.

The nature of drug information is that it is constantly evolving because of ongoing research and clinical experience and is often subject to interpretation. While great care has been taken to ensure the accuracy of the information presented, the reader is advised that the authors, editors, reviewers, contributors, and publishers cannot be responsible for the continued currency of the information or for any errors, omissions, or the application of this information, or for any consequences arising therefrom. Therefore, the author(s) and/or the publisher shall have no liability to any person or entity with regard to claims, loss, or damage caused, or alleged to be caused, directly or indirectly, by the use of information contained herein. Because of the dynamic nature of drug information, readers are advised that decisions regarding drug therapy must be based on the independent judgment of the clinician, changing information about a drug (eg, as reflected in the literature and manufacturer's most current product information), and changing medical practices. Therefore, this data is designed to be used in conjunction with other necessary information and is not designed to be solely relied upon by any user. The user of this data hereby and forever releases the authors of this data for any and all liability of any kind that might arise out of the use of this data. The editors are not responsible for any inaccuracy of quotation or for any false or misleading implication that may arise due to the text or formulas as used or due to the quotation of revisions no longer official.

The authors, editors, and contributors have written this book in their private capacities. No official support or endorsement by any federal or state agency or pharmaceutical company is intended or inferred.

The publishers have made every effort to trace the copyright holders for borrowed material. If they have inadvertently overlooked any, they will be pleased to make the necessary arrangements at the first opportunity.

If you have any suggestions or questions regarding any information presented in this data, please contact our drug information pharmacists at (330) 650-6506.

This manual was produced using the FormuLex™ Program — a complete publishing service of Lexi-Comp Inc.

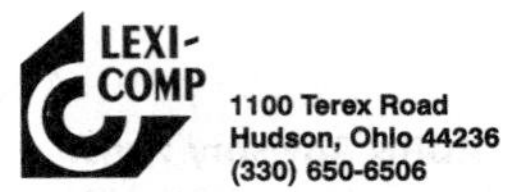

ISBN 1-59195-139-9

TABLE OF CONTENTS

TABLE OF CONTENTS *(Continued)*

ABOUT THE AORN ADVISORY PANEL

Rodney (Rod) Hicks, MSN, MPA

Mr Hicks is a nurse researcher and educator. He teaches pharmacology to advanced practice students at the Uniformed Services University of the Health Sciences in Bethesda, Maryland. Currently, he is a nurse researcher, focusing on safe medication use and he has published over 30 articles discussing medication errors. Mr Hicks's most recent work concentrated on medication errors across the perioperative environment. Findings of his work have been presented at several AORN and ASPAN conferences over the past few years.

Mr Hicks has a Master's of Science in Nursing in nursing administration and a Master's in Public Administration (MPA) from the University of Texas at Arlington. Currently, he is completing his PhD in Human Services with a concentration in Healthcare Administration from Capella University. He is nationally certified as a Family Nurse Practitioner.

Linda J. Wanzer, MSN

Ms Wanzer holds the academic rank of Assistant Professor at the Uniformed Services University of the Health Sciences in Bethesda, Maryland. As the Program Director for Perioperative Clinical Nurse Specialist Master's program, she is responsible for the development, implementation, and instruction of this national stand-alone Perioperative Clinical Nurse Specialist masters program. Ms Wanzer is a course coordinator for the Uniformed Services University's Applied Pharmacology for Advanced Nursing Practice and has facilitated student research in medication errors across the perioperative continuum.

Ms Wanzer has a Master's of Science in Nursing with a major in nursing administration and a minor in education from the Medical College of Georgia in Augusta. She is a Colonel in the United States Army and at Uniformed Services University of the Health Sciences and is nationally certified in Perioperative Nursing.

Cheryl A. Reilly, MSN

Ms Reilly has been practicing perioperative nursing for 26 years and has a diverse background in surgical patient care. For the past three years, she has been on faculty at the Uniformed Services University of the Health Sciences and has assisted with the development of and instruction for the Perioperative Clinical Nurse Specialist Master's Program. During this time, Ms Reilly has worked closely with students investigating and analyzing perioperative medication errors using US Pharmacopeia MedMARx data.

Ms Reilly obtained her Master's of Science in Nursing from the University of Texas Health Science Center in San Antonio as an Acute Care Clinical Nurse Specialist. She holds national certification in Perioperative Nursing and Nursing Administration. Ms Reilly is a Lieutenant Colonel in the United States Air Force and currently is the Operating Room Services Element Chief at Mike O'Callaghan Federal Hospital, Nellis AFB, Nevada.

Stella Harrington, BSN

Ms Harrington received her Bachelor of Science in Nursing, magna cum laude, from Northeastern University in Boston, Massachusetts. She currently practices as a perioperative nurse at Children's Hospital in Boston, MA and is nationally certified in Perioperative Nursing. She has been an active member of AORN at the local and national level. Ms Harrington has been a member of the Pediatric Specialty Assembly since its inception, serving as Chair and as a member of the governing council. She has recurring appointments to AORN's Presidential Commission on Patient Safety and received AORN's award for "Outstanding Achievement in Perioperative Clinical Practice" in 2005.

As a long-standing commitment, Ms Harrington has been involved with coordinating and participating as a volunteer on many medical/surgical missions throughout the world with various humanitarian organizations.

ABOUT THE AORN ADVISORY PANEL *(Continued)*

Sharon Giarrizzo-Wilson, RN, BSN/MS, AORN Content Advisory Editor

Ms Giarrizzo-Wilson has 22 years of perioperative nursing practice and has been involved with organization-wide strategic development for patient safety initiatives throughout her professional career. Ms Giarrizzo-Wilson has extensive experience in perioperative organizational design and management, staff development and education, quality and process improvement, infection control, clinical and professional consultation for perioperative nurses, ancillary hospital departments, and healthcare industry. Accomplishments include securing a federal sponsored grant for perioperative nurse training and publishing an article related to the process of training RN recruits for the O.R. She has completed multiple book reviews for the *AORN Journal* and the Nurse Review Board for the Nurses Book Society, is a frequent column contributor for the *AORN Journal*, and is highly sought out for interviews on perioperative patient care.

Ms Giarrizzo-Wilson received her BSN/MS degree in nursing administration and informatics from Northeastern University in Boston, Massachusetts and is nationally certified in Perioperative Nursing. She is currently employed at AORN as a Perioperative Nurse Consultant with designated responsibilities for patient safety, clinical consulting, and document and program development, including the AORN Safe Medication Administration Tool Kit.

ABOUT THE AUTHORS

Verna L. Baughman, MD

Dr Baughman is Professor of Anesthesiology and Neurosurgery at the University of Illinois at Chicago. She received her BA in 1968 from DePauw University, Greencastle, Indiana, with a major in both French and Biology. She then worked as a research editor/writer for the Encyclopaedia Britannica and as a hospital administrator. She attended Stritch School of Medicine at Loyola University, Chicago, receiving her medical degree in 1981. Following an internship and residency in Anesthesiology at Michael Reese Medical Center in Chicago, she spent a year as a Neuroanesthesia Research Fellow. Her interest in neuroanesthesia has dominated her laboratory research program, with a focus on stroke and the effects of various drug therapies in ameliorating neuronal damage from ischemia. She is also interested in the effects of estrogen and menopause in relation to cerebral ischemia.

Dr Baughman has to her credit over 100 publications including original research papers, textbook chapters, and editorials. She has been an active member of the editorial board for the Journal of Neurosurgical Anesthesia and Critical Care for sixteen years. She currently reviews papers for *Anesthesiology, Anesthesia & Analgesia, Journal of Clinical Anesthesia, Stroke* and *American Journal of Physiology.* She has been a visiting professor at many universities and a frequent lecturer at national meetings. Dr Baughman was cited in "Best Doctors in America" in 1995 and again in 1996.

Dr Baughman's interest in education is evidenced by consistently being voted by the resident staff as one of the best departmental teachers. She was selected to receive the 2001-2002 Excellence in Teaching Award, which recognizes quality teachers at the University of Illinois. In 2003 Dr. Baughman was honored as the first Distinguished Teacher of the Year by the Society of Neurosurgical Anesthesia and Critical Care. She is also a consultant to the pharmaceutical industry, evaluating new drugs and equipment. Dr Baughman is an active member of the American Society of Anesthesiologists, Society of Neurosurgical Anesthesia and Critical Care, International Anesthesia Research Society, and Stroke Council of the American Heart Association.

Mark F. Bonfiglio, BS, PharmD, RPh

Dr Bonfiglio received his bachelor's degrees and undergraduate training from the University of Toledo (BA in Biology/BS in Pharmacy) and his PharmD from the Ohio State University. He completed a residency in Critical Care Pharmacy at University Hospitals in Columbus, Ohio. On completion of his training, he worked for several years as a Clinical Specialist in Critical Care in the SUMMA Health System, followed by a position as Pharmacotherapy Specialist in Internal Medicine at Akron General Medical Center. In both of these positions he was concurrently employed by the College of Pharmacy at Ohio Northern University where he attained the rank of Associate Clinical Professor. In addition to his current responsibilities at Lexi-Comp, he has continued to remain active in science and healthcare education. He currently coordinates the Advanced Pharmacology course for the College of Nursing at Malone College, and serves as a Part-Time Faculty in the Department of Biological Sciences at Kent State University, serving as the primary lecturer for the Department's course in Immunology.

Dr Bonfiglio is currently the Director of the Medical Science Division of Lexi-Comp, Inc. He coordinates the development and maintenance of the core pharmacology database and serves as an author for several printed titles, including the *Drug Information Handbook for Advanced Practice Nursing* and *Drug Interactions Handbook.* He is also a contributing author to the *Pharmacogenomics Handbook.* Dr Bonfiglio maintains memberships in the Society for Critical Care Medicine (SCCM), the American Pharmacists Association (APhA), the American Society of Health-System Pharmacists (ASHP), the Ohio College of Clinical Pharmacy (OCCP), the American Society for Automation in Pharmacy (ASAP), and the American Association for the Advancement of Science (AAAS).

Andrew J. Donnelly, PharmD, MBA

Dr Donnelly received his Doctor of Pharmacy and Masters of Business Administration degrees from the University of Illinois. He has over 20 years of active pharmacy experience, with the majority concentrated in the areas of operating room pharmacy and anesthesiology. Dr. Donnelly is currently Director of Pharmacy at the University of Illinois Hospital at Chicago. In addition, he holds the appointment of Clinical Professor in the Department of Pharmacy Practice at the University of Illinois at Chicago College of Pharmacy.

Throughout his years of operating room/anesthesiology pharmacy practice, Dr. Donnelly has strived to expand the pharmacist's role in ensuring optimal patient outcome by

ABOUT THE AUTHORS *(Continued)*

developing methods to improve drug selection and use in the operating room setting. In recognition of this work, he was named a Fellow of the American Society of Health-System Pharmacists (FASHP). Dr Donnelly has published extensively in the areas of anesthesiology and operating room pharmacy and is frequently invited to speak at professional meetings on topics related to these areas.

Dr Donnelly is Associate Editor-in-Chief of *Anesthesia Today* and he serves on the editorial board of the *OR Pharmacy Services Bulletin.* He is an active member of the American Society of Health-System Pharmacists (ASHP); American Pharmacists Association (APhA); Society of Critical Care Medicine (SCCM); Operating Room Pharmacy Services Association; as well as various state and local pharmacy organizations.

Jeffrey P. Gonzales, PharmD, BCPS

Dr Gonzales received his Doctor of Pharmacy degree at Idaho State University in Pocatello, Idaho. He completed a Pharmacy Practice Residency at the University of Nebraska Medical Center, then went on to specialize with a Critical Care Residency at Detroit Receiving Hospital-Detroit Medical Center. Following his residency training, Dr Gonzales completed a Postdoctoral Fellowship in Critical Care at The University of Michigan College of Pharmacy, where he was the recipient of the 1999 American College of Clinical Pharmacy-Bayer Critical Care Fellowship Award.

Currently, Dr Gonzales is the Critical Care Clinical Specialist at The Cleveland Clinic Foundation, primarily practicing in the Medical Intensive Care Unit. His areas of interests and research are sedation, vasopressors, sepsis, and alterations in absorption in the critically ill population. He is a member of the Pharmacology Curriculum Committee, Cleveland Clinic Lerner College of Medicine at Case Western Reserve University. Dr Gonzales is a Board-Certified Pharmacotherapy Specialist (BCPS).

Dr Gonzales is an active member of the Society of Critical Care Medicine (SCCM), the Ohio College of Clinical Pharmacy (OCCP), the American College of Clinical Pharmacy (ACCP), and the American Society of Health-Systems Pharmacists (ASHP).

Brenda R. Lance, RN, MSN

Ms Lance received a diploma in nursing from Methodist Hospital School of Nursing in Lubbock, Texas. She also has earned bachelor's and master's degrees in nursing from Kent State University, Kent, Ohio.

Ms Lance's nursing experiences and expertise are numerous and varied. Her nursing career spans over 30 years, having worked in intensive care, emergency room, ambulatory care clinics, home health, and home infusion. She is currently the Program Development Director for Northcoast HealthCare Management Company and Northcoast Infusion Therapies located in Oakwood Village, Ohio.

In addition to many years of direct patient care experience, she is also certified in risk management, has extensive experience in Joint Commission on Accreditation of Healthcare Organizations standards and Medicare regulations for home health, and has been a military nurse for the past 30 years. She retired with the rank of Captain (0-6) from the U.S. Naval Reserve Nurse Corps.

Ms Lance is a member of the Sigma Theta Tau (National Honor Society of Nursing) and National Home Infusion Association.

Elizabeth A. Tomsik, Pharm.D, BCPS

Dr Tomsik received her bachelor's degree in pharmacy from the Albany College of Pharmacy and her Doctor of Pharmacy degree from the University of Sciences in Philadelphia. She completed a one-year residency at Truman Medical Center in Kansas City and went on to work at Hahnemann University Hospital for 2 years in the field of nutrition. She continued her work at Louis Stokes Veterans Affairs Medical Center in Cleveland for 12 years. Her areas of practice included intensive care, coronary care, nutrition support, and anticoagulation. She was actively involved in residency training and was in charge of the pharmacy residency program for many years. She held faculty appointments from Case Western Reserve University, College of Medicine and The University of Toledo, College of Pharmacy. She has been a Board Certified Pharmacotherapy Specialist since 1999.

Dr Tomsik has been with Lexi-Comp, Inc since 1999. She is actively involved in developing and maintaining the patient education series (LEXI-PALS™ and PEDI-PALS™), enhancing the database with particular focus on the areas of critical care and coronary care, and working as an active participant in the Medical Science Division at Lexi-Comp, Inc.

Dr Tomsik is a member of the Ohio College of Clinical Pharmacy and the American College of Clinical Pharmacy. She recently completed the Multidisciplinary Critical Care Review Course sponsored by the Society of Critical Care Medicine.

Beatrice B. Turkoski, RN, PhD

Dr Turkoski received her BSN from Alverno College in Wisconsin, an MS in Community Health Nursing from the University of Wisconsin-Milwaukee School of Nursing, and a PhD from the University of Wisconsin. Her extensive professional nursing experience includes several years as a clinician in critical care in Wisconsin and Israel, Director of Nursing, clinician, and researcher in gerontology and chronic adult illness in Wisconsin and Ohio, and clinical nurse specialist in family/community practice in Israel.

In her graduate faculty role at Kent State University College of Nursing, Dr Turkoski developed and teaches the Advanced Pharmacology course for graduate students in the Nurse Practitioner and Clinical Nurse Specialist programs. Her expertise in this area is highly regarded by both students and faculty. She also conducts continuing education programs and workshops in pharmacology and nursing practice, both in person and on the internet.

Dr Turkoski is an active member and past officer in several national and international professional organizations. She has made presentations at scientific conferences in the United States, Europe, China, Korea, Canada, and Israel. Dr Turkoski is also a frequent contributor to professional journals.

EDITORIAL ADVISORY PANEL

EDITORIAL ADVISORY PANEL *(Continued)*

Harold L. Crossley, DDS, PhD
Associate Professor of Pharmacology
Baltimore College of Dental Surgery
Dental School
University of Maryland Baltimore
Baltimore, Maryland

Wayne R. DeMott, MD
Consultant in Pathology and Laboratory Medicine
Shawnee Mission, Kansas

Samir Desai, MD
Assistant Professor of Medicine
Department of Medicine
Baylor College of Medicine
Houston, Texas
Staff Physician
Veterans Affairs Medical Center
Houston, Texas

Andrew J. Donnelly, PharmD, MBA
Director of Pharmacy
and
Clinical Professor of Pharmacy Practice
University of Illinois Medical Center at Chicago
Chicago, Illinois

Thom C. Dumsha, DDS
Associate Professor and Chair
Dental School
University of Maryland Baltimore
Baltimore, Maryland

Michael S. Edwards, PharmD, MBA
Assistant Director, Weinberg Pharmacy
Johns Hopkins Hospital
Baltimore, Maryland

Vicki L. Ellingrod, PharmD, BCPP
Associate Professor
University of Iowa
Iowa City, Iowa

Kelley K. Engle, BSPharm
Pharmacotherapy Specialist
Lexi-Comp, Inc
Hudson, Ohio

Margaret A. Fitzgerald, MS, APRN, BC, NP-C, FAANP
President
Fitzgerald Health Education Associates, Inc.
North Andover, Massachusetts
Family Nurse Practitioner
Greater Lawrence Family Health Center
Lawrence, Massachusetts

Matthew A. Fuller, PharmD, BCPS, BCPP, FASHP
Clinical Pharmacy Specialist, Psychiatry
Cleveland Department of Veterans Affairs Medical Center
Brecksville, Ohio
Associate Clinical Professor of Psychiatry
Clinical Instructor of Psychology
Case Western Reserve University
Cleveland, Ohio
Adjunct Associate Professor of Clinical Pharmacy
University of Toledo
Toledo, Ohio

David S. Jacobs, MD
President, Pathologists Chartered
Consultant in Pathology and Laboratory Medicine
Overland Park, Kansas

Polly E. Kintzel, PharmD, BCPS, BCOP
Clinical Pharmacy Specialist-Oncology
Spectrum Health
Grand Rapids, Michigan

Jill M. Kolesar, PharmD, FCCP, BCPS
Associate Professor of Pharmacy
University of Wisconsin
Madison, Wisconsin

Donna M. Kraus, PharmD, FAPhA
Associate Professor of Pharmacy Practice
Departments of Pharmacy Practice and Pediatrics
Pediatric Clinical Pharmacist
University of Illinois
Chicago, Illinois

Daniel L. Krinsky, RPh, MS
Director, Pharmacotherapy Sales and Marketing
Lexi-Comp, Inc
Hudson, Ohio

Kay Kyllonen, PharmD
Clinical Specialist
The Cleveland Clinic Children's Hospital
Cleveland, Ohio

Charles Lacy, RPh, PharmD, FCSHP
Vice President, Information Technologies
Professor, Pharmacy Practice
Professor, Business Leadership
University of Southern Nevada
Las Vegas, Nevada

Brenda R. Lance, RN, MSN
Program Development Director
Northcoast HealthCare Management Company
Northcoast Infusion Therapies
Oakwood Village, Ohio

Leonard L. Lance, RPh, BSPharm
Clinical Pharmacist
Lexi-Comp Inc
Hudson, Ohio

Jerrold B. Leikin, MD, FACP, FACEP, FACMT, FAACT
Director, Medical Toxicology
Evanston Northwestern Healthcare-OMEGA
Glenbrook Hospital
Glenview, Illinois
Associate Director
Toxikon Consortium at Cook County Hospital
Chicago, Illinois
Professor of Medicine
Pharmacology and Health Systems Management
Rush Medical College
Chicago, Ilinois
Professor of Medicine
Feinberg School of Medicine
Northwestern University
Chicago, Ilinois

Jeffrey D. Lewis, PharmD
Pharmacotherapy Specialist
Lexi-Comp, Inc
Hudson, Ohio

EDITORIAL ADVISORY PANEL *(Continued)*

Alpa Patel, PharmD
Clinical Specialist, Infectious Diseases
Johns Hopkins Hospital
Baltimore, Maryland

Luis F. Ramirez, MD
Adjunct Associate Professor of Psychiatry
Case Western Reserve University
Cleveland, Ohio

A.J. (Fred) Remillard, PharmD
Assistant Dean, Research and Graduate Affairs
College of Pharmacy and Nutrition
University of Saskatchewan
Saskatoon, Saskatchewan

Martha Sajatovic, MD
Associate Professor of Psychiatry
Case Western Reserve University
Cleveland, Ohio

Todd P. Semla, PharmD, BCPS, FCCP
Clinical Pharmacy Specialist
Department of Veterans Affairs
Pharmacy Benefits Management
Associate Professor of Clinical Psychiatry
Feinberg School of Medicine
Northwestern University
Chicago, Illinois

Francis G. Serio, DMD, MS
Professor & Chairman
Department of Periodontics
University of Mississippi
Jackson, Mississippi

Dominic A. Solimando, Jr, MA, FAPhA, FASHP, BCOP
Oncology Pharmacist
President, Oncology Pharmacy Services, Inc
Arlington, VA

Joni Lombardi Stahura, BS, PharmD, RPh
Pharmacotherapy Specialist
Lexi-Comp, Inc
Hudson, Ohio

Carol K. Taketomo, PharmD
Pharmacy Manager
Children's Hospital Los Angeles
Los Angeles, California

Mary Temple, PharmD
Pediatric Clinical Research Specialist
Hillcrest Hospital
Mayfield Heights, Ohio

Elizabeth A. Tomsik, PharmD, BCPS
Pharmacotherapy Specialist
Lexi-Comp, Inc
Hudson, Ohio

Beatrice B. Turkoski, RN, PhD
Associate Professor, Graduate Faculty
Advanced Pharmacology
College of Nursing
Kent State University
Kent, Ohio

EDITORIAL ADVISORY PANEL *(Continued)*

David M. Weinstein, PhD
Pharmacotherapy Specialist
Lexi-Comp, Inc.
Hudson, Ohio

Anne Marie Whelan, PharmD
College of Pharmacy
Dalhouise University
Halifax, Nova Scotia

Richard L. Wynn, PhD
Professor of Pharmacology
Baltimore College of Dental Surgery
Dental School
University of Maryland Baltimore
Baltimore, Maryland

PREFACE

Coordinating the unique complexities of the medication administration process within operative and procedural settings, the perioperative registered nurse is dedicated to the individualized needs and responses of the surgical patient. Having a reliable information source to assist with the numerous medications in perioperative patient care will support the clinician in safeguarding the patient at this vulnerable time. The *Perioperative Drug Information Handbook* is the one source for addressing the perioperative nurse's pharmaceutical information needs.

The resources included in this handbook are a result of requests from practicing perioperative registered nurses. The handbook is designed specifically for the perioperative nurse and contains information not readily available in other nursing drug reference books. Each phase of the perioperative encounter is addressed with emphasis on the special situations intrinsic to the perioperative patient care environment (eg, AORN medication guidance statements, anesthesia considerations per population, geriatric and pediatric considerations).

Individual drug monographs are concisely organized with the drug name in red. Each monograph also reviews basic pharmacokinetic and pharmacodynamic principles, contraindications, warnings, dosing guidelines, adverse reactions, and nutritional/herbal/ethanol interactions. Special topics sections and appendices allow quick reference to calculations and conversions, ACLS guidelines, latex allergy identification, lab values, common herbal supplements, preoperative assessment considerations, and postoperative management guidelines.

AORN is confident this premier issue of the *Perioperative Drug Information Handbook* will enhance safe medication administration practices and provide the resources needed. You are invited to provide suggestions to improve the quality of this text by completing the on-line user survey found on AORN's website (www.aorn.org).

ACKNOWLEDGMENTS

This handbook exists in its present form as the result of the concerted efforts of the following individuals: Robert D. Kerscher, publisher and president of Lexi-Comp, Inc; Mark Bonfiglio, PharmD, director of pharmacotherapy resources; Stacy S. Robinson, editorial manager; Leslie Jo Hoppes, pharmacology database manager; David C. Marcus, director of information systems; Tracey J. Henterly, graphic designer; and Matthew C. Kerscher, product manager.

Special acknowledgment to all Lexi-Comp staff for their contributions to this handbook.

Much of the material contained in this book was a result of pharmacy contributors throughout the United States and Canada. Lexi-Comp has assisted many medical institutions to develop hospital-specific formulary manuals that contain clinical drug information as well as dosing. Working with clinical pharmacists, hospital pharmacy and therapeutics committees, and hospital drug information centers, Lexi-Comp has developed an evolutionary drug database that reflects the practice of pharmacy in these major institutions.

In addition, the authors wish to thank their families, friends, and colleagues who supported them in their efforts to complete this handbook.

DESCRIPTION OF SECTIONS AND FIELDS

The *Drug Information Handbook for Perioperative Nursing, 1st Edition* is divided into six sections: Introductory Text, Alphabetical Listing of Drugs, Special Topics, Appendix, Pharmacologic Category Index, and Alphabetical Index.

Drug information is presented in a consistent format and provides the following:

Generic Name	U.S. adopted name
Pronunciation	Phonetic pronunciation of generic name
U.S. Brand Names	Trade names (manufacturer-specific) found in the United States. The symbol [DSC] appears after trade names that have been recently discontinued.
Synonyms	Other name(s) or accepted abbreviation(s) of the generic drug
Pharmacologic Category	Indicates one or more systematic classifications of the drug
Medication Safety Issues	In an effort to promote the safe use of medications, this field is intended to highlight possible sources of medication errors such as look-alike/sound-alike drugs or highly concentrated formulations which require vigilance on the part of healthcare professionals. In addition, medications which have been associated with severe consequences in the event of a medication error are also identified in this field.
Use	Description of FDA-approved indications of the drug
Unlabeled/Investigational Use	Information pertaining to non-FDA approved and investigational indications of the drug
Mechanism of Action	A brief description of how the drug works
Pharmacodynamics/Kinetics	The magnitude of a drug's effect depends on the drug concentration at the site of action. The pharmacodynamics are expressed in terms of onset of action and duration of action. Pharmacokinetics are expressed in terms of absorption, distribution (including appearance in breast milk and crossing of the placenta), protein binding, metabolism, bioavailability, half-life, time to peak serum concentration, and elimination.
Contraindications	Inappropriate use(s) of the drug or disease states and patient populations in which the drug should not be used, according to the FDA
Warnings/Precautions	Warnings include hazardous conditions related to use of the drug. Precautions include disease states or patient populations in which the drug should be used with caution.

DESCRIPTION OF SECTIONS AND FIELDS *(Continued)*

Drug Interactions	If a drug has demonstrated involvement with cytochrome P450 enzymes, the initial line of this field will identify the drug as an inhibitor, inducer, or substrate of specific isoenzymes (eg, CYP1A2). The remainder of the field presents a description of the interactions between the drug listed in the monograph and other drugs or drug classes. May include possible mechanisms and effect of combined therapy. May also include a strategy to manage the patient on combined therapy.
Nutritional/Herbal/Ethanol Interactions	Information regarding potential interactions with food, nutritional supplements (including herbal products and vitamins), ethanol, or cigarette smoking
Lab Interactions	Effect drug may have on assays during therapy
Adverse Reactions	Side effects are grouped by percentage of incidence (if known) and/or body system; in the interest of saving space, <1% effects are grouped only by percentage
Overdose/Toxicology	Comment or considerations with signs/ symptoms of excess drug ingestion
Dosing	The amount of drug to be typically given or taken during therapy; may include the following:
Adults	The recommended amount of drug to be given to adult patients
Adults and Elderly	This combined field is only used to indicate that no specific adjustments for elderly patients were identified. However, other issues should be considered (ie, renal or hepatic impairment). Also refer to Geriatric Considerations for additional information related to the elderly.
Elderly	A suggested amount of drug to be given to elderly patients which may include adjustments from adult dosing; lack of information in the monograph may imply that the drug is not used in the elderly patient or no specific adjustments could be identified
Pediatrics	Suggested amount of drug to be given to neonates, infants, and children
Renal Impairment	Suggested dosage adjustments or comments based on compromised renal function; may include dosing instructions for patients on dialysis
Hepatic Impairment	Suggested dosage adjustments or comments based on compromised liver function
Available Dosage Forms	A description of the product form(s), including strength and formulation (ie, tablet, capsule, injection, syrup, etc)
Nursing Guidelines	
Assessment	Monitoring guidelines
Monitoring Laboratory Tests	Suggested laboratory tests to monitor for safety and efficacy of the drug
Dietary Considerations	Includes information on how the medication should be taken relative to meals or food

Patient Education	Suggested items to discuss with the patient or caregiver when taking the medication; may include issues regarding contraception, self-monitoring, precautions, and administration
Geriatric Considerations	Comments or suggestions of drug use in elderly patients; may include monitoring, dose adjustments, precautions, or comments on appropriateness of use
Pregnancy Risk Factor	Indicates one or more of the five categories established by the FDA to indicate the potential of a systemically absorbed drug for causing birth defects
Pregnancy Issues	Comments related to safe drug administration during pregnancy, if appropriate
Lactation	Information regarding use of the drug while breast-feeding (where recommendation of American Academy of Pediatrics differs, notation is made); the following distinctions are made: Does not enter breast milk Enters breast milk (may include: /compatible, use caution, not recommended, contraindicated, or consult prescriber) Excretion in breast milk unknown (may include: /compatible, use caution, not recommended, contraindicated, or consult prescriber) Not indicated for use in women No data available (may include: /use caution)
Breast-Feeding Considerations	Provides further information relating to taking the drug while nursing
Perioperative/Anesthesia/ Other Concerns	This field provides a focused summary of some of the important issues concerning anesthesia and critical care applications relevant to the drug; other additional information may be included
Administration	
Oral I.M. I.V.	The administration field contains subfields by route regarding issues relative to appropriately giving a medication; includes suggestions on final drug concentrations and/or rates of infusion for parenteral medications and comments regarding the timing of drug administration relative to meals. Also see Compatibility.
Reconstitution	Includes comments on solution choice with time or conditions for the mixture to maintain full potency before administration
Compatibility	Provides information regarding stability of the drug in different solutions; known incompatibilities when admixed or coadministered with other drugs; and when it is administered through Y-site administration sets
Storage	Information relating to appropriate storage of the medication prior to opening the manufacturers original packaging; information is only given if recommendations are for storage at other than room temperature; includes storage requirements for reconstituted products
Related Information	Cross-reference to other pertinent drug information in this handbook

DESCRIPTION OF SECTIONS AND FIELDS *(Continued)*

Special Topics

This section is comprised of several text chapters dealing with various subjects and issues pertinent to the perioperative nurse.

Appendix

This section is an extensive appendix of useful information that includes abbreviations and measurements, laboratory information, perioperative information, herbals, and selected therapy guidelines.

Pharmacologic Category Index

Listing of the drugs by their unique pharmacologic category and includes cross-references to the monographs

Alphabetical Index

A comprehensive alphabetical listing of generic drug names, U.S. brand names, and synonyms.

FDA PREGNANCY CATEGORIES

Throughout this book there is a field labeled Pregnancy Risk Factor and the letter A, B, C, D, or X, immediately following, which signifies a category. The FDA has established these five categories to indicate the potential of a systemically-absorbed drug for causing birth defects. The key differentiation among the categories rests upon the reliability of documentation and the risk:benefit ratio. Category **X** is particularly notable, in that if any data exists that may implicate a drug as a teratogen, and the risk:benefit ratio is clearly negative, the drug is **contraindicated** during pregnancy.

These categories are summarized as follows:

A Controlled studies in pregnant women fail to demonstrate a risk to the fetus in the first trimester with no evidence of risk in later trimesters. The possibility of fetal harm appears remote.

B Either animal-reproduction studies have not demonstrated a fetal risk but there are no controlled studies in pregnant women, or animal-reproduction studies have shown an adverse effect (other than a decrease in fertility) that was not confirmed in controlled studies in women in the first trimester and there is no evidence of a risk in later trimesters.

C Either studies in animals have revealed adverse effects on the fetus (teratogenic or embryocidal effects or other) and there are no controlled studies in women, or studies in women and animals are not available. Drugs should be given only if the potential benefits justify the potential risk to the fetus.

D There is positive evidence of human fetal risk, but the benefits from use in pregnant women may be acceptable despite the risk (eg, if the drug is needed in a life-threatening situation or for a serious disease for which safer drugs cannot be used or are ineffective).

X Studies in animals or human beings have demonstrated fetal abnormalities or there is evidence of fetal risk based on human experience, or both, and the risk of the use of the drug in pregnant women clearly outweighs any possible benefit. The drug is contraindicated in women who are or may become pregnant.

FDA NAME DIFFERENTIATION PROJECT THE USE OF TALL-MAN LETTERS

Confusion between similar drug names is an important cause of medication errors. For years, The Institute For Safe Medication Practices (ISMP), has urged generic manufacturers to use a combination of large and small letters as well as bolding (ie, chlorpro**MAZINE** and chlorpro**PAMIDE**) to help distinguish drugs with look-alike names, especially when they share similar strengths. Recently the FDA's Division of Generic Drugs began to issue recommendation letters to manufacturers suggesting this novel way to label their products to help reduce this drug name confusion. Although this project has had marginal success, the method has successfully eliminated problems with products such as diphenhydr**AMINE** and dimenhy**DRINATE**. Hospitals should also follow suit by making similar changes in their own labels, preprinted order forms, computer screens and printouts, and drug storage location labels.

Lexi-Comp Medical Publishing will use "Tall-Man" letters for the drugs suggested by the FDA.

The following is a list of product names and recommended FDA revisions.

Drug Product	Recommended Revision
acetazolamide	aceta**ZOLAMIDE**
acetohexamide	aceto**HEXAMIDE**
bupropion	bu**PROP**ion
buspirone	bus**PIR**one
chlorpromazine	chlorpro**MAZINE**
chlorpropamide	chlorpro**PAMIDE**
clomiphene	clomi**PHENE**
clomipramine	clomi**PRAMINE**
cycloserine	cyclo**SERINE**
cyclosporine	cyclo**SPORINE**
daunorubicin	**DAUNO**rubicin
dimenhydrinate	dimenhy**DRINATE**
diphenhydramine	diphenhydr**AMINE**
dobutamine	**DOBUT**amine
dopamine	**DOP**amine
doxorubicin	**DOXO**rubicin
glipizide	glipi**ZIDE**
glyburide	gly**BURIDE**
hydralazine	hydr**ALAZINE**
hydroxyzine	hydr**OXY**zine
medroxyprogesterone	medroxy**PROGESTER**one
methylprednisolone	methyl**PREDNIS**olone
methyltestosterone	methyl**TESTOSTER**one
nicardipine	ni**CAR**dipine
nifedipine	**NIFE**dipine
prednisolone	predniso**LONE**
prednisone	predni**SONE**
sulfadiazine	sulfa**DIAZINE**
sulfisoxazole	sulfi**SOXAZOLE**
tolazamide	**TOLAZ**amide
tolbutamide	**TOLBUT**amide
vinblastine	vin**BLAS**tine
vincristine	vin**CRIS**tine

Institute for Safe Medication Practices. "New Tall-Man Lettering Will Reduce Mix-Ups Due to Generic Drug Name Confusion," *ISMP Medication Safety Alert*, September 19, 2001. Available at: http://www.ismp.org.

Institute for Safe Medication Practices. "Prescription Mapping, Can Improve Efficiency While Minimizing Errors With Look-Alike Products," *ISMP Medication Safety Alert*, October 6, 1999. Available at: http://www.ismp.org.

U.S. Pharmacopeia, "USP Quality Review: Use Caution-Avoid Confusion," March 2001, No. 76. Available at: http://www.usp.org.

SAFE WRITING PRACTICES

Health professionals and their support personnel frequently produce handwritten copies of information they see in print; therefore, such information is subjected to even greater possibilities for error or misinterpretation on the part of others. Thus, particular care must be given to how drug names and strengths are expressed when creating written healthcare documents.

The following are a few examples of safe writing rules suggested by the Institute for Safe Medication Practices, Inc.[1]

1. There should be a space between a number and its units as it is easier to read. There should be no periods after the abbreviations mg or mL.

Correct	Incorrect
10 mg	10mg
100 mg	100mg

2. Never place a decimal and a zero after a whole number (2 mg is correct and 2.0 mg is **incorrect**). If the decimal point is not seen because it falls on a line or because individuals are working from copies where the decimal point is not seen, this causes a tenfold overdose.
3. Just the opposite is true for numbers less than one. Always place a zero before a naked decimal (0.5 mL is correct, .5 mL is **incorrect**).
4. Never abbreviate the word unit. The handwritten U or u, looks like a 0 (zero), and may cause a tenfold overdose error to be made.
5. IU is not a safe abbreviation for international units. The handwritten IU looks like IV. Write out international units or use int. units.
6. Q.D. is not a safe abbreviation for once daily, as when the Q is followed by a sloppy dot, it looks like QID which means four times daily.
7. O.D. is not a safe abbreviation for once daily, as it is properly interpreted as meaning "right eye" and has caused liquid medications such as saturated solution of potassium iodide and Lugol's solution to be administered incorrectly. There is no safe abbreviation for once daily. It must be written out in full.
8. Do not use chemical names such as 6-mercaptopurine or 6-thioguanine, as sixfold overdoses have been given when these were not recognized as chemical names. The proper names of these drugs are mercaptopurine or thioguanine.
9. Do not abbreviate drug names (5FC, 6MP, 5-ASA, MTX, HCTZ, CPZ, PBZ, etc) as they are misinterpreted and cause error.
10. Do not use the apothecary system or symbols.
11. Do not abbreviate microgram as µg; instead use mcg as there is less likelihood of misinterpretation.
12. When writing an outpatient prescription, write a complete prescription. A complete prescription can prevent the prescriber, the pharmacist, and/or the patient from making a mistake and can eliminate the need for further clarification. The legible prescriptions should contain:
    a. patient's full name
    b. for pediatric or geriatric patients: their age (or weight where applicable)
    c. drug name, dosage form and strength; if a drug is new or rarely prescribed, print this information
    d. number or amount to be dispensed
    e. complete instructions for the patient, including the purpose of the medication
    f. when there are recognized contraindications for a prescribed drug, indicate to the pharmacist that you are aware of this fact (ie, when prescribing a potassium salt for a patient receiving an ACE inhibitor, write "K serum leveling being monitored")

[1]From "Safe Writing" by Davis NM, PharmD and Cohen MR, MS, Lecturers and Consultants for Safe Medication Practices, 1143 Wright Drive, Huntington Valley, PA 19006. Phone: (215) 947-7566.

SAFE HANDLING OF HAZARDOUS DRUGS

Due to their inherent toxicity, particularly mutagenicity and carcinogenicity, there is concern about the risks of long-term, low level exposure to a number of drugs, particularly antineoplastic agents. The possible risk to healthcare providers who are responsible for preparation and administration of such agents has been a subject of much debate, but few definite answers. Despite more than 20 years of research and literally thousands of publications on the topic, there is no definitive evidence of a causal relationship between prolonged exposure to low levels of antineoplastic agents in the workplace and development of malignancies. Neither is there conclusive evidence that such exposure is not hazardous. In the absence of convincing evidence that healthcare personnel are not at risk, prudence requires the presumption that there is some degree of risk, and employees should employ appropriate protective measures.

The potential for many antineoplastic agents to cause secondary malignancies in patients was identified in the 1960s and 1970s. Coupled with evidence of some drugs' carcinogenicity in animals, this information raised the question of possible adverse effects from prolonged low level exposure. In the late 1970s and 1980s, a large number of anecdotal reports of various side effects and adverse reactions in nurses, pharmacists, and pharmacy technicians involved in preparation and administration of antineoplastic therapy began to appear in the literature. These were followed by reports of increased urine mutagenicity, chromosome abnormalities, changes in immune function, and detectable blood or urine drug levels in personnel who routinely handled antineoplastic agents. As a result of these concerns, a number of groups issued guidelines intended to minimize exposure to antineoplastic agents in the workplace. By the end of the 1980s, a variety of organizations, including the Occupational Safety and Health Administration (OSHA), American Society of Hospital (now Health-System) Pharmacists (ASHP), the National Institutes of Health (NIH), and the National Study Commission on Cytotoxic Exposure had all issued documents addressing the proper handling of cytotoxic agents by healthcare personnel. Most of the early guidelines acknowledged the paucity and low quality of the available data, and recommended further research to define the actual risks.

During the remainder of the 1980s and 1990s, a number of studies and reports attempting to delineate the nature of the risk, and the appropriate safety measures to be taken were published. The vast majority of these were uncontrolled trials involving very small numbers of individuals, usually at a single institution. The nature and magnitude of the risk has never been properly delineated. Due to the nature of the problem, there has never been a large scale, prospective controlled trial to determine the efficacy of the various protective measures employed. As a result, there is no known threshold of safety for exposure to these agents; nor have any reliable monitoring techniques to assess exposure been developed. Most guidelines are therefore based on an assumption of "zero tolerance" - any exposure is hazardous, and must be avoided. Achieving the appropriate balance between necessary protection for personnel who must work with these agents and over-reaction to the threat remains a challenge.

Defining hazardous agents and identifying effective protective measures remains a problem. There is no agreement among various agencies as to the definition of a hazardous agent or which agents should be classified as hazardous. The Environmental Protection Agency (EPA), National Institute for Occupational Safety and Health (NIOSH), and American Society of Health-System Pharmacists all have guidelines for handling hazardous agents, but there is little agreement, and considerable variation among these guidelines. The EPA lists 723 chemicals as hazardous. Only eight are antineoplastic agents; an additional 16 non-antineoplastic agents are listed as hazardous. NIOSH has 60 drugs on its list (which it states is incomplete and "not all-inclusive"), including 13 nonantineoplastic agents. (see Tables 1 and 2 on the following pages). Some manufacturers also recommend special precautions for handling specific drugs (eg, mycophenolate, ganciclovir).

Table 1: Criteria for Defining Hazardous Agents

<table>
<tr><th>EPA</th><th>NIOSH</th><th>ASHP</th></tr>
<tr><td rowspan="5">Meets one of the following criteria:
Ignitability: Create fire under certain conditions or are spontaneously combustible and have a flash point <600°C

Corrosivity: Acids or bases (pH >2 or ≤12.5) capable of corroding metal containers

Reactivity: Unstable under "normal" conditions; can cause explosions, toxic fumes, gases, or vapors when mixed with water

Toxicity characteristic: When disposed of on land, contaminated liquid may drain or leach from the waste and pollute ground water</td><td>Designated as therapeutic category 10:00 (Antineoplastic Agent) in the American Hospital Formulary Service Drug Information</td><td>Genotoxic</td></tr>
<tr><td>Manufacturer suggests use of special techniques in handling administration, or disposal</td><td>Carcinogenic</td></tr>
<tr><td>Mutagenic</td><td>Teratogenic or impairs fertility</td></tr>
<tr><td>Carcinogenic</td><td>Causes serious organ or other toxic manifestation at low doses</td></tr>
<tr><td>Teratogenic or reproductive toxicant</td><td></td></tr>
<tr><td>OR</td><td>Acutely toxic to an organ system</td><td></td></tr>
<tr><td>Appears on one of the following lists:

F: Wastes from certain common or industrial manufacturing processes from nonspecific sources

K: Wastes from certain specific industries from specific sources

P: Wastes from pure or commercial grade formulations of certain specific unused chemicals

U: Wastes from pure or commercial grade formulations of certain specific unused chemicals</td><td>Investigational drugs</td><td></td></tr>
</table>

SAFE HANDLING OF HAZARDOUS DRUGS *(Continued)*

Table 2: Drugs Listed as Hazardous by EPA or NIOSH

EPA		NIOSH	
Antineoplastic	**Nonantineoplastic**	**Antineoplastic**	**Nonantineoplastic**
Arsenic Trioxide	Dichlorodifluoromethane	Altretamine	Anesthetic, agents
Chlorambucil	Diethylstilbesterol	Aminoglutethimide	Cyclosporine
Cyclophosphamide	Epinephrine	Azathioprine	Diethylstilbestrol
Daunomycin	Hexachlorophene	Asparaginase	Estradiol
Malphalan	Lindane	Bleomycin	Ethinyl Estradiol
Mitomycin	Nitroglycerin	Busulfan	Ganciclovir
Streptozocin	Paraldehyde	Carboplatin	Isotretinoin
Uracil Mustard	Phenacetin	Carmustine	Medroxyprogesterone
	Physostigmine	Chlorambucil	Nafarelin
	Physostigmine Salicylate	Chloramphenicol	Pentamidine
	Reserpine	Chlorozotocin	Plicamycin
	Resorcinol	Cisplatin	Ribavirin
	Saccharin	Cyclophosphamide	Testolactone
	Selenium Sulfide	Cytarabine	Vidarabine
	Trichloromono-fluoromethane	Dacarbazine	Zidovudine
	Warfarin	Dactinomycin	
		Daunorubicin	
		Doxorubicin	
		Estramustine	
		Etoposide	
		Floxuridine	
		Fluorouracil	
		Flutamide	
		Hydroxyurea	
		Idarubicin	
		Ifosfamide	
		Interferon A	
		Leuprolide	
		Levamisole	
		Lomustine	
		Mechlorethamine	
		Megestrol	
		Melphalan	
		Mercaptopurine	
		Methotrexate	
		Mitomycin	
		Mitotane	
		Mitoxantrone	
		Pipobroman	
		Procarbazine	
		Streptozocin	
		Tamoxifen	
		Thioguanine	
		Thiotepa	
		Uracil Mustard	
		Vinblastine	
		Vincristine	

In addition to the differences among the available guidelines, some criteria are extremely vague or broad, adding to the uncertainty. The NIOSH criterion "Acutely toxic to an organ system" could be applied to almost any drug. ASHP's "Causes serious organ or other toxic manifestation at low doses" could also apply to a large number of drugs not commonly considered "hazardous" to persons handling them. The EPA standard "Appears on one of the following lists" seems to be particularly subjective. Drugs appear on, and are removed from, the EPA lists in what appears a purely arbitrary manner. For example, cisplatin and dexamethasone have appeared on previous lists, but are not on the current one. Daunomycin and cyclophosphamide are listed as hazardous; other anthacyclines and ifosfamine are not. Inquiries to EPA have failed to identify why these changes were made; or why one drug in a class is considered hazardous, but other agents in that category are not.

Analysis of the problem has not completely clarified the risks. Rather, previously accepted practices are subject to question. A 1992 report on exposure of healthcare personnel to hazardous agents suggested that the standard biologic safety cabinets recommended for use when compounding hazardous drugs may not provided the desired level of protection. There is evidence suggesting rather than forming particles or aerosol droplets that could be trapped in a standard HEPA filter, some antineoplastic agents vaporize, yielding particles that cannot be trapped in the filter. This potential for vaporization may be a partial explanation for recent reports indicating detectable contamination of work surfaces in, and near, hazardous drug preparation areas. This information has led some institutions to begin investigating use of isolator cabinets and sealed preparation systems as replacements for the biologic cabinets.

A 1996 review of 64 studies of workplace exposure to cytotoxic drugs noted numerous methodologic flaws in study design and procedures. The report concluded the methods used to assess exposure in these studies were too nonspecific and insensitive to be reliable measures of exposure. One disturbing aspect of this is the fact that the studies and procedures found to be not sensitive enough to assess routine levels of exposure were the ones used as the basis for development of the existing handling guidelines.

Several studies have found containers have detectable amounts of drug residue on them when they arrive in the pharmacy. These reports raise the concern that exposure may be a hazard originating at least partially outside the pharmacy; and that additional procedures for decontaminating drug containers upon arrival at the pharmacy may be necessary.

Guidelines and institutional policies for minimizing exposure to hazardous materials have been based on the presumption that environmental exposure to hazardous drugs occurs through three mechanisms:

- **inhalation** of drug dust or aerosolized droplets
- **absorption** through the skin
- **ingestion** of contaminated food or drink

Accordingly, the existing recommendations are heavily weighted toward the use of physical barriers as the primary means of reducing exposure. Among the commonly employed precautions are:

- **Separation:** Hazardous agents are often prepared in a limited number of areas which are separated, to the extent possible, from other drug preparation areas. Almost all institutions have a separate biologic safety cabinet reserved solely for the preparation of antineoplastic agents. Many institutions have a separate "oncology" drug preparation area or satellite pharmacy.

- **Biologic safety cabinets:** Use of a Class IIA or B biologic safety cabinet for the preparation of hazardous agents. Recent reports have questioned the efficacy of these cabinets, and some institutions have adopted the use of Isolator® systems or special closed preparation systems for compounding hazardous agents.

- **Protective clothing:** Another almost universal precaution is the used of protective gloves, gowns, and eye protection while handling antineoplastic agents. If drug preparation is performed in a biologic safety cabinet equipped with a glass front, many institutions dispense with the requirement for wearing safety goggles.

- **Training:** Some of the early reports attributed lower, or undetectable, levels of exposure to hazardous drugs to the experience level, or skill at aseptic technique, of the individual worker. Many institutions require some degree of training before personnel are allowed to handle hazardous agents. Although most of the published guidelines

SAFE HANDLING OF HAZARDOUS DRUGS *(Continued)*

recommend personnel who handle hazardous agents have "appropriate" training and experience, none specify what should be included in such a program. Accordingly, the exact nature and length of the required training programs vary widely among institutions.

- **Monitoring:** Appropriate physical parameters for assessing exposure to hazardous drugs are not available. Although some institutions require periodic health monitoring, the definition of what constitutes an appropriate screening program is a matter of some debate. Attempts to monitor the existence of hazardous materials in the work area has been slightly more successful. Assessment of airborne drug levels and surface contamination, in preparation cabinets, "secure" work areas and areas outside the hazardous drug area has been reported. Additionally, techniques for using ultraviolet light to detect occult drug spills, and assess individual's handling technique have been reported. Most of these techniques have not been developed sufficiently to be used in routine practice, and are still limited to the research setting.
- **Decontamination:** Drug containers should be examined upon their arrival at the pharmacy. Containers that show signs of damage should be handled carefully, and may require quarantine and decontamination before being placed in stock. Consideration should be given to the possible need to quarantine and decontaminate all containers of hazardous agents as a routine precaution.

Selected Readings

American Society of Hospital Pharmacists, "ASHP Technical Assistance Bulletin on Handling Cytotoxic and Hazardous Drugs," *Am J Hosp Pharm*, 1990, 47:1033-49.

Baker ES and Connor TH, "Monitoring Occupational Exposure to Cancer Chemotherapy Drugs," *Am J Health Syst Pharm*, 1996, 53(22):2713-23.

Bos RP and Sessink PJ, "Biomonitoring of Occupational Exposures to Cytostatic Anticancer Drugs," *Rev Environ Health*, 1997, 12(1):43-58.

Connor TH, "Permeability of Nitrile Rubber, Latex, Polyurethane, and Neoprene Gloves to 18 Antineoplastic Drugs," *Am J Health Syst Pharm*, 1999, 56(23):2450-3.

Connor TH, Anderson RW, Sessink PJ, et al, "Surface Contamination With Antineoplastic Agents in Six Cancer Treatment Centers in Canada and the United States," *Am J Health Syst Pharm*, 1999, 56(14):1427-32.

Connor TH, Sessink PJ, Harrison BR, et al, "Surface Contamination of Chemotherapy Drug Vials and Evaluation of New Vial-Cleaning Techniques: Results of Three Studies," *Am J Health Syst Pharm*, 2005, 62(5):475-84.

"Preventing Occupational Exposure to Antineoplastic and Other Hazardous Drugs in Health Care Settings," Available at http://www.cdc.gov/niosh/docs/2004-165. Accessed February 6, 2005.

Sessink PJ, Anzion RB, Van den Broek PH, et al, "Detection of Contamination With Antineoplastic Agents in a Hospital Pharmacy Department," *Pharm Weekbl Sci*, 1992, 14(1):16-22.

Sessink PJ, Boer KA, Scheefhals AP, et al, "Occupational Exposure to Antineoplastic Agents at Several Departments in a Hospital. Environmental Contamination and Excretion of Cyclophosphamide and Ifosfamide in Urine of Exposed Workers," *Int Arch Occup Environ Health*, 1992, 64(2):105-12.

Sessink PJ and Bos RP, "Drugs Hazardous to Healthcare Workers. Evaluation of Methods for Monitoring Occupational Exposure to Cytostatic Drugs," *Drug Saf*, 1999, 20(4):347-59.

Solimando D and Wilson J, "Demonstration of Skin Fluorescence Following Exposure to Doxorubicin," *Cancer Nursing*, 1983, 6(4):313-5.

Sorsa M and Anderson D, "Monitoring of Occupational Exposure to Cytostatic Anticancer Agents," *Mutat Res*, 1996, 355(1-2):253-61.

Wilson J and Solimando D, "Aseptic Technique as a Safety Precaution in the Preparation of Antineoplastic Agents," *Hospital Pharmacy*, 1981, 16(11):575-81.

AORN GUIDANCE STATEMENT: SAFE MEDICATION PRACTICES IN PERIOPERATIVE SETTINGS ACROSS THE LIFE SPAN

Introduction

This guidance statement provides a framework for perioperative registered nurses to develop, implement, and evaluate safe medication management practices specific to the perioperative setting. This evidenced-based framework may be used to facilitate policy development and provide a foundation for the creation of quality improvement (QI)/process improvement (PI) monitors. It is the responsibility of individual healthcare organizations to develop a culture of medication safety. Proactively reviewing medication errors from the viewpoint of "systems failures" and "systems solutions" will help encourage a culture free from shame and blame.

Perioperative practice settings addressed by this document include traditional operating rooms, ambulatory surgery units, physicians' offices, cardiac catheterization suites, endoscopy suites, radiology departments, and all other areas where operative and invasive procedures may be performed. For the purpose of this document, the term O.R. is inclusive of all perioperative practice environments.

First published in May 2002, the current guidance statement has been reviewed and updated by AORN's Presidential Commission on Patient Safety, in collaboration with the United States Pharmacopeia (USP), to reflect current safe medication practices.

Background

The National Institute of Medicine report, To Err Is Human: Building a Better Health System, increased awareness of medication errors. The report noted that "medication errors account for one out of 131 outpatient deaths and one out of 854 inpatient deaths."[1] Medication errors can originate at any point in the medication use process and affect patients of all ages. Medication error poses a substantial threat to patients. The perioperative setting creates additional challenges for safe medication administration practices. Related factors affecting the medication process in the perioperative environment include

- the aseptic dispensing of medications onto the sterile field
- an intermediary to receive and transfer dispensed medications to the scrubbed licensed practitioner (eg, surgeon)
- time-sensitive conditions, and
- sensory distractions intrinsic to the environment

Specific concerns associated with medication errors in the perioperative setting include, but are not limited to,

- inconsistent practices to communicate current and previous medication regimes (ie, medication reconciliation)
- verbal orders delivered through surgical masks may be muffled and contribute to confusion in the medication order (eg, name, strength, and/or dose)
- incomplete, ambiguous, incorrect, or illegibly written or spoken orders
- inaccurate, illegible, or outdated surgical preference cards
- removal of the contents from the original manufacturer's packaging to aseptically deliver contents onto the sterile field
- limited knowledge of medications by scrubbed allied heath professionals receiving medications onto the sterile field
- inconsistent labeling of medications on and off the sterile field
- medication dispensed to the sterile field may be handled by multiple individuals before reaching the licensed individual administering the medication

AORN GUIDANCE STATEMENT: SAFE MEDICATION PRACTICES IN PERIOPERATIVE SETTINGS ACROSS THE LIFE SPAN *(Continued)*

- high-alert medications available in multiple dose forms and concentrations
- look-alike and sound-alike medications stored in close proximity
- patient care complexity requiring rapid perioperative interventions
- extended work hours leading to healthcare worker fatigue
- care is provided by multiple healthcare providers simultaneously, and
- multiple patient handoffs between care providers

The following guidance is offered to support perioperative registered nurses in the provision of safe perioperative patient care.

Guidance Statement

Healthcare organizations should identify in policy which people and/or job categories may participate in medication management and administration. Facility policy for safe medication practice should be based on the five "rights" of medication administration:

- the right patient
- the right medication
- the right dose
- the right time, and
- the right route

The five rights of safe medication practices should be a final check before the administration of any medication.

Healthcare organizations should develop standardized procedures for safe medication practices in the O.R. designed to include, but not limited to, the following.

- Ensure proper patient identification.
- Document all patient medications.
- Assess for medication(s) contraindications.
- Confirm weight-based dosing before administration.
- Establish dose limits.
- Minimize use of verbal orders to the extent possible.
- Manage medications off the sterile field.
- Deliver medications to the sterile field.
- Manage medications on the sterile field.
- Document all intraoperative medications.
- Monitor and document patient for effects of medications.
- Preserve all original medication/solution containers and delivery devices until the conclusion of the procedure.
- Continually evaluate the medication delivery process for patients within the surgical setting.
- Define procedures for the questioning of any medication order thought to be unclear or inappropriate.[2]

General Risk Reduction Strategies

The following risk reduction strategies offer guidance for the development of policies, procedures, and associated QI and PI monitoring tools and reporting processes related to safe medication handling in the O.R. The goal should be to meet or exceed the expectations for safe medication practice as outlined by published national patient safety initiatives (eg, the National Patient Safety Goals of the Joint Commission on Accreditation of Healthcare Organizations [JCAHO], guidelines of the Institute for Safe Medication Practices [ISMP] and USP).

Patient Identification

Minimize the potential for medication error related to incorrect identification of the patient through the establishment of standardized identification processes. Documentation of these processes may provide the necessary data to monitor outcomes for improvement.

- Consider the preoperative checklist as a permanent part of the patient care record.
- Perform patient identification using at least two patient identifiers, neither of which are to be the patient's room number.[3]
- Verification of patient identification should include information from the patient's identification (ID) band(s) or identification record when an ID band is not appropriate.
- Consider using the patient's date of birth as one means of identification (eg, pediatric population).
- Ensure that the contents of patient charts are verified for correct patient information.
- Imprints of patient information (eg, Addressograph stamp) on documents should be legible.
- Standardize forms should have patient identification in the same place on every page; duplexed pages should be identified on both sides in the same place.
- Identify in facility policy which people and/or job categories may participate in medication management and administration.

Accurate Medication List

Provider access to patient-specific information facilitates continuity of care and ensures that essential components for patient care decisions related to the medication management process are available. Readily accessible information should aid in the identification of risk related to medication allergy interaction, contraindication, and medication-medication or herbal-medication interaction. Documentation of this activity is an essential component of outcomes management in regard to patient safety.[4]

- Develop a consistent multidisciplinary approach for documenting the patient's medications using a standardized reconciliation sheet that is readily available for review before the procedure.[3]
- Actively involve the patient or authorized representative in the process of obtaining a complete list of the patient's current medications.[3]

Medication Contraindications

Whenever possible, written medication orders should be reviewed for appropriateness by a pharmacist before dispensing the medication. Concerns and issues related to medication, dose, frequency, route of administration, therapeutic duplication of the medication, its therapeutic class or chemical family, allergies, potential interactions, and contraindications are all elements of the review process.[4,5]

- Existing medication allergy information for each patient must be readily available and communicated to all members of the perioperative team.
- Allergy information may be obtained from patients, family members, legal guardians, and/or prior medical records.
- Healthcare organizations should provide readily available resources for perioperative personnel to identify medication class, nutrition and herbal supplement interactions (eg, calcium channel blockers and grapefruit), and associated medication class allergies (eg, amoxicillin and Keflex®).
- An organization-wide process should be in place to cross-reference patient drug allergy interactions, contraindication, and medication-medication/herbal-medication interaction potentials.[3]
  - Patient medications should be validated and cross-referenced during the medication-ordering phase of the medication delivery process.
  - Reference tools such as computer programs or charts should be used.

Accurate Dose Calculation

The patient's weight should be documented in both pounds and kilograms. Both mathematical formats provide a visual cue to eliminate discrepancies and to alert healthcare personnel to the proper numerical value used in weight calculations. Accurate weight measurement is critical for accurate dose calculation.[4] The medication dose calculation process should include, but is not limited to, the following.

- Accurately obtain weights on all patients before surgery.

AORN GUIDANCE STATEMENT: SAFE MEDICATION PRACTICES IN PERIOPERATIVE SETTINGS ACROSS THE LIFE SPAN *(Continued)*

- A facility-approved weight conversion chart (ie, pounds to kilograms) should be available for quick reference.
- Redesign patient care forms to clearly reflect weight in both pounds and kilograms.
- If there are discrepancies in weight or dose calculations, the patient should be reevaluated and the weight and dose recalculated.
- Medications ordered using weight-based dose schedules should be independently calculated and verified by two licensed individuals.
- Automate medication dosage calculations whenever possible.

Dose Limits

Healthcare organizations should identify high-risk and high-alert medications within the organization and develop processes to safeguard against error. Medications with narrow therapeutic ranges are considered at risk for error. Creating conversion charts targeting dose limits for high-risk medications will contribute to their safe use in surgery.[4]

- Dosage conversion charts or electronic aids should be used to calculate maximum dose limits, especially for high-alert medications.
- Separate weight-based conversion charts for children and adults should be developed for each of the major error-prone medications identified for that population at risk.

Verbal Orders

Verification of critical components of perioperative verbal orders, before the implementation of the order, affords an opportunity to confirm the accuracy of the verbal order.[3] Use of verbal and telephone orders should be limited.[2] When verbal orders are necessary, provide mechanisms to ensure accuracy, such as:

- Record the order in the patient's record according to facility policy as soon as feasible.[2,6]
- Perform a "read-back" of the written order.[2,6]
- Verbalize the read-back digit-by-digit (eg, say "one-two," not "twelve").[2,6]
- Allow only licensed healthcare providers to receive verbal orders.

Managing Medications Off the Sterile Field

Medications should be properly stored to ensure a process for safe and efficient delivery to the patient. Several key issues to consider are environmental conditions for storing medications to ensure product stability, look-alike and sound-alike medication storage, modification of the standard alphabetical medication storage system, and the care and handling of medical gases, reagents, and chemicals to eliminate catastrophic mistakes.[4]

- Standardize and limit the variation of strengths and concentrations of medications as much as possible.[3,4]
- Store medications safely with consideration given to separation of look-alikes and sound-alikes. This includes separating by generic name and packaging to the extent possible.[3,4,7]
- Limit the use of multidose vials whenever possible.[4,8,9]
- Include the facility pharmacist in formulating processes to determine when or if unused and unopened medications are allowed to be returned to the pharmacy.[4]
- Do not store medications alphabetically.[4]
- Label storage areas with both the medication's generic and brand names.
- Verify medication labels after medication retrieval and reconfirm with the written medication order.
- Label all medications, medication containers, and other solutions off the sterile field even if only one medication is involved.[3]

- At shift change or upon staff relief, all medications, medication labels, and the amount of medication administered should be verified concurrently by entering and exiting personnel.
- Discard any unlabeled solution or medication found in the O.R.
- Treat medical gases, chemicals, and reagents (eg, formalin, normal saline, Lugol's solution, radiopaque dyes, glutaraldehyde) in the O.R. with the same care and caution as medications.

Delivering Medications to the Sterile Field

Before administering any medication, a verification process should include a review of the product label for the medication name, strength, and expiration date. This review process should be accomplished in conjunction with an examination of the written medication order to confirm that the correct medication is to be administered. A visual inspection should be made for any indication that the medication was compromised during the storage process (eg, particulates, discoloration).[4]

- Confirm all medications listed on the physician's preference list with the surgeon before delivery to the sterile field.
- Orders with abbreviations, symbols, or acronyms should be clarified with the ordering clinician to minimize confusion or misinterpretation.
- Verify medication in its original container for the correct name, strength, dosage, and route with the surgeon's preference card or documented verbal order.
- Actively communicate the medication name, strength, dosage, and expiration date as the medication is passed to the sterile field.[4]
  - Verbally and visually confirm all medications delivered to the sterile field, including medication name, strength, dosage, and expiration date.[4]
  - Medications should be verified concurrently by the circulating registered nurse and scrub person.
  - If there is no designated scrub person, the circulating registered nurse should confirm the medication visually and verbally with the licensed professional performing the surgical procedure.
- Deliver one medication at a time onto the sterile field.
- Do not remove stoppers from vials for the purpose of pouring medications.
- Use commercially available sterile transfer devices when possible (eg, sterile vial spike, filter straw, plastic catheter).
- Reconfirm maximum dose limits.

Managing Medications on the Sterile Field

Communication is a vital key to the success of the medication delivery process.

- Verbally and visually confirm the medication (ie, medication name, strength, dosage, and expiration date) upon receipt from the circulating registered nurse even if only one medication is involved.[4]
- Label the medication container on the sterile field immediately before receipt of the medication. Avoid distractions and interruptions during the labeling process and while dispensing medications onto the sterile field.
- Label all medication containers and delivery devices with a minimum of the medication name, strength, and concentration when needed.[6]
- Verbally and visually confirm the medication name, strength, and dose by reading the medication label aloud while passing a medication to the licensed professional performing the procedure.[4]
- When patient hand-offs (eg, personnel relief) occur, the medication verification process should take place. The medication should be confirmed for accuracy (ie, product label reviewed for the medication name, strength, and expiration date) in conjunction with a review of the written medication order to validate that the correct medication is on the field.[3]
- Discard any solution or medication found on or off the sterile field without an identification label.

AORN GUIDANCE STATEMENT: SAFE MEDICATION PRACTICES IN PERIOPERATIVE SETTINGS ACROSS THE LIFE SPAN *(Continued)*

Documenting All Intraoperative Medications

A complete and accurate accounting of the medications and solutions used during the surgical encounter is essential to address medication-related issues that may arise during all phases of perioperative care.[4]

- Ensure that intraoperative documentation reflects all medications (including irrigation solutions, doses, and routes of administration) administered throughout the procedure.
- Document medication administration per organizational policy.
- Documentation should incorporate the Perioperative Nursing Data Set (PNDS). The expected outcome for safe medication practices is outcome O9, "The patient receives appropriate medication(s), safely administered during the perioperative period." This outcome falls within the domain of Safety (D1). The associated nursing diagnoses may include X29, "Risk for injury." The associated interventions leading to the desired outcome include I123, "Verifies allergies"; I8, "Administers prescribed medications and solutions"; and I51, "Evaluates response to medications."[10 (p 103-4)]

Monitoring Patients for Effects of Medications

Assessment and documentation of the patient's response to medication administration provides vital clues related to dose effectiveness and the presence of a potential medication-related adverse effect.[4]

- Continually assess, monitor, and document the patient's response to medication administered.[4,10 (p 104)]
- Policies and procedures should be developed for reporting and responding to medication errors and other adverse effects.
- Error reporting should occur in a nonpunitive culture.[3]

Retaining All Original Medication / Solution Containers and Delivery Devices

The practice of maintaining possession of medication containers and delivery devices until the patient leaves the O.R. is important in the event of a medication-related error or adverse reaction. A root cause analysis should be performed following any adverse event. Maintaining possession of these containers may facilitate the analysis.

Periodic Evaluation of the Medication Management Process

An essential step in the medication management process includes ongoing review. An established QI/PI program may identify failure points contributing to medication errors and may aid in improvements in patient safety.

- The QI/PI program should include a routine review and update of all preprinted order sheets, and facility-approved standing orders, including
  - medication choice
  - dose, and
  - delivery method
- Eliminate or minimize the use of problem-prone abbreviations, symbols, and acronyms.[11,12,13]

Additional Strategies for Medication Safety

1. Operationalize a process for the ongoing review of key elements of the medication delivery process known to contribute to medication errors, to include
   - prescribing
   - order processing
   - dispensing
   - administration, and
   - monitoring[14]

2. Provide O.R. personnel with appropriate and timely education related to medication safety procedures. Facilities should implement processes for validating perioperative medication competency covering all age-specific populations (eg, perioperative medication competencies in "AORN's safe medication administration tool kit").[15]
3. Use a competency checklist focused on the medication delivery process (eg, perioperative medication performance validation record in "AORN's safe medication administration tool kit").[15]
4. Establish outcomes, standards, and guidelines to monitor and manage institutional improvements in regard to medication safety, to include
   - the patient receives appropriate prescribed medication(s) safely administered during the perioperative period[10 (p 103)]
   - the patient demonstrates knowledge of medication management[10 (p 179)]
   - the patient demonstrates knowledge of pain management[10 (p 179)]
5. Modify work schedule requirements in surgical settings to minimize fatigue-induced errors.
6. Provide adequate lighting in dark environments (eg, endoscopy, minimally invasive procedures, ophthalmic procedures).
7. Initiate constraints and/or forcing functions to minimize risks related to medication management and administration.
   - Constraints are approaches that make a medication error difficult. Examples include dose limit protocols, automatic stop orders, triple-checking medications, and labeling all medication containers in the O.R.
   - Forcing functions are approaches that make a medication error impossible. Examples include removing certain medications (eg, cytotoxic agents, concentrations of saline higher than 0.9%) from the O.R.[3,16]
8. Adopt guidelines for unapproved abbreviations, acronyms, and symbols outlined in national patient safety initiatives.[11,12,13]
   - Care must be taken to decrease the risk for error and maximize patient safety by avoiding error-prone abbreviations and symbols known to cause confusion or lead to misinterpretation. Examples:
     - Use of the handwritten letter "U" for "units" can be mistaken for a zero.[11,12,13]
     - Zeros in combination with decimal points can lead to a 10-fold dosing error when the decimal point is not detected.[16]
   - A supplemental list or poster placed in the workplace outlining common abbreviation mistakes may help to focus attention on high-risk avoidance.[17]
   - Recommendations and guidance provided by the ISMP "List of error-prone abbreviations, symbols, and dose designations"; the USP "Potentially dangerous abbreviations"; and the JCAHO "Official 'Do Not Use' List" should be considered.
9. Ensure that current and reliable medication reference materials with age-specific guidelines are readily available to the perioperative team.
10. Provide pharmacy support for consultation regarding unusual medications and dosages.
11. Standardize institutional forms to aid communication and decrease confusion while enhancing productivity between healthcare providers.[3]

Footnotes

[1]Institute of Medicine, *To Err Is Human: Building a Safer Health System*, Committee on Quality of Heath Care in America, Kohn L, Corrigan J, and Donaldson M, eds, Washington, DC: National Academy Press, 2000, 27.

[2]"Council Recommendations to Reduce Medication Errors Associated With Verbal Medication Orders and Prescriptions," (Feb 20, 2001) National Coordinating Council for Medication Error Reporting and Prevention, http://www.nccmerp.org/council/council2001-02-20.html?USP (accessed 23 Jan 2006).

[3]"Facts About 2006 National Patient Safety Goals," Joint Commission on Accreditation of Healthcare Organizations, http://www.jcaho.org/accredited+organizations/patient+safety/06_npsg/06_facts.htm (accessed 23 Jan 2006).

AORN GUIDANCE STATEMENT: SAFE MEDICATION PRACTICES IN PERIOPERATIVE SETTINGS ACROSS THE LIFE SPAN *(Continued)*

[4]Rich DS, "New JCAHO Medication Management Standards for 2004," Am J Health-Sys Pharm, 61 (July 2004) 1349-58.
[5]"Therapeutic Duplication," Administration on Aging, http://www.homemeds.org/pdf_files/ProtocolUnnec.Therap_2.pdf (accessed 23 Jan 2006).
[6]"Joint Commission 2006 National Patient Safety Goals: Implementation Expectations," Joint Commission on Accreditation of Healthcare Organizations, http://www.jcaho.org/accredited+organizations/patient+safety/06_npsg_ie.pdf (accessed 23 Jan 2006).
[7]Joint Commission on Accreditation of Healthcare Organizations, "Look-Alike, Sound-Alike Drug Names," Sentinel Event Alert 19 (May 2001). Also available at http://www.jcaho.org/about+us/news+letters/sentinel+event+alert/sea_19.htm (accessed 23 Jan 2006).
[8]Institute for Safe Medication Practices, "Patient Safety Movement Calls for Reexamination of Multidose Vial Use," ISMP Medication Safety Alert (June 14, 2000). Also available at http://www.ismp.org/newsletters/acutecare/articles/20000614.asp (accessed 23 Jan 2006).
[9]Institute for Safe Medication Practices, "New Official Interpretation of JCAHO Standard Bars Access to Pharmacy After Hours," ISMP Medication Safety Alert (May 30, 2001). Also available at http://www.ismp.org/newsletters/acutecare articles/20010530.asp (accessed 23 Jan 2006).
[10]Beyea S, ed, Perioperative Nursing Data Set: The Perioperative Nursing Vocabulary, 2nd ed, Denver, CO: AORN, Inc, 2002, 103-4, 179.
[11]"The Official 'Do Not Use' List," Joint Commission on Accreditation of Healthcare Organizations, http://www.jcaho.org/accredited+organizations/patient+safety/dnu.htm (accessed 9 Oct 2005).
[12]United States Pharmacopeia, "Abbreviations Can Lead to Medication Errors," USP Quality Review No 80 (July 2004). Also available at http://www.usp.org/patientSafety/newsletters/qualityReview/qr802004-07-01.html (accessed 23 Jan 2006).
[13]"ISMP's List of Error-Prone Abbreviations, Symbols, and Dose Designations," Institute for Safe Medication Practices, http://www.ismp.org/tools/errorproneabbreviations.pdf (accessed 23 Jan 2006).
[14]"Frequently Asked Questions," Institute for Safe Medication Practices, http://www.ismp.org/faq.asp#Question_9 (accessed 9 Oct 2005).
[15]"AORN's Safe Medication Administration Tool Kit," AORN Online, http://www.aorn.org/toolkit/safemed (accessed 23 Jan 2006).
[16]Joint Commission on Accreditation of Healthcare Organizations, "High-Alert Medications and Patient Safety," Sentinel Event Alert 11 (Nov 19, 1999). Also available at http://www.jcaho.org/about+us/news+letters/sentinel+event+alert/sea_11.htm (accessed 23 Jan 2006).
[17]"Joint Commission Perspectives on Patient Safety: Maintaining Safety/Reducing Risk," Joint Commission Resources 2 (September 2002) 1-11.

Resources

Agency for Healthcare Research and Quality, http://www.ahrq.gov (accessed 29 Oct 2003).
Institute of Medicine, http://www.iom.edu (accessed 29 Oct 2003).
Institute for Safe Medication Practices, http://www.ismp.org (accessed 29 Oct 2003).
National Patient Safety Foundation, http://www.npsf.org (accessed 29 Oct 2003).
Partnership for Patient Safety, http://www.p4ps.org (accessed 29 Oct 2003).
The Leapfrog Group, http://www.leapfroggroup.org (accessed 29 Oct 2003).
The National Quality Forum, http://www.qualityforum.org (accessed 29 Oct 2003).
United States Pharmacopeia, http://www.usp.org (accessed 29 Aug 2005).

Originally published May 2002, *AORN Journal.*
Revised November 2003; published March 2004, *AORN Journal.*
Revised November 2005; scheduled for publication in the *AORN Journal* in 2006.

AORN GUIDANCE STATEMENT: "DO NOT USE" ABBREVIATIONS, ACRONYMS, DOSAGE DESIGNATIONS, AND SYMBOLS

Preamble

Confusing or easily misinterpreted abbreviations, acronyms, or symbols put caregivers at risk for making errors and compromising patient safety. Unintentional as an error may be, a misplaced decimal point, a "U" interpreted as a "0" (zero), QOD confused for QID, or AS misinterpreted as OS puts patients at risk for medical error with potential catastrophic results (eg, overdose, inadequate dose, omission due to laterality error, wrong medication administered, error in frequency of administration). Improving communication through reducing and standardizing abbreviations, acronyms, and symbols is a significant step toward reducing the occurrence of errors related to the inability to accurately read and interpret written medical orders and transcribed verbal orders.

The purpose of this guidance statement is to heighten the awareness of perioperative registered nurses concerning the dangers associated with the use of abbreviations, acronyms, and symbols, with the goal of eliminating their use in healthcare documentation. All perioperative settings should address the issue of error-prone abbreviations. These practice settings include, but are not limited to, hospital operating rooms, ambulatory surgery centers, preanesthesia and postanesthesia care units, cardiac catheterization departments, endoscopy suites, radiology departments, and all other areas where operative and other invasive procedures may be performed. Patient safety in the perioperative setting may be improved by focusing on communication among caregivers through the creation of a standardized list of "do-not-use" abbreviations, acronyms, and symbols.

Effective January 1, 2004, the Joint Commission on Accreditation of Healthcare Organizations (JCAHO) developed a list of dangerous abbreviations, acronyms, and symbols that are **not** to be used within accredited healthcare facilities. This requirement is intended as a means to improve communication among caregivers (see National Patient Safety Goal #2).[1] The Joint Commission's minimal list of required do-not-use abbreviations, acronyms, and symbols is the beginning of a process to assist organizations with the expansion of their error-prevention programs to improve safety for patients. The Joint Commission recommends that organizations limit the use of abbreviations initially by eliminating nine specific error-prone abbreviations from healthcare documentation. Seven additional error-prone abbreviations, acronyms, or symbols will be reviewed on an annual basis for inclusion on the official do-not-use list. Implementing this change in practice keeps an organization on a trajectory focused on patient safety as the number-one priority.

Guidance Statement

AORN recommends that all perioperative settings implement the Joint Commission's National Patient Safety Goal #2, adopt the minimum required list of do-not-use abbreviations, educate perioperative registered nurses regarding the removal of these items from all healthcare documentation, and monitor compliance with this activity. The following chart represents the Joint Commission's official list of do-not-use abbreviations, acronyms, and symbols, published January 1, 2004.

AORN GUIDANCE STATEMENT: "DO NOT USE" ABBREVIATIONS, ACRONYMS, DOSAGE DESIGNATIONS, AND SYMBOLS *(Continued)*

JCAHO's Required List of "Do-Not-Use" Abbreviations, Acronyms, and Symbols

Official "Do Not Use" List[1]

Do Not Use	Potential Problem	Use Instead
U (unit)	Mistaken for "0" (zero), the number "4" (four) or "cc"	Write "unit"
IU (International Unit)	Mistaken for IV (intravenous) or the number 10 (ten)	Write "International Unit"
Q.D., QD, q.d., qd (daily)	Mistaken for each other	Write "daily"
Q.O.D., QOD, q.o.d., qod (every other day)	Period after the Q mistaken for "I" and the "O" mistaken for "I"	Write "every other day"
Trailing zero (X.0 mg)[2]	Decimal point is missed	Write X mg
Lack of leading zero (.X mg)		Write 0.X mg
MS	Can mean morphine sulfate or magnesium sulfate	Write "morphine sulfate"
MSO_4 and $MgSO_4$	Confused for one another	Write "magnesium sulfate"

[1]Applies to all orders and all medication-related documentation that is handwritten (including free-text computer entry) or on preprinted forms.

[2]**Exception:** A "trailing zero" may be used only where required to demonstrate the level of precision of the value being reported, such as for laboratory results, imaging studies that report size of lesions, or catheter/tube sizes. It may not be used in medication orders or other medication-related documentation.

The minimum required list provided above is the first step in fulfilling JCAHO's National Patient Safety Goal #2. With the goal of eliminating all abbreviations from the healthcare setting, the Joint Commission is encouraging, but not mandating, each organization to voluntarily expand the above list with the addition of the do-not-use abbreviations, acronyms, and symbols identified as possible future inclusions to the "Official 'Do Not Use' List." Items in the following table have been identified by the Joint Commission, in concert with the Institute for Safe Medication Practice (ISMP), United States Pharmacopecia (USP), and the National Coordinating Council for Medication Error Reporting and Prevention (NCCMERP), to be considered annually as potential error-prone abbreviations to be included on the official do-not-use list.

Potential Additional "Do Not Use" Abbreviations, Acronyms, and Symbols

Additional Abbreviations, Acronyms, and Symbols

(For possible future inclusion in the Official "Do Not Use" List)

Do Not Use	Potential Problem	Use Instead
> (greater than) < (less than)	Misinterpreted as the number "7" (seven) or the letter "L" Confused for one another	Write "greater than" Write "less than"
Abbreviations for drug names	Misinterpreted due to similar abbreviations for multiple drugs	Write drug names in full
Apothecary units	Unfamiliar to many practitioners Confused with metric units	Use metric units
@	Mistaken for the number "2" (two)	Write "at"
cc	Mistaken for U (units) when poorly written	Write "mL" or "milliliters"
µg	Mistaken for mg (milligrams) resulting in one thousand-fold overdose	Write "mcg" or "micrograms"

Furthermore, AORN strongly recommends consideration be given to the selection of problem-prone, high-risk, high-volume abbreviations, acronyms, and symbols unique to the perioperative practice setting when augmenting the minimally required list of do-not-use items. At a minimum, abbreviations related to laterality should be eliminated from all documentation within the perioperative setting.

Error-Prone Abbreviation	Potential Problem	Preferred Term
L, R, Bil	Illegibility leads to confusion related to correct identification of laterality	Write out *left*, *right*, and *bilateral*

Further sources of information to help guide in the selection of do-not-use items may be derived from a review of problem-prone, high-risk, high-volume abbreviations, acronyms, and symbols found within handwritten, preprinted, and electronic forms of perioperative communication, such as

- surgical procedure list
- surgeon preference or procedure cards
- perioperative documentation (ie, preoperative, intraoperative, postoperative)
- progress notes
- specimen labeling
- consent
- history and physical
- surgical schedules
- staff orientation and competency materials
- patient teaching materials

Another strategy to improve communication among caregivers is a process to ensure that the signatures of the provider initiating the medical order and the caregiver transcribing the verbal order are legible. AORN suggests that all healthcare providers use block print and sign their names to all written and verbal orders. The extra step of block-printing the name affords the caregiver an opportunity to contact the provider if a question, concern, or issue were to arise related to the written order. If the caregiver is unable to read the written order, confusion or misinterpretation could result and lead to an adverse patient event.

This guidance statement reflects suggested minimal requirements to promote safety in patient care. It is not to be considered an all-inclusive listing of

AORN GUIDANCE STATEMENT: "DO NOT USE" ABBREVIATIONS, ACRONYMS, DOSAGE DESIGNATIONS, AND SYMBOLS *(Continued)*

error-prone abbreviations, acronyms, dosage designations, or symbols. It is the responsibility of the healthcare practitioner, in concert with the patient care organization, to ensure that documentation clearly and unambiguously reflects the individualized treatment of the patient.

Footnotes

[1]"National Patient Safety Goals," Joint Commission on Accreditation of Healthcare Organizations, http://www.jcaho.org/general+public/patient+safety/04_npsg.htm (2004) and http://www.jcaho.org/accredited +organizations/patient+safety/npsg.htm (2005-2006) (accessed 7 Sept 2005).
[2]"Official 'Do Not Use' List," Joint Commission on Accreditation of Healthcare Organizations, http://www.jcaho.org/accredited+organizations/patient+safety/dnu.htm (accessed 7 Sept 2005).

Additional Reading

Abbreviations Lists

Hicks RW, Cousins DD, and Williams RL, *Summary of Information Submitted to MEDMARX in the Year 2002: The Quest for Quality*, Rockville, MD: US Pharmacopecia Center for the Advancement of Patient Safety, 2003, 41-4.

Institute for Safe Medication Practices, "ISMP's List of Error-Prone Abbreviations, Symbols, and Dose Designations," *ISMP Medication Safety Alert 8 No 24* (November 27, 2003). Also available at http://www.ismp.org/PDF/ISMP Abbreviations.pdf or http://www.ismp.org/PDF/ErrorProne.pdf (accessed 8 Sept 2005).

Joint Commission on Accreditation of Healthcare Organizations, "Medication Errors Related to Potentially Dangerous Abbreviations," *Sentinel Event Alert 23* (September 2001). Also available at http://www.jcaho.org/about +us/news+letters/sentinel+event+alert/sea_23.htm (accessed 8 Sept 2005).

"New Joint Commission 'Do Not Use' List: Abbreviations, Acronyms, and Symbols," American Academy of Physical Medicine and Rehabilitation, http://www.aapmr.org/hpl/pracguide/jcahosymbols.htm (accessed 7 Sept 2005).

"Recommendations to Enhance Accuracy of Prescription Writing," (adopted Sept 4, 1996, revised June 2, 2005) National Coordinating Council for Medication Error Reporting and Prevention (NCCMERP), http://www.nccmerp.org/council/council1996-09-04.html (accessed 8 Sept 2005).

Implementation / Staff Education

Beyea SC, "Best Practices for Abbreviation Use," *AORN Journal*, 2004, 79(3):641-2.

"Five Dangerous Medical Abbreviations," *Ohioans First*, http://www.ohioansfirst.org/abbreviations/abbrev.htm (accessed 7 Sept 2005).

"Implementation Tips for Eliminating Dangerous Abbreviations," Joint Commission on Accreditation of Healthcare Organizations, http://www.jcaho.org/accredited+organizations/patient+safety/05+npsg/tips.htm (accessed 8 Sept 2005).

"Maximizing Patient Safety in the Medication Use Process: Practice Guidelines and Best Demonstrated Practices," Wisconsin Patient Safety Institute, http://www.wpsi.org/media/documents/pdf/Max_Pat_Saft_2002.pdf (accessed 31 Jan 2006).

"Patient Safety Program," US Department of Defense, http://patientsafety.satx.disa.mil (accessed 7 Sept 2005).

"Preventing Medical Errors: More on Dangerous Abbreviations," *Patient Safety News*, Show #25, March 2004, US Food and Drug Administration, http://www.accessdata.fda.gov/scripts/cdrh/cfdocs/psn/transcript.cfm?show=25 (accessed 31 Jan 2006).

Regional Medication Safety Program for Hospitals: Health Care Improvement Foundation. *Medication Safety Solutions Kit*, information available from Delaware Valley Healthcare Council, http://www.dvhc.org/safety/program/details.asp?ID=CQe3RU219Ngec94UQJ3g. Also available from ECRI, http://www.ecri.org/products_and_services/products/medication_safety/medsafetybrochure.pdf (accessed 7 Sept 2005).

Scheduled for publication in the *AORN Journal* in 2006.

COMMON SYMBOLS AND ABBREVIATIONS

Abbreviation	Meaning
°C	degrees Celsius (Centigrade)
<	less than
>	greater than
≤	less than or equal to
≥	greater than or equal to
µg	microgram
µmol	micromole
$\overline{aa}$, aa	of each
AAPC	antibiotic associated pseudomembranous colitis
ABG	arterial blood gas
ABMT	autologous bone marrow transplant
ac	before meals or food
ACE	angiotensin-converting enzyme
ACLS	advanced cardiac life support
ad	to, up to
a.d.	right ear
ADH	antidiuretic hormone
ad lib	at pleasure
AED	antiepileptic drug
AIDS	acquired immunodeficiency syndrome
a.l.	left ear
ALL	acute lymphoblastic leukemia
ALT	alanine aminotransferase (formerly called SGPT)
AM	morning
AML	acute myeloblastic leukemia
amp	ampul
amt	amount
ANA	antinuclear antibodies
ANC	absolute neutrophil count
ANLL	acute nonlymphoblastic leukemia
APTT	activated partial thromboplastin time
aq	water
aq. dest.	distilled water
a.s.	left ear
ASA (class I-IV)	American Society of Anesthesiology physical status classification of surgical patients according to their baseline health
	ASA I: Normal healthy patients
	ASA II: Patients having controlled disease states (eg, controlled hypertension)
	ASA III: Patients having a disease which compromises their organ function (eg, decompensated CHF, end stage renal failure)
	ASA IV: Patients who are extremely critically ill
ASAP	as soon as possible
AST	aspartate aminotransferase (formerly called SGOT)
a.u.	each ear
AUC	area under the curve (area under the serum concentration-time curve)
A-V	atrial-ventricular

COMMON SYMBOLS AND ABBREVIATIONS *(Continued)*

(continued)

Abbreviation	Meaning
bid	twice daily
bm	bowel movement
BMT	bone marrow transplant
bp	blood pressure
BPH	benign prostatic hyperplasia
BSA	body surface area
BUN	blood urea nitrogen
c	a gallon
$\bar{c}$	with
cal	calorie
cAMP	cyclic adenosine monophosphate
cap	capsule
CBC	complete blood count
cc	cubic centimeter
CHF	congestive heart failure
CI	cardiac index
Cl_{cr}	creatinine clearance
cm	centimeter
CMV	cytomegalovirus
CNS	central nervous system
comp	compound
cont	continue
COPD	chronic obstructive pulmonary disease
CSF	cerebrospinal fluid
CT	computed tomography
CVA	cerebral vascular accident
CVP	central venous pressure
d	day
D_5W	dextrose 5% in water
D_5/1/2NS	dextrose 5% in sodium chloride 0.45%
$D_{10}W$	dextrose 10% in water
d/c	discontinue
DIC	disseminated intravascular coagulation
dil	dilute
disp	dispense
div	divide
DL_{co}	pulmonary diffusion capacity for carbon monoxide
DNA	deoxyribonucleic acid
dtd	give of such a dose
DVT	deep vein thrombosis
ECHO	echocardiogram
ECMO	extracorporeal membrane oxygenation
EEG	electroencephalogram
EKG	electrocardiogram
elix, el	elixir
emp	as directed
ESR	erythrocyte sedimentation rate
et	and
E.T.	endotracheal

(continued)

Abbreviation	Meaning
ex aq	in water
f, ft	make, let be made
FDA	Food and Drug Administration
FEV_1	forced expiratory volume exhaled after 1 second
FSH	follicle-stimulating hormone
FVC	forced vital capacity
g	gram
G6PD	glucose-6-phosphate dehydrogenase
GA	gestational age
GABA	gamma-aminobutyric acid
GE	gastroesophageal
GI	gastrointestinal
gr	grain
gtt	a drop
GU	genitourinary
h	hour
HIV	human immunodeficiency virus
HPLC	high performance liquid chromatography
hs	at bedtime
IBW	ideal body weight
ICP	intracranial pressure
IgG	immune globulin G
I.M.	intramuscular
INR	international normalized ratio
int. unit	international units
I.O.	intraosseous
I & O	input and output
IOP	intraocular pressure
I.T.	intrathecal
I.V.	intravenous
IVH	intraventricular hemorrhage
IVP	intravenous push
JRA	juvenile rheumatoid arthritis
kcal	kilocalorie
kg	kilogram
L	liter
LDH	lactate dehydrogenase
LE	lupus erythematosus
LH	luteinizing hormone
liq	a liquor, solution
LP	lumbar puncture
LR	lactated Ringer's
M	mix
MAC	*Mycobacterium avium* complex
MAO	monoamine oxidase
MAP	mean arterial pressure
mcg	microgram
m. dict	as directed
mEq	milliequivalent
mg	milligram
MI	myocardial infarction

COMMON SYMBOLS AND ABBREVIATIONS *(Continued)*

(continued)

Abbreviation	Meaning
min	minute
mixt	a mixture
mL	milliliter
mm	millimeter
mo	month
mOsm	milliosmoles
MRI	magnetic resonance image
MRSA	methicillin-resistant *Staphylococcus aureus*
NCI	National Cancer Institute
ND	nasoduodenal
NF	National Formulary
ng	nanogram
NG	nasogastric
NMDA	n-methyl-d-aspartate
nmol	nanomole
no.	number
noc	in the night
non rep	do not repeat, no refills
NPO	nothing by mouth
NSAID	nonsteroidal anti-inflammatory drug
O, Oct	a pint
o.d.	right eye
o.l.	left eye
O.R.	operating room
o.s.	left eye
OTC	over-the-counter (nonprescription)
o.u.	each eye
PABA	para-aminobenzoic acid
PALS	pediatric advanced life support
pc, post cib	after meals
PCA	postconceptional age
PCP	*Pneumocystis carinii* pneumonia
PCWP	pulmonary capillary wedge pressure
PDA	patent ductus arteriosus
per	through or by
PIP	peak inspiratory pressure
PM	afternoon or evening
PNA	postnatal age
P.O.	by mouth
P.R.	rectally
prn	as needed
PSVT	paroxysmal supraventricular tachycardia
PT	prothrombin time
PTT	partial thromboplastin time
PUD	peptic ulcer disease
pulv	a powder
PVC	premature ventricular contraction
PVR	peripheral vascular resistance
q	every

(continued)

Abbreviation	Meaning
qad	every other day
qd	every day
qh	every hour
qid	four times a day
qod	every other day
qs	a sufficient quantity
qs ad, qsad	a sufficient quantity to make, add amount to equal
qty	quantity
qv	as much as you wish
RAP	right arterial pressure
RIA	radioimmunoassay
RNA	ribonucleic acid
Rx	take, a recipe
rep	let it be repeated
$\bar{s}$	without
S-A	sino-atrial
sa	according to art
sat	saturated
S_{cr}	serum creatinine
SIADH	syndrome of inappropriate antidiuretic hormone
sig	label, or let it be printed
SL	sublingual
SLE	systemic lupus erythematosus
sol	solution
solv	dissolve
$\overline{ss}$	one-half
sos	if there is need
stat	at once, immediately
supp	suppository
SubQ	subcutaneous
SVR	systemic vascular resistance
SVT	supraventricular tachycardia
SWI	sterile water for injection
syr	syrup
T_3	triiodothyronine
T_4	thyroxine
tab	tablet
tal	such
TIBC	total iron binding capacity
tid	three times a day
TPN	total parenteral nutrition
tr, tinct	tincture
trit	triturate
TSH	thyroid stimulating hormone
tsp	teaspoonful
TT	thrombin time
u.d., ut dict	as directed
ung	ointment
USAN	United States Adopted Names
USP	United States Pharmacopeia
UTI	urinary tract infection

COMMON SYMBOLS AND ABBREVIATIONS *(Continued)*

(continued)

Abbreviation	Meaning
V_d	volume of distribution
V_{dss}	volume of distribution at steady-state
VMA	vanillylmandelic acid
v.o.	verbal order
w.a.	while awake
w/w	weight for weight
x3	3 times
x4	4 times
y, yr	year

BASIC PHARMACOTHERAPEUTIC CONCEPTS

Safe and effective drug therapy requires an understanding of the basic principles of pharmacokinetics and pharmacodynamics and an awareness of how individual patient traits and lifestyles influence the actions and effects of drugs. A brief overview of basic concepts is discussed on the following pages.

1. Pharmacokinetics and Pharmacodynamics
2. Patient Factors That Influence Drug Therapy (pregnancy, age, weight, lifestyle)
3. Pharmacotherapeutics

PHARMACOKINETICS

The pharmacokinetics principles of absorption, distribution, and elimination govern how quickly a drug becomes available to the target organ and how long the drug will remain available.

Absorption

Absorption refers to how a drug progresses from the dosage form given into one bodily compartment into the blood stream to be distributed to the target site of action. The rate and degree of absorption depends on the formulation of the drug, the route of drug administration, and physiological variables. Drugs administered by the I.V. route require no absorption since they enter the circulatory system directly. Intramuscularly or subcutaneously administered drugs involve differing degrees of absorption. For instance, formulations in oil or microfine crystals (long-acting) have longer absorption times than other formulations and drugs administered into the deltoid muscle are absorbed faster than those administered into the gluteus muscle because of the increased blood flow in the deltoid muscle.

The oral route of drug administration is the preferred route for most drug therapy because it is more comfortable for the patient and usually safer and easier to use. The enteral route however, has a longer absorption time than other routes of absorption. This is, in part, related to the particular drug formulation (compressed tablet, extended release, repeat action). Anything that reduces systemic blood flow can reduce absorption rates, strenuous exercise decreases splanchnic blood flow as more blood is diverted to the muscles; pain and stress can also reduce blood flow in this area. Prolonged intestinal transit time (experienced with high-fat meals, solid food, anticholinergic drugs) may delay absorption rate, but increase the amount of total drug absorption. In addition, drug-drug interactions or drug-food interactions can reduce absorption; substances that significantly alter the gastric pH (eg, H_2-blockers, such as famotidine or proton pump inhibitors such as omeprazole, etc) can, in turn effect the absorption rates of some drugs. Absorption from the gastrointestinal tract may involve active transport across membranes. Some enzymes actually "pump" drug back into the GI lumen, opposing their absorption. One such enzyme is p-glycoprotein. Drugs which inhibit p-glycoprotein abolish this "pumping" action, and may lead to dramatic increases in the absorption of some drugs.

Orally administered drugs must pass through the portal system before they enter the systemic circulation. Many drugs undergo metabolic changes as they pass through the liver prior to reaching the systemic circulation. This means a substantial portion of the dose will never reach its target tissue (first-pass effect). The orally administered dose required to achieve a specific therapeutic response may, therefore be much larger than the dose for a route that bypasses portal circulation (parenteral or transdermal). Enterohepatic recycling (reabsorption) may occur with some drugs and may be a particular concern in some cases of toxicity. A few drugs (eg, digoxin, leflunomide, levothyroxine) re-enter the gastrointestinal tract (via excretion in the bile) from the bloodstream. They are then reabsorbed from the intestine and re-enter the circulatory system. Administration of substances, such as charcoal or cholestyramine resin (Questran®) or sodium polystyrene sulfonate (Kayexalate®), that bind the recycled drug in the GI tract, may be necessary to rapidly reduce the toxic serum levels of the recycled drug.

BASIC PHARMACOTHERAPEUTIC CONCEPTS *(Continued)*

Other routes of drug administration (eg, vaginal, rectal, topical, buccal, inhalation) all have positive and negative aspects of absorption. Advantages of drug absorption via these alternative sites include the ability to establish relatively high local concentrations of drugs at target tissues as well as the ability to bypass the "first-pass" metabolism of orally administered drugs. Drugs administered by inhalation must be formulated in microsized particles and are typically administered by nebulization or aerosolization in order to reach the terminal airways. Rectal absorption for systemic drugs is generally slow and administration of these drugs is often uncomfortable or painful. However, for some drugs and for some patients (for example, in severe nausea where oral medications cannot be administered), this is either the only route available or may be the route of choice. Topical absorption has the advantage of continuous absorption, although onset of action is generally slower than other forms of administration and degree of absorption may differ considerably depending on patient characteristics. Transdermal formulations have been designed to work together with the absorptive properties of the skin and may allow the delivery of a consistent rate of drug absorption for several days. Drugs for ophthalmic and otic administration are highly specific and are designed to produce high local concentrations, however healthcare professionals should also take the absorption properties and systemic effects of drugs administered by these routes into consideration.

Distribution

Distribution of an absorbed drug is dependent on several physical and/or chemical characteristics of the drug, including affinity for lipid or aqueous tissue and ability to permeate various tissue barriers (sometimes through the assistance of specific transport proteins), pH differences, blood flow, and degree of protein binding. The size and charge of the drug molecules will also help determine to which bodily compartment they are distributed. Drugs localize to specific tissues according to the combined properties of both drug and tissue. Drug concentrations can vary considerably between organs.

Drugs enter the system by one or another means of absorption, circulate (distribute) through the body via the circulatory system, interact with target receptors, and are excreted from the body in due course. When blood flow is impeded, the distribution of any substance in the blood is also impeded. Anything that alters the concentration of blood (eg, dehydration or edema) may also impact the distribution of drug molecules to the target site.

Albumin levels may also influence the distribution of some drugs that have a potential for binding to large proteins. Usually, the degree to which any drug binds to albumin remains predictable (eg, gentamicin <30% bound and warfarin >97% bound). Dosing recommendations are predicated on the idea that a certain level of unbound molecules remain "free" in the circulation when albumin levels are "normal." When disease states, nutritional status, or other drugs significantly change the amount of albumin available for binding or the ability to bind to this "carrier" protein, toxic serum levels of free (unbound) drug may occur.

Physiological barriers also influence distribution. One example is the blood-brain barrier that is a continuous network of cells with tight junctions that make the brain impermeable to some drugs according to their degree of water or lipid solubility. This makes the brain less accessible to drugs that are able to accumulate in other tissues (eg, many chemotherapeutic drugs and many antibiotics). In addition to this physical barrier, a substantial part of the ability of the brain to exclude certain chemicals is related to the presence of specialized transport proteins which actively "pump" these chemicals out of the CSF. Drugs which inhibit transport enzymes may influence the ability of drug to accumulate in tissues such as the brain.

Elimination via Metabolism

Elimination via metabolism is the process of biotransformation that occurs when a drug changes from its parent form to a more water-soluble form.

Some drugs are not metabolized and are excreted from the body unchanged (aminoglycosides, gabapentin). However, most drugs are metabolized in the liver, in tissues, in the gastric system, or in the lungs. The metabolites are most often inactive forms of the parent that are more water soluble than the parent drug and can therefore be excreted in the urine. In some instances, metabolism is required to convert a biologically inactive drug (prodrug) to an active form. Dopamine does not cross the blood-brain barrier; however, levodopa, an inactive precursor of dopamine, does cross the blood-brain barrier where it is metabolized to dopamine. In other cases, metabolism results in active metabolites (imipramine metabolizes to desipramine).

Hepatic metabolism is a result of specific enzymes and can be influenced by other drugs. In particular, enzymes belonging to the cytochrome P450 family are frequently involved in drug metabolism. Some drugs stimulate an increase in specific enzyme activity which increases the metabolism breakdown of other drugs; thereby decreasing the availability of the second drug (eg, phenobarbital induces the enzyme that metabolizes theophylline). Conversely, when a drug inhibits the enzyme activity necessary for metabolism of a second drug, toxic levels of the second drug can result (eg, cimetidine inhibits the enzyme that metabolizes theophylline; theophylline metabolism is inhibited thereby causing an elevated theophylline level). Much has been learned about the specific pathways by which certain drugs are metabolized, allowing more accurate prediction of potential interactions. Knowing that a drug is either an enzyme inhibitor or an enzyme inducer should cause a nurse monitoring drug effects to be alert for the effects of any other drugs that may be potentially affected.

Elimination via Excretion

Elimination via excretion is the process by which a drug or its metabolites is removed from the body.

Drugs can be eliminated through the lungs, kidneys, liver, skin, intestinal tract, or via excretory glands – in sweat, tears, saliva, or breast milk. Peritoneal dialysis or hemodialysis may also be used to remove drugs from the body.

Half-life is the time required for the blood levels of a drug to be diminished by one-half. This can be expressed as the percentage of the original concentration over time (eg, after one half-life 50% remains, after the second half-life 25%, third half-life 12.5%, etc). With normal functioning excretion, the half-life of a drug will help to determine spacing of dosing schedules. While a true half-life of a drug is specific to its persistence in an individual patient, it is a common practice to express this value as a population average measured in clinical trials. Because of this, it is important to recognize that the half-life in an individual patient can vary considerably, and may be substantially different in patients with organ dysfunction or deficiencies in metabolizing enzymes. For example, in the presence of decreased kidney function, elimination is slowed or delayed and more of the drug remains in the body than half-life figures from an otherwise healthy population would indicate. The actual half-life in these persons may be several times longer than the population average. Extended half-lives may result in higher drug accumulation. Elderly persons frequently have decreased kidney function as a part of the aging process – drugs excreted primarily via the kidneys thereby hold the potential for toxic levels for elderly persons when given in "normal" doses.

PHARMACODYNAMICS

Pharmacodynamics refers to the time course and relationships which determine how a drug brings about biophysical or biochemical changes.

Drug molecules must interact with specific receptors on target cell membranes in order to effect some biochemical or biophysical action. The drug-receptor interaction may alter or modify cellular function, at times activating new responses and/or previously unexpressed potential of the cell; however, drugs do not cause a new function in a cell or tissue. Action at the cellular level then impacts the tissue function in measurable or observable ways. For instance, insulin interacts with receptors to facilitate glucose transport across cellular membranes, this in turn causes a measurable increase in serum glucose levels; atropine blocks acetylcholine receptors, which results in a decrease in the effects of acetylcholine (anticholinergic response; see Pharmacologic Category Index). The effects of drug and receptor interactions may be desired (beneficial) or nonbeneficial (adverse or side effects).

Most drug molecules can only interact with specific receptors. These may be located within the cell or on cellular membranes for which they have an affinity in a "lock-and-key" type bond. Following interaction with a receptor, a sequence of events may occur within the cell. Pathways in the cell may be activated to alter the production or activity of the cellular enzymes. In some cases, this involves the

BASIC PHARMACOTHERAPEUTIC CONCEPTS *(Continued)*

activation of specific genes. Drugs that stimulate receptor actions are called agonists. Drugs that fit to receptors and prevent or inhibit cellular responses to other drugs or endogenous compounds are called antagonists. In some instances, antagonist action is desirable (eg, naloxone competes with opioids for opioid receptors and may be used to reverse an opioid overdose).

Some drugs are extremely specific for one kind of receptor and some drugs are less specific so that they nonselectively stimulate all of a particular class of receptors. For instance, epinephrine will stimulate all beta-adrenergic receptors resulting in stimulation of both cardiac tissue and pulmonary smooth muscle tissue whereas terbutaline is more selective for $beta_2$ adrenergic receptors and resulting action is primarily on the smooth muscle of the lungs.

Several factors may also influence the number of specific receptors (up-regulation or down-regulation) and their ability to couple with other drugs or endogenous substances. The changes in number of receptors (increase or decrease) or sensitivity may result in drug tolerance (eg, biogenic amines [antidepressants]). The rebound phenomena that follows abrupt withdrawal of some drugs is related to an increase in the availability of receptor sites as the drug is released from the receptor (ie, clonidine). Disease states can influence number and responsiveness of receptors (eg, thyroid hormones can increase the number of beta receptors and their sensitivity to catecholamines in cardiac muscle, which may account for the tachycardia of thyrotoxicosis). Age can decrease responsiveness to insulin. Pharmacodynamics are normally associated with changes in drug concentrations (pharmacokinetics). In other words, the concentration of available drug in systemic circulation as determined by pharmacokinetic properties (bioavailability, metabolism, and excretion) have direct influence on the degree of biophysical or biochemical changes effected by drugs or pharmacodynamics.

Ideally, the dose of a drug should achieve the desired response without the occurrence of adverse effects. Unfortunately, with some drugs, the onset of adverse effects occurs before therapeutic dosage levels can be reached. This precludes the use of this drug. Fortunately, many drugs have a fairly wide window of safety (eg, the relationship between effective dosing levels and adverse effects is wide enough so that adverse or toxic responses can be minimalized). Some drugs, however, have a very narrow therapeutic index (TI); the range between therapeutic effect and toxic response is very small. Drugs with a narrow TI should be monitored (physical assessment and/or serum drug levels) on a regular basis (eg, lithium, digoxin, phenytoin, theophylline, etc).

PATIENT FACTORS THAT INFLUENCE DRUG THERAPY

Many factors related to an individual patient, or a group of similar patients, can impact the pharmacokinetics of drugs and relate to adverse reactions.

Pregnancy / Lactation

The changes that occur during pregnancy may necessitate dosage changes for some drugs. Decreased gastric tract motility, increased blood volume, decreased protein binding sites, and increased glomerular filtration rates may alter the degree of anticipated pharmacotherapeutic response.

Primarily, the concern about drugs during pregnancy is the effect of drugs on the fetus, either teratogenic (causing birth defects) or systemic (causing addiction). Although many drugs cross the placenta, the type of drug, the concentration of that drug, and the gestational age at time of exposure of the fetus are primary determinants of fetal reaction. When prescribing or administering drugs to any childbearing age female, it is vital to ask when her last menstrual period was and, if necessary, to wait for the results of a pregnancy test before starting any drug therapy. Of course, it is best to avoid all drugs during pregnancy, however, in some cases, the physiological context (ie, cardiac output, renal blood flow, etc) may be altered enough to require the use of drugs that are not needed by the same woman when not pregnant.

Most systematically absorbed drugs have been assigned a pregnancy risk factor based on the drugs potential to cause birth defects. This permits an evaluation of the risk:benefit ratio when prescribing or administering drugs becomes necessary. Drugs in the risk factor class "A" are generally considered to be safe for use during pregnancy, class "X" drugs are never safe and are known to be positively teratogenic. See FDA Pregnancy Categories *on page 21*.

Contraception note: Many drugs will interact with and decrease the effect of oral contraceptives (eg, barbiturates, protease inhibitors, rifampin, and carbamazepine). When a second drug will decrease the effect of oral contraceptives, the patient needs to be educated about the necessity for using a "barrier" (nonhormonal) form of contraception. Barrier contraception (alone or in combination with some form of oral contraception) is often recommended for the patient who must take selected drugs with pregnancy risk factors "D" (idarubicin) or class "X" (isotretinoin).

Because many drugs and substances used by a mother appear in breast milk, care must be taken to evaluate the drug effects on the lactating woman and the infant. Some drugs are identified as being clearly contraindicated during lactation, others may cross into breast milk but adverse side effects on the fetus have not been identified, and for some drugs the administration times should be distanced from nursing time. Nurses should advise lactating women about the effects that drugs may have on the infant.

Age

All pharmacokinetics (absorption, distribution, metabolism, and excretion) are different in infants, young adults, and elderly patients. Elderly patients may have mildly decreased or severely decreased blood flow to all organs, gastric motility may be slowed, kidney function may be reduced, decreased nutrition may result in decreased albumin, and sedentary lifestyles may have an impact on drug response. Slower gastric motility means that absorption is slowed, resulting in longer time periods to clinical response. Decreased blood flow means that distribution is altered, resulting in decreased response or longer response time. Excretion may be altered with decreased glomerular filtration rates or slower gastric emptying which can result in increased levels of drug remaining in the system.

The ratio between total body water and total body fat also changes with age; older persons have decreased amounts of total body water and higher body fat. This aspect of aging also influences the blood concentration of some drugs. In a person with increased body fat, fat-soluble drugs are distributed to tissues more than to plasma; resulting in a longer response time as the drug must then be redistributed from tissue to plasma. The idiosyncratic response incidence also increases with an aging population. Responses to drugs may be both more exaggerated or diminished with the "usual" doses of some drugs.

In addition, and of major concern with elderly patients, is the incidence of poly-pharmacy; the increased numbers of drugs the patient may be taking. Older patients may have 2, 3, 4, or 5 (or more) chronic conditions for which they are taking medication. In addition, they may be seeing a different prescriber for each of these conditions. Often, it is a nurse who identifies and coordinates the care of these elderly patients, and the nurse must be aware of the possibility for increased incidence of adverse effects.

Body Weight / Build

Most "recommended" dosages of drugs are based on the average size, young or middle aged adult (usually males). Extremely obese or extremely thin patients may be prone to adverse effects as a result of "nonindividualized" prescribing. Serum creatinine is a breakdown product of skeletal muscle and its levels in the serum are frequently used to estimate renal function. Decreased muscle mass can result in reduced creatinine from muscle breakdown, leading to a serum creatinine, which is artificially low or appears normal. When dosing is based on estimated creatinine clearance (which is calculated based on the serum creatinine) rather than "actual" creatinine clearance, normal doses may be administered to patients with a diminished capacity for excretion, potentially leading to accumulation and toxicity. This is a particular problem in elderly and/or debilitated patients.

Smoking, Alcohol, Nutrition, and Hydration

Smoking has a direct impact on liver enzyme activity, blood flow, and the central nervous system. Excessive alcohol intake impacts liver enzymes, renal function, and has an additive effect with most antipsychotic, sedative, or anxiolytic medications, as well as altering responses to many other medications. Nutrition and hydration also play an important part in drug responses and possible adverse reactions. Poor

BASIC PHARMACOTHERAPEUTIC CONCEPTS *(Continued)*

hydration may result in reduced blood flow and excretion. Decreased or prolonged gastric motility can result in slowed excretion and/or prolonged absorption. Poor or inadequate nutrition may result in decreased protein available for binding.

It is vital that a patient's current habits are considered when prescribing, administering, or monitoring drug therapy, but in addition, patients must be aware of the need to inform their professional care provider that they have changed their smoking, alcohol, or dietary patterns. When dosage of theophylline is based on the fact that the patient is a smoker, the theophylline dosage must be adjusted to prevent overdose, if the patient quits smoking. When a patient is on warfarin, drastic increases in the amount of vitamin K intake through increased green leafy vegetables can dramatically alter the dose of warfarin.

Other Patient Factors That Influence Drug Response

- Genetic variations
- Differences in circadian patterns
- Disease states
- Psychological temperament

Genetic differences in enzymes may influence the effectiveness of therapy or the incidence of adverse effects (fast acetylators or slow acetylators). The emerging science of pharmacogenomics is devoted to the investigation of these genetic differences in drug response, and offers the hope of truly individualized therapy. Circadian rhythms differ among individuals and have an impact on absorption patterns, hormone secretion, or urinary excretion patterns. Disease states can and do change all aspects of pharmacokinetics. Cirrhosis can impair liver enzyme metabolism rate. Kidney disease will reduce excretion rates for many drugs. Abnormal thyroid function can influence drug metabolism. Diseases which affect blood circulation (eg, hypertension, CHF, Raynaud's phenomena, malignancies, etc) can have an impact on absorption, distribution, and excretion. Diabetes impacts the response to many drugs. Malnutrition, commonly associated with disease, can drastically reduce albumin levels.

See Therapeutic Nursing Management of Side Effects *on page 1908*

PHARMACOTHERAPEUTICS

Drug therapy is used for treatment of disease or symptoms of diseases (empiric, supportive, maintenance, or palliative), for prevention (immunization), and for diagnosis (iodine, barium). In some cases, drugs may be used to correct imbalances or improve regulation of excessive physiological responses.

Optimal drug therapy should be both effective and safe. It needs to be tailored to the patient and the problem (see Patient Factors That Influence Drug Therapy). Assessing the problem is the first step, this involves identifying the problem (eg, etiology, laboratory confirmation, subjective and objective symptoms, urgency, severity, and prognosis) and determining what is the goal of therapy. Identifying and assessing the various options require knowledge of what drug therapy is appropriate. These steps lead to clinical decision-making (eg, selecting the drug regimen that is appropriate to meet the goal for this patient).

While professionals responsible for prescribing medications usually select therapy, the implementing of therapy is often a responsibility of nurses, in collaboration with pharmacists. Implementing therapy includes not only the preparation and dispensing of the drug, but also the education of those individual(s) who will administer the drug: nurses, patients, and family members. A major aspect of the education of patients includes how to administer the drug, when to administer the drug, and any dietary or drug-related precautions.

Monitoring the results of that therapy is a major responsibility that involves the prescriber, pharmacist, nurse, patient, and other healthcare providers. A major aspect of monitoring is communicating the subjective and objective responses to the responsible prescriber. Patients, nurses, and other caregivers must know the anticipated results of drug therapy and how to assess and report possible adverse effects.

The design, implementation, and monitoring of drug therapy in an individual patient is a complex and time-consuming task, requiring participation of many members of the healthcare team. Several common types of problems may be encountered in drug therapy. These include omissions of potentially beneficial drugs from the regimen, duplications in therapy, selection/titration to the appropriate dosage, the identification and management of drug interactions, and the identification and management of adverse reactions. An awareness of these potential problems is essential to enhance the safety of drug therapy.

Drug Interactions

Drug interactions are a major concern in drug therapy. Interactions may occur between food and drugs or between different drugs (ie, over-the-counter drugs, herbals, home remedies, and prescription drugs). Careful assessment of **ALL** substances patients are using to treat themselves is imperative for safe drug therapy. Patients may not consider some of the substances they use to treat themselves as drugs and nurses may need to be highly sensitive and very aware when they discuss this subject with the patient.

The potential for drug interactions increases exponentially with the number of drugs a person is taking. Thus, the more illnesses a patient has, the more likely it is he/she will be taking multiple drugs, and the more likely he/she will be to experience drug interactions.

Drugs can interact with other drugs to produce additive effects (when combined they produce similar cumulative effects with a lesser dose of either drug than they would alone), synergistic effects (the combination produces a greater response than either alone), or antagonistic effect (one drug negates or reverses the effect of the other drug). Such interactions can be a result of altering the pharmacokinetics of the drugs involved; increasing or decreasing either the rate or the quantity in absorption, altering the distribution through competitive receptor binding, changing the metabolism by inducing or reducing actions of liver enzymes, altering blood flow, or excretion by altering renal clearance.

Food, alcohol, and cigarette smoking can interact with drugs. Absorption of some drugs is enhanced with high fat meals (griseofulvin) or by low protein or high carbohydrate meals (theophylline). Whereas, absorption of some drugs is slowed, rather than blocked, when the stomach is full and gastric transport is slowed. Other drugs can bind with food to impair or prevent absorption of food byproducts such as carbohydrates or vitamins (eg, cholestyramine, mineral oil). Some drugs, such as isotretinoin, are isomers of vitamins and dietary intake of vitamin A can cause overdose reactions.

Other foods can produce pharmacologic activity on their own and when the patient is also taking a medication that is designed to result in that same pharmacologic activity the result may be life-threatening. For instance, patients using a monoamine oxidase (MAO) inhibitor should avoid foods containing tyramines or tryptophan to prevent excess release of catecholamines resulting in severe potentially life-threatening effects.

Drugs can also impact the results of laboratory tests. This is the basis for instructions from the laboratory to "hold" certain medications prior to some laboratory tests.

Adverse Drug Reactions

Adverse reactions to drug therapy can range from mild to debilitating and life-threatening. Mild reactions may either be not severe enough to discontinue the drug or will disappear when the drug is discontinued. Severe or life-threatening reactions may require immediate discontinuance, treatment with other drugs, or dialysis. Adverse reactions may be related to the dosing, they may be inherent in the drug's primary actions, they may be iatrogenic to the drug, or they may be related to individual patient sensitivity or genetics.

Dose-related side effects can be addressed through careful dosage adjustment. Adverse effects associated with inherent properties of the drugs (constipation with opiates or some pain medications) can be addressed through appropriate interventions (ie, increasing fluids, fiber in diets, increased exercise, or stool softeners). Iatrogenic effects (ie, GI irritation and bleeding from aspirin or indomethacin, orthostatic hypotension from antihypertensives) can be reduced by taking a complete patient history, by patient administration and precaution education (eg, safe dose,

BASIC PHARMACOTHERAPEUTIC CONCEPTS *(Continued)*

time, diet, activity, etc), by prescribing another drug to address the anticipated iatrogenic response, or by choosing another drug for treatment. Thorough knowledge of the possible adverse effects, coupled with anticipatory action, will reduce the incidence of adverse side effects.

True allergic responses usually result from previous exposure to one drug or drugs with related chemical composition that sensitizes the patient's immune system. Careful drug histories and assessment of a patient's reported previous adverse responses will help in averting allergic reactions. Idiosyncratic responses are those that are specific to that patient and are generally unpredictable, although many times these are genetically determined.

ALPHABETICAL LISTING OF DRUGS

♦ 1370-999-397 *see* Anagrelide *on page 166*

Abacavir (a BAK a veer)

U.S. Brand Names Ziagen®

Synonyms Abacavir Sulfate; ABC

Pharmacologic Category Antiretroviral Agent, Reverse Transcriptase Inhibitor (Nucleoside)

Use Treatment of HIV infections in combination with other antiretroviral agents

Mechanism of Action Nucleoside reverse transcriptase inhibitor. Abacavir is a guanosine analogue which is phosphorylated to carbovir triphosphate which interferes with HIV viral RNA-dependent DNA polymerase resulting in inhibition of viral replication.

Pharmacodynamics/Kinetics

Absorption: Rapid and extensive absorption

Distribution: V_d: 0.86 L/kg

Protein binding: 50%

Metabolism: Hepatic via alcohol dehydrogenase and glucuronyl transferase to inactive carboxylate and glucuronide metabolites

Bioavailability: 83%

Half-life elimination: 1.5 hours

Time to peak: 0.7-1.7 hours

Excretion: Primarily urine (as metabolites, 1.2% as unchanged drug); feces (16% total dose)

Contraindications Hypersensitivity to abacavir (or carbovir) or any component of the formulation (do not rechallenge patients who have experienced hypersensitivity to abacavir); moderate-to-severe hepatic impairment

Warnings/Precautions Abacavir should always be used as a component of a multidrug regimen. Serious and sometimes fatal hypersensitivity reactions have occurred. **Patients exhibiting symptoms from two or more of the following: Fever, skin rash, constitutional symptoms (malaise, fatigue, aches), respiratory symptoms (eg, pharyngitis, dyspnea, cough), and GI symptoms (eg, abdominal pain, diarrhea, nausea, vomiting) should discontinue therapy immediately and call for medical attention. Abacavir should be permanently discontinued if hypersensitivity cannot be ruled out, even when other diagnoses are possible. Abacavir SHOULD NOT be restarted because more severe symptoms may occur within hours, including LIFE-THREATENING HYPOTENSION AND DEATH. Fatal hypersensitivity reactions have occurred following the reintroduction of abacavir in patients whose therapy was interrupted (ie, interruption in drug supply, temporary discontinuation while treating other conditions). Reactions occurred within hours. In some cases, signs of hypersensitivity may have been previously present, but attributed to other medical conditions (eg, acute onset respiratory diseases, gastroenteritis, reactions to other medications). If abacavir is restarted following an interruption in therapy, evaluate the patient for previously unsuspected symptoms of hypersensitivity. Do not restart if hypersensitivity is suspected or if hypersensitivity cannot be ruled out. To report these events on abacavir hypersensitivity, a registry has been established (1-800-270-0425).** Use with caution in patients with mild hepatic dysfunction (contraindicated in moderate-to-severe dysfunction). Lactic acidosis and severe hepatomegaly with steatosis (sometimes fatal) have occurred with antiretroviral nucleoside analogues; female gender, obesity, and prolonged treatment may increase the risk of hepatotoxicity.

Drug Interactions

Amprenavir: Abacavir increases the AUC of amprenavir.

Methadone: Abacavir may decrease the serum concentration of methadone (clearance increased 22%); in a minority of patients, methadone dosage increase may be required.

Ribavirin: Concomitant use of ribavirin and nucleoside analogues may increase the risk of developing lactic acidosis (includes adefovir, didanosine, lamivudine, stavudine, zalcitabine, zidovudine).

Nutritional/Herbal/Ethanol Interactions Ethanol: Ethanol may increase the risk of toxicity.

Adverse Reactions Hypersensitivity reactions (which may be fatal) occur in ~5% of patients (see Warnings/Precautions). Symptoms may include anaphylaxis, fever, rash (including erythema multiforme), fatigue, diarrhea, abdominal pain; respiratory symptoms (eg, pharyngitis, dyspnea, cough, adult respiratory distress syndrome, or respiratory failure); headache, malaise, lethargy, myalgia, myolysis, arthralgia, edema, paresthesia, nausea and vomiting, mouth ulcerations, conjunctivitis, lymphadenopathy, hepatic failure, and renal failure.

Note: Rates of adverse reactions were defined during combination therapy with other antiretrovirals (lamivudine and efavirenz **or** lamivudine and zidovudine). Only reactions which occurred at a higher frequency than in the comparator group are noted. Adverse reaction rates attributable to abacavir alone are not available.

>10%:
- Central nervous system: Headache (7% to 13%), fatigue and malaise (7% to 12%)
- Gastrointestinal: Nausea (7% to 19%, children 9%)

1% to 10%:
- Central nervous system: Depression (6%), dizziness (6%), fever (6%, children 9%), anxiety (5%), abnormal dreams (10%)
- Dermatologic: Rash (5% to 6%, children 7%)
- Gastrointestinal: Diarrhea (7%), vomiting (2% to 10%, children 9%), abdominal pain (6%)
- Hematologic: Thrombocytopenia (1%)
- Hepatic: AST increased (6%)
- Neuromuscular and skeletal: Musculoskeletal pain (5% to 6%)
- Respiratory: Bronchitis (4%), respiratory viral infection (5%)
- Miscellaneous: Hypersensitivity reactions (9%; may include reactions to other components of antiretroviral regimen), infection (EENT 5%)

<1% (Limited to important or life-threatening): Erythema multiforme, hepatotoxicity, lactic acidosis, pancreatitis, Stevens-Johnson syndrome, toxic epidermal necrolysis

Dosing

Adults & Elderly: HIV treatment: Oral: 300 mg twice daily or 600 mg once daily in combination with other antiretroviral agents

Pediatrics: HIV treatment: Oral: 3 months to 16 years: 8 mg/kg body weight twice daily (maximum: 300 mg twice daily) in combination with other antiretroviral agents

Hepatic Impairment:
- Mild dysfunction (Child-Pugh score 5-6): 200 mg twice daily (oral solution is recommended)
- Moderate-to-severe dysfunction: Use is contraindicated by the manufacturer

Available Dosage Forms

Solution, oral: 20 mg/mL (240 mL) [strawberry-banana flavor]
Tablet: 300 mg

Nursing Guidelines

Assessment: Assess closely for any previous exposure/allergy to abacavir prior to beginning treatment. Assess other prescriptions, OTC medications, or herbal products patient may be taking for potential interactions (see Drug Interactions) Patient must be closely monitored for any sign of hypersensitivity reaction (anaphylaxis, fever, rash, fatigue, diarrhea, abdominal pain; pharyngitis, dyspnea, cough, adult respiratory distress syndrome, or respiratory failure; headache, malaise, lethargy, myalgia, myolysis, arthralgia, edema, paresthesia, nausea and vomiting, mouth ulcerations, conjunctivitis, lymphadenopathy, hepatic failure, and renal failure). Hypersensitivity can occur within hours and may be fatal (see Warnings/Precautions). If hypersensitivity occurs, infusion should be stopped and prescriber notified. Assess effectiveness of therapy (decrease in infections and progress of disease [viral load and CD4 count]), adverse reactions (see Adverse Reactions). Teach patient proper use as part of combination drug regimen, possible side effects/interventions, and adverse symptoms to report (eg, signs and symptoms of hypersensitivity).

Dietary Considerations: May be taken with or without food.

Patient Education: Do not take any new medications during treatment without consulting prescriber. This drug will not cure HIV; use appropriate precautions to prevent spread to other persons. This drug is prescribed as one part of a multidrug combination; take exactly as directed, for full course of therapy. Maintain adequate hydration (2-3 L/day of fluids) unless advised by prescriber to restrict fluids. Avoid alcohol to decrease risk of hypersensitivity reaction. You may be susceptible to infection (avoid crowds and exposure to known infections and do not have any vaccinations without consulting prescriber). May cause dizziness or weakness (use caution when driving or engaging in tasks requiring alertness until response to drug is known); or nausea or vomiting (small frequent meals, frequent mouth care, chewing gum, or sucking lozenges may help). Report immediately symptoms of hypersensitivity (eg, fever; rash; fatigue

(Continued)

Abacavir *(Continued)*

or lethargy; persistent nausea, vomiting, diarrhea, or abdominal pain; mouth sores; sore throat, cough, difficulty breathing, headache, malaise, swelling of face, mouth or throat; numbness or loss of sensation; headache; loss of sensation, pain, tingling, or numbness in toes, feet, muscles or joints; swollen glands, alterations in urinary pattern; swelling of extremities or weight gain). If you are instructed to stop the medication, do not take this medication in the future. Do not restart without specific instruction by your prescriber. **Pregnancy/ breast-feeding precautions:** Inform prescriber if you are or intend to become pregnant. Do not breast-feed.

Pregnancy Risk Factor: C

Pregnancy Issues: It is not known if abacavir crosses the human placenta. Cases of lactic acidosis/hepatic steatosis syndrome have been reported in pregnant women receiving nucleoside analogues. It is not known if pregnancy itself potentiates this known side effect; however, pregnant women may be at increased risk of lactic acidosis and liver damage. Hepatic enzymes and electrolytes should be monitored frequently during the 3rd trimester of pregnancy in women receiving nucleoside analogues. The pharmacokinetics of abacavir during pregnancy are currently under study. The Perinatal HIV Guidelines Working Group considers abacavir to be an alternative NRTI in dual nucleoside combination regimens. Health professionals are encouraged to contact the antiretroviral pregnancy registry to monitor outcomes of pregnant women exposed to antiretroviral medications (1-800-258-4263 or www.APRegistry.com).

Lactation: Excretion in breast milk unknown/contraindicated

Breast-Feeding Considerations: HIV-infected mothers are discouraged from breast-feeding to decrease potential transmission of HIV.

Administration

Oral: May be administered with or without food.

Storage: Store oral solution and tablets at controlled room temperature of 20°C to 25°C (68°F to 77°F). Oral solution may be refrigerated; do not freeze.

Abacavir, Lamivudine, and Zidovudine

(a BAK a veer, la MI vyoo deen, & zye DOE vyoo deen)

U.S. Brand Names Trizivir®

Synonyms Azidothymidine, Abacavir, and Lamivudine; AZT, Abacavir, and Lamivudine; Compound S, Abacavir, and Lamivudine; Lamivudine, Abacavir, and Zidovudine; 3TC, Abacavir, and Zidovudine; ZDV, Abacavir, and Lamivudine; Zidovudine, Abacavir, and Lamivudine

Pharmacologic Category Antiretroviral Agent, Reverse Transcriptase Inhibitor (Nucleoside)

Use Treatment of HIV infection (either alone or in combination with other antiretroviral agents) in patients whose regimen would otherwise contain the components of Trizivir®

Mechanism of Action The combination of abacavir, lamivudine, and zidovudine is believed to act synergistically to inhibit reverse transcriptase via DNA chain termination after incorporation of the nucleoside analogue as well as to delay the emergence of mutations conferring resistance.

Pharmacodynamics/Kinetics Bioavailability studies of Trizivir® show no difference in AUC or C_{max} when compared to abacavir, lamivudine, and zidovudine given together as individual agents. See individual agents.

Contraindications Hypersensitivity to abacavir, lamivudine, zidovudine, or any component of the formulation. Do not rechallenge patients who have experienced hypersensitivity to abacavir (as Trizivir® or Ziagen®); life-threatening and fatal reactions have been reported.

Warnings/Precautions Fatal hypersensitivity reactions have occurred in patients taking abacavir (in Trizivir®). **Patients exhibiting symptoms of fever, skin rash, fatigue, respiratory symptoms (eg, pharyngitis, dyspnea, cough) and/or GI symptoms (eg, abdominal pain, nausea, vomiting, diarrhea) should discontinue therapy immediately and call for medical attention. Trizivir® should be permanently discontinued if hypersensitivity cannot be ruled out, even when other diagnoses are possible. Trizivir® SHOULD NOT be restarted because more severe symptoms may occur within hours, including LIFE-THREATENING HYPOTENSION AND DEATH. Fatal hypersensitivity reactions have occurred following the reintroduction of abacavir in patients whose therapy was interrupted (ie, interruption in drug supply, temporary**

discontinuation while treating other conditions). Reactions occurred within hours. In some cases, signs of hypersensitivity may have been previously present, but attributed to other medical conditions (eg, acute onset respiratory diseases, gastroenteritis, reactions to other medications). If Trizivir® is to be restarted following an interruption in therapy, first evaluate the patient for previously unsuspected symptoms of hypersensitivity. Do not restart if hypersensitivity is suspected or if hypersensitivity cannot be ruled out. To report these events on Trizivir® hypersensitivity, a registry has been established (1-800-270-0425). Trizivir®, as a fixed-dose combination tablet, should not be used in patients <40 kg or those requiring dosage adjustment; should not be used in patients with Cl_{cr} ≤50 mL/minute; not intended for use in pediatric patients; should not be administered concomitantly with abacavir, lamivudine, or zidovudine. Prior liver disease, prolonged use, and obesity may be risk factors for development of lactic acidosis and severe hepatomegaly with steatosis. Dose reductions may be required for zidovudine in patients with hepatic impairment. Trizivir® is a fixed-dose combination; it is not recommended (per manufacturer) in hepatic impairment. Use with caution in patients with bone marrow compromise; myopathy and myositis have been associated with prolonged use of zidovudine (in Trizivir®).

Drug Interactions See individual agents.

Adverse Reactions Fatal hypersensitivity reactions have occurred in patients taking abacavir (in Trizivir®). If Trizivir® is to be restarted following an interruption in therapy, first evaluate the patient for previously unsuspected symptoms of hypersensitivity. Do not restart if hypersensitivity is suspected or if hypersensitivity cannot be ruled out.

The following information is based on CNAAB3003 study data concerning effects noted in patients receiving abacavir, lamivudine, and zidovudine. See individual agent monographs for additional information.

>10%:

Endocrine & metabolic: Triglycerides increased (25%)

Gastrointestinal: Diarrhea (12%), nausea (47%), nausea and vomiting (16%), loss of appetite/anorexia (11%)

1% to 10%:

Central nervous system: Insomnia (7%)

Miscellaneous: Hypersensitivity (5% based on abacavir component)

Other (frequency unknown): GGT increased, pancreatitis

Postmarketing and/or case reports (limited to important or life-threatening): Redistribution/accumulation of body fat, anaphylaxis, cardiomyopathy, hepatic steatosis, lactic acidosis, Stevens-Johnson syndrome

Overdosage/Toxicology Symptoms of overdose with zidovudine include nausea, vomiting, headache, dizziness, drowsiness, lethargy, confusion, and hematologic changes. Myocardial degeneration has been documented in animals during long-term high-dose toxicology studies; clinical relevance is unknown. Peritoneal dialysis and hemodialysis have little to no effect on the removal of the components of Trizivir®.

Dosing

Adults: HIV treatment: Oral: 1 tablet twice daily. **Note:** Not recommended for patients <40 kg.

Elderly: Use with caution.

Pediatrics: HIV treatment: Adolescents: Refer to adult dosing (not recommended for patients <40 kg).

Renal Impairment: Cl_{cr} ≤50 mL/minute: Avoid use.

Hepatic Impairment: Use not recommended.

Available Dosage Forms Tablet [film coated]: Abacavir 300 mg, lamivudine 150 mg, and zidovudine 300 mg

Nursing Guidelines

Assessment: See individual agents.

Dietary Considerations: May be taken without regard to food or water.

Patient Education: This drug is not a cure for HIV infection, nor will it reduce the risk of transmission of HIV to others. Take exactly as prescribed without regard to food or water. Do not discontinue even if feeling better. You will need to have frequent blood tests to identify possible blood cell problems. You may experience headache, muscle pain, weakness, insomnia, unusual bleeding (eg, tarry stools, easy bruising, blood in stool, urine, or mouth), dizziness, or numbness; report these to your prescriber. **Note:** Trizivir® contains abacavir (also called Ziagen®). About 1 in 20 patients who take abacavir will have a serious

(Continued)

Abacavir, Lamivudine, and Zidovudine *(Continued)*

allergic reaction that can result in death if the drug is not stopped right away. You may be having this reaction if you get a skin rash or if you get one or more symptoms from at least two of the following groups: Fever; nausea, vomiting, diarrhea, stomach pain; extreme tiredness, achiness, general ill feeling; or sore throat, shortness of breath, cough. If you think you are having this reaction contact your prescriber immediately. If you stop Trizivir® because of this reaction, **never** take Trizivir® or Ziagen® (abacavir) again or you could die within hours. If you stop Trizivir® therapy for any other reason, consult your prescriber before restarting therapy. **Pregnancy/breast-feeding precautions:** Inform your prescriber if you are or intend to become pregnant. Breast-feeding is not recommended. HIV-infected mothers are discouraged from breast-feeding to decrease potential transmission of HIV.

Pregnancy Risk Factor: C

Pregnancy Issues: See individual agents.

Lactation: See individual agents.

Breast-Feeding Considerations: See individual agents.

Administration

Oral: Administer without regard to food or water.

Storage: Store at room temperature 25°C (77°F).

Related Information

Abacavir *on page 56*
Lamivudine *on page 999*
Zidovudine *on page 1732*

♦ Abacavir Sulfate *see* Abacavir *on page 56*
♦ Abbokinase® [DSC] *see* Urokinase *on page 1674*
♦ Abbott-43818 *see* Leuprolide *on page 1015*
♦ ABC *see* Abacavir *on page 56*

Abciximab (ab SIK si mab)

U.S. Brand Names ReoPro®

Synonyms C7E3; 7E3

Pharmacologic Category Antiplatelet Agent, Glycoprotein IIb/IIIa Inhibitor

Use Prevention of acute cardiac ischemic complications in patients at high risk for abrupt closure of the treated coronary vessel and patients at risk of restenosis; an adjunct with heparin to prevent cardiac ischemic complications in patients with unstable angina not responding to conventional therapy when a percutaneous coronary intervention (PCI) is scheduled within 24 hours

Unlabeled/Investigational Use Acute MI — combination regimen of abciximab (full dose), tenecteplase (half dose), and heparin (unlabeled dose)

Mechanism of Action Fab antibody fragment of the chimeric human-murine monoclonal antibody 7E3; this agent binds to platelet IIb/IIIa receptors, resulting in steric hindrance, thus inhibiting platelet aggregation

Pharmacodynamics/Kinetics Half-life elimination: ~30 minutes

Contraindications Hypersensitivity to abciximab, to murine proteins, or any component of the formulation; active internal hemorrhage or recent (within 6 weeks) clinically-significant GI or GU bleeding; history of cerebrovascular accident within 2 years or cerebrovascular accident with significant neurological deficit; clotting abnormalities or administration of oral anticoagulants within 7 days unless prothrombin time (PT) is ≤1.2 times control PT value; thrombocytopenia (<100,000 cells/µL); recent (within 6 weeks) major surgery or trauma; intracranial tumor, arteriovenous malformation, or aneurysm; severe uncontrolled hypertension; history of vasculitis; use of dextran before PTCA or intent to use dextran during PTCA; concomitant use of another parenteral GP IIb/IIIa inhibitor

Warnings/Precautions Administration of abciximab is associated with increased frequency of major bleeding complications, including retroperitoneal bleeding, pulmonary bleeding, spontaneous GI or GU bleeding, and bleeding at the arterial access. Risk may be increased with patients weighing <75 kilograms, elderly patients (>65 years of age), history of previous GI disease, and recent thrombolytic therapy. Avoid the creation of venous access at noncompressible sites.

The risk of major bleeds may increase with concurrent use of thrombolytics. Anticoagulation, such as with heparin, may contribute to the risk of bleeding. In serious, uncontrolled bleeding, abciximab and heparin should be stopped. Increased risk of hemorrhage during or following angioplasty is associated with unsuccessful PTCA, PTCA procedure >70 minutes duration, or PTCA performed within 12 hours of symptom onset for acute myocardial infarction.

Administration of abciximab may result in human antichimeric antibody formation that can cause hypersensitivity reactions (including anaphylaxis), thrombocytopenia, or diminished efficacy. Readministration of abciximab within 30 days or in patients with human antichimeric antibodies (HACA) increases the incidence and severity of thrombocytopenia.

Drug Interactions

Heparin and aspirin: Use with aspirin and heparin may increase bleeding over aspirin and heparin alone. However, aspirin and heparin were used concurrently in the majority of patients in the major clinical studies of abciximab.

Monoclonal antibodies: Allergic reactions may be increased in patients who have received diagnostic or therapeutic monoclonal antibodies due to the presence of HACA antibodies.

Thrombolytic agents theoretically may increase the risk of bleeding; use with caution.

Warfarin and oral anticoagulants: Risk of bleeding may be increased during concurrent therapy.

Other IIb/IIIa antagonists: Avoid concomitant use of other glycoprotein IIb/IIIa antagonists (see Contraindications).

Adverse Reactions As with all drugs which may affect hemostasis, bleeding is associated with abciximab. Hemorrhage may occur at virtually any site. Risk is dependent on multiple variables, including the concurrent use of multiple agents which alter hemostasis and patient susceptibility.

>10%:

Cardiovascular: Hypotension (14.4%), chest pain (11.4%)
Gastrointestinal: Nausea (13.6%)
Hematologic: Minor bleeding (4.0% to 16.8%)
Neuromuscular & skeletal: Back pain (17.6%)

1% to 10%:

Cardiovascular: Bradycardia (4.5%), peripheral edema (1.6%)
Central nervous system: Headache (6.45)
Gastrointestinal: Vomiting (7.3%), abdominal pain (3.1%)
Hematologic: Major bleeding (1.1% to 14%), thrombocytopenia: <100,000 cells/mm^3 (2.5% to 5.6%); <50,000 cells/mm^3 (0.4% to 1.7%)
Local: Injection site pain (3.6%)

<1% (Limited to important or life-threatening): Abnormal thinking, allergic reactions/anaphylaxis (possible), AV block, bronchospasm, bullous eruption, coma, confusion, diabetes mellitus, embolism, hyperkalemia, ileus, inflammation, intracranial hemorrhage, myalgia, nodal arrhythmia, pleural effusion, pulmonary embolism, prostatitis, pruritus, stroke, urinary retention, ventricular tachycardia, xerostomia

Overdosage/Toxicology Since abciximab is a platelet antiaggregate, patients who bleed following administration may be best treated with platelet infusions.

Dosing

Adults & Elderly:

Prevention of restenosis (patients at high risk for abrupt closure): I.V.: 0.25 mg/kg bolus administered 10-60 minutes before the start of intervention followed by an infusion of 0.125 mcg/kg/minute (maximum: 10 mcg/minute) for 12 hours

Patients with unstable angina not responding to conventional medical therapy and with planned percutaneous coronary intervention within 24 hours: I.V.: 0.25 mg/kg intravenous bolus followed by an 18- to 24-hour intravenous infusion of 10 mcg/minute, concluding 1 hour after the percutaneous coronary intervention.

Acute MI combination regimen (unlabeled): Half-dose tenecteplase (15-25 mg based on weight), abciximab 0.25 mg/kg bolus then 0.125 mcg/kg/minute (maximum: 10 mcg/minute) for 12 hours and heparin dosing as follows: Concurrent bolus of 40 units/kg (maximum: 3000 units), then 7 units/kg/hour (maximum: 800 units/hour) as continuous infusion. Adjust to aPTT target of 50-70 seconds.

Available Dosage Forms Injection, solution: 2 mg/mL (5 mL)

Nursing Guidelines

Assessment: Monitor vital signs and laboratory results prior to, during, and after therapy. Assess infusion insertion site and peripheral pulses during and after

(Continued)

Abciximab *(Continued)*

therapy. Observe and teach patient bleeding precautions (avoid invasive procedures and activities that could result in injury). Monitor closely for signs of excessive bleeding. Note breast-feeding caution.

Monitoring Laboratory Tests: Prothrombin time, activated partial thromboplastin time (aPTT), hemoglobin, hematocrit, platelet count, fibrinogen, fibrin split products, transfusion requirements, signs of hypersensitivity reactions, guaiac stools, Hemastix® urine. Platelet count should be monitored at baseline, 2-4 hours following bolus infusion, and at 24 hours (or prior to discharge, if before 24 hours). To minimize risk of bleeding:

Abciximab initiated 18-24 hours prior to PCI: Maintain aPTT between 60-85 seconds during the heparin/abciximab infusion period

During PCI: Maintain ACT between 200-300 seconds

Following PCI (if anticoagulation is maintained): Maintain aPTT between 50-75 seconds

Sheath removal should not occur until aPTT is ≤50 seconds or ACT ≤175 seconds.

Patient Education: This medication can only be administered I.V. You will have a tendency to bleed easily following this medication; use caution to prevent injury (use electric razor, soft toothbrush, and use caution with knives, needles, or anything sharp). If bleeding occurs, apply pressure to bleeding spot until bleeding stops completely. Report unusual bruising or bleeding; blood in urine, stool, or vomitus; bleeding gums; or vision changes. **Pregnancy/breast-feeding precautions:** Inform prescriber if you are or intend to become pregnant. Consult prescriber if breast-feeding.

Pregnancy Risk Factor: C

Lactation: Excretion in breast milk unknown/use caution

Perioperative/Anesthesia/Other Concerns: Platelet Effects: Abciximab has a long duration of action and platelet effects reverse slowly. It can take 24-48 hours for platelet function to return to normal after discontinuation of infusion making it difficult to use in patients likely to need CABG. Antiplatelet effects can be reversed with platelet transfusions. Platelet count monitoring is recommended 2-4 hours after initiation, and at 24 hours or prior to discharge, whichever is first. Acute profound thrombocytopenia with abciximab occurs within 24 hours of administration and may be treated by discontinuing the infusion (if still running) and administering platelets. Platelet counts should recover rapidly after discontinuation.

Administration

I.V.: Infuse at a rate of 17 mL/hour (10 mcg/minute) for 12 hours via pump. Abciximab is intended for coadministration with aspirin postangioplasty and heparin infused and weight adjusted to maintain a therapeutic bleeding time (eg, ACT 300-500 seconds). Solution must be filtered prior to administration. Do not shake the vial.

Reconstitution: After admixture, the prepared solution is stable for 12 hours.

Compatibility: Requires separate intravenous line; no incompatibilities have been observed with glass bottles or PVC bags.

Storage: Vials should be stored at 2°C to 8°C. Do not freeze or shake.

- Abelcet® *see* Amphotericin B (Lipid Complex) *on page 154*
- ABLC *see* Amphotericin B (Lipid Complex) *on page 154*
- Absorbable Cotton *see* Cellulose (Oxidized Regenerated) *on page 362*
- Absorbable Gelatin Sponge *see* Gelatin (Absorbable) *on page 801*
- Accolate® *see* Zafirlukast *on page 1730*
- AccuNeb™ *see* Albuterol *on page 96*
- Accupril® *see* Quinapril *on page 1446*
- Accutane® *see* Isotretinoin *on page 981*
- ACE *see* Captopril *on page 302*

Acebutolol (a se BYOO toe lole)

U.S. Brand Names Sectral®

Synonyms Acebutolol Hydrochloride

Pharmacologic Category Antiarrhythmic Agent, Class II; Beta Blocker With Intrinsic Sympathomimetic Activity

Medication Safety Issues

Sound-alike/look-alike issues:

Sectral® may be confused with Factrel®, Seconal®, Septra®

Use Treatment of hypertension, ventricular arrhythmias, angina

Mechanism of Action Competitively blocks $beta_1$-adrenergic receptors with little or no effect on $beta_2$-receptors except at high doses; exhibits membrane stabilizing and intrinsic sympathomimetic activity

Pharmacodynamics/Kinetics

Onset of action: 1-2 hours
Duration: 12-24 hours
Absorption: Oral: 40%
Protein binding: 5% to 15%
Metabolism: Extensive first-pass effect
Half-life elimination: 6-7 hours
Time to peak: 2-4 hours
Excretion: Feces (~55%); urine (35%)

Contraindications Hypersensitivity to beta-blocking agents; uncompensated congestive heart failure; cardiogenic shock; bradycardia or second- and third-degree heart block (except in patients with a functioning artificial pacemaker); sinus node dysfunction; pregnancy (2nd and 3rd trimesters)

Warnings/Precautions Abrupt withdrawal of drug **should be avoided.** May result in an exaggerated cardiac responsiveness such as tachycardia, hypertension, ischemia, angina, myocardial infarction, and sudden death. It is recommended that patients be gradually tapered off beta-blockers (over a 2-week period) rather than via abrupt discontinuation. Although acebutolol primarily blocks $beta_1$-receptors, high doses can result in $beta_2$-receptor blockage. Use with caution in diabetic patients. Beta-blockers may impair glucose tolerance, potentiate hypoglycemia, and/or mask symptoms of hypoglycemia in a diabetic patient. Use with caution in bronchospastic lung disease and renal dysfunction (especially the elderly). Beta-blockers with intrinsic sympathomimetic activity do not appear to be of benefit in CHF and should be avoided. See Dosage - Renal/Hepatic Impairment.

Drug Interactions Inhibits CYP2D6 (weak)

Alpha-blockers (prazosin, terazosin): Concurrent use of beta-blockers may increase risk of orthostasis.
Clonidine: Hypertensive crisis after or during withdrawal of either agent.
Drugs which slow AV conduction (digoxin): Effects may be additive with beta-blockers.
Glucagon: Acebutolol may blunt the hyperglycemic action of glucagon.
Insulin and oral hypoglycemics: Acebutolol masks the tachycardia from hypoglycemia.
NSAIDs (ibuprofen, indomethacin, naproxen, piroxicam) may reduce the antihypertensive effects of beta-blockers.
Salicylates may reduce the antihypertensive effects of beta-blockers.
Sulfonylureas: Beta-blockers may alter response to hypoglycemic agents.
Verapamil or diltiazem may have synergistic or additive pharmacological effects when taken concurrently with beta-blockers.

Nutritional/Herbal/Ethanol Interactions

Food: Peak serum acebutolol levels may be slightly decreased if taken with food.
Herb/Nutraceutical: Avoid dong quai if using for hypertension (has estrogenic activity). Avoid yohimbe, ginseng (may worsen hypertension).

Lab Interactions Increased triglycerides, potassium, uric acid, cholesterol (S), glucose, thyroxine (S); decreased HDL

Adverse Reactions

>10%: Central nervous system: Fatigue (11%)

1% to 10%:

- Cardiovascular: Chest pain (2%), edema (2%), bradycardia, hypotension, CHF
- Central nervous system: Headache (6%), dizziness (6%), insomnia (3%), depression (2%), abnormal dreams (2%), anxiety, hyperesthesia, hypoesthesia, impotence
- Dermatologic: Rash (2%), pruritus
- Gastrointestinal: Constipation (4%), diarrhea (4%), dyspepsia (4%), nausea (4%), flatulence (3%), vomiting, abdominal pain
- Genitourinary: Micturition frequency (3%), dysuria, nocturia, impotence (2%)
- Neuromuscular & skeletal: Arthralgia (2%), myalgia (2%), back pain, joint pain
- Ocular: Abnormal vision (2%), conjunctivitis, dry eyes, eye pain
- Respiratory: Dyspnea (4%), rhinitis (2%), cough (1%), pharyngitis, wheezing

<1% (Limited to important or life-threatening): AV block, exacerbation of pre-existing renal insufficiency, hepatotoxic reaction, impotence, lichen planus, pleurisy, pneumonitis, pulmonary granulomas, systemic lupus erythematosus, urinary retention, ventricular arrhythmia

(Continued)

Acebutolol *(Continued)*

Potential adverse effects (based on experience with other beta-blocking agents) include reversible mental depression, disorientation, catatonia, short-term memory loss, emotional lability, slightly clouded sensorium, laryngospasm, respiratory distress, allergic reactions, erythematous rash, agranulocytosis, purpura, thrombocytopenia, mesenteric artery thrombosis, ischemic colitis, alopecia, Peyronie's disease, claudication

Overdosage/Toxicology Symptoms of intoxication include cardiac disturbances, CNS toxicity, bronchospasm, hypoglycemia, and hyperkalemia. The most common cardiac symptoms include hypotension and bradycardia. Atrioventricular block, intraventricular conduction disturbances, cardiogenic shock, and asystole may occur with severe overdose, especially with membrane-depressant drugs (eg, propranolol). CNS effects include convulsions and coma. Respiratory arrest is commonly seen with propranolol and other membrane-depressant and lipid-soluble drugs. Treat symptomatically. Cardiac and hemodynamic monitoring may be necessary.

Dosing

Adults:

Angina, ventricular arrhythmia: Oral: 400-800 mg/day twice daily; maximum: 1200 mg/day

Hypertension: Oral: 400-800 mg/day twice daily; maximum: 1200 mg/day; usual dose range (JNC 7): 200-800 mg/day in 2 divided doses

Elderly: Oral: Initial: 200-400 mg/day; dose reduction due to age-related decrease in Cl_{cr} will be necessary; do not exceed 800 mg/day.

Renal Impairment:

Cl_{cr} 25-49 mL/minute/1.73 m^2: Reduce dose by 50%.

Cl_{cr} <25 mL/minute/1.73 m^2: Reduce dose by 75%.

Hepatic Impairment: Use with caution.

Available Dosage Forms Capsule, as hydrochloride: 200 mg, 400 mg

Nursing Guidelines

Assessment: Assess effectiveness and interactions of other medications patient may be taking. Assess results of laboratory tests, therapeutic effectiveness, and adverse response on a regular basis during therapy. When discontinuing therapy, taper dosage over 2 weeks. Assess knowledge/teach patient appropriate use, possible side effects (including altered glucose tolerance for patients with diabetes)/appropriate interventions, and adverse symptoms to report.

Dietary Considerations: May be taken without regard to meals.

Patient Education: Take exactly as directed; do not increase, decrease, or adjust dosage without consulting prescriber. May be taken without regard to meals. Take pulse daily, prior to medication, and follow prescriber's instruction about holding medication. Do not take with antacids. Do not use OTC medications such as cold remedies without consulting prescriber. If you have diabetes, monitor serum sugar closely (drug may alter glucose tolerance or mask signs of hypoglycemia). May cause fatigue, dizziness (use caution when driving or engaging in tasks that require alertness until response to drug is known); postural hypotension (use caution when changing position from lying or sitting to standing or when climbing stairs); or alteration in sexual performance (reversible). Report chest pain or palpitations, unresolved swelling of extremities or unusual weight gain, respiratory difficulty or new cough, skin rash, unresolved fatigue, unresolved constipation or diarrhea, unusual muscle weakness, or CNS disturbances. **Pregnancy/breast-feeding precautions:** Inform prescriber if you are pregnant. Consult prescriber if breast-feeding.

Geriatric Considerations: Geriatric patients may require dose reduction due to age-related increase in bioavailability and decrease in Cl_{cr}. Beta-adrenergic blocking drugs may result in a decreased response as compared to younger adults.

Pregnancy Risk Factor: B (manufacturer); D (2nd and 3rd trimesters - expert analysis)

Pregnancy Issues: Acebutolol crosses the placenta. Beta-blockers have been associated with persistent bradycardia, hypotension, and IUGR; IUGR is probably related to maternal hypertension. Available evidence suggests beta-blockers are generally safe during pregnancy (JNC 7). Cases of neonatal hypoglycemia have been reported following maternal use of beta-blockers at parturition or during breast-feeding. Monitor breast-fed infant for symptoms of beta-blockade.

Lactation: Enters breast milk/use caution

Breast-Feeding Considerations: Hypotension, bradycardia, and tachypnea have been reported in nursing infants.

Administration

Storage: Store at room temperature (~25°C/77°F). Protect from light and dispense in a light-resistant, tight container.

- ♦ Acebutolol Hydrochloride *see* Acebutolol *on page 62*
- ♦ Acephen® [OTC] *see* Acetaminophen *on page 65*
- ♦ Acetadote® *see* Acetylcysteine *on page 80*

Acetaminophen (a seet a MIN oh fen)

U.S. Brand Names Acephen® [OTC]; Aspirin Free Anacin® Maximum Strength [OTC]; Cetafen® [OTC]; Cetafen Extra® [OTC]; Comtrex® Sore Throat Maximum Strength [OTC]; ElixSure™ Fever/Pain [OTC]; FeverALL® [OTC]; Genapap® [OTC]; Genapap® Children [OTC]; Genapap® Extra Strength [OTC]; Genapap® Infant [OTC]; Genebs® [OTC]; Genebs® Extra Strength [OTC]; Mapap® [OTC]; Mapap® Arthritis [OTC]; Mapap® Children's [OTC]; Mapap® Extra Strength [OTC]; Mapap® Infants [OTC]; Redutemp® [OTC]; Silapap® Children's [OTC]; Silapap® Infants [OTC]; Tylenol® [OTC]; Tylenol® 8 Hour [OTC]; Tylenol® Arthritis Pain [OTC]; Tylenol® Children's [OTC]; Tylenol® Extra Strength [OTC]; Tylenol® Infants [OTC]; Tylenol® Junior [OTC]; Tylenol® Sore Throat [OTC]; Valorin [OTC]; Valorin Extra [OTC]

Synonyms APAP; N-Acetyl-P-Aminophenol; Paracetamol

Pharmacologic Category Analgesic, Miscellaneous

Medication Safety Issues

Sound-alike/look-alike issues:

Acephen® may be confused with AcipHex®

FeverALL® may be confused with Fiberall®

Tylenol® may be confused with atenolol, timolol, Tuinal®, Tylox®

Use Treatment of mild to moderate pain and fever (antipyretic/analgesic); does not have antirheumatic or anti-inflammatory effects

Mechanism of Action Inhibits the synthesis of prostaglandins in the central nervous system and peripherally blocks pain impulse generation; produces antipyresis from inhibition of hypothalamic heat-regulating center

Pharmacodynamics/Kinetics

Onset of action: <1 hour

Duration: 4-6 hours

Absorption: Incomplete; varies by dosage form

Protein binding: 8% to 43% at toxic doses

Metabolism: At normal therapeutic dosages, hepatic to sulfate and glucuronide metabolites, while a small amount is metabolized by CYP to a highly reactive intermediate (acetylimidoquinone) which is conjugated with glutathione and inactivated; at toxic doses (as little as 4 g daily) glutathione conjugation becomes insufficient to meet the metabolic demand causing an increase in acetylimidoquinone concentration, which may cause hepatic cell necrosis

Half-life elimination: Prolonged following toxic doses

Neonates: 2-5 hours

Adults: 1-3 hours (may be increased in elderly; however, this should not affect dosing)

Time to peak, serum: Oral: 10-60 minutes; may be delayed in acute overdoses

Excretion: Urine (2% to 5% unchanged; 55% as glucuronide metabolites; 30% as sulphate metabolites)

Contraindications Hypersensitivity to acetaminophen or any component of the formulation

Warnings/Precautions Limit dose to <4 g/day. May cause severe hepatic toxicity on acute overdose; in addition, chronic daily dosing in adults has resulted in liver damage in some patients. Use with caution in patients with alcoholic liver disease; consuming ≥3 alcoholic drinks/day may increase the risk of liver damage. Use caution in patients with known G6PD deficiency.

OTC labeling: When used for self-medication, patients should be instructed to contact healthcare provider if used for fever lasting >3 days or for pain lasting >10 days in adults or >5 days in children.

Drug Interactions Substrate (minor) of CYP1A2, 2A6, 2C8/9, 2D6, 2E1, 3A4; **Inhibits** CYP3A4 (weak)

(Continued)

Acetaminophen *(Continued)*

Decreased effect: Barbiturates, carbamazepine, hydantoins, rifampin, sulfinpyrazone may decrease the analgesic effect of acetaminophen. Cholestyramine may decrease acetaminophen absorption (separate dosing by at least 1 hour).

Increased toxicity: Barbiturates, carbamazepine, hydantoins, isoniazid, rifampin, sulfinpyrazone may increase the hepatotoxic potential of acetaminophen. Chronic ethanol abuse increases risk for acetaminophen toxicity; effect of warfarin may be enhanced.

Nutritional/Herbal/Ethanol Interactions

Ethanol: Excessive intake of ethanol may increase the risk of acetaminophen-induced hepatotoxicity. Avoid ethanol or limit to <3 drinks/day.

Food: Rate of absorption may be decreased when given with food.

Herb/Nutraceutical: St John's wort may decrease acetaminophen levels.

Lab Interactions Increased chloride, bilirubin, uric acid, glucose, ammonia (B), chloride (S), uric acid (S), alkaline phosphatase (S), chloride (S); decreased sodium, bicarbonate, calcium (S)

Adverse Reactions Frequency not defined.

Dermatologic: Rash

Endocrine & metabolic: May increase chloride, uric acid, glucose; may decrease sodium, bicarbonate, calcium

Hematologic: Anemia, blood dyscrasias (neutropenia, pancytopenia, leukopenia)

Hepatic: Bilirubin increased, alkaline phosphatase increased

Renal: Ammonia increased, nephrotoxicity with chronic overdose, analgesic nephropathy

Miscellaneous: Hypersensitivity reactions (rare)

Overdosage/Toxicology Symptoms of overdose include hepatic necrosis, transient azotemia, renal tubular necrosis with acute toxicity, anemia, and GI disturbances with chronic toxicity. Treatment consists of acetylcysteine 140 mg/kg orally (loading) followed by 70 mg/kg every 4 hours for 17 doses; therapy should be initiated based upon laboratory analysis suggesting a high probability of hepatotoxic potential. Activated charcoal is very effective at binding acetaminophen. Intravenous acetylcysteine should be reserved for patients unable to take oral forms.

Dosing

Adults & Elderly: Pain or fever: Oral, rectal: 325-650 mg every 4-6 hours or 1000 mg 3-4 times/day; do **not** exceed 4 g/day.

Pediatrics: Pain or fever: Oral, rectal: Children <12 years: 10-15 mg/kg/dose every 4-6 hours as needed; do **not** exceed 5 doses (2.6 g) in 24 hours; alternatively, the following doses may be used; see table.

Acetaminophen Dosing

Age	Dosage (mg)	Age	Dosage (mg)
0-3 mo	40	4-5 y	240
4-11 mo	80	6-8 y	320
1-2 y	120	9-10 y	400
2-3 y	160	11 y	480

Note: Higher rectal doses have been studied for use in preoperative pain control in children. However, specific guidelines are not available and dosing may be product dependent. The safety and efficacy of alternating acetaminophen and ibuprofen dosing has not been established.

Renal Impairment:

Cl_{cr} 10-50 mL/minute: Administer every 6 hours.

Cl_{cr} <10 mL/minute: Administer every 8 hours (metabolites accumulate).

Moderately dialyzable (20% to 50%)

Hepatic Impairment: Use with caution. Limited, low-dose therapy is usually well tolerated in hepatic disease/cirrhosis. However, cases of hepatotoxicity at daily acetaminophen dosages <4 g/day have been reported. Avoid chronic use in hepatic impairment.

Available Dosage Forms [DSC] = Discontinued product

Caplet (Cetafen Extra® Strength, Genapap® Extra Strength, Genebs® Extra Strength, Mapap® Extra Strength, Tylenol® Extra Strength): 500 mg

Caplet, extended release (Mapap® Arthritis, Tylenol® 8 Hour, Tylenol® Arthritis Pain): 650 mg

Capsule (Mapap® Extra Strength): 500 mg

Elixir: 160 mg/5 mL (120 mL, 480 mL, 3780 mL)
- Mapap® Children's: 160 mg/5 mL (120 mL) [alcohol free; contains benzoic acid and sodium benzoate; cherry flavor]

Gelcap (Mapap® Extra Strength, Tylenol® Extra Strength): 500 mg

Geltab (Mapap® Extra Strength, Tylenol® Extra Strength): 500 mg

Geltab, extended release (Tylenol® 8 Hour): 650 mg

Liquid, oral: 500 mg/15 mL (240 mL)
- Comtrex® Sore Throat Maximum Strength: 500 mg/15 mL (240 mL) [contains sodium benzoate; honey lemon flavor]
- Genapap® Children: 160 mg/5 mL (120 mL) [contains sodium benzoate; cherry and grape flavors]
- Silapap®: 160 mg/5 mL (120 mL, 240 mL, 480 mL) [sugar free; contains sodium benzoate; cherry flavor]
- Tylenol® Extra Strength: 500 mg/15 mL (240 mL) [contains sodium benzoate; cherry flavor]
- Tylenol® Sore Throat: 500 mg/15 mL (240 mL) [contains sodium benzoate; cherry and honey-lemon flavors]

Solution, oral drops: 80 mg/0.8 mL (15 mL) [droppers are marked at 0.4 mL (40 mg) and at 0.8 mL (80 mg)]
- Genapap® Infant: 80 mg/0.8 mL (15 mL) [fruit flavor]
- Silapap® Infant's: 80 mg/0.8 mL (15 mL, 30 mL) [contains sodium benzoate; cherry flavor]

Solution, oral: 160 mg/5 mL (120 mL, 480 mL)

Suppository, rectal: 120 mg, 325 mg, 650 mg
- Acephen®: 120 mg, 325 mg, 650 mg
- FeverALL®: 80 mg, 120 mg, 325 mg, 650 mg
- Mapap®: 125 mg, 650 mg

Suspension, oral:
- Mapap® Children's: 160 mg/5 mL (120 mL) [contains sodium benzoate; cherry flavor]
- Tylenol® Children's: 160 mg/5 mL (120 mL, 240 mL) [contains sodium benzoate; bubble gum yum, cherry blast, dye free cherry, grape splash, and very berry strawberry flavors]

Suspension, oral drops:
- Mapap® Infants 80 mg/0.8 mL (15 mL, 30 mL) [contains sodium benzoate; cherry flavor]
- Tylenol® Infants: 80 mg/0.8 mL (15 mL, 30 mL) [contains sodium benzoate; cherry, dye free cherry, and grape flavors]

Syrup, oral (ElixSure™ Fever/Pain): 160 mg/5 mL (120 mL) [bubble gum, cherry, and grape flavors]

Tablet: 325 mg, 500 mg
- Aspirin Free Anacin® Extra Strength, Genapap® Extra Strength, Genebs® Extra Strength, Mapap® Extra Strength, Redutemp®, Tylenol® Extra Strength, Valorin Extra: 500 mg
- Cetafen®, Genapap®, Genebs®, Mapap®, Tylenol®, Valorin: 325 mg

Tablet, chewable: 80 mg
- Genapap® Children: 80 mg [contains phenylalanine 6 mg/tablet; fruit and grape flavors]
- Mapap® Children's: 80 mg [contains phenylalanine 3 mg/tablet; bubble gum, fruit, and grape flavors]
- Mapap® Junior Strength: 160 mg [contains phenylalanine 12 mg/tablet; grape flavor]
- Tylenol® Children's: 80 mg [fruit and grape flavors contain phenylalanine 3 mg/tablet; bubble gum flavor contains phenylalanine 6 mg/tablet] [DSC]
- Tylenol® Junior: 160 mg [contains phenylalanine 6 mg/tablet; fruit and grape flavors] [DSC]

Tablet, orally-disintegrating:
- Tylenol® Children's Meltaways: 80 mg [bubble gum, grape, and watermelon flavors]
- Tylenol® Junior Meltaways: 160 mg [bubble gum and grape flavors]

Nursing Guidelines

Assessment: Assess patient for history of liver disease or ethanol abuse (acetaminophen and excessive ethanol may have adverse liver effects). Assess other medications patient may be taking for additive or adverse interactions. Assess knowledge/teach patient appropriate use. Teach patient to monitor for adverse reactions and appropriate interventions to reduce side effects.

Monitoring Laboratory Tests: Serum APAP levels with long-term use in patients with hepatic disease

(Continued)

Acetaminophen *(Continued)*

Dietary Considerations: Chewable tablets may contain phenylalanine (amount varies, ranges between 3-12 mg/tablet); consult individual product labeling.

Patient Education: Take exactly as directed; do not increase dose or frequency. Most adverse effects are related to excessive use. Take with food or milk. While using this medication, avoid or limit alcohol to <3 drinks/day and avoid other prescription or OTC medications that contain acetaminophen. Maintain adequate hydration (2-3 L/day of fluids) unless instructed to restrict fluid intake. This medication will not reduce inflammation; consult prescriber for anti-inflammatory, if needed. Report unusual bleeding (stool, mouth, urine) or bruising; unusual fatigue and weakness; change in elimination patterns; or change in color of urine or stool.

Pregnancy Risk Factor: B

Lactation: Enters breast milk/compatible

Perioperative/Anesthesia/Other Concerns: Avoid excessive doses of acetaminophen particularly in patients with a significant alcohol history or poor nutritional habits. The 2002 ACCM/SCCM guidelines for analgesia (critically-ill adult) recommend prescribing <2 g/day for patients with a significant alcohol history or those with malnutrition. Other patients may be limited to <4 g/day. Susceptibility to acetaminophen hepatotoxicity may be due to induction of hepatic enzymes caused by chronic alcohol ingestion, depletion of glutathione, malnutrition, and impaired glucuronidation caused by fasting.

Administration

Oral: Shake suspension well before pouring dose.

Storage: Do not freeze suppositories.

Related Information

Acute Postoperative Pain *on page 1742*

Acetaminophen and Codeine (a seet a MIN oh fen & KOE deen)

U.S. Brand Names Capital® and Codeine; Tylenol® With Codeine

Synonyms Codeine and Acetaminophen

Pharmacologic Category Analgesic, Narcotic

Medication Safety Issues

Sound-alike/look-alike issues:

Capital® may be confused with Capitrol®

Tylenol® may be confused with atenolol, timolol, Tuinal®, Tylox®

T3 is an error-prone abbreviation (mistaken as liothyronine)

Use Relief of mild to moderate pain

Mechanism of Action Inhibits the synthesis of prostaglandins in the central nervous system and peripherally blocks pain impulse generation; produces antipyresis from inhibition of hypothalamic heat-regulating center; binds to opiate receptors in the CNS, causing inhibition of ascending pain pathways, altering the perception of and response to pain; causes cough supression by direct central action in the medulla; produces generalized CNS depression. Caffeine (contained in some non-U.S. formulations) is a CNS stimulant; use with acetaminophen and codeine increases the level of analgesia provided by each agent.

Pharmacodynamics/Kinetics See individual agents.

Contraindications Hypersensitivity to acetaminophen, codeine, or any component of the formulation; significant respiratory depression (in unmonitored settings); acute or severe bronchial asthma; hypercapnia; paralytic ileus

Warnings/Precautions Use with caution in patients with hypersensitivity reactions to other phenanthrene derivative opioid agonists (morphine, hydrocodone, hydromorphone, levorphanol, oxycodone, oxymorphone); tablets contain metabisulfite which may cause allergic reactions. Tolerance or drug dependence may result from extended use.

Limit total acetaminophen dose to <4 g/day. May cause severe hepatic toxicity on acute overdose; in addition, chronic daily dosing in adults has resulted in liver damage in some patients. Use with caution in patients with alcoholic liver disease; consuming 3 alcoholic drinks/day may increase the risk of liver damage. Use caution in patients with known G6PD deficiency.

This combination should be used with caution in elderly or debilitated patients, hypotension, adrenocortical insufficiency, thyroid disorders, prostatic hyperplasia, urethral stricture, seizure disorder, CNS depression, head injury or increased intracranial pressure. Causes sedation; caution must be used in performing tasks which require alertness (eg, operating machinery or driving). Safety and efficacy in pediatric patients have not been established.

Note: Some non-U.S. formulations (including most Canadian formulations) may contain caffeine as an additional ingredient. Caffeine may cause CNS and cardiovascular stimulation, as well as GI irritation in high doses. Use with caution in patients with a history of peptic ulcer or GERD; avoid in patients with symptomatic cardiac arrhythmias.

Drug Interactions Acetaminophen: **Substrate** (minor) of CYP1A2, 2A6, 2C8/9, 2D6, 2E1, 3A4; **Inhibits** CYP3A4 (weak)

Increased toxicity: CNS depressants, phenothiazines, tricyclic antidepressants, guanabenz, MAO inhibitors (may also decrease blood pressure); effect of warfarin may be enhanced.

Nutritional/Herbal/Ethanol Interactions Ethanol: Excessive intake of ethanol may increase the risk of acetaminophen-induced hepatotoxicity. Avoid ethanol or limit to <3 drinks/day.

Adverse Reactions

>10%:

Central nervous system: Lightheadedness, dizziness, sedation
Gastrointestinal: Nausea, vomiting
Respiratory: Dyspnea

1% to 10%:

Central nervous system: Euphoria, dysphoria
Dermatologic: Pruritus
Gastrointestinal: Constipation, abdominal pain
Miscellaneous: Histamine release

<1% (Limited to important or life-threatening): Antidiuretic hormone release, biliary tract spasm, bradycardia, hypotension, intracranial pressure increased, physical and psychological dependence, respiratory depression, urinary retention

Overdosage/Toxicology

Symptoms of overdose include hepatic necrosis, blood dyscrasias, respiratory depression.

Acetylcysteine 140 mg/kg orally (loading) followed by 70 mg/kg every 4 hours for 17 doses; therapy should be initiated based upon laboratory analysis suggesting high probability of hepatotoxic potential.

Naloxone 2 mg I.V. (0.01 mg/kg for children) with repeat administration as necessary up to a total of 10 mg; can also be used to reverse the toxic effects of the opiate.

Activated charcoal is effective at binding certain chemicals, and this is especially true for acetaminophen (use within 2 hours of ingestion).

Dosing

Adults: Doses should be adjusted according to severity of pain and response of the patient. Adult doses ≥60 mg codeine fail to give commensurate relief of pain but merely prolong analgesia and are associated with an appreciably increased incidence of side effects.

Cough (Antitussive): Oral: Based on codeine (15-30 mg/dose) every 4-6 hours

Pain (Analgesic): Oral: Based on codeine (30-60 mg/dose) every 4-6 hours
1-2 tablets every 4 hours to a maximum of 12 tablets/24 hours

Elderly: Doses should be titrated to appropriate analgesic effect.

1 Tylenol® [#3] or 2 Tylenol® [#2] tablets every 4 hours; do **not** exceed 4 g/day acetaminophen.

Pediatrics:

Analgesic: Oral:

Codeine: 0.5-1 mg codeine/kg/dose every 4-6 hours

Acetaminophen: 10-15 mg/kg/dose every 4 hours up to a maximum of 2.6 g/24 hours for children <12 years

3-6 years: 5 mL 3-4 times/day as needed of elixir
7-12 years: 10 mL 3-4 times/day as needed of elixir
Children >12 years: 15 mL every 4 hours as needed of elixir

Renal Impairment: See individual monographs for Acetaminophen and Codeine.

Hepatic Impairment: Use with caution. Limited, low-dose therapy is usually well tolerated in hepatic disease/cirrhosis; however, cases of hepatotoxicity at daily acetaminophen dosages <4 g/day have been reported. Avoid chronic use in hepatic impairment.

(Continued)

Acetaminophen and Codeine *(Continued)*

Available Dosage Forms [DSC] = Discontinued product; [CAN] = Canadian brand name

Caplet:

ratio-Lenoltec No. 1 [CAN], Tylenol No. 1 [CAN]: Acetaminophen 300 mg, codeine phosphate, 8 mg and caffeine 15 mg [not available in the U.S.]

Tylenol No. 1 Forte [CAN]: Acetaminophen 500 mg, codeine phosphate 8 mg, and caffeine 15 mg [not available in the U.S.]

Elixir, oral [C-V]: Acetaminophen 120 mg and codeine phosphate 12 mg per 5 mL (5 mL, 10 mL, 12.5 mL, 15 mL, 120 mL, 480 mL) [contains alcohol 7%]

Tylenol® with Codeine [DSC]: Acetaminophen 120 mg and codeine phosphate 12 mg per 5 mL (480 mL) [contains alcohol 7%; cherry flavor]

Tylenol Elixir with Codeine [CAN]: Acetaminophen 160 mg and codeine phosphate 8 mg per 5 mL (500 mL) [contains alcohol 7%, sucrose 31%; cherry flavor; not available in the U.S.]

Suspension, oral [C-V] (Capital® and Codeine): Acetaminophen 120 mg and codeine phosphate 12 mg per 5 mL (480 mL) [alcohol free; fruit punch flavor]

Tablet [C-III]: Acetaminophen 300 mg and codeine phosphate 15 mg; acetaminophen 300 mg and codeine phosphate 30 mg; acetaminophen 300 mg and codeine phosphate 60 mg

ratio-Emtec [CAN], Triatec-30 [CAN]: Acetaminophen 300 mg and codeine phosphate 30 mg [not available in the U.S.]

ratio-Lenoltec No. 1 [CAN]: Acetaminophen 300 mg, codeine phosphate 8 mg, and caffeine 15 mg [not available in the U.S.]

ratio-Lenoltec No. 2 [CAN], Tylenol No. 2 with Codeine [CAN]: Acetaminophen 300 mg, codeine phosphate 15 mg, and caffeine 15 mg [not available in the U.S.]

ratio-Lenoltec No. 3 [CAN], Tylenol No. 3 with Codeine [CAN]: Acetaminophen 300 mg, codeine phosphate 30 mg, and caffeine 15 mg [not available in the U.S.]

ratio-Lenoltec No. 4 [CAN], Tylenol No. 4 with Codeine [CAN]: Acetaminophen 300 mg and codeine phosphate 60 mg [not available in the U.S.]

Triatec-8 [CAN]: Acetaminophen 325 mg, codeine phosphate 8 mg, and caffeine 30 mg [not available in the U.S.]

Triatec-8 Strong [CAN]: Acetaminophen 500 mg, codeine phosphate 8 mg, and caffeine 30 mg [not available in the U.S.]

Tylenol® with Codeine No. 3: Acetaminophen 300 mg and codeine phosphate 30 mg [contains sodium metabisulfite]

Tylenol® with Codeine No. 4: Acetaminophen 300 mg and codeine phosphate 60 mg [contains sodium metabisulfite]

Nursing Guidelines

Dietary Considerations: May be taken with food.

Patient Education: See individual agents. **Pregnancy/breast-feeding precautions:** Inform prescriber if you are or intend to become pregnant. Consult prescriber if breast-feeding.

Pregnancy Risk Factor: C

Lactation: Enters breast milk/use caution

♦ Acetaminophen and Hydrocodone *see* Hydrocodone and Acetaminophen *on page 867*

♦ Acetaminophen and Oxycodone *see* Oxycodone and Acetaminophen *on page 1286*

♦ Acetaminophen and Propoxyphene *see* Propoxyphene and Acetaminophen *on page 1427*

Acetaminophen and Tramadol

(a seet a MIN oh fen & TRA ma dole)

U.S. Brand Names Ultracet™

Synonyms APAP and Tramadol; Tramadol Hydrochloride and Acetaminophen

Pharmacologic Category Analgesic, Miscellaneous; Analgesic, Non-narcotic

Use Short-term (≤5 days) management of acute pain

Mechanism of Action

Based on **acetaminophen** component: Inhibits the synthesis of prostaglandins in the central nervous system and peripherally blocks pain impulse generation; produces antipyresis from inhibition of hypothalamic heat-regulating center

Based on **tramadol** component: Binds to μ-opiate receptors in the CNS causing inhibition of ascending pain pathways, altering the perception of and response to pain; also inhibits the reuptake of norepinephrine and serotonin, which also modifies the ascending pain pathway

Pharmacodynamics/Kinetics See individual agents.

Contraindications Hypersensitivity to acetaminophen, tramadol, opioids, or any component of the formulation; opioid-dependent patients; acute intoxication with ethanol, hypnotics, narcotics, centrally-acting analgesics, opioids, or psychotropic drugs; hepatic dysfunction

Warnings/Precautions Should be used only with extreme caution in patients receiving MAO inhibitors. Use with caution and reduce dosage when administering to patients receiving other CNS depressants. Seizures may occur when taken within the recommended dosage; risk is increased in patients receiving serotonin reuptake inhibitors (SSRIs or anorectics), tricyclic antidepressants, other cyclic compounds (including cyclobenzaprine, promethazine), neuroleptics, MAO inhibitors, or drugs which may lower seizure threshold. Patients with a history of seizures, or with a risk of seizures (head trauma, metabolic disorders, CNS infection, malignancy, or during alcohol/drug withdrawal) are also at increased risk. Do not use with ethanol or other acetaminophen- or tramadol-containing products.

Limit acetaminophen to <4 g/day. May cause severe hepatic toxicity in acute overdose; in addition, chronic daily dosing in adults has resulted in liver damage in some patients. Use with caution in patients with alcoholic liver disease; consuming ≥3 alcoholic drinks/day may increase the risk of liver damage. Use caution in patients with known G6PD deficiency.

Elderly patients and patients with chronic respiratory disorders may be at greater risk of adverse events. Use with caution in patients with increased intracranial pressure or head injury. Use tramadol with caution and reduce dosage in patients with renal dysfunction. Tolerance or drug dependence may result from extended use (withdrawal symptoms have been reported); abrupt discontinuation should be avoided. Tapering of dose at the time of discontinuation limits the risk of withdrawal symptoms. Safety and efficacy in pediatric patients have not been established.

Drug Interactions

Acetaminophen: **Substrate** (minor) of CYP1A2, 2A6, 2C8/9, 2D6, 2E1, 3A4; **Inhibits** CYP3A4 (weak)

Tramadol: **Substrate** of CYP2D6 (major), 3A4 (minor)

Amphetamines: May increase the risk of seizures with tramadol.

Anesthetic agents: May increase risk of CNS and respiratory depression; use together with caution and in reduced dosage.

Barbiturates: Barbiturates may increase the hepatotoxic effects of acetaminophen; in addition, acetaminophen levels may be lowered.

Carbamazepine: Carbamazepine decreases half-life of tramadol by 33% to 50%; also have increased risk of seizures; in addition, carbamazepine may increase the hepatotoxic effects and lower serum levels of acetaminophen; concomitant use is not recommended.

CYP2D6 inhibitors: May decrease the effects of tramadol. Example inhibitors include chlorpromazine, delavirdine, fluoxetine, miconazole, paroxetine, pergolide, quinidine, quinine, ritonavir, and ropinirole.

Digoxin: Rare reports of digoxin toxicity with concomitant tramadol use.

Hydantoin anticonvulsants: Phenytoin may increase the hepatotoxic effects of acetaminophen; in addition, acetaminophen levels may be lowered.

MAO inhibitors: May increase the risk of seizures. Use extreme caution.

Naloxone: May increase the risk of seizures (if administered in tramadol overdose).

Neuroleptic agents: May increase the risk of tramadol-associated seizures and may have additive CNS depressant effects.

Narcotics: May increase risk of CNS and respiratory depression; use together with caution and in reduced dosage.

Opioids: May increase the risk of seizures, and may have additive CNS depressant effects. Use together with caution and in reduced dosage.

Phenothiazines: May increase risk of CNS and respiratory depression; use together with caution and in reduced dosage.

(Continued)

Acetaminophen and Tramadol *(Continued)*

Rifampin: Rifampin may increase the clearance of acetaminophen.

Quinidine: May increase the tramadol serum concentrations by inhibiting CYP metabolism.

SSRIs: May increase the risk of seizures with tramadol by inhibiting CYP metabolism (citalopram, fluoxetine, paroxetine, sertraline).

Sulfinpyrazone: Sulfinpyrazone may increase the hepatotoxic effects of acetaminophen; in addition, acetaminophen levels may be lowered.

Tricyclic antidepressants: May increase the risk of seizures.

Warfarin: Acetaminophen and tramadol may lead to an elevation of prothrombin times; monitor.

Nutritional/Herbal/Ethanol Interactions

Ethanol: Avoid ethanol (increased liver toxicity with concomitant use).

Food: May delay time to peak plasma levels, however, the extent of absorption is not affected.

Herb/Nutraceutical:

Acetaminophen: Avoid St John's wort (may decrease acetaminophen levels).

Tramadol: Avoid valerian, St John's wort, kava kava, gotu kola (may increase CNS depression).

Adverse Reactions

1% to 10%:

Central nervous system: Somnolence (6%), dizziness (3%), insomnia (2%), anxiety, confusion, euphoria, fatigue, headache, nervousness, tremor

Dermatologic: Pruritus (2%), rash

Endocrine & metabolic: Hot flashes

Gastrointestinal: Constipation (6%), anorexia (3%), diarrhea (3%), nausea (3%), dry mouth (2%), abdominal pain, dyspepsia, flatulence, vomiting

Genitourinary: Prostatic disorder (2%)

Neuromuscular & skeletal: Weakness

Miscellaneous: Diaphoresis increased (4%)

<1% (Limited to important or life-threatening): Allergic reactions, amnesia, anaphylactoid reactions, anaphylaxis, arrhythmia, coma, depersonalization, drug abuse, dysphagia, dyspnea, emotional lability, hallucination, hepatitis, hypertonia, impotence, liver failure, migraine, muscle contractions (involuntary), oliguria, paresthesia, paroniria, pulmonary edema, rigors, seizure, serotonin syndrome, shivering, Stevens-Johnson syndrome, suicidal tendency, stupor, syncope, tinnitus, tongue edema, toxic epidermal necrolysis, urinary retention, urticaria, vertigo

A withdrawal syndrome may occur with abrupt discontinuation; includes anxiety, diarrhea, hallucinations (rare), nausea, pain, piloerection, rigors, sweating, and tremor. Uncommon discontinuation symptoms may include severe anxiety, panic attacks, or paresthesia.

Overdosage/Toxicology Symptoms of overdose include signs and symptoms from both acetaminophen and tramadol toxicity. Treatment should be symptom-directed and supportive.

Acetaminophen: Symptoms of overdose include hepatic necrosis, transient azotemia, renal tubular necrosis with acute toxicity, anemia, and GI disturbances with chronic toxicity. Treatment consists of acetylcysteine 140 mg/kg orally (loading), followed by 70 mg/kg every 4 hours for 17 doses; therapy should be initiated based upon laboratory analysis suggesting a high probability of hepatotoxic potential. Activated charcoal is very effective at binding acetaminophen. Intravenous acetylcysteine should be reserved for patients unable to take oral forms.

Tramadol: CNS and respiratory depression, coma, seizure, cardiac arrest, and death. Naloxone may be helpful, but may also increase risk of seizures.

Dosing

Adults & Elderly: Acute pain: Oral: Two tablets every 4-6 hours as needed for pain relief (maximum: 8 tablets/day); treatment should not exceed 5 days

Renal Impairment: Cl_{cr} <30 mL/minute: Maximum of 2 tablets every 12 hours. Treatment should not exceed 5 days.

Hepatic Impairment: Use is not recommended.

Available Dosage Forms Tablet: Acetaminophen 325 mg and tramadol hydrochloride 37.5 mg

Nursing Guidelines

Dietary Considerations: May be taken with or without food. Avoid use of ethanol and ethanol-containing products.

Patient Education: See individual agents. **Pregnancy/breast-feeding precautions:** Inform prescriber if you are or intend to become pregnant. Should not be used during pregnancy. Do not breast-feed.

Pregnancy Risk Factor: C

Pregnancy Issues: Tramadol has been shown to cross the placenta. Postmarketing reports following tramadol use during pregnancy include neonatal seizures, withdrawal syndrome, fetal death, and stillbirth. Not recommended for use during labor and delivery.

Lactation: Tramadol: Enters breast milk/contraindicated

Breast-Feeding Considerations: Not recommended for postdelivery analgesia in nursing mothers.

Administration

Storage: Store at controlled room temperature of 25°C (77°F).

◆ Acetaminophen, Butalbital, and Caffeine *see* Butalbital, Acetaminophen, and Caffeine *on page 280*

Acetaminophen, Dextromethorphan, and Pseudoephedrine

(a seet a MIN oh fen, deks troe meth OR fan, & soo doe e FED rin)

U.S. Brand Names Alka-Seltzer® Plus Flu Liqui-Gels® [OTC]; Comtrex® Non-Drowsy Cold and Cough Relief [OTC]; Contac® Severe Cold and Flu/ Non-Drowsy [OTC]; Infants' Tylenol® Cold Plus Cough Concentrated Drops [OTC]; Sudafed® Severe Cold [OTC]; Thera-Flu® Severe Cold Non-Drowsy [OTC] [DSC]; Triaminic® Cough and Sore Throat Formula [OTC]; Tylenol® Cold Day Non-Drowsy [OTC]; Tylenol® Flu Non-Drowsy Maximum Strength [OTC]; Vicks® DayQuil® Multi-Symptom Cold and Flu [OTC]

Synonyms Dextromethorphan, Acetaminophen, and Pseudoephedrine; Pseudoephedrine, Acetaminophen, and Dextromethorphan; Pseudoephedrine, Dextromethorphan, and Acetaminophen

Pharmacologic Category Antihistamine; Antitussive

Medication Safety Issues

Sound-alike/look-alike issues:

Sudafed® may be confused with Sufenta®

Thera-Flu® may be confused with Tamiflu®, Thera-Flur-N®

Tylenol® may be confused with atenolol, timolol, Tuinal®, Tylox®

Use Treatment of mild to moderate pain and fever; symptomatic relief of cough and congestion

Pharmacodynamics/Kinetics See individual agents.

Contraindications Hypersensitivity to acetaminophen, dextromethorphan, pseudoephedrine, or any component of the formulation

Drug Interactions

Acetaminophen: **Substrate** (minor) of CYP1A2, 2A6, 2C8/9, 2D6, 2E1, 3A4; **Inhibits** CYP3A4 (weak)

Dextromethorphan: **Substrate** of CYP2B6 (minor), 2C8/9 (minor), 2C19 (minor), 2D6 (major), 2E1 (minor), 3A4 (minor); **Inhibits** CYP2D6 (weak)

Also see individual agents.

Nutritional/Herbal/Ethanol Interactions Ethanol: Excessive intake of ethanol may increase the risk of acetaminophen-induced hepatotoxicity. Avoid ethanol or limit to <3 drinks/day.

Adverse Reactions See individual agents.

Dosing

Adults & Elderly:

Pain (Analgesic): Oral: Based on acetaminophen component: 325-650 mg every 4-7 hours as needed; do **not** exceed 4 g/day

Cough suppressant (Antitussive): Oral: Based on dextromethorphan component: 10-20 mg every 4-8 hours **or** 30 mg every 8 hours; do **not** exceed 120 mg/24 hours

Nasal congestion (Decongestant): Oral: Based on pseudoephedrine component: 60 mg every 4 hours (maximum: 360 mg/24 hours)

Product labeling:

Alka-Seltzer Plus® Cold and Flu Liqui-Gels®: Oral: 2 dose every 4 hours (maximum: 4 doses/24 hours)

Sudafed® Severe Cold, Thera-Flu® Non-Drowsy Maximum Strength (gelcap), Tylenol® Flu Non-Drowsy Maximum Strength: Oral: 2 doses every 6 hours (maximum: 8 doses/24 hours)

(Continued)

Acetaminophen, Dextromethorphan, and Pseudoephedrine *(Continued)*

Tylenol® Cold Non-Drowsy: Oral: 2 doses every 6 hours (maximum: 8 doses/24 hours)

Thera-Flu® Non-Drowsy Maximum Strength: Oral: 1 packet dissolved in hot water every 6 hours (maximum: 4 packets/24 hours)

Pediatrics:

Analgesic: Oral: Based on acetaminophen component: 10-15 mg/kg/dose every 4-6 hours as needed; do **not** exceed 5 doses/24 hours.

Cough suppressant: Oral: Based on dextromethorphan component:

Children 6-12 years: 15 mg every 6-8 hours; do **not** exceed 60 mg/24 hours

Children >12 years: Refer to adult dosing.

Decongestant: Oral: Based on pseudoephedrine component:

Children:

2-6 years: 15 mg every 4 hours (maximum: 90 mg/24 hours)

6-12 years: 30 mg every 4 hours (maximum: 180 mg/24 hours)

Children >12 years: Refer to adult dosing.

Product labeling:

Alka-Seltzer Plus® Cold and Flu Liqui-Gels®: Oral:

Children 6-12 years: 1 dose every 4 hours (maximum: 4 doses/24 hours)

Children >12 years: Refer to adult dosing.

Infants' Tylenol® Cold Plus Cough Concentrated Drops: Oral: Children 2-3 years (24-55 lb): 2 dropperfuls every 4-6 hours (maximum: 4 doses/24 hours)

Sudafed® Severe Cold, Thera-Flu® Non-Drowsy Maximum Strength (gelcap), Tylenol® Flu Non-Drowsy Maximum Strength: Oral: Children >12 years: Refer to adult dosing.

Tylenol® Cold Non-Drowsy: Oral:

Children 6-11 years: 1 dose every 6 hours (maximum: 4 doses/24 hours)

Children ≥12 years: Refer to adult dosing.

Thera-Flu® Non-Drowsy Maximum Strength: Oral: Children >12 years: Refer to adult dosing.

Hepatic Impairment: Use with caution. Limited, low-dose therapy usually well tolerated in hepatic disease/cirrhosis; however, cases of hepatotoxicity at daily acetaminophen dosages <4 g/day have been reported. Avoid chronic use in hepatic impairment.

Available Dosage Forms [DSC] = Discontinued product

Caplet:

Contac® Severe Cold and Flu/Non-Drowsy, Sudafed® Severe Cold, Tylenol® Cold Non-Drowsy: Acetaminophen 325 mg, dextromethorphan hydrobromide 15 mg, and pseudoephedrine hydrochloride 30 mg

Comtrex® Non-Drowsy Cold and Cough Relief: Acetaminophen 500 mg, dextromethorphan hydrobromide 15 mg, and pseudoephedrine hydrochloride 30 mg [contains benzoic acid]

Thera-Flu® Severe Cold Non-Drowsy: Acetaminophen 500 mg, dextromethorphan hydrobromide 15 mg, and pseudoephedrine hydrochloride 30 mg [contains lactose] [DSC]

Tylenol® Cold Day Non-Drowsy: Acetaminophen 325 mg dextromethorphan hydrobromide 15 mg, and pseudoephedrine hydrochloride 30 mg

Capsule, liquid:

Alka-Seltzer Plus® Flu Liqui-Gels®: Acetaminophen 325 mg, dextromethorphan hydrobromide 10 mg, and pseudoephedrine hydrochloride 30 mg

Vicks® DayQuil® Multi-Symptom Cold and Flu: Acetaminophen 250 mg, dextromethorphan hydrobromide 10 mg, and pseudoephedrine hydrochloride 30 mg

Gelcap:

Tylenol® Cold Day Non-Drowsy: Acetaminophen 325 mg dextromethorphan hydrobromide 15 mg, and pseudoephedrine hydrochloride 30 mg [contains benzyl alcohol]

Tylenol® Flu Non-Drowsy Maximum Strength: Acetaminophen 500 mg, dextromethorphan hydrobromide 15 mg, and pseudoephedrine hydrochloride 30 mg

Liquid:

Triaminic® Cough and Sore Throat Formula: Acetaminophen 160 mg, dextromethorphan hydrobromide 7.5 mg, and pseudoephedrine hydrochloride 15 mg per 5 mL (120 mL, 240 mL) [contains benzoic acid; grape flavor]

Vicks® DayQuil® Multi-Symptom Cold and Flu: Acetaminophen 325 mg, dextromethorphan hydrobromide 10 mg, and pseudoephedrine hydrochloride 30 mg per 15 mL (175 mL)

Powder for oral solution [packet] (Thera-Flu® Severe Cold Non-Drowsy): Acetaminophen 1000 mg, dextromethorphan hydrobromide 30 mg, and pseudoephedrine hydrochloride 60 mg [contains phenylalanine 17 mg/packet; lemon flavor] [DSC]

Suspension, oral drops (Infants' Tylenol® Cold Plus Cough Concentrated Drops): Acetaminophen 160 mg, dextromethorphan hydrobromide 5 mg, and pseudoephedrine hydrochloride 15 mg per 1.6 mL (15 mL) [1.6 mL = 2 dropperfuls] [cherry flavor]

Nursing Guidelines

Dietary Considerations: Thera-Flu® Severe Cold Non-Drowsy contains phenylalanine 17 mg/packet.

Related Information

Acetaminophen *on page 65*
Pseudoephedrine *on page 1436*

♦ Acetasol® HC *see* Acetic Acid, Propylene Glycol Diacetate, and Hydrocortisone *on page 78*

AcetaZOLAMIDE (a set a ZOLE a mide)

U.S. Brand Names Diamox® Sequels®

Pharmacologic Category Anticonvulsant, Miscellaneous; Carbonic Anhydrase Inhibitor; Diuretic, Carbonic Anhydrase Inhibitor; Ophthalmic Agent, Antiglaucoma

Medication Safety Issues

Sound-alike/look-alike issues:

AcetaZOLAMIDE may be confused with acetoHEXAMIDE
Diamox® Sequels® may be confused with Dobutrex®, Trimox®

Use Treatment of glaucoma (chronic simple open-angle, secondary glaucoma, preoperatively in acute angle-closure); drug-induced edema or edema due to congestive heart failure (adjunctive therapy); centrencephalic epilepsies (immediate release dosage form); prevention or amelioration of symptoms associated with acute mountain sickness

Unlabeled/Investigational Use Urine alkalinization; respiratory stimulant in COPD; metabolic alkalosis

Mechanism of Action Reversible inhibition of the enzyme carbonic anhydrase resulting in reduction of hydrogen ion secretion at renal tubule and an increased renal excretion of sodium, potassium, bicarbonate, and water to decrease production of aqueous humor; also inhibits carbonic anhydrase in central nervous system to retard abnormal and excessive discharge from CNS neurons

Pharmacodynamics/Kinetics

Onset of action: Capsule, extended release: 2 hours; I.V.: 2 minutes

Peak effect: Capsule, extended release: 8-12 hours; I.V.: 15 minutes; Tablet: 2-4 hours

Duration: Inhibition of aqueous humor secretion: Capsule, extended release: 18-24 hours; I.V.: 4-5 hours; Tablet: 8-12 hours

Distribution: Erythrocytes, kidneys; blood-brain barrier and placenta; distributes into milk (~30% of plasma concentrations)

Excretion: Urine (70% to 100% as unchanged drug)

Contraindications Hypersensitivity to acetazolamide, sulfonamides, or any component of the formulation; hepatic disease or insufficiency; decreased sodium and/or potassium levels; adrenocortical insufficiency, cirrhosis; hyperchloremic acidosis, severe renal disease or dysfunction; severe pulmonary obstruction; long-term use in noncongestive angle-closure glaucoma

Warnings/Precautions Use in impaired hepatic function may result in coma. Use with caution in patients with respiratory acidosis and diabetes mellitus. Impairment of mental alertness and/or physical coordination may occur. Chemical similarities are present among sulfonamides, sulfonylureas, carbonic anhydrase inhibitors, thiazides, and loop diuretics (except ethacrynic acid). Use in patients with sulfonamide allergy is specifically contraindicated in product labeling, however, a risk of cross-reaction exists in patients with allergy to any of these compounds; avoid use when previous reaction has been severe. Discontinue if signs of hypersensitivity are noted.

I.M. administration is painful because of the alkaline pH of the drug; use by this route is not recommended.

(Continued)

AcetaZOLAMIDE *(Continued)*

Drug may cause substantial increase in blood glucose in some diabetic patients; malaise and complaints of tiredness and myalgia are signs of excessive dosing and acidosis in the elderly.

Drug Interactions Inhibits CYP3A4 (weak)

Amphetamines: Urinary excretion of amphetamine may be decreased; magnitude and duration of effects may be enhanced.

Carbamazepine: May increase serum concentrations of carbamazepine.

Cyclosporine trough concentrations may be increased resulting in possible nephrotoxicity and neurotoxicity.

Flecainide: May decrease excretion of flecainide.

Lithium: Serum concentrations may be decreased by acetazolamide; monitor.

Memantine: May decrease excretion of memantine.

Methenamine: Urinary antiseptic effect may be prevented by acetazolamide.

Phenytoin: Serum concentrations of phenytoin may be increased; incidence of osteomalacia may be enhanced or increased in patients on chronic phenytoin therapy.

Primidone serum concentrations may be decreased; carbonic anhydrase inhibitors may enhance the adverse/toxic effects of primidone.

Quinidine: Urinary excretion of quinidine may be decreased and effects may be enhanced.

Salicylate use (high dose) may result in carbonic anhydrase inhibitor accumulation and toxicity including CNS depression and metabolic acidosis. Salicylate toxicity might also be enhanced.

Lab Interactions May cause false-positive results for urinary protein with Albustix®, Labstix®, Albutest®, Bumintest®. Interferes with HPLC theophylline assay and serum uric acid levels.

Adverse Reactions Frequency not defined.

Cardiovascular: Flushing

Central nervous system: Ataxia, confusion, convulsions, depression, dizziness, drowsiness, excitement, fatigue, fever, headache, malaise

Dermatologic: Allergic skin reactions, photosensitivity, Stevens-Johnson syndrome, toxic epidermal necrolysis, urticaria

Endocrine & metabolic: Electrolyte imbalance, growth retardation (children), hyperglycemia, hypoglycemia, hypokalemia, hyponatremia, metabolic acidosis

Gastrointestinal: Appetite decreased, diarrhea, melena, nausea, taste alteration, vomiting

Genitourinary: Crystalluria, glycosuria, hematuria, polyuria, renal failure

Hematologic: Agranulocytosis, aplastic anemia, leukopenia, thrombocytopenia, thrombocytopenic purpura

Hepatic: Cholestatic jaundice, fulminant hepatic necrosis, hepatic insufficiency, liver function tests abnormal

Local: Pain at injection site

Neuromuscular & skeletal: Flaccid paralysis, paresthesia

Ocular: Myopia

Otic: Hearing disturbance, tinnitus

Miscellaneous: Anaphylaxis

Overdosage/Toxicology Symptoms of overdose include low blood sugar, tingling of lips and tongue, nausea, yawning, confusion, agitation, tachycardia, sweating, convulsions, stupor, and coma. Hypoglycemia should be managed with 50 mL I.V. dextrose 50% followed immediately with a continuous infusion of 10% dextrose in water (administer at a rate sufficient enough to approach a serum glucose level of 100 mg/dL). The use of corticosteroids to treat hypoglycemia is controversial, however, adding 100 mg of hydrocortisone to the dextrose infusion may prove helpful. In certain instances, hemodialysis may be helpful.

Dosing

Adults: Note: I.M. administration is not recommended.

Glaucoma:

Chronic simple (open-angle): Oral: 250 mg 1-4 times/day or 500 mg sustained release capsule twice daily

Secondary, acute (closed-angle): I.V.: 250-500 mg, may repeat in 2-4 hours to a maximum of 1 g/day

Edema: Oral, I.V.: 250-375 mg once daily

Epilepsy: Oral: 8-30 mg/kg/day in 1-4 divided doses, not to exceed 1 g/day. **Note:** Sustained release capsule is not recommended for treatment of epilepsy.

Metabolic alkalosis (unlabeled use): I.V. 250 mg every 6 hours for 4 doses or 500 mg single dose; reassess need based upon acid-base status

Mountain sickness: Oral: 250 mg every 8-12 hours (or 500 mg extended release capsules every 12-24 hours). Therapy should begin 24-48 hours before and continue during ascent and for at least 48 hours after arrival at the high altitude.

Note: In situations of rapid ascent (such as rescue or military operations), 1000 mg/day is recommended.

Urine alkalinization (unlabeled use): Oral: 5 mg/kg/dose repeated 2-3 times over 24 hours

Respiratory stimulant in COPD (unlabeled use): Oral, I.V.: 250 mg twice daily

Elderly: Oral: Initial: 250 mg once or twice daily; use lowest effective dose possible.

Pediatrics: Note: I.M. administration is not recommended.

Glaucoma:

Oral: 8-30 mg/kg/day or 300-900 mg/m^2/day divided every 8 hours

I.V.: 20-40 mg/kg/24 hours divided every 6 hours, not to exceed 1 g/day

Edema: Oral, I.V.: 5 mg/kg or 150 mg/m^2 once every day

Epilepsy: Oral: Refer to adult dosing.

Renal Impairment:

Cl_{cr} 10-50 mL/minute: Administer every 12 hours.

Cl_{cr} <10 mL/minute: Avoid use (ineffective).

Moderately dialyzable (20% to 50%)

Available Dosage Forms

Capsule, sustained release (Diamox® Sequels®): 500 mg

Injection, powder for reconstitution: 500 mg

Tablet: 125 mg, 250 mg

Nursing Guidelines

Assessment: Assess allergy history prior to beginning therapy. Assess effectiveness and interactions of other medications patient may be taking. Monitor for signs of excessive dosing and acidosis (especially in elderly). Measure intraocular pressure at the beginning of therapy and periodically while on this medication. Assess results of laboratory tests, therapeutic effectiveness, and adverse response. Monitor growth in pediatric patients. Monitor blood glucose levels closely if diabetic. Assess knowledge/teach patient appropriate use, possible side effects/appropriate interventions, and adverse symptoms to report.

Monitoring Laboratory Tests: Intraocular pressure, serum electrolytes, periodic CBC with differential

Dietary Considerations: May be taken with food to decrease GI upset. May have additive effects with other folic acid antagonists. Sodium content of 500 mg injection: 47.2 mg (2.05 mEq).

Patient Education: Take as directed; do not chew or crush long-acting capsule (contents may be sprinkled on soft food). May be administered with food to decrease GI upset. You will need periodic ophthalmic examinations while taking this medication. You may experience drowsiness, dizziness, or weakness (use caution when driving or engaging in tasks that require alertness until response to drug is known); or nausea, loss of appetite, or altered taste (small, frequent meals, frequent mouth care, sucking lozenges, or chewing gum may help). Monitor serum glucose closely (may cause altered blood glucose in some patients with diabetes, or unusual response to some forms of glucose testing). You may experience increased sensitivity to sunlight (use sunblock, protective clothing, and avoid exposure to direct sunlight). Report unusual and persistent tiredness; numbness, burning, or tingling of extremities or around mouth, lips, or anus; muscle weakness; black stool; or excessive depression. **Pregnancy/breast-feeding precautions:** Inform prescriber if you are or intend to become pregnant. Consult prescriber if breast-feeding.

Geriatric Considerations: Malaise and complaints of tiredness and myalgia are signs of excessive dosing and acidosis in the elderly. Assess blood pressure (orthostatic hypotension can occur).

Pregnancy Risk Factor: C

Lactation: Enters breast milk/not recommended (AAP rates "compatible")

Administration

Reconstitution: Injection: Reconstitute with at least 5 mL sterile water to provide a solution containing not more than 100 mg/mL. Further dilute in D_5W or NS for I.V. infusion.

(Continued)

AcetaZOLAMIDE *(Continued)*

Compatibility: Stable in dextran 6% in D_5W, dextran 6% in NS, D_5LR, D_5NS, D_5½NS, D_5¼NS, D_5W, $D_{10}W$, LR, NS, ½NS

Compatibility when admixed: Incompatible with multivitamins

Storage:

Capsules, tablets: Store at controlled room temperature.

Injection: Store vial for injection (prior to reconstitution) at controlled room temperature. Stability of IVPB solution is 5 days at room temperature (25°C) and 44 days at refrigeration (5°C).

Acetic Acid (a SEE tik AS id)

U.S. Brand Names VoSol®

Synonyms Ethanoic Acid

Pharmacologic Category Otic Agent, Anti-infective; Topical Skin Product

Medication Safety Issues

Sound-alike/look-alike issues:

VoSol® may be confused with Vexol®

Use Irrigation of the bladder; treatment of superficial bacterial infections of the external auditory canal

Contraindications Hypersensitivity to acetic acid or any component of the formulation; during transurethral procedures

Warnings/Precautions Not for internal intake or I.V. infusion; topical use or irrigation use only. Use of irrigation in patients with mucosal lesions of urinary bladder may cause irritation. Systemic acidosis may result from absorption.

Adverse Reactions <1% (Limited to important or life-threatening): Hematuria, systemic acidosis, urologic pain

Dosing

Adults & Elderly:

Irrigation (**Note:** Dosage of an irrigating solution depends on the capacity or surface area of the structure being irrigated):

For continuous irrigation of the urinary bladder with 0.25% acetic acid irrigation, the rate of administration will approximate the rate of urine flow; usually 500-1500 mL/24 hours

For periodic irrigation of an indwelling urinary catheter to maintain patency, about 50 mL of 0.25% acetic acid irrigation is required

Otitis externa: Otic: Insert saturated wick; keep moist 24 hours; remove wick and instill 5 drops 3-4 times/day

Available Dosage Forms

Solution for irrigation: 0.25% (250 mL, 500 mL, 1000 mL)

Solution, otic (VōSol®): 2% [in propylene glycol] (15 mL)

Nursing Guidelines

Pregnancy Risk Factor: C

♦ Acetic Acid, Hydrocortisone, and Propylene Glycol Diacetate *see* Acetic Acid, Propylene Glycol Diacetate, and Hydrocortisone *on page 78*

Acetic Acid, Propylene Glycol Diacetate, and Hydrocortisone

(a SEE tik AS id, PRO pa leen GLY kole dye AS e tate, & hye droe KOR ti sone)

U.S. Brand Names Acetasol® HC; VoSol® HC

Synonyms Acetic Acid, Hydrocortisone, and Propylene Glycol Diacetate; Hydrocortisone, Acetic Acid, and Propylene Glycol Diacetate; Hydrocortisone, Propylene Glycol Diacetate, and Acetic Acid; Propylene Glycol Diacetate, Acetic Acid, and Hydrocortisone; Propylene Glycol Diacetate, Hydrocortisone, and Acetic Acid

Pharmacologic Category Otic Agent, Anti-infective

Use Treatment of superficial infections of the external auditory canal caused by organisms susceptible to the action of the antimicrobial, complicated by swelling

Drug Interactions Hydrocortisone: **Substrate** of CYP3A4 (minor); **Induces** CYP3A4 (weak)

Adverse Reactions Frequency not defined: Otic: Transient burning or stinging may be noticed occasionally when the solution is first instilled into the acutely inflamed ear

Dosing

Adults & Elderly: Otitis externa (superficial): Otic: Instill 4 drops in ear(s) 3-4 times/day

Pediatrics: Refer to adult dosing.

Available Dosage Forms Solution, otic drops: Acetic acid 2%, propylene glycol diacetate 3%, and hydrocortisone 1% (10 mL)

Nursing Guidelines

Assessment: Refer to Hydrocortisone monograph.

♦ **Acetoxymethylprogesterone** *see* MedroxyPROGESTERone *on page 1085*

Acetylcholine (a se teel KOE leen)

U.S. Brand Names Miochol-E®

Synonyms Acetylcholine Chloride

Pharmacologic Category Cholinergic Agonist; Ophthalmic Agent, Miotic

Medication Safety Issues

Sound-alike/look-alike issues:

Acetylcholine may be confused with acetylcysteine

Use Produces complete miosis in cataract surgery, keratoplasty, iridectomy, and other anterior segment surgery where rapid miosis is required

Mechanism of Action Causes contraction of the sphincter muscles of the iris, resulting in miosis and contraction of the ciliary muscle, leading to accommodation spasm

Pharmacodynamics/Kinetics

Onset of action: Rapid

Duration: ~10 minutes

Contraindications Hypersensitivity to acetylcholine chloride or any component of the formulation; acute iritis and acute inflammatory disease of the anterior chamber

Warnings/Precautions Systemic effects rarely occur but can cause problems for patients with acute cardiac failure, bronchial asthma, peptic ulcer, hyperthyroidism, GI spasm, urinary tract obstruction, and Parkinson's disease; open under aseptic conditions only.

Drug Interactions

Decreased effect possible with flurbiprofen and suprofen, ophthalmic.

Increased effect may be prolonged or enhanced in patients receiving tacrine.

Adverse Reactions Frequency not defined.

Cardiovascular: Bradycardia, hypotension, flushing

Central nervous system: Headache

Ocular: Distance vision altered, night vision decreased, transient lenticular opacities

Respiratory: Dyspnea

Miscellaneous: Diaphoresis

Overdosage/Toxicology Treatment includes flushing eyes with water or normal saline and supportive measures. If accidentally ingested, induce emesis or perform gastric lavage.

Dosing

Adults & Elderly: To produce miosis: Intraocular: 0.5-2 mL of 1% injection (5-20 mg) instilled into anterior chamber before or after securing one or more sutures

Available Dosage Forms Powder for intraocular solution, as chloride: 1:100 [10 mg/mL] (2 mL)

Nursing Guidelines

Patient Education: Do not touch dropper to eye. May sting on instillation. Use caution while driving at night or performing hazardous tasks.

Pregnancy Risk Factor: C

Pregnancy Issues: Acetylcholine is used primarily in the eye and there are no reports of its use in pregnancy. Because it is ionized at physiologic pH, transplacental passage would not be expected.

Perioperative/Anesthesia/Other Concerns: Systemic effects are rare after intraocular administration, but can occur. Caution should be used in patients with cardiovascular disease.

Administration

Reconstitution: Reconstitute immediately before use.

Storage: Prepare solution immediately before use and discard unused portion. Acetylcholine solutions are unstable.

♦ **Acetylcholine Chloride** *see* Acetylcholine *on page 79*

Acetylcysteine (a se teel SIS teen)

U.S. Brand Names Acetadote®; Mucomyst®

Synonyms Acetylcysteine Sodium; Mercapturic Acid; NAC; *N*-Acetylcysteine; *N*-Acetyl-L-cysteine

Pharmacologic Category Antidote; Mucolytic Agent

Medication Safety Issues

Sound-alike/look-alike issues:

Acetylcysteine may be confused with acetylcholine

Mucomyst® may be confused with Mucinex®

Use Adjunctive mucolytic therapy in patients with abnormal or viscid mucous secretions in acute and chronic bronchopulmonary diseases; pulmonary complications of surgery and cystic fibrosis; diagnostic bronchial studies; antidote for acute acetaminophen toxicity

Unlabeled/Investigational Use Prevention of radiocontrast-induced renal dysfunction (oral, I.V.); distal intestinal obstruction syndrome (DIOS, previously referred to as meconium ileus equivalent)

Mechanism of Action Exerts mucolytic action through its free sulfhydryl group which opens up the disulfide bonds in the mucoproteins thus lowering mucous viscosity. The exact mechanism of action in acetaminophen toxicity is unknown; thought to act by providing substrate for conjugation with the toxic metabolite.

Pharmacodynamics/Kinetics

Onset of action: Inhalation: 5-10 minutes

Duration: Inhalation: >1 hour

Distribution: 0.47 L/kg

Protein binding, plasma: 83%

Half-life elimination:

Reduced acetylcysteine: 2 hours

Total acetylcysteine: Adults: 5.5 hours; Newborns: 11 hours

Time to peak, plasma: Oral: 1-2 hours

Excretion: Urine

Contraindications Hypersensitivity to acetylcysteine or any component of the formulation

Warnings/Precautions

Inhalation: Since increased bronchial secretions may develop after inhalation, percussion, postural drainage, and suctioning should follow. If bronchospasm occurs, administer a bronchodilator; discontinue acetylcysteine if bronchospasm progresses.

Intravenous: Acute flushing and erythema have been reported; usually occurs within 30-60 minutes and may resolve spontaneously. Serious anaphylactoid reactions have also been reported. Acetylcysteine infusion may be interrupted until treatment of allergic symptoms is initiated; the infusion can then be carefully restarted. Treatment for anaphylactic reactions should be immediately available. Use caution with asthma or history of bronchospasm.

Acetaminophen overdose: The modified Rumack-Matthew nomogram allows for stratification of patients into risk categories based on the relationship between the serum acetaminophen level and time after ingestion. There are several situations where the nomogram is of limited use. Serum acetaminophen levels obtained prior to 4-hour postingestion are not interpretable; patients presenting late may have undetectable serum concentrations, but have received a lethal dose. The nomogram is less predictive in a chronic ingestion or in an overdose with an extended release product. Acetylcysteine should be administered for any signs of hepatotoxicity even if acetaminophen serum level is low or undetectable. The nomogram also does not take into account patients at higher risk of acetaminophen toxicity (eg, alcoholics, malnourished patients).

Drug Interactions Adsorbed by activated charcoal; clinical significance is minimal, though, once a pure acetaminophen ingestion requiring N-acetylcysteine is established; further charcoal dosing is unnecessary once the appropriate initial charcoal dose is achieved (5-10 g:g acetaminophen)

Adverse Reactions

Inhalation: Frequency not defined.

Central nervous system: Drowsiness, chills, fever

Gastrointestinal: Vomiting, nausea, stomatitis

Local: Irritation, stickiness on face following nebulization

Respiratory: Bronchospasm, rhinorrhea, hemoptysis

Miscellaneous: Acquired sensitization (rare), clamminess, unpleasant odor during administration

Intravenous:

>10%: Miscellaneous: Anaphylactoid reaction (~17%; reported as severe in 1% or moderate in 10% of patients within 15 minutes of first infusion; severe in 1% or mild-to-moderate in 6% to 7% of patients after 60-minute infusion)

1% to 10%:

- Cardiovascular: Angioedema (2% to 8%), vasodilation (1% to 6%), hypotension (1% to 4%), tachycardia (1% to 4%), syncope (1% to 3%), chest tightness (1%), flushing (1%)
- Central nervous system: Dysphoria (<1% to 2%)
- Dermatologic: Urticaria (2% to 7%), rash (1% to 5%), facial erythema (≤1%), palmar erythema (≤1%), pruritus (≤1% to 3%), pruritus with rash and vasodilation (2% to 9%)
- Gastrointestinal: Vomiting (<1% to 10%), nausea (1% to 10%), dyspepsia (≤1%)
- Neuromuscular & skeletal: Gait disturbance (<1% to 2%)
- Ocular: Eye pain (<1% to 3%)
- Otic: Ear pain (1%)
- Respiratory: Bronchospasm (1% to 6%), cough (1% to 4%), dyspnea (<1% to 3%), pharyngitis (1%), rhinorrhea (1%), rhonchi (1%), throat tightness (1%)
- Miscellaneous: Diaphoresis (≤1%)

Overdosage/Toxicology Treatment of acetylcysteine toxicity is usually aimed at reversing anaphylactoid symptoms or controlling nausea and vomiting. The use of epinephrine, antihistamines, and steroids may be beneficial.

Dosing

Adults & Elderly:

Acetaminophen poisoning:

Oral: 140 mg/kg; followed by 17 doses of 70 mg/kg every 4 hours; repeat dose if emesis occurs within 1 hour of administration; therapy should continue until acetaminophen levels are undetectable and there is no evidence of hepatotoxicity.

I.V. (Acetadote®): Loading dose is followed by 2 additional infusions: Initial maintenance dose of 50 mg/kg infused over 4 hours, followed by a second maintenance dose of 100 mg/kg infused over 16 hours. To avoid fluid overload in patients <40 kg and those requiring fluid restriction, decrease volume of D_5W proportionally.

Note: If commercial I.V. form is unavailable, the following dose has been reported using solution for oral inhalation (unlabeled): Loading dose: 140 mg/kg, followed by 70 mg/kg every 4 hours, for a total of 13 doses (loading dose and 48 hours of treatment); infuse each dose over 1 hour through a 0.2 micron Millipore filter (in-line).

Experts suggest that the duration of acetylcysteine administration may vary depending upon serial acetaminophen levels and liver function tests obtained during treatment. In general, patients without measurable acetaminophen levels and without significant LFT elevations (>3 times the ULN) can safely stop acetylcysteine after ≤24 hours of treatment. The patients who still have detectable levels of acetaminophen, and/or LFT elevations (>1000 units/L) continue to benefit from addition acetylcysteine administration

Adjuvant therapy in respiratory conditions:

Note: Patients should receive bronchodilator 15 minutes prior to dose.

Inhalation, nebulization (face mask, mouth piece, tracheostomy): Acetylcysteine 10% and 20% solution (Mucomyst®) (dilute 20% solution with sodium chloride or sterile water for inhalation); 10% solution may be used undiluted: 3-5 mL of 20% solution or 6-10 mL of 10% solution until nebulized given 3-4 times/day; dosing range: 1-10 mL of 20% solution or 2-20 mL of 10% solution every 2-6 hours

Inhalation, nebulization (tent, croupette): Dose must be individualized; may require up to 300 mL solution/treatment

Direct instillation:

- Into tracheostomy: 1-2 mL of 10% to 20% solution every 1-4 hours
- Through percutaneous intratracheal catheter: 1-2 mL of 20% or 2-4 mL of 10% solution every 1-4 hours via syringe attached to catheter

Diagnostic bronchogram: Nebulization or intratracheal: 1-2 mL of 20% solution or 2-4 mL of 10% solution administered 2-3 times prior to procedure

Prevention of radiocontrast-induced renal dysfunction (unlabeled use):
Oral: 600 mg twice daily for 2 days (beginning the day before the procedure);

(Continued)

Acetylcysteine *(Continued)*

may be given as powder in capsules, some centers use solution (diluted in cola beverage or juice). Hydrate patient with saline concurrently.

Pediatrics:

Acetaminophen poisoning: Refer to adult dosing.

Adjuvant therapy in respiratory conditions:

Note: Patients should receive an aerosolized bronchodilator 10-15 minutes prior to acetylcysteine

Inhalation, nebulization (face mask, mouth piece, tracheostomy): Acetylcysteine 10% and 20% solution (Mucomyst®) (dilute 20% solution with sodium chloride or sterile water for inhalation); 10% solution may be used undiluted.

Infants: 1-2 mL of 20% solution or 2-4 mL 10% solution until nebulized given 3-4 times/day

Children: Refer to adult dosing.

Inhalation, nebulization (tent, croupette): Children: Refer to adult dosing.

Available Dosage Forms

Injection, solution (Acetadote®): 20% [200 mg/mL] (30 mL) [contains disodium edetate]

Solution, as sodium (Mucomyst®): 10% [100 mg/mL] (4 mL, 10 mL, 30 mL); 20% [200 mg/mL] (4 mL, 10 mL, 30 mL)

Nursing Guidelines

Assessment: Instruct patient on appropriate use, adverse effects to report, and interventions to reduce side effects. Monitor pulmonary function and response to therapy. If giving I.V., monitor for possible anaphylactoid reactions and be prepared to treat appropriately if needed.

Monitoring Laboratory Tests: Acetaminophen overdose: AST, ALT, bilirubin, PT, serum creatinine, BUN, serum glucose, and electrolytes. Acetaminophen levels at ~4 hours postingestion (every 4-6 hours if extended release acetaminophen; plot on the nomogram) and every 4-6 hours to assess serum levels, and LFTs for possible hepatotoxicity.

Patient Education: Pulmonary treatment: Prepare solution (may dilute with sterile water to reduce concentrate from impeding nebulizer) and use as directed. Clear airway by coughing deeply before using aerosol. Wash face and face mask after treatment to remove any residual. You may experience drowsiness (use caution when driving), nausea, or vomiting (small, frequent meals may help). Report persistent chills or fever, adverse change in respiratory status, palpitations, or extreme anxiety or nervousness.

Pregnancy Risk Factor: B

Pregnancy Issues: Based on limited reports using acetylcysteine to treat acetaminophen overdose in pregnant women, acetylcysteine has been shown to cross the placenta and may provide protective levels in the fetus.

Lactation: Excretion in breast milk unknown/use caution

Perioperative/Anesthesia/Other Concerns: Intravenous acetylcysteine may be indicated over oral formulation in treatment of acetaminophen overdose for a restricted number of indications (oral cannot be tolerated; coingested toxin requires ongoing gastrointestinal decontamination; gastrointestinal tract nonfunctional; late presentation of acetaminophen overdose; neonatal toxicity from maternal overdose) (Yip, 1998). A commercially manufactured intravenous product is now available in the United States. If this formulation is unavailable, the product normally administered by inhalation can be administered intravenously. The inhalation preparation is sterile, but not labeled "pyrogen free." In Yip's retrospective case series, adverse reactions occurred in 4 (~5%) cases. Flushing, pruritus, and phlebitis were reported; one was labeled as an "anaphylactic reaction."

Bailey and McGuigan reviewed a retrospective case series of patients who received intravenous acetylcysteine and the literature to develop management guideline for anaphylactoid reactions (Bailey, 1998). Their recommendations for treatment of nonlife-threatening allergic reactions include reassessing the need for intravenous acetylcysteine, and administering diphenhydramine (1 mg/kg I.V.; maximum dose: 50 mg). If the acetylcysteine infusion was stopped initially and symptoms resolved, consider restarting infusion 1 hour after diphenhydramine's administration. Anaphylactoid reactions have also been reported with the commercial I.V. formulation. Monitor closely for allergic reactions. Be prepared to handle anaphylactoid reaction if it occurs.

Administration

Oral: For treatment of acetaminophen overdosage, administer orally as a 5% solution. Dilute the 20% solution 1:3 with a cola, orange juice, or other soft drink. Use within 1 hour of preparation. Unpleasant odor becomes less noticeable as treatment progresses. If patient vomits within 1 hour of dose, readminister.

I.V.: Intravenous formulation (Acetadote®): Administer loading dose 150 mg/kg over 15 minutes, followed by two separate maintenance infusions: 50 mg/kg over 4 hours followed by 100 mg/kg over 16 hours.

If not using commercially available I.V. formulation, use a 0.2-µ millipore filter (in-line).

Reconstitution:

Solution for injection (Acetadote®): To avoid fluid overload in patients <40 kg and those requiring fluid restriction, decrease volume of D_5W proportionally. Discard unused portion.

Loading dose: Dilute 150 mg/kg in D_5W 200 mL

Initial maintenance dose: Dilute 50 mg/kg in D_5W 500 mL

Second maintenance dose: Dilute 100 mg/kg in D_5W 1000 mL

Solution for inhalation (Mucomyst®): The 20% solution may be diluted with sodium chloride or sterile water; the 10% solution may be used undiluted.

Intravenous administration of solution for inhalation (unlabeled route): Using D_5W, dilute acetylcysteine 20% oral solution to a 3% solution.

Compatibility:

Inhalation: **Incompatible** with rubber and metals (particularly iron, copper, and nickel); do not mix with ampicillin, tetracycline, oxytetracycline, erythromycin

Intravenous: **Incompatible** with rubber and metals (particularly iron, copper, and nickel)

Storage:

Solution for injection (Acetadote®): Store vials at room temperature, 20°C to 25°C (68°F to 77°F). Following reconstitution with D_5W, solution is stable for 24 hours at room temperature.

Solution for inhalation (Mucomyst®): Store unopened vials at room temperature; once opened, store under refrigeration and use within 96 hours. A color change may occur in opened vials (light purple) and does not affect the safety or efficacy.

Related Information

Contrast Media Reactions, Premedication for Prophylaxis *on page 1911*

- Acetylcysteine Sodium *see* Acetylcysteine *on page 80*
- Acetylsalicylic Acid *see* Aspirin *on page 189*
- Achromycin *see* Tetracycline *on page 1613*
- Aciclovir *see* Acyclovir *on page 86*
- AcipHex® *see* Rabeprazole *on page 1457*

Acitretin (a si TRE tin)

U.S. Brand Names Soriatane®

Pharmacologic Category Retinoid-Like Compound

Medication Safety Issues

Sound-alike/look-alike issues:

Soriatane® may be confused with Loxitane®

Use Treatment of severe psoriasis

Pharmacodynamics/Kinetics Etretinate has been detected in serum for up to 3 years following therapy, possibly due to storage in adipose tissue.

Onset: May take 2-3 months for full effect; improvement may be seen within 8 weeks.

Absorption: Oral: ~72% absorbed when given with food

Protein binding: >99% bound, primarily to albumin

Metabolism: Metabolized to *cis*-acitretin; both compounds are further metabolized. Concomitant ethanol use leads to the formation of etretinate (active).

Half-life elimination: Acitretin: 49 hours (range: 33-96); *cis*-acitretin: 63 hours (range: 28-157); etretinate: 120 days (range: 84-168 days)

Excretion: Feces (34% to 54%); urine (16% to 53%)

Contraindications Hypersensitivity to acitretin, other retinoids, or any component of the formulation; patients who are pregnant or intend on becoming pregnant; ethanol ingestion; severe hepatic or renal dysfunction; chronically-elevated blood lipid levels; concomitant use with methotrexate or tetracycline

(Continued)

Acitretin *(Continued)*

Acitretin is contraindicated in females of childbearing potential unless all of the following conditions apply:

1) Patient has severe psoriasis unresponsive to other therapy or if clinical condition contraindicates other treatments.
2) Patient must have two negative urine or serum pregnancy tests prior to therapy.
3) Patient must commit to using two effective forms of birth control starting 1 month prior to acitretin treatment and for 3 years after discontinuation.
4) Patient is reliable in understanding and carrying out instructions.
5) Patient has received, and acknowledged, understanding of a careful oral and printed explanation of the hazards of fetal exposure to acitretin and the risk of possible contraception failure; this explanation may include showing a line drawing to the patient of an infant with the characteristic external deformities resulting from retinoid exposure during pregnancy. Patient must sign an agreement/informed consent document stating that she understands these risks and that she should not consume ethanol during therapy or for 2 months after discontinuation.
6) All patients (male and female) should not donate blood during and for 3 years following treatment with acitretin.

Warnings/Precautions Not for use by women who want to become pregnant; patient should not get pregnant for at least 3 years after discontinuation. All patients (male and female) should abstain from ethanol or ethanol-containing products during therapy and for 2 months after discontinuation. All patients should be advised not to donate blood during therapy or for 3 years following completion of therapy. Monitor for hepatotoxicity; discontinue if elevations of liver enzymes occur. Use with caution in patients at risk of hypertriglyceridemias. Rarely associated with pseudotumor cerebri. Discontinue if visual changes occur. May cause a decrease in night vision or decreased tolerance to contact lenses. All patients must be provided with a medication guide each time acitretin is dispensed. Female patients must also sign an informed consent prior to therapy. Safety and efficacy for pediatric patients have not been established; growth potential may be affected.

Drug Interactions

Ethanol: Etretinate (a retinoid with a much longer half-life) can be formed with concurrent use; contraindicated.

Methotrexate: The concomitant administration of methotrexate and etretinate has been associated with hepatitis, a similar increased hepatitis risk may be expected with the combined use of acitretin and methotrexate; concomitant use is contraindicated.

Progestins: Decreased contraceptive effect with concurrent use; use of "mini-pill" preparations are not recommended. Interactions with other progestational agents or hormonal contraceptives have not been established.

Sulfonylureas: Glucose-lowering effect may be potentiated. Effect seen with glibenclamide.

Tetracycline: Acitretin and tetracyclines may both cause increased intracranial pressure; concomitant use is contraindicated.

Vitamin A: Concomitant administration of vitamin A and other systemic retinoids must be avoided due to the risk of possible additive toxic effects.

Nutritional/Herbal/Ethanol Interactions Ethanol: Use leads to formation of etretinate, a teratogenic metabolite with a prolonged half-life; concomitant use of ethanol or ethanol-containing products is contraindicated.

Adverse Reactions

>10%:

Central nervous system: Hyperesthesia (10% to 25%)

Dermatologic: Cheilitis (>75%), alopecia (50% to 75%), skin peeling (50% to 75%), dry skin (25% to 50%), nail disorder (25% to 50%), pruritus (25% to 50%), erythematous rash (10% to 25%), skin atrophy (10% to 25%), sticky skin (10% to 25%), paronychia (10% to 25%)

Endocrine & metabolic: Hypercholesterolemia (25% to 50%), hypertriglyceridemia (50% to 75%), HDL decreased (25% to 50%), phosphorus increased (10% to 25%), potassium increased (10% to 25%), sodium increased (10% to 25%), magnesium increased/decreased (10% to 25%), fasting blood sugar increased (25% to 50%), fasting blood sugar decreased (10% to 25%)

Gastrointestinal: Xerostomia (10% to 25%)

Hematologic: Reticulocytes increased (25% to 50%), hematocrit decreased (10% to 25%), hemoglobin decreased (10% to 25%), WBC increased/

decreased (10% to 25%), haptoglobin increased (10% to 25%), neutrophils increased (10% to 25%)

Hepatic: Liver function tests increased (25% to 50%), alkaline phosphatase increased (10% to 25%), direct bilirubin increased (10% to 25%), GGTP increased (10% to 25%)

Neuromuscular & skeletal: Paresthesia (10% to 25%), arthralgia (10% to 25%), rigors (10% to 25%), CPK increased (25% to 50%), spinal hyperostosis progression (10% to 25%)

Ocular: Xerophthalmia (10% to 25%),

Renal: Uric acid increased (10% to 25%), acetonuria (10% to 25%), hematuria (10% to 25%), RBC in urine (10% to 25%)

Respiratory: Rhinitis (25% to 50%), epistaxis (10% to 25%)

1% to 10%:

Cardiovascular: Flushing, edema

Central nervous system: Headache, pain, depression, insomnia, somnolence, fatigue

Dermatologic: Skin odor, hair texture change, bullous eruption, dermatitis, diaphoresis increased, psoriasiform rash, purpura, pyogenic granuloma, rash, seborrhea, ulcers, fissures, sunburn

Endocrine & metabolic: Hot flashes, potassium decreased, phosphorus decreased, sodium decreased, calcium increased or decreased, chloride increased or decreased

Gastrointestinal: Gingival bleeding, gingivitis, saliva increased, stomatitis, thirst, ulcerative stomatitis, abdominal pain, diarrhea, nausea, taste disturbance, anorexia, appetite increased, tongue disorder

Hepatic: Total bilirubin increased

Neuromuscular & skeletal: Arthritis, back pain, hypertonia, myalgia, osteodynia, peripheral joint hyperostosis, Bell's palsy

Ocular: Blurred vision, blepharitis, conjunctivitis, night blindness, photophobia, corneal epithelial abnormality, eye pain, eyebrow or eyelash loss, diplopia, cataract

Otic: Earache, tinnitus

Renal: BUN increased, creatinine increased, glycosuria, proteinuria

Respiratory: Sinusitis

<1% (Limited to important or life-threatening): Anxiety, bleeding time increased, chest pain, cirrhosis, conjunctival hemorrhage, constipation, corneal ulceration, cyanosis, deafness, diplopia, dizziness, dyspepsia, dysphonia, dysuria, eczema, esophagitis, fever, furunculosis, gastritis, glossitis, gum hyperplasia, hair discoloration, hemorrhage, hepatic dysfunction, hepatitis, hyperkeratosis, hypertrichosis, hypoesthesia, impaired healing, intermittent claudication, itchy eyes, jaundice, leukorrhea, malaise, melena, MI, moniliasis, myopathy, nervousness, neuritis, pancreatitis, papilledema, peripheral ischemia, photosensitivity, pseudotumor cerebri, scleroderma, skin fragility or thinning, spinal hyperostosis (new lesion), stroke, taste loss, tendonitis, thromboembolism

Overdosage/Toxicology Symptoms of acute hypervitaminosis A (headache, vertigo) would be expected; vomiting has also been reported. Pregnancy test for women of childbearing age; counseling regarding potential for birth defects and appropriate contraceptive use.

Dosing

Adults & Elderly:

Psoriasis: Oral: Individualization of dosage is required to achieve maximum therapeutic response while minimizing side effects

Initial therapy: Therapy should be initiated at 25-50 mg/day, given as a single dose with the main meal

Maintenance: Doses of 25-50 mg/day may be given after initial response to treatment; the maintenance dose should be based on clinical efficacy and tolerability

Available Dosage Forms Capsule: 10 mg, 25 mg

Nursing Guidelines

Monitoring Laboratory Tests: Lipid profile (baseline and at 1- to 2-week intervals for 4-8 weeks); liver function tests (baseline, and at 1- to 2-week intervals until stable, then as clinically indicated); blood glucose in patients with diabetes

Dietary Considerations: Administer with food. Avoid ingestion of additional sources of exogenous vitamin A (in excess of RDA); use of ethanol and ethanol-containing products is contraindicated.

Patient Education: Take with food. Do not drink alcohol during therapy and for 2 months after discontinuation. Use contraception for 1 month before, during,

(Continued)

Acitretin *(Continued)*

and for 3 years after discontinuation. You may not be able to tolerate contact lenses during treatment. Do not donate blood during treatment and for 3 years after discontinuation. Avoid exposure to sunlight. Wear protective clothing and sunscreens. Avoid use of other vitamin A products. **Pregnancy/breast-feeding precautions:** Females: Use two effective forms of birth control. If you have had your tubes tied, then use an additional form of birth control. If you become pregnant, contact your prescriber immediately. Breast-feeding is not recommended.

Pregnancy Risk Factor: X

Lactation: Enters breast milk/not recommended

Breast-Feeding Considerations: Acitretin should not be given prior to or during nursing due to the potential for adverse effects in the nursing infant.

Administration

Storage: Store between 15°C to 25°C (59°F to 77°F). Protect from light. Avoid high temperatures and humidity.

- ♦ ACTH *see* Corticotropin *on page 450*
- ♦ ActHIB® *see Haemophilus* b Conjugate Vaccine *on page 837*
- ♦ Actifed® Cold and Allergy [OTC] *see* Triprolidine and Pseudoephedrine *on page 1670*
- ♦ Actimmune® *see* Interferon Gamma-1b *on page 952*
- ♦ Actiq® *see* Fentanyl *on page 712*
- ♦ Activase® *see* Alteplase *on page 117*
- ♦ Activated Dimethicone *see* Simethicone *on page 1533*
- ♦ Activated Ergosterol *see* Ergocalciferol *on page 627*
- ♦ Activated Methylpolysiloxane *see* Simethicone *on page 1533*
- ♦ Activella® *see* Estradiol and Norethindrone *on page 655*
- ♦ Acular® *see* Ketorolac *on page 990*
- ♦ Acular LS™ *see* Ketorolac *on page 990*
- ♦ Acular® PF *see* Ketorolac *on page 990*
- ♦ ACV *see* Acyclovir *on page 86*
- ♦ Acycloguanosine *see* Acyclovir *on page 86*

Acyclovir (ay SYE kloe veer)

U.S. Brand Names Zovirax®

Synonyms Aciclovir; ACV; Acycloguanosine

Pharmacologic Category Antiviral Agent

Medication Safety Issues

Sound-alike/look-alike issues:

Zovirax® may be confused with Zostrix®, Zyvox™

Use Treatment of genital herpes simplex virus (HSV), herpes labialis (cold sores), herpes zoster (shingles), HSV encephalitis, neonatal HSV, mucocutaneous HSV in immunocompromised patients, varicella-zoster (chickenpox)

Unlabeled/Investigational Use Prevention of HSV reactivation in HIV-positive patients; prevention of HSV reactivation in hematopoietic stem-cell transplant (HSCT); prevention of HSV reactivation during periods of neutropenia in patients with acute leukemia

Mechanism of Action Acyclovir is converted to acyclovir monophosphate by virus-specific thymidine kinase then further converted to acyclovir triphosphate by other cellular enzymes. Acyclovir triphosphate inhibits DNA synthesis and viral replication by competing with deoxyguanosine triphosphate for viral DNA polymerase and being incorporated into viral DNA.

Pharmacodynamics/Kinetics

Absorption: Oral: 15% to 30%

Distribution: V_d: 0.8 L/kg (63.6 L): Widely (eg, brain, kidney, lungs, liver, spleen, muscle, uterus, vagina, CSF)

Protein binding: 9% to 33%

Metabolism: Converted by viral enzymes to acyclovir monophosphate, and further converted to diphosphate then triphosphate (active form) by cellular enzymes

Bioavailability: Oral: 10% to 20% with normal renal function (bioavailability decreases with increased dose)

Half-life elimination: Terminal: Neonates: 4 hours; Children 1-12 years: 2-3 hours; Adults: 3 hours

Time to peak, serum: Oral: Within 1.5-2 hours

Excretion: Urine (62% to 90% as unchanged drug and metabolite)

Contraindications Hypersensitivity to acyclovir, valacyclovir, or any component of the formulation

Warnings/Precautions Use with caution in immunocompromised patients; thrombocytopenic purpura/hemolytic uremic syndrome (TTP/HUS) has been reported. Use caution in the elderly, pre-existing renal disease, or in those receiving other nephrotoxic drugs. Maintain adequate hydration during oral or intravenous therapy. Use I.V. preparation with caution in patients with underlying neurologic abnormalities, serious hepatic or electrolyte abnormalities, or substantial hypoxia.

Safety and efficacy of oral formulations have not been established in pediatric patients <2 years of age.

Chickenpox: Treatment should begin within 24 hours of appearance of rash; oral route not recommended for routine use in otherwise healthy children with varicella, but may be effective in patients at increased risk of moderate to severe infection (>12 years of age, chronic cutaneous or pulmonary disorders, long-term salicylate therapy, corticosteroid therapy).

Genital herpes: Physical contact should be avoided when lesions are present; transmission may also occur in the absence of symptoms. Treatment should begin with the first signs or symptoms.

Herpes labialis: For external use only to the lips and face; do not apply to eye or inside the mouth or nose. Treatment should begin with the first signs or symptoms.

Herpes zoster: Acyclovir should be started within 72 hours of appearance of rash to be effective.

Nutritional/Herbal/Ethanol Interactions Food: Does not affect absorption of oral acyclovir.

Adverse Reactions

Systemic: Oral:

>10%: Central nervous system: Malaise (12%)

1% to 10%:

Central nervous system: Headache (2%)

Gastrointestinal: Nausea (2% to 5%), vomiting (3%), diarrhea (2% to 3%)

Systemic: Parenteral:

1% to 10%:

Dermatologic: Hives (2%), itching (2%), rash (2%)

Gastrointestinal: Nausea/vomiting (7%)

Hepatic: Liver function tests increased (1% to 2%)

Local: Inflammation at injection site or phlebitis (9%)

Renal: BUN increased (5% to 10%), creatinine increased (5% to 10%), acute renal failure

Topical:

>10%: Dermatologic: Mild pain, burning, or stinging (ointment 30%)

1% to 10%: Dermatologic: Pruritus (ointment 4%), itching

All forms: <1% (Limited to important or life-threatening): Abdominal pain, aggression, agitation, alopecia, anaphylaxis, anemia, angioedema, anorexia, ataxia, coma, confusion, consciousness decreased, delirium, desquamation, diarrhea, disseminated intravascular coagulopathy, dizziness, dry lips, dysarthria, encephalopathy, erythema multiforme, fatigue, fever, gastrointestinal distress, hallucinations, hematuria, hemolysis, hepatitis, hyperbilirubinemia, hypotension, insomnia, jaundice, leukocytoclastic vasculitis, leukocytosis, leukopenia, local tissue necrosis (following extravasation), lymphadenopathy, mental depression, myalgia, neutrophilia, paresthesia, peripheral edema, photosensitization, pruritus, psychosis, renal failure, seizure, somnolence, sore throat, Stevens-Johnson syndrome, thrombocytopenia, thrombocytopenic purpura/hemolytic uremic syndrome (TTP/HUS), thrombocytosis, toxic epidermal necrolysis, tremor, urticaria, visual disturbances

Overdosage/Toxicology Overdoses of up to 20 g have been reported. Symptoms of overdose include agitation, seizures, somnolence, confusion, elevated serum creatinine, and renal failure. In the event of overdose, sufficient urine flow must be maintained to avoid drug precipitation within renal tubules. Hemodialysis has resulted in up to 60% reduction in serum acyclovir levels.

Dosing

Adults & Elderly: Note: Obese patients should be dosed using ideal body weight

(Continued)

Acyclovir *(Continued)*

Genital HSV:

I.V.: Immunocompetent: Initial episode, severe: 5 mg/kg every 8 hours for 5-7 days

Oral:

Initial episode: 200 mg every 4 hours while awake (5 times/day) for 10 days (per manufacturer's labeling); 400 mg 3 times/day for 5-10 days has also been reported

Recurrence: 200 mg every 4 hours while awake (5 times/day) for 5 days (per manufacturer's labeling; begin at earliest signs of disease); 400 mg 3 times/day for 5 days has also been reported

Chronic suppression: 400 mg twice daily or 200 mg 3-5 times/day, for up to 12 months followed by re-evaluation (per manufacturer's labeling); 400-1200 mg/day in 2-3 divided doses has also been reported

Topical: Immunocompromised: Ointment: Initial episode: ½" ribbon of ointment for a 4" square surface area every 3 hours (6 times/day) for 7 days

Herpes labialis (cold sores): Topical: Apply 5 times/day for 4 days

Herpes zoster (shingles):

Oral: Immunocompetent: 800 mg every 4 hours (5 times/day) for 7-10 days

I.V.: Immunocompromised: 10 mg/kg/dose or 500 mg/m²/dose every 8 hours for 7 days

HSV encephalitis: I.V.: 10 mg/kg/dose every 8 hours for 10 days (per manufacturer's labeling); 10-15 mg/kg/dose every 8 hours for 14-21 days also reported

Mucocutaneous HSV:

I.V.: Immunocompromised: 5 mg/kg/dose every 8 hours for 7 days (per manufacturer's labeling); dosing for up to 14 days also reported

Oral: Immunocompromised (unlabeled use): 400 mg 5 times a day for 7-14 days

Topical: Ointment: Nonlife-threatening, immunocompromised: ½" ribbon of ointment for a 4" square surface area every 3 hours (6 times/day) for 7 days

Varicella-zoster (chickenpox): Begin treatment within the first 24 hours of rash onset:

Oral: >40 kg (immunocompetent): 800 mg/dose 4 times a day for 5 days

I.V.: Immunocompromised (unlabeled use): 1500 mg/m²/day divided every 8 hours or 10 mg/kg/dose every 8 hours for 7-10 days

Prevention of HSV reactivation in HIV-positive patients, for use only when recurrences are frequent or severe (unlabeled use): Oral: 200 mg 3 times/day or 400 mg 2 times/day

Prevention of HSV reactivation in HSCT (unlabeled use): Note: Start at the beginning of conditioning therapy and continue until engraftment or until mucositis resolves (~30 days)

Oral: 200 mg 3 times/day

I.V.: 250 mg/m²/dose every 12 hours

Bone marrow transplant recipients (unlabeled use): I.V.: Allogeneic patients who are HSV and CMV seropositive: 500 mg/m²/dose (10 mg/kg) every 8 hours; for clinically-symptomatic CMV infection, consider replacing acyclovir with ganciclovir

Pediatrics: Note: Obese patients should be dosed using ideal body weight

Genital HSV:

I.V.: Children ≥12 years: Refer to adult dosing.

Oral:

Initial episode (unlabeled use): 40-80 mg/kg/day divided into 3-4 doses for 5-10 days (maximum: 1 g/day)

Chronic suppression (unlabeled use; limited data): 80 mg/kg/day in 3 divided doses (maximum: 1 g/day), re-evaluate after 12 months of treatment

Herpes labialis (cold sores): Topical: Children ≥12 years: Refer to adult dosing.

Herpes zoster (shingles): I.V.:

Children <12 years (immunocompromised): 20 mg/kg/dose every 8 hours for 7 days

Children ≥12 years: Refer to adult dosing.

HSV encephalitis: I.V.:

Children 3 months to 12 years: 20 mg/kg/dose every 8 hours for 10 days (per manufacturer's labeling); dosing for 14-21 days also reported

Children ≥12 years: Refer to adult dosing.

Mucocutaneous HSV: I.V.:

Children <12 years (immunocompromised): 10 mg/kg/dose every 8 hours for 7 days

Children ≥12 years: Refer to adult dosing.

Neonatal HSV: I.V.: Neonate: Birth to 3 months: 10 mg/kg/dose every 8 hours for 10 days (manufacturer's labeling); 15 mg/kg/dose or 20 mg/kg/dose every 8 hours for 14-21 days has also been reported

Varicella-zoster (chickenpox): Begin treatment within the first 24 hours of rash onset:

Oral:

Children ≥2 years and ≤40 kg (immunocompetent): 20 mg/kg/dose (up to 800 mg/dose) 4 times/day for 5 days

Children >40 kg: Refer to adult dosing.

I.V.:

Children <1 year (immunocompromised, unlabeled use): 10 mg/kg/dose every 8 hours for 7-10 days

Children ≥1 year: Refer to adult dosing.

Prevention of HSV reactivation in HIV-positive patients, for use only when recurrences are frequent or severe (unlabeled use): Oral: 80 mg/kg/day in 3-4 divided doses

Prevention of HSV reactivation in HSCT (unlabeled use): Note: Start at the beginning of conditioning therapy and continue until engraftment or until mucositis resolves (~30 days): I.V.: 250 mg/m^2/dose every 8 hours or 125 mg/m^2/dose every 6 hours

Bone marrow transplant recipients (unlabeled use): I.V.: Refer to adult dosing.

Renal Impairment:

Oral:

Cl_{cr} 10-25 mL/minute/1.73 m^2: Normal dosing regimen 800 mg every 4 hours: Administer 800 mg every 8 hours

Cl_{cr} <10 mL/minute/1.73 m^2:

Normal dosing regimen 200 mg every 4 hours, 200 mg every 8 hours, or 400 mg every 12 hours: Administer 200 mg every 12 hours

Normal dosing regimen 800 mg every 4 hours: Administer 800 mg every 12 hours

I.V.:

Cl_{cr} 25-50 mL/minute/1.73 m^2: Administer recommended dose every 12 hours

Cl_{cr} 10-25 mL/minute/1.73 m^2: Administer recommended dose every 24 hours

Cl_{cr} <10 mL/minute/1.73 m^2: Administer 50% of recommended dose every 24 hours

Hemodialysis: Administer dose after dialysis

Peritoneal dialysis: No supplemental dose needed

CAVH: 3.5 mg/kg/day

CVVHD/CVVH: Adjust dose based upon Cl_{cr} 30 mL/minute

Available Dosage Forms

Capsule: 200 mg

Cream, topical: 5% (2 g)

Injection, powder for reconstitution, as sodium: 500 mg, 1000 mg

Zovirax®: 500 mg

Injection, solution, as sodium [preservative free]: 25 mg/mL (20 mL, 40 mL); 50 mg/mL (10 mL, 20 mL)

Ointment, topical: 5% (15 g)

Suspension, oral: 200 mg/5 mL (480 mL) [banana flavor]

Tablet: 400 mg, 800 mg

Nursing Guidelines

Assessment: See Warnings/Precautions and Contraindications for use cautions. Assess potential for interactions with other prescriptions, OTC, or herbal medications patient may be taking (see Drug Interactions). **I.V.:** See Reconstitution and Compatibility; monitor closely during infusion. Assess results of laboratory tests (see below), therapeutic effects, and adverse responses (see Adverse Reactions and Overdose/Toxicology). Teach patient appropriate use (if self-administered), possible side effects/appropriate interventions, and adverse symptoms to report (see Patient Education).

Monitoring Laboratory Tests: Urinalysis, BUN, serum creatinine, liver enzymes, CBC

Dietary Considerations: May be taken with or without food. Acyclovir 500 mg injection contains sodium ~50 mg (~2 mEq).

(Continued)

Acyclovir *(Continued)*

Patient Education: Inform prescriber of all prescriptions, OTC medications, or herbal products you are taking, and any allergies you have. Do not take any new medication during therapy (including creams, lotions, or ointments) unless approved by prescriber. This is not a cure for herpes (recurrences tend to continually reappear every 3-6 months after original infection), nor will this medication reduce the risk of transmission to others when lesions are present; avoid sexual intercourse when visible lesions are present. Take as directed for full course of therapy; do not discontinue even if feeling better. Oral doses may be taken with food. Maintain adequate hydration (2-3 L/day of fluids) unless instructed to restrict fluid intake. May cause nausea or vomiting (small, frequent meals, frequent mouth care, sucking lozenges, or chewing gum may help); lightheadedness or dizziness (use caution when driving or engaging in tasks that require alertness until response to drug is known); or headache, fever, muscle pain (consult prescriber for approved analgesic). Report any change in urination (difficulty urinating, dark colored or concentrated urine); persistent lethargy; acute headache; severe nausea or vomiting; confusion or hallucinations; rash; or respiratory difficulty.

Topical: Apply as directed. Use gloves or finger cot when applying.

Geriatric Considerations: Calculate creatinine clearance. Dose adjustment may be necessary depending on renal function.

Pregnancy Risk Factor: B

Pregnancy Issues: Teratogenic effects were not observed in animal studies. Acyclovir has been shown to cross the human placenta. There are no adequate and well-controlled studies in pregnant women. Results from a pregnancy registry, established in 1984 and closed in 1999, did not find an increase in the number of birth defects with exposure to acyclovir when compared to those expected in the general population. However, due to the small size of the registry and lack of long-term data, the manufacturer recommends using during pregnancy with caution and only when clearly needed. Data from the pregnancy registry may be obtained from GlaxoSmithKline.

Lactation: Enters breast milk/use with caution (AAP rates "compatible")

Breast-Feeding Considerations: Nursing mothers with herpetic lesions near or on the breast should avoid breast-feeding. Limited data suggest exposure to the nursing infant of ~0.3 mg/kg/day following oral administration of acyclovir to the mother.

Administration

Oral: May be administered with or without food.

I.V.: For I.V. infusion only. Avoid rapid infusion. Infuse over 1 hour to prevent renal damage. Maintain adequate hydration of patient. Check for phlebitis and rotate infusion sites.

Reconstitution: Powder for injection: Reconstitute acyclovir 500 mg with SWFI 10 mL; do not use bacteriostatic water containing benzyl alcohol or parabens. For intravenous infusion, dilute to a final concentration of ≤7 mg/mL. Concentrations >10 mg/mL increase the risk of phlebitis.

Compatibility: Stable in D_5W, D_5NS, $D_5{}^1/_4NS$, $D_5{}^1/_2NS$, LR, NS

Incompatible with blood products and protein-containing solutions

Y-site administration: Incompatible with amifostine, amsacrine, aztreonam, cefepime, dobutamine, dopamine, fludarabine, foscarnet, gemcitabine, idarubicin, levofloxacin, ondansetron, piperacillin/tazobactam, sargramostim, vinorelbine

Compatibility when admixed: Incompatible with dobutamine, dopamine

Storage:

Capsule, tablet: Store at controlled room temperature of 15°C to 25°C (59°F to 77°F); protect from moisture.

Cream, suspension: Store at controlled room temperature of 15°C to 25°C (59°F to 77°F).

Ointment: Store at controlled room temperature of 15°C to 25°C (59°F to 77°F) in a dry place.

Injection: Store powder at controlled room temperature of 15°C to 25°C (59°F to 77°F). Reconstituted solutions remain stable for 12 hours at room temperature. Do not refrigerate reconstituted solutions as they may precipitate. Once diluted for infusion, use within 24 hours.

♦ **Adalat® CC** *see* NIFEdipine *on page 1227*

♦ **Adderall®** *see* Dextroamphetamine and Amphetamine *on page 507*

♦ **Adderall XR®** *see* Dextroamphetamine and Amphetamine *on page 507*

♦ ADEKs [OTC] *see* Vitamins (Multiple/Pediatric) *on page 1720*
♦ Adenocard® *see* Adenosine *on page 91*
♦ Adenoscan® *see* Adenosine *on page 91*

Adenosine (a DEN oh seen)

U.S. Brand Names Adenocard®; Adenoscan®

Synonyms 9-Beta-D-ribofuranosyladenine

Pharmacologic Category Antiarrhythmic Agent, Class IV; Diagnostic Agent

Use

Adenocard®: Treatment of paroxysmal supraventricular tachycardia (PSVT) including that associated with accessory bypass tracts (Wolff-Parkinson-White syndrome); when clinically advisable, appropriate vagal maneuvers should be attempted prior to adenosine administration; **not effective in atrial flutter, atrial fibrillation, or ventricular tachycardia**

Adenoscan®: Pharmacologic stress agent used in myocardial perfusion thallium-201 scintigraphy

Unlabeled/Investigational Use

Adenoscan®: Acute vasodilator testing in pulmonary artery hypertension

Mechanism of Action Slows conduction time through the AV node, interrupting the re-entry pathways through the AV node, restoring normal sinus rhythm

Pharmacodynamics/Kinetics

Onset of action: Rapid

Duration: Very brief

Metabolism: Blood and tissue to inosine then to adenosine monophosphate (AMP) and hypoxanthine

Half-life elimination: <10 seconds

Contraindications Hypersensitivity to adenosine or any component of the formulation; second- or third-degree AV block or sick sinus syndrome (except in patients with a functioning artificial pacemaker), atrial flutter, atrial fibrillation, and ventricular tachycardia (this drug is not effective in converting these arrhythmias to sinus rhythm). The manufacturer states that Adenoscan® should be avoided in patients with known or suspected bronchoconstrictive or bronchospastic lung disease.

Warnings/Precautions Adenosine decreases conduction through the AV node and may produce first-, second-, or third-degree heart block. Patients with pre-existing S-A nodal dysfunction may experience prolonged sinus pauses after adenosine; use caution in patients with first-degree AV block or bundle branch block; avoid use of adenosine for pharmacologic stress testing in patients with high-grade AV block or sinus node dysfunction (unless a functional pacemaker is in place). There have been reports of atrial fibrillation/flutter in patients with PSVT associated with accessory conduction pathways after adenosine. Rare, prolonged episodes of asystole have been reported, with fatal outcomes in some cases. Use caution in patients receiving other drugs which slow AV conduction (eg, digoxin, verapamil). Drugs which affect adenosine (theophylline, caffeine) should be withheld for five half-lives prior to adenosine use. Avoid dietary caffeine for 12-24 hours prior to pharmacologic stress testing.

Adenosine may also produce profound vasodilation with subsequent hypotension. When used as a bolus dose (PSVT), effects are generally self-limiting (due to the short half-life of adenosine). However, when used as a continuous infusion (pharmacologic stress testing), effects may be more pronounced and persistent, corresponding to continued exposure. Adenosine infusions should be used with caution in patients with autonomic dysfunction, stenotic valvular heart disease, pericarditis, pleural effusion, carotid stenosis (with cerebrovascular insufficiency), or uncorrected hypovolemia. Use caution in elderly patients; may be at increased risk of hemodynamic effects, bradycardia, and/or AV block.

A limited number of patients with asthma have received adenosine and have not experienced exacerbation of their asthma. Adenosine may cause bronchoconstriction in patients with asthma, and should be used cautiously in patients with obstructive lung disease not associated with bronchoconstriction (eg, emphysema, bronchitis).

Adenocard®: Transient AV block is expected. When used in PSVT, at the time of conversion to normal sinus rhythm, a variety of new rhythms may appear on the ECG. Administer as a rapid bolus, either directly into a vein or (if administered into an I.V. line), as close to the patient as possible (followed by saline flush).

Drug Interactions

Carbamazepine may increase heart block.

(Continued)

Adenosine *(Continued)*

Dipyridamole potentiates effects of adenosine; reduce dose of adenosine.

Theophylline and caffeine (methylxanthines) antagonize adenosine's effects; may require increased dose of adenosine.

Nutritional/Herbal/Ethanol Interactions Food: Avoid food or drugs with caffeine. Adenosine's therapeutic effect may be decreased if used concurrently with caffeine. Avoid dietary caffeine for 12-24 hours prior to pharmacologic stress testing.

Adverse Reactions Note: Frequency varies based on use; higher frequency of infusion-related effects, such as flushing and lightheadedness, were reported with continuous infusion (Adenoscan®).

>10%:

Cardiovascular: Facial flushing (18% to 44%)

Central nervous system: Headache (2% to 18%), lightheadedness (2% to 12%)

Neuromuscular & skeletal: Discomfort of neck, throat, jaw (<1% to 15%)

Respiratory: Dyspnea (12% to 28%), chest pressure/discomfort (7% to 40%)

1% to 10%:

Cardiovascular: Hypotension (<1% to 2%), AV block (infusion 6%; third degree <1%), ST segment depression (3%), palpitation, chest pain

Central nervous system: Dizziness, nervousness (2%), apprehension

Gastrointestinal: Nausea (3%)

Neuromuscular & skeletal: Upper extremity discomfort (up to 4%), numbness (up to 2%), paresthesia (up to 2%)

Respiratory: Hyperventilation

Miscellaneous: Diaphoresis

<1% (Limited to important or life-threatening): Asystole (prolonged), atrial fibrillation, back discomfort, bradycardia, bronchospasm, blurred vision, burning sensation, hypertension (transient), injection site reaction, intracranial pressure increased, metallic taste, pressure in groin, respiratory arrest, seizure, torsade de pointes, ventricular fibrillation, ventricular tachycardia

Overdosage/Toxicology Since adenosine half-life is <10 seconds, adverse effects are rapidly self-limiting. Treatment of prolonged effects requires individualization. To reverse the effects of Adenoscan®, administer theophylline 50-125 mg slow I.V. push.

Dosing

Adults:

Paroxysmal supraventricular tachycardia (Adenocard®): I.V. (rapid - over 1-2 seconds, via peripheral line): 6 mg; if not effective within 1-2 minutes, 12 mg may be given; may repeat 12 mg bolus if needed; maximum single dose: 12 mg.

Follow each I.V. bolus of adenosine with normal saline flush.

Note: Preliminary results in adults suggest adenosine may be administered via a central line at lower doses (ie, initial adult dose: 3 mg).

Pharmacologic stress agent (Adenoscan®): I.V.: Continuous I.V. infusion via peripheral line: 140 mcg/kg/minute for 6 minutes using syringe or columetric infusion pump; total dose: 0.84 mg/kg. Thallium-201 is injected at midpoint (3 minutes) of infusion.

Acute vasodilator testing (unlabeled use) (Adenoscan®): I.V.: Initial: 50 mcg/kg/minute increased by 50 mcg/kg/minute every 2 minutes to a maximum dose of 500 mcg/kg/minute; acutely assess vasodilator response

Elderly: Refer to adult dosing. Elderly may be more sensitive to effects of adenosine.

Pediatrics:

Paroxysmal supraventricular tachycardia (Adenocard®): Rapid I.V. push (over 1-2 seconds) via peripheral line: Infants and Children (manufacturer's recommendation):

Children <50 kg: 0.05-0.1 mg/kg. If conversion of PSVT does not occur within 1-2 minutes, may increase dose by 0.05-0.1 mg/kg. May repeat until sinus rhythm is established or to a maximum single dose of 0.3 mg/kg or 12 mg. Follow each dose with normal saline flush.

Children ≥50 kg: Refer to adult dosing.

Pediatric advanced life support (PALS): Treatment of SVT: I.V., I.O.: 0.1 mg/kg; if not effective, administer 0.2 mg/kg; maximum single dose: 12 mg. Follow each dose with normal saline flush.

Available Dosage Forms

Injection, solution [preservative free]: 3 mg/mL (2 mL)

Adenocard®: 3 mg/mL (2 mL, 4 mL)

Adenoscan®: 3 mg/mL (20 mL, 30 mL)

Nursing Guidelines

Assessment: Assess other medications patient may be taking for effectiveness and interactions. Requires use of infusion pump and continuous cardiac and hemodynamic monitoring during infusion. Monitor for adverse reactions. Note that adenosine could produce bronchoconstriction in patients with asthma.

Dietary Considerations: Avoid dietary caffeine for 12-24 hours prior to pharmacologic stress testing.

Patient Education: Adenosine is administered in emergencies, patient education should be appropriate to the situation.

Geriatric Considerations: Geriatric patients may be more sensitive to the effects of this medication.

Pregnancy Risk Factor: C

Lactation: Excretion in breast milk unknown

Perioperative/Anesthesia/Other Concerns: Short action is an advantage; has prolonged effects in patients taking dipyridamole or carbamazepine and in denervated transplanted hearts; adjust doses or choose alternative agent accordingly.

Adenosine acts via interruption of AV-nodal conduction and, when used for this purpose, requires administration as rapid intravenous push in increasing doses. Because of more direct access when administered through a central line, lower doses of adenosine may be tried in these situations. It is not uncommon to see heart block and sinus pause soon after adenosine administration. May aid in the identification of the arrhythmia by making the atrial fibrillation or flutter electrocardiographic morphology more apparent.

Administration

I.V.: For rapid bolus I.V. use only. Administer I.V. push over 1-2 seconds at a peripheral I.V. site as proximal as possible to trunk (ie, not in lower arm, hand, lower leg, or foot). If administered into an I.V. line, administer as close to the patient's heart as possible (followed by saline flush).

Compatibility: Stable in D_5LR, D_5W, LR, NS

Storage: Store at controlled room temperature of 15°C to 30°C (59°F to 86°F). Do **not** refrigerate; precipitation may occur (may dissolve by warming to room temperature).

Related Information

Management of Postoperative Arrhythmias *on page 1787*

- ♦ **ADH** *see* Vasopressin *on page 1691*
- ♦ **Adoxa™** *see* Doxycycline *on page 584*
- ♦ **Adrenalin®** *see* Epinephrine *on page 611*
- ♦ **Adrenaline** *see* Epinephrine *on page 611*
- ♦ **Adrenocorticotropic Hormone** *see* Corticotropin *on page 450*
- ♦ **ADR (error-prone abbreviation)** *see* DOXOrubicin *on page 576*
- ♦ **Adria** *see* DOXOrubicin *on page 576*
- ♦ **Adriamycin PFS®** *see* DOXOrubicin *on page 576*
- ♦ **Adriamycin RDF®** *see* DOXOrubicin *on page 576*
- ♦ **Adrucil®** *see* Fluorouracil *on page 745*
- ♦ **Advair Diskus®** *see* Fluticasone and Salmeterol *on page 765*
- ♦ **Advanced NatalCare®** *see* Vitamins (Multiple/Prenatal) *on page 1721*
- ♦ **Advate** *see* Antihemophilic Factor (Recombinant) *on page 170*
- ♦ **Advil® [OTC]** *see* Ibuprofen *on page 889*
- ♦ **Advil® Children's [OTC]** *see* Ibuprofen *on page 889*
- ♦ **Advil® Infants' [OTC]** *see* Ibuprofen *on page 889*
- ♦ **Advil® Junior [OTC]** *see* Ibuprofen *on page 889*
- ♦ **Advil® Migraine [OTC]** *see* Ibuprofen *on page 889*
- ♦ **Afeditab™ CR** *see* NIFEdipine *on page 1227*
- ♦ **A-Free Prenatal** *see* Vitamins (Multiple/Prenatal) *on page 1721*
- ♦ **Afrin® Extra Moisturizing [OTC]** *see* Oxymetazoline *on page 1290*
- ♦ **Afrin® Original [OTC]** *see* Oxymetazoline *on page 1290*
- ♦ **Afrin® Severe Congestion [OTC]** *see* Oxymetazoline *on page 1290*
- ♦ **Afrin® Sinus [OTC]** *see* Oxymetazoline *on page 1290*
- ♦ **$AgNO_3$** *see* Silver Nitrate *on page 1532*
- ♦ **Agrylin®** *see* Anagrelide *on page 166*
- ♦ **AH-chew® D [OTC]** *see* Phenylephrine *on page 1350*

- ♦ AHF (Recombinant) *see* Antihemophilic Factor (Recombinant) *on page 170*
- ♦ A-hydroCort *see* Hydrocortisone *on page 873*
- ♦ AK-Dilate® *see* Phenylephrine *on page 1350*
- ♦ AK-Fluor *see* Fluorescein Sodium *on page 742*
- ♦ Akne-Mycin® *see* Erythromycin *on page 634*
- ♦ AK-Pentolate® [DSC] *see* Cyclopentolate *on page 460*
- ♦ AK-Poly-Bac® *see* Bacitracin and Polymyxin B *on page 219*
- ♦ AK-Pred® *see* PrednisoLONE *on page 1399*
- ♦ AKTob® *see* Tobramycin *on page 1639*
- ♦ AK-Tracin® [DSC] *see* Bacitracin *on page 217*
- ♦ AK-Trol® *see* Neomycin, Polymyxin B, and Dexamethasone *on page 1211*
- ♦ Akwa Tears® [OTC] *see* Artificial Tears *on page 187*
- ♦ Alamag [OTC] *see* Aluminum Hydroxide and Magnesium Hydroxide *on page 122*
- ♦ Alamag Plus [OTC] *see* Aluminum Hydroxide, Magnesium Hydroxide, and Simethicone *on page 122*
- ♦ Alavert™ [OTC] *see* Loratadine *on page 1058*
- ♦ Alavert™ Allergy and Sinus [OTC] *see* Loratadine and Pseudoephedrine *on page 1060*
- ♦ Albumarc® *see* Albumin *on page 94*

Albumin (al BYOO min)

U.S. Brand Names Albumarc®; Albuminar®; Albutein®; Buminate®; Plasbumin®

Synonyms Albumin (Human); Normal Human Serum Albumin; Normal Serum Albumin (Human); Salt Poor Albumin; SPA

Pharmacologic Category Blood Product Derivative; Plasma Volume Expander, Colloid

Medication Safety Issues

Sound-alike/look-alike issues:

Albutein® may be confused with albuterol

Buminate® may be confused with bumetanide

Use Plasma volume expansion and maintenance of cardiac output in the treatment of certain types of shock or impending shock; may be useful for burn patients, ARDS, and cardiopulmonary bypass; other uses considered by some investigators (but not proven) are retroperitoneal surgery, peritonitis, and ascites; unless the condition responsible for hypoproteinemia can be corrected, albumin can provide only symptomatic relief or supportive treatment

Unlabeled/Investigational Use In cirrhotics, administered with diuretics to help facilitate diuresis; large volume paracentesis; volume expansion in dehydrated, mildly-hypotensive cirrhotics

Mechanism of Action Provides increase in intravascular oncotic pressure and causes mobilization of fluids from interstitial into intravascular space

Contraindications Hypersensitivity to albumin or any component of the formulation; patients with severe anemia or cardiac failure

Warnings/Precautions Use with caution in patients with hepatic or renal failure because of added protein load; rapid infusion of albumin solutions may cause vascular overload. All patients should be observed for signs of hypervolemia such as pulmonary edema. Use with caution in those patients for whom sodium restriction is necessary. Avoid 25% concentration in preterm infants due to risk of intraventricular hemorrhage. Nutritional supplementation is not an appropriate indication for albumin.

Drug Interactions ACE inhibitors: May have increased risk of atypical reactions; withhold ACEIs for at least 24 hours prior to plasma exchanges using large volumes of albumin

Adverse Reactions Frequency not defined.

Cardiovascular: CHF precipitation, edema, hyper-/hypotension, hypervolemia, tachycardia

Central nervous system: Chills, fever, headache

Dermatologic: Pruritus, rash, urticaria

Gastrointestinal: Nausea, vomiting

Respiratory: Bronchospasm, pulmonary edema

Miscellaneous: Anaphylaxis

Overdosage/Toxicology Symptoms of overdose include hypervolemia, congestive heart failure, and pulmonary edema.

Dosing

Adults & Elderly:

Note: Use **5%** solution in hypovolemic patients or intravascularly-depleted patients. Use **25%** solution in patients in whom fluid and sodium intake is restricted.

Usual dose: 25 g; initial dose may be repeated in 15-30 minutes if response is inadequate; no more than 250 g should be administered within 48 hours.

Hypoproteinemia: I.V.: 0.5-1 g/kg/dose; repeat every 1-2 days as calculated to replace ongoing losses.

Hypovolemia: I.V.: 0.5-1 g/kg/dose; repeat as needed; maximum: 6 g/kg/day.

Pediatrics:

Note: 5% should be used in hypovolemic patients or intravascularly-depleted patients. **25%** should be used in patients in whom fluid and sodium intake must be minimized.

Dose depends on condition of patient: Hypovolemia: I.V.: 0.5-1 g/kg/dose (10-20 mL/kg/dose of albumin 5%); maximum dose: 6 g/kg/day

Available Dosage Forms

Injection, solution, human: 5% [50 mg/mL] (50 mL, 250 mL, 500 mL); 25% [250 mg/mL] (50 mL, 100 mL)

Albumarc®: 5% [50 mg/mL] (250 mL, 500 mL); 25% [250 mg/mL] (50 mL, 100 mL)

Albuminar®: 5% [50 mg/mL] (50 mL, 250 mL, 500 mL, 1000 mL); 25% [250 mg/mL] (20 mL, 50 mL, 100 mL)

Albutein®, Buminate®: 5% [50 mg/mL]: (250 mL, 500 mL); 25% [250 mg/mL] (20 mL, 50 mL, 100 mL)

Plasbumin®: 5% [50 mg/mL] (50 mL, 250 mL, 500 mL); 25% [250 mg/mL] (20 mL, 50 mL, 100 mL)

Nursing Guidelines

Assessment: See Contraindications and Warnings/Precautions for use cautions. See Administration and Reconstitution for appropriate administration. Vital signs, central venous pressure, and fluid balance (intake/output) should be monitored closely during administration with frequent assessment for hypovolemia or fluid overload (see Adverse Reactions and Overdose/Toxicology). If adverse reactions (eg, fever, tachycardia, hypotension, or dyspnea) occur, infusion should be stopped and prescriber notified.

Monitoring Laboratory Tests: Hematocrit

Patient Education: Education is provided as appropriate for patient condition. This medication can only be administered intravenously. You will be monitored closely during the infusion. **Pregnancy precaution:** Inform prescriber if you are pregnant.

Pregnancy Risk Factor: C

Lactation: Excretion in breast milk unknown/compatible

Perioperative/Anesthesia/Other Concerns: An Australian/New Zealand group recently published results from their evaluation of resuscitation fluid (4% albumin versus normal saline) in a heterogeneous intensive care population (Finfer, 2004). They conducted this multicenter, randomized, double-blind trial to compare the effects of resuscitation fluid on mortality from any cause during the 28-day period after randomization. Patients were eligible for inclusion if the treating clinician judged that fluid resuscitation was required for intravascular fluid depletion as supported by one of the following criteria:

Heart rate >90 bpm,
Systolic BP <100 mm Hg,
Mean arterial BP <75 mm Hg,
Decrease of 40 mm Hg in systolic or mean arterial BP (as compared with baseline),
CVP <10 mm Hg,
PCWP <12 mm Hg,
Respiratory variation in systolic or mean BP >5 mm Hg,
Capillary refill time >1 second, or
Urine output <0.5 mL/kg for 1 hour

Patients were excluded for a variety of reasons, including ICU transfer following cardiac or liver transplantation surgery, or burn treatment. Almost 7000 patients were randomized; 3497 to albumin and 3500 to saline. Baseline characteristics were similar between the groups, except CVP pressure was slightly higher in the albumin group (9.0 in albumin versus 8.6 in saline). There was no significant mortality difference between groups (726 deaths in albumin group; 729 deaths

(Continued)

Albumin *(Continued)*

in saline group). There were no significant differences in secondary endpoints (length of stay in the ICU or hospital, days of mechanical ventilation, and days of renal replacement therapy). Similar outcomes resulted from use of either fluid for resuscitation in this patient population.

Administration

I.V.: For I.V. administration only. Use within 4 hours after opening vial; discard unused portion. In emergencies, may administer as rapidly as necessary to improve clinical condition. After initial volume replacement:

5%: Do not exceed 2-4 mL/minute in patients with normal plasma volume; 5-10 mL/minute in patients with hypoproteinemia

25%: Do not exceed 1 mL/minute in patients with normal plasma volume; 2-3 mL/minute in patients with hypoproteinemia

Reconstitution: If 5% human albumin is unavailable, it may be prepared by diluting 25% human albumin with 0.9% sodium chloride or 5% dextrose in water. Do not use sterile water to dilute albumin solutions, as this has been associated with hypotonic-associated hemolysis.

Compatibility: Stable in dextran 6% in D_5W, dextran 6% in NS, D_5LR, D_5NS, $D_5{}^1/_2NS$, $D_5{}^1/_4NS$, D_5W, $D_{10}W$, LR, NS, $^1/_2NS$; **incompatible** with sterile water

Y-site administration: Incompatible with midazolam, vancomycin, verapamil

Compatibility when admixed: Incompatible with verapamil

Storage: Store at a temperature ≤30°C (86°F); do not freeze. Do not use solution if it is turbid or contains a deposit; use within 4 hours after opening vial; discard unused portion.

♦ **Albuminar®** *see* Albumin *on page 94*

♦ **Albumin (Human)** *see* Albumin *on page 94*

♦ **Albutein®** *see* Albumin *on page 94*

Albuterol (al BYOO ter ole)

U.S. Brand Names AccuNeb™; Proventil®; Proventil® HFA; Proventil® Repetabs®; Ventolin® HFA; Volmax® [DSC]; VoSpire ER™

Synonyms Albuterol Sulfate; Salbutamol

Pharmacologic Category $Beta_2$-Adrenergic Agonist

Medication Safety Issues

Sound-alike/look-alike issues:

Albuterol may be confused with Albutein®, atenolol
Proventil® may be confused with Bentyl®, Prilosec® Prinivil®
Salbutamol may be confused with salmeterol
Ventolin® may be confused with phentolamine, Benylin®, Vantin®
Volmax® may be confused with Flomax®

Use Bronchodilator in reversible airway obstruction due to asthma or COPD; prevention of exercise-induced bronchospasm

Mechanism of Action Relaxes bronchial smooth muscle by action on $beta_2$-receptors with little effect on heart rate

Pharmacodynamics/Kinetics

Onset of action: Peak effect:

Nebulization/oral inhalation: 0.5-2 hours

CFC-propelled albuterol: 10 minutes

Ventolin® HFA: 25 minutes

Oral: 2-3 hours

Duration: Nebulization/oral inhalation: 3-4 hours; Oral: 4-6 hours

Metabolism: Hepatic to an inactive sulfate

Half-life elimination: Inhalation: 3.8 hours; Oral: 3.7-5 hours

Excretion: Urine (30% as unchanged drug)

Contraindications Hypersensitivity to albuterol, adrenergic amines, or any component of the formulation

Warnings/Precautions Optimize anti-inflammatory treatment before initiating maintenance treatment with albuterol. Do not use as a component of chronic therapy without an anti-inflammatory agent. Only the mildest forms of asthma (Step 1 and/or exercise-induced) would not require concurrent use based upon asthma guidelines. Patient must be instructed to seek medical attention in cases where acute symptoms are not relieved or a previous level of response is diminished. The need to increase frequency of use may indicate deterioration of asthma, and treatment must not be delayed.

Use caution in patients with cardiovascular disease (arrhythmia or hypertension or CHF), convulsive disorders, diabetes, glaucoma, hyperthyroidism, or hypokalemia. Beta agonists may cause elevation in blood pressure, heart rate, and result in CNS stimulation/excitation. $Beta_2$ agonists may increase risk of arrhythmia, increase serum glucose, or decrease serum potassium.

Do not exceed recommended dose; serious adverse events, including fatalities, have been associated with excessive use of inhaled sympathomimetics. Rarely, paradoxical bronchospasm may occur with use of inhaled bronchodilating agents; this should be distinguished from inadequate response. All patients should utilize a spacer device when using a metered-dose inhaler; in addition, face masks should be used in children <4 years of age.

Because of its minimal effect on $beta_1$-receptors and its relatively long duration of action, albuterol is a rational choice in the elderly when an inhaled beta agonist is indicated. Oral use should be avoided in the elderly due to adverse effects. Patient response may vary between inhalers that contain chlorofluorocarbons and those which are chlorofluorocarbon-free.

Drug Interactions **Substrate** of CYP3A4 (major)

Beta-adrenergic blockers (eg, propranolol) antagonize albuterol's effects; avoid concurrent use

CYP3A4 inducers: CYP3A4 inducers may decrease the levels/effects of albuterol. Example inducers include aminoglutethimide, carbamazepine, nafcillin, nevirapine, phenobarbital, phenytoin, and rifamycins.

Halothane may increase risk of malignant arrhythmias; avoid concurrent use

Inhaled ipratropium may increase duration of bronchodilation

MAO inhibitors may increase side effects; monitor heart rate and blood pressure

TCAs may increase side effects; monitor heart rate and blood pressure

Sympathomimetics may increase side effects; monitor heart rate and blood pressure

Nutritional/Herbal/Ethanol Interactions

Food: Avoid or limit caffeine (may cause CNS stimulation).

Herb/Nutraceutical: Avoid ephedra, yohimbe (may cause CNS stimulation).

Lab Interactions Increased renin (S), aldosterone (S)

Adverse Reactions Incidence of adverse effects is dependent upon age of patient, dose, and route of administration.

Cardiovascular: Angina, atrial fibrillation, chest discomfort, extrasystoles, flushing, hypertension, palpitation, tachycardia

Central nervous system: CNS stimulation, dizziness, drowsiness, headache, insomnia, irritability, lightheadedness, migraine, nervousness, nightmares, restlessness, sleeplessness, tremor

Dermatologic: Angioedema, erythema multiforme, rash, Stevens-Johnson syndrome, urticaria

Endocrine & metabolic: Hypokalemia, serum glucose increased, serum potassium decreased

Gastrointestinal: Diarrhea, dry mouth, gastroenteritis, nausea, unusual taste, vomiting, tooth discoloration

Genitourinary: Micturition difficulty

Neuromuscular & skeletal: Muscle cramps, weakness

Otic: Otitis media, vertigo

Respiratory: Asthma exacerbation, bronchospasm, cough, epistaxis, laryngitis, oropharyngeal drying/irritation, oropharyngeal edema

Miscellaneous: Allergic reaction, lymphadenopathy

Overdosage/Toxicology Symptoms of overdose include tachycardia, tremor, hypertension, angina, and seizures. Hypokalemia also may occur. Cardiac arrest and death may be associated with abuse of beta-agonist bronchodilators. Treatment includes immediate discontinuation and symptomatic and supportive therapies. Cautious use of beta-adrenergic blocking agents may be considered in severe cases.

Dosing

Adults:

Acute treatment of bronchospasm:

Inhalation: MDI 90 mcg/puff: 4-8 puffs every 20 minutes for up to 4 hours, then every 1-4 hours as needed

Nebulization: 2.5 mg, diluted to a total of 3 mL, 3-4 times/day over 5-15 minutes

NIH guidelines: 1.25-5 mg every 4-8 hours

(Continued)

Albuterol *(Continued)*

Bronchospasm in ICU patients (acute):

Nebulization: 2.5-5 mg every 20 minutes for 3 doses, then 2.5-10 mg every 1-4 hours as needed, **or** 10-15 mg/hour continuously

Chronic treatment of bronchospasm:

Inhalation: MDI 90 mcg/puff: 1-2 inhalations every 4-6 hours; maximum: 12 inhalations/day

NIH guidelines: 2 puffs 3-4 times a day as needed; may double dose for mild exacerbations

Oral:

Regular release: 2-4 mg/dose 3-4 times/day; maximum dose not to exceed 32 mg/day (divided doses)

Extended release: 8 mg every 12 hours; maximum dose not to exceed 32 mg/day (divided doses). A 4 mg dose every 12 hours may be sufficient in some patients, such as adults of low body weight.

Prophylaxis of exercise-induced bronchospasm: Inhalation: MDI 90 mcg/puff: 2 puffs 5-30 minutes prior to exercise

Elderly:

Inhalation: Refer to adult dosing.

Bronchospasm (treatment): Oral: 2 mg 3-4 times/day; maximum: 8 mg 4 times/day

Pediatrics:

Bronchospasm (acute):

Inhalation: MDI 90 mcg/puff:

Children ≤12 years: 4-8 puffs every 20 minutes for 3 doses, then every 1-4 hours; spacer/holding-chamber device should be used

Children >12 years: Refer to adult dosing.

Nebulization:

Children ≤12 years: Solution 0.5%: 0.15 mg/kg (minimum dose: 2.5 mg) every 20 minutes for 3 doses, then 0.15-0.3 mg/kg (up to 10 mg) every 1-4 hours as needed; may also use 0.5 mg/kg/hour by continuous infusion. Continuous nebulized albuterol at 0.3 mg/kg/hour has been used safely in the treatment of severe status asthmaticus in children; continuous nebulized doses of 3 mg/kg/hour ± 2.2 mg/kg/hour in children whose mean age was 20.7 months resulted in no cardiac toxicity; the optimal dosage for continuous nebulization remains to be determined.

Children >12 years: Refer to adult dosing.

Prophylaxis of exercise-induced bronchospasm:

Inhalation: MDI 90 mcg/puff:

Children ≤12 years: 1-2 puffs 5 minutes prior to exercise

Children >12 years: Refer to adult dosing.

Chronic treatment of bronchospasm:

Inhalation: MDI 90 mcg/puff: Children ≥4 years: Refer to adult dosing.

Oral:

Children: 2-6 years: 0.1-0.2 mg/kg/dose 3 times/day; maximum dose not to exceed 12 mg/day (divided doses)

Children: 6-12 years: 2 mg/dose 3-4 times/day; maximum dose not to exceed 24 mg/day (divided doses)

Extended release: 4 mg every 12 hours; maximum dose not to exceed 24 mg/day (divided doses)

Children >12 years: Refer to adult dosing.

Nebulization:

Children ≤12 years: 0.05 mg/kg every 4-6 hours; minimum dose: 1.25 mg, maximum dose: 2.5 mg

2-12 years: AccuNeb™: 0.63 mg or 1.25 mg 3-4 times/day, as needed, delivered over 5-15 minutes

Note: Use of the 0.5% solution should be used for bronchospasm (acute or treatment) in children <15 kg.

Children >40 kg, patients with more severe asthma, or children 11-12 years: May respond better with a 1.25 mg dose

Children >12 years: Refer to adult dosing.

Renal Impairment: Not removed by hemodialysis

Available Dosage Forms [DSC] = Discontinued product

Aerosol, oral (Proventil®): 90 mcg/dose (17 g) [200 doses]

Aerosol, oral, as sulfate [chlorofluorocarbon free]:

Proventil® HFA: 90 mcg/dose (6.7 g) [200 doses]

Ventolin® HFA: 90 mcg/dose (18 g) [200 doses]

Solution for oral inhalation, as sulfate: 0.083% (3 mL); 0.5% (20 mL)

AccuNeb™: 0.63 mg/3 mL (3 mL); 1.25 mg/3 mL (3 mL)

Proventil®: 0.083% (3 mL); 0.5% (20 mL)

Syrup, as sulfate: 2 mg/5 mL (480 mL)

Tablet, as sulfate: 2 mg, 4 mg

Tablet, extended release, as sulfate:

Proventil® Repetabs®: 4 mg

Volmax® [DSC], VoSpire ER™: 4 mg, 8 mg

Nursing Guidelines

Assessment: Assess effectiveness and interactions of other medications patient may be taking. Monitor vital signs, effectiveness of therapy, and adverse reactions at beginning of therapy and periodically with long-term use. Assess knowledge/teach patient appropriate use, interventions to reduce side effects, and adverse symptoms to report.

Monitoring Laboratory Tests: Arterial or capillary blood gases (if patients condition warrants); FEV_1, peak flow, and/or other pulmonary function tests; serum potassium, serum glucose (in selected patients)

Dietary Considerations: Oral forms should be administered with water 1 hour before or 2 hours after meals.

Patient Education: Use exactly as directed; do not use more often than recommended. Take oral medicine with water 1 hour before or 2 hours after meals. Maintain adequate hydration (2-3 L/day of fluids) unless instructed to restrict fluid intake. You may experience nervousness, dizziness, or fatigue (use caution when driving or engaging in hazardous activities until response to drug is known); dry mouth, unpleasant taste, stomach upset (frequent, small meals, frequent mouth care, chewing gum, or sucking lozenges may help); or difficulty urinating (always void before treatment). Report unresolved GI upset, dizziness or fatigue, vision changes, chest pain or palpitations, persistent inability to void, nervousness or insomnia, muscle cramping or tremor, or unusual cough.

Self-administered inhalation: Do not freeze. Shake canister before using. Sit when using medication. Close eyes when administering albuterol to avoid spray getting into eyes. Exhale slowly and completely through nose; inhale deeply through mouth while administering aerosol. Hold breath for 5-10 seconds after inhalation. Wait at least 1 full minute between inhalations. Wash mouthpiece between use. If more than one inhalation medication is used, use albuterol first and wait 5 minutes between medications. Prime inhaler prior to first use, and whenever the inhaler has not been used for more than 2 weeks, by releasing 4 test sprays into the air (away from face). Discard inhaler after labeled number of doses are used, even if the canister does not feel empty. **Ventolin® HFA:** Discard canister after 200 actuations or 3 months after removal from foil pouch, whichever comes first. Store with mouthpiece down. Do not allow metal canister to become wet.

Self-administered nebulizer: Wash hands before and after treatment. Wash and dry nebulizer after each treatment. Twist open the top of one unit-dose vial and squeeze contents into nebulizer reservoir. Connect nebulizer reservoir to the mouthpiece or face mask. Connect nebulizer to compressor. Sit in comfortable, upright position. Place mouthpiece in your mouth or put on face mask and turn on compressor. If face mask is used, avoid leakage around the mask to avoid mist getting into eyes which may cause vision problems. Breathe calmly and deeply until no more mist is formed in nebulizer (about 5 minutes). At this point, treatment is finished.

Volmax®: Tablets should be swallowed whole; do not crush or chew. Outer coating of tablet is not absorbed and may be found eliminated in stool.

Geriatric Considerations: Because of its minimal effect on $beta_1$-receptors and its relatively long duration of action, albuterol is a rational choice in the elderly when a beta agonist is indicated. Elderly patients may find it beneficial to utilize a spacer device when using a metered dose inhaler. The Ventolin Rotahaler® is an alternative for patients who have difficulty using the metered dose inhaler. Oral use should be avoided due to adverse effects.

Pregnancy Risk Factor: C

Pregnancy Issues: Albuterol crosses the placenta; tocolytic effects, fetal tachycardia, fetal hypoglycemia secondary to maternal hyperglycemia with oral or intravenous routes reported. Available evidence suggests safe use during pregnancy.

(Continued)

Albuterol *(Continued)*

Lactation: Excretion in breast milk unknown/use caution

Perioperative/Anesthesia/Other Concerns: Frequent use of inhaled beta agonists when used in patients with atrial fibrillation may counteract pharmacologic interventions directed at rate control. Inhaled beta agonists may be used to treat acute hyperkalemia in patients with renal failure.

Wait at least 1 minute between first and second puff of MDI. Because of its minimal effect on $beta_1$ receptors and its relatively long duration of action, albuterol is a rational choice in the elderly when a beta agonist is indicated. All patients should utilize a spacer device when using a metered-dose inhaler.

Administration

Oral: Do not crush or chew extended release tablets.

Reconstitution: Nebulization 0.5% solution: To prepare a 2.5 mg dose, dilute 0.5 mL of solution to a total of 3 mL with normal saline; also compatible with cromolyn or ipratropium nebulizer solutions.

Storage:

Syrup, nebulization 0.5% solution: Store at 2°C to 30°C (36°F to 86°F)

HFA aerosols: Store at 15°C to 25°C (59°F to 77°F)

Ventolin® HFA: Discard after using 200 actuations or 3 months after removal from protective pouch, whichever comes first. Store with mouthpiece down.

Inhalation solution: AccuNeb™: Store at 2°C to 25°C (36°F to 77°F). Do not use if solution changes color or becomes cloudy. Use within 1 week of opening foil pouch.

- ♦ **Albuterol and Ipratropium** *see* Ipratropium and Albuterol *on page 959*
- ♦ **Albuterol Sulfate** *see* Albuterol *on page 96*
- ♦ **Alcaine®** *see* Proparacaine *on page 1420*
- ♦ **Alcalak [OTC]** *see* Calcium Carbonate *on page 291*
- ♦ **Alcohol, Absolute** *see* Alcohol (Ethyl) *on page 100*
- ♦ **Alcohol, Dehydrated** *see* Alcohol (Ethyl) *on page 100*

Alcohol (Ethyl) (AL koe hol, ETH il)

U.S. Brand Names Lavacol® [OTC]

Synonyms Alcohol, Absolute; Alcohol, Dehydrated; Ethanol; Ethyl Alcohol; EtOH

Pharmacologic Category Antidote; Pharmaceutical Aid

Medication Safety Issues

Sound-alike/look-alike issues:

Ethanol may be confused with Ethyol®, Ethamolin®

Use Topical anti-infective; pharmaceutical aid; therapeutic neurolysis (nerve or ganglion block); replenishment of fluid and carbohydrate calories

Unlabeled/Investigational Use Antidote for ethylene glycol overdose; antidote for methanol overdose; treatment of fat occlusion of central venous catheters

Mechanism of Action When used to treat ethylene glycol or methanol toxicity, ethyl alcohol competitively inhibits their metabolism and decreases the formation of toxic metabolites.

Pharmacodynamics/Kinetics

Absorption: Oral: Rapid

Distribution: V_d: 0.6-0.7 L/kg; decreased in women

Metabolism: Hepatic (90% to 98%) to acetaldehyde or acetate

Half-life elimination: Rate: 15-20 mg/dL/hour (range: 10-34 mg/dL/hour); increased in alcoholics

Excretion: Kidneys and lungs (~2% unchanged)

Contraindications Hypersensitivity to ethyl alcohol or any component of the formulation; seizure disorder and diabetic coma; subarachnoid injection of dehydrated alcohol in patients receiving anticoagulants; pregnancy

Warnings/Precautions Ethyl alcohol is a flammable liquid and should be kept cool and away from any heat source. Proper positioning of the patient for neurolytic administration is essential to control localization of the injection of dehydrated alcohol (which is hypobaric) into the subarachnoid space; avoid extravasation. Not for SubQ administration. Do not administer simultaneously with blood due to the possibility of pseudoagglutination or hemolysis; may potentiate severe hypoprothrombic bleeding. Clinical evaluation and periodic lab determinations, including serum ethanol levels, are necessary to monitor effectiveness, changes in electrolyte concentrations, and acid-base balance (when used as an antidote).

Use with caution in diabetics (ethyl alcohol decreases blood sugar), hepatic impairment, patients with gout, shock, following cranial surgery, and in anticipated postpartum hemorrhage. Monitor blood glucose closely, particularly in children as treatment of ingestions is associated with hypoglycemia. Avoid extravasation during I.V. administration. Ethyl alcohol passes freely into breast milk at a level approximately equivalent to maternal serum level; minimize dermal exposure of ethyl alcohol in infants as significant systemic absorption and toxicity can occur.

Adverse Reactions Frequency not defined.

Central nervous system: Disorientation, encephalopathy, flushing, sedation, seizures (rare), vertigo

Endocrine & metabolic: Hypoglycemia

Genitourinary: Urinary retention

Local: Nerve and tissue destruction

Miscellaneous: Intoxication

Dosing

Adults & Elderly:

Treatment of methanol or ethylene glycol ingestion (unlabeled use): *Absolute ethanol (86 proof = 34 g EtoH/dL)/ethyl alcohol:* **Note:** Continue until methanol or ethylene glycol are no longer detected **or** <20 mg/dL and metabolic acidosis is corrected:

Oral: **Note:** Oral dosing is not recommended outside of a hospital setting:

Initial: 600 mg/kg [equivalent to 1.8 mL/kg using a 43% solution]

Maintenance dose:

Nondrinker: 66 mg/kg/hour [equivalent to 0.2 mL/kg/hour using a 43% solution]

Chronic drinker: 154 mg/kg/hour [equivalent to 0.46 mL/kg/hour using a 43% solution]

I.V.: Initial: 600 mg/kg [equivalent to 7.6 mL/kg using a 10% solution]

Maintenance dose:

Nondrinker: 66 mg/kg/hour [equivalent to 0.83 mL/kg/hour using a 10% solution]

Chronic drinker: 154 mg/kg/hour [equivalent to 1.96 mL/kg/hour using a 10% solution]

Treatment of fat occlusion of central venous catheters (unlabeled use): *Dehydrated alcohol injection:* I.V. (see institutional-based protocol for catheter clearance assessment, the following assessment is a general methodology): Up to 3 mL of ethanol 70% (maximum: 0.55 mL/kg); the volume to instill is equal to the internal volume of the catheter

Antiseptic: *Liquid denatured alcohol:* Topical: Apply 1-3 times/day as needed

Therapeutic neurolysis (nerve or ganglion block): *Dehydrated alcohol injection:* Intraneural: Dosage variable depending upon the site of injection (eg, trigeminal neuralgia: 0.05-0.5 mL as a single injection per interspace vs subarachnoid injection: 0.5-1 mL as a single injection per interspace); single doses >1.5 mL are seldom required

Replenishment of fluid and carbohydrate calories: *Dehydrated alcohol infusion:* Alcohol 5% and dextrose 5%: 1-2 L/day by slow infusion

Pediatrics:

Treatment of methanol or ethylene glycol ingestion (unlabeled use): *Absolute ethanol/ethyl alcohol:* Refer to adult dosing.

Treatment of fat occlusion of central venous catheters (unlabeled use): *Dehydrated alcohol injection:* Refer to adult dosing.

Antiseptic: *Liquid denatured alcohol:* Refer to adult dosing.

Renal Impairment: Treatment of methanol or ethylene glycol ingestion (unlabeled use): Absolute ethanol/ethyl alcohol: Dosage adjustment for hemodialysis: Maintenance dose:

Oral:

Nondrinker: 169 mg/kg/hour [equivalent to 0.5 mL/kg/hour using a 43% solution]

Chronic drinker: 257 mg/kg/hour [equivalent to 0.77 mL/kg/hour using a 43% solution]

I.V.:

Nondrinker: 169 mg/kg/hour [equivalent to 2.13 mL/kg/hour using a 10% solution]

Chronic drinker: 257 mg/kg/hour [equivalent to 3.26 mL/kg/hour using a 10% solution]

Available Dosage Forms

Infusion [in D_5W, dehydrated]: Alcohol 5% (1000 mL); alcohol 10% (1000 mL)

Injection, solution [dehydrated]: 98% (1 mL, 5 mL)

Liquid, topical [denatured] (Lavacol®): 70% (473 mL)

(Continued)

Alcohol (Ethyl) *(Continued)*

Nursing Guidelines

Monitoring Laboratory Tests: Antidotal therapy: Blood ethanol levels every 1-2 hours until steady state, then every 2-4 hours; blood glucose, electrolytes (including serum magnesium), arterial pH, blood gases, methanol or ethylene glycol blood levels

Pregnancy Risk Factor: C (D per expert opinion)/X (prolonged use or high doses at term)

Pregnancy Issues: Ethanol crosses the placenta, enters the fetal circulation, and has teratogenic effects in humans. The following withdrawal symptoms have been noted in the neonate following exposure to ethanol during pregnancy: Crying, hyperactivity, irritability, poor suck, tremors, seizures, poor sleeping pattern, hyperphagia, and diaphoresis. Fetal alcohol syndrome (FAS) is a term referring to a combination of physical, behavioral, and cognitive abnormalities resulting from ethanol exposure during fetal development. Since a "safe" amount of ethanol during pregnancy has not been determined, the AAP recommends those women who are pregnant or planning a pregnancy refrain from all ethanol intake. When used as an antidote during the second or third trimester, FAS is not likely to occur due to the short treatment period; use during the first trimester is controversial.

Lactation: Enters breast milk/use caution (AAP rates "compatible")

Breast-Feeding Considerations: Ethanol is found in breast milk. Drowsiness, diaphoresis, deep sleep, weakness, decreased linear growth, and abnormal weight gain have been reported in infants following large amounts of ethanol ingestion by the mother. Ingestion >1 g/kg/day decreases milk ejection reflex. The actual clearance of ethanol from breast milk is dependent upon the mother's weight and amount of ethanol consumed.

Perioperative/Anesthesia/Other Concerns:

Neurolytic block: Pain will occur after initial injection for a short period of time and will subside when neurolysis occurs. This agent will destroy nerve and should be administered when pain is from malignant origin only; administer carefully.

Methanol/ethylene glycol poisoning: Treatment involves inhibiting the formation of toxic metabolites by inhibiting alcohol dehydrogenase and/or urgent dialytic removal of these alcohols and their metabolites. Fomepizole and ethanol are both inhibitors of alcohol dehydrogenase and have been used to prevent toxicity. Currently, fomepizole is the drug of choice because of its ease of use and lack of CNS toxicity. When ethanol is used, a target serum level of 100-200 mg/dL is maintained during treatment. Patients are treated until serum levels of the poison (ethylene glycol/methanol) are <20 mg/dL.

Administration

Oral: Ethylene glycol or methanol poisoning: Dilute ethyl alcohol to 20% solution and administer hourly via NG tube; oral treatment is not recommended outside of a hospital setting

I.V.:

Ethylene glycol or methanol poisoning: Administer as a 10% solution in D_5W; initial dose should be administered over 1 hour

Treatment of occluded central venous catheter: Instill a 70% solution with a volume equal to the internal volume of the catheter; assess patency at 30-60 minutes (or per institutional protocol)

♦ **Aldactazide®** *see* Hydrochlorothiazide and Spironolactone *on page 865*

♦ **Aldactone®** *see* Spironolactone *on page 1566*

♦ **Aldroxicon I [OTC]** *see* Aluminum Hydroxide, Magnesium Hydroxide, and Simethicone *on page 122*

♦ **Aldroxicon II [OTC]** *see* Aluminum Hydroxide, Magnesium Hydroxide, and Simethicone *on page 122*

Alemtuzumab (ay lem TU zoo mab)

U.S. Brand Names Campath®

Synonyms C1H; Campath-1H; DNA-Derived Humanized Monoclonal Antibody; Humanized IgG1 Anti-CD52 Monoclonal Antibody

Pharmacologic Category Antineoplastic Agent, Monoclonal Antibody

Use Treatment of B-cell chronic lymphocytic leukemia (B-CLL)

Unlabeled/Investigational Use Treatment of refractory T-cell prolymphocytic leukemia (T-PLL); rheumatoid arthritis; graft-versus-host disease; multiple myeloma; preconditioning regimen for stem-cell transplantation and renal and liver transplantation; post-transplant rejection (renal)

Mechanism of Action Binds to CD52, a nonmodulating antigen present on the surface of B and T lymphocytes, a majority of monocytes, macrophages, NK cells, and a subpopulation of granulocytes. After binding to $CD52^+$ cells, an antibody-dependent lysis occurs.

Pharmacodynamics/Kinetics

Distribution: V_d: 0.18 L/kg

Metabolism: Clearance decreases with repeated dosing (due to loss of CD52 receptors in periphery), resulting in a sevenfold increase in AUC.

Half-life elimination: Initial: 11 hours; 6 days following repeated dosing

Contraindications Known type 1 hypersensitivity or anaphylactic reaction to alemtuzumab or any component of the formulation; hypersensitivity to another monoclonal antibody; active systemic infections; underlying immunodeficiency (eg, seropositive for HIV)

Warnings/Precautions Prophylactic therapy against PCP pneumonia and herpes viral infections is recommended upon initiation of therapy and for at least 2 months following last dose or until $CD4^+$ counts are ≥200 cells/μL. $CD4^+$ and $CD8^+$ lymphocyte counts may not return to baseline levels for more than 1 year. Serious and potentially fatal infusion-related reactions (acute respiratory distress syndrome, bronchospasm, cardiac arrest, cardiac arrhythmias, chills, fever, hypotension, myocardial infarction, pulmonary infiltrates, rash, rigors, shortness of breath, syncope) may occur; gradual escalation to the recommended maintenance dose is required at initiation and after interruption of therapy for ≥7 days to minimize infusion-related reactions. Severe, prolonged myelosuppression, autoimmune anemia, and autoimmune thrombocytopenia have occurred. Single doses >30 mg and cumulative weekly doses >90 mg are associated with an increased incidence of pancytopenia and should not be administered. Median duration of neutropenia is 21 days; median duration of thrombocytopenia is 21 days. Discontinue therapy during serious infection, serious hematologic or other serious toxicity until the event resolves. Permanently discontinue if autoimmune anemia or autoimmune thrombocytopenia occurs. Patients receiving blood products should only receive irradiated blood products due to the potential for GVHD during lymphopenia. Patients should not be immunized with live, viral vaccines during or recently after treatment. The ability to respond to any vaccine following therapy is unknown. Women of childbearing potential and men of reproductive potential should use effective contraceptive methods during treatment and for a minimum of 6 months following therapy. Safety and efficacy have not been established in pediatric patients.

Drug Interactions

Monoclonal antibodies: Allergic reactions may be increased in patients who have received diagnostic or therapeutic monoclonal antibodies due to the presence of HACA antibodies.

Vaccines: Avoid administration of live vaccines in immunosuppressive therapy.

Lab Interactions May interfere with diagnostic serum tests that utilize antibodies.

Adverse Reactions

>10%:

Cardiovascular: Hypotension (32%), peripheral edema (13%), hypertension (11%), tachycardia/SVT (11%)

Central nervous system: Fever (85%), fatigue (34%), headache (24%), dysthesias (15%), dizziness (12%)

Dermatologic: Rash (40%), urticaria (30%), pruritus (24%), herpes simplex (11%)

Gastrointestinal: Nausea (54%), vomiting (41%), anorexia (20%), diarrhea (22%), stomatitis/mucositis (14%), abdominal pain (11%)

Hematologic: Neutropenia (85%; grade 3/4: 64%; median duration: 28 days), anemia (80%; grade 3/4: 38%), thrombocytopenia (72%; grade 3/4: 50%; median duration: 21 days)

Neuromuscular & skeletal: Rigors (86%), skeletal muscle pain (24%), weakness (13%), myalgia (11%)

Respiratory: Dyspnea (26%), cough (25%), bronchitis/pneumonitis (21%), pneumonia (16%), pharyngitis (12%)

Miscellaneous: Infection (43% to 66%; incidence is lower if prophylaxis anti-infectives are utilized), diaphoresis (19%), sepsis (15%)

1% to 10%:

Cardiovascular: Chest pain (10%)

(Continued)

Alemtuzumab *(Continued)*

Central nervous system: Insomnia (10%), neutropenic fever (10%), malaise (9%), depression (7%), temperature change sensation (5%), somnolence (5%)
Dermatologic: Purpura (8%)
Gastrointestinal: Dyspepsia (10%), constipation (9%)
Hematologic: Pancytopenia/marrow hypoplasia (5% to 6%; grade 3/4: 3%), positive Coombs' test without hemolysis (2%), autoimmune thrombocytopenia (2%), autoimmune hemolytic anemia (1%)
Neuromuscular & skeletal: Back pain (10%), tremor (7%)
Respiratory: Bronchospasm (9%), epistaxis (7%), rhinitis (7%)
Miscellaneous: Moniliasis (8%)

<1% (Limited to important or life-threatening): Acidosis, acute renal failure, agranulocytosis, alkaline phosphatase increased, allergic reactions, anaphylactoid reactions, angina pectoris, angioedema, anuria, aphasia, ascites, asthma, atrial fibrillation, biliary pain, bone marrow aplasia, bronchitis, capillary fragility, cardiac arrest, cardiac failure, cellulitis, cerebral hemorrhage, cerebrovascular disorder, coagulation abnormality, coma, COPD, coronary artery disorder, cyanosis, deep vein thrombosis, disseminated intravascular coagulation, duodenal ulcer, fluid overload, gastrointestinal hemorrhage, hallucinations, haptoglobin decreased, hematemesis, hematoma, hematuria, hemolysis, hemolytic anemia, hemoptysis, hepatic failure, hepatocellular damage, hyperbilirubinemia, hyper-/hypoglycemia, hyper-/hypokalemia, hyperthyroidism, hypoalbuminemia, hyponatremia, hypovolemia, hypoxia, idiopathic thrombocytopenic purpura (ITP), interstitial pneumonitis, intestinal obstruction, intestinal perforation, intracranial hemorrhage, lymphadenopathy, lymphopenia, marrow depression, melena, meningitis, MI, optic neuropathy, osteomyelitis, otitis media, pancreatitis, paralysis, paralytic ileus, paroxysmal nocturnal hemoglobinuria-like monocytes, pericarditis, peritonitis, plasma cell dyscrasia, phlebitis, pleural effusion, pleurisy, pneumothorax, progressive multifocal leukoencephalopathy, pseudomembranous colitis, pulmonary edema, pulmonary embolism, pulmonary fibrosis, pulmonary infiltration, purpuric rash, renal dysfunction, respiratory alkalosis, respiratory depression, respiratory insufficiency, seizure (grand mal), splenic infarction, splenomegaly, subarachnoid hemorrhage, syncope, toxic nephropathy, thrombocythemia, thrombophlebitis, throat tightness, tumor lysis syndrome, ureteric obstruction, ventricular arrhythmia, ventricular tachycardia

Overdosage/Toxicology Symptoms are likely to be extensions of adverse events (may include hematologic toxicity, respiratory distress, bronchospasm, anuria, tumor lysis syndrome). Cumulative doses >90 mg/week have been associated with pancytopenia and severe (and occasionally fatal) ITP. Treatment is symptom-directed and supportive.

Dosing

Adults & Elderly:

B-CLL: I.V. infusion, SubQ (unlabeled route):
Initial: 3 mg/day; increase to 10 mg/day, then to 30 mg/day as tolerated
Maintenance: 30 mg/day 3 times/week on alternate days for up to 12 weeks

Note: Dose escalation is required; usually accomplished in 3-7 days. Do not exceed single doses >30 mg or cumulative doses >90 mg/week.

Available Dosage Forms [DSC] = Discontinued product
Injection, solution [ampul]: 10 mg/mL (3 mL) [DSC]
Injection, solution [vial]: 30 mg/mL (1 mL)

Nursing Guidelines

Assessment: See Warnings/Precautions and Contraindications for extensive use cautions. Note preinfusion medication instructions (see Administration). Monitor closely for alterations in blood pressure (especially in patients with heart disease or on antihypertensive medications) and/or infusion-related reactions during and for several hours following infusion. Assess knowledge/teach patient to monitor closely for postinfusion adverse reactions, appropriate interventions to reduce side effects, and symptoms to report (see Patient Education). Breast-feeding is contraindicated.

Monitoring Laboratory Tests: CBC and platelets; $CD4^+$ lymphocyte counts

Patient Education: This medication can only be administered I.V. During infusion, you will be closely monitored. You will need frequent laboratory tests during course of therapy. Do not use any prescription or OTC medications unless approved by your prescriber. Maintain adequate hydration (2-3 L/day of fluids) unless instructed to restrict fluid intake, and nutrition (small, frequent meals will help). You may experience abdominal pain, mouth sores, nausea, or vomiting (small, frequent meals, good mouth care with soft toothbrush or swabs, sucking lozenges or chewing gum, and avoidance of spicy or salty foods may help). Report unresolved GI problems, persistent fever, chills, muscle pain, skin rash, unusual bleeding or bruising, signs of infection (mouth sores, sore throat, white plaques in mouth or perianal area, burning on urination); swelling of extremities; respiratory difficulty; chest pain or palpitations; or other persistent adverse reactions. **Pregnancy/breast-feeding precautions:** Inform prescriber if you are or intend to become pregnant. Do not breast-feed.

Pregnancy Risk Factor: C

Pregnancy Issues: Human IgG is known to cross the placental barrier; therefore, alemtuzumab may also cross the barrier and cause fetal B- and T-lymphocyte depletion. Well-controlled human trials have not been done. Use during pregnancy only if the benefit to the mother outweighs the potential risk to the fetus.

Lactation: Excretion in breast milk unknown/contraindicated

Breast-Feeding Considerations: Human IgG is excreted in breast milk; therefore, alemtuzumab may also be excreted in milk. Breast-feeding should be discontinued during treatment and for at least 3 months following the last dose.

Administration

I.V.: Administer by I.V. infusion over 2 hours. Premedicate with diphenhydramine 50 mg and acetaminophen 650 mg 30 minutes before initiation of infusion. Hydrocortisone 200 mg has been effective in decreasing severe infusion-related events. Start anti-infective prophylaxis. Other drugs should not be added to or simultaneously infused through the same I.V. line. Do not give I.V. bolus or push.

Reconstitution: Gently invert the bag to mix the solution. Do not shake prior to use. Dilute with 100 mL NS or D_5W.

Compatibility: Medications should not be added to the solution or simultaneously infused through the same I.V. line.

Storage: Prior to dilution, store at 2°C to 8°C (36°F to 46°F). Do not freeze. Following dilution, use within 8 hours. Store at room temperature or refrigerate; protect from light.

Alendronate (a LEN droe nate)

U.S. Brand Names Fosamax®

Synonyms Alendronate Sodium

Pharmacologic Category Bisphosphonate Derivative

Medication Safety Issues

Sound-alike/look-alike issues:

Fosamax® may be confused with Flomax®

Use Treatment and prevention of osteoporosis in postmenopausal females; treatment of osteoporosis in males; Paget's disease of the bone in patients who are symptomatic, at risk for future complications, or with alkaline phosphatase ≥2 times the upper limit of normal; treatment of glucocorticoid-induced osteoporosis in males and females with low bone mineral density who are receiving a daily dosage ≥7.5 mg of prednisone (or equivalent)

Mechanism of Action A bisphosphonate which inhibits bone resorption via actions on osteoclasts or on osteoclast precursors; decreases the rate of bone resorption, leading to an indirect increase in bone mineral density. In Paget's disease, characterized by disordered resorption and formation of bone, inhibition of resorption leads to an indirect decrease in bone formation; but the newly-formed bone has a more normal architecture.

Pharmacodynamics/Kinetics

Distribution: 28 L (exclusive of bone)

Protein binding: ~78%

Metabolism: None

Bioavailability: Fasting: Female: 0.7%; Male: 0.6%; reduced 60% with food or drink

Half-life elimination: Exceeds 10 years

Excretion: Urine; feces (as unabsorbed drug)

Contraindications Hypersensitivity to alendronate, other bisphosphonates, or any component of the formulation; hypocalcemia; abnormalities of the esophagus which delay esophageal emptying such as stricture or achalasia; inability to stand

(Continued)

Alendronate *(Continued)*

or sit upright for at least 30 minutes; oral solution should not be used in patients at risk of aspiration

Warnings/Precautions Use caution in patients with renal impairment; hypocalcemia must be corrected before therapy initiation; ensure adequate calcium and vitamin D intake. May cause irritation to upper gastrointestinal mucosa. Esophagitis, esophageal ulcers, esophageal erosions, and esophageal stricture (rare) have been reported; risk increases in patients unable to comply with dosing instructions. Use with caution in patients with dysphagia, esophageal disease, gastritis, duodenitis, or ulcers (may worsen underlying condition).

Bisphosphonate therapy has been associated with osteonecrosis, primarily of the jaw; this has been observed mostly in cancer patients, but also in patients with postmenopausal osteoporosis and other diagnoses. Risk factors include a diagnosis of cancer, with concomitant chemotherapy, radiotherapy, or corticosteroids; anemia, coagulopathy, infection, or pre-existing dental disease. Symptoms included nonhealing extraction socket or an exposed jawbone. There are no data addressing whether discontinuation of therapy reduces the risk of developing osteonecrosis; however, as a precautionary measure, dental exams and preventative dentistry should be performed prior to placing patients with risk factors on chronic bisphosphonate therapy. Invasive dental procedures should be avoided during treatment.

Drug Interactions

Aspirin: Increased incidence of adverse GI effects when >10 mg alendronate is used in patients taking aspirin-containing products

Oral medications (especially those containing multivalent cations): May interfere with alendronate absorption; wait at least 30 minutes after taking alendronate before taking any oral medications

Ranitidine (by increasing gastric pH) can double the bioavailability of alendronate

Nutritional/Herbal/Ethanol Interactions Food: All food and beverages interfere with absorption. Coadministration with caffeine may reduce alendronate efficacy. Coadministration with dairy products may decrease alendronate absorption. Beverages (especially orange juice and coffee), food, and medications (eg, antacids, calcium, iron, and multivalent cations) may reduce the absorption of alendronate as much as 60%.

Lab Interactions Bisphosphonates may interfere with diagnostic imaging agents such as technetium-99m-diphosphonate in bone scans.

Adverse Reactions Note: Incidence of adverse effects (mostly GI) increases significantly in patients treated for Paget's disease at 40 mg/day.

>10%: Endocrine & metabolic: Hypocalcemia (transient, mild, 18%), hypophosphatemia (transient, mild, 10%)

1% to 10%:

Central nervous system: Headache (0.2% to 3%)

Gastrointestinal: Abdominal pain (1% to 7%), acid reflux (1% to 5%), dyspepsia (1% to 4%), nausea (1% to 4%), flatulence (0.2% to 4%), diarrhea (0.6% to 3%), constipation (0.3% to 3%), esophageal ulcer (0.1% to 2%), abdominal distension (0.2% to 1%), gastritis (0.2% to 1%), vomiting (0.2% to 1%), dysphagia (0.1% to 1%), gastric ulcer (1%), melena (1%)

Neuromuscular & skeletal: Musculoskeletal pain (0.4% to 4%), muscle cramps (0.2% to 1%)

<1% (Limited to important or life-threatening): Angioedema; bone, muscle, or joint pain (occasionally severe, considered incapacitating in rare cases); duodenal ulcer, esophageal erosions, esophageal perforation, esophageal stricture, esophagitis, hypocalcemia (symptomatic), hypersensitivity reactions, oropharyngeal ulceration, osteonecrosis (jaw), photosensitivity (rare), pruritus, rash, scleritis (rare), Stevens-Johnson syndrome, taste perversion, toxic epidermal necrolysis, urticaria, uveitis (rare)

Overdosage/Toxicology Symptoms of overdose include hypocalcemia, hypophosphatemia, and upper GI adverse affects (eg, upset stomach, heartburn, esophagitis, gastritis, or ulcer). Treat with milk or antacids to bind alendronate. Dialysis would not be beneficial.

Dosing

Adults & Elderly: Note: Patients treated with glucocorticoids and those with Paget's disease should receive adequate amounts of calcium and vitamin D.

Osteoporosis in postmenopausal females: Oral:

Prophylaxis: 5 mg once daily **or** 35 mg once weekly

Treatment: 10 mg once daily **or** 70 mg once weekly

Osteoporosis in males: Oral: 10 mg once daily **or** 70 mg once weekly

Osteoporosis secondary to glucocorticoids in males and females: Oral:
Treatment: 5 mg once daily; a dose of 10 mg once daily should be used in postmenopausal females who are not receiving estrogen.

Paget's disease of bone in males and females: Oral: 40 mg once daily for 6 months

Retreatment: Relapses during the 12 months following therapy occurred in 9% of patients who responded to treatment. Specific retreatment data are not available. Following a 6-month post-treatment evaluation period, treatment with alendronate may be considered in patients who have relapsed based on increases in serum alkaline phosphatase, which should be measured periodically. Retreatment may also be considered in those who failed to normalize their serum alkaline phosphatase.

Renal Impairment:

Cl_{cr} 35-60 mL/minute: None necessary.

Cl_{cr} <35 mL/minute: Alendronate is not recommended due to lack of experience.

Hepatic Impairment: No adjustment necessary.

Available Dosage Forms

Solution, oral, as monosodium trihydrate: 70 mg/75 mL [contains parabens; raspberry flavor]

Tablet, as sodium: 5 mg, 10 mg, 35 mg, 40 mg, 70 mg

Nursing Guidelines

Assessment: See Contraindications, Warnings/Precautions, and Dosing for use cautions. Assess results of laboratory tests (see below), therapeutic effectiveness, and adverse reactions (eg, hypocalcemia). Teach patient appropriate use and administration of medications (see Administration), lifestyle and dietary changes that will have a beneficial impact on Paget's disease or osteoporosis, possible side effects, interventions to reduce side effects, and adverse reactions to report. Note breast-feeding caution.

Monitoring Laboratory Tests: Alkaline phosphatase should be periodically measured; serum calcium and phosphorus; hormonal status (male and female) prior to therapy; bone mineral density (should be done prior to initiation of therapy and after 6-12 months of combined glucocorticoid and alendronate treatment)

Dietary Considerations: Ensure adequate calcium and vitamin D intake; however, wait at least 30 minutes after taking alendronate before taking any supplement. Must be taken with plain water first thing in the morning and at least 30 minutes before the first food or beverage of the day.

Patient Education: Inform prescriber of all prescriptions, OTC medications, or herbal products you are taking, and any allergies you have. Do not take any new medication during therapy unless approved by prescriber. Take as directed, with a full glass of water first thing in the morning and at least 30 minutes before the first food or beverage of the day. Wait at least 30 minutes after taking alendronate before taking anything else. Stay in sitting or standing position for 30 minutes following administration and until after the first food of the day to reduce potential for esophageal irritation. Consult prescriber to determine necessity of lifestyle changes (eg, decreased smoking, decreased alcohol intake, dietary supplements of calcium or vitamin D). May cause flatulence, bloating, nausea, or acid regurgitation; small, frequent meals may help. Report acute headache or gastric pain, unresolved GI upset, or acid stomach. **Pregnancy/breast-feeding precautions:** Inform prescriber if you are or intend to become pregnant. Consult prescriber if breast-feeding.

Geriatric Considerations: Since many elderly patients receive diuretics, evaluation of electrolyte status (calcium, phosphate, magnesium, potassium) may need to be done periodically due to the drug class (bisphosphonate). Should assure immobile patients are at least sitting up for 30 minutes after swallowing tablets. Drink a full glass of water with each dose.

Pregnancy Risk Factor: C

Pregnancy Issues: Safety and efficacy have not been established in pregnant women. Animal studies have shown delays in delivery and fetal/neonatal death (secondary to hypocalcemia). Bisphosphonates are incorporated into the bone matrix and gradually released over time. Theoretically, there may be a risk of fetal harm when pregnancy follows the completion of therapy. Based on limited case reports with pamidronate, serum calcium levels in the newborn may be altered if administered during pregnancy.

(Continued)

Alendronate *(Continued)*

Lactation: Excretion in breast milk unknown/use caution

Administration

Oral: Alendronate must be taken with plain water (tablets 6-8 oz; oral solution 2 oz) first thing in the morning and ≥30 minutes before the first food, beverage, or other medication of the day. Patients should be instructed to stay upright (not to lie down) for at least 30 minutes **and** until after first food of the day (to reduce esophageal irritation). Patients should receive supplemental calcium and vitamin D if dietary intake is inadequate.

Storage: Store tablets and oral solution at room temperature of 15°C to 30°C (59°F to 86°F). Keep in well-closed container.

- ♦ **Alendronate Sodium** *see* Alendronate *on page 105*
- ♦ **Aler-Cap [OTC]** *see* DiphenhydrAMINE *on page 546*
- ♦ **Aler-Dryl [OTC]** *see* DiphenhydrAMINE *on page 546*
- ♦ **Aler-Tab [OTC]** *see* DiphenhydrAMINE *on page 546*
- ♦ **Aleve® [OTC]** *see* Naproxen *on page 1203*
- ♦ **Alfenta®** *see* Alfentanil *on page 108*

Alfentanil (al FEN ta nil)

U.S. Brand Names Alfenta®

Synonyms Alfentanil Hydrochloride

Pharmacologic Category Analgesic, Narcotic

Medication Safety Issues

Sound-alike/look-alike issues:

Alfentanil may be confused with Anafranil®, fentanyl, remifentanil, sufentanil

Alfenta® may be confused with Sufenta®

Use Analgesic adjunct given by continuous infusion or in incremental doses in maintenance of anesthesia with barbiturate or N_2O or a primary anesthetic agent for the induction of anesthesia in patients undergoing general surgery in which endotracheal intubation and mechanical ventilation are required

Mechanism of Action Binds with stereospecific receptors at many sites within the CNS, increases pain threshold, alters pain perception, inhibits ascending pain pathways; is an ultra short-acting narcotic

Pharmacodynamics/Kinetics

Onset of action: Rapid

Duration (dose dependent): 30-60 minutes

Distribution: V_d: Newborns, premature: 1 L/kg; Children: 0.163-0.48 L/kg; Adults: 0.46 L/kg

Half-life elimination: Newborns, premature: 5.33-8.75 hours; Children: 40-60 minutes; Adults: 83-97 minutes

Contraindications Hypersensitivity to alfentanil hydrochloride, to narcotics, or any component of the formulation; increased intracranial pressure, severe respiratory depression

Warnings/Precautions Use with caution in patients with drug dependence, head injury, acute asthma and respiratory conditions; hypotension has occurred in neonates with respiratory distress syndrome; use caution when administering to patients with bradyarrhythmias; rapid I.V. infusion may result in skeletal muscle and chest wall rigidity, impaired ventilation, or respiratory distress/arrest; inject slowly over 3-5 minutes. Alfentanil may produce more hypotension compared to fentanyl, therefore, be sure to administer slowly and ensure patient has adequate hydration.

Drug Interactions Substrate of CYP3A4 (major)

Dextroamphetamine: May enhance the analgesic effect of morphine and other opiate agonists

Increased toxicity with CNS depressants (eg, benzodiazepines, barbiturates, tricyclic antidepressants), erythromycin, reserpine, beta-blockers

CYP3A4 inhibitors: May increase the levels/effects of alfentanil. Example inhibitors include azole antifungals, clarithromycin, diclofenac, doxycycline, erythromycin, imatinib, isoniazid, nefazodone, nicardipine, propofol, protease inhibitors, quinidine, telithromycin, and verapamil.

Adverse Reactions

>10%:

Cardiovascular: Bradycardia

Gastrointestinal: Nausea, vomiting

1% to 10%:
Cardiovascular: Orthostatic hypotension
Central nervous system: CNS depression
<1% (Limited to important or life-threatening): Biliary tract spasm, pruritus, respiratory depression, urinary retention

Overdosage/Toxicology Symptoms of overdose include miosis, respiratory depression, seizures, and CNS depression. Naloxone 2 mg I.V. (0.01 mg/kg for children) with repeat administration as necessary up to a total of 10 mg; may precipitate withdrawal.

Dosing

Adults & Elderly: Doses should be titrated to appropriate effects; wide range of doses is dependent upon desired degree of analgesia/anesthesia

Anesthesia: I.V.: Dose should be based on ideal body weight as follows (see table):

Alfentanil

Indication	Approx Duration of Anesthesia (min)	Induction Period (Initial Dose) (mcg/kg)	Maintenance Period (Increments/ Infusion)	Total Dose (mcg/kg)	Effects
Incremental injection	≤30	8-20	3-5 mcg/kg or 0.5-1 mcg/kg/min	8-40	Spontaneously breathing or assisted ventilation when required.
	30-60	20-50	5-15 mcg/kg	Up to 75	Assisted or controlled ventilation required. Attenuation of response to laryngoscopy and intubation.
Continuous infusion	>45	50-75	0.5-3 mcg/kg/min average infusion rate 1-1.5 mcg/kg/min	Dependent on duration of procedure	Assisted or controlled ventilation required. Some attenuation of response to intubation and incision, with intraoperative stability.
Anesthetic induction	>45	130-245	0.5-1.5 mcg/kg/min or general anesthetic	Dependent on duration of procedure	Assisted or controlled ventilation required. Administer slowly (over 3 minutes). Concentration of inhalation agents reduced by 30% to 50% for initial hour.

Pediatrics:
Children <12 years: Dose has not been established.
Children ≥12 years: Refer to adult dosing.

Available Dosage Forms Injection, solution, as hydrochloride [preservative free]: 500 mcg/mL (2 mL, 5 mL, 10 mL, 20 mL)

Nursing Guidelines

Pregnancy Risk Factor: C

Perioperative/Anesthesia/Other Concerns: Alfentanil may produce more muscle rigidity compared to fentanyl, therefore, be sure to administer slowly.

Administration

I.V.: Administer I.V. slowly over 3-5 minutes or by I.V. continuous infusion.

Compatibility: Stable in D_5W, NS, D_5LR, D_5NS

Y-site administration: Incompatible with amphotericin B cholesteryl sulfate complex, thiopental

Related Information

Narcotic / Opioid Analgesics *on page 1880*

- **Alfentanil Hydrochloride** *see* Alfentanil *on page 108*
- **Alka-Mints® [OTC]** *see* Calcium Carbonate *on page 291*
- **Alka-Seltzer® Plus Flu Liqui-Gels® [OTC]** *see* Acetaminophen, Dextromethorphan, and Pseudoephedrine *on page 73*
- **Allbee® C-800 [OTC]** *see* Vitamin B Complex Combinations *on page 1716*
- **Allbee® C-800 + Iron [OTC]** *see* Vitamin B Complex Combinations *on page 1716*
- **Allbee® with C [OTC]** *see* Vitamin B Complex Combinations *on page 1716*
- **Allegra®** *see* Fexofenadine *on page 723*
- **Allerfrim® [OTC]** *see* Triprolidine and Pseudoephedrine *on page 1670*

♦ **AllerMax® [OTC]** *see* DiphenhydrAMINE *on page 546*
♦ **Allfen Jr** *see* Guaifenesin *on page 834*
♦ **Almacone® [OTC]** *see* Aluminum Hydroxide, Magnesium Hydroxide, and Simethicone *on page 122*
♦ **Almacone Double Strength® [OTC]** *see* Aluminum Hydroxide, Magnesium Hydroxide, and Simethicone *on page 122*
♦ **Alophen® [OTC]** *see* Bisacodyl *on page 245*
♦ **Alora®** *see* Estradiol *on page 649*
♦ **Alphagan® P** *see* Brimonidine *on page 258*
♦ **Alph-E [OTC]** *see* Vitamin E *on page 1716*
♦ **Alph-E-Mixed [OTC]** *see* Vitamin E *on page 1716*

Alprazolam (al PRAY zoe lam)

U.S. Brand Names Alprazolam Intensol®; Niravam™; Xanax®; Xanax XR®

Pharmacologic Category Benzodiazepine

Medication Safety Issues

Sound-alike/look-alike issues:

Alprazolam may be confused with alprostadil, lorazepam, triazolam

Xanax® may be confused with Lanoxin®, Tenex®, Tylox®, Xopenex®, Zantac®, Zyrtec®

Use Treatment of anxiety disorder (GAD); panic disorder, with or without agoraphobia; anxiety associated with depression

Unlabeled/Investigational Use Anxiety in children

Mechanism of Action Binds to stereospecific benzodiazepine receptors on the postsynaptic GABA neuron at several sites within the central nervous system, including the limbic system, reticular formation. Enhancement of the inhibitory effect of GABA on neuronal excitability results by increased neuronal membrane permeability to chloride ions. This shift in chloride ions results in hyperpolarization (a less excitable state) and stabilization.

Pharmacodynamics/Kinetics

Distribution: V_d: 0.9-1.2 L/kg; enters breast milk

Protein binding: 80%

Metabolism: Hepatic via CYP3A4; forms two active metabolites (4-hydroxyalprazolam and α-hydroxyalprazolam)

Bioavailability: 90%

Half-life elimination:

Adults: 11.2 hours (range: 6.3-26.9)

Elderly: 16.3 hours (range: 9-26.9 hours)

Alcoholic liver disease: 19.7 hours (range: 5.8-65.3 hours)

Obesity: 21.8 hours (range: 9.9-40.4 hours)

Time to peak, serum: 1-2 hours

Excretion: Urine (as unchanged drug and metabolites)

Contraindications Hypersensitivity to alprazolam or any component of the formulation (cross-sensitivity with other benzodiazepines may exist); narrow-angle glaucoma; concurrent use with ketoconazole or itraconazole; pregnancy

Warnings/Precautions Rebound or withdrawal symptoms, including seizures, may occur 18 hours to 3 days following abrupt discontinuation or large decreases in dose (more common in patients receiving >4 mg/day or prolonged treatment). Dose reductions or tapering must be approached with extreme caution. Breakthrough anxiety may occur at the end of dosing interval. Use with caution in patients receiving concurrent CYP3A4 inhibitors, particularly when these agents are added to therapy. Has weak uricosuric properties, use with caution in renal impairment or predisposition to urate nephropathy. Use with caution in elderly or debilitated patients, patients with hepatic disease (including alcoholics), renal impairment, or obese patients.

Causes CNS depression (dose related) resulting in sedation, dizziness, confusion, or ataxia which may impair physical and mental capabilities. Patients must be cautioned about performing tasks which require mental alertness (eg, operating machinery or driving). Use with caution in patients receiving other CNS depressants or psychoactive agents. Effects with other sedative drugs or ethanol may be potentiated. Benzodiazepines have been associated with falls and traumatic injury and should be used with extreme caution in patients who are at risk of these events (especially the elderly). Use with caution in patients with respiratory disease or impaired gag reflex.

Use caution in patients with depression, particularly if suicidal risk may be present. Episodes of mania or hypomania have occurred in depressed patients treated with alprazolam. May cause physical or psychological dependence - use with caution in patients with a history of drug dependence. Acute withdrawal, including seizures, may be precipitated in patients after administration of flumazenil to patients receiving long-term benzodiazepine therapy.

Benzodiazepines have been associated with anterograde amnesia. Paradoxical reactions, including hyperactive or aggressive behavior, have been reported with benzodiazepines, particularly in adolescent/pediatric or psychiatric patients. Does not have analgesic, antidepressant, or antipsychotic properties.

Benzodiazepines have the potential to cause harm to the fetus, particularly when administered during the first trimester. In addition, withdrawal symptoms may occur in the neonate following *in utero* exposure. Use of alprazolam during pregnancy should be avoided. In addition, symptoms of withdrawal, lethargy, and loss of body weight have been reported in infants exposed to alprazolam and/or benzodiazepines while nursing; use during breast-feeding is not recommended.

Drug Interactions Substrate of CYP3A4 (major)

CNS depressants: Sedative effects and/or respiratory depression may be additive with CNS depressants. Includes ethanol, barbiturates, narcotic analgesics, and other sedative agents; monitor for increased effect.

CYP3A4 inducers: CYP3A4 inducers may decrease the levels/effects of alprazolam. Example inducers include aminoglutethimide, carbamazepine, nafcillin, nevirapine, phenobarbital, phenytoin, and rifamycins.

CYP3A4 inhibitors: May increase the levels/effects of alprazolam. Example inhibitors include azole antifungals, clarithromycin, diclofenac, doxycycline, erythromycin, imatinib, isoniazid, nefazodone, nicardipine, propofol, protease inhibitors, quinidine, telithromycin, and verapamil. Contraindicated with itraconazole and ketoconazole.

Fluoxetine: May increase plasma concentrations/effects of alprazolam.

Oral contraceptives: May increase serum levels/effects of alprazolam.

Theophylline: May partially antagonize some of the effects of benzodiazepines; monitor for decreased response; may require higher doses for sedation.

Tricyclic antidepressants: Plasma concentrations of imipramine and desipramine have been reported to be increased 31% and 20%, respectively, by concomitant administration; monitor.

Nutritional/Herbal/Ethanol Interactions

Cigarette smoking: May decrease alprazolam concentrations up to 50%.

Ethanol: Avoid ethanol (may increase CNS depression).

Food: Alprazolam serum concentration is unlikely to be increased by grapefruit juice because of alprazolam's high oral bioavailability. The C_{max} of the extended release formulation is increased by 25% when a high-fat meal is given 2 hours before dosing. T_{max} is decreased 30% when food is given immediately prior to dose. T_{max} is increased by 30% when food is given ≥1 hour after dose.

Herb/Nutraceutical: St John's wort may decrease alprazolam levels. Avoid valerian, St John's wort, kava kava, gotu kola (may increase CNS depression).

Lab Interactions Increased with alkaline phosphatase

Adverse Reactions

>10%:

- Central nervous system: Abnormal coordination, cognitive disorder, depression, drowsiness, fatigue, irritability, lightheadedness, memory impairment, sedation, somnolence
- Gastrointestinal: Appetite increased/decreased, constipation, salivation decreased, weight gain/loss, xerostomia
- Genitourinary: Micturition difficulty
- Neuromuscular & skeletal: Dysarthria

1% to 10%:

- Cardiovascular: Hypotension
- Central nervous system: Agitation, attention disturbance, confusion, depersonalization, derealization, disorientation, disinhibition, dizziness, dream abnormalities, fear, hallucinations, hypersomnia, nightmares, seizure, talkativeness
- Dermatologic: Dermatitis, pruritus, rash
- Endocrine & metabolic: Libido decreased/increased, menstrual disorders
- Gastrointestinal: Salivation increased
- Genitourinary: Incontinence
- Hepatic: Bilirubin increased, jaundice, liver enzymes increased
- Neuromuscular & skeletal: Arthralgia, ataxia, myalgia, paresthesia
- Ocular: Diplopia
- Respiratory: Allergic rhinitis, dyspnea

(Continued)

Alprazolam *(Continued)*

<1% (Limited to important or life-threatening): Amnesia, falls, galactorrhea, gynecomastia, hepatic failure, hepatitis, hyperprolactinemia, Stevens-Johnson syndrome

Overdosage/Toxicology Symptoms of overdose include somnolence, confusion, coma, and diminished reflexes. Treatment for benzodiazepine overdose is supportive. Flumazenil has been shown to selectively block the binding of benzodiazepines to CNS receptors, resulting in a reversal of benzodiazepine-induced sedation; however, its use may not reverse respiratory depression.

Dosing

Adults: Note: Treatment >4 months should be re-evaluated to determine the patient's continued need for the drug

Anxiety: Oral: *Immediate release:* Effective doses are 0.5-4 mg/day in divided doses; the manufacturer recommends starting at 0.25-0.5 mg 3 times/day; titrate dose upward; maximum: 4 mg/day

Anxiety associated with depression: Oral: *Immediate release:* Average dose required: 2.5-3 mg/day in divided doses

Ethanol withdrawal (unlabeled use): Oral: *Immediate release:* Usual dose: 2-2.5 mg/day in divided doses

Panic disorder: Oral:

Immediate release: Initial: 0.5 mg 3 times/day; dose may be increased every 3-4 days in increments ≤1 mg/day; many patients obtain relief at 2 mg/day, as much as 10 mg/day may be required

Extended release: 0.5-1 mg once daily; may increase dose every 3-4 days in increments ≤1 mg/day (range: 3-6 mg/day)

Switching from immediate release to extended release: Patients may be switched to extended release tablets by taking the total daily dose of the immediate release tablets and giving it once daily using the extended release preparation.

Dose reduction: Abrupt discontinuation should be avoided. Daily dose may be decreased by 0.5 mg every 3 days, however, some patients may require a slower reduction. If withdrawal symptoms occur, resume previous dose and discontinue on a less rapid schedule.

Elderly: Initial: 0.125-0.25 mg twice daily; increase by 0.125 mg/day as needed. The smallest effective dose should be used.

Immediate release: Initial 0.25 mg 2-3 times/day

Extended release: Initial: 0.5 mg once daily

Pediatrics:

Anxiety (unlabeled use): Oral: Immediate release: Initial: 0.005 mg/kg/dose or 0.125 mg/dose 3 times/day; increase in increments of 0.125-0.25 mg, up to a maximum of 0.02 mg/kg/dose or 0.06 mg/kg/day (0.375-3 mg/day)

Note: Treatment >4 months should be re-evaluated to determine the patient's continued need for the drug

Hepatic Impairment: Oral: Reduce dose by 50% to 60% or avoid in cirrhosis.

Available Dosage Forms

Solution, oral (Alprazolam Intensol®): 1 mg/mL (30 mL)

Tablet (Xanax®): 0.25 mg, 0.5 mg, 1 mg, 2 mg

Tablet, extended release (Xanax XR®): 0.5 mg, 1 mg, 2 mg, 3 mg

Tablet, orally-disintegrating (Niravam™): 0.25 mg, 0.5 mg, 1 mg, 2 mg [orange flavor]

Nursing Guidelines

Assessment: Assess other medications patient may be taking for effectiveness and interactions. Assess for signs of CNS depression. Assess for history of addiction; long-term use can result in dependence, abuse, or tolerance; periodically evaluate need for continued use. For inpatient use, institute safety measures and monitor effectiveness and adverse reactions. For outpatients, monitor therapeutic effectiveness and adverse reactions at beginning of therapy and periodically with long-term use. Taper dosage slowly when discontinuing. Assess knowledge/teach patient appropriate use, interventions to reduce side effects, and adverse symptoms to report.

Patient Education: Take exactly as directed; do not increase dose or frequency. Drug may cause physical and/or psychological dependence. Avoid alcohol and do not take other prescription or OTC medications (especially pain medications, sedatives, antihistamines, or hypnotics) without consulting prescriber. Do not stop medication or reduce dosage abruptly without consulting prescriber. Maintain adequate hydration (2-3 L/day of fluids) unless instructed to restrict fluid intake. You may experience drowsiness, lightheadedness, impaired coordination, dizziness, or blurred vision (use caution when driving or engaging in hazardous tasks until response to drug is known); nausea, vomiting, or dry mouth (small frequent meals, frequent mouth care, chewing gum, or sucking lozenges may help); constipation (increased exercise, fluids, fruit, and fiber may help); altered sexual drive or ability (reversible); or photosensitivity (use sunscreen, wear protective clothing and eyewear, and avoid direct sunlight). Report persistent CNS effects (eg, confusion, depression, increased sedation, excitation, headache, agitation, insomnia or nightmares, dizziness, fatigue, impaired coordination, changes in personality, or changes in cognition); changes in urinary pattern; muscle cramping, weakness, tremors, or rigidity; ringing in ears or visual disturbances; chest pain, palpitations, or rapid heartbeat; excessive perspiration; excessive GI symptoms (eg, cramping, constipation, vomiting, anorexia); or worsening of condition. **Pregnancy/breast-feeding precautions:** Do not get pregnant while taking this medication; use appropriate contraceptive measures as recommended by your prescriber. Breast-feeding is not recommended.

Geriatric Considerations: Due to short duration of action, it is considered to be a benzodiazepine of choice in the elderly.

Pregnancy Risk Factor: D

Pregnancy Issues: Benzodiazepines cross the placenta. The association between benzodiazepine exposure and malformations remains controversial. A number of types of malformation have been reported (oral cleft, inguinal hernia, cardiac defects, spina bifida, dysmorphic facial features, skeletal defects); however, confounding factors make a clear association difficult. Overall, the risk to the fetus may be low. Nonteratogenic effects (including neonatal flaccidity, respiratory and feeding problems, and withdrawal symptoms) during the postnatal period have also been reported with benzodiazepine use.

Lactation: Enters breast milk/not recommended (AAP rates "of concern")

Breast-Feeding Considerations: Symptoms of withdrawal, lethargy, and loss of body weight have been reported in infants exposed to alprazolam and/or benzodiazepines while nursing. Breast-feeding is not recommended.

Perioperative/Anesthesia/Other Concerns: Chronic use of this agent may increase the perioperative benzodiazepine dose needed to achieve desired effect; not intended for management of anxieties and minor distresses associated with everyday life. Treatment >4 months should be re-evaluated to determine the patient's need for the drug. Patients who become physically dependent on alprazolam tend to have a difficult time discontinuing it; withdrawal symptoms may be severe. To minimize withdrawal symptoms, taper dosage slowly; do not discontinue abruptly. Abrupt discontinuation after sustained use (generally >10 days) may cause withdrawal symptoms.

Administration

Oral:

Immediate release preparations: Can be administered sublingually with comparable onset and completeness of absorption.

Extended release tablet: Should be taken once daily in the morning; do not crush, break, or chew.

Orally-disintegrating tablets: Using dry hands, place tablet on tongue. If using one-half of tablet, immediately discard remaining half (may not remain stable). Administration with water is not necessary.

Storage:

Orally-disintegrating tablet: Store at room temperature of 20°C to 25°C (68°F to 77°F). Protect from moisture. Seal bottle tightly and discard any cotton packaged inside bottle.

♦ Alprazolam Intensol® *see* Alprazolam *on page 110*

Alprostadil (al PROS ta dill)

U.S. Brand Names Caverject®; Caverject® Impulse™; Edex®; Muse®; Prostin VR Pediatric®

Synonyms PGE_1; Prostaglandin E_1

Pharmacologic Category Prostaglandin

Medication Safety Issues

Sound-alike/look-alike issues:

Alprostadil may be confused with alprazolam

Use

Prostin VR Pediatric®: Temporary maintenance of patency of ductus arteriosus in neonates with ductal-dependent congenital heart disease until surgery can be

(Continued)

Alprostadil *(Continued)*

performed. These defects include cyanotic (eg, pulmonary atresia, pulmonary stenosis, tricuspid atresia, Fallot's tetralogy, transposition of the great vessels) and acyanotic (eg, interruption of aortic arch, coarctation of aorta, hypoplastic left ventricle) heart disease.

Caverject®: Treatment of erectile dysfunction of vasculogenic, psychogenic, or neurogenic etiology; adjunct in the diagnosis of erectile dysfunction

Edex®, Muse®: Treatment of erectile dysfunction of vasculogenic, psychogenic, or neurogenic etiology

Unlabeled/Investigational Use Investigational: Treatment of pulmonary hypertension in infants and children with congenital heart defects with left-to-right shunts

Mechanism of Action Causes vasodilation by means of direct effect on vascular and ductus arteriosus smooth muscle; relaxes trabecular smooth muscle by dilation of cavernosal arteries when injected along the penile shaft, allowing blood flow to and entrapment in the lacunar spaces of the penis (ie, corporeal veno-occlusive mechanism)

Pharmacodynamics/Kinetics

Onset of action: Rapid

Duration: <1 hour

Distribution: Insignificant following penile injection

Protein binding, plasma: 81% to albumin

Metabolism: ~75% by oxidation in one pass via lungs

Half-life elimination: 5-10 minutes

Excretion: Urine (90% as metabolites) within 24 hours

Contraindications Hypersensitivity to alprostadil or any component of the formulation; hyaline membrane disease or persistent fetal circulation and when a dominant left-to-right shunt is present; respiratory distress syndrome; conditions predisposing patients to priapism (sickle cell anemia, multiple myeloma, leukemia); patients with anatomical deformation of the penis, penile implants; use in men for whom sexual activity is inadvisable or contraindicated; pregnancy

Warnings/Precautions Use cautiously in neonates with bleeding tendencies; apnea may occur in 10% to 12% of neonates with congenital heart defects, especially in those weighing <2 kg at birth; apnea usually appears during the first hour of drug infusion.

When used in erectile dysfunction, priapism may occur; patient must be instructed to report to physician or seek immediate medical assistance if an erection persists for longer than 4 hours. Treat immediately to avoid penile tissue damage and permanent loss of potency; discontinue therapy if signs of penile fibrosis develop (penile angulation, cavernosal fibrosis, or Peyronie's disease). When used in erectile dysfunction (Muse®), syncope occurring within 1 hour of administration has been reported. The potential for drug-drug interactions may occur when Muse® is prescribed concomitantly with antihypertensives. Some lowering of blood pressure may occur without symptoms, and swelling of leg veins, leg pain, perineal pain, and rapid pulse have been reported in <2% of patients during in-clinic titration and home treatment.

Drug Interactions Risk of hypotension and syncope may be increased with antihypertensives.

Nutritional/Herbal/Ethanol Interactions Ethanol: Avoid concurrent use (vasodilating effect).

Adverse Reactions

Intraurethral:

>10%: Genitourinary: Penile pain, urethral burning

2% to 10%:

- Central nervous system: Headache, dizziness, pain
- Genitourinary: Vaginal itching (female partner), testicular pain, urethral bleeding (minor)

<2% (Limited to important or life-threatening): Tachycardia, perineal pain, leg pain

Intracavernosal injection:

>10%: Genitourinary: Penile pain

1% to 10%:

- Cardiovascular: Hypertension
- Central nervous system: Headache, dizziness
- Genitourinary: Prolonged erection (>4 hours, 4%), penile fibrosis, penis disorder, penile rash, penile edema
- Local: Injection site hematoma and/or bruising

<1% (Limited to important or life-threatening): Balanitis, injection site hemorrhage, priapism (0.4%)

Intravenous:

>10%:

Cardiovascular: Flushing

Central nervous system: Fever

Respiratory: Apnea

1% to 10%:

Cardiovascular: Bradycardia, hyper-/hypotension, tachycardia, cardiac arrest, edema

Central nervous system: Seizures, headache, dizziness

Endocrine & metabolic: Hypokalemia

Gastrointestinal: Diarrhea

Hematologic: Disseminated intravascular coagulation

Neuromuscular & skeletal: Back pain

Respiratory: Upper respiratory infection, flu syndrome, sinusitis, nasal congestion, cough

Miscellaneous: Sepsis, localized pain in structures other than the injection site

<1% (Limited to important or life-threatening): Anemia, anuria, bleeding, bradypnea, bronchial wheezing, cerebral bleeding, CHF, gastric regurgitation, hematuria, hyperbilirubinemia, hyperemia, hyperextension of neck, hyperirritability, hyperkalemia, hypoglycemia, hypothermia, jitteriness, lethargy, peritonitis, second degree heart block, shock, stiffness, supraventricular tachycardia, thrombocytopenia, ventricular fibrillation

Overdosage/Toxicology Symptoms of overdose when treating patent ductus arteriosus include apnea, bradycardia, hypotension, and flushing. If hypotension or pyrexia occurs, the infusion rate should be reduced until symptoms subside. Apnea or bradycardia requires drug discontinuation. If intracavernous overdose occurs, supervise until systemic effects have resolved or until penile detumescence has occurred.

Dosing

Adults & Elderly:

Erectile dysfunction:

Intracavernous (Caverject®, Edex®): Individualize dose by careful titration; doses >40 mcg (Edex®) or >60 mcg (Caverject®) are not recommended: Initial dose must be titrated in physician's office. Patient must stay in the physician's office until complete detumescence occurs; if there is no response, then the next higher dose may be given within 1 hour; if there is still no response, a 1-day interval before giving the next dose is recommended; increasing the dose or concentration in the treatment of impotence results in increasing pain and discomfort

Vasculogenic, psychogenic, or mixed etiology: Initiate dosage titration at 2.5 mcg, increasing by 2.5 mcg to a dose of 5 mcg and then in increments of 5-10 mcg depending on the erectile response until the dose produces an erection suitable for intercourse, not lasting >1 hour; if there is absolutely no response to initial 2.5 mcg dose, the second dose may be increased to 7.5 mcg, followed by increments of 5-10 mcg

Neurogenic etiology (eg, spinal cord injury): Initiate dosage titration at 1.25 mcg, increasing to a dose of 2.5 mcg and then 5 mcg; increase further in increments 5 mcg until the dose is reached that produces an erection suitable for intercourse, not lasting >1 hour

Maintenance: Once appropriate dose has been determined, patient may self-administer injections at a frequency of no more than 3 times/week with at least 24 hours between doses

Intraurethral (Muse® Pellet):

Initial: 125-250 mcg

Maintenance: Administer as needed to achieve an erection; duration of action is about 30-60 minutes; use only two systems per 24-hour period

Pediatrics:

Patent ductus arteriosus I.V.:

Prostin VR Pediatric®: I.V. continuous infusion into a large vein, or alternatively through an umbilical artery catheter placed at the ductal opening: 0.05-0.1 mcg/kg/minute with therapeutic response, rate is reduced to lowest effective dosage. With unsatisfactory response, rate is increased gradually; maintenance: 0.01-0.4 mcg/kg/minute.

(Continued)

Alprostadil *(Continued)*

Note: PGE_1 is usually given at an infusion rate of 0.1 mcg/kg/minute, but it is often possible to reduce the dosage to ½ or even ¹/₁₀ without losing the therapeutic effect. The mixing schedule is shown in the table.

Alprostadil

Add 1 Ampul (500 mcg) to:	Concentration (mcg/mL)	Infusion Rate	
		mL/min/kg Needed to Infuse 0.1 mcg/kg/min	mL/kg/24 h
250 mL	2	0.05	72
100 mL	5	0.02	28.8
50 mL	10	0.01	14.4
25 mL	20	0.005	7.2

Note: Therapeutic response is indicated by increased pH in those with acidosis or by an increase in oxygenation (PO_2) usually evident within 30 minutes.

Available Dosage Forms [DSC] = Discontinued product

Injection, powder for reconstitution:

Caverject®: 10 mcg, 20 mcg, 40 mcg [contains lactose; diluent contains benzyl alcohol]

Caverject® Impulse™: 10 mcg, 20 mcg [prefilled injection system; contains lactose; diluent contains benzyl alcohol]

Edex®: 10 mcg, 20 mcg, 40 mcg [contains lactose; diluent contains benzyl alcohol; also packaged in kits containing diluent, syringe, and alcohol swab]

Injection, solution: 500 mcg/mL (1 mL)

Caverject® [DSC]: 20 mcg/mL (2 mL)

Prostin VR Pediatric®: 500 mcg/mL (1 mL) [contains dehydrated alcohol]

Pellet, urethral (Muse®): 125 mcg, 250 mcg, 500 mcg, 1000 mcg

Nursing Guidelines

Assessment: Neonate: Monitor closely; apnea has occurred during first hour after administration. **Erectile dysfunction:** After individual dose titration is determined by physician, the Caverject® injection (or Muse®) is generally self-administered. Teach patient proper use if self-administered (appropriate injection technique and syringe/needle disposal), possible side effects/appropriate interventions, and adverse symptoms to report. **Pregnancy risk factor X:** See Pregnancy Issues.

Patient Education: Use only as directed, no more than 3 times/week, allowing 24 hours between injections. Avoid alcohol. Store in refrigerator and dilute with supplied diluent immediately before use. Use alternate sides of penis with each injection. Dispose of syringes and needle and single-dose vials in a safe manner (do not share medication, syringes, or needles). Note that the risk of transmitting blood-borne disease is increased with use of alprostadil injections since a small amount of bleeding at injection site is possible. Stop using and contact prescriber immediately if signs of priapism occur, erections last more than 4 hours, or you experience moderate to severe penile pain. Report penile problems (eg, nodules, new penile pain, rash, bruising, numbness, swelling, signs of infection, abnormal ejaculations); cardiac symptoms (hypo- or hypertension, chest pain, palpitations, irregular heartbeat); flushing, fever, flu-like symptoms; respiratory difficulty or wheezing; or other adverse reactions. Refer to prescriber every 3 months to ensure proper technique and for dosage evaluation. **Pregnancy precautions:** Consult prescriber about use of contraceptives. Do not give blood while taking this medication and for 1 month following discontinuance.

Geriatric Considerations: Elderly may have concomitant diseases which would contraindicate the use of alprostadil. Other forms of attaining penile tumescence are recommended.

Pregnancy Risk Factor: X/C (Muse®)

Pregnancy Issues: Alprostadil is embryotoxic in animal studies. It is not indicated for use in women. The manufacturer of Muse® recommends a condom barrier when being used during sexual intercourse with a pregnant women.

Lactation: Not indicated for use in women

Administration

Reconstitution:

Caverject® Impulse™: Provided as a dual-chamber syringe with diluent in one chamber. To mix, hold syringe with needle pointing upward and turn plunger clockwise; turn upside down several times to mix. Device can be set to deliver specified dose, each device can be set at various increments.

Caverject® powder: Use only the supplied diluent for reconstitution (ie, bacteriostatic/sterile water with benzyl alcohol 0.945%).

Edex®: Reconstitute with NS.

Storage:

Caverject® Impulse™: Store at controlled room temperature of 15°C to 30°C (59°F to 86°F). Following reconstitution, use within 24 hours and discard any unused solution.

Caverject® powder: The 5 mcg, 10 mcg, and 20 mcg vials should be stored at or below 25°C (77°F); The 40 mcg vial should be stored at 2°C to 8°C until dispensed. After dispensing, stable for up to 3 months at or below 25°C. Following reconstitution, all strengths should be stored at or below 25°C (77°F); do not refrigerate or freeze; use within 24 hours.

Caverject® solution: Prior to dispensing, store frozen at -20°C to -10°C (-4°F to -14°F). Once dispensed, may be stored frozen for up to 3 months, or under refrigeration at 2°C to 8°C (36°F to 46°F) for up to 7 days. Do not refreeze. Once removed from foil wrap, solution may be allowed to warm to room temperature prior to use. If not used immediately, solution should be discarded. Shake well prior to use.

Edex®: Store at controlled room temperature of 15°C to 30°C (59°F to 86°F); following reconstitution, use immediately and discard any unused solution.

Muse®: Refrigerate at 2°C to 8°C (36°F to 46°F); may be stored at room temperature for up to 14 days

Prostin VR Pediatric®: Refrigerate at 2°C to 8°C (36°F to 46°F). Prior to infusion, dilute with D_5W or NS; use within 24 hours.

- ♦ Altace® *see* Ramipril *on page 1459*
- ♦ Altachlore [OTC] *see* Sodium Chloride *on page 1545*
- ♦ Altafrin *see* Phenylephrine *on page 1350*
- ♦ Altamist [OTC] *see* Sodium Chloride *on page 1545*
- ♦ Altaryl [OTC] *see* DiphenhydrAMINE *on page 546*

Alteplase (AL te plase)

U.S. Brand Names Activase®; Cathflo™ Activase®

Synonyms Alteplase, Recombinant; Alteplase, Tissue Plasminogen Activator, Recombinant; tPA

Pharmacologic Category Thrombolytic Agent

Medication Safety Issues

Sound-alike/look-alike issues:

Alteplase may be confused with Altace®

"tPA" abbreviation should not be used when writing orders for this medication; has been misread as TNKase (tenecteplase)

Use Management of acute myocardial infarction for the lysis of thrombi in coronary arteries; management of acute massive pulmonary embolism (PE) in adults

Acute myocardial infarction (AMI): Chest pain ≥20 minutes, ≤12-24 hours; S-T elevation ≥0.1 mV in at least two ECG leads

Acute pulmonary embolism (APE): Age ≤75 years: Documented massive pulmonary embolism by pulmonary angiography or echocardiography or high probability lung scan with clinical shock

Cathflo™ Activase®: Restoration of central venous catheter function

Unlabeled/Investigational Use Acute peripheral arterial occlusive disease

Mechanism of Action Initiates local fibrinolysis by binding to fibrin in a thrombus (clot) and converts entrapped plasminogen to plasmin

Pharmacodynamics/Kinetics

Duration: >50% present in plasma cleared ~5 minutes after infusion terminated, ~80% cleared within 10 minutes

Excretion: Clearance: Rapidly from circulating plasma (550-650 mL/minute), primarily hepatic; >50% present in plasma is cleared within 5 minutes after the infusion is terminated, ~80% cleared within 10 minutes

Contraindications Hypersensitivity to alteplase or any component of the formulation

(Continued)

Alteplase *(Continued)*

Treatment of acute MI or PE: Active internal bleeding; history of CVA; recent intracranial or intraspinal surgery or trauma; intracranial neoplasm; arteriovenous malformation or aneurysm; known bleeding diathesis; severe uncontrolled hypertension

Treatment of acute ischemic stroke: Evidence of intracranial hemorrhage or suspicion of subarachnoid hemorrhage on pretreatment evaluation; recent (within 3 months) intracranial or intraspinal surgery; prolonged external cardiac massage; suspected aortic dissection; serious head trauma or previous stroke; history of intracranial hemorrhage; uncontrolled hypertension at time of treatment (eg, >185 mm Hg systolic or >110 mm Hg diastolic); seizure at the onset of stroke; active internal bleeding; intracranial neoplasm; arteriovenous malformation or aneurysm; known bleeding diathesis including but not limited to: current use of anticoagulants or an INR >1.7, administration of heparin within 48 hours preceding the onset of stroke and an elevated aPTT at presentation, platelet count <100,000/mm^3.

Other exclusion criteria (NINDS recombinant tPA study): Stroke or serious head injury within 3 months, major surgery or serious trauma within 2 weeks, GI or urinary tract hemorrhage within 3 weeks, aggressive treatment required to lower blood pressure, glucose level <50 mg/dL or >400 mg/dL, arterial puncture at a noncompressible site or lumbar puncture within 1 week, clinical presentation suggesting post-MI pericarditis, pregnancy

Warnings/Precautions Concurrent heparin anticoagulation may contribute to bleeding. Monitor all potential bleeding sites. Doses >150 mg are associated with increased risk of intracranial hemorrhage. Intramuscular injections and nonessential handling of the patient should be avoided. Venipunctures should be performed carefully and only when necessary. If arterial puncture is necessary, use an upper extremity vessel that can be manually compressed. If serious bleeding occurs, the infusion of alteplase and heparin should be stopped.

For the following conditions, the risk of bleeding is higher with use of thrombolytics and should be weighed against the benefits of therapy: Recent major surgery (eg, CABG, obstetrical delivery, organ biopsy, previous puncture of noncompressible vessels), cerebrovascular disease, recent gastrointestinal or genitourinary bleeding, recent trauma, hypertension (systolic BP >175 mm Hg and/or diastolic BP >110 mm Hg), high likelihood of left heart thrombus (eg, mitral stenosis with atrial fibrillation), acute pericarditis, subacute bacterial endocarditis, hemostatic defects including ones caused by severe renal or hepatic dysfunction, significant hepatic dysfunction, pregnancy, diabetic hemorrhagic retinopathy or other hemorrhagic ophthalmic conditions, septic thrombophlebitis or occluded AV cannula at seriously infected site, advanced age (eg, >75 years), patients receiving oral anticoagulants, any other condition in which bleeding constitutes a significant hazard or would be particularly difficult to manage because of location.

Coronary thrombolysis may result in reperfusion arrhythmias. Treatment of patients with acute ischemic stroke more than 3 hours after symptom onset is not recommended Treatment of patients with minor neurological deficit or with rapidly improving symptoms is not recommended.

Cathflo™ Activase®: When used to restore catheter function, use Cathflo™ cautiously in those patients with known or suspected catheter infections. Evaluate catheter for other causes of dysfunction before use. Avoid excessive pressure when instilling into catheter.

Drug Interactions

Aminocaproic acid (antifibrinolytic agent) may decrease effectiveness.

Drugs which affect platelet function (eg, NSAIDs, dipyridamole, ticlopidine, clopidogrel, IIb/IIIa antagonists) may potentiate the risk of hemorrhage; use with caution.

Heparin and aspirin: Use with aspirin and heparin may increase the risk of bleeding. However, aspirin and heparin were used concomitantly with alteplase in many patients in myocardial infarction or pulmonary embolism trials. This combination was prohibited in the NINDS tPA stroke trial.

Nitroglycerin may increase the hepatic clearance of alteplase, potentially reducing lytic activity (limited clinical information).

Warfarin or oral anticoagulants: Risk of bleeding may be increased during concurrent therapy.

Nutritional/Herbal/Ethanol Interactions Herb/Nutraceutical: Avoid cat's claw, dong quai, evening primrose, feverfew, red clover, horse chestnut, garlic, green tea, ginseng, ginkgo (all have additional antiplatelet activity).

Lab Interactions Altered results of coagulation and fibrinolytic agents

Adverse Reactions As with all drugs which may affect hemostasis, bleeding is the major adverse effect associated with alteplase. Hemorrhage may occur at virtually any site. Risk is dependent on multiple variables, including the dosage administered, concurrent use of multiple agents which alter hemostasis, and patient predisposition. Rapid lysis of coronary artery thrombi by thrombolytic agents may be associated with reperfusion-related atrial and/or ventricular arrhythmia. **Note:** Lowest rate of bleeding complications expected with dose used to restore catheter function.

1% to 10%:

Cardiovascular: Hypotension

Central nervous system: Fever

Dermatologic: Bruising (1%)

Gastrointestinal: GI hemorrhage (5%), nausea, vomiting

Genitourinary: GU hemorrhage (4%)

Hematologic: Bleeding (0.5% major, 7% minor: GUSTO trial)

Local: Bleeding at catheter puncture site (15.3%, accelerated administration)

<1% (Limited to important or life-threatening): Allergic reactions: Anaphylaxis, anaphylactoid reactions, laryngeal edema, rash, and urticaria (<0.02%); epistaxis; gingival hemorrhage; intracranial hemorrhage (0.4% to 0.87% when dose is ≤100 mg); pericardial hemorrhage; retroperitoneal hemorrhage

Additional cardiovascular events associated **with use in MI:** AV block, cardiogenic shock, heart failure, cardiac arrest, recurrent ischemia/infarction, myocardial rupture, electromechanical dissociation, pericardial effusion, pericarditis, mitral regurgitation, cardiac tamponade, thromboembolism, pulmonary edema, asystole, ventricular tachycardia, bradycardia, ruptured intracranial AV malformation, seizure, hemorrhagic bursitis, cholesterol crystal embolization

Additional events associated **with use in pulmonary embolism:** Pulmonary re-embolization, pulmonary edema, pleural effusion, thromboembolism

Additional events associated **with use in stroke:** Cerebral edema, cerebral herniation, seizure, new ischemic stroke

Overdosage/Toxicology Symptoms of overdose include increased incidence of intracranial bleeding.

Dosing

Adults & Elderly:

Coronary artery thrombi: I.V. Front loading dose (weight-based):

Patients >67 kg: Total dose: 100 mg over 1.5 hours; infuse 15 mg over 1-2 minutes. Infuse 50 mg over 30 minutes. See "Note."

Patients ≤67 kg: Total dose: 1.25 mg/kg; infuse 15 mg I.V. bolus over 1-2 minutes, then infuse 0.75 mg/kg (not to exceed 50 mg) over next 30 minutes, followed by 0.5 mg/kg over next 60 minutes (not to exceed 35 mg). See "Note."

Note: Concurrently, begin heparin 60 units/kg bolus (maximum: 4000 units) followed by continuous infusion of 12 units/kg/hour (maximum: 1000 units/hour) and adjust to aPTT target of 1.5-2 times the upper limit of control. Infuse remaining 35 mg of alteplase over the next hour.

Acute pulmonary embolism: I.V.: 100 mg over 2 hours.

Acute ischemic stroke: I.V.: Doses should be given within the first 3 hours of the onset of symptoms; recommended total dose: 0.9 mg/kg (maximum dose should not exceed 90 mg) infused over 60 minutes.

Load with 0.09 mg/kg (10% of the 0.9 mg/kg dose) as an I.V. bolus over 1 minute, followed by 0.81 mg/kg (90% of the 0.9 mg/kg dose) as a continuous infusion over 60 minutes. Heparin should not be started for 24 hours or more after starting alteplase for stroke.

Central venous catheter clearance: Intracatheter (Cathflo™ Activase® 1 mg/mL):

Patients <30 kg: 110% of the internal lumen volume of the catheter, not to exceed 2 mg/2 mL; retain in catheter for 0.5-2 hours; may instill a second dose if catheter remains occluded

Patients ≥30 kg: 2 mg (2 mL); retain in catheter for 0.5-2 hours; may instill a second dose if catheter remains occluded

Acute peripheral arterial occlusive disease (unlabeled use): Intra-arterial: 0.02-0.1 mg/kg/hour for up to 36 hours

Advisory Panel to the Society for Cardiovascular and Interventional Radiology on Thrombolytic Therapy recommendation: ≤2 mg/hour and subtherapeutic heparin (aPTT <1.5 times baseline)

(Continued)

Alteplase *(Continued)*

Pediatrics: Central venous catheter clearance: Intracatheter: Patients <30 kg: 110% of the internal lumen volume of the catheter, not to exceed 2 mg/2 mL; retain in catheter for 0.5-2 hours; may instill a second dose if catheter remains occluded

Available Dosage Forms Injection, powder for reconstitution, recombinant:
Activase®: 50 mg [29 million int. units]; 100 mg [58 million int. units]
Cathflo™ Activase®: 2 mg

Nursing Guidelines

Assessment: See Contraindications, Warnings/Precautions, and Dosing for use cautions. Assess potential for interactions with other prescriptions, OTC medications, or herbal products patient may be taking (especially those medications that may affect coagulation or platelet function - see Drug Interactions). See infusion specifics below. Vital signs, laboratory results (see below), and ECG should be monitored prior to, during, and after therapy. Arrhythmias may occur; antiarrhythmic drugs should be immediately available. Assess infusion site and monitor for hemorrhage every 10 minutes (or according to institutional policy) during therapy and for 1 hour following therapy (see Adverse Reactions and Overdose/Toxicology). Strict bedrest should be maintained and bleeding precautions should be instituted; avoid invasive procedures and activities that could cause trauma. Patient instructions determined by patient condition (see Patient Education). Note breast-feeding caution.

Monitoring Laboratory Tests: CBC, PTT

Patient Education: Inform prescriber of all prescriptions, OTC medications, or herbal products you are taking, and any allergies you have. This medication can only be administered by infusion; you will be monitored closely during and after treatment. You will have a tendency to bleed easily; use caution to prevent injury (use electric razor, soft toothbrush, and use caution with knives, needles, or anything sharp). Follow instructions for strict bedrest to reduce the risk of injury. If bleeding occurs, report immediately and apply pressure to bleeding spot until bleeding stops completely. Report unusual pain (acute headache, joint pain, chest pain); unusual bruising or bleeding; blood in urine, stool, or vomit; bleeding gums; vision changes; or respiratory difficulty. **Pregnancy/breast-feeding precautions:** Inform prescriber if you are or intend to become pregnant. Consult prescriber if breast-feeding.

Pregnancy Risk Factor: C

Lactation: Excretion in breast milk unknown/use caution

Perioperative/Anesthesia/Other Concerns: The Surgery Versus Thrombolysis for Ischemia of the Lower Extremity (STILE) trial (Ann Surg, 1994) compared surgery to intra-arterial thrombolytic therapy with either urokinase (250,000 units bolus, followed by 4000 units/minute for 4 hours, followed by 2000 units/minute for ≤36 hours) or alteplase (0.05 mg/kg/hour for ≤12 hours) in patients with acute (<14 days) or chronic peripheral arterial occlusive disease (PAOD). Patients with acute PAOD who received either fibrinolytic treatment had a shorter hospital stay and an improved amputation-free survival rate. There was no difference between alteplase or urokinase with regard to efficacy or bleeding events. A group from Stanford University recently did a retrospective comparison evaluating efficacy, safety, and cost of low-dose alteplase (<2 mg/hour) and subtherapeutic heparin to urokinase and therapeutic heparin for the treatment of PAOD or DVT (Sugimoto K, 2003). Efficacy was similar for both groups. The average dose of alteplase was 0.86 mg/hour and the dose of urokinase was 2250 units/minute. Alteplase infusions were shorter and less expensive than urokinase.

Administration

I.V.: Activase®: Acute MI: Accelerated infusion:

Bolus dose may be prepared by one of three methods:

1) removal of 15 mL reconstituted (1 mg/mL) solution from vial
2) removal of 15 mL from a port on the infusion line after priming
3) programming an infusion pump to deliver a 15 mL bolus at the initiation of infusion

Remaining dose may be administered as follows:

50 mg vial: Either PVC bag or glass vial and infusion set

100 mg vial: Insert spike end of the infusion set through the same puncture site created by transfer device and infuse from vial

If further dilution is desired, may be diluted in equal volume of 0.9% sodium chloride or D_5W to yield a final concentration of 0.5 mg/mL AD

Reconstitution:

Activase®:

50 mg vial: Use accompanying diluent (50 mL sterile water for injection); do not shake; final concentration: 1 mg/mL

100 mg vial: Use transfer set with accompanying diluent (100 mL vial of sterile water for injection); no vacuum is present in 100 mg vial; final concentration: 1 mg/mL

Cathflo™ Activase®: Add 2.2 mL SWFI to vial; do not shake. Final concentration: 1 mg/mL.

Compatibility: Stable in NS, SWFI; **incompatible** with bacteriostatic water

Y-site administration: Incompatible with dobutamine, dopamine, heparin, nitroglycerin

Compatibility when admixed: Incompatible with dobutamine, dopamine, heparin

Storage:

Activase®: The lyophilized product may be stored at room temperature (not to exceed 30°C/86°F), or under refrigeration; once reconstituted it should be used within 8 hours

Cathflo™ Activase®: Store lyophilized product in refrigerated. Once reconstituted, store at 2°C to 30°C (36°F to 86°F) and use within 8 hours.

♦ Alteplase, Recombinant *see* Alteplase *on page 117*

♦ Alteplase, Tissue Plasminogen Activator, Recombinant *see* Alteplase *on page 117*

♦ Altoprev™ *see* Lovastatin *on page 1070*

Aluminum Hydroxide and Magnesium Carbonate

(a LOO mi num hye DROKS ide & mag NEE zhum KAR bun nate)

U.S. Brand Names Gaviscon® Extra Strength [OTC]; Gaviscon® Liquid [OTC]

Synonyms Magnesium Carbonate and Aluminum Hydroxide

Pharmacologic Category Antacid

Use Temporary relief of symptoms associated with gastric acidity

Drug Interactions Decreased effect: Tetracyclines, digoxin, indomethacin, iron salts, isoniazid, allopurinol, benzodiazepines, corticosteroids, penicillamine, phenothiazines, ranitidine, ketoconazole, itraconazole

Adverse Reactions 1% to 10%:

Endocrine & metabolic: Hypermagnesemia, aluminum intoxication (prolonged use and concomitant renal failure), hypophosphatemia

Gastrointestinal: Constipation, diarrhea

Neuromuscular & skeletal: Osteomalacia

Dosing

Adults & Elderly: Dyspepsia, gastric acidity: Oral:

Liquid:

Gaviscon® Regular Strength: 15-30 mL 4 times/day after meals and at bedtime

Gaviscon® Extra Strength Relief: 15-30 mL 4 times/day after meals

Tablet (Gaviscon® Extra Strength Relief): Chew 2-4 tablets 4 times/day

Renal Impairment: Aluminum and/or magnesium may accumulate in renal impairment.

Available Dosage Forms

Liquid:

Gaviscon®: Aluminum hydroxide 31.7 mg and magnesium carbonate 119.3 mg per 5 mL (355 mL) [contains sodium 0.57 mEq/5 mL]

Gaviscon® Extra Strength: Aluminum hydroxide 84.6 mg and magnesium carbonate 79.1 mg per 5 mL (355 mL) [contains sodium 0.9 mEq/5 mL]

Tablet, chewable (Gaviscon® Extra Strength): Aluminum hydroxide 160 mg and magnesium carbonate 105 mg [contains sodium 1.3 mEq/tablet]

Nursing Guidelines

Dietary Considerations: Should be taken 1-3 hours after meals with water, milk or juice. Products contain sodium (0.57 mEq/5 mL regular strength liquid, 0.9 mEq/5 mL extra strength liquid, 1.3 mEq extra strength tablet).

Patient Education:

Liquid: Shake well. Do not use if you are on a sodium-restricted diet.

Tablet: Take tablets after meals and at bedtime, or as needed. Chew tablet, do not swallow whole. Follow tablets with 1/2 glass of water.

Aluminum Hydroxide and Magnesium Hydroxide

(a LOO mi num hye DROKS ide & mag NEE zhum hye DROK side)

U.S. Brand Names Alamag [OTC]; Maalox® TC (Therapeutic Concentrate) [OTC] [DSC]; Rulox; Rulox No. 1

Synonyms Magnesium Hydroxide and Aluminum Hydroxide

Pharmacologic Category Antacid

Medication Safety Issues

Sound-alike/look-alike issues:

Maalox® may be confused with Maox®, Monodox®

Use Antacid, hyperphosphatemia in renal failure

Drug Interactions Decreased effect: Tetracyclines, digoxin, indomethacin, iron salts, isoniazid, allopurinol, benzodiazepines, corticosteroids, penicillamine, phenothiazines, ranitidine, ketoconazole, itraconazole

Adverse Reactions

>10%: Gastrointestinal: Constipation, chalky taste, stomach cramps, fecal impaction

1% to 10%: Gastrointestinal: Nausea, vomiting, discoloration of feces (white speckles)

<1% (Limited to important or life-threatening): Hypomagnesemia, hypophosphatemia

Dosing

Adults & Elderly: Dyspepsia: Oral: 5-10 mL 4-6 times/day, between meals and at bedtime; may be used every hour for severe symptoms

Renal Impairment: Aluminum and/or magnesium may accumulate in renal impairment.

Available Dosage Forms [DSC] = Discontinued product

Suspension (Alamag, Rulox): Aluminum hydroxide 225 mg and magnesium hydroxide 200 mg per 5 mL (360 mL)

Suspension, high potency (Maalox® TC) [DSC]: Aluminum hydroxide 600 mg and magnesium hydroxide 300 mg per 5 mL (360 mL)

Tablet, chewable:

Alamag: Aluminum hydroxide 300 mg and magnesium hydroxide 150 mg

Rulox No. 1: Aluminum hydroxide 200 mg and magnesium hydroxide 200 mg

Nursing Guidelines

Dietary Considerations: Should be taken 1-3 hours after meals.

Patient Education: Notify prescriber if relief is not obtained or if signs of bleeding from GI tract occur.

Pregnancy Risk Factor: C

Aluminum Hydroxide, Magnesium Hydroxide, and Simethicone

(a LOO mi num hye DROKS ide, mag NEE zhum hye DROKS ide, & sye METH i kone)

U.S. Brand Names Alamag Plus [OTC]; Aldroxicon I [OTC]; Aldroxicon II [OTC]; Almacone® [OTC]; Almacone Double Strength® [OTC]; Gelusil® [OTC]; Maalox® [OTC]; Maalox® Max [OTC]; Mi-Acid [OTC]; Mi-Acid Maximum Strength [OTC]; Mintox Extra Strength [OTC]; Mintox Plus [OTC]; Mylanta® Liquid [OTC]; Mylanta® Maximum Strength Liquid [OTC]

Synonyms Magnesium Hydroxide, Aluminum Hydroxide, and Simethicone; Simethicone, Aluminum Hydroxide, and Magnesium Hydroxide

Pharmacologic Category Antacid; Antiflatulent

Medication Safety Issues

Sound-alike/look-alike issues:

Maalox® may be confused with Maox®, Monodox®

Mylanta® may be confused with Mynatal®

Use Temporary relief of hyperacidity associated with gas; may also be used for indications associated with other antacids

Drug Interactions Decreased effect: Tetracyclines, digoxin, indomethacin, iron salts, isoniazid, allopurinol, benzodiazepines, corticosteroids, penicillamine, phenothiazines, ranitidine, ketoconazole, itraconazole

Adverse Reactions

>10%: Gastrointestinal: Chalky taste, stomach cramps, constipation, bowel motility decreased, fecal impaction, hemorrhoids

1% to 10%: Gastrointestinal: Nausea, vomiting, discoloration of feces (white speckles)

<1% (Limited to important or life-threatening): Dehydration or fluid restriction, hypomagnesemia, hypophosphatemia

Dosing

Adults & Elderly: Dyspepsia, abdominal bloating: Oral: 10-20 mL or 2-4 tablets 4-6 times/day between meals and at bedtime; may be used every hour for severe symptoms

Renal Impairment: Aluminum and/or magnesium may accumulate in renal impairment.

Available Dosage Forms

Liquid: Aluminum hydroxide 200 mg, magnesium hydroxide 200 mg, and simethicone 20 mg per 5 mL (360 mL); aluminum hydroxide 400 mg, magnesium hydroxide 400 mg, and simethicone 40 mg per 5 mL (360 mL)

Aldroxicon I: Aluminum hydroxide 200 mg, magnesium hydroxide 200 mg, and simethicone 20 mg per 5 mL (30 mL)

Aldroxicon II: Aluminum hydroxide 400 mg, magnesium hydroxide 400 mg, and simethicone 40 mg per 5 mL (30 mL)

Almacone®: Aluminum hydroxide 200 mg, magnesium hydroxide 200 mg, and simethicone 20 mg per 5 mL (360 mL)

Almacone Double Strength®: Aluminum hydroxide 400 mg, magnesium hydroxide 400 mg, and simethicone 40 mg per 5 mL (360 mL)

Maalox®: Aluminum hydroxide 200 mg, magnesium hydroxide 200 mg, and simethicone 20 mg per 5 mL (360 mL, 770 mL) [lemon and mint flavors]

Maalox® Max: Aluminum hydroxide 400 mg, magnesium hydroxide 400 mg, and simethicone 40 mg per 5 mL (360 mL, 770 mL) [cherry, vanilla creme, and wild berry flavors]

Mi-Acid: Aluminum hydroxide 200 mg, magnesium hydroxide 200 mg, and simethicone 20 mg per 5 mL (360 mL)

Mi-Acid Maximum Strength: Aluminum hydroxide 400 mg, magnesium hydroxide 400 mg, and simethicone 40 mg per 5 mL (360 mL)

Mintox Extra Strength: Aluminum hydroxide 500 mg, magnesium hydroxide 450 mg, and simethicone 40 mg per 5 mL (360 mL) [lemon creme flavor]

Mylanta®: Aluminum hydroxide 200 mg, magnesium hydroxide 200 mg, and simethicone 20 mg per 5 mL (180 mL, 360 mL, 720 mL) [original, cherry, and mint flavors]

Mylanta® Maximum Strength: Aluminum hydroxide 400 mg, magnesium hydroxide 400 mg, and simethicone 40 mg per 5 mL (180 mL, 360 mL, 720 mL) [original, cherry, orange creme, and mint flavors]

Suspension (Alamag Plus): Aluminum hydroxide 225 mg, magnesium hydroxide 200 mg, and simethicone 25 mg per 5 mL (360 mL)

Tablet, chewable: Aluminum hydroxide 200 mg, magnesium hydroxide 200 mg, and simethicone 25 mg

Alamag Plus: Aluminum hydroxide 200 mg, magnesium hydroxide 200 mg, and simethicone 25 mg [cherry flavor]

Almacone®: Aluminum hydroxide 200 mg, magnesium hydroxide 200 mg, and simethicone 20 mg [peppermint flavor]

Gelusil®: Aluminum hydroxide 200 mg, magnesium hydroxide 200 mg, and simethicone 25 mg [peppermint flavor]

Mintox Plus: Aluminum hydroxide 200 mg, magnesium hydroxide 200 mg, and simethicone 25 mg

Nursing Guidelines

Dietary Considerations: Should be taken 1-3 hours after meals.

Patient Education: Dilute dose in water or juice; chew tablets thoroughly before swallowing with water; shake well; notify physician if relief is not obtained or if signs of bleeding from GI tract occur

Pregnancy Risk Factor: C

- **Aluminum Sucrose Sulfate, Basic** *see* Sucralfate *on page 1575*
- **Alupent®** *see* Metaproterenol *on page 1109*
- **Amaryl®** *see* Glimepiride *on page 813*
- **Ambien®** *see* Zolpidem *on page 1736*
- **Ambien CR™** *see* Zolpidem *on page 1736*
- **AmBisome®** *see* Amphotericin B (Liposomal) *on page 157*
- **Americaine® [OTC]** *see* Benzocaine *on page 232*
- **Americaine® Hemorrhoidal [OTC]** *see* Benzocaine *on page 232*
- **A-Methapred** *see* MethylPREDNISolone *on page 1140*
- **Amethocaine Hydrochloride** *see* Tetracaine *on page 1612*
- **Amethopterin** *see* Methotrexate *on page 1127*

♦ **Amicar®** *see* Aminocaproic Acid *on page 126*

♦ **Amidate®** *see* Etomidate *on page 694*

Amikacin (am i KAY sin)

U.S. Brand Names Amikin®

Synonyms Amikacin Sulfate

Pharmacologic Category Antibiotic, Aminoglycoside

Medication Safety Issues

Sound-alike/look-alike issues:

Amikacin may be confused with Amicar®, anakinra

Amikin® may be confused with Amicar®

Use Treatment of serious infections due to organisms resistant to gentamicin and tobramycin, including *Pseudomonas*, *Proteus*, *Serratia*, and other gram-negative bacilli (bone infections, respiratory tract infections, endocarditis, and septicemia); documented infection of mycobacterial organisms susceptible to amikacin

Mechanism of Action Inhibits protein synthesis in susceptible bacteria by binding to 30S ribosomal subunits

Pharmacodynamics/Kinetics

Absorption: I.M.: May be delayed in the bedridden patient

Distribution: Primarily into extracellular fluid (highly hydrophilic); penetrates blood-brain barrier when meninges inflamed; crosses placenta

Relative diffusion of antimicrobial agents from blood into CSF: Good only with inflammation (exceeds usual MICs)

CSF:blood level ratio: Normal meninges: 10% to 20%; Inflamed meninges: 15% to 24%

Half-life elimination (renal function and age dependent):

Infants: Low birth weight (1-3 days): 7-9 hours; Full-term >7 days: 4-5 hours

Children: 1.6-2.5 hours

Adults: Normal renal function: 1.4-2.3 hours; Anuria/end-stage renal disease: 28-86 hours

Time to peak, serum: I.M.: 45-120 minutes

Excretion: Urine (94% to 98%)

Contraindications Hypersensitivity to amikacin sulfate or any component of the formulation; cross-sensitivity may exist with other aminoglycosides; pregnancy

Warnings/Precautions Dose and/or frequency of administration must be monitored and modified in patients with renal impairment. Drug should be discontinued if signs of ototoxicity, nephrotoxicity, or hypersensitivity occur. Ototoxicity is proportional to the amount of drug given and the duration of treatment. Tinnitus or vertigo may be indications of vestibular injury and impending bilateral irreversible damage. Renal damage is usually reversible.

Drug Interactions

Decreased effect of aminoglycoside: High concentrations of penicillins and/or cephalosporins (*in vitro* data)

Increased toxicity of aminoglycoside: Indomethacin I.V., amphotericin, loop diuretics, vancomycin, enflurane, methoxyflurane; increased effect of neuromuscular-blocking agents and polypeptide antibiotics with administration of aminoglycosides

Lab Interactions Some penicillin derivatives may accelerate the degradation of aminoglycosides *in vitro*, leading to a potential underestimation of aminoglycoside serum concentration.

Adverse Reactions

1% to 10%:

Central nervous system: Neurotoxicity

Otic: Ototoxicity (auditory), ototoxicity (vestibular)

Renal: Nephrotoxicity

<1% (Limited to important or life-threatening): Allergic reaction, dyspnea, eosinophilia

Overdosage/Toxicology Symptoms of overdose include ototoxicity, nephrotoxicity, and neuromuscular toxicity. Treatment of choice, following a single acute overdose, appears to be maintenance of urine output of at least 3 mL/kg/hour during the acute treatment phase. Dialysis is of questionable value in enhancing aminoglycoside elimination. If required, hemodialysis is preferred over peritoneal dialysis in patients with normal renal function.

Dosing

Adults & Elderly: Individualization is critical because of the low therapeutic index

Note: Use of ideal body weight (IBW) for determining the mg/kg/dose appears to be more accurate than dosing on the basis of total body weight (TBW)

In morbid obesity, dosage requirement may best be estimated using a dosing weight of IBW + 0.4 (TBW - IBW)

Susceptible infections: I.M., I.V.: 5-7.5 mg/kg/dose every 8 hours

Adjustment: Initial and periodic peak and trough plasma drug levels should be determined, particularly in critically-ill patients with serious infections or in disease states known to significantly alter aminoglycoside pharmacokinetics (eg, cystic fibrosis, burns, or major surgery)

Note: Some clinicians suggest a daily dose of 15-20 mg/kg for all patients with normal renal function. This dose is at least as efficacious with similar, if not less, toxicity than conventional dosing.

Pediatrics: Infants and Children: Refer to adult dosing.

Renal Impairment: Individualization is critical because of the low therapeutic index. Some patients may require larger or more frequent doses if serum levels document the need (ie, cystic fibrosis or febrile granulocytopenic patients).

Cl_{cr} ≥60 mL/minute: Administer every 8 hours.

Cl_{cr} 40-60 mL/minute: Administer every 12 hours.

Cl_{cr} 20-40 mL/minute: Administer every 24 hours.

Cl_{cr} 10-20 mL/minute: Administer every 48 hours.

Cl_{cr} <10 mL/minute: Administer every 72 hours.

Dialyzable (50% to 100%)

Administer dose postdialysis or administer $^{2}/_{3}$ normal dose as a supplemental dose postdialysis and follow levels.

Peritoneal dialysis effects: Dose as for Cl_{cr} <10 mL/minute: Follow levels.

Continuous arteriovenous or venovenous hemodiafiltration effects: Dose as for Cl_{cr} 10-40 mL/minute: Follow levels.

Available Dosage Forms Injection, solution, as sulfate: 50 mg/mL (2 mL, 4 mL); 62.5 mg/mL (8 mL); 250 mg/mL (2 mL, 4 mL) [contains metabisulfite]

Nursing Guidelines

Assessment: Assess allergy history prior to beginning therapy. Assess potential for interactions with other prescriptions, OTC medications, or herbal products patient may be taking. Assess results of laboratory tests, therapeutic effectiveness, and adverse response. Monitor for ototoxicity, nephrotoxicity, neurotoxicity. Hearing and renal status should be assessed before, during, and after therapy. Teach patient possible side effects/appropriate interventions and adverse symptoms to report.

Monitoring Laboratory Tests: Perform culture and sensitivity testing prior to initiating therapy. Urinalysis, BUN, serum creatinine, appropriately timed peak and trough concentrations. Initial and periodic peak and trough plasma drug levels should be determined, particularly in critically-ill patients with serious infections or in disease states known to significantly alter aminoglycoside pharmacokinetics (eg, cystic fibrosis, burns, or major surgery). Aminoglycoside levels measured from blood taken from Silastic® central catheters can sometimes give falsely high readings (draw levels from alternate lumen or peripheral stick, if possible). Some penicillin derivatives may accelerate the degradation of aminoglycosides.

Dietary Considerations: Sodium content of 1 g: 29.9 mg (1.3 mEq)

Patient Education: Do not take any new medication during therapy unless approved by prescriber. This drug can only be administered by I.V. or I.M. injection. It is important to maintain adequate hydration (2-3 L/day of fluids) unless instructed to restrict fluid intake. Report immediately any change in hearing acuity, ringing or roaring in ears, alteration in balance, vertigo, feeling of fullness in head; pain, tingling, or numbness of any body part; or change in urinary pattern or decrease in urine. Report signs of opportunistic infection (eg, white plaques in mouth, vaginal discharge, unhealed sores, sore throat, unusual fever, chills); pain, redness, or swelling at injection site; or other adverse reactions. **Pregnancy precaution:** Inform prescriber if you are or intend to become pregnant.

Geriatric Considerations: Adjust dose based on renal function.

Pregnancy Risk Factor: D

Lactation: Enters breast milk/compatible

Breast-Feeding Considerations: No specific recommendations. However, aminoglycosides are not systemically available when taken orally. Therefore, the risk to the infant is minimal if ingested with breast milk.

(Continued)

Amikacin *(Continued)*

Administration

I.M.: Administer I.M. injection in large muscle mass. Administer around-the-clock to promote less variation in peak and trough serum levels. Do not mix with other drugs, administer separately.

I.V.: Infuse over 30-60 minutes.

Some penicillins (eg, carbenicillin, ticarcillin, and piperacillin) have been shown to inactivate *in vitro.* This has been observed to a greater extent with tobramycin and gentamicin, while amikacin has shown greater stability against inactivation. Concurrent use of these agents may pose a risk of reduced antibacterial efficacy *in vivo,* particularly in the setting of profound renal impairment. However, definitive clinical evidence is lacking. If combination penicillin/aminoglycoside therapy is desired in a patient with renal dysfunction, separation of doses (if feasible), and routine monitoring of aminoglycoside levels, CBC, and clinical response should be considered.

Compatibility: Stable in dextran 75 6% in NS, D_5LR, $D_5{}^1/_4NS$, $D_5{}^1/_3NS$, $D_5{}^1/_2NS$, D_5NS, $D_{10}NS$, D_5W, $D_{10}W$, $D_{20}W$, mannitol 20%, $^1/_4NS$, $^1/_2NS$, NS

Y-site administration: Incompatible with allopurinol, amphotericin B cholesteryl sulfate complex, hetastarch, propofol

Compatibility in syringe: Incompatible with heparin

Compatibility when admixed: Incompatible with amphotericin B, ampicillin, cefazolin, chlorothiazide, heparin, phenytoin, thiopental, vitamin B complex with C

Storage: Stable for 24 hours at room temperature and 2 days at refrigeration when mixed in D_5W, $D_5{}^1/_4NS$, $D_5{}^1/_2NS$, NS, LR.

- ♦ Amikacin Sulfate *see* Amikacin *on page 124*
- ♦ Amikin® *see* Amikacin *on page 124*
- ♦ Aminate Fe-90 *see* Vitamins (Multiple/Prenatal) *on page 1721*
- ♦ Aminobenzylpenicillin *see* Ampicillin *on page 160*

Aminocaproic Acid (a mee noe ka PROE ik AS id)

U.S. Brand Names Amicar®

Synonyms Epsilon Aminocaproic Acid

Pharmacologic Category Hemostatic Agent

Medication Safety Issues

Sound-alike/look-alike issues:

Amicar® may be confused with amikacin, Amikin®, Omacor®

Use Treatment of excessive bleeding from fibrinolysis

Unlabeled/Investigational Use Treatment of traumatic hyphema; control bleeding in thrombocytopenia; control oral bleeding in congenital and acquired coagulation disorders

Mechanism of Action Competitively inhibits activation of plasminogen to plasmin, also, a lesser antiplasmin effect

Pharmacodynamics/Kinetics

Onset of action: ~1-72 hours

Distribution: Widely through intravascular and extravascular compartments

V_d: Oral: 23 L, I.V.: 30 L

Metabolism: Minimally hepatic

Half-life elimination: 2 hours

Time to peak: Oral: Within 2 hours

Excretion: Urine (65% as unchanged drug, 11% as metabolite)

Contraindications Hypersensitivity to aminocaproic acid or any component of the formulation; disseminated intravascular coagulation (without heparin); evidence of an intravascular clotting process

Warnings/Precautions Avoid rapid I.V. administration; may induce hypotension, bradycardia, or arrhythmia. Aminocaproic acid may accumulate in patients with decreased renal function. Intrarenal obstruction may occur secondary to glomerular capillary thrombosis or clots in the renal pelvis and ureters. Do not use in hematuria of upper urinary tract origin unless possible benefits outweigh risks. Use with caution in patients with cardiac, renal, or hepatic disease. Do not administer without a definite diagnosis of laboratory findings indicative of hyperfibrinolysis. Inhibition of fibrinolysis may promote clotting or thrombosis; more likely due to the presence of DIC. Subsequently, use with great caution in patients with, or at risk for, veno-occlusive disease of the liver. Benzyl alcohol is used as a preservative in the injection, therefore, these products should not be used in the neonate. Do not administer with factor IX complex concentrates or anti-inhibitor coagulant complexes.

Drug Interactions Increased toxic effect with oral contraceptives, estrogens

Lab Interactions Increased potassium, creatine phosphokinase [CPK] (S)

Adverse Reactions Frequency not defined.

Cardiovascular: Arrhythmia, bradycardia, hypotension, peripheral ischemia, syncope, thrombosis

Central nervous system: Confusion, delirium, dizziness, fatigue, hallucinations, headache, intracranial hypertension, malaise, seizure, stroke

Dermatologic: Rash, pruritus

Gastrointestinal: Abdominal pain, anorexia, cramps, diarrhea, GI irritation, nausea

Genitourinary: Dry ejaculation

Hematologic: Agranulocytosis, bleeding time increased, leukopenia, thrombocytopenia

Neuromuscular & skeletal: CPK increased, myalgia, myositis, myopathy, rhabdomyolysis (rare), weakness

Ophthalmic: Watery eyes, vision decreased

Otic: Tinnitus

Renal: Failure (rare), myoglobinuria (rare)

Respiratory: Dyspnea, nasal congestion, pulmonary embolism

Overdosage/Toxicology Symptoms of overdose include acute renal failure, delirium, diarrhea, hepatic necrosis, nausea, seizures, transient hypotension, and thromboembolism. Aminocaproic acid may be removed by hemodialysis.

Dosing

Adults & Elderly:

Acute bleeding syndrome: Oral, I.V.: 4-5 g during the first hour, followed by 1 g/hour for 8 hours or until bleeding controlled (maximum daily dose: 30 g)

Control bleeding in thrombocytopenia (unlabeled use):

Initial: I.V.: 0.1 g/kg over 30-60 minutes

Maintenance: Oral: 1-3 g every 6 hours

Control oral bleeding in congenital and acquired coagulation disorder (unlabeled use): Oral: 50-60 mg/kg every 4 hours

Traumatic hyphema (unlabeled use): Oral: 100 mg/kg/dose every 4 hours (maximum daily dose: 30 g)

Pediatrics:

Acute bleeding syndrome (unlabeled use): Oral, I.V.: 100-200 mg/kg during the first hour, followed by continuous infusion at 33.3 mg/kg/hour or 100 mg/kg (oral or I.V.) every 6 hours

Traumatic hyphema (unlabeled use): Oral: Refer to adult dosing.

Renal Impairment: May accumulate in patients with decreased renal function.

Available Dosage Forms

Injection, solution: 250 mg/mL (20 mL) [contains benzyl alcohol]

Syrup: 1.25 g/5 mL (240 mL, 480 mL)

Amicar®: 1.25 g/5 mL (480 mL) [raspberry flavor]

Tablet [scored]: 500 mg, 1000 mg

Nursing Guidelines

Assessment: Monitor laboratory results on a regular basis during therapy. Monitor (teach patient to monitor and report) signs of adverse reactions (eg, bleeding, clotting, thromboembolism, hypotension, or CNS changes).

Monitoring Laboratory Tests: Fibrinogen, fibrin split products, creatine phosphokinase (with long-term therapy)

Patient Education: Take oral medication exactly as directed. This medication may cause dizziness and fatigue (use caution when driving or engaging in tasks that require alertness until response to drug is known); hypotension (use caution when rising from a lying or sitting position or climbing stairs); menstrual irregularities, increased body hair, or sexual dysfunction (should reverse when treatment is completed); or nausea or vomiting (small frequent meals, frequent mouth care, sucking lozenges, or chewing gum may help). Report immediately any chest pain; dyspnea; swelling; nosebleed; warmth, swelling, pain, or redness in calves; skin rash; muscle pain or weakness; ringing in ears; or acute abdominal cramping. **Pregnancy/breast-feeding precautions:** Inform prescriber if you are or intend to become pregnant. Consult prescriber if breast-feeding.

(Continued)

Aminocaproic Acid *(Continued)*

Pregnancy Risk Factor: C

Lactation: Excretion in breast milk unknown/use caution

Administration

I.V.: May be given over 30-60 minutes or by continuous infusion; rapid I.V. injection (IVP) should be avoided due to possible hypotension, bradycardia, and arrhythmia.

Reconstitution: Dilute I.V. solution (1 g/50 mL of diluent) with D_5W, 0.9% sodium chloride, or lactated Ringer's.

Compatibility: Stable in D_5W, NS

Storage: Store at 15°C to 30°C (59°F to 86°F).

Aminophylline (am in OFF i lin)

Synonyms Theophylline Ethylenediamine

Pharmacologic Category Theophylline Derivative

Medication Safety Issues

Sound-alike/look-alike issues:

Aminophylline may be confused with amitriptyline, ampicillin

Use Bronchodilator in reversible airway obstruction due to asthma or COPD; increase diaphragmatic contractility

Mechanism of Action Causes bronchodilatation, diuresis, CNS and cardiac stimulation, and gastric acid secretion by blocking phosphodiesterase which increases tissue concentrations of cyclic adenine monophosphate (cAMP) which in turn promote catecholamine stimulation of lipolysis, glycogenolysis, and gluconeogenesis and induce release of epinephrine from adrenal medulla cells

Pharmacodynamics/Kinetics

Theophylline:

Absorption: Oral: Dosage form dependent

Distribution: 0.45 L/kg based on ideal body weight

Protein binding: 40%, primarily to albumin

Metabolism: Children >1 year and Adults: Hepatic; involves CYP1A2, 2E1, and 3A4; forms active metabolites (caffeine and 3-methylxanthine)

Half-life elimination: Highly variable and dependent upon age, liver function, cardiac function, lung disease, and smoking history

Time to peak, serum:

Oral: Immediate release: 1-2 hours

I.V.: Within 30 minutes

Excretion: Children >3 months and Adults: 10% as unchanged urine

Contraindications Hypersensitivity to theophylline, ethylenediamine, or any component of the formulation

Warnings/Precautions If a patient develops signs and symptoms of theophylline toxicity, a serum level should be measured and subsequent doses held. Due to potential saturation of theophylline clearance at serum levels within (or in some patients less than) the therapeutic range, dosage adjustment should be made in small increments (maximum: 25% reduction). Due to wide interpatient variability, theophylline serum level measurements must be used to optimize therapy and prevent serious toxicity. Use caution with peptic ulcer, hyperthyroidism, seizure disorder, hypertension, or tachyarrhythmias.

Drug Interactions Substrate of CYP1A2 (major), 2E1 (minor), 3A4 (minor)

CYP1A2 inducers: May decrease the levels/effects of aminophylline. Example inducers include aminoglutethimide, carbamazepine, phenobarbital, and rifampin.

CYP1A2 inhibitors: May increase the levels/effects of aminophylline. Example inhibitors include amiodarone, ciprofloxacin, fluvoxamine, ketoconazole, norfloxacin, ofloxacin, and rofecoxib.

Nutritional/Herbal/Ethanol Interactions Food: Food does not appreciably affect absorption. Avoid extremes of dietary protein and carbohydrate intake. Changes in diet may affect the elimination of theophylline; charcoal-broiled foods may increase elimination, reducing half-life by 50%.

Adverse Reactions

Uncommon at serum theophylline concentrations ≤15 mcg/mL

1% to 10%:

Cardiovascular: Tachycardia

Central nervous system: Nervousness, restlessness

Gastrointestinal: Nausea, vomiting

<1% (Limited to important or life-threatening): Allergic reactions, gastric irritation, insomnia, irritability, skin rash, seizure, tremor

Dosing

Adults & Elderly:

Treatment of acute bronchospasm: I.V.:

Loading dose (in patients not currently receiving aminophylline or theophylline): 6 mg/kg (based on aminophylline) administered I.V. over 20-30 minutes; administration rate should not exceed 25 mg/minute (aminophylline)

Approximate I.V. maintenance dosages: Based upon **continuous infusions**; bolus dosing may be determined by multiplying the hourly infusion rate by 24 hours and dividing by the desired number of doses/day

Smoker: 0.8 mg/kg/hour

Nonsmoker: 0.5 mg/kg/hour

Older patients and patients with cor pulmonale: 0.3 mg/kg/hour

Patients with congestive heart failure: 0.1-0.2 mg/kg/hour

Dosage should be adjusted according to serum level measurements during the first 12- to 24-hour period.

Bronchodilator: Oral: Initial: 380 mg/day (equivalent to theophylline 300 mg/day) in divided doses every 6-8 hours; may increase dose after 3 days; maximum dose: 928 mg/day (equivalent to theophylline 800 mg/day)

Pediatrics:

Treatment of acute bronchospasm: I.V.:

Loading dose: Patients not currently receiving aminophylline or theophylline: 6 mg/kg (based on aminophylline) administered I.V. over 20-30 minutes; administration rate should not exceed 25 mg/minute (aminophylline)

Approximate I.V. maintenance dosages: Based upon **continuous infusions**; bolus dosing (often used in children <6 months of age) may be determined by multiplying the hourly infusion rate by 24 hours and dividing by the desired number of doses/day

6 weeks to 6 months: 0.5 mg/kg/hour

6 months to 1 year: 0.6-0.7 mg/kg/hour

1-9 years: 1 mg/kg/hour

9-16 years: Refer to adult dosing.

Dosage should be adjusted according to serum level measurements during the first 12- to 24-hour period.

Bronchodilator: Oral: Children ≥45 kg: Refer to adult dosing.

Available Dosage Forms [DSC] = Discontinued product

Injection, solution: 25 mg/mL (10 mL, 20 mL)

Liquid, oral [DSC]: 105 mg/5 mL (500 mL) [apricot flavor]

Tablet: 100 mg, 200 mg

Nursing Guidelines

Patient Education: Do not drink or eat large quantities of caffeine-containing beverages or food (colas, coffee, chocolate).

Pregnancy Risk Factor: C

Pregnancy Issues: Theophylline crosses the placenta; adverse effects may be seen in the newborn. Theophylline metabolism may change during pregnancy; monitor serum levels.

Lactation: Enters breast milk/compatible (AAP rates "compatible")

Breast-Feeding Considerations: Irritability may be observed in the nursing infant.

Administration

Oral: Should be administered around-the-clock rather than 4 times/day, 3 times/day, etc (ie, 12-6-12-6, not 9-1-5-9) to promote less variation in peak and trough serum levels.

I.M.: Not recommended

I.V.: Dilute with I.V. fluid to a concentration of 1 mg/mL and infuse over 20-30 minutes; maximum concentration: 25 mg/mL; maximum rate of infusion: 0.36 mg/kg/minute, and no greater than 25 mg/minute. I.M. administration is not recommended. Should be administered around-the-clock rather than 4 times/day, 3 times/day, etc (ie, 12-6-12-6, not 9-1-5-9) to promote less variation in peak and trough serum levels.

Compatibility: Stable in dextran 6% in D_5W, dextran 6% in NS, D_5LR, D_5NS, $D_5{}^1/_2NS$, $D_5{}^1/_4NS$, D_5W, $D_{10}W$, $D_{20}W$, LR, $^1/_2NS$, NS

Y-site administration: Incompatible with amiodarone, ciprofloxacin, clarithromycin, dobutamine, hydralazine, ondansetron, vinorelbine, warfarin

Compatibility in syringe: Incompatible with doxapram

(Continued)

Aminophylline *(Continued)*

Compatibility when admixed: Incompatible with atracurium, bleomycin, cefepime, ceftazidime, ceftriaxone, chlorpromazine, ciprofloxacin, clindamycin, dobutamine, doxorubicin, epinephrine, hydralazine, hydrocortisone sodium succinate with cephalothin sodium, hydroxyzine, insulin (regular), isoproterenol, levorphanol, meperidine, morphine, norepinephrine, papaverine with trimecaine, penicillin G potassium, pentazocine, prochlorperazine edisylate, prochlorperazine mesylate, promazine, promethazine, vitamin B complex with C

♦ 5-Aminosalicylic Acid *see* Mesalamine *on page 1105*

Amiodarone (a MEE oh da rone)

U.S. Brand Names Cordarone®; Pacerone®

Synonyms Amiodarone Hydrochloride

Pharmacologic Category Antiarrhythmic Agent, Class III

Medication Safety Issues

Sound-alike/look-alike issues:

Amiodarone may be confused with amiloride, amrinone

Cordarone® may be confused with Cardura®, Cordran®

High alert medication: The Institute for Safe Medication Practices (ISMP) includes this medication among its list of drugs which have a heightened risk of causing significant patient harm when used in error.

Use Management of life-threatening recurrent ventricular fibrillation (VF) or hemodynamically-unstable ventricular tachycardia (VT) refractory to other antiarrhythmic agents or in patients intolerant of other agents used for these conditions

Unlabeled/Investigational Use

Conversion of atrial fibrillation to normal sinus rhythm; maintenance of normal sinus rhythm

Prevention of postoperative atrial fibrillation during cardiothoracic surgery

Paroxysmal supraventricular tachycardia (SVT)

Control of rapid ventricular rate due to accessory pathway conduction in pre-excited atrial arrhythmias [ACLS guidelines]

After defibrillation and epinephrine in cardiac arrest with persistent ventricular tachycardia (VT) or ventricular fibrillation (VF) [ACLS guidelines]

Control of hemodynamically stable VT, polymorphic VT, or wide-complex tachycardia of uncertain origin [ACLS guidelines]

Mechanism of Action Class III antiarrhythmic agent which inhibits adrenergic stimulation, prolongs the action potential and refractory period in myocardial tissue; decreases AV conduction and sinus node function

Pharmacodynamics/Kinetics

Onset of action: Oral: 2 days to 3 weeks; I.V.: May be more rapid

Peak effect: 1 week to 5 months

Duration after discontinuing therapy: 7-50 days

Note: Mean onset of effect and duration after discontinuation may be shorter in children than adults

Distribution: V_d: 66 L/kg (range: 18-148 L/kg); crosses placenta; enters breast milk in concentrations higher than maternal plasma concentrations

Protein binding: 96%

Metabolism: Hepatic via CYP2C8 and 3A4 to active N-desethylamiodarone metabolite; possible enterohepatic recirculation

Bioavailability: Oral: ~50%

Half-life elimination: Terminal: 40-55 days (range: 26-107 days); shorter in children than adults

Excretion: Feces; urine (<1% as unchanged drug)

Contraindications Hypersensitivity to amiodarone, iodine, or any component of the formulation; severe sinus-node dysfunction; second- and third-degree heart block (except in patients with a functioning artificial pacemaker); bradycardia causing syncope (except in patients with a functioning artificial pacemaker); pregnancy

Warnings/Precautions Monitor for pulmonary toxicity, liver toxicity, or exacerbation of the arrhythmia (including torsade de pointes). Use very cautiously and with close monitoring in patients with thyroid or liver disease. May cause hyper- or hypothyroidism. Hyperthyroidism may aggravate or cause breakthrough arrhythmias. Significant heart block or sinus bradycardia can occur. Patients should be hospitalized when amiodarone is initiated. Amiodarone is a potent inhibitor of CYP enzymes and transport proteins (including p-glycoprotein), which may lead to increased serum concentrations/toxicity of a number of medications. Particular caution must be used when a drug with QT_c-prolonging potential relies on metabolism via these enzymes, since the effect of elevated concentrations may be additive with the effect of amiodarone. Carefully assess risk:benefit of coadministration of other drugs which may prolong QT_c interval. Correct electrolyte disturbances, especially hypokalemia or hypomagnesemia, prior to use and throughout therapy.

Pre-existing pulmonary disease does not increase risk of developing pulmonary toxicity, but if pulmonary toxicity develops then the prognosis is worse. Due to complex pharmacokinetics, it is difficult to predict when an arrhythmia or interaction with a subsequent treatment will occur following discontinuation of amiodarone. May cause optic neuropathy and/or optic neuritis, usually resulting in visual impairment. Corneal microdeposits occur in a majority of patients, and may cause visual disturbances in some patients (blurred vision, halos); these are not generally considered a reason to discontinue treatment.

May cause hypotension (infusion-rate related). Caution in surgical patients; may enhance hemodynamic effect of anesthetics; associated with increased risk of adult respiratory distress syndrome (ARDS) postoperatively. Injection contains benzyl alcohol, which has been associated with "gasping syndrome" in neonates. Safety and efficacy of amiodarone in children has not been fully established.

Drug Interactions Substrate of CYP1A2 (minor), 2C8/9 (major at low concentrations), 2C19 (minor), 2D6 (minor), 3A4 (major); **Inhibits** CYP1A2 (strong), 2A6 (moderate), 2B6 (weak), 2C8/9 (moderate), 2C19 (weak), 2D6 (moderate), 3A4 (moderate)

Note: Due to the long half-life of amiodarone, drug interactions may take 1 or more weeks to develop.

Anesthetics (halogenated, inhaled): Amiodarone enhances the myocardial depressant and conduction defects of inhalation anesthetics; monitor.

Azole antifungals: May prolong QT_c, potentially leading to malignant arrhythmias; use caution.

Beta-blockers may cause excessive AV block; monitor response.

Calcium channel blockers (diltiazem, verapamil): May cause excessive AV block; monitor.

Cimetidine: May increase amiodarone blood levels.

Cholestyramine: May decrease amiodarone blood levels.

Cisapride: May prolong QT_c interval potentially leading to malignant arrhythmias.

Clonazepam effects may be increased by amiodarone.

Cyclosporine: Serum levels may be increased by amiodarone; monitor.

CYP1A2 substrates: Amiodarone may increase the levels/effects of CYP1A2 substrates. Example substrates include aminophylline, fluvoxamine, mexiletine, mirtazapine, ropinirole, theophylline, and trifluoperazine.

CYP2A6 substrates: Amiodarone may increase the levels/effects of CYP2A6 substrates. Example substrates include dexmedetomidine and ifosfamide.

CYP2C8/9 inducers: May decrease the levels/effects of amiodarone. Example inducers include carbamazepine, phenobarbital, phenytoin, rifampin, rifapentine, and secobarbital.

CYP2C8/9 inhibitors: May increase the levels/effects of amiodarone. Example inhibitors include delavirdine, fluconazole, gemfibrozil, ketoconazole, nicardipine, NSAIDs, pioglitazone, and sulfonamides.

CYP2C8/9 substrates: Amiodarone may increase the levels/effects of CYP2C8/9 substrates. Example substrates include fluoxetine, glimepiride, glipizide, nateglinide, phenytoin, pioglitazone, rosiglitazone, sertraline, and warfarin.

CYP2D6 substrates: Amiodarone may increase the levels/effects of CYP2D6 substrates. Example substrates include amphetamines, selected beta-blockers, dextromethorphan, fluoxetine, lidocaine, mirtazapine, nefazodone, paroxetine, risperidone, ritonavir, thioridazine, tricyclic antidepressants, and venlafaxine.

CYP2D6 prodrug substrates: Amiodarone may decrease the levels/effects of CYP2D6 prodrug substrates. Example prodrug substrates include codeine, hydrocodone, oxycodone, and tramadol.

CYP3A4 inducers: CYP3A4 inducers may decrease the levels/effects of amiodarone. Example inducers include aminoglutethimide, carbamazepine, nafcillin, nevirapine, phenobarbital, phenytoin, and rifamycins.

CYP3A4 inhibitors: May increase the levels/effects of amiodarone. Example inhibitors include azole antifungals, clarithromycin, diclofenac, doxycycline,

(Continued)

Amiodarone *(Continued)*

erythromycin, imatinib, isoniazid, nefazodone, nicardipine, propofol, protease inhibitors, quinidine, telithromycin, and verapamil.

CYP3A4 substrates: Amiodarone may increase the levels/effects of CYP3A4 substrates. Example substrates include benzodiazepines, calcium channel blockers, ergot derivatives, mirtazapine, nateglinide, nefazodone, tacrolimus, and venlafaxine.

Digoxin levels may be increased by amiodarone; consider reducing digoxin dose by 50% and monitor digoxin blood levels closely.

Fentanyl: Concurrent use may lead to bradycardia, sinus arrest, and hypotension.

Flecainide blood levels may be increased; consider reducing flecainide dose by 25% to 33% with concurrent use.

Fluoroquinolones (sparfloxacin, gatifloxacin, moxifloxacin): May result in additional prolongation of the QT interval; concurrent use of sparfloxacin is contraindicated.

HMG-CoA reductase inhibitors (lovastatin, simvastatin, and others dependent on CYP3A4 metabolism): Amiodarone inhibits metabolism of lovastatin and/or simvastatin and may increase the risk of myopathy and rhabdomyolysis. Concurrent use of lovastatin or simvastatin is not recommended, but if unavoidable, dose of lovastatin should not exceed 40 mg/day. The dose of simvastatin should not exceed 20 mg/day; consider alternative HMG-CoA reductase inhibitor.

Lidocaine: Amiodarone may increase serum levels/toxicity of lidocaine. Sinus bradycardia may occur with concurrent use.

Macrolide antibiotics: May prolong QT_c, potentially leading to malignant arrhythmias. Use caution and evaluate risk:benefit.

Metoprolol blood levels may be increased; monitor response.

Phenytoin blood levels may be increased by amiodarone; amiodarone blood levels may be decreased by phenytoin.

Procainamide and NAPA plasma levels may be increased; consider reducing procainamide dosage by 25% with concurrent use.

Propranolol blood levels may be increased.

Protease inhibitors (amprenavir, indinavir, ritonavir): May increase amiodarone blood levels and toxicity; concurrent use is contraindicated.

QT_c interval prolonging agents (including but may not be limited to amitriptyline, bepridil, disopyramide, erythromycin, haloperidol, imipramine, quinidine, pimozide, procainamide, sotalol, and thioridazine): Effect/toxicity increased; use with caution.

Quinidine blood levels may be increased; monitor quinidine trough concentration.

Rifampin may decrease amiodarone blood levels.

Theophylline blood levels may be increased.

Thyroid supplements: Amiodarone may alter thyroid function; monitor closely.

Warfarin: Hypoprothrombinemic response increased. Monitor INR closely when amiodarone is initiated or discontinued. Reduce warfarin's dose by 1/3 to 1/2 when amiodarone is started.

Nutritional/Herbal/Ethanol Interactions

Food: Increases the rate and extent of absorption of amiodarone. Grapefruit juice increases bioavailability of oral amiodarone by 50% and decreases the conversion of amiodarone to N-DEA (active metabolite); altered effects are possible; use should be avoided during therapy.

Herb/Nutraceutical: St John's wort may decrease amiodarone levels or enhance photosensitization. Avoid ephedra (may worsen arrhythmia). Avoid dong quai.

Adverse Reactions In a recent meta-analysis, patients taking lower doses of amiodarone (152-330 mg daily for at least 12 months) were more likely to develop thyroid, neurologic, skin, ocular, and bradycardic abnormalities than those taking placebo (Vorperian, 1997). Pulmonary toxicity was similar in both the low dose amiodarone group and in the placebo group but there was a trend towards increased toxicity in the amiodarone group. Gastrointestinal and hepatic events were seen to a similar extent in both the low dose amiodarone group and placebo group. As the frequency of adverse events varies considerably across studies as a function of route and dose, a consolidation of adverse event rates is provided by Goldschlager, 2000.

Cardiovascular: Hypotension (I.V. 16%, refractory in rare cases)

Central nervous system (3% to 40%): Abnormal gait/ataxia, dizziness, fatigue, headache, malaise, impaired memory, involuntary movement, insomnia, poor coordination, peripheral neuropathy, sleep disturbances, tremor

Dermatologic: Photosensitivity (10% to 75%)
Endocrine & Metabolic: Hypothyroidism (1% to 22%)
Gastrointestinal: Nausea, vomiting, anorexia, and constipation (10% to 33%); AST or ALT level >2x normal (15% to 50%)
Ocular: Corneal microdeposits (>90%; causes visual disturbance in <10%)

1% to 10%:
Cardiovascular: CHF (3%), bradycardia (3% to 5%), AV block (5%), conduction abnormalities, SA node dysfunction (1% to 3%), cardiac arrhythmia, flushing, edema. Additional effects associated with I.V. administration include asystole, cardiac arrest, electromechanical dissociation, ventricular tachycardia, and cardiogenic shock.
Dermatologic: Slate blue skin discoloration (<10%)
Endocrine & metabolic: Hyperthyroidism (<3%), libido decreased
Gastrointestinal: Abdominal pain, abnormal salivation, abnormal taste (oral)
Hematologic: Coagulation abnormalities
Hepatic: Hepatitis and cirrhosis (<3%)
Local: Phlebitis (I.V., with concentrations >3 mg/mL)
Ocular: Visual disturbances (2% to 9%), halo vision (<5% occurring especially at night), optic neuritis (1%)
Respiratory: Pulmonary toxicity has been estimated to occur at a frequency between 2% and 7% of patients (some reports indicate a frequency as high as 17%). Toxicity may present as hypersensitivity pneumonitis; pulmonary fibrosis (cough, fever, malaise); pulmonary inflammation; interstitial pneumonitis; or alveolar pneumonitis. ARDS has been reported in up to 2% of patients receiving amiodarone, and postoperatively in patients receiving oral amiodarone.
Miscellaneous: Abnormal smell (oral)

<1% (Limited to important or life-threatening): Acute intracranial hypertension (I.V.), acute renal failure, agranulocytosis, alopecia, anaphylactic shock, angioedema, aplastic anemia, bone marrow granuloma, bronchiolitis obliterans organizing pneumonia (BOOP), bronchospasm, confusion, disorientation, dyspnea, encephalopathy, epididymitis (noninfectious), erectile dysfunction, erythema multiforme, exfoliative dermatitis, hallucination, hemolytic anemia, hemoptysis, hyperglycemia, hypertriglyceridemia, hypotension (oral), hypoxia, impotence, injection site reactions, leukocytoclastic vasculitis, muscle weakness, myopathy, neutropenia, optic neuropathy, pancreatitis, pancytopenia, parkinsonian symptoms, photophobia, pleuritis, proarrhythmia, pruritus, pseudotumor cerebri, pulmonary edema, QT interval increased, rash, renal impairment, renal insufficiency, SIADH, sinus arrest, spontaneous ecchymosis, Stevens-Johnson syndrome, thrombocytopenia, toxic epidermal necrolysis, vasculitis, ventricular fibrillation, wheezing

Overdosage/Toxicology Symptoms of overdose include extension of pharmacologic effects, sinus bradycardia and/or heart block, hypotension, and QT prolongation. Patients should be monitored for several days following ingestion. Intoxication with amiodarone necessitates ECG monitoring. Bradycardia may be atropine resistant. Injectable isoproterenol or a temporary pacemaker may be required. Dialysis is not beneficial.

Dosing

Adults & Elderly: Note: Lower loading and maintenance doses are preferable in women and all patients with low body weight.

Ventricular arrhythmias: Oral: 800-1600 mg/day in 1-2 doses for 1-3 weeks, then 600-800 mg/day in 1-2 doses for 1 month; maintenance: 400 mg/day; lower doses are recommended for supraventricular arrhythmias.

Breakthrough VF or VT: I.V.: 150 mg supplemental doses in 100 mL D_5W over 10 minutes

Pulseless VF or VT: I.V. push: Initial: 300 mg in 20-30 mL NS or D_5W; if VF or VT recurs, supplemental dose of 150 mg followed by infusion of 1 mg/minute for 6 hours, then 0.5 mg/minute (maximum daily dose: 2.1 g)

Note: When switching from I.V. to oral therapy, use the following as a guide:
<1 week I.V. infusion: 800-1600 mg/day
1- to 3-week I.V. infusion: 600-800 mg/day
>3 week I.V. infusion: 400 mg

Recommendations for conversion to intravenous amiodarone after oral administration: During long-term amiodarone therapy (ie, ≥4 months), the mean plasma-elimination half-life of the active metabolite of amiodarone is 61 days. Replacement therapy may not be necessary in such patients if oral therapy is discontinued for a period <2 weeks, since any changes in serum

(Continued)

Amiodarone *(Continued)*

amiodarone concentrations during this period may **not** be clinically significant.

Unlabeled uses:

Prophylaxis of atrial fibrillation following open heart surgery (unlabeled use): Note: A variety of regimens have been used in clinical trials, including oral and intravenous regimens:

Oral: 400 mg twice daily (starting in postop recovery) for up to 7 days. An alternative regimen of amiodarone 600 mg/day for 7 days prior to surgery, followed by 200 mg/day until hospital discharge has also been shown to decrease the risk of postoperative atrial fibrillation.

I.V.: 1000 mg infused over 24 hours (starting at postop recovery) for 2 days has been shown to reduce the risk of postoperative atrial fibrillation

Recurrent atrial fibrillation (unlabeled use): No standard regimen defined; examples of regimens include: Oral: Initial: 10 mg/kg/day for 14 days; followed by 300 mg/day for 4 weeks, followed by maintenance dosage of 100-200 mg/day (Roy D, 2000). Other regimens have been described and are used clinically (ie, 400 mg 3 times/day for 5-7 days, then 400 mg/day for 1 month, then 200 mg/day).

Stable VT or SVT (unlabeled use): I.V.: First 24 hours: 1050 mg according to following regimen

Step 1: 150 mg (100 mL) over first 10 minutes (mix 3 mL in 100 mL D_5W)

Step 2: 360 mg (200 mL) over next 6 hours (mix 18 mL in 500 mL D_5W): 1 mg/minute

Step 3: 540 mg (300 mL) over next 18 hours: 0.5 mg/minute

Note: After the first 24 hours: 0.5 mg/minute utilizing concentration of 1-6 mg/mL

Pediatrics:

Arrhythmias (unlabeled use):

Loading dose: Oral: 10-20 mg/kg/day in 1-2 doses for 4-14 days or until adequate control of arrhythmia or prominent adverse effects occur; alternative loading dose in children <1 year: 600-800 mg/1.73 m^2/day in 1-2 divided doses/day.

Maintenance dose: Oral: Dose may be reduced to 5 mg/kg/day for several weeks (or 200-400 mg/1.73 m^2/day given once daily); if no recurrence of arrhythmia, dose may be further reduced to 2.5 mg/kg/day; maintenance doses may be given 5-7 days/week.

Arrhythmias (unlabeled use, dosing based on limited data):

Loading dose: I.V.: 5 mg/kg over 30 minutes; may repeat up to 3 times if no response.

Maintenance dose: I.V.: 2-20 mg/kg/day (5-15 mcg/kg/minute) by continuous infusion.

Note: I.V. administration at low flow rates (potentially associated with use in pediatrics) may result in leaching of plasticizers (DEHP) from intravenous tubing. DEHP may adversely affect male reproductive tract development. Alternative means of dosing and administration (1 mg/kg aliquots) may need to be considered.

Pulseless VF or VT (PALS dosing): I.V.: 5 mg/kg rapid I.V. bolus or I.O.

Perfusing tachycardias (PALS dosing): I.V.: Loading dose: 5 mg/kg I.V. over 20-60 minutes or I.O.; may repeat up to maximum dose of 15 mg/kg/day

Renal Impairment:

Hemodialysis effects: Not removed by hemodialysis or peritoneal dialysis (0% to 5%); no supplemental doses required.

Hepatic Impairment: Dosage adjustment is probably necessary in substantial hepatic impairment. No specific guidelines available.

Available Dosage Forms

Injection, solution, as hydrochloride: 50 mg/mL (3 mL, 9 mL, 18 mL) [contains benzyl alcohol and polysorbate (Tween®) 80]

Cordarone®: 50 mg/mL (3 mL) [contains benzyl alcohol and polysorbate (Tween®) 80]

Tablet, as hydrochloride [scored]: 200 mg

Cordarone®: 200 mg

Pacerone®: 100 mg [not scored], 200 mg, 300 mg, 400 mg

Nursing Guidelines

Assessment: Assess other medications patient may be taking for effectiveness and interactions. Eye examinations should be performed periodically. Monitor cardiac status closely and assess for CNS changes. **I.V.:** Requires continuous cardiac/hemodynamic monitoring and observation for adverse reactions. **Oral:** Assess results of laboratory tests, therapeutic effectiveness, and symptoms of adverse effects at beginning of therapy and regularly during long-term therapy.

Monitoring Laboratory Tests: Thyroid function, pulmonary function, liver enzymes, serum electrolytes (potassium, magnesium)

Dietary Considerations: Administer consistently with regard to meals. Amiodarone contains iodine 37.3% by weight. Grapefruit juice is not recommended.

Patient Education: Emergency use: Patient condition will determine amount of patient education.

Oral: May be taken with food to reduce GI disturbance, but be consistent. Always take with food or always take without food. Do not change dosage or discontinue drug without consulting prescriber. Regular blood work, ophthalmic exams, and cardiac assessment will be necessary while taking this medication on a long-term basis. You may experience dizziness, weakness, or insomnia (use caution when driving, climbing stairs, or engaging in tasks requiring alertness until response to drug is known); hypotension (use caution when rising from sitting or lying position); nausea, vomiting, loss of appetite, stomach discomfort, or abnormal taste (small frequent meals, frequent mouth care, chewing gum, or sucking lozenges may help); photosensitivity (use sunscreen, wear protective clothing and eyewear, and avoid direct sunlight); or decreased libido (reversible). Report persistent dry cough or shortness of breath; chest pain, palpitations, irregular or slow heartbeat; unusual bruising or bleeding; blood in urine, feces (black stool), vomitus; warmth, swelling, pain in calves; muscle tremor, weakness, numbness, or changes in gait; skin rash or irritation; or changes in urinary patterns. **Pregnancy/breast-feeding precautions:** Do not get pregnant while taking this medication; use appropriate contraceptive measures. Do not breast-feed.

Geriatric Considerations: Elderly may be predisposed to toxicity (see Drug Interactions). Half-life may be prolonged due to decreased clearance (see Hepatic/Renal Impairment).

Pregnancy Risk Factor: D

Pregnancy Issues: May cause fetal harm when administered to a pregnant woman, leading to congenital goiter and hypo- or hyperthyroidism.

Lactation: Enters breast milk/not recommended (AAP rates "of concern")

Breast-Feeding Considerations: Hypothyroidism may occur in nursing infants. Both amiodarone and its active metabolite are excreted in human milk. Breast-feeding may lead to significant infant exposure and potential toxicity.

Perioperative/Anesthesia/Other Concerns:

Cardiac Arrest: The ARREST trial was a randomized, placebo-controlled trial evaluating amiodarone's efficacy in patients who had an out-of-hospital cardiac arrest with pulseless ventricular tachycardia or ventricular fibrillation. The primary endpoint was admission to the hospital with a spontaneous perfusing rhythm. Patients were randomized to receive 300 mg of intravenous amiodarone or placebo after being shocked >3 times, intubated, and receiving 1 mg of epinephrine. Ventricular fibrillation was the most common initial arrhythmia (88%). More patients in the amiodarone group were successfully resuscitated (44% amiodarone; 34% placebo; P=0.03) and admitted to the hospital, but mortality was similar in both groups (possibly due to sample size). More recently, the ALIVE trial compared amiodarone to lidocaine in out-of-hospital cardiac arrest victims whose ventricular fibrillation was resistant to three defibrillation attempts in addition to epinephrine and a fourth defibrillation attempt (Dorian, 2002). This was a randomized, double-blind comparison. Other inclusion criteria included ventricular fibrillation unrelated to trauma (or with other arrhythmias that converted to ventricular fibrillation) and recurrent ventricular fibrillation after successful initial defibrillation. The primary endpoint was the number of patients who were admitted to the hospital intensive care unit alive. Three hundred and forty-seven patients were enrolled. The initial amiodarone dose was 5 mg/kg and the lidocaine dose was 1.5 mg/kg. If ventricular fibrillation persisted after another shock, then the study drug could be administered again (amiodarone 2.5 mg/kg, lidocaine 1.5 mg/kg). Significantly more amiodarone patients (~23%) were admitted to the hospital alive than lidocaine patients (12%). The majority (>90%) of patients in the ALIVE trial had ventricular fibrillation as the initial arrhythmia. The authors concluded that intravenous amiodarone is superior to lidocaine in the treatment of shock-resistant, out-of-hospital ventricular fibrillation.

(Continued)

Amiodarone *(Continued)*

Adverse Events: Although adverse events are less common with 200 mg/day, amiodarone-induced pulmonary toxicity can occur and the patient must be monitored. Patients may present with very mild, nonspecific signs such as dyspnea on exertion or cough.

Administration

Oral: Administer consistently with regard to meals. Take in divided doses with meals if high daily dose or if GI upset occurs. If GI intolerance occurs with single-dose therapy, use twice daily dosing.

I.V.: Give I.V. therapy using an infusion pump at a concentration <2 mg/mL. Slow the infusion rate if hypotension develops. Infusions >2 hours must be administered in glass or polyolefin bottles. **Note:** I.V. administration at lower flow rates (potentially associated with use in pediatrics) and higher concentrations than recommended may result in leaching of plasticizers (DEHP) from intravenous tubing. DEHP may adversely affect male reproductive tract development. Alternative means of dosing and administration (1 mg/kg aliquots) may need to be considered. Use only volumetric infusion pump; use of drop counting may lead to under-dosing. Administer through I.V. line with in-line filter.

Compatibility:

Y-site administration: Incompatible with aminophylline, cefamandole, heparin, sodium bicarbonate

Compatibility in syringe: Incompatible with heparin

Compatibility when admixed: Incompatible with floxacillin

Storage: Store at room temperature; protect from light. When admixed in D_5W to a final concentration of 1-6 mg/mL, the solution is stable at room temperature for 24 hours in polyolefin or glass, or for 2 hours in PVC. Infusions >2 hours must be administered in glass or polyolefin bottles.

Related Information

Management of Postoperative Arrhythmias *on page 1787*

- **Amiodarone Hydrochloride** *see* Amiodarone *on page 130*
- **Amitone® [OTC]** *see* Calcium Carbonate *on page 291*

Amitriptyline (a mee TRIP ti leen)

U.S. Brand Names Elavil® [DSC]

Synonyms Amitriptyline Hydrochloride

Pharmacologic Category Antidepressant, Tricyclic (Tertiary Amine)

Medication Safety Issues

Sound-alike/look-alike issues:

Amitriptyline may be confused with aminophylline, imipramine, nortriptyline

Elavil® may be confused with Aldoril®, Eldepryl®, enalapril, Equanil®, Mellaril®, Oruvail®, Plavix®

Use Relief of symptoms of depression

Unlabeled/Investigational Use Analgesic for certain chronic and neuropathic pain; prophylaxis against migraine headaches; treatment of depressive disorders in children

Mechanism of Action Increases the synaptic concentration of serotonin and/or norepinephrine in the central nervous system by inhibition of their reuptake by the presynaptic neuronal membrane

Pharmacodynamics/Kinetics

Onset of action: Migraine prophylaxis: 6 weeks, higher dosage may be required in heavy smokers because of increased metabolism; Depression: 4-6 weeks, reduce dosage to lowest effective level

Distribution: Crosses placenta; enters breast milk

Metabolism: Hepatic to nortriptyline (active), hydroxy and conjugated derivatives; may be impaired in the elderly

Half-life elimination: Adults: 9-27 hours (average: 15 hours)

Time to peak, serum: ~4 hours

Excretion: Urine (18% as unchanged drug); feces (small amounts)

Contraindications Hypersensitivity to amitriptyline or any component of the formulation (cross-sensitivity with other tricyclics may occur); use of MAO inhibitors within past 14 days; acute recovery phase following myocardial infarction; concurrent use of cisapride

Warnings/Precautions Antidepressants increase the risk of suicidal thinking and behavior in children and adolescents with major depressive disorder (MDD) and other depressive disorders; consider risk prior to prescribing. Closely monitor for clinical worsening, suicidality, or unusual changes in behavior; the child's family or caregiver should be instructed to closely observe the patient and communicate condition with healthcare provider. Such observation would generally include at least weekly face-to-face contact with patients or their family members or caregivers during the first 4 weeks of treatment, then every other week visits for the next 4 weeks, then at 12 weeks, and as clinically indicated beyond 12 weeks. Additional contact by telephone may be appropriate between face-to-face visits. Adults treated with antidepressants should be observed similarly for clinical worsening and suicidality, especially during the initial few months of a course of drug therapy, or at times of dose changes, either increases or decreases. A medication guide should be dispensed with each prescription. **Amitriptyline is not FDA-approved for use in children <12 years of age.**

The possibility of a suicide attempt is inherent in major depression and may persist until remission occurs. Monitor for worsening of depression or suicidality, especially during initiation of therapy or with dose increases or decreases. Worsening depression and severe abrupt suicidality that are not part of the presenting symptoms may require discontinuation or modification of drug therapy. Use caution in high-risk patients during initiation of therapy. Prescriptions should be written for the smallest quantity consistent with good patient care. The patient's family or caregiver should be alerted to monitor patients for the emergence of suicidality and associated behaviors such as anxiety, agitation, panic attacks, insomnia, irritability, hostility, impulsivity, akathisia, hypomania, and mania; patients should be instructed to notify their healthcare provider if any of these symptoms or worsening depression occur.

May worsen psychosis in some patients or precipitate a shift to mania or hypomania in patients with bipolar disorder. Monotherapy in patients with bipolar disorder should be avoided. Patients presenting with depressive symptoms should be screened for bipolar disorder. **Amitriptyline is not FDA approved for the treatment of bipolar depression.**

Often causes drowsiness/sedation, resulting in impaired performance of tasks requiring alertness (eg, operating machinery or driving). Sedative effects may be additive with other CNS depressants and/or ethanol. The degree of sedation is very high relative to other antidepressants. May cause hyponatremia/SIADH. May increase the risks associated with electroconvulsive therapy. Consider discontinuing, when possible, prior to elective surgery. Therapy should not be abruptly discontinued in patients receiving high doses for prolonged periods.

May cause orthostatic hypotension; the risk of this problem is very high relative to other antidepressants. Use with caution in patients at risk of hypotension or in patients where transient hypotensive episodes would be poorly tolerated (cardiovascular disease or cerebrovascular disease). The degree of anticholinergic blockade produced by this agent is very high relative to other cyclic antidepressants; use with caution in patients with urinary retention, benign prostatic hyperplasia, narrow-angle glaucoma, xerostomia, visual problems, constipation, or a history of bowel obstruction. May alter glucose control - use with caution in patients with diabetes.

Use with caution in patients with a history of cardiovascular disease (including previous MI, stroke, tachycardia, or conduction abnormalities). The risk of conduction abnormalities with this agent is high relative to other antidepressants. May lower seizure threshold - use caution in patients with a previous seizure disorder or condition predisposing to seizures such as brain damage, alcoholism, or concurrent therapy with other drugs which lower the seizure threshold. Use with caution in hyperthyroid patients or those receiving thyroid supplementation. Use with caution in patients with hepatic or renal dysfunction and in elderly patients.

Drug Interactions **Substrate** of CYP1A2 (minor), 2B6 (minor), 2C8/9 (minor), 2C19 (minor), 2D6 (major), 3A4 (minor); **Inhibits** CYP1A2 (weak), 2C8/9 (weak), 2C19 (weak), 2D6 (weak), 2E1 (weak)

Altretamine: Concurrent use may cause orthostatic hypertension

Amphetamines: TCAs may enhance the effect of amphetamines; monitor for adverse CV effects

Anticholinergics: Combined use with TCAs may produce additive anticholinergic effects

Antihypertensives: Amitriptyline inhibits the antihypertensive response to bethanidine, clonidine, debrisoquin, guanadrel, guanethidine, guanabenz, guanfacine; monitor BP; consider alternate antihypertensive agent

Beta-agonists: When combined with TCAs may predispose patients to cardiac arrhythmias

(Continued)

Amitriptyline *(Continued)*

Bupropion: May increase the levels of tricyclic antidepressants; based on limited information, monitor response

Carbamazepine: Tricyclic antidepressants may increase carbamazepine levels; monitor

Cholestyramine and colestipol: May bind TCAs and reduce their absorption; monitor for altered response

Cisapride: May increase the risk of QT_c prolongation and/or arrhythmia; concurrent use is contraindicated

Clonidine: Abrupt discontinuation of clonidine may cause hypertensive crisis; amitriptyline may enhance the response (also see note on antihypertensives)

CNS depressants: Sedative effects may be additive with TCAs; monitor for increased effect; includes benzodiazepines, barbiturates, antipsychotics, ethanol, and other sedative medications

CYP2D6 inhibitors: May increase the levels/effects of amitriptyline; example inhibitors include chlorpromazine, delavirdine, fluoxetine, miconazole, paroxetine, pergolide, quinidine, quinine, ritonavir, and ropinirole

Epinephrine (and other direct alpha-agonists): Pressor response to I.V. epinephrine, norepinephrine, and phenylephrine may be enhanced in patients receiving TCAs. (**Note:** Effect is unlikely with epinephrine or levonordefrin dosages typically administered as infiltration in combination with local anesthetics.)

Fenfluramine: May increase tricyclic antidepressant levels/effects

Hypoglycemic agents (including insulin): TCAs may enhance the hypoglycemic effects of tolazamide, chlorpropamide, or insulin; monitor for changes in blood glucose levels; reported with chlorpropamide, tolazamide, and insulin

Levodopa: Tricyclic antidepressants may decrease the absorption (bioavailability) of levodopa; rare hypertensive episodes have also been attributed to this combination

Linezolid: Hyperpyrexia, hypertension, tachycardia, confusion, seizures, and **deaths have been reported** with agents which inhibit MAO (serotonin syndrome); this combination should be avoided

Lithium: Concurrent use with a TCA may increase the risk for neurotoxicity

MAO inhibitors: Hyperpyrexia, hypertension, tachycardia, confusion, seizures, and **deaths have been reported** (serotonin syndrome); this combination should be avoided

Methylphenidate: Metabolism of amitriptyline may be decreased

Phenothiazines: Serum concentrations of some TCAs may be increased; in addition, TCAs may increase concentration of phenothiazines; monitor for altered clinical response

QT_c prolonging agents: Concurrent use of tricyclic agents with other drugs which may prolong QT_c interval may increase the risk of potentially fatal arrhythmias; includes type Ia and type III antiarrhythmics agents, selected quinolones (sparfloxacin, gatifloxacin, moxifloxacin, grepafloxacin), cisapride, and other agents

Ritonavir: Combined use of high-dose tricyclic antidepressants with ritonavir may cause serotonin syndrome in HIV-positive patients; monitor

Sucralfate: Absorption of tricyclic antidepressants may be reduced with coadministration

Sympathomimetics, indirect-acting: Tricyclic antidepressants may result in a decreased sensitivity to indirect-acting sympathomimetics; includes dopamine and ephedrine; also see interaction with epinephrine (and direct-acting sympathomimetics)

Tramadol: Tramadol's risk of seizures may be increased with TCAs

Valproic acid: May increase serum concentrations/adverse effects of some tricyclic antidepressants

Warfarin (and other oral anticoagulants): Amitriptyline may increase the anticoagulant effect in patients stabilized on warfarin; monitor INR

Nutritional/Herbal/Ethanol Interactions

Ethanol: Avoid ethanol (may increase CNS depression).

Food: Grapefruit juice may inhibit the metabolism of some TCAs and clinical toxicity may result.

Herb/Nutraceutical: St John's wort may decrease amitriptyline levels. Avoid valerian, St John's wort, kava kava, gotu kola (may increase CNS depression).

Lab Interactions Amitriptyline may increase or decrease serum glucose levels, may elevate liver function tests, and may prolong conduction time.

Adverse Reactions Anticholinergic effects may be pronounced; moderate to marked sedation can occur (tolerance to these effects usually occurs).

Frequency not defined.

Cardiovascular: Orthostatic hypotension, tachycardia, ECG changes (nonspecific), AV conduction changes, cardiomyopathy (rare), MI, stroke, heart block, arrhythmia, syncope, hypertension, palpitation

Central nervous system: Restlessness, dizziness, insomnia, sedation, fatigue, anxiety, cognitive function impaired, seizure, extrapyramidal symptoms, coma, hallucinations, confusion, disorientation, coordination impaired, ataxia, headache, nightmares, hyperpyrexia

Dermatologic: Allergic rash, urticaria, photosensitivity, alopecia

Endocrine & metabolic: Syndrome of inappropriate ADH secretion

Gastrointestinal: Weight gain, xerostomia, constipation, paralytic ileus, nausea, vomiting, anorexia, stomatitis, peculiar taste, diarrhea, black tongue

Genitourinary: Urinary retention

Hematologic: Bone marrow depression, purpura, eosinophilia

Neuromuscular & skeletal: Numbness, paresthesia, peripheral neuropathy, tremor, weakness

Ocular: Blurred vision, mydriasis, ocular pressure increased

Otic: Tinnitus

Miscellaneous: Diaphoresis, withdrawal reactions (nausea, headache, malaise)

Postmarketing and/or case reports: Neuroleptic malignant syndrome (rare), serotonin syndrome (rare)

Overdosage/Toxicology Symptoms of overdose include agitation, confusion, hallucinations, urinary retention, hypothermia, hypotension, ventricular tachycardia, and seizures. Treatment is symptomatic and supportive. Alkalinization by sodium bicarbonate and/or hyperventilation may limit cardiac toxicity.

Dosing

Adults:

Depression:

Oral: 50-150 mg/day single dose at bedtime or in divided doses; dose may be gradually increased up to 300 mg/day.

I.M.: 20-30 mg 4 times/day

Chronic pain management (unlabeled use): Oral: Initial: 25 mg at bedtime; may increase as tolerated to 100 mg/day.

Migraine prophylaxis (unlabeled use): Oral: Initial: 10-25 mg at bedtime; usual dose: 150 mg; reported dosing ranges: 10-400 mg/day

Elderly: Depression: Oral: Initial: 10-25 mg at bedtime; dose should be increased in 10-25 mg increments every week if tolerated; dose range: 25-150 mg/day. See Renal/Hepatic Impairment.

Pediatrics:

Chronic pain management (unlabeled use): Oral: Initial: 0.1 mg/kg at bedtime, may advance as tolerated over 2-3 weeks to 0.5-2 mg/kg at bedtime

Depressive disorders:

Children (unlabeled use): Oral: Initial doses of 1 mg/kg/day given in 3 divided doses with increases to 1.5 mg/kg/day have been reported in a small number of children (n=9) 9-12 years of age; clinically, doses up to 3 mg/kg/day (5 mg/kg/day if monitored closely) have been proposed

Adolescents: Initial: 25-50 mg/day; may administer in divided doses; increase gradually to 100 mg/day in divided doses.

Migraine prophylaxis (unlabeled use): Oral: Initial: 0.25 mg/kg/day, given at bedtime; increase dose by 0.25 mg/kg/day to maximum 1 mg/kg/day. Reported dosing ranges: 0.1-2 mg/kg/day; maximum suggested dose: 10 mg.

Renal Impairment: Nondialyzable

Hepatic Impairment: Use with caution and monitor plasma levels and patient response.

Available Dosage Forms [DSC] = Discontinued product

Injection, as hydrochloride: 10 mg/mL (10 mL) [DSC]

Tablet, as hydrochloride: 10 mg, 25 mg, 50 mg, 75 mg, 100 mg, 150 mg

Nursing Guidelines

Assessment: Assess other medications patient may be taking for effectiveness and interactions. Assess for suicidal tendencies or unusual changes in behavior before beginning therapy and periodically thereafter. May cause physiological or psychological dependence, tolerance, or abuse; evaluate need for continued use periodically. Caution patients with diabetes; may alter serum glucose levels. Monitor therapeutic response and adverse reactions at beginning of therapy and periodically with long-term use. Taper dosage slowly when discontinuing. Teach patient appropriate use, interventions to reduce side effects, and adverse symptoms to report.

(Continued)

Amitriptyline *(Continued)*

Patient Education: Take exactly as directed; do not increase dose or frequency. It may take several weeks to achieve desired results. Restrict use of alcohol or caffeine; avoid grapefruit juice. Maintain adequate hydration (2-3 L/day of fluids) unless instructed to restrict fluid intake. If you have diabetes, monitor glucose levels closely; this medication may alter glucose levels. May turn urine blue-green (normal). May cause drowsiness, lightheadedness, impaired coordination, dizziness, or blurred vision (use caution when driving or engaging in tasks requiring alertness until response to drug is known); constipation (increased exercise, fluids, fruit, or fiber may help); urinary retention (void before taking medication); postural hypotension (use caution climbing stairs or when changing position from lying or sitting to standing); altered sexual drive or ability (reversible); or photosensitivity (use sunscreen, wear protective clothing and eyewear, and avoid direct sunlight). Report persistent CNS effects (eg, nervousness, restlessness, insomnia, headache, agitation, impaired coordination, changes in cognition); muscle cramping, weakness, tremors, or rigidity; ringing in ears or visual disturbances; chest pain, palpitations, or irregular heartbeat; blurred vision; or worsening of condition. **Pregnancy/breast-feeding precautions:** Do not get pregnant while taking this medication. Consult prescriber for appropriate contraceptive measures. Breast-feeding is not recommended.

Geriatric Considerations: The most anticholinergic and sedating of the antidepressants. Due to pronounced effects on the cardiovascular system (hypotension), many psychiatrists agree it is best to avoid in the elderly.

Pregnancy Risk Factor: C

Pregnancy Issues: Teratogenic effects have been observed in animal studies. Amitriptyline crosses the human placenta; CNS effects, limb deformities and developmental delay have been noted in case reports.

Lactation: Enters breast milk/not recommended (AAP rates "of concern")

Breast-Feeding Considerations: Generally, it is not recommended to breast-feed if taking antidepressants because of the long half-life, active metabolites, and the potential for side effects in the infant.

Perioperative/Anesthesia/Other Concerns: Plasma levels do not always correlate with clinical effectiveness. Desired therapeutic effect (for analgesia) may take as long as 1-3 weeks. When used for migraine headache prophylaxis, therapeutic effect may take as long as 6 weeks.

Tricyclic antidepressants affect conduction and have anticholinergic effects and, therefore, should be used with caution in patients with underlying cardiovascular disease. Therapy is relatively contraindicated in patients with conduction abnormalities or in patients with symptomatic hypotension. Heart block may be precipitated in patients with pre-existing conduction system disease. Cardiovascular signs of toxicity may include tachycardia, ventricular arrhythmia, impaired conduction, and shock.

Administration

I.V.: Do **not** administer I.V.

♦ **Amitriptyline Hydrochloride** *see* Amitriptyline *on page 136*

Amlodipine (am LOE di peen)

U.S. Brand Names Norvasc®

Synonyms Amlodipine Besylate

Pharmacologic Category Calcium Channel Blocker

Medication Safety Issues

Sound-alike/look-alike issues:

Amlodipine may be confused with amiloride

Norvasc® may be confused with Navane®, Norvir®, Vascor®

Use Treatment of hypertension; treatment of symptomatic chronic stable angina, vasospastic (Prinzmetal's) angina (confirmed or suspected); prevention of hospitalization due to angina with documented CAD (limited to patients without heart failure or ejection fraction <40%)

Mechanism of Action Inhibits calcium ion from entering the "slow channels" or select voltage-sensitive areas of vascular smooth muscle and myocardium during depolarization, producing a relaxation of coronary vascular smooth muscle and coronary vasodilation; increases myocardial oxygen delivery in patients with vasospastic angina

Pharmacodynamics/Kinetics

Onset of action: Antihypertensive: 30-50 minutes

Duration of antihypertensive effect: 24 hours
Absorption: Oral: Well absorbed
Distribution: V_d: 21 L/kg
Protein binding: 93% to 98%
Metabolism: Hepatic (>90%) to inactive metabolite
Bioavailability: 64% to 90%
Half-life elimination: 30-50 hours; increased with hepatic dysfunction
Time to peak, plasma: 6-12 hours
Excretion: Urine (10% as parent, 60% as metabolite)

Contraindications Hypersensitivity to amlodipine or any component of the formulation

Warnings/Precautions Increased angina and/or MI has occurred with initiation or dosage titration of calcium channel blockers. Use caution in severe aortic stenosis. Use caution in patients with severe hepatic impairment. Dosage titration should occur after 7-14 days on a given dose.

Drug Interactions **Substrate** of CYP3A4 (major); **Inhibits** CYP1A2 (moderate), 2A6 (weak), 2B6 (weak), 2C8/9 (weak), 2D6 (weak), 3A4 (weak)

Azole antifungals may inhibit calcium channel blocker metabolism; avoid this combination. Try an antifungal like terbinafine (if appropriate) or monitor closely for altered effect of the calcium channel blocker.

Calcium may reduce the calcium channel blocker's effects, particularly hypotension.

CYP1A2 substrates: Amlodipine may increase the levels/effects of CYP1A2 substrates. Example substrates include aminophylline, fluvoxamine, mexiletine, mirtazapine, ropinirole, theophylline, and trifluoperazine.

CYP3A4 inducers: CYP3A4 inducers may decrease the levels/effects of amlodipine. Example inducers include aminoglutethimide, carbamazepine, nafcillin, nevirapine, phenobarbital, phenytoin, and rifamycins.

CYP3A4 inhibitors: May increase the levels/effects of amlodipine. Example inhibitors include azole antifungals, clarithromycin, diclofenac, doxycycline, erythromycin, imatinib, isoniazid, nefazodone, nicardipine, propofol, protease inhibitors, quinidine, telithromycin, and verapamil.

Grapefruit juice: May modestly increase amlodipine levels.

Rifampin increases the metabolism of calcium channel blockers; adjust the dose of calcium channel blocker to maintain efficacy.

Sildenafil, tadalafil, vardenafil: Blood pressure-lowering effects are additive; use caution.

Nutritional/Herbal/Ethanol Interactions

Food: Grapefruit juice may modestly increase amlodipine levels.

Herb/Nutraceutical: St John's wort may decrease amlodipine levels. Avoid dong quai if using for hypertension (has estrogenic activity). Avoid ephedra, yohimbe, ginseng (may worsen hypertension). Avoid garlic (may have increased antihypertensive effects).

Adverse Reactions

>10%: Cardiovascular: Peripheral edema (2% to 15% dose related)

1% to 10%:

Cardiovascular: Flushing (1% to 3%), palpitation (1% to 4%)
Central nervous system: Headache (7%; similar to placebo 8%), dizziness (1% to 3%), fatigue (4%), somnolence (1% to 2%)
Dermatologic: Rash (1% to 2%), pruritus (1% to 2%)
Endocrine & metabolic: Male sexual dysfunction (1% to 2%)
Gastrointestinal: Nausea (3%), abdominal pain (1% to 2%), dyspepsia (1% to 2%), gingival hyperplasia
Neuromuscular & skeletal: Muscle cramps (1% to 2%), weakness (1% to 2%)
Respiratory: Dyspnea (1% to 2%), pulmonary edema (15% from PRAISE trial, CHF population)

<1% (Limited to important or life-threatening): Abnormal dreams, agitation alopecia, amnesia, anxiety, apathy, arrhythmia, ataxia, bradycardia, cardiac failure, cholestasis, depersonalization, depression, erythema multiforme, exfoliative dermatitis, extrapyramidal symptoms, gastritis, gynecomastia, hepatitis, hypotension, jaundice, leukocytoclastic vasculitis, migraine, nonthrombocytopenic purpura, paresthesia, peripheral ischemia, photosensitivity, postural hypotension, purpura, rash, skin discoloration, Stevens-Johnson syndrome, syncope, thrombocytopenia, tinnitus, transaminases increased, urticaria, weight loss, vertigo, xerophthalmia

Overdosage/Toxicology Primary cardiac symptoms of calcium channel blocker overdose include hypotension and bradycardia. Noncardiac symptoms include

(Continued)

Amlodipine *(Continued)*

confusion, stupor, nausea, vomiting, metabolic acidosis, and hyperglycemia. Treat other signs and symptoms symptomatically.

Dosing

Adults:

Hypertension: Oral: Initial dose: 5 mg once daily; maximum dose: 10 mg once daily. In general, titrate in 2.5 mg increments over 7-14 days. Usual dosage range (JNC 7): 2.5-10 mg once daily.

Angina: Oral: Usual dose: 5-10 mg; lower dose suggested in elderly or hepatic impairment; most patients require 10 mg for adequate effect.

Elderly: Dosing should start at the lower end of dosing range due to possible increased incidence of hepatic, renal, or cardiac impairment. Elderly patients also show decreased clearance of amlodipine.

Hypertension: Oral: 2.5 mg once daily

Angina: Oral: 5 mg once daily

Pediatrics: Hypertension: Oral: Children 6-17 years: 2.5-5 mg once daily

Hepatic Impairment:

Hypertension: Administer 2.5 mg once daily

Angina: Administer 5 mg once daily

Available Dosage Forms Tablet: 2.5 mg, 5 mg, 10 mg

Nursing Guidelines

Assessment: See Warnings/Precautions for use cautions. Assess potential for interactions with prescription, OTC medications, or herbal products patient may be taking (eg, nitrates or other drugs that effect blood pressure - see Drug Interactions). Assess therapeutic effectiveness and signs of adverse reactions at beginning of therapy, when changing dose, and periodically during long-term therapy (see Adverse Reactions and Overdose/Toxicology). Teach patient proper use, possible side effects/appropriate interventions, and adverse symptoms to report (see Patient Education). Note breast-feeding caution.

Dietary Considerations: May be taken without regard to meals.

Patient Education: Inform prescriber of all prescriptions, OTC medications, or herbal products you are taking, and any allergies you have. Do not take any new medication during therapy unless approved by prescriber. Take exactly as directed; do not alter dose or discontinue without consulting prescriber. May cause headache (if unrelieved, consult prescriber); nausea or vomiting (small, frequent meals, frequent mouth care, chewing gum or sucking lozenges may help); constipation (increased dietary bulk and fluids may help); or drowsiness (use caution when driving or engaging in tasks that require alertness until response to drug is known). Report unrelieved headache; vomiting, constipation; palpitations; peripheral or facial swelling; weight gain >5 lb/week; or respiratory changes. **Pregnancy/breast-feeding precautions:** Inform prescriber if you are or intend to become pregnant. Consult prescriber if breast-feeding.

Geriatric Considerations: Elderly or debilitated persons may experience a greater hypotensive response. Theoretically, constipation may be more of a problem with elderly.

Pregnancy Risk Factor: C

Lactation: Excretion in breast milk unknown/not recommended

Perioperative/Anesthesia/Other Concerns: Amlodipine may be used safely to treat hypertension and/or angina in patients with heart failure.

Administration

Oral: May be administered without regard to meals.

Storage: Store at room temperature of 15°C to 30°C (59°F to 86°F).

Amlodipine and Benazepril (am LOE di peen & ben AY ze pril)

U.S. Brand Names Lotrel®

Synonyms Benazepril Hydrochloride and Amlodipine Besylate

Pharmacologic Category Antihypertensive Agent, Combination

Use Treatment of hypertension

Mechanism of Action The mechanism through which benazepril lowers blood pressure is believed to be primarily suppression of the renin-angiotensin-aldosterone system; benazepril has an antihypertensive effect even in patients with low-renin hypertension; amlodipine is a dihydropyridine calcium antagonist that inhibits the transmembrane influx of calcium ions into vascular smooth muscle and cardiac muscle; amlodipine is a peripheral arterial vasodilator that acts directly on vascular smooth muscle to cause a reduction in peripheral vascular resistance and reduction in blood pressure

Pharmacodynamics/Kinetics See individual agents.

Contraindications Hypersensitivity to amlodipine, benazepril, other ACE inhibitors, or any component of the formulation; pregnancy (2nd and 3rd trimesters)

Warnings/Precautions Used as a replacement for separate dosing of components or combination therapy when response to single agent is suboptimal; the fixed combination is not indicated for initial treatment of hypertension; see individual monographs for additional warnings/precautions

Drug Interactions Amlodipine: **Substrate** of CYP3A4 (major); **Inhibits** CYP1A2 (moderate), 2A6 (weak), 2B6 (weak), 2C8/9 (weak), 2D6 (weak), 3A4 (weak)

Also see individual agents.

Adverse Reactions See individual agents.

Dosing

Adults: Hypertension: Oral: Dosage is individualized, given once daily.

Elderly: Initial dose: 2.5 mg (based on amlodipine component). Refer to adult dosing.

Renal Impairment: Cl_{cr} ≤30 mL/minute: Use of combination product is not recommended.

Hepatic Impairment: Initial dose: 2.5 mg based on amlodipine component.

Available Dosage Forms Capsule:

Amlodipine 2.5 mg and benazepril hydrochloride 10 mg
Amlodipine 5 mg and benazepril hydrochloride 10 mg
Amlodipine 5 mg and benazepril hydrochloride 20 mg
Amlodipine 10 mg and benazepril hydrochloride 20 mg

Nursing Guidelines

Assessment: See individual components listed in Related Information. **Pregnancy risk factor C/D** - see Pregnancy Risk Factor for use cautions. Assess knowledge/instruct patient on need to use appropriate contraceptive measures and the need to avoid pregnancy. Note breast-feeding caution.

Patient Education: See individual agents. **Pregnancy/breast-feeding precautions:** Inform prescriber if you are or intend to become pregnant. Consult prescriber if breast-feeding.

Pregnancy Risk Factor: C/D (2nd and 3rd trimesters)

Lactation:

Amlodipine: Excretion in breast milk unknown
Benazepril: Enters breast milk

Related Information

Amlodipine *on page 140*
Benazepril *on page 228*

♦ Amlodipine Besylate *see* Amlodipine *on page 140*

Ammonia Spirit (Aromatic) (a MOE nee ah SPEAR it, air oh MAT ik)

Synonyms Smelling Salts

Pharmacologic Category Respiratory Stimulant

Use Respiratory and circulatory stimulant; treatment of fainting

Contraindications Hypersensitivity to ammonia or any component of the formulation

Drug Interactions No data reported

Adverse Reactions 1% to 10%:

Gastrointestinal: Nausea, vomiting
Respiratory: Irritation to nasal mucosa, cough

Dosing

Adults & Elderly: Fainting: Inhalation: Used as "smelling salts" to treat or prevent fainting

Available Dosage Forms Solution for inhalation [ampul]: 1.7% to 2.1% (0.33 mL)

Nursing Guidelines

Pregnancy Risk Factor: C

Administration

Storage: Aromatic ammonia spirit should be protected from sunlight and stored at a temperature not exceeding 30°C.

♦ Amnesteem™ *see* Isotretinoin *on page 981*

Amoxicillin (a moks i SIL in)

U.S. Brand Names Amoxil®; DisperMox™; Moxilin®; Trimox®

Synonyms Amoxicillin Trihydrate; Amoxycillin; *p*-Hydroxyampicillin

Pharmacologic Category Antibiotic, Penicillin

Medication Safety Issues

Sound-alike/look-alike issues:

Amoxicillin may be confused with amoxapine, Amoxil®, Atarax®
Amoxil® may be confused with amoxapine, amoxicillin
Trimox® may be confused with Diamox®, Tylox®

Use Treatment of otitis media, sinusitis, and infections caused by susceptible organisms involving the respiratory tract, skin, and urinary tract; prophylaxis of bacterial endocarditis in patients undergoing surgical or dental procedures; as part of a multidrug regimen for *H. pylori* eradication

Unlabeled/Investigational Use Postexposure prophylaxis for anthrax exposure with documented susceptible organisms

Mechanism of Action Inhibits bacterial cell wall synthesis by binding to one or more of the penicillin-binding proteins (PBPs); which in turn inhibits the final transpeptidation step of peptidoglycan synthesis in bacterial cell walls, thus inhibiting cell wall biosynthesis. Bacteria eventually lyse due to ongoing activity of cell wall autolytic enzymes (autolysins and murein hydrolases) while cell wall assembly is arrested.

Pharmacodynamics/Kinetics

Absorption: Oral: Rapid and nearly complete; food does not interfere

Distribution: Widely to most body fluids and bone; poor penetration into cells, eyes, and across normal meninges

Pleural fluids, lungs, and peritoneal fluid; high urine concentrations are attained; also into synovial fluid, liver, prostate, muscle, and gallbladder; penetrates into middle ear effusions, maxillary sinus secretions, tonsils, sputum, and bronchial secretions; crosses placenta; low concentrations enter breast milk

CSF:blood level ratio: Normal meninges: <1%; Inflamed meninges: 8% to 90%

Protein binding: 17% to 20%

Metabolism: Partially hepatic

Half-life elimination:

Neonates, full-term: 3.7 hours
Infants and Children: 1-2 hours
Adults: Normal renal function: 0.7-1.4 hours
Cl_{cr} <10 mL/minute: 7-21 hours

Time to peak: Capsule: 2 hours; Suspension: 1 hour

Excretion: Urine (80% as unchanged drug); lower in neonates

Contraindications Hypersensitivity to amoxicillin, penicillin, or any component of the formulation

Warnings/Precautions In patients with renal impairment, doses and/or frequency of administration should be modified in response to the degree of renal impairment; a high percentage of patients with infectious mononucleosis have developed rash during therapy with amoxicillin; a low incidence of cross-allergy with other beta-lactams and cephalosporins exists

Drug Interactions

Allopurinol: Theoretically has an additive potential for amoxicillin rash

Aminoglycosides: May be synergistic against selected organisms

Methotrexate: Penicillins may increase the exposure to methotrexate during concurrent therapy; monitor.

Oral contraceptives: Anecdotal reports suggesting decreased contraceptive efficacy with penicillins have been refuted by more rigorous scientific and clinical data.

Probenecid, disulfiram: May increase levels of penicillins (amoxicillin)

Warfarin: Effects of warfarin may be increased

Lab Interactions Altered response to Benedict's reagent in Clinitest®

Some penicillin derivatives may accelerate the degradation of aminoglycosides *in vitro*, leading to a potential underestimation of aminoglycoside serum concentration.

Adverse Reactions Frequency not defined.

Central nervous system: Hyperactivity, agitation, anxiety, insomnia, confusion, convulsions, behavioral changes, dizziness

Dermatologic: Acute exanthematous pustulosis, erythematous maculopapular rash, erythema multiforme, Stevens-Johnson syndrome, exfoliative dermatitis, toxic epidermal necrolysis, hypersensitivity vasculitis, urticaria

Gastrointestinal: Nausea, vomiting, diarrhea, hemorrhagic colitis, pseudomembranous colitis, tooth discoloration (brown, yellow, or gray; rare)

Hematologic: Anemia, hemolytic anemia, thrombocytopenia, thrombocytopenia purpura, eosinophilia, leukopenia, agranulocytosis

Hepatic: AST (SGOT) and ALT (SGPT) increased, cholestatic jaundice, hepatic cholestasis, acute cytolytic hepatitis

Renal: Crystalluria

Overdosage/Toxicology Symptoms of penicillin overdose include neuromuscular hypersensitivity (eg, agitation, hallucinations, asterixis, encephalopathy, confusion, and seizures). Interstitial nephritis and/or crystalluria, possibly resulting in renal failure, may occur; hydration and diuresis may be beneficial. Electrolyte imbalance may occur if the preparation contains potassium or sodium salts, especially in renal failure. A study of 51 pediatric overdose victims suggests that ingestion of doses ≤250 mg/kg does not manifest significant clinical symptoms, and thus does not require gastric lavage. Hemodialysis may be helpful to aid in removal of the drug from blood; otherwise, treatment is symptom-directed and supportive.

Dosing

Adults & Elderly:

Usual dosage range: Oral: 250-500 mg every 8 hours or 500-875 mg twice daily

Ear, nose, throat, genitourinary tract or skin/skin structure infections:

Mild to moderate: 500 mg every 12 hours **or** 250 mg every 8 hours

Severe: 875 mg every 12 hours **or** 500 mg every 8 hours

Lower respiratory tract infections: 875 mg every 12 hours **or** 500 mg every 8 hours

Endocarditis prophylaxis: 2 g 1 hour before procedure

Peptic ulcer disease: Eradication of *Helicobacter pylori*: Oral: 1000 mg twice daily; requires combination therapy with at least one other antibiotic and an acid-suppressing agent (proton pump inhibitor or H_2 blocker)

Anthrax exposure (unlabeled use): Oral: **Note:** Postexposure prophylaxis only with documented susceptible organisms: 500 mg every 8 hours

Pediatrics:

Usual dosage range: Oral:

Children ≤3 months: 20-30 mg/kg/day divided every 12 hours

Children: >3 months and <40 kg: 20-50 mg/kg/day in divided doses every 8-12 hours

Ear, nose, throat, genitourinary tract, or skin/skin structure infections:

Oral: Children: >3 months and <40 kg:

Mild-to-moderate: 25 mg/kg/day in divided doses every 12 hours **or** 20 mg/kg/day in divided doses every 8 hours

Severe: 45 mg/kg/day in divided doses every 12 hours **or** 40 mg/kg/day in divided doses every 8 hours

Acute otitis media: Oral: Children: >3 months and <40 kg: 80-90 mg/kg/day divided every 12 hours

Lower respiratory tract infections: Oral: Children: >3 months and <40 kg: 45 mg/kg/day in divided doses every 12 hours **or** 40 mg/kg/day in divided doses every 8 hours

Subacute bacterial endocarditis prophylaxis: Oral: Children: >3 months and <40 kg: 50 mg/kg 1 hour before procedure

Anthrax exposure (unlabeled use): Oral: **Note:** Postexposure prophylaxis only with documented susceptible organisms:

<40 kg: 15 mg/kg every 8 hours

≥40 kg: 500 mg every 8 hours

Renal Impairment:

The 875 mg tablet should not be used in patients with Cl_{cr} <30 mL/minute.

Cl_{cr} 10-30 mL/minute: 250-500 mg every 12 hours

Cl_{cr} <10 mL/minute: 250-500 mg every 24 hours

Moderately dialyzable (20% to 50%) by hemodialysis or peritoneal dialysis; approximately 50 mg of amoxicillin per liter of filtrate is removed by continuous arteriovenous or venovenous hemofiltration. Dose as per Cl_{cr} <10 mL/minute guidelines.

Available Dosage Forms [DSC] = Discontinued product

Capsule, as trihydrate: 250 mg, 500 mg

Amoxil®: 250 mg [DSC], 500 mg

Moxilin®, Trimox®: 250 mg, 500 mg

(Continued)

Amoxicillin *(Continued)*

Powder for oral suspension, as trihydrate: 125 mg/5 mL (80 mL, 100 mL, 150 mL); 200 mg/5 mL (50 mL, 75 mL, 100 mL); 250 mg/5 mL (80 mL, 100 mL, 150 mL); 400 mg/5 mL (50 mL, 75 mL, 100 mL)

Amoxil®: 125 mg/5 mL (150 mL) [contains sodium benzoate; strawberry flavor] [DSC]; 200 mg/5 mL (5 mL, 50 mL, 75 mL, 100 mL) [contains sodium benzoate; bubble gum flavor]; 250 mg/5 mL (100 mL, 150 mL) [contains sodium benzoate; bubble gum flavor]; 400 mg/5 mL (5 mL, 50 mL, 75 mL, 100 mL) [contains sodium benzoate; bubble gum flavor]

Moxilin®: 250 mg/5 mL (100 mL, 150 mL)

Trimox®: 125 mg/5 mL (80 mL, 100 mL, 150 mL); 250 mg/5 mL (80 mL, 100 mL, 150 mL) [contains sodium benzoate; raspberry-strawberry flavor]

Powder for oral suspension, as trihydrate [drops] (Amoxil®): 50 mg/mL (15 mL [DSC], 30 mL) [bubble gum flavor]

Tablet, as trihydrate [film coated] (Amoxil®): 500 mg, 875 mg

Tablet, chewable, as trihydrate: 125 mg, 200 mg, 250 mg, 400 mg

Amoxil®: 200 mg [contains phenylalanine 1.82 mg/tablet; cherry banana peppermint flavor]; 400 mg [contains phenylalanine 3.64 mg/tablet; cherry banana peppermint flavor]

Tablet, for oral suspension, as trihydrate (DisperMox™): 200 mg [contains phenylalanine 5.6 mg; strawberry flavor]; 400 mg [contains phenylalanine 5.6 mg; strawberry flavor]; 600 mg [contains phenylalanine 11.23 mg; strawberry flavor]

Nursing Guidelines

Assessment: Assess for allergy history prior to starting therapy. See Contraindications and Warnings/Precautions for use cautions. Assess potential for interactions with other prescriptions, OTC medications, or herbal products patient may be taking (see Drug Interactions). Caution patients with diabetes about altered response to Clinitest®. Assess for therapeutic effectiveness and adverse reactions (eg, opportunistic infection: fever, chills, unhealed sores, white plaques in mouth or vagina, purulent vaginal discharge, fatigue - see Adverse Reactions and Overdose/Toxicology). Teach patient proper use, possible side effects/appropriate interventions, and adverse symptoms to report (see Patient Education).

Monitoring Laboratory Tests: Perform culture and sensitivity testing prior to initiating therapy.

Dietary Considerations: May be taken with food. Amoxil® chewable contains phenylalanine 1.82 mg per 200 mg tablet, phenylalanine 3.64 mg per 400 mg tablet. DisperMox™ contains phenylalanine 5.6 mg in each 200 mg and 400 mg tablet.

Patient Education: Inform prescriber of all prescriptions, OTC medications, or herbal products you are taking, and any allergies you have. Do not take any new medication during therapy unless approved by prescriber. Take entire prescription, even if you are feeling better. Take at equal intervals around-the-clock. May be taken with milk, juice, or food. If you have diabetes, drug may cause false test results with Clinitest® urine glucose monitoring; use of another type of glucose monitoring is preferable. May cause nausea or vomiting (small, frequent meals, frequent mouth care, sucking lozenges, or chewing gum may help). Report rash; unusual diarrhea; vaginal itching, burning, or pain; unresolved vomiting or constipation; fever or chills; abdominal pain; jaundice; unusual bruising or bleeding; or if condition being treated worsens or does not improve by the time prescription is completed.

Geriatric Considerations: Resistance to amoxicillin has been a problem in patients on frequent antibiotics or in nursing homes. Alternative antibiotics may be necessary in these populations. Consider renal function.

Pregnancy Risk Factor: B

Lactation: Enters breast milk/compatible

Administration

Oral: Administer around-the-clock to promote less variation in peak and trough serum levels. The appropriate amount of suspension may be mixed with formula, milk, fruit juice, water, ginger ale, or cold drinks; administer dose immediately after mixing.

DisperMox™: Dissolve 1 tablet in ~10 mL of water immediately before administration. Rinse container with additional water and drink entire contents to ensure that complete dose is taken. Do not chew or swallow tablet whole.

Some penicillins (eg, carbenicillin, ticarcillin, and piperacillin) have been shown to inactivate aminoglycosides *in vitro*. This has been observed to a greater extent with tobramycin and gentamicin, while amikacin has shown greater stability against inactivation. Concurrent use of these agents may pose a risk of reduced antibacterial efficacy *in vivo*, particularly in the setting of profound renal impairment. However, definitive clinical evidence is lacking. If combination penicillin/aminoglycoside therapy is desired in a patient with renal dysfunction, separation of doses (if feasible), and routine monitoring of aminoglycoside levels, CBC, and clinical response should be considered.

Reconstitution: DisperMox™: Dissolve 1 tablet in ~10 mL water immediately before use.

Storage: Amoxil®: Oral suspension remains stable for 14 days at room temperature or if refrigerated (refrigeration preferred); unit-dose antibiotic oral syringes are stable for 48 hours.

Amoxicillin and Clavulanate Potassium

(a moks i SIL in & klav yoo LAN ate poe TASS ee um)

U.S. Brand Names Augmentin®; Augmentin ES-600®; Augmentin XR™

Synonyms Amoxicillin and Clavulanic Acid; Clavulanic Acid and Amoxicillin

Pharmacologic Category Antibiotic, Penicillin

Medication Safety Issues

Sound-alike/look-alike issues:

Augmentin® may be confused with Azulfidine®

Use Treatment of otitis media, sinusitis, and infections caused by susceptible organisms involving the lower respiratory tract, skin and skin structure, and urinary tract; spectrum same as amoxicillin with additional coverage of beta-lactamase producing *B. catarrhalis*, *H. influenzae*, *N. gonorrhoeae*, and *S. aureus* (not MRSA). The expanded coverage of this combination makes it a useful alternative when amoxicillin resistance is present and patients cannot tolerate alternative treatments.

Mechanism of Action Clavulanic acid binds and inhibits beta-lactamases that inactivate amoxicillin resulting in amoxicillin having an expanded spectrum of activity. Amoxicillin inhibits bacterial cell wall synthesis by binding to one or more of the penicillin-binding proteins (PBPs); which in turn inhibits the final transpeptidation step of peptidoglycan synthesis in bacterial cell walls, thus inhibiting cell wall biosynthesis. Bacteria eventually lyse due to ongoing activity of cell wall autolytic enzymes (autolysins and murein hydrolases) while cell wall assembly is arrested.

Pharmacodynamics/Kinetics Amoxicillin pharmacokinetics are not affected by clavulanic acid.

Amoxicillin: See Amoxicillin monograph.

Clavulanic acid:

Metabolism: Hepatic

Excretion: Urine (30% to 40% as unchanged drug)

Contraindications Hypersensitivity to amoxicillin, clavulanic acid, penicillin, or any component of the formulation; history of cholestatic jaundice or hepatic dysfunction with amoxicillin/clavulanate potassium therapy; Augmentin XR™: severe renal impairment (Cl_{cr} <30 mL/minute) and hemodialysis patients

Warnings/Precautions Hypersensitivity reactions, including anaphylaxis (some fatal), have been reported. Prolonged use may result in superinfection, including *Pseudomembranous colitis*. In patients with renal impairment, doses and/or frequency of administration should be modified in response to the degree of renal impairment. High percentage of patients with infectious mononucleosis have developed rash during therapy. Incidence of diarrhea is higher than with amoxicillin alone. Use caution in patients with hepatic dysfunction. Hepatic dysfunction, although rare, is more common in elderly and/or males, and occurs more frequently with prolonged treatment, and may occur after therapy is complete. Due to differing content of clavulanic acid, not all formulations are interchangeable. Low incidence of cross-allergy with cephalosporins exists. Some products contain phenylalanine.

Drug Interactions

Allopurinol: Additive potential for amoxicillin rash

Aminoglycosides: May be synergistic against selected organisms

Methotrexate: Penicillins may increase the exposure to methotrexate during concurrent therapy; monitor.

Oral contraceptives: Anecdotal reports suggesting decreased contraceptive efficacy with penicillins have been refuted by more rigorous scientific and clinical data.

Probenecid: May increase levels of penicillins (amoxicillin); concomitant use not recommended.

(Continued)

Amoxicillin and Clavulanate Potassium *(Continued)*

Warfarin: Effects of warfarin may be increased

Lab Interactions Urinary glucose (Benedict's solution, Clinitest®, Fehling's solution)

Some penicillin derivatives may accelerate the degradation of aminoglycosides *in vitro*, leading to a potential underestimation of aminoglycoside serum concentration.

Augmentin® Product-Specific Considerations

Strength	Form	Consideration
125 mg	CT, S	q8h dosing
	S	For adults having difficulty swallowing tablets, 125 mg/5 mL suspension may be substituted for 500 mg tablet.
200 mg	CT, S	q12h dosing
	CT	Contains phenylalanine
	S	For adults having difficulty swallowing tablets, 200 mg/5 mL suspension may be substituted for 875 mg tablet.
250 mg	CT, S, T	q8h dosing
	CT	Contains phenylalanine
	T	Not for use in patients <40 kg
	CT, T	Tablet and chewable tablet are not interchangeable due to differences in clavulanic acid.
	S	For adults having difficulty swallowing tablets, 250 mg/5 mL suspension may be substituted for 500 mg tablet.
400 mg	CT, S	q12h dosing
	CT	Contains phenylalanine
	S	For adults having difficulty swallowing tablets, 400 mg/5 mL suspension may be substituted for 875 mg tablet.
500 mg	T	q8h or q12h dosing
600 mg	S	q12h dosing
		Contains phenylalanine
		Not for use in adults or children ≥40 kg
		600 mg/5 mL suspension is not equivalent to or interchangeable with 200 mg/5 mL or 400 mg/5 mL due to differences in clavulanic acid.
875 mg	T	q12h dosing; not for use in Cl_{cr} <30 mL/minute
1000 mg	XR	q12h dosing
		Not for use in children <16 years of age
		Not interchangeable with two 500 mg tablets
		Not for use if Cl_{cr} <30 mL/minute or hemodialysis

Legend: CT = chewable tablet, S = suspension, T = tablet, XR = extended release.

Adverse Reactions

>10%: Gastrointestinal: Diarrhea (3% to 34%; incidence varies upon dose and regimen used)

1% to 10%:

Dermatologic: Diaper rash, skin rash, urticaria

Gastrointestinal: Abdominal discomfort, loose stools, nausea, vomiting

Genitourinary: Vaginitis, vaginal mycosis

Miscellaneous: Moniliasis

<1% (Limited to important or life-threatening): Cholestatic jaundice, flatulence, headache, hepatic dysfunction, prothrombin time increased, thrombocytosis

Additional adverse reactions seen with **ampicillin-class antibiotics:** Agitation, agranulocytosis, alkaline phosphatase increased, anaphylaxis, anemia, angioedema, anxiety, behavioral changes, bilirubin increased, black "hairy" tongue, confusion, convulsions, crystalluria, dizziness, enterocolitis, eosinophilia, erythema multiforme, exanthematous pustulosis, exfoliative dermatitis, gastritis, glossitis, hematuria, hemolytic anemia, hemorrhagic colitis, indigestion, insomnia, hyperactivity, interstitial nephritis, leukopenia, mucocutaneous candidiasis, pruritus, pseudomembranous colitis, serum sickness-like reaction, Stevens-Johnson syndrome, stomatitis, transaminases increased, thrombocytopenia, thrombocytopenic purpura, tooth discoloration, toxic epidermal necrolysis

Overdosage/Toxicology Symptoms of overdose may include abdominal pain, diarrhea, drowsiness, rash, hyperactivity, stomach pain, and vomiting. Interstitial nephritis and/or crystalluria, possibly resulting in renal failure, may occur; hydration and diuresis may be beneficial. Electrolyte imbalance may occur, especially in renal failure. A study of 51 pediatric overdose victims suggests that ingestion of amoxicillin at doses ≤250 mg/kg do not manifest significant clinical symptoms, and thus do not require gastric lavage. Hemodialysis may be helpful to aid in removal of the drug from blood; otherwise, treatment is supportive or symptom-directed.

Dosing

Adults & Elderly: Note: Dose is based on the amoxicillin component; see "Augmentin® Product-Specific Considerations table" on previous page.

Susceptible infections: Oral: Children >40 kg and Adults: 250-500 mg every 8 hours or 875 mg every 12 hours

Acute bacterial sinusitis: Oral: Extended release tablet: Two 1000 mg tablets every 12 hours for 10 days

Community-acquired pneumonia: Oral: Extended release tablet: Two 1000 mg tablets every 12 hours for 7-10 days

Pediatrics: Note: Dose is based on the amoxicillin component; see "Augmentin® Product-Specific Considerations table" on previous page.

Susceptible infections: Oral: Infants <3 months: 30 mg/kg/day divided every 12 hours using the 125 mg/5 mL suspension

Otitis media (Augmentin® ES-600): Oral: Children ≥3 months and <40 kg: 90 mg/kg/day divided every 12 hours for 10 days in children with severe illness and when coverage for β-lactamase positive *H. influenzae* and *M. catarrhalis* is needed.

Lower respiratory tract infections, severe infections, sinusitis: Oral: Children ≥3 months and <40 kg: 45 mg/kg/day divided every 12 hours **or** 40 mg/kg/day divided every 8 hours

Less severe infections: Oral: Children ≥3 months and <40 kg: 25 mg/kg/day divided every 12 hours or 20 mg/kg/day divided every 8 hours

Children >40 kg: Refer to adult dosing.

Renal Impairment:

Cl_{cr} <30 mL/minute: Do not use 875 mg tablet or extended release tablets.

Cl_{cr} 10-30 mL/minute: 250-500 mg every 12 hours

Cl_{cr} <10 mL/minute: 250-500 every 24 hours

Hemodialysis: Moderately dialyzable (20% to 50%)

250-500 mg every 24 hours; administer dose during and after dialysis. Do not use extended release tablets.

Peritoneal dialysis: Moderately dialyzable (20% to 50%)

Amoxicillin: Administer 250 mg every 12 hours

Clavulanic acid: Dose for Cl_{cr} <10 mL/minute

Continuous arteriovenous or venovenous hemofiltration effects:

Amoxicillin: ~50 mg of amoxicillin/L of filtrate is removed

Clavulanic acid: Dose for Cl_{cr} <10 mL/minute

Available Dosage Forms

Powder for oral suspension: 200: Amoxicillin 200 mg and clavulanate potassium 28.5 mg per 5 mL (100 mL) [contains phenylalanine]; 400: Amoxicillin 400 mg and clavulanate potassium 57 mg per 5 mL (100 mL) [contains phenylalanine]; 600: Amoxicillin 600 mg and clavulanic potassium 42.9 mg per 5 mL (75 mL, 125 mL, 200 mL) [contains phenylalanine]

Augmentin®:

125: Amoxicillin 125 mg and clavulanate potassium 31.25 mg per 5 mL (75 mL, 100 mL, 150 mL) [banana flavor]

200: Amoxicillin 200 mg and clavulanate potassium 28.5 mg per 5 mL (50 mL, 75 mL, 100 mL) [contains phenylalanine 7 mg/5 mL; orange-raspberry flavor]

250: Amoxicillin 250 mg and clavulanate potassium 62.5 mg per 5 mL (75 mL, 100 mL, 150 mL) [orange flavor]

400: Amoxicillin 400 mg and clavulanate potassium 57 mg per 5 mL (50 mL, 75 mL, 100 mL) [contains phenylalanine 7 mg/5 mL; orange-raspberry flavor]

Augmentin ES-600®: Amoxicillin 600 mg and clavulanic potassium 42.9 mg per 5 mL (75 mL, 125 mL, 200 mL) [contains phenylalanine 7 mg/5 mL; strawberry cream flavor]

Tablet: 500: Amoxicillin trihydrate 500 mg and clavulanate potassium 125 mg; 875: Amoxicillin trihydrate 875 mg and clavulanate potassium 125 mg

Augmentin®:

250: Amoxicillin trihydrate 250 mg and clavulanate potassium 125 mg

(Continued)

Amoxicillin and Clavulanate Potassium *(Continued)*

500: Amoxicillin trihydrate 500 mg and clavulanate potassium 125 mg
875: Amoxicillin trihydrate 875 mg and clavulanate potassium 125 mg

Tablet, chewable: 200: Amoxicillin trihydrate 200 mg and clavulanate potassium 28.5 mg [contains phenylalanine]; 400: Amoxicillin trihydrate 400 mg and clavulanate potassium 57 mg [contains phenylalanine]

Augmentin®:

125: Amoxicillin trihydrate 125 mg and clavulanate potassium 31.25 mg [lemon-lime flavor]

200: Amoxicillin trihydrate 200 mg and clavulanate potassium 28.5 mg [contains phenylalanine 2.1 mg/tablet; cherry-banana flavor]

250: Amoxicillin trihydrate 250 mg and clavulanate potassium 62.5 mg [lemon-lime flavor]

400: Amoxicillin trihydrate 400 mg and clavulanate potassium 57 mg [contains phenylalanine 4.2 mg/tablet; cherry-banana flavor]

Tablet, extended release (Augmentin XR™): Amoxicillin 1000 mg and clavulanic acid 62.5 mg [contains potassium 29.3 mg (1.27 mEq) and sodium 12.6 mg (0.32 mEq)

Nursing Guidelines

Assessment: Assess for allergy history prior to starting therapy. See Contraindications and Warnings/Precautions for use cautions. Assess potential for interactions with other prescriptions, OTC medications, or herbal products patient may be taking (see Drug Interactions). Caution patients with diabetes about altered response to Clinitest®. Assess results of laboratory tests (see below), therapeutic effectiveness, and adverse reactions (eg, opportunistic infection: fever, chills, unhealed sores, white plaques in mouth or vagina, purulent vaginal discharge, fatigue - see Adverse Reactions and Overdose/Toxicology). Teach patient proper use, possible side effects/appropriate interventions, and adverse symptoms to report (see Patient Education). Note breast-feeding caution.

Monitoring Laboratory Tests: Renal, hepatic, and hematologic function periodically with prolonged therapy. Perform culture and sensitivity testing prior to initiating therapy.

Dietary Considerations: May be taken with meals or on an empty stomach; take with meals to increase absorption and decrease GI intolerance; may mix with milk, formula, or juice. Extended release tablets should be taken with food. Some products contain phenylalanine; avoid use in phenylketonurics. All dosage forms contain potassium.

Patient Education: Inform prescriber of all prescriptions, OTC medications, or herbal products you are taking, and any allergies you have. Do not take any new medication during therapy unless approved by prescriber. Take as directed, for as long as directed, even if you are feeling better. (For small children, bottles may contain more suspension than needed, take for number of days prescribed.) Take at equal intervals around-the-clock; may be taken with milk, juice, or food. Extended release tablets should be taken with food. If you have diabetes, drug may cause false test results with Clinitest® urine glucose monitoring; use of another type of glucose monitoring is preferable. May cause nausea or vomiting (small, frequent meals, frequent mouth care, sucking lozenges, or chewing gum may help). Report rash; unusual diarrhea; vaginal itching, burning, or pain; unresolved vomiting or constipation; fever or chills; abdominal pain; jaundice; unusual bruising or bleeding; or if condition being treated worsens or does not improve by the time prescription is completed. Some products contain phenylalanine. Avoid use in phenylketonurics. **Breast-feeding precaution:** Consult prescriber if breast-feeding.

Geriatric Considerations: Resistance to amoxicillin has been a problem in patients on frequent antibiotics or in nursing homes. However, expanded coverage of this combination makes it a useful alternative when amoxicillin resistance is present and patients cannot tolerate alternative treatments. Consider renal function. Considered one of the drugs of choice in the outpatient treatment of community-acquired pneumonia in older adults.

Pregnancy Risk Factor: B

Pregnancy Issues: Both amoxicillin and clavulanate potassium cross the human placenta. Teratogenic effects have not been reported. Use in women with premature rupture of fetal membranes may increase risk of necrotizing enterocolitis in neonates.

Lactation: Enters breast milk/use caution (AAP rates "compatible")

Breast-Feeding Considerations: The AAP considers amoxicillin to be "compatible" with breast-feeding.

Administration

Oral: Administer around-the-clock to promote less variation in peak and trough serum levels. Administer with food to decrease stomach upset; shake suspension well before use. Extended release tablets should be administered with food.

Some penicillins (eg, carbenicillin, ticarcillin, and piperacillin) have been shown to inactivate aminoglycosides *in vitro*. This has been observed to a greater extent with tobramycin and gentamicin, while amikacin has shown greater stability against inactivation. Concurrent use of these agents may pose a risk of reduced antibacterial efficacy *in vivo*, particularly in the setting of profound renal impairment. However, definitive clinical evidence is lacking. If combination penicillin/aminoglycoside therapy is desired in a patient with renal dysfunction, separation of doses (if feasible), and routine monitoring of aminoglycoside levels, CBC, and clinical response should be considered.

Reconstitution: Reconstitute powder for oral suspension with appropriate amount of water as specified on the bottle. Shake vigorously until suspended. Reconstituted oral suspension should be kept in refrigerator. Discard unused suspension after 10 days. Unit-dose antibiotic oral syringes are stable for 48 hours.

Storage:

Powder for oral suspension: Store dry powder at room temperature of 25°C (77°F).

Tablet: Store at room temperature of 25°C (77°F).

♦ **Amoxicillin and Clavulanic Acid** *see* Amoxicillin and Clavulanate Potassium *on page 147*

♦ **Amoxicillin Trihydrate** *see* Amoxicillin *on page 144*

♦ **Amoxil®** *see* Amoxicillin *on page 144*

♦ **Amoxycillin** *see* Amoxicillin *on page 144*

♦ **Amphadase™** *see* Hyaluronidase *on page 858*

♦ **Amphetamine and Dextroamphetamine** *see* Dextroamphetamine and Amphetamine *on page 507*

♦ **Amphocin®** *see* Amphotericin B (Conventional) *on page 151*

Amphotericin B (Conventional)

(am foe TER i sin bee con VEN sha nal)

U.S. Brand Names Amphocin®

Synonyms Amphotericin B Desoxycholate

Pharmacologic Category Antifungal Agent, Parenteral

Medication Safety Issues

Safety issues:

Conventional amphotericin formulations (Amphocin®, Fungizone®) may be confused with lipid-based formulations (AmBisome®, Abelcet®, Amphotec®).

Large overdoses have occurred when conventional formulations were dispensed inadvertently for lipid-based products. Single daily doses of conventional amphotericin formulation never exceed 1.5 mg/kg.

Use Treatment of severe systemic and central nervous system infections caused by susceptible fungi such as *Candida* species, *Histoplasma capsulatum*, *Cryptococcus neoformans*, *Aspergillus* species, *Blastomyces dermatitidis*, *Torulopsis glabrata*, and *Coccidioides immitis*; fungal peritonitis; irrigant for bladder fungal infections; used in fungal infection in patients with bone marrow transplantation, amebic meningoencephalitis, ocular aspergillosis (intraocular injection), candidal cystitis (bladder irrigation), chemoprophylaxis (low-dose I.V.), immunocompromised patients at risk of aspergillosis (intranasal/nebulized), refractory meningitis (intrathecal), coccidioidal arthritis (intra-articular/I.M.).

Low-dose amphotericin B has been administered after bone marrow transplantation to reduce the risk of invasive fungal disease.

Mechanism of Action Binds to ergosterol altering cell membrane permeability in susceptible fungi and causing leakage of cell components with subsequent cell death. Proposed mechanism suggests that amphotericin causes an oxidation-dependent stimulation of macrophages (Lyman, 1992).

Pharmacodynamics/Kinetics

Distribution: Minimal amounts enter the aqueous humor, bile, CSF (inflamed or noninflamed meninges), amniotic fluid, pericardial fluid, pleural fluid, and synovial fluid

Protein binding, plasma: 90%

Half-life elimination: Biphasic: Initial: 15-48 hours; Terminal: 15 days

(Continued)

Amphotericin B (Conventional) *(Continued)*

Time to peak: Within 1 hour following a 4- to 6-hour dose

Excretion: Urine (2% to 5% as biologically active form); ~40% eliminated over a 7-day period and may be detected in urine for at least 7 weeks after discontinued use

Contraindications Hypersensitivity to amphotericin or any component of the formulation

Warnings/Precautions Anaphylaxis has been reported with other amphotericin B-containing drugs. During the initial dosing, the drug should be administered under close clinical observation. Avoid use with other nephrotoxic drugs; drug-induced renal toxicity usually improves with interrupting therapy, decreasing dosage, or increasing dosing interval. Infusion reactions are most common 1-3 hours after starting the infusion and diminish with continued therapy. Use amphotericin B with caution in patients with decreased renal function. Pulmonary reactions may occur in neutropenic patients receiving leukocyte transfusions; separation of the infusions as much as possible is advised.

Drug Interactions

Increased nephrotoxicity: Aminoglycosides, cyclosporine, other nephrotoxic drugs

Potentiation of hypokalemia: Corticosteroids, corticotropin

Increased digitalis and neuromuscular-blocking agent toxicity due to hypokalemia

Decreased effect: Pharmacologic antagonism may occur with azole antifungal agents (eg, miconazole, ketoconazole)

Pulmonary toxicity has occurred with concomitant administration of amphotericin B and leukocyte transfusions

Lab Interactions Increased BUN (S), serum creatinine, alkaline phosphate, bilirubin; decreased magnesium, potassium (S)

Adverse Reactions

Systemic:

>10%:

Cardiovascular: Hypotension, tachypnea

Central nervous system: Fever, chills, headache (less frequent with I.T.), malaise

Endocrine & metabolic: Hypokalemia, hypomagnesemia

Gastrointestinal: Anorexia, nausea (less frequent with I.T.), vomiting (less frequent with I.T.), diarrhea, heartburn, cramping epigastric pain

Hematologic: Normochromic-normocytic anemia

Local: Pain at injection site with or without phlebitis or thrombophlebitis (incidence may increase with peripheral infusion of admixtures)

Neuromuscular & skeletal: Generalized pain, including muscle and joint pains (less frequent with I.T.)

Renal: Decreased renal function and renal function abnormalities including azotemia, renal tubular acidosis, nephrocalcinosis (>0.1 mg/mL)

1% to 10%:

Cardiovascular: Hypertension, flushing

Central nervous system: Delirium, arachnoiditis, pain along lumbar nerves (especially I.T. therapy)

Genitourinary: Urinary retention

Hematologic: Leukocytosis

Neuromuscular & skeletal: Paresthesia (especially with I.T. therapy)

<1% (Limited to important or life-threatening): Acute liver failure, agranulocytosis, anuria, bone marrow suppression, cardiac arrest, coagulation defects, convulsions, dyspnea, hearing loss, leukopenia, maculopapular rash, renal failure, renal tubular acidosis, thrombocytopenia, vision changes

Overdosage/Toxicology Symptoms of overdose include renal dysfunction, cardiac arrest, anemia, thrombocytopenia, granulocytopenia, fever, nausea, and vomiting. Treatment is supportive.

Dosing

Adults & Elderly:

Note: Premedication: For patients who experience infusion-related immediate reactions, premedicate with the following drugs 30-60 minutes prior to drug administration: NSAID (with or without diphenhydramine) **or** acetaminophen with diphenhydramine **or** hydrocortisone 50-100 mg. If the patient experiences rigors during the infusion, meperidine may be administered.

Test dose: I.V.: 1 mg infused over 20-30 minutes. Many clinicians believe a test dose is unnecessary.

Systemic fungal infections: I.V.: Maintenance dose: Usual: 0.25-1.5 mg/kg/day; 1-1.5 mg/kg over 4-6 hours every other day may be given once therapy is established. Aspergillosis, mucormycosis, rhinocerebral phycomycosis often require 1-1.5 mg/kg/day; do not exceed 1.5 mg/kg/day.

Duration of therapy varies with nature of infection: Usual duration is 4-12 weeks or cumulative dose of 1-4 g.

Meningitis, coccidioidal or cryptococcal: I.T.: Initial: 25-300 mcg every 48-72 hours; increase to 500 mcg to 1 mg as tolerated; maximum total dose: 15 mg has been suggested.

Cystitis (Candidal): Bladder irrigation: Irrigate with 50 mcg/mL solution instilled periodically or continuously for 5-10 days or until cultures are clear.

Bone marrow transplantation (prophylaxis): I.V.: Low-dose amphotericin B 0.1-0.25 mg/kg/day has been administered after bone marrow transplantation to reduce the risk of invasive fungal disease.

Note: Alternative routes of administration and extemporaneous preparations have been used when standard antifungal therapy is not available (eg, inhalation, intraocular injection, subconjunctival application, intracavitary administration into various joints and the pleural space).

Pediatrics:

Note: Premedication: For patients who experience infusion-related immediate reactions, premedicate with the following drugs 30-60 minutes prior to drug administration: NSAID (with or without diphenhydramine) **or** acetaminophen with diphenhydramine **or** hydrocortisone 50-100 mg. If the patient experiences rigors during the infusion, meperidine may be administered.

Test dose: I.V.: Infants and Children: 0.1 mg/kg/dose to a maximum of 1 mg; infuse over 30-60 minutes. Many clinicians believe a test dose is unnecessary.

Susceptible fungal infections: I.V.: Infants and Children: Maintenance dose: 0.25-1 mg/kg/day given once daily; infuse over 2-6 hours. Once therapy has been established, amphotericin B can be administered on an every-other-day basis at 1-1.5 mg/kg/dose; cumulative dose: 1.5-2 g over 6-10 weeks

Note: Duration of therapy varies with nature of infection: Usual duration is 4-12 weeks or cumulative dose of 1-4 g.

Meningitis, coccidioidal or cryptococcal: I.T.: Children: 25-100 mcg every 48-72 hours; increase to 500 mcg as tolerated

Renal Impairment:

If renal dysfunction is due to the drug, the daily total can be decreased by 50% or the dose can be given every other day. I.V. therapy may take several months.

Poorly dialyzed; no supplemental dose is necessary when using hemo- or peritoneal dialysis or CAVH/CAVHD.

Administration in dialysate: 1-2 mg/L of peritoneal dialysis fluid either with or without low-dose I.V. amphotericin B (a total dose of 2-10 mg/kg given over 7-14 days).

Available Dosage Forms Injection, powder for reconstitution, as desoxycholate: 50 mg

Nursing Guidelines

Assessment: See Contraindications, Warnings/Precautions, and Dosing for use cautions. Assess potential for interactions with other prescriptions, OTC medications, or herbal products patient may be taking (see Drug Interactions). See Administration and Compatibility prior to administering first dose. Assess results of laboratory tests (see below), therapeutic effectiveness, and adverse response (eg, anaphylactoid reactions, acute respiratory distress, hypokalemia, and nephrotoxicity - see Adverse Reactions and Overdose/Toxicology) frequently during therapy. Teach patient appropriate use (topical application or oral solution), possible side effects/appropriate interventions, and adverse symptoms to report (see Patient Education). Breast-feeding is contraindicated.

Monitoring Laboratory Tests: BUN and serum creatinine levels should be determined every other day when therapy is increased and at least weekly thereafter. Monitor serum electrolytes (especially potassium and magnesium), liver function, and CBC. Perform culture and sensitivity testing prior to initiating therapy.

Patient Education: Inform prescriber of all prescriptions, OTC medications, or herbal products you are taking, and any allergies you have. Do not take any new medication during therapy unless approved by prescriber. Take entire prescription, even if you are feeling better. Most skin lesions may take 1-3

(Continued)

Amphotericin B (Conventional) *(Continued)*

weeks of therapy; maintain good personal hygiene to reduce spread and recurrence of lesions. Maintain adequate hydration (2-3 L/day of fluids) unless instructed to restrict fluid intake. May cause nausea, vomiting, or anorexia (small, frequent meals, frequent mouth care, sucking lozenges, or chewing gum may help); generalized muscle or joint paint (consult prescriber for approved analgesic); or hypotension (use caution when rising from sitting or lying position or when climbing stairs). Report severe muscle cramping or weakness; chest pain or palpitations; CNS disturbances; skin rash; change in urinary patterns or difficulty voiding; black stool; unusual bruising or bleeding; or pain, redness, swelling at infusion site. **Breast-feeding precaution:** Do not breast-feed.

Geriatric Considerations: Caution should be exercised and renal function and desired effect monitored closely in older adults.

Pregnancy Risk Factor: B

Lactation: Excretion in breast milk unknown/contraindicated

Perioperative/Anesthesia/Other Concerns: Patients may be premedicated with acetaminophen and diphenhydramine 30 minutes prior to the amphotericin infusion. Meperidine (Demerol®) may help to reduce rigors. Avoid rapid injection (usually 4- to 6-hour infusion required). Dosage adjustments are not necessary with renal impairment. If decreased renal function is due to amphotericin, the daily dose can be decreased by 50% or the dose can be given every other day.

Hydrocortisone may be used in patients with severe or refractory infusion-related reactions. Bolus infusion of normal saline immediately preceding, or immediately preceding and following amphotericin B may reduce drug-induced nephrotoxicity. Risk of nephrotoxicity increases with amphotericin B doses >1 mg/kg/day. Infusion of admixtures more concentrated than 0.25 mg/mL should be limited to patients absolutely requiring volume restriction. Amphotericin B does not have a bacteriostatic constituent, subsequently admixture expiration is determined by sterility more than chemical stability.

Administration

I.V.: May be infused over 4-6 hours. For a patient who experiences chills, fever, hypotension, nausea, or other nonanaphylactic infusion-related reactions, premedicate with the following drugs 30-60 minutes prior to drug administration: A nonsteroidal (eg, ibuprofen, choline magnesium trisalicylate) with or without diphenhydramine **or** acetaminophen with diphenhydramine **or** hydrocortisone 50-100 mg. If the patient experiences rigors during the infusion, meperidine may be administered. Bolus infusion of normal saline immediately preceding, or immediately preceding and following amphotericin B may reduce drug-induced nephrotoxicity. Risk of nephrotoxicity increases with amphotericin B doses >1 mg/kg/day. Infusion of admixtures more concentrated than 0.25 mg/mL should be limited to patients absolutely requiring volume contraction.

Reconstitution: Add 10 mL of SWFI (without a bacteriostatic agent) to each vial of amphotericin B. Further dilute with 250-500 mL D_5W; final concentration should not exceed 0.1 mg/mL (peripheral infusion) or 0.25 mg/mL (central infusion).

Compatibility: Solution is **incompatible** with ampicillin, calcium gluconate, carbenicillin, cimetidine, dopamine, gentamicin, lidocaine, potassium chloride, sodium chloride, tetracycline, verapamil.

Storage: Store intact vials under refrigeration; protect from light. Reconstituted vials are stable, protected from light, for 24 hours at room temperature and 1 week when refrigerated. Parenteral admixtures are stable, protected from light, for 24 hours at room temperature and 2 days under refrigeration. Short-term exposure (<24 hours) to light during I.V. infusion does **not** appreciably affect potency.

♦ Amphotericin B Desoxycholate *see* Amphotericin B (Conventional) *on page 151*

Amphotericin B (Lipid Complex)

(am foe TER i sin bee LIP id KOM pleks)

U.S. Brand Names Abelcet®

Synonyms ABLC

Pharmacologic Category Antifungal Agent, Parenteral

Medication Safety Issues

Safety issues:

Lipid-based amphotericin formulations (Abelcet®) may be confused with conventional formulations (Amphocin®, Fungizone®)

Large overdoses have occurred when conventional formulations were dispensed inadvertently for lipid-based products. Single daily doses of conventional amphotericin formulation never exceed 1.5 mg/kg.

Use Treatment of aspergillosis or any type of progressive fungal infection in patients who are refractory to or intolerant of conventional amphotericin B therapy

Unlabeled/Investigational Use Effective in patients with serious *Candida* species infections

Mechanism of Action Binds to ergosterol altering cell membrane permeability in susceptible fungi and causing leakage of cell components with subsequent cell death. Proposed mechanism suggests that amphotericin causes an oxidation-dependent stimulation of macrophages.

Pharmacodynamics/Kinetics

Distribution: V_d: Increases with higher doses; reflects increased uptake by tissues (131 L/kg with 5 mg/kg/day)

Half-life elimination: ~24 hours

Excretion: Clearance: Increases with higher doses (5 mg/kg/day): 400 mL/hour/kg

Contraindications Hypersensitivity to amphotericin or any component of the formulation

Warnings/Precautions Anaphylaxis has been reported with other amphotericin B-containing drugs. Facilities for cardiopulmonary resuscitation should be available during administration due to the possibility of anaphylactic reaction. If severe respiratory distress occurs, the infusion should be immediately discontinued. During the initial dosing, the drug should be administered under close clinical observation. Acute reactions (including fever and chills) may occur 1-2 hours after starting an intravenous infusion. These reactions are usually more common with the first few doses and generally diminish with subsequent doses. Pulmonary reactions may occur in neutropenic patients receiving leukocyte transfusions; separation of the infusions as much as possible is advised.

Drug Interactions

Increased nephrotoxicity: Aminoglycosides, cyclosporine, other nephrotoxic drugs

Potentiation of hypokalemia: Corticosteroids, corticotropin

Increased digitalis and neuromuscular-blocking agent toxicity due to hypokalemia

Decreased effect: Pharmacologic antagonism may occur with azole antifungal agents (eg, miconazole, ketoconazole)

Pulmonary toxicity has occurred with concomitant administration of amphotericin B and leukocyte transfusions

Lab Interactions Increased BUN (S), serum creatinine, alkaline phosphate, bilirubin; decreased magnesium, potassium (S)

Adverse Reactions Nephrotoxicity and infusion-related hyperpyrexia, rigor, and chilling are reduced relative to amphotericin deoxycholate.

>10%:

- Central nervous system: Chills, fever
- Renal: Serum creatinine increased
- Miscellaneous: Multiple organ failure

1% to 10%:

- Cardiovascular: Hypotension, cardiac arrest
- Central nervous system: Headache, pain
- Dermatologic: Rash
- Endocrine & metabolic: Bilirubinemia, hypokalemia, acidosis
- Gastrointestinal: Nausea, vomiting, diarrhea, gastrointestinal hemorrhage, abdominal pain
- Renal: Renal failure
- Respiratory: Respiratory failure, dyspnea, pneumonia

Dosing

Adults & Elderly:

Note: Premedication: For patients who experience infusion-related immediate reactions, premedicate with the following drugs 30-60 minutes prior to drug administration: A nonsteroidal anti-inflammatory agent ± diphenhydramine **or** acetaminophen with diphenhydramine **or** hydrocortisone 50-100 mg. If the patient experiences rigors during the infusion, meperidine may be administered.

Usual dosage: I.V.: 2.5-5 mg/kg/day as a single infusion

Pediatrics: Refer to adult dosing.

Renal Impairment: The effects of renal impairment on drug pharmacokinetics or pharmacodynamics are currently unknown. The dose of amphotericin B lipid complex may be adjusted or drug administration may have to be interrupted in

(Continued)

Amphotericin B (Lipid Complex) *(Continued)*

patients with acute kidney dysfunction to reduce the magnitude of renal impairment.

Hemodialysis: Supplemental dose is not necessary.

Peritoneal dialysis: Supplemental dose is not necessary.

Continuous arteriovenous or venovenous hemofiltration: Supplemental dose is not necessary.

Available Dosage Forms Injection, suspension [preservative free]: 5 mg/mL (20 mL)

Nursing Guidelines

Assessment: See Warnings/Precautions, Contraindications, Dosing, and Administration for use cautions. Assess potential for interactions with other prescriptions, OTC medications, or herbal products patient may be taking (see Drug Interactions). See Administration prior to administering first infusion. Patient should be monitored closely for adverse response (eg, anaphylactoid reaction, hypokalemia, and nephrotoxicity - see Adverse Reactions and Overdose/Toxicology). Assess results of laboratory tests (see below) and therapeutic effectiveness frequently during therapy. Teach patient possible side effects/appropriate interventions and adverse symptoms to report (see Patient Education). Breast-feeding is contraindicated.

Monitoring Laboratory Tests: BUN and serum creatinine levels should be determined every other day while therapy is increased and at least weekly thereafter. Monitor serum electrolytes (especially potassium and magnesium), liver function, and CBC. Perform culture and sensitivity testing prior to initiating therapy.

Patient Education: Inform prescriber of all prescriptions, OTC medications, or herbal products you are taking, and any allergies you have. Do not take any new medication during therapy unless approved by prescriber. This medication can only be administered by infusion and therapy may last several weeks. Maintain good personal hygiene to reduce spread and recurrence of lesions. Maintain adequate hydration (2-3 L/day of fluids) unless instructed to restrict fluid intake. May cause postural hypotension (use caution when changing from lying or sitting position to standing or when climbing stairs); or nausea or vomiting (small, frequent meals, frequent mouth care, sucking lozenges, or chewing gum may help). Report chest pain or palpitations; CNS disturbances; skin rash; chills or fever; persistent nausea, vomiting, or abdominal pain; sore throat; excessive fatigue; swelling of extremities or unusual weight gain; respiratory difficulty; pain at infusion site; muscle cramping or weakness; or other adverse reactions. **Breast-feeding precaution:** Do not breast-feed.

Geriatric Considerations: Caution should be exercised and renal function and desired effect monitored closely in older adults.

Pregnancy Risk Factor: B

Lactation: Enters breast milk/contraindicated

Breast-Feeding Considerations: Due to limited data, consider discontinuing nursing during therapy.

Perioperative/Anesthesia/Other Concerns: This product is significantly more expensive than conventional amphotericin B. The incidence of nephrotoxicity with ABLC appears to be less when compared to conventional amphotericin B. The incidence of infusion-related reactions does not appear to be decreased with ABLC, but tolerance usually develops. Premedication may be considered to prevent/attenuate infusion-related adverse events. To prevent aggregation of the lipid products, it is important to shake the bag before hanging and once every 2 hours. *In vitro* experiments confirm that liposomal amphotericin B is at least as active as amphotericin B against clinical isolates of *Candida*, *Cryptococcus*, *Blastomyces*, and *Aspergillus*. Their activities also have appeared to be equal against *Fusarium*. Abelcet® may be restricted to patients who cannot tolerate or fail a standard amphotericin B formulation.

Administration

I.V.: For patients who experience nonanaphylactic infusion-related reactions, premedicate 30-60 minutes prior to drug administration with a nonsteroidal anti-inflammatory agent ± diphenhydramine **or** acetaminophen with diphenhydramine **or** hydrocortisone 50-100 mg. If the patient experiences rigors during the infusion, meperidine may be administered.

Invert infusion container several times prior to administration and every 2 hours during infusion.

Reconstitution: Shake vial gently to disperse yellow sediment at bottom of container. Dilute with D_5W to 1-2 mg/mL.

Compatibility: Do not admix or Y-site with any blood products, intravenous drugs, or intravenous fluids other than D_5W.

Storage: Intact vials should be stored at 2°C to 8°C (35°F to 46°F) and protected from exposure to light; do not freeze intact vials. Solutions for infusion are stable for 48 hours under refrigeration and 6 hours at room temperature.

Amphotericin B (Liposomal) (am foe TER i sin bee lye po SO mal)

U.S. Brand Names AmBisome®

Synonyms L-AmB

Pharmacologic Category Antifungal Agent, Parenteral

Medication Safety Issues

Safety issues:

Lipid-based amphotericin formulations (AmBisome®) may be confused with conventional formulations (Amphocin®, Fungizone®)

Large overdoses have occurred when conventional formulations were dispensed inadvertently for lipid-based products. Single daily doses of conventional amphotericin formulation never exceed 1.5 mg/kg.

Use Empirical therapy for presumed fungal infection in febrile, neutropenic patients; treatment of patients with *Aspergillus* species, *Candida* species, and/or *Cryptococcus* species infections refractory to amphotericin B desoxycholate, or in patients where renal impairment or unacceptable toxicity precludes the use of amphotericin B desoxycholate; treatment of cryptococcal meningitis in HIV-infected patients; treatment of visceral leishmaniasis

Unlabeled/Investigational Use Effective in patients with serious *Candida* species infections

Mechanism of Action Binds to ergosterol altering cell membrane permeability in susceptible fungi and causing leakage of cell components with subsequent cell death. Proposed mechanism suggests that amphotericin causes an oxidation-dependent stimulation of macrophages (Lyman, 1992).

Pharmacodynamics/Kinetics

Distribution: V_d: 131 L/kg

Half-life elimination: Terminal: 174 hours

Contraindications Hypersensitivity to amphotericin B or any component of the formulation unless, in the opinion of the treating physician, the benefit of therapy outweighs the risk

Warnings/Precautions Although amphotericin B (liposomal) has been shown to be significantly less toxic than amphotericin B desoxycholate, adverse events may still occur. Patients should be under close clinical observation during initial dosing. As with other amphotericin B-containing products, anaphylaxis has been reported. Facilities for cardiopulmonary resuscitation should be available during administration, and the drug should be administered by medically-trained personnel. Acute reactions (including fever and chills) may occur 1-2 hours after starting infusions; reactions are more common with the first few doses and generally diminish with subsequent doses. Immediately discontinue infusion if severe respiratory distress occurs; the patient should not receive further infusions. Safety and efficacy have not been established in patients <1 year of age.

Drug Interactions

Increased nephrotoxicity: Aminoglycosides, cyclosporine, other nephrotoxic drugs

Potentiation of hypokalemia: Corticosteroids, corticotropin

Increased digitalis and neuromuscular-blocking agent toxicity due to hypokalemia

Decreased effect: Pharmacologic antagonism may occur with azole antifungal agents (eg, miconazole, ketoconazole)

Pulmonary toxicity has occurred with concomitant administration of amphotericin B and leukocyte transfusions

Adverse Reactions Percentage of adverse reactions is dependent upon population studied and may vary with respect to premedications and underlying illness. Incidence of decreased renal function and infusion-related events are lower than rates observed with amphotericin B deoxycholate.

>10%:

Cardiovascular: Peripheral edema (15%), edema (12% to 14%), tachycardia (9% to 18%), hypotension (7% to 14%), hypertension (8% to 20%), chest pain (8% to 12%), hypervolemia (8% to 12%)

Central nervous system: Chills (29% to 48%), insomnia (17% to 22%), headache (9% to 20%), anxiety (7% to 14%), pain (14%), confusion (9% to 13%)

Dermatologic: Rash (5% to 25%), pruritus (11%)

(Continued)

Amphotericin B (Liposomal) *(Continued)*

Endocrine & metabolic: Hypokalemia (31% to 51%), hypomagnesemia (15% to 50%), hyperglycemia (8% to 23%), hypocalcemia (5% to 18%), hyponatremia (8% to 12%)
Gastrointestinal: Nausea (16% to 40%), vomiting (10% to 32%), diarrhea (11% to 30%), abdominal pain (7% to 20%), constipation (15%), anorexia (10% to 14%)
Hematologic: Anemia (27% to 48%), blood transfusion reaction (9% to 18%), leukopenia (15% to 17%), thrombocytopenia (6% to 13%)
Hepatic: Alkaline phosphatase increased (7% to 22%), BUN increased (7% to 21%), bilirubinemia (9% to 18%), ALT increased (15%), AST increased (13%), liver function tests abnormal (not specified) (4% to 13%)
Local: Phlebitis (9% to 11%)
Neuromuscular & skeletal: Weakness (6% to 13%), back pain (12%)
Renal: Creatinine increased (18% to 40%), hematuria (14%)
Respiratory: Dyspnea (18% to 23%), lung disorder (14% to 18%), cough increased (2% to 18%), epistaxis (8% to 15%), pleural effusion (12%), rhinitis (11%)
Miscellaneous: Sepsis (7% to 14%), infection (11% to 12%)

2% to 10% (Limited to important or life-threatening):
Cardiovascular: Arrhythmia, atrial fibrillation, bradycardia, cardiac arrest, cardiomegaly, postural hypotension
Central nervous system: Agitation, coma, convulsion, depression, dizziness (7% to 8%), hallucinations, malaise, somnolence
Dermatologic: Alopecia, rash, petechia, purpura, skin discoloration, urticaria
Endocrine & metabolic: Acidosis, hypernatremia (4%), hyperchloremia, hyperkalemia, hypermagnesemia, hyperphosphatemia, hypophosphatemia
Gastrointestinal: Gastrointestinal hemorrhage (10%), hematemesis, gum/oral hemorrhage, ileus, ulcerative stomatitis
Genitourinary: Vaginal hemorrhage
Hematologic: Coagulation disorder, hemorrhage, prothrombin decreased, thrombocytopenia
Hepatic: Hepatocellular damage, veno-occlusive liver disease
Local: Injection site inflammation
Neuromuscular & skeletal: Arthralgia, bone pain, dystonia, paresthesia, rigors, tremor
Ocular: Conjunctivitis, eye hemorrhage
Renal: Acute kidney failure, toxic nephropathy
Respiratory: Asthma, atelectasis, hemoptysis, pulmonary edema, respiratory alkalosis, respiratory failure, hypoxia (6% to 8%)
Miscellaneous: Allergic reaction, cell-mediated immunological reaction, flu-like syndrome, procedural complication (8% to 10%), diaphoresis (7%)

<1% (Limited to important or life-threatening): Agranulocytosis, angioedema, cyanosis/hypoventilation, erythema, hemorrhagic cystitis, pulmonary edema, urticaria

Overdosage/Toxicology The toxicity due to overdose has not been defined. Repeated daily doses up to 7.5 mg/kg have been administered in clinical trials with no reported dose-related toxicity. If overdosage should occur, cease administration immediately. Symptomatic supportive measures should be instituted. Particular attention should be given to monitoring renal function.

Dosing

Adults & Elderly:

Note: Premedication: For patients who experience chills, fever, hypotension, nausea, or other nonanaphylactic infusion-related immediate reactions, premedicate with the following drugs 30-60 minutes prior to drug administration: A nonsteroidal (eg, ibuprofen, choline magnesium trisalicylate) with or without diphenhydramine **or** acetaminophen with diphenhydramine **or** hydrocortisone 50-100 mg. If the patient experiences rigors during the infusion, meperidine may be administered.

Empiric therapy: I.V.: Recommended initial dose: 3 mg/kg/day

Systemic fungal infections (*Aspergillus*, *Candida*, *Cryptococcus*): I.V.: Recommended initial dose of 3-5 mg/kg/day

Cryptococcal meningitis in HIV-infected patients: I.V.: 6 mg/kg/day

Treatment of visceral leishmaniasis: I.V.:

Immunocompetent patients: 3 mg/kg/day on days 1-5, and 3 mg/kg/day on days 14 and 21; a repeat course may be given in patients who do not achieve parasitic clearance

Immunocompromised patients: 4 mg/kg/day on days 1-5, and 4 mg/kg/day on days 10, 17, 24, 31, and 38

Pediatrics: Refer to adult dosing.

Renal Impairment:

Dosing adjustment in renal impairment: None necessary; effects of renal impairment are not currently known.

Hemodialysis: Supplemental dose is not necessary.

Peritoneal dialysis effects: Supplemental dose is not necessary.

Continuous arteriovenous or venovenous hemofiltration: Supplemental dose is not necessary.

Available Dosage Forms Injection, powder for reconstitution: 50 mg

Nursing Guidelines

Assessment: Assess any history of previous reactions to amphotericin B. See Warnings/Precautions, Contraindications, and Dosing for use cautions. Assess potential for interactions with other prescriptions, OTC medications, or herbal products patient may be taking (see Drug Interactions). See Administration and Compatibility prior to administering first dose. Patient must be monitored closely for adverse reactions (see Adverse Reactions) during and for 2 hours following infusion. Assess results of laboratory tests (see below) during entire course of therapy. Teach patient interventions to reduce side effects, and adverse symptoms to report (see Patient Education). Breast-feeding is contraindicated.

Monitoring Laboratory Tests: BUN and serum creatinine levels should be determined every other day while therapy is increased and at least weekly thereafter. Serum potassium and magnesium should be monitored closely. Monitor electrolytes, liver function, hematocrit, and CBC regularly.

Patient Education: Inform prescriber of all prescriptions, OTC medications, or herbal products you are taking, and any allergies you have. Do not take any new medication during therapy unless approved by prescriber. This drug can only be administered intravenously. You will be monitored during infusion. Report immediately any chills, chest pain, respiratory difficulty, tightness in throat, or other adverse reaction. Personal hygiene is very important to help reduce the spread and recurrence of lesions. Most skin lesions require 1-3 weeks of therapy. Maintain adequate hydration (2-3 L/day of fluids) unless instructed to restrict fluid intake. May cause hypotension (use caution when changing from lying or sitting position to standing or when climbing stairs); or nausea or vomiting (small, frequent meals, frequent mouth care, sucking lozenges, or chewing gum may help). Report any hearing loss, skin rash, dizziness or weakness, muscle or bone pain, changes in color of urine or stool, persistent GI distress, alteration in voiding or bowel patterns, CNS disturbances, pain at injection site, or other adverse reactions. **Breast-feeding precaution:** Do not breast-feed.

Pregnancy Risk Factor: B

Lactation: Excretion in breast milk unknown/contraindicated

Perioperative/Anesthesia/Other Concerns: This product is significantly more expensive than conventional amphotericin B; Infectious Disease consult is recommended. AmBisome® is a true single bilayer liposomal drug delivery system. Liposomes are closed, spherical vesicles created by mixing specific proportions of amphophilic substances such as phospholipids and cholesterol so that they arrange themselves into multiple concentric bilayer membranes when hydrated in aqueous solutions. Single bilayer liposomes are then formed by microemulsification of multilamellar vesicles using a homogenizer. AmBisome® consists of these unilamellar bilayer liposomes with amphotericin B intercalated within the membrane. Due to the nature and quantity of amphophilic substances used, and the lipophilic moiety in the amphotericin B molecule, the drug is an integral part of the overall structure of the AmBisome® liposomes. AmBisome® contains true liposomes that are <100 nm in diameter.

Administration

I.V.: Should be administered by intravenous infusion, using a controlled infusion device, over a period of approximately 2 hours. Infusion time may be reduced to approximately 1 hour in patients in whom the treatment is well-tolerated. If the patient experiences discomfort during infusion, the duration of infusion may be increased. Administer at a rate of 2.5 mg/kg/hour. Discontinue if severe respiratory distress occurs.

For a patient who experiences chills, fever, hypotension, nausea, or other nonanaphylactic infusion-related reactions, premedicate with the following drugs, 30-60 minutes prior to drug administration: A nonsteroidal (eg, ibuprofen,

(Continued)

Amphotericin B (Liposomal) *(Continued)*

choline magnesium trisalicylate) with or without diphenhydramine **or** acetaminophen with diphenhydramine **or** hydrocortisone 50-100 mg. If the patient experiences rigors during the infusion, meperidine may be administered.

Reconstitution: Must be reconstituted using sterile water for injection, USP (without a bacteriostatic agent). Vials containing 50 mg of amphotericin B are prepared as follows.

1. Aseptically add 12 mL of sterile water for injection, USP to each vial to yield a preparation containing 4 mg amphotericin B/mL. **Caution:** Do not reconstitute with saline or add saline to the reconstituted concentration, or mix with other drugs. The use of any solution other than those recommended, or the presence of a bacteriostatic agent in the solution, may cause precipitation.

2. Immediately after the addition of water, **shake the vial vigorously** for 30 seconds to completely disperse the powder; it then forms a yellow, translucent suspension. Visually inspect the vial for particulate matter and continue shaking until completely dispersed.

Filtration and Dilution:

3. Calculate the amount of reconstituted (4 mg/mL) to be further diluted.

4. Withdraw this amount of reconstituted powder into a sterile syringe.

5. Attach the 5-micron filter, provided, to the syringe. Inject the syringe contents through the filter, into the appropriate amount of 5% dextrose injection. (Use only one filter per vial.)

6. Must be diluted with 5% dextrose injection to a final concentration of 1-2 mg/mL prior to administration. Lower concentrations (0.2-0.5 mg/mL) may be appropriate for infants and small children to provide sufficient volume for infusion. **Discard partially used vials.** Injection should commence within 6 hours of dilution with 5% dextrose injection. An in-line membrane filter may be used for the intravenous infusion, provided, **the mean pore diameter of the filter is not less than 1 micron.**

Storage: Unopened vials should be stored at temperatures ≤25°C (77°F).

Ampicillin (am pi SIL in)

U.S. Brand Names Principen®

Synonyms Aminobenzylpenicillin; Ampicillin Sodium; Ampicillin Trihydrate

Pharmacologic Category Antibiotic, Penicillin

Medication Safety Issues

Sound-alike/look-alike issues:

Ampicillin may be confused with aminophylline

Use Treatment of susceptible bacterial infections (nonbeta-lactamase-producing organisms); susceptible bacterial infections caused by streptococci, pneumococci, nonpenicillinase-producing staphylococci, *Listeria*, meningococci; some strains of *H. influenzae*, *Salmonella*, *Shigella*, *E. coli*, *Enterobacter*, and *Klebsiella*

Mechanism of Action Inhibits bacterial cell wall synthesis by binding to one or more of the penicillin-binding proteins (PBPs), which in turn inhibits the final transpeptidation step of peptidoglycan synthesis in bacterial cell walls, thus inhibiting cell wall biosynthesis. Bacteria eventually lyse due to ongoing activity of cell wall autolytic enzymes (autolysins and murein hydrolases) while cell wall assembly is arrested.

Pharmacodynamics/Kinetics

Absorption: Oral: 50%

Distribution: Bile, blister, and tissue fluids; penetration into CSF occurs with inflamed meninges only, good only with inflammation (exceeds usual MICs)

Normal meninges: Nil; Inflamed meninges: 5% to 10%

Protein binding: 15% to 25%

Half-life elimination:

Children and Adults: 1-1.8 hours

Anuria/end-stage renal disease: 7-20 hours

Time to peak: Oral: Within 1-2 hours

Excretion: Urine (~90% as unchanged drug) within 24 hours

Contraindications Hypersensitivity to ampicillin, any component of the formulation, or other penicillins

Warnings/Precautions Dosage adjustment may be necessary in patients with renal impairment. A low incidence of cross-allergy with other beta-lactams exists. High percentage of patients with infectious mononucleosis have developed rash during therapy with ampicillin. Appearance of a rash should be carefully evaluated to differentiate a nonallergic ampicillin rash from a hypersensitivity reaction. Ampicillin rash occurs in 5% to 10% of children receiving ampicillin and is a generalized dull red, maculopapular rash, generally appearing 3-14 days after the start of therapy. It normally begins on the trunk and spreads over most of the body. It may be most intense at pressure areas, elbows, and knees.

Drug Interactions

Allopurinol: Theoretically has an additive potential for ampicillin/amoxicillin rash

Aminoglycosides: May be synergistic against selected organisms

Methotrexate: Penicillins may increase the exposure to methotrexate during concurrent therapy; monitor.

Oral contraceptives: Anecdotal reports suggesting decreased contraceptive efficacy with penicillins have been refuted by more rigorous scientific and clinical data.

Probenecid, disulfiram: May increase levels of penicillins (ampicillin)

Warfarin: Effects of warfarin may be increased

Nutritional/Herbal/Ethanol Interactions Food: Food decreases ampicillin absorption rate; may decrease ampicillin serum concentration.

Lab Interactions Increased protein, positive Coombs' [direct]; alters result of urinary glucose (Benedict's solution, Clinitest®)

Some penicillin derivatives may accelerate the degradation of aminoglycosides *in vitro*, leading to a potential underestimation of aminoglycoside serum concentration.

Adverse Reactions Frequency not defined.

Central nervous system: Fever, penicillin encephalopathy, seizure

Dermatologic: Erythema multiforme, exfoliative dermatitis, rash, urticaria

Note: Appearance of a rash should be carefully evaluated to differentiate (if possible) nonallergic ampicillin rash from hypersensitivity reaction. Incidence is higher in patients with viral infection, *Salmonella* infection, lymphocytic leukemia, or patients that have hyperuricemia.

Gastrointestinal: Black hairy tongue, diarrhea, enterocolitis, glossitis, nausea, pseudomembranous colitis, sore mouth or tongue, stomatitis, vomiting

Hematologic: Agranulocytosis, anemia, hemolytic anemia, eosinophilia, leukopenia, thrombocytopenia purpura

Hepatic: AST increased

Renal: Interstitial nephritis (rare)

Respiratory: Laryngeal stridor

Miscellaneous: Anaphylaxis, serum sickness-like reaction

Overdosage/Toxicology Symptoms of penicillin overdose include neuromuscular hypersensitivity (eg, agitation, hallucinations, asterixis, encephalopathy, confusion, and seizures). Electrolyte imbalance may occur if the preparation contains potassium or sodium salts, especially in renal failure. Hemodialysis may be helpful to aid in removal of the drug from blood; otherwise, treatment is supportive or symptom-directed.

Dosing

Adults:

Usual dosage range:

Oral: 250-500 mg every 6 hours

I.M., I.V.: 250-500 mg every 6 hours

Sepsis/meningitis: I.M., I.V.: 150-250 mg/kg/24 hours divided every 3-4 hours (range: 6-12 g/day)

Endocarditis prophylaxis: I.M., I.V.:

Dental, oral, respiratory tract, or esophageal procedures: 2 g within 30 minutes prior to procedure in patients unable to take oral amoxicillin

Genitourinary and gastrointestinal tract (except esophageal) procedures:

High-risk patients: 2 g within 30 minutes prior to procedure, followed by ampicillin 1 g (or amoxicillin 1 g orally) 6 hours later; must be used in combination with gentamicin.

Moderate-risk patients: 2 g within 30 minutes prior to procedure.

Elderly: Administer usual adult dose unless renal function is markedly reduced.

Pediatrics:

Mild-to-moderate infections: Infants and Children:

I.M., I.V.: 100-150 mg/kg/day in divided doses every 6 hours (maximum: 2-4 g/day)

Oral: 50-100 mg/kg/day in doses divided every 6 hours (maximum: 2-4 g/day)

Severe infections/meningitis: Infants and Children: I.M., I.V.: 200-400 mg/kg/day in divided doses every 6 hours (maximum: 6-12 g/day)

(Continued)

Ampicillin *(Continued)*

Endocarditis prophylaxis: Infants and Children: I.M., I.V.:

Dental, oral, respiratory tract, or esophageal procedures: 50 mg/kg within 30 minutes prior to procedure in patients unable to take oral amoxicillin

Genitourinary and gastrointestinal tract (except esophageal) procedures:

High-risk patients: 50 mg/kg (maximum: 2 g) within 30 minutes prior to procedure, followed by ampicillin 25 mg/kg (or amoxicillin 25 mg/kg orally) 6 hours later; must be used in combination with gentamicin.

Moderate-risk patients: 50 mg/kg within 30 minutes prior to procedure.

Renal Impairment:

Cl_{cr} >50 mL/minute: Administer every 6 hours

Cl_{cr} 10-50 mL/minute: Administer every 6-12 hours

Cl_{cr} <10 mL/minute: Administer every 12-24 hours

Hemodialysis: Moderately dialyzable (20% to 50%); administer dose after dialysis

Peritoneal dialysis: Moderately dialyzable (20% to 50%)

Administer 250 mg every 12 hours

Continuous arteriovenous or venovenous hemofiltration effects: Dose as for Cl_{cr} 10-50 mL/minute; ~50 mg of ampicillin per liter of filtrate is removed

Available Dosage Forms

Capsule (Principen®): 250 mg, 500 mg

Injection, powder for reconstitution, as sodium: 125 mg, 250 mg, 500 mg, 1 g, 2 g, 10 g

Powder for oral suspension (Principen®): 125 mg/5 mL (100 mL, 200 mL); 250 mg/5 mL (100 mL, 200 mL)

Nursing Guidelines

Assessment: Assess for allergy history prior to starting therapy. See Contraindications, Warnings/Precautions, and Dosing for use cautions. Assess potential for interactions with other prescriptions, OTC medications, or herbal products patient may be taking (see Drug Interactions). Caution patients with diabetes about altered response to Clinitest®. Assess results of laboratory tests (see below), therapeutic effectiveness, and adverse reactions (eg, opportunistic infection: fever, chills, unhealed sores, white plaques in mouth or vagina, purulent vaginal discharge, fatigue - see Adverse Reactions and Overdose/Toxicology). Teach patient proper use, possible side effects/appropriate interventions, and adverse symptoms to report (see Patient Education).

Monitoring Laboratory Tests: Perform culture and sensitivity testing prior to initiating therapy.

Dietary Considerations: Take on an empty stomach 1 hour before or 2 hours after meals.

Sodium content of 5 mL suspension (250 mg/5 mL): 10 mg (0.4 mEq)

Sodium content of 1 g: 66.7 mg (3 mEq)

Patient Education: Inform prescriber of all prescriptions, OTC medications, or herbal products you are taking, and any allergies you have. Do not take any new medication during therapy unless approved by prescriber. Take entire prescription, even if you are feeling better. Take at equal intervals around-the-clock; preferably on an empty stomach with a full glass of water (1 hour before or 2 hours after meals). Maintain adequate hydration (2-3 L/day of fluids) unless instructed to restrict fluid intake. If you have diabetes, drug may cause false test results with Clinitest® urine glucose monitoring; use of another type of glucose monitoring is preferable. May cause nausea or vomiting (small, frequent meals, frequent mouth care, sucking lozenges, or chewing gum may help); or diarrhea (buttermilk, boiled milk, or yogurt may help). Report immediately any rash; swelling of face, tongue, mouth, or throat; or chest tightness. Report if condition being treated worsens or does not improve by the time prescription is completed.

Geriatric Considerations: See Drug Interactions and Renal Impairment. Adjust dose for renal impairment.

Pregnancy Risk Factor: B

Lactation: Enters breast milk/use caution

Administration

Oral: Administer around-the-clock to promote less variation in peak and trough serum levels. Administer on an empty stomach (ie, 1 hour prior to, or 2 hours after meals) to increase total absorption.

I.V.: Administer around-the-clock to promote less variation in peak and trough serum levels. Administer over 3-5 minutes (125-500 mg) or over 10-15 minutes

(1-2 g). More rapid infusion may cause seizures. Ampicillin and gentamicin should not be mixed in the same I.V. tubing.

Some penicillins (eg, carbenicillin, ticarcillin, and piperacillin) have been shown to inactivate aminoglycosides *in vitro*. This has been observed to a greater extent with tobramycin and gentamicin, while amikacin has shown greater stability against inactivation. Concurrent use of these agents may pose a risk of reduced antibacterial efficacy *in vivo*, particularly in the setting of profound renal impairment. However, definitive clinical evidence is lacking. If combination penicillin/aminoglycoside therapy is desired in a patient with renal dysfunction, separation of doses (if feasible), and routine monitoring of aminoglycoside levels, CBC, and clinical response should be considered.

Reconstitution: I.V.: Minimum volume: Concentration should not exceed 30 mg/mL due to concentration-dependent stability restrictions. Standard diluent: 500 mg/50 mL NS; 1 g/50 mL NS; 2 g/100 mL NS

Compatibility: Incompatible with D_5W, D_5NS, $D_{10}W$, fat emulsion 10%, hetastarch 6%, LR

Y-site administration: Incompatible with amphotericin B cholesteryl sulfate complex, epinephrine, fluconazole, hydralazine, midazolam, ondansetron, sargramostim, verapamil, vinorelbine

Compatibility in syringe: Incompatible with erythromycin lactobionate, gentamicin, hydromorphone, kanamycin, lincomycin, metoclopramide

Compatibility when admixed: Incompatible with amikacin, chlorpromazine, dopamine, gentamicin, hydralazine, prochlorperazine

Storage:

Oral: Oral suspension is stable for 7 days at room temperature or for 14 days under refrigeration.

I.V.: Solutions for I.M. or direct I.V. should be used within 1 hour. Solutions for I.V. infusion will be inactivated by dextrose at room temperature. If dextrose-containing solutions are to be used, the resultant solution will only be stable for 2 hours versus 8 hours in the 0.9% sodium chloride injection. D_5W has limited stability.

Stability of parenteral admixture in NS at room temperature (25°C) is 8 hours.

Stability of parenteral admixture in NS at refrigeration temperature (4°C) is 2 days.

Ampicillin and Sulbactam (am pi SIL in & SUL bak tam)

U.S. Brand Names Unasyn®

Synonyms Sulbactam and Ampicillin

Pharmacologic Category Antibiotic, Penicillin

Use Treatment of susceptible bacterial infections involved with skin and skin structure, intra-abdominal infections, gynecological infections; spectrum is that of ampicillin plus organisms producing beta-lactamases such as *S. aureus*, *H. influenzae*, *E. coli*, *Klebsiella*, *Acinetobacter*, *Enterobacter*, and anaerobes

Mechanism of Action The addition of sulbactam, a beta-lactamase inhibitor, to ampicillin extends the spectrum of ampicillin to include some beta-lactamase-producing organisms; inhibits bacterial cell wall synthesis by binding to one or more of the penicillin-binding proteins (PBPs), which in turn inhibits the final transpeptidation step of peptidoglycan synthesis in bacterial cell walls, thus inhibiting cell wall biosynthesis. Bacteria eventually lyse due to ongoing activity of cell wall autolytic enzymes (autolysins and murein hydrolases) while cell wall assembly is arrested.

Pharmacodynamics/Kinetics

Ampicillin: See Ampicillin monograph.

Sulbactam:

Distribution: Bile, blister, and tissue fluids

Protein binding: 38%

Half-life elimination: Normal renal function: 1-1.3 hours

Excretion: Urine (~75% to 85% as unchanged drug) within 8 hours

Contraindications Hypersensitivity to ampicillin, sulbactam, penicillins, or any component of the formulations

Warnings/Precautions Dosage adjustment may be necessary in patients with renal impairment. A low incidence of cross-allergy with other beta-lactams exists. High percentage of patients with infectious mononucleosis have developed rash during therapy with ampicillin. Appearance of a rash should be carefully evaluated to differentiate a nonallergic ampicillin rash from a hypersensitivity reaction. Ampicillin rash occurs in 5% to 10% of children receiving ampicillin and is a generalized dull red, maculopapular rash, generally appearing 3-14 days after the start of

(Continued)

Ampicillin and Sulbactam *(Continued)*

therapy. It normally begins on the trunk and spreads over most of the body. It may be most intense at pressure areas, elbows, and knees.

Drug Interactions

Allopurinol: Theoretically has an additive potential for ampicillin/amoxicillin rash

Aminoglycosides: May be synergistic against selected organisms

Methotrexate: Penicillins may increase the exposure to methotrexate during concurrent therapy; monitor.

Oral contraceptives: Anecdotal reports suggesting decreased contraceptive efficacy with penicillins have been refuted by more rigorous scientific and clinical data.

Probenecid, disulfiram: May increase levels of penicillins (ampicillin)

Warfarin: Effects of warfarin may be increased

Lab Interactions False-positive urinary glucose levels (Benedict's solution, Clinitest®); may cause temporary decreases in serum estrogens in pregnant women. Some penicillin derivatives may accelerate the degradation of aminoglycosides *in vitro*, leading to a potential underestimation of aminoglycoside serum concentration.

Adverse Reactions Also see Ampicillin monograph

>10%: Local: Pain at injection site (I.M.)

1% to 10%:

Dermatologic: Rash

Gastrointestinal: Diarrhea

Local: Pain at injection site (I.V.), thrombophlebitis

Miscellaneous: Allergic reaction (may include serum sickness, urticaria, bronchospasm, hypotension, etc)

<1% (Limited to important or life-threatening): Abdominal distension, candidiasis, chest pain, chills, dysuria, edema, epistaxis, erythema, facial swelling, fatigue, flatulence, glossitis, hairy tongue, headache, interstitial nephritis, itching, liver enzymes increased, malaise, mucosal bleeding, nausea, pseudomembranous colitis, seizure, substernal pain, throat tightness, thrombocytopenia, urine retention, vomiting

Overdosage/Toxicology Symptoms of penicillin overdose include neuromuscular hypersensitivity (eg, agitation, hallucinations, asterixis, encephalopathy, confusion, and seizures). Electrolyte imbalance may occur if the preparation contains potassium or sodium salts, especially in renal failure. Hemodialysis may be helpful to aid in removal of the drug from blood; otherwise, treatment is supportive or symptom-directed.

Dosing

Adults & Elderly: Note: Unasyn® (ampicillin/sulbactam) is a combination product. Dosage recommendations for Unasyn® are based on the ampicillin component.

Susceptible infections: I.M., I.V.: 1-2 g ampicillin (1.5-3 g Unasyn®) every 6 hours; maximum: 8 g ampicillin/day (12 g Unasyn®)

Pediatrics: Note: Unasyn® (ampicillin/sulbactam) is a combination product. Dosage recommendations for Unasyn® are based on the ampicillin component.

Mild-to-moderate infections: Children ≥1 year: I.V.: 100-150 mg ampicillin/kg/day (150-300 mg Unasyn®) divided every 6 hours; maximum: 8 g ampicillin/day (12 g Unasyn®)

Severe infections: Children ≥1 year: I.V.: 200-400 mg ampicillin/kg/day divided every 6 hours; maximum: 8 g ampicillin/day (12 g Unasyn®)

Renal Impairment:

Cl_{cr} 15-29 mL/minute: Administer every 12 hours

Cl_{cr} 5-14 mL/minute: Administer every 24 hours

Available Dosage Forms

Injection, powder for reconstitution: 1.5 g [ampicillin sodium 1 g and sulbactam sodium 0.5 g]; 3 g [ampicillin sodium 2 g and sulbactam sodium 1 g]; 15 g [ampicillin sodium 10 g and sulbactam sodium 5 g] [bulk package]

Unasyn®: 1.5 g [ampicillin sodium 1 g and sulbactam sodium 0.5 g]; 3 g [ampicillin sodium 2 g and sulbactam sodium 1 g]; 15 g [ampicillin sodium 10 g and sulbactam sodium 5 g] [bulk package]

Nursing Guidelines

Assessment: Assess for allergy history prior to starting therapy. See Contraindications, Warnings/Precautions, and Dosing for use cautions. Assess potential for interactions with other prescriptions, OTC medications, or herbal products patient may be taking (see Drug Interactions). Caution patients with diabetes about altered response to Clinitest®. Assess results of laboratory tests (see below), therapeutic effectiveness, and adverse reactions (eg, opportunistic infection: fever, chills, unhealed sores, white plaques in mouth or vagina, purulent vaginal discharge, fatigue - see Adverse Reactions and Overdose/Toxicology). Teach possible side effects/appropriate interventions and adverse symptoms to report (see Patient Education). Note breast-feeding caution.

Monitoring Laboratory Tests: Hematologic, renal, and hepatic function with prolonged therapy. Perform culture and sensitivity testing prior to initiating therapy.

Dietary Considerations: Sodium content of 1.5 g injection: 115 mg (5 mEq)

Patient Education: Inform prescriber of all prescriptions, OTC medications, or herbal products you are taking, and any allergies you have. Do not take any new medication during therapy unless approved by prescriber. This medication is administered by infusion/injection. Report immediately pain, redness, swelling, or burning at injection/infusion site or feelings of acute anxiety, chest tightness, or difficulty swallowing. Maintain adequate hydration (2-3 L/day of fluids) unless instructed to restrict fluid intake. If you have diabetes, drug may cause false test results with Clinitest® urine glucose monitoring; use of another type of glucose monitoring is preferable. May cause diarrhea (if persistent, consult prescriber for approved medication). Report rash or persistent, opportunistic infection (eg, fever, chills, unhealed sores, white plaques in mouth or vagina, purulent vaginal discharge, fatigue). **Breast-feeding precaution:** Consult prescriber if breast-feeding caution.

Geriatric Considerations: Adjust dose for renal function.

Pregnancy Risk Factor: B

Lactation: Enters breast milk/use caution

Administration

I.V.: Administer around-the-clock to promote less variation in peak and trough serum levels. Administer by slow injection over 10-15 minutes or I.V. over 15-30 minutes. Ampicillin and gentamicin should not be mixed in the same I.V. tubing.

Some penicillins (eg, carbenicillin, ticarcillin, and piperacillin) have been shown to inactivate aminoglycosides *in vitro*. This has been observed to a greater extent with tobramycin and gentamicin, while amikacin has shown greater stability against inactivation. Concurrent use of these agents may pose a risk of reduced antibacterial efficacy *in vivo*, particularly in the setting of profound renal impairment. However, definitive clinical evidence is lacking. If combination penicillin/aminoglycoside therapy is desired in a patient with renal dysfunction, separation of doses (if feasible), and routine monitoring of aminoglycoside levels, CBC, and clinical response should be considered.

Reconstitution: I.M. and direct I.V. administration: Use within 1 hour after preparation. Reconstitute with sterile water for injection or 0.5% or 2% lidocaine hydrochloride injection (I.M.). Sodium chloride 0.9% (NS) is the diluent of choice for I.V. piggyback use.

Compatibility: Stable in NS

Y-site administration: Incompatible with aminoglycosides (eg, gentamicin, tobramycin), amphotericin B cholesteryl sulfate complex, ciprofloxacin, idarubicin, ondansetron, sargramostim

Compatibility when admixed: Incompatible with aminoglycosides

Storage: Prior to reconstitution, store at ≤30°C (86°F). Solutions made in NS are stable up to 72 hours when refrigerated whereas dextrose solutions (same concentration) are stable for only 4 hours.

- Ampicillin Sodium *see* Ampicillin *on page 160*
- Ampicillin Trihydrate *see* Ampicillin *on page 160*
- Amrinone Lactate *see* Inamrinone *on page 902*

Amyl Nitrite (AM il NYE trite)

Synonyms Isoamyl Nitrite

Pharmacologic Category Antidote; Vasodilator

Use Coronary vasodilator in angina pectoris; adjunct in treatment of cyanide poisoning; produce changes in the intensity of heart murmurs

Mechanism of Action Relaxes vascular smooth muscle; decreased venous ratios and arterial blood pressure; reduces left ventricular work; decreases myocardial O_2 consumption; in cyanide poisoning, amyl nitrite converts hemoglobin to methemoglobin that binds with cyanide to form cyanate hemoglobin

Pharmacodynamics/Kinetics

Onset of action: Angina: Within 30 seconds

Duration: 3-15 minutes

(Continued)

Amyl Nitrite *(Continued)*

Contraindications Hypersensitivity to nitrates; severe anemia; head injury; angle-closure glaucoma; postural hypotension; head trauma or cerebral hemorrhage; pregnancy

Warnings/Precautions Use with caution in patients with increased intracranial pressure, low systolic blood pressure, and coronary artery disease.

Drug Interactions Increased toxicity: Ethanol

Adverse Reactions

1% to 10%:

Cardiovascular: Postural hypotension; cutaneous flushing of head, neck, and clavicular area; tachycardia

Central nervous system: Headache, restlessness

Gastrointestinal: Nausea, vomiting

<1% (Limited to important or life-threatening): Hemolytic anemia

Overdosage/Toxicology Symptoms of overdose include hypotension. Treatment includes general supportive measures.

Dosing

Adults & Elderly:

Angina: Inhalation: 1-6 inhalations from 1 crushed ampul; may repeat in 3-5 minutes

Cyanide poisoning: Inhalation: Inhale the vapor from a 0.3 mL crushed ampul every minute for 15-30 seconds until I.V. sodium nitrite infusion is available

Available Dosage Forms Vapor for inhalation [crushable glass perles]: 0.3 mL

Nursing Guidelines

Assessment: Monitor blood pressure and heart rate closely during and following therapy. **Pregnancy risk factor X.** Breast-feeding is not recommended.

Patient Education: When this drug is used in emergency situations, patient education should be appropriate to situation (ie, do not change positions or make any sudden moves without asking for assistance). If patient administered, lie down during administration, crush ampul in woven covering between fingers, and then hold under nose and inhale. May repeat in 3-5 minutes if necessary. If no relief after three doses, contact emergency services for immediate transport to the hospital. Vapors are highly flammable; do not use where vapors may ignite. **Pregnancy/breast-feeding precautions:** Inform prescriber if you are or intend to become pregnant, may cause severe fetal defects. Breast-feeding is not recommended.

Pregnancy Risk Factor: X

Lactation: Excretion in breast milk unknown/not recommended

Perioperative/Anesthesia/Other Concerns: Highly flammable - do not use where it might be ignited. Amyl nitrate is also used as a recreational drug during intercourse. However, when used in combination with phosphodiesterase-5 enzyme inhibitors, significant and profound hypotension may result.

Administration

Oral: Administer nasally. Keep patient lying down during administration. Crush ampul in woven covering between fingers and then hold under patient's nostrils for 15-30 seconds.

Storage: Store in cool place and protect from light.

Anagrelide (an AG gre lide)

U.S. Brand Names Agrylin®

Synonyms 1370-999-397; Anagrelide Hydrochloride; BL4162A; 6,7-Dichloro-1,5-Dihydroimidazo [2,1b] quinazolin-2(3H)-one Monohydrochloride

Pharmacologic Category Phospholipase A_2 Inhibitor

Use Treatment of essential thrombocythemia (ET) and thrombocythemia associated with chronic myelogenous leukemia (CML), polycythemia vera, and other myeloproliferative disorders

Mechanism of Action Anagrelide appears to inhibit cyclic nucleotide phosphodiesterase and the release of arachidonic acid from phospholipase, possibly by inhibiting phospholipase A_2. It also causes a dose-related reduction in platelet production, which results from decreased megakaryocyte hypermaturation. The drug disrupts the postmitotic phase of maturation.

Pharmacodynamics/Kinetics

Duration: 6-24 hours

Metabolism: Hepatic

Half-life elimination, plasma: 1.3 hours

Time to peak, serum: 1 hour

Excretion: Urine (<1% as unchanged drug)

Contraindications Hypersensitivity to anagrelide or any component of the formulation; severe hepatic impairment

Warnings/Precautions Use caution in patients with known or suspected heart disease; palpitations, orthostatic hypotension, and congestive heart failure have been reported. Use caution in patients with renal dysfunction (serum creatinine ≥2 mg/dL) or hepatic dysfunction (measures of liver function >1.5 times ULN).

Drug Interactions **Substrate** of CYP1A2 (minor)

Drotrecogin alfa: Antiplatelet agents may enhance the adverse/toxic effects of drotrecogin alfa.

NSAIDs: Concurrent use may enhance the adverse/toxic effects of antiplatelet agents.

Salicylates: Concurrent use may enhance the adverse/toxic effects of antiplatelet agents.

Treprostinil: Concurrent use may enhance the adverse/toxic effects of antiplatelet agents.

Nutritional/Herbal/Ethanol Interactions

Ethanol: May increase CNS adverse effects.

Food: No clinically significant effect on absorption.

Adverse Reactions

>10%:

Cardiovascular: Palpitations (27%), edema (other than peripheral: 21%)

Central nervous system: Headache (44%), dizziness (15%), pain (15%)

Gastrointestinal: Diarrhea (26%), nausea (17%), abdominal pain (16%)

Neuromuscular & skeletal: Weakness (23%)

Respiratory: Dyspnea (12%)

1% to 10%:

Cardiovascular: Angina, arrhythmias, cardiovascular disease, chest pain (8%), CHF, hypertension, orthostatic hypotension, peripheral edema (9%), syncope, tachycardia (7%), thrombosis, vasodilatation

Central nervous system: Amnesia, chills, confusion, depression, fever (9%), insomnia, malaise (6%), migraine, nervousness, somnolence

Dermatologic: Alopecia, photosensitivity, pruritus (6%), rash (8%), urticaria

Endocrine & skeletal: Dehydration

Gastrointestinal: Anorexia (8%), aphthous stomatitis, constipation, dyspepsia (5%), eructation, flatulence (10%), gastritis, GI distress, GI hemorrhage, melena, vomiting (10%)

Hematologic: Anemia, ecchymosis, hemorrhage, lymphadenoma, thrombocytopenia

Hepatic: Liver enzymes increased

Neuromuscular & skeletal: Arthralgia, back pain (6%), leg cramps, myalgia, paresthesia (6%)

Ocular: Amblyopia, diplopia, tinnitus, visual field abnormality

Renal: Dysuria, hematuria, renal failure

Respiratory: Asthma, bronchitis, cough (6%), epistaxis, pharyngitis (7%), pneumonia, rhinitis, sinusitis

Miscellaneous: Flu-like syndrome

Frequency not defined: Atrial fibrillation, cardiomegaly, cardiomyopathy, cerebrovascular accident, complete heart block, gastric/duodenal ulceration, leukocyte count increased, MI, pancreatitis, pericarditis, pericardial effusion, pleural effusion, pulmonary fibrosis, pulmonary infiltrates, pulmonary hypertension, seizure

Overdosage/Toxicology There are no reports of human overdosage with anagrelide. Platelet reduction from anagrelide therapy is dose-related; therefore, thrombocytopenia, which can potentially cause bleeding, is expected from overdosage. Should overdosage occur, cardiac and central nervous system toxicity can also be expected. In the case of overdosage, close clinical supervision of the patient is required; this especially includes monitoring of the platelet count for thrombocytopenia. Dosage should be decreased or stopped, as appropriate, until the platelet count returns to within the normal range. Upon discontinuation, platelet counts can be expected to rise in about 4 days.

Dosing

Adults & Elderly: Thrombocythemia (essential or secondary): Oral: 0.5 mg 4 times/day or 1 mg twice daily

Note: Maintain for ≥1 week, then adjust to the lowest effective dose to reduce and maintain platelet count <600,000/µL ideally to the normal range; the dose

(Continued)

Anagrelide *(Continued)*

must not be increased by >0.5 mg/day in any 1 week; maximum dose: 10 mg/day or 2.5 mg/dose

Pediatrics: Thrombocythemia (essential or secondary): Oral: Initial: 0.5 mg/day (range: 0.5 mg 1-4 times/day); see **"Note"** in adult dosing.

Hepatic Impairment:

Moderate impairment: Initial: 0.5 mg once daily; maintain for 1 week with careful monitoring of cardiovascular status

Severe impairment: Contraindicated

Available Dosage Forms Capsule: 0.5 mg, 1 mg

Nursing Guidelines

Monitoring Laboratory Tests: While the platelet count is being lowered (usually during the first 2 weeks of treatment), blood counts (hemoglobin, white blood cells), liver function test (AST, ALT), and renal function (serum creatinine, BUN) should be monitored. Platelet counts should be performed every 2 days during the first week of treatment and at least weekly until the maintenance dose is reached.

Patient Education: Before using this drug, tell your physician your entire medical history, including any allergies (especially drug allergies), heart, kidney, or liver disease. Limit alcohol intake, as it may aggravate side effects. To avoid dizziness and lightheadedness when rising from a seated or lying position, get up slowly. This medication should be used only when clearly needed during pregnancy. Discuss the risks and benefits with your physician. It is not known whether this drug is excreted into breast milk. It is recommended to discontinue the drug or to discontinue breast-feeding, taking into account the risk to the infant. Tell your physician and pharmacist of all nonprescription and prescription medications you may use, especially sucralfate. Do not share this medication with others. Laboratory tests will be done to monitor the effectiveness and possible side effects of this drug.

Pregnancy Risk Factor: C

Lactation: Excretion in breast milk unknown/not recommended

♦ Anagrelide Hydrochloride *see* Anagrelide *on page 166*
♦ Anaprox® *see* Naproxen *on page 1203*
♦ Anaprox® DS *see* Naproxen *on page 1203*
♦ Anaspaz® *see* Hyoscyamine *on page 886*

Anastrozole (an AS troe zole)

U.S. Brand Names Arimidex®

Synonyms ICI-D1033; ZD1033

Pharmacologic Category Aromatase Inhibitor

Use Treatment of locally-advanced or metastatic breast cancer (ER-positive or hormone receptor unknown) in postmenopausal women; treatment of advanced breast cancer in postmenopausal women with disease progression following tamoxifen therapy; adjuvant treatment of early ER-positive breast cancer in postmenopausal women

Mechanism of Action Potent and selective nonsteroidal aromatase inhibitor. By inhibiting aromatase, the conversion of androstenedione to estrone, and testosterone to estradiol, is prevented. Anastrozole causes an 85% decrease in estrone sulfate levels.

Pharmacodynamics/Kinetics

Onset of estradiol reduction: 24 hours (70% reduction; 80% after 2 weeks therapy)

Duration of estradiol reduction: 6 days

Absorption: Well absorbed (80%); not affected by food

Protein binding, plasma: 40%

Metabolism: Extensively hepatic (85%) via N-dealkylation, hydroxylation, and glucuronidation; primary metabolite inactive

Half-life elimination: 50 hours

Excretion: Feces (~75%); urine (10% as unchanged drug; 60% as metabolites)

Contraindications Hypersensitivity to anastrozole or any component of the formulation; pregnancy

Warnings/Precautions Use with caution in patients with hyperlipidemias; total cholesterol and LDL-cholesterol increase in patients receiving anastrozole; exclude pregnancy before initiating therapy. Anastrozole may be associated with a reduction in bone mineral density. Safety and efficacy in premenopausal women or pediatric patients have not been established.

Drug Interactions Inhibits CYP1A2 (weak), 2C8/9 (weak), 3A4 (weak)

Nutritional/Herbal/Ethanol Interactions Herb/Nutraceutical: Avoid black cohosh, hops, licorice, red clover, thyme, and dong quai.

Lab Interactions Lab test abnormalities: GGT, AST, ALT, alkaline phosphatase, total cholesterol, and LDL increased; threefold elevations of mean serum GGT levels have been observed among patients with liver metastases. These changes were likely related to the progression of liver metastases in these patients, although other contributing factors could not be ruled out. Mean serum total cholesterol levels increased by 0.5 mmol/L among patients.

Adverse Reactions

>10%:

Cardiovascular: Vasodilatation (25% to 36%), hypertension (5% to 13%)

Central nervous system: Mood disturbance (19%), pain (11% to 17%), headache (10% to 13%), depression (5% to 13%)

Dermatologic: Rash (6% to 11%)

Endocrine & metabolic: Hot flashes (12% to 36%)

Gastrointestinal: Nausea (11% to 19%), vomiting (8% to 13%)

Neuromuscular & skeletal: Weakness (16% to 19%), arthritis (17%), arthralgia (2% to 15%), back pain (10% to 12%), bone pain (6% to 11%), osteoporosis (11%)

Respiratory: Cough increased (8% to 11%), pharyngitis (6% to 14%)

1% to 10%:

Cardiovascular: Peripheral edema (5% to 10%), chest pain (5% to 7%), ischemic cardiovascular disease (4%), venous thromboembolic events (3% to 4%), ischemic cerebrovascular events (2%), angina (2%)

Central nervous system: Insomnia (6% to 10%), dizziness (8%), anxiety (6%), fever (2% to 5%), malaise (2% to 5%), confusion (2% to 5%), nervousness (2% to 5%), somnolence (2% to 5%), lethargy (1%)

Dermatologic: Alopecia (2% to 5%), pruritus (2% to 5%)

Endocrine & metabolic: Hypercholesterolemia (9%), breast pain (2% to 8%)

Gastrointestinal: Constipation (7% to 9%), abdominal pain (7% to 9%), diarrhea (7% to 9%), anorexia (5% to 7%), xerostomia (6%), dyspepsia (7%), weight gain (2% to 9%), weight loss (2% to 5%)

Genitourinary: Urinary tract infection (8%), vulvovaginitis (6%), pelvic pain (5%), vaginal bleeding (1% to 5%), vaginitis (4%), vaginal discharge (4%), vaginal hemorrhage (2% to 4%), leukorrhea (2% to 3%), vaginal dryness (2%)

Hematologic: Anemia (2% to 5%), leukopenia (2% to 5%)

Hepatic: Liver function tests increased (2% to 5%), alkaline phosphatase increased (2% to 5%), gamma GT increased (2% to 5%)

Local: Thrombophlebitis (2% to 5%)

Neuromuscular & skeletal: Fracture (10%), arthrosis (7%), paresthesia (5% to 7%), joint disorder (6%), myalgia (2% to 6%), neck pain (2% to 5%), hypertonia (3%)

Ocular: Cataracts (6%)

Respiratory: Dyspnea (8% to 10%), sinusitis (6%), bronchitis (5%), rhinitis (2% to 5%)

Miscellaneous: Lymph edema (10%), infection (2% to 9%), flu-like syndrome (2% to 7%), diaphoresis (2% to 5%), cyst (5%)

<1% (Limited to important or life-threatening): Anaphylaxis, angioedema, CVA, cerebral ischemia, cerebral infarct, endometrial cancer, erythema multiforme, joint pain, joint stiffness, MI, myocardial ischemia, pulmonary embolus, retinal vein thrombosis, Stevens-Johnson syndrome, urticaria

Overdosage/Toxicology Symptoms of overdose include severe irritation to the stomach (necrosis, gastritis, ulceration, and hemorrhage). There is no specific antidote; treatment must be symptomatic. Dialysis may be helpful because anastrozole is not highly protein bound.

Dosing

Adults & Elderly: Breast cancer: Oral (refer to individual protocols): 1 mg once daily

Renal Impairment: Dosage adjustment is not necessary.

Hepatic Impairment: Mild-to-moderate impairment: Plasma concentrations in subjects with stable hepatic cirrhosis were within the range concentrations in normal subjects across all clinical trials; therefore, no dosage adjustment required; however, patients should be monitored for side effects. Safety and efficacy in severe hepatic impairment have not been established.

Available Dosage Forms Tablet: 1 mg

(Continued)

Anastrozole *(Continued)*

Nursing Guidelines

Assessment: See Contraindications and Warnings/Precautions for use cautions. Assess potential for interactions with other prescriptions, OTC medications, or herbal products patient may be taking (see Drug Interactions). Assess results of laboratory results (see below), therapeutic effectiveness, and adverse reactions (see Adverse Reactions and Overdose/Toxicology) periodically during therapy. Teach patient proper use, possible side effects/appropriate interventions, and adverse symptoms to report (see Patient Education). **Pregnancy risk factor D** - determine that patient is not pregnant before beginning treatment. Instruct patients of childbearing age about appropriate barrier contraceptive measures. Note breast-feeding caution.

Monitoring Laboratory Tests: Bone mineral density; total cholesterol and LDL

Patient Education: Inform prescriber of all prescriptions, OTC medications, or herbal products you are taking, and any allergies you have. Do not take any new medication during therapy unless approved by prescriber. Take exactly as directed. Maintain adequate hydration (2-3 L/day of fluids) unless instructed to restrict fluid intake. May cause headache (consult prescriber for approved analgesic); drowsiness, dizziness, anxiety (use caution when driving or engaging in tasks that require alertness until response to drug is known); mild nausea or vomiting (small, frequent meals, frequent mouth care, chewing gum, or sucking lozenges may help); or increased pelvic, bone or tumor pain (may lessen with continued use; if not, consult prescriber for approved analgesic). Report rash; unresolved nausea or vomiting; pain or burning on urination; severe mood swings, confusion, anxiety; palpitations; flu-like symptoms; or respiratory difficulty. **Pregnancy/breast-feeding precautions:** Do not get pregnant while taking this medication. Consult prescriber for appropriate contraceptive measures. Consult prescriber if breast-feeding.

Pregnancy Risk Factor: D

Pregnancy Issues: Anastrozole can cause fetal harm when administered to a pregnant woman.

Lactation: Excretion in breast milk unknown/use caution

Administration

Storage: Store at 20°C to 25°C (68°F to 77°F).

- **Anbesol® [OTC]** *see* Benzocaine *on page 232*
- **Anbesol® Baby [OTC]** *see* Benzocaine *on page 232*
- **Anbesol® Cold Sore Therapy [OTC]** *see* Benzocaine *on page 232*
- **Anbesol® Jr. [OTC]** *see* Benzocaine *on page 232*
- **Anbesol® Maximum Strength [OTC]** *see* Benzocaine *on page 232*
- **Ancef®** *see* Cefazolin *on page 330*
- **Androderm®** *see* Testosterone *on page 1607*
- **AndroGel®** *see* Testosterone *on page 1607*
- **Anemagen™ OB** *see* Vitamins (Multiple/Prenatal) *on page 1721*
- **Anestacon®** *see* Lidocaine *on page 1033*
- **Aneurine Hydrochloride** *see* Thiamine *on page 1623*
- **Anexsia®** *see* Hydrocodone and Acetaminophen *on page 867*
- **Angiomax®** *see* Bivalirudin *on page 246*
- **Angiscein®** *see* Fluorescein Sodium *on page 742*
- **Anhydrous Glucose** *see* Dextrose *on page 511*
- **Anolor 300** *see* Butalbital, Acetaminophen, and Caffeine *on page 280*
- **Ansaid® [DSC]** *see* Flurbiprofen *on page 757*
- **Antara™** *see* Fenofibrate *on page 708*
- **AntibiOtic® Ear** *see* Neomycin, Polymyxin B, and Hydrocortisone *on page 1212*
- **Anti-CD20 Monoclonal Antibody** *see* Rituximab *on page 1484*
- **Antidiuretic Hormone** *see* Vasopressin *on page 1691*

Antihemophilic Factor (Recombinant)

(an tee hee moe FIL ik FAK tor ree KOM be nant)

U.S. Brand Names Advate; Helixate® FS; Kogenate® FS; Recombinate™; ReFacto®

Synonyms AHF (Recombinant); Factor VIII (Recombinant); rAHF

Pharmacologic Category Antihemophilic Agent

Use Management of hemophilia A (classic hemophilia) for patients in whom a deficiency in factor VIII has been demonstrated; prevention and control of bleeding episodes; perioperative management of hemophilia A; can be of significant therapeutic value in patients with acquired factor VIII inhibitors not exceeding 10 Bethesda units/mL

Mechanism of Action Protein (factor VIII) in normal plasma which is necessary for clot formation and maintenance of hemostasis; activates factor X in conjunction with activated factor IX; activated factor X converts prothrombin to thrombin, which converts fibrinogen to fibrin, and with factor XIII forms a stable clot

Pharmacodynamics/Kinetics Half-life elimination: Mean: 14-16 hours

Contraindications Hypersensitivity to mouse or hamster protein (Advate, Helixate® FS, Kogenate® FS); hypersensitivity to mouse, hamster, or bovine protein (Recombinate™, ReFacto®); hypersensitivity to any component of the formulation

Warnings/Precautions Monitor for signs of formation of antibodies to factor VIII; may occur at anytime but more common in young children with severe hemophilia. Monitor for allergic hypersensitivity reactions. Products vary by preparation method. Recombinate™ is stabilized using human albumin. Helixate® FS and Kogenate® FS are stabilized with sucrose.

Adverse Reactions <1% (Limited to important or life-threatening): Allergic reactions, anaphylaxis, angina pectoris, depersonalization, diaphoresis, dysgeusia, dyspnea, epistaxis, fever, headache, hot flashes, injection site reactions (burning, pruritus, erythema), nausea, pruritus, rash, somnolence, urticaria, vasodilation, venous catheter access complications, vomiting

Overdosage/Toxicology Massive doses of antihemophilic factor (human) have been reported to cause acute hemolytic anemia, increased bleeding tendency, or hyperfibrinogenemia. Occurrence is rare.

Dosing

Adults: Hemophilia: I.V.: Individualize dosage based on coagulation studies. performed prior to treatment and at regular intervals during treatment; 1 AHF unit is the activity present in 1 mL of normal pooled human plasma; dosage should be adjusted to actual vial size currently stocked in the pharmacy. (General guidelines presented; consult individual product labeling for specific dosing recommendations.)

Dosage based on desired factor VIII increase (%):

To calculate dosage needed based on desired factor VIII increase (%):

Body weight (kg) x 0.5 int. units/kg x desired factor VIII increase (%) = int. units factor VIII required

For example:

50 kg x 0.5 int. units/kg x 30 (% increase) = 750 int. units factor VIII

Dosage based on expected factor VIII increase (%):

It is also possible to calculate the **expected** % factor VIII increase:

(# int. units administered x 2%/int. units/kg) divided by body weight (kg) = expected % factor VIII increase

For example:

(1400 int. units x 2%/int. units/kg) divided by 70 kg = 40%

General guidelines:

Minor hemorrhage: Required peak postinfusion AHF level: 20% to 40% (10-20 int. units/kg); mild superficial or early hemorrhages may respond to a single dose; may repeat dose every 12-24 hours for 1-3 days until bleeding is resolved or healing achieved

Moderate hemorrhage/minor surgery: Required peak postinfusion AHF level: 30% to 60% (15-30 int. units/kg); repeat dose at 12-24 hours if needed; some products suggest continuing for ≥3 days until pain and disability are resolved

Severe/life-threatening hemorrhage: Required peak postinfusion AHF level: Initial dose: 80% to 100% (40-50 int. units/kg); maintenance dose: 40% to 50% (20-25 int. units/kg) every 8-12 hours until threat is resolved

Major surgery: Required peak pre- and postsurgery AHF level: ~100% (50 int. units/kg): Give first dose prior to surgery and repeat every 6-12 hours until healing complete (10-14 days)

Prophylaxis: May also be given on a regular schedule to prevent bleeding

If bleeding is not controlled with adequate dose, test for presence of inhibitor. It may not be possible or practical to control bleeding if inhibitor titers >10 Bethesda units/mL; antihemophilic factor (porcine) may be considered as an alternative.

(Continued)

Antihemophilic Factor (Recombinant) *(Continued)*

Elderly: Refer to adult dosing. Dosage should be individualized.

Pediatrics: Refer to adult dosing.

Available Dosage Forms Injection, powder for reconstitution, recombinant [preservative free]:

Advate: 250 int. units, 500 int. units, 1000 int. units, 1500 int. units [plasma/albumin free]

Helixate® FS, Kogenate® FS: 250 int. units, 500 int. units, 1000 int. units [contains sucrose 28 mg/vial]

Recombinate™: 250 int. units, 500 units, 1000 int. units [contains human albumin 12.5 mg/mL; packaging contains natural rubber latex]

ReFacto®: 250 int. units, 500 units, 1000 int. units, 2000 int. units [contains sucrose]

Nursing Guidelines

Assessment: See Contraindications, Warnings/Precautions, and Dosing for use cautions. Assess potential for interactions with other prescriptions, OTC medications, or herbal products patient may be taking (especially those medications that may affect coagulation or platelet function - see Drug Interactions). See infusion specifics below. During and after therapy, patient should be monitored closely (eg, vital signs, cardiac and CNS status) and observed for adverse reactions (eg, acute hypersensitivity reaction - see Adverse Reactions and Overdose/Toxicology). Note breast-feeding caution.

Monitoring Laboratory Tests: Development of circulating inhibitors; bleeding

Patient Education: Inform prescriber of all prescriptions, OTC medications, or herbal products you are taking, and any allergies you have. This medication can only be given intravenously. Immediately report any sudden-onset headache, rash, chest or back pain, wheezing or respiratory difficulties, hives, itching, low grade fever, stomach pain, nausea, or vomiting to prescriber. Wear identification indicating that you have a hemophilic condition. **Pregnancy/breast-feeding precautions:** Inform prescriber if you are pregnant. Consult prescriber if breast-feeding.

Pregnancy Risk Factor: C

Lactation: Excretion in breast milk unknown/use caution

Administration

I.V.: Infuse over 5-10 minutes (maximum: 10 mL/minute)

Advate: Infuse over ≤5 minutes (maximum: 10 mL/minute)

Reconstitution:

Gently agitate or rotate vial after adding diluent, do not shake vigorously.

Storage: Store under refrigeration, 2°C to 8°C (36°F to 46°F); avoid freezing. Use within 3 hours of reconstitution. Gently agitate or rotate vial after adding diluent, do not shake vigorously. Do not refrigerate after reconstitution, a precipitation may occur.

Advate: May also be stored at room temperature for up to 6 months.

Kogenate® FS: Avoid prolonged exposure to light during storage.

Recombinate™, ReFacto®: May also be stored at room temperature for up to 3 months; avoid prolonged exposure to light during storage.

If refrigerated, the dried concentrate and diluent should be warmed to room temperature before reconstitution.

Anti-inhibitor Coagulant Complex

(an tee-in HI bi tor coe AG yoo lant KOM pleks)

U.S. Brand Names Autoplex® T; Feiba VH®

Synonyms Coagulant Complex Inhibitor

Pharmacologic Category Antihemophilic Agent; Blood Product Derivative

Use Patients with factor VIII inhibitors who are to undergo surgery or those who are bleeding

Contraindications Disseminated intravascular coagulation; patients with normal coagulation mechanism

Warnings/Precautions Products are prepared from pooled human plasma; such plasma may contain the causative agents of viral diseases. Tests used to control efficacy such as aPTT, WBCT, and TEG do not correlate with clinical efficacy. Dosing to normalize these values may result in DIC. Identification of the clotting deficiency as caused by factor VIII inhibitors is essential prior to starting therapy. Use with extreme caution in patients with impaired hepatic function.

Lab Interactions Increased/decreased PT, PTT; increased fibrin split products; decreased WBCT, fibrin, platelets

Adverse Reactions <1% (Limited to important or life-threatening): Chills, disseminated intravascular coagulation, fever, headache, hypotension, rash, urticaria

Overdosage/Toxicology Rapid infusion may cause hypotension. Excessive administration can cause DIC.

Dosing

Adults & Elderly: Bleeding or surgery in patients with factor VIII inhibitors: I.V.: Dosage range: 25-100 factor VIII correctional units per kg depending on the severity of hemorrhage

Pediatrics: Refer to adult dosing.

Hepatic Impairment: Use with extreme caution.

Available Dosage Forms Injection, powder for reconstitution:

Autoplex® T: Each bottle is labeled with correctional units of factor VIII [with heparin 2 units/mL; packaging contains natural rubber latex]

Feiba VH®: Each bottle is labeled with correctional units of factor VIII [heparin free; packaging contains natural rubber latex]

Nursing Guidelines

Assessment: See Contraindications, Warnings/Precautions, and Dosing for use cautions. Assess potential for interactions with other prescriptions, OTC medications, or herbal products patient may be taking. **Caution:** See Monitoring Laboratory Tests. Vital signs, cardiac and hemodynamic status should be monitored during and after therapy (see Adverse Reactions and Overdose/Toxicology). If hypotension develops, the rate of infusion should be slowed and prescriber notified. Note breast-feeding caution.

Monitoring Laboratory Tests: Note: Tests used to control efficacy such as aPTT, WBCT, and TEG do not correlate with clinical efficacy. Dosing to normalize these values may result in DIC.

Patient Education: Inform prescriber of all prescriptions, OTC medications, or herbal products you are taking, and any allergies you have. This medication can only be given intravenously. Report sudden onset headache, rash, chest or back pain, wheezing or respiratory difficulties, hives, itching, or acute feelings of anxiety. Wear identification indicating that you have a hemophilic condition. **Pregnancy/breast-feeding precautions:** Inform prescriber if you are pregnant. Consult prescriber if breast-feeding.

Pregnancy Risk Factor: C

Lactation: Excretion in breast milk unknown/use caution

Administration

I.V.: I.V. push (maximum rate: 2 units/kg/minute or 2.5-7.5 mL/minutes).

Reconstitution: Do **not** shake or refrigerate after reconstitution. Use within 1-3 hours after reconstitution.

Storage: Store at 2°C to 8°C (36°F to 46°F)

Antithrombin III (an tee THROM bin three)

U.S. Brand Names Thrombate III®

Synonyms AT-III; Heparin Cofactor I

Pharmacologic Category Anticoagulant; Blood Product Derivative

Use Treatment of hereditary antithrombin III deficiency in connection with surgical or obstetrical procedures; thromboembolism

Unlabeled/Investigational Use Acquired antithrombin III deficiencies related to disseminated intravascular coagulation (DIC)

Mechanism of Action Antithrombin III is the primary physiologic inhibitor of *in vivo* coagulation. It is an alpha$_2$-globulin. Its principal actions are the inactivation of thrombin, plasmin, and other active serine proteases of coagulation, including factors IXa, Xa, XIa, XIIa, and VIIa. The inactivation of proteases is a major step in the normal clotting process. The strong activation of clotting enzymes at the site of every bleeding injury facilitates fibrin formation and maintains normal hemostasis. Thrombosis in the circulation would be caused by active serine proteases if they were not inhibited by antithrombin III after the localized clotting process. Patients with congenital deficiency are in a prethrombotic state, even if asymptomatic, as evidenced by elevated plasma levels of prothrombin activation fragment, which are normalized following infusions of antithrombin III concentrate.

Pharmacodynamics/Kinetics Half-life elimination: Biologic: 2.5 days (immunologic assay); 3.8 days (functional AT-III assay)

Contraindications Hypersensitivity to any component of the formulation

(Continued)

Antithrombin III *(Continued)*

Warnings/Precautions Product is prepared from pooled human plasma; may contain the causative agents of viral diseases.

Drug Interactions

Drotrecogin: Concurrent use may increase risk of bleeding.

Drugs which affect platelet function (eg, aspirin, NSAIDs, dipyridamole, ticlopidine, clopidogrel) may potentiate the risk of hemorrhage.

Heparin's anticoagulant effects are potentiated by antithrombin III; half-life of antithrombin III is decreased by heparin.

Thrombolytic agents increase the risk of hemorrhage.

Warfarin (and other oral anticoagulants) may increase the risk of bleeding with antithrombin III.

Adverse Reactions

1% to 10%: Central nervous system: Dizziness (2%)

<1% (Limited to important or life-threatening): Abdominal cramps, bowel fullness, chest pain, chest tightness, chills, cramps, fever, film over eye, foul taste, hematoma formation, hives, lightheadedness, nausea

Dosing

Adults & Elderly:

Antithrombin III deficiency:

Initial dose: Dosing is individualized based on pretherapy AT-III levels. The initial dose should raise antithrombin III levels (AT-III) to 120% and may be calculated based on the following formula:

Initial dosage (int. units) = [desired AT-III level % - baseline AT-III level %] x body weight (kg) divided by 1.4%/int. units/kg (eg, if a 70 kg adult patient had a baseline AT-III level of 57%, the initial dose would be (120% - 57%) x 70/1.4%/int. units/kg = 3150 int. units).

Maintenance dose: Subsequent dosing should be targeted to keep levels between 80% to 120% which may be achieved by administering 60% of the initial dose every 24 hours. Adjustments may be made by adjusting dose or interval. Maintain level within normal range for 2-8 days depending on type of surgery or procedure.

Available Dosage Forms Injection, powder for reconstitution [preservative free]: 500 int. units, 1000 int. units [contains heparin; packaged with diluent]

Nursing Guidelines

Assessment: Assess potential for interactions with other prescriptions, OTC medications, or herbal products patient may be taking (especially drugs affecting coagulation and platelet activity). Vital signs, cardiac status, and CNS status should be monitored during and after therapy. If tachycardia develops, infusion should be discontinued and prescriber notified.

Monitoring Laboratory Tests: Monitor antithrombin III levels (preinfusion and 20 minutes postinfusion for each dose); liver function tests

Dietary Considerations: Contains sodium 110-210 mEq/L

Patient Education: This medication can only be given intravenously. Report immediately any sudden onset headache; rash, itching, or hives; chest or back pain; or wheezing or respiratory difficulties. Wear identification indicating that you have an antithrombin III deficiency. **Breast-feeding precautions:** Consult prescriber if breast-feeding.

Pregnancy Risk Factor: B

Lactation: Excretion in breast milk unknown/use caution

Administration

I.V.: Infuse over 10-20 minutes.

Reconstitution: Reconstitute with sterile water for injection. Do not shake; swirl to mix to avoid foaming. Filter through sterile filter needle provided prior to administration.

Storage: Store vials under refrigeration at 2°C to 8°C (36°F to 46°F); avoid freezing. Bring to room temperature prior to reconstitution. Administer within 3 hours of mixing.

Antithymocyte Globulin (Equine)

(an te THY moe site GLOB yu lin, E kwine)

U.S. Brand Names Atgam®

Synonyms Antithymocyte Immunoglobulin; ATG; Horse Antihuman Thymocyte Gamma Globulin; Lymphocyte Immune Globulin

Pharmacologic Category Immunosuppressant Agent

Medication Safety Issues

Sound-alike/look-alike issues:

Atgam® may be confused with Ativan®

Use Prevention and treatment of acute renal allograft rejection; treatment of moderate to severe aplastic anemia in patients not considered suitable candidates for bone marrow transplantation

Unlabeled/Investigational Use Prevention and treatment of other solid organ allograft rejection; prevention of graft-versus-host disease following bone marrow transplantation

Mechanism of Action May involve elimination of antigen-reactive T lymphocytes (killer cells) in peripheral blood or alteration of T-cell function

Pharmacodynamics/Kinetics

Distribution: Poorly into lymphoid tissues; binds to circulating lymphocytes, granulocytes, platelets, bone marrow cells

Half-life elimination, plasma: 1.5-12 days

Excretion: Urine (~1%)

Contraindications Hypersensitivity to lymphocytic immune globulin, any component of the formulation, or other equine gamma globulins

Warnings/Precautions Must be administered via central line due to chemical phlebitis; should only be used by physicians experienced in immunosuppressive therapy or management of solid organ or bone marrow transplant patients. Adequate laboratory and supportive medical resources must be readily available in the facility for patient management; rash, dyspnea, hypotension, or anaphylaxis precludes further administration of the drug. Discontinue if severe and unremitting thrombocytopenia and/or leukopenia occur. Dose must be administered over at least 4 hours; patient may need to be pretreated with an antipyretic, antihistamine, and/or corticosteroid. Intradermal skin testing is recommended prior to first-dose administration.

Adverse Reactions

>10%:

Central nervous system: Fever, chills

Dermatologic: Pruritus, rash, urticaria

Hematologic: Leukopenia, thrombocytopenia

1% to 10%:

Cardiovascular: Bradycardia, chest pain, CHF, edema, encephalitis, hyper-/hypotension, myocarditis, tachycardia

Central nervous system: Agitation, headache, lethargy, lightheadedness, listlessness, seizure

Gastrointestinal: Diarrhea, nausea, stomatitis, vomiting

Hepatic: Hepatosplenomegaly, liver function tests abnormal

Local: Pain at injection site, phlebitis, thrombophlebitis, burning soles/palms

Neuromuscular & skeletal: Myalgia, back pain, arthralgia

Ocular: Periorbital edema

Renal: Abnormal renal function tests

Respiratory: Dyspnea, respiratory distress

Miscellaneous: Anaphylaxis, serum sickness, viral infection, night sweats, diaphoresis, lymphadenopathy

<1% (Limited to important or life-threatening): Acute renal failure, anemia, aplasia, confusion, cough, deep vein thrombosis, disorientation, dizziness, epigastric pain, faintness, GI bleeding, granulocytopenia, hemolysis, herpes simplex reactivation, hiccups, hyperglycemia, iliac vein obstruction, infection, kidney enlarged, laryngospasm, malaise, neutropenia, nosebleed, pancytopenia, paresthesia, pulmonary edema, renal artery thrombosis, serum sickness, toxic epidermal necrosis, vasculitis, weakness, wound dehiscence

Dosing

Adults & Elderly: Note: An intradermal skin test is recommended prior to administration of the initial dose of ATG; use 0.1 mL of a 1:1000 dilution of ATG in normal saline. A positive skin reaction consists of a wheal ≥10 mm in diameter. If a positive skin test occurs, the first infusion should be administered in a controlled environment with intensive life support immediately available. A systemic reaction precludes further administration of the drug. The absence of a reaction does **not** preclude the possibility of an immediate sensitivity reaction.

Note: Premedication with diphenhydramine, hydrocortisone, and is recommended prior to first dose.

Aplastic anemia protocol: I.V.: 10-20 mg/kg/day for 8-14 days, then give every other day for 7 more doses for a total of 21 doses in 28 days.

(Continued)

Antithymocyte Globulin (Equine) *(Continued)*

Renal allograft rejection, prevention: I.V.: 15 mg/kg/day for 14 days, then give every other day for 7 more doses for a total of 21 doses in 28 days; initial dose should be administered within 24 hours before or after transplantation.

Renal allograft rejection, treatment: I.V.: 10-15 mg/kg/day for 14 days, then give every other day for 7 more doses.

Pediatrics: Note: See adult dosing for notes on intradermal skin testing and premedication.

Aplastic anemia protocol: I.V.: 10-20 mg/kg/day for 8-14 days; then administer every other day for 7 more doses; addition doses may be given every other day for 21 total doses in 28 days.

Renal allograft: I.V.: 5-25 mg/kg/day

Available Dosage Forms Injection, solution: 50 mg/mL (5 mL)

Nursing Guidelines

Assessment: Assess for history of previous allergic reactions. Monitor vital signs during infusion and observe for adverse or allergic reactions. Teach patient adverse symptoms to report.

Monitoring Laboratory Tests: Lymphocyte profile, CBC with differential, platelet count

Patient Education: This medication can only be administered by infusion. You will be closely monitored during the infusion. Do not get up alone; ask for assistance if you must get up or change position. Do not have any vaccinations for the next 3 months without consulting prescriber. Immediately report chills; persistent dizziness or nausea; itching or stinging; acute back pain; chest pain, tightness, or rapid heartbeat; or respiratory difficulty. **Pregnancy/breast-feeding precautions:** Inform prescriber if you are pregnant. Consult prescriber if breast-feeding.

Pregnancy Risk Factor: C

Pregnancy Issues: Reproduction studies have not been conducted; use during pregnancy is not recommended. Women exposed to Atgam® during pregnancy may be enrolled in the National Transplantation Pregnancy Registry (877-955-6877).

Lactation: Excretion in breast milk unknown/use caution

Administration

I.V.: Infuse dose over at least 4 hours. Any severe systemic reaction to the skin test, such as generalized rash, tachycardia, dyspnea, hypotension, or anaphylaxis, should preclude further therapy. Epinephrine and resuscitative equipment should be nearby. Patient may need to be pretreated with an antipyretic, antihistamine, and/or corticosteroid. Mild itching and erythema can be treated with antihistamines. Infuse into a vascular shunt, arterial venous fistula, or high-flow central vein through a 0.2-1 micron in-line filter.

First dose: Premedicate with diphenhydramine orally 30 minutes prior to and hydrocortisone I.V. 15 minutes prior to infusion and acetaminophen 2 hours after start of infusion.

Reconstitution: Dilute into inverted bottle of sterile vehicle to ensure that undiluted lymphocyte immune globulin does not contact air. Gently rotate or swirl to mix. Final concentration should be 4 mg/mL. May be diluted in NS, $D_5$1/4NS, $D_5$1/2NS.

Storage: Ampuls must be refrigerated; do not freeze. Diluted solution is stable for 24 hours (including infusion time) at refrigeration.

Antithymocyte Globulin (Rabbit)

(an te THY moe site GLOB yu lin (RAB bit)

U.S. Brand Names Thymoglobulin®

Synonyms Antithymocyte Immunoglobulin; ATG

Pharmacologic Category Immune Globulin

Use Treatment of renal transplant acute rejection in conjunction with concomitant immunosuppression

Mechanism of Action May involve elimination of antigen-reactive T lymphocytes (killer cells) in peripheral blood or alteration of T-cell function

Pharmacodynamics/Kinetics Half-life elimination, plasma: 2-3 days

Contraindications History of allergy or anaphylaxis to rabbit proteins; acute viral illness

Warnings/Precautions Infusion may produce fever and chills. To minimize, the first dose should be infused over a minimum of 6 hours into a high-flow vein. Also, premedication with corticosteroids, acetaminophen, and/or an antihistamine and/or slowing the infusion rate may reduce reaction incidence and intensity.

Prolonged use or overdosage of Thymoglobulin® in association with other immunosuppressive agents may cause overimmunosuppression resulting in severe infections and may increase the incidence of lymphoma or post-transplant lymphoproliferative disease (PTLD) or other malignancies. Appropriate antiviral, antibacterial, antiprotozoal, and/or antifungal prophylaxis is recommended.

Thymoglobulin® should only be used by physicians experienced in immunosuppressive therapy for the treatment of renal transplant patients. Medical surveillance is required during the infusion. In rare circumstances, anaphylaxis has been reported with use. In such cases, the infusion should be terminated immediately. Medical personnel should be available to treat patients who experience anaphylaxis. Emergency treatment such as 0.3-0.5 mL aqueous epinephrine (1:1000 dilution) subcutaneously and other resuscitative measures including oxygen, intravenous fluids, antihistamines, corticosteroids, pressor amines, and airway management, as clinically indicated, should be provided. Thymoglobulin® or other rabbit immunoglobulins should not be administered again for such patients. Thrombocytopenia or neutropenia may result from cross-reactive antibodies and is reversible following dose adjustments.

Adverse Reactions

>10%:

- Cardiovascular: Hypertension, peripheral edema, tachycardia
- Central nervous system: Chills, fever, headache, pain, malaise
- Dermatologic: Rash
- Endocrine & metabolic: Hyperkalemia
- Gastrointestinal: Abdominal pain, diarrhea, nausea
- Hematologic: Leukopenia, thrombocytopenia
- Neuromuscular & skeletal: Weakness
- Respiratory: Dyspnea
- Miscellaneous: Systemic infection

1% to 10%: Central nervous system: Dizziness

Postmarketing and/or case reports: Anaphylaxis

Dosing

Adults & Elderly: Transplant rejection: I.V.: 1.5 mg/kg/day for 7-14 days

Dosage adjustment for toxicity:

WBC count 2000-3000 cells/mm^3 or platelet count 50,000-75,000 cells/mm^3: Reduce dose by 50%

WBC count <2000 cells/mm^3 or platelet count <50,000 cells/mm^3: Consider discontinuing treatment

Pediatrics: Refer to adult dosing.

Available Dosage Forms Injection, powder for reconstitution: 25 mg [packaged with diluent]

Nursing Guidelines

Pregnancy Risk Factor: C

Lactation: Excretion in breast milk unknown/use caution

Administration

I.V.: The first dose should be infused over at least 6 hours through a high-flow vein. Subsequent doses should be administered over at least 4 hours. Administer through an in-line 0.22 micron filter. Premedication with corticosteroids, acetaminophen, and/or an antihistamine may reduce infusion-related reactions.

Reconstitution: Allow vials to reach room temperature, then reconstitute using provided diluent. Rotate vial gently until dissolved. Prior to administration, further dilute one vial in 50 mL saline or dextrose (total volume is usually 50-500 mL depending on total number of vials needed per dose). Mix by gently inverting infusion bag once or twice.

Storage:

Store powder under refrigeration at 2°C to 8°C (36°F to 46°F); do not freeze. Protect from light. Reconstituted vials should be used within 4 hours. Use immediately following dilution for infusion.

♦ **Antithymocyte Immunoglobulin** *see* Antithymocyte Globulin (Rabbit) *on page 176*

♦ **Antivert®** *see* Meclizine *on page 1084*

♦ **Anucort-HC®** *see* Hydrocortisone *on page 873*

◆ **Anu-Med [OTC]** *see* Phenylephrine *on page 1350*
◆ **Anusol-HC®** *see* Hydrocortisone *on page 873*
◆ **Anusol® HC-1 [OTC]** *see* Hydrocortisone *on page 873*
◆ **Anzemet®** *see* Dolasetron *on page 563*
◆ **APAP** *see* Acetaminophen *on page 65*
◆ **APAP and Tramadol** *see* Acetaminophen and Tramadol *on page 70*
◆ **Apatate® [OTC]** *see* Vitamin B Complex Combinations *on page 1716*
◆ **Aphedrid™ [OTC]** *see* Triprolidine and Pseudoephedrine *on page 1670*
◆ **Apidra™** *see* Insulin Glulisine *on page 922*
◆ **Aplisol®** *see* Tuberculin Tests *on page 1673*
◆ **Aplonidine** *see* Apraclonidine *on page 178*

Apraclonidine (a pra KLOE ni deen)

U.S. Brand Names Iopidine®

Synonyms Aplonidine; Apraclonidine Hydrochloride; p-Aminoclonidine

Pharmacologic Category $Alpha_2$ Agonist, Ophthalmic

Medication Safety Issues

Sound-alike/look-alike issues:

Iopidine® may be confused with indapamide, iodine, Lodine®

Use Prevention and treatment of postsurgical intraocular pressure (IOP) elevation; short-term, adjunctive therapy in patients who require additional reduction of IOP

Mechanism of Action Apraclonidine is a potent alpha-adrenergic agent similar to clonidine; relatively selective for $alpha_2$-receptors but does retain some binding to $alpha_1$-receptors; appears to result in reduction of aqueous humor formation; its penetration through the blood-brain barrier is more polar than clonidine which reduces its penetration through the blood-brain barrier and suggests that its pharmacological profile is characterized by peripheral rather than central effects.

Pharmacodynamics/Kinetics

Onset of action: 1 hour

Peak effect: Decreased intraocular pressure: 3-5 hours

Absorption: Ocular: Systemically absorbed

Half-life elimination, systemic: 8 hours

Contraindications Hypersensitivity to apraclonidine, clonidine, or any component of the formulation; use with or within 14 days of MAO inhibitors

Warnings/Precautions IOP-lowering efficacy decreases over time in some patients. Most patients will experience decreased benefit from therapy lasting longer than 1 month. Closely monitor patients who develop exaggerated reductions in intraocular pressure. Use with caution in patients with cardiovascular disease, coronary insufficiency, recent myocardial infarction, cerebrovascular disease, history of vasovagal reactions, Raynaud's disease, thromboangiitis obliterans, depression, chronic renal failure, or severe renal or hepatic impairment.

Drug Interactions

Antihypertensive agents: Apraclonidine may reduce pulse and blood pressure, use systemic agents with caution.

Beta-blockers: Ophthalmic agents may have additive effect on IOP; apraclonidine may reduce pulse and blood pressure, use systemic agents with caution.

CNS depressants: May have additive CNS depression.

MAO inhibitors: Concomitant use is contraindicated.

Pilocarpine: Ophthalmic use may have additive effect on IOP.

Adverse Reactions

Ocular:

5% to 15%: Discomfort, hyperemia, pruritus

1% to 5%: Blanching, blurred vision, conjunctivitis, discharge, dry eye, foreign body sensation, lid edema, tearing

<1% (Limited to important or life-threatening): Abnormal vision, blepharitis, blepharoconjunctivitis, conjunctival edema, conjunctival follicles, corneal erosion, corneal infiltrate, corneal staining, edema, irritation, keratitis, keratopathy, lid disorder, lid erythema, lid margin crusting, lid retraction, lid scales, pain, photophobia

Other body systems:

1% to 10%: Gastrointestinal: Dry mouth (10%)

<3%:

Cardiovascular: Arrhythmia, chest pain, facial edema, peripheral edema

Central nervous system: Depression, dizziness, headache, insomnia, malaise, nervousness, somnolence

Dermatologic: Contact dermatitis, dermatitis

Gastrointestinal: Constipation, nausea, taste perversion

Neuromuscular & skeletal: Abnormal coordination, myalgia, paresthesia, weakness

Respiratory: Asthma, dry nose, dyspnea, parosmia, pharyngitis, rhinitis

Postmarketing and/or case reports: Allergic reactions, bradycardia

Overdosage/Toxicology Bradycardia, drowsiness, and hypothermia have been reported following ingestion of the ophthalmic solution.

Dosing

Adults & Elderly: Postsurgical intraocular pressure elevation (prevention/treatment): Ophthalmic:

0.5%: Instill 1-2 drops in the affected eye(s) 3 times/day

1%: Instill 1 drop in operative eye 1 hour prior to anterior segment laser surgery, second drop in eye immediately upon completion of procedure

Renal Impairment: Although the topical use of apraclonidine has not been studied in renal failure patients, structurally-related clonidine undergoes a significant increase in half-life in patients with severe renal impairment. Close monitoring of cardiovascular parameters in patients with impaired renal function is advised.

Hepatic Impairment: Close monitoring of cardiovascular parameters in patients with impaired liver function is advised because the systemic dosage form of clonidine is partially metabolized in the liver.

Available Dosage Forms Solution, ophthalmic, as hydrochloride: 0.5% (5 mL, 10 mL); 1% (0.1 mL) [contains benzalkonium chloride]

Nursing Guidelines

Assessment: See Contraindications, Warnings/Precautions, and Dosing for use cautions. Assess potential for interactions with other prescriptions, OTC medications, or herbal products patient may be taking (see Drug Interactions). Assess therapeutic response and adverse effects (see Adverse Reactions, and Overdose/Toxicology). Teach patient proper use, side effects/appropriate interventions, and symptoms to report (see Patient Education). Note breast-feeding caution.

Patient Education: For use in eyes only. May sting on instillation, do not touch dropper to eye. Visual acuity may be decreased after administration. Night vision may be decreased. Distance vision may be altered. Read package instructions for insertion. **Pregnancy/breast-feeding precautions:** Inform prescriber if you are or intend to become pregnancy. Consult prescriber if breast-feeding.

Pregnancy Risk Factor: C

Lactation: Excretion in breast milk unknown/use caution

Administration

Storage: Store between 2°C to 27°C (36°F to 80°F). Protect from freezing and light.

- Apraclonidine Hydrochloride *see* Apraclonidine *on page 178*
- Apresoline [DSC] *see* HydrALAZINE *on page 860*
- Apri® *see* Ethinyl Estradiol and Desogestrel *on page 675*
- Aprodine® [OTC] *see* Triprolidine and Pseudoephedrine *on page 1670*

Aprotinin (a proe TYE nin)

U.S. Brand Names Trasylol®

Pharmacologic Category Blood Product Derivative; Hemostatic Agent

Use Reduction or prevention of blood loss in patients undergoing coronary artery bypass surgery when a high risk of excessive bleeding exists, including open heart reoperation, pre-existing coagulopathies, operations on the great vessels, and when a patient's beliefs prohibit blood transfusions

Mechanism of Action Serine protease inhibitor; inhibits plasmin, kallikrein, and platelet activation producing antifibrinolytic effects; a weak inhibitor of plasma pseudocholinesterase. It also inhibits the contact phase activation of coagulation and preserves adhesive platelet glycoproteins making them resistant to damage from increased circulating plasmin or mechanical injury occurring during bypass.

Pharmacodynamics/Kinetics

Half-life elimination: 2.5 hours

Excretion: Urine

Contraindications Hypersensitivity to aprotinin or any component of the formulation

(Continued)

Aprotinin *(Continued)*

Warnings/Precautions Anaphylactic reactions are possible. Hypersensitivity reactions are more common with repeated use, especially when re-exposure is within 6 months. All patients should receive a test dose at least 10 minutes before loading dose. Patients with a history of allergic reactions to drugs or other agents may be more likely to develop a reaction.

Drug Interactions

Heparin and aprotinin prolong ACT. The ACT becomes a poor measure of adequate anticoagulation with the concurrent use of these drugs.

Fibrinolytic drugs may have poorer activity. Aprotinin blocks this fibrinolytic activity; avoid concurrent use.

Captopril's antihypertensive effects may be blocked; avoid concurrent use.

Lab Interactions Aprotinin prolongs whole blood clotting time of heparinized blood as determined by the Hemochrom® method or similar surface activation methods. Patients may require additional heparin even in the presence of activated clotting time levels that appear to represent adequate anticoagulation.

Adverse Reactions

1% to 10%:

Cardiovascular: Atrial fibrillation, MI, heart failure, atrial flutter, ventricular tachycardia, hypotension, supraventricular tachycardia

Central nervous system: Fever, mental confusion

Local: Phlebitis

Renal: Increased potential for postoperative renal dysfunction

Respiratory: Dyspnea, bronchoconstriction

<1% (Limited to important or life-threatening): Cerebral embolism, cerebrovascular events, convulsions, hemolysis, liver damage, pulmonary edema

Overdosage/Toxicology The maximum amount of aprotinin that can safely be given has not yet been determined. One case report of aprotinin overdose was associated with the development of hepatic and renal failure and eventually death. Autopsy demonstrated severe hepatic necrosis and extensive renal tubular and glomerular necrosis. The relationship between these findings and aprotinin remains unclear.

Dosing

Adults & Elderly:

Test dose: I.V.: **All** patients should receive a 1 mL I.V. test dose at least 10 minutes prior to the loading dose to assess the potential for allergic reactions. **Note:** To avoid physical incompatibility with heparin when adding to pump-prime solution, each agent should be added during recirculation to assure adequate dilution.

Limitation of blood loss: I.V.:

Regimen A (standard dose):

2 million units (280 mg) loading dose I.V. over 20-30 minutes

2 million units (280 mg) into pump prime volume

500,000 units/hour (70 mg/hour) I.V. during operation

Regimen B (low dose):

1 million units (140 mg) loading dose I.V. over 20-30 minutes

1 million units (140 mg) into pump prime volume

250,000 units/hour (35 mg/hour) I.V. during operation

Pediatrics: Refer to adult dosing.

Available Dosage Forms Injection, solution: 1.4 mg/mL [10,000 KIU/mL] (100 mL, 200 mL)

Nursing Guidelines

Assessment: Monitor infusion site carefully. Systemic hemodynamic monitoring is generally in effect when patients receive this drug. Continuous blood pressure monitoring is required. Sudden drops in blood pressure may occur. Observe for adequate fluid balance and adequate respiratory function.

Monitoring Laboratory Tests: Bleeding times, prothrombin time, activated clotting time, platelet count, red blood cell counts, hematocrit, hemoglobin, and fibrinogen degradation products; for toxicity also include renal function.

Patient Education: You will be unaware of the effects of this drug, however, you will be closely monitored at all times. **Breast-feeding precaution:** Consult prescriber if breast-feeding.

Pregnancy Risk Factor: B

Lactation: Excretion in breast milk unknown

Administration

I.V.: Administer through a central line. Infuse loading dose over 20-30 minutes, then continuous infusion at 50 mL/hour.

Compatibility: Incompatible with corticosteroids, heparin, tetracyclines, amino acid solutions, fat emulsion

Storage: Vials should be stored between 2°C and 25°C and protected from freezing.

- Aquachloral® Supprettes® *see* Chloral Hydrate *on page 368*
- AquaLase™ *see* Balanced Salt Solution *on page 224*
- Aquanil™ HC [OTC] *see* Hydrocortisone *on page 873*
- AquaSite® [OTC] *see* Artificial Tears *on page 187*
- Aquasol E® [OTC] *see* Vitamin E *on page 1716*
- Aquavit-E [OTC] *see* Vitamin E *on page 1716*
- Ara-C *see* Cytarabine *on page 477*
- Arabinosylcytosine *see* Cytarabine *on page 477*
- Aralen® *see* Chloroquine *on page 377*
- Aranesp® *see* Darbepoetin Alfa *on page 487*
- Aredia® *see* Pamidronate *on page 1298*

Argatroban (ar GA troh ban)

Pharmacologic Category Anticoagulant, Thrombin Inhibitor

Medication Safety Issues

Sound-alike/look-alike issues:

Argatroban may be confused with Aggrastat®

Use Prophylaxis or treatment of thrombosis in adults with heparin-induced thrombocytopenia; adjunct to percutaneous coronary intervention (PCI) in patients who have or are at risk of thrombosis associated with heparin-induced thrombocytopenia

Mechanism of Action A direct, highly-selective thrombin inhibitor. Reversibly binds to the active thrombin site of free and clot-associated thrombin. Inhibits fibrin formation; activation of coagulation factors V, VIII, and XIII; protein C; and platelet aggregation.

Pharmacodynamics/Kinetics

Onset of action: Immediate

Distribution: 174 mL/kg

Protein binding: Albumin: 20%; α_1-acid glycoprotein: 35%

Metabolism: Hepatic via hydroxylation and aromatization. Metabolism via CYP3A4/5 to four known metabolites plays a minor role. Unchanged argatroban is the major plasma component. Plasma concentration of metabolite M1 is 0% to 20% of the parent drug and is three- to fivefold weaker.

Half-life elimination: 39-51 minutes; Hepatic impairment: ≤181 minutes

Time to peak: Steady-state: 1-3 hours

Excretion: Feces (65%); urine (22%); low quantities of metabolites M2-4 in urine

Contraindications Hypersensitivity to argatroban or any component of the formulation; overt major bleeding

Warnings/Precautions Hemorrhage can occur at any site in the body. Extreme caution should be used when there is an increased danger of hemorrhage, such as severe hypertension, immediately following lumbar puncture, spinal anesthesia, major surgery (including brain, spinal cord, or eye surgery), congenital or acquired bleeding disorders, and gastrointestinal ulcers. Use caution in critically-ill patients; reduced clearance may require dosage reduction. Use caution with hepatic dysfunction. Concomitant use with warfarin will cause increased prolongation of the PT and INR greater than that of warfarin alone; alternative guidelines for monitoring therapy should be followed. Safety and efficacy for use with other thrombolytic agents has not been established. Discontinue all parenteral anticoagulants prior to starting therapy. Allow reversal of heparin's effects before initiation. Patients with hepatic dysfunction may require >4 hours to achieve full reversal of argatroban's anticoagulant effect following treatment. Avoid use during PCI in patients with elevations of ALT/AST (>3 times ULN); the use of argatroban in these patients has not been evaluated. Safety and efficacy in children <18 years of age have not been established.

Drug Interactions Substrate of CYP3A4 (minor)

Drugs which affect platelet function (eg, aspirin, NSAIDs, dipyridamole, ticlopidine, clopidogrel): May potentiate the risk of hemorrhage.

(Continued)

Argatroban *(Continued)*

Erythromycin: Concurrent therapy failed to demonstrate a significant effect on argatroban pharmacokinetics, indicating CYP3A4/5 is not a major route of argatroban metabolism.

Glycoprotein IIb/IIIa antagonists: Concurrent therapy has not been evaluated. An increased risk of bleeding would be expected.

Heparin: Sufficient time must pass after heparin therapy is discontinued; allow heparin's effect on the aPTT to decrease.

Thrombolytics: Safety and efficacy for concomitant use have not been established. May increase risk of bleeding. Intracranial bleeding has been reported.

Warfarin: Concomitant use with argatroban increases PT and INR greater than that of warfarin alone. Argatroban is commonly continued during the initiation of warfarin therapy to assure anticoagulation and to protect against possible transient hypercoagulability.

Adverse Reactions As with all anticoagulants, bleeding is the major adverse effect of argatroban. Hemorrhage may occur at virtually any site. Risk is dependent on multiple variables, including the intensity of anticoagulation and patient susceptibility.

>10%:

Cardiovascular: Chest pain (<1% to 15%), hypotension (7% to 11%)

Gastrointestinal: Gastrointestinal bleed (minor, 3% to 14%)

Genitourinary: Genitourinary bleed and hematuria (minor, 2% to 12%)

1% to 10%:

Cardiovascular: Cardiac arrest (6%), ventricular tachycardia (5%), bradycardia (5%), myocardial infarction (PCI: 4%), atrial fibrillation (3%), angina (2%), CABG-related bleeding (minor, 2%), myocardial ischemia (2%), cerebrovascular disorder (<1% to 2%), thrombosis (<1% to 2%)

Central nervous system: Fever (<1% to 7%), headache (5%), pain (5%), intracranial bleeding (1% to 4%)

Gastrointestinal: Nausea (5% to 7%), diarrhea (6%), vomiting (4% to 6%), abdominal pain (3% to 4%), bleeding (major, <1% to 2%)

Genitourinary: Urinary tract infection (5%)

Hematologic: Hemoglobin (<2 g/dL) and hematocrit (minor, 2% to 10%) decreased

Local: Bleeding at injection or access site (minor, 2% to 5%)

Neuromuscular & skeletal: Back pain (8%)

Renal: Abnormal renal function (3%)

Respiratory: Dyspnea (8% to 10%), cough (3% to 10%), hemoptysis (minor, <1% to 3%), pneumonia (3%)

Miscellaneous: Sepsis (6%), infection (4%)

<1% (Limited to important or life-threatening): Aortic stenosis, genitourinary bleeding and hematuria (major), GERD, hemoglobin/hematocrit decreased (major), limb and below-the-knee stump bleed, pulmonary edema, multisystem hemorrhage and DIC, retroperitoneal bleeding, vascular disorder

Overdosage/Toxicology No specific antidote is available. Treatment should be symptomatic and supportive. Discontinue or decrease infusion to control excessive anticoagulation with or without bleeding. Reversal of anticoagulant effects may be longer than 4 hours in patients with hepatic impairment. Hemodialysis may remove up to 20% of the drug; however, this is considered clinically insignificant.

Dosing

Adults & Elderly:

Prophylaxis of thrombosis (heparin-induced thrombocytopenia): I.V.:

Initial dose: 2 mcg/kg/minute

Maintenance dose: Measure aPTT after 2 hours, adjust dose until the steady-state aPTT is 1.5-3.0 times the initial baseline value, not exceeding 100 seconds; dosage should not exceed 10 mcg/kg/minute

Conversion to oral anticoagulant: Because there may be a combined effect on the INR when argatroban is combined with warfarin, loading doses of warfarin should not be used. Warfarin therapy should be started at the expected daily dose.

Patients receiving ≤2 mcg/kg/minute of argatroban: Argatroban therapy can be stopped when the combined INR on warfarin and argatroban is >4; repeat INR measurement in 4-6 hours; if INR is below therapeutic level, argatroban therapy may be restarted. Repeat procedure daily until desired INR on warfarin alone is obtained.

Patients receiving >2 mcg/kg/minute of argatroban: Reduce dose of argatroban to 2 mcg/kg/minute; measure INR for argatroban and warfarin 4-6 hours after dose reduction; argatroban therapy can be stopped when the combined INR on warfarin and argatroban is >4. Repeat INR measurement in 4-6 hours; if INR is below therapeutic level, argatroban therapy may be restarted. Repeat procedure daily until desired INR on warfarin alone is obtained.

Note: Critically-ill patients with normal hepatic function became excessively anticoagulated with FDA-approved or lower starting doses of argatroban (Reichert MG, 2003). Doses between 0.15-1.3 mcg/kg/minute were required to maintain aPTTs in the target range. Another report of a cardiac patient with anasarca secondary to acute renal failure had a reduction in argatroban clearance similar to patients with hepatic dysfunction (de Denus S, 2003). Reduced clearance may have been attributed to reduced perfusion to the liver. Consider reducing starting dose to 0.5-1 mcg/kg/minute in critically-ill patients who may have impaired hepatic perfusion (eg, patients requiring vasopressors, having decreased cardiac output, having fluid overload). In a retrospective review of critical care patients (Baghdasarian, 2004), patients with three organ system failure required 0.5 mcg/kg/minute. The mean argatroban dose of ICU patients was 0.9 mcg/kg/minute.

Percutaneous coronary intervention (PCI): I.V.:

Initial: Begin infusion of 25 mcg/kg/minute and administer bolus dose of 350 mcg/kg (over 3-5 minutes). ACT should be checked 5-10 minutes after bolus infusion; proceed with procedure if ACT >300 seconds. Following initial bolus:

ACT <300 seconds: Give an additional 150 mcg/kg bolus, and increase infusion rate to 30 mcg/kg/minute (recheck ACT in 5-10 minutes)

ACT >450 seconds: Decrease infusion rate to 15 mcg/kg/minute (recheck ACT in 5-10 minutes)

Once a therapeutic ACT (300-450 seconds) is achieved, infusion should be continued at this dose for the duration of the procedure.

If dissection, impending abrupt closure, thrombus formation during PCI, or inability to achieve ACT >300 sec: An additional bolus of 150 mcg/kg, followed by an increase in infusion rate to 40 mcg/kg/minute may be administered.

Note: Post-PCI anticoagulation, if required, may be achieved by continuing infusion at a reduced dose of 2-10 mcg/kg/minute, with close monitoring of aPTT.

Renal Impairment: Removal during hemodialysis and continuous venovenous hemofiltration is clinically insignificant. No dosage adjustment required.

Hepatic Impairment: Decreased clearance and increased elimination half-life are seen with hepatic impairment; dose should be reduced. Initial dose for moderate hepatic impairment is 0.5 mcg/kg/minute. **Note:** During PCI, avoid use in patients with elevations of ALT/AST (>3 times ULN); the use of argatroban in these patients has not been evaluated.

Available Dosage Forms Injection, solution: 100 mg/mL (2.5 mL) [contains dehydrated alcohol 1000 mg/mL]

Nursing Guidelines

Assessment: See Warnings/Precautions, Contraindications, and Drug Interactions for use cautions. Monitor therapeutic effectiveness (laboratory results) and adverse reactions (see Adverse Reactions) frequently during therapy. Observe bleeding precautions and teach patient interventions to reduce side effects and adverse reactions to report (see Patient Education). Breast-feeding is not recommended.

Monitoring Laboratory Tests: Hemoglobin, hematocrit

Patient Education: This medication can only be administered by intravenous infusion and you will be monitored with blood tests during therapy. You may have a tendency to bleed easily; use electric razor, brush teeth with soft brush, floss with waxed floss, avoid all scissors or sharp instruments (knives, needles, etc), and avoid injury or bruising. Report stomach cramping or pain; dark or bloody stools; blood in urine; acute headache or confusion; respiratory difficulty; nosebleed; or bleeding from gums. **Breast-feeding precaution:** Breast-feeding is not recommended.

Pregnancy Risk Factor: B

Lactation: Excretion in breast milk unknown/not recommended

Breast-Feeding Considerations: It is not known if argatroban is excreted in human milk. Because of the serious potential of adverse effects to the nursing

(Continued)

Argatroban *(Continued)*

infant, a decision to discontinue nursing or discontinue argatroban should be considered.

Perioperative/Anesthesia/Other Concerns: Argatroban achieves steady state rapidly (4-5 hours after initiating therapy) when administered I.V., with a predictable dose-response effect. PTTs generally remain stable at a given dose. Argatroban does not induce formation of antibodies that can alter its clearance, as is seen with lepirudin. Reduce dose in critically-ill patients, particularly those who may have impaired hepatic perfusion.

Administration

I.V.: Solution **must be diluted to 1 mg/mL** prior to administration.

Reconstitution: May be mixed with 0.9% sodium chloride injection, 5% dextrose injection, or lactated Ringer's injection. Do not mix with other medications. To prepare solution for I.V. administration, dilute each 250 mg vial with 250 mL of diluent. Mix by repeated inversion for one minute. Once mixed, final concentration should be 1 mg/mL. A slight but brief haziness may occur prior to mixing.

Compatibility: Stable in 0.9% NS, D_5W, LR

Y-site administration: Incompatible with other medications

Compatibility when admixed: Incompatible with other medications

Storage: Prior to use, store at 15°C to 30°C (59°F to 86°F). Protect from light. The prepared solution is stable for 24 hours at 15°C to 30°C (59°F to 86°F) in ambient indoor light. Do not expose to direct sunlight. Prepared solutions that are protected from light and kept at controlled room temperature of 20°C to 25°C (68°F to 77°F) or under refrigeration at 2°C to 8°C (36°F to 46°F) are stable for up to 96 hours.

♦ **8-Arginine Vasopressin** *see* Vasopressin *on page 1691*
♦ **Arimidex®** *see* Anastrozole *on page 168*
♦ **Aristocort®** *see* Triamcinolone *on page 1660*
♦ **Aristocort® A** *see* Triamcinolone *on page 1660*
♦ **Aristospan®** *see* Triamcinolone *on page 1660*
♦ **Arixtra®** *see* Fondaparinux *on page 770*

Arsenic Trioxide (AR se nik tri OKS id)

U.S. Brand Names Trisenox™

Synonyms NSC-706363

Pharmacologic Category Antineoplastic Agent, Miscellaneous

Use Induction of remission and consolidation in patients with acute promyelocytic leukemia (APL) which is specifically characterized by t(15;17) translocation or PML/RAR-alpha gene expression. Should be used only in those patients who have relapsed or are refractory to retinoid and anthracycline chemotherapy.

Orphan drug: Treatment of myelodysplastic syndrome; multiple myeloma; chronic myeloid leukemia (CML); acute myelocytic leukemia (AML)

Mechanism of Action Not fully understood; causes *in vitro* morphological changes and DNA fragmentation to NB4 human promyelocytic leukemia cells; also damages or degrades the fusion protein PML-RAR alpha

Pharmacodynamics/Kinetics

Metabolism: Hepatic; pentavalent arsenic is reduced to trivalent arsenic (active) by arsenate reductase; trivalent arsenic is methylated to monomethylarsinic acid, which is then converted to dimethylarsinic acid via methyltransferases

Excretion: Urine (as methylated metabolite); disposition not yet studied

Contraindications Hypersensitivity to arsenic or any component of the formulation; pregnancy

Warnings/Precautions The U.S. Food and Drug Administration (FDA) currently recommends that procedures for proper handling and disposal of antineoplastic agents be considered. For use only by physicians experienced with the treatment of acute leukemia. A baseline 12-lead ECG, serum electrolytes (potassium, calcium, magnesium), and creatinine should be obtained. Correct electrolyte abnormalities prior to treatment and monitor potassium and magnesium levels during therapy (potassium should stay >4 mEq/dL and magnesium >1.8 mg/dL). Correct QT_c >500 msec prior to treatment. Discontinue therapy and hospitalize patient if QT_c >500 msec, syncope, or irregular heartbeats develop during therapy. May prolong the QT interval. May lead to torsade de pointes or complete AV block. Risk factors for torsade de pointes include CHF, a history of torsade de pointes, pre-existing QT interval prolongation, patients taking potassium-wasting diuretics, and conditions which cause hypokalemia or hypomagnesemia. If possible, discontinue all medications known to prolong the QT interval. May cause retinoic-acid-acute promyelocytic leukemia (RA-APL) syndrome or APL differentiation syndrome (high-dose steroids have been used for treatment). May lead to the development of hyperleukocytosis. Use with caution in renal impairment. Safety and efficacy in children <5 years of age have not been established (limited experience with children 5-16 years of age).

Drug Interactions Use caution with medications causing hypokalemia or hypomagnesemia. Use caution with medications that prolong the QT interval; avoid concurrent use if possible.

Amphotericin B: Use with caution; can cause electrolyte abnormalities.

Diuretics: May cause electrolyte abnormalities; use with caution.

QT_c-prolonging agents: Concurrent use of arsenic trioxide with other drugs which may prolong QT_c interval may increase the risk of potentially-fatal arrhythmias; includes type Ia and type III antiarrhythmic agents, selected quinolones (sparfloxacin, gatifloxacin, moxifloxacin), cisapride, thioridazine, and other agents.

Nutritional/Herbal/Ethanol Interactions Herb/Nutraceutical: Avoid homeopathic products (arsenic is present in some homeopathic medications).

Adverse Reactions

>10%:

Cardiovascular: Tachycardia (55%), edema (40%), QT interval >500 msec (38%), chest pain (25%), hypotension (25%)

Central nervous system: Fatigue (63%), fever (63%), headache (60%), insomnia (43%), anxiety (30%), dizziness (23%), depression (20%), pain (15%)

Dermatologic: Dermatitis (43%), pruritus (33%), bruising (20%), dry skin (13%)

Endocrine & metabolic: Hypokalemia (50%), hyperglycemia (45%), hypomagnesemia (45%), hyperkalemia (18%)

Gastrointestinal: Nausea (75%), abdominal pain (58%), vomiting (58%), diarrhea (53%), sore throat (40%), constipation (28%), anorexia (23%), appetite decreased (15%), weight gain (13%)

Genitourinary: Vaginal hemorrhage (13%)

Hematologic: Leukocytosis (50%), APL differentiation syndrome (23%), thrombocytopenia (19%), anemia (14%), febrile neutropenia (13%)

Hepatic: ALT increased (20%), AST increased (13%)

Local: Injection site: Pain (20%), erythema (13%)

Neuromuscular & skeletal: Rigors (38%), arthralgia (33%), paresthesia (33%), myalgia (25%), bone pain (23%), back pain (18%), limb pain (13%), neck pain (13%), tremor (13%)

Respiratory: Cough (65%), dyspnea (53%), epistaxis (25%), hypoxia (23%), pleural effusion (20%), sinusitis (20%), postnasal drip (13%), upper respiratory tract infection (13%), wheezing (13%)

Miscellaneous: Herpes simplex (13%)

1% to 10% (Limited to important or life-threatening):

Cardiovascular: Hypotension (10%), flushing (10%), pallor (10%), palpitation (10%), facial edema (8%), abnormal ECG (not QT prolongation) (7%)

Central nervous system: Convulsion (8%), somnolence (8%), agitation (5%), coma (5%), confusion (5%)

Dermatologic: Erythema (10%), hyperpigmentation (8%), urticaria (8%), local exfoliation (5%)

Endocrine & metabolic: Hypocalcemia (10%), hypoglycemia (8%), petechia (8%), skin lesions (8%), acidosis (5%)

Gastrointestinal: Dyspepsia (10%), loose stools (10%), abdominal distension (8%), abdominal tenderness (8%), dry mouth (8%), fecal incontinence (8%), gastrointestinal hemorrhage (8%), hemorrhagic diarrhea (8%), oral blistering (8%), weight loss (8%), oral candidiasis (5%)

Genitourinary: Intermenstrual bleeding (8%), incontinence (5%)

Hematologic: Neutropenia (10%), DIC (8%), hemorrhage (8%), lymphadenopathy (8%)

Neuromuscular & skeletal: Weakness (10%)

Ocular: Blurred vision (10%), eye irritation (10%), dry eye (8%), eyelid edema (5%), painful eye (5%)

Otic: Earache (8%), tinnitus (5%)

Renal: Renal failure (8%), renal impairment (8%), oliguria (5%)

Respiratory: Crepitations (10%), breath sounds decreased (10%), rales (10%), hemoptysis (8%), rhonchi (8%), tachypnea (8%), nasopharyngitis (5%)

(Continued)

Arsenic Trioxide *(Continued)*

Miscellaneous: Diaphoresis increased (10%), injection site edema (10%), bacterial infection (8%), herpes zoster (8%), night sweats (8%), hypersensitivity (5%), sepsis (5%)

Overdosage/Toxicology Symptoms of arsenic toxicity include convulsions, muscle weakness, and confusion. Discontinue treatment and begin chelation therapy. One suggested adult protocol: Dimercaprol 3 mg/kg I.M. every 4 hours; continue until life-threatening toxicity has subsided. Follow with penicillamine 250 mg orally up to 4 times/day (total daily dose ≤1 g).

Dosing

Adults:

Antineoplastic:

Induction: I.V.: 0.15 mg/kg/day; administer daily until bone marrow remission; maximum induction: 60 doses

Consolidation: I.V.: 0.15 mg/kg/day starting 3-6 weeks after completion of induction therapy; maximum consolidation: 25 doses over 5 weeks

Elderly: Safety and efficacy have not been established. Clinical trials included patients ≤72 years of age. Use with caution due to the increased risk of renal impairment in the elderly.

Pediatrics: Children >5 years: Refer to adult dosing.

Renal Impairment: Safety and efficacy have not been established; use with caution due to renal elimination.

Hepatic Impairment: Safety and efficacy have not been established.

Available Dosage Forms Injection, solution [preservative free]: 1 mg/mL (10 mL)

Nursing Guidelines

Assessment: To be used only by physicians experienced with the treatment of acute leukemia. See Contraindications, Warnings/Precautions, and Dosing for use cautions. Assess potential for interactions with other prescriptions, OTC medications, or herbal products patient may be taking (especially anything that may cause hypokalemia or hypomagnesemia, or antiarrhythmic agents - see Drug Interactions). Assess results of laboratory tests (see below). Assess patient response at beginning and periodically during therapy (especially cardiac and electrolyte status - see Adverse Reactions and Overdose/Toxicology). Teach patient appropriate use and adverse symptoms to report (see Patient Education). **Pregnancy risk factor D** - determine that patient is not pregnant before beginning treatment. Teach patients of childbearing age appropriate use of barrier contraceptives. Breast-feeding is contraindicated.

Monitoring Laboratory Tests: Baseline then weekly 12-lead ECG, baseline then twice weekly serum electrolytes, hematologic and coagulation profiles at least twice weekly; more frequent monitoring may be necessary in unstable patients.

Patient Education: Inform prescriber of all prescriptions, OTC medications, or herbal products you are taking, and any allergies you have. Do not take any new medication during therapy unless approved by prescriber. This medication can only be administered by intravenous infusion. Report immediately any redness, swelling, pain, or burning at infusion site. May cause dizziness, fatigue, blurred vision (use caution when driving or engaging in tasks requiring alertness until response to drug is known); or nausea, vomiting, diarrhea, or decreased appetite (small, frequent meals, frequent mouth care, sucking lozenges, or chewing gum may help). Report immediately unexplained fever; respiratory difficulty; chest pain or palpitations; confusion, lightheadedness, or fainting; or other persistent adverse effects. **Pregnancy/breast-feeding precautions:** Inform prescriber if you are pregnant. Do not get pregnant while take this medication. Consult prescriber for appropriate contraceptive methods. Do not breast-feed.

Pregnancy Risk Factor: D

Lactation: Excretion in breast milk unknown/contraindicated

Administration

I.V.: Dilute in 100-250 mL D_5W or 0.9% sodium chloride. Does not contain a preservative; properly discard unused portion. Do not mix with other medications. Infuse over 1-2 hours. If acute vasomotor reactions occur, may infuse over a maximum of 4 hours. Does not require administration via a central venous catheter.

Storage: Store at room temperature, 25°C (77°F); do not freeze. Following dilution, stable for 24 hours at room temperature or 48 hours when refrigerated.

Artificial Tears (ar ti FISH il tears)

U.S. Brand Names Akwa Tears® [OTC]; AquaSite® [OTC]; Bion® Tears [OTC]; HypoTears [OTC]; HypoTears PF [OTC]; Isopto® Tears [OTC]; Liquifilm® Tears [OTC]; Moisture® Eyes [OTC]; Moisture® Eyes PM [OTC]; Murine® Tears [OTC]; Murocel® [OTC]; Nature's Tears® [OTC]; Nu-Tears® [OTC]; Nu-Tears® II [OTC]; OcuCoat® [OTC]; OcuCoat® PF [OTC]; Puralube® Tears [OTC]; Refresh® [OTC]; Refresh Plus® [OTC]; Refresh Tears® [OTC]; Teargen® [OTC]; Teargen® II [OTC]; Tearisol® [OTC]; Tears Again® [OTC]; Tears Naturale® [OTC]; Tears Naturale® Free [OTC]; Tears Naturale® II [OTC]; Tears Plus® [OTC]; Tears Renewed® [OTC]; Ultra Tears® [OTC]; Viva-Drops® [OTC]

Synonyms Hydroxyethylcellulose; Polyvinyl Alcohol

Pharmacologic Category Ophthalmic Agent, Miscellaneous

Medication Safety Issues

Sound-alike/look-alike issues:

Isopto® Tears may be confused with Isoptin®

Murocel® may be confused with Murocoll-2®

Use Ophthalmic lubricant; for relief of dry eyes and eye irritation

Warnings/Precautions Individual product formulations may include (as an active ingredient) benzalkonium chloride, polyvinyl alcohol, carboxymethylcellulose, hydroxymethylcellulose, hydroxypropyl methylcellulose, propylene glycol, dextran 70, or polysorbate 80. Refer to product labeling for specific ingredients.

Adverse Reactions 1% to 10%: Ocular: May cause mild stinging or temporary blurred vision

Dosing

Adults & Elderly: Ocular dryness/irritation: Ophthalmic: Use as needed to relieve symptoms, 1-2 drops into eye(s) 3-4 times/day

Pediatrics: Refer to adult dosing.

Available Dosage Forms Solution, ophthalmic: 15 mL and 30 mL dropper bottles

Nursing Guidelines

Patient Education: Wash hands thoroughly; if irritation or condition worsens or persists for longer than 3 days, discontinue use; do not touch tip of container to any surface; close immediately after use

Pregnancy Risk Factor: C

♦ ASA *see* Aspirin *on page 189*

♦ 5-ASA *see* Mesalamine *on page 1105*

♦ Asacol® *see* Mesalamine *on page 1105*

Ascorbic Acid (a SKOR bik AS id)

U.S. Brand Names C-500-GR™ [OTC]; Cecon® [OTC]; Cevi-Bid® [OTC]; C-Gram [OTC]; Dull-C® [OTC]; Vita-C® [OTC]

Synonyms Vitamin C

Pharmacologic Category Vitamin, Water Soluble

Use Prevention and treatment of scurvy and to acidify the urine

Unlabeled/Investigational Use Investigational: In large doses to decrease the severity of "colds"; dietary supplementation; a 20-year study was recently completed involving 730 individuals which indicates a possible decreased risk of death by stroke when ascorbic acid at doses ≥45 mg/day was administered

Mechanism of Action Not fully understood; necessary for collagen formation and tissue repair; involved in some oxidation-reduction reactions as well as other metabolic pathways, such as synthesis of carnitine, steroids, and catecholamines and conversion of folic acid to folinic acid

Pharmacodynamics/Kinetics

Absorption: Oral: Readily absorbed; an active process thought to be dose dependent

Distribution: Large

Metabolism: Hepatic via oxidation and sulfation

Excretion: Urine (with high blood levels)

Warnings/Precautions Diabetics and patients prone to recurrent renal calculi (eg, dialysis patients) should not take excessive doses for extended periods of time

Drug Interactions

Decreased effect:

Aspirin (decreases ascorbate levels, increases aspirin)

Fluphenazine (decreases fluphenazine levels)

Warfarin (decreased effect)

(Continued)

Ascorbic Acid *(Continued)*

Increased effect:
- Iron (absorption enhanced)
- Oral contraceptives (increased contraceptive effect)

Lab Interactions False-positive urinary glucose with cupric sulfate reagent, false-negative urinary glucose with glucose oxidase method; false-negative stool occult blood 48-72 hours after ascorbic acid ingestion

Adverse Reactions

1% to 10%: Renal: Hyperoxaluria (incidence dose related)

<1% (Limited to important or life-threatening): Dizziness, faintness, fatigue, flank pain, headache

Overdosage/Toxicology Symptoms of overdose include renal calculi, nausea, gastritis, and diarrhea. Diuresis with forced fluids may be useful following massive ingestion.

Dosing

Adults & Elderly:

Recommended daily allowance (RDA): Upper limit of intake should not exceed 2000 mg/day
- Male: 90 mg
- Female: 75 mg
  - Pregnant female:
    - ≤18 years: 80 mg; upper limit of intake should not exceed 1800 mg/day
    - 19-50 years: 85 mg; upper limit of intake should not exceed 2000 mg/day
  - Lactating female:
    - ≤18 years: 15 mg; upper limit of intake should not exceed 1800 mg/day
    - 19-50 years: 20 mg; upper limit of intake should not exceed 2000 mg/day
- Adult smoker: Add an additional 35 mg/day

Scurvy: Oral, I.M., I.V., SubQ: 100-250 mg 1-2 times/day for at least 2 weeks

Urinary acidification: Oral, I.V.: 4-12 g/day in 3-4 divided doses

Prevention and treatment of colds: Oral: 1-3 g/day

Dietary supplement: Oral: 50-200 mg/day

Pediatrics:

Recommended daily allowance (RDA):
- <6 months: 30 mg
- 6 months to 1 year: 35 mg
- 1-3 years: 40 mg
- 4-10 years: 45 mg
- 11-14 years: 50 mg
- >14 years: 60 mg

Scurvy: Oral, I.M., I.V., SubQ: Children: 100-300 mg/day in divided doses for at least 2 weeks

Urinary acidification: Oral, I.V.: Children: 500 mg every 6-8 hours

Dietary supplement: Oral: Children: 35-100 mg/day

Available Dosage Forms

Capsule: 500 mg, 1000 mg
- C-500-GR™: 500 mg

Capsule, timed release: 500 mg

Crystal (Vita-C®): 4 g/teaspoonful (100 g)

Injection, solution: 250 mg/mL (2 mL, 30 mL); 500 mg/mL (50 mL)
- Cenolate®: 500 mg/mL (1 mL, 2 mL) [contains sodium hydrosulfite]

Powder, solution (Dull-C®): 4 g/teaspoonful (100 g, 500 g)

Solution, oral (Cecon®): 90 mg/mL (50 mL)

Tablet: 100 mg, 250 mg, 500 mg, 1000 mg
- C-Gram: 1000 mg

Tablet, chewable: 100 mg, 250 mg, 500 mg [some products may contain aspartame]

Tablet, timed release: 500 mg, 1000 mg, 1500 mg
- Cevi-Bid®: 500 mg

Nursing Guidelines

Assessment: Assess effectiveness and interactions of other medications patient may be taking. Instruct patients with diabetes accordingly. Assess knowledge/teach patient appropriate administration according to formulation of drug and purpose for ascorbic acid therapy and adverse symptoms to report.

Monitoring Laboratory Tests: pH of urine when used as an acidifying agent

Dietary Considerations: Sodium content of 1 g: ~5 mEq

Patient Education: Take exactly as directed; do not take more than the recommended dose. Do not chew or crush extended release tablets. Take oral doses with 8 oz of water. If you have diabetes, use serum glucose monitoring method. Report pain on urination, faintness, or flank pain. **Pregnancy precaution:** Inform prescriber if you are or intend to become pregnant.

Geriatric Considerations: Minimum RDA for elderly is not established. Vitamin C is provided mainly in citrus fruits and tomatoes. The elderly, however, avoid citrus fruits due to cost and difficulty preparing (peeling). Daily replacement through a single multiple vitamin is recommended. Use of natural vitamin C or rose hips offers no advantages. Acidity may produce GI complaints.

Pregnancy Risk Factor: A/C (dose exceeding RDA recommendation)

Lactation: Enters breast milk/compatible

Administration

I.V.: Avoid rapid I.V. injection.

Compatibility: Stable in dextran 6% in D_5W, dextran 6% in NS, D_5LR, D_5NS, $D_5\frac{1}{2}NS$, $D_5\frac{1}{4}NS$, D_5W, $D_{10}W$, LR, ½NS, NS

Y-site administration: Incompatible with etomidate, thiopental

Compatibility in syringe: Incompatible with cefazolin, doxapram

Compatibility when admixed: Incompatible with bleomycin, chlorothiazide, nafcillin, sodium bicarbonate, theophylline

Storage: Injectable form should be stored under refrigeration (2°C to 8°C). Protect oral dosage forms from light. Rapidly oxidized when in solution in air and alkaline media.

- **Ascriptin® [OTC]** *see* Aspirin *on page 189*
- **Ascriptin® Extra Strength [OTC]** *see* Aspirin *on page 189*
- **Aspart Insulin** *see* Insulin Aspart *on page 916*
- **Aspercin [OTC]** *see* Aspirin *on page 189*
- **Aspercin Extra [OTC]** *see* Aspirin *on page 189*
- **Aspergum® [OTC]** *see* Aspirin *on page 189*

Aspirin (AS pir in)

U.S. Brand Names Ascriptin® [OTC]; Ascriptin® Extra Strength [OTC]; Aspercin [OTC]; Aspercin Extra [OTC]; Aspergum® [OTC]; Bayer® Aspirin [OTC]; Bayer® Aspirin Extra Strength [OTC]; Bayer® Aspirin Regimen Adult Low Strength [OTC]; Bayer® Aspirin Regimen Children's [OTC]; Bayer® Aspirin Regimen Regular Strength [OTC]; Bayer® Extra Strength Arthritis Pain Regimen [OTC]; Bayer® Plus Extra Strength [OTC]; Bayer® Women's Aspirin Plus Calcium [OTC]; Bufferin® [OTC]; Bufferin® Extra Strength [OTC]; Buffinol [OTC]; Buffinol Extra [OTC]; Easprin®; Ecotrin® [OTC]; Ecotrin® Low Strength [OTC]; Ecotrin® Maximum Strength [OTC]; Halfprin® [OTC]; St. Joseph® Adult Aspirin [OTC]; Sureprin 81™ [OTC]; ZORprin®

Synonyms Acetylsalicylic Acid; ASA

Pharmacologic Category Salicylate

Medication Safety Issues

Sound-alike/look-alike issues:

Aspirin may be confused with Afrin®, Asendin®
Ascriptin® may be confused with Aricept®
Ecotrin® may be confused with Akineton®, Edecrin®, Epogen®
Halfprin® may be confused with Halfan®, Haltran®
ZORprin® may be confused with Zyloprim®

Use Treatment of mild-to-moderate pain, inflammation, and fever; may be used as prophylaxis of myocardial infarction; prophylaxis of stroke and/or transient ischemic episodes; management of rheumatoid arthritis, rheumatic fever, osteoarthritis, and gout (high dose); adjunctive therapy in revascularization procedures (coronary artery bypass graft [CABG], percutaneous transluminal coronary angioplasty [PTCA], carotid endarterectomy), stent implantation

Unlabeled/Investigational Use Low doses have been used in the prevention of pre-eclampsia, complications associated with autoimmune disorders such as lupus or antiphospholipid syndrome

Mechanism of Action Inhibits prostaglandin synthesis, acts on the hypothalamus heat-regulating center to reduce fever, blocks prostaglandin synthetase action which prevents formation of the platelet-aggregating substance thromboxane A_2

Pharmacodynamics/Kinetics

Duration: 4-6 hours

(Continued)

Aspirin *(Continued)*

Absorption: Rapid

Distribution: V_d: 10 L; readily into most body fluids and tissues

Metabolism: Hydrolyzed to salicylate (active) by esterases in GI mucosa, red blood cells, synovial fluid, and blood; metabolism of salicylate occurs primarily by hepatic conjugation; metabolic pathways are saturable

Bioavailability: 50% to 75% reaches systemic circulation

Half-life elimination: Parent drug: 15-20 minutes; Salicylates (dose dependent): 3 hours at lower doses (300-600 mg), 5-6 hours (after 1 g), 10 hours with higher doses

Time to peak, serum: ~1-2 hours

Excretion: Urine (75% as salicyluric acid, 10% as salicylic acid)

Contraindications Hypersensitivity to salicylates, other NSAIDs, or any component of the formulation; asthma; rhinitis; nasal polyps; inherited or acquired bleeding disorders (including factor VII and factor IX deficiency); do not use in children (<16 years of age) for viral infections (chickenpox or flu symptoms), with or without fever, due to a potential association with Reye's syndrome; pregnancy (3rd trimester especially)

Warnings/Precautions Use with caution in patients with platelet and bleeding disorders, renal dysfunction, dehydration, erosive gastritis, or peptic ulcer disease. Heavy ethanol use (>3 drinks/day) can increase bleeding risks. Avoid use in severe renal failure or in severe hepatic failure. Discontinue use if tinnitus or impaired hearing occurs. Caution in mild-moderate renal failure (only at high dosages). Patients with sensitivity to tartrazine dyes, nasal polyps and asthma may have an increased risk of salicylate sensitivity. Surgical patients should avoid ASA if possible, for 1-2 weeks prior to surgery, to reduce the risk of excessive bleeding.

When used for self-medication (OTC labeling): Children and teenagers who have or are recovering from chickenpox or flu-like symptoms should not use this product. Changes in behavior (along with nausea and vomiting) may be an early sign of Reye's syndrome; patients should be instructed to contact their healthcare provider if these occur.

Drug Interactions Substrate of CYP2C8/9 (minor)

ACE inhibitors: The effects of ACE inhibitors may be blunted by aspirin administration, particularly at higher dosages.

Buspirone increases aspirin's free % *in vitro.*

Carbonic anhydrase inhibitors and corticosteroids have been associated with alteration in salicylate serum concentrations.

Heparin and low molecular weight heparins: Concurrent use may increase the risk of bleeding.

Methotrexate serum levels may be increased; consider discontinuing aspirin 2-3 days before high-dose methotrexate treatment or avoid concurrent use.

NSAIDs may increase the risk of gastrointestinal adverse effects and bleeding. Serum concentrations of some NSAIDs may be decreased by aspirin. Ibuprofen, and possibly other COX-1 inhibitors, may reduce the cardioprotective effects of aspirin. Avoid giving prior to aspirin therapy or on a regular basis in patients with CAD.

Platelet inhibitors (IIb/IIIa antagonists): Risk of bleeding may be increased.

Probenecid effects may be antagonized by aspirin.

Sulfonylureas: The effects of older sulfonylurea agents (tolazamide, tolbutamide) may be potentiated due to displacement from plasma proteins. This effect does not appear to be clinically significant for newer sulfonylurea agents (glyburide, glipizide, glimepiride).

Valproic acid may be displaced from its binding sites which can result in toxicity.

Verapamil may potentiate the prolongation of bleeding time associated with aspirin.

Warfarin and oral anticoagulants may increase the risk of bleeding.

Nutritional/Herbal/Ethanol Interactions

Ethanol: Avoid ethanol (may enhance gastric mucosal damage).

Food: Food may decrease the rate but not the extent of oral absorption.

- Folic acid: Hyperexcretion of folate; folic acid deficiency may result, leading to macrocytic anemia.
- Iron: With chronic aspirin use and at doses of 3-4 g/day, iron-deficiency anemia may result.
- Sodium: Hypernatremia resulting from buffered aspirin solutions or sodium salicylate containing high sodium content. Avoid or use with caution in CHF or any condition where hypernatremia would be detrimental.

Benedictine liqueur, prunes, raisins, tea, and gherkins: Potential salicylate accumulation.

Fresh fruits containing vitamin C: Displace drug from binding sites, resulting in increased urinary excretion of aspirin.

Herb/Nutraceutical: Avoid cat's claw, dong quai, evening primrose, feverfew, garlic, ginger, ginkgo, red clover, horse chestnut, green tea, ginseng (all have additional antiplatelet activity). Limit curry powder, paprika, licorice; may cause salicylate accumulation. These foods contain 6 mg salicylate/100 g. An ordinarily American diet contains 10-200 mg/day of salicylate.

Lab Interactions False-negative results for glucose oxidase urinary glucose tests (Clinistix®). Interferes with Gerhardt test, VMA determination; 5-HIAA, xylose tolerance test and T_3 and T_4.

Adverse Reactions As with all drugs which may affect hemostasis, bleeding is associated with aspirin. Hemorrhage may occur at virtually any site. Risk is dependent on multiple variables including dosage, concurrent use of multiple agents which alter hemostasis, and patient susceptibility. Many adverse effects of aspirin are dose related, and are extremely rare at low dosages. Other serious reactions are idiosyncratic, related to allergy or individual sensitivity. Accurate estimation of frequencies is not possible.

Central nervous system: Fatigue, insomnia, nervousness, agitation, confusion, dizziness, headache, lethargy, cerebral edema, hyperthermia, coma

Cardiovascular: Hypotension, tachycardia, dysrhythmias, edema

Dermatologic: Rash, angioedema, urticaria

Endocrine & metabolic: Acidosis, hyperkalemia, dehydration, hypoglycemia (children), hyperglycemia, hypernatremia (buffered forms)

Gastrointestinal: Nausea, vomiting, dyspepsia, epigastric discomfort, heartburn, stomach pain, gastrointestinal ulceration (6% to 31%), gastric erosions, gastric erythema, duodenal ulcers

Hematologic: Anemia, disseminated intravascular coagulation, prolongation of prothrombin times, coagulopathy, thrombocytopenia, hemolytic anemia, bleeding, iron-deficiency anemia

Hepatic: Hepatotoxicity, transaminases increased, hepatitis (reversible)

Neuromuscular & skeletal: Rhabdomyolysis, weakness, acetabular bone destruction (OA)

Otic: Hearing loss, tinnitus

Renal: Interstitial nephritis, papillary necrosis, proteinuria, renal failure (including cases caused by rhabdomyolysis), increased BUN, increased serum creatinine

Respiratory: Asthma, bronchospasm, dyspnea, laryngeal edema, hyperpnea, tachypnea, respiratory alkalosis, noncardiogenic pulmonary edema

Miscellaneous: Anaphylaxis, prolonged pregnancy and labor, stillbirths, low birth weight, peripartum bleeding, Reye's syndrome

Postmarketing and/or case reports: Colonic ulceration, esophageal stricture, esophagitis with esophageal ulcer, esophageal hematoma, oral mucosal ulcers (aspirin-containing chewing gum), coronary artery spasm, conduction defect and atrial fibrillation (toxicity), delirium, ischemic brain infarction, colitis, rectal stenosis (suppository), cholestatic jaundice, periorbital edema, rhinosinusitis

Overdosage/Toxicology Symptoms of overdose include tinnitus, headache, dizziness, confusion, metabolic acidosis, hyperpyrexia, hypoglycemia, and coma. Treatment should be based upon symptomatology.

Dosing

Adults & Elderly:

Analgesic and antipyretic: Oral, rectal: 325-650 mg every 4-6 hours up to 4 g/day

Anti-inflammatory: Oral: Initial: 2.4-3.6 g/day in divided doses; usual maintenance: 3.6-5.4 g/day; monitor serum concentrations

Acute myocardial infarction: 160-325 mg/day (have patient chew tablet if not taking aspirin before presentation)

Myocardial infarction prophylaxis: 75-325 mg/day; use of a lower aspirin dosage has been recommended in patients receiving ACE inhibitors

CABG: 75-325 mg/day starting 6 hours following procedure; if bleeding prevents administration at 6 hours after CABG, initiate as soon as possible

PTCA: Initial: 80-325 mg/day starting 2 hours before procedure; longer pretreatment durations (up to 24 hours) should be considered if lower dosages (80-100 mg) are used

Stent implantation: Oral: 325 mg 2 hours prior to implantation and 160-325 mg daily thereafter

Carotid endarterectomy: 81-325 mg/day preoperatively and daily thereafter

(Continued)

Aspirin *(Continued)*

Acute stroke: 160-325 mg/day, initiated within 48 hours (in patients who are not candidates for thrombolytics and are not receiving systemic anticoagulation)

Stroke prevention/TIA: 30-325 mg/day (dosages up to 1300 mg/day in 2-4 divided doses have been used in clinical trials)

Pre-eclampsia prevention (unlabeled use): 60-80 mg/day during gestational weeks 13-26 (patient selection criteria not established)

Pediatrics:

Analgesic and antipyretic: Oral, rectal: Children: 10-15 mg/kg/dose every 4-6 hours, up to a total of 4 g/day

Anti-inflammatory: Oral: Children: Initial: 60-90 mg/kg/day in divided doses; usual maintenance: 80-100 mg/kg/day divided every 6-8 hours; monitor serum concentrations

Antiplatelet effects: Oral: Children: Adequate pediatric studies have not been performed; pediatric dosage is derived from adult studies and clinical experience and is not well established; suggested doses have ranged from 3-5 mg/kg/day to 5-10 mg/kg/day given as a single daily dose. Doses are rounded to a convenient amount (eg, 1/2 of 80 mg tablet).

Mechanical prosthetic heart valves: Oral: Children: 6-20 mg/kg/day given as a single daily dose (used in combination with an oral anticoagulant in children who have systemic embolism despite adequate oral anticoagulation therapy (INR 2.5-3.5) and used in combination with low-dose anticoagulation (INR 2-3) and dipyridamole when full-dose oral anticoagulation is contraindicated)

Blalock-Taussig shunts: Oral: Children: 3-5 mg/kg/day given as a single daily dose

Kawasaki disease: Oral: Children: 80-100 mg/kg/day divided every 6 hours; monitor serum concentrations; after fever resolves: 3-5 mg/kg/day once daily; in patients without coronary artery abnormalities, give lower dose for at least 6-8 weeks or until ESR and platelet count are normal; in patients with coronary artery abnormalities, low-dose aspirin should be continued indefinitely

Antirheumatic: Oral: Children: 60-100 mg/kg/day in divided doses every 4 hours

Renal Impairment:

Cl_{cr} <10 mL/minute: Avoid use.

Dialyzable (50% to 100%)

Hepatic Impairment: Avoid use in severe liver disease.

Available Dosage Forms

Caplet:
- Bayer® Aspirin: 325 mg [film coated]
- Bayer® Aspirin Extra Strength: 500 mg [film coated]
- Bayer® Extra Strength Arthritis Pain Regimen: 500 mg [enteric coated]
- Bayer® Women's Aspirin Plus Calcium: 81 mg [contains elemental calcium 300 mg]

Caplet, buffered (Ascriptin® Extra Strength): 500 mg [contains aluminum hydroxide, calcium carbonate, and magnesium hydroxide]

Gelcap (Bayer® Aspirin Extra Strength): 500 mg

Gum (Aspergum®): 227 mg [cherry or orange flavor]

Suppository, rectal: 300 mg, 600 mg

Tablet: 325 mg
- Aspercin: 325 mg
- Aspercin Extra: 500 mg
- Bayer® Aspirin: 325 mg [film coated]

Tablet, buffered: 325 mg
- Ascriptin®: 325 mg [contains aluminum hydroxide, calcium carbonate, and magnesium hydroxide]
- Bayer® Plus Extra Strength: 500 mg [contains calcium carbonate]
- Bufferin®: 325 mg [contains citric acid]
- Bufferin® Extra Strength: 500 mg [contains citric acid]
- Buffinol: 325 mg [contains magnesium oxide]
- Buffinol Extra: 500 mg [contains magnesium oxide]

Tablet, chewable: 81 mg
- Bayer® Aspirin Regimen Children's Chewable: 81 mg [cherry, mint or orange flavor]
- St. Joseph® Adult Aspirin: 81 mg [orange flavor]

Tablet, controlled release (ZORprin®): 800 mg

Tablet, enteric coated: 81 mg, 325 mg, 500 mg, 650 mg

Bayer® Aspirin Regimen Adult Low Strength, Ecotrin® Low Strength, St. Joseph Adult Aspirin: 81 mg

Bayer® Aspirin Regimen Regular Strength, Ecotrin®: 325 mg

Easprin®: 975 mg

Ecotrin® Maximum Strength: 500 mg

Halfprin®: 81 mg, 162 mg

Sureprin 81™: 81 mg

Nursing Guidelines

Assessment: Do not use for persons with allergic reaction to salicylate or other NSAIDs. Assess other medications patient may be taking for additive or adverse interactions. Monitor therapeutic effectiveness and for signs of adverse reactions or overdose at beginning of therapy and periodically with long-term therapy. Assess knowledge/teach patient appropriate use. Teach patient to monitor for adverse reactions, adverse reactions to report, and appropriate interventions to reduce side effects.

Dietary Considerations: Take with food or large volume of water or milk to minimize GI upset.

Patient Education: If self-administered, use exactly as directed; do not increase dose or frequency. Adverse reactions can occur with overuse. Take with food or milk. Do not use aspirin with strong vinegar-like odor. Do not crush or chew extended release products. While using this medication, avoid alcohol, excessive amounts of vitamin C, or salicylate-containing foods (eg, curry powder, prunes, raisins, tea, or licorice), other prescription or OTC medications containing aspirin or salicylate, or other NSAIDs without consulting prescriber. Maintain adequate hydration (2-3 L/day of fluids) unless instructed to restrict fluid intake. You may experience nausea, vomiting, gastric discomfort (frequent mouth care, small frequent meals, sucking lozenges, or chewing gum may help); GI bleeding, ulceration, or perforation (can occur with or without pain); or discoloration of stool (pink/red). Stop taking aspirin and report ringing in ears; persistent stomach pain; unresolved nausea or vomiting; respiratory difficulty or shortness of breath; unusual bruising or bleeding (mouth, urine, stool); or skin rash. **Pregnancy/breast-feeding precautions:** Inform prescriber if you are or intend to become pregnant. Consult prescriber if breast-feeding.

Geriatric Considerations: Elderly are at high risk for adverse effects from NSAIDs. Elderly with GI complications can develop peptic ulceration and/or hemorrhage asymptomatically. The concomitant use of H_2 blockers and sucralfate is not effective as prophylaxis with the exception of NSAID-induced duodenal ulcers which may be prevented by the use of ranitidine. Misoprostol and proton pump inhibitors are the only prophylactic agents proven effective. Also, concomitant disease and drug use contribute to the risk for GI adverse effects. Use lowest effective dose for shortest period possible. Consider renal function decline with age. Use of NSAIDs can compromise existing renal function especially when Cl_{cr} is ≤30 mL/minute. Tinnitus may be a difficult and unreliable indication of toxicity due to age-related hearing loss or eighth cranial nerve damage. CNS adverse effects such as confusion, agitation, and hallucination are generally seen in overdose or high-dose situations, but elderly may demonstrate these adverse effects at lower doses than younger adults.

Pregnancy Risk Factor: C/D (full-dose aspirin in 3rd trimester - expert analysis)

Pregnancy Issues: Salicylates have been noted to cross the placenta and enter fetal circulation. Adverse effects reported in the fetus include mortality, intrauterine growth retardation, salicylate intoxication, bleeding abnormalities, and neonatal acidosis. Use of aspirin close to delivery may cause premature closure of the ductus arteriosus. Adverse effects reported in the mother include anemia, hemorrhage, prolonged gestation, and prolonged labor. Aspirin has been used for the prevention of pre-eclampsia; however, the ACOG currently recommends that it not be used in low-risk women. Low-dose aspirin is used to treat complications resulting from antiphospholipid syndrome in pregnancy (either primary or secondary to SLE). In general, low doses during pregnancy needed for the treatment of certain medical conditions have not been shown to cause fetal harm, however, discontinuing therapy prior to delivery is recommended. Use of safer agents for routine management of pain or headache should be considered.

Lactation: Enters breast milk/use caution

Breast-Feeding Considerations: Low amounts of aspirin can be found in breast milk. Milk/plasma ratios ranging from 0.03-0.3 have been reported. Peak

(Continued)

Aspirin *(Continued)*

levels in breast milk are reported to be at ~9 hours after a dose. Metabolic acidosis was reported in one infant following an aspirin dose of 3.9 g/day in the mother. The AAP states that aspirin should be used with caution while breast-feeding. The WHO considers occasional doses of aspirin to be compatible with breast-feeding, but to avoid long-term therapy and consider monitoring the infant for adverse effects. Other sources suggest avoiding aspirin while breast-feeding due to the theoretical risk of Reye's syndrome.

Perioperative/Anesthesia/Other Concerns:

Primary Prevention: The U.S. Preventive Services Task Force strongly recommends that clinicians discuss aspirin therapy for primary prevention of heart disease with adults who are at increased risk. The balance of benefits and harm is most favorable in patients at high risk for coronary heart disease (those with a 5-year risk ≥3%). Risk can be calculated at www.med-decisions.com. Adequate blood pressure control is necessary in hypertensive patients who are candidates for aspirin.

Secondary Prevention: In unstable angina, aspirin reduces the rate of refractory angina, nonfatal MI, and death. Aspirin reduces the rate of recurrent ischemia and infarction, stroke and death following MI. In patients who have acute coronary syndrome (ACS) but are not already receiving aspirin, the first dose may be chewed to rapidly establish a high blood level.

Administration

Oral: Do not crush sustained release or enteric coated tablet. Administer with food or a full glass of water to minimize GI distress. For acute myocardial infarction, have patient chew tablet.

Storage: Keep suppositories in refrigerator; do not freeze. Hydrolysis of aspirin occurs upon exposure to water or moist air, resulting in salicylate and acetate, which possess a vinegar-like odor. Do not use if a strong odor is present.

- **Aspirin and Hydrocodone** *see* Hydrocodone and Aspirin *on page 871*
- **Aspirin and Oxycodone** *see* Oxycodone and Aspirin *on page 1289*
- **Aspirin Free Anacin® Maximum Strength [OTC]** *see* Acetaminophen *on page 65*
- **Astelin®** *see* Azelastine *on page 210*
- **AsthmaNefrin®** *see* Epinephrine (Racemic/Dental) *on page 615*
- **Astramorph/PF™** *see* Morphine Sulfate *on page 1177*
- **AT-III** *see* Antithrombin III *on page 173*
- **Atacand®** *see* Candesartan *on page 299*
- **Atarax®** *see* HydrOXYzine *on page 884*

Atenolol (a TEN oh lole)

U.S. Brand Names Tenormin®

Pharmacologic Category Beta Blocker, $Beta_1$ Selective

Medication Safety Issues

Sound-alike/look-alike issues:

Atenolol may be confused with albuterol, Altenol®, timolol, Tylenol®

Tenormin® may be confused with Imuran®, Norpramin®, thiamine, Trovan®

Use Treatment of hypertension, alone or in combination with other agents; management of angina pectoris, postmyocardial infarction patients

Unlabeled/Investigational Use Acute ethanol withdrawal, supraventricular and ventricular arrhythmias, and migraine headache prophylaxis

Mechanism of Action Competitively blocks response to beta-adrenergic stimulation, selectively blocks $beta_1$-receptors with little or no effect on $beta_2$-receptors except at high doses

Pharmacodynamics/Kinetics

Onset of action: Peak effect: Oral: 2-4 hours

Duration: Normal renal function: 12-24 hours

Absorption: Incomplete

Distribution: Low lipophilicity; does not cross blood-brain barrier

Protein binding: 3% to 15%

Metabolism: Limited hepatic

Half-life elimination: Beta:

Neonates: ≤35 hours; Mean: 16 hours

Children: 4.6 hours; children >10 years may have longer half-life (>5 hours) compared to children 5-10 years (<5 hours)

Adults: Normal renal function: 6-9 hours, prolonged with renal impairment; End-stage renal disease: 15-35 hours

Excretion: Feces (50%); urine (40% as unchanged drug)

Contraindications Hypersensitivity to atenolol or any component of the formulation; sinus bradycardia; sinus node dysfunction; heart block greater than first-degree (except in patients with a functioning artificial pacemaker); cardiogenic shock; uncompensated cardiac failure; pulmonary edema; pregnancy

Warnings/Precautions Administer cautiously in compensated heart failure and monitor for a worsening of the condition (efficacy of atenolol in heart failure has not been established). Beta-blocker therapy should not be withdrawn abruptly (particularly in patients with CAD), but gradually tapered to avoid acute tachycardia, hypertension, and/or ischemia. Use caution with concurrent use of beta-blockers and either verapamil or diltiazem; bradycardia or heart block can occur. Avoid concurrent I.V. use of both agents. Beta-blockers should be avoided in patients with bronchospastic disease (asthma) and peripheral vascular disease (may aggravate arterial insufficiency). Atenolol, with B1 selectivity, has been used cautiously in bronchospastic disease with close monitoring. Use cautiously in diabetics - may mask hypoglycemic symptoms. May mask signs of thyrotoxicosis. May cause fetal harm when administered in pregnancy. Use cautiously in the renally impaired (dosage adjustment required). Use care with anesthetic agents which decrease myocardial function. Caution in myasthenia gravis.

Drug Interactions

Alpha-blockers (prazosin, terazosin): Concurrent use of beta-blockers may increase risk of orthostasis.

Ampicillin, in single doses of 1 gram, decrease atenolol's pharmacologic actions.

Antacids (magnesium-aluminum, calcium antacids or salts) may reduce the bioavailability of atenolol.

Clonidine: Hypertensive crisis after or during withdrawal of either agent.

Drugs which slow AV conduction (digoxin): Effects may be additive with beta-blockers.

Glucagon: Atenolol may blunt the hyperglycemic action of glucagon.

Insulin and oral hypoglycemics: Atenolol masks the tachycardia that usually accompanies hypoglycemia.

NSAIDs (ibuprofen, indomethacin, naproxen, piroxicam) may reduce the antihypertensive effects of beta-blockers.

Salicylates may reduce the antihypertensive effects of beta-blockers.

Sulfonylureas: Beta-blockers may alter response to hypoglycemic agents.

Verapamil or diltiazem may have synergistic or additive pharmacological effects when taken concurrently with beta-blockers.

Nutritional/Herbal/Ethanol Interactions

Food: Atenolol serum concentrations may be decreased if taken with food.

Herb/Nutraceutical: Avoid dong quai if using for hypertension (has estrogenic activity). Avoid ephedra, yohimbe, ginseng (may worsen hypertension). Avoid garlic (may have increased antihypertensive effect).

Lab Interactions Increased glucose; decreased HDL

Adverse Reactions

1% to 10%:

Cardiovascular: Persistent bradycardia, hypotension, chest pain, edema, heart failure, second- or third-degree AV block, Raynaud's phenomenon

Central nervous system: Dizziness, fatigue, insomnia, lethargy, confusion, mental impairment, depression, headache, nightmares

Gastrointestinal: Constipation, diarrhea, nausea

Genitourinary: Impotence

Miscellaneous: Cold extremities

<1% (Limited to important or life-threatening): Alopecia, dyspnea (especially with large doses), elevated liver enzymes, hallucinations, impotence, lupus syndrome, Peyronie's disease, positive ANA, psoriaform rash, psychosis, thrombocytopenia, wheezing

Overdosage/Toxicology Symptoms of toxicity include lethargy, respiratory drive disorder, wheezing, sinus pause and bradycardia. Additional effects associated with any beta-blocker are congestive heart failure, hypotension, bronchospasm, and hypoglycemia. Treatment includes removal of unabsorbed drug by induced emesis, gastric lavage, or administration of activated charcoal and symptomatic treatment of toxic responses. Atenolol can be removed by hemodialysis.

(Continued)

Atenolol *(Continued)*

Dosing

Adults & Elderly:

Hypertension:

Oral: 25-50 mg once daily, may increase to 100 mg/day. Doses >100 mg are unlikely to produce any further benefit.

I.V.: Dosages of 1.25-5 mg every 6-12 hours have been used in short-term management of patients unable to take oral enteral beta-blockers

Angina pectoris: Oral: 50 mg once daily, may increase to 100 mg/day. Some patients may require 200 mg/day.

Postmyocardial infarction:

I.V.: Early treatment: 5 mg slow I.V. over 5 minutes; may repeat in 10 minutes. If both doses are tolerated, may start oral atenolol 50 mg every 12 hours or 100 mg/day for 6-9 days postmyocardial infarction.

Oral: Follow I.V. dose with 100 mg/day or 50 mg twice daily for 6-9 days postmyocardial infarction.

Pediatrics:

Hypertension: Oral: Children: 0.8-1 mg/kg/dose given daily; range of 0.8-1.5 mg/kg/day; maximum dose: 2 mg/kg/day

Renal Impairment:

Cl_{cr} 15-35 mL/minute: Administer 50 mg/day maximum.

Cl_{cr} <15 mL/minute: Administer 50 mg every other day maximum.

Hemodialysis effects: Moderately dialyzable (20% to 50%) via hemodialysis. Administer dose postdialysis or administer 25-50 mg supplemental dose. Elimination is not enhanced with peritoneal dialysis. Supplemental dose is not necessary.

Available Dosage Forms

Injection, solution: 0.5 mg/mL (10 mL)

Tablet: 25 mg, 50 mg, 100 mg

Nursing Guidelines

Assessment: Assess potential for interactions with other prescriptions, OTC medications, or herbal products patient may be taking. I.V. administration requires cardiac and hemodynamic monitoring and hypotensive precautions. For oral administration, assess blood pressure and heart rate prior to and following first dose and any change in dosage. Assess therapeutic effectiveness and adverse effects (eg, CHF, edema, new cough, dyspnea, unresolved fatigue). Advise patients with diabetes to monitor glucose levels closely (beta-blockers may alter glucose tolerance). Do not discontinue abruptly; taper dose gradually. Teach patient appropriate use, possible side effects/interventions (hypotension precautions), and adverse symptoms to report.

Dietary Considerations: May be taken without regard to meals.

Patient Education: Do not take any new medication during therapy unless approved by prescriber. Take exactly as directed; with or without regard to meals; do not take with antacids. Do not adjust dosage or discontinue without consulting prescriber. Take pulse daily (prior to medication) and follow prescriber's instruction about holding medication. If you have diabetes, monitor serum sugar closely (drug may alter glucose tolerance or mask signs of hypoglycemia). May cause fatigue, dizziness, or postural hypotension (use caution when changing position from lying or sitting to standing, when driving, or climbing stairs until response to medication is known). Alteration in sexual performance (reversible); or constipation (increased dietary bulk and fluids and exercise may help). Report unresolved swelling of extremities, respiratory difficulty or new cough, unresolved fatigue, unusual weight gain, unresolved constipation, or unusual muscle weakness. **Pregnancy/breast-feeding precautions:** Do not get pregnant or cause a pregnancy (males) while using this medication. Consult prescriber for appropriate contraceptive measures. Consult prescriber if breast-feeding.

Geriatric Considerations: Due to alterations in the beta-adrenergic autonomic nervous system, beta-adrenergic blockade may result in less hemodynamic response than seen in younger adults.

Pregnancy Risk Factor: D

Pregnancy Issues: Atenolol crosses the placenta; beta-blockers have been associated with persistent bradycardia, hypotension, and IUGR; IUGR is probably related to maternal hypertension. Available evidence suggests beta-blockers are generally safe during pregnancy (JNC 7). Cases of neonatal hypoglycemia have been reported following maternal use of beta-blockers at parturition or during breast-feeding. Monitor breast-fed infant for symptoms of beta-blockade.

Lactation: Enters breast milk/use caution

Breast-Feeding Considerations: Symptoms of beta-blockade including cyanosis, hypothermia, and bradycardia have been reported in nursing infants.

Perioperative/Anesthesia/Other Concerns: Atenolol may mask signs and symptoms of hypoglycemia; may potentiate hypoglycemia in a diabetic patient.

Myocardial Infarction: Beta-blockers, in general without intrinsic sympathomimetic activity (ISA), have been shown to decrease morbidity and mortality when initiated in the acute treatment of myocardial infarction and continued long-term. In this setting, therapy should be avoided in patients with hypotension, cardiogenic shock, or heart block.

Surgery: Atenolol has also been shown to improve cardiovascular outcomes when used in the perioperative period in patients with underlying cardiovascular disease who are undergoing noncardiac surgery. Bisoprolol in high-risk patients undergoing vascular surgery reduced the perioperative incidence of death from cardiac causes and nonfatal myocardial infarction.

Withdrawal: Beta-blocker therapy should not be withdrawn abruptly, but gradually tapered to avoid acute tachycardia and hypertension.

Administration

I.V.: When administered acutely for cardiac treatment, monitor ECG and blood pressure. The injection can be administered undiluted or diluted with a compatible I.V. solution. May administer by rapid infusion (I.V. push) at a rate of 1 mg/minute or by slow infusion over ~30 minutes. Necessary monitoring for surgical patients who are unable to take oral beta-blockers (prolonged ileus) has not been defined. Some institutions require monitoring of baseline and postinfusion heart rate and blood pressure when a patient's response to beta-blockade has not been characterized (ie, the patient's initial dose or following a change in dose). Consult individual institutional policies and procedures.

Compatibility: Stable in D_5W, NS

Y-site administration: Incompatible with amphotericin B cholesteryl sulfate complex

Atenolol and Chlorthalidone (a TEN oh lole & klor THAL i done)

U.S. Brand Names Tenoretic®

Synonyms Chlorthalidone and Atenolol

Pharmacologic Category Antihypertensive Agent, Combination

Use Treatment of hypertension with a cardioselective beta-blocker and a diuretic

Pharmacodynamics/Kinetics See individual agents.

Drug Interactions See individual agents.

Adverse Reactions See individual agents.

Dosing

Adults & Elderly: Hypertension: Oral: Initial: 1 (50) tablet once daily, then individualize dose until optimal dose is achieved

Renal Impairment:

Cl_{cr} 15-35 mL/minute: Administer 50 mg/day.

Cl_{cr} <15 mL/minute: Administer 50 mg every other day.

Available Dosage Forms Tablet:

50: Atenolol 50 mg and chlorthalidone 25 mg

100: Atenolol 100 mg and chlorthalidone 25 mg

Nursing Guidelines

Assessment: See individual components listed in Related Information. **Pregnancy risk factor D** - determine that patient is not pregnant before beginning treatment. Instruct patients of childbearing age about appropriate barrier contraceptive measures. Note breast-feeding caution.

Dietary Considerations: Should be taken on empty stomach.

Patient Education: See individual agents. **Pregnancy/breast-feeding precautions:** Inform prescriber if you are or intend to become pregnant. Consult prescriber if breast-feeding.

Pregnancy Risk Factor: D

Lactation: Excretion in breast milk unknown

Related Information

Atenolol *on page 194*

Chlorthalidone *on page 383*

♦ **ATG** *see* Antithymocyte Globulin (Rabbit) *on page 176*

♦ Atgam® *see* Antithymocyte Globulin (Equine) *on page 174*
♦ Ativan® *see* Lorazepam *on page 1061*

Atorvastatin (a TORE va sta tin)

U.S. Brand Names Lipitor®

Pharmacologic Category Antilipemic Agent, HMG-CoA Reductase Inhibitor

Medication Safety Issues

Sound-alike/look-alike issues:

Lipitor® may be confused with Levatol®

Use Treatment of dyslipidemias or primary prevention of cardiovascular disease (atherosclerotic) as detailed below:

Primary prevention of cardiovascular disease (high-risk for CVD): To reduce the risk of MI or stroke in patients without evidence of heart disease who have multiple CVD risk factors or type 2 diabetes. Treatment reduces the risk for angina or revascularization procedures in patients with multiple risk factors.

Treatment of dyslipidemias: To reduce elevations in total cholesterol, LDL-C, apolipoprotein B, and triglycerides in patients with elevations of one or more components, and/or to increase HDL-C as present in Fredrickson type IIa, IIb, III, and IV hyperlipidemias; treatment of primary dysbetalipoproteinemia, homozygous familial hypercholesterolemia

Treatment of heterozygous familial hypercholesterolemia (HeFH) in adolescent patients (10-17 years of age, females >1 year postmenarche) having LDL-C ≥190 mg/dL or LDL ≥160 mg/dL with positive family history of premature cardiovascular disease (CVD) or with two or more CVD risk factors.

Mechanism of Action Inhibitor of 3-hydroxy-3-methylglutaryl coenzyme A (HMG-CoA) reductase, the rate limiting enzyme in cholesterol synthesis (reduces the production of mevalonic acid from HMG-CoA); this then results in a compensatory increase in the expression of LDL receptors on hepatocyte membranes and a stimulation of LDL catabolism

Pharmacodynamics/Kinetics

Onset of action: Initial changes: 3-5 days; Maximal reduction in plasma cholesterol and triglycerides: 2 weeks

Absorption: Rapid

Distribution: V_d: 318 L

Protein binding: ≥98%

Metabolism: Hepatic; forms active ortho- and parahydroxylated derivates and an inactive beta-oxidation product

Half-life elimination: Parent drug: 14 hours

Time to peak, serum: 1-2 hours

Excretion: Bile; urine (2% as unchanged drug)

Contraindications Hypersensitivity to atorvastatin or any component of the formulation; active liver disease; unexplained persistent elevations of serum transaminases; pregnancy; breast-feeding

Warnings/Precautions Secondary causes of hyperlipidemia should be ruled out prior to therapy. May cause hepatic dysfunction. Use with caution in patients who consume large amounts of ethanol or have a history of liver disease. Monitoring is recommended. Rhabdomyolysis with acute renal failure has occurred. Risk is dose-related and is increased with concurrent use of lipid-lowering agents which may cause rhabdomyolysis (gemfibrozil, fibric acid derivatives, or niacin at doses ≥1 g/day) or during concurrent use with potent CYP3A4 inhibitors (including amiodarone, clarithromycin, cyclosporine, erythromycin, itraconazole, ketoconazole, nefazodone, grapefruit juice in large quantities, verapamil, or protease inhibitors such as indinavir, nelfinavir, or ritonavir). Weigh the risk versus benefit when combining any of these drugs with atorvastatin. Discontinue in any patient experiencing an acute or serious condition predisposing to renal failure secondary to rhabdomyolysis. Safety and efficacy have not been established in patients <10 years of age or in premenarcheal girls.

Drug Interactions Substrate of CYP3A4 (major); **Inhibits** CYP3A4 (weak)

Antacids: Plasma concentrations may be decreased when given with magnesium-aluminum hydroxide containing antacids (reported with atorvastatin and pravastatin). Clinical efficacy is not altered, no dosage adjustment is necessary

Bile acid sequestrants (cholestyramine and colestipol): Reduce absorption of several HMG-CoA reductase inhibitors; separate administration times by at least 4 hours. Cholesterol-lowering effects are additive.

Cyclosporine: May increase serum concentrations of atorvastatin, increasing the risk of myopathy; monitor.

CYP3A4 inhibitors: May increase the levels/effects of atorvastatin. Example inhibitors include azole antifungals, clarithromycin, diclofenac, doxycycline, erythromycin, imatinib, isoniazid, nefazodone, nicardipine, propofol, protease inhibitors, quinidine, telithromycin, and verapamil.

Digoxin: Plasma concentrations of digoxin may be increased by ~20%; monitor.

Fibric acid derivatives (clofibrate and fenofibrate): May increase the risk of myopathy and rhabdomyolysis.

Grapefruit juice: May inhibit metabolism of atorvastatin via CYP3A4; more likely to occur with lovastatin or simvastatin; avoid high dietary intake of grapefruit juice

Niacin: May increase the risk of myopathy and rhabdomyolysis.

Nutritional/Herbal/Ethanol Interactions

Ethanol: Avoid excessive ethanol consumption (due to potential hepatic effects).

Food: Atorvastatin serum concentrations may be increased by grapefruit juice; avoid concurrent intake of large quantities (>1 quart/day). Red yeast rice contains an estimated 2.4 mg lovastatin per 600 mg rice.

Herb/Nutraceutical: St John's wort may decrease atorvastatin levels.

Adverse Reactions

>10%: Central nervous system: Headache (3% to 17%)

2% to 10%:

- Cardiovascular: Chest pain, peripheral edema
- Central nervous system: Insomnia, dizziness
- Dermatologic: Rash (1% to 4%)
- Gastrointestinal: Abdominal pain (up to 4%), constipation (up to 3%), diarrhea (up to 4%), dyspepsia (1% to 3%), flatulence (1% to 3%), nausea
- Genitourinary: Urinary tract infection
- Hepatic: Transaminases increased (2% to 3% with 80 mg/day dosing)
- Neuromuscular & skeletal: Arthralgia (up to 5%), arthritis, back pain (up to 4%), myalgia (up to 6%), weakness (up to 4%)
- Respiratory: Sinusitis (up to 6%), pharyngitis (up to 3%), bronchitis, rhinitis
- Miscellaneous: Infection (3% to 10%), flu-like syndrome (up to 3%), allergic reaction (up to 3%)

<2% (Limited to important or life-threatening): Alopecia, anaphylaxis, angina, angioneurotic edema, arrhythmia, bullous rash, cholestatic jaundice, deafness, dyspnea, erythema multiforme, esophagitis, facial paralysis, fatigue, glaucoma, gout, hepatitis, hyperkinesias, impotence, migraine, myasthenia, myopathy, myositis, nephritis, pancreatitis, paresthesia, peripheral neuropathy, petechiae, photosensitivity, postural hypotension, pruritus, rectal hemorrhage, rhabdomyolysis, somnolence, Stevens-Johnson syndrome, syncope, tendinous contracture, thrombocytopenia, tinnitus, torticollis, toxic epidermal necrolysis, urticaria, vaginal hemorrhage, vomiting

Overdosage/Toxicology Treatment is supportive.

Dosing

Adults & Elderly:

Hyperlipidemias: Oral: Initial: 10-20 mg once daily; patients requiring >45% reduction in LDL-C may be started at 40 mg once daily; range: 10-80 mg once daily

Note: Doses should be individualized according to the baseline LDL-cholesterol levels, the recommended goal of therapy, and patient response; adjustments should be made at intervals of 2-4 weeks

Primary prevention of CVD: Oral: 10 mg once daily

Pediatrics:

HeFH: Children 10-17 years (females >1 year postmenarche): Oral: 10 mg once daily (maximum: 20 mg/day)

Note: Doses should be individualized according to the baseline LDL-cholesterol levels, the recommended goal of therapy, and patient response; adjustments should be made at intervals of 2-4 weeks

Renal Impairment: No adjustment is necessary.

Hepatic Impairment: Decrease dosage with severe disease (eg, chronic alcoholic liver disease).

Available Dosage Forms Tablet: 10 mg, 20 mg, 40 mg, 80 mg

Nursing Guidelines

Assessment: See Contraindications and Warnings/Precautions for use cautions. Assess potential for interactions with other prescriptions, OTC medications, or herbal products patient may be taking (see Drug Interactions). Laboratory tests should be scheduled and results monitored prior to initiation and at regular intervals (see Monitoring Laboratory Tests). Assess for therapeutic response and adverse effects (see Adverse Reactions). Teach patient

(Continued)

Atorvastatin *(Continued)*

proper use, possible side effects/appropriate interventions, and adverse symptoms to report (see Patient Education). **Pregnancy risk factor X** - determine that patient is not pregnant before starting therapy. Do not give to childbearing age females unless capable of complying with effective contraceptive use. Breast-feeding is contraindicated.

Monitoring Laboratory Tests: Monitor lipid levels after 2-4 weeks; LFTs prior to initiation and 12 weeks after initiation or first dose or dose elevation, and periodically (semiannually) thereafter; CPK

Dietary Considerations: May take with food if desired; may take without regard to time of day. Before initiation of therapy, patients should be placed on a standard cholesterol-lowering diet for 3-6 months and the diet should be continued during drug therapy. Red yeast rice contains an estimated 2.4 mg lovastatin per 600 mg rice.

Patient Education: Inform prescriber of all prescriptions, OTC medications, or herbal products you are taking, and any allergies you have. Do not take any new medication during therapy unless approved by prescriber. May take without regard to food. Maintain adequate hydration (2-3 L/day of fluids) unless instructed to restrict fluid intake. You will need laboratory evaluation during therapy. May cause headache (consult prescriber for approved analgesic); diarrhea (buttermilk, boiled milk, or yogurt may help); euphoria, giddiness, or confusion (use caution when driving or engaging in tasks that require alertness until response to medication is known). Report unresolved diarrhea, unusual muscle cramping or weakness, changes in mood or memory, yellowing of skin or eyes, easy bruising or bleeding, or unusual fatigue. **Pregnancy/breast-feeding precautions:** Inform prescriber if you are pregnant. Do not get pregnant during therapy. Consult prescriber for instructions on appropriate contraceptive measures. This drug can cause severe fetal defects. Do not donate blood while taking this medication and for same period of time after discontinuing. Do not breast-feed.

Geriatric Considerations: Effective and well tolerated in elderly. The definition of and, therefore, when to treat hyperlipidemia in the elderly is a controversial issue. The National Cholesterol Education Program recommends that all adults maintain a plasma cholesterol <160 mg/dL. In elderly patients with one additional risk factor, goal LDL would decrease to <130 mg/dL. Pharmacologic treatment should be reserved for those who are unable to obtain a desirable plasma cholesterol concentration by diet alone and for whom the benefits of treatment are believed to outweigh the potential adverse effects, drug interactions, and cost of treatment.

Pregnancy Risk Factor: X

Pregnancy Issues: Cholesterol biosynthesis may be important in fetal development. Contraindicated in pregnancy. Administer to women of childbearing potential only when conception is highly unlikely and patients have been informed of potential hazards.

Lactation: Enters breast milk/contraindicated

Perioperative/Anesthesia/Other Concerns: Myopathy: Currently-marketed HMG-CoA reductase inhibitors appear to have a similar potential for causing myopathy. Incidence of severe myopathy is about 0.08% to 0.09%. The factors that increase risk include advanced age (especially >80 years), gender (occurs in women more frequently than men), small body frame, frailty, multisystem disease (eg, chronic renal insufficiency especially due to diabetes), multiple medications, **perioperative periods (higher risk when continued during hospitalization for major surgery)**, and drug interactions (use with caution or avoid).

Administration

Oral: May be administered with food if desired; may take without regard to time of day

Atracurium (a tra KYOO ree um)

U.S. Brand Names Tracrium®

Synonyms Atracurium Besylate

Pharmacologic Category Neuromuscular Blocker Agent, Nondepolarizing

Use Adjunct to general anesthesia to facilitate endotracheal intubation and to relax skeletal muscles during surgery; to facilitate mechanical ventilation in ICU patients; does not relieve pain or produce sedation

Mechanism of Action Blocks neural transmission at the myoneural junction by binding with cholinergic receptor sites

Pharmacodynamics/Kinetics

Onset of action (dose dependent): 2-3 minutes

Duration: Recovery begins in 20-35 minutes following initial dose of 0.4-0.5 mg/kg under balanced anesthesia; recovery to 95% of control takes 60-70 minutes

Metabolism: Undergoes ester hydrolysis and Hofmann elimination (nonbiologic process independent of renal, hepatic, or enzymatic function); metabolites have no neuromuscular blocking properties; laudanosine, a product of Hofmann elimination, is a CNS stimulant and can accumulate with prolonged use. Laudanosine is hepatically metabolized.

Half-life elimination: Biphasic: Adults: Initial (distribution): 2 minutes; Terminal: 20 minutes

Excretion: Urine (<5%)

Contraindications Hypersensitivity to atracurium besylate or any component of the formulation

Warnings/Precautions Reduce initial dosage and inject slowly (over 1-2 minutes) in patients in whom substantial histamine release would be potentially hazardous (eg, patients with clinically important cardiovascular disease); maintenance of an adequate airway and respiratory support is critical; certain clinical conditions may result in potentiation or antagonism of neuromuscular blockade:

Potentiation: Electrolyte abnormalities, severe hyponatremia, severe hypocalcemia, severe hypokalemia, hypermagnesemia, neuromuscular diseases, acidosis, acute intermittent porphyria, renal failure, hepatic failure

Antagonism: Alkalosis, hypercalcemia, demyelinating lesions, peripheral neuropathies, diabetes mellitus

Increased sensitivity in patients with myasthenia gravis, Eaton-Lambert syndrome; resistance in burn patients (>30% of body) for period of 5-70 days postinjury; resistance in patients with muscle trauma, denervation, immobilization, infection, chronic treatment with atracurium. Cross-sensitivity with other neuromuscular-blocking agents may occur; use extreme caution in patients with previous anaphylactic reactions. Bradycardia may be more common with atracurium than with other neuromuscular-blocking agents since it has no clinically significant effects on heart rate to counteract the bradycardia produced by anesthetics.

Drug Interactions

Prolonged neuromuscular blockade: Local anesthetics; calcium channel blockers; corticosteroids; antiarrhythmics (eg, quinidine or procainamide); antibiotics (eg, aminoglycosides, tetracyclines, vancomycin, clindamycin); immunosuppressants (eg, cyclosporine)

Increased sensitivity to muscle relaxants (eg, neuromuscular disorders such as myasthenia gravis or polymyositis)

Adverse Reactions Mild, rare, and generally suggestive of histamine release

1% to 10%: Cardiovascular: Flushing

<1%: Bronchial secretions, erythema, hives, itching, wheezing

Postmarketing and/or case reports: Allergic reaction, bradycardia, bronchospasm, dyspnea, hypotension, injection site reaction, seizure, acute quadriplegic myopathy syndrome (prolonged use), laryngospasm, myositis ossificans (prolonged use), tachycardia, urticaria

Causes of prolonged neuromuscular blockade: Excessive drug administration; cumulative drug effect, decreased metabolism/excretion (hepatic and/or renal impairment); accumulation of active metabolites; electrolyte imbalance (hypokalemia, hypocalcemia, hypermagnesemia, hypernatremia); hypothermia

Overdosage/Toxicology

Symptoms of overdose include respiratory depression and cardiovascular collapse.

Neostigmine 1-3 mg slow I.V. push in adults (0.5 mg in children) antagonizes the neuromuscular blockade, and should be administered with or immediately after atropine 1-1.5 mg I.V. push (adults). This may be especially useful in the presence of bradycardia.

Dosing

Adults & Elderly: For I.V. administration only (not to be used I.M.): Dose to effect; doses must be individualized due to interpatient variability; use ideal body weight for obese patients.

(Continued)

Atracurium *(Continued)*

Adjunct to surgical anesthesia (neuromuscular blockade):

I.V. (bolus): 0.4-0.5 mg/kg, then 0.08-0.1 mg/kg 20-45 minutes after initial dose to maintain neuromuscular block, followed by repeat doses of 0.08-0.1 mg/kg at 15- to 25-minute intervals

Initial dose after succinylcholine for intubation (balanced anesthesia): Adults: 0.2-0.4 mg/kg

Pretreatment/priming: I.V.: 10% of intubating dose given 3-5 minutes before initial dose

I.V. continuous infusion: Initial: 9-10 mcg/kg/minute at initial signs of recovery from bolus dose; block is usually maintained by a rate of 5-9 mcg/kg/minute under balanced anesthesia.

ICU neuromuscular blockade: I.V.: Initial (bolus) 0.4-0.5 mg/kg, followed by I.V. continuous infusion at an initial rate of 5-10 mcg/kg/min; block is usually maintained by rate of 11-13 mcg/kg/minute (rates for pediatric patients may be higher).

Pediatrics:

Adjunct to surgical anesthesia: I.V. (not to be used I.M.): Dose to effect; doses must be individualized due to interpatient variability; use ideal body weight for obese patients

Children 1 month to 2 years: Initial: 0.3-0.4 mg/kg followed by maintenance doses as needed to maintain neuromuscular blockade

Children >2 years: Refer to adult dosing.

Renal Impairment: No adjustment is necessary.

Hepatic Impairment: No adjustment is necessary.

Available Dosage Forms

Injection, as besylate: 10 mg/mL (10 mL) [contains benzyl alcohol]

Injection, as besylate [preservative free]: 10 mg/mL (5 mL)

Nursing Guidelines

Assessment: Only clinicians experienced in the use of neuromuscular-blocking drugs should administer and/or manage the use of atracurium. Dosage and rate of administration should be individualized and titrated to the desired effect, according to relevant clinical factors, premedication, concomitant medications, age, and general condition of the patient. Ventilatory support must be instituted and maintained until adequate respiratory muscle function and/or airway protection are assured. Assess other medications for effectiveness and safety. Other drugs that affect neuromuscular activity may increase/decrease neuromuscular block induced by atracurium. This drug does not cause anesthesia or analgesia; pain must be treated with appropriate analgesic agents. Continuous monitoring of vital signs, cardiac status, respiratory status, and degree of neuromuscular block (objective assessment with peripheral external nerve stimulator) is mandatory during infusion and until full muscle tone has returned. Muscle tone returns in a predictable pattern, starting with diaphragm, abdomen, chest, limbs, and finally muscles of the neck, face, and eyes. Safety precautions must be maintained until full muscle tone has returned. **Note:** It may take longer for return of muscle tone in obese or elderly patients or patients with renal or hepatic disease, myasthenia gravis, myopathy, other neuromuscular disease, dehydration, electrolyte imbalance, or severe acid/base imbalance. Provide appropriate patient teaching/support prior to and following administration.

Long-term use: Monitor fluid levels (intake and output) during and following infusion. Reposition patient and provide appropriate skin care, mouth care, and care of patient's eyes every 2-3 hours while sedated. Provide appropriate emotional and sensory support (auditory and environmental).

Monitoring Laboratory Tests: Renal function (serum creatinine, BUN) and liver function when in ICU

Patient Education: Patient will usually be unconscious prior to administration. Patient education should be appropriate to individual situation. Reassurance of constant monitoring and emotional support to reduce fear and anxiety should precede and follow administration. Following return of muscle tone, do not attempt to change position or rise from bed without assistance. Report immediately any skin rash or hives, pounding heartbeat, respiratory difficulty, or muscle tremors. **Pregnancy/breast-feeding precautions:** Inform prescriber if you are pregnant. Consult prescriber if breast-feeding.

Pregnancy Risk Factor: C

Lactation: Excretion in breast milk unknown/use caution

Perioperative/Anesthesia/Other Concerns: Atracurium is classified as an intermediate duration neuromuscular-blocking agent; does not appear to have a cumulative effect on the duration of blockade.

Critically-Ill Adult Patients: The 2002 ACCM/SCCM/ASHP clinical practice guidelines for sustained neuromuscular blockade in the adult critically-ill patient recommend:

Optimize sedatives and analgesics prior to initiation and monitor and adjust accordingly during course. Neuromuscular blockers do not relieve pain or produce sedation.

Protect patient's eyes from development of keratitis and corneal abrasion by administering ophthalmic ointment and taping eyelids closed or using eye patches. Reposition patient routinely to protect pressure points from breakdown. Address DVT prophylaxis.

Concurrent use of a neuromuscular blocker and corticosteroids appear to increase the risk of certain ICU myopathies; avoid or administer the corticosteroid at the lowest dose possible. Reassess need for neuromuscular blocker daily.

Using daily drug holidays (stopping neuromuscular-blocking agent until patient requires it again) may decrease the incidence of acute quadriplegic myopathy syndrome.

Tachyphylaxis can develop; switch to another neuromuscular blocker (taking into consideration the patient's organ function) if paralysis is still necessary.

Acidosis and severe hypothermia may delay the elimination of atracurium and cisatracurium.

Atracurium or cisatracurium is recommended for patients with significant hepatic or renal disease, due to organ-independent Hofmann elimination.

Monitor patients clinically and via "Train of Four" (TOF) testing with a goal of adjusting the degree of blockade to 1-2 twitches or based upon the patient's clinical condition.

Administration

I.M.: Not for I.M. injection due to tissue irritation.

I.V.: May be given undiluted as a bolus injection. Administration via infusion requires the use of an infusion pump. Use infusion solutions within 24 hours of preparation.

Compatibility: Stable in D_5W, NS, D_5NS; **incompatible** with LR

Y-site administration: Incompatible with diazepam, propofol, thiopental

Compatibility when admixed: Incompatible with aminophylline, cefazolin, heparin, quinidine gluconate, ranitidine, sodium nitroprusside

Storage: Refrigerate; unstable in alkaline solutions.

♦ Atracurium Besylate *see* Atracurium *on page 200*

♦ AtroPen® *see* Atropine *on page 203*

Atropine (A troe peen)

U.S. Brand Names AtroPen®; Atropine-Care®; Isopto® Atropine; Sal-Tropine™

Synonyms Atropine Sulfate

Pharmacologic Category Anticholinergic Agent; Anticholinergic Agent, Ophthalmic; Antidote; Antispasmodic Agent, Gastrointestinal; Ophthalmic Agent, Mydriatic

Use

Injection: Preoperative medication to inhibit salivation and secretions; treatment of symptomatic sinus bradycardia; AV block (nodal level); ventricular asystole; antidote for organophosphate pesticide poisoning

Ophthalmic: Produce mydriasis and cycloplegia for examination of the retina and optic disc and accurate measurement of refractive errors; uveitis

Oral: Inhibit salivation and secretions

Unlabeled/Investigational Use Pulseless electric activity, asystole, neuromuscular blockade reversal; treatment of nerve agent toxicity (chemical warfare) in combination with pralidoxime

Mechanism of Action Blocks the action of acetylcholine at parasympathetic sites in smooth muscle, secretory glands and the CNS; increases cardiac output, dries secretions, antagonizes histamine and serotonin

Pharmacodynamics/Kinetics

Onset of action: I.V.: Rapid

Absorption: Complete

(Continued)

Atropine *(Continued)*

Distribution: Widely throughout the body; crosses placenta; trace amounts enter breast milk; crosses blood-brain barrier

Metabolism: Hepatic

Half-life elimination: 2-3 hours

Excretion: Urine (30% to 50% as unchanged drug and metabolites)

Contraindications Hypersensitivity to atropine or any component of the formulation; narrow-angle glaucoma; adhesions between the iris and lens; tachycardia; obstructive GI disease; paralytic ileus; intestinal atony of the elderly or debilitated patient; severe ulcerative colitis; toxic megacolon complicating ulcerative colitis; hepatic disease; obstructive uropathy; renal disease; myasthenia gravis (unless used to treat side effects of acetylcholinesterase inhibitor); asthma; thyrotoxicosis; Mobitz type II block

Warnings/Precautions Heat prostration can occur in the presence of a high environmental temperature. Psychosis can occur in sensitive individuals. The elderly may be sensitive to side effects. Use caution in patients with myocardial ischemia. Use caution in hyperthyroidism, autonomic neuropathy, BPH, CHF, tachyarrhythmias, hypertension, and hiatal hernia associated with reflux esophagitis. Use with caution in children with spastic paralysis.

AtroPen®: There are no absolute contraindications for the use of atropine in organophosphate poisonings, however, use caution in those patients where the use of atropine would be otherwise contraindicated. Formulation for use by trained personnel only.

Drug Interactions

Drugs with anticholinergic activity (including phenothiazines and TCAs) may increase anticholinergic effects when used concurrently.

Sympathomimetic amines may cause tachyarrhythmias; avoid concurrent use.

Adverse Reactions Severity and frequency of adverse reactions are dose related and vary greatly; listed reactions are limited to significant and/or life-threatening.

Cardiovascular: Arrhythmia, flushing, hypotension, palpitation, tachycardia

Central nervous system: Ataxia, coma, delirium, disorientation, dizziness, drowsiness, excitement, fever, hallucinations, headache, insomnia, nervousness

Dermatologic: Anhidrosis, urticaria, rash, scarlatiniform rash

Gastrointestinal: Bloating, constipation, delayed gastric emptying, loss of taste, nausea, paralytic ileus, vomiting, xerostomia

Genitourinary: Urinary hesitancy, urinary retention

Neuromuscular & skeletal: Weakness

Ocular: Angle-closure glaucoma, blurred vision, cycloplegia, dry eyes, mydriasis, ocular tension increased

Respiratory: Dyspnea, laryngospasm, pulmonary edema

Miscellaneous: Anaphylaxis

Overdosage/Toxicology Symptoms of overdose include dilated, unreactive pupils; blurred vision; hot, dry flushed skin; dryness of mucous membranes; difficulty swallowing; foul breath; diminished or absent bowel sounds; urinary retention; tachycardia; hyperthermia; hypertension; and increased respiratory rate. For anticholinergic overdose with severe life-threatening symptoms, physostigmine 1-2 mg SubQ or I.V. slowly, may be given to reverse these effects.

Dosing

Adults: Doses <0.5 mg have been associated with paradoxical bradycardia.

Asystole:

I.V.: 1 mg; repeat in 3-5 minutes if asystole persists; total dose of 0.04 mg/kg.

Intratracheal: Administer 2-2.5 times the recommended I.V. dose; dilute in 10 mL NS or distilled water. **Note:** Absorption is greater with distilled water, but causes more adverse effects on PaO_2.

Inhibit salivation and secretions (preanesthesia):

I.M., I.V., SubQ: 0.4-0.6 mg 30-60 minutes preop and repeat every 4-6 hours as needed.

Oral: 0.4 mg, may repeat every 4-6 hours

Bradycardia: I.V.: 0.5-1 mg every 5 minutes, not to exceed a total of 3 mg or 0.04 mg/kg; may give intratracheal in 1 mg/10 mL dilution only, intratracheal dose should be 2-2.5 times the I.V. dose.

Neuromuscular blockade reversal: I.V.: 25-30 mcg/kg 30 seconds before neostigmine or 10 mcg/kg 30 seconds before edrophonium

Organophosphate or carbamate poisoning:

I.V.: 2 mg, followed by 2 mg every 15 minutes until adequate atropinization has occurred; initial doses of up to 6 mg may be used in life-threatening cases

I.M.: AtroPen®: Mild symptoms: Administer 2 mg as soon as exposure is known or suspected. If severe symptoms develop after first dose, 2 additional doses should be repeated in 10 minutes; do not administer more than 3 doses. Severe symptoms: Immediately administer three 2 mg doses.

Nerve agent toxicity management (unlabeled use): I.M.: See **Note**. Prehospital ("in the field") or hospital/emergency department: Mild-to-moderate symptoms: 2-4 mg; severe symptoms: 6 mg

Note: Pralidoxime is a component of the management of nerve agent toxicity; consult pralidoxime monograph for specific route and dose.

Prehospital ("in the field") management: Repeat atropine I.M. (2 mg) at 5-10 minute intervals until secretions have diminished and breathing is comfortable or airway resistance has returned to near normal.

Hospital management: Repeat atropine I.M. (2 mg) at 5-10 minute intervals until secretions have diminished and breathing is comfortable or airway resistance has returned to near normal.

Mydriasis, cycloplegia (preprocedure): Ophthalmic (1% solution): Instill 1-2 drops 1 hour before the procedure.

Uveitis: Ophthalmic:

1% solution: Instill 1-2 drops 4 times/day.

Ointment: Apply a small amount in the conjunctival sac up to 3 times/day. Compress the lacrimal sac by digital pressure for 1-3 minutes after instillation.

Elderly: Refer to adult dosing.

Nerve agent toxicity management (unlabeled use): I.M.: Elderly and frail patients: also see **"Note"** in adult dosing:

Prehospital ("in the field"): Mild-to-moderate symptoms: 1 mg; severe symptoms: 2-4 mg

Hospital/emergency department: Mild-to-moderate symptoms: 1 mg; severe symptoms: 2 mg

Pediatrics: Note: Doses <0.1 mg have been associated with paradoxical bradycardia.

Inhibit salivation and secretions (preanesthesia): Oral, I.M., I.V., SubQ: Neonates, Infants, and Children:

Children <5 kg: 0.02 mg/kg/dose 30-60 minutes preop then every 4-6 hours as needed. Use of a minimum dosage of 0.1 mg in neonates <5 kg will result in dosages >0.02 mg/kg. There is no documented minimum dosage in this age group.

Children >5 kg: 0.01-0.02 mg/kg/dose to a maximum 0.4 mg/dose 30-60 minutes preop; minimum dose: 0.1 mg

Alternate dosing:

3-7 kg (7-16 lb): 0.1 mg
8-11 kg (17-24 lb): 0.15 mg
11-18 kg (24-40 lb): 0.2 mg
18-29 kg (40-65 lb): 0.3 mg
>30 kg (>65 lb): 0.4 mg

Bradycardia: I.V., intratracheal: Neonates, Infants, and Children:

0.02 mg/kg, minimum dose 0.1 mg, maximum single dose: 0.5 mg in children and 1 mg in adolescents; may repeat in 5-minute intervals to a maximum total dose of 1 mg in children or 2 mg in adolescents. (**Note:** For intratracheal administration, the dosage must be diluted with normal saline to a total volume of 1-5 mL). When treating bradycardia in neonates, reserve use for those patients unresponsive to improved oxygenation and epinephrine.

Organophosphate or carbamate poisoning:

I.V.: Children: 0.03-0.05 mg/kg every 10-20 minutes until atropine effect, then every 1-4 hours for at least 24 hours

I.M. (AtroPen®): Children: Mild symptoms: Administer dose listed below as soon as exposure is known or suspected. If severe symptoms develop after first dose, 2 additional doses should be repeated in 10 minutes; do not administer more than 3 doses. Severe symptoms: Immediately administer 3 doses as follows:

<6.8 kg (15 lb): Use of **AtroPen® formulation not recommended**; administer atropine 0.05 mg/kg

6.8-18 kg (15-40 lb): 0.5 mg/dose

(Continued)

Atropine *(Continued)*

18-41 kg (40-90 lb): 1 mg/dose
>41 kg (>90 lb): 2 mg/dose

Nerve agent toxicity management (unlabeled use): I.M.: Infants and Children: See **"Note"** in adult dosing.

Prehospital ("in the field"):

Birth to <2 years: Mild-to-moderate symptoms: 0.05 mg/kg; severe symptoms: 0.1 mg/kg
2-10 years: Mild-to-moderate symptoms: 1 mg; severe symptoms: 2 mg
>10 years: Mild-to-moderate symptoms: 2 mg; severe symptoms: 4 mg

Hospital/emergency department:

Birth to <2 years: Mild-to-moderate symptoms: 0.05 mg/kg I.M. **or** 0.02 mg/kg I.V.; severe symptoms: 0.1 mg/kg I.M. **or** 0.02 mg/kg I.V.
2-10 years: Mild-to-moderate symptoms: 1 mg; severe symptoms: 2 mg
>10 years: Mild-to-moderate symptoms: 2 mg; severe symptoms: 4 mg

Available Dosage Forms

Injection, solution, as sulfate: 0.05 mg/mL (5 mL); 0.1 mg/mL (5 mL, 10 mL); 0.4 mg/mL (0.5 mL, 1 mL, 20 mL); 0.5 mg/mL (1 mL); 1 mg/mL (1 mL)
AtroPen® [prefilled autoinjector]: 0.5 mg/0.7 mL (0.7 mL); 1 mg/0.7 mL (0.7 mL); 2 mg/0.7 mL (0.7 mL)
Ointment, ophthalmic, as sulfate: 1% (3.5 g)
Solution, ophthalmic, as sulfate: 1% (5 mL, 15 mL)
Atropine-Care®: 1% (2 mL)
Isopto® Atropine: 1% (5 mL, 15 mL)
Tablet, as sulfate (Sal-Tropine™): 0.4 mg

Nursing Guidelines

Assessment: Assess other medications patient may be taking for effectiveness and interactions. Monitor for tachycardia, hypotension especially if cardiac problems are present. Be alert to the potential of heat prostration in the presence of high temperatures. Assess knowledge/teach patient appropriate use, interventions to reduce side effects, and adverse symptoms to report.

Patient Education: Take oral forms exactly as directed, 30 minutes before meals. Maintain adequate hydration (2-3 L/day of fluids) unless instructed to restrict fluid intake. Void before taking medication. You may experience dizziness, blurred vision, sensitivity to light (use caution when driving or engaging in tasks requiring alertness until response to drug is known); dry mouth, nausea, or vomiting (small frequent meals, frequent mouth care, sucking lozenges, or chewing gum may help); orthostatic hypotension (use caution when climbing stairs and when rising from lying or sitting position); constipation (increased exercise, fluids, fruit, or fiber may help; if not effective, consult prescriber); increased sensitivity to heat and decreased perspiration (avoid extremes of heat, reduce exercise in hot weather); or decreased milk if breast-feeding. Report hot, dry, flushed skin; blurred vision or vision changes; difficulty swallowing; chest pain, palpitations, or rapid heartbeat; painful or difficult urination; increased confusion, depression, or loss of memory; rapid or difficult respirations; muscle weakness or tremors; or eye pain.

Ophthalmic: Instill as often as recommended. Wash hands before using. Sit or lie down, open eye, look at ceiling, and instill prescribed amount of solution. Do not blink for 30 seconds, close eye and roll eye in all directions, and apply gentle pressure to inner corner of eye for 1-2 minutes. Do not let tip of applicator touch eye; do not contaminate tip of applicator (may cause eye infection, eye damage, or vision loss). Temporary stinging or blurred vision may occur.

Pregnancy/breast-feeding precautions: Inform prescriber if you are or intend to become pregnant. Consult prescriber if breast-feeding.

Geriatric Considerations: Anticholinergic agents are generally not well tolerated in the elderly and their use should be avoided when possible (see Warnings/Precautions, Adverse Reactions). In the elderly, anticholinergic agents should not be used as prophylaxis against extrapyramidal symptoms.

Pregnancy Risk Factor: C

Lactation: Enters breast milk (trace amounts)/use caution (AAP rates "compatible")

Breast-Feeding Considerations: Anticholinergic agents may suppress lactation.

Perioperative/Anesthesia/Other Concerns: Atropine, at usual recommended cardiovascular doses, causes blockade of muscarinic receptors at the cardiac SA-node and is parasympatholytic (ie, blocks vagal activity increasing heart rate). A dose 0.5-1 mg is recommended for the treatment of bradyarrhythmias. In administering atropine, it is important to recognize that lower doses (<0.5 mg) may have vagalmimetic effects (ie, increase vagal tone causing paradoxical bradycardia). A total dose of 3 mg (0.04 mg/kg) results in full vagal blockade in humans. In the absence of vascular access, atropine can be administered intratracheally.

Administration

I.M.: AtroPen®: Administer to outer thigh. May be given through clothing as long as pockets at the injection site are empty. Hold autoinjector in place for 10 seconds following injection; massage the injection site.

I.V.: Administer undiluted by rapid I.V. injection; slow injection may result in paradoxical bradycardia

Compatibility:

Y-site administration: Incompatible with thiopental

Compatibility in syringe: Incompatible with cimetidine/pentobarbital

Compatibility when admixed: Incompatible with floxacillin, metaraminol, methohexital, norepinephrine

Storage: Store injection at controlled room temperature of 15°C to 30°C (59°F to 86°F); avoid freezing. In addition, AtroPen® should be protected from light.

Related Information

Management of Postoperative Arrhythmias *on page 1787*

- Atropine-Care® *see* Atropine *on page 203*
- Atropine Sulfate *see* Atropine *on page 203*
- Atrovent® *see* Ipratropium *on page 957*
- Atrovent® HFA *see* Ipratropium *on page 957*
- A/T/S® *see* Erythromycin *on page 634*
- Augmentin® *see* Amoxicillin and Clavulanate Potassium *on page 147*
- Augmentin ES-600® *see* Amoxicillin and Clavulanate Potassium *on page 147*
- Augmentin XR™ *see* Amoxicillin and Clavulanate Potassium *on page 147*
- Autoplex® T *see* Anti-inhibitor Coagulant Complex *on page 172*
- Avagard™ [OTC] *see* Chlorhexidine Gluconate *on page 373*
- Avandamet™ *see* Rosiglitazone and Metformin *on page 1502*
- Avandia® *see* Rosiglitazone *on page 1500*
- Avapro® *see* Irbesartan *on page 960*
- Avelox® *see* Moxifloxacin *on page 1183*
- Avelox® I.V. *see* Moxifloxacin *on page 1183*
- Avinza® *see* Morphine Sulfate *on page 1177*
- Avitene® *see* Collagen Hemostat *on page 449*
- Avitene® Flour *see* Collagen Hemostat *on page 449*
- Avitene® Ultrafoam *see* Collagen Hemostat *on page 449*
- Avitene® UltraWrap™ *see* Collagen Hemostat *on page 449*
- Avonex® *see* Interferon Beta-1a *on page 947*
- Axid® *see* Nizatidine *on page 1240*
- Axid® AR [OTC] *see* Nizatidine *on page 1240*
- Ayr® Baby Saline [OTC] *see* Sodium Chloride *on page 1545*
- Ayr® Saline [OTC] *see* Sodium Chloride *on page 1545*
- Ayr® Saline No-Drip [OTC] *see* Sodium Chloride *on page 1545*
- Azactam® *see* Aztreonam *on page 215*
- Azasan® *see* Azathioprine *on page 207*

Azathioprine (ay za THYE oh preen)

U.S. Brand Names Azasan®; Imuran®

Synonyms Azathioprine Sodium

Pharmacologic Category Immunosuppressant Agent

Medication Safety Issues

Sound-alike/look-alike issues:

Azathioprine may be confused with azatadine, azidothymidine, Azulfidine®

Imuran® may be confused with Elmiron®, Enduron®, Imdur®, Inderal®, Tenormin®

Use Adjunctive therapy in prevention of rejection of kidney transplants; active rheumatoid arthritis

Unlabeled/Investigational Use Adjunct in prevention of rejection of solid organ (nonrenal) transplants; maintenance of remission in Crohn's disease

(Continued)

Azathioprine *(Continued)*

Mechanism of Action Azathioprine is an imidazolyl derivative of mercaptopurine; antagonizes purine metabolism and may inhibit synthesis of DNA, RNA, and proteins; may also interfere with cellular metabolism and inhibit mitosis. The 6-thioguanine nucleotides appear to mediate the majority of azathioprine's immunosuppressive and toxic effects.

Pharmacodynamics/Kinetics

Distribution: Crosses placenta

Protein binding: ~30%

Metabolism: Hepatic, to 6-mercaptopurine (6-MP), possibly by glutathione S-transferase (GST). Further metabolism of 6-MP (in the liver and GI tract), via three major pathways: Hypoxanthine guanine phosphoribosyltransferase (to 6-thioguanine-nucleotides, or 6-TGN), xanthine oxidase (to 6-thiouric acid), and thiopurine methyltransferase (TPMT), which forms 6-methylmercapotpurine (6-MMP).

Half-life elimination: Parent drug: 12 minutes; mercaptopurine: 0.7-3 hours; End-stage renal disease: Slightly prolonged

Time to peak, plasma: 1-2 hours (including metabolites)

Excretion: Urine (primarily as metabolites)

Contraindications Hypersensitivity to azathioprine or any component of the formulation; pregnancy

Warnings/Precautions Chronic immunosuppression increases the risk of neoplasia and serious infections. Azathioprine has mutagenic potential to both men and women and with possible hematologic toxicities; hematologic toxicities are dose-related and may be more severe with renal transplants undergoing rejection. Gastrointestinal toxicity may occur within the first several weeks of therapy and is reversible. Symptoms may include severe nausea, vomiting, diarrhea, rash, fever, malaise, myalgia, hypotension, and liver enzyme abnormalities. Use with caution in patients with liver disease, renal impairment; monitor hematologic function closely. Patients with genetic deficiency of thiopurine methyltransferase (TPMT) or concurrent therapy with drugs which may inhibit TPMT may be sensitive to myelosuppressive effects.

Drug Interactions

ACE inhibitors: Concomitant therapy may induce anemia and severe leukopenia.

Allopurinol: May increase serum levels of azathioprine's active metabolite (mercaptopurine). Decrease azathioprine dose to $^{1}/_{3}$ to $^{1}/_{4}$ of normal dose.

Aminosalicylates (olsalazine, mesalamine, sulfasalazine): May inhibit TPMT, increasing toxicity/myelosuppression of azathioprine. Use caution.

Warfarin: Effect may be decreased by azathioprine.

Nutritional/Herbal/Ethanol Interactions Herb/Nutraceutical: Avoid cat's claw, echinacea (have immunostimulant properties).

Adverse Reactions Frequency not defined; dependent upon dose, duration, and concomitant therapy.

Central nervous system: Fever, malaise

Dermatologic: Alopecia, rash

Gastrointestinal: Diarrhea, nausea, pancreatitis, vomiting

Hematologic: Bleeding, leukopenia, macrocytic anemia, pancytopenia, thrombocytopenia

Hepatic: Hepatotoxicity, hepatic veno-occlusive disease, steatorrhea

Neuromuscular & skeletal: Arthralgia, myalgia

Respiratory: Interstitial pneumonitis

Miscellaneous: Hypersensitivity reactions (rare), infection secondary to immunosuppression, neoplasia

Overdosage/Toxicology Symptoms of overdose include nausea, vomiting, diarrhea, and hematologic toxicity. Following initiation of essential overdose management, symptomatic and supportive treatment should be instituted. Dialysis has been reported to remove significant amounts of the drug and its metabolites, and should be considered as a treatment option in those patients who deteriorate despite established forms of therapy.

Dosing

Adults & Elderly: I.V. dose is equivalent to oral dose.

Renal transplantation: Oral, I.V.: Initial: 3-5 mg/kg/day usually given as a single daily dose, then 1-3 mg/kg/day maintenance

Rheumatoid arthritis: Oral:

Initial: 1 mg/kg/day given once daily or divided twice daily, for 6-8 weeks; increase by 0.5 mg/kg every 4 weeks until response or up to 2.5 mg/kg/day; an adequate trial should be a minimum of 12 weeks

Maintenance dose: Reduce dose by 0.5 mg/kg every 4 weeks until lowest effective dose is reached; optimum duration of therapy not specified; may be discontinued abruptly

Adjunctive management of severe recurrent aphthous stomatitis (unlabeled use): Oral: 50 mg once daily in conjunction with prednisone

Pediatrics: Renal transplantation, rheumatoid arthritis (unlabeled uses): Refer to adult dosing.

Renal Impairment:

Cl_{cr} 10-50 mL/minute: Administer 75% of normal dose.

Cl_{cr} <10 mL/minute: Administer 50% of normal dose.

Hemodialysis: Dialyzable (~45% removed in 8 hours)

Administer dose posthemodialysis: CAPD effects: Unknown; CAVH effects: Unknown

Available Dosage Forms

Injection, powder for reconstitution: 100 mg

Tablet [scored]: 50 mg

Azasan®: 75 mg, 100 mg

Imuran®: 50 mg

Nursing Guidelines

Assessment: Assess effectiveness and interactions of other medications patient may be taking. Assess results of laboratory tests, therapeutic effectiveness (according to purpose for use) and adverse reactions at beginning of therapy and periodically throughout therapy, especially opportunistic infection. Assess knowledge/teach patient appropriate use, interventions to reduce side effects, and adverse symptoms to report.

Monitoring Laboratory Tests: CBC, platelet counts, total bilirubin, liver function tests, TPMT genotyping or phenotyping

Dietary Considerations: May be taken with food.

Patient Education: Take as prescribed (may take in divided doses or with food if GI upset occurs). You will be susceptible to infection (avoid crowds and exposure to infection and do not have any vaccinations unless approved by prescriber). You may experience nausea, vomiting, loss of appetite (small frequent meals, frequent mouth care, chewing gum, or sucking lozenges may help). Report abdominal pain and unresolved GI upset (eg, persistent vomiting or diarrhea); unusual fever or chills; bleeding or bruising; sore throat, unhealed sores, or signs of infection; yellowing of skin or eyes; or change in color of urine or stool.

Rheumatoid arthritis: Response may not occur for up to 3 months; do not discontinue without consulting prescriber.

Organ transplant: Azathioprine will usually be prescribed with other antirejection medications.

Pregnancy/breast-feeding precautions: Do not get pregnant while taking this medication; use appropriate contraceptive measures. Breast-feeding is not recommended.

Geriatric Considerations: Immunosuppressive toxicity is increased in the elderly. Signs or symptoms of infection may differ in the elderly. Lethargy or confusion may be the first signs of infection.

Pregnancy Risk Factor: D

Pregnancy Issues: Azathioprine crosses the placenta in humans; congenital anomalies, immunosuppression and intrauterine growth retardation have been reported. There are no adequate and well-controlled studies in pregnant women. Azathioprine should not be used to treat arthritis during pregnancy; the potential benefit to the mother versus possible risk to the fetus should be considered when treating other disease states.

Lactation: Enters breast milk/not recommended

Breast-Feeding Considerations: Due to risk of immunosuppression, breast feeding is not recommended.

Administration

Oral: Administering tablets after meals or in divided doses may decrease adverse GI events.

I.V.: Can be administered IVP over 5 minutes at a concentration not to exceed 10 mg/mL **or** azathioprine can be further diluted with normal saline or D_5W and administered by intermittent infusion usually over 30-60 minutes; may be extended up to 8 hours.

Compatibility: Stable in neutral or acid solutions, but is hydrolyzed to mercaptopurine in alkaline solutions. Stable in D_5W, $^1/_2$NS, NS.

(Continued)

Azathioprine *(Continued)*

Storage:

Tablet: Store at room temperature of 15°C to 25°C (59°F to 77°F); protect from light

Powder for injection: Store at room temperature of 15°C to 25°C (59°F to 77°F) and protect from light. Parenteral admixture is stable at room temperature (25°C) for 24 hours, and stable under refrigeration (4°C) for 16 days.

♦ **Azathioprine Sodium** *see* Azathioprine *on page 207*

Azelastine (a ZEL as teen)

U.S. Brand Names Astelin®; Optivar®

Synonyms Azelastine Hydrochloride

Pharmacologic Category Antihistamine

Medication Safety Issues

Sound-alike/look-alike issues:

Optivar® may be confused with Optiray®

Use

Nasal spray: Treatment of the symptoms of seasonal allergic rhinitis such as rhinorrhea, sneezing, and nasal pruritus in children ≥5 years of age and adults; treatment of the symptoms of vasomotor rhinitis in children ≥12 years of age and adults

Ophthalmic: Treatment of itching of the eye associated with seasonal allergic conjunctivitis in children ≥3 years of age and adults

Mechanism of Action Competes with histamine for H_1-receptor sites on effector cells and inhibits the release of histamine and other mediators involved in the allergic response. When used intranasally, reduces hyper-reactivity of the airways; increases the motility of bronchial epithelial cilia, improving mucociliary transport

Pharmacodynamics/Kinetics

Onset of action: Peak effect: Nasal spray: 3 hours; Ophthalmic solution: 3 minutes

Duration: Nasal spray: 12 hours; Ophthalmic solution: 8 hours

Protein binding: 88%

Metabolism: Hepatic via CYP; active metabolite, desmethylazelastine

Bioavailability: Intranasal: 40%

Half-life elimination: 22 hours

Time to peak, serum: 2-3 hours

Contraindications Hypersensitivity to azelastine or any component of the formulation

Warnings/Precautions

Nasal spray: May cause drowsiness in some patients; instruct patient to use caution when driving or operating machinery. Effects may be additive with CNS depressants and/or ethanol.

Ophthalmic: Solution contains benzalkonium chloride; wait at least 10 minutes after instilling solution before inserting soft contact lenses. Do not use contact lenses if eyes are red.

Drug Interactions Substrate (minor) of CYP1A2, 2C19, 2D6, 3A4; **Inhibits** CYP2B6 (weak), 2C8/9 (weak), 2C19 (weak), 2D6 (weak), 3A4 (weak)

May cause additive sedation when concomitantly administered with other CNS depressant medications; cimetidine can increase the AUC and C_{max} of azelastine by as much as 65%

Nutritional/Herbal/Ethanol Interactions Ethanol: Avoid ethanol (may cause increased somnolence or fatigue).

Adverse Reactions

Nasal spray:

>10%:

Central nervous system: Headache (15%), somnolence (12%)

Gastrointestinal: Bitter taste (20%)

2% to 10%:

Central nervous system: Dizziness (2%), fatigue (2%)

Gastrointestinal: Nausea (3%), weight gain (2%), dry mouth (3%)

Respiratory: Nasal burning (4%), pharyngitis (4%), paroxysmal sneezing (3%), rhinitis (2%), epistaxis (2%)

<2% (Limited to important or life-threatening): Depression, anxiety, depersonalization, sleep disorder, ulcerative stomatitis, vomiting, bronchospasm, allergic reactions, anaphylactoid reaction, chest pain, dyspnea, involuntary muscle contractions, paresthesia, pruritus, rash, urinary retention

Ophthalmic:
>10%:
Central nervous system: Headache (15%)
Ocular: Transient burning/stinging (30%)
1% to 10%:
Central nervous system: Fatigue
Genitourinary: Bitter taste (10%)
Ocular: Conjunctivitis, eye pain, blurred vision (temporary)
Respiratory: Asthma, dyspnea, pharyngitis
Miscellaneous: Flu-like syndrome

Overdosage/Toxicology There have been no reported overdoses with azelastine; increased somnolence is likely to occur; supportive measures should be employed

Dosing
Adults & Elderly:
Seasonal allergic rhinitis, vasomotor rhinitis: Intranasal: 2 sprays (137 mcg/spray) each nostril twice daily
Seasonal allergic conjunctivitis: Ophthalmic: Instill 1 drop into affected eye(s) twice daily
Pediatrics:
Seasonal allergic rhinitis: Intranasal:
5-11 years: 1 spray each nostril twice daily
≥12 years: Refer to adult dosing.
Vasomotor rhinitis: Children ≥12 years: Refer to adult dosing.
Seasonal allergic conjunctivitis: Children ≥3 years: Ophthalmic: Refer to adult dosing.

Available Dosage Forms
Solution, intranasal spray, as hydrochloride (Astelin®): 1 mg/mL [137 mcg/spray] (17 mL, 30 mL) [contains benzalkonium chloride]
Solution, ophthalmic, as hydrochloride (Optivar®): 0.05% (6 mL) [contains benzalkonium chloride]

Nursing Guidelines
Patient Education: Avoid alcohol. **Pregnancy/breast-feeding precautions:** Inform prescriber if you are or intend to become pregnant. Consult prescriber if breast-feeding.

Nasal spray: Causes drowsiness and may impair ability to perform hazardous activities requiring mental alertness or physical coordination; avoid spraying in eyes. Do not use with other antihistamines unless instructed by prescriber. The delivery system must be primed prior to first use, and again if not used for more than 3 days.

Ophthalmic: Do not touch eyelids or surrounding area with tip of dropper; wait at least 10 minutes before inserting soft contact lenses. Do not use contacts if eyes are red.

Pregnancy Risk Factor: C
Lactation: Excretion in breast milk unknown/use caution

Administration
Storage:
Nasal spray: Store upright at controlled room temperature of 20°C to 25°C (68°F to 77°F); stable for 3 months after opening
Ophthalmic solution: Store upright between 2°C to 25°C (36°F to 77°F)

♦ **Azelastine Hydrochloride** *see* Azelastine *on page 210*
♦ **Azidothymidine** *see* Zidovudine *on page 1732*
♦ **Azidothymidine, Abacavir, and Lamivudine** *see* Abacavir, Lamivudine, and Zidovudine *on page 58*

Azithromycin (az ith roe MYE sin)

U.S. Brand Names Zithromax®; Zmax™
Synonyms Azithromycin Dihydrate; Zithromax® TRI-PAK™; Zithromax® Z-PAK®
Pharmacologic Category Antibiotic, Macrolide
Medication Safety Issues
Sound-alike/look-alike issues:
Azithromycin may be confused with erythromycin
Zithromax® may be confused with Zinacef®

Use Treatment of acute otitis media due to *H. influenzae*, *M. catarrhalis*, or *S. pneumoniae*; pharyngitis/tonsillitis due to *S. pyogenes*; treatment of mild-to-moderate upper and lower respiratory tract infections, infections of the
(Continued)

Azithromycin *(Continued)*

skin and skin structure, community-acquired pneumonia, pelvic inflammatory disease (PID), sexually-transmitted diseases (urethritis/cervicitis), pharyngitis/tonsillitis (alternative to first-line therapy), and genital ulcer disease (chancroid) due to susceptible strains of *C. trachomatis, M. catarrhalis, H. influenzae, S. aureus, S. pneumoniae, Mycoplasma pneumoniae*, and *C. psittaci*; acute bacterial exacerbations of chronic obstructive pulmonary disease (COPD) due to *H. influenzae, M. catarrhalis*, or *S. pneumoniae*; acute bacterial sinusitis

Unlabeled/Investigational Use Prevention of (or to delay onset of) or treatment of MAC in patients with advanced HIV infection; prophylaxis of bacterial endocarditis in patients who are allergic to penicillin and undergoing surgical or dental procedures; pertussis

Mechanism of Action Inhibits RNA-dependent protein synthesis at the chain elongation step; binds to the 50S ribosomal subunit resulting in blockage of transpeptidation

Pharmacodynamics/Kinetics

Absorption: Rapid

Distribution: Extensive tissue; distributes well into skin, lungs, sputum, tonsils, and cervix; penetration into CSF is poor; I.V.: 33.3 L/kg; Oral: 31.1 L/kg

Protein binding (concentration dependent): 7% to 51%

Metabolism: Hepatic

Bioavailability: 38%, decreased by 17% with extended release suspension; variable effect with food (increased with immediate or delayed release oral suspension,. unchanged with tablet)

Half-life elimination: Terminal: Immediate release: 68-72 hours; Extended release: 59 hours

Time to peak, serum: Immediate release: 2-3 hours; Extended release: 5 hours

Excretion: Biliary (major route); urine (6%)

Contraindications Hypersensitivity to azithromycin, other macrolide antibiotics, or any component of the formulation

Warnings/Precautions Use with caution in patients with hepatic dysfunction; hepatic impairment with or without jaundice has occurred chiefly in older children and adults; it may be accompanied by malaise, nausea, vomiting, abdominal colic, and fever; discontinue use if these occur. May mask or delay symptoms of incubating gonorrhea or syphilis, so appropriate culture and susceptibility tests should be performed prior to initiating azithromycin. Pseudomembranous colitis has been reported with use of macrolide antibiotics; use caution with renal dysfunction. Prolongation of the QT_c interval has been reported with macrolide antibiotics; use caution in patients at risk of prolonged cardiac repolarization. Safety and efficacy have not been established in children <6 months of age with acute otitis media, acute bacterial sinusitis, or community-acquired pneumonia, or in children <2 years of age with pharyngitis/tonsillitis. Suspensions (immediate release and extended release) are not interchangeable.

Drug Interactions **Substrate** of CYP3A4 (minor); **Inhibits** CYP3A4 (weak)

Cardiac glycosides: Macrolides may increase the serum concentrations of cardiac glycosides; monitor.

Colchicine: Macrolides may increase the adverse/toxic effects of colchicine.

Nelfinavir: May increase azithromycin serum levels; monitor for adverse effects.

Warfarin: Azithromycin and other macrolides may decrease metabolism, via CYP isoenzymes, of warfarin. Monitor for increased effects.

Nutritional/Herbal/Ethanol Interactions Food: Rate and extent of GI absorption may be altered depending upon the formulation. Azithromycin suspension, not tablet form, has significantly increased absorption (46%) with food.

Adverse Reactions

>10%: Gastrointestinal: Diarrhea (4% to 11%)

1% to 10%:

Central nervous system: Headache

Gastrointestinal: Nausea, abdominal pain, cramping, vomiting (especially with high single-dose regimens)

<1% (Limited to important or life-threatening): Acute renal failure, allergic reaction, aggressive behavior, anaphylaxis, angioedema, arrhythmia (including ventricular tachycardia), cholestatic jaundice, constipation, convulsion, deafness, dehydration, enteritis, erythema multiforme (rare), hearing loss, hepatic necrosis (rare), hepatitis, hypertrophic pyloric stenosis, hypotension, interstitial nephritis, leukopenia, LFTs increased, neutropenia, oral candidiasis, oral moniliasis, palpitations, pancreatitis, paresthesia, pruritus, pseudomembranous colitis, QT_c prolongation (rare), seizure, somnolence, Stevens-Johnson

syndrome (rare), syncope, taste perversion, thrombocytopenia, tinnitus, tongue discoloration (rare), torsade de pointes (rare), urticaria, vertigo

Overdosage/Toxicology Symptoms of overdose include nausea, vomiting, diarrhea, and prostration. Treatment is supportive and symptomatic.

Dosing

Adults & Elderly: Note: Extended release suspension (Zmax™) is not interchangeable with immediate release formulations. Use should be limited to approved indications. All doses are expressed as immediate release azithromycin unless otherwise specified.

Mild to moderate respiratory tract, skin, and soft tissue infections: Oral: 500 mg in a single loading dose on day 1 followed by 250 mg/day as a single dose on days 2-5

Alternative regimen: Bacterial exacerbation of COPD: 500 mg/day for a total of 3 days

Bacterial sinusitis: Oral: 500 mg/day for a total of 3 days

Extended release suspension (Zmax™): 2 g as a single dose

Community-acquired pneumonia: I.V.: 500 mg as a single dose for at least 2 days, follow I.V. therapy by the oral route with a single daily dose of 500 mg to complete a 7- to 10-day course of therapy.

Urethritis/cervicitis:

Due to *C. trachomatis*: Oral: 1 g as a single dose

Due to *N. gonorrhoeae*: Oral: 2 g as a single dose

Chancroid due to *H. ducreyi*: Oral: 1 g as a single dose

Pelvic inflammatory disease (PID): I.V.: 500 mg as a single dose for 1-2 days, follow I.V. therapy by the oral route with a single daily dose of 250 mg to complete a 7-day course of therapy.

Pertussis (CDC guidelines): 500 mg on day 1 followed by 250 mg/day on days 2-5 (maximum: 500 mg/day)

Prophylaxis for bacterial endocarditis (unlabeled use): Oral: 500 mg 1 hour prior to the procedure

Disseminated *M. avium* complex disease in patient with advanced HIV infection (unlabeled use):

Prophylaxis: Oral: 1200 mg once weekly (may be combined with rifabutin)

Treatment: Oral: 600 mg daily in combination with ethambutol 15 mg/kg

Pediatrics:

Note: Adolescents ≥16 years: Refer to adult dosing.

Community-acquired pneumonia: Oral: Children ≥6 months: 10 mg/kg on day 1 (maximum: 500 mg/day) followed by 5 mg/kg/day once daily on days 2-5 (maximum: 250 mg/day)

Bacterial sinusitis: Oral: Children ≥6 months: 10 mg/kg once daily for 3 days (maximum: 500 mg/day)

Otitis media: Oral: Children ≥6 months:

1-day regimen: 30 mg/kg as a single dose (maximum dose: 1500 mg)

3-day regimen: 10 mg/kg once daily for 3 days (maximum: 500 mg/day)

5-day regimen: 10 mg/kg on day 1 (maximum: 500 mg/day) followed by 5 mg/kg/day once daily on days 2-5 (maximum: 250 mg/day)

Pharyngitis, tonsillitis: Oral: Children ≥2 years: 12 mg/kg/day once daily for 5 days (maximum: 500 mg/day)

Pertussis (CDC guidelines):

Children <6 months: 10 mg/kg/day for 5 day

Children ≥6 months: 10 mg/kg on day 1 (maximum: 500 mg/day) followed by 5 mg/kg/day once daily on days 2-5 (maximum: 250 mg/day)

Disseminated *M. avium*-infected patients with acquired immunodeficiency syndrome (unlabeled use): Oral: 5 mg/kg/day once daily (maximum dose: 250 mg/day) or 20 mg/kg (maximum dose: 1200 mg) once weekly given alone or in combination with rifabutin

Treatment and secondary prevention of disseminated MAC (unlabeled use): Oral: 5 mg/kg/day once daily (maximum dose: 250 mg/day) in combination with ethambutol, with or without rifabutin

Prophylaxis for bacterial endocarditis (unlabeled use): Oral: 15 mg/kg 1 hour before procedure

Uncomplicated chlamydial urethritis or cervicitis (unlabeled use): Children ≥45 kg: 1 g as a single dose

Renal Impairment: Use caution in patients with Cl_{cr} <10 mL/minute

Hepatic Impairment: Use with caution due to potential for hepatotoxicity (rare). Specific guidelines for dosing in hepatic impairment have not been established.

(Continued)

Azithromycin *(Continued)*

Available Dosage Forms Note: Strength expressed as base

Injection, powder for reconstitution, as dihydrate (Zithromax®): 500 mg [contains sodium 114 mg (4.96 mEq) per vial]

Microspheres for oral suspension, extended release, as dihydrate (Zmax™): 2 g [single-dose bottle; contains sodium 148 mg per bottle; cherry and banana flavor]

Powder for oral suspension, immediate release, as dihydrate (Zithromax®): 100 mg/5 mL (15 mL) [contains sodium 3.7 mg/ 5 mL; cherry creme de vanilla and banana flavor]; 200 mg/5 mL (15 mL, 22.5 mL, 30 mL) [contains sodium 7.4 mg/ 5 mL; cherry creme de vanilla and banana flavor]; 1 g [single-dose packet; contains sodium 37 mg per packet; cherry creme de vanilla and banana flavor]

Tablet, as dihydrate:

Zithromax®: 250 mg [contains sodium 0.9 mg per tablet]; 500 mg [contains sodium 1.8 mg per tablet]; 600 mg [contains sodium 2.1 mg per tablet]

Zithromax® TRI-PAK™ [unit-dose pack]: 500 mg (3s)

Zithromax® Z-PAK® [unit-dose pack]: 250 mg (6s)

Tablet, as monohydrate: 250 mg, 500 mg, 600 mg

Nursing Guidelines

Assessment: Assess allergy history prior to beginning therapy. See Contraindications, Warnings/Precautions, and Dosing for use cautions. Assess potential for interactions with other prescriptions, OTC medications, or herbal products patient may be taking (see Drug Interactions). Assess results of laboratory tests (see below), therapeutic effectiveness, and adverse effects (see Adverse Reactions and Overdose/Toxicology). Instruct patients being treated for STDs about preventing transmission. Teach patient appropriate use, possible side effects/appropriate interventions, and adverse symptoms to report (see Patient Education). Note breast-feeding caution.

Monitoring Laboratory Tests: Liver function, CBC with differential. Perform culture and sensitivity testing prior to initiating therapy.

Dietary Considerations:

Oral suspension, immediate release, may be administered with or without food.

Oral suspension, extended release, should be taken on an empty stomach (at least 1 hour before or 2 hours following a meal).

Tablet may be administered with food to decrease GI effects.

Sodium content:

Injection: 114 mg (4.96 mEq) per vial

Oral suspension, immediate release: 3.7 mg per 100 mg/5 mL of constituted suspension; 7.4 mg per 200 mg/5 mL of constituted suspension; 37 mg per 1 g single-dose packet

Oral suspension, extended release: 148 mg per 2 g constituted suspension

Tablet: 0.9 mg/250 mg tablet; 1.8 mg/500 mg tablet; 2.1 mg/600 mg tablet

Patient Education: Do not take any new medication during therapy unless approved by prescriber. Take as directed. Take all of prescribed medication and do not discontinue until prescription is completed. Take extended release suspension 1 hour before or 2 hours after meals; immediate release suspension and tablets may be taken with or without food; tablet form may be taken with meals to decrease GI effects. Do not take with antacids that contain aluminum or magnesium. Maintain adequate hydration (2-3 L/day of fluids) unless instructed to restrict fluid intake. If taken to treat a sexually-transmitted disease, follow advice of prescriber related to sexual intercourse and preventing transmission. May cause transient abdominal distress, diarrhea, and headache. Report signs of additional infections (eg, sores in mouth or vagina, vaginal discharge, unresolved fever, severe vomiting, or loose or foul smelling stools). **Breast-feeding precaution:** Consult prescriber if breast-feeding.

Geriatric Considerations: Dosage adjustment does not appear to be necessary in the elderly. Considered one of the drugs of choice in the treatment of outpatient treatment of community-acquired pneumonia in older adults.

Pregnancy Risk Factor: B

Lactation: Enters breast milk/use caution

Breast-Feeding Considerations: Based on one case report, azithromycin has been shown to accumulate in breast milk.

Administration

Oral: Immediate release suspension and tablet may be taken without regard to food; extended release suspension should be taken on an empty stomach (at least 1 hour before or 2 hours following a meal), within 12 hours of reconstitution.

I.V.: Other medications should not be infused simultaneously through the same I.V. line.

Reconstitution: Injection: Prepare initiation solution by adding 4.8 mL of sterile water for injection to the 500 mg vial (resulting concentration: 100 mg/mL). Use of a standard syringe is recommended due to the vacuum in the vial (which may draw additional solution through an automated syringe).

The initial solution should be further diluted to a concentration of 1 mg/mL (500 mL) to 2 mg/mL (250 mL) in 0.9% sodium chloride, 5% dextrose in water, or lactated Ringer's. The diluted solution is stable for 24 hours at or below room temperature (30°C or 86°F) and for 7 days if stored under refrigeration (5°C or 41°F).

Compatibility: Other medications should not be infused simultaneously through the same I.V. line.

Storage:

Injection: Store intact vials of injection at room temperature. Reconstituted solution is stable for 24 hours when stored below 30°C/86°F.

Suspension, immediate release: Store dry powder below 30°C (86°F); following reconstitution, store at 5°C to 30°C (41°F to 86°F).

Suspension, extended release: Store dry powder below 30°C (86°F); following reconstitution, store at 15°C to 30°C (59°F to 86°F); do not freeze; should be consumed within 12 hours following reconstitution

Tablets: Store between 15°C to 30°C (59°F to 86°F).

- **Azithromycin Dihydrate** *see* Azithromycin *on page 211*
- **Azmacort®** *see* Triamcinolone *on page 1660*
- **AZO-Gesic® [OTC]** *see* Phenazopyridine *on page 1342*
- **AZO-Standard® [OTC]** *see* Phenazopyridine *on page 1342*
- **AZT, Abacavir, and Lamivudine** *see* Abacavir, Lamivudine, and Zidovudine *on page 58*
- **AZT (error-prone abbreviation)** *see* Zidovudine *on page 1732*
- **Azthreonam** *see* Aztreonam *on page 215*

Aztreonam (AZ tree oh nam)

U.S. Brand Names Azactam®

Synonyms Azthreonam

Pharmacologic Category Antibiotic, Miscellaneous

Medication Safety Issues

Sound-alike/look-alike issues:

Aztreonam may be confused with azidothymidine

Use Treatment of patients with urinary tract infections, lower respiratory tract infections, septicemia, skin/skin structure infections, intra-abdominal infections, and gynecological infections caused by susceptible gram-negative bacilli

Mechanism of Action Inhibits bacterial cell wall synthesis by binding to one or more of the penicillin binding proteins (PBPs); which in turn inhibits the final transpeptidation step of peptidoglycan synthesis in bacterial cell walls, thus inhibiting cell wall biosynthesis. Bacteria eventually lyse due to ongoing activity of cell wall autolytic enzymes (autolysins and murein hydrolases) while cell wall assembly is arrested. Monobactam structure makes cross-allergenicity with beta-lactams unlikely.

Pharmacodynamics/Kinetics

Absorption: I.M.: Well absorbed; I.M. and I.V. doses produce comparable serum concentrations

Distribution: Widely to most body fluids and tissues; crosses placenta; enters breast milk

V_d: Children: 0.2-0.29 L/kg; Adults: 0.2 L/kg

Relative diffusion of antimicrobial agents from blood into CSF: Good only with inflammation (exceeds usual MICs)

CSF:blood level ratio: Meninges: Inflamed: 8% to 40%; Normal: ~1%

Protein binding: 56%

Metabolism: Hepatic (minor %)

Half-life elimination:

Children 2 months to 12 years: 1.7 hours

Adults: Normal renal function: 1.7-2.9 hours

End-stage renal disease: 6-8 hours

Time to peak: I.M., I.V. push: Within 60 minutes; I.V. infusion: 1.5 hours

Excretion: Urine (60% to 70% as unchanged drug); feces (~13% to 15%)

(Continued)

Aztreonam *(Continued)*

Contraindications Hypersensitivity to aztreonam or any component of the formulation

Warnings/Precautions Rare cross-allergenicity to penicillins and cephalosporins has been reported. Use caution in renal impairment; dosing adjustment required.

Drug Interactions Avoid antibiotics that induce beta-lactamase production (cefoxitin, imipenem)

Lab Interactions Urine glucose (Clinitest®)

Adverse Reactions As reported in adults:

1% to 10%:

Dermatologic: Rash

Gastrointestinal: Diarrhea, nausea, vomiting

Local: Thrombophlebitis, pain at injection site

<1% (Limited to important or life-threatening): Abdominal cramps, abnormal taste, anaphylaxis, anemia, angioedema, aphthous ulcer, breast tenderness, bronchospasm, *C. difficile*-associated diarrhea, chest pain, confusion, diaphoresis, diplopia, dizziness, dyspnea, eosinophilia, erythema multiforme, exfoliative dermatitis, fever, flushing, halitosis, headache, hepatitis, hypotension, insomnia, jaundice, leukopenia, liver enzymes increased, muscular aches myalgia, neutropenia, numb tongue, pancytopenia, paresthesia, petechiae, pruritus, pseudomembranous colitis, purpura, seizure, sneezing, thrombocytopenia, tinnitus, toxic epidermal necrolysis, urticaria, vaginitis, vertigo, weakness, wheezing

Overdosage/Toxicology Symptoms of overdose include seizures. Treatment is supportive. If necessary, dialysis can reduce the drug concentration in the blood.

Dosing

Adults & Elderly:

Urinary tract infection: I.M., I.V.: 500 mg to 1 g every 8-12 hours

Moderately severe systemic infections:

I.M.: 1 g every 8-12 hours

I.V.: 1-2 g I.V. every 8-12 hours

Severe systemic or life-threatening infections (especially caused by *Pseudomonas aeruginosa*): I.V.: 2 g every 6-8 hours; maximum: 8 g/day

Pediatrics:

Susceptible infections: I.M., I.V.: Children >1 month:

Mild-to-moderate infections: 30 mg/kg every 8 hours

Moderate-to-severe infections: 30 mg/kg every 6-8 hours; maximum: 120 mg/kg/day (8 g/day)

Infection in children with cystic fibrosis: I.V.: Children >1 month: 50 mg/kg/dose every 6-8 hours (ie, up to 200 mg/kg/day); maximum: 8 g/day

Renal Impairment: Adults: Following initial dose, maintenance doses should be given as follows:

Cl_{cr} 10-30 mL/minute: 50% of usual dose at the usual interval

Cl_{cr} <10 mL/minute: 25% of usual dosage at the usual interval

Hemodialysis: Moderately dialyzable (20% to 50%); 1/8 of initial dose after each hemodialysis session (given in addition to the maintenance doses)

Peritoneal dialysis: Administer as for Cl_{cr} <10 mL/minute

Continuous arteriovenous or venovenous hemofiltration: Dose as for Cl_{cr} 10-30 mL/minute

Available Dosage Forms

Infusion [premixed]: 1 g (50 mL); 2 g (50 mL)

Injection, powder for reconstitution: 500 mg, 1 g, 2 g

Nursing Guidelines

Assessment: Assess allergy history before initiating therapy. See Contraindications, Warnings/Precautions, and Dosing for use cautions. I.V.: Note Administration, Reconstitution, and Compatibility. Assess therapeutic effectiveness and adverse response (see Adverse Reactions and Overdose/Toxicology). Caution patients with diabetes about altered response to Clinitest®. Teach patient possible side effects/appropriate interventions and adverse symptoms to report (see Patient Education). Note breast-feeding caution.

Monitoring Laboratory Tests: Obtain specimens for culture and sensitivity before the first dose.

Patient Education: Inform prescriber of all prescriptions, OTC medications, or herbal products you are taking, and any allergies you have. Do not take any new medication during therapy unless approved by prescriber. This medication can only be administered by injection or infusion. Report immediately any burning, pain, swelling, or redness at infusion/injection site. May cause nausea or GI distress (frequent mouth care, frequent small meals, sucking lozenges, or chewing gum may help relieve these symptoms). If you have diabetes, drug may cause false tests with Clinitest® urine glucose monitoring; use of another type of glucose monitoring is preferable. Report any persistent and unrelieved diarrhea or vomiting, pain at injection site, unresolved fever, unhealed or new sores in mouth or vagina, vaginal discharge, or acute onset of respiratory difficulty. **Breast-feeding precaution:** Consult prescriber if breast-feeding.

Geriatric Considerations: Adjust dose relative to renal function.

Pregnancy Risk Factor: B

Lactation: Enters breast milk/not recommended (AAP rates "compatible")

Breast-Feeding Considerations: Aztreonam is excreted in breast milk at levels <1% of the maternal serum concentration. The manufacturer recommends temporary discontinuation of nursing during therapy.

Perioperative/Anesthesia/Other Concerns: Although marketed as an agent similar to aminoglycosides, aztreonam is a monobactam antimicrobial with almost pure gram-negative aerobic activity. It cannot be used for gram-positive infections, whereas aminoglycosides are often used for synergy in gram-positive infections.

Administration

I.M.: Administer by deep injection into large muscle mass, such as upper outer quadrant of gluteus maximus or the lateral part of the thigh. Doses >1 g should be administered I.V.

I.V.: I.V. route is preferred for doses >1 g or in patients with severe life-threatening infections. Administer by IVP over 3-5 minutes or by intermittent infusion over 20-60 minutes at a final concentration not to exceed 20 mg/mL.

Reconstitution: Reconstituted solutions are colorless to light yellow straw and may turn pink upon standing without affecting potency. Use reconstituted solutions and I.V. solutions (in NS and D_5W) within 48 hours if kept at room temperature (25°C) or 7 days if kept in refrigerator (4°C).

I.M.: Reconstitute with at least 3 mL SWFI, sterile bacteriostatic water for injection, NS, or bacteriostatic sodium chloride.

I.V.:

Bolus injection: Reconstitute with 6-10 mL SWFI.

Infusion: Reconstitute to a final concentration ≤2%. Solution for infusion may be frozen at less than -2°C (less than -4°F) for up to 3 months. Thawed solution should be used within 24 hours if thawed at room temperature or within 72 hours if thawed under refrigeration. **Do not refreeze.**

Compatibility: Solution for infusion: Stable in D_5LR, $D_5{}^1\!/_4NS$, $D_5{}^1\!/_2NS$, D_5NS, D_5W, $D_{10}W$, mannitol 5%, mannitol 10%, LR, NS

Y-site administration: Incompatible with acyclovir, alatrofloxacin, amphotericin B, amphotericin B cholesteryl sulfate complex, amsacrine, chlorpromazine, daunorubicin, ganciclovir, lorazepam, metronidazole, mitomycin, mitoxantrone, prochlorperazine edisylate, streptozocin

Compatibility when admixed: Incompatible with metronidazole, nafcillin

Storage: Prior to reconstitution, store at room temperature. Avoid excessive heat.

♦ Azulfidine® *see* Sulfasalazine *on page 1586*

♦ Azulfidine® EN-tabs® *see* Sulfasalazine *on page 1586*

♦ B-D™ Glucose [OTC] *see* Dextrose *on page 511*

♦ BAC *see* Benzalkonium Chloride *on page 231*

♦ Baciguent® [OTC] *see* Bacitracin *on page 217*

♦ BaciiM® *see* Bacitracin *on page 217*

Bacitracin (bas i TRAY sin)

U.S. Brand Names AK-Tracin® [DSC]; Baciguent® [OTC]; BaciiM®

Pharmacologic Category Antibiotic, Miscellaneous; Antibiotic, Ophthalmic; Antibiotic, Topical

Medication Safety Issues

Sound-alike/look-alike issues:

Bacitracin may be confused with Bactrim®, Bactroban®

Use Treatment of susceptible bacterial infections mainly; has activity against gram-positive bacilli; due to toxicity risks, systemic and irrigant uses of bacitracin should be limited to situations where less toxic alternatives would not be effective

(Continued)

Bacitracin *(Continued)*

Unlabeled/Investigational Use Oral administration: Successful in antibiotic-associated colitis; has been used for enteric eradication of vancomycin-resistant enterococci (VRE)

Mechanism of Action Inhibits bacterial cell wall synthesis by preventing transfer of mucopeptides into the growing cell wall

Pharmacodynamics/Kinetics

Duration: 6-8 hours

Absorption: Poor from mucous membranes and intact or denuded skin; rapidly following I.M. administration; not absorbed by bladder irrigation, but absorption can occur from peritoneal or mediastinal lavage

Distribution: CSF: Nil even with inflammation

Protein binding, plasma: Minimal

Time to peak, serum: I.M.: 1-2 hours

Excretion: Urine (10% to 40%) within 24 hours

Contraindications Hypersensitivity to bacitracin or any component of the formulation; I.M. use is contraindicated in patients with renal impairment

Warnings/Precautions Prolonged use may result in overgrowth of nonsusceptible organisms; I.M. use may cause renal failure due to tubular and glomerular necrosis; **do not administer intravenously** because severe thrombophlebitis occurs

Drug Interactions Increased toxicity: Nephrotoxic drugs, neuromuscular blocking agents, and anesthetics (increases neuromuscular blockade)

Adverse Reactions 1% to 10%:

Cardiovascular: Hypotension, edema of the face/lips, tightness of chest

Central nervous system: Pain

Dermatologic: Rash, itching

Gastrointestinal: Anorexia, nausea, vomiting, diarrhea, rectal itching

Hematologic: Blood dyscrasias

Miscellaneous: Diaphoresis

Overdosage/Toxicology Symptoms of overdose include nephrotoxicity (parenteral), nausea, and vomiting (oral). Treatment is symptomatic and supportive.

Dosing

Adults & Elderly: Do not administer I.V.:

Antibiotic-associated colitis: Oral: 25,000 units 4 times/day for 7-10 days

VRE eradication (unlabeled use): Oral: 25,000 units 4 times/day for 7-10 days

Superficial dermal infection: Topical: Apply 1-5 times/day.

Ophthalmic infection: Ophthalmic (ointment): Instill 1/4" to 1/2" ribbon every 3-4 hours into conjunctival sac for acute infections, or 2-3 times/day for mild to moderate infections for 7-10 days.

Local irrigation: Solution: 50-100 units/mL in normal saline, lactated Ringer's, or sterile water for irrigation; soak sponges in solution for topical compresses 1-5 times/day or as needed during surgical procedures.

Pediatrics: Do not administer I.V.

Infants: I.M.:

≤2.5 kg: 900 units/kg/day in 2-3 divided doses

>2.5 kg: 1000 units/kg/day in 2-3 divided doses

Children: I.M.: 800-1200 units/kg/day divided every 8 hours

Available Dosage Forms [DSC] = Discontinued product

Injection, powder for reconstitution (BaciiM®): 50,000 units

Ointment, ophthalmic (AK-Tracin® [DSC]): 500 units/g (3.5 g)

Ointment, topical: 500 units/g (0.9 g, 15 g, 30 g, 120 g, 454 g)

Baciguent®: 500 units/g (15 g, 30 g)

Nursing Guidelines

Assessment: Do not administer I.V. Assess effectiveness and interactions of other medications patient may be taking (see Drug Interactions). **Oral, I.M.:** Monitor laboratory results, effectiveness of therapy, and adverse reactions (see Adverse Reactions). **Ophthalmic/topical:** Instruct patient on appropriate application and use, possible adverse reactions, and symptoms to report (see Patient Education). Note breast-feeding caution.

Monitoring Laboratory Tests: I.M.: Urinalysis, renal function

Patient Education: Oral/I.M.: Maintain adequate hydration (2-3 L/day of fluids) unless instructed to restrict fluid intake. Report rash, redness, or itching; change in urinary pattern; acute dizziness; swelling of face or lips; chest pain or tightness; acute nausea or vomiting; or loss of appetite (small, frequent meals or frequent mouth care may help).

Ophthalmic: Instill as many times per day as directed. Wash hands before using. Gently pull lower eyelid forward, instill prescribed amount of ointment into lower eyelid. Close eye and roll eyeball in all directions. May cause blurred vision; use caution when driving or engaging in tasks that require clear vision. Report any adverse reactions such as rash or itching, swelling of face or lips, burning or pain in eye, worsening of condition, or if condition does not improve.

Topical: Apply a thin film as many times as day as prescribed to the affected area. May cover with porous sterile bandage (avoid occlusive dressings). Do not use longer than 1 week unless advised by prescriber.

Pregnancy/breast-feeding precautions: Inform prescriber if you are or intend to become pregnant. Consult prescriber if breast-feeding.

Pregnancy Risk Factor: C

Lactation: Excretion in breast milk unknown/use caution

Administration

Oral: The injection formulation is extemporaneously prepared and flavored to improve palatability.

I.M.: For I.M. administration only. pH of urine should be kept >6 by using sodium bicarbonate. Bacitracin sterile powder should be dissolved in 0.9% sodium chloride injection containing 2% procaine hydrochloride. Do not use diluents containing parabens.

I.V.: Not for I.V. administration.

Reconstitution: For I.M. use only. Bacitracin sterile powder should be dissolved in 0.9% sodium chloride injection containing 2% procaine hydrochloride. Once reconstituted, bacitracin is stable for 1 week under refrigeration (2°C to 8°C). Sterile powder should be stored in the refrigerator. Do not use diluents containing parabens.

Bacitracin and Polymyxin B (bas i TRAY sin & pol i MIKS in bee)

U.S. Brand Names AK-Poly-Bac®; Betadine® First Aid Antibiotics + Moisturizer [OTC]; Polysporin® Ophthalmic; Polysporin® Topical [OTC]

Synonyms Polymyxin B and Bacitracin

Pharmacologic Category Antibiotic, Ophthalmic; Antibiotic, Topical

Medication Safety Issues

Sound-alike/look-alike issues:

Betadine® may be confused with Betagan®, betaine

Use Treatment of superficial infections caused by susceptible organisms

Mechanism of Action See individual monographs for Bacitracin and Polymyxin B

Pharmacodynamics/Kinetics See individual agents.

Drug Interactions No data reported

Adverse Reactions 1% to 10%: Local: Rash, itching, burning, anaphylactoid reactions, swelling, conjunctival erythema

Dosing

Adults & Elderly:

Ophthalmic infection: Ophthalmic (ointment): Instill 1/2" ribbon in the affected eye(s) every 3-4 hours for acute infections or 2-3 times/day for mild to moderate infections for 7-10 days.

Superficial dermal infection: Topical ointment/powder: Apply to affected area 1-4 times/day; may cover with sterile bandage if needed.

Pediatrics: Refer to adult dosing.

Available Dosage Forms

Ointment, ophthalmic (AK-Poly-Bac®, Polysporin®): Bacitracin 500 units and polymyxin B sulfate 10,000 units per g (3.5 g)

Ointment, topical [OTC]: Bacitracin 500 units and polymyxin B sulfate 10,000 units per g in white petrolatum (15 g, 30 g)

Betadine® First Aid Antibiotics + Moisturizer: Bacitracin 500 units and polymyxin B sulfate 10,000 units per g (14 g)

Polysporin®: Bacitracin 500 units and polymyxin B sulfate 10,000 units per g (15 g, 30 g)

Powder, topical (Polysporin®): Bacitracin 500 units and polymyxin B sulfate 10,000 units per g (10 g)

Nursing Guidelines

Assessment: See individual components listed in Related Information. Note breast-feeding caution.

(Continued)

Bacitracin and Polymyxin B *(Continued)*

Patient Education: See individual agents. **Pregnancy/breast-feeding precautions:** Inform prescriber if you are or intend to become pregnant. Consult prescriber if breast-feeding.

Pregnancy Risk Factor: C

Lactation: Excretion in breast milk unknown/use caution

Related Information

Bacitracin *on page 217*

Polymyxin B *on page 1380*

Bacitracin, Neomycin, and Polymyxin B

(bas i TRAY sin, nee oh MYE sin, & pol i MIKS in bee)

U.S. Brand Names Neosporin® Neo To Go® [OTC]; Neosporin® Ophthalmic Ointment [DSC]; Neosporin® Topical [OTC]

Synonyms Neomycin, Bacitracin, and Polymyxin B; Polymyxin B, Bacitracin, and Neomycin; Triple Antibiotic

Pharmacologic Category Antibiotic, Ophthalmic; Antibiotic, Topical

Use Helps prevent infection in minor cuts, scrapes and burns; short-term treatment of superficial external ocular infections caused by susceptible organisms

Mechanism of Action Refer to individual monographs for Bacitracin; Neomycin Sulfate; and Polymyxin B Sulfate

Pharmacodynamics/Kinetics See individual agents.

Contraindications Hypersensitivity to neomycin, polymyxin B, zinc bacitracin, or any component of the formulation; epithelial herpes simplex keratitis; mycobacterial or fungal infections; topical ointments for external use only

Warnings/Precautions

Ophthalmic ointment: Bacterial keratitis has been reported with the use of topical ophthalmic products in multiple-dose containers. Care should be taken to not contaminate the container.

Topical ointment: When used for self-medication (OTC use), patients should notify healthcare provider if needed for >1 week. Should not be used for self-medication on deep or puncture wounds, animal bites, or serious burns. Not for application to large areas of the body.

Drug Interactions No data reported

Adverse Reactions Frequency not defined.

Dermatologic: Reddening, allergic contact dermatitis

Local: Itching, failure to heal, swelling, irritation

Ophthalmic: Conjunctival edema

Miscellaneous: Anaphylaxis

Dosing

Adults & Elderly:

Ophthalmic infection: Ophthalmic ointment: Instill 1/2" into the conjunctival sac every 3-4 hours for 7-10 days for acute infections

Superficial dermal infection: Topical: Apply 1-3 times/day to infected area; may cover with sterile bandage if necessary.

Pediatrics: Refer to adult dosing.

Available Dosage Forms

Ointment, ophthalmic (Neosporin® [DSC]): Bacitracin 400 units, neomycin 3.5 mg, and polymyxin B 10,000 units per g (3.5 g)

Ointment, topical: Bacitracin 400 units, neomycin 3.5 mg, and polymyxin B 5000 units per g (0.9 g, 15 g, 30 g, 454 g)

Neosporin®: Bacitracin 400 units, neomycin 3.5 mg, and polymyxin B 5000 units per g (15 g, 30 g)

Neosporin® Neo To Go®: Bacitracin 400 units, neomycin 3.5 mg, and polymyxin B 5000 units per g (0.9 g)

Nursing Guidelines

Assessment: See individual components listed in Related Information. Note breast-feeding caution.

Patient Education: See individual agents. **Pregnancy/breast-feeding precautions:** Inform prescriber if you are or intend to become pregnant. Consult prescriber if breast-feeding.

Pregnancy Risk Factor: C

Lactation: Excretion in breast milk unknown/use caution

Related Information

Bacitracin *on page 217*

Neomycin *on page 1208*
Polymyxin B *on page 1208*

Bacitracin, Neomycin, Polymyxin B, and Hydrocortisone

(bas i TRAY sin, nee oh MYE sin, pol i MIKS in bee, & hye droe KOR ti sone)

U.S. Brand Names Cortisporin® Ointment

Synonyms Hydrocortisone, Bacitracin, Neomycin, and Polymyxin B; Neomycin, Bacitracin, Polymyxin B, and Hydrocortisone; Polymyxin B, Bacitracin, Neomycin, and Hydrocortisone

Pharmacologic Category Antibiotic, Ophthalmic; Antibiotic, Otic; Antibiotic, Topical; Corticosteroid, Ophthalmic; Corticosteroid, Otic; Corticosteroid, Topical

Use Prevention and treatment of susceptible inflammatory conditions where bacterial infection (or risk of infection) is present

Mechanism of Action Refer to individual monographs for Bacitracin, Neomycin, Polymyxin B, and Hydrocortisone

Pharmacodynamics/Kinetics See individual agents.

Contraindications Hypersensitivity to any component of the formulation; not for use in viral infections, fungal diseases, mycobacterial infections

Warnings/Precautions Prolonged use of corticosteroids may result in systemic effects. May suppress immune response, predisposing to secondary infections. May mask or enhance purulent infections; may increase severity of viral infections.

Ophthalmic ointment: Should never be directly introduced into the anterior chamber. May retard corneal healing. Prolonged use may result in ocular hypertension/glaucoma, corneal and scleral thinning, potentially resulting in perforation. Use with caution in glaucoma. Avoid use following ocular cataract surgery.

Drug Interactions Hydrocortisone: **Substrate** of CYP3A4 (minor); **Induces** CYP3A4 (weak)

Also see individual agents.

Adverse Reactions Frequency not defined.

Dermatologic: Rash, generalized itching

Ocular: Irritation

Respiratory: Apnea

Miscellaneous: Secondary infection

Dosing

Adults & Elderly:

Ophthalmic infection: Ophthalmic (ointment): Instill ½" ribbon to inside of lower lid every 3-4 hours until improvement occurs.

Superficial dermal infection: Topical: Apply sparingly 2-4 times/day.

Pediatrics: Refer to adult dosing.

Available Dosage Forms [DSC] = Discontinued product

Ointment, ophthalmic (Cortisporin® [DSC]): Bacitracin 400 units, neomycin sulfate 3.5 mg, polymyxin B 10,000 units, and hydrocortisone 10 mg per g (3.5 g)

Ointment, topical (Cortisporin®): Bacitracin 400 units, neomycin 3.5 mg, polymyxin B 5000 units, and hydrocortisone 10 mg per g (15 g)

Nursing Guidelines

Assessment: See individual components listed in Related Information. Note breast-feeding caution.

Patient Education: See individual agents. **Pregnancy/breast-feeding precautions:** Inform prescriber if you are or intend to become pregnant. Consult prescriber if breast-feeding.

Pregnancy Risk Factor: C

Lactation: Excretion in breast milk unknown/use caution

Administration

Storage: Store at controlled room temperature of 15°C to 25°C (59°F to 77°F).

Related Information

Bacitracin *on page 217*
Hydrocortisone *on page 873*
Neomycin *on page 1208*
Polymyxin B *on pag 1380*

Baclofen (BAK loe fen)

U.S. Brand Names Lioresal®

Pharmacologic Category Skeletal Muscle Relaxant

Medication Safety Issues

Sound-alike/look-alike issues:

Baclofen may be confused with Bactroban®

Lioresal® may be confused with lisinopril, Loniten®, Lotensin®

Use Treatment of reversible spasticity associated with multiple sclerosis or spinal cord lesions

Orphan drug: Intrathecal: Treatment of intractable spasticity caused by spinal cord injury, multiple sclerosis, and other spinal disease (spinal ischemia or tumor, transverse myelitis, cervical spondylosis, degenerative myelopathy)

Unlabeled/Investigational Use Intractable hiccups, intractable pain relief, bladder spasticity, trigeminal neuralgia, cerebral palsy, Huntington's chorea

Mechanism of Action Inhibits the transmission of both monosynaptic and polysynaptic reflexes at the spinal cord level, possibly by hyperpolarization of primary afferent fiber terminals, with resultant relief of muscle spasticity

Pharmacodynamics/Kinetics

Onset of action: 3-4 days

Peak effect: 5-10 days

Absorption (dose dependent): Oral: Rapid

Protein binding: 30%

Metabolism: Hepatic (15% of dose)

Half-life elimination: 3.5 hours

Time to peak, serum: Oral: Within 2-3 hours

Excretion: Urine and feces (85% as unchanged drug)

Contraindications Hypersensitivity to baclofen or any component of the formulation

Warnings/Precautions Use with caution in patients with seizure disorder or impaired renal function. Avoid abrupt withdrawal of the drug; abrupt withdrawal of intrathecal baclofen has resulted in severe sequelae (hyperpyrexia, obtundation, rebound/exaggerated spasticity, muscle rigidity, and rhabdomyolysis), leading to organ failure and some fatalities. Risk may be higher in patients with injuries at T-6 or above, history of baclofen withdrawal, or limited ability to communicate. Elderly are more sensitive to the effects of baclofen and are more likely to experience adverse CNS effects at higher doses.

Drug Interactions

Increased effect: Opiate analgesics, benzodiazepines, hypertensive agents

Increased toxicity: CNS depressants and ethanol (sedation), tricyclic antidepressants (short-term memory loss), clindamycin (neuromuscular blockade), guanabenz (sedation), MAO inhibitors (decrease blood pressure, CNS, and respiratory effects)

Nutritional/Herbal/Ethanol Interactions

Ethanol: Avoid ethanol (may increase CNS depression).

Herb/Nutraceutical: Avoid valerian, St John's wort, kava kava, gotu kola.

Lab Interactions Increased alkaline phosphatase, AST, glucose, ammonia (B); decreased bilirubin (S)

Adverse Reactions

>10%:

Central nervous system: Drowsiness, vertigo, dizziness, psychiatric disturbances, insomnia, slurred speech, ataxia, hypotonia

Neuromuscular & skeletal: Weakness

1% to 10%:

Cardiovascular: Hypotension

Central nervous system: Fatigue, confusion, headache

Dermatologic: Rash

Gastrointestinal: Nausea, constipation

Genitourinary: Polyuria

<1% (Limited to important or life-threatening): Chest pain, dyspnea, dysuria, enuresis, hematuria, impotence, inability to ejaculate, nocturia, palpitation, syncope, urinary retention; withdrawal reactions have occurred with abrupt discontinuation (particularly severe with intrathecal use).

Overdosage/Toxicology Symptoms of overdose include vomiting, muscle hypotonia, salivation, drowsiness, coma, seizures, and respiratory depression. Atropine has been used to improve ventilation, heart rate, blood pressure, and core body temperature. Treatment is symptom-directed and supportive.

For toxicity following intrathecal administration: For adults, administer physostigmine 2 mg I.M. or I.V. (not to exceed 1 mg/minute). For pediatric patients, administer physostigmine 0.02 mg/kg I.M. or I.V. (not to exceed 0.5 mg/minute). Consider withdrawal of 30-40 mL of CSF to reduce baclofen concentration. Abrupt withdrawal of intrathecal baclofen has resulted in severe sequelae (hyperpyrexia, obtundation, muscle rigidity, and rhabdomyolysis)

Dosing

Adults:

Spasticity:

Oral: 5 mg 3 times/day, may increase 5 mg/dose every 3 days to a maximum of 80 mg/day

Intrathecal:

Test dose: 50-100 mcg, doses >50 mcg should be given in 25 mcg increments, separated by 24 hours. A screening dose of 25 mcg may be considered in very small patients. Patients not responding to screening dose of 100 mcg should not be considered for chronic infusion/implanted pump.

Maintenance: After positive response to test dose, a maintenance intrathecal infusion can be administered via an implanted intrathecal pump. Initial dose via pump: Infusion at a 24-hourly rate dosed at twice the test dose. Avoid abrupt discontinuation.

Hiccups (unlabeled use): 10-20 mg 2-3 times/day

Elderly: Oral (the lowest effective dose is recommended): Initial: 5 mg 2-3 times/day, increasing gradually as needed; if benefits are not seen withdraw the drug slowly.

Pediatrics:

Spasticity:

Oral (avoid abrupt withdrawal of drug): Children:

2-7 years: Initial: 10-15 mg/24 hours divided every 8 hours; titrate dose every 3 days in increments of 5-15 mg/day to a maximum of 40 mg/day.

≥8 years: Maximum: 60 mg/day in 3 divided doses

Intrathecal: Refer to adult dosing.

Renal Impairment: May be necessary to reduce dosage; no specific guidelines have been established

Available Dosage Forms

Injection, solution, intrathecal [preservative free] (Lioresal®): 50 mcg/mL (1 mL); 500 mcg/mL (20 mL); 2000 mcg/mL (5 mL)

Tablet: 10 mg, 20 mg

Nursing Guidelines

Assessment: Assess effectiveness and interactions of other medications patient may be taking. Monitor effectiveness of therapy and adverse reactions at beginning of therapy and periodically with long-term use. Assess knowledge/teach patient appropriate use, interventions to reduce side effects, and adverse symptoms to report.

Patient Education: Take this drug as prescribed. Do not discontinue without consulting prescriber (abrupt discontinuation may cause hallucinations). Do not take any prescription or OTC sleep-inducing drugs, sedatives, or antispasmodics without consulting prescriber. Avoid alcohol use. You may experience transient drowsiness, lethargy, or dizziness; use caution when driving or engaging in tasks requiring alertness until response to drug is known. Frequent small meals or lozenges may reduce GI upset.

Intrathecal use: Keep scheduled pump refill visits; abrupt interruption can cause serious withdrawal symptoms. Report increased spasticity, itching, numbness, unresolved insomnia, painful urination, change in urinary patterns, constipation, high fever, or persistent confusion.

Pregnancy precaution: Inform prescriber if you are or intend to become pregnant.

Geriatric Considerations: The elderly are more sensitive to the effects of baclofen and are more likely to experience adverse CNS effects at higher doses. Two cases of encephalopathy were reported after inadvertent high doses (50 mg/day and 90 mg/day) were given to elderly patients.

Pregnancy Risk Factor: C

Lactation: Enters breast milk (small amounts)/compatible

Perioperative/Anesthesia/Other Concerns: Avoid abrupt withdrawal of the drug; abrupt withdrawal of intrathecal baclofen has resulted in severe sequelae (hyperpyrexia, obtundation, rebound/exaggerated spasticity, muscle rigidity,

(Continued)

Baclofen *(Continued)*

and rhabdomyolysis), leading to organ failure and some fatalities. Risk may be higher in patients with injuries at T-6 or above, history of baclofen withdrawal, or limited ability to communicate. Elderly are more sensitive to the effects of baclofen and are more likely to experience adverse CNS effects at higher doses.

Administration

Compatibility: Stable in sterile, preservative free NS

- ◆ BactoShield® CHG [OTC] *see* Chlorhexidine Gluconate *on page 373*
- ◆ Bactrim™ *see* Sulfamethoxazole and Trimethoprim *on page 1582*
- ◆ Bactrim™ DS *see* Sulfamethoxazole and Trimethoprim *on page 1582*
- ◆ Bactroban® *see* Mupirocin *on page 1187*
- ◆ Bactroban® Nasal *see* Mupirocin *on page 1187*
- ◆ Baking Soda *see* Sodium Bicarbonate *on page 1542*
- ◆ Balacet 325™ *see* Propoxyphene and Acetaminophen *on page 1427*

Balanced Salt Solution (BAL anced salt soe LOO shun)

U.S. Brand Names AquaLase™; BSS®; BSS Plus®

Pharmacologic Category Ophthalmic Agent, Miscellaneous

Use

AquaLase™, BSS®: Intraocular or extraocular irrigating solution

BSS® Plus: Intraocular irrigating solution

Warnings/Precautions For use during surgical procedures with an expected duration of ≤60 minutes. Use with caution in diabetic patients; intraoperative lens changes have been observed when undergoing vitrectomy procedure.

Adverse Reactions Frequency not defined.

Ocular: Bullous keratopathy, corneal clouding, corneal decompensation, corneal edema, corneal swelling, inflammatory reactions, lens changes

Dosing

Adults & Elderly: Ophthalmic irrigation: Based on standard for each surgical procedure

Available Dosage Forms

Solution, ophthalmic [irrigation; preservative free]: Sodium chloride 0.64%, potassium chloride 0.075%, calcium chloride 0.048%, magnesium chloride 0.03%, sodium acetate 0.39%, sodium citrate 0.17% (18 mL, 200 mL, 250 mL, 500 mL)

AquaLase™: Sodium chloride 0.64%, potassium chloride 0.075%, calcium chloride 0.048%, magnesium chloride 0.03%, sodium acetate 0.39%, sodium citrate 0.17% (90 mL)

BSS®: Sodium chloride 0.64%, potassium chloride 0.075%, calcium chloride 0.048%, magnesium chloride 0.03%, sodium acetate 0.39%, sodium citrate 0.17% (15 mL, 30 mL, 250 mL, 500 mL)

BSS Plus®: Sodium chloride 0.71%, potassium chloride 0.038%, calcium chloride 0.015%, magnesium chloride 0.02%, sodium phosphate 0.042%, sodium bicarbonate 0.21%, dextrose 0.092%, glutathione 0.018% (250 mL, 500 mL)

Nursing Guidelines

Patient Education: For the eye

Administration

Reconstitution: BSS Plus®: Prior to administration, add contents of the "Part II" vial to the contents of the "Part I" bottle. Mix gently and use within 6 hours.

Storage: Store between 2°C to 25°C (36°F to 77°F); do not freeze.

- ◆ Bancap HC® *see* Hydrocodone and Acetaminophen *on page 867*
- ◆ Band-Aid® Hurt-Free™ Antiseptic Wash [OTC] *see* Lidocaine *on page 1033*
- ◆ Banophen® [OTC] *see* DiphenhydrAMINE *on page 546*
- ◆ Banophen® Anti-Itch [OTC] *see* DiphenhydrAMINE *on page 546*
- ◆ Baridium® [OTC] *see* Phenazopyridine *on page 1342*

Basiliximab (ba si LIK si mab)

U.S. Brand Names Simulect®

Pharmacologic Category Monoclonal Antibody

Use Prophylaxis of acute organ rejection in renal transplantation

Mechanism of Action Chimeric (murine/human) monoclonal antibody which blocks the alpha-chain of the interleukin-2 (IL-2) receptor complex; this receptor is expressed on activated T lymphocytes and is a critical pathway for activating cell-mediated allograft rejection

Pharmacodynamics/Kinetics

Duration: Mean: 36 days (determined by IL-2R alpha saturation)
Distribution: Mean: V_d: Children: 5.2 ± 2.8 L; Adults: 8.6 ± 4.1 L
Half-life elimination: Children: 9.4 days; Adults: Mean: 7.2 days
Excretion: Clearance: Children: 20 mL/hour; Adults: Mean: 41 mL/hour

Contraindications Hypersensitivity basiliximab, murine proteins, or any component of the formulation

Warnings/Precautions To be used as a component of immunosuppressive regimen which includes cyclosporine and corticosteroids. Only physicians experienced in transplantation and immunosuppression should prescribe, and patients should receive the drug in a facility with adequate equipment and staff capable of providing the laboratory and medical support required for transplantation.

The incidence of lymphoproliferative disorders and/or opportunistic infections may be increased by immunosuppressive therapy. Severe hypersensitivity reactions, occurring within 24 hours, have been reported. Reactions, including anaphylaxis, have occurred both with the initial exposure and/or following re-exposure after several months. Use caution during re-exposure to a subsequent course of therapy in a patient who has previously received basiliximab. Discontinue the drug permanently if a reaction occurs. Medications for the treatment of hypersensitivity reactions should be available for immediate use. Treatment may result in the development of human antimurine antibodies (HAMA); however, limited evidence suggesting the use of muromonab-CD3 or other murine products is not precluded.

Drug Interactions Basiliximab is an immunoglobulin; specific drug interactions have not been evaluated, but are not anticipated

Vaccines: It is not known if the immune response to vaccines will be impaired during or following basiliximab therapy.

Adverse Reactions Administration of basiliximab did not appear to increase the incidence or severity of adverse effects in clinical trials. Adverse events were reported in 96% of both the placebo and basiliximab groups.

>10%:

- Cardiovascular: Peripheral edema, hypertension, atrial fibrillation
- Central nervous system: Fever, headache, insomnia, pain
- Dermatologic: Wound complications, acne
- Endocrine & metabolic: Hypokalemia, hyperkalemia, hyperglycemia, hyperuricemia, hypophosphatemia, hypercholesterolemia
- Gastrointestinal: Constipation, nausea, diarrhea, abdominal pain, vomiting, dyspepsia
- Genitourinary: Urinary tract infection
- Hematologic: Anemia
- Neuromuscular & skeletal: Tremor
- Respiratory: Dyspnea, infection (upper respiratory)
- Miscellaneous: Viral infection

3% to 10% (Limited to important or life-threatening):

- Cardiovascular: Chest pain, cardiac failure, hypotension, arrhythmia, tachycardia, edema, angina pectoris
- Central nervous system: Hypoesthesia, neuropathy, agitation, anxiety, depression
- Dermatologic: Cyst, hypertrichosis, pruritus, rash
- Endocrine & metabolic: Dehydration, diabetes mellitus, fluid overload, hypercalcemia, hyperlipidemia, hypoglycemia, hypomagnesemia, acidosis, hypertriglyceridemia, hypocalcemia, hyponatremia
- Gastrointestinal: GI hemorrhage, gingival hyperplasia, melena, esophagitis, ulcerative stomatitis
- Genitourinary: Impotence, genital edema, albuminuria, hematuria, renal tubular necrosis, urinary retention
- Hematologic: Hematoma, hemorrhage, thrombocytopenia, thrombosis, polycythemia, leukopenia
- Neuromuscular & skeletal: Arthralgia, arthropathy, paresthesia
- Ocular: Cataract, conjunctivitis, abnormal vision
- Respiratory: Bronchospasm, pulmonary edema
- Miscellaneous: Sepsis, infection, increased glucocorticoids

Postmarketing and/or case reports: Severe hypersensitivity reactions, including anaphylaxis, have been reported. Symptoms may include hypotension, tachycardia, cardiac failure, dyspnea, bronchospasm, pulmonary edema, urticaria, rash, pruritus, sneezing, capillary leak syndrome, and respiratory failure.

Overdosage/Toxicology There have been no reports of overdose.

(Continued)

Basiliximab *(Continued)*

Dosing

Adults & Elderly: Note: Patients previously administered basiliximab should only be re-exposed to a subsequent course of therapy with extreme caution.

Renal transplantation: I.V.: 20 mg within 2 hours prior to transplant surgery, followed by a second 20 mg dose 4 days after transplantation. The second dose should be withheld if complications occur (including severe hypersensitivity reactions or graft loss).

Pediatrics: Note: Patients previously administered basiliximab should only be re-exposed to a subsequent course of therapy with extreme caution.

Renal transplantation: I.V.:

Children <35 kg: 10 mg within 2 hours prior to transplant surgery, followed by a second 10 mg dose 4 days after transplantation; the second dose should be withheld if complications occur (including severe hypersensitivity reactions or graft loss)

Children ≥35 kg: Refer to adult dosing

Renal Impairment: No specific dosing adjustment is recommended.

Hepatic Impairment: No specific dosing adjustment is recommended.

Available Dosage Forms Injection, powder for reconstitution: 10 mg, 20 mg

Nursing Guidelines

Assessment: Monitor cardiorespiratory function, renal function, and adverse reactions during infusion and periodically following infusion. Be alert to opportunistic infections. Assess knowledge/teach patient possible side effects/interventions and adverse symptoms to report as inpatient or following discharge.

Patient Education: This medication, which may help to reduce transplant rejection, can only be given by infusion. You will be monitored and assessed closely during infusion and thereafter. It is important that you report any changes or problems for evaluation. You will be susceptible to infection (avoid crowds and exposure to infection). Frequent mouth care and small frequent meals may help counteract any GI effects you may experience and will help maintain adequate nutrition and fluid intake. Report any changes in urination; unusual bruising or bleeding; chest pain or palpitations; acute dizziness; respiratory difficulty; fever or chills; changes in cognition; rash; feelings of pain or numbness in extremities; severe GI upset or diarrhea; unusual back or leg pain or muscle tremors; vision changes; or any sign of infection (eg, chills, fever, sore throat, easy bruising or bleeding, mouth sores, unhealed sores, vaginal discharge). **Breast-feeding precaution:** Breast-feeding is not recommended.

Pregnancy Risk Factor: B (manufacturer)

Pregnancy Issues: IL-2 receptors play an important role in the development of the immune system. Use in pregnant women only when benefit exceeds potential risk to the fetus. Women of childbearing potential should use effective contraceptive measures before beginning treatment and for 4 months after completion of therapy with this agent.

Lactation: Excretion in breast milk unknown/not recommended

Breast-Feeding Considerations: It is not known whether basiliximab is excreted in human milk. Because many immunoglobulins are secreted in milk and the potential for serious adverse reactions exists, a decision should be made whether to discontinue nursing or discontinue the drug, taking into account the importance of the drug to the mother.

Administration

I.V.: For intravenous administration only. Infuse over 20-30 minutes.

Reconstitution: Reconstitute vials with sterile water for injection. Dilute reconstituted contents in normal saline or 5% dextrose.

Storage: Store vials under refrigeration 2°C to 8°C (36°F to 46°F). Reconstituted vials are stable under refrigeration for 24 hours, but only 4 hours at room temperature.

- **Bausch & Lomb® Computer Eye Drops [OTC]** *see* Glycerin *on page 826*
- **Bayer® Aspirin [OTC]** *see* Aspirin *on page 189*
- **Bayer® Aspirin Extra Strength [OTC]** *see* Aspirin *on page 189*
- **Bayer® Aspirin Regimen Adult Low Strength [OTC]** *see* Aspirin *on page 189*
- **Bayer® Aspirin Regimen Children's [OTC]** *see* Aspirin *on page 189*
- **Bayer® Aspirin Regimen Regular Strength [OTC]** *see* Aspirin *on page 189*
- **Bayer® Extra Strength Arthritis Pain Regimen [OTC]** *see* Aspirin *on page 189*

♦ Bayer® Plus Extra Strength [OTC] *see* Aspirin *on page 189*
♦ Bayer® Women's Aspirin Plus Calcium [OTC] *see* Aspirin *on page 189*
♦ BayGam® *see* Immune Globulin (Intramuscular) *on page 898*
♦ BayRho-D® Full-Dose *see* Rh_o(D) Immune Globulin *on page 1471*
♦ BayRho-D® Mini-Dose *see* Rh_o(D) Immune Globulin *on page 1471*
♦ BCNU *see* Carmustine *on page 318*
♦ B Complex Combinations *see* Vitamin B Complex Combinations *on page 1716*

Belladonna and Opium (bel a DON a & OH pee um)

U.S. Brand Names B&O Supprettes®

Synonyms Opium and Belladonna

Pharmacologic Category Analgesic Combination (Narcotic); Antispasmodic Agent, Urinary

Use Relief of moderate to severe pain associated with rectal or bladder tenesmus that may occur in postoperative states and neoplastic situations; pain associated with ureteral spasms not responsive to non-narcotic analgesics and to space intervals between injections of opiates

Mechanism of Action Anticholinergic alkaloids act primarily by competitive inhibition of the muscarinic actions of acetylcholine on structures innervated by postganglionic cholinergic neurons and on smooth muscle; resulting effects include antisecretory activity on exocrine glands and intestinal mucosa and smooth muscle relaxation. Contains many narcotic alkaloids including morphine; its mechanism for gastric motility inhibition is primarily due to this morphine content; it results in a decrease in digestive secretions, an increase in GI muscle tone, and therefore a reduction in GI propulsion.

Pharmacodynamics/Kinetics

Opium:

Onset of action: Within 30 minutes

Metabolism: Hepatic, with formation of glucuronide metabolites

Contraindications Glaucoma; severe renal or hepatic disease; bronchial asthma; respiratory depression; convulsive disorders; acute alcoholism; premature labor

Warnings/Precautions Usual precautions of opiate agonist therapy should be observed; infants <3 months of age are more susceptible to respiratory depression, use with caution and generally in reduced doses in this age group

Drug Interactions

Decreased effect: Phenothiazines

Increased effect/toxicity: CNS depressants, tricyclic antidepressants

Nutritional/Herbal/Ethanol Interactions Ethanol: Avoid ethanol (may increase sedation).

Lab Interactions Increased aminotransferase [ALT (SGPT)/AST (SGOT)] (S)

Adverse Reactions

>10%:

Dermatologic: Dry skin

Gastrointestinal: Constipation, dry throat, dry mouth

Local: Irritation at injection site

Respiratory: Dry nose

Miscellaneous: Diaphoresis (decreased)

1% to 10%:

Dermatologic: Increased sensitivity to light

Endocrine & metabolic: Decreased flow of breast milk

Gastrointestinal: Dysphagia

<1% (Limited to important or life-threatening): Ataxia, CNS depression, increased intraocular pain, loss of memory, orthostatic hypotension, respiratory depression, tachycardia, ventricular fibrillation

Overdosage/Toxicology Primary attention should be directed to ensuring adequate respiratory exchange. Opiate agonist-induced respiratory depression may be reversed with parenteral naloxone hydrochloride. Anticholinergic toxicity may be caused by strong binding of a belladonna alkaloid to cholinergic receptors. Physostigmine 1-2 mg given slowly SubQ or I.V. may be administered to reverse overdose with life-threatening effects.

Dosing

Adults & Elderly: Rectal/bladder tenesmus or ureteral spasm: Rectal: 1 suppository 1-2 times/day, up to 4 doses/day

Available Dosage Forms Suppository:

#15 A: Belladonna extract 16.2 mg and opium 30 mg

#16 A: Belladonna extract 16.2 mg and opium 60 mg

(Continued)

Belladonna and Opium *(Continued)*

Nursing Guidelines

Assessment: Assess other medications patient may be taking for additive or adverse interactions. Monitor therapeutic effectiveness, signs of overdose, and adverse effects at beginning of therapy and at regular intervals with long-term use. May cause physical and/or psychological dependence. For inpatients, implement safety measures. Assess knowledge/teach patient appropriate use if self-administered. Teach patient to monitor for adverse reactions, adverse reactions to report, and appropriate interventions to reduce side effects.

Patient Education: If self-administered, use exactly as directed; do not increase dose or frequency. Drug may cause physical and/or psychological dependence. While using this medication, do not use alcohol and other prescription or OTC medications (especially sedatives, tranquilizers, antihistamines, or pain medications) without consulting prescriber. Maintain adequate hydration (2-3 L/day of fluids) unless instructed to restrict fluid intake. May cause hypotension, dizziness, or drowsiness; use caution when driving, climbing stairs, or changing position (rising from sitting or lying to standing) or when engaging in tasks requiring alertness (until response to drug is known); dry mouth or throat (frequent mouth care, frequent sips of fluids, chewing gum, or sucking lozenges may help); constipation (increased exercise, fluids, fruit, or fiber may help; if unresolved, consult prescriber about use of stool softeners); photosensitivity (use sunscreen, wear protective clothing and eyewear, and avoid direct sunlight); or decreased perspiration (avoid extremes in temperature or excessive activity in hot environments). Report chest pain or palpitations; persistent dizziness; changes in mentation; changes in gait; blurred vision; shortness of breath or respiratory difficulty. **Pregnancy/breast-feeding precautions:** Inform prescriber if you are or intend to become pregnant. Consult prescriber if breast-feeding.

Pregnancy Risk Factor: C

Lactation: Excretion in breast milk unknown/use caution

Administration

Storage: Store at 15°C to 30°C; avoid freezing.

- ♦ **Benadryl® Allergy [OTC]** *see* DiphenhydrAMINE *on page 546*
- ♦ **Benadryl® Children's Allergy [OTC]** *see* DiphenhydrAMINE *on page 546*
- ♦ **Benadryl® Children's Allergy Fastmelt® [OTC]** *see* DiphenhydrAMINE *on page 546*
- ♦ **Benadryl® Dye-Free Allergy [OTC]** *see* DiphenhydrAMINE *on page 546*
- ♦ **Benadryl® Injection** *see* DiphenhydrAMINE *on page 546*
- ♦ **Benadryl® Itch Stopping [OTC]** *see* DiphenhydrAMINE *on page 546*
- ♦ **Benadryl® Itch Stopping Extra Strength [OTC]** *see* DiphenhydrAMINE *on page 546*

Benazepril (ben AY ze pril)

U.S. Brand Names Lotensin®

Synonyms Benazepril Hydrochloride

Pharmacologic Category Angiotensin-Converting Enzyme (ACE) Inhibitor

Medication Safety Issues

Sound-alike/look-alike issues:

Benazepril may be confused with Benadryl®

Lotensin® may be confused with Lioresal®, Loniten®, lovastatin

Use Treatment of hypertension, either alone or in combination with other antihypertensive agents

Mechanism of Action Competitive inhibition of angiotensin I being converted to angiotensin II, a potent vasoconstrictor, through the angiotensin I-converting enzyme (ACE) activity, with resultant lower levels of angiotensin II which causes an increase in plasma renin activity and a reduction in aldosterone secretion

Pharmacodynamics/Kinetics

Reduction in plasma angiotensin-converting enzyme (ACE) activity:

Onset of action: Peak effect: 1-2 hours after 2-20 mg dose

Duration: >90% inhibition for 24 hours after 5-20 mg dose

Reduction in blood pressure:

Peak effect: Single dose: 2-4 hours; Continuous therapy: 2 weeks

Absorption: Rapid (37%); food does not alter significantly; metabolite (benazeprilat) itself unsuitable for oral administration due to poor absorption

Distribution: V_d: ~8.7 L

Metabolism: Rapidly and extensively hepatic to its active metabolite, benazeprilat, via enzymatic hydrolysis; extensive first-pass effect

Half-life elimination: Benazeprilat: Effective: 10-11 hours; Terminal: Children: 5 hours, Adults: 22 hours

Time to peak: Parent drug: 0.5-1 hour

Excretion: Clearance: Nonrenal clearance (ie, biliary, metabolic) appears to contribute to the elimination of benazeprilat (11% to 12%), particularly patients with severe renal impairment; hepatic clearance is the main elimination route of unchanged benazepril

Dialysis: ~6% of metabolite removed in 4 hours of dialysis following 10 mg of benazepril administered 2 hours prior to procedure; parent compound not found in dialysate

Contraindications Hypersensitivity to benazepril or any component of the formulation; angioedema or serious hypersensitivity related to previous treatment with an ACE inhibitor; bilateral renal artery stenosis; patients with idiopathic or hereditary angioedema; pregnancy (2nd and 3rd trimesters)

Warnings/Precautions Anaphylactic reactions can occur. Angioedema can occur at any time during treatment (especially following first dose). Angioedema may involve head and neck (potentially affecting the airway) or the intestine (presenting with abdominal pain). Careful blood pressure monitoring with first dose (hypotension can occur especially in volume depleted patients). Dosage adjustment needed in renal impairment. Use with caution in hypovolemia; collagen vascular diseases; valvular stenosis (particularly aortic stenosis); hyperkalemia; or before, during, or immediately after anesthesia. Avoid rapid dosage escalation which may lead to renal insufficiency. Rare toxicities associated with ACE inhibitors include cholestatic jaundice (which may progress to hepatic necrosis) and neutropenia/agranulocytosis with myeloid hyperplasia. Hypersensitivity reactions may be seen during hemodialysis with high-flux dialysis membranes (eg, AN69). Deterioration in renal function can occur with initiation. Use with caution in unilateral renal artery stenosis and pre-existing renal insufficiency.

Drug Interactions

Alpha$_1$ blockers: Hypotensive effect increased.

Aspirin: The effects of ACE inhibitors may be blunted by aspirin administration, particularly at higher dosages and/or increase adverse renal effects.

Diuretics: Hypovolemia due to diuretics may precipitate acute hypotensive events or acute renal failure.

Insulin: Risk of hypoglycemia may be increased.

Lithium: Risk of lithium toxicity may be increased; monitor lithium levels.

NSAIDs: May attenuate hypertensive efficacy; effect has been seen with captopril and may occur with other ACE inhibitors; monitor blood pressure. May increase adverse renal effects.

Potassium-sparing diuretics or potassium supplements (amiloride, potassium, spironolactone, triamterene): Increased risk of hyperkalemia.

Trimethoprim (high dose) may increase the risk of hyperkalemia.

Nutritional/Herbal/Ethanol Interactions Herb/Nutraceutical: Avoid dong quai if using for hypertension (has estrogenic activity). Avoid ephedra, yohimbe, ginseng (may worsen hypertension). Avoid garlic (may have increased antihypertensive effect).

Adverse Reactions

1% to 10%:

Cardiovascular: Postural dizziness (1.5%)

Central nervous system: Headache (6.2%), dizziness (3.6%), fatigue (2.4%), somnolence (1.6%)

Endocrine & metabolic: Hyperkalemia (1%), increased uric acid

Gastrointestinal: Nausea (1.3%)

Renal: Increased serum creatinine (2%), worsening of renal function may occur in patients with bilateral renal artery stenosis or hypovolemia

Respiratory: Cough (1.2% to 10%)

<1% (Limited to important or life-threatening): Alopecia, angina, angioedema, asthma, dermatitis, dyspnea, hemolytic anemia, hypersensitivity, hypotension, impotence, insomnia, pancreatitis, paresthesia, photosensitivity, postural hypotension (0.3%), rash, shock, Stevens-Johnson syndrome, syncope, thrombocytopenia, vomiting

Eosinophilic pneumonitis, neutropenia, anaphylaxis, renal insufficiency and renal failure have been reported with other ACE inhibitors. In addition, a syndrome

(Continued)

Benazepril *(Continued)*

including fever, myalgia, arthralgia, interstitial nephritis, vasculitis, rash, eosinophilia, and elevated ESR has been reported to be associated with ACE inhibitors.

Overdosage/Toxicology Mild hypotension has been the primary toxic effect seen with acute overdose. Bradycardia may also occur. Hyperkalemia occurs even with therapeutic doses, especially in patients with renal insufficiency and those taking NSAIDs. Treatment is symptom-directed and supportive.

Dosing

Adults: Hypertension: Oral: Initial: 10 mg/day in patients not receiving a diuretic; 20-40 mg/day as a single dose or 2 divided doses; the need for twice-daily dosing should be assessed by monitoring peak (2-6 hours after dosing) and trough responses.

Note: Patients taking diuretics should have them discontinued 2-3 days prior to starting benazepril. If they cannot be discontinued, then initial dose should be 5 mg; restart after blood pressure is stabilized if needed.

Elderly: Oral: Initial: 5-10 mg/day in single or divided doses; usual range: 20-40 mg/day; adjust for renal function. Also see "Note" in adult dosing.

Pediatrics: Hypertension: Children ≥6 years: Oral: Initial: 0.2 mg/kg/day as monotherapy; dosing range: 0.1-0.6 mg/kg/day (maximum dose: 40 mg/day)

Renal Impairment:

Cl_{cr} <30 mL/minute:

Children: Use is not recommended.

Adults: Administer 5 mg/day initially; maximum daily dose: 40 mg.

Hemodialysis: Moderately dialyzable (20% to 50%); administer dose postdialysis or administer 25% to 35% supplemental dose.

Peritoneal dialysis: Supplemental dose is not necessary.

Available Dosage Forms Tablet, as hydrochloride: 5 mg, 10 mg, 20 mg, 40 mg

Nursing Guidelines

Assessment: See Contraindications, Warnings/Precautions, and Dosing for use cautions. Assess potential for interactions with other prescriptions, OTC medications, or herbal products patient may be taking (see Drug Interactions). Assess results of laboratory tests (see below), therapeutic effectiveness, and adverse response on a regular basis during therapy (see Adverse Reactions and Overdose/Toxicology). Teach patient proper use, possible side effects/appropriate interventions, and adverse symptoms to report (see Patient Education). **Pregnancy risk factor C/D** - see Pregnancy Risk Factor for use cautions. Instruct patient in appropriate use of contraceptives (see Pregnancy Issues).

Monitoring Laboratory Tests: CBC, renal function tests, electrolytes

Patient Education: Inform prescriber of all prescriptions, OTC medications, or herbal products you are taking, and any allergies you have. Do not take any new medication during therapy without consulting prescriber. Take exactly as directed; do not alter dose or discontinue without consulting prescriber. Take first dose at bedtime. Do not take potassium supplements or salt substitutes containing potassium without consulting prescriber. This drug does not eliminate need for diet or exercise regimen as recommended by prescriber. May cause dizziness, fainting, or lightheadedness (use caution when driving or engaging in tasks that require alertness until response to drug is known); postural hypotension (use caution when rising from lying or sitting position or climbing stairs); nausea, vomiting, abdominal pain, dry mouth, or transient loss of appetite (small, frequent meals, frequent mouth care, sucking lozenges, or chewing gum may help); report if these side effects persist. Report mouth sores; fever or chills; swelling of extremities, face, mouth, or tongue; respiratory difficulty or unusual cough; or other persistent adverse reactions. **Pregnancy precaution:** Inform prescriber if you are or intend to become pregnant. This drug should not be used in the 2nd or 3rd trimester of pregnancy. Consult prescriber for appropriate contraceptive measures.

Geriatric Considerations: Due to frequent decreases in glomerular filtration (also creatinine clearance) with aging, elderly patients may have exaggerated responses to ACE inhibitors. Differences in clinical response due to hepatic changes are not observed. ACE inhibitors may be preferred agents in elderly patients with congestive heart failure and diabetes mellitus. Diabetic proteinuria is reduced and insulin sensitivity is enhanced. In general, the side effect profile is favorable in elderly and causes little or no CNS confusion. Use lowest dose recommendations initially.

Pregnancy Risk Factor: C (1st trimester)/D (2nd and 3rd trimesters)

Pregnancy Issues: ACE inhibitors can cause fetal injury or death if taken during the 2nd or 3rd trimester. Discontinue ACE inhibitors as soon as pregnancy is detected.

Lactation: Enters breast milk/compatible

Perioperative/Anesthesia/Other Concerns: Aging patients with a decrease in glomerular filtration (also creatinine clearance), severe congestive heart failure, and renal failure may experience an exaggerated response with administration of ACE inhibitors. Diabetic proteinuria is reduced and insulin sensitivity is enhanced. In general, the side effect profile is favorable in elderly and causes little or no CNS confusion.

ACE inhibitors decrease morbidity and mortality in patients with asymptomatic and symptomatic left ventricular dysfunction. In this situation, they decrease hospitalizations for, and retard progression to, congestive heart failure. ACE inhibitors are also indicated in patients postmyocardial infarction in whom left ventricular ejection fraction is <40%. When used in patients with heart failure, the target dose or maximum tolerated dose, should be achieved, if possible. Lower daily doses of ACE inhibitors have not demonstrated the same cardioprotective effects. ACE inhibitors have renal protective effects in patients with proteinuria and possibly cardioprotective effects in high-risk patients.

ACE inhibitor therapy may elicit rapid increases in potassium and creatinine, especially when used in patients with bilateral renal artery stenosis. When ACE inhibition is introduced in patients with pre-existing diuretic therapy who are hypovolemic, the ACE inhibitor may induce acute hypotension. In those patients experiencing cough on an ACE inhibitor, the ACE inhibitor may be discontinued and, if necessary, angiotensin-receptor blocker therapy instituted. Concomitant NSAID therapy may attenuate blood pressure control; use of NSAIDs should be avoided or limited, with monitoring of blood pressure control. In the setting of heart failure, NSAID use may be associated with an increased risk for fluid accumulation and edema. Because of the potent teratogenic effects of ACE inhibitors, these drugs should be avoided, if possible, when treating women of childbearing potential not on effective birth control measures.

- ♦ Benazepril Hydrochloride *see* Benazepril *on page 228*
- ♦ Benazepril Hydrochloride and Amlodipine Besylate *see* Amlodipine and Benazepril *on page 142*
- ♦ Bentyl® *see* Dicyclomine *on page 526*
- ♦ Benza® [OTC] *see* Benzalkonium Chloride *on page 231*

Benzalkonium Chloride (benz al KOE nee um KLOR ide)

U.S. Brand Names Benza® [OTC]; HandClens® [OTC]; 3M™ Cavilon™ Skin Cleanser [OTC]; Ony-Clear [OTC] [DSC]; Zephiran® [OTC]

Synonyms BAC

Pharmacologic Category Antibiotic, Topical

Medication Safety Issues

Sound-alike/look-alike issues:

Benza® may be confused with Benzac®

Use Surface antiseptic and germicidal preservative

Adverse Reactions 1% to 10%: Hypersensitivity

Dosing

Adults & Elderly: Antiseptic: Topical: Thoroughly rinse anionic detergents and soaps from the skin or other areas prior to use of solutions because they reduce the antibacterial activity of BAC. To protect metal instruments stored in BAC solution, add crushed Anti-Rust Tablets, 4 tablets/quart, to antiseptic solution, change solution at least once weekly. Not to be used for storage of aluminum or zinc instruments, instruments with lenses fastened by cement, lacquered catheters, or some synthetic rubber goods.

Available Dosage Forms [DSC] = Discontinued product

Solution, topical:

Benza®: 1:750 (60 mL, 240 mL, 480 mL, 3840 mL)

HandClens®: 0.13% (120 mL, 480 mL, 800 mL)

Ony-Clear [DSC]: 1% (30 mL)

Zephiran®: 1:750 (240 mL, 3840 mL) [aqueous]

Solution, topical spray (3M™ Cavilon™ Skin Cleanser): 0.11% (240 mL)

(Continued)

Benzalkonium Chloride *(Continued)*

Nursing Guidelines

Pregnancy Risk Factor: C

♦ **Benzathine Benzylpenicillin** *see* Penicillin G Benzathine *on page 1330*

♦ **Benzathine Penicillin G** *see* Penicillin G Benzathine *on page 1330*

Benzocaine (BEN zoe kane)

U.S. Brand Names Americaine® [OTC]; Americaine® Hemorrhoidal [OTC]; Anbesol® [OTC]; Anbesol® Baby [OTC]; Anbesol® Cold Sore Therapy [OTC]; Anbesol® Jr. [OTC]; Anbesol® Maximum Strength [OTC]; Benzodent® [OTC]; Cepacol® Sore Throat [OTC]; Chiggerex® [OTC]; Chiggertox® [OTC]; Cylex® [OTC]; Dentapaine [OTC]; Dent's Extra Strength Toothache [OTC]; Dent's Maxi-Strength Toothache [OTC]; Dermoplast® Antibacterial [OTC]; Dermoplast® Pain Relieving [OTC]; Detane® [OTC]; Foille® [OTC]; HDA® Toothache [OTC]; Hurricaine® [OTC]; Ivy-Rid® [OTC]; Kanka® Soft Brush™ [OTC]; Lanacane® [OTC]; Lanacane® Maximum Strength [OTC]; Mycinettes® [OTC]; Orabase® with Benzocaine [OTC]; Orajel® Baby Daytime and Nighttime [OTC]; Orajel® Baby Teething [OTC]; Orajel® Baby Teething Nighttime [OTC]; Orajel® Denture Plus [OTC]; Orajel® Maximum Strength [OTC]; Orajel® Medicated Toothache [OTC]; Orajel® Mouth Sore [OTC]; Orajel® Multi-Action Cold Sore [OTC]; Orajel PM® [OTC]; Orajel® Ultra Mouth Sore [OTC]; Oticaine; Otocaine™; Outgro® [OTC]; Red Cross™ Canker Sore [OTC]; Rid-A-Pain Dental Drops [OTC]; Skeeter Stik [OTC]; Sting-Kill [OTC]; Tanac® [OTC]; Thorets [OTC]; Trocaine® [OTC]; Zilactin®-B [OTC]; Zilactin Toothache and Gum Pain® [OTC]

Synonyms Ethyl Aminobenzoate

Pharmacologic Category Local Anesthetic

Medication Safety Issues

Sound-alike/look-alike issues:

Orabase®-B may be confused with Orinase®

Use Temporary relief of pain associated with pruritic dermatosis, pruritus, minor burns, acute congestive and serous otitis media, swimmer's ear, otitis externa, bee stings, insect bites; mouth and gum irritations (toothache, minor sore throat pain, canker sores, dentures, orthodontia, teething, mucositis, stomatitis); sunburn, hemorrhoids; anesthetic lubricant for passage of catheters and endoscopic tubes

Mechanism of Action Ester local anesthetic blocks both the initiation and conduction of nerve impulses by decreasing the neuronal membrane's permeability to sodium ions, which results in inhibition of depolarization with resultant blockade of conduction

Pharmacodynamics/Kinetics

Absorption: Topical: Poor to intact skin; well absorbed from mucous membranes and traumatized skin

Metabolism: Hepatic (to a lesser extent) and plasma via hydrolysis by cholinesterase

Excretion: Urine (as metabolites)

Contraindications Hypersensitivity to benzocaine, other ester-type local anesthetics, or any component of the formulation; secondary bacterial infection of area; ophthalmic use; otic preparations are also contraindicated in the presence of perforated tympanic membrane

Warnings/Precautions Methemoglobinemia has been reported following topical use (rare); use caution in young children, the elderly, with application to inflamed areas or concomitant use with other medications known to cause this side effect.

When used for self-medication (OTC), notify healthcare provider if condition worsens or does not improve within 7 days, or if swelling, rash or fever develops. Do not use on open wounds. Avoid contact with the eyes.

Drug Interactions May antagonize actions of sulfonamides

Adverse Reactions Frequency not defined.

Hematologic: Methemoglobinemia

Local: Burning, contact dermatitis, edema, erythema, pruritus, rash, stinging, tenderness, urticaria

Miscellaneous: Hypersensitivity

Overdosage/Toxicology Methemoglobinemia has been reported with benzocaine in oral overdose. Treatment is primarily symptomatic and supportive; termination of anesthesia by pneumatic tourniquet inflation should be attempted when the agent is administered by infiltration or regional injection. Methemoglobinemia may be treated with methylene blue, 1-2 mg/kg I.V. infused over several minutes.

Seizures commonly respond to diazepam, while hypotension responds to I.V. fluids and Trendelenburg positioning. Bradyarrhythmias (when the heart rate is <60) can be treated with I.V., I.M., or SubQ atropine 15 mcg/kg. With the development of metabolic acidosis, I.V. sodium bicarbonate 0.5-2 mEq/kg and ventilatory assistance should be instituted.

Dosing

Adults & Elderly: Note: These are general dosing guidelines; Refer to specific product labeling for dosing instructions.

Bee stings, insect bites, minor burns, sunburn: Children ≥2 years and Adults: Topical 5% to 20%: Apply to affected area 3-4 times a day as needed. In cases of bee stings, remove stinger before treatment.

Lubricant for passage of catheters and instruments: Children ≥2 years and Adults: Topical 20%: Apply evenly to exterior of instrument prior to use.

Mouth and gum irritation: Children ≥2 years and Adults: Topical (oral) 10% to 20%: Apply thin layer to affected area up to 4 times daily

Sore throat: Children ≥5 years and Adults: Oral: Allow one lozenge (10-15 mg) to dissolve slowly in mouth; may repeat every 2 hours as needed

Hemorrhoids: Children ≥12 years and Adults: Rectal 5% to 20%: Apply externally to affected area up to 6 times daily

Otitis: Otic 20%: Adults: Instill 4-5 drops into external auditory canal; may repeat in 1-2 hours if needed

Pediatrics: Note: These are general dosing guidelines; Refer to specific product labeling for dosing instructions.

Teething pain: Children ≥4 months: Topical (oral): 7.5% to 10%: Apply to affected gum area up to 4 times daily

Children ≥2 years: Refer to adult dosing.

Available Dosage Forms

Aerosol, oral spray (Hurricaine®): 20% (60 mL) [dye free; cherry flavor]

Aerosol, topical spray:

- Americaine®: 20% (60 mL)
- Dermoplast® Antibacterial: 20% (83 mL) [contains aloe vera, benzethonium chloride, menthol]
- Dermoplast® Pain Relieving: 20% (60 mL, 83 mL) [contains menthol]
- Foille®: 5% (92 g) [contains chloroxylenol 0.63% and corn oil]
- Ivy-Rid®: 2% (83 mL)
- Lanacane® Maximum Strength: 20% (120 mL) [contains alcohol]
- Solarcaine®: 20% (120 mL) [contains triclosan 0.13%, alcohol 35%]

Combination package (Orajel® Baby Daytime and Nighttime):

- Gel, oral [Daytime Regular Formula]: 7.5% (5.3 g)
- Gel, oral [Nighttime Formula]: 10% (5.3 g)

Cream, oral:

- Benzodent®: 20% (7.5 g, 30 g)
- Orajel PM®: 20% (5.3 g, 7 g)

Cream, topical:

- Lanacane®: 6% (30 g, 60 g)
- Lanacane® Maximum Strength: 20% (30 g)

Gel, oral:

- Anbesol®: 10% (7.5 g) [contains benzyl alcohol; cool mint flavor]
- Anbesol® Baby: 7.5% (7.5 g) [contains benzoic acid; grape flavor]
- Anbesol® Jr.: 10% (7 g) [contains benzyl alcohol; bubble gum flavor]
- Anbesol® Maximum Strength: 20% (7.5 g, 10 g) [contains benzyl alcohol]
- Dentapaine: 20% (11 g) [contains clove oil]
- HDA® Toothache: 6.5% (15 mL) [contains benzyl alcohol]
- Hurricaine®: 20% (5 g) [dye free; wild cherry flavor]; (30 g) [dye free; mint, pina colada, watermelon, and wild cherry flavors]
- Kanka® Soft Brush™: 20% (2 mL) [packaged in applicator with brush tip]
- Orabase® with Benzocaine®: 20% (7 g) [contains ethyl alcohol 48%; mild mint flavor]
- Orajel®: 10% (5.3 g, 7 g, 9.4 g)
- Orajel® Baby Teething: 7.5% (9.4 g, 11.9 g) [cherry flavor]
- Orajel® Baby Teething Nighttime: 10% (5.3 g)
- Orajel® Denture Plus: 15% (9 g) [contains menthol 2%, ethyl alcohol 66.7%]
- Orajel® Maximum Strength: 20% (5.3 g, 7 g, 9.4 g, 11.9 g)
- Orajel® Mouth Sore: 20% (5.3 g, 9.4 g, 11.9 g) [contains benzalkonium chloride 0.02%, zinc chloride 0.1%]
- Orajel® Multi-Action Cold Sore: 20% (9.4 g) [contains allantoin 0.5%, camphor 3%, dimethicone 2%]

(Continued)

Benzocaine *(Continued)*

Orajel® Ultra Mouth Sore: 15% (9.4 g) [contains ethyl alcohol 66.7%, menthol 2%]
Zilactin®-B: 10% (7.5 g)
Gel, topical (Detane®): 7.5% (15 g)
Liquid, oral:
Anbesol®: 10% (9 mL) [cool mint flavor]
Anbesol® Maximum Strength: 20% (9 mL) [contains benzyl alcohol]
Hurricaine®: 20% (30 mL) [pina colada and wild cherry flavors]
Orajel® Baby Teething: 7.5% (13 mL) [very berry flavor]
Orajel® Maximum Strength: 20% (13 mL) [contains ethyl alcohol 44%, tartrazine]
Liquid, oral drop:
Dent's Maxi-Strength Toothache: 20% (3.7 mL) [contains alcohol 74%]
Rid-A-Pain Dental Drops: 6.3% (30 mL) [contains alcohol 70%]
Liquid, topical:
Chiggertox®: 2% (30 mL)
Outgro®: 20% (9 mL)
Skeeter Stik: 5% (14 mL) [contains menthol]
Tanac®: 10% (13 mL) [contains benzalkonium chloride]
Lozenge: 6 mg (18s) [contains menthol]; 15 mg (10s)
Cepacol® Sore Throat: 10 mg (18s) [contains cetylpyridinium, menthol; cherry, citrus, honey lemon, and menthol flavors]
Cepacol® Sore Throat: 10 mg (16s) [sugar free; contains cetylpyridinium, menthol; cherry and menthol flavors]
Cylex®: 15 mg [sugar free; contains cetylpyridinium chloride 5 mg; cherry flavor]
Mycinettes®: 15 mg (12s) [sugar free; contains sodium 9 mg; cherry or regular flavor]
Thorets: 18 mg (500s) [sugar free]
Trocaine®: 10 mg (40s, 400s)
Ointment, oral:
Anbesol® Cold Sore Therapy: 20% (7.1 g) [contains benzyl alcohol, allantoin, aloe, camphor, menthol, vitamin E]
Red Cross™ Canker Sore: 20% (7.5 g) [contains coconut oil]
Ointment, rectal (Americaine® Hemorrhoidal): 20% (30 g)
Ointment, topical:
Chiggerex®: 2% (50 g) [contains aloe vera]
Foille®: 5% (3.5 g, 14 g, 28 g) [contains chloroxylenol 0.1%, benzyl alcohol; corn oil base]
Pads, topical (Sting-Kill): 20% (8s) [contains menthol and tartrazine]
Paste, oral (Orabase® with Benzocaine): 20% (6 g)
Solution, otic drops (Oticaine, Otocaine™): 20% (15 mL)
Swabs, oral:
Hurricaine®: 20% (6s, 100s) [dye free; wild cherry flavor]
Orajel® Baby Teething: 7.5% (12s) [berry flavor]
Orajel® Medicated Mouth Sore, Orajel® Medicated Toothache: 20% (8s, 12s) [contains tartrazine]
Zilactin® Toothache and Gum Pain: 20% (8s) [grape flavor]
Swabs, topical (Sting-Kill): 20% (5s) [contains menthol and tartrazine]
Wax, oral (Dent's Extra Strength Toothache Gum): 20% (1 g)

Nursing Guidelines

Assessment: Monitor for effectiveness of application and adverse reactions. **Oral:** Use caution to prevent gagging or choking and avoid food or drink for 1 hour. Teach patient adverse reactions to report; use and teach appropriate interventions to promote safety.

Patient Education: Use as directed; do not overuse. Do not apply when infections are present and do not apply to large areas of broken skin. Do not eat or drink for 1 hour following oral application. Discontinue application and report if swelling of mouth, lips, tongue, or throat occurs; or if skin irritation occurs at application site. **Pregnancy/breast-feeding precautions:** Inform prescriber if you are pregnant. Consult prescriber if breast-feeding.

Pregnancy Risk Factor: C
Lactation: Excretion in breast milk unknown/use caution

Benzocaine, Butyl Aminobenzoate, Tetracaine, and Benzalkonium Chloride

(BEN zoe kane, BYOO til a meen oh BENZ oh ate, TET ra kane, & benz al KOE nee um KLOR ide)

U.S. Brand Names Cetacaine®

Synonyms Tetracaine Hydrochloride, Benzocaine Butyl Aminobenzoate, and Benzalkonium Chloride

Pharmacologic Category Local Anesthetic

Use Topical anesthetic to control pain or gagging

Adverse Reactions Dose related and may result from high plasma levels

1% to 10%:

Dermatologic: Contact dermatitis, angioedema

Local: Burning, stinging

<1% (Limited to important or life-threatening): Edema, methemoglobinemia (risk may be increased in infants), tenderness, urethritis, urticaria,

Dosing

Adults & Elderly: Local anesthetic: Topical: Apply to affected area for approximately 1 second

Available Dosage Forms

Aerosol, topical: Benzocaine 14%, butyl aminobenzoate 2%, tetracaine hydrochloride 2%, and benzalkonium chloride 0.5% (56 g) [also packaged in a kit with various sized cannulas]

Gel, topical: Benzocaine 14%, butyl aminobenzoate 2%, tetracaine hydrochloride 2%, and benzalkonium chloride 0.5% (29 g)

Liquid, topical: Benzocaine 14%, butyl aminobenzoate 2%, tetracaine hydrochloride 2%, and benzalkonium chloride 0.5% (56 mL)

Nursing Guidelines

Assessment: Instruct patient on appropriate precautions.

Patient Education: This spray may help control pain or gagging. If mouth or throat is numb, use caution with food and fluids. Your sensation to heat may be disturbed, your ability to swallow may be disturbed; use caution when swallowing to prevent choking. **Pregnancy precaution:** Inform prescriber if you are or intend to become pregnant.

Pregnancy Risk Factor: C
Lactation: For topical use

♦ Benzodent® [OTC] *see* Benzocaine *on page 232*

Benzoin (BEN zoin)

U.S. Brand Names TinBen® [OTC] [DSC]

Synonyms Gum Benjamin

Pharmacologic Category Antibiotic, Topical; Topical Skin Product

Use Protective application for irritations of the skin; sometimes used in boiling water as steam inhalants for their expectorant and their soothing action

Dosing

Adults & Elderly: Skin protectant: Topical: Apply 1-2 times/day

Pediatrics: Refer to adult dosing.

Available Dosage Forms [DSC] = Discontinued product

Tincture, USP: (15 mL, 60 mL, 120 mL, 480 mL, 4000 mL)

TinBen®: 120 mL [DSC]

Tincture, USP [spray]: 120 mL

Nursing Guidelines

Patient Education: For external use only

Benzonatate (ben ZOE na tate)

U.S. Brand Names Tessalon®

Pharmacologic Category Antitussive

Use Symptomatic relief of nonproductive cough

Mechanism of Action Tetracaine congener with antitussive properties; suppresses cough by topical anesthetic action on the respiratory stretch receptors

Pharmacodynamics/Kinetics

Onset of action: Therapeutic: 15-20 minutes

Duration: 3-8 hours

(Continued)

Benzonatate *(Continued)*

Contraindications Hypersensitivity to benzonatate, related compounds (such as tetracaine), or any component of the formulation

Drug Interactions No data reported

Adverse Reactions 1% to 10%:

Central nervous system: Sedation, headache, dizziness, mental confusion, visual hallucinations, vague "chilly" sensation

Dermatologic: Rash

Gastrointestinal: Constipation, nausea, vomiting, GI upset

Neuromuscular & skeletal: Numbness in chest

Ocular: Burning sensation in eyes

Respiratory: Nasal congestion

Overdosage/Toxicology Symptoms of overdose include restlessness, tremor, and CNS stimulation. Benzonatate's local anesthetic activity can reduce the patient's gag reflex and, therefore, may contradict the use of ipecac following ingestion. Treatment is supportive and symptomatic.

Dosing

Adults & Elderly: Cough: Oral: 100 mg 3 times/day or every 4 hours up to 600 mg/day

Pediatrics: Children >10 years: Refer to adult dosing.

Available Dosage Forms

Capsule: 100 mg

Tessalon®: 100 mg, 200 mg

Nursing Guidelines

Assessment: Monitor effectiveness of and adverse reactions (see Adverse Reactions) at beginning of therapy and periodically with long-term use. Assess knowledge/teach patient appropriate use, interventions to reduce side effects, and adverse symptoms to report (see Patient Education). Note breast-feeding caution.

Patient Education: Take only as prescribed; do not exceed prescribed dose or frequency. Do not break or chew capsule. Maintain adequate hydration (2-3 L/day of fluids) unless instructed to restrict fluid intake. Avoid use of other depressants, or sleep-inducing medications unless approved by prescriber. You may experience drowsiness, impaired coordination, blurred vision, or increased anxiety (use caution when driving or engaging in tasks requiring alertness until response to drug is known); or upset stomach or nausea (small, frequent meals, frequent mouth care, chewing gum, or sucking hard candy may help). Report persistent CNS changes (dizziness, sedation, tremor, or agitation); numbness in chest or feeling of chill; visual changes or burning in eyes; numbness of mouth or difficulty swallowing; or lack of improvement or worsening or condition. **Pregnancy/breast-feeding precautions:** Inform prescriber if you are or intend to become pregnant. Consult prescriber if breast-feeding.

Geriatric Considerations: No specific geriatric information is available about benzonatate. Avoid use in patients with impaired gag reflex or who cannot swallow the capsule whole.

Pregnancy Risk Factor: C

Lactation: Excretion in breast milk unknown

Administration

Oral: Swallow capsule whole (do not break or chew).

- **Benzylpenicillin Benzathine** *see* Penicillin G Benzathine *on page 1330*
- **Benzylpenicillin Potassium** *see* Penicillin G (Parenteral/Aqueous) *on page 1331*
- **Benzylpenicillin Sodium** *see* Penicillin G (Parenteral/Aqueous) *on page 1331*
- **9-Beta-D-ribofuranosyladenine** *see* Adenosine *on page 91*
- **Betadine® [OTC]** *see* Povidone-Iodine *on page 1392*
- **Betadine® First Aid Antibiotics + Moisturizer [OTC]** *see* Bacitracin and Polymyxin B *on page 219*
- **Betadine® Ophthalmic** *see* Povidone-Iodine *on page 1392*
- **Beta-HC®** *see* Hydrocortisone *on page 873*

Betaine Anhydrous (BAY ta een an HY drus)

U.S. Brand Names Cystadane®

Pharmacologic Category Homocystinuria, Treatment Agent

Medication Safety Issues

Sound-alike/look-alike issues:

Betaine may be confused with Betadine®

Use Orphan drug: Treatment of homocystinuria to decrease elevated homocysteine blood levels; included within the category of homocystinuria are deficiencies or defects in cystathionine beta-synthase (CBS), 5,10-methylenetetrahydrofolate reductase (MTHFR), and cobalamin cofactor metabolism (CBL).

Contraindications Hypersensitivity to betaine or any component of the formulation

Adverse Reactions Minimal; have included nausea, GI distress, and diarrhea

Dosing

Adults & Elderly: Treatment of homocystinuria: Oral: 6 g/day administered in divided doses of 3 g twice daily. Dosages of up to 20 g/day have been necessary to control homocysteine levels in some patients.

Dosage in all patients can be gradually increased until plasma homocysteine is undetectable or present only in small amounts

Pediatrics:

Treatment of homocystinuria: Oral:

Children <3 years: Dosage may be started at 100 mg/kg/day and then increased weekly by 100 mg/kg increments

Children ≥3 years: Refer to adult dosing.

Note: Dosage in all patients can be gradually increased until plasma homocysteine is undetectable or present only in small amounts.

Available Dosage Forms Powder for oral solution: 1 g/scoop (180 g) [1 scoop = 1.7 mL]

Nursing Guidelines

Patient Education: One level scoop is equivalent to 1 g of betaine anhydrous powder; use only the scoop provided; shake bottle lightly before opening, close cap tightly after use to protect from moisture; do not use if powder does not completely dissolve or gives a colored solution

Pregnancy Risk Factor: C

Betamethasone (bay ta METH a sone)

U.S. Brand Names Beta-Val®; Celestone®; Celestone® Soluspan®; Diprolene®; Diprolene® AF; Luxiq®; Maxivate®

Synonyms Betamethasone Dipropionate; Betamethasone Dipropionate, Augmented; Betamethasone Sodium Phosphate; Betamethasone Valerate; Flubenisolone

Pharmacologic Category Corticosteroid, Systemic; Corticosteroid, Topical

Medication Safety Issues

Sound-alike/look-alike issues:

Luxiq® may be confused with Lasix®

Use Inflammatory dermatoses such as seborrheic or atopic dermatitis, neurodermatitis, anogenital pruritus, psoriasis, inflammatory phase of xerosis

Mechanism of Action Controls the rate of protein synthesis, depresses the migration of polymorphonuclear leukocytes, fibroblasts, reverses capillary permeability, and lysosomal stabilization at the cellular level to prevent or control inflammation

Pharmacodynamics/Kinetics

Protein binding: 64%

Metabolism: Hepatic

Half-life elimination: 6.5 hours

Time to peak, serum: I.V.: 10-36 minutes

Excretion: Urine (<5% as unchanged drug)

Contraindications Hypersensitivity to betamethasone, other corticosteroids, or any component of the formulation; systemic fungal infections

Warnings/Precautions Topical use in patients ≤12 years of age is not recommended. May cause suppression of hypothalamic-pituitary-adrenal (HPA) axis, particularly in younger children or in patients receiving high doses for prolonged periods.

Very high potency topical products are not for treatment of rosacea, perioral dermatitis; not for use on face, groin, or axillae; not for use in a diapered area. Avoid concurrent use of other corticosteroids.

(Continued)

Betamethasone *(Continued)*

May suppress the immune system; patients may be more susceptible to infection. Use with caution in patients with systemic infections or ocular herpes simplex. Avoid exposure to chickenpox and measles.

Use with caution in patients with hypothyroidism, cirrhosis, ulcerative colitis; do not use occlusive dressings on weeping or exudative lesions and general caution with occlusive dressings should be observed; adverse effects may be increased. Discontinue if skin irritation or contact dermatitis should occur; do not use in patients with decreased skin circulation.

Drug Interactions **Inhibits** CYP3A4 (weak)

Phenytoin, phenobarbital, rifampin increase clearance of betamethasone.

Potassium-depleting diuretics increase potassium loss.

Skin test antigens, immunizations: Betamethasone may decrease response and increase potential infections.

Insulin or oral hypoglycemics: Betamethasone may increase blood glucose.

Nutritional/Herbal/Ethanol Interactions

Ethanol: Avoid ethanol (may enhance gastric mucosal irritation).

Food: Betamethasone interferes with calcium absorption.

Herb/Nutraceutical: Avoid cat's claw, echinacea (have immunostimulant properties).

Adverse Reactions

Systemic:

Cardiovascular: Congestive heart failure, edema, hyper-/hypotension

Central nervous system: Dizziness, headache, insomnia, intracranial pressure increased, lightheadedness, nervousness, pseudotumor cerebri, seizure, vertigo

Dermatologic: Ecchymoses, facial erythema, fragile skin, hirsutism, hyper-/hypopigmentation, impaired wound healing, perioral dermatitis (oral), petechiae, striae

Endocrine & metabolic: Amenorrhea, Cushing's syndrome, diabetes mellitus, growth suppression, hyperglycemia, hypokalemia, menstrual irregularities, pituitary-adrenal axis suppression, protein catabolism, sodium retention, water retention

Gastrointestinal: Abdominal distention, appetite increased, hiccups, indigestion, peptic ulcer, pancreatitis, ulcerative esophagitis

Local: Injection site reactions (intra-articular use), sterile abscess, Misc: Anaphylactoid reaction, diaphoresis, hypersensitivity, secondary infection

Neuromuscular & skeletal: Arthralgia, muscle atrophy, fractures, muscle weakness, myopathy, osteoporosis, necrosis (femoral and humeral heads)

Ocular: Cataracts, glaucoma, intraocular pressure increased

Topical:

Dermatologic: Acneiform eruptions, allergic dermatitis, burning, dry skin, erythema, folliculitis, hypertrichosis, irritation, miliaria, pruritus, skin atrophy, striae, vesiculation

Endocrine and metabolic effects have occasionally been reported with topical use.

Overdosage/Toxicology When consumed in high doses for prolonged periods, systemic hypercorticism and adrenal suppression may occur. In those cases, discontinuation of the corticosteroid should be done judiciously.

Dosing

Adults: Base dosage on severity of disease and patient response

Inflammatory conditions:

Oral: 2.4-4.8 mg/day in 2-4 doses; range: 0.6-7.2 mg/day

I.M.: Betamethasone sodium phosphate and betamethasone acetate: 0.6-9 mg/day (generally, $^1/_3$ to $^1/_2$ of oral dose) divided every 12-24 hours

Psoriasis (scalp): Topical (foam): Apply to the scalp twice daily, once in the morning and once at night.

Rheumatoid arthritis/osteoarthritis:

Intrabursal, intra-articular, intradermal: 0.25-2 mL

Intralesional:

Very large joints: 1-2 mL

Large joints: 1 mL

Medium joints: 0.5-1 mL

Small joints: 0.25-0.5 mL

Steroid-responsive dermatoses: Therapy should be discontinued when control is achieved; if no improvement is seen, reassessment of diagnosis may be necessary.

Gel, augmented formulation: Apply once or twice daily; rub in gently. **Note:** Do not exceed 2 weeks of treatment or 50 g/week.

Lotion: Apply a few drops twice daily

Augmented formulation: Apply a few drops once or twice daily; runb in gently. **Note:** Do not exceed 2 weeks of treatment or 50 mL/week.

Cream/ointment: Apply once or twice daily

Augmented formulation: Apply once or twice daily. **Note:** Do not exceed 2 weeks of treatment or 45 g/week.

Elderly: Refer to adult dosing. Use the lowest effective dose.

Pediatrics: Base dosage on severity of disease and patient response.

Inflammatory conditions: Note: Use lowest dose listed as initial dose for adrenocortical insufficiency (physiologic replacement).

I.M.: 0.0175-0.125 mg base/kg/day divided every 6-12 hours **or** 0.5-7.5 mg base/m^2/day divided every 6-12 hours

Oral: 0.0175-0.25 mg/kg/day divided every 6-8 hours **or** 0.5-7.5 mg/m^2/day divided every 6-8 hours

Topical: Children ≥13 years (use in children ≤12 years is not recommended): Use minimal amount for shortest period of time to avoid HPA axis suppression

Gel, augmented formulation: Apply once or twice daily; rub in gently. **Note:** Do not exceed 2 weeks of treatment or 50 g/week.

Lotion: Apply a few drops twice daily

Augmented formulation: Apply a few drops once or twice daily; rub in gently. **Note:** Do not exceed 2 weeks of treatment or 50 mL/week.

Cream/ointment: Apply one or twice daily.

Augmented formulation: Apply once or twice daily. **Note:** Do not exceed 2 weeks of treatment or 45 g/week.

Hepatic Impairment: Adjustments may be necessary in patients with liver failure because betamethasone is extensively metabolized in the liver

Available Dosage Forms [DSC] = Discontinued product

Note: Potency expressed as betamethasone base.

Cream, topical, as dipropionate: 0.05% (15 g, 45 g)

Maxivate®: 0.05% (45 g)

Cream, topical, as dipropionate augmented (Diprolene® AF): 0.05% (15 g, 50 g)

Cream, topical, as valerate (Beta-Val®): 0.1% (15 g, 45 g)

Foam, topical, as valerate (Luxiq®): 0.12% (50 g, 100 g, 150 g) [contains alcohol 60.4%]

Gel, topical, as dipropionate augmented: 0.05% (15 g, 50 g)

Injection, suspension (Celestone® Soluspan®): Betamethasone sodium phosphate 3 mg/mL and betamethasone acetate 3 mg/mL [6 mg/mL] (5 mL)

Lotion, topical, as dipropionate (Maxivate®): 0.05% (60 mL)

Lotion, topical, as dipropionate augmented (Diprolene®): 0.05% (30 mL, 60 mL)

Lotion, topical, as valerate (Beta-Val®): 0.1% (60 mL)

Ointment, topical, as dipropionate: 0.05% (15 g, 45 g)

Maxivate®: 0.05% (45 g)

Ointment, topical, as dipropionate augmented (Diprolene®): 0.05% (15 g, 50 g)

Ointment, topical, as valerate: 0.1% (15 g, 45 g)

Syrup, as base (Celestone®): 0.6 mg/5 mL (118 mL)

Nursing Guidelines

Assessment: Assess potential for interactions with other prescriptions, OTC medications, or herbal products patient may be taking. Assess therapeutic response and adverse effects according to indications for therapy, dose, route (systemic or topical), and duration of therapy. When used for long-term therapy (>10-14 days), do not discontinue abruptly; decrease dosage incrementally. Growth should be routinely monitored in pediatric patients. With systemic administration, caution patients with diabetes to monitor glucose levels closely (corticosteroids may alter glucose levels). Teach patient proper use (according to formulation), side effects/appropriate interventions, and symptoms to report.

Dietary Considerations: May be taken with food to decrease GI distress.

Patient Education: Do not take any new medication during therapy unless approved by prescriber. Take exactly as directed; do not increase dose or discontinue abruptly without consulting prescriber. Take oral medication with or after meals. Avoid alcohol and limit intake of caffeine or stimulants. Prescriber may recommend increased dietary vitamins, minerals, or iron. If you have diabetes, monitor glucose levels closely (antidiabetic medication may need to be adjusted). Inform prescriber if you are experiencing greater-than-normal levels of stress (medication may need adjustment). You may be more susceptible to infection (avoid crowds and exposure to infection and do not have any

(Continued)

Betamethasone *(Continued)*

vaccination without consulting prescriber). Some forms of this medication may cause GI upset (small frequent meals and frequent mouth care may help or oral medication may be taken with meals to reduce GI upset). Report promptly excessive nervousness or sleep disturbances; signs of infection (eg, sore throat, unhealed injuries); excessive growth of body hair or loss of skin color; vision changes; excessive or sudden weight gain (>3 lb/week); swelling of face or extremities; respiratory difficulty; muscle weakness; change in color of stools (tarry) or persistent abdominal pain; or worsening of condition or failure to improve.

Topical: For external use only. Do not use for eyes, mucous membranes, or open wounds. Use exactly as directed. Before using, wash and dry area gently. Apply in a thin layer (may rub in lightly). Apply light dressing (if necessary) to area being treated. Do not use occlusive dressing unless so advised by prescriber. Avoid prolonged or excessive use around sensitive tissues, genital, or rectal areas. Avoid exposing treated area to direct sunlight. Inform prescriber if condition worsens (redness, swelling, irritation, signs of infection, or open sores) or fails to improve.

Pregnancy/breast-feeding precautions: Inform prescriber if you are or intend to become pregnant. Consult prescriber if breast-feeding.

Geriatric Considerations: Because of the risk of adverse effects, systemic corticosteroids should be used cautiously in the elderly, in the smallest possible dose, and for the shortest possible time.

Pregnancy Risk Factor: C

Pregnancy Issues: There are no reports linking the use of betamethasone with congenital defects in the literature. Betamethasone is often used in patients with premature labor [26-34 weeks gestation] to stimulate fetal lung maturation.

Lactation: Excretion in breast milk unknown/use caution

Breast-Feeding Considerations: Systemic corticosteroids are excreted in human milk. The extent of topical absorption is variable. Use with caution while breast-feeding; do not apply to nipples.

Perioperative/Anesthesia/Other Concerns:

Neuromuscular Effects: ICU-acquired paresis was recently studied in 5 ICUs (3 medical and 2 surgical ICUs) at 4 French hospitals. All ICU patients without pre-existing neuromuscular disease admitted from March 1999 through June 2000 were evaluated (de Jonghe, 2002). Each patient had to be mechanically ventilated for ≥7 days and was screened daily for awakening. The first day the patient was considered awake was Study Day 1. Patients with severe muscle weakness on Study Day 7 were considered to have ICU-acquired paresis. Among the 95 patients who were evaluable, about 25% developed ICU-acquired paresis. Independent predictors included: female gender, the number of days with ≥2 organ dysfunction, and administration of corticosteroids. Further studies may be required to verify and characterize the association between the development of ICU-acquired paresis and use of corticosteroids. Concurrent use of a corticosteroid and muscle relaxant appear to increase the risk of certain ICU myopathies; avoid or administer the corticosteroid at the lowest dose possible.

Adrenal Insufficiency: Patients will often have steroid-induced adverse effects on glucose tolerance and lipid profiles. When discontinuing steroid therapy in patients on long-term steroid supplementation, it is important that the steroid therapy be discontinued gradually. Abrupt withdrawal may result in adrenal insufficiency with hypotension and hyperkalemia. Patients on long-term steroid supplementation will require higher corticosteroid doses when subject to stress (ie, trauma, surgery, severe infection). Guidelines for glucocorticoid replacement during various surgical procedures has been published (Salem, 1994; Coursin, 2002).

Septic Shock: A recent randomized, double-blind, placebo controlled trial assessed whether low dose corticosteroid administration could improve 28-day survival in patients with septic shock and relative adrenal insufficiency. Relative adrenal insufficiency was defined as an inappropriate response to corticotropin administration (increase of serum cortisol of ≤9 mcg/dL from baseline). Cortisol levels were drawn immediately before corticotropin administration and 30-60 minutes afterwards. Three hundred adult septic shock patients requiring mechanical ventilation and vasopressor support were randomized to either hydrocortisone (50 mg IVP every 6 hours) and fludrocortisone (50 mcg tablet daily via nasogastric tube) or matching placebos for 7 days. In patients who did not appropriately respond to corticotropin (nonresponders), there were significantly fewer deaths in the active treatment group. Vasopressor therapy was withdrawn more frequently in this subset of the active treatment group. Adverse events were similar in both groups. Patients who lack adrenal reserve and thus have relative adrenal insufficiency during the stress of septic shock may benefit from physiologic steroid replacement. However, there was a trend for increased mortality in patients who responded to the corticotropin test (increase serum cortisol >9 mcg/dL from baseline). These patients may not benefit from physiologic steroid replacement. Further study is required to better characterize the patient populations who may benefit.

Administration

Oral: Not for alternate day therapy; once daily doses should be given in the morning.

I.M.: Do **not** give injectable sodium phosphate/acetate suspension I.V.

- Betamethasone Dipropionate *see* Betamethasone *on page 237*
- Betamethasone Dipropionate, Augmented *see* Betamethasone *on page 237*
- Betamethasone Sodium Phosphate *see* Betamethasone *on page 237*
- Betamethasone Valerate *see* Betamethasone *on page 237*
- Betapace® *see* Sotalol *on page 1562*
- Betapace AF® *see* Sotalol *on page 1562*
- Betasept® [OTC] *see* Chlorhexidine Gluconate *on page 373*
- Betaseron® *see* Interferon Beta-1b *on page 950*
- Beta-Val® *see* Betamethasone *on page 237*

Betaxolol (be TAKS oh lol)

U.S. Brand Names Betoptic® S; Kerlone®

Synonyms Betaxolol Hydrochloride

Pharmacologic Category Beta Blocker, $Beta_1$ Selective

Medication Safety Issues

Sound-alike/look-alike issues:

Betaxolol may be confused with bethanechol, labetalol

Use Treatment of chronic open-angle glaucoma and ocular hypertension; management of hypertension

Mechanism of Action Competitively blocks $beta_1$-receptors, with little or no effect on $beta_2$-receptors; ophthalmic reduces intraocular pressure by reducing the production of aqueous humor

Pharmacodynamics/Kinetics

Onset of action: Ophthalmic: 30 minutes; Oral: 1-1.5 hours

Duration: Ophthalmic: ≥12 hours

Absorption: Ophthalmic: Some systemic; Oral: ~100%

Metabolism: Hepatic to multiple metabolites

Protein binding: Oral: 50%

Bioavailability: Oral: 89%

Half-life elimination: Oral: 12-22 hours

Time to peak: Ophthalmic: ~2 hours; Oral: 1.5-6 hours

Excretion: Urine

Contraindications Hypersensitivity to betaxolol or any component of the formulation; sinus bradycardia; heart block greater than first-degree (except in patients with a functioning artificial pacemaker); cardiogenic shock; uncompensated cardiac failure; pulmonary edema; pregnancy (2nd and 3rd trimester)

Warnings/Precautions Administer cautiously in compensated heart failure and monitor for a worsening of the condition. Beta-blocker therapy should not be withdrawn abruptly (particularly in patients with CAD), but gradually tapered to avoid acute tachycardia, hypertension, and/or ischemia. Use caution with concurrent use of beta-blockers and either verapamil or diltiazem; bradycardia or heart block can occur. Use caution in patients with PVD (can aggravate arterial insufficiency). In general, beta-blockers should be avoided in patients with bronchospastic disease. Betaxolol, with B1 selectivity, should be used cautiously in bronchospastic disease with close monitoring. Use cautiously in diabetics because it can mask prominent hypoglycemic symptoms. Can mask signs of thyrotoxicosis. Can cause fetal harm when administered in pregnancy. Dosage adjustment required in severe renal impairment and those on dialysis. Use care with anesthetic agents which decrease myocardial function.

(Continued)

Betaxolol *(Continued)*

Drug Interactions Substrate (major) of CYP1A2, 2D6; **Inhibits** CYP2D6 (weak)

Alpha-blockers (prazosin, terazosin): Concurrent use of beta-blockers may increase risk of orthostasis.

CYP1A2 inducers: May decrease the levels/effects of betaxolol. Example inducers include aminoglutethimide, carbamazepine, phenobarbital, and rifampin.

CYP1A2 inhibitors: May increase the levels/effects of betaxolol. Example inhibitors include amiodarone, ciprofloxacin, fluvoxamine, ketoconazole, norfloxacin, ofloxacin, and rofecoxib.

CYP2D6 inhibitors: May increase the levels/effects of betaxolol. Example inhibitors include chlorpromazine, delavirdine, fluoxetine, miconazole, paroxetine, pergolide, quinidine, quinine, ritonavir, and ropinirole.

Clonidine; Hypertensive crisis after or during withdrawal of either agent.

Drugs which slow AV conduction (digoxin): Effects may be additive with beta-blockers.

Glucagon: Betaxolol may blunt the hyperglycemic action of glucagon.

Insulin and oral hypoglycemics: May mask tachycardia from hypoglycemia.

NSAIDs (ibuprofen, indomethacin, naproxen, piroxicam) may reduce the antihypertensive effects of beta-blockers.

Salicylates may reduce the antihypertensive effects of beta-blockers.

Sulfonylureas: Beta-blockers may alter response to hypoglycemic agents.

Verapamil or diltiazem may have synergistic or additive pharmacological effects when taken concurrently with beta-blockers.

Nutritional/Herbal/Ethanol Interactions Herb/Nutraceutical: Avoid dong quai if using for hypertension (has estrogenic activity). Avoid ephedra, yohimbe, ginseng (may worsen hypertension). Avoid garlic (may have increased antihypertensive effect).

Adverse Reactions

Ophthalmic:

>10%: Ocular: Conjunctival hyperemia

1% to 10%:

Ocular: Anisocoria, corneal punctate keratitis, keratitis, corneal staining, decreased corneal sensitivity, eye pain, vision disturbances

Systemic:

>10%:

Central nervous system: Drowsiness, insomnia

Endocrine & metabolic: Decreased sexual ability

1% to 10%:

Cardiovascular: Bradycardia, palpitation, edema, CHF, reduced peripheral circulation

Central nervous system: Mental depression

Gastrointestinal: Diarrhea or constipation, nausea, vomiting, stomach discomfort

Respiratory: Bronchospasm

Miscellaneous: Cold extremities

<1% (Limited to important or life-threatening): Chest pain, thrombocytopenia

Overdosage/Toxicology Symptoms of significant overdose include bradycardia, hypotension, AV block, CHF, bronchospasm, hypoglycemia. Treat initially with fluids. Sympathomimetics (eg, epinephrine or dopamine), glucagon, or a pacemaker can be used to treat toxic bradycardia, asystole, and/or hypotension.

Dosing

Adults:

Glaucoma: Ophthalmic: Instill 1 drop twice daily.

Hypertension, angina: Oral: 5-10 mg/day; may increase dose to 20 mg/day after 7-14 days if desired response is not achieved

Elderly:

Ophthalmic: Refer to adult dosing.

Hypertension: Oral: Initial: 5 mg/day

Renal Impairment: Oral: Administer 5 mg/day; can increase every 2 weeks up to a maximum of 20 mg/day.

Cl_{cr} <10 mL/minute: Administer 50% of usual dose.

Available Dosage Forms

Solution, ophthalmic, as hydrochloride: 0.5% (5 mL, 10 mL, 15 mL) [contains benzalkonium chloride]

Suspension, ophthalmic, as hydrochloride (Betoptic® S): 0.25% (2.5 mL, 5 mL, 10 mL, 15 mL) [contains benzalkonium chloride]

Tablet, as hydrochloride (Kerlone®): 10 mg, 20 mg

Nursing Guidelines

Assessment: Assess potential for interactions with other prescriptions, OTC medications, or herbal products patient may be taking (especially products that affects cardiac function or blood pressure). Assess therapeutic response and adverse effects. Patients with diabetes should be cautioned that beta-blockers may mask prominent hypoglycemic symptoms. Teach patient proper use (according to formulation), side effects/appropriate interventions, and symptoms to report. Systemic absorption from ophthalmic instillation is minimal. Intraocular pressure should be measured periodically.

Monitoring Laboratory Tests: Ophthalmic: Intraocular pressure

Patient Education: Do not take any new medication during therapy unless approved by prescriber.

Oral: Use as directed and do not discontinue without consulting prescriber. May cause dizziness or blurred vision (use caution when driving or engaging in tasks requiring alertness until response to drug is known); or nausea or vomiting (small frequent meals, frequent mouth care, sucking lozenges, or chewing gum may help). If diabetic, may mask prominent hypoglycemic symptoms. Monitor blood glucose levels closely. Report chest pain, palpitations or irregular heartbeat; persistent GI upset (eg, nausea, vomiting, diarrhea, or constipation); unusual cough; respiratory difficulty; swelling or coolness of extremities; or unusual mental depression. **Pregnancy/breast-feeding precautions:** Inform prescriber if you are or intend to become pregnant. Consult prescriber if breast-feeding.

Ophthalmic: Shake suspension well before using. Tilt head back and instill in eye. Keep eye open; do not blink for 30 seconds. Apply gentle pressure to corner of eye for 1 minute. Wipe away excess from skin. Do not let tip of applicator touch eye; do not contaminate tip of applicator (may cause eye infection, eye damage, or vision loss). Report if condition does not improve or if you experience eye pain, vision changes, or other adverse eye response.

Geriatric Considerations: Oral: Due to alterations in the beta-adrenergic autonomic nervous system, beta-adrenergic blockade may result in less hemodynamic response than seen in younger adults.

Pregnancy Risk Factor: C (manufacturer); D (2nd and 3rd trimesters - expert analysis)

Lactation: Oral: Enters breast milk/use caution

Perioperative/Anesthesia/Other Concerns: Due to alterations in the autonomic nervous system, beta-blockade may result in less hemodynamic response in the elderly. Studies indicate that despite decreased sensitivity to the chronotropic effects of beta-blockade with age, there appears to be an increased myocardial sensitivity to the negative inotropic effect.

Myocardial Infarction: Beta-blockers, in general without intrinsic sympathomimetic activity (ISA), have been shown to decrease morbidity and mortality when initiated in the acute treatment of myocardial infarction and continued long-term. In this setting, therapy should be avoided in patients with hypotension, cardiogenic shock, or heart block.

Surgery: Atenolol has also been shown to improve cardiovascular outcomes when used in the perioperative period in patients with underlying cardiovascular disease who are undergoing noncardiac surgery. Bisoprolol in high-risk patients undergoing vascular surgery reduced the perioperative incidence of death from cardiac causes and nonfatal myocardial infarction.

Atrial Fibrillation: Beta-blocker therapy provides effective rate control in patients with atrial fibrillation.

Withdrawal: Beta-blocker therapy should not be withdrawn abruptly, but gradually tapered to avoid acute tachycardia and hypertension.

Administration

Storage: Avoid freezing.

♦ Betaxolol Hydrochloride *see* Betaxolol *on page 241*

♦ Betimol® *see* Timolol *on page 1633*

♦ Betoptic® S *see* Betaxolol *on page 241*

♦ Bextra® *[Withdrawn from Market]* *see* Valdecoxib *on page 1677*

♦ Biaxin® *see* Clarithromycin *on page 422*

♦ **Biaxin® XL** *see* Clarithromycin *on page 422*
♦ **Bicillin® L-A** *see* Penicillin G Benzathine *on page 1330*
♦ **Bicitra®** *see* Sodium Citrate and Citric Acid *on page 1548*
♦ **BiCNu®** *see* Carmustine *on page 318*

Bimatoprost (bi MAT oh prost)

U.S. Brand Names Lumigan®

Pharmacologic Category Ophthalmic Agent, Antiglaucoma; Prostaglandin, Ophthalmic

Use Reduction of intraocular pressure (IOP) in patients with open-angle glaucoma or ocular hypertension; should be used in patients who are intolerant of other IOP-lowering medications or failed treatment with another IOP-lowering medication

Mechanism of Action As a synthetic analog of prostaglandin with ocular hypotensive activity, bimatoprost decreases intraocular pressure by increasing the outflow of aqueous humor.

Pharmacodynamics/Kinetics

Onset of action: Reduction of IOP: ~4 hours

Peak effect: Maximum reduction of IOP: ~8-12 hours

Distribution: 0.67 L/kg

Protein binding: ~88%

Metabolism: Undergoes oxidation, N-demethylation, and glucuronidation after reaching systemic circulation; forms metabolites

Half-life elimination: I.V.: 45 minutes

Time to peak: 10 minutes

Excretion: Urine (67%); feces (25%)

Contraindications Hypersensitivity to bimatoprost or any component of the formulation

Warnings/Precautions May cause permanent changes in eye color (increases the amount of brown pigment in the iris), the eyelid skin, and eyelashes; long-term consequences and potential injury to eye are not known. In addition, may increase the length and/or number of eyelashes (may vary between eyes). Changes occur slowly and may not be noticeable for months or years. Bacterial keratitis, caused by inadvertent contamination of multiple-dose ophthalmic solutions, has been reported. Use caution in patients with intraocular inflammation, aphakic patients, pseudophakic patients with a torn posterior lens capsule, or patients with risk factors for macular edema. Contains benzalkonium chloride which may be adsorbed by contact lenses; remove contacts prior to administration and wait 15 minutes before reinserting. Safety and efficacy have not been determined in patients with renal impairment, angle closure, inflammatory or neovascular glaucoma. Safety and efficacy in pediatric patients have not been established.

Drug Interactions When using more than one ophthalmic product, wait at least 5 minutes between application of each medication

Latanoprost: Combination therapy may result in higher IOP than either agent alone.

Adverse Reactions

>10%: Ocular (15% to 45%): Conjunctival hyperemia, growth of eyelashes, ocular pruritus

1% to 10%:

Central nervous system: Headache (1% to 5%)

Dermatologic: Hirsutism (1% to 5%)

Hepatic: Abnormal liver function tests (1% to 5%)

Neuromuscular & skeletal: Weakness (1% to 5%)

Ocular:

3% to 10%: Blepharitis, burning, cataract, dryness, eyelid redness, eyelash darkening, foreign body sensation, irritation, pain, pigmentation of periocular skin, superficial punctate keratitis, visual disturbance

1% to 3%: Allergic conjunctivitis, asthenopia, conjunctival edema, discharge, increased iris pigmentation, photophobia, tearing

Respiratory: Upper respiratory tract infection (10%)

<1% (Limited to important or life-threatening): Bacterial keratitis (caused by inadvertent contamination of multiple-dose ophthalmic solutions), iritis, macular edema

Overdosage/Toxicology No information available; treatment is symptom-directed and supportive

Dosing

Adults & Elderly: Open-angle glaucoma or ocular hypertension: Ophthalmic: Instill 1 drop into affected eye(s) once daily in the evening; do not exceed once-daily dosing (may decrease IOP-lowering effect). If used with other topical ophthalmic agents, separate administration by at least 5 minutes.

Available Dosage Forms Solution, ophthalmic: 0.03% (2.5 mL, 5 mL, 7.5 mL) [contains benzalkonium chloride]

Nursing Guidelines

Assessment: Assess potential for interactions with other prescriptions, OTC medications, or herbal products patient may be taking. Assess therapeutic response and adverse effects. Teach patient proper use, side effects/appropriate interventions, and symptoms to report.

Patient Education: For use in eyes only. Wash hands before instilling. Sit or lie down to instill. Open eye, look at ceiling, and instill prescribed amount of solution. Apply gentle pressure to inner corner of eye. Do not let tip of applicator touch eye; do not contaminate tip of applicator (may cause eye infection, eye damage, or vision loss). Contact prescriber concerning continued use of drops if eye infection develops, trauma occurs to the eye, and prior to eye surgery. This product contains benzalkonium chloride which may be adsorbed by contact lenses; remove contacts prior to administration and wait 15 minutes before reinserting. May cause permanent changes in eye color (increases the amount of brown pigment in the iris), eyelid, and eyelashes. May also increase the length and/or number of eyelashes. Changes may occur slowly (months to years). May be used with other eye drops to lower intraocular pressure. If using more than one eye drop medicine, wait at least 5 minutes in between application of each medication. Notify prescriber if conjunctivitis or eyelid reactions occur with use of this product. **Pregnancy/breast-feeding precautions:** Inform prescriber if you are pregnant or breast-feeding.

Pregnancy Risk Factor: C

Lactation: Excretion in breast milk unknown/use caution

Administration

Storage: Store between 2°C to 25°C (36°F to 77°F).

- ♦ Biocef® *see* Cephalexin *on page 364*
- ♦ Biofed [OTC] *see* Pseudoephedrine *on page 1436*
- ♦ Biolon™ *see* Hyaluronate and Derivatives *on page 856*
- ♦ Bion® Tears [OTC] *see* Artificial Tears *on page 187*
- ♦ Bio-Statin® *see* Nystatin *on page 1249*
- ♦ Bisac-Evac™ [OTC] *see* Bisacodyl *on page 245*

Bisacodyl (bis a KOE dil)

U.S. Brand Names Alophen® [OTC]; Bisac-Evac™ [OTC]; Bisacodyl Uniserts® [OTC]; Correctol® Tablets [OTC]; Doxidan® *(reformulation)* [OTC]; Dulcolax® [OTC]; Femilax™ [OTC]; Fleet® Bisacodyl Enema [OTC]; Fleet® Stimulant Laxative [OTC]; Gentlax® [OTC] [DSC]; Modane Tablets® [OTC]; Veracolate [OTC]

Pharmacologic Category Laxative, Stimulant

Medication Safety Issues

Sound-alike/look-alike issues:

Doxidan® may be confused with doxepin

Modane® may be confused with Matulane®, Moban®

Use Treatment of constipation; colonic evacuation prior to procedures or examination

Mechanism of Action Stimulates peristalsis by directly irritating the smooth muscle of the intestine, possibly the colonic intramural plexus; alters water and electrolyte secretion producing net intestinal fluid accumulation and laxation

Pharmacodynamics/Kinetics

Onset of action: Oral: 6-10 hours; Rectal: 0.25-1 hour

Absorption: Oral, rectal: Systemic, <5%

Contraindications Hypersensitivity to bisacodyl or any component of the formulation; abdominal pain, obstruction, nausea or vomiting

Drug Interactions Decreased effect: Milk, antacids; decreased effect of warfarin

Nutritional/Herbal/Ethanol Interactions Food: Milk or dairy products may disrupt enteric coating, increasing stomach irritation.

Adverse Reactions <1% (Limited to important or life-threatening): Electrolyte and fluid imbalance (metabolic acidosis or alkalosis, hypocalcemia); mild abdominal cramps, nausea, rectal burning vertigo, vomiting

(Continued)

Bisacodyl *(Continued)*

Dosing

Adults & Elderly:

Relief of constipation:

Oral: 5-15 mg as single dose (up to 30 mg when complete evacuation of bowel is required)

Rectal: Suppository: 10 mg as single dose

Pediatrics:

Relief of constipation:

Oral: Children >6 years: 5-10 mg (0.3 mg/kg) at bedtime or before breakfast

Rectal (suppository): Children:

<2 years: 5 mg as a single dose

>2 years: 10 mg

Available Dosage Forms

Enema (Fleet® Bisacodyl Enema): 10 mg/30 mL (37 mL)

Suppository, rectal (Bisac-Evac™, Bisacodyl Uniserts®; Dulcolax®): 10 mg

Tablet, enteric coated (Alophen®; Bisac-Evac™, Correctol®, Dulcolax®, Femilax™, Fleet® Stimulant Laxative, Gentlax® [DSC], Modane®, Veracolate): 5 mg

Tablet, delayed release (Doxidan®): 5 mg

Nursing Guidelines

Dietary Considerations: Should not be administered within 1 hour of milk, any dairy products, or taking an antacid, to protect the coating; should be administered with glass of water on empty stomach for rapid effect.

Patient Education: Onset of action occurs 6-10 hours after oral dose or 15-60 minutes after a rectal dose; swallow tablets whole, do **not** crush or chew; do not take antacid or milk within 1 hour of taking drug

Pregnancy Risk Factor: C

Administration

Oral: Administered with glass of water on empty stomach for rapid effect. Do not administer within 1 hour of milk, any dairy products, or taking an antacid, to protect the coating.

- Bisacodyl Uniserts® [OTC] *see* Bisacodyl *on page 245*
- bis-chloronitrosourea *see* Carmustine *on page 318*
- Bistropamide *see* Tropicamide *on page 1672*

Bivalirudin (bye VAL i roo din)

U.S. Brand Names Angiomax®

Synonyms Hirulog

Pharmacologic Category Anticoagulant, Thrombin Inhibitor

Use Anticoagulant used in conjunction with aspirin for patients with unstable angina undergoing percutaneous transluminal coronary angioplasty (PTCA) or percutaneous coronary intervention (PCI) with provisional glycoprotein IIb/IIIa inhibitor; anticoagulant used in patients undergoing PCI with (or at risk of) heparin-induced thrombocytopenia (HIT) / thrombosis syndrome (HITTS)

Mechanism of Action Bivalirudin acts as a specific and reversible direct thrombin inhibitor; it binds to the catalytic and anionic exosite of both circulating and clot-bound thrombin. Catalytic binding site occupation functionally inhibits coagulant effects by preventing thrombin-mediated cleavage of fibrinogen to fibrin monomers, and activation of factors V, VIII and XIII. Shows linear dose- and concentration-dependent prolongation of ACT, aPTT, PT and TT.

Pharmacodynamics/Kinetics

Onset of action: Immediate

Duration: Coagulation times return to baseline ~1 hour following discontinuation of infusion

Distribution: 0.2 L/kg

Protein binding, plasma: Does not bind other than thrombin

Half-life elimination: Normal renal function: 25 minutes; Cl_{cr} 10-29 mL/minute: 57 minutes

Excretion: Urine, proteolytic cleavage

Contraindications Hypersensitivity to bivalirudin or any component of the formulation; active major bleeding

Warnings/Precautions Not for intramuscular use. Safety and efficacy have not been established in patients with unstable angina or acute coronary syndromes who are not undergoing PTCA or PCI. Increased risk of thrombus formation (some fatal) has been reported with bivalirudin use in gamma brachytherapy. As with all anticoagulants, bleeding may occur at any site and should be considered following an unexplained fall in blood pressure or hematocrit, or any unexplained symptom. Use with caution in patients with disease states associated with increased risk of bleeding. Safety and efficacy in pediatric patients have not been established.

Drug Interactions

Aspirin: May increase anticoagulant effect; all clinical trials included coadministration of aspirin

Other anticoagulants: May increase the risk of bleeding complications; monitor.

Treprostinil: May enhance the adverse/toxic effect of anticoagulants. Bleeding may occur.

Adverse Reactions As with all anticoagulants, bleeding is the major adverse effect of bivalirudin. Hemorrhage may occur at virtually any site. Risk is dependent on multiple variables, including the intensity of anticoagulation and patient susceptibility. Additional adverse effects are often related to idiosyncratic reactions, and the frequency is difficult to estimate.

Adverse reactions reported were generally less than those seen with heparin.

>10%:

- Cardiovascular: Hypotension (3% to 12%)
- Central nervous system: Pain (15%), headache (3% to 12%)
- Gastrointestinal: Nausea (3% to 15%)
- Neuromuscular & skeletal: Back pain (9% to 42%)

1% to 10%:

- Cardiovascular: Hypertension (6%), bradycardia (5%), angina (up to 5%)
- Central nervous system: Insomnia (7%), anxiety (6%), fever (5%), nervousness (5%)
- Gastrointestinal: Vomiting (6%), dyspepsia (5%), abdominal pain (5%)
- Genitourinary: Urinary retention (4%)
- Hematologic: Major hemorrhage (2% to 4%, compared to 4% to 9% with heparin); transfusion required (1% to 2%, compared to 2% to 6% with heparin), thrombocytopenia (<1% to 4%)
- Local: Injection site pain (3% to 8%)
- Neuromuscular & skeletal: Pelvic pain (6%)

<1% (Limited to important or life-threatening): Allergic reaction (including anaphylaxis), cerebral ischemia, confusion, facial paralysis, fatal bleeding, intracranial bleeding, kidney failure, pulmonary edema, retroperitoneal bleeding, syncope, thrombus formation (during PCI, including intracoronary brachytherapy), ventricular fibrillation

Overdosage/Toxicology Single bolus doses of up to 7.5 mg/kg have been reported without bleeding complications or other adverse events. Discontinue bivalirudin and monitor patients for signs of bleeding. Bivalirudin is hemodialyzable (~25% removed).

Dosing

Adults: Anticoagulant in patients undergoing PTCA/PCI or PCI with HITS/HITTS (treatment should be started just prior to procedure): Initial: Bolus: 0.75 mg/kg, followed by continuous infusion: 1.75 mg/kg/hour for the duration of procedure and up to 4 hours post-procedure if needed; determine ACT 5 minutes after bolus dose; may administer additional bolus of 0.3 mg/kg if necessary.

A glycoprotein IIb/IIIa inhibitor may be administered concomitantly during the procedure.

If needed, infusion may be continued beyond initial 4 hours at 0.2 mg/kg/hour for up to 20 hours.

Elderly: No dosage adjustment is needed in elderly patients with normal renal function. Puncture site hemorrhage and catheterization site hemorrhage were seen in more patients ≥65 years of age than in patients <65 years of age.

Renal Impairment: Infusion dose should be reduced based on degree of renal impairment. Initial bolus dose remains unchanged. Monitor activated coagulation time (ACT).

Cl_{cr} ≥30 mL/minute: No adjustment required

Cl_{cr} 10-29 mL/minute: Decrease infusion rate to 1 mg/kg/hour

Dialysis-dependent patients (off dialysis): Decrease infusion rate to 0.25 mg/kg/hour

Clearance of bivalirudin remains 1.8-fold greater than the glomerular filtration rate, regardless of the degree in renal impairment.

Hepatic Impairment: No adjustment necessary.

Available Dosage Forms Injection, powder for reconstitution: 250 mg

(Continued)

Bivalirudin *(Continued)*

Nursing Guidelines

Patient Education: This drug can only be administered by injection. You may have a tendency to bleed easily while taking this drug; brush teeth with soft brush, floss with waxed floss, use electric razor, avoid scissors or sharp knives, and potentially harmful activities. Report chest pain; unusual bleeding or bruising (bleeding gums, nosebleed, blood in urine, dark stool); pain in joints or back; or numbness, tingling, swelling, or pain at injection site. Inform prescriber if you are pregnant. Consult prescriber if breast-feeding.

Pregnancy Risk Factor: B

Pregnancy Issues: Although animal studies have not shown harm to the fetus, safety and efficacy for use in pregnant women have not been established. Bivalirudin is used in conjunction with aspirin, which may lead to maternal or fetal adverse effects, especially during the third trimester. Use during pregnancy only if clearly needed.

Lactation: Excretion in breast milk unknown/use caution

Perioperative/Anesthesia/Other Concerns:

Percutaneous Coronary Intervention (PCI): Compared with heparin, bivalirudin reduced the composite endpoint of death, myocardial infarction, or revascularization in patients undergoing PCI (Bittle, 2001). Bleeding complications were significantly decreased as well.

Heparin-induced thrombocytopenia (HIT): Because bivalirudin has no structural similarity to heparin, it may be safely administered to patients with HIT or heparin-induced thrombotic thrombocytopenia syndrome (HITTS) or a history of HIT or HITTS.

Administration

I.V.: For I.V. administration only.

Reconstitution: Reconstitute each 250 mg with 5 mL SWFI. Gently swirl to dissolve. Further dilution in D_5W or NS (50 mL to make 5 mg/mL solution **or** 500 mL to make 0.5 mg/mL solution) is required prior to infusion. Do not administer in same line with other medications.

Compatibility: Requires separate intravenous line. Stable in D_5W, NS, SWFI.

Y-site administration: Incompatible: Alteplase, amiodarone, amphotericin B, chlorpromazine, diazepam, dobutamine (concentration of 12.5 mg/mL), prochlorperazine, reteplase, streptokinase, vancomycin

Storage: Store unopened vials at 15°C to 30°C; following reconstitution, vials should be stored at 2°C to 8°C. Do not freeze. Final dilutions of 0.5 mg/mL or 5 mg/mL are stable at room temperature for up to 24 hours.

♦ **BL4162A** *see* Anagrelide *on page 166*

♦ **Black Draught Tablets [OTC]** *see* Senna *on page 1520*

♦ **Blenoxane®** *see* Bleomycin *on page 248*

♦ **Bleo** *see* Bleomycin *on page 248*

Bleomycin (blee oh MYE sin)

U.S. Brand Names Blenoxane®

Synonyms Bleo; Bleomycin Sulfate; BLM; NSC-125066

Pharmacologic Category Antineoplastic Agent, Antibiotic

Medication Safety Issues

Sound-alike/look-alike issues:

Bleomycin may be confused with Cleocin®

Use Treatment of squamous cell carcinomas, melanomas, sarcomas, testicular carcinoma, Hodgkin's lymphoma, and non-Hodgkin's lymphoma

Orphan drug: Sclerosing agent for malignant pleural effusion

Mechanism of Action Inhibits synthesis of DNA; binds to DNA leading to single- and double-strand breaks

Pharmacodynamics/Kinetics

Absorption: I.M. and intrapleural administration: 30% to 50% of I.V. serum concentrations; intraperitoneal and SubQ routes produce serum concentrations equal to those of I.V.

Distribution: V_d: 22 L/m²; highest concentrations in skin, kidney, lung, heart tissues; lowest in testes and GI tract; does not cross blood-brain barrier

Protein binding: 1%

Metabolism: Via several tissues including hepatic, GI tract, skin, pulmonary, renal, and serum

Half-life elimination: Biphasic (renal function dependent):
Normal renal function: Initial: 1.3 hours; Terminal: 9 hours
End-stage renal disease: Initial: 2 hours; Terminal: 30 hours
Time to peak, serum: I.M.: Within 30 minutes
Excretion: Urine (50% to 70% as active drug)

Contraindications Hypersensitivity to bleomycin sulfate or any component of the formulation; severe pulmonary disease; pregnancy

Warnings/Precautions The U.S. Food and Drug Administration (FDA) currently recommends that procedures for proper handling and disposal of antineoplastic agents be considered. Occurrence of pulmonary fibrosis is higher in elderly patients, patients receiving >400 units total lifetime dose or single doses >30 units, in smokers, and patients with prior radiation therapy or receiving concurrent oxygen. A severe idiosyncratic reaction consisting of hypotension, mental confusion, fever, chills and wheezing (similar to anaphylaxis) has been reported in 1% of lymphoma patients treated with bleomycin. Since these reactions usually occur after the first or second dose, careful monitoring is essential after these doses. Check lungs prior to each treatment for fine rales (1st sign). Follow manufacturer recommendations for administering O_2 during surgery to patients who have received bleomycin.

Drug Interactions
Cisplatin: May decrease bleomycin elimination
Digitalis glycosides: Bleomycin may decrease plasma levels of digoxin
Lomustine: Increased severity of leukopenia
Phenytoin: Results in decreased phenytoin levels

Adverse Reactions
>10%:
Cardiovascular: Raynaud's phenomenon
Dermatologic: Pain at the tumor site, phlebitis. About 50% of patients develop erythema, induration, hyperkeratosis, and peeling of the skin, particularly on the palmar and plantar surfaces of the hands and feet. Hyperpigmentation (50%), alopecia, nailbed changes may also occur. These effects appear dose related and reversible with discontinuation of the drug.
Gastrointestinal: Stomatitis and mucositis (30%), anorexia, weight loss
Respiratory: Tachypnea, rales, acute or chronic interstitial pneumonitis and pulmonary fibrosis (5% to 10%), hypoxia and death (1%). Symptoms include cough, dyspnea, and bilateral pulmonary infiltrates. The pathogenesis is not certain, but may be due to damage of pulmonary, vascular, or connective tissue. Response to steroid therapy is variable and somewhat controversial.
Miscellaneous: Acute febrile reactions (25% to 50%); anaphylactoid reactions characterized by hypotension, confusion, fever, chills, and wheezing. Onset may be immediate or delayed for several hours.
1% to 10%:
Dermatologic: Rash (8%), skin thickening, diffuse scleroderma, onycholysis
Miscellaneous: Acute anaphylactoid reactions
<1% (Limited to important or life-threatening): Angioedema, cerebrovascular accident, hepatotoxicity, MI, nausea, vomiting; Myelosuppressive (rare); Onset: 7 days, Nadir: 14 days, Recovery: 21 days

Overdosage/Toxicology Symptoms of overdose include chills, fever, pulmonary fibrosis, and hyperpigmentation. Treatment is supportive.

Dosing
Adults: Maximum cumulative lifetime dose: 400 units; refer to individual protocols; 1 unit = 1 mg; may be administered I.M., I.V., SubQ, or intracavitary.

Test dose for lymphoma patient: I.M., I.V., SubQ: 1-5 units of bleomycin before the first dose; monitor vital signs every 15 minutes; wait a minimum of 1 hour before administering remainder of dose.
Single agent therapy:
I.M./I.V./SubQ: Squamous cell carcinoma, lymphosarcoma, reticulum cell sarcoma, testicular carcinoma: 0.25-0.5 units/kg (10-20 units/m^2) 1-2 times/week
Continuous intravenous infusion: 15 units/m^2 over 24 hours/day for 4 days
Pleural sclerosing: Intracavitary: 60 units as a single infusion. Dose may be repeated at intervals of several days if fluid continues to accumulate (mix in 50-100 mL of D_5W, NS, or SWFI); may add lidocaine 100-200 mg to reduce local discomfort.

Elderly: Refer to adult dosing. Some recommend limiting the dose in the elderly to 40 units/m^2, maximum: 60 units.

(Continued)

Bleomycin *(Continued)*

Pediatrics: Refer to adult dosing.

Renal Impairment:

Cl_{cr} 10-50 mL/minute: Administer 75% of normal dose.

Cl_{cr} <10 mL/minute: Administer 50% of normal dose.

Available Dosage Forms Injection, powder for reconstitution, as sulfate: 15 units, 30 units

Nursing Guidelines

Assessment: See Contraindications and Warnings/Precautions for use cautions. Assess potential for interactions with other prescriptions, OTC medications, or herbal products patient may be taking (see Drug Interactions). Respiratory status should be monitored prior to each treatment (special attention to lymphoma patients - see Warnings/Precautions and Adverse Reactions) and prescriber notified of any changes. Test dose may be necessary (see Dosing). Infusion or injection site must be monitored closely to avoid extravasation. Assess results of laboratory tests (see below), therapeutic effectiveness, and adverse response (see Adverse Reactions and Overdose/Toxicology). Teach patient possible side effects/appropriate interventions and adverse symptoms to report (see Patient Education). **Pregnancy risk factor D** - determine that patient is not pregnant before beginning treatment. Instruct patients of childbearing age about appropriate contraceptive measures. Breast-feeding is not recommended.

Monitoring Laboratory Tests: Pulmonary function (total lung volume, forced vital capacity, carbon monoxide diffusion), renal function, chest x-ray, liver function

Patient Education: Inform prescriber of all prescriptions, OTC medications, or herbal products you are taking, and any allergies you have; do not take any new medications during treatment unless approved by prescriber. This medication can only be administered by injection or infusion; report immediately any redness, burning, pain, or swelling at injection/infusion site. May cause loss of appetite, nausea, or vomiting (small, frequent meals, sucking lozenges, or chewing gum may help); mouth sores (frequent mouth care with soft swabs and mouth rinses may help); fever or chills (will usually resolve); redness, peeling, or increased color of skin; or loss of hair (reversible after cessation of therapy). Report any change in respiratory status; respiratory difficulty; wheezing; air hunger; increased secretions; difficulty expectorating secretions; confusion; unresolved fever or chills; sores in mouth; vaginal itching, burning, or discharge; sudden onset of dizziness; acute headache; or burning, stinging, redness, or swelling at injection site. **Pregnancy/breast-feeding precautions:** Inform prescriber if you are pregnant. Do not get pregnant during or for 1 month following therapy. Consult prescriber for instruction on appropriate contraceptives. This drug may cause severe fetal defects. Breast-feeding is not recommended

Geriatric Considerations: Pulmonary toxicity has been reported more frequently in geriatric patients (>70 years of age).

Pregnancy Risk Factor: D

Lactation: Excretion in breast milk unknown/not recommended

Perioperative/Anesthesia/Other Concerns: The use of oxygen concentrations (>30%) in animals previously treated with bleomycin has been reported to promote pulmonary toxicity. Although this is still controversial, supplemental oxygen should be used judiciously in patients who have received bleomycin.

Administration

I.M.: May cause pain at injection site.

I.V.: May be an irritant. I.V. doses should be administered slowly (manufacturer recommends giving over a period of 10 minutes).

Reconstitution: Reconstitute powder with 1-5 mL BWFI or BNS which is stable at room temperature or under refrigeration for 28 days.

Standard I.V. dilution: Dose/50-1000 mL NS or D_5W

Stable for 96 hours at room temperature and 14 days under refrigeration.

Compatibility: Stable in NS

Compatibility when admixed: Incompatible with aminophylline, ascorbic acid injection, cefazolin, diazepam, hydrocortisone sodium succinate, methotrexate, mitomycin, nafcillin, penicillin G sodium, terbutaline

Storage: Refrigerate intact vials of powder; intact vials are stable for up to one month at 45°C

♦ **Bleomycin Sulfate** *see* Bleomycin *on page 248*

♦ **Bleph®-10** *see* Sulfacetamide *on page 1579*
♦ **Blephamide®** *see* Sulfacetamide and Prednisolone *on page 1581*
♦ **BLM** *see* Bleomycin *on page 248*
♦ **Blocadren®** *see* Timolol *on page 1633*
♦ **Bonine® [OTC]** *see* Meclizine *on page 1084*

Bortezomib (bore TEZ oh mib)

U.S. Brand Names Velcade®

Synonyms LDP-341; MLN341; PS-341

Pharmacologic Category Antineoplastic Agent; Proteasome Inhibitor

Use Treatment of multiple myeloma in patients who have had at least one prior therapy

Mechanism of Action Bortezomib inhibits proteasomes, enzyme complexes which regulate protein homeostasis within the cell. Specifically, it reversibly inhibits chymotrypsin-like activity at the 26S proteasome, leading to activation of signaling cascades, cell-cycle arrest and apoptosis.

Pharmacodynamics/Kinetics

Protein binding: ~83%

Metabolism: Hepatic via CYP 1A2, 2C9, 2C19, 2D6, 3A4; forms metabolites (inactive)

Half-life elimination: 9-15 hours

Contraindications Hypersensitivity to bortezomib, boron, mannitol, or any component of the formulation; pregnancy

Warnings/Precautions Hazardous agent - use appropriate precautions for handling and disposal. May cause peripheral neuropathy (usually sensory but may be mixed sensorimotor); risk may be increased with previous use of neurotoxic agents or pre-existing peripheral neuropathy; adjustment of dose and schedule may be required. May cause orthostatic/postural hypotension; use caution with dehydration, history of syncope or medications associated with hypotension. Has been associated with the development or exacerbation of congestive heart failure; use caution in patients with risk factors or existing heart disease. May cause tumor lysis syndrome; risk is increased in patients with large tumor burden prior to treatment. Hematologic toxicity with severe thrombocytopenia may occur; risk is increased in patients with pretreatment platelet counts <75,000 μL; frequent monitoring is required throughout treatment. Use caution with hepatic or renal impairment. Safety and efficacy have not been established in pediatric patients.

Drug Interactions Substrate of CYP1A2 (minor), 2C8/9 (minor), 2C19 (minor), 2D6 (minor), 3A4 (major); **Inhibits** CYP1A2 (weak), 2C8/9 (weak), 2C19 (moderate), 2D6 (weak), 3A4 (weak)

CYP2C19 substrates: Bortezomib may increase the levels/effects of CYP2C19 substrates. Example substrates include citalopram, diazepam, methsuximide, phenytoin, propranolol, and sertraline.

CYP3A4 inducers: CYP3A4 inducers may decrease the levels/effects of bortezomib. Example inducers include aminoglutethimide, carbamazepine, nafcillin, nevirapine, phenobarbital, phenytoin, and rifamycins.

CYP3A4 inhibitors: May increase the levels/effects of bortezomib. Example inhibitors include azole antifungals, clarithromycin, diclofenac, doxycycline, erythromycin, imatinib, isoniazid, nefazodone, nicardipine, propofol, protease inhibitors, quinidine, telithromycin, and verapamil.

Adverse Reactions

>10%:

Cardiovascular: Edema (25%), hypotension (12%)

Central nervous system: Pyrexia (35% to 36%), psychiatric disturbance (35%), headache (26% to 28%), insomnia (27%), dizziness (14% to 21%, excludes vertigo), anxiety (14%)

Dermatologic: Rash (18% to 21%), pruritus (11%)

Endocrine & metabolic: Dehydration (18%)

Gastrointestinal: Nausea (57% to 64%), diarrhea (51% to 57%), appetite decreased (43%), constipation (42% to 43%), vomiting (35% to 36%), abdominal pain (13% to 16%), abnormal taste (13%), dyspepsia (13%)

Hematologic: Thrombocytopenia (35% to 43%, Grade 3: 26% to 27%, Grade 4: 3%; Nadir: Day 11); anemia (26% to 32%, Grade 3: 9%); neutropenia (19% to 24%, Grade 3: 13%, Grade 4: 3%)

Neuromuscular & skeletal: Asthenic conditions (61% to 65%, Grade 3: 12% to 18% - includes fatigue, malaise, weakness); peripheral neuropathy (36% to

(Continued)

Bortezomib *(Continued)*

37%, Grade 3: 7% to 14%); arthralgia (14% to 26%); limb pain (26%); paresthesia and dysesthesia (23%), bone pain (16%), back pain (14%); muscle cramps (12% to 14%); myalgia (12% to 14%); rigors (11% to 12%)

Ocular: Blurred vision (11%)

Respiratory: Dyspnea (20% to 22%), upper respiratory tract infection (18%), cough (17% to 21%), lower respiratory infection (15%), nasopharyngitis (14%)

Miscellaneous: Herpes zoster (11% to 13%)

1% to 10%: Respiratory: Pneumonia (10%)

Frequency not defined (limited to significant and/or life-threatening): Acute respiratory distress syndrome, agitation, allergic reaction, anaphylaxis, ataxia, AV block, bacteremia, bradycardia, cardiogenic shock, cardiac tamponade, cerebral hemorrhage, CHF, cholestasis, coma, cranial palsy, deafness, deep venous thrombosis, disseminated intravascular coagulation, duodenitis (hemorrhagic), dysautonomia, embolism, gastritis (hemorrhagic), hematemesis, hematuria, hemoptysis, hemorrhagic cystitis, hepatitis, hydronephrosis, hypoxia, immune complex hypersensitivity, intestinal obstruction, intestinal perforation, ischemic colitis, MI, pancreatitis, paralytic ileus, paraplegia, pericardial effusion, pericarditis, pleural effusion, pneumonitis, portal vein thrombosis, proliferative glomerular nephritis, pulmonary edema, pulmonary embolism, pulmonary hypertension, psychosis, renal calculus, renal failure, seizure, septic shock, stroke, suicidal ideation, torsade de pointes, tumor lysis syndrome, ventricular tachycardia, vertigo

Overdosage/Toxicology In case of overdose, treatment should be symptom directed and supportive.

Dosing

Adults: Multiple myeloma: I.V.: 1.3 mg/m^2 twice weekly for 2 weeks on days 1, 4, 8, 11, every 21 days. Consecutive doses should be separated by at least 72 hours.

Renal Impairment: Specific guidelines are not available; studies did not include patients with Cl_{cr} <13 mL/minute and patients on hemodialysis. Monitor closely for toxicity.

Hepatic Impairment: Specific guidelines are not available; clearance may be decreased; monitor closely for toxicity.

Available Dosage Forms Injection, powder for reconstitution [preservative free]: 3.5 mg [contains mannitol 35 mg]

Nursing Guidelines

Assessment: Assess potential for interactions with other prescriptions, OTC medications, or herbal products patient may be taking. See Administration specifics. Assess results of laboratory tests, effectiveness of therapy, and adverse reactions on regular basis during therapy (eg, peripheral neuropathy, postural hypotension, dehydration, congestive heart failure, infections). Monitor for psychiatric disturbances. Teach patient possible side effects/appropriate interventions and adverse symptoms to report.

Monitoring Laboratory Tests: CBC

Patient Education: Do not take any new medication during therapy without consulting prescriber. This medication can only be administered intravenously; you will be monitored during and following infusion. Maintain adequate hydration (2-3 L/day of fluids) unless instructed to restrict fluid intake. May cause headache, dizziness (use caution when changing positions), anxiety, or fatigue (use caution when driving or engaging in hazardous tasks until response to drug is known); nausea, vomiting or abnormal taste (small frequent meals, frequent mouth care, chewing gum, or sucking lozenges may help) or diarrhea (boiled milk, yogurt, or buttermilk may help). Report immediately any chest pain, respiratory difficulty, itching, rash, acute headache, throat tightness, pain, redness, or swelling at infusion site. Report chest pain or shortness of breath, swelling in extremities, recent weight gain (>3-5 pounds/week), persistent headache; muscle, bone, or back pain; cramping or loss of sensation; changes in vision; psychiatric disturbances or other persistent adverse reactions. **Pregnancy/breast-feeding precautions:** Inform prescriber if you are pregnant. Do not get pregnant or cause a pregnancy (males) during therapy or for 1 month following therapy. Consult prescriber for instructions on appropriate nonhormonal contraceptive measures. This drug may cause fetal defects. Breast-feeding is not recommended.

Pregnancy Risk Factor: D

Pregnancy Issues: Adverse effects were observed in animal studies. Effective contraception is recommended for women of childbearing potential.

Lactation: Excretion in breast milk unknown/not recommended

Breast-Feeding Considerations: Breast-feeding should be avoided.

Administration

I.V.: Administer via rapid I.V. push (3-5 seconds).

Reconstitution: Dilute each 3.5 mg vial with 3.5 mL NS.

Storage: Prior to reconstitution, store at controlled room temperature, 15°C to 30°C (59°F to 86°F). Protect from light. Once reconstituted, may be stored at room temperature for up to 3 days, or under refrigeration for up to 5 days, in vial or syringe; protect from light.

♦ **B&O Supprettes®** *see* Belladonna and Opium *on page 227*

♦ **Botox®** *see* Botulinum Toxin Type A *on page 253*

♦ **Botox® Cosmetic** *see* Botulinum Toxin Type A *on page 253*

Botulinum Toxin Type A (BOT yoo lin num TOKS in type aye)

U.S. Brand Names Botox®; Botox® Cosmetic

Synonyms BTX-A

Pharmacologic Category Neuromuscular Blocker Agent, Toxin; Ophthalmic Agent, Toxin

Use Treatment of strabismus and blepharospasm associated with dystonia (including benign essential blepharospasm or VII nerve disorders in patients ≥12 years of age); cervical dystonia (spasmodic torticollis) in patients ≥16 years of age; temporary improvement in the appearance of lines/wrinkles of the face (moderate to severe glabellar lines associated with corrugator and/or procerus muscle activity) in adult patients ≤65 years of age; treatment of severe primary axillary hyperhidrosis in adults not adequately controlled with topical treatments

Orphan drug: Treatment of dynamic muscle contracture in pediatric cerebral palsy patients

Unlabeled/Investigational Use Treatment of oromandibular dystonia, spasmodic dysphonia (laryngeal dystonia) and other dystonias (ie, writer's cramp, focal task-specific dystonias); migraine treatment and prophylaxis

Mechanism of Action Botulinum A toxin is a neurotoxin produced by *Clostridium botulinum*, spore-forming anaerobic bacillus, which appears to affect only the presynaptic membrane of the neuromuscular junction in humans, where it prevents calcium-dependent release of acetylcholine and produces a state of denervation. Muscle inactivation persists until new fibrils grow from the nerve and form junction plates on new areas of the muscle-cell walls.

Pharmacodynamics/Kinetics

Onset of action (improvement):
- Blepharospasm: ~3 days
- Cervical dystonia: ~2 weeks
- Strabismus: ~1-2 days
- Reduction of glabellar lines (Botox® Cosmetic): 1-2 days, increasing in intensity during first week

Duration:
- Blepharospasm: ~3 months
- Cervical dystonia: <3 months
- Strabismus: ~2-6 weeks
- Primary axillary hyperhydrosis: 201 days (mean)
- Reduction of glabellar lines (Botox® Cosmetic): Up to 3 months

Absorption: Not expected to be present in peripheral blood at recommended doses

Time to peak:
- Blepharospasm: 1-2 weeks
- Cervical dystonia: ~6 weeks
- Strabismus: Within first week

Contraindications Hypersensitivity to albumin, botulinum toxin, or any component of the formulation; infection at the proposed injection site(s); pregnancy. Relative contraindications include diseases of neuromuscular transmission; coagulopathy including therapeutic anticoagulation; uncooperative patient

Warnings/Precautions Higher doses or more frequent administration may result in neutralizing antibody formation and loss of efficacy. Product contains albumin and may carry a remote risk of virus transmission. Use caution if there is inflammation, excessive weakness, or atrophy at the proposed injection site(s). Have

(Continued)

Botulinum Toxin Type A *(Continued)*

appropriate support in case of anaphylactic reaction. Use with caution in patients with neuromuscular diseases (such as myasthenia gravis), neuropathic disorders (such as amyotrophic lateral sclerosis), or patients taking aminoglycosides or other drugs that interfere with neuromuscular transmission. Ensure adequate contraception in women of childbearing years. Long-term effects of chronic therapy unknown.

Cervical dystonia: Dysphagia is common. It may be severe requiring alternative feeding methods. Risk factors include smaller neck muscle mass, bilateral injections into the sternocleidomastoid muscle or injections into the levator scapulae. Dysphasia may be associated with increased risk of upper respiratory infection.

Blepharospasm: Reduced blinking from injection of the orbicularis muscle can lead to corneal exposure and ulceration.

Strabismus: Retrobulbar hemorrhages may occur from needle penetration into orbit. Spatial disorientation, double vision, or past pointing may occur if one or more extraocular muscles are paralyzed. Covering the affected eye may help. Careful testing of corneal sensation, avoidance of lower lid injections, and treatment of epithelial defects necessary.

Primary axillary hyperhidrosis: Evaluate for secondary causes prior to treatment (eg, hyperthyroidism). Safety and efficacy for treatment of hyperhidrosis in other areas of the body have not been established.

Temporary reduction in glabellar lines: Do not use more frequently than every 3 months. Patients with marked facial asymmetry, ptosis, excessive dermatochalasis, deep dermal scarring, thick sebaceous skin, or the inability to substantially lessen glabellar lines by physically spreading them apart were excluded from clinical trials. Reduced blinking from injection of the orbicularis muscle can lead to corneal exposure and ulceration. Spatial disorientation, double vision, or past pointing may occur if one or more extraocular muscles are paralyzed.

Drug Interactions

Aminoglycosides: May increase neuromuscular blockade

Neuromuscular-blocking agents: May increase neuromuscular blockade

Other agents which may have neuromuscular-blocking activity: Calcium channel blockers, catecholamines, chloroquine, clindamycin, colistin, corticosteroids, digitalis glycosides, diuretics, inhalation anesthetics, lidocaine, lincomycin, magnesium salts, opioids, phenytoin, phenelzine, polymixin B, procainamide, propranolol, quinidine, tetracyclines

Adverse Reactions Adverse effects usually occur in 1 week and may last up to several months

>10%:

- Central nervous system: Headache (cervical dystonia up to 11%, reduction of glabellar lines up to 13%; can occur with other uses)
- Gastrointestinal: Dysphagia (cervical dystonia 19%)
- Neuromuscular & skeletal: Neck pain (cervical dystonia 11%)
- Ocular: Ptosis (blepharospasm 10% to 40%, strabismus 1% to 38%, reduction of glabellar lines 1% to 5%); vertical deviation (strabismus 17%)
- Respiratory: Upper respiratory infection (cervical dystonia 12%)

2% to 10%:

- Central nervous system: Anxiety (primary axillary hyperhydrosis); dizziness (cervical dystonia, reduction of glabellar lines); drowsiness (cervical dystonia); fever (cervical dystonia, primary axillary hyperhydrosis); speech disorder (cervical dystonia)
- Dermatologic: Nonaxillary sweating (primary axillary hyperhydrosis), pruritus (primary axillary hyperhydrosis)
- Gastrointestinal: Xerostomia (cervical dystonia), nausea (cervical dystonia, reduction of glabellar lines)
- Local: Injection site reaction
- Neuromuscular & skeletal: Back pain (cervical dystonia); facial pain (reduction of glabellar lines); hypertonia (cervical dystonia); weakness (cervical dystonia, reduction of glabellar lines)
- Ocular: Dry eyes (blepharospasm 6%), superficial punctate keratitis (blepharospasm 6%)
- Respiratory: Cough (cervical dystonia); infection (reduction of glabellar lines, primary axillary hyperhydrosis); pharyngitis (primary axillary hyperhydrosis); rhinitis (cervical dystonia)

Miscellaneous: Flu syndrome (cervical dystonia, reduction of glabellar lines, primary axillary hyperhydrosis)

<2%: Stiffness, diplopia (cervical dystonia, blepharospasm), ptosis (cervical dystonia), dyspnea (cervical dystonia), numbness (cervical dystonia), ectropion (blepharospasm), lagophthalmos (blepharospasm), facial weakness (blepharospasm), ecchymoses (blepharospasm), eyelid edema (blepharospasm), tearing (blepharospasm), photophobia (blepharospasm), entropion (blepharospasm)

Postmarketing and/or case reports: Allergic reactions, arrhythmia, erythema multiforme, MI, pruritus, psoriasiform eruption, skin rash, urticaria

Reported following treatment of cervical dystonia: Brachial plexopathy, dysphonia, aspiration

Reported following treatment of blepharospasm: Reduced blinking leading to corneal ulceration, corneal perforation, acute angle-closure glaucoma, focal facial paralysis, exacerbation of myasthenia gravis, syncope, vitreous hemorrhage

Reported following treatment of strabismus: Retrobulbar hemorrhage, ciliary ganglion damage, anterior segment eye ischemia

Reported following reduction of glabellar lines: Exacerbation of myasthenia gravis, retinal vein occlusion, abnormal hearing/hearing loss, glaucoma, vertigo with nystagmus

Overdosage/Toxicology Systemic weakness or muscle paralysis could occur for up to several weeks after overdose. Signs and symptoms of overdose are not apparent immediately. An antitoxin is available if there is immediate knowledge of an overdose or misinjection. Contact Allergan for additional information at (800) 433-8871 or (714) 246-5954. The antitoxin will not reverse toxin-induced muscle weakness already present.

Dosing

Adults & Elderly:

Cervical dystonia: I.M.: For dosing guidance, the mean dose is 236 units (25th to 75th percentile range 198-300 units) divided among the affected muscles in patients previously treated with botulinum toxin. Initial dose in previously untreated patients should be lower. Sequential dosing should be based on the patient's head and neck position, localization of pain, muscle hypertrophy, patient response, and previous adverse reactions. The total dose injected into the sternocleidomastoid muscles should be ≤100 units to decrease the occurrence of dysphagia.

Blepharospasm: I.M.: Initial dose: 1.25-2.5 units injected into the medial and lateral pretarsal orbicularis oculi of the upper and lower lid; dose may be increased up to twice the previous dose if the response from the initial dose lasted ≤2 months; maximum dose per site: 5 units; cumulative dose in a 30-day period: ≤200 units. Tolerance may occur if treatments are given more often than every 3 months, but the effect is not usually permanent.

Strabismus: I.M.:

Initial dose:

Vertical muscles and for horizontal strabismus <20 prism diopters: 1.25-2.5 units in any one muscle

Horizontal strabismus of 20-50 prism diopters: 2.5-5 units in any one muscle

Persistent VI nerve palsy >1 month: 1.5-2.5 units in the medial rectus muscle

Subsequent doses: Re-examine patients 7-14 days after each injection to assess the effect of that dose. Subsequent doses for patients experiencing incomplete paralysis of the target may be increased up to twice the previous administered dose. The maximum recommended dose as a single injection for any one muscle is 25 units. Do not administer subsequent injections until the effects of the previous dose are gone.

Primary axillary hyperhidrosis: Intradermal: 50 units/axilla. Injection area should be defined by standard staining techniques. Injections should be evenly distributed into multiple sites (10-15), administered in 0.1-0.2 mL aliquots, ~1-2 cm apart.

Reduction of glabellar lines: Adults ≤65 years: An effective dose is determined by gross observation of the patient's ability to activate the superficial muscles injected. The location, size and use of muscles may vary markedly among individuals. Inject 0.1 mL dose into each of five sites, two in each corrugator muscle and one in the procerus muscle (total dose 0.5 mL).

Pediatrics:

Blepharospasm/strabismus: Children ≥12 years: Refer to adult dosing.

Cervical dystonia: Children ≥16 years: Refer to adult dosing.

(Continued)

Botulinum Toxin Type A *(Continued)*

Renal Impairment: No adjustment is recommended.

Hepatic Impairment: No adjustment necessary.

Available Dosage Forms Injection, powder for reconstitution [preservative free]: *Clostridium botulinum* toxin type A 100 units [contains human albumin]

Nursing Guidelines

Patient Education: This medicine is given in a clinic or hospital setting by a prescriber. It is given as an injection. It is not a cure, but may be given on a periodic basis to help with spasms. Tell your prescriber if you have any nerve diseases or any infections where the shot might be given. Patients with blepharospasm may not have been very active. Start activity slowly and increase as you see how you feel. Call prescriber as soon as possible if you have trouble swallowing, speaking, or breathing. May have double vision or other problems where covering the eye with a patch may help. **Pregnancy/breast-feeding precautions:** Do not use in pregnancy and do not get pregnant while taking this drug. Use birth control that you can trust. Breast-feeding is not recommended.

Pregnancy Risk Factor: C (manufacturer)

Lactation: Excretion in breast milk unknown/not recommended

Administration

I.M.:

Cervical dystonia: Use 25-, 27-, or 30-gauge needle for superficial muscles and a longer 22-gauge needle for deeper musculature; electromyography may help localize the involved muscles

Blepharospasm: Use a 27- or 30-gauge needle without electromyography guidance. Avoid injecting near the levator palpebrae superioris (may decrease ptosis); avoid medial lower lid injections (may decrease diplopia). Apply pressure at the injection site to prevent ecchymosis in the soft eyelid tissues.

Strabismus injections: Must use surgical exposure or electromyographic guidance; use the electrical activity recorded from the tip of the injections needle as a guide to placement within the target muscle. Local anesthetic and ocular decongestant should be given before injection. The volume of injection should be 0.05-0.15 mL per muscle. Many patients will require additional doses because of inadequate response to initial dose.

Reduction of glabellar lines (Botox® Cosmetic): Use a 30-gauge needle. Ensure injected volume/dose is accurate and where feasible keep to a minimum. Avoid injection near the levator palpebrae superioris. Medial corrugator injections should be at least 1 cm above the bony supraorbital ridge. Do not inject toxin closer than 1 cm above the central eyebrow.

Reconstitution: Reconstitute with sterile normal saline without a preservative. Mix gently. After reconstitution, store in refrigerator (2°C to 8°C) and use within 4 hours (does not contain preservative). Do not freeze.

Botox®: Reconstitute vials with 1 mL of diluent to get 10 units per 0.1 mL; 2 mL of diluent to get 5 units per 0.1 mL; 4 mL of diluent to get 2.5 units per 0.1 mL; 8 mL of diluent to get 1.25 units per 0.1 mL.

Botox® Cosmetic: Reconstitute vials with 2.5 mL of diluent to get 0.4 units per 0.1 mL (20 units per 0.5 mL).

Storage: Store undiluted vials under refrigeration at 2°C to 8°C for up to 24 months. Administer within 4 hours after the vial is reconstituted.

♦ Breathe Right® Saline [OTC] *see* Sodium Chloride *on page 1545*
♦ Brethaire [DSC] *see* Terbutaline *on page 1604*
♦ Brethine® *see* Terbutaline *on page 1604*

Bretylium (bre TIL ee um)

Synonyms Bretylium Tosylate

Pharmacologic Category Antiarrhythmic Agent, Class III

Medication Safety Issues

Sound-alike/look-alike issues:

Bretylium may be confused with Brevibloc®

Use Treatment of ventricular tachycardia and fibrillation; treatment of other serious ventricular arrhythmias resistant to lidocaine

Mechanism of Action Class III antiarrhythmic; after an initial release of norepinephrine at the peripheral adrenergic nerve terminals, inhibits further release by postganglionic nerve endings in response to sympathetic nerve stimulation

Pharmacodynamics/Kinetics

Onset of action: I.M.: May require 2 hours; I.V.: 6-20 minutes

Peak effect: 6-9 hours

Duration: 6-24 hours
Protein binding: 1% to 6%
Metabolism: None
Half-life elimination: 7-11 hours; Mean: 4-17 hours; End-stage renal disease: 16-32 hours
Excretion: Urine (70% to 80% as unchanged drug) within 24 hours

Contraindications Hypersensitivity to bretylium or any component of the formulation; severe aortic stenosis; severe pulmonary hypertension

Warnings/Precautions Use only in areas where there is equipment and staff familiar with management of life-threatening arrhythmias. Use continuous cardiac and blood pressure monitoring. Keep patients supine (postural hypotension common). Initially, may see transient hypertension and increased frequency of arrhythmias. Adjust dose in patients with impaired renal function. Give to a pregnant woman only if clearly needed. Rapid I.V. administration may cause nausea and vomiting.

Drug Interactions

Increased toxicity when used with pressor catecholamines, and digitalis.
Agents which may prolong QT interval (including cisapride, tricyclic antidepressants, antipsychotics, erythromycin, Class Ia and Class III antiarrhythmics): Toxicity may be increased.
Quinolones: Risk of cardiotoxicity is increased with concurrent use of sparfloxacin, moxifloxacin, or gatifloxacin may increase toxicity due to the potential to prolong QT interval.
Sympathomimetic amines with initial use of bretylium may cause hypertension.
Digoxin toxicity may be aggravated by bretylium.

Adverse Reactions

>10%: Cardiovascular: Hypotension (both postural and supine)
1% to 10%: Gastrointestinal: Nausea, vomiting
<1% (Limited to important or life-threatening): Bradycardia, chest pain, dyspnea, flushing, increase in premature ventricular contractions (PVCs), nasal congestion, postural hypotension, renal impairment, respiratory depression, syncope, transient initial hypertension

Overdosage/Toxicology Symptoms of overdose include significant hypertension followed by severe hypotension. Administration of a short-acting hypotensive agent should be used for the hypertensive response. Treatment is symptomatic and supportive. Dialysis is not useful.

Dosing

Adults & Elderly: (**Note:** Patients should undergo defibrillation/cardioversion before and after bretylium doses as necessary.)

Immediate life-threatening ventricular arrhythmias, ventricular fibrillation, unstable ventricular tachycardia: I.V.: Initial: 5 mg/kg (undiluted) over 1 minute; if arrhythmia persists, give 10 mg/kg (undiluted) over 1 minute and repeat as necessary (usually at 15- to 30-minute intervals) up to a total dose of 30-35 mg/kg

Other life-threatening ventricular arrhythmias: I.M., I.V.:

Initial: 5-10 mg/kg, may repeat every 1-2 hours if arrhythmia persist; give I.V. dose (diluted) over 8-10 minutes

Maintenance dose: I.M.: 5-10 mg/kg every 6-8 hours; I.V. (diluted): 5-10 mg/kg every 6 hours; I.V. infusion (diluted): 1-2 mg/minute (little experience with doses >40 mg/kg/day)

Pediatrics: Note: Patients should undergo defibrillation/cardioversion before and after bretylium doses as necessary.

Arrhythmias:

Note: Not well established, although the following dosing has been suggested:

I.M.: Children: 2-5 mg/kg as a single dose

I.V.: Children: Acute ventricular fibrillation: Initial: 5 mg/kg, then attempt electrical defibrillation; repeat with 10 mg/kg if ventricular fibrillation persists at 15- to 30-minute intervals to maximum total of 30 mg/kg

Maintenance dose: I.M., I.V.: 5 mg/kg every 6 hours

Renal Impairment:

Cl_{cr} 10-50 mL/minute: Administer 25% to 50% of dose.
Cl_{cr} <10 mL/minute: Administer 25% of dose.
Not dialyzable

Available Dosage Forms [DSC] = Discontinued product

Injection, solution, as tosylate: 50 mg/mL (10 mL) [DSC]
(Continued)

Bretylium *(Continued)*

Injection, solution, as tosylate [premixed in D_5W]: 2 mg/mL (250 mL); 4 mg/mL (250 mL) [DSC]

Nursing Guidelines

Assessment: Assess other medications patient may be taking for effectiveness and interactions. **I.V.:** Requires use of infusion pump and continuous cardiac and hemodynamic monitoring. Be alert for adverse cardiovascular reactions. Patient education/instruction is according to patient condition.

Patient Education: Emergency use: Patient education is determined by patient condition. You may experience nausea or vomiting (call for assistance if this occurs, do not try to get out of bed or change position on your own). Report chest pain, acute dizziness, or respiratory difficulty immediately. **Breast-feeding precaution:** Consult prescriber if breast-feeding.

Geriatric Considerations: Elderly are particularly at risk of orthostatic hypotension. See Warnings/Precautions and Adverse Reactions.

Pregnancy Risk Factor: C

Lactation: Excretion in breast milk unknown

Perioperative/Anesthesia/Other Concerns: Bretylium has been removed from ACLS treatment algorithms/guidelines because of high occurrence of adverse events, the availability of safer agents, and its limited supply.

Administration

I.M.: I.M. injection in adults should not exceed 5 mL volume in any one site.

I.V.: 2 g/250 mL D_5W (infusion pump should be used for I.V. infusion)

Bolus, emergency: Infuse rapidly (1 minute).

Bolus, nonemergency: May be given over 8-10 minutes.

Suggested rate of I.V. infusion: 1-4 mg/minute.

1 mg/minute = 7 mL/hour
2 mg/minute = 15 mL/hour
3 mg/minute = 22 mL/hour
4 mg/minute = 30 mL/hour

Reconstitution: Standard diluent: 2 g/250 mL D_5W

Compatibility: Stable in D_5LR, D_5½NS, D_5NS, D_5W, mannitol 20%, LR, sodium bicarbonate 5%, NS

Y-site administration: Incompatible with amphotericin B cholesteryl sulfate complex, propofol, warfarin

Compatibility when admixed: Incompatible with phenytoin

Storage: The premix infusion should be stored at room temperature and protected from freezing.

♦ **Bretylium Tosylate** *see* Bretylium *on page 256*

♦ **Brevibloc®** *see* Esmolol *on page 643*

♦ **Brevital® Sodium** *see* Methohexital *on page 1125*

♦ **Bricanyl [DSC]** *see* Terbutaline *on page 1604*

Brimonidine (bri MOE ni deen)

U.S. Brand Names Alphagan® P

Synonyms Brimonidine Tartrate

Pharmacologic Category Alpha$_2$ Agonist, Ophthalmic; Ophthalmic Agent, Antiglaucoma

Medication Safety Issues

Sound-alike/look-alike issues:

Brimonidine may be confused with bromocriptine

Use Lowering of intraocular pressure (IOP) in patients with open-angle glaucoma or ocular hypertension

Mechanism of Action Selective agonism for alpha$_2$-receptors; causes reduction of aqueous humor formation and increased uveoscleral outflow

Pharmacodynamics/Kinetics

Onset of action: Peak effect: 2 hours

Metabolism: Hepatic

Half-life elimination: 2-3 hours

Time to peak, plasma: 0.5-2.5 hours

Excretion: Urine (74%)

Contraindications Hypersensitivity to brimonidine tartrate or any component of the formulation; during or within 14 days of MAO inhibitor therapy

Warnings/Precautions Exercise caution in treating patients with severe cardiovascular disease. Use with caution in patients with depression, cerebral or coronary insufficiency, Raynaud's phenomenon, orthostatic hypotension or thromboangiitis obliterans. Use with caution in patients with hepatic or renal impairment. May cause drowsiness or fatigue; use caution performing tasks which require alertness. Safety and efficacy in children <2 years of age have not been established.

Products may contain benzalkonium chloride which may be absorbed by contact lenses; remove contacts prior to administration and wait 15 minutes before reinserting. The IOP-lowering efficacy observed with brimonidine tartrate during the first of month of therapy may not always reflect the long term level of IOP reduction. Routinely monitor IOP.

Drug Interactions

Antihypertensives: Concomitant use may have additive effects

Cardiac glycosides: May increase effects

CNS depressants (eg, ethanol, barbiturates, opiates, sedatives, anesthetics): Concomitant use may have additive or potentiating effects.

MAO inhibitors: Concomitant use is contraindicated.

Pilocarpine: Additive decrease in intraocular pressure

Topical beta-blockers: Additive decreased intraocular pressure

Tricyclic antidepressants: Can affect the metabolism and uptake of circulating amines, resulting in decreased IOP-lowering effect of brimonidine.

Adverse Reactions Actual frequency of adverse reactions may be formulation dependant; percentages reported with Alphagan® P:

>10%: Ocular: Allergic conjunctivitis, conjunctival hyperemia, eye pruritus

1% to 10% (unless otherwise noted 1% to 4%):

Cardiovascular: Hypertension (5% to 9%), hypotension

Central nervous system: Dizziness, fatigue, headache, insomnia, somnolence

Dermatologic: Rash

Endocrine & metabolic: Hypercholesterolemia

Gastrointestinal: Xerostomia (5% to 9%), dyspepsia

Ocular: Burning sensation (5% to 9%), conjunctival folliculosis (5% to 9%), ocular allergic reaction (5% to 9%), visual disturbance (5% to 9%), blepharitis, blepharoconjunctivitis, blurred vision, cataract, conjunctival edema, conjunctival hemorrhage, conjunctivitis, dry eye, eye discharge, irritation, epiphora, eyelid disorder, eyelid edema, eyelid erythema, follicular conjunctivitis, foreign body sensation, keratitis, pain, photophobia, stinging, superficial punctate keratopathy, visual field defect, vitreous detachment, vitreous floaters, watery eyes, worsened visual acuity

Respiratory: Bronchitis, cough, dyspnea, pharyngitis, rhinitis, sinus infection, sinusitis

Miscellaneous: Allergic reaction, flu-like syndrome, infection

<1% (Limited to important or life-threatening): Bradycardia, corneal erosion, depression, hordeolum, iritis, keratoconjunctivitis sicca, miosis, nasal dryness, nausea, skin reactions, tachycardia, taste perversion; apnea, bradycardia, hypotension, hypotonia, and somnolence have been reported in infants

Overdosage/Toxicology No information is available on overdosage in humans. Treatment is supportive and symptomatic.

Dosing

Adults & Elderly: Glaucoma: Ophthalmic: Instill 1 drop in affected eye(s) 3 times/day (approximately every 8 hours)

Pediatrics: Children ≥2 years of age: Refer to adult dosing.

Available Dosage Forms

Solution, ophthalmic, as tartrate: 0.2% (5 mL, 10 mL, 15 mL) [may contain benzalkonium chloride]

Alphagan® P: 0.1% (5 mL, 10 mL, 15 mL) [contains Purite® as preservative]; 0.15% (5 mL, 10 mL, 15 mL) [contains Purite® as preservative]

Nursing Guidelines

Assessment: Assess potential for interactions with other prescriptions, OTC medications, or herbal products patient may be taking. Monitor intraocular pressure periodically. Assess therapeutic response and adverse effects. Teach patient proper use, side effects/appropriate interventions, and symptoms to report.

Patient Education: For use in eyes only. Wash hands before instilling. Sit or lie down to instill. Open eye, look at ceiling, and instill prescribed amount of solution. Apply gentle pressure to inner corner of eye. Do not let tip of applicator touch eyes; do not contaminate tip of applicator (may cause eye infection, eye

(Continued)

Brimonidine *(Continued)*

damage, or vision loss). Brimonidine tartrate may cause fatigue or drowsiness in some patients. Avoid engaging in hazardous activities due to potential for decreased mental alertness. Wait at least 15 minutes after instilling brimonidine tartrate before reinserting soft contact lenses. **Breast-feeding precaution:** Do not breast-feed.

Pregnancy Risk Factor: B

Lactation: Excretion in breast milk unknown/not recommended

Administration

Storage: Store between 15°C to 25°C (59°F to 77°F)

- ♦ Brimonidine Tartrate *see* Brimonidine *on page 258*
- ♦ Brioschi® [OTC] *see* Sodium Bicarbonate *on page 1542*
- ♦ BRL 43694 *see* Granisetron *on page 831*
- ♦ Broncho Saline® [OTC] *see* Sodium Chloride *on page 1545*
- ♦ Brontex® *see* Guaifenesin and Codeine *on page 835*
- ♦ BSS® *see* Balanced Salt Solution *on page 224*
- ♦ BSS Plus® *see* Balanced Salt Solution *on page 224*
- ♦ BTX-A *see* Botulinum Toxin Type A *on page 253*
- ♦ B-type Natriuretic Peptide (Human) *see* Nesiritide *on page 1216*
- ♦ Bubbli-Pred™ *see* PrednisoLONE *on page 1399*
- ♦ Budeprion™ SR *see* BuPROPion *on page 273*

Budesonide (byoo DES oh nide)

U.S. Brand Names Entocort™ EC; Pulmicort Respules®; Pulmicort Turbuhaler®; Rhinocort® Aqua®

Pharmacologic Category Corticosteroid, Inhalant (Oral); Corticosteroid, Nasal; Corticosteroid, Systemic

Use

Intranasal: Children ≥6 years of age and Adults: Management of symptoms of seasonal or perennial rhinitis

Nebulization: Children 12 months to 8 years: Maintenance and prophylactic treatment of asthma

Oral capsule: Treatment of active Crohn's disease (mild to moderate) involving the ileum and/or ascending colon; maintenance of remission (for up to 3 months) of Crohn's disease (mild to moderate) involving the ileum and/or ascending colon

Oral inhalation: Maintenance and prophylactic treatment of asthma; includes patients who require corticosteroids and those who may benefit from systemic dose reduction/elimination

Mechanism of Action Controls the rate of protein synthesis, depresses the migration of polymorphonuclear leukocytes, fibroblasts, reverses capillary permeability, and lysosomal stabilization at the cellular level to prevent or control inflammation

Pharmacodynamics/Kinetics

Onset of action: Respules®: 2-8 days; Rhinocort® Aqua®: ~10 hours; Turbuhaler®: 24 hours

Peak effect: Respules®: 4-6 weeks; Rhinocort® Aqua®: ~2 weeks; Turbuhaler®: 1-2 weeks

Distribution: 2.2-3.9 L/kg

Protein binding: 85% to 90%

Metabolism: Hepatic via CYP3A4 to two metabolites: 16-alpha-hydroxyprednisolone and 6 beta-hydroxybudesonide; minor activity

Bioavailability: Limited by high first-pass effect; Capsule: 9% to 21%; Respules®: 6%; Turbuhaler®: 6% to 13%; Nasal: 34%

Half-life elimination: 2-3.6 hours

Time to peak: Capsule: 0.5-10 hours (variable in Crohn's disease); Respules®: 10-30 minutes; Turbuhaler®: 1-2 hours; Nasal: 1 hour

Excretion: Urine (60%) and feces as metabolites

Contraindications Hypersensitivity to budesonide or any component of the formulation

Inhalation: Contraindicated in primary treatment of status asthmaticus, acute episodes of asthma; not for relief of acute bronchospasm

Warnings/Precautions May cause hypercorticism and/or suppression of hypothalamic-pituitary-adrenal (HPA) axis, particularly in younger children or in patients receiving high doses for prolonged periods. Particular care is required when patients are transferred from systemic corticosteroids to products with lower systemic bioavailability (ie, inhalation). May lead to possible adrenal insufficiency or withdrawal from steroids, including an increase in allergic symptoms. Patients receiving prolonged therapy of ≥20 mg per day of prednisone (or equivalent) may be most susceptible. Aerosol steroids do **not** provide the systemic steroid needed to treat patients having trauma, surgery, or infections.

Controlled clinical studies have shown that orally-inhaled and intranasal corticosteroids may cause a reduction in growth velocity in pediatric patients. (In studies of orally-inhaled corticosteroids, the mean reduction in growth velocity was approximately 1 centimeter per year [range 0.3-1.8 cm per year] and appears to be related to dose and duration of exposure.) To minimize the systemic effects of orally-inhaled and intranasal corticosteroids, each patient should be titrated to the lowest effective dose. Growth should be routinely monitored in pediatric patients.

May suppress the immune system, patients may be more susceptible to infection. Use with caution in patients with systemic infections or ocular herpes simplex. Avoid exposure to chickenpox and measles. Corticosteroids should be used with caution in patients with diabetes, hypertension, osteoporosis, peptic ulcer, glaucoma, cataracts, or tuberculosis. Use caution in hepatic impairment. Enteric-coated capsules should not be crushed or chewed.

Drug Interactions Substrate of CYP3A4 (major)

Cimetidine: Decreased clearance and increased bioavailability of budesonide

CYP3A4 inhibitors: Serum level and/or toxicity of budesonide may be increased; this effect was shown with ketoconazole, but not erythromycin. Other potential inhibitors include amiodarone, cimetidine, clarithromycin, delavirdine, diltiazem, dirithromycin, disulfiram, fluoxetine, fluvoxamine, grapefruit juice, indinavir, itraconazole, ketoconazole, nefazodone, nevirapine, propoxyphene, quinupristin-dalfopristin, ritonavir, saquinavir, telithromycin, verapamil, zafirlukast, zileuton.

Proton pump inhibitors (omeprazole, pantoprazole, rabeprazole): Theoretically, alteration of gastric pH may affect the rate of dissolution of enteric-coated capsules. Administration with omeprazole did not alter kinetics of budesonide capsules.

Salmeterol: The addition of salmeterol has been demonstrated to improve response to inhaled corticosteroids (as compared to increasing steroid dosage).

Nutritional/Herbal/Ethanol Interactions

Food: Grapefruit juice may double systemic exposure of orally-administered budesonide. Administration of capsules with a high-fat meal delays peak concentration, but does not alter the extent of absorption.

Herb/Nutraceutical: St John's wort may decrease budesonide levels.

Adverse Reactions Reaction severity varies by dose and duration; not all adverse reactions have been reported with each dosage form.

>10%:

- Central nervous system: Headache (up to 21%)
- Gastrointestinal: Nausea (up to 11%)
- Respiratory: Respiratory infection, rhinitis
- Miscellaneous: Symptoms of HPA axis suppression and/or hypercorticism may occur in >10% of patients following administration of dosage forms which result in higher systemic exposure (ie, oral capsule), but may be less frequent than rates observed with comparator drugs (prednisolone). These symptoms may be rare (<1%) following administration via methods which result in lower exposures (topical).

1% to 10%:

- Cardiovascular: Chest pain, edema, flushing, hypertension, palpitation, syncope, tachycardia
- Central nervous system: Dizziness, dysphonia, emotional lability, fatigue, fever, insomnia, migraine, nervousness, pain, vertigo
- Dermatologic: Acne, alopecia, bruising, contact dermatitis, eczema, hirsutism, pruritus, pustular rash, rash, striae
- Endocrine & metabolic: Adrenal insufficiency, hypokalemia, menstrual disorder
- Gastrointestinal: Abdominal pain, anorexia, diarrhea, dry mouth, dyspepsia, flatulence, gastroenteritis, oral candidiasis, taste perversion, vomiting, weight gain
- Genitourinary: Dysuria, hematuria, nocturia, pyuria
- Hematologic: Cervical lymphadenopathy, leukocytosis, purpura
- Hepatic: Alkaline increased
- Neuromuscular & skeletal: Arthralgia, back pain, fracture, hyperkinesis, hypertonia, myalgia, neck pain, weakness, paresthesia

(Continued)

Budesonide *(Continued)*

Ocular: Conjunctivitis, eye infection

Otic: Earache, ear infection, external ear infection

Respiratory: Bronchitis, bronchospasm, cough, epistaxis, nasal irritation, pharyngitis, sinusitis, stridor

Miscellaneous: Abscess, allergic reaction, c-reactive protein increased, erythrocyte sedimentation rate increased; fat distribution (moon face, buffalo hump); flu-like syndrome, herpes simplex, infection, moniliasis, viral infection, voice alteration

<1% (Limited to important or life-threatening): Aggressive reactions, alopecia, angioedema, avascular necrosis of the femoral head, benign intracranial hypertension, depression, dyspnea, growth suppression, hoarseness, hypersensitivity reactions (immediate and delayed; include rash, contact dermatitis, angioedema, bronchospasm), intermenstrual bleeding, irritability, nasal septum perforation, osteoporosis, psychosis, somnolence

Overdosage/Toxicology

Inhaled formulations: Symptoms of overdose include irritation and burning of the nasal mucosa, sneezing, intranasal and pharyngeal *Candida* infections, nasal ulceration, epistaxis, rhinorrhea, nasal stuffiness, headache.

When consumed in excessive quantities, systemic hypercorticism and adrenal suppression may occur, in those cases discontinuation and withdrawal of the corticosteroid should be done judiciously. Treatment should be symptomatic and supportive.

Dosing

Adults & Elderly:

Asthma: Inhalation: 1- to 4-inhalations twice daily using Pulmicort Turbuhaler® device; maintenance therapy may be gradually reduced to a single daily inhalation. See table.

Budesonide

Previous Therapy	Recommended Starting Dose	Highest Recommended Dose
Bronchodilators alone	200-400 mcg twice daily	400 mcg twice daily
Inhaled corticosteroids[1]	200-400 mcg twice daily	800 mcg twice daily
Oral corticosteroids	400-800 mcg twice daily	800 mcg twice daily

[1]In patients with mild-to-moderate asthma who are well controlled on inhaled corticosteroids, dosing with Pulmicort® Turbuhaler® 200 mcg or 400 mcg once daily may be considered. Pulmicort® Turbuhaler® can be administered once daily either in the morning or in the evening.

Crohn's disease (active): Oral: 9 mg once daily in the morning for up to 8 weeks; recurring episodes may be treated with a repeat 8-week course of treatment

Note: Patients receiving CYP3A4 inhibitors should be monitored closely for signs and symptoms of hypercorticism; dosage reduction may be required. If switching from oral prednisolone, prednisolone dosage should be tapered while budesonide (Entocort™ EC) treatment is initiated.

Crohn's disease, maintenance of remission: Following treatment of active disease (control of symptoms with CDAI <150), treatment may be continued at a dosage of 6 mg once daily for up to 3 months. If symptom control is maintained for 3 months, tapering of the dosage to complete cessation is recommended. Continued dosing beyond 3 months has not been demonstrated to result in substantial benefit.

Rhinitis: Nasal inhalation (Rhinocort® Aqua®): 64 mcg/day as a single 32 mcg spray in each nostril. Some patients who do not achieve adequate control may benefit from increased dosage. A reduced dosage may be effective after initial control is achieved.

Maximum dose: Children <12 years: 129 mcg/day; Adults: 256 mcg/day

Pediatrics:

Asthma:

Nasal inhalation: ≥6 years: Refer to adult dosing.

Oral inhalation: ≥6 years:

Previous therapy of bronchodilators alone: 200 mcg twice initially which may be increased up to 400 mcg twice daily

Previous therapy of inhaled corticosteroids: 200 mcg twice initially which may be increased up to 400 mcg twice daily

Previous therapy of oral corticosteroids: The highest recommended dose in children is 400 mcg twice daily

NIH Guidelines (NIH, 1997) (give in divided doses twice daily):

"Low" dose: 100-200 mcg/day

"Medium" dose: 200-400 mcg/day (1-2 inhalations/day)

"High" dose: >400 mcg/day (>2 inhalation/day)

Nebulization: Children 12 months to 8 years: Pulmicort Respules®: Titrate to lowest effective dose once patient is stable; start at 0.25 mg/day or use as follows:

Previous therapy of bronchodilators alone: 0.5 mg/day administered as a single dose or divided twice daily (maximum daily dose: 0.5 mg)

Previous therapy of inhaled corticosteroids: 0.5 mg/day administered as a single dose or divided twice daily (maximum daily dose: 1 mg)

Previous therapy of oral corticosteroids: 1 mg/day administered as a single dose or divided twice daily (maximum daily dose: 1 mg)

Hepatic Impairment: Monitor closely for signs and symptoms of hypercorticism; dosage reduction may be required.

Available Dosage Forms

Capsule, enteric coated (Entocort™ EC): 3 mg

Powder for oral inhalation (Pulmicort Turbuhaler®): 200 mcg/inhalation (104 g) [delivers ~160 mcg/inhalation; 200 metered doses]

Additional dosage strengths available in Canada: 100 mcg/inhalation, 400 mcg/inhalation

Suspension, nasal spray (Rhinocort® Aqua®): 32 mcg/inhalation (8.6 g) [120 metered doses]

Suspension for oral inhalation (Pulmicort Respules®): 0.25 mg/2 mL (30s), 0.5 mg/2 mL (30s)

Nursing Guidelines

Assessment: Monitor therapeutic effectiveness and adverse reactions. When changing from systemic steroids to inhalational steroids, taper reduction of systemic medication slowly (may take several months). Growth should be routinely monitored in pediatric patients. Assess knowledge/teach patient appropriate use, interventions to reduce side effects, and adverse symptoms to report.

Dietary Considerations: Avoid grapefruit juice when using oral capsules.

Patient Education: Use as directed; do not increase dosage or discontinue abruptly without consulting prescriber. May be more susceptible to infection; avoid exposure to chickenpox and measles unless immunity has been established. If exposure to measles or chickenpox occurs, notify your prescriber immediately. Report acute nervousness or inability to sleep; severe sneezing or nosebleed; respiratory difficulty, sore throat, hoarseness, or bronchitis; respiratory difficulty or bronchospasms; disturbed menstrual pattern; vision changes; loss of taste or smell perception; or worsening of condition or lack of improvement. **Pregnancy/breast-feeding precautions:** Inform prescriber if you are or intend to become pregnant. Consult prescriber if breast-feeding.

Oral capsule: Swallow whole; do not crush or chew capsule.

Inhalation/nebulization: This is not a bronchodilator and will not relieve acute asthma attacks. It may take several days for you to realize full effects of treatment. If you are also using an inhaled bronchodilator, wait 10 minutes before using this steroid aerosol. Take 5-10 deep breaths. Use inhaler on inspiration. Hold breath for 5-10 seconds after inhalation. Allow 1 full minute between inhalations. You may experience dizziness, anxiety, or blurred vision (rise slowly from sitting or lying position and use caution when driving or engaging in tasks requiring alertness until response to drug is known); or taste disturbance or aftertaste (frequent mouth care and mouth rinses may help). Rinse mouth with water following oral treatments to decrease risk of oral candidiasis (wash face if using a face mask).

Geriatric Considerations: Ensure that patients can correctly use nasal inhaler.

Pregnancy Risk Factor: C/B (Pulmicort Respules® and Turbuhaler®, Rhinocort® Aqua®)

Pregnancy Issues: There are no adequate and well-controlled studies in pregnant women; use only if potential benefit to the mother outweighs the possible risk to the fetus. Hypoadrenalism has been reported in infants.

(Continued)

Budesonide *(Continued)*

Lactation: Enters breast milk/use caution

Administration

Oral: Oral capsule: Capsule should be swallowed whole; do not crush or chew.

Storage:

Nebulizer: Store upright at 20°C to 25°C (68°F to 77°F) and protect from light. Do not refrigerate or freeze. Once aluminum package is opened, solution should be used within 2 weeks. Continue to protect from light.

Nasal inhaler: Store with valve up at 15°C to 30°C (59°F to 86°F). Use within 6 months after opening aluminum pouch. Protect from high humidity.

Nasal spray: Store with valve up at 20°C to 25°C (68°F to 77°F) and protect from light. Do not freeze.

- ♦ **Bufferin® [OTC]** *see* Aspirin *on page 189*
- ♦ **Bufferin® Extra Strength [OTC]** *see* Aspirin *on page 189*
- ♦ **Buffinol [OTC]** *see* Aspirin *on page 189*
- ♦ **Buffinol Extra [OTC]** *see* Aspirin *on page 189*

Bumetanide (byoo MET a nide)

U.S. Brand Names Bumex®

Pharmacologic Category Diuretic, Loop

Medication Safety Issues

Sound-alike/look-alike issues:

Bumetanide may be confused with Buminate®

Bumex® may be confused with Brevibloc®, Buprenex®, Permax®

Use Management of edema secondary to congestive heart failure or hepatic or renal disease including nephrotic syndrome; may be used alone or in combination with antihypertensives in the treatment of hypertension; can be used in furosemide-allergic patients

Mechanism of Action Inhibits reabsorption of sodium and chloride in the ascending loop of Henle and proximal renal tubule, interfering with the chloride-binding cotransport system, thus causing increased excretion of water, sodium, chloride, magnesium, phosphate and calcium; it does not appear to act on the distal tubule

Pharmacodynamics/Kinetics

Onset of action: Oral, I.M.: 0.5-1 hour; I.V.: 2-3 minutes

Duration: 4-6 hours

Distribution: V_d: 13-25 L/kg

Protein binding: 95%

Metabolism: Partially hepatic

Half-life elimination: Neonates: ~6 hours; Infants (1 month): ~2.4 hours; Adults: 1-1.5 hours

Excretion: Primarily urine (as unchanged drug and metabolites)

Contraindications Hypersensitivity to bumetanide, any component of the formulation, or sulfonylureas; anuria; patients with hepatic coma or in states of severe electrolyte depletion until the condition improves or is corrected; pregnancy (based on expert analysis)

Warnings/Precautions Adjust dose to avoid dehydration. In cirrhosis, avoid electrolyte and acid/base imbalances that might lead to hepatic encephalopathy. Ototoxicity is associated with I.V. rapid administration, renal impairment, excessive doses, and concurrent use of other ototoxins. Hypersensitivity reactions can rarely occur. Monitor fluid status and renal function in an attempt to prevent oliguria, azotemia, and reversible increases in BUN and creatinine. Close medical supervision of aggressive diuresis required. Watch for and correct electrolyte disturbances. Coadministration of antihypertensives may increase the risk of hypotension.

Chemical similarities are present among sulfonamides, sulfonylureas, carbonic anhydrase inhibitors, thiazides, and loop diuretics (except ethacrynic acid). Use in patients with sulfonylurea allergy is specifically contraindicated in product labeling, however, a risk of cross-reaction exists in patients with allergy to any of these compounds; avoid use when previous reaction has been severe.

Loop diuretics are potent diuretics; excess amounts can lead to profound diuresis with fluid and electrolyte loss; close medical supervision and dose evaluation is required; *in vitro* studies using pooled sera from critically-ill neonates have shown bumetanide to be a potent displacer of bilirubin; avoid use in neonates at risk for kernicterus.

Drug Interactions

ACE inhibitors: Hypotensive effects and/or renal effects are potentiated by hypovolemia.

Antidiabetic agents: Glucose tolerance may be decreased.

Antihypertensive agents: Hypotensive effects may be enhanced.

Cholestyramine or colestipol may reduce bioavailability of bumetanide.

Digoxin: Bumetanide-induced hypokalemia may predispose to digoxin toxicity; monitor potassium.

Indomethacin (and other NSAIDs) may reduce natriuretic and hypotensive effects of diuretics.

Lithium: Renal clearance may be reduced. Isolated reports of lithium toxicity have occurred; monitor lithium levels.

NSAIDs: Risk of renal impairment may increase when used in conjunction with diuretics.

Ototoxic drugs (aminoglycosides, cis-platinum): Concomitant use of bumetanide may increase risk of ototoxicity, especially in patients with renal dysfunction.

Peripheral adrenergic-blocking drugs or ganglionic blockers: Effects may be increased.

Salicylates (high-dose) with diuretics may predispose patients to salicylate toxicity due to reduced renal excretion or alter renal function.

Thiazides: Synergistic diuretic effects occur.

Nutritional/Herbal/Ethanol Interactions Herb/Nutraceutical: Avoid ephedra, yohimbe, ginseng (may worsen hypertension). Avoid dong quai if using for hypertension (has estrogenic activity). Avoid garlic (may have increased antihypertensive effect).

Adverse Reactions

>10%:

- Endocrine & metabolic: Hyperuricemia (18%), hypochloremia (15%), hypokalemia (15%)
- Renal: Azotemia (11%)

1% to 10%:

- Central nervous system: Dizziness (1%)
- Endocrine & metabolic: Hyponatremia (9%), hyperglycemia (7%), variations in phosphorus (5%), CO_2 content (4%), bicarbonate (3%), and calcium (2%)
- Neuromuscular & skeletal: Muscle cramps (1%)
- Otic: Ototoxicity (1%)
- Renal: Increased serum creatinine (7%)

<1% (Limited to important or life-threatening): Asterixis, dehydration, encephalopathy, hypernatremia, hypotension, impaired hearing, orthostatic hypotension, pruritus, rash, renal failure, vertigo, vomiting

Overdosage/Toxicology Symptoms of overdose include electrolyte depletion and volume depletion. Treatment is symptomatic and supportive.

Dosing

Adults:

Edema:

Oral: 0.5-2 mg/dose (maximum dose: 10 mg/day) 1-2 times/day

I.M., I.V.: 0.5-1 mg/dose; may repeat in 2-3 hours for up to 2 doses if needed (maximum dose: 10 mg/day)

Continuous I.V. infusion: Initial: 1 mg load then 0.5-2 mg/hour (ACC/AHA 2005 practice guidelines for chronic heart failure)

Hypertension: Oral: 0.5 mg daily (maximum dose: 5 mg/day)

Usual dosage range (JNC 7): 0.5-2 mg/day in 2 divided doses

Elderly: Initial: Oral: 0.5 mg once daily, increase as necessary.

Pediatrics: Edema (diuresis); Not FDA-approved for use in children <18 years of age:

<6 months: Dose not established

>6 months:

Oral: Initial: 0.015 mg/kg/dose once daily or every other day; maximum dose: 0.1 mg/kg/day

I.M., I.V.: Dose not established

Available Dosage Forms

Injection, solution: 0.25 mg/mL (2 mL, 4 mL, 10 mL) [contains benzyl alcohol]

Tablet (Bumex®): 0.5 mg, 1 mg, 2 mg

Nursing Guidelines

Assessment: See Contraindications and Warnings/Precautions for use cautions (especially with I.V. administration). Assess potential for interactions with other prescriptions, OTC medications, or herbal products patient may be

(Continued)

Bumetanide *(Continued)*

taking (see Drug Interactions). Blood pressure, weight, and fluid status should be monitored at beginning of therapy and periodically during therapy. Glucose levels for patients with diabetes should be monitored closely (glucose tolerance may be decreased by loop diuretics, requiring adjustment of hypoglycemic agents). Assess results of laboratory tests (see below), therapeutic effectiveness, and adverse effects (see Adverse Reactions and Overdose/Toxicology). Teach patient proper use, possible side effects/appropriate interventions, and adverse symptoms to report (see Patient Education). **Pregnancy risk factor C/D** - see Pregnancy Risk Factor for use cautions; benefits of use should outweigh possible risks. Note breast-feeding caution.

Monitoring Laboratory Tests: Serum electrolytes, renal function

Dietary Considerations: May require increased intake of potassium-rich foods.

Patient Education: Inform prescriber of all prescriptions, OTC medications, or herbal products you are taking, and any allergies you have. Do not take any new medication during therapy unless approved by prescriber. May be taken with food to reduce GI effects. If taking one dose daily, take single dose early in day; if taking twice daily, take last dose early in afternoon to prevent sleep interruptions. Include orange juice or bananas (or other sources of potassium-rich foods) in your daily diet but do not take supplemental potassium without consulting prescriber. If you have diabetes, monitor glucose levels closely (glucose tolerance may be decreased by loop diuretics) and notify prescriber of noted changes (hypoglycemic agent may need to be adjusted). May cause dizziness, hypotension, lightheadedness, or weakness (use caution when changing position from sitting or lying position, when driving, exercising, climbing stairs, or performing hazardous tasks until response to drug is known). Report palpitations or chest pain; swelling of ankles or feet, weight increase or decrease (>3 lb in any one day), increased fatigue, muscle cramps or trembling, and any changes in hearing. **Pregnancy/breast-feeding precautions:** Inform prescriber if you are or intend to become pregnant; contraceptives may be recommended. Consult prescriber if breast-feeding.

Geriatric Considerations: See Warnings/Precautions. Severe loss of sodium and/or increases in BUN can cause confusion. For any change in mental status in patients on bumetanide, monitor electrolytes and renal function.

Pregnancy Risk Factor: C (manufacturer); D (expert analysis)

Lactation: Excretion in breast milk unknown/use caution

Perioperative/Anesthesia/Other Concerns: If given the morning of surgery, it may render the patient volume depleted and blood pressure may be labile during general anesthesia.

Patients with impaired hepatic function must be monitored carefully, often requiring reduced doses. Larger doses may be necessary in patients with impaired renal function to obtain the same therapeutic response.

It is important that patients be closely followed for hypokalemia, hypomagnesemia, and volume depletion because of significant diuresis.

Administration

I.V.: Administer I.V. slowly, over 1-2 minutes; an alternate-day schedule or a 3-4 daily dosing regimen with rest periods of 1-2 days in between may be the most tolerable and effective regimen for the continued control of edema; reserve I.V. administration for those unable to take oral medications

Compatibility: Stable in D_5W, NS, LR

Y-site administration: Incompatible with midazolam

Compatibility when admixed: Incompatible with dobutamine, milrinone

Storage:

I.V.: Store vials at 15°C to 30°C (59°F to 86°F). Infusion solutions should be used within 24 hours after preparation; light sensitive, discoloration may occur when exposed to light.

Tablet: Store at 15°C to 30°C (59°F to 86°F).

♦ **Bumex®** *see* Bumetanide *on page 264*

♦ **Buminate®** *see* Albumin *on page 94*

Bupivacaine (byoo PIV a kane)

U.S. Brand Names Marcaine®; Marcaine® Spinal; Sensorcaine®; Sensorcaine®-MPF

Synonyms Bupivacaine Hydrochloride

Pharmacologic Category Local Anesthetic

Medication Safety Issues

Sound-alike/look-alike issues:

Bupivacaine may be confused with mepivacaine, ropivacaine

Marcaine® may be confused with Narcan®

Use Local anesthetic (injectable) for peripheral nerve block, infiltration, sympathetic block, caudal or epidural block, retrobulbar block

Mechanism of Action Blocks both the initiation and conduction of nerve impulses by decreasing the neuronal membrane's permeability to sodium ions, which results in inhibition of depolarization with resultant blockade of conduction

Pharmacodynamics/Kinetics

Onset of action: Anesthesia (route and dose dependent): 1-17 minutes

Duration (route and dose dependent): 2-9 hours

Protein binding: ~95%

Metabolism: Hepatic; forms metabolite (PPX)

Half-life elimination (age dependent): Neonates: 8.1 hours; Adults: 1.5-5.5 hours

Excretion: Urine (~6% unchanged)

Contraindications Hypersensitivity to bupivacaine hydrochloride, amide-type local anesthetics or any component of the formulation; obstetrical paracervical block anesthesia

Warnings/Precautions Use with caution in patients with hepatic impairment. Not recommended for use in children <12 years of age. The solution for spinal anesthesia should not be used in children <18 years of age. **Do not use solutions containing preservatives for caudal or epidural block.** Local anesthetics have been associated with rare occurrences of sudden respiratory arrest; convulsions due to systemic toxicity leading to cardiac arrest have also been reported, presumably following unintentional intravascular injection. The 0.75% is **not** recommended for obstetrical anesthesia. A test dose is recommended prior to epidural administration (prior to initial dose) and all reinforcing doses with continuous catheter technique. Use caution with cardiovascular dysfunction. Use caution in debilitated, elderly or acutely ill patients; dose reduction may be required.

Drug Interactions Substrate (minor) of CYP1A2, 2C19, 2D6, 3A4

Adverse Reactions Frequency not defined.

Cardiovascular: Cardiac arrest, hypotension, bradycardia, palpitation

Central nervous system: Seizures, restlessness, anxiety, dizziness

Gastrointestinal: Nausea, vomiting

Neuromuscular & skeletal: Weakness

Ocular: Blurred vision

Otic: Tinnitus

Respiratory: Apnea

Overdosage/Toxicology Treatment is symptomatic and supportive. Termination of anesthesia by pneumatic tourniquet inflation should be attempted when bupivacaine is administered by infiltration or regional injection. Treatment is symptomatic and supportive. Methemoglobinemia should be treated with methylene blue 1-2 mg/kg in a 1% sterile aqueous solution by I.V. push over 4-6 minutes, repeated up to a total dose of 7 mg/kg.

Dosing

Adults & Elderly: Note: Dose varies with procedure, depth of anesthesia, vascularity of tissues, duration of anesthesia and condition of patient. Do not use solutions containing preservatives for caudal or epidural block.

Local anesthesia: Infiltration: 0.25% infiltrated locally; maximum: 175 mg

Caudal block (preservative free): 15-30 mL of 0.25% or 0.5%

Epidural block (other than caudal block; preservative free): Administer in 3-5 mL increments, allowing sufficient time to detect toxic manifestations of inadvertent I.V. or I.T. administration: 10-20 mL of 0.25% or 0.5%

Surgical procedures requiring a high degree of muscle relaxation and prolonged effects **only**: 10-20 mL of 0.75% (**Note:** Not to be used in obstetrical cases)

Peripheral nerve block: 5 mL of 0.25 or 0.5%; maximum: 400 mg/day

Sympathetic nerve block: 20-50 mL of 0.25%

Retrobulbar anesthesia: 2-4 mL of 0.75%

Spinal anesthesia: Preservative free solution of 0.75% bupivacaine in 8.25% dextrose:

Lower extremity and perineal procedures: 1 mL

Lower abdominal procedures: 1.6 mL

(Continued)

Bupivacaine *(Continued)*

Normal vaginal delivery: 0.8 mL (higher doses may be required in some patients)

Cesarean section: 1-1.4 mL

Pediatrics: Note: Dose varies with procedure, depth of anesthesia, vascularity of tissues, duration of anesthesia and condition of patient. Do not use solutions containing preservatives for caudal or epidural block.

Caudal block, epidural block, local anesthesia: Children >12 years: Refer to adult dosing.

Peripheral or sympathetic nerve block: Children >12 years: Refer to adult dosing.

Retrobulbar anesthesia: Children >12 years: Refer to adult dosing.

Available Dosage Forms

Injection, solution, as hydrochloride [preservative free]: 0.25% [2.5 mg/mL] (10 mL, 20 mL, 30 mL, 50 mL); 0.5% [5 mg/mL] (10 mL, 20 mL, 30 mL); 0.75% [7.5 mg/mL] (10 mL, 20 mL, 30 mL)

Marcaine®: 0.25% [2.5 mg/mL] (10 mL, 30 mL); 0.5% [5 mg/mL] (10 mL, 30 mL); 0.75% [7.5 mg/mL] (10 mL, 30 mL)

Marcaine® Spinal: 0.75% [7.5 mg/mL] (2 mL) [in dextrose 8.25%]

Sensorcaine®-MPF: 0.25% [2.5 mg/mL] (10 mL, 30 mL); 0.5% [5 mg/mL] (10 mL, 30 mL); 0.75% [7.5 mg/mL] (10 mL, 30 mL)

Injection, solution, as hydrochloride (Marcaine®, Sensorcaine®): 0.25% [2.5 mg/mL] (50 mL); 0.5% [5 mg/mL] (50 mL) [contains methylparaben]

Nursing Guidelines

Assessment: Assess other medications patient may be taking for additive or adverse interactions. Monitor for effectiveness of anesthesia and adverse reactions. Monitor for return of sensation. Teach patient adverse reactions to report; use and teach appropriate interventions to promote safety.

Patient Education: This medication is given to reduce sensation in the injected area. You will experience decreased sensation to pain, heat, or cold in the area and/or decreased muscle strength (depending on area of application) until the effects wear off; use necessary caution to reduce incidence of possible injury until full sensation returns. If used in mouth, do not eat or drink until full sensation returns. Immediately report chest pain or palpitations; increased restlessness, anxiety, or dizziness; skeletal or muscle weakness; respiratory difficulty; ringing in ears; or vision changes. **Pregnancy/breast-feeding precautions:** Inform prescriber if you are pregnant. Do not breast-feed.

Pregnancy Risk Factor: C

Pregnancy Issues: Bupivacaine is approved for use at term in obstetrical anesthesia or analgesia. Bupivacaine 0.75% solutions have been associated with cardiac arrest following epidural anesthesia in obstetrical patients and use of this concentration is not recommended for this purpose. Use in obstetrical paracervical block anesthesia is contraindicated.

Lactation: Enters breast milk/not recommended

Administration

Compatibility: Stable in NS

Storage: Store at controlled room temperature of 15°C to 30°C (59°F to 86°F).

Related Information

Acute Postoperative Pain *on page 1742*

Local Anesthetics *on page 1854*

Bupivacaine and Epinephrine (byoo PIV a kane & ep i NEF rin)

U.S. Brand Names Marcaine® with Epinephrine; Sensorcaine®-MPF with Epinephrine; Sensorcaine® with Epinephrine

Synonyms Epinephrine Bitartrate and Bupivacaine Hydrochloride

Pharmacologic Category Local Anesthetic

Use Local anesthetic (injectable) for peripheral nerve block, infiltration, sympathetic block, caudal or epidural block, retrobulbar block

Mechanism of Action Local anesthetics bind selectively to the intracellular surface of sodium channels to block influx of sodium into the axon. As a result, depolarization necessary for action potential propagation and subsequent nerve function is prevented. The block at the sodium channel is reversible. When drug diffuses away from the axon, sodium channel function is restored and nerve propagation returns.

Epinephrine prolongs the duration of the anesthetic actions of bupivacaine by causing vasoconstriction (alpha adrenergic receptor agonist) of the vasculature surrounding the nerve axons. This prevents the diffusion of bupivacaine away from the nerves resulting in a longer retention in the axon

Pharmacodynamics/Kinetics Refer to bupivacaine monograph; epinephrine reduces the rate of absorption and peak plasma concentration of bupivacaine

Contraindications Hypersensitivity to bupivacaine, epinephrine, amide-type local anesthetics, or any component of the formulation

Warnings/Precautions Some commercially available formulations contain sodium metabisulfite, which may cause allergic-type reactions. Do not use solutions containing preservatives for caudal or epidural block. Local anesthetics have been associated with rare occurrences of sudden respiratory arrest; convulsions due to systemic toxicity leading to cardiac arrest have also been reported, presumably following unintentional intravascular injection. The 0.75% is not recommended for obstetrical anesthesia. A test dose is recommended prior to epidural administration and all reinforcing doses with continuous catheter technique. Use caution with cardiovascular dysfunction, hepatic impairment, or patients with compromised blood supply. Use caution in debilitated, elderly or acutely ill patients; dose reduction may be required. Not recommended for use in children <12 years of age.

Drug Interactions Bupivacaine: **Substrate** (minor) of CYP1A2, 2C19, 2D6, 3A4

Also see individual agents.

Adverse Reactions See individual agents.

Dosing

Adults & Elderly: Dose varies with procedure, depth of anesthesia, vascularity of tissues, duration of anesthesia, and condition of patient. Do not use solutions containing preservatives for caudal or epidural block.

Caudal block (preservative free): 15-30 mL of 0.25% or 0.5%

Epidural block (other than caudal block, preservative free):10-20 mL of 0.25% or 0.5%. Administer in 3-5 mL increments, allowing sufficient time to detect toxic manifestations of inadvertent I.V. or I.T. administration.

Surgical procedures requiring a high degree of muscle relaxation and prolonged effects only: 10-20 mL of 0.75% (**Note:** Not to be used in obstetrical cases)

Local anesthesia: Infiltration: 0.25% infiltrated locally (maximum: 175 mg of bupivacaine)

Peripheral nerve block: 5 mL of 0.25 or 0.5% (maximum: 400 mg/day of bupivacaine)

Retrobulbar anesthesia: 2-4 mL of 0.75%

Sympathetic nerve block: 20-50 mL of 0.25%

Infiltration and nerve block in maxillary and mandibular area: 9 mg (1.8 mL) of bupivacaine as a 0.5% solution with epinephrine 1:200,000 per injection site. A second dose may be administered if necessary to produce adequate anesthesia after allowing up to 10 minutes for onset. Up to a maximum of 90 mg of bupivacaine hydrochloride per dental appointment. The effective anesthetic dose varies with procedure, intensity of anesthesia needed, duration of anesthesia required, and physical condition of the patient; always use the lowest effective dose along with careful aspiration.

The following numbers of dental carpules (1.8 mL) provide the indicated amounts of bupivacaine hydrochloride 0.5% and vasoconstrictor (epinephrine 1:200,000): See table.

# of Cartridges (1.8 mL)	mg Bupivacaine (0.5%)	mg Vasoconstrictor (Epinephrine 1:200,000)
1	9	0.009
2	18	0.018
3	27	0.027
4	36	0.036
5	45	0.045
6	54	0.054
7	63	0.063
8	72	0.072
9	81	0.081
10	90	0.090

(Continued)

Bupivacaine and Epinephrine *(Continued)*

Note: Adult and children doses of bupivacaine hydrochloride with epinephrine cited from USP Dispensing Information (USP DI), 17th ed, The United States Pharmacopeial Convention, Inc, Rockville, MD, 1997, 134.

Pediatrics:

Children >12 years: Refer to adult dosing.

Available Dosage Forms

Injection, solution [preservative free]: Bupivacaine hydrochloride 0.25% and epinephrine bitartrate 1:200,000 (10 mL, 30 mL); bupivacaine hydrochloride 0.5% and epinephrine bitartrate 1:200,000 (10 mL, 30 mL)

Marcaine® with Epinephrine Preservative Free: Bupivacaine hydrochloride 0.25% and epinephrine bitartrate 1:200,000 (10 mL, 30 mL) [contains sodium metabisulfite]; bupivacaine hydrochloride 0.5% and epinephrine bitartrate 1:200,000 (1.8 mL, 3 mL, 10mL, 30 mL) [contains sodium metabisulfite]; bupivacaine hydrochloride 0.75% and epinephrine bitartrate 1:200,000 (30 mL) [contains sodium metabisulfite]

Sensorcaine® MPF with Epinephrine: Bupivacaine hydrochloride 0.25% and epinephrine bitartrate 1:200,000 (10 mL, 30 mL) [contains sodium metabisulfite]; bupivacaine hydrochloride 0.5% and epinephrine bitartrate 1:200,000 (10 mL, 30 mL) [contains sodium metabisulfite]

Injection, solution: Bupivacaine hydrochloride 0.25% and epinephrine bitartrate 1:200,000 (50 mL); bupivacaine hydrochloride 0.5% and epinephrine bitartrate 1:200,000 (50 mL)

Marcaine® with Epinephrine, Sensorcaine® with Epinephrine: Bupivacaine hydrochloride 0.25% and epinephrine bitartrate 1:200,000 (50 mL) [contains methylparaben]; bupivacaine hydrochloride 0.5% and epinephrine bitartrate 1:200,000 (50 mL) [contains methylparaben]

Nursing Guidelines

Pregnancy Risk Factor: C

Lactation: Enters breast milk/not recommended

Administration

Storage: Store at controlled room temperature of 15°C to 30°C (59° to 86°F) and protect from light. Do not autoclave.

♦ **Bupivacaine Hydrochloride** *see* Bupivacaine *on page 266*

♦ **Buprenex®** *see* Buprenorphine *on page 270*

Buprenorphine (byoo pre NOR feen)

U.S. Brand Names Buprenex®; Subutex®

Synonyms Buprenorphine Hydrochloride

Pharmacologic Category Analgesic, Narcotic

Medication Safety Issues

Sound-alike/look-alike issues:

Buprenex® may be confused with Brevibloc®, Bumex®

Use

Injection: Management of moderate to severe pain

Tablet: Treatment of opioid dependence

Unlabeled/Investigational Use Injection: Heroin and opioid withdrawal

Mechanism of Action Buprenorphine exerts its analgesic effect via high affinity binding to μ opiate receptors in the CNS; displays both agonist and antagonist activity

Pharmacodynamics/Kinetics

Onset of action: Analgesic: 10-30 minutes

Duration: 6-8 hours

Absorption: I.M., SubQ: 30% to 40%

Distribution: V_d: 97-187 L/kg

Protein binding: High

Metabolism: Primarily hepatic; extensive first-pass effect

Half-life elimination: 2.2-3 hours

Excretion: Feces (70%); urine (20% as unchanged drug)

Contraindications Hypersensitivity to buprenorphine or any component of the formulation

Warnings/Precautions An opioid-containing analgesic regimen should be tailored to each patient's needs and based upon the type of pain being treated (acute versus chronic), the route of administration, degree of tolerance for opioids (naive versus chronic user), age, weight, and medical condition. The optimal analgesic dose varies widely among patients. Doses should be titrated to pain relief/prevention.

May cause respiratory depression - use caution in patients with respiratory disease or pre-existing respiratory depression. Potential for drug dependency exists, abrupt cessation may precipitate withdrawal. Use caution in elderly, debilitated, or pediatric patients. Use with caution in patients with depression or suicidal tendencies, or in patients with a history of drug abuse. Tolerance, psychological and physical dependence may occur with prolonged use. Use with caution in patients with hepatic, pulmonary, or renal function impairment. May cause CNS depression, which may impair physical or mental abilities. Patients must be cautioned about performing tasks which require mental alertness (eg, operating machinery or driving). Effects with other sedative drugs or ethanol may be potentiated. Elderly may be more sensitive to CNS depressant and constipating effects. Use with caution in patients with head injury or increased ICP, biliary tract dysfunction, pancreatitis, patients with history of ileus or bowel obstruction, glaucoma, hyperthyroidism, adrenal insufficiency, prostatic hyperplasia, urinary stricture, CNS depression, toxic psychosis, alcoholism, delirium tremens, or kyphoscoliosis. Partial antagonist activity may precipitate acute narcotic withdrawal in opioid-dependent individuals. Tablets, which are used for induction treatment of opioid dependence, should not be started until effects of withdrawal are evident.

Drug Interactions Substrate of CYP3A4 (major); **Inhibits** CYP1A2 (weak), 2A6 (weak), 2C19 (weak), 2D6 (weak)

Cimetidine: May increase sedation from narcotic analgesics; however, histamine blockers may attenuate the cardiovascular response from histamine release associated with narcotic analgesics

CNS depressants: May produce additive respiratory and CNS depression; includes benzodiazepines, barbiturates, ethanol, and other sedatives. Respiratory and CV collapse was reported in a patient who received diazepam and buprenorphine.

CYP3A4 inducers: CYP3A4 inducers may decrease the levels/effects of buprenorphine. Example inducers include aminoglutethimide, carbamazepine, nafcillin, nevirapine, phenobarbital, phenytoin, and rifamycins.

CYP3A4 inhibitors: May increase the levels/effects of buprenorphine. Example inhibitors include azole antifungals, clarithromycin, diclofenac, doxycycline, erythromycin, imatinib, isoniazid, nefazodone, nicardipine, propofol, protease inhibitors, quinidine, and verapamil.

Naltrexone: May antagonize the effect of narcotic analgesics; concurrent use or use within 7-10 days of injection for pain relief is contraindicated

Nutritional/Herbal/Ethanol Interactions

Ethanol: Avoid ethanol (may increase CNS depression).

Herb/Nutraceutical: Avoid valerian, St John's wort, kava kava, gotu kola (may increase CNS depression).

Adverse Reactions

Injection:

>10%: Central nervous system: Sedation

1% to 10%:

Cardiovascular: Hypotension

Central nervous system: Respiratory depression, dizziness, headache

Gastrointestinal: Vomiting, nausea

Ocular: Miosis

Otic: Vertigo

Miscellaneous: Diaphoresis

<1% (Limited to important or life-threatening): Agitation, allergic reaction, apnea, appetite decreased, blurred vision, bradycardia, confusion, constipation, convulsion, coma, cyanosis, depersonalization, depression, diplopia, dyspnea, dysphoria, euphoria, fatigue, flatulence, flushing, hallucinations, hypertension, injection site reaction, malaise, nervousness, pallor, paresthesia, pruritus, psychosis, rash, slurred speech, tachycardia, tinnitus, tremor, urinary retention, urticaria, weakness, Wenckebach block, xerostomia

Tablet:

>10%:

Central nervous system: Headache (30%), pain (24%), insomnia (21% to 25%), anxiety (12%), depression (11%)

Gastrointestinal: Nausea (10% to 14%), abdominal pain (12%), constipation (8% to 11%)

Neuromuscular & skeletal: Back pain (14%), weakness (14%)

(Continued)

Buprenorphine *(Continued)*

Respiratory: Rhinitis (11%)

Miscellaneous: Withdrawal syndrome (19%; placebo 37%), infection (12% to 20%), diaphoresis (12% to 13%)

1% to 10%:

Central nervous system: Chills (6%), nervousness (6%), somnolence (5%), dizziness (4%), fever (3%)

Gastrointestinal: Vomiting (5% to 8%), diarrhea (5%), dyspepsia (3%)

Ocular: Lacrimation (5%)

Respiratory: Cough (4%), pharyngitis (4%)

Miscellaneous: Flu-like syndrome (6%)

Overdosage/Toxicology Symptoms of overdose include CNS depression, pinpoint pupils, hypotension, and bradycardia. Treatment is supportive. Naloxone may have limited effects in reversing respiratory depression; doxapram has also been used to stimulate respirations.

Dosing

Adults: Long-term use is not recommended

Note: These are guidelines and do not represent the maximum doses that may be required in all patients. Doses should be titrated to pain relief/prevention. In high-risk patients (eg, elderly, debilitated, presence of respiratory disease) and/or concurrent CNS depressant use, reduce dose by one-half. Buprenorphine has an analgesic ceiling.

Acute pain (moderate to severe):

I.M.: Initial: Opiate-naive: 0.3 mg every 6-8 hours as needed; initial dose (up to 0.3 mg) may be repeated once in 30-60 minutes after the initial dose if needed; usual dosage range: 0.15-0.6 mg every 4-8 hours as needed

Slow I.V.: Initial: Opiate-naive: 0.3 mg every 6-8 hours as needed; initial dose (up to 0.3 mg) may be repeated once in 30-60 minutes after the initial dose if needed

Heroin or opiate withdrawal (unlabeled use): I.M., slow I.V.: Variable; 0.1-0.4 mg every 6 hours

Opioid dependence: Sublingual:

Induction: Range: 12-16 mg/day (doses during an induction study used 8 mg on day 1, followed by 16 mg on day 2; induction continued over 3-4 days). Treatment should begin at least 4 hours after last use of heroin or short-acting opioid, preferably when first signs of withdrawal appear. Titrating dose to clinical effectiveness should be done as rapidly as possible to prevent undue withdrawal symptoms and patient drop-out during the induction period.

Maintenance: Target dose: 16 mg/day; range: 4-24 mg/day; patients should be switched to the buprenorphine/naloxone combination product for maintenance and unsupervised therapy

Elderly: Moderate to severe pain: I.M., slow I.V.: 0.15 mg every 6 hours; elderly patients are more likely to suffer from confusion and drowsiness compared to younger patients. **Long-term use is not recommended.**

Pediatrics:

Children 2-12 years: Moderate to severe pain: I.M., slow I.V.: 2-6 mcg/kg every 4-6 hours

Children ≥13 years: Management of moderate to severe pain or opioid dependence: Refer to adult dosing.

Available Dosage Forms

Injection, solution (Buprenex®): 0.3 mg/mL (1 mL)

Tablet, sublingual (Subutex®): 2 mg, 8 mg

Additional dosage strength available in Canada: 0.4 mg

Nursing Guidelines

Assessment: Assess other medications patient may be taking for possible additive or adverse interactions. Monitor for effectiveness of pain relief and adverse reactions or overdose (can cause respiratory depression) at beginning of therapy and at regular intervals with long-term use. For inpatients, implement safety measures. Assess knowledge/teach patient appropriate use (if self-administered). Teach patient to monitor and report adverse reactions and appropriate interventions to reduce side effects.

Monitoring Laboratory Tests: LFTs

Patient Education: If self-administered, use exactly as directed; do not increase dose or frequency. While using this medication, do not use alcohol and other prescription or OTC medications (especially sedatives, tranquilizers, antihistamines, or pain medications) without consulting prescriber. May cause dizziness, drowsiness, confusion, or blurred vision (use caution when driving, climbing stairs, rising from sitting or lying position, or engaging in tasks requiring alertness until response to drug is known). You may experience nausea or vomiting (frequent mouth care, small frequent meals, sucking lozenges, or chewing gum may help); or constipation (increased exercise, fluids, or dietary fruit and fiber may help). If constipation is unresolved, consult prescriber about use of stool softeners and/or laxatives. Report unresolved nausea or vomiting; respiratory difficulty or shortness of breath; excessive sedation or unusual weakness; or rapid heartbeat or palpitations. **Pregnancy/breast-feeding precautions:** Inform prescriber if you are or intend to become pregnant. Breast-feeding is not recommended.

Pregnancy Risk Factor: C

Pregnancy Issues: Withdrawal has been reported in infants of women receiving buprenorphine during pregnancy. Onset of symptoms ranged from day 1 to day 8 of life, most occurring on day 1.

Lactation: Enters breast milk/not recommended

Perioperative/Anesthesia/Other Concerns: Buprenorphine has a longer duration of action than either morphine or meperidine. It may precipitate withdrawal in narcotic-dependent patients. Buprenorphine is not readily reversed by naloxone. Avoid in labor.

Equivalent dosing: Buprenorphine 0.3 mg = morphine 10 mg or meperidine 75 mg I.M.

Administration

Oral: Sublingual: Tablet should be placed under the tongue until dissolved; should not be swallowed. If 2 or more tablets are needed per dose, all may be placed under the tongue at once, or 2 at a time; to ensure consistent bioavailability, subsequent doses should always be taken the same way.

I.V.: Administer slowly, over at least 2 minutes.

Compatibility: Injection:

Y-site administration: Incompatible with amphotericin B cholesteryl sulfate complex, doxorubicin liposome

Compatibility when admixed: Incompatible with diazepam, floxacillin, furosemide, lorazepam

Storage:

Injection: Protect from excessive heat of >40°C (>104°F) and light.

Tablet: Store at room temperature of 25°C (77°F).

Related Information

Narcotic / Opioid Analgesics *on page 1880*

♦ **Buprenorphine Hydrochloride** *see* Buprenorphine *on page 270*

♦ **Buproban™** *see* BuPROPion *on page 273*

BuPROPion (byoo PROE pee on)

U.S. Brand Names Budeprion™ SR; Buproban™; Wellbutrin®; Wellbutrin SR®; Wellbutrin XL™; Zyban®

Pharmacologic Category Antidepressant, Dopamine-Reuptake Inhibitor; Smoking Cessation Aid

Medication Safety Issues

Sound-alike/look-alike issues:

BuPROPion may be confused with busPIRone

Wellbutrin SR® may be confused with Wellbutrin XL™

Wellbutrin XL™ may be confused with Wellbutrin SR®

Zyban® may be confused with Zagam®

Use Treatment of depression; adjunct in smoking cessation

Unlabeled/Investigational Use Attention-deficit/hyperactivity disorder (ADHD)

Mechanism of Action Aminoketone antidepressant structurally different from all other marketed antidepressants; like other antidepressants the mechanism of bupropion's activity is not fully understood. Bupropion is a relatively weak inhibitor of the neuronal uptake of serotonin, norepinephrine, and dopamine, and does not inhibit monoamine oxidase. Metabolite inhibits the reuptake of norepinephrine. The primary mechanism of action is thought to be dopaminergic and/or noradrenergic.

Pharmacodynamics/Kinetics

Absorption: Rapid

Distribution: V_d: 19-21 L/kg

Protein binding: 82% to 88%

(Continued)

BuPROPion *(Continued)*

Metabolism: Extensively hepatic to 3 active metabolites: Hydroxybupropion, erythrohydrobupropion, threohydrobupropion (metabolite activity ranges from $^1/_5$ to $^1/_2$ potency of bupropion)

Bioavailability: 5% to 20% in animals

Half-life:

Distribution: 3-4 hours

Elimination: 21 ± 9 hours; Metabolites: Hydroxybupropion: 20 ± 5 hours; Erythrohydrobupropion: 33 ± 10 hours; Threohydrobupropion: 37 ± 13 hours

Time to peak, serum: Bupropion: ~3 hours; bupropion extended release: ~5 hours

Metabolites: Hydroxybupropion, erythrohydrobupropion, threohydrobupropion: 6 hours

Excretion: Urine (87%); feces (10%)

Contraindications Hypersensitivity to bupropion or any component of the formulation; seizure disorder; anorexia/bulimia; use of MAO inhibitors within 14 days; patients undergoing abrupt discontinuation of ethanol or sedatives (including benzodiazepines); patients receiving other dosage forms of bupropion

Warnings/Precautions Antidepressants increase the risk of suicidal thinking and behavior in children and adolescents with major depressive disorder (MDD) and other depressive disorders; consider risk prior to prescribing. Closely monitor for clinical worsening, suicidality, or unusual changes in behavior; the child's family or caregiver should be instructed to closely observe the patient and communicate condition with healthcare provider. Such observation would generally include at least weekly face-to-face contact with patients or their family members or caregivers during the first 4 weeks of treatment, then every other week visits for the next 4 weeks, then at 12 weeks, and as clinically indicated beyond 12 weeks. Additional contact by telephone may be appropriate between face-to-face visits. Adults treated with antidepressants should be observed similarly for clinical worsening and suicidality, especially during the initial few months of a course of drug therapy, or at times of dose changes, either increases or decreases. A medication guide should be dispensed with each prescription. **Bupropion is not FDA approved for use in children.**

The possibility of a suicide attempt is inherent in major depression and may persist until remission occurs. Monitor for worsening of depression or suicidality, especially during initiation of therapy or with dose increases or decreases. Worsening depression and severe abrupt suicidality that are not part of the presenting symptoms may require discontinuation or modification of drug therapy. Use caution in high-risk patients during initiation of therapy. Prescriptions should be written for the smallest quantity consistent with good patient care. The patient's family or caregiver should be alerted to monitor patients for the emergence of suicidality and associated behaviors such as anxiety, agitation, panic attacks, insomnia, irritability, hostility, impulsivity, akathisia, hypomania, and mania; patients should be instructed to notify their healthcare provider if any of these symptoms or worsening depression occur.

May worsen psychosis in some patients or precipitate a shift to mania or hypomania in patients with bipolar disorder. Monotherapy in patients with bipolar disorder should be avoided. Patients presenting with depressive symptoms should be screened for bipolar disorder. **Bupropion is not FDA approved for bipolar depression.**

When using immediate release tablets, seizure risk is increased at total daily dosage >450 mg, individual dosages >150 mg, or by sudden, large increments in dose. Data for the immediate-release formulation of bupropion revealed a seizure incidence of 0.4% in patients treated at doses in the 300-450 mg/day range. The estimated seizure incidence increases almost 10-fold between 450 mg and 600 mg per day. Data for the sustained release dosage form revealed a seizure incidence of 0.1% in patients treated at a dosage range of 100-300 mg/day, and increases to ~0.4% at the maximum recommended dose of 400 mg/day. The risk of seizures is increased in patients with a history of seizures, anorexia/bulimia, head trauma, CNS tumor, severe hepatic cirrhosis, abrupt discontinuation of sedative-hypnotics or ethanol, medications which lower seizure threshold (antipsychotics, antidepressants, theophyllines, systemic steroids), stimulants, or hypoglycemic agents. Discontinue and do not restart in patients experiencing a seizure. May cause CNS stimulation (restlessness, anxiety, insomnia) or anorexia. May increase the risks associated with electroconvulsive therapy. Consider discontinuing, when possible, prior to elective surgery. May cause weight loss; use caution in patients where weight loss is not desirable. The incidence of sexual dysfunction with bupropion is generally lower than with SSRIs.

Use caution in patients with cardiovascular disease, history of hypertension, or coronary artery disease; treatment-emergent hypertension (including some severe cases) has been reported, both with bupropion alone and in combination with nicotine transdermal systems. Use with caution in patients with hepatic or renal dysfunction and in elderly patients. Elderly patients may be at greater risk of accumulation during chronic dosing. May cause motor or cognitive impairment in some patients, use with caution if tasks requiring alertness such as operating machinery or driving are undertaken. Arthralgia, myalgia, and fever with rash and other symptoms suggestive of delayed hypersensitivity resembling serum sickness reported.

Drug Interactions **Substrate** of CYP1A2 (minor), 2A6 (minor), 2B6 (major), 2C8/9 (minor), 2D6 (minor), 2E1 (minor), 3A4 (minor); **Inhibits** CYP2D6 (weak)

Note: Seizure threshold-lowering agents: Use with caution in individuals receiving other agents that may lower seizure threshold (antipsychotics, antidepressants, fluoroquinolones, theophylline, abrupt discontinuation of benzodiazepines, systemic steroids)

Amantadine: Concurrent use appears to result in a higher incidence of adverse effects; use caution.

Cimetidine: May increase effect of bupropion (due to effect on bupropion metabolites)

CYP2B6 inducers: May decrease the levels/effects of bupropion. Example inducers include carbamazepine, nevirapine, phenobarbital, phenytoin, and rifampin.

CYP2B6 inhibitors: May increase the levels/effects of bupropion. Example inhibitors include desipramine, paroxetine, and sertraline.

Levodopa: Toxicity of bupropion is enhanced by levodopa

MAO inhibitors: Toxicity of bupropion is enhanced by MAO inhibitors (phenelzine); concurrent use is contraindicated

Nicotine: Treatment-emergent hypertension may occur; monitor BP in patients treated with bupropion and nicotine patch

Selegiline: When used in low doses (<10 mg/day), risk of interaction is theoretically lower than with nonselective MAO inhibitors

Tricyclic antidepressants: Serum levels may be increased by bupropion; in addition, these agents lower seizure threshold (see "Note")

Warfarin: Coadministration has resulted in altered PT/INR and thrombotic or hemorrhagic events. Monitor INR.

Nutritional/Herbal/Ethanol Interactions

Ethanol: Ethanol (may increase CNS depression).

Herb/Nutraceutical: Avoid valerian, St John's wort, SAMe, gotu kola, kava kava (may increase CNS depression).

Lab Interactions Decreased prolactin levels

Adverse Reactions Frequencies, when reported, reflect highest incidence reported with sustained release product.

>10%:

- Central nervous system: Dizziness (11%), headache (25%), insomnia (16%)
- Gastrointestinal: Nausea (18%), xerostomia (24%)
- Respiratory: Pharyngitis (11%)

1% to 10%:

- Cardiovascular: Arrhythmias, chest pain (4%), flushing, hypertension (may be severe), hypotension, palpitation (5%), syncope, tachycardia
- Central nervous system: Agitation (9%), anxiety (6%), confusion, depression, euphoria, hostility, irritability (2%), memory decreased (3%), migraine, nervousness (3%), sleep disturbance, somnolence (3%)
- Dermatologic: Pruritus (4%), rash (4%), sweating increased (5%), urticaria (1%)
- Endocrine & metabolic: Hot flashes, libido decreased, menstrual complaints
- Gastrointestinal: Abdominal pain, anorexia (3%), appetite increased, constipation (5%), diarrhea (7%), dyspepsia, dysphagia (2%), taste perversion (4%), vomiting (2%)
- Genitourinary: Urinary frequency (5%)
- Neuromuscular & skeletal: Arthralgia (4%), arthritis (2%), myalgia (6%), neck pain, paresthesia (2%), tremor (3%), twitching (2%)
- Ocular: Amblyopia (2%), blurred vision
- Otic: Auditory disturbance, tinnitus (6%)
- Respiratory: Cough increased (2%), sinusitis (1%)

(Continued)

BuPROPion *(Continued)*

Miscellaneous: Allergic reaction (including anaphylaxis, pruritus, urticaria), infection

Postmarketing and/or case reports (limited to important or life-threatening): Akinesia, amnesia, angioedema, aphasia, ataxia, atrioventricular block, bronchospasm, delirium, depersonalization, dysarthria, dyskinesia, dyspareunia, dystonia, edema, EEG abnormality, ejaculation abnormality, exfoliative dermatitis, extrapyramidal syndrome, gynecomastia, hallucinations, hepatitis, hostility, hyperkinesia, hypoglycemia, impotence, jaundice, leukopenia, maculopapular rash, manic reaction, myoclonus, neuralgia, neuropathy, nocturia, painful erection, pancreatitis, pancytopenia, paranoia, paresthesia, photosensitivity, postural hypotension, seizure, SIADH, suicidal ideation, tardive dyskinesia, thrombocytopenia, tongue edema, urinary incontinence, vaginitis, vertigo

Overdosage/Toxicology Symptoms of overdose include labored breathing, salivation, ataxia, and convulsions. Dialysis may be of limited value after drug absorption because of slow tissue-to-plasma diffusion. Treatment is symptomatic and supportive.

Dosing

Adults:

Depression: Oral:

Immediate release: 100 mg 3 times/day; begin at 100 mg twice daily; may increase to a maximum dose of 450 mg/day.

Sustained release: Initial: 150 mg/day in the morning; may increase to 150 mg twice daily by day 4 if tolerated; target dose: 300 mg/day given as 150 mg twice daily; maximum dose: 400 mg/day given as 200 mg twice daily.

Extended release: Initial: 150 mg/day in the morning; may increase as early as day 4 of dosing to 300 mg/day; maximum dose: 450 mg/day

Smoking cessation (Zyban®): Oral: Initiate with 150 mg once daily for 3 days; increase to 150 mg twice daily; treatment should continue for 7-12 weeks.

Elderly:

Depression: Oral: Initial: 37.5 mg of immediate release tablets twice daily or 100 mg/day of sustained release tablets; increase by 37.5-100 mg every 3-4 days as tolerated. **Note:** There is evidence that the elderly respond at 150 mg/day in divided doses, but some may require a higher dose.

Smoking cessation: Refer to adult dosing.

Pediatrics: ADHD (unlabeled use): Oral: Children and Adolescents: 1.4-6 mg/kg/day

Renal Impairment: Effect of renal disease on bupropion's pharmacokinetics has not been studied; elimination of the major metabolites of bupropion may be affected by reduced renal function. Patients with renal failure should receive a reduced dosage initially and be closely monitored.

Hepatic Impairment:

Mild to moderate hepatic impairment: Use with caution and/or reduced dose/frequency

Severe hepatic cirrhosis: Use with extreme caution; maximum dose:

Wellbutrin®: 75 mg/day;

Wellbutrin SR®: 100 mg/day or 150 mg every other day;

Wellbutrin XL™: 150 mg every other day

Zyban®: 150 mg every other day

Note: The mean AUC increased by ~1.5-fold for hydroxybupropion and ~2.5-fold for erythro/threohydrobupropion; median T_{max} was observed 19 hours later for hydroxybupropion, 31 hours later for erythro/threohydrobupropion; mean half-life for hydroxybupropion increased fivefold, and increased twofold for erythro/threohydrobupropion in patients with severe hepatic cirrhosis compared to healthy volunteers.

Available Dosage Forms

Tablet, as hydrochloride (Wellbutrin®): 75 mg, 100 mg

Tablet, extended release, as hydrochloride:

Buproban™: 150 mg [equivalent to Zyban®]

Budeprion™ SR: 100 mg [contains tartrazine; equivalent to Wellbutrin® SR], 150 mg [equivalent to Wellbutrin® SR]

Wellbutrin XL™: 150 mg, 300 mg

Tablet, sustained release, as hydrochloride: 100 mg, 150 mg [equivalent to Wellbutrin® SR], 150 mg [equivalent to Zyban®]

Wellbutrin® SR: 100 mg, 150 mg, 200 mg

Zyban®: 150 mg

Nursing Guidelines

Assessment: Assess other medications patient may be taking for effectiveness and interactions. Monitor therapeutic effectiveness and adverse reactions at beginning of therapy and periodically with long-term use. Monitor for clinical worsening and suicidality, especially at the beginning of therapy or when dose changes occur. Taper dosage slowly when discontinuing. Assess knowledge/ teach patient appropriate use, interventions to reduce side effects, and adverse symptoms to report.

Patient Education: Be aware that bupropion is marketed under different names and should not be taken together; Zyban® is for smoking cessation and Wellbutrin® is for treatment of depression. **Note:** Excessive use or abrupt discontinuation of alcohol or sedatives may alter seizure threshold.

Depression: Take as directed, in equally divided doses; do not take in larger dose or more often than recommended. Do not discontinue without consulting prescriber. Do not use alcohol or OTC medications not approved by prescriber. May cause drowsiness, clouded sensorium, headache, restlessness, or agitation (use caution when driving or engaging in tasks requiring alertness until response to drug is known); nausea, vomiting, or dry mouth (small, frequent meals, frequent mouth care, chewing gum, or sucking lozenges may help); constipation (increased exercise, fluids, fruit, or fiber may help); or impotence (reversible). Report persistent CNS effects (eg, agitation, confusion, anxiety, restlessness, insomnia, psychosis, hallucinations, seizures); suicidal ideation; muscle weakness or tremor; skin rash or irritation; chest pain or palpitations, abdominal pain or blood in stools; yellowing of skin or eyes; or respiratory difficulty, bronchitis, or unusual cough.

Smoking cessation: Use as directed; do not take extra doses. Do not combine nicotine patches with use of Zyban® unless approved by prescriber. May cause dry mouth and insomnia (these may resolve with continued use). Report any respiratory difficulty, unusual cough, dizziness, or muscle tremors.

Breast-feeding precaution: Breast-feeding is not recommended.

Geriatric Considerations: Limited data is available about the use of bupropion in the elderly. Two studies have found it equally effective when compared to imipramine. Its side effect profile (minimal anticholinergic and blood pressure effects) may make it useful in persons who do not tolerate traditional cyclic antidepressants.

Pregnancy Risk Factor: B

Lactation: Enters breast milk/not recommended (AAP rates "of concern")

Breast-Feeding Considerations: Generally, it is not recommended to breast-feed if taking antidepressants because of the long half-life, active metabolites, and the potential for side effects in the infant.

Perioperative/Anesthesia/Other Concerns: There are relatively few cardiovascular side effects compared to tricyclic antidepressants. However, several case reports include cardiovascular complications, including hypotension and MI. Use with caution in patients with recent MI or unstable angina. Recent information suggests that hypertension, in some cases severe and requiring acute treatment, has been reported in patients receiving bupropion alone, and especially when bupropion is used in conjunction with nicotine replacement therapy. Monitoring of blood pressure is recommended in patients receiving the combination of bupropion and nicotine replacement, particularly in those with hypertension and/or significant coronary artery disease.

Administration

Oral: May be taken without regard to meals. Zyban® and extended release tablets should be swallowed whole; do not crush, chew, or divide. The insoluble shell of the extended-release tablet may remain intact during GI transit and is eliminated in the feces. Wellbutrin® SR may be divided, but not crushed or chewed.

Storage: Store at controlled of 20°C to 25°C (68°F to 77°F).

- **Burnamycin [OTC]** *see* Lidocaine *on page 1033*
- **Burn Jel [OTC]** *see* Lidocaine *on page 1033*
- **Burn-O-Jel [OTC]** *see* Lidocaine *on page 1033*
- **BuSpar®** *see* BusPIRone *on page 278*

BusPIRone (byoo SPYE rone)

U.S. Brand Names BuSpar®

Synonyms Buspirone Hydrochloride

Pharmacologic Category Antianxiety Agent, Miscellaneous

Medication Safety Issues

Sound-alike/look-alike issues:

BusPIRone may be confused with buPROPion

Use Management of generalized anxiety disorder (GAD)

Unlabeled/Investigational Use Management of aggression in mental retardation and secondary mental disorders; major depression; potential augmenting agent for antidepressants; premenstrual syndrome

Mechanism of Action The mechanism of action of buspirone is unknown. Buspirone has a high affinity for serotonin 5-HT_{1A} and 5-HT_2 receptors, without affecting benzodiazepine-GABA receptors; buspirone has moderate affinity for dopamine D_2 receptors

Pharmacodynamics/Kinetics

Absorption: Oral: ~100%

Distribution: V_d: 5.3 L/kg

Protein binding: 95%

Metabolism: Hepatic via oxidation; extensive first-pass effect

Bioavailability: ~4%

Half-life elimination: Mean: 2.4 hours (range: 2-11 hours)

Time to peak, serum: Within 0.7-1.5 hours

Excretion: Urine: 65%; feces: 35%; ~1% dose excreted unchanged

Contraindications Hypersensitivity to buspirone or any component of the formulation

Warnings/Precautions Safety and efficacy not established in children <18 years of age; use in hepatic or renal impairment is not recommended; does not prevent or treat withdrawal from benzodiazepines. Low potential for cognitive or motor impairment. Use with MAO inhibitors may result in hypertensive reactions.

Drug Interactions Substrate of CYP2D6 (minor), 3A4 (major)

Calcium channel blockers: Diltiazem and verapamil may increase serum concentrations of buspirone; consider a dihydropyridine calcium channel blocker

CYP3A4 inducers: CYP3A4 inducers may decrease the levels/effects of buspirone. Example inducers include aminoglutethimide, carbamazepine, nafcillin, nevirapine, phenobarbital, phenytoin, and rifamycins.

CYP3A4 inhibitors: May increase the levels/effects of buspirone. Example inhibitors include azole antifungals, clarithromycin, diclofenac, doxycycline, erythromycin, imatinib, isoniazid, nefazodone, nicardipine, propofol, protease inhibitors, quinidine, telithromycin, and verapamil.

MAO inhibitors: Buspirone should not be used concurrently with an MAO inhibitor due to reports of increased blood pressure; includes classic MAO inhibitors and linezolid (due to ability to inhibit MAO)

Nefazodone: Concurrent use may increase risk of CNS adverse events. Limit buspirone initial dose (eg, 2.5 mg/day).

Selegiline: Theoretically, risk of interaction with selective MAO type B inhibitor would be less than with nonselective inhibitors; however, this combination is generally best avoided

SSRIs: Concurrent use of buspirone with SSRIs may cause serotonin syndrome. Some SSRIs may increase buspirone serum concentrations (see CYP3A4 inhibitors). Buspirone may increase the efficacy of fluoxetine in some patients; however, the anxiolytic activity of buspirone may be lost when combined with SSRIs (fluoxetine).

Trazodone: Concurrent use of buspirone with trazodone may cause serotonin syndrome

Nutritional/Herbal/Ethanol Interactions

Ethanol: Ethanol (may increase CNS depression).

Food: Food may decrease the absorption of buspirone, but it may also decrease the first-pass metabolism, thereby increasing the bioavailability of buspirone. Grapefruit juice may cause increased buspirone concentrations; avoid concurrent use.

Herb/Nutraceutical: St John's wort may decrease buspirone levels or increase CNS depression. Avoid valerian, gotu kola, kava kava (may increase CNS depression).

Lab Interactions Increased AST, ALT, growth hormone(s), prolactin (S)

Adverse Reactions

>10%: Central nervous system: Dizziness

1% to 10%:

Central nervous system: Drowsiness, EPS, serotonin syndrome, confusion, nervousness, lightheadedness, excitement, anger, hostility, headache

Dermatologic: Rash

Gastrointestinal: Diarrhea, nausea

Neuromuscular & skeletal: Muscle weakness, numbness, paresthesia, incoordination, tremor

Ocular: Blurred vision, tunnel vision

Miscellaneous: Diaphoresis, allergic reactions

Overdosage/Toxicology Symptoms of overdose include dizziness, drowsiness, pinpoint pupils, nausea, and vomiting. There is no known antidote for buspirone. Treatment is supportive.

Dosing

Adults: Anxiety disorders (GAD): Oral: 15 mg/day (7.5 mg twice daily); may increase in increments of 5 mg/day every 2-4 days to a maximum of 60 mg/day. Target dose for most people is 30 mg/day (15 mg twice daily).

Elderly: Oral: Initial: 5 mg twice daily, increase by 5 mg/day every 2-3 days as needed up to 20-30 mg/day; maximum daily dose: 60 mg/day (see Geriatric Considerations).

Pediatrics:

Generalized anxiety disorder (GAD): Oral: Children and Adolescents: Initial: 5 mg daily; increase in increments of 5 mg/day at weekly intervals as needed, to a maximum dose of 60 mg/day divided into 2-3 doses

Renal Impairment: Use in patients with severe renal impairment cannot be recommended.

Hepatic Impairment: Buspirone is metabolized by the liver and excreted by the kidneys. Patients with impaired hepatic or renal function demonstrated increased plasma levels and a prolonged half-life of buspirone. Therefore, use in patients with severe hepatic or renal impairment cannot be recommended.

Available Dosage Forms

Tablet, as hydrochloride: 5 mg, 7.5 mg, 10 mg, 15 mg, 30 mg

BuSpar®: 5 mg, 10 mg, 15 mg, 30 mg

Nursing Guidelines

Assessment: Assess other medications patient may be taking for effectiveness and interactions. Monitor therapeutic effectiveness and adverse reactions at beginning of therapy and periodically with long-term use. Assess knowledge/teach patient appropriate use, interventions to reduce side effects, and adverse symptoms to report..

Patient Education: Take only as directed; do not increase dose or take more often than prescribed. May take 2-3 weeks to see full effect; do not discontinue without consulting prescriber. Do not use alcohol or other prescription or OTC medications (especially pain medications, sedatives, antihistamines, or hypnotics) without consulting prescriber. Maintain adequate hydration (2-3 L/day of fluids) unless instructed to restrict fluid intake. You may experience drowsiness, lightheadedness, impaired coordination, dizziness, or blurred vision (use caution when driving or engaging in tasks requiring alertness until response to drug is known); or upset stomach, nausea (small frequent meals, frequent mouth care, chewing gum, or sucking lozenges may help). Report persistent vomiting; chest pain or rapid heartbeat; persistent CNS effects (eg, confusion, restlessness, anxiety, insomnia, excitation, headache, dizziness, fatigue, impaired coordination); or worsening of condition. **Breast-feeding precaution:** Breast-feeding is not recommended.

Geriatric Considerations: Because buspirone is less sedating than other anxiolytics, it may be a useful agent in geriatric patients when an anxiolytic is indicated.

Pregnancy Risk Factor: B

Lactation: Excretion in breast milk unknown/not recommended

Perioperative/Anesthesia/Other Concerns: Takes 2-3 weeks for full effect. Because of slow onset, not appropriate for "as needed" (prn) use or for brief, situational anxiety; not effective for severe anxiety; does not show cross-tolerance with benzodiazepines or other sedatives; less sedating than other anxiolytics; has shown little potential for abuse; needs continuous use; ineffective for benzodiazepine or ethanol withdrawal

◆ **Buspirone Hydrochloride** *see* BusPIRone *on page 278*

Butalbital, Acetaminophen, and Caffeine

(byoo TAL bi tal, a seet a MIN oh fen, & KAF een)

U.S. Brand Names Anolor 300; Dolgic® LQ; Dolgic® Plus; Esgic®; Esgic-Plus™; Fioricet®; Medigesic®; Repan®; Zebutal™

Synonyms Acetaminophen, Butalbital, and Caffeine

Pharmacologic Category Barbiturate

Medication Safety Issues

Sound-alike/look-alike issues:

Fioricet® may be confused with Fiorinal®, Lorcet®

Repan® may be confused with Riopan®

Use Relief of the symptomatic complex of tension or muscle contraction headache

Mechanism of Action

Butalbital is a short- to intermediate-acting barbiturate. Barbiturates depress the sensory cortex, decrease motor activity, alter cerebellar function, and produce drowsiness, sedation, hypnosis, and dose-dependent respiratory depression.

Acetaminophen inhibits the synthesis of prostaglandins in the central nervous system and peripherally blocks pain impulse generation; produces antipyresis from inhibition of hypothalamic heat-regulating center

Caffeine increases levels of 3'5' cyclic AMP by inhibiting phosphodiesterase; CNS stimulant which increases medullary respiratory center sensitivity to carbon dioxide, stimulates central inspiratory drive, and improves skeletal muscle contraction (diaphragmatic contractility)

Pharmacodynamics/Kinetics Also see individual monographs for Acetaminophen and Caffeine.

Absorption: Butalbital: Well absorbed

Protein binding: Butalbital: 45%

Half-life elimination: Butalbital: 35 hours

Excretion: Butalbital: Urine (59% to 88% as unchanged drug and metabolites)

Contraindications Hypersensitivity to butalbital, acetaminophen, caffeine, or any component of the formulation; porphyria

Warnings/Precautions Administer with caution, if at all, to patients who are mentally depressed, have suicidal tendencies, or a history of drug abuse. May be habit-forming; not recommended for extended use. Use caution with acute abdominal conditions, severe hepatic or renal impairment, or the elderly. Safety and efficacy in children <12 years of age have not been established.

Drug Interactions

Acetaminophen: **Substrate** (minor) of CYP1A2, 2A6, 2C8/9, 2D6, 2E1, 3A4; **Inhibits** CYP3A4 (weak)

Caffeine: **Substrate** of CYP1A2 (major), 2C8/9 (minor), 2D6 (minor), 2E1 (minor), 3A4 (minor); **Inhibits** CYP1A2 (weak), 3A4 (moderate)

See individual monographs for Acetaminophen and Caffeine. For butalbital, refer to Phenobarbital monograph.

Nutritional/Herbal/Ethanol Interactions Ethanol: Avoid ethanol (may increase CNS depression).

Lab Interactions Acetaminophen may produce false-positive test results for urinary 5-hydroxyindoleacetic acid.

Adverse Reactions Note: Specific percentages not reported.

Frequently observed:

Central nervous system: Dizziness, drowsiness, lightheadedness, sedation

Gastrointestinal: Abdominal pain, nausea, vomiting

Respiratory: Dyspnea

Miscellaneous: Intoxicated feeling

Infrequently observed:

Cardiovascular: Tachycardia

Central nervous system: Agitation, confusion, depression, euphoria, excitement, faintness, fever, headache, seizure

Dermatologic: Hyperhidrosis, pruritus

Endocrine & metabolic: Hot spells

Gastrointestinal: Constipation, dysphagia, heartburn, flatulence, xerostomia

Neuromuscular & skeletal: Leg pain, muscle fatigue, numbness, paresthesia

Ocular: Heavy eyelids

Otic: Earache, tinnitus

Renal: Diuresis

Respiratory: Nasal congestion

Miscellaneous: Allergic reaction, high energy, shaky feeling, sluggishness

Overdosage/Toxicology Symptoms of barbiturate overdose include unsteady gait, slurred speech, confusion, respiratory depression, hypotension, and coma. Treatment is supportive.

Symptoms of acetaminophen overdose include hepatic necrosis, transient azotemia, renal tubular necrosis with acute toxicity, anemia, and GI disturbances with chronic toxicity. Treatment consists of acetylcysteine. Therapy should be initiated based upon laboratory analysis suggesting a high probability of hepatotoxic potential. Activated charcoal is very effective at binding acetaminophen.

Dosing

Adults: Tension or muscle contraction headache: Oral: 1-2 tablets or capsules (or 15-30 mL elixir) every 4 hours; not to exceed 6 tablets or capsules (or 180 mL elixir) daily

Elderly: Not recommended for use in the elderly.

Renal Impairment: Dosage should be reduced.

Hepatic Impairment: Dosage should be reduced.

Available Dosage Forms

Capsule:

Anolor 300, Esgic®, Medigesic®: Butalbital 50 mg, caffeine 40 mg, and acetaminophen 325 mg

Dolgic® Plus: Butalbital 50 mg, caffeine 40 mg, and acetaminophen 750 mg

Esgic-Plus™, Zebutal™: Butalbital 50 mg, caffeine 40 mg, and acetaminophen 500 mg

Elixir (Dolgic® LQ): Butalbital 50 mg, caffeine 40 mg, and acetaminophen 325 mg per 15 mL (480 mL) [contains alcohol 7%; fruit flavor]

Tablet: Butalbital 50 mg, caffeine 40 mg, and acetaminophen 325 mg; butalbital 50 mg, caffeine 40 mg, and acetaminophen 500 mg

Esgic®, Fioricet®, Repan®: Butalbital 50 mg, caffeine 40 mg, and acetaminophen 325 mg

Nursing Guidelines

Assessment: Assess patient for history of liver disease or ethanol abuse. Assess other medications patient may be taking for additive or adverse interactions. Monitor therapeutic effectiveness. Assess knowledge/teach patient appropriate use, adverse reactions to report, and appropriate interventions to reduce side effects.

Patient Education: If self-administered, use exactly as directed; do not increase dose or frequency. Drug may cause physical and/or psychological dependence. Take with food or milk. While using this medication, do not use alcohol and other prescription or OTC medications (especially sedatives, tranquilizers, antihistamines, or pain medications) without consulting prescriber. Maintain adequate hydration (2-3 L/day of fluids) unless instructed to restrict fluid intake. May cause dizziness, lightheadedness, confusion, or drowsiness (use caution when driving, climbing stairs, or changing position - rising from sitting or lying to standing, or when engaging in tasks requiring alertness until response to drug is known); heartburn or epigastric discomfort (frequent mouth care, frequent sips of fluids, chewing gum, or sucking lozenges may help); or constipation (increased exercise, fluids, fruit, or fiber may help). Report chest pain or palpitations; persistent dizziness; confusion, nightmares, excitation, or changes in mentation; shortness of breath or respiratory difficulty; skin rash; unusual bleeding or bruising; or unusual fatigue and weakness.

Geriatric Considerations: Elderly may react to barbiturates with marked excitement, depression, and confusion.

Pregnancy Risk Factor: C

Pregnancy Issues: Reproduction studies have not been conducted with this combination. The FDA pregnancy classification for most other barbiturates is Category D. Withdrawal seizures were reported in an infant 2 days after birth following maternal use of a butalbital product during the last 2 months of pregnancy; butalbital levels were measured in the infants serum. In general, barbiturates cross the placenta and distribute in fetal tissue. Teratogenic effects have been reported with 1st trimester exposure. Exposure during the third trimester may lead to symptoms of acute withdrawal following delivery; symptoms may be delayed up to 14 days. Refer to individual monographs for specific information related to acetaminophen and caffeine.

Lactation: Enters breast milk/not recommended

Breast-Feeding Considerations: Specific data is not available for butalbital. Barbiturates, caffeine, and acetaminophen are excreted in breast milk. The manufacturer recommends discontinuing this medication or discontinuing nursing.

(Continued)

Butalbital, Acetaminophen, and Caffeine *(Continued)*

Administration

Storage: Store at room temperature below 30°C (86°F). Protect from moisture.

Related Information

Acetaminophen *on page 65*
Caffeine *on page 284*

Butorphanol (byoo TOR fa nole)

U.S. Brand Names Stadol®; Stadol® NS [DSC]

Synonyms Butorphanol Tartrate

Pharmacologic Category Analgesic, Narcotic

Medication Safety Issues

Sound-alike/look-alike issues:
Stadol® may be confused with Haldol®, sotalol

Use

Parenteral: Management of moderate to severe pain; preoperative medication; supplement to balanced anesthesia; management of pain during labor

Nasal spray: Management of moderate to severe pain, including migraine headache pain

Mechanism of Action Mixed narcotic agonist-antagonist with central analgesic actions; binds to opiate receptors in the CNS, causing inhibition of ascending pain pathways, altering the perception of and response to pain; produces generalized CNS depression

Pharmacodynamics/Kinetics

Onset of action: I.M.: 5-10 minutes; I.V.: <10 minutes; Nasal: Within 15 minutes
Peak effect: I.M.: 0.5-1 hour; I.V.: 4-5 minutes
Duration: I.M., I.V.: 3-4 hours; Nasal: 4-5 hours
Absorption: Rapid and well absorbed
Protein binding: 80%
Metabolism: Hepatic
Bioavailability: Nasal: 60% to 70%
Half-life elimination: 2.5-4 hours
Excretion: Primarily urine

Contraindications Hypersensitivity to butorphanol or any component of the formulation; avoid use in opiate-dependent patients who have not been detoxified, may precipitate opiate withdrawal; pregnancy (prolonged use or high doses at term)

Warnings/Precautions An opioid-containing analgesic regimen should be tailored to each patient's needs and based upon the type of pain being treated (acute versus chronic), the route of administration, degree of tolerance for opioids (naive versus chronic user), age, weight, and medical condition. The optimal analgesic dose varies widely among patients. Doses should be titrated to pain relief/prevention. May cause CNS depression, which may impair physical or mental abilities. Effects with other sedative drugs or ethanol may be potentiated. Use with caution in patients with hepatic/renal dysfunction. Tolerance or drug dependence may result from extended use. Concurrent use of sumatriptan nasal spray and butorphanol nasal spray may increase risk of transient high blood pressure.

Drug Interactions Increased toxicity: CNS depressants, phenothiazines, barbiturates, skeletal muscle relaxants, alfentanil, guanabenz, MAO inhibitors

Nutritional/Herbal/Ethanol Interactions

Ethanol: Avoid or limit ethanol (may increase CNS depression). Watch for sedation.

Herb/Nutraceutical: Avoid valerian, St John's wort, kava kava, gotu kola (may increase CNS depression).

Adverse Reactions

>10%:

- Central nervous system: Drowsiness (43%), dizziness (19%), insomnia (Stadol® NS)
- Gastrointestinal: Nausea/vomiting (13%)
- Respiratory: Nasal congestion (Stadol® NS)

1% to 10%:

- Cardiovascular: Vasodilation, palpitation
- Central nervous system: Lightheadedness, headache, lethargy, anxiety, confusion, euphoria, somnolence
- Dermatologic: Pruritus

Gastrointestinal: Anorexia, constipation, xerostomia, stomach pain, unpleasant aftertaste

Neuromuscular & skeletal: Tremor, paresthesia, weakness

Ocular: Blurred vision

Otic: Ear pain, tinnitus

Respiratory: Bronchitis, cough, dyspnea, epistaxis, nasal irritation, pharyngitis, rhinitis, sinus congestion, sinusitis, upper respiratory infection

Miscellaneous: Diaphoresis (increased)

<1% (Limited to important or life-threatening): Dependence (with prolonged use), depression, difficulty speaking (transient), dyspnea, hallucinations, hypertension, nightmares, paradoxical CNS stimulation, rash, respiratory depression, syncope, tinnitus, vertigo, withdrawal symptoms

Stadol® NS: Apnea, chest pain, convulsions, delusions, depressions, edema, hypertension, shallow breathing, tachycardia

Overdosage/Toxicology Symptoms of overdose include respiratory depression, cardiac and CNS depression. Treatment is supportive. Naloxone, 2 mg I.V. with repeat administration as necessary up to a total of 10 mg, can also be used to reverse toxic effects of the opiate.

Dosing

Adults: Note: These are guidelines and do not represent the maximum doses that may be required in all patients. Doses should be titrated to pain relief/prevention. Butorphanol has an analgesic ceiling.

Acute pain (moderate to severe):

I.M.: Initial: 2 mg, may repeat every 3-4 hours as needed; usual range: 1-4 mg every 3-4 hours as needed

I.V.: Initial: 1 mg, may repeat every 3-4 hours as needed; usual range: 0.5-2 mg every 3-4 hours as needed

Intranasal (spray) (includes use for migraine headache pain): Initial: 1 spray (~1 mg per spray) in 1 nostril; if adequate pain relief is not achieved within 60-90 minutes, an additional 1 spray in 1 nostril may be given; may repeat initial dose sequence in 3-4 hours after the last dose as needed

Note: In some clinical trials, an initial dose of 2 mg (as 2 doses 1 hour apart or 2 mg initially - 1 spray in each nostril) has been used, followed by 1 mg in 1 hour; side effects were greater at these dosages

Migraine: Nasal spray: Refer to "moderate to severe pain" indication

Preoperative medication: I.M.: 2 mg 60-90 minutes before surgery

Supplement to balanced anesthesia: I.V.: 2 mg shortly before induction and/or an incremental dose of 0.5-1 mg (up to 0.06 mg/kg), depending on previously administered sedative, analgesic, and hypnotic medications

Pain during labor (fetus >37 weeks gestation and no signs of fetal distress):

I.M., I.V.: 1-2 mg; may repeat in 4 hours

Note: Alternative analgesia should be used for pain associated with delivery or if delivery is anticipated within 4 hours

Elderly:

I.M., I.V.: 0.5-2 mg every 6-8 hours, increase as necessary

Nasal spray: Initial dose should not exceed 1 mg; after 90-120 minutes, assess whether a second dose is needed; may repeat in 3-4 hours.

Available Dosage Forms [DSC] Discontinued product

Injection, solution, as tartrate [preservative free] (Stadol®): 1 mg/mL (1 mL); 2 mg/mL (1 mL, 2 mL)

Injection, solution, as tartrate [with preservative] (Stadol®): 2 mg/mL (10 mL)

Solution, intranasal spray, as tartrate: 10 mg/mL (2.5 mL) [14-15 doses]

Stadol® NS [DSC]: 10 mg/mL (2.5 mL)

Nursing Guidelines

Assessment: Assess other medications patient may be taking for possible additive or adverse interactions. Monitor for effectiveness of pain relief, signs of overdose, vital signs, and adverse effects at beginning of therapy and at regular intervals with long-term use. For inpatients, implement safety measures. May cause physical and/or psychological dependence. Assess knowledge/teach patient appropriate use (if self-administered), adverse reactions to report, and appropriate interventions to reduce side effects.

Patient Education: If self-administered, use exactly as directed; do not increase dose or frequency. Drug may cause physical and/or psychological dependence. While using this medication, do not use alcohol and other prescription or OTC medications (especially sedatives, tranquilizers, antihistamines, or pain medications) without consulting prescriber. May cause dizziness, drowsiness, confusion, or blurred vision (use caution when driving, climbing

(Continued)

Butorphanol *(Continued)*

stairs, or changing position - rising from sitting or lying to standing, or when engaging in tasks requiring alertness until response to drug is known); nausea or vomiting, or loss of appetite (frequent mouth care, small frequent meals, sucking lozenges, or chewing gum may help). Report unresolved nausea or vomiting; respiratory difficulty or shortness of breath; restlessness, insomnia, euphoria, or nightmares; excessive sedation or unusual weakness; facial flushing, rapid heartbeat, or palpitations; urinary difficulty; or vision changes.

Nasal administration: Do not use more frequently than prescribed. Blow nose prior to administering. Follow directions on package insert. Insert nozzle of applicator gently into one nostril and exhale. With next breath, squeeze applicator once firmly and quickly once as you breath in. If adequate relief from headache is not achieved within 60-90 minutes, an additional 1 spray may be given. May be repeated in 3-4 hours following last dose, as needed. **Alternately:** Two sprays may be given - one spray in each nostril, if you are able to remain lying down (in the event of drowsiness or dizziness). Additional doses should not be taken for 3-4 hours. Avoid using simultaneously with intranasal migraine sprays. Separate by at least 30 minutes.

Pregnancy/breast-feeding precautions: Inform prescriber if you are or intend to become pregnant. If you are breast-feeding, take dose immediately after breast-feeding or 3-4 hours prior to next feeding.

Geriatric Considerations: Adjust dose for renal function in the elderly.

Pregnancy Risk Factor: C/D (prolonged use or high doses at term)

Lactation: Enters breast milk/use caution (AAP rates "compatible")

Perioperative/Anesthesia/Other Concerns: Butorphanol is a mixed agonist-antagonist opiate; may precipitate withdrawal in narcotic-dependent patients. Abrupt discontinuation after sustained use (generally >10 days) may cause withdrawal symptoms. This agent can potentially cause hallucinations.

Administration

Compatibility:

Y-site administration: Incompatible with amphotericin B cholesteryl sulfate complex, midazolam

Compatibility in syringe: Incompatible with dimenhydrinate, pentobarbital

Storage: Store at room temperature; protect from freezing.

Related Information

Narcotic / Opioid Analgesics *on page 1880*

- ♦ **Butorphanol Tartrate** *see* Butorphanol *on page 282*
- ♦ **B Vitamin Combinations** *see* Vitamin B Complex Combinations *on page 1716*
- ♦ **BW-430C** *see* Lamotrigine *on page 1002*
- ♦ **C1H** *see* Alemtuzumab *on page 102*
- ♦ **C2B8** *see* Rituximab *on page 1484*
- ♦ **C2B8 Monoclonal Antibody** *see* Rituximab *on page 1484*
- ♦ **C7E3** *see* Abciximab *on page 60*
- ♦ **C-500-GR™ [OTC]** *see* Ascorbic Acid *on page 187*
- ♦ **Cafcit®** *see* Caffeine *on page 284*
- ♦ **Caffedrine® [OTC]** *see* Caffeine *on page 284*

Caffeine (KAF een)

U.S. Brand Names Cafcit®; Caffedrine® [OTC]; Enerjets [OTC]; Lucidex [OTC]; No Doz® Maximum Strength [OTC]; Vivarin® [OTC]

Synonyms Caffeine and Sodium Benzoate; Caffeine Citrate; Sodium Benzoate and Caffeine

Pharmacologic Category Stimulant

Use

Caffeine citrate: Treatment of idiopathic apnea of prematurity

Caffeine and sodium benzoate: Treatment of acute respiratory depression (not a preferred agent)

Caffeine [OTC labeling]: Restore mental alertness or wakefulness when experiencing fatigue

Unlabeled/Investigational Use Caffeine and sodium benzoate: Treatment of spinal puncture headache; CNS stimulant; diuretic

Mechanism of Action Increases levels of 3'5' cyclic AMP by inhibiting phosphodiesterase; CNS stimulant which increases medullary respiratory center sensitivity to carbon dioxide, stimulates central inspiratory drive, and improves skeletal muscle contraction (diaphragmatic contractility); prevention of apnea may occur by competitive inhibition of adenosine

Pharmacodynamics/Kinetics

Distribution: V_d:

Neonates: 0.8-0.9 L/kg

Children >9 months to Adults: 0.6 L/kg

Protein binding: 17% (children) to 36% (adults)

Metabolism: Hepatic, via demethylation by CYP1A2. **Note:** In neonates, interconversion between caffeine and theophylline has been reported (caffeine levels are ~25% of measured theophylline after theophylline administration and ~3% to 8% of caffeine would be expected to be converted to theophylline)

Half-life elimination:

Neonates: 72-96 hours (range: 40-230 hours)

Children >9 months and Adults: 5 hours

Time to peak, serum: Oral: Within 30 minutes to 2 hours

Excretion:

Neonates ≤ month: 86% excreted unchanged in urine

Infants >1 month and Adults: In urine, as metabolites

Contraindications Hypersensitivity to caffeine or any component of the formulation; sodium benzoate is not for use in neonates

Warnings/Precautions Use with caution in patients with a history of peptic ulcer, gastroesophageal reflux, impaired renal or hepatic function, seizure disorders, or cardiovascular disease. Avoid use in patients with symptomatic cardiac arrhythmias, agitation, anxiety or tremor. Over-the-counter [OTC] products contain an amount of caffeine similar to one cup of coffee; limit the use of other caffeine-containing beverages or foods.

Caffeine citrate should not be interchanged with caffeine and sodium benzoate. Avoid use of products containing sodium benzoate in neonates; has been associated with a potentially fatal toxicity ("gasping syndrome") in neonates, including metabolic acidosis, respiratory distress, gasping respirations, seizures, intracranial hemorrhage, hypotension, and cardiovascular collapse. *In vitro* and animal studies have shown that benzoate also displaces bilirubin from protein-binding sites. Neonates receiving caffeine citrate should be closely monitored for the development of necrotizing enterocolitis. Caffeine serum levels should be closely monitored to optimize therapy and prevent serious toxicity.

Drug Interactions **Substrate** of CYP1A2 (major), 2C8/9 (minor), 2D6 (minor), 2E1 (minor), 3A4 (minor); **Inhibits** CYP1A2 (weak), 3A4 (moderate)

Benzodiazepines: Caffeine may diminish the sedative or anxiolytic effects of benzodiazepines.

CYP1A2 inducers: May decrease the levels/effects of caffeine. Example inducers include aminoglutethimide, carbamazepine, phenobarbital, and rifampin.

CYP1A2 inhibitors: May increase the levels/effects of caffeine. Example inhibitors include amiodarone, fluvoxamine, ketoconazole, and rofecoxib.

Quinolone antibiotics (specifically ciprofloxacin, norfloxacin, ofloxacin): May increase the levels/effects of caffeine.

Adverse Reactions Frequency not specified; primarily serum-concentration related.

Cardiovascular: Angina, arrhythmia (ventricular), chest pain, flushing, palpitation, sinus tachycardia, tachycardia (supraventricular), vasodilation

Central nervous system: Agitation, delirium, dizziness, hallucinations, headache, insomnia, irritability, psychosis, restlessness

Dermatologic: Urticaria

Gastrointestinal: Esophageal sphincter tone decreased, gastritis

Neuromuscular & skeletal: Fasciculations

Ocular: Intraocular pressure increased (>180 mg caffeine), miosis

Renal: Diuresis

Overdosage/Toxicology Symptoms may include CNS stimulation, tachyarrhythmias, and tremor. Treatment is symptomatic and supportive.

Dosing

Adults & Elderly:

Note: Caffeine citrate should not be interchanged with the caffeine sodium benzoate formulation.

Caffeine and sodium benzoate:

Respiratory depression: I.M., I.V.: 250 mg as a single dose; may repeat as needed. Maximum single dose should be limited to 500 mg; maximum amount in any 24-hour period should generally be limited to 2500 mg

(Continued)

Caffeine *(Continued)*

Spinal puncture headache (unlabeled use):

I.V.: 500 mg in 1000 mL NS infused over 1 hour, followed by 1000 mL NS infused over 1 hour; a second course of caffeine can be given for unrelieved headache pain in 4 hours.

Oral: 300 mg as a single dose

Stimulant/diuretic (unlabeled use): I.M., I.V.: 500 mg, maximum single dose: 1 g

OTC labeling (stimulant): Oral: 100-200 mg every 3-4 hours as needed

Pediatrics:

Note: Caffeine citrate should not be interchanged with the caffeine sodium benzoate formulation.

Caffeine citrate: Apnea of prematurity: Neonates: Oral, I.V.:

Loading dose: 10-20 mg/kg as caffeine citrate (5-10 mg/kg as caffeine base). If theophylline has been administered to the patient within the previous 3 days, a full or modified loading dose (50% to 75% of a loading dose) may be given.

Maintenance dose: 5 mg/kg/day as caffeine citrate (2.5 mg/kg/day as caffeine base) once daily starting 24 hours after the loading dose. Maintenance dose is adjusted based on patient's response and serum caffeine concentrations.

Caffeine and sodium benzoate: Stimulant:

I.M., I.V., SubQ: 8 mg/kg every 4 hours as needed

Oral: OTC labeling: Children ≥12 years: Refer to adult dosing.

Renal Impairment: No dosage adjustment required.

Available Dosage Forms

Caplet (Caffedrine®, Vivarin®): 200 mg [OTC]

Injection, solution, as citrate [preservative free] (Cafcit®): 20 mg/mL (3 mL) [equivalent to 10 mg/mL caffeine base]

Injection, solution [with sodium benzoate]: Caffeine 125 mg/mL and sodium benzoate 125 mg/mL (2 mL); caffeine 121 mg/mL and sodium benzoate 129 mg/mL (2 mL)

Lozenge: 75 mg [OTC; Hazelnut coffee or mochamint flavor]

Solution, oral, as citrate (Cafcit®): 20 mg/mL (3 mL) [equivalent to 10 mg/mL caffeine base]

Tablet:

Lucidex: 100 mg [OTC]

NoDoz® Maximum Strength, Vivarin®: 200 mg [OTC]

Nursing Guidelines

Assessment: Assess other prescription and OTC medications the patient may be taking to avoid duplications and interactions. Assess knowledge/teach patient appropriate use, side effects, and symptoms to report.

Patient Education: Take as directed. Do not exceed recommended dosage. Maintain adequate hydration (2-3 L/day of fluids) unless instructed to restrict fluid intake by prescriber. You may experience CNS stimulation, excitability, sensorium changes, flushing, dizziness, insomnia, or agitation. Report excessive excitability or nervousness, rapid heartbeat or palpitations, chest pain, or respiratory difficulty. **Pregnancy/breast-feeding precaution:** Inform prescriber if you are or intend to become pregnant. Consult prescriber if breast-feeding.

Pregnancy Risk Factor: C

Lactation: Enters breast milk/use caution (AAP rates "compatible")

Breast-Feeding Considerations: Irritability and poor sleeping patterns have been reported following maternal consumption of large amounts of caffeine. Moderate intake (2-3 cups/day) is considered to be compatible with breast-feeding.

Perioperative/Anesthesia/Other Concerns: Caffeine has 40% of the bronchodilatory activity of theophylline. Lithium blood levels may increase during caffeine withdrawal. Analgesia from transcutaneous electrical nerve stimulation may be lessened with concomitant caffeine use.

Administration

Oral: May be administered without regard to feedings or meals; may administer injectable formulation (caffeine citrate) orally

I.M.: Parenteral: **Caffeine and sodium benzoate:** May administer I.M. undiluted

I.V.: Parenteral:

Caffeine citrate: Infuse loading dose over at least 30 minutes; maintenance dose may be infused over at least 10 minutes; may administer without dilution or diluted with D_5W to 10 mg caffeine citrate/mL

Caffeine and sodium benzoate: I.V. as slow direct injection; for spinal headaches, dilute in 1000 mL NS and infuse over 1 hour; follow with 1000 mL NS, infuse over 1 hour; may administer I.M. undiluted

Storage: Store at 20°C to 25°C (68°F to 77°F).

♦ **Caffeine and Sodium Benzoate** *see* Caffeine *on page 284*
♦ **Caffeine Citrate** *see* Caffeine *on page 284*
♦ **Calan®** *see* Verapamil *on page 1702*
♦ **Calan® SR** *see* Verapamil *on page 1702*
♦ **Calcarb 600 [OTC]** *see* Calcium Carbonate *on page 291*
♦ **Calci-Chew® [OTC]** *see* Calcium Carbonate *on page 291*
♦ **Calciferol™** *see* Ergocalciferol *on page 627*
♦ **Calcijex®** *see* Calcitriol *on page 289*
♦ **Calci-Mix® [OTC]** *see* Calcium Carbonate *on page 291*

Calcitonin (kal si TOE nin)

U.S. Brand Names Fortical®; Miacalcin®

Synonyms Calcitonin (Salmon)

Pharmacologic Category Antidote; Hormone

Medication Safety Issues

Sound-alike/look-alike issues:

Calcitonin may be confused with calcitriol

Miacalcin® may be confused with Micatin®

Use Calcitonin (salmon): Treatment of Paget's disease of bone (osteitis deformans); adjunctive therapy for hypercalcemia; postmenopausal osteoporosis

Mechanism of Action Peptide sequence similar to human calcitonin; functionally antagonizes the effects of parathyroid hormone. Directly inhibits osteoclastic bone resorption; promotes the renal excretion of calcium, phosphate, sodium, magnesium and potassium by decreasing tubular reabsorption; increases the jejunal secretion of water, sodium, potassium, and chloride

Pharmacodynamics/Kinetics

Hypercalcemia:

Onset of action: ~2 hours

Duration: 6-8 hours

Absorption: Nasal: ~3% of I.M. level (range: 0.3% to 31%)

Distribution: Does not cross placenta

Half-life elimination: SubQ: 1.2 hours; Nasal: 43 minutes

Excretion: Urine (as inactive metabolites)

Contraindications Hypersensitivity to calcitonin salmon or any component of the formulation

Warnings/Precautions A skin test should be performed prior to initiating therapy of calcitonin salmon in patients with suspected sensitivity; have epinephrine immediately available for a possible hypersensitivity reaction. A detailed skin testing protocol is available from the manufacturers. Temporarily withdraw use of nasal spray if ulceration of nasal mucosa occurs. Safety and efficacy have not been established in pediatric patients.

Nutritional/Herbal/Ethanol Interactions Ethanol: Avoid ethanol (may increase risk of osteoporosis).

Adverse Reactions Unless otherwise noted, frequencies reported are with nasal spray.

>10%: Respiratory: Rhinitis (12%)

1% to 10%:

Cardiovascular: Flushing (nasal spray: <1%; injection: 2% to 5%), angina (1% to 3%), hypertension (1% to 3%)

Central nervous system: Depression (1% to 3%), dizziness (1% to 3%), fatigue (1% to 3%)

Dermatologic: Erythematous rash (1% to 3%)

Gastrointestinal: Abdominal pain (1% to 3%), constipation (1% to 3%), diarrhea (1% to 3%), dyspepsia (1% to 3%), nausea (injection: 10%; nasal spray: 1% to 3%)

Genitourinary: Cystitis (1% to 3%)

Hematologic: Lymphadenopathy (1% to 3%)

(Continued)

Calcitonin *(Continued)*

Local: Injection site reactions (injection: 10%)

Neuromuscular & skeletal: Back pain (5%), arthrosis (1% to 3%), myalgia (1% to 3%), paresthesia (1% to 3%)

Ocular: Conjunctivitis (1% to 3%), lacrimation abnormality (1% to 3%)

Respiratory: Bronchospasm (1% to 3%), sinusitis (1% to 3%), upper respiratory tract infection (1% to 3%)

Miscellaneous: Flu-like symptoms (1% to 3%), infection (1% to 3%)

<1% (Limited to important or life-threatening): Agitation, allergic reactions, alopecia, anaphylaxis, anemia, anorexia, anxiety, appetite increased, arthritis, blurred vision, bronchitis, bundle branch block, cerebrovascular accident, cholelithiasis, cough, diaphoresis, dry mouth, dyspnea, earache, eczema, fever, flatulence, gastritis, goiter, hearing loss, hematuria, hepatitis, hyperthyroidism, insomnia, migraine, myocardial infarction, neuralgia, nocturia, palpitation, parosmia, periorbital edema, pharyngitis, pneumonia, polymyalgia rheumatica, pruritus, pyelonephritis, rash, renal calculus, skin ulceration, stiffness, tachycardia, taste perversion, thirst, thrombophlebitis, tinnitus, vertigo, vitreous floater, vomiting, weight gain

Overdosage/Toxicology Symptoms of overdose include nausea, vomiting, hypocalcemia, and hypocalcemic tetany. Treat symptomatically.

Dosing

Adults & Elderly:

Paget's disease *(Miacalcin®)*: I.M., SubQ: Initial: 100 units/day; maintenance: 50 units/day or 50-100 units every 1-3 days

Hypercalcemia *(Miacalcin®)*: Initial: I.M., SubQ: 4 units/kg every 12 hours; may increase up to 8 units/kg every 12 hours to a maximum of every 6 hours

Postmenopausal osteoporosis:

Miacalcin®: I.M., SubQ: 100 units/every other day

Fortical®, Miacalcin®: Intranasal: 200 units (1 spray)/day

Available Dosage Forms

Injection, solution, calcitonin-salmon: (Miacalcin®): 200 int. units/mL (2 mL)

Solution, nasal spray, calcitonin-salmon:

Fortical®: 200 int. units/0.09 mL (3.7 mL) [rDNA origin; contains benzyl alcohol; delivers 30 doses, 200 units/actuation]

Miacalcin®: 200 int. units/0.09 mL (3.7 mL) [contains benzalkonium chloride; delivers 30 doses, 200 units/actuation]

Nursing Guidelines

Assessment: Skin test should be administered before initiating therapy (increased erythema or skin wheal indicates positive reaction and allergy). Assess potential for interactions with other prescriptions, OTC medications, or herbal products patient may be taking. Assess results of laboratory tests and patient response (eg, hypocalcemic tetany, hypercalcemia) at regular intervals during therapy. Teach appropriate administration (eg, subcutaneous or I.M. injections or nasal spray), dietary requirements (low calcium diet if used for hypercalcemia), possible side effects/appropriate interventions, and adverse symptoms to report.

Monitoring Laboratory Tests: Serum electrolytes and calcium, alkaline phosphatase and 24-hour urine collection for hydroxyproline excretion (Paget's disease); bone mineral density; height

Dietary Considerations: Adequate vitamin D and calcium intake is essential for preventing/treating osteoporosis. Patients with Paget's disease and hypercalcemia should follow a low calcium diet as prescribed.

Patient Education: Do not take any new medication during therapy unless approved by prescriber. If administered by injection, you or a significant other will be instructed on how to give the injections and dispose of syringes/needles (follow directions exactly). Keep drug vials in refrigerator; do not freeze. May cause increased warmth and flushing (this should only last about 1 hour after administration; taking drug in evening may minimize these discomforts). Report significant nasal irritation if using nasal spray. Immediately report twitching, muscle spasm, dark-colored urine, hives, significant skin rash, palpitations, or respiratory difficulty. **Pregnancy/breast-feeding precautions:** Inform prescriber if you are or intend to become pregnant. Consult prescriber if breast-feeding.

Geriatric Considerations: Calcitonin may be the drug of choice for postmenopausal women unable to take estrogens to increase bone density and reduce fractures. Calcium and vitamin D supplements should also be given. Calcitonin may also be effective in steroid-induced osteoporosis and other states associated with high bone turnover.

Pregnancy Risk Factor: C

Lactation: Excretion in breast milk unknown/not recommended

Breast-Feeding Considerations: Has been shown to decrease milk production in animals.

Administration

I.M.: Administer injection solution I.M. or SubQ; intramuscular route is recommended over the subcutaneous route when the volume of calcitonin to be injected exceeds 2 mL.

Reconstitution: Injection: NS has been recommended for the dilution to prepare a skin test in patients with suspected sensitivity.

Storage:

Injection: Store under refrigeration at 2°C to 8°C (36°F to 46°F); protect from freezing; NS has been recommended for the dilution to prepare a skin test in patients with suspected sensitivity

Nasal: Store unopened bottle under refrigeration at 2°C to 8°C (36°F to 46°F).

♦ Calcitonin (Salmon) *see* Calcitonin *on page 287*

Calcitriol (kal si TRYE ole)

U.S. Brand Names Calcijex®; Rocaltrol®

Synonyms 1,25 Dihydroxycholecalciferol

Pharmacologic Category Vitamin D Analog

Medication Safety Issues

Sound-alike/look-alike issues:

Calcitriol may be confused with calcifediol, Calciferol®, calcitonin

Dosage is expressed in mcg (micrograms), **not** mg (milligrams); rare cases of acute overdose have been reported

Use Management of hypocalcemia in patients on chronic renal dialysis; management of secondary hyperparathyroidism in moderate-to-severe chronic renal failure; management of hypocalcemia in hypoparathyroidism and pseudohypoparathyroidism

Unlabeled/Investigational Use Decrease severity of psoriatic lesions in psoriatic vulgaris; vitamin D resistant rickets

Mechanism of Action Promotes absorption of calcium in the intestines and retention at the kidneys thereby increasing calcium levels in the serum; decreases excessive serum phosphatase levels, parathyroid hormone levels, and decreases bone resorption; increases renal tubule phosphate resorption

Pharmacodynamics/Kinetics

Onset of action: ~2-6 hours

Duration: 3-5 days

Absorption: Oral: Rapid

Protein binding: 99.9%

Metabolism: Primarily to 1,24,25-trihydroxycholecalciferol and 1,24,25-trihydroxy ergocalciferol

Half-life elimination: 3-8 hours

Excretion: Primarily feces; urine (4% to 6%)

Contraindications Hypercalcemia; vitamin D toxicity; abnormal sensitivity to the effects of vitamin D; pregnancy (dose exceeding RDA)

Warnings/Precautions Adequate dietary (supplemental) calcium is necessary for clinical response to vitamin D. Monitor serum calcium and phosphate concentrations; avoid hypercalcemia; calcium-phosphate product (serum calcium times phosphorus) must not exceed 70. Immobilization or excessive dosage may increase risk of hypercalcemia and/or hypercalciuria. Maintain adequate hydration. Use caution in patients with malabsorption syndromes (efficacy may be limited and/or response may be unpredictable).

Drug Interactions Induces CYP3A4 (weak)

Cholestyramine, colestipol: May decrease absorption/effect of calcitriol.

Corticosteroids: May decrease hypercalcemic effect of calcitriol.

Digitalis: Risk of toxicity may be increased due to hypercalcemia from calcitriol. Monitor.

Magnesium-containing antacids: Toxicity may be increased by calcitriol. Avoid concurrent use.

Thiazide diuretics: May increase risk of hypercalcemia.

Lab Interactions Increased calcium, cholesterol, magnesium, BUN, AST, ALT, calcium (S), cholesterol (S); decreased alkaline phosphatase

(Continued)

Calcitriol *(Continued)*

Adverse Reactions

>10%: Endocrine & metabolic: Hypercalcemia (33%)

Frequency not defined:

Cardiovascular: Cardiac arrhythmia, hyper-/hypotension

Central nervous system: Headache, irritability, seizure (rare), somnolence, psychosis

Dermatologic: Pruritus, erythema multiforme

Endocrine & metabolic: Hypermagnesemia, hyperphosphatemia, polydipsia

Gastrointestinal: Anorexia, constipation, metallic taste, nausea, pancreatitis, vomiting, xerostomia

Hepatic: Elevated LFTs

Neuromuscular & skeletal: Bone pain, myalgia, dystrophy, soft tissue calcification

Ocular: Conjunctivitis, photophobia

Renal: Polyuria

Overdosage/Toxicology Toxicity rarely occurs from acute overdose. Symptoms of chronic overdose include hypercalcemia, hypercalciuria with weakness, altered mental status, GI upset, renal tubular injury, and occasionally cardiac arrhythmias. Following withdrawal of the drug, treatment consists of bed rest, liberal fluid intake, reduced calcium intake, and cathartic administration. Severe hypercalcemia requires I.V. hydration and forced diuresis. I.V. saline may increase excretion of calcium. Calcitonin, cholestyramine, prednisone, sodium EDTA, bisphosphonates, and mithramycin have all been used successfully to treat the more resistant cases of vitamin D-induced hypercalcemia. Use of peritoneal dialysis against a calcium-free dialysate has been reported.

Dosing

Adults & Elderly: Individualize dosage to maintain calcium levels of 9-10 mg/dL.

Renal failure:

Oral: 0.25 mcg/day or every other day (may require 0.5-1 mcg/day)

I.V.: 0.5 mcg (0.01 mcg/kg) 3 times/week; most doses in the range of 0.5-3 mcg (0.01-0.05 mcg/kg) 3 times/week

Hypoparathyroidism/pseudohypoparathyroidism: Oral: 0.5-2 mcg/day

Vitamin D-dependent rickets: Oral: 1 mcg once daily

Vitamin D-resistant rickets (familial hypophosphatemia): Oral: Initial: 0.015-0.02 mcg/kg once daily; maintenance: 0.03-0.06 mcg/kg once daily; maximum dose: 2 mcg once daily

Pediatrics: Individualize dosage to maintain calcium levels of 9-10 mg/dL.

Renal failure:

Children:

Oral: 0.25-2 mcg/day have been used (with hemodialysis); 0.014-0.041 mcg/kg/day (not receiving hemodialysis); increases should be made at 4- to 8-week intervals.

I.V.: 0.01-0.05 mcg/kg 3 times/week if undergoing hemodialysis

Hypoparathyroidism/pseudohypoparathyroidism: Oral (evaluate dosage at 2- to 4-week intervals):

Children:

<1 year: 0.04-0.08 mcg/kg once daily

1-5 years: 0.25-0.75 mcg once daily

Children >6 years: 0.5-2 mcg once daily

Vitamin D-dependent rickets: Refer to adult dosing.

Vitamin D-resistant rickets (familial hypophosphatemia): Refer to adult dosing.

Available Dosage Forms

Capsule (Rocaltrol®): 0.25 mcg, 0.5 mcg [each strength contains coconut oil]

Injection, solution: 1 mcg/mL (1 mL); 2 mcg/mL (2 mL)

Calcijex®: 1 mcg/mL (1 mL)

Solution, oral (Rocaltrol®): 1 mcg/mL (15 mL) [contains palm seed oil]

Nursing Guidelines

Assessment: Assess effectiveness and interactions of other medications patient may be taking. Assess results of laboratory tests, therapeutic effectiveness, and adverse effects at beginning of therapy and regularly with long-term use. Assess knowledge/teach patient appropriate use, appropriate nutritional counseling, possible side effects/interventions, and adverse symptoms to report.

Monitoring Laboratory Tests: Serum calcium and phosphorus, and renal function. The serum calcium times phosphate product should not be allowed to exceed 70.

Dietary Considerations: May be taken without regard to food. Give with meals to reduce GI problems.

Patient Education: Take exact dose as prescribed; do not increase dose. Maintain recommended diet and calcium supplementation. Avoid taking magnesium-containing antacids. You may experience nausea, vomiting, loss of appetite, or metallic taste (small frequent meals, frequent mouth care, chewing gum, or sucking lozenges may help); or hypotension (use caution when rising from sitting or lying position or when climbing stairs or bending over). Report chest pain or palpitations; acute headache; skin rash; change in vision or eye irritation; CNS changes; unusual weakness or fatigue; persistent nausea, vomiting, cramps, or diarrhea; or muscle or bone pain. **Pregnancy/ breast-feeding precautions:** Inform prescriber if you are or intend to become pregnant. Breast-feeding is not recommended.

Geriatric Considerations: Appetite and caloric requirements may decrease with advanced age. Assess diet for adequate nutrient intake with regard to vitamins and minerals. (Daily vitamin supplements are sometimes recommended). Persons >65 years of age have decreased absorption and may have decreased intake of vitamin D. This may require supplement with daily vitamin D intake, especially for those with high risk for osteoporosis.

Pregnancy Risk Factor: C (manufacturer); A/D (dose exceeding RDA recommendation) (expert analysis)

Lactation: Enters breast milk/not recommended

Administration

Oral: May be administered without regard to food. Give with meals to reduce GI problems.

I.V.: May be administered as a bolus dose I.V. through the catheter at the end of hemodialysis.

Compatibility: Stable in D_5W, NS, SWFI

Storage: Store in tight, light-resistant container. Calcitriol degrades upon prolonged exposure to light.

Calcium Carbonate (KAL see um KAR bun ate)

U.S. Brand Names Alcalak [OTC]; Alka-Mints® [OTC]; Amitone® [OTC]; Calcarb 600 [OTC]; Calci-Chew® [OTC]; Calci-Mix® [OTC]; Cal-Gest [OTC]; Cal-Mint [OTC]; Caltrate® 600 [OTC]; Children's Pepto [OTC]; Chooz® [OTC]; Florical® [OTC]; Mylanta® Children's [OTC]; Nephro-Calci® [OTC]; Os-Cal® 500 [OTC]; Oysco 500 [OTC]; Oyst-Cal 500 [OTC]; Titralac™ [OTC]; Titralac™ Extra Strength [OTC]; Tums® [OTC]; Tums® 500 [OTC]; Tums® E-X [OTC]; Tums® Extra Strength Sugar Free [OTC]; Tums® Smooth Dissolve [OTC]; Tums® Ultra [OTC]

Pharmacologic Category Antacid; Antidote; Calcium Salt; Electrolyte Supplement, Oral

Medication Safety Issues

Sound-alike/look-alike issues:

Florical® may be confused with Fiorinal®
Mylanta® may be confused with Mynatal®
Nephro-Calci® may be confused with Nephrocaps®
Os-Cal® may be confused with Asacol®

Use As an antacid, and treatment and prevention of calcium deficiency or hyperphosphatemia (eg, osteoporosis, osteomalacia, mild/moderate renal insufficiency, hypoparathyroidism, postmenopausal osteoporosis, rickets); has been used to bind phosphate

Mechanism of Action As dietary supplement, used to prevent or treat negative calcium balance; in osteoporosis, it helps to prevent or decrease the rate of bone loss. The calcium in calcium salts moderates nerve and muscle performance and allows normal cardiac function. Also used to treat hyperphosphatemia in patients with advanced renal insufficiency by combining with dietary phosphate to form insoluble calcium phosphate, which is excreted in feces. Calcium salts as antacids neutralize gastric acidity resulting in increased gastric an duodenal bulb pH; they additionally inhibit proteolytic activity of peptic if the pH is increased >4 and increase lower esophageal sphincter tone.

Pharmacodynamics/Kinetics

Absorption: Requires vitamin D; minimal unless chronic, high doses are given; calcium is absorbed in soluble, ionized form; solubility of calcium is increased in an acid environment

(Continued)

Calcium Carbonate *(Continued)*

Distribution: Crosses placenta; enters breast milk

Excretion: Primarily feces (as unabsorbed calcium); urine (20%)

Contraindications Hypercalcemia, renal calculi, hypophosphatemia; patients with suspected digoxin toxicity

Warnings/Precautions Calcium carbonate absorption is impaired in achlorhydria (common in elderly - use alternate salt, administer with food); administration is followed by increased gastric acid secretion within 2 hours of administration; while hypercalcemia and hypercalciuria may result when therapeutic replacement amounts are given for prolonged periods, they are most likely to occur in hypoparathyroid patients receiving high doses of vitamin D

Drug Interactions

Calcium channel blockers (eg, verapamil) effects may be diminished; monitor response.

Levothyroxine: Calcium carbonate (and possibly other calcium salts) may decrease T_4 absorption; separate dose from levothyroxine by at least 4 hours

Polystyrene sulfonate: Potassium-binding ability is reduced; avoid concurrent use.

Tetracycline, atenolol (and potentially other beta-blockers), iron, quinolone antibiotics, alendronate, sodium fluoride, and zinc absorption is significantly decreased; space administration times.

Thiazide diuretics can cause hypercalcemia; monitor response.

May potentiate digoxin toxicity. High doses of calcium with thiazide diuretics may result in milk-alkali syndrome and hypercalcemia.

Nutritional/Herbal/Ethanol Interactions

Ethanol: Avoid ethanol (may increase risk of osteoporosis).

Food: Food may increase calcium absorption. Calcium may decrease iron absorption. Bran, foods high in oxalates, or whole grain cereals may decrease calcium absorption.

Lab Interactions Increased calcium (S); decreased magnesium

Adverse Reactions Well tolerated

1% to 10%:

- Central nervous system: Headache
- Endocrine & metabolic: Hypophosphatemia, hypercalcemia
- Gastrointestinal: Constipation, laxative effect, acid rebound, nausea, vomiting, anorexia, abdominal pain, xerostomia, flatulence
- Miscellaneous: Milk-alkali syndrome with very high, chronic dosing and/or renal failure (headache, nausea, irritability, and weakness or alkalosis, hypercalcemia, renal impairment)

Overdosage/Toxicology

Acute single ingestions of calcium salts may produce mild gastrointestinal distress, but hypercalcemia or other toxic manifestations are extremely unlikely

Treatment is supportive

Dosing

Adults & Elderly: Dosage is in terms of elemental calcium:

Dietary Reference Intake:

Adults, Male/Female:

- 19-50 years: 1000 mg/day
- ≥51 years: 1200 mg/day

Female: Pregnancy: Same as for Adults, Male/Female

Female: Lactating: Same as for Adults, Male/Female

Hypocalcemia (dose depends on clinical condition and serum calcium level): Dose expressed in mg of **elemental calcium**: 1-2 g or more/day in 3-4 divided doses

Dietary supplementation: 500 mg to 2 g divided 2-4 times/day

Antacid: Dosage based on acid-neutralizing capacity of specific product; generally, 1-2 tablets or 5-10 mL every 2 hours; maximum: 7000 mg calcium carbonate per 24 hours; specific product labeling should be consulted

Osteoporosis: Adults >51 years: 1200 mg/day

Pediatrics: Dosage is in terms of elemental calcium:

Dietary Reference Intake:

- 0-6 months: 210 mg/day
- 7-12 months: 270 mg/day
- 1-3 years: 500 mg/day
- 4-8 years: 800 mg/day
- 9-19 years: 1300 mg/day

Hypocalcemia (dose depends on clinical condition and serum calcium level): Dose expressed in mg of **elemental calcium**

Neonates: 50-150 mg/kg/day in 4-6 divided doses; not to exceed 1 g/day

Children: 45-65 mg/kg/day in 4 divided doses

Antacid:

Children 2-5 years (24-47 lbs): Elemental calcium 161 mg as needed; maximum 483 mg per 24 hours

Children 6-11 years (48-95 lbs): Elemental calcium 322 mg as needed; maximum: 966 mg per 24 hours

Renal Impairment: Cl_{cr} <25 mL/minute: Dosage adjustments may be necessary depending on the serum calcium levels.

Available Dosage Forms

Capsule:

Calci-Mix®: 1250 mg [equivalent to elemental calcium 500 mg]

Florical®: 364 mg [equivalent to elemental calcium 145.6 mg; contains sodium fluoride 8.3 mg]

Powder: 1600 mg/teaspoonful (960 g)

Suspension, oral: 1250 mg/5 mL (5 mL, 500 mL) [equivalent to elemental calcium 500 mg/5 mL; mint flavor]

Tablet: 1250 mg [equivalent to elemental calcium 500 mg]; 1500 mg [equivalent to elemental calcium 600 mg]

Calcarb 600, Caltrate® 600, Nephro-Calci®: 1500 mg [equivalent to elemental calcium 600 mg]

Florical®: 364 mg [equivalent to elemental calcium 145.6 mg; contains sodium fluoride 8.3 mg]

Os-Cal® 500, Oysco 500, Oyst-Cal 500: 1250 mg [equivalent to elemental calcium 500 mg]

Tablet, chewable: 500 mg [equivalent to elemental calcium 200 mg]; 650 mg [equivalent to elemental calcium 260 mg]; 750 mg [equivalent to elemental calcium 300 mg]

Alcalak: 420 mg [equivalent to elemental calcium 168 mg]

Alka-Mints®: 850 mg [equivalent to elemental calcium 340 mg; assorted and spearmint flavors]

Amitone®: 420 mg [equivalent to elemental calcium 168 mg; spearmint flavor]

Cal-Gest: 500 mg [equivalent to elemental calcium 200 mg]

Calci-Chew®: 1250 mg [equivalent to elemental calcium 500 mg; cherry, lemon, and orange flavors]

Cal-Mint: 650 mg [equivalent to elemental calcium 260 mg; mint flavor]

Children's Pepto: 400 mg [equivalent to elemental calcium 161 mg; bubble gum or watermelon flavors]

Chooz®: 500 mg [equivalent to elemental calcium 200 mg; contains phenylalanine]

Mylanta® Children's: 400 mg [equivalent to elemental calcium 160 mg; bubble gum flavor]

Os-Cal® 500: 1250 mg [equivalent to elemental calcium 500 mg; Bavarian cream flavor]

Titralac™: 420 mg [equivalent to elemental calcium 168 mg; sugar free; mint flavor]

Titralac™ Extra Strength: 750 mg [equivalent to elemental calcium 300 mg; sugar free; mint flavor]

Tums®: 500 mg [equivalent to elemental calcium 200 mg; assorted fruit (contains tartrazine) and peppermint flavors]

Tums® E-X: 750 mg [equivalent to elemental calcium 300 mg; assorted fruit (contains tartrazine), fresh blend, tropical assorted fruit, wintergreen (contains tartrazine), and assorted berry flavors]

Tums® Extra Strength Sugar Free: 750 mg [equivalent to elemental calcium 300 mg; sugar free; contains phenylalanine <1 mg/tablet; orange cream flavor]

Tums® Smooth Dissolve: 750 mg [equivalent to elemental calcium 300 mg; assorted fruit (contains tartrazine) and peppermint flavors]

Tums® Ultra®: 1000 mg [equivalent to elemental calcium 400 mg; assorted mint, assorted berry, and tropical assorted berry (contains tartrazine) flavors]

Nursing Guidelines

Assessment: Assess other medications patient may be taking for effectiveness and interactions. Assess results of laboratory tests, therapeutic effect, and adverse/toxic effects. Assess knowledge/teach patient proper use, appropriate interventions to reduce side effects, and adverse symptoms to report.

(Continued)

Calcium Carbonate *(Continued)*

Dietary Considerations: As a dietary supplement, should be given with meals to increase absorption. May decrease iron absorption, so should be administered 1-2 hours before or after iron supplementation; limit intake of with bran, foods high in oxalates or whole grain cereals which may decrease calcium absorption.

Patient Education: Follow instructions for dosing. Take with a full glass of water or juice 1-2 hours before any iron supplements and 1-3 hours after meals or other medications. Avoid alcohol, other antacids, caffeine, or other calcium supplements, unless approved by prescriber. You may experience constipation (increased exercise, fluids, fiber, or fruit may help) or dry mouth (sucking lozenges or hard candy may help). Report severe, unresolved GI disturbances and unusual emotional liability (mood swings). **Pregnancy precaution:** Inform prescriber if you are or intend to become pregnant.

Calcium Carbonate and Magnesium Hydroxide

(KAL see um KAR bun ate & mag NEE zhum hye DROKS ide)

U.S. Brand Names Mi-Acid™ Double Strength [OTC]; Mylanta® Gelcaps® [OTC]; Mylanta® Supreme [OTC]; Mylanta® Ultra [OTC]; Rolaids® [OTC]; Rolaids® Extra Strength [OTC]

Synonyms Magnesium Hydroxide and Calcium Carbonate

Pharmacologic Category Antacid

Medication Safety Issues

Sound-alike/look-alike issues:

Mylanta® may be confused with Mynatal®

Use Hyperacidity

Pharmacodynamics/Kinetics See individual agents.

Drug Interactions See individual agents.

Dosing

Adults & Elderly: Hyperacidity: Oral: 2-4 tablets between meals, at bedtime, or as directed by healthcare provider

Available Dosage Forms

Gelcap (Mylanta® Gelcaps®): Calcium carbonate 550 mg and magnesium hydroxide 125 mg

Liquid (Mylanta® Supreme): Calcium carbonate 400 mg and magnesium hydroxide 135 mg per 5 mL (360 mL, 720 mL) [cherry flavor]

Tablet, chewable:

Mi-Acid™ Double Strength: Calcium carbonate 700 mg and magnesium hydroxide 300 mg

Mylanta® Ultra: Calcium carbonate 700 mg and magnesium hydroxide 300 mg [cherry créme and cool mint flavors]

Rolaids®: Calcium carbonate 550 mg and magnesium hydroxide 110 mg [sodium free; contains elemental calcium 220 mg and elemental magnesium 45 mg; original (peppermint), cherry, and spearmint flavors]

Rolaids® Extra Strength: Calcium carbonate 675 mg and magnesium hydroxide 135 mg [sodium free; contains elemental calcium 271 mg and elemental magnesium 56 mg, fruit flavor contains tartrazine; cool strawberry, fresh mint, fruit, and tropical fruit punch flavors]

Calcium Carbonate and Simethicone

(KAL see um KAR bun ate & sye METH i kone)

U.S. Brand Names Gas Ban™ [OTC]; Titralac® Plus [OTC]

Synonyms Simethicone and Calcium Carbonate

Pharmacologic Category Antacid; Antiflatulent

Use Relief of acid indigestion, heartburn

Pharmacodynamics/Kinetics See individual agents.

Drug Interactions See individual agents.

Dosing

Adults & Elderly: Hyperacidity, gas: Oral (OTC labeling): Two tablets every 2-3 hours as needed (maximum: 19 tablets/24 hours)

Available Dosage Forms Tablet, chewable:

Gas Ban™: Calcium carbonate 300 mg and simethicone 40 mg

Titralac® Plus: Calcium carbonate 420 mg and simethicone 21 mg [equivalent to elemental calcium 168 mg; sugar free; spearmint flavor]

Nursing Guidelines

Patient Education: Follow instructions for dosing. Take with a full glass of water or juice, 1-3 hours after other medications and 1-2 hours before any iron supplements. Avoid other antacids, caffeine, or other calcium supplements unless approved by prescriber. You may experience constipation (increased exercise, fluids, fruit, or fiber may help). Report severe, unresolved GI disturbances and unusual emotional lability (mood swings). **Pregnancy/breast-feeding precautions:** Inform prescriber if you are or intend to become pregnant. Consult prescriber if breast-feeding.

Pregnancy Risk Factor: C

Administration

Oral: Tablets may be chewed, swallowed whole, or allowed to melt in the mouth.

Calcium Chloride (KAL see um KLOR ide)

Pharmacologic Category Calcium Salt; Electrolyte Supplement, Parenteral

Use Cardiac resuscitation when epinephrine fails to improve myocardial contractions, cardiac disturbances of hyperkalemia, hypocalcemia, or calcium channel blocking agent toxicity; emergent treatment of hypocalcemic tetany, treatment of hypermagnesemia

Mechanism of Action Moderates nerve and muscle performance via action potential excitation threshold regulation

Pharmacodynamics/Kinetics

Distribution: Crosses placenta; enters breast milk

Excretion: Primarily feces (as unabsorbed calcium); urine (20%)

Contraindications In ventricular fibrillation during cardiac resuscitation, hypercalcemia, and in patients with risk of digitalis toxicity, renal or cardiac disease; not recommended in treatment of asystole and electromechanical dissociation; patients with suspected digoxin toxicity

Warnings/Precautions Avoid too rapid I.V. administration (<1 mL/minute) and extravasation; use with caution in digitalized patients, respiratory failure, or acidosis; hypercalcemia may occur in patients with renal failure, and frequent determination of serum calcium is necessary; avoid metabolic acidosis (ie, administer only 2-3 days then change to another calcium salt)

Drug Interactions

Calcium channel blockers (eg, verapamil) effects may be diminished; monitor response.

Levothyroxine: Calcium carbonate (and possibly other calcium salts) may decrease T_4 absorption; separate dose from levothyroxine by at least 4 hours

Thiazide diuretics can cause hypercalcemia; monitor response.

May potentiate digoxin toxicity. High doses of calcium with thiazide diuretics may result in milk-alkali syndrome and hypercalcemia.

Lab Interactions Increased calcium (S); decreased magnesium

Adverse Reactions <1% (Limited to important or life-threatening): Bradycardia, cardiac arrhythmia, coma, decreased serum magnesium, elevated serum amylase, erythema, hypercalcemia, hypercalciuria, hypotension, lethargy, mania, muscle weakness, syncope, tissue necrosis, vasodilation, ventricular fibrillation

Overdosage/Toxicology

Symptoms of overdose include lethargy, nausea, vomiting, coma

Following withdrawal of the drug, treatment consists of bed rest, liberal intake of fluids, reduced calcium intake, and cathartic administration. Severe hypercalcemia requires I.V. hydration and forced diuresis. Urine output should be monitored and maintained at >3 mL/kg/hour. I.V. saline and natriuretic agents (eg, furosemide) can quickly and significantly increase excretion of calcium.

Dosing

Adults & Elderly: Note: Calcium chloride has 3 times more elemental calcium than calcium gluconate. Calcium chloride is 27% elemental calcium; calcium gluconate is 9% elemental calcium. One gram of calcium chloride is equal to 270 mg of elemental calcium; one gram of calcium gluconate is equal to 90 mg of elemental calcium. Dosages are expressed in terms of the calcium chloride salt based on a solution concentration of 100 mg/mL (10%) containing 1.4 mEq (27.3 mg)/mL elemental calcium.

Cardiac arrest in the presence of hyperkalemia or hypocalcemia, magnesium toxicity, or calcium antagonist toxicity: I.V.: 2-4 mg/kg, repeated every 10 minutes if necessary

Hypocalcemia: I.V.: 500 mg to 1 g/dose repeated every 4-6 hours if needed

Hypocalcemic tetany: I.V.: 1 g over 10-30 minutes; may repeat after 6 hours

(Continued)

Calcium Chloride *(Continued)*

Hypocalcemia secondary to citrated blood transfusion: I.V.: 200-500 mg per 500 mL of citrated blood (infused into another vein)

Note: Routine administration of calcium, in the absence of signs/symptoms of hypocalcemia, is generally not recommended. A number of recommendations have been published seeking to address potential hypocalcemia during massive transfusion of citrated blood; however, many practitioners recommend replacement only as guided by clinical evidence of hypocalcemia and/or serial monitoring of ionized calcium.

Pediatrics: Note: Calcium chloride has 3 times more elemental calcium than calcium gluconate. Calcium chloride is 27% elemental calcium; calcium gluconate is 9% elemental calcium. One gram of calcium chloride is equal to 270 mg of elemental calcium; one gram of calcium gluconate is equal to 90 mg of elemental calcium. Dosages are expressed in terms of the calcium chloride salt based on a solution concentration of 100 mg/mL (10%) containing 1.4 mEq (27.3 mg)/mL elemental calcium.

Cardiac arrest in the presence of hyperkalemia or hypocalcemia, magnesium toxicity, or calcium antagonist toxicity: I.V.:

Infants and Children: 20 mg/kg; may repeat in 10 minutes if necessary

Adolescents: Refer to adult dosing.

Hypocalcemia: I.V.:

Children (manufacturer's recommendation): 2.7-5 mg/kg/dose every 4-6 hours

Alternative pediatric dosing: Infants and Children: 10-20 mg/kg/dose; repeat every 4-6 hours if needed

Hypocalcemic tetany: I.V.:

Neonates: Divided doses totaling approximately 170 mg/kg/24 hours

Infants and Children: 10 mg/kg over 5-10 minutes; may repeat after 6-8 hours or follow with an infusion with a maximum dose of 200 mg/kg/day; alternatively, higher doses of 35-50 mg/kg/dose repeated every 6-8 hours have been used

Hypocalcemia secondary to citrated blood transfusion: I.V.: Neonates, Infants, and Children: Give 32 mg (0.45 mEq **elemental** calcium) for each 100 mL citrated blood infused. See "**Note**" in adult dosing.

Renal Impairment: Cl_{cr} <25 mL/minute: Dosage adjustments may be necessary depending on the serum calcium levels.

Available Dosage Forms Injection, solution [preservative free]: 10% [100 mg/mL] (10 mL) [equivalent to elemental calcium 27.2 mg/mL, calcium 1.36 mEq/mL]

Nursing Guidelines

Patient Education: This medication can only be given intravenously. Do not make rapid postural changes while calcium is infusing. Report any feelings of excitation, chest pain, irregular or pounding heartbeat, vomiting, acute headache, or dizziness.

Pregnancy Risk Factor: C

Administration

Compatibility: Stable in most common intravenous infusion solutions

Compatibility when admixed: Incompatible with amphotericin B, chlorpheniramine

Y-site administration: Incompatible with amphotericin B cholesteryl sulfate complex, propofol, sodium bicarbonate

◆ **Calcium Disodium Edetate** *see* Edetate Calcium Disodium *on page 593*
◆ **Calcium Disodium Versenate®** *see* Edetate Calcium Disodium *on page 593*
◆ **Calcium EDTA** *see* Edetate Calcium Disodium *on page 593*

Calcium Gluconate (KAL see um GLOO koe nate)

Pharmacologic Category Calcium Salt; Electrolyte Supplement, Oral; Electrolyte Supplement, Parenteral

Medication Safety Issues

Sound-alike/look-alike issues:

Calcium gluconate may be confused with calcium glubionate

Use Treatment and prevention of hypocalcemia; treatment of tetany, cardiac disturbances of hyperkalemia, cardiac resuscitation when epinephrine fails to improve myocardial contractions, hypocalcemia, or calcium channel blocker toxicity; calcium supplementation

Unlabeled/Investigational Use Hydrofluoric acid (HF) burns

Mechanism of Action As dietary supplement, used to prevent or treat negative calcium balance; in osteoporosis, it helps to prevent or decrease the rate of bone loss. The calcium in calcium salts moderates nerve and muscle performance and allows normal cardiac function.

Pharmacodynamics/Kinetics

Absorption: Requires vitamin D; calcium is absorbed in soluble, ionized form; solubility of calcium is increased in an acid environment

Distribution: Primarily in bones and teeth; crosses placenta; enters breast milk

Protein binding: Primarily albumin

Excretion: Primarily feces (as unabsorbed calcium); urine (20%)

Contraindications Ventricular fibrillation during cardiac resuscitation; digitalis toxicity or suspected digoxin toxicity; hypercalcemia

Warnings/Precautions Injection solution is for I.V. use only; do not inject SubQ or I.M.; avoid too rapid I.V. administration and avoid extravasation. Use with caution in digitalized patients, severe hyperphosphatemia, respiratory failure or acidosis. May produce cardiac arrest. Hypercalcemia may occur in patients with renal failure, frequent determination of serum calcium is necessary. Use caution with renal disease. Solutions may contain aluminum; toxic levels may occur following prolonged administration in premature neonates or patients with renal dysfunction.

Drug Interactions

Bisphosphonate derivatives: Absorption may be decreased by calcium salts.

Calcium channel blockers (eg, verapamil) effects may be diminished; monitor response.

Digoxin: May potentiate digoxin toxicity.

Dobutamine: Calcium salts may diminish the therapeutic effect of dobutamine.

Levothyroxine: Calcium carbonate (and possibly other calcium salts) may decrease T_4 absorption; separate dose from levothyroxine by at least 4 hours

Phosphate supplements: Calcium salts may decrease the absorption of phosphate supplements.

Quinolone antibiotics: Calcium salts may decrease the absorption of quinolone antibiotics with oral administration of both agents.

Thiazide diuretics: Thiazide diuretics may decrease the excretion of calcium salts. Continued concomitant use can also result in metabolic alkalosis.

Lab Interactions Increased calcium (S); decreased magnesium

Adverse Reactions Frequency not defined.

I.V.:

- Cardiovascular: Arrhythmia, bradycardia, cardiac arrest, hypotension, vasodilation, and syncope may occur following rapid I.V. injection
- Central nervous system: Sense of oppression
- Gastrointestinal: Chalky taste
- Local: Abscess and necrosis following I.M. administration
- Neuromuscular & skeletal: Tingling sensation
- Miscellaneous: Heat waves

Postmarketing and/or case reports: Calcinosis cutis

Oral: Gastrointestinal: Constipation

Overdosage/Toxicology

Acute single oral ingestions of calcium salts may produce mild gastrointestinal distress, but hypercalcemia or other toxic manifestations are extremely unlikely. Symptoms of hypercalcemia include lethargy, nausea, vomiting, and coma.

Treatment is supportive. Severe hypercalcemia following parenteral overdose requires I.V. hydration. Urine output should be monitored and maintained at >3 mL/kg/hour. I.V. saline and natriuretic agents (eg, furosemide) can quickly and significantly increase excretion of calcium into urine.

Dosing

Adults & Elderly:

Dietary Reference Intake (expressed as elemental calcium):

Adults, Male/Female:

- 19-50 years: 1000 mg/day
- ≥51 years: 1200 mg/day

Female: Pregnancy: Same as for Adults, Male/Female

Female: Lactating: Same as for Adults, Male/Female

Dosage note: Calcium chloride has 3 times more elemental calcium than calcium gluconate. Calcium chloride is 27% elemental calcium; calcium gluconate is 9% elemental calcium. One gram of calcium chloride is equal to 270 mg of elemental calcium; one gram of calcium gluconate is equal to 90 mg of elemental calcium. The following dosages are expressed in terms of

(Continued)

Calcium Gluconate *(Continued)*

the calcium gluconate salt based on a solution concentration of 100 mg/mL (10%) containing 0.465 mEq (9.3 mg)/mL elemental calcium:

Hypocalcemia:

I.V.: 2-15 g/24 hours as a continuous infusion or in divided doses

Oral: 500 mg to 2 g 2-4 times/day

Osteoporosis/bone loss: Oral: 1000-1500 mg in divided doses/day

Hypocalcemia secondary to citrated blood infusion: I.V.: 500 mg to 1 g per 500 mL of citrated blood (infused into another vein). Single doses up to 2 g have also been recommended.

Note: Routine administration of calcium, in the absence of signs/symptoms of hypocalcemia, is generally not recommended. A number of recommendations have been published seeking to address potential hypocalcemia during massive transfusion of citrated blood; however, many practitioners recommend replacement only as guided by clinical evidence of hypocalcemia and/or serial monitoring of ionized calcium.

Hypocalcemic tetany: I.V.: 1-3 g/dose may be administered until therapeutic response occurs

Calcium antagonist toxicity, magnesium intoxication, or cardiac arrest in the presence of hyperkalemia or hypocalcemia: I.V.: 500-800 mg/dose (maximum: 3 g/dose)

Maintenance electrolyte requirements for TPN: I.V.: Daily requirements: 1.7-3.4 g/1000 kcal/24 hours

Pediatrics:

Dietary Reference Intake (expressed as elemental calcium):

0-6 months: 210 mg/day
7-12 months: 270 mg/day
1-3 years: 500 mg/day
4-8 years: 800 mg/day
9-18 years: 1300 mg/day

Dosage note: Calcium chloride has 3 times more elemental calcium than calcium gluconate. Calcium chloride is 27% elemental calcium; calcium gluconate is (9% elemental calcium). One gram of calcium chloride is equal to 270 mg of elemental calcium; one gram of calcium gluconate is equal to 90 mg of elemental calcium. The following dosages are expressed in terms of the calcium gluconate salt based on a solution concentration of 100 mg/mL (10%) containing 0.465 mEq (9.3 mg)/mL elemental calcium:

Hypocalcemia:

I.V.:

Neonates: 200-800 mg/kg/day as a continuous infusion or in 4 divided doses (maximum: 1 g/dose)

Infants and Children: 200-500 mg/kg/day as a continuous infusion or in 4 divided doses (maximum: 2-3 g/dose)

Oral: Children: 200-500 mg/kg/day divided every 6 hours

Hypocalcemia secondary to citrated blood infusion: I.V.: Neonates, Infants, and Children: Give 98 mg (0.45 mEq **elemental** calcium) for each 100 mL citrated blood infused. See "**Note**" in adult dosing.

Hypocalcemic tetany: I.V.:

Infants and Children: 100-200 mg/kg/dose over 5-10 minutes; may repeat every 6-8 hours **or** follow with an infusion of 500 mg/kg/day

Calcium antagonist toxicity, magnesium intoxication or cardiac arrest in the presence of hyperkalemia or hypocalcemia: I.V.: Infants and Children: 60-100 mg/kg/dose (maximum: 3 g/dose)

Renal Impairment: Cl_{cr} <25 mL/minute: Dosage adjustments may be necessary depending on the serum calcium levels.

Available Dosage Forms

Injection, solution [preservative free]: 10% [100 mg/mL] (10 mL, 50 mL, 100 mL, 200 mL) [equivalent to elemental calcium 9 mg/mL; calcium 0.46 mEq/mL]

Powder: 347 mg/tablespoonful (480 g)

Tablet: 500 mg [equivalent to elemental calcium 45 mg]; 650 mg [equivalent to elemental calcium 58.5 mg]; 975 mg [equivalent to elemental calcium 87.75 mg]

Nursing Guidelines

Assessment:

Assess other medications patient may be taking for effectiveness and interactions. Assess results of laboratory tests, therapeutic effect, and adverse/toxic effects. Assess knowledge/teach patient proper use, appropriate interventions to reduce side effects, and adverse symptoms to report. If administered I.V., monitor ECG, vital signs, and CNS. Observe infusion site closely. Avoid extravasation.

Patient Education: Do not take any new medication during therapy without consulting prescriber. Follow exact instructions for dosing. Take with a full glass of water or juice, 1-3 hours after other medications, and 1-2 hours before any approved iron supplements. Avoid alcohol, other antacids, caffeine, or other calcium supplements unless approved by prescriber. May cause constipation (increased exercise, fluids, fiber, or fruits may help) or dry mouth (frequent mouth care, chewing gum, or sucking lozenges may help). Report severe, unresolved GI disturbances and unusual emotional lability (mood swings). **Pregnancy precaution:** Inform prescriber if you are or intend to become pregnant.

Pregnancy Risk Factor: C

Lactation: Enters breast milk

Breast-Feeding Considerations: Endogenous calcium is excreted in breast milk.

Administration

I.M.: Not for I.M. or SubQ administration

I.V.: For I.V. administration only; administer slowly (~1.5 mL calcium gluconate 10% per minute) through a small needle into a large vein in order to avoid too rapid increased in serum calcium and extravasation

Compatibility: Stable in D_5LR, D_5NS, D_5W, $D_{10}W$, $D_{20}W$, LR, NS; **incompatible** in fat emulsion 10%

Y-site administration: Incompatible with amphotericin B cholesteryl sulfate complex, fluconazole, indomethacin

Compatibility in syringe: Incompatible with metoclopramide

Compatibility when admixed: Incompatible with amphotericin B, cefamandole, cefazolin, clindamycin, dobutamine, floxacillin, methylprednisolone sodium succinate

- **Calcium Leucovorin** *see* Leucovorin *on page 1013*
- **Caldecort® [OTC]** *see* Hydrocortisone *on page 873*
- **Cal-Gest [OTC]** *see* Calcium Carbonate *on page 291*
- **Cal-Mint [OTC]** *see* Calcium Carbonate *on page 291*
- **Cal-Nate™** *see* Vitamins (Multiple/Prenatal) *on page 1721*
- **Caltrate® 600 [OTC]** *see* Calcium Carbonate *on page 291*
- **Campath®** *see* Alemtuzumab *on page 102*
- **Campath-1H** *see* Alemtuzumab *on page 102*
- **Camphorated Tincture of Opium (error-prone synonym)** *see* Paregoric *on page 1312*
- **Camptosar®** *see* Irinotecan *on page 962*
- **Camptothecin-11** *see* Irinotecan *on page 962*
- **Canasa™** *see* Mesalamine *on page 1105*
- **Cancidas®** *see* Caspofungin *on page 324*

Candesartan (kan de SAR tan)

U.S. Brand Names Atacand®

Synonyms Candesartan Cilexetil

Pharmacologic Category Angiotensin II Receptor Blocker

Use Alone or in combination with other antihypertensive agents in treating essential hypertension; treatment of heart failure (NYHA class II-IV)

Mechanism of Action Candesartan is an angiotensin receptor antagonist. Angiotensin II acts as a vasoconstrictor. In addition to causing direct vasoconstriction, angiotensin II also stimulates the release of aldosterone. Once aldosterone is released, sodium as well as water are reabsorbed. The end result is an elevation in blood pressure. Candesartan binds to the AT1 angiotensin II receptor. This binding prevents angiotensin II from binding to the receptor thereby blocking the vasoconstriction and the aldosterone secreting effects of angiotensin II.

Pharmacodynamics/Kinetics

Onset of action: 2-3 hours

Peak effect: 6-8 hours

Duration: >24 hours

Distribution: V_d: 0.13 L/kg

Protein binding: 99%

Metabolism: To candesartan by the intestinal wall cells

Bioavailability: 15%

(Continued)

Candesartan *(Continued)*

Half-life elimination (dose dependent): 5-9 hours
Time to peak: 3-4 hours
Excretion: Urine (26%)
Clearance: Total body: 0.37 mL/kg/minute; Renal: 0.19 mL/kg/minute

Contraindications Hypersensitivity to candesartan or any component of the formulation; hypersensitivity to other A-II receptor antagonists; bilateral renal artery stenosis; pregnancy (2nd and 3rd trimesters)

Warnings/Precautions Avoid use or use a smaller dose in patients who are volume depleted; correct depletion first. May be associated with deterioration of renal function and/or increases in serum creatinine, particularly in patients dependent on renin-angiotensin-aldosterone system; deterioration may result in oliguria, acute renal failure, and progressive azotemia. Small increases in serum creatinine may occur following initiation; consider discontinuation only in patients with progressive and/or significant deterioration in renal function. Use with caution in unilateral renal artery stenosis, hepatic dysfunction, pre-existing renal insufficiency, or significant aortic/mitral stenosis. Use caution when initiating in heart failure; may need to adjust dose, and/or concurrent diuretic therapy, because of candesartan-induced hypotension. Although some properties may be shared between these agents, concurrent therapy with ACE inhibitor may be rational in selected patients.

Drug Interactions Substrate of CYP2C8/9 (minor); **Inhibits** CYP2C8/9 (weak)
Lithium: Risk of toxicity may be increased by candesartan; monitor lithium levels.
NSAIDs: May decrease angiotensin II antagonist efficacy; effect has been seen with losartan, but may occur with other medications in this class; monitor blood pressure
Potassium-sparing diuretics (amiloride, spironolactone, triamterene): May increase risk of hyperkalemia.
Potassium supplements: May increase the risk of hyperkalemia.
Trimethoprim (high dose): May increase the risk of hyperkalemia.

Nutritional/Herbal/Ethanol Interactions
Food: Food reduces the time to maximal concentration and increases the C_{max}.
Herb/Nutraceutical: Avoid dong quai if using for hypertension (has estrogenic activity). Avoid ephedra, yohimbe, ginseng (may worsen hypertension). Avoid garlic (may have increased antihypertensive effect).

Adverse Reactions
Cardiovascular: Angina, hypotension (CHF 19%), MI, palpitation, tachycardia
Central nervous system: Dizziness, lightheadedness, drowsiness, headache, vertigo, anxiety, depression, somnolence, fever
Dermatologic: Angioedema, rash
Endocrine & metabolic: Hyperglycemia, hyperkalemia (CHF <1% to 6%), hypertriglyceridemia, hyperuricemia
Gastrointestinal: Dyspepsia, gastroenteritis
Genitourinary: Hematuria
Neuromuscular & skeletal: Back pain, CPK increased, myalgia, paresthesia, weakness
Renal: Serum creatinine increased (up to 13% in patients with CHF with drug discontinuation required in 6%)
Respiratory: Dyspnea, epistaxis, pharyngitis, rhinitis, upper respiratory tract infection
Miscellaneous: Diaphoresis (increased)

<1%, postmarketing, and/or case reports: Abnormal hepatic function, agranulocytosis, anemia, hepatitis, hyponatremia, leukopenia, neutropenia, pruritus, renal failure, renal impairment, rhinitis, sinusitis, thrombocytopenia, urticaria; rhabdomyolysis has been reported (rarely) with angiotensin-receptor antagonists

Overdosage/Toxicology Symptoms of overdose include hypotension and tachycardia. Treatment is supportive.

Dosing

Adults & Elderly:

Hypertension: Oral: 4-32 mg once daily. Dosage must be individualized. Blood pressure response is dose-related over the range of 2-32 mg. The usual recommended starting dose is 16 mg once daily when it is used as monotherapy in patients who are not volume depleted. It can be administered once or twice daily with total daily doses ranging from 8-32 mg; larger doses do not appear to have a greater effect and there is relatively little experience with such doses.

Congestive heart failure: Oral: Initial: 4 mg once daily; double the dose at 2-week intervals, as tolerated; target dose: 32 mg

Note: In selected cases, concurrent therapy with an ACE inhibitor may provide additional benefit.

Hepatic Impairment: No initial dosage adjustment required in mild hepatic impairment. Consider initiation at lower dosages in moderate hepatic impairment (AUC increased by 145%). No data available concerning dosing in severe hepatic impairment.

Available Dosage Forms Tablet, as cilexetil: 4 mg, 8 mg, 16 mg, 32 mg

Nursing Guidelines

Assessment: See Contraindications, Warnings/Precautions, and Dosing for use cautions. Assess potential for interactions with other prescriptions, OTC medications, or herbal products patient may be taking (see Drug Interactions). Assess results of laboratory tests (see below) and patient response at beginning of therapy, when changing dose, and on a regular basis during long-term therapy (see Adverse Reactions and Overdose/Toxicology). Teach patient appropriate use, possible side effects/appropriate interventions, and adverse symptoms to report (see Patient Education). **Pregnancy risk factor C/D** - see Pregnancy Risk Factor for use cautions. Instruct patient of childbearing age about appropriate use of barrier contraceptives (see Pregnancy Issues). Breast-feeding is contraindicated.

Monitoring Laboratory Tests: Electrolytes, serum creatinine, BUN, urinalysis; in CHF, serum potassium during dose escalation and periodically thereafter

Patient Education: Inform prescriber of all prescriptions, OTC medications, or herbal products you are taking, and any allergies you have. Do not take any new medication during therapy unless approved by prescriber. Take exactly as directed and do not discontinue without consulting prescriber. Preferable to take on an empty stomach, 1 hour before or 2 hours after meals. This drug does not eliminate need for diet or exercise regimen as recommended by prescriber. May cause dizziness, fainting, or lightheadedness (use caution when driving or engaging in tasks that require alertness until response to drug is known); postural hypotension (use caution when rising from lying or sitting position or climbing stairs); nausea or vomiting (small, frequent meals, frequent mouth care, chewing gum, or sucking lozenges may help); or diarrhea (boiled milk, buttermilk, or yogurt may help). Report chest pain or palpitations; unusual weight gain or swelling of ankles and hands; persistent fatigue; unusual flu or cold symptoms or dry cough; respiratory difficulty; swelling of eyes, face, or lips; skin rash; muscle pain or weakness; unusual bleeding (blood in urine or stool, or from gums); or excessive sweating. **Pregnancy/breast-feeding precautions:** Inform prescriber if you are or intend to become pregnant. This drug should not be used in the 2nd or 3rd trimester of pregnancy. Consult prescriber for appropriate contraceptive measures if necessary. Do not breast-feed.

Geriatric Considerations: High concentrations occur in the elderly compared to younger subjects. AUC may be doubled in patients with renal impairment. No initial dose adjustment necessary since repeated dose did not demonstrate accumulation of drug or metabolites in elderly.

Pregnancy Risk Factor: C/D (2nd and 3rd trimesters)

Pregnancy Issues: The drug should be discontinued as soon as possible when pregnancy is detected. Drugs which act directly on renin-angiotensin can cause fetal and neonatal morbidity and death.

Lactation: Enters breast milk/contraindicated

Perioperative/Anesthesia/Other Concerns: The angiotensin II receptor antagonists appear to have similar indications as the ACE inhibitors. In heart failure, the angiotensin II antagonists are especially useful in providing an alternative therapy in those patients who have intractable cough in response to ACE inhibitor therapy. Candesartan has been studied as an alternative therapy in chronic heart failure patients who cannot tolerate an ACE-I (CHARM-Alternative) and as an added therapy in heart failure patients who are maintained on an ACE-I (CHARM-Added). In both studies the combined endpoint of cardiovascular death or heart failure hospitalizations was significantly improved over the placebo treated group. Similar to ACE inhibitors, pre-existing volume depletion caused by diuretic therapy may potentiate hypotension in response to angiotensin II antagonists. Concomitant NSAID therapy may attenuate blood pressure control; use of NSAIDs should be avoided or limited, with monitoring of blood pressure control. In the setting of heart failure, NSAID use may be associated with an increased risk for fluid accumulation and edema.

◆ **Candesartan Cilexetil** *see* Candesartan *on page 299*
◆ **Cankaid® [OTC]** *see* Carbamide Peroxide *on page 311*
◆ **Capital® and Codeine** *see* Acetaminophen and Codeine *on page 68*
◆ **Capoten®** *see* Captopril *on page 302*

Captopril (KAP toe pril)

U.S. Brand Names Capoten®

Synonyms ACE

Pharmacologic Category Angiotensin-Converting Enzyme (ACE) Inhibitor

Medication Safety Issues

Sound-alike/look-alike issues:

Captopril may be confused with Capitrol®, carvedilol

Use Management of hypertension; treatment of congestive heart failure, left ventricular dysfunction after myocardial infarction, diabetic nephropathy

Unlabeled/Investigational Use Treatment of hypertensive crisis, rheumatoid arthritis; diagnosis of anatomic renal artery stenosis, hypertension secondary to scleroderma renal crisis; diagnosis of aldosteronism, idiopathic edema, Bartter's syndrome, postmyocardial infarction for prevention of ventricular failure; increase circulation in Raynaud's phenomenon, hypertension secondary to Takayasu's disease

Mechanism of Action Competitive inhibitor of angiotensin-converting enzyme (ACE); prevents conversion of angiotensin I to angiotensin II, a potent vasoconstrictor; results in lower levels of angiotensin II which causes an increase in plasma renin activity and a reduction in aldosterone secretion

Pharmacodynamics/Kinetics

Onset of action: Peak effect: Blood pressure reduction: 1-1.5 hours after dose

Duration: Dose related, may require several weeks of therapy before full hypotensive effect

Absorption: 60% to 75%; reduced 30% to 40% by food

Protein binding: 25% to 30%

Metabolism: 50%

Half-life elimination (renal and cardiac function dependent):

Adults, healthy volunteers: 1.9 hours; Congestive heart failure: 2.06 hours; Anuria: 20-40 hours

Excretion: Urine (95%) within 24 hours

Contraindications Hypersensitivity to captopril or any component of the formulation; angioedema related to previous treatment with an ACE inhibitor; idiopathic or hereditary angioedema; bilateral renal artery stenosis; pregnancy (2nd or 3rd trimester)

Warnings/Precautions Anaphylactic reactions can occur. Angioedema can occur at any time during treatment (especially following first dose). Angioedema may involve head and neck (potentially affecting the airway) or the intestine (presenting with abdominal pain). Careful blood pressure monitoring with first dose (hypotension can occur especially in volume depleted patients). Dosage adjustment needed in renal impairment. Use with caution in hypovolemia; collagen vascular diseases; valvular stenosis (particularly aortic stenosis); hyperkalemia; or before, during, or immediately after anesthesia. Avoid rapid dosage escalation which may lead to renal insufficiency. Rare toxicities associated with ACE inhibitors include cholestatic jaundice (which may progress to hepatic necrosis) and neutropenia/agranulocytosis with myeloid hyperplasia. If patient has renal impairment then a baseline WBC with differential and serum creatinine should be evaluated and monitored closely during the first 3 months of therapy. Hypersensitivity reactions may be seen during hemodialysis with high-flux dialysis membranes (eg, AN69). Deterioration in renal function can occur with initiation. Use with caution in unilateral renal artery stenosis and pre-existing renal insufficiency.

Drug Interactions Substrate of CYP2D6 (major)

Allopurinol: Case reports (rare) indicate a possible increased risk of Stevens-Johnson syndrome when combined with captopril.

$Alpha_1$ blockers: Hypotensive effect increased.

Aspirin: The effects of ACE inhibitors may be blunted by aspirin administration, particularly at higher dosages (see Cardiovascular Considerations) and/or increase adverse renal effects.

CYP2D6 inhibitors: May increase the levels/effects of captopril. Example inhibitors include chlorpromazine, delavirdine, fluoxetine, miconazole, paroxetine, pergolide, quinidine, quinine, ritonavir, and ropinirole.

Diuretics: Hypovolemia due to diuretics may precipitate acute hypotensive events or acute renal failure.

Insulin: Risk of hypoglycemia may be increased.

Lithium: Risk of lithium toxicity may be increased; monitor lithium levels, especially the first 4 weeks of therapy.

Mercaptopurine: Risk of neutropenia may be increased.

NSAIDs: May attenuate hypertensive efficacy; effect has been seen with captopril and may occur with other ACE inhibitors; monitor blood pressure. May increase adverse renal effects.

Potassium-sparing diuretics (amiloride, potassium, spironolactone, triamterene): Increased risk of hyperkalemia.

Potassium supplements may increase the risk of hyperkalemia.

Trimethoprim (high dose) may increase the risk of hyperkalemia.

Nutritional/Herbal/Ethanol Interactions

Food: Captopril serum concentrations may be decreased if taken with food. Long-term use of captopril may result in a zinc deficiency which can result in a decrease in taste perception.

Herb/Nutraceutical: Avoid dong quai if using for hypertension (has estrogenic activity). Avoid ephedra, yohimbe, ginseng (may worsen hypertension). Avoid garlic (may have increased antihypertensive effect).

Lab Interactions Increased BUN, creatinine, potassium, positive Coombs' [direct]; decreased cholesterol (S); may cause false-positive results in urine acetone determinations using sodium nitroprusside reagent

Adverse Reactions

1% to 10%:

Cardiovascular: Hypotension (1% to 2.5%), tachycardia (1%), chest pain (1%), palpitation (1%)

Dermatologic: Rash (maculopapular or urticarial) (4% to 7%), pruritus (2%); in patients with rash, a positive ANA and/or eosinophilia has been noted in 7% to 10%.

Endocrine & metabolic: Hyperkalemia (1% to 11%)

Hematologic: Neutropenia may occur in up to 3.7% of patients with renal insufficiency or collagen-vascular disease.

Renal: Proteinuria (1%), increased serum creatinine, worsening of renal function (may occur in patients with bilateral renal artery stenosis or hypovolemia)

Respiratory: Cough (0.5% to 2%)

Miscellaneous: Hypersensitivity reactions (rash, pruritus, fever, arthralgia, and eosinophilia) have occurred in 4% to 7% of patients (depending on dose and renal function); dysgeusia - loss of taste or diminished perception (2% to 4%)

Frequency not defined:

Cardiovascular: Angioedema, cardiac arrest, cerebrovascular insufficiency, rhythm disturbances, orthostatic hypotension, syncope, flushing, pallor, angina, MI, Raynaud's syndrome, CHF

Central nervous system: Ataxia, confusion, depression, nervousness, somnolence

Dermatologic: Bullous pemphigus, erythema multiforme, Stevens-Johnson syndrome, exfoliative dermatitis

Endocrine & metabolic: Alkaline phosphatase increased, bilirubin increased, gynecomastia

Gastrointestinal: Pancreatitis, glossitis, dyspepsia

Genitourinary: Urinary frequency, impotence

Hematologic: Anemia, thrombocytopenia, pancytopenia, agranulocytosis

Hepatic: Jaundice, hepatitis, hepatic necrosis (rare), cholestasis, hyponatremia (symptomatic), transaminases increased

Neuromuscular & skeletal: Asthenia, myalgia, myasthenia

Ocular: Blurred vision

Renal: Renal insufficiency, renal failure, nephrotic syndrome, polyuria, oliguria

Respiratory: Bronchospasm, eosinophilic pneumonitis, rhinitis

Miscellaneous: Anaphylactoid reactions

Postmarketing and/or case reports: Alopecia, aplastic anemia, exacerbations of Huntington's disease, Guillain-Barré syndrome, hemolytic anemia, Kaposi's sarcoma, pericarditis, seizure (in premature infants), systemic lupus erythematosus. A syndrome which may include fever, myalgia, arthralgia, interstitial nephritis, vasculitis, rash, eosinophilia, and elevated ESR has been reported for captopril and other ACE inhibitors.

Overdosage/Toxicology Mild hypotension has been the primary toxic effect seen with acute overdose. Bradycardia may also occur. Hyperkalemia occurs

(Continued)

Captopril *(Continued)*

even with therapeutic doses, especially in patients with renal insufficiency and those taking NSAIDs. Treatment is symptom-directed and supportive.

Dosing

Adults & Elderly: Note: Dosage must be titrated according to patient's response

Acute hypertension (urgency/emergency): Oral: 12.5-25 mg, may repeat as needed (may be given sublingually but no therapeutic advantage demonstrated)

Hypertension: Oral: Initial: 12.5-25 mg 2-3 times/day; may increase by 12.5-25 mg/dose at 1- to 2-week intervals up to 50 mg 3 times/day. Maximum: 150 mg 3 times/day. Add diuretic before further dosage increases.

Usual dose range (JNC 7): 25-100 mg/day in 2 divided doses

Congestive heart failure: Oral:

Initial: 6.25-12.5 mg 3 times/day in conjunction with cardiac glycoside and diuretic therapy. Initial dose depends upon patient's fluid/electrolyte status.

Target: 50 mg 3 times/day

Prevention of LV dysfunction following MI: Oral: Initial: 6.25 mg; followed by 12.5 mg 3 times/day; increase to 25 mg 3 times/day over the next few days; following by gradual increase to a goal of 50 mg 3 times/day (Some dosage schedules increase the dosage more aggressively to achieve goal dosage within the first few days of initiation).

Diabetic nephropathy: Oral:

25 mg 3 times/day. May be taken with other antihypertensive therapy if required to further lower blood pressure.

Pediatrics: Note: Dosage must be titrated according to patient's response.

Hypertension: Oral:

Infants: Initial: 0.15-0.3 mg/kg/dose; titrate dose upward to maximum of 6 mg/kg/day in 1-4 divided doses; usual required dose: 2.5-6 mg/kg/day

Children: Initial: 0.5 mg/kg/dose; titrate upward to maximum of 6 mg/kg/day in 2-4 divided doses.

Older Children: Initial: 6.25-12.5 mg/dose every 12-24 hours; titrate upward to maximum of 6 mg/kg/day.

Adolescents: Initial: 12.5-25 mg/dose given every 8-12 hours; increase by 25 mg/dose to maximum of 450 mg/day.

Renal Impairment:

Cl_{cr} 10-50 mL/minute: Administer 75% of normal dose.

Cl_{cr} <10 mL/minute: Administer 50% of normal dose.

Note: Smaller dosages given every 8-12 hours are indicated in patients with renal dysfunction. Renal function and leukocyte count should be carefully monitored during therapy.

Hemodialysis effects: Moderately dialyzable (20% to 50%); administer dose postdialysis or administer 25% to 35% supplemental dose.

Peritoneal dialysis: Supplemental dose is not necessary.

Available Dosage Forms Tablet: 12.5 mg, 25 mg, 50 mg, 100 mg

Nursing Guidelines

Assessment: See Warnings/Precautions, Contraindications, and Dosing for use cautions. Assess potential for interactions with other prescriptions, OTC medications, or herbal products patient may be taking (especially anything that may impact fluid balance or cardiac status - see Drug Interactions). Assess results of laboratory tests (see below), therapeutic effectiveness, and adverse reactions on a regular basis during therapy (eg, hypovolemia, angioedema, postural hypotension - see Adverse Reactions and Overdose/Toxicology). Teach patient proper use, possible side effects/appropriate interventions, and adverse symptoms to report (see Patient Education). **Pregnancy risk factor C/D** - see Pregnancy Risk Factor for use cautions. Instruct patient in use of appropriate contraceptives (see Pregnancy Issues).

Monitoring Laboratory Tests: BUN, serum creatinine, urine dipstick for protein, CBC, electrolytes. If patient has renal impairment, a baseline WBC with differential and serum creatinine should be evaluated and monitored closely during the first 3 months of therapy.

Dietary Considerations: Should be taken at least 1 hour before or 2 hours after eating.

Patient Education: Inform prescriber of all prescriptions, OTC medications, or herbal products you are taking, and any allergies you have. Do not take any new medication during therapy unless approved by prescriber. Do not use potassium supplement or salt substitutes without consulting prescriber. Take exactly as directed; do not discontinue without consulting prescriber. Take first dose at bedtime. Take all doses on an empty stomach, 1 hour before or 2 hours after meals. This drug does not eliminate need for diet or exercise regimen as recommended by prescriber. May cause dizziness, fainting, or lightheadedness (use caution when driving or engaging in tasks that require alertness until response to drug is known); postural hypotension (use caution when rising from lying or sitting position or climbing stairs); or nausea, vomiting, abdominal pain, dry mouth, or transient loss of appetite (small, frequent meals, frequent mouth care, sucking lozenges, or chewing gum may help). Report chest pain or palpitations; mouth sores; fever or chills; swelling of extremities, face, mouth, or tongue; skin rash; numbness, tingling, or pain in muscles; respiratory difficulty or unusual cough; and other persistent adverse reactions. **Pregnancy precautions** Inform prescriber if you are or intend to become pregnant. This drug should not be used in the 2nd or 3rd trimester of pregnancy. Consult prescriber for appropriate contraceptive measures if necessary.

Geriatric Considerations: Due to frequent decreases in glomerular filtration (also creatinine clearance) with aging, elderly patients may have exaggerated responses to ACE inhibitors. Differences in clinical response due to hepatic changes are not observed.

Pregnancy Risk Factor: C (1st trimester)/D (2nd and 3rd trimesters)

Pregnancy Issues: ACE inhibitors can cause fetal injury or death if taken during the 2nd or 3rd trimester. Discontinue ACE inhibitors as soon as pregnancy is detected.

Lactation: Enters breast milk/not recommended (AAP rates "compatible")

Perioperative/Anesthesia/Other Concerns: Severe hypotension may occur in patients who are sodium and/or volume depleted.

ACE inhibitors are indicated in patients postmyocardial infarction in whom left ventricular ejection fraction is <40%. When used in patients with heart failure, the target dose of 50 mg 3 times/day should be achieved, if possible. Lower daily doses of ACE inhibitors have not demonstrated the same cardioprotective effects.

ACE inhibitor therapy may elicit rapid increases in potassium and creatinine, especially when used in patients with bilateral renal artery stenosis. When ACE inhibition is introduced in patients with pre-existing diuretic therapy who are hypovolemic, the ACE inhibitor may induce acute hypotension. Because of the potent teratogenic effects of ACE inhibitors, these drugs should be avoided, if possible, when treating women of childbearing potential not on effective birth control measures.

Administration

Oral: Unstable in aqueous solutions; to prepare solution for oral administration, mix prior to administration and use within 10 minutes.

♦ Carac™ *see* Fluorouracil *on page 745*

♦ Carafate® *see* Sucralfate *on page 1575*

Carbachol (KAR ba kole)

U.S. Brand Names Carbastat® [DSC]; Isopto® Carbachol; Miostat®

Synonyms Carbacholine; Carbamylcholine Chloride

Pharmacologic Category Cholinergic Agonist; Ophthalmic Agent, Antiglaucoma; Ophthalmic Agent, Miotic

Medication Safety Issues

Sound-alike/look-alike issues:

Isopto® Carbachol may be confused with Isopto® Carpine

Use Lowers intraocular pressure in the treatment of glaucoma; cause miosis during surgery

Mechanism of Action Synthetic direct-acting cholinergic agent that causes miosis by stimulating muscarinic receptors in the eye

Pharmacodynamics/Kinetics

Ophthalmic instillation:

Onset of action: Miosis: 10-20 minutes

Duration: Reduction in intraocular pressure: 4-8 hours

Intraocular administration:

Onset of action: Miosis: 2-5 minutes

Duration: 24 hours

Contraindications Hypersensitivity to carbachol or any component of the formulation; acute iritis, acute inflammatory disease of the anterior chamber

(Continued)

Carbachol *(Continued)*

Warnings/Precautions Use with caution in patients undergoing general anesthesia and in presence of corneal abrasion. Use caution with acute cardiac failure, asthma, peptic ulcer, hyperthyroidism, gastrointestinal spasm, urinary tract obstruction, and Parkinson's disease.

Drug Interactions Decreased effect of carbachol possible with topical NSAIDs

Adverse Reactions Frequency not defined.

Cardiovascular: Arrhythmia, flushing, hypotension, syncope
Central nervous system: Headache
Gastrointestinal: Abdominal cramps, diarrhea, epigastric distress, salivation, vomiting
Genitourinary: Urinary bladder tightness
Ocular: Bullous keratopathy, burning (transient), ciliary spasm, conjunctival injection, corneal clouding, irritation, postoperative iritis (following cataract extraction), retinal detachment, stinging (transient)
Respiratory: Asthma
Miscellaneous: Diaphoresis

Overdosage/Toxicology Symptoms of overdose include miosis, flushing, vomiting, bradycardia, bronchospasm, involuntary urination Atropine is the treatment of choice for intoxications manifesting with significant muscarinic symptoms. Atropine I.V. 1-2 mg every 5-60 minutes (or 0.04-0.08 mg/kg I.V. every 5-60 minutes if needed for children) should be repeated to control symptoms and then continued as needed for 1-2 days following the acute ingestion. Epinephrine 0.1-1 mg SubQ may be useful in reversing severe cardiovascular or pulmonary sequelae.

Dosing

Adults & Elderly:

Glaucoma: Ophthalmic: Instill 1-2 drops up to 3 times/day
Ophthalmic surgery (miosis): Intraocular: 0.5 mL instilled into anterior chamber before or after securing sutures

Available Dosage Forms [DSC] = Discontinued product

Solution, intraocular (Carbastat® [DSC], Miostat®): 0.01% (1.5 mL)
Solution, ophthalmic (Isopto® Carbachol): 1.5% (15 mL); 3% (30 mL) [contains benzalkonium chloride]

Nursing Guidelines

Patient Education: May sting on instillation. May cause headache, altered distance vision, and decreased night vision. **Pregnancy precaution:** Inform prescriber if you are or intend to become pregnant. Consult prescriber if breast-feeding.

Pregnancy Risk Factor: C

Lactation: Excretion in breast milk unknown/use caution

Administration

Storage:

Intraocular: Store at room temperature of 15°C to 30°C (59°F to 86°F)
Topical: Store at 8°C to 27°C (46°F to 80°F)

♦ **Carbacholine** *see* Carbachol *on page 305*

Carbamazepine (kar ba MAZ e peen)

U.S. Brand Names Carbatrol®; Epitol®; Equetro™; Tegretol®; Tegretol®-XR

Synonyms CBZ; SPD417

Pharmacologic Category Anticonvulsant, Miscellaneous

Medication Safety Issues

Sound-alike/look-alike issues:
Carbatrol® may be confused with Cartrol®
Epitol® may be confused with Epinal®
Tegretol®, Tegretol®-XR may be confused with Mebaral®, Tegrin®, Toprol-XL®, Toradol®, Trental®

Use

Carbatrol®, Tegretol®, Tegretol®-XR: Partial seizures with complex symptomatology (psychomotor, temporal lobe), generalized tonic-clonic seizures (grand mal), mixed seizure patterns, trigeminal neuralgia
Equetro™: Acute manic and mixed episodes associated with bipolar 1 disorder

Unlabeled/Investigational Use Treatment of resistant schizophrenia, ethanol withdrawal, restless leg syndrome, psychotic behavior associated with dementia, post-traumatic stress disorders

Mechanism of Action In addition to anticonvulsant effects, carbamazepine has anticholinergic, antineuralgic, antidiuretic, muscle relaxant, antimanic, antidepressive, and antiarrhythmic properties; may depress activity in the nucleus ventralis of the thalamus or decrease synaptic transmission or decrease summation of temporal stimulation leading to neural discharge by limiting influx of sodium ions across cell membrane or other unknown mechanisms; stimulates the release of ADH and potentiates its action in promoting reabsorption of water; chemically related to tricyclic antidepressants

Pharmacodynamics/Kinetics

Absorption: Slow

Distribution: V_d: Neonates: 1.5 L/kg; Children: 1.9 L/kg; Adults: 0.59-2 L/kg

Protein binding: Carbamazepine: 75% to 90%, may be decreased in newborns; Epoxide metabolite: 50%

Metabolism: Hepatic via CYP3A4 to active epoxide metabolite; induces hepatic enzymes to increase metabolism

Bioavailability: 85%

Half-life elimination:

Carbamazepine: Initial: 18-55 hours; Multiple doses: Children: 8-14 hours; Adults: 12-17 hours

Epoxide metabolite: Initial: 25-43 hours

Time to peak, serum: Unpredictable:

Immediate release: Suspension: 1.5 hour; tablet: 4-5 hours

Extended release: Carbatrol®, Equetro™: 12-26 hours (single dose), 4-8 hours (multiple doses); Tegretol®-XR: 3-12 hours

Excretion: Urine 72% (1% to 3% as unchanged drug); feces (28%)

Contraindications Hypersensitivity to carbamazepine, tricyclic antidepressants, or any component of the formulation; bone marrow depression; with or within 14 days of MAO inhibitor use; pregnancy

Warnings/Precautions Administer carbamazepine with caution to patients with history of cardiac damage, hepatic or renal disease; potentially fatal blood cell abnormalities have been reported following treatment; patients with a previous history of adverse hematologic reaction to any drug may be at increased risk; early detection of hematologic change is important; advise patients of early signs and symptoms including fever, sore throat, mouth ulcers, infections, easy bruising, petechial or purpuric hemorrhage. Prescriptions should be written for the smallest quantity consistent with good patient care. The smallest effective dose is suggested for use in bipolar disorder to reduce the risk for overdose; high-risk patients should be monitored. Actuation of latent psychosis is possible.

Carbamazepine is not effective in absence, myoclonic or akinetic seizures; exacerbation of certain seizure types have been seen after initiation of carbamazepine therapy in children with mixed seizure disorders. Abrupt discontinuation is not recommended in patients being treated for seizures. Dizziness or drowsiness may occur; caution should be used when performing tasks which require alertness (operating machinery or driving) until the effects are known. Coadministration of carbamazepine and delavirdine may lead to loss of virologic response and possible resistance. Elderly may have increased risk of SIADH-like syndrome. Carbamazepine has mild anticholinergic activity; use with caution in patients with increased intraocular pressure (monitor closely), or sensitivity to anticholinergic effects (urinary retention, constipation). Severe dermatologic reactions, including Lyell and Stevens-Johnson syndromes, although rarely reported, have resulted in fatalities. Drug should be discontinued if there are any signs of hypersensitivity.

Drug Interactions **Substrate** of CYP2C8/9 (minor), 3A4 (major); **Induces** CYP1A2 (strong), 2B6 (strong), 2C8/9 (strong), 2C19 (strong), 3A4 (strong)

Acetaminophen: Carbamazepine may enhance hepatotoxic potential of acetaminophen; risk is greater in acetaminophen overdose

Antimalarial drugs (chloroquine, mefloquine): Concomitant use with carbamazepine may reduce seizure control by lowering plasma levels. Monitor.

Antipsychotics: Carbamazepine may enhance the metabolism (decrease the efficacy) of antipsychotics; monitor for altered response; dose adjustment may be needed

Barbiturates: May reduce serum concentrations of carbamazepine; monitor

Benzodiazepines: Serum concentrations and effect of benzodiazepines may be reduced by carbamazepine; monitor for decreased effect

Calcium channel blockers: Diltiazem and verapamil may increase carbamazepine levels, due to enzyme inhibition (see below); other calcium channel blockers (felodipine) may be decreased by carbamazepine due to enzyme induction

(Continued)

Carbamazepine *(Continued)*

Chlorpromazine: **Note:** Carbamazepine suspension is incompatible with chlorpromazine solution. Schedule carbamazepine suspension at least 1-2 hours apart from other liquid medicinals.

Corticosteroids: Metabolism may be increased by carbamazepine

Cyclosporine (and other immunosuppressants): Carbamazepine may enhance the metabolism of immunosuppressants, decreasing its clinical effect; includes both cyclosporine and tacrolimus.

CYP1A2 substrates: Carbamazepine may decrease the levels/effects of CYP1A2 substrates. Example substrates include aminophylline, estrogens, fluvoxamine, mirtazapine, ropinirole, and theophylline.

CYP2B6 substrates: Carbamazepine may decrease the levels/effects of CYP2B6 substrates. Example substrates include bupropion, efavirenz, promethazine, selegiline, and sertraline.

CYP2C8/9 substrates: Carbamazepine may decrease the levels/effects of CYP2C8/9 substrates. Example substrates include amiodarone, fluoxetine, glimepiride, glipizide, losartan, nateglinide, phenytoin, pioglitazone, rosiglitazone, sertraline, sulfonamides, warfarin, and zafirlukast.

CYP2C19 substrates: Carbamazepine may decrease the levels/effects of CYP2C19 substrates. Example substrates include citalopram, diazepam, methsuximide, phenytoin, propranolol, proton pump inhibitors, sertraline, and voriconazole.

CYP3A4 inducers: CYP3A4 inducers may decrease the levels/effects of carbamazepine. Example inducers include aminoglutethimide, nafcillin, nevirapine, phenobarbital, phenytoin, and rifamycins. Carbamazepine may induce its own metabolism.

CYP3A4 inhibitors: May increase the levels/effects of carbamazepine. Example inhibitors include azole antifungals, clarithromycin, diclofenac, doxycycline, erythromycin, imatinib, isoniazid, nefazodone, nicardipine, propofol, protease inhibitors, quinidine, telithromycin, and verapamil.

CYP3A4 substrates: Carbamazepine may decrease the levels/effects of CYP3A4 substrates. Example substrates include benzodiazepines, calcium channel blockers, clarithromycin, cyclosporine, erythromycin, estrogens, mirtazapine, nateglinide, nefazodone, nevirapine, protease inhibitors, tacrolimus, and venlafaxine.

Danazol: May increase serum concentrations of carbamazepine; monitor

Delavirdine: May lead to loss of virologic response and possible resistance.

Doxycycline: Carbamazepine may enhance the metabolism of doxycycline, decreasing its clinical effect

Ethosuximide: Serum levels may be reduced by carbamazepine

Felbamate: May increase carbamazepine levels and toxicity (increased epoxide metabolite concentrations); carbamazepine may decrease felbamate levels due to enzyme induction

Immunosuppressants: Carbamazepine may enhance the metabolism of immunosuppressants, decreasing its clinical effect; includes both cyclosporine and tacrolimus

Isoniazid: May increase the serum concentrations and toxicity of carbamazepine; in addition, carbamazepine may increase the hepatic toxicity of isoniazid (INH)

Isotretinoin: May decrease the effect of carbamazepine

Lamotrigine: Increases the epoxide metabolite of carbamazepine resulting in toxicity; carbamazepine increases the metabolism of lamotrigine

Lithium: Neurotoxicity may result in patients receiving concurrent carbamazepine

Loxapine: May increase concentrations of epoxide metabolite and toxicity of carbamazepine

Methadone: Carbamazepine may enhance the metabolism of methadone resulting in methadone withdrawal

Methylphenidate: concurrent use of carbamazepine may reduce the therapeutic effect of methylphenidate; limited documentation; monitor for decreased effect

Neuromuscular blocking agents, nondepolarizing: Effects may be of shorter duration when administered to patients receiving carbamazepine

Oral contraceptives: Metabolism may be increased by carbamazepine, resulting in a loss of efficacy

Phenytoin: Carbamazepine levels may be decreased by phenytoin. Metabolism of phenytoin may be altered by carbamazepine; phenytoin levels may be increased or decreased.

SSRIs: Metabolism may be increased by carbamazepine (due to enzyme induction)

Theophylline: Serum levels may be reduced by carbamazepine

Thioridazine: **Note:** Carbamazepine suspension is incompatible with thioridazine liquid. Schedule carbamazepine suspension at least 1-2 hours apart from other liquid medicinals.

Thyroid: Serum levels may be reduced by carbamazepine

Tramadol: Tramadol's risk of seizures may be increased with TCAs (carbamazepine may be associated with similar risk due to chemical similarity to TCAs)

Tricyclic antidepressants: May increase serum concentrations of carbamazepine; carbamazepine may decrease concentrations of tricyclics due to enzyme induction

Valproic acid: Serum levels may be reduced by carbamazepine; carbamazepine levels may also be altered by valproic acid

Warfarin: Carbamazepine may inhibit the hypoprothrombinemic effects of oral anticoagulants via increased metabolism; this combination should generally be avoided

Nutritional/Herbal/Ethanol Interactions

Ethanol: Avoid ethanol (may increase CNS depression).

Food: Carbamazepine serum levels may be increased if taken with food. Carbamazepine serum concentration may be increased if taken with grapefruit juice; avoid concurrent use.

Herb/Nutraceutical: Avoid evening primrose (seizure threshold decreased). Avoid valerian, St John's wort, kava kava, gotu kola (may increase CNS depression).

Lab Interactions May interact with some pregnancy tests; increased BUN, AST, ALT, bilirubin, alkaline phosphatase (S); decreased calcium, T_3, T_4, sodium (S)

Adverse Reactions Frequency not defined, unless otherwise specified.

Cardiovascular: Arrhythmias, AV block, bradycardia, chest pain (bipolar use), CHF, edema, hyper-/hypotension, lymphadenopathy, syncope, thromboembolism, thrombophlebitis

Central nervous system: Amnesia (bipolar use), anxiety (bipolar use), aseptic meningitis (case report), ataxia (bipolar use 15%), confusion, depression (bipolar use), dizziness (bipolar use 44%), fatigue, headache (bipolar use 22%), sedation, slurred speech, somnolence (bipolar use 32%)

Dermatologic: Alopecia, alterations in skin pigmentation, erythema multiforme, exfoliative dermatitis, photosensitivity reaction, pruritus (bipolar use 8%), purpura, rash, Stevens-Johnson syndrome, toxic epidermal necrolysis, urticaria

Endocrine & metabolic: Chills, fever, hyponatremia, syndrome of inappropriate ADH secretion (SIADH)

Gastrointestinal: Abdominal pain, anorexia, constipation, diarrhea, dyspepsia (bipolar use), gastric distress, nausea (bipolar use 29%), pancreatitis, vomiting (bipolar use 18%), xerostomia (bipolar use)

Genitourinary: Azotemia, impotence, renal failure, urinary frequency, urinary retention

Hematologic: Acute intermittent porphyria, agranulocytosis, aplastic anemia, bone marrow suppression, eosinophilia, leukocytosis, leukopenia, pancytopenia, thrombocytopenia

Hepatic: Abnormal liver function tests, hepatic failure, hepatitis, jaundice

Neuromuscular & skeletal: Back pain, pain (bipolar use 12%), peripheral neuritis, weakness

Ocular: Blurred vision, conjunctivitis, lens opacities, nystagmus

Otic: Hyperacusis, tinnitus

Miscellaneous: Diaphoresis, hypersensitivity (including multiorgan reactions, may include disorders mimicking lymphoma, eosinophilia, hepatosplenomegaly, vasculitis); infection (bipolar use 12%)

Overdosage/Toxicology Symptoms of overdose include dizziness ataxia, drowsiness, nausea, vomiting, tremor, agitation, nystagmus, urinary retention, dysrhythmias, coma, seizures, twitches, respiratory depression, and neuromuscular disturbances. Severe cardiac complications occur with very high doses. Activated charcoal is effective at binding carbamazepine. Other treatment is supportive and symptomatic.

Dosing

Adults: Dosage must be adjusted according to patient's response and serum concentrations. Administer tablets (chewable or conventional) in 2-3 divided doses daily and suspension in 4 divided doses daily. Oral:

Epilepsy: Initial: 200 mg twice daily (tablets, extended release tablets, or extended release capsules) or 100 mg of suspension 4 times/day (400 mg daily); increase by up to 200 mg/day at weekly intervals using a twice daily

(Continued)

Carbamazepine *(Continued)*

regimen of extended release tablets or capsules, or a 3-4 times/day regimen of other formulations until optimal response and therapeutic levels are achieved; usual dose: 800-1200 mg/day

Maximum recommended dose: 1600 mg/day; however, some patients have required up to 1.6-2.4 g/day

Trigeminal or glossopharyngeal neuralgia: Oral: Initial: 100 mg twice daily with food, gradually increasing in increments of 100 mg twice daily as needed

Maintenance: Usual: 400-800 mg daily in 2 divided doses; maximum dose: 1200 mg/day

Bipolar disorder (Equetro™): Oral: Initial: 400 mg/day in divided doses, twice daily; may adjust by 200 mg daily increments; maximum dose: 1600 mg/day

Elderly: 100 mg 1-2 times daily, increase in increments of 100 mg/day at weekly intervals until therapeutic level is achieved; usual dose: 400-1000 mg/day

Pediatrics: Dosage must be adjusted according to patient's response and serum concentrations. Administer tablets (chewable or conventional) in 2-3 divided doses daily and suspension in 4 divided doses daily.

Epilepsy: Oral:

Children <6 years: Initial: 10-20 mg/kg/day divided twice or 3 times daily as tablets or 4 times/day as suspension; increase dose every week until optimal response and therapeutic levels are achieved

Maintenance dose: Divide into 3-4 doses daily (tablets or suspension); maximum recommended dose: 35 mg/kg/day

Children 6-12 years: Initial: 100 mg twice daily (tablets or extended release tablets) or 50 mg of suspension 4 times/day (200 mg/day); increase by up to 100 mg/day at weekly intervals using a twice daily regimen of extended release tablets or 3-4 times daily regimen of other formulations until optimal response and therapeutic levels are achieved

Maintenance: Usual: 400-800 mg/day; maximum recommended dose: 1000 mg/day

Note: Children <12 years who receive ≥400 mg/day of carbamazepine may be converted to extended release capsules (Carbatrol®) using the same total daily dosage divided twice daily

Children >12 years: Refer to adult dosing.

Maximum recommended doses:

Children 12-15 years: 1000 mg/day

Children >15 years: 1200 mg/day

Available Dosage Forms

Capsule, extended release (Carbatrol®, Equetro™): 100 mg, 200 mg, 300 mg

Suspension, oral: 100 mg/5 mL (10 mL, 450 mL)

Tegretol®: 100 mg/5 mL (450 mL) [citrus vanilla flavor]

Tablet (Epitol®, Tegretol®): 200 mg

Tablet, chewable (Tegretol®): 100 mg

Tablet, extended release (Tegretol®-XR): 100 mg, 200 mg, 400 mg

Nursing Guidelines

Assessment: Assess effectiveness and interactions of other medications patient may be taking. Monitor therapeutic effectiveness, laboratory values, and adverse reactions at beginning of therapy and periodically with long-term use. Taper dosage slowly when discontinuing. Observe and teach seizure/safety precautions. Monitor for mental and CNS changes, excessive sedation (especially when initiating or increasing therapy), suicide ideation. Baseline and periodic eye exams (slit lamp, funduscopy, and tonometry) are recommended. Assess knowledge/teach patient appropriate use, interventions to reduce side effects, and adverse symptoms to report.

Monitoring Laboratory Tests: CBC with platelet count, reticulocytes, serum iron, liver function tests, urinalysis, BUN, serum carbamazepine levels, thyroid function tests, serum sodium

Dietary Considerations: Drug may cause GI upset, take with large amount of water or food to decrease GI upset. May need to split doses to avoid GI upset.

Patient Education: Take exactly as directed; do not increase dose or frequency or discontinue without consulting prescriber. Do not use extended release tablets which have been damaged or crushed. While using this medication, do not use alcohol and other prescription or OTC medications (especially pain medications, sedatives, antihistamines, or hypnotics) without consulting prescriber. Maintain adequate hydration (2-3 L/day of fluids) unless instructed to restrict fluid intake. You may experience drowsiness, dizziness, or blurred vision (use caution when driving or engaging in tasks requiring alertness until response to drug is known); or nausea, vomiting, loss of appetite, or dry mouth (small frequent meals, frequent mouth care, chewing gum, or sucking lozenges may help). Wear identification of epileptic status and medications. Report CNS changes, mentation changes, or changes in cognition; muscle cramping, weakness, tremors, sore throat, mouth ulcers, swollen glands, jaundice, changes in gait; persistent GI symptoms (cramping, constipation, vomiting, anorexia); rash or skin irritations; unusual bruising or bleeding (mouth, urine, stool); or worsening of seizure activity, or loss of seizure control. **Pregnancy/breast-feeding precautions:** Inform prescriber if you are or intend to become pregnant. Breast-feeding is not recommended.

Geriatric Considerations: Elderly may have increased risk of SIADH-like syndrome.

Pregnancy Risk Factor: D

Pregnancy Issues: Crosses the placenta. Dysmorphic facial features, cranial defects, cardiac defects, spina bifida, IUGR, and multiple other malformations have been reported. Epilepsy itself, number of medications, genetic factors, or a combination of these probably influence the teratogenicity of anticonvulsant therapy. Benefit:risk ratio usually favors continued use during pregnancy.

Lactation: Enters breast milk/not recommended (AAP rates "compatible")

Breast-Feeding Considerations: Carbamazepine and its metabolites are found in breast milk. The manufacturer does not recommend use while breast-feeding. However, AAP rates this medication "compatible" in breast-feeding. However, AAP rates this medication as "compatible" with breast-feeding.

Perioperative/Anesthesia/Other Concerns: Carbamazepine is not effective in absence, myoclonic or akinetic seizures; exacerbation of certain seizure types has been seen after initiation of carbamazepine therapy in children with mixed seizure disorders. Elderly may have increase risk of SIADH-like syndrome and psychosis. Simultaneous administration of carbamazepine suspension with other liquids can precipitate the drug.

Administration

Oral:

Suspension: Must be given on a 3-4 times/day schedule versus tablets which can be given 2-4 times/day. When carbamazepine suspension has been combined with chlorpromazine or thioridazine solutions a precipitate forms which may result in loss of effect. Therefore, it is recommended that the carbamazepine suspension dosage form not be administered at the same time with other liquid medicinal agents or diluents. Since a given dose of suspension will produce higher peak levels than the same dose given as the tablet form, patients given the suspension should be started on lower doses and increased slowly to avoid unwanted side effects. Should be administered with meals.

Extended release capsule (Carbatrol®, Equetro™): Consists of three different types of beads: Immediate release, extended-release, and enteric release. The bead types are combined in a ratio to allow twice daily dosing. May be opened and contents sprinkled over food such as a teaspoon of applesauce; may be administered with or without food; do not crush or chew.

Extended release tablet: Should be inspected for damage. Damaged extended release tablets (without release portal) should not be administered. Should be administered with meals; swallow whole, do not crush or chew.

Related Information

Perioperative Management of Patients on Antiseizure Medication *on page 1801*

Carbamide Peroxide (KAR ba mide per OKS ide)

U.S. Brand Names Cankaid® [OTC]; Debrox® [OTC]; Dent's Ear Wax [OTC]; E•R•O [OTC]; Gly-Oxide® [OTC]; Murine® Ear Wax Removal System [OTC]; Orajel® Perioseptic® Spot Treatment [OTC]

Synonyms Urea Peroxide

Pharmacologic Category Anti-inflammatory, Locally Applied; Otic Agent, Cerumenolytic

Use Relief of minor inflammation of gums, oral mucosal surfaces and lips including canker sores and dental irritation; emulsify and disperse ear wax

Mechanism of Action Carbamide peroxide releases hydrogen peroxide which serves as a source of nascent oxygen upon contact with catalase; deodorant

(Continued)

Carbamide Peroxide *(Continued)*

action is probably due to inhibition of odor-causing bacteria; softens impacted cerumen due to its foaming action

Pharmacodynamics/Kinetics Onset of action: ~24 hours

Contraindications Hypersensitivity to carbamide peroxide or any component of the formulation; otic preparation should not be used in patients with a perforated tympanic membrane; ear drainage, ear pain or rash in the ear

Warnings/Precautions

Oral: With prolonged use of oral carbamide peroxide, there is a potential for overgrowth of opportunistic organisms; damage to periodontal tissues; delayed wound healing; should not be used for longer than 7 days; not for OTC use in children <2 years of age

Otic: Do not use if ear drainage or discharge, ear pain, irritation, or rash in ear; should not be used for longer than 4 days; not for OTC use in children <12 years of age

Drug Interactions No data reported

Adverse Reactions Frequency not defined.

Dermatologic: Rash

Local: Irritation, redness

Miscellaneous: Superinfection

Dosing

Adults & Elderly:

Minor inflammation of gums, oral mucosal surfaces and lips: Topical: Oral solution (should not be used for >7 days): Apply several drops undiluted on affected area 4 times/day after meals and at bedtime; expectorate after 2-3 minutes **or** place 10 drops onto tongue, mix with saliva, swish for several minutes, expectorate

Ear wax removal: Otic: Tilt head sideways and instill 5-10 drops twice daily up to 4 days, tip of applicator should not enter ear canal; keep drops in ear for several minutes by keeping head tilted and placing cotton in ear

Pediatrics:

Relief of minor inflammation of gums, oral mucosal surfaces and lips: Topical: Children ≥2 years: Refer to adult dosing.

Ear wax removal: Otic:

Children <12 years: Tilt head sideways and individualize the dose according to patient size; 3 drops (range: 1-5 drops) twice daily for up to 4 days, tip of applicator should not enter ear canal. Keep drops in ear for several minutes by keeping head tilted and placing cotton in ear.

Children ≥12 years: Refer to adult dosing.

Available Dosage Forms

Solution, oral: 10% (60 mL)

Cankaid®: 10% (22 mL) [in anhydrous glycerol]

Gly-Oxide®: 10% (15 mL, 60 mL) [contains glycerin]

Orajel® Perioseptic® Spot Treatment: 15% (13.3 mL) [contains anhydrous glycerin]

Solution, otic: 6.5% (15 mL)

Debrox®: 6.5% (15 mL, 30 mL) [contains propylene glycol]

Dent's Ear Wax: 6.5% (3.7 mL) [contains glycerin]

E•R•O: 6.5% (15 mL)

Murine® Ear Wax Removal System: 6.5% (15 mL) [contains alcohol 6.3% and glycerin]

Nursing Guidelines

Patient Education: Contact physician if dizziness or otic redness, rash, irritation, tenderness, pain, drainage, or discharge develop; do not drink or rinse mouth for 5 minutes after oral use of gel

Pregnancy Risk Factor: C

Administration

Storage: Protect from excessive heat and direct sunlight.

- ♦ **Carbamylcholine Chloride** *see* Carbachol *on page 305*
- ♦ **Carbastat® [DSC]** *see* Carbachol *on page 305*
- ♦ **Carbatrol®** *see* Carbamazepine *on page 306*
- ♦ **Carbocaine®** *see* Mepivacaine *on page 1101*
- ♦ **Carbolic Acid** *see* Phenol *on page 1347*

Carboplatin (KAR boe pla tin)

U.S. Brand Names Paraplatin®

Synonyms CBDCA

Pharmacologic Category Antineoplastic Agent, Alkylating Agent

Medication Safety Issues

Sound-alike/look-alike issues:

Carboplatin may be confused with cisplatin

Paraplatin® may be confused with Platinol®

Use Treatment of ovarian cancer

Unlabeled/Investigational Use Lung cancer, head and neck cancer, endometrial cancer, esophageal cancer, bladder cancer, breast cancer, cervical cancer, CNS tumors, germ cell tumors, osteogenic sarcoma, and high-dose therapy with stem cell/bone marrow support

Mechanism of Action Carboplatin is an alkylating agent which covalently binds to DNA; possible cross-linking and interference with the function of DNA

Pharmacodynamics/Kinetics

Distribution: V_d: 16 L/kg; Into liver, kidney, skin, and tumor tissue

Protein binding: 0%; platinum is 30% irreversibly bound

Metabolism: Minimally hepatic to aquated and hydroxylated compounds

Half-life elimination: Terminal: 22-40 hours; Cl_{cr} >60 mL/minute: 2.5-5.9 hours

Excretion: Urine (~60% to 90%) within 24 hours

Contraindications History of severe allergic reaction to cisplatin, carboplatin, other platinum-containing formulations, mannitol, or any component of the formulation; pregnancy

Warnings/Precautions Hazardous agent — use appropriate precautions for handling and disposal. High doses have resulted in severe abnormalities of liver function tests. Bone marrow suppression, which may be severe, and vomiting are dose related; reduce dosage in patients with bone marrow suppression and impaired renal function. Increased risk of allergic reactions in patients previously exposed to platinum therapy. When administered as sequential infusions, taxane derivatives (docetaxel, paclitaxel) should be administered before the platinum derivatives (carboplatin, cisplatin) to limit myelosuppression and to enhance efficacy.

Drug Interactions

Increased toxicity: Nephrotoxic drugs; aminoglycosides increase risk of ototoxicity

Docetaxel, paclitaxel (taxane derivatives): When administered as sequential infusions, taxane derivatives should be administered before platinum derivatives to limit myelosuppression and to enhance efficacy.

Nutritional/Herbal/Ethanol Interactions Herb/Nutraceutical: Avoid black cohosh, dong quai in estrogen-dependent tumors.

Adverse Reactions

>10%:

Dermatologic: Alopecia

Endocrine & metabolic: Hypomagnesemia, hypokalemia, hyponatremia, hypocalcemia; less severe than those seen after cisplatin (usually asymptomatic)

Gastrointestinal: Nausea, vomiting, stomatitis

Hematologic: Myelosuppression (dose related and dose-limiting); thrombocytopenia (37% to 80%); leukopenia (27% to 38%)

Nadir: ~21 days following a single dose

Hepatic: Alkaline phosphatase increased, AST increased (usually mild and reversible)

Otic: Hearing loss at high tones (above speech ranges, up to 19%); clinically-important ototoxicity is not usually seen

Renal: BUN and/or creatinine increased

1% to 10%:

Gastrointestinal: Diarrhea, anorexia

Hematologic: Hemorrhagic complications

Local: Pain at injection site

Neuromuscular & skeletal: Peripheral neuropathy (4% to 6%; up to 10% in older and/or previously-treated patients)

Otic: Ototoxicity

<1% (Limited to important or life-threatening): Neurotoxicity, anaphylaxis, hypertension, malaise, nephrotoxicity (uncommon), rash, secondary malignancies, urticaria

BMT:

Dermatologic: Alopecia

Endocrine & metabolic: Hypokalemia, hypomagnesemia

(Continued)

Carboplatin *(Continued)*

Gastrointestinal: Nausea, vomiting, mucositis

Hepatic: Elevated liver function tests

Renal: Nephrotoxicity

Overdosage/Toxicology Symptoms of overdose include bone marrow suppression and hepatic toxicity. Treatment is symptomatic and supportive.

Dosing

Adults & Elderly: Refer to individual protocols: **Note:** Doses are usually determined by the AUC using the Calvert formula.

IVPB, I.V. infusion, intraperitoneal:

Autologous BMT: I.V.: 1600 mg/m^2 (total dose) divided over 4 days

Ovarian cancer: 300-360 mg/m^2 I.V. every 3-4 weeks

Pediatrics: Refer to individual protocols: **Note:** Doses are usually determined by the AUC using the Calvert formula.

IVPB, I.V. infusion, intraperitoneal:

Solid tumor: 300-600 mg/m^2 once every 4 weeks

Brain tumor: 175 mg/m^2 weekly for 4 weeks every 6 weeks, with a 2-week recovery period between courses

Renal Impairment:

No guidelines are available.

Hepatic Impairment: No guidelines are available.

Available Dosage Forms

Injection, powder for reconstitution: 50 mg, 150 mg, 450 mg

Injection, solution: 10 mg/mL (5 mL, 15 mL, 45 mL, 60 mL)

Nursing Guidelines

Assessment: See Contraindications, Warnings/Precautions, and Dosing for use cautions. Assess potential for interactions with other prescriptions, OTC medications, or herbal products patient may be taking (especially anything that is ototoxic or nephrotoxic - see Drug Interactions). Administer antiemetic prior to therapy. See Administration, Reconstitution, and Compatibility for infusion specifics. Observe bleeding precautions. Assess results of laboratory tests (see below), therapeutic effectiveness, and adverse response (see Adverse Reactions and Overdose/Toxicology) prior to initiating therapy and on a regular basis throughout therapy. Teach patient (or caregiver) possible side effects/appropriate interventions and adverse symptoms to report (see Patient Education). **Pregnancy risk factor D** - determine that patient is not pregnant before beginning treatment. Instruct patients of childbearing age or males who may have intercourse with women of childbearing age about appropriate contraceptive measures during therapy and for 1 month following therapy. Breast-feeding is contraindicated.

Monitoring Laboratory Tests: CBC with differential and platelet count, serum electrolytes, creatinine clearance, liver function

Patient Education: Inform prescriber of all prescriptions, OTC medications, or herbal products you are taking, and any allergies you have. Do not take any new medication during therapy unless approved by healthcare provider. This medicine can only be administered by I.V. Report immediately any redness, burning, pain, or swelling at infusion site. It is important that you maintain adequate nutrition (small, frequent meals may help) and adequate hydration (2-3 L/day of fluids) unless instructed to restrict fluid intake. You will be susceptible to infection (avoid crowds and exposure to infection and do not have any vaccinations without consulting prescriber). May cause nausea and vomiting (small, frequent meals, frequent mouth care, chewing gum, or sucking lozenges may help - if unresolved, consult prescriber for antiemetic); mouth sores (use soft toothbrush or cotton swabs for mouth care); or loss of hair (reversible). Report chest pain or palpitations; sore throat, fever, chills, unusual fatigue; unusual bruising/bleeding; respiratory difficulty; numbness, pain, or tingling in extremities; muscle cramps or twitching; change in hearing acuity; or other persistent adverse effects. **Pregnancy/breast-feeding precautions:** Inform prescriber if you are pregnant. Do not get pregnant during or for 1 month following therapy. Male: Do not cause a female to become pregnant. Male/female: Consult prescriber for instruction on appropriate contraceptive measures. This drug may cause severe fetal defects. Do not breast-feed.

Geriatric Considerations: Peripheral neuropathy is more frequent in patients >65 years of age.

Pregnancy Risk Factor: D

Lactation: Excretion in breast milk unknown/contraindicated

Administration

I.V.: Administer over 15 minutes, up to 24 hours. May also be administered intraperitoneally. When administered as sequential infusions, taxane derivatives (docetaxel, paclitaxel) should be administered before platinum derivatives to limit myelosuppression and to enhance efficacy.

Reconstitution: Reconstitute powder to yield a final concentration of 10 mg/mL; reconstituted carboplatin 10 mg/mL should be further diluted to a final concentration of 0.5-2 mg/mL with D_5W or NS for administration

Compatibility: Stable in D_5¼NS, D_5½NS, D_5NS, D_5W, NS

Y-site administration: Incompatible with amphotericin B cholesteryl sulfate complex

Compatibility when admixed: Incompatible with fluorouracil, mesna

Storage: Store intact vials at room temperature of 15°C to 30°C (59°F to 86°F); protect from light. Further dilution to a concentration as low as 0.5 mg/mL is stable at room temperature (25°C) or under refrigeration for 8 days in D_5W.

Powder for reconstitution: Reconstituted to a final concentration of 10 mg/mL is stable for 5 days at room temperature (25°C).

Solution for injection: Multidose vials are stable for up to 14 days after opening when stored at room temperature.

♦ **Carboprost** *see* Carboprost Tromethamine *on page 315*

Carboprost Tromethamine (KAR boe prost tro METH a meen)

U.S. Brand Names Hemabate®

Synonyms Carboprost

Pharmacologic Category Abortifacient; Prostaglandin

Use Termination of pregnancy and refractory postpartum uterine bleeding

Unlabeled/Investigational Use Investigational: Hemorrhagic cystitis

Mechanism of Action Carboprost tromethamine is a prostaglandin similar to prostaglandin F_2 alpha (dinoprost) except for the addition of a methyl group at the C-15 position. This substitution produces longer duration of activity than dinoprost; carboprost stimulates uterine contractility which usually results in expulsion of the products of conception and is used to induce abortion between 13-20 weeks of pregnancy. Hemostasis at the placentation site is achieved through the myometrial contractions produced by carboprost.

Contraindications Hypersensitivity to carboprost tromethamine or any component of the formulation; acute pelvic inflammatory disease; pregnancy

Warnings/Precautions Use with caution in patients with history of asthma, hypotension or hypertension, cardiovascular, adrenal, renal or hepatic disease, anemia, jaundice, diabetes, epilepsy or compromised uteri

Drug Interactions Increased toxicity: Oxytocic agents

Adverse Reactions

>10%: Gastrointestinal: Diarrhea, vomiting, nausea

1% to 10%:

Cardiovascular: Flushing

Central nervous system: Dizziness, headache

Gastrointestinal: Stomach cramps

<1% (Limited to important or life-threatening): Abnormal taste, asthma, bladder spasms, blurred vision, bradycardia or tachycardia, breast tenderness, cough, drowsiness, dry mouth, dystonia, fever, hiccups, hematemesis, hyper-/hypotension, myalgia, nervousness, respiratory distress, septic shock, vasovagal syndrome, vertigo

Dosing

Adults & Elderly:

Abortion: I.M.: 250 mcg to start, 250 mcg at 1½-hour to 3½-hour intervals depending on uterine response; a 500 mcg dose may be given if uterine response is not adequate after several 250 mcg doses; do not exceed 12 mg total dose.

Refractory postpartum uterine bleeding: I.M.: Initial: 250 mcg; may repeat at 15- to 90-minute intervals to a total dose of 2 mg

Hemorrhagic cystitis: Bladder irrigation (refer to individual protocols): [0.4-1.0 mg/dL as solution] 50 mL instilled into bladder 4 times/day for 1 hour

Available Dosage Forms Injection, solution: Carboprost 250 mcg and tromethamine 83 mcg per mL (1 mL) [contains benzyl alcohol]

(Continued)

Carboprost Tromethamine *(Continued)*

Nursing Guidelines

Assessment: Premedication with an antiemetic should be considered. Monitor effectiveness and adverse reactions. Assess for complete expulsion of uterine contents (fetal tissue). Assess knowledge/instruct patient on adverse symptoms to report. **Pregnancy risk factor X.**

Patient Education: This medication is used to stimulate expulsion of uterine contents (fetal tissue) or stimulate uterine contractions to reduce uterine bleeding. Report increased blood loss, acute abdominal cramping, foul-smelling vaginal discharge, or persistent elevation of temperature. Increased temperature (elevated temperature) may occur 1-16 hours after therapy and last for several hours. **Pregnancy precaution:** If being treated for hemorrhagic cystitis, inform prescriber if you are pregnant.

Pregnancy Risk Factor: X

Lactation: Excretion in breast milk unknown/opportunity for use is minimal

Administration

I.M.: Give deep I.M.; rotate site if repeat injections are required.

I.V.: Do not inject I.V.; may result in bronchospasm, hypertension, vomiting, and anaphylaxis.

Reconstitution: Bladder irrigation: Dilute immediately prior to administration in NS; stability unknown.

Storage: Refrigerate ampuls.

♦ **Carbose D** *see* Carboxymethylcellulose *on page 316*

Carboxymethylcellulose (kar boks ee meth il SEL yoo lose)

U.S. Brand Names Refresh Liquigel™ [OTC]; Refresh Plus® [OTC]; Refresh Tears® [OTC]; Tears Again® Gel Drops™ [OTC]; Tears Again® Night and Day™ [OTC]; Theratears®

Synonyms Carbose D; Carboxymethylcellulose Sodium

Pharmacologic Category Ophthalmic Agent, Miscellaneous

Use Artificial tear substitute

Dosing

Adults & Elderly: Dry eyes: Ophthalmic: Instill 1-2 drops into eye(s) 3-4 times/day

Available Dosage Forms

Gel, ophthalmic, as sodium (Tears Again® Night and Day™): 1.5% (3.5 g)

Solution ophthalmic, as sodium:

- Refresh Liquigel™: 1% (15 mL) [liquid gel formulation]
- Refresh Plus®: 0.5% (0.4 mL) [preservative free; available in packages of 30 or 50]
- Refresh Tears®: 0.5% (15 mL)
- Tears Again® Gel Drops™: 0.7% (15 mL)
- Theratears®: 0.25% (0.6 mL [preservative free], 15 mL)

♦ **Carboxymethylcellulose Sodium** *see* Carboxymethylcellulose *on page 316*
♦ **Cardene®** *see* NiCARdipine *on page 1220*
♦ **Cardene® I.V.** *see* NiCARdipine *on page 1220*
♦ **Cardene® SR** *see* NiCARdipine *on page 1220*
♦ **Cardizem®** *see* Diltiazem *on page 540*
♦ **Cardizem® CD** *see* Diltiazem *on page 540*
♦ **Cardizem® LA** *see* Diltiazem *on page 540*
♦ **Cardizem® SR [DSC]** *see* Diltiazem *on page 540*
♦ **Cardura®** *see* Doxazosin *on page 574*
♦ **CareNate™ 600** *see* Vitamins (Multiple/Prenatal) *on page 1721*
♦ **Carimune™ NF** *see* Immune Globulin (Intravenous) *on page 899*
♦ **Carisoprodate** *see* Carisoprodol *on page 316*

Carisoprodol (kar eye soe PROE dole)

U.S. Brand Names Soma®

Synonyms Carisoprodate; Isobamate

Pharmacologic Category Skeletal Muscle Relaxant

Use Skeletal muscle relaxant

Mechanism of Action Precise mechanism is not yet clear, but many effects have been ascribed to its central depressant actions

Pharmacodynamics/Kinetics

Onset of action: ~30 minutes

Duration: 4-6 hours

Distribution: Crosses placenta; high concentrations enter breast milk

Metabolism: Hepatic

Half-life elimination: 8 hours

Excretion: Urine

Contraindications Hypersensitivity to carisoprodol, meprobamate or any component of the formulation; acute intermittent porphyria

Warnings/Precautions May cause CNS depression, which may impair physical or mental abilities. Effects with other sedative drugs or ethanol may be potentiated. Use with caution in patients with hepatic/renal dysfunction. Tolerance or drug dependence may result from extended use.

Drug Interactions **Substrate** of CYP2C19 (major)

Increased toxicity: Ethanol, CNS depressants, phenothiazines

CYP2C19 inhibitors: May increase the levels/effects of carisoprodol. Example inhibitors include delavirdine, fluconazole, fluvoxamine, gemfibrozil, isoniazid, omeprazole, and ticlopidine.

Nutritional/Herbal/Ethanol Interactions Ethanol: Avoid ethanol (may increase CNS depression).

Adverse Reactions

>10%: Central nervous system: Drowsiness

1% to 10%:

- Cardiovascular: Tachycardia, tightness in chest, flushing of face, syncope
- Central nervous system: Mental depression, allergic fever, dizziness, lightheadedness, headache, paradoxical CNS stimulation
- Dermatologic: Angioedema, dermatitis (allergic)
- Gastrointestinal: Nausea, vomiting, stomach cramps
- Neuromuscular & skeletal: Trembling
- Ocular: Burning eyes
- Respiratory: Dyspnea
- Miscellaneous: Hiccups

<1% (Limited to important or life-threatening): Aplastic anemia, clumsiness, eosinophilia, erythema multiforme, leukopenia, rash, urticaria

Overdosage/Toxicology Symptoms of overdose include CNS depression, stupor, coma, shock, and respiratory depression. Treatment is supportive.

Dosing

Adults: Muscle spasm (including spasm associated with acute temporomandibular joint pain): Oral: 350 mg 3-4 times/day; take last dose at bedtime; compound: 1-2 tablets 4 times/day

Elderly: Not recommended for use in the elderly (see Geriatric Considerations).

Available Dosage Forms Tablet: 350 mg

Nursing Guidelines

Assessment: Assess effectiveness and interactions of other medications patient may be taking. Monitor effectiveness of therapy (according to rationale for therapy) and adverse reactions. Monitor for excessive drowsiness at beginning of therapy and periodically with long-term use. Do not discontinue abruptly; taper dosage slowly (withdrawal symptoms may occur). Assess knowledge/teach patient appropriate use, interventions to reduce side effects, and adverse symptoms to report.

Patient Education: Take exactly as directed with food. Do not increase dose or discontinue without consulting prescriber. Do not use alcohol, prescriptive or OTC antidepressants, sedatives, and pain medications without consulting prescriber. You may experience drowsiness, dizziness, lightheadedness (avoid driving or engaging in tasks requiring alertness until response to drug is known); nausea, vomiting, or cramping (small frequent meals, frequent mouth care, or sucking hard candy may help); or postural hypotension (change position slowly when rising from sitting or lying or when climbing stairs). Report excessive drowsiness or mental agitation; palpitations, rapid heartbeat, chest pain; skin rash; muscle cramping or tremors; or respiratory difficulty. **Pregnancy/breast-feeding precautions:** Inform prescriber if you are or intend to become pregnant. Breast-feeding is not recommended.

Geriatric Considerations: Because of the risk of orthostatic hypotension and CNS depression, avoid or use with caution in the elderly. Not considered a drug of choice in the elderly.

(Continued)

Carisoprodol *(Continued)*

Pregnancy Risk Factor: C

Lactation: Enters breast milk (high concentrations)/not recommended

Administration

Oral: Give with food to decrease GI upset.

♦ Carmol® Scalp *see* Sulfacetamide *on page 1579*

Carmustine (kar MUS teen)

U.S. Brand Names BiCNu®; Gliadel®

Synonyms BCNU; bis-chloronitrosourea; Carmustinum; NSC-409962; WR-139021

Pharmacologic Category Antineoplastic Agent; Antineoplastic Agent, Alkylating Agent (Nitrosourea); Antineoplastic Agent, DNA Adduct-Forming Agent; Antineoplastic Agent, DNA Binding Agent

Medication Safety Issues

Sound-alike/look-alike issues:

Carmustine may be confused with lomustine

Use

Injection: Treatment of brain tumors (glioblastoma, brainstem glioma, medulloblastoma, astrocytoma, ependymoma, and metastatic brain tumors), multiple myeloma, Hodgkin's disease, non-Hodgkin's lymphomas, melanoma, lung cancer, colon cancer

Wafer (implant): Adjunct to surgery in patients with recurrent glioblastoma multiforme; adjunct to surgery and radiation in patients with high-grade malignant glioma

Mechanism of Action Interferes with the normal function of DNA by alkylation and cross-linking the strands of DNA, and by possible protein modification

Pharmacodynamics/Kinetics

Distribution: Readily crosses blood-brain barrier producing CSF levels equal to 15% to 70% of blood plasma levels; enters breast milk; highly lipid soluble

Metabolism: Rapidly hepatic

Half-life elimination: Biphasic: Initial: 1.4 minutes; Secondary: 20 minutes (active metabolites: plasma half-life of 67 hours)

Excretion: Urine (~60% to 70%) within 96 hours; lungs (6% to 10% as CO_2)

Contraindications Hypersensitivity to carmustine or any component of the formulation; myelosuppression; pregnancy

Warnings/Precautions The U.S. Food and Drug Administration (FDA) currently recommends that procedures for proper handling and disposal of antineoplastic agents be considered. Administer with caution to patients with depressed platelet, leukocyte or erythrocyte counts, renal or hepatic impairment. Diluent contains significant amounts of ethanol; use caution with aldehyde dehydrogenase-2 deficiency or history of "alcohol flushing syndrome." Do not give courses more frequently than every 6 week.

Drug Interactions

Cimetidine: Reported to cause bone marrow suppression

Ethanol: Diluent for infusion contains alcohol; avoid concurrent use of medications that inhibit aldehyde dehydrogenase-2 or cause disulfiram-like reactions.

Etoposide: Reported to cause severe hepatic dysfunction with hyperbilirubinemia, ascites, and thrombocytopenia

Nutritional/Herbal/Ethanol Interactions Ethanol: Avoid ethanol.

Adverse Reactions

>10%:

Cardiovascular: Hypotension is associated with **high-dose** administration secondary to the high content of the diluent

Central nervous system: Dizziness, ataxia; Wafers: Seizures (54%) postoperatively

Dermatologic: Hyperpigmentation of skin

Gastrointestinal: Nausea and vomiting occur within 2-4 hours after drug injection; dose related

Emetic potential:

<200 mg: Moderately high (60% to 90%)

≥200 mg: High (>90%)

Time course of nausea/vomiting: Onset: 2-6 hours; Duration: 4-6 hours

Hematologic: Myelosuppressive: Delayed, occurs 4-6 weeks after administration and is dose related; usually persists for 1-2 weeks; thrombocytopenia is usually more severe than leukopenia. Myelofibrosis and preleukemic syndromes have been reported.

WBC: Moderate

Platelets: Severe

Onset: 14 days

Nadir: 21-35 days

Recovery: 42-50 days

Local: Burning at injection site

Irritant chemotherapy: Pain at injection site

Ocular: Ocular toxicity, and retinal hemorrhages

1% to 10%:

Dermatologic: Facial flushing is probably due to the alcohol used in reconstitution, alopecia

Gastrointestinal: Stomatitis, diarrhea, anorexia

Hematologic: Anemia

<1% (Limited to important or life-threatening): Reversible toxicity; increased LFTs in 20%; fibrosis occurs mostly in patients treated with prolonged total doses >1400 mg/m^2 or with bone marrow transplantation doses; risk factors include a history of lung disease, concomitant bleomycin, or radiation therapy; PFTs should be conducted prior to therapy and monitored; patients with predicted FVC or DLCO <70% are at a higher risk; azotemia; decrease in kidney size; renal failure

BMT:

Cardiovascular: Hypotension (infusion-related), arrhythmia (infusion-related)

Central nervous system: Encephalopathy, ethanol intoxication, seizure, fever

Endocrine & metabolic: Hyperprolactinemia and hypothyroidism in patients with brain tumors treated with radiation

Gastrointestinal: Severe nausea and vomiting

Hepatic: Hepatitis, hepatic veno-occlusive disease

Pulmonary: Dyspnea

Overdosage/Toxicology Symptoms of overdose include nausea, vomiting, thrombocytopenia, and leukopenia. Treatment is symptomatic and supportive.

Dosing

Adults & Elderly: Refer to individual protocols.

Usual dosage (per manufacturer labeling): I.V.: 150-200 mg/m^2 every 6 weeks as a single dose or divided into daily injections on 2 successive days

Alternative regimens:

75-120 mg/m^2 days 1 and 2 every 6-8 weeks **or**

50-80 mg/m^2 days 1,2,3 every 6-8 weeks

Primary brain cancer:

150-200 mg/m^2 every 6-8 weeks as a single dose **or**

75-120 mg/m^2 days 1 and 2 every 6-8 weeks **or**

20-65 mg/m^2 every 4-6 weeks **or**

0.5-1 mg/kg every 4-6 weeks **or**

40-80 mg/m^2/day for 3 days every 6-8 weeks

Autologous BMT: I.V.: ALL OF THE FOLLOWING DOSES ARE FATAL WITHOUT BMT

Combination therapy: Up to 300-900 mg/m^2

Single-agent therapy: Up to 1200 mg/m^2 (fatal necrosis is associated with doses >2 g/m^2)

Glioblastoma multiforme (recurrent), malignant glioma: Implantation (wafer): Up to 8 wafers may be placed in the resection cavity (total dose 62.6 mg); should the size and shape not accommodate 8 wafers, the maximum number of wafers allowed should be placed

Pediatrics: Refer to individual protocols: Children: I.V.: 200-250 mg/m^2 every 4-6 weeks as a single dose

Hepatic Impairment: Dosage adjustment may be necessary; however, no specific guidelines are available.

Available Dosage Forms

Injection, powder for reconstitution (BiCNu®): 100 mg [packaged with 3 mL of absolute alcohol as diluent]

Wafer (Gliadel®): 7.7 mg (8s)

Nursing Guidelines

Assessment: See Contraindications, Warnings/Precautions, and Dosing for use cautions. Assess potential for interactions with other prescriptions, OTC medications, or herbal products patient may be taking (see Drug Interactions). Administer antiemetic prior to therapy. See Administration, Compatibility, and Reconstitution information. Infusion site should be monitored closely to prevent

(Continued)

Carmustine *(Continued)*

extravasation (acute cellulitis may occur - see Extravasation Management) and bleeding precautions must be observed. Assess results of laboratory tests (see below), therapeutic response, and adverse effects (see Adverse Reactions and Overdose/Toxicology) regularly during therapy. Teach patient or caregiver proper use (appropriate injection technique and syringe/needle disposal), possible side effects/appropriate interventions, and adverse symptoms to report (see Patient Education). **Pregnancy risk factor D** - determine that patient is not pregnant before beginning treatment. Instruct females of childbearing age or males who may have intercourse with females of childbearing age about appropriate contraceptive measures during and for 1 month following therapy. Breast-feeding is contraindicated.

Monitoring Laboratory Tests: CBC with differential, platelet count, pulmonary function, liver and renal function

Patient Education: Inform prescriber of all prescriptions, OTC medications, or herbal products you are taking, and any allergies you have. Do not take any new medication during therapy unless approved by prescriber. This medication can only be administered by I.V. Report immediately any pain, burning, swelling at infusion site. Limit oral intake for 4-6 hours before therapy to reduce potential for nausea/vomiting. It is important that you maintain adequate nutrition between treatments (small, frequent meals may help) and adequate hydration (2-3 L/day of fluids) unless instructed to restrict fluid intake. You will be susceptible to infection (avoid crowds and exposure to infection and do not have any vaccinations without consulting prescriber). May cause nausea, vomiting, or anorexia (small, frequent meals, frequent mouth care, chewing gum, or sucking lozenges may help - if nausea/vomiting are severe, request antiemetic); mouth sores (use soft toothbrush or cotton swabs for mouth care); hyperpigmentation of skin and loss of hair (reversible); or sensitivity to sunlight (use sunblock, wear protective clothing and dark glasses, and avoid direct exposure to sunlight). Report chest pain or palpitations; sore throat, fever, chills, unusual fatigue; unusual bruising/bleeding; change in color of urine or stool; respiratory difficulty; change in visual acuity; or pain, redness, or swelling at injection site. **Pregnancy/breast-feeding precautions:** Inform prescriber if you are pregnant. Do not get pregnant or cause a pregnancy (males) during therapy or for 1 month following therapy. Consult prescriber for instruction on appropriate contraceptive measures. This drug may cause severe fetal defects. Do not breast-feed.

Pregnancy Risk Factor: D

Pregnancy Issues: Carmustine can cause fetal harm if administered to a pregnant woman.

Lactation: Excretion in breast milk unknown/contraindicated

Breast-Feeding Considerations: It is not known if carmustine is excreted in human breast milk. Due to potential harm to infant, breast-feeding is not recommended.

Administration

I.V.: Irritant (alcohol-based diluent). Injection: Significant absorption to PVC containers - should be administered in either glass or Excel® container. I.V. infusion over 1-2 hours is recommended; infusion through a free-flowing saline or dextrose infusion, or administration through a central catheter can alleviate venous pain/irritation

High-dose carmustine: Maximum rate of infusion of $\leq$3 mg/m^2/minute to avoid excessive flushing, agitation, and hypotension; infusions should run over at least 2 hours; some investigational protocols dictate shorter infusions.

Fatal doses if not followed by bone marrow or peripheral stem cell infusions.

Reconstitution: Injection: Initially, dilute with 3 mL of absolute alcohol. Further dilute with SWFI to a concentration of 3.3 mg/mL.

Compatibility: Stable in NS

Y-site administration: Incompatible with allopurinol

Compatibility when admixed: Incompatible with sodium bicarbonate

Storage:

Injection: Store intact vials under refrigeration; vials are stable for 36 days at room temperature. Reconstituted solutions are stable for 8 hours at room temperature (25°C) and 24 hours under refrigeration (2°C to 8°C) and protected from light. Further dilution in D_5W or NS is stable for 8 hours at room temperature (25°C) and 48 hours under refrigeration (4°C) in glass or Excel® protected from light.

Wafer: Store at or below -20°C (-4°F). May be kept at room temperature for up to 6 hours.

♦ **Carmustinum** *see* Carmustine *on page 318*

♦ **Cartia XT™** *see* Diltiazem *on page 540*

Carvedilol (KAR ve dil ole)

U.S. Brand Names Coreg®

Pharmacologic Category Beta Blocker With Alpha-Blocking Activity

Medication Safety Issues

Sound-alike/look-alike issues:

Carvedilol may be confused with captopril, carteolol

Use Mild to severe heart failure of ischemic or cardiomyopathic origin (usually in addition to standardized therapy); left ventricular dysfunction following myocardial infarction (MI); management of hypertension

Unlabeled/Investigational Use Angina pectoris

Mechanism of Action As a racemic mixture, carvedilol has nonselective beta-adrenoreceptor and alpha-adrenergic blocking activity. No intrinsic sympathomimetic activity has been documented. Associated effects in hypertensive patients include reduction of cardiac output, exercise- or beta agonist-induced tachycardia, reduction of reflex orthostatic tachycardia, vasodilation, decreased peripheral vascular resistance (especially in standing position), decreased renal vascular resistance, reduced plasma renin activity, and increased levels of atrial natriuretic peptide. In CHF, associated effects include decreased pulmonary capillary wedge pressure, decreased pulmonary artery pressure, decreased heart rate, decreased systemic vascular resistance, increased stroke volume index, and decreased right arterial pressure (RAP).

Pharmacodynamics/Kinetics

Onset of action: 1-2 hours

Peak antihypertensive effect: ~1-2 hours

Absorption: Rapid; food decreases rate but not extent of absorption; administration with food minimizes risks of orthostatic hypotension

Distribution: V_d: 115 L

Protein binding: >98%, primarily to albumin

Metabolism: Extensively hepatic, via **CYP2C9, 2D6,** 3A4, and 2C19 (2% excreted unchanged); three active metabolites (4-hydroxyphenyl metabolite is 13 times more potent than parent drug for beta-blockade); first-pass effect; plasma concentrations in the elderly and those with cirrhotic liver disease are 50% and 4-7 times higher, respectively

Bioavailability: 25% to 35%

Half-life elimination: 7-10 hours

Excretion: Primarily feces

Contraindications Hypersensitivity to carvedilol or any component of the formulation; patients with decompensated cardiac failure requiring intravenous inotropic therapy; bronchial asthma or related bronchospastic conditions; second- or third-degree AV block, sick sinus syndrome, and severe bradycardia (except in patients with a functioning artificial pacemaker); cardiogenic shock; severe hepatic impairment; pregnancy (2nd and 3rd trimesters)

Warnings/Precautions Initiate cautiously and monitor for possible deterioration in patient status (including symptoms of CHF). Adjustment of other medications (ACE inhibitors and/or diuretics) may be required. In severe chronic heart failure, trial patients were excluded if they had cardiac-related rales, ascites, or a serum creatinine >2.8 mg/dL. Congestive heart failure patients may experience a worsening of renal function; risks include ischemic disease, diffuse vascular disease, underlying renal dysfunction; systolic BP <100 mm Hg. Patients should be advised to avoid driving or other hazardous tasks during initiation of therapy due to the risk of syncope. Avoid abrupt discontinuation (may exacerbate underlying condition), particularly in patients with coronary artery disease; dose should be tapered over 1-2 weeks with close monitoring.

Manufacturer recommends discontinuation of therapy if liver injury occurs (confirmed by laboratory testing). Use caution in patients with PVD (can aggravate arterial insufficiency). Use caution with concurrent use of verapamil or diltiazem; bradycardia or heart block can occur. Use caution in patients with bronchospastic disease. Use cautiously in diabetics because it can mask prominent hypoglycemic symptoms. May mask signs of thyrotoxicosis. Use care with

(Continued)

Carvedilol *(Continued)*

anesthetic agents that decrease myocardial function. Safety and efficacy in children <18 years of age have not been established.

Drug Interactions Substrate of CYP1A2 (minor), 2C8/9 (major), 2D6 (major), 2E1 (minor), 3A4 (minor)

Alpha-blockers (prazosin, terazosin): Concurrent use of beta-blockers may increase risk of orthostasis.

Beta-agonists: Beta-blockers may counteract desired effects of beta-agonists.

Calcium channel blockers (nondihydropyridine): May enhance hypotensive effects of beta-blockers.

Cimetidine: May increase carvedilol serum levels.

CYP2C8/9 inducers: May decrease the levels/effects of carvedilol. Example inducers include carbamazepine, phenobarbital, phenytoin, rifampin, rifapentine, and secobarbital.

CYP2C8/9 inhibitors: May increase the levels/effects of carvedilol. Example inhibitors include delavirdine, fluconazole, gemfibrozil, ketoconazole, nicardipine, NSAIDs, pioglitazone, and sulfonamides.

CYP2D6 inhibitors: May increase the levels/effects of carvedilol. Example inhibitors include chlorpromazine, delavirdine, fluoxetine, miconazole, paroxetine, pergolide, quinidine, quinine, ritonavir, and ropinirole.

Digoxin: Carvedilol may increase the serum levels of digoxin.

Disopyramide: May exacerbate heart failure or enhance bradycardic effect of beta-blockers.

Drugs which slow AV conduction (digoxin): Effects may be additive with beta-blockers.

Insulin and oral hypoglycemics: Carvedilol may mask symptoms of hypoglycemia.

NSAIDs (ibuprofen, indomethacin, naproxen, piroxicam) may reduce the antihypertensive effects of beta-blockers.

Rifampin: May increase the metabolism of carvedilol.

Salicylates: May reduce the antihypertensive effects of beta-blockers.

SSRIs: May decrease the metabolism of carvedilol.

Sulfonylureas: Beta blockers may alter response to hypoglycemic agents.

Verapamil, diltiazem: May have synergistic or additive pharmacological effects when taken concurrently with beta-blockers.

Nutritional/Herbal/Ethanol Interactions Herb/Nutraceutical: Avoid dong quai if using for hypertension (has estrogenic activity). Avoid ephedra, yohimbe, ginseng (may worsen hypertension). Avoid garlic (may have increased antihypertensive effect).

Lab Interactions Increased hepatic enzymes, BUN, NPN, alkaline phosphatase; decreased HDL

Adverse Reactions Note: Frequency ranges include data from hypertension and heart failure trials. Higher rates of adverse reactions have generally been noted in patients with CHF. However, the frequency of adverse effects associated with placebo is also increased in this population. Events occurring at a frequency > placebo in clinical trials.

>10%:
- Cardiovascular: Hypotension (9% to 20%)
- Central nervous system: Dizziness (6% to 32%), fatigue (4% to 24%)
- Endocrine & metabolic: Hyperglycemia (5% to 12%), weight gain (10% to 12%)
- Gastrointestinal: Diarrhea (2% to 12%)
- Neuromuscular & skeletal: Weakness (11%)

1% to 10%:
- Cardiovascular: Bradycardia (2% to 10%), hypertension (3%), AV block (3%), angina (2% to 6%), postural hypotension (2%), syncope (3% to 8%), dependent edema (4%), palpitation, peripheral edema (1% to 7%), generalized edema (5% to 6%)
- Central nervous system: Headache (5% to 8%), fever (3%), paresthesia (2%), somnolence (2%), insomnia (2%), malaise, hypoesthesia, vertigo
- Endocrine & metabolic: Alkaline phosphatase increased, gout (6%), hypercholesterolemia (4%), dehydration (2%), hyperkalemia (3%), hypervolemia (2%), hypertriglyceridemia (1%), hyperuricemia, hypoglycemia, hyponatremia
- Gastrointestinal: Nausea (4% to 9%), vomiting (6%), melena, periodontitis
- Genitourinary: Hematuria (3%), impotence
- Hematologic: Thrombocytopenia (1% to 2%), decreased prothrombin, purpura
- Hepatic: Transaminases increased
- Neuromuscular & skeletal: Back pain (2% to 7%), arthralgia (6%), myalgia (3%), muscle cramps

Ocular: Blurred vision (3% to 5%), lacrimation

Renal: Increased BUN (6%), abnormal renal function, albuminuria, glycosuria, increased creatinine (3%), kidney failure

Respiratory: Rhinitis (2%), increased cough (5%)

Miscellaneous: Injury (3% to 6%), allergy, sudden death

<1% (Limited to important or life-threatening): Aggravated depression, anaphylactoid reaction, anemia, aplastic anemia (rare, all events occurred in patients receiving other medications capable of causing this effect); asthma, AV block (complete), bronchospasm, bundle branch block, cholestatic jaundice, convulsion, diabetes mellitus, erythema multiforme, exfoliative dermatitis, GI hemorrhage, interstitial pneumonitis, leukopenia, migraine, myocardial ischemia, neuralgia, pancytopenia, peripheral ischemia, pulmonary edema, Stevens-Johnson syndrome, toxic epidermal necrolysis, urinary incontinence

Overdosage/Toxicology Symptoms of intoxication include cardiac disturbances, CNS toxicity, bronchospasm, hypoglycemia, and hyperkalemia. The most common cardiac symptoms include hypotension and bradycardia. Atrioventricular block, intraventricular conduction disturbances, cardiogenic shock, and asystole may occur with severe overdose, especially with membrane-depressant drugs (eg, propranolol). CNS effects include convulsions, coma, and respiratory arrest (commonly seen with propranolol and other membrane-depressant and lipid-soluble drugs). Treatment is symptom-directed and supportive. Carvedilol does not appear to be significantly cleared by hemodialysis.

Dosing

Adults & Elderly: Reduce dosage if heart rate drops to <55 beats/minute.

Hypertension: Oral: 6.25 mg twice daily; if tolerated, dose should be maintained for 1-2 weeks, then increased to 12.5 mg twice daily. Dosage may be increased to a maximum of 25 mg twice daily after 1-2 weeks. Maximum dose: 50 mg/day

Congestive heart failure: Oral: 3.125 mg twice daily for 2 weeks; if this dose is tolerated, may increase to 6.25 mg twice daily. Double the dose every 2 weeks to the highest dose tolerated by patient. (Prior to initiating therapy, other heart failure medications should be stabilized and fluid retention minimized.)

Maximum recommended dose: Oral:

Mild to moderate heart failure:

<85 kg: 25 mg twice daily

>85 kg: 50 mg twice daily

Severe heart failure: Oral: 25 mg twice daily

Left ventricular dysfunction following MI: Initial 3.125-6.25 mg twice daily; increase dosage incrementally (ie, from 6.25 to 12.5 mg twice daily) at intervals of 3-10 days, based on tolerance, to a target dose of 25 mg twice daily. **Note**: Should be initiated only after patient is hemodynamically stable and fluid retention has been minimized.

Angina pectoris (unlabeled use): Oral: 25-50 mg twice daily

Renal Impairment: None necessary

Hepatic Impairment: Use is contraindicated in severe liver dysfunction.

Available Dosage Forms Tablet: 3.125 mg, 6.25 mg, 12.5 mg, 25 mg

Nursing Guidelines

Assessment: Assess potential for interactions with other prescriptions, OTC medications, or herbal products patient may be taking (especially anything that will effect blood pressure). Blood pressure and heart rate should be assessed prior to and following first doses and any change in dose. Caution patients with diabetes to monitor glucose levels closely (beta-blockers may alter glucose tolerance). Assess results of laboratory tests, therapeutic effectiveness (eg, reduction of hypertension or angina), and adverse response (eg, CHF). Teach patient proper use, possible side effects/appropriate interventions, and adverse symptoms to report.

Monitoring Laboratory Tests: Renal studies, BUN, liver function

Dietary Considerations: Should be taken with food to minimize the risk of orthostatic hypotension.

Patient Education: Do not take any new medication during therapy unless approved by prescriber. Take exactly as directed. Do not alter dose or discontinue without consulting prescriber. Take pulse daily, prior to taking medication; follow prescriber's instruction about holding medication. If you have diabetes, monitor serum glucose closely (drug may alter glucose tolerance or mask signs of hypoglycemia). You may experience fatigue, dizziness, or postural hypotension (use caution when changing position from lying or sitting to standing,

(Continued)

Carvedilol *(Continued)*

driving, or climbing stairs until response to medication is known); alteration in sexual performance (reversible); or diarrhea (buttermilk, boiled milk, or yogurt may help). Report unresolved swelling of extremities; respiratory difficulty or new cough; unresolved fatigue; unusual weight gain (>5 lb/week); unresolved constipation or diarrhea; or unusual muscle weakness. **Pregnancy/breast-feeding precautions:** Inform prescriber if you are pregnant. Do not get pregnant while taking this medications. Consult prescriber for appropriate contraceptive use. Do not breast-feed.

Geriatric Considerations: Due to alterations in the beta-adrenergic autonomic nervous system, beta-adrenergic blockade may result in less hemodynamic response than seen in younger adults. In U.S. trials conducted by the manufacturer, hypertension patients who were elderly (>65%) had a higher incidence of dizziness (8.8% vs 6%) than seen in younger patients. No other differences noted between young and old in these trials.

Pregnancy Risk Factor: C (manufacturer); D (2nd and 3rd trimesters - expert analysis)

Pregnancy Issues: No data available on whether carvedilol crosses the placenta; beta-blockers have been associated with persistent bradycardia, hypotension, and IUGR; IUGR probably related to maternal hypertension. Cases of neonatal hypoglycemia have been reported following maternal use of beta-blockers at parturition or during breast-feeding. Use during pregnancy only if the potential benefit justifies the risk.

Lactation: Excretion in breast milk unknown/contraindicated

Perioperative/Anesthesia/Other Concerns:

Withdrawal: Beta-blocker therapy should not be withdrawn abruptly, but gradually tapered to avoid acute tachycardia and hypertension.

Heart Failure: Carvedilol is a nonselective beta-blocker with alpha-blocking and antioxidant properties.

Administration

Oral: Administer with food.

Storage: Store at 30°C (86°F).

♦ Casanthranol and Docusate *see* Docusate and Casanthranol *on page 561*

Caspofungin (kas poe FUN jin)

U.S. Brand Names Cancidas®

Synonyms Caspofungin Acetate

Pharmacologic Category Antifungal Agent, Parenteral

Use Treatment of invasive *Aspergillus* infections in patients who are refractory or intolerant of other therapy; treatment of candidemia and other *Candida* infections (intra-abdominal abscesses, esophageal, peritonitis, pleural space); empirical treatment for presumed fungal infections in febrile neutropenic patient

Mechanism of Action Inhibits synthesis of β(1,3)-D-glucan, an essential component of the cell wall of susceptible fungi. Highest activity in regions of active cell growth. Mammalian cells do not require β(1,3)-D-glucan, limiting potential toxicity.

Pharmacodynamics/Kinetics

Protein binding: 97% to albumin

Metabolism: Slowly, via hydrolysis and *N*-acetylation as well as by spontaneous degradation, with subsequent metabolism to component amino acids. Overall metabolism is extensive.

Half-life elimination: Beta (distribution): 9-11 hours; Terminal: 40-50 hours

Excretion: Urine (41% as metabolites, 1% to 9% unchanged) and feces (35% as metabolites)

Contraindications Hypersensitivity to caspofungin or any component of the formulation

Warnings/Precautions Has not been studied as initial therapy for invasive *Aspergillus*. Concurrent use of cyclosporine should be limited to patients for whom benefit outweighs risk, due to a high frequency of hepatic transaminase elevations observed during concurrent use. Limited data are available concerning treatment durations longer than 4 weeks; however, treatment appears to be well tolerated. Use caution in hepatic impairment; dosage reduction required in moderate impairment. Safety and efficacy in pediatric patients have not been established.

Drug Interactions

Cyclosporine: Concurrent administration may increase caspofungin concentrations. Serum hepatic transaminases may be increased. Limit use to patients for whom benefit outweighs risk.

Rifampin: May decrease caspofungin concentrations. Caspofungin dose should be 70 mg daily during concomitant therapy.

Tacrolimus: Caspofungin may decrease blood concentrations of tacrolimus; monitor.

Adverse Reactions

>10%:

- Central nervous system: Headache (up to 11%), fever (3% to 26%), chills (up to 14%)
- Endocrine & metabolic: Hypokalemia (4% to 11%)
- Hematologic: Hemoglobin decreased (1% to 12%)
- Hepatic: Serum alkaline phosphatase (3% to 11%) increased, transaminases increased (up to 13%)
- Local: Infusion site reactions (2% to 12%), phlebitis/thrombophlebitis (up to 16%)

1% to 10%:

- Cardiovascular: Flushing (2% to 3%), facial edema (up to 3%), hypertension (1% to 2%), tachycardia (1% to 2%), hypotension (1%)
- Central nervous system: Dizziness (2%), pain (1% to 5%), insomnia (1%)
- Dermatologic: Rash (<1% to 6%), pruritus (1% to 3%), erythema (1% to 2%)
- Gastrointestinal: Nausea (2% to 6%), vomiting (1% to 4%), abdominal pain (1% to 4%), diarrhea (1% to 4%), anorexia (1%)
- Hematologic: Eosinophils increased (3%), neutrophils decreased (2% to 3%), WBC decreased (5% to 6%), anemia (up to 4%), platelet count decreased (2% to 3%)
- Hepatic: Bilirubin increased (3%)
- Local: Induration (up to 3%)
- Neuromuscular & skeletal: Myalgia (up to 3%), paresthesia (1% to 3%), tremor (≤2%)
- Renal: Nephrotoxicity (8%)*, proteinuria (5%), hematuria (2%), serum creatinine increased (<1% to 4%), urinary WBCs increased (up to 8%), urinary RBCs increased (1% to 4%), blood urea nitrogen increased (1%)
- *Nephrotoxicity defined as serum creatinine ≥2X baseline value or ≥1 mg/dL in patients with serum creatinine above ULN range (patients with Cl_{cr} <30 mL/minute were excluded)
- Miscellaneous: Flu-like syndrome (3%), diaphoresis (up to 3%)

<1% (Limited to important or life-threatening): Adult respiratory distress syndrome (ARDS), anaphylaxis, hepatic dysfunction, pulmonary edema, renal insufficiency; histamine-mediated reaction (including facial swelling, bronchospasm, sensation of warmth) have been reported

Overdosage/Toxicology No experience with overdosage has been reported. Caspofungin is not dialyzable. Treatment is symptomatic and supportive.

Dosing

Adults & Elderly: Note: Duration of caspofungin treatment should be determined by patient status and clinical response. Empiric therapy should be given until neutropenia resolves. In patients with positive cultures, treatment should continue until 14 days after last positive culture. In neutropenic patients, treatment should be given at least 7 days after both signs and symptoms of infection **and** neutropenia resolve.

Empiric therapy: Initial dose: 70 mg on day 1; subsequent dosing: 50 mg/day; may increase up to 70 mg/day if tolerated, but clinical response is inadequate.

Invasive *Aspergillus*, candidiasis: I.V.: Initial dose: 70 mg on day 1; subsequent dosing: 50 mg/day

Esophageal candidiasis: I.V.: 50 mg/day; **Note:** The majority of patients studied for this indication also had oropharyngeal involvement.

Dosage adjustment with concomitant use of an enzyme inducer:

Patients receiving rifampin: 70 mg caspofungin daily

Patients receiving carbamazepine, dexamethasone, efavirenz, nevirapine, or phenytoin (and possibly other enzyme inducers) may require an increased daily dose of caspofungin (70 mg/day).

Pediatrics: Safety and efficacy in pediatric patients have not been established.

Renal Impairment: No specific dosage adjustment is required; supplemental dose is not required following dialysis.

(Continued)

Caspofungin *(Continued)*

Hepatic Impairment:

Mild hepatic insufficiency (Child-Pugh score 5-6): No adjustment necessary.

Moderate hepatic insufficiency (Child-Pugh score 7-9): 35 mg/day; initial 70 mg loading dose should still be administered in treatment of invasive infections.

Severe hepatic insufficiency (Child-Pugh score >9): No clinical experience.

Available Dosage Forms Injection, powder for reconstitution, as acetate: 50 mg [contains sucrose 39 mg], 70 mg [contains sucrose 54 mg]

Nursing Guidelines

Assessment: See Warnings/Precautions, Contraindications, and Dosing for use cautions. Assess therapeutic effectiveness and adverse reactions (eg, headache, hypokalemia, cardiovascular changes - see Adverse Reactions). See Administration for specific infusion directions. Teach patient possible side effects, appropriate interventions, and adverse symptoms to report (see Patient Education). Note breast-feeding caution.

Patient Education: Inform prescriber of all prescriptions, OTC medications, or herbal products you are taking, and any allergies you have. This medication can only be administered by infusion. Report immediately any pain, burning, or swelling at infusion site, or any signs of allergic reaction (eg, respiratory difficulty or swallowing, back pain, chest tightness, rash, hives, or swelling of lips or mouth). Report nausea, vomiting, abdominal pain, or diarrhea. **Pregnancy/breast-feeding precautions:** Inform prescriber if you are or intend to become pregnant. Consult prescriber if breast-feeding.

Pregnancy Risk Factor: C

Lactation: Excretion in breast milk unknown/use caution

Administration

I.V.: Infuse slowly, over 1 hour. Do not coadminister with other medications.

Reconstitution: Bring refrigerated vial to room temperature. Reconstitute vials using 0.9% sodium chloride for injection, SWFI, or bacteriostatic water for injection. Mix gently until clear solution is formed; do not use if cloudy or contains particles. Solution should be further diluted with 0.9%, 0.45%, or 0.225% sodium chloride or LR. Do not mix with dextrose-containing solutions. Do not coadminister with other medications.

Compatibility: Do not mix with dextrose-containing solutions or coadminister with other medications.

Storage: Store vials at 2°C to 8°C (36°F to 46°F). Reconstituted solution may be stored at less than 25°C (77°F) for 1 hour prior to preparation of infusion solution. Infusion solutions may be stored at less than 25°C (77°F) and should be used within 24 hours; up to 48 hours if stored at 2°C to 8°C (36°F to 46°F).

- ♦ **Caspofungin Acetate** *see* Caspofungin *on page 324*
- ♦ **Castellani Paint Modified [OTC]** *see* Phenol *on page 1347*
- ♦ **Cataflam®** *see* Diclofenac *on page 521*
- ♦ **Catapres®** *see* Clonidine *on page 433*
- ♦ **Catapres-TTS®** *see* Clonidine *on page 433*
- ♦ **Cathflo™ Activase®** *see* Alteplase *on page 117*
- ♦ **Caverject®** *see* Alprostadil *on page 113*
- ♦ **Caverject® Impulse™** *see* Alprostadil *on page 113*
- ♦ **CBDCA** *see* Carboplatin *on page 313*
- ♦ **CBZ** *see* Carbamazepine *on page 306*
- ♦ **2-CdA** *see* Cladribine *on page 420*
- ♦ **CDDP** *see* Cisplatin *on page 412*
- ♦ **Cecon® [OTC]** *see* Ascorbic Acid *on page 187*
- ♦ **CEE** *see* Estrogens (Conjugated/Equine) *on page 661*

Cefaclor (SEF a klor)

U.S. Brand Names Raniclor™

Pharmacologic Category Antibiotic, Cephalosporin (Second Generation)

Medication Safety Issues

Sound-alike/look-alike issues:

Cefaclor may be confused with cephalexin

Use Treatment of susceptible bacterial infections including otitis media, lower respiratory tract infections, acute exacerbations of chronic bronchitis, pharyngitis and tonsillitis, urinary tract infections, skin and skin structure infections

Mechanism of Action Inhibits bacterial cell wall synthesis by binding to one or more of the penicillin-binding proteins (PBPs) which in turn inhibits the final transpeptidation step of peptidoglycan synthesis in bacterial cell walls, thus inhibiting cell wall biosynthesis. Bacteria eventually lyse due to ongoing activity of cell wall autolytic enzymes (autolysins and murein hydrolases) while cell wall assembly is arrested.

Pharmacodynamics/Kinetics

Absorption: Well absorbed, acid stable

Distribution: Widely throughout the body and reaches therapeutic concentration in most tissues and body fluids, including synovial, pericardial, pleural, peritoneal fluids; bile, sputum, and urine; bone, myocardium, gallbladder, skin and soft tissue; crosses placenta; enters breast milk

Protein binding: 25%

Metabolism: Partially hepatic

Half-life elimination: 0.5-1 hour; prolonged with renal impairment

Time to peak: Capsule: 60 minutes; Suspension: 45 minutes

Excretion: Urine (80% as unchanged drug)

Contraindications Hypersensitivity to cefaclor, any component of the formulation, or other cephalosporins

Warnings/Precautions Modify dosage in patients with severe renal impairment. Prolonged use may result in superinfection. Use with caution in patients with a history of penicillin allergy especially IgE-mediated reactions (eg, anaphylaxis, urticaria). Beta-lactamase-negative, ampicillin-resistant (BLNAR) strains of *H. influenzae* should be considered resistant to cefaclor. Extended release tablets are not approved for use in children <16 years of age.

Drug Interactions

Aminoglycosides: May be additive to nephrotoxicity.

Furosemide: May be additive to nephrotoxicity.

Probenecid: May decrease cephalosporin elimination.

Nutritional/Herbal/Ethanol Interactions

Food: Cefaclor serum levels may be decreased slightly if taken with food. The bioavailability of cefaclor extended release tablets is decreased 23% and the maximum concentration is decreased 67% when taken on an empty stomach.

Lab Interactions Positive direct Coombs', false-positive urinary glucose test using cupric sulfate (Benedict's solution, Clinitest®, Fehling's solution), false-positive serum or urine creatinine with Jaffé reaction

Adverse Reactions

1% to 10%:

- Dermatologic: Rash (maculopapular, erythematous, or morbilliform) (1% to 2%)
- Gastrointestinal: Diarrhea (3%)
- Genitourinary: Vaginitis (2%)
- Hematologic: Eosinophilia (2%)
- Hepatic: Transaminases increased (3%)
- Miscellaneous: Moniliasis (2%)

<1% (Limited to important or life-threatening): Agitation, agranulocytosis, anaphylaxis, angioedema, aplastic anemia, arthralgia, cholestatic jaundice, CNS irritability, confusion, dizziness, hallucinations, hemolytic anemia, hepatitis, hyperactivity, insomnia, interstitial nephritis, nausea, nervousness, neutropenia, paresthesia, PT prolonged, pruritus, pseudomembranous colitis, seizure, serum-sickness, somnolence, Stevens-Johnson syndrome, thrombocytopenia, toxic epidermal necrolysis, urticaria, vomiting

Reactions reported with other cephalosporins include abdominal pain, cholestasis, fever, hemorrhage, renal dysfunction, superinfection, toxic nephropathy

Overdosage/Toxicology Symptoms of overdose include diarrhea, epigastric distress, nausea, and vomiting. Many beta-lactam containing antibiotics have the potential to cause neuromuscular hyperirritability or seizures. Hemodialysis may be helpful to aid in removal of the drug from blood; otherwise, treatment is supportive and symptom-directed.

Dosing

Adults & Elderly: Susceptible infection: Oral: Dosing range: 250-500 mg every 8 hours

Pediatrics: Susceptible infections: Oral: Children >1 month: Dosing range: 20-40 mg/kg/day divided every 8-12 hours; maximum dose: 1 g/day

Otitis media: 40 mg/kg/day divided every 12 hours

Pharyngitis: 20 mg/kg/day divided every 12 hours

Renal Impairment:

Cl_{cr} 10-50 mL/minute: Administer 50% to 100% of dose

(Continued)

Cefaclor *(Continued)*

Cl_{cr} <10 mL/minute: Administer 50% of dose

Hemodialysis: Moderately dialyzable (20% to 50%)

Available Dosage Forms

Capsule: 250 mg, 500 mg

Powder for oral suspension: 125 mg/5 mL (75 mL, 150 mL); 187 mg/5 mL (50 mL, 100 mL); 250 mg/5 mL (75 mL, 150 mL); 375 mg/5 mL (50 mL, 100 mL)

Tablet, chewable (Raniclor™): 125 mg [contains phenylalanine 2.8 mg; fruity flavor], 187 mg [contains phenylalanine 4.2 mg; fruity flavor], 250 mg [contains phenylalanine 5.6 mg; fruity flavor], 375 mg [contains phenylalanine 8.4 mg; fruity flavor]

Nursing Guidelines

Assessment: See Contraindications, Warnings/Precautions, and Dosing for use cautions. Assess potential for interactions with other prescriptions, OTC medications, or herbal products patient may be taking, and allergies they may have (eg, nephrotoxicity - see Drug Interactions). Assess results of laboratory tests (see below), therapeutic response, and adverse effects (hypersensitivity can occur days after therapy is started - see Adverse Reactions and Overdose/Toxicology). Advise patients with diabetes about use of Clinitest®. Teach patient proper use, possible side effects/appropriate interventions, and adverse symptoms to report (eg, nephrotoxicity, opportunistic infection: fever, malaise, rash, diarrhea, itching, fever, chills, or increased cough - see Patient Education). Note breast-feeding caution.

Monitoring Laboratory Tests: Perform culture and sensitivity studies prior to initiating drug therapy; renal function

Dietary Considerations: Capsule, chewable tablet, and suspension may be taken with or without food. Raniclor™ contains phenylalanine 2.8 mg/cefaclor 125 mg.

Patient Education: Inform prescriber of all prescriptions, OTC medications, or herbal products you are taking, and any allergies you have. Do not take any new medication during therapy unless approved by prescriber. Take as directed, at regular intervals around-the-clock (with or without food). Chilling oral suspension improves flavor (do not freeze). Maintain adequate hydration (2-3 L/day of fluids) unless instructed to restrict fluid intake. Complete full course of medication, even if you feel better. May cause false test results with Clinitest®; use of another type of testing is preferable. May cause diarrhea (yogurt, boiled milk, or buttermilk may help). Report rash; respiratory difficulty or swallowing; persistent nausea, vomiting, or abdominal pain; changes in urinary pattern or pain on urination; opportunistic infection (eg, vaginal itching or drainage; sores in mouth; blood in stool or urine, vaginal itching or drainage, unusual fever or chills); or CNS changes (eg, irritability, agitation, nervousness, insomnia, hallucinations). **Breast-feeding precaution:** Consult prescriber if breast-feeding.

Pregnancy Risk Factor: B

Lactation: Enters breast milk/use caution

Breast-Feeding Considerations: Theoretically, drug absorbed by nursing infant may change bowel flora or affect fever work-up result. Small amounts can be detected in breast milk (trace amounts after 1 hour, increasing to 0.16 mcg/mL at 5 hours). **Note:** As a class, cephalosporins are used to treat bacterial infections in infants.

Administration

Oral: Administer around-the-clock to promote less variation in peak and trough serum levels.

Chewable tablet: Should be chewed before swallowing; should not be swallowed whole.

Oral suspension: Shake well before using.

Storage: Store at controlled room temperature. Refrigerate suspension after reconstitution. Discard after 14 days. Do not freeze.

Related Information

Cephalosporins by Generation *on page 1858*

Cefadroxil (sef a DROKS il)

U.S. Brand Names Duricef®

Synonyms Cefadroxil Monohydrate

Pharmacologic Category Antibiotic, Cephalosporin (First Generation)

Use Treatment of susceptible bacterial infections, including those caused by group A beta-hemolytic *Streptococcus*; prophylaxis against bacterial endocarditis in patients who are allergic to penicillin and undergoing surgical or dental procedures

Mechanism of Action Inhibits bacterial cell wall synthesis by binding to one or more of the penicillin-binding proteins (PBPs) which in turn inhibits the final transpeptidation step of peptidoglycan synthesis in bacterial cell walls, thus inhibiting cell wall biosynthesis. Bacteria eventually lyse due to ongoing activity of cell wall autolytic enzymes (autolysins and murein hydrolases) while cell wall assembly is arrested.

Pharmacodynamics/Kinetics

Absorption: Rapid and well absorbed

Distribution: Widely throughout the body and reaches therapeutic concentrations in most tissues and body fluids, including synovial, pericardial, pleural, and peritoneal fluids; bile, sputum, and urine; bone, myocardium, gallbladder, skin and soft tissue; crosses placenta; enters breast milk

Protein binding: 20%

Half-life elimination: 1-2 hours; Renal failure: 20-24 hours

Time to peak, serum: 70-90 minutes

Excretion: Urine (>90% as unchanged drug)

Contraindications Hypersensitivity to cefadroxil, other cephalosporins, or any component of the formulation

Warnings/Precautions Modify dosage in patients with severe renal impairment; prolonged use may result in superinfection; use with caution in patients with a history of penicillin allergy especially IgE-mediated reactions (eg, anaphylaxis, angioedema, urticaria). May cause antibiotic-associated colitis or colitis secondary to *C. difficile*.

Drug Interactions

Increased effect: Probenecid may decrease cephalosporin elimination

Increased toxicity: Furosemide, aminoglycosides may be a possible additive to nephrotoxicity

Nutritional/Herbal/Ethanol Interactions Food: Concomitant administration with food, infant formula, or cow's milk does **not** significantly affect absorption.

Lab Interactions Positive direct Coombs', false-positive urinary glucose test using cupric sulfate (Benedict's solution, Clinitest®, Fehling's solution), false-positive serum or urine creatinine with Jaffé reaction

Adverse Reactions

1% to 10%: Gastrointestinal: Diarrhea

<1% (Limited to important or life-threatening): Abdominal pain, agranulocytosis, anaphylaxis, angioedema, arthralgia, cholestasis, dyspepsia, erythema multiforme, fever, nausea, neutropenia, pruritus, pseudomembranous colitis, rash (maculopapular and erythematous), serum sickness, Stevens-Johnson syndrome, thrombocytopenia, transaminases increased, urticaria, vaginitis, vomiting

Reactions reported with other cephalosporins include abdominal pain, aplastic anemia, BUN increased, creatinine increased, eosinophilia, hemolytic anemia, hemorrhage, pancytopenia, prolonged prothrombin time, renal dysfunction, seizure, superinfection, toxic epidermal necrolysis, toxic nephropathy

Overdosage/Toxicology Symptoms of overdose include neuromuscular hypersensitivity and convulsions. Many beta-lactam containing antibiotics have the potential to cause neuromuscular hyperirritability or convulsive seizures. Hemodialysis may be helpful to aid in removal of the drug from blood; otherwise, treatment is supportive or symptom-directed.

Dosing

Adults & Elderly:

Susceptible infections: Oral: 1-2 g/day in 2 divided doses

Prophylaxis against bacterial endocarditis: Oral: 2 g 1 hour prior to the procedure

Pediatrics:

Susceptible infections: Oral: Children: 30 mg/kg/day divided twice daily up to a maximum of 2 g/day

Prophylaxis against bacterial endocarditis: Oral: Children: 50 mg/kg 1 hour prior to the procedure

(Continued)

Cefadroxil *(Continued)*

Renal Impairment:

Cl_{cr} 10-25 mL/minute: Administer every 24 hours.

Cl_{cr} <10 mL/minute: Administer every 36 hours.

Available Dosage Forms

Capsule, as monohydrate: 500 mg

Powder for oral suspension, as monohydrate: 250 mg/5 mL (50 mL, 100 mL); 500 mg/5 mL (75 mL, 100 mL) [contains sodium benzoate; orange-pineapple flavor]

Tablet, as monohydrate: 1 g

Nursing Guidelines

Assessment: Assess for previous allergy history prior to therapy. See Contraindications and Warnings/Precautions for use cautions. Assess potential for interactions with other prescriptions, OTC medications, or herbal products patient may be taking (eg, anticoagulants - see Drug Interactions). Assess results of laboratory tests (see below), therapeutic response, and adverse response (eg, hypersensitivity can occur several days after therapy is started - see Adverse Reactions). Advise patients with diabetes about use of Clinitest®. Teach patient proper use, possible side effects/appropriate interventions, and adverse symptoms to report (eg, nephrotoxicity, opportunistic infection - see Patient Education). Note breast-feeding caution.

Monitoring Laboratory Tests: Perform culture and sensitivity studies prior to initiating drug therapy; renal function

Patient Education: Inform prescriber of all prescriptions, OTC medications, or herbal products you are taking, and any allergies you have. Do not take any new medication during therapy unless approved by prescriber. Take as directed, at regular intervals around-the-clock (with or without food). Chilling oral suspension improves flavor (do not freeze). Do not chew or crush extended release tablets. Maintain adequate hydration (2-3 L/day of fluids) unless instructed to restrict fluid intake. Complete full course of medication, even if you feel better. May cause false test results with Clinitest®; use of another type of glucose testing is preferable. May cause diarrhea (yogurt, boiled milk, or buttermilk may help). Report changes in urinary pattern or pain on urination; opportunistic infection (eg, vaginal itching or drainage; sores in mouth; blood in urine or stool; unusual fever or chills); or nausea, vomiting, or abdominal pain. **Breast-feeding precaution:** Consult prescriber if breast-feeding.

Geriatric Considerations: Adjust dose for renal function in the elderly.

Pregnancy Risk Factor: B

Lactation: Enters breast milk (small amounts)/use caution (AAP rates "compatible")

Breast-Feeding Considerations: Theoretically, drug absorbed by nursing infant may change bowel flora or affect fever work-up result. **Note:** As a class, cephalosporins are used to treat infections in infants.

Administration

Oral: Administer around-the-clock to promote less variation in peak and trough serum levels.

Reconstitution: Refrigerate suspension after reconstitution. Discard after 14 days.

Related Information

Cephalosporins by Generation *on page 1858*

♦ **Cefadroxil Monohydrate** *see* Cefadroxil *on page 329*

Cefazolin (sef A zoe lin)

U.S. Brand Names Ancef®

Synonyms Cefazolin Sodium

Pharmacologic Category Antibiotic, Cephalosporin (First Generation)

Medication Safety Issues

Sound-alike/look-alike issues:

Cefazolin may be confused with cefprozil, cephalexin, cephalothin

Kefzol® may be confused with Cefzil®

Use Treatment of respiratory tract, skin and skin structure, genital, urinary tract, biliary tract, bone and joint infections, and septicemia due to susceptible gram-positive cocci (except enterococcus); some gram-negative bacilli including *E. coli*, *Proteus*, and *Klebsiella* may be susceptible; perioperative prophylaxis

Unlabeled/Investigational Use Prophylaxis against bacterial endocarditis

Mechanism of Action Inhibits bacterial cell wall synthesis by binding to one or more of the penicillin-binding proteins (PBPs) which in turn inhibits the final

transpeptidation step of peptidoglycan synthesis in bacterial cell walls, thus inhibiting cell wall biosynthesis. Bacteria eventually lyse due to ongoing activity of cell wall autolytic enzymes (autolysins and murein hydrolases) while cell wall assembly is arrested.

Pharmacodynamics/Kinetics

Distribution: Widely into most body tissues and fluids including gallbladder, liver, kidneys, bone, sputum, bile, pleural, and synovial; CSF penetration is poor; crosses placenta; enters breast milk

Protein binding: 74% to 86%

Metabolism: Minimally hepatic

Half-life elimination: 90-150 minutes; prolonged with renal impairment

Time to peak, serum: I.M.: 0.5-2 hours

Excretion: Urine (80% to 100% as unchanged drug)

Contraindications Hypersensitivity to cefazolin sodium, any component of the formulation, or other cephalosporins

Warnings/Precautions Modify dosage in patients with severe renal impairment; prolonged use may result in superinfection; use with caution in patients with a history of penicillin allergy especially IgE-mediated reactions (eg, anaphylaxis, angioedema, urticaria). May cause antibiotic-associated colitis or colitis secondary to *C. difficile*.

Drug Interactions

Aminoglycosides: Aminoglycosides increase nephrotoxic potential.

Probenecid: High-dose probenecid decreases clearance.

Warfarin: Cefazolin may increase the hypothrombinemic response to warfarin (due to alteration of GI microbial flora).

Lab Interactions Positive direct Coombs', false-positive urinary glucose test using cupric sulfate (Benedict's solution, Clinitest®, Fehling's solution), false-positive serum or urine creatinine with Jaffé reaction

Some penicillin derivatives may accelerate the degradation of aminoglycosides *in vitro*, leading to a potential underestimation of aminoglycoside serum concentration.

Adverse Reactions Frequency not defined.

Central nervous system: Fever, seizure

Dermatologic: Rash, pruritus, Stevens-Johnson syndrome

Gastrointestinal: Diarrhea. nausea, vomiting, abdominal cramps, anorexia, pseudomembranous colitis, oral candidiasis

Genitourinary: Vaginitis

Hepatic: Transaminases increased, hepatitis

Hematologic: Eosinophilia, neutropenia, leukopenia, thrombocytopenia, thrombocytosis

Local: Pain at injection site, phlebitis

Renal: BUN increased, serum creatinine increased, renal failure

Miscellaneous: Anaphylaxis

Reactions reported with other cephalosporins include toxic epidermal necrolysis, abdominal pain, cholestasis, superinfection, toxic nephropathy, aplastic anemia, hemolytic anemia, hemorrhage, prolonged prothrombin time, pancytopenia

Overdosage/Toxicology Symptoms of overdose include neuromuscular hypersensitivity and convulsions. Many beta-lactam containing antibiotics have the potential to cause neuromuscular hyperirritability or convulsive seizures. Hemodialysis may be helpful to aid in the removal of drug from blood; otherwise, treatment is supportive or symptom-directed.

Dosing

Adults & Elderly:

Usual dosage range: I.M., I.V.: 1-2 g every 8 hours, depending on severity of infection; maximum: 12 g/day

Mild-to-moderate infections: 500 mg to 1 g every 6-8 hours

Mild infection with gram-positive cocci: 250-500 mg every 8 hours

Perioperative prophylaxis: 1 g given 30 minutes prior to surgery (repeat with 500 mg to 1 g during prolonged surgery); followed by 500 mg to 1 g every 6-9 hours for 24 hours postop

Pneumococcal pneumonia: 500 mg every 12 hours

Severe infection: 1-2 g every 6 hours

Prophylaxis against bacterial endocarditis (unlabeled use): 1 g 30 minutes before procedure

UTI (uncomplicated): 1 g every 12 hours

(Continued)

Cefazolin *(Continued)*

Pediatrics:

Usual dosage range: I.M., I.V.: Children >1 month: 25-100 mg/kg/day divided every 6-8 hours; maximum: 6 g/day

Prophylaxis against bacterial endocarditis (unlabeled use): Infants and Children: 25 mg/kg 30 minutes before procedure; maximum dose: 1 g

Renal Impairment:

Cl_{cr} 10-30 mL/minute: Administer every 12 hours.

Cl_{cr} <10 mL/minute: Administer every 24 hours.

Moderately dialyzable (20% to 50%); administer dose postdialysis or administer supplemental dose of 0.5-1 g after dialysis.

Peritoneal dialysis: Administer 0.5 g every 12 hours.

Continuous arteriovenous or venovenous hemofiltration: Dose as for Cl_{cr} 10-30 mL/minute. Removes 30 mg of cefazolin per liter of filtrate per day.

Available Dosage Forms [DSC] = Discontinued product

Infusion [premixed in D_5W]: 500 mg (50 mL); 1 g (50 mL)

Injection, powder for reconstitution: 500 mg, 1 g, 10 g, 20 g

Ancef®: 1 g; 10 g [DSC]

Nursing Guidelines

Assessment: Assess for previous allergy history prior to therapy. See Contraindications and Warnings/Precautions for use cautions. Assess potential for interactions with other prescriptions, OTC medications, or herbal products patient may be taking (see Drug Interactions). Assess results of laboratory tests (see below), therapeutic response, and adverse effects (see Adverse Reactions and Overdose/Toxicology). Advise patients with diabetes about use of Clinitest®. Teach patient possible side effects, interventions to reduce side effects and adverse symptoms to report (eg, opportunistic infection - see Patient Education). Note breast-feeding caution.

Monitoring Laboratory Tests: Perform culture and sensitivity studies prior to initiating drug therapy; renal function

Dietary Considerations: Sodium content of 1 g: 48 mg (2 mEq)

Patient Education: Inform prescriber of all prescriptions, OTC medications, or herbal products you are taking, and any allergies you have. Do not take any new medication during therapy unless approved by prescriber. This medication is administered by injection or infusion. Report immediately any redness, swelling, burning, or pain at injection/infusion site; rash or hives; or respiratory difficulty, chest pain, or difficulty swallowing. Maintain adequate hydration (2-3 L/day of fluids) unless instructed to restrict fluid intake. If you have diabetes, drug may cause false test results with Clinitest® urine glucose monitoring; use of another type of glucose monitoring is preferable. May cause diarrhea (yogurt, boiled milk, or buttermilk may help). Report severe, unresolved diarrhea; opportunistic infection (vaginal itching or drainage; sores in mouth; blood in stool or urine; unusual fever or chills); or respiratory difficulty. **Breast-feeding precautions:** Consult prescriber if breast-feeding.

Geriatric Considerations: Adjust dose for renal function.

Pregnancy Risk Factor: B

Lactation: Enters breast milk (small amounts)/use caution (AAP rates "compatible")

Breast-Feeding Considerations: Theoretically, drug absorbed by nursing infant may change bowel flora or affect fever work-up result. **Note:** As a class, cephalosporins are used to treat infections in infants.

Administration

I.M.: Inject deep I.M. into large muscle mass.

I.V.: Inject direct I.V. over 5 minutes. Infuse intermittent infusion over 30-60 minutes.

Some penicillins (eg, carbenicillin, ticarcillin and piperacillin) have been shown to inactivate aminglycosides *in vitro*. This has been observed to a greater extent with tobramycin and gentamicin, while amikacin has shown greater stability against inactivation. Concurrent use of these agents may pose a risk of reduced antibacterial efficacy *in vivo*, particularly in the setting of profound renal impairment. However, definitive clinical evidence is lacking. If combination penicillin/aminoglycoside therapy is desired in a patient with renal dysfunction, separation of doses (if feasible), and routine monitoring of aminoglycoside levels, CBC, and clinical response should be considered.

Reconstitution: Dilute large vial with 2.5 mL SWFI; 10 g vial may be diluted with 45 mL to yield 1 g/5 mL or 96 mL to yield 1 g/10 mL. May be injected or further dilution for I.V. administration in 50-100 mL compatible solution. Standard diluent is 1 g/50 mL D_5W or 2 g/50 mL D_5W.

Compatibility: Stable in D_5W, D_5LR, $D_5 1/4NS$, $D_5 1/2NS$, D_5NS, $D_{10}W$,LR, NS

Y-site administration: Incompatible with amphotericin B cholesteryl sulfate complex, idarubicin, pentamidine, vinorelbine

Compatibility in syringe: Incompatible with ascorbic acid injection, cimetidine, lidocaine

Compatibility when admixed: Incompatible with amikacin, amobarbital, atracurium, bleomycin, calcium gluconate, clindamycin with gentamicin, colistimethate, kanamycin, pentobarbital, polymyxin B sulfate, ranitidine

Storage: Store intact vials at room temperature and protect from temperatures exceeding 40°C. Reconstituted solutions of cefazolin are light yellow to yellow. Protection from light is recommended for the powder and for the reconstituted solutions. Reconstituted solutions are stable for 24 hours at room temperature and for 10 days under refrigeration. Stability of parenteral admixture at room temperature (25°C) is 48 hours. Stability of parenteral admixture at refrigeration temperature (4°C) is 14 days.

DUPLEX™: Store at 20°C to 25°C (68°F to 77°F); excursions permitted to 15°C to 30°C (59°F to 86°F) prior to activation. Following activation, stable for 24 hours at room temperature and for 7 days under refrigeration.

Related Information

Cephalosporins by Generation *on page 1858*

Prevention of Wound Infection and Sepsis in Surgical Patients *on page 1830*

♦ **Cefazolin Sodium** *see* Cefazolin *on page 330*

Cefdinir (SEF di ner)

U.S. Brand Names Omnicef®

Synonyms CFDN

Pharmacologic Category Antibiotic, Cephalosporin (Third Generation)

Use Treatment of community-acquired pneumonia, acute exacerbations of chronic bronchitis, acute bacterial otitis media, acute maxillary sinusitis, pharyngitis/tonsillitis, and uncomplicated skin and skin structure infections.

Mechanism of Action Inhibits bacterial cell wall synthesis by binding to one or more of the penicillin-binding proteins (PBPs) which in turn inhibits the final transpeptidation step of peptidoglycan synthesis in bacterial cell walls, thus inhibiting cell wall biosynthesis. Bacteria eventually lyse due to ongoing activity of cell wall autolytic enzymes (autolysins and murein hydrolases) while cell wall assembly is arrested.

Pharmacodynamics/Kinetics

Distribution: V_d:

Children 6 months to 12 years: 0.29-1.05 L/kg

Adults: 0.06-0.64 L/kg

Protein binding: 60% to 70%

Metabolism: Minimally hepatic

Bioavailability: Capsule: 16% to 21%; suspension 25%

Half-life elimination: 100 minutes

Excretion: Primarily urine

Contraindications Hypersensitivity to cefdinir, other cephalosporins, related antibiotics, or any component of the formulation

Warnings/Precautions Administer cautiously to penicillin-sensitive patients, especially IgE-mediated reactions (eg, anaphylaxis, urticaria). There is evidence of partial cross-allergenicity and cephalosporins cannot be assumed to be an absolutely safe alternative to penicillin in the penicillin-allergic patient. Serum sickness-like reactions have been reported. Signs and symptoms occur after a few days of therapy and resolve a few days after drug discontinuation with no serious sequelae. Pseudomembranous colitis occurs; consider its diagnosis in patients who develop diarrhea with antibiotic use. Use caution with renal dysfunction; dose adjustment may be required.

Drug Interactions

Antacids: May reduce the rate and extent of cefdinir absorption; separate dosing by 2 hours.

Iron: May reduce the rate and extent of cefdinir absorption. Separate dosing by 2 hours. May be administered with iron fortified infant formula.

Probenecid: May increase the effects of cefdinir by decreasing renal elimination. Peak plasma levels of cefdinir are increased by 54% and half-life is prolonged by 50%.

(Continued)

Cefdinir *(Continued)*

Adverse Reactions

>10%: Gastrointestinal: Diarrhea (8% to 15%)

1% to 10%:

Central nervous system: Headache (2%)

Dermatologic: Rash (≤3%)

Gastrointestinal: Nausea (≤3%), abdominal pain (≤1%), vomiting (≤1%)

Genitourinary: Vaginal moniliasis (≤4%), urine leukocytes increased (2%), urine protein increased (1% to 2%), vaginitis (≤1%)

Hematologic: Eosinophils increased (1%)

Hepatic: Alkaline phosphatase increased (≤1%), platelets increased (1%)

Renal: Microhematuria (1%)

Miscellaneous: Lymphocytes increased (≤2%), GGT increased (1%), lactate dehydrogenase increased (≤1%), bicarbonate decreased (≤1%), lymphocytes decreased (≤1%), PMN changes (≤1%)

<1% (Limited to important or life-threatening): Allergic vasculitis, anaphylaxis, anorexia, bloody diarrhea, cardiac failure, chest pain, cholestasis, coagulation disorder, constipation, cutaneous moniliasis, disseminated intravascular coagulation, enterocolitis (acute), eosinophilic pneumonia, erythema multiforme, erythema nodosum, exfoliative dermatitis, facial edema, fulminant hepatitis, granulocytopenia, hemolytic anemia, hemorrhagic colitis, hepatic failure, hepatitis (acute), hyperkinesia, hypertension, idiopathic thrombocytopenia purpura, ileus, interstitial pneumonia (idiopathic), involuntary movement, jaundice, laryngeal edema, leukopenia, loss of consciousness, maculopapular rash, melena, MI, nephropathy, pancytopenia, pruritus, pseudomembranous colitis, renal failure (acute), respiratory failure (acute), rhabdomyolysis, serum sickness, shock, Stevens-Johnson syndrome, thrombocytopenia, toxic epidermal necrolysis, upper GI bleed, weakness, xerostomia

Reactions reported with other cephalosporins include dizziness, fever, encephalopathy, asterixis, neuromuscular excitability, seizure, aplastic anemia, interstitial nephritis, toxic nephropathy, angioedema, hemorrhage, prolonged PT, and superinfection

Overdosage/Toxicology After acute overdose, most agents cause only nausea, vomiting, and diarrhea, although neuromuscular hypersensitivity and seizures are possible, especially in patients with renal insufficiency. Hemodialysis may be helpful to aid in the removal of the drug from the blood but not usually indicated, otherwise most treatment is supportive or symptom-directed following GI decontamination.

Dosing

Adults & Elderly:

Community-acquired pneumonia, uncomplicated skin and skin structure infections: Oral: 300 mg twice daily for 10 days

Acute exacerbations of chronic bronchitis, pharyngitis/tonsillitis: Oral: 300 mg twice daily for 5-10 days **or** 600 mg once daily for 10 days

Acute maxillary sinusitis: Oral: 300 mg twice daily **or** 600 mg once daily for 10 days

Pediatrics:

Children 6 months to 12 years:

Acute bacterial otitis media, pharyngitis/tonsillitis: Oral: 7 mg/kg/dose twice daily for 5-10 days **or** 14 mg/kg/dose once daily for 10 days (maximum: 600 mg/day)

Acute maxillary sinusitis: Oral: 7 mg/kg/dose twice daily **or** 14 mg/kg/dose once daily for 10 days (maximum: 600 mg/day)

Uncomplicated skin and skin structure infections: Oral: 7 mg/kg/dose twice daily for 10 days (maximum: 600 mg/day)

Children >12 years: Refer to adult dosing.

Renal Impairment:

Children: 7 mg/kg once daily (maximum: 300 mg/day)

Adults: 300 mg once daily

Available Dosage Forms

Capsule: 300 mg

Powder for oral suspension: 125 mg/5 mL (60 mL, 100 mL) [contains sodium benzoate and sucrose 2.86 g/5 mL; strawberry flavor]; 250 mg/5 mL (60 mL, 100 mL) [contains sodium benzoate and sucrose 2.86 g/5 mL; strawberry flavor]

Nursing Guidelines

Assessment: Assess results of culture/sensitivity tests and patient's allergy history prior to therapy. Assess potential for interactions with other pharmacological agents patient may be taking (eg, anticoagulants). Assess therapeutic response and adverse effects. Teach patient proper use, possible side effects/appropriate interventions, and adverse symptoms to report (eg, opportunistic infection, hypersensitivity).

Monitoring Laboratory Tests: Perform culture and sensitivity studies prior to initiating drug therapy; renal function

Dietary Considerations: Suspension contains sucrose 2.86 g/5 mL

Patient Education: Take as directed, at regular intervals around-the-clock (with or without food). Chilling oral suspension improves flavor (do not freeze). Complete full course of medication, even if you feel better. Maintain adequate hydration (2-3 L/day of fluids) unless instructed to restrict fluid intake. May cause diarrhea (yogurt, boiled milk, or buttermilk may help); or nausea, vomiting, flatulence (small frequent meals, frequent mouth care, chewing gum, or sucking lozenges may help). Report rash; breathing or swallowing difficulty; persistent diarrhea, nausea, vomiting, or abdominal pain; changes in urinary pattern or pain on urination; opportunistic infection (eg, vaginal itching or drainage; sores in mouth; blood in stool or urine, unusual fever or chills); CNS changes (eg, irritability, agitation, nervousness, insomnia, hallucinations); or other adverse reactions. **Breast-feeding precaution:** Consult prescriber if breast-feeding.

Pregnancy Risk Factor: B

Lactation: Excretion in breast milk unknown/use caution

Breast-Feeding Considerations: Following a single 600 mg dose, cefdinir was not detected in breast milk; information following multiple doses is not available.

Administration

Oral: Twice daily doses should be given every 12 hours. May be taken with or without food. The suspension should be shaken well before each administration.

Reconstitution: Oral suspension should be mixed with 38 mL water for the 60 mL bottle and 63 mL of water for the 120 mL bottle.

Storage: Capsules and unmixed powder should be stored at room temperature of 25°C (77°F). After mixing, the suspension can be stored at room temperature of 25°C (77°F) for 10 days.

Related Information

Cephalosporins by Generation *on page 1858*

Cefditoren (sef de TOR en)

U.S. Brand Names Spectracef™

Synonyms Cefditoren Pivoxil

Pharmacologic Category Antibiotic, Cephalosporin

Use Treatment of acute bacterial exacerbation of chronic bronchitis or community-acquired pneumonia (due to susceptible organisms including *Haemophilus influenzae*, *Haemophilus parainfluenzae*, *Streptococcus pneumoniae*-penicillin susceptible only, *Moraxella catarrhalis*); pharyngitis or tonsillitis (*Streptococcus pyogenes*); and uncomplicated skin and skin-structure infections (*Staphylococcus aureus* - not MRSA, *Streptococcus pyogenes*)

Mechanism of Action Inhibits bacterial cell wall synthesis by binding to one or more of the penicillin binding proteins (PBPs); which in turn inhibits the final transpeptidation step of peptidoglycan synthesis in bacterial cell walls, thus inhibiting cell wall biosynthesis. Bacteria eventually lyse due to ongoing activity of cell wall autolytic enzymes (autolysins and murein hydrolases) while cell wall assembly is arrested.

Pharmacodynamics/Kinetics

Distribution: 9.3 ± 1.6 L

Protein binding: 88% (*in vitro*), primarily to albumin

Metabolism: Cefditoren pivoxil is hydrolyzed to cefditoren (active) and pivalate

Bioavailability: ~14% to 16%, increased by moderate to high-fat meal

Half-life elimination: 1.6 ± 0.4 hours

Time to peak: 1.5-3 hours

Excretion: Urine (as cefditoren and pivaloylcarnitine)

Contraindications Hypersensitivity to cefditoren, other cephalosporins, milk protein, or any component of the formulation; carnitine deficiency

(Continued)

Cefditoren *(Continued)*

Warnings/Precautions Use with caution in patients with a history of penicillin allergy, especially IgE-mediated reactions (eg, anaphylaxis, urticaria). May cause antibiotic-associated colitis or colitis secondary to *C. difficile*. Prolonged use may result in superinfection. Caution in individuals with seizure disorders. Use caution in patients with renal or hepatic impairment; modify dosage in patients with severe renal impairment. Cefditoren causes renal excretion of carnitine; do not use in patients with carnitine deficiency; not for long-term therapy due to the possible development of carnitine deficiency over time. May prolong prothrombin time; use with caution in patients with a history of bleeding disorder. Cefditoren tablets contain sodium caseinate, which may cause hypersensitivity reactions in patients with milk protein hypersensitivity; this does not affect patients with lactose intolerance. Safety and efficacy have not been established in children <12 years of age.

Drug Interactions

Probenecid: Serum concentration of cefditoren may be increased.
Warfarin: Prothrombin time may be prolonged by cefditoren; monitor.

Nutritional/Herbal/Ethanol Interactions Food: Moderate- to high-fat meals increase bioavailability and maximum plasma concentration.

Lab Interactions May induce a positive direct Coomb's test. May cause a false-negative ferricyanide test; Glucose oxidase or hexokinase methods recommended for blood/plasma glucose determinations. False-positive urine glucose test when using copper reduction based assays (eg, Clinitest®).

Adverse Reactions

>10%: Gastrointestinal: Diarrhea (11% to 15%)

1% to 10%:

- Central nervous system: Headache (2% to 3%)
- Endocrine & metabolic: Glucose increased (1% to 2%)
- Gastrointestinal: Nausea (4% to 6%), abdominal pain (2%), dyspepsia (1% to 2%), vomiting (1%)
- Genitourinary: Vaginal moniliasis (3% to 6%)
- Hematologic: Hematocrit decreased (2%)
- Renal: Hematuria (3%), urinary white blood cells increased (2%)

<1% (Limited to important or life-threatening): Acute renal failure, allergic reaction, arthralgia, eosinophilic pneumonia, increased BUN, coagulation time increased, interstitial pneumonia, positive direct Coombs' test, pseudomembranous colitis, rash, thrombocytopenia albumin decreased, asthma, calcium decreased, fungal infection, hyperglycemia, interstitial pneumonia, leukopenia, leukorrhea, potassium increased, sodium decreased, thrombocythemia, thrombocytopenia, white blood cell increase/decrease

Additional adverse effects seen with cephalosporin antibiotics: Anaphylaxis, aplastic anemia, cholestasis, erythema multiforme, hemorrhage, hemolytic anemia, renal dysfunction, reversible hyperactivity, serum sickness-like reaction, Stevens-Johnson syndrome, toxic epidermal necrolysis, toxic nephropathy

Overdosage/Toxicology Specific information not available. General symptoms of cephalosporin overdose may include nausea, vomiting, epigastric distress, diarrhea, and seizures. Treatment should be symptom-directed and supportive. Hemodialysis may be helpful (removes ~30% from circulation).

Dosing

Adults & Elderly:

Acute bacterial exacerbation of chronic bronchitis: Oral: 400 mg twice daily for 10 days

Community-acquired pneumonia: Oral: 400 mg twice daily for 14 days

Pharyngitis, tonsillitis, uncomplicated skin and skin structure infections: Oral: 200 mg twice daily for 10 days

Pediatrics: Children ≥12 years: Refer to adult dosing.

Renal Impairment:

Cl_{cr} 30-49 mL/minute/1.73 m^2: Maximum dose: 200 mg twice daily
Cl_{cr} <30 mL/minute/1.73 m^2: Maximum dose: 200 mg once daily
End-stage renal disease: Appropriate dosing not established

Hepatic Impairment:

Mild or moderate impairment: Adjustment not required
Severe impairment (Child-Pugh class C): Specific guidelines not available

Available Dosage Forms Tablet, as pivoxil: 200 mg [equivalent to cefditoren; contains sodium caseinate]

Nursing Guidelines

Assessment: Assess for previous allergy history prior to therapy. See Contraindications, Warnings/Precautions, and Dosing for use cautions. Assess potential for interactions with other prescriptions, OTC medications, and herbal products patient may be taking (see Drug Interactions). Assess therapeutic effectiveness and adverse reactions (see Adverse Reactions and Overdose/Toxicology). Teach patient proper use, possible side effects/appropriate interventions, and adverse symptoms to report (see Patient Education). Note breast-feeding caution.

Monitoring Laboratory Tests: Perform culture and sensitivity studies prior to initiating drug therapy; renal function

Dietary Considerations: Cefditoren should be taken with meals. Plasma carnitine levels are decreased during therapy (39% with 200 mg dosing, 63% with 400 mg dosing); normal concentrations return within 7-10 days after treatment is discontinued.

Patient Education: Inform prescriber of all prescriptions, OTC medications, or herbal products you are taking, and any allergies you have. Do not take any new medication during therapy without consulting prescriber. Take as directed, at regular intervals around-the-clock, with food. Maintain adequate hydration (2-3 L/day of fluids unless instructed to restrict fluid intake). Complete full course of medication, even if you feel better. If you have diabetes, monitor glucose levels closely; may cause false test results with Clinitest® urine glucose monitoring; use of another type of glucose monitoring is preferable. May cause diarrhea (yogurt, buttermilk, or boiled milk may help); or nausea or vomiting (small, frequent meals, frequent mouth care, sucking lozenges, or chewing gum may help). Report severe, unresolved diarrhea; opportunistic infection (vaginal itching or drainage, sores in mouth, or unusual fever or chills); unusual bleeding or bruising; change in urinary pattern; or rash. **Breast-feeding precaution:** Consult prescriber if breast-feeding.

Pregnancy Risk Factor: B

Lactation: Excretion in breast milk unknown/use caution

Administration

Oral: Should be taken with meals.

Storage: Store at controlled room temperature of 15°C to 30°C (59°F to 86°F). Protect from light and moisture.

♦ **Cefditoren Pivoxil** *see* Cefditoren *on page 335*

Cefepime (SEF e pim)

U.S. Brand Names Maxipime®

Synonyms Cefepime Hydrochloride

Pharmacologic Category Antibiotic, Cephalosporin (Fourth Generation)

Use Treatment of uncomplicated and complicated urinary tract infections, including pyelonephritis caused by typical urinary tract pathogens; monotherapy for febrile neutropenia; uncomplicated skin and skin structure infections caused by *Streptococcus pyogenes*; moderate to severe pneumonia caused by pneumococcus, *Pseudomonas aeruginosa*, and other gram-negative organisms; complicated intra-abdominal infections (in combination with metronidazole). Also active against methicillin-susceptible staphylococci, *Enterobacter* sp, and many other gram-negative bacilli.

Children 2 months to 16 years: Empiric therapy of febrile neutropenia patients, uncomplicated skin/soft tissue infections, pneumonia, and uncomplicated/complicated urinary tract infections.

Mechanism of Action Inhibits bacterial cell wall synthesis by binding to one or more of the penicillin-binding proteins (PBPs) which in turn inhibits the final transpeptidation step of peptidoglycan synthesis in bacterial cell walls, thus inhibiting cell wall biosynthesis. Bacteria eventually lyse due to ongoing activity of cell wall autolytic enzymes (autolysis and murein hydrolases) while cell wall assembly is arrested.

Pharmacodynamics/Kinetics

Absorption: I.M.: Rapid and complete

Distribution: V_d: Adults: 14-20 L; penetrates into inflammatory fluid at concentrations ~80% of serum levels and into bronchial mucosa at levels ~60% of those reached in the plasma; crosses blood-brain barrier

Protein binding, plasma: 16% to 19%

Metabolism: Minimally hepatic

Half-life elimination: 2 hours

Time to peak: 0.5-1.5 hours

Excretion: Urine (85% as unchanged drug)

(Continued)

Cefepime *(Continued)*

Contraindications Hypersensitivity to cefepime, any component of the formulation, or other cephalosporins

Warnings/Precautions Modify dosage in patients with severe renal impairment; prolonged use may result in superinfection; use with caution in patients with a history of penicillin or cephalosporin allergy, especially IgE-mediated reactions (eg, anaphylaxis, urticaria). May cause antibiotic-associated colitis or colitis secondary to *C. difficile*.

Drug Interactions

Increased effect: High-dose probenecid decreases clearance

Increased toxicity: Aminoglycosides increase nephrotoxic potential

Lab Interactions Positive direct Coombs', false-positive urinary glucose test using cupric sulfate (Benedict's solution, Clinitest®, Fehling's solution), false-positive serum or urine creatinine with Jaffé reaction

Adverse Reactions

>10%: Hematologic: Positive Coombs' test without hemolysis

1% to 10%:

- Central nervous system: Fever (1%), headache (1%)
- Dermatologic: Rash, pruritus
- Gastrointestinal: Diarrhea, nausea, vomiting
- Local: Pain, erythema at injection site

<1% (Limited to important or life-threatening): Agranulocytosis, anaphylactic shock, anaphylaxis, coma, encephalopathy, hallucinations, leukopenia, myoclonus, neuromuscular excitability, neutropenia, seizure, thrombocytopenia

Other reactions with cephalosporins include aplastic anemia, erythema multiforme, hemolytic anemia, hemorrhage, pancytopenia, prolonged PT, renal dysfunction, Stevens-Johnson syndrome, superinfection, toxic epidermal necrolysis, toxic nephropathy, vaginitis

Overdosage/Toxicology Symptoms of overdose include neuromuscular hypersensitivity and CNS toxicity (including hallucinations, confusion, seizures, and coma). Many beta-lactam containing antibiotics have the potential to cause neuromuscular hyperirritability or convulsive seizures. Hemodialysis may be helpful to aid in removal of the drug from blood; otherwise, treatment is supportive and symptom-directed.

Dosing

Adults & Elderly:

Susceptible infections: I.V.: 1-2 g every 12 hours for 7-10 days; higher doses or more frequent administration may be required in pseudomonal infections

Urinary tract infections, mild to moderate: I.V., I.M.: 500-1000 mg every 12 hours

Febrile neutropenia: I.V.: 2 g every 8 hours for 7 days or until neutropenia resolves

Pediatrics:

Febrile neutropenia: I.V.: Children >2 months of age: 50 mg/kg every 8 hours for 7-10 days

Uncomplicated skin/soft tissue infections, pneumonia, and complicated/ uncomplicated UTI: I.V.: Children >2 months of age: 50 mg/kg twice daily

Renal Impairment:

Adjustment of recommended maintenance schedule is required:

Normal dosing schedule: 500 mg every 12 hours
- Cl_{cr} 30-60 mL/minute: 500 mg every 24 hours
- Cl_{cr} 11-29 mL/minute: 500 mg every 24 hours
- Cl_{cr} <11 mL/minute: 250 mg every 24 hours

Normal dosing schedule: 1 g every 12 hours
- Cl_{cr} 30-60 mL/minute: 1 g every 24 hours
- Cl_{cr} 11-29 mL/minute: 500 mg every 24 hours
- Cl_{cr} <11 mL/minute: 250 mg every 24 hours

Normal dosing schedule: 2 g every 12 hours
- Cl_{cr} 30-60 mL/minute: 2 g every 24 hours
- Cl_{cr} 11-29 mL/minute: 1 g every 24 hours
- Cl_{cr} <11 mL/minute: 500 mg every 24 hours

Normal dosing schedule: 2 g every 8 hours
- Cl_{cr} 30-60 mL/minute: 2 g every 12 hours
- Cl_{cr} 11-29 mL/minute: 2 g every 24 hours
- Cl_{cr} <11 mL/minute: 1 g every 24 hours

Hemodialysis effects: Initial: 1 g (single dose) on day 1. Maintenance: 500 mg once daily (1 g once daily in febrile neutropenic patients). Dosage should be administered after dialysis on dialysis days.

Peritoneal dialysis effects: Removed to a lesser extent than hemodialysis; administer 250 mg every 48 hours.

Continuous arteriovenous hemofiltration: Dose as for Cl_{cr} >30 mL/minute.

Available Dosage Forms Injection, powder for reconstitution, as hydrochloride: 500 mg, 1 g, 2 g

Nursing Guidelines

Assessment: Assess for previous allergy history prior to therapy. See Contraindications, Warnings/Precautions, and Dosing for use cautions. Assess potential for interactions with other prescriptions, OTC medications, or herbal products patient may be taking (see Drug Interactions). Assess results of laboratory tests (see below), therapeutic response and adverse effects (see Adverse Reactions and Overdose/Toxicology). Advise patients with diabetes about use of Clinitest®. Teach patient proper use, possible side effects/appropriate interventions, and adverse symptoms to report (eg, nephrotoxicity, opportunistic infection - see Patient Education). Note breast-feeding caution.

Monitoring Laboratory Tests: Perform culture and sensitivity studies prior to initiating drug therapy; renal function

Patient Education: Inform prescriber of all prescriptions, OTC medications, or herbal products you are taking, and any allergies you have. Do not take any new medication during therapy unless approved by prescriber. This medication is administered by infusion or injection. Report immediately any redness, swelling, burning, or pain at injection/infusion site; itching or hives; difficulty swallowing or breathing. Maintain adequate hydration (2-3 L/day of fluids unless instructed to restrict fluid intake). May cause false test results with Clinitest®; use of another type of glucose testing is preferable. May cause diarrhea (yogurt, boiled milk, or buttermilk may help); nausea, and vomiting (small, frequent meals, frequent mouth care, chewing gum, or sucking lozenges may help). Report unresolved diarrhea; opportunistic infection (vaginal itching or drainage; sores in mouth; blood in stool or urine; unusual fever or chills); or respiratory difficulty. **Breast-feeding precaution:** Consult prescriber if breast-feeding.

Geriatric Considerations: Adjust dose for changes in renal function.

Pregnancy Risk Factor: B

Lactation: Enters breast milk/use caution

Breast-Feeding Considerations: Theoretically, drug absorbed by nursing infant may change bowel flora or affect fever work-up result. **Note:** As a class, cephalosporins are used to treat infections in infants.

Administration

I.M.: Inject deep I.M. into large muscle mass.

I.V.: Inject direct I.V. over 5 minutes. Infuse intermittent infusion over 30-60 minutes.

Compatibility: Stable in D_5LR, D_5NS, D_5W, $D_{10}W$, NS, bacteriostatic water, SWFI

Y-site administration: Incompatible with acyclovir, amphotericin B, amphotericin B cholesteryl sulfate complex, chlordiazepoxide, chlorpromazine, cimetidine, ciprofloxacin, cisplatin, dacarbazine, daunorubicin, diazepam, diphenhydramine, dobutamine, dopamine, doxorubicin, droperidol, enalaprilat, etoposide, etoposide phosphate, famotidine, filgrastim, floxuridine, ganciclovir, haloperidol, hydroxyzine, idarubicin, ifosfamide, magnesium sulfate, mannitol, mechlorethamine, meperidine, metoclopramide, mitomycin, mitoxantrone, morphine, nalbuphine, ofloxacin, ondansetron, plicamycin, prochlorperazine edisylate, promethazine, streptozocin, vancomycin, vinblastine, vincristine

Compatibility when admixed: Incompatible with aminophylline, gentamicin, netilmicin, tobramycin, vancomycin

Related Information

Cephalosporins by Generation *on page 1858*

♦ **Cefepime Hydrochloride** *see* Cefepime *on page 337*

♦ **Cefizox®** *see* Ceftizoxime *on page 351*

♦ **Cefotan® [DSC]** *see* Cefotetan *on page 342*

Cefotaxime (sef oh TAKS eem)

U.S. Brand Names Claforan®

Synonyms Cefotaxime Sodium

Pharmacologic Category Antibiotic, Cephalosporin (Third Generation)

Medication Safety Issues

Sound-alike/look-alike issues:

Cefotaxime may be confused with cefoxitin, ceftizoxime, cefuroxime

Use Treatment of susceptible infection in respiratory tract, skin and skin structure, bone and joint, urinary tract, gynecologic as well as septicemia, and documented or suspected meningitis. Active against most gram-negative bacilli (not *Pseudomonas*) and gram-positive cocci (not enterococcus). Active against many penicillin-resistant pneumococci.

Mechanism of Action Inhibits bacterial cell wall synthesis by binding to one or more of the penicillin-binding proteins (PBPs) which in turn inhibits the final transpeptidation step of peptidoglycan synthesis in bacterial cell walls, thus inhibiting cell wall biosynthesis. Bacteria eventually lyse due to ongoing activity of cell wall autolytic enzymes (autolysins and murein hydrolases) while cell wall assembly is arrested.

Pharmacodynamics/Kinetics

Distribution: Widely to body tissues and fluids including aqueous humor, ascitic and prostatic fluids, bone; penetrates CSF best when meninges are inflamed; crosses placenta; enters breast milk

Metabolism: Partially hepatic to active metabolite, desacetylcefotaxime

Half-life elimination:

Cefotaxime: Premature neonates <1 week: 5-6 hours; Full-term neonates <1 week: 2-3.4 hours; Adults: 1-1.5 hours; prolonged with renal and/or hepatic impairment

Desacetylcefotaxime: 1.5-1.9 hours; prolonged with renal impairment

Time to peak, serum: I.M.: Within 30 minutes

Excretion: Urine (as unchanged drug and metabolites)

Contraindications Hypersensitivity to cefotaxime, any component of the formulation, or other cephalosporins

Warnings/Precautions Modify dosage in patients with severe renal impairment; prolonged use may result in superinfection; a potentially life-threatening arrhythmia has been reported in patients who received a rapid bolus injection via central line. Use caution in patients with colitis; minimize tissue inflammation by changing infusion sites when needed. Use with caution in patients with a history of penicillin allergy especially IgE-mediated reactions (eg, anaphylaxis, urticaria). May cause antibiotic-associated colitis or colitis secondary to *C. difficile.*

Drug Interactions

Increased effect: Probenecid may decrease cephalosporin elimination

Increased toxicity: Furosemide, aminoglycosides may be a possible additive to nephrotoxicity

Lab Interactions Positive direct Coombs', false-positive urinary glucose test using cupric sulfate (Benedict's solution, Clinitest®, Fehling's solution), false-positive serum or urine creatinine with Jaffé reaction

Adverse Reactions

1% to 10%:

Dermatologic: Rash, pruritus

Gastrointestinal: Diarrhea, nausea, vomiting, colitis

Local: Pain at injection site

<1% (Limited to important or life-threatening): Anaphylaxis, arrhythmia (after rapid I.V. injection via central catheter), BUN increased, candidiasis, creatinine increased, eosinophilia, erythema multiforme, fever, headache, interstitial nephritis, neutropenia, phlebitis, pseudomembranous colitis, Stevens-Johnson syndrome, thrombocytopenia, transaminases increased, toxic epidermal necrolysis, urticaria, vaginitis

Reactions reported with other cephalosporins include agranulocytosis, aplastic anemia, cholestasis, hemolytic anemia, hemorrhage, pancytopenia, renal dysfunction, seizure, superinfection, toxic nephropathy.

Overdosage/Toxicology Symptoms of overdose include neuromuscular hypersensitivity and convulsions. Many beta-lactam containing antibiotics have the potential to cause neuromuscular hyperirritability or convulsive seizures. Hemodialysis may be helpful to aid in removal of the drug from blood; otherwise, treatment is supportive or symptom-directed.

Dosing

Adults & Elderly:

Gonorrhea: I.M.: 1 g as a single dose

Uncomplicated infections: I.M., I.V.: 1 g every 12 hours

Moderate/severe infections: I.M., I.V.: 1-2 g every 8 hours

Infections commonly needing higher doses (eg, septicemia): I.V.: 2 g every 6-8 hours

Life-threatening infections: I.V.: 2 g every 4 hours

Preop: I.M., I.V.: 1 g 30-90 minutes before surgery

C-section: 1 g as soon as the umbilical cord is clamped, then 1 g I.M., I.V. at 6- and 12-hours intervals.

Pediatrics:

Susceptible infections: I.M., I.V.: Infants and Children 1 month to 12 years: <50 kg: 50-180 mg/kg/day in divided doses every 4-6 hours

Meningitis: 200 mg/kg/day in divided doses every 6 hours

Children >12 years: Refer to adult dosing.

Renal Impairment:

Cl_{cr} 10-50 mL/minute: Administer every 8-12 hours.

Cl_{cr} <10 mL/minute: Administer every 24 hours.

Moderately dialyzable (20% to 50%)

Continuous arteriovenous hemofiltration: 1 g every 12 hours.

Hepatic Impairment: Moderate dosage reduction is recommended in severe liver disease.

Available Dosage Forms

Infusion, as sodium [premixed in D_5W]: 1 g (50 mL); 2 g (50 mL)

Injection, powder for reconstitution, as sodium: 500 mg, 1 g, 2 g, 10 g, 20 g

Claforan®: 500 mg, 1 g, 2 g, 10 g [contains sodium 50.5 mg (2.2 mEq) per cefotaxime 1 g]

Nursing Guidelines

Assessment: Assess for previous allergy history prior to therapy. See Contraindications and Warnings/Precautions for use cautions (eg, arrhythmia, colitis). Assess potential for interactions with other prescriptions, OTC medications, or herbal products patient may be taking (eg, nephrotoxicity - see Drug Interactions). Assess results of laboratory tests (eg, hypoprothrombinemia - see Monitoring Laboratory Tests and Overdose/Toxicology), therapeutic response, and adverse effects (see Adverse Reactions). Advise patients with diabetes about use of Clinitest®. Teach patient possible side effects/appropriate interventions and adverse symptoms to report (eg, nephrotoxicity, opportunistic infection - see Patient Education). Note breast-feeding caution.

Monitoring Laboratory Tests: Perform culture and sensitivity studies prior to initiating drug therapy; CBC with differential (especially with long courses); renal function

Dietary Considerations: Sodium content of 1 g: 50.5 mg (2.2 mEq)

Patient Education: Inform prescriber of all prescriptions, OTC medications, or herbal products you are taking, and any allergies you have. Do not take any new medication during therapy unless approved by prescriber. This medication is administered by injection or infusion. Report immediately any redness, swelling, burning, or pain at injection/infusion site; chest pain, palpitations, respiratory difficulty or swallowing; or itching or hives. Maintain adequate hydration (2-3 L/day of fluids) unless instructed to restrict fluid intake. May cause false test results with Clinitest®; use of another type of glucose testing is preferable. May cause diarrhea (yogurt, boiled milk, or buttermilk may help); GI distress or nausea (small, frequent meals, frequent oral care, chewing gum, or sucking lozenges may help). Report unresolved diarrhea; opportunistic infection (vaginal itching or drainage; sores in mouth; blood in stool or urine; easy bleeding or bruising, unusual fever or chills); or respiratory difficulty. **Breast-feeding precaution:** Consult prescriber if breast-feeding.

Geriatric Considerations: Adjust dose for renal function.

Pregnancy Risk Factor: B

Lactation: Enters breast milk/use caution (AAP rates "compatible")

Breast-Feeding Considerations: Theoretically, drug absorbed by nursing infant may change bowel flora or affect fever work-up result. **Note:** As a class, cephalosporins are used to treat infections in infants.

Administration

I.M.: Inject deep I.M. into large muscle mass.

I.V.: Inject direct I.V. over 3-5 minutes. Infuse intermittent infusion over 30 minutes.

(Continued)

Cefotaxime *(Continued)*

Reconstitution: Reconstituted solution is stable for 12-24 hours at room temperature and 7-10 days when refrigerated and for 13 weeks when frozen; for I.V. infusion in NS or D_5W, solution is stable for 24 hours at room temperature, 5 days when refrigerated, or 13 weeks when frozen in Viaflex® plastic containers; thawed solutions previously of frozen premixed bags are stable for 24 hours at room temperature or 10 days when refrigerated.

Compatibility: Stable in D_5¼NS, D_5½NS, D_5NS, D_5W, $D_{10}W$, LR, NS

Y-site administration: Incompatible with allopurinol, filgrastim, fluconazole, gemcitabine, hetastarch, pentamidine

Compatibility in syringe: Incompatible with doxapram

Compatibility when admixed: Incompatible with aminoglycosides, aminophylline, sodium bicarbonate

Related Information

Cephalosporins by Generation *on page 1858*

♦ Cefotaxime Sodium *see* Cefotaxime *on page 340*

Cefotetan (SEF oh tee tan)

U.S. Brand Names Cefotan® [DSC]

Synonyms Cefotetan Disodium

Pharmacologic Category Antibiotic, Cephalosporin (Second Generation)

Medication Safety Issues

Sound-alike/look-alike issues:

Cefotetan may be confused with cefoxitin, Ceftin®

Cefotan® may be confused with Ceftin®

Use Surgical prophylaxis; intra-abdominal infections and other mixed infections; respiratory tract, skin and skin structure, bone and joint, urinary tract and gynecologic as well as septicemia; active against gram-negative enteric bacilli including *E. coli*, *Klebsiella*, and *Proteus*; less active against staphylococci and streptococci than first generation cephalosporins, but active against anaerobes including *Bacteroides fragilis*

Mechanism of Action Inhibits bacterial cell wall synthesis by binding to one or more of the penicillin-binding proteins (PBPs) which in turn inhibits the final transpeptidation step of peptidoglycan synthesis in bacterial cell walls, thus inhibiting cell wall biosynthesis. Bacteria eventually lyse due to ongoing activity of cell wall autolytic enzymes (autolysins and murein hydrolases) while cell wall assembly is arrested.

Pharmacodynamics/Kinetics

Distribution: Widely to body tissues and fluids including bile, sputum, prostatic, peritoneal; low concentrations enter CSF; crosses placenta; enters breast milk

Protein binding: 76% to 90%

Half-life elimination: 3-5 hours

Time to peak, serum: I.M.: 1.5-3 hours

Excretion: Primarily urine (as unchanged drug); feces (20%)

Contraindications Hypersensitivity to cefotetan, any component of the formulation, or other cephalosporins; previous cephalosporin-associated hemolytic anemia

Warnings/Precautions Modify dosage in patients with severe renal impairment; prolonged use may result in superinfection; although cefotetan contains the methyltetrazolethiol side chain, bleeding has not been a significant problem; use with caution in patients with a history of penicillin allergy especially IgE-mediated reactions (eg, anaphylaxis, urticaria). Cefotetan has been associated with a higher risk of hemolytic anemia relative to other cephalosporins (approximately threefold); monitor carefully during use and consider cephalosporin-associated immune anemia in patients who have received cefotetan within 2-3 weeks (either as treatment or prophylaxis). May cause antibiotic-associated colitis or colitis secondary to *C. difficile*.

Drug Interactions

Ethanol: Disulfiram-like reaction may occur if ethanol is consumed by a patient taking cefotetan.

Probenecid: May increase cefotetan plasma levels.

Warfarin: Cefotetan may increase risk of bleeding in patients receiving warfarin.

Nutritional/Herbal/Ethanol Interactions Ethanol: Avoid ethanol (may cause a disulfiram-like reaction).

Lab Interactions Positive direct Coombs', false-positive urinary glucose test using cupric sulfate (Benedict's solution, Clinitest®, Fehling's solution), false-positive serum or urine creatinine with Jaffé reaction

Adverse Reactions

1% to 10%:

Gastrointestinal: Diarrhea (1%)

Hepatic: Transaminases increased (1%)

Miscellaneous: Hypersensitivity reactions (1%)

<1%: Anaphylaxis, urticaria, rash, pruritus, pseudomembranous colitis, nausea, vomiting, eosinophilia, thrombocytosis, agranulocytosis, hemolytic anemia, leukopenia, thrombocytopenia, prolonged PT, bleeding, elevated BUN, elevated creatinine, nephrotoxicity, phlebitis, fever

Reactions reported with other cephalosporins include seizure, Stevens-Johnson syndrome, toxic epidermal necrolysis, renal dysfunction, toxic nephropathy, cholestasis, aplastic anemia, hemolytic anemia, hemorrhage, pancytopenia, agranulocytosis, colitis, superinfection

Overdosage/Toxicology Symptoms of overdose include neuromuscular hypersensitivity and convulsions. Many beta-lactam containing antibiotics have the potential to cause neuromuscular hyperirritability or convulsive seizures. Hemodialysis may be helpful to aid in removal of the drug from blood; otherwise, treatment is supportive or symptom-directed.

Dosing

Adults & Elderly:

Susceptible infections: I.M., I.V.: 1-6 g/day in divided doses every 12 hours; usual dose: 1-2 g every 12 hours for 5-10 days; 1-2 g may be given every 24 hours for urinary tract infection

Pelvic inflammatory disease: I.V.: 2 g every 12 hours; used in combination with doxycycline

Preoperative prophylaxis: I.M., I.V.: 1-2 g 30-60 minutes prior to surgery; when used for cesarean section, dose should be given as soon as umbilical cord is clamped

Pediatrics:

Severe infections (unlabeled use): I.M., I.V.: 20-40 mg/kg/dose every 12 hours; maximum: 6 g/day

Preoperative prophylaxis (unlabeled use): I.M., I.V.: 40 mg/kg 30-60 minutes prior to surgery

Pelvic inflammatory disease: Adolescents: I.V.: Refer to adult dosing.

Renal Impairment: I.M., I.V.:

Cl_{cr} 10-30 mL/minute: Administer every 24 hours

Cl_{cr} <10 mL/minute: Administer every 48 hours

Hemodialysis: Dialyzable (5% to 20%); administer 1/4 the usual dose every 24 hours on days between dialysis; administer 1/2 the usual dose on the day of dialysis.

Continuous arteriovenous or venovenous hemodiafiltration effects: Administer 750 mg every 12 hours

Available Dosage Forms [DSC] = Discontinued product

Infusion [premixed iso-osmotic solution]: 1 g (50 mL); 2 g (50 mL) [contains sodium 80 mg/g (3.5 mEq/g)] [DSC]

Injection, powder for reconstitution: 1 g, 2 g [contains sodium 80 mg/g (3.5 mEq/g)] [DSC]

Nursing Guidelines

Assessment: Assess for previous allergy history prior to therapy. See Contraindications, Warnings/Precautions, and Dosing for use cautions. Assess potential for interactions with other prescriptions, OTC medications, or herbal products patient may be taking (see Drug Interactions). Assess results of laboratory tests (see Effects on Lab Values and Monitoring Laboratory Tests). Monitor for therapeutic response and adverse effects (eg, hemolytic anemia, hypoprothrombinemia, and bleeding - see Adverse Reactions and Overdose/Toxicology). Advise patients with diabetes about use of Clinitest® (may cause false-positive test). Teach patient possible side effects/appropriate interventions and adverse symptoms to report (eg, nephrotoxicity, opportunistic infection, hypersensitivity reaction - see Patient Education). Note breast-feeding caution.

Monitoring Laboratory Tests: Prothrombin time; perform culture and sensitivity studies prior to initiating drug therapy; renal function

Dietary Considerations: Contains sodium of 80 mg (3.5 mEq) per cefotetan 1 g

(Continued)

Cefotetan *(Continued)*

Patient Education: Inform prescriber of all prescriptions, OTC medications, or herbal products you are using and any allergies you have. Do not take any new medication during therapy unless approved by prescriber. This medication is administered by injection or infusion. Report immediately any redness, swelling, burning, or pain at injection/infusion site, or immediately report any itching, hives, difficulty swallowing or respiratory difficulty. Maintain adequate hydration (2-3 L/day of fluids) unless instructed to restrict fluid intake. Avoid alcohol during therapy and for 72 hours after last dose (may cause severe disulfiram-like reactions). May cause false test results with Clinitest®; use of another type of glucose testing is preferable. May cause diarrhea (yogurt, boiled milk, or buttermilk may help). Report severe, unresolved diarrhea; opportunistic infection (vaginal itching or drainage; sores in mouth; blood or mucus in stool or urine; easy bleeding or bruising, unusual fever or chills); unusual persistent weakness or fatigue; rash; respiratory difficulty. **Breast-feeding precaution:** Consult prescriber if breast-feeding.

Geriatric Considerations: Cefotetan has not been studied in the elderly. Adjust dose for renal function in the elderly.

Pregnancy Risk Factor: B

Lactation: Enters breast milk (small amounts)/use caution

Breast-Feeding Considerations: Theoretically, drug absorbed by nursing infant may change bowel flora or affect fever work-up result. **Note:** As a class, cephalosporins are used to treat infections in infants.

Administration

I.M.: Inject deep I.M. into large muscle mass.

I.V.: Inject direct I.V. over 3-5 minutes. Infuse intermittent infusion over 30 minutes.

Reconstitution: Reconstituted solution is stable for 24 hours at room temperature and 96 hours when refrigerated. For I.V. infusion in NS or D_5W solution and after freezing, thawed solution is stable for 24 hours at room temperature or 96 hours when refrigerated. Frozen solution is stable for 12 weeks.

Compatibility: Stable in D_5W, NS

Y-site administration: Incompatible with promethazine, vinorelbine

Compatibility in syringe: Incompatible with doxapram, promethazine

Compatibility when admixed: Incompatible with gentamicin, heparin, tetracyclines

Related Information

Cephalosporins by Generation *on page 1858*
Prevention of Wound Infection and Sepsis in Surgical Patients *on page 1830*

♦ **Cefotetan Disodium** *see* Cefotetan *on page 342*

Cefoxitin (se FOKS i tin)

U.S. Brand Names Mefoxin®

Synonyms Cefoxitin Sodium

Pharmacologic Category Antibiotic, Cephalosporin (Second Generation)

Medication Safety Issues

Sound-alike/look-alike issues:

Cefoxitin may be confused with cefotaxime, cefotetan, Cytoxan®
Mefoxin® may be confused with Lanoxin®

Use Less active against staphylococci and streptococci than first generation cephalosporins, but active against anaerobes including *Bacteroides fragilis*; active against gram-negative enteric bacilli including *E. coli*, *Klebsiella*, and *Proteus*; used predominantly for respiratory tract, skin and skin structure, bone and joint, urinary tract and gynecologic as well as septicemia; surgical prophylaxis; intra-abdominal infections and other mixed infections; indicated for bacterial *Eikenella corrodens* infections

Mechanism of Action Inhibits bacterial cell wall synthesis by binding to one or more of the penicillin-binding proteins (PBPs) which in turn inhibits the final transpeptidation step of peptidoglycan synthesis in bacterial cell walls, thus inhibiting cell wall biosynthesis. Bacteria eventually lyse due to ongoing activity of cell wall autolytic enzymes (autolysins and murein hydrolases) while cell wall assembly is arrested.

Pharmacodynamics/Kinetics

Distribution: Widely to body tissues and fluids including pleural, synovial, ascitic, bile; poorly penetrates into CSF even with inflammation of the meninges; crosses placenta; small amounts enter breast milk

Protein binding: 65% to 79%
Half-life elimination: 45-60 minutes; significantly prolonged with renal impairment
Time to peak, serum: I.M.: 20-30 minutes
Excretion: Urine (85% as unchanged drug)

Contraindications Hypersensitivity to cefoxitin, any component of the formulation, or other cephalosporins

Warnings/Precautions Use with caution in patients with history of colitis; cefoxitin may increase resistance of organisms by inducing beta-lactamase; modify dosage in patients with severe renal impairment; prolonged use may result in superinfection; use with caution in patients with a history of penicillin allergy especially IgE-mediated reactions (eg, anaphylaxis, urticaria). May cause antibiotic-associated colitis or colitis secondary to *C. difficile*.

Drug Interactions

Increased effect: Probenecid may decrease cephalosporin elimination
Increased toxicity: Aminoglycosides and furosemide may increase nephrotoxic potential

Lab Interactions Positive direct Coombs', false-positive urinary glucose test using cupric sulfate (Benedict's solution, Clinitest®, Fehling's solution), false-positive serum or urine creatinine with Jaffé reaction

Adverse Reactions

1% to 10%: Gastrointestinal: Diarrhea
<1% (Limited to important or life-threatening): Anaphylaxis, angioedema, bone marrow suppression, BUN increased, creatinine increased, dyspnea, eosinophilia, exacerbation of myasthenia gravis, exfoliative dermatitis, fever, hemolytic anemia, hypotension, interstitial nephritis, jaundice, leukopenia, nausea, nephrotoxicity (with aminoglycosides), phlebitis, prolonged PT, pruritus, pseudomembranous colitis, rash, thrombocytopenia, thrombophlebitis, toxic epidermal necrolysis, transaminases increased, urticaria, vomiting
Other reactions with cephalosporins include agranulocytosis, aplastic anemia, cholestasis, colitis, erythema multiforme, hemolytic anemia, hemorrhage, pancytopenia, renal dysfunction, seizure, serum-sickness reactions, Stevens-Johnson syndrome, superinfection, toxic nephropathy, vaginitis

Overdosage/Toxicology Symptoms of overdose include neuromuscular hypersensitivity and convulsions. Many beta-lactam containing antibiotics have the potential to cause neuromuscular hyperirritability or convulsive seizures. Hemodialysis may be helpful to aid in removal of the drug from blood; otherwise, treatment is supportive or symptom-directed.

Dosing

Adults & Elderly: Susceptible infections: I.M., I.V.: 1-2 g every 6-8 hours (I.M. injection is painful); up to 12 g/day

Pediatrics: Infants >3 months and Children:

Mild to moderate infection: I.M., I.V.: 80-100 mg/kg/day in divided doses every 4-6 hours

Severe infection: I.M., I.V.: 100-160 mg/kg/day in divided doses every 4-6 hours

Maximum dose: 12 g/day

Renal Impairment: I.M., I.V.:

Cl_{cr} 30-50 mL/minute: Administer 1-2 g every 8-12 hours
Cl_{cr} 10-29 mL/minute: Administer 1-2 g every 12-24 hours
Cl_{cr} 5-9 mL/minute: Administer 0.5-1 g every 12-24 hours
Cl_{cr} <5 mL/minute: Administer 0.5-1 g every 24-48 hours
Hemodialysis: Moderately dialyzable (20% to 50%); administer a loading dose of 1-2 g after each hemodialysis; maintenance dose as noted above based on Cl_{cr}
Continuous arteriovenous or venovenous hemodiafiltration effects: Dose as for Cl_{cr} 10-50 mL/minute

Available Dosage Forms

Infusion, as sodium [premixed iso-osmotic solution]: 1 g (50 mL); 2 g (50 mL) [contains sodium 53.8 mg/g (2.3 mEq/g)]
Injection, powder for reconstitution, as sodium: 1 g, 2 g, 10 g [contains sodium 53.8 mg/g (2.3 mEq/g)]

Nursing Guidelines

Assessment: Assess for previous allergy history prior to therapy. See Contraindications and Warnings/Precautions for use cautions (eg, colitis). Assess potential for interactions with other prescriptions, OTC medications, or herbal products patient may be taking (see Drug Interactions). Assess results of laboratory tests (eg, hypoprothrombinemia), therapeutic response, and

(Continued)

Cefoxitin *(Continued)*

adverse effects (see Adverse Reactions and Overdose/Toxicology). Advise patients with diabetes about use of Clinitest®. Teach patient possible side effects/appropriate interventions and adverse symptoms to report (eg, nephrotoxicity, opportunistic infection - see Patient Education). Note breast-feeding caution.

Monitoring Laboratory Tests: Prothrombin times; perform culture and sensitivity studies prior to initiating drug therapy; renal function

Dietary Considerations: Sodium content of 1 g: 53 mg (2.3 mEq)

Patient Education: Inform prescriber of all prescriptions, OTC medications, herbal products you are taking, and any allergies you have. Do not take any new medication during therapy unless approved by prescriber. This medication is administered by injection or infusion. Report immediately any redness, swelling, burning, or pain at injection/infusion site; chest pain, palpitations, respiratory difficulty or swallowing; itching or hives. Maintain adequate hydration (2-3 L/day of fluids) unless instructed to restrict fluid intake. May cause false test results with Clinitest®; use of another type of glucose testing is preferable. May cause diarrhea (yogurt, boiled milk, or buttermilk may help). Report unresolved diarrhea; opportunistic infection (vaginal itching or drainage, sores in mouth, blood in urine or stool, easy bleeding or bruising, unusual fever or chills); rash; or respiratory difficulty. **Breast-feeding precaution:** Consult prescriber if breast-feeding.

Geriatric Considerations: Adjust dose for renal function in the elderly.

Pregnancy Risk Factor: B

Lactation: Enters breast milk (small amounts)/use caution (AAP rates "compatible")

Breast-Feeding Considerations: Theoretically, drug absorbed by nursing infant may change bowel flora or affect fever work-up result. **Note:** As a class, cephalosporins are used to treat infections in infants.

Administration

I.M.: Inject deep I.M. into large muscle mass.

I.V.: Can be administered IVP over 3-5 minutes at a maximum concentration of 100 mg/mL or I.V. intermittent infusion over 10-60 minutes at a final concentration for I.V. administration not to exceed 40 mg/mL

Reconstitution: Reconstitute vials with SWFI, bacteriostatic water for injection, NS, or D_5W. For I.V. infusion, solutions may be further diluted in NS, $D_5{}^1\!/_4NS$, $D_5{}^1\!/_2NS$, D_5NS, D_5W, $D_{10}W$, LR, D_5LR, mannitol 10%, or sodium bicarbonate 5%.

Compatibility: Stable in D_5LR, $D_5{}^1\!/_4NS$, $D_5{}^1\!/_2NS$, D_5NS, D_5W, $D_{10}W$, LR, NS, mannitol 10%, sodium bicarbonate 5%

Y-site administration: Incompatible with filgrastim, gatifloxacin, hetastarch, pentamidine

Compatibility when admixed: Incompatible with ranitidine

Storage: Reconstituted solution is stable for 6 hours at room temperature or 7 days when refrigerated; I.V. infusion in NS or D_5W solution is stable for 18 hours at room temperature or 48 hours when refrigerated. Premixed frozen solution, when thawed, is stable for 24 hours at room temperature or 21 days when refrigerated.

Related Information

Cephalosporins by Generation *on page 1858*
Prevention of Wound Infection and Sepsis in Surgical Patients *on page 1830*

♦ **Cefoxitin Sodium** *see* Cefoxitin *on page 344*

Cefprozil (sef PROE zil)

U.S. Brand Names Cefzil®

Pharmacologic Category Antibiotic, Cephalosporin (Second Generation)

Medication Safety Issues

Sound-alike/look-alike issues:

Cefprozil may be confused with cefazolin, cefuroxime
Cefzil® may be confused with Cefol®, Ceftin®, Kefzol®

Use Treatment of otitis media and infections involving the respiratory tract and skin and skin structure; active against methicillin-sensitive staphylococci, many streptococci, and various gram-negative bacilli including *E. coli*, some *Klebsiella*, *P. mirabilis*, *H. influenzae*, and *Moraxella*.

Mechanism of Action Inhibits bacterial cell wall synthesis by binding to one or more of the penicillin-binding proteins (PBPs) which in turn inhibits the final

transpeptidation step of peptidoglycan synthesis in bacterial cell walls, thus inhibiting cell wall biosynthesis. Bacteria eventually lyse due to ongoing activity of cell wall autolytic enzymes (autolysins and murein hydrolases) while cell wall assembly is arrested.

Pharmacodynamics/Kinetics

Absorption: Well absorbed (94%)

Distribution: Low amounts enter breast milk

Protein binding: 35% to 45%

Half-life elimination: Normal renal function: 1.3 hours

Time to peak, serum: Fasting: 1.5 hours

Excretion: Urine (61% as unchanged drug)

Contraindications Hypersensitivity to cefprozil, any component of the formulation, or other cephalosporins

Warnings/Precautions Modify dosage in patients with severe renal impairment; prolonged use may result in superinfection; use with caution in patients with a history of penicillin allergy especially IgE-mediated reactions (eg, anaphylaxis, urticaria). May cause antibiotic-associated colitis or colitis secondary to *C. difficile*.

Drug Interactions

Increased effect: Probenecid may decrease cephalosporin elimination

Increased toxicity: Aminoglycosides and furosemide may increase nephrotoxic potential

Nutritional/Herbal/Ethanol Interactions Food: Food delays cefprozil absorption.

Lab Interactions Positive direct Coombs', false-positive urinary glucose test using cupric sulfate (Benedict's solution, Clinitest®, Fehling's solution), false-positive serum or urine creatinine with Jaffé reaction

Adverse Reactions

1% to 10%:

- Central nervous system: Dizziness (1%)
- Dermatologic: Diaper rash (1.5%)
- Gastrointestinal: Diarrhea (2.9%), nausea (3.5%), vomiting (1%), abdominal pain (1%)
- Genitourinary: Vaginitis, genital pruritus (1.6%)
- Hepatic: Transaminases increased (2%)
- Miscellaneous: Superinfection

<1% (Limited to important or life-threatening): Anaphylaxis, angioedema, arthralgia, BUN increased, cholestatic jaundice, confusion, creatinine increased, eosinophilia, erythema multiforme, fever, headache, hyperactivity, insomnia, leukopenia, pseudomembranous colitis, rash, serum sickness, somnolence, Stevens-Johnson syndrome, thrombocytopenia, urticaria

Other reactions with cephalosporins include agranulocytosis, aplastic anemia, colitis, hemolytic anemia, hemorrhage, interstitial nephritis, pancytopenia, renal dysfunction, seizure, superinfection, toxic epidermal necrolysis, toxic nephropathy, vaginitis

Overdosage/Toxicology Symptoms of overdose include neuromuscular hypersensitivity and convulsions. Many beta-lactam containing antibiotics have the potential to cause neuromuscular hyperirritability or convulsive seizures. Hemodialysis may be helpful to aid in removal of the drug from blood; otherwise, treatment is supportive or symptom-directed.

Dosing

Adults & Elderly:

Pharyngitis/tonsillitis: Oral: 500 mg every 24 hours for 10 days

Uncomplicated skin and skin structure infections: Oral: 250 mg every 12 hours, or 500 mg every 12-24 hours for 10 days

Secondary bacterial infection of acute bronchitis or acute bacterial exacerbation of chronic bronchitis: Oral: 500 mg every 12 hours for 10 days

Pediatrics:

Otitis media: Oral: Children >6 months to 12 years: 15 mg/kg every 12 hours for 10 days

Pharyngitis/tonsillitis: Oral: Children:

- 2-12 years: 7.5 -15 mg/kg/day divided every 12 hours for 10 days (administer for >10 days if due to *S. pyogenes*); maximum: 1 g/day
- >13 years: Refer to adult dosing.

Uncomplicated skin and skin structure infections: Oral:

- 2-12 years: 20 mg/kg every 24 hours for 10 days; maximum: 1 g/day
- >13 years: Refer to adult dosing.

(Continued)

Cefprozil *(Continued)*

Renal Impairment:

Cl_{cr} <30 mL/minute: Reduce dose by 50%.

Hemodialysis effects: 55% is removed by hemodialysis.

Available Dosage Forms

Powder for oral suspension, as anhydrous: 125 mg/5 mL (50 mL, 75 mL, 100 mL); 250 mg/5 mL (50 mL, 75 mL, 100 mL) [contains phenylalanine 28 mg/5 mL and sodium benzoate; bubble gum flavor]

Tablet, as anhydrous: 250 mg, 500 mg

Nursing Guidelines

Assessment: Assess for previous allergy history prior to therapy. See Contraindications, Warnings/Precautions, and Dosing for use cautions. Assess potential for interactions with other prescriptions, OTC medications, or herbal products patient may be taking (see Drug Interactions). Assess results of laboratory tests (see below), therapeutic response, and adverse effects (see Adverse Reactions and Overdose/Toxicology). Advise patients with diabetes about use of Clinitest®. Teach patient proper use, possible side effects/appropriate interventions, and adverse symptoms to report (eg, nephrotoxicity, opportunistic infection - see Patient Education). **Pregnancy risk factor C/D** - benefits of use should outweigh risks. Note breast-feeding caution.

Monitoring Laboratory Tests: Perform culture and sensitivity studies prior to initiating drug therapy; renal function

Dietary Considerations: May be taken with food. Oral suspension contains phenylalanine 28 mg/5 mL.

Patient Education: Inform prescriber of all prescriptions, OTC medications, or herbal products you are taking, and any allergies you have. Do not take any new medication during therapy unless approved by prescriber. Take as directed, at regular intervals around-the-clock (with or without food). Chilling oral suspension improves flavor (do not freeze). Maintain adequate hydration (2-3 L/day of fluids) unless instructed to restrict fluid intake. Complete full course of medication, even if you feel better. May cause false test results with Clinitest®; use of another type of glucose testing is preferable. May cause dizziness (use caution when driving or engaging in potentially hazardous tasks until response to drug is known); nausea or vomiting (small, frequent meals, frequent mouth care, sucking lozenges, or chewing gum may help); or diarrhea (yogurt, boiled milk, or buttermilk may help). Report changes in urinary pattern (decreased output); vaginal burning, itching, or drainage; unresolved diarrhea; or opportunistic infection (vaginal itching or drainage, sores in mouth, blood in urine or stool, unusual fever or chills). **Breast-feeding precaution:** Consult prescriber if breast-feeding.

Geriatric Considerations: Has not been studied exclusively in the elderly. Adjust dose for estimated renal function.

Pregnancy Risk Factor: B

Lactation: Enters breast milk/use caution (AAP rates "compatible")

Breast-Feeding Considerations: Theoretically, drug absorbed by nursing infant may change bowel flora or affect fever work-up result. **Note:** As a class, cephalosporins are used to treat infections in infants.

Administration

Oral: Administer around-the-clock to promote less variation in peak and trough serum levels. Chilling the reconstituted oral suspension improves flavor (do not freeze).

Related Information

Cephalosporins by Generation *on page 1858*

Ceftazidime (SEF tay zi deem)

U.S. Brand Names Ceptaz® [DSC]; Fortaz®; Tazicef®

Pharmacologic Category Antibiotic, Cephalosporin (Third Generation)

Medication Safety Issues

Sound-alike/look-alike issues:

Ceftazidime may be confused with ceftizoxime

Ceptaz® may be confused with Septra®

Tazicef® may be confused with Tazidime®

Tazidime® may be confused with Tazicef®

Use Treatment of documented susceptible *Pseudomonas aeruginosa* infection and infections due to other susceptible aerobic gram-negative organisms; empiric therapy of a febrile, granulocytopenic patient

Mechanism of Action Inhibits bacterial cell wall synthesis by binding to one or more of the penicillin-binding proteins (PBPs) which in turn inhibits the final transpeptidation step of peptidoglycan synthesis in bacterial cell walls, thus inhibiting cell wall biosynthesis. Bacteria eventually lyse due to ongoing activity of cell wall autolytic enzymes (autolysins and murein hydrolases) while cell wall assembly is arrested.

Pharmacodynamics/Kinetics

Distribution: Widely throughout the body including bone, bile, skin, CSF (higher concentrations achieved when meninges are inflamed), endometrium, heart, pleural and lymphatic fluids

Protein binding: 17%

Half-life elimination: 1-2 hours, prolonged with renal impairment; Neonates <23 days: 2.2-4.7 hours

Time to peak, serum: I.M.: ~1 hour

Excretion: Urine (80% to 90% as unchanged drug)

Contraindications Hypersensitivity to ceftazidime, any component of the formulation, or other cephalosporins

Warnings/Precautions Modify dosage in patients with severe renal impairment; prolonged use may result in superinfection; use with caution in patients with a history of penicillin allergy especially IgE-mediated reactions (eg, anaphylaxis, urticaria). May cause antibiotic-associated colitis or colitis secondary to *C. difficile*.

Drug Interactions

Increased effect: Probenecid may decrease cephalosporin elimination; aminoglycosides: *in vitro* studies indicate additive or synergistic effect against some strains of Enterobacteriaceae and *Pseudomonas aeruginosa*

Increased toxicity: Aminoglycosides and furosemide may increase nephrotoxic potential

Lab Interactions Positive direct Coombs', false-positive urinary glucose test using cupric sulfate (Benedict's solution, Clinitest®, Fehling's solution), false-positive serum or urine creatinine with Jaffé reaction

Adverse Reactions

1% to 10%:

Gastrointestinal: Diarrhea (1%)

Local: Pain at injection site (1%)

Miscellaneous: Hypersensitivity reactions (2%)

<1% (Limited to important or life-threatening): Anaphylaxis, angioedema, asterixis, BUN increased, candidiasis, creatinine increased, dizziness, encephalopathy, eosinophilia, erythema multiforme, fever, headache, hemolytic anemia, hyperbilirubinemia, jaundice, leukopenia, myoclonus, nausea, neuromuscular excitability, paresthesia, phlebitis, pruritus, pseudomembranous colitis, rash, Stevens-Johnson syndrome, thrombocytosis, toxic epidermal necrolysis, transaminases increased, vaginitis, vomiting

Other reactions with cephalosporins include agranulocytosis, aplastic anemia, cholestasis, colitis, hemolytic anemia, hemorrhage, interstitial nephritis, pancytopenia, prolonged PT, renal dysfunction, seizure, serum-sickness reactions, superinfection, toxic nephropathy, urticaria

Overdosage/Toxicology Symptoms of overdose include neuromuscular hypersensitivity and convulsions. Many beta-lactam containing antibiotics have the potential to cause neuromuscular hyperirritability or convulsive seizures. Hemodialysis may be helpful to aid in removal of the drug from blood; otherwise, treatment is supportive or symptom-directed.

Dosing

Adults:

Bone and joint infections: I.V.: 2 g every 12 hours

Cystic fibrosis, lung infection caused by *Pseudomonas* spp: I.V.: 30-50 mg/kg every 8 hours (maximum 6 g/day)

Intra-abdominal or gynecologic infection: I.V.: 2 g every 8 hours

Meningitis: I.V.: 2 g every 8 hours

Pneumonia: I.V.:

Uncomplicated: 500 mg to 1 g every 8 hours

Complicated or severe: 2 g every 8 hours

Skin and soft tissue infections: I.V., I.M.: 500 mg to 1 g every 8 hours

Severe, life-threatening infection (especially in immunocompromised host): I.V.: 2 g every 8 hours

Urinary tract infections: I.V., I.M.:

Uncomplicated: 250 mg every 12 hours

(Continued)

Ceftazidime *(Continued)*

Complicated: 500 mg every 8-12 hours

Elderly: I.M., I.V.: Dosage should be based on renal function with a dosing interval not more frequent then every 12 hours.

Pediatrics: Susceptible infections: I.V.:

Children 1 month to 12 years: 30-50 mg/kg/dose every 8 hours; maximum dose: 6 g/day (higher doses reserved for immunocompromised patients, cystic fibrosis, or meningitis)

Children ≥12 years: Refer to adult dosing.

Renal Impairment:

Cl_{cr} 30-50 mL/minute: Administer every 12 hours

Cl_{cr} 10-30 mL/minute: Administer every 24 hours

Cl_{cr} <10 mL/minute: Administer every 48-72 hours

Hemodialysis: Dialyzable (50% to 100%)

Continuous arteriovenous or venovenous hemodiafiltration effects: Dose as for Cl_{cr} 30-50 mL/minute

Available Dosage Forms [DSC] = Discontinued product

Infusion, as sodium [premixed iso-osmotic solution] (Fortaz®): 1 g (50 mL); 2 g (50 mL)

Injection, powder for reconstitution:

Ceptaz® [DSC]: 10 g [L-arginine formulation]

Fortaz®: 500 mg, 1 g, 2 g, 6 g [contains sodium carbonate]

Tazicef®: 1 g, 2 g, 6 g [contains sodium carbonate]

Nursing Guidelines

Assessment: Assess for previous allergy history prior to therapy. See Contraindications and Warnings/Precautions for use cautions. Assess potential for interactions with other prescriptions, OTC medications, or herbal products patient may be taking (eg, nephrotoxicity - see Drug Interactions). Assess results of laboratory tests (see below), therapeutic response, and adverse effects (see Adverse Reactions and Overdose/Toxicology). Advise patients with diabetes about use of Clinitest®. Teach patient possible side effects/appropriate interventions and adverse symptoms to report (eg, opportunistic infection - see Patient Education). Note breast-feeding caution.

Monitoring Laboratory Tests: Perform culture and sensitivity studies prior to initiating drug therapy; renal function

Dietary Considerations: Sodium content of 1 g: 2.3 mEq

Patient Education: Inform prescriber of all prescriptions, OTC medications, or herbal products you are taking, and any allergies you have. Do not take any new medication during therapy unless approved by prescriber. This medication is administered by infusion or injection. Report immediately any redness, swelling, burning, or pain at injection/infusion site; itching or hives; or difficulty swallowing or breathing. Maintain adequate hydration (2-3 L/day of fluids) unless instructed to restrict fluid intake. May cause false test results with Clinitest®; use of another type of glucose testing is preferable. May cause diarrhea (yogurt, boiled milk, or buttermilk may help). Report unresolved diarrhea; opportunistic infection (vaginal itching or drainage; sores in mouth; blood, pus, or mucus in stool or urine); easy bleeding or bruising; rash; or respiratory difficulty. **Breast-feeding precaution:** Consult prescriber if breast-feeding.

Geriatric Considerations: Changes in renal function associated with aging and corresponding alterations in pharmacokinetics result in every 12-hour dosing being an adequate dosing interval. Adjust dose based on renal function.

Pregnancy Risk Factor: B

Lactation: Enters breast milk (small amounts)/use caution (AAP rates "compatible")

Breast-Feeding Considerations: Theoretically, drug absorbed by nursing infant may change bowel flora or affect fever work-up result. **Note:** As a class, cephalosporins are used to treat infections in infants.

Administration

I.M.: Inject deep I.M. into large mass muscle.

I.V.: Ceftazidime can be administered IVP over 3-5 minutes or I.V. intermittent infusion over 15-30 minutes.

Reconstitution: Reconstituted solution and I.V. infusion in NS or D_5W solution are stable for 24 hours at room temperature, 10 days when refrigerated, or 12 weeks when frozen. After freezing, thawed solution is stable for 24 hours at room temperature or 4 days when refrigerated. After mixing for 96 hours refrigerated.

Compatibility: Stable in D_5NS, D_5W, NS, SWFI

Y-site administration: Incompatible with alatrofloxacin, amphotericin B cholesteryl sulfate complex, amsacrine, doxorubicin liposome, fluconazole, idarubicin, midazolam, pentamidine, warfarin

Compatibility when admixed: Incompatible with aminoglycosides in same bottle/bag, aminophylline, ranitidine

Related Information

Cephalosporins by Generation *on page 1858*

♦ Ceftin® *see* Cefuroxime *on page 356*

Ceftizoxime (sef ti ZOKS eem)

U.S. Brand Names Cefizox®

Synonyms Ceftizoxime Sodium

Pharmacologic Category Antibiotic, Cephalosporin (Third Generation)

Medication Safety Issues

Sound-alike/look-alike issues:

Ceftizoxime may be confused with cefotaxime, ceftazidime, cefuroxime

Use Treatment of susceptible bacterial infection, mainly respiratory tract, skin and skin structure, bone and joint, urinary tract and gynecologic, as well as septicemia; active against many gram-negative bacilli (not *Pseudomonas*), some gram-positive cocci (not *Enterococcus*), and some anaerobes

Mechanism of Action Inhibits bacterial cell wall synthesis by binding to one or more of the penicillin-binding proteins (PBPs) which in turn inhibits the final transpeptidation step of peptidoglycan synthesis in bacterial cell walls, thus inhibiting cell wall biosynthesis. Bacteria eventually lyse due to ongoing activity of cell wall autolytic enzymes (autolysins and murein hydrolases) while cell wall assembly is arrested.

Pharmacodynamics/Kinetics

Distribution: V_d: 0.35-0.5 L/kg; widely into most body tissues and fluids including gallbladder, liver, kidneys, bone, sputum, bile, pleural and synovial fluids; has good CSF penetration; crosses placenta; small amounts enter breast milk

Protein binding: 30%

Half-life elimination: 1.6 hours; Cl_{cr} <10 mL/minute: 25 hours

Time to peak, serum: I.M.: 0.5-1 hour

Excretion: Urine (as unchanged drug)

Contraindications Hypersensitivity to ceftizoxime, any component of the formulation, or other cephalosporins

Warnings/Precautions Modify dosage in patients with severe renal impairment, prolonged use may result in superinfection; use with caution in patients with a history of penicillin allergy, especially IgE-mediated reactions (eg, anaphylaxis, urticaria). May cause antibiotic-associated colitis or colitis secondary to *C. difficile*.

Drug Interactions

Increased effect: Probenecid may decrease cephalosporin elimination

Increased toxicity: Aminoglycosides and furosemide may increase nephrotoxic potential

Lab Interactions Positive direct Coombs', false-positive urinary glucose test using cupric sulfate (Benedict's solution, Clinitest®, Fehling's solution), false-positive serum or urine creatinine with Jaffé reaction

Adverse Reactions

1% to 10%:

Central nervous system: Fever

Dermatologic: Rash, pruritus

Hematologic: Eosinophilia, thrombocytosis

Hepatic: Alkaline phosphatase increased, transaminases increased

Local: Pain, burning at injection site

<1% (Limited to important or life-threatening): Anaphylaxis, anemia, bilirubin increased, BUN increased, creatinine increased, diarrhea, injection site reactions, leukopenia, nausea, neutropenia, numbness, paresthesia, phlebitis, thrombocytopenia, vaginitis, vomiting

Other reactions reported with cephalosporins include agranulocytosis, angioedema, aplastic anemia, asterixis, candidiasis, cholestasis, colitis, encephalopathy, erythema multiforme, hemolytic anemia, hemorrhage, interstitial nephritis, neuromuscular excitability, pancytopenia, prolonged PT, pseudomembranous colitis, renal dysfunction, seizure, serum-sickness reactions, Stevens-Johnson syndrome, superinfection, toxic epidermal necrolysis, toxic nephropathy

(Continued)

Ceftizoxime *(Continued)*

Overdosage/Toxicology Symptoms of overdose include neuromuscular hypersensitivity and convulsions. Many beta-lactam containing antibiotics have the potential to cause neuromuscular hyperirritability or convulsive seizures. Hemodialysis may be helpful to aid in removal of the drug from blood; otherwise, treatment is supportive or symptom-directed.

Dosing

Adults & Elderly: Susceptible infections: I.M., I.V.: 1-2 g every 8-12 hours, up to 2 g every 4 hours or 4 g every 8 hours for life-threatening infections

Pediatrics: Susceptible infections: I.M., I.V.: Children ≥6 months: 150-200 mg/kg/day divided every 6-8 hours (maximum of 12 g/24 hours)

Renal Impairment:

Cl_{cr} 50-79 mL/minute: Administer 500-1500 mg every 8 hours.

Cl_{cr} 5-49 mL/minute: Administer 250-1000 mg every 12 hours.

Cl_{cr} 0-4 mL/minute: Administer 500-1000 mg every 48 hours or 250-500 mg every 24 hours.

Moderately dialyzable (20% to 50%)

Continuous arteriovenous hemofiltration: Dose as for Cl_{cr} 10-50 mL/minute.

Available Dosage Forms

Infusion [premixed iso-osmotic solution]: 1 g (50 mL); 2 g (50 mL)

Injection, powder for reconstitution: 1 g, 2 g, 10 g

Nursing Guidelines

Assessment: Assess for previous allergy history prior to therapy. See Contraindications and Warnings/Precautions for use cautions. Assess potential for interactions with other prescriptions, OTC medications, or herbal products patient may be taking (eg, nephrotoxicity - see Drug Interactions). Assess results of laboratory tests (see below), therapeutic response, and adverse effects (see Adverse Reactions and Overdose/Toxicology). Advise patients with diabetes about use of Clinitest®. Teach patient possible side effects/appropriate interventions and adverse symptoms to report (see Patient Education). Note breast-feeding caution.

Monitoring Laboratory Tests: Perform culture and sensitivity studies prior to initiating drug therapy; renal function

Dietary Considerations: Sodium content of 1 g: 60 mg (2.6 mEq)

Patient Education: Inform prescriber of all prescriptions, OTC medications, or herbal products you are taking, and any allergies you have. Do not take any new medication during therapy unless approved by prescriber. This medication is administered by infusion or injection. Report immediately any redness, swelling, burning, or pain at injection/infusion site; itching or hives; or difficulty swallowing or breathing. Maintain adequate hydration (2-3 L/day of fluids) unless instructed to restrict fluid intake. May cause false test results with Clinitest®; use of another type of glucose testing is preferable. Report opportunistic infection (vaginal itching or drainage; sores in mouth; blood, pus, or mucus in stool or urine; or easy bleeding or bruising). **Breast-feeding precaution:** Consult prescriber if breast-feeding.

Geriatric Considerations: Adjust dose for renal function in the elderly.

Pregnancy Risk Factor: B

Lactation: Enters breast milk (small amounts)/use caution

Breast-Feeding Considerations: Theoretically, drug absorbed by nursing infant may change bowel flora or affect fever work-up result. **Note:** As a class, cephalosporins are used to treat infections in infants.

Administration

I.M.: Inject deep I.M. into large muscle mass.

I.V.: Inject direct I.V. over 3-5 minutes. Infuse intermittent infusion over 30 minutes.

Reconstitution: Reconstituted solution is stable for 24 hours at room temperature and 96 hours when refrigerated. For I.V. infusion in NS or D_5W, solution is stable for 24 hours at room temperature, 96 hours when refrigerated or 12 weeks when frozen. After freezing, thawed solution is stable for 24 hours at room temperature or 10 days when refrigerated.

Compatibility: Stable in D_5¼NS, D_5½NS, D_5NS, D_5W, $D_{10}W$, LR, NS, sodium bicarbonate 5%

Y-site administration: Incompatible with filgrastim

Related Information

Cephalosporins by Generation *on page 1858*

♦ **Ceftizoxime Sodium** *see* Ceftizoxime *on page 351*

Ceftriaxone (sef trye AKS one)

U.S. Brand Names Rocephin®

Synonyms Ceftriaxone Sodium

Pharmacologic Category Antibiotic, Cephalosporin (Third Generation)

Medication Safety Issues

Sound-alike/look-alike issues:

Rocephin® may be confused with Roferon®

Use Treatment of lower respiratory tract infections, acute bacterial otitis media, skin and skin structure infections, bone and joint infections, intra-abdominal and urinary tract infections, pelvic inflammatory disease (PID), uncomplicated gonorrhea, bacterial septicemia, and meningitis; used in surgical prophylaxis

Unlabeled/Investigational Use Treatment of chancroid, epididymitis, complicated gonococcal infections; sexually-transmitted diseases (STD); periorbital or buccal cellulitis; salmonellosis or shigellosis; atypical community-acquired pneumonia; Lyme disease; used in chemoprophylaxis for high-risk contacts and persons with invasive meningococcal disease; sexual assault

Mechanism of Action Inhibits bacterial cell wall synthesis by binding to one or more of the penicillin-binding proteins (PBPs) which in turn inhibits the final transpeptidation step of peptidoglycan synthesis in bacterial cell walls, thus inhibiting cell wall biosynthesis. Bacteria eventually lyse due to ongoing activity of cell wall autolytic enzymes (autolysins and murein hydrolases) while cell wall assembly is arrested.

Pharmacodynamics/Kinetics

Absorption: I.M.: Well absorbed

Distribution: Widely throughout the body including gallbladder, lungs, bone, bile, CSF (higher concentrations achieved when meninges are inflamed); crosses placenta; enters amniotic fluid and breast milk

Protein binding: 85% to 95%

Half-life elimination: Normal renal and hepatic function: 5-9 hours

Time to peak, serum: I.M.: 1-2 hours

Excretion: Urine (33% to 65% as unchanged drug); feces

Contraindications Hypersensitivity to ceftriaxone sodium, any component of the formulation, or other cephalosporins; **do not use in hyperbilirubinemic neonates**, particularly those who are premature since ceftriaxone is reported to displace bilirubin from albumin binding sites

Warnings/Precautions Modify dosage in patients with severe renal impairment, prolonged use may result in superinfection. Use with caution in patients with a history of penicillin allergy, especially IgE-mediated reactions (eg, anaphylaxis, urticaria). May cause antibiotic-associated colitis or colitis secondary to *C. difficile.* Discontinue in patients with signs and symptoms of gallbladder disease.

Drug Interactions

Coumarin derivative (eg, dicumarol, warfarin): Cephalosporins may increase the anticoagulant effect of coumarin derivatives.

Uricosuric agents (eg, probenecid, sulfinpyrazone): Uricosuric agents may decrease the excretion of cephalosporin; monitor for toxic effects.

Lab Interactions Positive direct Coombs', false-positive urinary glucose test using cupric sulfate (Benedict's solution, Clinitest®, Fehling's solution), false-positive serum or urine creatinine with Jaffé reaction

Adverse Reactions

1% to 10%:

Dermatologic: Rash (2%)

Gastrointestinal: Diarrhea (3%)

Hematologic: Eosinophilia (6%), thrombocytosis (5%), leukopenia (2%)

Hepatic: Transaminases increased (3.1% to 3.3%)

Local: Pain, induration at injection site (I.V. 1%); warmth, tightness, induration (5% to 17%) following I.M. injection

Renal: Increased BUN (1%)

<1% (Limited to important or life-threatening): Agranulocytosis, allergic pneumonitis, anaphylaxis, anemia, basophilia, bronchospasm, candidiasis, chills, colitis, diaphoresis, dizziness, dysgeusia, flushing, gallstones, glycosuria, headache, hematuria, hemolytic anemia, jaundice, leukocytosis, lymphocytosis, lymphopenia, monocytosis, nausea, nephrolithiasis, neutropenia, phlebitis, prolonged or decreased PT, pruritus, pseudomembranous colitis, renal precipitations, renal stones, seizure, serum sickness, thrombocytopenia, urinary casts, vaginitis, vomiting; increased alkaline phosphatase, bilirubin, and creatinine

(Continued)

Ceftriaxone *(Continued)*

Reactions reported with other cephalosporins include angioedema, aplastic anemia, asterixis, cholestasis, encephalopathy, erythema multiforme, hemorrhage, interstitial nephritis, neuromuscular excitability, pancytopenia, paresthesia, renal dysfunction, Stevens-Johnson syndrome, superinfection, toxic epidermal necrolysis, toxic nephropathy

Overdosage/Toxicology Symptoms of overdose include neuromuscular hypersensitivity and convulsions. Many beta-lactam containing antibiotics have the potential to cause neuromuscular hyperirritability or convulsive seizures. Hemodialysis may be helpful to aid in removal of the drug from blood; otherwise, treatment is supportive or symptom-directed.

Dosing

Adults & Elderly:

Dosage range: Usual dose: 1-2 g every 12-24 hours, depending on the type and severity of infection

Meningitis:I.V.: 2 g every 12 hours for 7-14 days (longer courses may be necessary for selected organisms

Chemoprophylaxis for high-risk contacts and persons with invasive meningococcal disease (unlabeled use): I.M.: 250 mg in a single dose

Epididymitis, acute (unlabeled use): I.M.: 250 mg in a single dose

Gonococcal conjunctivitis, complicated (unlabeled use): I.M.: 1 g in a single dose

Gonococcal endocarditis (unlabeled use): I.M., I.V.: 1-2 g every 12 hours for at least 28 days

Gonococcal infection, disseminated (unlabeled use): I.M., I.V.: 1 g once daily for 7 days

Gonococcal infection, uncomplicated: I.M.: 125-250 mg in a single dose

PID: I.M.: 250 mg in a single dose

Surgical prophylaxis: I.V.: 1 g 30 minutes to 2 hours before surgery

Pediatrics:

Dosage range: Infants and Children: Usual dose: I.M., I.V.:

Mild-to-moderate infections: 50-75 mg/kg/day in 1-2 divided doses every 12-24 hours (maximum: 2 g/day); continue until at least 2 days after signs and symptoms of infection have resolved

Serious infections: 80-100 mg/kg/day in 1-2 divided doses (maximum: 4 g/day)

Gonococcal infection, uncomplicated: I.M.: 125 mg in a single dose

Gonococcal conjunctivitis, complicated (unlabeled use): I.M.:

<45 kg: 50 mg/kg in a single dose (maximum: 1 g)

>45 kg: 1 g in a single dose

Gonococcal endocarditis (unlabeled use):

<45 kg: I.M., I.V.: 50 mg/kg/day every 12 hours (maximum: 2 g/day) for at least 28 days

>45 kg: I.V.: 1-2 g every 12 hours, for at least 28 days

Gonococcal infection, disseminated (unlabeled use): I.M., I.V.:

<45 kg: 25-50 mg/kg once daily (maximum: 1 g)

>45 kg: 1 g once daily for 7 days

Meningitis: I.M., I.V.:

Uncomplicated: Loading dose of 100 mg/kg (maximum: 4 g), followed by 100 mg/kg/day divided every 12-24 hours (maximum: 4 g/day); usual duration of treatment is 7-14 days

Gonococcal, complicated:

<45 kg: 50 mg/kg/day given every 12 hours (maximum: 2 g/day); usual duration of treatment is 10-14 days

>45 kg: I.V.: 1-2 g every 12 hours; usual duration of treatment is 10-14 days

Otitis media: I.M., I.V.:

Acute: 50 mg/kg in a single dose (maximum: 1 g)

Persistent or relapsing (unlabeled use): 50 mg/kg once daily for 3 days

STD, sexual assault (unlabeled uses): 125 mg in a single dose

Chemoprophylaxis for high-risk contacts and persons with invasive meningococcal disease (unlabeled use):

Children ≤15 years: I.M.: 125 mg in a single dose

Children >15 years: Refer to adult dosing.

Epididymitis, acute: Children >8 years (≥45 kg) and Adolescents (unlabeled use): I.M.: 125 mg in a single dose

Renal Impairment:

No adjustment is necessary.

Not dialyzable (0% to 5%)

Administer dose postdialysis.

Peritoneal dialysis effects: Administer 750 mg every 12 hours.

Continuous arteriovenous or venovenous hemofiltration: Removes 10 mg of ceftriaxone of liter of filtrate per day.

Hepatic Impairment: No adjustment necessary.

Available Dosage Forms Note: Contains sodium 83 mg (3.6 mEq) per ceftriaxone 1 g

Infusion [premixed in dextrose]: 1 g (50 mL); 2 g (50 mL)

Injection, powder for reconstitution: 250 mg, 500 mg, 1 g, 2 g, 10 g

Nursing Guidelines

Assessment: Assess for previous allergy history prior to therapy. See Contraindications, Warnings/Precautions, and Dosing for use cautions. See Administration (I.V. and I.M.) specifics below. Assess potential for interactions with other prescriptions, OTC medications, or herbal products patient may be taking (eg, nephrotoxicity - see Drug Interactions). Assess results of laboratory tests (see below) therapeutic response, and adverse effects (see Adverse Reactions and Overdose/Toxicology). Advise patients with diabetes about use of Clinitest®. Teach patient possible side effects/appropriate interventions and adverse symptoms to report (see Patient Education). Note breast-feeding caution.

Monitoring Laboratory Tests: Prothrombin times; perform culture and sensitivity studies prior to initiating drug therapy.

Dietary Considerations: Sodium contents: 83 mg (3.6 mEq) per ceftriaxone 1 g

Patient Education: Inform prescriber of all prescriptions, OTC medications, or herbal products you are taking, and any allergies you have. Do not take any new medication during therapy unless approved by prescriber. This medication is administered by infusion or injection. Report immediately any redness, swelling, burning or pain at injection/infusion site; rash, itching, or hives; or difficulty swallowing or breathing. Maintain adequate hydration (2-3 L/day of fluids) unless instructed to restrict fluid intake. May cause false test results with Clinitest®; use of another type of glucose testing is preferable. May cause diarrhea (yogurt, boiled milk, or buttermilk may help). Report unresolved diarrhea; opportunistic infection (vaginal itching or drainage; sores in mouth; blood, pus, or mucus in stool or urine); easy bleeding or bruising; unusual fever or chills; rash; or respiratory difficulty. **Breast-feeding precaution:** Consult prescriber if breast-feeding.

Geriatric Considerations: No adjustment for changes in renal function necessary.

Pregnancy Risk Factor: B

Lactation: Enters breast milk/use caution (AAP rates "compatible")

Breast-Feeding Considerations: Theoretically, drug absorbed by nursing infant may change bowel flora or affect fever work-up result. **Note:** As a class, cephalosporins are used to treat infections in infants.

Administration

I.M.: Inject deep I.M. into large muscle mass; a concentration of 250 mg/mL or 350 mg/mL is recommended for all vial sizes except the 250 mg size (250 mg/mL is suggested); can be diluted with 1:1 water and 1% lidocaine for I.M. administration

I.V.: Do not admix with aminoglycosides in same bottle/bag. Infuse intermittent infusion over 30 minutes.

Reconstitution:

I.M. injection: Vials should be reconstituted with appropriate volume of diluent (including D_5W, NS, or 1% lidocaine) to make a final concentration of 250 mg/mL or 350 mg/mL.

Volume to add to create a **250 mg/mL** solution:

250 mg vial: 0.9 mL

500 mg vial: 1.8 mL

1 g vial: 3.6 mL

2 g vial: 7.2 mL

Volume to add to create a **350 mg/mL** solution:

500 mg vial: 1.0 mL

1 g vial: 2.1 mL

2 g vial: 4.2 mL

I.V. infusion: Infusion is prepared in two stages: Initial reconstitution of powder, followed by dilution to final infusion solution.

(Continued)

Ceftriaxone *(Continued)*

Vials: Reconstitute powder with appropriate I.V. diluent (including SWFI, D_5W, NS) to create an initial solution of ~100 mg/mL. Recommended volume to add:

250 mg vial: 2.4 mL

500 mg vial: 4.8 mL

1 g vial: 9.6 mL

2 g vial: 19.2 mL

Note: After reconstitution of powder, further dilution into a volume of compatible solution (eg, 50-100 mL of D_5W or NS) is recommended.

Piggyback bottle: Reconstitute powder with appropriate I.V. diluent (D_5W or NS) to create a resulting solution of ~100 mg/mL. Recommended initial volume to add:

1 g bottle:10 mL

2 g bottle: 20 mL

Note: After reconstitution, to prepare the final infusion solution, further dilution to 50 mL or 100 mL volumes with the appropriate I.V. diluent (including D_5W or NS) is recommended.

Compatibility: Stable in D_5W with KCl 10 mEq, D_5¼NS with KCl 20 mEq, D_5½ NS, D_5W, $D_{10}W$, NS, mannitol 5%, mannitol 10%, sodium bicarbonate 5%, bacteriostatic water, SWFI

Y-site administration: Incompatible with alatrofloxacin, amphotericin B cholesteryl sulfate complex, amsacrine, filgrastim, fluconazole, labetalol, pentamidine, vinorelbine

Compatibility when admixed: Incompatible with aminophylline, clindamycin, linezolid, theophylline

Storage:

Powder for injection: Prior to reconstitution, store at room temperature of 25°C (77°F); protect from light.

Premixed solution (manufacturer premixed): Store at -20°C; once thawed, solutions are stable for 3 days at room temperature of 25°C (77°F) or for 21 days refrigerated at 5°C (41°F). Do not refreeze.

Stability of reconstituted solutions:

10-40 mg/mL: Reconstituted in D_5W or NS: Stable for 2 days at room temperature of 25°C (77°F) or for 10 days when refrigerated at 5°C (41°F).

100 mg/mL:

Reconstituted in D_5W or NS: Stable for 2 days at room temperature of 25°C (77°F) or for 10 days when refrigerated at 5°C (41°F). Stable for 26 weeks when frozen at -20°C. Once thawed, solutions are stable for 2 days at room temperature of 25°C (77°F) or for 10 days when refrigerated at 5°C (41°F); does not apply to manufacturer's premixed bags. Do not refreeze.

Reconstituted in lidocaine 1% solution: Stable for 24 hours at room temperature of 25°C (77°F) or for 10 days when refrigerated at 5°C (41°F).

250-350 mg/mL: Reconstituted in D_5W, NS, lidocaine 1% solution, or SWFI: Stable for 24 hours at room temperature of 25°C (77°F) or for 3 days when refrigerated at 5°C (41°F).

Related Information

Cephalosporins by Generation *on page 1858*

♦ Ceftriaxone Sodium *see* Ceftriaxone *on page 353*

Cefuroxime (se fyoor OKS eem)

U.S. Brand Names Ceftin®; Zinacef®

Synonyms Cefuroxime Axetil; Cefuroxime Sodium

Pharmacologic Category Antibiotic, Cephalosporin (Second Generation)

Medication Safety Issues

Sound-alike/look-alike issues:

Cefuroxime may be confused with cefotaxime, cefprozil, ceftizoxime, deferoxamine

Ceftin® may be confused with Cefotan®, cefotetan, Cefzil®, Cipro®

Zinacef® may be confused with Zithromax®

Use Treatment of infections caused by staphylococci, group B streptococci, *H. influenzae* (type A and B), *E. coli*, *Enterobacter*, *Salmonella*, and *Klebsiella*; treatment of susceptible infections of the lower respiratory tract, otitis media, urinary tract, skin and soft tissue, bone and joint, sepsis and gonorrhea

Mechanism of Action Inhibits bacterial cell wall synthesis by binding to one or more of the penicillin-binding proteins (PBPs) which in turn inhibits the final transpeptidation step of peptidoglycan synthesis in bacterial cell walls, thus inhibiting cell wall biosynthesis. Bacteria eventually lyse due to ongoing activity of cell wall autolytic enzymes (autolysins and murein hydrolases) while cell wall assembly is arrested.

Pharmacodynamics/Kinetics

Absorption: Oral (cefuroxime axetil): Increases with food

Distribution: Widely to body tissues and fluids; crosses blood-brain barrier; therapeutic concentrations achieved in CSF even when meninges are not inflamed; crosses placenta; enters breast milk

Protein binding: 33% to 50%

Bioavailability: Tablet: Fasting: 37%; Following food: 52%

Half-life elimination: Adults: 1-2 hours; prolonged with renal impairment

Time to peak, serum: I.M.: ~15-60 minutes; I.V.: 2-3 minutes

Excretion: Urine (66% to 100% as unchanged drug)

Contraindications Hypersensitivity to cefuroxime, any component of the formulation, or other cephalosporins

Warnings/Precautions Modify dosage in patients with severe renal impairment, prolonged use may result in superinfection; use with caution in patients with a history of penicillin allergy, especially IgE-mediated reactions (eg, anaphylaxis, urticaria). May cause antibiotic-associated colitis or colitis secondary to *C. difficile.* May be associated with increased INR, especially in nutritionally-deficient patients, prolonged treatment, hepatic or renal disease. Tablets and oral suspension are not bioequivalent (do not substitute on a mg-per-mg basis).

Drug Interactions

Increased effect: High-dose probenecid decreases clearance

Increased toxicity: Aminoglycosides increase nephrotoxic potential

Nutritional/Herbal/Ethanol Interactions Food: Bioavailability is increased with food; cefuroxime serum levels may be increased if taken with food or dairy products.

Lab Interactions Positive direct Coombs', false-positive urinary glucose test using cupric sulfate (Benedict's solution, Clinitest®, Fehling's solution), false-positive serum or urine creatinine with Jaffé reaction

Adverse Reactions

1% to 10%:

Hematologic: Eosinophilia (7%), decreased hemoglobin and hematocrit (10%)

Hepatic: Increased transaminases (4%), increased alkaline phosphatase (2%)

Local: Thrombophlebitis (1.7%)

<1% (Limited to important or life-threatening): Anaphylaxis, angioedema, BUN increased, cholestasis, colitis, creatinine increased, diarrhea, dizziness, erythema multiforme, fever, GI bleeding, hemolytic anemia, headache, hepatitis, interstitial nephritis, jaundice, leukopenia, nausea, neutropenia, pain at injection site, pancytopenia, prolonged PT/INR, pseudomembranous colitis, rash, seizure, Stevens-Johnson syndrome, stomach cramps, thrombocytopenia, toxic epidermal necrolysis, vaginitis, vomiting

Other reactions with cephalosporins include agranulocytosis, aplastic anemia, asterixis, colitis, encephalopathy, hemorrhage, neuromuscular excitability, serum-sickness reactions, superinfection, toxic nephropathy

Overdosage/Toxicology Symptoms of overdose include neuromuscular hypersensitivity and convulsions. Many beta-lactam containing antibiotics have the potential to cause neuromuscular hyperirritability or convulsive seizures. Hemodialysis may be helpful to aid in removal of the drug from blood; otherwise, treatment is supportive or symptom-directed.

Dosing

Adults & Elderly: Note: Cefuroxime axetil film-coated tablets and oral suspension are not bioequivalent and are not substitutable on a mg/mg basis.

Acute bacterial maxillary sinusitis: Oral: 250 mg twice daily for 10 days

Bronchitis, acute (and exacerbations of chronic bronchitis):

Oral: 250-500 mg every 12 hours for 10 days

I.V.: 500-750 mg every 8 hours (complete therapy with oral dosing)

Gonococcal infection, uncomplicated:

Oral: 1 g as a single dose

I.M.: 1.5 g as a single dose (administered at two different sites along with 1 g oral probenecid)

Gonococcal infection, disseminated: I.M., I.V.: 750 mg every 8 hours

Lyme disease (early): Oral: 500 mg twice daily for 20 days

(Continued)

Cefuroxime *(Continued)*

Pharyngitis, tonsillitis: Oral: 250 mg twice daily for 10 days
Skin/skin structure infection, uncomplicated:
Oral: 250-500 mg every 12 hours for 10 days
I.M., I.V.: 750 mg every 8 hours
Urinary tract infection, uncomplicated:
Oral: 125-250 mg twice daily for 7-10 days
I.V., I.M.: 750 mg every 8 hours
Pneumonia, uncomplicated: I.M., I.V.: 750 mg every 8 hours
Severe or complicated infections: I.M., I.V.: 1.5 g every 8 hours (up to 1.5 g every 6 hours in life-threatening infections)
Surgical prophylaxis: I.V.: 1.5 g 30 minutes to 1 hour before procedure; 750 mg every 8 hours I.M. when procedure is prolonged
Open heart surgery: I.V.: 1.5 g at the induction of anesthesia and every 12 hours thereafter to a total of 6 g is recommended

Pediatrics: Note: Cefuroxime axetil film-coated tablets and oral suspension are not bioequivalent and are not substitutable on a mg/mg basis.

Children ≥3 months to 12 years:
Pharyngitis, tonsillitis:
Oral:
Suspension: 20 mg/kg/day (maximum: 500 mg/day) in 2 divided doses for 10 days
Tablet: 125 mg every 12 hours for 10 days
I.M., I.V.: 75-150 mg/kg/day divided every 8 hours; maximum dose: 6 g/day
Acute otitis media, impetigo:
Oral:
Suspension: 30 mg/kg/day (maximum: 1 g/day) in 2 divided doses
Tablet: 250 mg every 12 hours
I.M., I.V.: 75-150 mg/kg/day divided every 8 hours; maximum dose: 6 g/day
Meningitis: NOT recommended (doses of 200-240 mg/kg/day divided every 6-8 hours have been used); maximum dose: 9 g/day
Acute bacterial maxillary sinusitis: Oral:
Suspension: 30 mg/kg/day in 2 divided doses for 10 days; maximum dose: 1 g/day
Tablet: 250 mg twice daily for 10 days
Children ≥13 years: Refer to adult dosing.

Renal Impairment:
Cl_{cr} 10-20 mL/minute: Administer every 12 hours.
Cl_{cr} <10 mL/minute: Administer every 24 hours.
Hemodialysis: Dialyzable (25%)
Note: Cefuroxime axetil film-coated tablets and oral suspension are not bioequivalent and are not substitutable on a mg/mg basis.
Continuous arteriovenous or venovenous hemodiafiltration effects: Dose as for Cl_{cr} 10-20 mL/minute.

Available Dosage Forms

Infusion, as sodium [premixed] (Zinacef®): 750 mg (50 mL); 1.5 g (50 mL) [contains sodium 4.8 mEq (111 mg) per 750 mg]
Injection, powder for reconstitution, as sodium (Zinacef®): 750 mg, 1.5 g, 7.5 g [contains sodium 4.8 mEq (111 mg) per 750 mg]
Powder for oral suspension, as axetil (Ceftin®): 125 mg/5 mL (100 mL) [contains phenylalanine 11.8 mg/5 mL; tutti-frutti flavor]; 250 mg/5 mL (50 mL, 100 mL) [contains phenylalanine 25.2 mg/5 mL; tutti-frutti flavor]
Tablet, as axetil (Ceftin®): 250 mg, 500 mg

Nursing Guidelines

Assessment: Assess for previous allergy history prior to therapy. See Contraindications, Warnings/Precautions and Dosing for use cautions. Assess potential for interactions with other prescriptions, OTC medications, or herbal products patient may be taking (eg, nephrotoxicity - see Drug Interactions). Assess results of laboratory tests (see below), therapeutic response, and adverse reactions (see Adverse Reactions and Overdose/Toxicology). Advise patients with diabetes about use of Clinitest®. Teach patient proper use, possible side effects/appropriate interventions, and adverse symptoms to report (see Patient Education). Note breast-feeding caution.

Monitoring Laboratory Tests: Perform culture and sensitivity studies prior to initiating therapy; renal function

Dietary Considerations: May be taken with food.
Zinacef®: Sodium content: 4.8 mEq (111 mg) per 750 mg

Ceftin®: Powder for oral suspension 125 mg/5 mL contains phenylalanine 11.8 mg/5 mL; 250 mg/5 mL contains phenylalanine 25.2 mg/5 mL.

Patient Education: Inform prescriber of all prescriptions, OTC medications, or herbal products you are taking, and any allergies you have. Do not take any new medication during therapy unless approved by prescriber. If administered by injection or infusion, report immediately any swelling, redness, or pain at injection/infusion site; respiratory difficulty or swallowing; chest pain; or rash. Oral suspension should be taken as directed, at regular intervals around-the-clock (with or without food); complete full course of medication, even if you feel better. Chilling suspension improves flavor (do not freeze). Maintain adequate hydration (2-3 L/day of fluids) unless instructed to restrict fluid intake. May cause false test results with Clinitest®; use of another type of glucose testing is preferable. Report unusual bruising or bleeding; or opportunistic infection (vaginal itching or drainage, sores in mouth, blood in urine or stool).

Breast-feeding precaution: Consult prescriber if breast-feeding.

Geriatric Considerations: Adjust dose for renal function in the elderly. Considered one of the drugs of choice for outpatient treatment of community-acquired pneumonia in the older adult.

Pregnancy Risk Factor: B

Lactation: Enters breast milk/use caution

Breast-Feeding Considerations: Theoretically, drug absorbed by nursing infant may change bowel flora or affect fever work-up result. **Note:** As a class, cephalosporins are used to treat infections in infants.

Administration

Oral: Administer around-the-clock to promote less variation in peak and trough serum levels. Oral suspension: Administer with food. Shake well before use.

I.M.: Inject deep I.M. into large muscle mass.

I.V.: Inject direct I.V. over 3-5 minutes. Infuse intermittent infusion over 15-30 minutes.

Reconstitution:

Injectable: Reconstituted solution is stable for 24 hours at room temperature and 48 hours when refrigerated. I.V. infusion in NS or D_5W solution is stable for 24 hours at room temperature, 7 days when refrigerated, or 26 weeks when frozen. After freezing, thawed solution is stable for 24 hours at room temperature or 21 days when refrigerated.

Oral suspension: Store in refrigerator or at room temperature. Discard after 10 days.

Compatibility: Stable in $D_5{}^1/_4NS$, $D_5{}^1/_2NS$, D_5NS, D_5W, $D_{10}W$, LR, NS

Y-site administration: Incompatible with clarithromycin, filgrastim, fluconazole, midazolam, vinorelbine

Compatibility in syringe: Incompatible with doxapram

Compatibility when admixed: Incompatible with aminoglycosides, sodium bicarbonate

Related Information

Cephalosporins by Generation *on page 1858*

Prevention of Wound Infection and Sepsis in Surgical Patients *on page 1830*

- **Cefuroxime Axetil** *see* Cefuroxime *on page 356*
- **Cefuroxime Sodium** *see* Cefuroxime *on page 356*
- **Cefzil®** *see* Cefprozil *on page 346*
- **Celebrex®** *see* Celecoxib *on page 359*

Celecoxib (se le KOKS ib)

U.S. Brand Names Celebrex®

Pharmacologic Category Nonsteroidal Anti-inflammatory Drug (NSAID), COX-2 Selective

Medication Safety Issues

Sound-alike/look-alike issues:

Celebrex® may be confused with Celexa™, cerebra, Cerebyx®

Use Relief of the signs and symptoms of osteoarthritis, ankylosing spondylitis, and rheumatoid arthritis; management of acute pain; treatment of primary dysmenorrhea; decreasing intestinal polyps in familial adenomatous polyposis (FAP). **Note:** The Notice of Compliance for the use of celecoxib in FAP has been suspended by Health Canada.

Mechanism of Action Inhibits prostaglandin synthesis by decreasing the activity of the enzyme, cyclooxygenase-2 (COX-2), which results in decreased formation

(Continued)

Celecoxib *(Continued)*

of prostaglandin precursors. Celecoxib does not inhibit cyclooxygenase-1 (COX-1) at therapeutic concentrations.

Pharmacodynamics/Kinetics

Distribution: V_d (apparent): 400 L

Protein binding: 97% to albumin

Metabolism: Hepatic via CYP2C9; forms inactive metabolites

Bioavailability: Absolute: Unknown

Half-life elimination: 11 hours (fasted)

Time to peak: 3 hours

Excretion: Urine (27% as metabolites, <3% as unchanged drug); feces (57%)

Contraindications Hypersensitivity to celecoxib, sulfonamides, aspirin, other NSAIDs, or any component of the formulation; perioperative pain in the setting of coronary artery bypass surgery (CABG); pregnancy (3rd trimester)

Warnings/Precautions NSAIDs are associated with an increased risk of adverse cardiovascular events, including MI, and new onset or worsening of pre-existing hypertension. Risk may be increased with duration of use or pre-existing cardiovascular risk-factors or disease. Carefully evaluate individual cardiovascular risk profiles prior to prescribing. Use caution with fluid retention, CHF, cerebrovascular disease, ischemic heart disease, or hypertension.

NSAIDs may increase risk of gastrointestinal irritation, ulceration, bleeding, and perforation. These events may occur at any time during therapy and without warning. Use caution with a history of GI disease (bleeding or ulcers), concurrent therapy with aspirin, anticoagulants and/or corticosteroids, smoking, use of alcohol, the elderly or debilitated patients.

Use the lowest effective dose for the shortest duration of time, consistent with individual patient goals, to reduce risk of cardiovascular or GI adverse events. Alternate therapies should be considered for patients at high risk.

NSAIDs may cause serious skin adverse events including exfoliative dermatitis, Stevens-Johnson syndrome (SJS), and toxic epidermal necrolysis (TEN). Anaphylactoid reactions may occur, even without prior exposure; patients with 'aspirin triad' (bronchial asthma, aspirin intolerance, rhinitis) may be at increased risk. Do not use in patients who experience bronchospasm, asthma, rhinitis, or urticaria with NSAID or aspirin therapy.

Use with caution in patients with dehydration, decreased renal or hepatic function. Use of NSAIDs can compromise existing renal function especially when Cl_{cr} <30 mL/minute. Not recommended for use in severe renal or hepatic impairment.

Anaphylactoid reactions may occur, even with no prior exposure to celecoxib. Use caution in patients with known or suspected deficiency of cytochrome P450 isoenzyme 2C9. Safety and efficacy have not been established in patients <18 years of age.

Drug Interactions **Substrate** (minor) of CYP2C8/9, 3A4; **Inhibits** CYP2D6 (weak)

ACE inhibitors: Antihypertensive effect may be diminished by celecoxib.

Aminoglycosides: Celecoxib may decrease excretion; monitor levels.

Aspirin: Low-dose aspirin may be used with celecoxib, however, monitor for GI complications.

Beta-blockers: Antihypertensive effect may be diminished by celecoxib.

Bile acid sequestrants: May decrease absorption of NSAIDs.

Cyclosporine: NSAIDs may increase levels/nephrotoxicity of cyclosporine.

Fluconazole: Fluconazole increases celecoxib concentrations twofold. Lowest dose of celecoxib should be used.

Hydralazine: Antihypertensive effect may be diminished by celecoxib.

Lithium: Plasma levels of lithium are increased by ~17% when used with celecoxib. Monitor lithium levels closely when treatment with celecoxib is started or withdrawn.

Loop diuretics (bumetanide, furosemide, torsemide): Natriuretic effect of furosemide and other loop diuretics may be decreased by celecoxib.

Methotrexate: Severe bone marrow suppression, aplastic anemia, and GI toxicity have been reported with concomitant NSAID therapy. Selective COX-2 inhibitors appear to have a lower risk of this toxicity, however, caution is warranted.

Thiazide diuretics: Natriuretic effects of thiazide diuretics may be decreased by celecoxib.

Vancomycin: Celecoxib may decrease excretion; monitor levels.

Warfarin: Bleeding events (including rare intracranial hemorrhage in association with increased prothrombin time) have been reported with concomitant use. Monitor closely, especially in the elderly.

Nutritional/Herbal/Ethanol Interactions

Ethanol: Avoid ethanol (increased GI irritation).

Food: Peak concentrations are delayed and AUC is increased by 10% to 20% when taken with a high-fat meal.

Adverse Reactions

>10%: Central nervous system: Headache (15.8%)

2% to 10%:

Cardiovascular: Peripheral edema (2.1%)

Central nervous system: Insomnia (2.3%), dizziness (2%)

Dermatologic: Skin rash (2.2%)

Gastrointestinal: Dyspepsia (8.8%), diarrhea (5.6%), abdominal pain (4.1%), nausea (3.5%), flatulence (2.2%)

Neuromuscular & skeletal: Back pain (2.8%)

Respiratory: Upper respiratory tract infection (8.1%), sinusitis (5%), pharyngitis (2.3%), rhinitis (2%)

Miscellaneous: Accidental injury (2.9%)

<2%, postmarketing, and/or case reports (limited to important or life-threatening): Acute renal failure, agranulocytosis, albuminuria, allergic reactions, alopecia, anaphylactoid reactions, angioedema, aplastic anemia, arthralgia, aseptic meningitis, ataxia, bronchospasm, cerebrovascular accident, CHF, colitis, conjunctivitis, cystitis, deafness, diabetes mellitus, dyspnea, dysuria, ecchymosis, erythema multiforme, esophageal perforation, esophagitis, exfoliative dermatitis, flu-like syndrome, gangrene, gastroenteritis, gastroesophageal reflux, gastrointestinal bleeding, glaucoma, hematuria, hepatic failure, hepatitis, hypertension, hypoglycemia, hypokalemia, hyponatremia, interstitial nephritis, intestinal perforation, intracranial hemorrhage (fatal in association with warfarin), jaundice, leukopenia, melena, migraine, myalgia, MI, neuralgia, neuropathy, pancreatitis, pancytopenia, paresthesia, photosensitivity, prostate disorder, pulmonary embolism, rash, renal calculi, sepsis, Stevens-Johnson syndrome, stomatitis, sudden death, syncope, thrombophlebitis, tinnitus, toxic epidermal necrolysis, urticaria, vaginal bleeding, vaginitis, vasculitis, ventricular fibrillation, vertigo, vomiting

Overdosage/Toxicology Doses up to 2400 mg/day for up to 10 days have been reported without serious toxicity. Symptoms of overdose may include epigastric pain, drowsiness, lethargy, nausea, and vomiting; gastrointestinal bleeding may occur. Rare manifestations include hypertension, respiratory depression, coma, and acute renal failure. Treatment is symptomatic and supportive. Forced diuresis, hemodialysis and/or urinary alkalinization may not be useful.

Dosing

Adults:

Osteoarthritis: Oral: 200 mg/day as a single dose or in divided dose twice daily

Ankylosing spondylitis: 200 mg/day as a single dose or in divided doses twice daily; if no effect after 6 weeks, may increase to 400 mg/day. If no response following 6 weeks of treatment with 400 mg/day, consider discontinuation and alternative treatment.

Rheumatoid arthritis: Oral: 100-200 mg twice daily

Familial adenomatous polyposis: Oral: 400 mg twice daily

Acute pain or primary dysmenorrhea: Oral: Initial dose: 400 mg, followed by an additional 200 mg if needed on day 1; maintenance dose: 200 mg twice daily as needed

Elderly: Refer to adult dosing. No specific adjustment is recommended. However, the AUC in elderly patients may be increased by 50% as compared to younger subjects. Use the lowest recommended dose in patients weighing <50 kg.

Renal Impairment: No specific dosage adjustment is recommended. Not recommended in patients with advanced renal disease.

Hepatic Impairment: Reduced dosage is recommended (AUC may be increased by 40% to 180%). Decrease dose by 50% in patients with moderate hepatic impairment (Child-Pugh class B).

Available Dosage Forms Capsule: 100 mg, 200 mg, 400 mg

Nursing Guidelines

Assessment: Evaluate cardiac risk and potential for GI bleeding prior to prescribing this medication. Assess effectiveness and interactions of other medications patient may be taking (ie, monitor patients taking lithium closely).

(Continued)

Celecoxib *(Continued)*

Assess allergy history (aspirin, NSAIDs, salicylates). Monitor blood pressure at the beginning of therapy and periodically during use. Monitor effectiveness of therapy. Assess knowledge/teach patient appropriate use, possible side effects/interventions, and adverse symptoms to report.

Dietary Considerations: Lower doses (200 mg twice daily) may be taken without regard to meals. Larger doses should be taken with food to improve absorption.

Patient Education: Do not take more than recommended dose. May be taken with food to reduce GI upset. Do not take with antacids. Avoid alcohol, aspirin, and OTC medication unless approved by prescriber. You may experience dizziness, confusion, or blurred vision (avoid driving or engaging in tasks requiring alertness until response to drug is known); anorexia, nausea, vomiting, taste disturbance, gastric distress (small frequent meals, frequent mouth care, sucking lozenges, or chewing gum may help). GI bleeding, ulceration, or perforation can occur with or without pain. It is unclear whether celecoxib has rates of these events which are similar to nonselective NSAIDs. Stop taking medication and report immediately stomach pain or cramping; unusual bleeding or bruising (blood in vomitus, stool, or urine). Report persistent insomnia; skin rash; unusual fatigue, muscle pain, tremors, or weakness; sudden weight gain or edema; chest pain; shortness of breath; changes in hearing (ringing in ears) or vision; changes in urination pattern; or respiratory difficulty. **Pregnancy/breast-feeding precautions:** Inform your prescriber if you are or intend to become pregnant. This drug should not be used in the 3rd trimester of pregnancy. Breast-feeding is not recommended.

Geriatric Considerations: The elderly are at increased risk for adverse effects from NSAIDs. As many as 60% of elderly can develop peptic ulceration and/or hemorrhage asymptomatically. CNS adverse effects such as confusion, agitation, and hallucination are generally seen in overdose or high-dose situations; however, elderly patients may demonstrate these adverse effects at lower doses than younger adults. The elderly are also at increased risk of renal toxicity.

Pregnancy Risk Factor: C/D (3rd trimester)

Pregnancy Issues: In late pregnancy, this drug may cause premature closure of the ductus arteriosus.

Lactation: Enters breast milk/not recommended (contraindicated in Canadian labeling)

Breast-Feeding Considerations: Based on limited data, celecoxib has been found to be excreted in milk; a decision should be made whether to discontinue nursing or discontinue the drug, taking into account the importance of the drug to the mother.

Perioperative/Anesthesia/Other Concerns: Celecoxib does not inhibit platelets or prolong bleeding time.

Administration

Storage: Store at controlled room temperature of 25°C (77°F).

- Celestone® *see* Betamethasone *on page 237*
- Celestone® Soluspan® *see* Betamethasone *on page 237*
- Celexa® *see* Citalopram *on page 416*
- CellCept® *see* Mycophenolate *on page 1188*
- Cellugel® *see* Hydroxypropyl Methylcellulose *on page 883*

Cellulose (Oxidized Regenerated)

(SEL yoo lose, OKS i dyzed re JEN er aye ted)

U.S. Brand Names Surgicel®; Surgicel® Fibrillar; Surgicel® NuKnit

Synonyms Absorbable Cotton; Oxidized Regenerated Cellulose

Pharmacologic Category Hemostatic Agent

Medication Safety Issues

Sound-alike/look-alike issues:

Surgicel® may be confused with Serentil®

Use Hemostatic; temporary packing for the control of capillary, venous, or small arterial hemorrhage

Mechanism of Action Cellulose, oxidized regenerated is saturated with blood at the bleeding site and swells into a brownish or black gelatinous mass which aids in the formation of a clot. When used in small amounts, it is absorbed from the sites of implantation with little or no tissue reaction. In addition to providing hemostasis, oxidized regenerated cellulose also has been shown *in vitro* to have bactericidal properties.

Pharmacodynamics/Kinetics Absorption: 7-14 days

Contraindications Hypersensitivity to any component of the formulation; implantation into bone defects; hemorrhage from large arteries; nonhemorrhagic oozing; use as an adhesion product

Warnings/Precautions Pain, numbness, or paralysis have been reported if used near a bony or neural space and left inside patient; use minimum amount necessary to achieve hemostasis. Remove as much of agent as possible after hemostasis is achieved. Do not leave in a contaminated or infected space. Always remove completely following hemostasis if applied in proximity to foramina in bone, areas of bony confine, the spinal cord or optic nerve and chasm; product may swell and exert unwanted pressure. The material should not be moistened before insertion since the hemostatic effect is greater when applied dry. The material should not be impregnated with anti-infective agents. Its hemostatic effect is not enhanced by the addition of thrombin.

Drug Interactions No data reported

Adverse Reactions Frequency not defined.

Central nervous system: Headache

Respiratory: Nasal burning or stinging, sneezing (rhinological procedures)

Miscellaneous: Encapsulation of fluid, foreign body reactions (with or without) infection

Postmarketing and/or case reports: Numbness, pain, paralysis

Dosing

Adults & Elderly: Bleeding: Topical: Minimal amounts of the fabric strip are laid on the bleeding site or held firmly against the tissues until hemostasis occurs; remove excess material

Available Dosage Forms

Fabric, fibrous (Surgicel® Fibrillar):
- 1" x 2" (10s)
- 2" x 4" (10s)
- 4" x 4" (10s)

Fabric, knitted (Surgicel® NuKnit):
- 1" x 1" (24s)
- 1" x 3½" (10s)
- 3" x 4" (24s)
- 6" x 9" (10s)

Fabric, sheer weave (Surgicel®):
- ½" x 2" (24s)
- 2" x 3" (24s)
- 2" x 14" (24s)
- 4" x 8" (24s)

Nursing Guidelines

Pregnancy Risk Factor: No data reported

Administration

Storage: Store at controlled room temperature. Inactivated by autoclaving; do not resterilize. Do not use if package is damaged. Do not reuse after opening.

- ♦ **Cenestin®** *see* Estrogens (Conjugated A/Synthetic) *on page 658*
- ♦ **Centany™** *see* Mupirocin *on page 1187*
- ♦ **Centrum® [OTC]** *see* Vitamins (Multiple/Oral) *on page 1720*
- ♦ **Centrum® Kids Jimmy Neutron® Complete [OTC]** *see* Vitamins (Multiple/Pediatric) *on page 1720*
- ♦ **Centrum® Kids Jimmy Neutron® Extra C [OTC]** *see* Vitamins (Multiple/Pediatric) *on page 1720*
- ♦ **Centrum® Kids Rugrats™ Complete [OTC]** *see* Vitamins (Multiple/Pediatric) *on page 1720*
- ♦ **Centrum® Kids Rugrats™ Extra C [OTC]** *see* Vitamins (Multiple/Pediatric) *on page 1720*
- ♦ **Centrum® Kids Rugrats™ Extra Calcium [OTC]** *see* Vitamins (Multiple/Pediatric) *on page 1720*
- ♦ **Centrum® Performance™ [OTC]** *see* Vitamins (Multiple/Oral) *on page 1720*
- ♦ **Centrum® Silver® [OTC]** *see* Vitamins (Multiple/Oral) *on page 1720*
- ♦ **Cepacol® Antibacterial Mouthwash [OTC]** *see* Cetylpyridinium *on page 368*
- ♦ **Cepacol® Antibacterial Mouthwash Gold [OTC]** *see* Cetylpyridinium *on page 368*
- ♦ **Cepacol® Sore Throat [OTC]** *see* Benzocaine *on page 232*

♦ Cepastat® [OTC] *see* Phenol *on page 1347*
♦ Cepastat® Extra Strength [OTC] *see* Phenol *on page 1347*

Cephalexin (sef a LEKS in)

U.S. Brand Names Biocef®; Keflex®; Panixine DisperDose™

Synonyms Cephalexin Monohydrate

Pharmacologic Category Antibiotic, Cephalosporin (First Generation)

Medication Safety Issues

Sound-alike/look-alike issues:

Cephalexin may be confused with cefaclor, cefazolin, cephalothin, ciprofloxacin

Use Treatment of susceptible bacterial infections including respiratory tract infections, otitis media, skin and skin structure infections, bone infections and genitourinary tract infections, including acute prostatitis; alternative therapy for acute bacterial endocarditis prophylaxis

Mechanism of Action Inhibits bacterial cell wall synthesis by binding to one or more of the penicillin-binding proteins (PBPs) which in turn inhibits the final transpeptidation step of peptidoglycan synthesis in bacterial cell walls, thus inhibiting cell wall biosynthesis. Bacteria eventually lyse due to ongoing activity of cell wall autolytic enzymes (autolysins and murein hydrolases) while cell wall assembly is arrested.

Pharmacodynamics/Kinetics

Absorption: Delayed in young children

Distribution: Widely into most body tissues and fluids, including gallbladder, liver, kidneys, bone, sputum, bile, and pleural and synovial fluids; CSF penetration is poor; crosses placenta; enters breast milk

Protein binding: 6% to 15%

Half-life elimination: Adults: 0.5-1.2 hours; prolonged with renal impairment

Time to peak, serum: ~1 hour

Excretion: Urine (80% to 100% as unchanged drug) within 8 hours

Contraindications Hypersensitivity to cephalexin, any component of the formulation, or other cephalosporins

Warnings/Precautions Modify dosage in patients with severe renal impairment, prolonged use may result in superinfection; use with caution in patients with a history of penicillin allergy, especially IgE-mediated reactions (eg, anaphylaxis, urticaria). May cause antibiotic-associated colitis or colitis secondary to *C. difficile*.

Drug Interactions

Aminoglycosides: Increase nephrotoxic potential.

Probenecid: High-dose probenecid decreases clearance of cephalexin.

Nutritional/Herbal/Ethanol Interactions Food: Peak antibiotic serum concentration is lowered and delayed, but total drug absorbed is not affected. Cephalexin serum levels may be decreased if taken with food.

Lab Interactions Positive direct Coombs', false-positive urinary glucose test using cupric sulfate (Benedict's solution, Clinitest®, Fehling's solution), false-positive serum or urine creatinine with Jaffé reaction

Adverse Reactions Frequency not defined.

Central nervous system: Agitation, confusion, dizziness, fatigue, hallucinations, headache

Dermatologic: Angioedema, erythema multiforme (rare), rash, Stevens-Johnson syndrome (rare), toxic epidermal necrolysis (rare), urticaria

Gastrointestinal: Abdominal pain, diarrhea, dyspepsia, gastritis, nausea (rare), pseudomembranous colitis, vomiting (rare)

Genitourinary: Genital pruritus, genital moniliasis, vaginitis, vaginal discharge

Hematologic: Eosinophilia, neutropenia, thrombocytopenia

Hepatic: AST/ALT increased, cholestatic jaundice (rare), transient hepatitis (rare)

Neuromuscular & skeletal: Arthralgia, arthritis, joint disorder

Renal: Interstitial nephritis (rare)

Miscellaneous: Allergic reactions

Overdosage/Toxicology Symptoms of overdose include epigastric distress, diarrhea, hematuria, nausea, and vomiting. Many beta-lactam containing antibiotics have the potential to cause neuromuscular hyperirritability or seizures. Hemodialysis may be helpful to aid in removal of the drug from blood; otherwise, treatment is supportive and symptom-directed.

Dosing

Adults & Elderly:

Dosing range: Oral: 250-1000 mg every 6 hours; maximum: 4 g/day

Streptococcal pharyngitis, skin and skin structure infections: Oral: 500 mg every 12 hours

Uncomplicated cystitis: Oral: 500 mg every 12 hours for 7-14 days

Prophylaxis of bacterial endocarditis (dental, oral, respiratory tract, or esophageal procedures): Oral: 2 g 1 hour prior to procedure

Pediatrics:

Usual dose: Oral: Children >1 year: Dosing range: 25-50 mg/kg/day every 6-8 hours; more severe infections: 50-100 mg/kg/day in divided doses every 6-8 hours; maximum: 4 g/24 hours

Otitis media: 75-100 mg/kg/day in 4 divided doses

Streptococcal pharyngitis, skin and skin structure infections: 25-50 mg/kg/day divided every 12 hours

Uncomplicated cystitis: Children >15 years: Refer to adult dosing.

Prophylaxis of bacterial endocarditis (dental, oral, respiratory tract, or esophageal procedures): 50 mg/kg 1 hour prior to procedure (maximum: 2 g)

Renal Impairment:

Cl_{cr} <10 mL/minute: Adults: 250-500 mg every 12 hours

Hemodialysis: Moderately dialyzable (20% to 50%)

Available Dosage Forms

Capsule: 250 mg, 500 mg

Biocef®: 500 mg

Keflex®: 250 mg, 500 mg

Powder for oral suspension: 125 mg/5 mL (100 mL, 200 mL); 250 mg/5 mL (100 mL, 200 mL)

Biocef®: 125 mg/5 mL (100 mL); 250 mg/5 mL (100 mL)

Keflex®: 125 mg/5 mL (100 mL, 200 mL); 250 mg/5 mL (100 mL, 200 mL)

Tablet, for oral suspension (Panixine DisperDose™): 125 mg [contains phenylalanine 2.8 mg; peppermint flavor], 250 mg [contains phenylalanine 5.6 mg; peppermint flavor]

Nursing Guidelines

Assessment: Assess for previous allergy history prior to therapy. See Contraindications, Warnings/Precautions, and Dosing for use cautions. Assess potential for interactions with other prescriptions, OTC medications, or herbal products patient may be taking (see Drug Interactions). Assess results of laboratory tests (see below), therapeutic response, and adverse reactions (see Adverse Reactions and Overdose/Toxicology). Advise patients with diabetes about use of Clinitest®. Teach patient proper use, possible side effects/appropriate interventions, and adverse symptoms to report (see Patient Education). Note breast-feeding caution.

Monitoring Laboratory Tests: Renal, hepatic, and hematologic function periodically with prolonged therapy; perform culture and sensitivity studies prior to initiating drug therapy.

Dietary Considerations: Take without regard to food. If GI distress, take with food. Panixine DisperDose™ contains phenylalanine 2.8 mg/cephalexin 125 mg.

Patient Education: Inform prescriber of all prescriptions, OTC medications, or herbal products you are taking, and any allergies you have. Do not take any new medication during therapy unless approved by prescriber. Take as directed, at regular intervals around-the-clock (with or without food). Chilling oral suspension improves flavor (do not freeze). Maintain adequate hydration (2-3 L/day of fluids) unless instructed to restrict fluid intake. Complete full course of medication, even if you feel better. May cause false test results with Clinitest®; use of another type of glucose testing is preferable. May cause diarrhea (buttermilk, boiled milk, or yogurt may help). Report unresolved diarrhea; unusual bruising or bleeding; changes in urinary pattern; or opportunistic infection (vaginal itching or drainage, sores in mouth, blood in urine or stool). **Breast-feeding precaution:** Consult prescriber if breast-feeding.

Geriatric Considerations: Adjust dose for renal function.

Pregnancy Risk Factor: B

Lactation: Enters breast milk (small amounts)/use caution

Breast-Feeding Considerations: Theoretically, drug absorbed by nursing infant may change bowel flora or affect fever work-up result. Cephalexin levels can be detected in breast milk, reaching a maximum concentration 4 hours after a single oral dose and gradually decreasing by 8 hours after administration. **Note:** As a class, cephalosporins are used to treat bacterial infections in infants.

(Continued)

Cephalexin *(Continued)*

Administration

Oral: Take without regard to food. If GI distress, take with food. Give around-the-clock to promote less variation in peak and trough serum levels.

Panixine DisperDose™: Tablets should be mixed in ~10 mL of water immediately prior to administration. Drink entire solution, then rinse glass with additional water and drink contents to ensure entire dose has been taken. Tablets should not be chewed or swallowed whole.

Reconstitution: Tablets for oral suspension (Panixine DisperDose™): Tablets must be dissolved in ~10 mL water prior to administration.

Storage: Refrigerate suspension after reconstitution; discard after 14 days. Tablets for suspension should be used immediately after dissolving.

Related Information

Cephalosporins by Generation *on page 1858*

- **Cephalexin Monohydrate** *see* Cephalexin *on page 364*
- **Ceptaz® [DSC]** *see* Ceftazidime *on page 348*
- **Cerebyx®** *see* Fosphenytoin *on page 781*
- **C.E.S.** *see* Estrogens (Conjugated/Equine) *on page 661*
- **Cesia™** *see* Ethinyl Estradiol and Desogestrel *on page 675*
- **Cetacaine®** *see* Benzocaine, Butyl Aminobenzoate, Tetracaine, and Benzalkonium Chloride *on page 235*
- **Cetacort®** *see* Hydrocortisone *on page 873*
- **Cetafen® [OTC]** *see* Acetaminophen *on page 65*
- **Cetafen Extra® [OTC]** *see* Acetaminophen *on page 65*
- **Ceta-Plus®** *see* Hydrocodone and Acetaminophen *on page 867*

Cetirizine (se TI ra zeen)

U.S. Brand Names Zyrtec®

Synonyms Cetirizine Hydrochloride; P-071; UCB-P071

Pharmacologic Category Antihistamine

Medication Safety Issues

Sound-alike/look-alike issues:

Zyrtec® may be confused with Serax®, Xanax®, Zantac®, Zyprexa®

Use Perennial and seasonal allergic rhinitis and other allergic symptoms including urticaria; chronic idiopathic urticaria

Mechanism of Action Competes with histamine for H_1-receptor sites on effector cells in the gastrointestinal tract, blood vessels, and respiratory tract

Pharmacodynamics/Kinetics

Onset of action: 15-30 minutes
Absorption: Rapid
Protein binding, plasma: Mean: 93%
Metabolism: Limited hepatic
Half-life elimination: 8 hours
Time to peak, serum: 1 hour
Excretion: Urine (70%); feces (10%)

Contraindications Hypersensitivity to cetirizine, hydroxyzine, or any component of the formulation

Warnings/Precautions Cetirizine should be used cautiously in patients with hepatic or renal dysfunction and the elderly. Use in breast-feeding women is not recommended. May cause drowsiness, use caution performing tasks which require alertness (eg, operating machinery or driving). Safety and efficacy in pediatric patients <6 months of age have not been established.

Drug Interactions Substrate of CYP3A4 (minor)

Increased toxicity: CNS depressants, anticholinergics

Nutritional/Herbal/Ethanol Interactions Ethanol: Avoid ethanol (may increase CNS depression).

Adverse Reactions

>10%: Central nervous system: Headache (children 11% to 14%, placebo 12%), somnolence (adults 14%, children 2% to 4%)

2% to 10%:

Central nervous system: Insomnia (children 9%, adults <2%), fatigue (adults 6%), malaise (4%), dizziness (adults 2%)

Gastrointestinal: Abdominal pain (children 4% to 6%), dry mouth (adults 5%), diarrhea (children 2% to 3%), nausea (children 2% to 3%, placebo 2%), vomiting (children 2% to 3%)

Respiratory: Epistaxis (children 2% to 4%, placebo 3%), pharyngitis (children 3% to 6%, placebo 3%), bronchospasm (children 2% to 3%, placebo 2%)

<2% (Limited to important or life-threatening; as reported in adults and/or children): Aggressive reaction, anaphylaxis, angioedema, ataxia, chest pain, confusion, convulsions, depersonalization, depression, edema, fussiness, hallucinations, hemolytic anemia, hepatitis, hypertension, hypotension (severe), irritability, liver function abnormal, nervousness, ototoxicity, palpitation, paralysis, paresthesia, photosensitivity, rash, suicidal ideation, suicide, taste perversion, tongue discoloration, tongue edema, tremor, visual field defect, weakness

Overdosage/Toxicology Symptoms of overdose may include somnolence, restlessness, or irritability. Treatment is symptomatic and supportive. Cetirizine is not removed by dialysis.

Dosing

Adults: Perennial or seasonal allergic rhinitis, chronic urticaria: Oral: 5-10 mg once daily, depending upon symptom severity

Elderly: Oral: Initial: 5 mg once daily; may increase to 10 mg/day

Note: Manufacturer recommends 5 mg/day in patients ≥77 years of age.

Pediatrics:

Perennial allergic rhinitis, chronic urticaria: Oral: Children:

6-12 months: 2.5 mg once daily

12 months to <2 years: 2.5 mg once daily; may increase to 2.5 mg every 12 hours if needed

Perennial or seasonal allergic rhinitis, chronic urticaria: Oral: Children:

2-5 years: Initial: 2.5 mg once daily; may be increased to 2.5 mg every 12 hours **or** 5 mg once daily

≥6 years Refer to adult dosing.

Renal Impairment:

Children <6 years: Cetirizine use not recommended.

Children 6-11 years: <2.5 mg once daily

Children ≥12 and Adults:

Cl_{cr} 11-31 mL/minute or hemodialysis: Administer 5 mg once daily

Cl_{cr} <11 mL/minute, not on dialysis: Cetirizine use not recommended.

Hepatic Impairment:

Children <6 years: Cetirizine use not recommended.

Children 6-11 years: <2.5 mg once daily

Children ≥12 and Adults: Administer 5 mg once daily

Available Dosage Forms

Syrup, as hydrochloride: 5 mg/5 mL (120 mL, 480 mL) [banana-grape flavor]

Tablet, as hydrochloride: 5 mg, 10 mg

Tablet, chewable, as hydrochloride: 5 mg, 10 mg [grape flavor]

Nursing Guidelines

Assessment: Assess effectiveness and interactions of other medications patient may be taking. Monitor effectiveness of therapy and adverse reactions at beginning of therapy and periodically with long-term use. Assess knowledge/teach patient appropriate use, interventions to reduce side effects, and adverse symptoms to report. Breast-feeding is not recommended.

Dietary Considerations: May be taken with or without food.

Patient Education: Take as directed; do not exceed recommended dose. Avoid use of other depressants, alcohol, or sleep-inducing medications unless approved by prescriber. You may experience drowsiness or dizziness (use caution when driving or engaging in tasks requiring alertness until response to drug is known); or dry mouth (frequent small meals, frequent mouth care, chewing gum, or sucking hard candy may help). Report persistent sedation, confusion, or agitation; persistent nausea or vomiting; changes in urinary pattern; blurred vision; chest pain or palpitations; persistent headaches; or lack of improvement or worsening of condition. **Breast-feeding precaution:** Breast-feeding is not recommended.

(Continued)

Cetirizine *(Continued)*

Geriatric Considerations: Adjust dose for renal function.

Pregnancy Risk Factor: B

Lactation: Enters breast milk/not recommended

Administration

Oral: May be administered with or without food.

Storage:

Syrup: Store at room temperature of 15°C to 30°C (59°F to 86°F), or under refrigeration at 2°C to 8°C (36°F to 46°F).

Tablet: Store at room temperature of 15°C to 30°C (59°F to 86°F).

♦ Cetirizine Hydrochloride *see* Cetirizine *on page 366*

Cetylpyridinium (SEE til peer i DI nee um)

U.S. Brand Names Cepacol® Antibacterial Mouthwash [OTC]; Cepacol® Antibacterial Mouthwash Gold [OTC]; DiabetAid Gingivitis Mouth Rinse [OTC]

Synonyms Cetylpyridinium Chloride; CPC

Pharmacologic Category Antiseptic, Oral Mouthwash

Use Antiseptic to aid in the prevention and reduction of plaque and gingivitis, and to freshen breath

Contraindications Hypersensitivity to cetylpyridinium or any component of the formulation

Warnings/Precautions Not labeled for OTC use in children <6 years of age.

Adverse Reactions Frequency not defined: Gastrointestinal: Tooth and tongue staining, oral irritation

Dosing

Adults & Elderly: Antiseptic: Oral (OTC labeling): Rinse or gargle to freshen mouth; may be used before or after brushing

Pediatrics: Antiseptic: Children ≥6 years: Refer to adult dosing.

Available Dosage Forms Liquid, as chloride, oral [mouthwash/gargle]:

Cepacol® Antibacterial Mouthwash Gold: 0.05% (120 mL, 360 mL, 720 mL, 960 mL) [contains alcohol 14% and tartrazine; original flavor]

Cepacol® Antibacterial Mouthwash: 0.05% (120 mL, 360 mL, 720 mL, 960 mL) [contains alcohol 14% and tartrazine; mint flavor]

DiabetAid Gingivitis Mouth Rinse: 0.1% (480 mL) [sugar free]

Nursing Guidelines

Pregnancy Risk Factor: C

♦ Cetylpyridinium Chloride *see* Cetylpyridinium *on page 368*
♦ Cevi-Bid® [OTC] *see* Ascorbic Acid *on page 187*
♦ CFDN *see* Cefdinir *on page 333*
♦ CG *see* Chorionic Gonadotropin (Human) *on page 387*
♦ C-Gram [OTC] *see* Ascorbic Acid *on page 187*
♦ Cheracol® [OTC] *see* Phenol *on page 1347*
♦ Cheratussin AC *see* Guaifenesin and Codeine *on page 835*
♦ CHG *see* Chlorhexidine Gluconate *on page 373*
♦ Chiggerex® [OTC] *see* Benzocaine *on page 232*
♦ Chiggertox® [OTC] *see* Benzocaine *on page 232*
♦ Children's Pepto [OTC] *see* Calcium Carbonate *on page 291*
♦ Children's Vitamins *see* Vitamins (Multiple/Pediatric) *on page 1720*
♦ Chirocaine® [DSC] *see* Levobupivacaine *on page 1023*
♦ Chloral *see* Chloral Hydrate *on page 368*

Chloral Hydrate (KLOR al HYE drate)

U.S. Brand Names Aquachloral® Supprettes®; Somnote™

Synonyms Chloral; Hydrated Chloral; Trichloroacetaldehyde Monohydrate

Pharmacologic Category Hypnotic, Nonbenzodiazepine

Use Short-term sedative and hypnotic (<2 weeks), sedative/hypnotic for diagnostic procedures; sedative prior to EEG evaluations

Mechanism of Action Central nervous system depressant effects are due to its active metabolite trichloroethanol, mechanism unknown

Pharmacodynamics/Kinetics

Onset of action: Peak effect: 0.5-1 hour

Duration: 4-8 hours

Absorption: Oral, rectal: Well absorbed

Distribution: Crosses placenta; negligible amounts enter breast milk

Metabolism: Rapidly hepatic to trichloroethanol (active metabolite); variable amounts hepatically and renally to trichloroacetic acid (inactive)

Half-life elimination: Active metabolite: 8-11 hours

Excretion: Urine (as metabolites); feces (small amounts)

Contraindications Hypersensitivity to chloral hydrate or any component of the formulation; hepatic or renal impairment; gastritis or ulcers; severe cardiac disease

Warnings/Precautions Use with caution in patients with porphyria; use with caution in neonates, drug may accumulate with repeated use, prolonged use in neonates associated with hyperbilirubinemia; tolerance to hypnotic effect develops, therefore, not recommended for use >2 weeks; taper dosage to avoid withdrawal with prolonged use; trichloroethanol (TCE), a metabolite of chloral hydrate, is a carcinogen in mice; there is no data in humans. Chloral hydrate is considered a second line hypnotic agent in the elderly. Recent interpretive guidelines from the Centers for Medicare and Medicaid Services (CMS) discourage the use of chloral hydrate in residents of long-term care facilities.

Drug Interactions

CNS depressants: Sedative effects and/or respiratory depression with chloral hydrate may be additive with other CNS depressants; monitor for increased effect; includes ethanol, sedatives, antidepressants, narcotic analgesics, and benzodiazepines

Furosemide: Diaphoresis, flushing, and hypertension have occurred in patients who received I.V. furosemide within 24 hours after administration of chloral hydrate; consider using a benzodiazepine

Phenytoin: Half-life may be decreased by chloral hydrate; limited documentation (small, single-dose study); monitor

Warfarin: Effect of oral anticoagulants may be increased by chloral hydrate; monitor INR; warfarin dosage may require adjustment. Chloral hydrate's metabolite may displace warfarin from its protein binding sites resulting in an increase in the hypoprothrombinemic response to warfarin.

Nutritional/Herbal/Ethanol Interactions

Ethanol: Avoid ethanol (may increase CNS depression).

Herb/Nutraceutical: Avoid valerian, St John's wort, kava kava, gotu kola (may increase CNS depression).

Lab Interactions False-positive urine glucose using Clinitest® method; may interfere with fluorometric urine catecholamine and urinary 17-hydroxycorticosteroid tests

Adverse Reactions Frequency not defined.

Central nervous system: Ataxia, disorientation, sedation, excitement (paradoxical), dizziness, fever, headache, confusion, lightheadedness, nightmares, hallucinations, drowsiness, "hangover" effect

Dermatologic: Rash, urticaria

Gastrointestinal: Gastric irritation, nausea, vomiting, diarrhea, flatulence

Hematologic: Leukopenia, eosinophilia, acute intermittent porphyria

Miscellaneous: Physical and psychological dependence may occur with prolonged use of large doses

Overdosage/Toxicology Symptoms of overdose include hypotension, respiratory depression, coma, hypothermia, and cardiac arrhythmias. Treatment is supportive and symptomatic.

Dosing

Adults:

Sedation, anxiety: Oral, rectal: 250 mg 3 times/day

Hypnotic: Oral, rectal: 500-1000 mg at bedtime or 30 minutes prior to procedure, not to exceed 2 g/24 hours

Discontinuation: Withdraw gradually over 2 weeks if patient has been maintained on high doses for prolonged period of time. Do not stop drug abruptly.

Elderly: Hypnotic: Initial: Oral: 250 mg at bedtime; adjust for renal impairment. See Geriatric Considerations.

Pediatrics:

Sedation, anxiety: Oral, rectal: 5-15 mg/kg/dose every 8 hours, maximum: 500 mg/dose

Prior to EEG: Oral, rectal: 20-25 mg/kg/dose, 30-60 minutes prior to EEG; may repeat in 30 minutes to maximum of 100 mg/kg or 2 g total

Hypnotic: Oral, rectal: 20-40 mg/kg/dose up to a maximum of 50 mg/kg/24 hours or 1 g/dose or 2 g/24 hours

(Continued)

Chloral Hydrate *(Continued)*

Conscious sedation: Oral: 50-75 mg/kg/dose 30-60 minutes prior to procedure; may repeat 30 minutes after initial dose if needed, to a total maximum dose of 120 mg/kg or 1 g total

Discontinuation: Withdraw gradually over 2 weeks if patient has been maintained on high doses for prolonged period of time. Do not stop drug abruptly.

Renal Impairment:

Cl_{cr} <50 mL/minute: Avoid use.

Hemodialysis effects: Supplemental dose is not necessary; dialyzable (50% to 100%).

Hepatic Impairment: Avoid use in patients with severe hepatic impairment.

Available Dosage Forms

Capsule (Somnote™): 500 mg

Suppository, rectal (Aquachloral® Supprettes®): 325 mg [contains tartrazine], 650 mg

Syrup: 500 mg/5 mL (480 mL) [contains sodium benzoate]

Nursing Guidelines

Assessment: For short-term use. Assess effectiveness and interactions of other medications patient may be taking. Assess for history of addiction; long-term use can result in dependence, abuse, or tolerance. Monitor for excessive sedation. Evaluate periodically for need for continued use (symptoms of dependence may resemble alcoholism, but usually there is more gastritis). After long-term use, taper dosage slowly when discontinuing. For inpatient use, institute safety measures and monitor effectiveness and adverse reactions. For outpatients, monitor for effectiveness of therapy and adverse reactions at beginning of therapy and periodically with long-term use. Assess knowledge/ teach patient appropriate use, interventions to reduce side effects, and adverse symptoms to report.

Patient Education: Use exactly as directed; do not increase dose or frequency or discontinue without consulting prescriber. Drug may cause physical and/or psychological dependence. While using this medication, do not use alcohol and other prescription or OTC medications (especially, pain medications, sedatives, antihistamines, or hypnotics) without consulting prescriber. Maintain adequate hydration (2-3 L/day of fluids) unless instructed to restrict fluid intake. You may experience drowsiness, dizziness, or blurred vision (use caution when driving or engaging in tasks requiring alertness until response to drug is known); nausea, vomiting, unpleasant taste (small frequent meals, frequent mouth care, chewing gum, or sucking lozenges may help); or diarrhea (buttermilk, boiled milk, yogurt may help). Report skin rash or irritation, CNS changes (confusion, depression, increased sedation, excitation, headache, insomnia, or nightmares), unresolved GI distress, chest pain or palpitations, or ineffectiveness of medication. **Pregnancy precaution:** Inform prescriber if you are or intend to become pregnant.

Geriatric Considerations: Chloral hydrate is considered a second- or third-line hypnotic agent in the elderly. Interpretive guidelines from the Centers for Medicare and Medicaid Services (CMS) discourage the use of chloral hydrate in residents of long-term care facilities.

Pregnancy Risk Factor: C

Lactation: Enters breast milk/compatible

Administration

Oral: Chilling the syrup may help to mask unpleasant taste. Do not crush capsule (contains drug in liquid form). Gastric irritation may be minimized by diluting dose in water or other oral liquid.

Storage: Sensitive to light. Exposure to air causes volatilization. Store in light-resistant, airtight container.

Chloramphenicol (klor am FEN i kole)

U.S. Brand Names Chloromycetin® Sodium Succinate

Pharmacologic Category Antibiotic, Miscellaneous

Medication Safety Issues

Sound-alike/look-alike issues:

Chloromycetin® may be confused with chlorambucil, Chlor-Trimeton®

Use Treatment of serious infections due to organisms resistant to other less toxic antibiotics or when its penetrability into the site of infection is clinically superior to other antibiotics to which the organism is sensitive; useful in infections caused by

Bacteroides, *H. influenzae*, *Neisseria meningitidis*, *Salmonella*, and *Rickettsia*; active against many vancomycin-resistant enterococci

Mechanism of Action Reversibly binds to 50S ribosomal subunits of susceptible organisms preventing amino acids from being transferred to growing peptide chains thus inhibiting protein synthesis

Pharmacodynamics/Kinetics

Distribution: To most tissues and body fluids; readily crosses placenta; enters breast milk

CSF:blood level ratio: Normal meninges: 66%; Inflamed meninges: >66%

Protein binding: 60%

Metabolism: Extensively hepatic (90%) to inactive metabolites, principally by glucuronidation; chloramphenicol sodium succinate is hydrolyzed by esterases to active base

Half-life elimination

Normal renal function: 1.6-3.3 hours

End-stage renal disease: 3-7 hours

Cirrhosis: 10-12 hours

Excretion: Urine (5% to 15%)

Contraindications Hypersensitivity to chloramphenicol or any component of the formulation

Warnings/Precautions Serious and fatal blood dyscrasias have occurred after both short-term and prolonged therapy including reports associated with topical treatment. Should not be used when less potentially toxic agents are effective; prolonged use may result in superinfection. Use with caution in patients with impaired renal or hepatic function and in neonates; reduce dose with impaired liver function; use with care in patients with glucose 6-phosphate dehydrogenase deficiency.

Drug Interactions **Inhibits** CYP2C8/9 (weak), 3A4 (weak)

Decreased effect: Phenobarbital and rifampin may decrease concentration of chloramphenicol

Increased toxicity: Chloramphenicol inhibits the metabolism of chlorpropamide, phenytoin, oral anticoagulants

Nutritional/Herbal/Ethanol Interactions Food: May decrease intestinal absorption of vitamin B_{12} may have increased dietary need for riboflavin, pyridoxine, and vitamin B_{12}.

Lab Interactions May cause false-positive results in urine glucose tests when using cupric sulfate (Benedict's solution, Clinitest®).

Adverse Reactions

Three (3) major toxicities associated with chloramphenicol include:

Aplastic anemia, an idiosyncratic reaction which can occur with any route of administration; usually occurs 3 weeks to 12 months after initial exposure to chloramphenicol

Bone marrow suppression is thought to be dose related with serum concentrations >25 mcg/mL and reversible once chloramphenicol is discontinued; anemia and neutropenia may occur during the first week of therapy

Gray syndrome is characterized by circulatory collapse, cyanosis, acidosis, abdominal distention, myocardial depression, coma, and death; reaction appears to be associated with serum levels ≥50 mcg/mL; may result from drug accumulation in patients with impaired hepatic or renal function

Additional adverse reactions, frequency not defined:

Central nervous system: Confusion, delirium, depression, fever, headache

Dermatologic: Angioedema, rash, urticaria

Gastrointestinal: Diarrhea, enterocolitis, glossitis, nausea, stomatitis, vomiting

Hematologic: Granulocytopenia, hypoplastic anemia, pancytopenia, thrombocytopenia

Ocular: Optic neuritis

Miscellaneous: Anaphylaxis, hypersensitivity reactions

Overdosage/Toxicology Symptoms of overdose include anemia, metabolic acidosis, hypotension, and hypothermia. Treatment is supportive.

Dosing

Adults & Elderly: Systemic infections: I.V.: 50-100 mg/kg/day in divided doses every 6 hours; maximum daily dose: 4 g/day.

Pediatrics:

Meningitis: I.V.: Infants >30 days and Children: 50-100 mg/kg/day divided every 6 hours

Other infections: I.V.: Infants >30 days and Children: 50-75 mg/kg/day divided every 6 hours; maximum daily dose: 4 g/day

(Continued)

Chloramphenicol *(Continued)*

Renal Impairment: Slightly dialyzable (5% to 20%) via hemo- and peritoneal dialysis; no supplemental doses are needed in dialysis or continuous arteriovenous or venovenous hemofiltration.

Hepatic Impairment: Avoid use in severe liver impairment as increased toxicity may occur.

Available Dosage Forms Injection, powder for reconstitution: 1 g [contains sodium ~52 mg/g (2.25 mEq/g)]

Nursing Guidelines

Assessment: Assess effectiveness and interactions of other medications patient may be taking (see Drug Interactions). Assess results of laboratory tests (see below), therapeutic effectiveness, and adverse reactions (see Adverse Reactions). Assess knowledge/teach patient appropriate use appropriate for form prescribed, interventions to reduce side effects, and adverse symptoms to report (see Patient Education). Breast-feeding is not recommended.

Monitoring Laboratory Tests: CBC with reticulocyte and platelet counts, periodic liver and renal function, serum drug concentration; culture and sensitivity prior to initiating therapy

Dietary Considerations: May have increased dietary need for riboflavin, pyridoxine, and vitamin B_{12}. Sodium content of 1 g injection: ~52 mg (2.25 mEq).

Patient Education: I.V.: You may experience a bitter taste during administration, this will pass.

If you have diabetes, drug may cause false test results with Clinitest® glucose monitoring; use alternative glucose monitoring. This drug may interfere with effectiveness of oral contraceptives. You may experience nausea, vomiting (small, frequent meals, frequent mouth care, sucking lozenges, or chewing gum may help). Report persistent rash, diarrhea; pain, burning, or numbness of extremities; petechiae; sore throat; fatigue; unusual bleeding or bruising; vaginal itching or discharge; mouth sores; yellowing of skin or eyes; dark urine or stool discoloration (blue); CNS disturbances (nightmares, acute headache); lack of improvement or worsening of condition.

Pregnancy/breast-feeding precautions: Inform prescriber if you are or intend to become pregnant. Breast-feeding is not recommended.

Geriatric Considerations: Chloramphenicol has not been studied in the elderly. It is not necessary to adjust the dose based upon the decrease in renal function associated with age. Chloramphenicol should be reserved for serious infections and the oral form avoided.

Pregnancy Risk Factor: C

Pregnancy Issues: Embryotoxic and teratogenic in animals, but there are no adequate and well-controlled trials in pregnant women. Has been shown to cross placental barrier.

Lactation: Enters breast milk/not recommended (AAP rates "of concern")

Breast-Feeding Considerations: Excreted in breast milk. Not recommended due to potential bone marrow suppression to the infant.

Administration

I.V.: Do not administer I.M.; can be administered IVP over at least 1 minute at a concentration of 100 mg/mL, or I.V. intermittent infusion over 15-30 minutes at a final concentration for administration of ≤20 mg/mL.

Compatibility: Stable in dextran 6% in dextrose, dextran 6% in NS, D_5LR, $D_5{}^1/_4NS$, $D_5{}^1/_2NS$, D_5NS, D_5W, $D_{10}W$, fat emulsion 10%, LR, $^1/_2NS$, NS

Y-site administration: Incompatible with fluconazole

Compatibility in syringe: Incompatible with glycopyrrolate, metoclopramide

Compatibility when admixed: Incompatible with chlorpromazine, hydroxyzine, phenytoin, polymyxin B sulfate, prochlorperazine edisylate, prochlorperazine mesylate, promethazine, vancomycin

Storage: Store at room temperature prior to reconstitution; reconstituted solutions remain stable for 30 days; use only clear solutions; frozen solutions remain stable for 6 months

◆ **ChloraPrep® [OTC]** *see* Chlorhexidine Gluconate *on page 373*
◆ **Chloraseptic® Gargle [OTC]** *see* Phenol *on page 1347*
◆ **Chloraseptic® Mouth Pain [OTC]** *see* Phenol *on page 1347*
◆ **Chloraseptic® Rinse [OTC]** *see* Phenol *on page 1347*
◆ **Chloraseptic® Spray [OTC]** *see* Phenol *on page 1347*

♦ Chloraseptic® Spray for Kids [OTC] *see* Phenol *on page 1347*

Chlorhexidine Gluconate (klor HEKS i deen GLOO koe nate)

U.S. Brand Names Avagard™ [OTC]; BactoShield® CHG [OTC]; Betasept® [OTC]; ChloraPrep® [OTC]; Dyna-Hex® [OTC]; Hibiclens® [OTC]; Hibistat® [OTC]; Operand® Chlorhexidine Gluconate [OTC]; Peridex®; PerioChip®; PerioGard®

Synonyms CHG; 3M™ Avagard™ [OTC]

Pharmacologic Category Antibiotic, Oral Rinse; Antibiotic, Topical

Medication Safety Issues

Sound-alike/look-alike issues:

Peridex® may be confused with Precedex™

Use Skin cleanser for surgical scrub, cleanser for skin wounds, preoperative skin preparation, germicidal hand rinse, and as antibacterial dental rinse. Chlorhexidine is active against gram-positive and gram-negative organisms, facultative anaerobes, aerobes, and yeast.

Orphan drug: Peridex®: Oral mucositis with cytoreductive therapy when used for patients undergoing bone marrow transplant

Mechanism of Action The bactericidal effect of chlorhexidine is a result of the binding of this cationic molecule to negatively charged bacterial cell walls and extramicrobial complexes. At low concentrations, this causes an alteration of bacterial cell osmotic equilibrium and leakage of potassium and phosphorous resulting in a bacteriostatic effect. At high concentrations of chlorhexidine, the cytoplasmic contents of the bacterial cell precipitate and result in cell death.

Pharmacodynamics/Kinetics

Topical hand sanitizer (Avagard™): Duration of antimicrobial protection: 6 hours

Oral rinse (Peridex®, PerioGard®):

Absorption: ~30% retained in the oral cavity following rinsing and slowly released into oral fluids; poorly absorbed

Time to peak, plasma: Oral rinse: Detectable levels not present after 12 hours

Excretion: Feces (~90%); urine (<1%)

Contraindications Hypersensitivity to chlorhexidine gluconate or any component of the formulation

Warnings/Precautions

Oral: Staining of oral surfaces (mucosa, teeth, tooth restorations, dorsum of tongue) may occur; may be visible as soon as 1 week after therapy begins and is more pronounced when there is a heavy accumulation of unremoved plaque and when teeth fillings have rough surfaces. Stain does not have a clinically adverse effect, but because removal may not be possible, patient with frontal restoration should be advised of the potential permanency of the stain.

Topical: For topical use only. Keep out of eyes and ears. May stain fabric. There have been case reports of anaphylaxis following chlorhexidine disinfection. Not for preoperative preparation of face or head; avoid contact with meninges.

Drug Interactions No data reported

Adverse Reactions

Oral:

>10%: Increase of tartar on teeth, changes in taste. Staining of oral surfaces (mucosa, teeth, dorsum of tongue) may be visible as soon as 1 week after therapy begins and is more pronounced when there is a heavy accumulation of unremoved plaque and when teeth fillings have rough surfaces. Stain does not have a clinically adverse effect but because removal may not be possible, patient with frontal restoration should be advised of the potential permanency of the stain.

1% to 10%: Gastrointestinal: Tongue irritation, oral irritation

<1% (Limited to important or life-threatening): Dyspnea, facial edema, nasal congestion

Topical: Skin erythema and roughness, dryness, sensitization, allergic reactions

Overdosage/Toxicology Symptoms of oral overdose include gastric distress, nausea, or signs of ethanol intoxication

Dosing

Adults & Elderly:

Oral rinse (Peridex®, PerioGard®):

Floss and brush teeth, completely rinse toothpaste from mouth and swish 15 mL (one capful) undiluted oral rinse around in mouth for 30 seconds, then expectorate. Caution patient not to swallow the medicine and instruct not to eat for 2-3 hours after treatment. (Cap on bottle measures 15 mL.)

(Continued)

Chlorhexidine Gluconate *(Continued)*

Treatment of gingivitis: Oral prophylaxis: Swish for 30 seconds with 15 mL chlorhexidine, then expectorate; repeat twice daily (morning and evening). Patient should have a re-evaluation followed by a dental prophylaxis every 6 months.

Periodontal chip: One chip is inserted into a periodontal pocket with a probing pocket depth ≥5 mm. Up to 8 chips may be inserted in a single visit. Treatment is recommended every 3 months in pockets with a remaining depth ≥5 mm. If dislodgment occurs 7 days or more after placement, the subject is considered to have had the full course of treatment. If dislodgment occurs within 48 hours, a new chip should be inserted. The chip biodegrades completely and does not need to be removed. Patients should avoid dental floss at the site of PerioChip® insertion for 10 days after placement because flossing might dislodge the chip.

Insertion of periodontal chip: Pocket should be isolated and surrounding area dried prior to chip insertion. The chip should be grasped using forceps with the rounded edges away from the forceps. The chip should be inserted into the periodontal pocket to its maximum depth. It may be maneuvered into position using the tips of the forceps or a flat instrument.

Cleanser:

Surgical scrub: Scrub 3 minutes and rinse thoroughly, wash for an additional 3 minutes

Hand sanitizer (Avagard™): Dispense 1 pumpful in palm of one hand; dip fingertips of opposite hand into solution and work it under nails. Spread remainder evenly over hand and just above elbow, covering all surfaces. Repeat on other hand. Dispense another pumpful in each hand and reapply to each hand up to the wrist. Allow to dry before gloving.

Hand wash: Wash for 15 seconds and rinse

Hand rinse: Rub 15 seconds and rinse

Available Dosage Forms

Chip, for periodontal pocket insertion (PerioChip®): 2.5 mg

Liquid, topical [surgical scrub]:

Avagard™: 1% (500 mL) [contains ethyl alcohol and moisturizers]

BactoShield® CHG: 2% (120 mL, 480 mL, 750 mL, 1000 mL, 3800 mL); 4% (120 mL, 480 mL, 750 mL, 1000 mL, 3800 mL) [contains isopropyl alcohol]

Betasept®: 4% (120 mL, 240 mL, 480 mL, 960 mL, 3840 mL) [contains isopropyl alcohol]

ChloraPrep®: 2% (0.67 mL, 1.5 mL, 3 mL, 10.5 mL) [contains isopropyl alcohol 70%; prefilled applicator]

Dyna-Hex®: 2% (120 mL, 960 mL, 3840 mL); 4% (120 mL, 960 mL, 3840 mL)

Hibiclens®: 4% (15 mL, 120 mL, 240 mL, 480 mL, 960 mL, 3840 mL) [contains isopropyl alcohol]

Operand® Chlorhexidine Gluconate: 2% (120 mL); 4% (120 mL, 240 mL, 480 mL, 960 mL, 3840 mL) [contains isopropyl alcohol]

Liquid, oral rinse: 0.12% (480 mL)

Peridex®: 0.12% (480 mL) [contains alcohol 11.6%]

PerioGard®: 0.12% (480 mL) [contains alcohol 11.6%; mint flavor]

Pad [prep pad] (Hibistat®): 0.5% (50s) [contains isopropyl alcohol]

Sponge/Brush (BactoShield® CHG): 4% per sponge/brush [contains isopropyl alcohol]

Nursing Guidelines

Patient Education:

Oral rinse: Do not swallow, do not rinse after use; may cause reduced taste perception which is reversible; may cause discoloration of teeth

Periodontal chip: Avoid dental floss at the site of the chip insertion for 10 days after placement because flossing might dislodge the chip.

Topical: For external use only.

Pregnancy Risk Factor: B

Administration

Oral: Periodontal chip insertion: Pocket should be isolated and surrounding area dried prior to chip insertion. The chip should be grasped using forceps with the rounded edges away from the forceps. The chip should be inserted into the periodontal pocket to its maximum depth. It may be maneuvered into position using the tips of the forceps or a flat instrument. The chip biodegrades completely and does not need to be removed. Patients should avoid dental floss at the site of PerioChip® insertion for 10 days after placement because flossing might dislodge the chip.

Compatibility: Avagard™: Hand lotions and gel hand sanitizers are incompatible. The thickeners used in these products (eg, carbomer) react to form an insoluble salt and cause loss of antibacterial action.

Storage: Store at room temperature

Avagard™: Avoid excessive heat. Ethanol-containing products are flammable; keep away from flames or fire.

♦ Chlormeprazine *see* Prochlorperazine *on page 1412*

♦ 2-Chlorodeoxyadenosine *see* Cladribine *on page 420*

♦ Chloromag® *see* Magnesium Chloride *on page 1074*

♦ Chloromycetin® Sodium Succinate *see* Chloramphenicol *on page 370*

Chloroprocaine (klor oh PROE kane)

U.S. Brand Names Nesacaine®; Nesacaine®-MPF

Synonyms Chloroprocaine Hydrochloride

Pharmacologic Category Local Anesthetic

Medication Safety Issues

Sound-alike/look-alike issues:

Nesacaine® may be confused with Neptazane®

Use Infiltration anesthesia and peripheral and epidural anesthesia

Mechanism of Action Chloroprocaine HCl is benzoic acid, 4-amino-2-chloro-2-(diethylamino) ethyl ester monohydrochloride. Chloroprocaine is an ester-type local anesthetic, which stabilizes the neuronal membranes and prevents initiation and transmission of nerve impulses thereby affecting local anesthetic actions. Local anesthetics including chloroprocaine, reversibly prevent generation and conduction of electrical impulses in neurons by decreasing the transient increase in permeability to sodium. The differential sensitivity generally depends on the size of the fiber; small fibers are more sensitive than larger fibers and require a longer period for recovery. Sensory pain fibers are usually blocked first, followed by fibers that transmit sensations of temperature, touch, and deep pressure. High concentrations block sympathetic somatic sensory and somatic motor fibers. The spread of anesthesia depends upon the distribution of the solution. This is primarily dependent on the volume of drug injected.

Pharmacodynamics/Kinetics

Onset of action: 6-12 minutes

Duration: 30-60 minutes

Distribution: V_d: Depends upon route of administration; high concentrations found in highly perfused organs such as liver, lungs, heart, and brain

Metabolism: Plasma cholinesterases

Excretion: Urine

Contraindications Hypersensitivity to chloroprocaine, other ester type anesthetics, or any component of the formulation; myasthenia gravis; do not use for subarachnoid administration

Warnings/Precautions Use with caution in patients with hepatic impairment. **Do not use solutions containing preservatives for caudal or epidural block.** Local anesthetics have been associated with rare occurrences of sudden respiratory arrest; seizures due to systemic toxicity leading to cardiac arrest have also been reported, presumably following unintentional intravascular injection. A test dose is recommended prior to epidural administration (prior to initial dose) and all reinforcing doses with continuous catheter technique.

Drug Interactions

PABA (from ester-type anesthetics) may inhibit sulfonamides.

Adverse Reactions

Frequency not defined.

Cardiovascular: Bradycardia, cardiac arrest, hypotension, ventricular arrhythmia

Central nervous system: Anxiety, dizziness, restlessness, tinnitus, unconsciousness

Dermatologic: Angioneurotic edema, erythema, pruritus, urticaria

Ocular: Blurred vision

Respiratory: Respiratory arrest

Miscellaneous: Allergic reactions, anaphylactoid reactions

<1% (Limited to important or life-threatening): Seizure (0.1%)

Overdosage/Toxicology Symptoms may include anxiety, blurred vision, bradyarrhythmias, CNS depression, dizziness, drowsiness, metabolic acidosis, methemoglobinemia, restlessness, seizures, and tremors. Treatment is symptomatic and supportive. Termination of anesthesia by pneumatic tourniquet inflation

(Continued)

Chloroprocaine *(Continued)*

should be attempted when chloroprocaine is administered by infiltration or regional injection.

Dosing

Adults & Elderly: Dosage varies with anesthetic procedure, the area to be anesthetized, the vascularity of the tissues, depth of anesthesia required, degree of muscle relaxation required, and duration of anesthesia; range.

Maximum single dose (without epinephrine): 11 mg/kg; maximum dose: 800 mg

Maximum single dose (with epinephrine): 14 mg/kg; maximum dose: 1000 mg

Infiltration and peripheral nerve block:

Mandibular: 2%: 2-3 mL; total dose 40-60 mg

Infraorbital: 2%: 0.5-1 mL; total dose 10-20 mg

Brachial plexus: 2%; 30-40 mL; total dose 600-800 mg

Digital (without epinephrine): 1%; 3-4 mL; total dose: 30-40 mg

Pudendal: 2%; 10 mL each side; total dose: 400 mg

Paracervical: 1%; 3 mL per each of four sites

Caudal block: Preservative-free: 2% or 3%: 15-25 mL; may repeat at 40-60 minute intervals

Lumbar epidural block: Preservative-free: 2% or 3%: 2-2.5 mL per segment; usual total volume: 15-25 mL; may repeat with doses that are 2-6 mL less than initial dose every 40-50 minutes.

Pediatrics: Dosage varies with anesthetic procedure, the area to be anesthetized, the vascularity of the tissues, depth of anesthesia required, degree of muscle relaxation required, and duration of anesthesia; range.

Children >3 years (normally developed): Maximum dose (without epinephrine): 11 mg/kg; for infiltration, concentrations of 0.5% to 1% are recommended; for nerve block, concentrations of 1% to 1.5% are recommended

Available Dosage Forms

Injection, solution, as hydrochloride (Nesacaine®): 1% (30 mL); 2% (30 mL) [contains disodium EDTA and methylparaben]

Injection, solution, as hydrochloride (Nesacaine®-MPF) [preservative free]: 2% (20 mL); 3% (20 mL)

Nursing Guidelines

Assessment: Monitor for effectiveness of anesthesia, and adverse reactions. Monitor for return of sensation. Teach patient adverse reactions to report; use and teach appropriate interventions to promote safety.

Patient Education: This medication is given to reduce sensation in the injected area. You will experience decreased sensation to pain, heat, or cold in the area and/or decreased muscle strength (depending on area of application) until the effects wear off; use necessary caution to reduce incidence of possible injury until full sensation returns. Immediately report chest pain or palpitations; increased restlessness, confusion, anxiety, or dizziness; respiratory difficulty; chills, shivering, or tremors; ringing in ears; or vision changes. **Pregnancy/breast-feeding precautions:** Inform prescriber if you are pregnant. Consult prescriber if breast-feeding.

Pregnancy Risk Factor: C

Lactation: Excretion in breast milk unknown/use caution

Perioperative/Anesthesia/Other Concerns: Termination of anesthesia by pneumatic tourniquet inflation should be attempted when the agent is administered by infiltration or regional injection. Seizures commonly respond to diazepam, midazolam, or thiopental, while hypotension responds to I.V. fluids and Trendelenburg positioning. Bradyarrhythmias (when the heart rate is <60) can be treated with I.V., I.M., or SubQ atropine 15 mcg/kg. With the development of metabolic acidosis, I.V. sodium bicarbonate 0.5-2 mEq/kg and ventilatory assistance should be instituted.

Administration

Reconstitution: Dilute with NS. To prepare 1:200,000 epinephrine-chloroprocaine HCl injection, add 0.1 mL of a 1:1000 epinephrine injection to 20 mL of preservative free chloroprocaine.

Storage: Store at 15°C to 30°C (59°F to 86°F); protect from light and freezing. Discard Nesacaine®-MPF following single use.

Related Information

Local Anesthetics *on page 1854*

♦ **Chloroprocaine Hydrochloride** *see* Chloroprocaine *on page 375*

Chloroquine (KLOR oh kwin)

U.S. Brand Names Aralen®

Synonyms Chloroquine Phosphate

Pharmacologic Category Aminoquinoline (Antimalarial)

Use Suppression or chemoprophylaxis of malaria; treatment of uncomplicated or mild to moderate malaria; extraintestinal amebiasis

Unlabeled/Investigational Use Rheumatoid arthritis; discoid lupus erythematosus

Mechanism of Action Binds to and inhibits DNA and RNA polymerase; interferes with metabolism and hemoglobin utilization by parasites; inhibits prostaglandin effects; chloroquine concentrates within parasite acid vesicles and raises internal pH resulting in inhibition of parasite growth; may involve aggregates of ferriprotoporphyrin IX acting as chloroquine receptors causing membrane damage; may also interfere with nucleoprotein synthesis

Pharmacodynamics/Kinetics

Duration: Small amounts may be present in urine months following discontinuation of therapy

Absorption: Oral: Rapid (~89%)

Distribution: Widely in body tissues (eg, eyes, heart, kidneys, liver, lungs) where retention prolonged; crosses placenta; enters breast milk

Metabolism: Partially hepatic

Half-life elimination: 3-5 days

Time to peak, serum: 1-2 hours

Excretion: Urine (~70% as unchanged drug); acidification of urine increases elimination

Contraindications Hypersensitivity to chloroquine or any component of the formulation; retinal or visual field changes

Warnings/Precautions Use with caution in patients with liver disease, G6PD deficiency, alcoholism or in conjunction with hepatotoxic drugs. May exacerbate psoriasis or porphyria. Retinopathy (irreversible) has occurred with long or high-dose therapy; discontinue drug if any abnormality in the visual field or if muscular weakness develops during treatment. Use caution in patients with pre-existing auditory damage; discontinue immediately if hearing defects are noted. Use caution in patients with seizure disorders.

Drug Interactions **Substrate** (major) of CYP2D6, 3A4; **Inhibits** CYP2D6 (moderate)

Ampicillin: Chloroquine may reduce the absorption of ampicillin; separate administration by 2 hours.

Antacids and kaolin: Chloroquine and other 4-aminoquinolones may be decreased due to GI binding with kaolin or magnesium trisilicate.

Cimetidine: Cimetidine increases levels of chloroquine and probably other 4-aminoquinolones.

Cyclosporine: Chloroquine may increase cyclosporine concentrations; monitor.

CYP2D6 inhibitors: May increase the levels/effects of chloroquine. Example inhibitors include chlorpromazine, delavirdine, fluoxetine, miconazole, paroxetine, pergolide, quinidine, quinine, ritonavir, and ropinirole.

CYP2D6 substrates: Chloroquine may increase the levels/effects of CYP2D6 substrates. Example substrates include amphetamines, selected beta-blockers, dextromethorphan, fluoxetine, lidocaine, mirtazapine, nefazodone, paroxetine, risperidone, ritonavir, thioridazine, tricyclic antidepressants, and venlafaxine.

CYP2D6 prodrug substrates: Chloroquine may decrease the levels/effects of CYP2D6 prodrug substrates. Example prodrug substrates include codeine, hydrocodone, oxycodone, and tramadol.

CYP3A4 inducers: CYP3A4 inducers may decrease the levels/effects of chloroquine. Example inducers include aminoglutethimide, carbamazepine, nafcillin, nevirapine, phenobarbital, phenytoin, and rifamycins.

CYP3A4 inhibitors: May increase the levels/effects of chloroquine. Example inhibitors include azole antifungals, clarithromycin, diclofenac, doxycycline, erythromycin, imatinib, isoniazid, nefazodone, nicardipine, propofol, protease inhibitors, quinidine, telithromycin, and verapamil.

Praziquantel: Chloroquine may decrease praziquantel concentrations.

Nutritional/Herbal/Ethanol Interactions Ethanol: Avoid ethanol (may increase GI irritation).

Adverse Reactions Frequency not defined.

Cardiovascular: Hypotension (rare), ECG changes (rare; including T-wave inversion), cardiomyopathy

(Continued)

Chloroquine *(Continued)*

Central nervous system: Fatigue, personality changes, headache, psychosis, seizure, delirium, depression

Dermatologic: Pruritus, hair bleaching, pleomorphic skin eruptions, lichen planus eruptions, alopecia, mucosal pigmentary changes (blue-black), photosensitivity

Gastrointestinal: Nausea, diarrhea, vomiting, anorexia, stomatitis, abdominal cramps

Hematologic: Aplastic anemia, agranulocytosis (reversible), neutropenia, thrombocytopenia

Neuromuscular & skeletal: Rare cases of myopathy, neuromyopathy, proximal muscle atrophy, and depression of deep tendon reflexes have been reported

Ocular: Retinopathy (including irreversible changes in some patients long-term or high-dose therapy), blurred vision

Otic: Nerve deafness, tinnitus, reduced hearing (risk increased in patients with pre-existing auditory damage)

Overdosage/Toxicology Symptoms of overdose include headache, visual changes, cardiovascular collapse, shock, seizures, abdominal cramps, vomiting, cyanosis, methemoglobinemia, leukopenia, and respiratory and cardiac arrest. Following initial measures (immediate GI decontamination), treatment is supportive and symptomatic.

Dosing

Adults & Elderly:

Malaria, suppression or prophylaxis: Oral: 500 mg/week (300 mg base) on the same day each week; begin 1-2 weeks prior to exposure; continue for 4-6 weeks after leaving endemic area; if suppressive therapy is not begun prior to exposure, double the initial loading dose to 1 g (600 mg base) and administer in 2 divided doses 6 hours apart, followed by the usual dosage regimen.

Malaria, acute attack: Oral: 1 g (600 mg base) on day 1, followed by 500 mg (300 mg base) 6 hours later, followed by 500 mg (300 mg base) on days 2 and 3.

Extraintestinal amebiasis: Oral: 1 g/day (600 mg base) for 2 days followed by 500 mg/day (300 mg base) for at least 2-3 weeks.

Rheumatoid arthritis, lupus erythematosus (unlabeled uses): Oral: 250 mg (150 mg base) once daily; reduce dosage following maximal response (taper to discontinue after response in lupus); generally requires 3-6 weeks. **Note:** Not considered first-line agent.

Pediatrics:

Malaria, suppression or prophylaxis: Oral: Administer 5 mg base/kg/week on the same day each week (not to exceed 300 mg base/dose); begin 1-2 weeks prior to exposure; continue for 4-6 weeks after leaving endemic area; if suppressive therapy is not begun prior to exposure, double the initial loading dose to 10 mg base/kg and administer in 2 divided doses 6 hours apart, followed by the usual dosage regimen

Malaria, acute attack: Oral: 10 mg/kg (base) on day 1, followed by 5 mg/kg (base) 6 hours later and 5 mg/kg (base) on days 2 and 3

Extraintestinal amebiasis: Oral: 10 mg/kg (base) once daily for 2-3 weeks (up to 300 mg base/day)

Renal Impairment:

Cl_{cr} <10 mL/minute: Administer 50% of dose.

Hemodialysis effects: Minimally removed by hemodialysis

Available Dosage Forms

Tablet, as phosphate: 250 mg [equivalent to 150 mg base]; 500 mg [equivalent to 300 mg base]

Aralen®: 500 mg [equivalent to 300 mg base]

Nursing Guidelines

Assessment: See Contraindications, Warnings/Precautions, and Dosing for use cautions. Assess potential for interactions with other prescriptions, OTC medications, or herbal products patient may be taking (see Drug Interactions). Assess results of laboratory tests (see below), therapeutic effectiveness (according to purpose for use), and adverse response (see Adverse Reactions and Overdose/Toxicology) regularly during long-term therapy. Teach patient appropriate use, possible side effects/appropriate interventions, and adverse symptoms to report (see Patient Education). See Lactation for breast-feeding considerations.

Monitoring Laboratory Tests: Periodic CBC

Dietary Considerations: May be taken with meals to decrease GI upset.

Patient Education: Inform prescriber of all prescriptions, OTC medications, or herbal products you are taking, and any allergies you have. Do not take any new medication during therapy unless approved by prescriber. It is important to complete full course of therapy, which may take up to 6 months for full effect. May be taken with meals to decrease GI upset and bitter aftertaste. Avoid alcohol. You should have regular ophthalmic exams (every 4-6 months) if using this medication over extended periods. May cause skin discoloration (blue/black), hair bleaching, or skin rash. If you have psoriasis, may cause exacerbation. May turn urine black/brown (normal). May cause headache (if persistent, consult prescriber for analgesic); nausea, vomiting, or loss of appetite (small, frequent meals, frequent mouth care, sucking lozenges, or chewing gum may help); or increased sensitivity to sunlight (wear dark glasses and protective clothing, use sunblock, and avoid direct exposure to sunlight). Report vision changes; rash or itching; persistent diarrhea or GI disturbances; change in hearing acuity or ringing in the ears; chest pain or palpitation; CNS changes; unusual fatigue, easy bruising or bleeding; or any other persistent adverse reactions. **Pregnancy/breast-feeding precautions:** Inform prescriber if you are or intend to become pregnant. Consult prescriber if breast-feeding.

Pregnancy Risk Factor: C

Pregnancy Issues: There are no adequate and well-controlled studies using chloroquine during pregnancy. However, based on clinical experience and because malaria infection in pregnant women may be more severe than in nonpregnant women, chloroquine prophylaxis may be considered in areas of chloroquine-sensitive *P. falciparum* malaria. Pregnant women should be advised not to travel to areas of *P. falciparum* resistance to chloroquine.

Lactation: Enters breast milk/not recommended (AAP considers "compatible")

Administration

Oral: Chloroquine phosphate tablets have also been mixed with chocolate syrup or enclosed in gelatin capsules to mask the bitter taste.

Storage: Store tablets at 25°C (77°F). Excursions permitted at 15°C to 30°C (59°F to 86°F).

◆ Chloroquine Phosphate *see* Chloroquine *on page 377*

ChlorproMAZINE (klor PROE ma zeen)

U.S. Brand Names Thorazine® [DSC]

Synonyms Chlorpromazine Hydrochloride; CPZ

Pharmacologic Category Antipsychotic Agent, Typical, Phenothiazine

Medication Safety Issues

Sound-alike/look-alike issues:

ChlorproMAZINE may be confused with chlorproPAMIDE, clomiPRAMINE, prochlorperazine, promethazine

Thorazine® may be confused with thiamine, thioridazine

Use Control of mania; treatment of schizophrenia; control of nausea and vomiting; relief of restlessness and apprehension before surgery; acute intermittent porphyria; adjunct in the treatment of tetanus; intractable hiccups; combativeness and/or explosive hyperexcitable behavior in children 1-12 years of age and in short-term treatment of hyperactive children

Unlabeled/Investigational Use Management of psychotic disorders

Mechanism of Action Chlorpromazine is an aliphatic phenothiazine antipsychotic which blocks postsynaptic mesolimbic dopaminergic receptors in the brain; exhibits a strong alpha-adrenergic blocking effect and depresses the release of hypothalamic and hypophyseal hormones; believed to depress the reticular activating system, thus affecting basal metabolism, body temperature, wakefulness, vasomotor tone, and emesis

Pharmacodynamics/Kinetics

Onset of action: I.M.: 15 minutes; Oral: 30-60 minutes

Absorption: Rapid

Distribution: V_d: 20 L/kg; crosses the placenta; enters breast milk

Protein binding: 92% to 97%

Metabolism: Extensively hepatic to active and inactive metabolites

Bioavailability: 20%

Half-life, biphasic: Initial: 2 hours; Terminal: 30 hours

Excretion: Urine (<1% as unchanged drug) within 24 hours

(Continued)

ChlorproMAZINE *(Continued)*

Contraindications Hypersensitivity to chlorpromazine or any component of the formulation (cross-reactivity between phenothiazines may occur); severe CNS depression; coma

Warnings/Precautions Highly sedating, use with caution in disorders where CNS depression is a feature. Use with caution in Parkinson's disease. Caution in patients with hemodynamic instability; bone marrow suppression; predisposition to seizures, subcortical brain damage, severe cardiac, hepatic, renal, or respiratory disease. Esophageal dysmotility and aspiration have been associated with antipsychotic use - use with caution in patients at risk of aspiration pneumonia (ie, Alzheimer's disease). Caution in breast cancer or other prolactin-dependent tumors (may elevate prolactin levels). May alter temperature regulation or mask toxicity of other drugs due to antiemetic effects. May alter cardiac conduction - life-threatening arrhythmias have occurred with therapeutic doses of neuroleptics. May cause orthostatic hypotension - use with caution in patients at risk of this effect or those who would tolerate transient hypotensive episodes (cerebrovascular disease, cardiovascular disease, or other medications which may predispose). Significant hypotension may occur, particularly with parenteral administration. Injection contains sulfites and benzyl alcohol.

Phenothiazines may cause anticholinergic effects (confusion, agitation, constipation, xerostomia, blurred vision, urinary retention). Therefore, they should be used with caution in patients with decreased gastrointestinal motility, urinary retention, BPH, xerostomia, or visual problems. Conditions which also may be exacerbated by cholinergic blockade include narrow-angle glaucoma (screening is recommended) and worsening of myasthenia gravis. Relative to other neuroleptics, chlorpromazine has a moderate potency of cholinergic blockade.

May cause extrapyramidal symptoms, including pseudoparkinsonism, acute dystonic reactions, akathisia, and tardive dyskinesia (risk of these reactions is low-moderate relative to other neuroleptics). May be associated with neuroleptic malignant syndrome (NMS) or pigmentary retinopathy.

Drug Interactions **Substrate** of CYP1A2 (minor), 2D6 (major), 3A4 (minor); **Inhibits** CYP2D6 (strong), 2E1 (weak)

Acetylcholinesterase inhibitors (central): May increase the risk of antipsychotic-related extrapyramidal symptoms; monitor.

Aluminum salts: May decrease the absorption of phenothiazines; monitor

Amphetamines: Efficacy may be diminished by antipsychotics; in addition, amphetamines may increase psychotic symptoms; avoid concurrent use

Anticholinergics: May inhibit the therapeutic response to phenothiazines and excess anticholinergic effects may occur; includes benztropine, trihexyphenidyl, biperiden, and drugs with significant anticholinergic activity (TCAs, antihistamines, disopyramide)

Antihypertensives: Concurrent use of phenothiazines with an antihypertensive may produce additive hypotensive effects (particularly orthostasis)

Bromocriptine: Phenothiazines inhibit the ability of bromocriptine to lower serum prolactin concentrations

CNS depressants: Sedative effects may be additive with phenothiazines; monitor for increased effect; includes barbiturates, benzodiazepines, narcotic analgesics, ethanol and other sedative agents

CYP2D6 inhibitors: May increase the levels/effects of chlorpromazine. Example inhibitors include delavirdine, fluoxetine, miconazole, paroxetine, pergolide, quinidine, quinine, ritonavir, and ropinirole.

CYP2D6 substrates: Chlorpromazine may increase the levels/effects of CYP2D6 substrates. Example substrates include amphetamines, selected beta-blockers, dextromethorphan, fluoxetine, lidocaine, mirtazapine, nefazodone, paroxetine, risperidone, ritonavir, thioridazine, tricyclic antidepressants, and venlafaxine.

CYP2D6 prodrug substrates: Chlorpromazine may decrease the levels/effects of CYP2D6 prodrug substrates. Example prodrug substrates include codeine, hydrocodone, oxycodone, and tramadol.

Epinephrine: Chlorpromazine (and possibly other low potency antipsychotics) may diminish the pressor effects of epinephrine

Guanethidine and guanadrel: Antihypertensive effects may be inhibited by chlorpromazine

Levodopa: Chlorpromazine may inhibit the antiparkinsonian effect of levodopa; avoid this combination

Lithium: Chlorpromazine may produce neurotoxicity with lithium; this is a rare effect

Metoclopramide: May increase extrapyramidal symptoms (EPS) or risk.
Phenytoin: May reduce serum levels of phenothiazines; phenothiazines may increase phenytoin serum levels
Propranolol: Serum concentrations of phenothiazines may be increased; propranolol also increases phenothiazine concentrations
Polypeptide antibiotics: Rare cases of respiratory paralysis have been reported with concurrent use of phenothiazines
QT_c-prolonging agents: Effects on QT_c interval may be additive with phenothiazines, increasing the risk of malignant arrhythmias; includes type Ia antiarrhythmics, TCAs, and some quinolone antibiotics (sparfloxacin, moxifloxacin and gatifloxacin)
Sulfadoxine-pyrimethamine: May increase phenothiazine concentrations
Tricyclic antidepressants: Concurrent use may produce increased toxicity or altered therapeutic response
Trazodone: Phenothiazines and trazodone may produce additive hypotensive effects
Valproic acid: Serum levels may be increased by phenothiazines

Nutritional/Herbal/Ethanol Interactions

Ethanol: Avoid ethanol (may increase CNS depression).
Herb/Nutraceutical: Avoid St John's wort (may decrease chlorpromazine levels, increase photosensitization, or enhance sedative effect). Avoid dong quai (may enhance photosensitization). Avoid kava kava, gotu kola, valerian (may increase CNS depression).

Lab Interactions False-positives for phenylketonuria, amylase, uroporphyrins, urobilinogen. May cause false-positive pregnancy test.

Adverse Reactions Frequency not defined.

Cardiovascular: Postural hypotension, tachycardia, dizziness, nonspecific QT changes
Central nervous system: Drowsiness, dystonias, akathisia, pseudoparkinsonism, tardive dyskinesia, neuroleptic malignant syndrome, seizure
Dermatologic: Photosensitivity, dermatitis, skin pigmentation (slate gray)
Endocrine & metabolic: Lactation, breast engorgement, false-positive pregnancy test, amenorrhea, gynecomastia, hyper- or hypoglycemia
Gastrointestinal: Xerostomia, constipation, nausea
Genitourinary: Urinary retention, ejaculatory disorder, impotence
Hematologic: Agranulocytosis, eosinophilia, leukopenia, hemolytic anemia, aplastic anemia, thrombocytopenic purpura
Hepatic: Jaundice
Ocular: Blurred vision, corneal and lenticular changes, epithelial keratopathy, pigmentary retinopathy

Overdosage/Toxicology Symptoms of overdose include deep sleep, coma, extrapyramidal symptoms, abnormal involuntary muscle movements, and hypotension. Following initiation of essential overdose management, toxic symptom treatment and supportive treatment should be initiated. Neuroleptics often cause extrapyramidal symptoms (eg, dystonic reactions) requiring management with anticholinergic agents such as benztropine mesylate 1-2 mg for adult patients (oral, I.M., I.V.) or diphenhydramine 25-50 mg (oral, I.M., I.V.) may be effective.

Dosing

Adults:

Schizophrenia/psychoses:

Oral: Range: 30-800 mg/day in 1-4 divided doses, initiate at lower doses and titrate as needed; usual dose: 200 mg/day; some patients may require 1-2 g/day
I.M., I.V.: Initial: 25 mg, may repeat (25-50 mg) in 1-4 hours, gradually increase to a maximum of 400 mg/dose every 4-6 hours until patient is controlled; usual dose: 300-800 mg/day

Intractable hiccups: Oral, I.M.: 25-50 mg 3-4 times/day

Nausea and vomiting:

Oral: 10-25 mg every 4-6 hours
I.M., I.V.: 25-50 mg every 4-6 hours

Elderly:

Behavioral symptoms associated with dementia: Initial: 10-25 mg 1-2 times/day; increase at 4- to 7-day intervals by 10-25 mg/day. Increase dose intervals (eg, twice daily, 3 times/day) as necessary to control behavior response or side effects; maximum daily dose: 800 mg; gradual increases (titration) may prevent some side effects or decrease their severity.
Other indications: Refer to adult dosing.

(Continued)

ChlorproMAZINE *(Continued)*

Pediatrics:

Schizophrenia/psychoses: Children ≥6 months:

Oral: 0.5-1 mg/kg/dose every 4-6 hours; older children may require 200 mg/day or higher.

I.M., I.V.: 0.5-1 mg/kg/dose every 6-8 hours; maximum dose for <5 years (22.7 kg): 40 mg/day; maximum for 5-12 years (22.7-45.5 kg): 75 mg/day

Nausea and vomiting: Children ≥6 months:

Oral: 0.5-1 mg/kg/dose every 4-6 hours as needed

I.M., I.V.: 0.5-1 mg/kg/dose every 6-8 hours; maximum dose for <5 years (22.7 kg): 40 mg/day; maximum for 5-12 years (22.7-45.5 kg): 75 mg/day

Renal Impairment: Not dialyzable (0% to 5%)

Hepatic Impairment: Avoid use in severe hepatic dysfunction.

Available Dosage Forms

Injection, solution, as hydrochloride: 25 mg/mL (10 mL) [contains benzyl alcohol, sodium bisulfite, and sodium sulfite]

Tablet, as hydrochloride: 10 mg, 25 mg, 50 mg, 100 mg, 200 mg

Nursing Guidelines

Assessment: Assess other medications patient is taking for effectiveness and interactions. Review ophthalmic exam and monitor laboratory results, therapeutic effectiveness, and adverse reactions at beginning of therapy and periodically with long-term use. **I.V./I.M.:** Significant hypotension may occur. Initiate at lower doses (see Dosing) and taper dosage slowly when discontinuing. Assess knowledge/teach patient appropriate use, interventions to reduce side effects, and adverse symptoms to report. **Note:** Chlorpromazine may cause false-positive pregnancy test.

Monitoring Laboratory Tests: Lipid profile, fasting blood glucose/Hgb A_{1c}; BMI

Patient Education: Use exactly as directed; do not increase dose or frequency. Do not discontinue without consulting prescriber. Tablets may be taken with food. Do not take within 2 hours of any antacid. Store away from light. Avoid alcohol or caffeine and other prescription or OTC medications not approved by prescriber. Maintain adequate hydration (2-3 L/day of fluids) unless instructed to restrict fluid intake. May turn urine red-brown (normal). You may experience excess drowsiness, lightheadedness, dizziness, or blurred vision (use caution driving or when engaging in tasks requiring alertness until response to drug is known); dry mouth, upset stomach, nausea, vomiting, anorexia (small frequent meals, frequent mouth care, sucking lozenges, or chewing gum may help); constipation (increased exercise, fluids, fruit, or fiber may help); postural hypotension (use caution climbing stairs or when changing position from lying or sitting to standing); urinary retention (void before taking medication); ejaculatory dysfunction (reversible); decreased perspiration (avoid strenuous exercise in hot environments); or photosensitivity (use sunscreen, wear protective clothing and eyewear, and avoid direct sunlight). Report persistent CNS effects (trembling fingers, altered gait or balance, excessive sedation, seizures, unusual movements, anxiety, abnormal thoughts, confusion, personality changes); chest pain, palpitations, rapid heartbeat, or severe dizziness; unresolved urinary retention or changes in urinary pattern; altered menstrual pattern, change in libido, swelling or pain in breasts (male or female); vision changes, skin rash, irritation, or changes in color of skin (gray-blue); or worsening of condition. **Pregnancy/breast-feeding precautions:** Inform prescriber if you are or intend to become pregnant. Breast-feeding is not recommended.

Geriatric Considerations: See Warnings/Precautions, Adverse Reactions, and Overdose/Toxicology. Elderly patients have an increased risk of adverse response to side effects or adverse reactions to antipsychotics.

Pregnancy Risk Factor: C

Lactation: Enters breast milk/not recommended (AAP rates "of concern")

Breast-Feeding Considerations: Drowsiness and lethargy have been reported in nursing infants; galactorrhea has been reported in mother.

Administration

I.V.: Direct of intermittent infusion: Infuse 1 mg or portion thereof over 1 minute. **Note:** Avoid skin contact with solution; may cause contact dermatitis.

Reconstitution: Dilute injection (1 mg/mL) with NS for I.V. administration.

Compatibility: Stable in dextran 6% in dextrose, dextran 6% in NS, D_5LR, $D_5{}^1/_4NS$, $D_5{}^1/_2NS$, D_5NS, D_5W, $D_{10}W$, LR, $^1/_2NS$, NS

Y-site administration: Incompatible with allopurinol, amifostine, amphotericin B cholesteryl sulfate complex, aztreonam, cefepime, etoposide phosphate, fludarabine, furosemide, linezolid, melphalan, methotrexate, paclitaxel, piperacillin/tazobactam, sargramostim

Compatibility in syringe: Incompatible with cimetidine, dimenhydrinate, heparin, pentobarbital, thiopental

Compatibility when admixed: Incompatible with aminophylline, amphotericin B, ampicillin, chloramphenicol, chlorothiazide, floxacillin, furosemide, methohexital, penicillin G potassium, penicillin G sodium, phenobarbital

Storage: Injection: Protect from light. A slightly yellowed solution does not indicate potency loss, but a markedly discolored solution should be discarded. Diluted injection (1 mg/mL) with NS and stored in 5 mL vials remains stable for 30 days.

♦ **Chlorpromazine Hydrochloride** *see* ChlorproMAZINE *on page 379*

Chlorthalidone (klor THAL i done)

U.S. Brand Names Thalitone®

Synonyms Hygroton

Pharmacologic Category Diuretic, Thiazide

Use Management of mild to moderate hypertension when used alone or in combination with other agents; treatment of edema associated with congestive heart failure or nephrotic syndrome. Recent studies have found chlorthalidone effective in the treatment of isolated systolic hypertension in the elderly.

Mechanism of Action Sulfonamide-derived diuretic that inhibits sodium and chloride reabsorption in the cortical-diluting segment of the ascending loop of Henle

Pharmacodynamics/Kinetics

Onset of action: Peak effect: 2-6 hours

Duration of action: 24-72 hours

Absorption: 65%

Distribution: Crosses placenta; enters breast milk

Metabolism: Hepatic

Half-life elimination: 35-55 hours; may be prolonged with renal impairment; Anuria: 81 hours

Excretion: Urine (~50% to 65% as unchanged drug)

Contraindications Hypersensitivity to chlorthalidone or any component of the formulation; cross-sensitivity with other thiazides or sulfonamides; anuria; renal decompensation; pregnancy

Warnings/Precautions Use with caution in patients with hypokalemia, renal disease, hepatic disease, gout, lupus erythematosus, or diabetes mellitus. Use with caution in severe renal diseases. Correct hypokalemia before initiating therapy. Chemical similarities are present among sulfonamides, sulfonylureas, carbonic anhydrase inhibitors, thiazides, and loop diuretics (except ethacrynic acid). Use in patients with thiazide or sulfonamide allergy is specifically contraindicated in product labeling, however, a risk of cross-reaction exists in patients with allergy to any of these compounds; avoid use when previous reaction has been severe.

Drug Interactions

ACE inhibitors: Increased hypotension if aggressively diuresed with a thiazide diuretic.

Beta-blockers increase hyperglycemic effects of thiazides in type 2 diabetes mellitus (noninsulin dependent, NIDDM)

Cyclosporine and thiazides can increase the risk of gout or renal toxicity; avoid concurrent use.

Digoxin toxicity can be exacerbated if a thiazide induces hypokalemia or hypomagnesemia.

Lithium toxicity can occur by reducing renal excretion of lithium; monitor lithium concentration and adjust as needed.

Neuromuscular blocking agents can prolong blockade; monitor serum potassium and neuromuscular status.

NSAIDs can decrease the efficacy of thiazides reducing the diuretic and antihypertensive effects.

Nutritional/Herbal/Ethanol Interactions Herb/Nutraceutical: Avoid dong quai if using for hypertension (has estrogenic activity). Avoid dong quai, St John's Wort (may also cause photosensitization). Avoid ephedra, yohimbe, ginseng (may worsen hypertension).

(Continued)

Chlorthalidone *(Continued)*

Lab Interactions Increased creatine phosphokinase [CPK] (S), ammonia (B), amylase (S), calcium (S), chloride (S), cholesterol (S), glucose, acid (S); decreased chloride (S), magnesium, potassium (S), sodium (S)

Adverse Reactions

1% to 10%:

Dermatologic: Photosensitivity

Endocrine & metabolic: Hypokalemia

Gastrointestinal: Anorexia, epigastric distress

<1% (Limited to important or life-threatening): Agranulocytosis, aplastic anemia, cholecystitis, cutaneous vasculitis, gout, hypercalcemia, hyperglycemia, hyponatremia, leukopenia, necrotizing angiitis, pancreatitis, paresthesia, purpura, rash, thrombocytopenia, urticaria, vasculitis, vomiting

Overdosage/Toxicology Symptoms of overdose include hypermotility, diuresis, lethargy, confusion, muscle weakness, and coma. Treatment is supportive.

Dosing

Adults:

Hypertension: Oral: 25-100 mg/day or 100 mg 3 times/week; usual dosage range (JNC 7): 12.5-25 mg/day

Edema: Initial: 50-100 mg/day or 100 mg on alternate days; maximum dose: 200 mg/day

Heart failure-associated edema: 12.5-25 mg once daily; maximum daily dose: 100 mg (ACC/AHA 2005 Heart Failure Guidelines)

Elderly: Oral: Initial: 12.5-25 mg/day or every other day; there is little advantage to using doses >25 mg/day.

Pediatrics: Oral: Children (nonapproved): 2 mg/kg/dose 3 times/week or 1-2 mg/kg/day

Renal Impairment: Cl_{cr} <10 mL/minute: Avoid use. Ineffective with low GFR (Aronoff G, 2002)

Note: ACC/AHA 2005 Heart Failure Guidelines suggest that thiazides lose their efficacy when Cl_{cr} <40 mL/minute

Available Dosage Forms

Tablet: 25 mg, 50 mg, 100 mg

Thalitone®: 15 mg

Nursing Guidelines

Assessment: Assess allergy history prior to beginning therapy. See Contraindications and Warnings/Precautions for use cautions. Assess potential for interactions with other prescriptions, OTC medications, or herbal products patient may be taking (see Drug Interactions). Assess results of laboratory tests (see below) on a regular basis throughout therapy. Assess therapeutic effectiveness and adverse response (eg, blood pressure, fluid status, and electrolyte balance - see Adverse Reactions and Overdose/Toxicology) regularly during long-term therapy. Caution patients with diabetes to monitor glucose levels (may reduce effect of oral hypoglycemics). Teach patient proper use, possible side effects/ appropriate interventions, and adverse symptoms to report (see Patient Education). **Pregnancy risk factor B/D** - see Pregnancy Risk Factor for use cautions; benefits of use should outweigh possible risks. Note breast-feeding caution.

Monitoring Laboratory Tests: Serum electrolytes, renal function

Dietary Considerations: This product may cause a potassium loss; your healthcare provider may prescribe a potassium supplement, another medication to help prevent the potassium loss, or recommend that you eat foods high in potassium, especially citrus fruits; do not change your diet on your own while taking this medication, especially if you are taking potassium supplements or medications to reduce potassium loss; too much potassium can be as harmful as too little.

Patient Education: Inform prescriber of all prescriptions, OTC medications, or herbal products you are taking, and any allergies you have. Do not take any new medication during therapy unless approved by prescriber. Take once-daily dose in morning or last of daily doses early in the day to avoid night-time disturbances. You may need to make dietary changes; follow dietary suggestions of prescriber (see Dietary Considerations). If using oral hypoglycemics, monitor glucose levels closely (this medication may reduce effect of oral hypoglycemics); contact prescriber with any major changes. May cause sensitivity to sunlight (use sunblock, wear protective clothing, and avoid direct sunlight); or anorexia or GI distress (small, frequent meals, frequent mouth care, chewing gum, or sucking lozenges may help). Report muscle twitching or cramps; nausea or vomiting; confusion; numbness of extremities; loss of appetite or GI distress; severe rash, redness, or itching of skin; chest pain or palpitations; or respiratory difficulty. **Pregnancy/breast-feeding precautions:** Do not get pregnant while taking this medication. Consult prescriber for appropriate contraceptive measures. Consult prescriber if breast-feeding.

Geriatric Considerations: Studies have found chlorthalidone effective in the treatment of isolated systolic hypertension in the elderly.

Pregnancy Risk Factor: B (manufacturer); D (expert analysis)

Lactation: Enters breast milk/use caution (AAP rates "compatible")

♦ Chlorthalidone and Atenolol *see* Atenolol and Chlorthalidone *on page 197*

Choline Magnesium Trisalicylate

(KOE leen mag NEE zhum trye sa LIS i late)

U.S. Brand Names Trilisate® [DSC]

Synonyms Tricosal

Pharmacologic Category Salicylate

Use Management of osteoarthritis, rheumatoid arthritis, and other arthritis; acute painful shoulder

Mechanism of Action Inhibits prostaglandin synthesis; acts on the hypothalamus heat-regulating center to reduce fever; blocks the generation of pain impulses

Pharmacodynamics/Kinetics

Onset of action: Peak effect: ~2 hours

Absorption: Stomach and small intestines

Distribution: Readily into most body fluids and tissues; crosses placenta; enters breast milk

Half-life elimination (dose dependent): Low dose: 2-3 hours; High dose: 30 hours

Time to peak, serum: ~2 hours

Contraindications Hypersensitivity to salicylates, other nonacetylated salicylates, other NSAIDs, or any component of the formulation; bleeding disorders; pregnancy (3rd trimester)

Warnings/Precautions Salicylate salts may not inhibit platelet aggregation and, therefore, should not be substituted for aspirin in the prophylaxis of thrombosis. Use with caution in patients with impaired renal function, dehydration, erosive gastritis, asthma, or peptic ulcer. Discontinue use 1 week prior to surgical procedures. Children and teenagers who have or are recovering from chickenpox or flu-like symptoms should not use this product. Changes in behavior (along with nausea and vomiting) may be an early sign of Reye's syndrome; patients should be instructed to contact their healthcare provider if these occur.

Elderly are a high-risk population for adverse effects from NSAIDs. As many as 60% of elderly can develop peptic ulceration and/or hemorrhage asymptomatically. Use lowest effective dose for shortest period possible. Tinnitus or impaired hearing may indicate toxicity. Tinnitus may be a difficult and unreliable indication of toxicity due to age-related hearing loss or eighth cranial nerve damage. CNS adverse effects may be observed in the elderly at lower doses than younger adults.

Drug Interactions

ACE inhibitors: Effects of ACE inhibitors may be decreased by concurrent therapy with NSAIDs.

Antacids: Concomitant use may lead to decreased salicylate concentration.

Warfarin: Concomitant use may increase the hypoprothrombinemic effect of warfarin.

Nutritional/Herbal/Ethanol Interactions

Ethanol: Avoid ethanol (may enhance gastric mucosal irritation).

Food: May decrease the rate but not the extent of oral absorption.

Herb/Nutraceutical: Avoid cat's claw, dong quai, evening primrose, feverfew, garlic, ginger, ginkgo, red clover, horse chestnut, green tea, ginseng (all have additional antiplatelet activity). Limit curry powder, paprika, licorice, Benedictine liqueur, prunes, raisins, tea, and gherkins; may cause salicylate accumulation. These foods contain 6 mg salicylate/100 g.

Lab Interactions False-negative results for glucose oxidase urinary glucose tests (Clinistix®); false-positives using the cupric sulfate method (Clinitest®); also, interferes with Gerhardt test (urinary ketone analysis), VMA determination; 5-HIAA, xylose tolerance test, and T_3 and T_4; increased PBI; increased uric acid

Adverse Reactions

<20%:

Gastrointestinal: Nausea, vomiting, diarrhea, heartburn, dyspepsia, epigastric pain, constipation

(Continued)

Choline Magnesium Trisalicylate *(Continued)*

Otic: Tinnitus

<2%:

Central nervous system: Headache, lightheadedness, dizziness, drowsiness, lethargy

Otic: Hearing impairment

<1%: Anorexia, asthma, BUN and creatinine increased, bruising, confusion, duodenal ulceration, dysgeusia, edema, epistaxis, erythema multiforme, esophagitis, hallucinations, hearing loss (irreversible), hepatic enzymes increased, gastric ulceration, occult bleeding, pruritus, rash, weight gain

Overdosage/Toxicology Symptoms of overdose include tinnitus, vomiting, acute renal failure, hyperthermia, irritability, seizures, coma, and metabolic acidosis. For acute ingestion, determine serum salicylate levels 6 hours after ingestion. Nomograms, such as the "Done" nomogram, may be helpful for estimating the severity of aspirin poisoning and directing treatment using serum salicylate levels. Treatment is based upon symptomatology.

Dosing

Adults & Elderly: Arthritis, pain: Oral (based on total salicylate content): 500 mg to 1.5 g 2-3 times/day **or** 3 g at bedtime; usual maintenance dose: 1-4.5 g/day

Pediatrics: Children: Oral (based on total salicylate content): <37 kg: 50 mg/kg/day given in 2 divided doses; 2250 mg/day for heavier children

Renal Impairment: Avoid use in severe renal impairment.

Available Dosage Forms

Liquid: 500 mg/5 mL (240 mL) [choline salicylate 293 mg and magnesium salicylate 362 mg per 5 mL; cherry cordial flavor]

Tablet: 500 mg [choline salicylate 293 mg and magnesium salicylate 362 mg]; 750 mg [choline salicylate 440 mg and magnesium salicylate 544 mg]; 1000 mg [choline salicylate 587 mg and magnesium salicylate 725 mg]

Nursing Guidelines

Assessment: Do not use for persons with allergic reaction to salicylates or other NSAIDs. Assess other medications patient may be taking for additive or adverse interactions. Monitor for effectiveness of pain relief. Monitor for signs of adverse reactions or overdose at beginning of therapy and periodically during long-term therapy. Assess knowledge/teach patient appropriate use. Teach patient to monitor for adverse reactions, adverse reactions to report, and appropriate interventions to reduce side effects.

Monitoring Laboratory Tests: Serum magnesium with high-dose therapy or in patients with impaired renal function, serum salicylate levels, renal function

Dietary Considerations: Take with food or large volume of water or milk to minimize GI upset. Liquid may be mixed with fruit juice just before drinking. Hypermagnesemia resulting from magnesium salicylate; avoid or use with caution in renal insufficiency.

Patient Education: Use exactly as directed; do not increase dose or frequency. Adverse reactions can occur with overuse. Take with food or milk. While using this medication, do not use alcohol, excessive amounts of vitamin C, or salicylate-containing foods (curry powder, prunes, raisins, tea, or licorice), other prescription or OTC medications containing aspirin or salicylate, or other NSAIDs without consulting prescriber. Maintain adequate hydration (2-3 L/day of fluids) unless instructed to restrict fluid intake. You may experience nausea, vomiting, gastric discomfort (frequent mouth care, small frequent meals, sucking lozenges, or chewing gum may help). GI bleeding, ulceration, or perforation can occur with or without pain. Stop taking medication and report ringing in ears; persistent stomach pain; unresolved nausea or vomiting; respiratory difficulty or shortness of breath; or unusual bruising or bleeding (mouth, urine, stool); or skin rash. **Pregnancy/breast-feeding precautions:** Inform prescriber if you are or intend to become pregnant. Consult prescriber if breast-feeding.

Geriatric Considerations: Elderly are at high risk for adverse effects from nonsteroidal anti-inflammatory agents. As much as 60% of elderly can develop peptic ulceration and/or hemorrhage asymptomatically.

Pregnancy Risk Factor: C/D (3rd trimester)

Pregnancy Issues: Animal reproduction studies have not been conducted. Due to the known effects of other salicylates (closure of ductus arteriosus), use during late pregnancy should be avoided.

Lactation: Enters breast milk/use caution

Breast-Feeding Considerations: Excreted in breast milk; peak levels occur 9-12 hours after dose. Use caution if used during breast-feeding.

Perioperative/Anesthesia/Other Concerns: Salicylate salts do not inhibit platelet aggregation and, therefore, should not be substituted for aspirin in the prophylaxis of thrombosis.

Administration

Oral: Liquid may be mixed with fruit juice just before drinking. Do not administer with antacids. Take with a full glass of water and remain in an upright position for 15-30 minutes after administration.

Storage: Store at controlled room temperature of 15°C to 30°C (59°F to 86°F).

Chondroitin Sulfate and Sodium Hyaluronate

(kon DROY tin SUL fate & SOW de um hye al yoor ON ate)

U.S. Brand Names Viscoat®

Synonyms Sodium Hyaluronate-Chrondroitin Sulfate

Pharmacologic Category Ophthalmic Agent, Viscoelastic

Use Surgical aid in anterior segment procedures, protects corneal endothelium and coats intraocular lens thus protecting it

Mechanism of Action Functions as a tissue lubricant and is thought to play an important role in modulating the interactions between adjacent tissues

Pharmacodynamics/Kinetics

Absorption: Intravitreous injection: Diffusion occurs slowly

Excretion: By Canal of Schlemm

Contraindications Hypersensitivity to hyaluronate

Warnings/Precautions Product is extracted from avian tissues and contains minute amounts of protein, potential risks of hypersensitivity may exist. Intraocular pressure may be elevated as a result of pre-existing glaucoma, compromised outflow and by operative procedures and sequelae including enzymatic zonulysis, absence of an iridectomy, trauma to filtration structures and by blood and lenticular remnants in the anterior chamber. Monitor IOP, especially during the immediate postoperative period.

Lab Interactions False-negative results for Clinistix® urine test; false-positive results with Clinitest®

Adverse Reactions 1% to 10%: Ocular: Increased intraocular pressure

Dosing

Adults & Elderly: Surgical aid: Ophthalmic: Carefully introduce (using a 27-gauge needle or cannula) into anterior chamber after thoroughly cleaning the chamber with a balanced salt solution

Available Dosage Forms Solution, ophthalmic: Sodium chondroitin 4% and sodium hyaluronate 3% (0.5 mL)

Nursing Guidelines

Pregnancy Risk Factor: C

Administration

Storage: Store at 2°C to 8°C (36°F to 46°F). Do not freeze.

♦ Chooz® [OTC] *see* Calcium Carbonate *on page 291*

♦ Choriogonadotropin Alfa *see* Chorionic Gonadotropin (Recombinant) *on page 389*

Chorionic Gonadotropin (Human)

(kor ee ON ik goe NAD oh troe pin, HYU man)

U.S. Brand Names Novarel™; Pregnyl®

Synonyms CG; hCG

Pharmacologic Category Ovulation Stimulator

Use Induces ovulation and pregnancy in anovulatory, infertile females; treatment of hypogonadotropic hypogonadism, prepubertal cryptorchidism; spermatogenesis induction with follitropin alfa or follitropin beta

Mechanism of Action Stimulates production of gonadal steroid hormones by causing production of androgen by the testis; as a substitute for luteinizing hormone (LH) to stimulate ovulation

Pharmacodynamics/Kinetics

Half-life elimination: Biphasic: Initial: 11 hours; Terminal: 23 hours

Excretion: Urine (as unchanged drug) within 3-4 days

Contraindications Hypersensitivity to chorionic gonadotropin or any component of the formulation; precocious puberty, prostatic carcinoma or similar neoplasms

(Continued)

Chorionic Gonadotropin (Human) *(Continued)*

Warnings/Precautions Use with caution in asthma, seizure disorders, migraine, cardiac or renal disease; **not** effective in the treatment of obesity

Drug Interactions No data reported

Adverse Reactions

1% to 10%:

- Central nervous system: Mental depression, fatigue
- Endocrine & metabolic: Pelvic pain, ovarian cysts, enlargement of breasts, precocious puberty
- Local: Pain at the injection site
- Neuromuscular & skeletal: Premature closure of epiphyses

<1% (Limited to important or life-threatening): Gynecomastia, headache, irritability, ovarian hyperstimulation syndrome, peripheral edema, restlessness

Dosing

Adults & Elderly:

Use with menotropins to stimulate spermatogenesis: I.M.: 5000 units 3 times/week for 4-6 months. With the beginning of menotropins therapy, hCG dose is continued at 2000 units 2 times/week.

Induction of ovulation and pregnancy: I.M.: 5000-10,000 units 1 day following last dose of menotropins

Spermatogenesis induction: Male: I.M.: Initial: 1500 int. units twice weekly to normalize serum testosterone levels. If no response in 8 weeks, increase dose to 3000 int. units twice weekly. After normalization of testosterone levels, combine with follitropin beta (Follistim®). Continue hCG at same dose used to normalize testosterone levels. Treatment response was noted at up to 12 months.

Pediatrics:

Prepubertal cryptorchidism: I.M.: Children: 1000-2000 units/m^2/dose 3 times/week for 3 weeks **or** 4000 units 3 times/week for 3 weeks **or** 5000 units every second day for 4 injections **or** 500 units 3 times/week for 4-6 weeks

Hypogonadotropic hypogonadism: I.M.: Children: 500-1000 units 3 times/week for 3 weeks, followed by the same dose twice weekly for 3 weeks **or** 1000-2000 units 3 times/week **or** 4000 units 3 times/week for 6-9 months; reduce dosage to 2000 units 3 times/week for additional 3 months.

Available Dosage Forms

Injection, powder for reconstitution: 10,000 units [packaged with diluent; diluent contains benzyl alcohol and mannitol]

- Novarel™: 10,000 units [packaged with diluent; diluent contains benzyl alcohol and mannitol]
- Pregnyl®: 10,000 units [packaged with diluent; diluent contains benzyl alcohol]

Nursing Guidelines

Assessment: Assess therapeutic effectiveness (according to purpose for use) and adverse response regularly during long-term therapy. Teach patient proper use if self-administered (appropriate injection technique and syringe/needle disposal), possible side effects/appropriate interventions, and adverse symptoms to report.

Patient Education: This medication can only be administered by injection. If self-administered, follow instruction for reconstitution, injection, and needle disposal. Use exactly as directed; do not alter dosage or miss a dose. May cause headache, depression, irritability, or restlessness (use caution when driving or engaging in potentially hazardous tasks until response to drug is known). Contact prescriber if symptoms are severe or do not resolve with use. Contact prescriber if breasts swell; if you experience swelling of legs or feet; or if there is pain, redness, or swelling at injection site. **Pregnancy/breast-feeding precautions:** Inform prescriber if you are or intend to become pregnant. Consult prescriber if breast-feeding.

Pregnancy Risk Factor: C

Lactation: Excretion in breast milk unknown/unlikely to be used

Administration

I.M.: I.M. administration only

Reconstitution: Following reconstitution with the provided diluent, solutions are stable for 30-90 days, depending on the specific preparation, when stored at 2°C to 15°C.

Chorionic Gonadotropin (Recombinant)

(kor ee ON ik goe NAD oh troe pin ree KOM be nant)

U.S. Brand Names Ovidrel®

Synonyms Choriogonadotropin Alfa; r-hCG

Pharmacologic Category Gonadotropin; Ovulation Stimulator

Use As part of an assisted reproductive technology (ART) program, induces ovulation in infertile females who have been pretreated with follicle stimulating hormones (FSH); induces ovulation and pregnancy in infertile females when the cause of infertility is functional

Mechanism of Action Luteinizing hormone analogue produced by recombinant DNA techniques; stimulates rupture of the ovarian follicle once follicular development has occurred.

Pharmacodynamics/Kinetics

Distribution: V_d: 5.9 ± 1 L

Bioavailability: 40%

Half-life elimination: Initial: 4 hours; Terminal: 29 hours

Time to peak: 12-24 hours

Excretion: Urine (10% of dose)

Contraindications Hypersensitivity to hCG preparations or any component of the formulation; primary ovarian failure; uncontrolled thyroid or adrenal dysfunction; uncontrolled organic intracranial lesion (ie, pituitary tumor); abnormal uterine bleeding, ovarian cyst or enlargement of undetermined origin; sex hormone dependent tumors; pregnancy

Warnings/Precautions For use by infertility specialists; may cause ovarian hyperstimulation syndrome (OHSS); if severe, treatment should be discontinued and patient should be hospitalized. OHSS results in a rapid (<24 hours to 7 days) accumulation of fluid in the peritoneal cavity, thorax, and possibly the pericardium, which may become more severe if pregnancy occurs; monitor for ovarian enlargement; use may lead to multiple births; risk of arterial thromboembolism with hCG products; safety and efficacy in pediatric and geriatric patients have not been established.

Drug Interactions Specific drug interaction studies have not been conducted

Lab Interactions May interfere with interpretation of pregnancy tests; may cross-react with radioimmunoassay of luteinizing hormone and other gonadotropins

Adverse Reactions

2% to 10%:

Endocrine & metabolic: Ovarian cyst (3%), ovarian hyperstimulation (<2% to 3%)

Gastrointestinal: Abdominal pain (3% to 4%), nausea (3%), vomiting (3%)

Local: Injection site: Pain (8%), bruising (3% to 5%), reaction (<2% to 3%), inflammation (<2% to 2%)

Miscellaneous: Postoperative pain (5%)

<2% (Limited to important or life-threatening): Abdominal enlargement, albuminuria, back pain, breast pain, cardiac arrhythmia, cervical carcinoma, cervical lesion, cough, diarrhea, dizziness, dysuria, ectopic pregnancy, emotional lability, fever, flatulence, genital herpes, genital moniliasis, headache, heart murmur, hiccups, hot flashes, hyperglycemia, insomnia, intermenstrual bleeding, leukocytosis, leukorrhea, malaise, paresthesia, pharyngitis, pruritus, rash, upper respiratory tract infection, urinary incontinence, urinary tract infection, vaginal hemorrhage, vaginitis

In addition, the following have been reported with menotropin therapy: Adnexal torsion, hemoperitoneum, mild to moderate ovarian enlargement, pulmonary and vascular complications. Ovarian neoplasms have also been reported (rare) with multiple drug regimens used for ovarian induction (relationship not established).

Dosing

Adults: Assisted reproductive technologies (ART) and ovulation induction in females: SubQ: 250 mcg given 1 day following the last dose of follicle stimulating agent. Use only after adequate follicular development has been determined. Hold treatment when there is an excessive ovarian response.

Elderly: Safety and efficacy have not been established.

Renal Impairment: Safety and efficacy have not been established.

Hepatic Impairment: Safety and efficacy have not been established.

Available Dosage Forms [DSC] = Discontinued product

Injection, powder for reconstitution: 285 mcg [packaged with 1 mL SWFI; delivers 250 mcg r-hCG following reconstitution] [DSC]

(Continued)

Chorionic Gonadotropin (Recombinant) *(Continued)*

Injection, solution: 257.5 mcg/0.515 mL (0.515 mL) [prefilled syringe; delivers 250 mcg r-hCG/0.5 mL]

Nursing Guidelines

Assessment: For use only under the supervision/direction of an infertility physician. Monitor for adverse reactions. Teach patient proper use if self-administered (storage, reconstitution, injection technique, needle/syringe disposal; recommend return demonstration), monitoring requirements, interventions to reduce side effects, and adverse reactions to report. **Pregnancy risk factor X:** Determine that patient is not pregnant before beginning treatment and monitor ovulation closely during treatment.

Patient Education: Note that there is a risk of multiple births associated with treatment. This drug must be administered exactly as scheduled (1 day following last dose of follicle stimulating agent); maintain a calendar of treatment days. Follow administration directions exactly. Keep all ultrasound and laboratory appointments as instructed by prescriber. Avoid strenuous exercise, especially those with pelvic involvement. You may experience nausea, vomiting, or GI upset (small frequent meals, frequent mouth care, sucking lozenges, or chewing gum may help), hot flashes (cool clothes, cool room, adequate rest may help) if persistent consult prescriber. Report immediately any persistent abdominal pain, vomiting, or acute pelvic pain; chest pain or palpitations; shortness of breath; or urinary tract or vaginal infection or urinary incontinence. **Pregnancy/breast-feeding precautions:** Do not take this medicine if you are pregnant and report to prescriber immediately if you suspect you are pregnant. Consult prescriber if breast-feeding.

Pregnancy Risk Factor: X

Pregnancy Issues: Ectopic pregnancy, premature labor, postpartum fever, and spontaneous abortion have been reported in clinical trials. Congenital abnormalities have also been observed, however, the incidence is similar during natural conception.

Lactation: Excretion in breast milk unknown/use caution

Administration

Reconstitution: Powder for reconstitution: Mix vial with 1 mL sterile water for injection. Gently mix by rotating vial to dissolve powder; do not shake. Use immediately following reconstitution.

Storage:

Powder for reconstitution: Store in original package under refrigeration or at room temperature of 2°C to 25°C (36°F to 77°F). Protect from light.

Prefilled syringe: Prior to dispensing, store at 2°C to 8°C (36°F to 46°F). Patient may store at 25°C (77°F) for up to 30 days. Protect from light.

♦ **Chromagen® OB** *see* Vitamins (Multiple/Prenatal) *on page 1721*

Ciclopirox (sye kloe PEER oks)

U.S. Brand Names Loprox®; Penlac®

Synonyms Ciclopirox Olamine

Pharmacologic Category Antifungal Agent, Topical

Medication Safety Issues

Sound-alike/look-alike issues:

Loprox® may be confused with Lonox®

Use

Cream/suspension: Treatment of tinea pedis (athlete's foot), tinea cruris (jock itch), tinea corporis (ringworm), cutaneous candidiasis, and tinea versicolor (pityriasis)

Gel: Treatment of tinea pedis (athlete's foot), tinea corporis (ringworm); seborrheic dermatitis of the scalp

Lacquer (solution): Topical treatment of mild-to-moderate onychomycosis of the fingernails and toenails due to *Trichophyton rubrum* (not involving the lunula) and the immediately-adjacent skin

Shampoo: Treatment of seborrheic dermatitis of the scalp

Mechanism of Action Inhibiting transport of essential elements in the fungal cell disrupting the synthesis of DNA, RNA, and protein

Pharmacodynamics/Kinetics

Absorption: Cream, solution: <2% through intact skin; increased with gel; <5% with lacquer

Distribution: Scalp application: To epidermis, corium (dermis), including hair, hair follicles, and sebaceous glands

Protein binding: 94% to 98%
Half-life elimination: Biologic: 1.7 hours (solution); elimination: 5.5 hours (gel)
Excretion: Urine (gel: 3% to 10%); feces (small amounts)

Contraindications Hypersensitivity to ciclopirox or any component of the formulation; avoid occlusive wrappings or dressings

Warnings/Precautions For external use only; avoid contact with eyes; nail lacquer is for topical use only and has not been studied in conjunction with systemic therapy or in patients with type 1 diabetes mellitus (insulin dependent, IDDM).

Drug Interactions No data reported

Adverse Reactions
>10%: Local: Burning sensation (gel: 34%; ≤1% with other forms)
1% to 10%:
Central nervous system: Headache
Dermatologic: Erythema, nail disorder, pruritus, rash
Local: Irritation, redness, or pain
<1% (Limited to important or life-threatening): Alopecia, dry skin, facial edema

Dosing

Adults & Elderly:

Tinea pedis, tinea cruris, tinea corporis, cutaneous candidiasis, and tinea versicolor: Cream/lotion/suspension: Apply twice daily, gently massage into affected areas; if no improvement after 4 weeks of treatment, re-evaluate the diagnosis

Tinea pedis, tinea corporis, seborrheic dermatitis of the scalp: Gel: Apply twice daily, gently massage into affected areas and surrounding skin; if no improvement after 4 weeks of treatment, re-evaluate diagnosis

Seborrheic dermatitis of the scalp: Shampoo: Apply to wet hair, lather, and leave in place ~3 minute; rinse. Repeat twice weekly for 4 weeks; allow a minimum of 3 days between applications.

Onychomycosis of the fingernails and toenails: Lacquer (solution): Apply to adjacent skin and affected nails daily (as a part of a comprehensive management program for onychomycosis). Remove with alcohol every 7 days.

Pediatrics:

Tinea pedis, tinea cruris, tinea corporis, cutaneous candidiasis, and tinea versicolor: Children >10 years: Refer to adult dosing.

Seborrheic dermatitis of the scalp: Children >16 years: Refer to adult dosing.

Onychomycosis of the fingernails and toenails: Children ≥12 years: Refer to adult dosing.

Available Dosage Forms
Cream, as olamine (Loprox®): 0.77% (15 g, 30 g, 90 g)
Gel (Loprox®): 0.77% (30 g, 45 g, 100 g)
Shampoo (Loprox®): 1% (120 mL)
Solution, topical [nail lacquer] (Penlac®): 8% (6.6 mL)
Suspension, topical, as olamine (Loprox®): 0.77% (30 mL, 60 mL)

Nursing Guidelines

Patient Education: Avoid contact with eyes; if sensitivity or irritation occurs, discontinue use

Pregnancy Risk Factor: B

Lactation: Excretion in breast milk unknown/use caution

Administration

Storage:
Cream, suspension: Store between 5°C to 25°C (41°F to 77°F).
Lacquer (solution): Store at room temperature of 15°C to 30°C (59°F to 86°F). Protect from light. Flammable; keep away from heat and flame.
Gel, shampoo: Store at room temperature of 15°C to 30°C (59°F to 86°F).

♦ **Ciclopirox Olamine** *see* Ciclopirox *on page 390*

Cidofovir (si DOF o veer)

U.S. Brand Names Vistide®

Pharmacologic Category Antiviral Agent

Use Treatment of cytomegalovirus (CMV) retinitis in patients with acquired immunodeficiency syndrome (AIDS). **Note:** Should be administered with probenecid.

Mechanism of Action Cidofovir is converted to cidofovir diphosphate which is the active intracellular metabolite; cidofovir diphosphate suppresses CMV replication by selective inhibition of viral DNA synthesis. Incorporation of cidofovir into growing viral DNA chain results in reductions in the rate of viral DNA synthesis.
(Continued)

Cidofovir *(Continued)*

Pharmacodynamics/Kinetics The following pharmacokinetic data is based on a combination of cidofovir administered with probenecid:

Distribution: V_d: 0.54 L/kg; does not cross significantly into CSF

Protein binding: <6%

Metabolism: Minimal; phosphorylation occurs intracellularly

Half-life elimination, plasma: ~2.6 hours

Excretion: Urine

Contraindications Hypersensitivity to cidofovir; history of clinically-severe hypersensitivity to probenecid or other sulfa-containing medications; serum creatinine >1.5 mg/dL; Cl_{cr} <55 mL/minute; urine protein ≥100 mg/dL (≥2+ proteinuria); use with or within 7 days of nephrotoxic agents; direct intraocular injection

Warnings/Precautions Dose-dependent nephrotoxicity requires dose adjustment or discontinuation if changes in renal function occur during therapy (eg, proteinuria, glycosuria, decreased serum phosphate, uric acid or bicarbonate, and elevated creatinine); neutropenia and ocular hypotony have also occurred; safety and efficacy have not been established in children or the elderly; administration must be accompanied by oral probenecid and intravenous saline prehydration; prepare admixtures in a class two laminar flow hood, wearing protective gear; dispose of cidofovir as directed

Drug Interactions

Nephrotoxic agents: Drugs with nephrotoxic potential (eg, amphotericin B, aminoglycosides, foscarnet, and I.V. pentamidine) should not be used with or within 7 days of cidofovir therapy.

Zidovudine: Due to concomitant probenecid administration, temporarily discontinue or decrease zidovudine dose by 50% on the day of cidofovir administration only.

Adverse Reactions

>10%:

- Central nervous system: Chills, fever, headache, pain
- Dermatologic: Alopecia, rash
- Gastrointestinal: Nausea, vomiting, diarrhea, anorexia
- Hematologic: Anemia, neutropenia
- Neuromuscular & skeletal: Weakness
- Ocular: Intraocular pressure decreased, iritis, ocular hypotony, uveitis
- Renal: Creatinine increased, proteinuria, renal toxicity
- Respiratory: Cough, dyspnea
- Miscellaneous: Infection, oral moniliasis, serum bicarbonate decreased

1% to 10%:

- Renal: Fanconi syndrome
- Respiratory: Pneumonia

<1%: Hepatic failure, metabolic acidosis, pancreatitis

Frequency not defined (limited to important or life-threatening reactions):

- Cardiovascular: Cardiomyopathy, cardiovascular disorder, CHF, edema, postural hypotension, shock, syncope, tachycardia
- Central nervous system: Agitation, amnesia, anxiety, confusion, convulsion, dizziness, hallucinations, insomnia, malaise, vertigo
- Dermatologic: Photosensitivity reaction, skin discoloration, urticaria
- Endocrine & metabolic: Adrenal cortex insufficiency
- Gastrointestinal: Abdominal pain, aphthous stomatitis, colitis, constipation, dysphagia, fecal incontinence, gastritis, GI hemorrhage, gingivitis, melena, proctitis, splenomegaly, stomatitis, tongue discoloration
- Genitourinary: Urinary incontinence
- Hematologic: Hypochromic anemia, leukocytosis, leukopenia, lymphadenopathy, lymphoma-like reaction, pancytopenia, thrombocytopenia, thrombocytopenic purpura
- Hepatic: Hepatomegaly, hepatosplenomegaly, jaundice, liver function tests abnormal, liver damage, liver necrosis
- Local: Injection site reaction
- Neuromuscular & skeletal: Tremor
- Ocular: Amblyopia, blindness, cataract, conjunctivitis, corneal lesion, diplopia, vision abnormal
- Otic: Hearing loss
- Miscellaneous: Allergic reaction, sepsis

Overdosage/Toxicology Hemodialysis and hydration may reduce drug plasma concentrations. Probenecid may assist in decreasing active tubular secretion.

Dosing

Adults & Elderly: Treatment of cytomegalovirus (CMV) retinitis: I.V.:

Induction treatment: 5 mg/kg once weekly for 2 consecutive weeks

Maintenance treatment: 5 mg/kg administered once every 2 weeks

Note: Probenecid must be administered orally with each dose of cidofovir.

Probenecid dose: 2 g 3 hours prior to cidofovir dose, 1 g 2 hours and 8 hours after completion of the infusion; patients should also receive 1 L of normal saline intravenously prior to each infusion of cidofovir; saline should be infused over 1-2 hours.

Renal Impairment:

Changes in renal function during therapy: If the creatinine increases by 0.3-0.4 mg/dL, reduce the cidofovir dose to 3 mg/kg; discontinue therapy for increases ≥0.5 mg/dL or development of ≥3+ proteinuria

Pre-existing renal impairment: Use is contraindicated with serum creatinine >1.5 mg/dL, Cl_{cr} <55 mL/minute, or urine protein ≥100 mg/dL (≥2+ proteinuria)

Available Dosage Forms Injection, solution [preservative free]: 75 mg/mL (5 mL)

Nursing Guidelines

Assessment: See Contraindications, Warnings/Precautions, and Dosing for use cautions. Assess potential for interactions with other prescriptions, OTC medications, or herbal products patient may be taking (eg, nephrotoxicity - see Drug Interactions). See Dosing, Administration, and Reconstitution directions. Infusion site should be monitored closely to avoid extravasation. Assess results of laboratory tests with each dose (see below), therapeutic effectiveness, and adverse response (see Adverse Reactions and Overdose/Toxicology) regularly during therapy. For patients with diabetes, serum glucose should be monitored closely (may cause hyperglycemia). Teach patient possible side effects/appropriate interventions and adverse symptoms to report (see Patient Education). Breast-feeding is contraindicated.

Monitoring Laboratory Tests: Serum creatinine, serum bicarbonate, acid-base status, urine protein, WBC should be monitored with each dose; monitor intraocular pressure frequently.

Patient Education: Inform prescriber of all prescriptions, OTC medications, or herbal products you are taking, and any allergies you have. Do not take any new medication during therapy unless approved by prescriber. This drug can only be administered I.V. Report immediately any pain, stinging, swelling at infusion site. You may be more susceptible to infection (avoid crowds and exposure to infection and do not have any vaccinations without consulting prescriber). May cause hair loss (reversible); headache, anxiety, confusion (use caution when driving or engaging in tasks that require alertness until response to drug is known); diarrhea (buttermilk or yogurt may help); nausea, heartburn, or vomiting (small, frequent meals, frequent mouth care, sucking lozenges, or chewing gum may help); constipation (increased exercise, fluids, fruit, or fiber may help); or postural hypotension (use caution changing from lying to sitting or standing position and when climbing stairs). Report severe unresolved vomiting, constipation, or diarrhea; chills, fever, signs of infection; respiratory difficulty or unusual coughing; palpitations, chest pain, or syncope; CNS changes (eg, hallucinations, depression, excessive sedation, amnesia, seizures, insomnia); vision changes; or other severe side effects. **Pregnancy/breast-feeding precautions:** Inform prescriber if you are pregnant and do not get pregnant while taking this medicine. Consult prescriber for appropriate contraceptives. Do not breast-feed.

Geriatric Considerations: Since elderly individuals frequently have reduced kidney function, particular attention should be paid to assessing renal function before and frequently during administration.

Pregnancy Risk Factor: C

Pregnancy Issues: Cidofovir was shown to be teratogenic and embryotoxic in animal studies, some at doses which also produced maternal toxicity. Reduced testes weight and hypospermia were also noted in animal studies. There are no adequate and well-controlled studies in pregnant women; use during pregnancy only if the potential benefit to the mother outweighs the possible risk to the fetus. Women of childbearing potential should use effective contraception during therapy and for 1 month following treatment. Males should use a barrier contraceptive during therapy and for 3 months following treatment.

(Continued)

Cidofovir *(Continued)*

Lactation: Excretion in breast milk unknown/contraindicated

Breast-Feeding Considerations: The CDC recommends **not** to breast-feed if diagnosed with HIV to avoid postnatal transmission of the virus.

Administration

I.V.: For I.V. infusion only. Infuse over 1 hour. Hydrate with 1 L of 0.9% NS I.V. prior to cidofovir infusion; a second liter may be administered over a 1- to 3-hour period immediately following infusion, if tolerated

Reconstitution: Dilute dose in NS 100 mL prior to infusion.

Compatibility: Stable in $D_5{}^1\!/_4$NS, D_5W, NS

Storage: Store at controlled room temperature 20°C to 25°C (68°F to 77°F). Store admixtures under refrigeration for ≤24 hours. Cidofovir infusion admixture should be administered within 24 hours of preparation at room temperature or refrigerated. Admixtures should be allowed to equilibrate to room temperature prior to use.

Cilostazol (sil OH sta zol)

U.S. Brand Names Pletal®

Synonyms OPC-13013

Pharmacologic Category Antiplatelet Agent; Phosphodiesterase Enzyme Inhibitor

Medication Safety Issues

Sound-alike/look-alike issues:

Pletal® may be confused with Plendil®

Use Symptomatic management of peripheral vascular disease, primarily intermittent claudication

Unlabeled/Investigational Use Treatment of acute coronary syndromes and for graft patency improvement in percutaneous coronary interventions with or without stenting

Mechanism of Action Cilostazol and its metabolites are inhibitors of phosphodiesterase III. As a result, cyclic AMP is increased leading to reversible inhibition of platelet aggregation and vasodilation. Other effects of phosphodiesterase III inhibition include increased cardiac contractility, accelerated AV nodal conduction, increased ventricular automaticity, heart rate, and coronary blood flow.

Pharmacodynamics/Kinetics

Onset of action: 2-4 weeks; may require up to 12 weeks

Protein binding: 97% to 98%

Metabolism: Hepatic via CYP3A4 (primarily), 1A2, 2C19, and 2D6; at least one metabolite has significant activity

Half-life elimination: 11-13 hours

Excretion: Urine (74%) and feces (20%) as metabolites

Contraindications Hypersensitivity to cilostazol or any component of the formulation; heart failure (of any severity)

Warnings/Precautions Use with caution in patients receiving other platelet aggregation inhibitors or in patients with thrombocytopenia. Discontinue therapy if thrombocytopenia or leukopenia occur, progression to agranulocytosis (reversible) has been reported when cilostazol was not immediately stopped. When cilostazol and clopidogrel are used concurrently, manufacturer recommends checking bleeding times. Withhold for at least 4-6 half-lives prior to elective surgical procedures. Use with caution in patients receiving CYP3A4 inhibitors (eg, ketoconazole or erythromycin) or CYP2C19 inhibitors (eg, omeprazole); use with caution in severe underlying heart disease. Use caution in moderate to severe hepatic impairment. Use cautiously in severe renal impairment (Cl_{cr} <25 mL/minute). Safety and efficacy in pediatric patients have not been established.

Drug Interactions Substrate of CYP1A2 (minor), 2C19 (major), 2D6 (minor), 3A4 (major)

Antifungal agents (imidazole): May decrease the metabolism, via CYP isoenzymes, of cilostazol. Manufacturer recommends a reduced dose of cilostazole during concurrent therapy.

CYP2C19 inhibitors may increase the levels/effects of cilostazol. Example inhibitors include delavirdine, fluconazole, fluvoxamine, gemfibrozil, isoniazid, omeprazole, and ticlopidine.

CYP3A4 inhibitors may increase the levels/effects of cilostazol. Example inhibitors include azole antifungals, clarithromycin, diclofenac, doxycycline, erythromycin, imatinib, isoniazid, nefazodone, nicardipine, propofol, protease inhibitors, quinidine, telithromycin, and verapamil.

Drotrecogin alfa: Antiplatelet agents may enhance the adverse/toxic effect of drotrecogin alfa. Bleeding may occur.

Macrolide antibiotics: May decrease the metabolism, via CYP isoenzymes, of cilostazol. Examples include clarithromycin, erythromycin, telithromycin. The manufacturer recommends considering a reduced dose (50 mg twice daily) during coadministration of these agents.

Nonsteroidal anti-inflammatory agents: May enhance the adverse/toxic effect of antiplatelet agents. An increased risk of bleeding may occur.

Omeprazole: May enhance the adverse/toxic effect of cilostazol. The manufacturer recommends considering a reduced dose (50 mg twice daily) during coadministration of omeprazole.

Salicylates: Antiplatelet agents such as cilostazol may enhance the adverse/toxic effect of salicylates. Increased risk of bleeding may result.

Treprostinil: May enhance the adverse/toxic effect of antiplatelet agents such as cilostazol. Bleeding may occur.

Nutritional/Herbal/Ethanol Interactions Food: Taking cilostazol with a high-fat meal may increase peak concentration by 90%. Avoid concurrent ingestion of grapefruit juice due to the potential to inhibit CYP3A4.

Adverse Reactions

>10%:

Central nervous system: Headache (27% to 34%)

Gastrointestinal: Abnormal stools (12% to 15%), diarrhea (12% to 19%)

Respiratory: Rhinitis (7% to 12%)

Miscellaneous: Infection (10% to 14%)

2% to 10%:

Cardiovascular: Peripheral edema (7% to 9%), palpitation (5% to 10%), tachycardia (4%)

Central nervous system: Dizziness (9% to 10%), vertigo (up to 3%)

Gastrointestinal: Dyspepsia (6%), nausea (6% to 7%), abdominal pain (4% to 5%), flatulence (2% to 3%)

Neuromuscular & skeletal: Back pain (6% to 7%), myalgia (2% to 3%)

Respiratory: Pharyngitis (7% to 10%), cough (3% to 4%)

<2% (Limited to important or life-threatening): Agranulocytosis, anemia, asthma, atrial fibrillation, atrial flutter, blindness, bursitis, cardiac arrest, cerebral infarction/ischemia, cholelithiasis, colitis, CHF, cystitis, diabetes mellitus, duodenal ulcer, duodenitis, esophageal hemorrhage, esophagitis, extradural hematoma, gout, granulocytopenia, hemorrhage, hepatic dysfunction, hypotension, leukopenia, myocardial infarction/ischemia, neuralgia, nodal arrhythmia, periodontal abscess, peptic ulcer, pneumonia, polycythemia, postural hypotension, QT_c prolongation, rectal hemorrhage, retinal hemorrhage, retroperitoneal hemorrhage, Stevens-Johnson syndrome, subdural hematoma, supraventricular tachycardia, syncope, thrombocytopenia, thrombosis, torsade de pointes, ventricular tachycardia

Overdosage/Toxicology Experience with overdosage in humans is limited. Headache, diarrhea, hypotension, tachycardia, and/or cardiac arrhythmias may occur. Treatment is symptomatic and supportive. Hemodialysis is unlikely to be of value. In some animal models, high-dose or long-term administration was associated with a variety of cardiovascular lesions, including endocardial hemorrhage, hemosiderin deposition and left ventricular fibrosis, coronary arteritis, and periarteritis.

Dosing

Adults & Elderly: Peripheral vascular disease: Oral: 100 mg twice daily taken at least 30 minutes before or 2 hours after breakfast and dinner; dosage should be reduced to 50 mg twice daily during concurrent therapy with inhibitors of CYP3A4 or CYP2C19 (see Drug Interactions).

Available Dosage Forms Tablet: 50 mg, 100 mg

Nursing Guidelines

Assessment: Assess effectiveness and interactions of other medications patient may be taking. Monitor effectiveness of therapy and adverse reactions at beginning of therapy and periodically with long-term use. Assess knowledge/teach patient appropriate use, interventions to reduce side effects, and adverse symptoms to report.

Dietary Considerations: It is best to take cilostazol 30 minutes before or 2 hours after meals.

Patient Education: Use exactly as directed; do not discontinue without consulting prescriber. Beneficial effect may take between 2-12 weeks. Take on empty stomach (30 minutes before or 2 hours after meals). Do not take with

(Continued)

Cilostazol *(Continued)*

grapefruit juice. You may experience nervousness, dizziness, or fatigue (use caution when driving or engaging in tasks requiring alertness until response to treatment is known); nausea, vomiting, or flatulence (small frequent meals, frequent mouth care, chewing gum or sucking hard candy may help); or postural hypotension (change position slowly when rising from sitting or lying position or climbing stairs). Report chest pain, palpitations, unusual heartbeat, or swelling of extremities; unusual bleeding; unresolved GI upset or pain; dizziness, nervousness, sleeplessness, or fatigue; muscle cramping or tremor; unusual cough; or other adverse effects. **Pregnancy/breast-feeding precautions:** Inform prescriber if you are or intend to become pregnant. Breast-feeding is not recommended.

Pregnancy Risk Factor: C

Pregnancy Issues: In animal studies, abnormalities of the skeletal, renal and cardiovascular system were increased. In addition, the incidence of stillbirth and decreased birth weights were increased.

Lactation: Excretion in breast milk unknown/not recommended

Breast-Feeding Considerations: It is not known whether cilostazol is excreted in human milk. Because of the potential risk to nursing infants, a decision to discontinue the drug or discontinue nursing should be made.

Perioperative/Anesthesia/Other Concerns: In some animal models, high-dose or long-term administration was associated with a variety of cardiovascular lesions, including endocardial hemorrhage, hemosiderin deposition and left ventricular fibrosis, coronary arteritis, and periarteritis.

♦ **Ciloxan®** *see* Ciprofloxacin *on page 400*

Cimetidine (sye MET i deen)

U.S. Brand Names Tagamet®; Tagamet® HB 200 [OTC]

Pharmacologic Category Histamine H_2 Antagonist

Medication Safety Issues

Sound-alike/look-alike issues:

Cimetidine may be confused with simethicone

Use Short-term treatment of active duodenal ulcers and benign gastric ulcers; long-term prophylaxis of duodenal ulcer; gastric hypersecretory states; gastroesophageal reflux; prevention of upper GI bleeding in critically-ill patients; labeled for OTC use for prevention or relief of heartburn, acid indigestion, or sour stomach

Unlabeled/Investigational Use Part of a multidrug regimen for *H. pylori* eradication to reduce the risk of duodenal ulcer recurrence

Mechanism of Action Competitive inhibition of histamine at H_2-receptors of the gastric parietal cells resulting in reduced gastric acid secretion, gastric volume and hydrogen ion concentration reduced

Pharmacodynamics/Kinetics

Onset of action: 1 hour

Duration: 6 hours

Distribution: Crosses placenta; enters breast milk

Protein binding: 20%

Metabolism: Partially hepatic

Bioavailability: 60% to 70%

Half-life elimination: Neonates: 3.6 hours; Children: 1.4 hours; Adults: Normal renal function: 2 hours

Time to peak, serum: Oral: 1-2 hours

Excretion: Primarily urine (as unchanged drug); feces (some)

Contraindications Hypersensitivity to cimetidine, any component of the formulation, or other H_2 antagonists

Warnings/Precautions Reversible confusional states, usually clearing within 3-4 days after discontinuation, have been linked to use. Increased age (>50 years) and renal or hepatic impairment are thought to be associated. Dosage should be adjusted in renal/hepatic impairment or in patients receiving drugs metabolized through the P450 system.

Use of over the counter (OTC) cimetidine should not occur by individuals experiencing painful swallowing, vomiting with blood, or bloody or black stools; medical attention should be sought. A physician should be consulted prior to use when pain in the stomach, shoulder, arms or neck is present; if heartburn has occurred for >3 months; or if unexplained weight loss, or nausea and vomiting occur. Frequent wheezing, shortness of breath, lightheadedness, or sweating, especially with chest pain or heartburn, should also be reported. Consultation of a healthcare provider should occur by patients if also taking theophylline, phenytoin, or warfarin; if heartburn or stomach pain continues or worsens; or if use is required for >14 days. Pregnant or breast-feeding women should speak to a healthcare provider before use. OTC cimetidine is not approved for use in patients <12 years of age.

Drug Interactions Inhibits CYP1A2 (moderate), 2C8/9 (weak), 2C19 (moderate), 2D6 (moderate), 2E1 (weak), 3A4 (moderate)

Note: There are many potential interactions. Listed are the most significant ones.

Alfentanil: Increased serum concentration; monitor for toxicity.

Amiodarone's serum concentration is increased; avoid concurrent use.

Benzodiazepine's (except lorazepam, oxazepam, temazepam) serum concentration is increased; consider alternative H_2 antagonist or monitor for benzodiazepine toxicity.

Beta-blockers (except atenolol, betaxolol, bisoprolol, nadolol, penbutolol) effects may be increased; use a renally-eliminated beta-blocker or alternative H_2 antagonist.

Calcium channel blockers serum concentration is increased; monitor for toxicity.

Carbamazepine's plasma concentrations may increase transiently (1 week). Monitor for carbamazepine toxicity or use an alternative H_2 antagonist.

Carmustine's myelotoxicity is increased; avoid concurrent use.

Cefpodoxime's and cefuroxime's oral absorption may be reduced by increased pH; consider alternative antibiotic.

Cisapride's bioavailability is increased; avoid concurrent use.

Citalopram's serum concentration is increased; use an alternative H_2 antagonist or adjust citalopram's dose.

Cyclosporine's serum concentration may increase; monitor cyclosporine levels.

CYP1A2 substrates: Cimetidine may increase the levels/effects of CYP1A2 substrates. Example substrates include aminophylline, fluvoxamine, mexiletine, mirtazapine, ropinirole, theophylline, and trifluoperazine.

CYP2C19 substrates: Cimetidine may increase the levels/effects of CYP2C19 substrates. Example substrates include citalopram, diazepam, methsuximide, phenytoin, propranolol, and sertraline.

CYP2D6 substrates: Cimetidine may increase the levels/effects of CYP2D6 substrates. Example substrates include amphetamines, selected beta-blockers, dextromethorphan, fluoxetine, lidocaine, mirtazapine, nefazodone, paroxetine, risperidone, ritonavir, thioridazine, tricyclic antidepressants, and venlafaxine.

CYP2D6 prodrug substrates: Cimetidine may decrease the levels/effects of CYP2D6 prodrug substrates. Example prodrug substrates include codeine, hydrocodone, oxycodone, and tramadol.

CYP3A4 substrates: Cimetidine may increase the levels/effects of CYP3A4 substrates. Example substrates include benzodiazepines, calcium channel blockers, cyclosporine, mirtazapine, nateglinide, nefazodone, sildenafil (and other PDE-5 inhibitors), tacrolimus, and venlafaxine. Selected benzodiazepines (midazolam and triazolam), cisapride, ergot alkaloids, selected HMG-CoA reductase inhibitors (lovastatin and simvastatin), and pimozide are generally contraindicated with strong CYP3A4 inhibitors.

Delavirdine's absorption is decreased; avoid concurrent use with H_2 antagonists.

Flecainide's serum concentration is increased, especially in patients with renal failure.

Ketoconazole, fluconazole, itraconazole (especially capsule): Decreased serum concentration; avoid concurrent use with H_2 antagonists.

Lidocaine's serum concentration is increased; use alternative H_2 antagonist.

Melphalan's serum concentration may be decreased; monitor for reduced efficacy.

Meperidine: Increased serum concentration; monitor for toxicity.

Moricizine's serum concentration is increased; monitor for toxicity.

Paroxetine's serum concentration is increased.

Phenytoin toxicity; avoid concurrent use.

Propafenone's serum concentration is increased; monitor for toxicity.

Quinolones: Renal elimination of quinolone antibiotics may be decreased.

Tacrine's plasma concentration is increased; consider alternative H_2 antagonist.

TCAs serum concentration is increased; consider alternative H_2 antagonist or monitor for TCAs toxicity.

Theophylline's serum concentration is increased; consider alternative H_2 antagonist.

(Continued)

Cimetidine *(Continued)*

Warfarin's INR is increased; cimetidine's effect is dose-related. Use an alternative H_2 antagonist if possible or monitor INR closely and adjust warfarin dose as needed.

Nutritional/Herbal/Ethanol Interactions

Ethanol: Avoid ethanol (may enhance gastric mucosal irritation).

Food: Cimetidine may increase serum caffeine levels if taken with caffeine. Cimetidine peak serum levels may be decreased if taken with food.

Herb/Nutraceutical: St John's wort may decrease cimetidine levels.

Lab Interactions Increased creatinine (S), AST, ALT

Adverse Reactions

1% to 10%:

Central nervous system: Headache, dizziness, agitation, drowsiness

Gastrointestinal: Diarrhea, nausea, vomiting

<1% (Limited to important or life-threatening): Agranulocytosis, AST and ALT increased, bradycardia, creatinine increased, hypotension, neutropenia, tachycardia, thrombocytopenia

Overdosage/Toxicology Treatment is symptomatic and supportive. There is no reported experience with intentional overdose. Reported ingestion of 20 g have had transient side effects seen with recommended doses. Animal data has shown respiratory failure, tachycardia, muscle tremor, vomiting, restlessness, hypotension, salivation, emesis, and diarrhea.

Dosing

Adults & Elderly:

Short-term treatment of active ulcers:

Oral: 300 mg 4 times/day or 800 mg at bedtime or 400 mg twice daily for up to 8 weeks

I.M., I.V.: 300 mg every 6 hours or 37.5 mg/hour by continuous infusion; I.V. dosage should be adjusted to maintain an intragastric pH ≥5

Note: *Patients with active bleeding:* Give cimetidine as a continuous infusion (see above)

Duodenal ulcer prophylaxis: Oral: 400-800 mg at bedtime

Gastric hypersecretory conditions: Oral, I.M., I.V.: 300-600 mg every 6 hours; dosage not to exceed 2.4 g/day

Peptic ulcer disease eradication of *Helicobacter pylori* (unlabeled use): Oral: 400 mg twice daily; requires combination therapy with antibiotics

Heartburn, acid indigestion, sour stomach (OTC labeling): Oral: 200 mg up to twice daily; may take 30 minutes prior to eating foods or beverages expected to cause heartburn or indigestion

Pediatrics:

Oral, I.M., I.V.: 20-40 mg/kg/day in divided doses every 6 hours

Heartburn, acid indigestion, sour stomach (OTC labeling): Children ≥12 years: Oral: Refer to adult dosing.

Renal Impairment:

Cl_{cr} 10-50 mL/minute: Administer 50% of normal dose.

Cl_{cr} <10 mL/minute: Administer 25% of normal dose.

Slightly dialyzable (5% to 20%)

Hepatic Impairment: Usual dose is safe in mild liver disease but use with caution and in reduced dosage in severe liver disease. Increased risk of CNS toxicity in cirrhosis suggested by enhanced penetration of CNS.

Available Dosage Forms

Infusion, as hydrochloride [premixed in NS]: 300 mg (50 mL)

Injection, solution, as hydrochloride: 150 mg/mL (2 mL, 8 mL) [8 mL size contains benzyl alcohol]

Liquid, oral, as hydrochloride: 300 mg/5 mL (240 mL, 480 mL) [contains alcohol 2.8%; mint-peach flavor]

Tablet: 200 mg [OTC], 300 mg, 400 mg, 800 mg

Tagamet®: 300 mg, 400 mg

Tagamet® HB 200: 200 mg

Nursing Guidelines

Assessment: See Contraindications, Warnings/Precautions, and Dosing for use cautions. Assess potential for interactions with other prescriptions, OTC medications, or herbal products patient may be taking (see Drug Interactions). See I.V. specifics. Assess results of laboratory tests, therapeutic effectiveness, and adverse effects (eg, changes in CNS, especially in elderly patients - see Adverse Reactions and Overdose/Toxicology) regularly during therapy. Teach patient proper use possible side effects/appropriate interventions, and adverse symptoms to report (see Patient Education).

Monitoring Laboratory Tests: CBC, gastric pH, occult blood with GI bleeding; monitor renal function to correct dose.

Patient Education: Inform prescriber of all prescriptions, OTC medications, or herbal products you are taking, and any allergies you have. Do not take any new medication during therapy unless approved by prescriber. Take with meals. Do not increase dose or frequency without consulting prescriber. Limit xanthine-containing foods and beverages which may decrease iron absorption. To be effective, continue to take for the prescribed time (possibly 4-8 weeks) even though symptoms may have improved. Smoking decreases the effectiveness of cimetidine (stop smoking if possible). Avoid alcohol and caffeine. May cause headache, dizziness, agitation (use caution when driving or engaging in any potentially hazardous tasks until response to drug is known); nausea or vomiting (small, frequent meals, frequent mouth care, chewing gum, or sucking lozenges may help); or diarrhea (buttermilk, boiled milk, or yogurt may help). Report persistent diarrhea; black tarry stools or coffee ground-like emesis; dizziness, confusion, or agitation; rash; unusual bleeding or bruising; sore throat; or fever.

Geriatric Considerations: Patients diagnosed with PUD should be evaluated for *Helicobacter pylori.* When H_2-blockers are indicated, they are the preferred drugs for treating PUD in the elderly due to cost and ease of administration and reduced side effects.

Pregnancy Risk Factor: B

Lactation: Enters breast milk/compatible

Perioperative/Anesthesia/Other Concerns: Cimetidine has extensive drug interactions, particularly with antiarrhythmics (lidocaine, phenytoin, procainamide, quinidine) and may also increase the likelihood of theophylline and cyclosporine toxicity. Because of inhibition of warfarin metabolism, cimetidine may increase INR in patients on anticoagulation therapy.

Administration

Oral: Give with meals so that the drug's peak effect occurs at the proper time (peak inhibition of gastric acid secretion occurs at 1 and 3 hours after dosing in fasting subjects and approximately 2 hours in nonfasting subjects. This correlates well with the time food is no longer in the stomach offering a buffering effect). Stagger doses of antacids with cimetidine.

I.V.: May be administered as a slow I.V. push or preferably as an I.V. intermittent or I.V. continuous infusion. Administer each 300 mg (or fraction thereof) over a minimum of 5 minutes when giving I.V. push. Give intermittent infusion over 15-30 minutes for each 300 mg dose. Intermittent infusions are administered over 15-30 minutes at a final concentration not to exceed 6 mg/mL; for patients with an active bleed, preferred method of administration is continuous infusion.

Reconstitution: Stability at room temperature for prepared bags is 7 days. Stable in parenteral nutrition solutions for up to 7 days when protected from light.

Compatibility: Stable in D_5LR, $D_5{}^1/_4NS$, $D_5{}^1/_2NS$, D_5NS, D_5W, $D_{10}W$, $D_{10}NS$, LR, sodium bicarbonate 5%, NS

Y-site administration: Incompatible with allopurinol, amphotericin B cholesteryl sulfate complex, amsacrine, cefepime, indomethacin, warfarin

Compatibility in syringe: Incompatible with atropine/pentobarbital, cefamandole, cefazolin, chlorpromazine, ioxaglate meglumine and ioxaglate sodium, pentobarbital, secobarbital

Compatibility when admixed: Incompatible with amphotericin B, barbiturates

Storage: Intact vials of cimetidine should be stored at room temperature and protected from light. Cimetidine may precipitate from solution upon exposure to cold but can be redissolved by warming without degradation.

Stability at room temperature for premixed bags: Manufacturer expiration dating and out of overwrap stability: 15 days.

♦ **Cipro®** *see* Ciprofloxacin *on page 400*

Ciprofloxacin (sip roe FLOKS a sin)

U.S. Brand Names Ciloxan®; Cipro®; Cipro® XR; Proquin® XR

Synonyms Ciprofloxacin Hydrochloride

Pharmacologic Category Antibiotic, Ophthalmic; Antibiotic, Quinolone

Medication Safety Issues

Sound-alike/look-alike issues:

Ciprofloxacin may be confused with cephalexin

Ciloxan® may be confused with cinoxacin, Cytoxan®

Cipro® may be confused with Ceftin®

Use

Children: Complicated urinary tract infections and pyelonephritis due to *E. coli*. **Note:** Although effective, ciprofloxacin is not the drug of first choice in children.

Children and adults: To reduce incidence or progression of disease following exposure to aerolized *Bacillus anthracis*. Ophthalmologically, for superficial ocular infections (corneal ulcers, conjunctivitis) due to susceptible strains

Adults: Treatment of the following infections when caused by susceptible bacteria: Urinary tract infections; acute uncomplicated cystitis in females; chronic bacterial prostatitis; lower respiratory tract infections (including acute exacerbations of chronic bronchitis); acute sinusitis; skin and skin structure infections; bone and joint infections; complicated intra-abdominal infections (in combination with metronidazole); infectious diarrhea; typhoid fever due to *Salmonella typhi* (eradication of chronic typhoid carrier state has not been proven); uncomplicated cervical and urethra gonorrhea (due to *N. gonorrhoeae*); nosocomial pneumonia; empirical therapy for febrile neutropenic patients (in combination with piperacillin)

Unlabeled/Investigational Use Acute pulmonary exacerbations in cystic fibrosis (children); cutaneous/gastrointestinal/oropharyngeal anthrax (treatment, children and adults); disseminated gonococcal infection (adults); chancroid (adults); prophylaxis to *Neisseria meningitidis* following close contact with an infected person

Mechanism of Action Inhibits DNA-gyrase in susceptible organisms; inhibits relaxation of supercoiled DNA and promotes breakage of double-stranded DNA

Pharmacodynamics/Kinetics

Absorption: Oral: Immediate release tablet: Rapid (~50% to 85%)

Distribution: V_d: 2.1-2.7 L/kg; tissue concentrations often exceed serum concentrations especially in kidneys, gallbladder, liver, lungs, gynecological tissue, and prostatic tissue; CSF concentrations: 10% of serum concentrations (noninflamed meninges), 14% to 37% (inflamed meninges); crosses placenta; enters breast milk

Protein binding: 20% to 40%

Metabolism: Partially hepatic; forms 4 metabolites (limited activity)

Half-life elimination: Children: 2.5 hours; Adults: Normal renal function: 3-5 hours

Time to peak: Oral:

Immediate release tablet: 0.5-2 hours

Extended release tablet: Cipro® XR: 1-2.5 hours, Proquin® XR: 3.5-8.7 hours

Excretion: Urine (30% to 50% as unchanged drug); feces (15% to 43%)

Contraindications Hypersensitivity to ciprofloxacin, any component of the formulation, or other quinolones

Warnings/Precautions CNS stimulation may occur (tremor, restlessness, confusion, and very rarely hallucinations or seizures). Use with caution in patients with known or suspected CNS disorder. Prolonged use may result in superinfection. Tendon inflammation and/or rupture have been reported with ciprofloxacin and other quinolone antibiotics. Risk may be increased with concurrent corticosteroids, particularly in the elderly. Discontinue at first sign of tendon inflammation or pain. Adverse effects, including those related to joints and/or surrounding tissues, are increased in pediatric patients. Rare cases of peripheral neuropathy may occur.

Severe hypersensitivity reactions, including anaphylaxis, have occurred with quinolone therapy. Quinolones may exacerbate myasthenia gravis, use with caution (rare, potentially life-threatening weakness of respiratory muscles may occur). Use caution in renal impairment. Avoid excessive sunlight; may cause moderate-to-severe phototoxicity reactions.

Drug Interactions Inhibits CYP1A2 (strong), 3A4 (weak)

Caffeine: Ciprofloxacin may decrease the metabolism of caffeine

Corticosteroids: Concurrent use may increase the risk of tendon rupture, particularly in elderly patients (overall incidence rare).

CYP1A2 substrates: Ciprofloxacin may increase the levels/effects of CYP1A2 substrates. Example substrates include aminophylline, fluvoxamine, mexiletine, mirtazapine, ropinirole, and trifluoperazine.

Foscarnet: Concomitant use with ciprofloxacin has been associated with an increased risk of seizures.

Glyburide: Quinolones may increase the effect of glyburide. Monitor

Metal cations (aluminum, calcium, iron, magnesium, and zinc) bind quinolones in the gastrointestinal tract and inhibit absorption. Concurrent administration of most antacids, oral electrolyte supplements, quinapril, sucralfate, some didanosine formulations (chewable/buffered tablets and pediatric powder for oral suspension), and other highly-buffered oral drugs, should be avoided. Ciprofloxacin should be administered 2 hours before or 6 hours after these agents.

Methotrexate: Ciprofloxacin may decrease renal secretion of methotrexate; monitor.

Phenytoin: Ciprofloxacin may decrease phenytoin levels; monitor.

Probenecid: May decrease renal secretion of quinolones.

Ropivacaine: Ciprofloxacin may decrease the metabolism of ropivacaine.

Theophylline: Serum levels may be increased by ciprofloxacin; in addition, CNS stimulation/seizures may occur at lower theophylline serum levels due to additive CNS effects.

Warfarin: The hypoprothrombinemic effect of warfarin may be enhanced by ciprofloxacin; monitor INR.

Nutritional/Herbal/Ethanol Interactions

Food: Food decreases rate, but not extent, of absorption. Ciprofloxacin serum levels may be decreased if taken with dairy products or calcium-fortified juices. Ciprofloxacin may increase serum caffeine levels if taken with caffeine.

Enteral feedings may decrease plasma concentrations of ciprofloxacin probably by >30% inhibition of absorption. Ciprofloxacin should not be administered with enteral feedings. The feeding would need to be discontinued for 1-2 hours prior to and after ciprofloxacin administration. Nasogastric administration produces a greater loss of ciprofloxacin bioavailability than does nasoduodenal administration.

Herb/Nutraceutical: Avoid dong quai, St John's wort (may also cause photosensitization).

Adverse Reactions

1% to 10%:

Central nervous system: Neurologic events (children 2%, includes dizziness, insomnia, nervousness, somnolence); fever (children 2%); headache (I.V. administration); restlessness (I.V. administration)

Dermatologic: Rash (children 2%, adults 1%)

Gastrointestinal: Nausea (children/adults 3%); diarrhea (children 5%, adults 2%); vomiting (children 5%, adults 1%); abdominal pain (children 3%, adults <1%); dyspepsia (children 3%)

Hepatic: ALT/AST increased (adults 1%)

Local: Injection site reactions (I.V. administration)

Respiratory: Rhinitis (children 3%)

<1% (Limited to important or life-threatening): Abnormal gait, acute renal failure, agitation, agranulocytosis, albuminuria, allergic reactions, anaphylactic shock, anaphylaxis, anemia, angina pectoris, angioedema, anorexia, anosmia, arthralgia, ataxia, atrial flutter, bone marrow depression (life-threatening), breast pain, bronchospasm, candidiasis, candiduria, cardiopulmonary arrest, cerebral thrombosis, chills, cholestatic jaundice, chromatopsia, confusion, constipation, crystalluria (particularly in alkaline urine), cylindruria, delirium, depersonalization, depression, dizziness, drowsiness, dyspepsia (adults), dysphagia, dyspnea, edema, eosinophilia, erythema multiforme, erythema nodosum, exfoliative dermatitis, fever (adults), fixed eruption, flatulence, gastrointestinal bleeding, hallucinations, headache (oral), hematuria, hemolytic anemia, hepatic failure, hepatic necrosis, hyperesthesia, hyperglycemia, hyperpigmentation, hyper-/hypotension, hypertonia, insomnia, interstitial nephritis, intestinal perforation, irritability, jaundice, joint pain, laryngeal edema, lightheadedness, lymphadenopathy, malaise, manic reaction, methemoglobinemia, MI, migraine, moniliasis, myalgia, myasthenia gravis, myoclonus, nephritis, nightmares, nystagmus, orthostatic hypotension, palpitation, pancreatitis, pancytopenia (life-threatening or fatal), paranoia, paresthesia, peripheral neuropathy, petechia, photosensitivity, prolongation of PT/INR, pseudomembranous colitis, psychosis, pulmonary edema, renal calculi, seizure; serum cholesterol, glucose, triglycerides increased; serum sickness-like reactions, Stevens-Johnson syndrome, syncope, tachycardia, taste loss, tendon rupture,

(Continued)

Ciprofloxacin *(Continued)*

tendonitis, thrombophlebitis, tinnitus, torsade de pointes, toxic epidermal necrolysis (Lyell's syndrome), tremor, twitching, urethral bleeding, vaginal candidiasis, vaginitis, vasculitis, ventricular ectopy, visual disturbance, weakness

Overdosage/Toxicology Symptoms of overdose include acute renal failure and seizures. Treatment is supportive and should include adequate hydration and renal function monitoring. Magnesium or calcium containing antacids may be given to decrease absorption of oral ciprofloxacin. Only a small amount of ciprofloxacin (<10%) is removed from the body after hemodialysis or peritoneal dialysis.

Dosing

Adults: Note: Extended release tablets and immediate release formulations are not interchangeable. Unless otherwise specified, oral dosing reflects the use of immediate release formulations.

Urinary tract infection:

Acute uncomplicated: Oral: Immediate release formulation: 250 mg every 12 hours for 3 days

Acute uncomplicated pyelonephritis: Oral: Extended release formulation (Cipro® XR): 1000 mg every 24 hours for 7-14 days

Uncomplicated/acute cystitis: Oral: Extended release formulation (Cipro® XR, Proquin® XR): 500 mg every 24 hours for 3 days

Mild/moderate:

Oral: Immediate release formulation: 250 mg every 12 hours for 7-14 days

I.V.: 200 mg every 12 hours for 7-14 days

Severe/complicated:

Oral:

Immediate release formulation: 500 mg every 12 hours for 7-14 days

Extended release formulation (Cipro® XR): 1000 mg every 24 hours for 7-14 days

I.V.: 400 mg every 12 hours for 7-14 days

Lower respiratory tract, skin/skin structure infections:

Oral: 500-750 mg twice daily for 7-14 days depending on severity and susceptibility

I.V.:

Mild/moderate: 400 mg every 12 hours for 7-14 days

Severe/complicated: 400 mg every 8 hours for 7-14 days

Nosocomial pneumonia (mild to moderate to severe): I.V.: 400 mg every 8 hours for 10-14 days

Bone/joint infections:

Oral: 500-750 mg twice daily for 4-6 weeks, depending on severity and susceptibility

I.V.:

Mild/moderate: 400 mg every 12 hours for 4-6 weeks

Severe/complicated: 400 mg every 8 hours for 4-6 weeks

Infectious diarrhea: Oral: 500 mg every 12 hours for 5-7 days

Intra-abdominal (in combination with metronidazole):

Oral: 500 mg every 12 hours for 7-14 days

I.V.: 400 mg every 12 hours for 7-14 days

Febrile neutropenia (with piperacillin): I.V.: 400 mg every 8 hours for 7-14 days

Typhoid fever: Oral: 500 mg every 12 hours for 10 days

Gonococcal infections:

Urethral/cervical gonococcal infections: Oral: 250-500 mg as a single dose (CDC recommends concomitant doxycycline or azithromycin due to developing resistance; avoid use in Asian or Western Pacific travelers)

Disseminated gonococcal infection (CDC guidelines): Oral: 500 mg twice daily to complete 7 days of therapy (initial treatment with ceftriaxone 1 g I.M./I.V. daily for 24-48 hours after improvement begins)

Chancroid (CDC guidelines): Oral: 500 mg twice daily for 3 days

Sinusitis (acute):

Oral: 500 mg every 12 hours for 10 days

I.V.: 400 mg every 12 hours for 10 days

Prostatitis (chronic, bacterial):

Oral: 500 mg every 12 hours for 28 days

I.V.: 400 mg every 12 hours for 28 days

Anthrax:

Inhalational (postexposure prophylaxis):

Oral: 500 mg every 12 hours for 60 days

I.V.: 400 mg every 12 hours for 60 days

Cutaneous (treatment, CDC guidelines): Oral: Immediate release formulation: 500 mg every 12 hours for 60 days. **Note:** In the presence of systemic involvement, extensive edema, lesions on head/neck, refer to I.V. dosing for treatment of inhalational/gastrointestinal/oropharyngeal anthrax.

Inhalational/gastrointestinal/oropharyngeal (treatment, CDC guidelines): I.V.: 400 mg every 12 hours. **Note:** Initial treatment should include two or more agents predicted to be effective (per CDC recommendations). Agents suggested for use in conjunction with ciprofloxacin or doxycycline include rifampin, vancomycin, imipenem, penicillin, ampicillin, chloramphenicol, clindamycin, and clarithromycin. May switch to oral antimicrobial therapy when clinically appropriate. Continue combined therapy for 60 days.

Bacterial conjunctivitis:

Ophthalmic solution: Instill 1-2 drops in eye(s) every 2 hours while awake for 2 days and 1-2 drops every 4 hours while awake for the next 5 days

Ophthalmic ointment: Apply a 1/2" ribbon into the conjunctival sac 3 times/day for the first 2 days, followed by a 1/2" ribbon applied twice daily for the next 5 days

Corneal ulcer: Ophthalmic solution: Instill 2 drops into affected eye every 15 minutes for the first 6 hours, then 2 drops into the affected eye every 30 minutes for the remainder of the first day. On day 2, instill 2 drops into the affected eye hourly. On days 3-14, instill 2 drops into affected eye every 4 hours. Treatment may continue after day 14 if re-epithelialization has not occurred.

Elderly: Refer to adult dosing. Adjust dose carefully based on renal function.

Pediatrics: See Warnings/Precautions. **Note:** Extended release tablets and immediate release formulations are not interchangeable. Unless otherwise specified, oral dosing reflects the use of immediate release formulations.

Complicated urinary tract infection or pyelonephritis: Children 1-17 years:

Oral: 20-30 mg/kg/day in 2 divided doses (every 12 hours) for 10-21 days; maximum: 1.5 g/day

I.V.: 6-10 mg/kg every 8 hours for 10-21 days (maximum: 400 mg/dose)

Cystic fibrosis (unlabeled use): Children 5-17 years:

Oral: 40 mg/kg/day divided every 12 hours administered following 1 week of I.V. therapy has been reported in a clinical trial; total duration of therapy: 10-21 days

I.V.: 30 mg/kg/day divided every 8 hours for 1 week, followed by oral therapy, has been reported in a clinical trial

Anthrax:

Inhalational (postexposure prophylaxis):

Oral: 15 mg/kg/dose every 12 hours for 60 days; maximum: 500 mg/dose

I.V.: 10 mg/kg/dose every 12 hours for 60 days; do **not** exceed 400 mg/dose (800 mg/day)

Cutaneous (treatment, CDC guidelines): Oral: 10-15 mg/kg every 12 hours for 60 days (maximum: 1 g/day); amoxicillin 80 mg/kg/day divided every 8 hours is an option for completion of treatment after clinical improvement. **Note:** In the presence of systemic involvement, extensive edema, lesions on head/neck, refer to I.V. dosing for treatment of inhalational/gastrointestinal/oropharyngeal anthrax.

Inhalational/gastrointestinal/oropharyngeal (treatment, CDC guidelines): I.V.: Initial: 10-15 mg/kg every 12 hours for 60 days (maximum: 500 mg/dose); switch to oral therapy when clinically appropriate; refer to Adults dosing for notes on combined therapy and duration

Bacterial conjunctivitis:

Ophthalmic solution: Children >1 year: Refer to adult dosing.

Ophthalmic ointment: Children >2 years: Refer to adult dosing.

Corneal ulcer: Children >1 year: Refer to adult dosing.

Renal Impairment: Adults:

Cl_{cr} 30-50 mL/minute: Oral: Administer 250-500 mg every 12 hours.

Cl_{cr} <30 mL/minute: Acute uncomplicated pyelonephritis or complicated UTI: Oral: Extended release formulation: 500 mg every 24 hours

Cl_{cr} 5-29 mL/minute:

Oral: Administer 250-500 mg every 18 hours.

I.V.: Administer 200-400 mg every 18-24 hours.

(Continued)

Ciprofloxacin *(Continued)*

Dialysis: Only small amounts of ciprofloxacin are removed by hemo- or peritoneal dialysis (<10%); usual dose: Oral: 250-500 mg every 24 hours following dialysis.

Continuous arteriovenous or venovenous hemodiafiltration effects: Administer 200-400 mg I.V. every 12 hours.

Available Dosage Forms [DSC] = Discontinued product

Infusion, [premixed in D_5W] (Cipro®): 200 mg (100 mL); 400 mg (200 mL) [latex free]

Injection, solution (Cipro®): 10 mg/mL (20 mL, 40 mL, 120 mL [DSC])

Microcapsules for oral suspension (Cipro®): 250 mg/5 mL (100 mL); 500 mg/5 mL (100 mL) [strawberry flavor]

Ointment, ophthalmic, as hydrochloride (Ciloxan®): 3.33 mg/g [0.3% base] (3.5 g)

Solution, ophthalmic, as hydrochloride (Ciloxan®): 3.5 mg/mL [0.3% base] (2.5 mL, 5 mL, 10 mL) [contains benzalkonium chloride]

Tablet: 250 mg, 500 mg, 750 mg

Cipro®: 100 mg, 250 mg, 500 mg, 750 mg

Tablet, extended release:

Cipro® XR: 500 mg [equivalent to ciprofloxacin hydrochloride 287.5 mg and ciprofloxacin base 212.6 mg]; 1000 mg [equivalent to ciprofloxacin hydrochloride 574.9 mg and ciprofloxacin base 425.2 mg]

Proquin® XR: 500 mg

Nursing Guidelines

Assessment: See Contraindications, Warnings/Precautions and Dosing for use cautions. Assess potential for interactions with other prescriptions, OTC medications, or herbal products patient may be taking, and any allergies they may have (see Drug Interactions). **I.V.:** See Administration, Reconstitution, and Compatibility for specific directions. Assess results of laboratory tests (see below), therapeutic effectiveness, and adverse effects (eg, changes in CNS, especially in elderly patients - see Adverse Reactions and Overdose/Toxicology) regularly during therapy. Teach patient proper use (appropriate for formulation), possible side effects/appropriate interventions, and adverse symptoms to report (see Patient Education). Breast-feeding is contraindicated.

Monitoring Laboratory Tests: CBC, renal and hepatic function during prolonged therapy; patients receiving concurrent ciprofloxacin, theophylline, or cyclosporine should have serum theophylline or cyclosporine levels monitored. Culture and sensitivity specimen should be taken prior to initiating therapy.

Dietary Considerations:

Food: Drug may cause GI upset; take without regard to meals (manufacturer prefers that immediate release tablet is taken 2 hours after meals). Extended release tablet may be taken with meals that contain dairy products (calcium content <800 mg), but not with dairy products alone.

Dairy products, calcium-fortified juices, oral multivitamins, and mineral supplements: Absorption of ciprofloxacin is decreased by divalent and trivalent cations. The manufacturer states that the usual dietary intake of calcium (including meals which include dairy products) has not been shown to interfere with ciprofloxacin absorption. Immediate release ciprofloxacin and Cipro® XR may be taken 2 hours before or 6 hours after, and Proquin® XR may be taken 4 hours before or 6 hours after, any of these products.

Caffeine: Patients consuming regular large quantities of caffeinated beverages may need to restrict caffeine intake if excessive cardiac or CNS stimulation occurs.

Patient Education: Do not take any new medication during therapy unless approved by prescriber.

Infusion: Report immediately any redness, burning, or swelling at infusion site; tightness or swelling in mouth or throat, difficulty swallowing, difficulty breathing, skin rash, rapid heartbeat or palpitations, or onset of other adverse response.

Oral: Take exactly as directed, (at least 2 hours before or 6 hours after antacids or other drug products containing calcium, iron, or zinc). Extended release tablet may be taken with meals containing dairy products, but not with dairy products alone; do not crush, split, or chew extended release tablet. Swallow oral suspension; do not chew microcapsules. Shake bottle vigorously with each use. Take entire prescription, even if feeling better. Maintain adequate hydration to avoid concentrated urine and crystal formation (2-3 L/day) unless instructed to restrict fluid intake. You may experience nausea, vomiting, or anorexia (small frequent meals, frequent mouth care, sucking lozenges, or chewing gum may help); or increased sensitivity to sunlight (use sunscreen, wear protective clothing and dark glasses, and avoid direct exposure to sunlight). If signs of inflammation or tendon pain occur, discontinue use immediately and report to prescriber. If signs of allergic reaction (eg, itching, urticaria, respiratory difficulty, facial edema, difficulty swallowing, loss of consciousness, tingling, chest pain, palpitations) occur, discontinue use immediately and report to prescriber. Report unusual fever or chills, vaginal itching or foul-smelling vaginal discharge, easy bruising or bleeding, or tendon or muscle pain.

Ophthalmic: Use exactly as directed. Wash hands prior to instilling eye medication. Do not touch dropper to eye or any other surface. Do not wear contact lenses while using this medication (check with prescriber before using again). Tilt head back, look upward and pull lower eyelid down to make a pouch. Drop prescribed number of drops directly into eye. Close eye, place one finger at corner of eye near nose and apply gentle pressure. Do not blink or rub eye. If also using ointment, use drops before ointment. Use for exact time as prescribed, do not discontinue even if symptoms disappear. May cause temporary stinging or burning. Report persistent eye discomfort, itching, redness, unusual tearing, feeling as if something is in your eye, blurred vision, eye pain, worsening vision, a bad taste in your mouth, sensitivity to light, skin rash, difficulty breathing, or worsening of symptoms.

Pregnancy/breast-feeding precautions: Inform prescriber if you are or intend to become pregnant. Do not breast-feed.

Geriatric Considerations: Ciprofloxacin should not be used as first-line therapy unless the culture and sensitivity findings show resistance to usual therapy. The interactions with caffeine and theophylline can result in serious toxicity in the elderly. Adjust dose for renal function.

Pregnancy Risk Factor: C

Pregnancy Issues: Ciprofloxacin crosses the placenta and concentrates in amniotic fluid; maternal serum levels may be decreased during pregnancy. Reports of arthropathy (observed in immature animals and reported rarely in humans) have limited the use of fluoroquinolones in pregnancy. According to the FDA, the Teratogen Information System concluded that therapeutic doses during pregnancy are unlikely to produce substantial teratogenic risk, but data are insufficient to say that there is no risk. Since safer alternatives are usually available, quinolones should generally be avoided in pregnancy. When considering treatment for life-threatening infection and/or prolonged duration of therapy, the potential risk to the fetus must be balanced against the severity of the potential illness.

Lactation: Enters breast milk/not recommended (AAP rates "compatible")

Breast-Feeding Considerations: Ciprofloxacin is excreted in breast milk; however, the exposure to the infant is considered small and one source suggests that the decision to breast-feed be independent of the need for the antibiotic in the mother. Another source recommends the mother wait 48 hours after the last dose of ciprofloxacin to continue nursing. The manufacturer recommends to discontinue nursing or to discontinue ciprofloxacin.

Perioperative/Anesthesia/Other Concerns: Ciprofloxacin may increase theophylline levels resulting in relevant cardiovascular side effects, including tachycardia.

Administration

Oral: May administer with food to minimize GI upset; avoid antacid use; maintain proper hydration and urine output. Administer immediate release ciprofloxacin and Cipro® XR at least 2 hours before or 6 hours after, and Proquin® XR at least 4 hours before or 6 hours after antacids or other products containing calcium, iron, or zinc (including dairy products or calcium-fortified juices). Separate oral administration from drugs which may impair absorption (see Drug Interactions).

Oral suspension: Should not be administered through feeding tubes (suspension is oil-based and adheres to the feeding tube). Patients should avoid chewing on the microcapsules.

Nasogastric/orogastric tube: Crush immediate-release tablet and mix with water. Flush feeding tube before and after administration. Hold tube feedings at least 1 hour before and 2 hours after administration.

Tablet, extended release: Do not crush, split, or chew. May be administered with meals containing dairy products (calcium content <800 mg), but not with

(Continued)

Ciprofloxacin *(Continued)*

dairy products alone. Proquin® XR should be administered with a main meal of the day; evening meal is preferred

I.V.: Administer by slow I.V. infusion over 60 minutes into a large vein.

Reconstitution: Injection, vial: May be diluted with NS, D_5W, SWFI, $D_{10}W$, $D_5$1/4NS, $D_5$1/2NS, LR.

Compatibility: Stable in $D_5$1/4NS, $D_5$1/2NS, D_5W, $D_{10}W$, LR, NS

Y-site administration: Incompatible with aminophylline, ampicillin/sulbactam, cefepime, dexamethasone sodium phosphate, furosemide, heparin, hydrocortisone sodium succinate, methylprednisolone sodium succinate, phenytoin, propofol, sodium phosphates, warfarin

Compatibility when admixed: Incompatible with aminophylline, clindamycin, floxacillin, heparin

Storage:

Injection:

Premixed infusion: Store between 5°C to 25°C (41°F to 77°F). Protect from light. Avoid freezing.

Vial: Store between 5°C to 30°C (41°F to 86°F). Protect from light. Avoid freezing. Diluted solutions of 0.5-2 mg/mL are stable for up to 14 days refrigerated or at room temperature.

Ophthalmic solution/ointment: Store at 36°F to 77°F (2°C to 25°C). Protect from light.

Microcapsules for oral suspension: Prior to reconstitution, store below 25°C (77°F). Protect from freezing. Following reconstitution, store below 30°C (86°F) for up to 14 days. Protect from freezing.

Tablet:

Immediate release: Store below 30°C (86°F).

Extended release: Store at room temperature of 15°C to 30°C (59°F to 86°F).

Related Information

Prevention of Wound Infection and Sepsis in Surgical Patients *on page 1830*

◆ **Ciprofloxacin Hydrochloride** *see* Ciprofloxacin *on page 400*

◆ **Cipro® XR** *see* Ciprofloxacin *on page 400*

Cisapride (SIS a pride)

U.S. Brand Names Propulsid®

Pharmacologic Category Gastrointestinal Agent, Prokinetic

Medication Safety Issues

Sound-alike/look-alike issues:

Propulsid® may be confused with propranolol

Use Treatment of nocturnal symptoms of gastroesophageal reflux disease (GERD); has demonstrated effectiveness for gastroparesis, refractory constipation, and nonulcer dyspepsia

Mechanism of Action Enhances the release of acetylcholine at the myenteric plexus. *In vitro* studies have shown cisapride to have serotonin-4 receptor agonistic properties which may increase gastrointestinal motility and cardiac rate; increases lower esophageal sphincter pressure and lower esophageal peristalsis; accelerates gastric emptying of both liquids and solids.

Pharmacodynamics/Kinetics

Onset of action: 0.5-1 hour

Protein binding: 97.5% to 98%

Metabolism: Extensively hepatic to norcisapride

Bioavailability: 35% to 40%

Half-life elimination: 6-12 hours

Excretion: Urine and feces (<10%)

Contraindications

Hypersensitivity to cisapride or any component of the formulations; GI hemorrhage, mechanical obstruction, GI perforation, or other situations when GI motility stimulation is dangerous

Serious cardiac arrhythmias including ventricular tachycardia, ventricular fibrillation, torsade de pointes, and QT prolongation have been reported in patients taking cisapride with other drugs that inhibit CYP3A4. Some of these events have been fatal. Concomitant oral or intravenous administration of the following drugs with cisapride may lead to elevated cisapride blood levels and is contraindicated:

Antibiotics: Oral or I.V. erythromycin, clarithromycin, troleandomycin

Antidepressants: Nefazodone

Antifungals: Oral or I.V. fluconazole, itraconazole, miconazole, oral ketoconazole

Protease inhibitors: Indinavir, ritonavir, amprenavir, atazanavir

Cisapride is also contraindicated for patients with a prolonged electrocardiographic QT intervals (QT_c >450 msec), a history of QT_c prolongation, or known family history of congenital long QT syndrome; clinically significant bradycardia, renal failure, history of ventricular arrhythmias, ischemic heart disease, and congestive heart failure; uncorrected electrolyte disorders (hypokalemia, hypomagnesemia); respiratory failure; and concomitant medications known to prolong the QT interval and increase the risk of arrhythmia, such as certain antiarrhythmics, certain antipsychotics, certain antidepressants, bepridil, sparfloxacin, and terodiline. The preceding lists of drugs are not comprehensive. Cisapride should not be used in patients with uncorrected hypokalemia or hypomagnesemia or who might experience rapid reduction of plasma potassium such as those administered potassium-wasting diuretics and/or insulin in acute settings.

Warnings/Precautions Safety and effectiveness in children have not been established.

On March 24, 2000 the FDA announced that the manufacturer of cisapride would voluntarily withdraw its product from the U.S. market on July 14, 2000. This decision was based on 341 reports of heart rhythm abnormalities including 80 reports of deaths. The company will continue to make the drug available to patients who meet specific clinical eligibility criteria for a limited-access protocol (contact 1-800-JANSSEN). Serious cardiac arrhythmias including ventricular tachycardia, ventricular fibrillation, torsade de pointes, and QT prolongation have been reported in patients taking this drug. Many of these patients also took drugs expected to increase cisapride blood levels by inhibiting the cytochrome P450 3A4 enzymes that metabolize cisapride. These drugs include clarithromycin, erythromycin, troleandomycin, nefazodone, fluconazole, itraconazole, ketoconazole, indinavir and ritonavir. Some of these events have been fatal. Cisapride is contraindicated in patients taking any of these drugs. **QT prolongation, torsade de pointes (sometimes with syncope), cardiac arrest and sudden death have been reported in patients taking cisapride without the above-mentioned contraindicated drugs.** Most patients had disorders that may have predisposed them to arrhythmias with cisapride. Cisapride is contraindicated for those patients with: history of prolonged electrocardiographic QT intervals; renal failure; history of ventricular arrhythmias, ischemic heart disease, and CHF; uncorrected electrolyte disorders (hypokalemia, hypomagnesemia); respiratory failure; and concomitant medications known to prolong the QT interval and increase the risk of arrhythmia, such as certain antiarrhythmics, including those of Class 1A (such as quinidine and procainamide) and Class III (such as sotalol); tricyclic antidepressants (such as amitriptyline); certain tetracyclic antidepressants (such as maprotiline); certain antipsychotic medications (such as certain phenothiazines and sertindole), protease inhibitors, bepridil, sparfloxacin and terodiline. (The preceding lists of drugs are not comprehensive.) Recommended doses of cisapride should not be exceeded.

Patients should have a baseline ECG and an electrolyte panel (magnesium, calcium, potassium) prior to initiating cisapride (see Contraindications). Potential benefits should be weighed against risks prior administration of cisapride to patients who have or may develop prolongation of cardiac conduction intervals, particularly QT_c. These include patients with conditions that could predispose them to the development of serious arrhythmias, such as multiple organ failure, COPD, apnea and advanced cancer. Cisapride should not be used in patients with uncorrected hypokalemia or hypomagnesemia, such as those with severe dehydration, vomiting or malnutrition, or those taking potassium-wasting diuretics. Cisapride should not be used in patients who might experience rapid reduction of plasma potassium, such as those administered potassium-wasting diuretics and/or insulin in acute settings.

Drug Interactions Substrate of CYP1A2 (minor), 2A6 (minor), 2B6 (minor), 2C8/9 (minor), 2C19 (minor), 3A4 (major); **Inhibits** CYP2D6 (weak), 3A4 (weak)

Azole antifungals (fluconazole, itraconazole, ketoconazole, miconazole) increase cisapride's concentration. Pre-existing cardiovascular disease or electrolyte imbalances increase the risk of malignant arrhythmias; concurrent use is contraindicated.

Bepridil increases the risk of malignant arrhythmias; concurrent use is contraindicated

(Continued)

Cisapride *(Continued)*

Cimetidine increases the bioavailability of cisapride; use an alternative H_2 antagonist

Class Ia (quinidine, procainamide) and Class III (amiodarone, sotalol) antiarrhythmics increase the risk of malignant arrhythmias; concurrent use is contraindicated

CYP3A4 inhibitors: May increase the levels/effects of cisapride. Example inhibitors include azole antifungals, clarithromycin, diclofenac, doxycycline, erythromycin, imatinib, isoniazid, nefazodone, nicardipine, propofol, protease inhibitors, quinidine, telithromycin, and verapamil. Concurrent use of azole antifungals, clarithromycin, erythromycin, nefazodone, and protease inhibitors is contraindicated.

Grapefruit juice may increase the bioavailability of cisapride; concomitant use should be avoided.

Macrolides (clarithromycin, erythromycin, troleandomycin) increase serum concentrations of cisapride. Risk of arrhythmias; concurrent use is contraindicated.

Nefazodone and maprotiline may increase the risk of malignant arrhythmias; concurrent use is contraindicated

Phenothiazines (prochlorperazine, promethazine) may increase the risk of malignant arrhythmias; concurrent use is contraindicated

Pimozide may prolong the QT interval; concurrent use is contraindicated.

Protease inhibitors (amprenavir, atazanavir, indinavir, nelfinavir, ritonavir) increase cisapride's concentration. Increased risk of malignant arrhythmias; concurrent use is contraindicated.

Quinolone antibiotics: Sparfloxacin, gatifloxacin, moxifloxacin increase the risk of malignant arrhythmias; concurrent use is contraindicated

Sertindole may increase the risk of malignant arrhythmias; concurrent use is contraindicated

TCAs increase the risk of malignant arrhythmias; concurrent use is contraindicated

Warfarin: Isolated cases of increased INR; monitor closely

Nutritional/Herbal/Ethanol Interactions

Ethanol: Avoid ethanol (may increase CNS depression).

Food: Coadministration of grapefruit juice with cisapride increases the bioavailability of cisapride and concomitant use should be avoided.

Herb/Nutraceutical: St John's wort may decrease cisapride levels.

Adverse Reactions

>10%:

Central nervous system: Headache

Gastrointestinal: Diarrhea (dose dependent)

1% to 10%:

Cardiovascular: Tachycardia

Central nervous system: Extrapyramidal effects, somnolence, fatigue, insomnia, anxiety

Dermatologic: Rash

Gastrointestinal: Abdominal cramping, constipation, nausea

Respiratory: Sinusitis, rhinitis, cough, upper respiratory tract infection, increased incidence of viral infection

<1% (Limited to important or life-threatening): Apnea, bronchospasm, gynecomastia, hyperprolactinemia, methemoglobinemia, photosensitivity, psychiatric disturbances, seizure (have been reported only in patients with a history of seizure)

Dosing

Adults & Elderly: GERD or gastrointestinal dysmotility: Oral: Initial: 5-10 mg 4 times/day at least 15 minutes before meals and at bedtime; in some patients the dosage will need to be increased to 20 mg to obtain a satisfactory result.

Pediatrics: Gastrointestinal dysmotility: Oral: Children: 0.15-0.3 mg/kg/dose 3-4 times/day; maximum: 10 mg/dose

Hepatic Impairment: Initiate at 50% usual dose.

Nursing Guidelines

Assessment: See Contraindications and Warnings/Precautions for use cautions and limitations. Assess potential for interactions with other prescriptions, OTC medications, or herbal products patient may be taking (see Drug Interactions). Assess results of laboratory tests (eg, ECG, electrolyte balance and renal function), therapeutic effectiveness, and adverse response (see Adverse Reactions and

Overdose/Toxicology) regularly during therapy. Teach patient proper use, possible side effects/appropriate interventions, and adverse symptoms to report (see Patient Education). Note breast-feeding caution.

Monitoring Laboratory Tests: A 12-lead ECG should be performed prior to administration of cisapride. Treatment with cisapride should not be initiated if the QT_c value exceeds 450 milliseconds. Serum electrolytes (potassium, calcium, and magnesium) and creatinine should be assessed prior to administration of cisapride and whenever conditions develop that may affect electrolyte balance or renal function.

Patient Education: It is absolutely vital that you inform prescriber of all prescriptions, OTC medications, or herbal products you are taking, and any allergies you have. Do not take any new medication during therapy unless approved by prescriber. Take before meals. Avoid alcohol and grapefruit juice. May cause increased sedation, headache, anxiety (use caution when driving or engaging in hazardous tasks until response to drug is known). Immediately report rapid heartbeat, palpitations, chest pain, or tightness. Report severe abdominal pain, prolonged diarrhea, weight loss, extreme fatigue, or other persistent adverse effects. **Pregnancy/breast-feeding precautions:** Inform prescriber if you are or intend to become pregnant. Consult prescriber if breast-feeding.

Geriatric Considerations: Steady-state serum concentrations are higher than those in younger adults; however, the therapeutic dose and pharmacologic effects are the same as those in younger adults and no adjustment in dose recommended for elderly.

Pregnancy Risk Factor: C

Lactation: Enters breast milk/use caution (AAP rates "compatible")

Perioperative/Anesthesia/Other Concerns:

IMPORTANT NOTE: On March 24, 2000, the FDA announced that the manufacturer of cisapride would voluntarily withdraw its product from the U.S. market on July 14, 2000. This decision was based on 341 reports of heart rhythm abnormalities including 80 reports of deaths. The company will continue to make the drug available to patients who meet specific clinical eligibility criteria for a limited-access protocol (contact 1-800-JANSSEN).

The potential for arrhythmogenic effects may also increase secondary to significant drug interactions (see Drug Interactions).

In the absence of a known disease or drug contraindication, all patients should have a 12-lead ECG and an electrolyte panel (potassium, calcium, and magnesium) completed prior to initiating cisapride therapy. Serum electrolytes and 12-lead ECG should be again evaluated within the first 48 hours of therapy and periodically thereafter. Patients on diuretic and cisapride therapies should be monitored more closely for the development of hypokalemia, hypocalcemia, and hypomagnesemia. Cisapride therapy should be stopped and the patient monitored closely in patients who develop hypokalemia, hypocalcemia, hypomagnesemia, or QT prolongation (QT_c >450 milliseconds).

Cisatracurium (sis a tra KYOO ree um)

U.S. Brand Names Nimbex®

Synonyms Cisatracurium Besylate

Pharmacologic Category Neuromuscular Blocker Agent, Nondepolarizing

Medication Safety Issues

Sound-alike/look-alike issues:

Nimbex® may be confused with Revex®

Use Adjunct to general anesthesia to facilitate endotracheal intubation and to relax skeletal muscles during surgery; to facilitate mechanical ventilation in ICU patients; does not relieve pain or produce sedation

Mechanism of Action Blocks neural transmission at the myoneural junction by binding with cholinergic receptor sites

Pharmacodynamics/Kinetics

Onset of action: I.V.: 2-3 minutes

Peak effect: 3-5 minutes

Duration: Recovery begins in 20-35 minutes when anesthesia is balanced; recovery is attained in 90% of patients in 25-93 minutes

Metabolism: Undergoes rapid nonenzymatic degradation in the bloodstream (Hofmann elimination), additional metabolism occurs via ester hydrolysis; some active metabolites

(Continued)

Cisatracurium *(Continued)*

Half-life elimination: 22-29 minutes

Contraindications Hypersensitivity to cisatracurium besylate or any component of the formulation

Warnings/Precautions Maintenance of an adequate airway and respiratory support is critical; certain clinical conditions may result in potentiation or antagonism of neuromuscular blockade:

Potentiation: Electrolyte abnormalities, severe hyponatremia, severe hypocalcemia, severe hypokalemia, hypermagnesemia, neuromuscular diseases, acidosis, acute intermittent porphyria, renal failure, hepatic failure

Antagonism: Alkalosis, hypercalcemia, demyelinating lesions, peripheral neuropathies, diabetes mellitus

Increased sensitivity in patients with myasthenia gravis, Eaton-Lambert syndrome; resistance in burn patients (>30% of body) for period of 5-70 days postinjury; resistance in patients with muscle trauma, denervation, immobilization, infection. Cross-sensitivity with other neuromuscular-blocking agents may occur; use extreme caution in patients with previous anaphylactic reactions. Bradycardia may be more common with cisatracurium than with other neuromuscular-blocking agents since it has no clinically significant effects on heart rate to counteract the bradycardia produced by anesthetics.

Drug Interactions

Prolonged neuromuscular blockade:

Inhaled anesthetics:

Halothane has only a marginal effect, enflurane and isoflurane increase the potency and prolong duration of neuromuscular blockade induced by cisatracurium

Dosage should be reduced by 30% to 40% in patients receiving isoflurane or enflurane

Local anesthetics

Lithium

Magnesium salts

Antiarrhythmics (eg, quinidine or procainamide)

Antibiotics (eg, aminoglycosides, tetracyclines, vancomycin, clindamycin)

Resistance to neuromuscular blockade: Chronic phenytoin or carbamazepine

Adverse Reactions <1%: Effects are minimal and transient, bradycardia and hypotension, flushing, pruritus, rash, bronchospasm, acute quadriplegic myopathy syndrome (prolonged use), myositis ossificans (prolonged use)

Overdosage/Toxicology

Symptoms of overdose include respiratory depression and cardiovascular collapse.

Neostigmine 1-3 mg slow I.V. push in adults (0.5 mg in children) antagonizes the neuromuscular blockade, and should be administered with or immediately after atropine 1-1.5 mg I.V. push (adults). This may be especially useful in the presence of bradycardia.

Dosing

Adults & Elderly: Neuromuscular blockade: I.V. (not to be used I.M.):

Operating room administration:

Intubating doses: 0.15-0.2 mg/kg as components of propofol/nitrous oxide/oxygen induction-intubation technique. (**Note:** May produce generally good or excellent conditions for tracheal intubation in 1.5-2 minutes with clinically effective duration of action during propofol anesthesia of 55-61 minutes.) Initial dose after succinylcholine for intubation: 0.1 mg/kg; maintenance dose: 0.03 mg/kg 40-60 minutes after initial dose, then at ~20-minute intervals based on clinical criteria.

Continuous infusion: After an initial bolus, a diluted solution can be given by continuous infusion for maintenance of neuromuscular blockade during extended surgery; adjust the rate of administration according to the patient's response as determined by peripheral nerve stimulation. An initial infusion rate of 3 mcg/kg/minute may be required to rapidly counteract the spontaneous recovery of neuromuscular function; thereafter, a rate of 1-2 mcg/kg/minute should be adequate to maintain continuous neuromuscular block in the 89% to 99% range in most pediatric and adult patients. Consider reduction of the infusion rate by 30% to 40% when administering during stable isoflurane, enflurane, sevoflurane, or desflurane anesthesia. Spontaneous recovery from neuromuscular blockade following discontinuation of infusion of cisatracurium may be expected to proceed at a rate comparable to that following single bolus administration.

Intensive care unit administration: Follow the principles for infusion in the operating room. At initial signs of recovery from bolus dose, begin the infusion at a dose of 3 mcg/kg/minute and adjust rates accordingly; dosage ranges of 0.5-10 mcg/kg/minute have been reported. If patient is allowed to recover from neuromuscular blockade, readministration of a bolus dose may be necessary to quickly re-establish neuromuscular block prior to reinstituting the infusion. See table.

Cisatracurium Besylate Infusion Chart

Drug Delivery Rate (mcg/kg/min)	Infusion Rate (mL/kg/min) 0.1 mg/mL (10 mg/100 mL)	Infusion Rate (mL/kg/min) 0.4 mg/mL (40 mg/100 mL)
1	0.01	0.0025
1.5	0.015	0.00375
2	0.02	0.005
3	0.03	0.0075
5	0.05	0.0125

Pediatrics: Neuromuscular blockade:

Operating room administration:

Children 2-12 years: I.V. (Not to be used I.M.)

Intubating doses: 0.1 mg over 5-15 seconds during either halothane or opioid anesthesia. (**Note:** When given during stable opioid nitrous oxide/oxygen anesthesia, 0.1 mg/kg produces maximum neuromuscular block in an average of 2.8 minutes and clinically effective block for 28 minutes.)

Continuous infusion: Refer to adult dosing.

Intensive care unit administration: Refer to adult dosing.

Renal Impairment: Because slower times to onset of complete neuromuscular block were observed in renal dysfunction patients, extending the interval between the administration of cisatracurium and intubation attempt may be required to achieve adequate intubation conditions.

Available Dosage Forms

Injection, solution: 2 mg/mL (5 mL); 10 mg/mL (20 mL)

Injection, solution: 2 mg/mL (10 mL) [contains benzyl alcohol]

Nursing Guidelines

Assessment: Only clinicians experienced in the use of neuromuscular blocking drugs should administer and/or manage the use of cisatracurium. Dosage and rate of administration should be individualized and titrated to the desired effect, according to relevant clinical factors, premedication, concomitant medications, age, and general condition of the patient. Ventilatory support must be instituted and maintained until adequate respiratory muscle function and/or airway protection are assured. Assess other medications for effectiveness and safety. Other drugs that affect neuromuscular activity may increase/decrease neuromuscular block induced by cisatracurium. This drug does not cause anesthesia or analgesia; pain must be treated with appropriate analgesic agents. Continuous monitoring of vital signs, cardiac status, respiratory status, and degree of neuromuscular block (objective assessment with peripheral external nerve stimulator) is mandatory during infusion and until full muscle tone has returned. Muscle tone returns in a predictable pattern, starting with diaphragm, abdomen, chest, limbs, and finally muscles of the neck, face, and eyes. Safety precautions must be maintained until full muscle tone has returned. **Note:** It may take longer for return of muscle tone in obese or elderly patients or patients with renal or hepatic disease, myasthenia gravis, myopathy, other neuromuscular disease, dehydration, electrolyte imbalance, or severe acid/base imbalance. Provide appropriate patient teaching/support prior to and following administration.

Long-term use: Monitor fluid levels (intake and output) during and following infusion. Reposition patient and provide appropriate skin care, mouth care, and care of patient's eyes every 2-3 hours while sedated. Provide appropriate emotional and sensory support (auditory and environmental).

Note breast-feeding caution.

Patient Education: Patient will usually be unconscious prior to administration. Patient education should be appropriate to individual situation. Reassurance of constant monitoring and emotional support to reduce fear and anxiety should precede and follow administration. Following return of muscle tone, do not

(Continued)

Cisatracurium *(Continued)*

attempt to change position or rise from bed without assistance. Report immediately any skin rash or hives, pounding heartbeat, respiratory difficulty, or muscle tremors. **Breast-feeding precaution:** Consult prescriber if breast-feeding.

Pregnancy Risk Factor: B

Lactation: Excretion in breast milk unknown/use caution

Perioperative/Anesthesia/Other Concerns: Cisatracurium is classified as an intermediate duration neuromuscular-blocking agent; does not appear to have a cumulative effect on the duration of blockade; neuromuscular-blocking potency is 3 times that of atracurium.

Critically-Ill Adult Patients: The 2002 ACCM/SCCM/ASHP clinical practice guidelines for sustained neuromuscular blockade in the adult critically-ill patient recommend:

Optimize sedatives and analgesics prior to initiation and monitor and adjust accordingly during course. Neuromuscular blockers do not relieve pain or produce sedation.

Protect patient's eyes from development of keratitis and corneal abrasion by administering ophthalmic ointment and taping eyelids closed or using eye patches. Reposition patient routinely to protect pressure points from breakdown. Address DVT prophylaxis.

Concurrent use of a neuromuscular blocker and corticosteroids appear to increase the risk of certain ICU myopathies; avoid or administer the corticosteroid at the lowest dose possible. Reassess need for neuromuscular blocker daily.

Using daily drug holidays (stopping neuromuscular-blocking agent until patient requires it again) may decrease the incidence of acute quadriplegic myopathy syndrome.

Tachyphylaxis can develop; switch to another neuromuscular blocker (taking into consideration the patient's organ function) if paralysis is still necessary.

Acidosis and severe hypothermia may delay the elimination of atracurium and cisatracurium.

Atracurium or cisatracurium is recommended for patients with significant hepatic or renal disease, due to organ-independent Hofmann elimination.

Monitor patients clinically and via "Train of Four" (TOF) testing with a goal of adjusting the degree of blockade to 1-2 twitches or based upon the patient's clinical condition.

Administration

I.M.: Not for I.M. injection, too much tissue irritation.

I.V.: Administer I.V. only. The use of a peripheral nerve stimulator will permit the most advantageous use of cisatracurium, minimize the possibility of overdosage or underdosage and assist in the evaluation of recovery.

Give undiluted as a bolus injection. Continuous administration requires the use of an infusion pump.

Compatibility: Stable in D_5W, NS, D_5NS

Y-site administration: Incompatible with amphotericin B cholesteryl sulfate complex, cefoperazone

Compatibility when admixed: Incompatible with ketorolac, propofol

Storage: Refrigerate intact vials at 2°C to 8°C/36°F to 46°F. Use vials within 21 days upon removal from the refrigerator to room temperature (25°C to 77°F). Dilutions of 0.1-0.2 mg/mL in 0.9% sodium chloride or dextrose 5% in water are stable for up to 24 hours at room temperature.

◆ **Cisatracurium Besylate** *see* Cisatracurium *on page 409*

Cisplatin (SIS pla tin)

U.S. Brand Names Platinol®-AQ [DSC]

Synonyms CDDP

Pharmacologic Category Antineoplastic Agent, Alkylating Agent

Medication Safety Issues

Sound-alike/look-alike issues:

Cisplatin may be confused with carboplatin

Platinol®-AQ may be confused with Paraplatin®, Patanol®, Plaquenil®

Doses >100 mg/m² once every 3-4 weeks are rarely used and should be verified with the prescriber.

Use Treatment of bladder, testicular, and ovarian cancer

Unlabeled/Investigational Use Treatment of head and neck, breast, gastric, lung, esophageal, cervical, prostate and small cell lung cancer; Hodgkin's and non-Hodgkin's lymphoma; neuroblastoma; sarcomas, myeloma, melanoma, mesothelioma, and osteosarcoma

Mechanism of Action Inhibits DNA synthesis by the formation of DNA cross-links; denatures the double helix; covalently binds to DNA bases and disrupts DNA function; may also bind to proteins; the *cis*-isomer is 14 times more cytotoxic than the *trans*-isomer; both forms cross-link DNA but cis-platinum is less easily recognized by cell enzymes and, therefore, not repaired. Cisplatin can also bind two adjacent guanines on the same strand of DNA producing intrastrand cross-linking and breakage.

Pharmacodynamics/Kinetics

Distribution: I.V.: Rapidly into tissue; high concentrations in kidneys, liver, ovaries, uterus, and lungs

Protein binding: >90%

Metabolism: Nonenzymatic; inactivated (in both cell and bloodstream) by sulfhydryl groups; covalently binds to glutathione and thiosulfate

Half-life elimination: Initial: 20-30 minutes; Beta: 60 minutes; Terminal: ~24 hours; Secondary half-life: 44-73 hours

Excretion: Urine (>90%); feces (10%)

Contraindications Hypersensitivity to cisplatin, other platinum-containing compounds, or any component of the formulation (anaphylactic-like reactions have been reported); pre-existing renal insufficiency; myelosuppression; hearing impairment; pregnancy

Warnings/Precautions Hazardous agent - use appropriate precautions for handling and disposal. Doses >100 mg/m^2 once every 3-4 weeks are rarely used and should be verified with the prescriber. All patients should receive adequate hydration, with or without diuretics, prior to and for 24 hours after cisplatin administration. Reduce dosage in renal impairment. Cumulative renal toxicity may be severe. Elderly patients may be more susceptible to nephrotoxicity; select dose cautiously and monitor closely. Dose-related toxicities include myelosuppression, nausea, and vomiting. Ototoxicity, especially pronounced in children, is manifested by tinnitus or loss of high frequency hearing and occasionally, deafness. **Serum magnesium, as well as other electrolytes, should be monitored both before and within 48 hours after cisplatin therapy.** When administered as sequential infusions, taxane derivatives (docetaxel, paclitaxel) should be administered before platinum derivatives (carboplatin, cisplatin).

Drug Interactions

Amifostine: Theoretically inactivates drug systemically; has been used clinically to reduce nephrotoxicity and neutropenia associated with administration of cisplatin.

Bleomycin: Delayed bleomycin elimination with decreased glomerular filtration rate.

Ethacrynic acid: Has resulted in severe ototoxicity in animals.

Sodium thiosulfate: Theoretically inactivates drug systemically; has been used clinically to reduce systemic toxicity with intraperitoneal administration of cisplatin.

Taxane derivatives (docetaxel, paclitaxel): When administered as sequential infusions, taxane derivatives should be administered before platinum derivatives to limit myelosuppression and to enhance efficacy.

Nutritional/Herbal/Ethanol Interactions Herb/Nutraceutical: Avoid black cohosh, dong quai in estrogen-dependent tumors.

Adverse Reactions

>10%:

- Central nervous system: Neurotoxicity: Peripheral neuropathy is dose- and duration-dependent.
- Dermatologic: Mild alopecia
- Gastrointestinal: Nausea and vomiting (76% to 100%)
- Hematologic: Myelosuppression (25% to 30%; mild with moderate doses, mild to moderate with high-dose therapy)
  - WBC: Mild
  - Platelets: Mild
  - Onset: 10 days
  - Nadir: 14-23 days
  - Recovery: 21-39 days
- Hepatic: Liver enzymes increased
- Renal: Nephrotoxicity (acute renal failure and chronic renal insufficiency)

(Continued)

Cisplatin *(Continued)*

Otic: Ototoxicity (10% to 30%; manifested as high frequency hearing loss; ototoxicity is especially pronounced in children)

1% to 10%:

Gastrointestinal: Diarrhea

Local: Tissue irritation

<1% (Limited to important or life-threatening): Anaphylactic reaction, arrhythmias, blurred vision, bradycardia, cerebral blindness, hemolytic anemia, liver enzymes increased, mild alopecia, mouth sores, optic neuritis, papilledema

BMT:

Central nervous system: Peripheral and autonomic neuropathy, ototoxicity

Endocrine & metabolic: Hypokalemia, hypomagnesemia

Gastrointestinal: Highly emetogenic

Hematologic: Myelosuppression

Renal: Acute renal failure, increased serum creatinine, azotemia

Miscellaneous: Transient pain at tumor, transient autoimmune disorders

Overdosage/Toxicology Symptoms of overdose include severe myelosuppression, intractable nausea and vomiting, kidney and liver failure, deafness, ocular toxicity, and neuritis. Overdose may be fatal. There is no known antidote. Hemodialysis appears to have little effect. Treatment is symptom-directed and supportive.

Dosing

Adults & Elderly:

Advanced bladder cancer: 50-70 mg/m^2 every 3-4 weeks

Head and neck cancer (unlabeled use): 100-120 mg/m^2 every 3-4 weeks

Malignant pleural mesothelioma in combination with pemetrexed (unlabeled use): 75 mg/m^2 on day 1 of each 21-day cycle; see Pemetrexed monograph for additional details

Metastatic ovarian cancer: 75-100 mg/m^2 every 3-4 weeks

Intraperitoneal: Cisplatin has been administered intraperitoneal with systemic sodium thiosulfate for ovarian cancer; doses up to 90-270 mg/m^2 have been administered and retained for 4 hours before draining

Testicular cancer: 10-20 mg/m^2/day for 5 days repeated every 3-4 weeks

High dose BMT: Continuous I.V.: 55 mg/m^2/24 hours for 72 hours; total dose: 165 mg/m^2

Pediatrics: Refer to individual protocols. **VERIFY ANY CISPLATIN DOSE EXCEEDING 100 mg/m^2 PER COURSE.**

Unlabeled pediatric uses:

Intermittent dosing schedule: 37-75 mg/m^2 once every 2-3 weeks or 50-100 mg/m^2 over 4-6 hours, once every 21-28 days

Daily dosing schedule: 15-20 mg/m^2/day for 5 days every 3-4 weeks

Osteogenic sarcoma or neuroblastoma: 60-100 mg/m^2 on day 1 every 3-4 weeks

Recurrent brain tumors: 60 mg/m^2 once daily for 2 consecutive days every 3-4 weeks

Bone marrow/blood cell transfusion: Continuous Infusion: High dose: 55 mg/m^2/day for 72 hours; total dose = 165 mg/m^2

Renal Impairment: Note: The manufacturer(s) recommend that repeat courses of cisplatin should not be given until serum creatinine is <1.5 mg/100 mL and/or BUN is <25 mg/100 mL. There is no FDA-approved renal dosing adjustment guideline; the following guidelines have been used by some clinicians:

Kintzel, 1995:

Cl_{cr} 46-60 mL/minute: Reduce dose by 25%

Cl_{cr} 31-45 mL/minute: Reduce dose by 50%

Cl_{cr} <30 mL/minute: Consider use of alternative drug

Aronoff, 1999:

Cl_{cr} 10-50 mL/minute: Administer 75% of dose

Cl_{cr} <10 mL/minute: Administer 50% of dose

Hemodialysis: Partially cleared by hemodialysis.

Administer dose posthemodialysis.

CAPD effects: Unknown

CAVH effects: Unknown

Available Dosage Forms [DSC] = Discontinued product

Injection, solution: 1 mg/mL (50 mL, 100 mL, 200 mL)

Platinol®-AQ: 1 mg/mL (50 mL, 100 mL) [contains sodium 9 mg/mL] [DSC]

Nursing Guidelines

Assessment: See Contraindications, Warnings/Precautions, and Dosing for extensive use cautions. Assess potential for interactions with other prescriptions, OTC medications, or herbal products patient may be taking (especially anything that is ototoxic or nephrotoxic - see Drug Interactions). Patient should be well hydrated prior to and for 24 hours following infusion. Administer antiemetic prior to each treatment and as needed between infusions. See detailed infusion specifics; infusion site must be monitored closely to reduce potential for extravasation (see Administration). Assess results of laboratory tests (see below), auditory evaluation, therapeutic effectiveness, and adverse response (see Adverse Reactions and Overdose/Toxicology) prior to each treatment and regularly during therapy. Teach patient (or caregiver) possible side effects/appropriate interventions (eg, importance of adequate hydration) and adverse symptoms to report (see Patient Education). **Pregnancy risk factor D** - determine that patient is not pregnant before beginning treatment. Instruct patients of childbearing age about appropriate contraceptive measures. See Lactation for breast-feeding considerations.

Monitoring Laboratory Tests: Renal function (serum creatinine, BUN, Cl_{cr}); electrolytes (particularly magnesium, calcium, potassium) before and within 48 hours after cisplatin therapy; liver function periodically, CBC with differential and platelet count, urinalysis

Dietary Considerations: Sodium content: 9 mg/mL (equivalent to 0.9% sodium chloride solution)

Patient Education: Inform prescriber of all prescriptions, OTC medications, or herbal products you are taking, and any allergies you have. Do not take any new medication during therapy unless approved by prescriber. This medication can only be administered by I.V. and numerous side-effects can occur. Report immediately any burning, pain, itching, or redness at infusion site. It is important that you maintain adequate hydration (2-3 L/day of fluids) unless instructed to restrict fluid intake, and adequate nutrition (small, frequent meals may help) and. May cause severe nausea or vomiting that can be delayed for up to 48 hours after infusion and last for 1 week (consult prescriber for appropriate antiemetic medication); mouth sores (use soft toothbrush or cotton swabs for mouth care); or loss of hair (reversible). You will be susceptible to infection (avoid crowds and exposure to infection and do not have any vaccinations without consulting prescriber). Report promptly any loss of hearing; rash or hives; respiratory difficulty or swallowing; fever or chills; chest pain or palpitations; unusual fatigue; unusual bruising/bleeding; numbness, pain or tingling in extremities; muscle cramps or twitching; pain, redness; swelling at infusion site; or any other unusual symptoms. **Pregnancy/breast-feeding precautions:** Inform prescriber if you are pregnant. Do not get pregnant during therapy. Consult prescriber for instruction on appropriate contraceptive measures. This drug may cause severe fetal defects. Consult prescriber if breast-feeding.

Pregnancy Risk Factor: D

Pregnancy Issues: Animal studies have demonstrated teratogenicity and embryotoxicity. There are no adequate and well-controlled studies in pregnant women. Women of childbearing potential should be advised to avoid pregnancy. If used in pregnancy, or if patient becomes pregnant during treatment, the patient should be apprised of potential hazard to the fetus.

Lactation: Enters breast milk/contraindicated

Perioperative/Anesthesia/Other Concerns:

Nephrotoxicity: Related to elimination, protein binding, and uptake of cisplatin. Two types of nephrotoxicity: Acute renal failure and chronic renal insufficiency.

Acute renal failure and azotemia is a dose-dependent process and can be minimized with proper administration and prophylaxis. Damage to the proximal tubules by unbound cisplatin is suspected to cause the toxicity. It is manifested as increased BUN/creatinine, oliguria, protein wasting, and potassium, calcium, and magnesium wasting.

Chronic renal dysfunction can develop in patients receiving multiple courses of cisplatin. Slow release of tissue-bound cisplatin may contribute to chronic nephrotoxicity. Manifestations of this toxicity are varied, and can include sodium and water wasting, nephropathy, hyperuricemia, decreased Cl_{cr}, and magnesium wasting.

Recommendations for minimizing nephrotoxicity include:

Prepare cisplatin in saline-containing vehicles.

Infuse dose over 24 hours.

(Continued)

Cisplatin *(Continued)*

Vigorously hydrate patient (125-150 mL/hour) before, during, and after cisplatin administration.
Simultaneously administer either mannitol or furosemide.
Pretreat with amifostine.
Avoid other nephrotoxic agents (aminoglycosides, amphotericin, etc).

Neurotoxicity: Peripheral neuropathy is dose- and duration-dependent. The mechanism is through axonal degeneration with subsequent damage to the long sensory nerves. Toxicity can first be noted at cumulative doses of 200 mg/m^2, with measurable toxicity at cumulative doses >350 mg/m^2. This process is irreversible and progressive with continued therapy.

Anaphylactic Reaction: Occurs within minutes after intravenous or intraperitoneal administration; can be controlled with epinephrine, antihistamines, and steroids.

Administration

I.V.: Irritant. Perform pretreatment hydration (see Dosage).

I.V.: Rate of administration has varied from a 15- to 120-minute infusion, 1 mg/minute infusion, 6- to 8-hour infusion, 24-hour infusion, or per protocol. Maximum rate of infusion: 1 mg/minute in patients with CHF.

When administered as sequential infusions, taxane derivatives (docetaxel, paclitaxel) should be administered before platinum derivatives to limit myelosuppression and to enhance efficacy.

Reconstitution: Further dilutions in NS, D_5/0.45% NaCl or D_5/NS to a concentration of 0.05-2 mg/mL are stable for 72 hours at 4°C to 25°C. The infusion solution should have a final sodium chloride concentration of ≥0.2%.

Compatibility: Stable in D_5¼NS, D_5½NS, D_5NS, ¼NS, ⅓NS, ½NS, NS; **incompatible** with sodium bicarbonate 5%

Y-site administration: Incompatible with amifostine, amphotericin B cholesteryl sulfate complex, cefepime, piperacillin/tazobactam, thiotepa

Compatibility when admixed: Incompatible with fluorouracil, mesna, thiotepa

Storage: Store intact vials at room temperature 15°C to 25°C (59°F to 77°F) and protect from light. Do not refrigerate solution as a precipitate may form. Further dilution **stability is dependent on the chloride ion concentration** and should be mixed in solutions of NS (at least 0.3% NaCl). After initial entry into the vial, solution is stable for 28 days protected from light or for at least 7 days under fluorescent room light at room temperature.

♦ **13-*cis*-Retinoic Acid** *see* Isotretinoin *on page 981*

Citalopram (sye TAL oh pram)

U.S. Brand Names Celexa®

Synonyms Citalopram Hydrobromide; Nitalapram

Pharmacologic Category Antidepressant, Selective Serotonin Reuptake Inhibitor

Medication Safety Issues

Sound-alike/look-alike issues:

Celexa™ may be confused with Celebrex®, Cerebra®, Cerebyx®, Zyprexa®

Use Treatment of depression

Unlabeled/Investigational Use Treatment of dementia, smoking cessation, ethanol abuse, obsessive-compulsive disorder (OCD) in children, diabetic neuropathy

Mechanism of Action A bicyclic phthalane derivative, citalopram selectively inhibits serotonin reuptake in the presynaptic neurons

Pharmacodynamics/Kinetics

Distribution: V_d: 12 L/kg
Protein binding, plasma: ~80%
Metabolism: Extensively hepatic, including CYP, to N-demethylated, N-oxide, and deaminated metabolites
Bioavailability: 80%
Half-life elimination: 24-48 hours; average 35 hours (doubled with hepatic impairment)
Time to peak, serum: 1-6 hours, average within 4 hours
Excretion: Urine (10% as unchanged drug)

Note: Clearance was decreased, while AUC and half-life were significantly increased in elderly patients and in patients with hepatic impairment. Mild to moderate renal impairment may reduce clearance (17%) and prolong half-life of citalopram. No pharmacokinetic information is available concerning patients with severe renal impairment.

Contraindications Hypersensitivity to citalopram or any component of the formulation; hypersensitivity or other adverse sequelae during therapy with other SSRIs; concomitant use with MAO inhibitors or within 2 weeks of discontinuing MAO inhibitors.

Warnings/Precautions

Major psychiatric warnings:

- Antidepressants increase the risk of suicidal thinking and behavior in children and adolescents with major depressive disorder (MDD) and other depressive disorders; consider risk prior to prescribing.
- Closely monitor for clinical worsening, suicidality, or unusual changes in behavior; the child's family or caregiver should be instructed to closely observe the patient and communicate condition with healthcare provider. **Citalopram is not FDA approved for use in children.**
- Adults treated with antidepressants should be observed similarly for clinical worsening and suicidality, especially during the initial few months of a course of drug therapy, or at times of dose changes, either increases or decreases. A medication guide should be dispensed with each prescription.
- The possibility of a suicide attempt is inherent in major depression and may persist until remission occurs. Worsening depression and severe abrupt suicidality that are not part of the presenting symptoms may require discontinuation or modification of drug therapy. Use caution in high-risk patients during initiation of therapy.
- Prescriptions should be written for the smallest quantity consistent with good patient care. The patient's family or caregiver should be alerted to monitor patients for the emergence of suicidality and associated behaviors such as anxiety, agitation, panic attacks, insomnia, irritability, hostility, impulsivity, akathisia, hypomania, and mania; patients should be instructed to notify their healthcare provider if any of these symptoms or worsening depression or psychosis occur.
- May worsen psychosis in some patients or precipitate a shift to mania or hypomania in patients with bipolar disorder. Monotherapy in patients with bipolar disorder should be avoided. Patients presenting with depressive symptoms should be screened for bipolar disorder. **Citalopram is not FDA approved for the treatment of bipolar depression.**

Key adverse effects:

- Anticholinergic effects: Relatively devoid of these side effects.
- CNS depression: Has a low potential to impair cognitive or motor performance; caution operating hazardous machinery or driving.
- SIADH and hyponatremia: Has been associated with the development of SIADH; hyponatremia has been reported rarely, predominately in the elderly

Concurrent disease:

- Hepatic impairment: Use caution; clearance is decreased and plasma concentrations are increased; a lower dosage may be needed.
- Platelet aggregation: May impair platelet aggregation, resulting in bleeding.
- Renal impairment: Use caution; clearance is decreased and plasma concentrations are increased; a lower dosage may be needed.
- Sexual dysfunction: May cause or exacerbate sexual dysfunction.

Concurrent drug therapy:

- Anticoagulants/Antiplatelets: Use caution with concomitant use of NSAIDs, ASA, or other drugs that affect coagulation; the risk of bleeding is potentiated.
- CNS depressants: Use caution with concomitant therapy.
- MAO inhibitors: Potential for severe reaction when used with MAO inhibitors; autonomic instability, coma, death, delirium, diaphoresis, hyperthermia, mental status changes/agitation, muscular rigidity, myoclonus, neuroleptic malignant syndrome features, and seizures may occur.

Special populations:

- Elderly: Use caution in elderly patients.
- Pregnancy: Use caution in pregnant patients; high doses of citalopram have been associated with teratogenicity in animals.

Special notes:

- Electroconvulsive therapy: May increase the risks associated with electroconvulsive therapy; consider discontinuing, when possible, prior to ECT treatment.
- Withdrawal syndrome: May cause dysphoric mood, irritability, agitation, dizziness, sensory disturbances, anxiety, confusion, headache, lethargy,

(Continued)

Citalopram *(Continued)*

emotional lability, insomnia, hypomania, tinnitus, and seizures. Upon discontinuation of citalopram therapy, gradually taper dose. If intolerable symptoms occur following a decrease in dosage or upon discontinuation of therapy, then resuming the previous dose with a more gradual taper should be considered.

Drug Interactions **Substrate** of CYP2C19 (major), 2D6 (minor), 3A4 (major); **Inhibits** CYP1A2 (weak), 2B6 (weak), 2C19 (weak), 2D6 (weak)

Aspirin: Concomitant use of citalopram and NSAIDs, aspirin, or other drugs affecting coagulation has been associated with an increased risk of bleeding; monitor.

Beta-blockers: Citalopram may increase levels of some beta-blockers (see Carvedilol and Metoprolol); monitor carefully

Buspirone: Concurrent use of citalopram with buspirone may cause serotonin syndrome; avoid concurrent use

Carbamazepine: May enhance the metabolism of citalopram

Carvedilol: Serum concentrations may be increased; monitor carefully for increased carvedilol effect (hypotension and bradycardia)

Cimetidine: May inhibit the metabolism of citalopram

CYP2C19 inducers: May decrease the levels/effects of citalopram. Example inducers include aminoglutethimide, carbamazepine, phenytoin, and rifampin.

CYP2C19 inhibitors: May increase the levels/effects of citalopram. Example inhibitors include delavirdine, fluconazole, fluvoxamine, gemfibrozil, isoniazid, omeprazole, and ticlopidine.

CYP3A4 inducers: CYP3A4 inducers may decrease the levels/effects of citalopram. Example inducers include aminoglutethimide, carbamazepine, nafcillin, nevirapine, phenobarbital, phenytoin, and rifamycins.

CYP3A4 inhibitors: May increase the levels/effects of citalopram. Example inhibitors include azole antifungals, clarithromycin, diclofenac, doxycycline, erythromycin, imatinib, isoniazid, nefazodone, nicardipine, propofol, protease inhibitors, quinidine, telithromycin, and verapamil.

Linezolid: Hyperpyrexia, hypertension, tachycardia, confusion, seizures, and **deaths have been reported** with agents which inhibit MAO (serotonin syndrome); this combination should be avoided

MAO inhibitors: Hyperpyrexia, hypertension, tachycardia, confusion, seizures, and **deaths have been reported** with MAO inhibitors (serotonin syndrome); this combination should be avoided

Meperidine: Combined use theoretically may increase the risk of serotonin syndrome

Metoprolol: Citalopram may increase plasma levels of metoprolol; monitor for increased effect

Moclobemide: Concurrent use of citalopram with moclobemide may cause serotonin syndrome; avoid concurrent use

Nefazodone: Concurrent use of citalopram with nefazodone may cause serotonin syndrome

NSAIDs: Concomitant use of citalopram and NSAIDs, aspirin, or other drugs affecting coagulation has been associated with an increased risk of bleeding; monitor.

Ritonavir: Combined use of citalopram with ritonavir may cause serotonin syndrome in HIV-positive patients; monitor

Selegiline: Concurrent use with citalopram has been reported to cause serotonin syndrome; as an MAO type B inhibitor, the risk of serotonin syndrome may be less than with nonselective MAO inhibitors, and reports indicate that this combination has been well tolerated in Parkinson's patients

Serotonin reuptake inhibitors: Concurrent use with other reuptake inhibitors may increase the risk of serotonin syndrome

Sibutramine: May increase the risk of serotonin syndrome with SSRIs

Sumatriptan (and other serotonin agonists): Concurrent use may result in toxicity; weakness, hyper-reflexia, and incoordination have been observed with sumatriptan and SSRIs. In addition, concurrent use may theoretically increase the risk of serotonin syndrome; includes sumatriptan, naratriptan, rizatriptan, and zolmitriptan.

Tramadol: Concurrent use of citalopram with tramadol may cause serotonin syndrome; avoid concurrent use

Trazodone: Concurrent use of citalopram with trazodone may cause serotonin syndrome

Venlafaxine: Combined use with citalopram may increase the risk of serotonin syndrome

Nutritional/Herbal/Ethanol Interactions

Ethanol: Avoid ethanol (may increase CNS depression).

Herb/Nutraceutical: Avoid valerian, St John's wort, SAMe, kava kava, and gotu kola (may increase CNS depression).

Adverse Reactions

>10%:

Central nervous system: Somnolence, insomnia
Gastrointestinal: Nausea, xerostomia
Miscellaneous: Diaphoresis

<10%:

Central nervous system: Anxiety, anorexia, agitation, yawning
Dermatologic: Rash, pruritus
Endocrine & metabolic: Sexual dysfunction
Gastrointestinal: Diarrhea, dyspepsia, vomiting, abdominal pain, weight gain
Neuromuscular & skeletal: Tremor, arthralgia, myalgia
Respiratory: Cough, rhinitis, sinusitis

<1%, Postmarketing, and/or case reports (limited to important or life-threatening): Acute renal failure, anaphylaxis, angioedema, delirium, dyskinesia, epidermal necrolysis, erythema multiforme, hemolytic anemia, hepatic necrosis, neuroleptic malignant syndrome (NMS), pancreatitis, priapism, QT prolonged, rhabdomyolysis, serotonin syndrome, SIADH, ventricular arrhythmia, torsade de pointes, withdrawal syndrome

Overdosage/Toxicology Symptoms of overdose include dizziness, nausea, vomiting, sweating, tremor, somnolence, and sinus tachycardia. Rare symptoms have included amnesia, confusion, coma, seizures, hyperventilation, and ECG changes (including QT_c prolongation, ventricular arrhythmia, and torsade de pointes). Management is supportive and symptomatic.

Dosing

Adults: Depression: Oral: Initial: 20 mg/day, generally with an increase to 40 mg/day; doses of more than 40 mg are not usually necessary. Should a dose increase be necessary, it should occur in 20 mg increments at intervals of no less than 1 week. Maximum dose: 60 mg/day.

Elderly: Oral: Initial dose: 10-20 mg once daily. Increase dose to 40 mg/day only in nonresponders.

Pediatrics: Children and Adolescents: OCD (unlabeled use): Oral: 10-40 mg/day

Renal Impairment: None necessary in mild-moderate renal impairment; best avoided in severely impaired renal function (Cl_{cr} <20 mL/minute).

Hepatic Impairment: Reduce dosage in those with hepatic impairment.

Available Dosage Forms

Solution, oral: 10 mg/5 mL (240 mL) [alcohol free, sugar free; peppermint flavor]

Tablet: 10 mg, 20 mg, 40 mg

Nursing Guidelines

Assessment: Assess other medications patient may be taking for possible interaction (especially MAO inhibitors, P450 inhibitors, and other CNS active agents). Monitor for effectiveness of therapy and adverse reactions. Assess mental status for depression, suicidal ideation, anxiety, social functioning, mania, or panic attack. Assess knowledge/teach patient appropriate use, interventions to reduce side effects (eg, hypotensive precautions), and adverse symptoms to report.

Monitoring Laboratory Tests: Liver function tests and CBC with continued therapy

Dietary Considerations: May be taken without regard to food.

Patient Education: It may take up to 3 weeks to see therapeutic effects from this medication. Take as directed; do not alter dose or frequency without consulting prescriber. May be taken with or without food. Avoid alcohol, caffeine, and CNS stimulants. Avoid use of aspirin or other NSAIDs unless approved by prescriber (may increase risk of bleeding). You may experience sexual dysfunction (reversible). May cause dizziness, anxiety, or blurred vision (rise slowly from sitting or lying position and use caution when driving or engaging in tasks requiring alertness until response to drug is known); or nausea or dry mouth (small frequent meals, frequent mouth care, chewing gum, or sucking lozenges may help). Report confusion or impaired concentration, thoughts of suicide, severe headache, palpitations, rash, insomnia or nightmares, changes in personality, muscle weakness or tremors, altered gait pattern, signs and symptoms of respiratory infection, or excessive perspiration.

(Continued)

Citalopram *(Continued)*

Pregnancy/breast-feeding precautions: Inform prescriber if you are or intend to become pregnant. Do not breast-feed.

Geriatric Considerations: Clearance was decreased, while AUC and half-life were significantly increased in elderly patients and in patients with hepatic impairment. Mild to moderate renal impairment may reduce clearance of citalopram (17% reduction noted in trials). No pharmacokinetic information is available concerning patients with severe renal impairment.

Pregnancy Risk Factor: C

Pregnancy Issues: Teratogenic effects have been observed in animal studies. Nonteratogenic effects including respiratory distress, cyanosis, apnea, seizures, temperature instability, feeding difficulty, vomiting, hypoglycemia, hypo- or hypertonia, hyper-reflexia, jitteriness, irritability, constant crying, and tremor have been reported in the neonate immediately following delivery after exposure late in the third trimester. Adverse effects may be due to toxic effects of SSRI or drug discontinuation. In some cases, may present clinically as serotonin syndrome. There are no adequate and well-controlled studies in pregnant women. Use during pregnancy only if the potential benefit to the mother outweighs the possible risk to the fetus. If treatment during pregnancy is required, consider tapering therapy during the third trimester.

Lactation: Enters breast milk/contraindicated

Breast-Feeding Considerations: Citalopram is excreted in human milk. Excessive somnolence, decreased feeding, and weight loss have been reported in breast-fed infants. A decision should be made whether to continue or discontinue nursing or discontinue the drug.

Administration

Storage: Store below 25°C.

- **Citalopram Hydrobromide** *see* Citalopram *on page 416*
- **Citracal® Prenatal Rx** *see* Vitamins (Multiple/Prenatal) *on page 1721*
- **Citrate of Magnesia** *see* Magnesium Citrate *on page 1075*
- **Citrovorum Factor** *see* Leucovorin *on page 1013*
- **CI-719** *see* Gemfibrozil *on page 804*

Cladribine (KLA dri been)

U.S. Brand Names Leustatin®

Synonyms 2-CdA; 2-Chlorodeoxyadenosine

Pharmacologic Category Adjuvant, Radiosensitizing Agent; Antineoplastic Agent, Antimetabolite; Antineoplastic Agent, Antimetabolite (Purine Antagonist)

Medication Safety Issues

Sound-alike/look-alike issues:

Leustatin® may be confused with lovastatin

Use Treatment of hairy cell leukemia, chronic lymphocytic leukemia (CLL), chronic myelogenous leukemia (CML)

Unlabeled/Investigational Use Non-Hodgkin's lymphomas, progressive multiple sclerosis

Mechanism of Action A purine nucleoside analogue; prodrug which is activated via phosphorylation by deoxycytidine kinase to a 5'-triphosphate derivative. This active form incorporates into DNA to result in the breakage of DNA strand and shutdown of DNA synthesis. This also results in a depletion of nicotinamide adenine dinucleotide and adenosine triphosphate (ATP). Cladribine is cell-cycle nonspecific.

Pharmacodynamics/Kinetics

Absorption: Oral: 55%; SubQ: 100%; Rectal: 20%

Distribution: V_d: 4.52 ± 2.82 L/kg

Protein binding, plasma: 20%

Metabolism: Hepatic; 5′-triphosphate moiety-active

Half-life elimination: Biphasic: Alpha: 25 minutes; Beta: 6.7 hours; Terminal, mean: Normal renal function: 5.4 hours

Excretion: Urine (21% to 44%)

Clearance: Estimated systemic: 640 mL/hour/kg

Contraindications Hypersensitivity to cladribine or any component of the formulation; pregnancy

Warnings/Precautions The U.S. Food and Drug Administration (FDA) currently recommends that procedures for proper handling and disposal of antineoplastic agents be considered. Use with caution in patients with pre-existing hematologic or immunologic abnormalities.

Nutritional/Herbal/Ethanol Interactions Ethanol: Avoid ethanol (due to GI irritation).

Adverse Reactions

>10%:

Allergic: Fever (70%), chills (18%); skin reactions (erythema, itching) at the catheter site (18%)

Central nervous system: Fatigue (17%), headache (13%)

Dermatologic: Rash

Hematologic: Myelosuppression, common, dose-limiting; leukopenia (70%); anemia (37%); thrombocytopenia (12%)

Nadir: 5-10 days

Recovery: 4-8 weeks

1% to 10%:

Cardiovascular: Edema, tachycardia

Central nervous system: Dizziness; pains; chills; malaise; severe infection, possibly related to thrombocytopenia

Dermatologic: Pruritus, erythema

Gastrointestinal: Nausea, mild to moderate, usually not seen at doses <0.3 mg/kg/day; constipation; abdominal pain

Neuromuscular & skeletal: Myalgia, arthralgia, weakness

Renal: Renal failure at high (>0.3 mg/kg/day) doses

Miscellaneous: Diaphoresis, delayed herpes zoster infection, tumor lysis syndrome

<1% (Limited to important or life-threatening): Paraparesis, quadriplegia (reported at high doses); increased risk of opportunistic infection

Dosing

Adults & Elderly: Refer to individual protocols.

Hairy cell leukemia: I.V. Continuous infusion:

0.09-0.1 mg/kg/day days 1-7; may be repeated every 28-35 days **or**

3.4 mg/m^2/day SubQ days 1-7

Chronic lymphocytic leukemia: I.V. Continuous infusion:

0.1 mg/kg/day days 1-7 **or**

0.028-0.14 mg/kg/day as a 2-hour infusion days 1-5

Chronic myelogenous leukemia: I.V. 15 mg/m^2/day as a 1-hour infusion days 1-5; if no response increase dose to 20 mg/m^2/day in the second course.

Pediatrics: Refer to individual protocols.

Acute leukemias: 6.2-7.5 mg/m^2/day continuous infusion for days 1-5; maximum tolerated dose was 8.9 mg/m^2/day.

Available Dosage Forms Injection, solution [preservative free]: 1 mg/mL (10 mL)

Nursing Guidelines

Assessment: See Contraindications, Warnings/Precautions, and Dosing for extensive use cautions. See Administration, Compatibility, and Reconstitution information. Assess results of laboratory tests (see below), therapeutic effectiveness, and adverse response (see Adverse Reactions) prior to therapy, regularly during therapy, and following therapy (patients should be considered immunosuppressed for up to 1 year after cladribine therapy). Teach patient (or caregiver) possible side effects/appropriate interventions and adverse symptoms to report (see Patient Education). **Pregnancy risk factor D** - determine that patient is not pregnant before beginning treatment. Instruct patients of childbearing age about appropriate contraceptive measures. Breast-feeding is contraindicated.

Monitoring Laboratory Tests: Liver and renal function tests, CBC with differential, platelets, uric acid

Patient Education: Inform prescriber of all prescriptions, OTC medications, or herbal products you are taking, and any allergies you have. Do not take any new medication during therapy unless approved by prescriber. This drug can only be administered by infusion. It is important to maintain adequate hydration (2-3 L/day of fluids) unless instructed to restrict fluid intake, and nutrition during therapy (small, frequent meals may help). You will be more susceptible to infection during therapy and for up to 1 year following therapy (avoid crowds and exposure to infection and do not have any vaccinations without consulting prescriber). May cause nausea or vomiting (small, frequent meals, frequent mouth care, sucking lozenges, or chewing gum may help); muscle weakness or pain (consult prescriber for mild analgesics); or mouth sores (use frequent mouth care with soft toothbrush or cotton swabs and frequent mouth rinses).

(Continued)

Cladribine *(Continued)*

Report immediately rash, unusual excessive fatigue, and/or signs of infection. Report rapid heartbeat or palpitations; unusual bruising or bleeding; persistent GI disturbances; diarrhea or constipation; yellowing of eyes or skin; change in color of urine or stool; swelling, warmth, or pain in extremities; or difficult respirations. **Pregnancy/breast-feeding precautions:** Do not get pregnant while taking this medication. Consult prescriber for appropriate contraceptive measures. Do not breast-feed until prescriber advises it is safe.

Pregnancy Risk Factor: D

Lactation: Enters breast milk/contraindicated

Administration

I.V.: Administer as a 1- to 2-hour infusion or by continuous infusion

Reconstitution: Solutions for 7-day infusion should be prepared in bacteriostatic NS.

Compatibility: Stable in NS; **incompatible** with D_5W

Storage: Store intact vials under refrigeration 2°C to 8°C (36°F to 46°F). Dilutions in 500 mL NS are stable for 72 hours. Stable in PVC containers for 24 hours at room temperature of 15°C to 30°C (59°F to 86°F) and 7 days in Pharmacia Deltec® cassettes.

♦ Claforan® *see* Cefotaxime *on page 340*

♦ Claravis™ *see* Isotretinoin *on page 981*

Clarithromycin (kla RITH roe mye sin)

U.S. Brand Names Biaxin®; Biaxin® XL

Pharmacologic Category Antibiotic, Macrolide

Medication Safety Issues

Sound-alike/look-alike issues:

Clarithromycin may be confused with erythromycin

Use

Children:

Pharyngitis/tonsillitis, acute maxillary sinusitis, uncomplicated skin/skin structure infections, and mycobacterial infections

Acute otitis media (*H. influenzae, M. catarrhalis*, or *S. pneumoniae*)

Prevention of disseminated mycobacterial infections due to MAC disease in patients with advanced HIV infection

Adults:

Pharyngitis/tonsillitis due to susceptible *S. pyogenes*

Acute maxillary sinusitis and acute exacerbation of chronic bronchitis due to susceptible *H. influenzae, M. catarrhalis*, or *S. pneumoniae*

Community-acquired pneumonia due to susceptible *H. influenzae, H. parainfluenzae, Mycoplasma pneumoniae, S. pneumoniae,* or *Chlamydia pneumoniae* (TWAR)

Uncomplicated skin/skin structure infections due to susceptible *S. aureus, S. pyogenes*

Disseminated mycobacterial infections due to *M. avium* or *M. intracellulare*

Prevention of disseminated mycobacterial infections due to *M. avium* complex (MAC) disease (eg, patients with advanced HIV infection)

Duodenal ulcer disease due to *H. pylori* in regimens with other drugs including amoxicillin and lansoprazole or omeprazole, ranitidine bismuth citrate, bismuth subsalicylate, tetracycline, and/or an H_2 antagonist

Alternate antibiotic for prophylaxis of bacterial endocarditis in patients who are allergic to penicillin and undergoing surgical or dental procedures

Unlabeled/Investigational Use Pertussis

Mechanism of Action Exerts its antibacterial action by binding to 50S ribosomal subunit resulting in inhibition of protein synthesis. The 14-OH metabolite of clarithromycin is twice as active as the parent compound against certain organisms.

Pharmacodynamics/Kinetics

Absorption: Highly stable in presence of gastric acid (unlike erythromycin); food delays but does not affect extent of absorption

Distribution: Widely into most body tissues except CNS

Metabolism: Partially hepatic via CYP3A4; converted to 14-OH clarithromycin (active metabolite)

Bioavailability: 50%

Half-life elimination: Clarithromycin: 3-7 hours; 14-OH-clarithromycin: 5-9 hours

Time to peak: 2-4 hours

Excretion: Primarily urine

Clearance: Approximates normal GFR

Contraindications Hypersensitivity to clarithromycin, erythromycin, or any macrolide antibiotic; use with ergot derivatives, pimozide, cisapride; combination with ranitidine bismuth citrate should not be used in patients with history of acute porphyria or Cl_{cr} <25 mL/minute

Warnings/Precautions Dosage adjustment required with severe renal impairment, decreased dosage or prolonged dosing interval may be appropriate; antibiotic-associated colitis has been reported with use of clarithromycin. Macrolides (including clarithromycin) have been associated with rare QT prolongation and ventricular arrhythmias, including torsade de pointes. The extended release formulation consists of drug within a nondeformable matrix; following drug release/absorption, the matrix/shell is expelled in the stool. The use of nondeformable products in patients with known stricture/narrowing of the GI tract has been associated with symptoms of obstruction. Safety and efficacy in children <6 months of age have not been established.

Drug Interactions **Substrate** of CYP3A4 (major); **Inhibits** CYP1A2 (weak), 3A4 (strong)

Alfentanil (and possibly other narcotic analgesics): Serum levels may be increased by clarithromycin; monitor for increased effect.

Benzodiazepines (those metabolized by CYP3A4, including alprazolam, midazolam, triazolam): Serum levels may be increased by clarithromycin; somnolence and confusion have been reported.

Bromocriptine: Serum levels may be increased by clarithromycin; monitor for increased effect.

Buspirone: Serum levels may be increased by clarithromycin; monitor.

Calcium channel blockers (felodipine, verapamil, and potentially others metabolized by CYP3A4): Serum levels may be increased by clarithromycin; monitor.

Carbamazepine: Serum levels may be increased by clarithromycin; monitor.

Cilostazol: Serum levels may be increased by clarithromycin; monitor.

Cisapride: Serum levels may be increased by clarithromycin; serious arrhythmias have occurred; concurrent use contraindicated.

Clopidogrel: Therapeutic effect may be decreased by clarithromycin; monitor.

Clozapine: Serum levels may be increased by clarithromycin; monitor.

Colchicine: Serum levels/toxicity may be increased by clarithromycin; monitor. Avoid use, if possible.

Cyclosporine: Serum levels may be increased by clarithromycin; monitor serum levels.

CYP3A4 inducers: CYP3A4 inducers may decrease the levels/effects of clarithromycin. Example inducers include aminoglutethimide, carbamazepine, nafcillin, nevirapine, phenobarbital, phenytoin, and rifamycins.

CYP3A4 inhibitors: May increase the levels/effects of clarithromycin. Example inhibitors include azole antifungals, diclofenac, doxycycline, erythromycin, imatinib, isoniazid, nefazodone, nicardipine, propofol, protease inhibitors, quinidine, telithromycin, and verapamil.

CYP3A4 substrates: Clarithromycin may increase the levels/effects of CYP3A4 substrates. Example substrates include benzodiazepines, calcium channel blockers, mirtazapine, nateglinide, nefazodone, tacrolimus, and venlafaxine. Selected benzodiazepines (midazolam and triazolam), cisapride, ergot alkaloids, selected HMG-CoA reductase inhibitors (lovastatin and simvastatin), and pimozide are generally contraindicated with strong CYP3A4 inhibitors.

Delavirdine: Serum levels may be increased by clarithromycin; monitor.

Digoxin: Serum levels may be increased by clarithromycin; digoxin toxicity and potentially fatal arrhythmias have been reported; monitor digoxin levels.

Disopyramide: Serum levels may be increased by clarithromycin; in addition, QT_c prolongation and risk of malignant arrhythmia may be increased; avoid combination.

Ergot alkaloids: Concurrent use may lead to acute ergot toxicity (severe peripheral vasospasm and dysesthesia).

Fluconazole: Increases clarithromycin levels and AUC by ~25%

HMG-CoA reductase inhibitors (atorvastatin, lovastatin, and simvastatin); Clarithromycin may increase serum levels of "statins" metabolized by CYP3A4, increasing the risk of myopathy/rhabdomyolysis (does not include fluvastatin and pravastatin). Switch to pravastatin/fluvastatin or suspend treatment during course of clarithromycin therapy.

Methylprednisolone: Serum levels may be increased by clarithromycin; monitor.

Phenytoin: Serum levels may be increased by clarithromycin; other evidence suggested phenytoin levels may be decreased in some patients; monitor.

(Continued)

Clarithromycin *(Continued)*

Pimozide: Serum levels may be increased, leading to malignant arrhythmias; concomitant use is contraindicated.

Protease inhibitors (amprenavir, nelfinavir, and ritonavir): May increase serum levels of clarithromycin.

QT_c-prolonging agents: Concomitant use may increase the risk of malignant arrhythmias.

Quinidine: Serum levels may be increased by clarithromycin; in addition, the risk of QT_c prolongation and malignant arrhythmias may be increased during concurrent use.

Quinolone antibiotics (sparfloxacin, gatifloxacin, or moxifloxacin): Concurrent use may increase the risk of malignant arrhythmias.

Rifabutin: Serum levels may be increased by clarithromycin; monitor.

Sildenafil, tadalafil, vardenafil: Serum levels may be increased by clarithromycin. Do not exceed single sildenafil doses of 25 mg in 48 hours, a single tadalafil dose of 10 mg in 72 hours, or a single vardenafil dose of 2.5 mg in 24 hours.

Tacrolimus: Serum levels may be increased by clarithromycin; monitor serum concentration.

Theophylline: Serum levels may be increased by clarithromycin; monitor.

Thioridazine: Risk of QT_c prolongation and malignant arrhythmias may be increased.

Valproic acid (and derivatives): Serum levels may be increased by clarithromycin; monitor.

Vinblastine (and vincristine): Serum levels may be increased by clarithromycin.

Warfarin: Effects may be potentiated; monitor INR closely and adjust warfarin dose as needed or choose another antibiotic

Zidovudine: Peak levels (but not AUC) of zidovudine may be increased; other studies suggest levels may be decreased.

Zopiclone: Serum levels may be increased by clarithromycin; monitor.

Nutritional/Herbal/Ethanol Interactions

Food: Delays absorption; total absorption remains unchanged.

Herb/Nutraceutical: St John's wort may decrease clarithromycin levels.

Adverse Reactions

1% to 10%:

- Central nervous system: Headache (adults and children 2%)
- Dermatologic: Rash (children 3%)
- Gastrointestinal: Abnormal taste (adults 3% to 7%), diarrhea (adults 3% to 6%; children 6%), vomiting (children 6%), nausea (adults 3%), heartburn (adults 2%), abdominal pain (adults 2%; children 3%), dyspepsia 2%
- Hepatic: Prothrombin time increased (1%)
- Renal: BUN increased (4%)

<1% (Limited to important or life-threatening): *Clostridium difficile* colitis, alkaline phosphatase increased, anaphylaxis, anorexia, anxiety, behavioral changes, bilirubin increased, confusion, disorientation, dizziness, dyspnea, glossitis, hallucinations, hearing loss (reversible), hepatic dysfunction, hepatic failure, hepatitis, hypoglycemia, insomnia, interstitial nephritis, jaundice, leukopenia, manic behavior, neuromuscular blockade (case reports), neutropenia, nightmares, oral moniliasis, pancreatitis, psychosis, QT prolongation, seizure, serum creatinine increased, smell alteration, Stevens-Johnson syndrome, stomatitis, thrombocytopenia, tinnitus, tongue discoloration, tooth discoloration, torsade de pointes, toxic epidermal necrolysis, transaminases increased, tremor, urticaria, ventricular tachycardia, ventricular arrhythmia, vertigo

Overdosage/Toxicology Symptoms of overdose include nausea, vomiting, diarrhea, prostration, reversible pancreatitis, hearing loss with or without tinnitus, or vertigo. Treatment includes symptomatic and supportive care. Dialysis not likely to benefit.

Dosing

Adults & Elderly:

Usual dose: Oral: 250-500 mg every 12 hours **or** 1000 mg (two 500 mg extended release tablets) once daily for 7-14 days

Upper respiratory tract: Oral: 250-500 mg every 12 hours for 10-14 days

Pharyngitis/tonsillitis: 250 mg every 12 hours for 10 days

Acute maxillary sinusitis: 500 mg every 12 hours **or** 1000 mg (two 500 mg extended release tablets) once daily for 14 days

Lower respiratory tract: Oral: 250-500 mg every 12 hours for 7-14 days

Acute exacerbation of chronic bronchitis due to:

M. catarrhalis and *S. pneumoniae*: 250 mg every 12 hours for 7-14 days**or** 1000 mg (two 500 mg extended release tablets) once daily for 7 days

H. influenzae: 500 mg every 12 hours for 7-14 days or 1000 mg (two 500 mg extended release tablets) for 7 days

H. parainfluenzae: 500 mg every 12 hours for 7 days or 1000 mg (two 500 mg extended release tablets) for 7 days

Pneumonia due to:

C. pneumoniae, *M. pneumoniae*, and *S. pneumoniae*: 250 mg every 12 hours for 7-14 days **or** 1000 mg (two 500 mg extended release tablets) once daily for 7 days

H. influenzae: 250 mg every 12 hours for 7 days **or** 1000 mg (two 500 mg extended release tablets) once daily for 7 days

Mycobacterial infection (prevention and treatment): Oral: 500 mg twice daily (use with other antimycobacterial drugs, eg, ethambutol, clofazimine, or rifampin)

Pertussis (CDC guidelines): 500 mg twice daily for 7 days

Prophylaxis of bacterial endocarditis: Oral: 500 mg 1 hour prior to procedure

Uncomplicated skin and skin structure: Oral: 250 mg every 12 hours for 7-14 days

Peptic ulcer disease: Eradication of *Helicobacter pylori*: Oral: Dual or triple combination regimen with bismuth subsalicylate, tetracycline, clarithromycin, and an H_2-receptor; or combination of omeprazole and clarithromycin; 500 mg every 8-12 hours for 10-14 days

Pediatrics: Oral:

Children ≥1 months: **Pertussis (CDC guidelines):**15 mg/kg/day divided every 12 hours for 7 days; maximum: 1 g/day

Children ≥6 months: 15 mg/kg/day divided every 12 hours for 10 days

Community-acquired pneumonia, sinusitis, bronchitis, skin infections: 15 mg/kg/day divided every 12 hours for 10 days

Mycobacterial infection (prevention and treatment): 7.5 mg/kg twice daily, up to 500 mg twice daily. **Note:** Safety of clarithromycin for MAC not studied in children <20 months.

Prophylaxis of bacterial endocarditis: 15 mg/kg 1 hour before procedure (maximum dose: 500 mg)

Renal Impairment:

Cl_{cr} <30 mL/minute: Half the normal dose or double the dosing interval.

In combination with ritonavir:

Cl_{cr} 30-60 mL/minute: Reduce dose by 50%.

Cl_{cr} <30 mL/minute: Reduce dose by 75%.

Hepatic Impairment: No dosing adjustment is needed as long as renal function is normal.

Available Dosage Forms

Granules for oral suspension (Biaxin®): 125 mg/5 mL (50 mL, 100 mL); 250 mg/5 mL (50 mL, 100 mL) [fruit punch flavor]

Tablet [film coated] (Biaxin®): 250 mg, 500 mg

Tablet, extended release [film coated] (Biaxin® XL): 500 mg

Nursing Guidelines

Assessment: Assess results of culture and sensitivity tests and patient's allergy history prior to therapy. Assess potential for interactions with other pharmacological agents or herbal products patient may be taking (eg, drugs that affect or are affected by CYP3A4 enzyme activity; see Drug Interactions). Assess therapeutic effectiveness (according to purpose for use) and adverse reactions. Teach patient proper use, possible side effects/appropriate interventions, and adverse symptoms to report.

Monitoring Laboratory Tests: Perform culture and sensitivity studies prior to initiating drug therapy.

Dietary Considerations: May be taken with or without meals; may be taken with milk. Biaxin® XL should be taken with food.

Patient Education: Do not take any new medication during therapy unless approved by prescriber. Take full course of therapy even if feeling better; do not discontinue without consulting prescriber. Tablets or suspension may be taken with or without food or milk. Extended release tablets should be taken with food. Do not crush or chew extended release tablets. Do not refrigerate oral suspension (more palatable at room temperature). Maintain adequate hydration (2-3 L/day of fluids) unless instructed to restrict fluid intake. May cause nausea, heartburn, or abnormal taste (small frequent meals, frequent mouth care,

(Continued)

Clarithromycin *(Continued)*

chewing gum or sucking lozenges may help); diarrhea (buttermilk, boiled milk, or yogurt may help); or headache or abdominal cramps (consult prescriber for analgesic). Report rapid heartbeat or palpitations, persistent fever or chills, easy bruising or bleeding, joint pain, severe persistent diarrhea, skin rash, sores in mouth, foul-smelling urine, or respiratory difficulty. **Pregnancy/breast-feeding precautions:** Inform prescriber if you are or intend to become pregnant. Consult prescriber if breast-feeding.

Geriatric Considerations: Considered one of the drugs of choice in the outpatient treatment of community-acquired pneumonia in older adults. After doses of 500 mg every 12 hours for 5 days, 12 healthy elderly had significantly increased C_{max} and C_{min}, elimination half-lives of clarithromycin and 14-OH clarithromycin compared to 12 healthy young subjects. These changes were attributed to a significant decrease in renal clearance. At a dose of 1000 mg twice daily, 100% of 13 older adults experienced an adverse event compared to only 10% taking 500 mg twice daily.

Pregnancy Risk Factor: C

Pregnancy Issues: There are no adequate and well-controlled studies in pregnant women. Due to adverse fetal effects reported in animal studies, the manufacturer recommends that clarithromycin not be used in a pregnant woman unless there are no alternatives to therapy.

Lactation: Excretion in breast milk unknown/use caution

Breast-Feeding Considerations: Erythromycins may be taken while breast-feeding. Use caution.

Administration

Oral: Clarithromycin may be given with or without meals. Give every 12 hours rather than twice daily to avoid peak and trough variation.

Biaxin® XL: Should be given with food. Do not crush or chew extended release tablet.

Reconstitution: Reconstituted oral suspension should not be refrigerated because it might gel. Microencapsulated particles of clarithromycin in suspension is stable for 14 days when stored at room temperature.

Storage: Store tablets and granules for oral suspension at controlled room temperature.

- **Claritin® [OTC]** *see* Loratadine *on page 1058*
- **Claritin-D® 12-Hour [OTC]** *see* Loratadine and Pseudoephedrine *on page 1060*
- **Claritin-D® 24-Hour [OTC]** *see* Loratadine and Pseudoephedrine *on page 1060*
- **Claritin® Hives Relief [OTC]** *see* Loratadine *on page 1058*
- **Clavulanic Acid and Amoxicillin** *see* Amoxicillin and Clavulanate Potassium *on page 147*
- **Cleocin®** *see* Clindamycin *on page 426*
- **Cleocin HCl®** *see* Clindamycin *on page 426*
- **Cleocin Pediatric®** *see* Clindamycin *on page 426*
- **Cleocin Phosphate®** *see* Clindamycin *on page 426*
- **Cleocin T®** *see* Clindamycin *on page 426*
- **Climara®** *see* Estradiol *on page 649*
- **Clindagel®** *see* Clindamycin *on page 426*
- **ClindaMax™** *see* Clindamycin *on page 426*

Clindamycin (klin da MYE sin)

U.S. Brand Names Cleocin®; Cleocin HCl®; Cleocin Pediatric®; Cleocin Phosphate®; Cleocin T®; Clindagel®; ClindaMax™; Clindesse™; Clindets®; Evoclin™

Synonyms Clindamycin Hydrochloride; Clindamycin Palmitate; Clindamycin Phosphate

Pharmacologic Category Antibiotic, Lincosamide

Medication Safety Issues

Sound-alike/look-alike issues:

Cleocin® may be confused with bleomycin, Clinoril®, Lincocin®

Use Treatment against aerobic and anaerobic streptococci (except enterococci), most staphylococci, *Bacteroides* sp and *Actinomyces*; bacterial vaginosis (vaginal cream, vaginal suppository); pelvic inflammatory disease (I.V.); topically in treatment of severe acne; vaginally for *Gardnerella vaginalis*

Unlabeled/Investigational Use May be useful in PCP; alternate treatment for toxoplasmosis

Mechanism of Action Reversibly binds to 50S ribosomal subunits preventing peptide bond formation thus inhibiting bacterial protein synthesis; bacteriostatic or bactericidal depending on drug concentration, infection site, and organism

Pharmacodynamics/Kinetics

Absorption: Topical: ~10%; Oral: Rapid (90%)

Distribution: High concentrations in bone and urine; no significant levels in CSF, even with inflamed meninges; crosses placenta; enters breast milk

Metabolism: Hepatic

Bioavailability: Topical: <1%

Half-life elimination: Neonates: Premature: 8.7 hours; Full-term: 3.6 hours; Adults: 1.6-5.3 hours (average: 2-3 hours)

Time to peak, serum: Oral: Within 60 minutes; I.M.: 1-3 hours

Excretion: Urine (10%) and feces (~4%) as active drug and metabolites

Contraindications Hypersensitivity to clindamycin or any component of the formulation; previous pseudomembranous colitis; regional enteritis, ulcerative colitis

Warnings/Precautions Dosage adjustment may be necessary in patients with severe hepatic dysfunction; can cause severe and possibly fatal colitis; discontinue drug if significant diarrhea, abdominal cramps, or passage of blood and mucus occurs. Vaginal products may weaken latex or rubber condoms, or contraceptive diaphragms. Barrier contraceptives are not recommended concurrently or for 3-5 days (depending on the product) following treatment. Some dosage forms contain benzyl alcohol or tartrazine. Use caution in atopic patients.

Drug Interactions Increased duration of neuromuscular blockade from tubocurarine, pancuronium

Nutritional/Herbal/Ethanol Interactions

Food: Peak concentrations may be delayed with food.

Herb/Nutraceutical: St John's wort may decrease clindamycin levels.

Adverse Reactions

Systemic:

>10%: Gastrointestinal: Diarrhea, abdominal pain

1% to 10%:

- Cardiovascular: Hypotension
- Dermatologic: Urticaria, rash, Stevens-Johnson syndrome
- Gastrointestinal: Pseudomembranous colitis, nausea, vomiting
- Local: Thrombophlebitis, sterile abscess at I.M. injection site
- Miscellaneous: Fungal overgrowth, hypersensitivity

<1% (Limited to important or life-threatening): Granulocytopenia, neutropenia, polyarthritis, renal dysfunction (rare), thrombocytopenia

Topical:

>10%: Dermatologic: Dryness, burning, itching, scaliness, erythema, or peeling of skin (lotion, solution); oiliness (gel, lotion)

1% to 10%: Central nervous system: Headache

<1% (Limited to important or life-threatening): Pseudomembranous colitis, nausea, vomiting, diarrhea (severe), abdominal pain, folliculitis, hypersensitivity reactions

Vaginal:

>10%: Genitourinary: Fungal vaginosis, vaginitis or vulvovaginal pruritus (from *Candida albicans*)

1% to 10%:

- Central nervous system: Back pain, headache
- Gastrointestinal: Constipation, diarrhea
- Genitourinary: Urinary tract infection
- Respiratory: Nasopharyngitis
- Miscellaneous: Fungal infection

<1% (Limited to important or life-threatening): Atrophic vaginitis, bladder infection, bladder spasm, cervical dysplasia, diarrhea, dizziness, epistaxis, erythema, fever, hypersensitivity, hyperthyroidism, local edema, menstrual disorder, nausea, pain, palpable lymph node, pruritus, pyelonephritis, pyrexia, rash, sciatica, stomach cramps, upper respiratory urticaria, uterine cervical disorder, uterine spasm, vaginal burning, vertigo, vomiting, vulvar erythema, vulvar laceration, wheezing

Overdosage/Toxicology Symptoms of overdose include diarrhea, nausea, and vomiting. Treatment is supportive.

(Continued)

Clindamycin *(Continued)*

Dosing

Adults & Elderly:

Usual dose:

Oral: 150-450 mg/dose every 6-8 hours; maximum dose: 1.8 g/day

I.M., I.V.: 1.2-1.8 g/day in 2-4 divided doses; maximum dose: 4.8 g/day

Pelvic inflammatory disease: *I.V.:* 900 mg every 8 hours with gentamicin 2 mg/kg, then 1.5 mg/kg every 8 hours; continue after discharge with doxycycline 100 mg twice daily to complete 14 days of total therapy

Pneumonia due to *Pneumocystis carinii* (unlabeled use):

Oral: 300-450 mg 4 times/day with primaquine

I.M., I.V.: 1200-2400 mg/day with pyrimethamine

I.V.: 600 mg 4 times/day with primaquine

Acne: *Topical:*

Gel, pledget, lotion, solution: Apply a thin film twice daily

Foam (Evoclin™): Apply once daily

Bacterial vaginosis: *Intravaginal:*

Suppositories: Insert one ovule (100 mg clindamycin) daily into vagina at bedtime for 3 days

Cream:

Cleocin®: One full applicator inserted intravaginally once daily before bedtime for 3 or 7 consecutive days in nonpregnant patients or for 7 consecutive days in pregnant patients

Clindesse™: One full applicator inserted intravaginally as a single dose at anytime during the day in nonpregnant patients

Prevention of bacterial endocarditis in patients unable to take amoxicillin (unlabeled use): *Oral:* 600 mg 1 hour before procedure with no follow-up dose needed; for patients allergic to penicillin and unable to take oral medications: 600 mg I.V. within 30 minutes before procedure

Orofacial infections: 150-450 mg every 6 hours for at least 7 days; maximum dose: 1.8 g/day

Patients with prosthesis allergic to penicillin: *Oral:* 600 mg 1 hour before procedure; for patients with prosthesis allergic to penicillin and unable to take oral medication: I.V.: 600 mg 1 hour before procedure

Pediatrics:

Usual dose:

Oral: Infants and Children: 8-20 mg/kg/day as hydrochloride; 8-25 mg/kg/day as palmitate in 3-4 divided doses; minimum dose of palmitate: 37.5 mg 3 times/day

I.M., I.V.:

<1 month: 15-20 mg/kg/day

>1 month: 20-40 mg/kg/day in 3-4 divided doses

Prevention of bacterial endocarditis (unlabeled use): *Oral:* Children: 20 mg/kg 1 hour before procedure with no follow-up dose needed; for patients allergic to penicillin and unable to take oral medications: 20 mg/kg I.V. within 30 minutes before procedure

Orofacial infections: 8-25 mg/kg in 3-4 equally divided doses

Acne: *Topical:* Children ≥12 years: Refer to adult dosing.

Babesiosis: *Oral:* 20-40 mg/kg divided every 8 hours for 7 days plus quinine

Hepatic Impairment:
Systemic use: Adjustment is recommended in patients with severe hepatic disease.

Available Dosage Forms Note: Strength is expressed as base

Capsule, as hydrochloride: 150 mg, 300 mg

Cleocin HCl®: 75 mg [contains tartrazine], 150 mg [contains tartrazine], 300 mg

Cream, vaginal, as phosphate:

Cleocin®: 2% (40 g) [contains benzyl alcohol and mineral oil; packaged with 7 disposable applicators]

Clindesse™: 2% (5 g) [contains mineral oil; prefilled single disposable applicator]

Foam, topical, as phosphate (Evoclin™): 1% (50 g, 100 g) [contains ethanol 58%]

Gel, topical, as phosphate: 1% [10 mg/g] (30 g, 60 g)

Cleocin T®: 1% [10 mg/g] (30 g, 60 g)

Clindagel®: 1% [10 mg/g] (40 mL, 75 mL)

ClindaMax™: 1% (30 g, 60 g)

Granules for oral solution, as palmitate (Cleocin Pediatric®): 75 mg/5 mL (100 mL) [cherry flavor]

Infusion, as phosphate [premixed in D_5W] (Cleocin Phosphate®): 300 mg (50 mL); 600 mg (50 mL); 900 mg (50 mL)

Injection, solution, as phosphate (Cleocin Phosphate®): 150 mg/mL (2 mL, 4 mL, 6 mL, 60 mL) [contains benzyl alcohol and disodium edetate 0.5 mg]

Lotion, as phosphate (Cleocin T®, ClindaMax™): 1% [10 mg/mL] (60 mL)

Pledgets, topical: 1% (60s) [contains alcohol]

Clindets®: 1% (69s) [contains isopropyl alcohol 52%]

Cleocin T®: 1% (60s) [contains isopropyl alcohol 50%]

Solution, topical, as phosphate (Cleocin T®): 1% [10 mg/mL] (30 mL, 60 mL) [contains isopropyl alcohol 50%]

Suppository (ovule), vaginal, as phosphate (Cleocin®): 100 mg (3s) [contains oleaginous base; single reusable applicator]

Nursing Guidelines

Assessment: Assess previous allergy history prior to beginning therapy. See Contraindications, Warnings/Precautions, and Drug Interactions for use cautions. **I.V.:** Monitor cardiac status and blood pressure. Keep patient recumbent after infusion until blood pressure is stabilized. Assess results of laboratory tests (see below) and patient response according to dose, route of administration, and purpose of therapy (see Adverse Reactions and Overdose/Toxicology). Teach patient proper use, possible side effects/appropriate interventions, and adverse symptoms to report (eg, severe diarrhea, opportunistic infection - see Patient Education).

Monitoring Laboratory Tests: CBC, liver and renal function periodically with prolonged therapy

Dietary Considerations: May be taken with food.

Patient Education:

I.M., I.V.: Report any burning, pain, swelling, or redness at infusion or injection site.

Oral: Take as directed. Take each dose with a full glass of water. Complete full prescription, even if feeling better. If a dose is missed, take as soon as possible, but do not double doses. Report immediately any diarrhea, bloody stools, abdominal pain or cramping (do not use antidiarrheals without consulting prescriber). You may experience headache (consult prescriber for appropriate analgesic); nausea or vomiting (small, frequent meals, frequent mouth care, chewing gum, or sucking lozenges may help). Report dizziness, skin redness or rash; fever, chills, unusual bruising, bleeding, or signs of infection (plaques on tongue, vaginal itching or discharge); other persistent adverse effects, or no improvement.

Topical, foam: Wash hands thoroughly or wear gloves. Do not dispense directly onto hands or face (foam will begin to melt on contact with warm skin). Dispense an amount the will cover the affected area directly into the cap or onto a cool surface. If can seems warm or foam seems runny, run can under cold water. Pick up small amounts of foam with fingertips and gently massage into affected areas until foam disappears. Wash hands thoroughly. Wait 30 minutes before shaving or applying make-up.

Topical gel, lotion, or solution: Wash hands thoroughly before applying or wear gloves. Apply thin film of gel, lotion, or solution to affected area. May apply porous dressing. Wash hands thoroughly. Wait 30 minutes before shaving or applying make-up. Report persistent burning, swelling, itching, excessive dryness, or worsening of condition.

Vaginal: Wash hands before using. At bedtime, gently insert full applicator into vagina and expel cream. Wash applicator with soap and water following use. Remain lying down for 30 minutes following administration. Avoid intercourse during therapy. Report adverse reactions (dizziness, nausea, vomiting, stomach cramps, or headache) or lack of improvement or worsening of condition.

Geriatric Considerations: Elderly patients are often at a higher risk for developing serious colitis and require close monitoring.

Pregnancy Risk Factor: B

Lactation: Enters breast milk/compatible

Perioperative/Anesthesia/Other Concerns: Clindamycin may increase the duration of neuromuscular blockade after anesthesia. In adults, clindamycin injection can usually be dosed effectively on an every-8-hour basis.

(Continued)

Clindamycin *(Continued)*

Administration

Oral: Administer oral dosage form with a full glass of water to minimize esophageal ulceration. Give around-the-clock to promote less variation in peak and trough serum levels.

I.M.: Deep I.M. sites, rotate sites. Do not exceed 600 mg in a single injection.

I.V.: **Never administer as bolus**; administer by I.V. intermittent infusion over at least 10-60 minutes, at a rate **not** to exceed 30 mg/minute (not exceed 1200 mg/hour); final concentration for administration should not exceed 18 mg/mL

Compatibility: Stable in D_5LR, D_5½NS, D_5NS, D_5W, D_{10}W, LR, NS

Y-site administration: Incompatible with allopurinol, filgrastim, fluconazole, idarubicin

Compatibility in syringe: Incompatible with tobramycin

Compatibility when admixed: Incompatible with aminophylline, barbiturates, calcium gluconate, ceftriaxone, ciprofloxacin, gentamicin with cefazolin, magnesium sulfate, phenytoin

Storage:

Capsule: Store at room temperature of 20°C to 25°C (68°F to 77°F).

Cream: Store at room temperature.

Foam: Store at room temperature of 20°C to 25°C (68°F to 77°F). Avoid fire, flame, or smoking during or following application.

Gel: Store at room temperature.

Clindagel®: Do not store in direct sunlight.

I.V.: Infusion solution in NS or D_5W solution is stable for 16 days at room temperature.

Lotion: Store at room temperature of 20°C to 25°C (68°F to 77°F).

Oral solution: Do not refrigerate reconstituted oral solution (it will thicken). Following reconstitution, oral solution is stable for 2 weeks at room temperature of 20°C to 25°C (68°F to 77°F).

Ovule: Store at room temperature of 15°C to 30°C (68°F to 77°F).

Pledget: Store at room temperature.

Topical solution: Store at room temperature of 20°C to 25°C (68°F to 77°F).

Related Information

Prevention of Wound Infection and Sepsis in Surgical Patients *on page 1830*

- ♦ **Clindamycin Hydrochloride** *see* Clindamycin *on page 426*
- ♦ **Clindamycin Palmitate** *see* Clindamycin *on page 426*
- ♦ **Clindamycin Phosphate** *see* Clindamycin *on page 426*
- ♦ **Clindesse™** *see* Clindamycin *on page 426*
- ♦ **Clindets®** *see* Clindamycin *on page 426*

Clonazepam (kloe NA ze pam)

U.S. Brand Names Klonopin®

Pharmacologic Category Benzodiazepine

Medication Safety Issues

Sound-alike/look-alike issues:

Clonazepam may be confused with clofazimine, clonidine, clorazepate, clozapine, lorazepam

Klonopin® may be confused with clofazimine, clonidine, clorazepate, clozapine, lorazepam

Use Alone or as an adjunct in the treatment of petit mal variant (Lennox-Gastaut), akinetic, and myoclonic seizures; petit mal (absence) seizures unresponsive to succimides; panic disorder with or without agoraphobia

Unlabeled/Investigational Use Restless legs syndrome; neuralgia; multifocal tic disorder; parkinsonian dysarthria; bipolar disorder; adjunct therapy for schizophrenia

Mechanism of Action The exact mechanism is unknown, but believed to be related to its ability to enhance the activity of GABA; suppresses the spike-and-wave discharge in absence seizures by depressing nerve transmission in the motor cortex

Pharmacodynamics/Kinetics

Onset of action: 20-60 minutes

Duration: Infants and young children: 6-8 hours; Adults: ≤12 hours

Absorption: Well absorbed

Distribution: Adults: V_d: 1.5-4.4 L/kg

Protein binding: 85%

Metabolism: Extensively hepatic via glucuronide and sulfate conjugation

Half-life elimination: Children: 22-33 hours; Adults: 19-50 hours

Time to peak, serum: 1-3 hours; Steady-state: 5-7 days

Excretion: Urine (<2% as unchanged drug); metabolites excreted as glucuronide or sulfate conjugates

Contraindications Hypersensitivity to clonazepam or any component of the formulation (cross-sensitivity with other benzodiazepines may exist); significant liver disease; narrow-angle glaucoma; pregnancy

Warnings/Precautions Use with caution in elderly or debilitated patients, patients with hepatic disease (including alcoholics), or renal impairment. Use with caution in patients with respiratory disease or impaired gag reflex or ability to protect the airway from secretions (salivation may be increased). Worsening of seizures may occur when added to patients with multiple seizure types. Concurrent use with valproic acid may result in absence status. Monitoring of CBC and liver function tests has been recommended during prolonged therapy.

Causes CNS depression (dose-related) resulting in sedation, dizziness, confusion, or ataxia which may impair physical and mental capabilities. Patients must be cautioned about performing tasks which require mental alertness (eg, operating machinery or driving). Use with caution in patients receiving other CNS depressants or psychoactive agents. Effects with other sedative drugs or ethanol may be potentiated. Benzodiazepines have been associated with falls and traumatic injury and should be used with extreme caution in patients who are at risk of these events (especially the elderly).

Use caution in patients with depression, particularly if suicidal risk may be present. Use with caution in patients with a history of drug dependence. Benzodiazepines have been associated with dependence and acute withdrawal symptoms, including seizures, on discontinuation or reduction in dose. Acute withdrawal, including seizures, may be precipitated in patients after administration of flumazenil to patients receiving long-term benzodiazepine therapy.

Benzodiazepines have been associated with anterograde amnesia. Paradoxical reactions, including hyperactive or aggressive behavior, have been reported with benzodiazepines, particularly in adolescent/pediatric or psychiatric patients. Does not have analgesic, antidepressant, or antipsychotic properties.

Drug Interactions **Substrate** of CYP3A4 (major)

CNS depressants: Sedative effects and/or respiratory depression may be additive with CNS depressants; includes ethanol, barbiturates, narcotic analgesics, and other sedative agents; monitor for increased effect

CYP3A4 inducers: CYP3A4 inducers may decrease the levels/effects of clonazepam. Example inducers include aminoglutethimide, carbamazepine, nafcillin, nevirapine, phenobarbital, phenytoin, and rifamycins.

CYP3A4 inhibitors: May increase the levels/effects of clonazepam. Example inhibitors include azole antifungals, clarithromycin, diclofenac, doxycycline, erythromycin, imatinib, isoniazid, nefazodone, nicardipine, propofol, protease inhibitors, quinidine, telithromycin, and verapamil.

Disulfiram: Disulfiram may inhibit the metabolism of clonazepam; monitor for increased benzodiazepine effect

Levodopa: Therapeutic effects may be diminished in some patients following the addition of a benzodiazepine; limited/inconsistent data

Oral contraceptives: May decrease the clearance of some benzodiazepines (those which undergo oxidative metabolism); monitor for increased benzodiazepine effect

Theophylline: May partially antagonize some of the effects of benzodiazepines; monitor for decreased response; may require higher doses for sedation

Valproic acid: The combined use of clonazepam and valproic acid has been associated with absence seizures

Nutritional/Herbal/Ethanol Interactions

Ethanol: Avoid ethanol (may increase CNS depression).

Food: Clonazepam serum concentration is unlikely to be increased by grapefruit juice because of clonazepam's high oral bioavailability.

Herb/Nutraceutical: St John's wort may decrease clonazepam levels. Avoid valerian, St John's wort, kava kava, gotu kola (may increase CNS depression).

Adverse Reactions Reactions reported in patients with seizure and/or panic disorder. Frequency not defined.

Cardiovascular: Edema (ankle or facial), palpitation

Central nervous system: Amnesia, ataxia (seizure disorder ~30%; panic disorder 5%), behavior problems (seizure disorder ~25%), coma, confusion, depression, dizziness, drowsiness (seizure disorder ~50%), emotional lability, fatigue, fever, hallucinations, headache, hypotonia, hysteria, insomnia, intellectual

(Continued)

Clonazepam *(Continued)*

ability reduced, memory disturbance, nervousness; paradoxical reactions (including aggressive behavior, agitation, anxiety, excitability, hostility, irritability, nervousness, nightmares, sleep disturbance, vivid dreams); psychosis, slurred speech, somnolence (panic disorder 37%), suicidal attempt, vertigo

Dermatologic: Hair loss, hirsutism, skin rash

Endocrine & metabolic: Dysmenorrhea, libido increased/decreased

Gastrointestinal: Abdominal pain, anorexia, appetite increased/decreased, coated tongue, constipation, dehydration, diarrhea, gastritis, gum soreness, nausea, weight changes (loss/gain), xerostomia

Genitourinary: Colpitis, dysuria, ejaculation delayed, enuresis, impotence, micturition frequency, nocturia, urinary retention, urinary tract infection

Hematologic: Anemia, eosinophilia, leukopenia, thrombocytopenia

Hepatic: Alkaline phosphatase increased (transient), hepatomegaly, transaminases increased (transient)

Neuromuscular & skeletal: Choreiform movements, coordination abnormal, dysarthria, muscle pain, muscle weakness, myalgia, tremor

Ocular: Blurred vision, eye movements abnormal, diplopia, nystagmus

Respiratory: Chest congestion, cough, bronchitis, hypersecretions, pharyngitis, respiratory depression, respiratory tract infection, rhinitis, rhinorrhea, shortness of breath, sinusitis

Miscellaneous: Allergic reaction, aphonia, dysdiadochokinesis, encopresis, "glassy-eyed" appearance, hemiparesis, lymphadenopathy

Overdosage/Toxicology May produce somnolence, confusion, ataxia, diminished reflexes, or coma. Treatment for benzodiazepine overdose is supportive. Flumazenil has been shown to selectively block the binding of benzodiazepines to CNS receptors, resulting in a reversal of benzodiazepine-induced CNS depression, but not respiratory depression.

Dosing

Adults:

Seizure disorders: Oral:

Initial daily dose not to exceed 1.5 mg given in 3 divided doses; may increase by 0.5-1 mg every third day until seizures are controlled or adverse effects seen (maximum: 20 mg/day)

Usual maintenance dose: 0.05-0.2 mg/kg; do not exceed 20 mg/day

Panic disorder: Oral: 0.25 mg twice daily; increase in increments of 0.125-0.25 mg twice daily every 3 days; target dose: 1 mg/day (maximum: 4 mg/day)

Discontinuation of treatment: To discontinue, treatment should be withdrawn gradually. Decrease dose by 0.125 mg twice daily every 3 days until medication is completely withdrawn.

Elderly: Refer to adult dosing. Initiate with low doses and observe closely.

Pediatrics:

Seizure disorders (see Use): Oral:

Children <10 years or 30 kg:

Initial daily dose: 0.01-0.03 mg/kg/day (maximum: 0.05 mg/kg/day) given in 2-3 divided doses; increase by no more than 0.5 mg every third day until seizures are controlled or adverse effects seen.

Usual maintenance dose: 0.1-0.2 mg/kg/day divided 3 times/day; not to exceed 0.2 mg/kg/day.

Children >10 years or 30 kg: Refer to adult dosing.

Renal Impairment: Hemodialysis: Supplemental dose is not necessary.

Available Dosage Forms

Tablet: 0.5 mg, 1 mg, 2 mg

Tablet, orally-disintegrating [wafer]: 0.125 mg, 0.25 mg, 0.5 mg, 1 mg, 2 mg

Nursing Guidelines

Assessment: Assess effectiveness and interactions of other medications patient may be taking. Assess for signs of CNS depression. Assess for history of addiction; long-term use can result in dependence, abuse, or tolerance; periodically evaluate need for continued use. For inpatient use, institute safety measures and monitor effectiveness and adverse reactions. For outpatients, monitor therapeutic effectiveness and adverse reactions at beginning of therapy and periodically with long-term use. Taper dosage slowly when discontinuing. Assess knowledge/teach patient seizure precautions (if administered for seizures), appropriate use, interventions to reduce side effects, and adverse symptoms to report.

Monitoring Laboratory Tests: Renal function

Patient Education: Take exactly as directed; do not increase dose or frequency. Drug may cause physical and/or psychological dependence. While using this medication, do not use alcohol and other prescription or OTC medications (especially pain medications, sedatives, antihistamines, or hypnotics) without consulting prescriber. Maintain adequate hydration (2-3 L/day of fluids) unless instructed to restrict fluid intake. You may experience drowsiness, dizziness, or blurred vision (use caution when driving or engaging in tasks requiring alertness until response to drug is known); nausea, vomiting, loss of appetite, or dry mouth (small frequent meals, frequent mouth care, chewing gum, or sucking lozenges may help); or constipation (increased exercise, fluids, fruit, or fiber may help). If medication is used to control seizures, wear identification that you are taking an antiepileptic medication. Report excessive drowsiness, dizziness, fatigue, or impaired coordination; CNS changes (confusion, depression, increased sedation, excitation, headache, agitation, insomnia, or nightmares) or changes in cognition; respiratory difficulty or shortness of breath; changes in urinary pattern, changes in sexual activity; muscle cramping, weakness, tremors, or rigidity; ringing in ears or visual disturbances, excessive perspiration, or excessive GI symptoms (cramping, constipation, vomiting, anorexia); worsening of seizure activity, or loss of seizure control. **Pregnancy/ breast-feeding precautions:** Inform prescriber if you are or intend to become pregnant. Breast-feeding is not recommended.

Geriatric Considerations: Hepatic clearance may be decreased allowing accumulation of active drug. Also, metabolites of clonazepam are renally excreted and may accumulate in the elderly as renal function declines with age. Observe for signs of CNS and pulmonary toxicity.

Pregnancy Risk Factor: D

Pregnancy Issues: Benzodiazepines cross the placenta. The association between benzodiazepine exposure and malformations remains controversial. A number of types of malformation have been reported (oral cleft, inguinal hernia, cardiac defects, spina bifida, dysmorphic facial features, skeletal defects); however, confounding factors make a clear association difficult. Overall, the risk to the fetus may be low. Nonteratogenic effects (including neonatal flaccidity, respiratory and feeding problems, and withdrawal symptoms) during the postnatal period have also been reported with benzodiazepine use.

Lactation: Enters breast milk/not recommended

Breast-Feeding Considerations: Clonazepam enters breast milk; clinical effects on the infant include CNS depression, respiratory depression reported (no recommendation from the AAP).

Perioperative/Anesthesia/Other Concerns: Ethosuximide or valproic acid may be preferred for treatment of absence (petit mal) seizures. Flumazenil, a competitive benzodiazepine antagonist at the CNS receptor site, reverses benzodiazepine-induced CNS depression. Abrupt discontinuation after sustained use (generally >10 days) may cause withdrawal symptoms.

Administration

Oral: Orally-disintegrating tablet: Open pouch and peel back foil on the blister; do not push tablet through foil. Use dry hands to remove tablet and place in mouth. May be swallowed with or without water. Use immediately after removing from package.

Clonidine (KLON i deen)

U.S. Brand Names Catapres®; Catapres-TTS®; Duraclon™

Synonyms Clonidine Hydrochloride

Pharmacologic Category Alpha$_2$-Adrenergic Agonist

Medication Safety Issues

Sound-alike/look-alike issues:

Clonidine may be confused with Clomid®, clomiPHENE, clonazepam, clozapine, Klonopin™, Loniten®, quinidine

Catapres® may be confused with Cataflam®, Cetapred®, Combipres®

Transdermal patch may contain conducting metal (eg, aluminum); remove patch prior to MRI.

Use Management of mild to moderate hypertension; either used alone or in combination with other antihypertensives

Orphan drug: Duraclon™: For continuous epidural administration as adjunctive therapy with intraspinal opiates for treatment of cancer pain in patients tolerant to or unresponsive to intraspinal opiates

(Continued)

Clonidine *(Continued)*

Unlabeled/Investigational Use Heroin or nicotine withdrawal; severe pain; dysmenorrhea; vasomotor symptoms associated with menopause; ethanol dependence; prophylaxis of migraines; glaucoma; diabetes-associated diarrhea; impulse control disorder, attention-deficit/hyperactivity disorder (ADHD), clozapine-induced sialorrhea

Mechanism of Action Stimulates alpha$_2$-adrenoceptors in the brain stem, thus activating an inhibitory neuron, resulting in reduced sympathetic outflow from the CNS, producing a decrease in peripheral resistance, renal vascular resistance, heart rate, and blood pressure; epidural clonidine may produce pain relief at spinal presynaptic and postjunctional alpha$_2$-adrenoceptors by preventing pain signal transmission; pain relief occurs only for the body regions innervated by the spinal segments where analgesic concentrations of clonidine exist

Pharmacodynamics/Kinetics

Onset of action: Oral: 0.5-1 hour; Transdermal: Initial application: 2-3 days

Duration: 6-10 hours

Distribution: V_d: Adults: 2.1 L/kg; highly lipid soluble; distributes readily into extravascular sites

Protein binding: 20% to 40%

Metabolism: Extensively hepatic to inactive metabolites; undergoes enterohepatic recirculation

Bioavailability: 75% to 95%

Half-life elimination: Adults: Normal renal function: 6-20 hours; Renal impairment: 18-41 hours

Time to peak: 2-4 hours

Excretion: Urine (65%, 32% as unchanged drug); feces (22%)

Contraindications Hypersensitivity to clonidine hydrochloride or any component of the formulation

Warnings/Precautions Gradual withdrawal is needed (over 1 week for oral, 2-4 days with epidural) if drug needs to be stopped. Patients should be instructed about abrupt discontinuation (causes rapid increase in BP and symptoms of sympathetic overactivity). In patients on both a beta-blocker and clonidine where withdrawal of clonidine is necessary, withdraw the beta-blocker first and several days before clonidine. Then slowly decrease clonidine.

Use with caution in patients with severe coronary insufficiency; conduction disturbances; recent MI, CVA, or chronic renal insufficiency. Caution in sinus node dysfunction. Discontinue within 4 hours of surgery then restart as soon as possible after. Clonidine injection should be administered via a continuous epidural infusion device. Epidural clonidine is not recommended for perioperative, obstetrical, or postpartum pain. It is not recommended for use in patients with severe cardiovascular disease or hemodynamic instability. In all cases, the epidural may lead to cardiovascular instability (hypotension, bradycardia). Transdermal patch may contain conducting metal (eg, aluminum); remove patch prior to MRI. Due to the potential for altered electrical conductivity, remove transdermal patch before cardioversion or defibrillation. Clonidine cause significant CNS depression and xerostomia. Caution in patients with pre-existing CNS disease or depression. Elderly may be at greater risk for CNS depressive effects, favoring other agents in this population.

Drug Interactions

Antipsychotics: Concurrent use with antipsychotics (especially low potency) or nitroprusside may produce additive hypotensive effects

Beta-blockers: May potentiate bradycardia in patients receiving clonidine and may increase the rebound hypertension of withdrawal; discontinue beta-blocker several days before clonidine is tapered

CNS depressants: Sedative effects may be additive; monitor for increased effect; includes barbiturates, benzodiazepines, narcotic analgesics, ethanol, and other sedative agents

Cyclosporine: Clonidine may increase cyclosporine (and perhaps tacrolimus) serum concentrations; cyclosporine dosage adjustment may be needed

Hypoglycemic agents: Clonidine may decrease the symptoms of hypoglycemia; monitor patients receiving antidiabetic agents

Levodopa: Effects may be reduced by clonidine in some patients with Parkinson's disease (limited documentation); monitor

Local anesthetics: Epidural clonidine may prolong the sensory and motor blockade of local anesthetics

Mirtazapine: Antihypertensive effects of clonidine may be antagonized by mirtazapine (hypertensive urgency has been reported following addition of mirtazapine to clonidine); in addition, mirtazapine may potentially enhance the hypertensive response associated with abrupt clonidine withdrawal. Avoid this combination; consider an alternative agent.

Narcotic analgesics: May potentiate hypotensive effects of clonidine

Tricyclic antidepressants: Antihypertensive effects of clonidine may be antagonized by tricyclic antidepressants; in addition, tricyclic antidepressants may enhance the hypertensive response associated with abrupt clonidine withdrawal; avoid this combination; consider an alternative agent

Verapamil: Concurrent administration may be associated with hypotension and AV block in some patients (limited documentation); monitor

Nutritional/Herbal/Ethanol Interactions

Ethanol: Avoid ethanol (may increase CNS depression).

Herb/Nutraceutical: Avoid dong quai if using for hypertension (has estrogenic activity). Avoid ephedra, yohimbe, ginseng (may worsen hypertension). Avoid valerian, St John's wort, kava kava, gotu kola (may increase CNS depression).

Lab Interactions Increased sodium (S), transient serum glucose; decreased catecholamines (U); positive Coombs'

Adverse Reactions Incidence of adverse events is not always reported.

>10%:

Central nervous system: Drowsiness (35% oral, 12% transdermal), dizziness (16% oral, 2% transdermal)

Dermatologic: Transient localized skin reactions characterized by pruritus, and erythema (15% to 50% transdermal)

Gastrointestinal: Dry mouth (40% oral, 25% transdermal)

Neuromuscular & skeletal: Weakness (10% transdermal)

1% to 10%:

Cardiovascular: Orthostatic hypotension (3% oral)

Central nervous system: Headache (1% oral, 5% transdermal), sedation (3% transdermal), fatigue (6% transdermal), lethargy (3% transdermal), insomnia (2% transdermal), nervousness (3% oral, 1% transdermal), mental depression (1% oral)

Dermatologic: Rash (1% oral), allergic contact sensitivity (5% transdermal), localized vesiculation (7%), hyperpigmentation (5% at application site), edema (3%), excoriation (3%), burning (3%), throbbing, blanching (1%), papules (1%), and generalized macular rash (1%) has occurred in patients receiving transdermal clonidine.

Endocrine & metabolic: Sodium and water retention, sexual dysfunction (3% oral, 2% transdermal), impotence (3% oral, 2% transdermal), weakness (10% transdermal)

Gastrointestinal: Nausea (5% oral, 1% transdermal), vomiting (5% oral), anorexia and malaise (1% oral), constipation (10% oral, 1% transdermal), dry throat (2% transdermal), taste disturbance (1% transdermal), weight gain (1% oral)

Genitourinary: Nocturia (1% oral)

Hepatic: Liver function test (mild abnormalities, 1% oral)

Miscellaneous: Withdrawal syndrome (1% oral)

<1% (Limited to important or life-threatening): Abdominal pain, agitation, alopecia, angioedema, AV block, behavioral changes, blurred vision, bradycardia, chest pain, CHF, contact dermatitis (transdermal), CVA, delirium, depression, dryness of the eyes, ECG abnormalities, gynecomastia, hallucinations, hepatitis, increased sensitivity to ethanol, localized hypo- or hyperpigmentation (transdermal), nightmares, orthostatic symptoms, pseudo-obstruction, rash, Raynaud's phenomenon, syncope, tachycardia, thrombocytopenia, urinary retention, urticaria, vomiting, withdrawal syndrome

Overdosage/Toxicology Symptoms of overdose include bradycardia, CNS depression, hypothermia, diarrhea, respiratory depression, and apnea. Treatment is supportive and symptomatic. Naloxone may be utilized in treating CNS depression and/or apnea and should be given I.V., 0.4-2 mg, with repeated doses as needed up to a total of 10 mg, or as an infusion.

Dosing

Adults:

Acute hypertension (urgency): Oral: Initial 0.1-0.2 mg; may be followed by additional doses of 0.1 mg every hour, if necessary, to a maximum total dose of 0.6 mg

Unlabeled route of administration: Sublingual clonidine 0.1-0.2 mg twice daily may be effective in patients unable to take oral medication

(Continued)

Clonidine *(Continued)*

Hypertension:

Oral: Initial dose: 0.1 mg twice daily (maximum recommended dose: 2.4 mg/day); usual dose range (JNC 7): 0.1-0.8 mg/day in 2 divided doses

Transdermal: Apply once every 7 days; for initial therapy start with 0.1 mg and increase by 0.1 mg at 1- to 2-week intervals (dosages >0.6 mg do not improve efficacy); usual dose range (JNC 7): 0.1-0.3 mg once weekly

Note: If transitioning from oral to transdermal, overlap oral for 1-2 days. Transdermal route takes 2-3 days to achieve therapeutic effects.

Conversion from oral to transdermal:

Day 1: Place Catapres-TTS® 1; administer 100% of oral dose.
Day 2: Administer 50% of oral dose.
Day 3: Administer 25% of oral dose.
Day 4: Patch remains, no further oral supplement necessary.

Nicotine withdrawal symptoms: 0.1 mg twice daily to maximum of 0.4 mg/day for 3-4 weeks

Pain management: Epidural infusion: Starting dose: 30 mcg/hour; titrate as required for relief of pain or presence of side effects; minimal experience with doses >40 mcg/hour; should be considered an adjunct to intraspinal opiate therapy

Elderly: Oral: Initial: 0.1 mg once daily at bedtime, increase gradually as needed.

Pediatrics:

Hypertension: Oral: Initial: 5-10 mcg/kg/day in divided doses every 8-12 hours; increase gradually at 5- to 7-day intervals to 25 mcg/kg/day in divided doses every 6 hours; maximum: 0.9 mg/day.

Clonidine tolerance test (growth hormone release from pituitary): Oral: 0.15 mg/m^2 or 4 mcg/kg as single dose

ADHD (unlabeled use): Oral: Initial: 0.05 mg/day, increase every 3-7 days by 0.05 mg/day to 3-5 mcg/kg/day given in divided doses 3-4 times/day; maximum dose: 0.3-0.4 mg/day

Pain management: Epidural infusion: Reserved for patients with severe intractable pain, unresponsive to other analgesics or epidural or spinal opiates: Initial: 0.5 mcg/kg/hour; adjust with caution, based on clinical effect

Renal Impairment:

Cl_{cr} <10 mL/minute: Administer 50% to 75% of normal dose initially.

Not dialyzable (0% to 5%) via hemo- or peritoneal dialysis; supplemental dose is not necessary.

Available Dosage Forms

Injection, epidural solution, as hydrochloride [preservative free] (Duraclon™): 100 mcg/mL (10 mL); 500 mcg/mL (10 mL)

Patch, transdermal [once-weekly patch]:

Catapres-TTS®-1: 0.1 mg/24 hours (4s)
Catapres-TTS®-2: 0.2 mg/24 hours (4s)
Catapres-TTS®-3: 0.3 mg/24 hours (4s)

Tablet, as hydrochloride (Catapres®): 0.1 mg, 0.2 mg, 0.3 mg

Nursing Guidelines

Assessment: Use with caution and monitor closely in presence of pre-existing cardiovascular disease, hemodynamic instability, CNS disease, or depression. Assess potential for interactions with other pharmacological agents or herbal products patient may be taking (eg, potential for additive hypotension, bradycardia, CNS depression). Monitor results of laboratory tests, therapeutic effectiveness (according to purpose for use), and adverse response regularly during therapy. Advise patients using oral hypoglycemic agents or insulin to check glucose levels closely; clonidine may decrease the symptoms of hypoglycemia. When discontinuing, monitor blood pressure and taper dose slowly over 1 week or more. Teach patient proper use, possible side effects/appropriate interventions, and adverse symptoms to report.

Monitoring Laboratory Tests: Liver function tests

Dietary Considerations: Hypertensive patients may need to decrease sodium and calories in diet.

Patient Education: Do not take anything new (especially cough or cold remedies and sleep or stay-awake medications that might affect blood pressure) during treatment unless approved by prescriber. Take as directed, at bedtime. If using patch, check daily for correct placement. Do not skip doses or discontinue without consulting prescriber (this drug must be discontinued on a specific schedule to prevent serious adverse effects). Follow dietary restrictions as recommended by prescriber. This medication may cause drowsiness, dizziness, or impaired judgment (use caution when driving or engaging in tasks that require alertness until response is known); decreased libido or sexual function (will resolve when drug is discontinued); postural hypotension (use caution when rising from sitting or lying position or when climbing stairs); constipation (increase roughage, bulk in diet); or dry mouth or nausea (frequent mouth care or sucking lozenges may help). Report difficulty, pain, or burning on urination; increased nervousness or depression; sudden weight gain (weigh yourself in the same clothes at the same time of day once a week); unusual or persistent swelling of ankles, feet, or extremities; wet cough or respiratory difficulty; chest pain or palpitations; muscle weakness, fatigue, or pain; or other persistent side effects. **Pregnancy/breast-feeding precautions:** Inform prescriber if you are or intend to become pregnant. Breast-feeding is not recommended.

Geriatric Considerations: Because of its potential CNS adverse effects, clonidine may not be considered a drug of choice in the elderly. If the decision is to use clonidine, adjust dose based on response and adverse reactions.

Pregnancy Risk Factor: C

Pregnancy Issues: Clonidine crosses the placenta. Caution should be used with this drug due to the potential of rebound hypertension with abrupt discontinuation.

Lactation: Enters breast milk/not recommended

Breast-Feeding Considerations: Enters breast milk; AAP has NO RECOMMENDATION.

Perioperative/Anesthesia/Other Concerns: Abrupt withdrawal from clonidine therapy should be avoided. Clonidine patch has provided an important alternative to frequent daily dosing; may be used in patients unable to take oral medication. Transdermal therapy takes 2-3 days for therapeutic effects.

Administration

Oral: Do not discontinue clonidine abruptly. if needed, gradually reduce dose over 2-4 days to avoid rebound hypertension.

♦ Clonidine Hydrochloride *see* Clonidine *on page 433*

Clopidogrel (kloh PID oh grel)

U.S. Brand Names Plavix®

Synonyms Clopidogrel Bisulfate

Pharmacologic Category Antiplatelet Agent

Medication Safety Issues

Sound-alike/look-alike issues:

Plavix® may be confused with Elavil®, Paxil®

Use Reduce atherosclerotic events (myocardial infarction, stroke, vascular deaths) in patients with atherosclerosis documented by recent myocardial infarction (MI), recent stroke, or established peripheral arterial disease; acute coronary syndrome (unstable angina or non-Q-wave MI) managed medically or through PCI (with or without stent)

Unlabeled/Investigational Use In aspirin-allergic patients, prevention of coronary artery bypass graft closure (saphenous vein)

Mechanism of Action Blocks the ADP receptors, which prevent fibrinogen binding at that site and thereby reduce the possibility of platelet adhesion and aggregation

Pharmacodynamics/Kinetics

Onset of action: Inhibition of platelet aggregation detected: 2 hours after 300 mg administered; after second day of treatment with 50-100 mg/day

Peak effect: 50-100 mg/day: Bleeding time: 5-6 days; Platelet function: 3-7 days

Absorption: Well absorbed

Metabolism: Extensively hepatic via hydrolysis; biotransformation primarily to carboxyl acid derivative (inactive). The active metabolite that inhibits platelet aggregation has not been isolated.

Half-life elimination: ~8 hours

Time to peak, serum: ~1 hour

Excretion: Urine

Contraindications Hypersensitivity to clopidogrel or any component of the formulation; active pathological bleeding such as PUD or intracranial hemorrhage; coagulation disorders

Warnings/Precautions Use with caution in patients who may be at risk of increased bleeding, including patients with peptic ulcer disease, trauma, or surgery. Consider discontinuing 5 days before elective surgery. Use caution in concurrent treatment with other antiplatelet drugs; bleeding risk is increased. Use

(Continued)

Clopidogrel *(Continued)*

with caution in patients with severe liver disease (experience is limited). Cases of thrombotic thrombocytopenic purpura (usually occurring within the first 2 weeks of therapy) have been reported; urgent referral to a hematologist is required.

Drug Interactions **Substrate** (minor) of CYP1A2, 3A4; **Inhibits** CYP2C8/9 (weak)

Anticoagulants or other antiplatelet agents may increase the risk of bleeding. Use with heparin in acute coronary syndrome is clinically accepted.

Aspirin: Clopidogrel may increase the antiplatelet effect of aspirin; bleeding time is not prolonged relative to clopidogrel alone. Concurrent use is accepted in clinical practice (particularly in ACS treatment).

Atorvastatin: Atorvastatin may attenuate the effects of clopidogrel; monitor.

Drotrecogin alfa may increase the risk of bleeding.

Macrolide antibiotics: CYP3A4-inhibiting macrolides may attenuate the effects of clopidogrel. These include clarithromycin, erythromycin, and troleandomycin. Monitor.

NSAIDs: Concurrent use with clopidogrel may increase gastrointestinal effects, including GI blood loss. NSAID use was excluded in ACS trial (CURE).

Rifampin: Rifampin may increase the effects of clopidogrel; monitor.

Thrombolytics may increase the risk of bleeding.

Nutritional/Herbal/Ethanol Interactions Herb/Nutraceutical: Avoid cat's claw, dong quai, evening primrose, feverfew, garlic, ginger, ginkgo, red clover, horse chestnut, green tea, ginseng (all have additional antiplatelet activity).

Adverse Reactions As with all drugs which may affect hemostasis, bleeding is associated with clopidogrel. Hemorrhage may occur at virtually any site. Risk is dependent on multiple variables, including the concurrent use of multiple agents which alter hemostasis and patient susceptibility.

>10%: Gastrointestinal: The overall incidence of gastrointestinal events (including abdominal pain, vomiting, dyspepsia, gastritis and constipation) has been documented to be 27% compared to 30% in patients receiving aspirin.

3% to 10%:

- Cardiovascular: Chest pain (8%), edema (4%), hypertension (4%)
- Central nervous system: Headache (3% to 8%), dizziness (2% to 6%), depression (4%), fatigue (3%), general pain (6%)
- Dermatologic: Rash (4%), pruritus (3%)
- Endocrine & metabolic: Hypercholesterolemia (4%)
- Gastrointestinal: Abdominal pain (2% to 6%), dyspepsia (2% to 5%), diarrhea (2% to 5%), nausea (3%)
- Genitourinary: Urinary tract infection (3%)
- Hematologic: Bleeding (major 4%; minor 5%), purpura (5%), epistaxis (3%)
- Hepatic: Liver function test abnormalities (<3%; discontinued in 0.11%)
- Neuromuscular & skeletal: Arthralgia (6%), back pain (6%)
- Respiratory: Dyspnea (5%), rhinitis (4%), bronchitis (4%), cough (3%), upper respiratory infection (9%)
- Miscellaneous: Flu-like syndrome (8%)

1% to 3%:

- Cardiovascular: Atrial fibrillation, cardiac failure, palpitation, syncope
- Central nervous system: Fever, insomnia, vertigo, anxiety
- Dermatologic: Eczema
- Endocrine & metabolic: Gout, hyperuricemia
- Gastrointestinal: Constipation, GI hemorrhage, vomiting
- Genitourinary: Cystitis
- Hematologic: Hematoma, anemia
- Neuromuscular & skeletal: Arthritis, leg cramps, neuralgia, paresthesia, weakness
- Ocular: Cataract, conjunctivitis

<1% (Limited to important or life-threatening): Acute liver failure, agranulocytosis, allergic reaction, anaphylactoid reaction, angioedema, aplastic anemia, bilirubinemia, bronchospasm, bullous eruption, erythema multiforme, fatty liver, fever, granulocytopenia, hematuria, hemoptysis, hemothorax, hepatitis, hypersensitivity, hypochromic anemia, interstitial pneumonitis, intracranial hemorrhage (0.4%), ischemic necrosis, leukopenia, lichen planus, maculopapular rash, menorrhagia, neutropenia (0.05%), ocular hemorrhage, pancreatitis, pancytopenia, pulmonary hemorrhage, purpura, retroperitoneal bleeding, serum sickness, Stevens-Johnson syndrome, stomatitis, thrombocytopenia, thrombotic thrombocytopenic purpura (TTP), toxic epidermal necrolysis, urticaria, vasculitis

Overdosage/Toxicology

Symptoms of acute toxicity include vomiting, prostration, difficulty breathing, and gastrointestinal hemorrhage. Only one case of overdose with clopidogrel has been reported to date, no symptoms were reported with this case and no specific treatments were required.

Based on its pharmacology, platelet transfusions may be an appropriate treatment when attempting to reverse the effects of clopidogrel. After decontamination, treatment is symptomatic and supportive.

Dosing

Adults & Elderly:

Recent MI, recent stroke, or established arterial disease: Oral: 75 mg once daily

Acute coronary syndrome: Oral: Initial: 300 mg loading dose, followed by 75 mg once daily (in combination with aspirin 75-325 mg once daily). **Note:** A loading dose of 600 mg has been used in some investigations; limited research exists comparing the two doses.

Prevention of coronary artery bypass graft closure (saphenous vein): Aspirin-allergic patients (unlabeled use): Oral: Loading dose: 300 mg 6 hours following procedure; maintenance: 50-100 mg/day

Renal Impairment: No adjustment is necessary.

Hepatic Impairment: Dose adjustment may be necessary for patients with moderate to severe hepatic disease.

Available Dosage Forms Tablet [film coated]: 75 mg

Nursing Guidelines

Assessment: Assess effectiveness or interactions of other medications patient may be taking. Clopidogrel is a P450 enzyme inhibitor. Monitor for unusual bleeding. Monitor therapeutic effectiveness and instruct patient what symptoms to report.

Monitoring Laboratory Tests: Hemoglobin and hematocrit periodically

Dietary Considerations: May be taken without regard to meals.

Patient Education: Take as directed. May cause headache or dizziness; use caution when driving or engaging in tasks that require alertness until response to drug is known. It may take longer than usual to stop bleeding. Small frequent meals, frequent mouth care, sucking lozenges, or chewing gum may reduce nausea or vomiting. Mild analgesics may reduce arthralgia or back pain. Inform physicians and dentists that you are taking this medication prior to scheduling any surgery or dental procedure. Report immediately unusual or acute chest pain or respiratory difficulties; skin rash; unresolved bleeding, diarrhea, or GI distress; nosebleed; or acute headache. **Breast-feeding precaution:** Breast-feeding is not recommended.

Geriatric Considerations: Plasma levels of the primary clopidogrel metabolite were significantly higher in the elderly (≥75 years). This was not associated with changes in bleeding time or platelet aggregation. No dosage adjustment is recommended.

Pregnancy Risk Factor: B

Lactation: Excretion in breast milk unknown/not recommended

Perioperative/Anesthesia/Other Concerns: Withhold clopidogrel for 5-7 days prior to elective CABG surgery.

Administration

Storage: Store at 25°C (77°F); excursions permitted to 15°C to 3°C (59°F to 86°F).

♦ **Clopidogrel Bisulfate** *see* Clopidogrel *on page 437*

Clotrimazole (kloe TRIM a zole)

U.S. Brand Names Cruex® Cream [OTC]; Gyne-Lotrimin® 3 [OTC]; Lotrimin® AF Athlete's Foot Cream [OTC]; Lotrimin® AF Athlete's Foot Solution [OTC]; Lotrimin® AF Jock Itch Cream [OTC]; Mycelex®; Mycelex®-7 [OTC]; Mycelex® Twin Pack [OTC]

Pharmacologic Category Antifungal Agent, Oral Nonabsorbed; Antifungal Agent, Topical; Antifungal Agent, Vaginal

Medication Safety Issues

Sound-alike/look-alike issues:

Clotrimazole may be confused with co-trimoxazole

Lotrimin® may be confused with Lotrisone®, Otrivin®

Mycelex® may be confused with Myoflex®

(Continued)

Clotrimazole *(Continued)*

Use Treatment of susceptible fungal infections, including oropharyngeal candidiasis, dermatophytoses, superficial mycoses, and cutaneous candidiasis, as well as vulvovaginal candidiasis; limited data suggest that clotrimazole troches may be effective for prophylaxis against oropharyngeal candidiasis in neutropenic patients

Mechanism of Action Binds to phospholipids in the fungal cell membrane altering cell wall permeability resulting in loss of essential intracellular elements

Pharmacodynamics/Kinetics

Absorption: Topical: Negligible through intact skin

Time to peak, serum:

Oral topical (troche): Salivary levels occur within 3 hours following 30 minutes of dissolution time

Vaginal cream: High vaginal levels: 8-24 hours

Vaginal tablet: High vaginal levels: 1-2 days

Excretion: Feces (as metabolites)

Contraindications Hypersensitivity to clotrimazole or any component of the formulation

Warnings/Precautions Clotrimazole should not be used for treatment of systemic fungal infection; safety and effectiveness of clotrimazole lozenges (troches) in children <3 years of age have not been established; when using topical formulation, avoid contact with eyes

Drug Interactions Inhibits CYP1A2 (weak), 2A6 (weak), 2B6 (weak), 2C8/9 (weak), 2C19 (weak), 2D6 (weak), 2E1 (weak), 3A4 (moderate)

CYP3A4 substrates: Clotrimazole may increase the levels/effects of CYP3A4 substrates. Example substrates include benzodiazepines, calcium channel blockers, cyclosporine, mirtazapine, nateglinide, nefazodone, sildenafil (and other PDE-5 inhibitors), tacrolimus, and venlafaxine. Selected benzodiazepines (midazolam and triazolam), cisapride, ergot alkaloids, selected HMG-CoA reductase inhibitors (lovastatin and simvastatin), and pimozide are generally contraindicated with strong CYP3A4 inhibitors.

Adverse Reactions

Oral:

>10%: Hepatic: Abnormal liver function tests

1% to 10%:

Gastrointestinal: Nausea and vomiting may occur in patients on clotrimazole troches

Local: Mild burning, irritation, stinging to skin or vaginal area

Vaginal:

1% to 10%: Genitourinary: Vulvar/vaginal burning

<1% (Limited to important or life-threatening): Burning or itching of penis of sexual partner; polyuria; vulvar itching, soreness, edema, or discharge

Dosing

Adults & Elderly:

Oropharyngeal candidiasis: Oral:

Prophylaxis: 10 mg troche dissolved 3 times/day for the duration of chemotherapy or until steroids are reduced to maintenance levels

Treatment: 10 mg troche dissolved slowly 5 times/day for 14 consecutive days

Dermatophytosis, cutaneous candidiasis: Topical (cream, solution): Apply twice daily; if no improvement occurs after 4 weeks of therapy, re-evaluate diagnosis.

Vulvovaginal candidiasis: Intravaginal:

Cream (1%): Insert 1 applicatorful of 1% vaginal cream daily (preferably at bedtime) for 7 consecutive days.

Cream (2%): Insert 1 applicatorful of 2% vaginal cream daily (preferably at bedtime) for 3 consecutive days.

Tablet: Insert 100 mg/day for 7 days or 500 mg single dose.

Dermatologic infection (superficial): Topical (cream, solution): Apply to affected area twice daily (morning and evening) for 7 consecutive days.

Pediatrics:

Oropharyngeal candidiasis: Children >3 years: Refer to adult dosing.

Vaginal, Topical infections: Children >12 years: Refer to adult dosing.

Available Dosage Forms

Combination pack (Mycelex®-7): Vaginal tablet 100 mg (7s) and vaginal cream 1% (7 g)

Cream, topical: 1% (15 g, 30 g, 45 g)

Cruex®: 1% (15 g)
Lotrimin® AF Athlete's Foot: 1% (12 g, 24 g)
Lotrimin® AF Jock Itch: 1% (12 g)
Cream, vaginal: 2% (21 g)
Mycelex®-7: 1% (45 g)
Solution, topical: 1% (10 mL, 30 mL)
Lotrimin® AF Athlete's Foot: 1% (10 mL)
Tablet, vaginal (Gyne-Lotrimin® 3): 200 mg (3s)
Troche (Mycelex®): 10 mg

Nursing Guidelines

Assessment: Monitor laboratory values, effectiveness of treatment, and adverse reactions. Assess knowledge/teach patient appropriate use, interventions to reduce side effects, and adverse symptoms to report. Assess for opportunistic infection.

Monitoring Laboratory Tests: Periodic liver function during oral therapy with clotrimazole troche

Patient Education:

Oral (troche): Do not swallow oral medication whole; allow to dissolve slowly in mouth. You may experience nausea or vomiting (small frequent meals, frequent mouth care, chewing gum, or sucking lozenges may help). Report signs of opportunistic infection (eg, white plaques in mouth, fever, chills, perianal itching, vaginal itching or discharge, fatigue, unhealed wounds or sores).

Topical: Avoid contact with eyes. Wash hands before applying or wear gloves. Apply thin film to affected area. May apply porous dressing. Report persistent burning, swelling, itching, worsening of condition, or lack of response to therapy.

Vaginal: Wash hands before using. Insert full applicator into vagina gently and expel cream, or insert tablet into vagina, at bedtime. Wash applicator with soap and water following use. Remain lying down for 30 minutes following administration. Avoid intercourse during therapy (sexual partner may experience penile burning or itching). Report adverse reactions (eg, vulvar itching, frequent urination), worsening of condition, or lack of response to therapy. Contact prescriber if symptoms do not improve within 3 days or you do not feel well within 7 days. Do not use tampons until therapy is complete. Contact prescriber immediately if you experience abdominal pain, fever, or foul-smelling discharge.

Pregnancy/breast-feeding precautions: Inform prescriber if you are pregnant. Consult prescriber if breast-feeding.

Geriatric Considerations: Localized fungal infections frequently follow broad spectrum antimicrobial therapy. Specifically, oral and vaginal infections due to *Candida*.

Pregnancy Risk Factor: B (topical); C (troches)

Lactation: Excretion in breast milk unknown

Administration

Oral: Troche: Allow to dissolve slowly over 15-30 minutes.

♦ Coagulant Complex Inhibitor *see* Anti-inhibitor Coagulant Complex *on page 172*
♦ Coagulation Factor VIIa *see* Factor VIIa (Recombinant) *on page 700*

Cocaine (koe KANE)

Synonyms Cocaine Hydrochloride

Pharmacologic Category Local Anesthetic

Use Topical anesthesia for mucous membranes

Mechanism of Action Ester local anesthetic blocks both the initiation and conduction of nerve impulses by decreasing the neuronal membrane's permeability to sodium ions, which results in inhibition of depolarization with resultant blockade of conduction; interferes with the uptake of norepinephrine by adrenergic nerve terminals producing vasoconstriction

Pharmacodynamics/Kinetics Following topical administration to mucosa:

Onset of action: ~1 minute
Peak effect: ~5 minutes
Duration (dose dependent): ≥30 minutes; cocaine metabolites may appear in urine of neonates up to 5 days after birth due to maternal cocaine use shortly before birth
Absorption: Well absorbed through mucous membranes; limited by drug-induced vasoconstriction; enhanced by inflammation
Distribution: Enters breast milk
(Continued)

Cocaine *(Continued)*

Metabolism: Hepatic; major metabolites are ecgonine methyl ester and benzoyl ecgonine

Half-life elimination: 75 minutes

Excretion: Primarily urine (<10% as unchanged drug and metabolites)

Contraindications Hypersensitivity to cocaine or any component of the topical solution; ophthalmologic anesthesia (causing sloughing of the corneal epithelium); pregnancy (nonmedicinal use)

Warnings/Precautions For topical use only. Limit to office and surgical procedures only. Resuscitative equipment and drugs should be immediately available when any local anesthetic is used. Debilitated, elderly patients, acutely ill patients, and children should be given reduced doses consistent with their age and physical status. Use caution in patients with severely traumatized mucosa and sepsis in the region of the proposed application. Use with caution in patients with cardiovascular disease or a history of cocaine abuse. In patients being treated for cardiovascular complication of cocaine abuse, avoid beta-blockers for treatment.

Drug Interactions **Substrate** of CYP3A4 (major); **Inhibits** CYP2D6 (strong), 3A4 (weak)

Beta-blockers potentiate cocaine-induced coronary vasoconstriction (potentiate alpha-adrenergic effect of cocaine); avoid concurrent use.

CYP2D6 substrates: Cocaine may increase the levels/effects of CYP2D6 substrates. Example substrates include amphetamines, selected beta-blockers, dextromethorphan, fluoxetine, lidocaine, mirtazapine, nefazodone, paroxetine, risperidone, ritonavir, thioridazine, tricyclic antidepressants, and venlafaxine.

CYP2D6 prodrug substrates: Cocaine may decrease the levels/effects of CYP2D6 prodrug substrates. Example prodrug substrates include codeine, hydrocodone, oxycodone, and tramadol.

CYP3A4 inhibitors: May increase the levels/effects of cocaine. Example inhibitors include azole antifungals, clarithromycin, diclofenac, doxycycline, erythromycin, imatinib, isoniazid, nefazodone, nicardipine, propofol, protease inhibitors, quinidine, telithromycin, and verapamil.

Sympathomimetic amines may cause malignant arrhythmias; avoid concurrent use.

Adverse Reactions

>10%:

Central nervous system: CNS stimulation
Gastrointestinal: Loss of taste perception
Respiratory: Rhinitis, nasal congestion
Miscellaneous: Loss of smell

1% to 10%:

Cardiovascular: Heart rate (decreased) with low doses, tachycardia with moderate doses, hypertension, cardiomyopathy, cardiac arrhythmia, myocarditis, QRS prolongation, Raynaud's phenomenon, cerebral vasculitis, thrombosis, fibrillation (atrial), flutter (atrial), sinus bradycardia, CHF, pulmonary hypertension, sinus tachycardia, tachycardia (supraventricular), arrhythmia (ventricular), vasoconstriction

Central nervous system: Fever, nervousness, restlessness, euphoria, excitation, headache, psychosis, hallucinations, agitation, seizure, slurred speech, hyperthermia, dystonic reactions, cerebral vascular accident, vasculitis, clonic-tonic reactions, paranoia, sympathetic storm

Dermatologic: Skin infarction, pruritus, madarosis

Gastrointestinal: Nausea, anorexia, colonic ischemia, spontaneous bowel perforation

Genitourinary: Priapism, uterine rupture

Hematologic: Thrombocytopenia

Neuromuscular & skeletal: Chorea (extrapyramidal), paresthesia, tremor, fasciculations

Ocular: Mydriasis (peak effect at 45 minutes; may last up to 12 hours), sloughing of the corneal epithelium, ulceration of the cornea, iritis, chemosis

Renal: Myoglobinuria, necrotizing vasculitis

Respiratory: Tachypnea, nasal mucosa damage (when snorting), hyposmia, bronchiolitis obliterans organizing pneumonia

Miscellaneous: "Washed-out" syndrome

Overdosage/Toxicology Symptoms of overdose include anxiety, excitement, confusion, nausea, vomiting, headache, rapid pulse, irregular respiration, delirium, fever, seizures, respiratory arrest, hallucinations, dilated pupils, muscle spasms, sensory aberrations, and cardiac arrhythmias.

Fatal dose: Oral: 500 mg to 1.2 g; severe toxic effects have occurred with doses as low as 20 mg.

Since no specific antidote for cocaine exists, serious toxic effects are treated symptomatically.

Dosing

Adults: Topical application (ear, nose, throat, bronchoscopy): Dosage depends on the area to be anesthetized, tissue vascularity, technique of anesthesia, and individual patient tolerance; the lowest dose necessary to produce adequate anesthesia should be used; concentrations of 1% to 10% are used (not to exceed 1 mg/kg). Use reduced dosages for children, elderly, or debilitated patients.

Elderly: Refer to adult dosing; use with caution.

Available Dosage Forms

Powder, as hydrochloride: 1 g, 5 g, 25 g

Solution, topical, as hydrochloride: 4% [40 mg/mL] (4 mL, 10 mL); 10% [100 mg/mL] (4 mL, 10 mL)

Nursing Guidelines

Assessment: Assess other medications patient may be taking for interactions. Monitor adverse effects and teach patient adverse symptoms to report. **Pregnancy risk factor C/X (if nonmedicinal use).** Breast-feeding is contraindicated.

Patient Education: When used orally, do not take anything by mouth until full sensation returns. **Ocular:** Use caution when driving or engaging in tasks that require alert vision (mydriasis may last for several hours). At time of use or immediately thereafter, report any unusual cardiovascular, CNS, or respiratory symptoms. Following use, report skin irritation or eruption; alterations in vision, eye pain, or irritation; persistent GI effects; muscle or skeletal tremors, numbness, or rigidity; urinary or genital problems; or persistent fatigue. **Pregnancy/breast-feeding precautions:** Inform prescriber if you are pregnant. Do not breast-feed.

Pregnancy Risk Factor: C/X (nonmedicinal use)

Lactation: Enters breast milk/contraindicated

Breast-Feeding Considerations: Irritability, vomiting, diarrhea, tremors, and seizures have been reported in nursing infants.

Perioperative/Anesthesia/Other Concerns: Cocaine may also be associated with cerebral vascular accidents in young patients without any previous risk factors.

Administration

Storage: Store in well-closed, light-resistant containers.

Related Information

Local Anesthetics *on page 1854*

Substance Abuse and Anesthesia *on page 1832*

♦ Cocaine Hydrochloride *see* Cocaine *on page 441*

Codeine (KOE deen)

Synonyms Codeine Phosphate; Codeine Sulfate; Methylmorphine

Pharmacologic Category Analgesic, Narcotic; Antitussive

Medication Safety Issues

Sound-alike/look-alike issues:

Codeine may be confused with Cardene®, Cophene®, Cordran®, iodine, Lodine®

Use Treatment of mild to moderate pain; antitussive in lower doses; dextromethorphan has equivalent antitussive activity but has much lower toxicity in accidental overdose

Mechanism of Action Binds to opiate receptors in the CNS, causing inhibition of ascending pain pathways, altering the perception of and response to pain; causes cough supression by direct central action in the medulla; produces generalized CNS depression

Pharmacodynamics/Kinetics

Onset of action: Oral: 0.5-1 hour; I.M.: 10-30 minutes

Peak effect: Oral: 1-1.5 hours; I.M.: 0.5-1 hour

Duration: 4-6 hours

Absorption: Oral: Adequate

Distribution: Crosses placenta; enters breast milk

Protein binding: 7%

Metabolism: Hepatic to morphine (active)

(Continued)

Codeine *(Continued)*

Half-life elimination: 2.5-3.5 hours

Excretion: Urine (3% to 16% as unchanged drug, norcodeine, and free and conjugated morphine)

Contraindications Hypersensitivity to codeine or any component of the formulation; pregnancy (prolonged use or high doses at term)

Warnings/Precautions An opioid-containing analgesic regimen should be tailored to each patient's needs and based upon the type of pain being treated (acute versus chronic), the route of administration, degree of tolerance for opioids (naive versus chronic user), age, weight, and medical condition. The optimal analgesic dose varies widely among patients. Doses should be titrated to pain relief/prevention.

Use with caution in patients with hypersensitivity reactions to other phenanthrene derivative opioid agonists (morphine, hydrocodone, hydromorphone, levorphanol, oxycodone, oxymorphone); respiratory diseases including asthma, emphysema, COPD, or severe liver or renal insufficiency; some preparations contain sulfites which may cause allergic reactions; tolerance or drug dependence may result from extended use

Not recommended for use for cough control in patients with a productive cough; not recommended as an antitussive for children <2 years of age; the elderly may be particularly susceptible to the CNS depressant and confusion as well as constipating effects of narcotics

Not approved for I.V. administration (although this route has been used clinically). If given intravenously, must be given slowly and the patient should be lying down. Rapid intravenous administration of narcotics may increase the incidence of serious adverse effects, in part due to limited opportunity to assess response prior to administration of the full dose. Access to respiratory support should be immediately available

Drug Interactions **Substrate** of CYP2D6 (major), 3A4 (minor); **Inhibits** CYP2D6 (weak)

CYP2D6 inhibitors: May decrease the effects of codeine. Example inhibitors include chlorpromazine, delavirdine, fluoxetine, miconazole, paroxetine, pergolide, quinidine, quinine, ritonavir, and ropinirole.

Decreased effect with cigarette smoking

Increased toxicity: CNS depressants, phenothiazines, TCAs, other narcotic analgesics, guanabenz, MAO inhibitors, neuromuscular blockers

Nutritional/Herbal/Ethanol Interactions

Ethanol: Avoid or limit ethanol (may increase CNS depression).

Herb/Nutraceutical: St John's wort may decrease codeine levels. Avoid valerian, St John's wort, kava kava, gotu kola (may increase CNS depression).

Lab Interactions Increased aminotransferase [ALT (SGPT)/AST (SGOT)] (S)

Adverse Reactions

>10%:

- Central nervous system: Drowsiness
- Gastrointestinal: Constipation

1% to 10%:

- Cardiovascular: Tachycardia or bradycardia, hypotension
- Central nervous system: Dizziness, lightheadedness, false feeling of well being, malaise, headache, restlessness, paradoxical CNS stimulation, confusion
- Dermatologic: Rash, urticaria
- Gastrointestinal: Dry mouth, anorexia, nausea, vomiting
- Hepatic: Transaminases increased
- Genitourinary: Decreased urination, ureteral spasm
- Local: Burning at injection site
- Neuromuscular & skeletal: Weakness
- Ocular: Blurred vision
- Respiratory: Dyspnea
- Miscellaneous: Physical and psychological dependence, histamine release

<1% (Limited to important or life-threatening): Convulsions, hallucinations, insomnia, mental depression, nightmares

Overdosage/Toxicology Symptoms of overdose include CNS and respiratory depression, GI cramping, and constipation. Naloxone, 2 mg I.V. with repeat administration as necessary up to a total of 10 mg, can also be used to reverse toxic effects of the opiate.

Dosing

Adults & Elderly: Note: These are guidelines and do not represent the maximum doses that may be required in all patients. Doses should be titrated to pain relief/prevention. Doses >1.5 mg/kg body weight are not recommended.

Pain management (analgesic):

Oral, regular release: 30 mg every 4-6 hours as needed; patients with prior opiate exposure may require higher initial doses. Usual range: 15-120 mg every 4-6 hours as needed

Oral, controlled release formulation (Codeine Contin®, not available in U.S.): 50-300 mg every 12 hours. **Note:** A patient's codeine requirement should be established using prompt release formulations; conversion to long acting products may be considered when chronic, continuous treatment is required. Higher dosages should be reserved for use only in opioid-tolerant patients.

I.M., SubQ: 30 mg every 4-6 hours as needed; patients with prior opiate exposure may require higher initial doses. Usual range: 15-120 mg every 4-6 hours as needed; more frequent dosing may be needed

Cough (antitussive): Oral (for nonproductive cough): 10-20 mg/dose every 4-6 hours as needed; maximum: 120 mg/day

Pediatrics: Note: These are guidelines and do not represent the maximum doses that may be required in all patients. Doses should be titrated to pain relief/prevention. Doses >1.5 mg/kg body weight are not recommended.

Analgesic: Oral, I.M., SubQ: Children: 0.5-1 mg/kg/dose every 4-6 hours as needed; maximum: 60 mg/dose

Antitussive: Oral (for nonproductive cough): Children: 1-1.5 mg/kg/day in divided doses every 4-6 hours as needed: Alternative dose according to age:

2-6 years: 2.5-5 mg every 4-6 hours as needed; maximum: 30 mg/day

6-12 years: 5-10 mg every 4-6 hours as needed; maximum: 60 mg/day

Renal Impairment:

Cl_{cr} 10-50 mL/minute: Administer 75% of dose.

Cl_{cr} <10 mL/minute: Administer 50% of dose.

Hepatic Impairment: Dosing adjustment is probably necessary in hepatic insufficiency.

Available Dosage Forms

Injection, as phosphate: 15 mg/mL (2 mL); 30 mg/mL (2 mL) [contains sodium metabisulfite]

Solution, oral, as phosphate: 15 mg/5 mL (5 mL, 500 mL) [strawberry flavor]

Tablet, controlled release (Codeine Contin®) [not available in U.S.]: 50 mg, 100 mg, 150 mg, 200 mg

Tablet, as phosphate: 30 mg, 60 mg

Tablet, as sulfate: 15 mg, 30 mg, 60 mg

Nursing Guidelines

Assessment: Assess other medications patient may be taking for possible additive or adverse interactions. Monitor for effectiveness of pain relief, for signs of overdose, vital signs and CNS status, and adverse reactions at beginning of therapy and at regular intervals with long-term use. May cause physical and/or psychological dependence. For inpatients, implement safety measures. Assess knowledge/teach patient appropriate use (if self-administered). Teach patient to monitor for adverse reactions, adverse reactions to report, and appropriate interventions to reduce side effects.

Patient Education: If self-administered, use exactly as directed; do not increase dose or frequency. Drug may cause physical and/or psychological dependence. While using this medication, do not use alcohol and other prescription or OTC medications (especially sedatives, tranquilizers, antihistamines, or pain medications) without consulting prescriber. Maintain adequate hydration (2-3 L/day of fluids) unless instructed to restrict fluid intake. May cause dizziness, drowsiness, confusion, agitation, impaired coordination, or blurred vision (use caution when driving, climbing stairs, or changing position - rising from sitting or lying to standing, or when engaging in tasks requiring alertness until response to drug is known); nausea or vomiting, or loss of appetite (frequent mouth care, small frequent meals, sucking lozenges, or chewing gum may help); or constipation (increased exercise, fluids, fruit, or fiber may help; if unresolved, consult prescriber about use of stool softeners). Report confusion, insomnia, excessive nervousness, excessive sedation or drowsiness, or shakiness; acute GI upset; respiratory difficulty or shortness of breath; facial flushing, rapid heartbeat, or palpitations; urinary difficulty; unusual

(Continued)

Codeine *(Continued)*

muscle weakness; or vision changes. **Pregnancy/breast-feeding precautions:** Inform prescriber if you are or intend to become pregnant. If you are breast-feeding, take medication immediately after breast-feeding or 3-4 hours prior to next feeding.

Geriatric Considerations: The elderly may be particularly susceptible to CNS depression and confusion as well as the constipating effects of narcotics.

Pregnancy Risk Factor: C/D (prolonged use or high doses at term)

Lactation: Enters breast milk/use caution (AAP rates "compatible")

Perioperative/Anesthesia/Other Concerns: The 2002 ACCM/SCCM guidelines for analgesia (critically-ill adult) recommend against using codeine because of its lack of potency, histamine release (may cause hypotension), potential accumulation of active metabolites. The guidelines recommend fentanyl in patients who need immediate pain relief because of its rapid onset of action; fentanyl or hydromorphone is preferred in patients who are hypotensive or have renal dysfunction. Morphine or hydromorphone is recommended for intermittent, scheduled therapy. Both have a longer duration of action requiring less frequent administration.

Administration

Storage: Store injection between 15°C to 30°C, avoid freezing. Do not use if injection is discolored or contains a precipitate. Protect injection from light.

Related Information

Acute Postoperative Pain *on page 1742*
Narcotic / Opioid Analgesics *on page 1880*

- ♦ **Codeine and Acetaminophen** *see* Acetaminophen and Codeine *on page 68*
- ♦ **Codeine and Guaifenesin** *see* Guaifenesin and Codeine *on page 835*
- ♦ **Codeine Phosphate** *see* Codeine *on page 443*
- ♦ **Codeine Sulfate** *see* Codeine *on page 443*
- ♦ **Co-Gesic®** *see* Hydrocodone and Acetaminophen *on page 867*
- ♦ **Colace® [OTC]** *see* Docusate *on page 560*
- ♦ **Colace® Adult/Children Suppositories [OTC]** *see* Glycerin *on page 826*
- ♦ **Colace® Infant/Children Suppositories [OTC]** *see* Glycerin *on page 826*

Colchicine (KOL chi seen)

Pharmacologic Category Colchicine

Medication Safety Issues

High alert medication: The Institute for Safe Medication Practices (ISMP) includes this medication among its list of drugs which have a heightened risk of causing significant patient harm when used in error.

Use Treatment of acute gouty arthritis attacks and prevention of recurrences of such attacks

Unlabeled/Investigational Use Primary biliary cirrhosis; management of familial Mediterranean fever; pericarditis

Mechanism of Action Decreases leukocyte motility, decreases phagocytosis in joints and lactic acid production, thereby reducing the deposition of urate crystals that perpetuates the inflammatory response

Pharmacodynamics/Kinetics

Onset of action: Oral: Pain relief: ~12 hours if adequately dosed

Distribution: Concentrates in leukocytes, kidney, spleen, and liver; does not distribute in heart, skeletal muscle, and brain

Protein binding: 10% to 31%

Metabolism: Partially hepatic via deacetylation

Half-life elimination: 12-30 minutes; End-stage renal disease: 45 minutes

Time to peak, serum: Oral: 0.5-2 hours, declining for the next 2 hours before increasing again due to enterohepatic recycling

Excretion: Primarily feces; urine (10% to 20%)

Contraindications Hypersensitivity to colchicine or any component of the formulation; severe renal, gastrointestinal, hepatic, or cardiac disorders; blood dyscrasias; pregnancy (parenteral)

Warnings/Precautions Use with caution in debilitated patients or elderly patients; use caution in patients with mild-to-moderate cardiac, GI, renal, or liver disease. Severe local irritation can occur following SubQ or I.M. administration. Dosage reduction is recommended in patients who develop weakness or gastrointestinal symptoms (anorexia, diarrhea, nausea, vomiting) related to drug therapy.

Intravenous: Use only with extreme caution; potential for serious, life-threatening complications. Should not be administered to patients with renal insufficiency, hepatobiliary obstruction, patients >70 years of age, or recent oral colchicine use. Should be reserved for hospitalized patients who are under the care of a physician experienced in the use of intravenous colchicine.

Drug Interactions **Substrate** of CYP3A4 (major); **Induces** CYP2C8/9 (weak), 2E1 (weak), 3A4 (weak)

Cyclosporine: Concurrent use with colchicine may increase toxicity of colchicine.

CYP3A4 inhibitors: May increase the levels/effects of colchicine. Example inhibitors include azole antifungals, diclofenac, doxycycline, imatinib, isoniazid, nefazodone, nicardipine, propofol, protease inhibitors, quinidine, telithromycin, and verapamil.

Macrolide antibiotics (clarithromycin, erythromycin, troleandomycin): May decrease the metabolism of colchicine resulting in severe colchicine toxicity. Avoid, if possible.

Telithromycin: May decrease the metabolism of colchicine resulting in colchicine toxicity. Avoid, if possible.

Verapamil: May increase colchicine toxicity (especially nephrotoxicity).

Nutritional/Herbal/Ethanol Interactions

Ethanol: Avoid ethanol.

Food: Cyanocobalamin (vitamin B_{12}): Malabsorption of the substrate. May result in macrocytic anemia or neurologic dysfunction.

Herb/Nutraceutical: Vitamin B_{12} absorption may be decreased by colchicine.

Lab Interactions May cause false-positive results in urine tests for erythrocytes or hemoglobin

Adverse Reactions

>10%: Gastrointestinal: Nausea, vomiting, diarrhea, abdominal pain

1% to 10%:

Dermatologic: Alopecia

Gastrointestinal: Anorexia

<1% (Limited to important or life-threatening): Agranulocytosis, aplastic anemia, arrhythmia (with intravenous administration), bone marrow suppression, hepatotoxicity

Overdosage/Toxicology Symptoms of overdose include acute nausea, vomiting, abdominal pain, shock, kidney damage, muscle weakness, burning in throat, watery to bloody diarrhea, hypotension, anuria, cardiovascular collapse, delirium, convulsions, and respiratory paralysis. Treatment includes gastric lavage and measures to prevent shock, hemodialysis or peritoneal dialysis. Atropine and morphine may relieve abdominal pain.

Dosing

Adults:

Familial Mediterranean fever (unlabeled use): Prophylaxis: Oral: 1-2 mg daily in divided doses (occasionally reduced to 0.6 mg/day in patients with GI intolerance)

Gouty arthritis:

Prophylaxis of acute attacks: Oral: 0.6 mg twice daily; initial and/or subsequent dosage may be decreased (ie, 0.6 mg once daily) in patients at risk of toxicity or in those who are intolerant (including weakness, loose stools, or diarrhea); range: 0.6 mg every other day to 0.6 mg 3 times/day

Acute attacks:

Oral: Initial: 0.6-1.2 mg, followed by 0.6 every 1-2 hours; some clinicians recommend a maximum of 3 doses; more aggressive approaches have recommended a maximum dose of up to 6 mg. Wait at least 3 days before initiating another course of therapy

I.V.: Initial: 1-2 mg, then 0.5 mg every 6 hours until response, not to exceed total dose of 4 mg. If pain recurs, it may be necessary to administer additional daily doses. The amount of colchicine administered intravenously in an acute treatment period (generally ~1 week) should not exceed a total dose of 4 mg. Do not administer more colchicine by any route for at least 7 days after a full course of I.V. therapy.

Note: Many experts would avoid use because of potential for serious, life-threatening complications. Should not be administered to patients with renal insufficiency, hepatobiliary obstruction, patients >70 years of age, or recent oral colchicine use. Should be reserved for hospitalized patients who are under the care of a physician experienced in the use of intravenous colchicine.

(Continued)

Colchicine *(Continued)*

Surgery: Gouty arthritis, prophylaxis of recurrent attacks: Oral: 0.6 mg/day or every other day; patients who are to undergo surgical procedures may receive 0.6 mg 3 times/day for 3 days before and 3 days after surgery

Primary biliary cirrhosis (unlabeled use): Oral: 0.6 mg twice daily

Pericarditis (unlabeled use): Oral: 0.6 mg twice daily

Elderly: Refer to adult dosing. Reduce maintenance/prophylactic dose by 50% in individuals >70 years.

Pediatrics: Prophylaxis of familial Mediterranean fever (unlabeled use): Oral:

Children ≤5 years: 0.5 mg/day

Children >5 years: 1-1.5 mg/day in 2-3 divided doses

Renal Impairment:

Gouty arthritis, acute attacks: Oral: Specific dosing recommendations not available from the manufacturer:

Prophylaxis:

Cl_{cr} 35-49 mL/minute: 0.6 mg once daily

Cl_{cr} 10-34 mL/minute: 0.6 mg every 2-3 days

Cl_{cr} <10 mL/minute: Avoid chronic use of colchicine. Use in serious renal impairment is contraindicated by the manufacturer.

Treatment: Cl_{cr} <10 mL/minute: Use in serious renal impairment is contraindicated by the manufacturer. If a decision is made to use colchicine, decrease dose by 75%.

Peritoneal dialysis: Supplemental dose is not necessary

Hepatic Impairment: Avoid in hepatobiliary dysfunction and in patients with hepatic disease.

Available Dosage Forms

Injection, solution: 0.5 mg/mL (2 mL)

Tablet: 0.6 mg

Nursing Guidelines

Assessment: Assess effectiveness and interactions of other medications patient may be taking. **I.V.:** Monitor therapeutic effectiveness, laboratory values, and adverse reactions at beginning of therapy and periodically with long-term use. Assess knowledge/teach patient appropriate use, interventions to reduce side effects, and adverse symptoms to report.

Monitoring Laboratory Tests: CBC and renal function on a regular basis

Dietary Considerations: May need to supplement with vitamin B_{12}.

Patient Education: Take as directed; do not exceed recommended dosage. Consult prescriber about a low-purine diet. Maintain adequate hydration (2-3 L/day of fluids) unless instructed to restrict fluid intake. Do not use alcohol or aspirin-containing medication without consulting prescriber. You may experience nausea, vomiting, or anorexia (small frequent meals, frequent mouth care, chewing gum, or sucking lozenges may help); hair loss (reversible). Stop medication and report to prescriber if severe vomiting, watery or bloody diarrhea, or abdominal pain occurs. Report muscle tremors or weakness; fatigue; easy bruising or bleeding; yellowing of eyes or skin; or pale stool or dark urine. **Pregnancy/breast-feeding precautions:** Inform prescriber if you are or intend to become pregnant. Consult prescriber if breast-feeding.

Geriatric Considerations: Colchicine appears to be more toxic in the elderly, particularly in the presence of renal, gastrointestinal, or cardiac disease. The most predictable oral side effects are (gastrointestinal) vomiting, abdominal pain, and nausea. If colchicine is stopped at this point, other more severe adverse effects may be avoided, such as bone marrow suppression, peripheral neuritis, etc.

Pregnancy Risk Factor: C (oral); D (parenteral)

Lactation: Enters breast milk/use caution (AAP rates "compatible")

Administration

Oral: Administer tablet orally with water and maintain adequate fluid intake.

I.V.: Injection should be made over 2-5 minutes into tubing of free-flowing I.V. with compatible fluid. Do not administer I.M. or SubQ; severe local irritation can occur following SubQ or I.M. administration. Extravasation can cause tissue irritation.

Compatibility: I.V. colchicine is **incompatible** with dextrose or I.V. solutions with preservatives.

Storage: Protect tablets from light.

♦ **Colistin, Neomycin, Hydrocortisone, and Thonzonium** *see* Neomycin, Colistin, Hydrocortisone, and Thonzonium *on page 1210*

♦ Collagen *see* Collagen Hemostat *on page 449*
♦ Collagen Absorbable Hemostat *see* Collagen Hemostat *on page 449*

Collagen Hemostat (KOL la jen HEE moe stat)

U.S. Brand Names Avitene®; Avitene® Flour; Avitene® Ultrafoam; Avitene® UltraWrap™; EndoAvitene®; Helistat®; Helitene®; Instat™; Instat™ MCH; SyringeAvitene™

Synonyms Collagen; Collagen Absorbable Hemostat; MCH; Microfibrillar Collagen Hemostat

Pharmacologic Category Hemostatic Agent

Medication Safety Issues

Sound-alike/look-alike issues:

Avitene® may be confused with Ativan®

Over 100 reports of paralysis or other neural deficits have been received by the FDA, attributable to collagen hemostat-associated neuronal impingement; see Warnings/Precautions

Use Adjunct to hemostasis when control of bleeding by ligature is ineffective or impractical

Mechanism of Action Collagen hemostat is an absorbable topical hemostatic agent prepared from purified bovine corium collagen and shredded into fibrils. Physically, microfibrillar collagen hemostat yields a large surface area. Chemically, it is collagen with hydrochloric acid noncovalently bound to some of the available amino groups in the collagen molecules. When in contact with a bleeding surface, collagen hemostat attracts platelets which adhere to its fibrils and undergo the release phenomenon. This triggers aggregation of the platelets into thrombi in the interstices of the fibrous mass, initiating the formation of a physiologic platelet plug.

Pharmacodynamics/Kinetics

Onset: Hemostasis: 2-5 minutes

Absorption: ≥8 weeks

Contraindications Hypersensitivity to any component of the formulation; products of bovine origin; closure of skin incisions, contaminated wounds; application to bone surfaces to which prosthetic materials are attached with methylmethacrylate adhesives

Warnings/Precautions Pain, numbness, or paralysis have been reported if used near a bony or neural space and left inside patient; use minimum amount necessary to achieve hemostasis. Remove as much of agent as possible after hemostasis is achieved. Do not leave in a contaminated or infected space. Fragments of MCH may pass through filters of blood scavenging systems; avoid reintroduction of blood from operative sites treated with MCH. Not intended to treat systemic coagulation disorders. Not for use when origin of bleeding is unknown.

Drug Interactions No data reported

Adverse Reactions Frequency not defined.

Miscellaneous: Adhesion formation, allergic reaction, edema, foreign body reaction, hematoma, inflammation, potentiation of infection

Postmarketing and/or case reports: Numbness, pain, paralysis, subgaleal seroma; alveolalgia and transient laryngospasm with dental use

Dosing

Adults & Elderly: Hemostasis: Topical: Apply dry directly to source of bleeding; remove excess material after ~10-15 minutes

Available Dosage Forms

Pad (Instat™) [bovine derived]: 1 inch x 2 inch (24s); 3 inch x 4 inch (24s)

Powder:

Avitene® Flour [microfibrillar product, bovine derived]: 0.5 g, 1 g, 5 g

Helitene® [bovine derived]: 0.5 g, 1 g

Instat™ MCH [microfibrillar product, bovine derived]: 0.5 g, 1 g

SyringeAvitene™ [microfibrillar product, bovine derived, prefilled syringe]: 1 g

Sheet:

Avitene® [microfibrillar product, bovine derived, nonwoven web]: 35 mm x 35 mm (1s); 70 mm x 35 mm (6s, 12s); 70 mm x 70 mm (6s, 12s)

EndoAvitene® [microfibrillar product, bovine derived, preloaded applicator]: 5 mm diameter (6s); 10 mm diameter (6s)

Sponge:

Avitene® Ultrafoam [microfibrillar product, bovine derived]: 2 cm x 6.25 cm x 7 mm (12s); 8 cm x 6.25 cm x 1 cm (6s); 8 cm x 12.5 cm x 1 cm (6s); 8 cm x 12.5 cm x 3 mm (6s)

(Continued)

Collagen Hemostat *(Continued)*

Avitene® UltraWrap™ [microfibrillar product, bovine derived]: 8 cm x 12.5 cm (6s)

Helistat® [bovine derived]: 0.5 inch x 1 inch x 7 mm (18s) [packaged as 3 strips of 6 sponges]; 3 inch x 4 inch x 5 inch (10s)

Administration

Storage: Store at controlled room temperature. Inactivated by autoclaving; do not resterilize. Do not use if package is damaged. Do not reuse after opening.

- ♦ **Colocort®** *see* Hydrocortisone *on page 873*
- ♦ **Coly-Mycin® S** *see* Neomycin, Colistin, Hydrocortisone, and Thonzonium *on page 1210*
- ♦ **CombiPatch®** *see* Estradiol and Norethindrone *on page 655*
- ♦ **Combivent®** *see* Ipratropium and Albuterol *on page 959*
- ♦ **Commit™ [OTC]** *see* Nicotine *on page 1223*
- ♦ **Compazine** *see* Prochlorperazine *on page 1412*
- ♦ **Compound E** *see* Cortisone *on page 451*
- ♦ **Compound F** *see* Hydrocortisone *on page 873*
- ♦ **Compound S** *see* Zidovudine *on page 1732*
- ♦ **Compound S, Abacavir, and Lamivudine** *see* Abacavir, Lamivudine, and Zidovudine *on page 58*
- ♦ **Compoz® Nighttime Sleep Aid [OTC]** *see* DiphenhydrAMINE *on page 546*
- ♦ **Compro™** *see* Prochlorperazine *on page 1412*
- ♦ **Comtrex® Non-Drowsy Cold and Cough Relief [OTC]** *see* Acetaminophen, Dextromethorphan, and Pseudoephedrine *on page 73*
- ♦ **Comtrex® Sore Throat Maximum Strength [OTC]** *see* Acetaminophen *on page 65*
- ♦ **Concerta®** *see* Methylphenidate *on page 1137*
- ♦ **Conray®** *see* Iothalamate Meglumine *on page 956*
- ♦ **Conray® 30** *see* Iothalamate Meglumine *on page 956*
- ♦ **Conray® 43** *see* Iothalamate Meglumine *on page 956*
- ♦ **Contac® Severe Cold and Flu/Non-Drowsy [OTC]** *see* Acetaminophen, Dextromethorphan, and Pseudoephedrine *on page 73*
- ♦ **Contact® Cold [OTC]** *see* Pseudoephedrine *on page 1436*
- ♦ **Copaxone®** *see* Glatiramer Acetate *on page 812*
- ♦ **Copegus®** *see* Ribavirin *on page 1475*
- ♦ **Copolymer-1** *see* Glatiramer Acetate *on page 812*
- ♦ **Cordarone®** *see* Amiodarone *on page 130*
- ♦ **Coreg®** *see* Carvedilol *on page 321*
- ♦ **Corlopam®** *see* Fenoldopam *on page 711*
- ♦ **Correctol® Tablets [OTC]** *see* Bisacodyl *on page 245*
- ♦ **Cortaid® Intensive Therapy [OTC]** *see* Hydrocortisone *on page 873*
- ♦ **Cortaid® Maximum Strength [OTC]** *see* Hydrocortisone *on page 873*
- ♦ **Cortaid® Sensitive Skin [OTC]** *see* Hydrocortisone *on page 873*
- ♦ **Cortef®** *see* Hydrocortisone *on page 873*
- ♦ **Corticool® [OTC]** *see* Hydrocortisone *on page 873*

Corticotropin (kor ti koe TROE pin)

U.S. Brand Names H.P. Acthar® Gel

Synonyms ACTH; Adrenocorticotropic Hormone; Corticotropin, Repository

Pharmacologic Category Corticosteroid, Systemic

Use Acute exacerbations of multiple sclerosis; diagnostic aid in adrenocortical insufficiency, severe muscle weakness in myasthenia gravis

Cosyntropin is preferred over corticotropin for diagnostic test of adrenocortical insufficiency (cosyntropin is less allergenic and test is shorter in duration)

Mechanism of Action Stimulates the adrenal cortex to secrete adrenal steroids (including hydrocortisone, cortisone), androgenic substances, and a small amount of aldosterone

Contraindications Hypersensitivity to corticotropin or any component of the formulation; scleroderma; osteoporosis; systemic fungal infections; ocular herpes simplex; peptic ulcer

Drug Interactions

Decreased effect: Can antagonize the effect of anticholinesterases (eg, neostigmine) in patients with myasthenia gravis

Decreased corticotropin levels with barbiturates

Adverse Reactions Frequency not defined.

Central nervous system: Insomnia, nervousness
Dermatologic: Hirsutism
Endocrine & metabolic: Diabetes mellitus
Gastrointestinal: Increased appetite, indigestion
Neuromuscular & skeletal: Arthralgia
Ocular: Cataracts
Respiratory: Epistaxis

Dosing

Adults & Elderly:

Acute exacerbation of multiple sclerosis: I.M.: 80-120 units/day for 2-3 weeks

Repository injection: I.M., SubQ: 40-80 units every 24-72 hours

Pediatrics:

Anti-inflammatory/immunosuppressant: I.M.: 0.8 units/kg/day or 25 units/m^2/day divided every 12-24 hours

Infantile spasms: Various regimens have been used. Some neurologists recommend low-dose ACTH (5-40 units/day) for short periods (1-6 weeks), while others recommend larger doses of ACTH (40-160 units/day) for long periods of treatment (3-12 months). Well designed comparative dosing studies are needed. Example of low dose regimen:

Initial: I.M.: 20 units/day for 2 weeks, if patient responds, taper and discontinue; if patient does not respond, increase dose to 30 units/day for 4 weeks then taper and discontinue

Usual dosage range: I.M.: 20-40 units/day or 5-8 units/kg/day in 1-2 divided doses; range: 5-160 units/day

Note: Oral prednisone (2 mg/kg/day) was as effective as I.M. ACTH gel (20 units/day) in controlling infantile spasms

Available Dosage Forms Injection, gelatin: 80 units/mL (5 mL)

Nursing Guidelines

Dietary Considerations: May increase renal loss of potassium, calcium, zinc, and vitamin C; may need to increase dietary intake or give supplements.

Patient Education: Do not abruptly discontinue the medication; your physician may want you to follow a low salt/potassium rich diet; tell physician you are using this drug before having skin tests, before surgery, or emergency treatment if you get a serious infection or injury

Pregnancy Risk Factor: C

Administration

Storage: Store in the refrigerator. Warm gel before administration.

♦ Corticotropin, Repository *see* Corticotropin *on page 450*
♦ Cortifoam® *see* Hydrocortisone *on page 873*
♦ Cortisol *see* Hydrocortisone *on page 873*

Cortisone (KOR ti sone)

Synonyms Compound E; Cortisone Acetate

Pharmacologic Category Corticosteroid, Systemic

Medication Safety Issues

Sound-alike/look-alike issues:

Cortisone may be confused with Cortizone®

Use Management of adrenocortical insufficiency

Mechanism of Action Decreases inflammation by suppression of migration of polymorphonuclear leukocytes and reversal of increased capillary permeability

Pharmacodynamics/Kinetics

Onset of action: Peak effect: Oral: ~2 hours; I.M.: 20-48 hours
Duration: 30-36 hours
Absorption: Slow
Distribution: Muscles, liver, skin, intestines, and kidneys; crosses placenta; enters breast milk
Metabolism: Hepatic to inactive metabolites
Half-life elimination: 0.5-2 hours; End-stage renal disease: 3.5 hours
Excretion: Urine and feces

Contraindications Hypersensitivity to cortisone acetate or any component of the formulation; serious infections, except septic shock or tuberculous meningitis; administration of live virus vaccines; pregnancy

(Continued)

Cortisone *(Continued)*

Warnings/Precautions Use with caution in patients with hypothyroidism, cirrhosis, hypertension, CHF, ulcerative colitis, thromboembolic disorders, osteoporosis, convulsive disorders, peptic ulcer, diabetes mellitus, myasthenia gravis; prolonged therapy (>5 days) of pharmacologic doses of corticosteroids may lead to hypothalamic-pituitary-adrenal suppression, the degree of adrenal suppression varies with the degree and duration of glucocorticoid therapy; this must be taken into consideration when taking patients off steroids

Drug Interactions

Decreased effect:

- Barbiturates, phenytoin, rifampin may decrease cortisone effects
- Live virus vaccines
- Anticholinesterase agents may decrease effect
- Cortisone may decrease warfarin effects
- Cortisone may decrease effects of salicylates

Increased effect: Estrogens (increase cortisone effects)

Increased toxicity:

- Cortisone + NSAIDs may increase ulcerogenic potential
- Cortisone may increase potassium deletion due to diuretics

Nutritional/Herbal/Ethanol Interactions Food: Limit caffeine intake.

Adverse Reactions

>10%:

- Central nervous system: Insomnia, nervousness
- Gastrointestinal: Increased appetite, indigestion

1% to 10%:

- Dermatologic: Hirsutism
- Endocrine & metabolic: Diabetes mellitus
- Neuromuscular & skeletal: Arthralgia
- Ocular: Cataracts, glaucoma
- Respiratory: Epistaxis

<1% (Limited to important or life-threatening): Alkalosis, Cushing's syndrome, delirium, edema, euphoria, fractures, hallucinations, hypersensitivity reactions, hypertension, hypokalemia, muscle wasting, myalgia, osteoporosis, pancreatitis, peptic ulcer, pituitary-adrenal axis suppression, pseudotumor cerebri, psychoses, seizure, skin atrophy, ulcerative esophagitis

Overdosage/Toxicology When consumed in excessive quantities for prolonged periods, systemic hypercorticism and adrenal suppression may occur; in those cases, discontinuation and withdrawal of the corticosteroid should be done judiciously. Cushingoid changes from continued administration of large doses results in moon face, central obesity, striae, hirsutism, acne, ecchymoses, hypertension, osteoporosis, myopathy, sexual dysfunction, diabetes, hyperlipidemia, peptic ulcer, increased susceptibility to infection, and electrolyte and fluid imbalance.

Dosing

Adults & Elderly: If possible, administer glucocorticoids before 9 AM to minimize adrenocortical suppression; dosing depends upon the condition being treated and the response of the patient. **Note:** Supplemental doses may be warranted during times of stress in the course of withdrawing therapy

Anti-inflammatory or immunosuppressive: Oral: 25-300 mg/day in divided doses every 12-24 hours

Physiologic replacement: Oral: 25-35 mg/day

Pediatrics: If possible, administer glucocorticoids before 9 AM to minimize adrenocortical suppression; dosing depends upon the condition being treated and the response of the patient. **Note:** Supplemental doses may be warranted during times of stress in the course of withdrawing therapy

Anti-inflammatory or immunosuppressive: Oral: 2.5-10 mg/kg/day **or** 20-300 mg/m^2/day in divided doses every 6-8 hours

Physiologic replacement: Oral: 0.5-0.75 mg/kg/day **or** 20-25 mg/m^2/day in divided doses every 8 hours

Renal Impairment:

Hemodialysis: Supplemental dose is not necessary.

Peritoneal dialysis: Supplemental dose is not necessary.

Available Dosage Forms Tablet, as acetate: 25 mg

Nursing Guidelines

Dietary Considerations: May need diet with increased potassium, pyridoxine, vitamin C, vitamin D, folate, calcium, and phosphorus and decreased sodium; may be taken with food to decrease GI distress.

Patient Education: Take oral formulation as directed, with food or milk in the morning. Do not take more than prescribed or discontinue without consulting prescriber. Maintain adequate nutritional intake; consult prescriber for possibility of special dietary instructions. If you have diabetes, monitor serum glucose closely and notify prescriber of any changes; this medication can alter hypoglycemic requirements. Inform prescriber if you are experiencing unusual stress; dosage may need to be adjusted. You will be susceptible to infection (avoid crowds and exposure to infection). You may experience insomnia or nervousness; use caution when driving or engaging in tasks requiring alertness until response to drug is known. Report excessive or sudden weight gain, swelling of extremities, respiratory difficulty, muscle pain or weakness, change in menstrual pattern, vision changes, signs of hyperglycemia, signs of infection (eg, fever, chills, mouth sores, perianal itching, vaginal discharge), other persistent side effects, or worsening of condition. **Pregnancy/breast-feeding precautions:** Do not get pregnant while taking this medication; use appropriate contraceptive measures. Consult prescriber if breast-feeding.

Pregnancy Risk Factor: D

Lactation: Enters breast milk/use caution

Administration

Oral: Insoluble in water.

- ♦ **Cortisone Acetate** *see* Cortisone *on page 451*
- ♦ **Cortisporin® Cream** *see* Neomycin, Polymyxin B, and Hydrocortisone *on page 1212*
- ♦ **Cortisporin® Ointment** *see* Bacitracin, Neomycin, Polymyxin B, and Hydrocortisone *on page 221*
- ♦ **Cortisporin® Ophthalmic** *see* Neomycin, Polymyxin B, and Hydrocortisone *on page 1212*
- ♦ **Cortisporin® Otic** *see* Neomycin, Polymyxin B, and Hydrocortisone *on page 1212*
- ♦ **Cortisporin®-TC** *see* Neomycin, Colistin, Hydrocortisone, and Thonzonium *on page 1210*
- ♦ **Cortizone®-10 Maximum Strength [OTC]** *see* Hydrocortisone *on page 873*
- ♦ **Cortizone®-10 Plus Maximum Strength [OTC]** *see* Hydrocortisone *on page 873*
- ♦ **Cortizone®-10 Quick Shot [OTC]** *see* Hydrocortisone *on page 873*
- ♦ **Cosopt®** *see* Dorzolamide and Timolol *on page 569*
- ♦ **Co-Trimoxazole** *see* Sulfamethoxazole and Trimethoprim *on page 1582*
- ♦ **Coumadin®** *see* Warfarin *on page 1723*
- ♦ **Covera-HS®** *see* Verapamil *on page 1702*
- ♦ **Cozaar®** *see* Losartan *on page 1066*
- ♦ **CPC** *see* Cetylpyridinium *on page 368*
- ♦ **CPM** *see* Cyclophosphamide *on page 462*
- ♦ **CPT-11** *see* Irinotecan *on page 962*
- ♦ **CPZ** *see* ChlorproMAZINE *on page 379*
- ♦ **Creon®** *see* Pancrelipase *on page 1301*
- ♦ **Crolom®** *see* Cromolyn *on page 453*
- ♦ **Cromoglycic Acid** *see* Cromolyn *on page 453*

Cromolyn (KROE moe lin)

U.S. Brand Names Crolom®; Gastrocrom®; Intal®; NasalCrom® [OTC]; Opticrom®

Synonyms Cromoglycic Acid; Cromolyn Sodium; Disodium Cromoglycate; DSCG

Pharmacologic Category Mast Cell Stabilizer

Medication Safety Issues

Sound-alike/look-alike issues:

Intal® may be confused with Endal®

NasalCrom® may be confused with Nasacort®, Nasalide®

Use

Inhalation: May be used as an adjunct in the prophylaxis of allergic disorders, including asthma; prevention of exercise-induced bronchospasm

Nasal: Prevention and treatment of seasonal and perennial allergic rhinitis

Oral: Systemic mastocytosis

Ophthalmic: Treatment of vernal keratoconjunctivitis, vernal conjunctivitis, and vernal keratitis

Unlabeled/Investigational Use Oral: Food allergy, treatment of inflammatory bowel disease

(Continued)

Cromolyn *(Continued)*

Mechanism of Action Prevents the mast cell release of histamine, leukotrienes and slow-reacting substance of anaphylaxis by inhibiting degranulation after contact with antigens

Pharmacodynamics/Kinetics

Onset: Response to treatment:

Nasal spray: May occur at 1-2 weeks

Ophthalmic: May be seen within a few days; treatment for up to 6 weeks is often required

Oral: May occur within 2-6 weeks

Absorption:

Inhalation: ~8% reaches lungs upon inhalation; well absorbed

Oral: <1% of dose absorbed

Half-life elimination: 80-90 minutes

Time to peak, serum: Inhalation: ~15 minutes

Excretion: Urine and feces (equal amounts as unchanged drug); exhaled gases (small amounts)

Contraindications Hypersensitivity to cromolyn or any component of the formulation; acute asthma attacks

Warnings/Precautions Severe anaphylactic reactions may occur rarely; cromolyn is a prophylactic drug with no benefit for acute situations; caution should be used when withdrawing the drug or tapering the dose as symptoms may reoccur; use with caution in patients with a history of cardiac arrhythmias. Transient burning or stinging may occur with ophthalmic use. Dosage of oral product should be decreased with hepatic or renal dysfunction.

Drug Interactions Corticosteroids: Ophthalmic preparation may be used with ophthalmic corticosteroids

Adverse Reactions

Inhalation: >10%: Gastrointestinal: Unpleasant taste in mouth

Nasal:

>10%: Respiratory: Increase in sneezing, burning, stinging, or irritation inside of nose

1% to 10%:

Central nervous system: Headache

Gastrointestinal: Unpleasant taste

Respiratory: Hoarseness, cough, postnasal drip

<1% (Limited to important or life-threatening): Anaphylactic reactions, epistaxis

Ophthalmic: Frequency not defined:

Ocular: Conjunctival injection, dryness around the eye, edema, eye irritation, immediate hypersensitivity reactions, itchy eyes, puffy eyes, styes, rash, watery eyes

Respiratory: Dyspnea

Systemic: Frequency not defined:

Cardiovascular: Angioedema, chest pain, edema, flushing, palpitation, premature ventricular contractions, tachycardia

Central nervous system: Anxiety, behavior changes, convulsions, depression, dizziness, fatigue, hallucinations, headache, irritability, insomnia, lethargy, migraine, nervousness, hypoesthesia, postprandial lightheadedness, psychosis

Dermatologic: Erythema, photosensitivity, pruritus, purpura, rash, urticaria

Gastrointestinal: Abdominal pain, constipation, diarrhea, dyspepsia, dysphagia, esophagospasm, flatulence, glossitis, nausea, stomatitis, unpleasant taste, vomiting

Genitourinary: Dysuria, urinary frequency

Hematologic: Neutropenia, pancytopenia, polycythemia

Hepatic: Liver function test abnormal

Local: Burning

Neuromuscular & skeletal: Arthralgia, leg stiffness, leg weakness, myalgia, paresthesia

Otic: Tinnitus

Respiratory: Dyspnea, pharyngitis

Miscellaneous: Lupus erythematosus

Overdosage/Toxicology Symptoms of overdose include bronchospasm, laryngeal edema, and dysuria. Treat symptomatically.

Dosing

Adults & Elderly:

Allergic rhinitis (treatment and prophylaxis): Nasal: Instill 1 spray in each nostril 3-4 times/day

Asthma: For chronic control of asthma, taper frequency to the lowest effective dose (ie, 4 times/day to 3 times/day to twice daily). **Note:** Not effective for immediate relief of symptoms in acute asthmatic attacks; must be used at regular intervals for 2-4 weeks to be effective.

Nebulization solution: Initial: 20 mg 4 times/day; usual dose: 20 mg 3-4 times/day

Metered spray: Initial: 2 inhalations 4 times/day; usual dose: 2-4 inhalations 3-4 times/day

Prophylaxis of bronchospasm (allergen- or exercise-induced):

Note: Administer 10-15 minutes prior to exercise or allergen exposure but no longer than 1 hour before:

Nebulization solution: Single dose of 20 mg

Metered spray: Single dose of 2 inhalations

Conjunctivitis and keratitis: Ophthalmic: 1-2 drops in each eye 4-6 times/day

Mastocytosis: Oral: 200 mg 4 times/day; given ½ hour prior to meals and at bedtime. If control of symptoms is not seen within 2-3 weeks, dose may be increased to a maximum 40 mg/kg/day

Food allergy and inflammatory bowel disease (unlabeled use): Oral: Initial dose: 200 mg 4 times/day; may double the dose if effect is not satisfactory within 2-3 weeks; up to 400 mg 4 times/day

Pediatrics:

Allergic rhinitis (treatment and prophylaxis): Nasal: Children ≥2 years: Refer to adult dosing.

Asthma: Inhalation:

Note: For chronic control of asthma, taper frequency to the lowest effective dose (ie, 4 times/day to 3 times/day to twice daily):

Nebulization solution: Children >2 years: Initial: 20 mg 4 times/day; usual dose: 20 mg 3-4 times/day

Metered spray:

Children 5-12 years: Initial: 2 inhalations 4 times/day; usual dose: 1-2 inhalations 3-4 times/day

Children ≥12 years: Refer to adult dosing.

Prevention of allergen- or exercise-induced bronchospasm:

Note: Administer 10-15 minutes prior to exercise or allergen exposure but no longer than 1 hour before:

Nebulization solution: Children >2 years: Refer to adult dosing.

Metered spray: Children >5 years: Single dose of 2 inhalations

Systemic mastocytosis: Oral:

Children 2-12 years: 100 mg 4 times/day; not to exceed 40 mg/kg/day; given ½ hour prior to meals and at bedtime

Children >12 years: Refer to adult dosing.

Food allergy and inflammatory bowel disease (unlabeled use): Oral:

Children <2 years: Not recommended

Children 2-12 years: Initial dose: 100 mg 4 times/day; may double the dose if effect is not satisfactory within 2-3 weeks; not to exceed 40 mg/kg/day

Children >12 years: Refer to adult dosing.

Note: Once desired effect is achieved, dose may be tapered to lowest effective dose

Renal Impairment: Specific guidelines not available; consider lower dose of oral product.

Hepatic Impairment: Specific guidelines not available; consider lower dose of oral product.

Available Dosage Forms

Aerosol, for oral inhalation, as sodium (Intal®): 800 mcg/inhalation (8.1 g) [112 metered inhalations; 56 doses], (14.2 g) [200 metered inhalations; 100 doses]

Solution for nebulization, as sodium (Intal®): 20 mg/2 mL (60s, 120s)

Solution, intranasal spray, as sodium (NasalCrom®): 40 mg/mL (13 mL, 26 mL) [5.2 mg/inhalation; contains benzalkonium chloride]

Solution, ophthalmic, as sodium (Crolom®, Opticrom®): 4% (10 mL) [contains benzalkonium chloride]

Solution, oral, as sodium (Gastrocrom®): 100 mg/5 mL (96s)

Nursing Guidelines

Assessment: This is prophylactic therapy, not to be used for acute situations. Assess results of laboratory tests (long-term use) and adverse reactions.

(Continued)

Cromolyn *(Continued)*

Assess knowledge/teach patient appropriate use, interventions to reduce side effects, and adverse symptoms to report.

Monitoring Laboratory Tests: Periodic pulmonary function

Dietary Considerations: Oral: Should be taken at least 30 minutes before meals.

Patient Education: Oral: Use as directed; do not increase dosage or discontinue abruptly without consulting prescriber. Take at least 30 minutes before meals. You may experience dizziness or nervousness (use caution when driving or engaging in tasks requiring alertness until response to drug is known); diarrhea (boiled milk, yogurt, or buttermilk may help); or headache or muscle pain (mild analgesic may offer relief). Report persistent insomnia; skin rash or irritation; abdominal pain or difficulty swallowing; unusual cough, bronchospasm, or respiratory difficulty; decreased urination; or if condition worsens or fails to improve. **Breast-feeding precaution:** Consult prescriber if breast-feeding.

Nebulizer: Store nebulizer solution away from light. Prepare nebulizer according to package instructions. Clear as much mucus as possible before use. Rinse mouth following each use to prevent opportunistic infection and reduce unpleasant aftertaste. Report if symptoms worsen or condition fails to improve.

Nasal: Instill 1 spray into each nostril 3-4 times a day. You may experience unpleasant taste (rinsing mouth and frequent oral care may help); or headache (mild analgesic may help). Report increased sneezing, burning, stinging, or irritation inside of nose; sore throat, hoarseness, nosebleed; anaphylactic reaction (skin rash, fever, chills, backache, respiratory difficulty, chest pain); or worsening of condition or lack of improvement.

Ophthalmic: For ophthalmic use only. Wash hands before using. Tilt head back and look upward. Put drops of suspension inside lower eyelid. Close eye and roll eyeball in all directions. Do not blink for ½ minute. Apply gentle pressure to inner corner of eye for 30 seconds. Do not let tip of applicator touch eye; do not contaminate tip of applicator (may cause eye infection, eye damage, or vision loss). Do not share medication with anyone else. Temporary stinging or blurred vision may occur. Inform prescriber if condition worsens or fails to improve or if you experience eye pain, redness, burning, watering, dryness, double vision, puffiness around eye, vision changes, or other adverse eye response; or worsening of condition or lack of improvement. Do not wear contact lenses during treatment.

Geriatric Considerations: Assess the patient's ability to empty capsules via the Spinhaler®. Older persons often have difficulty with inhaled and ophthalmic dosage forms.

Pregnancy Risk Factor: B

Pregnancy Issues: Available evidence suggests safe use during pregnancy.

Lactation: Excretion in breast milk unknown/use caution

Breast-Feeding Considerations: No data available on whether cromolyn enters into breast milk or clinical effects on the infant.

Administration

Oral: Oral solution: Open ampul and squeeze contents into glass of water; stir well. Administer at least 30 minutes before meals and at bedtime.

Compatibility: Nebulizer solution is **compatible** with metaproterenol sulfate, isoproterenol hydrochloride, 0.25% isoetharine hydrochloride, epinephrine hydrochloride, terbutaline sulfate, and 20% acetylcysteine solution for at least 1 hour after their admixture.

Storage: Store at room temperature of 15°C to 30°C (59°F to 86°F); protect from light. Do not use oral solution if solution becomes discolored or forms a precipitate.

- **Cromolyn Sodium** *see* Cromolyn *on page 453*
- **Crosseal™** *see* Fibrin Sealant Kit *on page 724*
- **Cruex® Cream [OTC]** *see* Clotrimazole *on page 439*
- **Crystalline Penicillin** *see* Penicillin G (Parenteral/Aqueous) *on page 1331*
- **Crystal Violet** *see* Gentian Violet *on page 811*
- **CsA** *see* CycloSPORINE *on page 465*
- **CTX** *see* Cyclophosphamide *on page 462*
- **Cutivate®** *see* Fluticasone *on page 760*

◆ CyA *see* CycloSPORINE *on page 465*

Cyanocobalamin (sye an oh koe BAL a min)

U.S. Brand Names Nascobal®; Twelve Resin-K

Synonyms Vitamin B_{12}

Pharmacologic Category Vitamin, Water Soluble

Use Treatment of pernicious anemia; vitamin B_{12} deficiency due to malabsorption diseases, inadequaste secretion of intrinisic factor, and inadequate utilization of B_{12} (eg, during neoplastic treatment); increased B_{12} requirements due to pregnancy, thyrotoxicosis, hemorrhage, malignancy, liver or kidney disease

Mechanism of Action Coenzyme for various metabolic functions, including fat and carbohydrate metabolism and protein synthesis, used in cell replication and hematopoiesis

Pharmacodynamics/Kinetics

Absorption: Oral: Variable from the terminal ileum; requires the presence of calcium and gastric "intrinsic factor" to transfer the compound across the intestinal mucosa

Distribution: Principally stored in the liver and bone marrow, also stored in the kidneys and adrenals

Protein binding: To transcobalamin II

Metabolism: Converted in tissues to active coenzymes, methylcobalamin and deoxyadenosylcobalamin

Bioavailability: Intranasal:

- Gel: 8.9% (relative to I.M.)
- Solution: 6.1% (relative to I.M.)

Contraindications Hypersensitivity to cyanocobalamin or any component of the formulation, cobalt; hereditary optic nerve atrophy (Leber's disease)

Warnings/Precautions I.M. route used to treat pernicious anemia; vitamin B_{12} deficiency for >3 months results in irreversible degenerative CNS lesions; treatment of vitamin B_{12} megaloblastic anemia may result in severe hypokalemia, sometimes fatal, due to intracellular potassium shift upon anemia resolution. B_{12} deficiency masks signs of polycythemia vera; vegetarian diets may result in B_{12} deficiency; pernicious anemia occurs more often in gastric carcinoma than in general population. Patients with Leber's disease may suffer rapid optic atrophy when treated with vitamin B_{12}; an intradermal test dose of parenteral B_{12} is recommended prior to administration of intranasal product in patients suspected of cyanocobalamin sensitivity; do not use folic acid as substitute for vitamin B_{12} in preventing anemia, as progression of spinal cord degeneration may occur; some parenteral products contain aluminum: use caution in neonates and patients with renal impairment.

Drug Interactions Neomycin, colchicine, anticonvulsants, and metformin may decrease oral absorption of B_{12}, chloramphenicol may decrease B_{12} effects

Nutritional/Herbal/Ethanol Interactions Ethanol: Heavy consumption may impair vitamin B_{12} absorption.

Lab Interactions Methotrexate, pyrimethamine, and most antibiotics invalidate folic acid and vitamin B_{12} diagnostic microbiological blood assays

Adverse Reactions

>10%:

- Cardiovascular: Peripheral vascular disease
- Central nervous system: Headache (2% to 11%)

1% to 10%:

- Central nervous system: Anxiety, dizziness, pain, nervousness, hypoesthesia
- Dermatologic: Itching
- Gastrointestinal: Sore throat, nausea and vomiting, dyspepsia, diarrhea
- Neuromuscular & skeletal: Weakness (1% to 4%), back pain, arthritis, myalgia, paresthesia, abnormal gait, incoordination
- Respiratory: Dyspnea, rhinitis
- Miscellaneous: Infection

Frequency not defined: Peripheral vascular thrombosis, urticaria, anaphylaxis, CHF, pulmonary edema, polycythemia vera, transient exanthema

Dosing

Adults & Elderly:

Recommended daily allowance (RDA): 2.4 mcg/day

- Pregnancy: 2.6 mcg/day
- Lactation: 2.8 mcg/day

Vitamin B_{12} deficiency:

- Intranasal: 500 mcg in one nostril once weekly

(Continued)

Cyanocobalamin *(Continued)*

Oral: 250 mcg/day

I.M., deep SubQ: Initial: 30 mcg/day for 5-10 days; maintenance: 100-200 mcg/month

Pernicious anemia: I.M., deep SubQ (administer concomitantly with folic acid if needed, 1 mg/day for 1 month): 100 mcg/day for 6-7 days; if improvement, administer same dose on alternate days for 7 doses, then every 3-4 days for 2-3 weeks; once hematologic values have returned to normal, maintenance dosage: 100 mcg/month. **Note:** Alternative dosing of 1000 mcg/day for 5 days (followed by 500-1000 mcg/month) has been used.

Hematologic remission (without evidence of nervous system involvement):

Intranasal gel: 500 mcg in one nostril once weekly

Oral: 1000-2000 mcg/day

I.M., SubQ: 100-1000 mcg/month

Schilling test: I.M.: 1000 mcg

Pediatrics:

Recommended daily allowance (RDA): 0.9-2.4 mcg/day

Vitamin B_{12} deficiency:

Intranasal: 500 mcg in one nostril once weekly

Oral: 250 mcg/day

I.M., deep SubQ: Dosage in children not well established: 0.2 mcg/kg for 2 days, followed by 1000 mcg/day for 2-7 days, followed by 100 mcg/week for one month; for malabsorptive causes of B_{12} deficiency, monthly maintenance doses of 100 mcg have been recommended **or** as an alternative 100 mcg/day for 10-15 days, then once or twice weekly for several months

Pernicious anemia: I.M., deep SubQ (administer concomitantly with folic acid if needed, 1 mg/day for 1 month): 30-50 mcg/day for 2 or more weeks (to a total dose of 1000-5000 mcg), then follow with 100 mcg/month as maintenance dosage

Available Dosage Forms

Gel, intranasal (Nascobal®): 500 mcg/0.1 mL (2.3 mL) [contains benzalkonium chloride; delivers 8 doses]

Injection, solution: 1000 mcg/mL (1 mL, 10 mL, 30 mL) [may contain benzyl alcohol and/or aluminum]

Lozenge [OTC]: 100 mcg, 250 mcg, 500 mcg

Solution, intranasal spray (Nascobal®): 500 mcg/0.1 mL actuation (2.3 mL) [contains benzalkonium chloride; delivers 8 doses]

Tablet [OTC]: 50 mcg, 100 mcg, 250 mcg, 500 mcg, 1000 mcg, 5000 mcg

Twelve Resin-K: 1000 mcg [may be used as oral, sublingual, or buccal]

Tablet, extended release [OTC]: 1500 mcg

Tablet, sublingual [OTC]: 2500 mcg

Nursing Guidelines

Assessment: Assess effectiveness and interactions of other medications patient may be taking. Assess results of laboratory tests at beginning of therapy and periodically with long-term therapy. Teach patient proper use (injection technique and needle disposal), appropriate nutritional counseling, and adverse symptoms to report.

Monitoring Laboratory Tests: Erythrocyte and reticulocyte count, hemoglobin, hematocrit; monitor potassium concentrations during early therapy

Dietary Considerations: Vegetarian diets may result in vitamin B_{12} deficiency; use intranasal product at least 1 hour before or after ingestion of hot foods or liquids due to increased nasal secretions

Patient Education: Use exactly as directed. Pernicious anemia may require monthly injections for life. Report skin rash; swelling, pain, or redness of extremities; or acute persistent diarrhea. **Pregnancy precaution:** Inform prescriber if you are pregnant.

Geriatric Considerations: There exists evidence that people, particularly elderly whose serum cobalamin concentrations <500 pg/mL, should receive replacement parenteral therapy.

Pregnancy Risk Factor: A/C (dose exceeding RDA recommendation); C (intranasal)

Lactation: Enters breast milk/compatible

Administration

Oral: Not recommended due to variable absorption; however, oral therapy of 1000-2000 mcg/day has been effective for anemia if I.M./SubQ routes refused or not tolerated.

I.M.: I.M. or deep SubQ are preferred routes of administration.

I.V.: Not recommended

Compatibility: Stable in dextran 6% in dextrose, dextran 6% in NS, D_5LR, $D_5{}^1/_4NS$, $D_5{}^1/_2NS$, D_5NS, D_5W, $D_{10}W$, $D_{10}NS$, LR, $^1/_2NS$, NS

Compatibility when admixed: Incompatible with chlorpromazine, phytonadione, prochlorperazine edisylate, warfarin

Storage: Injection: Clear pink to red solutions are stable at room temperature. Protect from light.

♦ Cyclessa® *see* Ethinyl Estradiol and Desogestrel *on page 675*

Cyclobenzaprine (sye kloe BEN za preen)

U.S. Brand Names Flexeril®

Synonyms Cyclobenzaprine Hydrochloride

Pharmacologic Category Skeletal Muscle Relaxant

Medication Safety Issues

Sound-alike/look-alike issues:

Cyclobenzaprine may be confused with cycloSERINE, cyproheptadine

Flexeril® may be confused with Floxin®

Use Treatment of muscle spasm associated with acute painful musculoskeletal conditions

Mechanism of Action Centrally-acting skeletal muscle relaxant pharmacologically related to tricyclic antidepressants; reduces tonic somatic motor activity influencing both alpha and gamma motor neurons

Pharmacodynamics/Kinetics

Onset of action: ~1 hour

Duration: 12-24 hours

Absorption: Complete

Metabolism: Hepatic via CYP3A4, 1A2, and 2D6; may undergo enterohepatic recirculation

Bioavailability: 33% to 55%

Half-life elimination: 18 hours (range: 8-37 hours)

Time to peak, serum: 3-8 hours

Excretion: Urine (as inactive metabolites); feces (as unchanged drug)

Contraindications Hypersensitivity to cyclobenzaprine or any component of the formulation; do not use concomitantly or within 14 days of MAO inhibitors; hyperthyroidism; congestive heart failure; arrhythmias; acute recovery phase of MI

Warnings/Precautions Cyclobenzaprine shares the toxic potentials of the tricyclic antidepressants and the usual precautions of tricyclic antidepressant therapy should be observed; use with caution in patients with urinary hesitancy, angle-closure glaucoma, hepatic impairment, or in the elderly. Do not use concomitantly or within 14 days after MAO inhibitors; combination may cause hypertensive crisis, severe convulsions. Safety and efficacy have not been established in patients <15 years of age.

Drug Interactions Substrate of CYP1A2 (major), 2D6 (minor), 3A4 (minor)

Anticholinergics: Because of cyclobenzaprine's anticholinergic action, use with caution in patients receiving these agents.

CNS depressants: Effects may be enhanced by cyclobenzaprine.

CYP1A2 inhibitors: May increase the levels/effects of cyclobenzaprine. Example inhibitors include amiodarone, ciprofloxacin, fluvoxamine, ketoconazole, norfloxacin, ofloxacin, and rofecoxib.

Guanethidine: Antihypertensive effect of guanethidine may be decreased; effect seen with tricyclic antidepressants.

MAO inhibitors: Do not use concomitantly or within 14 days after MAO inhibitors.

Tramadol: May increase risk of seizure; effect seen with tricyclic antidepressants and tramadol.

Nutritional/Herbal/Ethanol Interactions

Ethanol: Avoid ethanol (may increase CNS depression).

Herb/Nutraceutical: Avoid valerian, kava kava, gotu kola (may increase CNS depression).

Adverse Reactions

>10%:

Central nervous system: Drowsiness (29% to 39%), dizziness (1% to 11%)

Gastrointestinal: Xerostomia (21% to 32%)

1% to 10%:

Central nervous system: Fatigue (1% to 6%), confusion (1% to 3%), headache (1% to 3%), irritability (1% to 3%), mental acuity decreased (1% to 3%), nervousness (1% to 3%)

(Continued)

Cyclobenzaprine *(Continued)*

Gastrointestinal: Abdominal pain (1% to 3%), constipation (1% to 3%), diarrhea (1% to 3%), dyspepsia (1% to 3%), nausea (1% to 3%)
Neuromuscular & skeletal: Muscle weakness (1% to 3%)
Ocular: Blurred vision (1% to 3%)
Respiratory: Pharyngitis (1% to 3%)

<1% (Limited to important or life-threatening): Ageusia, agitation, anaphylaxis, angioedema, anorexia, arrhythmia, cholestasis, diplopia, facial edema, gastritis, hallucinations, hepatitis (rare), hypertonia, hypotension, insomnia, jaundice, liver function tests abnormal, malaise, palpitation, paresthesia, pruritus, psychosis, rash, seizure, tachycardia, thinking abnormal, tinnitus, tongue edema, tremor, urinary frequency, urinary retention, urticaria, vertigo, vomiting

Overdosage/Toxicology Symptoms of overdose include troubled breathing, drowsiness, syncope, seizures, tachycardia, hallucinations, and vomiting. Following initiation of essential overdose management, treatment is supportive and symptomatic.

Dosing

Adults: Muscle spasm (including spasms associated with acute temporomandibular joint pain): Oral: Initial: 5 mg 3 times/day; may increase to 10 mg 3 times/day if needed. Do not use longer than 2-3 weeks.

Elderly: Plasma concentrations and adverse effects are increased in older patients. See Geriatric Considerations.

Hepatic Impairment:
Mild: 5 mg 3 times/day; use with caution and titrate slowly.
Moderate to severe: Use not recommended.

Available Dosage Forms

Tablet, as hydrochloride: 10 mg
Flexeril®: 5 mg, 10 mg [film coated]

Nursing Guidelines

Assessment: Assess effectiveness and interactions of other medications patient may be taking. Monitor effectiveness of therapy (according to rationale for therapy) and adverse reactions at beginning and periodically during therapy. Assess knowledge/teach patient appropriate use, interventions to reduce side effects (postural hypotension precautions), and adverse symptoms to report.

Patient Education: Take exactly as directed. Do not increase dose or discontinue without consulting prescriber. Do not use alcohol, prescriptive or OTC antidepressants, sedatives, or pain medications without consulting prescriber. You may experience drowsiness, dizziness, lightheadedness (avoid driving or engaging in tasks that require alertness until response to drug is known); or urinary retention (void before taking medication). Report excessive drowsiness or mental agitation, chest pain, skin rash, swelling of mouth/face, difficulty speaking, ringing in ears, or blurred vision. **Breast-feeding precaution:** Breast-feeding is not recommended.

Geriatric Considerations: High doses in the elderly caused drowsiness and dizziness; therefore, use the lowest dose possible. Because cyclobenzaprine causes anticholinergic effects, it may not be the skeletal muscle relaxant of choice in the elderly.

Pregnancy Risk Factor: B

Lactation: Excretion in breast milk unknown/not recommended

Administration

Storage: Store at room temperature 25°C (77°F); excursions permitted to 15°C to 30°C (59°F to 86°F).

- ♦ **Cyclobenzaprine Hydrochloride** *see* Cyclobenzaprine *on page 459*
- ♦ **Cyclogyl®** *see* Cyclopentolate *on page 460*
- ♦ **Cyclomydril®** *see* Cyclopentolate and Phenylephrine *on page 461*

Cyclopentolate (sye kloe PEN toe late)

U.S. Brand Names AK-Pentolate® [DSC]; Cyclogyl®; Cylate®

Synonyms Cyclopentolate Hydrochloride

Pharmacologic Category Anticholinergic Agent, Ophthalmic

Use Diagnostic procedures requiring mydriasis and cycloplegia

Mechanism of Action Prevents the muscle of the ciliary body and the sphincter muscle of the iris from responding to cholinergic stimulation, causing mydriasis and cycloplegia

Pharmacodynamics/Kinetics

Onset of action: Peak effect: Cycloplegia: 25-75 minutes; Mydriasis: 30-60 minutes

Duration: ≤24 hours

Contraindications Hypersensitivity to cyclopentolate or any component of the formulation; narrow-angle glaucoma

Warnings/Precautions 2% solution may result in psychotic reactions and behavioral disturbances in children, usually occurring approximately 30-45 minutes after instillation; use with caution in elderly patients and other patients who may be predisposed to increased intraocular pressure

Drug Interactions Decreased effect of carbachol, cholinesterase inhibitors

Adverse Reactions 1% to 10%:

Cardiovascular: Tachycardia

Central nervous system: Restlessness, hallucinations, psychosis, hyperactivity, seizure, incoherent speech, ataxia

Dermatologic: Burning sensation

Ocular: Increase in intraocular pressure, loss of visual accommodation

Miscellaneous: Allergic reaction

Overdosage/Toxicology Antidote, if needed, is pilocarpine

Dosing

Adults & Elderly: Diagnostic aid (mydriasis and cycloplegia): Ophthalmic: Instill 1 drop of 1% followed by another drop in 5 minutes; 2% solution in heavily pigmented iris

Pediatrics: Diagnostic aid (mydriasis and cycloplegia): Ophthalmic:

Neonates and Infants: **Note:** Cyclopentolate and phenylephrine combination formulation is the preferred agent for use in neonates and infants due to lower cyclopentolate concentration and reduced risk for systemic reactions

Children: Instill 1 drop of 0.5%, 1%, or 2% in eye followed by 1 drop of 0.5% or 1% in 5 minutes, if necessary

Available Dosage Forms [DSC] = Discontinued product

Solution, ophthalmic, as hydrochloride: 1% (2 mL, 15 mL)

AK-Pentolate® [DSC], Cylate®: 1% (2 mL, 15 mL) [contains benzalkonium chloride]

Cyclogyl®: 0.5% (15 mL); 1% (2 mL, 5 mL, 15 mL); 2% (2 mL, 5 mL, 15 mL) [contains benzalkonium chloride]

Nursing Guidelines

Patient Education: May cause blurred vision and increased sensitivity to light

Pregnancy Risk Factor: C

Cyclopentolate and Phenylephrine

(sye kloe PEN toe late & fen il EF rin)

U.S. Brand Names Cyclomydril®

Synonyms Phenylephrine and Cyclopentolate

Pharmacologic Category Ophthalmic Agent, Antiglaucoma

Use Induce mydriasis greater than that produced with cyclopentolate HCl alone

Pharmacodynamics/Kinetics See individual agents.

Drug Interactions See individual agents.

Dosing

Adults & Elderly: Diagnostic aid (mydriasis and cycloplegia): Ophthalmic: Instill 1 drop into the eye every 5-10 minutes, for up to 3 doses, approximately 40-50 minutes before the examination

Pediatrics: Diagnostic aid: Ophthalmic: Neonates, Infants, Children: Refer to adult dosing.

Available Dosage Forms Solution, ophthalmic: Cyclopentolate hydrochloride 0.2% and phenylephrine hydrochloride 1% (2 mL, 5 mL) [contains benzalkonium chloride]

Nursing Guidelines

Patient Education: May cause blurred vision and increased sensitivity to light

Pregnancy Risk Factor: C

♦ **Cyclopentolate Hydrochloride** *see* Cyclopentolate *on page 460*

Cyclophosphamide (sye kloe FOS fa mide)

U.S. Brand Names Cytoxan®

Synonyms CPM; CTX; CYT; NSC-26271

Pharmacologic Category Antineoplastic Agent, Alkylating Agent

Medication Safety Issues

Sound-alike/look-alike issues:

Cyclophosphamide may be confused with cycloSPORINE, ifosfamide

Cytoxan® may be confused with cefoxitin, Centoxin®, Ciloxan®, cytarabine, CytoGam®, Cytosar®, Cytosar-U®, Cytotec®

Use

Oncologic: Treatment of Hodgkin's and non-Hodgkin's lymphoma, Burkitt's lymphoma, chronic lymphocytic leukemia (CLL), chronic myelocytic leukemia (CML), acute myelocytic leukemia (AML), acute lymphocytic leukemia (ALL), mycosis fungoides, multiple myeloma, neuroblastoma, retinoblastoma, rhabdomyosarcoma, Ewing's sarcoma; breast, testicular, endometrial, ovarian, and lung cancers, and in conditioning regimens for bone marrow transplantation

Nononcologic: Prophylaxis of rejection for kidney, heart, liver, and bone marrow transplants, severe rheumatoid disorders, nephrotic syndrome, Wegener's granulomatosis, idiopathic pulmonary hemosideroses, myasthenia gravis, multiple sclerosis, systemic lupus erythematosus, lupus nephritis, autoimmune hemolytic anemia, idiopathic thrombocytic purpura (ITP), macroglobulinemia, and antibody-induced pure red cell aplasia

Mechanism of Action Cyclophosphamide is an alkylating agent that prevents cell division by cross-linking DNA strands and decreasing DNA synthesis. It is a cell cycle phase nonspecific agent. Cyclophosphamide also possesses potent immunosuppressive activity. Cyclophosphamide is a prodrug that must be metabolized to active metabolites in the liver.

Pharmacodynamics/Kinetics

Absorption: Oral: Well absorbed

Distribution: V_d: 0.48-0.71 L/kg; crosses placenta; crosses into CSF (not in high enough concentrations to treat meningeal leukemia)

Protein binding: 10% to 56%

Metabolism: Hepatic to active metabolites acrolein, 4-aldophosphamide, 4-hydroperoxycyclophosphamide, and nor-nitrogen mustard

Bioavailability: >75%

Half-life elimination: 4-8 hours

Time to peak, serum: Oral: ~1 hour

Excretion: Urine (<30% as unchanged drug, 85% to 90% as metabolites)

Contraindications Hypersensitivity to cyclophosphamide or any component of the formulation; pregnancy

Warnings/Precautions Hazardous agent - use appropriate precautions for handling and disposal. Dosage adjustment needed for renal or hepatic failure.

Drug Interactions Substrate of CYP2A6 (minor), 2B6 (major), 2C8/9 (minor), 2C19 (minor), 3A4 (major); **Inhibits** CYP3A4 (weak); **Induces** CYP2B6 (weak), 2C8/9 (weak)

Allopurinol may cause increase in bone marrow depression and may result in significant elevations of cyclophosphamide cytotoxic metabolites.

Anesthetic agents: Cyclophosphamide reduces serum pseudocholinesterase concentrations and may prolong the neuromuscular blocking activity of succinylcholine; use with caution with halothane, nitrous oxide, and succinylcholine.

Chloramphenicol results in prolonged cyclophosphamide half-life to increase toxicity.

CYP2B6 inducers: May increase the levels/effects of acrolein (the active metabolite of cyclophosphamide). Example inducers include carbamazepine, nevirapine, phenobarbital, phenytoin, and rifampin.

CYP2B6 inhibitors: May decrease the levels/effects of acrolein (the active metabolite of cyclophosphamide). Example inhibitors include desipramine, paroxetine, and sertraline.

CYP3A4 inducers: CYP3A4 inducers may increase the levels/effects of acrolein (the active metabolite of cyclophosphamide). Example inducers include aminoglutethimide, carbamazepine, nafcillin, nevirapine, phenobarbital, phenytoin, and rifamycins.

CYP3A4 inhibitors: May decrease the levels/effects of acrolein (the active metabolite of cyclophosphamide). Example inhibitors include azole antifungals, ciprofloxacin, clarithromycin, diclofenac, doxycycline, erythromycin, imatinib, isoniazid, nefazodone, nicardipine, propofol, protease inhibitors, quinidine, and verapamil.

Digoxin: Cyclophosphamide may decrease digoxin serum levels.
Doxorubicin: Cyclophosphamide may enhance cardiac toxicity of anthracyclines.
Tetrahydrocannabinol results in enhanced immunosuppression in animal studies.
Thiazide diuretics: Leukopenia may be prolonged.

Nutritional/Herbal/Ethanol Interactions Herb/Nutraceutical: Avoid black cohosh, dong quai in estrogen-dependent tumors.

Lab Interactions Increased uric acid in serum and urine; false-positive Pap test; suppression of some skin tests

Adverse Reactions

>10%:
- Dermatologic: Alopecia (40% to 60%) but hair will usually regrow although it may be a different color and/or texture. Hair loss usually begins 3-6 weeks after the start of therapy.
- Endocrine & metabolic: Fertility: May cause sterility; interferes with oogenesis and spermatogenesis; may be irreversible in some patients; gonadal suppression (amenorrhea)
- Gastrointestinal: Nausea and vomiting, usually beginning 6-10 hours after administration; anorexia, diarrhea, mucositis, and stomatitis are also seen
- Genitourinary: Severe, potentially fatal acute hemorrhagic cystitis (7% to 40%)
- Hematologic: Thrombocytopenia and anemia are less common than leukopenia
  - Onset: 7 days
  - Nadir: 10-14 days
  - Recovery: 21 days

1% to 10%:
- Cardiovascular: Facial flushing
- Central nervous system: Headache
- Dermatologic: Skin rash
- Renal: SIADH may occur, usually with doses >50 mg/kg (or 1 g/m^2); renal tubular necrosis, which usually resolves with discontinuation of the drug, is also reported
- Respiratory: Nasal congestion occurs when I.V. doses are administered too rapidly; patients experience runny eyes, rhinorrhea, sinus congestion, and sneezing during or immediately after the infusion.

<1% (Limited to important or life-threatening): High-dose therapy may cause cardiac dysfunction manifested as CHF; cardiac necrosis or hemorrhagic myocarditis has occurred rarely, but may be fatal. Cyclophosphamide may also potentiate the cardiac toxicity of anthracyclines. Other adverse reactions include anaphylactic reactions, darkening of skin/fingernails, dizziness, hemorrhagic colitis, hemorrhagic ureteritis, hepatotoxicity, hyperuricemia, hypokalemia, jaundice, neutrophilic eccrine hidradenitis, radiation recall, renal tubular necrosis, secondary malignancy (eg, bladder carcinoma), Stevens-Johnson syndrome, toxic epidermal necrolysis; interstitial pneumonitis and pulmonary fibrosis are occasionally seen with high doses

BMT:
- Cardiovascular: Heart failure, cardiac necrosis, pericardial tamponade
- Endocrine & metabolic: Hyponatremia
- Hematologic: Methemoglobinemia
- Gastrointestinal: Severe nausea and vomiting
- Miscellaneous: Hemorrhagic cystitis, secondary malignancy

Overdosage/Toxicology Symptoms of overdose include myelosuppression, alopecia, nausea, and vomiting. Treatment is supportive.

Dosing

Adults: Refer to individual protocols.

Usual dose:

Oral: 50-100 mg/m^2/day as continuous therapy or 400-1000 mg/m^2 in divided doses over 4-5 days as intermittent therapy

I.V.:
- Single doses: 400-1800 mg/m^2 (30-50 mg/kg) per treatment course (1-5 days) which can be repeated at 2- to 4-week intervals
- Continuous daily doses: 60-120 mg/m^2 (1-2.5 mg/kg) per day

JRA/vasculitis: I.V.: 10 mg/kg every 2 weeks

High dose BMT:

I.V.:
- 60 mg/kg/day for 2 days (total dose: 120 mg/kg)
- 50 mg/kg/day for 4 days (total dose: 200 mg/kg)
- 1.8 g/m^2/day for 4 days (total dose: 7.2 g/m^2)

Continuous I.V.:
- 1.5 g/m^2/24 hours for 96 hours (total dose: 6 g/m^2)

(Continued)

Cyclophosphamide *(Continued)*

1875 mg/m^2/24 hours for 72 hours (total dose: 5625 mg/m^2)

Note: Duration of infusion is 1-24 hours; generally combined with other high-dose chemotherapeutic drugs, lymphocyte immune globulin, or total body irradiation (TBI).

Nephrotic syndrome: Oral: 2-3 mg/kg/day every day for up to 12 weeks when corticosteroids are unsuccessful

Elderly: Refer to individual protocols: Initial and maintenance for induction: 1-2 mg/kg/day; adjust for renal clearance.

Pediatrics: Refer to individual protocols. Children:

Chemotherapy: Refer to adult dosing.

SLE: I.V.: 500-750 mg/m^2 every month; maximum dose: 1 g/m^2

JRA/vasculitis: I.V.: Refer to adult dosing.

Nephrotic syndrome: Refer to adult dosing.

Renal Impairment: A large fraction of cyclophosphamide is eliminated by hepatic metabolism; some authors recommend no dose adjustment unless severe renal insufficiency (Cl_{cr} <20 mL/minute).

Cl_{cr} >10 mL/minute: Administer 100% of normal dose.

Cl_{cr} <10 mL/minute: Administer 75% of normal dose.

Hemodialysis effects: Moderately dialyzable (20% to 50%)
Administer dose posthemodialysis

CAPD effects: Unknown

CAVH effects: Unknown

Hepatic Impairment: The pharmacokinetics of cyclophosphamide are not significantly altered in the presence of hepatic insufficiency. No dosage adjustments are recommended.

Available Dosage Forms

Injection, powder for reconstitution (Cytoxan®): 500 mg, 1 g, 2 g [contains mannitol 75 mg per cyclophosphamide 100 mg]

Tablet (Cytoxan®): 25 mg, 50 mg

Nursing Guidelines

Assessment: See Warnings/Precautions, Contraindications, and Dosing for extensive use cautions. Assess potential for interactions with other prescriptions, OTC medications, or herbal products patient may be taking (eg, increased nephrotoxicity - see Drug Interactions). For I.V. specifics, see I.V. below. Infusion site must be monitored to prevent extravasation. Assess results of laboratory tests (see below), therapeutic effectiveness (according to purpose for use), and adverse response (see Adverse Reactions and Overdose/Toxicology) prior to each infusion and regularly during therapy. Teach patient (or caregiver) proper use (oral), possible side effects/appropriate interventions (eg, importance of adequate hydration), and adverse symptoms to report (see Patient Education). **Pregnancy risk factor D** - determine that patient is not pregnant before beginning treatment. Instruct patients of childbearing age about appropriate contraceptive measures. Breast-feeding is contraindicated.

Monitoring Laboratory Tests: CBC with differential, platelet count, ESR, BUN, UA, serum electrolytes, serum creatinine

Dietary Considerations: Tablets should be administered during or after meals.

Patient Education: Inform prescriber of all prescriptions, OTC medications, or herbal products you are taking, and any allergies you have. Do not take any new medication during therapy unless approved by prescriber. Take exactly as directed, during or after meals; do not take at night. Maintain adequate hydration (2-3 L/day of fluids) unless instructed to restrict fluid intake and void frequently to reduce incidence of bladder irritation. You will be more susceptible to infection (avoid crowds and exposure to infection and do not have any vaccinations without consulting prescriber). May cause loss of hair (reversible, although regrowth hair may be different color or texture); fertility or amenorrhea; nausea or vomiting (small, frequent meals, good mouth care, chewing gum, or sucking lozenges may help - if persistent consult prescriber for antiemetic); headache (consult prescriber for analgesic); nasal congestion or cold symptoms (consult prescriber for decongestant); or mouth sores (use soft toothbrush or cotton swab for oral care). Report any difficulty or pain with urination; chest pain, rapid heartbeat, or palpitations; easy bruising or bleeding; unusual rash; persistent nausea or vomiting; menstrual irregularities; swelling of extremities; respiratory difficulty; or unusual fatigue. **Pregnancy/breast-feeding precautions:** Inform prescriber if you are pregnant. Do not get pregnant during therapy. Consult prescriber for instruction on appropriate contraceptive measures. This drug may cause severe fetal defects. Do not breast-feed.

Geriatric Considerations: Toxicity to immunosuppressives is increased in the elderly. Start with lowest recommended adult doses. Signs of infection, such as fever and WBC rise, may not occur. Lethargy and confusion may be more prominent signs of infection; adjust dose for renal function in the elderly.

Pregnancy Risk Factor: D

Lactation: Enters breast milk/contraindicated

Administration

Oral: Tablets are not scored and should not be cut or crushed; should be administered during or after meals.

I.V.: I.P., intrapleurally, IVPB, or continuous intravenous infusion; I.V. infusions may be administered over 1-24 hours. Doses >500 mg to approximately 2 g may be administered over 20-30 minutes.

To minimize bladder toxicity, increase normal fluid intake during and for 1-2 days after cyclophosphamide dose. Most adult patients will require a fluid intake of at least 2 L/day. High-dose regimens should be accompanied by vigorous hydration with or without mesna therapy.

Reconstitution: Reconstitute vials with SWI, NS, or D_5W to a concentration of 20 mg/mL.

Compatibility: Stable in D_5LR, D_5NS, D_5W, LR, 1/2NS, NS

Y-site administration: Incompatible with amphotericin B cholesteryl sulfate complex

Storage: Store intact vials of powder at room temperature of (25°C to 35°C). Reconstituted solutions are stable for 24 hours at room temperature (25°C) and 6 days under refrigeration (5°C). Further dilutions in D_5W or NS are stable for 24 hours at room temperature (25°C) and 6 days at refrigeration (5°C).

♦ **Cyclosporin A** *see* CycloSPORINE *on page 465*

CycloSPORINE (SYE kloe spor een)

U.S. Brand Names Gengraf®; Neoral®; Restasis™; Sandimmune®

Synonyms CsA; CyA; Cyclosporin A

Pharmacologic Category Immunosuppressant Agent

Medication Safety Issues

Sound-alike/look-alike issues:

CycloSPORINE may be confused with cyclophosphamide, Cyklokapron®, cycloSERINE

Gengraf® may be confused with Prograf®

Neoral® may be confused with Neurontin®, Nizoral®

Sandimmune® may be confused with Sandostatin®

Use Prophylaxis of organ rejection in kidney, liver, and heart transplants, has been used with azathioprine and/or corticosteroids; severe, active rheumatoid arthritis (RA) not responsive to methotrexate alone; severe, recalcitrant plaque psoriasis in nonimmunocompromised adults unresponsive to or unable to tolerate other systemic therapy

Ophthalmic emulsion (Restasis™): Increase tear production when suppressed tear production is presumed to be due to keratoconjunctivitis sicca-associated ocular inflammation (in patients not already using topical anti-inflammatory drugs or punctal plugs)

Unlabeled/Investigational Use Short-term, high-dose cyclosporine as a modulator of multidrug resistance in cancer treatment; allogenic bone marrow transplants for prevention and treatment of graft-versus-host disease; also used in some cases of severe autoimmune disease (ie, SLE, myasthenia gravis) that are resistant to corticosteroids and other therapy; focal segmental glomerulosclerosis

Mechanism of Action Inhibition of production and release of interleukin II and inhibits interleukin II-induced activation of resting T-lymphocytes.

Pharmacodynamics/Kinetics

Absorption:

Ophthalmic emulsion: Serum concentrations not detectable.

Oral:

Cyclosporine (non-modified): Erratic and incomplete; dependent on presence of food, bile acids, and GI motility; larger oral doses are needed in pediatrics due to shorter bowel length and limited intestinal absorption

Cyclosporine (modified): Erratic and incomplete; increased absorption, up to 30% when compared to cyclosporine (non-modified); less dependent on

(Continued)

CycloSPORINE *(Continued)*

food, bile acids, or GI motility when compared to cyclosporine (non-modified)

Distribution: Widely in tissues and body fluids including the liver, pancreas, and lungs; crosses placenta; enters breast milk

V_{dss}: 4-6 L/kg in renal, liver, and marrow transplant recipients (slightly lower values in cardiac transplant patients; children <10 years have higher values)

Protein binding: 90% to 98% to lipoproteins

Metabolism: Extensively hepatic via CYP; forms at least 25 metabolites; extensive first-pass effect following oral administration

Bioavailability: Oral:

Cyclosporine (non-modified): Dependent on patient population and transplant type (<10% in adult liver transplant patients and as high as 89% in renal transplant patients); bioavailability of Sandimmune® capsules and oral solution are equivalent; bioavailability of oral solution is ~30% of the I.V. solution

Children: 28% (range: 17% to 42%); gut dysfunction common in BMT patients and oral bioavailability is further reduced

Cyclosporine (modified): Bioavailability of Neoral® capsules and oral solution are equivalent:

Children: 43% (range: 30% to 68%)

Adults: 23% greater than with cyclosporine (non-modified) in renal transplant patients; 50% greater in liver transplant patients

Half-life elimination: Oral: May be prolonged in patients with hepatic impairment and shorter in pediatric patients due to the higher metabolism rate

Cyclosporine (non-modified): Biphasic: Alpha: 1.4 hours; Terminal: 19 hours (range: 10-27 hours)

Cyclosporine (modified): Biphasic: Terminal: 8.4 hours (range: 5-18 hours)

Time to peak, serum: Oral:

Cyclosporine (non-modified): 2-6 hours; some patients have a second peak at 5-6 hours

Cyclosporine (modified): Renal transplant: 1.5-2 hours

Excretion: Primarily feces; urine (6%, 0.1% as unchanged drug and metabolites)

Contraindications Hypersensitivity to cyclosporine or any component of the formulation. Rheumatoid arthritis and psoriasis: Abnormal renal function, uncontrolled hypertension, malignancies. Concomitant treatment with PUVA or UVB therapy, methotrexate, other immunosuppressive agents, coal tar, or radiation therapy are also contraindications for use in patients with psoriasis. Ophthalmic emulsion is contraindicated in patients with active ocular infections.

Warnings/Precautions Dose-related risk of nephrotoxicity and hepatotoxicity; monitor renal function and adjust dose appropriately. Use caution with other potentially nephrotoxic drugs (eg, acyclovir, aminoglycoside antibiotics, amphotericin B, ciprofloxacin). Increased risk of lymphomas, other malignancies, infection. May cause hypertension. Use caution when changing dosage forms; products are not equally interchangeable. Cyclosporine (modified): Refers to the capsule dosage formulation of cyclosporine in an aqueous dispersion (previously referred to as "microemulsion"). Cyclosporine (modified) has increased bioavailability as compared to cyclosporine (non-modified) and cannot be used interchangeably without close monitoring. Monitor cyclosporine concentrations closely following the addition, modification, or deletion of other medications; live, attenuated vaccines may be less effective; use should be avoided.

Transplant patients: May cause significant hyperkalemia and hyperuricemia. May cause seizures, particularly if used with high-dose corticosteroids. Encephalopathy has been reported, predisposing factors include hypertension, hypomagnesemia, hypocholesterolemia, high-dose corticosteroids, high cyclosporine serum concentration, and graft-versus-host disease; may be more common in patients with liver transplant. To avoid toxicity or possible organ rejection, make dose adjustments based on cyclosporine blood concentrations. Adjustment of dose should only be made under the direct supervision of an experienced physician. Anaphylaxis has been reported with I.V. use; reserve for patients who cannot take oral form.

Psoriasis: Patients should avoid excessive sun exposure; safety and efficacy in children <18 have not been established

Rheumatoid arthritis: Safety and efficacy for use in juvenile rheumatoid arthritis have not been established. If receiving other immunosuppressive agents, radiation or UV therapy, concurrent use of cyclosporine is not recommended.

Ophthalmic emulsion: Has not been studied in patients with a history of herpes keratitis. Safety and efficacy have not been established in patients <16 years of age.

Products may contain corn oil, castor oil, ethanol, or propylene glycol; injection also contains Cremophor® EL (polyoxyethylated castor oil), which has been associated with rare anaphylactic reactions.

Drug Interactions **Substrate** of CYP3A4 (major); **Inhibits** CYP2C8/9 (weak), 3A4 (moderate)

Allopurinol: Increases cyclosporine concentrations by inhibiting cyclosporine metabolism

Antibiotics: Concomitant use may potentiate renal dysfunction (seen with gentamicin, tobramycin, vancomycin, trimethoprim and sulfamethoxazole); increased cyclosporine concentrations by inhibiting cyclosporine metabolism (seen with clarithromycin, erythromycin, and norfloxacin); may decrease cyclosporine concentrations by inducing cyclosporine metabolism (seen with nafcillin, and rifampin); may decrease immunosuppressant effects (seen with ciprofloxacin); CNS disturbances, seizures (seen with imipenem)

Anticonvulsants: May decrease cyclosporine concentrations by inducing cyclosporine metabolism (seen with carbamazepine, phenobarbital, and phenytoin)

Antineoplastics: Concomitant use may potentiate renal dysfunction (seen with melphalan)

Antifungals: Concomitant use may potentiate renal dysfunction (seen with amphotericin B, ketoconazole); increase cyclosporine concentrations by inhibiting cyclosporine metabolism (seen with fluconazole, itraconazole, and ketoconazole)

Bromocriptine: Increases cyclosporine concentrations by inhibiting cyclosporine metabolism

Calcineurin inhibitors (cyclosporine, tacrolimus): Concurrent therapy may increase the risk of HUS/TTP/TMA.

Calcium channel blockers (diltiazem, nicardipine, verapamil): Increase cyclosporine concentrations by inhibiting cyclosporine metabolism. Nifedipine has been reported to increase the risk of gingival hyperplasia.

Colchicine: May potentiate renal dysfunction.

CYP3A4 inducers: CYP3A4 inducers may decrease the levels/effects of cyclosporine. Example inducers include aminoglutethimide, carbamazepine, nafcillin, nevirapine, phenobarbital, phenytoin, and rifamycins.

CYP3A4 inhibitors: May increase the levels/effects of cyclosporine. Example inhibitors include azole antifungals, clarithromycin, diclofenac, doxycycline, erythromycin, imatinib, isoniazid, nefazodone, nicardipine, propofol, protease inhibitors, quinidine, telithromycin, and verapamil.

CYP3A4 substrates: Cyclosporine may increase the levels/effects of CYP3A4 substrates. Example substrates include benzodiazepines, calcium channel blockers, cyclosporine, mirtazapine, nateglinide, nefazodone, sildenafil (and other PDE-5 inhibitors), tacrolimus, and venlafaxine. Selected benzodiazepines (midazolam and triazolam), cisapride, ergot alkaloids, selected HMG-CoA reductase inhibitors (lovastatin and simvastatin), and pimozide are generally contraindicated with strong CYP3A4 inhibitors.

Danazol: Increases cyclosporine concentrations by inhibiting cyclosporine metabolism

Digoxin: Decreased clearance and decreased volume of distribution of digoxin; severe digitalis toxicity has been observed

Diuretics, potassium-sparing: Concomitant use may lead to hyperkalemia

Fibric acid derivatives: May increase the risk of renal dysfunction and may alter CSA concentrations; monitor.

Glucocorticoids: Increase cyclosporine concentrations by inhibiting cyclosporine metabolism, seen with methylprednisolone. Decreased clearance of prednisolone and convulsions observed when used with cyclosporine.

H_2 blockers: Concomitant use may potentiate renal dysfunction (seen with cimetidine, ranitidine)

HMG-CoA reductase inhibitors: Cyclosporine may increase levels/effects of HMG-CoA reductase inhibitors, resulting in myalgias, rhabdomyolysis, acute renal failure; dosage adjustments of HMG-CoA reductase inhibitors are recommended.

Imatinib: May increase cyclosporine serum concentrations.

Immunosuppressives: Concomitant use may potentiate renal dysfunction (seen with tacrolimus, muromonab-CD3)

Metoclopramide: Increases cyclosporine concentrations by inhibiting cyclosporine metabolism

(Continued)

CycloSPORINE *(Continued)*

Methotrexate: Cyclosporine increases plasma levels of methotrexate and decreases plasma levels of its metabolite; monitor closely for signs of toxicity

Minoxidil: Concomitant use may lead to severe hypertrichosis

NSAIDs: Concomitant use may potentiate renal dysfunction, especially in dehydrated patients (seen with diclofenac, naproxen, sulindac). In addition, diclofenac plasma levels are doubled when given with cyclosporine; the lowest possible dose of diclofenac should be used. Monitor serum creatinine.

Octreotide: May decrease cyclosporine concentrations by inducing cyclosporine metabolism

Oral contraceptives (hormonal): May increase serum levels of cyclosporine; monitor for signs of toxicity

Orlistat: May decrease absorption of cyclosporine; avoid concomitant use.

Prednisolone: Cyclosporine may increase serum levels/effects of prednisolone.

Protease inhibitors: Formal interaction studies have not been done; protease inhibitors are known to induce CYP3A4; use caution when using cyclosporine with indinavir, nelfinavir, ritonavir, or saquinavir

Rifabutin: Formal interaction studies have not been done; rifabutin is known to increase the metabolism of medications via CYP3A4.

Sirolimus: Cyclosporine (modified) may increase serum levels/effects; monitor. Concurrent therapy may increase the risk of HUS/TTP/TMA.

Sulfinpyrazone: May decrease cyclosporine levels; monitor.

Ticlopidine: May decrease cyclosporine concentrations by inducing cyclosporine metabolism

Vaccines: Vaccination may be less effective; avoid use of live vaccines during therapy.

Voriconazole: Cyclosporine serum concentrations may be increased; monitor serum concentrations and renal function. Decrease cyclosporine dosage by 50% when initiating voriconazole.

Nutritional/Herbal/Ethanol Interactions

Food: Grapefruit juice increases absorption; unsupervised use should be avoided.

Herb/Nutraceutical: Avoid St John's wort; as an enzyme inducer, it may increase the metabolism of and decrease plasma levels of cyclosporine; organ rejection and graft loss have been reported. Avoid cat's claw, echinacea (have immunostimulant properties).

Lab Interactions Specific whole blood, HPLC assay for cyclosporine may be falsely elevated if sample is drawn from the same line through which dose was administered (even if flush has been administered and/or dose was given hours before).

Adverse Reactions Adverse reactions reported with systemic use, including rheumatoid arthritis, psoriasis, and transplantation (kidney, liver, and heart). Percentages noted include the highest frequency regardless of indication/dosage. Frequencies may vary for specific conditions or formulation.

>10%:

Cardiovascular: Hypertension (8% to 53%), edema (5% to 14%)

Central nervous system: Headache (2% to 25%)

Dermatologic: Hirsutism (21% to 45%), hypertrichosis (5% to 19%)

Endocrine & metabolic: Triglycerides increased (15%), female reproductive disorder (9% to 11%)

Gastrointestinal: Nausea (23%), diarrhea (3% to 13%), gum hyperplasia (2% to 16%), abdominal discomfort (<1% to 15%), dyspepsia (2% to 12%)

Neuromuscular & skeletal: Tremor (7% to 55%), paresthesia (1% to 11%), leg cramps/muscle contractions (2% to 12%)

Renal: Renal dysfunction/nephropathy (10% to 38%), creatinine increased (16% to ≥50%)

Respiratory: Upper respiratory infection (1% to 14%)

Miscellaneous: Infection (3% to 25%)

1% to 10%:

Cardiovascular: Chest pain (4% to 6%), arrhythmia (2% to 5%), abnormal heart sounds, cardiac failure, flushes (<1% to 5%), MI, peripheral ischemia

Central nervous system: Dizziness (8%), pain (6%), convulsions (1% to 5%), insomnia (4%), psychiatric events (4% to 5%), pain (3% to 4%), depression (1% to 6%), migraine (2% to 3%), anxiety, confusion, fever, hypoesthesia, emotional lability, impaired concentration, insomnia, lethargy, malaise, nervousness, paranoia, somnolence, vertigo

Dermatologic: Hypertrichosis (5% to 7%), purpura (3% to 4%), acne (1% to 6%), brittle fingernails, hair breaking, abnormal pigmentation, angioedema, cellulitis, dermatitis, dry skin, eczema, folliculitis, keratosis, pruritus, rash, skin disorder, skin malignancies, urticaria

Endocrine & metabolic: Gynecomastia (<1% to 4%), menstrual disorder (1% to 3%), breast fibroadenosis, breast pain, hyper-/hypoglycemia, diabetes mellitus, goiter, hot flashes, hyperkalemia, hyperuricemia, libido increased/decreased

Gastrointestinal: Vomiting (2% to 10%), flatulence (5%), gingivitis (up to 4%), cramps (up to 4%), anorexia, constipation, dry mouth, dysphagia, enanthema, eructation, esophagitis, gastric ulcer, gastritis, gastroenteritis, gastrointestinal bleeding (upper), gingival bleeding, glossitis, mouth sores, peptic ulcer, pancreatitis, swallowing difficulty, salivary gland enlargement, taste perversion, tongue disorder, tooth disorder, weight loss/gain

Genitourinary: Leukorrhea (1%), abnormal urine, micturition increased, micturition urgency, nocturia, polyuria, pyelonephritis, urinary incontinence, uterine hemorrhage

Hematologic: Leukopenia (<1% to 6%), anemia, bleeding disorder, clotting disorder, platelet disorder, red blood cell disorder, thrombocytopenia

Hepatic: Hepatotoxicity (<1% to 7%), hyperbilirubinemia

Neuromuscular & skeletal: Arthralgia (1% to 6%), bone fracture, joint dislocation, joint pain, muscle pain, mylagia, neuropathy, stiffness, synovial cyst, tendon disorder, tingling, weakness

Ocular: Abnormal vision, cataract, conjunctivitis, eye pain, visual disturbance

Otic: Deafness, hearing loss, tinnitus, vestibular disorder

Renal: BUN increased, hematuria, renal abscess

Respiratory: Sinusitis (<1% to 7%), bronchospasm (up to 5%), cough (3% to 5%), pharyngitis (3% to 5%), dyspnea (1% to 5%), rhinitis (up to 5%), abnormal chest sounds, epistaxis, respiratory infection, pneumonia (up to 1%)

Miscellaneous: Flu-like symptoms (8% to 10%), lymphoma (<1% to 6% reported in transplant), abscess, allergic reactions, bacterial infection, carcinoma, diaphoresis increased, fungal infection, herpes simplex, herpes zoster, hiccups, lymphadenopathy, moniliasis, night sweats, tonsillitis, viral infection

Postmarketing and/or case reports (any indication): Anaphylaxis/anaphylactoid reaction (possibly associated with Cremophor® EL vehicle in injection formulation), benign intracranial hypertension, cholesterol increased, death (due to renal deterioration), encephalopathy, gout, hyperbilirubinemia, hyperkalemia, hypomagnesemia (mild), impaired consciousness, neurotoxicity, papilloedema, pulmonary edema (noncardiogenic), uric acid increased

Ophthalmic emulsion (Restasis™):

>10%: Ocular: Burning (17%)

1% to 10%: Ocular: Hyperemia (conjunctival 5%), eye pain, pruritus, stinging

Overdosage/Toxicology Symptoms of overdose include hepatotoxicity, nephrotoxicity, nausea, vomiting, tremor. CNS secondary to direct action of the drug may not be reflected in serum concentrations, may be more predictable by renal magnesium loss. Forced emesis may be beneficial if done within 2 hours of ingestion of cyclosporine capsules (modified). Treatment is symptomatic and supportive. Cyclosporine is not dialyzable.

Dosing

Adults: Note: Neoral® and Sandimmune® are not bioequivalent and cannot be used interchangeably

Newly-transplanted patients: Adjunct therapy with corticosteroids is recommended. Initial dose should be given 4-12 hours prior to transplant or may be given postoperatively; adjust initial dose to achieve desired plasma concentration.

Oral: Dose is dependent upon type of transplant and formulation:

Cyclosporine (modified):

Renal: 9 ± 3 mg/kg/day, divided twice daily

Liver: 8 ± 4 mg/kg/day, divided twice daily

Heart: 7 ± 3 mg/kg/day, divided twice daily

Cyclosporine (non-modified): Initial dose: 15 mg/kg/day as a single dose (range 14-18 mg/kg); lower doses of 10-14 mg/kg/day have been used for renal transplants. Continue initial dose daily for 1-2 weeks; taper by 5% per week to a maintenance dose of 5-10 mg/kg/day; some renal transplant patients may be dosed as low as 3 mg/kg/day

(Continued)

CycloSPORINE *(Continued)*

Note: When using the non-modified formulation, cyclosporine levels may increase in liver transplant patients when the T-tube is closed; dose may need decreased

I.V.: Manufacturer's labeling: Cyclosporine (non-modified): Initial dose: 5-6 mg/kg/day as a single dose ($^1/_3$ the oral dose), infused over 2-6 hours; use should be limited to patients unable to take capsules or oral solution; patients should be switched to an oral dosage form as soon as possible

Note: Many transplant centers administer cyclosporine as "divided dose" infusions (in 2-3 doses/day) or as a continuous (24-hour) infusion; dosages range from 3-7.5 mg/kg/day. Specific institutional protocols should be consulted.

Note: Conversion to cyclosporine (modified) from cyclosporine (non-modified): Start with daily dose previously used and adjust to obtain preconversion cyclosporine trough concentration. Plasma concentrations should be monitored every 4-7 days and dose adjusted as necessary, until desired trough level is obtained. When transferring patients with previously poor absorption of cyclosporine (non-modified), monitor trough levels at least twice weekly (especially if initial dose exceeds 10 mg/kg/day); high plasma levels are likely to occur.

Rheumatoid arthritis: Oral: Cyclosporine (modified): Initial dose: 2.5 mg/kg/day, divided twice daily; salicylates, NSAIDs, and oral glucocorticoids may be continued (refer to Drug Interactions); dose may be increased by 0.5-0.75 mg/kg/day if insufficient response is seen after 8 weeks of treatment; additional dosage increases may be made again at 12 weeks (maximum dose: 4 mg/kg/day). Discontinue if no benefit is seen by 16 weeks of therapy.

Note: Increase the frequency of blood pressure monitoring after each alteration in dosage of cyclosporine. Cyclosporine dosage should be decreased by 25% to 50% in patients with no history of hypertension who develop sustained hypertension during therapy and, if hypertension persists, treatment with cyclosporine should be discontinued.

Psoriasis: Oral: Cyclosporine (modified): Initial dose: 2.5 mg/kg/day, divided twice daily; dose may be increased by 0.5 mg/kg/day if insufficient response is seen after 4 weeks of treatment; additional dosage increases may be made every 2 weeks if needed (maximum dose: 4 mg/kg/day). Discontinue if no benefit is seen by 6 weeks of therapy. Once patients are adequately controlled, the dose should be decreased to the lowest effective dose. Doses <2.5 mg/kg/day may be effective. Treatment longer than 1 year is not recommended.

Note: Increase the frequency of blood pressure monitoring after each alteration in dosage of cyclosporine. Cyclosporine dosage should be decreased by 25% to 50% in patients with no history of hypertension who develop sustained hypertension during therapy and, if hypertension persists, treatment with cyclosporine should be discontinued.

Focal segmental glomerulosclerosis: Initial: 3 mg/kg/day divided every 12 hours

Autoimmune diseases: 1-3 mg/kg/day

Keratoconjunctivitis sicca: Ophthalmic: Instill 1 drop in each eye every 12 hours

Elderly: Refer to adult dosing (**Note:** Sandimmune® and Neoral® are not bioequivalent and cannot be used interchangeably without physician supervision).

Pediatrics: Transplant: Refer to adult dosing; children may require, and are able to tolerate, larger doses than adults.

Renal Impairment: For severe psoriasis:

Serum creatinine levels ≥25% above pretreatment levels: Take another sample within 2 weeks; if the level remains ≥25% above pretreatment levels, decrease dosage of cyclosporine (modified) by 25% to 50%. If two dosage adjustments do not reverse the increase in serum creatinine levels, treatment should be discontinued.

Serum creatinine levels ≥50% above pretreatment levels: Decrease cyclosporine dosage by 25% to 50%. If two dosage adjustments do not reverse the increase in serum creatinine levels, treatment should be discontinued.

Hemodialysis: Supplemental dose is not necessary.

Peritoneal dialysis: Supplemental dose is not necessary.

Hepatic Impairment: Dosage adjustment is probably necessary; monitor levels closely

Available Dosage Forms

Capsule, soft gel, modified: 25 mg, 100 mg [contains castor oil, ethanol]

Gengraf®: 25 mg, 100 mg [contains ethanol, castor oil, propylene glycol]

Neoral®: 25 mg, 100 mg [contains dehydrated ethanol, corn oil, castor oil, propylene glycol]

Capsule, soft gel, non-modified (Sandimmune®): 25 mg, 100 mg [contains dehydrated ethanol, corn oil]

Emulsion, ophthalmic [preservative free, single-use vial] (Restasis™): 0.05% (0.4 mL) [contains glycerin, castor oil, polysorbate 80, carbomer 1342; 32 vials/box]

Injection, solution, non-modified (Sandimmune®): 50 mg/mL (5 mL) [contains Cremophor® EL (polyoxyethylated castor oil), ethanol]

Solution, oral, modified:

Gengraf®: 100 mg/mL (50 mL) [contains castor oil, propylene glycol]

Neoral®: 100 mg/mL (50 mL) [contains dehydrated ethanol, corn oil, castor oil, propylene glycol]

Solution, oral, non-modified (Sandimmune®): 100 mg/mL (50 mL) [contains olive oil, ethanol]

Nursing Guidelines

Assessment: Assess effectiveness and interactions of other medications patient may be taking. Monitor kidney and hepatic function closely. Assess results of laboratory tests, therapeutic effectiveness, and adverse reactions at beginning of therapy and periodically throughout therapy. **I.V.:** Monitor closely for first 30-60 minutes of infusion and frequently thereafter to assess for adverse reactions. **Oral:** Teach patient appropriate administration, possible side effects, and symptoms to report.

Monitoring Laboratory Tests: Cyclosporine levels, serum electrolytes, renal function, hepatic function

Dietary Considerations: Administer this medication consistently with relation to time of day and meals.

Patient Education: Oral: Take dose at the same time each day. You will be susceptible to infection (avoid crowds and exposure to infection and do not have any vaccinations without consulting prescriber). Practice good oral hygiene to reduce gum inflammation; see a dentist regularly during treatment. Report severe headache; unusual hair growth or deepening of voice; mouth sores or swollen gums; persistent nausea, vomiting, or abdominal pain; muscle pain or cramping; tremors; unusual swelling of extremities, weight gain, or change in urination; or chest pain or rapid heartbeat. Increase in blood pressure or damage to the kidney is possible. Your prescriber will need to monitor you closely. Do not change one brand of cyclosporine for another; any changes must be done by your prescriber. If you are taking this medication for psoriasis, your risk of cancer may be increased when taking additional medications. **Solution:** Diluting oral solution improves flavor. Dilute Neoral® with orange juice or apple juice. Dilute Sandimmune® with milk, chocolate milk, or orange juice. Avoid changing what you mix with your cyclosporine. Mix thoroughly and drink at once. Use syringe provided to measure dose. Mix in a glass container (do not use plastic or styrofoam) and rinse container with more juice/milk to ensure total dose is taken. Do not rinse syringe before or after use (may cause dose variation). **Pregnancy/breast-feeding precautions:** Inform prescriber if you are or intend to become pregnant. Do not breast-feed.

Pregnancy Risk Factor: C

Pregnancy Issues: Cyclosporine crosses the placenta. Based on clinical use, premature births and low birth weight were consistently observed. Use only if the benefit to the mother outweighs the possible risks to the fetus.

Lactation: Enters breast milk/contraindicated

Administration

Oral: Oral solution: Do not administer liquid from plastic or styrofoam cup. May dilute Neoral® oral solution with orange juice or apple juice. May dilute Sandimmune® oral solution with milk, chocolate milk, or orange juice. Avoid changing diluents frequently. Mix thoroughly and drink at once. Use syringe provided to measure dose. Mix in a glass container and rinse container with more diluent to ensure total dose is taken. Do not rinse syringe before or after use (may cause dose variation).

I.V.: The manufacturer recommends that following dilution, intravenous admixture be administered over 2-6 hours. However, many transplant centers administer as divided doses (2-3 doses/day) or as a 24-hour continuous infusion.

(Continued)

CycloSPORINE *(Continued)*

Patients should be under continuous observation for at least the first 30 minutes of the infusion, and should be monitored frequently thereafter.

Reconstitution:

Sandimmune® injection: Injection should be further diluted [1 mL (50 mg) of concentrate in 20-100 mL of D_5W or NS] for administration by intravenous infusion. Light protection is not required for intravenous admixtures of cyclosporine.

Stability of injection of parenteral admixture at room temperature (25°C) is 6 hours in PVC; 24 hours in Excel®, PAB® containers, or glass.

Polyoxyethylated castor oil (Cremophor® EL) surfactant in cyclosporine injection may leach phthalate from PVC containers such as bags and tubing. The actual amount of diethylhexyl phthalate (DEHP) plasticizer leached from PVC containers and administration sets may vary in clinical situations, depending on surfactant concentration, bag size, and contact time.

Compatibility: Stable in D_5W, fat emulsion 10%, fat emulsion 20%, NS

Y-site administration: Incompatible with amphotericin B cholesteryl sulfate complex

Compatibility when admixed: Incompatible with magnesium sulfate

Storage:

Capsule: Store at controlled room temperature

Injection: Store at controlled room temperature; do not refrigerate. Ampuls should be protected from light.

Ophthalmic emulsion: Store at 15°C to 25°C (59°F to 77°F). Vials are single-use; discard immediately following administration.

Oral solution: Store at controlled room temperature; do not refrigerate. Use within 2 months after opening; should be mixed in glass containers.

♦ Cylate® *see* Cyclopentolate *on page 460*

♦ Cylex® [OTC] *see* Benzocaine *on page 232*

Cyproheptadine (si proe HEP ta deen)

Synonyms Cyproheptadine Hydrochloride; Periactin

Pharmacologic Category Antihistamine

Medication Safety Issues

Sound-alike/look-alike issues:

Cyproheptadine may be confused with cyclobenzaprine

Periactin may be confused with Perative®, Percodan®, Persantine®

Use Perennial and seasonal allergic rhinitis and other allergic symptoms including urticaria

Unlabeled/Investigational Use Appetite stimulation, blepharospasm, cluster headaches, migraine headaches, Nelson's syndrome, pruritus, schizophrenia, spinal cord damage associated spasticity, and tardive dyskinesia

Mechanism of Action A potent antihistamine and serotonin antagonist, competes with histamine for H_1-receptor sites on effector cells in the gastrointestinal tract, blood vessels, and respiratory tract

Pharmacodynamics/Kinetics

Absorption: Completely

Metabolism: Almost completely hepatic

Excretion: Urine (>50% primarily as metabolites); feces (~25%)

Contraindications Hypersensitivity to cyproheptadine or any component of the formulation; narrow-angle glaucoma; bladder neck obstruction; acute asthmatic attack; stenosing peptic ulcer; GI tract obstruction; concurrent use of MAO inhibitors; avoid use in premature and term newborns due to potential association with SIDS

Warnings/Precautions Do not use in neonates, safety and efficacy have not been established in children <2 years of age; symptomatic prostate hypertrophy; antihistamines are more likely to cause dizziness, excessive sedation, syncope, toxic confusion states, and hypotension in the elderly. In case reports, cyproheptadine has promoted weight gain in anorexic adults, though it has not been specifically studied in the elderly. All cases of weight loss or decreased appetite should be adequately assessed.

Drug Interactions

Cyproheptadine may potentiate the effect of CNS depressants.

MAO inhibitors may cause hallucinations when taken with cyproheptadine.

Nutritional/Herbal/Ethanol Interactions Ethanol: Avoid ethanol (may increase CNS sedation).

Lab Interactions Diagnostic antigen skin tests; increased amylases (S); decreased fasting glucose (S)

Adverse Reactions

>10%:

Central nervous system: Slight to moderate drowsiness

Respiratory: Thickening of bronchial secretions

1% to 10%:

Central nervous system: Headache, fatigue, nervousness, dizziness

Gastrointestinal: Appetite stimulation, nausea, diarrhea, abdominal pain, dry mouth

Neuromuscular & skeletal: Arthralgia

Respiratory: Pharyngitis

<1% (Limited to important or life-threatening): Bronchospasm, CNS stimulation, depression, epistaxis, hemolytic anemia, hepatitis, leukopenia, sedation, seizure, thrombocytopenia

Overdosage/Toxicology Symptoms of overdose include CNS depression or stimulation, dry mouth, flushed skin, fixed and dilated pupils, and apnea. There is no specific treatment for antihistamine overdose. Clinical toxicity is due to blockade of cholinergic receptors. For anticholinergic overdose with severe life-threatening symptoms, physostigmine 1-2 mg I.V. slowly, may be given to reverse these effects.

Dosing

Adults:

Appetite stimulation (including anorexia nervosa): Oral: 2 mg 4 times/day; may be increased gradually over a 3-week period to 8 mg 4 times/day

Allergic conditions: Oral: 4-20 mg/day divided every 8 hours (not to exceed 0.5 mg/kg/day)

Cluster headaches: Oral: 4 mg 4 times/day

Migraine headaches: Oral: 4-8 mg 3 times/day

Spasticity associated with spinal cord damage: Oral: 4 mg at bedtime; increase by a 4 mg dose every 3-4 days; average daily dose: 16 mg in divided doses; not to exceed 36 mg/day

Elderly: Oral: Initial: 4 mg twice daily

Pediatrics:

Allergic conditions: Oral: Children: 0.25 mg/kg/day or 8 mg/m^2/day in 2-3 divided doses **or**

2-6 years: 2 mg every 8-12 hours (not to exceed 12 mg/day)

7-14 years: 4 mg every 8-12 hours (not to exceed 16 mg/day)

Migraine headaches: 4 mg 2-3 times/day

Spasticity associated with spinal cord damage: Oral: Children ≥12 years: Refer to adult dosing.

Appetite stimulation (including anorexia nervosa): Children >13 years: Refer to adult dosing.

Hepatic Impairment: Dosage should be reduced in patients with significant hepatic dysfunction.

Available Dosage Forms

Syrup, as hydrochloride: 2 mg/5 mL (473 mL) [contains alcohol 5%; mint flavor]

Tablet, as hydrochloride: 4 mg

Nursing Guidelines

Assessment: Assess effectiveness and interactions of other medications patient may be taking. Monitor weight periodically. Monitor effectiveness of therapy and adverse reactions (eg, excess anticholinergic effects) at beginning of therapy and periodically with long-term use. Assess knowledge/teach patient appropriate use, interventions to reduce side effects, and adverse symptoms to report.

Patient Education: Take as directed; do not exceed recommended dose. Avoid use of other depressants, alcohol, or sleep-inducing medications unless approved by prescriber. You may experience drowsiness or dizziness (use caution when driving or engaging in tasks requiring alertness until response to drug is known); or dry mouth, nausea, or abdominal pain (small frequent meals, frequent mouth care, chewing gum, or sucking hard candy may help). Report persistent sedation, confusion, or agitation; changes in urinary pattern; blurred vision; chest pain or palpitations; sore throat respiratory difficulty or expectorating (thick secretions); significant change in weight; or lack of improvement or worsening or condition. **Breast-feeding precaution:** Do not breast-feed.

(Continued)

Cyproheptadine *(Continued)*

Geriatric Considerations: Elderly may not tolerate anticholinergic effects.

Pregnancy Risk Factor: B

Lactation: Excretion in breast milk unknown/contraindicated

Perioperative/Anesthesia/Other Concerns: May stimulate appetite; in case reports, cyproheptadine has promoted weight gain in anorexic adults.

♦ Cyproheptadine Hydrochloride *see* Cyproheptadine *on page 472*

Cyproterone and Ethinyl Estradiol

(sye PROE ter one & ETH in il es tra DYE ole)

Synonyms Ethinyl Estradiol and Cyproterone Acetate

Pharmacologic Category Acne Products; Estrogen and Progestin Combination

Use Treatment of females with severe acne, unresponsive to other therapies, with associated symptoms of androgenization (including mild hirsutism or seborrhea). **Should not be used solely for contraception;** however, will provide reliable contraception if taken as recommended for approved indications.

Mechanism of Action

Ethinyl estradiol: Estrogens are responsible for the development and maintenance of the female reproductive system and secondary sexual characteristics. Estrogens modulate the pituitary secretion of gonadotropins, luteinizing hormone, and follicle-stimulating hormone through a negative feedback system. Estrogen increases levels of sex hormone-binding globulin (SHBG) and may reduce unbound androgen levels. Ethinyl estradiol is a synthetic derivative of estradiol. The addition of the ethinyl group prevents rapid degradation by the liver.

Cyproterone: Steroidal compound with antiandrogenic, antigonadotropic and progestin-like activity.

Pharmacodynamics/Kinetics

Cyproterone:

Absorption: Rapid and complete

Metabolism: Hepatic; some metabolites have activity

Half-life elimination: 38 hours

Time to peak: 3-4 hours

Excretion: As metabolites: Urine (35%), feces

Contraindications Hypersensitivity to ethinyl estradiol, cyproterone, or any component of the formulation; history of or current thrombophlebitis or venous thromboembolic disorders (including DVT, PE); active or recent (within 1 year) arterial thromboembolic disease (eg, stroke, MI); cerebral vascular disease, coronary artery disease, valvular heart disease with complications, severe hypertension; diabetes mellitus with vascular involvement; severe headache with focal neurological symptoms; known or suspected breast carcinoma, endometrial cancer, estrogen-dependent neoplasms, undiagnosed abnormal genital bleeding; hepatic dysfunction or tumor, cholestatic jaundice of pregnancy, jaundice with prior combination hormonal contraceptive use; major surgery with prolonged immobilization; heavy smoking (≥15 cigarettes/day) in patients >35 years of age; ocular lesions resulting from vascular disease; history of otosclerosis with deterioration during pregnancy; pregnancy

Warnings/Precautions Should not be prescribed solely for its contraceptive properties (secondary nonhormonal contraception recommended in patients who may not adhere to dosing). May increase the risk of thromboembolism; users appear to have an elevated risk relative to users of oral contraceptives in some published studies. Should not be used in combination with other oral contraceptives.

The combination of cyproterone and ethinyl estradiol shares many of the risks of oral contraceptive agents. The risk of cardiovascular side effects with oral contraceptives increases in women who smoke cigarettes, especially those who are >35 years of age; women who use combination estrogen/progestin therapy should be strongly advised not to smoke. May lead to increased risk of myocardial infarction, use with caution in patients with risk factors for coronary artery disease. May have a dose-related risk of vascular disease, hypertension, and gallbladder disease.

Avoid use in hypertensive women. The use of combination oral contraceptive therapy has been associated with a slight increase in frequency of breast cancer, however, studies are not consistent. May cause glucose intolerance. Use with caution in patients with renal disease, conditions that may be aggravated by fluid retention, depression, or history of migraine.

Drug Interactions Ethinyl estradiol: **Substrate** of CYP2C8/9 (minor), 3A4 (major), 3A5-7 (minor); **Inhibits** CYP1A2 (weak), 2B6 (weak), 2C19 (weak), 3A4 (weak)

Acetaminophen: May increase plasma concentration of synthetic estrogens, possibly by inhibiting conjugation. Combination hormonal contraceptives may also decrease the plasma concentration of acetaminophen.

Acitretin: Interferes with the contraceptive effect of microdosed progestin-containing "minipill" preparations. The effect on other progestational contraceptives (eg, implants, injectables) is unknown.

Aminoglutethimide: May increase CYP metabolism of progestins leading to possible decrease in contraceptive effectiveness. Use of a nonhormonal contraceptive product is recommended.

Antibiotics (ampicillin, tetracycline): Pregnancy has been reported following concomitant use, however, pharmacokinetic studies have not shown consistent effects with these antibiotics on plasma concentrations of synthetic steroids. Use of a nonhormonal contraceptive product is recommended.

Anticoagulants: Combination hormonal contraceptives may increase or decrease the effects of coumarin derivatives. Combination hormonal contraceptives may also increase risk of thromboembolic disorders

Anticonvulsants (carbamazepine, felbamate, phenobarbital, phenytoin, topiramate): Increase the metabolism of ethinyl estradiol and/or some progestins, leading to possible decrease in contraceptive effectiveness. Use of a nonhormonal contraceptive product is recommended.

Ascorbic acid: Doses of ascorbic acid (vitamin C) 1 g/day have been reported to increase plasma concentration of synthetic estrogens by ~47%, possibly by inhibiting conjugation; clinical implications are unclear.

Benzodiazepines: Combination hormonal contraceptives may decrease the clearance of some benzodiazepines (alprazolam, chlordiazepoxide, diazepam) and increase the clearance of others (lorazepam, oxazepam, temazepam)

Clofibric acid: Combination hormonal contraceptives may increase the clearance of clofibric acid.

Cyclosporine: Combination hormonal contraceptives may inhibit the metabolism of cyclosporine, leading to increased plasma concentrations; monitor cyclosporine.

CYP3A4 inducers: May decrease the levels/effects of estrogens. Example inducers include aminoglutethimide, carbamazepine, nafcillin, nevirapine, phenobarbital, phenytoin, and rifamycins.

Griseofulvin: Griseofulvin may induce the metabolism of combination hormonal contraceptives causing menstrual changes; pregnancies have been reported. Use of barrier form of contraception is suggested while on griseofulvin therapy.

Morphine: Combination hormonal contraceptives may increase the clearance of morphine.

Non-nucleoside reverse transcriptase inhibitors (NNRTIs): Nevirapine may decrease plasma levels of combination hormonal contraceptives; use of a nonhormonal contraceptive product is recommended. No data for delavirdine; incomplete data for efavirenz.

Prednisolone: Ethinyl estradiol may inhibit the metabolism of prednisolone, leading to increased plasma concentrations.

Protease inhibitors: Amprenavir, lopinavir, nelfinavir, and ritonavir have been shown to decrease plasma levels of combination hormonal contraceptives; use of a nonhormonal contraceptive product is recommended. Indinavir has been shown to increase plasma levels of combination hormonal contraceptives. No data for saquinavir.

Rifampin: Rifampin increases the metabolism of ethinyl estradiol and some progestins (norethindrone) resulting in decreased contraceptive effectiveness and increased menstrual irregularities. Use of a nonhormonal contraceptive product is recommended.

Salicylic acid: Combination hormonal contraceptives may increase the clearance of salicylic acid.

Selegiline: Combination hormonal contraceptives may increase the serum concentration of selegiline.

Theophylline: Ethinyl estradiol may inhibit the metabolism of theophylline, leading to increased plasma concentrations.

Tricyclic antidepressants (amitriptyline, imipramine, nortriptyline): Metabolism may be inhibited by combination hormonal contraceptives, increasing plasma levels of antidepressant; use caution.

Troglitazone: Troglitazone decreases the serum concentration of ethinyl estradiol and norethindrone by ~30%, leading to possible reduction in contraceptive

(Continued)

Cyproterone and Ethinyl Estradiol *(Continued)*

effectiveness. The effect of troglitazone on other hormonal combinations is unknown.

Nutritional/Herbal/Ethanol Interactions

Food: CNS effects of caffeine may be enhanced if combination hormonal contraceptives are used concurrently with caffeine. Grapefruit juice increases ethinyl estradiol concentrations and would be expected to increase progesterone serum levels as well; clinical implications are unclear.

Herb/Nutraceutical: St John's wort may decrease the effectiveness of combination hormonal contraceptives by inducing hepatic enzymes. Avoid dong quai and black cohosh (have estrogen activity). Avoid saw palmetto, red clover, ginseng.

Adverse Reactions Note: This listing reflects reactions reported with combination hormonal contraceptives. Percentages specific to this combination are identified in parentheses.

Cardiovascular: Arterial thromboembolism, cerebral hemorrhage, cerebral thrombosis, edema (2%), hypertension, mesenteric thrombosis, MI

Note: The frequency of venous thromboembolism in users of cyproterone and ethinyl estradiol has been estimated to be from 1.2 to 9.9 events per 10,000 women-years. The incidence of these events in nonusers of any oral contraceptive has been estimated to be 0.5 to 1 event per 10,000 women-years, and increases to 4 events per 10,000 women-years for users of low-dose estrogen combinations.

Central nervous system: Headache (5%), depression (3%), dizziness (1%), nervousness (4%), migraine, premenstrual syndrome, stroke

Dermatologic: Chloasma (4%), acne, erythema multiforme, erythema nodosum, hirsutism, loss of scalp hair, melasma (may persist), rash (allergic)

Endocrine & metabolic: Dysmenorrhea (10%), breast tenderness (7%), libido changes (3%), sex hormone-binding globulins (SHBG) increased, amenorrhea, breakthrough bleeding, breast enlargement, breast secretion, carbohydrate intolerance, lactation decreased (postpartum), glucose tolerance decreased, menstrual flow changes, spotting, temporary infertility (following discontinuation), thyroid-binding globulin increased, triglycerides increased

Gastrointestinal: Nausea (2%), abdominal cramps, appetite changes, bloating, cholestasis, colitis, gallbladder disease, jaundice, vomiting, weight gain/loss

Genitourinary: Cervical erosion changes, cervical secretion changes, cystitis-like syndrome, vaginal candidiasis, vaginitis

Hematologic: Antithrombin III decreased, folate levels decreased, hemolytic uremic syndrome, norepinephrine-induced platelet aggregability increased, porphyria, prothrombin increased; factors VII, VIII, IX, and X increased

Hepatic: Benign liver tumors, Budd-Chiari syndrome, cholestatic jaundice, hepatic adenomas

Local: Thrombophlebitis

Ocular: Cataracts, change in corneal curvature (steepening), contact lens intolerance, optic neuritis, retinal thrombosis

Renal: Impaired renal function

Respiratory: Pulmonary thromboembolism

Miscellaneous: Hemorrhagic eruption

Overdosage/Toxicology Toxicity is unlikely following single exposures of excessive doses. May cause withdrawal bleeding in females. Any treatment following emesis and charcoal administration should be supportive and symptomatic.

Dosing

Adults: Female: Acne: Oral: One tablet daily for 21 days, followed by 7 days off; first cycle should begin on the first day of menstrual flow. Discontinue therapy 3-4 cycles after symptoms have resolved.

Renal Impairment: Specific guidelines not available; use with caution.

Hepatic Impairment: Contraindicated in hepatic impairment or active liver disease.

Available Dosage Forms Tablet: Cyproterone acetate 2 mg and ethinyl estradiol 0.35 mg [orange tablets] (21s)

Nursing Guidelines

Monitoring Laboratory Tests: Pap smear, pregnancy; lipid profiles in patients being treated for hyperlipidemias

Pregnancy Risk Factor: X

Pregnancy Issues: Pregnancy should be ruled out prior to treatment and discontinued if pregnancy occurs. In general, the use of combination hormonal contraceptives when inadvertently taken early in pregnancy have not been associated with teratogenic effects. Due to increased risk of thromboembolism postpartum, combination hormonal contraceptives should not be started earlier than 4-6 weeks following delivery.

Lactation: Enters breast milk/not recommended

Administration

Oral: Administer at the same time each day.

Storage: Store at controlled room temperature of 25°C (77°F).

- **Cystadane®** *see* Betaine Anhydrous *on page 237*
- **Cysto-Conray® II** *see* Iothalamate Meglumine *on page 956*
- **Cystografin®** *see* Diatrizoate Meglumine *on page 513*
- **Cystografin® Dilute** *see* Diatrizoate Meglumine *on page 513*
- **Cystospaz®** *see* Hyoscyamine *on page 886*
- **Cystospaz-M® [DSC]** *see* Hyoscyamine *on page 886*
- **CYT** *see* Cyclophosphamide *on page 462*

Cytarabine (sye TARE a been)

U.S. Brand Names Cytosar-U®

Synonyms Arabinosylcytosine; Ara-C; Cytarabine Hydrochloride; Cytosine Arabinosine Hydrochloride; NSC-63878

Pharmacologic Category Antineoplastic Agent, Antimetabolite

Medication Safety Issues

Sound-alike/look-alike issues:

Cytarabine may be confused with Cytadren®, Cytosar®, Cytoxan®, vidarabine

Cytosar-U® may be confused with cytarabine, Cytovene®, Cytoxan®, Neosar®

Use Cytarabine is one of the most active agents in leukemia; also active against lymphoma, meningeal leukemia, and meningeal lymphoma; has little use in the treatment of solid tumors

Mechanism of Action Inhibition of DNA synthesis. Cytosine gains entry into cells by a carrier process, and then must be converted to its active compound, aracytidine triphosphate. Cytosine is a purine analog and is incorporated into DNA; however, the primary action is inhibition of DNA polymerase resulting in decreased DNA synthesis and repair. The degree of cytotoxicity correlates linearly with incorporation into DNA; therefore, incorporation into the DNA is responsible for drug activity and toxicity. Cytarabine is specific for the S phase of the cell cycle.

Pharmacodynamics/Kinetics

Distribution: V_d: Total body water; widely and rapidly since it enters the cells readily; crosses blood-brain barrier with CSF levels of 40% to 50% of plasma level

Metabolism: Primarily hepatic; aracytidine triphosphate is the active moiety; about 86% to 96% of dose is metabolized to inactive uracil arabinoside

Half-life elimination: Initial: 7-20 minutes; Terminal: 0.5-2.6 hours

Excretion: Urine (~80% as metabolites) within 24-36 hours

Contraindications Hypersensitivity to cytarabine or any component of the formulation

Warnings/Precautions The U.S. Food and Drug Administration (FDA) currently recommends that procedures for proper handling and disposal of antineoplastic agents be considered. Use with caution in patients with impaired renal and hepatic function.

Drug Interactions

Methotrexate: When administered prior to cytarabine, may enhance the efficacy and toxicity of cytarabine. Some combination treatment regimens (eg, hyper-CVAD) have been designed to take advantage of this interaction.

Decreased effect of gentamicin, flucytosine; decreases digoxin oral tablet absorption

Increased toxicity: Alkylating agents and radiation; purine analogs

Adverse Reactions

>10%:

High-dose therapy toxicities: Cerebellar toxicity, conjunctivitis (make sure the patient is on steroid eye drops during therapy), corneal keratitis, hyperbilirubinemia, pulmonary edema, pericarditis, and tamponade

Central nervous system: Seizures (when given I.T.), cerebellar toxicity (ataxia, dysarthria, and dysdiadochokinesia; dose related)

Dermatologic: Oral/anal ulceration, rash

Gastrointestinal: Nausea, vomiting, anorexia, stomatitis, mucositis

(Continued)

Cytarabine *(Continued)*

Emetic potential:
<500 mg: Moderately low (10% to 30%)
500 mg to 1500 mg: Moderately high (60% to 90%)
>1-1.5 g: High (>90%)
Time course of nausea/vomiting: Onset: 1-3 hours; Duration: 3-8 hours
Hematologic: Bleeding, leukopenia, thrombocytopenia
Myelosuppressive: Occurs within the first week of treatment and lasts for 10-14 days; primarily manifested as granulocytopenia, but anemia can also occur
WBC: Severe
Platelets: Severe
Onset (days): 4-7
Nadir (days): 14-18
Recovery (days): 21-28
Hepatic: Hepatic dysfunction, mild jaundice, transaminases increased
1% to 10%:
Cardiovascular: Cardiomegaly
Central nervous system: Dizziness, headache, somnolence, confusion, neuritis, malaise
Dermatologic: Skin freckling, itching, alopecia, cellulitis at injection site
Endocrine & metabolic: Hyperuricemia or uric acid nephropathy
Gastrointestinal: Esophagitis, diarrhea
Genitourinary: Urinary retention
Hematologic: Megaloblastic anemia
Hepatic: Hepatotoxicity
Local: Thrombophlebitis
Neuromuscular & skeletal: Myalgia, bone pain, peripheral neuropathy
Respiratory: Syndrome of sudden respiratory distress progressing to pulmonary edema, pneumonia
Miscellaneous: Sepsis
<1% (Limited to important or life-threatening): Pancreatitis

BMT:
Dermatologic: Rash, desquamation may occur following cytarabine and TBI
Gastrointestinal: Severe nausea and vomiting, mucositis, diarrhea
Neurologic:
Cerebellar toxicity: Nystagmus, dysarthria, dysdiadochokinesia, slurred speech
Cerebral toxicity: Somnolence, confusion
Ocular: Photophobia, excessive tearing, blurred vision, local discomfort, chemical conjunctivitis
Respiratory: Noncardiogenic pulmonary edema (onset 22-27 days following completion of therapy)

Overdosage/Toxicology Symptoms of overdose include myelosuppression, megaloblastosis, nausea, vomiting, respiratory distress, and pulmonary edema. A syndrome of sudden respiratory distress progressing to pulmonary edema and cardiomegaly has been reported following high doses. Treatment is symptomatic and supportive.

Dosing

Adults & Elderly: I.V. bolus, IVPB, and continuous intravenous infusion doses of cytarabine are very different. Bolus doses are relatively well tolerated since the drug is rapidly metabolized. Continuous infusion uniformly results in myelosuppression. Refer to individual protocols.

Induction remission:
I.V.: 200 mg/m^2/day for 5 days at 2-week intervals
100-200 mg/m^2/day for 5- to 10-day therapy course or every day until remission
I.T.: 5-75 mg/m^2 every 2-7 days until CNS findings normalize

Maintenance remission:
I.V.: 70-200 mg/m^2/day for 2-5 days at monthly intervals
I.M., SubQ: 1-1.5 mg/kg single dose for maintenance at 1- to 4-week intervals

High-dose therapies for leukemia/lymphoma:
Doses as high as 1-3 g/m^2 have been used for refractory or secondary leukemias or refractory non-Hodgkin's lymphoma.
Doses of 1-3 g/m^2 every 12 hours for up to 12 doses have been used

Bone marrow transplant: 1.5 g/m^2 continuous infusion over 48 hours

Pediatrics: I.V. bolus, IVPB, and CIV doses of cytarabine are very different. Bolus doses are relatively well tolerated since the drug is rapidly metabolized; bolus doses are associated with greater gastrointestinal and neurotoxicity; continuous infusion uniformly results in myelosuppression. Refer to individual protocols.

Induction remission:

I.V.: 200 mg/m²/day for 5 days at 2-week intervals

100-200 mg/m²/day for 5- to 10-day therapy course or every day until remission

I.T.: 5-75 mg/m² every 4 days until CNS findings normalize

or

<1 year: 20 mg

1-2 years: 30 mg

2-3 years: 50 mg

>3 years: 70 mg

Maintenance remission: Refer to adult dosing.

Renal Impairment: In one study, 76% of patients with a Cl_{cr} <60 mL/minute experienced neurotoxicity. Dosage adjustment of high-dose therapy should be considered in patients with renal insufficiency.

Hepatic Impairment: Dose may need to be adjusted in patients with liver failure since cytarabine is partially detoxified in the liver.

Available Dosage Forms

Injection, powder for reconstitution: 100 mg, 500 mg, 1 g, 2 g

Injection, solution: 20 mg/mL (5 mL, 25 mL, 50 mL); 100 mg/mL (20 mL)

Nursing Guidelines

Assessment: See Contraindications, Warnings/Precautions, and Dosing for use cautions. Assess potential for interactions with other prescriptions, OTC medications, or herbal products patient may be taking (see Drug Interactions). See Administration, Dosing, Reconstitution, and Compatibility for specifics. Premedicate with antiemetic; especially with larger doses. Conjunctivitis is prevented and treated with saline or corticosteroid eye drops. Assess results of laboratory tests (see below) and adverse response (see Adverse Reactions and Overdose/Toxicology) prior to therapy and on a regular basis throughout therapy. Teach patient possible side effects/appropriate interventions (eg, importance of adequate hydration) and adverse symptoms to report (see Patient Education). **Pregnancy risk factor D** - determine that patient is not pregnant before beginning treatment. Instruct patients of childbearing age about appropriate contraceptive measures. Breast-feeding is not recommended.

Monitoring Laboratory Tests: Liver function, CBC with differential and platelet count, serum creatinine, BUN, serum uric acid

Patient Education: Inform prescriber of all prescriptions, OTC medications, or herbal products you are taking, and any allergies you have. Do not take any new medication during therapy unless approved by prescriber. This drug can only be given by infusion or injection. Report immediately any redness, swelling, burning, or pain at injection/infusion site. Maintain adequate hydration (2-3 L/day of fluids) unless instructed to restrict fluid intake. You will be more susceptible to infection (avoid crowds and exposure to infection and do not have any vaccinations without consulting prescriber). May cause nausea, vomiting or loss of appetite (small, frequent meals, frequent mouth care, sucking lozenges, or chewing gum may help - if ineffective, consult prescriber for antiemetic medication); diarrhea (buttermilk, boiled milk, or yogurt may help - if persistent, consult with prescriber); mouth sores (use soft toothbrush or cotton swabs for oral care); or dizziness, headache, or confusion (use caution when driving or engaging in potentially hazardous tasks until response to drug is known). Report immediately any signs of CNS changes, change in gait, respiratory distress or respiratory difficulty, easy bruising or bleeding, persistent GI upset, yellowing of eyes or skin, change in color of urine or blackened stool, or any other persistent adverse effects. **Pregnancy/breast-feeding precautions:** Inform prescriber if you are pregnant. Consult prescriber for instruction on appropriate contraceptive measures. This drug may cause severe fetal defects. Breast-feeding is not recommended.

Pregnancy Risk Factor: D

Pregnancy Issues: Cytarabine is teratogenic in animal studies. Limb and ear defects have been noted in case reports when cytarabine has been used during pregnancy. The following have also been noted in the neonate: Pancytopenia, WBC depression, electrolyte abnormalities, prematurity, low birth weight,

(Continued)

Cytarabine *(Continued)*

decreased hematocrit or platelets. Risk to the fetus is decreased if therapy is avoided during the 1st trimester; however, women of childbearing potential should be advised of the potential risks.

Lactation: Excretion in breast milk unknown/not recommended

Administration

I.V.: Can be administered I.M., I.V. infusion, I.T., or SubQ at a concentration not to exceed 100 mg/mL. I.V. may be administered either as a bolus, IVPB (high doses of >500 mg/m^2), or continuous intravenous infusion (doses of 100-200 mg/m^2). High-dose regimens are usually administered by I.V. infusion over 1-3 hours or as I.V. continuous infusion.

Reconstitution: Reconstitute powder with bacteriostatic water for injection. High-dose regimens are usually administered by I.V. infusion over 1-3 hours or as I.V. continuous infusion; for I.T. use, reconstitute with preservative free saline or preservative free lactated Ringer's solution

Standard I.V. infusion dilution: Dose/250-1000 mL D_5W or NS.

Standard intrathecal dilutions: Dose/3-5 mL lactated Ringer's ± methotrexate (12 mg) ± hydrocortisone (15-50 mg)

Note: Solutions containing bacteriostatic agents should not be used for the preparation of either high doses or intrathecal doses of cytarabine; may be used for I.M., SubQ, and low-dose (100-200 mg/m^2) I.V. solution.

Compatibility: Stable in D_5LR, $D_5{}^1/_4NS$, D_5NS, $D_{10}NS$, D_5W, LR, NS

Y-site administration: Incompatible with allopurinol, amphotericin B cholesteryl sulfate complex, ganciclovir

Compatibility when admixed: Incompatible with fluorouracil, gentamicin, heparin, insulin (regular), nafcillin, oxacillin, penicillin G sodium

Storage:

Powder for reconstitution: Store intact vials of powder at room temperature 15°C to 30°C (59°F to 86°F). Reconstituted solutions are for up to 8 days at room temperature.

Solution: Prior to dilution, store at room temperature, 15°C to 30°C (59°F to 86°F); protect from light.

♦ **Cytarabine Hydrochloride** *see* Cytarabine *on page 477*
♦ **Cytosar-U®** *see* Cytarabine *on page 477*
♦ **Cytosine Arabinosine Hydrochloride** *see* Cytarabine *on page 477*
♦ **Cytotec®** *see* Misoprostol *on page 1166*
♦ **Cytovene®** *see* Ganciclovir *on page 794*
♦ **Cytoxan®** *see* Cyclophosphamide *on page 462*
♦ **Cytra-2** *see* Sodium Citrate and Citric Acid *on page 1548*
♦ **D_5W** *see* Dextrose *on page 511*
♦ **$D_{10}W$** *see* Dextrose *on page 511*
♦ **$D_{25}W$** *see* Dextrose *on page 511*
♦ **$D_{30}W$** *see* Dextrose *on page 511*
♦ **$D_{40}W$** *see* Dextrose *on page 511*
♦ **$D_{50}W$** *see* Dextrose *on page 511*
♦ **$D_{60}W$** *see* Dextrose *on page 511*
♦ **$D_{70}W$** *see* Dextrose *on page 511*

Daclizumab (dac KLYE zue mab)

U.S. Brand Names Zenapax®

Pharmacologic Category Immunosuppressant Agent

Use Part of an immunosuppressive regimen (including cyclosporine and corticosteroids) for the prophylaxis of acute organ rejection in patients receiving renal transplant

Unlabeled/Investigational Use Graft-versus-host disease; prevention of organ rejection after heart transplant

Mechanism of Action Daclizumab is a chimeric (90% human, 10% murine) monoclonal IgG antibody produced by recombinant DNA technology. Daclizumab inhibits immune reactions by binding and blocking the alpha-chain of the interleukin-2 receptor (CD25) located on the surface of activated lymphocytes.

Pharmacodynamics/Kinetics

Distribution: V_d:

Adults: Central compartment: 0.031 L/kg; Peripheral compartment: 0.043 L/kg

Children: Central compartment: 0.067 L/kg; Peripheral compartment: 0.047 L/kg

Half-life elimination (estimated): Adults: Terminal: 20 days; Children: 13 days

Contraindications Hypersensitivity to daclizumab or any component of the formulation

Warnings/Precautions Patients on immunosuppressive therapy are at increased risk for infectious complications and secondary malignancies. Long-term effects of daclizumab on immune function are unknown. Severe hypersensitivity reactions have been rarely reported; anaphylaxis has been observed on initial exposure and following re-exposure; medications for the management of severe allergic reaction should be available for immediate use. Anti-idiotype antibodies have been measured in patients that have received daclizumab (adults 14%; children 34%); detection of antibodies may be influenced by multiple factors and may therefore be misleading.

In cardiac transplant patients, the combined use of daclizumab, cyclosporine, mycophenolate mofetil, and corticosteroids has been associated with an increased mortality. Higher mortality may be associated with the use of antilymphocyte globulin and a higher incidence of severe infections.

Drug Interactions

Immunosuppressants: The combined use of daclizumab, cyclosporine, mycophenolate mofetil, and corticosteroids has been associated with an increased mortality in a population of cardiac transplant recipients, particularly in patients who received antilymphocyte globulin and in patients with severe infections.

Adverse Reactions Although reported adverse events are frequent, when daclizumab is compared with placebo the incidence of adverse effects is similar between the two groups. Many of the adverse effects reported during clinical trial use of daclizumab may be related to the patient population, transplant procedure, and concurrent transplant medications. Diarrhea, fever, postoperative pain, pruritus, respiratory tract infection, urinary tract infection, and vomiting occurred more often in children than adults.

≥5%:

- Cardiovascular: Chest pain, edema, hyper-/hypotension, tachycardia, thrombosis
- Central nervous system: Dizziness, fatigue, fever, headache, insomnia, pain, post-traumatic pain, tremor
- Dermatologic: Acne, cellulitis, wound healing impaired
- Gastrointestinal: Abdominal distention, abdominal pain, constipation, diarrhea, dyspepsia, epigastric pain, nausea, pyrosis, vomiting
- Genitourinary: Dysuria
- Hematologic: Bleeding
- Neuromuscular & skeletal: Back pain, musculoskeletal pain
- Renal: Oliguria, renal tubular necrosis
- Respiratory: Cough, dyspnea, pulmonary edema
- Miscellaneous: Lymphocele, wound infection

≥2% to <5%:

- Central nervous system: Anxiety, depression, shivering
- Dermatologic: Hirsutism, pruritus, rash
- Endocrine & metabolic: Dehydration, diabetes mellitus, fluid overload
- Gastrointestinal: Flatulence, gastritis, hemorrhoids
- Genitourinary: Urinary retention, urinary tract bleeding
- Local: Application site reaction
- Neuromuscular & skeletal: Arthralgia, leg cramps, myalgia, weakness
- Ocular: Vision blurred
- Renal: Hydronephrosis, renal damage, renal insufficiency
- Respiratory: Atelectasis, congestion, hypoxia, pharyngitis, pleural effusion, rales, rhinitis
- Miscellaneous: Night sweats, prickly sensation, diaphoresis

<1% (Limited to important or life-threatening): Severe hypersensitivity reactions (rare): Anaphylaxis, bronchospasm, cardiac arrest, cytokine release syndrome, hypotension, laryngeal edema, pulmonary edema, pruritus, urticaria

Overdosage/Toxicology Overdose has not been reported.

Dosing

Adults:

Note: Daclizumab is used adjunctively with other immunosuppressants (eg, cyclosporine, corticosteroids, mycophenolate mofetil, and azathioprine).

(Continued)

Daclizumab *(Continued)*

Immunoprophylaxis against acute renal allograft rejection: I.V.: 1 mg/kg infused over 15 minutes within 24 hours before transplantation (day 0), then every 14 days for 4 additional doses

Treatment of graft-versus-host disease (unlabeled use, limited data): I.V.: 0.5-1.5 mg/kg, repeat same dosage for transient response. Repeat doses have been administered 11-48 days following the initial dose.

Prevention of organ rejection after heart transplant (unlabeled use): 1 mg/kg up to a maximum of 100 mg; administer within 12 hours after heart transplant and on days 8, 22, 36, and 50 post-transplant

Elderly: Refer to adult dosing. Use with caution.

Pediatrics: Refer to adult dosing.

Renal Impairment: No dosage adjustment needed.

Hepatic Impairment: No data available for patients with severe impairment.

Available Dosage Forms Injection, solution [preservative free]: 5 mg/mL (5 mL)

Nursing Guidelines

Assessment: Assess potential for interactions with other prescriptions, OTC medications, or herbal products patient may be taking. Assess cardiorespiratory and renal function (fluid overload) and adverse reactions during infusion and periodically between infusions. Be alert to the possibility of the development of infection or malignancies. **Note:** Hypersensitivity reactions can occur; medications for immediate treatment of severe allergic reactions should be available for immediate use. Teach patient possible side effects/appropriate interventions and adverse symptoms to report.

Patient Education: This medication, which may help transplant rejection, can only be administered by infusion. You will be monitored closely during infusion. Report immediately any respiratory or swallowing difficulty; tightness in jaw or throat; chest pain; or rash, pain, burning, redness, or swelling at infusion site. You will be more susceptible to infection (avoid crowds and exposure to infection and do not have any vaccinations without consulting prescriber). Maintain adequate hydration (2-3 L/day of fluids) unless instructed to restrict fluid intake and nutrition (small frequent meals may be advisable). May cause headache, dizziness, fatigue (use caution when driving or engaging in tasks that require alertness until response to drug is known): back pain, leg cramps, or musculoskeletal pain (consult prescriber for approved analgesic); or nausea, vomiting, dyspepsia, or abdominal discomfort (good mouth care, small frequent meals, chewing gum, or sucking lozenges may help). Report changes in urinary pattern; unusual bleeding or bruising; chest pain or palpitations; persistent dizziness, tremors, or headache; respiratory difficulty or unusual cough; rash; opportunistic infection (vaginal itching or drainage, sores in mouth, unusual fever or chills); or other persistent adverse effects. **Pregnancy/breast-feeding precautions:** Inform prescriber if you are or intend to become pregnant. Consult prescriber if breast-feeding.

Pregnancy Risk Factor: C

Pregnancy Issues: Animal reproduction studies have not been conducted. Generally, IgG molecules cross the placenta. Do not use during pregnancy unless the potential benefit to the mother outweighs the possible risk to the fetus. Women of childbearing potential should use effective contraception before, during, and for 4 months following treatment.

Lactation: Excretion in breast milk unknown/use caution

Administration

I.V.: For I.V. administration following dilution. Daclizumab solution should be administered within 4 hours of preparation if stored at room temperature; infuse over a 15-minute period via a peripheral or central vein.

Reconstitution: Dose should be further diluted in 50 mL 0.9% sodium chloride solution. When mixing, gently invert bag to avoid foaming; do not shake. Do not use if solution is discolored. Diluted solution is stable for 24 hours at 4°C or for 4 hours at room temperature.

Compatibility: Do not mix with other medications or infuse other medications through same I.V. line.

Storage: Refrigerate vials at 2°C to 8°C (36°F to 46°F). Do not shake or freeze; protect undiluted solution against direct sunlight.

♦ **Dakin's Solution** *see* Sodium Hypochlorite Solution *on page 1549*

♦ **Dalmane®** *see* Flurazepam *on page 754*

♦ **d-Alpha-Gems™ [OTC]** *see* Vitamin E *on page 1716*

♦ ***d*-Alpha Tocopherol** *see* Vitamin E *on page 1716*

Dalteparin (dal TE pa rin)

U.S. Brand Names Fragmin®

Pharmacologic Category Low Molecular Weight Heparin

Use Prevention of deep vein thrombosis which may lead to pulmonary embolism, in patients requiring abdominal surgery who are at risk for thromboembolism complications (eg, patients >40 years of age, obesity, patients with malignancy, history of deep vein thrombosis or pulmonary embolism, and surgical procedures requiring general anesthesia and lasting >30 minutes); prevention of DVT in patients undergoing hip-replacement surgery; patients immobile during an acute illness; acute treatment of unstable angina or non-Q-wave myocardial infarction; prevention of ischemic complications in patients on concurrent aspirin therapy

Unlabeled/Investigational Use Active treatment of deep vein thrombosis

Mechanism of Action Low molecular weight heparin analog with a molecular weight of 4000-6000 daltons; the commercial product contains 3% to 15% heparin with a molecular weight <3000 daltons, 65% to 78% with a molecular weight of 3000-8000 daltons and 14% to 26% with a molecular weight >8000 daltons; while dalteparin has been shown to inhibit both factor Xa and factor IIa (thrombin), the antithrombotic effect of dalteparin is characterized by a higher ratio of antifactor Xa to antifactor IIa activity (ratio = 4)

Pharmacodynamics/Kinetics

Onset of action: 1-2 hours

Duration: >12 hours

Half-life elimination (route dependent): 2-5 hours

Time to peak, serum: 4 hours

Contraindications Hypersensitivity to dalteparin or any component of the formulation; thrombocytopenia associated with a positive *in vitro* test for antiplatelet antibodies in the presence of dalteparin; hypersensitivity to heparin or pork products; patients with active major bleeding; patients with unstable angina or non-Q-wave MI undergoing regional anesthesia; not for I.M. or I.V. use

Warnings/Precautions **Patients with recent or anticipated neuraxial anesthesia (epidural or spinal anesthesia) are at risk of spinal or epidural hematoma and subsequent paralysis.** Consider risk versus benefit prior to neuraxial anesthesia. Risk is increased by concomitant agents which may alter hemostasis, as well as traumatic or repeated epidural or spinal puncture. Patient should be observed closely for bleeding if dalteparin is administered during or immediately following diagnostic lumbar puncture, epidural anesthesia, or spinal anesthesia.

Not to be used interchangeably (unit for unit) with heparin or any other low molecular weight heparins. Use with caution in patients with known hypersensitivity to methylparaben or propylparaben. Use with caution in patients with history of heparin-induced thrombocytopenia. Monitor platelet count closely. Rare thrombocytopenia may occur. Consider discontinuation of dalteparin in any patient developing significant thrombocytopenia. Monitor patient closely for signs or symptoms of bleeding. Certain patients are at increased risk of bleeding. Risk factors include bacterial endocarditis; congenital or acquired bleeding disorders; active ulcerative or angiodysplastic GI diseases; severe uncontrolled hypertension; hemorrhagic stroke; or use shortly after brain, spinal, or ophthalmology surgery; in patient treated concomitantly with platelet inhibitors; recent GI bleeding; thrombocytopenia or platelet defects; severe liver disease; hypertensive or diabetic retinopathy; or in patients undergoing invasive procedures.

Use with caution in patients with severe renal failure (has not been studied). Safety and efficacy in pediatric patients have not been established. Rare cases of thrombocytopenia with thrombosis have occurred. Multidose vials contain benzyl alcohol and should not be used in pregnant women. Heparin can cause hyperkalemia by affecting aldosterone. Similar reactions could occur with LMWHs. Monitor for hyperkalemia.

Drug Interactions

Drugs which affect platelet function (eg, aspirin, NSAIDs, dipyridamole, ticlopidine, clopidogrel) may potentiate the risk of hemorrhage.

Thrombolytic agents increase the risk of hemorrhage.

Warfarin: Risk of bleeding may be increased during concurrent therapy. Dalteparin is commonly continued during the initiation of warfarin therapy to assure anticoagulation and to protect against possible transient hypercoagulability.

Nutritional/Herbal/Ethanol Interactions Herb/Nutraceutical: Avoid cat's claw, dong quai, evening primrose, garlic, ginseng (all have additional antiplatelet activity).

(Continued)

Dalteparin *(Continued)*

Lab Interactions Increased AST, ALT levels

Adverse Reactions

1% to 10%:

Hematologic: Bleeding (3% to 5%), wound hematoma (0.1% to 3%)

Local: Pain at injection site (up to 12%), injection site hematoma (0.2% to 7%)

<1% (Limited to important or life-threatening): Allergic reaction (fever, pruritus, rash, injection site reaction, bullous eruption), anaphylactoid reaction, gastrointestinal bleeding, injection site hematoma, operative site bleeding, skin necrosis, thrombocytopenia (including heparin-induced thrombocytopenia). Spinal or epidural hematomas can occur following neuraxial anesthesia or spinal puncture, resulting in paralysis. Risk is increased in patients with indwelling epidural catheters or concomitant use of other drugs affecting hemostasis, osteoporosis (3-6 month use).

Dosing

Adults & Elderly:

Abdominal surgery (DVT prophylaxis):

Low-to-moderate DVT risk: SubQ: 2500 int. units 1-2 hours prior to surgery, then once daily for 5-10 days postoperatively

High DVT risk: SubQ: 5000 int. units 1-2 hours prior to surgery and then once daily for 5-10 days postoperatively

Total hip surgery (DVT prophylaxis): SubQ: **Note:** Three treatment options are currently available. Dose is given for 5-10 days, although up to 14 days of treatment have been tolerated in clinical trials:

Postoperative start:

Initial: 2500 int. units 4-8 hours* after surgery

Maintenance: 5000 int. units once daily; start at least 6 hours after post-surgical dose

Preoperative (starting day of surgery):

Initial: 2500 int. units within 2 hours before surgery

Adjustment: 2500 int. units 4-8 hours* after surgery

Maintenance: 5000 int. units once daily; start at least 6 hours after post-surgical dose

Preoperative (starting evening prior to surgery):

Initial: 5000 int. units 10-14 hours before surgery

Adjustment: 5000 int. units 4-8 hours* after surgery

Maintenance: 5000 int. units once daily, allowing 24 hours between doses.

***Note:** Dose may be delayed if hemostasis is not yet achieved.

Unstable angina or non-Q-wave myocardial infarction: SubQ: 120 int. units/kg body weight (maximum dose: 10,000 int. units) every 12 hours for 5-8 days with concurrent aspirin therapy. Discontinue dalteparin once patient is clinically stable.

Immobility/acute illness (DVT prophylaxis): 5000 int. units once daily

Available Dosage Forms

Injection, solution [multidose vial]: Antifactor Xa 10,000 int. units per 1 mL (9.5 mL) [contains benzyl alcohol]; antifactor Xa 25,000 units per 1 mL (3.8 mL) [contains benzyl alcohol]

Injection, solution [preservative free; prefilled syringe]: Antifactor Xa 2500 int. units per 0.2 mL (0.2 mL); antifactor Xa 5000 int. units per 0.2 mL (0.2 mL); antifactor Xa 7500 int. units per 0.3 mL (0.3 mL); antifactor Xa 10,000 int. units per 1 mL (1 mL)

Nursing Guidelines

Assessment: See Contraindications, Warnings/Precautions, and Dosing for use cautions. Assess potential for interactions with other prescriptions, OTC medications, or herbal products patient may be taking (especially anything that will impact coagulation or platelet aggregation - see Drug Interactions). Assess results of laboratory tests (see below), therapeutic effectiveness (according to purpose for use), and adverse response (eg, thrombolytic reactions - see Adverse Reactions and Overdose/Toxicology). Teach patient possible side effects/appropriate interventions and adverse symptoms to report (see Patient Education). Note breast-feeding caution.

Monitoring Laboratory Tests: Periodic CBC including platelet count, stool occult blood; monitoring of PT and PTT is not necessary.

Patient Education: Inform prescriber of all prescriptions, OTC medications, or herbal products you are taking, and any allergies you have. Do not take any new medication during therapy unless approved by prescriber. This drug can only be administered by injection. You may have a tendency to bleed easily while taking this drug (brush teeth with soft brush, use waxed dental floss, use electric razor, avoid scissors or sharp knives and potentially harmful activities). Report unusual fever; unusual bleeding or bruising (bleeding gums, nosebleed, blood in urine, dark stool); pain in joints or back; severe head pain; skin rash; or redness, swelling, or pain at injection site. **Breast-feeding precaution:** Consult prescriber if breast-feeding.

Pregnancy Risk Factor: B

Pregnancy Issues: Multiple-dose vials contain benzyl alcohol (avoid in pregnant women due to association with fetal syndrome in premature infants).

Lactation: Excretion in breast milk unknown/use caution

Perioperative/Anesthesia/Other Concerns: Many critically-ill and surgery patients require preventive measures for venous thromboembolism. LMWHs compare favorably to unfractionated heparin in the prevention and treatment of venous thromboembolism. LMWHs are associated with less thrombocytopenia, compared to heparin, and do not require routine therapeutic monitoring.

Obesity/Renal Dysfunction: There is no consensus for adjusting/correcting the weight-based dosage of LMWH for patients who are morbidly obese. Monitoring of antifactor Xa concentration 4 hours after injection may be warranted. Patients who have a reduction in calculated creatinine clearance are at risk of accumulated anticoagulant effect when they are treated with certain LMWHs. All LMWHs may not behave the same in patients with renal dysfunction. Some clinicians monitor anti-Xa levels for patients with Cl_{cr} <30 mL/minute.

Administration

I.M.: Do not give I.M.

Storage: Store at temperatures 20°C to 25°C (68°F to 77°F).

♦ Damason-P® *see* Hydrocodone and Aspirin *on page 871*
♦ Dantrium® *see* Dantrolene *on page 485*

Dantrolene (DAN troe leen)

U.S. Brand Names Dantrium®

Synonyms Dantrolene Sodium

Pharmacologic Category Skeletal Muscle Relaxant

Medication Safety Issues

Sound-alike/look-alike issues:

Dantrium® may be confused with danazol, Daraprim®

Use Treatment of spasticity associated with spinal cord injury, stroke, cerebral palsy, or multiple sclerosis; treatment of malignant hyperthermia

Unlabeled/Investigational Use Neuroleptic malignant syndrome (NMS)

Mechanism of Action Acts directly on skeletal muscle by interfering with release of calcium ion from the sarcoplasmic reticulum; prevents or reduces the increase in myoplasmic calcium ion concentration that activates the acute catabolic processes associated with malignant hyperthermia

Pharmacodynamics/Kinetics

Absorption: Oral: Slow and incomplete

Metabolism: Hepatic

Half-life elimination: 8.7 hours

Excretion: Feces (45% to 50%); urine (25% as unchanged drug and metabolites)

Contraindications Active hepatic disease; should not be used where spasticity is used to maintain posture or balance

Warnings/Precautions Use with caution in patients with impaired cardiac function or impaired pulmonary function; has potential for hepatotoxicity; overt hepatitis has been most frequently observed between the third and twelfth month of therapy; hepatic injury appears to be greater in females and in patients >35 years of age

Drug Interactions Substrate of CYP3A4 (major)

CYP3A4 inducers: CYP3A4 inducers may decrease the levels/effects of dantrolene. Example inducers include aminoglutethimide, carbamazepine, nafcillin, nevirapine, phenobarbital, phenytoin, and rifamycins.

CYP3A4 inhibitors: May increase the levels/effects of dantrolene. Example inhibitors include azole antifungals, clarithromycin, diclofenac, doxycycline, erythromycin, imatinib, isoniazid, nefazodone, nicardipine, propofol, protease inhibitors, quinidine, telithromycin, and verapamil.

Increased toxicity: Estrogens (hepatotoxicity), CNS depressants (sedation), MAO inhibitors, phenothiazines, clindamycin (increased neuromuscular blockade), verapamil (hyperkalemia and cardiac depression), warfarin, clofibrate, and tolbutamide

(Continued)

Dantrolene *(Continued)*

Nutritional/Herbal/Ethanol Interactions

Ethanol: Avoid ethanol (may increase CNS depression).

Herb/Nutraceutical: Avoid valerian, St John's wort, kava kava, gotu kola (may increase CNS depression).

Lab Interactions Increased aminotransferase [ALT (SGPT)/AST (SGOT)] (S), alkaline phosphatase, LDH, BUN, and total serum bilirubin

Adverse Reactions

>10%:

Central nervous system: Drowsiness, dizziness, lightheadedness, fatigue
Dermatologic: Rash
Gastrointestinal: Diarrhea (mild), vomiting
Neuromuscular & skeletal: Muscle weakness

1% to 10%:

Cardiovascular: Pleural effusion with pericarditis
Central nervous system: Chills, fever, headache, insomnia, nervousness, mental depression
Gastrointestinal: Diarrhea (severe), constipation, anorexia, stomach cramps
Ocular: Blurred vision
Respiratory: Respiratory depression

<1% (Limited to important or life-threatening): Confusion, hepatic necrosis, hepatitis, seizure

Overdosage/Toxicology Symptoms of overdose include CNS depression, hypotension, nausea, and vomiting. For decontamination, lavage with activated charcoal and administer a cathartic. Do not use ipecac. Other treatment is supportive and symptomatic.

Dosing

Adults & Elderly:

Spasticity: Oral: 25 mg/day to start, increase frequency to 2-4 times/day, then increase dose by 25 mg every 4-7 days to a maximum of 100 mg 2-4 times/day or 400 mg/day

Malignant hyperthermia:

Preoperative prophylaxis:

Oral: 4-8 mg/kg/day in 4 divided doses, begin 1-2 days prior to surgery with last dose 3-4 hours prior to surgery

I.V.: 2.5 mg/kg ~1¼ hours prior to anesthesia and infused over 1 hour with additional doses as needed and individualized

Crisis: I.V.: 2.5 mg/kg; may repeat dose up to cumulative dose of 10 mg/kg; if physiologic and metabolic abnormalities reappear, repeat regimen

Postcrisis follow-up: Oral: 4-8 mg/kg/day in 4 divided doses for 1-3 days; I.V. dantrolene may be used when oral therapy is not practical; individualize dosage beginning with 1 mg/kg or more as the clinical situation dictates

Neuroleptic malignant syndrome (unlabeled use): I.V.: 1 mg/kg; may repeat dose up to maximum cumulative dose of 10 mg/kg, then switch to oral dosage

Pediatrics:

Spasticity: Oral: Initial: 0.5 mg/kg/dose twice daily, increase frequency to 3-4 times/day at 4- to 7-day intervals, then increase dose by 0.5 mg/kg to a maximum of 3 mg/kg/dose 2-4 times/day up to 400 mg/day

Malignant hyperthermia: Refer to adult dosing.

Available Dosage Forms

Capsule, as sodium: 25 mg, 50 mg, 100 mg

Injection, powder for reconstitution, as sodium: 20 mg [contains mannitol 3 g]

Nursing Guidelines

Assessment: Assess effectiveness and interactions of other medications patient may be taking. **I.V.:** Monitor vital signs, cardiac function, respiratory status, and I.V. site (extravasation very irritating to tissues). Monitor effectiveness of therapy and adverse reactions at beginning and periodically during therapy. Assess knowledge/teach patient appropriate use, interventions to reduce side effects, and adverse symptoms to report.

Monitoring Laboratory Tests: Liver function for potential hepatotoxicity

Patient Education: Take exactly as directed. Do not increase dose or discontinue without consulting prescriber. Do not use alcohol, prescriptive or OTC antidepressants, sedatives, or pain medications without consulting prescriber. You may experience drowsiness, dizziness, lightheadedness (avoid driving or engaging in tasks that require alertness until response to drug is known); nausea or vomiting (small frequent meals, frequent mouth care, or sucking hard candy may help); or diarrhea (buttermilk, boiled milk, or yogurt may help). Report excessive confusion; drowsiness or mental agitation; chest pain, palpitations, or respiratory difficulty; skin rash; or vision changes. **Pregnancy/breast-feeding precautions:** Inform prescriber if you are or intend to become pregnant. Breast-feeding is not recommended.

Pregnancy Risk Factor: C

Lactation: Excretion in breast milk unknown/not recommended

Administration

I.V.: Therapeutic or emergency dose can be administered with rapid continuous I.V. push. Follow-up doses should be administered over 2-3 minutes.

Reconstitution: Reconstitute vial by adding 60 mL of sterile water for injection USP (**not bacteriostatic water for injection**). Protect from light. Use within 6 hours. Avoid glass bottles for I.V. infusion.

♦ Dantrolene Sodium *see* Dantrolene *on page 485*

Darbepoetin Alfa (dar be POE e tin AL fa)

U.S. Brand Names Aranesp®

Synonyms Erythropoiesis Stimulating Protein

Pharmacologic Category Colony Stimulating Factor; Growth Factor; Recombinant Human Erythropoietin

Medication Safety Issues

Sound-alike/look-alike issues:

Darbepoetin alfa may be confused with epoetin alfa

Use Treatment of anemia associated with chronic renal failure (CRF), including patients on dialysis (ESRD) and patients not on dialysis; anemia associated with chemotherapy for nonmyeloid malignancies

Mechanism of Action Induces erythropoiesis by stimulating the division and differentiation of committed erythroid progenitor cells; induces the release of reticulocytes from the bone marrow into the bloodstream, where they mature to erythrocytes. There is a dose response relationship with this effect. This results in an increase in reticulocyte counts followed by a rise in hematocrit and hemoglobin levels. When administered SubQ or I.V., darbepoetin's half-life is ~3 times that of epoetin alfa concentrations.

Pharmacodynamics/Kinetics

Onset of action: Increased hemoglobin levels not generally observed until 2-6 weeks after initiating treatment

Absorption: SubQ: Slow

Distribution: V_d: 0.06 L/kg

Bioavailability: CRF: SubQ: ~37% (range: 30% to 50%)

Half-life elimination: CRF: Terminal: I.V.: 21 hours, SubQ: 49 hours; **Note:** Half-life is ~3 times as long as epoetin alfa

Time to peak: SubQ: CRF: 34 hours (range: 24-72 hours); Cancer: 90 hours (range: 71-123 hours)

Contraindications Hypersensitivity to darbepoetin or any component of the formulation (including polysorbate 80 and/or albumin); uncontrolled hypertension

Warnings/Precautions Erythropoietic therapies may be associated with an increased risk of cardiovascular and/or neurologic events in chronic renal failure. Darbepoetin alfa should be managed carefully; avoid hemoglobin increases >1 g/dL in any 2-week period, and do not exceed a target level of 12 g/dL. Prior to and during therapy, iron stores must be evaluated. Supplemental iron is recommended if serum ferritin <100 mcg/mL or serum transferrin saturation <20%. In cancer patients, the risk of thrombotic events (eg, pulmonary emboli, thrombophlebitis, thrombosis) was increased by erythropoietic therapy.

Use with caution in patients with hypertension or with a history of seizures. If hypertension is difficult to control, reduce or hold darbepoetin alpha. **Not** recommended for acute correction of severe anemia or as a substitute for transfusion. Consider discontinuing in patients who receive a renal transplant.

Prior to treatment, correct or exclude deficiencies of vitamin B_{12} and/or folate, as well as other factors which may impair erythropoiesis (aluminum toxicity, inflammatory conditions, infections). Poor response should prompt evaluation of these potential factors, as well as possible malignant processes, occult blood loss, hemolysis, and/or bone marrow fibrosis. Pure red cell aplasia (PRCA) with associated neutralizing antibodies to erythropoietin has been reported, predominantly in patients with CRF. Patients with loss of response to darbepoetin alfa should be evaluated. Discontinue treatment in patients with PRCA secondary to neutralizing antibodies to erythropoietin.

(Continued)

Darbepoetin Alfa *(Continued)*

Due to the delayed onset of erythropoiesis, darbepoetin is of no value in the acute treatment of anemia. Safety and efficacy in patients with underlying hematologic diseases have not been established, including porphyria, thalassemia, hemolytic anemia, and sickle cell disease. Risk of thrombosis, including pulmonary embolism, increased in cancer patients. Do not shake solution; vigorous shaking may denature darbepoetin alfa, rendering it biologically inactive. Safety and efficacy in pediatric patients have not been established.

Drug Interactions No data available

Nutritional/Herbal/Ethanol Interactions Ethanol: Should be avoided due to adverse effects on erythropoiesis.

Adverse Reactions Note: Frequency of adverse events cited in patients with CRF or cancer and may be, in part, a reflection of population in which the drug is used and/or associated with dialysis procedures.

>10%:

- Cardiovascular: Hypertension (4% to 23%), hypotension (22%), edema (21%), peripheral edema (11%)
- Central nervous system: Fatigue (9% to 33%), fever (9% to 19%), headache (12% to 16%), dizziness (8% to 14%)
- Gastrointestinal: Diarrhea (16% to 22%), constipation (5% to 18%), vomiting (15%), nausea (14%), abdominal pain (12%)
- Neuromuscular & skeletal: Myalgia (8% to 21%), arthralgia (11% to 13%)
- Respiratory: Upper respiratory infection (14%), dyspnea (12%)
- Miscellaneous: Infection (27%)

1% to 10%:

- Cardiovascular: Arrhythmia (10%), angina/chest pain (6% to 8%), fluid overload (6%), CHF (6%), thrombosis (6%), MI (2%)
- Central nervous system: Seizure (<1% to 1%), stroke (1%), TIA (1%)
- Dermatologic: Pruritus (8%), rash (7%)
- Endocrine & metabolic: Dehydration (5%)
- Local: Injection site pain (7%)
- Neuromuscular & skeletal: Back pain (8%), weakness (5%), limb pain (10%)
- Respiratory: Cough (10%), bronchitis (6%), pulmonary embolism (1%)
- Miscellaneous: Vascular access thrombosis (8%; annualized rate 0.22 events per patient year), death (7%), vascular access infection (6%), influenza-like symptoms (6%), vascular access hemorrhage (6%)
- Postmarketing and/or case reports: Pure red cell aplasia, severe anemia (with or without other cytopenias)

Overdosage/Toxicology The maximum amount of darbepoetin which may be safely administered has not been determined. However, cardiovascular and neurologic adverse events have been correlated to excessive and/or rapid rise in hemoglobin. Phlebotomy may be performed if clinically indicated.

Dosing

Adults & Elderly:

Correction of anemia associated with CRF: I.V., SubQ:

Manufacturer recommended dosing: Initial: 0.45 mcg/kg once weekly; titrate to response; some patients may respond to doses given once every 2 weeks

Unlabeled dosing:

Every 2-weeks: 0.75 mcg/kg every 2 weeks (Toto, 2004)

or

Every 4-weeks: 0.75 mcg/kg every 2 weeks; once titrated, multiply dose by 2 and give every 4 weeks (Jadoul, 2004).

Anemia associated with chemotherapy: SubQ:

Manufacturer recommended dosing: Initial: 2.25 mcg/kg once weekly; with inadequate response: 4.5 mcg/kg once weekly

Unlabeled dosing:

Every 2-weeks:

Initial: 200 mcg every 2 weeks; inadequate response: 300 mcg every 2 weeks (Thames, 2003)

or

Initial: 3 mcg/kg every 2 weeks; inadequate response: 5 mcg/kg every 2 weeks (Vadhan-Raj, 2003)

or

Every 3-weeks (front load): Initial: 4.5 mcg/kg every week until desired Hgb obtained; maintenance: 4.5 mcg/kg (or titrated dose) every 3 weeks (Hesketh, 2004)

or

Initial: 325 mcg every week until desired Hgb obtained; maintenance: 325 mcg every 3 weeks (Hesketh, 2004)

Treatment goals: **Note:** Titration may be required to limit rises of Hgb to <1 g/dL over any 2-week interval and to reach a Hgb concentration not to exceed 12 g/dL.

Inadequate response: Increase dose; refer to individual dosing regimens for adjustment when Hgb increase <1 g/dL after 4-6 weeks

Excessive response: Hold dose and/or decrease dose by 25%

Decrease dose by 25% when Hgb increases >1 g/dL in any 2-week period **or** Hgb increases and approaches 12 g/dL in any 2-week period

Hold dose, then decrease dose by 25% when Hgb increases despite previous dose decrease (hold until Hgb decreases) **or** when Hgb ≥13 g/dL (hold until Hgb ≤12 g/dL)

Conversion from epoetin alfa to darbepoetin alfa: See table.

Conversion From Epoetin Alfa to Darbepoetin Alfa

Previous Dosage of Epoetin Alfa (units/week)	Darbepoetin Alfa Dosage (mcg/week)	Darbepoetin Alfa Dosage (mcg/every 2 weeks)
<2500	6.25	12.5
2500-4999	12.5	25
5000-10,999	25	50
11,000-17,999	40	80
18,000-33,999	60	120
34,000-89,999	100	200
≥90,000	200	400

Note: In patients receiving epoetin alfa 2-3 times per week, darbepoetin alfa is administered once weekly. In patients receiving epoetin alfa once weekly, darbepoetin alfa is administered once every 2 weeks.

Renal Impairment: Dosage requirements for patients with chronic renal failure who do not require dialysis may be lower than in dialysis patients. Monitor patients closely during the time period in which a dialysis regimen is initiated, dosage requirement may increase.

Available Dosage Forms

Injection, solution, with human albumin 2.5 mg/mL [preservative free, single-dose vial]: 25 mcg/mL (1 mL); 40 mcg/mL (1 mL); 60 mcg/mL (1 mL); 100 mcg/mL (1 mL); 150 mcg/0.75 mL (0.75 mL); 200 mcg/mL (1 mL); 300 mcg/mL (1 mL)

Injection, solution, with human albumin 2.5 mg/mL [preservative free, prefilled syringe]: 25 mcg/0.42 mL (0.42 mL); 40 mcg/0.4 mL (0.4 mL); 60 mcg/0.3 mL (0.3 mL); 100 mcg/0.5 mL (0.5 mL); 200 mcg/0.4 mL (0.4 mL); 300 mcg/0.6 mL (0.6 mL); 500 mcg/mL (1 mL)

Nursing Guidelines

Assessment: Assess potential for interactions with other prescriptions, OTC medications, or herbal products patient may be taking (eg, nutritional or supplemental iron). Monitor blood pressure and be alert for signs of fluid retention. Assess GI function. Assess results of laboratory tests prior to and during therapy. Assess therapeutic effectiveness and adverse response on a regular basis during therapy. Teach patient proper use if self-administered (appropriate injection technique and syringe/needle disposal), possible side effects/appropriate interventions, and adverse symptoms to report.

Monitoring Laboratory Tests: Hemoglobin (weekly); prior to and during therapy, iron stores must be evaluated (supplemental iron is recommended in any patient with a serum ferritin <100 mcg/mL or serum transferrin saturation <20%)

Dietary Considerations: Supplemental iron intake may be required in patients with low iron stores.

Patient Education: Do not take any new medication during therapy without consulting prescriber. This medication can only be administered by infusion or injection (if self-administered, follow exact directions for injection and needle disposal). You will need frequent blood tests to determine appropriate dosage. Avoid alcohol and do not make significant changes in your dietary iron without consulting prescriber. Check your blood pressure as frequently as recommended and report any significant changes. May cause nausea or vomiting (small frequent meals, frequent mouth care, sucking lozenges, or chewing gum

(Continued)

Darbepoetin Alfa *(Continued)*

may help); diarrhea (boiled milk, buttermilk, or yogurt may help); constipation (increased dietary fruit, fiber, fluids, and increased exercise may help); or dizziness, fatigue, or headache (use caution when driving or engaging in tasks that require alertness until response to drug is known). Report signs of edema (swollen extremities, respiratory difficulty); sudden onset of acute headache, back pain, or chest pain; muscle tremors or weakness; cough or signs of respiratory infection; or other adverse effects. **Pregnancy/breast-feeding precautions:** Inform prescriber if you are or intend to become pregnant. Consult prescriber if breast-feeding.

Pregnancy Risk Factor: C

Lactation: Excretion in breast milk unknown/use caution

Perioperative/Anesthesia/Other Concerns: Recently, a prospective, randomized, double-blind, placebo-controlled, multicenter trial was performed in critically-ill patients (Corwin, 2002) assessing the efficacy of recombinant human erythropoietin in reducing red blood cell transfusions. Patients were enrolled from December 1998 through June 2001. Over thirteen hundred ICU (medical, surgical, or medical/surgical) patients were randomized to receive placebo or 40,000 units of erythropoietin subcutaneously on ICU day 3 and then weekly for patients who remained in the hospital. Each patient's physician determined the need for red blood cell transfusion. The mean baseline hemoglobin was 9.97 g/dL in each group. Patients receiving erythropoietin were less likely to receive transfusions. The mean number of units transfused per patient in the placebo group was 3 and in the erythropoietin group was 2.4. The erythropoietin group had a 19% reduction in total units of red blood cells transfused. Mortality and adverse clinical events were not significantly different between groups. The authors concluded that weekly administration of erythropoietin in critically-ill patients reduces red blood cell transfusions and increases hemoglobin. The authors also suggest that further study is needed to determine whether use of erythropoietin results in improved clinical outcomes. In addition, data on cost effectiveness would be helpful.

A restrictive transfusion approach (Hebert, 1999) was described in a transfusion trial that was published after Corwin's trial was underway. Hebert and his group evaluated a restrictive transfusion strategy (transfuse if hemoglobin <7 g/dL to maintain between 7 and 9 g/dL) versus a liberal strategy (transfuse if hemoglobin <10 g/dL to maintain between 10 and 12 g/dL). The restrictive approach to transfusion was at least as effective as, and possibly superior to, a liberal transfusion policy in critically-ill patients. The exception to this may be patients with acute myocardial infarction and unstable angina.

Administration

I.V.: May be administered by SubQ or I.V. injection. Do not shake; vigorous shaking may denature darbepoetin alfa, rendering it biologically inactive. Do not dilute or administer in conjunction with other drug solutions. Discard any unused portion of the vial; do not pool unused portions. Discontinue immediately if signs/symptoms of anaphylaxis occur.

Compatibility: Do not dilute or administer with other solutions.

Storage: Store at 2°C to 8°C (36°F to 46°F). Do not freeze or shake. Protect from light.

- **Darvocet A500™** *see* Propoxyphene and Acetaminophen *on page 1427*
- **Darvocet-N® 50** *see* Propoxyphene and Acetaminophen *on page 1427*
- **Darvocet-N® 100** *see* Propoxyphene and Acetaminophen *on page 1427*
- **Darvon®** *see* Propoxyphene *on page 1425*
- **Darvon-N®** *see* Propoxyphene *on page 1425*
- **DDAVP®** *see* Desmopressin *on page 492*
- **ddI** *see* Didanosine *on page 528*
- **1-Deamino-8-D-Arginine Vasopressin** *see* Desmopressin *on page 492*
- **Debrox® [OTC]** *see* Carbamide Peroxide *on page 311*
- **Decadron®** *see* Dexamethasone *on page 495*
- **Decadron® Phosphate [DSC]** *see* Dexamethasone *on page 495*
- **Deep Sea [OTC]** *see* Sodium Chloride *on page 1545*
- **Dehydrobenzperidol** *see* Droperidol *on page 590*
- **Delatestryl®** *see* Testosterone *on page 1607*
- **Delestrogen®** *see* Estradiol *on page 649*
- **Delta-9-tetrahydro-cannabinol** *see* Dronabinol *on page 588*

Desflurane (DES flure ane)

U.S. Brand Names Suprane®

Pharmacologic Category General Anesthetic, Inhalation

Medication Safety Issues

Sound-alike/look-alike issues:

Desflurane may be confused with Desferal®

Use Maintenance of general anesthesia

Pharmacodynamics/Kinetics

Onset of action: 1-2 minutes

Duration: Emergence time: Depends on blood concentration when desflurane is discontinued

The rate of change of anesthetic concentration in the lung is more rapid with desflurane because of its low blood/gas solubility (0.42), which is similar to nitrous oxide.

Metabolism: Hepatic (0.02%)

Excretion: Exhaled gases

Contraindications Hypersensitivity to desflurane or any component of the formulation; severe hypotension; known or suspected history of malignant hyperthermia; children; patients at risk for CAD; patients in whom an increase in heart rate or blood pressure is undesirable

Warnings/Precautions Decrease in blood pressure is dose dependent, due to peripheral vasodilation, with maintenance of cardiac output. Abrupt increases in inspired concentration >1 MAC can produce a transient increase in blood pressure and heart rate due to increased plasma catecholamine levels. Hepatic blood flow is decreased. Respiration is depressed as is hypoxic pulmonary vasoconstriction, which may lead to increased pulmonary shunt. Hypoxemia-induced increase in ventilation is abolished at low desflurane concentration. It dilates the cerebral vasculature and may, in certain conditions, increase intracranial pressure. Desflurane triggers malignant hyperthermia in humans, and therefore, should not be used on patients susceptible to malignant hyperthermia. Desflurane can produce elevated carbon monoxide levels in the presence of a dry carbon dioxide absorbent within the circle breathing system of an anesthetic machine.

(Continued)

Desflurane *(Continued)*

Drug Interactions Excessive hypotension may occur when combined with antihypertensive drugs. Potentiates the action of nondepolarizing neuromuscular blocking agents. Concurrent use of opioids and/or benzodiazepines decreases the MAC of desflurane.

Adverse Reactions The pungency of desflurane produces laryngospasm, cough, breath holding, increased secretions, and apnea making inhalation induction difficult.

Frequency not defined:

Cardiovascular: Hypotension, myocardial depression, tachycardia, bradycardia, hypertension

Central nervous system: Emergence delirium

Gastrointestinal: Nausea, vomiting

Respiratory: Respiratory depression/arrest, hypoxemia

Miscellaneous: Shivering

Dosing

Adults: Inhalation: The minimum alveolar concentration (MAC), the concentration at which 50% of patients do not respond to surgical incision, ranges from 6.0% (45 years of age) to 7.3% (25 years of age). The concentration at which amnesia and loss of awareness occur (MAC - awake) is 2.4%. Surgical levels of anesthesia are achieved with concentrations between 2.5% to 8.5%.

Note: Because of the higher vapor pressure of desflurane, its vaporizer is heated in order to deliver a constant concentration

Elderly: MAC is reduced (5.2% at 70 years of age).

Pediatrics: Anesthesia maintenance: Children: Surgical levels of anesthesia range between 5.2% to 10%

Note: Because of the higher vapor pressure of desflurane, its vaporizer is heated in order to deliver a constant concentration

Available Dosage Forms Liquid, for inhalation: 240 mL

Nursing Guidelines

Pregnancy Risk Factor: B

Perioperative/Anesthesia/Other Concerns: Use of desflurane for induction of general anesthesia is not recommended due to its irritant properties and unpleasant odor which may cause breath holding and coughing.

Related Information

Inhalational Anesthetics *on page 1850*

Desmopressin (des moe PRES in)

U.S. Brand Names DDAVP®; Stimate™

Synonyms 1-Deamino-8-D-Arginine Vasopressin; Desmopressin Acetate

Pharmacologic Category Antihemophilic Agent; Hemostatic Agent; Vasopressin Analog, Synthetic

Use

Injection: Treatment of diabetes insipidus; control of bleeding in hemophilia A, and mild-to-moderate classic von Willebrand disease (type I)

Tablet, nasal solution: Treatment of diabetes insipidus; primary nocturnal enuresis

Mechanism of Action Enhances reabsorption of water in the kidneys by increasing cellular permeability of the collecting ducts; possibly causes smooth muscle constriction with resultant vasoconstriction; raises plasma levels of von Willebrand factor and factor VIII

Pharmacodynamics/Kinetics

Intranasal administration:

Onset of increased factor VIII activity: 30 minutes (dose related)

Peak effect 1.5 hours

Bioavailability: 3.2%

I.V. infusion:

Onset of increased factor VIII activity: 30 minutes (dose related)

Peak effect: 1.5-2 hours

Half-life elimination: Terminal: 3 hours (up to 9 hours in renal dysfunction)

Excretion: Urine

Oral tablet:

Onset of action: ADH: ~1 hour

Peak effect: 4-7 hours

Bioavailability: 5% compared to intranasal; 0.16% compared to I.V.

Half-life elimination: 1.5-2.5 hours

Contraindications Injection, tablet: Hypersensitivity to desmopressin or any component of the formulation

Nasal solution: Hypersensitivity to desmopressin or any component of the formulation; moderate to severe renal impairment (Cl_{cr}<50 mL/minute)

Warnings/Precautions Fluid intake should be adjusted downward in the elderly and very young patients to decrease the possibility of water intoxication and hyponatremia. Avoid overhydration especially when drug is used for its hemostatic effect. Use may rarely lead to extreme decreases in plasma osmolality, resulting in seizures and coma. Use caution with cystic fibrosis or other conditions associated with fluid and electrolyte imbalance due to potential hyponatremia. Use caution with coronary artery insufficiency or hypertensive cardiovascular disease; may increase or decrease blood pressure leading to changes in heart rate. Consider switching from nasal to intravenous solution if changes in the nasal mucosa (scarring, edema) occur leading to unreliable absorption. Use caution in patients predisposed to thrombus formation; thrombotic events (acute cerebrovascular thrombosis, acute myocardial infarction) have occurred (rare). Injection is not for use in hemophilia B, severe classic von Willebrand disease (type IIB), or in patients with factor VIII antibodies. In general, the injection is also not recommended for use in patients with ≤5% factor VIII activity level, although it may be considered in selected patients with activity levels between 2% and 5%. Some patients may demonstrate a change in response after long-term therapy (>6 months) characterized as decreased response or a shorter duration of response.

Drug Interactions

Demeclocycline: May decrease response to endogenous antidiuretic hormone (ADH). Use caution.

Chlorpropamide: May increase response to ADH. Use caution.

Fludrocortisone: May increase response to ADH. Use caution.

Lithium: May decrease response to ADH. Use caution.

Nutritional/Herbal/Ethanol Interactions Ethanol: Avoid ethanol (may decrease antidiuretic effect).

Adverse Reactions Frequency not defined (may be dose or route related).

Cardiovascular: Acute cerebrovascular thrombosis, acute MI, blood pressure increased/decreased, chest pain, edema, facial flushing, palpitation

Central nervous system: Agitation, chills, coma, dizziness, headache, insomnia, somnolence

Dermatologic: Rash

Endocrine & metabolic: Hyponatremia, water intoxication

Gastrointestinal: Abdominal cramps, dyspepsia, nausea, sore throat, vomiting

Genitourinary: Balanitis, vulval pain

Local: Injection: Burning pain, erythema, and swelling at the injection site

Ocular: Conjunctivitis, eye edema, lacrimation disorder

Respiratory: Cough, nasal congestion, epistaxis, rhinitis

Miscellaneous: Allergic reactions (rare), anaphylaxis (rare)

Overdosage/Toxicology Symptoms of overdose include drowsiness, headache, confusion, anuria, and water intoxication. In case of overdose, decrease or discontinue desmopressin.

Dosing

Adults & Elderly:

Diabetes insipidus:

I.V., SubQ: 2-4 mcg/day (0.5-1 mL) in 2 divided doses or 1/10 of the maintenance intranasal dose

Intranasal (100 mcg/mL nasal solution): 10-40 mcg/day (0.1-0.4 mL) divided 1-3 times/day; adjust morning and evening doses separately for an adequate diurnal rhythm of water turnover. **Note:** The nasal spray pump can only deliver doses of 10 mcg (0.1 mL) or multiples of 10 mcg (0.1 mL); if doses other than this are needed, the rhinal tube delivery system is preferred.

Oral: Initial: 0.05 mg twice daily; total daily dose should be increased or decreased as needed to obtain adequate antidiuresis (range: 0.1-1.2 mg divided 2-3 times/day)

Nocturnal enuresis:

Intranasal (using 100 mcg/mL nasal solution): Initial: 20 mcg (0.2 mL) at bedtime; range: 10-40 mcg; it is recommended that ½ of the dose be given in each nostril. For 10 mcg dose, administer in one nostril. **Note:** The nasal spray pump can only deliver doses of 10 mcg (0.1 mL) or multiples of 10 mcg (0.1 mL); if doses other than this are needed, the rhinal tube delivery system is preferred.

(Continued)

Desmopressin *(Continued)*

Oral: 0.2 mg at bedtime; dose may be titrated up to 0.6 mg to achieve desired response. Patients previously on intranasal therapy can begin oral tablets 24 hours after the last intranasal dose.

Hemophilia A and mild-to-moderate von Willebrand disease (type I):

I.V.: 0.3 mcg/kg by slow infusion, begin 30 minutes before procedure

Nasal spray: Using high concentration spray (1.5 mg/mL): <50 kg: 150 mcg (1 spray); >50 kg: 300 mcg (1 spray each nostril); repeat use is determined by the patient's clinical condition and laboratory work. If using preoperatively, administer 2 hours before surgery.

Pediatrics:

Diabetes insipidus:

Intranasal (using 100 mcg/mL nasal solution):

Children 3 months to 12 years: Initial: 5 mcg/day (0.05 mL/day) divided 1-2 times/day; range: 5-30 mcg/day (0.05-0.3 mL/day) divided 1-2 times/day; adjust morning and evening doses separately for an adequate diurnal rhythm of water turnover; doses <10 mcg should be administered using the rhinal tube system

Children >12 years: Refer to adult dosing.

Oral: Children ≥4 years: Initial: 0.05 mg twice daily; total daily dose should be increased or decreased as needed to obtain adequate antidiuresis (range: 0.1-1.2 mg divided 2-3 times/day)

Hemophilia A and von Willebrand disease (type I):

I.V.: >3 months: 0.3 mcg/kg by slow infusion; may repeat dose if needed; begin 30 minutes before procedure

Intranasal: ≥11 months: Refer to adult dosing.

Nocturnal enuresis:

Children ≥6 years:

Intranasal (using 100 mcg/mL nasal solution): Initial: 20 mcg (0.2 mL) at bedtime; range: 10-40 mcg; it is recommended that ½ of the dose be given in each nostril. **Note:** The nasal spray pump can only deliver doses of 10 mcg (0.1 mL) or multiples of 10 mcg (0.1 mL); if doses other than this are needed, the rhinal tube delivery system is preferred. For 10 mcg dose, administer in one nostril.

Oral: 0.2 mg at bedtime. Dose may be titrated up to 0.6 mg to achieve desired response. Patients previously on intranasal therapy can begin oral tablets 24 hours after the last intranasal dose.

Children >12 years: Refer to adult dosing.

Available Dosage Forms

Injection, solution, as acetate (DDAVP®): 4 mcg/mL (1 mL, 10 mL)
Solution, intranasal, as acetate (DDAVP®): 100 mcg/mL (2.5 mL) [with rhinal tube]
Solution, intranasal spray, as acetate: 100 mcg/mL (5 mL) [delivers 10 mcg/spray]
DDAVP®: 100 mcg/mL (5 mL) [delivers 10 mcg/spray]
Stimate™: 1.5 mg/mL (2.5 mL) [delivers 150 mcg/spray]
Tablet, as acetate (DDAVP®): 0.1 mg, 0.2 mg

Nursing Guidelines

Assessment: See Contraindications, Warnings/Precautions, Drug Interactions, and Dosing for use cautions. Assess results of laboratory tests according to purpose for use (see above), therapeutic effectiveness, and adverse reactions (see Adverse Reactions and Overdose/Toxicology) on a regular basis throughout therapy. Teach patient proper use (if self-administered), possible side effects/appropriate interventions, and adverse symptoms to report (see Patient Education). Note breast-feeding caution.

Monitoring Laboratory Tests:

Diabetes insipidus: Fluid intake, urine volume, specific gravity, plasma and urine osmolality, serum electrolytes

Hemophilia A: Factor VIII coagulant activity, Factor VIII ristocetin cofactor activity, and Factor VIII antigen levels, aPTT

Von Willebrand disease: Factor VIII coagulant activity, Factor VIII ristocetin cofactor activity, and Factor VIII von Willebrand antigen levels, bleeding time

Nocturnal enuresis: Serum electrolytes if used for >7 days

Patient Education: Inform prescriber of all prescriptions, OTC medications, or herbal products you are taking, and any allergies you have. Do not take any new medication during therapy unless approved by prescriber. Use specific product as directed. Avoid alcohol.

Diabetes insipidus: Avoid overhydration. Weigh yourself daily at the same time in the same clothes. Report increased weight or swelling of extremities. If using intranasal product, inspect nasal membranes regularly. Report swelling or increased nasal congestion.

All uses: Report unresolved headache, respiratory difficulty, acute heartburn or nausea, abdominal cramping, or vulval pain. **Breast-feeding precaution:** Consult prescriber if breast-feeding.

Geriatric Considerations: Elderly patients should be cautioned not to increase their fluid intake beyond that sufficient to satisfy their thirst in order to avoid water intoxication and hyponatremia.

Pregnancy Risk Factor: B

Lactation: Excretion in breast milk unknown/use caution

Perioperative/Anesthesia/Other Concerns: If desmopressin I.V. is given preoperatively, administer 30 minutes prior to surgery.

Administration

I.V.: Dilute in 0.9% sodium chloride and infuse over 15-30 minutes; dose should be diluted in 10 mL NS for children ≤10 kg; 50 mL NS for adults and children >10 kg

Storage:

DDAVP®:

Tablet, nasal spray: Store at controlled room temperature of 20°C to 25°C (68°F to 77°F). Keep nasal spray in upright position.

Rhinal tube: Store refrigerated at 2°C to 8°C (36°F to 46°F). May store at room temperature for up to 3 weeks.

Injection: Store refrigerated at 2°C to 8°C (36°F to 46°F).

Stimate™: Store refrigerated at 2°C to 8°C (36°F to 46°F). May store at room temperature for up to 3 weeks.

- Desmopressin Acetate *see* Desmopressin *on page 492*
- Desogen® *see* Ethinyl Estradiol and Desogestrel *on page 675*
- Desogestrel and Ethinyl Estradiol *see* Ethinyl Estradiol and Desogestrel *on page 675*
- Desyrel® *see* Trazodone *on page 1657*
- Detane® [OTC] *see* Benzocaine *on page 232*
- Detemir Insulin *see* Insulin Detemir *on page 919*
- Detrol® *see* Tolterodine *on page 1646*
- Detrol® LA *see* Tolterodine *on page 1646*
- Dex4 Glucose [OTC] *see* Dextrose *on page 511*
- Dexacidin® [DSC] *see* Neomycin, Polymyxin B, and Dexamethasone *on page 1211*
- Dexacine™ [DSC] *see* Neomycin, Polymyxin B, and Dexamethasone *on page 1211*

Dexamethasone (deks a METH a sone)

U.S. Brand Names Decadron®; Decadron® Phosphate [DSC]; Dexamethasone Intensol®; DexPak® TaperPak®; Maxidex®

Synonyms Dexamethasone Sodium Phosphate

Pharmacologic Category Anti-inflammatory Agent; Anti-inflammatory Agent, Ophthalmic; Antiemetic; Corticosteroid, Ophthalmic; Corticosteroid, Systemic; Corticosteroid, Topical

Medication Safety Issues

Sound-alike/look-alike issues:

Dexamethasone may be confused with desoximetasone

Decadron® may be confused with Percodan®

Maxidex® may be confused with Maxzide®

Use Systemically and locally for chronic swelling; allergic, hematologic, neoplastic, and autoimmune diseases; may be used in management of cerebral edema, septic shock, as a diagnostic agent, antiemetic

Unlabeled/Investigational Use General indicator consistent with depression; diagnosis of Cushing's syndrome

Mechanism of Action Decreases inflammation by suppression of neutrophil migration, decreased production of inflammatory mediators, and reversal of increased capillary permeability; suppresses normal immune response. Dexamethasone's mechanism of antiemetic activity is unknown.

Pharmacodynamics/Kinetics

Onset of action: Acetate: Prompt

Duration of metabolic effect: 72 hours; acetate is a long-acting repository preparation

(Continued)

Dexamethasone *(Continued)*

Metabolism: Hepatic

Half-life elimination: Normal renal function: 1.8-3.5 hours; Biological half-life: 36-54 hours

Time to peak, serum: Oral: 1-2 hours; I.M.: ~8 hours

Excretion: Urine and feces

Contraindications Hypersensitivity to dexamethasone or any component of the formulation; active untreated infections; ophthalmic use in viral, fungal, or tuberculosis diseases of the eye

Warnings/Precautions Use with caution in patients with hypothyroidism, cirrhosis, hypertension, CHF, ulcerative colitis, or thromboembolic disorders. Corticosteroids should be used with caution in patients with diabetes, osteoporosis, peptic ulcer, glaucoma, cataracts, or tuberculosis. Use caution following acute MI (corticosteroids have been associated with myocardial rupture). Use caution in hepatic impairment. Because of the risk of adverse effects, systemic corticosteroids should be used cautiously in the elderly in the smallest possible effective dose for the shortest duration.

May cause suppression of hypothalamic-pituitary-adrenal (HPA) axis, particularly in younger children or in patients receiving high doses for prolonged periods. Symptoms of adrenocortical insufficiency in suppressed patients may result from rapid discontinuation/withdrawal; deficits in HPA response may persist for months following discontinuation and require supplementation during metabolic stress. Patients receiving 20 mg/day of prednisone (or equivalent) may be most susceptible. Particular care is required when patients are transferred from systemic corticosteroids to inhaled products due to possible adrenal insufficiency or exacerbation of underlying disease, including an increase in allergic symptoms. Fatalities have occurred due to adrenal insufficiency in asthmatic patients during and after transfer from systemic corticosteroids to aerosol steroids; aerosol steroids do **not** provide the systemic steroid needed to treat patients having trauma, surgery, or infections. Dexamethasone does not provide adequate mineralocorticoid activity in adrenal insufficiency (may be employed as a single dose while cortisol assays are performed). Dexamethasone does not cross-react with cortisol assays.

Controlled clinical studies have shown that orally-inhaled and intranasal corticosteroids may cause a reduction in growth velocity in pediatric patients. (In studies of orally-inhaled corticosteroids, the mean reduction in growth velocity was ~1 cm per year [range 0.3-1.8 cm per year] and appears to be related to dose and duration of exposure). The growth of pediatric patients receiving inhaled corticosteroids, should be monitored routinely (eg, via stadiometry). To minimize the systemic effects of orally-inhaled and intranasal corticosteroids, each patient should be titrated to the lowest effective dose.

May suppress the immune system; patients may be more susceptible to infection. Use with caution in patients with systemic infections or ocular herpes simplex. Avoid exposure to chickenpox and measles.

Drug Interactions **Substrate** of CYP3A4 (minor); **Induces** CYP2A6 (weak), 2B6 (weak), 2C8/9 (weak), 3A4 (weak)

Aminoglutethimide: May reduce the serum levels/effects of dexamethasone; likely via induction of microsomal isoenzymes.

Antacids: May increase the absorption of corticosteroids; separate administration by 2 hours.

Anticholinesterases: Concurrent use may lead to severe weakness in patients with myasthenia gravis.

Azole antifungals: May increase the serum levels of corticosteroids; monitor.

Bile acid sequestrants: May reduce the absorption of corticosteroids; separate administration by 2 hours.

Calcium channel blockers (nondihydropyridine): May increase the serum levels of corticosteroids; monitor.

Cyclosporine: Corticosteroids may increase the serum levels of cyclosporine. In addition, cyclosporine may increase levels of corticosteroids

Estrogens: May increase the serum levels of corticosteroids; monitor.

Fluoroquinolones: Concurrent use may increase the risk of tendon rupture, particularly in elderly patients (overall incidence rare).

Isoniazid: Serum concentrations may be decreased by corticosteroids.

Neuromuscular-blocking agents: Concurrent use with corticosteroids may increase the risk of myopathy.

Nonsteroidal anti-inflammatory drugs (NSAIDs): Concurrent use with corticosteroids may lead to an increased incidence of gastrointestinal adverse effects; use caution.

Phenytoin: Dexamethasone may decrease serum levels/effects of phenytoin; monitor.

Salicylates: Salicylates may increase the gastrointestinal adverse effects of corticosteroids.

Thalidomide: Concurrent use with corticosteroids may increase the risk of selected adverse effects (toxic epidermal necrolysis and DVT); use caution

Vaccines, toxoids: Corticosteroids may suppress the response to vaccinations. The use of live vaccines is contraindicated in immunosuppressed patients. In patients receiving high doses of systemic corticosteroids for ≥14 days, wait at least 1 month between discontinuing steroid therapy and administering immunization.

Warfarin: Corticosteroids may lead to a reduction in warfarin effect; monitor.

Nutritional/Herbal/Ethanol Interactions

Ethanol: Avoid ethanol (may enhance gastric mucosal irritation).

Food: Dexamethasone interferes with calcium absorption. Limit caffeine.

Herb/Nutraceutical: Avoid cat's claw, echinacea (have immunostimulant properties).

Adverse Reactions Frequency not defined.

Cardiovascular: Edema, hypertension, arrhythmia, cardiomyopathy, myocardial rupture (post-MI), syncope, thromboembolism, thrombophlebitis, vasculitis

Central nervous system: Insomnia, nervousness, vertigo, seizure, psychosis, pseudotumor cerebri (usually following discontinuation), headache, mood swings, delirium, hallucinations, euphoria

Dermatologic: Hirsutism, acne, skin atrophy, bruising, hyperpigmentation, pruritus (generalized), perianal pruritus (following I.V. injection), urticaria

Endocrine & metabolic: Diabetes mellitus, adrenal suppression, hyperlipidemia, Cushing's syndrome, pituitary-adrenal axis suppression, growth suppression, glucose intolerance, gynecomastia, hypokalemia, alkalosis, amenorrhea, sodium and water retention, hyperglycemia, hypercalciuria, weight gain

Gastrointestinal: Appetite increased, indigestion, peptic ulcer, nausea, vomiting, abdominal distention, ulcerative esophagitis, pancreatitis, intestinal perforation

Genitourinary: Altered (increased or decreased) spermatogenesis

Hematologic: Transient leukocytosis

Hepatic: Transaminases increased, hepatomegaly

Neuromuscular & skeletal: Arthralgia, muscle weakness, osteoporosis, fractures, myopathy (particularly in conjunction with neuromuscular disease or neuromuscular blocking agents), tendon rupture, vertebral compression fractures, neuropathy, neuritis, parasthesia

Ocular: Cataracts, glaucoma, exophthalmos, intraocular pressure increased

Miscellaneous: Infections, anaphylactoid reaction, anaphylaxis, angioedema, avascular necrosis, secondary malignancy, Kaposi's sarcoma, intractable hiccups, impaired wound healing, abnormal fat deposition, moon face

Topical: <1%: Itching, dryness, folliculitis, hypertrichosis, acneiform eruptions, hypopigmentation, perioral dermatitis, allergic contact dermatitis, skin maceration, skin atrophy, striae, miliaria, local burning, irritation. secondary infection

Overdosage/Toxicology When consumed in high doses over prolonged periods, systemic hypercorticism and adrenal suppression may occur. In these cases, discontinuation of the corticosteroid should be done judiciously.

Dosing

Adults:

Anti-inflammatory:

Oral, I.M., I.V. (injections should be given as sodium phosphate): 0.75-9 mg/day in divided doses every 6-12 hours

Intra-articular, intralesional, or soft tissue (as sodium phosphate): 0.4-6 mg/day

Extubation or airway edema: Oral, I.M., I.V. (injections should be given as sodium phosphate): 0.5-2 mg/kg/day in divided doses every 6 hours beginning 24 hours prior to extubation and continuing for 4-6 doses afterwards

Antiemetic:

Prophylaxis: Oral, I.V.: 10-20 mg 15-30 minutes before treatment on each treatment day

Continuous infusion regimen: Oral or I.V.: 10 mg every 12 hours on each treatment day

Mildly emetogenic therapy: Oral, I.M., I.V.: 4 mg every 4-6 hours

(Continued)

Dexamethasone *(Continued)*

Delayed nausea/vomiting: Oral: 4-10 mg 1-2 times/day for 2-4 days **or**
8 mg every 12 hours for 2 days; then
4 mg every 12 hours for 2 days **or**
20 mg 1 hour before chemotherapy; then
10 mg 12 hours after chemotherapy; then
8 mg every 12 hours for 4 doses; then
4 mg every 12 hours for 4 doses

Ophthalmic anti-inflammatory:

Ophthalmic ointment: Apply thin coating into conjunctival sac 3-4 times/day; gradually taper dose to discontinue.

Ophthalmic suspension: Instill 2 drops into conjunctival sac every hour during the day and every other hour during the night; gradually reduce dose to every 3-4 hours, then to 3-4 times/day.

Steroid-responsive dermatoses: Topical: Apply 1-4 times/day. Therapy should be discontinued when control is achieved; if no improvement is seen, reassessment of diagnosis may be necessary.

Chemotherapy: Oral, I.V.: 40 mg every day for 4 days, repeated every 4 weeks (VAD regimen)

Cerebral edema: I.V. 10 mg stat, 4 mg I.M./I.V. (should be given as sodium phosphate) every 6 hours until response is maximized, then switch to oral regimen, then taper off if appropriate; dosage may be reduced after 24 days and gradually discontinued over 5-7 days

Dexamethasone suppression test (depression indicator) (unlabeled use): Oral: 1 mg at 11 PM, draw blood at 8 AM the following day for plasma cortisol determination

Cushing's syndrome, diagnostic: Oral: 1 mg at 11 PM, draw blood at 8 AM; greater accuracy for Cushing's syndrome may be achieved by the following:

Dexamethasone 0.5 mg by mouth every 6 hours for 48 hours (with 24-hour urine collection for 17-hydroxycorticosteroid excretion)

Differentiation of Cushing's syndrome due to ACTH excess from Cushing's due to other causes: Oral: Dexamethasone 2 mg every 6 hours for 48 hours (with 24-hour urine collection for 17-hydroxycorticosteroid excretion)

Multiple sclerosis (acute exacerbation): Oral: 30 mg/day for 1 week, followed by 4-12 mg/day for 1 month

Treatment of shock:

Addisonian crisis/shock (ie, adrenal insufficiency/responsive to steroid therapy): I.V. (given as sodium phosphate): 4-10 mg as a single dose, which may be repeated if necessary

Unresponsive shock (ie, unresponsive to steroid therapy): I.V. (given as sodium phosphate): 1-6 mg/kg as a single I.V. dose or up to 40 mg initially followed by repeat doses every 2-6 hours while shock persists

Physiological replacement: Oral, I.M., I.V. (should be given as sodium phosphate): 0.03-0.15 mg/kg/day **or** 0.6-0.75 mg/m^2/day in divided doses every 6-12 hours

Elderly: Refer to adult dosing. Use cautiously in the elderly in the smallest possible dose.

Pediatrics:

Antiemetic (prior to chemotherapy): I.V. (should be given as sodium phosphate): 5-20 mg given 15-30 minutes before treatment

Anti-inflammatory and/or immunosuppressant: Oral, I.M., I.V. (injections should be given as sodium phosphate): 0.08-0.3 mg/kg/day **or** 2.5-10 mg/m^2/day in divided doses every 6-12 hours

Extubation or airway edema: Oral, I.M., I.V. (injections should be given as sodium phosphate): 0.5-2 mg/kg/day in divided doses every 6 hours beginning 24 hours prior to extubation and continuing for 4-6 doses afterwards

Cerebral edema: I.V. (should be given as sodium phosphate): Loading dose: 1-2 mg/kg/dose as a single dose; maintenance: 1-1.5 mg/kg/day (maximum: 16 mg/day) in divided doses every 4-6 hours for 5 days then taper for 5 days, then discontinue

Bacterial meningitis in infants and children >2 months: I.V. (should be given as sodium phosphate): 0.6 mg/kg/day in 4 divided doses every 6 hours for the first 4 days of antibiotic treatment; start dexamethasone at the time of the first dose of antibiotic

Physiologic replacement: Oral, I.M., I.V.: 0.03-0.15 mg/kg/day or 0.6-0.75 mg/m^2/day in divided doses every 6-12 hours

Ophthalmic inflammation: Refer to adult dosing.

Renal Impairment: Hemodialysis or peritoneal dialysis: Supplemental dose is not necessary.

Available Dosage Forms [DSC] = Discontinued product

Elixir, as base: 0.5 mg/5 mL (240 mL) [contains alcohol 5%; raspberry flavor]

Injection, solution, as sodium phosphate: 4 mg/mL (1 mL, 5 mL, 10 mL, 25 mL, 30 mL); 10 mg/mL (1 mL, 10 mL)

Decadron® Phosphate: 4 mg/mL (5 mL, 25 mL); 24 mg/mL (5 mL) [contains sodium bisulfite] [DSC]

Ointment, ophthalmic, as sodium phosphate: 0.05% (3.5 g)

Solution, ophthalmic, as sodium phosphate: 0.1% (5 mL)

Solution, oral: 0.5 mg/5 mL (500 mL) [cherry flavor]

Solution, oral concentrate (Dexamethasone Intensol®): 1 mg/mL (30 mL) [contains alcohol 30%]

Suspension, ophthalmic (Maxidex®): 0.1% (5 mL, 15 mL)

Tablet: 0.25 mg, 0.5 mg, 0.75 mg, 1 mg, 1.5 mg, 2 mg, 4 mg, 6 mg [some 0.5 mg tablets may contain tartrazine]

Decadron®: 0.5 mg, 0.75 mg, 4 mg

DexPak® TaperPak®: 1.5 mg [51 tablets on taper dose card]

Nursing Guidelines

Assessment: Assess potential for interactions with other prescriptions, OTC medications, or herbal products patient may be taking. Assess results of laboratory tests, therapeutic response, and adverse effects, according to indications for therapy, dose, route, and duration of therapy. When used for long-term therapy (>10-14 days), do not discontinue abruptly; decrease dosage incrementally. With systemic administration, caution patients with diabetes to monitor glucose levels closely (corticosteroids may alter glucose levels). Teach patient proper use (according to formulation), side effects/appropriate interventions, and symptoms to report.

Monitoring Laboratory Tests: Hemoglobin, occult blood loss, serum potassium, glucose

Dexamethasone suppression test, overnight: 8 AM cortisol <6 mg/100 mL (dexamethasone 1 mg). Plasma cortisol determination should be made on the day after giving dose.

Dietary Considerations: May be taken with meals to decrease GI upset. May need diet with increased potassium, pyridoxine, vitamin C, vitamin D, folate, calcium, and phosphorus.

Patient Education: Do not take any new medication during therapy unless approved by prescriber. Take exactly as directed, do not increase dose or discontinue abruptly without consulting prescriber.

Oral: Take with or after meals. Avoid alcohol and limit intake of caffeine or stimulants. Prescriber may recommend increased dietary vitamins, minerals, or iron. If you have diabetes, monitor glucose levels closely (antidiabetic medication may need to be adjusted). Inform prescriber if you are experiencing greater-than-normal levels of stress (medication may need adjustment). You may be more susceptible to infection (avoid crowds and persons with contagious or infective conditions and do not have any vaccinations unless approved by prescriber). Some forms of this medication may cause GI upset (small frequent meals and frequent mouth care may help). Report promptly excessive nervousness or sleep disturbances; signs of infection (eg, sore throat, unhealed injuries); excessive growth of body hair or loss of skin color; vision changes; excessive or sudden weight gain (>3 lb/week); swelling of face or extremities; respiratory difficulty; muscle weakness; tarry stool, persistent abdominal pain; worsening of condition or failure to improve. **Pregnancy/breast-feeding precautions:** Inform prescriber if you are or intend to become pregnant. Consult prescriber if breast-feeding.

Ophthalmic: For use in eyes only. Wash hands before using. Lie down or tilt your head back and look upward. Put drops of suspension or apply thin ribbon of ointment inside lower eyelid. Close eye and roll eyeball in all directions. Do not blink for ½ minute. Apply gentle pressure to inner corner of eye for 30 seconds. Do not use any other eye preparation for at least 10 minutes. Do not let tip of applicator touch eye; do not contaminate tip of applicator (may cause eye infection, eye damage, or vision loss). Do not share medication with anyone else. Wear sunglasses when in sunlight; you may be more sensitive to bright light. Inform prescriber if condition worsens, fails to improve, or if you experience eye pain, disturbances of vision, or other adverse eye response.

(Continued)

Dexamethasone *(Continued)*

Topical: For external use only. Do not use for eyes, mucous membranes, or open wounds. Use exactly as directed and for no longer than the period prescribed. Before using, wash and dry area gently. Apply in thin layer (may rub in lightly). Apply light dressing (if necessary) to area being treated. Do not use occlusive dressing unless so advised by prescriber. Avoid exposing treated area to sunlight (severe sunburn may occur). Inform prescriber if condition worsens (swelling, redness, irritation, pain, open sores) or fails to improve.

Geriatric Considerations: Because of the risk of adverse effects, systemic corticosteroids should be used cautiously in the elderly in the smallest possible dose, and for the shortest possible time.

Pregnancy Risk Factor: C

Pregnancy Issues: Dexamethasone has been used in patients with premature labor (26-34 weeks gestation) to stimulate fetal lung maturation. Effects on the fetus: Crosses the placenta; transient leukocytosis has been reported. Available evidence suggests safe use during pregnancy.

Lactation: Excretion in breast milk unknown

Perioperative/Anesthesia/Other Concerns: Dexamethasone is a long-acting corticosteroid with minimal sodium-retaining potential. Corticosteroids and muscle relaxants appear to trigger some types of ICU myopathy; avoid or administer at the lowest dose possible.

Patients will often have steroid-induced adverse effects on glucose tolerance and lipid profiles. In discontinuing steroid therapy in patients on long-term steroid supplementation, it is important that the steroid therapy be discontinued gradually. Abrupt withdrawal may result in adrenal insufficiency with hypotension and hyperkalemia. Patients on long-term steroid supplementation will require higher corticosteroid doses when subject to stress (ie, trauma, surgery, severe infection).

Oral and intravenous steroid therapy in patients with heart failure should be administered cautiously with special attention given to signs and symptoms of fluid retention.

Administration

Oral: Administer oral formulation with meals to decrease GI upset.

I.M.: Acetate injection is **not** for I.V. use.

I.V.: Administer as a 5-10 minute bolus; rapid injection is associated with a high incidence of perianal discomfort.

Reconstitution: Injection should be diluted in 50-100 mL NS or D_5W.

Compatibility: Stable in D_5W, NS

Y-site administration: Incompatible with ciprofloxacin, idarubicin, midazolam, topotecan

Compatibility in syringe: Incompatible with doxapram, glycopyrrolate

Compatibility when admixed: Incompatible with daunorubicin, diphenhydramine with lorazepam and metoclopramide, metaraminol, vancomycin

Storage: Injection solution: Store at room temperature; protect from light and freezing.

Stability of injection of parenteral admixture at room temperature (25°C): 24 hours

Stability of injection of parenteral admixture at refrigeration temperature (4°C): 2 days; protect from light and freezing

Related Information

Postoperative Nausea and Vomiting *on page 1807*

- **Dexamethasone and Tobramycin** *see* Tobramycin and Dexamethasone *on page 1643*
- **Dexamethasone Intensol®** *see* Dexamethasone *on page 495*
- **Dexamethasone, Neomycin, and Polymyxin B** *see* Neomycin, Polymyxin B, and Dexamethasone *on page 1211*
- **Dexamethasone Sodium Phosphate** *see* Dexamethasone *on page 495*
- **Dexasporin** *see* Neomycin, Polymyxin B, and Dexamethasone *on page 1211*
- **Dexedrine®** *see* Dextroamphetamine *on page 505*
- **Dexferrum®** *see* Iron Dextran Complex *on page 966*

Dexmedetomidine (deks MED e toe mi deen)

U.S. Brand Names Precedex™

Synonyms Dexmedetomidine Hydrochloride

Pharmacologic Category $Alpha_2$-Adrenergic Agonist; Sedative

Medication Safety Issues

Sound-alike/look-alike issues:

Precedex™ may be confused with Peridex®

Use Sedation of initially intubated and mechanically ventilated patients during treatment in an intensive care setting; duration of infusion should not exceed 24 hours

Unlabeled/Investigational Use Unlabeled uses include premedication prior to anesthesia induction with thiopental; relief of pain and reduction of opioid dose following laparoscopic tubal ligation; as an adjunct anesthetic in ophthalmic surgery; treatment of shivering; premedication to attenuate the cardiostimulatory and postanesthetic delirium of ketamine

Mechanism of Action Selective $alpha_2$-adrenoceptor agonist with sedative properties; $alpha_1$ activity was observed at high doses or after rapid infusions

Pharmacodynamics/Kinetics

Onset of action: Rapid

Distribution: V_{ss}: Approximately 118 L; rapid

Protein binding: 94%

Metabolism: Hepatic via glucuronidation and CYP2A6

Half-life elimination: 6 minutes; Terminal: 2 hours

Excretion: Urine (95%); feces (4%)

Contraindications Hypersensitivity to dexmedetomidine or any component of the formulation; use outside of an intensive care setting

Warnings/Precautions Should be administered only by persons skilled in management of patients in intensive care setting. Patients should be continuously monitored. Episodes of bradycardia, hypotension, and sinus arrest have been associated with dexmedetomidine when administered rapidly I.V. (eg, bolus administration) or to patients with high vagal tone. Use caution in patients with heart block, severe ventricular dysfunction, hypovolemia, diabetes, chronic hypertension, and in the elderly. Use with caution in patients receiving vasodilators or drugs which decrease heart rate. If medical intervention is required, treatment may include stopping or decreasing the infusion; increasing the rate of I.V. fluid administration, use of pressor agents, and elevation of the lower extremities. Transient hypertension has been primarily observed during the dose in association with the initial peripheral vasoconstrictive effects of dexmedetomidine. Treatment of this is not generally necessary; however, reduction of infusion rate may be desirable.

Drug Interactions **Substrate** of CYP2A6 (major); **Inhibits** CYP1A2 (weak), 2C8/9 (weak), 2D6 (strong), 3A4 (weak)

CYP2A6 inhibitors: May increase the levels/effects of dexmedetomidine. Example inhibitors include isoniazid, methoxsalen, and miconazole.

CYP2D6 substrates: Dexmedetomidine may increase the levels/effects of CYP2D6 substrates. Example substrates include amphetamines, selected beta-blockers, dextromethorphan, fluoxetine, lidocaine, mirtazapine, nefazodone, paroxetine, risperidone, ritonavir, thioridazine, tricyclic antidepressants, and venlafaxine.

CYP2D6 prodrug substrates: Dexmedetomidine may decrease the levels/effects of CYP2D6 prodrug substrates. Example prodrug substrates include codeine, hydrocodone, oxycodone, and tramadol.

Hypotension and/or bradycardia may be increased by vasodilators and heart rate-lowering agents.

Adverse Reactions

>10%:

Cardiovascular: Hypotension (30%)

Gastrointestinal: Nausea (11%)

1% to 10%:

Cardiovascular: Bradycardia (8%), atrial fibrillation (7%)

Central nervous system: Pain (3%)

Hematologic: Anemia (3%), leukocytosis (2%)

Renal: Oliguria (2%)

Respiratory: Hypoxia (6%), pulmonary edema (2%), pleural effusion (3%)

Miscellaneous: Infection (2%), thirst (2%)

Overdosage/Toxicology In reports of overdosages where the blood concentration was 13 times the upper boundary of the therapeutic range, first-degree AV

(Continued)

Dexmedetomidine *(Continued)*

block and second degree heart block occurred. No hemodynamic compromise was noted with the AV block and the heart block resolved spontaneously within one minute. Two patients who received a 2 mcg/kg loading dose over 10 minutes experienced bradycardia and/or hypotension. One patient who received a loading dose of undiluted dexmedetomidine (19.4 mcg/kg) had cardiac arrest and was successfully resuscitated.

Dosing

Adults:

ICU sedation: I.V.: Initial: Loading infusion of 1 mcg/kg over 10 minutes, followed by a maintenance infusion of 0.2-0.7 mcg/kg/hour (individualized and titrated to desired clinical effect); not indicated for infusions lasting >24 hours

Note: Solution must be diluted prior to administration.

Elderly: Refer to adult dosing. Dosage reduction may need to be considered. No specific guidelines available. Dose selections should be cautious, at the low end of dosage range; titration should be slower, allowing adequate time to evaluate response.

Renal Impairment: Dosage reduction may need to be considered.

Hepatic Impairment: Dosage reduction may need to be considered. No specific guidelines available.

Available Dosage Forms Injection, solution [preservative free]: 100 mcg/mL (2 mL)

Nursing Guidelines

Assessment: Administration should be managed by professionals experienced in anesthesia. Dosage and rate of administration should be individualized and titrated to the desired effect, according to relevant clinical factors, premedication, concomitant medications, age, and general condition of patient. Assess other medications for effectiveness and safety. Other drugs that cause CNS depression may increase CNS depression induced by dexmedetomidine (monitor and adjust dosage as necessary). Continuous monitoring of vital signs, cardiac and respiratory status, and level of sedation is mandatory during infusion and until full consciousness is regained. Safety precautions must be maintained until patient is fully alert. Dexmedetomidine is an anesthetic; pain must be treated with appropriate analgesic agents. Do not discontinue abruptly (may result in rapid awakening associated with anxiety, agitation, and resistance to mechanical ventilation). Titrate infusion rate so patient awakes slowly. Monitor fluid levels (intake and output) during and following infusion. Reposition patient and provide appropriate skin, mouth, and eye care every 2-3 hours, while sedated. Provide appropriate emotional and sensory support (auditory and environmental).

Patient Education: This is an anesthetic. Patient education should be appropriate to individual situation. Following return of consciousness, do not attempt to change position or rise from bed without assistance. Report immediately any pounding or unusual heartbeat, respiratory difficulty, or acute dizziness. **Pregnancy/breast-feeding precautions:** Inform prescriber if you are pregnant. Consult prescriber if breast-feeding.

Pregnancy Risk Factor: C

Lactation: Excretion in breast milk unknown/use caution

Perioperative/Anesthesia/Other Concerns: Unlabeled uses include premedication prior to anesthesia induction with thiopental (0.33-0.67 mcg/kg); relief of pain and reduction of opioid dose following laparoscopic tubal ligation; as an adjunct anesthetic in ophthalmic surgery; treatment of shivering; and premedication (2.5 mcg/kg) to attenuate the cardiostimulatory and postanesthetic delirium of ketamine.

Dexmedetomidine has not been reported to cause respiratory depression. Assess the patient for pain during infusion; the sedation produced by this agent is not equivalent to analgesia. Adequate pain management should be addressed.

Dexmedetomidine should not be coadministered through the same I.V. catheter with plasma or blood products (physical compatibility not established). It is compatible with lactated Ringer's, 5% dextrose in water, 0.9% sodium chloride in water, 20% mannitol, thiopental, etomidate, vecuronium, pancuronium, succinylcholine, atracurium, mivacurium, fentanyl, and a plasma substitute. Dexmedetomidine may adsorb to some types of natural rubber; administration components made with synthetic or coated natural rubber gaskets are recommended.

In a prospective, observational study of 12 ventilator-dependent patients, dexmedetomidine was assessed as a sedative. Patients received a loading dose infusion of 1 mcg/kg over 10 minutes followed by the manufacturer's recommended infusion rate (0.2-0.7 mcg/kg/hour) for up to 7 days. Some patients required higher maintenance infusion rates than recommended by the manufacturer. Mean infusion rate was 1 ± 0.7 mcg/kg/hour. The maximum rate was 2.5 mcg/kg/hour. Adverse cardiovascular events were most frequently related to the initial loading infusion. These investigators suggest using a lower loading infusion. Higher maintenance infusions may be required in some patients. Patients did not go through a withdrawal syndrome when the infusion was discontinued (Venn, 2003).

The package insert suggests that there is a potential for withdrawal with symptoms such as nervousness, agitation, headaches, and rapid rise in blood pressure.

Administration

I.V.: Administer using a controlled infusion device. Must be diluted in 0.9% sodium chloride solution to achieve the required concentration prior to administration. Advisable to use administration components made with synthetic or coated natural rubber gaskets. Parenteral products should be inspected visually for particulate matter and discoloration prior to administration.

Compatibility: Stable in D_5W, LR, 0.9% NS, 20% mannitol, plasma substitute

May adsorb to certain types of natural rubber; use components made with synthetic or coated natural rubber gaskets whenever possible.

♦ **Dexmedetomidine Hydrochloride** *see* Dexmedetomidine *on page 501*

♦ **DexPak® TaperPak®** *see* Dexamethasone *on page 495*

Dextran (DEKS tran)

U.S. Brand Names Gentran®; LMD®

Synonyms Dextran 40; Dextran 70; Dextran, High Molecular Weight; Dextran, Low Molecular Weight

Pharmacologic Category Plasma Volume Expander

Medication Safety Issues

Sound-alike/look-alike issues:

Dextran may be confused with Dexatrim®, Dexedrine®

Use Blood volume expander used in treatment of shock or impending shock when blood or blood products are not available; dextran 40 is also used as a priming fluid in cardiopulmonary bypass and for prophylaxis of venous thrombosis and pulmonary embolism in surgical procedures associated with a high risk of thromboembolic complications

Mechanism of Action Produces plasma volume expansion by virtue of its highly colloidal starch structure, similar to albumin

Pharmacodynamics/Kinetics

Onset of action: Minutes to 1 hour (depending upon the molecular weight polysaccharide administered)

Excretion: Urine (~75%) within 24 hours

Contraindications Hypersensitivity to dextran or any component of the formulation; marked hemostatic defects (thrombocytopenia, hypofibrinogenemia) of all types including those caused by drugs; marked cardiac decompensation; renal disease with severe oliguria or anuria

Warnings/Precautions Hypersensitivity reactions have been reported (dextran 40 rarely causes a reaction), usually early in the infusion. Monitor closely during infusion initiation for signs or symptoms of a hypersensitivity reaction. Dextran 1 is indicated for prophylaxis of serious anaphylactic reactions to dextran infusions. Administration can cause fluid or solute overload. Use caution in patients with fluid overload. Use with caution in patients with active hemorrhage. Use caution in patients receiving corticosteroids. Renal failure has been reported. Fluid status including urine output should be monitored closely. Exercise care to prevent a depression of hematocrit <30% (can cause hemodilution). Observe for signs of bleeding.

Drug Interactions

Abciximab: Dextran may enhance the anticoagulant effect of abciximab. Avoid concurrent use.

Adverse Reactions <1% (Limited to important or life-threatening): Mild hypotension, tightness of chest, wheezing

(Continued)

Dextran *(Continued)*

Overdosage/Toxicology Symptoms of overdose include fluid overload, pulmonary edema, increased bleeding time, and decreased platelet function. Treatment is supportive. Blood products containing clotting factors may be necessary.

Dosing

Adults:

Volume expansion/shock:

Children: Total dose should not exceed 20 mL/kg during first 24 hours

Adults: 500-1000 mL at a rate of 20-40 mL/minute; maximum daily dose: 20 mL/kg for first 24 hours; 10 mL/kg/day thereafter; therapy should not be continued beyond 5 days

Pump prime (Dextran 40): Varies with the volume of the pump oxygenator; generally, the 10% solution is added in a dose of 1-2 g/kg

Prophylaxis of venous thrombosis/pulmonary embolism (Dextran 40): Begin during surgical procedure and give 50-100 g on the day of surgery; an additional 50 g (500 mL) should be administered every 2-3 days during the period of risk (up to 2 weeks postoperatively); usual maximum infusion rate for nonemergency use: 4 mL/minute

Elderly: Use with extreme caution in patients with renal or hepatic impairment.

Pediatrics: Treatment of shock or impending shock (when blood or blood products are not available): I.V. (requires an infusion pump): Children: Total dose should not be >20 mL/kg during first 24 hours

Renal Impairment: Use with extreme caution.

Hepatic Impairment: Use with extreme caution.

Available Dosage Forms

Infusion [premixed in D_5W; high molecular weight]: 6% Dextran 70 (500 mL)

Infusion [premixed in D_5W; low molecular weight] (Gentran®, LMD®): 10% Dextran 40 (500 mL)

Infusion [premixed in $D_{10}W$; high molecular weight]: 32% Dextran 70 (500 mL)

Infusion [premixed in NS; high molecular weight] (Gentran®): 6% Dextran 70 (500 mL)

Infusion [premixed in NS; low molecular weight] (Gentran®, LMD®): 10% Dextran (500 mL)

Nursing Guidelines

Assessment: See Contraindications, Warnings/Precautions, Drug Interactions, and Dosing for use cautions. See Administration and Compatibility. Fluid status, vital signs, and CVP should be monitored during first minute of infusion, every 5-15 minutes for first hour, and periodically thereafter (see Adverse Reactions and Overdose/Toxicology). Patient teaching should be appropriate to patient condition (see Patient Education). Note breast-feeding caution.

Monitoring Laboratory Tests: Hemoglobin and hematocrit, electrolytes, serum protein

Patient Education: Since this medication is generally used in emergency situations, patient education should be appropriate to patient condition.

Pregnancy Risk Factor: C

Lactation: Excretion in breast milk unknown

Perioperative/Anesthesia/Other Concerns: Dextran should be used with extreme caution in patients with restrictive cardiovascular disease and renal or hepatic impairment. Patients should be observed closely during the first several minutes of the infusion in case anaphylactoid reaction occurs.

Dextran 40 is known as low molecular weight dextran (LMD®) and has an average molecular weight of 40,000.

Dextran 75 has an average molecular weight of 75,000.

Dextran 70 has an average molecular weight of 70,000.

Administration

I.V.: For I.V. infusion only (use an infusion pump). Infuse initial 500 mL at a rate of 20-40 mL/minute if hypervolemic. Reduce rate for additional infusion to 4 mL/minute. **Observe patients closely for anaphylactic reaction.**

Compatibility: Dextran 40 is stable in D_5W, NS

Solution **incompatible** with other drugs

To prevent coagulation of blood, flush tubing well or change I.V. tubing before infusing blood after dextran.

Compatibility when admixed: Incompatible with amoxicillin

Storage: Store at room temperature. Discard partially used containers.

♦ **Dextran 40** *see* Dextran *on page 503*
♦ **Dextran 70** *see* Dextran *on page 503*
♦ **Dextran, High Molecular Weight** *see* Dextran *on page 503*
♦ **Dextran, Low Molecular Weight** *see* Dextran *on page 503*

Dextroamphetamine (deks troe am FET a meen)

U.S. Brand Names Dexedrine®; Dextrostat®

Synonyms Dextroamphetamine Sulfate

Pharmacologic Category Stimulant

Medication Safety Issues

Sound-alike/look-alike issues:

Dexedrine® may be confused with dextran, Excedrin®

Use Narcolepsy; attention-deficit/hyperactivity disorder (ADHD)

Unlabeled/Investigational Use Exogenous obesity; depression; abnormal behavioral syndrome in children (minimal brain dysfunction)

Mechanism of Action Blocks reuptake of dopamine and norepinephrine from the synapse, thus increases the amount of circulating dopamine and norepinephrine in cerebral cortex to reticular activating system; inhibits the action of monoamine oxidase and causes catecholamines to be released. Peripheral actions include elevated blood pressure, weak bronchodilator, and respiratory stimulant action.

Pharmacodynamics/Kinetics

Onset of action: 1-1.5 hours

Distribution: V_d: Adults: 3.5-4.6 L/kg; distributes into CNS; mean CSF concentrations are 80% of plasma; enters breast milk

Metabolism: Hepatic via CYP monooxygenase and glucuronidation

Half-life elimination: Adults: 10-13 hours

Time to peak, serum: T_{max}: Immediate release: 3 hours; sustained release: 8 hours

Excretion: Urine (as unchanged drug and inactive metabolites)

Contraindications Hypersensitivity or idiosyncrasy to dextroamphetamine or other sympathomimetic amines. Patients with advanced arteriosclerosis, symptomatic cardiovascular disease, moderate to severe hypertension (stage II or III), hyperthyroidism, glaucoma, diabetes mellitus, agitated states, patients with a history of drug abuse, and during or within 14 days following MAO inhibitor therapy. Stimulant medications are contraindicated for use in children with attention-deficit/hyperactivity disorders and concomitant Tourette's syndrome or tics.

Warnings/Precautions Use with caution in patients with bipolar disorder, cardiovascular disease, seizure disorders, insomnia, porphyria, mild hypertension (stage I), or history of substance abuse. May exacerbate symptoms of behavior and thought disorder in psychotic patients. Stimulants may unmask tics in individuals with coexisting Tourette's syndrome. Potential for drug dependency exists - avoid abrupt discontinuation in patients who have received for prolonged periods. Use in weight reduction programs only when alternative therapy has been ineffective. Products may contain tartrazine - use with caution in potentially sensitive individuals. Stimulant use in children has been associated with growth suppression.

Drug Interactions Substrate of CYP2D6 (major)

Acidifiers: Very large doses of potassium acid phosphate or ammonium chloride may increase the renal elimination of amphetamines due to urinary acidification

Alkalinizers: Large doses of sodium bicarbonate or other alkalinizers may increase renal tubular reabsorption (decreased elimination) and diminish the effect of amphetamine; includes potassium or sodium citrate and acetate

Antipsychotics: Efficacy of amphetamines may be decreased by antipsychotics; in addition, amphetamines may induce an increase in psychotic symptoms in some patients

CYP2D6 inhibitors: May increase the levels/effects of dextroamphetamine. Example inhibitors include chlorpromazine, delavirdine, fluoxetine, miconazole, paroxetine, pergolide, quinidine, quinine, ritonavir, and ropinirole.

Furazolidone: Amphetamines may induce hypertensive episodes in patients receiving furazolidone

Guanethidine: Amphetamines inhibit the antihypertensive response to guanethidine; probably also may occur with guanadrel

MAO inhibitors: Severe hypertensive episodes have occurred with amphetamine when used in patients receiving MAO inhibitors; concurrent use or use within 14 days is contraindicated.

Norepinephrine: Amphetamines enhance the pressor response to norepinephrine

(Continued)

Dextroamphetamine *(Continued)*

Sibutramine: Concurrent use of sibutramine and amphetamines may cause severe hypertension and tachycardia; use is contraindicated with SSRIs; amphetamines may increase the potential for serotonin syndrome when used concurrently with selective serotonin reuptake inhibitors (including fluoxetine, fluvoxamine, paroxetine, and sertraline)

Tricyclic antidepressants: Concurrent of amphetamines with TCAs may result in hypertension and CNS stimulation; avoid this combination

Nutritional/Herbal/Ethanol Interactions

Ethanol: Avoid ethanol (may increase CNS depression).

Food: Dextroamphetamine serum levels may be altered if taken with acidic food, juices, or vitamin C.

Herb/Nutraceutical: Avoid ephedra (may cause hypertension or arrhythmias).

Adverse Reactions Frequency not defined.

Cardiovascular: Palpitations, tachycardia, hypertension, cardiomyopathy

Central nervous system: Overstimulation, euphoria, dyskinesia, dysphoria, exacerbation of motor and phonic tics, restlessness, insomnia, dizziness, headache, psychosis, Tourette's syndrome

Dermatologic: Rash, urticaria

Endocrine & metabolic: Changes in libido

Gastrointestinal: Diarrhea, constipation, anorexia, weight loss, xerostomia, unpleasant taste

Genitourinary: Impotence

Neuromuscular & skeletal: Tremor

Overdosage/Toxicology Symptoms of overdose include restlessness, tremor, confusion, hallucinations, panic, dysrhythmias, nausea, and vomiting. There is no specific antidote for dextroamphetamine intoxication and treatment is primarily supportive. Hyperactivity and agitation usually respond to reduced sensory input; however, with extreme agitation, haloperidol (2-5 mg I.M. for adults) may be required.

Dosing

Adults:

Narcolepsy: Oral: Initial: 10 mg/day, may increase at 10 mg increments in weekly intervals until side effects appear; maximum: 60 mg/day

Exogenous obesity (short-term adjunct): Oral: 5-30 mg/day in divided doses of 5-10 mg 30-60 minutes before meals

Elderly: Refer to adult dosing; start at lowest dose. Use with caution.

Pediatrics:

Narcolepsy: Oral: Children 6-12 years: Initial: 5 mg/day, may increase at 5 mg increments in weekly intervals until side effects appear; maximum dose: 60 mg/day

Attention-deficit/hyperactivity disorder (ADHD): Oral:

Children 3-5 years: Initial: 2.5 mg/day given every morning; increase by 2.5 mg/day in weekly intervals until optimal response is obtained, usual range: 0.1-0.5 mg/kg/dose every morning with maximum of 40 mg/day

Children ≥6 years: 5 mg once or twice daily; increase in increments of 5 mg/day at weekly intervals until optimal response is reached, usual range: 0.1-0.5 mg/kg/dose every morning (5-20 mg/day) with maximum of 40 mg/day

Available Dosage Forms

Capsule, sustained release, as sulfate: 5 mg, 10 mg, 15 mg

Dexedrine® Spansule®: 5 mg, 10 mg, 15 mg

Tablet, as sulfate: 5 mg, 10 mg

Dexedrine®: 5 mg [contains tartrazine]

Dextrostat®: 5 mg, 10 mg [contains tartrazine]

Nursing Guidelines

Assessment: Assess effectiveness and interactions of other medications patient may be taking. Assess for history of psychopathology, homicidal or suicidal tendencies, or addiction; long-term use can result in dependence, abuse, or tolerance. Periodically evaluate the need for continued use. Monitor therapeutic effectiveness, vital signs, and adverse reactions at start of therapy, when changing dosage, and at regular intervals during therapy. Monitor serum glucose closely in patients with diabetes (amphetamines may alter antidiabetic requirements). Taper dosage slowly when discontinuing. Assess knowledge/teach patient appropriate use, possible side effects, and symptoms to report.

Dietary Considerations: Should be taken 30 minutes before meals and at least 6 hours before bedtime.

Patient Education: Take exactly as directed; do not increase dose or frequency without consulting prescriber. Drug may cause physical and/or psychological dependence. Take early in day to avoid sleep disturbance, 30 minutes before meals. Avoid alcohol, caffeine, or OTC medications that act as stimulants. You may experience restlessness, false sense of euphoria, or impaired judgment (use caution when driving or engaging in tasks requiring alertness until response to drug is known); dry mouth (frequent mouth care, sucking lozenges, or chewing gum may help); nausea or vomiting (small frequent meals, frequent mouth care may help); constipation (increased exercise, fluids, fruit, or fiber may help); diarrhea (buttermilk, boiled milk, or yogurt may help); or altered libido (reversible). Patients with diabetes need to monitor serum glucose closely (may alter antidiabetic medication requirements). Report chest pain, palpitations, or irregular heartbeat; extreme fatigue or depression; CNS changes (aggressiveness, restlessness, euphoria, sleep disturbances); severe unremitting abdominal distress or cramping; blackened stool; changes in sexual activity; or blurred vision. **Pregnancy/breast-feeding precautions:** Inform prescriber if you are or intend to become pregnant. Do not breast-feed.

Pregnancy Risk Factor: C

Lactation: Enters breast milk/contraindicated

Administration

Oral: Do not crush sustained release drug product. Administer as single dose in morning or as divided doses with breakfast and lunch. Should be administered 30 minutes before meals and at least 6 hours before bedtime.

Storage: Protect from light.

Dextroamphetamine and Amphetamine

(deks troe am FET a meen & am FET a meen)

U.S. Brand Names Adderall®; Adderall XR®

Synonyms Amphetamine and Dextroamphetamine

Pharmacologic Category Stimulant

Medication Safety Issues

Sound-alike/look-alike issues:

Adderall® may be confused with Inderal®

Use Attention-deficit/hyperactivity disorder (ADHD); narcolepsy

Mechanism of Action Blocks reuptake of dopamine and norepinephrine from the synapse, thus increases the amount of circulating dopamine and norepinephrine in cerebral cortex to reticular activating system; inhibits the action of monoamine oxidase and causes catecholamines to be released. Peripheral actions include elevation of blood pressure, weak bronchodilation, and respiratory stimulation.

Pharmacodynamics/Kinetics

Onset: 30-60 minutes

Duration: 4-6 hours

Absorption: Well-absorbed

Distribution: V_d: Adults: 3.5-4.6 L/kg; concentrates in breast milk (avoid breast-feeding); distributes into CNS, mean CSF concentrations are 80% of plasma

Half-life elimination:

Children 6-12 years: d-amphetamine: 9 hours; l-amphetamine: 11 hours

Adolescents 13-17 years: d-amphetamine: 11 hours; l-amphetamine: 13-14 hours

Adults: d-amphetamine: 10 hours; l-amphetamine: 13 hours

Metabolism: Hepatic via cytochrome P450 monooxygenase and glucuronidation

Time to peak: T_{max}: Adderall®: 3 hours; Adderall XR®: 7 hours

Excretion: Urine (highly dependent on urinary pH); 70% of a single dose is eliminated within 24 hours; excreted as unchanged amphetamine (30%, may range from ~1% in alkaline urine to ~75% in acidic urine), benzoic acid, hydroxyamphetamine, hippuric acid, norephedrine, and *p*-hydroxynorephedrine

Contraindications Hypersensitivity to dextroamphetamine, amphetamine, or any component of the formulation; advanced arteriosclerosis; symptomatic cardiovascular disease; moderate to severe hypertension; hyperthyroidism; hypersensitivity or idiosyncrasy to the sympathomimetic amines; glaucoma; agitated states; patients with a history of drug abuse; with or within 14 days following MAO inhibitor (hypertensive crisis)

Warnings/Precautions Amphetamine has a high abuse potential; prolonged use may lead to dependency. Avoid use in patients with structural cardiac abnormalities; has been associated with sudden death. Use caution in patients with hypertension (including mildly hypertensive patients); sustained increases in blood

(Continued)

Dextroamphetamine and Amphetamine *(Continued)*

pressure may require dosage reduction or antihypertensive therapy. Amphetamines may impair the ability to engage in potentially hazardous activities. In psychotic children, amphetamines may exacerbate symptoms of behavior disturbance and thought disorder. Stimulants may unmask tics in individuals with coexisting Tourette's syndrome. Appetite suppresson may occur; monitor weight during therapy, particularly in children. Not recommended for children <3 years of age. Avoid abrupt discontinuation.

Drug Interactions

Dextroamphetamine: **Substrate** of CYP2D6 (major)

Amphetamine: **Substrate** of CYP2D6 (major); **Inhibits** CYP2D6 (weak)

Acidifiers (urinary): Very large doses of potassium acid phosphate or ammonium chloride may increase the renal elimination of amphetamines due to urinary acidification. Acidification of the urine may increase risk of acute renal failure in the presence of myoglobinuria.

Alkalinizers (urinary): Large doses of sodium bicarbonate or other alkalinizers may increase renal tubular reabsorption (decreased elimination) and potentiate the effect of amphetamine; includes potassium or sodium citrate and acetate

Antihypertensive agents: Amphetamines may antagonize the hypotensive effect.

Antipsychotics: Efficacy of amphetamines may be decreased by antipsychotics.

CYP2D6 inhibitors: May increase the levels/effects of amphetamine and dextroamphetamine. Example inhibitors include chlorpromazine, delavirdine, fluoxetine, miconazole, paroxetine, pergolide, quinidine, quinine, ritonavir, and ropinirole.

Ethosuximide: Absorption of ethosuximide may de delayed.

Furazolidone: Amphetamines may induce hypertensive episodes in patients receiving furazolidone

Guanethidine: Amphetamines inhibit the antihypertensive response to guanethidine; probably also may occur with guanadrel

Lithium: Inhibits anorectic and stimulant effects of amphetamines.

MAO inhibitors: Severe hypertensive episodes have occurred with amphetamine when used in patients receiving MAO inhibitors; use with or within 14 days is contraindicated

Meperidine: Analgesic effects of meperidine may be potentiated.

Norepinephrine: Amphetamines enhance the pressor response to norepinephrine

Phenobarbital: Absorption of phenobarbital may be delayed; may have synergistic anticonvulsant action.

Phenytoin: Absorption of phenytoin may be delayed; may have synergistic anticonvulsant action.

SSRIs: Increase sensitivity to amphetamines; amphetamines may increase risk of serotonin syndrome.

Tricyclic antidepressants: Concurrent of amphetamines with TCAs may result in hypertension and CNS stimulation; avoid this combination

Nutritional/Herbal/Ethanol Interactions

Ethanol: Avoid ethanol (may increase CNS depression).

Food: Dextroamphetamine serum levels may be altered if taken with acidic food, juices, or vitamin C. Avoid caffeine.

Herb/Nutraceutical: Avoid ephedra (may cause hypertension or arrhythmias).

Lab Interactions Increased corticosteroid levels (greatest in evening); may interfere with urinary steroid testing

Adverse Reactions

As reported with Adderall XR®:

>10%:

- Central nervous system: Insomnia (12% to 27%), headache (up to 26% in adults)
- Gastrointestinal: Appetite decreased (22% to 36%), abdominal pain (11% to 14%), dry mouth (2% to 35%), weight loss (4% to 11%)

1% to 10%:

- Cardiovascular: Palpitation (2% to 4%), tachycardia (up to 6% in adults)
- Central nervous system: Emotional lability (2% to 9%), agitation (up to 8% in adults), anxiety (8%), dizziness (2% to 7%), nervousness (6%), fever (5%), somnolence (2% to 4%)
- Dermatologic: Photosensitization (2% to 4%)
- Endocrine & metabolic: Dysmenorrhea (2% to 4%), impotence (2% to 4%), libido decreased (2% to 4%)
- Gastrointestinal: Nausea (2% to 8%), vomiting (2% to 7%), diarrhea (2% to 6%), constipation (2% to 4%), dyspepsia (2% to 4%)

Neuromuscular & skeletal: Twitching (2% to 4%), weakness (2% to 6%)

Respiratory: Dyspnea (2% to 4%)

Miscellaneous: Diaphoresis (2% to 4%), infection (2% to 4%), speech disorder (2% to 4%)

<1% (Limited to important or life-threatening): MI, seizure, stroke, sudden death

Adverse reactions reported with other amphetamines include: Cardiomyopathy, dyskinesia, dysphoria, euphoria, exacerbation of motor and phonic tics, exacerbation of Tourette's syndrome, headache, hypertension, overstimulation, palpitation, psychosis, rash, restlessness, tachycardia, tremor, urticaria

Overdosage/Toxicology Manifestations of overdose vary widely. Symptoms of central stimulation are usually followed by fatigue and depression. Cardiovascular and gastrointestinal symptoms are also reported. Treatment is symptomatic and supportive. Chlorpromazine may be used to antagonize CNS effects.

Dosing

Adults & Elderly: Note: Use lowest effective individualized dose; administer first dose as soon as awake; use intervals of 4-6 hours between additional doses.

ADHD: Oral:

Adderall®: Initial: 5 mg once or twice daily; increase daily dose in 5 mg increments at weekly intervals until optimal response is obtained; usual maximum dose: 40 mg/day given in 1-3 divided doses per day.

Adderall XR®: Initial: 20 mg once daily in the morning; higher doses (up to 60 mg once daily) have been evaluated; however, there is not adequate evidence that higher doses afforded additional benefit,

Narcolepsy: *Adderall®*: Oral: Initial: 10 mg/day; increase daily dose in 10 mg increments at weekly intervals until optimal response is obtained; maximum dose: 60 mg/day given in 1-3 divided doses per day.

Pediatrics:

Note: Use lowest effective individualized dose; administer first dose as soon as awake

ADHD: Oral:

Children: <3 years: Not recommended.

Children: 3-5 years (Adderall®): Initial 2.5 mg/day given every morning; increase daily dose in 2.5 mg increments at weekly intervals until optimal response is obtained; maximum dose: 40 mg/day given in 1-3 divided doses per day. Use intervals of 4-6 hours between additional doses.

Children: ≥6 years:

Adderall®: Initial: 5 mg once or twice daily; increase daily dose in 5 mg increments at weekly intervals until optimal response is obtained; usual maximum dose: 40 mg/day given in 1-3 divided doses per day. Use intervals of 4-6 hours between additional doses.

Adderall XR®: 5-10 mg once daily in the morning; if needed, may increase daily dose in 5-10 mg increments at weekly intervals (maximum dose: 30 mg/day)

Adolescents 13-17 years (Adderall XR®): 10 mg once daily in the morning ; maybe increased to 20 mg/day after 1 week if symptoms are not controlled; higher doses (up to 60 mg)/day have been evaluated; however, there is not adequate evidence that higher doses afforded additional benefit.

Narcolepsy: *Adderall®*: Oral:

Children: 6-12 years: Initial: 5 mg/day; increase daily dose in 5 mg increments at weekly intervals until optimal response is obtained; maximum dose: 60 mg/day given in 1-3 divided doses per day.

Children >12 years: Refer to adult dosing.

Available Dosage Forms

Capsule, extended release (Adderall XR®):

5 mg [dextroamphetamine sulfate 1.25 mg, dextroamphetamine saccharate 1.25 mg, amphetamine aspartate monohydrate 1.25 mg, amphetamine sulfate 1.25 mg (equivalent to amphetamine base 3.1 mg)]

10 mg [dextroamphetamine sulfate 2.5 mg, dextroamphetamine saccharate 2.5 mg, amphetamine aspartate monohydrate 2.5 mg, amphetamine sulfate 2.5 mg (equivalent to amphetamine base 6.3 mg)]

15 mg [dextroamphetamine sulfate 3.75 mg, dextroamphetamine saccharate 3.75 mg, amphetamine aspartate monohydrate 3.75 mg, amphetamine sulfate 3.75 mg (equivalent to amphetamine base 9.4 mg)]

(Continued)

Dextroamphetamine and Amphetamine *(Continued)*

20 mg [dextroamphetamine sulfate 5 mg, dextroamphetamine saccharate 5 mg, amphetamine aspartate monohydrate 5 mg, amphetamine sulfate 5 mg (equivalent to amphetamine base 12.5 mg)]

25 mg [dextroamphetamine sulfate 6.25 mg, dextroamphetamine saccharate 6.25 mg, amphetamine aspartate monohydrate 6.25 mg, amphetamine sulfate 6.25 mg (equivalent to amphetamine base 15.6 mg)]

30 mg [dextroamphetamine sulfate 7.5 mg, dextroamphetamine saccharate 7.5 mg, amphetamine aspartate monohydrate 7.5 mg, amphetamine sulfate 7.5 mg (equivalent to amphetamine base 18.8 mg)]

Tablet (Adderall®):

5 mg [dextroamphetamine sulfate 1.25 mg, dextroamphetamine saccharate 1.25 mg, amphetamine aspartate 1.25 mg, amphetamine sulfate 1.25 mg (equivalent to amphetamine base 3.13 mg)]

7.5 mg [dextroamphetamine 1.875 mg, dextroamphetamine saccharate 1.875 mg, amphetamine aspartate 1.875 mg, amphetamine sulfate 1.875 mg (equivalent to amphetamine base 4.7 mg)]

10 mg [dextroamphetamine sulfate 2.5 mg, dextroamphetamine saccharate 2.5 mg, amphetamine aspartate 2.5 mg, amphetamine sulfate 2.5 mg (equivalent to amphetamine base 6.3 mg)]

12.5 mg [dextroamphetamine sulfate 3.125 mg, dextroamphetamine saccharate 3.125 mg, amphetamine aspartate 3.125 mg, amphetamine sulfate 3.125 mg (equivalent to amphetamine base 7.8 mg)]

15 mg [dextroamphetamine sulfate 3.75 mg, dextroamphetamine saccharate 3.75 mg, amphetamine aspartate 3.75 mg, amphetamine sulfate 3.75 mg (equivalent to amphetamine base 9.4 mg)]

20 mg [dextroamphetamine sulfate 5 mg, dextroamphetamine saccharate 5 mg, amphetamine aspartate 5 mg, amphetamine sulfate 5 mg (equivalent to amphetamine base 12.6 mg)]

30 mg [dextroamphetamine sulfate 7.5 mg, dextroamphetamine saccharate 7.5 mg, amphetamine aspartate 7.5 mg, amphetamine sulfate 7.5 mg (equivalent to amphetamine base 18.8 mg)]

Nursing Guidelines

Assessment: Assess effectiveness and interactions of other medications patient may be taking. Assess for history of psychopathology, homicidal or suicidal tendencies, or addiction; long-term use can result in dependence, abuse, or tolerance. Periodically evaluate the need for continued use. Monitor therapeutic effectiveness, blood pressure, vital signs, and adverse reactions at start of therapy, when changing dosage, and at regular intervals during therapy. Monitor serum glucose closely in patients with diabetes (amphetamines may alter antidiabetic requirements). Taper dosage slowly when discontinuing. Assess knowledge/teach patient appropriate use, possible side effects, and symptoms to report.

Patient Education: Take exactly as directed; do not increase dose or frequency without consulting prescriber. Drug may cause physical and/or psychological dependence. Take early in the day to avoid sleep disturbance. If you miss a dose, take it as soon as you can. If it is almost time for your next dose, do not take double dose. Avoid alcohol, caffeine, or OTC medications that act as stimulants. You may experience restlessness, headaches, false sense of euphoria, or impaired judgment (use caution when driving or engaging in tasks requiring alertness until response to drug is known); dry mouth (frequent mouth care, sucking lozenges, or chewing gum may help); decreased appetite; nausea or vomiting (small frequent meals, frequent mouth care may help); constipation (increased exercise, fluids, fruit, or fiber may help); diarrhea (buttermilk, boiled milk, or yogurt may help); altered libido (reversible); or altered acuity of taste or smell. Patients with diabetes need to monitor serum glucose closely (may alter antidiabetic medication requirements). Report increased respirations, chest pain, palpitations, or irregular heartbeat; extreme fatigue or depression; CNS changes (aggressiveness, restlessness, euphoria, sleep disturbances); severe unremitting abdominal distress or cramping; blackened stool; changes in sexual activity; or blurred vision. **Pregnancy/breast-feeding precautions:** Inform prescriber if you are pregnant. Do not breast-feed.

Pregnancy Risk Factor: C

Pregnancy Issues: Use during pregnancy may lead to increased risk of premature delivery and low birth weight. Infants may experience symptoms of withdrawal. Teratogenic effects were reported when taken during the 1st trimester.

Lactation: Enters breast milk/contraindicated

Administration

Oral:

Adderall®: To avoid insomnia, last daily dose should be administered no less than 6 hours before retiring.

Adderall XR®: Should be given by noon. Capsule may be swallowed whole or it may be opened and the contents sprinkled on applesauce. Applesauce should be consumed immediately without chewing. Do not divide the contents of the capsule.

Storage: Store at controlled room temperature of 15°C to 30°C (59°F to 86°F)

- ♦ **Dextroamphetamine Sulfate** *see* Dextroamphetamine *on page 505*
- ♦ **Dextromethorphan, Acetaminophen, and Pseudoephedrine** *see* Acetaminophen, Dextromethorphan, and Pseudoephedrine *on page 73*
- ♦ **Dextropropoxyphene** *see* Propoxyphene *on page 1425*

Dextrose (DEKS trose)

U.S. Brand Names B-D™ Glucose [OTC]; Dex4 Glucose [OTC]; Enfamil® Glucose; Glutol™ [OTC]; Glutose™ [OTC]; Insta-Glucose® [OTC]

Synonyms Anhydrous Glucose; Dextrose Monohydrate; D_5W; $D_{10}W$; $D_{25}W$; $D_{30}W$; $D_{40}W$; $D_{50}W$; $D_{60}W$; $D_{70}W$; Glucose; Glucose Monohydrate; Glycosum

Pharmacologic Category Antidote, Hypoglycemia; Intravenous Nutritional Therapy

Medication Safety Issues

Sound-alike/look-alike issues:

Glutose™ may be confused with Glutofac®

Use

Oral: Treatment of hypoglycemia

5% and 10% solutions: Peripheral infusion to provide calories and fluid replacement

25% (hypertonic) solution: Treatment of acute symptomatic episodes of hypoglycemia in infants and children to restore depressed blood glucose levels; adjunctive treatment of hyperkalemia when combined with insulin

50% (hypertonic) solution: Treatment of insulin-induced hypoglycemia (hyperinsulinemia or insulin shock) and adjunctive treatment of hyperkalemia in adolescents and adults

≥10% solutions: Infusion after admixture with amino acids for nutritional support

Mechanism of Action Dextrose, a monosaccharide, is a source of calories and fluid for patients unable to obtain an adequate oral intake; may decrease body protein and nitrogen losses; promotes glycogen deposition in the liver. When used in the treatment of hyperkalemia (combined with insulin), dextrose stimulates the uptake of potassium by cells, especially in muscle tissue, lowering serum potassium.

Pharmacodynamics/Kinetics

Onset of action: Treatment of hypoglycemia: Oral: 10 minutes

Maximum effect: Treatment of hyperkalemia: I.V.: 30 minutes

Absorption: Rapidly from the small intestine by an active mechanism

Metabolism: Metabolized to carbon dioxide and water

Time to peak, serum: Oral: 40 minutes

Contraindications Hypersensitivity to corn or corn products; diabetic coma with hyperglycemia; hypertonic solutions in patients with intracranial or intraspinal hemorrhage; patients with delirium tremens and dehydration; patients with anuria, hepatic coma, or glucose-galactose malabsorption syndrome

Warnings/Precautions Hypertonic solutions (>10%) may cause thrombosis if infused via peripheral veins; administer hypertonic solutions via a central venous catheter. Rapid administration of hypertonic solutions may produce significant hyperglycemia, glycosuria, and shifts in electrolytes; this may result in dehydration, hyperosmolar syndrome, coma, and death especially in patients with chronic uremia or carbohydrate intolerance. Excessive or rapid dextrose administration in very low birth weight infants has been associated with increased serum osmolality and possible intracerebral hemorrhage.

Use with caution in patients with diabetes. Hyperglycemia and glycosuria may be functions of the rate of administration of dextrose; to minimize these effects, reduce the rate of infusion; addition of insulin may be necessary. Administration of potassium free I.V. dextrose solutions may result in significant hypokalemia, particularly if highly concentrated dextrose solutions are used; monitor closely and/or add potassium to dextrose solutions for patients with adequate renal

(Continued)

Dextrose *(Continued)*

function. Abrupt withdrawal of dextrose solution may be associated with rebound hypoglycemia. An unexpected rise in blood glucose level in an otherwise stable patient may be an early symptom of infection. Do not use oral forms in unconscious patients

Parenteral dextrose solutions contain aluminum which may accumulate to toxic levels with prolonged administration particularly in patients with impaired renal function. Patients with impaired renal function including premature neonates who receive aluminum at >4-5 mcg/kg/day accumulate aluminum at levels associated with CNS and bone toxicity.

Drug Interactions Corticosteroids

Adverse Reactions Frequency not defined. **Note:** Most adverse effects are associated with excessive dosage or rate of infusion.

Cardiovascular: Venous thrombosis, phlebitis, hypovolemia, hypervolemia, dehydration, edema

Central nervous system: Fever, mental confusion, unconsciousness, hyperosmolar syndrome

Endocrine & metabolic: Hyperglycemia, hypokalemia, acidosis, hypophosphatemia, hypomagnesemia

Genitourinary: Polyuria, glycosuria, ketonuria

Gastrointestinal: Polydipsia, nausea, diarrhea (oral)

Local: Pain, vein irritation, tissue necrosis

Respiratory: Tachypnea, pulmonary edema

Dosing

Adults:

Treatment of hypoglycemia: Doses may be repeated in severe cases

Oral: 10-20 g as single dose; repeat in 10 minutes if necessary

I.V.: 10-25 g (40-100 mL of 25% solution or 20-50 mL of 50% solution)

Treatment of hyperkalemia: I.V. (in combination with insulin): 25-50 g dextrose (250-500 mL $D_{10}W$) combined with 10 units regular insulin administered over 30-60 minutes; repeat as needed or as an alternative 25 g dextrose (50 mL $D_{50}W$) combined with 5-10 units regular insulin infused over 5 minutes; repeat as needed

Note: More rapid infusions (<30 minutes) may be associated with hyperglycemia and hyperosmolality and will exacerbate hyperkalemia; avoid use in patients who are already hyperglycemic

Pediatrics:

Treatment of hypoglycemia: Doses may be repeated in severe cases

Oral: Children >2 years: Refer to adult dosing.

I.V.:

Infants ≤6 months: 0.25-0.5 g/kg/dose (1-2 mL/kg/dose of 25% solution); maximum: 25 g/dose

Infants >6 months and Children: 0.5-1 g/kg/dose (2-4 mL/kg/dose of 25% solution); maximum: 25 g/dose

Adolescents: Refer to adult dosing.

Treatment of hyperkalemia: I.V. (in combination with insulin):

Infants and Children: 0.5-1 g/kg (using 25% or 50% solution) combined with regular insulin 1 unit for every 4-5 g dextrose given; infuse over 2 hours (infusions as short as 30 minutes have been recommended); repeat as needed

Adolescents: Refer to adult dosing.

Available Dosage Forms

Gel, as 40% dextrose:

Glutose™: 40% (15 g, 45 g)

Insta-Glucose®: 40% (30 g)

Infusion, as 2.5% dextrose: 1000 mL

Infusion, as 5% dextrose: 25 mL, 50 mL, 100 mL, 150 mL, 250 mL, 500 mL, 1000 mL

Infusion, as 10% dextrose: 3 mL, 5 mL, 250 mL, 500 mL, 1000 mL

Infusion, as 20% dextrose: 500 mL, 1000 mL

Infusion, as 25% dextrose: 10 mL

Infusion, as 30% dextrose: 500 mL, 1000 mL

Infusion, as 40% dextrose: 500 mL, 1000 mL

Infusion, as 50% dextrose: 50 mL, 500 mL, 1000 mL, 2000 mL

Infusion, as 60% dextrose: 500 mL, 1000 mL

Infusion, as 70% dextrose: 70 mL, 500 mL, 1000 mL, 2000 mL

Solution, oral:

Enfamil® Glucose: 5% (90 mL) [5 g dextrose/100 mL]; 10% (90 mL) [10 g dextrose/100 mL]

Glutol™: 55% (180 mL) [100 g dextrose/180 mL]

Tablet, chewable:

B-D™ Glucose: 5 g

Dex4 Glucose: 4 g

Nursing Guidelines

Monitoring Laboratory Tests: Blood and urine sugar, serum electrolytes

Pregnancy Risk Factor: C/A (oral)

Administration

Oral: Must be swallowed to be absorbed (see Warnings)

I.V.: Not for SubQ or I.M. administration; dilute concentrated dextrose solutions for peripheral venous administration to a maximum concentration of 12.5%; in emergency situations, 25% dextrose has been used peripherally; for direct I.V. infusion, infuse at a maximum rate of 200 mg/kg over 1 minute; continuous infusion rates very with tolerance and range from 4.5-15 mg/kg/minute; hyperinsulinemic neonates may require up to 15-25 mg/kg/minute infusion rates

Storage: Stable at room temperature. Protect from freezing and extreme heat. Store oral dextrose in airtight containers.

- Dextrose Monohydrate *see* Dextrose *on page 511*
- Dextrostat® *see* Dextroamphetamine *on page 505*
- DHE *see* Dihydroergotamine *on page 537*
- D.H.E. 45® *see* Dihydroergotamine *on page 537*
- DHPG Sodium *see* Ganciclovir *on page 794*
- Diabeta *see* GlyBURIDE *on page 820*
- DiabetAid Gingivitis Mouth Rinse [OTC] *see* Cetylpyridinium *on page 368*
- Diabetic Tussin C® *see* Guaifenesin and Codeine *on page 835*
- Diabetic Tussin® EX [OTC] *see* Guaifenesin *on page 834*
- Diaβeta® *see* GlyBURIDE *on page 820*
- Diaminocyclohexane Oxalatoplatinum *see* Oxaliplatin *on page 1275*
- Diamode [OTC] *see* Loperamide *on page 1056*
- Diamox® Sequels® *see* AcetaZOLAMIDE *on page 75*
- Diastat® *see* Diazepam *on page 515*
- Diastat® AcuDial™ *see* Diazepam *on page 515*

Diatrizoate Meglumine (dye a tri ZOE ate MEG loo meen)

U.S. Brand Names Cystografin®; Cystografin® Dilute; Hypaque-Cysto™; Hypaque™ Meglumine; Reno-30®; Reno-60®; Reno-Dip®

Pharmacologic Category Iodinated Contrast Media; Radiological/Contrast Media, Ionic

Use

Solution for instillation: Retrograde cystourethrography; retrograde or ascending pyelography

Solution for injection: Arthrography, cerebral angiography, direct cholangiography, discography, drip infusion pyelography, excretory urography, peripheral arteriography, splenoportography, venography; contrast enhancement of computed tomographic head imaging

Contraindications Hypersensitivity to diatrizoate or any component of the formulation; solutions for instillation should not be used for intravascular injection; solutions for injection are not for intrathecal use

Refer to product labeling for procedure-specific contraindications.

Available Dosage Forms

Solution, for instillation:

Cystografin®: Diatrizoate meglumine 30% (100 mL, 300 mL) [provides organically-bound iodine 141 mg/mL; contains edetate disodium]

Cystografin® Dilute: Diatrizoate meglumine 18% (300 mL) [provides organically-bound iodine 85 mg/mL; contains edetate disodium]

Reno-30®: Diatrizoate meglumine 30% (50 mL) [provides organically-bound iodine 141 mg/mL; contains edetate disodium]

Solution, for instillation [preservative free] (Hypaque-Cysto™): Diatrizoate meglumine 30% (250 mL) [provides organically-bound iodine 141 mg/mL; contains edetate calcium disodium]

(Continued)

Diatrizoate Meglumine *(Continued)*

Solution, injection:

Hypaque™ Meglumine: Diatrizoate meglumine 60% (50 mL, 100 mL, 150 mL, 200 mL) [provides organically-bound iodine 282 mg/mL; contains edetate calcium disodium]

Reno-60®: Diatrizoate meglumine 60% (10 mL, 50 mL, 100 mL, 150 mL) [provides organically-bound iodine 282 mg/mL; contains edetate disodium, sodium 0.91 mg (0.04 mEq)/mL]

Reno-Dip®: Diatrizoate meglumine 30% (300 mL) [provides organically-bound iodine 141 mg/mL; contains edetate disodium, sodium 0.049 mg (0.002 mEq)/mL]

Nursing Guidelines

Pregnancy Risk Factor: C

Pregnancy Issues: Animal reproduction studies have not been conducted. Diatrizoate salts cross the placenta and may enter fetal circulation. Abnormal neonatal opacification of the small intestine and colon have been reported in the newborn 4-6 days after delivery. In general, iodinated contrast media agents are avoided during pregnancy unless essential for diagnosis.

Lactation: Enters breast milk/use caution

Breast-Feeding Considerations: Diatrizoate salts are reported to be excreted in human milk

Diatrizoate Meglumine and Diatrizoate Sodium

(dye a tri ZOE ate MEG loo meen & dye a tri ZOE ate SOW dee um)

U.S. Brand Names Gastrografin®; Hypaque™-76; MD-76®R; MD-Gastroview®; RenoCal-76®; Renografin®-60

Synonyms Diatrizoate Sodium and Diatrizoate Meglumine

Pharmacologic Category Iodinated Contrast Media; Radiological/Contrast Media, Ionic

Use

Oral/rectal: Examination of GI tract; adjunct to contrast enhancement in computed tomography of the torso

Injection: Angiocardiography, aortography, central venography, cerebral angiography, cholangiography, digital arteriography, excretory urography, nephrotomography, peripheral angiography, peripheral arteriography, renal arteriography, renal venography, splenoportography, visceral arteriography; contrast enhancement of computed tomographic imaging

Contraindications Hypersensitivity to diatrizoate or any component of the formulation; injection is not intended for intrathecal use

Refer to product labeling for procedure-specific contraindications.

Warnings/Precautions Use caution with history of previous reaction to contrast dye or iodine. Solutions may be hypertonic and may cause mucosal irritation and intraluminal water movement resulting in laxative effect; use caution with children or debilitated patients; monitor hydration and electrolyte status. Use caution with thyroid dysfunction; hyperthyroidism has been reported.

Lab Interactions Thyroid function tests (protein bound iodine uptake studies) may be inaccurate for up to 1 year after administration; may cause false low trypsin values (determined spectrophotometrically).

Adverse Reactions Frequency not defined.

Cardiovascular: Tachyarrhythmia

Dermatologic: Urticaria

Gastrointestinal: Diarrhea, nausea, vomiting

Respiratory: Dyspnea, hypoxia

Miscellaneous: Anaphylaxis

Overdosage/Toxicology Potential for hypotension, hypovolemia, or shock; maintain I.V. access for rehydration; monitor and support symptomatically.

Dosing

Adults & Elderly:

Radiographic exam of GI tract segments:

Oral: 30-90 mL

Rectal enema: Dilute 240 mL in 1000 mL tap water

Tomography: Oral: 25-77 mL in 1000 mL tap water 15-30 minutes prior to imaging

Pediatrics: Radiographic exam of GI tract segments:

Oral:

Children <5 years: 30 mL, dilute 1:1 (if <10 kg or debilitated, dilute 1:3)

Children 5-10 years: 60 mL, dilute 1:1 (if <10 kg or debilitated, dilute 1:3)

Rectal enema:

Children <5 years: Dilute 1:5 in tap water

Children >5 years: Dilute 90 mL in 500 mL tap water

Available Dosage Forms

Solution, injection:

Hypaque™-76: Diatrizoate meglumine 66% and diatrizoate sodium 10% (50 mL, 200 mL) [provides organically-bound iodine 370 mg/mL; contains edetate calcium disodium, sodium 3.68 (0.16 mEq)/mL]

MD-76®R: Diatrizoate meglumine 66% and diatrizoate sodium 10% (50 mL, 100 mL, 150 mL, 200 mL) [provides organically-bound iodine 370 mg/mL; contains edetate calcium disodium, sodium 3.65 mg (0.16 mEq)/mL]

RenoCal-76®: Diatrizoate meglumine 66% and diatrizoate sodium 10% (50 mL, 100 mL, 150 mL, 200 mL) [provides organically-bound iodine 370 mg/mL; contains edetate calcium disodium, sodium 3.69 mg (0.16 mEq)/mL]

Renografin®-60: Diatrizoate meglumine 520 mg and diatrizoate sodium 80 mg per mL (10 mL, 50 mL, 100 mL) [provides organically-bound iodine 292.5 mg/mL; contains edetate disodium, sodium 3.76 mg (0.16 mEq)/mL]

Solution, oral/rectal:

Gastrografin®: Diatrizoate meglumine 660 mg and diatrizoate sodium 100 mg per mL (30 mL, 120 mL) [provides organically-bound iodine 367 mg/mL; contains edetate disodium, sodium 4.8 mg (0.21 mEq)/mL; lemon flavor]

MD-Gastroview®: Diatrizoate meglumine 660 mg and diatrizoate sodium 100 mg per mL (25 mL, 120 mL, 240 mL) [provides organically-bound iodine 367 mg/mL; contains edetate disodium, sodium 4.8 mg (0.21 mEq)/mL; lemon-vanilla flavor]

Nursing Guidelines

Pregnancy Risk Factor: B/C (manufacturer dependent)

Pregnancy Issues: Diatrizoate salts cross the placenta and may enter fetal circulation. Abnormal neonatal opacification of the small intestine and colon have been reported in the newborn 4-6 days after delivery. In general, iodinated contrast media agents are avoided during pregnancy unless essential for diagnosis.

Lactation: Enters breast milk/use caution

Breast-Feeding Considerations: Diatrizoate salts are reported to be excreted in human milk. One manufacturer recommends bottle feedings for 24 hours following administration.

Administration

Oral: May be diluted 1:1 with water, carbonated beverage, milk, or mineral oil for children and cachectic elderly; for very young (<10kg) and debilitated children, dilute 1:3 in water.

Storage: Store at 20°C to 25°C (68°F to 77°F). Protect from light.

- **Diatrizoate Sodium and Diatrizoate Meglumine** *see* Diatrizoate Meglumine and Diatrizoate Sodium *on page 514*
- **Diatx™** *see* Vitamin B Complex Combinations *on page 1716*
- **DiatxFe™** *see* Vitamin B Complex Combinations *on page 1716*

Diazepam (dye AZ e pam)

U.S. Brand Names Diastat®; Diastat® AcuDial™; Diazepam Intensol®; Valium®

Pharmacologic Category Benzodiazepine

Medication Safety Issues

Sound-alike/look-alike issues:

Diazepam may be confused with diazoxide, Ditropan®, lorazepam

Valium® may be confused with Valcyte™

Use Management of anxiety disorders, ethanol withdrawal symptoms; skeletal muscle relaxant; treatment of convulsive disorders

Orphan drug: Viscous solution for rectal administration: Management of selected, refractory epilepsy patients on stable regimens of antiepileptic drugs (AEDs) requiring intermittent use of diazepam to control episodes of increased seizure activity

Unlabeled/Investigational Use Panic disorders; preoperative sedation, light anesthesia, amnesia

Mechanism of Action Binds to stereospecific benzodiazepine receptors on the postsynaptic GABA neuron at several sites within the central nervous system, including the limbic system, reticular formation. Enhancement of the inhibitory effect of GABA on neuronal excitability results by increased neuronal membrane (Continued)

Diazepam *(Continued)*

permeability to chloride ions. This shift in chloride ions results in hyperpolarization (a less excitable state) and stabilization.

Pharmacodynamics/Kinetics

I.V.: Status epilepticus:

Onset of action: Almost immediate

Duration: 20-30 minutes

Absorption: Oral: 85% to 100%, more reliable than I.M.

Protein binding: 98%

Metabolism: Hepatic

Half-life elimination: Parent drug: Adults: 20-50 hours; increased half-life in neonates, elderly, and those with severe hepatic disorders; Active major metabolite (desmethyldiazepam): 50-100 hours; may be prolonged in neonates

Contraindications Hypersensitivity to diazepam or any component of the formulation (cross-sensitivity with other benzodiazepines may exist); narrow-angle glaucoma; not for use in children <6 months of age (oral, rectal gel) or <30 days of age (parenteral); pregnancy

Warnings/Precautions Diazepam has been associated with increasing the frequency of grand mal seizures. Withdrawal has also been associated with an increase in the seizure frequency. Use with caution with drugs which may decrease diazepam metabolism. Use with caution in elderly or debilitated patients, patients with hepatic disease (including alcoholics), or renal impairment. Active metabolites with extended half-lives may lead to delayed accumulation and adverse effects. Use with caution in patients with respiratory disease or impaired gag reflex.

Acute hypotension, muscle weakness, apnea, and cardiac arrest have occurred with parenteral administration. Acute effects may be more prevalent in patients receiving concurrent barbiturates, narcotics, or ethanol. Appropriate resuscitative equipment and qualified personnel should be available during administration and monitoring. Avoid use of the injection in patients with shock, coma, or acute ethanol intoxication. Intra-arterial injection or extravasation of the parenteral formulation should be avoided. Parenteral formulation contains propylene glycol, which has been associated with toxicity when administered in high dosages. Administration of rectal gel should only be performed by individuals trained to recognize characteristic seizure activity for which the product is indicated, and capable of monitoring response to determine need for additional medical intervention.

Causes CNS depression (dose-related) resulting in sedation, dizziness, confusion, or ataxia which may impair physical and mental capabilities. Patients must be cautioned about performing tasks which require mental alertness (eg, operating machinery or driving). Use with caution in patients receiving other CNS depressants or psychoactive agents. Effects with other sedative drugs or ethanol may be potentiated. The dosage of narcotics should be reduced by approximately 1/3 when diazepam is added. Benzodiazepines have been associated with falls and traumatic injury and should be used with extreme caution in patients who are at risk of these events (especially the elderly).

Use caution in patients with depression, particularly if suicidal risk may be present. Use with caution in patients with a history of drug dependence. Benzodiazepines have been associated with dependence and acute withdrawal symptoms on discontinuation or reduction in dose. Acute withdrawal, including seizures, may be precipitated in patients after administration of flumazenil to patients receiving long-term benzodiazepine therapy.

Diazepam has been associated with anterograde amnesia. Paradoxical reactions, including hyperactive or aggressive behavior, have been reported with benzodiazepines, particularly in adolescent/pediatric or psychiatric patients. Does not have analgesic, antidepressant, or antipsychotic properties.

Drug Interactions **Substrate** of CYP1A2 (minor), 2B6 (minor), 2C8/9 (minor), 2C19 (major), 3A4 (major); **Inhibits** CYP2C19 (weak), 3A4 (weak)

CNS depressants: Sedative effects and/or respiratory depression may be additive with CNS depressants; includes ethanol, barbiturates, narcotic analgesics, and other sedative agents; monitor for increased effect

CYP2C19 inducers: May decrease the levels/effects of diazepam. Example inducers include aminoglutethimide, carbamazepine, phenytoin, and rifampin.

CYP2C19 inhibitors: May increase the levels/effects of diazepam. Example inhibitors include delavirdine, fluconazole, fluvoxamine, gemfibrozil, isoniazid, omeprazole, and ticlopidine.

CYP3A4 inducers: CYP3A4 inducers may decrease the levels/effects of diazepam. Example inducers include aminoglutethimide, carbamazepine, nafcillin, nevirapine, phenobarbital, phenytoin, and rifamycins.

CYP3A4 inhibitors: May increase the levels/effects of diazepam. Example inhibitors include azole antifungals, clarithromycin, diclofenac, doxycycline, erythromycin, imatinib, isoniazid, nefazodone, nicardipine, propofol, protease inhibitors, quinidine, telithromycin, and verapamil.

Levodopa: Therapeutic effects may be diminished in some patients following the addition of a benzodiazepine; limited/inconsistent data

Oral contraceptives: May decrease the clearance of some benzodiazepines (those which undergo oxidative metabolism); monitor for increased benzodiazepine effect

Theophylline: May partially antagonize some of the effects of benzodiazepines; monitor for decreased response; may require higher doses for sedation

Nutritional/Herbal/Ethanol Interactions

Ethanol: Avoid ethanol (may increase CNS depression).

Food: Diazepam serum levels may be increased if taken with food. Diazepam effect/toxicity may be increased by grapefruit juice; avoid concurrent use.

Herb/Nutraceutical: St John's wort may decrease diazepam levels. Avoid valerian, St John's wort, kava kava, gotu kola (may increase CNS depression).

Lab Interactions False-negative urinary glucose determinations when using Clinistix® or Diastix®

Adverse Reactions Frequency not defined. Adverse reactions may vary by route of administration.

Cardiovascular: Hypotension, vasodilatation

Central nervous system: Agitation, amnesia, anxiety, ataxia, confusion, depression, dizziness, drowsiness, emotional lability, euphoria, fatigue, headache, incoordination, insomnia, memory impairment, paradoxical excitement or rage, seizure, slurred speech, somnolence, vertigo

Dermatologic: Rash

Endocrine & metabolic: Changes in libido

Gastrointestinal: Changes in salivation, constipation, diarrhea, nausea

Genitourinary: Incontinence, urinary retention

Hepatic: Jaundice

Local: Phlebitis, pain with injection

Neuromuscular & skeletal: Dysarthria, tremor, weakness

Ocular: Blurred vision, diplopia

Respiratory: Apnea, asthma, decrease in respiratory rate

Overdosage/Toxicology Symptoms of overdose include somnolence, confusion, coma, hypoactive reflexes, dyspnea, hypotension, slurred speech, or impaired coordination. Treatment for benzodiazepine overdose is supportive. Flumazenil has been shown to selectively block the binding of benzodiazepines to CNS receptors, resulting in a reversal of benzodiazepine-induced CNS depression, but not respiratory depression.

Dosing

Adults: Note: Oral absorption is more reliable than I.M.

Anticonvulsant (acute treatment): Rectal gel: 0.2 mg/kg. **Note:** Dosage should be rounded upward to the next available dose, 2.5, 5, 10, 12.5, 15, 17.5, and 20 mg/dose; dose may be repeated in 4-12 hours if needed; do not use for more than 5 episodes per month or more than one episode every 5 days.

Anxiety/sedation/skeletal muscle relaxation:

Oral: 2-10 mg 2-4 times/day

I.M., I.V.: 2-10 mg, may repeat in 3-4 hours if needed

Sedation in the ICU patient: I.V.: 0.03-0.1 mg/kg every 30 minutes to 6 hours

Status epilepticus: I.V.: 5-10 mg every 10-20 minutes, up to 30 mg in an 8-hour period; may repeat in 2-4 hours if necessary

Rapid tranquilization of agitated patient (administer every 30-60 minutes): Oral: 5-10 mg; average total dose for tranquilization: 20-60 mg

Elderly: Oral absorption is more reliable than I.M..

Oral: Initial:

Anxiety: 1-2 mg 1-2 times/day; increase gradually as needed, rarely need to use >10 mg/day.

Skeletal muscle relaxant: 2-5 mg 2-4 times/day

Rectal gel: Due to the increased half-life in elderly and debilitated patients, consider reducing dose.

(Continued)

Diazepam *(Continued)*

Pediatrics:

Conscious sedation for procedures:

Oral:

Children: 0.2-0.3 mg/kg (maximum dose: 10 mg) 45-60 minutes prior to procedure

Adolescents: 10 mg

I.V.: Adolescents: 5 mg; may repeat with 2.5 mg if needed

Febrile seizure prophylaxis: Oral: Children: 1 mg/kg/day divided every 8 hours; initiate therapy at first sign of fever and continue for 24 hours after fever is gone

Sedation or muscle relaxation or anxiety:

Oral: Children: 0.12-0.8 mg/kg/day in divided doses every 6-8 hours

I.M., I.V.: Children: 0.04-0.3 mg/kg/dose every 2-4 hours to a maximum of 0.6 mg/kg within an 8-hour period if needed

Status epilepticus:

I.V.:

Infants >30 days and Children <5 years: 0.05-0.3 mg/kg/dose given over 3-5 minutes, every 15-30 minutes to a maximum total dose of 5 mg **or** 0.2-0.5 mg/dose every 2-5 minutes to a maximum total dose of 5 mg; repeat in 2-4 hours as needed

Children ≥5 years: 0.05-0.3 mg/kg/dose given over 3-5 minutes, every 15-30 minutes to a maximum total dose of 10 mg **or** 1 mg/dose every 2-5 minutes to a maximum of 10 mg; repeat in 2-4 hours as needed

Rectal: 0.5 mg/kg/dose then 0.25 mg/kg/dose in 10 minutes if needed

Anticonvulsant (acute treatment): Rectal gel:

Infants <6 months: Not recommended

Children <2 years: Safety and efficacy have not been studied

Children 2-5 years: 0.5 mg/kg

Children 6-11 years: 0.3 mg/kg

Children ≥12 years: Refer to adult dosing.

Note: Dosage should be rounded upward to the next available dose, 2.5, 5, 10, 12.5, 15, 17.5, and 20 mg/dose; dose may be repeated in 4-12 hours if needed; do not use for more than 5 episodes per month or more than one episode every 5 days.

Muscle spasm associated with tetanus: I.V., I.M.:

Infants >30 days: 1-2 mg/dose every 3-4 hours as needed

Children ≥5 years: 5-10 mg/dose every 3-4 hours as needed

Renal Impairment: Hemodialysis effects: Not dialyzable (0% to 5%); supplemental dose is **not** necessary.

Hepatic Impairment: Reduce dose by 50% in cirrhosis and avoid in severe/acute liver disease.

Available Dosage Forms

Gel, rectal:

Diastat®: Pediatric rectal tip [4.4 cm]: 5 mg/mL (2.5 mg, 5 mg) [contains ethyl alcohol 10%, sodium benzoate, benzyl alcohol 1.5%; twin pack]

Diastat® AcuDial™ delivery system:

10 mg: Pediatric/adult rectal tip [4.4 cm]: 5 mg/mL (delivers set doses of 5 mg, 7.5 mg, and 10 mg) [contains ethyl alcohol 10%, sodium benzoate, benzyl alcohol 1.5%; twin pack]

20 mg: Adult rectal tip [6 cm]: 5 mg/mL (delivers set doses of 10 mg, 12.5 mg, 15 mg, 17.5 mg, and 20 mg) [contains ethyl alcohol 10%, sodium benzoate, benzyl alcohol 1.5%; twin pack]

Injection, solution: 5 mg/mL (2 mL, 10 mL) [may contain benzyl alcohol, sodium benzoate, benzoic acid]

Solution, oral: 5 mg/5 mL (5 mL, 500 mL) [wintergreen-spice flavor]

Solution, oral concentrate (Diazepam Intensol®): 5 mg/mL (30 mL)

Tablet (Valium®): 2 mg, 5 mg, 10 mg

Nursing Guidelines

Assessment: Assess effectiveness and interactions of other medications patient may be taking. Assess for history of addiction; long-term use can result in dependence, abuse, or tolerance; periodically evaluate need for continued use. Monitor blood pressure, CNS status. For inpatient use, institute safety measures and monitor effectiveness and adverse reactions. For outpatients, monitor therapeutic effectiveness and adverse reactions at beginning of therapy and periodically with long-term use. Taper dosage slowly when discontinuing. Assess knowledge/teach patient seizure precautions (if administered for seizures), appropriate use, interventions to reduce side effects, and adverse symptoms to report.

Patient Education: Take exactly as directed; do not increase dose or frequency. Drug may cause physical and/or psychological dependence. While using this medication, do not use alcohol and other prescription or OTC medications (especially pain medications, sedatives, antihistamines, or hypnotics) without consulting prescriber. Maintain adequate hydration (2-3 L/day of fluids) unless instructed to restrict fluid intake. You may experience drowsiness, dizziness, or blurred vision (use caution when driving or engaging in tasks requiring alertness until response to drug is known); nausea, vomiting, loss of appetite, or dry mouth (small frequent meals, frequent mouth care, chewing gum, or sucking lozenges may help); constipation (increased exercise, fluids, fruit, or fiber may help). If medication is used to control seizures, wear identification that you are taking an antiepileptic medication. Report CNS changes (confusion, depression, increased sedation, excitation, headache, agitation, insomnia or nightmares, dizziness, fatigue, or impaired coordination) or changes in cognition; respiratory difficulty or shortness of breath; changes in urinary pattern; changes in sexual activity; muscle cramping, weakness, tremors, or rigidity; ringing in ears or visual disturbances; excessive perspiration; excessive GI symptoms (cramping, constipation, vomiting, anorexia); or worsening of seizure activity or loss of seizure control. **Pregnancy/breast-feeding precautions:** Do not get pregnant while taking this medication; use appropriate contraceptive measures. Do not breast-feed.

Geriatric Considerations: Due to its long-acting metabolite, diazepam is not considered a drug of choice in the elderly. Long-acting benzodiazepines have been associated with falls in the elderly. Interpretive guidelines from the Centers for Medicare and Medicaid Services (CMS) strongly discourage the use of this agent in residents of long-term care facilities.

Pregnancy Risk Factor: D

Pregnancy Issues: Benzodiazepines cross the placenta. The association between benzodiazepine exposure and malformations remains controversial. A number of types of malformation have been reported (oral cleft, inguinal hernia, cardiac defects, spina bifida, dysmorphic facial features, skeletal defects); however, confounding factors make a clear association difficult. Overall, the risk to the fetus may be low. Nonteratogenic effects (including neonatal flaccidity, respiratory and feeding problems, and withdrawal symptoms) during the postnatal period have also been reported with benzodiazepine use.

Lactation: Enters breast milk/contraindicated (AAP rates "of concern")

Breast-Feeding Considerations: Clinical effects on the infant include sedation; AAP reports that USE MAY BE OF CONCERN.

Perioperative/Anesthesia/Other Concerns:

Oral absorption more reliable than intramuscular. Intensol® should be diluted before use. Diazepam does not have any analgesic effects. Chronic use of this agent may increase the perioperative benzodiazepine dose needed to achieve desired effect. Abrupt discontinuation after sustained use (generally >10 days) may cause withdrawal symptoms. Hypotension may result in orthostatic lightheadedness or syncope. Benzodiazepines, as a class, may depress respiration. The 2002 ACCM/SCCM guidelines for the sustained use of sedatives and analgesics in critically-ill adults recommend diazepam or midazolam for rapid sedation of acutely-agitated patients.

Status Epilepticus: A randomized, double-blind trial (Treiman D, 1998) evaluated the efficacy of four treatments in overt status epilepticus. Treatment arms were designed based upon accepted practices of North American neurologists. The treatments were: 1) lorazepam 0.1 mg/kg, 2) diazepam 0.15 mg/kg followed by phenytoin 18 mg/kg, 3) phenytoin 18 mg/kg alone, and 4) phenobarbital 15 mg/kg. Treatment was considered successful if the seizures were terminated (clinically and by EEG) within 20 minutes of start of therapy without seizure recurrence within 60 minutes from the start of therapy. Patients who failed the first treatment received a second and a third, if necessary. Patients did not receive randomized treatments after the first one but the treating physician remained blinded. Treatment success: Lorazepam 64.9%, phenobarbital 58.2%, diazepam/phenytoin 55.8%, and phenytoin alone 43.6%. Using an "intention-to-treat" analysis, there was no statistical difference between the groups. Results of subsequent treatments in patients who failed the first therapy indicated that response rate significantly dropped regardless of treatment. Aggregate response rate to the second treatment was 7.0% and third treatment 2.3%.

(Continued)

Diazepam *(Continued)*

Administration

Oral: Intensol® should be diluted before use.

I.V.: Continuous infusion is not recommended because of precipitation in I.V. fluids and absorption of drug into infusion bags and tubing. In children, do not exceed 1-2 mg/minute IVP; in adults 5 mg/minute.

Reconstitution: Most stable at pH 4-8, hydrolysis occurs at pH <3.

Compatibility: Do not mix I.V. product with other medications.

Y-site administration: Incompatible with amphotericin B cholesteryl sulfate complex, atracurium, cefepime, diltiazem, fluconazole, foscarnet, gatifloxacin, heparin, heparin with hydrocortisone sodium succinate, hydromorphone, linezolid, meropenem, pancuronium, potassium chloride, propofol, vecuronium, vitamin B complex with C

Compatibility in syringe: Incompatible with doxapram, glycopyrrolate, heparin, hydromorphone, nalbuphine, sufentanil

Compatibility when admixed: Incompatible with bleomycin, buprenorphine, dobutamine, doxorubicin, floxacillin, fluorouracil, furosemide

Storage:

Protect parenteral dosage form from light; potency is retained for up to 3 months when kept at room temperature.

Rectal gel: Store at 25°C (77°F); excursion permitted to 15°C to 30°C (59°F to 86°F).

Related Information

Conscious Sedation *on page 1779*
Intravenous Anesthetic Agents *on page 1853*
Perioperative Management of Patients on Antiseizure Medication *on page 1801*

♦ Diazepam Intensol® *see* Diazepam *on page 515*

Dibucaine (DYE byoo kane)

U.S. Brand Names Nupercainal® [OTC]

Pharmacologic Category Local Anesthetic

Use Fast, temporary relief of pain and itching due to hemorrhoids, minor burns

Mechanism of Action Local anesthetics bind selectively to the intracellular surface of sodium channels to block influx of sodium into the axon. As a result, depolarization necessary for action potential propagation and subsequent nerve function is prevented. The block at the sodium channel is reversible. When drug diffuses away from the axon, sodium channel function is restored and nerve propagation returns.

Pharmacodynamics/Kinetics

Onset of action: ~15 minutes

Duration: 2-4 hours

Absorption: Poor through intact skin; well absorbed through mucous membranes and excoriated skin

Contraindications Hypersensitivity to amide-type anesthetics, ophthalmic use

Drug Interactions No data reported

Adverse Reactions 1% to 10%:

Dermatologic: Angioedema, contact dermatitis

Local: Burning

Dosing

Adults & Elderly: Local pain (local anesthetic): Topical: Apply gently to the affected areas; no more than 30 g for adults or 7.5 g for children should be used in any 24-hour period

Pediatrics: Children: Topical: Refer to adult dosing.

Available Dosage Forms

Ointment: 1% (30 g, 454 g)

Nupercainal®: 1% (30 g, 60g) [contains sodium bisulfite]

Nursing Guidelines

Patient Education: If condition worsens or if symptoms persist for >7 days, stop using and consult a physician; wash hands after use

Pregnancy Risk Factor: C

Breast-Feeding Considerations: No data reported; however, topical administration is probably compatible.

Administration

Storage: Darkens on light exposure.

♦ 6,7-Dichloro-1,5-Dihydroimidazo [2,1b] quinazolin-2(3H)-one Monohydrochloride *see* Anagrelide *on page 166*

Diclofenac (dye KLOE fen ak)

U.S. Brand Names Cataflam®; Solaraze®; Voltaren®; Voltaren Ophthalmic®; Voltaren®-XR

Synonyms Diclofenac Potassium; Diclofenac Sodium

Pharmacologic Category Nonsteroidal Anti-inflammatory Drug (NSAID); Nonsteroidal Anti-inflammatory Drug (NSAID), Ophthalmic; Nonsteroidal Anti-inflammatory Drug (NSAID), Oral

Medication Safety Issues

Sound-alike/look-alike issues:

Diclofenac may be confused with Diflucan®, Duphalac®

Cataflam® may be confused with Catapres®

Voltaren® may be confused with tramadol, Ultram®, Verelan®

Use

Immediate release: Ankylosing spondylitis; primary dysmenorrhea; acute and chronic treatment of rheumatoid arthritis, osteoarthritis

Delayed-release tablets: Acute and chronic treatment of rheumatoid arthritis, osteoarthritis, ankylosing spondylitis

Extended-release tablets: Chronic treatment of osteoarthritis, rheumatoid arthritis

Ophthalmic solution: Postoperative inflammation following cataract extraction; temporary relief of pain and photophobia in patients undergoing corneal refractive surgery

Topical gel: Actinic keratosis (AK) in conjunction with sun avoidance

Unlabeled/Investigational Use Juvenile rheumatoid arthritis

Mechanism of Action Inhibits prostaglandin synthesis by decreasing the activity of the enzyme, cyclooxygenase, which results in decreased formation of prostaglandin precursors. Mechanism of action for the treatment of AK has not been established.

Pharmacodynamics/Kinetics

Onset of action: Cataflam® is more rapid than sodium salt (Voltaren®) because it dissolves in the stomach instead of the duodenum

Absorption: Topical gel: 10%

Protein binding: 99% to albumin

Metabolism: Hepatic to several metabolites

Half-life elimination: 2 hours

Time to peak, serum: Cataflam®: ~1 hour; Voltaren®: ~2 hours

Excretion: Urine (65%); feces (35%)

Contraindications Hypersensitivity to diclofenac, aspirin, other NSAIDs, or any component of the formulation; perioperative pain in the setting of coronary artery bypass surgery (CABG); pregnancy (3rd trimester)

Warnings/Precautions NSAIDs are associated with an increased risk of adverse cardiovascular events, including MI, stroke, and new onset or worsening of pre-existing hypertension. Risk may be increased with duration of use or pre-existing cardiovascular risk factors or disease. Carefully evaluate individual cardiovascular risk profiles prior to prescribing. Use caution with fluid retention, CHF, or hypertension.

Use of NSAIDs can compromise existing renal function. Renal toxicity can occur in patient with impaired renal function, dehydration, heart failure, liver dysfunction, those taking diuretics and ACEI, and the elderly. Rehydrate patient before starting therapy. Monitor renal function closely. Use caution in patients with advanced renal disease.

NSAIDs may increase risk of gastrointestinal irritation, ulceration, bleeding, and perforation. These events may occur at any time during therapy and without warning. Use caution with a history of GI disease (bleeding or ulcers), concurrent therapy with aspirin, anticoagulants and/or corticosteroids, smoking, use of alcohol, the elderly or debilitated patients.

Use the lowest effective dose for the shortest duration of time, consistent with individual patient goals, to reduce risk of cardiovascular or GI adverse events. Alternate therapies should be considered for patients at high risk.

NSAIDs may cause serious skin adverse events including exfoliative dermatitis, Stevens-Johnson syndrome (SJS), and toxic epidermal necrolysis (TEN). (Continued)

Diclofenac *(Continued)*

Anaphylactoid reactions may occur, even without prior exposure; patients with "aspirin triad" (bronchial asthma, aspirin intolerance, rhinitis) may be at increased risk. Do not use in patients who experience bronchospasm, asthma, rhinitis, or urticaria with NSAID or aspirin therapy.

Use with caution in patients with decreased hepatic function. Closely monitor patients with any abnormal LFT. Severe hepatic reactions (eg, fulminant hepatitis, liver failure) have occurred with NSAID use, rarely; discontinue if signs or symptoms of liver disease develop, or if systemic manifestations occur.

The elderly are at increased risk for adverse effects (especially peptic ulceration, CNS effects, renal toxicity) from NSAIDs even at low doses.

Withhold for at least 4-6 half-lives prior to surgical or dental procedures.

Topical gel should not be applied to the eyes, open wounds, infected areas, or to exfoliative dermatitis. Monitor patients for 1 year following application of ophthalmic drops for corneal refractive procedures. Patients using ophthalmic drops should not wear soft contact lenses. Ophthalmic drops may slow/delay healing or prolong bleeding time following surgery.

Drug Interactions Substrate (minor) of CYP1A2, 2B6, 2C8/9, 2C19, 2D6, 3A4; **Inhibits** CYP1A2 (moderate), 2C8/9 (weak), 2E1 (weak), 3A4 (strong)

ACE inhibitors: Antihypertensive effects may be decreased by concurrent therapy with NSAIDs; monitor blood pressure

Angiotensin II antagonists: Antihypertensive effects may be decreased by concurrent therapy with NSAIDs; monitor blood pressure

Anticoagulants (warfarin, heparin, LMWHs) in combination with NSAIDs can cause increased risk of bleeding.

Other antiplatelet drugs (ticlopidine, clopidogrel, aspirin, abciximab, dipyridamole, eptifibatide, tirofiban) can cause an increased risk of bleeding.

Cholestyramine and colestipol reduce the bioavailability of diclofenac; separate administration times.

Corticosteroids may increase the risk of GI ulceration; avoid concurrent use.

Cyclosporine: NSAIDs may increase serum creatinine, potassium, blood pressure, and cyclosporine levels; monitor cyclosporine levels and renal function carefully.

CYP1A2 substrates: Diclofenac may increase the levels/effects of CYP1A2 substrates. Example substrates include aminophylline, fluvoxamine, mexiletine, mirtazapine, ropinirole, theophylline, and trifluoperazine.

CYP3A4 substrates: Diclofenac may increase the levels/effects of CYP3A4 substrates. Example substrates include benzodiazepines, calcium channel blockers, mirtazapine, nateglinide, nefazodone, tacrolimus, and venlafaxine. Selected benzodiazepines (midazolam and triazolam), cisapride, ergot alkaloids, selected HMG-CoA reductase inhibitors (lovastatin and simvastatin), and pimozide are generally contraindicated with strong CYP3A4 inhibitors.

Gentamicin and amikacin serum concentrations are increased by indomethacin in premature infants. Results may apply to other aminoglycosides and NSAIDs.

Hydralazine's antihypertensive effect is decreased; avoid concurrent use.

Lithium levels can be increased; avoid concurrent use if possible or monitor lithium levels and adjust dose. Sulindac may have the least effect. When NSAID is stopped, lithium will need adjustment again.

Loop diuretics efficacy (diuretic and antihypertensive effect) is reduced. Indomethacin reduces this efficacy, however, it may be anticipated with any NSAID.

Methotrexate: Severe bone marrow suppression, aplastic anemia, and GI toxicity have been reported with concomitant NSAID therapy. Avoid use during moderate or high-dose methotrexate (increased and prolonged methotrexate levels). NSAID use during low-dose treatment of rheumatoid arthritis has not been fully evaluated; extreme caution is warranted.

Thiazides antihypertensive effects are decreased; avoid concurrent use.

Verapamil plasma concentration is decreased by diclofenac; avoid concurrent use.

Warfarin's INRs may be increased by piroxicam. Other NSAIDs may have the same effect depending on dose and duration. Monitor INR closely. Use the lowest dose of NSAIDs possible and for the briefest duration.

Nutritional/Herbal/Ethanol Interactions

Ethanol: Avoid ethanol (may enhance gastric mucosal irritation).

Herb/Nutraceutical: Avoid alfalfa, anise, bilberry, bladderwrack, bromelain, cat's claw, celery, coleus, cordyceps, dong quai, evening primrose, feverfew, fenugreek, garlic, ginger, ginkgo biloboa, red clover, horse chestnut, grapeseed, green tea, ginseng, guggul, horse chestnut seed, horseradish, licorice, prickly ash, red clover, reishi, SAMe, sweet clover, turmeric, white willow (all have additional antiplatelet activity).

Adverse Reactions

>10%:

Local: Application site reactions (gel): Pruritus (31% to 52%), rash (35% to 46%), contact dermatitis (19% to 33%), dry skin (25% to 27%), pain (15% to 26%), exfoliation (6% to 24%), paresthesia (8% to 20%)

Ocular: Ophthalmic drops (incidence may be dependent upon indication): Lacrimation (30%), keratitis (28%), elevated IOP (15%), transient burning/stinging (15%)

1% to 10%:

Central nervous system: Headache (7%), dizziness (3%)

Dermatologic: Pruritus (1% to 3%), rash (1% to 3%)

Endocrine & metabolic: Fluid retention (1% to 3%)

Gastrointestinal: Abdominal cramps (3% to 9%), abdominal pain (3% to 9%), constipation (3% to 9%), diarrhea (3% to 9%), flatulence (3% to 9%), indigestion (3% to 9%), nausea (3% to 9%), abdominal distention (1% to 3%), peptic ulcer/GI bleed (0.6% to 2%)

Hepatic: Increased ALT/AST (2%)

Local: Application site reactions (gel): Edema (4%)

Ocular: Ophthalmic drops: Abnormal vision, acute elevated IOP, blurred vision, conjunctivitis, corneal deposits, corneal edema, corneal opacity, corneal lesions, discharge, eyelid swelling, injection, iritis, irritation, itching, lacrimation disorder, ocular allergy

Otic: Tinnitus (1% to 3%)

<1% (Limited to important or life-threatening): Oral dosage forms: Acute renal failure, agranulocytosis, allergic purpura, alopecia, anaphylactoid reactions, anaphylaxis, angioedema, aplastic anemia, aseptic meningitis, asthma, bullous eruption, cirrhosis, CHF, eosinophilia, erythema multiforme major, GI hemorrhage, hearing loss, hemolytic anemia, hepatic necrosis, hepatitis, hepatorenal syndrome, interstitial nephritis, jaundice, laryngeal edema, leukopenia, nephrotic syndrome, pancreatitis, papillary necrosis, photosensitivity, purpura, Stevens-Johnson syndrome, swelling of lips and tongue, thrombocytopenia, urticaria, visual changes, vomiting

Overdosage/Toxicology Symptoms of overdose include acute renal failure, vomiting, drowsiness, and leukocytosis. Management of NSAID intoxication is supportive and symptomatic.

Dosing

Adults & Elderly:

Analgesia/primary dysmenorrhea: Oral: Starting dose: 50 mg 3 times/day; maximum dose: 150 mg/day

Rheumatoid arthritis: Oral: 150-200 mg/day in 2-4 divided doses (100 mg/day of sustained release product)

Osteoarthritis: Oral: 100-150 mg/day in 2-3 divided doses (100-200 mg/day of sustained release product)

Ankylosing spondylitis: Oral: 100-125 mg/day in 4-5 divided doses

Cataract surgery: Ophthalmic: Instill 1 drop into affected eye 4 times/day beginning 24 hours after cataract surgery and continuing for 2 weeks

Corneal refractive surgery: Ophthalmic: Instill 1-2 drops into affected eye within the hour prior to surgery, within 15 minutes following surgery, and then continue for 4 times/day, up to 3 days

Actinic keratosis (AK): Topical (gel): Apply gel to lesion area twice daily for 60-90 days

Renal Impairment: Monitor closely in patients with significant renal impairment.

Hepatic Impairment: No adjustment necessary.

Available Dosage Forms

Gel, as sodium (Solaraze®): 30 mg/g (50 g)

Solution, ophthalmic, as sodium (Voltaren Ophthalmic®): 0.1% (2.5 mL, 5 mL)

Tablet, as potassium (Cataflam®): 50 mg

Tablet, delayed release, enteric coated, as sodium (Voltaren®): 25 mg, 50 mg, 75 mg

Tablet, extended release, as sodium (Voltaren®-XR): 100 mg

Nursing Guidelines

Assessment: Evaluate cardiac risk and potential for GI bleeding prior to prescribing this medication. Assess other medications patient may be taking for effectiveness and interactions. Monitor blood pressure at the beginning of

(Continued)

Diclofenac *(Continued)*

therapy and periodically during use. Assess results of laboratory tests, therapeutic effectiveness, and adverse reactions (systemic or ophthalmic) at beginning of therapy and periodically throughout therapy. Schedule ophthalmic evaluations for patients who develop eye complaints during long-term NSAID therapy. Assess knowledge/teach patient appropriate use (oral, ophthalmic, gel), interventions to reduce side effects, and adverse symptoms to report.

Monitoring Laboratory Tests: CBC, liver enzymes, urine output and BUN/serum creatinine in patients receiving diuretics, occult blood loss

Dietary Considerations: May be taken with food to decrease GI distress.

Diclofenac potassium = Cataflam®; potassium content: 5.8 mg (0.15 mEq) per 50 mg tablet

Patient Education: Oral: Take this medication exactly as directed; do not increase dose without consulting prescriber. Do not crush or chew tablets. Take with 8 oz of water, along with food or milk products to reduce GI distress. Maintain adequate hydration (2-3 L/day of fluids) unless instructed to restrict fluid intake. Avoid alcohol, aspirin and aspirin-containing medication, or any other anti-inflammatory medications unless consulting prescriber. You may experience dizziness, nervousness, or headache (use caution when driving or engaging in tasks requiring alertness until response to drug is known); nausea, vomiting, dry mouth, or heartburn (small frequent meals, frequent mouth care, sucking lozenges, or chewing gum may help); or constipation (increased exercise, fluids, fruit, or fiber may help). GI bleeding, ulceration, or perforation can occur with or without pain; discontinue medication and contact prescriber if persistent abdominal pain or cramping, or blood in stool occurs. Report chest pain or palpitations; breathlessness or respiratory difficulty; unusual bruising/bleeding or blood in urine, stool, mouth, or vomitus; unusual fatigue; skin rash or itching; jaundice, unusual weight gain, or swelling of extremities; change in urinary pattern; change in vision or hearing (ringing in ears). **Pregnancy/breast-feeding precautions:** Consult prescriber if you are pregnant. This drug should not be used in the 3rd trimester of pregnancy. Consult prescriber if you are breast-feeding.

Ophthalmic: For ophthalmic use only. Apply prescribed amount as often as directed. Wash hands before using. Tilt head back and look upward. Gently pull down lower lid and put drop(s) in inner corner of eye. Do not let tip of applicator touch eye; do not contaminate tip of applicator (may cause eye infection, eye damage, or vision loss). Close eye and roll eyeball in all directions. Do not blink for 1/2minute. Apply gentle pressure to inner corner of eye for 30 seconds. Wipe away excess from skin around eye. Do not use any other eye preparation for at least 10 minutes. Do not share medication with anyone else. May cause sensitivity to bright light (dark glasses may help); temporary stinging or blurred vision may occur. Inform prescriber if you experience eye pain, redness, burning, watering, dryness, double vision, puffiness around eye, vision changes, other adverse eye response, worsening of condition, or lack of improvement.

Gel: This preparation is for topical use only. Treatment may take up to 3 months. Do not use more often than recommended; use at regular intervals. Wash hands before and after use. Follow directions on prescription label. Gently apply enough of the gel to cover the lesion. Advise prescriber if you are using any other skin preparations. Avoid direct sunlight and sunlamps while using this medication. You may experience dry skin, itching, peeling, swelling, or tingling at site of application. If severe skin reaction develops, stop applications and notify your prescriber at once.

Geriatric Considerations: The elderly are at increased risk for adverse effects from NSAIDs. As many as 60% of elderly can develop peptic ulceration and/or hemorrhage asymptomatically. CNS adverse effects such as confusion, agitation, and hallucination are generally seen in overdose or high-dose situations; however, elderly patients may demonstrate these adverse effects at lower doses than younger adults. The elderly are also at increased risk of renal toxicity.

Pregnancy Risk Factor: B (topical); C (oral)/D (3rd trimester)

Pregnancy Issues: Safety and efficacy in pregnant women have not been established. Exposure late in pregnancy may lead to premature closure of the ductus arteriosus and may inhibit uterine contractions.

Lactation: Excretion in breast milk unknown/not recommended

Perioperative/Anesthesia/Other Concerns: The 2002 ACCM/SCCM guidelines for analgesia (critically-ill adult) suggest that NSAIDs may be used in combination with opioids in select patients for pain management. Concern about adverse events (increased risk of renal dysfunction, altered platelet function and gastrointestinal irritation) limits its use in patients who have other underlying risks for these events.

In short-term use, NSAIDs vary considerably in their effect on blood pressure. When NSAIDs are used in patients with hypertension, appropriate monitoring of blood pressure responses should be completed and the duration of therapy, when possible, kept short. The use of NSAIDs in the treatment of patients with congestive heart failure may be associated with an increased risk for fluid accumulation and edema; may precipitate renal failure in dehydrated patients.

Administration

Oral: Do not crush tablets. Administer with food or milk to avoid gastric distress. Take with full glass of water to enhance absorption.

Storage: Store above 30°C (86°F); protect from moisture, store in tight container.

- **Diclofenac Potassium** *see* Diclofenac *on page 521*
- **Diclofenac Sodium** *see* Diclofenac *on page 521*

Dicloxacillin (dye kloks a SIL in)

Synonyms Dicloxacillin Sodium

Pharmacologic Category Antibiotic, Penicillin

Use Treatment of systemic infections such as pneumonia, skin and soft tissue infections, and osteomyelitis caused by penicillinase-producing staphylococci

Mechanism of Action Inhibits bacterial cell wall synthesis by binding to one or more of the penicillin binding proteins (PBPs); which in turn inhibits the final transpeptidation step of peptidoglycan synthesis in bacterial cell walls, thus inhibiting cell wall biosynthesis. Bacteria eventually lyse due to ongoing activity of cell wall autolytic enzymes (autolysins and murein hydrolases) while cell wall assembly is arrested.

Pharmacodynamics/Kinetics

Absorption: 35% to 76%; rate and extent reduced by food

Distribution: Throughout body with highest concentrations in kidney and liver; CSF penetration is low; crosses placenta; enters breast milk

Protein binding: 96%

Half-life elimination: 0.6-0.8 hour; slightly prolonged with renal impairment

Time to peak, serum: 0.5-2 hours

Excretion: Feces; urine (56% to 70% as unchanged drug); prolonged in neonates

Contraindications Hypersensitivity to dicloxacillin, penicillin, or any component of the formulation

Warnings/Precautions Monitor PT if patient concurrently on warfarin; elimination of drug is slow in neonates; use with caution in patients allergic to cephalosporins

Drug Interactions Induces CYP3A4 (weak)

Methotrexate: Penicillins may increase the exposure to methotrexate during concurrent therapy; monitor.

Oral contraceptives: Anecdotal reports suggesting decreased contraceptive efficacy with penicillins have been refuted by more rigorous scientific and clinical data.

Probenecid, disulfiram: May increase levels of penicillins (dicloxacillin)

Warfarin: Concurrent use may decrease effect of warfarin

Nutritional/Herbal/Ethanol Interactions Food: Decreases drug absorption rate; decreases drug serum concentration.

Lab Interactions Positive Coombs' test [direct]

Adverse Reactions

1% to 10%: Gastrointestinal: Nausea, diarrhea, abdominal pain

<1% (Limited to important or life-threatening): Agranulocytosis, eosinophilia, hemolytic anemia, hepatotoxicity, hypersensitivity, interstitial nephritis, leukopenia, neutropenia, prolonged PT, pseudomembranous colitis, rash (maculopapular to exfoliative), seizure with extremely high doses and/or renal failure, serum sickness-like reactions, thrombocytopenia, vaginitis, vomiting

Overdosage/Toxicology Symptoms of penicillin overdose include neuromuscular hypersensitivity (eg, agitation, hallucinations, asterixis, encephalopathy, confusion, and seizures). Electrolyte imbalance may occur if the preparation contains potassium or sodium salts, especially in renal failure. Hemodialysis may be helpful to aid in removal of the drug from blood; otherwise, treatment is supportive or symptom-directed.

(Continued)

Dicloxacillin *(Continued)*

Dosing

Adults & Elderly: Susceptible infections: Oral: 125-500 mg every 6 hours

Pediatrics: Use in newborns is not recommended.

Susceptible infections: Oral:

Children <40 kg: 12.5-25 mg/kg/day divided every 6 hours; doses of 50-100 mg/kg/day in divided doses every 6 hours have been used for therapy of osteomyelitis

Children >40 kg: 125-250 mg every 6 hours

Renal Impairment:

Dosage adjustment is not necessary.

Not dialyzable (0% to 5%); supplemental dose is not necessary.

Peritoneal dialysis effects: Supplemental dose is not necessary.

Continuous arteriovenous or venovenous hemofiltration: Supplemental dose is not necessary.

Available Dosage Forms Capsule: 250 mg, 500 mg

Nursing Guidelines

Assessment: Assess allergy history prior to beginning therapy. See Contraindications and Warnings/Precautions for use cautions. Assess potential for interactions with other prescriptions, OTC medications, or herbal products patient may be taking (see Drug Interactions). Assess results of laboratory tests (see below), therapeutic effectiveness, and adverse reactions (see Adverse Reactions and Overdose/Toxicology) on a regular basis throughout therapy. Teach patient proper use, possible side effects/appropriate interventions, and adverse symptoms to report (see Patient Education). Note breast-feeding caution.

Monitoring Laboratory Tests: Perform culture and sensitivity studies prior to initiating therapy.

Dietary Considerations: Administer on an empty stomach 1 hour before or 2 hours after meals. Sodium content of 250 mg capsule: 13 mg (0.6 mEq)

Patient Education: Inform prescriber of all prescriptions, OTC medications, or herbal products you are taking, and any allergies you have. Do not take any new medication during therapy unless approved by prescriber. Take medication as directed, with a large glass of water 1 hour before or 2 hours after meals. Take at regular intervals around-the-clock and take for length of time prescribed. If you have diabetes, drug may cause false test results with Clinitest® urine glucose monitoring; use of another type of glucose monitoring is preferable. May cause some gastric distress (small, frequent meals may help) and diarrhea (if this persists, consult prescriber). Report fever, vaginal itching, sores in the mouth, loose foul-smelling stools, yellowing of skin or eyes, or change in color of urine or stool. **Breast-feeding precaution:** Consult prescriber if breast-feeding.

Pregnancy Risk Factor: B

Lactation: Excretion in breast milk unknown (probably similar to penicillin G)

Breast-Feeding Considerations: No data reported; however, other penicillins may be taken while breast-feeding.

Administration

Oral: Administer 1 hour before or 2 hours after meals. Administer around-the-clock to promote less variation in peak and trough serum levels.

♦ **Dicloxacillin Sodium** *see* Dicloxacillin *on page 525*

Dicyclomine (dye SYE kloe meen)

U.S. Brand Names Bentyl®

Synonyms Dicyclomine Hydrochloride; Dicycloverine Hydrochloride

Pharmacologic Category Anticholinergic Agent

Medication Safety Issues

Sound-alike/look-alike issues:

Dicyclomine may be confused with diphenhydrAMINE, doxycycline, dyclonine

Bentyl® may be confused with Aventyl®, Benadryl®, Bontril®, Cantil®, Proventil®, Trental®

Use Treatment of functional disturbances of GI motility such as irritable bowel syndrome

Unlabeled/Investigational Use Urinary incontinence

Mechanism of Action Blocks the action of acetylcholine at parasympathetic sites in smooth muscle, secretory glands and the CNS

Pharmacodynamics/Kinetics

Onset of action: 1-2 hours

Duration: ≤4 hours
Absorption: Oral: Well absorbed
Metabolism: Extensive
Half-life elimination: Initial: 1.8 hours; Terminal: 9-10 hours
Excretion: Urine (small amounts as unchanged drug)

Contraindications Hypersensitivity to any anticholinergic drug; narrow-angle glaucoma; myasthenia gravis; should not be used in infants <6 months of age

Warnings/Precautions Use with caution in patients with hepatic or renal disease, ulcerative colitis, hyperthyroidism, cardiovascular disease, hypertension, tachycardia, GI obstruction, obstruction of the urinary tract. The elderly are at increased risk for anticholinergic effects, confusion and hallucinations.

Drug Interactions

Decreased effect: Phenothiazines, anti-Parkinson's drugs, haloperidol, sustained release dosage forms; decreased effect with antacids

Increased toxicity: Anticholinergics, amantadine, narcotic analgesics, type I antiarrhythmics, antihistamines, phenothiazines, TCAs

Nutritional/Herbal/Ethanol Interactions Ethanol: Avoid ethanol (may increase CNS depression).

Adverse Reactions Adverse reactions are included here that have been reported for pharmacologically similar drugs with anticholinergic/antispasmodic action

Cardiovascular: Syncope, tachycardia, palpitation

Central nervous system: Dizziness, lightheadedness, tingling, headache, drowsiness, nervousness, numbness, mental confusion and/or excitement, dyskinesia, lethargy, speech disturbance, insomnia

Dermatologic: Rash, urticaria, itching, and other dermal manifestations; severe allergic reaction or drug idiosyncrasies including anaphylaxis

Endocrine & metabolic: Suppression of lactation

Gastrointestinal: Xerostomia, nausea, vomiting, constipation, bloated feeling, abdominal pain, taste loss, anorexia

Genitourinary: Urinary hesitancy, urinary retention, impotence

Neuromuscular & skeletal: Weakness

Ocular: Blurred vision, diplopia, mydriasis, cycloplegia, increased ocular tension

Respiratory: Dyspnea, apnea, asphyxia, nasal stuffiness or congestion, sneezing, throat congestion

Miscellaneous: Decreased diaphoresis

Overdosage/Toxicology Symptoms of overdose include CNS stimulation followed by depression, confusion, delusions, nonreactive pupils, tachycardia, and hypertension. Unilateral numbness, cold fingertips, abdominal and flank pain have also been described as symptoms of toxicity.

Dosing

Adults: Gastrointestinal motility disorders/irritable bowel:

Oral: Begin with 80 mg/day in 4 equally divided doses, then increase up to 160 mg/day

I.M. **(should not be used I.V.)**: 80 mg/day in 4 divided doses (20 mg/dose)

Elderly: 10-20 mg 4 times/day; increasing as necessary to 160 mg/day

Pediatrics: Oral:

Infants >6 months: 5 mg/dose 3-4 times/day
Children: 10 mg/dose 3-4 times/day

Available Dosage Forms

Capsule, as hydrochloride: 10 mg
Injection, solution, as hydrochloride: 10 mg/mL (2 mL)
Syrup, as hydrochloride: 10 mg/5 mL (480 mL)
Tablet, as hydrochloride: 20 mg

Nursing Guidelines

Assessment: See Contraindications and Warnings/Precautions for use cautions. Assess potential for interactions with other prescriptions, OTC medications, or herbal products patient may be taking (see Drug Interactions). Assess effectiveness of therapy and adverse response (see Adverse Reactions and Overdose/Toxicology - eg, anticholinergic response). Teach patient proper use, possible side effects/appropriate interventions, and adverse symptoms to report (see Patient Education). Breast-feeding is contraindicated.

Patient Education: Inform prescriber of all prescriptions, OTC medications, or herbal products you are taking, and any allergies you have. Do not take any new medication during therapy unless approved by prescriber (especially antihistamines, sleeping aids, or antidepressants). Take as directed before meals; do not increase dose and do not discontinue without consulting prescriber. Avoid alcohol. Void before taking medication. This drug may impair mental

(Continued)

Dicyclomine *(Continued)*

alertness (use caution when driving or engaging in tasks that require alertness until response to drug is known); or constipation (increased exercise, fluids, fruit, or fiber may help). Report excessive and persistent anticholinergic effects (blurred vision, headache, flushing, tachycardia, nervousness, dizziness, insomnia, mental confusion or excitement, dry mouth, altered taste perception, dysphagia, palpitations, bradycardia, urinary hesitancy or retention, impotence, decreased sweating); change in color of urine or stools; or irritation or redness at injection site. **Breast-feeding precaution:** Do not breast-feed.

Geriatric Considerations: Long-term use of antispasmodics should be avoided in the elderly. The potential for a toxic reaction is greater than the potential benefit. In addition, the anticholinergic effects of dicyclomine are not well tolerated in the elderly.

Pregnancy Risk Factor: B

Lactation: Enters breast milk/contraindicated

Administration

Oral: Administer 30-60 minutes before a meal.

I.M.: Administer as I.M. injection only.

I.V.: Do not administer I.V.

Storage: Protect from light.

♦ **Dicyclomine Hydrochloride** *see* Dicyclomine *on page 526*
♦ **Dicycloverine Hydrochloride** *see* Dicyclomine *on page 526*
♦ **Di-Dak-Sol** *see* Sodium Hypochlorite Solution *on page 1549*

Didanosine (dye DAN oh seen)

U.S. Brand Names Videx®; Videx® EC

Synonyms ddI; Dideoxyinosine

Pharmacologic Category Antiretroviral Agent, Reverse Transcriptase Inhibitor (Nucleoside)

Medication Safety Issues

Sound-alike/look-alike issues:
Videx® may be confused with Lidex®

Use Treatment of HIV infection; always to be used in combination with at least two other antiretroviral agents

Mechanism of Action Didanosine, a purine nucleoside (adenosine) analog and the deamination product of dideoxyadenosine (ddA), inhibits HIV replication *in vitro* in both T cells and monocytes. Didanosine is converted within the cell to the mono-, di-, and triphosphates of ddA. These ddA triphosphates act as substrate and inhibitor of HIV reverse transcriptase substrate and inhibitor of HIV reverse transcriptase thereby blocking viral DNA synthesis and suppressing HIV replication.

Pharmacodynamics/Kinetics

Absorption: Subject to degradation by acidic pH of stomach; some formulations are buffered to resist acidic pH; ≤50% reduction in peak plasma concentration is observed in presence of food. Delayed release capsules contain enteric-coated beadlets which dissolve in the small intestine.

Distribution: V_d: Children: 35.6 L/m²; Adults: 1.08 L/kg

Protein binding: <5%

Metabolism: Has not been evaluated in humans; studies conducted in dogs show extensive metabolism with allantoin, hypoxanthine, xanthine, and uric acid being the major metabolites found in urine

Bioavailability: 42%

Half-life elimination:

Children and Adolescents: 0.8 hour

Adults: Normal renal function: 1.5 hours; active metabolite, ddATP, has an intracellular half-life >12 hours *in vitro*; Renal impairment: 2.5-5 hours

Time to peak: Buffered tablets: 0.67 hours; Delayed release capsules: 2 hours

Excretion: Urine (~55% as unchanged drug)

Clearance: Total body: Averages 800 mL/minute

Contraindications Hypersensitivity to didanosine or any component of the formulation

Warnings/Precautions Pancreatitis (sometimes fatal) has been reported, incidence is dose related. Risk factors for developing pancreatitis include a previous history of the condition, concurrent cytomegalovirus or *Mycobacterium avium-intracellulare* infection, and concomitant use of stavudine, pentamidine, or co-trimoxazole. Discontinue didanosine if clinical signs of pancreatitis occur.

Lactic acidosis, symptomatic hyperlactatemia, and severe hepatomegaly with steatosis (sometimes fatal) have occurred with antiretroviral nucleoside analogues, including didanosine. Hepatotoxicity may occur even in the absence of marked transaminase elevations; suspend therapy in any patient developing clinical/laboratory findings which suggest hepatotoxicity. Pregnant women may be at increased risk of lactic acidosis and liver damage.

Peripheral neuropathy occurs in ~20% of patients receiving the drug. Retinal changes (including retinal depigmentation) and optic neuritis have been reported in adults and children using didanosine. Patients should undergo retinal examination every 6-12 months. Use with caution in patients with decreased renal or hepatic function, phenylketonuria, sodium-restricted diets, or with edema, CHF, or hyperuricemia. Twice-daily dosing is the preferred dosing frequency for didanosine tablets. Didanosine delayed release capsules are indicated for once-daily use.

Drug Interactions Drugs whose absorption depends on the level of acidity in the stomach (such as ketoconazole, itraconazole, and dapsone) should be administered at least 2 hours prior to the buffered formulations of didanosine (not affected by delayed release capsules)

Decreased effect: Buffered formulations of didanosine (tablets, pediatric oral solution) may decrease absorption of quinolones or tetracyclines, separate dosing by 2 hours; didanosine should be held during PCP treatment with pentamidine; didanosine may decrease levels of indinavir

Increased toxicity: Concomitant administration of other drugs (including hydroxyurea) which have the potential to cause peripheral neuropathy or pancreatitis may increase the risk of these toxicities

Allopurinol: May increase didanosine concentration; avoid concurrent use

Antacids: Concomitant use with buffered tablet or pediatric didanosine solution may potentiate adverse effects of aluminum- or magnesium-containing antacids

Ganciclovir: May increase didanosine concentration; monitor

Hydroxyurea: May precipitate didanosine-induced pancreatitis if added to therapy; concomitant use is not recommended

Methadone: May decrease didanosine concentration; monitor

Ribavirin: Coadministration may increase exposure to didanosine and/or its active metabolite, increasing the risk or severity of didanosine toxicities, including pancreatitis, lactic acidosis, and peripheral neuropathy. Coadministration of ribavirin with didanosine should be undertaken with caution, and patients should be monitored closely for didanosine-related toxicities; suspend therapy if signs or symptoms of toxicity are noted.

Tenofovir: Coadministration may increase exposure to didanosine and/or its active metabolite increasing the risk or severity of didanosine toxicities, including pancreatitis, hyperglycemia, lactic acidosis, and peripheral neuropathy. Some patients have experienced reduced CD4 cell counts and/or decreased virologic response. Coadministration of tenofovir with didanosine should be undertaken with caution, and patients should be monitored closely for didanosine-related toxicities; specific dosing adjustment is recommended; suspend therapy if signs or symptoms of toxicity are noted.

Nutritional/Herbal/Ethanol Interactions

Ethanol: Avoid ethanol (increases risk of pancreatitis).

Food: Decreases AUC and C_{max}. Didanosine serum levels may be decreased by 55% if taken with food.

Adverse Reactions As reported in monotherapy studies; risk of toxicity may increase when combined with other agent.

>10%:

Gastrointestinal: Increased amylase (15% to 17%), abdominal pain (7% to 13%), diarrhea (19% to 28%)

Neuromuscular & skeletal: Peripheral neuropathy (17% to 20%)

1% to 10%:

Dermatologic: Rash, pruritus

Endocrine & metabolic: Increased uric acid

Gastrointestinal: Pancreatitis; patients >65 years of age had a higher frequency of pancreatitis than younger patients

Hepatic: Increased SGOT, increased SGPT, increased alkaline phosphatase

Postmarketing and/or case reports: Alopecia, anaphylactoid reaction, anemia, anorexia, arthralgia, diabetes mellitus, granulocytopenia, hepatitis, hyperlactatemia (symptomatic), hypersensitivity, lactic acidosis/hepatomegaly, leukopenia, liver failure, myalgia, myopathy, neuritis, optic renal impairment,

(Continued)

Didanosine *(Continued)*

pain, retinal depigmentation, rhabdomyolysis, seizure, thrombocytopenia, weakness

Overdosage/Toxicology Chronic overdose may cause pancreatitis, peripheral neuropathy, diarrhea, hyperuricemia, and hepatic impairment. There is no known antidote for didanosine overdose. Treatment is symptomatic.

Dosing

Adults: Treatment of HIV infection: Oral (administer on an empty stomach): Oral:

Note: Preferred dosing frequency is twice daily for didanosine tablets

Chewable tablets, powder for oral solution:

<60 kg: 125 mg twice daily or 250 mg once daily

≥60 kg: 200 mg twice daily or 400 mg once daily

Note: Adults should receive 2-4 tablets per dose for adequate buffering and absorption; tablets should be chewed or dispersed (in 1 ounce of water).

Delayed release capsule (Videx® EC):

<60 kg: 250 mg once daily

≥60 kg; 400 mg once daily

Dosing adjustment with tenofovir (didanosine tablets or delayed release capsules; based on tenofovir product labeling):

<60 kg: 200 mg once daily

≥60 kg: 250 mg once daily

Elderly: Refer to adult dosing. Elderly patients have a higher frequency of pancreatitis (10% versus 5% in younger patients); monitor renal function and dose accordingly.

Pediatrics:

Treatment of HIV infection: Oral (administer on an empty stomach):

Children:

2 weeks to 8 months: 100 mg/m² twice daily is recommended by the manufacturer; 50 mg/m² may be considered in infants 2 weeks to 4 months

>8 months: 120 mg/m² twice daily; dosing range: 90-150 mg/m² twice daily; patients with CNS disease may require higher dose

Note: At least 2 tablets per dose should be administered for adequate buffering and absorption; tablets should be chewed or dispersed (in 1 ounce of water).

Adolescents: Refer to adult dosing.

Renal Impairment: See table.

Recommended Dose (mg) of Didanosine by Body Weight

Creatinine Clearance (mL/min)	≥60 kg		<60 kg	
	Tablet[1] (mg)	Delayed Release Capsule (mg)	Tablet[1] (mg)	Delayed Release Capsule (mg)
≥60	400 daily or 200 twice daily	400 daily	250 daily or 125 twice daily	250 daily
30-59	200 daily or 100 twice daily	200 daily	150 daily or 75 twice daily	125 daily
10-29	150 daily	125 daily	100 daily	125 daily
<10	100 daily	125 daily	75 daily	See footnote 2.

[1]Chewable/dispersible buffered tablet; 2 tablets must be taken with each dose; different strengths of tablets may be combined to yield the recommended dose.

[2]Not suitable for use in patients <60 kg with Cl_{cr} <10 mL/minute; use alternate formulation.

Patients requiring hemodialysis or CAPD: Dose per Cl_{cr} 10 mL/minute

Hepatic Impairment: Should be considered; monitor for toxicity.

Available Dosage Forms

Capsule, delayed release: 200 mg, 250 mg, 400 mg

Videx® EC: 125 mg, 200 mg, 250 mg, 400 mg

Powder for oral solution, pediatric (Videx®): 2 g, 4 g [makes 10 mg/mL solution after final mixing]

Tablet, buffered, chewable/dispersible (Videx®): 25 mg, 50 mg, 100 mg, 150 mg, 200 mg [all strengths contain phenylalanine 36.5 mg/tablet; orange flavor]

Nursing Guidelines

Assessment: See Contraindications, Warnings/Precautions, and Dosing for use cautions. Assess potential for interactions with other prescriptions, OTC medications, or herbal products patient may be taking (see Drug Interactions).

Assess results of laboratory tests (see below), therapeutic response, and adverse reactions (eg, peripheral neuropathy, CNS changes, pancreatitis, opportunistic infection - see Adverse Reactions and Overdose/Toxicology) on a regular basis throughout therapy. Teach patient proper use (see Administration, Storage, and Reconstitution), possible side effects/appropriate interventions, and adverse symptoms to report (see Patient Education). Breast-feeding is contraindicated.

Monitoring Laboratory Tests: Serum potassium, uric acid, creatinine, hemoglobin, CBC with neutrophil, platelet count, CD4 cells, liver function, amylase; viral load

Dietary Considerations:

Videx® EC: Take on an empty stomach; administer at least 1 hour before or 2 hours after eating

Chewable/dispersible tablet: Take on an empty stomach, 30 minutes before or 2 hours after eating. Chew well or mix in water; if mixed in water, may add 2 tablespoons (1 oz) apple juice for flavor. Do not use other juices. Each chewable tablet contains 36.5 mg phenylalanine and 8.6 mEq magnesium. Sodium content of buffered tablets: 264.5 mg (11.5 mEq).

Patient Education: Inform prescriber of all prescriptions, OTC medications, or herbal products you are taking, and any allergies you have. Do not take any new medication during therapy unless approved by prescriber. This drug will not cure HIV; use appropriate precautions to prevent spread of HIV to other persons. Take as directed, 1 hour before or 2 hours after meals. Avoid alcohol. Chew tablets thoroughly. Maintain adequate hydration (2-3 L/day of fluids) unless instructed to restrict fluid intake. A dilated retinal eye exam is recommended every 6-12 months while on this therapy. You may be susceptible to infection (avoid crowds and exposure to infection and do not have any vaccinations without consulting prescriber). May cause dizziness or weakness (use caution when driving or engaging in tasks requiring alertness until response to drug is known); nausea or vomiting (small, frequent meals, frequent mouth care, chewing gum, or sucking lozenges may help); diarrhea (boiled milk, yogurt, or buttermilk may help); or headache, back or joint pain (mild analgesics may offer relief). Report immediately any loss of sensation, numbness, or tingling in fingers, toes, or feet; persistent unresolved abdominal distress (nausea, vomiting, diarrhea); or signs of infection (burning on urination, perineal itching, white plaques in mouth, unhealed sores, persistent sore throat or cough). **Pregnancy/breast-feeding precautions:** Inform prescriber if you are or intend to become pregnant. Do not breast-feed.

Geriatric Considerations: Since the elderly often have a creatinine clearance <60 mL/minute, monitor closely for adverse reactions and adjust dose accordingly to maintain efficacy (CD4 counts).

Pregnancy Risk Factor: B

Pregnancy Issues: Cases of fatal and nonfatal lactic acidosis, with or without pancreatitis, have been reported in pregnant women. It is not known if pregnancy itself potentiates this known side effect; however, pregnant women may be at increased risk of lactic acidosis and liver damage. Hepatic enzymes and electrolytes should be monitored frequently during the 3rd trimester of pregnancy. Use during pregnancy only if the potential benefit to the mother outweighs the potential risk of this complication. Didanosine has been shown to cross the placenta. Pharmacokinetics are not significantly altered during pregnancy; dose adjustments are not needed. The Perinatal HIV Guidelines Working Group considers didanosine to be an alternative NRTI in dual nucleoside combination regimens; use with stavudine only if no other alternatives are available. Health professionals are encouraged to contact the antiretroviral pregnancy registry to monitor outcomes of pregnant women exposed to antiretroviral medications (1-800-258-4263 or www.APRegistry.com).

Lactation: Excretion in breast milk unknown/contraindicated

Breast-Feeding Considerations: HIV-infected mothers are discouraged from breast-feeding to decrease potential transmission of HIV.

Administration

Oral:

Chewable/dispersible buffered tablets: The 200 mg tablet should only be used in once-daily dosing. At least 2 tablets, but no more than 4 tablets, should be taken together to allow adequate buffering. Tablets may be chewed or dispersed prior to consumption. To disperse, dissolve in 1 oz water, stir until uniform dispersion is formed, and drink immediately. May also add 1 oz of

(Continued)

Didanosine *(Continued)*

clear apple juice to initial dispersion if additional flavor is needed. The apple juice dilution is stable for 1 hour at room temperature.

Pediatric powder for oral solution: Prior to dispensing, the powder should be mixed with purified water USP to an initial concentration of 20 mg/mL and then further diluted with an appropriate antacid suspension to a final mixture of 10 mg/mL. Stable for 30 days under refrigeration. Shake well prior to use.

Reconstitution: Unbuffered powder for oral solution must be reconstituted and mixed with an equal volume of antacid at time of preparation.

Storage: Tablets and delayed release capsules should be stored in tightly closed bottles at 15°C to 30°C. Undergoes rapid degradation when exposed to an acidic environment. Tablets dispersed in water are stable for 1 hour at room temperature. Reconstituted pediatric solution is stable for 30 days if refrigerated.

- ♦ **Dideoxyinosine** *see* Didanosine *on page 528*
- ♦ **Diflucan®** *see* Fluconazole *on page 734*
- ♦ **Digitek®** *see* Digoxin *on page 532*

Digoxin (di JOKS in)

U.S. Brand Names Digitek®; Lanoxicaps®; Lanoxin®

Pharmacologic Category Antiarrhythmic Agent, Class IV; Cardiac Glycoside

Medication Safety Issues

Sound-alike/look-alike issues:

Digoxin may be confused with Desoxyn®, doxepin

Lanoxin® may be confused with Lasix®, Levoxyl®, Levsinex®, Lomotil®, Lonox®, Mefoxin®, Xanax®

Use Treatment of congestive heart failure and to slow the ventricular rate in tachyarrhythmias such as atrial fibrillation, atrial flutter, and supraventricular tachycardia (paroxysmal atrial tachycardia); cardiogenic shock

Mechanism of Action

Congestive heart failure: Inhibition of the sodium/potassium ATPase pump which acts to increase the intracellular sodium-calcium exchange to increase intracellular calcium leading to increased contractility

Supraventricular arrhythmias: Direct suppression of the AV node conduction to increase effective refractory period and decrease conduction velocity - positive inotropic effect, enhanced vagal tone, and decreased ventricular rate to fast atrial arrhythmias. Atrial fibrillation may decrease sensitivity and increase tolerance to higher serum digoxin concentrations.

Pharmacodynamics/Kinetics

Onset of action: Oral: 1-2 hours; I.V.: 5-30 minutes

Peak effect: Oral: 2-8 hours; I.V.: 1-4 hours

Duration: Adults: 3-4 days both forms

Absorption: By passive nonsaturable diffusion in the upper small intestine; food may delay, but does not affect extent of absorption

Distribution:

Normal renal function: 6-7 L/kg

V_d: Extensive to peripheral tissues, with a distinct distribution phase which lasts 6-8 hours; concentrates in heart, liver, kidney, skeletal muscle, and intestines. Heart/serum concentration is 70:1. Pharmacologic effects are delayed and do not correlate well with serum concentrations during distribution phase.

Hyperthyroidism: Increased V_d

Hyperkalemia, hyponatremia: Decreased digoxin distribution to heart and muscle

Hypokalemia: Increased digoxin distribution to heart and muscles

Concomitant quinidine therapy: Decreased V_d

Chronic renal failure: 4-6 L/kg

Decreased sodium/potassium ATPase activity - decreased tissue binding

Neonates, full-term: 7.5-10 L/kg

Children: 16 L/kg

Adults: 7 L/kg, decreased with renal disease

Protein binding: 30%; in uremic patients, digoxin is displaced from plasma protein binding sites

Metabolism: Via sequential sugar hydrolysis in the stomach or by reduction of lactone ring by intestinal bacteria (in ~10% of population, gut bacteria may metabolize up to 40% of digoxin dose); metabolites may contribute to therapeutic and toxic effects of digoxin; metabolism is reduced with CHF

Bioavailability: Oral (formulation dependent): Elixir: 75% to 85%; Tablet: 70% to 80%

Half-life elimination (age, renal and cardiac function dependent):

Neonates: Premature: 61-170 hours; Full-term: 35-45 hours

Infants: 18-25 hours

Children: 35 hours

Adults: 38-48 hours

Adults, anephric: 4-6 days

Half-life elimination: Parent drug: 38 hours; Metabolites: Digoxigenin: 4 hours; Monodigitoxoside: 3-12 hours

Time to peak, serum: Oral: ~1 hour

Excretion: Urine (50% to 70% as unchanged drug)

Contraindications Hypersensitivity to digoxin or any component of the formulation; hypersensitivity to cardiac glycosides (another may be tried); history of toxicity; ventricular tachycardia or fibrillation; idiopathic hypertrophic subaortic stenosis; constrictive pericarditis; amyloid disease; second- or third-degree heart block (except in patients with a functioning artificial pacemaker); Wolff-Parkinson-White syndrome and atrial fibrillation concurrently

Warnings/Precautions Withdrawal in CHF patients may lead to recurrence of CHF symptoms. Some arrhythmias that digoxin is used to treat may be exacerbated in digoxin toxicity. Sinus nodal disease may be worsened. Adjust doses in renal impairment and when verapamil, quinidine or amiodarone are added to a patient on digoxin. Correct hypokalemia and hypomagnesemia before initiating therapy. Calcium, especially when administered rapidly I.V., can produce serious arrhythmias. Atrial arrhythmias associated with hypermetabolic states are very difficult to treat. Rate control in atrial fibrillation may be better in a sedentary patient than an active one. Use with caution in acute MI (within 6 months). Serum concentration monitoring should be done before the next dose (patient can hold AM dose for blood test) for an accurate assessment. Reduce or hold dose 1-2 days before elective electrical cardioversion.

Drug Interactions Substrate of CYP3A4 (minor)

Amiloride may reduce the inotropic response to digoxin.

Amiodarone reduces renal and nonrenal clearance of digoxin and may have additive effects on heart rate. Reduce digoxin dose by 50% with start of amiodarone.

Benzodiazepines (alprazolam, diazepam) have been associated with isolated reports of digoxin toxicity.

Beta-blocking agents (propranolol) may have additive effects on heart rate.

Calcium preparations: Rare cases of acute digoxin toxicity have been associated with parenteral calcium (bolus) administration.

Carvedilol may increase digoxin blood levels in addition to potentiating its effects on heart rate.

Cholestyramine, colestipol, kaolin-pectin may reduce digoxin absorption. Separate administration.

Cyclosporine may increase digoxin levels, possibly due to reduced renal clearance.

Erythromycin, clarithromycin, and tetracyclines may increase digoxin (not capsule form) blood levels in a subset of patients.

Indomethacin has been associated with isolated reports of increased digoxin blood levels/toxicity.

Itraconazole may increase digoxin blood levels in some patients; monitor.

Levothyroxine (and other thyroid supplements) may decrease digoxin blood levels.

Metoclopramide may reduce the absorption of digoxin tablets.

Moricizine may increase the toxicity of digoxin (mechanism undefined).

Penicillamine has been associated with reductions in digoxin blood levels

Propafenone increases digoxin blood levels. Effects are highly variable; monitor closely.

Propylthiouracil (and methimazole) may increase digoxin blood levels by reducing thyroid hormone.

Quinidine increases digoxin blood levels substantially. Effect is variable (33% to 50%). Monitor digoxin blood levels/effect closely. Reduce digoxin dose by 50% with start of quinidine. Other related agents (hydroxychloroquine, quinine) should be used with caution.

Spironolactone may interfere with some digoxin assays, but may also increase blood levels directly. However, spironolactone may attenuate the inotropic effect of digoxin. Monitor effects of digoxin closely.

(Continued)

Digoxin *(Continued)*

Succinylcholine administration to patients on digoxin has been associated with an increased risk of arrhythmias.

Verapamil diltiazem, bepridil, and nitrendipine increased serum digoxin concentrations. Other calcium channel blocking agents do not appear to share this effect. Reduce digoxin's dose with the start of verapamil.

Drugs which cause hypokalemia (thiazide and loop diuretics, amphotericin B): Hypokalemia may potentiate digoxin toxicity.

These medications have been associated with reduced digoxin blood levels which appear to be of limited clinical significance: Aminoglutethimide, aminosalicylic acid, aluminum-containing antacids, sucralfate, sulfasalazine, neomycin, ticlopidine.

These medications have been associated with increased digoxin blood levels which appear to be of limited clinical significance: Famciclovir, flecainide, ibuprofen, fluoxetine, nefazodone, cimetidine, famotidine, ranitidine, omeprazole, trimethoprim.

Nutritional/Herbal/Ethanol Interactions

Food: Digoxin peak serum levels may be decreased if taken with food. Meals containing increased fiber (bran) or foods high in pectin may decrease oral absorption of digoxin.

Herb/Nutraceutical: Avoid ephedra (risk of cardiac stimulation). Avoid natural licorice (causes sodium and water retention and increases potassium loss).

Adverse Reactions Incidence of reactions are not always reported.

Cardiovascular: Heart block; first-, second- (Wenckebach), or third-degree heart block; asystole; atrial tachycardia with block; AV dissociation; accelerated junctional rhythm; ventricular tachycardia or ventricular fibrillation; PR prolongation; ST segment depression

Central nervous system: Visual disturbances (blurred or yellow vision), headache (3.2%), dizziness (4.9%), apathy, confusion, mental disturbances (4.1%), anxiety, depression, delirium, hallucinations, fever

Dermatologic: Maculopapular rash (1.6%); erythematous, scarlatiniform, papular, vesicular, or bullous rash; urticaria; pruritus; facial, angioneurotic, or laryngeal edema; shedding of fingernails or toenails; alopecia

Gastrointestinal: Nausea (3.2%), vomiting (1.6%), diarrhea (3.2%), abdominal pain

Neuromuscular & skeletal: Weakness

<1% (Limited to important or life-threatening): Abdominal pain, anorexia, eosinophilia, gynecomastia, hemorrhagic necrosis of the intestines, increased plasma estrogen and decreased serum luteinizing hormone in men and postmenopausal women and decreased plasma testosterone in men, intestinal ischemia, palpitation, sexual dysfunction, thrombocytopenia, unifocal or multiform ventricular premature contractions (especially bigeminy or trigeminy), vaginal cornification

Any arrhythmia seen in a child on digoxin should be considered as digoxin toxicity. The gastrointestinal and central nervous system symptoms are not frequently seen in children.

Overdosage/Toxicology Manifested by a wide variety of signs and symptoms difficult to distinguish from effects associated with cardiac disease. Nausea and vomiting are common early signs of toxicity and may precede or follow evidence of cardiotoxicity. Other symptoms include anorexia, diarrhea, abdominal discomfort, headache, weakness, drowsiness, visual disturbances, mental depression, confusion, restlessness, disorientation, seizures, and hallucinations. Cardiac abnormalities include ventricular tachycardia, unifocal or multifocal PVCs (bigeminal, trigeminal), paroxysmal nodal rhythms, AV dissociation, excessive slowing of the pulse, AV block of varying degree, P-R prolongation, S-T depression, and occasional atrial fibrillation. Ventricular fibrillation is a common cause of death (alterations in cardiac rate and rhythm can result in any type of known arrhythmia).

Antidote: Life-threatening digoxin toxicity is treated with Digibind®. Administer potassium except in cases of complete heart block or renal failure. Digitalis-induced arrhythmias not responsive to potassium may be treated with phenytoin or lidocaine. Cholestyramine and colestipol may decrease absorption. Other agents to consider, based on ECG and clinical assessment, include atropine, quinidine, procainamide, and propranolol. **Note:** Other antiarrhythmics appear more dangerous to use in toxicity.

Dosing

Adults:

Note: When changing from oral (tablets or liquid) or I.M. to I.V. therapy, dosage should be reduced by 20% to 25%.

Atrial dysrhythmias (rate control), CHF:

Initial: Total digitalizing dose: Give 1/2 of the total digitalizing dose (TDD) in the initial dose, then give 1/4 of the TDD in each of two subsequent doses at 9- to 12-hour intervals. Obtain ECG 6 hours after each dose to assess potential toxicity.

Oral: 0.75-1.5 mg

I.V. or I.M.: 0.5-1 mg

Daily maintenance dose: Give once daily to children >10 years of age and adults.

Oral: 0.125-0.5 mg

I.V. or I.M.: 0.1-0.4 mg

Elderly: Dose is based on lean body weight and normal renal function for age. Decrease dose in patients with decreased renal function (see Dosing in Renal Impairment).

Pediatrics: Atrial dysrhythmias (rate control), CHF: When changing from oral (tablets or liquid) or I.M. to I.V. therapy, dosage should be reduced by 20% to 25%. See table.

Dosage Recommendations for Digoxin

Age	Total Digitalizing Dose[2] (mcg/kg[1])		Daily Maintenance Dose[3] (mcg/kg[1])	
	P.O.	I.V. or I.M.	P.O.	I.V. or I.M.
Preterm infant[1]	20-30	15-25	5-7.5	4-6
Full-term infant[1]	25-35	20-30	6-10	5-8
1 mo - 2 y[1]	35-60	30-50	10-15	7.5-12
2-5 y[1]	30-40	25-35	7.5-10	6-9
5-10 y[1]	20-35	15-30	5-10	4-8
>10 y[1]	10-15	8-12	2.5-5	2-3

[1]Based on lean body weight and normal renal function for age. Decrease dose in patients with ↓ renal function; digitalizing dose often not recommended in infants and children.

[2]Give one-half of the total digitalizing dose (TDD) in the initial dose, then give one-quarter of the TDD in each of two subsequent doses at 8- to 12-hour intervals. Obtain ECG 6 hours after each dose to assess potential toxicity.

[3]Divided every 12 hours in infants and children <10 years of age. Given once daily to children >10 years of age and adults.

Renal Impairment:

Cl_{cr} 10-50 mL/minute: Administer 25% to 75% of dose or every 36 hours.

Cl_{cr} <10 mL/minute: Administer 10% to 25% of dose or every 48 hours.

Reduce loading dose by 50% in ESRD.

Not dialyzable (0% to 5%)

Available Dosage Forms [DSC] = Discontinued product

Capsule (Lanoxicaps®): 50 mcg [DSC], 100 mcg, 200 mcg [contains ethyl alcohol]

Elixir: 50 mcg/mL (2.5 mL, 5 mL, 60 mL) [contains alcohol 10%; lime flavor]

Lanoxin® (pediatric): 50 mcg/mL (60 mL) [contains alcohol 10%; lime flavor] [DSC]

Injection: 250 mcg/mL (1 mL, 2 mL) [contains alcohol 10% and propylene glycol 40%]

Lanoxin®: 250 mcg/mL (2 mL) [contains alcohol 10% and propylene glycol 40%]

Injection, pediatric: 100 mcg/mL (1 mL) [contains alcohol 10% and propylene glycol 40%]

Tablet: 125 mcg, 250 mcg

Digitek®, Lanoxin®: 125 mcg, 250 mcg

Nursing Guidelines

Assessment: Closely assess effects and interactions with other prescriptions, OTC medications, or herbal products patient may be taking. Assess results of laboratory tests (when beginning or changing dosage, especially with I.V. administration and when patients are receiving diuretics or amphotericin). Monitor therapeutic effectiveness and adverse reactions at beginning of therapy, periodically throughout therapy, or when changing dosage. Monitor for signs of digoxin toxicity. **I.V.:** Monitor ECG continuously. **Oral:** Monitor apical

(Continued)

Digoxin *(Continued)*

pulse before administering any dose. Assess knowledge/teach patient appropriate use, adverse reactions to report, and appropriate interventions to reduce side effects.

Monitoring Laboratory Tests:

When to draw serum digoxin concentrations: Digoxin serum levels should be drawn **at least 4 hours after an intravenous dose** and **at least 6 hours after an oral dose (optimally 12-24 hours after a dose).**

Initiation of therapy:

If a loading dose is given: Digoxin serum concentration may be drawn within 12-24 hours after the initial loading dose administration. Levels drawn this early may confirm the relationship of digoxin plasma levels and response but are of little value in determining maintenance doses.

If a loading dose is not given: Digoxin serum concentration should be obtained after 3-5 days of therapy.

Maintenance monitoring:

Trough concentrations should be followed just prior to the next dose or at a minimum of 4 hours after an I.V. dose and at least 6 hours after an oral dose.

Digoxin serum concentrations should be obtained within 5-7 days (approximate time to steady-state) after any dosage changes. Continue to obtain digoxin serum concentrations 7-14 days after any change in maintenance dose. **Note:** In patients with end-stage renal disease, it may take 15-20 days to reach steady-state.

Patients who are receiving potassium-depleting medications such as diuretics, should be monitored for potassium, magnesium, and calcium levels.

Digoxin serum concentrations should be obtained whenever any of the following conditions occur:

Questionable patient compliance or to evaluate clinical deterioration following an initial good response

Changing renal function

Suspected digoxin toxicity

Initiation or discontinuation of therapy with drugs (amiodarone, quinidine, verapamil) which potentially interact with digoxin; if quinidine therapy is started; digoxin levels should be drawn within the first 24 hours after starting quinidine therapy, then 7-14 days later or empirically skip one day's digoxin dose and decrease the daily dose by 50%.

Any disease changes (hypothyroidism)

Dietary Considerations: Maintain adequate amounts of potassium in diet to decrease risk of hypokalemia (hypokalemia may increase risk of digoxin toxicity).

Patient Education: Take as directed; do not discontinue without consulting prescriber. Maintain adequate dietary intake of potassium (do not increase without consulting prescriber). Adequate dietary potassium will reduce risk of digoxin toxicity. Take pulse at the same time each day; follow prescriber instructions for holding medication if pulse is <50. Notify prescriber of acute changes in pulse. Report loss of appetite, nausea, vomiting, persistent diarrhea, swelling of extremities, palpitations, 'yellowing' or blurred vision, mental confusion or depression, or unusual fatigue. **Pregnancy precaution:** Inform prescriber if you are or intend to become pregnant.

Geriatric Considerations: Elderly may develop exaggerated serum/tissue concentrations due to age-related alterations in clearance and pharmacodynamic differences. Elderly are at risk for toxicity due to age-related changes.

Pregnancy Risk Factor: C

Lactation: Enters breast milk (small amounts)/compatible

Perioperative/Anesthesia/Other Concerns: Elderly are at risk for toxicity due to age-related changes; volume of distribution is diminished significantly; half-life is increased as a result of decreased total body clearance. Digoxin toxicity may be potentiated in patients with hypokalemia, hypomagnesemia, and hypercalcemia. Digoxin may also rapidly approach toxic levels in patients with renal failure. For patients with renal failure, the loading dose is unchanged but maintenance doses may be adjusted and levels should be monitored very carefully. Signs of digoxin toxicity include both brady- and tachyarrhythmias. Bidirectional VT induced by digitalis toxicity indicates imminent development of ventricular fibrillation.

Digoxin has been used for many years in treatment of heart failure. Digoxin therapy is associated with a decrease in frequency in hospitalizations for exacerbations of heart failure. Digoxin use for ventricular rate control in patients with atrial fibrillation is a particularly useful strategy in those patients with coexisting systolic dysfunction. While digoxin may control ventricular response rate for atrial fibrillation at rest, the medication is less effective for rate control during exercise.

Administration

I.M.: Inject no more than 2 mL per injection site. May cause intense pain.

I.V.: Inject slowly 1-5 minutes for undiluted form. May dilute up to fourfold with SWI, D_5W, or NS.

Compatibility: Stable in $D_5{}^1/_2NS$ with KCl 20 mEq, D_5W, $D_{10}W$, LR, $^1/_2NS$, NS, and SWFI (when diluted fourfold or greater)

Y-site administration: Incompatible with amphotericin B cholesteryl sulfate complex, fluconazole, foscarnet, propofol

Compatibility in syringe: Incompatible with doxapram

Compatibility when admixed: Incompatible with dobutamine

Storage: Protect elixir and injection from light.

Related Information

Management of Postoperative Arrhythmias *on page 1787*

Dihydroergotamine (dye hye droe er GOT a meen)

U.S. Brand Names D.H.E. 45®; Migranal®

Synonyms DHE; Dihydroergotamine Mesylate

Pharmacologic Category Ergot Derivative

Use Treatment of migraine headache with or without aura; injection also indicated for treatment of cluster headaches

Unlabeled/Investigational Use Adjunct for DVT prophylaxis for hip surgery, for orthostatic hypotension, xerostomia secondary to antidepressant use, and pelvic congestion with pain

Mechanism of Action Ergot alkaloid alpha-adrenergic blocker directly stimulates vascular smooth muscle to vasoconstrict peripheral and cerebral vessels; also has effects on serotonin receptors

Pharmacodynamics/Kinetics

Onset of action: 15-30 minutes

Duration: 3-4 hours

Distribution: V_d: 14.5 L/kg

Protein binding: 93%

Metabolism: Extensively hepatic

Half-life elimination: 1.3-3.9 hours

Time to peak, serum: I.M.: 15-30 minutes

Excretion: Primarily feces; urine (10% mostly as metabolites)

Contraindications Hypersensitivity to dihydroergotamine or any component of the formulation; high-dose aspirin therapy; uncontrolled hypertension, ischemic heart disease, angina pectoris, history of MI, silent ischemia, or coronary artery vasospasm including Prinzmetal's angina; hemiplegic or basilar migraine; peripheral vascular disease; sepsis; severe hepatic or renal dysfunction; following vascular surgery; avoid use within 24 hours of sumatriptan, zolmitriptan, other serotonin agonists, or ergot-like agents; avoid during or within 2 weeks of discontinuing MAO inhibitors; ergot alkaloids are contraindicated with potent inhibitors of CYP3A4 (includes protease inhibitors, azole antifungals, and some macrolide antibiotics); pregnancy

Warnings/Precautions Do not give to patients with risk factors for CAD until a cardiovascular evaluation has been performed; if evaluation is satisfactory, the healthcare provider should administer the first dose and cardiovascular status should be periodically evaluated. May cause vasospastic reactions; persistent vasospasm may lead to gangrene or death in patients with compromised circulation. Discontinue if signs of vasoconstriction develop. Rare reports of increased blood pressure in patients without history of hypertension. Rare reports of adverse cardiac events (acute MI, life-threatening arrhythmias, death) have been reported following use of the injection. Cerebral hemorrhage, subarachnoid hemorrhage, and stroke have also occurred following use of the injection. Not for prolonged use. Pleural and peritoneal fibrosis have been reported with prolonged daily use. Cardiac valvular fibrosis has also been associated with ergot alkaloids. Safety and efficacy in pediatric patients have not been established.

(Continued)

Dihydroergotamine *(Continued)*

Drug Interactions **Substrate** of CYP3A4 (major); **Inhibits** CYP3A4 (weak)

Antifungals, azole derivatives (itraconazole, ketoconazole) increase levels of ergot alkaloids by inhibiting CYP3A4 metabolism, resulting in toxicity; concomitant use is contraindicated.

Antipsychotics: May diminish the effects of dihydroergotamine (due to dopamine antagonism); these combinations should generally be avoided.

Beta blockers: severe peripheral vasoconstriction has been reported with concomitant use of beta blockers and ergot derivatives. Monitor.

CYP3A4 inhibitors: May increase the levels/effects of dihydroergotamine. Example inhibitors include azole antifungals, clarithromycin, diclofenac, doxycycline, erythromycin, imatinib, isoniazid, nefazodone, nicardipine, propofol, protease inhibitors, quinidine, telithromycin, and verapamil. Ergot alkaloids are contraindicated with potent CYP3A4 inhibitors.

Heparin: When given with heparin, dihydroergotamine I.M. leads to hematoma at the injection site; combined administration not recommended.

Macrolide antibiotics: Erythromycin, clarithromycin, and troleandomycin may increase levels of ergot alkaloids by inhibiting CYP3A4 metabolism, resulting in toxicity (ischemia, vasospasm); concomitant use is contraindicated.

MAO inhibitors: The serotonergic effects of ergot derivatives may be increased by MAO inhibitors. Monitor for signs and symptoms of serotonin syndrome.

Metoclopramide: May diminish the effects of dihydroergotamine (due to dopamine antagonism); concurrent therapy should generally be avoided.

Nitroglycerin: May increase bioavailability of dihydroergotamine, decrease antianginal effects of nitrate; may need to decrease dose of dihydroergotamine. Monitor.

Protease inhibitors (ritonavir, amprenavir, atazanavir, indinavir, nelfinavir, and saquinavir) increase blood levels of ergot alkaloids by inhibiting CYP3A4 metabolism, acute ergot toxicity has been reported; concomitant use is contraindicated.

Serotonin agonists: Concurrent use with dihydroergotamine may increase the risk of serotonin syndrome (includes buspirone, SSRIs, TCAs, nefazodone, sumatriptan, and trazodone).

Sibutramine: May cause serotonin syndrome; concurrent use with ergot alkaloids is contraindicated.

Sumatriptan and other serotonin 5-HT_1 receptor agonists: Prolong vasospastic reactions; do not use sumatriptan or ergot-containing drugs within 24 hours of each other.

Vasoconstrictors: Concomitant use with peripheral vasoconstrictors may cause synergistic elevation of blood pressure; use is contraindicated.

Adverse Reactions

>10%: Nasal spray: Respiratory: Rhinitis (26%)

1% to 10%: Nasal spray:

- Central nervous system: Dizziness (4%), somnolence (3%)
- Endocrine & metabolic: Hot flashes (1%)
- Gastrointestinal: Nausea (10%), taste disturbance (8%), vomiting (4%), diarrhea (2%)
- Local: Application site reaction (6%)
- Neuromuscular & skeletal: Weakness (1%), stiffness (1%)
- Respiratory: Pharyngitis (3%)

<1% (Limited to important or life-threatening): Injection and nasal spray: Cerebral hemorrhage, coronary artery vasospasm, hypertension, MI, paresthesia, peripheral cyanosis, peripheral ischemia, rash, stroke, subarachnoid hemorrhage, ventricular fibrillation, ventricular tachycardia. Pleural and retroperitoneal fibrosis have been reported following prolonged use of the injection; cardiac valvular fibrosis has been associated with ergot alkaloids.

Overdosage/Toxicology Symptoms of overdose include peripheral ischemia, paresthesia, headache, nausea, and vomiting. Treatment is supportive. Activated charcoal is effective at binding ergot alkaloids.

Dosing

Adults:

Migraine, cluster headache:

I.M., SubQ: 1 mg at first sign of headache; repeat hourly to a maximum dose of 3 mg total; maximum dose: 6 mg/week

I.V.: 1 mg at first sign of headache; repeat hourly up to a maximum dose of 2 mg total; maximum dose: 6 mg/week

Intranasal: 1 spray (0.5 mg) of nasal spray should be administered into each nostril; if needed, repeat after 15 minutes, up to a total of 4 sprays. **Note:** Do not exceed 3 mg (6 sprays) in a 24-hour period and no more than 8 sprays in a week.

Elderly: Refer to adult dosing. Patients >65 years of age were not included in controlled clinical studies.

Renal Impairment: Contraindicated in severe renal impairment

Hepatic Impairment: Dosage reductions are probably necessary but specific guidelines are not available; contraindicated in severe hepatic dysfunction.

Available Dosage Forms

Injection, solution, as mesylate (D.H.E. 45®): 1 mg/mL (1 mL) [contains ethanol 94%]

Solution, intranasal spray, as mesylate (Migranal®): 4 mg/mL [0.5 mg/spray] (1 mL) [contains caffeine 10 mg/mL]

Nursing Guidelines

Assessment: Assess potential for interactions with other prescriptions, OTC medications, or herbal products patient may be taking. Assess therapeutic response and adverse effects on a regular basis. Teach patient proper use for either nasal spray or injection (storage, administration, injection technique, and syringe/needle disposal), possible side effects/appropriate interventions, and adverse symptoms to report. **Pregnancy risk factor X:** Determine that patient is not pregnant before starting therapy. Do not give to women of childbearing age, unless patient is capable of complying with contraceptive use. Breast-feeding is contraindicated.

Patient Education: Take this drug as rapidly as possible when first symptoms occur. May cause rare feelings of numbness or tingling of fingers, toes, or face (use caution and avoid injury) or drowsiness (use caution when driving or engaging in potentially hazardous tasks until response to drug is known). Report heart palpitations, severe nausea or vomiting, and severe numbness of fingers or toes.

Nasal spray: Follow directions for use on package insert. Wait 15 minutes between inhalations. Use no more than 4 inhalations (2 mg) for a single administration; do not use >3 mg (6 sprays) in a 24-hour period and no more than 8 sprays in a week.

I.M.: Follow directions for injections and needle disposal.

Pregnancy/breast-feeding precautions: Inform prescriber if you are pregnant. Consult prescriber for instruction on appropriate contraceptive measures. This drug may cause severe fetal defects. Do not breast-feed.

Geriatric Considerations: Monitor cardiac and peripheral effects closely in the elderly since they often have cardiovascular disease and peripheral vascular impairment (ie, diabetes mellitus, PVD) that will complicate therapy and monitoring for adverse effects.

Pregnancy Risk Factor: X

Pregnancy Issues: Dihydroergotamine is oxytocic and should not be used during pregnancy.

Lactation: May be excreted in breast milk/contraindicated

Breast-Feeding Considerations: Ergot derivatives inhibit prolactin and it is known that ergotamine is excreted in breast milk (vomiting, diarrhea, weak pulse, and unstable blood pressure have been reported in nursing infants). It is not known if dihydroergotamine would also cause these effects, however, it is likely that it is excreted in human breast milk. Do not use in nursing women.

Administration

Storage:

Injection: Store below 25°C (77°F), do not refrigerate or freeze; protect from heat and light

Nasal spray: Prior to use, store below 25°C (77°F), do not refrigerate or freeze; once spray applicator has been prepared, use within 8 hours; discard any unused solution

- ♦ **Dihydroergotamine Mesylate** *see* Dihydroergotamine *on page 537*
- ♦ **Dihydrohydroxycodeinone** *see* Oxycodone *on page 1284*
- ♦ **Dihydromorphinone** *see* Hydromorphone *on page 879*
- ♦ **1,25 Dihydroxycholecalciferol** *see* Calcitriol *on page 289*
- ♦ **Dihydroxydeoxynorvinkaleukoblastine** *see* Vinorelbine *on page 1713*
- ♦ **Dilacor® XR** *see* Diltiazem *on page 540*
- ♦ **Dilantin®** *see* Phenytoin *on page 1354*

♦ **Dilatrate®-SR** *see* Isosorbide Dinitrate *on page 976*
♦ **Dilaudid®** *see* Hydromorphone *on page 879*
♦ **Dilaudid-HP®** *see* Hydromorphone *on page 879*
♦ **Diltia XT®** *see* Diltiazem *on page 540*

Diltiazem (dil TYE a zem)

U.S. Brand Names Cardizem®; Cardizem® CD; Cardizem® LA; Cardizem® SR [DSC]; Cartia XT™; Dilacor® XR; Diltia XT®; Taztia XT™; Tiazac®

Synonyms Diltiazem Hydrochloride

Pharmacologic Category Calcium Channel Blocker

Medication Safety Issues

Sound-alike/look-alike issues:

Diltiazem may be confused with Dilantin®

Cardizem® may be confused with Cardene®, Cardene SR®, Cardizem CD®, Cardizem SR®, cardiem

Cartia XT™ may be confused with Procardia XL®

Tiazac® may be confused with Tigan®, Ziac®

Use

Oral: Essential hypertension; chronic stable angina or angina from coronary artery spasm

Injection: Atrial fibrillation or atrial flutter; paroxysmal supraventricular tachycardia (PSVT)

Unlabeled/Investigational Use Investigational: Therapy of Duchenne muscular dystrophy

Mechanism of Action Inhibits calcium ion from entering the "slow channels" or select voltage-sensitive areas of vascular smooth muscle and myocardium during depolarization, producing a relaxation of coronary vascular smooth muscle and coronary vasodilation; increases myocardial oxygen delivery in patients with vasospastic angina

Pharmacodynamics/Kinetics

Onset of action: Oral: Immediate release tablet: 30-60 minutes

Absorption: 70% to 80%

Distribution: V_d: 3-13 L/kg; enters breast milk

Protein binding: 70% to 80%

Metabolism: Hepatic; extensive first-pass effect; following single I.V. injection, plasma concentrations of N-monodesmethyldiltiazem and desacetyldiltiazem are typically undetectable; however, these metabolites accumulate to detectable concentrations following 24-hour constant rate infusion. N-monodesmethyldiltiazem appears to have 20% of the potency of diltiazem; desacetyldiltiazem is about 25% to 50% as potent as the parent compound.

Bioavailability: Oral: ~40%

Half-life elimination: Immediate release tablet: 3-4.5 hours, may be prolonged with renal impairment

Time to peak, serum: Immediate release tablet: 2-4 hours

Excretion: Urine and feces (primarily as metabolites)

Contraindications Hypersensitivity to diltiazem or any component of the formulation; sick sinus syndrome; second- or third-degree AV block (except in patients with a functioning artificial pacemaker); hypotension (systolic <90 mm Hg); acute MI and pulmonary congestion

Warnings/Precautions Concomitant use with beta-blockers or digoxin can result in conduction disturbances. Avoid concurrent I.V. use of diltiazem and a beta-blocker. Use caution in left ventricular dysfunction (can exacerbate condition). Symptomatic hypotension can occur. Use with caution in hepatic or renal dysfunction.

Drug Interactions **Substrate** of CYP2C8/9 (minor), 2D6 (minor), 3A4 (major); **Inhibits** CYP2C8/9 (weak), 2D6 (weak), 3A4 (moderate)

Alfentanil's plasma concentration is increased. Fentanyl and sufentanil may be affected similarly.

Amiodarone use may lead to bradycardia, other conduction delays, and decreased cardiac output; monitor closely if using together.

Azole antifungals may inhibit the calcium channel blocker's metabolism; avoid this combination. Try an antifungal like terbinafine (if appropriate) or monitor closely for altered effect of the calcium channel blocker.

Benzodiazepines (midazolam, triazolam) plasma concentrations are increased by diltiazem; monitor for prolonged CNS depression.

Beta-blockers may have increased pharmacodynamic interactions with diltiazem (see Warnings/Precautions).

Buspirone: Diltiazem may increase serum levels of buspirone; monitor.

Calcium may reduce the calcium channel blocker's effects, particularly hypotension.

Carbamazepine's serum concentration is increased and toxicity may result; avoid this combination.

Cimetidine reduced diltiazem's metabolism; consider an alternative H_2 antagonist.

Cyclosporine's serum concentrations are increased by diltiazem; avoid the combination. Use another calcium channel blocker or monitor cyclosporine trough levels and renal function closely.

CYP3A4 inducers: CYP3A4 inducers may decrease the levels/effects of diltiazem. Example inducers include aminoglutethimide, carbamazepine, nafcillin, nevirapine, phenobarbital, phenytoin, and rifamycins.

CYP3A4 inhibitors: May increase the levels/effects of diltiazem. Example inhibitors include azole antifungals, clarithromycin, diclofenac, doxycycline, erythromycin, imatinib, isoniazid, nefazodone, nicardipine, propofol, protease inhibitors, quinidine, telithromycin, and verapamil.

CYP3A4 substrates: Diltiazem may increase the levels/effects of CYP3A4 substrates. Example substrates include benzodiazepines, calcium channel blockers, cyclosporine, mirtazapine, nateglinide, nefazodone, sildenafil (and other PDE-5 inhibitors), tacrolimus, and venlafaxine. Selected benzodiazepines (midazolam and triazolam), cisapride, ergot alkaloids, selected HMG-CoA reductase inhibitors (lovastatin and simvastatin), and pimozide are generally contraindicated with strong CYP3A4 inhibitors.

Digoxin's serum concentration can be increased in some patients; monitor for increased effects of digoxin.

HMG-CoA reductase inhibitors (atorvastatin, lovastatin, simvastatin): Serum concentration will likely be increased; consider pravastatin/fluvastatin or a second generation dihydropyridine calcium channel blocker as an alternative.

Lithium neurotoxicity may result when diltiazem is added; monitor lithium levels.

Moricizine's serum concentration is increased; monitor clinical response closely.

Nafcillin decreases plasma concentration of diltiazem; avoid this combination.

Nitroprusside's dose required reduction in patients started on diltiazem; monitor blood pressure.

Protease inhibitor like amprenavir and ritonavir may increase diltiazem's serum concentration.

Quinidine: Diltiazem may increase serum levels of quinidine. Dosage adjustment may be required.

Rifampin increases the metabolism of calcium channel blockers; adjust the dose of the calcium channel blocker to maintain efficacy or consider an alternative to rifampin.

Sildenafil, tadalafil, vardenafil: Blood pressure-lowering effects may be additive; use caution.

Tacrolimus's serum concentrations are increased by diltiazem; avoid the combination. Use another calcium channel blocker or monitor tacrolimus trough levels and renal function closely.

Nutritional/Herbal/Ethanol Interactions

Ethanol: Avoid ethanol (may increase risk of hypotension or vasodilation).

Food: Diltiazem serum levels may be elevated if taken with food. Serum concentrations were not altered by grapefruit juice in small clinical trials.

Herb/Nutraceutical: St John's wort may decrease diltiazem levels. Avoid dong quai if using for hypertension (has estrogenic activity). Avoid ephedra (may worsen arrhythmia or hypertension). Avoid yohimbe, ginseng (may worsen hypertension). Avoid garlic (may have increased antihypertensive effect).

Adverse Reactions Note: Frequencies represent ranges for various dosage forms. Patients with impaired ventricular function and/or conduction abnormalities may have higher incidence of adverse reactions.

>10%:

Cardiovascular: Edema (2% to 15%)

Central nervous system: Headache (5% to 12%)

2% to 10%:

Cardiovascular: AV block (first degree 2% to 8%), edema (lower limb, 2% to 8%), pain (6%), bradycardia (2% to 6%), hypotension (<2% to 4%), vasodilation (2% to 3%), extrasystoles (2%), flushing (1% to 2%), palpitation (1% to 2%)

Central nervous system: Dizziness (3% to 10%), nervousness (2%)

Dermatologic: Rash (1% to 4%)

Endocrine & metabolic: Gout (1% to 2%)

(Continued)

Diltiazem *(Continued)*

Gastrointestinal: Dyspepsia (1% to 6%), constipation (<2% to 4%), vomiting (2%), diarrhea (1% to 2%)

Local: Injection site reactions: Burning, itching (4%)

Neuromuscular & skeletal: Weakness (1% to 4%), myalgia (2%)

Respiratory: Rhinitis (<2% to 10%), pharyngitis (2% to 6%), dyspnea (1% to 6%), bronchitis (1% to 4%), sinus congestion (1% to 2%)

<2% (Limited to important or life-threatening): Alkaline phosphatase increased, allergic reaction, amblyopia, amnesia, arrhythmia, AV block (second or third degree), bundle branch block, CHF, depression, dysgeusia, extrapyramidal symptoms, gingival hyperplasia, hemolytic anemia, petechiae, photosensitivity, SGOT increased, SGPT increased, Stevens-Johnson syndrome, syncope, tachycardia, thrombocytopenia, tremor, toxic epidermal necrolysis

Overdosage/Toxicology Primary cardiac symptoms of calcium blocker overdose include hypotension and bradycardia. Noncardiac symptoms include confusion, stupor, nausea, vomiting, metabolic acidosis, and hyperglycemia.

Following initial gastric decontamination, if possible, repeated calcium administration may promptly reverse depressed cardiac contractility (but not sinus node depression or peripheral vasodilation). Glucagon, epinephrine, and amrinone may treat refractory hypotension. Glucagon and epinephrine also increase heart rate (outside the U.S., 4-aminopyridine may be available as an antidote). Dialysis and hemoperfusion are not effective in enhancing elimination although repeat-dose activated charcoal may serve as an adjunct with sustained-release preparations.

Dosing

Adults:

Angina: Oral:

Capsule, extended release (Cardizem® CD, Cartia XT™, Dilacor® XR, Diltia XT®, Tiazac®): Initial: 120-180 mg once daily (maximum dose: 480 mg/day)

Tablet, extended release (Cardizem® LA): 180 mg once daily; may increase at 7- to 14-day intervals (maximum recommended dose: 360 mg/day)

Tablet, immediate release (Cardizem®): Usual starting dose: 30 mg 4 times/day; usual range: 180-360 mg/day

Hypertension: Oral:

Capsule, extended release (Cardizem® CD, Cartia XT™, Dilacor® XR, Diltia XT®, Tiazac®): Initial: 180-240 mg once daily; dose adjustment may be made after 14 days; usual dose range (JNC 7): 180-420 mg/day; Tiazac®: usual dose range: 120-540 mg/day

Capsule, sustained release (Cardizem® SR): Initial: 60-120 mg twice daily; dose adjustment may be made after 14 days; usual range: 240-360 mg/day

Tablet, extended release (Cardizem® LA): Initial: 180-240 mg once daily; dose adjustment may be made after 14 days; usual dose range (JNC 7): 120-540 mg/day

Atrial fibrillation, atrial flutter, PSVT: I.V.:

Initial bolus dose: 0.25 mg/kg actual body weight over 2 minutes (average adult dose: 20 mg)

Repeat bolus dose (may be administered after 15 minutes if the response is inadequate): 0.35 mg/kg actual body weight over 2 minutes (average adult dose: 25 mg)

Continuous infusion (requires an infusion pump; infusions >24 hours or infusion rates >15 mg/hour are not recommended): Initial infusion rate of 10 mg/hour; rate may be increased in 5 mg/hour increments up to 15 mg/hour as needed; some patients may respond to an initial rate of 5 mg/hour.

If diltiazem injection is administered by continuous infusion for >24 hours, the possibility of decreased diltiazem clearance, prolonged elimination half-life, and increased diltiazem and/or diltiazem metabolite plasma concentrations should be considered.

Conversion from I.V. diltiazem to oral diltiazem: Start oral approximately 3 hours after bolus dose.

Oral dose (mg/day) is approximately equal to [rate (mg/hour) x 3 + 3] x 10.

3 mg/hour = 120 mg/day
5 mg/hour = 180 mg/day
7 mg/hour = 240 mg/day
11 mg/hour = 360 mg/day

Elderly: Refer to adult dosing. **Note:** Patients ≥60 years may respond to a lower initial dose (eg, 120 mg once daily using extended release capsule)

Pediatrics:

Children: Minimal information available; some centers use the following:

Hypertension: Oral: Initial: 1.5-2 mg/kg/day in 3-4 divided doses; maximum dose: 3.5 mg/kg/day

Note: Doses up to 8 mg/kg/day given in 4 divided doses have been used for investigational therapy of Duchenne muscular dystrophy

Adolescents: Refer to adult dosing.

Renal Impairment: Use with caution as diltiazem is extensively metabolized by the liver and excreted in the kidneys and bile. Not removed by hemo- or peritoneal dialysis; supplemental dose is not necessary.

Hepatic Impairment: Use with caution as diltiazem is extensively metabolized by the liver and excreted in the kidneys and bile.

Available Dosage Forms [DSC] = Discontinued product

Capsule, extended release, as hydrochloride [once-daily dosing]: 120 mg, 180 mg, 240 mg, 300 mg

Cardizem® CD: 120 mg, 180 mg, 240 mg, 300 mg, 360 mg

Cartia XT™: 120 mg, 180 mg, 240 mg, 300 mg

Dilacor® XR, Diltia XT®: 120 mg, 180 mg, 240 mg

Taztia XT™: 120 mg, 180 mg, 240 mg, 300 mg, 360 mg

Tiazac®: 120 mg, 180 mg, 240 mg, 300 mg, 360 mg, 420 mg

Capsule, sustained release, as hydrochloride [twice-daily dosing] (Cardizem® SR [DSC]): 60 mg, 90 mg, 120 mg

Injection, solution, as hydrochloride: 5 mg/mL (5 mL, 10 mL, 25 mL)

Injection, powder for reconstitution, as hydrochloride (Cardizem®): 25 mg

Tablet, as hydrochloride (Cardizem®): 30 mg, 60 mg, 90 mg, 120 mg

Tablet, extended release, as hydrochloride (Cardizem® LA): 120 mg, 180 mg, 240 mg, 300 mg, 360 mg, 420 mg

Nursing Guidelines

Assessment: See Contraindications, Warnings/Precautions, and Dosing for use cautions. Assess potential for interactions with other prescriptions, OTC medications, or herbal products patient may be taking (see Drug Interactions). I.V. requires use of infusion pump and continuous cardiac and hemodynamic monitoring. Assess results of laboratory tests, therapeutic effectiveness, and adverse reactions (see Warnings/Precautions, Adverse Reactions, and Overdose/Toxicology) when beginning therapy, when changing dose, and periodically during long-term therapy. Teach patient appropriate use (oral), interventions to reduce side effects, and adverse symptoms to report (see Patient Education). See Lactation for breast-feeding considerations.

Monitoring Laboratory Tests: Liver function tests

Patient Education: Inform prescriber of all prescriptions, OTC medications, or herbal products you are taking, and any allergies you have. Do not take any new medication during therapy unless approved by prescriber. Oral: Take as directed; do not alter dosage or discontinue therapy without consulting prescriber. Do not crush or chew extended release form. Avoid (or limit) alcohol and caffeine. May cause dizziness or lightheadedness (use caution when driving or engaging in tasks requiring alertness until response to drug is known); nausea or vomiting (small, frequent meals, frequent mouth care, chewing gum, or sucking lozenges may help); constipation (increased exercise, fluids, fruit, or fiber may help); or diarrhea (buttermilk, boiled milk, or yogurt may help). Report chest pain, palpitations, irregular heartbeat; unusual cough, respiratory difficulty; swelling of extremities; muscle tremors or weakness; confusion or acute lethargy; skin rash; or other adverse reactions. **Pregnancy/breast-feeding precautions:** Inform prescriber if you are or intend to become pregnant. Consult prescriber if breast-feeding.

Geriatric Considerations: Elderly may experience a greater hypotensive response.

Pregnancy Risk Factor: C

Pregnancy Issues: Teratogenic and embryotoxic effects have been demonstrated in small animals.

Lactation: Enters breast milk/not recommended (AAP considers "compatible")

Breast-Feeding Considerations: Freely diffuses into breast milk; however, the AAP considers diltiazem to be **compatible** with breast-feeding. Available evidence suggest safe use during breast-feeding.

Perioperative/Anesthesia/Other Concerns: Diltiazem may be administered intravenously in the acute setting to attain ventricular rate control in patients with atrial fibrillation or flutter. Patients who respond, defined in general as at

(Continued)

Diltiazem *(Continued)*

least a 20% decrease in ventricular response rate or attaining a rate <100 beats/minute, can be continued on oral therapy to maintain control. It is important to consider the potential drug interaction with digoxin, as these agents are both used in this setting. Intravenous diltiazem may be administered safely for up to 24 hours in patients with left ventricular dysfunction.

Administration

Oral: Do not crush long acting dosage forms.

Tiazac®: Capsules may be opened and sprinkled on a spoonful of applesauce. Applesauce should be swallowed without chewing, followed by drinking a glass of water.

I.V.: Bolus doses given over 2 minutes with continuous ECG and blood pressure monitoring. Continuous infusion should be via infusion pump.

Compatibility: Stable in D_5½NS, D_5W, NS

Y-site administration: Incompatible with diazepam, furosemide, phenytoin, rifampin, thiopental

Storage:

Capsule, tablet: Store at controlled room temperature.

Solution for injection: Store in refrigerator at 2°C to 8°C (36°F to 46°F). May be stored at room temperature for up to one month; do not freeze. Following dilution with $D_5$1/2NS, D_5W, or NS, solution is stable for 24 hours at room temperature or under refrigeration.

Related Information

Management of Postoperative Arrhythmias *on page 1787*

♦ Diltiazem Hydrochloride *see* Diltiazem *on page 540*

DimenhyDRINATE (dye men HYE dri nate)

U.S. Brand Names Dramamine® [OTC]; TripTone® [OTC]

Pharmacologic Category Antihistamine

Medication Safety Issues

Sound-alike/look-alike issues:

DimenhyDRINATE may be confused with diphenhydrAMINE

Use Treatment and prevention of nausea, vertigo, and vomiting associated with motion sickness

Mechanism of Action Competes with histamine for H_1-receptor sites on effector cells in the gastrointestinal tract, blood vessels, and respiratory tract; blocks chemoreceptor trigger zone, diminishes vestibular stimulation, and depresses labyrinthine function through its central anticholinergic activity

Pharmacodynamics/Kinetics

Onset of action: Oral: ~15-30 minutes

Absorption: Oral: Well absorbed

Contraindications Hypersensitivity to dimenhydrinate or any component

Warnings/Precautions Causes sedation, caution must be used in performing tasks which require alertness (eg, operating machinery or driving). Sedative effects of CNS depressants or ethanol are potentiated. Use with caution in patients with angle-closure glaucoma, pyloroduodenal obstruction (including stenotic peptic ulcer), urinary tract obstruction (including bladder neck obstruction and symptomatic prostatic hyperplasia), hyperthyroidism, increased intraocular pressure, and cardiovascular disease (including hypertension and tachycardia). May cause paradoxical excitation in pediatric patients, and can result in hallucinations, coma, and death in overdose.

Drug Interactions

Increased effect/toxicity with CNS depressants, anticholinergics, TCAs, MAO inhibitors

Increased toxicity of antibiotics, especially aminoglycosides (ototoxicity)

Nutritional/Herbal/Ethanol Interactions Ethanol: Avoid ethanol (may increase CNS depression).

Adverse Reactions

>10%:

Central nervous system: Slight to moderate drowsiness

Respiratory: Thickening of bronchial secretions

1% to 10%:

Central nervous system: Headache, fatigue, nervousness, dizziness

Gastrointestinal: Appetite increase, weight gain, nausea, diarrhea, abdominal pain, xerostomia

Neuromuscular & skeletal: Arthralgia

Respiratory: Pharyngitis

Dosing

Adults & Elderly: Motion sickness (prevention/treatment): Oral: 50-100 mg every 4-6 hours, not to exceed 400 mg/day

Pediatrics: Motion sickness (prevention/treatment): Oral:

2-5 years: 12.5-25 mg every 6-8 hours, maximum: 75 mg/day

6-12 years: 25-50 mg every 6-8 hours, maximum: 150 mg/day

Available Dosage Forms

Caplet (TripTone®): 50 mg

Tablet (Dramamine®): 50 mg

Tablet, chewable (Dramamine®): 50 mg [contains phenylalanine 1.5 mg/tablet and tartrazine; orange flavor]

Nursing Guidelines

Dietary Considerations: May be taken with food or water.

Patient Education: May cause drowsiness, may impair judgment and coordination; avoid alcohol; drink plenty of fluids for dry mouth and to prevent constipation

Pregnancy Risk Factor: B

Related Information

Postoperative Nausea and Vomiting *on page 1807*

- Dimetapp® 12-Hour Non-Drowsy Extentabs® [OTC] *see* Pseudoephedrine *on page 1436*
- Dimetapp® Children's ND [OTC] [DSC] *see* Loratadine *on page 1058*
- Dimetapp® Decongestant Infant [OTC] *see* Pseudoephedrine *on page 1436*

Dimethyl Sulfoxide (dye meth il sul FOKS ide)

U.S. Brand Names Rimso®-50

Synonyms DMSO

Pharmacologic Category Urinary Tract Product

Use Symptomatic relief of interstitial cystitis

Drug Interactions Inhibits CYP2C8/9 (weak), 2C19 (weak)

Increased toxicity with sulindac

Adverse Reactions

>10%: Gastrointestinal: Garlic-like breath

1% to 10%:

Central nervous system: Headache, sedation

Gastrointestinal: Nausea, vomiting

Local: Local dermatitis

Ocular: Burning eyes

Dosing

Adults & Elderly: Interstitial cystitis: Not for I.M. or I.V. administration; only for bladder instillation. Instill 50 mL of solution directly into bladder and allow to remain for 15 minutes. Repeat in 2 weeks or until symptoms are relieved, then increase intervals between treatments.

Available Dosage Forms Solution, intravesical: 50% [500 mg/mL] (50 mL)

Nursing Guidelines

Assessment: For bladder instillation only. Assess knowledge/teach patient interventions to reduce side effects and adverse symptoms to report.

Patient Education: This medication is only for use as a bladder instillation. Maintain adequate hydration (2-3 L/day of fluids) unless instructed to restrict fluid intake. Report persistent adverse reactions. **Pregnancy/breast-feeding precautions:** Inform prescriber if you are or intend to become pregnant. Note breast-feeding caution.

Pregnancy Risk Factor: C

Lactation: Excretion in breast milk unknown

- Diocto® [OTC] *see* Docusate *on page 560*
- Diocto C® [DSC] [OTC] *see* Docusate and Casanthranol *on page 561*
- Dioctyl Calcium Sulfosuccinate *see* Docusate *on page 560*
- Dioctyl Sodium Sulfosuccinate *see* Docusate *on page 560*
- Diovan® *see* Valsartan *on page 1684*
- Diovan HCT® *see* Valsartan and Hydrochlorothiazide *on page 1687*
- Diphen® [OTC] *see* DiphenhydrAMINE *on page 546*
- Diphen® AF [OTC] *see* DiphenhydrAMINE *on page 546*
- Diphenhist [OTC] *see* DiphenhydrAMINE *on page 546*

DiphenhydrAMINE (dye fen HYE dra meen)

U.S. Brand Names Aler-Cap [OTC]; Aler-Dryl [OTC]; Aler-Tab [OTC]; AllerMax® [OTC]; Altaryl [OTC]; Banophen® [OTC]; Banophen® Anti-Itch [OTC]; Benadryl® Allergy [OTC]; Benadryl® Children's Allergy [OTC]; Benadryl® Children's Allergy Fastmelt® [OTC]; Benadryl® Dye-Free Allergy [OTC]; Benadryl® Injection; Benadryl® Itch Stopping [OTC]; Benadryl® Itch Stopping Extra Strength [OTC]; Compoz® Nighttime Sleep Aid [OTC]; Dermamycin® [OTC]; Dermarest® Insect Bite [OTC]; Dermarest® Plus [OTC]; Diphen® [OTC]; Diphen® AF [OTC]; Diphenhist [OTC]; Dytan™; Genahist® [OTC]; Hydramine® [OTC]; Nytol® Quick Caps [OTC]; Nytol® Quick Gels [OTC]; Q-Dryl [OTC]; Quenalin [OTC]; Siladryl® Allergy [OTC]; Siladryl® DAS [OTC]; Silphen® [OTC]; Simply Sleep® [OTC]; Sleep-ettes D [OTC]; Sleepinal® [OTC]; Sominex® [OTC]; Sominex® Maximum Strength [OTC]; Triaminic® Thin Strips™ Cough and Runny Nose [OTC]; Twilite® [OTC]; Unisom® Maximum Strength SleepGels® [OTC]

Synonyms Diphenhydramine Citrate; Diphenhydramine Hydrochloride; Diphenhydramine Tannate

Pharmacologic Category Antihistamine

Medication Safety Issues

Sound-alike/look-alike issues:

DiphenhydrAMINE may be confused with desipramine, dicyclomine, dimenhyDRINATE

Benadryl® may be confused with benazepril, Bentyl®, Benylin®, Caladryl®

Use Symptomatic relief of allergic symptoms caused by histamine release which include nasal allergies and allergic dermatosis; can be used for mild nighttime sedation; prevention of motion sickness and as an antitussive; has antinauseant and topical anesthetic properties; treatment of antipsychotic-induced extrapyramidal symptoms

Mechanism of Action Competes with histamine for H_1-receptor sites on effector cells in the gastrointestinal tract, blood vessels, and respiratory tract; anticholinergic and sedative effects are also seen

Pharmacodynamics/Kinetics

Onset of action: Maximum sedative effect: 1-3 hours

Duration: 4-7 hours

Protein binding: 78%

Metabolism: Extensively hepatic; smaller degrees in pulmonary and renal systems; significant first-pass effect

Bioavailability: Oral: 40% to 60%

Half-life elimination: 2-8 hours; Elderly: 13.5 hours

Time to peak, serum: 2-4 hours

Excretion: Urine (as unchanged drug)

Contraindications Hypersensitivity to diphenhydramine or any component of the formulation; acute asthma; not for use in neonates

Warnings/Precautions Causes sedation, caution must be used in performing tasks which require alertness (eg, operating machinery or driving). Sedative effects of CNS depressants or ethanol are potentiated. Use with caution in patients with angle-closure glaucoma, pyloroduodenal obstruction (including stenotic peptic ulcer), urinary tract obstruction (including bladder neck obstruction and symptomatic prostatic hyperplasia), hyperthyroidism, increased intraocular pressure, and cardiovascular disease (including hypertension and tachycardia). Diphenhydramine has high sedative and anticholinergic properties, so it may not be considered the antihistamine of choice for prolonged use in the elderly. May cause paradoxical excitation in pediatric patients, and can result in hallucinations, coma, and death in overdose. Some preparations contain sodium bisulfite; syrup formulations may contain alcohol. Some preparations contain soy protein; patients with soy protein or peanut allergies should avoid.

Drug Interactions **Inhibits** CYP2D6 (moderate)

Amantadine, rimantadine: Central and/or peripheral anticholinergic syndrome can occur when administered with amantadine or rimantadine

Anticholinergic agents: Central and/or peripheral anticholinergic syndrome can occur when administered with narcotic analgesics, phenothiazines and other antipsychotics (especially with high anticholinergic activity), tricyclic antidepressants, quinidine and some other antiarrhythmics, and antihistamines

Atenolol: Drugs with high anticholinergic activity may increase the bioavailability of atenolol (and possibly other beta-blockers); monitor for increased effect

Cholinergic agents: Drugs with high anticholinergic activity may antagonize the therapeutic effect of cholinergic agents; includes donepezil, rivastigmine, and tacrine

CNS depressants: Sedative effects may be additive with CNS depressants; includes ethanol, benzodiazepines, barbiturates, narcotic analgesics, and other sedative agents; monitor for increased effect

CYP2D6 substrates: Diphenhydramine may increase the levels/effects of CYP2D6 substrates. Example substrates include amphetamines, selected beta-blockers, dextromethorphan, fluoxetine, lidocaine, mirtazapine, nefazodone, paroxetine, risperidone, ritonavir, thioridazine, tricyclic antidepressants, and venlafaxine.

CYP2D6 prodrug substrates: Diphenhydramine may decrease the levels/effects of CYP2D6 prodrug substrates. Example prodrug substrates include codeine, hydrocodone, oxycodone, and tramadol.

Digoxin: Drugs with high anticholinergic activity may decrease gastric degradation and increase the amount of digoxin absorbed by delaying gastric emptying

Ethanol: Syrup should not be given to patients taking drugs that can cause disulfiram reactions (ie, metronidazole, chlorpropamide) due to high alcohol content

Levodopa: Drugs with high anticholinergic activity may increase gastric degradation and decrease the amount of levodopa absorbed by delaying gastric emptying

Neuroleptics: Drugs with high anticholinergic activity may antagonize the therapeutic effects of neuroleptics

Nutritional/Herbal/Ethanol Interactions

Ethanol: Avoid ethanol (may increase CNS depression).

Herb/Nutraceutical: Avoid valerian, St John's wort, kava kava, gotu kola (may increase CNS depression).

Lab Interactions May suppress the wheal and flare reactions to skin test antigens.

Adverse Reactions Frequency not defined.

Cardiovascular: Hypotension, palpitation, tachycardia

Central nervous system: Sedation, sleepiness, dizziness, disturbed coordination, headache, fatigue, nervousness, paradoxical excitement, insomnia, euphoria, confusion

Dermatologic: Photosensitivity, rash, angioedema, urticaria

Gastrointestinal: Nausea, vomiting, diarrhea, abdominal pain, xerostomia, appetite increase, weight gain, dry mucous membranes, anorexia

Genitourinary: Urinary retention, urinary frequency, difficult urination

Hematologic: Hemolytic anemia, thrombocytopenia, agranulocytosis

Neuromuscular & skeletal: Tremor, paresthesia

Ocular: Blurred vision

Respiratory: Thickening of bronchial secretions

Overdosage/Toxicology Symptoms of overdose include CNS stimulation or depression; overdose may result in death in infants and children. There is no specific treatment for antihistamine overdose. Clinical toxicity is due to blockade of cholinergic receptors. For anticholinergic overdose with life-threatening symptoms, physostigmine 1-2 mg SubQ or I.V. slowly may be given to reverse these effects.

Dosing

Adults:

Minor allergic rhinitis or motion sickness: Oral: 25-50 mg every 4-6 hours; maximum: 300 mg/day

Moderate to severe allergic reactions:

Oral: 25-50 mg every 4 hours, not to exceed 400 mg/day

I.M., I.V.: 10-50 mg in a single dose every 2-4 hours, not to exceed 400 mg/day

Night-time sleep aid: Oral: 50 mg at bedtime

Dystonic reaction: I.M., I.V.: 50 mg in a single dose; may repeat in 20-30 minutes if necessary

Allergic dermatosis: Topical: For external application, not longer than 7 days

Elderly: Initial: 25 mg 2-3 times/day increasing as needed

Pediatrics:

Treatment of dystonic reactions and moderate to severe allergic reactions: Oral, I.M., I.V.: 5 mg/kg/day or 150 mg/m^2/day in divided doses every 6-8 hours, not to exceed 300 mg/day

Minor allergic rhinitis or motion sickness: Oral, I.M., I.V.:

2 to <6 years: 6.25 mg every 4-6 hours; maximum: 37.5 mg/day

6 to <12 years: 12.5-25 mg every 4-6 hours; maximum: 150 mg/day

≥12 years: 25-50 mg every 4-6 hours; maximum: 300 mg/day

(Continued)

DiphenhydrAMINE *(Continued)*

Night-time sleep aid: 30 minutes before bedtime: Oral, I.M., I.V.:

2 to <12 years: 1 mg/kg/dose; maximum: 50 mg/dose

≥12 years: 50 mg

Antitussive: Oral, I.M., I.V.:

2 to <6 years: 6.25 mg every 4 hours; maximum 37.5 mg/day

6 to <12 years: 12.5 mg every 4 hours; maximum 75 mg/day

≥12 years: 25 mg every 4 hours; maximum 150 mg/day

Available Dosage Forms

Caplet, as hydrochloride: 25 mg, 50 mg

Aler-Dryl, AllerMax®, Compoz® Nighttime Sleep Aid, Sleep-ettes D, Sominex® Maximum Strength, Twilite®: 50 mg

Simply Sleep®, Nytol® Quick Caps: 25 mg

Capsule, as hydrochloride: 25 mg, 50 mg

Aler-Cap, Banophen®, Benadryl® Allergy, Diphen®, Diphenhist, Genahist®, Q-Dryl: 25 mg

Sleepinal®: 50 mg

Capsule, softgel, as hydrochloride: 50 mg

Benadryl® Dye-Free Allergy: 25 mg [dye-free]

Compoz® Nighttime Sleep Aid, Nytol® Quick Gels, Sleepinal®, Unisom® Maximum Strength SleepGels®: 50 mg

Captab, as hydrochloride (Diphenhist®): 25 mg

Cream, as hydrochloride: 2% (30 g) [contains zinc acetate 0.1%]

Banophen® Anti-Itch: 2% (30 g) [contains zinc acetate 0.1%]

Benadryl® Itch Stopping: 1% (30 g) [contains zinc acetate 0.1%]

Benadryl® Itch Stopping Extra Strength: 2% (30 g) [contains zinc acetate 0.1%]

Diphenhist®: 2% (30 g) [contains zinc acetate 0.1%]

Elixir, as hydrochloride:

Altaryl: 12.5 mg/5 mL (120 mL, 480 mL, 3840 mL) [cherry flavor]

Banophen®: 12.5 mg/5 mL (120 mL)

Diphen AF: 12.5 mg/5 mL (120 mL, 240 mL, 480 mL) [alcohol free; cherry flavor]

Q-Dryl: 12.5 mg/5 mL (480 mL) [alcohol free]

Gel, topical, as hydrochloride:

Benadryl® Itch Stopping Extra Strength: 2% (120 mL)

Dermarest® Plus: 2% (28 g, 42 g) [contains menthol 1%]

Injection, solution, as hydrochloride: 50 mg/mL (1 mL)

Benadryl®: 50 mg/mL (1 mL, 10 mL)

Liquid, as hydrochloride:

AllerMax®: 12.5 mg/5 mL (120 mL)

Benadryl® Allergy: 12.5 mg/5 mL (120 mL, 240 mL) [alcohol free; contains sodium benzoate; cherry flavor]

Benadryl® Dye-Free Allergy: 12.5 mg/5 mL (120 mL) [alcohol free, dye free, sugar free; contains sodium benzoate; bubble gum flavor]

Genahist®: 12.5 mg/5 mL (120 mL) [alcohol free, sugar free; contains sodium benzoate; cherry flavor]

Hydramine®: 12.5 mg/5 mL (120 mL, 480 mL) [alcohol free]

Q-Dryl: 12.5 mg/5 mL (120 mL) [alcohol free; cherry flavor]

Quenalin: 12.5 mg/5 mL (120 mL) [fruit flavor]

Siladryl® Allergy: 12.5 mg/5 mL (120 mL, 240 mL, 480 mL) [alcohol free, sugar free; black cherry flavor]

Siladryl® DAS: 12.5 mg/5 mL (120 mL) [alcohol free, dye free, sugar free; black cherry flavor]

Liquid, topical, as hydrochloride [stick] (Benadryl® Itch Stopping Extra Strength): 2% (14 mL) [contains zinc acetate 0.1% and alcohol]

Solution, oral, as hydrochloride:

Banophen®: 12.5 mg/5mL (480 mL) [sugar free]

Diphenhist: 12.5 mg/5 mL (120 mL, 480 mL) [alcohol free; contains sodium benzoate]

Solution, topical, as hydrochloride [spray]:

Benadryl® Itch Stopping Extra Strength: 2% (60 mL) [contains zinc acetate 0.1% and alcohol]

Dermamycin®, Dermarest® Insect Bite: 2% (60 mL) [contains menthol 1%]

Strips, oral, as hydrochloride (Triaminic® Thin Strips™ Cough and Runny Nose): 12. 5 mg (16s) [grape flavor]

Suspension, as tannate (Dytan™): 25 mg/5 mL (120 mL) [strawberry flavor]

Syrup, as hydrochloride (Silphen® Cough): 12.5 mg/5 mL (120 mL, 240 mL, 480 mL) [contains alcohol; 5%; strawberry flavor]

Tablet, as hydrochloride: 25 mg, 50 mg

Aler-Tab, Benadryl® Allergy, Genahist®, Sleepinal®, Sominex®: 25 mg

Tablet, chewable, as hydrochloride (Benadryl® Children's Allergy): 12.5 mg [contains phenylalanine 4.2 mg/tablet; grape flavor]

Tablet, chewable, as tannate (Dytan™): 25 mg [contains phenylalanine; strawberry flavor]

Tablet, orally-disintegrating, as citrate (Benadryl® Children's Allergy Fastmelt®): 19 mg [equivalent to diphenhydramine hydrochloride 12.5 mg; contains phenylalanine 4.5 mg/tablet and soy protein isolate; cherry flavor]

Nursing Guidelines

Assessment: Assess effectiveness and interactions of other medications patient may be taking. Monitor effectiveness of therapy and adverse reactions at beginning of therapy and periodically with long-term use. Assess knowledge/teach patient appropriate use, interventions to reduce side effects, and adverse symptoms to report.

Dietary Considerations: Tablet:

Chewable, as hydrochloride: Contains phenylalanine 4.2 mg per 12.5 mg tablet

Chewable, as tannate: Contains phenylalanine 1.5 mg per 25 mg tablet

Orally-disintegrating, as citrate: Contains phenylalanine 4.5 mg per 19 mg [equivalent to diphenhydramine hydrochloride 12.5 mg] tablet; contains soy protein isolate (contraindicated in patients with soy protein allergies; use caution in peanut allergic individuals, ~10% are estimated to also have soy protein allergies)

Patient Education: Take as directed; do not exceed recommended dose. Avoid use of other depressants, alcohol, or sleep-inducing medications unless approved by prescriber. You may experience drowsiness or dizziness (use caution when driving or engaging in tasks requiring alertness until response to drug is known); or dry mouth, nausea, or vomiting (small frequent meals, frequent mouth care, chewing gum, or sucking hard candy may help). Report persistent sedation, confusion, or agitation; changes in urinary pattern; blurred vision; sore throat, respiratory difficulty, or expectorating (thick secretions); or lack of improvement or worsening or condition. **Breast-feeding precaution:** Do not breast-feed.

Geriatric Considerations: Diphenhydramine has high sedative and anticholinergic properties, so it may not be considered the antihistamine of choice for prolonged use in the elderly. Its use as a sleep aid is discouraged due to its anticholinergic effects.

Pregnancy Risk Factor: B

Lactation: Enters breast milk/contraindicated

Breast-Feeding Considerations: Infants may be more sensitive to the effects of antihistamines.

Perioperative/Anesthesia/Other Concerns: Diphenhydramine's use as a sleep aid is discouraged due to its anticholinergic effects.

Administration

Compatibility: Stable in dextran 6% in dextrose, dextran 6% in NS, D_5LR, $D_5{}^1/_4NS$, $D_5{}^1/_2NS$, D_5NS, D_5W, $D_{10}W$, fat emulsion 10%, LR, $^1/_2NS$, NS

Y-site administration: Incompatible with allopurinol, amphotericin B cholesteryl sulfate complex, cefepime, foscarnet

Compatibility in syringe: Incompatible with diatrizoate meglumine 52% and diatrizoate sodium 8%, diatrizoate sodium 60%, haloperidol, iodipamide meglumine, iodipamide meglumine 52%, ioxaglate meglumine 39.3% and ioxaglate sodium 19.6%, pentobarbital, thiopental

Compatibility when admixed: Incompatible with amobarbital, amphotericin B, dexamethasone sodium phosphate with lorazepam and metoclopramide, iodipamide meglumine, phenytoin, phenobarbital, thiopental

Storage: Protect injection from light.

Related Information

Contrast Media Reactions, Premedication for Prophylaxis *on page 1911*

Postoperative Nausea and Vomiting *on page 1807*

◆ **Diphenhydramine Citrate** *see* DiphenhydrAMINE *on page 546*

◆ **Diphenhydramine Hydrochloride** *see* DiphenhydrAMINE *on page 546*

◆ **Diphenhydramine Tannate** *see* DiphenhydrAMINE *on page 546*

◆ **Diphenylhydantoin** *see* Phenytoin *on page 1354*

- **Diphtheria and Tetanus Toxoids and Acellular Pertussis Adsorbed, Hepatitis B (Recombinant) and Inactivated Poliovirus Vaccine Combined** *see* Diphtheria, Tetanus Toxoids, Acellular Pertussis, Hepatitis B (Recombinant), and Poliovirus (Inactivated) Vaccine *on page 550*
- **Diphtheria CRM_{197} Protein** *see* Pneumococcal Conjugate Vaccine (7-Valent) *on page 1376*
- **Diphtheria CRM_{197} Protein Conjugate** *see Haemophilus* b Conjugate Vaccine *on page 837*

Diphtheria, Tetanus Toxoids, Acellular Pertussis, Hepatitis B (Recombinant), and Poliovirus (Inactivated) Vaccine

(dif THEER ee a, TET a nus TOKS oyds, ay CEL yoo lar per TUS sis, hep a TYE tis bee ree KOM be nant, & POE lee oh VYE rus vak SEEN, in ak ti VAY ted vak SEEN)

U.S. Brand Names Pediarix™

Synonyms Diphtheria and Tetanus Toxoids and Acellular Pertussis Adsorbed, Hepatitis B (Recombinant) and Inactivated Poliovirus Vaccine Combined

Pharmacologic Category Vaccine

Use Combination vaccine for the active immunization against diphtheria, tetanus, pertussis, hepatitis B virus (all known subtypes), and poliomyelitis (caused by poliovirus types 1, 2, and 3)

Mechanism of Action Promotes active immunity to diphtheria, tetanus, pertussis, hepatitis B and poliovirus (types 1, 2 and 3) by inducing production of specific antibodies and antitoxins.

Pharmacodynamics/Kinetics Onset of action: Immune response observed to all components 1 month following the 3-dose series

Contraindications Hypersensitivity to diphtheria and tetanus toxoids, pertussis, hepatitis B, poliovirus vaccine, yeast, neomycin, polymyxin B, or any component of the vaccine; encephalopathy occurring within 7 days of a previous pertussis vaccine not (not attributable to another identifiable cause); progressive neurologic disorders (including infantile spasms, uncontrolled epilepsy, or progressive encephalopathy)

Warnings/Precautions Immediate treatment for anaphylactic/anaphylactoid reaction should be available during vaccine use. Infants born of HB_sAg-positive mothers should receive monovalent hepatitis B vaccine and hepatitis B immune globulin; infants born of HB_sAg-unknown mothers should receive monovalent hepatitis B vaccine; use of combination product in these patients to complete the hepatitis B vaccination series has not been studied. Use caution if one or more has occurred following the use of whole-cell DTP or a vaccine containing acellular pertussis: Temperature ≥40.5°C (≥105°F) within 48 hours not due to an identifiable cause; collapse or shock-like state within 48 hours; persistent, inconsolable crying that occurs within 48 hours and lasts ≥3 hours; seizures with or without fever that occur within 3 days. Use caution if Guillain-Barré syndrome occurs within 6 weeks of prior vaccination with tetanus toxoid. Defer administration during moderate or severe illness with or without fever. Antipyretics should be administered at the time of and for 24 hours following vaccination to patients at high risk for seizures. Use caution with bleeding disorders. Not for use as a booster dose following the 3-dose primary series. Safety and efficacy have not been established for use in children <6 weeks or adults and children ≥7 years of age.

Drug Interactions

Diphtheria antitoxin: May be administered concomitantly at separate sites.

Haemophilus influenzae type b vaccine (Hib): May be administered concomitantly at separate sites.

Immunosuppressant medications or therapies (antimetabolites, alkylating agents, cytotoxic drugs, corticosteroids, irradiation): The effect of the vaccine may be decreased; consider deferring vaccination for 3 months after immunosuppressant therapy is discontinued.

Pneumococcal conjugate vaccine: May be administered concomitantly at separate sites.

Tetanus immune globulin: May be administered concomitantly at separate sites.

Adverse Reactions All serious adverse reactions must be reported to the U.S. Department of Health and Human Services (DHHS) Vaccine Adverse Event Reporting System (VAERS) 1-800-822-7967.

As reported in a U.S. lot Consistency Study:

>10%:

Central nervous system:

Sleeping increased (28% to 47%, grade 3: <1% to 2%)

Restlessness (28% to 30%, grade 3: ≤1%)

Fever ≥100.4°F (26% to 31%); >103.1°F (<1%); incidence of fever is higher than reported with separately administered vaccines

Gastrointestinal: Appetite decreased (19% to 22%, grade 3: <1%)

Local: Injection site:

Redness (25% to 36%, >20 mm: ≤1%)

Pain (23% to 30%, grade 3: ≤1%)

Swelling (15% to 22%; >20 mm: 1%)

Miscellaneous: Fussiness (57% to 64%; grade 3: 2% to 3%)

Refer to individual product monographs for additional adverse reactions, including postmarketing and case reports.

Dosing

Pediatrics:

Immunization: I.M.: 0.5 mL; repeat in 6-8 week intervals (preferably 8-week intervals) for a total of 3 doses. Vaccination usually begins at 2 months, but may be started as early as 6 weeks of age.

Use in children previously vaccinated with one or more component, and who are also scheduled to receive all vaccine components:

Hepatitis B vaccine: Infants born of HB_sAg-negative mothers who received 1 dose of hepatitis B vaccine at birth may be given Pediarix™ (safety data limited); use in infants who received more than 1 dose of hepatitis B vaccine has not been studied. Infants who received 1 or more doses of hepatitis B vaccine (recombinant) may be given Pediarix™ to complete the hepatitis B series (safety and efficacy not established).

Diphtheria and tetanus toxoids, and acellular pertussis vaccine (DTaP): Infants previously vaccinated with 1 or 2 doses of Infanrix® may use Pediarix™ to complete the first 3 doses of the series (safety and efficacy not established); use of Pediarix™ to complete DTaP vaccination started with products other than Infanrix® is not recommended.

Inactivated polio vaccine (IPV): Infants previously vaccinated with 1 or 2 doses of IPV may use Pediarix™ to complete the first 3 doses of the series (safety and efficacy not established).

Available Dosage Forms Injection, suspension [single-dose]: Diphtheria toxoid 25 Lf, tetanus toxoid 10 Lf, inactivated PT 25 mcg, FHA 25 mcg, pertactin 8 mcg, HB_sAg 10 mcg, poliovirus type 1 40 DU, poliovirus type 2 8 DU, and poliovirus type 3 32 DU per 0.5 mL [contains neomycin sulfate ≤0.05 ng/0.5 mL, polymyxin B ≤0.01 ng/0.5 mL, and yeast protein ≤5%; packaged in vials or prefilled syringes; the needleless prefilled syringes contain dry natural latex rubber in the tip cap and plunger]

Nursing Guidelines

Assessment: Children who are moderately to severely ill (with or without fever) should not get this vaccination until they have recovered. Assess any hypersensitivity history prior to administering. Treatment for anaphylactic/anaphylactoid reaction should be available during vaccine use. See Contraindications, Warnings/Precautions, Dosing, and Administration for specific use cautions. Before administering, see Drug Interactions. Antipyretics should be administered at time of and for 24 hours following vaccination to patients at high-risk for seizures. **Note:** All serious adverse reactions must be reported the the US DHHS (see Adverse Reactions). Record date of administration, name of manufacturer, lot number, and administering person's name, title, and address into patient's permanent medical record. Teach caregiver possible side effects/ appropriate interventions, and adverse symptoms to report (see Patient Education).

Patient Education: Children who are moderately to severely ill (with or without fever) should not get this vaccination until they have recovered. Inform prescriber of all previous allergic reactions and any other medications being used. Three doses will be required for effective immunity; consult prescriber for appropriate schedule of vaccinations. May cause increased sleeping, restlessness, fussiness, decreased appetite, or fever (use antipyretic if directed by prescriber, or consult prescriber for appropriate antipyretic). May cause some redness, pain, or swelling at injection site; consult prescriber if excessive or

(Continued)

Diphtheria, Tetanus Toxoids, Acellular Pertussis, Hepatitis B (Recombinant), and Poliovirus (Inactivated) Vaccine *(Continued)*

persistent. Notify prescriber immediately of any excessive or persistent reactions (eg, fever >105°F within 48 hours, inconsolable crying that occurs within 48 hours and lasts 3 hours, seizures that occur within 3 days).

Pregnancy Risk Factor: C

Breast-Feeding Considerations: Not indicated for use by patients ≥7 years of age.

Administration

I.M.: For I.M. use only; do not administer I.V. or SubQ. Shake well prior to use; do not use unless a homogeneous, turbid, white suspension forms. Administer in the anterolateral aspects of the thigh or the deltoid muscle of the upper arm. Do not inject in the gluteal area (suboptimal hepatitis B immune response) or where there may be a major nerve trunk. Do not administer additional vaccines or immunoglobulins at the same site, or using the same syringe.

For patients at risk of hemorrhage following intramuscular injection, the ACIP recommends "it should be administered intramuscularly if, in the opinion of the physician familiar with the patients bleeding risk, the vaccine can be administered with reasonable safety by this route. If the patient receives antihemophilia or other similar therapy, intramuscular vaccination can be scheduled shortly after such therapy is administered. A fine needle (23 gauge or smaller) can be used for the vaccination and firm pressure applied to the site (without rubbing) for at least 2 minutes. The patient should be instructed concerning the risk of hematoma from the injection."

Federal law requires that the date of administration, name of the vaccine manufacturer, lot number of vaccine, and the administering person's name, title, and address be entered into the patient's permanent medical record.

Compatibility: Do not mix with other vaccines or injections.

Storage: Store under refrigeration of 2°C to 8°C (36°F to 46°F). Do not freeze; discard if frozen.

- ♦ **Diphtheria Toxoid Conjugate** *see Haemophilus* b Conjugate Vaccine *on page 837*
- ♦ **Diprivan®** *see* Propofol *on page 1421*
- ♦ **Diprolene®** *see* Betamethasone *on page 237*
- ♦ **Diprolene® AF** *see* Betamethasone *on page 237*
- ♦ **Dipropylacetic Acid** *see* Valproic Acid and Derivatives *on page 1680*
- ♦ **Disodium Cromoglycate** *see* Cromolyn *on page 453*
- ♦ ***d*-Isoephedrine Hydrochloride** *see* Pseudoephedrine *on page 1436*

Disopyramide (dye soe PEER a mide)

U.S. Brand Names Norpace®; Norpace® CR

Synonyms Disopyramide Phosphate

Pharmacologic Category Antiarrhythmic Agent, Class Ia

Medication Safety Issues

Sound-alike/look-alike issues:

Disopyramide may be confused with desipramine, dipyridamole

Norpace® may be confused with Norpramin®

Use Suppression and prevention of unifocal and multifocal atrial and premature, ventricular premature complexes, coupled ventricular tachycardia; effective in the conversion of atrial fibrillation, atrial flutter, and paroxysmal atrial tachycardia to normal sinus rhythm and prevention of the recurrence of these arrhythmias after conversion by other methods

Unlabeled/Investigational Use Hypertrophic obstructive cardiomyopathy (HOCM)

Mechanism of Action Class Ia antiarrhythmic: Decreases myocardial excitability and conduction velocity; reduces disparity in refractory between normal and infarcted myocardium; possesses anticholinergic, peripheral vasoconstrictive, and negative inotropic effects

Pharmacodynamics/Kinetics

Onset of action: 0.5-3.5 hours

Duration: 1.5-8.5 hours

Absorption: 60% to 83%

Protein binding (concentration dependent): 20% to 60%

Metabolism: Hepatic to inactive metabolites

Half-life elimination: Adults: 4-10 hours; prolonged with hepatic or renal impairment

Excretion: Urine (40% to 60% as unchanged drug); feces (10% to 15%)

Contraindications Hypersensitivity to disopyramide or any component of the formulation; cardiogenic shock; pre-existing second- or third-degree heart block (except in patients with a functioning artificial pacemaker); congenital QT syndrome; sick sinus syndrome

Warnings/Precautions Monitor and adjust dose to prevent QT_c prolongation. Watch for proarrhythmic effects. May precipitate or exacerbate CHF. Due to significant anticholinergic effects, do not use in patients with urinary retention, BPH, glaucoma, or myasthenia gravis. Reduce dosage in renal or hepatic impairment. The extended release form is not recommended for Cl_{cr} <40 mL/minute. In patients with atrial fibrillation or flutter, block the AV node before initiating. Use caution in Wolff-Parkinson-White syndrome or bundle branch block. Correct hypokalemia before initiating therapy. Hypokalemia may worsen toxicity. Monitor closely for hypotension during the initiation of therapy. Avoid concurrent use with other medications with prolong QT interval or decrease myocardial contractility.

Drug Interactions **Substrate** of CYP3A4 (major)

Beta-blockers may cause additive/excessive negative inotropic activity.

CYP3A4 inducers: CYP3A4 inducers may decrease the levels/effects of disopyramide. Example inducers include aminoglutethimide, carbamazepine, nafcillin, nevirapine, phenobarbital, phenytoin, and rifamycins.

CYP3A4 inhibitors: May increase the levels/effects of disopyramide. Example inhibitors include azole antifungals, clarithromycin, diclofenac, doxycycline, erythromycin, imatinib, isoniazid, nefazodone, nicardipine, propofol, protease inhibitors, quinidine, telithromycin, and verapamil.

Erythromycin and clarithromycin increase disopyramide blood levels; may cause QRS widening and/or QT interval prolongation.

Procainamide, quinidine, propafenone, or flecainide can cause increased/excessive negative inotropic effects or prolonged conduction.

Drugs which may prolong the QT interval (amiodarone, amitriptyline, bepridil, cisapride, disopyramide, erythromycin, haloperidol, imipramine, pimozide, quinidine, sotalol, and thioridazine) may be additive with disopyramide; use with caution.

Sparfloxacin, gatifloxacin, and moxifloxacin may result in additional prolongation of the QT interval; concurrent use is contraindicated.

Nutritional/Herbal/Ethanol Interactions

Ethanol: Avoid ethanol (may increase CNS depression).

Herb/Nutraceutical: St John's wort may decrease disopyramide levels. Avoid ephedra (may worsen arrhythmia).

Adverse Reactions The most common adverse effects are related to cholinergic blockade. The most serious adverse effects of disopyramide are hypotension and CHF.

>10%:

Gastrointestinal: Xerostomia (32%), constipation (11%)

Genitourinary: Urinary hesitancy (14% to 23%)

1% to 10%:

Cardiovascular: CHF, hypotension, cardiac conduction disturbance, edema, syncope, chest pain

Central nervous system: Fatigue, headache, malaise, dizziness, nervousness

Dermatologic: Rash, generalized dermatoses, pruritus

Endocrine & metabolic: Hypokalemia, elevated cholesterol, elevated triglycerides

Gastrointestinal: Dry throat, nausea, abdominal distension, flatulence, abdominal bloating, anorexia, diarrhea, vomiting, weight gain

Genitourinary: Urinary retention, urinary frequency, urinary urgency, impotence (1% to 3%)

Neuromuscular & skeletal: Muscle weakness, muscular pain

Ocular: Blurred vision, dry eyes

Respiratory: Dyspnea

<1% (Limited to important or life-threatening): Agranulocytosis, AV block, cholestatic jaundice, depression, dysuria, creatinine increased, gynecomastia, hepatotoxicity, hypoglycemia, BUN increased, insomnia, new or worsened arrhythmia (proarrhythmic effect), paresthesia, psychotic reaction, respiratory distress, thrombocytopenia, transaminases increased. Rare cases of lupus

(Continued)

Disopyramide *(Continued)*

have been reported (generally in patients previously receiving procainamide), peripheral neuropathy, psychosis, toxic cutaneous blisters

Overdosage/Toxicology Has a low toxic:therapeutic ratio and may easily produce fatal intoxication (acute toxic dose: 1 g in adults). Symptoms of overdose include sinus bradycardia, sinus node arrest or asystole, P-R, QRS, or QT interval prolongation, torsade de pointes (polymorphous ventricular tachycardia) and depressed myocardial contractility, which along with alpha-adrenergic or ganglionic blockade, may result in hypotension and pulmonary edema. Other effects are anticholinergic (dry mouth, dilated pupils, and delirium), as well as seizures, coma, and respiratory arrest.

Treatment is symptomatic and effects usually respond to conventional therapies. **Note:** Do not use other Type 1A or 1C antiarrhythmic agents to treat ventricular tachycardia. Sodium bicarbonate may treat wide QRS intervals or hypotension. Markedly impaired conduction or high degree AV block, unresponsive to bicarbonate, indicates consideration of a pacemaker.

Dosing

Adults & Elderly:

Dysrhythmia: Oral:

<50 kg: 100 mg every 6 hours or 200 mg every 12 hours (controlled release)

>50 kg: 150 mg every 6 hours or 300 mg every 12 hours (controlled release); if no response, may increase to 200 mg every 6 hours; maximum dose required for patients with severe refractory ventricular tachycardia is 400 mg every 6 hours.

Hypertrophic obstructive cardiomyopathy (unlabeled use): Oral: Initial: Controlled release: 200 mg twice daily. If symptoms do not improve, increase by 100 mg/day at 2-week intervals to a maximum daily dose of 600 mg.

Pediatrics: Antiarrhythmic: Oral:

<1 year: 10-30 mg/kg/24 hours in 4 divided doses

1-4 years: 10-20 mg/kg/24 hours in 4 divided doses

4-12 years: 10-15 mg/kg/24 hours in 4 divided doses

12-18 years: 6-15 mg/kg/24 hours in 4 divided doses

Renal Impairment: Oral: 100 mg (nonsustained release) given at the following intervals, based on creatinine clearance (mL/minute):

Cl_{cr} 30-40 mL/minute: Administer every 8 hours

Cl_{cr} 15-30 mL/minute: Administer every 12 hours

Cl_{cr} <15 mL/minute: Administer every 24 hours

or alter the dose as follows:

Cl_{cr} 30-<40 mL/minute: Reduce dose 50%

Cl_{cr} 15-30 mL/minute: Reduce dose 75%

Not dialyzable (0% to 5%) by hemo- or peritoneal methods; supplemental dose is not necessary.

Hepatic Impairment: Administer 100 mg every 6 hours or 200 mg every 12 hours (controlled release).

Available Dosage Forms

Capsule (Norpace®): 100 mg, 150 mg

Capsule, controlled release (Norpace® CR): 100 mg, 150 mg

Nursing Guidelines

Assessment: Assess other medications patient may be taking for effectiveness and interactions. Assess results of laboratory tests, therapeutic effectiveness, and adverse reactions when beginning therapy, when titrating dosage, and periodically during long-term therapy. **Note:** Disopyramide has a low toxic:therapeutic ratio and overdose may easily produce severe and life threatening reactions. Assess knowledge/teach patient appropriate use, interventions to reduce side effects, and adverse symptoms to report.

Monitoring Laboratory Tests: ECG, disopyramide drug level

Dietary Considerations: Should be taken on an empty stomach.

Patient Education: Take as directed, at regular intervals around-the-clock on an empty stomach. Do not alter dosage or discontinue therapy without consulting prescriber. Do not crush or chew extended release form. Avoid (or limit) alcohol and caffeine. You may experience dizziness or blurred vision (use caution when driving or engaging in tasks requiring alertness until response to drug is known); or dry mouth (frequent mouth care or sucking on lozenges may help). Report any change in urinary pattern or difficulty urinating; chest pain, palpitations, irregular heartbeat; unusual cough, respiratory difficulty, swelling of extremities; muscle tremors or weakness; confusion or acute lethargy; or skin rash. **Pregnancy precaution:** Inform prescriber if you are or intend to become pregnant.

Geriatric Considerations: Due to changes in total clearance (decreased) in the elderly, monitor closely. The anticholinergic action may be intolerable and require discontinuation. Monitor for CNS anticholinergic effects (confusion, agitation, hallucinations, etc). **Note:** Dose needs to be altered with Cl_{cr} <40 mL/minute which may be found frequently in the elderly.

Pregnancy Risk Factor: C

Lactation: Enters breast milk/compatible

Perioperative/Anesthesia/Other Concerns: In patients with pre-existing cardiovascular disease, the incidence of proarrhythmic effects and mortality may be increased with Class Ia antiarrhythmic agents. Disopyramide has significant anticholinergic effects which also limits its role in patients with cardiovascular disease.

Administration

Oral: Do not break or chew controlled release capsules. Administer around-the-clock to promote less variation in peak and trough serum levels.

♦ **Disopyramide Phosphate** *see* Disopyramide *on page 552*
♦ **DisperMox™** *see* Amoxicillin *on page 144*
♦ **Ditropan®** *see* Oxybutynin *on page 1281*
♦ **Ditropan® XL** *see* Oxybutynin *on page 1281*
♦ **Divalproex Sodium** *see* Valproic Acid and Derivatives *on page 1680*
♦ ***dl*-Alpha Tocopherol** *see* Vitamin E *on page 1716*
♦ ***D*-Mannitol** *see* Mannitol *on page 1079*
♦ **DMSO** *see* Dimethyl Sulfoxide *on page 545*
♦ **DNA-Derived Humanized Monoclonal Antibody** *see* Alemtuzumab *on page 102*

DOBUTamine (doe BYOO ta meen)

Synonyms Dobutamine Hydrochloride

Pharmacologic Category Adrenergic Agonist Agent

Medication Safety Issues

Sound-alike/look-alike issues:

DOBUTamine may be confused with DOPamine

Use Short-term management of patients with cardiac decompensation

Unlabeled/Investigational Use Positive inotropic agent for use in myocardial dysfunction of sepsis

Mechanism of Action Stimulates $beta_1$-adrenergic receptors, causing increased contractility and heart rate, with little effect on $beta_2$- or alpha-receptors

Pharmacodynamics/Kinetics

Onset of action: I.V.: 1-10 minutes

Peak effect: 10-20 minutes

Metabolism: In tissues and hepatically to inactive metabolites

Half-life elimination: 2 minutes

Excretion: Urine (as metabolites)

Contraindications Hypersensitivity to dobutamine or sulfites (some contain sodium metabisulfate), or any component of the formulation; idiopathic hypertrophic subaortic stenosis (IHSS)

Warnings/Precautions May increase heart rate. Patients with atrial fibrillation may experience an increase in ventricular response. An increase in blood pressure is more common, but occasionally a patient may become hypotensive. May exacerbate ventricular ectopy. If needed, correct hypovolemia first to optimize hemodynamics. Ineffective in the presence of mechanical obstruction such as severe aortic stenosis. Use caution post-MI (can increase myocardial oxygen demand). Use cautiously in the elderly starting at lower end of the dosage range.

Drug Interactions

Beta-blockers (nonselective ones) may increase hypertensive effect; avoid concurrent use.

Cocaine may cause malignant arrhythmias; avoid concurrent use.

Guanethidine can increase the pressor response; be aware of the patient's drug regimen.

MAO inhibitors potentiate hypertension and hypertensive crisis; avoid concurrent use.

Methyldopa can increase the pressor response; be aware of patient's drug regimen.

Reserpine increases the pressor response; be aware of patient's drug regimen.

TCAs increase the pressor response; be aware of patient's drug regimen.

(Continued)

DOBUTamine *(Continued)*

Lab Interactions May affect serum assay of chloramphenicol.

Adverse Reactions Incidence of adverse events is not always reported.

Cardiovascular: Increased heart rate, increased blood pressure, increased ventricular ectopic activity, hypotension, premature ventricular beats (5%, dose related), anginal pain (1% to 3%), nonspecific chest pain (1% to 3%), palpitation (1% to 3%)

Central nervous system: Fever (1% to 3%), headache (1% to 3%), paresthesia

Endocrine & metabolic: Slight decrease in serum potassium

Gastrointestinal: Nausea (1% to 3%)

Hematologic: Thrombocytopenia (isolated cases)

Local: Phlebitis, local inflammatory changes and pain from infiltration, cutaneous necrosis (isolated cases)

Neuromuscular & skeletal: Mild leg cramps

Respiratory: Dyspnea (1% to 3%)

Overdosage/Toxicology Symptoms of overdose include fatigue, nervousness, tachycardia, hypertension, and arrhythmias. Reduce rate of administration or discontinue infusion until condition stabilizes.

Dosing

Adults & Elderly: Cardiac decompensation: I.V. infusion: 2.5-20 mcg/kg/minute; maximum: 40 mcg/kg/minute, titrate to desired response; see table.

Infusion Rates of Various Dilutions of Dobutamine

Desired Delivery Rate (mcg/kg/min)	Infusion Rate (mL/kg/min)	
	500 mcg/mL[1]	1000 mcg/mL[2]
2.5	0.005	0.0025
5.0	0.01	0.005
7.5	0.015	0.0075
10.0	0.02	0.01
12.5	0.025	0.0125
15.0	0.03	0.015

[1]500 mg per liter or 250 mg per 500 mL of diluent.

[2]1000 mg per liter or 250 mg per 250 mL of diluent.

Pediatrics: Cardiac decompensation: Refer to adult dosing.

Available Dosage Forms

Infusion, as hydrochloride [premixed in dextrose]: 1 mg/mL (250 mL, 500 mL); 2 mg/mL (250 mL); 4 mg/mL (250 mL)

Injection, solution, as hydrochloride: 12.5 mg/mL (20 mL, 40 mL, 100 mL) [contains sodium bisulfite]

Nursing Guidelines

Assessment: Assess other medications patient may be taking for effectiveness and interactions. Infusion pump and continuous cardiac and hemodynamic monitoring are required. Monitor therapeutic effectiveness and adverse reactions. Instruct patient on adverse symptoms to report.

Monitoring Laboratory Tests: Serum glucose, renal function

Patient Education: When administered in emergencies, patient education should be appropriate to the situation. If patient is aware, instruct to promptly report chest pain, palpitations, rapid heartbeat, headache, nervousness, or restlessness, nausea or vomiting, or respiratory difficulty. **Breast-feeding precaution:** Consult prescriber if breast-feeding.

Geriatric Considerations: Beneficial hemodynamic effects have been demonstrated in elderly patients; however, significant hypotension may occur more frequently in elderly patients; monitor closely.

Pregnancy Risk Factor: B

Pregnancy Issues: Since dobutamine has not been given to pregnant women, benefits of use should outweigh the risks.

Lactation: Excretion in breast milk unknown

Perioperative/Anesthesia/Other Concerns: Septic Shock: Septic patients who have been adequately fluid resuscitated and have an adequate mean arterial pressure but low cardiac index (<2.5 L/minute/m^2) may require dobutamine. Dobutamine may help reverse tissue hypoperfusion by increasing cardiac output. Increasing cardiac output beyond the normal range has not been shown in clinical trials to improve patient outcome.

Early goal-directed therapy in the treatment of severe sepsis and septic shock provides significant survival benefits to this subset of patients. About 14% of the patients in the early goal-directed group received dobutamine. The early goal-directed patients received significantly more fluid, red-cell transfusions, and inotropic support during the initial 6 hours of their visit (Rivers E, 2001).

Administration

I.V.: Always administer via infusion device; administer into large vein.

Reconstitution: Remix solution every 24 hours. Store reconstituted solution under refrigeration for 48 hours or 6 hours at room temperature. Pink discoloration of solution indicates slight oxidation but **no** significant loss of potency. Stability of parenteral admixture at room temperature (25°C) is 48 hours; at refrigeration (4°C) stability is 7 days.

Standard adult diluent: 250 mg/500 mL D_5W; 500 mg/500 mL D_5W

Compatibility: Do not give through same I.V. line as heparin, hydrocortisone sodium succinate, cefazolin, or penicillin. **Incompatible** with heparin, cefazolin, penicillin, and in alkaline solutions (sodium bicarbonate).

Stable in D_5LR, $D_5{}^1/_2NS$, D_5NS, D_5W, $D_{10}W$, LR, $^1/_2NS$, NS, mannitol 20%; **incompatible** with sodium bicarbonate 5%

Y-site administration: Incompatible with acyclovir, alatrofloxacin, alteplase, aminophylline, amphotericin B cholesteryl sulfate complex, cefepime, foscarnet, indomethacin, phytonadione, piperacillin/tazobactam, thiopental, warfarin

Compatibility in syringe: Incompatible with doxapram

Compatibility when admixed: Incompatible with acyclovir, alteplase, aminophylline, bumetanide, calcium gluconate, diazepam, digoxin, floxacillin, furosemide, insulin (regular), magnesium sulfate, phenytoin, potassium phosphates, sodium bicarbonate

♦ **Dobutamine Hydrochloride** *see* DOBUTamine *on page 555*

Docetaxel (doe se TAKS el)

U.S. Brand Names Taxotere®

Synonyms NSC-628503; RP-6976

Pharmacologic Category Antineoplastic Agent, Natural Source (Plant) Derivative

Medication Safety Issues

Sound-alike/look-alike issues:

Taxotere® may be confused with Taxol®

Use Treatment of locally-advanced or metastatic breast cancer; adjuvant treatment of operable node-positive breast cancer (in combination with doxorubicin and cyclophosphamide); treatment of locally-advanced or metastatic nonsmall cell lung cancer (NSCLC) in combination with cisplatin in treatment of patients who have not previously received chemotherapy for unresected NSCLC; treatment of prostate cancer (hormone refractory, metastatic)

Unlabeled/Investigational Use Investigational: Treatment of gastric, pancreatic, head and neck, and ovarian cancers, soft tissue sarcoma, and melanoma

Mechanism of Action Docetaxel promotes the assembly of microtubules from tubulin dimers, and inhibits the depolymerization of tubulin which stabilizes microtubules in the cell. This results in inhibition of DNA, RNA, and protein synthesis. Most activity occurs during the M phase of the cell cycle.

Pharmacodynamics/Kinetics Exhibits linear pharmacokinetics at the recommended dosage range

Distribution: Extensive extravascular distribution and/or tissue binding; V_d: 80-90 L/m^2, V_{dss}: 113 L (mean steady state)

Protein binding: 94%, primarily to alpha$_1$-acid glycoprotein, albumin, and lipoproteins

Metabolism: Hepatic; oxidation via CYP3A4 to metabolites

Half-life elimination: Alpha, beta, gamma: 4 minutes, 36 minutes, and 10-18 hours, respectively

Excretion: Feces (75%); urine (6%); ~80% within 48 hours

Clearance: Total body: Mean: 21 L/hour/m^2

Contraindications Hypersensitivity to docetaxel or any component of the formulation; pre-existing bone marrow suppression (neutrophils <1500 cells/mm^3); pregnancy

Warnings/Precautions Use caution in hepatic disease; avoid use in patients with AST/ALT >1.5 times ULN in conjunction in conjunction with alkaline phosphatase >2.5 ULN. Early studies reported severe hypersensitivity reactions characterized

(Continued)

Docetaxel *(Continued)*

by hypotension, bronchospasms, or minor reactions characterized by generalized rash/erythema. The overall incidence was 25% in patients who did not receive premedication. Incidence reduced to 2.2% in patients who receive premedication. Patients should be premedicated with a steroid to prevent hypersensitivity reactions and fluid retention.

Fluid retention syndrome characterized by pleural effusions, ascites, edema, and weight gain (2-15 kg) has also been reported. It has not been associated with cardiac, pulmonary, renal, hepatic, or endocrine dysfunction. The incidence and severity of the syndrome increase sharply at cumulative doses ≥400 mg/m^2.

Neutropenia was the dose-limiting toxicity; however, this rarely resulted in treatment delays and prophylactic colony stimulating factors have not been routinely used. Patients with increased liver function tests experienced more episodes of neutropenia with a greater number of severe infections. Patients with an absolute neutrophil count <1500 cells/mm^3 should not receive docetaxel.

Docetaxel preparation should be performed in a Class II laminar flow biologic safety cabinet. Personnel should be wearing surgical gloves and a closed front surgical gown with knit cuffs. Appropriate safety equipment is recommended for preparation, administration, and disposal of antineoplastics. If docetaxel contacts the skin, wash and flush thoroughly with water. Contains Polysorbate 80®; diluent contains ethanol.

When administered as sequential infusions, taxane derivatives (docetaxel, paclitaxel) should be administered before platinum derivatives (carboplatin, cisplatin) to limit myelosuppression and to enhance efficacy.

Drug Interactions Substrate of CYP3A4 (major); **Inhibits** CYP3A4 (weak)

Carboplatin, cisplatin (platinum derivatives): When administered as sequential infusions, taxane derivatives should be administered before platinum derivatives to limit myelosuppression.

CYP3A4 inducers: CYP3A4 inducers may decrease the levels/effects of docetaxel. Example inducers include aminoglutethimide, carbamazepine, nafcillin, nevirapine, phenobarbital, phenytoin, and rifamycins.

CYP3A4 inhibitors: May increase the levels/effects of docetaxel. Example inhibitors include azole antifungals, clarithromycin, diclofenac, doxycycline, erythromycin, imatinib, isoniazid, nefazodone, nicardipine, propofol, protease inhibitors, quinidine, telithromycin, and verapamil.

Nutritional/Herbal/Ethanol Interactions

Ethanol: Avoid ethanol (due to GI irritation).

Herb/Nutraceutical: St John's wort may decrease docetaxel levels.

Adverse Reactions Note: Frequencies cited for nonsmall cell lung cancer and breast cancer treatment. Exact frequency may vary based on tumor type, prior and/or current treatment, premedication, and dosage of docetaxel.

>10%:

Cardiovascular: Fluid retention, including peripheral edema, pleural effusion, and ascites (33% to 47%); may be more common at cumulative doses ≥400 mg/m^2. Up to 64% in breast cancer patients with dexamethasone premedication.

Dermatologic: Alopecia (56% to 76%); nail disorder (11% to 31%, banding, onycholysis, hypo- or hyperpigmentation)

Gastrointestinal: Mucositis/stomatitis (26% to 42%, severe in 6% to 7%), may be dose-limiting (premedication may reduce frequency and severity); nausea and vomiting (40% to 80%, severe in 1% to 5%); diarrhea (33% to 43%)

Hematologic: Myelosuppression, neutropenia (75% to 85%), thrombocytopenia, anemia

Onset: 4-7 days

Nadir: 5-9 days

Recovery: 21 days

Hepatic: Transaminases increased (18%)

Neuromuscular & skeletal: Myalgia (3% to 21%); neurosensory changes (paresthesia, dysesthesia, pain) noted in 23% to 49% (severe in up to 6%). Motor neuropathy (including weakness) noted in as many as 16% of lung cancer patients (severe in up to 5%). Neuropathy may be more common at higher cumulative docetaxel dosages or with prior cisplatin therapy.

Ocular: Epiphora associated with canalicular stenosis (up to 77% with weekly administration; up to 1% with every-3-week administration)

Miscellaneous: Hypersensitivity reactions (6% to 13%; angioedema, rash, flushing, fever, hypotension); frequency substantially reduced by premedication with dexamethasone starting one day prior to docetaxel administration.

1% to 10%:

Cardiovascular: Hypotension (3%)

Dermatologic: Rash and skin eruptions (6%)

Gastrointestinal: Taste perversion (6%)

Hepatic: Bilirubin increased (9%)

Neuromuscular & skeletal: Arthralgia (3% to 9%)

Miscellaneous: Infusion site reactions (up to 4%)

<1% (Limited to important or life-threatening): Arrhythmias, atrial fibrillation, acute respiratory distress syndrome (ARDS), confusion, deep vein thrombosis, dehydration, erythema multiforme, gastrointestinal hemorrhage, gastrointestinal obstruction, gastrointestinal perforation, hand and foot syndrome, hepatitis, ileus, interstitial pneumonia, ischemic colitis, lacrimal duct obstruction, loss of consciousness (transient), MI, neutropenic enterocolitis, pulmonary edema, pulmonary embolism, pulmonary fibrosis, radiation recall, seizure, Stevens-Johnson syndrome, toxic epidermal necrolysis, visual disturbances (transient)

Dosing

Adults & Elderly: Refer to individual protocols:

Breast cancer:

Locally-advanced or metastatic: I.V.: 60-100 mg/m^2 every 3 weeks; patients initially started at 60 mg/m^2 who do not develop toxicity may tolerate higher doses

Operable, node-positive (adjuvant treatment): 75 mg/m^2 every 3 weeks for 6 courses

Nonsmall-cell lung cancer: I.V.: 75 mg/m^2 every 3 weeks

Prostate cancer:: I.V.: 75 mg/m^2 every 3 weeks; prednisone (5 mg twice daily) is administered continuously

Pediatrics: Children ≥16 years: Refer to adult dosing.

Hepatic Impairment: Total bilirubin ≥ the upper limit of normal (ULN), or AST (SGOT)/ALT (SGPT) >1.5 times ULN concomitant with alkaline phosphatase >2.5 times ULN: Docetaxel **should not be administered**.

Available Dosage Forms Injection, solution [concentrate]: 20 mg/0.5 mL (0.5 mL, 2 mL) [contains Polysorbate 80®; diluent contains ethanol 13%]

Nursing Guidelines

Assessment: Assess potential for interactions with other pharmacological agents or herbal products patient may be taking (eg, drugs that may increase or decrease levels/effects of docetaxel). **Caution:** Severe hypersensitivity reactions have been reported; premedication with dexamethasone may be advisable. Patient should be monitored continuously during infusion; dosing adjustment may be necessary. Assess results of laboratory tests, therapeutic response, and adverse effects (eg, neutropenia, severe fluid retention, pleural effusion, opportunistic infections, anemia) prior to each infusion and on a regular basis throughout therapy. Teach patient possible side effects/appropriate interventions and adverse symptoms to report.

Monitoring Laboratory Tests: CBC with differential and platelet count; liver function especially bilirubin, AST, ALT, and alkaline phosphatase

Patient Education: Do not take any new medication during therapy unless approved by prescriber. This medication can only be administered by infusion; report immediately any pain, burning, swelling, or redness at infusion site, difficulty breathing or swallowing, chest pain, or sudden chills. It is important to maintain adequate hydration (2-3 L/day of fluids) unless instructed to restrict fluid intake and adequate nutrition (small frequent meals may help). You will be more susceptible to infection (avoid crowds and exposure to infection and do not have any vaccinations without consulting prescriber). May cause nausea or vomiting (small frequent meals, frequent mouth care, sucking lozenges, or chewing gum may help); loss of hair (reversible); or diarrhea (buttermilk, boiled milk, or yogurt may help; if unresolved, contact prescriber for medication relief). Report immediately swelling of extremities, respiratory difficulty, unusual weight gain, abdominal distention, chest pain, palpitations, fever, chills, unusual bruising or bleeding, signs of infection, excessive fatigue, or rash. **Pregnancy/breast-feeding precautions:** Inform prescriber if you are pregnant. Do not get pregnant while taking this drug. Consult prescriber for appropriate contraceptives. Do not breast-feed.

(Continued)

Docetaxel *(Continued)*

Pregnancy Risk Factor: D

Pregnancy Issues: Docetaxel was found to be embryotoxic and fetotoxic in animal studies. A pregnancy registry is available for all cancers diagnosed during pregnancy at Cooper Health (856-757-7876).

Lactation: Excretion in breast milk unknown/contraindicated

Breast-Feeding Considerations: The manufacturer recommends discontinuing nursing prior to treatment.

Administration

I.V.: Irritant.

Premedication with corticosteroids is recommended to prevent hypersensitivity reactions and pulmonary/peripheral edema.

Administer I.V. infusion over 1-hour through nonsorbing (nonpolyvinylchloride) tubing; in-line filter is not necessary. When administered as sequential infusions, taxane derivatives should be administered before platinum derivatives (cisplatin, carboplatin) to limit myelosuppression and to enhance efficacy.

Reconstitution: Intact vials of solution should be diluted with 13% (w/w) ethanol/water to a final concentration of 10 mg/mL. Mix by repeated inversions; do not shake. Docetaxel dose should then be further diluted with NS or D_5W to a final concentration of 0.3-0.74 mg/mL and must be prepared in a glass bottle, polypropylene, or polyolefin plastic bag to prevent leaching of plasticizers.

Compatibility: Stable in D_5W, NS

Y-site administration: Incompatible with amphotericin B, doxorubicin liposome, methylprednisolone sodium succinate, nalbuphine

Storage: Intact vials should be stored at 2°C to 25°C (36°F to 77°F) and protected from light. Freezing does not adversely affect the product. Vials should be stored at room temperature for approximately 5 minutes before using. Following initial dilution, solution is stable for 8 hours at room temperature or under refrigeration. Following second dilution, the manufacturer recommends using within 4 hours. According to other references, the final diluted solutions are stable for up to 4 weeks at room temperature 15°C to 25°C (59°F to 77°F) in polyolefin containers. (Thiesen J, 1999).

Docusate (DOK yoo sate)

U.S. Brand Names Colace® [OTC]; Diocto® [OTC]; Docusoft-S™ [OTC]; DOK™ [OTC]; DOS® [OTC]; D-S-S® [OTC]; Dulcolax® Stool Softener [OTC]; Enemeez® [OTC]; Fleet® Sof-Lax® [OTC]; Genasoft® [OTC]; Phillips'® Stool Softener Laxative [OTC]; Silace [OTC]; Surfak® [OTC]

Synonyms Dioctyl Calcium Sulfosuccinate; Dioctyl Sodium Sulfosuccinate; Docusate Calcium; Docusate Potassium; Docusate Sodium; DOSS; DSS

Pharmacologic Category Stool Softener

Medication Safety Issues

Sound-alike/look-alike issues:

Docusate may be confused with Doxinate®

Colace® may be confused with Calan®

Surfak® may be confused with Surbex®

Use Stool softener in patients who should avoid straining during defecation and constipation associated with hard, dry stools; prophylaxis for straining (Valsalva) following myocardial infarction. A safe agent to be used in elderly; some evidence that doses <200 mg are ineffective; stool softeners are unnecessary if stool is well hydrated or "mushy" and soft; shown to be ineffective used long-term.

Unlabeled/Investigational Use Ceruminolytic

Mechanism of Action Reduces surface tension of the oil-water interface of the stool resulting in enhanced incorporation of water and fat allowing for stool softening

Pharmacodynamics/Kinetics

Onset of action: 12-72 hours

Excretion: Feces

Contraindications Hypersensitivity to docusate or any component of the formulation; concomitant use of mineral oil; intestinal obstruction, acute abdominal pain, nausea, or vomiting

Warnings/Precautions Prolonged, frequent or excessive use may result in dependence or electrolyte imbalance

Lab Interactions Decreased potassium (S), chloride (S)

Adverse Reactions 1% to 10%:

Gastrointestinal: Intestinal obstruction, diarrhea, abdominal cramping

Miscellaneous: Throat irritation

Overdosage/Toxicology Symptoms of overdose include abdominal cramps, diarrhea, fluid loss, and hypokalemia. Treatment is symptomatic.

Dosing

Adults & Elderly: Note: Docusate salts are interchangeable; the amount of sodium, calcium, or potassium per dosage unit is clinically insignificant.

Stool softener:

Oral: 50-500 mg/day in 1-4 divided doses

Rectal: Add 50-100 mg of docusate liquid to enema fluid (saline or water); give as retention or flushing enema

Pediatrics: Note: Docusate salts are interchangeable; the amount of sodium, calcium, or potassium per dosage unit is clinically insignificant.

Stool softener:

Oral:

Infants and Children <3 years: 10-40 mg/day in 1-4 divided doses

Children:

3-6 years: 20-60 mg/day in 1-4 divided doses

6-12 years: 40-150 mg/day in 1-4 divided doses

Adolescents: Refer to adult dosing.

Rectal: Older Children: Refer to adult dosing.

Available Dosage Forms

Capsule, as calcium (Surfak®): 240 mg

Capsule, as sodium: 100 mg, 250 mg

Colace®: 50 mg [contains sodium 3 mg], 100 mg [contains sodium 5 mg]

Docusoft-S™: 100 mg [contains sodium 5 mg]

DOK™, Genasoft®: 100 mg

DOS®, D-S-S®: 100 mg, 250 mg

Dulcolax® Stool Softener: 100 mg [contains sodium 5 mg]

Phillips'® Stool Softener Laxative: 100 mg [contains sodium 5.2 mg]

Enema, rectal, as sodium (Enemeez®): 283 mg/5 mL 5 mL

Gelcap, as sodium (Fleet® Sof-Lax®): 100 mg

Liquid, as sodium: 150 mg/15 mL (480 mL)

Colace®: 150 mg/15 mL (30 mL) [contains sodium 1 mg/mL]

Diocto®: 150 mg/15 mL (480 mL) [vanilla flavor]

Silace: 150 mg/15 mL (480 mL) [lemon-vanilla flavor]

Syrup, as sodium: 60 mg/15 mL (480 mL)

Colace®, Diocto®: 60 mg/15 mL (480 mL) [alcohol free, sugar free; contains sodium 36 mg/5 mL]

Silace: 20 mg/5 mL (480 mL) [peppermint flavor]

Nursing Guidelines

Assessment: See Contraindications, Warnings/Precautions, and Drug Interactions for use cautions. Monitor for effectiveness and instruct patient in proper use, side effects/appropriate interventions, and adverse effects to report.

Dietary Considerations: Should be taken with a full glass of water, milk, or fruit juice.

Patient Education: Docusate should be taken with a full glass of water, milk, or fruit juice. Do not use if abdominal pain, nausea, or vomiting are present. Laxative use should be used for a short period of time (<1 week). Prolonged use may result in abuse, dependence, as well as fluid and electrolyte loss. Report bleeding or if constipation occurs. **Pregnancy precaution:** Inform prescriber if you are or intend to become pregnant.

Geriatric Considerations: A safe agent to be used in the elderly. Some evidence that doses <200 mg are ineffective.

Pregnancy Risk Factor: C

Lactation: Excretion in breast milk unknown/compatible

Administration

Oral: Docusate liquid should be given with milk, or fruit juice, to mask the bitter taste. Capsules should be administered with a full glass of water, milk, or fruit juice.

Docusate and Casanthranol (DOK yoo sate & ka SAN thra nole)

U.S. Brand Names Diocto C® [DSC] [OTC]; Docusoft Plus™ [DSC] [OTC]; Doxidan® [DSC] [OTC]; Fleet® Sof-Lax® Overnight [DSC] [OTC]; Genasoft® Plus [DSC] [OTC]; Peri-Colace® [DSC] [OTC]

(Continued)

Docusate and Casanthranol *(Continued)*

Synonyms Casanthranol and Docusate; DSS With Casanthranol

Pharmacologic Category Laxative/Stool Softener

Medication Safety Issues

Sound-alike/look-alike issues:

Doxidan® may be confused with doxepin

Use Treatment of constipation generally associated with dry, hard stools and decreased intestinal motility

Adverse Reactions 1% to 10%:

Dermatologic: Rash

Gastrointestinal: Intestinal obstruction, diarrhea, abdominal cramping, throat irritation

Dosing

Adults & Elderly: Stool softener/cathartic: Oral: 1-2 capsules or 15-30 mL syrup at bedtime, may be increased to 2 capsules or 30 mL twice daily or 3 capsules at bedtime

Pediatrics: Stool softener/cathartic: Oral: 5-15 mL of syrup at bedtime or 1 capsule at bedtime

Available Dosage Forms [DSC] = Discontinued product

Capsule (Docusoft Plus™, Doxidan®, Fleet® Sof-Lax® Overnight, Genasoft® Plus, Peri-Colace®): Docusate sodium 100 mg and casanthranol 30 mg [DSC]

Syrup (Diocto C®, Peri-Colace®): Docusate sodium 60 mg and casanthranol 30 mg per 15 mL (480 mL) [contains alcohol] [DSC]

Nursing Guidelines

Patient Education: Adults: Take with a full glass of water; patients should assure proper dietary fiber and fluid intake with adequate exercise if medically appropriate; do not use if abdominal pain, nausea, or vomiting are present; laxative use should be used for a short period of time (<1 week); prolonged use may result in abuse, dependence, as well as fluid and electrolyte loss; notify physician if bleeding occurs or if constipation is not relieved

Pregnancy Risk Factor: C

Administration

Storage: Store in tight, light-resistant containers.

Docusate and Senna (DOK yoo sate & SEN na)

U.S. Brand Names Peri-Colace® *(reformulation)* [OTC]; Senokot-S® [OTC]

Synonyms Senna and Docusate; Senna-S

Pharmacologic Category Laxative, Stimulant; Stool Softener

Medication Safety Issues

Sound-alike/look-alike issues:

Senokot® may be confused with Depakote®

Use Short-term treatment of constipation

Unlabeled/Investigational Use Evacuate the colon for bowel or rectal examinations; management/prevention of opiate-induced constipation

Mechanism of Action Docusate is a stool softener; sennosides are laxatives

Contraindications Hypersensitivity to any component; intestinal obstruction; acute intestinal inflammation (eg, Crohn's disease); ulcerative colitis; appendicitis; abdominal pain of unknown origin; concurrent use of mineral oil; pregnancy (per Commission E for senna)

Warnings/Precautions Not recommended for over-the-counter (OTC) use in patients experiencing stomach pain, nausea, vomiting, or a sudden change in bowel movements which lasts >2 weeks. OTC labeling does not recommend for use longer than 1 week. Not recommended for OTC use in children <2 years of age.

Adverse Reactions Frequency not defined.

Gastrointestinal: Nausea, vomiting, diarrhea, abdominal cramps

Genitourinary: Urine discoloration (red/brown)

Dosing

Adults: Constipation: OTC ranges: Oral: Initial: 2 tablets (17.2 mg sennosides plus 100 mg docusate) once daily (maximum: 4 tablets twice daily)

Elderly: Constipation: OTC ranges: Oral: Consider half the initial dose in older, debilitated patients

Pediatrics: Constipation: OTC ranges: Oral: Children:

2-6 years: Initial: 4.3 mg sennosides plus 25 mg docusate ($^1/_2$ tablet) once daily (maximum: 1 tablet twice daily)

6-12 years: Initial: 8.6 sennosides plus 50 mg docusate (1 tablet) once daily (maximum: 2 tablets twice daily)

≥12 years: Refer to adult dosing.

Available Dosage Forms

Tablet: Docusate sodium 50 mg and sennosides 8.6 mg

Peri-Colace® (reformulation): Docusate sodium 50 mg and sennosides 8.6 mg

Senokot-S®: Docusate sodium 50 mg and sennosides 8.6 mg [sugar free; contains sodium 3 mg/tablet]

Nursing Guidelines

Dietary Considerations: Senokot-S®: Sodium content: 3 mg per tablet

Administration

Oral: Once-daily doses should be taken at bedtime.

- Docusate Calcium *see* Docusate *on page 560*
- Docusate Potassium *see* Docusate *on page 560*
- Docusate Sodium *see* Docusate *on page 560*
- Docusoft Plus™ [DSC] [OTC] *see* Docusate and Casanthranol *on page 561*
- Docusoft-S™ [OTC] *see* Docusate *on page 560*
- DOK™ [OTC] *see* Docusate *on page 560*

Dolasetron (dol A se tron)

U.S. Brand Names Anzemet®

Synonyms Dolasetron Mesylate; MDL 73,147EF

Pharmacologic Category Antiemetic; Selective 5-HT_3 Receptor Antagonist

Medication Safety Issues

Sound-alike/look-alike issues:

Anzemet® may be confused with Aldomet®

Dolasetron may be confused with granisetron, ondansetron, palonosetron

Use Prevention of nausea and vomiting associated with emetogenic cancer chemotherapy; prevention of postoperative nausea and vomiting; treatment of postoperative nausea and vomiting (injectable form only)

Not recommended for treatment of existing chemotherapy-induced emesis (CIE).

Mechanism of Action Selective serotonin receptor (5-HT_3) antagonist, blocking serotonin both peripherally (primary site of action) and centrally at the chemoreceptor trigger zone

Pharmacodynamics/Kinetics

Absorption: Rapid and complete

Distribution: 5.8 L/kg

Protein binding: Hydrodolasetron: 69% to 77% (50 bound to $alpha_1$-acid glycoprotein)

Metabolism: Hepatic; reduction by carbonyl reductase to hydrodolasetron (active metabolite); further metabolized by CYP3A and flavin monooxygenase

Bioavailability: 75%

Half-life elimination: Dolasetron: 10 minutes; hydrodolasetron: 6-8 hours

Time to peak, plasma: 1 hour

Excretion: Urine ~67% (61% active metabolite); feces ~33%

Contraindications Hypersensitivity to dolasetron or any component of the formulation

Warnings/Precautions Administer with caution in patients who have or may develop prolongation of cardiac conduction intervals, particularly QT_c intervals. These include patients with hypokalemia or hypomagnesemia, patients taking diuretics with potential for inducing electrolyte abnormalities, patients with congenital QT syndrome, patients taking antiarrhythmic drugs or other drugs which lead to QT prolongation, and cumulative high-dose anthracycline therapy. Safety and efficacy in children <2 years of age have not been established.

Drug Interactions Substrate (minor) of CYP2C8/9, 3A4; **Inhibits** CYP2D6 (weak)

Apomorphine: Due to reports of profound hypotension during concomitant therapy with ondansetron, the manufacturer of apomorphine contraindicates its use with all 5-HT_3 antagonists.

QT_c-prolonging agents (includes but may not be limited to amitriptyline, bepridil, disopyramide, erythromycin, haloperidol, imipramine, quinidine, pimozide, procainamide, sotalol, and thioridazine): Effect/toxicity of dolasetron and other QT_c-prolonging agents may be increased; use with caution.

Nutritional/Herbal/Ethanol Interactions Herb/Nutraceutical: St John's wort may decrease dolasetron levels.

(Continued)

Dolasetron *(Continued)*

Adverse Reactions Adverse events may vary according to indication

>10%:

Central nervous system: Headache (7% to 24%)
Gastrointestinal: Diarrhea (2% to 12%)

1% to 10%:

Cardiovascular: Bradycardia (5%), hypotension (5%), hypertension (2% to 3%), tachycardia (2% to 3%)
Central nervous system: Dizziness (1% to 6%), fatigue (3% to 6%), fever (3% to 5%), chills/shivering (1% to 2%), sedation (2%)
Dermatological: Pruritus (3% to 4%)
Gastrointestinal: Dyspepsia (2% to 3%), abdominal pain (3%)
Hepatic: Abnormal hepatic function (4%)
Neuromuscular & skeletal: Pain (3%)
Renal: Oliguria (1% to 3%), urinary retention (2%)

<1% (Limited to important or life-threatening): Abnormal vision, abnormal dreaming, acute renal failure, anaphylactic reaction, anemia, anorexia, ataxia, bronchospasm, confusion, constipation, diaphoresis increased, dyspnea, , edema, epistaxis, GGT increased, hematuria, hyperbilirubinemia, ischemia (peripheral), local injection site reaction, pancreatitis, photophobia, polyuria; prolonged P-R, QRS, and QT_c intervals; prothrombin time increased, purpura/ hematoma, rash, sleep disorder, syncope, taste perversion, thrombocytopenia, thrombophlebitis/phlebitis, tinnitus, urticaria

Overdosage/Toxicology Prolongation of QT, AV block, severe hypotension, and dizziness have been reported. Treatment is supportive, and continuous ECG monitoring (telemetry) is recommended.

Dosing

Adults & Elderly:

Nausea and vomiting associated with cancer chemotherapy:
Oral:100 mg single dose 1 hour prior to chemotherapy
I.V.: 1.8 mg/kg or 100 mg 30 minutes prior to chemotherapy

Postoperative nausea and vomiting:
Prevention:
Oral: 100 mg within 2 hours before surgery (doses of 25-200 mg have been used)
I.V.: 12.5 mg ~15 minutes before stopping anesthesia
Treatment: I.V. (only): 12.5 mg as soon as needed

Pediatrics:

Nausea and vomiting prophylaxis, chemotherapy-induced (including initial and repeat courses): Children 2-16 years:
Oral: 1.8 mg/kg within 1 hour before chemotherapy; maximum: 100 mg/dose
I.V.: 1.8 mg/kg ~30 minutes before chemotherapy; maximum: 100 mg/dose

Postoperative nausea and vomiting: Children 2-16 years:
Prevention:
Oral: 1.2 mg/kg within 2 hours before surgery; maximum: 100 mg/dose
I.V.: 0.35 mg/kg (maximum: 12.5 mg) ~15 minutes before stopping anesthesia
Treatment: I.V. (only): 0.35 mg/kg as soon as needed

Available Dosage Forms

Injection, solution, as mesylate: 20 mg/mL (0.625 mL) [single-use ampul, Carpuject®, or vial]; 20 mg/mL (5 mL) [single-use vial]; 20 mg/mL (25 mL) [multidose vial]
Tablet, as mesylate: 50 mg, 100 mg

Nursing Guidelines

Assessment: See Contraindications and Warnings/Precautions for use cautions. Assess potential for interactions with other prescriptions, OTC medications, or herbal products patient may be taking (see Drug Interactions). Assess therapeutic effectiveness and adverse reactions (see Adverse Reactions and Overdose/Toxicology, eg, cardiac abnormalities) on a regular basis. Teach patient possible side effects/appropriate interventions and adverse symptoms to report (see Patient Education). Note breast-feeding caution.

Patient Education: Inform prescriber of all prescriptions, OTC medications, or herbal products you are taking, and any allergies you have. This drug is given to reduce the incidence of nausea and vomiting. May cause headache, drowsiness, or dizziness (request assistance when getting up or changing position and do not perform activities requiring alertness). Report immediately any chest pain, rapid heartbeat, or palpitations; unusual pain, chills, or fever; severe headache or diarrhea; chest pain, palpitations, or tightness; swelling of throat or feeling of tightness in throat; or difficulty urinating. **Breast-feeding precaution:** Consult prescriber if breast-feeding.

Pregnancy Risk Factor: B

Lactation: Excretion in breast milk unknown/use caution

Perioperative/Anesthesia/Other Concerns: Oral administration of the intravenous solution is equivalent to tablets.

Administration

Oral: Dolasetron injection may be diluted in apple or apple-grape juice and taken orally; this dilution is stable for 2 hours at room temperature.

I.V.: I.V. injection may be given either undiluted IVP over 30 seconds or diluted in 50 mL of compatible fluid and infused over 15 minutes. Line should be flushed, prior to and after, dolasetron administration.

Reconstitution: Dilute in 50-100 mL of a compatible solution.

Compatibility: Stable in 0.9% NS, D_5W, D_5W and 0.45% NS, D_5W and LR, LR, and 10% mannitol injection

Storage: Store intact vials and tablets at room temperature. Protect from light. Stock solution (20 mg/mL) drawn into syringes is stable for 8 months at room temperature. After dilution, I.V. dolasetron is stable under normal lighting conditions at room temperature for 24 hours or under refrigeration for 48 hours with the following **compatible** intravenous fluids: 0.9% sodium chloride injection, 5% dextrose injection, 5% dextrose and 0.45% sodium chloride injection, 5% dextrose and lactated Ringer's injection, lactated Ringer's injection, and 10% mannitol injection

Related Information

Postoperative Nausea and Vomiting *on page 1807*

♦ **Dolasetron Mesylate** *see* Dolasetron *on page 563*

♦ **Dolgic® LQ** *see* Butalbital, Acetaminophen, and Caffeine *on page 280*

♦ **Dolgic® Plus** *see* Butalbital, Acetaminophen, and Caffeine *on page 280*

♦ **Dolophine®** *see* Methadone *on page 1115*

DOPamine (DOE pa meen)

Synonyms Dopamine Hydrochloride; Intropin

Pharmacologic Category Adrenergic Agonist Agent

Medication Safety Issues

Sound-alike/look-alike issues:

DOPamine may be confused with DOBUTamine, Dopram®

Use Adjunct in the treatment of shock (eg, MI, open heart surgery, renal failure, cardiac decompensation) which persists after adequate fluid volume replacement

Unlabeled/Investigational Use Symptomatic bradycardia or heart block unresponsive to atropine or pacing

Mechanism of Action Stimulates both adrenergic and dopaminergic receptors, lower doses are mainly dopaminergic stimulating and produce renal and mesenteric vasodilation, higher doses also are both dopaminergic and $beta_1$-adrenergic stimulating and produce cardiac stimulation and renal vasodilation; large doses stimulate alpha-adrenergic receptors

Pharmacodynamics/Kinetics

Children: Dopamine has exhibited nonlinear kinetics in children; with medication changes, may not achieve steady-state for ~1 hour rather than 20 minutes

Onset of action: Adults: 5 minutes

Duration: Adults: <10 minutes

Metabolism: Renal, hepatic, plasma; 75% to inactive metabolites by monoamine oxidase and 25% to norepinephrine

Half-life elimination: 2 minutes

Excretion: Urine (as metabolites)

Clearance: Neonates: Varies and appears to be age related; clearance is more prolonged with combined hepatic and renal dysfunction

Contraindications Hypersensitivity to sulfites (commercial preparation contains sodium bisulfite); pheochromocytoma; ventricular fibrillation

Warnings/Precautions Use with caution in patients with cardiovascular disease or cardiac arrhythmias or patients with occlusive vascular disease. Correct hypovolemia and electrolytes when used in hemodynamic support. May cause increases in HR and arrhythmia. Avoid infiltration - may cause severe tissue necrosis. Use with caution in post-MI patients.

(Continued)

DOPamine *(Continued)*

Drug Interactions

Beta-blockers (nonselective ones) may increase hypertensive effect; avoid concurrent use.

Cocaine may cause malignant arrhythmias; avoid concurrent use.

Guanethidine's hypotensive effects may only be partially reversed; may need to use a direct-acting sympathomimetic.

MAO inhibitors potentiate hypertension and hypertensive crisis; avoid concurrent use.

Methyldopa can increase the pressor response; be aware of patient's drug regimen.

Reserpine increases the pressor response; be aware of patient's drug regimen.

TCAs increase the pressor response; be aware of patient's drug regimen.

Adverse Reactions Frequency not defined.

Most frequent:

- Cardiovascular: Ectopic beats, tachycardia, anginal pain, palpitation, hypotension, vasoconstriction
- Central nervous system: Headache
- Gastrointestinal: Nausea and vomiting
- Respiratory: Dyspnea

Infrequent:

- Cardiovascular: Aberrant conduction, bradycardia, widened QRS complex, ventricular arrhythmia (high dose), gangrene (high dose), hypertension
- Central nervous system: Anxiety
- Endocrine & metabolic: Piloerection, serum glucose increased (usually not above normal limits)
- Local: Extravasation of dopamine can cause tissue necrosis and sloughing of surrounding tissues
- Ocular: Intraocular pressure increased, dilated pupils
- Renal: Azotemia, polyuria

Overdosage/Toxicology Symptoms of overdose include severe hypertension, cardiac arrhythmias, acute renal failure. Treat symptomatically.

Important: Antidote for peripheral ischemia: To prevent sloughing and necrosis in ischemic areas, the area should be infiltrated as soon as possible with 10-15 mL of saline solution containing 5-10 mg of Regitine (brand of phentolamine), an adrenergic blocking agent. A syringe with a fine hypodermic needle should be used, and the solution liberally infiltrated throughout the ischemic area. Sympathetic blockade with phentolamine causes immediate and conspicuous local hyperemic changes if the area is infiltrated within 12 hours. Therefore, phentolamine should be given as soon as possible after extravasation is noted.

Dosing

Adults & Elderly:

Hemodynamic support: I.V. infusion: 1-5 mcg/kg/minute up to 50 mcg/kg/minute, titrate to desired response; infusion may be increased by 1-4 mcg/kg/minute at 10- to 30-minute intervals until optimal response is obtained

Note: If dosages >20-30 mcg/kg/minute are needed, a more direct-acting vasopressor may be more beneficial (ie, epinephrine, norepinephrine).

Hemodynamic effects of dopamine are dose dependent:

- Low-dose: 1-5 mcg/kg/minute, increased renal blood flow and urine output
- Intermediate-dose: 5-15 mcg/kg/minute, increased renal blood flow, heart rate, cardiac contractility, and cardiac output
- High-dose: >15 mcg/kg/minute, alpha-adrenergic effects begin to predominate, vasoconstriction, increased blood pressure

Pediatrics: Hemodynamic support: I.V. infusion:

Children: 1-20 mcg/kg/minute, maximum: 50 mcg/kg/minute continuous infusion, titrate to desired response.

Available Dosage Forms

Infusion, as hydrochloride [premixed in D_5W]: 0.8 mg/mL (250 mL, 500 mL); 1.6 mg/mL (250 mL, 500 mL); 3.2 mg/mL (250 mL)

Injection, solution, as hydrochloride: 40 mg/mL (5 mL, 10 mL); 80 mg/mL (5 mL); 160 mg/mL (5 mL) [contains sodium metabisulfite]

Nursing Guidelines

Assessment: Assess other medications patient may be taking for effectiveness and interactions. Infusion pump, continuous cardiac and hemodynamic monitoring, and frequent assessment of I.V. site is required for inpatient therapy. Low-dose home infusion therapy requires frequent monitoring of cardiac and renal status and adverse reactions. Monitor therapeutic effectiveness and adverse reactions. Instruct patient on adverse symptoms to report.

Monitoring Laboratory Tests: Serum glucose, renal function

Patient Education: When administered in emergencies, patient education should be appropriate to the situation. If patient is aware, instruct to promptly report chest pain, palpitations, rapid heartbeat, headache, nervousness or restlessness, nausea or vomiting, or respiratory difficulty.

Geriatric Considerations: Has not been specifically studied in the elderly.

Pregnancy Risk Factor: C

Lactation: Excretion in breast milk unknown

Perioperative/Anesthesia/Other Concerns:

Low-Dose Dopamine: There is no clear evidence that low-dose dopamine confers any renal benefit. The 1999 ACCM/SCCM Practice Parameters for Hemodynamic Support of Sepsis in Adult Patients recommends against the use of low doses of dopamine to maintain renal function. Low-dose dopamine may increase renal blood flow in some patients requiring norepinephrine. Kellum and Decker (2001) reviewed 58 studies in a meta-analysis focused on determining if low-dose dopamine reduced the severity of acute renal failure, the need for dialysis, or mortality in critically-ill patients. They concluded that the use of low-dose dopamine for the treatment or prevention of acute renal failure cannot be justified. A more recent randomized, double-blind, placebo-controlled trial came to a similar conclusion (Australian and New Zealand Intensive Care Society Clinical Trials Group, 2000). This study enrolled over 300 ICU patients with clinical evidence of renal dysfunction. They were randomized to low-dose dopamine (2 mcg/kg/minute) or placebo. The investigators found no difference in serum creatinine, renal replacement therapy, intensive care length of stay, hospital stay, or mortality between the groups.

Septic Shock: In septic shock, dopamine is effective in increasing mean arterial pressure in patients who remain hypotensive after adequate volume expansion. Undesirable effects include tachycardia; increased pulmonary shunt, and decreased P_aO_2. As catecholamine stores are depleted, tachyphylaxis may occur. The 1999 ACCM/SCCM Practice Parameters for Hemodynamic Support of Sepsis in Adult Patients recommends either dopamine or norepinephrine as vasopressor therapy. Norepinephrine has a wider dosage range than dopamine.

Administration

I.V.: Vesicant. **Must be diluted prior to use**. Do not discontinue suddenly - sudden discontinuation may lead to marked hypotension.

Compatibility: Stable in D_5LR, $D_5{}^1/_2NS$, D_5NS, D_5W, $D_{10}W$, LR, mannitol 20%, NS; **incompatible** with sodium bicarbonate 5%, and alkaline solutions or iron salts.

Y-site administration: Incompatible with acyclovir, alteplase, amphotericin B cholesteryl sulfate complex, cefepime, indomethacin, insulin (regular), thiopental

Compatibility when admixed: Incompatible with acyclovir, alteplase, amphotericin B, ampicillin, metronidazole with sodium bicarbonate, penicillin G potassium

Storage: Protect from light. Solutions that are darker than slightly yellow should not be used.

♦ **Dopamine Hydrochloride** *see* DOPamine *on page 565*

♦ **Dopram®** *see* Doxapram *on page 572*

♦ **Doryx®** *see* Doxycycline *on page 584*

Dorzolamide (dor ZOLE a mide)

U.S. Brand Names Trusopt®

Synonyms Dorzolamide Hydrochloride

Pharmacologic Category Carbonic Anhydrase Inhibitor; Ophthalmic Agent, Antiglaucoma

Use Lowers intraocular pressure in patients with ocular hypertension or open-angle glaucoma

Mechanism of Action Reversible inhibition of the enzyme carbonic anhydrase resulting in reduction of hydrogen ion secretion at renal tubule and an increased renal excretion of sodium, potassium, bicarbonate, and water to decrease production of aqueous humor; also inhibits carbonic anhydrase in central nervous system to retard abnormal and excessive discharge from CNS neurons

(Continued)

Dorzolamide *(Continued)*

Pharmacodynamics/Kinetics

Onset of action: Peak effect: 2 hours

Duration: 8-12 hours

Absorption: Topical: Reaches systemic circulation where it accumulates in RBCs during chronic dosing as a result of binding to CA-11

Distribution: In RBCs during chronic administration

Protein binding: 33%

Metabolism: To N-desethyl metabolite (less potent than parent drug)

Half-life elimination: Terminal RBC: 147 days; washes out of RBCs nonlinearly, resulting in a rapid decline of drug concentration initially, followed by a slower elimination phase with a half-life of about 4 months

Excretion: Urine (as unchanged drug and metabolite, N-desethyl)

Contraindications Hypersensitivity to dorzolamide or any component of the formulation

Warnings/Precautions Although administered topically, systemic absorption occurs. Similar adverse reactions attributed to sulfonamides may occur with topical administration. Chemical similarities are present among sulfonamides, sulfonylureas, carbonic anhydrase inhibitors, thiazides, and loop diuretics (except ethacrynic acid). In patients with allergy to one of these compounds, a risk of cross-reaction exists; avoid use when previous reaction has been severe.

Because dorzolamide and its metabolite are excreted predominantly by the kidney, it is not recommended for use in patients with severe renal impairment (Cl_{cr} <30 mL/minute); use with caution in patients with hepatic impairment. Local ocular adverse effects (conjunctivitis and lid reactions) were reported with chronic administration. Many resolved with discontinuation of drug therapy. If such reactions occur, discontinue dorzolamide. Choriodal detachment has been reported after filtration procedures.

Contains benzalkonium chloride which may be absorbed by soft contact lenses. Dorzolamide should not be administered while wearing soft contact lenses. Safety and efficacy have not been established in children <2 years of age.

Drug Interactions Substrate (minor) of CYP2C8/9, 3A4

Salicylates: High-dose salicylate therapy may result in carbonic anhydrase inhibitor accumulation and toxicity including CNS depression and metabolic acidosis; avoid use if possible.

Adverse Reactions

>10%:

Gastrointestinal: Bitter taste following administration (25%)

Ocular: Burning, stinging or discomfort immediately following administration (33%); superficial punctate keratitis (10% to 15%); signs and symptoms of ocular allergic reaction (10%)

1% to 5%: Ocular: Blurred vision, conjunctivitis, dryness, lid reactions, photophobia, tearing

<1% (Limited to important or life-threatening): Allergic reaction (systemic), angioedema, bronchospasm, choriodal detachment (following filtration procedures), fatigue, headache, iridocyclitis (rare), nausea, paresthesia, rash (rare), urolithiasis, weakness, xerostomia

Overdosage/Toxicology

Symptoms of overdose include electrolyte imbalance, development of an acidotic state and possible CNS effects. Treatment should be symptom-directed and supportive.

Dosing

Adults & Elderly: Reduction of intraocular pressure: Ophthalmic: Instill 1 drop in the affected eye(s) 3 times/day

Pediatrics: Refer to adult dosing.

Available Dosage Forms Solution, ophthalmic, as hydrochloride: 2% (5 mL, 10 mL) [contains benzalkonium chloride]

Nursing Guidelines

Assessment: Assess potential for interactions with other prescriptions, OTC medications, or herbal products patient may be taking. Assess therapeutic response and adverse effects. Teach patient proper use, side effects/appropriate interventions, and symptoms to report.

Patient Education: For use in eyes only. If serious or unusual reactions or signs of hypersensitivity occur, discontinue use of the product. If any ocular reactions, particularly conjunctivitis and lid reactions, discontinue use and notify prescriber. If an intercurrent ocular condition (eg, trauma, ocular surgery, infection) occur, immediately seek your prescriber's advice concerning the continued use of the present multidose container. Avoid allowing the tip of the dispensing container to contact the eye or surrounding structures. Take out contact lenses before using medicine. Lenses can be replaced 15 minutes after medicine is given. **Pregnancy precaution:** Inform prescriber if you are pregnant.

Pregnancy Risk Factor: C

Lactation: Excretion in breast milk unknown/not recommended

Administration

Storage: Store at room temperature (25°C).

Dorzolamide and Timolol (dor ZOLE a mide & TYE moe lole)

U.S. Brand Names Cosopt®

Synonyms Timolol and Dorzolamide

Pharmacologic Category Beta-Adrenergic Blocker; Carbonic Anhydrase Inhibitor

Use Reduction of intraocular pressure in patients with ocular hypertension or open-angle glaucoma

Pharmacodynamics/Kinetics See individual agents.

Contraindications Hypersensitivity to dorzolamide, timolol, or any component of the formulation; sinus bradycardia, sinus node dysfunction, heart block greater than first degree (except in patients with a functioning artificial pacemaker); cardiogenic shock; uncompensated cardiac failure; bronchospastic disease or asthma; severe COPD. Also see individual agents.

Warnings/Precautions Contains a sulfonamide moiety; use with caution in patients allergic to sulfa. Not recommended for use in patients with severe renal impairment (Cl_{cr} <30 mL/minute). Use with caution in patients with hepatic impairment. Local ocular adverse effects (conjunctivitis and lid reactions) were reported with chronic administration; many resolved upon discontinuation of drug therapy. Choroidal detachment has been reported after filtration procedures.

Use with caution in heart failure and monitor for a worsening of the condition; discontinue if worsening cardiovascular function. Gradually taper therapy (particularly in patients with CAD) to avoid acute cardiovascular reactions (eg, tachycardia, hypertension, and/or ischemia). Use caution with concurrent verapamil or diltiazem; bradycardia or heart block can occur. Beta-blockers can aggravate symptoms in patients with PVD. Avoid use in patients with bronchospastic disease. May mask prominent hypoglycemic symptoms; use with caution in diabetics. May mask signs of thyrotoxicosis. Use care with anesthetic agents which decrease myocardial function. Can worsen myasthenia gravis.

Product contains benzalkonium chloride which may be absorbed by soft contact lenses; do not administer while wearing soft contact lenses.

Also see individual agents.

Drug Interactions

Dorzolamide: **Substrate** (minor) of CYP2C8/9, 3A4

Timolol: **Substrate** of CYP2D6 (major); **Inhibits** CYP2D6 (weak)

Also see individual agents.

Adverse Reactions Percentages as reported with combination product. Also see individual agents.

>5%:

Gastrointestinal: Taste perversion (≤30%)

Ocular: Burning/stinging (≤30%), conjunctival hyperemia (5% to 15%), blurred vision (5% to 15%), superficial punctuate keratitis (5% to 15%), itching (5% to 15%)

1% to 5%:

Cardiovascular: Hypertension

Central nervous system: Dizziness, headache

Gastrointestinal: Abdominal pain, dyspepsia, nausea

Genitourinary: UTI

Neuromuscular & skeletal: Back pain

Ocular: Blepharitis, cloudy vision, conjunctival discharge, conjunctival edema, conjunctival follicles, conjunctivitis, corneal erosion, corneal staining, cortical lens opacity, dryness, eye debris, eye/eyelid discharge, eye/eyelid pain, eye debris, eye/eyelid discharge, eye/eyelid pain, tearing, eyelid edema, eyelid erythema, foreign body sensation, glaucomatous cupping, lens nucleus discoloration, lens opacity, post-capsular cataract, tearing, visual field defect, vitreous detachment

Respiratory: Bronchitis, cough, sinusitis, URTI

(Continued)

Dorzolamide and Timolol *(Continued)*

Miscellaneous: Flu

<1%, postmarketing, and/or case reports: Bradycardia, cardiac failure, cerebral vascular accident, chest pain, choroidal detachment, depression, diarrhea, dyspnea, heart block, hypotension, iridocyclitis, MI, nasal congestion, paresthesia, photophobia, respiratory failure, skin rash, urolithiasis, vomiting, xerostomia

Overdosage/Toxicology

Symptoms of overdose may include electrolyte imbalance, cardiac effects (eg, bradycardia), acidosis, CNS effects, and respiratory effects (eg, bronchospasm). Treatment should be symptom-directed and supportive. Also refer to individual agents.

Dosing

Adults & Elderly: Ocular hypertension or open-angle glaucoma: Ophthalmic: Instill 1 drop in affected eye(s) twice daily

Pediatrics:

Ocular hypertension or open-angle glaucoma:Ophthalmic: Children ≥2 years: Refer to adult dosing.

Available Dosage Forms Solution, ophthalmic: Dorzolamide hydrochloride 2% (as base) and timolol maleate 0.5% (as base) (5 mL, 10 mL) [contains benzalkonium chloride]

Nursing Guidelines

Patient Education: See individual agents.

Pregnancy Risk Factor: C

Lactation:

Excreted in breast milk (timolol)/not recommended

Breast-Feeding Considerations:

Timolol is excreted in breast milk following oral and ophthalmic administration, and is considered compatible by the AAP. However, it is unknown whether dorzolamide is also excreted. Therefore, use of the combination product during lactation cannot be recommended at this time.

Administration

Storage: Store at 15°C to 30°C (59°F to 86°F). Protect from light.

♦ Dorzolamide Hydrochloride *see* Dorzolamide *on page 567*
♦ DOS® [OTC] *see* Docusate *on page 560*
♦ DOSS *see* Docusate *on page 560*

Doxacurium (doks a KYOO ri um)

U.S. Brand Names Nuromax®

Synonyms Doxacurium Chloride

Pharmacologic Category Neuromuscular Blocker Agent, Nondepolarizing

Medication Safety Issues

Sound-alike/look-alike issues:

Doxacurium may be confused with doxapram, DOXOrubicin

Use Adjunct to general anesthesia to facilitate endotracheal intubation and to relax skeletal muscles during surgery; to facilitate mechanical ventilation in ICU patients; does not relieve pain or produce sedation; the characteristics of this agent make it especially useful in procedures requiring careful maintenance of hemodynamic stability for prolonged periods

Mechanism of Action Prevents depolarization of muscle membrane and subsequent muscle contraction by acting as a competitive antagonist to acetylcholine at the alpha subunits of the nicotinic cholinergic receptors on the motor endplates in skeletal muscle, also interferes with the mobilization of acetylcholine presynaptically; the neuromuscular blockade can be pharmacologically reversed with an anticholinesterase agent (neostigmine, edrophonium, pyridostigmine)

Pharmacodynamics/Kinetics

Onset of action: 5-11 minutes

Duration: 30 minutes (range: 12-54 minutes)

Protein binding: 30%

Excretion: Primarily urine and feces (as unchanged drug); recovery time prolonged in elderly

Contraindications Hypersensitivity to doxacurium or any component of the formulation

Warnings/Precautions Use with caution in the elderly, effects and duration are more variable; product contains benzyl alcohol, use with caution in newborns; use with caution in patients with renal or hepatic impairment; certain clinical conditions may result in potentiation or antagonism of neuromuscular blockade:

Potentiation: Electrolyte abnormalities, severe hyponatremia, severe hypocalcemia, severe hypokalemia, hypermagnesemia, neuromuscular diseases, acidosis, acute intermittent porphyria, renal failure, hepatic failure

Antagonism: Alkalosis, hypercalcemia, demyelinating lesions, peripheral neuropathies, diabetes mellitus

Increased sensitivity in patients with myasthenia gravis, Eaton-Lambert syndrome; resistance in burn patients (>30% of body) for period of 5-70 days postinjury; resistance in patients with muscle trauma, denervation, immobilization, infection; does not counteract bradycardia produced by anesthetics/vagal stimulation. Cross-sensitivity with other neuromuscular-blocking agents may occur; use extreme caution in patients with previous anaphylactic reactions.

Drug Interactions

Decreased effect: Phenytoin, carbamazepine (decreases neuromuscular blockade)

Increased effect: Magnesium, lithium

Prolonged neuromuscular blockade: Corticosteroids, inhaled anesthetics, local anesthetics, calcium channel blockers; antiarrhythmics (eg, quinidine or procainamide); antibiotics (eg, aminoglycosides, tetracyclines, vancomycin, clindamycin); immunosuppressants (eg, cyclosporine)

Adverse Reactions <1% (Limited to important or life-threatening): Acute quadriplegic myopathy syndrome (prolonged use), diplopia, fever, hypotension, myositis ossificans (prolonged use), respiratory insufficiency and apnea, skeletal muscle weakness, urticaria, wheezing; **produces little, if any, histamine release**,

Overdosage/Toxicology

Overdosage is manifested by prolonged neuromuscular blockage.

Treatment is supportive; reverse blockade with neostigmine, pyridostigmine, or edrophonium.

Dosing

Adults & Elderly: Administer I.V.; dose to effect; doses will vary due to interpatient variability; use ideal body weight for obese patients.

Surgery (adjunct to anesthesia): I.V.: 0.05-0.08 mg/kg with thiopental/narcotic or 0.025 mg/kg after initial dose of succinylcholine for intubation; initial maintenance dose of 0.005-0.01 mg/kg after 100-160 minutes followed by repeat doses every 30-45 minutes

Pretreatment/priming: I.V.: 10% of intubating dose given 3-5 minutes before initial dose

Neuromuscular blockade in the ICU : I.V.: 0.05 mg/kg bolus followed by 0.025 mg/kg every 2-3 hours or 0.25-0.75 mcg/kg/minute once initial recovery from bolus dose observed

Pediatrics: Note: Administer I.V.; dose to effect; doses will vary due to interpatient variability; use ideal body weight for obese patients

Surgery (adjunct to anesthesia): Children >2 years: I.V.: Initial: 0.03-0.05 mg/kg followed by maintenance doses of 0.005-0.01 mg/kg after 30-45 minutes

Renal Impairment: Reduce initial dose and titrate carefully as duration may be prolonged.

Available Dosage Forms Injection, solution, as chloride: 1 mg/mL (5 mL) [contains benzyl alcohol]

Nursing Guidelines

Assessment: Only clinicians experienced in the use of neuromuscular-blocking drugs should administer and/or manage the use of doxacurium. Dosage and rate of administration should be individualized and titrated to the desired effect, according to relevant clinical factors, premedication, concomitant medications, age, and general condition of the patient. Ventilatory support must be instituted and maintained until adequate respiratory muscle function and/or airway protection are assured. Assess other medications for effectiveness and safety. Other drugs that affect neuromuscular activity may increase/decrease neuromuscular block induced by doxacurium. This drug does not cause anesthesia or analgesia; pain must be treated with appropriate analgesic agents. Continuous monitoring of vital signs, cardiac status, respiratory status, and degree of neuromuscular block (objective assessment with peripheral external nerve stimulator) is mandatory during infusion and until full muscle tone has returned. Muscle tone returns in a predictable pattern, starting with diaphragm, abdomen, chest,

(Continued)

Doxacurium *(Continued)*

limbs, and finally muscles of the neck, face, and eyes. Safety precautions must be maintained until full muscle tone has returned. **Note:** It may take longer for return of muscle tone in obese or elderly patients or patients with renal or hepatic disease, myasthenia gravis, myopathy, other neuromuscular disease, dehydration, electrolyte imbalance, or severe acid/base imbalance. Provide appropriate patient teaching/support prior to and following administration.

Long-term use: Monitor fluid levels (intake and output) during and following infusion. Reposition patient and provide appropriate skin care, mouth care, and care of patient's eyes every 2-3 hours while sedated. Provide appropriate emotional and sensory support (auditory and environmental).

Patient Education: Patient will usually be unconscious prior to administration. Patient education should be appropriate to individual situation. Reassurance of constant monitoring and emotional support to reduce fear and anxiety should precede and follow administration. Following return of muscle tone, do not attempt to change position or rise from bed without assistance. Report immediately any skin rash or hives, pounding heartbeat, respiratory difficulty, or muscle tremors. **Pregnancy precaution:** Inform prescriber if you are pregnant.

Pregnancy Risk Factor: C

Perioperative/Anesthesia/Other Concerns: Doxacurium is classified as a long-acting nondepolarizing, neuromuscular blocker with virtually no cardiovascular side effects; characteristics of this agent make it especially useful in procedures requiring careful maintenance of hemodynamic stability for prolonged periods; reduce dosage in renal impairment.

Critically-Ill Adult Patients: The 2002 ACCM/SCCM/ASHP clinical practice guidelines for sustained neuromuscular blockade in the adult critically-ill patient recommend:

Optimize sedatives and analgesics prior to initiation and monitor and adjust accordingly during course. Neuromuscular blockers do not relieve pain or produce sedation.

Protect patient's eyes from development of keratitis and corneal abrasion by administering ophthalmic ointment and taping eyelids closed or using eye patches. Reposition patient routinely to protect pressure points from breakdown. Address DVT prophylaxis.

Concurrent use of a neuromuscular blocker and corticosteroids appear to increase the risk of certain ICU myopathies; avoid or administer the corticosteroid at the lowest dose possible. Reassess need for neuromuscular blocker daily.

Using daily drug holidays (stopping neuromuscular-blocking agent until patient requires it again) may decrease the incidence of acute quadriplegic myopathy syndrome.

Tachyphylaxis can develop; switch to another neuromuscular blocker (taking into consideration the patient's organ function) if paralysis is still necessary.

Atracurium or cisatracurium is recommended for patients with significant hepatic or renal disease, due to organ-independent Hofmann elimination.

Monitor patients clinically and via "Train of Four" (TOF) testing with a goal of adjusting the degree of blockade to 1-2 twitches or based upon the patient's clinical condition.

Administration

I.V.: May be given rapid I.V. injection undiluted or via a continuous infusion using an infusion pump. Use infusion solutions within 24 hours of preparation.

Compatibility: Stable in D_5LR, D_5NS, D_5W, LR, NS

Storage: Stable for 24 hours at room temperature when diluted, up to 0.1 mg/mL in dextrose 5% or normal saline.

♦ Doxacurium Chloride *see* Doxacurium *on page 570*

Doxapram (DOKS a pram)

U.S. Brand Names Dopram®

Synonyms Doxapram Hydrochloride

Pharmacologic Category Respiratory Stimulant; Stimulant

Medication Safety Issues

Sound-alike/look-alike issues:

Doxapram may be confused with doxacurium, doxazosin, doxepin, Doxinate®, DOXOrubicin

Dopram® may be confused with DOPamine

Use Respiratory and CNS stimulant for respiratory depression secondary to anesthesia, drug-induced CNS depression; acute hypercapnia secondary to COPD

Mechanism of Action Stimulates respiration through action on respiratory center in medulla or indirectly on peripheral carotid chemoreceptors

Pharmacodynamics/Kinetics

Onset of action: Respiratory stimulation: I.V.: 20-40 seconds

Peak effect: 1-2 minutes

Duration: 5-12 minutes

Half-life elimination, serum: Adults: Mean: 3.4 hours

Contraindications Hypersensitivity to doxapram or any component of the formulation; cardiovascular disease, cerebral edema, cerebral vascular accident, epilepsy, head injury, hyperthyroidism, mechanical disorders of ventilation, mechanical ventilation or neuromuscular blockade, pheochromocytoma, pulmonary embolism, or severe hypertension

Warnings/Precautions Adequate airway required; consider airway protection in case of vomiting. Rapid infusion may result in hemolysis. Solution contains benzyl alcohol; not for use in neonates. If patient has received anesthesia with a volatile agent known to sensitize the myocardium to catecholamines, avoid use of doxapram until anesthetic has been eliminated. Use with caution in hepatic or renal dysfunction. Use with caution in patients with cerebral disease; lowered pCO_2 induced by hyperventilation produces cerebral vasoconstriction and decreased circulation. Use with caution in treating pulmonary disease; a pressor effect on pulmonary circulation may result in a fall in arterial pO_2. May cause severe CNS toxicity, seizures. Doxapram is neither a nonspecific CNS depressant antagonist nor an opiate antagonist. Resuscitative equipment (in addition to anticonvulsants and oxygen) should be readily available. Safety and efficacy have not been established in children <12 years of age.

Drug Interactions

Inhaled anesthetics: Halothane, cyclopropane, and enflurane may sensitize the myocardium to catecholamine and epinephrine which is released at the initiation of doxapram, hence, separate discontinuation of anesthetics and start of doxapram until the volatile agent has been excreted.

MAO inhibitors: May increase increase hypertensive effect when used with doxapram.

Sympathomimetics: May increase hypertensive effect when used with doxapram.

Adverse Reactions Frequency not defined.

Cardiovascular: Arrhythmia, blood pressure increased, chest pain, chest tightness, flushing, heart rate changes, T waves lowered, ventricular tachycardia, ventricular fibrillation

Central nervous system: Apprehension, Babinski turns positive, disorientation, dizziness, hallucinations, headache, hyperactivity, pyrexia, seizure

Dermatologic: Burning sensation, pruritus

Gastrointestinal: Defecation urge, diarrhea, nausea, vomiting

Genitourinary: Spontaneous voiding, urinary retention

Hematologic: Hematocrit decreased, hemoglobin decreased, hemolysis, red blood cell count decreased

Local: Phlebitis

Neuromuscular & skeletal: Clonus, deep tendon reflexes increase, fasciculations, involuntary muscle movement, muscle spasm, paresthesia

Ocular: Pupillary dilatation

Renal: Albuminuria, BUN increased

Respiratory: Bronchospasm, cough, dyspnea, hiccups, hyperventilation, laryngospasm, rebound hypoventilation, tachypnea

Miscellaneous: Diaphoresis

Overdosage/Toxicology Symptoms of overdose include excessive increases in blood pressure, tachycardia, arrhythmias, muscle spasticity, dyspnea, agitation, confusion, sweating, cough, and enhanced deep tendon reflexes. Supportive care is the preferred treatment. Seizures are unlikely and can be treated with benzodiazepines. Doxapram is not dialyzable.

Dosing

Adults & Elderly:

Respiratory depression following anesthesia:

Intermittent injection: Initial: 0.5-1 mg/kg; may repeat at 5-minute intervals (only in patients who demonstrate initial response); maximum total dose: 2 mg/kg

I.V. infusion: Initial: 5 mg/minute until adequate response or adverse effects seen; decrease to 1-3 mg/minute; maximum total dose: 4 mg/kg

(Continued)

Doxapram *(Continued)*

Drug-induced CNS depression:

Intermittent injection: Initial: Priming dose of 1-2 mg/kg; repeat after 5 minutes; may repeat at 1-2 hour intervals (until sustained consciousness); maximum 3 g/day. May repeat in 24 hours if necessary.

I.V. infusion: Initial: Priming dose of 1-2 mg/kg repeated in 5 minutes. If no response, wait 1-2 hours and repeat. If some stimulation is noted, initiate infusion at 1-3 mg/minute (depending on size of patient/depth of CNS depression); suspend infusion if patient begins to awaken. Infusion should not be continued for >2 hours. May reinstitute infusion as described above, including bolus, after rest interval of 30 minutes to 2 hours; maximum: 3 g/day

Acute hypercapnia secondary to COPD: I.V. infusion: Initial: Initiate infusion at 1-2 mg/minute (depending on size of patient/depth of CNS depression); may increase to maximum rate of 3 mg/minute; infusion should not be continued for >2 hours. Monitor arterial blood gases prior to initiation of infusion and at 30-minute intervals during the infusion (to identify possible development of acidosis/CO_2 retention). Additional infusions are not recommended (per manufacturer).

Available Dosage Forms Injection, solution, as hydrochloride: 20 mg/mL (20 mL) [contains benzyl alcohol]

Nursing Guidelines

Patient Education: This drug is generally used in an emergency. Teaching should be appropriate to patient education. Someone will be observing response at all times. **Breast-feeding precaution:** Consult prescriber if breast-feeding.

Pregnancy Risk Factor: B

Lactation: Excretion in breast milk unknown/use caution

Perioperative/Anesthesia/Other Concerns: Because of doxapram's transient effect, doxapram should not be used as a drug of choice to treat anesthesia-induced respiratory depression. Initial studies suggest a therapeutic range of at least 1.5 mg/L. Toxicity becomes frequent at serum levels >5 mg/L.

Administration

I.V.: Avoid rapid infusion.

Reconstitution:

Drug-induced CNS depression or post-anesthesia: Mix doxapram 250 mg in 250 mL of D_5W, $D_{10}W$, or NS

COPD-associated hypercapnia: Mix doxapram 400 mg in 180 mL of D_5W, $D_{10}W$, or NS (final concentration: 2 mg/mL)

Compatibility: Stable in D_5W, $D_{10}W$, NS

Compatibility in syringe: Incompatible with aminophylline, ascorbic acid injection, cefoperazone, cefotaxime, cefotetan, cefuroxime, dexamethasone sodium phosphate, diazepam, digoxin, dobutamine, folic acid, furosemide, hydrocortisone sodium phosphate, hydrocortisone sodium succinate, ketamine, methylprednisolone sodium succinate, minocycline, thiopental, ticarcillin

Compatibility when admixed: Incompatible with aminophylline, sodium bicarbonate, thiopental

Storage: Store at 20°C to 25°C (68°F to 77°F).

♦ **Doxapram Hydrochloride** *see* Doxapram *on page 572*

Doxazosin (doks AY zoe sin)

U.S. Brand Names Cardura®

Synonyms Doxazosin Mesylate

Pharmacologic Category Alpha$_1$ Blocker

Medication Safety Issues

Sound-alike/look-alike issues:

Doxazosin may be confused with doxapram, doxepin, DOXOrubicin

Cardura® may be confused with Cardene®, Cordarone®, Cordran®, Coumadin®, K-Dur®, Ridaura®

Use Treatment of hypertension alone or in conjunction with diuretics, cardiac glycosides, ACE inhibitors, or calcium antagonists (particularly appropriate for those with hypertension and other cardiovascular risk factors such as hypercholesterolemia and diabetes mellitus); treatment of urinary outflow obstruction and/or obstructive and irritative symptoms associated with benign prostatic hyperplasia (BPH), particularly useful in patients with troublesome symptoms who are unable or unwilling to undergo invasive procedures, but who require rapid symptomatic relief; can be used in combination with finasteride

Mechanism of Action Competitively inhibits postsynaptic alpha-adrenergic receptors which results in vasodilation of veins and arterioles and a decrease in total peripheral resistance and blood pressure; approximately 50% as potent on a weight by weight basis as prazosin

Pharmacodynamics/Kinetics Not significantly affected by increased age

Duration: >24 hours

Metabolism: Extensively hepatic

Half-life elimination: 22 hours

Time to peak, serum: 2-3 hours

Excretion: Feces (63%); urine (9%)

Contraindications Hypersensitivity to quinazolines (prazosin, terazosin), doxazosin, or any component of the formulation; concurrent use with phosphodiesterase-5 (PDE-5) inhibitors including sildenafil (>25 mg), tadalafil, or vardenafil

Warnings/Precautions Can cause significant orthostatic hypotension and syncope, especially with first dose. Prostate cancer should be ruled out before starting for BPH. May need dosage adjustment in severe hepatic dysfunction. Anticipate a similar effect if therapy is interrupted for a few days, if dosage is rapidly increased, or if another antihypertensive drug is introduced.

Drug Interactions

ACE inhibitors: Hypotensive effect may be increased.

Beta-blockers: Hypotensive effect may be increased.

Calcium channel blockers: Hypotensive effect may be increased.

NSAIDs may reduce antihypertensive efficacy.

Sildenafil, tadalafil, vardenafil: Blood pressure-lowering effects are additive. Use of tadalafil or vardenafil is contraindicated by the manufacturer. Use sildenafil with extreme caution (dose ≤25 mg).

Nutritional/Herbal/Ethanol Interactions Herb/Nutraceutical: Avoid dong quai if using for hypertension (has estrogenic activity). Avoid ephedra, yohimbe, ginseng (may worsen hypertension). Avoid saw palmetto when used for BPH (due to limited experience with this combination). Avoid garlic (may have increased antihypertensive effect).

Lab Interactions Increased urinary VMA 17%, norepinephrine metabolite 42%

Adverse Reactions Note: "Combination therapy" refers to doxazosin and finasteride.

>10%:

- Cardiovascular: Postural hypotension (combination therapy 18%)
- Central nervous system: Dizziness (16% to 19%; combination therapy 23%), headache (10% to 14%)
- Endocrine & metabolic: Impotence (combination therapy 23%), libido decreased (combination therapy 12%)
- Genitourinary: Ejaculation disturbances (combination therapy 14%)
- Neuromuscular & skeletal: Weakness (combination therapy 17%)

1% to 10%:

- Cardiovascular: Orthostatic hypotension (dose related; 0.3% up to 10%), edema (3% to 4%), hypotension (2%), palpitation (1% to 2%), chest pain (1% to 2%), arrhythmia (1%), syncope (2%), flushing (1%)
- Central nervous system: Fatigue (8% to 12%), somnolence (3% to 5%), nervousness (2%), pain (2%), vertigo (2%), insomnia (1%), anxiety (1%), paresthesia (1%), movement disorder (1%), ataxia (1%), hypertonia (1%), depression (1%), weakness (1%)
- Dermatologic: Rash (1%), pruritus (1%)
- Endocrine & metabolic: Sexual dysfunction (2%)
- Gastrointestinal: Abdominal pain (2%), diarrhea (2%), dyspepsia (1% to 2%), nausea (2% to 3%), xerostomia (1% to 2%), constipation (1%), flatulence (1%)
- Genitourinary: Urinary tract infection (1%), impotence (1%), polyuria (2%), incontinence (1%)
- Neuromuscular & skeletal: Back pain (2%), arthritis (1%), muscle weakness (1%), myalgia (1%), muscle cramps (1%)
- Ocular: Abnormal vision (1% to 2%), conjunctivitis (1%)
- Otic: Tinnitus (1%)
- Respiratory: Rhinitis (3%), dyspnea (1% to 3%), respiratory disorder (1%), epistaxis (1%)
- Miscellaneous: Diaphoresis increased (1%), flu-like syndrome (1%)

<1% (Limited to important or life-threatening): Agitation, alopecia, amnesia, angina, bronchospasm, cataplexy, depersonalization, eczema, emotional

(Continued)

Doxazosin *(Continued)*

lability, enuresis, fecal incontinence, fever, gout, hot flashes, impaired concentration, infection, leukopenia, MI, paranoia, paresis, peripheral ischemia, photophobia, purpura, renal calculus, rigors, stroke, syncope, systemic lupus erythematosus, urticaria

Overdosage/Toxicology Symptoms of overdose include severe hypotension, drowsiness, and tachycardia. Treatment is supportive and symptomatic.

Dosing

Adults: Hypertension or urinary outflow obstruction: Oral: 1 mg once daily in morning or evening; may be increased to 2 mg once daily; thereafter titrate upwards, if needed, over several weeks, balancing therapeutic benefit with doxazosin-induced postural hypotension; maximum dose for **hypertension**: 16 mg/day, for **BPH**: 8 mg/day (goal: 4-8 mg/day)

Elderly: Oral: Initial: 0.5 mg once daily

Available Dosage Forms Tablet: 1 mg, 2 mg, 4 mg, 8 mg

Nursing Guidelines

Assessment: See Contraindications and Warnings/Precautions for use cautions. Assess potential for interactions with other prescriptions, OTC medications, or herbal products patient may be taking (see Drug Interactions). Assess results of laboratory tests (see below), therapeutic effectiveness, and adverse reactions (see Adverse Reactions and Overdose/Toxicology) at beginning of therapy and on a regular basis with long-term therapy. When discontinuing, monitor blood pressure and taper dose slowly over 1 week or more. Teach patient proper use, possible side effects/appropriate interventions, and adverse symptoms to report (see Patient Education). Note breast-feeding caution.

Monitoring Laboratory Tests: White blood count

Patient Education: Inform prescriber of all prescriptions, OTC medications, or herbal products you are taking, and any allergies you have. Do not take any new medication during therapy unless approved by prescriber. Take as directed, at bedtime. Do not skip dose or discontinue without consulting prescriber. Follow recommended diet and exercise program. May cause drowsiness, dizziness, or impaired judgment (use caution when driving or engaging in tasks that require alertness until response to drug is known); postural hypotension (use caution when rising from sitting or lying position or when climbing stairs); or dry mouth or nausea (frequent mouth care or sucking lozenges may help). Report increased nervousness or depression; sudden weight gain (weigh yourself in the same clothes at the same time of day once a week); unusual or persistent swelling of ankles, feet, or extremities; palpitations or rapid heartbeat; muscle weakness, fatigue, or pain; or other persistent side effects. **Pregnancy/breast-feeding precautions:** Inform prescriber if you are or intend to become pregnant. Consult prescriber if breast-feeding.

Geriatric Considerations: Adverse reactions such as dry mouth and urinary problems can be particularly bothersome in the elderly.

Pregnancy Risk Factor: C

Lactation: Excretion in breast milk unknown

Administration

Oral: Syncope may occur usually within 90 minutes of the initial dose.

♦ **Doxazosin Mesylate** *see* Doxazosin *on page 574*

♦ **Doxidan® [DSC] [OTC]** *see* Docusate and Casanthranol *on page 561*

♦ **Doxidan®** ***(reformulation)*** **[OTC]** *see* Bisacodyl *on page 245*

♦ **Doxil®** *see* DOXOrubicin (Liposomal) *on page 580*

DOXOrubicin (doks oh ROO bi sin)

U.S. Brand Names Adriamycin PFS®; Adriamycin RDF®; Rubex®

Synonyms ADR (error-prone abbreviation); Adria; Doxorubicin Hydrochloride; Hydroxydaunomycin Hydrochloride; Hydroxyldaunorubicin Hydrochloride; NSC-123127

Pharmacologic Category Antineoplastic Agent, Anthracycline

Medication Safety Issues

Sound-alike/look-alike issues:

DOXOrubicin may be confused with dactinomycin, DAUNOrubicin, doxacurium, doxapram, doxazosin, epirubicin, idarubicin

Adriamycin PFS® may be confused with achromycin, Aredia®, Idamycin®

Rubex® may be confused with Robaxin®

Conventional formulations (Adriamycin PFS®, Adriamycin RDF®, Rubex®) may be confused with liposomal formulations (DaunoXome®, Doxil®)

ADR is an error-prone abbreviation

Use Treatment of leukemias, lymphomas, multiple myeloma, osseous and nonosseous sarcomas, mesotheliomas, germ cell tumors of the ovary or testis, and carcinomas of the head and neck, thyroid, lung, breast, stomach, pancreas, liver, ovary, bladder, prostate, uterus, and neuroblastoma

Mechanism of Action Inhibition of DNA and RNA synthesis by intercalation between DNA base pairs by inhibition of topoisomerase II and by steric obstruction. Doxorubicin intercalates at points of local uncoiling of the double helix. Although the exact mechanism is unclear, it appears that direct binding to DNA (intercalation) and inhibition of DNA repair (topoisomerase II inhibition) result in blockade of DNA and RNA synthesis and fragmentation of DNA. Doxorubicin is also a powerful iron chelator; the iron-doxorubicin complex can bind DNA and cell membranes and produce free radicals that immediately cleave the DNA and cell membranes.

Pharmacodynamics/Kinetics

Absorption: Oral: Poor (<50%)

Distribution: V_d: 25 L/kg; to many body tissues, particularly liver, spleen, kidney, lung, heart; does not distribute into the CNS; crosses placenta

Protein binding, plasma: 70%

Metabolism: Primarily hepatic to doxorubicinol (active), then to inactive aglycones, conjugated sulfates, and glucuronides

Half-life elimination:

Distribution: 10 minutes

Elimination: Doxorubicin: 1-3 hours; Metabolites: 3-3.5 hours

Terminal: 17-30 hours

Male: 54 hours; Female: 35 hours

Excretion: Feces (~40% to 50% as unchanged drug); urine (~3% to 10% as metabolites, 1% doxorubicinol, <1% Adriamycin aglycones, and unchanged drug)

Clearance: Male: 113 L/hour; Female: 44 L/hour

Contraindications Hypersensitivity to doxorubicin or any component of the formulation; congestive heart failure or arrhythmias; previous therapy with high cumulative doses of doxorubicin and/or daunorubicin; pre-existing bone marrow suppression; pregnancy

Warnings/Precautions The U.S. Food and Drug Administration (FDA) currently recommends that procedures for proper handling and disposal of antineoplastic agents be considered. Use with caution in patients who have received radiation therapy or in the presence of hepatobiliary dysfunction; reduce dosage in patients who are receiving radiation therapy simultaneously. Administration of live vaccines to immunosuppressed patients may be hazardous.

Total dose should not exceed 550 mg/m^2 or 450 mg/m^2 in patients with previous or concomitant treatment with daunorubicin, cyclophosphamide, or irradiation of the cardiac region; irreversible myocardial toxicity may occur as total dosage approaches 550 mg/m^2. A baseline cardiac evaluation (ECG, LVEF, +/- ECHO) is recommended, especially in patients with risk factors for increased cardiac toxicity and in pediatric patients. Pediatric patients are at increased risk for delayed cardiotoxicity. Reduce dose in patients with impaired hepatic function; severe myelosuppression is also possible. Secondary acute myelogenous leukemia may occur following treatment.

I.V. use only. Doxorubicin is a potent vesicant; if extravasation occurs, severe tissue damage leading to ulceration and necrosis, and pain may occur.

Drug Interactions **Substrate** (major) of CYP2D6, 3A4; **Inhibits** CYP2B6 (moderate), 2D6 (weak), 3A4 (weak)

Allopurinol may enhance the antitumor activity of doxorubicin (animal data only).

Cyclophosphamide enhances the cardiac toxicity of doxorubicin by producing additional myocardial cell damage.

Cyclosporine may decrease clearance of parent and metabolite and may induce coma or seizures and enhance hematologic toxicity.

CYP2B6 substrates: Doxorubicin may increase the levels/effects of CYP2B6 substrates. Example substrates include bupropion, promethazine, propofol, selegiline, and sertraline.

CYP2D6 inhibitors: May increase the levels/effects of doxorubicin. Example inhibitors include chlorpromazine, delavirdine, fluoxetine, miconazole, paroxetine, pergolide, quinidine, quinine, ritonavir, and ropinirole.

(Continued)

DOXOrubicin *(Continued)*

CYP3A4 inducers: CYP3A4 inducers may decrease the levels/effects of doxorubicin. Example inducers include aminoglutethimide, carbamazepine, nafcillin, nevirapine, phenobarbital, phenytoin, and rifamycins.

CYP3A4 inhibitors: May increase the levels/effects of doxorubicin. Example inhibitors include azole antifungals, clarithromycin, diclofenac, doxycycline, erythromycin, imatinib, isoniazid, nefazodone, nicardipine, propofol, protease inhibitors, quinidine, telithromycin, and verapamil.

Digoxin: Doxorubicin may decrease plasma levels and effectiveness of digoxin.

Mercaptopurine increases toxicities.

Paclitaxel reduces doxorubicin clearance and increases toxicity if administered prior to doxorubicin.

Phenobarbital increases elimination (decreases effect) of doxorubicin.

Phenytoin: Doxorubicin may decrease plasma levels and effectiveness of phenytoin.

Progesterone: High doses of progesterone enhance toxicity (neutropenia and thrombocytopenia).

Streptozocin greatly enhances leukopenia and thrombocytopenia.

Verapamil alters the cellular distribution of doxorubicin and may result in increased cell toxicity by inhibition of the P-glycoprotein pump. Based on mouse studies, cardiotoxicity may be enhanced by verapamil.

Zidovudine: Doxorubicin may decrease the antiviral activity of zidovudine.

Nutritional/Herbal/Ethanol Interactions Herb/Nutraceutical: St John's wort may decrease doxorubicin levels. Avoid black cohosh, dong quai in estrogen-dependent tumors.

Adverse Reactions

>10%:

Cardiovascular: Transient ECG abnormalities (supraventricular tachycardia, S-T wave changes, atrial or ventricular extrasystoles); generally asymptomatic and self-limiting. CHF, dose related, may be delayed for 7-8 years after treatment. Cumulative dose, mediastinal/pericardial radiation therapy, cardiovascular disease, age, and use of cyclophosphamide (or other cardiotoxic agents) all increase the risk.

Recommended maximum cumulative doses:

No risk factors: 550 mg/m^2

Concurrent radiation: 450 mg/m^2

Note: Regardless of cumulative dose, if the left ventricular ejection fraction is <30% to 40%, the drug is usually not given.

Dermatologic: Alopecia

Gastrointestinal: Acute nausea and vomiting (21% to 55%), mucositis, ulceration, and necrosis of the colon, anorexia, and diarrhea, stomatitis, esophagitis

Genitourinary: Discoloration of urine (red)

Hematologic: Myelosuppression, leukopenia (75%), dose-limiting toxicity

WBC: Moderate

Platelets: Moderate

Onset (days): 7

Nadir (days): 10-14

Recovery (days): 21-28

Local: **Vesicant chemotherapy**

1% to 10%:

Cardiovascular: Acute: Arrhythmias, heart block, pericarditis-myocarditis, facial flushing; Delayed: CHF (related to cumulative dose; usually a maximum total lifetime dose of 450-550 mg/m^2; possibly higher if given by continuous infusion)

Dermatologic: Hyperpigmentation of nail beds, erythematous streaking along the vein if administered rapidly

Endocrine & metabolic: Hyperuricemia

<1% (Limited to important or life-threatening):

Pediatric patients may be at increased risk of later neoplastic disease, particularly acute myeloid leukemia (pediatric patients). Prepubertal growth failure may result from intensive chemotherapy regimens.

Radiation recall: Noticed in patients who have had prior irradiation; reactions include redness, warmth, erythema, and dermatitis in the radiation port. Can progress to severe desquamation and ulceration. Occurs 5-7 days after doxorubicin administration; local therapy with topical corticosteroids and cooling have given the best relief.

Overdosage/Toxicology Symptoms of overdose include myelosuppression, nausea, vomiting, and myocardial toxicity. Treatment of acute overdose consists of treatment of the severely myelosuppressed patient with hospitalization, antibiotics, platelet and granulocyte transfusions, and symptomatic treatment of mucositis.

Dosing

Adults & Elderly: Refer to individual protocols.

Usual or typical dose: I.V.: 60-75 mg/m^2 as a single dose, repeat every 21 days **or** other dosage regimens like 20-30 mg/m^2/day for 2-3 days, repeat in 4 weeks **or** 20 mg/m^2 once weekly.

Note: The lower dose regimen should be given to patients with decreased bone marrow reserve, prior therapy or marrow infiltration with malignant cells.

Pediatrics: Refer to individual protocols. Usual/typical dosages: I.V.:

Children:

35-75 mg/m^2 as a single dose, repeat every 21 days **or**

20-30 mg/m^2 once weekly **or**

60-90 mg/m^2 given as a continuous infusion over 96 hours every 3-4 weeks

Renal Impairment:

Adjustments are not required.

Hemodialysis effects: Supplemental dose is not necessary.

Hepatic Impairment:

ALT/AST 2-3 times ULN: Administer 75% of dose

ALT/AST >3 times ULN **or** bilirubin 1.2-3 mg/dL (20-51 μmol/L): Administer 50% of dose

Bilirubin 3.1-5 mg/dL (51-85 μmol/L): Administer 25% of dose

Bilirubin >5 mg/dL (85 μmol/L): Do not administer

Available Dosage Forms

Injection, powder for reconstitution, as hydrochloride: 10 mg, 20 mg, 50 mg [contains lactose]

Adriamycin RDF®: 10 mg, 20 mg, 50 mg, 150 mg [contains lactose; rapid dissolution formula]

Rubex®: 50 mg, 100 mg [contains lactose]

Injection, solution, as hydrochloride [preservative free]: 2 mg/mL (5 mL, 10 mL, 25 mL, 100 mL)

Adriamycin PFS® [preservative free]: 2 mg/mL (5 mL, 10 mL, 25 mL, 37.5 mL, 100 mL)

Nursing Guidelines

Assessment: See Contraindications, Warnings/Precautions, and Dosing for use cautions. Assess potential for interactions with other prescriptions, OTC medications, or herbal products patient may be taking (see Drug Interactions). See Administration, Dosing, Reconstitution, and Compatibility for administration specifics. Premedication with antiemetic is recommended (especially with larger doses). Infusion site must be closely monitored; extravasation can cause sloughing or tissue necrosis (see Extravasation Management). Assess results of laboratory tests (see below), therapeutic effectiveness, and adverse response (see Adverse Reactions and Overdose/Toxicology) prior to each treatment and on a regular basis throughout therapy. Teach patient possible side effects/appropriate interventions (eg, importance of adequate hydration) and adverse symptoms to report (see Patient Education). **Pregnancy risk factor D** - determine that patient is not pregnant before beginning treatment. Instruct patients of childbearing age on appropriate contraceptive measures. Breast-feeding is contraindicated.

Monitoring Laboratory Tests: CBC with differential, platelet count, cardiac and liver function

Patient Education: Inform prescriber of all prescriptions, OTC medications, or herbal products you are taking, and any allergies you have. Do not take any new medication during therapy unless approved by prescriber. This medication can only be administered intravenously. Report immediately any swelling, pain, burning, or redness at infusion site. Maintain adequate nutrition (small, frequent meals may help). You will be more susceptible to infection (avoid crowds and exposure to infection and do not have any vaccinations without consulting prescriber). May cause nausea or vomiting (small, frequent meals, frequent mouth care, sucking lozenges, or chewing gum may help); diarrhea (buttermilk, boiled milk, or yogurt may help); loss of hair (reversible); or darker yellow urine (normal). Report immediately chest pain, swelling of extremities, respiratory difficulty, palpitations, or rapid heartbeat. Report unresolved nausea, vomiting,

(Continued)

DOXOrubicin *(Continued)*

or diarrhea; alterations in urinary pattern (increased or decreased); opportunistic infection (fever, chills, unusual bruising or bleeding fatigue, purulent vaginal discharge, unhealed mouth sores); abdominal pain or blood in stools; excessive fatigue; or yellowing of eyes or skin. **Pregnancy/breast-feeding precautions:** Inform prescriber if you are pregnant. Do not get pregnant while taking this medication or for 1 month following therapy. Consult prescriber for appropriate barrier contraceptives. Do not breast-feed.

Pregnancy Risk Factor: D

Pregnancy Issues: Advise patients to avoid becoming pregnant (females) and to avoid causing pregnancy (males).

Lactation: Enters breast milk/contraindicated

Administration

I.V.: Vesicant. Administer I.V. push over 1-2 minutes or IVPB. Infusion via central venous line recommended.

Reconstitution: Reconstitute lyophilized powder with NS to a final concentration of 2 mg/mL as follows. Reconstituted solution is stable for 7 days at room temperature (25°C) and 15 days under refrigeration (5°C) when protected from light.

Further dilution in D_5W or NS is stable for 48 hours at room temperature (25°C) when protected from light.

Unstable in solutions with a pH <3 or >7. Avoid aluminum needles as precipitation or decomposition (darkening of solution) may occur; protect from direct sunlight.

Standard I.V. dilution:

I.V. push: Dose/syringe (concentration: 2 mg/mL)

Syringes are stable for 7 days at room temperature (25°C) and 15 days under refrigeration (5°C) when protected from light.

IVPB: Dose/50-100 mL D_5W or NS

IVPB solutions are stable for 48 hours at room temperature (25°C) when protected from light.

Compatibility: Stable in D_5W, LR, NS

Y-site administration: Incompatible with allopurinol, amphotericin B cholesteryl sulfate complex, cefepime, ganciclovir, piperacillin/tazobactam, propofol

Compatibility in syringe: Incompatible with furosemide, heparin

Compatibility when admixed: Incompatible with aminophylline, diazepam, fluorouracil

Storage: Store intact vials of solution under refrigeration at 2°C to 8°C and protected from light. Store intact vials of lyophilized powder at room temperature (15°C to 30°C).

♦ **Doxorubicin Hydrochloride** *see* DOXOrubicin *on page 576*

♦ **Doxorubicin Hydrochloride (Liposomal)** *see* DOXOrubicin (Liposomal) *on page 580*

DOXOrubicin (Liposomal) (doks oh ROO bi sin lip pah SOW mal)

U.S. Brand Names Doxil®

Synonyms Doxorubicin Hydrochloride (Liposomal)

Pharmacologic Category Antineoplastic Agent, Anthracycline

Medication Safety Issues

Sound-alike/look-alike issues:

DOXOrubicin may be confused with dactinomycin, DAUNOrubicin, doxacurium, doxapram, doxazosin, epirubicin, idarubicin

Doxil® may be confused with Doxy®, Paxil®

Liposomal formulations (Doxil®) may be confused with conventional formulations (Adriamycin PFS®, Adriamycin RDF®, Cerubidine®, Rubex®).

Use Treatment of AIDS-related Kaposi's sarcoma, breast cancer, ovarian cancer, solid tumors

Mechanism of Action Doxorubicin inhibits DNA and RNA synthesis by intercalating between DNA base pairs causing steric obstruction and inhibits topoisomerase-II at the point of DNA cleavage. Doxorubicin is also a powerful iron chelator. The iron-doxorubicin complex can bind DNA and cell membranes, producing free hydroxyl (OH) radicals that cleave DNA and cell membranes. Active throughout entire cell cycle.

Pharmacodynamics/Kinetics

Distribution: V_{dss}: 2.8 L/m^2

Protein binding, plasma: Unknown; nonliposomal doxorubicin 70%

Half-life elimination: Terminal: Distribution: 4.7-5.2 hours, Elimination: 44-55 hours

Metabolism: Hepatic and in plasma to doxorubicinol and the sulfate and glucuronide conjugates of 4-demethyl,7-deoxyaglycones

Excretion: Urine (5% as doxorubicin or doxorubicinol)

Clearance: Mean: 0.041 L/hour/m^2

Contraindications Hypersensitivity to doxorubicin, other anthracyclines, or any component of the formulation; breast-feeding, pregnancy

Warnings/Precautions The U.S. Food and Drug Administration (FDA) currently recommends that procedures for proper handling and disposal of antineoplastic agents be considered.

Doxorubicin is associated with dose-related myocardial damage leading to congestive heart failure. Doxorubicin and liposomal doxorubicin should be used cautiously in patients with high cumulative doses of anthracyclines, anthracenediones, and cyclophosphamide. Caution should also be used in patients with previous thoracic radiation or who have pre-existing cardiac disease. Total cumulative doses of anthracyclines, including liposomal doxorubicin and anthracenediones should not exceed 550 mg/m^2 or 400 mg/m^2 in patients with previous or concomitant treatment (with daunorubicin, cyclophosphamide, or irradiation of the cardiac region); irreversible myocardial toxicity may occur at these doses. Symptoms of anthracycline-induced CHF and/or cardiomyopathy may be delayed in onset (up to 7-8 years in some cases). For I.V. use only; local tissue irritation will result if extravasation occurs; reduce dose in patients with impaired hepatic function; severe myelosuppression is also possible. Acute infusion reactions may occur, some may be serious/life-threatening. Liposomal formulations of doxorubicin should not be substituted for doxorubicin hydrochloride on a mg-per-mg basis.

Hand-foot syndrome (palmar-plantar erythrodysesthesia) has been reported in up to 51% of patients with ovarian cancer (and significantly lower frequency in patients with Kaposi's sarcoma). May occur early in treatment, but is usually seen after 2-3 treatment cycles. Dosage modification may be required. In severe cases, treatment discontinuation may be required.

Drug Interactions **Substrate** (major) of CYP2D6, 3A4; **Inhibits** CYP2B6 (moderate), 2D6 (weak), 3A4 (weak)

Allopurinol may enhance the antitumor activity of doxorubicin (animal data only).

Cyclophosphamide enhances the cardiac toxicity of doxorubicin by producing additional myocardial cell damage.

Cyclosporine may decrease clearance of parent and metabolite and may induce coma or seizures and enhance hematologic toxicity.

CYP2B6 substrates: Doxorubicin may increase the levels/effects of CYP2B6 substrates. Example substrates include bupropion, promethazine, propofol, selegiline, and sertraline.

CYP2D6 inhibitors: May increase the levels/effects of doxorubicin. Example inhibitors include chlorpromazine, delavirdine, fluoxetine, miconazole, paroxetine, pergolide, quinidine, quinine, ritonavir, and ropinirole.

CYP3A4 inducers: CYP3A4 inducers may decrease the levels/effects of doxorubicin. Example inducers include aminoglutethimide, carbamazepine, nafcillin, nevirapine, phenobarbital, phenytoin, and rifamycins.

CYP3A4 inhibitors: May increase the levels/effects of doxorubicin. Example inhibitors include azole antifungals, clarithromycin, diclofenac, doxycycline, erythromycin, imatinib, isoniazid, nefazodone, nicardipine, propofol, protease inhibitors, quinidine, telithromycin, and verapamil.

Doxorubicin may decrease plasma levels and effectiveness of digoxin and phenytoin.

Mercaptopurine increases toxicities.

Paclitaxel reduces doxorubicin clearance and increases toxicity if administered prior to doxorubicin.

Phenobarbital increases elimination (decreases effect) of doxorubicin.

Progesterone: High doses of progesterone enhance toxicity (neutropenia and thrombocytopenia).

Streptozocin greatly enhances leukopenia and thrombocytopenia.

Verapamil alters the cellular distribution of doxorubicin and may result in increased cell toxicity by inhibition of the P-glycoprotein pump. Based on mouse studies, cardiotoxicity may be enhanced by verapamil.

Zidovudine: Doxorubicin may decrease the antiviral activity of zidovudine.

Nutritional/Herbal/Ethanol Interactions

Ethanol: Avoid ethanol (due to GI irritation).

(Continued)

DOXOrubicin (Liposomal) *(Continued)*

Herb/Nutraceutical: St John's wort may decrease doxorubicin levels. Avoid black cohosh, dong quai in estrogen-dependent tumors.

Adverse Reactions

>10%:

Cardiovascular: Peripheral edema (up to 11%)

Central nervous system: Fever (8% to 12%), headache (up to 11%), pain (up to 21%)

Dermatologic: Alopecia (9% to 19%); palmar-plantar erythrodysesthesia/hand-foot syndrome (up to 51% in ovarian cancer, 4% in Kaposi's sarcoma), rash (up to 29% in ovarian cancer, up to 5% in Kaposi's sarcoma)

Gastrointestinal: Stomatitis (5% to 41%), vomiting (8% to 33%), nausea (18% to 46%), mucositis (up to 14%), constipation (up to 30%), anorexia (up to 20%), diarrhea (5% to 21%), dyspepsia (up to 12%), intestinal obstruction (up to 11%)

Hematologic: Myelosuppression, neutropenia (12% to 62%), leukopenia (36%), thrombocytopenia (13% to 65%), anemia (6% to 74%)

Onset: 7 days

Nadir: 10-14 days

Recovery: 21-28 days

Neuromuscular & skeletal: Weakness (7% to 40%), back pain (up to 12%)

Respiratory: Pharyngitis (up to 16%), dyspnea (up to 15%)

1% to 10%:

Cardiovascular: Cardiac arrest, chest pain, edema, hypotension, pallor, tachycardia, vasodilation

Central nervous system: Agitation, anxiety, chills, confusion, depression, dizziness, emotional lability, insomnia, somnolence, vertigo

Dermatologic: Acne, dry skin (6%), dermatitis, furunculosis, herpes simplex/zoster, maculopapular rash, pruritus, rash, skin discoloration, vesiculobullous rash

Endocrine & metabolic: Dehydration, hyperbilirubinemia, hyperglycemia, hypocalcemia, hypokalemia, hyponatremia

Gastrointestinal: Abdomen enlarged, ascites, cachexia, dyspepsia, dysphagia, esophagitis, flatulence, gingivitis, glossitis, ileus, mouth ulceration, rectal bleeding, taste perversion, weight loss, xerostomia

Genitourinary: Cystitis, dysuria, leukorrhea, pelvic pain, polyuria, urinary incontinence, urinary tract infection, urinary urgency, vaginal bleeding

Hematologic: Ecchymosis, hemolysis, prothrombin time increased

Hepatic: ALT increased

Local: Thrombophlebitis

Neuromuscular & skeletal: Arthralgia, hypertonia, myalgia, neuralgia, neuritis (peripheral), neuropathy, paresthesia (up to 10%), pathological fracture,

Ocular: Conjunctivitis, dry eyes, retinitis

Otic: Ear pain

Renal: Albuminuria, hematuria

Respiratory: Apnea, cough increased (up to 10%), epistaxis, pleural effusion, pneumonia, rhinitis, sinusitis

Miscellaneous: Allergic reaction; infusion-related reactions (bronchospasm, chest tightness, chills, dyspnea, facial edema, flushing, headache, hypotension, pruritus); moniliasis, diaphoresis

<1% (Limited to important or life-threatening): Abscess, acute brain syndrome, abnormal vision, anaphylactic or anaphylactoid reaction, asthma, blindness, bone pain, BUN increased, bundle branch block, cardiomegaly, cellulitis, colitis, creatinine increased, cryptococcosis, diabetes mellitus, erythema multiforme, erythema nodosum, eosinophilia, eye pain, flu-like syndrome, glucosuria, heart arrest, hematuria, hemiplegia, hemorrhage, hepatic failure, hepatitis, hepatosplenomegaly, hypercalcemia, hyperkalemia, hypernatremia, hyperuricemia, hyperventilation, hypoglycemia, hypokinesia, hypolipidemia, hypomagnesemia, hyponatremia, hypophosphatemia, hypoproteinemia, hypothermia, injection site hemorrhage, injection site pain, jaundice, ketosis, lactic dehydrogenase increased, kidney failure, lymphadenopathy, lymphangitis, migraine, myositis, optic neuritis, otitis media, palpitation, pancreatitis, pericardial effusion, petechia, pleural effusion, pneumothorax, radiation injury, sclerosing cholangitis, seizure, sepsis, skin necrosis, skin ulcer, syncope, thrombophlebitis, thromboplastin decreased, thrombosis, tinnitus, urticaria, visual field defect, ventricular arrhythmia, weight gain

Overdosage/Toxicology Symptoms of overdose include increases in mucositis, leukopenia, and thrombocytopenia. For acute overdose, treatment of the severely myelosuppressed patient consists of hospitalization, antibiotics, hematopoietic growth factors, platelet and granulocyte transfusion, and symptomatic treatment of mucositis.

Dosing

Adults & Elderly: Refer to individual protocols.

AIDS-KS: I.V.: 20 mg/m^2 every 3 weeks

Breast cancer: I.V.: 20-80 mg/m^2/dose every 8 weeks

Ovarian cancer: I.V.: 50 mg/m^2/dose every 4 weeks

Solid tumors: I.V.: 50-60 mg/m^2/dose every 3-4 weeks

Hepatic Impairment:

ALT/AST 2-3 times ULN: Administer 75% of dose

ALT/AST >3 times ULN **or** bilirubin 1.2-3 mg/dL (20-51 μmol/L): Administer 50% of dose

Bilirubin 3.1-5 mg/dL (51-85 μmol/L): Administer 25% of dose

Bilirubin >5 mg/dL (85 μmol/L): Do not administer

Available Dosage Forms Injection, solution, as hydrochloride: 2 mg/mL (10 mL, 25 mL)

Nursing Guidelines

Assessment: See Contraindications, Warnings/Precautions, and Dosing for use cautions. Assess potential for interactions with other prescriptions, OTC medications, or herbal products patient may be taking (see Drug Interactions). See Administration, Dosing, Reconstitution, and Compatibility for administration specifics. Premedication with antiemetic is recommended - especially with larger doses. Infusion site must be closely monitored. Assess results of laboratory tests (see below), therapeutic response, and adverse reactions (see Adverse Reactions and Overdose/Toxicology) prior to each treatment and on a regular basis throughout therapy. Teach patient possible side effects/appropriate interventions (eg, importance of adequate hydration) and adverse symptoms to report (see Patient Education). **Pregnancy risk factor D** - determine that patient is not pregnant before beginning treatment. Instruct patients of childbearing age on appropriate contraceptive measures. Breast-feeding is contraindicated.

Monitoring Laboratory Tests: CBC with differential, platelet count, echocardiogram, liver function

Patient Education: Inform prescriber of all prescriptions, OTC medications, or herbal products you are taking, and any allergies you have. Do not take any new medication during therapy unless approved by prescriber. This medication can only be administered by infusion. Report immediately any swelling, pain, burning, or redness at infusion site. Avoid alcohol. It is important to maintain adequate hydration (2-3 L/day of fluids) unless instructed to restrict fluid intake, and adequate nutrition (small, frequent meals may help). You will be more susceptible to infection (avoid crowds and exposure to infection and do not have any vaccinations without consulting prescriber). May cause nausea or vomiting (small, frequent meals, frequent mouth care, sucking lozenges, or chewing gum may help); diarrhea (buttermilk, boiled milk, or yogurt may help); loss of hair (reversible); or red-pink urine (normal). Report immediately chest pain, swelling of extremities, respiratory difficulty, palpitations, or rapid heartbeat. Report unresolved nausea, vomiting, or diarrhea; alterations in urinary pattern (increased or decreased); opportunistic infection (fever, chills, unusual bruising or bleeding fatigue, purulent vaginal discharge, unhealed mouth sores); abdominal pain or blood in stools; excessive fatigue; or yellowing of eyes or skin. **Pregnancy/breast-feeding precautions:** Do not get pregnant while taking this medication or for 1 month following therapy. Consult prescriber for appropriate contraceptives. Do not breast-feed.

Pregnancy Risk Factor: D

Pregnancy Issues: Advise patients to avoid becoming pregnant (females) and to avoid causing pregnancy (males).

Lactation: Excretion in breast milk unknown/contraindicated

Administration

I.V.: Irritant. May be administered IVPB over 30 minutes; manufacturer recommends administering at initial rate of 1 mg/minute to minimize risk of infusion reactions until the absence of a reaction has been established, then increase the infusion rate for completion over 1 hour. Do not administer as a bolus injection or undiluted solution. **Do not administer intramuscular or subcutaneous. Do not use with in-line filters.**

(Continued)

DOXOrubicin (Liposomal) *(Continued)*

Reconstitution: Doses Doxil® ≤90 mg must be diluted in 250 mL of D_5W prior to administration. Doses >90 mg should be diluted in 500 mL D_5W.

Compatibility: Stable in D_5W

Y-site administration: Incompatible with amphotericin B, amphotericin B cholesteryl sulfate complex, buprenorphine, cefoperazone, ceftazidime, docetaxel, fluorouracil, furosemide, heparin, hydroxyzine, mannitol, meperidine, metoclopramide, mitoxantrone, morphine, ofloxacin, paclitaxel, piperacillin/tazobactam, promethazine, sodium bicarbonate

Storage: Store intact vials of solution under refrigeration (2°C to 8°C); avoid freezing. Prolonged freezing may adversely affect liposomal drug products, however, short-term freezing (<1 month) does not appear to have a deleterious effect. Diluted doxorubicin hydrochloride liposome injection may be refrigerated at 2°C to 8°C or at room temperature; administer within 24 hours. **Do not use with in-line filters.**

♦ Doxy-100® *see* Doxycycline *on page 584*

Doxycycline (doks i SYE kleen)

U.S. Brand Names Adoxa™; Doryx®; Doxy-100®; Monodox®; Periostat®; Vibramycin®; Vibra-Tabs®

Synonyms Doxycycline Calcium; Doxycycline Hyclate; Doxycycline Monohydrate

Pharmacologic Category Antibiotic, Tetracycline Derivative

Medication Safety Issues

Sound-alike/look-alike issues:

Doxycycline may be confused with dicyclomine, doxepin, doxylamine

Doxy-100® may be confused with Doxil®

Monodox® may be confused with Maalox®

Use Principally in the treatment of infections caused by susceptible *Rickettsia*, *Chlamydia*, and *Mycoplasma*; alternative to mefloquine for malaria prophylaxis; treatment for syphilis, uncomplicated *Neisseria gonorrhoeae*, *Listeria*, *Actinomyces israelii*, and *Clostridium* infections in penicillin-allergic patients; used for community-acquired pneumonia and other common infections due to susceptible organisms; anthrax due to *Bacillus anthracis,* including inhalational anthrax (postexposure); treatment of infections caused by uncommon susceptible gram-negative and gram-positive organisms including *Borrelia recurrentis*, *Ureaplasma urealyticum*, *Haemophilus ducreyi*, *Yersinia pestis*, *Francisella tularensis*, *Vibrio cholerae*, *Campylobacter fetus*, *Brucella* spp, *Bartonella bacilliformis*, and *Calymmatobacterium granulomatis*

Unlabeled/Investigational Use Sclerosing agent for pleural effusion injection; vancomycin-resistant enterococci (VRE)

Mechanism of Action Inhibits protein synthesis by binding with the 30S and possibly the 50S ribosomal subunit(s) of susceptible bacteria; may also cause alterations in the cytoplasmic membrane

Periostat® capsules (proposed mechanism): Has been shown to inhibit collagenase activity *in vitro.* Also has been noted to reduce elevated collagenase activity in the gingival crevicular fluid of patients with periodontal disease. Systemic levels do not reach inhibitory concentrations against bacteria.

Pharmacodynamics/Kinetics

Absorption: Oral: Almost complete; reduced by food or milk by 20%

Distribution: Widely into body tissues and fluids including synovial, pleural, prostatic, seminal fluids, and bronchial secretions; saliva, aqueous humor, and CSF penetration is poor; readily crosses placenta; enters breast milk

Protein binding: 90%

Metabolism: Not hepatic; partially inactivated in GI tract by chelate formation

Half-life elimination: 12-15 hours (usually increases to 22-24 hours with multiple doses); End-stage renal disease: 18-25 hours

Time to peak, serum: 1.5-4 hours

Excretion: Feces (30%); urine (23%)

Contraindications Hypersensitivity to doxycycline, tetracycline or any component of the formulation; children <8 years of age, except in treatment of anthrax (including inhalational anthrax postexposure prophylaxis); severe hepatic dysfunction; pregnancy

Warnings/Precautions Do not use during pregnancy - use of tetracyclines during tooth development may cause permanent discoloration of the teeth and enamel hypoplasia; prolonged use may result in superinfection, including oral or vaginal candidiasis; photosensitivity reaction may occur with this drug; avoid prolonged exposure to sunlight or tanning equipment. Avoid in children ≤8 years of age.

Additional specific warnings for Periostat®: Effectiveness has not been established in patients with coexistent oral candidiasis; use with caution in patients with a history or predisposition to oral candidiasis

Drug Interactions **Substrate** of CYP3A4 (major); **Inhibits** CYP3A4 (moderate)

Antacids (containing aluminum, calcium, or magnesium): Decreased absorption of tetracyclines

Anticoagulants: Tetracyclines may decrease plasma thrombin activity; monitor

Barbiturates: Decreased half-life of doxycycline

Carbamazepine: Decreased half-life of doxycycline

CYP3A4 inducers: CYP3A4 inducers may decrease the levels/effects of doxycycline. Example inducers include aminoglutethimide, carbamazepine, nafcillin, nevirapine, phenobarbital, phenytoin, and rifamycins.

CYP3A4 substrates: Doxycycline may increase the levels/effects of CYP3A4 substrates. Example substrates include benzodiazepines, calcium channel blockers, mirtazapine, nateglinide, nefazodone, tacrolimus, and venlafaxine. Selected benzodiazepines (midazolam and triazolam), cisapride, ergot alkaloids, selected HMG-CoA reductase inhibitors (lovastatin and simvastatin), and pimozide are generally contraindicated with strong CYP3A4 inhibitors.

Iron-containing products: Decreased absorption of tetracyclines

Methoxyflurane: Concomitant use may cause fatal renal toxicity.

Oral contraceptives: Anecdotal reports suggesting decreased contraceptive efficacy with tetracyclines have been refuted by more rigorous scientific and clinical data.

Phenytoin: Decreased half-life of doxycycline

Nutritional/Herbal/Ethanol Interactions

Ethanol: Chronic ethanol ingestion may reduce the serum concentration of doxycycline.

Food: Doxycycline serum levels may be slightly decreased if taken with food or milk. Administration with iron or calcium may decrease doxycycline absorption. May decrease absorption of calcium, iron, magnesium, zinc, and amino acids.

Herb/Nutraceutical: St John's wort may decrease doxycycline levels. Avoid dong quai, St John's wort (may also cause photosensitization).

Lab Interactions False-negative urine glucose using Clinistix®

Adverse Reactions Frequency not defined.

Cardiovascular: Intracranial hypertension, pericarditis

Dermatologic: Angioneurotic edema, exfoliative dermatitis (rare), photosensitivity, rash, urticaria

Endocrine & metabolic: Brown/black discoloration of thyroid gland (no dysfunction reported)

Gastrointestinal: Anorexia, diarrhea, dysphagia, enterocolitis, esophagitis (rare), esophageal ulcerations (rare), glossitis, inflammatory lesions in anogenital region, tooth discoloration (children)

Hematologic: Eosinophilia, hemolytic anemia, neutropenia, thrombocytopenia

Renal: Increased BUN

Miscellaneous: Anaphylactoid purpura, anaphylaxis, bulging fontanels (infants), SLE exacerbation

Note: Adverse effects in clinical trials with Periostat® occurring at a frequency more than 1% greater than placebo included nausea, dyspepsia, joint pain, diarrhea, menstrual cramp, and pain.

Overdosage/Toxicology Symptoms of overdose include nausea, anorexia, and diarrhea. Treatment is supportive.

Dosing

Adults & Elderly:

Usual dosage range: Oral, I.V.: 100-200 mg/day in 1-2 divided doses

Acute gonococcal infection (PID) in combination with another antibiotic: 100 mg every 12 hours until improved, followed by 100 mg orally twice daily to complete 14 days

Community-acquired pneumonia, bronchitis: Oral, I.V.: 100 mg twice daily

Uncomplicated chlamydial infections: Oral: 100 mg twice daily for ≥7 days

Endometritis, salpingitis, parametritis, or peritonitis: 100 mg I.V. twice daily with cefoxitin 2 g every 6 hours for 4 days and for ≥48 hours after patient improves; then continue with oral therapy 100 mg twice daily to complete a 10- to 14-day course of therapy

Sclerosing agent for pleural effusion injection (unlabeled use): 500 mg as a single dose in 30-50 mL of NS or SWI

(Continued)

Doxycycline *(Continued)*

Lyme disease: Oral: 100 mg twice daily for 14-21 days

Syphilis:

Early syphilis: Oral, I.V.: 200 mg/day in divided doses for 14 days

Late syphilis: Oral, I.V.: 200 mg/day in divided doses for 28 days

Periodontitis: Oral (Periostat®): 20 mg twice daily as an adjunct following scaling and root planing; may be administered for up to 9 months. Safety beyond 12 months of treatment and efficacy beyond 9 months of treatment have not been established.

Anthrax:

Inhalational (postexposure prophylaxis): Oral, I.V. (use oral route when possible): 100 mg every 12 hours for 60 days (*MMWR*, 2001, 50:889-93); **Note:** Preliminary recommendation, FDA review and update is anticipated.

Cutaneous (treatment): Oral: 100 mg every 12 hours for 60 days. **Note:** In the presence of systemic involvement, extensive edema, lesions on head/neck, refer to I.V. dosing for treatment of inhalational/gastrointestinal/oropharyngeal anthrax

Inhalational/gastrointestinal/oropharyngeal (treatment): I.V.: Initial: 100 mg every 12 hours; switch to oral therapy when clinically appropriate; some recommend initial loading dose of 200 mg, followed by 100 mg every 8-12 hours (*JAMA*, 1997, 278:399-411).

Note: Initial treatment should include two or more agents predicted to be effective (per CDC recommendations). Agents suggested for use in conjunction with doxycycline or ciprofloxacin include rifampin, vancomycin, imipenem, penicillin, ampicillin, chloramphenicol, clindamycin, and clarithromycin. May switch to oral antimicrobial therapy when clinically appropriate. Continue combined therapy for 60 days.

Pediatrics:

Usual dosage range:

Children ≥8 years (<45 kg): Oral, I.V.: 2-5 mg/kg/day in 1-2 divided doses, not to exceed 200 mg/day

Children >8 years (>45 kg): Oral, I.V.: Refer to adult dosing.

Anthrax:

Inhalational (postexposure prophylaxis) (MMWR, 2001, 50:889-93): Oral, I.V. (use oral route when possible):

≤8 years: 2.2 mg/kg every 12 hours for 60 days

>8 years and ≤45 kg: 2.2 mg/kg every 12 hours for 60 days

>8 years and >45 kg: 100 mg every 12 hours for 60 days

Cutaneous (treatment): Oral: See dosing for "Inhalational (postexposure prophylaxis)"

Note: In the presence of systemic involvement, extensive edema, and/or lesions on head/neck, doxycycline should initially be administered I.V.

Inhalational/gastrointestinal/oropharyngeal (treatment): I.V.: Refer to dosing for inhalational anthrax (postexposure prophylaxis); switch to oral therapy when clinically appropriate.

Note: Initial treatment should include two or more agents predicted to be effective (per CDC recommendations). Agents suggested for use in conjunction with doxycycline or ciprofloxacin include rifampin, vancomycin, imipenem, penicillin, ampicillin, chloramphenicol, clindamycin, and clarithromycin. May switch to oral antimicrobial therapy when clinically appropriate. Continue combined therapy for 60 days

Renal Impairment: No adjustment necessary.

Not dialyzable; 0% to 5% by hemo- and peritoneal methods or by continuous arteriovenous or venovenous hemofiltration; supplemental dose is not necessary.

Available Dosage Forms [DSC] = Discontinued product

Capsule, as hyclate: 50 mg, 100 mg

Vibramycin®: 100 mg

Capsule, as monohydrate (Monodox®): 50 mg, 100 mg

Capsule, coated pellets, as hyclate (Doryx®): 75 mg, 100 mg [DSC]

Injection, powder for reconstitution, as hyclate (Doxy-100®): 100 mg

Powder for oral suspension, as monohydrate (Vibramycin®): 25 mg/5 mL (60 mL) [raspberry flavor]

Syrup, as calcium (Vibramycin®): 50 mg/5 mL (480 mL) [contains sodium metabisulfite; raspberry-apple flavor]

Tablet, as hyclate: 100 mg

Periostat®: 20 mg

Vibra-Tabs®: 100 mg

Tablet, as monohydrate:

Adoxa™: 50 mg, 75 mg, 100 mg

Adoxa® Pak™ 1/75 [unit-dose pack]: 75 mg (31s)

Adoxa® Pak™ 1/100 [unit-dose pack]: 100 mg (31s)

Adoxa® Pak™ 1/150 [unit-dose pack]: 150 mg (30s)

Adoxa® Pak™ 2/100 [unit-dose pack]: 100 mg (60s)

Tablet, delayed-release coated pellets, as hyclate (Doryx®): 75 mg [contains sodium 4.5 mg (0.196 mEq)], 100 mg [contains sodium 6 mg (0.261 mEq)]

Nursing Guidelines

Assessment: See Contraindications, Warnings/Precautions, and Dosing for use cautions. Assess potential for interactions with other prescriptions, OTC medications, or herbal products patient may be taking (see Drug Interactions and Nutritional/Ethanol Interactions). **For I.V. infusion,** see Administration, Dosing, Reconstitution, and Compatibility. Infusion site must be closely monitored; extravasation can be very irritating to veins (see I.V. Detail). Assess results of laboratory tests (see Monitoring Laboratory Tests), therapeutic effectiveness, and adverse response (see Adverse Reactions and Overdose/Toxicology) on a regular basis throughout therapy. Advise patients with diabetes about use of Clinistix®. Teach patient appropriate use/administration (oral), possible side effects, interventions to reduce side effects (eg, importance of adequate hydration) and adverse symptoms to report (see Patient Education). **Pregnancy risk factor D** - determine that patient is not pregnant before beginning treatment. Instruct patients of childbearing age on appropriate contraceptive measures. Breast-feeding is not recommended.

Monitoring Laboratory Tests: Perform culture and sensitivity testing prior to initiating therapy.

Dietary Considerations:

Take with food if gastric irritation occurs. While administration with food may decrease GI absorption of doxycycline by up to 20%, administration on an empty stomach is not recommended due to GI intolerance. Of currently available tetracyclines, doxycycline has the least affinity for calcium.

Doryx® 75 mg and 100 mg tablets contain sodium 4.5 mg and 6 mg, respectively.

Patient Education: Inform prescriber of all prescriptions, OTC medications, or herbal products you are taking, and any allergies you have. If administered by infusion, report immediately any acute back pain, difficulty breathing or swallowing, chest tightness, pain, redness, or swelling at infusion site. Oral: Do not take any new medication during therapy unless approved by prescriber. Take entire prescription as directed, even if you are feeling better. Take each oral dose with food or a full glass of water to reduce stomach upset. Avoid alcohol and maintain adequate hydration (2-3 L/day of fluids) unless instructed to restrict fluid intake. If you have diabetes, drug may cause false test results with Clinistix® urine glucose monitoring; use of another form of glucose monitoring is preferable. You may be very sensitive to sunlight (use sunblock, wear protective clothing and eyewear, or avoid exposure to direct sunlight). May cause lightheadedness, dizziness, or drowsiness (use caution when driving or engaging in tasks that require alertness until response to drug is known); nausea or vomiting (small, frequent meals, frequent mouth care, sucking lozenges, or chewing gum may help); or diarrhea (buttermilk, boiled milk, or yogurt may help). Report skin rash or itching; easy bruising or bleeding; yellowing of skin or eyes; pale stool or dark urine; unhealed mouth sores; vaginal itching or discharge; fever, chills, or unusual cough. **Pregnancy/breast-feeding precautions:** Inform prescriber if you are pregnant. Do not get pregnant while taking this medication. Consult prescriber for appropriate barrier contraceptive measures. Breast-feeding is not recommended.

Pregnancy Risk Factor: D

Pregnancy Issues: Exposure during the last half or pregnancy causes permanent yellow-gray-brown discoloration of the teeth. Tetracyclines also form a complex in bone-forming tissue, leading to a decreased fibula growth rate when given to premature infants. According to the FDA, the Teratogen Information System concluded that therapeutic doses during pregnancy are unlikely to produce substantial teratogenic risk, but data are insufficient to say that there is no risk. In general, reports of exposure have been limited to short durations of therapy in the first trimester. When considering treatment for life-threatening infection and/or prolonged duration of therapy (such as in anthrax), the potential risk to the fetus must be balanced against the severity of the potential illness.

(Continued)

Doxycycline *(Continued)*

Lactation: Enters breast milk/not recommended

Administration

Oral: May give with meals to decrease GI upset. Capsule and tablet: Administer with at least 8 ounces of water and have patient sit up for at least 30 minutes after taking to reduce the risk of esophageal irritation and ulceration.

Doryx® capsules and tablets are bioequivalent. Doryx® capsules may be opened and contents sprinkled on applesauce. Applesauce should be swallowed immediately; do not chew. Follow with 8 ounces of water. Applesauce should not be hot and should be soft enough to swallow without chewing.

I.V.: Infuse slowly, usually over 1-4 hours. Avoid extravasation.

Reconstitution: I.V. infusion: Following reconstitution with sterile water for injection, dilute to a final concentration of 0.1-1 mg/mL using a compatible solution. Protect from light. Stability varies based on solution.

Compatibility: Stable in NS, D_5W, LR, D_5LR

Y-site administration: Incompatible with allopurinol, heparin, piperacillin/ tazobactam

Storage: Capsule, tablet: Store at controlled room temperature 15°C to 30°C (59°F to 86°F). Protect from light.

Related Information

Prevention of Wound Infection and Sepsis in Surgical Patients *on page 1830*

- **Doxycycline Calcium** *see* Doxycycline *on page 584*
- **Doxycycline Hyclate** *see* Doxycycline *on page 584*
- **Doxycycline Monohydrate** *see* Doxycycline *on page 584*
- **DPA** *see* Valproic Acid and Derivatives *on page 1680*
- **DPH** *see* Phenytoin *on page 1354*
- **Dramamine® [OTC]** *see* DimenhyDRINATE *on page 544*
- **Dramamine® Less Drowsy Formula [OTC]** *see* Meclizine *on page 1084*
- **Drisdol®** *see* Ergocalciferol *on page 627*

Dronabinol (droe NAB i nol)

U.S. Brand Names Marinol®

Synonyms Delta-9-tetrahydro-cannabinol; Delta-9 THC; Tetrahydrocannabinol; THC

Pharmacologic Category Antiemetic; Appetite Stimulant

Medication Safety Issues

Sound-alike/look-alike issues:

Dronabinol may be confused with droperidol

Use Chemotherapy-associated nausea and vomiting refractory to other antiemetic; AIDS-related anorexia

Unlabeled/Investigational Use

Cancer-related anorexia

Mechanism of Action Unknown, may inhibit endorphins in the emetic center, suppress prostaglandin synthesis, and/or inhibit medullary activity through an unspecified cortical action

Pharmacodynamics/Kinetics

Onset of action: Within 1 hour

Peak effect: 2-4 hours

Duration: 24 hours (appetite stimulation)

Absorption: Oral: 90% to 95%; 10% to 20% of dose gets into systemic circulation

Distribution: V_d: 10 L/kg; dronabinol is highly lipophilic and distributes to adipose tissue

Protein binding: 97% to 99%

Metabolism: Hepatic to at least 50 metabolites, some of which are active; 11-hydroxy-delta-9-tetrahydrocannabinol (11-OH-THC) is the major metabolite; extensive first-pass effect

Half-life elimination: Dronabinol: 25-36 hours (terminal); Dronabinol metabolites: 44-59 hours

Time to peak, serum: 0.5-4 hours

Excretion: Feces (50% as unconjugated metabolites, 5% as unchanged drug); urine (10% to 15% as acid metabolites and conjugates)

Contraindications Hypersensitivity to dronabinol, cannabinoids, or any component of the formulation, or marijuana; should be avoided in patients with a history of schizophrenia

Warnings/Precautions Use with caution in patients with heart disease, hepatic disease, or seizure disorders. Reduce dosage in patients with severe hepatic impairment. May cause additive CNS effects with sedatives, hypnotics or other psychoactive agents; patients must be cautioned about performing tasks which require mental alertness (eg, operating machinery or driving).

May have potential for abuse; drug is psychoactive substance in marijuana; use caution in patients with a history of substance abuse. May cause withdrawal symptoms upon abrupt discontinuation. Use with caution in patients with mania, depression, or schizophrenia; careful psychiatric monitoring is recommended.

Drug Interactions CNS depressants: Sedative effects may be additive with CNS depressants; includes barbiturates, narcotic analgesics, and other sedative agents; monitor for increased effect

Nutritional/Herbal/Ethanol Interactions

Ethanol: Avoid ethanol (may increase CNS depression).

Food: Administration with high-lipid meals may increase absorption.

Herb/Nutraceutical: St John's wort may decrease dronabinol levels.

Lab Interactions Decreased FSH, LH, growth hormone, testosterone

Adverse Reactions

>10%:

Central nervous system: Drowsiness (48%), sedation (53%), confusion (30%), dizziness (21%), detachment, anxiety, difficulty concentrating, mood change

Gastrointestinal: Appetite increased (when used as an antiemetic), xerostomia (38% to 50%)

1% to 10%:

Cardiovascular: Orthostatic hypotension, tachycardia

Central nervous system: Ataxia (4%), depression (7%), headache, vertigo, hallucinations (5%), memory lapse (4%)

Neuromuscular & skeletal: Paresthesia, weakness

<1% (Limited to important or life-threatening): Diaphoresis, diarrhea, myalgia, nightmares, syncope, tinnitus

Overdosage/Toxicology Symptoms of overdose may include tachycardia, hyper- or hypotension, behavioral disturbances, lethargy, panic reactions, seizures or motor incoordination. Benzodiazepines may be helpful for agitative behavior; Trendelenburg position and hydration may be helpful for hypotensive effects. For other manifestations, treatment should be symptom-directed and supportive.

Dosing

Adults & Elderly:

Antiemetic: Oral: 5 mg/m^2 1-3 hours before chemotherapy, then give 5 mg/m^2/dose every 2-4 hours after chemotherapy for a total of 4-6 doses/day; dose may be increased up to a maximum of 15 mg/m^2/dose if needed (dosage may be increased by 2.5 mg/m^2 increments).

Appetite stimulant (AIDS-related): Oral: Initial: 2.5 mg twice daily (before lunch and dinner); titrate up to a maximum of 20 mg/day.

Pediatrics: Antiemetic: Oral: Refer to adult dosing.

Hepatic Impairment: Usual dose should be reduced in patients with severe liver failure.

Available Dosage Forms Capsule, gelatin: 2.5 mg, 5 mg, 10 mg [contains sesame oil]

Nursing Guidelines

Assessment: See Contraindications, Warnings/Precautions, and Dosing for use cautions. Assess potential for interactions with other prescriptions, OTC medications, or herbal products patient may be taking (see Drug Interactions). Assess effectiveness of therapy and adverse response (eg, severe psychotic reactions). This drug is the psychoactive substance in marijuana (see Adverse Reactions and Overdose/Toxicology). Teach patient appropriate use, possible side effects/appropriate interventions, and adverse symptoms to report (see Patient Education). Breast-feeding is contraindicated.

Dietary Considerations: Capsules contain sesame oil.

Patient Education: Inform prescriber of all prescriptions, OTC medications, or herbal products you are taking, and any allergies you have. Do not take any new medication during therapy unless approved by prescriber (especially barbiturates, and benzodiazepines). Take exactly as directed; do not increase dose or take more often than prescribed. Avoid alcohol. May cause psychotic reaction, impaired coordination or judgment, faintness, dizziness, or drowsiness (do

(Continued)

Dronabinol *(Continued)*

not drive or engage in activities that require alertness and coordination until response to drug is known); or clumsiness, unsteadiness, or muscular weakness (change position slowly and use caution when climbing stairs). Report excessive or persistent CNS changes (euphoria, anxiety, depression, memory lapse, bizarre though patterns, excitability, inability to control thoughts or behavior, fainting); respiratory difficulties; rapid heartbeat; or other adverse reactions. **Pregnancy/breast-feeding precautions:** Inform prescriber if you are or intend to become pregnant. Do not breast-feed.

Pregnancy Risk Factor: C

Lactation: Enters breast milk/contraindicated

Administration

Storage: Store under refrigeration (or in a cool environment) between 8°C and 15°C (46°F and 59°F). Protect from freezing.

Droperidol (droe PER i dole)

U.S. Brand Names Inapsine®

Synonyms Dehydrobenzperidol

Pharmacologic Category Antiemetic; Antipsychotic Agent, Typical

Medication Safety Issues

Sound-alike/look-alike issues:

Droperidol may be confused with dronabinol

Inapsine® may be confused with Nebcin®

Use Antiemetic in surgical and diagnostic procedures; preoperative medication in patients when other treatments are ineffective or inappropriate

Mechanism of Action Droperidol is a butyrophenone antipsychotic; antiemetic effect is a result of blockade of dopamine stimulation of the chemoreceptor trigger zone. Other effects include alpha-adrenergic blockade, peripheral vascular dilation, and reduction of the pressor effect of epinephrine resulting in hypotension and decreased peripheral vascular resistance; may also reduce pulmonary artery pressure

Pharmacodynamics/Kinetics

Onset of action: Peak effect: Parenteral: ~30 minutes

Duration: Parenteral: 2-4 hours, may extend to 12 hours

Absorption: I.M.: Rapid

Distribution: Crosses blood-brain barrier and placenta

V_d: Children: ~0.25-0.9 L/kg; Adults: ~2 L/kg

Protein binding: Extensive

Metabolism: Hepatic, to *p*-fluorophenylacetic acid, benzimidazolone, *p*-hydroxypiperidine

Half-life elimination: Adults: 2.3 hours

Excretion: Urine (75%, <1% as unchanged drug); feces (22%, 11% to 50% as unchanged drug)

Contraindications Hypersensitivity to droperidol or any component of the formulation; known or suspected QT prolongation, including congenital long QT syndrome (prolonged QT_c is defined as >440 msec in males or >450 msec in females)

Warnings/Precautions May alter cardiac conduction. Cases of QT prolongation and torsade de pointes, including some fatal cases, have been reported. Use extreme caution in patients with bradycardia (<50 bpm), cardiac disease, concurrent MAOI therapy, Class I and Class III antiarrhythmics or other drugs known to prolong QT interval, and electrolyte disturbances (hypokalemia or hypomagnesemia), including concomitant drugs which may alter electrolytes (diuretics).

Use with caution in patients with seizures, bone marrow suppression, or severe liver disease. May be sedating, use with caution in disorders where CNS depression is a feature. Caution in patients with hemodynamic instability, predisposition to seizures, subcortical brain damage, renal or respiratory disease. Esophageal dysmotility and aspiration have been associated with antipsychotic use - use with caution in patients at risk of pneumonia (ie, Alzheimer's disease). Caution in breast cancer or other prolactin-dependent tumors (may elevate prolactin levels). May alter temperature regulation or mask toxicity of other drugs due to antiemetic effects. May cause orthostatic hypotension - use with caution in patients at risk of this effect or those who would tolerate transient hypotensive episodes (cerebrovascular disease, cardiovascular disease, or other medications which may predispose). Significant hypotension may occur; injection contains benzyl alcohol; injection also contains sulfites which may cause allergic reaction.

May cause anticholinergic effects (confusion, agitation, constipation, xerostomia, blurred vision, urinary retention). Therefore, they should be used with caution in patients with decreased gastrointestinal motility, urinary retention, BPH, xerostomia, or visual problems. Conditions which also may be exacerbated by cholinergic blockade include narrow-angle glaucoma (screening is recommended) and worsening of myasthenia gravis. Relative to other neuroleptics, droperidol has a low potency of cholinergic blockade.

May cause extrapyramidal symptoms, including pseudoparkinsonism, acute dystonic reactions, akathisia, and tardive dyskinesia (risk of these reactions is high relative to other neuroleptics). May be associated with neuroleptic malignant syndrome (NMS) or pigmentary retinopathy. Safety in children <6 months of age has not been established.

Drug Interactions

Acetylcholinesterase inhibitors (central): May increase the risk of antipsychotic-related extrapyramidal symptoms; monitor.

CNS depressants: Sedative effects may be additive with other CNS depressants; monitor for increased effect; includes benzodiazepines, barbiturates, antipsychotics, ethanol, opiates, and other sedative medications

Cyclobenzaprine: Droperidol and cyclobenzaprine may have an additive effect on prolonging the QT interval; based on limited documentation; monitor

Inhalation anesthetics: Droperidol in combination with certain forms of induction anesthesia may produce peripheral vasodilitation and hypotension

Metoclopramide: May increase extrapyramidal symptoms (EPS) or risk.

Potassium- or magnesium-depleting agents: May increase the risk of serious arrhythmias with droperidol; includes many diuretics, aminoglycosides, cyclosporine, supraphysiologic doses of corticosteroids with mineralocorticoid effects, laxatives, and amphotericin B; monitor serum potassium and magnesium levels closely.

Propofol: An increased incidence of postoperative nausea and vomiting have been reported following coadministration

QT_c-prolonging agents: May result in additive effects on cardiac conduction, potentially resulting in malignant or lethal arrhythmias; concurrent use is contraindicated. Includes cisapride, Class I and Class III antiarrhythmics (amiodarone, dofetilide, procainamide, quinidine, sotalol), pimozide, some quinolone antibiotics (moxifloxacin, sparfloxacin, gatifloxacin), tricyclic antidepressants, and some phenothiazines (mesoridazine, thioridazine).

Adverse Reactions

>10%:

Cardiovascular: QT_c prolongation (dose dependent)

Central nervous system: Restlessness, anxiety, extrapyramidal symptoms, dystonic reactions, pseudoparkinsonian signs and symptoms, tardive dyskinesia, seizure, altered central temperature regulation, sedation, drowsiness

Endocrine & metabolic: Swelling of breasts

Gastrointestinal: Weight gain, constipation

1% to 10%:

Cardiovascular: Hypotension (especially orthostatic), tachycardia, abnormal T waves with prolonged ventricular repolarization, hypertension

Central nervous system: Hallucinations, persistent tardive dyskinesia, akathisia

Gastrointestinal: Nausea, vomiting

Genitourinary: Dysuria

<1% (Limited to important or life-threatening): Adynamic ileus, agranulocytosis, alopecia, arrhythmia, cholestatic jaundice, decreased visual acuity (may be irreversible), heat stroke, hyperpigmentation, laryngospasm, leukopenia, neuroleptic malignant syndrome (NMS), obstructive jaundice, photosensitivity (rare), priapism, rash, respiratory depression, retinal pigmentation, tardive dystonia, torsade de pointes, urinary retention, ventricular tachycardia

Overdosage/Toxicology Symptoms of overdose include hypotension, tachycardia, hallucinations, and extrapyramidal symptoms. Following initiation of essential overdose management, toxic symptom treatment and supportive treatment should be initiated. Prolonged QT interval, seizures, and arrhythmias have been reported.

Dosing

Adults & Elderly: Titrate carefully to desired effect: Nausea and vomiting: I.M., I.V.: Initial: 2.5 mg; additional doses of 1.25 mg may be administered to achieve desired effect; administer additional doses with caution

(Continued)

Droperidol *(Continued)*

Pediatrics: Titrate carefully to desired effect: Children 2-12 years: Nausea and vomiting: I.M., I.V.: 0.05-0.06 mg/kg (maximum initial dose: 0.1 mg/kg); additional doses may be repeated to achieve effect; administer additional doses with caution

Available Dosage Forms Injection, solution: 2.5 mg/mL (1 mL, 2 mL)

Nursing Guidelines

Assessment: Assess other medications the patient may be taking for effectiveness and interactions. Monitor vital signs; cardiac and respiratory status on a frequent basis and especially immediately following administration and for several hours afterward. Monitor for extrapyramidal symptoms for 24-48 hours after therapy. Teach and use safety precautions until the patient is stable. Teach adverse reactions to report.

Monitoring Laboratory Tests: To identify QT prolongation, a 12-lead ECG prior to use is recommended; ECG monitoring for 2-3 hours following administration is recommended. Lipid profile, fasting blood glucose/Hgb A_{1c}, serum magnesium and potassium; BMI

Patient Education: This drug may cause you to feel very sleepy; do not attempt to get up without assistance. May cause orthostatic hypotension (use caution when changing position from lying or sitting to standing). You may experience constipation, (increasing exercise, fluids, fruit/fiber may help). Immediately report any respiratory difficulty, confusion, loss of thought processes, or palpitations. **Pregnancy/breast-feeding precautions:** Inform prescriber if you are pregnant. Consult prescriber if breast-feeding.

Geriatric Considerations: Use of droperidol in the elderly may result in severe and often irreversible undesirable effects. Before initiating antipsychotic therapy, the clinician should investigate possible reversible causes.

Pregnancy Risk Factor: C

Lactation: Excretion in breast milk unknown

Perioperative/Anesthesia/Other Concerns: May cause hypotension and reflex tachycardia; this is more pronounced when the drug is given intravenously. Warnings concerning QT prolongation have altered recommendations concerning perioperative use and monitoring. Baseline 12-lead ECG screening is recommended, and continued ECG monitoring for 2-3 hours postadministration is advised. Use should be limited to patients in whom alternatives are unacceptable. Droperidol does not possess analgesic effects and has little or no amnesic properties.

Administration

I.V.: Administer I.M. or I.V.; I.V. should be administered as a rapid IVP (over 30-60 seconds); for I.V. infusion, dilute in 50-100 mL NS or D_5W. ECG monitoring for 2-3 hours after administration is recommended.

Compatibility: Stable in D_5W, LR, NS

Y-site administration: Incompatible with allopurinol, amphotericin B cholesteryl sulfate complex, cefepime, fluorouracil, foscarnet, furosemide, leucovorin, nafcillin, piperacillin/tazobactam

Compatibility in syringe: Incompatible with fluorouracil, furosemide, heparin, leucovorin, methotrexate, ondansetron, pentobarbital

Storage: Droperidol ampuls/vials should be stored at room temperature and protected from light. Solutions diluted in NS or D_5W are stable at room temperature for up to 7 days.

Related Information

Postoperative Nausea and Vomiting *on page 1807*

- ♦ **Drospirenone and Ethinyl Estradiol** *see* Ethinyl Estradiol and Drospirenone *on page 680*
- ♦ **DSCG** *see* Cromolyn *on page 453*
- ♦ **D-Ser(Bu[t])[6],Azgly[10]-LHRH** *see* Goserelin *on page 829*
- ♦ **D-S-S® [OTC]** *see* Docusate *on page 560*
- ♦ **DSS With Casanthranol** *see* Docusate and Casanthranol *on page 561*
- ♦ **DTO (error-prone abbreviation)** *see* Opium Tincture *on page 1272*
- ♦ **Duet®** *see* Vitamins (Multiple/Prenatal) *on page 1721*
- ♦ **Duet™ DHA** *see* Vitamins (Multiple/Prenatal) *on page 1721*
- ♦ **Dulcolax® [OTC]** *see* Bisacodyl *on page 245*
- ♦ **Dulcolax® Milk of Magnesia [OTC]** *see* Magnesium Hydroxide *on page 1076*
- ♦ **Dulcolax® Stool Softener [OTC]** *see* Docusate *on page 560*
- ♦ **Dull-C® [OTC]** *see* Ascorbic Acid *on page 187*

- DuoNeb™ *see* Ipratropium and Albuterol *on page 959*
- DuP 753 *see* Losartan *on page 1066*
- Duraclon™ *see* Clonidine *on page 433*
- Duragesic® *see* Fentanyl *on page 712*
- Duramist® Plus [OTC] *see* Oxymetazoline *on page 1290*
- Duramorph® *see* Morphine Sulfate *on page 1177*
- Duration® [OTC] *see* Oxymetazoline *on page 1290*
- Duricef® *see* Cefadroxil *on page 329*
- Dyazide® *see* Hydrochlorothiazide and Triamterene *on page 866*
- Dygase *see* Pancrelipase *on page 1301*
- DynaCirc® [DSC] *see* Isradipine *on page 984*
- DynaCirc® CR *see* Isradipine *on page 984*
- Dyna-Hex® [OTC] *see* Chlorhexidine Gluconate *on page 373*
- Dytan™ *see* DiphenhydrAMINE *on page 546*
- 7E3 *see* Abciximab *on page 60*
- EarSol® HC *see* Hydrocortisone *on page 873*
- Easprin® *see* Aspirin *on page 189*
- EC-Naprosyn® *see* Naproxen *on page 1203*
- Econopred® Plus *see* PrednisoLONE *on page 1399*
- Ecotrin® [OTC] *see* Aspirin *on page 189*
- Ecotrin® Low Strength [OTC] *see* Aspirin *on page 189*
- Ecotrin® Maximum Strength [OTC] *see* Aspirin *on page 189*
- Edathamil Disodium *see* Edetate Disodium *on page 595*

Edetate Calcium Disodium

(ED e tate KAL see um dye SOW dee um)

U.S. Brand Names Calcium Disodium Versenate®

Synonyms Calcium Disodium Edetate; Calcium EDTA

Pharmacologic Category Chelating Agent

Use Treatment of symptomatic acute and chronic lead poisoning or for symptomatic patients with high blood lead levels; used as an aid in the diagnosis of lead poisoning; possibly useful in poisoning by zinc, manganese, and certain heavy radioisotopes

Mechanism of Action Calcium is displaced by divalent and trivalent heavy metals, forming a nonionizing soluble complex that is excreted in urine

Pharmacodynamics/Kinetics

Onset of action: Chelation of lead: I.V.: 1 hour

Absorption: I.M., SubQ: Well absorbed

Distribution: Into extracellular fluid; minimal CSF penetration

Half-life elimination, plasma: I.M.: 1.5 hours; I.V.: 20 minutes

Excretion: Urine (as metal chelates or unchanged drug); decreased GFR decreases elimination

Contraindications Severe renal disease, anuria

Warnings/Precautions Potentially nephrotoxic; renal tubular acidosis and fatal nephrosis may occur, especially with high doses; ECG changes may occur during therapy; do not exceed recommended daily dose; avoid rapid I.V. infusion in the management of lead encephalopathy, may increase intracranial pressure to lethal levels. If anuria, increasing proteinuria, or hematuria occurs during therapy, discontinue calcium EDTA. Minimize nephrotoxicity by adequate hydration, establishment of good urine output, avoidance of excessive doses, and limitation of continuous administration to ≤5 days.

Drug Interactions Decreased effect: Do not use simultaneously with zinc insulin preparations; do not mix in the same syringe with dimercaprol

Lab Interactions If calcium EDTA is given as a continuous I.V. infusion, stop the infusion for at least 1 hour before blood is drawn for lead concentration to avoid a falsely elevated value

Adverse Reactions Frequency not defined.

Cardiovascular: Arrhythmias, ECG changes, hypotension

Central nervous system: Chills, fever, headache

Dermatologic: Cheilosis, skin lesions

Endocrine & metabolic: Hypercalcemia

Gastrointestinal: Anorexia, GI upset, nausea, vomiting

Hematologic: Anemia, bone marrow suppression (transient)

Hepatic: Liver function test increased (mild)

(Continued)

Edetate Calcium Disodium *(Continued)*

Local: Thrombophlebitis following I.V. infusion (when concentration >5 mg/mL), pain at injection site following I.M. injection

Neuromuscular & skeletal: Arthralgia, numbness, tremor, paresthesia

Ocular: Lacrimation

Renal: Renal tubular necrosis, microscopic hematuria, proteinuria

Respiratory: Nasal congestion, sneezing

Miscellaneous: Zinc deficiency

Dosing

Adults & Elderly: Several regimens have been recommended:

Diagnosis of lead poisoning: Mobilization test (not recommended by AAP guidelines): I.M., I.V.:

500 mg/m^2/dose

Note: Urine is collected for 24 hours after first EDTA dose and analyzed for lead content; if the ratio of mcg of lead in urine to mg calcium EDTA given is >1, then test is considered positive; for convenience, an 8-hour urine collection may be done after a single 50 mg/kg I.M. (maximum dose: 1 g) or 500 mg/m^2 I.V. dose; a positive test occurs if the ratio of lead excretion to mg calcium EDTA >0.5-0.6.

Treatment of lead poisoning (Regimen is specific for route):

Symptoms of lead encephalopathy and/or blood lead level >70 mcg/dL: Treat 5 days; give in conjunction with dimercaprol; wait a minimum of 2 days with no treatment before considering a repeat course:

I.M.: 250 mg/m^2/dose every 4 hours

I.V.: 50 mg/kg/day as 24-hour continuous I.V. infusion **or** 1-1.5 g/m^2 I.V. as either an 8- to 24-hour infusion or divided into 2 doses every 12 hours

Symptomatic lead poisoning without encephalopathy OR asymptomatic with blood lead level >70 mcg/dL: Treat 3-5 days; treatment with dimercaprol is recommended until the blood lead level concentration <50 mcg/dL:

I.M.: 167 mg/m^2 every 4 hours

I.V.: 1 g/m^2 as an 8- to 24-hour infusion or divided every 12 hours

Adults with lead nephropathy: An alternative dosing regimen reflecting the reduction in renal clearance is based upon the serum creatinine. Refer to the following:

Dose of Ca EDTA based on serum creatinine:

S_{cr} ≤2 mg/dL: 1 g/m^2/day for 5 days*

S_{cr} 2-3 mg/dL: 500 mg/m^2/day for 5 days*

S_{cr} 3-4 mg/dL: 500 mg/m^2/dose every 48 hours for 3 doses*

S_{cr} >4 mg/dL: 500 mg/m^2/week*

*Repeat these regimens monthly until lead excretion is reduced toward normal.

Pediatrics: Several regimens have been recommended:

Diagnosis of lead poisoning: Mobilization test (not recommended by AAP guidelines): I.M., I.V.:

Children: 500 mg/m^2/dose (maximum dose: 1 g) as a single dose or divided into 2 doses

Note: Urine is collected for 24 hours after first EDTA dose and analyzed for lead content; if the ratio of mcg of lead in urine to mg calcium EDTA given is >1, then test is considered positive; for convenience, an 8-hour urine collection may be done after a single 50 mg/kg I.M. (maximum dose: 1 g) or 500 mg/m^2 I.V. dose; a positive test occurs if the ratio of lead excretion to mg calcium EDTA >0.5-0.6.

Treatment of lead poisoning: Children: Refer to adult dosing.

Asymptomatic children with blood lead level 45-69 mcg/dL: I.V.: 25 mg/kg/day for 5 days as an 8- to 24-hour infusion or divided into 2 doses every 12 hours

Note: Depending upon the blood lead level, additional courses may be necessary; repeat at least 2-4 days and preferably 2-4 weeks apart.

Available Dosage Forms Injection, solution: 200 mg/mL (5 mL)

Nursing Guidelines

Patient Education: You will most likely require frequent blood tests and monitoring during therapy. Report pain at injection/infusion site, palpitations, or difficulty urinating. You must remain supine for a period of time following treatment, change position slowly, ask for assistance if you must get up. Inform prescriber if you are pregnant. Do not breast-feed.

Pregnancy Risk Factor: B

Administration

Compatibility: Stable in D_5W, NS; **incompatible** with $D_{10}W$, LR

Compatibility when admixed: Incompatible with amphotericin B, hydralazine

Edetate Disodium (ED e tate dye SOW dee um)

U.S. Brand Names Endrate®

Synonyms Edathamil Disodium; EDTA; Sodium Edetate

Pharmacologic Category Chelating Agent

Use Emergency treatment of hypercalcemia; control digitalis-induced cardiac dysrhythmias (ventricular arrhythmias)

Mechanism of Action Chelates with divalent or trivalent metals to form a soluble complex that is then eliminated in urine

Pharmacodynamics/Kinetics

Metabolism: None

Half-life elimination: 20-60 minutes

Time to peak: I.V.: 24-48 hours

Excretion: Following chelation: Urine (95%); chelates within 24-48 hours

Contraindications Severe renal failure or anuria

Warnings/Precautions Use of this drug is recommended only when the severity of the clinical condition justifies the aggressive measures associated with this type of therapy; use with caution in patients with renal dysfunction, intracranial lesions, seizure disorders, coronary or peripheral vascular disease

Drug Interactions Increased effect of insulin (edetate disodium may decrease blood glucose concentrations and reduce insulin requirements in diabetic patients treated with insulin)

Adverse Reactions Rapid I.V. administration or excessive doses may cause a sudden drop in serum calcium concentration which may lead to hypocalcemic tetany, seizure, arrhythmia, and death from respiratory arrest. Do **not** exceed recommended dosage and rate of administration.

1% to 10%: Gastrointestinal: Nausea, vomiting, abdominal cramps, diarrhea

<1% (Limited to important or life-threatening): Acute tubular necrosis, anemia, arrhythmia, back pain, chills, death from respiratory arrest, dermatologic lesions, eruptions, fever, headache, hypokalemia, hypomagnesemia, muscle cramps, nephrotoxicity, pain at the site of injection, paresthesia may occur, seizure, tetany, thrombophlebitis, transient hypotension

Overdosage/Toxicology

Symptoms of overdose include hypotension, dysrhythmias, tetany, seizures

Treatment includes immediate I.V. calcium salts for hypocalcemia related adverse reactions; replace calcium cautiously in patients on digitalis

Dosing

Adults & Elderly:

Hypercalcemia: I.V.: 50 mg/kg/day over 3 or more hours to a maximum of 3 g/24 hours; a suggested regimen of 5 days followed by 2 days without drug and repeated courses up to 15 total doses

Digitalis-induced arrhythmias: I.V.: 15 mg/kg/hour (maximum dose: 60 mg/kg/day) as continuous infusion

Pediatrics:

Hypercalcemia: I.V.: 40-70 mg/kg/day slow infusion over 3-4 hours or more to a maximum of 3 g/24 hours; administer for 5 days and allow 5 days between courses of therapy.

Digitalis-induced arrhythmias: I.V.: Children: Refer to adult dosing.

Available Dosage Forms Injection, solution: 150 mg/mL (20 mL)

Nursing Guidelines

Dietary Considerations: Sodium content of 1 g: 5.4 mEq

Patient Education: Patient education and instruction will be determined by patient condition and ability to understand. You will require frequent blood tests and monitoring during this infusion. You must remain supine during infusion and for a period of time following treatment; change position slowly and ask for assistance if you must get up. Immediately report any respiratory difficulty, chest pain, or irregular heartbeat; headache, abdominal cramps, chills, back pain, or muscle rigidity or cramping; or pain at injection/infusion site. Inform prescriber if you are pregnant.

Pregnancy Risk Factor: C

Administration

Compatibility: Stable in dextran 6% in dextrose, dextran 6% in NS, $D_5{}^1/_4NS$, $D_5{}^1/_2NS$, D_5NS, D_5W, $D_{10}W$, $D_{10}NS$, $^1/_2NS$, NS

♦ Edex® see Alprostadil on page 113

Edrophonium (ed roe FOE nee um)

U.S. Brand Names Enlon®; Reversol®

Synonyms Edrophonium Chloride

Pharmacologic Category Antidote; Cholinergic Agonist; Diagnostic Agent

Use Diagnosis of myasthenia gravis; differentiation of cholinergic crises from myasthenia crises; reversal of nondepolarizing neuromuscular blockers; adjunct treatment of respiratory depression caused by curare overdose

Mechanism of Action Inhibits destruction of acetylcholine by acetylcholinesterase. This facilitates transmission of impulses across myoneural junction and results in increased cholinergic responses such as miosis, increased tonus of intestinal and skeletal muscles, bronchial and ureteral constriction, bradycardia, and increased salivary and sweat gland secretions.

Pharmacodynamics/Kinetics

Onset of action: I.M.: 2-10 minutes; I.V.: 30-60 seconds

Duration: I.M.: 5-30 minutes: I.V.: 10 minutes

Distribution: V_d: 1.1 L/kg

Half-life elimination: 1.8 hours

Contraindications Hypersensitivity to edrophonium, sulfites, or any component of the formulation; GI or GU obstruction

Warnings/Precautions Use with caution in patients with bronchial asthma and those receiving a cardiac glycoside; atropine sulfate should always be readily available as an antagonist. Overdosage can cause cholinergic crisis which may be fatal. I.V. atropine should be readily available for treatment of cholinergic reactions.

Drug Interactions

Decreased effect: Atropine, nondepolarizing muscle relaxants, procainamide, quinidine

Increased effect: Succinylcholine, digoxin, I.V. acetazolamide, neostigmine, physostigmine

Lab Interactions Increased aminotransferase [ALT (SGPT)/AST (SGOT)] (S), amylase (S)

Adverse Reactions Frequency not defined.

Cardiovascular: Arrhythmias (especially bradycardia), hypotension, decreased carbon monoxide, tachycardia, AV block, nodal rhythm, nonspecific ECG changes, cardiac arrest, syncope, flushing

Central nervous system: Convulsions, dysarthria, dysphonia, dizziness, loss of consciousness, drowsiness, headache

Dermatologic: Skin rash, thrombophlebitis (I.V.), urticaria

Gastrointestinal: Hyperperistalsis, nausea, vomiting, salivation, diarrhea, stomach cramps, dysphagia, flatulence

Genitourinary: Urinary urgency

Neuromuscular & skeletal: Weakness, fasciculations, muscle cramps, spasms, arthralgia

Ocular: Small pupils, lacrimation

Respiratory: Increased bronchial secretions, laryngospasm, bronchiolar constriction, respiratory muscle paralysis, dyspnea, respiratory depression, respiratory arrest, bronchospasm

Miscellaneous: Diaphoresis (increased), anaphylaxis, allergic reactions

Overdosage/Toxicology Symptoms of overdose include muscle weakness, nausea, vomiting, miosis, bronchospasm, and respiratory paralysis. Maintain an adequate airway. For muscarinic symptoms, the antidote is atropine 0.4-0.5 mg I.V. repeated every 3-10 minutes (initial doses as high as 1.2 mg have been administered). Skeletal muscle effects of edrophonium are not alleviated by atropine.

Dosing

Adults & Elderly: Usually administered I.V., however, if not possible, I.M. or SubQ may be used.

Diagnosis of Myasthenia gravis:

I.V.: 2 mg test dose administered over 15-30 seconds; 8 mg given 45 seconds later if no response is seen. Test dose may be repeated after 30 minutes.

I.M.: Initial: 10 mg; if no cholinergic reaction occurs, give 2 mg 30 minutes later to rule out false-negative reaction.

Titration of oral anticholinesterase therapy: 1-2 mg given 1 hour after oral dose of anticholinesterase; if strength improves, an increase in neostigmine or pyridostigmine dose is indicated.

Differentiation of cholinergic from myasthenic crisis: I.V.: 1 mg; may repeat after 1 minute. **Note:** Intubation and controlled ventilation may be required if patient has cholinergic crisis.

Reversal of nondepolarizing neuromuscular blocking agents (neostigmine with atropine usually preferred): I.V.: 10 mg over 30-45 seconds; may repeat every 5-10 minutes up to 40 mg.

Termination of paroxysmal atrial tachycardia: I.V. rapid injection: 5-10 mg

Pediatrics: Usually administered I.V., however, if not possible, I.M. or SubQ may be used:

Infants:

I.M.: 0.5-1 mg

I.V.: Initial: 0.1 mg, followed by 0.4 mg if no response; total dose = 0.5 mg

Children:

Diagnosis: Initial: 0.04 mg/kg over 1 minute followed by 0.16 mg/kg if no response, to a maximum total dose of 5 mg for children <34 kg, or 10 mg for children >34 kg **or**

Alternative dosing (manufacturer's recommendation):

≤34 kg: 1 mg; if no response after 45 seconds, repeat dosage in 1 mg increments every 30-45 seconds, up to a total of 5 mg

>34 kg: 2 mg; if no response after 45 seconds, repeat dosage in 1 mg increments every 30-45 seconds, up to a total of 10 mg

I.M.:

<34 kg: 1 mg

>34 kg: 5 mg

Titration of oral anticholinesterase therapy: 0.04 mg/kg once given 1 hour after oral intake of the drug being used in treatment. If strength improves, an increase in neostigmine or pyridostigmine dose is indicated.

Renal Impairment: Dose may need to be reduced in patients with chronic renal failure.

Available Dosage Forms Injection, solution, as chloride:

Enlon®: 10 mg/mL (15 mL) [contains sodium sulfite]

Reversol®: 10 mg/mL (10 mL) [contains sodium sulfite]

Nursing Guidelines

Assessment: Administration of edrophonium for MG diagnosis is supervised by a neurologist and use as a neuromuscular blocking agent is supervised by an anesthesiologist. Patient must be monitored closely during and following procedure, especially for cholinergic crisis; keep atropine at hand for antidote. Patients receiving the medication for MG testing will have been advised by their neurologist about drug effects. Those patients receiving medication for neuromuscular block will be unaware of drug effects. Patient should never be left alone until all drug effects and the possibility of cholinergic crisis have passed.

Patient Education: Pregnancy/breast-feeding precautions: Inform prescriber if you are or intend to become pregnant. Consult prescriber if breast-feeding.

Geriatric Considerations: Many elderly will have diseases which may influence the use of edrophonium. Also, many elderly will need doses reduced 50% due to creatinine clearances in the 10-50 mL/minute range (common in the aged). Side effects or concomitant disease may warrant use of pyridostigmine.

Pregnancy Risk Factor: C

Lactation: Excretion in breast milk unknown

Perioperative/Anesthesia/Other Concerns: Atropine should be administered along with edrophonium when reversing the effects of nondepolarizing agents to antagonize the cholinergic effects at the muscarinic receptors, especially bradycardia; important to recognize the difference in dose for diagnosis of myasthenia gravis versus reversal of muscle relaxant, a much larger dose is needed for desired effect of reversal of muscle paralysis

♦ **Edrophonium Chloride** *see* Edrophonium *on page 596*

♦ **EDTA** *see* Edetate Disodium *on page 595*

♦ **E.E.S.®** *see* Erythromycin *on page 634*

Efavirenz (e FAV e renz)

U.S. Brand Names Sustiva®

Pharmacologic Category Antiretroviral Agent, Reverse Transcriptase Inhibitor (Non-nucleoside)

(Continued)

Efavirenz *(Continued)*

Use Treatment of HIV-1 infections in combination with at least two other antiretroviral agents

Mechanism of Action As a non-nucleoside reverse transcriptase inhibitor, efavirenz has activity against HIV-1 by binding to reverse transcriptase. It consequently blocks the RNA-dependent and DNA-dependent DNA polymerase activities including HIV-1 replication. It does not require intracellular phosphorylation for antiviral activity.

Pharmacodynamics/Kinetics

Absorption: Increased by fatty meals

Distribution: CSF concentrations exceed free fraction in serum

Protein binding: >99%, primarily to albumin

Metabolism: Hepatic via CYP3A4 and 2B6; may induce its own metabolism

Half-life elimination: Single dose: 52-76 hours; Multiple doses: 40-55 hours

Time to peak: 3-8 hours

Excretion: Feces (16% to 41% primarily as unchanged drug); urine (14% to 34% as metabolites)

Contraindications Clinically-significant hypersensitivity to efavirenz or any component of the formulation; concurrent use of cisapride, midazolam, triazolam, voriconazole, or ergot alkaloids (includes dihydroergotamine, ergotamine, ergonovine, methylergonovine); pregnancy

Warnings/Precautions Do not use as single-agent therapy; avoid pregnancy; women of childbearing potential should undergo pregnancy testing prior to initiation of therapy; use caution with other agents metabolized by cytochrome P450 isoenzyme 3A4 (see Contraindications); use caution with history of mental illness/drug abuse (predisposition to psychological reactions); may cause CNS and psychiatric symptoms, which include impaired concentration, dizziness or drowsiness (avoid potentially hazardous tasks such as driving or operating machinery if these effects are noted); serious psychiatric side effects have been associated with efavirenz, including severe depression, suicide, paranoia, and mania; discontinue if severe rash (involving blistering, desquamation, mucosal involvement or fever) develops. Children are more susceptible to development of rash; prophylactic antihistamines may be used. Caution in patients with known or suspected hepatitis B or C infection (monitoring of liver function is recommended); hepatic impairment. Persistent elevations of serum transaminases >5 times the upper limit of normal should prompt evaluation - benefit of continued therapy should be weighed against possible risk of hepatotoxicity. Concomitant use with St John's wort is not recommended.

Drug Interactions Substrate (major) of CYP2B6, 3A4; **Inhibits** CYP2C8/9 (moderate), 2C19 (moderate), 3A4 (moderate); **Induces** CYP2B6 (weak), 3A4 (strong)

Amprenavir: AUC of amprenavir may be decreased by 36%.

Atazanavir: Serum concentration of atazanavir may be reduced by efavirenz; dosage adjustment of atazanavir is recommended.

Benzodiazepines: Toxicity of some benzodiazepines may be increased by efavirenz; concurrent use of midazolam and triazolam is contraindicated.

Cisapride: Toxicity is significantly increased by efavirenz; concurrent use is contraindicated.

Clarithromycin: Serum concentrations of clarithromycin are decreased by efavirenz, clinical significance unknown; rash reported with concomitant use (46%); azithromycin or other alternative agent should be considered.

CYP2B6 inducers: May decrease the levels/effects of efavirenz. Example inducers include carbamazepine, nevirapine, phenobarbital, phenytoin, and rifampin.

CYP2C8/9 substrates: Efavirenz may increase the levels/effects of CYP2C8/9 substrates. Example substrates include fluoxetine, glimepiride, glipizide, nateglinide, phenytoin, pioglitazone, rosiglitazone, sertraline, and warfarin.

CYP2C19 substrates: Efavirenz may increase the levels/effects of CYP2C19 substrates. Example substrates include citalopram, diazepam, methsuximide, phenytoin, propranolol, and sertraline.

CYP3A4 inducers: CYP3A4 inducers may decrease the levels/effects of efavirenz. Example inducers include aminoglutethimide, carbamazepine, nafcillin, nevirapine, phenobarbital, phenytoin, and rifamycins.

CYP3A4 substrates: Efavirenz may alter the levels/effects of CYP3A4 substrates. Example substrates include benzodiazepines, calcium channel blockers, ergot derivatives, mirtazapine, nateglinide, nefazodone, tacrolimus, and venlafaxine.

Ergot alkaloids (dihydroergotamine, ergotamine, ergonovine, methylergonovine): Toxicity is significantly increased by efavirenz; concurrent use is contraindicated.

Estrogens (ethinyl estradiol): Serum concentrations of ethinyl estradiol. are increased by efavirenz; clinical significance not known, barrier contraception is recommended.

Indinavir: AUC of indinavir is decreased by 31%; dose of indinavir should be increased.

Lopinavir/ritonavir: Serum concentration of lopinavir are decreased; increase dosage of lopinavir/ritonavir to 533 mg/133 mg twice daily.

Methadone: Serum concentrations of methadone are decreased by efavirenz; stable patients should be monitored for withdrawal.

Nelfinavir: AUC of nelfinavir is increased by 20%.

Rifabutin: Serum concentrations of rifabutin are decreased by efavirenz; rifabutin dose should be increased.

Rifampin: Serum concentrations of efavirenz are decreased by rifampin.

Ritonavir: AUC of both agents are increased by ~20%; associated with increased adverse effects and laboratory abnormalities; monitoring of liver enzymes is recommended.

Saquinavir: AUC of saquinavir is decreased by ~60%; do not use saquinavir as sole protease inhibitor.

Sertraline: Serum concentrations may be decreased by efavirenz.

St John's wort: Specific drug interaction studies have not been conducted; serum concentrations of efavirenz are expected to significantly decrease.

Voriconazole: Serum levels may be reduced by efavirenz; concurrent use is contraindicated.

Warfarin: Serum concentrations of warfarin may be increased or decreased; monitor.

Nutritional/Herbal/Ethanol Interactions

Ethanol: Avoid ethanol (hepatic and CNS adverse effects).

Food: Avoid high-fat meals (increase the absorption of efavirenz).

Herb/Nutraceutical: St John's wort may decrease efavirenz serum levels. Avoid concurrent use.

Lab Interactions False-positive test for cannabinoids have been reported when the CEDIA DAU Multilevel THC assay is used. False-positive results with other assays for cannabinoids have not been observed.

Adverse Reactions

>10%:

Central nervous system: Dizziness* (2% to 28%), depression (1% to 16%), insomnia (6% to 16%), anxiety (1% to 11%), pain* (1% to 13%)

Dermatologic: Rash* (NCI grade 1: 9% to 11%, NCI grade 2: 15% to 32%, NCI grade 3 or 4: <1%); 26% experienced new rash vs 17% in control groups; up to 46% of pediatric patients experience rash (median onset: 8 days)

Endocrine & metabolic: HDL increased (25% to 35%), total cholesterol increased (20% to 40%)

Gastrointestinal: Diarrhea* (3% to 14%), nausea* (2% to 12%)

1% to 10%:

Central nervous system: Impaired concentration (2% to 8%), headache* (2% to 7%), somnolence (2% to 7%), fatigue (2% to 7%), abnormal dreams (1% to 6%), nervousness (2% to 6%), severe depression (2%), hallucinations (1%)

Dermatologic: Pruritus (1% to 9%)

Gastrointestinal: Vomiting* (6% to 7%), dyspepsia (3%), abdominal pain (1% to 3%), anorexia (1% to 2%)

Miscellaneous: Diaphoresis increased (1% to 2%)

*Adverse effect reported in ≥10% of patients 3-16 years of age

<1% (Limited to important or life-threatening): Aggressive reaction, agitation, allergic reaction, body fat accumulation/redistribution, convulsions, liver failure, manic reaction, neuropathy, paranoid reaction, Stevens-Johnson syndrome, suicide, visual abnormality

Overdosage/Toxicology Increased central nervous system symptoms and involuntary muscle contractions have been reported in accidental overdose. Treatment is supportive. Activated charcoal may enhance elimination; dialysis is unlikely to remove the drug.

Dosing

Adults & Elderly: Dosing at bedtime is recommended to limit central nervous system effects; should not be used as single-agent therapy.

HIV infection (as part of combination): Oral: 600 mg once daily

(Continued)

Efavirenz *(Continued)*

Pediatrics: Dosing at bedtime is recommended to limit central nervous system effects; should not be used as single-agent therapy. Dosage is based on body weight.

HIV infection (as part of combination): Oral: Children ≥3 years:

10 kg to <15 kg: 200 mg once daily
15 kg to <20 kg: 250 mg once daily
20 kg to <25 kg: 300 mg once daily
25 kg to <32.5 kg: 350 mg once daily
32.5 kg to <40 kg: 400 mg once daily
≥40 kg: 600 mg once daily

Renal Impairment: No adjustment is necessary.

Hepatic Impairment: Limited clinical experience - use with caution.

Available Dosage Forms

Capsule: 50 mg, 100 mg, 200 mg
Tablet: 600 mg

Nursing Guidelines

Assessment: Do not use as single-agent therapy. See Warnings/Precautions for use cautions (eg, mental illness, hepatic disease or impairment). Assess potential for interactions with other pharmacological agents or herbal products patient may be taking (eg, increased risk for CNS depression, or toxicities; see Drug Interactions). Assess results of laboratory test, therapeutic effectiveness (CD4 counts and viral load), and adverse reactions (CNS changes, rash, increased lipid levels; see Adverse Reactions) on a regular basis throughout therapy. Teach patient proper use, possible side effects/appropriate interventions, and adverse symptoms to report (see Patient Education).

Monitoring Laboratory Tests: Monitor serum transaminases (discontinuation of treatment should be considered for persistent elevations greater than five times the upper limit of normal), cholesterol, and triglycerides.

Dietary Considerations: Should be taken on an empty stomach.

Patient Education: Do not take any new medication during therapy unless approved by prescriber. This drug is not a cure for HIV nor has it been found to reduce transmission of HIV. Take as directed, on an empty stomach (1 hour before or 2 hours after eating). This drug is usually used in combination with other medications; maintain recommended schedule of all medications. Maintain adequate hydration (2-3 L/day of fluids) unless instructed to restrict fluid intake. Avoid alcohol (may cause undesirable reactions). May cause dizziness, anxiety, tremor, impaired coordination, inability to concentrate (use caution when driving or engaging in tasks requiring alertness until response to drug is known); nausea or vomiting (small frequent meals, good mouth care, chewing gum, or sucking lozenges may help; consult prescriber if nausea or vomiting persists); or diarrhea (buttermilk, boiled milk, or yogurt may help). Report CNS changes (acute headache, abnormal dreams, sleepiness or fatigue, seizures, hallucinations, amnesia, emotional lability, confusion); muscle pain, weakness, tremors, numbness; rash; or other unusual effects. **Pregnancy/breast-feeding precautions:** Inform prescriber if you are or intend to become pregnant. Do not breast-feed.

Pregnancy Risk Factor: D

Pregnancy Issues: Teratogenic effects have been observed in Primates receiving efavirenz. Severe CNS defects have been reported in infants following efavirenz exposure in the first trimester. Pregnancy should be avoided and alternate therapy should be considered in women of childbearing potential. Women of childbearing potential should undergo pregnancy testing prior to initiation of efavirenz. Barrier contraception should be used in combination with other (hormonal) methods of contraception. If therapy with efavirenz is administered during pregnancy, avoid use during the first trimester. Health professionals are encouraged to contact the antiretroviral pregnancy registry to monitor outcomes of pregnant women exposed to antiretroviral medications (1-800-258-4263 or www.APRegistry.com).

Lactation: Excretion is breast milk unknown/contraindicated

Breast-Feeding Considerations: HIV-infected mothers are discouraged from breast-feeding to decrease potential transmission of HIV.

Administration

Oral: Administer on an empty stomach. Capsules may be opened and added to liquids or small amounts of food.

Storage: Store below 25°C (77°F).

♦ Effexor® *see* Venlafaxine *on page 1697*
♦ Effexor® XR *see* Venlafaxine *on page 1697*
♦ Eflone® [DSC] *see* Fluorometholone *on page 743*
♦ Efudex® *see* Fluorouracil *on page 745*
♦ E-Gems® [OTC] *see* Vitamin E *on page 1716*
♦ E-Gems Elite® [OTC] *see* Vitamin E *on page 1716*
♦ E-Gems Plus® [OTC] *see* Vitamin E *on page 1716*
♦ Elavil® [DSC] *see* Amitriptyline *on page 136*
♦ Eldepryl® *see* Selegiline *on page 1517*
♦ Eligard® *see* Leuprolide *on page 1015*
♦ Elixophyllin® *see* Theophylline *on page 1619*
♦ ElixSure™ Congestion [OTC] *see* Pseudoephedrine *on page 1436*
♦ ElixSure™ Fever/Pain [OTC] *see* Acetaminophen *on page 65*
♦ ElixSure™ IB [OTC] *see* Ibuprofen *on page 889*
♦ Ellence® *see* Epirubicin *on page 615*
♦ Eloxatin™ *see* Oxaliplatin *on page 1275*
♦ EMLA® *see* Lidocaine and Prilocaine *on page 1042*
♦ ENA 713 *see* Rivastigmine *on page 1487*

Enalapril (e NAL a pril)

U.S. Brand Names Vasotec®

Synonyms Enalaprilat; Enalapril Maleate

Pharmacologic Category Angiotensin-Converting Enzyme (ACE) Inhibitor

Medication Safety Issues

Sound-alike/look-alike issues:

Enalapril may be confused with Anafranil®, Elavil®, Eldepryl®, nafarelin, ramipril

Use Management of mild to severe hypertension; treatment of congestive heart failure, left ventricular dysfunction after myocardial infarction

Unlabeled/Investigational Use

Unlabeled: Hypertensive crisis, diabetic nephropathy, rheumatoid arthritis, diagnosis of anatomic renal artery stenosis, hypertension secondary to scleroderma renal crisis, diagnosis of aldosteronism, idiopathic edema, Bartter's syndrome, postmyocardial infarction for prevention of ventricular failure

Investigational: Severe congestive heart failure in infants, neonatal hypertension, acute pulmonary edema

Mechanism of Action Competitive inhibitor of angiotensin-converting enzyme (ACE); prevents conversion of angiotensin I to angiotensin II, a potent vasoconstrictor; results in lower levels of angiotensin II which causes an increase in plasma renin activity and a reduction in aldosterone secretion

Pharmacodynamics/Kinetics

Onset of action: Oral: ~1 hour

Duration: Oral: 12-24 hours

Absorption: Oral: 55% to 75%

Protein binding: 50% to 60%

Metabolism: Prodrug, undergoes hepatic biotransformation to enalaprilat

Half-life elimination:

Enalapril: Adults: Healthy: 2 hours; Congestive heart failure: 3.4-5.8 hours

Enalaprilat: Infants 6 weeks to 8 months old: 6-10 hours; Adults: 35-38 hours

Time to peak, serum: Oral: Enalapril: 0.5-1.5 hours; Enalaprilat (active): 3-4.5 hours

Excretion: Urine (60% to 80%); some feces

Contraindications Hypersensitivity to enalapril or enalaprilat; angioedema related to previous treatment with an ACE inhibitor; patients with idiopathic or hereditary angioedema; bilateral renal artery stenosis; pregnancy (2nd and 3rd trimesters)

Warnings/Precautions Anaphylactic reactions can occur. Angioedema can occur at any time during treatment (especially following first dose). Angioedema may involve head and neck (potentially affecting the airway) or the intestine (presenting with abdominal pain). Careful blood pressure monitoring with first dose (hypotension can occur especially in volume depleted patients). Dosage adjustment needed in renal impairment. Use with caution in hypovolemia; collagen vascular diseases; valvular stenosis (particularly aortic stenosis); hyperkalemia; or before, during, or immediately after anesthesia. Avoid rapid dosage escalation which may lead to renal insufficiency.

(Continued)

Enalapril *(Continued)*

Rare toxicities associated with ACE inhibitors include cholestatic jaundice (which may progress to hepatic necrosis) and neutropenia/agranulocytosis with myeloid hyperplasia. Hypersensitivity reactions may be seen during hemodialysis with high-flux dialysis membranes (eg, AN69). Hyperkalemia may rarely occur. If patient has renal impairment then a baseline WBC with differential and serum creatinine should be evaluated and monitored closely during the first 3 months of therapy. Use with caution in unilateral renal artery stenosis and pre-existing renal insufficiency.

Drug Interactions Substrate of CYP3A4 (major)

Alpha$_1$ blockers: Hypotensive effect increased.

Aspirin: The effects of ACE inhibitors may be blunted by aspirin administration, particularly at higher dosages (see Cardiovascular Considerations) and/or increase adverse renal effects.

CYP3A4 inducers: CYP3A4 inducers may decrease the levels/effects of enalapril. Example inducers include aminoglutethimide, carbamazepine, nafcillin, nevirapine, phenobarbital, phenytoin, and rifamycins.

Diuretics: Hypovolemia due to diuretics may precipitate acute hypotensive events or acute renal failure.

Insulin: Risk of hypoglycemia may be increased.

Lithium: Risk of lithium toxicity may be increased; monitor lithium levels, especially in the first 4 weeks of therapy.

Mercaptopurine: Risk of neutropenia may be increased.

NSAIDs: May attenuate hypertensive efficacy; effect has been seen with captopril and may occur with other ACE inhibitors; monitor blood pressure. May increase risk of renal adverse effects.

Potassium-sparing diuretics (amiloride, spironolactone, triamterene): Increased risk of hyperkalemia.

Potassium supplements may increase the risk of hyperkalemia.

Trimethoprim (high dose) may increase the risk of hyperkalemia.

Nutritional/Herbal/Ethanol Interactions Herb/Nutraceutical: St John's wort may decrease enalapril levels. Avoid dong quai if using for hypertension (has estrogenic activity). Avoid ephedra, yohimbe, ginseng (may worsen hypertension). Avoid natural licorice (causes sodium and water retention and increases potassium loss). Avoid garlic (may have increased antihypertensive effect).

Lab Interactions Positive Coombs' [direct]; may cause false-positive results in urine acetone determinations using sodium nitroprusside reagent

Adverse Reactions Note: Frequency ranges include data from hypertension and heart failure trials. Higher rates of adverse reactions have generally been noted in patients with CHF. However, the frequency of adverse effects associated with placebo is also increased in this population.

1% to 10%:

- Cardiovascular: Hypotension (0.9% to 6.7%), chest pain (2%), syncope (0.5% to 2%), orthostasis (2%), orthostatic hypotension (2%)
- Central nervous system: Headache (2% to 5%), dizziness (4% to 8%), fatigue (2% to 3%)
- Dermatologic: Rash (1.5%)
- Gastrointestinal: Abnormal taste, abdominal pain, vomiting, nausea, diarrhea, anorexia, constipation
- Neuromuscular & skeletal: Weakness
- Renal: Increased serum creatinine (0.2% to 20%), worsening of renal function (in patients with bilateral renal artery stenosis or hypovolemia)
- Respiratory (1% to 2%): Bronchitis, cough, dyspnea

<1% (Limited to important or life-threatening): Agranulocytosis, alopecia, angina pectoris, angioedema, ataxia, bronchospasm, cardiac arrest, cerebral vascular accident, depression, erythema multiforme, exfoliative dermatitis, giant cell arteritis, gynecomastia, hallucinations, hemolysis with G6PD, Henoch-Schönlein purpura, hepatitis, ileus, impotence, jaundice, lichen-form reaction, MI, neutropenia, ototoxicity, pancreatitis, paresthesia, pemphigus, pemphigus foliaceus, photosensitivity, psychosis, pulmonary edema, sicca syndrome, Stevens-Johnson syndrome, systemic lupus erythematosus, toxic epidermal necrolysis, toxic pustuloderma, vertigo. Worsening of renal function may occur in patients with bilateral renal artery stenosis or in hypovolemic patients. A syndrome which may include fever, myalgia, arthralgia, interstitial nephritis, vasculitis, rash, eosinophilia and positive ANA, and elevated ESR has been reported for enalapril and other ACE inhibitors.

Overdosage/Toxicology Mild hypotension has been the primary toxic effect seen with acute overdose. Bradycardia may also occur. Hyperkalemia occurs even with therapeutic doses, especially in patients with renal insufficiency and those taking NSAIDs. Following initiation of essential overdose management, toxic symptom treatment and supportive treatment should be initiated.

Dosing

Adults & Elderly: Use lower listed initial dose in patients with hyponatremia, hypovolemia, severe congestive heart failure, decreased renal function, or in those receiving diuretics.

Asymptomatic left ventricular dysfunction: Oral: 2.5 mg twice daily, titrated as tolerated to 20 mg/day

Hypertension:

Oral: 2.5-5 mg/day then increase as required, usually at 1- to 2-week intervals; usual dose range (JNC 7): 2.5-40 mg/day in 1-2 divided doses. **Note:** Initiate with 2.5 mg if patient is taking a diuretic which cannot be discontinued. May add a diuretic if blood pressure cannot be controlled with enalapril alone.

I.V. (Enalaprilat): 1.25 mg/dose, given over 5 minutes every 6 hours; doses as high as 5 mg/dose every 6 hours have been tolerated for up to 36 hours. **Note:** If patients are concomitantly receiving diuretic therapy, begin with 0.625 mg I.V. over 5 minutes; if the effect is not adequate after 1 hour, repeat the dose and administer 1.25 mg at 6-hour intervals thereafter; if adequate, administer 0.625 mg I.V. every 6 hours.

Heart failure:

Oral: Initial: 2.5 mg once or twice daily (usual range: 5-40 mg/day in 2 divided doses). Titrate slowly at 1- to 2-week intervals. Target dose: 10-20 mg twice daily (ACC/AHA 2005 Heart Failure Guidelines)

I.V.: Avoid I.V. administration in patients with unstable heart failure or those suffering acute myocardial infarction.

Conversion from I.V. to oral therapy if not concurrently on diuretics: 5 mg once daily; subsequent titration as needed; if concurrently receiving diuretics and responding to 0.625 mg I.V. every 6 hours, initiate with 2.5 mg/day.

Pediatrics:

Hypertension: Oral: Children 1 month to 16 years: Initial: 0.08 mg/kg (up to 5 mg) once daily; adjust dosage based on patient response; doses >0.58 mg/kg (40 mg) have not been evaluated in pediatric patients

Heart failure (non-FDA approved):

Infants and Children:

Oral (Enalapril): Initial: 0.1 mg/kg/day in 1-2 divided doses; increase as required over 2 weeks to maximum of 0.5 mg/kg/day; mean dose required for CHF improvement in 39 children (9 days to 17 years) was 0.36 mg/kg/day; investigationally, select individuals have been treated with doses up to 0.94 mg/kg/day

I.V. (Enalaprilat): 5-10 mcg/kg/dose administered every 8-24 hours (as determined by blood pressure readings); monitor patients carefully; select patients may require higher doses

Adolescents: Refer to adult dosing.

Renal Impairment:

Oral: Enalapril: Hypertension:

Cl_{cr} 30-80 mL/minute: Administer 5 mg/day titrated upwards to maximum of 40 mg.

Cl_{cr} <30 mL/minute: Administer 2.5 mg day titrated upward until blood pressure is controlled up to a maximum of 40 mg.

For heart failure patients with sodium <130 mEq/L or serum creatinine >1.6 mg/dL, initiate dosage with 2.5 mg/day, increasing to twice daily as needed; increase further in increments of 2.5 mg/dose at >4-day intervals to a maximum daily dose of 40 mg.

I.V.: Enalaprilat:

Cl_{cr} >30 mL/minute: Initiate with 1.25 mg every 6 hours and increase dose based on response.

Cl_{cr} <30 mL/minute: Initiate with 0.625 mg every 6 hours and increase dose based on response.

Moderately dialyzable (20% to 50%)

Administer dose postdialysis (eg, 0.625 mg I.V. every 6 hours) or administer 20% to 25% supplemental dose following dialysis; Clearance: 62 mL/minute

Peritoneal dialysis effects: Supplemental dose is not necessary, although some removal of drug occurs.

(Continued)

Enalapril *(Continued)*

Hepatic Impairment: Hydrolysis of enalapril to enalaprilat may be delayed and/or impaired in patients with severe hepatic impairment, but the pharmacodynamic effects of the drug do not appear to be significantly altered. No dosage adjustment is necessary.

Available Dosage Forms

Injection, solution, as enalaprilat: 1.25 mg/mL (1 mL, 2 mL) [contains benzyl alcohol]

Tablet, as maleate (Vasotec®): 2.5 mg, 5 mg, 10 mg, 20 mg

Nursing Guidelines

Assessment: See Contraindications, Warnings/Precautions, and Dosing for use cautions. Assess potential for interactions with other prescriptions, OTC medications, or herbal products patient may be taking (especially anything that may impact fluid balance or cardiac status - see Drug Interactions). **Infusion:** See Administration details. Assess results of laboratory tests (see below), therapeutic effectiveness, and adverse response on a regular basis during therapy (eg, hypovolemia, angioedema, postural hypotension - see Adverse Reactions and Overdose/Toxicology). Teach patient appropriate use, possible side effects/appropriate interventions, and adverse symptoms to report (see Patient Education). **Pregnancy risk factor C/D** - see Pregnancy Risk Factor for use cautions. Instruct patient in appropriate use of barrier contraceptives. Danger of use during pregnancy must outweigh risk to fetus - see Pregnancy Issues.

Monitoring Laboratory Tests: CBC, renal function tests, electrolytes. If patient has renal impairment then a baseline WBC with differential and serum creatinine should be evaluated and monitored closely during the first 3 months of therapy.

Dietary Considerations: Limit salt substitutes or potassium-rich diet.

Patient Education: Inform prescriber of all prescriptions, OTC medications, or herbal products you are taking, and any allergies you have. Do not take any new medication during therapy unless approved by prescriber. Do not use potassium supplement or salt substitutes without consulting prescriber. Take exactly as directed; do not discontinue without consulting prescriber. Take first dose at bedtime. Take all doses on an empty stomach, 1 hour before or 2 hours after meals. This drug does not eliminate need for diet or exercise regimen as recommended by prescriber. May cause dizziness, fainting, or lightheadedness (use caution when driving or engaging in tasks that require alertness until response to drug is known); postural hypotension (use caution when rising from lying or sitting position or climbing stairs); or nausea, vomiting, abdominal pain, dry mouth, or transient loss of appetite (small, frequent meals, frequent mouth care, sucking lozenges, or chewing gum may help). Report persistent nausea and vomiting; chest pain or palpitations; mouth sores; fever or chills; swelling of extremities, face, mouth, or tongue; skin rash; numbness, tingling, or pain in muscles; respiratory difficulty or unusual cough; or other persistent adverse reactions. **Pregnancy precaution:** Inform prescriber if you are or intend to become pregnant. This drug should not be used in the 2nd or 3rd trimester of pregnancy. Consult prescriber for appropriate contraceptive measures if necessary.

Geriatric Considerations: Due to frequent decreases in glomerular filtration (also creatinine clearance) with aging, elderly patients may have exaggerated responses to ACE inhibitors.

Pregnancy Risk Factor: C (1st trimester)/D (2nd and 3rd trimesters)

Pregnancy Issues: ACE inhibitors can cause fetal injury or death if taken during the 2nd or 3rd trimester. Discontinue ACE inhibitors as soon as pregnancy is detected.

Lactation: Enters breast milk/not recommended (AAP rates "compatible")

Perioperative/Anesthesia/Other Concerns: Severe hypotension may occur in patients who are sodium and/or volume depleted, initiate lower doses and monitor closely when starting therapy in these patients

ACE inhibitors decrease morbidity and mortality in patients with asymptomatic and symptomatic left ventricular dysfunction. In this situation, they decrease hospitalizations for, and retard progression to, congestive heart failure. ACE inhibitors are also indicated in patients postmyocardial infarction in whom left ventricular ejection fraction is <40%. When used in patients with heart failure, the target dose of 10 mg twice daily should be achieved, if possible. Lower daily doses of ACE inhibitors have not demonstrated the same cardioprotective effects.

ACE inhibitor therapy may elicit rapid increases in potassium and creatinine, especially when used in patients with bilateral renal artery stenosis. When ACE inhibition is introduced in patients with pre-existing diuretic therapy who are hypovolemic, the ACE inhibitor may induce acute hypotension.

Administration

I.V.: Give direct IVP over at least 5 minutes or dilute up to 50 mL and infuse.

Reconstitution: Enalaprilat: I.V. is stable for 24 hours at room temperature in D_5W or NS.

Compatibility: Stable in dextran 40 10% in dextrose, D_5LR, D_5NS, D_5W, hetastarch 6%, NS

Y-site administration: Incompatible with amphotericin B, amphotericin B cholesteryl sulfate complex, cefepime, phenytoin

Storage: Enalaprilat: Clear, colorless solution which should be stored at <30°C.

Related Information

Postoperative Hypertension *on page 1815*

- Enalaprilat *see* Enalapril *on page 601*
- Enalapril Maleate *see* Enalapril *on page 601*
- Enbrel® *see* Etanercept *on page 673*
- EndoAvitene® *see* Collagen Hemostat *on page 449*
- Endocet® *see* Oxycodone and Acetaminophen *on page 1286*
- Endodan® *see* Oxycodone and Aspirin *on page 1289*
- Endrate® *see* Edetate Disodium *on page 595*
- Enemeez® [OTC] *see* Docusate *on page 560*
- Enerjets [OTC] *see* Caffeine *on page 284*
- Enfamil® Glucose *see* Dextrose *on page 511*
- Enlon® *see* Edrophonium *on page 596*

Enoxaparin (ee noks a PA rin)

U.S. Brand Names Lovenox®

Synonyms Enoxaparin Sodium

Pharmacologic Category Low Molecular Weight Heparin

Medication Safety Issues

Sound-alike/look-alike issues:

Lovenox® may be confused with Lotronex®, Protonix®

High alert medication: The Institute for Safe Medication Practices (ISMP) includes this medication among its list of drugs which have a heightened risk of causing significant patient harm when used in error.

Use

DVT Treatment (acute): Inpatient treatment (patients with and without pulmonary embolism) and outpatient treatment (patients without pulmonary embolism)

DVT prophylaxis: Following hip or knee replacement surgery, abdominal surgery, or in medical patients with severely-restricted mobility during acute illness in patients at risk of thromboembolic complications

Note: High-risk patients include those with one or more of the following risk factors: >40 years of age, obesity, general anesthesia lasting >30 minutes, malignancy, history of deep vein thrombosis or pulmonary embolism

Unstable angina and non-Q-wave myocardial infarction (to prevent ischemic complications)

Unlabeled/Investigational Use Prophylaxis and treatment of thromboembolism in children

Mechanism of Action Standard heparin consists of components with molecular weights ranging from 4000-30,000 daltons with a mean of 16,000 daltons. Heparin acts as an anticoagulant by enhancing the inhibition rate of clotting proteases by antithrombin III impairing normal hemostasis and inhibition of factor Xa. Low molecular weight heparins have a small effect on the activated partial thromboplastin time and strongly inhibit factor Xa. Enoxaparin is derived from porcine heparin that undergoes benzylation followed by alkaline depolymerization. The average molecular weight of enoxaparin is 4500 daltons which is distributed as (≤20%) 2000 daltons (≥68%) 2000-8000 daltons, and (≤15%) >8000 daltons. Enoxaparin has a higher ratio of antifactor Xa to antifactor IIa activity than unfractionated heparin.

Pharmacodynamics/Kinetics

Onset of action: Peak effect: SubQ: Antifactor Xa and antithrombin (antifactor IIa): 3-5 hours

Duration: 40 mg dose: Antifactor Xa activity: ~12 hours

(Continued)

Enoxaparin *(Continued)*

Metabolism: Hepatic, to lower molecular weight fragments (little activity)
Protein binding: Does not bind to heparin binding proteins
Half-life elimination, plasma: 2-4 times longer than standard heparin, independent of dose; based on anti-Xa activity: 4.5-7 hours
Excretion: Urine (40% of dose; 10% as active fragments)

Contraindications Hypersensitivity to enoxaparin, heparin, or any component of the formulation; thrombocytopenia associated with a positive *in vitro* test for antiplatelet antibodies in the presence of enoxaparin; hypersensitivity to pork products; active major bleeding; not for I.M. or I.V. use

Warnings/Precautions **Patients with recent or anticipated neuraxial anesthesia (epidural or spinal anesthesia) are at risk of spinal or epidural hematoma and subsequent paralysis.** Consider risk versus benefit prior to neuraxial anesthesia; risk is increased by concomitant agents which may alter hemostasis, as well as traumatic or repeated epidural or spinal puncture. Patient should be observed closely for bleeding if enoxaparin is administered during or immediately following diagnostic lumbar puncture, epidural anesthesia, or spinal anesthesia.

Not recommended for thromboprophylaxis in patients with prosthetic heart valves (especially pregnant women). Not to be used interchangeably (unit for unit) with heparin or any other low molecular weight heparins. Use caution in patients with history of heparin-induced thrombocytopenia. Monitor patient closely for signs or symptoms of bleeding. Certain patients are at increased risk of bleeding. Risk factors include bacterial endocarditis; congenital or acquired bleeding disorders; active ulcerative or angiodysplastic GI diseases; severe uncontrolled hypertension; hemorrhagic stroke; use shortly after brain, spinal, or ophthalmology surgery; patients treated concomitantly with platelet inhibitors; recent GI bleeding; thrombocytopenia or platelet defects; severe liver disease; hypertensive or diabetic retinopathy; or in patients undergoing invasive procedures. Monitor platelet count closely. Rare cases of thrombocytopenia have occurred. Manufacturer recommends discontinuation of therapy if platelets are <100,000/mm^3. Risk of bleeding may be increased in women <45 kg and in men <57 kg. Use caution in patients with renal failure; dosage adjustment needed if Cl_{cr} <30 mL/minute. Safety and efficacy in pediatric patients have not been established. Use with caution in the elderly (delayed elimination may occur). Heparin can cause hyperkalemia by affecting aldosterone. Similar reactions could occur with LMWHs. Monitor for hyperkalemia. Multiple-dose vials contain benzyl alcohol (use caution in pregnant women).

Drug Interactions

Drugs which affect platelet function (eg, aspirin, NSAIDs, dipyridamole, ticlopidine, clopidogrel) may potentiate the risk of hemorrhage.
Thrombolytic agents increase the risk of hemorrhage.
Warfarin: Risk of bleeding may be increased during concurrent therapy. Enoxaparin is commonly continued during the initiation of warfarin therapy to assure anticoagulation and to protect against possible transient hypercoagulability.

Nutritional/Herbal/Ethanol Interactions Herb/Nutraceutical: Avoid cat's claw, dong quai, evening primrose, feverfew, garlic, ginger, ginkgo, red clover, horse chestnut, green tea, ginseng (all have additional antiplatelet activity).

Lab Interactions Increased AST, ALT levels

Adverse Reactions As with all anticoagulants, bleeding is the major adverse effect of enoxaparin. Hemorrhage may occur at virtually any site. Risk is dependent on multiple variables. At the recommended doses, single injections of enoxaparin do not significantly influence platelet aggregation or affect global clotting time (ie, PT or aPTT).

1% to 10%:
- Central nervous system: Fever (5% to 8%), confusion, pain
- Dermatologic: Erythema, bruising
- Gastrointestinal: Nausea (3%), diarrhea
- Hematologic: Hemorrhage (5% to 13%), thrombocytopenia (2%), hypochromic anemia (2%)
- Hepatic: Increased ALT/AST
- Local: Injection site hematoma (9%), local reactions (irritation, pain, ecchymosis, erythema)

<1% (Limited to important or life-threatening): Allergic reaction, anaphylactoid reaction, eczematous plaques, hyperlipidemia, hypersensitivity cutaneous vasculitis, hypertriglyceridemia, itchy erythematous patches. pruritus, purpura, skin necrosis, thrombocytosis, urticaria, vesicobullous rash. Retroperitoneal or

intracranial bleed (some fatal). Spinal or epidural hematomas can occur following neuraxial anesthesia or spinal puncture, resulting in paralysis. Risk is increased in patients with indwelling epidural catheters or concomitant use of other drugs affecting hemostasis. Cases of heparin-induced thrombocytopenia with thrombosis (some complicated by organ infarction, limb ischemia, or death) have been reported. Prosthetic valve thrombosis, including fatal cases, has been reported in pregnant women receiving enoxaparin as thromboprophylaxis.

Overdosage/Toxicology Symptoms of overdose include hemorrhage. Protamine sulfate has been used to reverse effects (protamine 1 mg neutralizes enoxaparin 1 mg). Monitor aPTT 2-4 hours after first infusion; consider readministration of protamine (50% of original dose). Note: anti-Xa activity is never completely neutralized (maximum of 60% to 75%). Avoid overdose of protamine.

Dosing

Adults:

DVT prophylaxis: SubQ:

Hip replacement surgery:

Twice-daily dosing: 30 mg twice daily, with initial dose within 12-24 hours after surgery, and every 12 hours until risk of DVT has diminished or the patient is adequately anticoagulated on warfarin.

Once-daily dosing: 40 mg once daily, with initial dose within 9-15 hours before surgery, and daily until risk of DVT has diminished or the patient is adequately anticoagulated on warfarin.

Knee replacement surgery: 30 mg twice daily, with initial dose within 12-24 hours after surgery, and every 12 hours until risk of DVT has diminished (usually 7-10 days).

Abdominal surgery: 40 mg once daily, with initial dose given 2 hours prior to surgery; continue until risk of DVT has diminished (usual 7-10 days).

Medical patients with severely-restricted mobility during acute illness: 40 mg once daily; continue until risk of DVT has diminished

DVT treatment (acute): SubQ: **Note:** Start warfarin within 72 hours and continue enoxaparin until INR is between 2.0 and 3.0 (usually 7 days).

Inpatient treatment (with or without pulmonary embolism): 1 mg/kg/dose every 12 hours or 1.5 mg/kg once daily.

Outpatient treatment (without pulmonary embolism): 1 mg/kg/dose every 12 hours.

Unstable angina or non-Q-wave MI: SubQ: 1 mg/kg twice daily in conjunction with oral aspirin therapy (100-325 mg once daily); continue until clinical stabilization (a minimum of at least 2 days)

Elderly: SubQ: Increased incidence of bleeding with doses of 1.5 mg/kg/day or 1 mg/kg every 12 hours. Injection-associated bleeding and serious adverse reactions are also increased in the elderly. Careful attention should be paid to elderly patients <45 kg.

Pediatrics: Thromboembolism (unlabeled use): SubQ:

Infants <2 months: Initial:

Prophylaxis: 0.75 mg/kg every 12 hours

Treatment: 1.5 mg/kg every 12 hours

Infants >2 months and Children ≤18 years: Initial:

Prophylaxis: 0.5 mg/kg every 12 hours

Treatment: 1 mg/kg every 12 hours

Maintenance: See **Dosage Titration** table:

Enoxaparin Pediatric Dosage Titration

Antifactor Xa	Dose Titration	Time to Repeat Antifactor Xa Level
<0.35 units/mL	Increase dose by 25%	4 h after next dose
0.35-0.49 units/mL	Increase dose by 10%	4 h after next dose
0.5-1 unit/mL	Keep same dosage	Next day, then 1 wk later, then monthly (4 h after dose)
1.1-1.5 units/mL	Decrease dose by 20%	Before next dose
1.6-2 units/mL	Hold dose for 3 h and decrease dose by 30%	Before next dose, then 4 h after next dose
>2 units/mL	Hold all doses until antifactor Xa is 0.5 units/mL, then decrease dose by 40%	Before next dose and every 12 h until antifactor Xa <0.5 units/mL

Modified from Monagle P, Michelson AD, Bovill E, et al, "Antithrombotic Therapy in Children," *Chest*, 2001, 119:344S-70S.

(Continued)

Enoxaparin *(Continued)*

Renal Impairment:

Cl_{cr} ≥30 mL/minute: No specific adjustment recommended (per manufacturer); monitor closely for bleeding.

Cl_{cr} <30 mL/minute:

DVT prophylaxis in abdominal surgery, hip replacement, knee replacement, or in medical patients during acute illness: SubQ: 30 mg once daily

DVT treatment (inpatient or outpatient treatment in conjunction with warfarin): SubQ: 1 mg/kg once daily

Unstable angina, non-Q-wave MI (with ASA): SubQ: 1 mg/kg once daily

Dialysis: Enoxaparin has not been FDA approved for use in dialysis patients. It's elimination is primarily via the renal route. Serious bleeding complications have been reported with use in patients who are dialysis dependent or have severe renal failure. LMWH administration at fixed doses without monitoring has greater unpredictable anticoagulant effects in patients with chronic kidney disease. If used, dosages should be reduced and anti-Xa activity frequently monitored, as accumulation may occur with repeated doses. Many clinicians would not use enoxaparin in this population especially without timely anti-Xa activity assay results.

Hemodialysis: Supplemental dose is not necessary.

Peritoneal dialysis: Significant drug removal is unlikely based on physiochemical characteristics.

Available Dosage Forms

Injection, solution, as sodium [graduated prefilled syringe; preservative free]: 60 mg/0.6 mL (0.6 mL); 80 mg/0.8 mL (0.8 mL); 100 mg/mL (1 mL); 120 mg/0.8 mL (0.8 mL); 150 mg/mL (1 mL)

Injection, solution, as sodium [multidose vial]: 100 mg/mL (3 mL) [contains benzyl alcohol]

Injection, solution, as sodium [prefilled syringe; preservative free]: 30 mg/0.3 mL (0.3 mL); 40 mg/0.4 mL (0.4 mL)

Nursing Guidelines

Assessment: See Contraindications, Warnings/Precautions, and Dosing for use cautions. Assess potential for interactions with other prescriptions, OTC medications, or herbal products patient may be taking (especially anything that may impact fluid balance or cardiac status - see Drug Interactions). See Administration specifics. Assess results of laboratory tests (see below), therapeutic effectiveness, and adverse response on a regular basis during therapy (eg, hypovolemia, angioedema, postural hypotension - see Adverse Reactions and Overdose/Toxicology). Teach patient proper use if self-administered (appropriate injection technique and syringe/needle disposal), possible side effects/appropriate interventions, and adverse symptoms to report (see Patient Education). See Pregnancy Issues. Note breast-feeding caution.

Monitoring Laboratory Tests: Platelets, occult blood, anti-Xa activity, if available; the monitoring of PT and/or aPTT is not necessary.

Patient Education: Inform prescriber of all prescriptions, OTC medications, or herbal products you are taking, and any allergies you have. Do not take any new medication during therapy without consulting prescriber. This drug can only be administered by injection. If self-administered, follow exact directions for injection and needle disposal. You may have a tendency to bleed easily while taking this drug (brush teeth with soft brush, use waxed dental floss, use electric razor, avoid scissors or sharp knives, and potentially harmful activities). Report chest pain; persistent constipation; persistent erection; unusual bleeding or bruising (bleeding gums, nosebleed, blood in urine, dark stool); pain in joints or back; or redness, swelling, burning, or pain at injection site. **Pregnancy/breast-feeding precautions:** Inform prescriber if you are pregnant. Consult prescriber if breast-feeding.

Geriatric Considerations: No specific recommendations.

Pregnancy Risk Factor: B

Pregnancy Issues: There are no adequate and well-controlled studies using enoxaparin in pregnant women. Postmarketing reports include congenital abnormalities (cause and effect not established) and also fetal death when used in pregnant women. In addition, prosthetic valve thrombosis, including fatal cases, has been reported in pregnant women receiving enoxaparin as thromboprophylaxis. Multiple-dose vials contain benzyl alcohol; use caution in pregnant women.

Lactation: Excretion in breast milk unknown/use caution

Breast-Feeding Considerations: This drug has a high molecular weight that would minimize excretion in breast milk and is inactivated by the GI tract which further reduces the risk to the infant.

Perioperative/Anesthesia/Other Concerns: Many critically-ill and surgical patients require preventative measures for venous thromboembolism. Low molecular weight heparins (LMWHs) compare favorably to unfractionated heparin in the prevention and treatment of venous thromboembolism. LMWHs are associated with less thrombocytopenia, compared to heparin, and do not require routine therapeutic monitoring.

Obesity/Renal Dysfunction: There is no consensus for adjusting/correcting the weight-based dosage of LMWH for patients who are morbidly obese. Monitoring of antifactor Xa concentration 4 hours after injection may be warranted. Patients who have a reduction in calculated creatinine clearance are at risk of accumulated anticoagulant effect when they are treated with certain LMWHs. All LMWHs may not behave the same in patients with renal dysfunction. Some clinicians monitor anti-Xa levels in patients with Cl_{cr} <30 mL/minute.

Administration

Compatibility: Stable in NS

Storage: Store at 15°C to 25°C (59°F to 77°F). Do not freeze. Do not mix with other injections or infusions.

♦ Enoxaparin Sodium *see* Enoxaparin *on page 605*
♦ Entocort™ EC *see* Budesonide *on page 260*
♦ Entsol® [OTC] *see* Sodium Chloride *on page 1545*

Ephedrine (e FED rin)

U.S. Brand Names Pretz-D® [OTC]

Synonyms Ephedrine Sulfate

Pharmacologic Category Alpha/Beta Agonist

Medication Safety Issues

Sound-alike/look-alike issues:

Ephedrine may be confused with Epifrin®, epinephrine

Use Treatment of bronchial asthma, nasal congestion, acute bronchospasm, idiopathic orthostatic hypotension

Mechanism of Action Releases tissue stores of epinephrine and thereby produces an alpha- and beta-adrenergic stimulation; longer-acting and less potent than epinephrine

Pharmacodynamics/Kinetics

Onset of action: Oral: Bronchodilation: 0.25-1 hour

Duration: Oral: 3-6 hours

Distribution: Crosses placenta; enters breast milk

Metabolism: Minimally hepatic

Half-life elimination: 2.5-3.6 hours

Excretion: Urine (60% to 77% as unchanged drug) within 24 hours

Contraindications Hypersensitivity to ephedrine or any component of the formulation; cardiac arrhythmias; angle-closure glaucoma; concurrent use of other sympathomimetic agents

Warnings/Precautions Blood volume depletion should be corrected before ephedrine therapy is instituted; use caution in patients with unstable vasomotor symptoms, diabetes, hyperthyroidism, prostatic hyperplasia, or a history of seizures; also use caution in the elderly and those patients with cardiovascular disorders such as coronary artery disease, arrhythmias, and hypertension. Ephedrine may cause hypertension resulting in intracranial hemorrhage. Long-term use may cause anxiety and symptoms of paranoid schizophrenia. Avoid as a bronchodilator; generally not used as a bronchodilator since new $beta_2$ agents are less toxic. Use with caution in the elderly, since it crosses the blood-brain barrier and may cause confusion.

Drug Interactions

Alpha- and beta-adrenergic-blocking agents decrease ephedrine vasopressor effects.

Cardiac glycosides or general anesthetics may increase cardiac stimulation.

MAO inhibitors or atropine may increase blood pressure

Sympathomimetic agents: Additive cardiostimulation with other sympathomimetic agents.

Theophylline may lead to cardiostimulation.

(Continued)

Ephedrine *(Continued)*

Nutritional/Herbal/Ethanol Interactions Herb/Nutraceutical: Avoid ephedra, yohimbe (may cause CNS stimulation).

Lab Interactions Can cause a false-positive amphetamine EMIT assay

Adverse Reactions Frequency not defined.

Cardiovascular: Hypertension, tachycardia, palpitation, elevation or depression of blood pressure, unusual pallor, chest pain, arrhythmia

Central nervous system: CNS stimulating effects, nervousness, anxiety, apprehension, fear, tension, agitation, excitation, restlessness, irritability, insomnia, hyperactivity, dizziness, headache

Gastrointestinal: Xerostomia, nausea, anorexia, GI upset, vomiting

Genitourinary: Painful urination

Neuromuscular & skeletal: Trembling, tremor (more common in the elderly), weakness

Respiratory: Dyspnea

Miscellaneous: Diaphoresis (increased)

Overdosage/Toxicology Symptoms of overdose include dysrhythmias, CNS excitation, respiratory depression, vomiting, and convulsions. There is no specific antidote for ephedrine intoxication and treatment is primarily supportive.

Dosing

Adults & Elderly:

Asthma, nasal congestion, acute bronchospasm, idiopathic orthostatic hypotension:

I.M., SubQ: 25-50 mg, parenteral adult dose should not exceed 150 mg in 24 hours

I.V.: 5-25 mg/dose slow I.V. push repeated after 5-10 minutes as needed, then every 3-4 hours not to exceed 150 mg/24 hours

Nasal congestion: Nasal spray: 2-3 sprays into each nostril, not more frequently than every 4 hours

Pediatrics:

Bronchospasm, nasal congestion:

Oral, SubQ: 3 mg/kg/day or 25-100 mg/m^2/day in 4-6 divided doses every 4-6 hours

I.M., slow I.V. push: 0.2-0.3 mg/kg/dose every 4-6 hours

Nasal congestion: Nasal spray:

Children 6-12 years: 1-2 sprays into each nostril, not more frequently than every 4 hours

Children ≥12 years: Refer to adult dosing.

Available Dosage Forms

Capsule, as sulfate: 25 mg

Injection, solution, as sulfate: 50 mg/mL (1 mL, 10 mL)

Solution, intranasal spray, as sulfate (Pretz-D®): 0.25% (50 mL)

Nursing Guidelines

Assessment: Assess other medications patient may be taking for effectiveness and interactions. Monitor therapeutic effectiveness and adverse reactions when initiating therapy and at regular intervals with long-term therapy. Assess knowledge/teach patient appropriate use, interventions to reduce side effects, and adverse symptoms to report.

Patient Education: Use this medication exactly as directed; do not take more than recommended dosage. Avoid other stimulant prescriptive or OTC medications to avoid serious overdose reactions. Store this medication away from light. You may experience dizziness, blurred vision, restlessness (use caution when driving or engaging in tasks requiring alertness until response to drug is known); or difficulty urinating (empty bladder immediately before taking this medication). Report excessive nervousness or excitation, inability to sleep, facial flushing, pounding heartbeat, muscle tremors or weakness, chest pain or palpitations, bronchial irritation or coughing, or increased sweating. **Pregnancy/breast-feeding precautions:** Inform prescriber if you are or intend to become pregnant. Breast-feeding is not recommended.

Geriatric Considerations: Oral formulation was recently removed from the market; avoid as a bronchodilator. Use caution since it crosses the blood-brain barrier and may cause confusion (see Warnings/Precautions, Adverse Reactions).

Pregnancy Risk Factor: C

Lactation: Enters breast milk/not recommended

Perioperative/Anesthesia/Other Concerns: For I.V. administration, give the undiluted injection slowly. Additional I.V. doses may be given every 5-10 minutes if needed. Do not exceed adult parenteral dose of 150 mg/24 hours. Do not exceed pediatric dose of 3 mg/kg/24 hours. Use the smallest effective dose.

Administration

I.V.: Do not administer unless solution is clear.

Compatibility: Stable in dextran 6% in dextrose, dextran 6% in NS, D_5LR, $D_5 1/4NS$, $D_5 1/2NS$, D_5NS, D_5W, $D_{10}W$, LR, 1/2NS, NS

Y-site administration: Incompatible with thiopental

Compatibility in syringe: Incompatible with thiopental

Compatibility when admixed: Incompatible with hydrocortisone sodium succinate, pentobarbital, phenobarbital

Storage: Protect all dosage forms from light.

Related Information

Contrast Media Reactions, Premedication for Prophylaxis *on page 1911*
Postoperative Nausea and Vomiting *on page 1807*

♦ Ephedrine Sulfate *see* Ephedrine *on page 609*

Epinephrine (ep i NEF rin)

U.S. Brand Names Adrenalin®; EpiPen®; EpiPen® Jr; Primatene® Mist [OTC]; Twinject™

Synonyms Adrenaline; Epinephrine Bitartrate; Epinephrine Hydrochloride

Pharmacologic Category Alpha/Beta Agonist; Antidote

Medication Safety Issues

Sound-alike/look-alike issues:

Epinephrine may be confused with ephedrine
Epifrin® may be confused with ephedrine, EpiPen®
EpiPen® may be confused with Epifrin®

Medication errors have occurred due to confusion with epinephrine products expressed as ratio strengths (eg, 1:1000 vs 1:10,000).

Epinephrine 1:1000 = 1 mg/mL and is most commonly used SubQ.
Epinephrine 1:10,000 = 0.1 mg/mL and is used I.V.

Use Treatment of bronchospasms, anaphylactic reactions, cardiac arrest; added to local anesthetics to decrease systemic absorption, increase duration of action, and decrease toxicity of the local anesthetic

Unlabeled/Investigational Use ACLS guidelines: Ventricular fibrillation (VF) or pulseless ventricular tachycardia (VT) unresponsive to initial defibrillatory shocks; pulseless electrical activity, asystole, hypotension unresponsive to volume resuscitation; symptomatic bradycardia or heart block unresponsive to atropine or pacing

Mechanism of Action Stimulates alpha-, $beta_1$-, and $beta_2$-adrenergic receptors resulting in relaxation of smooth muscle of the bronchial tree, cardiac stimulation, and dilation of skeletal muscle vasculature; small doses can cause vasodilation via $beta_2$-vascular receptors; large doses may produce constriction of skeletal and vascular smooth muscle

Pharmacodynamics/Kinetics

Onset of action: Bronchodilation: SubQ: ~5-10 minutes; Inhalation: ~1 minute

Distribution: Crosses placenta

Metabolism: Taken up into the adrenergic neuron and metabolized by monoamine oxidase and catechol-o-methyltransferase; circulating drug hepatically metabolized

Excretion: Urine (as inactive metabolites, metanephrine, and sulfate and hydroxy derivatives of mandelic acid, small amounts as unchanged drug)

Contraindications Hypersensitivity to epinephrine or any component of the formulation; cardiac arrhythmias; angle-closure glaucoma

Warnings/Precautions Use with caution in elderly patients, patients with diabetes mellitus, cardiovascular diseases (angina, tachycardia, myocardial infarction), thyroid disease, or cerebral arteriosclerosis, Parkinson's; some products contain sulfites as preservatives. Rapid I.V. infusion may cause death from cerebrovascular hemorrhage or cardiac arrhythmias. Oral inhalation of epinephrine is **not** the preferred route of administration.

Drug Interactions Increased toxicity: Increased cardiac irritability if administered concurrently with halogenated inhalational anesthetics, beta-blocking agents, alpha-blocking agents

(Continued)

Epinephrine *(Continued)*

Nutritional/Herbal/Ethanol Interactions Herb/Nutraceutical: Avoid ephedra, yohimbe (may cause CNS stimulation).

Lab Interactions Increased bilirubin (S), catecholamines (U), glucose, uric acid (S)

Adverse Reactions Frequency not defined.

Cardiovascular: Tachycardia (parenteral), pounding heartbeat, flushing, hypertension, pallor, chest pain, increased myocardial oxygen consumption, cardiac arrhythmia, sudden death, angina, vasoconstriction

Central nervous system: Nervousness, anxiety, restlessness, headache, dizziness, lightheadedness, insomnia

Gastrointestinal: Nausea, vomiting, xerostomia, dry throat

Genitourinary: Acute urinary retention in patients with bladder outflow obstruction

Neuromuscular & skeletal: Weakness, trembling

Ocular: Precipitation of or exacerbation of narrow-angle glaucoma, transient stinging, burning, eye pain, allergic lid reaction, ocular irritation

Renal: Decreased renal and splanchnic blood flow

Respiratory: Wheezing, dyspnea

Miscellaneous: Diaphoresis (increased)

Overdosage/Toxicology Symptoms of overdose include hypertension, which may result in subarachnoid hemorrhage and hemiplegia; arrhythmias; unusually large pupils; pulmonary edema; renal failure; and metabolic acidosis. There is no specific antidote for epinephrine intoxication and treatment is primarily supportive.

Dosing

Adults & Elderly:

Asystole:

I.V.: 1 mg every 3-5 minutes; if this approach fails, higher doses of epinephrine (up to 0.2 mg/kg) may be used, but are not recommended (Class Indeterminate; 2000 ACLS guidelines)

Intratracheal: Administer 2-2.5 times the recommended I.V. dose; dilute in 10 mL NS or distilled water. **Note:** Absorption is greater with distilled water, but causes more adverse effects on PaO_2.

Bronchospasm:

I.M., SubQ (1:1000): 0.1-0.5 mg every 10-15 minutes to 4 hours

Suspension (1:200): SubQ: 0.1-0.3 mL (0.5-1.5 mg)

I.V.: 0.1-0.25 mg (single dose maximum: 1 mg)

Nebulization: Instill 8-15 drops into nebulizer reservoirs; administer 1-3 inhalations 4-6 times/day.

Hypotension (refractory to dopamine/dobutamine): Continuous I.V. infusion: Initial: 1 mcg/minute (range: 1-10 mcg/minute); titrate to desired effect; severe cardiac dysfunction may require doses >10 mcg/minute (up to 0.1 mcg/kg/minute)

Hypersensitivity reaction: I.M., SubQ: 0.2-0.5 mg every 20 minutes to 4 hours (single dose maximum: 1 mg)

Nasal congestion: Intranasal: Apply locally as drops or spray or with sterile swab.

Pediatrics:

Bronchodilator:

SubQ: Infants and Children: 10 mcg/kg (0.01 mL/kg of **1:1000**) (single doses not to exceed 0.5 mg) **or** suspension (1:200): 0.005 mL/kg/dose (0.025 mg/kg/dose) to a maximum of 0.15 mL (0.75 mg for single dose) every 8-12 hours

Nebulization: Infants and Children: 0.25-0.5 mL of 2.25% **racemic epinephrine** solution diluted in 3 mL normal saline, or L-epinephrine at an equivalent dose; racemic epinephrine 10 mg = 5 mg L-epinephrine; use lower end of dosing range for younger infants.

Bradycardia:

I.V.: 0.01 mg/kg (0.1 mL/kg of **1:10,000** solution) every 3-5 minutes as needed (maximum: 1 mg/10 mL)

Intratracheal: 0.1 mg/kg (0.1 mL/kg of **1:1000** solution every 3-5 minutes); doses as high as 0.2 mg/kg may be effective

Asystole or pulseless arrest:

I.V. or intraosseous: Initial dose: 0.01 mg/kg (0.1 mL/kg of a **1:10,000** solution). Subsequent doses: 0.1 mg/kg (0.1 mL/kg of a **1:1000** solution); doses as high as 0.2 mg/kg may be effective; repeat every 3-5 minutes.

Intratracheal: 0.1 mg/kg (0.1 mL/kg of a **1:1000** solution); doses as high as 0.2 mg/kg may be effective.

Hypersensitivity reaction: SubQ: 0.01 mg/kg every 15 minutes for 2 doses then every 4 hours as needed (single doses not to exceed 0.5 mg)

Refractory hypotension (refractory to dopamine/dobutamine): Continuous I.V. infusions of 0.1-1 mcg/kg/minute; titrate dosage to desired effect.

Nasal congestion: Intranasal: Children ≥6 years: Apply locally as drops or spray or with sterile swab.

Available Dosage Forms

Aerosol for oral inhalation (Primatene® Mist): 0.22 mg/inhalation (15 mL, 22.5 mL) [contains CFCs]

Injection, solution [prefilled auto injector]:

EpiPen®: 0.3 mg/0.3 mL [1:1000] (2 mL) [contains sodium metabisulfite; available as single unit or in double-unit pack with training unit]

EpiPen® Jr: 0.15 mg/0.3 mL [1:2000] (2 mL) [contains sodium metabisulfite; available as single unit or in double-unit pack with training unit]

Twinject™: 0.15 mg/0.15 mL [1:1000] (1.1 mL) [contains sodium bisulfite; two 0.15 mg doses per injector]; 0.3 mg/0.3 mL [1:1000] (1.1 mL) [contains sodium bisulfite; two 0.3 mg doses per injector]

Injection, solution, as hydrochloride: 0.1 mg/mL [1:10,000] (10 mL); 1 mg/mL [1:1000] (1 mL) [products may contain sodium metabisulfite]

Adrenalin®: 1 mg/mL [1:1000] (1 mL, 30 mL) [contains sodium bisulfite]

Solution for oral inhalation, as hydrochloride (Adrenalin®): 1% [10 mg/mL, 1:100] (7.5 mL) [contains sodium bisulfite]

Nursing Guidelines

Assessment: Assess other medications patient may be taking for effectiveness and interactions. Monitor therapeutic effectiveness (according to purpose for use) and adverse reactions. Monitor vital signs. Assess knowledge/teach patient appropriate use, interventions to reduce side effects, and adverse symptoms to report. I.V. central line with infusion pump and continuous cardiac/hemodynamic monitoring is necessary.

Patient Education: Use this medication exactly as directed; do not take more than recommended dosage. Avoid other stimulant prescriptive or OTC medications to avoid serious overdose reactions. You may experience dizziness, blurred vision, restlessness (use caution when driving or engaging in tasks requiring alertness until response to drug is known); or difficulty urinating (empty bladder immediately before taking this medication). Report excessive nervousness or excitation, inability to sleep, facial flushing, pounding heartbeat, muscle tremors or weakness, chest pain or palpitations, bronchial irritation or coughing, or increased sweating.

Aerosol: Use aerosol or nebulizer as per instructions. Clear as much mucus as possible before use. Rinse mouth following each use. If more than one inhalation is necessary, wait 1 minute between inhalations. May cause restlessness or nervousness; use caution when driving or engaging in hazardous activities until response to medication is known. Report persistent nervousness, restlessness, sleeplessness, palpitations, tachycardia, chest pain, muscle tremors, dizziness, flushing, or if breathing difficulty persists.

Nasal: Instill 1 spray into each nostril 3-4 times a day. Report if symptoms worsen or nasal passages become irritated.

Pregnancy/breast-feeding precautions: Inform prescriber if you are or intend to become pregnant. Consult prescriber if breast-feeding.

Geriatric Considerations: The use of epinephrine in the treatment of acute exacerbations of asthma was studied in older adults. A dose of 0.3 mg SubQ every 20 minutes for three doses was well tolerated in older patients with no history of angina or recent myocardial infarction. There was no significant difference in the incidence of ventricular arrhythmias in older adults versus younger adults.

Pregnancy Risk Factor: C

Pregnancy Issues: Crosses the placenta. Reported association with malformations in 1 study; may be secondary to severe maternal disease.

Lactation: Excretion in breast milk unknown

Perioperative/Anesthesia/Other Concerns:

Septic Shock: Epinephrine's use may be limited by its effects on renal and gastric blood flow and its propensity to increase lactic acid concentrations.

Cardiac Arrest: Epinephrine can be given by endotracheal route during cardiac resuscitation. High-intravenous dose epinephrine (0.1 mg/kg) has not shown to improve survival or neurological outcomes. May have more

(Continued)

Epinephrine *(Continued)*

postresuscitation complications than survivors who receive standard dose epinephrine. Eight randomized clinical studies (>9000 patients) have found no improvement in survival to hospital discharge or neurological outcomes compared with standard epinephrine.

A prospective, multicenter, double-blind randomized, controlled trial evaluated the efficacy of vasopressin or epinephrine when administered to adult patients who suffered an out-of-hospital cardiac arrest (Wenzel V, 2004). For inclusions, patients presented with ventricular fibrillation, pulseless electrical activity, or asystole. They were excluded if they were successfully defibrillated without the administration of a vasopressor, had a terminal illness or had a DNR order, a lack of intravenous access, hemorrhagic shock, pregnancy, cardiac arrest due to trauma, or were <18 years of age. Eligible patients were randomized to intravenous vasopressin (40 units) or epinephrine (1 mg). Each patient received an injection of the study drug, if spontaneous circulation was not restored in 3 minutes they received a second dose (same amount) of the same study drug. If there was no response, the managing physician had the option of giving epinephrine. Patients with ventricular fibrillation were randomized after the first three attempts at defibrillation failed; all others were randomized immediately. The primary endpoint was survival to hospital admission; the secondary endpoint was survival to hospital discharge. Five hundred and eighty-nine patients were randomized to vasopressin and five hundred and ninety-seven patients were randomized to epinephrine. There was no significant difference in the rate of hospital admission between the vasopressin group and the epinephrine group if they had ventricular fibrillation (46.2% vs 43% respectively, p: 0.48) or pulseless electrical activity (33.7% vs 30.5% respectively, p: 0.65). Patients with asystole responded significantly better to vasopressin; having higher rates of hospital admission (29% vs 20.3% in the epinephrine group, p: 0.02) and hospital discharge (4.7% vs 1.5% in the epinephrine group, p: 0.04). Patients who failed vasopressin therapy and received additional epinephrine had significant improvement in survival to hospital admission (25.7% vs 16.4% in the epinephrine group, p: 0.002) and discharge (6.2% vs 1.7%, p: 0.002). Similar patients who were randomized to epinephrine and failed to respond did not improve with additional epinephrine. Cerebral performance among all patients who survived to discharge was similar in both groups. In this trial, vasopressin was superior to epinephrine in patients with asystole. Vasopressin followed by epinephrine may be more effective than epinephrine alone in refractory out-of-hospital cardiac arrest.

A small in-hospital cardiac arrest study evaluated the efficacy of vasopressin or epinephrine in 200 patients. These investigators did not find any differences between the two treatment groups with regard to survival, discharge, or cerebral performance (Stiell I, 2001).

Administration

I.M.: I.M. administration into the buttocks should be avoided.

I.V.: Central line administration only. I.V. infusions require an infusion pump.

Endotracheal: Doses (2-2.5 times the I.V. dose) should be diluted to 10 mL with NS or distilled water prior to administration.

Epinephrine can be administered SubQ, I.M., I.V.

Reconstitution:

Standard diluent: 1 mg/250 mL NS

Preparation of adult I.V. infusion: Dilute 1 mg in 250 mL of D_5W or NS (4 mcg/mL). Administer at an initial rate of 1 mcg/minute and increase to desired effects. At 20 mcg/minute pure alpha effects occur.

1 mcg/minute: 15 mL/hour

2 mcg/minute: 30 mL/hour

3 mcg/minute: 45 mL/hour, etc

Stability of injection of parenteral admixture at room temperature (25°C) or refrigeration (4°C) is 24 hours.

Compatibility: Stable in dextran 6% in dextrose, dextran 6% in NS, D_5LR, $D_5{}^1/_4NS$, $D_5{}^1/_2NS$, D_5NS, D_5W, $D_{10}W$, $D_{10}NS$, LR, NS; **incompatible** with sodium bicarbonate 5%

Y-site administration: Incompatible with ampicillin, thiopental

Compatibility when admixed: Incompatible with aminophylline, hyaluronidase, mephentermine, sodium bicarbonate

Storage: Epinephrine is sensitive to light and air. Protection from light is recommended. Oxidation turns drug pink, then a brown color. **Solutions should not be used if they are discolored or contain a precipitate.**

- **Epinephrine and Lidocaine** *see* Lidocaine and Epinephrine *on page 1039*
- **Epinephrine Bitartrate** *see* Epinephrine *on page 611*
- **Epinephrine Bitartrate and Bupivacaine Hydrochloride** *see* Bupivacaine and Epinephrine *on page 268*
- **Epinephrine Hydrochloride** *see* Epinephrine *on page 611*

Epinephrine (Racemic/Dental) (ep i NEF rin, ra SEE mik)

U.S. Brand Names AsthmaNefrin®; microNefrin®; S-2®; Vaponefrin®

Pharmacologic Category Alpha/Beta Agonist; Vasoconstrictor

Medication Safety Issues

Sound-alike/look-alike issues:

Epifrin® may be confused with ephedrine, EpiPen®

Pharmacodynamics/Kinetics

Onset of action: Bronchodilation: SubQ: 5-10 minutes; Inhalation: ~1 minute

Absorption: Oral: None

Contraindications

Refer to Epinephrine monograph

Warnings/Precautions

Refer to Epinephrine monograph

Drug Interactions Refer to Epinephrine monograph

Adverse Reactions Refer to Epinephrine monograph

Available Dosage Forms Solution for oral inhalation (AsthmaNefrin®, microNefrin®, S-2®): Racepinephrine 2.25% [epinephrine base 1.125%] (7.5 mL, 15 mL, 30 mL)

- **EpiPen®** *see* Epinephrine *on page 611*
- **EpiPen® Jr** *see* Epinephrine *on page 611*
- **Epipodophyllotoxin** *see* Etoposide *on page 695*

Epirubicin (ep i ROO bi sin)

U.S. Brand Names Ellence®

Synonyms Pidorubicin; Pidorubicin Hydrochloride

Pharmacologic Category Antineoplastic Agent, Anthracycline

Medication Safety Issues

Sound-alike/look-alike issues:

Epirubicin may be confused with DOXOrubicin, DAUNOrubicin, idarubicin

Ellence® may be confused with Elase®

Use Adjuvant therapy for primary breast cancer

Mechanism of Action Epirubicin is an anthracycline antibiotic. Epirubicin is known to inhibit DNA and RNA synthesis by steric obstruction after intercalating between DNA base pairs; active throughout entire cell cycle. Intercalation triggers DNA cleavage by topoisomerase II, resulting in cytocidal activity. Epirubicin also inhibits DNA helicase, and generates cytotoxic free radicals.

Pharmacodynamics/Kinetics

Distribution: V_{ss} 21-27 L/kg

Protein binding: 77% to albumin

Metabolism: Extensively via hepatic and extrahepatic (including RBCs) routes

Half-life elimination: Triphasic; Mean terminal: 33 hours

Excretion: Feces; urine (lesser extent)

Contraindications Hypersensitivity to epirubicin, other anthracyclines, or anthracenediones; severe myocardial insufficiency, severe arrhythmias; recent myocardial infarction; severe hepatic dysfunction; baseline neutrophil count 1500 cells/mm^3; previous anthracycline treatment up to maximum cumulative dose; pregnancy

Warnings/Precautions Hazardous agent - use appropriate precautions for handling and disposal. The primary toxicity is myelosuppression; severe thrombocytopenia or anemia may occur. Thrombophlebitis and thromboembolic phenomena (including pulmonary embolism) have occurred.

Potential cardiotoxicity, particularly in patients who have received prior anthracyclines, prior radiotherapy to the mediastinal/pericardial area, or who have pre-existing cardiac disease, may occur. Acute toxicity (primarily arrhythmias) and delayed toxicity (CHF) have been described. Delayed toxicity usually develops late in the course of therapy or within 2-3 months after completion,

(Continued)

Epirubicin *(Continued)*

however, events with an onset of several months to years after termination of treatment have been described. The risk of delayed cardiotoxicity increases more steeply at dosages above 900 mg/m^2, and this dose should be exceeded only with extreme caution. Toxicity may be additive with other anthracyclines or anthracenediones, and may be increased in pediatric patients. Regular monitoring of LVEF and discontinuation at the first sign of impairment is recommended especially in patients with risk factors or impaired cardiac function.

Reduce dosage and use with caution in mild to moderate hepatic impairment or in severe renal dysfunction (serum creatinine >5 mg/dL). May cause tumor lysis syndrome or radiation recall. Treatment with anthracyclines may increase the risk of secondary leukemias. For I.V. administration only, severe local tissue necrosis will result if extravasation occurs. Epirubicin is emetogenic. Women ≥70 years of age should be especially monitored for toxicity; women of childbearing age should be advised to avoid becoming pregnant.

Drug Interactions Cimetidine increased the AUC of epirubicin by 50%.

Nutritional/Herbal/Ethanol Interactions

Ethanol: Avoid ethanol (due to GI irritation).

Herb/Nutraceutical: St John's wort may decrease doxorubicin levels. Avoid black cohosh, dong quai in estrogen-dependent tumors.

Adverse Reactions

>10%:

- Central nervous system: Lethargy (1% to 46%)
- Dermatologic: Alopecia (69% to 95%)
- Endocrine & metabolic: Amenorrhea (69% to 72%), hot flashes (5% to 39%)
- Gastrointestinal: Nausea, vomiting (83% to 92%), mucositis (9% to 59%), diarrhea (7% to 25%)
- Hematologic: Leukopenia (49% to 80%; Grade 3 and 4: 1.5% to 58.6%), neutropenia (54% to 80%), anemia (13% to 72%), thrombocytopenia (5% to 49%)
- Local: Injection site reactions (3% to 20%)
- Ocular: Conjunctivitis (1% to 15%)
- Miscellaneous: Infection (15% to 21%)

1% to 10%:

- Cardiovascular: CHF (0.4% to 1.5%), decreased LVEF (asymptomatic) (1.4% to 2.1%); recommended maximum cumulative dose: 900 mg/m^2
- Central nervous system: Fever (1% to 5%)
- Dermatologic: Rash (1% to 9%), skin changes (0.7% to 5%)
- Gastrointestinal: Anorexia (2% to 3%)

Other reactions (percentage not specified): Acute lymphoid leukemia, acute myelogenous leukemia (0.3% at 3 years, 0.5% at 5 years, 0.6% at 8 years), anaphylaxis, hypersensitivity, photosensitivity reaction, premature menopause in women, pulmonary embolism, radiation recall, skin and nail hyperpigmentation, thromboembolic phenomena, thrombophlebitis, transaminases increased, urticaria

Overdosage/Toxicology Symptoms of overdose are generally extensions of known cytotoxic effects, including myelosuppression, mucositis, gastrointestinal bleeding, lactic acidosis, multiple organ failure, and death. Treatment is supportive.

Dosing

Adults: I.V.: 100-120 mg/m^2 once weekly every 3-4 weeks **or** 50-60 mg/m^2 days 1 and 8 every 3-4 weeks

Breast cancer:

- CEF-120: 60 mg/m^2 on days 1 and 8 every 28 days for 6 cycles
- FEC-100: 100 mg/m^2 on day 1 every 21 days for 6 cycles
- **Note:** Note: Patients receiving 120 mg/m^2/cycle as part of combination therapy should also receive prophylactic therapy with sulfamethoxazole/trimethoprim or a fluoroquinolone.

Dosage modifications:

- Delay day 1 dose until platelets are ≥100,000/mm^3, ANC ≥1500/mm^3, and nonhematologic toxicities have recovered to ≤grade 1
- Reduce day 1 dose in subsequent cycles to 75% of previous day 1 dose if patient experiences nadir platelet counts <50,000/mm^3, ANC <250/mm^3, neutropenic fever, or grade 3/4 nonhematologic toxicity during the previous cycle
- For divided doses (day 1 and day 8), reduce day 8 dose to 75% of day 1 dose if platelet counts are 75,000-100,000/mm^3 and ANC is 1000-1499/mm^3;

omit day 8 dose if platelets are <75,000/mm^3, ANC <1000/mm^3, or grade 3/4 nonhematologic toxicity

Dosage adjustment in bone marrow dysfunction: Heavily-treated patients, patients with pre-existing bone marrow depression or neoplastic bone marrow infiltration: Lower starting doses (75-90 mg/mm^2) should be considered.

Elderly: Plasma clearance of epirubicin in elderly female patients was noted to be reduced by 35%. Although no initial dosage reduction is specifically recommended, particular care should be exercised in monitoring toxicity and adjusting subsequent dosage in elderly patients (particularly females >70 years of age).

Renal Impairment: Severe renal impairment (serum creatinine >5 mg/dL): Lower doses should be considered.

Hepatic Impairment:

Bilirubin 1.2-3 mg/dL or AST 2-4 times the upper limit of normal: 50% of recommended starting dose.

Bilirubin >3 mg/dL or AST >4 times the upper limit of normal: 25% of recommended starting dose.

Available Dosage Forms Injection, solution [preservative free]: 2 mg/mL (25 mL, 100 mL)

Nursing Guidelines

Assessment: This drug should be administered only under the supervision of a physician experienced in the use of chemotherapy. See Contraindications, Warnings/Precautions, and Dosing for use cautions. See Administration, Dosing, Reconstitution, and Compatibility for administration specifics. Premedication with an antiemetic may be ordered (emetogenic). Infusion site must be monitored closely to prevent extravasation (see Administration). Assess results of laboratory tests (see below) and patient response (see Adverse Reactions and Overdose/Toxicology) prior to each treatment and on a regular basis throughout therapy. Teach patient possible side effects/appropriate interventions (eg, importance of adequate hydration) and adverse symptoms to report (see Patient Education). **Pregnancy risk factor D** - determine that patient is not pregnant before beginning treatment. Instruct patients of childbearing age on appropriate barrier contraceptive measures. Breast-feeding is contraindicated.

Monitoring Laboratory Tests: CBC with differential and platelet count, liver function tests, renal function, ECG, and left ventricular ejection fraction (baseline and repeated measurement). The method used for assessment of LVEF (echocardiogram or MUGA) should be consistent during routine monitoring.

Patient Education: Inform prescriber of all prescriptions, OTC medications, or herbal products you are taking, and any allergies you have. Do not take any new medication during therapy unless approved by prescriber. This medication can only be administered by infusion. Report immediately any swelling, pain, burning, or redness at infusion site. Avoid alcohol. Maintain adequate hydration (2-3 L/day of fluids) unless instructed to restrict fluid intake, and adequate nutrition (small, frequent meals may help). You will be more susceptible to infection (avoid crowds and exposure to infection and do not have any vaccinations without consulting prescriber). May cause nausea or vomiting (small, frequent meals, frequent mouth care, sucking lozenges, or chewing gum may help); diarrhea (buttermilk, boiled milk, or yogurt may help); loss of hair (reversible); hyperpigmentation of skin or nails; mouth sores (frequent mouth care, soft toothbrush may help); or changes in menstrual cycle (consult prescriber). Report chest pain, swelling of extremities, palpitations, or rapid heartbeat; respiratory difficulty or unusual cough; unresolved nausea, vomiting, or diarrhea; alterations in urinary pattern (increased or decreased); opportunistic infection (fever, chills, unusual bruising or bleeding, fatigue, purulent vaginal discharge, unhealed mouth sores); skin rash; abdominal pain; blood in urine or stool; or other unresolved reactions. **Pregnancy/breast-feeding precautions:** Do not get pregnant while taking this medication and for 1 month following therapy. Consult prescriber for appropriate barrier contraceptives. Do not breast-feed.

Pregnancy Risk Factor: D

Pregnancy Issues: Epirubicin is mutagenic and carcinogenic. If a pregnant woman is treated with epirubicin, or if a woman becomes pregnant while receiving this drug, she should be informed of the potential hazard to the fetus. Women of childbearing potential should be advised to avoid becoming pregnant.

(Continued)

Epirubicin *(Continued)*

Lactation: Excretion in breast milk unknown/contraindicated

Breast-Feeding Considerations: Excretion in human breast milk is unknown, however, other anthracyclines are excreted. Breast-feeding is contraindicated.

Administration

I.V.: Administer I.V. into the tubing of a freely-flowing intravenous infusion (0.9% sodium chloride or 5% glucose solution) over 3-5 minutes.

Compatibility: Stable in D_5W, LR, NS; **incompatible** with any solution of alkaline pH

Incompatible with heparin, fluorouracil

Compatibility in syringe: Incompatible with fluorouracil, ifosfamide with mesna, any solution of alkaline pH

Storage: Store refrigerated (2°C to 8°C/36°F to 46°F). Protect from light. Solution should be used within 24 hours of penetrating the rubber stopper.

♦ Epitol® *see* Carbamazepine *on page 306*
♦ Epivir® *see* Lamivudine *on page 999*
♦ Epivir-HBV® *see* Lamivudine *on page 999*
♦ EPO *see* Epoetin Alfa *on page 618*

Epoetin Alfa (e POE e tin AL fa)

U.S. Brand Names Epogen®; Procrit®

Synonyms EPO; Erythropoietin; *r*HuEPO-α

Pharmacologic Category Colony Stimulating Factor

Medication Safety Issues

Sound-alike/look-alike issues:

Epoetin alfa may be confused with darbepoetin alfa

Use Treatment of anemia related to HIV therapy, chronic renal failure, antineoplastic therapy; reduction of allogeneic blood transfusion for elective, noncardiac, nonvascular surgery

Unlabeled/Investigational Use Anemia associated with rheumatic disease; hypogenerative anemia of Rh hemolytic disease; sickle cell anemia; acute renal failure; Gaucher's disease; Castleman's disease; paroxysmal nocturnal hemoglobinuria; anemia of critical illness (limited documentation); anemia of prematurity

Mechanism of Action Induces erythropoiesis by stimulating the division and differentiation of committed erythroid progenitor cells; induces the release of reticulocytes from the bone marrow into the bloodstream, where they mature to erythrocytes. There is a dose response relationship with this effect. This results in an increase in reticulocyte counts followed by a rise in hematocrit and hemoglobin levels.

Pharmacodynamics/Kinetics

Onset of action: Several days

Peak effect: 2-3 weeks

Distribution: V_d: 9 L; rapid in the plasma compartment; concentrated in liver, kidneys, and bone marrow

Metabolism: Some degradation does occur

Bioavailability: SubQ: ~21% to 31%; intraperitoneal epoetin: 3% (a few patients)

Half-life elimination: Circulating: Chronic renal failure: 4-13 hours; Healthy volunteers: 20% shorter

Time to peak, serum: SubQ: Chronic renal failure: 5-24 hours

Excretion: Feces (majority); urine (small amounts, 10% unchanged in normal volunteers)

Contraindications Hypersensitivity to albumin (human) or mammalian cell-derived products; uncontrolled hypertension

Warnings/Precautions Use caution with history of seizures or hypertension; blood pressure should be controlled prior to start of therapy and monitored closely throughout treatment. Excessive rate of rise of hematocrit may be possibly associated with the exacerbation of hypertension or seizures; decrease the epoetin dose if the hemoglobin increase exceeds 1 g/dL in any 2-week period. Use caution in patients at risk for thrombosis or with history of cardiovascular disease. Increased mortality has occurred when aggressive dosing is used in CHF or anginal patients undergoing hemodialysis. One study demonstrated that when patients were targeted for a hematocrit of 42% versus a less aggressive 30%, mortality was higher (35% versus 29%).

Pure red cell aplasia (PRCA) with neutralizing antibodies to erythropoietin has been reported in limited patients treated with recombinant products; may occur more in patients with CRF. Patients should be evaluated for any loss of effect to therapy and treatment discontinued with evidence of PRCA. Response to therapy may be limited by multiple factors.

Prior to and during therapy iron stores must be evaluated. Iron supplementation should be given during therapy. Use caution with porphyria. Not recommended for acute correction of severe anemia or as a substitute for transfusion.

Serum EPO levels can be ordered routinely from Clinical Chemistry (red top serum separator tube).

Adverse Reactions Note: Adverse drug reaction incidences vary based on condition being treated and dose administered.

>10%:
- Cardiovascular: Edema, hypertension
- Central nervous system: Fever, headache, insomnia
- Dermatologic: Pruritus, rash
- Gastrointestinal: Dyspepsia, nausea, vomiting
- Local: Injection site reaction
- Neuromuscular & skeletal: Arthralgia, paresthesia, weakness
- Respiratory: Congestion, cough, dyspnea, upper respiratory infection

1% to 10%:
- Cardiovascular: Chest pain
- Central nervous system: Fatigue, seizure
- Gastrointestinal: Diarrhea
- Hematologic: Clotted access, deep vein thrombosis

<1% (Limited to important or life-threatening): Allergic reaction, CVA, flu-like syndrome, hyperkalemia, hypersensitivity reactions, MI, myalgia, pulmonary embolism, pure red cell aplasia, severe anemia (with or without other cytopenias), tachycardia, thrombosis, TIA

Overdosage/Toxicology Symptoms of overdose include erythrocytosis. Maintain adequate airway and provide other supportive measures and agents for treating anaphylaxis when the I.V. drug is given.

Dosing

Adults & Elderly: Individuals with anemia due to iron deficiency, sickle cell disease, autoimmune hemolytic anemia, and bleeding, generally have appropriate endogenous EPO levels to drive erythropoiesis and would not ordinarily be candidates for EPO therapy.

Chronic renal failure patients: I.V., SubQ: Initial dose: 50-100 units/kg 3 times/week

Titration: Reduce dose by 25% when hemoglobin approaches 12 g/dL **or** when hemoglobin increases 1 g/dL in any 2-week period. Increase dose by 25% if hemoglobin does not increase by 2 g/dL after 8 weeks of therapy and hemoglobin is below suggested target range; suggested target hemoglobin range: 10-12 g/dL.

Maintenance dose: Individualize to target range; limit additional dosage increases to every 4 weeks (or longer)

Dialysis patients: Median dose: 75 units/kg 3 times/week

Nondialysis patients: Median dose: 75-150 units/kg

Zidovudine-treated, HIV-infected patients (patient with erythropoietin levels >500 mU/mL is unlikely to respond): I.V., SubQ: 100 units/kg 3 times/week for 8 weeks

Increase dose by 50-100 units/kg 3 times/week if response is not satisfactory in terms of reducing transfusion requirements or increasing hemoglobin after 8 weeks of therapy. Evaluate response every 4-8 weeks thereafter and adjust the dose accordingly by 50-100 units/kg increments 3 times/week. If patient has not responded satisfactorily to a 300 unit/kg dose 3 times/week, a response to higher doses is unlikely. Stop dose if hemoglobin exceeds 13 g/dL and resume treatment at a 25% dose reduction when hemoglobin drops to 12 g/dL.

Cancer patients on chemotherapy: Treatment of patients with erythropoietin levels >200 mU/mL is **not recommended**. SubQ:

150 units/kg 3 times/week or 40,000 units once weekly; commonly used doses range from 10,000 units 3 times/week to 40,000-60,000 units once weekly.

Dose adjustment: If response is not satisfactory after a sufficient period of evaluation (8 weeks of 3 times/week and 4 weeks of once-weekly therapy), the dose may be increased every 4 weeks (or longer) up to 300 units/kg 3 times/week, **or** when dosed weekly, increased all at once to 60,000 units

(Continued)

Epoetin Alfa *(Continued)*

weekly. If patient does not respond, a response to higher doses is unlikely. Stop dose when hemoglobin drops to 12 g/dL; reduce dose by 25% if hemoglobin increases by 1 g/dL in any 2-week period.

Alternative dose (unlabeled dosing): Initial dose: 60,000 units once weekly for 8 weeks. **Dose adjustment:** If patient does not respond, a response to higher doses is unlikely. If response is adequate (hemoglobin increases >2 g/dL after 8 weeks), begin maintenance dose of 120,000 units, to be given once every 3 weeks. During any point of initial or maintenance therapy, if the hemoglobin increases 1.3 g/dL in a 2-week period, decrease dose to 40,000 units once weekly. Stop dose if hemoglobin exceeds 15 g/dL and resume treatment at 20,000 units once-weekly when hemoglobin drops to 13 g/dL (Patton, 2003).

Surgery patients: Prior to initiating treatment, obtain a hemoglobin to establish that is >10 mg/dL or ≤13 mg/dL: SubQ: Initial dose: 300 units/kg/day for 10 days before surgery, on the day of surgery, and for 4 days after surgery

Alternative dose: 600 units/kg in once weekly doses (21, 14, and 7 days before surgery) plus a fourth dose on the day of surgery

Anemia of critical illness (unlabeled use): SubQ: 40,000 units once weekly

Pediatrics:

Anemia of prematurity (unlabeled use): Infants: I.V., SubQ: Dosing range: 500-1250 units/kg/week; commonly used dose: 250 units/kg 3 times/week; supplement with oral iron therapy 3-8 mg/kg/day

Chronic renal failure patients: I.V., SubQ: Initial dose: 50 units/kg 3 times/ week

Dosage adjustment: Reduce dose by 25% when hemoglobin approaches 12 g/dL **or** when hemoglobin increases 1 g/dL in any 2-week period. Increase dose by 25% if hemoglobin does not increase by 2 g/dL after 8 weeks of therapy and hemoglobin is below suggested target range; suggested target hemoglobin range: 10-12 g/dL

Maintenance dose: Individualize to target range; limit additional dosage increases to every 4 weeks (or longer)

Dialysis patients: Median dose: 167 units/kg/week **or** 76 units/kg 2-3 times/ week

Nondialysis patients: Dosing range: 50-250 units/kg 1-3 times/week

Zidovudine-treated, HIV-infected patients (patient with erythropoietin levels >500 mU/mL is unlikely to respond): I.V., SubQ: Initial dose: Reported dosing range: 50-400 units/kg 2-3 times/week

Cancer patients on chemotherapy: Treatment of patients with erythropoietin levels >200 mU/mL is **not recommended**: I.V., SubQ: Dosing range: 25-300 units/kg 3-7 times/week; commonly reported initial dose: 150 units/kg

Dosage adjustment: If response is not satisfactory after a sufficient period of evaluation (8 weeks), the dose may be increased every 4 weeks (or longer) up to 300 units/kg 3 times/week. If patient does not respond, a response to higher doses is unlikely. Stop dose if hemoglobin exceeds 13 g/dL and resume treatment at a 25% dose reduction when hemoglobin drops to 12 g/ dL; reduce dose by 25% if hemoglobin increases by 1 g/dL in any 2-week period, or if hemoglobin approaches 12 g/dL.

Renal Impairment:

Dialysis patient: Usually administered as I.V. bolus 3 times/week. While administration is independent of the dialysis procedure, it may be administered into the venous line at the end of the dialysis procedure to obviate the need for additional venous access.

Chronic renal failure patients not on dialysis: May be given either as an I.V. or SubQ injection.

Hemodialysis: Supplemental dose is not necessary.

Peritoneal dialysis: Supplemental dose is not necessary.

Available Dosage Forms

Injection, solution [preservative free]: 2000 units/mL (1 mL); 3000 units/mL (1 mL); 4000 units/mL (1 mL); 10,000 units/mL (1 mL); 40,000 units/mL (1 mL) [contains human albumin]

Injection, solution [with preservative]: 10,000 units/mL (2 mL); 20,000 units/mL (1 mL) [contains human albumin and benzyl alcohol]

Nursing Guidelines

Assessment: See Contraindications, Warnings/Precautions, and Dosing for use cautions. Assess potential for interactions with other prescriptions, OTC medications, or herbal products patient may be taking (see Drug Interactions, eg, nutritional or supplemental iron). See Administration specifics. I.V. lines should be monitored for possible clotting. Assess results of laboratory tests (see below), therapeutic effectiveness, and adverse response (eg, hypovolemia, angioedema, postural hypotension - see Adverse Reactions and Overdose/ Toxicology) on a regular basis during therapy. Teach patient proper use if self-administered (appropriate injection technique and syringe/needle disposal), possible side effects/appropriate interventions, and adverse symptoms to report (see Patient Education). Note breast-feeding caution.

Monitoring Laboratory Tests: Hematocrit should be determined twice weekly until stabilization within the target range (30% to 36%), and twice weekly for at least 2-6 weeks after a dose increase. See table.

Test	Initial Phase Frequency	Maintenance Phase Frequency
Hematocrit/hemoglobin	2 x/week	2-4 x/month
Blood pressure	3 x/week	3 x/week
Serum ferritin	Monthly	Quarterly
Transferrin saturation	Monthly	Quarterly
Serum chemistries including CBC with differential, creatinine, blood urea nitrogen, potassium, phosphorous	Regularly per routine	Regularly per routine

Patient Education: Inform prescriber of all prescriptions, OTC medications, or herbal products you are taking, and any allergies you have. Do not take any new medication during therapy without consulting prescriber. If self-administered, follow exact directions for injection and needle disposal. You will require frequent blood tests to determine appropriate dosage. Do not make significant changes in your dietary iron without consulting prescriber. Report signs or symptoms of edema (eg, swollen extremities, respiratory difficulty, rapid weight gain); onset of severe headache; acute back pain; chest pain; or muscular tremors or seizure activity. **Pregnancy/breast-feeding precautions:** Inform prescriber if you are or intend to become pregnant. Consult prescriber if breast-feeding.

Geriatric Considerations: There is limited information about the use of epoetin alfa in the elderly. Endogenous erythropoietin secretion has been reported to be decreased in older adults with normocytic or iron-deficiency anemias or those with a serum hemoglobin concentration <12 g/dL; one study did not find such a relationship in the elderly with chronic anemia. A blunted erythropoietin response to anemia has been reported in patients with cancer, rheumatoid arthritis, and AIDS.

Pregnancy Risk Factor: C

Pregnancy Issues: Epoetin alpha has been shown to have adverse effects in rats when given in doses 5 times the human dose. Use only if potential benefit justifies the potential risk to the fetus.

Lactation: Excretion in breast milk unknown/use caution

Breast-Feeding Considerations: When administered enterally to neonates (mixed with human milk or infant formula), *r*HuEPO-α did not significantly increase serum EPO concentrations. If passage via breast milk does occur, risk to a nursing infant appears low.

Perioperative/Anesthesia/Other Concerns: Recently a prospective, randomized, double-blind, placebo-controlled, multicenter trial was performed with critically-ill patients (Corwin HL, 2002), assessing the efficacy of recombinant human erythropoietin in reducing red blood cell transfusions. Patients were enrolled from December 1998 through June 2001. Over 1300 ICU (medical, surgical, or medical/surgical) patients were randomized to receive placebo or 40,000 units of erythropoietin subcutaneously on ICU day 3 and then weekly for patients who remained in the hospital. Inclusion criteria included ICU stay for 3 days, age >18 years, and hematocrit <38%. Exclusion criteria included acute ischemic heart disease. Each patient's physician determined the need for red blood cell transfusion. Results: The mean baseline hemoglobin was 9.97 g/dL in each group. Patients receiving erythropoietin were less likely to receive transfusions. The median number of units transfused per patient in the placebo group was 2 and in the erythropoietin group was 1 (P <0.001). The erythropoietin group had a 19% reduction in total units of red blood cells

(Continued)

Epoetin Alfa *(Continued)*

transfused per days alive (P=0.04; confidence interval [CI] 0.79-0.83). Mortality and adverse clinical events were not significantly different between groups. The authors concluded that weekly administration of erythropoietin in critically-ill patients reduces red blood cell transfusions and increases hemoglobin. The authors also suggest that further study is needed to determine whether use of erythropoietin results in improved clinical outcomes. In addition, data on cost effectiveness would be helpful.

A restrictive transfusion approach (Hebert PC, 1999) was described in a transfusion trial that was published after Corwin's trial was underway. Hebert and his group evaluated a restrictive transfusion strategy (transfuse if hemoglobin <7 g/dL to maintain between 7 and 9 g/dL) versus a liberal strategy (transfuse if hemoglobin <10 g/dL to maintain between 10 and 12 g/dL). Inclusion criteria included anticipated ICU stay >24 hours, hemoglobin ≤9 g/dL with 72 hours of ICU admission, and euvolemia after initial treatment. Exclusion criteria included chronic anemia, active bleeding, or admission after a routine cardiac surgical procedure. The restrictive approach to transfusion was at least as effective as and possibly superior to a liberal transfusion policy in critically-ill patients. The exception to this may be patients with acute myocardial infarction and unstable angina.

Administration

I.V.: I.V. (not recommended; I.V. administration may require up to 40% more drug as SubQ/I.M. administration to achieve the same therapeutic result)

Patients with CRF on dialysis: May be administered I.V. bolus into the venous line after dialysis.

Patients with CRF not on dialysis: May be administered I.V. or SubQ

Reconstitution: Prior to SubQ administration, preservative free solutions may be mixed with bacteriostatic NS containing benzyl alcohol 0.9% in a 1:1 ratio. Dilutions of 1:10 in $D_{10}W$ with human albumin 0.05% or 0.1% are stable for 24 hours.

Compatibility: Stable in $D_{10}W$ with albumin 0.05%, $D_{10}W$ with albumin 0.1%; **incompatible** with $D_{10}W$ with albumin 0.01%, $D_{10}W$, NS

Storage: Vials should be stored at 2°C to 8°C (36°F to 46°F); **do not freeze or shake**.

Single-dose 1 mL vial contains no preservative: Use one dose per vial; do not re-enter vial; discard unused portions.

Single-dose vials (except 40,000 units/mL vial) are stable for 2 weeks at room temperature; single-dose 40,000 units/mL vial is stable for 1 week at room temperature.

Multidose 1 mL or 2 mL vial contains preservative; store at 2°C to 8°C after initial entry and between doses; discard 21 days after initial entry.

Multidose vials (with preservative) are stable for 1 week at room temperature.

Prefilled syringes containing the 20,000 units/mL formulation with preservative are stable for 6 weeks refrigerated (2°C to 8°C).

♦ **Epogen®** *see* Epoetin Alfa *on page 618*

Epoprostenol (e poe PROST en ole)

U.S. Brand Names Flolan®

Synonyms Epoprostenol Sodium; PGI_2; PGX; Prostacyclin

Pharmacologic Category Prostaglandin

Use Treatment of idiopathic pulmonary arterial hypertension [IPAH]; pulmonary hypertension associated with the scleroderma spectrum of disease [SSD] in NYHA Class III and Class IV patients who do not respond adequately to conventional therapy

Mechanism of Action Epoprostenol is also known as prostacyclin and PGI_2. It is a strong vasodilator of all vascular beds. In addition, it is a potent endogenous inhibitor of platelet aggregation. The reduction in platelet aggregation results from epoprostenol's activation of intracellular adenylate cyclase and the resultant increase in cyclic adenosine monophosphate concentrations within the platelets. Additionally, it is capable of decreasing thrombogenesis and platelet clumping in the lungs by inhibiting platelet aggregation.

Pharmacodynamics/Kinetics

Metabolism: Rapidly hydrolyzed; subject to some enzymatic degradation; forms one active metabolite and 13 inactive metabolites

Half-life elimination: 6 minutes

Excretion: Urine (84%); feces (4%)

Contraindications Hypersensitivity to epoprostenol or to structurally-related compounds; chronic use in patients with CHF due to severe left ventricular systolic dysfunction; patients who develop pulmonary edema during dose initiation

Warnings/Precautions Abrupt interruptions or large sudden reductions in dosage may result in rebound pulmonary hypertension; some patients with primary pulmonary hypertension have developed pulmonary edema during dose ranging, which may be associated with pulmonary veno-occlusive disease; during chronic use, unless contraindicated, anticoagulants should be coadministered to reduce the risk of thromboembolism

Drug Interactions

Antihypertensive agents: The hypotensive effects of epoprostenol may be exacerbated by other vasodilators, diuretics, or by using acetate in dialysis fluids.

Antiplatelet agents (aspirin, IIb/IIIa antagonists, clopidogrel, ticlopidine): Risk of bleeding may be increased

Digoxin: Serum levels may be increased; clearance decreased by 15%; monitor

Furosemide: Serum levels may be increased; clinical significance low; clearance decreased by 13%

Heparin (including low molecular weight heparins): Risk of bleeding may be increased

Warfarin: Risk of bleeding may be increased

Adverse Reactions

Note: Adverse events reported during dose initiation and escalation include flushing (58%), headache (49%), nausea/vomiting (32%), hypotension (16%), anxiety/nervousness/agitation (11%), chest pain (11%); abdominal pain, back pain, bradycardia, diaphoresis, dizziness, dyspepsia, dyspnea, hypesthesia/paresthesia, musculoskeletal pain, and tachycardia are also reported. The following adverse events have been reported during chronic administration for IPAH. Although some may be related to the underlying disease state, anxiety, diarrhea, flu-like symptoms, flushing, headache, jaw pain, nausea, nervousness, and vomiting the following are clearly contributed to epoprostenol.

>10%:

Cardiovascular: Chest pain (67%), palpitation (63%), flushing (42%), tachycardia (35%), arrhythmia (27%), hemorrhage (19%), bradycardia (15%)

Central nervous system: Dizziness (83%), headache (83%), chills/fever/sepsis/flu-like symptoms (25%), anxiety/nervousness/tremor (21%)

Gastrointestinal: Nausea/vomiting (67%), diarrhea (37%)

Genitourinary: Weight loss (27%)

Local: Injection-site reactions: Infection (21%), pain (13%)

Neuromuscular & skeletal: Weakness (87%), jaw pain (54%), myalgia (44%), musculoskeletal pain (35%; predominantly involving legs and feet), hypesthesia/hyperparesthesia/paresthesia (12%)

Respiratory: Dyspnea (90%)

1% to 10%:

Cardiovascular: Supraventricular tachycardia (8%), cerebrovascular accident (4%)

Central nervous system: Convulsion (4%)

Dermatologic: Rash (10%; conventional therapy 13%), pruritus (4%)

Endocrine & metabolic: Hypokalemia (6%)

Gastrointestinal: Constipation (6%), weight gain (6%)

Neuromuscular & skeletal: Arthralgia (6%)

Ocular: Amblyopia (8%), vision abnormality (4%)

Respiratory: Epistaxis (4%), pleural effusion (4%)

<1% (Limited to important or life-threatening): Anemia, ascites, hypersplenism, hyperthyroidism, pancytopenia, splenomegaly, thrombocytopenia

Overdosage/Toxicology Symptoms of overdose include headache, hypotension, tachycardia, nausea, vomiting, diarrhea, and flushing. If any of these symptoms occur, reduce the infusion rate until symptoms subside. If symptoms do not subside, consider drug discontinuation. No fatal events have been reported following overdose with epoprostenol. Long-term overdose may lead to high output cardiac failure.

Dosing

Adults & Elderly: IPAH or SSD: I.V.: Initial: 1-2 ng/kg/minute, increase dose in increments of 1-2 ng/kg/minute every 15 minutes or longer until dose-limiting side effects are noted or tolerance limit to epoprostenol is observed

(Continued)

Epoprostenol *(Continued)*

Dose adjustment:

Increase dose in 1-2 ng/kg/minute increments at intervals of at least 15 minutes if symptoms persist or recur following improvement. In clinical trials, dosing increases occurred at intervals of 24-48 hours.

Decrease dose in 2 ng/kg/minute decrements at intervals of at least 15 minutes in case of dose-limiting pharmacologic events. Avoid abrupt withdrawal or sudden large dose reductions.

Lung transplant: In patients receiving lung transplants, epoprostenol was tapered after the initiation of cardiopulmonary bypass.

Pediatrics: Unlabeled use; refer to adult dosing.

Available Dosage Forms Injection, powder for reconstitution, as sodium: 0.5 mg, 1.5 mg [provided with 50 mL sterile diluent]

Nursing Guidelines

Assessment: Institutional: Continuous pulmonary and hemodynamic arterial monitoring, protimes. **Noninstitutional:** Avoid sudden rate reduction or abrupt withdrawal or interruption of therapy. When adjustment in rate is made, monitor blood pressure (standing and supine) and pulse for several hours to ensure tolerance to new rate. Monitor for bleeding. Monitor (or teach appropriate caregiver or patient to monitor) vital signs on 3 times/day basis. Monitor for improved pulmonary function and improved quality of life. Be alert for any infusion pump malfunction. Assess for signs of overdose (eg, hypoxia, flushing, tachycardia, fever, chills, anxiety, acute headache, tremor, vomiting, diarrhea).

Patient Education: Therapy on this drug will probably be prolonged, possibly for years. You may experience mild headache, nausea or vomiting, and some muscular pains (use of a mild analgesia may be recommended by your prescriber). Report immediately any signs or symptoms of acute or severe headache, back pain, increased difficult breathing, flushing, fever or chills, any unusual bleeding or bruising, or any onset of unresolved diarrhea. **Breast-feeding precaution:** Consult prescriber if breast-feeding.

Pregnancy Risk Factor: B

Pregnancy Issues: Teratogenic effects were not reported in animal studies. There are no adequate and well-controlled studies in pregnant women. Pregnant women with IPAH are encouraged to avoid pregnancy.

Lactation: Excretion in breast milk unknown/use caution

Administration

I.V.:

The ambulatory infusion pump should be small and lightweight, be able to adjust infusion rates in 2 ng/kg/minute increments, have occlusion, end of infusion, and low battery alarms, have ± 6% accuracy of the programmed rate, and have positive continuous or pulsatile pressure with intervals ≤3 minutes between pulses. The reservoir should be made of polyvinyl chloride, polypropylene, or glass. The infusion pump used in the most recent clinical trial was CADD-1 HFX 5100 (Pharmacia Deltec).

Reconstitution: Reconstitute only with provided sterile diluent. See table.

Preparation of Epoprostenol Infusion

To make 100 mL of solution with concentration:	Directions
3000 ng/mL	Dissolve one 0.5 mg vial with 5 mL supplied diluent, withdraw 3 mL, and add to sufficient diluent to make a total of 100 mL.
5000 ng/mL	Dissolve one 0.5 mg vial with 5 mL supplied diluent, withdraw entire vial contents, and add a sufficient volume of diluent to make a total of 100 mL.
10,000 ng/mL	Dissolve two 0.5 mg vials each with 5 mL supplied diluent, withdraw entire vial contents, and add a sufficient volume of diluent to make a total of 100 mL.
15,000 ng/mL	Dissolve one 1.5 mg vial with 5 mL supplied diluent, withdraw entire vial contents, and add a sufficient volume of diluent to make a total of 100 mL.

Compatibility: Do not mix or administer with any other drugs prior to or during administration.

Storage: Prior to use, store vials at 15°C to 25°C (59°F to 77°F); protect from light, do not freeze. Following reconstitution, solution must be stored under refrigeration at 2°C to 8°C (36°F to 46°F) if not used immediately; protect from light, do not freeze; discard if refrigerated for >48 hours. During use, a single reservoir of solution may be used at room temperature for a total duration of 8 hours, or used with a cold pouch for administration up to 24 hours. Cold packs should be changed every 12 hours.

♦ Epoprostenol Sodium *see* Epoprostenol *on page 622*
♦ Epsilon Aminocaproic Acid *see* Aminocaproic Acid *on page 126*
♦ Epsom Salts *see* Magnesium Sulfate *on page 1077*
♦ Eptacog Alfa (Activated) *see* Factor VIIa (Recombinant) *on page 700*

Eptifibatide (ep TIF i ba tide)

U.S. Brand Names Integrilin®

Synonyms Intrifiban

Pharmacologic Category Antiplatelet Agent, Glycoprotein IIb/IIIa Inhibitor

Use Treatment of patients with acute coronary syndrome (unstable angina/non-Q wave myocardial infarction [UA/NQMI]), including patients who are to be managed medically and those undergoing percutaneous coronary intervention (PCI including angioplasty, intracoronary stenting)

Mechanism of Action Eptifibatide is a cyclic heptapeptide which blocks the platelet glycoprotein IIb/IIIa receptor, the binding site for fibrinogen, von Willebrand factor, and other ligands. Inhibition of binding at this final common receptor reversibly blocks platelet aggregation and prevents thrombosis.

Pharmacodynamics/Kinetics

Onset of action: Within 1 hour

Duration: Platelet function restored ~4 hours following discontinuation

Protein binding: ~25%

Half-life elimination: 2.5 hours

Excretion: Primarily urine (as eptifibatide and metabolites); significant renal impairment may alter disposition of this compound

Clearance: Total body: 55-58 mL/kg/hour; Renal: ~50% of total in healthy subjects

Contraindications Hypersensitivity to eptifibatide or any component of the product; active abnormal bleeding or a history of bleeding diathesis within the previous 30 days; history of CVA within 30 days or a history of hemorrhagic stroke; severe hypertension (systolic blood pressure >200 mm Hg or diastolic blood pressure >110 mm Hg) not adequately controlled on antihypertensive therapy; major surgery within the preceding 6 weeks; current or planned administration of another parenteral GP IIb/IIIa inhibitor; thrombocytopenia; dependency on renal dialysis

Warnings/Precautions Bleeding is the most common complication. Most major bleeding occurs at the arterial access site where the cardiac catheterization was done. When bleeding can not be controlled with pressure, discontinue infusion and heparin. Use caution in patients with hemorrhagic retinopathy or with other drugs that affect hemostasis. Concurrent use with thrombolytics has not been established as safe. Minimize other procedures including arterial and venous punctures, I.M. injections, nasogastric tubes, etc. Sheath should not be removed unless the aPTT <45 sec or the ACT <150 sec. Use caution in renal dysfunction (estimated Cl_{cr} <50 mL/minute); dosage adjustment required. Safety and efficacy in pediatric patients have not been determined.

Drug Interactions

Cephalosporins which contain the MTT side chain may theoretically increase the risk of hemorrhage

Drotrecogin alfa: Antiplatelet agents (eg, eptifibatide) may enhance the adverse/toxic effect of drotrecogin alfa; bleeding may occur.

Drugs which affect platelet function (eg, aspirin, NSAIDs, dipyridamole, ticlopidine, clopidogrel) may potentiate the risk of hemorrhage; use with caution

Heparin and aspirin: Use with aspirin and heparin may increase bleeding over aspirin and heparin alone. However, aspirin and heparin were used concurrently in the majority of patients in the major clinical studies of eptifibatide

Thrombolytic agents theoretically may increase the risk of hemorrhage; use with caution

Warfarin and oral anticoagulants: Risk of bleeding may be increased during concurrent therapy

Other IIb/IIIa antagonists: Avoid concomitant use of other glycoprotein IIb/IIIa antagonists (see Contraindications)

(Continued)

Eptifibatide *(Continued)*

Nutritional/Herbal/Ethanol Interactions Herb/Nutraceutical: Avoid alfalfa, anise, bilberry, bladderwrack, bromelain, cat's claw, celery, coleus, cordyceps, dong quai, evening primrose oil, fenugreek, feverfew, garlic, ginger, ginkgo biloba, ginseng (American), ginseng (Panax), ginseng (Siberian), grape seed, green tea, guggul, horse chestnut seed, horseradish, licorice, prickly ash, red clover, reishi, same (s-adenosylmethionine), sweet clover, turmeric, and white willow (all have additional antiplatelet activity).

Adverse Reactions Bleeding is the major drug-related adverse effect. Access site is often primary source of bleeding complications. Incidence of bleeding is also related to heparin intensity. Patients weighing <70 kg may have an increased risk of major bleeding.

>10%: Hematologic: Bleeding (major: 1% to 11%; minor: 3% to 14%; transfusion required: 2% to 13%)

1% to 10%:

- Cardiovascular: Hypotension (up to 7%)
- Hematologic: Thrombocytopenia (1% to 3%)
- Local: Injection site reaction

<1% (Limited to important or life-threatening): Acute profound thrombocytopenia, anaphylaxis, fatal bleeding events, GI hemorrhage, intracranial hemorrhage (0.5% to 0.7%), pulmonary hemorrhage, stroke

Overdosage/Toxicology Two cases of human overdose have been reported; neither case was eventful or associated with major bleeding. Symptoms of overdose in animal studies include loss of righting reflex, dyspnea, ptosis, decreased muscle tone, and petechial hemorrhage. Treatment is supportive. Dialysis may be beneficial.

Dosing

Adults:

Acute coronary syndrome: I.V.: Bolus of 180 mcg/kg (maximum: 22.6 mg) over 1-2 minutes, begun as soon as possible following diagnosis, followed by a continuous infusion of 2 mcg/kg/minute (maximum: 15 mg/hour) until hospital discharge or initiation of CABG surgery, up to 72 hours. Concurrent aspirin and heparin therapy (target aPTT 50-70 seconds) are recommended.

Percutaneous coronary intervention (PCI) with or without stenting: I.V.: Bolus of 180 mcg/kg (maximum: 22.6 mg) administered immediately before the initiation of PCI, followed by a continuous infusion of 2 mcg/kg/minute (maximum: 15 mg/hour). A second 180 mcg/kg bolus (maximum: 22.6 mg) should be administered 10 minutes after the first bolus. Infusion should be continued until hospital discharge or for up to 18-24 hours, whichever comes first. Concurrent aspirin (160-325 mg 1-24 hours before PCI and daily thereafter) and heparin therapy (ACT 200-300 seconds during PCI) are recommended. Heparin infusion after PCI is discouraged. In patients who undergo coronary artery bypass graft surgery, discontinue infusion prior to surgery.

Elderly: Refer to adult dosing. No dosing adjustment for the elderly appears to be necessary; adjust carefully to renal function.

Renal Impairment: Dialysis is a contraindication to use.

Acute coronary syndrome: Cl_{cr} <50 mL/minute: Use 180 mcg/kg bolus (maximum: 22.6 mg) and 1 mcg/kg/minute infusion (maximum: 7.5 mg/hour)

Percutaneous coronary intervention (PCI) with or without stenting: Cl_{cr} <50 mL/minute: Use 180 mcg/kg bolus (maximum: 22.6 mg) administered immediately before the initiation of PCI and followed by a continuous infusion of 1 mcg/kg/minute (maximum: 7.5 mg/hour). A second 180 mcg/kg (maximum: 22.6 mg) bolus should be administered 10 minutes after the first bolus.

Available Dosage Forms Injection, solution: 0.75 mg/mL (100 mL); 2 mg/mL (10 mL, 100 mL)

Nursing Guidelines

Assessment: Assess other medications for possible interactions or additive effects. Monitor vital signs and laboratory results prior to, during, and after therapy. Monitor closely for signs of excessive/unusual bleeding. Observe and teach patient bleeding precautions and adverse reactions to report.

Monitoring Laboratory Tests: Laboratory tests at baseline and monitoring during therapy: Hematocrit and hemoglobin, platelet count, serum creatinine, PT/aPTT (maintain aPTT between 50-70 seconds unless PCI is to be performed), and ACT with PCI (maintain ACT between 200-300 seconds during PCI). Prior to sheath removal, the aPTT or ACT should be checked (do not remove unless aPTT is <45 seconds or the ACT <150 seconds).

Patient Education: Emergency use may dictate depth of patient education. This medication can only be administered intravenously. You will have a tendency to bleed easily following this medication. Use caution to prevent injury (use electric razor, use soft toothbrush, use caution with sharps). If bleeding occurs, apply pressure to bleeding spot until bleeding stops completely. Report unusual bruising or bleeding (eg, blood in urine, stool, or vomitus, bleeding gums), dizziness or vision changes, or back pain. **Breast-feeding precaution:** Breast-feeding is not recommended.

Pregnancy Risk Factor: B

Lactation: Excretion in breast milk unknown/use caution

Perioperative/Anesthesia/Other Concerns: Eptifibatide has a short duration of action and hemostasis is restored within about 4 hours after discontinuation in patients with normal renal function. Acute profound thrombocytopenia has been associated with eptifibatide use. (Nagge J, 2003; Rezkalla SH, 2003; Salengro E, 2003)

Administration

I.V.: Do not shake vial. Administer bolus doses by I.V. push over 1-2 minutes. Begin continuous infusion immediately following bolus administration; administer directly from the 100 mL vial.

Compatibility: Stable in NS (infusion may contain up to 60 mEq/L KCl), NS/D_5W (infusion may contain up to 60 mEq/L KCl)

Storage: Vials should be stored refrigerated at 2°C to 8°C (36°F to 46°F). Vials can be kept at room temperature for 2 months. Protect from light until administration. Do not use beyond the expiration date. Discard any unused portion left in the vial.

♦ Equalizer Gas Relief [OTC] *see* Simethicone *on page 1533*

♦ Equetro™ *see* Carbamazepine *on page 306*

Ergocalciferol (er goe kal SIF e role)

U.S. Brand Names Calciferol™; Drisdol®

Synonyms Activated Ergosterol; Viosterol; Vitamin D_2

Pharmacologic Category Vitamin D Analog

Medication Safety Issues

Sound-alike/look-alike issues:

Calciferol™ may be confused with calcitriol

Drisdol® may be confused with Drysol™

Use Treatment of refractory rickets, hypophosphatemia, hypoparathyroidism; dietary supplement

Mechanism of Action Stimulates calcium and phosphate absorption from the small intestine, promotes secretion of calcium from bone to blood; promotes renal tubule phosphate resorption

Pharmacodynamics/Kinetics

Onset of action: Peak effect: ~1 month following daily doses

Absorption: Readily; requires bile

Metabolism: Inactive until hydroxylated hepatically and renally to calcifediol and then to calcitriol (most active form)

Contraindications Hypersensitivity to ergocalciferol or any component of the formulation; hypercalcemia; malabsorption syndrome; evidence of vitamin D toxicity

Warnings/Precautions Administer with extreme caution in patients with impaired renal function, heart disease, renal stones, or arteriosclerosis; must administer concomitant calcium supplementation; maintain adequate fluid intake; avoid hypercalcemia; renal function impairment with secondary hyperparathyroidism. Use as a dietary supplement is recommended for all breast-fed or nonbreast-fed infants receiving <500 mL/day of vitamin D-fortified formula, and in adults and children receiving <500 mL/day of vitamin D-fortified milk and who do not get regular sun exposure.

Drug Interactions

Decreased effect: Cholestyramine, colestipol, mineral oil may decrease oral absorption

Increased effect: Thiazide diuretics may increase vitamin D effects

Increased toxicity: Cardiac glycosides may increase toxicity

Adverse Reactions Generally well tolerated

Frequency not defined: Cardiac arrhythmia, hypertension (late), irritability, headache, psychosis (rare), somnolence, hyperthermia (late), pruritus, decreased libido (late), hypercholesterolemia, mild acidosis (late), polydipsia (late),

(Continued)

Ergocalciferol *(Continued)*

nausea, vomiting, anorexia, pancreatitis, metallic taste, weight loss (rare), xerostomia, constipation, polyuria (late), increased BUN (late), increased LFTs (late), bone pain, myalgia, weakness, conjunctivitis, photophobia (late), vascular/nephrocalcinosis (rare)

Overdosage/Toxicology Symptoms of chronic overdose include hypercalcemia, weakness, fatigue, lethargy, and anorexia. Following withdrawal of the drug and oral decontamination, treatment consists of bedrest, liberal intake of fluids, reduced calcium intake, and cathartic administration. Severe hypercalcemia requires I.V. hydration and forced diuresis with I.V. furosemide. Urine output should be monitored and maintained at >3 mL/kg/hour during the acute treatment phase. I.V. saline can quickly and significantly increase excretion of calcium into urine. Calcitonin, mithramycin, and bisphosphonates have all been used successfully to treat the more resistant cases of vitamin D-induced hypercalcemia.

Dosing

Adults: Oral dosing is preferred; I.M. therapy is required with GI, liver, or biliary disease associated with malabsorption.

Dietary supplementation (each 1 mcg = 40 int. units): Oral:

18-50 years: 5 mcg/day (200 int. units/day)

51-70 years: 10 mcg/day (400 int. units/day)

Familial phosphatemia: 10,000-80,000 int. units/day and phosphorus 1-2 g/day

Renal failure: Oral: 500 mcg/day (20,000 int. units)

Hypoparathyroidism: Oral: 625 mcg to 5 mg/day (25,000-200,000 int. units) and calcium supplements

Vitamin D-dependent rickets: Oral: 250 mcg to 1.5 mg/day (10,000-60,000 int. units)

Nutritional rickets and osteomalacia: Oral:

With normal absorption: 25-125 mcg/day (1000-5000 int. units)

With malabsorption: 250-7500 mcg/day (10,000-300,000 int. units)

Vitamin D-resistant rickets: Oral: 250-1500 mcg/day (10,000-60,000 int. units) with phosphate supplements

Elderly: Refer to adult dosing (see Geriatric Considerations

Dietary supplementation (each 1 mcg = 40 int. units): >70 years: Oral: 15 mcg/day (600 int. units/day)

Pediatrics: Oral dosing is preferred; I.M. therapy is required with GI, liver, or biliary disease associated with malabsorption.

Dietary supplementation (each mcg = 40 int. units): Infants and Children: 5 mcg/day (200 int. units/day)

Renal failure: Children: 100-1000 mcg/day (4000-40,000 int. units)

Hypoparathyroidism: Children: 1.25-5 mg/day (50,000-200,000 int. units) and calcium supplements

Vitamin D-dependent rickets: Children: 75-125 mcg/day (3000-5000 int. units); maximum: 1500 mcg/day

Nutritional rickets and osteomalacia:

Children with normal absorption: 25-125 mcg/day (1000-5000 int. units)

Children with malabsorption: 250-625 mcg/day (10,000-25,000 int. units)

Vitamin D-resistant rickets: Children: Initial: 1000-2000 mcg/day (40,000-80,000 int. units) with phosphate supplements; daily dosage is increased at 3- to 4-month intervals in 250-500 mcg (10,000-20,000 int. units) increments

Familial hypophosphatemia: 10,000-80,000 units daily plus 1-2 g/day elemental phosphorus

Available Dosage Forms [DSC] = Discontinued product

Capsule (Drisdol®): 50,000 int. units [1.25 mg; contains tartrazine and soybean oil]

Injection, solution (Calciferol™): 500,000 int. units/mL [12.5 mg/mL] (1 mL) [contains sesame oil] [DSC]

Liquid, drops (Calciferol™, Drisdol®): 8000 int. units/mL [200 mcg/mL] (60 mL) [OTC]

Nursing Guidelines

Assessment: Assess effectiveness and interactions of other medications patient may be taking. Assess results of laboratory tests, therapeutic effectiveness, and adverse effects at beginning of therapy and regularly with long-term use. Teach patient proper use if self-administered (appropriate injection technique and syringe/needle disposal), appropriate nutritional counseling, possible side effects/interventions, and adverse symptoms to report.

Monitoring Laboratory Tests: Serum calcium, BUN, phosphorus every 1-2 weeks

Patient Education: Take exact dose prescribed; do not take more than recommended. Your prescriber may recommend a special diet; do not increase calcium intake without consulting prescriber. Avoid magnesium supplements or magnesium-containing antacids. You may experience nausea, vomiting, or metallic taste (small frequent meals, frequent mouth care, or sucking hard candy may help). Report chest pain or palpitations; acute headache, dizziness, or feeling of weakness; unresolved nausea or vomiting; persistent metallic taste; unrelieved muscle or bone pain; or CNS irritability. **Pregnancy precaution:** Inform prescriber if you are pregnant.

Geriatric Considerations: Recommended daily allowances (RDA) have not been developed for persons >65 years of age. Vitamin D, folate, and B_{12} (cyanocobalamin) have decreased absorption with age, but the clinical significance is yet unknown. Calorie requirements decrease with age and therefore, nutrient density must be increased to ensure adequate nutrient intake, including vitamins and minerals. Therefore, the use of a daily supplement with a multiple vitamin with minerals is recommended. Elderly consume less vitamin D, absorption may be decreased and many elderly have decreased sun exposure; therefore, elderly >70 years of age should receive supplementation with 600 units (15 mcg)/day. This is a recommendation of particular need to those with high risk for osteoporosis.

Pregnancy Risk Factor: A/C (dose exceeding RDA recommendation)

Lactation: Enters breast milk/compatible

Administration

I.M.: Parenteral injection is for I.M. use only.

Storage: Protect from light.

♦ Ergomar® *see* Ergotamine *on page 629*

Ergotamine (er GOT a meen)

U.S. Brand Names Ergomar®

Synonyms Ergotamine Tartrate

Pharmacologic Category Ergot Derivative

Use Abort or prevent vascular headaches, such as migraine, migraine variants, or so-called "histaminic cephalalgia"

Mechanism of Action Has partial agonist and/or antagonist activity against tryptaminergic, dopaminergic and alpha-adrenergic receptors depending upon their site; is a highly active uterine stimulant; it causes constriction of peripheral and cranial blood vessels and produces depression of central vasomotor centers

Pharmacodynamics/Kinetics

Absorption: Oral: Erratic; enhanced by caffeine coadministration

Metabolism: Extensively hepatic

Time to peak, serum: 0.5-3 hours

Half-life elimination: 2 hours

Excretion: Feces (90% as metabolites)

Contraindications Hypersensitivity to ergotamine or any component of the formulation; peripheral vascular disease; hepatic or renal disease; coronary artery disease; hypertension; sepsis; ergot alkaloids are contraindicated with strong inhibitors of CYP3A4 (includes protease inhibitors, azole antifungals, and some macrolide antibiotics); pregnancy

Warnings/Precautions Avoid prolonged administration or excessive dosage because of the danger of ergotism (intense vasoconstriction), gangrene, cardiac valvular fibrosis, retroperitoneal and/or pleuropulmonary fibrosis. Patients who take ergotamine for extended periods of time may experience withdrawal symptoms and rebound headache when ergotamine is discontinued. May be harmful due to reduction in cerebral blood flow; may precipitate angina, myocardial infarction, or aggravate intermittent claudication; therefore, not considered a drug of choice in the elderly.

Concomitant use with medications considered to be "strong" CYP3A4 inhibitors has been associated with acute ergot toxicity; use caution with inhibitors of CYP3A4 enzymes.

(Continued)

Ergotamine *(Continued)*

Drug Interactions Substrate of CYP3A4 (major); Inhibits CYP3A4 (weak)

Antifungals, azole derivatives (itraconazole, ketoconazole) increase levels of ergot alkaloids by inhibiting CYP3A4 metabolism, resulting in toxicity; concomitant use is contraindicated.

Antipsychotics: May diminish the effects of ergotamine (due to dopamine antagonism); these combinations should generally be avoided.

Beta blockers: severe peripheral vasoconstriction has been reported with concomitant use of beta blockers and ergot derivatives. Monitor.

CYP3A4 inhibitors: May increase the levels/effects of ergotamine. Example inhibitors include azole antifungals, clarithromycin, diclofenac, doxycycline, erythromycin, imatinib, isoniazid, nefazodone, nicardipine, propofol, protease inhibitors, quinidine, telithromycin, and verapamil. Ergot alkaloids are contraindicated with potent CYP3A4 inhibitors.

Macrolide antibiotics: Erythromycin, clarithromycin, and troleandomycin may increase levels of ergot alkaloids by inhibiting CYP3A4 metabolism, resulting in toxicity (ischemia, vasospasm); concomitant use is contraindicated.

MAO inhibitors: The serotonergic effects of ergot derivatives may be increased by MAO inhibitors. Monitor for signs and symptoms of serotonin syndrome.

Metoclopramide: May diminish the effects of ergotamine (due to dopamine antagonism); concurrent therapy should generally be avoided.

Protease inhibitors (ritonavir, amprenavir, atazanavir, indinavir, nelfinavir, and saquinavir) increase blood levels of ergot alkaloids by inhibiting CYP3A4 metabolism, acute ergot toxicity has been reported; concomitant use is contraindicated.

Sibutramine: May cause serotonin syndrome; concurrent use with ergot alkaloids is contraindicated.

Serotonin agonists: Concurrent use with ergotamine may increase the risk of serotonin syndrome (includes buspirone, SSRIs, TCAs, nefazodone, sumatriptan, and trazodone).

Sumatriptan and other serotonin 5-HT_1 receptor agonists: Prolong vasospastic reactions; do not use sumatriptan or ergot-containing drugs within 24 hours of each other.

Vasoconstrictors: Concomitant use of some ergot derivatives and peripheral vasoconstrictors may cause synergistic elevation of blood pressure; use is contraindicated.

Nutritional/Herbal/Ethanol Interactions Food: Avoid tea, cola, and coffee (caffeine may increase GI absorption of ergotamine). Grapefruit juice may cause increased blood levels of ergotamine, leading to increased toxicity.

Adverse Reactions Frequency not defined.

Cardiovascular: Absence of pulse, bradycardia, cardiac valvular fibrosis, cyanosis, edema, ECG changes, gangrene, hypertension, ischemia, precordial distress and pain, tachycardia, vasospasm

Central nervous system: Vertigo

Dermatologic: Itching

Gastrointestinal: Nausea, vomiting

Genitourinary: Retroperitoneal fibrosis

Neuromuscular & skeletal: Muscle pain, numbness, paresthesia, weakness

Respiratory: Pleuropulmonary fibrosis

Miscellaneous: Cold extremities

Overdosage/Toxicology Symptoms of overdose include vasospastic effects, nausea, vomiting, lassitude, impaired mental function, hypotension, hypertension, unconsciousness, seizures, shock, and death. Treatment includes general supportive therapy. Activated charcoal is effective at binding ergot alkaloids. Vasodilators should be used with caution to avoid exaggerating any pre-existing hypotension.

Dosing

Adults: Migraine: Sublingual: One tablet under tongue at first sign, then 1 tablet every 30 minutes if needed; maximum dose: 3 tablets/24 hours, 5 tablets/week

Elderly: See Geriatric Considerations.

Available Dosage Forms Tablet, sublingual: Ergotamine tartrate 2 mg

Nursing Guidelines

Assessment: Assess potential for interactions with other prescriptions, OTC medications, or herbal products patient may be taking. Assess therapeutic effectiveness and adverse response on a regular basis during therapy. Teach patient proper use, possible side effects/appropriate interventions, and adverse symptoms to report. **Pregnancy risk factor X:** Determine that patient is not pregnant before beginning treatment. Do not give to women of childbearing unless woman is capable of complying with contraceptive measures 1 month prior to therapy, during therapy, and for 1 month following therapy. Instruct patient on appropriate contraceptive measures. Breast-feeding is not recommended.

Patient Education: Do not take any new medication during therapy without consulting prescriber. Take this drug as directed; do not increase dose or use more often than prescribed. If relief is not obtained, contact your prescriber. Avoid products that contain caffeine (eg, tea, coffee, colas, cocoa); caffeine increases GI absorption of ergotamines. May cause drowsiness (avoid activities requiring alertness until effects of medication are known); mild nausea or vomiting (consult prescriber for approved antiemetic); or mild weakness or numbness of extremities (avoid activities that may have a potential for injury). Inspect your extremities for coldness, numbness, or injury. Report immediately any extreme numbness, pain, tingling or weakness in extremities (toes, fingers); severe unresolved nausea or vomiting; or respiratory difficulty or irregular heartbeat. **Pregnancy/breast-feeding precautions:** Inform prescriber if you are pregnant. Do not get pregnant 1 month before, during, or for 1 month following therapy. Consult prescriber for instruction on appropriate contraceptive measures. This drug may cause severe fetal defects. Do not donate blood during or for 1 month following therapy (same reason). Breast-feeding is not recommended.

Geriatric Considerations: Not recommended for use in the elderly. May be harmful due to reduction in cerebral blood flow. May precipitate angina, myocardial infarction, or aggravate intermittent claudication (see Contraindications and Warnings/Precautions).

Pregnancy Risk Factor: X

Pregnancy Issues: May cause prolonged constriction of the uterine vessels and/or increased myometrial tone leading to reduced placental blood flow. This has contributed to fetal growth retardation in animals. Ergotamine also has oxytocic effects.

Lactation: Enters breast milk/not recommended

Breast-Feeding Considerations: Ergotamine is excreted in breast milk and may cause vomiting, diarrhea, weak pulse, and unstable blood pressure in the nursing infant. Consider discontinuing the drug or discontinuing nursing.

Administration

Oral: Do not crush sublingual tablets.

Storage: Store sublingual tablet at room temperature. Protect from light and heat.

♦ **Ergotamine Tartrate** *see* Ergotamine *on page 629*

Ertapenem (er ta PEN em)

U.S. Brand Names Invanz®

Synonyms Ertapenem Sodium; L-749,345; MK0826

Pharmacologic Category Antibiotic, Carbapenem

Medication Safety Issues

Sound-alike/look-alike issues:

Invanz® may be confused with Avinza™

Use Treatment of the following moderate-severe infections: Complicated intra-abdominal infections, complicated skin and skin structure infections (including diabetic foot infections without osteomyelitis), complicated UTI (including pyelonephritis), acute pelvic infections, and community-acquired pneumonia. Antibacterial coverage includes aerobic gram-positive organisms, aerobic gram-negative organisms, anaerobic organisms.

Note: Methicillin-resistant *Staphylococcus*, *Enterococcus* spp, penicillin-resistant strains of *Streptococcus pneumoniae*, beta-lactamase-positive strains of *Haemophilus influenzae* are **resistant** to ertapenem, as are most *Pseudomonas aeruginosa*.

Mechanism of Action Inhibits bacterial cell wall synthesis by binding to one or more of the penicillin binding proteins; which in turn inhibits the final transpeptidation step of peptidoglycan synthesis in bacterial cell walls, thus inhibiting cell wall biosynthesis. Bacteria eventually lyse due to ongoing activity of cell wall autolytic enzymes (autolysins and murein hydrolases) while cell wall assembly is arrested.

Pharmacodynamics/Kinetics

Absorption: I.M.: Almost complete

(Continued)

Ertapenem *(Continued)*

Distribution: V_{dss}:
  Children 3 months to 12 years: 0.2 L/kg
  Children 13-17 years: 0.16 L/kg
  Adults: 0.12 L/kg
Protein binding (concentration dependent): 85% at 300 mcg/mL, 95% at <100 mcg/mL
Metabolism: Hydrolysis to inactive metabolite
Bioavailability: I.M.: 90%
Half-life elimination:
  Children 3 months to 12 years: 2.5 hours
  Children ≥13 years and Adults: 4 hours
Time to peak: I.M.: 2.3 hours
Excretion: Urine (80% as unchanged drug and metabolite); feces (10%)

Contraindications Hypersensitivity to ertapenem, other carbapenems, or any component of the formulation; anaphylactic reactions to beta-lactam antibiotics. If using intramuscularly, known hypersensitivity to local anesthetics of the amide type (lidocaine is the diluent).

Warnings/Precautions Use caution with renal impairment. Dosage adjustment required in patients with moderate-to-severe renal dysfunction; elderly patients often require lower doses (based upon renal function). Prolonged use may result in superinfection. Has been associated with CNS adverse effects, including confusional states and seizures; use caution with CNS disorders (eg, brain lesions, history of seizures). Serious hypersensitivity reactions, including anaphylaxis, have been reported (some without a history of previous allergic reactions to beta-lactams). Doses for I.M. administration are mixed with lidocaine; consult Lidocaine *on page 1033* for information associated with Warnings/Precautions. Safety and efficacy in patients <3 months of age have not been established.

Drug Interactions
Probenecid: Serum concentrations of ertapenem may be increased; use caution.
Valproic acid: Ertapenem may decrease valproic acid serum concentrations to subtherapeutic levels; monitor.

Adverse Reactions Note: Percentages reported in adults.

1% to 10%:
  Cardiovascular: Swelling/edema (3%), chest pain (1%), hypertension (0.7% to ≤2%), hypotension (1% to 2%), tachycardia (1% to 2%)
  Central nervous system: Headache (6% to 7%), altered mental status (ie, agitation, confusion, disorientation, decreased mental acuity, changed mental status, somnolence, stupor) (3% to 5%), fever (2% to 5%), insomnia (3%), dizziness (2%), fatigue (1%), anxiety (0.8% to ≤1%)
  Dermatologic: Rash (2% to 3%), pruritus (1% to 2%), erythema (1% to 2%)
  Gastrointestinal: Diarrhea (9% to 10%), nausea (6% to 9%), abdominal pain (4%), vomiting (4%), constipation (3% to 4%), acid regurgitation (1% to 2%), dyspepsia (1%), oral candidiasis (0.1% to ≤1%)
  Genitourinary: Vaginitis (1% to 3%)
  Hematologic: Platelet count increased (4% to 7%), eosinophils increased (1% to 2%)
  Hepatic: Hepatic enzyme elevations (7% to 9%), alkaline phosphatase increase (4% to 7%)
  Local: Infused vein complications (5% to 7%), phlebitis/thrombophlebitis (2%), extravasation (0.7% to ≤2%)
  Neuromuscular & skeletal: Leg pain (0.4% to 1%)
  Respiratory: Dyspnea (1% to 3%), cough (1% to 2%), pharyngitis (0.7% to ≤1%), rales/rhonchi (0.5% to ≤1%), respiratory distress (0.2% to ≤1%)

<1% (Limited to important or life-threatening): Anaphylaxis, arrhythmia, asthma, asystole, atrial fibrillation, bradycardia, cardiac arrest, cholelithiasis, epistaxis, gastrointestinal hemorrhage, gout, hallucinations, heart failure, heart murmur, hypoxemia, ileus, pancreatitis, pseudomembranous colitis, pyloric stenosis, seizure (0.5%), subdural hemorrhage, syncope, urticaria, ventricular tachycardia, vertigo

Overdosage/Toxicology Treatment is symptom-directed and supportive. Ertapenem is removed by hemodialysis (plasma clearance increased by 30% following 4-hour session).

Dosing

Adults & Elderly: Note: I.V. therapy may be administered for up to 14 days; I.M. for up to 7 days

Intra-abdominal infection: I.M., I.V.: 1 g/day for 5-14 days

Skin and skin structure infections (including diabetic foot infections): I.M., I.V.: 1 g/day for 7-14 days

Community-acquired pneumonia: I.M., I.V.: 1 g/day; duration of total antibiotic treatment: 10-14 days*

Urinary tract infections/pyelonephritis: I.M., I.V.: 1 g/day; duration of total antibiotic treatment: 10-14 days*

Acute pelvic infections: I.M., I.V.: 1 g/day for 3-10 days

*Duration includes possible switch to appropriate oral therapy after at least 3 days of parenteral treatment, once clinical improvement demonstrated.

Pediatrics: Note: I.V. therapy may be administered for up to 14 days; I.M. therapy for up to 7 days

Children 3 months to 12 years:

Intra-abdominal infection: I.M., I.V.: 15 mg/kg twice daily (maximum: 1 g/day) for 5-14 days

Skin and skin structure infections: I.M., I.V.: 15 mg/kg twice daily (maximum: 1 g/day) for 7-14 days

Community-acquired pneumonia: I.M., I.V.: 15 mg/kg twice daily (maximum: 1 g/day); duration of total antibiotic treatment: 10-14 days*

Urinary tract infections/pyelonephritis: I.M., I.V.: 15 mg/kg twice daily (maximum: 1 g/day); duration of total antibiotic treatment: 10-14 days*

Acute pelvic infections: I.M., I.V.: 15 mg/kg twice daily (maximum: 1 g/day) for 3-10 days

Children ≥13 years: Refer to adult dosing.

*Duration includes possible switch to appropriate oral therapy after at least 3 days of parenteral treatment, once clinical improvement demonstrated.

Renal Impairment:

Children: No data available for pediatric patients with renal insufficiency.

Adults: Cl_{cr} <30 mL/minute and ESRD: 500 mg/day

Hemodialysis: When the daily dose is given within 6 hours prior to hemodialysis, a supplementary dose of 150 mg is required following hemodialysis.

Hepatic Impairment: Adjustments cannot be recommended (lack of experience and research in this patient population).

Available Dosage Forms Injection, powder for reconstitution: 1 g [contains sodium 137 mg/g (~6 mEq/g)]

Nursing Guidelines

Assessment: Assess results of culture and sensitivity tests and patient history of previous allergies or adverse drug reactions. Use caution in presence of impaired renal function; CNS disorder. See Administration for specific infusion/injection directions. Monitor closely for adverse reactions, especially CNS adverse effects (history of seizures, head injuries, or other CNS events increases risk). Teach patient interventions to reduce side effects and adverse symptoms to report.

Dietary Considerations: Sodium content: 137 mg (~6 mEq) per gram of ertapenem

Patient Education: This medication can only be administered intravenously or by intramuscular injections; report warmth, swelling, irritation at infusion or injection site. Maintain adequate hydration (2-3 L/day of fluids) unless instructed to restrict fluid intake, and nutrition. Report unresolved nausea or vomiting (small, frequent meals, frequent mouth care, and sucking hard candy may help). Report immediately any CNS changes (eg, dizziness, disorientation, visual disturbances, headaches, confusion, or seizures). Report prolonged GI effects, diarrhea, vomiting, abdominal pain; change in respirations or respiratory difficulty; chest pain or palpitations; skin rash; foul-smelling vaginal discharge; or white plaques in mouth. **Breast-feeding precaution:** Consult prescriber if breast-feeding.

Pregnancy Risk Factor: B

Lactation: Enters breast milk/use caution

Breast-Feeding Considerations: The concentration in human breast milk within 24 hours of last dose (1 g I.V. for 3-10 days) ranged from <0.13 mcg/mL (lower limit of quantitation) to 0.38 mcg/mL. Five days after discontinuation of therapy, the ertapenem level was undetectable in 80% (4 of 5 women) and below the lower limit of quantitation in 20% (1 of 5 women).

Administration

I.M.: Avoid injection into a blood vessel. Make sure patient does not have an allergy to lidocaine or another anesthetic of the amide type. Administer by deep I.M. injection into a large muscle mass (eg, gluteal muscle or lateral part of the

(Continued)

Ertapenem *(Continued)*

thigh). Do not administer I.M. preparation or drug reconstituted for I.M. administration intravenously.

I.V.: Infuse over 30 minutes

Reconstitution:

I.M.: Reconstitute 1 g vial with 3.2 mL of 1% lidocaine HCl injection (without epinephrine). Shake well.

I.V.: Reconstitute 1 g vial with 10 mL of water for injection, 0.9% sodium chloride injection, or bacteriostatic water for injection. Shake well. For adults, transfer dose to 50 mL of 0.9% sodium chloride injection; for children, dilute dose with NS to a final concentration of ≤20 mg/mL.

Compatibility: Do not mix with other medications or use diluents containing dextrose.

Storage: Before reconstitution store at ≤25°C (77°F).

I.M.: Use within 1 hour after preparation.

I.V.: Reconstituted I.V. solution may be stored at room temperature and used within 6 hours **or** refrigerated, stored for up to 24 hours and used within 4 hours after removal from refrigerator. Do not freeze.

- Ertapenem Sodium *see* Ertapenem *on page 631*
- Eryc® *see* Erythromycin *on page 634*
- Eryderm® *see* Erythromycin *on page 634*
- Erygel® *see* Erythromycin *on page 634*
- EryPed® *see* Erythromycin *on page 634*
- Ery-Tab® *see* Erythromycin *on page 634*
- Erythrocin® *see* Erythromycin *on page 634*

Erythromycin (er ith roe MYE sin)

U.S. Brand Names Akne-Mycin®; A/T/S®; E.E.S.®; Eryc®; Eryderm®; Erygel®; EryPed®; Ery-Tab®; Erythrocin®; PCE®; Romycin®; Staticin® [DSC]; Theramycin Z®; T-Stat® [DSC]

Synonyms Erythromycin Base; Erythromycin Estolate; Erythromycin Ethylsuccinate; Erythromycin Gluceptate; Erythromycin Lactobionate; Erythromycin Stearate

Pharmacologic Category Antibiotic, Macrolide; Antibiotic, Ophthalmic; Antibiotic, Topical; Topical Skin Product; Topical Skin Product, Acne

Medication Safety Issues

Sound-alike/look-alike issues:

Erythromycin may be confused with azithromycin, clarithromycin, Ethmozine®
Akne-Mycin® may be confused with AK-Mycin®
E.E.S.® may be confused with DES®
Eryc® may be confused with Emcyt®, Ery-Tab®
Ery-Tab® may be confused with Eryc®
Erythrocin® may be confused with Ethmozine®

Use

Systemic: Treatment of susceptible bacterial infections including *S. pyogenes*, some *S. pneumoniae*, some *S. aureus*, *M. pneumoniae*, *Legionella pneumophila*, diphtheria, pertussis, chancroid, *Chlamydia*, erythrasma, *N. gonorrhoeae*, *E. histolytica*, syphilis and nongonococcal urethritis, and *Campylobacter* gastroenteritis; used in conjunction with neomycin for decontaminating the bowel

Ophthalmic: Treatment of superficial eye infections involving the conjunctiva or cornea; neonatal ophthalmia

Topical: Treatment of acne vulgaris

Unlabeled/Investigational Use Systemic: Treatment of gastroparesis

Mechanism of Action Inhibits RNA-dependent protein synthesis at the chain elongation step; binds to the 50S ribosomal subunit resulting in blockage of transpeptidation

Pharmacodynamics/Kinetics

Absorption: Oral: Variable but better with salt forms than with base form; 18% to 45%; ethylsuccinate may be better absorbed with food

Distribution: Crosses placenta; enters breast milk

Relative diffusion from blood into CSF: Minimal even with inflammation

CSF:blood level ratio: Normal meninges: 1% to 12%; Inflamed meninges: 7% to 25%

Protein binding: 75% to 90%

Metabolism: Hepatic via demethylation

Half-life elimination: Peak: 1.5-2 hours; End-stage renal disease: 5-6 hours
Time to peak, serum: Base: 4 hours; Ethylsuccinate: 0.5-2.5 hours; delayed with food due to differences in absorption
Excretion: Primarily feces; urine (2% to 15% as unchanged drug)

Contraindications Hypersensitivity to erythromycin or any component of the formulation

Systemic: Pre-existing liver disease (erythromycin estolate); concomitant use with ergot derivatives, pimozide, or cisapride

Warnings/Precautions Systemic: Use caution with hepatic impairment with or without jaundice has occurred, it may be accompanied by malaise, nausea, vomiting, abdominal colic, and fever; discontinue use if these occur; avoid using erythromycin lactobionate in neonates since formulations may contain benzyl alcohol which is associated with toxicity in neonates; observe for superinfections. Use in infants has been associated with infantile hypertrophic pyloric stenosis (IHPS). Macrolides have been associated with rare QT prolongation and ventricular arrhythmias, including torsade de pointes. Elderly may be at increased risk of adverse events, including hearing loss and/or torsade de pointes when dosage ≥4 g/day, particularly if concurrent renal/hepatic impairment.

Drug Interactions Substrate of CYP2B6 (minor), 3A4 (major); **Inhibits** CYP1A2 (weak), 3A4 (moderate)

Alfentanil (and possibly other narcotic analgesics): Serum levels may be increased by erythromycin; monitor for increased effect.

Antipsychotic agents (particularly mesoridazine and thioridazine): Risk of QT_c prolongation and malignant arrhythmias may be increased.

Benzodiazepines (those metabolized by CYP3A4, including alprazolam and triazolam): Serum levels may be increased by erythromycin; somnolence and confusion have been reported.

Bromocriptine: Serum levels may be increased by erythromycin; monitor for increased effect.

Buspirone: Serum levels may be increased by erythromycin; monitor.

Calcium channel blockers (felodipine, verapamil, and potentially others metabolized by CYP3A4): Serum levels may be increased by erythromycin; monitor.

Carbamazepine: Serum levels may be increased by erythromycin; monitor.

Cilostazol: Serum levels may be increased by erythromycin.

Cisapride: Serum levels may be increased by erythromycin; serious arrhythmias have occurred; concurrent use contraindicated.

Clindamycin (and lincomycin): Use with erythromycin may result in pharmacologic antagonism; manufacturer recommends avoiding this combination.

Clozapine: Serum levels may be increased by erythromycin; monitor.

Colchicine: serum levels/toxicity may be increased by erythromycin; monitor. Avoid use, if possible.

Cyclosporine: Serum levels may be increased by erythromycin; monitor serum levels.

CYP3A4 inducers: CYP3A4 inducers may decrease the levels/effects of erythromycin. Example inducers include aminoglutethimide, carbamazepine, nafcillin, nevirapine, phenobarbital, phenytoin, and rifamycins.

CYP3A4 inhibitors: May increase the levels/effects of erythromycin. Example inhibitors include azole antifungals, clarithromycin, diclofenac, doxycycline, imatinib, isoniazid, nefazodone, nicardipine, propofol, protease inhibitors, quinidine, telithromycin, and verapamil.

CYP3A4 substrates: Erythromycin may increase the levels/effects of CYP3A4 substrates. Example substrates include benzodiazepines, calcium channel blockers, cyclosporine, mirtazapine, nateglinide, nefazodone, sildenafil (and other PDE-5 inhibitors), tacrolimus, and venlafaxine. Selected benzodiazepines (midazolam and triazolam), cisapride, ergot alkaloids, selected HMG-CoA reductase inhibitors (lovastatin and simvastatin), and pimozide are generally contraindicated with strong CYP3A4 inhibitors.

Delavirdine: Serum levels of erythromycin may be increased; also, serum levels of delavirdine may increased by erythromycin (low risk); monitor.

Digoxin: Serum levels may be increased by erythromycin; monitor digoxin levels.

Disopyramide: Serum levels may be increased by erythromycin; in addition, QT_c prolongation and risk of malignant arrhythmia may be increased; avoid combination.

Ergot alkaloids: Concurrent use may lead to acute ergot toxicity (severe peripheral vasospasm and dysesthesia).

HMG-CoA reductase inhibitors (atorvastatin, lovastatin, and simvastatin); Erythromycin may increase serum levels of "statins" metabolized by CYP3A4, increasing the risk of myopathy/rhabdomyolysis (does not include fluvastatin

(Continued)

Erythromycin *(Continued)*

and pravastatin). Switch to pravastatin/fluvastatin or suspend treatment during course of erythromycin therapy.

Loratadine: Serum levels may be increased by erythromycin; monitor.

Methylprednisolone: Serum levels may be increased by erythromycin; monitor.

Neuromuscular-blocking agents: May be potentiated by erythromycin (case reports).

Phenytoin: Serum levels may be increased by erythromycin; other evidence suggested phenytoin levels may be decreased in some patients; monitor.

Pimozide: Serum levels may be increased, leading to malignant arrhythmias; concomitant use is contraindicated.

Protease inhibitors (amprenavir, nelfinavir, and ritonavir): May increase serum levels of erythromycin.

QT_c-prolonging agents: Concomitant use may increase the risk of malignant arrhythmias.

Quinidine: Serum levels may be increased by erythromycin; in addition, the risk of QT_c prolongation and malignant arrhythmias may be increased during concurrent use.

Quinolone antibiotics (sparfloxacin, gatifloxacin, and moxifloxacin): Concurrent use may increase the risk of malignant arrhythmias.

Rifabutin: Serum levels may be increased by erythromycin; monitor.

Sildenafil, tadalafil, vardenafil: Serum concentration may be substantially increased by erythromycin. Do not exceed single sildenafil doses of 25 mg in 48 hours, a single tadalafil dose of 10 mg in 72 hours, or a single vardenafil dose of 2.5 mg in 24 hours.

Tacrolimus: Serum levels may be increased by erythromycin; monitor serum concentration.

Theophylline: Serum levels may be increased by erythromycin; monitor.

Valproic acid (and derivatives): Serum levels may be increased by erythromycin; monitor.

Vinblastine (and vincristine): Serum levels may be increased by erythromycin.

Warfarin: Effects may be potentiated; monitor INR closely and adjust warfarin dose as needed or choose another antibiotic.

Zafirlukast: Serum levels may be decreased by erythromycin; monitor.

Zopiclone: Serum levels may be increased by erythromycin; monitor.

Nutritional/Herbal/Ethanol Interactions

Ethanol: Avoid ethanol (may decrease absorption of erythromycin or enhance ethanol effects).

Food: Increased drug absorption with meals; erythromycin serum levels may be altered if taken with food.

Herb/Nutraceutical: St John's wort may decrease erythromycin levels.

Lab Interactions False-positive urinary catecholamines

Adverse Reactions

Systemic:

Cardiovascular: Ventricular arrhythmia, QT_c prolongation, torsade de pointes (rare), ventricular tachycardia (rare)

Central nervous system: Headache (8%), pain (2%), fever, seizure

Dermatitis: Rash (3%), pruritus (1%)

Gastrointestinal: Abdominal pain (8%), cramping, nausea (8%), oral candidiasis, vomiting (3%), diarrhea (7%), dyspepsia (2%), flatulence (2%), anorexia, pseudomembranous colitis, hypertrophic pyloric stenosis (including cases in infants or IHPS), pancreatitis

Hematologic: Eosinophilia (1%)

Hepatic: Cholestatic jaundice (most common with estolate), increased liver function tests (2%)

Local: Phlebitis at the injection site, thrombophlebitis

Neuromuscular & skeletal: Weakness (2%)

Respiratory: Dyspnea (1%), cough (3%)

Miscellaneous: Hypersensitivity reactions, allergic reactions

Topical: 1% to 10%: Dermatologic: Erythema, desquamation, dryness, pruritus

Overdosage/Toxicology Symptoms of overdose include nausea, vomiting, diarrhea, prostration, reversible pancreatitis, hearing loss with or without tinnitus or vertigo. Care is general and supportive only.

Dosing

Adults & Elderly:

Usual dosage range:

Oral: (**Note:** Due to differences in absorption, 400 mg erythromycin ethylsuccinate produces the same serum levels as 250 mg erythromycin base, sterate or estolate)

Base: 30-50 mg/kg/day in 2-4 divided doses; do not exceed 2 g/day

Estolate: 30-50 mg/kg/day in 2-4 divided doses; do not exceed 2 g/day

Ethylsuccinate: 30-50 mg/kg/day in 2-4 divided doses; do not exceed 3.2 g/day

Stearate: 30-50 mg/kg/day in 2-4 divided doses; do not exceed 2 g/day

I.V.: Lactobionate: 15-20 mg/kg/day divided every 6 hours or 500 mg to 1 g every 6 hours, or given as a continuous infusion over 24 hours (maximum: 4 g/24 hours)

Ophthalmic infection: Ophthalmic: Instill ½" (1.25 cm) 2-6 times/day depending on the severity of the infection

Dermatologic infection: Topical: Apply over the affected area twice daily after the skin has been thoroughly washed and patted dry

Indication-specific dosing:

Cervicitis: Oral: 500 mg 4 times/day for 7 days

Chancroid (unlabeled use; not a preferred agent): Oral: 500 mg 4 times/day for 7 days

Community-acquired pneumonia, bronchitis: Oral, I.V.: 500-1000 mg 4 times/day for 10-14 days. If *Legionella* is suspected/confirmed, 750-1000 mg 4 times/day for 21 days or more may be recommended. **Note:** Other macrolides and/or fluoroquinolones may be preferred and better tolerated.

Lymphogranuloma venereum: Oral: 500 mg 4 times/day for 21 days

Nongonococcal urethritis (recurrent): Oral: CDC Guidelines for the Treatment of Sexually Transmitted Diseases recommendation: Metronidazole (2 g as a single dose) plus 7 days of erythromycin base (500 mg 4 times/day) or erythromycin ethylsuccinate (800 mg 4 times/day)

Pertussis (CDC guidelines): Oral: 500 mg every 6 hours for 14 days

Preop bowel preparation (unlabeled use): Oral: 1 g erythromycin base at 1, 2, and 11 PM on the day before surgery combined with mechanical cleansing of the large intestine and oral neomycin

Gastrointestinal prokinetic (unlabeled use): Oral: Erythromycin has been used as a prokinetic agent to improve gastric emptying time and intestinal motility. In adults, 200 mg was infused I.V. initially followed by 250 mg orally 3 times/day 30 minutes before meals. Lower dosages have been used in some trials.

Pediatrics:

Prophylaxis of neonatal gonococcal or chlamydial conjunctivitis: Neonates: Ophthalmic: 0.5-1 cm ribbon of ointment should be instilled into each conjunctival sac

Usual dosage range: Infants and Children:

Oral: **Note:** Due to differences in absorption, 400 mg erythromycin ethylsuccinate produces the same serum levels as 250 mg erythromycin base, stearate or estolate).

Base: 30-50 mg/kg/day in 2-4 divided doses; do not exceed 2 g/day

Estolate: 30-50 mg/kg/day in 2-4 divided doses; do not exceed 2 g/day

Ethylsuccinate: 30-50 mg/kg/day in 2-4 divided doses; do not exceed 3.2 g/day

Stearate: 30-50 mg/kg/day in 2-4 divided doses; do not exceed 2 g/day

I.V. (as lactobionate): 15-50 mg/kg/day divided every 6 hours, not to exceed 4 g/day

Indication-specific dosing:

Acne vulgaris (unlabeled use): Adolescents: Oral: 250-1500 mg/day in 2 divided doses; therapy may be continued for 4-6 weeks at lowest possible dose

Pharyngitis: Oral: 40 mg/kg/day in 2 doses; maximum: 1600 mg/day; short-course therapy for 5 days may be considered

Pertussis (CDC guidelines): Oral: 40-50 mg/kg/day in 4 divided doses for 14 days; maximum 2 g/day (not preferred agent for infants <1 month

Preop bowel preparation: Oral: 20 mg/kg erythromycin base at 1, 2, and 11 PM on the day before surgery combined with mechanical cleansing of the large intestine and oral neomycin

Ophthalmic infection: Ophthalmic: Refer to adult dosing.

Topical: Refer to adult dosing.

(Continued)

Erythromycin *(Continued)*

Renal Impairment: Slightly dialyzable (5% to 20%); supplemental dose is not necessary in hemo- or peritoneal dialysis or in continuous arteriovenous or venovenous hemofiltration.

Available Dosage Forms [DSC] = Discontinued product; [CAN] = Canadian brand name

Capsule, delayed release, enteric-coated pellets, as base (Eryc®): 250 mg
Gel, topical: 2% (30 g, 60 g)
A/T/S®: 2% (30 g) [contains alcohol 92%]
Erygel®: 2% (30 g, 60 g) [contains alcohol 92%]
Granules for oral suspension, as ethylsuccinate (E.E.S.®): 200 mg/5 mL (100 mL, 200 mL) [cherry flavor]
Injection, powder for reconstitution, as lactobionate (Erythrocin®): 500 mg, 1 g
Ointment, ophthalmic: 0.5% [5 mg/g] (1 g, 3.5 g)
Romycin®: 0.5% [5 mg/g] (3.5 g)
Ointment, topical (Akne-Mycin®): 2% (25 g)
Powder for oral suspension, as ethylsuccinate (EryPed®): 200 mg/5 mL (100 mL, 200 mL) [fruit flavor]; 400 mg/5 mL (100 mL, 200 mL) [banana flavor]
Powder for oral suspension, as ethylsuccinate [drops] (EryPed®): 100 mg/2.5 mL (50 mL) [fruit flavor]
Solution, topical: 2% (60 mL)
A/T/S®: 2% (60 mL) [contains alcohol 66%]
Eryderm®, T-Stat® [DSC], Theramycin Z®: 2% (60 mL) [contain alcohol]
Sans Acne® [CAN]: 2% (60 mL) [contains ethyl alcohol 44%; not available in U.S.]
Staticin®: 1.5% (60 mL) [DSC]
Suspension, oral, as estolate: 125 mg/5 mL (480 mL); 250 mg/5 mL (480 mL)
Suspension, oral, as ethylsuccinate: 200 mg/5 mL (480 mL); 400 mg/5 mL (480 mL)
E.E.S.®: 200 mg/5 mL (100 mL, 480 mL) [fruit flavor]; 400 mg/5 mL (100 mL, 480 mL) [orange flavor]
Swab (T-Stat® [DSC]): 2% (60s)
Tablet, chewable, as ethylsuccinate (EryPed®): 200 mg [fruit flavor] [DSC]
Tablet, delayed release, enteric coated, as base (Ery-Tab®): 250 mg, 333 mg, 500 mg
Tablet [film coated], as base: 250 mg, 500 mg
Tablet [film coated], as ethylsuccinate (E.E.S.®): 400 mg
Tablet [film coated], as stearate: 250 mg
Erythrocin®: 250 mg, 500 mg
Tablet [polymer-coated particles], as base (PCE®): 333 mg, 500 mg

Nursing Guidelines

Assessment: Assess for previous allergy history prior to therapy. See Contraindications and Warnings/Precautions for use cautions. Assess potential for interactions with other prescriptions, OTC medications, or herbal products patient may be taking (see Drug Interactions). Note infusion specifics. Assess therapeutic effectiveness and adverse reactions (see Adverse Reactions and Overdose/Toxicology). Teach patient proper use (according to formulation and purpose for use), possible side effects/appropriate interventions, and adverse symptoms to report (see Patient Education).

Monitoring Laboratory Tests: Perform culture and sensitivity studies prior to initiating drug therapy.

Dietary Considerations: Systemic: Drug may cause GI upset; may take with food.

Patient Education: Inform prescriber of all prescriptions, OTC medications, or herbal products you are taking, and any allergies you have. Do not take any new medication during therapy. Take as directed, around-the-clock, with a full glass of water (not juice or milk); may take with food to reduce GI upset. Do not chew or crush extended release capsules or tablets. Take complete prescription even if you are feeling better. Avoid alcohol (may cause adverse response). May cause nausea, vomiting, or mouth sores (small, frequent meals, frequent mouth care may help). Report immediately and unusual malaise, nausea, vomiting, abdominal colic, or fever; skin rash or itching; easy bruising or bleeding; vaginal itching or discharge; watery or bloody diarrhea; yellowing of skin or eyes, pale stool or dark urine; white plaques, sores, or fuzziness in mouth; or any change in hearing.

Geriatric Considerations: Dose of erythromycin does not need to be adjusted in the elderly unless there is severe renal impairment or hepatic dysfunction.

Elderly patients may be at an increased risk for torsade de pointes. Risk of ototoxicity may be increased in elderly, particularly when dose is ≥4 g/day in conjunction with renal or hepatic impairment.

Pregnancy Risk Factor: B

Lactation: Enters breast milk/use caution (AAP considers "compatible")

Perioperative/Anesthesia/Other Concerns: Erythromycin, when used with drugs that affect the QT interval (eg, cisapride, ergot derivatives, pimozide) or when administered to patients with a prolonged QT interval, may further increase the QT interval and the risk of torsade de pointes (proarrhythmias).

Administration

Oral: Do not crush enteric coated drug product. GI upset, including diarrhea, is common. May be administered with food to decrease GI upset. Do not give with milk or acidic beverages.

I.V.: Infuse 1 g over 20-60 minutes.

Reconstitution: Erythromycin lactobionate should be reconstituted with sterile water for injection without preservatives to avoid gel formation. I.V. form has the longest stability in NS and should be prepared in this base solution whenever possible. Do not use D_5W as a diluent unless sodium bicarbonate is added to solution. If I.V. must be prepared in D_5W, 0.5 mL of the 8.4% sodium bicarbonate solution should be added per each 100 mL of D_5W.

Stability of parenteral admixture at room temperature (25°C) and at refrigeration temperature (4°C) is 24 hours.

Standard diluent: 500 mg/250 mL D_5W/NS; 750 mg/250 mL D_5W/NS; 1 g/250 mL D_5W/NS.

Compatibility: Erythromycin lactobionate: Stable in NS; **incompatible** with D_5LR, $D_{10}W$

Y-site administration: Incompatible with fluconazole

Compatibility in syringe: Incompatible with ampicillin, heparin

Compatibility when admixed: Incompatible with colistimethate, floxacillin, furosemide, heparin, metaraminol, metoclopramide, riboflavin, vitamin B complex with C

Storage:

Injection: Reconstituted solution is stable for 2 weeks when refrigerated or for 24 hours at room temperature. Erythromycin I.V. infusion solution is stable at pH 6-8; stability of lactobionate is pH dependent; I.V. form has longest stability in NS. Stability of parenteral admixture at room temperature (25°C) and at refrigeration temperature (4°C) is 24 hours.

Granules for oral suspension: After mixing, store under refrigeration and use within 10 days.

Powder for oral suspension: Refrigerate to preserve taste. Erythromycin ethylsuccinate may be stored at room temperature if used within 14 days. EryPed® drops should be used within 35 days following reconstitution; may store at room temperature or under refrigeration.

Topical and ophthalmic formulations: Store at room temperature.

Related Information

Prevention of Wound Infection and Sepsis in Surgical Patients *on page 1830*

- **Erythromycin Base** *see* Erythromycin *on page 634*
- **Erythromycin Estolate** *see* Erythromycin *on page 634*
- **Erythromycin Ethylsuccinate** *see* Erythromycin *on page 634*
- **Erythromycin Gluceptate** *see* Erythromycin *on page 634*
- **Erythromycin Lactobionate** *see* Erythromycin *on page 634*
- **Erythromycin Stearate** *see* Erythromycin *on page 634*
- **Erythropoiesis Stimulating Protein** *see* Darbepoetin Alfa *on page 487*
- **Erythropoietin** *see* Epoetin Alfa *on page 618*

Escitalopram (es sye TAL oh pram)

U.S. Brand Names Lexapro®

Synonyms Escitalopram Oxalate; Lu-26-054; S-Citalopram

Pharmacologic Category Antidepressant, Selective Serotonin Reuptake Inhibitor

Use Treatment of major depressive disorder; generalized anxiety disorders (GAD)

Mechanism of Action Escitalopram is the S-enantiomer of the racemic derivative citalopram, which selectively inhibits the reuptake of serotonin with little to no effect on norepinephrine or dopamine reuptake. It has no or very low affinity for

(Continued)

Escitalopram *(Continued)*

$5\text{-}HT_{1\text{-}7}$, alpha- and beta-adrenergic, $D_{1\text{-}5}$, $H_{1\text{-}3}$, $M_{1\text{-}5}$, and benzodiazepine receptors. Escitalopram does not bind or has low affinity for Na^+, K^+, Cl^-, and Ca^{++} ion channels.

Pharmacodynamics/Kinetics

Protein binding: 56% to plasma proteins

Metabolism: Hepatic via CYP2C19 and 3A4 to an active metabolite, S-desmethylcitalopram (S-DCT; 1/7 the activity); S-DCT is metabolized to S-didesmethylcitalopram (S-DDCT; active; 1/27 the activity) via CYP2D6

Half-life elimination: Escitalopram: 27-32 hours; S-desmethylcitalopram: 59 hours

Time to peak: Escitalopram: 5 ± 1.5 hours; S-desmethylcitalopram: 14 hours

Excretion: Urine (Escitalopram: 8%; S-DCT: 10%)

Clearance: Total body: 37-40 L/hour; Renal: Escitalopram: 2.7 L/hour; S-desmethylcitalopram: 6.9 L/hour

Contraindications Hypersensitivity to escitalopram, citalopram, or any component of the formulation; concomitant use or within 2 weeks of MAO inhibitors

Warnings/Precautions

Major psychiatric warnings:

- Antidepressants increase the risk of suicidal thinking and behavior in children and adolescents with major depressive disorder (MDD) and other depressive disorders; consider risk prior to prescribing.
- Closely monitor for clinical worsening, suicidality, or unusual changes in behavior; the child's family or caregiver should be instructed to closely observe the patient and communicate condition with healthcare provider. **Escitalopram is not FDA approved for use in children.**
- Adults treated with antidepressants should be observed similarly for clinical worsening and suicidality, especially during the initial few months of a course of drug therapy, or at times of dose changes, either increases or decreases. A medication guide should be dispensed with each prescription.
- The possibility of a suicide attempt is inherent in major depression and may persist until remission occurs. Worsening depression and severe abrupt suicidality that are not part of the presenting symptoms may require discontinuation or modification of drug therapy. Use caution in high-risk patients during initiation of therapy.
- Prescriptions should be written for the smallest quantity consistent with good patient care. The patient's family or caregiver should be alerted to monitor patients for the emergence of suicidality and associated behaviors such as anxiety, agitation, panic attacks, insomnia, irritability, hostility, impulsivity, akathisia, hypomania, and mania; patients should be instructed to notify their healthcare provider if any of these symptoms or worsening depression or psychosis occur.
- May worsen psychosis in some patients or precipitate a shift to mania or hypomania in patients with bipolar disorder. Monotherapy in patients with bipolar disorder should be avoided. Patients presenting with depressive symptoms should be screened for bipolar disorder. **Escitalopram is not FDA approved for the treatment of bipolar depression.**

Key adverse effects:

- Anticholinergic effects: Relatively devoid of these side effects.
- CNS depression: Has a low potential to impair cognitive or motor performance; caution operating hazardous machinery or driving.
- SIADH and hyponatremia: Has been associated with the development of SIADH; hyponatremia has been reported rarely, predominately in the elderly

Concurrent disease:

- Hepatic impairment: Use caution; clearance is decreased and plasma concentrations are increased; a lower dosage may be needed.
- Platelet aggregation: May impair platelet aggregation, resulting in bleeding.
- Renal impairment: Use caution; clearance is decreased and plasma concentrations are increased; a lower dosage may be needed.
- Seizure disorders: Use caution with a previous seizure disorder or condition predisposing to seizures such as brain damage or alcoholism.
- Sexual dysfunction: May cause or exacerbate sexual dysfunction.

Concurrent drug therapy:

- Agents which lower seizure threshold: Concurrent therapy with other drugs which lower the seizure threshold.
- Anticoagulants/Antiplatelets: Use caution with concomitant use of NSAIDs, ASA, or other drugs that affect coagulation; the risk of bleeding is potentiated.
- CNS depressants: Use caution with concomitant therapy.

- MAO inhibitors: Potential for severe reaction when used with MAO inhibitors; autonomic instability, coma, death, delirium, diaphoresis, hyperthermia, mental status changes/agitation, muscular rigidity, myoclonus, neuroleptic malignant syndrome features, and seizures may occur.

Special populations:

- Elderly: Use caution in elderly patients.
- Pregnancy: Use caution in pregnant patients; high doses of citalopram have been associated with teratogenicity in animals.

Special notes:

- Electroconvulsive therapy: May increase the risks associated with electroconvulsive therapy; consider discontinuing, when possible, prior to ECT treatment.
- Withdrawal syndrome: May cause dysphoric mood, irritability, agitation, dizziness, sensory disturbances, anxiety, confusion, headache, lethargy, emotional lability, insomnia, hypomania, tinnitus, and seizures. Upon discontinuation of venlafaxine therapy, gradually taper dose. If intolerable symptoms occur following a decrease in dosage or upon discontinuation of therapy, then resuming the previous dose with a more gradual taper should be considered.

Drug Interactions Substrate (major) of CYP2C19, 3A4; **Inhibits** CYP2D6 (weak)

Aspirin: Concomitant use of escitalopram and NSAIDs, aspirin, or other drugs affecting coagulation has been associated with an increased risk of bleeding; monitor.

Buspirone: Concurrent use of citalopram with buspirone may cause serotonin syndrome; avoid concurrent use.

Cimetidine: May inhibit the metabolism of citalopram.

CYP2C19 inducers: May decrease the levels/effects of escitalopram. Example inducers include aminoglutethimide, carbamazepine, phenytoin, and rifampin.

CYP2C19 inhibitors: May increase the levels/effects of escitalopram. Example inhibitors include delavirdine, fluconazole, fluvoxamine, gemfibrozil, isoniazid, omeprazole, and ticlopidine.

CYP3A4 inducers: CYP3A4 inducers may decrease the levels/effects of escitalopram. Example inducers include aminoglutethimide, carbamazepine, nafcillin, nevirapine, phenobarbital, phenytoin, and rifamycins.

CYP3A4 inhibitors: May increase the levels/effects of escitalopram. Example inhibitors include azole antifungals, clarithromycin, diclofenac, doxycycline, erythromycin, imatinib, isoniazid, nefazodone, nicardipine, propofol, protease inhibitors, quinidine, telithromycin, and verapamil.

Desipramine: Escitalopram may increase desipramine levels.

Linezolid: Hyperpyrexia, hypertension, tachycardia, confusion, seizures, and deaths have been reported with agents which inhibit MAO (serotonin syndrome); this combination should be avoided.

MAO inhibitors: Hyperpyrexia, hypertension, tachycardia, confusion, seizures, and deaths have been reported with MAO inhibitors (serotonin syndrome); this combination should be avoided.

Meperidine: Combined use theoretically may increase the risk of serotonin syndrome.

Metoprolol: Escitalopram may increase plasma levels of metoprolol; monitor for increased effect.

Moclobemide: Concurrent use of citalopram with moclobemide may cause serotonin syndrome; avoid concurrent use.

Nefazodone: Concurrent use of citalopram with nefazodone may cause serotonin syndrome.

NSAIDs: Concomitant use of escitalopram and NSAIDs, aspirin, or other drugs affecting coagulation has been associated with an increased risk of bleeding; monitor.

Selegiline: Concurrent use with citalopram has been reported to cause serotonin syndrome; as an MAO type B inhibitor, the risk of serotonin syndrome may be less than with nonselective MAO inhibitors, and reports indicate that this combination has been well tolerated in Parkinson's patients.

SSRIs: Concurrent use with other reuptake inhibitors may increase the risk of serotonin syndrome.

Sibutramine: May increase the risk of serotonin syndrome with SSRIs.

Sumatriptan (and other serotonin agonists): Concurrent use may result in toxicity; weakness, hyper-reflexia, and incoordination have been observed with sumatriptan and SSRIs. In addition, concurrent use may theoretically increase the risk of serotonin syndrome; includes sumatriptan, naratriptan, rizatriptan, and zolmitriptan.

(Continued)

Escitalopram *(Continued)*

Tramadol: Concurrent use of citalopram with tramadol may cause serotonin syndrome; avoid concurrent use.

Trazodone: Concurrent use of citalopram with trazodone may cause serotonin syndrome.

Venlafaxine: Combined use with citalopram may increase the risk of serotonin syndrome.

Warfarin: Use with caution; may increase risk of bleeding.

Nutritional/Herbal/Ethanol Interactions

Ethanol: Avoid ethanol (may increase CNS depression).

Herb/Nutraceutical: Avoid valerian, St John's wort, SAMe, kava kava, and gotu kola (may increase CNS depression).

Adverse Reactions

>10%:

Central nervous system: Headache (24%), somnolence (6% to 13%), insomnia (9% to 12%)

Gastrointestinal: Nausea (15%)

Genitourinary: Ejaculation disorder (9% to 14%)

1% to 10%:

Cardiovascular: Chest pain, hypertension, palpitation

Central nervous system: Dizziness (5%), fatigue (5% to 8%), dreaming abnormal, concentration impaired, fever, irritability, lethargy, lightheadedness, migraine, vertigo, yawning

Dermatologic: Rash

Endocrine & metabolic: Libido decreased (3% to 7%), anorgasmia (2% to 6%), hot flashes, menstrual cramps, menstrual disorder

Gastrointestinal: Diarrhea (8%), xerostomia (6% to 9%), appetite decreased (3%), constipation (3% to 5%), indigestion (3%), abdominal pain (2%), abdominal cramps, appetite increased, flatulence, gastroenteritis, gastroesophageal reflux, heartburn, toothache, vomiting, weight gain/loss

Genitourinary: Impotence (3%), urinary tract infection, urinary frequency

Neuromuscular & skeletal: Arthralgia, limb pain, muscle cramp, myalgia, neck/shoulder pain, paresthesia, tremor

Ocular: Blurred vision

Otic: Earache, tinnitus

Respiratory: Rhinitis (5%), sinusitis (3%), bronchitis, cough, nasal or sinus congestion, sinus headache

Miscellaneous: Diaphoresis (4% to 5%), flu-like syndrome (5%), allergy

<1% (Limited to important or life-threatening): Acute renal failure, aggression, akathisia, allergic reaction, anaphylaxis, anemia, angioedema, anxiety attack, apathy, atrial fibrillation, auditory hallucination, bradycardia, carbohydrate craving, chest tightness, choreoathetosis, confusion, decreased prothrombin, delirium, depersonalization, depression aggravated, depression, dyskinesia, ecchymosis, ECG abnormal, emotional lability, epidermal necrolysis, erythema multiforme, excitability, grand mal seizure, hallucination, hemolytic anemia, hepatic necrosis, hepatitis, hypercholesterolemia, hyperglycemia, hyper-reflexia, increased bilirubin, malaise, muscle contractions (involuntary), muscle weakness, nystagmus, pancreatitis, panic reaction, priapism, prolactinemia, pulmonary embolism, QT prolonged, rhabdomyolysis, serotonin syndrome, SIADH, spontaneous abortion, suicidal tendency, suicide attempt, syncope, tachycardia, taste alteration, thrombocytopenia, thrombosis, tics, torsade de pointes, ventricular arrhythmia, vision abnormal, visual disturbance, weakness, withdrawal syndrome

Overdosage/Toxicology Treatment should be symptom-directed and supportive.

Dosing

Adults: Depression, GAD: Oral: Initial: 10 mg/day; dose may be increased to 20 mg/day after at least 1 week

Elderly: Depression: Oral: 5-10 mg/day; doses may be increased by 5-10 mg/day after at least 1 week.

Renal Impairment:

Mild to moderate impairment: No dosage adjustment needed.

Severe impairment: Cl_{cr} <20 mL/minute: Use caution.

Hepatic Impairment: 10 mg/day

Available Dosage Forms

Solution, oral: 1 mg/mL (240 mL) [peppermint flavor]

Tablet: 5 mg, 10 mg, 20 mg

Note: Cipralex® [CAN] is available only in 10 mg and 20 mg strengths.

Nursing Guidelines

Assessment: Assess potential for interactions with other prescriptions, OTC medications, or herbal products patient may be taking (eg, MAO inhibitors and other SSRIs). Assess therapeutic effectiveness and adverse reactions at the beginning of therapy and on a regular basis throughout therapy (eg, suicidal ideation, mania, hypomania, anxiety, or panic attacks). Teach patient proper use, possible side effects, interventions to reduce side effects, and adverse symptoms to report.

Dietary Considerations: May be taken with or without food.

Patient Education: Do not take any new medication during therapy without consulting prescriber. Take exactly as directed; do not alter dose or discontinue without consulting prescriber (effects of medication may take up to 3 weeks to occur). Avoid other stimulants: caffeine or alcohol. May cause dizziness, lightheadedness, insomnia, impaired concentration, headache (use caution when driving or engaging in tasks requiring alertness until response to drug is known); nausea, vomiting, loss or increase of appetite, indigestion, or heartburn (small frequent meals, frequent mouth care, sucking lozenges, or chewing gum may help); constipation (increased dietary fluid, fruit, fiber, and increased exercise may help); sexual dysfunction (reversible when drug is discontinued); hot flashes or menstrual cramps; or muscle pain, cramps, or tremor (consult prescriber for approved analgesia). Report immediately any CNS changes such as increased depression, confusion, impaired concentration, severe headache, insomnia, nightmares, irritability, acute anxiety, panic attacks, or thoughts of suicide; persistent GI changes; chest pain or palpitations; blurred vision or vision changes; ringing in ears; unusual cough; or other persistent adverse effects. **Pregnancy/breast-feeding precautions:** Inform prescriber if you are or intend to become pregnant. Breast-feeding is not recommended.

Pregnancy Risk Factor: C

Pregnancy Issues: Teratogenic effects have been reported in animal studies. Nonteratogenic effects including respiratory distress, cyanosis, apnea, seizures, temperature instability, feeding difficulty, vomiting, hypoglycemia, hypo- or hypertonia, hyper-reflexia, jitteriness, irritability, constant crying, and tremor have been reported in the neonate immediately following delivery after exposure late in the third trimester. Adverse effects may be due to toxic effects of SSRI or drug discontinuation. In some cases, may present clinically as serotonin syndrome. There are no adequate and well-controlled studies in pregnant women. Use during pregnancy only if the potential benefit to the mother outweighs the possible risk to the fetus. If treatment during pregnancy is required, consider tapering therapy during the third trimester.

Lactation: Enters breast milk/not recommended

Breast-Feeding Considerations: Escitalopram is excreted in human milk. Excessive somnolence, decreased feeding and weight loss have been reported in breast-fed infants. A decision should be made whether to continue or discontinue nursing or discontinue the drug.

Administration

Oral: Administer once daily (morning or evening), with or without food.

Storage: Store at 25°C (77°F).

- **Escitalopram Oxalate** *see* Escitalopram *on page 639*
- **Esclim®** *see* Estradiol *on page 649*
- **Eserine Salicylate** *see* Physostigmine *on page 1361*
- **Esgic®** *see* Butalbital, Acetaminophen, and Caffeine *on page 280*
- **Esgic-Plus™** *see* Butalbital, Acetaminophen, and Caffeine *on page 280*
- **Eskalith® [DSC]** *see* Lithium *on page 1052*
- **Eskalith CR®** *see* Lithium *on page 1052*

Esmolol (ES moe lol)

U.S. Brand Names Brevibloc®

Synonyms Esmolol Hydrochloride

Pharmacologic Category Antiarrhythmic Agent, Class II; Beta Blocker, $Beta_1$ Selective

Medication Safety Issues

Sound-alike/look-alike issues:

Esmolol may be confused with Osmitrol®

Brevibloc® may be confused with bretylium, Brevital®, Bumex®, Buprenex®

(Continued)

Esmolol *(Continued)*

Use Treatment of supraventricular tachycardia (SVT) and atrial fibrillation/flutter (control ventricular rate); treatment of tachycardia and/or hypertension (especially intraoperative or postoperative); treatment of noncompensatory sinus tachycardia

Unlabeled/Investigational Use In children, for SVT and postoperative hypertension

Mechanism of Action Class II antiarrhythmic: Competitively blocks response to beta$_1$-adrenergic stimulation with little or no effect of beta$_2$-receptors except at high doses, no intrinsic sympathomimetic activity, no membrane stabilizing activity

Pharmacodynamics/Kinetics

Onset of action: Beta-blockade: I.V.: 2-10 minutes (quickest when loading doses are administered)

Duration of hemodynamic effects: 10-30 minutes; prolonged following higher cumulative doses, extended duration of use

Protein binding: 55%

Metabolism: In blood by red blood cell esterases

Half-life elimination: Adults: 9 minutes; elimination of metabolite decreases with end stage renal disease

Excretion: Urine (~69% as metabolites, 2% unchanged drug)

Contraindications Hypersensitivity to esmolol or any component of the formulation; sinus bradycardia; heart block greater than first degree (except in patients with a functioning artificial pacemaker); cardiogenic shock; bronchial asthma (relative); uncompensated cardiac failure; hypotension; pregnancy (2nd and 3rd trimesters)

Warnings/Precautions Hypotension is common; patients need close blood pressure monitoring. Administer cautiously in compensated heart failure and monitor for a worsening of the condition. Use caution in patients with PVD (can aggravate arterial insufficiency). Use caution with concurrent use of beta-blockers and either verapamil or diltiazem; bradycardia or heart block can occur. Avoid concurrent I.V. use of both agents. Use beta-blockers cautiously in patients with bronchospastic disease; monitor pulmonary status closely. Use cautiously in diabetics because it can mask prominent hypoglycemic symptoms. Can mask signs of thyrotoxicosis. Can cause fetal bradycardia when administered in the 3rd trimester of pregnancy or at delivery. Use caution in patients with renal dysfunction (active metabolite retained). Do not use in the treatment of hypertension associated with vasoconstriction related to hypothermia. Concentrations >10 mg/mL or infusion into small veins or through a butterfly catheter should be avoided (can cause thrombophlebitis). Extravasation can lead to skin necrosis and sloughing.

Drug Interactions

Acetylcholinesterase Inhibitors: May enhance the bradycardic effect of beta-blockers.

Alpha/beta agonists (direct acting): Beta blockers may enhance the vasopressor effect of alpha/beta agonists (direct-acting). Epinephrine used as a local anesthetic for dental procedures will not likely cause clinically-relevant problems.

Alpha$_1$-blockers: Beta blockers may enhance the orthostatic effect of alpha$_1$ blockers. The risk associated with ophthalmic products is probably less than systemic products.

Alpha$_2$ agonists: Beta blockers may enhance the rebound hypertensive effect of alpha$_2$ agonists. This effect can occur when the alpha$_2$ agonist is abruptly withdrawn.

Amiodarone: May enhance the bradycardic effect of beta-blockers. Possibly to the point of cardiac arrest. Consider therapy modification.

Beta$_2$ agonists: May diminish the bradycardic effect of beta-blockers (beta$_1$ selective); of concern with high doses of some beta-blockers.

Calcium channel blockers (nondihydropyridine): May enhance the hypotensive effect of beta-blockers. Bradycardia and signs of heart failure have also been reported.

Cardiac glycosides: Beta-blockers may enhance the bradycardic effect of cardiac glycosides.

Disopyramide; May enhance the bradycardic effect of beta-blockers. Use caution if coadministering disopyramide and a beta-blocker (especially if both are I.V.).

Insulin preparations: Beta-blockers may enhance the hypoglycemic effect of insulin preparations.

NSAIDs: May diminish the antihypertensive effect of beta-blockers.

Sulfonylureas: Beta-blockers may enhance the hypoglycemic effect of sulfonylureas. Cardioselective beta-blockers (eg, esmolol) may be safer than nonselective beta-blockers. All beta-blockers appear to mask tachycardia as an initial symptom of hypoglycemia.

Lab Interactions Increased cholesterol (S), glucose

Adverse Reactions

>10%:

Cardiovascular: Asymptomatic hypotension (dose-related: 25% to 38%), symptomatic hypotension (dose-related: 12%)

Miscellaneous: Diaphoresis (10%)

1% to 10%:

Cardiovascular: Peripheral ischemia (1%)

Central nervous system: Dizziness (3%), somnolence (3%), confusion (2%), headache (2%), agitation (2%), fatigue (1%)

Gastrointestinal: Nausea (7%), vomiting (1%)

Local: Pain on injection (8%), infusion site reaction

<1% (Limited to important or life-threatening): Alopecia, bronchospasm, chest pain, CHF, depression, dyspnea, edema, exfoliative dermatitis, heart block, infusion site reactions, paresthesia, pruritus, pulmonary edema, rigors, seizure, severe bradycardia/asystole (rare), skin necrosis (from extravasation), syncope, thrombophlebitis, urinary retention

Overdosage/Toxicology Symptoms of overdose include hypotension, bradycardia, bronchospasm, congestive heart failure, and heart block. Initially, a decrease/discontinuation of the esmolol infusion and administration of fluids may be the best treatment for hypotension. Sympathomimetics (eg, epinephrine or dopamine), glucagon, or an anticholinergic or a pacemaker can be used to treat the toxic bradycardia, asystole, and/or hypotension.

Dosing

Adults & Elderly: Infusion requires an infusion pump (must be adjusted to individual response and tolerance):

Intraoperative tachycardia and/or hypertension (immediate control): I.V.: Initial bolus: 80 mg (~1 mg/kg) over 30 seconds, followed by a 150 mcg/kg/minute infusion, if necessary. Adjust infusion rate as needed to maintain desired heart rate and/or blood pressure, up to 300 mcg/kg/minute.

For control of postoperative hypertension, as many as one-third of patients may require higher doses (250-300 mcg/kg/minute) to control blood pressure; the safety of doses >300 mcg/kg/minute has not been studied.

Supraventricular tachycardia or gradual control of postoperative tachycardia/hypertension: I.V.: Loading dose: 500 mcg/kg over 1 minute; follow with a 50 mcg/kg/minute infusion for 4 minutes; response to this initial infusion rate may be a rough indication of the responsiveness of the ventricular rate.

Infusion may be continued at 50 mcg/kg/minute or, if the response is inadequate, titrated upward in 50 mcg/kg/minute increments (increased no more frequently than every 4 minutes) to a maximum of 200 mcg/kg/minute.

Note: To achieve more rapid response, following the initial loading dose and 50 mcg/kg/minute infusion, rebolus with a second 500 mcg/kg loading dose over 1 minute, and increase the maintenance infusion to 100 mcg/kg/minute for 4 minutes. If necessary, a third (and final) 500 mcg/kg loading dose may be administered, prior to increasing to an infusion rate of 150 mcg/minute. After 4 minutes of the 150 mcg/kg/minute infusion, the infusion rate may be increased to a maximum rate of 200 mcg/kg/minute (without a bolus dose).

Supraventricular tachycardias (SVT); usual dose range: Usual dosage range: 50-200 mcg/kg/minute with average dose of 100 mcg/kg/minute.

Guidelines for transfer to oral therapy (beta blocker, calcium channel blocker):

Infusion should be reduced by 50% 30 minutes following the first dose of the alternative agent

Manufacturer suggests following the second dose of the alternative drug, patient's response should be monitored and if control is adequate for the first hours, esmolol may be discontinued.

Pediatrics:

Supraventricular tachycardias (unlabeled use): I.V.: A limited amount of information regarding esmolol use in pediatric patients is currently available. Some centers have utilized doses of 100-500 mcg/kg given over 1 minute for control of supraventricular tachycardias.

(Continued)

Esmolol *(Continued)*

Postoperative hypertension (unlabeled use): I.V.: Loading doses of 500 mcg/kg/minute over 1 minute with maximal doses of 50-250 mcg/kg/minute (mean = 173) have been used in addition to nitroprusside to treat postoperative hypertension after coarctation of aorta repair.

Renal Impairment: Not removed by hemo- or peritoneal dialysis. Supplemental dose is not necessary.

Available Dosage Forms

Infusion [premixed in sodium chloride; preservative free] (Brevibloc®): 2000 mg (100 mL) [20 mg/mL; double strength]; 2500 mg (250 mL) [10 mg/mL]

Injection, solution, as hydrochloride: 10 mg/mL (10 mL) [premixed in sodium chloride]

Brevibloc®: 10 mg/mL (10 mL) [alcohol free; premixed in sodium chloride]; 20 mg/mL (5 mL, 100 mL) [alcohol free; double strength; premixed in sodium chloride]; 250 mg/mL (10 mL) [contains alcohol 25%, propylene glycol 25%; concentrate]

Nursing Guidelines

Assessment: Assess other medications patient may be taking for effectiveness and interactions. Requires continuous cardiac, hemodynamic, and infusion site monitoring (extravasation). If diabetic, may mask signs of hypoglycemia. Monitor blood sugars closely. Monitor therapeutic effectiveness and adverse reactions.

Patient Education: Esmolol is administered in emergencies, patient education should be appropriate to the situation. **Pregnancy/breast-feeding precautions:** Inform prescriber if you are pregnant. Consult prescriber if breast-feeding.

Geriatric Considerations: Due to alterations in the beta-adrenergic autonomic nervous system, beta-adrenergic blockade may result in less hemodynamic response than seen in younger adults.

Pregnancy Risk Factor: C (manufacturer); D (2nd and 3rd trimesters - expert analysis)

Lactation: Excretion in breast milk unknown/use with caution

Perioperative/Anesthesia/Other Concerns: Esmolol 250 mg/mL contains propylene glycol 258 mg/mL (25% v/v).

This agent is also used to blunt sympathetic response during intubation, in "at-risk" patients such as those with coronary artery disease (CAD), angina, uncontrolled hypertension, and hyperthyroidism. Esmolol may lose $beta_1$-specificity after higher doses. It should be used with caution in patients with pulmonary disease and diabetes.

Esmolol provides an important mechanism for close titration of rate control in patients with atrial fibrillation; may also be beneficial in allowing close blood pressure control. Esmolol should only be administered in intensive care or closely monitored situations. Potential adverse effects include hypotension and bradyarrhythmias (usually short-lived due to short half-life of 9 minutes).

Administration

I.V.: The 250 mg/mL ampul is **not** for direct I.V. injection, but rather must first be diluted to a final concentration of 10 mg/mL (ie, 2.5 g in 250 mL or 5 g in 500 mL). Concentrations >10 mg/mL or infusion into small veins or through a butterfly catheter should be avoided (can cause thrombophlebitis).

Compatibility: Stable in D_5LR, $D_5{}^1/_2NS$, D_5NS, D_5W, D_5W with KCl 40 mEq/L, LR, $^1/_2NS$, NS, sodium bicarbonate 5%

Y-site administration: Incompatible with amphotericin B cholesteryl sulfate complex, furosemide, warfarin

Compatibility when admixed: Incompatible with diazepam, procainamide, sodium bicarbonate, thiopental

Storage: Clear, colorless to light yellow solution which should be stored at 15°C to 30°C (59°F to 85°F); protect from freezing and excessive heat.

Related Information

Management of Postoperative Arrhythmias *on page 1787*
Postoperative Hypertension *on page 1815*

♦ **Esmolol Hydrochloride** *see* Esmolol *on page 643*

Esomeprazole (es oh ME pray zol)

U.S. Brand Names Nexium®

Synonyms Esomeprazole Magnesium

Pharmacologic Category Proton Pump Inhibitor; Substituted Benzimidazole

Use

Oral: Short-term (4-8 weeks) treatment of erosive esophagitis; maintaining symptom resolution and healing of erosive esophagitis; treatment of symptomatic gastroesophageal reflux disease (GERD); as part of a multidrug regimen for *Helicobacter pylori* eradication in patients with duodenal ulcer disease (active or history of within the past 5 years); prevention of gastric ulcers associated with continuous NSAID therapy

I.V.: Short-term (≤10 weeks) treatment of gastroesophageal reflux disease (GERD) when oral therapy is not possible or appropriate

Mechanism of Action Proton pump inhibitor suppresses gastric acid secretion by inhibition of the H^+/K^+-ATPase in the gastric parietal cell

Pharmacodynamics/Kinetics

Distribution: V_{dss}: 16 L

Protein binding: 97%

Metabolism: Hepatic via CYP2C19 and 3A4 enzymes to hydroxy, desmethyl, and sulfone metabolites (all inactive)

Bioavailability: 90% with repeat dosing

Half-life elimination: 1-1.5 hours

Time to peak: 1.5 hours

Excretion: Urine (80%); feces (20%)

Contraindications Hypersensitivity to esomeprazole, substituted benzimidazoles (ie, lansoprazole, omeprazole, pantoprazole, rabeprazole), or any component of the formulation

Warnings/Precautions Relief of symptoms does not preclude the presence of a gastric malignancy. Atrophic gastritis (by biopsy) has been noted with long-term omeprazole therapy; this may also occur with esomeprazole. No reports of enterochromaffin-like (ECL) cell carcinoids, dysplasia, or neoplasia has occurred. Safety and efficacy in pediatric patients have not been established.

Drug Interactions Substrate of CYP2C19 (major), 3A4 (minor)

Benzodiazepines metabolized by oxidation (eg, diazepam, midazolam, triazolam): Esomeprazole and omeprazole may increase levels of benzodiazepines metabolized by oxidation.

Carbamazepine: Esomeprazole and omeprazole may increase carbamazepine levels. Carbamazepine may decrease the effects of esomeprazole.

CYP2C19 inducers: May decrease the levels/effects of esomeprazole. Example inducers include aminoglutethimide, carbamazepine, phenytoin, and rifampin.

Iron salts: Esomeprazole may decrease the absorption of orally-administered iron salts.

Itraconazole and ketoconazole: Proton pump inhibitors may decrease the absorption of itraconazole and ketoconazole.

Protease inhibitors: Proton pump inhibitors may decrease absorption of some protease inhibitors (atazanavir and indinavir).

Nutritional/Herbal/Ethanol Interactions Food: Absorption is decreased by 43% to 53% when taken with food.

Adverse Reactions Unless otherwise specified, percentages represent adverse reactions identified in clinical trials evaluating the intravenous formulation.

>10%: Central nervous system: Headache (I.V. 11%)

1% to 10%:

Central nervous system: Dizziness (3%), headache (oral 4% to 6%)

Dermatologic: Pruritus (≤1%)

Gastrointestinal: Flatulence (10%), nausea (6%), abdominal pain (6%; oral 4%), diarrhea (4%), xerostomia (4%), dyspepsia (<1% to 6%), constipation (3%)

Local: Injection site reaction (2%)

Respiratory: Sinusitis (≤2%), respiratory infection (1%)

<1% (Limited to important or life-threatening): Allergic reactions, anaphylaxis, angina, angioedema, arthritis, asthma, confusion, depression, dyspnea; edema (facial, larynx, peripheral, tongue); erythema multiforme, goiter, hematuria, hypertension, hypertonia, hyponatremia, impotence, hepatitis, jaundice, migraine, myalgia, pancreatitis, paresthesia, polymyalgia rheumatica, rash, Stevens-Johnson syndrome, thrombocytopenia, toxic epidermal necrolysis, ulcerative stomatitis, urticaria, vertigo

(Continued)

Esomeprazole *(Continued)*

Overdosage/Toxicology Symptoms of overdose may include confusion, drowsiness, blurred vision, tachycardia, nausea, sweating, headache or dry mouth. Treatment is symptom-directed and supportive; not dialyzable.

Dosing

Adults & Elderly:

Healing of erosive esophagitis: Oral: 20-40 mg once daily for 4-8 weeks; may consider an additional 4-8 weeks of treatment if patient is not healed

Maintenance of healing of erosive esophagitis: Oral: 20 mg once daily; clinical trials evaluated therapy for ≤6 months

Symptomatic gastroesophageal reflux: Oral: 20 mg once daily for 4 weeks; may consider an additional 4 weeks of treatment if symptoms do not resolve

Treatment of GERD (short-term): I.V.: 20 mg or 40 mg once daily for ≤10 days; change to oral therapy as soon as appropriate

Peptic ulcer disease: Eradication of *Helicobacter pylori*: Oral: 40 mg once daily; requires combination therapy

Prevention of NSAID-induced gastric ulcers: 20-40 mg once daily for up to 6 months

Renal Impairment: No adjustment is necessary.

Hepatic Impairment:

Mild-to-moderate hepatic impairment (Child-Pugh Class A or B): No dosage adjustment needed.

Severe hepatic impairment (Child-Pugh Class C): Dose should not exceed 20 mg/day.

Available Dosage Forms

Capsule, delayed release: 20 mg, 40 mg

Injection, powder for reconstitution: 20 mg, 40 mg [contains edetate sodium]

Nursing Guidelines

Assessment: Assess other medications patient may be taking for effectiveness and interactions (especially those dependent on cytochrome P450 metabolism or those dependent on an acid environment for absorption). Monitor effectiveness of therapeutic effectiveness and adverse reactions at beginning of therapy and periodically throughout therapy. Assess knowledge/teach appropriate use of this medication, interventions to reduce side effects, and adverse symptoms to report.

Monitoring Laboratory Tests: Susceptibility testing is recommended in patients who fail *H. pylori* eradication regimen (esomeprazole, clarithromycin, and amoxicillin).

Dietary Considerations: Take at least 1 hour before meals; best if taken before breakfast. The contents of the capsule may be mixed in applesauce or water; pellets also remain intact when exposed to orange juice, apple juice, and yogurt.

Patient Education: Take as directed, 1 hour before eating at same time each day. Swallow capsule whole; do not crush or chew. If you cannot swallow capsule whole, open capsule, mix contents with 1 tablespoon of applesauce, and swallow immediately; do not chew mixture. Do not store for future use. You may experience headache; constipation (increased exercise, fluids, fruit, or fiber may help); diarrhea (boiled milk, yogurt, or buttermilk may help); or abdominal pain (should diminish with use). Report persistent headache, diarrhea, constipation, abdominal pain, changes in urination or pain on urination, chest pain or palpitations, changes in respiratory status, CNS changes, persistent muscular aches or pain, ringing in ears or visual changes, or other adverse reactions. **Breast-feeding precaution:** Breast-feeding is not recommended.

Pregnancy Risk Factor: B

Lactation: Excretion in breast milk unknown/not recommended

Breast-Feeding Considerations: Esomeprazole excretion into breast milk has not been studied. However, omeprazole is excreted in breast milk, and therefore considered likely that esomeprazole is similarly excreted; breast-feeding is not recommended..

Perioperative/Anesthesia/Other Concerns: The contents of the capsule remain intact when exposed to tap water, orange juice, apple juice, and yogurt.

For administration into a nasogastric tube: Open capsule and place intact granules into a 60 mL syringe; mix with 50 mL of water. Replace plunger and shake vigorously for 15 seconds. Do not administer if pellets dissolve or disintegrate. After administration, flush nasogastric tube with additional water. Use suspension immediately after preparation.

Administration

Oral: Capsule should be swallowed whole and taken at least 1 hour before eating (best if taken before breakfast). For patients with difficulty swallowing, open capsule and mix contents with 1 tablespoon of applesauce. Swallow immediately; mixture should not be chewed or warmed. The mixture should not be stored for future use.

I.V.:

May be administered by injection (≥3 minutes) or infusion (10-30 minutes). Flush line prior to and after administration with NS, LR, or D_5W.

Reconstitution: Powder for injection:

For I.V. injection: Reconstitute powder with 5 mL NS.

For I.V. infusion: Initially reconstitute powder with 5 mL of NS, LR, or D_5W, then further dilute to a final volume of 50 mL.

Storage: Capsule: Store at 15°C to 30°C (59°F to 86°F). Keep container tightly closed.

Powder for injection: Store at 15°C to 30°C (59°F to 86°F). Protect from light. Following reconstitution, solution for injection prepared in NS, and solution for infusion prepared in NS or LR should be used within 12 hours. Following reconstitution, solution for infusion prepared in D_5W should be used within 6 hours. Refrigeration is not required following reconstitution.

♦ Esomeprazole Magnesium *see* Esomeprazole *on page 647*
♦ Ester-E™ [OTC] *see* Vitamin E *on page 1716*
♦ Esterified Estrogens *see* Estrogens (Esterified) *on page 669*
♦ Estrace® *see* Estradiol *on page 649*
♦ Estraderm® *see* Estradiol *on page 649*

Estradiol (es tra DYE ole)

U.S. Brand Names Alora®; Climara®; Delestrogen®; Depo®-Estradiol; Esclim®; Estrace®; Estraderm®; Estrasorb™; Estring®; EstroGel®; Femring™; Femtrace®; Gynodiol®; Menostar™; Vagifem®; Vivelle®; Vivelle-Dot®

Synonyms Estradiol Acetate; Estradiol Cypionate; Estradiol Hemihydrate; Estradiol Transdermal; Estradiol Valerate

Pharmacologic Category Estrogen Derivative

Medication Safety Issues

Sound-alike/look-alike issues:

Alora® may be confused with Aldara™

Estraderm® may be confused with Testoderm®

Transdermal patch may contain conducting metal (eg, aluminum); remove patch prior to MRI.

Use Treatment of moderate-to-severe vasomotor symptoms associated with menopause; treatment of vulvar and vaginal atrophy; hypoestrogenism (due to hypogonadism, castration, or primary ovarian failure); prostatic cancer (palliation), breast cancer (palliation), osteoporosis (prophylaxis); abnormal uterine bleeding due to hormonal imbalance; postmenopausal urogenital symptoms of the lower urinary tract (urinary urgency, dysuria)

Mechanism of Action Estrogens are responsible for the development and maintenance of the female reproductive system and secondary sexual characteristics. Estradiol is the principle intracellular human estrogen and is more potent than estrone and estriol at the receptor level; it is the primary estrogen secreted prior to menopause. Following menopause, estrone and estrone sulfate are more highly produced. Estrogens modulate the pituitary secretion of gonadotropins, luteinizing hormone, and follicle-stimulating hormone through a negative feedback system; estrogen replacement reduces elevated levels of these hormones in postmenopausal women.

Pharmacodynamics/Kinetics

Absorption: Oral, topical: Well absorbed

Distribution: Crosses placenta; enters breast milk

Protein binding: 37% to sex hormone-binding globulin; 61% to albumin

Metabolism: Hepatic via oxidation and conjugation in GI tract; hydroxylated via CYP3A4 to metabolites; first-pass effect; enterohepatic recirculation; reversibly converted to estrone and estriol

Excretion: Primarily urine (as metabolites estrone and estriol); feces (small amounts)

Contraindications Hypersensitivity to estradiol or any component of the formulation; undiagnosed abnormal vaginal bleeding; history of or current thrombophlebitis or venous thromboembolic disorders (including DVT, PE); active or recent

(Continued)

Estradiol *(Continued)*

(within 1 year) arterial thromboembolic disease (eg, stroke, MI); carcinoma of the breast, except in appropriately selected patients being treated for metastatic disease; estrogen-dependent tumor; hepatic dysfunction or disease; porphyria; pregnancy

Warnings/Precautions

Cardiovascular-related considerations: Estrogens with or without progestin should not be used to prevent coronary heart disease. Use caution with cardiovascular disease or dysfunction. May increase the risks of hypertension, myocardial infarction (MI), stroke, pulmonary emboli (PE), and deep vein thrombosis; incidence of these effects was shown to be significantly increased in postmenopausal women using conjugated equine estrogens (CEE) in combination with medroxyprogesterone acetate (MPA). Nonfatal MI, PE, and thrombophlebitis have also been reported in males taking high doses of CEE (eg, for prostate cancer). Estrogen compounds are generally associated with lipid effects such as increased HDL-cholesterol and decreased LDL-cholesterol. Triglycerides may also be increased; use with caution in patients with familial defects of lipoprotein metabolism. Whenever possible, estrogens should be discontinued at least 4 weeks prior to and for 2 weeks following elective surgery associated with an increased risk of thromboembolism or during periods of prolonged immobilization.

Neurological considerations: The risk of dementia may be increased in postmenopausal women; increased incidence was observed in women ≥65 years of age taking CEE in combination with MPA.

Cancer-related considerations: Unopposed estrogens may increase the risk of endometrial carcinoma in postmenopausal women. Estrogens may exacerbate endometriosis. Malignant transformation of residual endometrial implants has been reported post-hysterectomy with estrogen only therapy. Consider adding a progestin in women with residual endometriosis post-hysterectomy. Estrogens may increase the risk of breast cancer. An increased risk of invasive breast cancer was observed in postmenopausal women using CEE in combination with MPA; a smaller increase in risk was seen with estrogen therapy alone in observational studies. An increase in abnormal mammograms has also been reported with estrogen and progestin therapy. Estrogen use may lead to severe hypercalcemia in patients with breast cancer and bone metastases; discontinue estrogen if hypercalcemia occurs.

Estrogens may cause retinal vascular thrombosis; discontinue permanently if papilledema or retinal vascular lesions are observed on examination. Use with caution in patients with diseases which may be exacerbated by fluid retention, including asthma, epilepsy, migraine, diabetes or renal dysfunction. Use with caution in patients with a history of severe hypocalcemia, SLE, hepatic hemangiomas, endometriosis, and gallbladder disease. Use caution with history of cholestatic jaundice associated with past estrogen use or pregnancy. Safety and efficacy in pediatric patients have not been established. Prior to puberty, estrogens may cause premature closure of the epiphyses, premature breast development in girls or gynecomastia in boys. Vaginal bleeding and vaginal cornification may also be induced in girls.

Before prescribing estrogen therapy to postmenopausal women, the risks and benefits must be weighed for each patient. Women should be informed of these risks and benefits, as well as possible effects of progestin when added to estrogen therapy. Estrogens with or without progestin should be used for shortest duration possible consistent with treatment goals. Conduct periodic risk:benefit assessments.

When used solely for prevention of osteoporosis in women at significant risk, nonestrogen treatment options should be considered. When used solely for the treatment of vulvar and vaginal atrophy, topical vaginal products should be considered. Use caution applying topical products to severely atrophic vaginal mucosa. Absorption of topical emulsion is increased by application of sunscreen; do not apply both products within close proximity of each other. Application of gel formulation with sunscreen has not been evaluated. Transdermal patch may contain conducting metal (eg, aluminum); remove patch prior to MRI.

Drug Interactions Substrate of CYP1A2 (major), 2A6 (minor), 2B6 (minor), 2C8/9 (minor), 2C19 (minor), 2D6 (minor), 2E1 (minor), 3A4 (major); **Inhibits** CYP1A2 (weak); **Induces** CYP3A4 (weak)

Anticoagulants: Increase potential for thromboembolic events

Corticosteroids: Estrogens may enhance the effects of hydrocortisone and prednisone.

CYP1A2 inducers: May decrease the levels/effects of estradiol. Example inducers include aminoglutethimide, carbamazepine, phenobarbital, and rifampin.

CYP3A4 inducers: CYP3A4 inducers may decrease the levels/effects of estradiol. Example inducers include aminoglutethimide, carbamazepine, nafcillin, nevirapine, phenobarbital, phenytoin, and rifamycins.

Nutritional/Herbal/Ethanol Interactions

Ethanol: Avoid ethanol (routine use increases estrogen level and risk of breast cancer). Ethanol may also increase the risk of osteoporosis.

Food: Folic acid absorption may be decreased

Herb/Nutraceutical: St John's wort may decrease estradiol levels. Avoid black cohosh, dong quai (has estrogenic activity). Avoid red clover, saw palmetto, ginseng.

Lab Interactions Increased Prothrombin and factors VII, VIII, IX, X; increased platelet aggregability, thyroid-binding globulin, total thyroid hormone (T_4), serum triglycerides/phospholipids; decreased antithrombin III, serum folate concentration

Adverse Reactions Frequency not defined.

Cardiovascular: Edema, hypertension, MI, venous thromboembolism

Central nervous system: Anxiety, dizziness, epilepsy exacerbation, headache, irritability, mental depression, migraine, mood disturbances, nervousness

Dermatologic: Chloasma, erythema multiforme, erythema nodosum, hemorrhagic eruption, hirsutism, loss of scalp hair, melasma, rash, pruritus

Endocrine & metabolic: Breast enlargement, breast tenderness, libido (changes in), increased thyroid-binding globulin, increased total thyroid hormone (T_4), increased serum triglycerides/phospholipids, increased HDL-cholesterol, decreased LDL-cholesterol, impaired glucose tolerance, hypercalcemia

Gastrointestinal: Abdominal cramps, abdominal pain, bloating, cholecystitis, cholelithiasis, diarrhea, flatulence, gallbladder disease, nausea, pancreatitis, vomiting, weight gain/loss

Genitourinary: Alterations in frequency and flow of menses, changes in cervical secretions, endometrial cancer, increased size of uterine leiomyomata, Pap smear suspicious, vaginal candidiasis

Vaginal: Trauma from applicator insertion may occur in women with severely atrophic vaginal mucosa

Hematologic: Aggravation of porphyria, antithrombin III and antifactor Xa decreased, levels of fibrinogen increased, platelet aggregability increased and platelet count; increased prothrombin and factors VII, VIII, IX, X

Hepatic: Cholestatic jaundice

Local: Transdermal patches: Burning, erythema, irritation, thrombophlebitis

Neuromuscular & skeletal: Chorea, back pain

Ocular: Intolerance to contact lenses, steeping of corneal curvature

Respiratory: Pulmonary thromboembolism

Miscellaneous: Anaphylactoid/anaphylactic reactions, carbohydrate intolerance

Postmarketing and/or case reports: Vivelle®: Liver function tests increased (rare), leg pain

Overdosage/Toxicology Symptoms of overdose include fluid retention, jaundice, thrombophlebitis, nausea, and vomiting. Toxicity is unlikely following single exposure of excessive doses. Treatment following emesis and charcoal administration should be supportive and symptomatic.

Dosing

Adults & Elderly: All dosage needs to be adjusted based upon the patient's response:

Atrophic vaginitis, vulvar/vaginal atrophy:

Intravaginal:

Vaginal cream: Atrophic vaginitis, kraurosis vulvae: Insert 2-4 g/day for 2 weeks then gradually reduce to ½ the initial dose for 2 weeks followed by a maintenance dose of 1 g 1-3 times/week

Vaginal ring:

Postmenopausal vaginal atrophy, urogenital symptoms (Estring®): 2 mg intravaginally; following insertion, ring should remain in place for 90 days

Vulvar/vaginal atrophy (Femring™): 0.05 mg intravaginally; following insertion, ring should remain in place for 3 months; dose may be increased to 0.1 mg if needed

(Continued)

Estradiol *(Continued)*

Vaginal tablets (Vagifem®); Atrophic vaginitis: Initial: Insert 1 tablet once daily for 2 weeks; maintenance: Insert 1 tablet twice weekly. Attempts to discontinue or taper medication should be made at 3- to 6-month intervals

Topical gel: Vulvar/vaginal atrophy: 1.25 g/day applied at the same time each day

Transdermal: Refer to product-specific dosing (below)

Breast cancer (females; inoperable, progressing): Oral: 10 mg 3 times/day for at least 3 months

Hypogonadism:

Oral: 1-2 mg/day in a cyclic regimen for 3 weeks on drug, then 1 week off drug

I.M.: Cypionate: 1.5-2 mg monthly; Valerate: 10-20 mg every 4 weeks

Transdermal: Refer to product-specific dosing (below)

Osteoporosis prevention (females):

Oral: 0.5 mg/day in a cyclic regimen (3 weeks on and 1 week off of drug)

Transdermal: Refer to product-specific dosing (below)

Prostate cancer:

I.M. (valerate): ≥30 mg or more every 1-2 weeks

Oral (androgen-dependent, inoperable, progressing): 10 mg 3 times/day for at least 3 months

Vasomotor symptoms (moderate-severe) associated with menopause:

Oral (in addition to I.M. dosing): 1-2 mg daily, adjusted as necessary to limit symptoms. Administrations should be cyclic (3 weeks on, 1 week off). Patients should be re-evaluated at 3-6 month intervals to determine if treatment is still necessary

I.M.: Cypionate: 1-5 mg every 3-4 weeks; Valerate: 10-20 mg every 4 weeks

Topical emulsion: 3.84 g applied once daily in the morning

Topical gel: 1.25 g/day applied at the same time each day

Vaginal ring (Femring™): 0.05 mg intravaginally; following insertion, ring should remain in place for 3 months; dose may be increased to 0.1 mg if needed

Transdermal: See product-specific dosing (below)

Transdermal product-specific dosing:

Note: Indicated dose may be used continuously in patients without an intact uterus. May be given continuously or cyclically (3 weeks on, 1 week off) in patients with an intact uterus **(exception - Menostar™, see specific dosing instructions).** When changing patients from oral to transdermal therapy, start transdermal patch 1 week after discontinuing oral hormone (may begin sooner if symptoms reappear within 1 week):

Transdermal once-weekly patch:

Moderate to severe vasomotor symptoms associated with menopause (Climara®): Apply 0.025 mg/day patch once weekly. Adjust dose as necessary to control symptoms. Patients should be re-evaluated at 3- to 6-month intervals to determine if treatment is still necessary.

Prevention of osteoporosis in postmenopausal women:

Climara®: Apply patch once weekly; minimum effective dose 0.025 mg/day; adjust dosage based on response to therapy as indicated by biological markers and bone mineral density.

Menostar™: Apply patch once weekly. In women with a uterus, also administer a progestin for 14 days every 6-12 months.

Transdermal twice-weekly patch (Alora®, Esclim®, Estraderm®, Vivelle®):

Moderate to severe vasomotor symptoms associated with menopause, vulvar/vaginal atrophy, female hypogonadism: Titrate to lowest dose possible to control symptoms, adjusting initial dose after the first month of therapy; re-evaluate therapy at 3- to 6-month intervals to taper or discontinue medication:

Alora®, Esclim®, Estraderm®, Vivelle-Dot®: Apply 0.05 mg patch twice weekly

Vivelle®: Apply 0.0375 mg patch twice weekly

Prevention of osteoporosis in postmenopausal women:

Alora®, Vivelle®, Vivelle-Dot®: Apply 0.025 mg patch twice weekly, increase dose as necessary

Estraderm®: Apply 0.05 mg patch twice weekly

Available Dosage Forms

Cream, vaginal (Estrace®): 0.1 mg/g (12 g) [refill tube]: 0.1 mg/g (42.5 g) [tube with applicator]

Emulsion, topical, as hemihydrate (Estrasorb™): 2.5 mg/g (56s) [each pouch contains 4.35 mg estradiol hemihydrate; contents of two pouches delivers estradiol 0.05 mg/day]

Gel, topical (EstroGel®): 0.06% (93 g) [pump; delivers estradiol 0.75 mg/1.25 g; 64 doses]

Injection, oil, as cypionate (Depo®-Estradiol): 5 mg/mL (5 mL) [contains chlorobutanol; in cottonseed oil]

Injection, oil, as valerate (Delestrogen®):
- 10 mg/mL (5 mL) [contains chlorobutanol; in sesame oil]
- 20 mg/mL (5 mL) [contains benzyl alcohol; in castor oil]
- 40 mg/mL (5 mL) [contains benzyl alcohol; in castor oil]

Ring, vaginal, as base (Estring®): 2 mg [total estradiol 2 mg; releases 7.5 mcg/day over 90 days] (1s)

Ring, vaginal, as acetate (Femring™): 0.05 mg [total estradiol 12.4 mg; releases 0.05 mg/day over 3 months] (1s); 0.1 mg [total estradiol 24.8 mg; releases 0.1 mg/day over 3 months] (1s)

Tablet, oral, as acetate (Femtrace®): 0.45 mg, 0.9 mg, 1.8 mg

Tablet, oral, micronized: 0.5 mg, 1 mg, 2 mg
- Estrace®: 0.5 mg, 1 mg, 2 mg [2 mg tablets contain tartrazine]
- Gynodiol®: 0.5 mg, 1 mg, 1.5 mg, 2 mg

Tablet, vaginal, as base (Vagifem®): 25 mcg [contains lactose]

Transdermal system: 0.025 mg/24 hours [once-weekly patch]; 0.05 mg/24 hours (4s) [once-weekly patch]; 0.075 mg/24 hours [once-weekly patch]; 0.1 mg/24 hours (4s) [once-weekly patch]
- Alora® [twice-weekly patch]:
  - 0.025 mg/24 hours [9 cm^2, total estradiol 0.77 mg] (8s)
  - 0.05 mg/24 hours [18 cm^2, total estradiol 1.5 mg] (8s, 24s)
  - 0.075 mg/24 hours [27 cm^2, total estradiol 2.3 mg] (8s)
  - 0.1 mg/24 hours [36 cm^2, total estradiol 3.1 mg] (8s)
- Climara® [once-weekly patch]:
  - 0.025 mg/24 hours [6.5 cm^2, total estradiol 2.04 mg] (4s)
  - 0.0375 mg/24 hours [9.375 cm^2, total estradiol 2.85 mg] (4s)
  - 0.05 mg/24 hours [12.5 cm^2, total estradiol 3.8 mg] (4s)
  - 0.06 mg/24 hours [15 cm^2, total estradiol 4.55 mg] (4s)
  - 0.075 mg/24 hours [18.75 cm^2, total estradiol 5.7 mg] (4s)
  - 0.1 mg/24 hours [25 cm^2, total estradiol 7.6 mg] (4s)
- Esclim® [twice-weekly patch]:
  - 0.025 mg/day [11 cm^2, total estradiol 5 mg] (8s)
  - 0.0375 mg/day [16.5 cm^2, total estradiol 7.5 mg] (8s)
  - 0.05 mg/day [22 cm^2, total estradiol 10 mg] (8s)
  - 0.075 mg/day [33 cm^2, total estradiol 15 mg] (8s)
  - 0.1 mg/day [44 cm^2, total estradiol 20 mg] (8s)
- Estraderm® [twice-weekly patch]:
  - 0.05 mg/24 hours [10 cm^2, total estradiol 4 mg] (8s)
  - 0.1 mg/24 hours [20 cm^2, total estradiol 8 mg] (8s)
- Menostar™ [once-weekly patch]: 0.014 mg/24 hours [3.25 cm^2, total estradiol 1 mg] (4s)
- Vivelle® [twice-weekly patch]:
  - 0.05 mg/24 hours [14.5 cm^2, total estradiol 4.33 mg] (8s)
  - 0.1 mg/24 hours [29 cm^2, total estradiol 8.66 mg] (8s)
- Vivelle-Dot® [twice-weekly patch]:
  - 0.025 mg/day [2.5 cm^2, total estradiol 0.39 mg] (8s)
  - 0.0375 mg/day [3.75 cm^2, total estradiol 0.585 mg] (8s)
  - 0.05 mg/day [5 cm^2, total estradiol 0.78 mg] (8s)
  - 0.075 mg/day [7.5 cm^2, total estradiol 1.17 mg] (8s)
  - 0.1 mg/day [10 cm^2, total estradiol 1.56 mg] (8s)

Nursing Guidelines

Assessment: Assess potential for interactions with other pharmacological agents or herbal products patient may be taking (eg, increased or decreased levels/effects of estradiol or increased potential for toxicity or thrombolic events). Assess results of annual gynecological exam, therapeutic effectiveness (dependent on rationale for use), need for continued therapy, and adverse effects (eg, thromboembolism, hypertension, edema, CNS changes) on a regular basis during therapy. **Note:** Before prescribing estrogen therapy to postmenopausal women, the risks and benefits must be weighed for each

(Continued)

Estradiol *(Continued)*

patient. Women should be informed of these risks and benefits, as well as possible effects of progestin when added to estrogen therapy. Estrogens with or without progestin should be used for shortest duration possible consistent with treatment goals and periodic assessment of risk:benefit should be made. Caution patients with diabetes to monitor glucose levels closely (may impair glucose tolerance). Teach patient proper use and application (according to formulation), possible side effects/appropriate interventions, and adverse symptoms to report. Remind patient about the importance of frequent self-breast exams and the need for annual gynecological exam. **Pregnancy risk factor X:** Determine that patient is not pregnant before starting therapy. Do not give to females of childbearing age unless patient is capable of complying with contraceptive use. Advise patient about contraceptive measures as appropriate.

Monitoring Laboratory Tests: Yearly Papanicolaou smear, mammogram. Adequate diagnostic measures, including endometrial sampling, if indicated, should be performed to rule out malignancy in all cases of undiagnosed abnormal vaginal bleeding.

Dietary Considerations: Ensure adequate calcium and vitamin D intake when used for the prevention of osteoporosis.

Patient Education: Do not take any new medication during therapy without consulting prescriber. Use/apply exactly as directed and maintain prescribed cycles or term as prescribed. Routine use of alcohol may increase estrogen level and risk of breast cancer. Annual gynecologic and regular self-breast exams are important. If you have diabetes, monitor glucose levels closely (may impair glucose tolerance). You may experience nausea, vomiting or abdominal pain (small, frequent meals may help); dizziness or mental depression (use caution when driving); rash; hair loss; headache; or breast pain, increased/decreased libido, or enlargement/tenderness of breasts. difficult/painful menstrual cycles. Report unusual swelling of extremities; sudden acute pain in legs or calves, chest, or abdomen; shortness of breath; severe headache or vomiting; sudden blindness; weakness or numbness of arm or leg; unusual vaginal bleeding; yellowing of skin or eyes; unusual bruising or bleeding, or other persistent adverse reactions. You may become intolerant to wearing contact lenses, notify prescriber if this occurs. **Pregnancy/breast-feeding precautions:** Inform prescriber if you are pregnant. Do not get pregnant while taking this medication. Consult prescriber for appropriate contraceptive measures. This medication may cause fetal defects and should not be used during pregnancy. Consult prescriber if breast-feeding.

Transdermal patch: Apply to clean dry skin. Do not apply transdermal patch to breasts. Apply to trunk of body (preferably abdomen). Rotate application sites. Aerosol topical corticosteroids may reduce allergic skin reaction; report persistent skin reaction.

Intravaginal cream: Insert high in vagina. Wash hands and applicator before and after use.

Topical emulsion: Contents of 2 pouches are applied one at time to each thigh and rubbed into thigh and calf. Excess on hands should be applied to buttocks. Wash hands with soap and water after application. Allow skin to dry before covering legs with clothes. Do not apply sunscreen soon after or before applying emulsion. Do not apply to red or irritated skin.

Topical gel: Apply dose to one arm (alternate arms daily) at the same time each day. Spread thinly from waist to shoulder. Allow to dry for 5 minutes prior to dressing. Wash hands with soap and water after application. Do not apply to red or irritated skin. Do not apply to breast.

Vaginal ring: Wash hands thoroughly before removing ring from pouch. In position that is comfortable for insertion (may be lying on your back with knees bent and resting apart), hold ring between thumb and forefinger and press sides together. Insert compressed ring gently into your vagina and push ring toward lower back. If the ring feels uncomfortable you may need to push ring further into vagina. If ring falls out, it may be washed with warm water and reinserted. Ring should be removed and replaced every 3 months.

Geriatric Considerations: Before prescribing estrogen therapy to postmenopausal women, the risks and benefits must be weighed for each patient. Data in women 80 years and older is minimal and it is unclear if reduced risk is applicable to women in this age group. Women should be informed of risks and benefits, as well as possible side effects and the return of menstrual bleeding (when cycled with a progestin), and should be involved in the prescribing options. Oral therapy may be more convenient for vaginal atrophy and urinary incontinence.

Pregnancy Risk Factor: X

Pregnancy Issues: Estrogens are not indicated for use during pregnancy or immediately postpartum. Increased risk of fetal reproductive tract disorders and other birth defects have been observed with diethylstilbestrol (DES); do not use during pregnancy.

Lactation: Enters breast milk/use caution

Breast-Feeding Considerations: The AAP considers ethinyl estradiol, an estrogen derivative, to be "usually compatible" with breast-feeding. Estrogen has been shown to decrease the quantity and quality of human milk; use only if clearly needed; monitor the growth of the infant closely.

Administration

I.M.: Injection for intramuscular administration only.

♦ Estradiol Acetate *see* Estradiol *on page 649*

Estradiol and Norethindrone (es tra DYE ole & nor eth IN drone)

U.S. Brand Names Activella®; CombiPatch®

Synonyms Norethindrone and Estradiol

Pharmacologic Category Estrogen and Progestin Combination

Medication Safety Issues

Transdermal patch may contain conducting metal (eg, aluminum); remove patch prior to MRI.

Use Women with an intact uterus:

Tablet: Treatment of moderate-to-severe vasomotor symptoms associated with menopause; treatment of vulvar and vaginal atrophy; prophylaxis for postmenopausal osteoporosis

Transdermal patch: Treatment of moderate-to-severe vasomotor symptoms associated with menopause; treatment of vulvar and vaginal atrophy; treatment of hypoestrogenism due to hypogonadism, castration, or primary ovarian failure

Pharmacodynamics/Kinetics

Activella®:

Bioavailability: Estradiol: 50%; Norethindrone: 100%

Half-life elimination: Estradiol: 12-14 hours; Norethindrone: 8-11 hours

Time to peak: Estradiol: 5-8 hours

See individual agents.

Contraindications Hypersensitivity to estrogens, progestins, or any components; carcinoma of the breast; estrogen-dependent tumor; undiagnosed abnormal vaginal bleeding; history of or current thrombophlebitis or venous thromboembolic disorders (including DVT, PE); active or recent (within 1 year) arterial thromboembolic disease (eg, stroke, MI); hysterectomy; hepatic dysfunction or disease; pregnancy

Warnings/Precautions

Cardiovascular-related considerations: Estrogens with or without progestin should not be used to prevent coronary heart disease. Use caution with cardiovascular disease or dysfunction. May increase the risks of hypertension, myocardial infarction (MI), stroke, pulmonary emboli (PE), and deep vein thrombosis; incidence of these effects was shown to be significantly increased in postmenopausal women using conjugated equine estrogens (CEE) in combination with medroxyprogesterone acetate (MPA). Nonfatal MI, PE, and thrombophlebitis have also been reported in males taking high doses of CEE (eg, for prostate cancer). Estrogen compounds are generally associated with lipid effects such as increased HDL-cholesterol and decreased LDL-cholesterol. Triglycerides may also be increased; use with caution in patients with familial defects of lipoprotein metabolism. Whenever possible, combination hormonal contraceptives should be discontinued at least 4 weeks prior to and for 2 weeks following elective surgery associated with an increased risk of thromboembolism or during periods of prolonged immobilization.

Neurological considerations: The risk of dementia may be increased in postmenopausal women; increased incidence was observed in women ≥65 years of age taking CEE in combination with MPA.

Cancer-related considerations: Unopposed estrogens may increase the risk of endometrial carcinoma in postmenopausal women. Estrogens may exacerbate endometriosis. Malignant transformation of residual endometrial implants has been reported post-hysterectomy with estrogen only therapy. Estrogens may

(Continued)

Estradiol and Norethindrone *(Continued)*

increase the risk of breast cancer. An increased risk of invasive breast cancer was observed in postmenopausal women using CEE in combination with MPA; a smaller increase in risk was seen with estrogen therapy alone in observational studies. An increase in abnormal mammograms has also been reported with estrogen and progestin therapy. Estrogen use may lead to severe hypercalcemia in patients with breast cancer and bone metastases; discontinue estrogen if hypercalcemia occurs.

Estrogens may cause retinal vascular thrombosis; discontinue permanently if papilledema or retinal vascular lesions are observed on examination. Use with caution in patients with diseases which may be exacerbated by fluid retention, including asthma, epilepsy, migraine, diabetes or renal dysfunction. Use with caution in patients with a history of severe hypocalcemia, SLE, hepatic hemangiomas, porphyria, endometriosis, and gallbladder disease. Use caution with history of cholestatic jaundice associated with past estrogen use or pregnancy. Safety and efficacy in pediatric patients have not been established.

Before prescribing estrogen therapy to postmenopausal women, the risks and benefits must be weighed for each patient. Women should be informed of these risks and benefits, as well as possible effects of progestin when added to estrogen therapy. Estrogens with or without progestin should be used for shortest duration possible consistent with treatment goals. Conduct periodic risk:benefit assessments.

When used solely for prevention of osteoporosis in women at significant risk, nonestrogen treatment options should be considered. When used solely for the treatment of vulvar and vaginal atrophy, topical vaginal products should be considered.

Transdermal patch may contain conducting metal (eg, aluminum); remove patch prior to MRI.

Drug Interactions

Estradiol: **Substrate** of CYP1A2 (major), 2A6 (minor), 2B6 (minor), 2C8/9 (minor), 2C19 (minor), 2D6 (minor), 2E1 (minor), 3A4 (major); **Inhibits** CYP1A2 (weak); **Induces** CYP3A4 (weak)

Norethindrone: **Substrate** of CYP3A4 (major); **Induces** CYP2C19 (weak)

Also see individual agents.

Nutritional/Herbal/Ethanol Interactions

Ethanol: Avoid ethanol (routine use increases estrogen level and risk of breast cancer). Ethanol may also increase the risk of osteoporosis.

Food: Folic acid absorption may be decreased

Herb/Nutraceutical: St John's wort may decrease estradiol levels. Avoid black cohosh, dong quai (has estrogenic activity). Avoid red clover, saw palmetto, ginseng.

Adverse Reactions Frequency not defined.

Cardiovascular: Altered blood pressure, cardiovascular accident, edema, venous thromboembolism

Central nervous system: Dizziness, fatigue, headache, insomnia, mental depression, migraine, nervousness

Dermatologic: Chloasma, erythema multiforme, erythema nodosum, hemorrhagic eruption, hirsutism, itching, loss of scalp hair, melasma, pruritus, skin rash

Endocrine & metabolic: Breast enlargement, breast tenderness, breast pain, libido (changes in)

Gastrointestinal: Abdominal pain, bloating, changes in appetite, flatulence, gallbladder disease, nausea, pancreatitis, vomiting, weight gain/loss

Genitourinary: Alterations in frequency and flow of menses, changes in cervical secretions, cystitis-like syndrome, increased size of uterine leiomyomata, premenstrual-like syndrome, vaginal candidiasis, vaginitis

Hematologic: Aggravation of porphyria

Hepatic: Cholestatic jaundice

Local: Application site reaction (transdermal patch)

Neuromuscular & skeletal: Arthralgia, back pain, chorea, myalgia, weakness

Ocular: Intolerance to contact lenses, steeping of corneal curvature

Respiratory: Pharyngitis, pulmonary thromboembolism, rhinitis

Miscellaneous: Allergic reactions, carbohydrate intolerance, flu-like syndrome

Dosing

Adults & Elderly:

Hypoestrogenism: Transdermal (patch):

Continuous combined regimen: Apply one patch twice weekly

Continuous sequential regimen: Apply estradiol-only patch for first 14 days of cycle, followed by one CombiPatch® applied twice weekly for the remaining 14 days of a 28-day cycle.

Osteoporosis, prevention in postmenopausal females (Activella®): Oral: 1 tablet daily

Menopause (moderate to severe vasomotor symptoms); vulvar and vaginal atrophy:

Oral (Activella®): 1 tablet daily

Transdermal (patch):

Continuous combined regimen: Apply one patch twice weekly

Continuous sequential regimen: Apply estradiol-only patch for first 14 days of cycle, followed by one CombiPatch® applied twice weekly for the remaining 14 days of a 28-day cycle.

Transdermal patch, combination pack (product-specific dosing for Canadian formulation):

Estalis®: Continuous combined regimen: Apply a new patch twice weekly during a 28-day cycle

Estalis-Sequi®: Continuous sequential regimen: Apply estradiol-only patch (Vivelle®) for first 14 days, followed by one Estalis® patch applied twice weekly during the last 14 days of a 28-day cycle

Note: In women previously receiving oral estrogens, initiate upon reappearance of menopausal symptoms following discontinuation of oral therapy.

Available Dosage Forms [CAN] = Canadian brand name

Combination pack (Estalis-Sequi® [CAN; not available in U.S.]):

140/50:

Transdermal system (Vivelle®): Estradiol 50 mcg per day (4s) [14.5 sq cm; total estradiol 4.33 mg]

Transdermal system (Estalis®): Norethindrone acetate 140 mcg and estradiol 50 mcg per day (4s) [9 sq cm; total norethindrone acetate 2.7 mg, total estradiol 0.62 mg; not available in U.S.]

250/50:

Transdermal system (Vivelle®): Estradiol 50 mcg per day (4s) [14.5 sq cm; total estradiol 4.33 mg]

Transdermal system (Estalis®): Norethindrone acetate 250 mcg and estradiol 50 mcg per day (4s) [16 sq cm; total norethindrone acetate 4.8 mg, total estradiol 0.51 mg; not available in U.S.]

Tablet (Activella®): Estradiol 1 mg and norethindrone acetate 0.5 mg (28s)

Transdermal system:

CombiPatch®:

0.05/0.14: Estradiol 0.05 mg and norethindrone acetate 0.14 mg per day (8s) [9 sq cm]

0.05/0.25: Estradiol 0.05 mg and norethindrone acetate 0.25 mg per day (8s) [16 sq cm]

Estalis® [CAN]:

140/50: Norethindrone acetate 140 mcg and estradiol 50 mcg per day (8s) [9 sq cm; total norethindrone acetate 2.7 mg, total estradiol 0.62 mg; not available in U.S.]

250/50 Norethindrone acetate 250 mcg and estradiol 50 mcg per day (8s) [16 sq cm; total norethindrone acetate 4.8 mg, total estradiol 0.51 mg; not available in U.S.]

Nursing Guidelines

Assessment: Assess potential for interactions with other prescriptions, OTC medications, or herbal products patient may be taking. Assess results of annual gynecological exam (eg, Pap smear, mammogram), therapeutic effectiveness (dependent on rationale for use), and adverse effects (eg, thromboembolism, hypertension, edema, CNS changes) on a regular basis during therapy. **Note:** Before prescribing estrogen therapy to postmenopausal women, the risks and benefits must be weighed for each patient. Women should be informed of these risks and benefits, as well as possible effects of progestin when added to estrogen therapy. Caution patients with diabetes to monitor glucose levels closely (may impair glucose tolerance). Teach patient appropriate administration/use according to formulation, possible side effects, interventions to reduce side effects, adverse symptoms to report, importance of frequent self-breast

(Continued)

Estradiol and Norethindrone *(Continued)*

exams, and need for annual gynecological exam. **Pregnancy risk factor X:** Determine that patient is not pregnant before starting therapy.

Patient Education: Do not take any new medication during therapy without consulting prescriber. Use/apply exactly as directed and maintain prescribed cycles or term as prescribed. Avoid routine use of alcohol (ethanol may increase the risk of breast cancer or osteoporosis). Annual gynecologic and regular self-breast exams are important. If you have diabetes, monitor glucose levels closely (may impair glucose tolerance). You may experience nausea, vomiting or abdominal pain (small frequent meals may help); dizziness or mental depression (use caution when driving); rash; hair loss; headache; or breast pain, increased/decreased libido, or enlargement/tenderness of breasts, difficult/painful menstrual cycles. Report significant swelling of extremities; sudden acute pain in legs or calves, chest, or abdomen; shortness of breath; severe headache or vomiting; sudden blindness; weakness or numbness of arm or leg; unusual vaginal bleeding; yellowing of skin or eyes; unusual bruising or bleeding, or other persistent adverse reactions. You may become intolerant to wearing contact lenses, notify prescriber if this occurs. **Pregnancy/breast-feeding precautions:** Inform prescriber if you are pregnant. Do not get pregnant while taking this medication. This medication may cause fetal defects and should not be used during pregnancy. Consult prescriber if breast-feeding.

Pregnancy Risk Factor: X

Pregnancy Issues: Estrogens/progestins should not be used during pregnancy.

Estrogens: Increased risk of fetal reproductive tract disorders and other birth defects; do not use during pregnancy.

Progestins: Associated with fetal genital abnormalities when used during the 1st trimester; not recommended for use during pregnancy.

Lactation: Enters breast milk/use caution

- **Estradiol Cypionate** *see* Estradiol *on page 649*
- **Estradiol Hemihydrate** *see* Estradiol *on page 649*
- **Estradiol Transdermal** *see* Estradiol *on page 649*
- **Estradiol Valerate** *see* Estradiol *on page 649*
- **Estrasorb™** *see* Estradiol *on page 649*
- **Estring®** *see* Estradiol *on page 649*
- **EstroGel®** *see* Estradiol *on page 649*
- **Estrogenic Substances, Conjugated** *see* Estrogens (Conjugated/Equine) *on page 661*

Estrogens (Conjugated A/Synthetic)

(ES troe jenz, KON joo gate ed, aye, sin THET ik)

U.S. Brand Names Cenestin®

Pharmacologic Category Estrogen Derivative

Medication Safety Issues

Sound-alike/look-alike issues:

Cenestin® may be confused with Senexon®

Use Treatment of moderate to severe vasomotor symptoms of menopause; treatment of vulvar and vaginal atrophy

Mechanism of Action Conjugated A/synthetic estrogens contain a mixture of 9 synthetic estrogen substances, including sodium estrone sulfate, sodium equilin sulfate, sodium 17 alpha-dihydroequilin, sodium 17 alpha-estradiol and sodium 17 beta-dihydroequilin. Estrogens are responsible for the development and maintenance of the female reproductive system and secondary sexual characteristics. Estradiol is the principle intracellular human estrogen and is more potent than estrone and estriol at the receptor level; it is the primary estrogen secreted prior to menopause. Following menopause, estrone and estrone sulfate are more highly produced. Estrogens modulate the pituitary secretion of gonadotropins, luteinizing hormone, and follicle-stimulating hormone through a negative feedback system; estrogen replacement reduces elevated levels of these hormones in postmenopausal women.

Pharmacodynamics/Kinetics

Absorption: Readily absorbed

Protein-binding: Sex hormone-binding globulin (SHBG) and albumin

Metabolism: Hepatic to metabolites

Time to peak: 4-16 hours

Excretion: Urine

Contraindications Hypersensitivity to estrogens or any component of the formulation; undiagnosed abnormal vaginal bleeding; history of or current thrombophlebitis or venous thromboembolic disorders (including DVT, PE); active or recent (within 1 year) arterial thromboembolic disease (eg, stroke, MI); carcinoma of the breast; estrogen-dependent tumor; hepatic dysfunction or disease; pregnancy

Warnings/Precautions

Cardiovascular-related considerations: Estrogens with or without progestin should not be used to prevent coronary heart disease. Use caution with cardiovascular disease or dysfunction. May increase the risks of hypertension, myocardial infarction (MI), stroke, pulmonary emboli (PE), and deep vein thrombosis; incidence of these effects was shown to be significantly increased in postmenopausal women using conjugated equine estrogens (CEE) in combination with medroxyprogesterone acetate (MPA). Nonfatal MI, PE, and thrombophlebitis have also been reported in males taking high doses of CEE (eg, for prostate cancer). Estrogen compounds are generally associated with lipid effects such as increased HDL-cholesterol and decreased LDL-cholesterol. Triglycerides may also be increased; use with caution in patients with familial defects of lipoprotein metabolism. Whenever possible, estrogens should be discontinued at least 4 weeks prior to and for 2 weeks following elective surgery associated with an increased risk of thromboembolism or during periods of prolonged immobilization.

Neurological considerations: The risk of dementia may be increased in postmenopausal women; increased incidence was observed in women ≥65 years of age taking CEE in combination with MPA.

Cancer-related considerations: Unopposed estrogens may increase the risk of endometrial carcinoma in postmenopausal women. Estrogens may exacerbate endometriosis. Malignant transformation of residual endometrial implants has been reported post-hysterectomy with estrogen only therapy. Consider adding a progestin in women with residual endometriosis post-hysterectomy. Estrogens may increase the risk of breast cancer. An increased risk of invasive breast cancer was observed in postmenopausal women using CEE in combination with MPA; a smaller increase in risk was seen with estrogen therapy alone in observational studies. An increase in abnormal mammograms has also been reported with estrogen and progestin therapy. Estrogen use may lead to severe hypercalcemia in patients with breast cancer and bone metastases; discontinue estrogen if hypercalcemia occurs.

Estrogens may cause retinal vascular thrombosis; discontinue permanently if papilledema or retinal vascular lesions are observed on examination. Use with caution in patients with diseases which may be exacerbated by fluid retention, including asthma, epilepsy, migraine, diabetes or renal dysfunction. Use with caution in patients with a history of severe hypocalcemia, SLE, hepatic hemangiomas, porphyria, endometriosis, and gallbladder disease. Use caution with history of cholestatic jaundice associated with past estrogen use or pregnancy. Safety and efficacy in pediatric patients have not been established. Prior to puberty, estrogens may cause premature closure of the epiphyses, premature breast development in girls or gynecomastia in boys. Vaginal bleeding and vaginal cornification may also be induced in girls.

Before prescribing estrogen therapy to postmenopausal women, the risks and benefits must be weighed for each patient. Women should be informed of these risks and benefits, as well as possible effects of progestin when added to estrogen therapy. Estrogens with or without progestin should be used for shortest duration possible consistent with treatment goals. Conduct periodic risk:benefit assessments.

When used solely for prevention of osteoporosis in women at significant risk, nonestrogen treatment options should be considered. When used solely for the treatment of vulvar and vaginal atrophy, topical vaginal products should be considered.

Drug Interactions

Based on estradiol and estrone: **Substrate** of CYP1A2 (major), 2A6 (minor), 2B6 (minor), 2C8/9 (minor), 2C19 (minor), 2D6 (minor), 2E1 (minor), 3A4 (major); **Inhibits** CYP1A2 (weak); **Induces** CYP3A4 (weak)

Anticoagulants: Increase potential for thromboembolic events.

Corticosteroids: Estrogens may enhance the effects of hydrocortisone and prednisone.

CYP1A2 inducers: May decrease the levels/effects of estrogens. Example inducers include aminoglutethimide, carbamazepine, phenobarbital, and rifampin.

(Continued)

Estrogens (Conjugated A/Synthetic) *(Continued)*

CYP3A4 inducers: CYP3A4 inducers may decrease the levels/effects of estrogens. Example inducers include aminoglutethimide, carbamazepine, nafcillin, nevirapine, phenobarbital, phenytoin, and rifamycins.

Nutritional/Herbal/Ethanol Interactions

Ethanol: Avoid ethanol (routine use increases estrogen level and risk of breast cancer).

Food: Grapefruit juice may increase estrogen levels, leading to increased adverse effects.

Herb/Nutraceutical: St John's wort may decrease levels. Avoid black cohosh, dong quai (has estrogenic activity). Avoid red clover, saw palmetto, ginseng (due to potential hormonal effects).

Lab Interactions Pathologist should be advised of estrogen/progesterone therapy when specimens are submitted. Reduced response to metyrapone test observed with conjugated estrogens (equine).

Adverse Reactions Adverse effects associated with estrogen therapy; frequency not defined

Cardiovascular: Edema, hypertension, venous thromboembolism

Central nervous system: Dizziness, headache, mental depression, migraine

Dermatologic: Chloasma, erythema multiforme, erythema nodosum, hemorrhagic eruption, hirsutism, loss of scalp hair, melasma

Endocrine & metabolic: Breast enlargement, breast tenderness, libido (changes in), thyroid-binding globulin increased, total thyroid hormone (T_4) increased, serum triglycerides/phospholipids increased, HDL-cholesterol increased, LDL-cholesterol decreased, impaired glucose tolerance, hypercalcemia

Gastrointestinal: Abdominal cramps, bloating, cholecystitis, cholelithiasis, gallbladder disease, nausea, pancreatitis, vomiting, weight gain/loss

Genitourinary: Alterations in frequency and flow of menses, changes in cervical secretions, endometrial cancer, increased size of uterine leiomyomata, vaginal candidiasis

Hematologic: Aggravation of porphyria, antithrombin III and antifactor Xa decreased, levels of fibrinogen decreased, platelet aggregability and platelet count increased; prothrombin and factors VII, VIII, IX, X increased

Hepatic: Cholestatic jaundice

Neuromuscular & skeletal: Chorea

Ocular: Intolerance to contact lenses, steeping of corneal curvature

Respiratory: Pulmonary thromboembolism

Miscellaneous: Carbohydrate intolerance

Overdosage/Toxicology Symptoms of overdose include nausea and vomiting; withdrawal bleeding may occur in females. Toxicity is unlikely following single exposures of excessive doses, any treatment following emesis and charcoal administration should be supportive and symptomatic.

Dosing

Adults: The lowest dose that will control symptoms should be used. Medication should be discontinued as soon as possible.

Menopause, moderate to severe vasomotor symptoms: Oral: 0.45 mg/day; may be titrated up to 1.25 mg/day; attempts to discontinue medication should be made at 3- to 6-month intervals

Vulvar and vaginal atrophy: Oral: 0.3 mg/day

Elderly: Refer to adult dosing. A higher incidence of stroke and invasive breast cancer were observed in women >75 years in a WHI substudy using conjugated equine estrogen.

Available Dosage Forms Tablet: 0.3 mg, 0.45 mg, 0.625 mg, 0.9 mg, 1.25 mg

Nursing Guidelines

Assessment: Assess potential for interactions with other pharmacological agents or herbal products patient may be taking (eg, increased potential for decreased levels/effects or increased potential for toxicity or thrombolic events). Assess results of annual gynecological exam, therapeutic effectiveness (dependent on rationale for use), need for continued treatment, and adverse effects (eg, thromboembolism, hypertension, edema, CNS changes) on a regular basis during therapy. **Note:** Before prescribing estrogen therapy to postmenopausal women, the risks and benefits must be weighed for each patient. Women should be informed of these risks and benefits, as well as possible effects of progestin when added to estrogen therapy. Estrogens with or without progestin should be used for shortest duration possible consistent with treatment goals and periodic assessment of risk:benefit should be made. Caution patients with diabetes to monitor glucose levels closely (may impair glucose tolerance). Teach patient proper use, possible side effects/appropriate interventions, and adverse symptoms to report. Remind patient about the importance of frequent self-breast exams and the need for annual gynecological exam. **Pregnancy risk factor X:** Determine that patient is not pregnant before starting therapy. Do not give to females of childbearing age unless patient is capable of complying with contraceptive use. Advise patient about contraceptive measures as appropriate.

Monitoring Laboratory Tests: Yearly Papanicolaou smear, mammogram. Adequate diagnostic measures, including endometrial sampling, if indicated, should be performed to rule out malignancy in all cases of undiagnosed abnormal vaginal bleeding.

Patient Education: Do not take any new medication during therapy without consulting prescriber. Take exactly as directed and maintain prescribed cycles or term as prescribed. Routine use of alcohol may increase estrogen level and risk of breast cancer. Annual gynecologic and regular self-breast exams are important. If you have diabetes, monitor glucose levels closely (may impair glucose tolerance). You may experience nausea, vomiting or abdominal pain (small, frequent meals may help); dizziness or mental depression (use caution when driving); rash; hair loss; headache; or breast pain, increased/decreased libido, or enlargement/tenderness of breasts. difficult/painful menstrual cycles. Report significant swelling of extremities; sudden acute pain in legs or calves, chest, or abdomen; shortness of breath; severe headache or vomiting; sudden blindness; weakness or numbness of arm or leg; unusual vaginal bleeding; yellowing of skin or eyes; unusual bruising or bleeding, or other persistent adverse reactions. You may become intolerant to wearing contact lenses, notify prescriber if this occurs. **Pregnancy/breast-feeding precautions:** Inform prescriber if you are pregnant. Do not get pregnant while taking this medication. Consult prescriber for appropriate contraceptive measures. This medication may cause fetal defects and should not be used during pregnancy. Consult prescriber if breast-feeding.

Pregnancy Risk Factor: X

Lactation: Enters breast milk/use caution

Administration

Storage: Store at room temperature of 25°C (77°F).

Estrogens (Conjugated/Equine)

(ES troe jenz KON joo gate ed, EE kwine)

U.S. Brand Names Premarin®

Synonyms CEE; C.E.S.; Estrogenic Substances, Conjugated

Pharmacologic Category Estrogen Derivative

Medication Safety Issues

Sound-alike/look-alike issues:

Premarin® may be confused with Primaxin®, Provera®, Remeron®

Use Treatment of moderate to severe vasomotor symptoms associated with menopause; treatment of vulvar and vaginal atrophy; hypoestrogenism (due to hypogonadism, castration, or primary ovarian failure); prostatic cancer (palliation); breast cancer (palliation); osteoporosis (prophylaxis, postmenopausal women at significant risk only); abnormal uterine bleeding

Unlabeled/Investigational Use Uremic bleeding

Mechanism of Action Conjugated estrogens contain a mixture of estrone sulfate, equilin sulfate, 17 alpha-dihydroequilin, 17 alpha-estradiol and 17 beta-dihydroequilin. Estrogens are responsible for the development and maintenance of the female reproductive system and secondary sexual characteristics. Estradiol is the principle intracellular human estrogen and is more potent than estrone and estriol at the receptor level; it is the primary estrogen secreted prior to menopause. Following menopause, estrone and estrone sulfate are more highly produced. Estrogens modulate the pituitary secretion of gonadotropins, luteinizing hormone, and follicle-stimulating hormone through a negative feedback system; estrogen replacement reduces elevated levels of these hormones in postmenopausal women.

Pharmacodynamics/Kinetics

Absorption: Well absorbed

Metabolism: Hepatic via CYP3A4; estradiol is converted to estrone and estriol; also undergoes enterohepatic recirculation; estrone sulfite is the main metabolite in postmenopausal women

Excretion: Urine (primarily estriol, also as estradiol, estrone, and conjugates

(Continued)

Estrogens (Conjugated/Equine) *(Continued)*

Contraindications Hypersensitivity to estrogens or any component of the formulation; undiagnosed abnormal vaginal bleeding; history of or current thrombophlebitis or venous thromboembolic disorders (including DVT, PE); active or recent (within 1 year) arterial thromboembolic disease (eg, stroke, MI); carcinoma of the breast (except in appropriately selected patients being treated for metastatic disease); estrogen-dependent tumor; hepatic dysfunction or disease; pregnancy

Warnings/Precautions

Cardiovascular-related considerations: Estrogens with or without progestin should not be used to prevent coronary heart disease. Use caution with cardiovascular disease or dysfunction. May increase the risks of hypertension, myocardial infarction (MI), stroke, pulmonary emboli (PE), and deep vein thrombosis; incidence of these effects was shown to be significantly increased in postmenopausal women using conjugated equine estrogens (CEE) in combination with medroxyprogesterone acetate (MPA). Nonfatal MI, PE, and thrombophlebitis have also been reported in males taking high doses of CEE (eg, for prostate cancer). Estrogen compounds are generally associated with lipid effects such as increased HDL-cholesterol and decreased LDL-cholesterol. Triglycerides may also be increased; use with caution in patients with familial defects of lipoprotein metabolism. Whenever possible, estrogens should be discontinued at least 4 weeks prior to and for 2 weeks following elective surgery associated with an increased risk of thromboembolism or during periods of prolonged immobilization.

Neurological considerations: The risk of dementia may be increased in postmenopausal women; increased incidence was observed in women ≥65 years of age taking CEE in combination with MPA.

Cancer-related considerations: Unopposed estrogens may increase the risk of endometrial carcinoma in postmenopausal women. Estrogens may exacerbate endometriosis. Malignant transformation of residual endometrial implants has been reported post-hysterectomy with estrogen only therapy. Consider adding a progestin in women with residual endometriosis post-hysterectomy. Estrogens may increase the risk of breast cancer. An increased risk of invasive breast cancer was observed in postmenopausal women using CEE in combination with MPA; a smaller increase in risk was seen with estrogen therapy alone in observational studies. An increase in abnormal mammograms has also been reported with estrogen and progestin therapy. Estrogen use may lead to severe hypercalcemia in patients with breast cancer and bone metastases; discontinue estrogen if hypercalcemia occurs.

Estrogens may cause retinal vascular thrombosis; discontinue permanently if papilledema or retinal vascular lesions are observed on examination. Use with caution in patients with diseases which may be exacerbated by fluid retention, including asthma, epilepsy, migraine, diabetes or renal dysfunction. Use with caution in patients with a history of severe hypocalcemia, SLE, hepatic hemangiomas, porphyria, endometriosis, and gallbladder disease. Use caution with history of cholestatic jaundice associated with past estrogen use or pregnancy. Safety and efficacy in pediatric patients have not been established. Prior to puberty, estrogens may cause premature closure of the epiphyses, premature breast development in girls or gynecomastia in boys. Vaginal bleeding and vaginal cornification may also be induced in girls.

Before prescribing estrogen therapy to postmenopausal women, the risks and benefits must be weighed for each patient. Women should be informed of these risks and benefits, as well as possible effects of progestin when added to estrogen therapy. Estrogens with or without progestin should be used for shortest duration possible consistent with treatment goals. Conduct periodic risk:benefit assessments.

When used solely for prevention of osteoporosis in women at significant risk, nonestrogen treatment options should be considered. When used solely for the treatment of vulvar and vaginal atrophy, topical vaginal products should be considered. Use caution applying topical products to severely atrophic vaginal mucosa.

Drug Interactions

Based on estradiol and estrone: **Substrate** of CYP1A2 (major), 2A6 (minor), 2B6 (minor), 2C8/9 (minor), 2C19 (minor), 2D6 (minor), 2E1 (minor), 3A4 (major); **Inhibits** CYP1A2 (weak); **Induces** CYP3A4 (weak)

Anticoagulants: Increase potential for thromboembolic events

Corticosteroids: Estrogens may enhance the effects of hydrocortisone and prednisone.

CYP1A2 inducers: May decrease the levels/effects of estrogens. Example inducers include aminoglutethimide, carbamazepine, phenobarbital, and rifampin.

CYP3A4 inducers: CYP3A4 inducers may decrease the levels/effects of estrogens. Example inducers include aminoglutethimide, carbamazepine, nafcillin, nevirapine, phenobarbital, phenytoin, and rifamycins.

Nutritional/Herbal/Ethanol Interactions

Ethanol: Avoid ethanol (routine use increases estrogen level and risk of breast cancer). Ethanol may also increase the risk of osteoporosis.

Food: Folic acid absorption may be decreased.

Herb/Nutraceutical: St John's wort may decrease levels. Avoid black cohosh, dong quai (has estrogenic activity). Avoid red clover, saw palmetto, ginseng (due to potential hormonal effects).

Lab Interactions Increased Prothrombin and factors VII, VIII, IX, X; increased platelet aggregability, thyroid-binding globulin, total thyroid hormone (T_4), serum triglycerides/phospholipids; decreased antithrombin III, serum folate concentration

Adverse Reactions

Note: Percentages reported in postmenopausal women.

>10%:

- Central nervous system: Headache (26% to 32%; placebo 28%)
- Endocrine & metabolic: Breast pain (7% to 12%; placebo 9%)
- Gastrointestinal: Abdominal pain (15% to 17%)
- Genitourinary: Vaginal hemorrhage (2% to 14%)
- Neuromuscular & skeletal: Back pain (13% to 14%)

1% to 10%:

- Central nervous system: Nervousness (2% to 5%)
- Endocrine & metabolic: Leukorrhea (4% to 7%)
- Gastrointestinal: Flatulence (6% to 7%)
- Genitourinary: Vaginitis (5% to 7%), vaginal moniliasis (5% to 6%)
- Neuromuscular & skeletal: Weakness (7% to 8%), leg cramps (3% to 7%)

In addition, the following have been reported with estrogen and/or progestin therapy:

Cardiovascular: Edema, hypertension, MI, stroke, venous thromboembolism

Central nervous system: Dizziness, epilepsy exacerbation, headache, irritability, mental depression, migraine, mood disturbances, nervousness

Dermatologic: Angioedema, chloasma, erythema multiforme, erythema nodosum, hemorrhagic eruption, hirsutism, loss of scalp hair, melasma, pruritus, rash, urticaria

Endocrine & metabolic: Breast cancer, breast enlargement, breast tenderness, libido (changes in), increased thyroid-binding globulin, increased total thyroid hormone (T_4), increased serum triglycerides/phospholipids, increased HDL-cholesterol, decreased LDL-cholesterol, impaired glucose tolerance, hypercalcemia, hypocalcemia

Gastrointestinal: Abdominal cramps, bloating, cholecystitis, cholelithiasis, gallbladder disease, nausea, pancreatitis, vomiting, weight gain/loss

Genitourinary: Alterations in frequency and flow of menses, changes in cervical secretions, endometrial cancer, endometrial hyperplasia, increased size of uterine leiomyomata, vaginal candidiasis

Hematologic: Aggravation of porphyria, decreased antithrombin III and antifactor Xa, increased levels of fibrinogen, increased platelet aggregability and platelet count; increased prothrombin and factors VII, VIII, IX, X

Hepatic: Cholestatic jaundice, hepatic hemangiomas enlarged

Neuromuscular & skeletal: Arthralgias, chorea, leg cramps

Local: Thrombophlebitis

Ocular: Intolerance to contact lenses, retinal vascular thrombosis, steeping of corneal curvature

Respiratory: Asthma exacerbation, pulmonary thromboembolism

Miscellaneous: Anaphylactoid/anaphylactic reactions, carbohydrate intolerance

Overdosage/Toxicology Toxicity is unlikely following single exposures of excessive doses, any treatment following emesis and charcoal administration should be supportive and symptomatic. Effects noted after large doses include headache, nausea, and vomiting. Bleeding may occur in females.

(Continued)

Estrogens (Conjugated/Equine) *(Continued)*

Dosing

Adults:

Breast cancer palliation, metastatic disease in selected patients (male and female): Oral: 10 mg 3 times/day for at least 3 months

Uremic bleeding (unlabeled use): I.V.: 0.6 mg/kg/day for 5 days

Androgen-dependent prostate cancer palliation (males): Oral: 1.25-2.5 mg 3 times/day

Prevention of postmenopausal osteoporosis: Oral: Initial: 0.3 mg/day, cyclically* or daily, depending on medical assessment of patient. Dose may be adjusted based on bone mineral density and clinical response. The lowest effective dose should be used.

Menopause (moderate to severe vasomotor symptoms): Oral: Initial: 0.3 mg/day. May be given cyclically* or daily, depending on medical assessment of patient. The lowest dose that will control symptoms should be used. Medication should be discontinued as soon as possible.

Vulvar and vaginal atrophy: Oral: Initial: 0.3 mg/day. The lowest dose that will control symptoms should be used. May be given cyclically* or daily, depending on medical assessment of patient. Medication should be discontinued as soon as possible.

Vaginal cream: Intravaginal: $^1/_2$ to 2 g/day given cyclically*

Female hypogonadism: Oral: 0.3-0.625 mg/day given cyclically*; dose may be titrated in 6- to 12-month intervals; progestin treatment should be added to maintain bone mineral density once skeletal maturity is achieved.

Female castration, primary ovarian failure: Oral: 1.25 mg/day given cyclically*; adjust according to severity of symptoms and patient response. For maintenance, adjust to the lowest effective dose.

Abnormal uterine bleeding:

Acute/heavy bleeding:

Oral (unlabeled route): 1.25 mg, may repeat every 4 hours for 24 hours, followed by 1.25 mg once daily for 7-10 days

I.M., I.V.: 25 mg, may repeat in 6-12 hours if needed

Note: Treatment should be followed by a low-dose oral contraceptive; medroxyprogesterone acetate along with or following estrogen therapy can also be given

Nonacute/lesser bleeding: Oral (unlabeled route): 1.25 mg once daily for 7-10 days

***Cyclic administration:** Either 3 weeks on, 1 week off **or** 25 days on, 5 days off

Elderly: Refer to adult dosing. A higher incidence of stroke and breast cancer was observed in women >75 years in a WHI substudy.

Pediatrics: Adolescents: Refer to adult dosing.

Hepatic Impairment:

Mild to moderate liver impairment: Dosage reduction of estrogens is recommended.

Severe liver impairment: **Not recommended.**

Available Dosage Forms

Cream, vaginal: 0.625 mg/g (42.5 g)

Injection, powder for reconstitution: 25 mg [contains lactose 200 mg; diluent contains benzyl alcohol]

Tablet: 0.3 mg, 0.45 mg, 0.625 mg, 0.9 mg, 1.25 mg

Nursing Guidelines

Assessment: Assess potential for interactions with other pharmacological agents or herbal products patient may be taking (eg, increased potential for decreased levels/effects or increased potential for toxicity or thrombolic events). Assess results of annual gynecological exam, therapeutic effectiveness (dependent on rationale for use), need for continued therapy, and adverse effects (eg, thromboembolism, hypertension, edema, CNS changes) on a regular basis during therapy. **Note:** Before prescribing estrogen therapy to postmenopausal women, the risks and benefits must be weighed for each patient. Women should be informed of these risks and benefits, as well as possible effects of progestin when added to estrogen therapy. Estrogens with or without progestin should be used for shortest duration possible consistent with treatment goals and periodic assessment of risk:benefit should be made. Caution patients with diabetes to monitor glucose levels closely (may impair glucose tolerance). Teach patient proper use, possible side effects/appropriate interventions, and adverse symptoms to report. Remind patient about the importance of frequent self-breast exams and the need for annual gynecological exam. **Pregnancy risk factor X:** Determine that patient is not pregnant before starting therapy. Do not give to females of childbearing age unless patient is capable of complying with contraceptive use. Advise patient about appropriate contraceptive measures as appropriate.

Monitoring Laboratory Tests: Yearly physical examination that includes blood pressure and Papanicolaou smear. Adequate diagnostic measures, including endometrial sampling, if indicated, should be performed to rule out malignancy in all cases of undiagnosed abnormal vaginal bleeding.

Dietary Considerations: Ensure adequate calcium and vitamin D intake when used for the prevention of osteoporosis. Powder for reconstitution for injection (25 mg) contains lactose 200 mg.

Patient Education: Do not take any new medication during therapy without consulting prescriber. Use/apply exactly as directed and maintain prescribed cycles or term as prescribed. Routine use of alcohol may increase estrogen level and risk of breast cancer. Annual gynecologic exams and regular self-breast exams are important. If you have diabetes, monitor glucose levels closely (may impair glucose tolerance). You may experience nausea, vomiting or abdominal pain (small, frequent meals may help); dizziness or mental depression (use caution when driving); rash; hair loss; headache; or breast pain, increased/decreased libido, enlargement/tenderness of breasts; difficult/painful menstrual cycles. Report significant swelling of extremities; sudden acute pain in legs or calves, chest, or abdomen; shortness of breath; severe headache or vomiting; sudden blindness; weakness or numbness of arm or leg; unusual vaginal bleeding; yellowing of skin or eyes; unusual bruising or bleeding, or other persistent adverse reactions. You may become intolerant to wearing contact lenses, notify prescriber if this occurs. **Pregnancy/breast-feeding precautions:** Inform prescriber if you are pregnant. Do not get pregnant while taking this medication. Consult prescriber for appropriate contraceptive measures. This medication may cause fetal defects and should not be used during pregnancy. Consult prescriber if breast-feeding.

Geriatric Considerations: Before prescribing estrogen therapy to postmenopausal women, the risks and benefits must be weighed for each patient. Data in women 80 years and older is minimal and it is unclear if reduced risk is applicable to women in this age group. Women should be informed of risks and benefits, as well as possible side effects and the return of menstrual bleeding (when cycled with a progestin), and should be involved in prescribing options. Oral therapy may be more convenient for vaginal atrophy and urinary incontinence.

Pregnancy Risk Factor: X

Pregnancy Issues: Increased risk of fetal reproductive tract disorders and other birth defects; do not use during pregnancy.

Lactation: Enters breast milk/use caution

Breast-Feeding Considerations: The AAP considers ethinyl estradiol, an estrogen derivative, to be "usually compatible" with breast-feeding. Estrogen has been shown to decrease the quantity and quality of human milk. Use only if clearly needed. Monitor the growth of the infant closely.

Administration

Oral: Give at bedtime to minimize adverse effects.

I.M.: May be administered intramuscularly.

I.V.: Administer I.V. doses slowly to avoid a flushing reaction.

Reconstitution: Injection: Reconstitute using provided diluent; do not shake violently.

Compatibility: Stable in D_5W and NS

Compatibility when admixed: Incompatible with ascorbic acid

Storage:

Injection: Refrigerate at 2°C to 8°C (36°F to 46°F) prior to reconstitution. Following reconstitution, solution may be stored under refrigeration for up to 60 days. Do not use if darkening or precipitation occurs.

Tablets, vaginal cream: Store at room temperature (25°C).

Estrogens (Conjugated/Equine) and Medroxyprogesterone

(ES troe jenz KON joo gate ed/EE kwine & me DROKS ee proe JES te rone)

U.S. Brand Names Premphase®; Prempro™

Synonyms Medroxyprogesterone and Estrogens (Conjugated); MPA and Estrogens (Conjugated)

(Continued)

Estrogens (Conjugated/Equine) and Medroxyprogesterone *(Continued)*

Pharmacologic Category Estrogen and Progestin Combination

Medication Safety Issues

Sound-alike/look-alike issues:

Premphase® may be confused with Prempro™

Prempro™ may be confused with Premphase®

Use Women with an intact uterus: Treatment of moderate to severe vasomotor symptoms associated with menopause; treatment of atrophic vaginitis; osteoporosis (prophylaxis)

Mechanism of Action

Conjugated estrogens contain a mixture of estrone sulfate, equilin sulfate, 17 alpha-dihydroequilin, 17 alpha-estradiol, and 17 beta-dihydroequilin. Estrogens are responsible for the development and maintenance of the female reproductive system and secondary sexual characteristics. Estradiol is the principle intracellular human estrogen and is more potent than estrone and estriol at the receptor level; it is the primary estrogen secreted prior to menopause. Following menopause, estrone and estrone sulfate are more highly produced. Estrogens modulate the pituitary secretion of gonadotropins, luteinizing hormone, and follicle-stimulating hormone through a negative feedback system; estrogen replacement reduces elevated levels of these hormones in postmenopausal women.

MPA inhibits gonadotropin production which then prevents follicular maturation and ovulation. In women with adequate estrogen, MPA transforms a proliferative endometrium into a secretory endometrium; when administered with conjugated estrogens, reduces the incidence of endometrial hyperplasia and risk of adenocarcinoma.

Pharmacodynamics/Kinetics See individual agents.

Contraindications Hypersensitivity to conjugated estrogens, medroxyprogesterone (MPA), or any component of the formulation; undiagnosed abnormal vaginal bleeding; history of or current thrombophlebitis or venous thromboembolic disorders (including DVT, PE); active or recent (within 1 year) arterial thromboembolic disease (eg, stroke, MI); carcinoma of the breast; estrogen-dependent tumor; hepatic dysfunction or disease; pregnancy

Warnings/Precautions

Cardiovascular-related considerations: Estrogens with or without progestin should not be used to prevent coronary heart disease. Use caution with cardiovascular disease or dysfunction. May increase the risks of hypertension, myocardial infarction (MI), stroke, pulmonary emboli (PE), and deep vein thrombosis; incidence of these effects was shown to be significantly increased in postmenopausal women using conjugated equine estrogens (CEE) in combination with medroxyprogesterone acetate (MPA). Nonfatal MI, PE, and thrombophlebitis have also been reported in males taking high doses of CEE (eg, for prostate cancer). Estrogen compounds are generally associated with lipid effects such as increased HDL-cholesterol and decreased LDL-cholesterol. Triglycerides may also be increased; use with caution in patients with familial defects of lipoprotein metabolism. Whenever possible, combination hormonal contraceptives should be discontinued at least 4 weeks prior to and for 2 weeks following elective surgery associated with an increased risk of thromboembolism or during periods of prolonged immobilization.

Neurological considerations: The risk of dementia may be increased in postmenopausal women; increased incidence was observed in women ≥65 years of age taking CEE in combination with MPA.

Cancer-related considerations: Unopposed estrogens may increase the risk of endometrial carcinoma in postmenopausal women. Estrogens may exacerbate endometriosis. Malignant transformation of residual endometrial implants has been reported post-hysterectomy with estrogen only therapy. Estrogens may increase the risk of breast cancer. An increased risk of invasive breast cancer was observed in postmenopausal women using CEE in combination with MPA; a smaller increase in risk was seen with estrogen therapy alone in observational studies. An increase in abnormal mammograms has also been reported with estrogen and progestin therapy. Estrogen use may lead to severe hypercalcemia in patients with breast cancer and bone metastases; discontinue estrogen if hypercalcemia occurs.

Estrogens may cause retinal vascular thrombosis; discontinue permanently if papilledema or retinal vascular lesions are observed on examination. Use with caution in patients with diseases which may be exacerbated by fluid retention, including asthma, epilepsy, migraine, diabetes or renal dysfunction. Use with caution in patients with a history of severe hypocalcemia, SLE, hepatic hemangiomas, porphyria, endometriosis, and gallbladder disease. Use caution with history of cholestatic jaundice associated with past estrogen use or pregnancy. Safety and efficacy in pediatric patients have not been established. Prior to puberty, estrogens may cause premature closure of the epiphyses, premature breast development in girls or gynecomastia in boys. Vaginal bleeding and vaginal cornification may also be induced in girls.

Before prescribing estrogen therapy to postmenopausal women, the risks and benefits must be weighed for each patient. Women should be informed of these risks and benefits, as well as possible effects of progestin when added to estrogen therapy. Estrogens with or without progestin should be used for shortest duration possible consistent with treatment goals. Conduct periodic risk:benefit assessments.

When used solely for prevention of osteoporosis in women at significant risk, nonestrogen treatment options should be considered. When used solely for the treatment of vulvar and vaginal atrophy, topical vaginal products should be considered.

Drug Interactions

Based on estradiol and estrone: **Substrate** of CYP1A2 (major), 2A6 (minor), 2B6 (minor), 2C8/9 (minor), 2C19 (minor), 2D6 (minor), 2E1 (minor), 3A4 (major); **Inhibits** CYP1A2 (weak); **Induces** CYP3A4 (weak)

Medroxyprogesterone: **Substrate** of CYP3A4 (major); **Induces** CYP3A4 (weak)

See individual agents.

Nutritional/Herbal/Ethanol Interactions

Ethanol: Avoid ethanol (routine use increases estrogen level and risk of breast cancer). Ethanol may also increase the risk of osteoporosis.

Food: Folic acid absorption may be decreased.

Herb/Nutraceutical: St John's wort may decrease levels. Avoid black cohosh, dong quai (has estrogenic activity). Avoid red clover, saw palmetto, ginseng (due to potential hormonal effects).

Lab Interactions Accelerated PT, partial thromboplastin time, and platelet aggregation time; increased platelet count; increased HDL; increased factors II, VII antigen, VIII coagulant activity, IX, X, XII, XII-X complex, II-VII-X complex, and beta-thromboglobulin; increased levels of fibrinogen and fibrinogen activity; increased plasminogen antigen and activity; increased thyroid-binding globulin; increased triglycerides; impaired glucose tolerance; reduced response to metyrapone test; reduced serum folate concentration; other binding proteins may be elevated; decreased LDL; decreased levels of antifactor Xa and antithrombin III; decreased antithrombin III activity

Adverse Reactions

>10%:

Central nervous system: Headache (28% to 37%), pain (11% to 13%), depression (6% to 11%)

Endocrine & metabolic: Breast pain (32% to 38%), dysmenorrhea (8% to 13%)

Gastrointestinal: Abdominal pain (16% to 23%), nausea (9% to 11%)

Neuromuscular & skeletal: Back pain (13% to 16%)

Respiratory: Pharyngitis (11% to 13%)

Miscellaneous: Infection (16% to 18%), flu-like syndrome (10% to 13%)

1% to 10%:

Cardiovascular: Peripheral edema (3% to 4%)

Central nervous system: Dizziness (3% to 5%)

Dermatologic: Pruritus (5% to 10%), rash (4% to 6%)

Endocrine & metabolic: Leukorrhea (5% to 9%)

Gastrointestinal: Flatulence (8% to 9%), diarrhea (5% to 6%), dyspepsia (5% to 6%)

Genitourinary: Vaginitis (5% to 7%), cervical changes (4% to 5%), vaginal hemorrhage (1% to 3%)

Neuromuscular & skeletal: Weakness (6% to 10%), arthralgia (7% to 9%), leg cramps (3% to 5%), hypertonia (3% to 4%)

Respiratory: Sinusitis (7% to 8%), rhinitis (6% to 8%)

Additional adverse effects reported with conjugated estrogens and/or progestins (limited): Abnormal vaginal bleeding, amenorrhea, anaphylactoid reactions, anaphylaxis, breast enlargement/tenderness, cerebral embolism/thrombosis,

(Continued)

Estrogens (Conjugated/Equine) and Medroxyprogesterone *(Continued)*

cholecystitis, cholelithiasis, cholestatic jaundice, chorea, coagulation factor changes, contact lens intolerance, decreased carbohydrate tolerance, endometrial hyperplasia, erythema multiforme, erythema nodosum, HDL-cholesterol increased, hirsutism, hypertension, increase in size of uterine leiomyomata, gallbladder disease, libido changes, LDL-cholesterol decreased, migraine, optic neuritis, pancreatitis, pulmonary embolism, retinal thrombosis, thrombophlebitis, triglycerides increased, urticaria

Overdosage/Toxicology Effects noted after large doses include nausea, vomiting; withdrawal bleeding may occur in females. Treatment should be supportive and symptomatic.

Dosing

Adults:

Treatment of moderate to severe vasomotor symptoms associated with menopause or treatment of atrophic vaginitis in females with an intact uterus: (Note: The lowest dose that will control symptoms should be used; medication should be discontinued as soon as possible): Oral:

Premphase®: One maroon conjugated estrogen 0.625 mg tablet daily on days 1 through 14 and one light blue conjugated estrogen 0.625 mg/MPA 5 mg tablet daily on days 15 through 28; re-evaluate patients at 3- and 6-month intervals to determine if treatment is still necessary; monitor patients for signs of endometrial cancer; rule out malignancy if unexplained vaginal bleeding occurs

Prempro™: One conjugated estrogen 0.3 mg/MPA 1.5 mg tablet daily; re-evaluate at 3-and 6-month intervals to determine if therapy is still needed; dose may be increased to a maximum of one conjugated estrogen 0.625 mg/MPA 5 mg tablet daily in patients with bleeding or spotting, once malignancy has been ruled out

Osteoporosis prophylaxis in females with an intact uterus: Oral:

Premphase®: One maroon conjugated estrogen 0.625 tablet daily on days 1 through 14 and one light blue conjugated estrogen 0.625 mg/MPA 5 mg tablet daily on days 15 through 28; monitor patients for signs of endometrial cancer; rule out malignancy if unexplained vaginal bleeding occurs

Prempro™: One conjugated estrogen 0.3 mg/MPA 1.5 mg tablet daily; dose may be increased to one conjugated estrogen 0.625 mg/MPA 5 mg tablet daily; in patients with bleeding or spotting, once malignancy has been ruled out

Elderly: Refer to adult dosing. A higher incidence of stroke and breast cancer was observed in women >75 years in a WHI substudy.

Available Dosage Forms Tablet:

Premphase® [therapy pack contains 2 separate tablet formulations]: Conjugated estrogens 0.625 mg [14 maroon tablets] and conjugated estrogen 0.625 mg/medroxyprogesterone acetate 5 mg [14 light blue tablets] (28s)

Prempro™:

0.3/1.5: Conjugated estrogens 0.3 mg and medroxyprogesterone acetate 1.5 mg (28s)

0.45/1.5: Conjugated estrogens 0.45 mg and medroxyprogesterone acetate 1.5 mg (28s)

0.625/2.5: Conjugated estrogens 0.625 mg and medroxyprogesterone acetate 2.5 mg (28s)

0.625/5: Conjugated estrogens 0.625 mg and medroxyprogesterone acetate 5 mg (28s)

Nursing Guidelines

Assessment: Assess potential for interactions with other prescriptions, OTC medications, or herbal products patient may be taking. Assess results of annual gynecological exam (eg, Pap smear and mammogram), therapeutic effectiveness (dependent on rationale for use), and adverse effects (eg, thromboembolism, hypertension, edema, CNS changes) on a regular basis during therapy. **Note:** Before prescribing estrogen therapy to postmenopausal women, the risks and benefits must be weighed for each patient. Women should be informed of these risks and benefits, as well as possible effects of progestin when added to estrogen therapy. Caution patients with diabetes to monitor glucose levels closely (may impair glucose tolerance). Teach patient appropriate administration/use according to formulation, possible side effects, interventions to reduce side effects, adverse symptoms to report, importance of frequent self-breast exams, and need for annual gynecological exam. **Pregnancy risk factor X:** Determine that patient is not pregnant before starting therapy.

Monitoring Laboratory Tests: Serum cholesterol, HDL, LDL triglycerides

Dietary Considerations: Administration with food decreases nausea, administer with food. Ensure adequate calcium and vitamin D intake when used for the prevention of osteoporosis.

Patient Education: Do not take any new medication during therapy without consulting prescriber. Take exactly as directed and maintain prescribed cycles or term as prescribed. Avoid routine use of alcohol (ethanol may increase the risk of breast cancer or osteoporosis). Annual gynecologic and regular self-breast exams are important. If you have diabetes, monitor glucose levels closely (may impair glucose tolerance). You may experience nausea, vomiting or abdominal pain (small frequent meals may help); dizziness or mental depression (use caution when driving); rash; hair loss; headache; or breast pain, increased/decreased libido, or enlargement/tenderness of breasts, difficult/painful menstrual cycles. Report significant swelling of extremities; sudden acute pain in legs or calves, chest, or abdomen; shortness of breath; severe headache or vomiting; sudden blindness; weakness or numbness of arm or leg; unusual vaginal bleeding; yellowing of skin or eyes; unusual bruising or bleeding, or other persistent adverse reactions. You may become intolerant to wearing contact lenses, notify prescriber if this occurs. **Pregnancy/breast-feeding precautions:** Inform prescriber if you are pregnant. Do not get pregnant while taking this medication. This medication may cause fetal defects and should not be used during pregnancy.

Pregnancy Risk Factor: X

Pregnancy Issues:

Estrogens: Increased risk of fetal reproductive tract disorders and other birth defects; do not use during pregnancy.

Progestins: Associated with fetal genital abnormalities when used during the 1st trimester; not recommended for use during pregnancy.

Lactation:

Estrogens: Enters breast milk/use caution

Progestins: Enters breast milk/use caution

Breast-Feeding Considerations: The AAP considers ethinyl estradiol, an estrogen derivative, to be "usually compatible" with breast-feeding. Estrogen has been shown to decrease the quantity and quality of human milk. Monitor the growth of the infant closely. The AAP considers medroxyprogesterone to be "usually compatible" with breast-feeding.

Administration

Storage: Store at room temperature 20°C to 25°C (68°F to 77°F).

Estrogens (Esterified) (ES troe jenz, es TER i fied)

U.S. Brand Names Menest®

Synonyms Esterified Estrogens

Pharmacologic Category Estrogen Derivative

Medication Safety Issues

Sound-alike/look-alike issues:

Estratab® may be confused with Estratest®, Estratest® H.S.

Use Treatment of moderate to severe vasomotor symptoms associated with menopause; treatment of vulvar and vaginal atrophy; hypoestrogenism (due to hypogonadism, castration, or primary ovarian failure); prostatic cancer (palliation); breast cancer (palliation); osteoporosis (prophylaxis, in women at significant risk only)

Mechanism of Action Esterified estrogens contain a mixture of estrogenic substances; the principle component is estrone. Preparations contain 75% to 85% sodium estrone sulfate and 6% to 15% sodium equilin sulfate such that the total is not <90%. Estrogens are responsible for the development and maintenance of the female reproductive system and secondary sexual characteristics. Estradiol is the principle intracellular human estrogen and is more potent than estrone and estriol at the receptor level; it is the primary estrogen secreted prior to menopause. In males and following menopause in females, estrone and estrone sulfate are more highly produced. Estrogens modulate the pituitary secretion of gonadotropins, luteinizing hormone, and follicle-stimulating hormone through a negative feedback system; estrogen replacement reduces elevated levels of these hormones.

Pharmacodynamics/Kinetics

Absorption: Readily

(Continued)

Estrogens (Esterified) *(Continued)*

Metabolism: Rapidly hepatic to estrone sulfate, conjugated and unconjugated metabolites; first-pass effect

Excretion: Urine (as unchanged drug and as glucuronide and sulfate conjugates)

Contraindications Hypersensitivity to estrogens or any component of the formulation; undiagnosed abnormal vaginal bleeding; history of or current thrombophlebitis or venous thromboembolic disorders (including DVT, PE); active or recent (within 1 year) arterial thromboembolic disease (eg, stroke, MI); carcinoma of the breast, except in appropriately selected patients being treated for metastatic disease; estrogen-dependent tumor; hepatic dysfunction or disease; pregnancy

Warnings/Precautions

Cardiovascular-related considerations: Estrogens with or without progestin should not be used to prevent coronary heart disease. Use caution with cardiovascular disease or dysfunction. May increase the risks of hypertension, myocardial infarction (MI), stroke, pulmonary emboli (PE), and deep vein thrombosis; incidence of these effects was shown to be significantly increased in postmenopausal women using conjugated equine estrogens (CEE) in combination with medroxyprogesterone acetate (MPA). Nonfatal MI, PE, and thrombophlebitis have also been reported in males taking high doses of CEE (eg, for prostate cancer). Estrogen compounds are generally associated with lipid effects such as increased HDL-cholesterol and decreased LDL-cholesterol. Triglycerides may also be increased; use with caution in patients with familial defects of lipoprotein metabolism. Whenever possible, estrogens should be discontinued at least 4 weeks prior to and for 2 weeks following elective surgery associated with an increased risk of thromboembolism or during periods of prolonged immobilization.

Neurological considerations: The risk of dementia may be increased in postmenopausal women; increased incidence was observed in women ≥65 years of age taking CEE in combination with MPA.

Cancer-related considerations: Unopposed estrogens may increase the risk of endometrial carcinoma in postmenopausal women. Estrogens may exacerbate endometriosis. Malignant transformation of residual endometrial implants has been reported post-hysterectomy with estrogen only therapy. Consider adding a progestin in women with residual endometriosis post-hysterectomy. Estrogens may increase the risk of breast cancer. An increased risk of invasive breast cancer was observed in postmenopausal women using CEE in combination with MPA; a smaller increase in risk was seen with estrogen therapy alone in observational studies. An increase in abnormal mammograms has also been reported with estrogen and progestin therapy. Estrogen use may lead to severe hypercalcemia in patients with breast cancer and bone metastases; discontinue estrogen if hypercalcemia occurs.

Estrogens may cause retinal vascular thrombosis; discontinue permanently if papilledema or retinal vascular lesions are observed on examination. Use with caution in patients with diseases which may be exacerbated by fluid retention, including asthma, epilepsy, migraine, diabetes or renal dysfunction. Use with caution in patients with a history of severe hypocalcemia, SLE, hepatic hemangiomas, porphyria, endometriosis, and gallbladder disease. Use caution with history of cholestatic jaundice associated with past estrogen use or pregnancy. Safety and efficacy in pediatric patients have not been established. Prior to puberty, estrogens may cause premature closure of the epiphyses, premature breast development in girls or gynecomastia in boys. Vaginal bleeding and vaginal cornification may also be induced in girls.

Before prescribing estrogen therapy to postmenopausal women, the risks and benefits must be weighed for each patient. Women should be informed of these risks and benefits, as well as possible effects of progestin when added to estrogen therapy. Estrogens with or without progestin should be used for shortest duration possible consistent with treatment goals. Conduct periodic risk:benefit assessments.

When used solely for prevention of osteoporosis in women at significant risk, nonestrogen treatment options should be considered. When used solely for the treatment of vulvar and vaginal atrophy, topical vaginal products should be considered.

Drug Interactions Based on estrone: **Substrate** of CYP1A2 (major), 2B6 (minor), 2C8/9 (minor), 2E1 (minor), 3A4 (major)

Anticoagulants: Increases potential for thromboembolic events with anticoagulants

Corticosteroids: Estrogens may enhance the effects of hydrocortisone and prednisone.

CYP1A2 inducers: May decrease the levels/effects of estrogens. Example inducers include aminoglutethimide, carbamazepine, phenobarbital, and rifampin.

CYP3A4 inducers: CYP3A4 inducers may decrease the levels/effects of estrogens. Example inducers include aminoglutethimide, carbamazepine, nafcillin, nevirapine, phenobarbital, phenytoin, and rifamycins.

Nutritional/Herbal/Ethanol Interactions

Ethanol: Avoid ethanol (routine use increases estrogen level and risk of breast cancer). Ethanol may also increase the risk of osteoporosis.

Food: Folic acid absorption may be decreased.

Herb/Nutraceutical: St John's wort may decrease levels. Avoid black cohosh, dong quai (has estrogenic activity). Avoid red clover, saw palmetto, ginseng (due to potential hormonal effects).

Lab Interactions Endocrine function test may be altered; increased prothrombin and factors VII, VIII, IX, X; increased platelet aggregability, thyroid-binding globulin, total thyroid hormone (T_4), serum triglycerides/phospholipids; decreased antithrombin III, serum folate concentration

Adverse Reactions

Cardiovascular: Edema, hypertension, venous thromboembolism

Central nervous system: Dizziness, headache, mental depression, migraine

Dermatologic: Chloasma, erythema multiforme, erythema nodosum, hemorrhagic eruption, hirsutism, loss of scalp hair, melasma

Endocrine & metabolic: Breast enlargement, breast tenderness, libido (changes in), increased thyroid-binding globulin, increased total thyroid hormone (T_4), increased serum triglycerides/phospholipids, increased HDL-cholesterol, decreased LDL-cholesterol, impaired glucose tolerance, hypercalcemia

Gastrointestinal: Abdominal cramps, bloating, cholecystitis, cholelithiasis, gallbladder disease, nausea, pancreatitis, vomiting, weight gain/loss

Genitourinary: Alterations in frequency and flow of menses, changes in cervical secretions, endometrial cancer, increased size of uterine leiomyomata, vaginal candidiasis

Hematologic: Aggravation of porphyria, decreased antithrombin III and antifactor Xa, increased levels of fibrinogen, increased platelet aggregability and platelet count; increased prothrombin and factors VII, VIII, IX, X

Hepatic: Cholestatic jaundice

Neuromuscular & skeletal: Chorea

Ocular: Intolerance to contact lenses, steeping of corneal curvature

Respiratory: Pulmonary thromboembolism

Miscellaneous: Carbohydrate intolerance

Overdosage/Toxicology Toxicity is unlikely following single exposures of excessive doses, any treatment following emesis and charcoal administration should be supportive and symptomatic. Effects noted after large doses include headache, nausea, and vomiting. Bleeding may occur in females.

Dosing

Adults:

Prostate cancer (palliation): Oral: 1.25-2.5 mg 3 times/day

Female hypogonadism: Oral: 2.5-7.5 mg of estrogen daily for 20 days followed by a 10-day rest period. Administer cyclically (3 weeks on and 1 week off). If bleeding does not occur by the end of the 10-day period, repeat the same dosing schedule; the number of courses dependent upon the responsiveness of the endometrium. If bleeding occurs before the end of the 10-day period, begin an estrogen-progestin cyclic regimen of 2.5-7.5 mg esterified estrogens daily for 20 days. During the last 5 days of estrogen therapy, give an oral progestin. If bleeding occurs before regimen is concluded, discontinue therapy and resume on the fifth day of bleeding.

Menopause, moderate to severe vasomotor symptoms: Oral: 1.25 mg/day administered cyclically (3 weeks on and 1 week off). If patient has not menstruated within the last 2 months or more, cyclic administration is started arbitrary. If the patient is menstruating, cyclical administration is started on day 5 of the bleeding. For short-term use only and should be discontinued as soon as possible. Re-evaluate at 3- to 6-month intervals for tapering or discontinuation of therapy.

Atopic vaginitis and kraurosis vulvae: Oral: 0.3 to ≥1.25 mg/day, depending on the tissue response of the individual patient. Administer cyclically. For short-term use only and should be discontinued as soon as possible.

(Continued)

Estrogens (Esterified) *(Continued)*

Re-evaluate at 3- to 6-month intervals for tapering or discontinuation of therapy.

Breast cancer (palliation): Oral: 10 mg 3 times/day for at least 3 months

Osteoporosis in postmenopausal women: Oral: Initial: 0.3 mg/day and increase to a maximum daily dose of 1.25 mg/day; initiate therapy as soon as possible after menopause; cyclically or daily, depending on medical assessment of patient. Monitor patients with an intact uterus for signs of endometrial cancer; rule out malignancy if unexplained vaginal bleeding occurs

Female castration and primary ovarian failure: Oral: 1.25 mg/day, cyclically. Adjust dosage upward or downward, according to the severity of symptoms and patient response. For maintenance, adjust dosage to lowest level that will provide effective control.

Elderly: Refer to adult dosing. A higher incidence of stroke and invasive breast cancer were observed in women >75 years in a WHI substudy using conjugated equine estrogen.

Hepatic Impairment:

Mild to moderate liver impairment: Dosage reduction of estrogens is recommended.

Severe liver impairment: **Not recommended.**

Available Dosage Forms Tablet: 0.3 mg, 0.625 mg, 1.25 mg, 2.5 mg

Nursing Guidelines

Assessment: Assess potential for interactions with other pharmacological agents or herbal products patient may be taking (eg, increased potential for decreased levels/effects or increased potential for toxicity or thrombolic events). Assess results of annual gynecological exam, therapeutic effectiveness (dependent on rationale for use), need for continued treatment, and adverse effects (eg, thromboembolism, hypertension, edema, CNS changes) on a regular basis during therapy. **Note:** Before prescribing estrogen therapy to postmenopausal women, the risks and benefits must be weighed for each patient. Women should be informed of these risks and benefits, as well as possible effects of progestin when added to estrogen therapy. Estrogens with or without progestin should be used for shortest duration possible consistent with treatment goals and periodic assessment of risk:benefit should be made. Caution patients with diabetes to monitor glucose levels closely (may impair glucose tolerance). Teach patient proper use, possible side effects/appropriate interventions, and adverse symptoms to report. Remind patient about the importance of frequent self-breast exams and the need for annual gynecological exam. **Pregnancy risk factor X:** Determine that patient is not pregnant before starting therapy. Do not give to females of childbearing age unless patient is capable of complying with contraceptive use. Advise patient about contraceptive measures as appropriate.

Monitoring Laboratory Tests: Yearly Papanicolaou smear, mammogram. Adequate diagnostic measures, including endometrial sampling, if indicated, should be performed to rule out malignancy in all cases of undiagnosed abnormal vaginal bleeding.

Dietary Considerations: Should be taken with food at same time each day. Ensure adequate calcium and vitamin D intake when used for the prevention of osteoporosis.

Patient Education: Do not take any new medication during therapy without consulting prescriber. Take exactly as directed and maintain prescribed cycles or term as prescribed. Routine use of alcohol may increase estrogen level and risk of breast cancer. Annual gynecologic and regular self-breast exams are important. If you have diabetes, monitor glucose levels closely (may impair glucose tolerance). You may experience nausea, vomiting or abdominal pain (small, frequent meals may help); dizziness or mental depression (use caution when driving); rash; hair loss; headache; or breast pain, increased/decreased libido, or enlargement/tenderness of breasts. difficult/painful menstrual cycles. Report significant swelling of extremities; sudden acute pain in legs or calves, chest, or abdomen; shortness of breath; severe headache or vomiting; sudden blindness; weakness or numbness of arm or leg; unusual vaginal bleeding; yellowing of skin or eyes; unusual bruising or bleeding, or other persistent adverse reactions. You may become intolerant to wearing contact lenses, notify prescriber if this occurs. **Pregnancy/breast-feeding precautions:** Inform prescriber if you are pregnant. Do not get pregnant while taking this medication. Consult prescriber for appropriate contraceptive measures. This medication may cause fetal defects and should not be used during pregnancy. Consult prescriber if breast-feeding.

Pregnancy Risk Factor: X

Pregnancy Issues: Increased risk of fetal reproductive tract disorders and other birth defects; do not use during pregnancy.

Lactation: Enters breast milk/use caution

Breast-Feeding Considerations: The AAP considers ethinyl estradiol, an estrogen derivative, to be "usually compatible" with breast-feeding. Estrogen has been shown to decrease the quantity and quality of human milk; use only if clearly needed; monitor the growth of the infant closely.

Administration

Storage: Store below 30°C (86°F); protect from moisture

Etanercept (et a NER sept)

U.S. Brand Names Enbrel®

Pharmacologic Category Antirheumatic, Disease Modifying; Tumor Necrosis Factor (TNF) Blocking Agent

Use Treatment of moderately- to severely-active rheumatoid arthritis, moderately- to severely-active polyarticular juvenile arthritis (in patients with inadequate response to at least one disease-modifying antirheumatic drug), psoriatic arthritis, active ankylosing spondylitis (AS); moderate-to-severe chronic plaque psoriasis

Mechanism of Action Etanercept is a recombinant DNA-derived protein composed of tumor necrosis factor receptor (TNFR) linked to the Fc portion of human IgG1. Etanercept binds tumor necrosis factor (TNF) and blocks its interaction with cell surface receptors. TNF plays an important role in the inflammatory processes and the resulting joint pathology of rheumatoid arthritis (RA), polyarticular-course juvenile arthritis (JRA), ankylosing spondylitis (AS), and plaque psoriasis.

Pharmacodynamics/Kinetics

Onset of action: ~2-3 weeks

Half-life elimination: 115 hours (range: 98-300 hours)

Time to peak: 72 hours (range: 48-96 hours)

Excretion: Clearance: Children: 45.9 mL/hour/m^2; Adults: 89 mL/hour (52 mL/hour/m^2)

Contraindications Hypersensitivity to etanercept or any component of the formulation; patients with sepsis (mortality may be increased); active infections (including chronic or local infection)

Warnings/Precautions Etanercept may affect defenses against infections and malignancies. Safety and efficacy in patients with immunosuppression or chronic infections have not been evaluated. Rare cases of tuberculosis have been reported. Rare reactivation of hepatitis B has occurred in chronic virus carriers; evaluate prior to initiation and during treatment. Discontinue administration if patient develops a serious infection. Do not start drug in patients with an active infection. Use caution in patients predisposed to infection, such as poorly-controlled diabetes.

Impact on the development and course of malignancies is not fully defined. As compared to the general population, an increased risk of lymphoma has been noted in clinical trials; however, rheumatoid arthritis has been previously associated with an increased rate of lymphoma. Etanercept is not recommended for use in patients with Wegener's granulomatosis who are receiving immunosuppressive therapy. Treatment may result in the formation of autoimmune antibodies; cases of autoimmune disease have not been described. Non-neutralizing antibodies to etanercept may also be formed. Rarely, a reversible lupus-like syndrome has occurred. The safety of etanercept has not been studied in children <4 years of age.

Use caution in patients with pre-existing or recent-onset demyelinating CNS disorders (rare cases described in postmarketing experience). Use caution in patients with CHF; has been associated with worsening and new-onset CHF. Use caution in patients with a history of significant hematologic abnormalities; has been associated with pancytopenia and aplastic anemia (rare cases in postmarketing experience). Patients must be advised to seek medical attention if they develop signs and symptoms suggestive of blood dyscrasias. Discontinue if significant hematologic abnormalities are confirmed.

Allergic reactions may occur (<2%), but anaphylaxis has not been observed. If an anaphylactic reaction or other serious allergic reaction occurs, administration of etanercept should be discontinued immediately and appropriate therapy initiated.

(Continued)

Etanercept *(Continued)*

Patients should be brought up to date with all immunizations before initiating therapy. Live vaccines should not be given concurrently. No data are available concerning secondary transmission of live vaccines in patients receiving etanercept. Patients with a significant exposure to varicella virus should temporarily discontinue etanercept. Treatment with varicella zoster immune globulin should be considered.

Drug Interactions Specific drug interaction studies have not been conducted with etanercept.

Anakinra: An increased rate of serious infections has been noted with concurrent therapy, without additional improvement in American College of Rheumatology (ACR) response criteria.

Cyclophosphamide: May increase the risk of noncutaneous solid malignancy when used with etanercept. Concurrent therapy is not recommended.

Vaccines: Live vaccines should not be given during therapy.

Adverse Reactions

>10%:

Central nervous system: Headache (17%)

Local: Injection site reaction (14% to 37%)

Respiratory: Respiratory tract infection (upper, 29%, other than upper 38%), rhinitis (12%)

Miscellaneous: Infection (35%), positive ANA (11%), positive antidouble-stranded DNA antibodies (15% by RIA, 3% by *Crithidia luciliae* assay)

≥3% to 10%:

Central nervous system: Dizziness (7%)

Dermatologic: Rash (5%)

Gastrointestinal: Abdominal pain (5%), dyspepsia (4%), nausea (9%), vomiting (3%)

Neuromuscular & skeletal: Weakness (5%)

Respiratory: Pharyngitis (7%), respiratory disorder (5%), sinusitis (3%), cough (6%)

<3% (Limited to important or life-threatening): Allergic reactions, alopecia, angioedema, aplastic anemia, appendicitis, bursitis, cerebral ischemia, chest pain, cholecystitis, CHF, coagulopathy, deep vein thrombosis; demyelinating CNS disorders (suggestive of multiple sclerosis, transverse myelitis, or optic neuritis); depression, fever, flushing, flu syndrome, gastrointestinal hemorrhage, heart failure, hyper-/hypotension, infection (serious), intestinal perforation, leukopenia, lupus-like syndrome, lymphadenopathy, malignancies (including lymphoma), membranous glomerulopathy, MI, mouth ulcer, multiple sclerosis, myocardial ischemia, neutropenia, optic neuritis, pancreatitis, pancytopenia, paresthesia, polymyositis, pruritus, pulmonary disease, pulmonary embolism, renal calculus, sarcoidosis, seizure, stroke, thrombocytopenia, thrombophlebitis, transaminases increased, tuberculosis, urticaria, vasculitis (cutaneous), weight gain

Pediatric patients (JRA): The percentages of patients reporting abdominal pain (17%) and vomiting (13%) were higher than in adult RA. Two patients developed varicella infection associated with aseptic meningitis which resolved without complications (see Warnings/Precautions).

Overdosage/Toxicology No dose-limiting toxicities have been observed during clinical trials. Single I.V. doses up to 60 mg/m^2 have been administered to healthy volunteers in an endotoxemia study without evidence of dose-limiting toxicities.

Dosing

Adults:

Rheumatoid arthritis, psoriatic arthritis, ankylosing spondylitis: SubQ:

Once-weekly dosing: 50 mg once weekly

Twice-weekly dosing: 25 mg given twice weekly (individual doses should be separated by 72-96 hours)

Note: If the physician determines that it is appropriate, patients may self-inject after proper training in injection technique.

Elderly: SubQ: Although greater sensitivity of some elderly patients cannot be ruled out, no overall differences in safety or effectiveness were observed.

Pediatrics:

Juvenile rheumatoid arthritis: Children 4-17 years: SubQ:

Once-weekly dosing: 0.8 mg/kg (maximum: 50 mg/dose) once weekly

Twice-weekly dosing: 0.4 mg/kg (maximum: 25 mg/dose) twice weekly (individual doses should be separated by 72-96 hours)

Available Dosage Forms

Injection, powder for reconstitution: 25 mg [diluent contains benzyl alcohol; packaging may contain dry natural rubber (latex)]

Injection, solution: 50 mg/mL (0.98 mL) [prefilled syringe with 27-gauge ½ inch needle]

Nursing Guidelines

Assessment: Monitor for signs and symptoms of infection. Assess for liver dysfunction. Monitor effectiveness of therapy (eg, pain, range of motion, mobility, ADL function, inflammation). Assess knowledge/teach patient appropriate administration (injection technique and needle disposal if self-administered), possible side effects/interventions, and adverse symptoms to report.

Patient Education: If self-injecting, follow instructions for injection and disposal of needles exactly. If redness, swelling, or irritation appears at the injection site, contact prescriber. Do not have any vaccinations while using this medication without consulting prescriber first. You may experience headache or dizziness (use caution when driving or engaging in tasks requiring alertness until response to drug is known). If stomach pain or cramping; unusual bleeding or bruising; persistent fever; paleness; blood in vomitus, stool, or urine occurs, stop medication and contact prescriber **immediately**. Also immediately report skin rash, unusual muscle or bone weakness, or signs of respiratory flu or other infection (eg, chills, fever, sore throat, easy bruising or bleeding, mouth sores, unhealed sores). **Breast-feeding precaution:** Breast-feeding is not recommended.

Pregnancy Risk Factor: B

Lactation: Excretion in breast milk unknown/not recommended

Breast-Feeding Considerations: It is not known whether etanercept is excreted in human milk or absorbed systemically after ingestion. Because many immunoglobulins are excreted in human milk, and because of the potential for serious adverse reactions in nursing infants from Enbrel®, a decision should be made whether to discontinue nursing or to discontinue the drug.

Administration

Reconstitution: Reconstitute aseptically with 1 mL sterile bacteriostatic water for injection, USP (supplied). Do not filter reconstituted solution during preparation or administration. **Note:** The needle cover of the diluent syringe may contain dry natural rubber (latex), which should not be handled by persons sensitive to this substance. Swirl to mix; do not shake or vigorously agitate.

Storage: The prefilled syringe or dose tray containing etanercept (sterile powder) must be refrigerated at 2°C to 8°C (36°F to 46°F). Do not freeze. Reconstituted solutions of etanercept should be administered as soon as possible after reconstitution. If not administered immediately after reconstitution, etanercept may be stored in the vial at 2°C to 8°C (36°F to 46°F) for up to 14 days.

♦ Ethanoic Acid *see* Acetic Acid *on page 78*

♦ Ethanol *see* Alcohol (Ethyl) *on page 100*

♦ Ethinyl Estradiol and Cyproterone Acetate *see* Cyproterone and Ethinyl Estradiol *on page 474*

Ethinyl Estradiol and Desogestrel

(ETH in il es tra DYE ole & des oh JES trel)

U.S. Brand Names Apri®; Cesia™; Cyclessa®; Desogen®; Kariva™; Mircette®; Ortho-Cept®; Reclipsen™; Solia™; Velivet™

Synonyms Desogestrel and Ethinyl Estradiol; Ortho Cept

Pharmacologic Category Contraceptive; Estrogen and Progestin Combination

Medication Safety Issues

Sound-alike/look-alike issues:

Ortho-Cept® may be confused with Ortho-Cyclen®

Use Prevention of pregnancy

Unlabeled/Investigational Use Treatment of hypermenorrhea (menorrhagia); pain associated with endometriosis; dysmenorrhea; dysfunctional uterine bleeding

Mechanism of Action Combination hormonal contraceptives inhibit ovulation via a negative feedback mechanism on the hypothalamus, which alters the normal pattern of gonadotropin secretion of a follicle-stimulating hormone (FSH) and luteinizing hormone by the anterior pituitary. The follicular phase FSH and midcycle surge of gonadotropins are inhibited. In addition, combination hormonal (Continued)

Ethinyl Estradiol and Desogestrel *(Continued)*

contraceptives produce alterations in the genital tract, including changes in the cervical mucus, rendering it unfavorable for sperm penetration even if ovulation occurs. Changes in the endometrium may also occur, producing an unfavorable environment for nidation. Combination hormonal contraceptive drugs may alter the tubal transport of the ova through the fallopian tubes. Progestational agents may also alter sperm fertility.

Pharmacodynamics/Kinetics

Desogestrel:

Absorption: Rapid and complete

Protein binding: Etonogestrel (active metabolite): 98%, primarily to sex hormone-binding globulin

Metabolism: Hepatic via CYP2C9 to active metabolite etonogestrel (3-keto-desogestrel); etonogestrel metabolized via CYP3A4

Half-life elimination: 37.1 hours

Excretion: Urine and feces (as metabolites)

Contraindications Hypersensitivity to ethinyl estradiol, etonogestrel, desogestrel, or any component of the formulation; history of or current thrombophlebitis or venous thromboembolic disorders (including DVT, PE); active or recent (within 1 year) arterial thromboembolic disease (eg, stroke, MI); cerebral vascular disease, coronary artery disease, valvular heart disease with complications, severe hypertension; diabetes mellitus with vascular involvement; severe headache with focal neurological symptoms; known or suspected breast carcinoma, endometrial cancer, estrogen-dependent neoplasms, undiagnosed abnormal genital bleeding; hepatic dysfunction or tumor, cholestatic jaundice of pregnancy, jaundice with prior combination hormonal contraceptive use; major surgery with prolonged immobilization; heavy smoking (≥15 cigarettes/day) in patients >35 years of age; pregnancy

Warnings/Precautions Combination hormonal contraceptives do not protect against HIV infection or other sexually-transmitted diseases. The risk of cardiovascular side effects increases in women who smoke cigarettes, especially those who are >35 years of age; women who use combination hormonal contraceptives should be strongly advised not to smoke. Combination hormonal contraceptives may lead to increased risk of myocardial infarction, use with caution in patients with risk factors for coronary artery disease. May increase the risk of thromboembolism. Whenever possible, combination hormonal contraceptives should be discontinued at least 4 weeks prior to and for 2 weeks following elective surgery associated with an increased risk of thromboembolism or during periods of prolonged immobilization. Combination hormonal contraceptives may have a dose-related risk of vascular disease, hypertension, and gallbladder disease. Women with hypertension or renal disease should be encouraged to use another form of contraception. The use of combination hormonal contraceptives has been associated with a slight increase in frequency of breast cancer, however, studies are not consistent. Combination hormonal contraceptives may cause glucose intolerance. Retinal thrombosis has been reported (rarely). Use caution in conditions that may be aggravated by fluid retention, depression, or history of migraine. Not for use prior to menarche.

The minimum dosage combination of estrogen/progestin that will effectively treat the individual patient should be used. New patients should be started on products containing ≤0.035 mg of estrogen per tablet.

Drug Interactions

Ethinyl estradiol: **Substrate** of CYP2C8/9 (minor), 3A4 (major), 3A5-7 (minor); **Inhibits** CYP1A2 (weak), 2B6 (weak), 2C19 (weak), 3A4 (weak)

Desogestrel: **Substrate** of CYP2C19 (major)

Acetaminophen: May increase plasma concentration of synthetic estrogens, possibly by inhibiting conjugation. Combination hormonal contraceptives may also decrease the plasma concentration of acetaminophen.

Acitretin: Interferes with the contraceptive effect of microdosed progestin-containing "minipill" preparations. The effect on other progestational contraceptives (eg, implants, injectables) is unknown.

Aminoglutethimide: May increase CYP metabolism of progestins leading to possible decrease in contraceptive effectiveness. Use of a nonhormonal contraceptive product is recommended.

Antibiotics (ampicillin, tetracycline): Pregnancy has been reported following concomitant use, however, pharmacokinetic studies have not shown consistent effects with these antibiotics on plasma concentrations of synthetic steroids. Use of a nonhormonal contraceptive product is recommended.

Anticoagulants: Combination hormonal contraceptives may increase or decrease the effects of coumarin derivatives. Combination hormonal contraceptives may also increase risk of thromboembolic disorders

Anticonvulsants (carbamazepine, felbamate, phenobarbital, phenytoin, topiramate): Increase the metabolism of ethinyl estradiol and/or some progestins, leading to possible decrease in contraceptive effectiveness. Use of a nonhormonal contraceptive product is recommended.

Ascorbic acid: Doses of ascorbic acid (vitamin C) 1 g/day have been reported to increase plasma concentration of synthetic estrogens by ~47%, possibly by inhibiting conjugation; clinical implications are unclear.

Atorvastatin: Atorvastatin increases the AUC for norethindrone and ethinyl estradiol.

Benzodiazepines: Combination hormonal contraceptives may decrease the clearance of some benzodiazepines (alprazolam, chlordiazepoxide, diazepam) and increase the clearance of others (lorazepam, oxazepam, temazepam)

Clofibric acid: Combination hormonal contraceptives may increase the clearance of clofibric acid.

Cyclosporine: Combination hormonal contraceptives may inhibit the metabolism of cyclosporine, leading to increased plasma concentrations; monitor cyclosporine.

CYP2C19 inducers: May decrease the levels/effects of desogestrel. Example inducers include aminoglutethimide, carbamazepine, phenytoin, and rifampin.

CYP3A4 inducers: CYP3A4 inducers may decrease the levels/effects of ethinyl estradiol. Example inducers include aminoglutethimide, carbamazepine, nafcillin, nevirapine, phenobarbital, phenytoin, and rifamycins.

Griseofulvin: Griseofulvin may induce the metabolism of combination hormonal contraceptives causing menstrual changes; pregnancies have been reported. Use of barrier form of contraception is suggested while on griseofulvin therapy.

Morphine: Combination hormonal contraceptives may increase the clearance of morphine.

Non-nucleoside reverse transcriptase inhibitors (NNRTIs): Nevirapine may decrease plasma levels of combination hormonal contraceptives; use of a nonhormonal contraceptive product is recommended. No data for delavirdine; incomplete data for efavirenz.

Prednisolone: Ethinyl estradiol may inhibit the metabolism of prednisolone, leading to increased plasma concentrations.

Protease inhibitors: Amprenavir, lopinavir, nelfinavir, and ritonavir have been shown to decrease plasma levels of combination hormonal contraceptives; use of a nonhormonal contraceptive product is recommended. Indinavir has been shown to increase plasma levels of combination hormonal contraceptives. No data for saquinavir.

Repaglinide: Increased level of ethinyl estradiol when combined with levonorgestrel.

Rifampin: Rifampin increases the metabolism of ethinyl estradiol and some progestins (norethindrone) resulting in decreased contraceptive effectiveness and increased menstrual irregularities. Use of a nonhormonal contraceptive product is recommended.

Salicylic acid: Combination hormonal contraceptives may increase the clearance of salicylic acid.

Selegiline: Combination hormonal contraceptives may increase the serum concentration of selegiline.

Theophylline: Ethinyl estradiol may inhibit the metabolism of theophylline, leading to increased plasma concentrations.

Tricyclic antidepressants (amitriptyline, imipramine, nortriptyline): Metabolism may be inhibited by combination hormonal contraceptives, increasing plasma levels of antidepressant; use caution.

Troglitazone: Troglitazone decreases the serum concentration of ethinyl estradiol and norethindrone by ~30%, leading to possible reduction in contraceptive effectiveness.

Nutritional/Herbal/Ethanol Interactions

Food: CNS effects of caffeine may be enhanced if combination hormonal contraceptives are used concurrently with caffeine. Grapefruit juice increases ethinyl estradiol concentrations and would be expected to increase progesterone serum levels as well; clinical implications are unclear.

Herb/Nutraceutical: St John's wort may decrease the effectiveness of combination hormonal contraceptives by inducing hepatic enzymes. Avoid dong quai and black cohosh (have estrogen activity). Avoid saw palmetto, red clover, ginseng.

(Continued)

Ethinyl Estradiol and Desogestrel *(Continued)*

Lab Interactions Increased platelet aggregation, thyroid-binding globulin, total thyroid hormone (T_4), serum triglycerides/phospholipids; decreased antithrombin III, serum folate concentration

Adverse Reactions Frequency not defined.

Cardiovascular: Arterial thromboembolism, cerebral hemorrhage, cerebral thrombosis, edema, hypertension, mesenteric thrombosis, MI

Central nervous system: Depression, dizziness, headache, migraine, nervousness, premenstrual syndrome, stroke

Dermatologic: Acne, erythema multiforme, erythema nodosum, hirsutism, loss of scalp hair, melasma (may persist), rash (allergic)

Endocrine & metabolic: Amenorrhea, breakthrough bleeding, breast enlargement, breast secretion, breast tenderness, carbohydrate intolerance, lactation decreased (postpartum), glucose tolerance decreased, libido changes, menstrual flow changes, sex hormone-binding globulins (SHBG) increased, spotting, temporary infertility (following discontinuation), thyroid-binding globulin increased, triglycerides increased

Gastrointestinal: Abdominal cramps, appetite changes, bloating, cholestasis, colitis, gallbladder disease, jaundice, nausea, vomiting, weight gain/loss

Genitourinary: Cervical erosion changes, cervical secretion changes, cystitis-like syndrome, vaginal candidiasis, vaginitis

Hematologic: Antithrombin III decreased, folate levels decreased, hemolytic uremic syndrome, norepinephrine induced platelet aggregability increased, porphyria, prothrombin increased; factors VII, VIII, IX, and X increased

Hepatic: Benign liver tumors, Budd-Chiari syndrome, cholestatic jaundice, hepatic adenomas

Local: Thrombophlebitis

Ocular: Cataracts, change in corneal curvature (steepening), contact lens intolerance, optic neuritis, retinal thrombosis

Renal: Impaired renal function

Respiratory: Pulmonary thromboembolism

Miscellaneous: Hemorrhagic eruption

Overdosage/Toxicology Toxicity is unlikely following single exposures of excessive doses. May cause withdrawal bleeding in females. Any treatment following emesis and charcoal administration should be supportive and symptomatic.

Dosing

Adults: Female: Contraception: Oral:

Schedule 1 (Sunday starter): Dose begins on first Sunday after onset of menstruation; if the menstrual period starts on Sunday, take first tablet that very same day. **With a Sunday start, an additional method of contraception should be used until after the first 7 days of consecutive administration.**

For 21-tablet package: Dosage is 1 tablet daily for 21 consecutive days, followed by 7 days off of the medication; a new course begins on the 8th day after the last tablet is taken.

For 28-tablet package: Dosage is 1 tablet daily without interruption.

Schedule 2 (Day 1 starter): Dose starts on first day of menstrual cycle taking 1 tablet daily.

For 21-tablet package: Dosage is 1 tablet daily for 21 consecutive days, followed by 7 days off of the medication; a new course begins on the 8th day after the last tablet is taken.

For 28-tablet package: Dosage is 1 tablet daily without interruption.

If all doses have been taken on schedule and one menstrual period is missed, continue dosing cycle. If two consecutive menstrual periods are missed, pregnancy test is required before new dosing cycle is started.

Missed doses **monophasic formulations** (refer to package insert for complete information):

One dose missed: Take as soon as remembered or take 2 tablets next day

Two consecutive doses missed in the first 2 weeks: Take 2 tablets as soon as remembered or 2 tablets next 2 days. **An additional method of contraception should be used for 7 days after missed dose.**

Two consecutive doses missed in week 3 or three consecutive doses missed at any time: Schedule 1 (Sunday starter): Continue to take 1 tablet daily until Sunday, then discard the rest of the pack, and a new pack is started that same day. Schedule 2 (Day 1 starter): Current pack should be discarded, and a new pack started that same day. **An additional method of contraception should be used for 7 days after missed dose.**

Missed doses **biphasic/triphasic formulations** (refer to package insert for complete information):

One dose missed: Take as soon as remembered or take 2 tablets next day.

Two consecutive doses missed in week 1 or week 2 of the pack: Take 2 tablets as soon as remembered and 2 tablets the next day. Resume taking 1 tablet daily until the pack is empty. **An additional method of contraception should be used for 7 days after a missed dose.**

Two consecutive doses missed in week 3 of the pack; **an additional method of contraception must be used for 7 days after a missed dose**:

Schedule 1 (Sunday starter): Take 1 tablet every day until Sunday. Discard the remaining pack and start a new pack of pills on the same day.

Schedule 2 (Day 1 starter): Discard the remaining pack and start a new pack the same day.

Three or more consecutive doses missed; **an additional method of contraception must be used for 7 days after a missed dose**:

Schedule 1 (Sunday starter): Take 1 tablet every day until Sunday; on Sunday, discard the pack and start a new pack.

Schedule 2 (Day 1 starter): Discard the remaining pack and begin new pack of tablets starting on the same day.

Pediatrics: Female: Contraception: Oral: See adult dosing; not to be used prior to menarche.

Renal Impairment: Specific guidelines not available; use with caution and monitor blood pressure closely. Consider other forms of contraception.

Hepatic Impairment: Contraindicated in patients with hepatic impairment.

Available Dosage Forms

Tablet, low-dose formulations:

Kariva™:

Day 1-21: Ethinyl estradiol 0.02 mg and desogestrel 0.15 mg [21 white tablets]

Day 22-23: 2 inactive light green tablets

Day 24-28: Ethinyl estradiol 0.01 mg [5 light blue tablets] (28s)

Mircette®:

Day 1-21: Ethinyl estradiol 0.02 mg and desogestrel 0.15 mg [21 white tablets]

Day 22-23: 2 inactive green tablets

Day 24-28: Ethinyl estradiol 0.01 mg [5 yellow tablets] (28s)

Tablet, monophasic formulations:

Apri® 28: Ethinyl estradiol 0.03 mg and desogestrel 0.15 mg [21 rose tablets and 7 white inactive tablets] (28s)

Desogen®, Reclipsen™, Solia™: Ethinyl estradiol 0.03 mg and desogestrel 0.15 mg [21 white tablets and 7 green inactive tablets] (28s)

Ortho-Cept® 28: Ethinyl estradiol 0.03 mg and desogestrel 0.15 mg [21 orange tablets and 7 green inactive tablets] (28s)

Tablet, triphasic formulations:

Cesia™, Cyclessa®:

Day 1-7:Ethinyl estradiol 0.025 mg and desogestrel 0.1 mg [7 light yellow tablets]

Day 8-14: Ethinyl estradiol 0.025 mg and desogestrel 0.125 mg [7 orange tablets]

Day 14-21: Ethinyl estradiol 0.025 mg and desogestrel 0.15 mg [7 red tablets]

Day 21-28: 7 green inactive tablets (28s)

Velivet™:

Day 1-7: Ethinyl estradiol 0.025 mg and desogestrel 0.1 mg [7 beige tablets]

Day 8-14: Ethinyl estradiol 0.025 mg and desogestrel 0.125 mg [7 orange tablets]

Day 14-21: Ethinyl estradiol 0.025 mg and desogestrel 0.15 mg [7 pink tablets]

Day 21-28: 7 white inactive tablets (28s)

Nursing Guidelines

Assessment: Monitor blood pressure on a regular basis. Assess for adverse reactions and potential drug interactions. Assess knowledge/teach importance of regular (monthly) blood pressure checks and annual physical assessment, Pap smear, and vision assessment. Teach importance of maintaining prescribed schedule of dosing. **Pregnancy risk factor X:** Do not use if patient is pregnant.

(Continued)

Ethinyl Estradiol and Desogestrel *(Continued)*

Dietary Considerations: Should be taken at same time each day.

Patient Education: Oral contraceptives do not protect against HIV infection or other sexually-transmitted diseases. Take exactly as directed by prescriber (see package insert). You are at risk of becoming pregnant if doses are missed. Detailed and complete information on dosing and missed doses can be found in the package insert. Be aware that some medications may reduce the effectiveness of oral contraceptives; an alternate form of contraception may be needed. Check all medicines (prescription and over-the-counter), herbal and alternative products with prescriber. It is important that you check your blood pressure monthly (same day each month) and that you have an annual physical assessment, Pap smear, and vision exam while taking this medication. Avoid smoking while taking this medication; smoking increases risk of adverse effects, including thromboembolic events and heart attacks. You may experience loss of appetite (small frequent meals will help); or constipation (increased exercise, fluids, fruit, fiber, or stool softeners may help). If you have diabetes, use accurate serum glucose testing to identify any changes in glucose tolerance; notify prescriber of significant changes so antidiabetic medication can be adjusted if necessary. Report immediately pain or muscle soreness; warmth, swelling, pain, or redness in calves; shortness of breath; sudden loss of vision; unresolved leg/foot swelling; change in menstrual pattern (unusual bleeding, amenorrhea, breakthrough spotting); breast tenderness that does not go away; acute abdominal cramping; signs of vaginal infection (drainage, pain, itching); CNS changes (blurred vision, confusion, acute anxiety, or unresolved depression); or significant weight gain (>5 lb/week). Notify prescriber of changes in contact lens tolerance. **Pregnancy/breast-feeding precautions:** This medication should not be used during pregnancy. If you suspect you may become pregnant, contact prescriber immediately.

Pregnancy Risk Factor: X

Pregnancy Issues: Pregnancy should be ruled out prior to treatment and discontinued if pregnancy occurs. In general, the use of combination hormonal contraceptives when inadvertently taken early in pregnancy have not been associated with teratogenic effects. Due to increased risk of thromboembolism postpartum, combination hormonal contraceptives should not be started earlier than 4-6 weeks following delivery.

Lactation: Enters breast milk/not recommended (AAP rates "compatible")

Breast-Feeding Considerations: Jaundice and breast enlargement in the nursing infant have been reported following the use of combination hormonal contraceptives. May decrease the quality and quantity of breast milk; a nonhormonal form of contraception is recommended.

Administration

Oral: Administer at the same time each day.

Storage: Store at controlled room temperature of 25°C (77°F).

Ethinyl Estradiol and Drospirenone

(ETH in il es tra DYE ole & droh SPYE re none)

U.S. Brand Names Yasmin®

Synonyms Drospirenone and Ethinyl Estradiol

Pharmacologic Category Contraceptive; Estrogen and Progestin Combination

Use Prevention of pregnancy

Unlabeled/Investigational Use Treatment of hypermenorrhea (menorrhagia); pain associated with endometriosis; dysmenorrhea; dysfunctional uterine bleeding

Mechanism of Action Combination oral contraceptives inhibit ovulation via a negative feedback mechanism on the hypothalamus, which alters the normal pattern of gonadotropin secretion of a follicle-stimulating hormone (FSH) and luteinizing hormone by the anterior pituitary. The follicular phase FSH and midcycle surge of gonadotropins are inhibited. In addition, oral contraceptives produce alterations in the genital tract, including changes in the cervical mucus, rendering it unfavorable for sperm penetration even if ovulation occurs. Changes in the endometrium may also occur, producing an unfavorable environment for nidation. Oral contraceptive drugs may alter the tubal transport of the ova through the fallopian tubes. Progestational agents may also alter sperm fertility. Drospirenone is a spironolactone analogue with antimineralocorticoid and antiandrogenic activity.

Pharmacodynamics/Kinetics

Drospirenone:

Distribution: 4 L/kg

Protein binding: Serum proteins (excluding sex hormone-binding globulin and corticosteroid binding globulin): 97%

Metabolism: To inactive metabolites; minor metabolism hepatically via CYP3A4

Bioavailability: 76%

Half-life elimination: 30 hours

Time to peak: 1-3 hours

Excretion: Urine and feces

Contraindications Hypersensitivity to ethinyl estradiol, drospirenone, or to any component of the formulation; history of or current thrombophlebitis or venous thromboembolic disorders (including DVT, PE); active or recent (within 1 year) arterial thromboembolic disease (eg, stroke, MI); cerebral vascular disease, coronary artery disease, severe hypertension; diabetes with vascular involvement; headache with focal neurological symptoms; known or suspected breast carcinoma, endometrial cancer, estrogen-dependent neoplasms, undiagnosed abnormal genital bleeding; renal insufficiency, hepatic dysfunction or tumor, adrenal insufficiency, cholestatic jaundice of pregnancy, jaundice with prior oral contraceptive use; heavy smoking (≥15 cigarettes/day) in patients >35 years of age; pregnancy

Warnings/Precautions Oral contraceptives do not protect against HIV infection or other sexually-transmitted diseases. The risk of cardiovascular side effects increases in women who smoke cigarettes, especially those who are >35 years of age; women who use oral contraceptives should be strongly advised not to smoke. Oral contraceptives may lead to increased risk of myocardial infarction, use with caution in patients with risk factors for coronary artery disease. May increase the risk of thromboembolism. Whenever possible, combination hormonal contraceptives should be discontinued at least 4 weeks prior to and for 2 weeks following elective surgery associated with an increased risk of thromboembolism or during periods of prolonged immobilization. Oral contraceptives may have a dose-related risk of vascular disease (decreases HDL), hypertension, and gallbladder disease; a preparation with the lowest effective estrogen/progesterone combination should be used. Women with high blood pressure should be encouraged to use another form of contraception. Oral contraceptives may cause glucose intolerance. Retinal thrombosis has been reported (rarely) with oral contraceptive use. Use with caution in patients with conditions that may be aggravated by fluid retention, depression, or patients with history of migraine. Not for use prior to menarche.

Drospirenone has antimineralocorticoid activity that may lead to hyperkalemia in patients with renal insufficiency, hepatic dysfunction, or adrenal insufficiency. Use caution with medications that may increase serum potassium.

Drug Interactions

Ethinyl estradiol: **Substrate** of CYP2C8/9 (minor), 3A4 (major), 3A5-7 (minor); **Inhibits** CYP1A2 (weak), 2B6 (weak), 2C19 (weak), 3A4 (weak)

Drospirenone: **Substrate** of CYP3A4 (minor); **Inhibits** CYP1A2 (weak), 2C8/9 (weak), 2C19 (weak), 3A4 (weak)

ACE inhibitors: Potential for hyperkalemia with concomitant use; monitor serum potassium during first cycle

Acetaminophen: May increase plasma concentration of synthetic estrogens, possibly by inhibiting conjugation. Oral contraceptives may also decrease the plasma concentration of acetaminophen.

Aldosterone antagonists: Potential for hyperkalemia with concomitant use; monitor serum potassium during first cycle

Aminoglutethimide: May increase CYP metabolism of progestins.

Angiotensin II receptor antagonists: Potential for hyperkalemia with concomitant use; monitor serum potassium during first cycle

Antibiotics (ampicillin, griseofulvin, tetracycline): Pregnancy has been reported following concomitant use, however, pharmacokinetic studies have not shown consistent effects with these antibiotics on plasma concentrations of synthetic steroids.

Anticoagulants: Oral contraceptives may increase or decrease the effects of coumarin derivatives.

Anticonvulsants (carbamazepine, felbamate, phenobarbital, phenytoin, topiramate): Increase the metabolism of ethinyl estradiol and/or some progestins, leading to possible decrease in contraceptive effectiveness.

(Continued)

Ethinyl Estradiol and Drospirenone *(Continued)*

Ascorbic acid: May increase plasma concentration of synthetic estrogens, possibly by inhibiting conjugation.

Atorvastatin: Atorvastatin increases the AUC for norethindrone and ethinyl estradiol.

Cyclosporine: Ethinyl estradiol may inhibit the metabolism of cyclosporine, leading to increased plasma concentrations.

CYP3A4 inducers: May decrease the levels/effects of estrogens. Example inducers include aminoglutethimide, carbamazepine, nafcillin, nevirapine, phenobarbital, phenytoin, and rifamycins.

Clofibric acid: Oral contraceptives may increase the clearance of clofibric acid.

Heparin: Potential for hyperkalemia with concomitant use; monitor serum potassium during first cycle

Morphine: Oral contraceptives may increase the clearance of morphine

NSAIDs: Potential for hyperkalemia with concomitant use when taken daily, long term; monitor serum potassium during first cycle

Phenylbutazone: May decrease contraceptive effectiveness and increase menstrual irregularities.

Potassium-sparing diuretics: Potential for hyperkalemia with concomitant use; monitor serum potassium during first cycle

Prednisolone: Ethinyl estradiol may inhibit the metabolism of prednisolone, leading to increased plasma concentrations.

Rifampin: Rifampin increases the metabolism of ethinyl estradiol and some progestins (norethindrone), resulting in decreased contraceptive effectiveness and increased menstrual irregularities.

Ritonavir: May decrease the serum concentration of estrogens, leading to decreased effectiveness.

Salicylic acid: Oral contraceptives may increase the clearance of salicylic acid.

Selegiline: Oral contraceptives may increase the serum concentration of selegiline.

Temazepam: Oral contraceptives may increase the clearance of temazepam.

Theophylline: Ethinyl estradiol may inhibit the metabolism of theophylline, leading to increased plasma concentrations.

Nutritional/Herbal/Ethanol Interactions

Food: CNS effects of caffeine may be enhanced if oral contraceptives are used concurrently with caffeine. Grapefruit juice increases ethinyl estradiol concentrations; clinical implications are unclear.

Herb/Nutraceutical: St John's wort may decrease the effectiveness of oral contraceptives by inducing hepatic enzymes; may also result in breakthrough bleeding.

Adverse Reactions

>1%:

Central nervous system: Depression, dizziness, emotional lability, headache, migraine, nervousness

Dermatologic: Acne, pruritus, rash

Endocrine & metabolic: Amenorrhea, dysmenorrhea, intermenstrual bleeding, menstrual irregularities

Gastrointestinal: Abdominal pain, diarrhea, gastroenteritis, nausea, vomiting

Genitourinary: Cystitis, leukorrhea, vaginal moniliasis, vaginitis

Neuromuscular & skeletal: Back pain, weakness

Respiratory: Bronchitis, pharyngitis, sinusitis, upper respiratory infection

Miscellaneous: Allergic reaction, flu-like syndrome, infection

Adverse reactions reported with other oral contraceptives: Appetite changes, antithrombin III decreased, arterial thromboembolism, benign liver tumors, breast changes, Budd-Chiari syndrome, carbohydrate intolerance, cataracts, cerebral hemorrhage, cerebral thrombosis, cervical changes, change in corneal curvature (steepening), cholestatic jaundice, colitis, contact lens intolerance, decreased lactation (postpartum), deep vein thrombosis, diplopia, edema, erythema multiforme, erythema nodosum; factors VII, VIII, IX, X increased; folate serum concentrations decreased, gallbladder disease, glucose intolerance, hemorrhagic eruption, hemolytic uremic syndrome, hepatic adenomas, hirsutism, hypercalcemia, hypertension, hyperglycemia, libido changes, melasma, mesenteric thrombosis, MI, papilledema, platelet aggregability increased, porphyria, premenstrual syndrome, proptosis, prothrombin increased, pulmonary thromboembolism, renal function impairment, retinal thrombosis, sex hormone-binding globulin increased, thrombophlebitis, thyroid-binding globulin increased, total thyroid hormone (T_4) increased, triglycerides/phospholipids increased, vaginal candidiasis, weight changes

Overdosage/Toxicology May cause nausea; withdrawal bleeding may occur in females. Due to antimineralocorticoid properties of drospirenone, monitor potassium and sodium serum concentrations and evidence of metabolic acidosis.

Dosing

Adults: Female: Contraception: Oral: Dosage is 1 tablet daily for 28 consecutive days. Dose should be taken at the same time each day, either after the evening meal or at bedtime. Dosing may be started on the first day of menstrual period (Day 1 starter) or on the first Sunday after the onset of the menstrual period (Sunday starter).

Day 1 starter: Dose starts on first day of menstrual cycle taking 1 tablet daily.

Sunday starter: Dose begins on first Sunday after onset of menstruation; if the menstrual period starts on Sunday, take first tablet that very same day. **With a Sunday start, an additional method of contraception should be used until after the first 7 days of consecutive administration.**

If all doses have been taken on schedule and one menstrual period is missed, continue dosing cycle. If two consecutive menstrual periods are missed, pregnancy test is required before new dosing cycle is started.

If doses have been missed during the first 3 weeks and the menstrual period is missed, pregnancy should be ruled out prior to continuing treatment.

Missed doses (monophasic formulations) (refer to package insert for complete information):

One dose missed: Take as soon as remembered or take 2 tablets next day

Two consecutive doses missed in the first 2 weeks: Take 2 tablets as soon as remembered or 2 tablets next 2 days. **An additional method of contraception should be used for 7 days after missed dose.**

Two consecutive doses missed in week 3 or three consecutive doses missed at any time: **An additional method of contraception must be used for 7 days after a missed dose.**

Day 1 starter: Current pack should be discarded, and a new pack should be started that same day.

Sunday starter: Continue dose of 1 tablet daily until Sunday, then discard the rest of the pack, and a new pack should be started that same day.

Any number of doses missed in week 4: Continue taking one pill each day until pack is empty; no back-up method of contraception is needed

Pediatrics: Female: Contraception: Oral: Refer to adult dosing; not to be used prior to menarche.

Renal Impairment: Contraindicated in patients with renal dysfunction (Cl_{cr} ≤50 mL/minute).

Hepatic Impairment: Contraindicated in patients with hepatic dysfunction.

Available Dosage Forms Tablet: Ethinyl estradiol 0.03 mg and drospirenone 3 mg [21 yellow active tablets and 7 white inactive tablets] (28s)

Nursing Guidelines

Assessment: Monitor or teach patient to monitor blood pressure on a regular (monthly) basis, and the importance of annual physical examinations (including Pap smear and vision exam). Assess knowledge/teach patient the importance of maintaining prescribed schedule of dosing, possible side effects, appropriate interventions, and adverse reactions to report. **Pregnancy risk factor X:** Determine patient is not pregnant prior to prescribing.

Patient Education: Take exactly as directed by prescriber (see package insert). An additional form of contraception should be used until after the first 7 consecutive days of administration. You are at risk of becoming pregnant if doses are missed. If you miss a dose, take as soon as possible or double the dose the next day. If two or more consecutive doses are missed, contact prescriber for restarting directions. Detailed and complete information on dosing and missed doses can be found in the package insert. If any number of doses are missed in week 4, continue taking one pill each day until pack is empty; no back-up method of contraception is needed. Be aware that some medications may reduce the effectiveness of oral contraceptives; an alternate form of contraception may be needed (see Drug Interactions). It is important that you check your blood pressure monthly (on same day each month) and report any increased blood pressure to prescriber. Have an annual physical assessment, Pap smear, and vision exam while taking this medication. Avoid smoking while taking this medication; smoking increases risk of adverse effects, including thromboembolic events and heart attacks. You may experience loss of appetite (small frequent meals will help); or constipation (increased exercise, fluids, fruit, fiber,

(Continued)

Ethinyl Estradiol and Drospirenone *(Continued)*

or stool softeners may help). If you have diabetes, you should use accurate serum glucose testing to identify any changes in glucose tolerance; notify prescriber of significant changes so antidiabetic medication can be adjusted if necessary. Report immediately pain or muscle soreness; warmth, swelling, pain, or redness in calves; shortness of breath; sudden loss of vision; unresolved leg/foot swelling or weight gain (>5 lb); change in menstrual pattern (unusual bleeding, amenorrhea, breakthrough spotting); breast tenderness that does not go away; acute abdominal cramping; signs of vaginal infection (drainage, pain, itching); CNS changes (blurred vision, confusion, acute anxiety, or unresolved depression); or other persistent adverse effects. **Pregnancy/breast-feeding precautions:** Inform prescriber if you are pregnant. Breast-feeding is not recommended.

Pregnancy Risk Factor: X

Pregnancy Issues: In general, the use of oral contraceptives when inadvertently taken early in pregnancy have not been associated with teratogenic effects. Esophageal atresia was reported in one infant with a single-cycle exposure to ethinyl estradiol and drospirenone *in utero* (association not known). Pregnancy should be ruled out prior to treatment and discontinued if pregnancy occurs. Due to increased risk of thromboembolism postpartum, do not start oral contraceptives earlier than 4-6 weeks following delivery.

Lactation: Enters breast milk/not recommended

Breast-Feeding Considerations: The amount of drospirenone excreted in breast milk is ~0.02%, resulting in a maximum of ~3 mcg/day drospirenone to the infant. Jaundice and breast enlargement in the nursing infant have been reported following the use of other oral contraceptives. In addition, may decrease the quality and quantity of breast milk. Other forms of contraception are recommended while breast-feeding.

Administration

Oral: To be taken at the same time each day, either after the evening meal or at bedtime

Storage: Store at 25°C (77°F).

♦ **Ethinyl Estradiol and NGM** *see* Ethinyl Estradiol and Norgestimate *on page 689*

Ethinyl Estradiol and Norelgestromin

(ETH in il es tra DYE ole & nor el JES troe min)

U.S. Brand Names Ortho Evra®

Synonyms Norelgestromin and Ethinyl Estradiol; Ortho-Evra

Pharmacologic Category Contraceptive; Estrogen and Progestin Combination

Medication Safety Issues

Transdermal patch may contain conducting metal (eg, aluminum); remove patch prior to MRI.

Use Prevention of pregnancy

Mechanism of Action Combination hormonal contraceptives inhibit ovulation via a negative feedback mechanism on the hypothalamus, which alters the normal pattern of gonadotropin secretion of a follicle-stimulating hormone (FSH) and luteinizing hormone by the anterior pituitary. The follicular phase FSH and midcycle surge of gonadotropins are inhibited. In addition, combination hormonal contraceptives produce alterations in the genital tract, including changes in the cervical mucus, rendering it unfavorable for sperm penetration even if ovulation occurs. Changes in the endometrium may also occur, producing an unfavorable environment for nidation. Combination hormonal contraceptive drugs may alter the tubal transport of the ova through the fallopian tubes. Progestational agents may also alter sperm fertility.

Pharmacodynamics/Kinetics

Ortho Evra®:

Absorption: Topical: Equivalent when applied to abdomen, buttock, upper outer arm, and upper torso

Ethinyl estradiol and norelgestromin: Rapid; reaches plateau by ~48 hours. Absorption of ethinyl estradiol may be increased with heat exposure due to sauna, whirlpool, or treadmill.

The amount of ethinyl estradiol absorbed is 20 mcg/day and results in greater exposure than produced by oral ethinyl estradiol 20 mcg. In contrast, peak levels of ethinyl estradiol are higher in women taking oral tablets.

Protein binding: Norelgestromin: >97% to albumin

Metabolism: Topical:

Ethinyl estradiol: First-pass effect avoided; forms metabolites

Norelgestromin: Hepatic to norgestrel and others; first-pass effect avoided

Bioavailability: Ethinyl estradiol: ~60% greater using the topical patch when compared to oral tablets.

Half-life elimination: Topical:

Ethinyl estradiol: 17 hours

Norelgestromin: 28 hours

Excretion: Ethinyl estradiol and norelgestromin: Urine and feces

Contraindications Hypersensitivity to ethinyl estradiol, norelgestromin, or any component of the formulation; history of or current thrombophlebitis or venous thromboembolic disorders (including DVT, PE); active or recent (within 1 year) arterial thromboembolic disease (eg, stroke, MI); cerebral vascular disease, coronary artery disease, valvular heart disease with complications, severe hypertension; diabetes mellitus with vascular involvement; severe headache with focal neurological symptoms; known or suspected breast carcinoma, endometrial cancer, estrogen-dependent neoplasms, undiagnosed abnormal genital bleeding; hepatic dysfunction or tumor, cholestatic jaundice of pregnancy, jaundice with prior combination hormonal contraceptive use; major surgery with prolonged immobilization; heavy smoking (≥15 cigarettes/day) in patients >35 years of age; pregnancy

Warnings/Precautions Combination hormonal contraceptives do not protect against HIV infection or other sexually-transmitted diseases. The risk of cardiovascular side effects increases in women who smoke cigarettes, especially those who are >35 years of age; women who use combination hormonal contraceptives should be strongly advised not to smoke. Combination hormonal contraceptives may lead to increased risk of myocardial infarction, use with caution in patients with risk factors for coronary artery disease. May increase the risk of thromboembolism. Whenever possible, combination hormonal contraceptives should be discontinued at least 4 weeks prior to and for 2 weeks following elective surgery associated with an increased risk of thromboembolism or during periods of prolonged immobilization. Combination hormonal contraceptives may have a dose-related risk of vascular disease, hypertension, and gallbladder disease. Women with hypertension or renal disease should be encouraged to use a nonhormonal form of contraception. The use of combination hormonal contraceptives has been associated with a slight increase in frequency of breast cancer, however, studies are not consistent. Combination hormonal contraceptives may cause glucose intolerance. Retinal thrombosis has been reported (rarely). Use caution with conditions that may be aggravated by fluid retention, depression, or history of migraine. Not for use prior to menarche.

The combination hormonal contraceptive patch may have adverse effects similar to those associated with oral contraceptive products. The topical patch may be less effective in patients weighing ≥90 kg (198 lb) and an increased incidence of pregnancy has been reported in this population; consider another form of contraception. Transdermal patch may contain conducting metal (eg, aluminum); remove patch prior to MRI. The amount of ethinyl estradiol absorbed from the patch results in greater exposure than achieved if administered orally. The increased estrogen exposure from the topical patch should be balanced against the potential for pregnancy if compliance using an oral contraceptive tablet is poor; the difference in risk of serious adverse effects between the two dosage forms is not known. Variability in actual estrogen exposure may be greater in women using the topical patch when compared to women using the oral tablet. The minimum dosage combination of estrogen/progestin that will effectively treat the individual patient should be used.

Drug Interactions

Ethinyl estradiol: **Substrate** of CYP2C8/9 (minor), 3A4 (major), 3A5-7 (minor); **Inhibits** CYP1A2 (weak), 2B6 (weak), 2C19 (weak), 3A4 (weak)

Norelgestromin: **Substrate** of CYP3A4 (minor)

Interactions seen with oral contraceptive agents are likely to occur with the contraceptive patch; reported interactions include:

Acetaminophen: May increase plasma concentration of synthetic estrogens, possibly by inhibiting conjugation. Combination hormonal contraceptives may also decrease the plasma concentration of acetaminophen.

Acitretin: Interferes with the contraceptive effect of microdosed progestin-containing "minipill" preparations. The effect on other progestational contraceptives (eg, implants, injectables) is unknown.

(Continued)

Ethinyl Estradiol and Norelgestromin *(Continued)*

Aminoglutethimide: May increase CYP metabolism of progestins leading to possible decrease in contraceptive effectiveness. Use of a nonhormonal contraceptive product is recommended.

Antibiotics (ampicillin, tetracycline): Pregnancy has been reported following concomitant use, however, pharmacokinetic studies have not shown consistent effects with these antibiotics on plasma concentrations of synthetic steroids. Use of a nonhormonal contraceptive product is recommended.

Anticoagulants: Combination hormonal contraceptives may increase or decrease the effects of coumarin derivatives. Combination hormonal contraceptives may also increase risk of thromboembolic disorders

Anticonvulsants (carbamazepine, felbamate, phenobarbital, phenytoin, topiramate): Increase the metabolism of ethinyl estradiol and/or some progestins, leading to possible decrease in contraceptive effectiveness. Use of a nonhormonal contraceptive product is recommended.

Ascorbic acid: Doses of ascorbic acid (vitamin C) 1 g/day have been reported to increase plasma concentration of synthetic estrogens by ~47%, possibly by inhibiting conjugation; clinical implications are unclear.

Atorvastatin: Atorvastatin increases the AUC for norethindrone and ethinyl estradiol.

Benzodiazepines: Combination hormonal contraceptives may decrease the clearance of some benzodiazepines (alprazolam, chlordiazepoxide, diazepam) and increase the clearance of others (lorazepam, oxazepam, temazepam)

Clofibric acid: Combination hormonal contraceptives may increase the clearance of clofibric acid.

Cyclosporine: Combination hormonal contraceptives may inhibit the metabolism of cyclosporine, leading to increased plasma concentrations; monitor cyclosporine levels

CYP3A4 inducers: CYP3A4 inducers may decrease the levels/effects of ethinyl estradiol. Example inducers include aminoglutethimide, carbamazepine, nafcillin, nevirapine, phenobarbital, phenytoin, and rifamycins.

Griseofulvin: Griseofulvin may induce the metabolism of combination hormonal contraceptives causing menstrual changes; pregnancies have been reported. Use of barrier form of contraception is suggested while on griseofulvin therapy.

Morphine: Combination hormonal contraceptives may increase the clearance of morphine.

Non-nucleoside reverse transcriptase inhibitors (NNRTIs): Nevirapine may decrease plasma levels of combination hormonal contraceptives; use of a nonhormonal contraceptive product is recommended. No data for delavirdine; incomplete data for efavirenz

Prednisolone: Ethinyl estradiol may inhibit the metabolism of prednisolone, leading to increased plasma concentrations.

Protease inhibitors: Amprenavir, lopinavir, nelfinavir, and ritonavir have been shown to decrease plasma levels of combination hormonal contraceptives; use of a nonhormonal contraceptive product is recommended. Indinavir has been shown to increase plasma levels of combination hormonal contraceptives. No data for saquinavir.

Rifampin: Rifampin increases the metabolism of ethinyl estradiol and some progestins (norethindrone) resulting in decreased contraceptive effectiveness and increased menstrual irregularities. Use of a nonhormonal contraceptive product is recommended.

Salicylic acid: Combination hormonal contraceptives may increase the clearance of salicylic acid.

Selegiline: Combination hormonal contraceptives may increase the serum concentration of selegiline.

Theophylline: Ethinyl estradiol may inhibit the metabolism of theophylline, leading to increased plasma concentrations.

Tricyclic antidepressants (amitriptyline, imipramine, nortriptyline): Metabolism may be inhibited by combination hormonal contraceptives, increasing plasma levels of antidepressant; use caution.

Troglitazone: Troglitazone decreases the serum concentrations of ethinyl estradiol and norethindrone by ~30%, leading to possible reduction in contraceptive effectiveness.

Nutritional/Herbal/Ethanol Interactions

Food: CNS effects of caffeine may be enhanced if combination hormonal contraceptives are used concurrently with caffeine. Grapefruit juice increases ethinyl estradiol concentrations and would be expected to increase progesterone serum levels as well; clinical implications are unclear.

Herb/Nutraceutical: St John's wort may decrease the effectiveness of combination hormonal contraceptives by inducing hepatic enzymes. Avoid dong quai and black cohosh (have estrogen activity). Avoid saw palmetto, red clover, ginseng.

Adverse Reactions The following reactions have been reported with the contraceptive patch. Adverse reactions associated with oral combination hormonal contraceptive agents are also likely to appear with the topical contraceptive patch (frequency difficult to anticipate). Refer to individual **oral** contraceptive monographs for additional information.

9% to 22%: Abdominal pain, application site reaction, breast symptoms, headache, menstrual cramps, nausea, upper respiratory infection

Overdosage/Toxicology Overdosage is unlikely due to the design of the patch. Toxicity from oral combination hormonal contraceptives is unlikely following single exposures of excessive doses. May cause withdrawal bleeding in females. If overdose is suspected, patch should be removed and treatment should be symptomatic and supportive.

Dosing

Adults: Female: Contraception: Topical:

Apply one patch each week for 3 weeks (21 total days); followed by one week that is patch-free. Each patch should be applied on the same day each week ("patch change day") and only one patch should be worn at a time. No more than 7 days should pass during the patch-free interval.

Schedule 1 (Sunday starter): Dose begins on first Sunday after onset of menstruation; if the menstrual period starts on Sunday, apply one patch that very same day. **With a Sunday start, an additional method of contraception (nonhormonal) should be used until after the first 7 days of consecutive administration.** Each patch change will then occur on Sunday.

Schedule 2 (Day 1 starter): Dose starts on first day of menstrual cycle, applying one patch during the first 24 hours of menstrual cycle. No back-up method of contraception is needed as long as the patch is applied on the first day of cycle. Each patch change will then occur on that same day of the week.

Additional dosing considerations:

No bleeding during patch-free week/missed menstrual period: If patch has been applied as directed, continue treatment on usual "patch change day". If used correctly, no bleeding during patch-free week does not necessarily indicate pregnancy. However, if no withdrawal bleeding occurs for 2 consecutive cycles, pregnancy should be ruled out. If patch has not been applied as directed, and one menstrual period is missed, pregnancy should be ruled out prior to continuing treatment.

If a patch becomes partially or completely detached for <24 hours: Try to reapply to same place, or replace with a new patch immediately. Do not reapply if patch is no longer sticky, if it is sticking to itself or another surface, or if it has material sticking to it.

If a patch becomes partially or completely detached for >24 hours (or time period is unknown): Apply a new patch and use this day of the week as the new "patch change day" from this point on. **An additional method of contraception (nonhormonal) should be used until after the first 7 days of consecutive administration.**

Switching from oral contraceptives: Apply first patch on the first day of withdrawal bleeding. If there is no bleeding within 5 days of taking the last active tablet, pregnancy must first be ruled out. If patch is applied later than the first day of bleeding, **an additional method of contraception (nonhormonal) should be used until after the first 7 days of consecutive administration**

Use after childbirth: Therapy should not be started <4 weeks after childbirth. Pregnancy should be ruled out prior to treatment if menstrual periods have not restarted. **An additional method of contraception (nonhormonal) should be used until after the first 7 days of consecutive administration.**

Use after abortion or miscarriage: Therapy may be started immediately if abortion/miscarriage occur within the first trimester. If therapy is not started within 5 days, follow instructions for first time use. If abortion/miscarriage occur during the second trimester, therapy should not be started for at least 4 weeks. Follow directions for use after childbirth.

(Continued)

Ethinyl Estradiol and Norelgestromin *(Continued)*

Pediatrics: Female: Contraception: Topical: Refer to adult dosing; not to be used prior to menarche.

Renal Impairment: Specific guidelines not available; use with caution and monitor blood pressure closely. Consider other forms of contraception

Hepatic Impairment: Contraindicated in patients with hepatic impairment.

Available Dosage Forms Note: The formulation available in Canada differs from the U.S. product in both composition and the manufacturing process (although delivery rates appear similar).

Patch, transdermal: Ethinyl estradiol 0.75 mg and norelgestromin 6 mg [releases ethinyl estradiol 20 mcg and norelgestromin 150 mcg per day] (1s, 3s)

Canadian Formulation:

Patch, transdermal: Ethinyl estradiol 0.6 mg and norelgestromin 6 mg [releases ethinyl estradiol 20 mcg and norelgestromin 150 mcg per day] (1s, 3s)

Nursing Guidelines

Patient Education: Topical contraceptive patches do not protect against HIV or other sexually-transmitted diseases. Use exactly as directed by prescriber (also see package insert), always applying patch on same day of each week. You are at risk of becoming pregnant if doses are missed. Detailed and complete information on dosing and missed doses can be found in the package insert. Be aware that some medications may reduce the effectiveness of contraceptives; an alternate form of contraception may be needed. Check all medicines (prescription and OTC), herbal, and alternative products with prescriber. It is important that you check your blood pressure monthly (on same day each month) and that you have an annual physical assessment, Pap smear, and vision assessment while taking this medication. Avoid smoking while taking this medication; smoking increases risk of adverse effects, including thromboembolic events and heart attacks. You may experience loss of appetite (small, frequent meals will help); or constipation (increased exercise, fluids, fruit, fiber, or stool softeners may help). If you have diabetes, use accurate serum glucose testing to identify any changes in glucose tolerance; notify prescriber of significant changes so antidiabetic medication can be adjusted if necessary. Report immediately pain or muscle soreness; warmth, swelling, pain, or redness in calves; shortness of breath; sudden loss of vision; unresolved leg/foot swelling; change in menstrual pattern (unusual bleeding, amenorrhea, breakthrough spotting); breast tenderness that does not go away; acute abdominal cramping; signs of vaginal infection (drainage, pain, itching); CNS changes (blurred vision, confusion, acute anxiety, or unresolved depression); or significant weight gain (>5 lb/week). Notify prescriber of changes in contact lens tolerance. **Pregnancy/breast-feeding precautions:** This medication should not be used during pregnancy. If you suspect you may become pregnant, contact prescriber immediately. Breast-feeding is not recommended.

New patches should be applied on the same day each week. Apply to clean, dry, intact and healthy skin on the buttock, abdomen, upper arm or upper torso. Avoid areas that will be rubbed by tight clothing. Do not apply to the breasts or to skin that is red, irritated, or cut. Do not apply make-up, creams, lotions, powders, or other topical products to the skin where the patch will be placed. Remove the patch and the plastic liner from the foil pouch, being careful not to remove the clear liner when removing the patch. Apply patch by first peeling back half of the clear protective liner. Avoid touching surface of patch. Apply patch to skin and remove the rest of the liner. Press patch down firmly onto skin using palm of the hand; apply pressure for 10 seconds. When changing the patch each week, the new patch may be applied in the same anatomic area but should be applied to a new spot in that area. Do not use supplemental adhesives or wraps to hold patch into place.

If a patch becomes partially or completely detached for <24 hours: Try to reapply to same place, or replace with a new patch immediately. Do not reapply if patch is no longer sticky, if it is sticking to itself or another surface, or if it has material sticking to it.

Disposing of patch: Because the used patch contains some active hormones, fold it in half so that it sticks to itself before throwing it away.

Pregnancy Risk Factor: X

Pregnancy Issues: Pregnancy should be ruled out prior to treatment and discontinued if pregnancy occurs. In general, the use of combination hormonal contraceptives when inadvertently taken early in pregnancy have not been associated with teratogenic effects. Due to increased risk of thromboembolism postpartum, combination hormonal contraceptives should not be started earlier than 4-6 weeks following delivery.

Lactation: Enters breast milk/not recommended (AAP rates "compatible")

Breast-Feeding Considerations: Jaundice and breast enlargement in the nursing infant have been reported following the use of combination hormonal contraceptives. May decrease the quality and quantity of breast milk; a nonhormonal form of contraception is recommended.

Administration

Storage: Store at controlled room temperature of 25°C (77°F). Do not refrigerate or freeze.

Ethinyl Estradiol and Norgestimate

(ETH in il es tra DYE ole & nor JES ti mate)

U.S. Brand Names MonoNessa™; Ortho-Cyclen®; Ortho Tri-Cyclen®; Ortho Tri-Cyclen® Lo; Previfem™; Sprintec™; TriNessa™; Tri-Previfem™; Tri-Sprintec™

Synonyms Ethinyl Estradiol and NGM; Norgestimate and Ethinyl Estradiol; Ortho Cyclen; Ortho Tri Cyclen

Pharmacologic Category Contraceptive; Estrogen and Progestin Combination

Medication Safety Issues

Sound-alike/look-alike issues:

Ortho-Cyclen® may be confused with Ortho-Cept®

Use Prevention of pregnancy; treatment of acne

Unlabeled/Investigational Use Treatment of hypermenorrhea (menorrhagia); pain associated with endometriosis; dysmenorrhea; dysfunctional uterine bleeding

Mechanism of Action Combination hormonal contraceptives inhibit ovulation via a negative feedback mechanism on the hypothalamus, which alters the normal pattern of gonadotropin secretion of a follicle-stimulating hormone (FSH) and luteinizing hormone by the anterior pituitary. The follicular phase FSH and midcycle surge of gonadotropins are inhibited. In addition, combination hormonal contraceptives produce alterations in the genital tract, including changes in the cervical mucus, rendering it unfavorable for sperm penetration even if ovulation occurs. Changes in the endometrium may also occur, producing an unfavorable environment for nidation. Combination hormonal contraceptive drugs may alter the tubal transport of the ova through the fallopian tubes. Progestational agents may also alter sperm fertility.

Pharmacodynamics/Kinetics

Norgestimate:

Absorption: Well absorbed

Protein binding: To albumin and sex hormone-binding globulin (SHBG); SHBG capacity is affected by plasma ethinyl estradiol levels

Metabolism: Hepatic; forms 17-deacetylnorgestimate (major active metabolite) and other metabolites

Half-life elimination: 17-deacetylnorgestimate: 12-30 hours

Excretion: Urine and feces

Contraindications Hypersensitivity to ethinyl estradiol, norgestimate, or any component of the formulation; history of or current thrombophlebitis or venous thromboembolic disorders (including DVT, PE); active or recent (within 1 year) arterial thromboembolic disease (eg, stroke, MI); cerebral vascular disease, coronary artery disease, valvular heart disease with complications, severe hypertension; severe headache with focal neurological symptoms; known or suspected breast carcinoma, endometrial cancer, estrogen-dependent neoplasms, undiagnosed abnormal genital bleeding; hepatic dysfunction or tumor, cholestatic jaundice of pregnancy, jaundice with prior combination hormonal contraceptive use; heavy smoking (≥15 cigarettes/day) in patients >35 years of age; pregnancy

Warnings/Precautions Combination hormonal contraceptives do not protect against HIV infection or other sexually-transmitted diseases. The risk of cardiovascular side effects increases in women who smoke cigarettes, especially those who are >35 years of age; women who use combination hormonal contraceptives should be strongly advised not to smoke. Combination hormonal contraceptives may lead to increased risk of myocardial infarction, use with caution in patients with risk factors for coronary artery disease. May increase the risk of thromboembolism. Whenever possible, combination hormonal contraceptives should be discontinued at least 4 weeks prior to and for 2 weeks following elective surgery associated with an increased risk of thromboembolism or during periods of prolonged immobilization. Combination hormonal contraceptives may have a

(Continued)

Ethinyl Estradiol and Norgestimate *(Continued)*

dose-related risk of vascular disease, hypertension, and gallbladder disease. Women with hypertension or renal disease should be encouraged to use a nonhormonal form of contraception. The use of combination hormonal contraceptives has been associated with a slight increase in frequency of breast cancer, however, studies are not consistent. Combination hormonal contraceptives may cause glucose intolerance. Retinal thrombosis has been reported (rarely). Use caution with conditions that may be aggravated by fluid retention, depression, or history of migraine. Not for use prior to menarche.

The minimum dosage combination of estrogen/progestin that will effectively treat the individual patient should be used. New patients should be started on products containing ≤0.035 mg of estrogen per tablet.

Acne: For use only in females ≥15 years, who also desire combination hormonal contraceptive therapy, are unresponsive to topical treatments, and have no contraindications to combination hormonal contraceptive use.

Drug Interactions Ethinyl estradiol: **Substrate** of CYP2C8/9 (minor), 3A4 (major), 3A5-7 (minor); **Inhibits** CYP1A2 (weak), 2B6 (weak), 2C19 (weak), 3A4 (weak)

Acetaminophen: May increase plasma concentration of synthetic estrogens, possibly by inhibiting conjugation. Combination hormonal contraceptives may also decrease the plasma concentration of acetaminophen.

Acitretin: Interferes with the contraceptive effect of microdosed progestin-containing "minipill" preparations. The effect on other progestational contraceptives (eg, implants, injectables) is unknown.

Aminoglutethimide: May increase CYP metabolism of progestins leading to possible decrease in contraceptive effectiveness. Use of a nonhormonal contraceptive product is recommended.

Antibiotics (ampicillin, tetracycline): Pregnancy has been reported following concomitant use, however, pharmacokinetic studies have not shown consistent effects with these antibiotics on plasma concentrations of synthetic steroids. Use of a nonhormonal contraceptive product is recommended.

Anticoagulants: Combination hormonal contraceptives may increase or decrease the effects of coumarin derivatives. Combination hormonal contraceptives may also increase risk of thromboembolic disorders

Anticonvulsants (carbamazepine, felbamate, phenobarbital, phenytoin, topiramate): Increase the metabolism of ethinyl estradiol and/or some progestins, leading to possible decrease in contraceptive effectiveness. Use of a nonhormonal contraceptive product is recommended.

Ascorbic acid: Doses of ascorbic acid (vitamin C) 1 g/day have been reported to increase plasma concentration of synthetic estrogens by ~47%, possibly by inhibiting conjugation; clinical implications are unclear.

Atorvastatin: Atorvastatin increases the AUC for norethindrone and ethinyl estradiol.

Benzodiazepines: Combination hormonal contraceptives may decrease the clearance of some benzodiazepines (alprazolam, chlordiazepoxide, diazepam) and increase the clearance of others (lorazepam, oxazepam, temazepam)

Clofibric acid: Combination hormonal contraceptives may increase the clearance of clofibric acid.

Cyclosporine: Combination hormonal contraceptives may inhibit the metabolism of cyclosporine, leading to increased plasma concentrations; monitor cyclosporine levels

CYP3A4 inducers: CYP3A4 inducers may decrease the levels/effects of ethinyl estradiol. Example inducers include aminoglutethimide, carbamazepine, nafcillin, nevirapine, phenobarbital, phenytoin, and rifamycins.

Griseofulvin: Griseofulvin may induce the metabolism of combination hormonal contraceptives causing menstrual changes; pregnancies have been reported. Use of barrier form of contraception is suggested while on griseofulvin therapy.

Morphine: Combination hormonal contraceptives may increase the clearance of morphine.

Non-nucleoside reverse transcriptase inhibitors (NNRTIs): Nevirapine may decrease plasma levels of combination hormonal contraceptives; use of a nonhormonal contraceptive product is recommended. No data for delavirdine; incomplete data for efavirenz

Prednisolone: Ethinyl estradiol may inhibit the metabolism of prednisolone, leading to increased plasma concentrations.

Protease inhibitors: Amprenavir, lopinavir, nelfinavir, and ritonavir have been shown to decrease plasma levels of combination hormonal contraceptives; use of a nonhormonal contraceptive product is recommended. Indinavir has been shown to increase plasma levels of combination hormonal contraceptives. No data for saquinavir.

Rifampin: Rifampin increases the metabolism of ethinyl estradiol and some progestins (norethindrone) resulting in decreased contraceptive effectiveness and increased menstrual irregularities. Use of a nonhormonal contraceptive product is recommended.

Salicylic acid: Combination hormonal contraceptives may increase the clearance of salicylic acid.

Selegiline: Combination hormonal contraceptives may increase the serum concentration of selegiline.

Theophylline: Ethinyl estradiol may inhibit the metabolism of theophylline, leading to increased plasma concentrations.

Tricyclic antidepressants (amitriptyline, imipramine, nortriptyline): Metabolism may be inhibited by combination hormonal contraceptives, increasing plasma levels of antidepressant; use caution.

Nutritional/Herbal/Ethanol Interactions

Food: CNS effects of caffeine may be enhanced if combination hormonal contraceptives are used concurrently with caffeine. Grapefruit juice increases ethinyl estradiol concentrations and would be expected to increase progesterone serum levels as well; clinical implications are unclear.

Herb/Nutraceutical: St John's wort may decrease the effectiveness of combination hormonal contraceptives by inducing hepatic enzymes. Avoid dong quai and black cohosh (have estrogen activity). Avoid saw palmetto, red clover, ginseng.

Lab Interactions Increased amylase (S), cholesterol (S), iron (B), sodium (S), thyroxine (S); decreased calcium (S), protein, prothrombin time

Adverse Reactions Frequency not defined.

Cardiovascular: Arterial thromboembolism, cerebral hemorrhage, cerebral thrombosis, edema, hypertension, mesenteric thrombosis, MI

Central nervous system: Depression, dizziness, headache, migraine, nervousness, premenstrual syndrome, stroke

Dermatologic: Acne, erythema multiforme, erythema nodosum, hirsutism, loss of scalp hair, melasma (may persist), rash (allergic)

Endocrine & metabolic: Amenorrhea, breakthrough bleeding, breast enlargement, breast secretion, breast tenderness, carbohydrate intolerance, lactation decreased (postpartum), glucose tolerance decreased, libido changes, menstrual flow changes, sex hormone-binding globulins (SHBG) increased, spotting, temporary infertility (following discontinuation), thyroid-binding globulin increased, triglycerides increased

Gastrointestinal: Abdominal cramps, appetite changes, bloating, cholestasis, colitis, gallbladder disease, jaundice, nausea, vomiting, weight gain/loss

Genitourinary: Cervical erosion changes, cervical secretion changes, cystitis-like syndrome, vaginal candidiasis, vaginitis

Hematologic: Antithrombin III decreased, folate levels decreased, hemolytic uremic syndrome, norepinephrine induced platelet aggregability increased, porphyria, prothrombin increased; factors VII, VIII, IX, and X increased

Hepatic: Benign liver tumors, Budd-Chiari syndrome, cholestatic jaundice, hepatic adenomas

Local: Thrombophlebitis

Ocular: Cataracts, change in corneal curvature (steepening), contact lens intolerance, optic neuritis, retinal thrombosis

Renal: Impaired renal function

Respiratory: Pulmonary thromboembolism

Miscellaneous: Hemorrhagic eruption

Overdosage/Toxicology Toxicity is unlikely following single exposures of excessive doses. May cause withdrawal bleeding in females. Any treatment following emesis and charcoal administration should be supportive and symptomatic.

Dosing

Adults: Female:

Acne (Ortho Tri-Cyclen®): Oral: Refer to dosing for contraception

Contraception: Oral:

Schedule 1 (Sunday starter): Dose begins on first Sunday after onset of menstruation; if the menstrual period starts on Sunday, take first tablet that very same day. **With a Sunday start, an additional method of contraception should be used until after the first 7 days of consecutive administration.**

(Continued)

Ethinyl Estradiol and Norgestimate *(Continued)*

For 21-tablet package: Dosage is 1 tablet daily for 21 consecutive days, followed by 7 days off of the medication; a new course begins on the 8th day after the last tablet is taken.

For 28-tablet package: Dosage is 1 tablet daily without interruption.

Schedule 2 (Day 1 starter): Dose starts on first day of menstrual cycle taking 1 tablet daily.

For 21-tablet package: Dosage is 1 tablet daily for 21 consecutive days, followed by 7 days off of the medication; a new course begins on the 8th day after the last tablet is taken.

For 28-tablet package: Dosage is 1 tablet daily without interruption.

If all doses have been taken on schedule and one menstrual period is missed, continue dosing cycle. If two consecutive menstrual periods are missed, pregnancy test is required before new dosing cycle is started.

Missed doses **monophasic formulations** (refer to package insert for complete information):

One dose missed: Take as soon as remembered or take 2 tablets next day

Two consecutive doses missed in the first 2 weeks: Take 2 tablets as soon as remembered or 2 tablets next 2 days. **An additional method of contraception should be used for 7 days after missed dose.**

Two consecutive doses missed in week 3 or three consecutive doses missed at any time: **An additional method of contraception must be used for 7 days after a missed dose:**

Schedule 1 (Sunday starter): Continue dose of 1 tablet daily until Sunday, then discard the rest of the pack, and a new pack should be started that same day.

Schedule 2 (Day 1 starter): Current pack should be discarded, and a new pack should be started that same day.

Missed doses **biphasic/triphasic formulations** (refer to package insert for complete information):

One dose missed: Take as soon as remembered or take 2 tablets next day.

Two consecutive doses missed in week 1 or week 2 of the pack: Take 2 tablets as soon as remembered and 2 tablets the next day. Resume taking 1 tablet daily until the pack is empty. **An additional method of contraception must be used for 7 days after a missed dose.**

Two consecutive doses missed in week 3 of the pack. **An additional method of contraception must be used for 7 days after a missed dose.**

Schedule 1 (Sunday starter): Take 1 tablet every day until Sunday. Discard the remaining pack and start a new pack of pills on the same day.

Schedule 2 (Day 1 starter): Discard the remaining pack and start a new pack the same day.

Three or more consecutive doses missed. **An additional method of contraception must be used for 7 days after a missed dose.**

Schedule 1 (Sunday starter): Take 1 tablet every day until Sunday; on Sunday, discard the pack and start a new pack.

Schedule 2 (Day 1 starter): Discard the remaining pack and begin new pack of tablets starting on the same day.

Pediatrics: Female:

Acne: Oral: Children ≥15 years; refer to adult dosing for contraception

Contraception: Oral: Refer to adult dosing; not to be used prior to menarche.

Renal Impairment: Specific guidelines not available; use with caution and monitor blood pressure closely. Consider other forms of contraception.

Hepatic Impairment: Contraindicated in patients with hepatic impairment.

Available Dosage Forms

Tablet, monophasic formulations:

MonoNessa™, Ortho-Cyclen®: Ethinyl estradiol 0.035 mg and norgestimate 0.25 mg [21 blue tablets and 7 green inactive tablets] (28s)

Previfem™: Ethinyl estradiol 0.035 mg and norgestimate 0.25 mg [21 blue tablets and 7 teal inactive tablets] (28s)

Sprintec™: Ethinyl estradiol 0.035 mg and norgestimate 0.25 mg [21 blue tablets and 7 white inactive tablets] (28s)

Tablet, triphasic formulations:

Ortho Tri-Cyclen®, TriNessa™:

Day 1-7: Ethinyl estradiol 0.035 mg and norgestimate 0.18 mg [7 white tablets]

Day 8-14: Ethinyl estradiol 0.035 mg and norgestimate 0.215 mg [7 light blue tablets]

Day 15-21: Ethinyl estradiol 0.035 mg and norgestimate 0.25 mg [7 blue tablets]

Day 22-28: 7 green inactive tablets (28s)

Tri-Previfem™:

Day 1-7: Ethinyl estradiol 0.035 mg and norgestimate 0.18 mg [7 white tablets]

Day 8-14: Ethinyl estradiol 0.035 mg and norgestimate 0.215 mg [7 light blue tablets]

Day 15-21: Ethinyl estradiol 0.035 mg and norgestimate 0.25 mg [7 blue tablets]

Day 22-28: 7 teal inactive tablets (28s)

Tri-Sprintec™:

Day 1-7: Ethinyl estradiol 0.035 mg and norgestimate 0.18 mg [7 gray tablets]

Day 8-14: Ethinyl estradiol 0.035 mg and norgestimate 0.215 mg [7 light blue tablets]

Day 15-21: Ethinyl estradiol 0.035 mg and norgestimate 0.25 mg [7 blue tablets]

Day 22-28: 7 white inactive tablets (28s)

Ortho Tri-Cyclen® Lo:

Day 1-7: Ethinyl estradiol 0.025 mg and norgestimate 0.18 mg [7 white tablets]

Day 8-14: Ethinyl estradiol 0.025 mg and norgestimate 0.215 mg [7 light blue tablets]

Day 15-21: Ethinyl estradiol 0.025 mg and norgestimate 0.25 mg [7 dark blue tablets]

Day 22-28: 7 green inactive tablets (28s)

Nursing Guidelines

Assessment: Assess for adverse reactions and potential drug interactions. Emphasize importance of regular (monthly) blood pressure checks and annual physical assessment, Pap smear, and vision assessment. Teach importance of maintaining prescribed schedule of dosing. **Pregnancy risk factor X:** Do not use if patient is pregnant.

Dietary Considerations: Should be taken at same time each day.

Patient Education: Oral contraceptives do not protect against HIV or other sexually-transmitted diseases. Take exactly as directed by prescriber (also see package insert). You are at risk of becoming pregnant if doses are missed. Detailed and complete information on dosing and missed doses can be found in the package insert. Be aware that some medications may reduce the effectiveness of oral contraceptives; an alternate form of contraception may be needed. Check all medicines (prescription and OTC), herbal, and alternative products with prescriber. It is important that you check your blood pressure monthly (on same day each month) and that you have an annual physical assessment, Pap smear, and vision assessment while taking this medication. Avoid smoking while taking this medication; smoking increases risk of adverse effects, including thromboembolic events and heart attacks. You may experience loss of appetite (small frequent meals will help); or constipation (increased exercise, fluids, fruit, fiber, or stool softeners may help). If you have diabetes, use accurate serum glucose testing to identify any changes in glucose tolerance; notify prescriber of significant changes so antidiabetic medication can be adjusted if necessary. Report immediately pain or muscle soreness; warmth, swelling, pain, or redness in calves; shortness of breath; sudden loss of vision; unresolved leg/ foot swelling; change in menstrual pattern (unusual bleeding, amenorrhea, breakthrough spotting); breast tenderness that does not go away; acute abdominal cramping; signs of vaginal infection (drainage, pain, itching); CNS changes (blurred vision, confusion, acute anxiety, or unresolved depression); or significant weight gain (>5 lb/week). Notify prescriber of changes in contact lens tolerance. **Pregnancy/breast-feeding precautions:** This medication should not be used during pregnancy. If you suspect you may become pregnant, contact prescriber immediately. Consult prescriber if breast-feeding.

Pregnancy Risk Factor: X

Pregnancy Issues: Pregnancy should be ruled out prior to treatment and discontinued if pregnancy occurs. In general, the use of combination hormonal contraceptives when inadvertently taken early in pregnancy have not been associated with teratogenic effects. Due to increased risk of thromboembolism postpartum, combination hormonal contraceptives should not be started earlier than 4-6 weeks following delivery.

(Continued)

Ethinyl Estradiol and Norgestimate *(Continued)*

Lactation: Enters breast milk/not recommended (AAP rates "compatible")

Breast-Feeding Considerations: Jaundice and breast enlargement in the nursing infant have been reported following the use of combination hormonal contraceptives. May decrease the quality and quantity of breast milk; a nonhormonal form of contraception is recommended.

Administration

Oral: Administer at the same time each day.

Storage: Store at controlled room temperature of 25°C (77°F).

- Ethoxynaphthamido Penicillin Sodium *see* Nafcillin *on page 1194*
- Ethyl Alcohol *see* Alcohol (Ethyl) *on page 100*
- Ethyl Aminobenzoate *see* Benzocaine *on page 232*
- Ethyl Esters of Omega-3 Fatty Acids *see* Omega-3-Acid Ethyl Esters *on page 1263*
- EtOH *see* Alcohol (Ethyl) *on page 100*

Etomidate (e TOM i date)

U.S. Brand Names Amidate®

Pharmacologic Category General Anesthetic

Medication Safety Issues

Sound-alike/look-alike issues:

Etomidate may be confused with etidronate

Use Induction and maintenance of general anesthesia

Unlabeled/Investigational Use Sedation for diagnosis of seizure foci

Mechanism of Action Ultrashort-acting nonbarbiturate hypnotic (benzylimidazole) used for the induction of anesthesia; chemically, it is a carboxylated imidazole which produces a rapid induction of anesthesia with minimal cardiovascular effects; produces EEG burst suppression at high doses

Pharmacodynamics/Kinetics

Onset of action: 30-60 seconds

Peak effect: 1 minute

Duration: 3-5 minutes; terminated by redistribution

Distribution: V_d: 2-4.5 L/kg

Protein binding: 76%;

Metabolism: Hepatic and plasma esterases

Half-life elimination: Terminal: 2.6 hours

Contraindications Hypersensitivity to etomidate or any component of the formulation

Warnings/Precautions Etomidate inhibits 11-B-hydroxylase, an enzyme important in adrenal steroid production. A single induction dose blocks the normal stress-induced increase in adrenal cortisol production for 4-8 hours, up to 24 hours in elderly and debilitated patients. Continuous infusion of etomidate for sedation in the ICU may increase mortality because patients may not be able to respond to stress. No problem has been identified with a single dose for induction of anesthesia. Consider exogenous corticosteroid replacement in patients undergoing severe stress.

Drug Interactions

Fentanyl: Decreases etomidate elimination

Verapamil: May increase the anesthetic and respiratory depressant effects of etomidate

Adverse Reactions

>10%:

Gastrointestinal: Nausea, vomiting on emergence from anesthesia

Local: Pain at injection site (30% to 80%)

Neuromuscular & skeletal: Myoclonus (33%), transient skeletal movements, uncontrolled eye movements

1% to 10%: Hiccups

<1% (Limited to important or life-threatening): Apnea, arrhythmia, bradycardia, decreased cortisol synthesis, hypertension, hyperventilation, hypotension, hypoventilation, laryngospasm, tachycardia

Overdosage/Toxicology Symptoms of overdose include respiratory arrest and coma. Treatment is supportive.

Dosing

Adults & Elderly: Anesthesia: I.V.: Initial: 0.2-0.6 mg/kg over 30-60 seconds for induction of anesthesia; maintenance: 5-20 mcg/kg/minute

Pediatrics: Children >10 years: Refer to adult dosing.

Available Dosage Forms Injection, solution: 2 mg/mL (10 mL, 20 mL) [contains propylene glycol 35% v/v]

Nursing Guidelines

Assessment:

Assess other medications patient may be taking for effectiveness and interactions. Assess results of laboratory tests, therapeutic effect, and adverse/toxic effects, particularly for signs of adrenal insufficiency (including hypotension, hyperkalemia). Monitor respiratory status (for conscious sedation, includes pulse oximetry), cardiovascular status, CNS status (when used for procedures monitor sedation score); cardiac monitor and blood pressure monitor required. Infusion site should be monitored closely due to potential irritation (see Administration).

Pregnancy Risk Factor: C

Perioperative/Anesthesia/Other Concerns: Etomidate 2 mg/mL contains propylene glycol 362.6 mg/mL (35% v/v).

Etomidate decreases cerebral metabolism and cerebral blood flow while maintaining perfusion pressure; can enhance somatosensory evoked potential recordings. Premedication with opioids or benzodiazepines can decrease myoclonus. Etomidate is a relatively safe anesthetic for use in patients with stable cardiovascular disease.

Administration

I.V.: Administer I.V. push over 30-60 seconds. Solution is highly irritating; avoid administration into small vessels; in some cases, preadministration of lidocaine may be considered.

Compatibility: Y-site administration: Incompatible with ascorbic acid, vecuronium

Storage: Store at room temperature.

Related Information

Intravenous Anesthetic Agents *on page 1853*

Etoposide (e toe POE side)

U.S. Brand Names Toposar®; VePesid®

Synonyms Epipodophyllotoxin; VP-16; VP-16-213

Pharmacologic Category Antineoplastic Agent, Podophyllotoxin Derivative

Medication Safety Issues

Sound-alike/look-alike issues:

Etoposide may be confused with teniposide

VePesid® may be confused with Versed

Use Treatment of lymphomas, ANLL, lung, testicular, bladder, and prostate carcinoma, hepatoma, rhabdomyosarcoma, uterine carcinoma, neuroblastoma, mycosis fungoides, Kaposi's sarcoma, histiocytosis, gestational trophoblastic disease, Ewing's sarcoma, Wilms' tumor, and brain tumors

Mechanism of Action Etoposide does not inhibit microtubular assembly. It has been shown to delay transit of cells through the S phase and arrest cells in late S or early G_2 phase. The drug may inhibit mitochondrial transport at the NADH dehydrogenase level or inhibit uptake of nucleosides into HeLa cells. Etoposide is a topoisomerase II inhibitor and appears to cause DNA strand breaks.

Pharmacodynamics/Kinetics

Absorption: Oral: 25% to 75%; significant inter- and intrapatient variation

Distribution: Average V_d: 3-36 L/m^2; poor penetration across the blood-brain barrier; CSF concentrations <10% of plasma concentrations

Protein binding: 94% to 97%

Metabolism: Hepatic to hydroxy acid and cislactone metabolites

Half-life elimination: Terminal: 4-15 hours; Children: Normal renal/hepatic function: 6-8 hours

Time to peak, serum: Oral: 1-1.5 hours

Excretion:

Children: Urine (≤55% as unchanged drug)

Adults: Urine (42% to 67%; 8% to 35% as unchanged drug) within 24 hours; feces (up to 16%)

Contraindications Hypersensitivity to etoposide or any component of the formulation; **intrathecal administration**; pregnancy

Warnings/Precautions The U.S. Food and Drug Administration (FDA) currently recommends that procedures for proper handling and disposal of antineoplastic

(Continued)

Etoposide *(Continued)*

agents be considered. Severe myelosuppression with resulting infection or bleeding may occur. Dosage should be adjusted in patients with hepatic or renal impairment.

Etoposide preparation should be performed in a Class II laminar flow biologic safety cabinet. Personnel should be wearing surgical gloves and a closed front surgical gown with knit cuffs. Appropriate safety equipment is recommended for preparation, administration, and disposal of antineoplastics. If etoposide contacts the skin, wash and flush thoroughly with water.

Drug Interactions **Substrate** of CYP1A2 (minor), 2E1 (minor), 3A4 (major); **Inhibits** CYP2C8/9 (weak), 3A4 (weak)

Calcium antagonists: Increases the rate of VP-16-induced DNA damage and cytotoxicity *in vitro*.

Carmustine: Reports of frequent hepatic dysfunction with hyperbilirubinemia, ascites, and thrombocytopenia.

Cyclosporine: Additive cytotoxic effects on tumor cells.

CYP3A4 inducers: CYP3A4 inducers may decrease the levels/effects of etoposide. Example inducers include aminoglutethimide, carbamazepine, nafcillin, nevirapine, phenobarbital, phenytoin, and rifamycins.

CYP3A4 inhibitors: May increase the levels/effects of etoposide. Example inhibitors include azole antifungals, clarithromycin, diclofenac, doxycycline, erythromycin, imatinib, isoniazid, nefazodone, nicardipine, propofol, protease inhibitors, quinidine, telithromycin, and verapamil.

Methotrexate: Alteration of methotrexate transport has been found as a slow efflux of methotrexate and its polyglutamated form out of the cell, leading to intercellular accumulation of methotrexate.

Warfarin may elevate prothrombin time with concurrent use.

Nutritional/Herbal/Ethanol Interactions

Ethanol: Avoid ethanol (may increase GI irritation).

Food: Administration of food does not affect GI absorption with doses ≤200 mg of injection.

Herb/Nutraceutical: St John's wort may decrease etoposide levels.

Adverse Reactions

>10%:

Dermatologic: Alopecia (reversible)

Gastrointestinal: Diarrhea, nausea, vomiting severe mucositis (with BMT doses), anorexia

Emetic potential: Moderately low (10% to 30%)

Hematologic: Anemia, leukopenia

WBC: Mild to severe

Platelets: Mild

Onset (days): 10

Nadir (days): granulocytes 7-14 days; platelets 9-16 days

Recovery (days): 21-28

1% to 10%:

Cardiovascular: Hypotension: Related to drug infusion time; may be related to vehicle used in the I.V. preparation (polysorbate 80 plus polyethylene glycol). Best to administer the drug over 1 hour.

Central nervous system: Unusual fatigue

Gastrointestinal: Stomatitis, diarrhea, abdominal pain, hepatitic dysfunction

<1% (Limited to important or life-threatening): Tachycardia, neurotoxicity, peripheral neuropathy, toxic hepatitis (with high-dose therapy), flushing and bronchospasm (may be prevented by pretreatment with corticosteroids and antihistamines)

Irritant, thrombophlebitis has been reported

BMT:

Cardiovascular: Hypotension (infusion-related)

Dermatologic: Skin lesions resembling Stevens-Johnson syndrome, alopecia

Endocrine & metabolic: Metabolic acidosis

Gastrointestinal: Severe nausea and vomiting, mucositis

Hepatic: Hepatitis

Miscellaneous: Secondary malignancy, ethanol intoxication

Overdosage/Toxicology Symptoms of overdose include bone marrow suppression, leukopenia, thrombocytopenia, nausea, and vomiting. Treatment is supportive.

Dosing

Adults & Elderly: Refer to individual protocols.

Small cell lung cancer:

Oral: Twice the I.V. dose rounded to the nearest 50 mg given once daily if total dose ≤400 mg or in divided doses if >400 mg

I.V.: 35 mg/m²/day for 4 days or 50 mg/m²/day for 5 days every 3-4 weeks total dose ≤400 mg/day or in divided doses if >400 mg/day

IVPB: 200-250 mg/m² repeated every 7 weeks

Continuous intravenous infusion: 500 mg/m² over 24 hours every 3 weeks

Testicular cancer:

IVPB: 50-100 mg/m²/day for 5 days repeated every 3-4 weeks

I.V.: 100 mg/m² every other day for 3 doses repeated every 3-4 weeks

BMT/relapsed leukemia: *I.V.:* 2.4-3.5 g/m² or 25-70 mg/kg administered over 4-36 hours

BMT high dose: *I.V.:* 750-2400 mg/m²; 10-60 mg/kg; duration of infusion is 1-4 hours to 24 hours; generally combined with other high-dose chemotherapeutic drugs or total body irradiation (TBI).

Pediatrics: Refer to individual protocols.

Children: I.V.: 60-120 mg/m²/day for 3-5 days every 3-6 weeks

AML: I.V.:

Remission induction: 150 mg/m²/day for 2-3 days for 2-3 cycles

Intensification or consolidation: 250 mg/m²/day for 3 days, courses 2-5

Brain tumor: I.V.: 150 mg/m²/day on days 2 and 3 of treatment course

Neuroblastoma: I.V.: 100 mg/m²/day over 1 hour on days 1-5 of cycle; repeat cycle every 4 weeks

BMT conditioning regimen used in patients with rhabdomyosarcoma or neuroblastoma: I.V. continuous infusion: 160 mg/m²/day for 4 days

Conditioning regimen for allogenic BMT: I.V.: 60 mg/kg/dose as a single dose

Renal Impairment:

Cl_{cr} 10-50 mL/minute: Administer 75% of normal dose.

Cl_{cr} <10 mL minute: Administer 50% of normal dose.

Hemodialysis effects: Supplemental dose is not necessary.

CAPD effects: Unknown

CAVH effects: Unknown

Hepatic Impairment:

Bilirubin 1.5-3 mg/dL or AST 60-180 units: Reduce dose by 50%.

Bilirubin >3 mg/dL or AST >180 units: Reduce by 75%.

Available Dosage Forms [DSC] = Discontinued product

Capsule, softgel (VePesid®): 50 mg

Injection, solution: 20 mg/mL (5 mL, 25 mL, 50 mL) [may contain benzyl alcohol or alcohol]

Toposar®: 20 mg/mL (5 mL, 10 mL, 25 mL) [contains benzyl alcohol]

VePesid®: 20 mg/mL (5 mL, 7.5 mL, 25 mL, 50 mL) [contains benzyl alcohol and alcohol 30%] [DSC]

Nursing Guidelines

Assessment: See Contraindications, Warnings/Precautions, and Dosing for use cautions. Assess potential for interactions with other prescriptions, OTC medications, or herbal products patient may be taking (see Drug Interactions). See specific Administration, Dosing, Reconstitution, and Compatibility directions. Infusion site should be monitored closely to prevent extravasation (see Administration). Assess results of laboratory tests (see below), therapeutic effectiveness, and adverse response (see Adverse Reactions) prior to each treatment and on a regular basis throughout therapy. Teach patient possible side effects/appropriate interventions and adverse symptoms to report (see Patient Education). **Pregnancy risk factor D** - determine that patient is not pregnant before beginning treatment. Instruct patients of childbearing age about appropriate barrier contraceptive measures. Breast-feeding is contraindicated.

Monitoring Laboratory Tests: CBC with differential, platelet count, bilirubin, renal function

Patient Education: Inform prescriber of all prescriptions, OTC medications, or herbal products you are taking, and any allergies you have. Do not take any new medication during therapy unless approved by prescriber. This medication may be administered by infusion. Report immediately any swelling, pain, burning, or redness at infusion site. Avoid alcohol. It is important to maintain adequate hydration (2-3 L/day of fluids) unless instructed to restrict fluid intake, and adequate nutrition (small, frequent meals may help). You will be more susceptible to infection (avoid crowds and exposure to infection and do not

(Continued)

Etoposide *(Continued)*

have any vaccinations without consulting prescriber). May cause nausea or vomiting (small, frequent meals, frequent mouth care, sucking lozenges, or chewing gum may help); diarrhea (buttermilk, boiled milk, or yogurt may help); loss of hair (reversible); or mouth sores (use soft toothbrush or cotton swabs for oral care and rinse mouth frequently). Report immediately chest pain, swelling of extremities, respiratory difficulty, palpitations, or rapid heartbeat. Report extreme fatigue, pain or numbness in extremities, severe GI upset or diarrhea, bleeding or bruising, fever, chills, sore throat, vaginal discharge, respiratory difficulty, yellowing of eyes or skin, or any changes in color of urine or stool. **Pregnancy/breast-feeding precautions:** Do not get pregnant while taking this medication. Consult prescriber for appropriate contraceptive measures to use during and for 1 month following therapy. Do not breast-feed.

Pregnancy Risk Factor: D

Lactation: Enters breast milk/contraindicated

Administration

Oral: If necessary, the injection may be used for oral administration. Mix with orange juice, apple juice, or lemonade to a concentration of 0.4 mg/mL or less, and use within a 3-hour period.

I.M.: Do not administer I.M. or SubQ (severe tissue necrosis).

I.V.: Irritant. Administer lower doses IVPB over at least 30 minutes to minimize the risk of hypotensive reactions.

Reconstitution: VP-16 should be further diluted in D_5W or NS for administration. Diluted solutions have concentration-dependent stability: More concentrated solutions have shorter stability times.

At room temperature in D_5W or NS in polyvinyl chloride, the concentration is stable as follows:

0.2 mg/mL: 96 hours
0.4 mg/mL: 48 hours
0.6 mg/mL: 8 hours
1 mg/mL: 2 hours
2 mg/mL: 1 hour
20 mg/mL (undiluted): 24 hours

Standard I.V. dilution:

Lower dose regimens (<1 g/dose):

Doses may be diluted in 100-1000 mL of D_5W or NS

If the concentration is less than or equal to 0.6 mg/mL, the bag should be mixed with the appropriate expiration dating.

If the concentration is >0.6 mg/mL, the concentration is highly unstable and a syringe of undiluted etoposide accompanied with the appropriate volume of diluent will be sent to the nursing unit to be mixed at the bedside just prior to administration.

High-dose regimens (>1g/dose):

Total dose should be drawn into an empty Viaflex® container and the appropriate amount of diluent (for a final concentration of 1 mg/mL) will be sent.

Use the **2-Channel Pump Method**: Instill all of the etoposide dose into one Viaflex® container (concentration = 20 mg/mL). Infuse this into one channel (Baxter Flow-Guard 6300 Dual Channel Volumetric Infusion Pump - or any 2-channel infusion pump that does not require a "hard" plastic cassette). Infuse the indicated diluent (ie, D_5W or NS) at a rate of at least 20 times the infusion rate of the etoposide to simulate a 1 mg/mL concentration in the line. The etoposide should be Y-sited into the port most proximal to the patient. A 0.22 micron filter should be attached to the line after the Y-site and before entry into the patient.

Compatibility: Stable in D_5W, LR

Y-site administration: Incompatible with cefepime, filgrastim, idarubicin

Storage: Store intact vials of injection at room temperature and protected from light. Injection solution contains polyethylene glycol vehicle with absolute alcohol. Store oral capsules under refrigeration. Capsules are stable for 3 months at room temperature.

- Euflexxa™ *see* Hyaluronate and Derivatives *on page 856*
- Evac-U-Gen [OTC] *see* Senna *on page 1520*
- Evoclin™ *see* Clindamycin *on page 426*
- Exelon® *see* Rivastigmine *on page 1487*

♦ ex-lax® [OTC] *see* Senna *on page 1520*
♦ ex-lax® Maximum Strength [OTC] *see* Senna *on page 1520*

Ezetimibe (ez ET i mibe)

U.S. Brand Names Zetia™

Pharmacologic Category Antilipemic Agent, 2-Azetidinone

Medication Safety Issues

Sound-alike/look-alike issues:

Zetia™ may be confused with Zestril®

Use Use in combination with dietary therapy for the treatment of primary hypercholesterolemia (as monotherapy or in combination with HMG-CoA reductase inhibitors); homozygous sitosterolemia; homozygous familial hypercholesterolemia (in combination with atorvastatin or simvastatin)

Mechanism of Action Inhibits absorption of cholesterol at the brush border of the small intestine, leading to a decreased delivery of cholesterol to the liver, reduction of hepatic cholesterol stores and an increased clearance of cholesterol from the blood; decreases total C, LDL-cholesterol (LDL-C), ApoB, and triglycerides (TG) while increasing HDL-cholesterol (HDL-C).

Pharmacodynamics/Kinetics

Protein binding: >90% to plasma proteins

Metabolism: Undergoes conjugation in the small intestine and liver; forms metabolite (active); may undergo enterohepatic recycling

Bioavailability: Variable

Half-life: 22 hours (ezetimibe and metabolite)

Time to peak, plasma: 4-12 hours

Excretion: Feces (78%, 69% as ezetimibe); urine (11%, 9% as metabolite)

Contraindications Hypersensitivity to ezetimibe or any component of the formulation

Warnings/Precautions Secondary causes of hyperlipidemia should be ruled out prior to therapy. Use caution with renal or mild hepatic impairment; not recommended for use with moderate or severe hepatic impairment. Safety and efficacy have not been established in patients <10 years of age.

Drug Interactions

Bile acid sequestrants (cholestyramine): May decrease ezetimibe bioavailability; administer ≥2 hours before or ≥4 hours after bile acid sequestrants

Cyclosporine: Ezetimibe serum levels may be increased. Ezetimibe may also increase serum levels of cyclosporine. Monitor.

Fibric acid derivatives: May increase serum concentrations of ezetimibe; safety and efficacy of concomitant use not established

Adverse Reactions

1% to 10%:

Cardiovascular: Chest pain (3%), dizziness (3%), fatigue (2%)

Central nervous system: Headache (8%)

Gastrointestinal: Diarrhea (3% to 4%), abdominal pain (3%)

Neuromuscular & skeletal: Arthralgia (4%)

Respiratory: Sinusitis (4% to 5%), pharyngitis (2% to 3%, placebo 2%)

Postmarketing and/or case reports: Cholecystitis, cholelithiasis, CPK increased, hepatitis, hypersensitivity reactions (including angioedema and rash), myalgia, myopathy, nausea, pancreatitis, rhabdomyolysis, thrombocytopenia, transaminases increased

Overdosage/Toxicology Doses of up to 50 mg/day were well-tolerated. Treatment should be symptom-directed and supportive.

Dosing

Adults & Elderly:

Hyperlipidemias: Oral: 10 mg/day

Sitosterolemia: Oral: 10 mg/day

Pediatrics: Hyperlipidemias: Children ≥10 years: Refer to adult dosing.

Renal Impairment: Bioavailability increased with severe impairment; no dosing adjustment recommended.

Hepatic Impairment: Bioavailability increased with hepatic impairment

Mild impairment (Child-Pugh score 5-6): No dosing adjustment necessary.

Moderate to severe impairment (Child-Pugh score 7-15): Use of ezetimibe not recommended.

Available Dosage Forms Tablet: 10 mg [capsule shaped]

(Continued)

Ezetimibe *(Continued)*

Nursing Guidelines

Assessment: See Contraindications, Warnings/Precautions, and Dosing for use cautions. Assess potential for interactions with other prescriptions, OTC medications, or herbal products patient may be taking (see Drug Interactions). Assess results of laboratory tests prior to and periodically during therapy (see Monitoring Laboratory Tests), therapeutic effectiveness, and adverse response at beginning of and at regular intervals during therapy (see Adverse Reactions and Overdose/Toxicology). Teach patient proper use, possible side effects/appropriate interventions, and adverse reactions to report (see Patient Education). Breast-feeding is not recommended.

Monitoring Laboratory Tests: Total cholesterol profile prior to therapy, and when clinically indicated and/or periodically thereafter

Dietary Considerations: May be taken without regard to meals. Before initiation of therapy, patients should be placed on a standard cholesterol-lowering diet for 6 weeks and the diet should be continued during drug therapy.

Patient Education: Inform prescriber of all prescriptions, OTC medications, or herbal products you are taking, and any allergies you have. Do not take any new medication during therapy without consulting prescriber. Take at the same time of day, without regard for meals. Take 2 hours before or 4 hours after bile acid binding agents (ie, Questran®). This medication does not replace the need for dietary and exercise recommendations of prescriber. May cause headache, dizziness, or fatigue (use caution when driving or engaged in potentially hazardous tasks until response to drug is known); diarrhea (boiled milk, buttermilk, or yogurt may help); abdominal pain. Report any severe or persistent side effects (eg, chest pain; muscle, skeletal, or joint pain; increased perspiration).

Pregnancy/breast-feeding precautions: Inform prescriber if you are or intend to become pregnant. Breast-feeding is not recommended.

Pregnancy Risk Factor: C

Lactation: Excretion in breast milk unknown/not recommended

Administration

Oral: May be administered without regard to meals. May be taken at the same time as HMG-CoA reductase inhibitors. Administer ≥2 hours before or ≥4 hours after bile acid sequestrants.

Storage: Store at controlled room temperature of 15°C to 30°C (59°F to 86°F). Protect from moisture.

♦ **E•R•O [OTC]** *see* Carbamide Peroxide *on page 311*

♦ **Factor VIII (Recombinant)** *see* Antihemophilic Factor (Recombinant) *on page 170*

Factor VIIa (Recombinant) (FAK ter SEV en ree KOM be nant)

U.S. Brand Names NovoSeven®

Synonyms Coagulation Factor VIIa; Eptacog Alfa (Activated); rFVIIa

Pharmacologic Category Antihemophilic Agent; Blood Product Derivative

Medication Safety Issues

Sound-alike/look-alike issues:

NovoSeven® may be confused with Novacet®

Use Treatment of bleeding episodes and prevention of bleeding in surgical interventions in patients with hemophilia A or B with inhibitors to factor VIII or factor IX and in patients with congenital factor VII deficiency

Mechanism of Action Recombinant factor VIIa, a vitamin K-dependent glycoprotein, promotes hemostasis by activating the extrinsic pathway of the coagulation cascade. It replaces deficient activated coagulation factor VII, which complexes with tissue factor and may activate coagulation factor X to Xa and factor IX to IXa. When complexed with other factors, coagulation factor Xa converts prothrombin to thrombin, a key step in the formation of a fibrin-platelet hemostatic plug.

Pharmacodynamics/Kinetics

Distribution: V_d: 103 mL/kg (78-139)

Half-life elimination: 2.3 hours (1.7-2.7)

Excretion: Clearance: 33 mL/kg/hour (27-49)

Contraindications Hypersensitivity to factor VII or any component of the formulation; hypersensitivity to mouse, hamster, or bovine proteins

Warnings/Precautions Patients should be monitored for signs and symptoms of activation of the coagulation system or thrombosis. Thrombotic events may be increased in patients with disseminated intravascular coagulation (DIC), advanced atherosclerotic disease, sepsis, crush injury, or concomitant treatment with prothrombin complex concentrates. Decreased dosage or discontinuation is warranted in confirmed DIC. Efficacy with prolonged infusions and data evaluating this agent's long-term adverse effects are limited.

Adverse Reactions

1% to 10%:

Cardiovascular: Hypertension

Central nervous system: Fever

Hematologic: Hemorrhage, decreased plasma fibrinogen

Neuromuscular & skeletal: Hemarthrosis

<1% (Limited to important or life-threatening): Abnormal renal function, allergic reaction, anaphylactic reaction, arterial thrombosis, arthrosis, bradycardia, cerebral infarction and/or ischemia, coagulation disorder, consumptive coagulopathy, decreased therapeutic response, deep vein thrombosis, disseminated intravascular coagulation (DIC), edema, fibrinolysis increased, gastrointestinal bleeding, headache, hypersensitivity, hypotension, injection-site reactions, intracranial hemorrhage, localized phlebitis, MI, myocardial ischemia, pain, pneumonia, prothrombin decreased, pruritus, pulmonary embolism, purpura, rash, splenic hematoma, thrombophlebitis, thrombosis, vomiting

Overdosage/Toxicology Experience with overdose in humans is limited; an increased risk of thrombotic events may occur in overdosage. Treatment is symptomatic and supportive.

Dosing

Adults & Elderly: Hemophilia A or B with inhibitors: For I.V. administration only:

Bleeding episodes: 90 mcg/kg every 2 hours until hemostasis is achieved or until the treatment is judged ineffective. The dose and interval may be adjusted based upon the severity of bleeding and the degree of hemostasis achieved. For patients experiencing severe bleeds, dosing should be continued at 3- to 6-hour intervals after hemostasis has been achieved and the duration of dosing should be minimized.

Surgical interventions: 90 mcg/kg immediately before surgery, repeat at 2-hour intervals for the duration of surgery. Continue every 2 hours for 48 hours, then every 2-6 hours until healed for minor surgery; continue every 2 hours for 5 days, then every 4 hours until healed for major surgery.

Congenital factor VII deficiency: Bleeding episodes and surgical interventions: 15-30 mcg/kg every 4-6 hours until hemostasis. Doses as low as 10 mcg/kg have been effective.

Pediatrics: Refer to adult dosing.

Available Dosage Forms Injection, powder for reconstitution [preservative free]: 1.2 mg, 2.4 mg, 4.8 mg [latex free; contains sodium 0.44 mEq/mg rFVIIa, polysorbate 80]

Nursing Guidelines

Assessment: See Contraindications, Warnings/Precautions, and Dosing for use cautions. Assess potential for interactions with other prescriptions, OTC medications, herbal products patient may be taking - especially those medications that may affect coagulation or platelet function (see Drug Interactions). See infusion specifics. Assess results of laboratory tests (see below). During and after therapy patient should be monitored closely (eg, vital signs, cardiac and CNS status, and adverse reactions (eg, acute hypersensitivity reaction) - see Adverse Reactions and Overdose/Toxicology). Provide patient education according to patient condition.

Monitoring Laboratory Tests: Although the prothrombin time, aPTT, and factor VII clotting activity have no correlation with achieving hemostasis, these parameters may be useful as adjunct tests to evaluate efficacy and guide dose or interval adjustments

Dietary Considerations: Contains sodium 0.44 mEq/mg rFVIIa

Patient Education: This medication can only be administered I.V. Report swelling, pain, burning, or itching at infusion site. Report acute headache, visual changes, pain in joints or muscles, respiratory difficulty, chills, back pain, dizziness, nausea, or other unusual effects. **Pregnancy precaution:** Inform prescriber if you are or intend to become pregnant.

(Continued)

Factor VIIa (Recombinant) *(Continued)*

Pregnancy Risk Factor: C

Lactation: Excretion in breast milk unknown/compatible

Administration

I.V.: I.V. administration only; bolus over 2-5 minutes; administer within 3 hours after reconstitution

Reconstitution:

Prior to reconstitution, bring vials to room temperature. Reconstitute each vial to a final concentration of 0.6 mg/mL as follows:

1.2 mg vial: 2.2 mL sterile water

2.4 mg vial: 4.3 mL sterile water

4.8 mg vial: 8.5 mL sterile water

Add diluent along wall of vial, do not inject directly into powder. Gently swirl until dissolved.

Storage: Store under refrigeration (2°C to 8°C/36°F to 46°F). Protect from light. Reconstituted solutions may be stored at room temperature or under refrigeration, but must be infused within 3 hours of reconstitution.

Famotidine (fa MOE ti deen)

U.S. Brand Names Fluxid™; Pepcid®; Pepcid® AC [OTC]

Pharmacologic Category Histamine H_2 Antagonist

Use Therapy and treatment of duodenal ulcer, gastric ulcer, control gastric pH in critically-ill patients, symptomatic relief in gastritis, gastroesophageal reflux, active benign ulcer, and pathological hypersecretory conditions

OTC labeling: Relief of heartburn, acid indigestion, and sour stomach

Unlabeled/Investigational Use Part of a multidrug regimen for *H. pylori* eradication to reduce the risk of duodenal ulcer recurrence

Mechanism of Action Competitive inhibition of histamine at H_2 receptors of the gastric parietal cells, which inhibits gastric acid secretion

Pharmacodynamics/Kinetics

Onset of action: GI: Oral: Within 1-3 hour

Duration: 10-12 hours

Protein binding: 15% to 20%

Bioavailability: Oral: 40% to 50%

Half-life elimination:

Injection, oral suspension, tablet: 2.5-3.5 hours; prolonged with renal impairment; Oliguria: 20 hours

Orally-disintegrating tablet: 2.5-5 hours

Time to peak, serum: Oral: ~1-3 hours

Excretion: Urine (as unchanged drug)

Contraindications Hypersensitivity to famotidine, other H_2 antagonists, or any component of the formulation

Warnings/Precautions Modify dose in patients with renal impairment; chewable tablets contain phenylalanine; multidose vials contain benzyl alcohol

OTC labeling: When used for self-medication, patients should be instructed not to use if they have difficulty swallowing, have vomiting with blood, or bloody or black stools. Not for use with other acid reducers.

Drug Interactions

Cefpodoxime: Histamine H_2 antagonists may decrease the absorption of cefpodoxime; separate oral doses by at least 2 hours. Risk: Moderate

Cefuroxime: Histamine H_2 antagonists may decrease the absorption of cefuroxime; separate oral doses by at least 2 hours. Risk: Moderate

Cyclosporine: Histamine H_2 antagonists may increase the serum concentration of cyclosporine; monitor

Delavirdine: Delavirdine's absorption is decreased; avoid concurrent use with H_2 antagonists

Itraconazole: Histamine H_2 antagonists may decrease the absorption of itraconazole; monitor

Ketoconazole: Histamine H_2 antagonists may decrease the absorption of ketoconazole; monitor

Nutritional/Herbal/Ethanol Interactions

Ethanol: Avoid ethanol (may cause gastric mucosal irritation).

Food: Famotidine bioavailability may be increased if taken with food.

Adverse Reactions

Note: Agitation and vomiting have been reported in up to 14% of pediatric patients <1 year of age.

1% to 10%:

Central nervous system: Dizziness (1%), headache (5%)

Gastrointestinal: Constipation (1%), diarrhea (2%)

<1% (Limited to important or life-threatening): Abdominal discomfort, acne, agranulocytosis, allergic reaction, alopecia, anaphylaxis, angioedema, anorexia, arrhythmia, AST/ALT increased, bradycardia, bronchospasm, BUN/creatinine increased, drowsiness, fatigue, fever, hypertension, insomnia, jaundice, neutropenia, palpitation, paresthesia, proteinuria, pruritus, psychic disturbances, rash, seizure, tachycardia, thrombocytopenia, toxic epidermal necrolysis, urticaria, vomiting, weakness

Overdosage/Toxicology Symptoms of overdose include hypotension, tachycardia, vomiting, and drowsiness. Treatment is symptomatic and supportive.

Dosing

Adults & Elderly:

Duodenal ulcer: Oral: Acute therapy: 40 mg/day at bedtime for 4-8 weeks; maintenance therapy: 20 mg/day at bedtime

Gastric ulcer: Oral: Acute therapy: 40 mg/day at bedtime

Hypersecretory conditions: Oral: Initial: 20 mg every 6 hours, may increase in increments up to 160 mg every 6 hours

GERD: Oral: 20 mg twice daily for 6 weeks

Esophagitis and accompanying symptoms due to GERD: Oral: 20 mg or 40 mg twice daily for up to 12 weeks

Peptic ulcer disease: Eradication of *Helicobacter pylori* (unlabeled use): Oral: 40 mg once daily; requires combination therapy with antibiotics

Patients unable to take oral medication: I.V.: 20 mg every 12 hours

Heartburn, indigestion, sour stomach: OTC labeling: Oral: 10-20 mg every 12 hours; dose may be taken 15-60 minutes before eating foods known to cause heartburn

Pediatrics: Treatment duration and dose should be individualized

Peptic ulcer: 1-16 years:

Oral: 0.5 mg/kg/day at bedtime or divided twice daily (maximum dose: 40 mg/day); doses of up to 1 mg/kg/day have been used in clinical studies

I.V.: 0.25 mg/kg every 12 hours (maximum dose: 40 mg/day); doses of up to 0.5 mg/kg have been used in clinical studies

GERD: Oral:

<3 months: 0.5 mg/kg once daily

3-12 months: 0.5 mg/kg twice daily

1-16 years: 1 mg/kg/day divided twice daily (maximum dose: 40 mg twice daily); doses of up to 2 mg/kg/day have been used in clinical studies

Heartburn, indigestion, sour stomach: OTC labeling: Oral: Children ≥12 years: Refer to adult dosing.

Renal Impairment: Cl_{cr} <50 mL/minute: Manufacturer recommendation: Administer 50% of dose **or** increase the dosing interval to every 36-48 hours (to limit potential CNS adverse effects).

Available Dosage Forms [DSC] = Discontinued product

Gelcap (Pepcid® AC): 10 mg

Infusion [premixed in NS] (Pepcid®): 20 mg (50 mL)

Injection, solution: 10 mg/mL (4 mL, 20 mL, 50 mL) [contains benzyl alcohol]

Pepcid®: 10 mg/mL (4 mL [DSC], 20 mL)

Injection, solution [preservative free] (Pepcid®): 10 mg/mL (2 mL)

Powder for oral suspension (Pepcid®): 40 mg/5 mL (50 mL) [contains sodium benzoate; cherry-banana-mint flavor]

Tablet: 10 mg [OTC], 20 mg, 40 mg

Pepcid®: 20 mg, 40 mg [film coated]

Pepcid® AC: 10 mg, 20 mg

Tablet, chewable (Pepcid® AC): 10 mg [contains phenylalanine 1.4 mg/tablet; mint flavor]

Tablet, orally-disintegrating (Fluxid™): 20 mg, 40 mg [cherry flavor]

Nursing Guidelines

Assessment: See Contraindications and Warnings/Precautions for use cautions. Assess potential for interactions with other prescriptions, OTC medications, or herbal products patient may be taking (see Drug Interactions). Assess result of laboratory tests (see below) and patient response (see Adverse Reactions) prior to each treatment and on a regular basis throughout therapy. **I.V.:** See Administration specifics. Teach patient proper use, possible side effects/appropriate interventions, and adverse symptoms to report (see Patient Education). Breast-feeding is not recommended.

(Continued)

Famotidine *(Continued)*

Dietary Considerations: Phenylalanine content: Pepcid® AC chewable: Each 10 mg tablet contains phenylalanine 1.4 mg

Patient Education: Inform prescriber of all prescriptions, OTC medications, or herbal products you are taking, and any allergies you have. Do not take any new medication during therapy without consulting prescriber. Take as directed; do not alter dose or frequency or discontinue without consulting prescriber. May cause some drowsiness or dizziness (use caution when driving or engaging in tasks that require alertness until response to drug is known); constipation (increased exercise, fluids, fruit, or fiber may help); or diarrhea (buttermilk, boiled milk, or yogurt may help). Report acute headache, unresolved constipation or diarrhea, palpitations, black tarry stools, abdominal pain, rash, worsening of condition being treated, or recurrence of symptoms after therapy is completed.

Orally-disintegrating tablet: Do not break tablet.

Oral suspension: Shake well before use.

OTC: Do not use for more than 14 days unless recommended by prescriber.

Breast-feeding precaution: Breast-feeding is not recommended.

Geriatric Considerations: H_2 blockers are the preferred drugs for treating PUD in the elderly due to cost and ease of administration. They are no less or more effective than any other therapy. Famotidine is one of the preferred agents (due to side effects, drug interaction profile, and pharmacokinetics). Treatment for PUD in the elderly is recommended for 12 weeks since their lesions are typically larger; therefore, take longer to heal. Always adjust dose based upon creatinine clearance, since slight accumulation may result in CNS side effects, mainly confusion.

Pregnancy Risk Factor: B

Lactation: Enters breast milk/not recommended

Breast-Feeding Considerations: Famotidine is concentrated in breast milk, but to a lesser degree than cimetidine or ranitidine; some sources prefer its use if one of these agents is needed.

Administration

Oral:

Suspension: Shake vigorously before use. May be taken with or without food.

Tablet: May be taken with or without food.

Orally-disintegrating tablet: Place tablet on tongue with dry hands; tablet dissolves rapidly in saliva. May be taken with or without liquid or food. Do not break tablet.

I.V.:

I.V. push: Inject over at least 2 minutes

Solution for infusion: Administer over 15-30 minutes

Reconstitution: Solution for injection:

I.V. push: Dilute famotidine with NS (or another compatible solution) to a total of 5-10 mL (some centers also administer undiluted).

Infusion: Dilute with D_5W 100 mL or another compatible solution.

Compatibility: Stable in D_5W, $D_{10}W$, LR, fat emulsion 10%, NS, sodium bicarbonate 5%

Y-site administration: Incompatible with alatrofloxacin, amphotericin B cholesteryl sulfate complex, cefepime, piperacillin/tazobactam

Storage:

Oral:

Powder for oral suspension: Prior to mixing, dry powder should be stored at room temperature of 25°C (77°F). Reconstituted oral suspension is stable for 30-days at room temperature. Do not freeze.

Tablet: Store at 20°C (77°F); excursions permitted between 15°C to 30°C (59°F to 86°F). Protect from moisture.

Orally-disintegrating tablet: Store at 20°C to 25°C (68°F to 77°F); excursions permitted between 15°C to 30°C (59°F to 86°F). Protect from moisture.

I.V.:

Solution for injection: Prior to use, store at 2°C to 8°C (36°F to 46°F). If solution freezes, allow to solubilize at room temperature.

I.V. push: Following reconstitution, solutions for I.V. push should be used immediately, or may be stored in refrigerator and used within 48 hours.

Infusion: Following reconstitution, solutions for infusion are stable for 7 days at room temperature.

Solution for injection, premixed bags: Store at room temperature of 25°C (77°F). Avoid excessive heat.

Fat Emulsion (fat e MUL shun)

U.S. Brand Names Intralipid®; Liposyn® III

Synonyms Intravenous Fat Emulsion

Pharmacologic Category Caloric Agent

Use Source of calories and essential fatty acids for patients requiring parenteral nutrition of extended duration

Mechanism of Action Essential for normal structure and function of cell membranes

Pharmacodynamics/Kinetics

Metabolism: Undergoes lipolysis to free fatty acids which are utilized by reticuloendothelial cells

Half-life elimination: 0.5-1 hour

Contraindications Hypersensitivity to fat emulsion or any component of the formulation; severe egg or legume (soybean) allergies; pathologic hyperlipidemia, lipoid nephrosis pancreatitis with hyperlipemia

Warnings/Precautions Use caution in patients with severe liver damage, pulmonary disease, anemia, or blood coagulation disorder; use with caution in jaundiced, premature, and low birth weight children. Some formulations may contain aluminum which may accumulate following prolonged administration in renally-impaired patients. Premature neonates are particularly at risk of accumulation/toxicity from aluminum. To avoid hyperlipidemia and/or fat deposition, do not exceed recommended daily doses,

Adverse Reactions Frequency not defined.

Cardiovascular: Cyanosis, flushing, chest pain

Central nervous system: Headache, dizziness

Endocrine & metabolic: Hyperlipemia, hypertriglyceridemia

Gastrointestinal: Nausea, vomiting, diarrhea

Hematologic: Hypercoagulability, thrombocytopenia in neonates (rare)

Hepatic: Hepatomegaly, pancreatitis

Local: Thrombophlebitis

Respiratory: Dyspnea

Miscellaneous: Sepsis, diaphoresis, brown pigment deposition in the reticuloendothelial system (significance unknown)

Overdosage/Toxicology Rapid administration results in fluid or fat overload causing dilution of serum electrolytes, overhydration, pulmonary edema, impaired pulmonary diffusion capacity, and metabolic acidosis. Treatment is supportive.

Dosing

Adults & Elderly:

Caloric source: I.V. (fat emulsion should not exceed 60% of the total daily calories): Initial: 1 g/kg/day, increase by 0.5-1 g/kg/day to a maximum of 2.5 g/kg/day of 10% and 3 g/kg/day of 20%; maximum rate of infusion: 0.25 g/kg/hour (1.25 mL/kg/hour of 20% solution); do not exceed 50 mL/hour (20%) or 100 mL/hour (10%)

Prevention of fatty acid deficiency (8% to 10% of total caloric intake): I.V.:

0.5-1 g/kg/24 hours

500 mL twice weekly at rate of 1 mL/minute for 30 minutes, then increase to 500 mL over 4-6 hours

Note: May be used on a daily basis as a caloric source in TPN

Pediatrics:

Caloric source: I.V. (fat emulsion should not exceed 60% of the total daily calories):

Premature Infants: Initial dose: 0.25-0.5 g/kg/day, increase by 0.25-0.5 g/kg/day to a maximum of 3 g/kg/day depending on needs/nutritional goals; limit to 1 g/kg/day if on phototherapy; maximum rate of infusion: 0.15 g/kg/hour (0.75 mL/kg/hour of 20% solution)

Infants and Children: Initial dose: 0.5-1 g/kg/day, increase by 0.5 g/kg/day to a maximum of 3 g/kg/day depending on needs/nutritional goals; maximum rate of infusion: 0.25 g/kg/hour (1.25 mL/kg/hour of 20% solution)

Adolescents: Refer to adult dosing.

Prevention of essential fatty acid deficiency (8% to 10% of total caloric intake): I.V.: 0.5-1 g/kg/24 hours

Children: 5-10 mL/kg/day at 0.1 mL/minute then up to 100 mL/hour

(Continued)

Fat Emulsion *(Continued)*

Available Dosage Forms Injection, emulsion [soybean oil]:

Intralipid®: 10% [100 mg/mL] (100 mL, 250 mL, 500 mL); 20% [200 mg/mL] (50 mL, 100 mL, 250 mL, 500 mL, 1000 mL); 30% [300 mg/mL] (500 mL)

Liposyn® III: 10% [100 mg/mL] (200 mL, 500 mL); 20% [200 mg/mL] (200 mL, 500 mL); 30% [300 mg/mL] (500 mL)

Nursing Guidelines

Assessment: Assess for allergy to eggs prior to initiating therapy (pruritic urticaria can occur in patients allergic to eggs). Inspect emulsion before administering. Do not administer if oil separation or oiliness is noted. Monitor closely for allergic reactions, fluid overload, thrombosis or sepsis.

Monitoring Laboratory Tests: Serum triglycerides before initiation of therapy and at least weekly during therapy. Frequent (some advise daily) platelet counts should be performed in neonatal patients receiving parenteral lipids.

Patient Education: Report pain at infusion site, respiratory difficulty, chest pain, calf pain, or excessive sweating. **Pregnancy precaution:** Inform prescriber if you are pregnant

Pregnancy Risk Factor: C

Lactation: Excretion in breast milk unknown/compatible

Administration

I.V.: At the onset of therapy, the patient should be observed for any immediate allergic reactions such as dyspnea, cyanosis, and fever. Infuse for 10-15 minutes at a slower rate. Infuse 10% at 1 mL/minute. If no untoward effects, may increase rate to 500 mL over 4-6 hours. Infuse 20% at 0.5 mL/minute initially; increase to rate of 250 mL over 4-6 hours.

Storage: May be stored at room temperature. Do not store partly used bottles for later use. Do not use if emulsion appears to be oiling out.

♦ Feiba VH® *see* Anti-inhibitor Coagulant Complex *on page 172*

Felodipine (fe LOE di peen)

U.S. Brand Names Plendil®

Pharmacologic Category Calcium Channel Blocker

Medication Safety Issues

Sound-alike/look-alike issues:

Plendil® may be confused with Isordil®, pindolol, Pletal®, Prilosec®, Prinivil®

Use Treatment of hypertension

Mechanism of Action Inhibits calcium ions from entering the "slow channels" or select voltage-sensitive areas of vascular smooth muscle and myocardium during depolarization, producing a relaxation of coronary vascular smooth muscle and coronary vasodilation; increases myocardial oxygen delivery in patients with vasospastic angina

Pharmacodynamics/Kinetics

Onset of action: Antihypertensive: 2-5 hours

Duration of antihypertensive effect: 24 hours

Absorption: 100%; Absolute: 20% due to first-pass effect

Protein binding: >99%

Metabolism: Hepatic; CYP3A4 substrate (major); extensive first-pass effect

Half-life elimination: Immediate release: 11-16 hours

Excretion: Urine (70% as metabolites); feces 10%

Contraindications Hypersensitivity to felodipine, any component of the formulation, or other calcium channel blocker

Warnings/Precautions Watch for hypotension and syncope (can rarely occur). Reflex tachycardia may occur. Use caution in patients with heart failure particularly with concurrent beta-blocker use. Elderly patients and patients with hepatic impairment should start off with a lower dose. Peripheral edema is the most common side effect (occurs within 2-3 weeks of starting therapy). Use caution in hepatic impairment. Safety and efficacy in children have not been established. Dosage titration should occur after 14 days on a given dose.

Drug Interactions Substrate of CYP3A4 (major); **Inhibits** CYP2C8/9 (weak), 2D6 (weak), 3A4 (weak)

Azole antifungals may inhibit calcium channel blocker's metabolism; avoid this combination. Try an antifungal like terbinafine (if appropriate) or monitor closely for altered effect of the calcium channel blocker.

Beta-blockers may have increased pharmacokinetic or pharmacodynamic interactions with felodipine.

Calcium may reduce the calcium channel blocker's effects, particularly hypotension.

Carbamazepine significantly reduces felodipine's bioavailability; avoid this combination.

Cimetidine may inhibit felodipine metabolism (AUC increased by 50%); use caution and monitor for potential hypotension.

Cyclosporine increases felodipine's serum concentration; avoid the combination or reduce dose of felodipine and monitor blood pressure.

CYP3A4 inducers: CYP3A4 inducers may decrease the levels/effects of felodipine. Example inducers include aminoglutethimide, carbamazepine, nafcillin, nevirapine, phenobarbital, phenytoin, and rifamycins.

CYP3A4 inhibitors: May increase the levels/effects of felodipine. Example inhibitors include azole antifungals, clarithromycin, diclofenac, doxycycline, erythromycin, imatinib, isoniazid, nefazodone, nicardipine, propofol, protease inhibitors, quinidine, telithromycin, and verapamil.

Erythromycin decreases felodipine's metabolism; coadministration results in a twofold increase in the AUC and half-life of felodipine; monitor for hypotension.

Nafcillin decreases plasma concentration of felodipine; avoid this combination.

Rifampin increases the metabolism of the calcium channel blocker; adjust the dose of the calcium channel blocker to maintain efficacy.

Sildenafil, tadalafil, vardenafil: Blood pressure-lowering effects may be additive; use caution.

Tacrolimus: Felodipine may increase tacrolimus serum levels; monitor.

Nutritional/Herbal/Ethanol Interactions

Ethanol: Increases felodipine's absorption; watch for a greater hypotensive effect.

Food: Increased therapeutic and vasodilator side effects, including severe hypotension and myocardial ischemia, may occur if felodipine is taken with grapefruit juice; avoid concurrent use. High-fat/carbohydrate meals will increase C_{max} by 60%; grapefruit juice will increase C_{max} by twofold.

Herb/Nutraceutical: St John's wort may decrease felodipine levels. Avoid dong quai if using for hypertension (has estrogenic activity). Avoid ephedra, yohimbe, ginseng (may worsen hypertension). Avoid garlic (may have increased antihypertensive effect).

Adverse Reactions

>10%: Central nervous system: Headache (11% to 15%)

2% to 10%: Cardiovascular: Peripheral edema (2% to 17%), tachycardia (0.4% to 2.5%), flushing (4% to 7%)

<1% (Limited to important or life-threatening): Angina, angioedema, anxiety, arrhythmia, CHF, CVA, libido decreased, depression, dizziness, gingival hyperplasia, dyspnea, dysuria, gynecomastia, hypotension, impotence, insomnia, irritability, leukocytoclastic vasculitis, MI, nervousness, paresthesia, somnolence, syncope, urticaria, vomiting

Overdosage/Toxicology Primary cardiac symptoms of calcium blocker overdose include hypotension and bradycardia. Noncardiac symptoms include confusion, stupor, nausea, vomiting, metabolic acidosis, and hyperglycemia. Treat symptomatically.

Dosing

Adults: Hypertension: Oral: 5-10 mg once daily; increase by 5 mg at 2-week intervals, as needed, to a maximum of 20 mg/day; usual dose range (JNC 7): 2.5-20 mg once daily.

Elderly: Oral: Initial 2.5 mg/day

Hepatic Impairment: Initial: 2.5 mg/day; monitor blood pressure

Available Dosage Forms Tablet, extended release: 2.5 mg, 5 mg, 10 mg

Nursing Guidelines

Assessment: See Warnings/Precautions for use cautions. Assess potential for interactions with prescription, OTC medications, or herbal products patient may be taking (eg, beta blockers or other drugs that effect blood pressure - see Drug Interactions). Assess for therapeutic effectiveness and signs/symptoms of adverse reactions at beginning of therapy, when changing dosage, and periodically throughout long-term therapy (see Adverse Reactions and Overdose/Toxicology). When discontinuing, taper gradually (over 2 weeks). Teach patient proper use, possible side effects/interventions, and adverse symptoms to report (see Patient Education). Note breast-feeding caution.

Dietary Considerations: Should be taken without food.

Patient Education: Inform prescriber of all prescriptions, OTC medications, or herbal products you are using and any allergies you have. Do not take any new

(Continued)

Felodipine *(Continued)*

medication during therapy unless approved by prescriber. Take exactly as directed, without food. Avoid concurrent grapefruit juice and alcohol (may cause hypotension). Swallow whole, do not crush or chew. Do not alter dose or stop taking without consulting prescriber. May cause headache (consult prescriber for analgesic); nausea or vomiting (small, frequent meals, frequent mouth care, chewing gum, or sucking lozenges may help); constipation (increased dietary bulk and fluids may help); or drowsiness (use caution when driving or engaging in tasks that require alertness until response to drug is known). Report irregular heartbeat, chest pain or palpitations; persistent headache; vomiting; constipation; peripheral or facial swelling; weight gain >5 lb/week; dyspnea or respiratory changes. **Pregnancy/breast-feeding precautions:** Inform prescriber if you are or intend to become pregnant. Consult prescriber if breast-feeding.

Geriatric Considerations: Elderly may experience a greater hypotensive response. Theoretically, constipation may be more of a problem in the elderly.

Pregnancy Risk Factor: C

Pregnancy Issues: Potentially, calcium channel blockers may prolong labor. There are no adequate or well-controlled studies in pregnant women.

Lactation: Excretion in breast milk unknown/not recommended

Administration

Oral: Do not crush or chew extended release tablets; swallow whole.

◆ **Femilax™ [OTC]** *see* Bisacodyl *on page 245*

◆ **Femring™** *see* Estradiol *on page 649*

◆ **Femtrace®** *see* Estradiol *on page 649*

Fenofibrate (fen oh FYE brate)

U.S. Brand Names Antara™; Lofibra™; TriCor®; Triglide™

Synonyms Procetofene; Proctofene

Pharmacologic Category Antilipemic Agent, Fibric Acid

Use Adjunct to dietary therapy for the treatment of adults with elevations of serum triglyceride levels (types IV and V hyperlipidemia); adjunct to dietary therapy for the reduction of low density lipoprotein cholesterol (LDL-C), total cholesterol (total-C), triglycerides, and apolipoprotein B (apo B) in adult patients with primary hypercholesterolemia or mixed dyslipidemia (Fredrickson types IIa and IIb)

Mechanism of Action Fenofibric acid is believed to increase VLDL catabolism by enhancing the synthesis of lipoprotein lipase; as a result of a decrease in VLDL levels, total plasma triglycerides are reduced by 30% to 60%; modest increase in HDL occurs in some hypertriglyceridemic patients

Pharmacodynamics/Kinetics

Absorption: Increased when taken with meals

Distribution: Widely to most tissues

Protein binding: >99%

Metabolism: Tissue and plasma via esterases to active form, fenofibric acid; undergoes inactivation by glucuronidation hepatically or renally

Half-life elimination: 16-23 hours

Time to peak: 3-8 hours

Excretion: Urine (60% as metabolites); feces (25%); hemodialysis has no effect on removal of fenofibric acid from plasma

Contraindications Hypersensitivity to fenofibrate or any component of the formulation; hepatic or severe renal dysfunction including primary biliary cirrhosis and unexplained persistent liver function abnormalities; pre-existing gallbladder disease

Warnings/Precautions Hepatic transaminases can become significantly elevated (dose-related); hepatocellular, chronic active, and cholestatic hepatitis have been reported. Regular monitoring of liver function tests is required. May cause cholelithiasis. Use caution with warfarin; adjustments in warfarin therapy may be required. Use caution with HMG-CoA reductase inhibitors (may lead to myopathy, rhabdomyolysis). Therapy should be withdrawn if an adequate response is not obtained after 2 months of therapy at the maximal daily dose. May cause mild to moderate decreases in hemoblogin, hematocrit and WBC upon initiation of therapy which usually stabilizes with long-term therapy. Rare hypersensitivity reactions may occur. Dose adjustment is required for renal impairment and elderly patients. Safety and efficacy in children have not been established.

Drug Interactions Substrate of CYP3A4 (minor); **Inhibits** (weak) CYP1A6, 2C9, 2C19

Bile acid sequestrants: May decrease absorption of fenofibrate; administer fenofibrate at least 1 hour before or 4-6 hours after a bile acid binding resin.

Ezetimibe: Fibric acid derivatives may increase serum concentrations of ezetimibe.

HMG-CoA reductase inhibitors (atorvastatin, fluvastatin, lovastatin, pravastatin, rosuvastatin, simvastatin): May increase the risk of myopathy and rhabdomyolysis. The manufacturer warns against concomitant use. However, combination therapy with statins has been used in some patients with resistant hyperlipidemias (with great caution).

Sulfonylureas: Fibric acid derivatives may enhance the hypoglycemic effects of sulfonylureas.

Warfarin: Increased anticoagulant response; monitor INRs closely when fenofibrate is initiated or discontinued.

Adverse Reactions

1% to 10%:

Gastrointestinal: Abdominal pain (5%), constipation (2%)

Hepatic: Liver function tests abnormal (8%), ALT/AST increased (3%), creatine phosphokinase increased (3%)

Neuromuscular & skeletal: Back pain (3%)

Respiratory: Respiratory disorder (6%), rhinitis (2%)

Frequency not defined:

Cardiovascular: Angina pectoris, arrhythmia, atrial fibrillation, cardiovascular disorder, chest pain, coronary artery disorder, edema, electrocardiogram abnormality, extrasystoles, hyper-/hypotension, MI, palpitation, peripheral edema, peripheral vascular disorder, phlebitis, tachycardia, varicose veins, vasodilatation

Central nervous system: Anxiety, depression, dizziness, fever, headache, insomnia, malaise, nervousness, neuralgia, pain, somnolence, vertigo

Dermatologic: Acne, alopecia, bruising, contact dermatitis, eczema, fungal dermatitis, maculopapular rash, nail disorder, photosensitivity reaction, pruritus, skin ulcer, Stevens-Johnson syndrome, toxic epidermal necrolysis, urticaria

Endocrine & metabolic: Diabetes mellitus, gout, gynecomastia, hypoglycemia, hyperuricemia, libido decreased

Gastrointestinal: Anorexia, appetite increased, colitis, diarrhea, dry mouth, duodenal ulcer, dyspepsia, eructation, esophagitis, flatulence, gastroenteritis, gastritis, gastrointestinal disorder, nausea, peptic ulcer, rectal disorder, rectal hemorrhage, tooth disorder, vomiting, weight gain/loss

Genitourinary: Cystitis, dysuria, prostatic disorder, libido decreased, pregnancy (unintended), urinary frequency, urolithiasis, vaginal moniliasis

Hematologic: Agranulocytosis, anemia, eosinophilia, leukopenia, lymphadenopathy, thrombocytopenia

Hepatic: Cholelithiasis, cholecystitis, fatty liver deposits

Neuromuscular & skeletal: Arthralgia, arthritis, arthrosis, bursitis, hypertonia, joint disorder, leg cramps, muscle pain, myalgia, myasthenia, myopathy, myositis, paresthesia, rhabdomyolysis, tenderness, tenosynovitis, weakness

Ocular: Abnormal vision, amblyopia, cataract, conjunctivitis, eye disorder, refraction disorder

Otic: Ear pain, otitis media

Renal: Creatinine increased, kidney function abnormality

Respiratory: Asthma, bronchitis, cough increased, dyspnea, laryngitis, pharyngitis, pneumonia, sinusitis

Miscellaneous: Allergic reaction, cyst, diaphoresis, hernia, herpes simplex, herpes zoster, hypersensitivity reaction, infection

Overdosage/Toxicology Symptoms of overdose include nausea, vomiting, diarrhea, and GI distress. Treatment is supportive. Hemodialysis has no effect on removal of fenofibric acid from the plasma.

Dosing

Adults:

Hypertriglyceridemia: Oral: Initial:

Antara™: 43-130 mg/day

Lofibra™: 67 mg/day with meals, up to 200 mg/day

TriCor®: 48 mg/day, up to 145 mg/day

Previously dosed as 54 mg/day with meals (up to 160 mg/day) using the old tablet formulation

Triglide™: 50-160 mg/day

(Continued)

Fenofibrate *(Continued)*

Hypercholesterolemia or mixed hyperlipidemia: Oral:
Antara™: 130 mg/day
Lofibra™: 200 mg/day with meals
TriCor®: 145 mg/day
Previously dosed as 160 mg/day with meals using the old tablet formulation
Triglide™: 160 mg/day

Elderly: Oral: Initial:
Antara™: 43 mg/day
Lofibra™: 67 mg/day
TriCor®: 48 mg/day
Triglide™: 50 mg/day

Renal Impairment: Monitor renal function and lipid panel before adjusting. Decrease dose or increase dosing interval for patients with renal failure: Initial:
Antara™: 43 mg/day
Lofibra™: 67 mg/day
TriCor®: 48 mg/day
Triglide™: 50 mg/day

Available Dosage Forms [DSC] = Discontinued product

Capsule [micronized]:
Antara™: 43 mg, 87 mg, 130 mg
Lofibra™: 67 mg, 134 mg, 200 mg

Tablet :
TriCor®: 54 mg [DSC], 160 mg [DSC]
TriCor® [new formulation]: 48 mg, 145 mg
Triglide™: 50 mg, 160 mg

Nursing Guidelines

Assessment: Use caution and monitor closely in presence of hepatic or renal dysfunction, gallbladder disease, and advanced age. Assess potential for interactions with other pharmacological agents the patient may be taking (eg, increased risk of myopathy and rhabdomyolysis). Assess result of laboratory tests and patient response on a regular basis throughout therapy (eg, arrhythmias, gastrointestinal upset, CNS changes, hypoglycemia, myalgia). Teach patient possible side effects/appropriate interventions and adverse symptoms to report.

Monitoring Laboratory Tests: Total serum cholesterol and triglyceride concentration and CLDL, LDL, and HDL levels should be measured periodically; if only marginal changes are noted in 6-8 weeks, the drug should be discontinued. Serum transaminases should be measured every 3 months; if ALT values increase >100 units/L, therapy should be discontinued. Monitor LFTs prior to initiation, at 6 and 12 weeks after initiation or first dose, then periodically thereafter.

Dietary Considerations:
Lofibra™: Take with meals.
Antara™, TriCor®, Triglide™: May be taken with or without food.

Patient Education: Do not take any new medication during therapy without consulting prescriber. Take as directed with food. Do not change dosage, dosage form, or frequency without consulting prescriber. Maintain diet and exercise program as prescribed. If you are a diabetic taking a sulfonylurea, monitor blood sugars closely; this medication may alter the effects of your antidiabetic medication. May cause mild GI disturbances (eg, gas, diarrhea, constipation, nausea); inform prescriber if these are severe. Report immediately unusual muscle pain or weakness, skin rash or irritation, insomnia, persistent dizziness; chest pain or palpitations; difficult respirations; or any other persistent adverse effects. **Pregnancy/breast-feeding precautions:** Inform prescriber if you are or intend to become pregnant. Breast-feeding is not recommended.

Pregnancy Risk Factor: C

Pregnancy Issues: Although teratogenicity and mutagenicity tests in animals have been negative, significant risk has been identified with clofibrate. Use should be avoided, if possible, in pregnant women since the neonatal glucuronide conjugation pathways are immature.

Lactation: Excretion in breast milk unknown/not recommended

Breast-Feeding Considerations: Tumor formation was observed in animal studies; nursing is not recommended if the medication cannot be discontinued.

Administration

Oral: 6-8 weeks of therapy is required to determine efficacy.

Lofibra™: Administer with meals.

Antara™, TriCor®, Triglide™: May be administered with or without food.

Storage: Store at controlled room temperature. Protect from moisture.

Fenoldopam (fe NOL doe pam)

U.S. Brand Names Corlopam®

Synonyms Fenoldopam Mesylate

Pharmacologic Category Dopamine Agonist

Use Treatment of severe hypertension (up to 48 hours in adults), including in patients with renal compromise; short-term (up to 4 hours) blood pressure reduction in pediatric patients

Mechanism of Action A selective postsynaptic dopamine agonist (D_1-receptors) which exerts hypotensive effects by decreasing peripheral vasculature resistance with increased renal blood flow, diuresis, and natriuresis; 6 times as potent as dopamine in producing renal vasodilitation; has minimal adrenergic effects

Pharmacodynamics/Kinetics

Onset of action: I.V.: 10 minutes

Duration: I.V.: 1 hour

Distribution: V_d: 0.6 L/kg

Half-life elimination: I.V.: Children: 3-5 minutes; Adults: ~5 minutes

Metabolism: Hepatic via methylation, glucuronidation, and sulfation; the 8-sulfate metabolite may have some activity; extensive first-pass effect

Excretion: Urine (90%); feces (10%)

Contraindications Hypersensitivity of fenoldopam or any component of the formulation

Warnings/Precautions Use caution in patients with glaucoma or intraocular hypertension. A dose-related tachycardia can occur, especially at infusion rates >0.1 mcg/kg/minute. Use caution in angina patients (can increase myocardial oxygen demand with tachycardia). Close monitoring of blood pressure is necessary (hypotension can occur). Monitor for hypokalemia at intervals of 6 hours during infusion. For continuous infusion only (no bolus doses). The effects of hemodialysis on the pharmacokinetics of fenoldopam have not been evaluated. Use caution with increased intracranial pressure. Contains sulfites; may cause allergic reaction in susceptible individuals.

Drug Interactions

Concurrent acetaminophen may increase fenoldopam levels (30% to 70%).

Beta-blockers increase the risk of hypotension. Avoid concurrent use; if used concurrently, close monitoring is recommended.

Adverse Reactions Frequency not always defined.

Cardiovascular: Angina, asymptomatic T wave flattening on ECG, chest pain, edema, facial flushing (>5%), fibrillation (atrial), flutter (atrial), hypotension (>5%), tachycardia

Central nervous system: Dizziness, headache (>5%)

Endocrine & metabolic: Hypokalemia

Gastrointestinal: Abdominal pain/fullness, diarrhea, nausea (>5%), vomiting, xerostomia

Local: Injection site reactions

Ocular: Intraocular pressure (increased), blurred vision

Hepatic: Increases in portal pressure in cirrhotic patients

Dosing

Adults & Elderly: Hypertension, severe: I.V.: Initial: 0.1-0.3 mcg/kg/minute (lower initial doses may be associated with less reflex tachycardia); may be increased in increments of 0.05-0.1 mcg/kg/minute every 15 minutes until target blood pressure is reached; the maximal infusion rate reported in clinical studies was 1.6 mcg/kg/minute

Pediatrics: Hypertension, severe: I.V.: Initial: 0.2 mcg/kg/minute; may be increased to dosages of 0.3-0.5 mcg/kg/minute every 20-30 minutes (maximum dose: 0.8 mcg/kg/minute); limited to short-term (4 hours) use

Renal Impairment: No guidelines are available.

Available Dosage Forms Injection, solution: 10 mg/mL (1 mL, 2 mL) [contains sodium metabisulfite and propylene glycol]

(Continued)

Fenoldopam *(Continued)*

Nursing Guidelines

Pregnancy Risk Factor: B

Lactation: Excretion in breast milk unknown/use caution

Perioperative/Anesthesia/Other Concerns: Suitable for use in patients whose condition is unstable or rapidly changing because the effects of the drug are predictable and easily reversible; it has been found to safely control blood pressure in patients with a variety of pre-existing conditions including kidney disease, liver disease, and heart failure. (Clinical benefit other than blood pressure reduction has not been established.) Dosage adjustment is not required in any of these situations. The drug is quickly metabolized into inactive substances before it is excreted. Unlike the situation with some other intravenous antihypertensives, the patient does not need an arterial line for blood pressure monitoring; a blood pressure cuff is sufficient. Since the drug induces natriuresis, diuresis, and increased creatinine clearance, it may have an advantage over nitroprusside, especially in patients with severe renal insufficiency and in volume-overloaded patients.

Contrast Nephropathy: Fenoldopam is ineffective in the prevention of contrast-induced nephropathy.

Administration

I.V.: For I.V. infusion using an infusion pump.

Reconstitution: Must be diluted prior to infusion; compatible with NS or D_5W. Final dilution for children is 60 mcg/mL and for adults is 40 mcg/mL.

Storage: Store at 2°C to 30°C (35°F to 86°F). Following dilution, store at room temperature and use solution within 24 hours.

Related Information

Postoperative Hypertension *on page 1815*

♦ **Fenoldopam Mesylate** *see* Fenoldopam *on page 711*

Fentanyl (FEN ta nil)

U.S. Brand Names Actiq®; Duragesic®; Sublimaze®

Synonyms Fentanyl Citrate

Pharmacologic Category Analgesic, Narcotic; General Anesthetic

Medication Safety Issues

Sound-alike/look-alike issues:

Fentanyl may be confused with alfentanil, sufentanil

New patch dosage form of Duragesic®-12 actually delivers 12.5 mcg/hour of fentanyl. Use caution, as orders may be written as "Duragesic 12.5" which can be erroneously interpreted as a 125 mcg dose.

Transdermal patch may contain conducting metal (eg, aluminum); remove patch prior to MRI.

Use

Injection: Sedation, relief of pain, preoperative medication, adjunct to general or regional anesthesia

Transdermal: Management of moderate-to-severe chronic pain

Transmucosal (Actiq®): Management of breakthrough cancer pain

Mechanism of Action Binds with stereospecific receptors at many sites within the CNS, increases pain threshold, alters pain reception, inhibits ascending pain pathways

Pharmacodynamics/Kinetics

Onset of action: Analgesic: I.M.: 7-15 minutes; I.V.: Almost immediate; Transmucosal: 5-15 minutes

Peak effect: Transmucosal: Analgesic: 20-30 minutes

Duration: I.M.: 1-2 hours; I.V.: 0.5-1 hour; Transmucosal: Related to blood level; respiratory depressant effect may last longer than analgesic effect

Absorption: Transmucosal: Rapid, ~25% from the buccal mucosa; 75% swallowed with saliva and slowly absorbed from GI tract

Distribution: Highly lipophilic, redistributes into muscle and fat

Metabolism: Hepatic, primarily via CYP3A4

Bioavailability: Transmucosal: ~50% (range: 36% to 71%)

Half-life elimination: 2-4 hours; Transmucosal: 6.6 hours (range: 5-15 hours); Transdermal: 17 hours (half-life is influenced by absorption rate)

Time to peak: Transdermal: 24-72 hours

Excretion: Urine (primarily as metabolites, 10% as unchanged drug)

Contraindications Hypersensitivity to fentanyl or any component of the formulation; increased intracranial pressure; severe respiratory disease or depression including acute asthma (unless patient is mechanically ventilated); paralytic ileus; severe liver or renal insufficiency; pregnancy (prolonged use or high doses near term)

Transmucosal lozenges (Actiq®) or transdermal patches must not be used in patients who are not opioid tolerant. Patients are considered opioid-tolerant if they are taking at least 60 mg morphine/day, 30 mg oral oxycodone/day, 8 mg oral hydromorphone/day, 25 mcg transdermal fentanyl/hour, or an equivalent dose of another opioid for ≥1 week. Transdermal patches are not for use in acute pain, mild pain, intermittent pain, or postoperative pain management.

Warnings/Precautions An opioid-containing analgesic regimen should be tailored to each patient's needs and based upon the type of pain being treated (acute versus chronic), the route of administration, degree of tolerance for opioids (naive versus chronic user), age, weight, and medical condition. The optimal analgesic dose varies widely among patients. Doses should be titrated to pain relief/prevention. When using with other CNS depressants, reduce dose of one or both agents. Fentanyl shares the toxic potentials of opiate agonists, and precautions of opiate agonist therapy should be observed; use with caution in patients with bradycardia; rapid I.V. infusion may result in skeletal muscle and chest wall rigidity leading to respiratory distress and/or apnea, bronchoconstriction, laryngospasm; inject slowly over 3-5 minutes. Tolerance or drug dependence may result from extended use. Use caution in patients with a history of drug dependence or abuse. The elderly may be particularly susceptible to the CNS depressant and constipating effects of narcotics. Use extreme caution in patients with COPD or other chronic respiratory conditions.

Actiq® should be used only for the care of cancer patients and is intended for use by specialists who are knowledgeable in treating cancer pain. For patients who have received transmucosal product within 6-12 hours, it is recommended that if other narcotics are required, they should be used at starting doses 1/4 to 1/3 those usually recommended. Actiq® preparations contain an amount of medication that can be fatal to children. Keep all units out of the reach of children and discard any open units properly. Patients and caregivers should be counseled on the dangers to children including the risk of exposure to partially-consumed units.

Topical patches: Serious or life-threatening hypoventilation may occur, even in opioid-tolerant patients. Serum fentanyl concentrations may increase approximately one-third for patients with a body temperature of 40°C secondary to a temperature-dependent increase in fentanyl release from the system and increased skin permeability. Avoid exposure of application site to direct external heat sources. Patients who experience adverse reactions should be monitored for at least 24 hours after removal of the patch. Transdermal patch may contain conducting metal (eg, aluminum); remove patch prior to MRI. Safety and efficacy of transdermal system have been limited to children ≥2 years of age who are opioid tolerant.

Drug Interactions **Substrate** of CYP3A4 (major); **Inhibits** CYP3A4 (weak)

CNS depressants: Increased sedation with CNS depressants, phenothiazines

CYP3A4 inhibitors: May increase the levels/effects of fentanyl. Potentially fatal respiratory depression may occur when a potent inhibitor is used in a patient receiving chronic fentanyl (eg, transdermal). Example inhibitors include azole antifungals, clarithromycin, diclofenac, doxycycline, erythromycin, imatinib, isoniazid, nefazodone, nicardipine, propofol, protease inhibitors, quinidine, telithromycin, and verapamil.

MAO inhibitors: Not recommended to use Actiq® within 14 days. Severe and unpredictable potentiation by MAO inhibitors has been reported with opioid analgesics.

Nutritional/Herbal/Ethanol Interactions

Ethanol: Avoid ethanol (may increase CNS depression).

Food: Glucose may cause hyperglycemia.

Herb/Nutraceutical: St John's wort may decrease fentanyl levels. Avoid valerian, St John's wort, kava kava, gotu kola (may increase CNS depression).

Adverse Reactions

>10%:

Cardiovascular: Hypotension, bradycardia

Central nervous system: CNS depression, confusion, drowsiness, sedation

Gastrointestinal: Nausea, vomiting, constipation, xerostomia

Neuromuscular & skeletal: Chest wall rigidity (high dose I.V.), weakness

Ocular: Miosis

(Continued)

Fentanyl *(Continued)*

Respiratory: Respiratory depression
Miscellaneous: Diaphoresis

1% to 10%:

Cardiovascular: Cardiac arrhythmia, edema, orthostatic hypotension, hypertension, syncope

Central nervous system: Abnormal dreams, abnormal thinking, agitation, amnesia, dizziness, euphoria, fatigue, fever, hallucinations, headache, insomnia, nervousness, paranoid reaction

Dermatologic: Erythema, papules, pruritus, rash

Gastrointestinal: Abdominal pain, anorexia, biliary tract spasm, diarrhea, dyspepsia, flatulence

Local: Application site reaction

Neuromuscular & skeletal: Abnormal coordination, abnormal gait, back pain, paresthesia, rigors, tremor

Respiratory: Apnea, bronchitis, dyspnea, hemoptysis, pharyngitis, rhinitis, sinusitis, upper respiratory infection

Miscellaneous: Hiccups, flu-like syndrome, speech disorder

<1% (Limited to important or life-threatening): Abdominal distention, ADH release, amblyopia, anorgasmia, aphasia, bladder pain, blurred vision, bradycardia, bronchospasm, circulatory depression, CNS excitation or delirium, cold/clammy skin, convulsions, dental caries (Actiq®), depersonalization, dysesthesia, ejaculatory difficulty, exfoliative dermatitis, gum line erosion (Actiq®), hyper-/hypotonia, hostility, laryngospasm, libido decreased, oliguria, paradoxical dizziness, physical and psychological dependence with prolonged use, polyuria, pustules, stertorous breathing, stupor, tachycardia, tooth loss (Actiq®), urinary tract spasm, urticaria, vertigo, weight loss

Overdosage/Toxicology Symptoms of overdose include CNS depression, respiratory depression, and miosis; muscle and chest wall rigidity (may require nondepolarizing skeletal muscle relaxant). Treatment is supportive. Naloxone, 2 mg I.V. with repeat administration as necessary up to a total of 10 mg, can also be used to reverse toxic effects of the opiate. Patients who experience adverse reactions during use of transdermal fentanyl should be monitored for at least 24 hours after removal of the patch.

Dosing

Adults: Note: These are guidelines and do not represent the maximum doses that may be required in all patients. Doses should be titrated to pain relief/prevention. Monitor vital signs routinely. Single I.M. doses have a duration of 1-2 hours, single I.V. doses last 0.5-1 hour.

Sedation for minor procedures/analgesia: I.V.: 25-50 mcg; may repeat every 3-5 minutes to desired effect or adverse event; maximum dose of 500 mcg/4 hours; higher doses are used for major procedures

Surgery:

Premedication: I.M., slow I.V.: 25-100 mcg/dose 30-60 minutes prior to surgery

Adjunct to regional anesthesia: Slow I.V.: 25-100 mcg/dose over 1-2 minutes. **Note:** An I.V. should be in place with regional anesthesia so the I.M. route is rarely used but still maintained as an option in the package labeling.

Adjunct to general anesthesia: Slow I.V.:

Low dose: 0.5-2 mcg/kg/dose depending on the indication. For example, 0.5 mcg/kg will provide analgesia or reduce the amount of propofol needed for laryngeal mask airway insertion with minimal respiratory depression. However, to blunt the hemodynamic response to intubation 2 mcg/kg is often necessary.

Moderate dose: Initial: 2-15 mcg/kg/dose; maintenance (bolus or infusion): 1-2 mcg/kg/hour. Discontinuing fentanyl infusion 30-60 minutes prior to the end of surgery will usually allow adequate ventilation upon emergence from anesthesia. For "fast-tracking" and early extubation following major surgery, total fentanyl doses are limited to 10-15 mcg/kg.

High dose: **Note:** High-dose (20-50 mcg/kg/dose) fentanyl is rarely used, but is still maintained in the package labeling.

Acute pain management:

Severe: I.M, I.V.: 50-100 mcg/dose every 1-2 hours as needed; patients with prior opiate exposure may tolerate higher initial doses

Patient-controlled analgesia (PCA): I.V.: Usual concentration: 10 mcg/mL

Demand dose: Usual: 10 mcg; range: 10-50 mcg

Lockout interval: 5-8 minutes

Breakthrough cancer pain: Transmucosal: Actiq® dosing should be individually titrated to provide adequate analgesia with minimal side effects. For patients who are tolerant to and currently receiving opioid therapy for persistent cancer pain. Initial starting dose: 200 mcg; the second dose may be started 15 minutes after completion of the first dose. Consumption should be limited to 4 units/day or less. Patients needing more than 4 units/day should have the dose of their long-term opioid re-evaluated.

Chronic pain management: Opioid-tolerant patients: Transdermal:

Initial: To convert patients from oral or parenteral opioids to transdermal formulation, a 24-hour analgesic requirement should be calculated (based on prior opiate use). Using the tables, the appropriate initial dose can be determined. The initial fentanyl dosage may be approximated from the 24-hour morphine dosage and titrated to minimize adverse effects and provide analgesia. Change patch every 72 hours.

Titration: Short-acting agents may be required until analgesic efficacy is established and/or as supplements for "breakthrough" pain. The amount of supplemental doses should be closely monitored. Appropriate dosage increases may be based on daily supplemental dosage using the ratio of 45 mg/24 hours of oral morphine to a 12.5 mcg/hour increase in fentanyl dosage.

Frequency of adjustment: The dosage should not be titrated more frequently than every 3 days after the initial dose or every 6 days thereafter. Patients should wear a consistent fentanyl dosage through two applications (6 days) before dosage increase based on supplemental opiate dosages can be estimated.

Frequency of application: The majority of patients may be controlled on every 72-hour administration; however, a small number of patients require every 48-hour administration.

Dose conversion guidelines for transdermal fentanyl[1] (see tables below and on next page)

Dosing Conversion Guidelines[1,2]

Current Analgesic	Daily Dosage (mg/day)			
Morphine (I.M./ I.V.)	10-22	23-37	38-52	53-67
Oxycodone (oral)	30-67	67.5-112	112.5-157	157.5-202
Oxycodone (I.M./ I.V.)	15-33	33.1-56	56.1-78	78.1-101
Codeine (oral)	150-447	448-747	748-1047	1048-1347
Hydromorphone (oral)	8-17	17.1-28	28.1-39	39.1-51
Hydromorphone (I.V.)	1.5-3.4	3.5-5.6	5.7-7.9	8-10
Meperidine (I.M.)	75-165	166-278	279-390	391-503
Methadone (oral)	20-44	45-74	75-104	105-134
Methadone (I.M.)	10-22	23-37	38-52	53-67
Fentanyl transdermal recommended dose (mcg/h)	**25 mcg/h**	**50 mcg/h**	**75 mcg/h**	**100 mcg/h**

[1] The table should NOT be used to convert from transdermal fentanyl to other opioid analgesics. Rather, following removal of the patch, titrate the dose of the new opioid until adequate analgesia is achieved.

[2] Duragesic® product insert, Janssen Pharmaceutica, Feb 2005.

(Continued)

Fentanyl *(Continued)*

Recommended Initial Duragesic® Dose Based Upon Daily Oral Morphine Dose[1]

Oral 24-Hour Morphine (mg/d)	Duragesic® Dose (mcg/h)
60-134[2]	25
135-224	50
225-314	75
315-404	100
405-494	125
495-584	150
585-674	175
675-764	200
765-854	225
855-944	250
945-1034	275
1035-1124	300

[1] The table should NOT be used to convert from transdermal fentanyl to other opioid analgesics. Rather, following removal of the patch, titrate the dose of the new opioid until adequate analgesia is achieved.
[2]Pediatric patients initiating therapy on a 25 mcg/hour Duragesic® system should be opioid-tolerant and receiving at least 60 mg oral morphine equivalents per day.

Opioid Analgesics Initial Oral Dosing Commonly Used for Severe Pain

Drug	Equianalgesic Dose (mg)		Initial Oral Dose	
	Oral[1]	Parenteral[2]	Children (mg/kg)	Adults (mg)
Buprenorphine	—	0.4	—	—
Butorphanol	—	2	—	—
Hydromorphone	7.5	1.5	0.06	4-8
Levorphanol	4 (acute) 1 (chronic)	2 (acute) 1 (chronic)	0.04	2-4
Meperidine	300	75	Not Recommended	
Methadone	10	5	0.2	0.2
Morphine	30	10	0.3	15-30
Nalbuphine	—	10	—	—
Pentazocine	50	30	—	—
Oxycodone	20	—	0.3	10-20
Oxymorphone	1	—	—	—

From "Principles of Analgesic Use in the Treatment of Acute Pain and Cancer Pain," *Am Pain Soc*, Fifth Ed.

[1]Elderly: Starting dose should be lower for this population group

[2]Standard parenteral doses for acute pain in adults; can be used to doses for I.V. infusions and repeated small I.V. boluses. Single I.V. boluses, use half the I.M. dose. Children >6 months: I.V. dose = parenteral equianalgesic dose x weight (kg)/100

Elderly: Elderly have been found to be twice as sensitive as younger patients to the effects of fentanyl. A wide range of doses may be used. When choosing a dose, take into consideration the following patient factors: age, weight, physical status, underlying disease states, other drugs used, type of anesthesia used, and the surgical procedure to be performed.

Transmucosal: Dose should be reduced to 2.5-5 mcg/kg. Suck on lozenge vigorously approximately 20-40 minutes before the start of procedure.

Pediatrics: Note: These are guidelines and do not represent the maximum doses that may be required in all patients. Doses should be titrated to pain relief/prevention. Monitor vital signs routinely. Single I.M. doses have a duration of 1-2 hours, single I.V. doses last 0.5-1 hour.

Sedation for minor procedures/analgesia:

Children 1-12 years: I.M., I.V.: 1-2 mcg/kg/dose; may repeat at 30- to 60-minute intervals. **Note:** Children 18-36 months of age may require 2-3 mcg/kg/dose

Children >12 years: Refer to adult dosing.

Continuous sedation/analgesia: Children 1-12 years: Initial I.V. bolus: 1-2 mcg/kg; then 1-3 mcg/kg/hour to a maximum dose of 5 mcg/kg/hour

Chronic pain management: Children ≥2 years (opioid-tolerant patients): Transdermal: Refer to adult dosing.

Hepatic Impairment: Fentanyl kinetics may be altered in hepatic disease.

Available Dosage Forms

Infusion [premixed in NS]: 0.05 mg (10 mL); 1 mg (100 mL); 1.25 mg (250 mL); 2 mg (100 mL); 2.5 mg (250 mL)

Injection, solution, as citrate [preservative free]: 0.05 mg/mL (2 mL, 5 mL, 10 mL, 20 mL, 30 mL, 50 mL)

Sublimaze®: 0.05 mg/mL (2 mL, 5 mL, 10 mL, 20 mL)

Lozenge, oral transmucosal, as citrate (Actiq®): 200 mcg, 400 mcg, 600 mcg, 800 mcg, 1200 mcg, 1600 mcg [mounted on a plastic radiopaque handle; raspberry flavor]

Transdermal system: 25 mcg/hour [6.25 cm^2] (5s); 50 mcg/hour [12.5 cm^2] (5s); 75 mcg/hour [18.75 cm^2]; 100 mcg/hour [25 cm^2] (5s)

Duragesic®: 12 [delivers 12.5 mcg/hour; 5 cm^2] (5s); 25 [delivers 25 mcg/hour; 10 cm^2] (5s); 50 [delivers 50 mcg/hour; 20 cm^2] (5s); 75 [delivers 75 mcg/hour; 30 cm^2]; 100 [delivers 100 mcg/hour; 40 cm^2] (5s)

Nursing Guidelines

Assessment: Assess other medications patient may be taking for additive or adverse interactions. Monitor therapeutic effectiveness and signs of adverse or overdose reactions. Monitor blood pressure, CNS and respiratory status, and degree of sedation at beginning of therapy and at regular intervals with long-term use. Monitor closely for 24 hours after transdermal product is removed. Order safety precautions for inpatient use. May cause physical and/or psychological dependence. Assess knowledge/teach patient appropriate use (if self-administered), adverse reactions to report, and appropriate interventions to reduce side effects.

Dietary Considerations: Actiq® contains 2 g sugar per unit.

Patient Education: While using this medication, do not use alcohol and other prescription or OTC medications (especially sedatives, tranquilizers, antihistamines, or pain medications) without consulting prescriber. If using Actiq® oral transmucosal, you may be at risk for dental carries due to the sugar content. Maintain good oral hygiene. If using patch, avoid exposing application site to external heat sources (eg, heating pad, electric blanket, hot tub, heat lamp). Maintain adequate hydration (2-3 L/day of fluids) unless instructed to restrict fluid intake. May cause hypotension, dizziness, drowsiness, impaired coordination, or blurred vision (use caution when driving, climbing stairs, or changing position - rising from sitting or lying to standing, or when engaging in tasks requiring alertness until response to drug is known); nausea or vomiting (frequent mouth care, small frequent meals, chewing gum, or sucking lozenges may help); or constipation (increased exercise, fluids, fruit, or fiber may help; if unresolved, consult prescriber about use of stool softeners). Report acute dizziness, chest pain, slow or rapid heartbeat, acute headache; confusion or changes in mentation; changes in voiding frequency or amount; swelling of extremities or unusual weight gain; shortness of breath or respiratory difficulty; or vision changes. **Pregnancy/breast-feeding precautions:** Inform prescriber if you are or intend to become pregnant. Consult prescriber if breast-feeding.

Transdermal: Apply to clean, dry skin, immediately after removing from package. Firmly press in place and hold for 30 seconds.

Transmucosal (Actiq®): Contains an amount of medication that can be fatal to children. Keep all units out of the reach of children and discard any open units properly. Actiq® Welcome Kits are available which contain educational materials, safe storage, and disposal instructions.

Geriatric Considerations: The elderly may be particularly susceptible to the CNS depressant and constipating effects of narcotics; therefore, use with caution.

Pregnancy Risk Factor: C/D (prolonged use or high doses at term)

Pregnancy Issues: Fentanyl crosses the placenta and has been used safely during labor. Chronic use during pregnancy has shown detectable serum levels in the newborn with mild opioid withdrawal (case report).

(Continued)

Fentanyl *(Continued)*

Lactation: Enters breast milk/not recommended (AAP rates "compatible")

Breast-Feeding Considerations: Fentanyl is excreted in low concentrations into breast milk. Breast-feeding is considered acceptable following single doses to the mother; however, no information is available when used long-term.

Perioperative/Anesthesia/Other Concerns: When developing a therapeutic plan for pain control, scheduled, intermittent opioid dosing or continuous infusion is preferred over the "as needed" regimen. The 2002 ACCM/SCCM guidelines for analgesia (critically-ill adult) recommend fentanyl in patients who need immediate pain relief because of its rapid onset of action. Repeated doses or a continuous infusion of fentanyl may cause accumulation. Fentanyl or hydromorphone is preferred in patients who are hypotensive or have renal dysfunction. Morphine or hydromorphone is recommended for intermittent, scheduled therapy. Both have a longer duration of action requiring less frequent administration. Fentanyl is great to prevent pain during a procedure and can be dosed intermittently for such an application. Prolonged analgesia requires an infusion.

Fentanyl is 50-100 times as potent as morphine; morphine 10 mg I.M. is equivalent to fentanyl 0.1-0.2 mg I.M.; fentanyl has less hypotensive effects than morphine due to lack of histamine release. However, fentanyl may cause rigidity with high doses. If the patient has required high-dose analgesia or has used for a prolonged period (~7 days), taper dose to prevent withdrawal; monitor for signs and symptoms of withdrawal.

Administration

I.V.: Muscular rigidity may occur with rapid I.V. administration.

Compatibility: Stable in D_5W, NS

Compatibility in syringe: Incompatible with pentobarbital

Compatibility when admixed: Incompatible with fluorouracil, methohexital, pentobarbital, thiopental

Storage:

Injection formulation: Store at controlled room temperature of 15°C to 25°C (59°F to 86°F). Protect from light.

Transdermal: Do not store above 25°C (77°F).

Transmucosal: Store at controlled room temperature of 15°C to 30°C (59°F to 86°F).

Related Information

Acute Postoperative Pain *on page 1742*

Conscious Sedation *on page 1779*

- **Fentanyl Citrate** *see* Fentanyl *on page 712*
- **Feosol® [OTC]** *see* Ferrous Sulfate *on page 721*
- **Feratab® [OTC]** *see* Ferrous Sulfate *on page 721*
- **Fer-Gen-Sol [OTC]** *see* Ferrous Sulfate *on page 721*
- **Fergon® [OTC]** *see* Ferrous Gluconate *on page 720*
- **Fer-In-Sol® [OTC]** *see* Ferrous Sulfate *on page 721*
- **Fer-Iron® [OTC]** *see* Ferrous Sulfate *on page 721*

Ferric Gluconate (FER ik GLOO koe nate)

U.S. Brand Names Ferrlecit®

Synonyms Sodium Ferric Gluconate

Pharmacologic Category Iron Salt

Medication Safety Issues

Sound-alike/look-alike issues:

Ferrlecit® may be confused with Ferralet®

Use Repletion of total body iron content in patients with iron-deficiency anemia who are undergoing hemodialysis in conjunction with erythropoietin therapy

Mechanism of Action Supplies a source to elemental iron necessary to the function of hemoglobin, myoglobin and specific enzyme systems; allows transport of oxygen via hemoglobin

Pharmacodynamics/Kinetics Half-life elimination: Bound: 1 hour

Contraindications Hypersensitivity to ferric gluconate or any component of the formulation; use in any anemia not caused by iron deficiency; heart failure (of any severity); iron overload

Warnings/Precautions Potentially serious hypersensitivity reactions may occur. Fatal immediate hypersensitivity reactions have occurred with other iron carbohydrate complexes. Avoid rapid administration. Flushing and transient hypotension may occur. May augment hemodialysis-induced hypotension. Use with caution in elderly patients. Safety and efficacy in children <6 years of age have not been established. Contains benzyl alcohol; do not use in neonates.

Drug Interactions

Chloramphenicol: Chloramphenicol may diminish the therapeutic effects of ferric gluconate injection

Iron preparations, oral: Ferric gluconate injection may reduce the absorption of oral iron preparations

Adverse Reactions Major adverse reactions include hypotension and hypersensitivity reactions. Hypersensitivity reactions have included pruritus, chest pain, hypotension, nausea, abdominal pain, flank pain, fatigue and rash.

1% to 10%:

Cardiovascular: Hypotension (serious hypotension in 1%), chest pain, hypertension, syncope, tachycardia, angina, MI, pulmonary edema, hypovolemia, peripheral edema

Central nervous system: Headache, fatigue, fever, malaise, dizziness, paresthesia, insomnia, agitation, somnolence, pain

Dermatologic: Pruritus, rash

Endocrine & metabolic: Hyperkalemia, hypoglycemia, hypokalemia

Gastrointestinal: Abdominal pain, nausea, vomiting, diarrhea, rectal disorder, dyspepsia, flatulence, melena

Genitourinary: Urinary tract infection

Hematologic: Anemia, abnormal erythrocytes, lymphadenopathy

Local: Injection site reactions, injection site pain

Neuromuscular & skeletal: Weakness, back pain, leg cramps, myalgia, arthralgia, paresthesia

Ocular: Blurred vision, conjunctivitis

Respiratory: Dyspnea, cough, rhinitis, upper respiratory infection, pneumonia

Miscellaneous: Hypersensitivity reactions, infection, rigors, chills, flu-like syndrome, sepsis, carcinoma, diaphoresis (increased)

<1% (Limited to important or life-threatening): Dry mouth, epigastric pain, groin pain, hemorrhage, hypertonia, nervousness

Overdosage/Toxicology Symptoms of iron overdose include CNS toxicity, acidosis, hepatic and renal impairment, hematemesis, and lethargy. A serum iron level ≥300 mcg/mL requires treatment due to severe toxicity. Treatment is generally symptomatic and supportive, but severe overdoses may be treated with deferoxamine. Deferoxamine may be administered I.V. (80 mg/kg over 24 hours) or I.M. (40-90 mg/kg every 8 hours). Usual toxic dose of elemental iron: ≥35 mg/kg.

Dosing

Adults & Elderly: Note: A test dose of 2 mL diluted in 50 mL 0.9% sodium chloride over 60 minutes was previously recommended (not in current manufacturer labeling).

Repletion of iron in hemodialysis patients: I.V.: 125 mg elemental iron per 10 mL (either by I.V. infusion or slow I.V. injection). Most patients will require a cumulative dose of 1 g elemental iron over approximately 8 sequential dialysis treatments to achieve a favorable response.

Pediatrics: Repletion of iron in hemodialysis patients: I.V.: Children ≥6 years: 1.5 mg/kg (maximum: 125 mg/dose) diluted in NS 25 mL, administered over 60 minutes at 8 sequential dialysis sessions

Available Dosage Forms Injection, solution: Elemental iron 12.5 mg/mL (5 mL) [contains benzyl alcohol and sucrose 20%]

Nursing Guidelines

Assessment: Assess results of test dose, infusion rate, effectiveness of therapy (laboratory results), and adverse reactions at beginning of therapy and periodically during therapy. Monitor blood pressure during infusion. Hypotension can occur. Be alert to the potential for hypersensitivity reactions. Assess knowledge/teach patient adverse symptoms to report.

Monitoring Laboratory Tests: Hemoglobin and hematocrit, serum ferritin, iron saturation

Patient Education: This medication will be administered by I.V. in conjunction with your dialysis treatment. Report chest pain, rapid heartbeat, or palpitations; respiratory difficulty; headache, dizziness, agitation, or inability to sleep; nausea, vomiting, abdominal or flank pain; or skin rash, itching, or redness. **Breast-feeding precaution:** Consult prescriber if breast-feeding.

(Continued)

Ferric Gluconate *(Continued)*

Pregnancy Risk Factor: B

Lactation: Excretion in breast milk unknown/use caution

Administration

I.V.:

Adults: May be diluted prior to administration; avoid rapid administration. Infusion rate should not exceed 2.1 mg/minute. If administered undiluted, infuse slowly at a rate of up to 12.5 mg/minute.

Reconstitution: For I.V. infusion, dilute 10 mL ferric gluconate in 0.9% sodium chloride (children: 25 mL NS, adults: 100 mL NS); use immediately after dilution. Do **not** mix with parenteral nutrition solutions or other medications.

Compatibility: Stable in NS

Do not mix with parenteral nutrition solutions or other medications.

Storage: Store at 20°C to 25°C (68°F to 77°F).

♦ Ferrlecit® *see* Ferric Gluconate *on page 718*

Ferrous Gluconate (FER us GLOO koe nate)

U.S. Brand Names Fergon® [OTC]

Synonyms Iron Gluconate

Pharmacologic Category Iron Salt

Use Prevention and treatment of iron-deficiency anemias

Mechanism of Action Replaces iron found in hemoglobin, myoglobin, and enzymes; allows the transportation of oxygen via hemoglobin

Pharmacodynamics/Kinetics Onset of action: Hematologic response: Oral: 3-10 days; peak reticulocytosis occurs in 5-10 days, and hemoglobin values increase in ~2-4 weeks

Contraindications Hypersensitivity to iron salts or any component of the formulation; hemochromatosis, hemolytic anemia

Warnings/Precautions Administration of iron for >6 months should be avoided except in patients with continued bleeding, menorrhagia, or repeated pregnancies; avoid in patients with peptic ulcer, enteritis, or ulcerative colitis. Anemia in the elderly is often caused by "anemia of chronic disease" or associated with inflammation rather than blood loss. Iron stores are usually normal or increased, with a serum ferritin >50 ng/mL and a decreased total iron binding capacity. Hence, the "anemia of chronic disease" is not secondary to iron deficiency but the inability of the reticuloendothelial system to reclaim available iron stores.

Drug Interactions

Antacids and H_2 blockers (cimetidine): Concurrent administration may decrease iron absorption.

Chloramphenicol: Response to iron therapy may be delayed.

Levodopa, methyldopa, penicillamine: Iron may decrease absorption when given at the same time.

Quinolones: Absorption may be decreased due to formation of a ferric ion-quinolone complex

Tetracyclines: Absorption of oral preparation of iron and tetracyclines are decreased when both of these drugs are given together

Vitamin C: Concurrent administration of ≥200 mg vitamin C per 30 mg elemental iron increases absorption of oral iron.

Nutritional/Herbal/Ethanol Interactions Food: Cereals, dietary fiber, tea, coffee, eggs, and milk may decrease absorption.

Lab Interactions False-positive for blood in stool by the guaiac test

Adverse Reactions

>10%: Gastrointestinal: Stomach cramping, constipation, nausea, vomiting, dark stools

1% to 10%:

Gastrointestinal: Heartburn, diarrhea, staining of teeth

Genitourinary: Discoloration of urine

<1% (Limited to important or life-threatening): Contact irritation

Overdosage/Toxicology

Symptoms of overdose include acute GI irritation; erosion of GI mucosa, hepatic and renal impairment, coma, hematemesis, lethargy, acidosis

Following treatment for fluid losses, metabolic acidosis, and shock, a severe iron overdose may be treated with deferoxamine. Deferoxamine may be administered I.V. (80 mg/kg over 24 hours) or I.M. (40-90 mg/kg every 8 hours). Usual toxic dose of elemental iron: ≥35 mg/kg.

Dosing

Adults & Elderly: (Dose expressed in terms of elemental iron):

Treatment of iron deficiency anemia: Oral: 60 mg twice daily up to 60 mg 4 times/day

Prophylaxis of iron deficiency: Oral: 60 mg/day

Pediatrics: (Dose expressed in terms of elemental iron):

Treatment of severe iron-deficiency anemia: Oral: 4-6 mg Fe/kg/day in 3 divided doses

Treatment of mild-to-moderate iron-deficiency anemia: Oral: 3 mg Fe/kg/day in 1-2 divided doses

Prophylaxis: Oral: 1-2 mg Fe/kg/day

Available Dosage Forms

Tablet: 246 mg [elemental iron 28 mg]; 300 mg [elemental iron 34 mg]; 325 mg [elemental iron 36 mg]

Fergon®: 240 mg [elemental iron 27 mg]

Nursing Guidelines

Monitoring Laboratory Tests: Serum iron, total iron binding capacity, reticulocyte count, hemoglobin

Dietary Considerations: Should be taken with water or juice on an empty stomach; may be administered with food to prevent irritation; however, not with cereals, dietary fiber, tea, coffee, eggs, or milk.

Elemental iron content of ferrous gluconate: 12%

Patient Education: May color stool black. Take between meals for maximum absorption; take with food if GI upset occurs. Do not take with milk or antacids. Keep out of reach of children.

Pregnancy Risk Factor: A

Administration

Oral: Administer 2 hours before or 4 hours after antacids. Administration of iron preparations to premature infants with vitamin E deficiency may cause increased red cell hemolysis and hemolytic anemia, therefore, vitamin E deficiency should be corrected if possible.

Ferrous Sulfate (FER us SUL fate)

U.S. Brand Names Feosol® [OTC]; Feratab® [OTC]; Fer-Gen-Sol [OTC]; Fer-In-Sol® [OTC]; Fer-Iron® [OTC]; Slow FE® [OTC]

Synonyms $FeSO_4$; Iron Sulfate

Pharmacologic Category Iron Salt

Medication Safety Issues

Sound-alike/look-alike issues:

Feosol® may be confused with Feostat®, Fer-In-Sol®

Fer-In-Sol® may be confused with Feosol®

Slow FE® may be confused with Slow-K®

Use Prevention and treatment of iron-deficiency anemias

Mechanism of Action Replaces iron, found in hemoglobin, myoglobin, and other enzymes; allows the transportation of oxygen via hemoglobin

Pharmacodynamics/Kinetics

Onset of action: Hematologic response: Oral: ~3-10 days

Peak effect: Reticulocytosis: 5-10 days; hemoglobin increases within 2-4 weeks

Absorption: Iron is absorbed in the duodenum and upper jejunum; in persons with normal serum iron stores, 10% of an oral dose is absorbed; this is increased to 20% to 30% in persons with inadequate iron stores. Food and achlorhydria will decrease absorption

Protein binding: To transferrin

Excretion: Urine, sweat, sloughing of the intestinal mucosa, and menses

Contraindications Hypersensitivity to iron salts or any component of the formulation; hemochromatosis, hemolytic anemia

Warnings/Precautions Administration of iron for >6 months should be avoided except in patients with continued bleeding, menorrhagia, or repeated pregnancies; avoid in patients with peptic ulcer, enteritis, or ulcerative colitis. Anemia in the elderly is often caused by "anemia of chronic disease" or associated with inflammation rather than blood loss. Iron stores are usually normal or increased, with a serum ferritin >50 ng/mL and a decreased total iron binding capacity. Hence, the "anemia of chronic disease" is not secondary to iron deficiency but the inability of the reticuloendothelial system to reclaim available iron stores.

Drug Interactions

Antacids and H_2 blockers (cimetidine): Concurrent administration may decrease iron absorption.

Chloramphenicol: Response to iron therapy may be delayed.

(Continued)

Ferrous Sulfate *(Continued)*

Levodopa, methyldopa, penicillamine: Iron may decrease absorption when given at the same time.

Quinolones: Absorption may be decreased due to formation of a ferric ion-quinolone complex

Tetracyclines: Absorption of oral preparation of iron and tetracyclines are decreased when both of these drugs are given together

Vitamin C: Concurrent administration of ≥200 mg vitamin C per 30 mg elemental iron increases absorption of oral iron.

Nutritional/Herbal/Ethanol Interactions Food: Cereals, dietary fiber, tea, coffee, eggs, and milk may decrease absorption.

Lab Interactions False-positive for blood in stool by the guaiac test

Adverse Reactions

>10%: Gastrointestinal: GI irritation, epigastric pain, nausea, dark stools, vomiting, stomach cramping, constipation

1% to 10%:

Gastrointestinal: Heartburn, diarrhea

Genitourinary: Discoloration of urine

Miscellaneous: Liquid preparations may temporarily stain the teeth

<1% (Limited to important or life-threatening): Contact irritation

Overdosage/Toxicology

Symptoms of overdose include acute GI irritation; erosion of GI mucosa, hepatic and renal impairment, coma, hematemesis, lethargy, acidosis

Following treatment for fluid losses, metabolic acidosis, and shock, a severe iron overdose may be treated with deferoxamine. Deferoxamine may be administered I.V. (80 mg/kg over 24 hours) or I.M. (40-90 mg/kg every 8 hours). Usual toxic dose of elemental iron: ≥35 mg/kg.

Dosing

Adults & Elderly: Dose expressed in terms of ferrous sulfate:

Treatment of iron deficiency anemia: Oral: 300 mg twice daily up to 300 mg 4 times/day or 250 mg (extended release) 1-2 times/day

Prophylaxis of iron deficiency: Oral: 300 mg/day

Pediatrics: Dosage expressed in terms of elemental iron:

Treatment of severe iron-deficiency anemia: Oral: 4-6 mg Fe/kg/day in 3 divided doses

Treatment of mild-to-moderate iron-deficiency anemia: Oral: 3 mg Fe/kg/day in 1-2 divided doses

Prophylaxis: Oral: 1-2 mg Fe/kg/day up to a maximum of 15 mg/day

Available Dosage Forms

Elixir: 220 mg/5 mL (480 mL) [elemental iron 44 mg/5 mL; contains alcohol]

Liquid, oral drops: 75 mg/0.6 mL (50 mL) [elemental iron 15 mg/0.6 mL]

Fer-Gen-Sol: 75 mg/0.6 mL (50 mL) [elemental iron 15 mg/0.6 mL]

Fer-In-Sol®: 75 mg/0.6 mL (50 mL) [elemental iron 15 mg/0.6 mL; contains alcohol 0.2% and sodium bisulfite]

Fer-Iron®: 75 mg/0.6 mL (50 mL) [elemental iron 15 mg/0.6 mL]

Tablet: 324 mg [elemental iron 65 mg]; 325 mg [elemental iron 65 mg]

Feratab®: 300 mg [elemental iron 60 mg]

Tablet, exsiccated (Feosol®): 200 mg [elemental iron 65 mg]

Tablet, exsiccated, timed release (Slow FE®): 160 mg [elemental iron 50 mg]

Nursing Guidelines

Assessment: Assess therapeutic response and adverse effects. May cause GI irritation. Monitor GI function (observe for epigastric pain, nausea, dark stools, vomiting, stomach cramping, constipation).

Monitoring Laboratory Tests: Serum iron, total iron binding capacity, reticulocyte count, hemoglobin

Dietary Considerations: Should be taken with water or juice on an empty stomach; may be administered with food to prevent irritation; however, not with cereals, dietary fiber, tea, coffee, eggs, or milk.

Elemental iron content of iron salts in ferrous sulfate is 20% (ie, 300 mg ferrous sulfate is equivalent to 60 mg ferrous iron)

Patient Education: May color stool black. Take between meals for maximum absorption; take with food if GI upset occurs. Do not take with milk or antacids. You may experience constipation; increasing exercise, fluids, fruit/fiber may help. Keep out of reach of children.

Pregnancy Risk Factor: A

◆ $FeSO_4$ *see* Ferrous Sulfate *on page 721*
◆ FeverALL® [OTC] *see* Acetaminophen *on page 65*

Fexofenadine (feks oh FEN a deen)

U.S. Brand Names Allegra®

Synonyms Fexofenadine Hydrochloride

Pharmacologic Category Antihistamine, Nonsedating

Medication Safety Issues

Sound-alike/look-alike issues:

Allegra® may be confused with Viagra®

Use Relief of symptoms associated with seasonal allergic rhinitis; treatment of chronic idiopathic urticaria

Mechanism of Action Fexofenadine is an active metabolite of terfenadine and like terfenadine it competes with histamine for H_1-receptor sites on effector cells in the gastrointestinal tract, blood vessels and respiratory tract; it appears that fexofenadine does not cross the blood brain barrier to any appreciable degree, resulting in a reduced potential for sedation

Pharmacodynamics/Kinetics

Onset of action: 60 minutes

Duration: Antihistaminic effect: ≥12 hours

Protein binding: 60% to 70%, primarily albumin and $alpha_1$-acid glycoprotein

Metabolism: Minimal (~5%)

Half-life elimination: 14.4 hours

Time to peak, serum: ~2.6 hours

Excretion: Feces (~80%) and urine (~11%) as unchanged drug

Contraindications Hypersensitivity to fexofenadine or any component of the formulation

Warnings/Precautions Safety and effectiveness in children <6 years of age have not been established.

Drug Interactions **Substrate** of CYP3A4 (minor); **Inhibits** CYP2D6 (weak)

Antacids (containing aluminum or magnesium): AUC of fexofenadine was decreased by 41% and C_{max} by 43% with concomitant administration; separate administration is recommended.

Erythromycin: Levels of fexofenadine are increased (82% higher); not associated with increased adverse effects and no difference in QT_c intervals.

Ketoconazole: Levels of fexofenadine are increased (135% higher); not associated with increased adverse effects and no difference in QT_c intervals.

Nutritional/Herbal/Ethanol Interactions

Ethanol: Avoid ethanol (although limited with fexofenadine, may increase risk of sedation).

Food: Fruit juice (apple, grapefruit, orange, pineapple) may decrease bioavailability of fexofenadine by ~36%.

Herb/Nutraceutical: St John's wort may decrease fexofenadine levels.

Adverse Reactions

>10%: Central nervous system: Headache (5% to 11%)

1% to 10%:

Central nervous system: Fever (2%), dizziness (2%), pain (2%), drowsiness (1%), fatigue (1%)

Endocrine & metabolic: Dysmenorrhea (2%)

Gastrointestinal: Nausea (2%), dyspepsia (1% to 5%)

Neuromuscular & skeletal: Back pain (2% to 3%), myalgia (3%)

Otic: Otitis media (2%)

Respiratory: Cough (4%), upper respiratory tract infection (2% to 4%), nasopharyngitis (2%)

Miscellaneous: Viral infection (3%)

<1% (Limited to important or life-threatening): Hypersensitivity reactions (anaphylaxis, angioedema, dyspnea, flushing, pruritus, rash, urticaria); insomnia, nervousness, sleep disorders, paroniria

Overdosage/Toxicology Limited information from overdose describes dizziness, drowsiness, and dry mouth. Not effectively removed by hemodialysis. Doses up to 690 mg twice daily were administered for 1 month without significant adverse effects. Treatment is supportive.

Dosing

Adults:

Allergic rhinitis, idiopathic urticaria: Oral: 60 mg twice daily **or** 180 mg once daily

(Continued)

Fexofenadine *(Continued)*

Elderly: Starting dose: 60 mg once daily; adjust for renal impairment.

Pediatrics: Allergic rhinitis, idiopathic urticaria:

Children 6-11 years: Oral: 30 mg twice daily

Children ≥12 years: Refer to adult dosing.

Renal Impairment: Cl_{cr} <80 mL/minute:

Children 6-11 years: Initial: 30 mg once daily

Children ≥12 years and Adults: Initial: 60 mg once daily

Not effectively removed by hemodialysis

Available Dosage Forms Tablet, as hydrochloride: 30 mg, 60 mg, 180 mg

Nursing Guidelines

Assessment: Assess effectiveness and interactions of other medications patient may be taking. Monitor effectiveness of therapy and adverse reactions at beginning of therapy and periodically with long-term use. Assess knowledge/teach patient appropriate use, interventions to reduce side effects, and adverse symptoms to report.

Patient Education: Take as directed; do not exceed recommended dose. Store at room temperature in a dry place. If taking antacids, separate administration of antacid and this medication. Avoid use of other depressants, alcohol, or sleep-inducing medications unless approved by prescriber. You may experience mild drowsiness or dizziness (use caution when driving or engaging in tasks requiring alertness until response to drug is known); or nausea (small frequent meals, frequent mouth care, chewing gum, or sucking hard candy may help). Report persistent sedation or drowsiness, menstrual irregularities, or lack of improvement or worsening or condition. **Pregnancy/breast-feeding precautions:** Inform prescriber if you are or intend to become pregnant. Consult prescriber if breast-feeding.

Geriatric Considerations: Plasma levels in the elderly are generally higher than those observed in other age groups. Once daily dosing is recommended when starting therapy in elderly patients or patients with decreased renal function.

Pregnancy Risk Factor: C

Lactation: Excretion in breast milk unknown/use caution (AAP rates "compatible")

Administration

Oral: Administer with water.

Storage: Store at controlled room temperature of 20°C to 25°C (68°F to 77°F). Protect from excessive moisture.

♦ **Fexofenadine Hydrochloride** *see* Fexofenadine *on page 723*

♦ **Fiberall®** *see* Psyllium *on page 1438*

Fibrin Sealant Kit (FI brin SEEL ent kit)

U.S. Brand Names Crosseal™; Tisseel® VH

Synonyms FS

Pharmacologic Category Hemostatic Agent

Use

Crosseal™: Adjunct to hemostasis in liver surgery

Tisseel® VH: Adjunct to hemostasis in cardiopulmonary bypass surgery and splenic injury (due to blunt or penetrating trauma to the abdomen) when the control of bleeding by conventional surgical techniques is ineffective or impractical; adjunctive sealant for closure of colostomies; hemostatic agent in heparinized patients undergoing cardiopulmonary bypass

Mechanism of Action Formation of a biodegradable adhesive is done by duplicating the last step of the coagulation cascade, the formation of fibrin from fibrinogen. Fibrinogen is the main component of the sealant solution. The solution also contains thrombin, which transforms fibrinogen from the sealer protein solution into fibrin, and fibrinolysis inhibitor (aprotinin), which prevents the premature degradation of fibrin. When mixed as directed, a viscous solution forms that sets into an elastic coagulum.

Pharmacodynamics/Kinetics Onset of action:

Crosseal™: Time to hemostasis: 5.3 minutes

Tisseel® VH: Time to hemostasis: 5 minutes (65% of patients); Final prepared sealant: 70% strength: ~10 minutes; Full strength: ~2 hours

Contraindications Hypersensitivity to any component of the formulations in the kit; massive and brisk arterial bleeding

Crosseal™: Hypersensitivity to human blood products; not for use in surgical situations where contact with CSF or dura mater may occur

Tisseel® VH: Hypersensitivity to human blood products or bovine protein

Warnings/Precautions For topical use only; do not inject into a vessel or tissue. Components of the kit made from human plasma may potentially transmit disease. Any infection suspected of being transmitted by this product should be reported to the manufacturer.

Tisseel® VH: Do not apply to wound surface containing alcohol, iodine, or heavy-metal ions. Do not use with oxycellulose-containing preparations. Safety and efficacy in pediatric patients have not been established.

Drug Interactions

Alcohol, heavy-metal ions, iodine: May denature the sealer protein and thrombin solution in the Tisseel® VH kit; wound surface should be cleaned to remove these products prior to application of fibrin sealant

Oxycellulose preparations: Reduce efficacy of Tisseel®; do not use as a carrier

Adverse Reactions No adverse events were reported in clinical trials. Anaphylactoid or anaphylactic reactions have occurred with other plasma-derived products.

Dosing

Adults & Elderly: Adjunct to hemostasis: Apply topically; actual dose is based on size of surface to be covered:

Crosseal™: To cover a layer of 1 mm thickness:

Maximum area to be sealed: 20 cm^2
Required size of Crosseal™ kit: 1 mL
Maximum area to be sealed: 40 cm^2
Required size of Crosseal™ kit: 2 mL
Maximum area to be sealed: 100 cm^2
Required size of Crosseal™ kit: 5 mL

Note: If hemostatic effect is not complete, apply a second layer.

Tisseel® VH:

Maximum area to be sealed: 4 cm^2
Required size of Tisseel® VH kit: 0.5 mL
Maximum area to be sealed: 8 cm^2
Required size of Tisseel® VH kit: 1 mL
Maximum area to be sealed: 16 cm^2
Required size of Tisseel® VH kit: 2 mL
Maximum area to be sealed: 40 cm^2
Required size of Tisseel® VH kit: 5 mL

Apply in thin layers to avoid excess formation of granulation tissue and slow absorption of the sealant. Following application, hold the sealed parts in the desired position for 3-5 minutes. To prevent sealant from adhering to gloves or surgical instruments, wet them with saline prior to contact.

Pediatrics: Adjunct to hemostasis: Topical (Crosseal™): Refer to adult dosing.

Available Dosage Forms Topical: Kit [each kit contains]:

Crosseal™: Fibrinogen 40-60 mg/mL [human; also contains tranexamic acid]; thrombin 800-1200 int. units/mL [human; also contains human albumin and mannitol]; spray application device (1 mL, 2 mL, 5 mL)

Tisseel® VH: Fibrinogen 75-115 mg/mL [sealer protein concentrate, human]; aprotinin 3000 KIU/mL [fibrinolysis inhibitor solution, bovine]; thrombin 500 int. units/mL [human]; calcium chloride solution 40 micromoles/mL (0.5 mL, 1 mL, 2 mL, 5 mL)

Nursing Guidelines

Pregnancy Risk Factor: C

Administration

Reconstitution: Tisseel® VH solution may be prepared by reconstituting the freeze-dried sealer protein concentrate using the Fibrinotherm® (preferred method), a water bath, or an incubator. The thrombin solution is prepared separately. The two solutions are then transferred to the sterile field and applied to the affected area using the Duploject® syringe system. Application must be done within 4 hours of preparing the solution. Total reconstitution time may take up to 40 minutes.

To reconstitute the sealer protein: Fibrinotherm® method: The Fibrinotherm® is a combined heating and stirring device that can be obtained from the manufacturer. After removing the caps from the sealer concentrate and the fibrinolysis inhibitor solution, disinfect with a germicidal solution that does **not** contain iodine. Turn on the stirring switch of the Fibrinotherm® and insert each vial into the appropriate openings. Turn on the heating switch. The vials will

(Continued)

Fibrin Sealant Kit *(Continued)*

automatically preheat at 37°C for 10 minutes. Transfer the fibrinolysis inhibitor solution into the vial of sealer protein concentrate. Use the adapter to insert the vial into the largest opening of the Fibrinotherm®. Stir contents for 8-10 minutes. If total dissolution has not occurred within 20 minutes, discard and prepare a fresh kit. If not used promptly, keep the solution at 37°C. Stir again shortly before drawing up solution.

Preparation of thrombin solution: After removing the caps from the calcium chloride and thrombin vials, disinfect with a germicidal solution that does **not** contain iodine. Add the calcium chloride to the thrombin vial. Swirl briefly. Keep the prepared solution at 37°C until use.

Note: Prior to application, the sealer protein solution and the thrombin solution should be transferred to a sterile field. To do this, the scrub nurse should withdraw the solution into the provided syringes, while the circulating nurse holds the vials. Withdraw solutions slowly to reduce the possible formation of large air bubbles.

Preparation of the final solution: The two resulting solutions are then placed into the Duploject® system, comprised of two identical disposable syringes, provided in the kit. The syringes have a common plunger, which allows equal volumes of both solutions to be fed through a joining piece, mixed, and ejected through a common application needle. Both syringes should contain equal volumes of solution. Do not expel any air bubbles (may clog). If the application process is interrupted, immediately prior to resuming application, replace the needle with one of the 3 spare needles provided in the kit. Discard any remaining solution.

Storage:

Crosseal™: Store frozen at or below -18°C; unopened vials may be stored at 2°C to 8°C (35°F to 46°F) for up to 30 days or up to 24 hours at room temperature. Store device at room temperature. Vials should be thawed prior to use.

Tisseel® VH: Store at 2°C to 8°C (35°F to 46°F).

♦ Fibro-XL [OTC] *see* Psyllium *on page 1438*
♦ Fibro-Lax [OTC] *see* Psyllium *on page 1438*

Filgrastim (fil GRA stim)

U.S. Brand Names Neupogen®

Synonyms G-CSF; Granulocyte Colony Stimulating Factor

Pharmacologic Category Colony Stimulating Factor

Medication Safety Issues

Sound-alike/look-alike issues:

Neupogen® may be confused with Epogen®, Neumega®, Nutramigen®

Use Stimulation of granulocyte production in patients with malignancies, including myeloid malignancies; receiving myelosuppressive therapy associated with a significant risk of neutropenia; severe chronic neutropenia (SCN); receiving bone marrow transplantation (BMT); undergoing peripheral blood progenitor cell (PBPC) collection

Mechanism of Action Stimulates the production, maturation, and activation of neutrophils; filgrastim activates neutrophils to increase both their migration and cytotoxicity. See table.

Comparative Effects — Filgrastim vs Sargramostim

Proliferation/Differentiation	Filgrastim	Sargramostim
Neutrophils	Yes	Yes
Eosinophils	No	Yes
Macrophages	No	Yes
Neutrophil migration	Enhanced	Inhibited

Pharmacodynamics/Kinetics

Onset of action: ~24 hours; plateaus in 3-5 days

Duration: ANC decreases by 50% within 2 days after discontinuing filgrastim; white counts return to the normal range in 4-7 days; peak plasma levels can be maintained for up to 12 hours

Absorption: SubQ: 100%

Distribution: V_d: 150 mL/kg; no evidence of drug accumulation over a 11- to 20-day period
Metabolism: Systemically degraded
Half-life elimination: 1.8-3.5 hours
Time to peak, serum: SubQ: 2-6 hours

Contraindications Hypersensitivity to filgrastim, *E. coli*-derived proteins, or any component of the formulation; concurrent myelosuppressive chemotherapy or radiation therapy

Warnings/Precautions Do not use filgrastim in the period 24 hours before to 24 hours after administration of cytotoxic chemotherapy because of the potential sensitivity of rapidly dividing myeloid cells to cytotoxic chemotherapy. Precaution should be exercised in the usage of filgrastim in any malignancy with myeloid characteristics. Filgrastim can potentially act as a growth factor for any tumor type, particularly myeloid malignancies. Tumors of nonhematopoietic origin may have surface receptors for filgrastim.

Allergic-type reactions have occurred in patients receiving the parent compound, filgrastim (G-CSF) with first or later doses. Reactions tended to occur more frequently with intravenous administration and within 30 minutes of infusion. Rare cases of splenic rupture or adult respiratory distress syndrome have been reported in association with filgrastim; patients must be instructed to report left upper quadrant pain or shoulder tip pain or respiratory distress. Use caution in patients with sickle cell diseases; sickle cell crises have been reported following filgrastim therapy.

Adverse Reactions Effects are generally mild and dose related

>10%:
- Central nervous system: Neutropenic fever, fever
- Dermatologic: Alopecia
- Gastrointestinal: Nausea, vomiting, diarrhea, mucositis, splenomegaly (more common in patients who prolonged (>14 days) treatment, usually subclinical)
- Neuromuscular & skeletal: Medullary bone pain (24%)

1% to 10%:
- Cardiovascular: Chest pain, fluid retention
- Central nervous system: Headache
- Dermatologic: Skin rash
- Gastrointestinal: Anorexia, stomatitis, constipation
- Hematologic: Leukocytosis
- Local: Pain at injection site
- Neuromuscular & skeletal: Weakness
- Respiratory: Dyspnea, cough, sore throat

<1% (Limited to important or life-threatening): Pericarditis, thrombophlebitis, transient supraventricular arrhythmia

Overdosage/Toxicology No clinical adverse effects have been seen with high doses producing ANC >10,000/mm³.

Dosing

Adults & Elderly: Refer to individual protocols.

Note: Dosing should be based on actual body weight (even in morbidly obese patients). Rounding doses to the nearest vial size often enhances patient convenience and reduces costs without compromising clinical response.

Myelosuppressive therapy: I.V., SubQ: 5 mcg/kg/day - doses may be increased by 5 mcg/kg according to the duration and severity of the neutropenia.

Bone marrow transplantation: I.V., SubQ: 5-10 mcg/kg/day - doses may be increased by 5 mcg/kg according to the duration and severity of neutropenia; recommended steps based on neutrophil response:

When ANC >1000/mm³ for 3 consecutive days: Reduce filgrastim dose to 5 mcg/kg/day.

If ANC remains >1000/mm³ for 3 more consecutive days: Discontinue filgrastim.

If ANC decreases to <1000/mm³: Resume at 5 mcg/kg/day.

If ANC decreases <1000/mm³ during the 5 mcg/kg/day dose: Increase filgrastim to 10 mcg/kg/day and follow the above steps.

Peripheral blood progenitor cell (PBPC) collection: I.V., SubQ: 10 mcg/kg/day **or** 5-8 mcg/kg twice daily in donors. The optimal timing and duration of growth factor stimulation has not been determined.

Severe chronic neutropenia: SubQ:

Congenital: 6 mcg/kg twice daily

Idiopathic/cyclic: 5 mcg/kg/day

(Continued)

Filgrastim *(Continued)*

Pediatrics: Children: Refer to adult dosing.

Available Dosage Forms

Injection, solution [preservative free]: 300 mcg/mL (1 mL, 1.6 mL) [vial; contains sodium 0.035 mg/mL and sorbitol]

Injection, solution [preservative free]: 600 mcg/mL (0.5 mL, 0.8 mL) [prefilled Singleject® syringe; contains sodium 0.035 mg/mL and sorbitol]

Nursing Guidelines

Assessment: Assess for hypersensitivity to *E. coli* products prior to beginning therapy. Assess potential for interactions with pharmacological agents the patient may be taking that may potentiate the release of neutrophils. Assess results of CBC and platelet counts twice weekly during therapy. Monitor therapeutic effectiveness and signs/symptoms of adverse reactions at beginning of therapy and periodically throughout therapy (eg, allergic-type reactions have occurred in patients receiving G-CSF with first or later doses). If self-administered, teach patient (or caregiver) proper storage, administration, and syringe/needle disposal. Teach patient (or caregiver) possible side effects/ appropriate interventions and adverse symptoms to report.

Monitoring Laboratory Tests: CBC and platelet count should be obtained twice weekly. Leukocytosis (white blood cell counts ≥100,000/mm^3) has been observed in ~2% of patients receiving filgrastim at doses >5 mcg/kg/day. Monitor platelets and hematocrit regularly.

Dietary Considerations: Injection solution contains sodium 0.035 mg/mL and sorbitol.

Patient Education: Do not take any new medication during therapy unless approved by prescriber. If self-administered, follow directions for proper storage and administration of SubQ medication. Never reuse syringes or needles. May cause bone pain (request analgesic); nausea or vomiting (small, frequent meals may help); hair loss (reversible); or sore mouth (frequent mouth care with soft toothbrush or cotton swab may help). Report immediately any respiratory difficulty or pain in left shoulder, chest or back. Report unusual fever or chills; unhealed sores; severe bone pain; pain, redness, or swelling at injection site; unusual swelling of extremities; or chest pain and palpitations. **Pregnancy/ breast-feeding precautions:** Inform prescriber if you are or intend to become pregnant. Consult prescriber if breast-feeding.

Pregnancy Risk Factor: C

Lactation: Excretion in breast milk unknown/use caution

Perioperative/Anesthesia/Other Concerns:

Reimbursement Hotline: 1-800-272-9376

Professional Services [AMGEN]: 1-800-77-AMGEN

Administration

I.V.: May be administered undiluted by SubQ injection. May also be administered by I.V. bolus over 15-30 minutes in D_5W, or by continuous SubQ or I.V. infusion. Do not administer earlier than 24 hours after cytotoxic chemotherapy.

Reconstitution:

Do not dilute with saline at any time; product may precipitate. Filgrastim may be diluted in dextrose 5% in water to a concentration 5-15 mcg/mL for I.V. infusion administration (minimum concentration: 5 mcg/mL). Dilution to <5 mcg/ mL is not recommended. Concentrations 5-15 mcg/mL require addition of albumin (final concentration of 2 mg/mL) to the bag to prevent absorption to plastics.

Compatibility: Standard diluent: ≥375 mcg/25 mL D_5W. Stable in D_5W; **incompatible** with NS

Y-site administration: Incompatible with amphotericin B, cefepime, cefoperazone, cefotaxime, cefoxitin, ceftizoxime, ceftriaxone, cefuroxime, clindamycin, dactinomycin, etoposide, fluorouracil, furosemide, heparin, mannitol, methylprednisolone sodium succinate, metronidazole, mitomycin, piperacillin, prochlorperazine edisylate, thiotepa

Storage: Intact vials and prefilled syringes should be stored under refrigeration at 2°C to 8°C (36°F to 46°F) and protected from direct sunlight. Filgrastim should be protected from freezing and temperatures >30°C to avoid aggregation. If inadvertently frozen, thaw in a refrigerator and use within 24 hours; do not use if frozen >24 hours or frozen more than once. The solution should not be shaken since bubbles and/or foam may form. If foaming occurs, the solution should be left undisturbed for a few minutes until bubbles dissipate.

Filgrastim vials and prefilled syringes are stable for 7 days at 9°C to 30°C (47°F to 86°F), however, the manufacturer recommends discarding after 24 hours because of microbiological concerns. The product is packaged without a preservative.

Undiluted filgrastim is stable for 24 hours at 15°C to 30°C and for 2 weeks at 2°C to 8°C (36°F to 46°F) in tuberculin syringes. However, the manufacturer recommends to use immediately because of concern for bacterial contamination.

Filgrastim diluted for I.V. infusion (5-15 mcg/mL) is stable for 7 days at 2°C to 8°C (36°F to 46°F). Compatible with glass bottles, PVC and polyolefin I.V. bags, and polypropylene syringes when diluted in 5% dextrose or 5% dextrose with albumin.

Finasteride (fi NAS teer ide)

U.S. Brand Names Propecia®; Proscar®

Pharmacologic Category 5 Alpha-Reductase Inhibitor

Medication Safety Issues

Sound-alike/look-alike issues:

Proscar® may be confused with ProSom®, Prozac®, Psorcon®

Use

Propecia®: Treatment of male pattern hair loss in **men only**. Safety and efficacy were demonstrated in men between 18-41 years of age.

Proscar®: Treatment of symptomatic benign prostatic hyperplasia (BPH); can be used in combination with an alpha blocker, doxazosin

Unlabeled/Investigational Use Adjuvant monotherapy after radical prostatectomy in the treatment of prostatic cancer; female hirsutism

Mechanism of Action Finasteride is a competitive inhibitor of both tissue and hepatic 5-alpha reductase. This results in inhibition of the conversion of testosterone to dihydrotestosterone and markedly suppresses serum dihydrotestosterone levels

Pharmacodynamics/Kinetics

Onset of action: 3-6 months of ongoing therapy

Duration:

After a single oral dose as small as 0.5 mg: 65% depression of plasma dihydrotestosterone levels persists 5-7 days

After 6 months of treatment with 5 mg/day: Circulating dihydrotestosterone levels are reduced to castrate levels without significant effects on circulating testosterone; levels return to normal within 14 days of discontinuation of treatment

Distribution: V_{dss}: 76 L

Protein binding: 90%

Metabolism: Hepatic via CYP3A4; two active metabolites (<20% activity of finasteride)

Bioavailability: Mean: 63%

Half-life elimination, serum: Elderly: 8 hours; Adults: 6 hours (3-16)

Time to peak, serum: 2-6 hours

Excretion: Feces (57%) and urine (39%) as metabolites

Contraindications Hypersensitivity to finasteride or any component of the formulation; pregnancy; not for use in children

Warnings/Precautions Hazardous agent - use appropriate precautions for handling and disposal. A minimum of 6 months of treatment may be necessary to determine whether an individual will respond to finasteride. Use with caution in those patients with hepatic dysfunction. Carefully monitor patients with a large residual urinary volume or severely diminished urinary flow for obstructive uropathy. These patients may not be candidates for finasteride therapy.

Drug Interactions Substrate of CYP3A4 (minor)

Nutritional/Herbal/Ethanol Interactions

Herb/Nutraceutical: St John's wort may decrease finasteride levels. Avoid saw palmetto (concurrent use has not been adequately studied).

Adverse Reactions Note: "Combination therapy" refers to finasteride and doxazosin.

>10%:

Endocrine & metabolic: Impotence (19%; combination therapy 23%), libido decreased (10%; combination therapy 12%)

Neuromuscular & skeletal: Weakness (5%; combination therapy 17%)

(Continued)

Finasteride *(Continued)*

1% to 10%:

Cardiovascular: Postural hypotension (9%; combination therapy 18%), edema (1%, combination therapy 3%)

Central nervous system: Dizziness (7%; combination therapy 23%), somnolence (2%; combination therapy 3%)

Genitourinary: Ejaculation disturbances (7%; combination therapy 14%), decreased volume of ejaculate

Endocrine & metabolic: Gynecomastia (2%)

Respiratory: Dyspnea (1%; combination therapy 2%), rhinitis (1%; combination therapy 2%)

<1%, postmarketing and/or case reports: Hypersensitivity (pruritus, rash, urticaria, swelling of face/lips); breast tenderness, breast enlargement, breast cancer (males), prostate cancer (high grade), testicular pain

Dosing

Adults & Elderly:

Benign prostatic hyperplasia (Proscar®): Oral: 5 mg/day as a single dose; clinical responses occur within 12 weeks to 6 months of initiation of therapy; long-term administration is recommended for maximal response

Male pattern baldness (Propecia®): Oral: 1 mg daily

Female hirsutism (unlabeled use): Oral: 5 mg/day

Renal Impairment: No adjustment is necessary.

Hepatic Impairment: Use with caution in patients with liver function abnormalities because finasteride is metabolized extensively in the liver

Available Dosage Forms Tablet [film coated]:

Propecia®: 1 mg

Proscar®: 5 mg

Nursing Guidelines

Assessment: See Contraindications, Warnings/Precautions, and Dosing for use cautions. Assess potential for interactions with prescription, OTC medications, or herbal products patient may be taking (see Drug Interactions). Assess therapeutic effectiveness and signs/symptoms of adverse reactions (see Adverse Reactions and Overdose/Toxicology). Teach patient proper use, possible side effects/appropriate interventions and adverse symptoms to report (see Patient Education). **Pregnancy risk factor X** - instruct patient on absolute need for barrier contraceptives. Women of childbearing age should not touch or handle broken tablets.

Monitoring Laboratory Tests: Finasteride does not interfere with free PSA levels.

Patient Education: Inform prescriber of all prescriptions, OTC medications, or herbal products you are taking, and any allergies you have. Do not take any new medication during therapy unless approved by prescriber. Results of therapy may take several months. Take with or without meals. May cause decreased libido or impotence during therapy. Report any increase in urinary volume or voiding patterns occurs. Report changes in breast condition (pain, lumps, or nipple discharge) in male and female patients. **Pregnancy precautions:** This drug will cause fetal abnormalities - use barrier contraceptives and do not allow women of childbearing age to touch or handle broken or crushed tablets.

Geriatric Considerations: Clearance of finasteride is decreased in the elderly, but no dosage reductions are necessary.

Pregnancy Risk Factor: X

Lactation: Excretion in breast milk unknown/contraindicated

Breast-Feeding Considerations: Not indicated for use in women.

Perioperative/Anesthesia/Other Concerns: Finasteride may be useful in men with moderately symptomatic BPH who either refuse prostatectomy or are poor surgical candidates. Currently, there is no way to predict which men will respond to finasteride. Treatment with finasteride does not alter the ratio of free to total PSA, which is used to detect prostatic cancer.

Administration

Oral: Administration with food may delay the rate and reduce the extent of oral absorption. Women of childbearing age should not touch or handle broken tablets.

Storage: Store below 30°C (86°F). Protect from light.

♦ **Fioricet®** *see* Butalbital, Acetaminophen, and Caffeine *on page 280*

♦ **First® Testosterone** *see* Testosterone *on page 1607*

- ♦ **First® Testosterone MC** *see* Testosterone *on page 1607*
- ♦ **Fisalamine** *see* Mesalamine *on page 1105*
- ♦ **Fish Oil** *see* Omega-3-Acid Ethyl Esters *on page 1263*
- ♦ **FK506** *see* Tacrolimus *on page 1593*
- ♦ **Flagyl®** *see* Metronidazole *on page 1154*
- ♦ **Flagyl ER®** *see* Metronidazole *on page 1154*
- ♦ **Flagyl® I.V. RTU™** *see* Metronidazole *on page 1154*
- ♦ **Flarex®** *see* Fluorometholone *on page 743*

Flecainide (fle KAY nide)

U.S. Brand Names Tambocor™

Synonyms Flecainide Acetate

Pharmacologic Category Antiarrhythmic Agent, Class Ic

Medication Safety Issues

Sound-alike/look-alike issues:

Flecainide may be confused with fluconazole

Tambocor™ may be confused with tamoxifen

Use Prevention and suppression of documented life-threatening ventricular arrhythmias (eg, sustained ventricular tachycardia); controlling symptomatic, disabling supraventricular tachycardias in patients without structural heart disease in whom other agents fail

Mechanism of Action Class Ic antiarrhythmic; slows conduction in cardiac tissue by altering transport of ions across cell membranes; causes slight prolongation of refractory periods; decreases the rate of rise of the action potential without affecting its duration; increases electrical stimulation threshold of ventricle, His-Purkinje system; possesses local anesthetic and moderate negative inotropic effects

Pharmacodynamics/Kinetics

Absorption: Oral: Rapid

Distribution: Adults: V_d: 5-13.4 L/kg

Protein binding: $Alpha_1$ glycoprotein: 40% to 50%

Metabolism: Hepatic

Bioavailability: 85% to 90%

Half-life elimination: Infants: 11-12 hours; Children: 8 hours; Adults: 7-22 hours, increased with congestive heart failure or renal dysfunction; End-stage renal disease: 19-26 hours

Time to peak, serum: ~1.5-3 hours

Excretion: Urine (80% to 90%, 10% to 50% as unchanged drug and metabolites)

Contraindications Hypersensitivity to flecainide or any component of the formulation; pre-existing second- or third-degree AV block or with right bundle branch block when associated with a left hemiblock (bifascicular block) (except in patients with a functioning artificial pacemaker); cardiogenic shock; coronary artery disease (based on CAST study results); concurrent use of ritonavir or amprenavir

Warnings/Precautions Not recommend for patients with chronic atrial fibrillation. A worsening or new arrhythmia may occur (proarrhythmic effect). Use caution in heart failure (may precipitate or exacerbate CHF). Dose-related increases in PR, QRS, and QT intervals occur. Use with caution in sick sinus syndrome or with permanent pacemakers or temporary pacing wires (can increase endocardial pacing thresholds). Pre-existing hypokalemia or hyperkalemia should be corrected before initiation (can alter drug's effect). Cautious use in significant hepatic impairment.

Drug Interactions Substrate of CYP1A2 (minor), 2D6 (major); **Inhibits** CYP2D6 (weak)

Amiodarone increases in flecainide plasma levels; consider reducing flecainide dose by 25% to 33% with concurrent use.

Amprenavir and ritonavir may increase cardiotoxicity of flecainide (decrease metabolism).

Cimetidine may decrease flecainide's metabolism; monitor cardiac status or use an alternative H_2 antagonist.

CYP2D6 inhibitors: May increase the levels/effects of flecainide. Example inhibitors include chlorpromazine, delavirdine, fluoxetine, miconazole, paroxetine, pergolide, quinidine, quinine, ritonavir, and ropinirole.

Digoxin's serum concentration may increase slightly.

Propranolol (and possibly other beta-blockers) increases flecainide blood levels, and propranolol blood levels are increased with concurrent use; monitor for excessive negative inotropic effects.

(Continued)

Flecainide *(Continued)*

Quinidine may decrease flecainide's metabolism; monitor cardiac status.
Urinary alkalinizers (antacids, sodium bicarbonate, acetazolamide) may increase flecainide blood levels.

Nutritional/Herbal/Ethanol Interactions Food: Clearance may be decreased in patients following strict vegetarian diets due to urinary pH ≥8. Dairy products (milk, infant formula, yogurt) may interfere with the absorption of flecainide in infants; there is one case report of a neonate (GA 34 weeks PNA >6 days) who required extremely large doses of oral flecainide when administered every 8 hours with feedings ("milk feeds"); changing the feedings from "milk feeds" to 5% glucose feeds alone resulted in a doubling of the flecainide serum concentration and toxicity.

Adverse Reactions

>10%:
Central nervous system: Dizziness (19% to 30%)
Ocular: Visual disturbances (16%)
Respiratory: Dyspnea (~10%)

1% to 10%:
Cardiovascular: Palpitations (6%), chest pain (5%), edema (3.5%), tachycardia (1% to 3%), proarrhythmic (4% to 12%), sinus node dysfunction (1.2%), syncope
Central nervous system: Headache (4% to 10%), fatigue (8%), nervousness (5%) additional symptoms occurring at a frequency between 1% and 3%: fever, malaise, hypoesthesia, paresis, ataxia, vertigo, somnolence, tinnitus, anxiety, insomnia, depression
Dermatologic: Rash (1% to 3%)
Gastrointestinal: Nausea (9%), constipation (1%), abdominal pain (3%), anorexia (1% to 3%), diarrhea (0.7% to 3%)
Neuromuscular & skeletal: Tremor (5%), weakness (5%), paresthesia (1%)
Ocular: Diplopia (1% to 3%), blurred vision

<1% (Limited to important or life-threatening): Alopecia, alters pacing threshold, amnesia, angina, AV block, bradycardia, bronchospasm, CHF, corneal deposits, depersonalization, euphoria, exfoliative dermatitis, granulocytopenia, heart block, increased P-R, leukopenia, metallic taste, neuropathy, paradoxical increase in ventricular rate in atrial fibrillation/flutter, paresthesia, photophobia, pneumonitis, pruritus, QRS duration, swollen lips/tongue/mouth, tardive dyskinesia, thrombocytopenia, urinary retention, urticaria, ventricular arrhythmia

Overdosage/Toxicology Flecainide has a narrow therapeutic index and severe toxicity may occur slightly above the therapeutic range, especially if combined with other antiarrhythmic drugs. (Acute single ingestion of twice the daily therapeutic dose is life-threatening). Symptoms of overdose include increase in P-R, QRS, or QT intervals and amplitude of the T wave, AV block, bradycardia, hypotension, ventricular arrhythmias (monomorphic or polymorphic ventricular tachycardia), and asystole. Other symptoms include dizziness, blurred vision, headache, and GI upset. Treatment is supportive.

Dosing

Adults & Elderly:

Life-threatening ventricular arrhythmias: Oral:
Initial: 100 mg every 12 hours; increase by 50-100 mg/day (given in 2 doses/day) every 4 days; maximum: 400 mg/day
For patients receiving 400 mg/day who are not controlled and have trough concentrations <0.6 mcg/mL, dosage may be increased to 600 mg/day.

Prevention of paroxysmal supraventricular arrhythmias: Oral:
Note: In patients with disabling symptoms but no structural heart disease
Initial: 50 mg every 12 hours; increase by 50 mg twice daily at 4-day intervals; maximum: 300 mg/day

Pediatrics:

Life-threatening ventricular arrhythmias: Oral: Children:
Initial: 3 mg/kg/day or 50-100 mg/m^2/day in 3 divided doses
Usual maintenance: 3-6 mg/kg/day or 100-150 mg/m^2/day in 3 divided doses; up to 11 mg/kg/day or 200 mg/m^2/day for uncontrolled patients with subtherapeutic levels

Renal Impairment:

Cl_{cr} <10 mL/minute: Decrease usual dose by 25% to 50% in severe renal impairment.
Not dialyzable (0% to 5%) via hemo- or peritoneal dialysis; no supplemental dose is necessary.

Hepatic Impairment: Monitoring of plasma levels is recommended because half-life is significantly increased. When transferring from another antiarrhythmic agent, allow for 2-4 half-lives of the agent to pass before initiating flecainide therapy.

Available Dosage Forms Tablet, as acetate: 50 mg, 100 mg, 150 mg

Nursing Guidelines

Assessment: Assess other medications patient may be taking for effectiveness and interactions. Monitor cardiac status. Assess results of laboratory tests, therapeutic effectiveness, and adverse reactions when beginning therapy, when titrating dosage, and periodically during long-term therapy. **Note:** Flecainide has a low toxic:therapeutic ratio and overdose may easily produce severe and life-threatening reactions. Assess knowledge/teach patient appropriate use, interventions to reduce side effects, and adverse symptoms to report.

Monitoring Laboratory Tests: Periodic serum concentrations, especially in patients with renal or hepatic impairment

Patient Education: Take exactly as directed, around-the-clock. Do not discontinue without consulting prescriber. You will require frequent monitoring while taking this medication. You may experience lightheadedness, nervousness, dizziness, visual disturbances (use caution when driving or engaging in tasks requiring alertness until response to drug is known); or nausea, vomiting, or loss of appetite (small frequent meals may help). Report palpitations, chest pain, excessively slow or rapid heartbeat; acute nervousness, headache, or fatigue; unusual weight gain; unusual cough; respiratory difficulty; swelling of hands or ankles; or muscle tremor, numbness, or weakness. **Pregnancy precaution:** Inform prescriber if you are or intend to become pregnant.

Pregnancy Risk Factor: C

Lactation: Enters breast milk/compatible

Perioperative/Anesthesia/Other Concerns: Based on adverse outcomes noted with flecainide in the CAST trial, the FDA recommends that use of flecainide be limited to patients with life-threatening ventricular arrhythmias.

Administration

Oral: Administer around-the-clock to promote less variation in peak and trough serum levels.

- ♦ **Flecainide Acetate** *see* Flecainide *on page 731*
- ♦ **Fleet® Accu-Prep® [OTC]** *see* Sodium Phosphates *on page 1549*
- ♦ **Fleet® Babylax® [OTC]** *see* Glycerin *on page 826*
- ♦ **Fleet® Bisacodyl Enema [OTC]** *see* Bisacodyl *on page 245*
- ♦ **Fleet® Enema [OTC]** *see* Sodium Phosphates *on page 1549*
- ♦ **Fleet® Glycerin Suppositories [OTC]** *see* Glycerin *on page 826*
- ♦ **Fleet® Glycerin Suppositories Maximum Strength [OTC]** *see* Glycerin *on page 826*
- ♦ **Fleet® Liquid Glycerin Suppositories [OTC]** *see* Glycerin *on page 826*
- ♦ **Fleet® Phospho-Soda® [OTC]** *see* Sodium Phosphates *on page 1549*
- ♦ **Fleet® Sof-Lax® [OTC]** *see* Docusate *on page 560*
- ♦ **Fleet® Sof-Lax® Overnight [DSC] [OTC]** *see* Docusate and Casanthranol *on page 561*
- ♦ **Fleet® Stimulant Laxative [OTC]** *see* Bisacodyl *on page 245*
- ♦ **Fletcher's® Castoria® [OTC]** *see* Senna *on page 1520*
- ♦ **Flexeril®** *see* Cyclobenzaprine *on page 459*
- ♦ **Flintstones® Complete [OTC]** *see* Vitamins (Multiple/Pediatric) *on page 1720*
- ♦ **Flintstones® Plus Calcium [OTC]** *see* Vitamins (Multiple/Pediatric) *on page 1720*
- ♦ **Flintstones® Plus Extra C [OTC]** *see* Vitamins (Multiple/Pediatric) *on page 1720*
- ♦ **Flintstones® Plus Iron [OTC]** *see* Vitamins (Multiple/Pediatric) *on page 1720*
- ♦ **Flolan®** *see* Epoprostenol *on page 622*
- ♦ **Flomax®** *see* Tamsulosin *on page 1598*
- ♦ **Flonase®** *see* Fluticasone *on page 760*
- ♦ **Florical® [OTC]** *see* Calcium Carbonate *on page 291*
- ♦ **Florinef®** *see* Fludrocortisone *on page 737*
- ♦ **Flovent® [DSC]** *see* Fluticasone *on page 760*
- ♦ **Flovent® HFA** *see* Fluticasone *on page 760*
- ♦ **Floxin®** *see* Ofloxacin *on page 1255*
- ♦ **Floxin Otic Singles** *see* Ofloxacin *on page 1255*
- ♦ **Fluarix™** *see* Influenza Virus Vaccine *on page 913*

♦ Flubenisolone *see* Betamethasone *on page 237*

Fluconazole (floo KOE na zole)

U.S. Brand Names Diflucan®

Pharmacologic Category Antifungal Agent, Oral; Antifungal Agent, Parenteral

Medication Safety Issues

Sound-alike/look-alike issues:

Fluconazole may be confused with flecainide

Diflucan® may be confused with diclofenac, Diprivan®, disulfiram

Use Treatment of candidiasis (vaginal, oropharyngeal, esophageal, urinary tract infections, peritonitis, pneumonia, and systemic infections); cryptococcal meningitis; antifungal prophylaxis in allogeneic bone marrow transplant recipients

Mechanism of Action Interferes with cytochrome P450 activity, decreasing ergosterol synthesis (principal sterol in fungal cell membrane) and inhibiting cell membrane formation

Pharmacodynamics/Kinetics

Distribution: Widely throughout body with good penetration into CSF, eye, peritoneal fluid, sputum, skin, and urine

Relative diffusion blood into CSF: Adequate with or without inflammation (exceeds usual MICs)

CSF:blood level ratio: Normal meninges: 70% to 80%; Inflamed meninges: >70% to 80%

Protein binding, plasma: 11% to 12%

Bioavailability: Oral: >90%

Half-life elimination: Normal renal function: ~30 hours

Time to peak, serum: Oral: 1-2 hours

Excretion: Urine (80% as unchanged drug)

Contraindications Hypersensitivity to fluconazole, other azoles, or any component of the formulation; concomitant administration with cisapride

Warnings/Precautions Should be used with caution in patients with renal and hepatic dysfunction or previous hepatotoxicity from other azole derivatives. Patients who develop abnormal liver function tests during fluconazole therapy should be monitored closely and discontinued if symptoms consistent with liver disease develop. Use caution in patients at risk of proarrhythmias.

Drug Interactions Inhibits CYP1A2 (weak), 2C8/9 (strong), 2C19 (strong), 3A4 (moderate)

Benzodiazepines (metabolized by oxidation, eg, alprazolam, triazolam, midazolam, diazepam) serum concentrations are increased by fluconazole which may cause increased CNS sedation. Consider a benzodiazepine not metabolized by CYP3A4 or another antifungal.

Caffeine's metabolism is decreased; monitor for tachycardia, nervousness, and anxiety.

Calcium channel blockers may have increased serum concentrations; consider another agent instead of a calcium channel blocker, another antifungal, or reduce the dose of the calcium channel blocker. Monitor blood pressure.

Cisapride's serum concentration is increased which may lead to malignant arrhythmias; concurrent use is contraindicated.

Cyclosporine's serum concentration is increased; monitor cyclosporine's serum concentration and renal function.

CYP2C8/9 substrates: Fluconazole may increase the levels/effects of CYP2C8/9 substrates. Example substrates include amiodarone, fluoxetine, glimepiride, glipizide, nateglinide, phenytoin, pioglitazone, rosiglitazone, sertraline, and warfarin.

CYP2C19 substrates: Fluconazole may increase the levels/effects of CYP2C19 substrates. Example substrates include citalopram, diazepam, methsuximide, phenytoin, propranolol, and sertraline.

CYP3A4 substrates: Fluconazole may increase the levels/effects of CYP3A4 substrates. Example substrates include benzodiazepines, calcium channel blockers, cyclosporine, mirtazapine, nateglinide, nefazodone, sildenafil (and other PDE-5 inhibitors), tacrolimus, and venlafaxine. Selected benzodiazepines (midazolam and triazolam), cisapride, ergot alkaloids, selected HMG-CoA reductase inhibitors (lovastatin and simvastatin), and pimozide are generally contraindicated with strong CYP3A4 inhibitors.

HMG-CoA reductase inhibitors (except pravastatin and fluvastatin) have increased serum concentrations; switch to pravastatin/fluvastatin or monitor for development of myopathy.

Losartan's active metabolite is reduced in concentration; consider another antihypertensive agent unaffected by the azole antifungals, another antifungal, or monitor blood pressure closely.

Phenytoin's serum concentration is increased; monitor phenytoin levels and adjust dose as needed.

Rifampin decreases fluconazole's serum concentration; monitor infection status.

Tacrolimus's serum concentration is increased; monitor tacrolimus's serum concentration and renal function.

Warfarin's effects are increased; monitor INR and adjust warfarin's dose as needed.

Adverse Reactions Frequency not always defined.

Cardiovascular: Angioedema, pallor, QT prolongation, torsade de pointes

Central nervous system: Headache (2% to 13%), seizure, dizziness

Dermatologic: Rash (2%), alopecia, toxic epidermal necrolysis, Stevens-Johnson syndrome

Endocrine & metabolic: Hypercholesterolemia, hypertriglyceridemia, hypokalemia

Gastrointestinal: Nausea (4% to 7%), vomiting (2%), abdominal pain (2% to 6%), diarrhea (2% to 3%), taste perversion, dyspepsia

Hematologic: Agranulocytosis, leukopenia, neutropenia, thrombocytopenia

Hepatic: Hepatic failure (rare), hepatitis, cholestasis, jaundice, increased ALT/AST, increased alkaline phosphatase

Respiratory: Dyspnea

Miscellaneous: Anaphylactic reactions (rare)

Overdosage/Toxicology Symptoms of overdose include decreased lacrimation, salivation, respiration and motility, urinary incontinence, and cyanosis. Treatment includes supportive measures. A 3-hour hemodialysis will remove 50%.

Dosing

Adults & Elderly: The daily dose of fluconazole is the same for both oral and I.V. administration

Usual dosage range: 200-400 mg daily; duration and dosage depends on severity of infection

Indication-specific dosing:

Candidiasis:

Candidemia, primary therapy, non-neutropenic: 400-800 mg/day for 14 days after last positive blood culture and resolution of signs/symptoms

Alternate therapy: 800 mg/day with amphotericin B for 4-7 days followed by 800 mg/day for 14 days after last positive blood culture and resolution of signs/symptoms

Candidemia, secondary, neutropenic: 6-12 mg/kg/day for 14 days after last positive blood culture and resolution of signs/symptoms

Chronic, disseminated: 6 mg/kg/day for 3-6 months

Oropharyngeal (long-term suppression): 200 mg/day; chronic therapy is recommended in immunocompromised patients with history of oropharyngeal candidiasis (OPC)

Osteomyelitis: 6 mg/kg/day for 6-12 months

Esophageal: 200 mg on day 1, then 100-200 mg/day for 2-3 weeks after clinical improvement

Prophylaxis in bone marrow transplant: 400 mg/day; begin 3 days before onset of neutropenia and continue for 7 days after neutrophils >1000 cells/mm^3

Urinary: 200 mg/day for 1-2 weeks

Vaginal: 150 mg as a single dose

Coccidiomycosis: 400 mg/day; doses of 800-1000 mg/day have been used for meningeal disease; usual duration of therapy ranges from 3-6 months for primary uncomplicated infections and up to 1 year for pulmonary (chronic and diffuse) infection

Endocarditis, prosthetic valve, early: 6-12 mg/kg/day for 6 weeks after valve replacement

Endophthalmitis: 6-12 mg/kg/day or 400-800 mg/day for 6-12 weeks after surgical intervention. **Note:** *C. krusei* and *C. galbrata* infection acquired exogenously should be treated with voriconazole.

Meningitis, cryptococcal: 400-800 mg/day for 10-12 weeks or with flucytosine 100-150 mg/day for 6 weeks; maintenance: 200-400 mg/day

Pneumonia, cryptococcal (mild-to-moderate): 200-400 mg/day for 6-12 months (life-long in HIV-positive patients)

Pediatrics: The daily dose of fluconazole is the same for oral and I.V. administration

(Continued)

Fluconazole *(Continued)*

Usual dosage ranges:

Neonates: First 2 weeks of life, especially premature neonates: Same dose as older children every 72 hours

Children: Loading dose: 6-12 mg/kg; maintenance: 3-12 mg/kg/day; duration and dosage depends on severity of infection

Indication-specific dosing:

Candidiasis:

Oropharyngeal: Loading dose: 6 mg/kg; maintenance: 3 mg/kg/day for 2 weeks

Esophageal: Loading dose: 6 mg/kg; maintenance: 3-12 mg/kg/day for 21 days and at least 2 weeks following resolution of symptoms

Systemic infection: 6 mg/kg every 12 hours for 28 days

Meningitis, cryptococcal: Loading dose: 12 mg/kg; maintenance: 6-12 mg/kg/day for 10-12 weeks following negative CSF culture; relapse suppression: 6 mg/kg/day

Renal Impairment:

No adjustment for vaginal candidiasis single-dose therapy

For multiple dosing, administer usual load then adjust daily doses

Cl_{cr} ≤50 mL/minute (no dialysis): Administer 50% of recommended dose or administer every 48 hours.

Hemodialysis: 50% is removed by hemodialysis; administer 100% of daily dose (according to indication) after each dialysis treatment.

Continuous arteriovenous or venovenous hemofiltration: Dose as for Cl_{cr} 10-50 mL/minute.

Available Dosage Forms

Infusion [premixed in sodium chloride]: 2 mg/mL (100 mL, 200 mL)

Diflucan® [premixed in sodium chloride or dextrose] 2 mg/mL (100 mL, 200 mL)

Powder for oral suspension (Diflucan®): 10 mg/mL (35 mL); 40 mg/mL (35 mL) [contains sodium benzoate; orange flavor]

Tablet (Diflucan®): 50 mg, 100 mg, 150 mg, 200 mg

Nursing Guidelines

Assessment: Assess allergy history prior to beginning therapy. See Contraindications, Warnings/Precautions, and Dosing for use cautions. Assess potential for interactions with other prescriptions, OTC medications, and herbal products patient may be taking (see Drug Interactions). See specific Administration and Compatibility directions. Assess results of laboratory tests (see below), therapeutic effectiveness, and adverse response (see Adverse Reactions) on a regular basis throughout therapy. Teach patient use, possible side effects/ appropriate interventions, and adverse symptoms to report (see Patient Education). Note breast-feeding caution.

Monitoring Laboratory Tests: Culture prior to beginning therapy, periodic liver function (AST, ALT, alkaline phosphatase) and renal function, potassium

Dietary Considerations: Take with or without regard to food.

Patient Education: Inform prescriber of all prescriptions, OTC medications, or herbal products you are taking, and any allergies you have. Do not take any new medication during therapy unless approved by prescriber. Take as directed, around-the-clock. Take full course of medication as ordered. Take with or without food. Follow good hygiene measures to prevent reinfection. Frequent blood tests may be required. Maintain adequate hydration (2-3 L/day of fluids) unless instructed to restrict fluid intake. May cause headache, dizziness, drowsiness (use caution when driving or engaging in tasks that require alertness until response to drug is known); or nausea, vomiting, or diarrhea (small, frequent meals, frequent mouth care, sucking lozenges, or chewing gum may help). Report skin rash, redness, or irritation; persistent GI upset; urinary pattern changes; excessively dry eyes or mouth; or changes in color of stool or urine. **Pregnancy/breast-feeding precautions:** Inform prescriber if you are or intend to become pregnant. Consult prescriber if breast-feeding.

Geriatric Considerations: Dose may need adjustment based on changes of renal function.

Pregnancy Risk Factor: C

Pregnancy Issues: When used in high doses, fluconazole is teratogenic in animal studies. Following exposure during the first trimester, case reports have noted similar malformations in humans when used in higher doses (400 mg/ day) over extended periods of time. Use of lower doses (150 mg as a single dose or 200 mg/day) may have less risk; however, additional data is needed. Use during pregnancy only if the potential benefit to the mother outweighs any potential risk to the fetus.

Lactation: Enters breast/not recommended (AAP rates "compatible")

Breast-Feeding Considerations: Fluconazole is found in breast milk at concentration similar to plasma.

Perioperative/Anesthesia/Other Concerns: Do not use if cloudy or precipitated. If administered by I.V. infusion, give over 1-2 hours.

Administration

I.M.: For I.V. only; do not administer I.M. or SubQ

I.V.: Do not exceed 200 mg/hour when giving I.V. infusion

Compatibility: Stable in D_5W, LR, NS

Y-site administration: Incompatible with amphotericin B, amphotericin B cholesteryl sulfate complex, ampicillin, calcium gluconate, cefotaxime, ceftazidime, ceftriaxone, cefuroxime, chloramphenicol, clindamycin, co-trimoxazole, diazepam, digoxin, erythromycin lactobionate, furosemide, haloperidol, hydroxyzine, imipenem/cilastatin, pentamidine, piperacillin, ticarcillin

Compatibility when admixed: Incompatible with co-trimoxazole

Storage:

Powder for oral suspension: Store dry powder at ≤30°C (86°F). Following reconstitution, store at 5°C to 30°C (41°F to 86°F). Discard unused portion after 2 weeks. Do not freeze.

Injection: Store injection in glass at 5°C to 30°C (41°F to 86°F). Store injection in Viaflex® at 5°C to 25°C (41°F to 77°F). Protect from freezing. Do not unwrap unit until ready for use.

Fludrocortisone (floo droe KOR ti sone)

U.S. Brand Names Florinef®

Synonyms 9α-Fluorohydrocortisone Acetate; Fludrocortisone Acetate; Fluohydrisone Acetate; Fluohydrocortisone Acetate

Pharmacologic Category Corticosteroid, Systemic

Medication Safety Issues

Sound-alike/look-alike issues:

Florinef® may be confused with Fiorinal®

Use Partial replacement therapy for primary and secondary adrenocortical insufficiency in Addison's disease; treatment of salt-losing adrenogenital syndrome

Mechanism of Action Promotes increased reabsorption of sodium and loss of potassium from renal distal tubules

Pharmacodynamics/Kinetics

Absorption: Rapid and complete

Protein binding: 42%

Metabolism: Hepatic

Half-life elimination, plasma: 30-35 minutes; Biological: 18-36 hours

Time to peak, serum: ~1.7 hours

Contraindications Hypersensitivity to fludrocortisone or any component of the formulation; systemic fungal infections

Warnings/Precautions Taper dose gradually when therapy is discontinued; use with caution with Addison's disease, sodium retention and potassium loss

Drug Interactions Decreased effect:

Anticholinesterases effects are antagonized

Decreased corticosteroid effects by rifampin, barbiturates, and hydantoins

Decreased salicylate levels

Adverse Reactions Frequency not defined.

Cardiovascular: Hypertension, edema, CHF

Central nervous system: Convulsions, headache, dizziness

Dermatologic: Acne, rash, bruising

Endocrine & metabolic: Hypokalemic alkalosis, suppression of growth, hyperglycemia, HPA suppression

Gastrointestinal: Peptic ulcer

Neuromuscular & skeletal: Muscle weakness

Ocular: Cataracts

Miscellaneous: Diaphoresis, anaphylaxis (generalized)

Overdosage/Toxicology Symptoms of overdose include hypertension, edema, hypokalemia, excessive weight gain. When consumed in excessive quantities, systemic hypercorticism and adrenal suppression may occur. In those cases, discontinuation of the corticosteroid should be done judiciously.

(Continued)

Fludrocortisone *(Continued)*

Dosing

Adults & Elderly: Mineralocorticoid deficiency: Oral: 0.05-0.2 mg/day with ranges of 0.1 mg 3 times/week to 0.2 mg/day

Pediatrics: Mineralocorticoid deficiency: Oral: Infants and Children: 0.05-0.1 mg/day

Available Dosage Forms Tablet, as acetate: 0.1 mg

Nursing Guidelines

Assessment: Assess effectiveness and interactions of other medications patient may be taking. Monitor for effectiveness of therapy and adverse reactions according to dose and length of therapy. Assess knowledge/teach patient appropriate use, possible side effects/interventions, and adverse symptoms to report (eg, opportunistic infection, adrenal suppression). Instruct patients with diabetes to monitor serum glucose levels closely; corticosteroids can alter glycemic response. Dose may need to be increased if patient is experiencing higher than normal levels of stress. When discontinuing, taper dose and frequency slowly.

Monitoring Laboratory Tests: Serum electrolytes, serum renin activity

Dietary Considerations: Systemic use of mineralocorticoids/corticosteroids may require a diet with increased potassium, vitamins A, B_6, C, D, folate, calcium, zinc, and phosphorus, and decreased sodium. With fludrocortisone, a decrease in dietary sodium is often not required as the increased retention of sodium is usually the desired therapeutic effect.

Patient Education: Take exactly as directed. Do not take more than prescribed dose and do not discontinue abruptly; consult prescriber. Take with or after meals. Take once-a-day dose with food in the morning. Limit intake of caffeine or stimulants. Maintain adequate nutrition; consult prescriber for possibility of special dietary recommendations. If you have diabetes, monitor serum glucose closely and notify prescriber of changes; this medication can alter glycemic response. Notify prescriber if you are experiencing higher than normal levels of stress; medication may need adjustment. Periodic ophthalmic examinations will be necessary with long-term use. You will be susceptible to infection (avoid crowds and exposure to infection). You may experience insomnia or nervousness; use caution when driving or engaging in tasks requiring alertness until response to drug is known. Report weakness, change in menstrual pattern, vision changes, signs of hyperglycemia, signs of infection (eg, fever, chills, mouth sores, perianal itching, vaginal discharge), other persistent side effects, or worsening of condition. **Pregnancy/breast-feeding precautions:** Inform prescriber if you are or intend to become pregnant. Consult prescriber if breast-feeding.

Geriatric Considerations: The most common use of fludrocortisone in the elderly is orthostatic hypotension that is unresponsive to more conservative measures. Attempt nonpharmacologic measures (hydration, support stockings etc) before starting drug therapy.

Pregnancy Risk Factor: C

Lactation: Excretion in breast milk unknown

Perioperative/Anesthesia/Other Concerns: In patients with salt-losing forms of congenital adrenogenital syndrome, use along with cortisone or hydrocortisone. Fludrocortisone 0.1 mg has sodium retention activity equal to DOCA® 1 mg.

Adrenal Insufficiency: Patients on long-term steroid supplementation will require higher corticosteroid doses when subject to stress (ie, trauma, surgery, severe infection). This agent has significant mineralocorticoid activity with consequent hemodynamic effects. Fludrocortisone has been used to treat severe orthostatic hypotension. Abrupt withdrawal may result in adrenal insufficiency with hypotension and hyperkalemia. A recent randomized, double-blind, placebo controlled trial assessed whether low dose corticosteroid administration could improve 28-day survival in patients with septic shock and acquired adrenal insufficiency. A lack of adrenal reserves is defined by an increase in serum cortisol of ≤9 mcg/dL in response to corticotropin administration. Cortisol levels were drawn immediately before corticotropin administration and 30 to 60 minutes afterwards. Three hundred adult septic shock patients requiring mechanical ventilation and vasopressor support were randomized to either hydrocortisone (50 mg IVP every 6 hours) and fludrocortisone (50 mcg tablet daily via nasogastric tube) or matching placebos for 7 days. Patients included had severe sepsis requiring vasopressor support and mechanical ventilation. In patients who did not appropriately respond to corticotropin (nonresponders), there were significantly fewer deaths in the active treatment group. Vasopressor therapy was withdrawn more frequently in this subset of the active treatment group. Adverse events were similar in both groups. Patients who lack adrenal reserve and thus have acquired adrenal insufficiency during the stress of septic shock may benefit from physiologic steroid replacement. Further study is required to better characterize the patient populations who may benefit.

Administration

Oral: Administration in conjunction with a glucocorticoid is preferable.

♦ Fludrocortisone Acetate *see* Fludrocortisone *on page 737*

Flumazenil (FLOO may ze nil)

U.S. Brand Names Romazicon®

Pharmacologic Category Antidote

Use Benzodiazepine antagonist; reverses sedative effects of benzodiazepines used in conscious sedation and general anesthesia; treatment of benzodiazepine overdose

Mechanism of Action Competitively inhibits the activity at the benzodiazepine recognition site on the GABA/benzodiazepine receptor complex. Flumazenil does not antagonize the CNS effect of drugs affecting GABA-ergic neurons by means other than the benzodiazepine receptor (ethanol, barbiturates, general anesthetics) and does not reverse the effects of opioids

Pharmacodynamics/Kinetics

Onset of action: 1-3 minutes; 80% response within 3 minutes

Peak effect: 6-10 minutes

Duration: Resedation: ~1 hour; duration related to dose given and benzodiazepine plasma concentrations; reversal effects of flumazenil may wear off before effects of benzodiazepine

Distribution: Initial V_d: 0.5 L/kg; V_{dss} 0.77-1.6 L/kg

Protein binding: 40% to 50%

Metabolism: Hepatic; dependent upon hepatic blood flow

Half-life elimination: Adults: Alpha: 7-15 minutes; Terminal: 41-79 minutes

Excretion: Feces; urine (0.2% as unchanged drug)

Contraindications Hypersensitivity to flumazenil, benzodiazepines, or any component of the formulation; patients given benzodiazepines for control of potentially life-threatening conditions (eg, control of intracranial pressure or status epilepticus); patients who are showing signs of serious cyclic-antidepressant overdosage

Warnings/Precautions Benzodiazepine reversal may result in seizures in some patients. Patients who may develop seizures include patients on benzodiazepines for long-term sedation, tricyclic antidepressant overdose patients, concurrent major sedative-hypnotic drug withdrawal, recent therapy with repeated doses of parenteral benzodiazepines, myoclonic jerking or seizure activity prior to flumazenil administration. Flumazenil does not reverse respiratory depression/hypoventilation or cardiac depression. Resedation occurs more frequently in patients where a large single dose or cumulative dose of a benzodiazepine is administered along with a neuromuscular blocking agent and multiple anesthetic agents. Flumazenil should be used with caution in the intensive care unit because of increased risk of unrecognized benzodiazepine dependence in such settings. Should not be used to diagnose benzodiazepine-induced sedation. Reverse neuromuscular blockade before considering use. Flumazenil does not antagonize the CNS effects of other GABA agonists (such as ethanol, barbiturates, or general anesthetics); nor does it reverse narcotics. Use with caution in patients with a history of panic disorder; may provoke panic attacks. Use caution in drug and ethanol-dependent patients; these patients may also be dependent on benzodiazepines. Not recommended for treatment of benzodiazepine dependence. Use with caution in head injury patients. Use caution in patients with mixed drug overdoses; toxic effects of other drugs taken may emerge once benzodiazepine effects are reversed. Flumazenil does not consistently reverse amnesia; patient may not recall verbal instructions after procedure. Use caution in severe hepatic dysfunction and in patients relying on a benzodiazepine for seizure control. Safety and efficacy have not been established in children >1 year of age.

Drug Interactions

Nonbenzodiazepine hypnotics (zaleplon, zolpidem, zopiclone): Flumazenil reverses the effects of these hypnotics.

Adverse Reactions

>10%: Gastrointestinal: Vomiting, nausea

(Continued)

Flumazenil *(Continued)*

1% to 10%:

Cardiovascular: Palpitations

Central nervous system: Headache, anxiety, nervousness, insomnia, abnormal crying, euphoria, depression, agitation, dizziness, emotional lability, ataxia, depersonalization, increased tears, dysphoria, paranoia, fatigue, vertigo

Endocrine & metabolic: Hot flashes

Gastrointestinal: Xerostomia

Local: Pain at injection site

Neuromuscular & skeletal: Tremor, weakness, paresthesia

Ocular: Abnormal vision, blurred vision

Respiratory: Dyspnea, hyperventilation

Miscellaneous: Diaphoresis

<1% (Limited to important or life-threatening): Bradycardia, chest pain, confusion, fear, generalized convulsions, hypertension, junctional tachycardia, panic attacks, tachycardia, ventricular tachycardia, withdrawal syndrome

Overdosage/Toxicology Excessively high doses may cause anxiety, agitation, increased muscle tone, hyperesthesia and seizures.

Dosing

Adults: See table.

Flumazenil

Adult dosage for **reversal of conscious sedation and general anesthesia:**	
Initial dose	0.2 mg intravenously over 15 seconds
Repeat doses	If desired level of consciousness is not obtained, 0.2 mg may be repeated at 1-minute intervals.
Maximum total cumulative dose	1 mg (usual dose: 0.6-1 mg) **In the event of resedation:** Repeat doses may be given at 20-minute intervals with maximum of 1 mg/dose and 3 mg/hour.
Adult dosage for **suspected benzodiazepine overdose:**	
Initial dose	0.2 mg intravenously over 30 seconds; if the desired level of consciousness is not obtained, 0.3 mg can be given over 30 seconds
Repeat doses	0.5 mg over 30 seconds repeated at 1-minute intervals
Maximum total cumulative dose	3 mg (usual dose: 1-3 mg) Patients with a partial response at 3 mg may require additional titration up to a total dose of 5 mg. If a patient has not responded 5 minutes after cumulative dose of 5 mg, the major cause of sedation is not likely due to benzodiazepines. **In the event of resedation:** May repeat doses at 20-minute intervals with maximum of 1 mg/dose and 3 mg/hour.

Resedation: Repeated doses may be given at 20-minute intervals as needed; repeat treatment doses of 1 mg (at a rate of 0.5 mg/minute) should be given at any time and no more than 3 mg should be given in any hour. After intoxication with high doses of benzodiazepines, the duration of a single dose of flumazenil is not expected to exceed 1 hour; if desired, the period of wakefulness may be prolonged with repeated low intravenous doses of flumazenil, or by an infusion of 0.1-0.4 mg/hour. Most patients with benzodiazepine overdose will respond to a cumulative dose of 1-3 mg and doses >3 mg do not reliably produce additional effects. Rarely, patients with a partial response at 3 mg may require additional titration up to a total dose of 5 mg. **If a patient has not responded 5 minutes after receiving a cumulative dose of 5 mg, the major cause of sedation is not likely to be due to benzodiazepines.**

Elderly: Refer to adult dosing. No differences in safety or efficacy have been reported; however, increased sensitivity may occur in some elderly patients.

Pediatrics:

Reversal of benzodiazepine when used in conscious sedation or general anesthesia: I.V.: Initial dose: 0.01 mg/kg (maximum dose: 0.2 mg) given over 15 seconds; may repeat 0.01 mg/kg (maximum dose: 0.2 mg) after 45 seconds, and then every minute (maximum: 4 doses) to a maximum of total cumulative dose of 0.05 mg/kg or 1 mg, whichever is lower; usual total dose: 0.08-1 mg (mean: 0.65 mg).

Renal Impairment: Not significantly affected by renal failure (Cl_{cr} <10 mL/minute) or hemodialysis beginning 1 hour after drug administration.

Hepatic Impairment: Initial dose of flumazenil used for initial reversal of benzodiazepine effects is not changed; however, subsequent doses in liver disease patients should be reduced in amount or frequency.

Available Dosage Forms Injection, solution: 0.1 mg/mL (5 mL, 10 mL) [contains edetate sodium]

Nursing Guidelines

Assessment: Assess level of consciousness frequently. Monitor vital signs and airway closely. ECG monitoring and oxygenation via pulse oximetry is highly recommended. Observe continually for resedation, respiratory depression, preseizure activity, or other residual benzodiazepine effects. May require pain medication sooner after reversal. Assess for nausea and vomiting.

Patient Education: Flumazenil does not consistently reverse amnesia. Do not engage in activities requiring alertness for 18-24 hours after discharge. Avoid alcohol or OTC medications for 24 hours after receiving this medication, unless approved by prescriber. Resedation may occur in patients on long-acting benzodiazepines (such as diazepam). **Pregnancy/breast-feeding precautions:** Inform prescriber if you are or intend to become pregnant. Consult prescriber if breast-feeding.

Pregnancy Risk Factor: C

Lactation: Excretion in breast milk unknown/use caution

Perioperative/Anesthesia/Other Concerns: Flumazenil does **not** antagonize the CNS effects of other GABA agonists (such as ethanol, barbiturates, or general anesthetics), nor does it reverse narcotics.

Administration

I.V.: Administer in freely-running I.V. into large vein. Inject over 15 seconds for conscious sedation and general anesthesia and over 30 seconds for overdose.

Reconstitution: For I.V. use only. Once drawn up in the syringe or mixed with solution use within 24 hours. Discard any unused solution after 24 hours.

Compatibility: Stable in D_5W, LR, NS

Storage: Store at 15°C to 30°C (59°F to 86°F).

Related Information

Conscious Sedation *on page 1779*

♦ **fluMist®** *see* Influenza Virus Vaccine *on page 913*

Fluocinonide (floo oh SIN oh nide)

U.S. Brand Names Lidex®; Lidex-E®; Vanos™

Pharmacologic Category Corticosteroid, Topical

Medication Safety Issues

Sound-alike/look-alike issues:

Fluocinonide may be confused with flunisolide, fluocinolone

Lidex® may be confused with Lasix®, Videx®, Wydase®

Use Anti-inflammatory, antipruritic; treatment of plaque-type psoriasis (up to 10% of body surface area) [high-potency topical corticosteroid]

Mechanism of Action Fluorinated topical corticosteroid considered to be of high potency. The mechanism of action for all topical corticosteroids is not well defined, however, is felt to be a combination of three important properties: anti-inflammatory activity, immunosuppressive properties, and antiproliferative actions.

Pharmacodynamics/Kinetics

Absorption: Dependent on strength of product, amount applied, and nature of skin at application site; ranges from ~1% in areas of thick stratum corneum (palms, soles, elbows, etc) to 36% in areas of thin stratum corneum (face, eyelids, etc); increased in areas of skin damage, inflammation, or occlusion

Distribution: Throughout local skin; absorbed drug into muscle, liver, skin, intestines, and kidneys

Metabolism: Primarily in skin; small amount absorbed into systemic circulation is primarily hepatic to inactive compounds

Excretion: Urine (primarily as glucuronide and sulfate, also as unconjugated products); feces (small amounts as metabolites)

Contraindications Hypersensitivity to fluocinonide or any component of the formulation; viral, fungal, or tubercular skin lesions, herpes simplex

Warnings/Precautions Adverse systemic effects may occur when used on large areas of the body, denuded areas, for prolonged periods of time, with an occlusive dressing, and/or in infants or small children. Pediatric patients may be more susceptible to HPA axis suppression. Lower-strength cream (0.05%) may be used cautiously on face or opposing skin surfaces that may rub or touch (eg, skin

(Continued)

Fluocinonide *(Continued)*

folds of the groin, axilla, and breasts); higher-strength (0.1%) should not be used on the face, groin, or axillae. Use of the 0.1% cream for >2 weeks or in patients <18 years of age is not recommended.

Drug Interactions No data reported. Concomitant use with other corticosteroids (by any route) may increase the risk of HPA axis suppression.

Adverse Reactions Frequency not defined.

Cardiovascular: Intracranial hypertension

Dermatologic: Acne, allergic dermatitis, contact dermatitis, dry skin, folliculitis, hypertrichosis, hypopigmentation, maceration of the skin, miliaria, perioral dermatitis, pruritus, skin atrophy, striae, telangiectasia

Endocrine & metabolic: Cushing's syndrome, growth retardation, HPA suppression, hyperglycemia

Local: Burning, irritation

Renal: Glycosuria

Miscellaneous: Secondary infection

Dosing

Adults & Elderly:

Pruritus and inflammation: Topical (0.5% cream): Apply thin layer to affected area 2-4 times/day depending on the severity of the condition. Therapy should be discontinued when control is achieved; if no improvement is seen, reassessment of diagnosis may be necessary.

Plaque-type psoriasis (Vanos™): Topical (0.1% cream): Apply a thin layer once or twice daily to affected areas (limited to <10% of body surface area). **Note:** Not recommended for use >2 consecutive weeks or >60 g/week total exposure. Discontinue when control is achieved.

Pediatrics: Refer to adult dosing.

Available Dosage Forms

Cream, anhydrous, emollient (Lidex®): 0.05% (15 g, 30 g, 60 g)

Cream, aqueous, emollient (Lidex-E®): 0.05% (15 g, 30 g, 60 g)

Cream (Vanos™): 0.1% (30 g, 60 g)

Gel (Lidex®): 0.05% (15 g, 30 g, 60 g)

Ointment (Lidex®): 0.05% (15 g, 30 g, 60 g)

Solution (Lidex®): 0.05% (60 mL) [contains alcohol 35%]

Nursing Guidelines

Assessment: Assess potential for interactions with other prescriptions, OTC medications, or herbal products patient may be taking. Assess patient response. Teach patient proper use (according to formulation), side effects/appropriate interventions, and symptoms to report.

Patient Education: For external use only. Do not use for eyes, mucous membranes, or open wounds. Use exactly as directed and for no longer than the period prescribed. Before using, wash and dry area gently. Apply in a thin layer (may rub in lightly). Apply light dressing (if necessary) to area being treated. Do not use occlusive dressing unless so advised by prescriber. Avoid prolonged or excessive use around sensitive tissues, genital, or rectal areas. Avoid exposing treated area to direct sunlight. Inform prescriber if condition worsens (redness, swelling, irritation, signs of infection, or open sores) or fails to improve. **Pregnancy precaution:** Inform prescriber if you are or intend to become pregnant

Pregnancy Risk Factor: C

♦ **Fluohydrisone Acetate** *see* Fludrocortisone *on page 737*

♦ **Fluohydrocortisone Acetate** *see* Fludrocortisone *on page 737*

♦ **Fluor-I-Strip®** *see* Fluorescein Sodium *on page 742*

♦ **Fluor-I-Strip-AT®** *see* Fluorescein Sodium *on page 742*

Fluorescein Sodium (FLURE e seen SOW dee um)

U.S. Brand Names AK-Fluor; Angiscein®; Fluorescite®; Fluorets®; Fluor-I-Strip®; Fluor-I-Strip-AT®; Ful-Glo®

Synonyms Soluble Fluorescein

Pharmacologic Category Diagnostic Agent

Use Demonstrates defects of corneal epithelium; diagnostic aid in ophthalmic angiography

Mechanism of Action Yellow, water soluble, dibasic acid xanthine dye which penetrates any break in epithelial barrier to permit rapid penetration

Contraindications Hypersensitivity to fluorescein or any other component of the formulation; do not use with soft contact lenses, as this will cause them to discolor; pregnancy (parenteral product)

Warnings/Precautions Use with caution in patients with history of hypersensitivity, allergies, or asthma; avoid extravasation; should not be used in patients with soft contact lenses, will cause them to discolor

Adverse Reactions

1% to 10%:

Dermatologic: Burning sensation

Local: Temporary stinging

<1% (Limited to important or life-threatening): Basilar artery ischemia, cardiac arrest, GI distress, headache, hypotension, nausea, severe shock, syncope, thrombophlebitis, vomiting

Dosing

Adults & Elderly:

Diagnostic aid: Ophthalmic:

Solution: Instill 1-2 drops of 2% solution and allow a few seconds for staining; wash out excess with sterile water or irrigating solution

Strips: Moisten strip with sterile water. Place moistened strip at the fornix into the lower cul-de-sac close to the punctum. For best results, patient should close lid tightly over strip until desired amount of staining is obtained. Patient should blink several times after application.

Removal of foreign bodies, sutures or tonometry (Fluress®): Instill 1 or 2 drops (single instillations) into each eye before operating

Deep ophthalmic anesthesia (Fluress®): Instill 2 drops into each eye every 90 seconds up to 3 doses

Angiography: Injection: Prior to use, perform intradermal skin test; have epinephrine 1:1000, an antihistamine, and oxygen available

Adults: 500-750 mg injected rapidly into antecubital vein

Pediatrics:

Diagnostic aid: Ophthalmic: Refer to adult dosing.

Angiography: I.V.: Prior to use, perform intradermal skin test; have epinephrine 1:1000, an antihistamine, and oxygen available.

Children: 3.5 mg/lb (7.5 mg/kg) injected rapidly into antecubital vein

Available Dosage Forms

Injection, solution:

AK-Fluor, Fluorescite®: 10% (5 mL); 25% (2 mL)

Angiscein®: 10% (5 mL)

Strip, ophthalmic:

Fluorets®, Fluor-I-Strip-AT®: 1 mg

Fluor-I-Strip®: 9 mg

Ful-Glo®: 0.6 mg

Nursing Guidelines

Patient Education: Do not replace soft contact lenses for at least 1 hour, flush eye before replacing; skin discoloration may last 6-12 hours, urine 24-36 hours if given systemically

Pregnancy Risk Factor: C (topical); X (parenteral)

♦ Fluorescite® *see* Fluorescein Sodium *on page 742*

♦ Fluorets® *see* Fluorescein Sodium *on page 742*

♦ 9α-Fluorohydrocortisone Acetate *see* Fludrocortisone *on page 737*

Fluorometholone (flure oh METH oh lone)

U.S. Brand Names Eflone® [DSC]; Flarex®; Fluor-Op® [DSC]; FML®; FML® Forte

Pharmacologic Category Corticosteroid, Ophthalmic

Use Treatment of steroid-responsive inflammatory conditions of the eye

Mechanism of Action Decreases inflammation by suppression of migration of polymorphonuclear leukocytes and reversal of increased capillary permeability

Pharmacodynamics/Kinetics Absorption: Into aqueous humor with slight systemic absorption

Contraindications Hypersensitivity to fluorometholone or any component of the formulation; viral diseases of the cornea and conjunctiva (including epithelial herpes simplex keratitis, vaccinia and varicella); mycobacterial or fungal infections of the eye; untreated eye infections which may be masked/enhanced by a steroid

Warnings/Precautions Not recommended in children <2 years of age; prolonged use may result in glaucoma, elevated intraocular pressure, or other ocular

(Continued)

Fluorometholone *(Continued)*

damage; may exacerbate severity of viral infections, use caution in patients with history of herpes simplex; re-evaluate after 2 days if symptoms have not improved; may delay healing following cataract surgery; some products contain sulfites

Drug Interactions No data reported

Adverse Reactions

Ocular: Anterior uveitis, burning upon application, cataract formation, conjunctival hyperemia, conjunctivitis, corneal ulcers, glaucoma with optic nerve damage, perforation of the globe, secondary ocular infection (bacterial, fungal, viral), intraocular pressure elevation, visual acuity and field defects, keratitis, mydriasis, stinging upon application, delayed wound healing

Miscellaneous: Systemic hypercorticoidism (rare) and taste perversion have also been reported

Overdosage/Toxicology When consumed in high doses over prolonged periods, systemic hypercorticism and adrenal suppression may occur. In those cases, discontinuation of the corticosteroid should be done judiciously.

Dosing

Adults & Elderly:

Occular inflammation: Ophthalmic:

Ointment: Apply small amount (~$^1/_2$ inch ribbon) to conjunctival sac every 4 hours in severe cases; 1-3 times/day in mild to moderate cases.

Solution: Instill 1-2 drops into conjunctival sac every hour during day, every 2 hours at night until favorable response is obtained, then use 1 drop every 4 hours; for mild to moderate inflammation, instill 1-2 drops into conjunctival sac 2-4 times/day.

Note: Re-evaluate therapy if improvement is not seen within 2 days; use care not to discontinue prematurely; in chronic conditions, gradually decrease dosing frequency prior to discontinuing treatment.

Pediatrics: Children >2 years: Refer to adult dosing.

Available Dosage Forms [DSC] = Discontinued product

Ointment, ophthalmic, as base (FML®): 0.1% (3.5 g)

Suspension, ophthalmic, as base: (5 mL, 10 mL, 15 mL)

Fluor-Op®: 0.1% (5 mL, 10 mL, 15 mL) [contains benzalkonium chloride and polyvinyl alcohol] [DSC]

FML®: 0.1% (5 mL, 10 mL, 15 mL) [contains benzalkonium chloride]

FML® Forte: 0.25% (2 mL, 5 mL, 10 mL, 15 mL) [contains benzalkonium chloride]

Suspension, ophthalmic, as acetate:

Eflone®: 0.1% (5 mL, 10 mL) [DSC]

Flarex®: 0.1% (5 mL, 10 mL) [contains benzalkonium chloride]

Nursing Guidelines

Assessment: Monitor intraocular pressure in patients with glaucoma or when used for ≥10 days; monitor for presence of secondary infections (including the development of fungal infections and exacerbation of viral infections). Assess knowledge/teach patient appropriate use, interventions to reduce side effects, and adverse symptoms to report.

Patient Education: For ophthalmic use only. Apply prescribed amount as often as directed. Wash hands before using. Wipe away excess from skin around eye. Do not use any other eye preparation for at least 10 minutes. Do not touch tip of applicator to eye or any other surface. Do not share medication with anyone else. May cause sensitivity to bright light (dark glasses may help); temporary stinging or blurred vision may occur. Do not wear contacts during administration and for 15 minutes after. Inform prescriber if you experience eye pain, redness, burning, watering, dryness, double vision, puffiness around eye, vision changes, or other adverse eye response; worsening of condition or lack of improvement. **Pregnancy/breast-feeding precautions:** Inform prescriber if you are pregnant. Consult prescriber if breast-feeding.

Ointment: Gently squeeze the tube to apply to inside of lower lid. Close eye for 1-2 minutes and roll eyeball in all directions.

Suspension: Shake well before using. Tilt head back and look upward. Gently pull down lower lid and put drop(s) in inner corner of eye. Close eye and roll eyeball in all directions. Do not blink for 30 seconds. Apply gentle pressure to inner corner of eye for 30 seconds.

Pregnancy Risk Factor: C

Lactation: Excretion in breast milk unknown/use caution

Administration

Storage: Store at room temperature.

- Fluor-Op® [DSC] *see* Fluorometholone *on page 743*
- Fluoroplex® *see* Fluorouracil *on page 745*

Fluorouracil (flure oh YOOR a sil)

U.S. Brand Names Adrucil®; Carac™; Efudex®; Fluoroplex®

Synonyms 5-Fluorouracil; FU; 5-FU

Pharmacologic Category Antineoplastic Agent, Antimetabolite

Medication Safety Issues

Sound-alike/look-alike issues:

Fluorouracil may be confused with flucytosine

Efudex® may be confused with Efidac (Efidac 24®), Eurax®

Use Treatment of carcinomas of the breast, colon, head and neck, pancreas, rectum, or stomach; topically for the management of actinic or solar keratoses and superficial basal cell carcinomas

Mechanism of Action A pyrimidine antimetabolite that interferes with DNA synthesis by blocking the methylation of deoxyuridylic acid; fluorouracil inhibits thymidylate synthetase (TS), or is incorporated into RNA. The reduced folate cofactor is required for tight binding to occur between the 5-FdUMP and TS.

Pharmacodynamics/Kinetics

Duration: ~3 weeks

Distribution: V_d: ~22% of total body water; penetrates extracellular fluid, CSF, and third space fluids (eg, pleural effusions and ascitic fluid)

Metabolism: Hepatic (90%); via a dehydrogenase enzyme; FU must be metabolized to be active

Bioavailability: <75%, erratic and undependable

Half-life elimination: Biphasic: Initial: 6-20 minutes; two metabolites, FdUMP and FUTP, have prolonged half-lives depending on the type of tissue

Excretion: Lung (large amounts as CO_2); urine (5% as unchanged drug) in 6 hours

Contraindications Hypersensitivity to fluorouracil or any component of the formulation; poor nutritional status; depressed bone marrow function; thrombocytopenia; potentially serious infections; major surgery within the previous month; dihydropyrimidine dehydrogenase (DPD) enzyme deficiency; pregnancy

Warnings/Precautions The U.S. Food and Drug Administration (FDA) currently recommends that procedures for proper handling and disposal of antineoplastic agents be considered. Use with caution in patients with impaired kidney or liver function. The drug should be discontinued if intractable vomiting or diarrhea, precipitous falls in leukocyte or platelet counts, stomatitis, hemorrhage, or myocardial ischemia occurs. Use with caution in patients who have had high-dose pelvic radiation or previous use of alkylating agents. Palmar-plantar erythrodysesthesia (hand-foot) syndrome has been associated with use. Safety and efficacy have not been established in pediatric patients.

Administration to patients with a genetic deficiency of dihydropyrimidine dehydrogenase (DPD) has been associated with diarrhea, neutropenia, and neurotoxicity. Systemic toxicity normally associated with parenteral administration has also been associated with topical use, particularly in patients with DPD. Discontinue if symptoms of DPD occur. Avoid topical application to mucous membranes due to potential for local inflammation and ulceration. The use of occlusive dressings with topical preparations may increase the severity of inflammation in nearby skin areas. Avoid exposure to ultraviolet rays during and immediately following therapy.

Drug Interactions Warfarin: May increase aPTT and bleeding time; monitor

Nutritional/Herbal/Ethanol Interactions

Ethanol: Avoid ethanol (due to GI irritation).

Herb/Nutraceutical: Avoid black cohosh, dong quai in estrogen-dependent tumors.

Adverse Reactions Toxicity depends on route and duration of infusion. **Note:** Systemic toxicity normally associated with parenteral administration (including neutropenia, neurotoxicity, and gastrointestinal toxicity) has been associated with topical use particularly in patients with a genetic deficiency of dihydropyrimidine dehydrogenase (DPD).

(Continued)

Fluorouracil *(Continued)*

>10%:

Dermatologic: Dermatitis, pruritic maculopapular rash, alopecia

Gastrointestinal (route and schedule dependent): Heartburn, nausea, vomiting, anorexia, stomatitis, esophagitis, anorexia, stomatitis, diarrhea

Emetic potential:

<1000 mg: Moderately low (10% to 30%)

≥1000 mg: Moderate (30% to 60%)

Hematologic: Leukopenia; Myelosuppressive (tends to be more pronounced in patients receiving bolus dosing of FU):

WBC: Moderate

Platelets: Mild to moderate

Onset (days): 7-10

Nadir (days): 14

Recovery (days): 21

Local: **Irritant chemotherapy**

1% to 10%:

Dermatologic: Dry skin

Gastrointestinal: GI ulceration

<1% (Limited to important or life-threatening): Cardiac enzyme abnormalities, chest pain, coagulopathy, dyspnea, ECG changes similar to ischemic changes, hepatotoxicity; hyperpigmentation of nailbeds, face, hands, and veins used in infusion; hypotension, palmar-plantar syndrome (hand-foot syndrome), photosensitization

Cerebellar ataxia, headache, somnolence, ataxia are seen primarily in intracarotid arterial infusions for head and neck tumors.

Topical: Note: Systemic toxicity normally associated with parenteral administration (including neutropenia, neurotoxicity, and gastrointestinal toxicity) has been associated with topical use particularly in patients with a genetic deficiency of dihydropyrimidine dehydrogenase (DPD).

Overdosage/Toxicology Symptoms of overdose include myelosuppression, nausea, vomiting, diarrhea, and alopecia. No specific antidote exists. Monitor hematologically for at least 4 weeks. Treatment is supportive.

Dosing

Adults & Elderly:

Refer to individual protocols.

I.V. bolus: 500-600 mg/m^2 every 3-4 weeks **or**
425 mg/m^2 on days 1-5 every 4 weeks

Continuous I.V. infusion: 1000 mg/m^2/day for 4-5 days every 3-4 weeks **or**
2300-2600 mg/m^2 on day 1 every week **or**
300-400 mg/m^2/day **or**
225 mg/m^2/day for 5-8 weeks (with radiation therapy)

Actinic keratoses: Topical:

Carac™: Apply thin film to lesions once daily for up to 4 weeks, as tolerated

Efudex®: Apply to lesions twice daily for 2-4 weeks; complete healing may not be evident for 1-2 months following treatment

Fluoroplex®: Apply to lesions twice daily for 2-6 weeks

Superficial basal cell carcinoma: Topical: Efudex® 5%: Apply to affected lesions twice daily for 3-6 weeks; treatment may be continued for up to 10-12 weeks

Pediatrics: Refer to adult dosing.

Renal Impairment: Hemodialysis: Administer dose following hemodialysis.

Hepatic Impairment: Bilirubin >5 mg/dL: Omit use.

Available Dosage Forms

Cream, topical:

Carac™: 0.5% (30 g)

Efudex®: 5% (25 g, 40 g)

Fluoroplex®: 1% (30 g) [contains benzyl alcohol]

Injection, solution: 50 mg/mL (10 mL, 20 mL, 50 mL, 100 mL)

Adrucil®: 50 mg/mL (10 mL, 50 mL, 100 mL)

Solution, topical (Efudex®): 2% (10 mL); 5% (10 mL)

Nursing Guidelines

Assessment: Note specific Warnings/Precautions for use cautions. Assess potential for interactions with other pharmacological agents or herbal products the patient may be taking (see Drug Interactions). Assess results of laboratory tests prior to each infusion and regularly with all formulations, including topical use. Assess patient response (eg, cardiovascular, respiratory, and renal function; see Adverse Reactions and Overdose/Toxicology) prior to each infusion and on a regular basis throughout therapy. **Note:** The drug should be discontinued if intractable vomiting or diarrhea, precipitous fall in leukocyte or platelet counts, or myocardial ischemia occurs. Teach patient proper use (oral or topical application), possible side effects/appropriate interventions (eg, importance of adequate hydration), and adverse symptoms to report (see Patient Education). **Pregnancy risk factor D/X:** Determine that patient is not pregnant before starting therapy. Do not give to females of childbearing age unless patient is capable of complying with contraceptive use. Male/female: Advise patient about contraceptive measures as appropriate.

Monitoring Laboratory Tests: CBC with differential, platelet count, renal and liver function

Dietary Considerations: Increase dietary intake of thiamine.

Patient Education: Do not take any new medication during therapy without consulting prescriber. Avoid excessive alcohol (may increase gastrointestinal irritation). Maintain adequate hydration (2-3 L/day of fluids) unless instructed to restrict fluid intake and nutrition (small frequent meals may help). May cause sensitivity to sunlight (use sunblock, wear protective clothing, and avoid direct sunlight); susceptibility to infection (avoid crowds and exposure to infection); nausea, vomiting, diarrhea, or loss of appetite (small frequent meals may help; request medication); weakness, lethargy, dizziness, decreased vision (use caution when driving or engaging in tasks requiring alertness until response to drug is known); or headache (request medication). Report signs and symptoms of infection (eg, fever, chills, sore throat, burning urination, vaginal itching or discharge, fatigue, mouth sores); bleeding (eg, black or tarry stools, easy bruising, unusual bleeding); vision changes; unremitting nausea, vomiting, or abdominal pain; CNS changes; respiratory difficulty; chest pain or palpitations; severe skin reactions to topical application; or any other adverse reactions.

Topical: Use as directed; do not overuse. Wash hands thoroughly before and after applying medication. Avoid contact with eyes, nostrils, and mouth. Avoid occlusive dressings; use a porous dressing. May cause local reaction (pain, burning, or swelling), if severe contact prescriber.

Oral solution: May be mixed in water, grape juice, or carbonated beverage. It is generally best to drink undiluted solution, then rinse the mouth. CocaCola® has been recommended as the 'best chaser' for oral fluorouracil.

Pregnancy/breast-feeding precautions: Inform prescriber if you are pregnant. Do not get pregnant during or for 1 month following therapy. Male: Do not cause a pregnancy. Male/female: Consult prescriber for instruction on appropriate contraceptive measures. This drug may cause severe fetal defects. Breast-feeding is not recommended.

Pregnancy Risk Factor: D (injection); X (topical)

Pregnancy Issues: There are no adequate and well-controlled studies in pregnant women, however, fetal defects and miscarriages have been reported following use of topical and intravenous products. Use is contraindicated during pregnancy.

Lactation: Excretion in breast milk unknown/not recommended

Administration

Oral: I.V. formulation may be given orally mixed in water, grape juice, or carbonated beverage. It is generally best to drink undiluted solution, then rinse the mouth. CocaCola® has been recommended as the "best chaser" for oral fluorouracil.

I.V.: Irritant. Direct I.V. push injection (50 mg/mL solution needs no further dilution) or by I.V. infusion. Toxicity may be reduced by giving the drug as a constant infusion. Bolus doses may be administered by slow IVP or IVPB.

Reconstitution: Further dilution in D_5W or NS at concentrations of 0.5-10 mg/mL are stable for 72 hours at 4°C to 25°C.

Compatibility: Stable in D_5LR, D_5W, NS

Incompatible with concentrations >25 mg/mL of fluorouracil and >2 mg/mL of leucovorin (precipitation occurs)

Y-site administration: Incompatible with amphotericin B cholesteryl sulfate complex, droperidol, filgrastim, ondansetron, topotecan, vinorelbine

Compatibility in syringe: Incompatible with droperidol, epirubicin

Compatibility when admixed: Incompatible with carboplatin, cisplatin, cytarabine, diazepam, doxorubicin, fentanyl, leucovorin, metoclopramide, morphine

(Continued)

Fluorouracil *(Continued)*

Storage:

Injection: Store intact vials at room temperature and protect from light; slight discoloration does not usually denote decomposition. If exposed to cold, a precipitate may form; **gentle** heating to 60°C will dissolve the precipitate without impairing the potency; solutions in 50-1000 mL NS or D_5W, or undiluted solutions in syringes are stable for 72 hours at room temperature.

Topical: Store at controlled room temperature of 15°C to 30°C (59°F to 86°F).

♦ 5-Fluorouracil *see* Fluorouracil *on page 745*

Fluoxetine (floo OKS e teen)

U.S. Brand Names Prozac®; Prozac® Weekly™; Sarafem®

Synonyms Fluoxetine Hydrochloride

Pharmacologic Category Antidepressant, Selective Serotonin Reuptake Inhibitor

Medication Safety Issues

Sound-alike/look-alike issues:

Fluoxetine may be confused with duloxetine, fluvastatin

Prozac® may be confused with Prilosec®, Proscar®, ProSom®, ProStep®

Sarafem® may be confused with Serophene®

Use Treatment of major depressive disorder; treatment of binge-eating and vomiting in patients with moderate-to-severe bulimia nervosa; obsessive-compulsive disorder (OCD); premenstrual dysphoric disorder (PMDD); panic disorder with or without agoraphobia

Unlabeled/Investigational Use Selective mutism

Mechanism of Action Inhibits CNS neuron serotonin reuptake; minimal or no effect on reuptake of norepinephrine or dopamine; does not significantly bind to alpha-adrenergic, histamine, or cholinergic receptors

Pharmacodynamics/Kinetics

Absorption: Well absorbed; delayed 1-2 hours with weekly formulation

Protein binding: 95%

Metabolism: Hepatic to norfluoxetine (active; equal to fluoxetine)

Half-life elimination: Adults:

Parent drug: 1-3 days (acute), 4-6 days (chronic), 7.6 days (cirrhosis)

Metabolite (norfluoxetine): 9.3 days (range: 4-16 days), 12 days (cirrhosis)

Due to long half-life, resolution of adverse reactions after discontinuation may be slow

Time to peak: 6-8 hours

Excretion: Urine (10% as norfluoxetine, 2.5% to 5% as fluoxetine)

Note: Weekly formulation results in greater fluctuations between peak and trough concentrations of fluoxetine and norfluoxetine compared to once-daily dosing (24% daily/164% weekly; 17% daily/43% weekly, respectively). Trough concentrations are 76% lower for fluoxetine and 47% lower for norfluoxetine than the concentrations maintained by 20 mg once-daily dosing. Steady-state fluoxetine concentrations are ~50% lower following the once-weekly regimen compared to 20 mg once daily. Average steady-state concentrations of once-daily dosing were highest in children ages 6 to <13 (fluoxetine 171 ng/mL; norfluoxetine 195 ng/mL), followed by adolescents ages 13 to <18 (fluoxetine 86 ng/mL; norfluoxetine 113 ng/mL); concentrations were considered to be within the ranges reported in adults (fluoxetine 91-302 ng/mL; norfluoxetine 72-258 ng/mL).

Contraindications Hypersensitivity to fluoxetine or any component of the formulation; patients currently receiving MAO inhibitors, thioridazine, or mesoridazine

Note: MAO inhibitor therapy must be stopped for 14 days before fluoxetine is initiated. Treatment with MAO inhibitors, thioridazine, or mesoridazine should not be initiated until 5 weeks after the discontinuation of fluoxetine.

Warnings/Precautions

Major psychiatric warnings:

- Antidepressants increase the risk of suicidal thinking and behavior in children and adolescents with major depressive disorder (MDD) and other depressive disorders; consider risk prior to prescribing.
- Closely monitor for clinical worsening, suicidality, or unusual changes in behavior; the child's family or caregiver should be instructed to closely observe the patient and communicate condition with healthcare provider. **Fluoxetine is not FDA approved for use in children.**
- Adults treated with antidepressants should be observed similarly for clinical worsening and suicidality, especially during the initial few months of a course

of drug therapy, or at times of dose changes, either increases or decreases. A medication guide should be dispensed with each prescription.

- The possibility of a suicide attempt is inherent in major depression and may persist until remission occurs. Worsening depression and severe abrupt suicidality that are not part of the presenting symptoms may require discontinuation or modification of drug therapy. Use caution in high-risk patients during initiation of therapy.
- Prescriptions should be written for the smallest quantity consistent with good patient care. The patient's family or caregiver should be alerted to monitor patients for the emergence of suicidality and associated behaviors such as anxiety, agitation, panic attacks, insomnia, irritability, hostility, impulsivity, akathisia, hypomania, and mania; patients should be instructed to notify their healthcare provider if any of these symptoms or worsening depression or psychosis occur.
- May worsen psychosis in some patients or precipitate a shift to mania or hypomania in patients with bipolar disorder. Monotherapy in patients with bipolar disorder should be avoided. Patients presenting with depressive symptoms should be screened for bipolar disorder. **Fluoxetine is not FDA approved for the treatment of bipolar depression.**

Key adverse effects:

- Allergic events and rash: Fluoxetine use has been associated with occurrences of significant rash and allergic events, including vasculitis, lupus-like syndrome, laryngospasm, anaphylactoid reactions, and pulmonary inflammatory disease.
- Anticholinergic effects: Relatively devoid of these side effects
- CNS depression: Has a low potential to impair cognitive or motor performance; caution operating hazardous machinery or driving.
- CNS effects: May cause insomnia, anxiety, nervousness or anorexia.
- SIADH and hyponatremia: Has been associated with the development of SIADH; hyponatremia has been reported rarely, predominately in the elderly.

Concurrent disease:

- Diabetes: May alter glycemic control in patients with diabetes.
- Hepatic impairment: Use caution; clearance is decreased and plasma concentrations are increased; a lower dosage may be needed.
- Platelet aggregation: May impair platelet aggregation, resulting in bleeding.
- Renal impairment: Use caution; clearance is decreased and plasma concentrations are increased; a lower dosage may be needed.
- Seizure disorders: Use caution with a previous seizure disorder or condition predisposing to seizures such as brain damage or alcoholism.
- Sexual dysfunction: May cause or exacerbate sexual dysfunction.
- Weight loss: May cause weight loss. Use caution in patients where weight loss is undesirable.

Concurrent drug therapy:

- Agents which lower seizure threshold: Concurrent therapy with other drugs which lower the seizure threshold.
- Anticoagulants/Antiplatelets: Use caution with concomitant use of NSAIDs, ASA, or other drugs that affect coagulation; the risk of bleeding is potentiated.
- CNS depressants: Use caution with concomitant therapy.
- MAO inhibitors: Potential for severe reaction when used with MAO inhibitors; autonomic instability, coma, death, delirium, diaphoresis, hyperthermia, mental status changes/agitation, muscular rigidity, myoclonus, neuroleptic malignant syndrome features, and seizures may occur.
- Thioridazine: Fluoxetine may elevate plasma levels of thioridazine; increasing risk of QTc interval prolongation; this may lead to serious ventricular arrhythmias such as torsade de pointes-type arrhythmias and sudden death. **Use is contraindicated.**

Special populations:

- Elderly: Use caution in elderly patients.

Special notes:

- Electroconvulsive therapy: May increase the risks associated with electroconvulsive therapy; consider discontinuing, when possible, prior to ECT treatment.
- Long half-life: Due to the long half-life of fluoxetine and its metabolites, the effects and interactions noted may persist for prolonged periods following discontinuation.
- Withdrawal syndrome: May cause dysphoric mood, irritability, agitation, dizziness, sensory disturbances, anxiety, confusion, headache, lethargy,

(Continued)

Fluoxetine *(Continued)*

emotional lability, insomnia, hypomania, tinnitus, and seizures. Upon discontinuation of venlafaxine therapy, gradually taper dose. If intolerable symptoms occur following a decrease in dosage or upon discontinuation of therapy, then resuming the previous dose with a more gradual taper should be considered.

Drug Interactions Substrate of CYP1A2 (minor), 2B6 (minor), 2C8/9 (major), 2C19 (minor), 2D6 (major), 2E1 (minor), 3A4 (minor); **Inhibits** CYP1A2 (moderate), 2B6 (weak), 2C8/9 (weak), 2C19 (moderate), 2D6 (strong), 3A4 (weak)

Amphetamines: SSRIs may increase the sensitivity to amphetamines, and amphetamines may increase the risk of serotonin syndrome.

Benzodiazepines: Fluoxetine may inhibit the metabolism of alprazolam and diazepam resulting in elevated serum levels; monitor for increased sedation and psychomotor impairment.

Beta-blockers: Fluoxetine may inhibit the metabolism of metoprolol and propranolol resulting in cardiac toxicity; monitor for bradycardia, hypotension, and heart failure if combination is used; not established for all beta-blockers (unlikely with atenolol or nadolol due to renal elimination).

Buspirone: Fluoxetine inhibits the reuptake of serotonin; combined use with a serotonin agonist (buspirone) may cause serotonin syndrome.

Carbamazepine: Fluoxetine may inhibit the metabolism of carbamazepine resulting in increased carbamazepine levels and toxicity; monitor for altered carbamazepine response.

Carvedilol: Serum concentrations may be increased; monitor carefully for increased carvedilol effect (hypotension and bradycardia).

Clozapine: Fluoxetine may increase serum levels of clozapine; levels may increase by 76%; monitor for increased effect/toxicity.

Cyclosporine: Fluoxetine may increase serum levels of cyclosporine (and possibly tacrolimus); monitor.

CYP1A2 substrates: Fluoxetine may increase the levels/effects of CYP1A2 substrates. Example substrates include aminophylline, fluvoxamine, mexiletine, mirtazapine, ropinirole, theophylline, and trifluoperazine.

CYP2C8/9 inducers: May decrease the levels/effects of fluoxetine. Example inducers include carbamazepine, phenobarbital, phenytoin, rifampin, rifapentine, and secobarbital.

CYP2C8/9 inhibitors: May increase the levels/effects of fluoxetine. Example inhibitors include delavirdine, fluconazole, gemfibrozil, ketoconazole, nicardipine, NSAIDs, pioglitazone, and sulfonamides.

CYP2C19 substrates: Fluoxetine may increase the levels/effects of CYP2C19 substrates. Example substrates include citalopram, diazepam, methsuximide, phenytoin, propranolol, and sertraline.

CYP2D6 inhibitors: May increase the levels/effects of fluoxetine. Example inhibitors include chlorpromazine, delavirdine, miconazole, paroxetine, pergolide, quinidine, quinine, ritonavir, and ropinirole.

CYP2D6 substrates: Fluoxetine may increase the levels/effects of CYP2D6 substrates. Example substrates include amphetamines, selected beta-blockers, dextromethorphan, lidocaine, mirtazapine, nefazodone, paroxetine, risperidone, ritonavir, thioridazine, tricyclic antidepressants, and venlafaxine.

CYP2D6 prodrug substrates: Fluoxetine may decrease the levels/effects of CYP2D6 prodrug substrates. Example prodrug substrates include codeine, hydrocodone, oxycodone, and tramadol.

Cyproheptadine: May inhibit the effects of serotonin reuptake inhibitors (fluoxetine); monitor for altered antidepressant response; cyproheptadine acts as a serotonin agonist.

Dextromethorphan: Fluoxetine inhibits the metabolism of dextromethorphan; visual hallucinations occurred in a patient receiving this combination; monitor for serotonin syndrome.

Digoxin: Fluoxetine may increase serum levels of digoxin; monitor.

Haloperidol: Fluoxetine may inhibit the metabolism of haloperidol and cause extrapyramidal symptoms (EPS); monitor patients for EPS if combination is utilized.

HMG-CoA reductase inhibitors: Fluoxetine may inhibit the metabolism of lovastatin and simvastatin resulting in myositis and rhabdomyolysis; these combinations are best avoided.

Lithium: Reports of both increased and decreased lithium levels when used concomitantly with fluoxetine. Patients receiving fluoxetine and lithium have developed neurotoxicity. If combination is used; monitor lithium levels and for neurotoxicity.

Loop diuretics: Fluoxetine may cause hyponatremia; additive hyponatremic effects may be seen with combined use of a loop diuretic (bumetanide, furosemide, torsemide); monitor for hyponatremia.

MAO inhibitors: Combined use of fluoxetine with nonselective MAOIs (ie, isocarboxazid, phenelzine) is contraindicated; fatal reactions have been reported; wait 5 weeks after stopping fluoxetine before starting an MAO inhibitor and 2 weeks after stopping an MAO inhibitor before starting fluoxetine.

Meperidine: Combined use with fluoxetine theoretically may increase the risk of serotonin syndrome.

Mesoridazine: Fluoxetine may inhibit the metabolism of mesoridazine, resulting in increased plasma levels and increasing the risk of QT_c interval prolongation. This may lead to serious ventricular arrhythmias, such as torsade de pointes-type arrhythmias and sudden death. Do not use concurrently. Wait at least 5 weeks after discontinuing fluoxetine prior to starting mesoridazine.

Nefazodone: May increase the risk of serotonin syndrome with SSRIs; monitor.

NSAIDs: Concomitant use of fluoxetine and NSAIDs, aspirin, or other drugs affecting coagulation has been associated with an increased risk of bleeding; monitor.

Phenytoin: Fluoxetine inhibits the metabolism of phenytoin and may result in phenytoin toxicity; monitor for phenytoin toxicity (ataxia, confusion, dizziness, nystagmus, involuntary muscle movement).

Propafenone: Serum concentrations and/or toxicity may be increased by fluoxetine; avoid concurrent administration.

Ritonavir: Combined use of fluoxetine with ritonavir may cause serotonin syndrome in HIV-positive patients; monitor.

Selegiline: Fluoxetine has been reported to cause mania or hypertension when combined with selegiline; this combination is best avoided. Concurrent use with SSRIs has also been reported to cause serotonin syndrome. As a MAO type B inhibitor, the risk of serotonin syndrome may be less than with nonselective MAO inhibitors.

Sibutramine: May increase the risk of serotonin syndrome with SSRIs; avoid coadministration.

SSRIs: Fluoxetine inhibits the reuptake of serotonin; combined use with other drugs which inhibit the reuptake may cause serotonin syndrome.

Sumatriptan (and other serotonin agonists): Concurrent use may result in toxicity; weakness, hyper-reflexia, and incoordination have been observed with sumatriptan and SSRIs. In addition, concurrent use may theoretically increase the risk of serotonin syndrome; includes sumatriptan, naratriptan, rizatriptan, and zolmitriptan.

Sympathomimetics: May increase the risk of serotonin syndrome with SSRIs.

Thioridazine: Fluoxetine may inhibit the metabolism of thioridazine, resulting in increased plasma levels and increasing the risk of QT_c interval prolongation. This may lead to serious ventricular arrhythmias, such as torsade de pointes-type arrhythmias and sudden death. Do not use together. Wait at least 5 weeks after discontinuing fluoxetine prior to starting thioridazine.

Tramadol: Fluoxetine combined with tramadol (serotonergic effects) may cause serotonin syndrome; monitor.

Trazodone: Fluoxetine may inhibit the metabolism of trazodone resulting in increased toxicity; monitor.

Tricyclic antidepressants: Fluoxetine inhibits the metabolism of tricyclic antidepressants (amitriptyline, desipramine, imipramine, nortriptyline) resulting is elevated serum levels; if combination is warranted, a low dose of TCA (10-25 mg/day) should be utilized.

Tryptophan: Fluoxetine inhibits the reuptake of serotonin; combination with tryptophan, a serotonin precursor, may cause agitation and restlessness; this combination is best avoided.

Valproic acid: Fluoxetine may increase serum levels of valproic acid; monitor.

Venlafaxine: Fluoxetine may increase the risk of serotonin syndrome.

Warfarin: Fluoxetine may alter the hypoprothrombinemic response to warfarin; monitor.

Nutritional/Herbal/Ethanol Interactions

Ethanol: Avoid ethanol (may increase CNS depression). Depressed patients should avoid/limit intake.

Herb/Nutraceutical: Avoid valerian, St John's wort, kava kava, gotu kola (may increase CNS depression).

Lab Interactions Increased albumin in urine

(Continued)

Fluoxetine *(Continued)*

Adverse Reactions Percentages listed for adverse effects as reported in placebo-controlled trials and were generally similar in adults and children; actual frequency may be dependent upon diagnosis and in some cases the range presented may be lower than or equal to placebo for a particular disorder.

>10%:

Central nervous system: Insomnia (10% to 33%), headache (21%), anxiety (6% to 15%), nervousness (8% to 14%), somnolence (5% to 17%)

Endocrine & metabolic: Libido decreased (1% to 11%)

Gastrointestinal: Nausea (12% to 29%), diarrhea (8% to 18%), anorexia (4% to 11%), xerostomia (4% to 12%)

Neuromuscular & skeletal: Weakness (7% to 21%), tremor (3% to 13%)

Respiratory: Pharyngitis (3% to 11%), yawn (<1% to 11%)

1% to 10%:

Cardiovascular: Vasodilation (1% to 5%), fever (2%), chest pain, hemorrhage, hypertension, palpitation

Central nervous system: Dizziness (9%), dream abnormality (1% to 5%), thinking abnormality (2%), agitation, amnesia, chills, confusion, emotional lability, sleep disorder

Dermatologic: Rash (2% to 6%), pruritus (4%)

Endocrine & metabolic: Ejaculation abnormal (<1% to 7%), impotence (<1% to 7%)

Gastrointestinal: Dyspepsia (6% to 10%), constipation (5%), flatulence (3%), vomiting (3%), weight loss (2%), appetite increased, taste perversion, weight gain

Genitourinary: Urinary frequency

Ocular: Vision abnormal (2%)

Otic: Ear pain, tinnitus

Respiratory: Sinusitis (1% to 6%)

Miscellaneous: Flu-like syndrome (3% to 10%), diaphoresis (2% to 8%)

<1% (Limited to important or life-threatening): Allergies, alopecia, anaphylactoid reactions, angina, arrhythmia, asthma, cataract, CHF, cholelithiasis, cholestatic jaundice, colitis, dyskinesia, dysphagia, eosinophilic pneumonia, erythema nodosum, esophagitis, euphoria, exfoliative dermatitis, extrapyramidal symptoms (rare), gout, hallucinations, hepatic failure/necrosis, hemorrhage, hyperprolactinemia, immune-related hemolytic anemia, laryngospasm, lupus-like syndrome, MI, neuroleptic malignant syndrome (NMS), optic neuritis, pancreatitis, pancytopenia, photosensitivity reaction, postural hypotension, priapism, pulmonary embolism, pulmonary hypertension, QT prolongation, renal failure, serotonin syndrome, Stevens-Johnson syndrome, syncope, thrombocytopenia, thrombocytopenic purpura, vasculitis, ventricular tachycardia (including torsade de pointes)

Overdosage/Toxicology Among 633 adult patients who overdosed on fluoxetine alone, 34 resulted in a fatal outcome. Symptoms of overdose include ataxia, sedation, coma, and ECG abnormalities (QT prolongation, torsade de pointes). Respiratory depression may occur, especially with coingestion of ethanol or other drugs. Seizures rarely occur. Treatment is supportive.

Dosing

Adults:

Depression, OCD, PMDD, bulimia: 20 mg/day in the morning; may increase after several weeks by 20 mg/day increments; maximum: 80 mg/day; doses >20 mg may be given once daily or divided twice daily. **Note:** Lower doses of 5-10 mg/day have been used for initial treatment.

Usual dosage range:

Depression: 20-40 mg/day; patients maintained on Prozac® 20 mg/day may be changed to Prozac® Weekly™ 90 mg/week, starting dose 7 days after the last 20 mg/day dose

Obsessive compulsive disorder (OCD): 40-80 mg/day

Premenstrual dysphoric disorder (Sarafem™): 20 mg/day continuously, **or** 20 mg/day starting 14 days prior to menstruation and through first full day of menses (repeat with each cycle)

Bulimia nervosa: 60-80 mg/day

Panic disorder: Initial: 10 mg/day; after 1 week, increase to 20 mg/day; may increase after several weeks; doses >60 mg/day have not been evaluated

Elderly: Oral: Some patients may require an initial dose of 10 mg/day with dosage increases of 10 mg and 20 mg every several weeks as tolerated; should not be taken at night unless patient experiences sedation.

Pediatrics:

Depression: Oral: 8-18 years: 10-20 mg/day; lower-weight children can be started at 10 mg/day, may increase to 20 mg/day after 1 week if needed

OCD: Oral: 7-18 years: Initial: 10 mg/day; in adolescents and higher-weight children, dose may be increased to 20 mg/day after 2 weeks. Range: 10-60 mg/day

Selective mutism (unlabeled use): Oral:

<5 years: No dosing information available

5-18 years: Initial: 5-10 mg/day; titrate upwards as needed (usual maximum dose: 60 mg/day)

Renal Impairment:

Single dose studies: Pharmacokinetics of fluoxetine and norfluoxetine were similar among subjects with all levels of impaired renal function, including anephric patients on chronic hemodialysis.

Chronic administration: Additional accumulation of fluoxetine or norfluoxetine may occur in patients with severely impaired renal function.

Not removed by hemodialysis; use of lower dose or less frequent dosing is not usually necessary.

Hepatic Impairment: Elimination half-life of fluoxetine is prolonged in patients with hepatic impairment. A lower dose or less frequent dosing of fluoxetine should be used in these patients.

Cirrhosis patient: Administer a lower dose or less frequent dosing interval.
Compensated cirrhosis without ascites: Administer 50% of normal dose.

Available Dosage Forms [DSC] = Discontinued product

Capsule, as hydrochloride: 10 mg, 20 mg, 40 mg

Prozac®: 10 mg, 20 mg, 40 mg

Sarafem®: 10 mg, 20 mg

Capsule, delayed release, as hydrochloride (Prozac® Weekly™): 90 mg

Solution, oral, as hydrochloride (Prozac®): 20 mg/5 mL (120 mL) [contains alcohol 0.23% and benzoic acid; mint flavor]

Tablet, as hydrochloride: 10 mg, 20 mg

Prozac® [scored]: 10 mg [DSC]

Nursing Guidelines

Assessment: Assess other medications patient may be taking for effectiveness and interactions. Assess results of laboratory tests, therapeutic effectiveness, and adverse reactions at beginning of therapy and periodically with long-term use. Taper dosage slowly when discontinuing. Assess mental status for depression, suicidal ideation, anxiety, social functioning, mania, or panic attack. Assess knowledge/teach patient appropriate use, interventions to reduce side effects and adverse symptoms to report.

Monitoring Laboratory Tests: Baseline liver and renal function before beginning drug therapy

Dietary Considerations: May be taken with or without food.

Patient Education: Take exactly as directed; do not increase dose or frequency. It may take 2-3 weeks to achieve desired results. Take once-a-day dose in the morning to reduce incidence of insomnia. Avoid alcohol, caffeine, and other prescription or OTC medications not approved by prescriber. Maintain adequate hydration (2-3 L/day of fluids) unless instructed to restrict fluid intake. You may experience drowsiness, lightheadedness, impaired coordination, dizziness, or blurred vision (use caution when driving or engaging in tasks requiring alertness until response to drug is known); constipation (increased exercise, fluids, fruit, or fiber may help); anorexia (maintain regular dietary intake to avoid excessive weight loss); or postural hypotension (use caution when climbing stairs or changing position from lying or sitting to standing). If you have diabetes, monitor serum glucose closely (may cause hypoglycemia). Report persistent CNS effects (nervousness, restlessness, insomnia, anxiety, excitation, suicide ideation, headache, sedation); thoughts of suicide; rash or skin irritation; muscle cramping, tremors, or change in gait; respiratory depression or respiratory difficulty; or worsening of condition. **Pregnancy/breast-feeding precautions:** Inform prescriber if you are pregnant. Breast-feeding is not recommended.

Geriatric Considerations: Fluoxetine's favorable side effect profile makes it a useful alternative to the traditional tricyclic antidepressants. Its potential stimulating and anorexic effects may be bothersome to some patients. Has not been shown to be superior in efficacy to the traditional tricyclic antidepressants or other SSRIs. The long half-life in the elderly makes it less attractive compared to other SSRIs. Data from a clinical trial comparing fluoxetine to tricyclics

(Continued)

Fluoxetine *(Continued)*

suggests that fluoxetine is significantly less effective than nortriptyline in hospitalized elderly patients with unipolar major affective disorder, especially those with melancholia and concurrent cardiovascular diseases. As with other SSRIs, fluoxetine has been associated with hyponatremia in elderly patients.

Pregnancy Risk Factor: C

Pregnancy Issues: Fluoxetine crosses the placenta. Nonteratogenic effects including respiratory distress, cyanosis, apnea, seizures, temperature instability, feeding difficulty, vomiting, hypoglycemia, hypo- or hypertonia, hyper-reflexia, jitteriness, irritability, constant crying, and tremor have been reported in the neonate immediately following delivery after exposure to other SSRIs late in the third trimester. Adverse effects may be due to toxic effects of SSRI or drug discontinuation. In some cases, may present clinically as serotonin syndrome. There are no adequate and well-controlled studies in pregnant women. Use during pregnancy only if the potential benefit to the mother outweighs the possible risk to the fetus. If treatment during pregnancy is required, consider tapering SSRI therapy during the third trimester.

Lactation: Enters breast milk/not recommended (AAP rates "of concern")

Breast-Feeding Considerations: Colic, irritability, slow weight gain, feeding and sleep disorders have been reported in nursing infants.

Perioperative/Anesthesia/Other Concerns: SSRIs are relatively safe compared to other antidepressants in patients with cardiovascular disease.

Buspirone and cyproheptadine, may be useful in treatment of sexual dysfunction during treatment with a selective serotonin reuptake inhibitor.

Weekly capsules are a delayed release formulation containing enteric-coated pellets of fluoxetine hydrochloride, equivalent to 90 mg fluoxetine. Therapeutic equivalence of weekly formulation with daily formulation for delaying time to relapse has not been established.

Administration

Storage: All dosage forms should be stored at controlled room temperature of 15°C to 30°C (50°F to 86°F); oral liquid should be dispensed in a light-resistant container

♦ **Fluoxetine Hydrochloride** *see* Fluoxetine *on page 748*

Flurazepam (flure AZ e pam)

U.S. Brand Names Dalmane®

Synonyms Flurazepam Hydrochloride

Pharmacologic Category Hypnotic, Benzodiazepine

Medication Safety Issues

Sound-alike/look-alike issues:

Flurazepam may be confused with temazepam

Dalmane® may be confused with Demulen®, Dialume®

Use Short-term treatment of insomnia

Mechanism of Action Binds to stereospecific benzodiazepine receptors on the postsynaptic GABA neuron at several sites within the central nervous system, including the limbic system, reticular formation. Enhancement of the inhibitory effect of GABA on neuronal excitability results by increased neuronal membrane permeability to chloride ions. This shift in chloride ions results in hyperpolarization (a less excitable state) and stabilization.

Pharmacodynamics/Kinetics

Onset of action: Hypnotic: 15-20 minutes

Peak effect: 3-6 hours

Duration: 7-8 hours

Metabolism: Hepatic to N-desalkylflurazepam (active)

Half-life elimination: Desalkylflurazepam:

Adults: Single dose: 74-90 hours; Multiple doses: 111-113 hours

Elderly (61-85 years): Single dose: 120-160 hours; Multiple doses: 126-158 hours

Contraindications Hypersensitivity to flurazepam or any component of the formulation (cross-sensitivity with other benzodiazepines may exist); narrow-angle glaucoma; pregnancy

Warnings/Precautions Use with caution in elderly or debilitated patients, patients with hepatic disease (including alcoholics), or renal impairment. Active metabolites with extended half-lives may lead to delayed accumulation and adverse effects. Use with caution in patients with respiratory disease, or impaired gag reflex. Avoid use in patients with sleep apnea.

Causes CNS depression (dose-related) resulting in sedation, dizziness, confusion, or ataxia which may impair physical and mental capabilities. Patients must be cautioned about performing tasks which require mental alertness (eg, operating machinery or driving). Use with caution in patients receiving other CNS depressants or psychoactive agents. Effects with other sedative drugs or ethanol may be potentiated. Benzodiazepines have been associated with falls and traumatic injury and should be used with extreme caution in patients who are at risk of these events (especially the elderly).

Use caution in patients with depression, particularly if suicidal risk may be present. Use with caution in patients with a history of drug dependence. Benzodiazepines have been associated with dependence and acute withdrawal symptoms on discontinuation or reduction in dose (may occur after as little as 10 days of use). Acute withdrawal, including seizures, may be precipitated in patients after administration of flumazenil to patients receiving long-term benzodiazepine therapy.

As a hypnotic, should be used only after evaluation of potential causes of sleep disturbance. Failure of sleep disturbance to resolve after 7-10 days may indicate psychiatric or medical illness. A worsening of insomnia or the emergence of new abnormalities of thought or behavior may represent unrecognized psychiatric or medical illness and requires immediate and careful evaluation.

Benzodiazepines have been associated with anterograde amnesia. Paradoxical reactions, including hyperactive or aggressive behavior have been reported with benzodiazepines, particularly in adolescent/pediatric or psychiatric patients. Does not have analgesic, antidepressant, or antipsychotic properties.

Drug Interactions **Substrate** of CYP3A4 (major); **Inhibits** CYP2E1 (weak)

CNS depressants: Sedative effects and/or respiratory depression may be additive with CNS depressants; includes ethanol, barbiturates, narcotic analgesics, and other sedative agents; monitor for increased effect

CYP3A4 inducers: CYP3A4 inducers may decrease the levels/effects of flurazepam. Example inducers include aminoglutethimide, carbamazepine, nafcillin, nevirapine, phenobarbital, phenytoin, and rifamycins.

CYP3A4 inhibitors: May increase the levels/effects of flurazepam. Example inhibitors include azole antifungals, clarithromycin, diclofenac, doxycycline, erythromycin, imatinib, isoniazid, nefazodone, nicardipine, propofol, protease inhibitors, quinidine, telithromycin, and verapamil.

Levodopa: Therapeutic effects may be diminished in some patients following the addition of a benzodiazepine; limited/inconsistent data

Oral contraceptives: May decrease the clearance of some benzodiazepines (those which undergo oxidative metabolism); monitor for increased benzodiazepine effect

Theophylline: May partially antagonize some of the effects of benzodiazepines; monitor for decreased response; may require higher doses for sedation

Nutritional/Herbal/Ethanol Interactions

Ethanol: Avoid ethanol (may increase CNS depression).

Food: Serum levels and response to flurazepam may be increased by grapefruit juice, but unlikely because of flurazepam's high oral bioavailability.

Herb/Nutraceutical: Avoid valerian, St John's wort, kava kava, gotu kola (may increase CNS depression).

Lab Interactions Elevated alkaline phosphatase, AST, ALT, and bilirubin (total and direct)

Adverse Reactions Frequency not defined.

Cardiovascular: Palpitations, chest pain

Central nervous system: Drowsiness, ataxia, lightheadedness, memory impairment, depression, headache, hangover effect, confusion, nervousness, dizziness, falling, apprehension, irritability, euphoria, slurred speech, restlessness, hallucinations, paradoxical reactions, talkativeness

Dermatologic: Rash, pruritus

Gastrointestinal: Xerostomia, constipation, increased/excessive salivation, heartburn, upset stomach, nausea, vomiting, diarrhea, increased or decreased appetite, bitter taste, weight gain/loss

Hematologic: Euphoria, granulocytopenia

Hepatic: Elevated SGOT/SGPT, total bilirubin, alkaline phosphatase; cholestatic jaundice

Neuromuscular & skeletal: Dysarthria, body/joint pain, reflex slowing, weakness

(Continued)

Flurazepam *(Continued)*

Ocular: Blurred vision, burning eyes, difficulty focusing

Otic: Tinnitus

Respiratory: Apnea, dyspnea

Miscellaneous: Diaphoresis, drug dependence

Overdosage/Toxicology Symptoms of overdose include respiratory depression, hypoactive reflexes, unsteady gait, and hypotension. Treatment for benzodiazepine overdose is supportive. Flumazenil has been shown to selectively block the binding of benzodiazepines to CNS receptors, resulting in a reversal of benzodiazepine-induced CNS depression. Respiratory depression may not be reversed.

Dosing

Adults: Insomnia (short-term treatment): Oral: 15-30 mg at bedtime

Elderly: Oral: 15 mg at bedtime. Avoid use if possible.

Pediatrics: Hypnotic: Oral:

≤15 years: Dose not established

>15 years: 15 mg at bedtime

Available Dosage Forms Capsule, as hydrochloride: 15 mg, 30 mg

Nursing Guidelines

Assessment: For short-term use. Assess effectiveness and interactions of other medications patient may be taking. Assess for history of addiction; long-term use can result in dependence, abuse, or tolerance. Evaluate periodically for need for continued use. Monitor for CNS changes. After long-term use, taper dosage slowly when discontinuing. For inpatient use, institute safety measures and monitor effectiveness and adverse reactions. For outpatients, monitor therapeutic effectiveness and adverse reactions at beginning of therapy and periodically with long-term use. Assess knowledge/teach patient appropriate use, interventions to reduce side effects, and adverse symptoms to report. **Pregnancy risk factor X:** Determine that patient is not pregnant before starting therapy. Do not give to sexually-active female patients unless capable of complying with contraceptive use.

Patient Education: Use exactly as directed; do not increase dose or frequency or discontinue without consulting prescriber. Drug may cause physical and/or psychological dependence. May take with food to decrease GI upset. While using this medication, do not use alcohol or other prescription or OTC medications (especially, pain medications, sedatives, antihistamines, or hypnotics) without consulting prescriber. Maintain adequate hydration (2-3 L/day of fluids) unless instructed to restrict fluid intake. You may experience drowsiness, dizziness, lightheadedness, or blurred vision (use caution when driving or engaging in tasks requiring alertness until response to drug is known); dry mouth, nausea, or vomiting (small frequent meals, frequent mouth care, chewing gum, or sucking lozenges may help); difficulty urinating (void before taking medication); or altered libido (resolves when medication is discontinued). Report CNS changes (confusion, depression, increased sedation, excitation, headache, abnormal thinking, insomnia, or nightmares, memory impairment, impaired coordination); muscle pain or weakness; respiratory difficulty; persistent dizziness, chest pain, or palpitations; alterations in normal gait; vision changes; ringing in ears; or ineffectiveness of medication. **Pregnancy/breast-feeding precautions:** Inform prescriber if you are pregnant. Do not get pregnant during or for 1 month following therapy. Consult prescriber for instruction on appropriate contraceptive measures. This drug may cause severe fetal defects. Breast-feeding is not recommended.

Geriatric Considerations: Due to its long-acting metabolite, flurazepam is not considered a drug of choice in the elderly. Long-acting benzodiazepines have been associated with falls in the elderly. Interpretive guidelines from the Centers for Medicare and Medicaid Services (CMS) discourage the use of this agent in residents of long-term care facilities.

Pregnancy Risk Factor: X

Pregnancy Issues: Benzodiazepines cross the placenta. The association between benzodiazepine exposure and malformations remains controversial. A number of types of malformation have been reported (oral cleft, inguinal hernia, cardiac defects, spina bifida, dysmorphic facial features, skeletal defects); however, confounding factors make a clear association difficult. Overall, the risk to the fetus may be low. Nonteratogenic effects (including neonatal flaccidity, respiratory and feeding problems, and withdrawal symptoms) during the postnatal period have also been reported with benzodiazepine use.

Lactation: Excretion in breast milk unknown/not recommended

Perioperative/Anesthesia/Other Concerns: Chronic use of this agent may increase the perioperative benzodiazepine dose needed to achieve desired effect. Abrupt discontinuation after sustained use (generally >10 days) may cause withdrawal symptoms.

Administration

Oral: Give 30 minutes to 1 hour before bedtime on an empty stomach with full glass of water. May be taken with food if GI distress occurs.

Storage: Store in light-resistant containers.

♦ Flurazepam Hydrochloride *see* Flurazepam *on page 754*

Flurbiprofen (flure BI proe fen)

U.S. Brand Names Ansaid® [DSC]; Ocufen®

Synonyms Flurbiprofen Sodium

Pharmacologic Category Nonsteroidal Anti-inflammatory Drug (NSAID), Ophthalmic; Nonsteroidal Anti-inflammatory Drug (NSAID), Oral

Medication Safety Issues

Sound-alike/look-alike issues:

Flurbiprofen may be confused with fenoprofen

Ansaid® may be confused with Asacol®, Axid®

Ocufen® may be confused with Ocuflox®, Ocupress®

Use

Oral: Treatment of rheumatoid arthritis and osteoarthritis

Ophthalmic: Inhibition of intraoperative miosis

Mechanism of Action Inhibits prostaglandin synthesis by decreasing the activity of the enzyme, cyclooxygenase, which results in decreased formation of prostaglandin precursors

Pharmacodynamics/Kinetics

Onset of action: ~1-2 hours

Distribution: V_d: 0.12 L/kg

Protein binding: 99%, primarily albumin

Metabolism: Hepatic via CYP2C9; forms metabolites

Half-life elimination: 5.7 hours

Time to peak: 1.5 hours

Excretion: Urine

Contraindications Hypersensitivity to flurbiprofen, aspirin, other NSAIDs, or any component of the formulation; perioperative pain in the setting of coronary artery bypass surgery (CABG); dendritic keratitis; pregnancy (3rd trimester)

Warnings/Precautions NSAIDs are associated with an increased risk of adverse cardiovascular events, including MI, stroke, and new onset or worsening of pre-existing hypertension. Risk may be increased with duration of use or pre-existing cardiovascular risk-factors or disease. Carefully evaluate individual cardiovascular risk profiles prior to prescribing. Use caution with fluid retention, CHF, or hypertension.

Use of NSAIDs can compromise existing renal function. Renal toxicity can occur in patient with impaired renal function, dehydration, heart failure, liver dysfunction, those taking diuretics and ACEI, and the elderly. Rehydrate patient before starting therapy. Monitor renal function closely. Use caution in patients with advanced renal disease.

NSAIDs may increase risk of gastrointestinal irritation, ulceration, bleeding, and perforation. These events may occur at any time during therapy and without warning. Use caution with a history of GI disease (bleeding or ulcers), concurrent therapy with aspirin, anticoagulants and/or corticosteroids, smoking, use of alcohol, the elderly or debilitated patients.

Use the lowest effective dose for the shortest duration of time, consistent with individual patient goals, to reduce risk of cardiovascular or GI adverse events. Alternate therapies should be considered for patients at high risk.

NSAIDs may cause serious skin adverse events including exfoliative dermatitis, Stevens-Johnson syndrome (SJS), and toxic epidermal necrolysis (TEN). Anaphylactoid reactions may occur, even without prior exposure; patients with "aspirin triad" (bronchial asthma, aspirin intolerance, rhinitis) may be at increased risk. Do not use in patients who experience bronchospasm, asthma, rhinitis, or urticaria with NSAID or aspirin therapy.

Use with caution in patients with decreased hepatic function. Closely monitor patients with any abnormal LFT. Severe hepatic reactions (eg, fulminant hepatitis,

(Continued)

Flurbiprofen *(Continued)*

liver failure) have occurred with NSAID use, rarely; discontinue if signs or symptoms of liver disease develop, or if systemic manifestations occur.

The elderly are at increased risk for adverse effects (especially peptic ulceration, CNS effects, renal toxicity) from NSAIDs even at low doses.

Withhold for at least 4-6 half-lives prior to surgical or dental procedures. Safety and efficacy have not been established in children <18 years of age.

Drug Interactions Substrate of CYP2C8/9 (minor); **Inhibits** CYP2C8/9 (strong)

ACE inhibitors: Antihypertensive effects may be decreased by concurrent therapy with NSAIDs; monitor blood pressure.

Angiotensin II antagonists: Antihypertensive effects may be decreased by concurrent therapy with NSAIDs; monitor blood pressure.

Anticoagulants (warfarin, heparin, LMWHs) in combination with NSAIDs can cause increased risk of bleeding.

Antiplatelet drugs (ticlopidine, clopidogrel, aspirin, abciximab, dipyridamole, eptifibatide, tirofiban) can cause an increased risk of bleeding.

Cholestyramine and colestipol reduce the bioavailability of some NSAIDs; separate administration times.

Corticosteroids may increase the risk of GI ulceration; avoid concurrent use.

Cyclosporine: NSAIDs may increase serum creatinine, potassium, blood pressure, and cyclosporine levels; monitor cyclosporine levels and renal function carefully.

CYP2C8/9 substrates: Flurbiprofen may increase the levels/effects of CYP2C8/9 substrates. Example substrates include amiodarone, fluoxetine, glimepiride, glipizide, nateglinide, phenytoin, pioglitazone, rosiglitazone, sertraline, and warfarin.

Gentamicin and amikacin serum concentrations are increased by indomethacin in premature infants. Results may apply to other aminoglycosides and NSAIDs.

Hydralazine's antihypertensive effect is decreased; avoid concurrent use.

Lithium levels can be increased; avoid concurrent use if possible or monitor lithium levels and adjust dose. Sulindac may have the least effect. When NSAID is stopped, lithium will need adjustment again.

Loop diuretics efficacy (diuretic and antihypertensive effect) is reduced. Indomethacin reduces this efficacy, however, it may be anticipated with any NSAID.

Methotrexate: Severe bone marrow suppression, aplastic anemia, and GI toxicity have been reported with concomitant NSAID therapy. Avoid use during moderate or high-dose methotrexate (increased and prolonged methotrexate levels). NSAID use during low-dose treatment of rheumatoid arthritis has not been fully evaluated; extreme caution is warranted.

Thiazides antihypertensive effects are decreased; avoid concurrent use.

Warfarin's INRs may be increased by piroxicam. Other NSAIDs may have the same effect depending on dose and duration. Monitor INR closely. Use the lowest dose of NSAIDs possible and for the briefest duration.

Verapamil plasma concentration is decreased by some NSAIDs; avoid concurrent use.

Nutritional/Herbal/Ethanol Interactions

Ethanol: Avoid ethanol (may enhance gastric mucosal irritation).

Food: Food may decrease the rate but not the extent of absorption.

Herb/Nutraceutical: Avoid alfalfa, anise, bilberry, bladderwrack, bromelain, cat's claw, celery, coleus, cordyceps, dong quai, evening primrose, feverfew, fenugreek, garlic, ginger, ginkgo biloboa, red clover, horse chestnut, grapeseed, green tea, ginseng, guggul, horse chestnut seed, horseradish, licorice, prickly ash, red clover, reishi, SAMe, sweet clover, turmeric, white willow (all have additional antiplatelet activity).

Adverse Reactions

Ophthalmic: Frequency not defined: Ocular: Slowing of corneal wound healing, mild ocular stinging, itching and burning, ocular irritation, fibrosis, miosis, mydriasis, bleeding tendency increased

Oral:

>1%:

Cardiovascular: Edema

Central nervous system: Amnesia, anxiety, depression, dizziness, headache, insomnia, malaise, nervousness, somnolence

Dermatologic: Rash

Gastrointestinal: Abdominal pain, constipation, diarrhea, dyspepsia, flatulence, GI bleeding, nausea, vomiting, weight changes

Hepatic: Liver enzymes elevated

Neuromuscular & skeletal: Reflexes increased, tremor, vertigo, weakness

Ocular: Vision changes

Otic: Tinnitus

Respiratory: Rhinitis

<1% (Limited to important or life-threatening): Anaphylactic reaction, anemia, angioedema, asthma, bruising, cerebrovascular ischemia, CHF, confusion, eczema, eosinophilia, epistaxis, exfoliative dermatitis, fever, gastric/peptic ulcer, hematocrit decreased, hematuria, hemoglobin decreased, hepatitis, hypertension, hyperuricemia, interstitial nephritis, jaundice, leukopenia, paresthesia, parosmia, photosensitivity, pruritus, purpura, renal failure, stomatitis, thrombocytopenia, toxic epidermal necrolysis, urticaria, vasodilation

Overdosage/Toxicology Symptoms of overdose include apnea, metabolic acidosis, coma, nystagmus, leukocytosis, and renal failure. Management of NSAID intoxication is supportive and symptomatic. Since many NSAIDs undergo enterohepatic cycling, multiple doses of charcoal may be needed to reduce the potential for delayed toxicities.

Dosing

Adults & Elderly:

Rheumatoid arthritis and osteoarthritis: Oral: 200-300 mg/day in 2-, 3-, or 4 divided doses; do not administer more than 100 mg for any single dose; maximum: 300 mg/day

Management of postoperative dental pain: 100 mg every 12 hours

Ophthalmic anti-inflammatory/surgical aid: Ophthalmic: Instill 1 drop every 30 minutes, beginning 2 hours prior to surgery (total of 4 drops in each affected eye)

Available Dosage Forms [DSC] = Discontinued product

Solution, ophthalmic, as sodium (Ocufen®): 0.03% (2.5 mL) [contains thimerosal]

Tablet: 50 mg, 100 mg

Ansaid®: 50 mg, 100 mg [DSC]

Nursing Guidelines

Assessment: Evaluate cardiac risk and potential for GI bleeding prior to prescribing this medication. **Assess for allergic reaction to salicylate or other NSAIDs**. Assess effectiveness and interactions of other medications patient may be taking. Monitor blood pressure at the beginning of therapy and periodically during use. Monitor therapeutic response and adverse reactions at beginning of therapy and periodically throughout therapy. Assess knowledge/teach patient proper use, appropriate interventions to reduce side effects, and adverse symptoms to report.

Dietary Considerations: Tablet may be taken with food, milk, or antacid to decrease GI effects.

Patient Education: Oral: Take this medication exactly as directed; do not increase dose without consulting prescriber. Do not crush tablets. Take with food or milk to reduce GI distress. Maintain adequate hydration (2-3 L/day of fluids) unless instructed to restrict fluid intake. Do not use alcohol, aspirin or aspirin-containing medication, or any other anti-inflammatory medications without consulting prescriber. You may experience drowsiness, dizziness, nervousness, or headache (use caution when driving or engaging in tasks requiring alertness until response to drug is known); anorexia, nausea, vomiting, or heartburn (small frequent meals, frequent mouth care, sucking lozenges, or chewing gum may help); fluid retention (weigh yourself weekly and report unusual (3-5 lb/week) weight gain). GI bleeding, ulceration, or perforation can occur with or without pain; discontinue medication and contact prescriber if persistent abdominal pain or cramping, or blood in stool occurs. Report breathlessness, respiratory difficulty, or unusual cough; chest pain, rapid heartbeat, palpitations; unusual bruising/bleeding; blood in urine, stool, mouth, or vomitus; swollen extremities; skin rash or itching; acute fatigue; or hearing changes (ringing in ears). **Pregnancy/breast-feeding precautions:** Inform prescriber if you are or intend to become pregnant. This drug should not be used in the 3rd trimester of pregnancy. Breast-feeding is not recommended.

Ophthalmic: Wash hands before instilling. Sit or lie down to instill. Open eye, look at ceiling, and instill prescribed amount of medication. Close eye and roll eye in all directions, and apply gentle pressure to inner corner of eye. Do not let tip of applicator touch eye; do not contaminate tip of applicator (may cause eye infection, eye damage, or vision loss). Use protective dark eyewear until healed; avoid direct sunlight. Temporary stinging or burning may occur. Report

(Continued)

Flurbiprofen *(Continued)*

persistent pain, burning, redness, vision changes, swelling, itching, or worsening of condition.

Geriatric Considerations: Elderly are at high risk for adverse effects from NSAIDs. As much as 60% of elderly can develop peptic ulceration and/or hemorrhage asymptomatically. The concomitant use of H_2 blockers, omeprazole, and sucralfate is not effective as prophylaxis with the exception of NSAID-induced duodenal ulcers which may be prevented by the use of ranitidine. Misoprostol is the only prophylactic agent proven effective. Also, concomitant disease and drug use contribute to the risk for GI adverse effects. Use lowest effective dose for shortest period possible. Consider renal function decline with age. Use of NSAIDs can compromise existing renal function especially when Cl_{cr} is ≤30 mL/minute. Tinnitus may be a difficult and unreliable indication of toxicity due to age-related hearing loss or eighth cranial nerve damage. CNS adverse effects such as confusion, agitation, and hallucination are generally seen in overdose or high-dose situations, but elderly may demonstrate these adverse effects at lower doses than younger adults.

Pregnancy Risk Factor: C/D (3rd trimester)

Lactation: Enters breast milk/not recommended

Perioperative/Anesthesia/Other Concerns: The 2002 ACCM/SCCM guidelines for analgesia (critically-ill adult) suggest that NSAIDs may be used in combination with opioids in select patients for pain management. Concern about adverse events (increased risk of renal dysfunction, altered platelet function and gastrointestinal irritation) limits its use in patients who have other underlying risks for these events.

In short-term use, NSAIDs vary considerably in their effect on blood pressure. When NSAIDs are used in patients with hypertension, appropriate monitoring of blood pressure responses should be completed and the duration of therapy, when possible, kept short. The use of NSAIDs in the treatment of patients with congestive heart failure may be associated with an increased risk for fluid accumulation and edema; may precipitate renal failure in dehydrated patients.

Administration

Oral: Take with a full glass of water.

♦ Flurbiprofen Sodium *see* Flurbiprofen *on page 757*

Fluticasone (floo TIK a sone)

U.S. Brand Names Cutivate®; Flonase®; Flovent® [DSC]; Flovent® HFA

Synonyms Fluticasone Propionate

Pharmacologic Category Corticosteroid, Inhalant (Oral); Corticosteroid, Nasal; Corticosteroid, Topical; Corticosteroid, Topical (Medium Potency)

Medication Safety Issues

Sound-alike/look-alike issues:

Cutivate® may be confused with Ultravate®

Use

Inhalation: Maintenance treatment of asthma as prophylactic therapy. It is also indicated for patients requiring oral corticosteroid therapy for asthma to assist in total discontinuation or reduction of total oral dose

Intranasal: Management of seasonal and perennial allergic rhinitis and nonallergic rhinitis

Topical: Relief of inflammation and pruritus associated with corticosteroid-responsive dermatoses; atopic dermatitis

Mechanism of Action Fluticasone belongs to a new group of corticosteroids which utilizes a fluorocarbothioate ester linkage at the 17 carbon position; extremely potent vasoconstrictive and anti-inflammatory activity; has a weak HPA inhibitory potency when applied topically, which gives the drug a high therapeutic index. The effectiveness of inhaled fluticasone is due to its direct local effect. The mechanism of action for all topical corticosteroids is believed to be a combination of three important properties: anti-inflammatory activity, immunosuppressive properties, and antiproliferative actions.

Pharmacodynamics/Kinetics

Onset: Flovent® HFA: Maximal benefit may take 1-2 weeks or longer

Absorption:

Topical cream: 5% (increased with inflammation)

Oral inhalation: Absorbed systemically (DISKUS®: ~18%) primarily via lungs, minimal GI absorption (<1%) due to presystemic metabolism

Distribution: 4.2 L/kg

Protein binding: 91%

Metabolism: Hepatic via CYP3A4 to 17β-carboxylic acid (negligible activity)

Bioavailability: Nasal: ≤2%; Oral inhalation: (~18% to 21%)

Excretion: Feces (as parent drug and metabolites); urine (<5% as metabolites)

Contraindications Hypersensitivity to fluticasone or any component of the formulation; primary treatment of status asthmaticus or acute bronchospasm

Topical: Do not use if infection is present at treatment site, in the presence of skin atrophy, or for the treatment of rosacea or perioral dermatitis

Warnings/Precautions May cause hypercorticism or suppression of hypothalamic-pituitary-adrenal (HPA) axis, particularly in younger children or in patients receiving high doses for prolonged periods. HPA axis suppression may lead to adrenal crisis. Fluticasone may cause less HPA axis suppression than therapeutically equivalent oral doses of prednisone. Particular care is required when patients are transferred from systemic corticosteroids to inhaled products due to possible adrenal insufficiency or withdrawal from steroids, including an increase in allergic symptoms. Patients receiving 20 mg per day of prednisone (or equivalent) may be most susceptible. Concurrent use of ritonavir (and potentially other strong inhibitors of CYP3A4) may increase fluticasone levels and effects on HPA suppression.

Controlled clinical studies have shown that orally-inhaled and intranasal corticosteroids may cause a reduction in growth velocity in pediatric patients. (In studies of orally-inhaled corticosteroids, the mean reduction in growth velocity was approximately 1 centimeter per year [range 0.3-1.8 cm per year] and appears to be related to dose and duration of exposure.) To minimize the systemic effects of orally-inhaled and intranasal corticosteroids, each patient should be titrated to the lowest effective dose. The risk of growth velocity reduction with intranasal administration of fluticasone may be very low; in a small, placebo-controlled study, no statistically-significant reduction was observed.

May suppress the immune system, patients may be more susceptible to infection. Use with caution, if at all, in patients with systemic infections, active or quiescent tuberculosis infection, or ocular herpes simplex. Avoid exposure to chickenpox and measles.

Supplemental steroids (oral or parenteral) may be needed during stress or severe asthma attacks. Rare cases of vasculitis (Churg-Strauss syndrome) or other eosinophilic conditions can occur.

Inhalation: Not to be used in status asthmaticus or for the relief of acute bronchospasm. Flovent® Diskus® [CAN] contain lactose; very rare anaphylactic reactions have been reported in patients with severe milk protein allergy.

Topical: May also cause suppression of HPA axis, especially when used on large areas of the body, denuded areas, for prolonged periods of time or with an occlusive dressing. Pediatric patients may be more susceptible to systemic toxicity.

Drug Interactions **Substrate** of CYP3A4 (major)

Azole antifungals: May increase the levels/effects of fluticasone.

CYP3A4 inhibitors: May increase the levels/effects of fluticasone. Example inhibitors include azole antifungals, clarithromycin, diclofenac, doxycycline, erythromycin, imatinib, isoniazid, nefazodone, nicardipine, propofol, protease inhibitors, quinidine, telithromycin, and verapamil.

Protease inhibitors: May increase the levels/effects of fluticasone. Avoid concurrent use with ritonavir.

Ritonavir: May increase serum levels (due to CYP3A4 inhibition) and the potential for steroid-related adverse effects (eg, Cushing syndrome, adrenal suppression). Avoid concurrent use.

Salmeterol: The addition of salmeterol has been demonstrated to improve response to inhaled corticosteroids (as compared to increasing steroid dosage).

Nutritional/Herbal/Ethanol Interactions Herb/Nutraceutical: In theory, St John's wort may decrease serum levels of fluticasone by inducing CYP3A4 isoenzymes.

Adverse Reactions

>10%:

Central nervous system: Headache (5% to 16%)

Respiratory: Upper respiratory tract infection (16% to 18%)

1% to 10%:

Cardiovascular: Chest symptoms (1% to 3%)

Central nervous system (all 1% to 3%): Dizziness, fever, migraine, pain

(Continued)

Fluticasone *(Continued)*

Dermatologic: Dry skin (7%), skin burning/stinging (2% to 5%), pruritus (3%), skin irritation (3%), viral skin infection (1% to 3%), exacerbation of eczema (2%), excoriation (2%), dryness (1%), numbness of fingers (1%)

Gastrointestinal: Nausea/vomiting (3% to 5%); all others (1% to 3%): abdominal pain, diarrhea, dyspepsia, gastrointestinal infection (viral), gastrointestinal discomfort/pain, hyposalivation

Genitourinary: Urinary tract infection (1% to 3%)

Neuromuscular & skeletal (all 1% to 3%): Musculoskeletal pain, muscle pain, muscle stiffness/tightness/rigidity

Respiratory: Throat irritation (8% to 10%), pharyngitis (6% to 8%), epistaxis (6% to 7%), sinusitis/sinus infection (4% to 7%), asthma symptoms (3% to 7%), cough (4% to 6%), bronchitis (1% to 6%), hoarseness/dysphonia (2% to 6%), upper respiratory tract inflammation (2% to 5%), nasal burning/irritation (2% to 3%), blood in nasal mucous (1% to 3%), runny nose (1% to 3%), rhinitis (1% to 3%), throat infection (1% to 3%), rhinorrhea/postnasal drip (1% to 3%), nasal sinus disorder (1% to 3%), laryngitis (1% to 3%)

Miscellaneous: Oral candidiasis (2% to 5%), aches and pains (1% to 3%), flu-like symptoms (1% to 3%)

<1%, postmarketing and/or case reports: Aggression, agitation, anaphylaxis/anaphylactoid reactions, angioedema, anxiety, aphonia, arthralgia, asthma exacerbation, anxiety, blurred vision, bronchospasm (immediate and delayed), cataracts, chest tightness, Churg-Strauss syndrome, conjunctivitis, contusion, Cushingoid features, cutaneous hypersensitivity, depression, dry throat, dry/irritated eyes, dyspnea, ecchymoses, edema (face and tongue), eosinophilia, fatigue, glaucoma, growth velocity reduction in children/adolescents, hoarseness, HPA axis suppression, hyperactivity/irritability (primarily children), hyperglycemia, hypersensitivity reactions (immediate and delayed), intraocular pressure increased, malaise, nasal septal perforation (rare), nasal ulcer, oropharyngeal edema, osteoporosis, paradoxical bronchospasm, pneumonia, rash, restlessness, sleep disorder, smell alterations, sore throat, taste perversion, urticaria, voice changes, weight gain, wheezing

Reported with other topical corticosteroids (in decreasing order of occurrence): Irritation, folliculitis, acneiform eruptions, hypopigmentation, perioral dermatitis, allergic contact dermatitis, secondary infection, skin atrophy, striae, miliaria, pustular psoriasis from chronic plaque psoriasis

Overdosage/Toxicology When consumed in high doses over prolonged periods, systemic hypercorticism and adrenal suppression may occur. In those cases, discontinuation of the corticosteroid should be done judiciously.

Dosing

Adults & Elderly:

Asthma: Inhalation, oral: **Note:** Titrate to the lowest effective dose once asthma stability is achieved

Flovent®, Flovent® HFA: Manufacturers labeling: Dosing based on previous therapy

Bronchodilator alone: Recommended starting dose: 88 mcg twice daily; highest recommended dose: 440 mcg twice daily

Inhaled corticosteroids: Recommended starting dose: 88-220 mcg twice daily; highest recommended dose: 440 mcg twice daily; a higher starting dose may be considered in patients previously requiring higher doses of inhaled corticosteroids

Oral corticosteroids:

Recommended starting dose:

Flovent®: 880 mcg twice daily

Flovent® HFA: 440 mcg twice daily

Highest recommended dose: 880 mcg twice daily; starting dose is patient dependent. In patients on chronic oral corticosteroids therapy, reduce prednisone dose no faster than 2.5-5 mg/day on a weekly basis; begin taper after 1 week of fluticasone therapy

NIH Asthma Guidelines (administer in divided doses twice daily).

"Low" dose: 88-264 mcg/day

"Medium" dose: 264-660 mcg/day

"High" dose: >660 mcg/day

Flovent® Diskus® [CAN]:

Mild asthma: 100-250 mcg twice daily

Moderate asthma: 250-500 mcg twice daily

Severe asthma: 500 mcg twice daily; may increase to 1000 mcg twice daily in very severe patients requiring high doses of corticosteroids

Corticosteroid-responsive dermatoses: Topical: Cream, lotion, ointment: Apply sparingly to affected area twice daily. If no improvement is seen within 2 weeks, reassessment of diagnosis may be necessary.

Atopic dermatitis: Topical: Cream, lotion: Apply sparingly to affected area once or twice daily. If no improvement is seen within 2 weeks, reassessment of diagnosis may be necessary.

Rhinitis: Intranasal: Initial: 2 sprays (50 mcg/spray) per nostril once daily; may also be divided into 100 mcg twice a day. After the first few days, dosage may be reduced to 1 spray per nostril once daily for maintenance therapy. Dosing should be at regular intervals.

Pediatrics:

Asthma: Inhalation, oral:

Flovent®, Flovent® HFA:

Children <12 years (unlabeled use): NIH Asthma Guidelines (administer in divided doses twice daily):

"Low" dose: 88-176 mcg/day

"Medium" dose: 176-440 mcg/day

"High" dose: >440 mcg/day

Children ≥12 years: Refer to adult dosing.

Flovent® Diskus® [CAN]:

Children 4-16 years: Usual starting dose: 50-100 mcg twice daily; may increase to 200 mcg twice daily in patients not adequately controlled; titrate to the lowest effective dose once asthma stability is achieved

Children ≥16 years: Refer to adult dosing.

Corticosteroid-responsive dermatoses: Topical: Children ≥3 months: Cream: Apply sparingly to affected area twice daily. If no improvement is seen within 2 weeks, reassessment of diagnosis may be necessary. **Note:** Safety and efficacy of treatment >4 weeks duration have not been established.

Atopic dermatitis: Topical:

Children ≥3 months: Cream: Apply sparingly to affected area 1-2 times/day. If no improvement is seen within 2 weeks, reassessment of diagnosis may be necessary.

Children ≥1 year: Lotion: Apply sparingly to affected area once daily.

Note: Safety and efficacy of treatment >4 weeks duration have not been established.

Rhinitis: Intranasal: Children ≥4 years and Adolescents: Initial: 1 spray (50 mcg/spray) per nostril once daily; patients not adequately responding or patients with more severe symptoms may use 2 sprays (100 mcg) per nostril. Depending on response, dosage may be reduced to 100 mcg daily. Total daily dosage should not exceed 2 sprays in each nostril (200 mcg)/day. Dosing should be at regular intervals.

Hepatic Impairment: Fluticasone is primarily cleared in the liver. Fluticasone plasma levels may be increased in patients with hepatic impairment, use with caution; monitor.

Available Dosage Forms [DSC] = Discontinued product; [CAN] = Canadian brand name

Aerosol for oral inhalation, as propionate [contains CFCs] (Flovent®):

44 mcg/inhalation (7.9 g) [60 metered doses], (13 g) [120 metered doses] [DSC]

110 mcg/inhalation (7.9 g) [60 metered doses], (13 g) [120 metered doses] [DSC]

220 mcg/inhalation (7.9 g) [60 metered doses], (13 g) [120 metered doses] [DSC]

Aerosol for oral inhalation, as propionate [CFC free] (Flovent® HFA):

44 mcg/inhalation (10.6 g) [120 metered doses]

110 mcg/inhalation (12 g) [120 metered doses]

220 mcg/inhalation (12 g) [120 metered doses]

Cream, as propionate (Cutivate®): 0.05% (15 g, 30 g, 60 g)

Lotion, as propionate (Cutivate®): 0.05% (60 mL)

Ointment, as propionate (Cutivate®): 0.005% (15 g, 30 g, 60 g)

Powder for oral inhalation, as propionate [prefilled blister pack] (Flovent® Diskus®) [CAN; not available in the United States]:

50 mcg (28s, 60s) [delivers 46 mcg per inhalation; contains lactose]

100 mcg (28s, 60s) [delivers 94 mcg per inhalation; contains lactose]

250 mcg (28s, 60s) [delivers 235 mcg per inhalation; contains lactose]

(Continued)

Fluticasone *(Continued)*

500 mcg (28s, 60s) [contains lactose]

Suspension, intranasal spray, as propionate (Flonase®): 50 mcg/inhalation (16 g) [120 metered doses]

Nursing Guidelines

Assessment: Monitor effectiveness of therapy and adverse reactions at beginning of therapy and periodically with long-term use. May take as long as 2 weeks before full benefit of medication is known. Assess knowledge/teach patient appropriate use, interventions to reduce side effects, and adverse symptoms to report. Monitor for possible eosinophilic conditions (including Churg-Strauss syndrome); growth (adolescents and children); and signs/symptoms of HPA axis suppression/adrenal insufficiency.

Dietary Considerations: Flovent® Diskus® [CAN] contains lactose; very rare anaphylactic reactions have been reported with Flovent® Rotadisk® in patients with severe milk protein allergy.

Patient Education: Use as directed; do not overuse and use only for length of time prescribed. Although you may see improvement within a few hours of use, the full benefit of the medication may not be achieved for several days. Do not change the prescribed dosage without consulting prescriber. Avoid exposure to chickenpox or measles. If exposed, inform your prescriber as soon as possible. **Pregnancy/breast-feeding precautions:** Inform prescriber if you are or intend to become pregnant. Consult prescriber if breast-feeding.

Metered-dose inhalation: Sit when using. Take deep breaths for 3-5 minutes, and clear nasal passages before administration (use decongestant as needed). Hold breath for 5-10 seconds after use, and wait 1-3 minutes between inhalations. Follow package insert instructions for use. Do not exceed maximum dosage. If also using inhaled bronchodilator, use before fluticasone. Rinse mouth and throat after use to reduce aftertaste and prevent candidiasis.

Nasal spray: Shake gently before use. Use at regular intervals, no more frequently than directed. Report unusual cough or spasm; persistent nasal bleeding, burning, or irritation; or worsening of condition.

Powder for oral inhalation: Flovent® Diskus® [CAN]: Do not attempt to take device apart. Do not use with a spacer device. Do not exhale into the Diskus®, use in a level horizontal position. Do not wash the mouthpiece.

Topical: For external use only. Apply thin film to affected area only; rub in lightly. Do not apply occlusive covering unless advised by prescriber. Wash hand thoroughly after use; avoid contact with eyes. Notify prescriber if skin condition persists or worsens. Do not use for treatment of diaper dermatitis or under diapers or plastic pants.

Geriatric Considerations: No specific information for the elderly patient is available.

Pregnancy Risk Factor: C

Pregnancy Issues: There are no adequate and well-controlled studies using inhaled fluticasone in pregnant women. Oral corticosteroid use has shown animals to be more prone to teratogenic effects than humans. Due to the natural increase in corticosteroid production during pregnancy, most women may require a lower steroid dose; use with caution.

Lactation: Excretion in breast milk unknown/use caution

Breast-Feeding Considerations: Systemic corticosteroids are excreted in human milk. The extent of topical absorption is variable. Use with caution while breast-feeding; do not apply to nipples.

Administration

Storage:

Nasal spray: Store between 4°C to 30°C (39°F to 86°F).

Oral inhalation: Flovent®, Flovent® HFA: Store at 15°C to 30°C (59°F to 86°F). Store with mouthpiece down.

Powder for oral inhalation: Flovent® Diskus® [CAN]: Store between 2°C to 30°C in a dry place away from direct frost, heat, or sunlight. Do not store in a damp environment (eg, bathroom).

Topical, cream: Store at 15°C to 30°C (59°F to 86°F).

Cutivate® lotion: Store at 15°C to 30°C (59°F to 86°F). Do not refrigerate.

Cutivate® cream, ointment: Store at 2°C to 30°C (36°F to 86°F).

Fluticasone and Salmeterol (floo TIK a sone & sal ME te role)

U.S. Brand Names Advair Diskus®

Synonyms Salmeterol and Fluticasone

Pharmacologic Category Beta$_2$-Adrenergic Agonist; Corticosteroid, Inhalant (Oral)

Medication Safety Issues

Sound-alike/look-alike issues:

Advair may be confused with Advicor®

Use Maintenance treatment of asthma in adults and children ≥4 years; **not** for use for relief of acute bronchospasm; maintenance treatment of COPD associated with chronic bronchitis

Mechanism of Action Combination of fluticasone (corticosteroid) and salmeterol (long-acting beta$_2$ agonist) designed to improve pulmonary function and control over what is produced by either agent when used alone. Because fluticasone and salmeterol act locally in the lung, plasma levels do not predict therapeutic effect.

Fluticasone: The mechanism of action for all topical corticosteroids is believed to be a combination of three important properties: Anti-inflammatory activity, immunosuppressive properties, and antiproliferative actions. Fluticasone has extremely potent vasoconstrictive and anti-inflammatory activity.

Salmeterol: Relaxes bronchial smooth muscle by selective action on beta$_2$-receptors with little effect on heart rate

Pharmacodynamics/Kinetics

Advair Diskus®:

Onset of action: 30-60 minutes

Peak effect: ≥1 week for full effect

Duration: 12 hours

See individual agents.

Contraindications Hypersensitivity to fluticasone, salmeterol, or any component of the formulation; status asthmaticus; acute episodes of asthma

Warnings/Precautions Not indicated for treatment of acute symptoms of asthma. Not for use in patients with rapidly deteriorating or life-threatening episodes of asthma. Fatalities have been reported. Do not use in conjunction with other long-acting beta$_2$ agonist inhalers. Do not exceed recommended dosage; short-acting beta$_2$ agonist should be used for acute symptoms and symptoms occurring between treatments. Do not use to transfer patients from oral corticosteroid therapy. Immediate hypersensitivity reactions (urticaria, angioedema, rash, bronchospasm) have been reported. Rare cases of vasculitis (Churg-Strauss syndrome) have been reported with fluticasone use.

May cause hypercorticism or suppression of hypothalamic-pituitary-adrenal (HPA) axis, particularly in younger children or in patients receiving high doses for prolonged periods. HPA axis suppression may lead to adrenal crisis. Withdrawal and discontinuation of a corticosteroid should be done slowly and carefully. Particular care is required when patients are transferred from systemic corticosteroids to inhaled products due to possible adrenal insufficiency or withdrawal from steroids, including an increase in allergic symptoms. Patients receiving 20 mg per day of prednisone (or equivalent) may be most susceptible. Concurrent use of ritonavir (and potentially other strong inhibitors of CYP3A4) may increase fluticasone levels and effects on HPA suppression. Fatalities have occurred due to adrenal insufficiency in asthmatic patients during and after transfer from systemic corticosteroids to aerosol steroids; aerosol steroids do **not** provide the systemic steroid needed to treat patients having trauma, surgery, or infections. May suppress the immune system; use with caution in patients with systemic infections or ocular herpes simplex. Avoid exposure to chickenpox and measles.

Controlled clinical studies have shown that orally-inhaled and intranasal corticosteroids may cause a reduction in growth velocity in pediatric patients. (In studies of orally-inhaled corticosteroids, the mean reduction in growth velocity was ~1 cm per year [range 0.3-1.8 cm per year] and appears to be related to dose and duration of exposure.) Long-term use may affect bone mineral density in adults. To minimize the systemic effects of orally-inhaled and intranasal corticosteroids, each patient should be titrated to the lowest effective dose.

Beta agonists may cause elevation in blood pressure, heart rate, and result in CNS excitement. Use caution in patients with cardiovascular disease (arrhythmia or hypertension or CHF), convulsive disorders, diabetes, glaucoma, hyperthyroidism, or hypokalemia. May increase risk of arrhythmia and may increase

(Continued)

Fluticasone and Salmeterol *(Continued)*

serum glucose or decrease serum potassium concentrations. In a large, randomized clinical trial (SMART), salmeterol was associated with a small, but statistically significant increase in asthma-related deaths (when added to usual asthma therapy); risk may be greater in African-American patients versus Caucasians. The elderly may be at greater risk of cardiovascular side effects. Safety and efficacy have not been established in children <4 years of age.

Powder for oral inhalation contains lactose; very rare anaphylactic reactions have been reported in patients with severe milk protein allergy.

Drug Interactions Fluticasone: **Substrate** of CYP3A4 (major)

Beta-adrenergic blockers (eg, propranolol): Decreased effect of salmeterol component and may cause bronchospasm in asthmatics; use with caution.

$Beta_2$-agonists (long-acting): Should not be coadministered with fluticasone/salmeterol combination.

Diuretics (loop, thiazide): Hypokalemia from diuretics may be worsened by beta-agonists (dose related); use with caution.

CYP3A4 inhibitors: May increase levels and/or effects of fluticasone. Example inhibitors include azole antifungals, ciprofloxacin, clarithromycin, diclofenac, doxycycline, erythromycin, imatinib, isoniazid, nefazodone, nicardipine, propofol, protease inhibitors, quinidine, telithromycin, and verapamil.

MAO inhibitors, tricyclic antidepressants: Increased toxicity (cardiovascular); wait at least 2 weeks after discontinuing these agents to start fluticasone/salmeterol.

Ritonavir: May increase serum levels (due to CYP3A4 inhibition) and the potential for steroid-related adverse effects (eg, Cushing syndrome, adrenal suppression). Avoid concurrent use.

Adverse Reactions Percentages reported in patients with asthma

>10%:

Central nervous system: Headache (12% to 13%)

Endocrine & metabolic: Serum glucose increased, serum potassium decreased

Respiratory: Pharyngitis (10% to 13%), upper respiratory tract infection (21% to 27%)

>3% to 10%:

Gastrointestinal: Diarrhea (2% to 4%), GI pain/discomfort (1% to 4%), oral candidiasis (1% to 4%), nausea/vomiting (4% to 6%)

Neuromuscular & skeletal: Musculoskeletal pain (2% to 4%)

Respiratory: Bronchitis (2% to 8%), cough (3% to 6%), hoarseness/dysphonia (2% to 5%), sinusitis (4% to 5%), upper respiratory tract inflammation (6% to 7%), viral respiratory tract infection (4%)

1% to 3%:

Cardiovascular: Chest symptoms, fluid retention, palpitation

Central nervous system: Compressed nerve syndromes, hypnagogic effects, pain, sleep disorders, tremor

Dermatologic: Hives, skin flakiness/ichthyosis, urticaria, viral skin infection

Gastrointestinal: Appendicitis, constipation, dental discomfort/pain, gastrointestinal disorder, gastrointestinal infection, gastrointestinal signs and symptoms (nonspecified), oral discomfort/pain, oral erythema/rash, oral ulcerations, unusual taste, viral GI infection (0% to 3%)

Hematologic: Contusions/hematomas, lymphatic signs and symptoms (nonspecified)

Hepatic: Abnormal liver function tests

Neuromuscular & skeletal: Arthralgia, articular rheumatism, bone/cartilage disorders, fractures, muscle injuries, muscle stiffness, tightness/rigidity

Ocular: Conjunctivitis, eye redness, keratitis

Otic: Ear signs and symptoms (nonspecified)

Respiratory: Blood in nasal mucosa, congestion, ear/nose/throat infection, lower respiratory tract infection, lower respiratory signs and symptoms (nonspecified), nasal irritation, nasal signs and symptoms (nonspecified), nasal sinus disorders, pneumonia, rhinitis, rhinorrhea/post nasal drip, sneezing, wheezing

Miscellaneous: Allergies/allergic reactions, bacterial infection, burns, candidiasis (0% to 3%), sweat/sebum disorders, sweating, viral infection, wounds and lacerations

<1% (Limited to important or life-threatening): Aphonia, arrhythmia, bronchospasm (paradoxical), Cushing syndrome, cataracts, depression, dysmenorrhea, eosinophilic conditions, glaucoma, growth velocity reduction (in children/adolescents), hypercorticism, hyperglycemia, hypersensitivity reaction (immediate and delayed), hypokalemia, hypothyroidism, influenza, laryngeal spasm/

irritation, osteoporosis, paradoxical tracheitis, paresthesia, photodermatitis, rare cases of vasculitis (Churg-Strauss syndrome), restlessness, stridor, syncope, ventricular tachycardia, vulvovaginitis, xerostomia

Overdosage/Toxicology Symptoms of overdose include tachycardia, tremor, hypertension, angina, and seizures. Hypokalemia also may occur. Cardiac arrest and death may be associated with abuse of beta-agonist bronchodilators. Treatment includes immediate discontinuation and symptomatic and supportive therapies. Cautious use of beta-adrenergic blocking agents may be considered in severe cases.

Dosing

Adults & Elderly: Do not use to transfer patients from systemic corticosteroid therapy

COPD: Oral inhalation: Fluticasone 250 mcg/salmeterol 50 mcg twice daily, 12 hours apart

Asthma (maintenance): Oral inhalation: One inhalation twice daily, morning and evening, 12 hours apart

Note: Advair Diskus® is available in 3 strengths, initial dose prescribed should be based upon previous asthma therapy. Dose should be increased after 2 weeks if adequate response is not achieved. Patients should be titrated to lowest effective dose once stable. (Because each strength contains salmeterol 50 mcg/inhalation, dose adjustments should be made by changing inhaler strength. No more than 1 inhalation of any strength should be taken more than twice a day). Maximum dose: Fluticasone 500 mcg/salmeterol 50 mcg, one inhalation twice daily.

Patients not currently on inhaled corticosteroids: Fluticasone 100 mcg/salmeterol 50 mcg

Patients currently using inhaled beclomethasone dipropionate:

≤420 mcg/day: Fluticasone 100 mcg/salmeterol 50 mcg
462-840 mcg/day: Fluticasone 250 mcg/salmeterol 50 mcg

Patients currently using inhaled budesonide:

≤400 mcg/day: Fluticasone 100 mcg/salmeterol 50 mcg
800-1200 mcg/day: Fluticasone 250 mcg/salmeterol 50 mcg
1600 mcg/day: Fluticasone 500 mcg/salmeterol 50 mcg

Patients currently using inhaled flunisolide:

≤1000 mcg/day: Fluticasone 100 mcg/salmeterol 50 mcg
1250-2000 mcg/day: Fluticasone 250 mcg/salmeterol 50 mcg

Patients currently using inhaled fluticasone propionate aerosol:

≤176 mcg/day: Fluticasone 100 mcg/salmeterol 50 mcg
440 mcg/day: Fluticasone 250 mcg/salmeterol 50 mcg
660-880 mcg/day: Fluticasone 500 mcg/salmeterol 50 mcg

Patients currently using inhaled fluticasone propionate powder:

≤200 mcg/day: Fluticasone 100 mcg/salmeterol 50 mcg
500 mcg/day: Fluticasone 250 mcg/salmeterol 50 mcg
1000 mcg/day: Fluticasone 500 mcg/salmeterol 50 mcg

Patients currently using inhaled triamcinolone acetonide:

≤1000 mcg/day: Fluticasone 100 mcg/salmeterol 50 mcg
1100-1600 mcg/day: Fluticasone 250 mcg/salmeterol 50 mcg

Pediatrics: Asthma: Oral inhalation:

Children 4-11 years: Fluticasone 100 mcg/salmeterol 50 mcg twice daily, 12 hours apart

Children ≥12 years: Refer to adult dosing.

Hepatic Impairment: Fluticasone is cleared by hepatic metabolism. No dosing adjustment suggested. Use with caution in patients with impaired liver function.

Available Dosage Forms Powder for oral inhalation:

100/50: Fluticasone propionate 100 mcg and salmeterol xinafoate 50 mcg (28s, 60s) [contains lactose]

250/50: Fluticasone propionate 250 mcg and salmeterol xinafoate 50 mcg (28s, 60s) [contains lactose]

500/50: Fluticasone propionate 500 mcg and salmeterol xinafoate 50 mcg (28s, 60s) [contains lactose]

Nursing Guidelines

Assessment: See individual components listed in Related Information. Note breast-feeding caution

Monitoring Laboratory Tests: FEV_1, peak flow, and/or other pulmonary function tests; serum glucose, serum potassium

(Continued)

Fluticasone and Salmeterol *(Continued)*

Dietary Considerations: Powder for oral inhalation contains lactose; very rare anaphylactic reactions have been reported in patients with severe milk protein allergy.

Patient Education: See individual components listed in Related Information. **Pregnancy/breast-feeding precautions:** Inform prescriber if you are or intend to become pregnant. Consult prescriber if breast-feeding.

Pregnancy Risk Factor: C

Pregnancy Issues: There are no adequate and well-controlled studies of fluticasone and/or salmeterol in pregnant women. Use only during pregnancy if the potential benefit to the mother outweighs the potential risk to the fetus. The use of fluticasone and/or salmeterol have not been studied in nursing women.

Lactation:

Fluticasone: Excretion in breast milk unknown/use caution
Salmeterol: Enters breast milk/use caution

Perioperative/Anesthesia/Other Concerns: Inhaled steroid therapy, usually used for chronic obstructive lung disease; has the important advantage of having minimal systemic effects. Beta-agonists may induce increases in heart rate. This should be considered in patients with resting tachycardia. Frequent use of inhaled beta-agonists when used in patients with atrial fibrillation may counteract pharmacologic interventions directed at ventricular rate control. It may take ≥1 week to see full benefits from treatment. This agent is not to be used for the relief of acute attacks.

Administration

Storage: Store at 20°C to 25°C (68°F to 77°F). Store in a dry place out of direct heat or sunlight. Keep out of reach of children. Diskus® device should be discarded 1 month after removal from foil pouch, or when dosing indicator reads "zero," whichever comes first. Device is not reusable.

Related Information

Fluticasone *on page 760*
Salmeterol *on page 1507*

- **Fluticasone Propionate** *see* Fluticasone *on page 760*
- **Fluvirin®** *see* Influenza Virus Vaccine *on page 913*
- **Fluxid™** *see* Famotidine *on page 702*
- **Fluzone®** *see* Influenza Virus Vaccine *on page 913*
- **FML®** *see* Fluorometholone *on page 743*
- **FML® Forte** *see* Fluorometholone *on page 743*
- **Foille® [OTC]** *see* Benzocaine *on page 232*
- **Folacin** *see* Folic Acid *on page 768*
- **Folate** *see* Folic Acid *on page 768*

Folic Acid (FOE lik AS id)

Synonyms Folacin; Folate; Pteroylglutamic Acid

Pharmacologic Category Vitamin, Water Soluble

Medication Safety Issues

Sound-alike/look-alike issues:

Folic acid may be confused with folinic acid

Use Treatment of megaloblastic and macrocytic anemias due to folate deficiency; dietary supplement to prevent neural tube defects

Mechanism of Action Folic acid is necessary for formation of a number of coenzymes in many metabolic systems, particularly for purine and pyrimidine synthesis; required for nucleoprotein synthesis and maintenance in erythropoiesis; stimulates WBC and platelet production in folate deficiency anemia

Pharmacodynamics/Kinetics

Onset of effect: Peak effect: Oral: 0.5-1 hour
Absorption: Proximal part of small intestine

Contraindications Hypersensitivity to folic acid or any component of the formulation

Warnings/Precautions Not appropriate for monotherapy with pernicious, aplastic, or normocytic anemias when anemia is present with vitamin D deficiency. Doses >0.1 mg/day may obscure pernicious anemia with continuing irreversible nerve damage progression. Resistance to treatment may occur with depressed hematopoiesis, alcoholism, deficiencies of other vitamins. Injection contains benzyl alcohol (1.5%) as preservative (use care in administration to neonates).

Drug Interactions

Phenytoin: Folic acid may decrease phenytoin concentrations

Raltitrexed: Folic acid may diminish the therapeutic effect of raltitrexed

Lab Interactions Falsely low serum concentrations may occur with the *Lactobacillus casei* assay method in patients on anti-infectives (eg, tetracycline).

Adverse Reactions Frequency not defined.

Allergic reaction, bronchospasm, flushing (slight), malaise (general), pruritus, rash

Dosing

Adults:

Anemia: Oral, I.M., I.V., SubQ: 0.4 mg/day

Pregnant and lactating women: 0.8 mg/day

RDA: Expressed as dietary folate equivalents: 400 mcg/day

Prevention of neural tube defects: Oral:

Females of childbearing potential: 400 mcg/day

Females at high risk or with family history of neural tube defects: 4 mg/day

Elderly: Refer to adults dosing. Vitamin B_{12} deficiency must be ruled out before initiating folate therapy due to frequency of combined nutritional deficiencies: RDA requirements (1999): 400 mcg/day (0.4 mg) minimum.

Pediatrics:

Anemia: Oral, I.M., I.V., SubQ:

Infants: 0.1 mg/day

Children <4 years: Up to 0.3 mg/day

Children >4 years and Adults: Refer to adult dosing.

RDA: Expressed as dietary folate equivalents: Oral: Children:

1-3 years: 150 mcg/day

4-8 years: 200 mcg/day

9-13 years: 300 mcg/day

≥14 years: Refer to adult dosing.

Available Dosage Forms

Injection, solution, as sodium folate: 5 mg/mL (10 mL) [contains benzyl alcohol]

Tablet: 0.4 mg, 0.8 mg, 1 mg

Nursing Guidelines

Assessment: Assess potential for interactions with other prescriptions, OTC medications, or herbal products patient may be taking. Assess therapeutic effectiveness and adverse response on a regular basis throughout therapy. Teach patient proper use, possible side effects/appropriate interventions, and adverse symptoms to report.

Dietary Considerations: As of January 1998, the FDA has required manufacturers of enriched flour, bread, corn meal, pasta, rice and other grain products to add folic acid to their products. The intent is to help decrease the risk of neural tube defects by increasing folic acid intake. Other foods which contain folic acid include dark green leafy vegetables, citrus fruits and juices, and lentils.

Patient Education: Do not take any new medication during therapy unless approved by prescriber. Take exactly as prescribed. Toxicity can occur from elevated doses. Increased intake of foods high in folic acid (eg, dried beans, nuts, bran, vegetables, fruits) may be recommended by prescriber. Excessive use of alcohol increases requirement for folic acid. May turn urine more intensely yellow. Report skin rash. **Pregnancy precaution:** Inform prescriber if you are pregnant..

Geriatric Considerations: Elderly frequently have combined nutritional deficiencies. Must rule out vitamin B_{12} deficiency before initiating folate therapy. Elderly RDA requirements from 1999 RDA are 400 mcg minimum (0.4 mg). Elderly, due to decreased nutrient intake, may benefit from daily intake of a multiple vitamin with minerals.

Pregnancy Risk Factor: A

Lactation: Enters breast milk/compatible

Administration

Oral: A diluted solution for oral administration may be prepared by diluting 1 mL of folic acid injection (5 mg/mL), with 49 mL sterile water for injection. Resulting solution is 0.1 mg folic acid per 1 mL.

I.M.: May also be administered by deep I.M. injection.

I.V.: May also be administered by I.V. injection by diluting 1 mL of folic acid injection (5 mg/mL), with 49 mL sterile water for injection. Resulting solution is 0.1 mg folic acid per 1 mL.

(Continued)

Folic Acid *(Continued)*

Compatibility: Stable in D_5W, $D_{20}W$, NS, fat emulsion 10%; **incompatible** with $D_{40}W$, $D_{50}W$

Compatibility in syringe: Incompatible with doxapram

Compatibility when admixed: Incompatible with calcium gluconate

♦ Folinic Acid *see* Leucovorin *on page 1013*

Fondaparinux (fon da PARE i nuks)

U.S. Brand Names Arixtra®

Synonyms Fondaparinux Sodium

Pharmacologic Category Factor Xa Inhibitor

Use Prophylaxis of deep vein thrombosis (DVT) in patients undergoing surgery for hip replacement, knee replacement, hip fracture (including extended prophylaxis following hip fracture surgery), or abdominal surgery (in patients at risk for thromboembolic complications); treatment of acute pulmonary embolism (PE); treatment of acute DVT without PE

Mechanism of Action Fondaparinux is a synthetic pentasaccharide that causes an antithrombin III-mediated selective inhibition of factor Xa. Neutralization of factor Xa interrupts the blood coagulation cascade and inhibits thrombin formation and thrombus development.

Pharmacodynamics/Kinetics

Absorption: Rapid and complete

Distribution: V_d: 7-11 L; mainly in blood

Protein binding: ≥94% to antithrombin III

Bioavailability: 100%

Half-life elimination: 17-21 hours; prolonged with worsening renal impairment

Time to peak: 2-3 hours

Excretion: Urine (as unchanged drug); decreased clearance in patients <50 kg

Contraindications Hypersensitivity to fondaparinux or any component of the formulation; severe renal impairment (Cl_{cr} <30 mL/minute); body weight <50 kg (prophylaxis); active major bleeding; bacterial endocarditis; thrombocytopenia associated with a positive *in vitro* test for antiplatelet antibody in the presence of fondaparinux

Warnings/Precautions Patients with recent or anticipated neuraxial anesthesia (epidural or spinal anesthesia) are at risk of spinal or epidural hematoma and subsequent paralysis. Consider risk versus benefit prior to neuraxial anesthesia; risk is increased by concomitant agents which may alter hemostasis, as well as traumatic or repeated epidural or spinal puncture. Patient should be observed closely for bleeding if administered during or immediately following diagnostic lumbar puncture, epidural anesthesia, or spinal anesthesia.

Not to be used interchangeably (unit-for-unit) with heparin, low molecular weight heparins (LMWHs), or heparinoids. Use caution in patients with moderate renal dysfunction (Cl_{cr} 30-50 mL/minute). Patients with serum creatinine >2 mg/dL were excluded from clinical trials. Periodically monitor renal function; discontinue if severe dysfunction or labile function develops.

Use caution in conditions with increased risk of hemorrhage such as congenital or acquired bleeding disorders; active ulcerative or angiodysplastic gastrointestinal disease; hemorrhagic stroke; shortly after brain, spinal, or ophthalmologic surgery; or in patients taking platelet inhibitors. Risk of major bleeding may be increased if initial dose is administered earlier then recommended (initiation recommended at 6-8 hours following surgery). Discontinue agents that may enhance the risk of hemorrhage if possible. If thrombocytopenia occurs, discontinue fondaparinux. Use caution in the elderly, patients with a history of heparin-induced thrombocytopenia, patients with a bleeding diathesis, uncontrolled hypertension, recent gastrointestinal ulceration, diabetic retinopathy, and hemorrhage. Use caution in patients <50 kg who are being treated for DVT/PE; fondaparinux clearance may be decreased. Safety and efficacy in pediatric patients have not been established.

Drug Interactions

Anticoagulants: May enhance the effects of other anticoagulants.

Antiplatelet agents (including abciximab, anagrelide, cilostazol, clopidogrel, dipyridamole, eptifibatide, ticlopidine, tirofiban): May enhance the anticoagulant effect of fondaparinux.

Drotrecogin alfa: May enhance the bleeding potential with drotrecogin alfa.

NSAIDs: May enhance the anticoagulant effect of fondaparinux.

Salicylates: May enhance the anticoagulant effect of fondaparinux.

Thrombolytic agents: Increase the risk of hemorrhage.

Nutritional/Herbal/Ethanol Interactions Herb/Nutraceutical: Avoid alfalfa, anise, bilberry, bladderwrack, bromelain, cat's claw, celery, coleus, cordyceps, dong quai, evening primrose oil, fenugreek, feverfew, garlic, ginger, ginkgo biloba, ginseng (American/Panax/Siberian), grape seed, green tea, guggul, horse chestnut seed, horseradish, licorice, prickly ash, red clover, reishi, sweet clover, turmeric, white willow (all possess anticoagulant or antiplatelet activity and as such, may enhance the anticoagulant effects of fondaparinux).

Lab Interactions International standards of heparin or LMWH are not the appropriate calibrators for antifactor Xa activity of fondaparinux.

Adverse Reactions As with all anticoagulants, bleeding is the major adverse effect. Hemorrhage may occur at any site. Risk appears increased by a number of factors including renal dysfunction, age (>75 years), and weight (<50 kg).

>10%:

- Central nervous system: Fever (4% to 14%)
- Gastrointestinal: Nausea (11%)
- Hematologic: Anemia (20%)

1% to 10%:

- Cardiovascular: Edema (9%), hypotension (4%), confusion (3%)
- Central nervous system: Insomnia (5%), dizziness (4%), headache (2% to 5%), pain (2%)
- Dermatologic: Rash (8%), purpura (4%), bullous eruption (3%)
- Endocrine & metabolic: Hypokalemia (1% to 4%)
- Gastrointestinal: Constipation (5% to 9%), vomiting (6%), diarrhea (3%), dyspepsia (2%)
- Genitourinary: Urinary tract infection (4%), urinary retention (3%)
- Hematologic: Moderate thrombocytopenia (50,000-100,000/mm^3: 3%), major bleeding (1% to 3%), minor bleeding (2% to 4%), hematoma (3%); risk of major bleeding increased as high as 5% in patients receiving initial dose <6 hours following surgery
- Hepatic: SGOT increased (2%), SGPT increased (3%)
- Local: Injection site reaction (bleeding, rash, pruritus)
- Miscellaneous: Wound drainage increased (5%)

<1% (Limited to important or life-threatening): Hepatic enzymes increased, severe thrombocytopenia (<50,000/mm^3)

Overdosage/Toxicology Treatment is symptom-directed and supportive. Hemodialysis may increase clearance by 20%.

Dosing

Adults & Elderly:

DVT prophylaxis: SubQ: Adults ≥50 kg: 2.5 mg once daily. **Note:** Initiate dose after hemostasis has been established, 6-8 hours postoperatively.

Usual duration: 5-9 days (up to 10 days following abdominal surgery or up to 11 days following hip replacement or knee replacement).

Extended prophylaxis is recommended following hip fracture surgery (has been tolerated for up to 32 days).

Acute DVT/PE treatment: SubQ: **Note:** Concomitant treatment with warfarin sodium should be initiated as soon as possible, usually within 72 hours:

<50 kg: 5 mg once daily

50-100 kg: 7.5 mg once daily

>100 kg: 10 mg once daily

Usual duration: 5-9 days (has been administered up to 26 days)

Renal Impairment:

Cl_{cr} 30-50 mL/minute: Use caution

Cl_{cr} <30 mL/minute: Contraindicated

Available Dosage Forms Injection, solution, as sodium [preservative free]: 2.5 mg/0.5 mL (0.5 mL); 5 mg/0.4mL (0.4 mL); 7.5 mg/0.6 mL (0.6 mL); 10 mg/0.8 mL (0.8 mL) [prefilled syringe]

Nursing Guidelines

Assessment: Assess potential for interactions with other prescriptions, OTC medications, or herbal products patient may be taking (especially anything that will affect coagulation or platelet function). Assess closely for bleeding; bleeding precautions should be observed. Assess results of laboratory tests, therapeutic effectiveness, and adverse response regularly during therapy. Teach patient possible side effects/appropriate interventions (eg, bleeding precautions) and adverse symptoms to report.

Monitoring Laboratory Tests: CBC, platelet count, serum creatinine; stool occult blood tests

(Continued)

Fondaparinux *(Continued)*

Patient Education: Do not take any new medication during therapy without consulting prescriber. This drug can only be administered by injection. Report pain, burning, redness, or swelling at injection site. You may have a tendency to bleed easily while taking this drug (brush teeth with soft brush, floss with waxed floss, use electric razor, avoid scissors or sharp knives, and avoid potentially harmful activities). May cause nausea or vomiting (small frequent meals, frequent mouth care, chewing gum, or sucking lozenges may help); or dizziness, headache, insomnia (use caution when driving or engaging in tasks that require alertness until response to drug is known). Report unusual bleeding or bruising (bleeding gums, nosebleed, blood in urine, dark stool); pain in joints or back; CNS changes (fever, severe headache, confusion); unusual fever; persistent nausea or GI upset; changes in urinary pattern; or other persistent adverse response. **Breast-feeding precaution:** Consult prescriber if breast-feeding.

Geriatric Considerations: Patients studied for DVT prophylaxis following elective knee or hip fracture surgery averaged 67.5 and 77 years of age, respectively. Use with caution in patients with estimated or actual creatinine clearance between 30-50 mL/minute. Contraindicated in patients whose Cl_{cr} <30 mL/minute.

Pregnancy Risk Factor: B

Pregnancy Issues: Reproductive animal studies have not shown fetal harm. Based on case reports, small amounts of fondaparinux have been detected in the umbilical cord following multiple doses during pregnancy. There are no adequate and well-controlled studies in pregnant women; use only if clearly needed.

Lactation: Excretion in breast milk unknown/use caution

Administration

I.M.: Do not administer I.M.

Compatibility: Do not mix with other injections or infusions.

Storage: Store at 15°C to 30°C (59°F to 86°F).

- ♦ **Fondaparinux Sodium** *see* Fondaparinux *on page 770*
- ♦ **Foradil® Aerolizer™** *see* Formoterol *on page 772*
- ♦ **Forane®** *see* Isoflurane *on page 971*

Formoterol (for MOH te rol)

U.S. Brand Names Foradil® Aerolizer™

Synonyms Formoterol Fumarate

Pharmacologic Category $Beta_2$-Adrenergic Agonist

Medication Safety Issues

Sound-alike/look-alike issues:

Foradil® may be confused with Toradol®

Foradil® capsules for inhalation are for administration via Aerolizer™ inhaler and are not for oral use.

Use Maintenance treatment of asthma and prevention of bronchospasm in patients ≥5 years of age with reversible obstructive airway disease, including patients with symptoms of nocturnal asthma, who require regular treatment with inhaled, short-acting $beta_2$ agonists; maintenance treatment of bronchoconstriction in patients with COPD; prevention of exercise-induced bronchospasm in patients ≥5 years of age

Note: Oxeze® is also approved in Canada for acute relief of symptoms ("on demand" treatment) in patients ≥6 years of age.

Mechanism of Action Relaxes bronchial smooth muscle by selective action on $beta_2$ receptors with little effect on heart rate. Formoterol has a long-acting effect.

Pharmacodynamics/Kinetics

Onset: Within 3 minutes

Peak effect: 80% of peak effect within 15 minutes

Duration: Improvement in FEV_1 observed for 12 hours in most patients

Absorption: Rapidly into plasma

Protein binding: 61% to 64% *in vitro* at higher concentrations than achieved with usual dosing

Metabolism: Hepatic via direct glucuronidation and O-demethylation; CYP2D6, CYP2C8/9, CYP2C19, CYP2A6 involved in O-demethylation

Half-life elimination: ~10-14 hours

Time to peak: Maximum improvement in FEV_1 in 1-3 hours

Excretion:

Children 5-12 years: Urine (7% to 9% as direct glucuronide metabolites, 6% as unchanged drug)

Adults: Urine (15% to 18% as direct glucuronide metabolites, 10% as unchanged drug)

Contraindications Hypersensitivity to adrenergic amines, formoterol, or any component of the formulation

Note: The approved U.S. labeling lists the need for acute bronchodilation as a contraindication; however, a formulation (Oxeze®) is approved for acute treatment in other countries (ie, Canada).

Warnings/Precautions Optimize anti-inflammatory treatment before initiating maintenance treatment with formoterol. Do not use as a component of chronic therapy without an anti-inflammatory agent. Patient must be instructed to seek medical attention in cases where acute symptoms are not relieved by rapid-onset beta-agonist or when a previous level of response is diminished. Treatment must not be delayed. Rarely, paradoxical bronchospasm may occur with use of inhaled bronchodilating agents; this should be distinguished from inadequate response.

Acute episodes should be treated with rapid-onset $beta_2$ agonist. The approved U.S. labeling states that formoterol is not meant to relieve acute asthmatic symptoms. Although, a formulation of formoterol (Oxeze®) is approved for acute treatment outside the U.S. (ie, Canada).

Do not exceed recommended dose; serious adverse events (including fatalities) have been associated with excessive use of inhaled sympathomimetics. $Beta_2$ agonists may increase risk of arrhythmias, decrease serum potassium, prolong QT_c interval, or increase serum glucose. These effects may be exacerbated in hypoxemia. Use caution in patients with cardiovascular disease (arrhythmia or hypertension or CHF), convulsive disorders, diabetes, glaucoma, hyperthyroidism, or hypokalemia. Beta agonists may cause elevation in blood pressure, heart rate, and result in CNS stimulation/excitation. Safety and efficacy have not been established in children <5 years of age.

Drug Interactions Substrate (minor) of CYP2A6, 2C8/9, 2C19, 2D6

Adrenergic agonist: Additive adrenergic stimulation may occur with concurrent use

Antidepressants, tricyclic: Concurrent use may potentiate cardiovascular side effects

Beta blockers: May block therapeutic effects of formoterol; may produce bronchospasm. If use is necessary, cautiously consider a cardioselective beta-blocker. Monitor closely.

Corticosteroids: May potentiate hypokalemia

Diuretics (thiazide or loops): May potentiate hypokalemia

MAO inhibitors: Concurrent use may potentiate cardiovascular side effects.

QT_c-prolonging agents: Concurrent use may potentiate cardiovascular side effects; includes dofetilide, type Ia antiarrhythmics (quinidine, procainamide), pimozide, some quinolone antibiotics (moxifloxacin, sparfloxacin, gatifloxacin), sotalol, mesoridazine, and thioridazine

Theophylline derivatives: May potentiate hypokalemia

Adverse Reactions Children are more likely to have infection, inflammation, abdominal pain, nausea, and dyspepsia.

>10%:

Endocrine & metabolic: Serum glucose increased, serum potassium decreased

Miscellaneous: Viral infection (17%)

1% to 10%:

Cardiovascular: Chest pain (2%)

Central nervous system: Tremor (2%), dizziness (2%), insomnia (2%), dysphonia (1%)

Dermatologic: Rash (1%)

Respiratory: Bronchitis (5%), infection (3%), dyspnea (2%), tonsillitis (1%)

<1% (Limited to important or life-threatening): Anaphylactic reactions (severe hypotension, angioedema), asthma exacerbation

Overdosage/Toxicology Symptoms of overdose include tachycardia, tremor, hypertension, angina, and seizures. Hypokalemia also may occur. Cardiac arrest and death may be associated with abuse of beta-agonist bronchodilators. Treatment includes immediate discontinuation and symptomatic and supportive therapies. Cautious use of beta-adrenergic blocking agents may be considered in severe cases.

(Continued)

Formoterol *(Continued)*

Dosing

Adults & Elderly:

Asthma (maintenance): Inhalation: 12 mcg capsule every 12 hours

Oxeze® (CAN): **Note:** Not labeled for use in the U.S.: Inhalation: 6 mcg or 12 mcg every 12 hours. Maximum dose: Children: 24 mcg/day; Adults: 48 mcg/day

Exercise-induced bronchospasm: Inhalation: 12 mcg capsule at least 15 minutes before exercise on an "as needed" basis; additional doses should not be used for another 12 hours. **Note:** If already using for asthma maintenance then should not use additional doses for exercise-induced bronchospasm.

Oxeze® (CAN): **Note:** Not labeled for use in the U.S.: Children ≥6 years and Adults: Inhalation: 6 mcg or 12 mcg at least 15 minutes before exercise.

COPD (maintenance): Inhalation: 12 mcg capsule every 12 hours

Acute ("on demand") relief of bronchoconstriction: *Indication for Oxeze® approved in Canada:* 6 mcg or 12 mcg as a single dose (maximum dose: 72 mcg in any 24-hour period). The prolonged use of high dosages (48 mcg/day for ≥3 consecutive days) may be a sign of suboptimal control, and should prompt the re-evaluation of therapy.

Pediatrics:

Asthma maintenance: Inhalation: Children ≥5 years: Refer to adult dosing.

Exercise-induced bronchospasm: Inhalation: Children ≥5 years: Refer to adult dosing.

Acute "on demand" treatment of bronchospasm (Oxeze® [CAN]): Inhalation: Refer to adult dosing.

Renal Impairment: Not studied

Available Dosage Forms [CAN] = Canadian brand name

Aerosol, oral (Oxeze® [CAN]): 6 mcg/dose (60 doses), 12 mcg/dose (60 doses) [contains lactose 600 mcg/dose]

Powder for oral inhalation, as fumarate [capsule]: 12 mcg (12s, 60s) [contains lactose 25 mg]

Nursing Guidelines

Assessment: Assess other medications patient may be taking for effectiveness and interactions. Monitor therapeutic effectiveness and adverse reactions at beginning of therapy and periodically throughout period of therapy. Assess knowledge/teach appropriate use of medication, interventions to reduce side effects, and adverse symptoms to report.

Monitoring Laboratory Tests: FEV_1, peak flow, and/or other pulmonary function tests; serum potassium, serum glucose (in selected patients)

Patient Education: Do not swallow capsules; this medication can only be used in the Aerolizer™ Inhaler. Use exactly as directed and do not use more often than recommended. Store capsules in blister and do not remove from blister until ready for treatment. Maintain adequate hydration (2-3 L/day of fluids) unless instructed to restrict fluid intake. It is recommended that you wear identification (Med-Alert bracelet) if you have an asthmatic condition. You may experience nervousness, dizziness, or insomnia (use caution when driving or engaging in hazardous activities until response to medication is known); dry mouth, nausea, or GI discomfort (small frequent meals, good mouth care, sucking lozenges, or chewing gum may help); or difficulty voiding (always void before treatment). Report any unresolved GI upset, nervousness or dizziness, muscle cramping, chest pain or palpitations, skin rash, signs of infection, unusual cough, or worsening of condition. **Pregnancy/breast-feeding precautions:** Inform prescriber if you are or intend to become pregnant. Consult prescriber if breast-feeding.

Administration: Follow directions for use and storage of inhaler exactly. Wash hands prior to treatment and sit in comfortable position for treatment. Remove capsule from foil blister immediately before treatment and place capsule in the capsule-chamber in the base of the Aerolizer™ Inhaler. Press both buttons once only and then release. Hold inhaler in a level, horizontal position, exhale fully (do not exhale into inhaler). Tilt head slightly back and inhale from inhaler rapidly, steadily, and deeply. Hold breath as long as possible. If any powder remains in capsule, exhale and inhale again. Repeat until capsule is empty. Throw away empty capsule. Do not use a spacer with Aerolizer™. Do not wash inhaler; store in dry place.

Pregnancy Risk Factor: C

Pregnancy Issues: There are no adequate and well-controlled studies in pregnant women. Use only if benefit outweighs risk to the fetus. Beta agonists interfere with uterine contractility so use during labor only if benefit outweighs risk to the fetus.

Lactation: Excretion in breast milk unknown/use caution

Administration

Storage: Prior to dispensing, store in refrigerator at 2°C to 8°C (36°F to 46°F); after dispensing, store at room temperature at 20°C to 25°C (68°F to 77°F). Protect from heat and moisture. Capsules should always be stored in the blister and only removed immediately before use. Always check expiration date. Use within 4 months of purchase date or product expiration date, whichever comes first.

- Formoterol Fumarate *see* Formoterol *on page 772*
- Formulation R™ [OTC] *see* Phenylephrine *on page 1350*
- 5-Formyl Tetrahydrofolate *see* Leucovorin *on page 1013*
- Fortamet™ *see* Metformin *on page 1112*
- Fortaz® *see* Ceftazidime *on page 348*
- Fortical® *see* Calcitonin *on page 287*
- Fosamax® *see* Alendronate *on page 105*

Foscarnet (fos KAR net)

U.S. Brand Names Foscavir®

Synonyms PFA; Phosphonoformate; Phosphonoformic Acid

Pharmacologic Category Antiviral Agent

Use

Treatment of herpes virus infections suspected to be caused by acyclovir-resistant (HSV, VZV) or ganciclovir-resistant (CMV) strains; this occurs almost exclusively in immunocompromised persons (eg, with advanced AIDS) who have received prolonged treatment for a herpes virus infection

Treatment of CMV retinitis in persons with AIDS

Unlabeled/Investigational Use Other CMV infections in persons unable to tolerate ganciclovir; may be given in combination with ganciclovir in patients who relapse after monotherapy with either drug

Mechanism of Action Pyrophosphate analogue which acts as a noncompetitive inhibitor of many viral RNA and DNA polymerases as well as HIV reverse transcriptase. Similar to ganciclovir, foscarnet is a virostatic agent. Foscarnet does not require activation by thymidine kinase.

Pharmacodynamics/Kinetics

Distribution: Up to 28% of cumulative I.V. dose may be deposited in bone

Metabolism: Biotransformation does not occur

Half-life elimination: ~3 hours

Excretion: Urine (≤28% as unchanged drug)

Contraindications Hypersensitivity to foscarnet or any component of the formulation; Cl_{cr} <0.4 mL/minute/kg during therapy

Warnings/Precautions Renal impairment occurs to some degree in the majority of patients treated with foscarnet; renal impairment may occur at any time and is usually reversible within 1 week following dose adjustment or discontinuation of therapy, however, several patients have died with renal failure within 4 weeks of stopping foscarnet; therefore, renal function should be closely monitored. Foscarnet is deposited in teeth and bone of young, growing animals; it has adversely affected tooth enamel development in rats; safety and effectiveness in children have not been studied. Imbalance of serum electrolytes or minerals occurs in 6% to 18% of patients (hypocalcemia, low ionized calcium, hypo- or hyperphosphatemia, hypomagnesemia or hypokalemia).

Patients with a low ionized calcium may experience perioral tingling, numbness, paresthesias, tetany, and seizures. Seizures have been experienced by up to 10% of AIDS patients. Risk factors for seizures include a low baseline absolute neutrophil count (ANC), impaired baseline renal function and low total serum calcium. Some patients who have experienced seizures have died, while others have been able to continue or resume foscarnet treatment after their mineral or electrolyte abnormality has been corrected, their underlying disease state treated, or their dose decreased. Foscarnet has been shown to be mutagenic *in vitro* and in mice at very high doses. Information on the use of foscarnet is lacking in the elderly; dose adjustments and proper monitoring must be performed because of the decreased renal function common in older patients.

(Continued)

Foscarnet *(Continued)*

Drug Interactions Increased toxicity:

Ciprofloxacin: Concurrent use with ciprofloxacin increases seizure potential

Cyclosporine: Acute renal failure (reversible) has been reported with cyclosporine due most likely to toxic synergistic effect

Nephrotoxic drugs (amphotericin B, I.V. pentamidine, aminoglycosides, etc): Should be avoided, if possible, to minimize additive renal risk with foscarnet

Pentamidine: Increases hypocalcemia

Ritonavir, saquinavir: Increased risk of renal impairment has been associated with concurrent use with foscarnet

Adverse Reactions

>10%:

Central nervous system: Fever, headache, seizure

Endocrine & metabolic: Electrolyte disorders (hyper- or hypocalcemia; hyper- or hypomagnesemia, hyper- or hypophosphatemia, or hypokalemia)

Gastrointestinal: Nausea, diarrhea, vomiting

Hematologic: Anemia

Renal: Nephrotoxicity (abnormal renal function, decreased creatinine clearance)

1% to 10%:

Central nervous system: Seizures (in up to 10% of HIV patients), fatigue, malaise, dizziness, hypoesthesia, depression, confusion, anxiety

Dermatologic: Rash

Gastrointestinal: Anorexia

Hematologic: Granulocytopenia, leukopenia

Local: Injection site pain

Neuromuscular & skeletal: Paresthesia, involuntary muscle contractions, rigors, neuropathy (peripheral), weakness

Ocular: Vision abnormalities

Respiratory: Coughing, dyspnea

Miscellaneous: Sepsis, diaphoresis (increased)

<1% (Limited to important or life-threatening): Arrhythmias, ascites, bradycardia, cardiac failure, cerebral edema, cholecystitis, cholelithiasis, hepatitis, hepatosplenomegaly, leg edema, peripheral edema, substernal chest pain, syncope, vocal cord paralysis

Overdosage/Toxicology Symptoms of overdose include seizures, renal dysfunction, perioral or limb paresthesia, and hypocalcemia. Treatment is supportive.

Dosing

Adults & Elderly:

CMV retinitis: I.V.:

Induction treatment: 60 mg/kg/dose every 8 hours for 14-21 days

Maintenance therapy: 90-120 mg/kg/day as a single infusion

Acyclovir-resistant HSV induction treatment: I.V.: 40 mg/kg/dose every 8-12 hours for 14-21 days

Pediatrics: Adolescents: Refer to adult dosing.

Renal Impairment: See tables below and on next page.

Induction Dosing of Foscarnet in Patients With Abnormal Renal Function

Cl_{cr} (mL/min/kg)	HSV Equivalent to 40 mg/kg q12h	HSV Equivalent to 40 mg/kg q8h	CMV Equivalent to 60 mg/kg q8h	CMV Equivalent to 90 mg/kg q12h
<0.4	Not recommended	Not recommended	Not recommended	Not recommended
≥0.4-0.5	20 mg/kg every 24 hours	35 mg/kg every 24 hours	50 mg/kg every 24 hours	50 mg/kg every 24 hours
>0.5-0.6	25 mg/kg every 24 hours	40 mg/kg every 24 hours	60 mg/kg every 24 hours	60 mg/kg every 24 hours
>0.6-0.8	35 mg/kg every 24 hours	25 mg/kg every 12 hours	40 mg/kg every 12 hours	80 mg/kg every 24 hours
>0.8-1.0	20 mg/kg every 12 hours	35 mg/kg every 12 hours	50 mg/kg every 12 hours	50 mg/kg every 12 hours
>1.0-1.4	30 mg/kg every 12 hours	30 mg/kg every 8 hours	45 mg/kg every 8 hours	70 mg/kg every 12 hours
>1.4	40 mg/kg every 12 hours	40 mg/kg every 8 hours	60 mg/kg every 8 hours	90 mg/kg every 12 hours

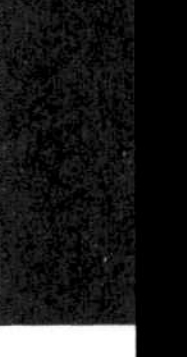

Maintenance Dosing of Foscarnet in Patients With Abnormal Renal Function

Cl_{cr} (mL/min/kg)	CMV	CMV
	Equivalent to 90 mg/kg q24h	Equivalent to 120 mg/kg q24h
<0.4	Not recommended	Not recommended
≥0.4-0.5	50 mg/kg every 48 hours	65 mg/kg every 48 hours
>0.5-0.6	60 mg/kg every 48 hours	80 mg/kg every 48 hours
>0.6-0.8	80 mg/kg every 48 hours	105 mg/kg every 48 hours
>0.8-1.0	50 mg/kg every 24 hours	65 mg/kg every 24 hours
>1.0-1.4	70 mg/kg every 24 hours	90 mg/kg every 24 hours
>1.4	90 mg/kg every 24 hours	120 mg/kg every 24 hours

Available Dosage Forms [DSC] = Discontinued product

Injection, solution: 24 mg/mL (250 mL [DSC], 500 mL)

Nursing Guidelines

Assessment: See Contraindications, Warnings/Precautions, Drug Interactions, and Dosing for use cautions. Assess potential for interactions with other prescriptions, OTC medications, or herbal products patient may be taking (see Drug Interactions). See Administration, Reconstitution, and Compatibility for specific directions. Assess results of laboratory tests (see below), therapeutic effectiveness, and adverse response (eg, nephrotoxicity, electrolyte imbalance, seizures - see Adverse Reactions and Overdose/Toxicology). Teach patient possible side effects/appropriate interventions and adverse symptoms to report (see Patient Education). Breast-feeding is contraindicated.

Monitoring Laboratory Tests: Renal function, CBC, electrolytes, calcium, magnesium

Patient Education: Inform prescriber of all prescriptions, OTC medications, or herbal products you are taking, and any allergies you have. Do not take any new medication during therapy unless approved by prescriber. Foscarnet is not a cure for the disease; progression may occur during or following therapy. While on therapy, it is important to maintain adequate hydration (2-3 L/day of fluids) unless instructed to restrict fluid intake, and nutrition (small, frequent meals may help). Regular dental check-ups are recommended. May cause dizziness or confusion (use caution when driving or engaging in tasks that require alertness until response to drug is known); nausea and vomiting (small, frequent meals, frequent mouth care, chewing gum or sucking lozenges may help); or diarrhea (buttermilk, boiled milk, or yogurt may help). Report any change in sensorium or seizures; unresolved diarrhea or vomiting; unusual fever, chills, sore throat, unhealed sores, swollen lymph glands; or malaise. **Pregnancy/breast-feeding precautions:** Inform prescriber if you are pregnant. Barrier contraceptives are recommended to reduce transmission of disease. Do not breast-feed.

Geriatric Considerations: Information on the use of foscarnet is lacking in the elderly. Dose adjustments and proper monitoring must be performed because of the decreased renal function common in older patients.

Pregnancy Risk Factor: C

Lactation: Excretion in breast milk unknown/contraindicated

Breast-Feeding Considerations: The CDC recommends **not** to breast-feed if diagnosed with HIV to avoid postnatal transmission of the virus.

Administration

I.V.: Use an infusion pump, at a rate not exceeding 1 mg/kg/minute. Adult induction doses of 60 mg/kg are administered over 1 hour. Adult maintenance doses of 90-120 mg/kg are infused over 2 hours.

Reconstitution: Foscarnet should be diluted in D_5W or NS and transferred to PVC containers. It is stable for 24 hours at room temperature or refrigeration. For peripheral line administration, foscarnet **must** be diluted to 12 mg/mL with D_5W or NS. For central line administration, foscarnet may be administered undiluted.

Compatibility: Stable in D_5W, NS; **incompatible** with LR, dextrose 30%, TPN, I.V. solutions containing calcium, magnesium, or vancomycin

(Continued)

Foscarnet *(Continued)*

Y-site administration: Incompatible with acyclovir, amphotericin B, diazepam, digoxin, diphenhydramine, dobutamine, droperidol, ganciclovir, haloperidol, leucovorin, midazolam, pentamidine, prochlorperazine edisylate, promethazine, trimetrexate

Storage: Foscarnet injection is a clear, colorless solution. It should be stored at room temperature and protected from temperatures >40°C and from freezing.

♦ Foscavir® *see* Foscarnet *on page 775*

Fosinopril (foe SIN oh pril)

U.S. Brand Names Monopril®

Synonyms Fosinopril Sodium

Pharmacologic Category Angiotensin-Converting Enzyme (ACE) Inhibitor

Medication Safety Issues

Sound-alike/look-alike issues:

Fosinopril may be confused with lisinopril

Monopril® may be confused with Accupril®, minoxidil, moexipril, Monoket®, Monurol™, ramipril

Use Treatment of hypertension, either alone or in combination with other antihypertensive agents; treatment of congestive heart failure, left ventricular dysfunction after myocardial infarction

Mechanism of Action Competitive inhibitor of angiotensin-converting enzyme (ACE); prevents conversion of angiotensin I to angiotensin II, a potent vasoconstrictor; results in lower levels of angiotensin II which causes an increase in plasma renin activity and a reduction in aldosterone secretion; a CNS mechanism may also be involved in hypotensive effect as angiotensin II increases adrenergic outflow from CNS; vasoactive kallikreins may be decreased in conversion to active hormones by ACE inhibitors, thus reducing blood pressure

Pharmacodynamics/Kinetics

Onset of action: 1 hour

Duration: 24 hours

Absorption: 36%

Protein binding: 95%

Metabolism: Prodrug, hydrolyzed to its active metabolite fosinoprilat by intestinal wall and hepatic esterases

Bioavailability: 36%

Half-life elimination, serum (fosinoprilat): 12 hours

Time to peak, serum: ~3 hours

Excretion: Urine and feces (as fosinoprilat and other metabolites in roughly equal proportions, 45% to 50%)

Contraindications Hypersensitivity to fosinopril or any component of the formulation; angioedema related to previous treatment with an ACE inhibitor; idiopathic or hereditary angioedema; bilateral renal artery stenosis; pregnancy (2nd and 3rd trimesters)

Warnings/Precautions Anaphylactic reactions can occur. Angioedema can occur at any time during treatment (especially following first dose). Angioedema may involve head and neck (potentially affecting the airway) or the intestine (presenting with abdominal pain). Careful blood pressure monitoring (hypotension can occur especially in volume depleted patients). Dosage adjustment needed in severe renal impairment (Cl_{cr} <10 mL/minute). Use with caution in hypovolemia; collagen vascular diseases; valvular stenosis (particularly aortic stenosis); hyperkalemia; or before, during, or immediately after anesthesia. Avoid rapid dosage escalation which may lead to renal insufficiency. Rare toxicities associated with ACE inhibitors include cholestatic jaundice (which may progress to hepatic necrosis) and neutropenia/agranulocytosis with myeloid hyperplasia. Hypersensitivity reactions may be seen during hemodialysis with high-flux dialysis membranes (eg, AN69). Hyperkalemia may rarely occur. If patient has renal impairment, then a baseline WBC with differential and serum creatinine should be evaluated and monitored closely during initial therapy. Use with caution in unilateral renal artery stenosis and pre-existing renal insufficiency.

Drug Interactions

Alpha$_1$ blockers: Hypotensive effect increased.

Antacids (aluminum hydroxide, magnesium hydroxide and simethicone): Absorption of fosinopril impaired; separate dose by 2 hours.

Aspirin: The effects of ACE inhibitors may be blunted by aspirin administration, particularly at higher dosages (see Cardiovascular Considerations) and/or increase adverse renal effects.

Diuretics: Hypovolemia due to diuretics may precipitate acute hypotensive events or acute renal failure.

Insulin: Risk of hypoglycemia may be increased.

Lithium: Risk of lithium toxicity may be increased; monitor lithium levels, especially the first 4 weeks of therapy.

Mercaptopurine: Risk of neutropenia may be increased.

NSAIDs: May attenuate hypertensive efficacy; effect has been seen with captopril and may occur with other ACE inhibitors; monitor blood pressure. May increase risk of adverse renal effects.

Potassium-sparing diuretics (amiloride, spironolactone, triamterene): Increased risk of hyperkalemia.

Potassium supplements may increase the risk of hyperkalemia.

Trimethoprim (high dose) may increase the risk of hyperkalemia.

Nutritional/Herbal/Ethanol Interactions Herb/Nutraceutical: Avoid dong quai if using for hypertension (has estrogenic activity). Avoid ephedra, garlic, yohimbe, ginseng (may worsen hypertension).

Lab Interactions Positive Coombs' (direct); may cause false-positive results in urine acetone determinations using sodium nitroprusside reagent; may cause false low serum digoxin levels with the Digi-Tab RIA kit for digoxin.

Adverse Reactions Note: Frequency ranges include data from hypertension and heart failure trials. Higher rates of adverse reactions have generally been noted in patients with CHF. However, the frequency of adverse effects associated with placebo is also increased in this population.

>10%: Central nervous system: Dizziness (1.6% to 11.9%)

1% to 10%:

- Cardiovascular: Orthostatic hypotension (1.4% to 1.9%), palpitation (1.4%)
- Central nervous system: Dizziness (1% to 2%; up to 12% in CHF patients), headache (3.2%), fatigue (1% to 2%)
- Endocrine & metabolic: Hyperkalemia (2.6%)
- Gastrointestinal: Diarrhea (2.2%), nausea/vomiting (1.2% to 2.2%)
- Hepatic: Transaminases increased
- Neuromuscular & skeletal: Musculoskeletal pain (<1% to 3.3%), noncardiac chest pain (<1% to 2.2%), weakness (1.4%)
- Renal: Increased serum creatinine, worsening of renal function (in patients with bilateral renal artery stenosis or hypovolemia)
- Respiratory: Cough (2.2% to 9.7%)
- Miscellaneous: Upper respiratory infection (2.2%)

>1% but ≤ frequency in patients receiving placebo: Sexual dysfunction, fever, flu-like syndrome, dyspnea, rash, headache, insomnia

<1% (Limited to important or life-threatening): Anaphylactoid reaction, angina, angioedema, arthralgia, bronchospasm, cerebral infarction, cerebrovascular accident, gout, hepatitis, hepatomegaly, myalgia, MI, pancreatitis, paresthesia, photosensitivity, pleuritic chest pain, pruritus, rash, renal insufficiency, shock, sudden death, syncope, TIA, tinnitus, urticaria, vertigo. In a small number of patients, a symptom complex of cough, bronchospasm, and eosinophilia has been observed with fosinopril.

Other events reported with ACE inhibitors: Acute renal failure, agranulocytosis, anemia, aplastic anemia, bullous pemphigus, cardiac arrest, eosinophilic pneumonitis, exfoliative dermatitis, gynecomastia, hemolytic anemia, hepatic failure, jaundice, neutropenia, pancytopenia, Stevens-Johnson syndrome, symptomatic hyponatremia, thrombocytopenia. In addition, a syndrome which may include fever, myalgia, arthralgia, interstitial nephritis, vasculitis, rash, eosinophilia and positive ANA, and elevated ESR has been reported for other ACE inhibitors.

Overdosage/Toxicology Mild hypotension has been the primary toxic effect seen with acute overdose. Bradycardia may also occur; hyperkalemia occurs even with therapeutic doses, especially in patients with renal insufficiency and those taking NSAIDs. Treatment is symptom-directed and supportive.

Dosing

Adults & Elderly:

Hypertension: Oral: Initial: 10 mg/day; increase to a maximum dose of 80 mg/day. Most patients are maintained on 20-40 mg/day. May need to divide the dose into two if trough effect is inadequate. Discontinue the diuretic, if

(Continued)

Fosinopril *(Continued)*

possible 2-3 days before initiation of therapy. Resume diuretic therapy carefully, if needed.

Heart failure: Oral: Initial: 10 mg/day (5 mg if renal dysfunction present) and increase, as needed, to a maximum of 40 mg once daily over several weeks. Usual dose: 20-40 mg/day. If hypotension, orthostasis, or azotemia occurs during titration, consider decreasing concomitant diuretic dose, if any.

Pediatrics: Hypertension: Children >50 kg: Oral: Initial: 5-10 mg once daily

Renal Impairment: None needed since hepatobiliary elimination compensates adequately diminished renal elimination.

Hemodialysis: Moderately dialyzable (20% to 50%)

Hepatic Impairment: Decrease dose and monitor effects

Available Dosage Forms Tablet, as sodium: 10 mg, 20 mg, 40 mg

Nursing Guidelines

Assessment: See Contraindications, Warnings/Precautions, and Dosing for use cautions. Assess potential for interactions with other prescriptions, OTC medications, or herbal products patient may be taking (especially anything that may impact fluid balance or cardiac status - see Drug Interactions). Assess results of laboratory tests (see below), therapeutic effectiveness, and adverse response on a regular basis during therapy (eg, anaphylactic reactions, hypovolemia, angioedema, postural hypotension - see Adverse Reactions and Overdose/Toxicology). Teach patient appropriate use, possible side effects/appropriate interventions, and adverse symptoms to report (see Patient Education). **Pregnancy risk factor C/D** - see Pregnancy Risk Factor for use cautions. Instruct patient in appropriate use of barrier contraceptives. Danger of use during pregnancy must outweigh risk to fetus - see Pregnancy Issues. Breast-feeding is not recommended.

Monitoring Laboratory Tests: CBC, renal function tests, electrolytes. If patient has renal impairment, a baseline WBC with differential and serum creatinine should be evaluated and monitored closely during initial therapy.

Dietary Considerations: Should not take a potassium salt supplement without the advice of healthcare provider.

Patient Education: Inform prescriber of all prescriptions, OTC medications, or herbal products you are taking, and any allergies you have. Do not take any new medication during therapy unless approved by prescriber. Do not use potassium supplement or salt substitutes without consulting prescriber. Take exactly as directed; do not discontinue without consulting prescriber. This drug does not eliminate need for diet or exercise regimen as recommended by prescriber. May cause dizziness, fainting, or lightheadedness (use caution when driving or engaging in tasks that require alertness until response to drug is known); postural hypotension (use caution when rising from lying or sitting position or climbing stairs); or nausea, vomiting, abdominal pain, dry mouth, or loss of appetite (small, frequent meals, frequent mouth care, sucking lozenges, or chewing gum may help) - report if these persist. Report chest pain or palpitations; mouth sores; fever or chills; swelling of extremities, face, mouth, or tongue; skin rash; numbness, tingling, or pain in muscles; respiratory difficulty; unusual cough; or other persistent adverse reactions. **Pregnancy/breast-feeding precautions:** Inform prescriber if you are or intend to become pregnant. This drug should not be used in the 2nd or 3rd trimester of pregnancy. Consult prescriber for appropriate contraceptive measures if necessary. Breast-feeding is not recommended.

Geriatric Considerations: Due to frequent decreases in glomerular filtration (also creatinine clearance) with aging, elderly patients may have exaggerated responses to ACE inhibitors. Differences in clinical response due to hepatic changes are not observed. ACE inhibitors may be preferred agents in elderly patients with congestive heart failure and diabetes mellitus. Diabetic proteinuria is reduced and insulin sensitivity is enhanced. In general, the side effect profile is favorable in the elderly and causes little or no CNS confusion; use lowest dose recommendations initially.

Pregnancy Risk Factor: C (1st trimester)/D (2nd and 3rd trimesters)

Pregnancy Issues: ACE inhibitors can cause fetal injury or death if taken during the 2nd or 3rd trimester. Discontinue ACE inhibitors as soon as pregnancy is detected.

Lactation: Enters breast milk/not recommended

Perioperative/Anesthesia/Other Concerns: ACE inhibitor therapy may elicit rapid increases in potassium and creatinine, especially when used in patients with bilateral renal artery stenosis. When ACE inhibition is introduced in patients with pre-existing diuretic therapy who are hypovolemic, the ACE inhibitor may induce acute hypotension. Concomitant NSAID therapy may attenuate blood pressure control; use of NSAIDs should be avoided or limited, with monitoring of blood pressure control. Because of the potent teratogenic effects of ACE inhibitors, these drugs should be avoided, if possible, when treating women of childbearing potential not on effective birth control measures.

ACE inhibitors decrease morbidity and mortality in patients with asymptomatic and symptomatic left ventricular dysfunction. ACE inhibitors are also indicated in patients postmyocardial infarction in whom left ventricular ejection fraction is <40%. ACE inhibitors have renal protective effects in patients with proteinuria and possibly cardioprotective effects in high-risk patients.

Administration

Storage: Store at 25°C (77°F); excursions permitted to 15°C to 30°C (59°F to 86°F). Protect from moisture by keeping bottle tightly closed.

♦ **Fosinopril Sodium** *see* Fosinopril *on page 778*

Fosphenytoin (FOS fen i toyn)

U.S. Brand Names Cerebyx®

Synonyms Fosphenytoin Sodium

Pharmacologic Category Anticonvulsant, Hydantoin

Medication Safety Issues

Sound-alike/look-alike issues:

Cerebyx® may be confused with Celebrex®, Celexa™, Cerezyme®

Use Used for the control of generalized convulsive status epilepticus and prevention and treatment of seizures occurring during neurosurgery; indicated for short-term parenteral administration when other means of phenytoin administration are unavailable, inappropriate or deemed less advantageous (the safety and effectiveness of fosphenytoin in this use has not been systematically evaluated for more than 5 days)

Mechanism of Action Diphosphate ester salt of phenytoin which acts as a water soluble prodrug of phenytoin; after administration, plasma esterases convert fosphenytoin to phosphate, formaldehyde and phenytoin as the active moiety; phenytoin works by stabilizing neuronal membranes and decreasing seizure activity by increasing efflux or decreasing influx of sodium ions across cell membranes in the motor cortex during generation of nerve impulses

Pharmacodynamics/Kinetics Also refer to Phenytoin monograph for additional information.

Protein binding: Fosphenytoin: 95% to 99% to albumin; can displace phenytoin and increase free fraction (up to 30% unbound) during the period required for conversion of fosphenytoin to phenytoin

Metabolism: Fosphenytoin is rapidly converted via hydrolysis to phenytoin; phenytoin is metabolized in the liver and forms metabolites

Bioavailability: I.M.: Fosphenytoin: 100%

Half-life elimination:

Fosphenytoin: 15 minutes

Phenytoin: Variable (mean: 12-29 hours); kinetics of phenytoin are saturable

Time to peak: Conversion to phenytoin: Following I.V. administration (maximum rate of administration): 15 minutes; following I.M. administration, peak phenytoin levels are reached in 3 hours

Excretion: Phenytoin: Urine (as inactive metabolites)

Contraindications Hypersensitivity to phenytoin, other hydantoins, or any component of the formulation; patients with sinus bradycardia, sinoatrial block, second- and third-degree AV block, or Adams-Stokes syndrome; occurrence of rash during treatment (should not be resumed if rash is exfoliative, purpuric, or bullous); treatment of absence seizures

Warnings/Precautions Doses of fosphenytoin are expressed as their phenytoin sodium equivalent (PE). Antiepileptic drugs should not be abruptly discontinued. Hypotension may occur, especially after I.V. administration at high doses and high rates of administration. Administration of phenytoin has been associated with atrial and ventricular conduction depression and ventricular fibrillation. Careful cardiac monitoring is needed when administering I.V. loading doses of fosphenytoin. Acute hepatotoxicity associated with a hypersensitivity syndrome characterized by fever, skin eruptions, and lymphadenopathy has been reported to occur within the first 2 months of treatment. Discontinue if skin rash or lymphadenopathy occurs. Use with caution in patients with hypotension, severe

(Continued)

Fosphenytoin *(Continued)*

myocardial insufficiency, diabetes mellitus, porphyria, hypoalbuminemia, hypothyroidism, fever, or hepatic or renal dysfunction.

Drug Interactions As phenytoin: **Substrate** of CYP2C8/9 (major), 2C19 (major), 3A4 (minor); **Induces** CYP2B6 (strong), 2C8/9 (strong), 2C19 (strong), 3A4 (strong)

Acetaminophen: Phenytoin may enhance the hepatotoxic potential of acetaminophen overdoses

Acetazolamide: Concurrent use with phenytoin may result in an increased risk of osteomalacia

Acyclovir: May decrease phenytoin serum levels; limited documentation; monitor

Allopurinol: May increase phenytoin serum concentrations; monitor

Antiarrhythmics: Phenytoin may increase the metabolism of antiarrhythmics, decreasing their clinical effect; includes disopyramide, propafenone, and quinidine; amiodarone also may increase phenytoin concentrations (see CYP inhibitors)

Anticonvulsants: Phenytoin may increase the metabolism of anticonvulsants; includes barbiturates, carbamazepine, ethosuximide, felbamate, lamotrigine, tiagabine, topiramate, and zonisamide; does not appear to affect gabapentin or levetiracetam; felbamate and gabapentin may increase phenytoin levels; monitor

Antineoplastics: Several chemotherapeutic agents have been associated with a decrease in serum phenytoin levels; includes cisplatin, bleomycin, carmustine, methotrexate, and vinblastine; monitor phenytoin serum levels. Limited evidence also suggest that enzyme-inducing anticonvulsant therapy may reduce the effectiveness of some chemotherapy regimens (specifically in ALL). Teniposide and methotrexate may be cleared more rapidly in these patients.

Antipsychotics: Phenytoin may enhance the metabolism (decrease the efficacy) of antipsychotics; monitor for altered response; dose adjustment may be needed; also see note on clozapine

Benzodiazepines: Phenytoin may decrease the serum concentrations of some benzodiazepines; monitor for decreased benzodiazepine effect

Beta-blockers: Metabolism of beta-blockers may be increased and clinical effect decreased; atenolol and nadolol are unlikely to interact given their renal elimination

Calcium channel blockers: Phenytoin may enhance the metabolism of calcium channel blockers, decreasing their clinical effect; calcium channel blockers (diltiazem, nifedipine) have been reported to increase phenytoin levels (case report); monitor

Capecitabine: May increase the serum concentrations of phenytoin; monitor

Chloramphenicol: Phenytoin may increase the metabolism of chloramphenicol and chloramphenicol may inhibit phenytoin metabolism; monitor for altered response

Cimetidine: May increase the serum concentrations of phenytoin; monitor.

Ciprofloxacin: Case reports indicate ciprofloxacin may increase or decrease serum phenytoin concentrations; monitor

Clozapine: May decrease phenytoin serum concentrations; monitor

CNS depressants: Sedative effects may be additive with other CNS depressants; monitor for increased effect; includes ethanol, barbiturates, sedatives, antidepressants, narcotic analgesics, and benzodiazepines

Corticosteroids: Phenytoin may increase the metabolism of corticosteroids, decreasing their clinical effect; also see dexamethasone

Cyclosporine and tacrolimus: Levels may be decreased by phenytoin; monitor

CYP2B6 substrates: Phenytoin may decrease the levels/effects of CYP2B6 substrates. Example substrates include bupropion, efavirenz, promethazine, selegiline, and sertraline.

CYP2C8/9 inducers: May decrease the levels/effects of phenytoin. Example inducers include carbamazepine, phenobarbital, rifampin, rifapentine, and secobarbital.

CYP2C8/9 inhibitors: May increase the levels/effects of phenytoin. Example inhibitors include delavirdine, fluconazole, gemfibrozil, ketoconazole, nicardipine, NSAIDs, pioglitazone, and sulfonamides.

CYP2C8/9 substrates: Phenytoin may decrease the levels/effects of CYP2C8/9 substrates. Example substrates include amiodarone, fluoxetine, glimepiride, glipizide, losartan, nateglinide, phenytoin, pioglitazone, rosiglitazone, sertraline, sulfonamides, warfarin, and zafirlukast.

CYP2C19 inducers: May decrease the levels/effects of phenytoin. Example inducers include aminoglutethimide, carbamazepine, phenytoin, and rifampin.

CYP2C19 inhibitors: May increase the levels/effects of phenytoin. Example inhibitors include delavirdine, fluconazole, fluvoxamine, gemfibrozil, isoniazid, omeprazole, and ticlopidine.

CYP2C19 substrates: Phenytoin may decrease the levels/effects of CYP2C19 substrates. Example substrates include citalopram, diazepam, methsuximide, phenytoin, propranolol, proton pump inhibitors, sertraline, and voriconazole

CYP3A4 substrates: Phenytoin may decrease the levels/effects of CYP3A4 substrates. Example substrates include benzodiazepines, calcium channel blockers, clarithromycin, cyclosporine, erythromycin, estrogens, mirtazapine, nateglinide, nefazodone, nevirapine, protease inhibitors, tacrolimus, and venlafaxine

Dexamethasone: May decrease serum phenytoin due to increased metabolism; monitor

Digoxin: Effects and/or levels of digitalis glycosides may be decreased by phenytoin

Disulfiram: May increase serum phenytoin concentrations; monitor

Dopamine: Phenytoin (I.V.) may increase the effect of dopamine (enhanced hypotension)

Doxycycline: Phenytoin may enhance the metabolism of doxycycline, decreasing its clinical effect; higher dosages may be required

Estrogens: Phenytoin may increase the metabolism of estrogens, decreasing their clinical effect; monitor

Folic acid: Replacement of folic acid has been reported to increase the metabolism of phenytoin, decreasing its serum concentrations and/or increasing seizures

HMG-CoA reductase inhibitors: Phenytoin may increase the metabolism of these agents, reducing their clinical effect; monitor

Itraconazole: Phenytoin may decrease the effect of itraconazole

Levodopa: Phenytoin may inhibit the anti-Parkinson effect of levodopa

Lithium: Concurrent use of phenytoin and lithium has resulted in lithium intoxication

Methadone: Phenytoin may enhance the metabolism of methadone resulting in methadone withdrawal

Methylphenidate: May increase serum phenytoin concentrations; monitor

Metronidazole: May increase the serum concentrations of phenytoin; monitor.

Neuromuscular-blocking agents: Duration of effect may be decreased by phenytoin

Omeprazole: May increase serum phenytoin concentrations; monitor

Oral contraceptives: Phenytoin may enhance the metabolism of oral contraceptives, decreasing their clinical effect; an alternative method of contraception should be considered

Primidone: Phenytoin enhances the conversion of primidone to phenobarbital resulting in elevated phenobarbital serum concentrations

Quetiapine: Serum concentrations may be substantially reduced by phenytoin, potentially resulting in a loss of efficacy; limited documentation; monitor

SSRIs: May increase phenytoin serum concentrations; fluoxetine and fluvoxamine are known to inhibit metabolism via CYP enzymes; sertraline and paroxetine have also been shown to increase concentrations in some patients; monitor

Theophylline: Phenytoin may increase metabolism of theophylline derivatives and decrease their clinical effect; theophylline may also increase phenytoin concentrations

Thyroid hormones (including levothyroxine): Phenytoin may alter the metabolism of thyroid hormones, reducing its effect; there is limited documentation of this interaction, but monitoring should be considered

Ticlopidine: May increase serum phenytoin concentrations and/or toxicity; monitor

Tricyclic antidepressants: Phenytoin may increase metabolism of tricyclic antidepressants and decrease their clinical effect; sedative effects may be additive; tricyclics may also increase phenytoin concentrations

Topiramate: Phenytoin may decrease serum levels of topiramate; topiramate may increase the effect of phenytoin

Trazodone: Serum levels of phenytoin may be increased; limited documentation; monitor

Trimethoprim: May increase serum phenytoin concentrations; monitor

(Continued)

Fosphenytoin *(Continued)*

Valproic acid (and sulfisoxazole): May displace phenytoin from binding sites; valproic acid may increase, decrease, or have no effect on phenytoin serum concentrations

Vigabatrin: May reduce phenytoin serum concentrations; monitor

Warfarin: Phenytoin transiently increased the hypothrombinemia response to warfarin initially; this is followed by an inhibition of the hypoprothrombinemic response

Nutritional/Herbal/Ethanol Interactions

Ethanol:

Acute use: Avoid or limit ethanol (inhibits metabolism of phenytoin); watch for sedation.

Chronic use: Avoid or limit ethanol (stimulates metabolism of phenytoin).

Lab Interactions May decrease serum concentrations of thyroxine; may produce artifactually low results in dexamethasone or metyrapone tests; may cause increase serum concentrations of glucose, alkaline phosphatase, and gamma glutamyl transpeptidase (GGT)

Adverse Reactions The more important adverse clinical events caused by the I.V. use of fosphenytoin or phenytoin are cardiovascular collapse and/or central nervous system depression. Hypotension can occur when either drug is administered rapidly by the I.V. route. Do not exceed a rate of 150 mg phenytoin equivalent/minute when administering fosphenytoin.

The adverse clinical events most commonly observed with the use of fosphenytoin in clinical trials were nystagmus, dizziness, pruritus, paresthesia, headache, somnolence, and ataxia. Paresthesia and pruritus were seen more often following fosphenytoin (versus phenytoin) administration and occurred more often with I.V. fosphenytoin than with I.M. administration. These events were dose- and rate-related (doses ≥15 mg/kg at a rate of 150 mg/minute). These sensations, generally described as itching, burning, or tingling are usually not at the infusion site. The location of the discomfort varied with the groin mentioned most frequently. The paresthesia and pruritus were transient events that occurred within several minutes of the start of infusion and generally resolved within 10 minutes after completion of infusion.

Transient pruritus, tinnitus, nystagmus, somnolence, and ataxia occurred 2-3 times more often at doses ≥15 mg/kg and rates ≥150 mg/minute.

I.V. administration (maximum dose/rate):

>10%:

Central nervous system: Nystagmus, dizziness, somnolence, ataxia

Dermatologic: Pruritus

1% to 10%:

Cardiovascular: Hypotension, vasodilation, tachycardia

Central nervous system: Stupor, incoordination, paresthesia, extrapyramidal syndrome, tremor, agitation, hypoesthesia, dysarthria, vertigo, brain edema, headache

Gastrointestinal: Nausea, tongue disorder, dry mouth, vomiting

Neuromuscular & skeletal: Pelvic pain, muscle weakness, back pain

Ocular: Diplopia, amblyopia

Otic: Tinnitus, deafness

Miscellaneous: Taste perversion

I.M. administration (substitute for oral phenytoin):

1% to 10%:

Central nervous system: Nystagmus, tremor, ataxia, headache, incoordination, somnolence, dizziness, paresthesia, reflexes decreased

Dermatologic: Pruritus

Gastrointestinal: Nausea, vomiting

Hematologic/lymphatic: Ecchymosis

Neuromuscular & skeletal: Muscle weakness

<1% (Limited to important or life-threatening): Acidosis, acute hepatic failure, acute hepatotoxicity, alkalosis, anemia, atrial flutter, bundle branch block, cardiac arrest, cardiomegaly, cerebral hemorrhage, cerebral infarct, CHF, cyanosis, dehydration, hyperglycemia, hyperkalemia, hypertension, hypochromic anemia, hypokalemia, hypophosphatemia, ketosis, leukocytosis, leukopenia, lymphadenopathy, palpitation, postural hypotension, pulmonary embolus, QT interval prolongation, sinus bradycardia, syncope, thrombocytopenia, thrombophlebitis, ventricular extrasystoles

Overdosage/Toxicology Symptoms of fosphenytoin overdose include bradycardia, asystole, cardiac arrest, hypotension, vomiting, metabolic acidosis, and lethargy. Treatment is supportive for hypotension.

Dosing

Adults:

The dose, concentration in solutions, and infusion rates for fosphenytoin are expressed as phenytoin sodium equivalents (PE); fosphenytoin should always be prescribed and dispensed in phenytoin sodium equivalents (PE)

Status epilepticus: I.V.: Loading dose: 15-20 mg PE/kg I.V. administered at 100-150 mg PE/minute

Nonemergent loading and maintenance dosing: I.V. or I.M.:

Loading dose: 10-20 mg PE/kg I.V. or I.M. (maximum I.V. rate: 150 mg PE/minute)

Initial daily maintenance dose: 4-6 mg PE/kg/day I.V. or I.M.

Substitution for oral phenytoin therapy: I.M. or I.V.: May be substituted for oral phenytoin sodium at the same total daily dose; however, Dilantin® capsules are ~90% bioavailable by the oral route; phenytoin, supplied as fosphenytoin, is 100% bioavailable by both the I.M. and I.V. routes; for this reason, plasma phenytoin concentrations may increase when I.M. or I.V. fosphenytoin is substituted for oral phenytoin sodium therapy; in clinical trials I.M. fosphenytoin was administered as a single daily dose utilizing either 1 or 2 injection sites; some patients may require more frequent dosing

Elderly: Phenytoin clearance is decreased in geriatric patients; lower doses may be required. In addition, older adults may have lower serum albumin which may increase the free fraction and, therefore, pharmacologic response. Refer to adult dosing.

Pediatrics:

Note: The dose, concentration in solutions, and infusion rates for fosphenytoin are expressed as phenytoin sodium equivalents (PE); fosphenytoin should always be prescribed and dispensed in phenytoin sodium equivalents (PE).

Infants and Children (unlabeled use): I.V.:

Loading dose: 10-20 mg PE/kg for the treatment of generalized convulsive status epilepticus.

Maintenance dosing: Phenytoin dosing guidelines in pediatric patients are used when dosing fosphenytoin using doses in PE equal to the phenytoin doses (ie, phenytoin 1 mg = fosphenytoin 1 PE); maintenance doses may be started 8-12 hours after a loading dose

Renal Impairment: Free phenytoin levels should be monitored closely in patients with renal disease or in those with hypoalbuminemia; furthermore, fosphenytoin clearance to phenytoin may be increased without a similar increase in phenytoin clearance in these patients leading to increase frequency and severity of adverse events.

Hepatic Impairment: Phenytoin clearance may be substantially reduced in cirrhosis and plasma level monitoring with dose adjustment advisable. Free phenytoin levels should be monitored closely in patients with hepatic disease or in those with hypoalbuminemia; furthermore, fosphenytoin clearance to phenytoin may be increased without a similar increase in phenytoin clearance in these patients leading to increase frequency and severity of adverse events.

Available Dosage Forms Injection, solution, as sodium: 75 mg/mL [equivalent to phenytoin sodium 50 mg/mL] (2 mL, 10 mL)

Nursing Guidelines

Assessment: Assess all other medications patient may be taking. Continuous monitoring is essential during infusion and for 30 minutes following infusion. Monitor closely for adverse or overdose reactions during and following infusion.

Monitoring Laboratory Tests: Serum phenytoin, renal function, albumin

Dietary Considerations: Provides phosphate 0.0037 mmol/mg PE fosphenytoin

Patient Education: Patients may not be in a position to evaluate their response. If conscious or alert, advise patient to report signs or symptoms of palpitations, racing or falling heartbeat, respiratory difficulty, acute faintness, or CNS disturbances (eg, somnolence, ataxia), and visual disturbances. **Pregnancy precaution:** Inform prescriber if you are pregnant.

Geriatric Considerations: No significant changes in fosphenytoin pharmacokinetics with age have been noted. Phenytoin clearance is decreased in the

(Continued)

Fosphenytoin *(Continued)*

elderly and lower doses may be needed. Elderly may have reduced hepatic clearance due to age decline in Phase I metabolism. Elderly may have low albumin which will increase free fraction and, therefore, pharmacologic response. Monitor closely in those who are hypoalbuminemic. Free fraction measurements advised, also elderly may display a higher incidence of adverse effects (cardiovascular) when using the I.V. loading regimen; therefore, recommended to decrease loading I.V. dose to 25 mg/minute.

Pregnancy Risk Factor: D

Pregnancy Issues: Fosphenytoin is the prodrug of phenytoin. Refer to Phenytoin monograph for additional information.

Lactation: Excretion in breast milk unknown/not recommended

Breast-Feeding Considerations: Fosphenytoin is the prodrug of phenytoin. It is not known if fosphenytoin is excreted in breast milk prior to conversion to phenytoin. Refer to Phenytoin monograph for additional information.

Perioperative/Anesthesia/Other Concerns: Fosphenytoin 1.5 mg is approximately equivalent to phenytoin 1 mg.

Fosphenytoin is compatible with all diluents; does not require propylene glycol or ethanol for solubility. Since there is no precipitation problem with fosphenytoin, no I.V. filter is required. Formaldehyde production is not expected to be clinically consequential (about 200 mg) if used for 1 week. As with phenytoin, fosphenytoin, when given I.V., can cause marked and dramatic hypotension and reflex tachycardia. Fosphenytoin administration is safer, in that the risk of hypotension may be somewhat less, and there are no adverse effects of extravasation. Avoid rapid I.V. infusion of fosphenytoin (infusion rates >150 mg of phenytoin equivalent per minute). Pruritus can be severe, requiring discontinuation of infusion.

Administration

I.M.: I.M. may be administered as a single daily dose using either 1 or 2 injection sites.

I.V.: Rates of infusion:

Children: 1-3 mg PE/kg/minute

Adults: Should not exceed 150 mg PE/minute

Reconstitution: Must be diluted to concentrations 1.5-25 mg PE/mL, in normal saline or D_5W, for I.V. infusion

Compatibility: Stable in D_5LR, $D_5{}^1/_2NS$, D_5W, $D_{10}W$, hetastarch 6% in NS, mannitol 20%, LR, NS

Y-site administration: Incompatible with midazolam

Storage: Refrigerate at 2°C to 8°C (36°F to 46°F). Do not store at room temperature for more than 48 hours. Do not use vials that develop particulate matter.

Related Information

Perioperative Management of Patients on Antiseizure Medication *on page 1801*

- ♦ **Fosphenytoin Sodium** *see* Fosphenytoin *on page 781*
- ♦ **Fragmin®** *see* Dalteparin *on page 483*
- ♦ **Frusemide** *see* Furosemide *on page 786*
- ♦ **FS** *see* Fibrin Sealant Kit *on page 724*
- ♦ **FU** *see* Fluorouracil *on page 745*
- ♦ **5-FU** *see* Fluorouracil *on page 745*
- ♦ **Ful-Glo®** *see* Fluorescein Sodium *on page 742*
- ♦ **Furadantin®** *see* Nitrofurantoin *on page 1232*

Furosemide (fyoor OH se mide)

U.S. Brand Names Lasix®

Synonyms Frusemide

Pharmacologic Category Diuretic, Loop

Medication Safety Issues

Sound-alike/look-alike issues:

Furosemide may be confused with torsemide

Lasix® may be confused with Esidrix®, Lanoxin®, Lidex®, Lomotil®, Luvox®, Luxiq®

Use Management of edema associated with congestive heart failure and hepatic or renal disease; alone or in combination with antihypertensives in treatment of hypertension

Mechanism of Action Inhibits reabsorption of sodium and chloride in the ascending loop of Henle and distal renal tubule, interfering with the chloride-binding cotransport system, thus causing increased excretion of water, sodium, chloride, magnesium, and calcium

Pharmacodynamics/Kinetics

Onset of action: Diuresis: Oral: 30-60 minutes; I.M.: 30 minutes; I.V.: ~5 minutes

Peak effect: Oral: 1-2 hours

Duration: Oral: 6-8 hours; I.V.: 2 hours

Absorption: Oral: 60% to 67%

Protein binding: >98%

Metabolism: Minimally hepatic

Half-life elimination: Normal renal function: 0.5-1.1 hours; End-stage renal disease: 9 hours

Excretion: Urine (Oral: 50%, I.V.: 80%) within 24 hours; feces (as unchanged drug); nonrenal clearance prolonged in renal impairment

Contraindications Hypersensitivity to furosemide, any component, or sulfonylureas; anuria; patients with hepatic coma or in states of severe electrolyte depletion until the condition improves or is corrected

Warnings/Precautions Adjust dose to avoid dehydration. In cirrhosis, avoid electrolyte and acid/base imbalances that might lead to hepatic encephalopathy. Ototoxicity is associated with rapid I.V. administration, renal impairment, excessive doses, and concurrent use of other ototoxins. Hypersensitivity reactions can rarely occur. Monitor fluid status and renal function in an attempt to prevent oliguria, azotemia, and reversible increases in BUN and creatinine. Close medical supervision of aggressive diuresis required. Monitor closely for electrolyte imbalances particularly hypokalemia. Watch for and correct electrolyte disturbances. Coadministration of antihypertensives may increase the risk of hypotension. Avoid use of medications in which the toxicity is enhanced by hypokalemia (including quinolones with QT prolongation).

Chemical similarities are present among sulfonamides, sulfonylureas, carbonic anhydrase inhibitors, thiazides, and loop diuretics (except ethacrynic acid). Use in patients with sulfonylurea allergy is specifically contraindicated in product labeling, however, a risk of cross-reaction exists in patients with allergy to any of these compounds; avoid use when previous reaction has been severe.

Drug Interactions

ACE inhibitors: Hypotensive effects and/or renal effects are potentiated by hypovolemia.

Antidiabetic agents: Glucose tolerance may be decreased.

Antihypertensive agents: Hypotensive effects may be enhanced.

Cephaloridine or cephalexin: Nephrotoxicity may occur.

Cholestyramine or colestipol may reduce bioavailability of furosemide.

Digoxin: Furosemide-induced hypokalemia may predispose to digoxin toxicity. Monitor potassium.

Fibric acid derivatives: Blood levels of furosemide and fibric acid derivatives (ie, clofibrate and fenofibrate) may be increased during concurrent dosing (particularly in hypoalbuminemia). Limited documentation; monitor for increased effect/toxicity.

Indomethacin (and other NSAIDs) may reduce natriuretic and hypotensive effects of furosemide.

Lithium: Renal clearance may be reduced. Isolated reports of lithium toxicity have occurred; monitor lithium levels.

Metformin may decrease furosemide concentrations.

Metformin blood levels may be increased by furosemide.

NSAIDs: Risk of renal impairment may increase when used in conjunction with furosemide.

Ototoxic drugs (aminoglycosides, cis-platinum): Concomitant use of furosemide may increase risk of ototoxicity, especially in patients with renal dysfunction.

Peripheral adrenergic-blocking drugs or ganglionic blockers: Effects may be increased.

Phenobarbital or phenytoin may reduce diuretic response to furosemide.

Salicylates (high-dose) with furosemide may predispose patients to salicylate toxicity due to reduced renal excretion or alter renal function.

Succinylcholine: Action may be potentiated by furosemide.

Sucralfate may limit absorption of furosemide, effects may be significantly decreased; separate oral administration by 2 hours.

Thiazides: Synergistic diuretic effects occur.

(Continued)

Furosemide *(Continued)*

Tubocurarine: The skeletal muscle-relaxing effect may be attenuated by furosemide.

Nutritional/Herbal/Ethanol Interactions

Food: Furosemide serum levels may be decreased if taken with food.

Herb/Nutraceutical: Avoid dong quai if using for hypertension (has estrogenic activity). Avoid ephedra, yohimbe, ginseng (may worsen hypertension). Limit intake of natural licorice. Avoid garlic (may have increased antihypertensive effect).

Adverse Reactions Frequency not defined.

Cardiovascular: Orthostatic hypotension, necrotizing angiitis, thrombophlebitis, chronic aortitis, acute hypotension, sudden death from cardiac arrest (with I.V. or I.M. administration)

Central nervous system: Paresthesias, vertigo, dizziness, lightheadedness, headache, blurred vision, xanthopsia, fever, restlessness

Dermatologic: Exfoliative dermatitis, erythema multiforme, purpura, photosensitivity, urticaria, rash, pruritus, cutaneous vasculitis

Endocrine & metabolic: Hyperglycemia, hyperuricemia, hypokalemia, hypochloremia, metabolic alkalosis, hypocalcemia, hypomagnesemia, gout, hyponatremia

Gastrointestinal: Nausea, vomiting, anorexia, oral and gastric irritation, cramping, diarrhea, constipation, pancreatitis, intrahepatic cholestatic jaundice, ischemia hepatitis

Genitourinary: Urinary bladder spasm, urinary frequency

Hematological: Aplastic anemia (rare), thrombocytopenia, agranulocytosis (rare), hemolytic anemia, leukopenia, anemia, purpura

Neuromuscular & skeletal: Muscle spasm, weakness

Otic: Hearing impairment (reversible or permanent with rapid I.V. or I.M. administration), tinnitus, reversible deafness (with rapid I.V. or I.M. administration)

Renal: Vasculitis, allergic interstitial nephritis, glycosuria, fall in glomerular filtration rate and renal blood flow (due to overdiuresis), transient rise in BUN

Miscellaneous: Anaphylaxis (rare), exacerbate or activate systemic lupus erythematosus

Overdosage/Toxicology Symptoms of overdose include electrolyte depletion, volume depletion, hypotension, dehydration, and circulatory collapse. Treatment is supportive.

Dosing

Adults:

Edema, CHF, or hypertension (diuresis):

Oral: 20-80 mg/dose initially increased in increments of 20-40 mg/dose at intervals of 6-8 hours; usual maintenance dose interval is twice daily or every day

Usual dosage range for hypertension (JNC 7): 20-80 mg/day in 2 divided doses

I.M., I.V.: 20-40 mg/dose, may be repeated in 1-2 hours as needed and increased by 20 mg/dose with each succeeding dose up to 1000 mg/day; usual dosing interval: 6-12 hours. **Note:** ACC/AHA 2005 guidelines for chronic congestive heart failure recommend a maximum single dose of 160-200 mg.

Continuous I.V. infusion: Initial I.V. bolus dose of 0.1 mg/kg followed by continuous I.V. infusion doses of 0.1 mg/kg/hour doubled every 2 hours to a maximum of 0.4 mg/kg/hour if urine output is <1 mL/kg/hour have been found to be effective and result in a lower daily requirement of furosemide than with intermittent dosing. Other studies have used 20-160 mg/hour continuous I.V. infusion. **Note:** ACC/AHA 2005 guidelines for chronic congestive heart failure recommend 40 mg I.V. load then 10-40 mg/hour infusion.

Refractory heart failure: Oral, I.V.: Doses up to 8 g/day have been used.

Elderly: Oral, I.M., I.V.: Initial: 20 mg/day; increase slowly to desired response.

Pediatrics:

Edema, CHF, or hypertension (diuresis): Infants and Children:

Oral: 1-2 mg/kg/dose increased in increments of 1 mg/kg/dose with each succeeding dose until a satisfactory effect is achieved to a maximum of 6 mg/kg/dose no more frequently than 6 hours

I.M., I.V.: 1 mg/kg/dose, increasing by each succeeding dose at 1 mg/kg/dose at intervals of 6-12 hours until a satisfactory response up to 6 mg/kg/dose

Renal Impairment:

Acute renal failure: Doses up to 1-3 g/day may be necessary to initiate desired response; avoid use in oliguric states.

Not removed by hemo- or peritoneal dialysis; supplemental dose is not necessary.

Hepatic Impairment: Diminished natriuretic effect with increased sensitivity to hypokalemia and volume depletion in cirrhosis. Monitor effects, particularly with high doses.

Available Dosage Forms

Injection, solution: 10 mg/mL (2 mL, 4 mL, 8 mL, 10 mL)

Solution, oral: 10 mg/mL (60 mL, 120 mL) [orange flavor]; 40 mg/5 mL (5 mL, 500 mL) [pineapple-peach flavor]

Tablet (Lasix®): 20 mg, 40 mg, 80 mg

Nursing Guidelines

Assessment: Assess for allergy to sulfonylurea before beginning therapy. See Contraindications, Warnings/Precautions, and Dosing for use cautions. Assess potential for interactions with other prescriptions, OTC medications, or herbal products patient may be taking (especially anything that may impact fluid balance or increase potential for ototoxicity or hypotension- see Drug Interactions). **I.V.:** See specific directions below. Assess results of laboratory tests, therapeutic effectiveness, and adverse response on a regular basis during therapy (eg, dehydration, electrolyte imbalance, postural hypotension - see Adverse Reactions and Overdose/Toxicology). Caution patients with diabetes about closely monitoring glucose levels (glucose tolerance may be decreased). Teach patient appropriate use, possible side effects/appropriate interventions, and adverse symptoms to report (see Patient Education). Note breast-feeding caution.

Monitoring Laboratory Tests: Serum electrolytes, renal function

Dietary Considerations: May cause a potassium loss; potassium supplement or dietary changes may be required. Administer on an empty stomach. May be administered with food or milk if GI distress occurs. Do not mix with acidic solutions.

Patient Education: Inform prescriber of all prescriptions, OTC medications, or herbal products you are taking, and any allergies you have. Do not take any new medication during therapy unless approved by prescriber. Take as directed with food or milk (to reduce GI distress) early in the day (daily), or if twice daily, take last dose in late afternoon in order to avoid sleep disturbance and achieve maximum therapeutic effect. Keep medication in original container, away from light; do not use discolored medication. Follow dietary advice of prescriber; include bananas or orange juice or other potassium-rich foods in daily diet. Do not take potassium supplements without advice of prescriber. Weigh yourself each day, at the same time, in the same clothes when beginning therapy and weekly on long-term therapy. Report unusual or unanticipated weight gain or loss. May cause dizziness, blurred vision, or drowsiness (use caution when driving or engaging in tasks that require alertness until response to drug is known); postural hypotension (use caution when rising from lying or sitting position or when climbing stairs); or sensitivity to sunlight (use sunblock or wear protective clothing and sunglasses). Report signs of edema (eg, weight gains, swollen ankles, feet or hands), trembling, numbness or fatigue, cramping or muscle weakness, palpitations, unresolved nausea or vomiting, or change in hearing. **Pregnancy/breast-feeding precautions:** Inform prescriber if you are or intend to become pregnant. Consult prescriber if breast-feeding.

Geriatric Considerations: Severe loss of sodium and/or increase in BUN can cause confusion. For any change in mental status in patients on furosemide, monitor electrolytes and renal function.

Pregnancy Risk Factor: C

Pregnancy Issues: Crosses the placenta. Increased fetal urine production, electrolyte disturbances reported. Generally, use of diuretics during pregnancy is avoided due to risk of decreased placental perfusion.

Lactation: Enters breast milk/use caution

Breast-Feeding Considerations: Crosses into breast milk; may suppress lactation. AAP has NO RECOMMENDATION.

Perioperative/Anesthesia/Other Concerns: It is important that patients be closely followed for hypokalemia, hypomagnesemia, and volume depletion because of significant diuresis. If given the morning of surgery, it may render

(Continued)

Furosemide *(Continued)*

the patient volume depleted and blood pressure may be labile during general anesthesia.

Administration

I.V.: Replace parenteral therapy with oral therapy as soon as possible. I.V. injections should be given slowly. In adults, undiluted direct I.V. injections may be administered at a rate of 40 mg over 1-2 minutes; maximum rate of administration for IVPB or continuous infusion: 4 mg/minute. In children, a maximum rate of 0.5 mg/kg/minute has been recommended.

Reconstitution: I.V. infusion solution mixed in NS or D_5W solution is stable for 24 hours at room temperature. May also be diluted for infusion 1-2 mg/mL (maximum: 10 mg/mL) over 10-15 minutes (following infusion rate parameters).

Compatibility: Stable in D_5LR, D_5NS, D_5W, $D_{10}W$, $D_{20}W$, mannitol 20%, LR, NS

Y-site administration: Incompatible with alatrofloxacin, amiodarone, amsacrine, chlorpromazine, ciprofloxacin, clarithromycin, diltiazem, droperidol, esmolol, filgrastim, fluconazole, gatifloxacin, gemcitabine, gentamicin, hydralazine, idarubicin, levofloxacin, metoclopramide, midazolam, milrinone, netilmicin, nicardipine, ondansetron, quinidine gluconate, thiopental, vecuronium, vinblastine, vincristine, vinorelbine

Compatibility in syringe: Incompatible with doxapram, doxorubicin, droperidol, metoclopramide, milrinone, vinblastine, vincristine

Compatibility when admixed: Incompatible with buprenorphine, chlorpromazine, diazepam, dobutamine, erythromycin lactobionate, isoproterenol, meperidine, metoclopramide, netilmicin, prochlorperazine edisylate, promethazine

Storage: Furosemide injection should be stored at controlled room temperature and protected from light. Exposure to light may cause discoloration. Do not use furosemide solutions if they have a yellow color. Refrigeration may result in precipitation or crystallization, however, resolubilization at room temperature or warming may be performed without affecting the drugs stability.

Gabapentin (GA ba pen tin)

U.S. Brand Names Neurontin®

Pharmacologic Category Anticonvulsant, Miscellaneous

Medication Safety Issues

Sound-alike/look-alike issues:

Neurontin® may be confused with Neoral®, Noroxin®

Use Adjunct for treatment of partial seizures with and without secondary generalized seizures in patients >12 years of age with epilepsy; adjunct for treatment of partial seizures in pediatric patients 3-12 years of age; management of postherpetic neuralgia (PHN) in adults

Unlabeled/Investigational Use Social phobia; chronic pain

Mechanism of Action Exact mechanism of action is not known, but does have properties in common with other anticonvulsants; although structurally related to GABA, it does not interact with GABA receptors, but does not bind to a voltage-gated calcium channel, inhibiting neuronal calcium influx.

Pharmacodynamics/Kinetics

Absorption: 50% to 60% from proximal small bowel by L-amino transport system

Distribution: V_d: 0.6-0.8 L/kg

Protein binding: <3%

Bioavailability: Inversely proportional to dose due to saturable absorption:

- 900 mg/day: 60%
- 1200 mg/day: 47%
- 2400 mg/day: 34%
- 3600 mg/day: 33%
- 4800 mg/day: 27%

Half-life elimination: 5-7 hours; anuria 132 hours; during dialysis 3.8 hours

Excretion: Proportional to renal function; urine (as unchanged drug)

Contraindications Hypersensitivity to gabapentin or any component of the formulation

Warnings/Precautions Avoid abrupt withdrawal, may precipitate seizures; use cautiously in patients with severe renal dysfunction; male rat studies demonstrated an association with pancreatic adenocarcinoma (clinical implication unknown). May cause CNS depression, which may impair physical or mental abilities. Patients must be cautioned about performing tasks which require mental alertness (eg, operating machinery or driving). Effects with other sedative drugs or ethanol may be potentiated. Pediatric patients (3-12 years of age) have shown increased incidence of CNS-related adverse effects, including emotional lability, hostility, thought disorder, and hyperkinesia. Safety and efficacy in children <3 years of age have not been established.

Drug Interactions CNS depressants: Sedative effects may be additive with CNS depressants; includes ethanol, barbiturates, narcotic analgesics, and other sedative agents. Monitor for increased effect.

Nutritional/Herbal/Ethanol Interactions

Ethanol: Avoid ethanol (may increase CNS depression).

Food: Does not change rate or extent of absorption.

Herb/Nutraceutical: Avoid evening primrose (seizure threshold decreased). Avoid valerian, St John's wort, kava kava, gotu kola (may increase CNS depression).

Lab Interactions False positives have been reported with the Ames N-Multistix SG® dipstick test for urine protein

Adverse Reactions As reported in patients >12 years of age, unless otherwise noted in children (3-12 years)

>10%:

Central nervous system: Somnolence (20%; children 8%), dizziness (17% to 28%; children 3%), ataxia (13%), fatigue (11%)

Miscellaneous: Viral infection (children 11%)

1% to 10%:

Cardiovascular: Peripheral edema (2% to 8%), vasodilatation (1%)

Central nervous system: Fever (children 10%), hostility (children 8%), emotional lability (children 4%), fatigue (children 3%), headache (3%), ataxia (3%), abnormal thinking (2% to 3%; children 2%), amnesia (2%), depression (2%), dysarthria (2%), nervousness (2%), abnormal coordination (1% to 2%), twitching (1%), hyperesthesia (1%)

Dermatologic: Pruritus (1%), rash (1%)

Endocrine & metabolic: Hyperglycemia (1%)

Gastrointestinal: Diarrhea (6%), nausea/vomiting (3% to 4%; children 8%), abdominal pain (3%), weight gain (adults and children 2% to 3%), dyspepsia (2%), flatulence (2%), dry throat (2%), xerostomia (2% to 5%), constipation (2% to 4%), dental abnormalities (2%), appetite stimulation (1%)

Genitourinary: Impotence (2%)

Hematologic: Leukopenia (1%), decreased WBC (1%)

Neuromuscular & skeletal: Tremor (7%), weakness (6%), hyperkinesia (children 3%), abnormal gait (2%), back pain (2%), myalgia (2%), fracture (1%)

Ocular: Nystagmus (8%), diplopia (1% to 6%), blurred vision (3% to 4%), conjunctivitis (1%)

Otic: Otitis media (1%)

Respiratory: Rhinitis (4%), bronchitis (children 3%), respiratory infection (children 3%), pharyngitis (1% to 3%), cough (2%)

Miscellaneous: Infection (5%)

Postmarketing and additional clinical reports (limited to important or life-threatening): Acute renal failure, anemia, angina, angioedema, aphasia, arrhythmias (various), aspiration pneumonia, blindness, bradycardia, bronchospasm, cerebrovascular accident, CNS tumors, coagulation defect, colitis, Cushingoid appearance, dyspnea, encephalopathy, facial paralysis, fecal incontinence, glaucoma, glycosuria, heart block, hearing loss, hematemesis, hematuria, hemiplegia, hemorrhage, hepatitis, hepatomegaly, hyper-/hypotension, hyperlipidemia, hyper-/hypothyroidism, hyper-/hypoventilation, gastroenteritis, heart failure, leukocytosis, liver function tests increased, local myoclonus, lymphadenopathy, lymphocytosis, meningismus, MI, migraine, nephrosis, nerve palsy, non-Hodgkin's lymphoma, ovarian failure, pulmonary thrombosis, pericardial rub, pulmonary embolus, pericardial effusion, pericarditis, pancreatitis, peptic ulcer, purpura, paresthesia, palpitation, peripheral vascular disorder, pneumonia, psychosis, renal stone, retinopathy, skin necrosis, status epilepticus, subdural hematoma, syncope, tachycardia, thrombocytopenia, thrombophlebitis

Overdosage/Toxicology Acute oral overdoses of up to 49 g have been reported; double vision, slurred speech, drowsiness, lethargy, and diarrhea were observed. Patients recovered with supportive care. Decontaminate using lavage/activated charcoal with cathartic. Multiple dosing of activated charcoal may be useful; hemodialysis may be useful.

Dosing

Adults:

Anticonvulsant: Oral:

Initial: 300 mg 3 times/day, if necessary the dose may be increased up to 1800 mg/day

(Continued)

Gabapentin *(Continued)*

Maintenance: 900-1800 mg/day administered in 3 divided doses; doses of up to 2400 mg/day have been tolerated in long-term clinical studies; up to 3600 mg/day has been tolerated in short-term studies

Note: If gabapentin is discontinued or if another anticonvulsant is added to therapy, it should be done slowly over a minimum of 1 week.

Chronic pain (unlabeled use): Oral: 300-1800 mg/day given in 3 divided doses has been the most common dosage range

Postoperative pain (unlabeled use): 300-1200 mg 1-2 hours before surgery

Postherpetic neuralgia: Day 1: 300 mg, Day 2: 300 mg twice daily, Day 3: 300 mg 3 times/day; dose may be titrated as needed for pain relief (range: 1800-3600 mg/day, daily doses >1800 mg do not generally show greater benefit)

Elderly: Studies in elderly patients have shown a decrease in clearance as age increases. This is most likely due to age-related decreases in renal function; dose reductions may be needed.

Pediatrics:

Anticonvulsant: Oral

Children 3-12 years: Initial: 10-15 mg/kg/day in 3 divided doses; titrate to effective dose over ~3 days; dosages of up to 50 mg/kg/day have been tolerated in clinical studies

Children 3-4 years: Effective dose: 40 mg/kg/day in 3 divided doses

Children ≥5-12 years: Effective dose: 25-35 mg/kg/day in 3 divided doses

Children >12 years: Refer to adult dosing.

Note: If gabapentin is discontinued or if another anticonvulsant is added to therapy, it should be done slowly over a minimum of 1 week

Renal Impairment: Children ≥12 years and Adults: See table.

Hemodialysis: Dialyzable

Gabapentin Dosing Adjustments in Renal Impairment

Creatinine Clearance (mL/min)	Daily Dose Range
≥60	300-1200 mg tid
>30-59	200-700 mg bid
>15-29	200-700 mg daily
15[1]	100-300 mg daily
Hemodialysis[2]	125-350 mg

[1]Cl_{cr}<15 mL/minute: Reduce daily dose in proportion to creatinine clearance.

[2]Single supplemental dose administered after each 4 hours of hemodialysis

Available Dosage Forms

Capsule (Neurontin®): 100 mg, 300 mg, 400 mg

Solution, oral (Neurontin®): 250 mg/5 mL (480 mL) [cool strawberry anise flavor]

Tablet: 100 mg, 300 mg, 400 mg

Neurontin®: 600 mg, 800 mg

Nursing Guidelines

Assessment: Assess effectiveness and interactions of other medications patient may be taking. Monitor therapeutic effectiveness, laboratory values, and adverse reactions at beginning of therapy and periodically with long-term use. Assess for CNS depression. Taper dosage slowly when discontinuing. Assess knowledge/teach patient safety and seizure precautions, appropriate use, interventions to reduce side effects, and adverse symptoms to report.

Monitoring Laboratory Tests: Monitor serum levels of concomitant anticonvulsant therapy. Routine monitoring of gabapentin levels is not mandatory.

Dietary Considerations: May be taken without regard to meals.

Patient Education: Take exactly as directed; do not increase dose or frequency. It may take 2-3 weeks to achieve desired results; may cause physical and/or psychological dependence. If prescribed once-a-day, take dose at bedtime. If taking antacids, take at least 2 hours after antacids. Do not stop medication abruptly, may lead to increased seizure activity. Avoid alcohol, caffeine, and other prescription or OTC medications not approved by prescriber. Maintain adequate hydration (2-3 L/day of fluids) unless instructed to restrict fluid intake. You may experience drowsiness, lightheadedness, impaired coordination, dizziness, or blurred vision (use caution when driving or engaging in tasks requiring alertness until response to drug is known); nausea, vomiting, or anorexia (small frequent meals, frequent mouth care, chewing gum, or sucking lozenges may help); constipation (increased exercise, fluids, fruit, or fiber may help); diarrhea (buttermilk, yogurt, or boiled milk may help); postural hypotension (use caution when climbing stairs or changing position from lying or sitting to standing); or decreased sexual function or libido (reversible). Report persistent CNS effects (nervousness, restlessness, insomnia, anxiety, excitation, headache, sedation, seizures, mania, abnormal thinking); rash or skin irritation; muscle cramping, tremors, or change in gait; chest pain or palpitations; change in urinary pattern; or worsening of condition. **Pregnancy/breast-feeding precautions:** Inform prescriber if you are or intend to become pregnant. Breast-feeding is not recommended.

Geriatric Considerations: No clinical studies to specifically evaluate this drug in the elderly have been performed; however, in premarketing studies, patients >65 years of age did not demonstrate any difference in side effect profiles from younger adults. Since gabapentin is eliminated renally, dose **must** be adjusted for creatinine clearance in the elderly patient.

Pregnancy Risk Factor: C

Pregnancy Issues: No data on crossing the placenta; there have been reports of normal pregnancy outcomes, as well as respiratory distress, pyloric stenosis, and inguinal hernia following 1st trimester exposure to gabapentin plus carbamazepine; epilepsy itself, number of medications, genetic factors, or a combination of these probably influence the teratogenicity of anticonvulsant therapy. Use during pregnancy only if the potential benefit to the mother outweighs the potential risk to the fetus.

Lactation: Enters breast milk/use caution

Breast-Feeding Considerations: Gabapentin is excreted in human breast milk. A nursed infant could be exposed to ~1 mg/kg/day of gabapentin; the effect on the child is not known. Use in breast-feeding women only if the benefits to the mother outweigh the potential risk to the infant.

Perioperative/Anesthesia/Other Concerns: CSF level is 20% of blood concentration. Gabapentin is not recommended for children <3 years of age.

Administration

Oral: Administer first dose on first day at bedtime to avoid somnolence and dizziness. Dosage must be adjusted for renal function; when given 3 times daily, the maximum time between doses should not exceed 12 hours.

Storage: Store at 25°C (77°F); excursions permitted to 15°C to 30°C (59°F to 86°F).

Gadoteridol (gad oh TER i dol)

U.S. Brand Names ProHance®

Synonyms Gd-HP-DO3A

Pharmacologic Category Radiological/Contrast Media, Nonionic

Use Contrast medium for magnetic resonance imaging (MRI)

Available Dosage Forms Injection, solution:

ProHance® [preservative free; vial]: 279.3 mg/mL (5 mL, 10 mL, 15 mL, 20 mL, 50 mL) [contains calteridol calcium 0.23 mg/mL and tromethamine 1.21 mg/mL]

ProHance® [preservative free; prefilled syringe]: 279.3 mg/mL (10 mL, 17 mL) [contains calteridol calcium 0.23 mg/mL and tromethamine 1.21 mg/mL]

ProHance® Multipack™ [preservative free; pharmacy bulk package]: 279.3 mg/mL (50 mL) [contains calteridol calcium 0.23 mg/mL and tromethamine 1.21 mg/mL]

Nursing Guidelines

Pregnancy Risk Factor: C

Lactation: Excretion in breast milk unknown/use caution

- **Gamma E-Gems® [OTC]** *see* Vitamin E *on page 1716*
- **Gamma-E Plus [OTC]** *see* Vitamin E *on page 1716*
- **Gammagard® Liquid** *see* Immune Globulin (Intravenous) *on page 899*
- **Gammagard® S/D** *see* Immune Globulin (Intravenous) *on page 899*
- **Gamma Globulin** *see* Immune Globulin (Intramuscular) *on page 898*
- **Gammar®-P I.V.** *see* Immune Globulin (Intravenous) *on page 899*
- **Gamunex®** *see* Immune Globulin (Intravenous) *on page 899*

Ganciclovir (gan SYE kloe veer)

U.S. Brand Names Cytovene®; Vitrasert®

Synonyms DHPG Sodium; GCV Sodium; Nordeoxyguanosine

Pharmacologic Category Antiviral Agent

Medication Safety Issues

Sound-alike/look-alike issues:

Cytovene® may be confused with Cytosar®, Cytosar-U®

Use

Parenteral: Treatment of CMV retinitis in immunocompromised individuals, including patients with acquired immunodeficiency syndrome; prophylaxis of CMV infection in transplant patients

Oral: Alternative to the I.V. formulation for maintenance treatment of CMV retinitis in immunocompromised patients, including patients with AIDS, in whom retinitis is stable following appropriate induction therapy and for whom the risk of more rapid progression is balanced by the benefit associated with avoiding daily I.V. infusions.

Implant: Treatment of CMV retinitis

Unlabeled/Investigational Use May be given in combination with foscarnet in patients who relapse after monotherapy with either drug

Mechanism of Action Ganciclovir is phosphorylated to a substrate which competitively inhibits the binding of deoxyguanosine triphosphate to DNA polymerase resulting in inhibition of viral DNA synthesis

Pharmacodynamics/Kinetics

Distribution: V_d: 15.26 L/1.73 m^2; widely to all tissues including CSF and ocular tissue

Protein binding: 1% to 2%

Bioavailability: Oral: Fasting: 5%; Following food: 6% to 9%; Following fatty meal: 28% to 31%

Half-life elimination: 1.7-5.8 hours; prolonged with renal impairment; End-stage renal disease: 5-28 hours

Excretion: Urine (80% to 99% as unchanged drug)

Contraindications Hypersensitivity to ganciclovir, acyclovir, or any component of the formulation; absolute neutrophil count <500/mm^3; platelet count <25,000/mm^3

Warnings/Precautions Hazardous agent - use appropriate precautions for handling and disposal. Dosage adjustment or interruption of ganciclovir therapy may be necessary in patients with neutropenia and/or thrombocytopenia and patients with impaired renal function. Use with extreme caution in children since long-term safety has not been determined and due to ganciclovir's potential for long-term carcinogenic and adverse reproductive effects; ganciclovir may adversely affect spermatogenesis and fertility; due to its mutagenic potential, contraceptive precautions for female and male patients need to be followed during and for at least 90 days after therapy with the drug; take care to administer only into veins with good blood flow.

Drug Interactions

Decreased effect: Didanosine: A decrease in steady-state ganciclovir AUC may occur

Increased toxicity:

- Immunosuppressive agents may increase cytotoxicity of ganciclovir
- Imipenem/cilastatin may increase seizure potential
- Zidovudine: Oral ganciclovir increased the AUC of zidovudine, although zidovudine decreases steady state levels of ganciclovir. Since both drugs have the potential to cause neutropenia and anemia, some patients may not tolerate concomitant therapy with these drugs at full dosage.
- Probenecid: The renal clearance of ganciclovir is decreased in the presence of probenecid
- Didanosine levels are increased with concurrent ganciclovir
- Other nephrotoxic drugs (eg, amphotericin and cyclosporine) may have additive nephrotoxicity with ganciclovir

Adverse Reactions

>10%:

- Central nervous system: Fever (38% to 48%)
- Dermatologic: Rash (15% oral, 10% I.V.)
- Gastrointestinal: Abdominal pain (17% to 19%), diarrhea (40%), nausea (25%), anorexia (15%), vomiting (13%)
- Hematologic: Anemia (20% to 25%), leukopenia (30% to 40%)

1% to 10%:

- Central nervous system: Confusion, neuropathy (8% to 9%), headache (4%)

Dermatologic: Pruritus (5%)
Hematologic: Thrombocytopenia (6%), neutropenia with ANC <500/mm^3 (5% oral, 14% I.V.)
Neuromuscular & skeletal: Paresthesia (6% to 10%), weakness (6%)
Ocular: Retinal detachment (8% oral, 11% I.V.; relationship to ganciclovir not established)
Miscellaneous: Sepsis (4% oral, 15% I.V.)
<1% (Limited to important or life-threatening): Alopecia, arrhythmia, ataxia, bronchospasm, coma, dyspnea, encephalopathy, eosinophilia, exfoliative dermatitis, extrapyramidal symptoms, hemorrhage, nervousness, pancytopenia, psychosis, renal failure, seizure, SIADH, Stevens-Johnson syndrome, torsade de pointes, urticaria, visual loss

Overdosage/Toxicology Symptoms of overdose include neutropenia, vomiting, hypersalivation, bloody diarrhea, cytopenia, and testicular atrophy. Treatment is supportive. Hemodialysis removes 50% of the drug. Hydration may be of some benefit.

Dosing

Adults & Elderly: Dosing is based on total body weight.

CMV retinitis:

I.V. (slow infusion):

Induction therapy: 5 mg/kg/dose every 12 hours for 14-21 days followed by maintenance therapy

Maintenance therapy: 5 mg/kg/day as a single daily dose for 7 days/week or 6 mg/kg/day for 5 days/week

Oral: 1000 mg 3 times/day with food **or** 500 mg 6 times/day with food

Ocular implant: Intravitreally: One implant for 5- to 8-month period; following depletion of ganciclovir, as evidenced by progression of retinitis, implant may be removed and replaced

Prevention of CMV disease in patients with advanced HIV infection and normal renal function: Oral: 1000 mg 3 times/day with food

Prevention of CMV disease in transplant patients: Same initial and maintenance dose as CMV retinitis except duration of initial course is 7-14 days, duration of maintenance therapy is dependent on clinical condition and degree of immunosuppression

Pediatrics: CMV retinitis: Children >3 months: Refer to adult dosing.

Renal Impairment:

I.V. (Induction):

Cl_{cr} 50-69 mL/minute: Administer 2.5 mg/kg/dose every 12 hours.
Cl_{cr} 25-49 mL/minute: Administer 2.5 mg/kg/dose every 24 hours.
Cl_{cr} 10-24 mL/minute: Administer 1.25 mg/kg/dose every 24 hours.
Cl_{cr} <10 mL/minute: Administer 1.25 mg/kg/dose 3 times/week following hemodialysis.

I.V. (Maintenance):

Cl_{cr} 50-69 mL/minute: Administer 2.5 mg/kg/dose every 24 hours.
Cl_{cr} 25-49 mL/minute: Administer 1.25 mg/kg/dose every 24 hours.
Cl_{cr} 10-24 mL/minute: Administer 0.625 mg/kg/dose every 24 hours
Cl_{cr} <10 mL/minute: Administer 0.625 mg/kg/dose 3 times/week following hemodialysis.

Oral:

Cl_{cr} 50-69 mL/minute: Administer 1500 mg/day or 500 mg 3 times/day.
Cl_{cr} 25-49 mL/minute: Administer 1000 mg/day or 500 mg twice daily.
Cl_{cr} 10-24 mL/minute: Administer 500 mg/day.
Cl_{cr} <10 mL/minute: Administer 500 mg 3 times/week following hemodialysis.

Hemodialysis effects: Dialyzable (50%) following hemodialysis; administer dose postdialysis. During peritoneal dialysis, dose as for Cl_{cr} <10 mL/minute. During continuous arteriovenous or venovenous hemofiltration, administer 2.5 mg/kg/dose every 24 hours.

Available Dosage Forms

Capsule: 250 mg, 500 mg
Cytovene®: 250 mg, 500 mg [DSC]
Implant, intravitreal (Vitrasert®): 4.5 mg [released gradually over 5-8 months]
Injection, powder for reconstitution, as sodium (Cytovene®): 500 mg

Nursing Guidelines

Assessment: See Contraindications, Warnings/Precautions, Drug Interactions, and Dosing for use cautions. Assess potential for interactions with other prescriptions, OTC medications, or herbal products patient may be taking (see Drug Interactions). **I.V.:** See Administration, Reconstitution, and Compatibility.

(Continued)

Ganciclovir *(Continued)*

Assess results of laboratory tests (see Monitoring Lab Tests), therapeutic effectiveness, and adverse response (eg, paresthesia, neutropenia, anemia, nephrotoxicity, retinal detachment - see Adverse Reactions and Overdose/ Toxicology). Teach possible side effects/appropriate interventions and adverse symptoms to report (see Patient Education). **Pregnancy risk factor C** - ganciclovir may adversely affect spermatogenesis and fertility. Due to its mutagenic potential, contraceptive precautions for both female and male patients need to be followed during and for at least 90 days after therapy with the drug. Instruct patients in appropriate barrier contraceptive measures. Breast-feeding is contraindicated.

Monitoring Laboratory Tests: CBC with differential and platelet count, serum creatinine before beginning therapy and on a regular basis thereafter; liver function tests

Dietary Considerations: Sodium content of 500 mg vial: 46 mg

Patient Education: Inform prescriber of all prescriptions, OTC medications, or herbal products you are taking, and any allergies you have. Do not take any new medication during therapy unless approved by prescriber. Ganciclovir is not a cure for CMV retinitis. For oral administration, take as directed and maintain adequate hydration (2-3 L/day of fluids) unless instructed to restrict fluid intake. You will need frequent blood tests and regular ophthalmic exams while taking this drug. You may experience increased susceptibility to infection (avoid crowds and exposure to infection and do not have any vaccinations without consulting prescriber). You may experience confusion or headache (use cautions when driving or engaging in potentially hazardous tasks until response to drug is known); nausea, vomiting, or anorexia (small, frequent meals, frequent mouth care, chewing gum, or sucking lozenges may help); diarrhea (buttermilk, boiled milk, or yogurt may help); or photosensitivity (use sunscreen, wear protective clothing and eyewear, and avoid direct sunlight). Report rash, infection (fever, chills, unusual bleeding or bruising, infection, or unhealed sores or white plaques in mouth); abdominal pain; tingling, weakness, or pain in extremities; any vision changes; or pain, redness, swelling at injection site. **Pregnancy/breast-feeding precautions**: Inform prescriber if you are pregnant. Males and females should use appropriate barrier contraceptive measures during and for 60-90 days following end of therapy. Consult prescriber for appropriate barrier contraceptive measures. Do not breast-feed.

Geriatric Considerations: Adjust dose based upon renal function.

Pregnancy Risk Factor: C

Lactation: Excretion in breast milk unknown/contraindicated

Breast-Feeding Considerations: The CDC recommends **not** to breast-feed if diagnosed with HIV to avoid postnatal transmission of the virus.

Administration

Oral: Should be administered with food.

I.V.: Should not be administered by I.M., SubQ, or rapid IVP. Administer by slow I.V. infusion over at least 1 hour. Too rapid infusion can cause increased toxicity and excessive plasma levels.

Reconstitution: Reconstitute powder with unpreserved sterile water not bacteriostatic water because parabens may cause precipitation. Dilute in 250-1000 mL D_5W or NS to a concentration ≤10 mg/mL for infusion. Reconstituted solution is stable for 12 hours at room temperature, however, conflicting data indicates that reconstituted solution is stable for 60 days under refrigeration (4°C). Stability of parenteral admixture at room temperature (25°C) and at refrigeration temperature (4°C) is 5 days.

Compatibility: Stable in D_5W, LR, NS; **incompatible** with paraben preserved bacteriostatic water for injection (may cause precipitation)

Y-site administration: Incompatible with aldesleukin, amifostine, amsacrine, aztreonam, cefepime, cytarabine, doxorubicin, fludarabine, foscarnet, gemcitabine, ondansetron, piperacillin/tazobactam, sargramostim, vinorelbine

Storage: Intact vials should be stored at room temperature and protected from temperatures >40°C.

- **Ganidin NR** *see* Guaifenesin *on page 834*
- **Gani-Tuss® NR** *see* Guaifenesin and Codeine *on page 835*
- **Garamycin** *see* Gentamicin *on page 807*
- **Gas-X® [OTC]** *see* Simethicone *on page 1533*
- **Gas-X® Extra Strength [OTC]** *see* Simethicone *on page 1533*

- ♦ Gas-X® Maximum Strength [OTC] *see* Simethicone *on page 1533*
- ♦ GasAid [OTC] *see* Simethicone *on page 1533*
- ♦ Gas Ban™ [OTC] *see* Calcium Carbonate and Simethicone *on page 294*
- ♦ Gastrocrom® *see* Cromolyn *on page 453*
- ♦ Gastrografin® *see* Diatrizoate Meglumine and Diatrizoate Sodium *on page 514*

Gatifloxacin (gat i FLOKS a sin)

U.S. Brand Names Tequin®; Zymar™

Pharmacologic Category Antibiotic, Ophthalmic; Antibiotic, Quinolone

Use

Oral, I.V.: Treatment of the following infections when caused by susceptible bacteria: Acute bacterial exacerbation of chronic bronchitis; acute sinusitis; community-acquired pneumonia including pneumonia caused by multi-drug-resistant *S. pneumoniae* (MDRSP); uncomplicated skin and skin structure infection; uncomplicated urinary tract infections (cystitis); complicated urinary tract infections; pyelonephritis; uncomplicated urethral and cervical gonorrhea; acute, uncomplicated rectal infections in women

Ophthalmic: Bacterial conjunctivitis

Mechanism of Action Gatifloxacin is a DNA gyrase inhibitor, and also inhibits topoisomerase IV. DNA gyrase (topoisomerase II) is an essential bacterial enzyme that maintains the superhelical structure of DNA. DNA gyrase is required for DNA replication and transcription, DNA repair, recombination, and transposition; inhibition is bactericidal.

Pharmacodynamics/Kinetics

Absorption: Oral: Well absorbed; Ophthalmic: Not measurable

Distribution: V_d: 1.5-2.0 L/kg; concentrates in alveolar macrophages and lung parenchyma

Protein binding: 20%

Metabolism: Only 1%; no interaction with CYP

Bioavailability: 96%

Half-life elimination: 7.1-13.9 hours; ESRD/CAPD: 30-40 hours

Time to peak: Oral: 1 hour

Excretion: Urine (70% as unchanged drug, <1% as metabolites); feces (5%)

Contraindications Hypersensitivity to gatifloxacin, other quinolone antibiotics, or any component of the formulation

Warnings/Precautions Use with caution in patients with significant bradycardia or acute myocardial ischemia. May prolong QT interval (concentration related). Use caution in patients with known prolongation of QT interval, uncorrected hypokalemia, or concurrent administration of other medications known to prolong the QT interval (including Class Ia and Class III antiarrhythmics, cisapride, erythromycin, antipsychotics, and tricyclic antidepressants). May cause increased CNS stimulation, increased intracranial pressure, convulsions, or psychosis. Use with caution in individuals at risk of seizures (CNS disorders or concurrent therapy with medications which may lower seizure threshold). Discontinue in patients who experience significant CNS adverse effects (dizziness, hallucinations, suicidal ideation or actions). Use caution in renal dysfunction (dosage adjustment required) and in severe hepatic insufficiency (no data available). Serious disruptions in glucose regulation (including hyperglycemia and severe hypoglycemia) may occur, usually (but not always) in patients with diabetes. Hypoglycemia may be more prevalent in the initial 3 days of therapy while a greater risk of hyperglycemia may be present after the initial 3 days (particularly days 4-10). Monitor closely and discontinue if hyper- or hypoglycemia occur. Tendon inflammation and/or rupture has been reported with this and other quinolone antibiotics. Risk may be increased with concurrent corticosteroids, particularly in the elderly. Discontinue at first signs or symptoms of tendon or pain.

Severe hypersensitivity reactions, including anaphylaxis, have occurred with quinolone therapy. If an allergic reaction occurs (itching, urticaria, dyspnea, facial edema, loss of consciousness, tingling, cardiovascular collapse) discontinue drug immediately. Prolonged use may result in superinfection; pseudomembranous colitis may occur and should be considered in all patients who present with diarrhea. Quinolones may exacerbate myasthenia gravis, use with caution (rare, potentially life-threatening weakness of respiratory muscles may occur). May cause peripheral neuropathy (rare); discontinue if symptoms of sensory or sensorimotor neuropathy occur. Do not inject ophthalmic solution subconjunctivally or introduce directly into the anterior chamber of the eye.

(Continued)

Gatifloxacin *(Continued)*

Safety and efficacy for ophthalmic use have not been established in children <1 year of age. Safety and efficacy for systemic use have not been established in patients <18 years of age.

Drug Interactions

Corticosteroids: Concurrent use may increase the risk of tendon rupture, particularly in elderly patients (overall incidence rare).

Hypoglycemic agents: Gatifloxacin may alter glucose control in patients receiving hypoglycemic agents with or without insulin. Cases of severe disturbances (including symptomatic hypoglycemia) have been reported, typically within 1-3 days of gatifloxacin initiation.

Metal cations (aluminum, calcium, iron, magnesium, and zinc) bind quinolones in the gastrointestinal tract and inhibit absorption. Concurrent administration of most antacids (not calcium carbonate), oral electrolyte supplements, quinapril, sucralfate, some didanosine formulations (chewable/buffered tablets and pediatric powder for oral suspension), and other highly-buffered oral drugs, should be avoided. Gatifloxacin should be administered 4 hours before these agents.

Probenecid: May decrease renal secretion of quinolones.

QT_c-prolonging agents: Effects may be additive with gatifloxacin. Use caution with Class Ia and Class III antiarrhythmics, erythromycin, cisapride, antipsychotics, and cyclic antidepressants.

Warfarin: The hypoprothrombinemic effect of warfarin may be enhanced by some quinolone antibiotics; monitor INR.

Nutritional/Herbal/Ethanol Interactions Herb/Nutraceutical: Avoid dong quai, St John's wort (may also cause photosensitization).

Adverse Reactions

Systemic therapy:

3% to 10%:

Central nervous system: Headache (3%), dizziness (3%)

Gastrointestinal: Nausea (8%), diarrhea (4%)

Genitourinary: Vaginitis (6%)

Local: Injection site reactions (5%)

0.1% to 3%: Abdominal pain, abnormal dreams, abnormal vision, agitation, alkaline phosphatase increased, allergic reaction, anorexia, anxiety, arthralgia, back pain, chest pain, chills, confusion, constipation, diaphoresis, dry skin, dyspepsia, dyspnea, dysuria, facial edema, fever, flatulence, gastritis, glossitis, hematuria, hyperglycemia, hypertension, insomnia, leg cramps, mouth ulceration, nervousness, oral candidiasis, palpitation, paresthesia, peripheral edema, pharyngitis, pruritus, rash, serum amylase increased, serum bilirubin increased, serum transaminases increased, somnolence, stomatitis, taste perversion, thirst, tinnitus, tremor, weakness, vasodilation, vertigo, vomiting

<0.1% (Limited to important or life-threatening): Abnormal thinking, acute renal failure, anaphylactic reaction, angioneurotic edema, arthritis, asthenia, ataxia, bone pain, bradycardia, breast pain, bronchospasm, cheilitis, colitis, cyanosis, depersonalization, depression, diabetes mellitus, dysphagia, ear pain, ecchymosis, edema, epistaxis, ethanol intolerance, euphoria, eye pain, gastrointestinal hemorrhage, gingivitis, halitosis, hallucination, hematemesis, hematuria, hepatitis, hostility, hyperesthesia, hypertonia, hyperventilation, hypoglycemia, increased INR, increased prothrombin time, lymphadenopathy, maculopapular rash, metrorrhagia, migraine, myalgia, myasthenia, neck pain, nonketotic hyperglycemia, pancreatitis, panic attacks, paranoia, parosmia, peripheral neuropathy, photophobia, pseudomembranous colitis, psychosis, ptosis, rectal hemorrhage, seizure, severe hyper-/hypoglycemia, Stevens-Johnson syndrome, stress, syncope, tachycardia, taste disturbance, tendon rupture, rupture, thrombocytopenia, torsade de pointes, tongue edema, vesiculobullous rash

Ophthalmic therapy:

5% to 10%: Ocular: Conjunctival irritation, keratitis, lacrimation increased, papillary conjunctivitis

1% to 4%:

Central nervous system: Headache

Gastrointestinal: Taste disturbance

Ocular: Chemosis, conjunctival hemorrhage, discharge, dry eye, edema, irritation, pain, visual acuity decreased

Overdosage/Toxicology Potential symptoms of overdose may include CNS excitation, seizures, QT prolongation, and arrhythmias (including torsade de pointes). Patients should be monitored by continuous ECG in the event of an overdose. Management is supportive and symptomatic. Not removed by dialysis.

Dosing

Adults & Elderly:

Acute sinusitis: Oral, I.V.: 400 mg every 24 hours for 10 days

Bacterial conjunctivitis: Ophthalmic:

Days 1 and 2: Instill 1 drop into affected eye(s) every 2 hours while awake (maximum: 8 times/day)

Days 3-7: Instill 1 drop into affected eye(s) up to 4 times/day while awake

Community-acquired pneumonia: Oral, I.V.: 400 mg every 24 hours for 7-14 days

COPD (acute bacterial exacerbation): Oral, I.V.: 400 mg every 24 hours for 5 days

Uncomplicated skin/skin structure infections: Oral, I.V.: 400 mg every 24 hours for 7-10 days

Urinary tract infections (uncomplicated or cystitis): Oral, I.V.: 400 mg single dose or 200 mg every 24 hours for 3 days

Urinary tract infections (complicated): Oral, I.V.: 400 mg every 24 hours for 7-10 days

Pyelonephritis: Oral, I.V.: 400 mg every 24 hours for 7-10 days

Gonorrhea (uncomplicated urethral infection in men, cervical or rectal gonorrhea in women): Oral, I.V.: 400 mg single dose

Pediatrics: Bacterial conjunctivitis: Children ≥1 year: Ophthalmic: Refer to adult dosing.

Renal Impairment: Creatinine clearance <40 mL/minute (or patients on hemodialysis/CAPD) should receive an initial dose of 400 mg, followed by a subsequent dose of 200 mg every 24 hours. Patients receiving single-dose or 3-day therapy for appropriate indications do not require dosage adjustment. Administer after hemodialysis.

Hepatic Impairment: No dosage adjustment is required in mild-moderate hepatic disease. No data are available in severe hepatic impairment (Child-Pugh Class C).

Available Dosage Forms

Injection, infusion [premixed in D_5W] (Tequin®): 200 mg (100 mL); 400 mg (200 mL)

Injection, solution [preservative free] (Tequin®): 10 mg/mL (40 mL)

Solution, ophthalmic (Zymar™): 0.3% (2.5 mL, 5 mL) [contains benzalkonium chloride]

Tablet (Tequin®): 200 mg, 400 mg

Tequin® Teq-paq™ [unit-dose pack]: 400 mg (5s)

Nursing Guidelines

Assessment: Assess allergy history before initiating therapy. See Contraindications, Warnings/Precautions, and Dosing for use cautions. Assess potential for interactions with other prescriptions, OTC medications, or herbal products patient may be taking (see Drug Interactions). **I.V.:** See Administration, Reconstitution, and Compatibility. Patient must be monitored closely during and after infusion for immediate allergic reaction. Assess results of laboratory tests (see below), therapeutic effectiveness, and adverse effects (eg, changes in CNS, especially in elderly patients - see Adverse Reactions and Overdose/Toxicology) regularly during therapy. Teach patient appropriate use (oral/ophthalmic), possible side effects/appropriate interventions, and adverse symptoms to report (see Patient Education). Breast-feeding is not recommended.

Monitoring Laboratory Tests: WBC

Dietary Considerations: May take tablets with or without food, milk, or calcium supplements. Gatifloxacin should be taken 4 hours before supplements (including multivitamins) containing iron, zinc, or magnesium.

Patient Education: Inform prescriber of all prescriptions, OTC medications, or herbal products you are taking, and any allergies you have. Do not take any new medication during therapy without consulting prescriber. **Pregnancy/breast-feeding precautions:** Inform prescriber if you are or intend to be pregnant. Do not breast-feed while taking this medication.

I.V.: Report any redness, pain, itching, burning, or signs of irritation at infusion site; swelling of mouth, lips, or tongue, back pain, tendon pain; dizziness, abnormal thinking, or anxiety

Ophthalmic: Tilt head back and instill drops in affected eye at often as directed for length of time prescribed. Do not allow touch dropper to any surface,

(Continued)

Gatifloxacin *(Continued)*

including the eyes or hands. Apply light pressure to the inside corner of the eye (near the nose) after each drop. Do not wear contact lenses if being treated for a bacterial eye infection. May cause some temporary stinging, burning, itching, redness or tearing; eyelid swelling or itching, or a bad taste in you mouth after instillation. Report persistent pain, burning, swelling, or visual disturbances.

Oral: Take exactly as directed with or without food. Avoid alcohol. Take 4 hours before antacids or mineral supplements (iron, magnesium, or zinc). Do not miss a dose (take a missed dose as soon as possible unless it is almost time for next dose). Take entire prescription even if feeling better. Maintain adequate hydration (2-3 L/day of fluids, unless instructed to restrict fluids). May cause nausea, vomiting, taste perversion (small, frequent meals, good mouth care, chewing gum, or sucking hard candy may help); headache, dizziness, insomnia, anxiety (use caution when driving or engaging in tasks requiring alertness until response is known). Report immediately any CNS changes (dizziness, insomnia, hallucinations, suicidal ideation or actions); rash or itching; respiratory difficulty or swallowing; tendon pain; swelling of mouth, lips, tongue, or throat; chest pain or tightness; or back pain. Report changes in voiding pattern, vaginal itching, burning, or discharge; vision changes or hearing; abnormal bruising or bleeding or blood in urine; or other adverse reactions.

Pregnancy Risk Factor: C

Pregnancy Issues: Reports of arthropathy (observed in immature animals and reported rarely in humans) have limited the use of fluoroquinolones during pregnancy. Gatifloxacin has been show to be fetotoxic in animal studies. There are no adequate and well-controlled studies in pregnant women. Based on limited data, quinolones are not expected to be a major human teratogen. Although quinolone antibiotics should not be used as first-line agents during pregnancy, when considering treatment for life-threatening infection and/or prolonged duration of therapy, the potential risk to the fetus must be balanced against the severity of the potential illness.

Lactation: Excretion in breast milk unknown/use caution

Breast-Feeding Considerations: Other quinolones are known to be excreted in breast milk. The manufacturer recommends using caution if gatifloxacin is administered while nursing.

Perioperative/Anesthesia/Other Concerns: Gatifloxacin causes a dose-dependent QT prolongation. Coadministration of gatifloxacin with other drugs that also prolong the QT interval or induce bradycardia (eg, beta-blockers, amiodarone) should be done cautiously. Careful consideration should be given in the use of gatifloxacin in patients with cardiovascular disease, particularly in those with conduction abnormalities.

Administration

Oral: May be administered with or without food, milk, or calcium supplements. Gatifloxacin should be taken 4 hours before supplements (including multivitamins) containing iron, zinc, or magnesium.

I.V.: For I.V. infusion only. Concentrated injection (10 mg/mL) must be diluted to 2 mg/mL prior to administration. No further dilution is required for premixed 100 mL and 200 mL solutions. Infuse over 60 minutes. Avoid rapid or bolus infusions.

Reconstitution:

Solution for injection: Single-use vials must be diluted to a concentration of 2 mg/mL prior to administration; may be diluted with D_5W, NS, D_5NS, D_5LR, 5% sodium bicarbonate, or Plasma-Lyte® 56 and D_5W. Do not dilute with SWFI (a hypertonic solution results).

Compatibility: Stable in D_5LR, D_5W, D_5NS, 5% dextrose or 0.45% sodium chloride containing up to 20 mEq/L potassium chloride, M/6 sodium lactate, NS, Plasma-Lyte® 56/5% dextrose injection, 5% sodium bicarbonate injection; **incompatible** with SWFI (results in a hypertonic solution)

Y-site administration: Incompatible with amphotericin B, amphotericin B cholesteryl sulfate complex, cefoperazone, cefoxitin, diazepam, furosemide, heparin, phenytoin, piperacillin, piperacillin/tazobactam, potassium phosphates, vancomycin

Storage:

Ophthalmic solution: Store between 15°C to 25°C (59°F to 77°F). Do not freeze.

Solution for injection: Store at 25°C (77°F). Do not freeze. Following dilution, stable for 14 days when stored between 20°C to 25°C or 2° to 8°C. Diluted solutions (except those prepared in 5% sodium bicarbonate) may also be frozen for up to 6 months when stored at -25°C to -10°C (-13°F to 14°F). Solutions may then be thawed at room temperature and should be used within 14 days (store between 20°C to 25°C or 2°C to 8°C). Do not refreeze.

Tablet: Store at 25°C (77°F).

Related Information

Prevention of Wound Infection and Sepsis in Surgical Patients *on page 1830*

- Gaviscon® Extra Strength [OTC] *see* Aluminum Hydroxide and Magnesium Carbonate *on page 121*
- Gaviscon® Liquid [OTC] *see* Aluminum Hydroxide and Magnesium Carbonate *on page 121*
- G-CSF *see* Filgrastim *on page 726*
- G-CSF (PEG Conjugate) *see* Pegfilgrastim *on page 1320*
- GCV Sodium *see* Ganciclovir *on page 794*
- Gd-HP-DO3A *see* Gadoteridol *on page 793*

Gelatin (Absorbable) (JEL a tin, ab SORB a ble)

U.S. Brand Names Gelfilm®; Gelfoam®

Synonyms Absorbable Gelatin Sponge

Pharmacologic Category Hemostatic Agent

Use Adjunct to provide hemostasis in surgery; open prostatic surgery

Contraindications Should not be used in closure of skin incisions since they may interfere with the healing of skin edges

Warnings/Precautions Do not sterilize by heat; do not use in the presence of infection

Drug Interactions No data reported

Adverse Reactions 1% to 10%: Local: Infection and abscess formation

Dosing

Adults & Elderly: Hemostasis: Local: Apply packs or sponges dry or saturated with sodium chloride. When applied dry, hold in place with moderate pressure. When applied wet, squeeze to remove air bubbles. The powder is applied as a paste prepared by adding approximately 4 mL of sterile saline solution to the powder.

Pediatrics: Refer to adult dosing.

Available Dosage Forms

Film, ophthalmic (Gelfilm®): 25 mm x 50 mm (6s)
Film, topical (Gelfilm®): 100 mm x 125 mm (1s)
Powder, topical (Gelfoam®): 1 g
Sponge, dental (Gelfoam®): Size 4 (12s)
Sponge, topical (Gelfoam®):
- Size 50 (4s)
- Size 100 (6s)
- Size 200 (6s)
- Size 2 cm (1s)
- Size 6 cm (6s)
- Size 12-7 mm (12s)

Nursing Guidelines

Pregnancy Risk Factor: No data reported

- Gelfilm® *see* Gelatin (Absorbable) *on page 801*
- Gelfoam® *see* Gelatin (Absorbable) *on page 801*
- Gelusil® [OTC] *see* Aluminum Hydroxide, Magnesium Hydroxide, and Simethicone *on page 122*

Gemcitabine (jem SITE a been)

U.S. Brand Names Gemzar®

Synonyms Gemcitabine Hydrochloride

Pharmacologic Category Antineoplastic Agent, Antimetabolite (Pyrimidine Antagonist)

Medication Safety Issues

Sound-alike/look-alike issues:

Gemzar® may be confused with Zinecard®

Use

Adenocarcinoma of the pancreas: First-line therapy in locally-advanced (nonresectable stage II or stage III) or metastatic (stage IV) adenocarcinoma of the pancreas

Breast cancer: First-line therapy in metastatic breast cancer

(Continued)

Gemcitabine *(Continued)*

Nonsmall-cell lung cancer: First-line therapy in locally-advanced (stage IIIA or IIIB) or metastatic (stage IV) nonsmall-cell lung cancer

Unlabeled/Investigational Use Bladder cancer, ovarian cancer

Mechanism of Action A pyrimidine antimetabolite that inhibits DNA synthesis by inhibition of DNA polymerase and ribonucleotide reductase, specific for the S-phase of the cycle.

Pharmacodynamics/Kinetics

Distribution: Infusions <70 minutes: 50 L/m^2; Long infusion times: 370 L/m^2

Protein binding: Low

Metabolism: Hepatic, metabolites: di- and triphosphates (active); uridine derivative (inactive)

Half-life elimination:

Gemcitabine: Infusion time ≤1 hour: 32-94 minutes; infusion time 3-4 hours: 4-10.5 hours

Metabolite (gemcitabine triphosphate), terminal phase: 1.7-19.4 hours

Time to peak, plasma: 30 minutes

Excretion: Urine (99%, 92% to 98% as intact drug or inactive uridine metabolite); feces (<1%)

Contraindications Hypersensitivity to gemcitabine or any component of the formulation; pregnancy

Warnings/Precautions Hazardous agent — use appropriate precautions for handling and disposal. Prolongation of the infusion time >60 minutes and more frequent than weekly dosing have been shown to increase toxicity. Gemcitabine can suppress bone marrow function manifested by leukopenia, thrombocytopenia and anemia, and myelosuppression is usually the dose-limiting toxicity. Gemcitabine may cause fever in the absence of clinical infection. Pulmonary toxicity has occurred; discontinue if severe. Use with caution in patients with pre-existing renal or hepatic impairment. Safety and efficacy have not been established with radiation therapy or in pediatric patients.

Drug Interactions No confirmed interactions have been reported. No specific drug interaction studies have been conducted.

Nutritional/Herbal/Ethanol Interactions Ethanol: Avoid ethanol (due to GI irritation).

Adverse Reactions Percentages reported with single-agent therapy for pancreatic cancer and other malignancies.

>10%:

Central nervous system: Pain (42% to 48%; grades 3 and 4: <1% to 9%), fever (38% to 41%; grades 3 and 4: ≤2%), somnolence (11%; grades 3 and 4: <1%). Fever was reported to occur in the absence of infection in pancreatic cancer treatment.

Dermatologic: Rash (28% to 30%; grades 3 and 4: <1%), alopecia (15% to 16%; grades 3 and 4: <1%). Rash in pancreatic cancer treatment was typically a macular or finely-granular maculopapular pruritic eruption of mild-to-moderate severity involving the trunk and extremities.

Gastrointestinal: Nausea and vomiting (69% to 71%; grades 3 and 4: 1% to 13%), constipation (23% to 31%; grades 3 and 4: <1% to 3%), diarrhea (19% to 30%; grades 3 and 4: ≤3%), stomatitis (10% to 11%; grades 3 and 4: <1%)

Hematologic: Anemia (73% to 68%; grades 3 and 4: 1% to 8%), leukopenia (62% to 64%; grades 3 and 4: <1% to 9%), neutropenia (61% to 63%; grades 3 and 4: 6% to 19%), thrombocytopenia (24% to 36%; grades 3 and 4: <1% to 7%), hemorrhage (4% to 17%; grades 3 or 4: <1%). Myelosuppression may be the dose-limiting toxicity with pancreatic cancer

Hepatic: Transaminases increased (68% to 78%; grades 3 and 4: 1% to 12%), alkaline phosphatase increased (55% to 77%; grades 3 and 4: 2% to 16%), bilirubin increased (13% to 26%; grades 3 or 4: <1% to 6%). Serious hepatotoxicity was reported rarely in pancreatic cancer treatment.

Renal: Proteinuria (32% to 45%; grades 3 and 4: <1%), hematuria (23% to 35%; grades 3 and 4: <1%), BUN increased (15% to 16%; grades 3 and 4: 0%)

Respiratory: Dyspnea (10% to 23%; grades 3 and 4: <1% to 3%)

Miscellaneous: Infection (10% to 16%; grades 3 or 4: <1% to 2%)

1% to 10%:

Local: Injection site reactions (4%)

Neuromuscular & skeletal: Paresthesias (10%)

Renal: Creatinine increased (6% to 8%)

Respiratory: Bronchospasm (<2%)

<1% (Limited to important or life-threatening): Anaphylactoid reaction, hemolytic uremic syndrome. Reported with single-agent use or with combination therapy, all reported rarely: Arrhythmias, cellulitis, CHF, gangrene, liver failure, MI, parenchymal toxicity, vascular toxicity

Overdosage/Toxicology Symptoms of overdose include myelosuppression, paresthesia, and severe rash. The principle toxicities were seen when a single dose as high as 5700 mg/m^2 was administered by I.V. infusion over 30 minutes every 2 weeks. Monitor blood counts and administer supportive therapy as needed.

Dosing

Adults & Elderly: Refer to individual protocols. **Note**: Prolongation of the infusion time >60 minutes and administration more frequently than once weekly have been shown to increase toxicity. I.V.:

Pancreatic cancer: Initial: 1000 mg/m^2 over 30 minutes once weekly for up to 7 weeks followed by 1 week rest; subsequent cycles once weekly for 3 consecutive weeks out of every 4 weeks.

Dose adjustment: Patients who complete an entire cycle of therapy may have the dose in subsequent cycles increased by 25% as long as the absolute granulocyte count (AGC) nadir is >1500 x 10^6/L, platelet nadir is >100,000 x 10^6/L, and nonhematologic toxicity is less than WHO Grade 1. If the increased dose is tolerated (with the same parameters) the dose in subsequent cycles may again be increased by 20%.

Nonsmall cell lung cancer:

28-day cycle: 1000 mg/m^2 over 30 minutes on days 1, 8, 15; repeat every 28 days

or

21-day cycle: 1250 mg/m^2 over 30 minutes on days 1, 8; repeat every 21 days

Breast cancer: 1250 mg/m^2 over 30 minutes on days 1 and 8 of each 21-day cycle

Bladder cancer (unlabeled use): 1000 mg/m^2 once weekly for 3 weeks; repeat cycle every 4 weeks

Ovarian cancer (unlabeled use): 1000 mg/m^2 once weekly for 3 weeks; repeat cycle every 4 weeks

Renal Impairment: Use with caution; has not been studied in patients with significant renal dysfunction.

Hepatic Impairment: Use with caution; gemcitabine has not been studied in patients with significant hepatic dysfunction.

Available Dosage Forms Injection, powder for reconstitution, as hydrochloride: 200 mg, 1 g

Nursing Guidelines

Assessment: See Contraindications, Warnings/Precautions, and Dosing for use cautions. See specific Administration, Reconstitution, and Storage directions. Assess results of laboratory tests (see below), therapeutic effectiveness, and adverse response (see Adverse Reactions and Overdose/Toxicology) prior to each treatment and on a regular basis throughout therapy. Teach patient possible side effects/appropriate interventions and adverse symptoms to report (see Patient Education). **Pregnancy risk factor D** - determine that patient is not pregnant before beginning treatment. Instruct patients of childbearing age on appropriate barrier contraceptive measures. Breast-feeding is contraindicated.

Monitoring Laboratory Tests: Monitor CBC, including differential and platelet count, prior to each dose. Renal and hepatic function should be performed prior to initiation of therapy and periodically thereafter.

Patient Education: Inform prescriber of all prescriptions, OTC medications, or herbal products you are taking, and any allergies you have. Do not take any new medication during therapy unless approved by prescriber. This drug can only be administered by infusion. During therapy, do not use alcohol. Maintain adequate hydration (2-3 L/day of fluids) unless instructed to restrict fluid intake, and nutrition (small, frequent meals may help). You will be more susceptible to infection (avoid crowds and exposure to infection and do not have any vaccinations without consulting prescriber). You may experience fatigue, lethargy, somnolence (use caution when driving or engaging in potentially hazardous tasks until response to drug is known); nausea or vomiting (small, frequent meals, frequent mouth care, sucking lozenges, or chewing gum may help); loss of hair (reversible); mouth sores (frequent mouth care and use of a soft toothbrush or cotton swabs may help); or diarrhea (buttermilk, boiled milk, or yogurt

(Continued)

Gemcitabine *(Continued)*

may help reduce diarrhea). This drug may cause sterility. Report extreme fatigue; severe GI upset or diarrhea; bleeding or bruising; fever, chills, sore throat; vaginal discharge; signs of fluid retention (swelling extremities, respiratory difficulty, unusual weight gain); yellowing of skin or eyes; change in color of urine or stool; or muscle or skeletal pain or weakness. **Pregnancy/ breast-feeding precautions**: Inform prescriber if you are pregnant. Do not get pregnant while taking this medication. Consult prescriber for appropriate barrier contraceptives measures. This drug may cause severe fetal birth defects. Do not breast-feed.

Geriatric Considerations: Clearance is affected by age. There is no evidence; however, that unusual dose adjustment is necessary in patients older than 65 years of age. In general, adverse reaction rates were similar to patients older and younger than 65 years. Grade 3/4 thrombocytopenia was more common in the elderly.

Pregnancy Risk Factor: D

Pregnancy Issues: It is embryotoxic causing fetal malformations (cleft palate, incomplete ossification, fused pulmonary artery, absence of gallbladder) in animals. There are no studies in pregnant women. If patient becomes pregnant she should be informed of risks.

Lactation: Excretion in breast milk unknown/contraindicated

Administration

I.V.: Administer over 30 minutes. **Note**: Prolongation of the infusion time >60 minutes has been shown to increase toxicity.

Reconstitution: Reconstitute the 200 mg vial with preservative free 0.9% NaCl 5 mL or the 1000 mg vial with preservative free 0.9% NaCl 25 mL. Resulting solution is ~38 mg/mL, but is variable. Dilute with 50-500 mL 0.9% sodium chloride injection or D_5W to concentrations as low as 0.1 mg/mL.

Compatibility: Stable in D_5W, NS

Y-site administration: Incompatible with acyclovir, amphotericin B, cefoperazone, cefotaxime, furosemide, ganciclovir, imipenem/cilastatin, irinotecan, methotrexate, methylprednisolone sodium succinate, mitomycin, piperacillin, piperacillin/tazobactam, prochlorperazine edisylate

Storage: Store intact vials at room temperature (20°C to 25°C/68°F to 77°F). Reconstituted vials and infusion solutions diluted in 0.9% sodium chloride are stable up to 24 hours. Do not refrigerate.

♦ **Gemcitabine Hydrochloride** *see* Gemcitabine *on page 801*

Gemfibrozil (jem FI broe zil)

U.S. Brand Names Lopid®

Synonyms CI-719

Pharmacologic Category Antilipemic Agent, Fibric Acid

Medication Safety Issues

Sound-alike/look-alike issues:

Lopid® may be confused with Levbid®, Lodine®, Lorabid®, Slo-bid™

Use Treatment of hypertriglyceridemia in types IV and V hyperlipidemia for patients who are at greater risk for pancreatitis and who have not responded to dietary intervention

Mechanism of Action The exact mechanism of action of gemfibrozil is unknown, however, several theories exist regarding the VLDL effect; it can inhibit lipolysis and decrease subsequent hepatic fatty acid uptake as well as inhibit hepatic secretion of VLDL; together these actions decrease serum VLDL levels; increases HDL-cholesterol; the mechanism behind HDL elevation is currently unknown

Pharmacodynamics/Kinetics

Onset of action: May require several days

Absorption: Well absorbed

Protein binding: 99%

Metabolism: Hepatic via oxidation to two inactive metabolites; undergoes enterohepatic recycling

Half-life elimination: 1.4 hours

Time to peak, serum: 1-2 hours

Excretion: Urine (70% primarily as conjugated drug); feces (6%)

Contraindications Hypersensitivity to gemfibrozil or any component of the formulation; significant hepatic or renal dysfunction; primary biliary cirrhosis; pre-existing gallbladder disease

Warnings/Precautions Possible increased risk of malignancy and cholelithiasis. No evidence of cardiovascular mortality benefit. Anemia and leukopenia have been reported. Elevations in serum transaminases can be seen. Discontinue if lipid response not seen. Be careful in patient selection; this is not a first- or second-line choice. Other agents may be more suitable. Adjustments in warfarin therapy may be required with concurrent use. Use caution when combining gemfibrozil with HMG-CoA reductase inhibitors (may lead to myopathy, rhabdomyolysis). Renal function deterioration has been seen when used in patients with a serum creatinine >2.0 mg/dL. Safety and efficacy in pediatric patients have not been established.

Drug Interactions **Substrate** of CYP3A4 (minor); **Inhibits** CYP1A2 (moderate), 2C8/9 (strong), 2C19 (strong)

Bexarotene's serum concentration is significantly increased; avoid concurrent use.

Chlorpropamide: May increase risk of hypoglycemia.

Cyclosporine's blood levels may be reduced; monitor cyclosporine levels and renal function.

CYP1A2 substrates: Gemfibrozil may increase the levels/effects of CYP1A2 substrates. Example substrates include aminophylline, fluvoxamine, mexiletine, mirtazapine, ropinirole, theophylline, and trifluoperazine.

CYP2C8/9 substrates: Gemfibrozil may increase the levels/effects of CYP2C8/9 substrates. Example substrates include amiodarone, fluoxetine, glimepiride, glipizide, nateglinide, phenytoin, pioglitazone, rosiglitazone, sertraline, and warfarin.

CYP2C19 substrates: Gemfibrozil may increase the levels/effects of CYP2C19 substrates. Example substrates include citalopram, diazepam, methsuximide, phenytoin, propranolol, and sertraline.

Furosemide: Increased blood levels of both in hypoalbuminemia.

Glyburide (and possibly other sulfonylureas): The hypoglycemic effects may be increased.

HMG-CoA reductase inhibitors (atorvastatin, fluvastatin, lovastatin, pravastatin, simvastatin) may increase the risk of myopathy and rhabdomyolysis. The manufacturer warns against the concurrent use of lovastatin (if unavoidable, limit lovastatin to <20 mg/day). Combination therapy with statins has been used in some patients with resistant hyperlipidemias (with great caution).

Repaglinide: Gemfibrozil may increase the serum concentration of repaglinide (prolonged, severe hypoglycemia has been reported). The addition of itraconazole may augment the effects of gemfibrozil on repaglinide. Consider alternative therapy.

Rifampin: Decreased gemfibrozil blood levels.

Warfarin: Hypoprothrombinemic response increased; monitor INRs closely when gemfibrozil is initiated or discontinued.

Nutritional/Herbal/Ethanol Interactions Ethanol: Avoid ethanol to decrease triglycerides.

Adverse Reactions

>10%: Gastrointestinal: Dyspepsia (20%)

1% to 10%:

Central nervous system: Fatigue (4%), vertigo (2%), headache (1%)

Dermatologic: Eczema (2%), rash (2%)

Gastrointestinal: Abdominal pain (10%), diarrhea (7%), nausea/vomiting (3%), constipation (1%)

<1% (Limited to important or life-threatening): Alopecia, anaphylaxis, angioedema, bone marrow hypoplasia, cataracts, cholelithiasis, cholecystitis, depression, dermatomyositis/polymyositis, drug-induced lupus-like syndrome, eosinophilia, exfoliative dermatitis, hypokalemia, impotence, intracranial hemorrhage, jaundice, laryngeal edema, leukopenia, myasthenia, myopathy, nephrotoxicity, pancreatitis, paresthesia, peripheral neuritis, photosensitivity, positive ANA, rash, Raynaud's phenomenon, retinal edema, rhabdomyolysis, seizure, syncope, thrombocytopenia, urticaria, vasculitis

Overdosage/Toxicology Symptoms of overdose include abdominal pain, diarrhea, nausea, and vomiting. Treatment is supportive.

Dosing

Adults & Elderly: Hyperlipidemia/hypertriglyceridemia: Oral: 1200 mg/day in 2 divided doses, 30 minutes before breakfast and dinner

Renal Impairment: Hemodialysis effects: Not removed by hemodialysis; supplemental dose is not necessary.

Available Dosage Forms Tablet [film coated]: 600 mg

(Continued)

Gemfibrozil *(Continued)*

Nursing Guidelines

Assessment: See Contraindications, Warnings/Precautions, and Dosing for use cautions. Assess potential for interactions with other prescriptions, OTC medications, or herbal products patient may be taking (see Drug Interactions). Assess results of laboratory tests (see Monitoring Lab Tests), therapeutic effectiveness, and patient response (see Adverse Reactions and Overdose/Toxicology). Teach possible proper use, side effects/appropriate interventions, and adverse symptoms to report (see Patient Education). Breast-feeding is contraindicated.

Monitoring Laboratory Tests: Serum cholesterol, LFTs

Dietary Considerations: Before initiation of therapy, patients should be placed on a standard cholesterol-lowering diet for 3-6 months and the diet should be continued during drug therapy.

Patient Education: Inform prescriber of all prescriptions, OTC medications, or herbal products you are taking, and any allergies you have. Do not take any new medication during therapy unless approved by prescriber. Should be taken 30 minutes before meals. Take with milk or meals if GI upset occurs. Avoid alcohol. Follow dietary recommendations of prescriber. You will need check-ups and blood work to assess effectiveness of therapy. You may experience loss of appetite and flatulence (small, frequent meals may help); or diarrhea (buttermilk, boiled milk, or yogurt may help). Report severe stomach pain, nausea, vomiting; headache; persistent diarrhea; or vision changes. **Pregnancy/breast-feeding precautions**: Inform prescriber if you are or intend to become pregnant. Do not breast-feed.

Geriatric Considerations: Gemfibrozil is the drug of choice for the treatment of hypertriglyceridemia and hypoalphaproteinemia in the elderly; it is usually well tolerated; myositis may be more common in patients with poor renal function.

Pregnancy Risk Factor: C

Lactation: Excretion in breast milk unknown/contraindicated

Perioperative/Anesthesia/Other Concerns: Gemfibrozil increases HDL, decreases total cholesterol and triglycerides. A recent study (HIT), showed that gemfibrozil therapy resulted in a significant reduction in the risk of major cardiovascular events in patients with low HDL-cholesterol. These findings suggest that the rate of coronary events is reduced by raising HDL-cholesterol levels and lowering triglyceride levels. The treatment of low HDL in the general population, is not established.

- **Gemzar®** *see* Gemcitabine *on page 801*
- **Genac® [OTC]** *see* Triprolidine and Pseudoephedrine *on page 1670*
- **Genahist® [OTC]** *see* DiphenhydrAMINE *on page 546*
- **Genapap® [OTC]** *see* Acetaminophen *on page 65*
- **Genapap® Children [OTC]** *see* Acetaminophen *on page 65*
- **Genapap® Extra Strength [OTC]** *see* Acetaminophen *on page 65*
- **Genapap® Infant [OTC]** *see* Acetaminophen *on page 65*
- **Genaphed® [OTC]** *see* Pseudoephedrine *on page 1436*
- **Genasal [OTC]** *see* Oxymetazoline *on page 1290*
- **Genasoft® [OTC]** *see* Docusate *on page 560*
- **Genasoft® Plus [DSC] [OTC]** *see* Docusate and Casanthranol *on page 561*
- **Genasyme® [OTC]** *see* Simethicone *on page 1533*
- **Genebs® [OTC]** *see* Acetaminophen *on page 65*
- **Genebs® Extra Strength [OTC]** *see* Acetaminophen *on page 65*
- **Genfiber® [OTC]** *see* Psyllium *on page 1438*
- **Gengraf®** *see* CycloSPORINE *on page 465*
- **Genoptic® [DSC]** *see* Gentamicin *on page 807*
- **Genotropin®** *see* Somatropin *on page 1555*
- **Genotropin Miniquick®** *see* Somatropin *on page 1555*
- **Genpril® [OTC]** *see* Ibuprofen *on page 889*
- **Gentak®** *see* Gentamicin *on page 807*

Gentamicin (jen ta MYE sin)

U.S. Brand Names Genoptic® [DSC]; Gentak®

Synonyms Garamycin; Gentamicin Sulfate

Pharmacologic Category Antibiotic, Aminoglycoside; Antibiotic, Ophthalmic; Antibiotic, Topical

Medication Safety Issues

Sound-alike/look-alike issues:

Gentamicin may be confused with kanamycin

Garamycin® may be confused with kanamycin, Terramycin®

Use Treatment of susceptible bacterial infections, normally gram-negative organisms including *Pseudomonas*, *Proteus*, *Serratia*, and gram-positive *Staphylococcus*; treatment of bone infections, respiratory tract infections, skin and soft tissue infections, as well as abdominal and urinary tract infections, endocarditis, and septicemia; used topically to treat superficial infections of the skin or ophthalmic infections caused by susceptible bacteria; prevention of bacterial endocarditis prior to dental or surgical procedures

Mechanism of Action Interferes with bacterial protein synthesis by binding to 30S and 50S ribosomal subunits resulting in a defective bacterial cell membrane

Pharmacodynamics/Kinetics

Absorption: Oral: None

Distribution: Crosses placenta

V_d: Increased by edema, ascites, fluid overload; decreased with dehydration

Neonates: 0.4-0.6 L/kg

Children: 0.3-0.35 L/kg

Adults: 0.2-0.3 L/kg

Relative diffusion from blood into CSF: Minimal even with inflammation

CSF:blood level ratio: Normal meninges: Nil; Inflamed meninges: 10% to 30%

Protein binding: <30%

Half-life elimination:

Infants: <1 week old: 3-11.5 hours; 1 week to 6 months old: 3-3.5 hours

Adults: 1.5-3 hours; End-stage renal disease: 36-70 hours

Time to peak, serum: I.M.: 30-90 minutes; I.V.: 30 minutes after 30-minute infusion

Excretion: Urine (as unchanged drug)

Clearance: Directly related to renal function

Contraindications Hypersensitivity to gentamicin or other aminoglycosides

Warnings/Precautions Not intended for long-term therapy due to toxic hazards associated with extended administration; pre-existing renal insufficiency, vestibular or cochlear impairment, myasthenia gravis, hypocalcemia, conditions which depress neuromuscular transmission

Parenteral aminoglycosides have been associated with significant nephrotoxicity or ototoxicity; the ototoxicity may be directly proportional to the amount of drug given and the duration of treatment; tinnitus or vertigo are indications of vestibular injury and impending hearing loss; renal damage is usually reversible

Drug Interactions

Increased toxicity:

Aminoglycosides may potentiate the effects of neuromuscular-blocking agents.

Penicillins, cephalosporins, amphotericin B, loop diuretics may increase nephrotoxic potential

Decreased effect: Gentamicin's efficacy reduced when given concurrently with carbenicillin, ticarcillin, or piperacillin to patients with severe renal impairment (inactivation). Separate administration.

Lab Interactions

Some penicillin derivatives may accelerate the degradation of aminoglycosides *in vitro*, leading to a potential underestimation of aminoglycoside serum concentration.

Adverse Reactions

>10%:

Central nervous system: Neurotoxicity (vertigo, ataxia)

Neuromuscular & skeletal: Gait instability

Otic: Ototoxicity (auditory), ototoxicity (vestibular)

Renal: Nephrotoxicity, decreased creatinine clearance

1% to 10%:

Cardiovascular: Edema

Dermatologic: Skin itching, reddening of skin, rash

(Continued)

Gentamicin *(Continued)*

<1% (Limited to important or life-threatening): Agranulocytosis, allergic reaction, dyspnea, granulocytopenia, photosensitivity, pseudomotor cerebri, thrombocytopenia

Overdosage/Toxicology Symptoms of overdose include ototoxicity, nephrotoxicity, and neuromuscular toxicity. Serum level monitoring is recommended. The treatment of choice, following a single acute overdose, appears to be maintenance of urine output of at least 3 mL/kg/hour during the acute treatment phase. Dialysis is of questionable value in enhancing aminoglycoside elimination.

Dosing

Adults & Elderly: Individualization is **critical** because of the low therapeutic index.

Use of ideal body weight (IBW) for determining the mg/kg/dose appears to be more accurate than dosing on the basis of total body weight (TBW). In morbid obesity, dosage requirement may best be estimated using a dosing weight of IBW + 0.4 (TBW - IBW).

Initial and periodic plasma drug levels (eg, peak and trough with conventional dosing) should be determined, particularly in critically-ill patients with serious infections or in disease states known to significantly alter aminoglycoside pharmacokinetics (eg, cystic fibrosis, burns, or major surgery).

Usual dosage ranges:

I.M., I.V.:

Conventional: 1-2.5 mg/kg/dose every 8-12 hours; to ensure adequate peak concentrations early in therapy, higher initial dosage may be considered in selected patients when extracellular water is increased (edema, septic shock, postsurgical, or trauma)

Once daily: 4-7 mg/kg/dose once daily; some clinicians recommend this approach for all patients with normal renal function; this dose is at least as efficacious with similar, if not less, toxicity than conventional dosing

Intrathecal: 4-8 mg/day

Ophthalmic:

Ointment: Instill 1/2" (1.25 cm) 2-3 times/day to every 3-4 hours

Solution: Instill 1-2 drops every 2-4 hours, up to 2 drops every hour for severe infections

Topical: Apply 3-4 times/day to affected area

Indication-specific dosing: I.M., I.V.:

Brucellosis: 240 mg (I.M.) daily or 5 mg/kg (I.V.) daily for 7 days; either regimen recommended in combination with doxycycline

Cholangitis: 4-6 mg/kg once daily with ampicillin

Diverticulitis (complicated): 1.5-2 mg/kg every 8 hours (with ampicillin and metronidazole)

Endocarditis prophylaxis: Dental, oral, upper respiratory procedures, GI/GU procedures: 1.5 mg/kg with ampicillin (50 mg/kg) 30 minutes prior to procedure

Endocarditis or synergy (for Gram-positive infections): 1 mg/kg every 8 hours (with ampicillin)

Meningitis, Listeria species: 5-7 mg/kg/day (with penicillin) for 1 week

Meningitis, neonatal:

0-7 days of age: <2000 g: 2.5 mg/kg every 18-24 hours; >2000 g: 2.5 mg/kg every 12 hours

8-28 days of age: <2000 g: 2.5 mg/kg every 8-12 hours; >2000 g: 2.5 mg/kg every 8 hours

Pelvic inflammatory disease: Loading dose: 2 mg/kg, then 1.5 mg/kg every 8 hours

Alternate therapy: 4.5 mg/kg once daily

Plague (Yersinia pestis): Treatment: 5 mg/kg/day, followed by postexposure prophylaxis with doxycycline

Pneumonia, hospital- or ventilator-associated: 7 mg/kg/day (with antipseudomonal beta-lactam or carbapenem)

Tularemia: 5 mg/kg/day divided every 8 hours for 1-2 weeks

Urinary tract infection: 1.5 mg/kg/dose every 8 hours

Pediatrics: Individualization is **critical** because of the low therapeutic index.

Use of ideal body weight (IBW) for determining the mg/kg/dose appears to be more accurate than dosing on the basis of total body weight (TBW). In morbid obesity, dosage requirement may best be estimated using a dosing weight of IBW + 0.4 (TBW - IBW).

Initial and periodic plasma drug levels (eg, peak and trough with conventional dosing) should be determined, particularly in critically-ill patients with serious infections or in disease states known to significantly alter aminoglycoside pharmacokinetics (eg, cystic fibrosis, burns, or major surgery).

Usual dosage ranges: I.M., I.V.:

Infants and Children <5 years: 2.5 mg/kg/dose every 8 hours*

Children ≥5 years: 2-2.5 mg/kg/dose every 8 hours*

***Note:** Higher individual doses and/or more frequent intervals (eg, every 6 hours) may be required in selected clinical situations (cystic fibrosis) or serum levels document the need

CNS infections: Intrathecal: See adult dosing.

Ophthalmic, Dermatologic infections: See adult dosing.

Indication-specific dosing: See adult dosing.

Renal Impairment:

Conventional dosing:

Cl_{cr} ≥60 mL/minute: Administer every 8 hours

Cl_{cr} 40-60 mL/minute: Administer every 12 hours

Cl_{cr} 20-40 mL/minute: Administer every 24 hours

Cl_{cr} <20 mL/minute: Loading dose, then monitor levels

High-dose therapy: Interval may be extended (eg, every 48 hours) in patients with moderate renal impairment (Cl_{cr} 30-59 mL/minute) and/or adjusted based on serum level determinations.

Hemodialysis: Dialyzable; removal by hemodialysis: 30% removal of aminoglycosides occurs during 4 hours of HD; administer dose after dialysis and follow levels

Removal by continuous ambulatory peritoneal dialysis (CAPD):

Administration via CAPD fluid:

Gram-negative infection: 4-8 mg/L (4-8 mcg/mL) of CAPD fluid

Gram-positive infection (eg, synergy): 3-4 mg/L (3-4 mcg/mL) of CAPD fluid

Administration via I.V., I.M. route during CAPD: Dose as for Cl_{cr} <10 mL/minute and follow levels

Removal via continuous arteriovenous or venovenous hemofiltration: Dose as for Cl_{cr} 10-40 mL/minute and follow levels

Hepatic Impairment: Monitor plasma concentrations.

Available Dosage Forms [DSC] = Discontinued product

Cream, topical, as sulfate: 0.1% (15 g, 30 g)

Infusion, as sulfate [premixed in NS]: 40 mg (50 mL); 60 mg (50 mL, 100 mL); 70 mg (50 mL); 80 mg (50 mL, 100 mL); 90 mg (100 mL); 100 mg (50 mL, 100 mL); 120 mg (100 mL)

Injection, solution, as sulfate [ADD-Vantage® vial]: 10 mg/mL (6 mL, 8 mL, 10 mL)

Injection, solution, as sulfate: 40 mg/mL (2 mL, 20 mL) [may contain sodium metabisulfite]

Injection, solution, pediatric, as sulfate: 10 mg/mL (2 mL) [may contain sodium metabisulfite]

Injection, solution, pediatric, as sulfate [preservative free]: 10 mg/mL (2 mL)

Ointment, ophthalmic, as sulfate (Gentak®): 0.3% [3 mg/g] (3.5 g)

Ointment, topical, as sulfate: 0.1% (15 g, 30 g)

Solution, ophthalmic, as sulfate: 0.3% (5 mL, 15 mL) [contains benzalkonium chloride]

Genoptic®: 0.3% (1 mL) [contains benzalkonium chloride] [DSC]

Gentak®: 0.3% (5 mL; 15 mL [DSC]) [contains benzalkonium chloride]

Nursing Guidelines

Assessment: Assess effectiveness and interactions of other medications patient may be taking. Assess kidney function and hearing before, during, and following therapy. **Note:** This medication has a very low TI. Monitor for decreased renal function, ototoxicity, and neurotoxicity. Perform hearing tests prior to initiating treatment and periodically during therapy (>2 weeks) if at high risk. Monitor therapeutic effectiveness, laboratory values and adverse reactions at beginning of therapy and periodically throughout therapy. Assess knowledge/teach patient appropriate use, interventions to reduce side effects, and adverse symptoms to report.

Monitoring Laboratory Tests: Urinalysis, BUN, serum creatinine, plasma gentamicin levels (as appropriate to dosing method). Peak levels are drawn 30 minutes after the end of a 30-minute infusion or 1 hour after initiation of infusion or I.M. injection. The trough is drawn just before the next dose. Levels are typically obtained after the third dose in conventional dosing. Perform culture and sensitivity studies prior to initiating therapy to determine the causative

(Continued)

Gentamicin *(Continued)*

organism and its susceptibility to gentamicin. Some penicillin derivatives may accelerate the degradation of aminoglycosides.

Dietary Considerations: Calcium, magnesium, potassium: Renal wasting may cause hypocalcemia, hypomagnesemia, and/or hypokalemia.

Patient Education: Take exactly as directed and when prescribed. Drink adequate amounts of water (2-3 L/day) unless instructed to restrict fluid intake. You may experience headaches, ringing in ears, dizziness, blurred vision (use caution when driving or engaging in tasks requiring alertness until response to drug is known); GI upset, loss of appetite (small frequent meals and frequent mouth care may help); or photosensitivity (use sunscreen wear protective clothing and eyewear, and avoid direct sunlight). Report severe headache, changes in hearing acuity, ringing in ears, change in balance, changes in urine pattern, respiratory difficulty, rash, fever, unhealed sores, sores in mouth, vaginal drainage, muscle or bone pain, change in gait, or worsening of condition. **Pregnancy/breast-feeding precautions:** Inform prescriber if you are or intend to become pregnant. Consult prescriber if breast-feeding.

Ophthalmic: Wash hands before instilling. Sit or lie down to instill. Open eye, look at ceiling, and instill prescribed amount of solution; for ointment, pull lower lid down gently, instill thin ribbon of ointment inside lid. Close eye and roll eye in all directions, and apply gentle pressure to inner corner of eye. Do not let tip of applicator touch eye; do not contaminate tip of applicator (may cause eye infection, eye damage, or vision loss). Temporary stinging or blurred vision may occur. Report persistent pain, burning, vision changes, swelling, itching, or worsening of condition.

Topical: Apply thin film of ointment to affected area as often as recommended. May apply porous dressing. Report persistent burning, swelling, itching, worsening of condition, or lack of response to therapy.

Geriatric Considerations: Aminoglycosides are important therapeutic interventions for susceptible organisms and as empiric therapy in seriously ill patients. Their use is not without risk of toxicity, however. Additional studies comparing high-dose, once-daily aminoglycosides to traditional dosing regimens in the elderly are needed before once-daily aminoglycoside dosing can be routinely adopted to this patient population.

Pregnancy Risk Factor: C

Lactation: Enters breast milk (small amounts)/use caution (AAP rates "compatible")

Breast-Feeding Considerations: No data reported; however, gentamicin is not absorbed orally and other aminoglycosides may be taken while breast-feeding.

Perioperative/Anesthesia/Other Concerns: Gentamicin is the only aminoglycoside that is commercially available in a preservative-free solution for injection.

Administration

I.M.: Administer by deep I.M. route if possible. Slower absorption and lower peak concentrations, probably due to poor circulation in the atrophic muscle, may occur following I.M. injection; in paralyzed patients, suggest I.V. route.

I.V.: Some penicillins (eg, carbenicillin, ticarcillin and piperacillin) have been shown to inactivate aminglycosides *in vitro*. This has been observed to a greater extent with tobramycin and gentamicin, while amikacin has shown greater stability against inactivation. Concurrent use of these agents may pose a risk of reduced antibacterial efficacy *in vivo*, particularly in the setting of profound renal impairment. However, definitive clinical evidence is lacking. If combination penicillin/aminoglycoside therapy is desired in a patient with renal dysfunction, separation of doses (if feasible), and routine monitoring of aminoglycoside levels, CBC, and clinical response should be considered.

Reconstitution: I.V. infusion solutions mixed in NS or D_5W solution are stable for 24 hours at room temperature and refrigeration.

Premixed bag: Manufacturer expiration date; remove from overwrap stability: 30 days

Compatibility: Stable in dextran 40, D_5W, $D_{10}W$, mannitol 20%, LR, NS; **incompatible** with fat emulsion 10%

Y-site administration: Incompatible with allopurinol, amphotericin B cholesteryl sulfate complex, cefamandole, furosemide, heparin, hetastarch, idarubicin, indomethacin, iodipamide meglumine, phenytoin, propofol, warfarin

Compatibility in syringe: Incompatible with ampicillin, cefamandole, heparin

Compatibility when admixed: Incompatible with amphotericin B, ampicillin, cefamandole, cefazolin with clindamycin, cefepime, heparin, nafcillin, ticarcillin

Storage: Gentamicin is a colorless to slightly yellow solution which should be stored between 2°C to 30°C, but refrigeration is not recommended.

Related Information

Prevention of Wound Infection and Sepsis in Surgical Patients *on page 1830*

♦ Gentamicin Sulfate *see* Gentamicin *on page 807*

♦ GenTeal® [OTC] *see* Hydroxypropyl Methylcellulose *on page 883*

♦ GenTeal® Mild [OTC] *see* Hydroxypropyl Methylcellulose *on page 883*

Gentian Violet (JEN shun VYE oh let)

Synonyms Crystal Violet; Methylrosaniline Chloride

Pharmacologic Category Antibiotic, Topical; Antifungal Agent, Topical

Use Treatment of cutaneous or mucocutaneous infections caused by *Candida albicans* and other superficial skin infections

Mechanism of Action Topical antiseptic/germicide effective against some vegetative gram-positive bacteria, particularly *Staphylococcus* sp, and some yeast; it is much less effective against gram-negative bacteria and is ineffective against acid-fast bacteria

Contraindications Hypersensitivity to gentian violet or any component of the formulation; ulcerated areas; porphyria

Warnings/Precautions Infants should be turned face down after application to minimize amount of drug swallowed; may result in tattooing of the skin when applied to granulation tissue; solution is for external use only; avoid contact with eyes

Drug Interactions No data reported

Adverse Reactions Frequency not defined.

Dermatologic: Vesicle formation

Gastrointestinal: Esophagitis, ulceration of mucous membranes

Local: Burning, irritation

Respiratory: Laryngitis, laryngeal obstruction, tracheitis

Miscellaneous: Sensitivity reactions

Overdosage/Toxicology Signs and symptoms: Laryngeal obstruction

Dosing

Adults & Elderly:

Superficial skin or mucocutaneous infection: Topical: Apply 0.5% to 2% locally with cotton to lesion 2-3 times/day for 3 days, do not swallow and avoid contact with eyes

Vaginal infection: Intravaginal: Insert one tampon for 3-4 hours once or twice daily for 12 days

Pediatrics: Superficial skin or mucocutaneous infection: Refer to adult dosing.

Available Dosage Forms Solution, topical: 1% (30 mL); 2% (30 mL)

Nursing Guidelines

Patient Education: Drug stains skin and clothing purple; do not apply to an ulcerative lesion; may result in "tattooing" of the skin.

Pregnancy Risk Factor: C

♦ Gentlax® [OTC] [DSC] *see* Bisacodyl *on page 245*

♦ Gentran® *see* Dextran *on page 503*

♦ Geriation [OTC] *see* Vitamins (Multiple/Oral) *on page 1720*

♦ Geritol Complete® [OTC] *see* Vitamins (Multiple/Oral) *on page 1720*

♦ Geritol Extend® [OTC] *see* Vitamins (Multiple/Oral) *on page 1720*

♦ Geritol® Tonic [OTC] *see* Vitamins (Multiple/Oral) *on page 1720*

♦ German Measles Vaccine *see* Rubella Virus Vaccine (Live) *on page 1505*

♦ Gevrabon® [OTC] *see* Vitamin B Complex Combinations *on page 1716*

♦ GG *see* Guaifenesin *on page 834*

♦ GI87084B *see* Remifentanil *on page 1467*

♦ Glargine Insulin *see* Insulin Glargine *on page 920*

Glatiramer Acetate (gla TIR a mer AS e tate)

U.S. Brand Names Copaxone®

Synonyms Copolymer-1

Pharmacologic Category Biological, Miscellaneous

Medication Safety Issues

Sound-alike/look-alike issues:

Copaxone® may be confused with Compazine®

Use Treatment of relapsing-remitting type multiple sclerosis; studies indicate that it reduces the frequency of attacks and the severity of disability; appears to be most effective for patients with minimal disability

Mechanism of Action Glatiramer is a mixture of random polymers of four amino acids; L-alanine, L-glutamic acid, L-lysine and L-tyrosine, the resulting mixture is antigenically similar to myelin basic protein, which is an important component of the myelin sheath of nerves; glatiramer is thought to suppress T-lymphocytes specific for a myelin antigen, it is also proposed that glatiramer interferes with the antigen-presenting function of certain immune cells opposing pathogenic T-cell function

Pharmacodynamics/Kinetics

Distribution: Small amounts of intact and partial hydrolyzed drug enter lymphatic circulation

Metabolism: SubQ: Large percentage hydrolyzed locally

Contraindications Previous hypersensitivity to any component of the copolymer formulation, glatiramer acetate, or mannitol

Warnings/Precautions For SubQ use only, **not for I.V. administration**. Glatiramer acetate is antigenic, and may possibly lead to the induction of untoward host responses. Systemic postinjection reactions occur in a substantial percentage of patients (~10% in premarketing studies). Safety and efficacy have not been established in patients <18 years of age.

Adverse Reactions Reported in >2% of patients in placebo-controlled trials:

>10%:

Cardiovascular: Chest pain (21%), vasodilation (27%), palpitation (17%)

Central nervous system: Pain (28%), vasodilation (27%), anxiety (23%)

Dermatologic: Pruritus (18%), rash (18%), diaphoresis (15%)

Gastrointestinal: Nausea (22%), diarrhea (12%)

Local: Injection site reactions: Pain (73%), erythema (66%), inflammation (49%), pruritus (40%), mass (27%), induration (13%), welt (11%)

Neuromuscular & skeletal: Weakness (41%), arthralgia (24%), hypertonia (22%), back pain (16%)

Respiratory: Dyspnea (19%), rhinitis (14%)

Miscellaneous: Infection (50%), flu-like syndrome (19%), lymphadenopathy (12%)

1% to 10%:

Cardiovascular: Peripheral edema (7%), facial edema (6%), edema (3%), tachycardia (5%), hypertension (1%), syncope (5%)

Central nervous system: Fever (8%), vertigo (6%), migraine (5%), agitation (4%), chills (4%), confusion (2%), nervousness (2%), speech disorder (2%), abnormal dreams (1%), emotional lability (1%), stupor (1%)

Dermatologic: Bruising (8%), erythema (4%), urticaria (4%), skin nodule (2%), eczema, herpes zoster, pustular rash, skin atrophy

Endocrine & metabolic: Dysmenorrhea (6%), amenorrhea (1%), menorrhagia (1%), vaginal hemorrhage (1%)

Gastrointestinal: Anorexia (8%), vomiting (6%), gastrointestinal disorder (5%), gastroenteritis (3%), weight gain (3%), oral moniliasis (1%), ulcerative stomatitis (1%), salivary gland enlargement

Genitourinary: Urinary urgency (10%), vaginal moniliasis (8%), hematuria (1%), impotence (1%)

Local: Injection site reactions: Hemorrhage (5%), urticaria (5%), edema (1%), atrophy (1%), abscess (1%), hypersensitivity (1%)

Neuromuscular & skeletal: Tremor (7%), foot drop (3%)

Ocular: Eye disorder (4%), nystagmus (2%), visual field defect (1%)

Otic: Ear pain (7%)

Respiratory: Bronchitis (9%), laryngismus (5%)

Miscellaneous: Neck pain (8%), bacterial infection (5%), herpes simplex (4%), cyst (2%)

<1% (Limited to important or life-threatening): Anaphylactoid reaction, angina, angioedema, aphasia, arrhythmia, blindness, carcinoma (breast, bladder, lung), cardiomyopathy, cholecystitis, cholelithiasis, cirrhosis, coma, CHF, corneal

ulcer, esophageal ulcer, esophagitis, ethanol intolerance, gastrointestinal hemorrhage, GI carcinoma, glaucoma, gout, hallucinations, hematemesis, hepatitis, hepatomegaly, hypotension, leukopenia, lupus erythematosus, mania, meningitis, MI, neuralgia, optic neuritis, pancreatitis, pancytopenia, paraplegia, pericardial effusion, photosensitivity, postural hypotension, priapism, pulmonary embolism, rash, renal failure, rheumatoid arthritis, seizure, sepsis, serum sickness, splenomegaly, stomatitis, stroke, suicide attempt, thrombocytopenia, thrombosis

Overdosage/Toxicology Well tolerated; no serious toxicities can be anticipated

Dosing

Adults & Elderly: Multiple sclerosis (relapsing-remitting): SubQ: 20 mg daily

Available Dosage Forms Injection, solution [preservative free]: 20 mg/mL (1 mL) [prefilled syringe; contains mannitol; packaged with alcohol pads]

Nursing Guidelines

Assessment: Assess potential for interactions with other prescriptions, OTC medications, or herbal products patient may be taking. Assess effectiveness and adverse response (eg, postinjection reactions — self-resolving flushing, chest tightness, dyspnea, palpitations). Teach patient proper use (reconstitution, injection technique, and syringe/needle disposal), possible side effects/ appropriate interventions, and adverse symptoms to report.

Patient Education: This drug will not cure MS, but may help relieve the severity and frequency of attacks. This drug can only be given by subcutaneous injection; your prescriber will instruct you in how to prepare the medication, proper injection technique, and syringe/needle disposal. If using prefilled glass syringe, use **only** the auto*ject*® 2 *for glass syringe* device (not the original Copaxone® autoject). Do not stop or change doses without consulting your prescriber. May cause a transient reaction after injection, including flushing, chest tightness, dyspnea, or palpitations (usually last 30 minutes or less). May cause weakness, dizziness, confusion, nervousness, or anxiety (use caution when driving or engaging in tasks requiring alertness until response to drug is known); or nausea or vomiting (frequent mouth care and sucking on lozenges may help). Report chest pain or pounding heartbeat; persistent diarrhea or GI upset; infection (vaginal itching or drainage, sores in mouth, unusual fever or chills) or flu-like symptoms (swollen glands, chills, excessive sweating); bruising, rash, or skin irritation; joint pain or neck pain; swelling of puffiness of face; vision changes or ear pain; unusual cough or respiratory difficulty; alterations in menstrual pattern; skin depression, hard lump, redness, pain, or swelling at injection site; or any other persistent adverse reactions. **Breast-feeding precaution:** Consult prescriber if breast-feeding.

Pregnancy Risk Factor: B

Lactation: Excretion in breast milk unknown/use caution

Administration

Storage: Store in refrigerator at 2°C to 8°C (36°F to 46°F); excursions to room temperature for up to 1 week do not have a negative impact on potency.

◆ **Gliadel®** *see* Carmustine *on page 318*

◆ **Glibenclamide** *see* GlyBURIDE *on page 820*

Glimepiride (GLYE me pye ride)

U.S. Brand Names Amaryl®

Pharmacologic Category Antidiabetic Agent, Sulfonylurea

Medication Safety Issues

Sound-alike/look-alike issues:

Glimepiride may be confused with glipiZIDE

Amaryl® may be confused with Altace®, Amerge®, Reminyl®

Use Management of type 2 diabetes mellitus (noninsulin dependent, NIDDM) as an adjunct to diet and exercise to lower blood glucose; may be used in combination with metformin or insulin in patients whose hyperglycemia cannot be controlled by diet and exercise in conjunction with a single oral hypoglycemic agent

Mechanism of Action Stimulates insulin release from the pancreatic beta cells; reduces glucose output from the liver; insulin sensitivity is increased at peripheral target sites

Pharmacodynamics/Kinetics

Onset of action: Peak effect: Blood glucose reductions: 2-3 hours

Duration: 24 hours

Absorption: 100%; delayed when given with food

Distribution: V_d: 8.8 L

(Continued)

Glimepiride *(Continued)*

Protein binding: >99.5%

Metabolism: Hepatic oxidation via CYP2C9 to M1 metabolite (~33% activity of parent compound); further oxidative metabolism to inactive M2 metabolite

Half-life elimination: 5-9 hours

Time to peak, plasma: 2-3 hours

Excretion: Urine (60%, 80% to 90% M1 and M2); feces (40%, 70% M1 and M2)

Contraindications Hypersensitivity to glimepiride, any component of the formulation, or sulfonamides; diabetic ketoacidosis (with or without coma)

Warnings/Precautions All sulfonylurea drugs are capable of producing severe hypoglycemia. Hypoglycemia is more likely to occur when caloric intake is deficient, after severe or prolonged exercise, when ethanol is ingested, or when more than one glucose-lowering drug is used.

Chemical similarities are present among sulfonamides, sulfonylureas, carbonic anhydrase inhibitors, thiazides, and loop diuretics (except ethacrynic acid). Use in patients with sulfonamide allergy is specifically contraindicated in product labeling, however, a risk of cross-reaction exists in patients with allergy to any of these compounds; avoid use when previous reaction has been severe.

Product labeling states oral hypoglycemic drugs may be associated with an increased cardiovascular mortality as compared to treatment with diet alone or diet plus insulin. Data to support this association are limited, and several studies, including a large prospective trial (UKPDS) have not supported an association. Safety and efficacy in pediatric patients have not been established.

Drug Interactions Substrate of CYP2C8/9 (major)

Beta blockers: Beta blockers may enhance the effects of sulfonylureas.

Chloramphenicol: Chloramphenicol may increase the effects of sulfonylureas.

Cimetidine: Cimetidine may increase the effects of glimepiride.

Cyclosporine: Sulfonylureas may increase the levels of cyclosporine.

CYP2C8/9 inducers: May decrease the levels/effects of glimepiride. Example inducers include carbamazepine, phenobarbital, phenytoin, rifampin, rifapentine, and secobarbital.

CYP2C8/9 inhibitors: May increase the levels/effects of glimepiride. Example inhibitors include delavirdine, fluconazole, gemfibrozil, ketoconazole, nicardipine, NSAIDs, pioglitazone, and sulfonamides.

Ethanol: Sulfonylureas may induce a disulfiram-like reaction.

Fibric acid derivatives: May increase the hypoglycemic effects of sulfonylureas; monitor.

Fluconazole: Fluconazole may increase the levels of sulfonylureas.

Hyperglycemia-producing agents: Certain drugs tend to produce hyperglycemia and may lead to loss of control. These drugs include the thiazides and other diuretics, corticosteroids, phenothiazines, thyroid products, estrogens, oral contraceptives, phenytoin, nicotinic acid, sympathomimetics, and isoniazid.

Pegvisomant: Pegvisomant may increase the effects of sulfonylureas.

Rifampin: Rifampin may decrease the effects of sulfonylureas.

Salicylates: Salicylates may increase the effects of sulfonylureas.

Sulfonamides: Sulfonamides may increase the effects of sulfonylureas.

Tricyclic antidepressants: TCAs may increase the effects of sulfonylureas.

Nutritional/Herbal/Ethanol Interactions

Ethanol: Caution with ethanol (may cause hypoglycemia).

Herb/Nutraceutical: Caution with chromium, garlic, gymnema (may cause hypoglycemia).

Adverse Reactions

1% to 10%:

- Central nervous system: Dizziness (2%), headache (2%)
- Endocrine & metabolic: Hypoglycemia (1% to 2%)
- Gastrointestinal: Nausea (1%)
- Neuromuscular & skeletal: Weakness (2%)

<1% or frequency not defined: Agranulocytosis, anorexia, aplastic anemia, cholestatic jaundice, constipation, diarrhea, disulfiram-like reaction, diuretic effect, edema, epigastric fullness, gastrointestinal pain, erythema, heartburn, hemolytic anemia, hepatitis, hypoglycemia, hyponatremia, leukopenia, liver function tests abnormal, nausea, pancytopenia, photosensitivity, porphyria cutanea tarda, pruritus, rash (morbilliform or maculopapular), SIADH, thrombocytopenia, urticaria, vasculitis (allergic), visual accommodation changes (early treatment), vomiting

Overdosage/Toxicology Symptoms of overdose include low blood sugar, tingling of lips and tongue, nausea, yawning, confusion, agitation, tachycardia, sweating, convulsions, stupor, and coma. Intoxication with sulfonylureas can cause hypoglycemia and are best managed with glucose administration (oral for milder hypoglycemia or by injection in more severe forms). Patients should be monitored for a minimum of 24-48 hours after ingestion.

Dosing

Adults:

Type 2 diabetes: Oral:

Initial: 1-2 mg once daily, administered with breakfast or the first main meal

Adjustment: Allow several days between dose titrations: usual maintenance dose: 1-4 mg once daily; after a dose of 2 mg once daily, increase in increments of 2 mg at 1- to 2-week intervals based upon the patient's blood glucose response to a maximum of 8 mg once daily. If inadequate response to maximal dose, combination therapy with metformin may be considered.

Combination with insulin therapy:

Note: Fasting glucose level for instituting combination therapy is in the range of >150 mg/dL in plasma or serum depending on the patient)

Initial: 8 mg once daily with the first main meal

Adjustment: After starting with low-dose insulin, upward adjustments of insulin can be done approximately weekly as guided by frequent measurements of fasting blood glucose. Once stable, combination-therapy patients should monitor their capillary blood glucose on an ongoing basis, preferably daily.

Conversion from therapy with long half-life agents: Observe patient carefully for 1-2 weeks when converting from a longer half-life agent (eg, chlorpropamide) to glimepiride due to overlapping hypoglycemic effects.

Elderly: Initial: 1 mg/day; dose titration and maintenance dosing should be conservative to avoid hypoglycemia

Pediatrics: Type 2 diabetes: Oral: Children 10-18 years (unlabeled use): Initial: 1 mg once daily; maintenance: 1-4 mg once daily

Renal Impairment: Cl_{cr} <22 mL/minute: Initial starting dose should be 1 mg and dosage increments should be based on fasting blood glucose levels.

Available Dosage Forms Tablet: 1 mg, 2 mg, 4 mg

Nursing Guidelines

Assessment: Assess any allergies prior to beginning therapy. Assess potential for interactions with other prescriptions, OTC medications, or herbal products patient may be taking. Assess results of laboratory tests, therapeutic effectiveness, and adverse response at regular intervals during therapy. Teach patient proper use (or refer patient to diabetic educator for instruction), possible side effects/appropriate interventions, and adverse symptoms to report.

Monitoring Laboratory Tests: Urine for glucose and ketones, fasting blood glucose, hemoglobin A_{1c}, fructosamine

Dietary Considerations: Administer with breakfast or the first main meal of the day. Dietary modification based on ADA recommendations is a part of therapy. Decreases blood glucose concentration. Hypoglycemia may occur. Must be able to recognize symptoms of hypoglycemia (palpitations, sweaty palms, lightheadedness).

Patient Education: Do not take any new medication during therapy unless approved by prescriber. This medication is used to control diabetes; it is not a cure. Monitor glucose as recommended by prescriber. Other important components of treatment plan may include prescribed diet and exercise regimen (consult prescriber or diabetic educator). Always carry quick source of sugar with you. Take exactly as directed with breakfast or the first main meal of the day. Do not change dose or discontinue without consulting prescriber. Avoid alcohol while taking this medication; could cause severe reaction. Do not take other medication within 2 hours of this medication unless advised by prescriber. If you experience hypoglycemic reaction, contact prescriber immediately. You may experience side effects during first weeks of therapy (eg, headache, nausea); consult prescriber if these persist. Report severe or persistent side effects (eg, hypoglycemia: palpitations, sweaty palms, lightheadedness; extended vomiting or flu-like symptoms; skin rash; easy bruising or bleeding; or change in color of urine or stool). **Pregnancy/breast-feeding precautions:** Inform prescriber if you are or intend to become pregnant. Do not breast-feed.

Geriatric Considerations: Rapid and prolonged hypoglycemia (>12 hours) despite hypertonic glucose injections have been reported; age, hepatic, and

(Continued)

Glimepiride *(Continued)*

renal impairment are independent risk factors for hypoglycemia; dosage titration should be made at weekly intervals. How "tightly" a geriatric patient's blood glucose should be controlled is controversial; however, a fasting blood sugar <150 mg/dL is now an acceptable end point. Such a decision should be based on the patient's functional and cognitive status, how well they recognize hypoglycemic or hyperglycemic symptoms, and how to respond to them and their other disease states.

Pregnancy Risk Factor: C

Pregnancy Issues: Abnormal blood glucose levels are associated with a higher incidence of congenital abnormalities. Insulin is the drug of choice for the control of diabetes mellitus during pregnancy.

Lactation: Excretion in breast milk unknown/contraindicated

Administration

Oral: Administer once daily with breakfast or first main meal of the day. Patients who are NPO may need to have their dose held to avoid hypoglycemia.

Related Information

Perioperative Management of the Diabetic Patient *on page 1794*

GlipiZIDE (GLIP i zide)

U.S. Brand Names Glucotrol®; Glucotrol® XL

Synonyms Glydiazinamide

Pharmacologic Category Antidiabetic Agent, Sulfonylurea

Medication Safety Issues

Sound-alike/look-alike issues:

GlipiZIDE may be confused with glimepiride, glyBURIDE
Glucotrol® may be confused with Glucophage®, Glucotrol® XL, glyBURIDE
Glucotrol® XL may be confused with Glucotrol®

Use Management of type 2 diabetes mellitus (noninsulin dependent, NIDDM)

Mechanism of Action Stimulates insulin release from the pancreatic beta cells; reduces glucose output from the liver; insulin sensitivity is increased at peripheral target sites

Pharmacodynamics/Kinetics

Onset of action: Peak effect: Blood glucose reductions: 1.5-2 hours
Duration: 12-24 hours
Absorption: Delayed with food
Protein binding: 92% to 99%
Metabolism: Hepatic with metabolites
Half-life elimination: 2-4 hours
Excretion: Urine (60% to 80%, 91% to 97% as metabolites); feces (11%)

Contraindications Hypersensitivity to glipizide or any component of the formulation, other sulfonamides; type 1 diabetes mellitus (insulin dependent, IDDM)

Warnings/Precautions Use with caution in patients with severe hepatic disease.

Chemical similarities are present among sulfonamides, sulfonylureas, carbonic anhydrase inhibitors, thiazides, and loop diuretics (except ethacrynic acid). Use in patients with sulfonamide allergy is specifically contraindicated in product labeling, however, a risk of cross-reaction exists in patients with allergy to any of these compounds; avoid use when previous reaction has been severe.

The extended release formulation consists of drug within a nondeformable matrix; following drug release/absorption, the matrix/shell is expelled in the stool. The use of nondeformable products in patients with known stricture/narrowing of the GI tract has been associated with symptoms of obstruction. Avoid use of extended release tablets (Glucotrol® XL) in patients with severe gastrointestinal narrowing or esophageal dysmotility.

Product labeling states oral hypoglycemic drugs may be associated with an increased cardiovascular mortality as compared to treatment with diet alone or diet plus insulin. Data to support this association are limited, and several studies, including a large prospective trial (UKPDS) have not supported an association.

Drug Interactions Substrate of 2C8/9 (major)

Anabolic steroids may increase hypoglycemic effect; monitor blood glucose.
ACE inhibitors may increase hypoglycemic effect; monitor blood glucose.
Beta-blockers decrease hypoglycemic effect, mask most hypoglycemic symptoms, decrease glycogenolysis; avoid use in diabetics with frequent hypoglycemic episodes.
Cholestyramine decreases glipizide's absorption; separate administration times.

Corticosteroids cause hyperglycemia; adjustment of hypoglycemic agent may be necessary.

Cyclosporine serum concentration is increased; monitor cyclosporine levels and renal function.

CYP2C8/9 inducers: May decrease the levels/effects of glipizide. Example inducers include carbamazepine, phenobarbital, phenytoin, rifampin, rifapentine, and secobarbital.

CYP2C8/9 inhibitors: May increase the levels/effects of glipizide. Example inhibitors include delavirdine, fluconazole, gemfibrozil, ketoconazole, nicardipine, NSAIDs, pioglitazone, and sulfonamides.

Ethanol (large amounts) decreases hypoglycemic effect; avoid concurrent use; rare disulfiram reaction.

H_2 antagonists, antacids, oral sodium bicarbonate may increase the hypoglycemic effect; monitor glucose response.

Rifampin may decrease hypoglycemic effects of glipizide; monitor blood glucose.

Tacrolimus serum concentrations may be increased; monitor tacrolimus serum concentrations and renal function.

Nutritional/Herbal/Ethanol Interactions

Ethanol: Caution with ethanol (may cause hypoglycemia or rare disulfiram reaction).

Food: A delayed release of insulin may occur if glipizide is taken with food. Immediate release tablets should be administered 30 minutes before meals to avoid erratic absorption.

Herb/Nutraceutical: Caution with chromium, garlic, gymnema (may cause hypoglycemia).

Adverse Reactions Frequency not defined.

Cardiovascular: Edema, syncope

Central nervous system: Anxiety, depression, dizziness, headache, insomnia, nervousness

Dermatologic: Rash, urticaria, photosensitivity, pruritus

Endocrine & metabolic: Hypoglycemia, hyponatremia, SIADH (rare)

Gastrointestinal: Anorexia, nausea, vomiting, diarrhea, epigastric fullness, constipation, heartburn, flatulence

Hematologic: Blood dyscrasias, aplastic anemia, hemolytic anemia, bone marrow suppression, thrombocytopenia, agranulocytosis

Hepatic: Cholestatic jaundice, hepatic porphyria

Neuromuscular & skeletal: Arthralgia, leg cramps, myalgia, tremor

Ocular: Blurred vision

Renal: Diuretic effect (minor)

Miscellaneous: Diaphoresis, disulfiram-like reaction

Postmarketing and/or case reports: Abdominal pain

Overdosage/Toxicology Symptoms of overdose include low blood sugar, tingling of lips and tongue, nausea, yawning, confusion, agitation, tachycardia, sweating, convulsions, stupor, and coma. Intoxication with sulfonylureas can cause hypoglycemia and are best managed with glucose administration (oral for milder hypoglycemia or by injection in more severe forms).

Dosing

Adults:

Type 2 diabetes: Oral (allow several days between dose titrations): Initial: 5 mg/day; adjust dosage at 2.5-5 mg daily increments as determined by blood glucose response at intervals of several days.

Immediate release tablet: Maximum recommended once-daily dose: 15 mg; maximum recommended total daily dose: 40 mg

Extended release tablet (Glucotrol® XL): Maximum recommended dose: 20 mg

When transferring from insulin to glipizide:

Current insulin requirement ≤20 units: Discontinue insulin and initiate glipizide at usual dose

Current insulin requirement >20 units: Decrease insulin by 50% and initiate glipizide at usual dose; gradually decrease insulin dose based on patient response. Several days should elapse between dosage changes.

Elderly: Initial: 2.5 mg/day; increase by 2.5-5 mg/day at 1- to 2-week intervals.

Renal Impairment: Cl_{cr} <10 mL/minute: Some investigators recommend not using.

Hepatic Impairment: Initial dosage should be 2.5 mg/day.

Available Dosage Forms

Tablet (Glucotrol®): 5 mg, 10 mg

(Continued)

GlipiZIDE *(Continued)*

Tablet, extended release: 5 mg, 10 mg

(Glucotrol® XL): 2.5 mg, 5 mg, 10 mg

Nursing Guidelines

Assessment: Assess potential for interactions with other prescriptions, OTC medications, or herbal products patient may be taking, and any allergies they may have. Assess results of laboratory tests, therapeutic effects, and adverse response (eg, hypoglycemia) at regular intervals during therapy. Teach patient proper use (or refer patient to diabetic educator for instruction), possible side effects/appropriate interventions, and adverse symptoms to report.

Monitoring Laboratory Tests: Urine for glucose and ketones, fasting blood glucose, hemoglobin A_{1c}, fructosamine

Dietary Considerations: Take immediate release tablets 30 minutes before meals; extended release tablets should be taken with breakfast. Dietary modification based on ADA recommendations is a part of therapy. Decreases blood glucose concentration. Hypoglycemia may occur. Must be able to recognize symptoms of hypoglycemia (palpitations, sweaty palms, lightheadedness).

Patient Education: Do not take any new medication during therapy unless approved by prescriber. This medication is used to control diabetes; it is not a cure. Monitor glucose as recommended by prescriber. Other important components of treatment plan may include prescribed diet and exercise regimen (consult prescriber or diabetic educator). Always carry quick source of sugar with you. Take exactly as directed. Immediate release tablets should be taken 30 minutes before meals, at the same time each day. Extended release tablets should be taken with breakfast. Do not chew or crush extended release tablets. Do not change dose or discontinue without consulting prescriber. Avoid alcohol while taking this medication; could cause severe reaction. Do not take other medication within 2 hours of this medication unless advised by prescriber. If you experience hypoglycemic reaction, contact prescriber immediately. You may experience more sensitivity to sunlight (use sunscreen, wear protective clothing and eyewear, and avoid direct sunlight); or headache or nausea (consult prescriber if these persist). Report severe or persistent side effects (eg, hypoglycemia: palpitations, sweaty palms, lightheadedness; extended vomiting; diarrhea or constipation; flu-like symptoms; skin rash; easy bruising or bleeding; or change in color of urine or stool). **Pregnancy/breast-feeding precautions:** Inform prescriber if you are or intend to become pregnant. Breast-feeding is not recommended

Geriatric Considerations: Glipizide is a useful agent since there are few drug to drug interactions and elimination of the active drug is not dependent upon renal function. How "tightly" a geriatric patient's blood glucose should be controlled is controversial; however, a fasting blood sugar <150 mg/dL is now an acceptable end point. Such a decision should be based on the patient's functional and cognitive status, how well they recognize hypoglycemic or hyperglycemic symptoms, and how to respond to them and their other disease states.

Pregnancy Risk Factor: C

Pregnancy Issues: Crosses the placenta. Abnormal blood glucose levels are associated with a higher incidence of congenital abnormalities. Insulin is the drug of choice for the control of diabetes mellitus during pregnancy. If glipizide is used during pregnancy, discontinue and change to insulin at least 1 month prior to delivery to decrease prolonged hypoglycemia in the neonate.

Lactation: Excretion in breast milk unknown/not recommended

Breast-Feeding Considerations: Due to risk of neonatal hypoglycemia, breast-feeding is not recommended. Discontinue nursing or consider switching to insulin if diet alone does not control blood glucose.

Perioperative/Anesthesia/Other Concerns: The possibility of higher doses of sulfonylureas eliciting an increase in cardiovascular events, because of their effects on blocking potassium sensitive ATP channels, has been raised. Longer-term prospective trials of sulfonylurea therapy, such as the UKPDS, do not reveal any increased cardiovascular mortality.

Administration

Oral: Administer immediate release tablets 30 minutes before a meal to achieve greatest reduction in postprandial hyperglycemia. Extended release tablets should be given with breakfast. Patients who are NPO may need to have their dose held to avoid hypoglycemia.

Related Information

Perioperative Management of the Diabetic Patient *on page 1794*

♦ GlucaGen® *see* Glucagon *on page 819*
♦ GlucaGen® Diagnostic Kit *see* Glucagon *on page 819*
♦ GlucaGen® HypoKit™ *see* Glucagon *on page 819*

Glucagon (GLOO ka gon)

U.S. Brand Names GlucaGen®; GlucaGen® Diagnostic Kit; GlucaGen® HypoKit™; Glucagon Diagnostic Kit [DSC]; Glucagon Emergency Kit

Synonyms Glucagon Hydrochloride

Pharmacologic Category Antidote; Diagnostic Agent

Medication Safety Issues

Sound-alike/look-alike issues:

Glucagon may be confused with Glaucon®

Use Management of hypoglycemia; diagnostic aid in radiologic examinations to temporarily inhibit GI tract movement

Unlabeled/Investigational Use Used with some success as a cardiac stimulant in management of severe cases of beta-adrenergic blocking agent overdosage; treatment of myocardial depression due to calcium channel blocker overdose

Mechanism of Action Stimulates adenylate cyclase to produce increased cyclic AMP, which promotes hepatic glycogenolysis and gluconeogenesis, causing a raise in blood glucose levels

Pharmacodynamics/Kinetics

Onset of action: Peak effect: Blood glucose levels: Parenteral:

I.V.: 5-20 minutes

I.M.: 30 minutes

SubQ: 30-45 minutes

Duration: Hyperglycemia: 60-90 minutes

Metabolism: Primarily hepatic; some inactivation occurring renally and in plasma

Half-life elimination, plasma: 3-10 minutes

Contraindications Hypersensitivity to glucagon or any component of the formulation; insulinoma; pheochromocytoma

Warnings/Precautions Use caution with prolonged fasting, starvation, adrenal insufficiency or chronic hypoglycemia; levels of glucose stores in liver may be decreased. Following response to therapy, oral carbohydrates should be administered to prevent hypoglycemia.

Drug Interactions Oral anticoagulant: Hypoprothrombinemic effects may be increased possibly with bleeding; effect seen with glucagon doses of 50 mg administered over 1-2 days

Nutritional/Herbal/Ethanol Interactions Glucagon depletes glycogen stores.

Adverse Reactions Frequency not defined.

Cardiovascular: Hypotension (up to 2 hours after GI procedures), hypertension, tachycardia

Gastrointestinal: Nausea, vomiting (high incidence with rapid administration of high doses)

Miscellaneous: Hypersensitivity reactions, anaphylaxis

Overdosage/Toxicology Symptoms include hypokalemia, nausea and vomiting, inhibition of GI tract motility, decreased blood pressure, tachycardia

Dosing

Adults & Elderly:

Hypoglycemia or insulin shock therapy: I.M., I.V., SubQ: 1 mg; may repeat in 20 minutes as needed

Note: If patient fails to respond to glucagon, I.V. dextrose must be given.

Beta-blocker overdose, calcium channel blocker overdose (unlabeled use): I.V.: 5-10 mg over 1 minutes followed by an infusion of 1-10 mg/hour. The following has also been reported for beta-blocker overdose: 3-10 mg or initially 0.5-5 mg bolus followed by continuous infusion 1-5 mg/hour

Diagnostic aid: I.M., I.V.: 0.25-2 mg 10 minutes prior to procedure

Pediatrics:

Hypoglycemia or insulin shock therapy: I.M., I.V., SubQ:

Children <20 kg: 0.5 mg or 20-30 mcg/kg/dose; repeated in 20 minutes as needed

Children ≥20 kg: Refer to adult dosing.

Note: If patient fails to respond to glucagon, I.V. dextrose must be given.

Available Dosage Forms Injection, powder for reconstitution, as hydrochloride:

GlucaGen®: 1 mg [equivalent to 1 unit; contains lactose 107 mg]

(Continued)

Glucagon *(Continued)*

GlucaGen® Diagnostic Kit: 1 mg [equivalent to 1 unit; contains lactose 107 mg; packaged with sterile water]
GlucaGen® HypoKit™: 1 mg [equivalent to 1 unit; contains lactose 107 mg; packaged with prefilled syringe containing sterile water]
Glucagon®: 1 mg [equivalent to 1 unit; contains lactose 49 mg]
Glucagon Diagnostic Kit, Glucagon Emergency Kit: 1 mg [equivalent to 1 unit; contains lactose 49 mg; packaged with diluent syringe containing glycerin 12 mg/mL and water for injection]

Nursing Guidelines

Assessment: Arouse patient from hypoglycemic or insulin shock as soon as possible and administer carbohydrates. Evaluate insulin dosage and patient's ability to administer appropriate dose. Instruct patient (or significant other) in appropriate administration procedures for emergency use of glucagon. If home glucose monitoring device is available, check blood sugar as soon as possible.

Monitoring Laboratory Tests: Blood glucose

Dietary Considerations: Administer carbohydrates to patient as soon as possible after response to treatment.

Patient Education: Identify appropriate support person to administer glucagon if necessary. Follow prescribers instructions for administering glucagon. Review diet, insulin administration, and testing procedures with prescriber or diabetic educator.

Pregnancy Risk Factor: B

Lactation: Excretion in breast milk unknown/compatible

Perioperative/Anesthesia/Other Concerns: 1 unit = 1 mg

Administration

I.V.: Bolus may be associated with nausea and vomiting. Continuous infusions may be used in beta-blocker overdose/toxicity.

Reconstitution: Reconstitute powder for injection by adding 1 mL of sterile diluent to a vial containing 1 unit of the drug, to provide solutions containing 1 mg of glucagon/mL. Gently roll vial to dissolve. If dose to be administered is <2 mg of the drug, then use only the diluent provided by the manufacturer. If >2 mg, use sterile water for injection. Use immediately after reconstitution. May be kept at 5°C for up to 48 hours if necessary.

Storage: Prior to reconstitution, store at controlled room temperature of 20°C to 25° (69°F to 77°F). Do not freeze.

- **Glucagon Diagnostic Kit [DSC]** *see* Glucagon *on page 819*
- **Glucagon Emergency Kit** *see* Glucagon *on page 819*
- **Glucagon Hydrochloride** *see* Glucagon *on page 819*
- **Glucophage®** *see* Metformin *on page 1112*
- **Glucophage® XR** *see* Metformin *on page 1112*
- **Glucose** *see* Dextrose *on page 511*
- **Glucose Monohydrate** *see* Dextrose *on page 511*
- **Glucotrol®** *see* GlipiZIDE *on page 816*
- **Glucotrol® XL** *see* GlipiZIDE *on page 816*
- **Glucovance®** *see* Glyburide and Metformin *on page 823*
- **Glulisine Insulin** *see* Insulin Glulisine *on page 922*
- **Glutofac®-MX** *see* Vitamins (Multiple/Oral) *on page 1720*
- **Glutofac®-ZX** *see* Vitamins (Multiple/Oral) *on page 1720*
- **Glutol™ [OTC]** *see* Dextrose *on page 511*
- **Glutose™ [OTC]** *see* Dextrose *on page 511*
- **Glybenclamide** *see* GlyBURIDE *on page 820*
- **Glybenzcyclamide** *see* GlyBURIDE *on page 820*

GlyBURIDE (GLYE byoor ide)

U.S. Brand Names Diaβeta®; Glynase® PresTab®; Micronase®

Synonyms Diabeta; Glibenclamide; Glybenclamide; Glybenzcyclamide

Pharmacologic Category Antidiabetic Agent, Sulfonylurea

Medication Safety Issues

Sound-alike/look-alike issues:
GlyBURIDE may be confused with glipiZIDE, Glucotrol®
Diaβeta® may be confused with Diabinese®, Zebeta®
Micronase® may be confused with microK®, miconazole, Micronor®

Use Management of type 2 diabetes mellitus (noninsulin dependent, NIDDM)

Unlabeled/Investigational Use Alternative to insulin in women for the treatment of gestational diabetes (11-33 weeks gestation)

Mechanism of Action Stimulates insulin release from the pancreatic beta cells; reduces glucose output from the liver; insulin sensitivity is increased at peripheral target sites

Pharmacodynamics/Kinetics

Onset of action: Serum insulin levels begin to increase 15-60 minutes after a single dose

Duration: ≤24 hours

Protein binding, plasma: >99%

Metabolism: To one moderately active and several inactive metabolites

Half-life elimination: 5-16 hours; may be prolonged with renal or hepatic impairment

Time to peak, serum: Adults: 2-4 hours

Excretion: Feces (50%) and urine (50%) as metabolites

Contraindications Hypersensitivity to glyburide, any component of the formulation, or other sulfonamides; type 1 diabetes mellitus (insulin dependent, IDDM), diabetic ketoacidosis with or without coma

Warnings/Precautions Elderly: Rapid and prolonged hypoglycemia (>12 hours) despite hypertonic glucose injections have been reported; age and hepatic and renal impairment are independent risk factors for hypoglycemia; dosage titration should be made at weekly intervals. Use with caution in patients with renal and hepatic impairment, malnourished or debilitated conditions, or adrenal or pituitary insufficiency.

Chemical similarities are present among sulfonamides, sulfonylureas, carbonic anhydrase inhibitors, thiazides, and loop diuretics (except ethacrynic acid). Use in patients with sulfonamide allergy is specifically contraindicated in product labeling, however, a risk of cross-reaction exists in patients with allergy to any of these compounds; avoid use when previous reaction has been severe.

Product labeling states oral hypoglycemic drugs may be associated with an increased cardiovascular mortality as compared to treatment with diet alone or diet plus insulin. Data to support this association are limited, and several studies, including a large prospective trial (UKPDS) have not supported an association.

Drug Interactions **Inhibits** CYP3A4 (weak)

Decreased effect: Thiazides may decrease effectiveness of glyburide

Increased effect: Possible interaction between glyburide and fluoroquinolone antibiotics has been reported resulting in a potentiation of hypoglycemic action of glyburide

Increased toxicity:

- Since this agent is highly protein bound, the toxic potential is increased when given concomitantly with other highly protein bound drugs (ie, phenylbutazone, oral anticoagulants, hydantoins, salicylates, NSAIDs, beta-blockers, sulfonamides) - increase hypoglycemic effect
- Ethanol increases disulfiram reactions
- Phenylbutazone can increase hypoglycemic effects
- Certain drugs tend to produce hyperglycemia and may lead to loss of control (ie, thiazides and other diuretics, corticosteroids, phenothiazines, thyroid products, estrogens, oral contraceptives, phenytoin, nicotinic acid, sympathomimetics, calcium channel blocking drugs, and isoniazid)

Possible interactions between glyburide and coumarin derivatives have been reported that may either potentiate or weaken the effects of coumarin derivatives

Nutritional/Herbal/Ethanol Interactions

Ethanol: Caution with ethanol (may cause hypoglycemia).

Herb/Nutraceutical: Caution with chromium, garlic, gymnema (may cause hypoglycemia).

Adverse Reactions Frequency not defined.

Central nervous system: Headache, dizziness

Dermatologic: Pruritus, rash, urticaria, photosensitivity reaction

Endocrine & metabolic: Hypoglycemia, hyponatremia (SIADH reported with other sulfonylureas)

Gastrointestinal: Nausea, epigastric fullness, heartburn, constipation, diarrhea, anorexia

Genitourinary: Nocturia

Hematologic: Leukopenia, thrombocytopenia, hemolytic anemia, aplastic anemia, bone marrow suppression, agranulocytosis

Hepatic: Cholestatic jaundice, hepatitis

(Continued)

GlyBURIDE *(Continued)*

Neuromuscular & skeletal: Arthralgia, paresthesia
Ocular: Blurred vision
Renal: Diuretic effect (minor)

Overdosage/Toxicology Symptoms of overdose include severe hypoglycemia, seizures, cerebral damage, tingling of lips and tongue, nausea, yawning, confusion, agitation, tachycardia, sweating, convulsions, stupor, and coma. Intoxication with sulfonylureas can cause hypoglycemia and is best managed with glucose administration (oral for milder hypoglycemia or by injection in more severe forms).

Dosing

Adults:

Type 2 diabetes: Oral:

Note: Regular tablets cannot be used interchangeably with micronized tablet formulations

Regular tablets (Diaβeta®, Micronase®):

Initial: 2.5-5 mg/day, administered with breakfast or the first main meal of the day. In patients who are more sensitive to hypoglycemic drugs, start at 1.25 mg/day.

Adjustment: Increase in increments of no more than 2.5 mg/day at weekly intervals based on the patient's blood glucose response

Maintenance: 1.25-20 mg/day given as single or divided doses; maximum: 20 mg/day

Micronized tablets (Glynase® PresTab®):

Initial: 1.5-3 mg/day, administered with breakfast or the first main meal of the day in patients who are more sensitive to hypoglycemic drugs, start at 0.75 mg/day. Increase in increments of no more than 1.5 mg/day in weekly intervals based on the patient's blood glucose response.

Maintenance: 0.75-12 mg/day given as a single dose or in divided doses. Some patients (especially those receiving >6 mg/day) may have a more satisfactory response with twice-daily dosing.

Elderly: Regular tablets (Diaβeta®, Micronase®): Oral: Initial: 1.25-2.5 mg/day, increase by 1.25-2.5 mg/day every 1-3 weeks. Refer to adult dosing.

Renal Impairment: Cl_{cr} <50 mL/minute: Not recommended

Hepatic Impairment: Use conservative initial and maintenance doses and avoid use in severe disease.

Available Dosage Forms [DSC] = Discontinued product

Tablet (Diaβeta®, Micronase®): 1.25 mg, 2.5 mg, 5 mg
Tablet, micronized: 1.5 mg, 3 mg, 6 mg
Glynase® PresTab®: 1.5 mg [DSC], 3 mg, 6 mg

Nursing Guidelines

Assessment: Assess allergy history prior to beginning therapy. Assess potential for interactions with other prescriptions, OTC medications, or herbal products patient may be taking. Assess results of laboratory tests, therapeutic effectiveness, and adverse response (eg, hypoglycemia) at regular intervals during therapy. Teach patient proper use (or refer patient to diabetic educator) for instruction, possible side effects/appropriate interventions, and adverse symptoms to report.

Monitoring Laboratory Tests: Fasting blood glucose, hemoglobin A_{1c}, fructosamine

Dietary Considerations: Should be taken with meals at the same time each day. Dietary modification based on ADA recommendations is a part of therapy. Decreases blood glucose concentration. Hypoglycemia may occur. Must be able to recognize symptoms of hypoglycemia (palpitations, sweaty palms, lightheadedness).

Patient Education: Do not take any new medication during therapy unless approved by prescriber. This medication is used to control diabetes; it is not a cure. Monitor glucose as recommended by prescriber. Other important components of treatment plan may include prescribed diet and exercise regimen (consult prescriber or diabetic educator). If you experience hypoglycemic reaction, contact prescriber immediately. Always carry quick source of sugar with you. Take exactly as directed, 30 minutes before meal(s) at the same time each day. Do not change dose or discontinue without consulting prescriber. Avoid alcohol while taking this medication; could cause severe reaction. Do not take other medication within 2 hours of this medication unless advised by prescriber. You may experience more sensitivity to sunlight (use sunscreen, wear protective clothing and eyewear, and avoid direct sunlight); headache; or nausea (consult prescriber if these persist). Report severe or persistent side effects; hypoglycemia (palpitations, sweaty palms, lightheadedness); extended vomiting, diarrhea, or constipation; flu-like symptoms; skin rash; easy bruising or bleeding; or change in color of urine or stool. **Pregnancy/breast-feeding precautions:** Inform prescriber if you are or intend to become pregnant. Do not breast-feed.

Geriatric Considerations: Rapid and prolonged hypoglycemia (>12 hours) despite hypertonic glucose injections have been reported; age, hepatic, and renal impairment are independent risk factors for hypoglycemia; conservative initial dosing and slow titration are required to avoid hypoglycemic reactions; dosage titration should be made at weekly intervals.

Pregnancy Risk Factor: C

Pregnancy Issues: Glyburide was not found to significantly cross the placenta *in vitro.* Studies have shown glyburide to be an acceptable alternative to insulin when treatment is needed for gestational diabetes. However, one retrospective study comparing glyburide to insulin noted an increased risk of preeclampsia in women taking glyburide and a higher rate of phototherapy in neonates. Insulin is the drug of choice for the control of diabetes mellitus during pregnancy.

Lactation: Does not enter breast milk/ use caution

Breast-Feeding Considerations: Based on data from 11 women, glyburide was not detected in breast milk following a single-dose study (5 mg or 10 mg/dose), or a daily-dose study (5 mg/day). Hypoglycemia was not observed in the 3 nursing infants who were wholly breast fed.

Perioperative/Anesthesia/Other Concerns: The possibility of higher doses of sulfonylureas eliciting an increase in cardiovascular events, because of their effects on blocking potassium sensitive ATP channels, has been raised. Longer-term prospective trials of sulfonylurea therapy, such as the UKPDS, do not reveal any increased cardiovascular mortality.

Administration

Oral: Administer with meals at the same time each day. Patients who are anorexic or NPO may need to have their dose held to avoid hypoglycemia.

Related Information

Perioperative Management of the Diabetic Patient *on page 1794*

Glyburide and Metformin (GLYE byoor ide & met FOR min)

U.S. Brand Names Glucovance®

Synonyms Glyburide and Metformin Hydrochloride; Metformin and Glyburide

Pharmacologic Category Antidiabetic Agent, Biguanide; Antidiabetic Agent, Sulfonylurea

Use Initial therapy for management of type 2 diabetes mellitus (noninsulin dependent, NIDDM). Second-line therapy for management of type 2 diabetes (NIDDM) when hyperglycemia cannot be managed with a sulfonylurea or metformin; combination therapy with a thiazolidinedione may be required to achieve additional control.

Mechanism of Action The combination of glyburide and metformin is used to improve glycemic control in patients with type 2 diabetes mellitus by using two different, but complementary, mechanisms of action:

Glyburide: Stimulates insulin release from the pancreatic beta cells; reduces glucose output from the liver; insulin sensitivity is increased at peripheral target sites

Metformin: Decreases hepatic glucose production, decreasing intestinal absorption of glucose and improves insulin sensitivity (increases peripheral glucose uptake and utilization)

Pharmacodynamics/Kinetics

Glucovance®:

Bioavailability: 18% with 2.5 mg glyburide/500 mg metformin dose; 7% with 5 mg glyburide/500 mg metformin dose; bioavailability is greater than that of Micronase® brand of glyburide and therefore not bioequivalent

Time to peak: 2.75 hours when taken with food

Glyburide: See Glyburide monograph.

Metformin: This component of Glucovance® is bioequivalent to metformin coadministration with glyburide.

Contraindications Hypersensitivity to glyburide or other sulfonamides, metformin, or any component of the formulation; renal disease or renal dysfunction (serum creatinine ≥1.5 mg/dL in males or ≥1.4 mg/dL in females, or abnormal creatinine clearance which may also result from conditions such as cardiovascular collapse, acute myocardial infarction, and septicemia); acute or chronic

(Continued)

Glyburide and Metformin *(Continued)*

metabolic acidosis with or without coma (including diabetic ketoacidosis); congestive heart failure requiring pharmacologic treatment

Note: Temporarily discontinue in patients undergoing radiologic studies in which intravascular iodinated contrast materials are utilized.

Warnings/Precautions Age, hepatic and renal impairment are independent risk factors for hypoglycemia. Use with caution in patients with hepatic impairment, malnourished or debilitated conditions, or adrenal or pituitary insufficiency. Use caution in patients with renal impairment. Lactic acidosis is a rare, but potentially severe consequence of therapy with metformin. Withhold therapy in hypoxemia, dehydration, or sepsis. The risk of lactic acidosis is increased in any patient with CHF requiring pharmacologic management. This risk is particularly high during acute or unstable CHF because of the risk of hypoperfusion and hypoxemia.

Metformin is substantially excreted by the kidney. The risk of accumulation and lactic acidosis increases with the degree of impairment of renal function. Patients with renal function below the limit of normal for their age should not receive metformin. In elderly patients, renal function should be monitored regularly; should not be used in any patient ≥80 years of age unless measurement of creatinine clearance verifies normal renal function. Use of concomitant medications that may affect renal function (ie, affect tubular secretion) may also affect metformin disposition. Metformin should be suspended in patients with dehydration and/or prerenal azotemia. Therapy should be suspended for any surgical procedures (resume only after normal intake resumed and normal renal function is verified).Intravascular iodinated contrast materials used for radiologic studies are associated with alteration of renal function and may increase risk of lactic acidosis. Discontinue Glucovance® at the time of or prior to the procedure and withhold for 48 hours subsequent to the procedure; reinstitute only after renal function has been re-evaluated and found to be normal.

Chemical similarities are present among sulfonamides, sulfonylureas, carbonic anhydrase inhibitors, thiazides, and loop diuretics (except ethacrynic acid). Use in patients with sulfonamide allergy is specifically contraindicated in product labeling, however a risk of cross-reaction exists in patients with allergy to any of these compounds; avoid use when previous reaction has been severe.

Product labeling states oral hypoglycemic drugs may be associated with an increased cardiovascular mortality as compared to treatment with diet alone or diet plus insulin. Data to support this association are limited, and several studies, including a large prospective trial (UKPDS), have not supported an association.

Drug Interactions Also see individual agents.

Decreased effect: Drugs that tend to produce hyperglycemia (eg, diuretics, corticosteroids, phenothiazines, thyroid products, estrogens, oral contraceptives, phenytoin, nicotinic acid, sympathomimetics, calcium channel blocking drugs, isoniazid) may lead to a loss of glycemic control

Nutritional/Herbal/Ethanol Interactions

Ethanol: May cause hypoglycemia; incidence of lactic acidosis may be increased; a disulfiram-like reaction characterized by flushing, headache, nausea, vomiting, sweating, or tachycardia has been reported with sulfonylureas; avoid or limit use.

Food: Metformin decreases absorption of vitamin B_{12}. Metformin decreases absorption of folic acid.

Adverse Reactions See individual agents.

Overdosage/Toxicology

Glyburide: Symptoms of overdose include severe hypoglycemia, seizures, cerebral damage, tingling of lips and tongue, nausea, yawning, confusion, agitation, tachycardia, sweating, convulsions, stupor, and coma. Intoxications with sulfonylureas can cause hypoglycemia and are best managed with glucose administration (orally for milder hypoglycemia or by injection in more severe forms).

Metformin: Hypoglycemia (10% of cases) or lactic acidosis (~32% of cases) may occur. Hemodialysis may be used in suspected cases of overdose.

Dosing

Adults: Note: Dose must be individualized. All doses should be taken with a meal. Twice daily dosage should be taken with the morning and evening meals. Dosages expressed as glyburide/metformin components.

Type 2 diabetes: Oral:

No prior treatment with sulfonylurea or metformin: Initial: 1.25 mg/250 mg once daily with a meal; patients with Hb A_{1c} >9% or fasting plasma glucose

(FPG) >200 mg/dL may start with 1.25 mg/250 mg twice daily. Adjustment: Dosage may be increased in increments of 1.25 mg/250 mg, at intervals of not less than 2 weeks; maximum daily dose: 10 mg/2000 mg (limited experience with higher doses)

Previously treated with a sulfonylurea or metformin alone: Initial: 2.5 mg/500 mg or 5 mg/500 mg twice daily; increase in increments no greater than 5 mg/500 mg; maximum daily dose: 20 mg/2000 mg

Note: When switching patients previously on a sulfonylurea and metformin together, do not exceed the daily dose of glyburide (or glyburide equivalent) or metformin.

Combination with thiazolidinedione: May be combined with a thiazolidinedione in patients with an inadequate response to glyburide/metformin therapy, however the risk of hypoglycemia may be increased.

Elderly: Refer to adult dosing. Adjust carefully to renal function. Should not be used in patients ≥80 years of age unless renal function is verified as normal.

Available Dosage Forms Tablet [film coated]:

1.25 mg/250 mg: Glyburide 1.25 mg and metformin hydrochloride 250 mg

2.5 mg/500 mg: Glyburide 2.5 mg and metformin hydrochloride 500 mg

5 mg/500 mg: Glyburide 5 mg and metformin hydrochloride 500 mg

Nursing Guidelines

Assessment: See individual components listed in Related Information. **Pregnancy risk factor B/C** - see Pregnancy Risk Factor for use cautions; benefits of use should outweigh possible risks. Note breast-feeding caution.

Dietary Considerations: May cause GI upset; take with food to decrease GI upset. Dietary modification based on ADA recommendations is a part of therapy. Decreases blood glucose concentration. Hypoglycemia may occur. Must be able to recognize symptoms of hypoglycemia (palpitations, sweaty palms, lightheadedness). Monitor for signs and symptoms of vitamin B_{12} deficiency. Monitor for signs and symptoms of folic acid deficiency.

Patient Education: See individual agents. **Pregnancy/breast-feeding precautions:** Inform prescriber if you are or intend to become pregnant. Consult prescriber if breast-feeding.

Geriatric Considerations: Conservative doses are recommended in the elderly due to potentially decreased renal function. **Do not titrate to maximum dose**. Should not be used in patients ≥80 years of age unless renal function is verified as normal.

Pregnancy Risk Factor: B (manufacturer); C (expert analysis)

Pregnancy Issues: Abnormal blood glucose levels during pregnancy may be associated with an increased incidence of congenital abnormalities. Insulin is the drug of choice for the control of diabetes mellitus during pregnancy. Use glyburide/metformin during pregnancy only if clearly needed.

Glyburide: Crosses the placenta. Hypoglycemia, ear defects reported; other malformations reported but may have been secondary to poor maternal glucose control/diabetes.

Metformin: May partially cross the placenta.

Severe prolonged hypoglycemia has been reported in neonates whose mothers were taking sulfonylureas at the time of delivery. If the decision has been made to use glyburide/metformin during pregnancy, it should be discontinued at least 2 weeks prior to delivery.

Lactation: No data available/use caution

Breast-Feeding Considerations: No data available for glyburide, however, other sulfonylureas are excreted in breast milk. It is possible that hypoglycemia may occur in a nursing infant.

Administration

Oral: All doses should be administered with a meal. Twice-daily dosing should be administered with the morning and evening meals. Patients who are anorexic or NPO may need to have their dose held to avoid hypoglycemia.

Storage: Store at 25°C (77°F).

Related Information

GlyBURIDE *on page 820*
Metformin *on page 1112*

♦ **Glyburide and Metformin Hydrochloride** *see* Glyburide and Metformin *on page 823*

Glycerin (GLIS er in)

U.S. Brand Names Bausch & Lomb® Computer Eye Drops [OTC]; Colace® Adult/Children Suppositories [OTC]; Colace® Infant/Children Suppositories [OTC]; Fleet® Babylax® [OTC]; Fleet® Glycerin Suppositories [OTC]; Fleet® Glycerin Suppositories Maximum Strength [OTC]; Fleet® Liquid Glycerin Suppositories [OTC]; Osmoglyn® [DSC]; Sani-Supp® [OTC]

Synonyms Glycerol

Pharmacologic Category Laxative, Osmotic; Ophthalmic Agent, Miscellaneous

Use Constipation; reduction of intraocular pressure; reduction of corneal edema; glycerin has been administered orally to reduce intracranial pressure

Mechanism of Action Osmotic dehydrating agent which increases osmotic pressure; draws fluid into colon and thus stimulates evacuation

Pharmacodynamics/Kinetics

Onset of action:

Decrease in intraocular pressure: Oral: 10-30 minutes

Reduction of intracranial pressure: Oral: 10-60 minutes

Constipation: Suppository: 15-30 minutes

Peak effect:

Decrease in intraocular pressure: Oral: 60-90 minutes

Reduction of intracranial pressure: Oral: 60-90 minutes

Duration:

Decrease in intraocular pressure: Oral: 4-8 hours

Reduction of intracranial pressure: Oral: ~2-3 hours

Absorption: Oral: Well absorbed; Rectal: Poorly absorbed

Half-life elimination, serum: 30-45 minutes

Adverse Reactions Frequency not defined.

Central nervous system: Dizziness, headache

Endocrine & metabolic: Hyperglycemia

Gastrointestinal: Diarrhea, nausea, tenesmus, vomiting

Local: Pain, rectal irritation, cramping pain

Miscellaneous: Thirst

Dosing

Adults & Elderly:

Constipation: Rectal: 1 adult suppository 1-2 times/day as needed or 5-15 mL as an enema

Reduction of intracranial pressure: Oral: 1.5 g/kg/day divided every 4 hours; 1 g/kg/dose every 6 hours has also been used

Reduction of corneal edema: Ophthalmic solution: Instill 1-2 drops in eye(s) prior to examination OR for lubricant effect, instill 1-2 drops in eye(s) every 3-4 hours

Reduction of intraocular pressure: Oral: 1-1.8 g/kg 1-1½ hours preoperatively; additional doses may be administered at 5-hour intervals

Pediatrics:

Constipation: Rectal:

Children <6 years: 1 infant suppository 1-2 times/day as needed or 2-5 mL as an enema

Children >6 years: Refer to adult dosing.

Reduction of intraocular pressure: Refer to adult dosing.

Reduction of intracranial pressure: Refer to adult dosing.

Reduction of corneal edema: Refer to adult dosing.

Available Dosage Forms [DSC] = Discontinued product

Solution, ophthalmic, sterile (Bausch & Lomb® Computer Eye Drops): 1% (15 mL) [contains benzalkonium chloride]

Solution, oral (Osmoglyn®): 50% (220 mL) [lime flavor] [DSC]

Solution, rectal:

Fleet® Babylax®: 2.3 g/2.3 mL (4 mL) [6 units per box]

Fleet® Liquid Glycerin Suppositories: 5.6 g/5.5 mL (7.5 mL) [4 units per box]

Suppository, rectal: 82.5% (12s, 25s) [pediatric size]; 82.5% (12s, 24s, 25s, 50s, 100s) [adult size]

Colace® Adult/Children: 2.1 g (12s, 24s, 48s, 100s)

Colace® Infant/Children: 1.2 g (12s, 24s)

Fleet® Glycerin Suppositories: 1 g (12s) [pediatric size]; 2g (12s, 24s, 50s) [adult size]

Fleet® Glycerin Suppositories Maximum Strength: 3g (18s) [adult size]

Sani-Supp®: 82.5% (10s, 25s) [pediatric size]; 82.5% (10s, 25s, 50s) [adult size]

Nursing Guidelines

Patient Education: Do not use if experiencing abdominal pain, nausea, or vomiting

Pregnancy Risk Factor: C

- Glycerol *see* Glycerin *on page 826*
- Glycerol Guaiacolate *see* Guaifenesin *on page 834*
- Glyceryl Trinitrate *see* Nitroglycerin *on page 1234*

Glycopyrrolate (glye koe PYE roe late)

U.S. Brand Names Robinul®; Robinul® Forte

Synonyms Glycopyrronium Bromide

Pharmacologic Category Anticholinergic Agent

Use Inhibit salivation and excessive secretions of the respiratory tract preoperatively; reversal of neuromuscular blockade; control of upper airway secretions; adjunct in treatment of peptic ulcer

Mechanism of Action Blocks the action of acetylcholine at parasympathetic sites in smooth muscle, secretory glands, and the CNS

Pharmacodynamics/Kinetics

Onset of action: Oral: 50 minutes; I.M.: 15-30 minutes; I.V.: ~1 minute

Peak effect: Oral: ~1 hour; I.M.: 30-45 minutes

Duration: Vagal effect: 2-3 hours; Inhibition of salivation: Up to 7 hours; Anticholinergic: Oral: 8-12 hours

Absorption: Oral: Poor and erratic

Distribution: V_d: 0.2-0.62 L/kg

Metabolism: Hepatic (minimal)

Bioavailability: ~10%

Half-life elimination: Infants: 22-130 minutes; Children 19-99 minutes; Adults: ~30-75 minutes

Excretion: Urine (as unchanged drug, I.M.: 80%, I.V.: 85%); bile (as unchanged drug)

Contraindications Hypersensitivity to glycopyrrolate or any component of the formulation; severe ulcerative colitis, toxic megacolon complicating ulcerative colitis, paralytic ileus, obstructive disease of GI tract, intestinal atony in the elderly or debilitated patient; unstable cardiovascular status in acute hemorrhage; narrow-angle glaucoma; acute hemorrhage; tachycardia; obstructive uropathy; myasthenia gravis

Warnings/Precautions Use caution in elderly, patients with autonomic neuropathy, hepatic or renal disease, ulcerative colitis (may precipitate/aggravate toxic megacolon), hyperthyroidism, CAD, CHF, arrhythmias, tachycardia, BPH, or hiatal hernia with reflux. Use of anticholinergics in gastric ulcer treatment may cause a delay in gastric emptying due to antral statis. Caution should be used in individuals demonstrating decreased pigmentation (skin and iris coloration, dark versus light) since there has been some evidence that these individuals have an enhanced sensitivity to the anticholinergic response. May cause drowsiness, eye sensitivity to light, or blurred vision; caution should be used when performing tasks which require mental alertness, such as driving. The risk of heat stroke with this medication may be increased during exercise or hot weather. Infants, patients with Down syndrome, and children with spastic paralysis or brain damage may be hypersensitive to antimuscarine effects. Product packaging may contain latex. Injection contains benzyl alcohol (associated with gasping syndrome in neonates). Not recommended for use in children <12 years of age for the management of peptic ulcer or <16 years for preanesthetic use.

Drug Interactions

Anticholinergic agents: Effects of other anticholinergic agents or medications with anticholinergic activity may be increased by glycopyrrolate.

Potassium chloride: Severity of potassium chloride-induced gastrointestinal lesions (when potassium is given in a wax matrix formulation, eg, Klor-Con®) may be increased by glycopyrrolate.

Pramlinitide: May enhance the anticholinergic effects of anticholinergics. These effects are specific to the GI tract.

Adverse Reactions Frequency not defined. **Note:** Includes adverse effects which may occur as an extension of the pharmacologic action of anticholinergics (including glycopyrrolate) and adverse effects reported postmarketing with glycopyrrolate.

Cardiovascular: Arrhythmias, cardiac arrest, heart block, hyper-/hypotension, malignant hyperthermia, palpitation, QT_c interval prolongation, tachycardia

(Continued)

Glycopyrrolate *(Continued)*

Central nervous system: Confusion, dizziness, drowsiness, excitement, headache, insomnia, nervousness, seizures

Dermatologic: Dry skin, pruritus, sensitivity to light increased

Endocrine & metabolic: Lactation suppression

Gastrointestinal: Bloated feeling, constipation, loss of taste, nausea, vomiting, xerostomia

Genitourinary: Impotence, urinary hesitancy, urinary retention

Local: Irritation at injection site

Neuromuscular & skeletal: Weakness

Ocular: Blurred vision, cycloplegia, mydriasis, ocular tension increased, photophobia, sensitivity to light increased

Respiratory: Respiratory depression

Miscellaneous: Anaphylactoid reactions, diaphoresis decreased, hypersensitivity reactions

Overdosage/Toxicology

Symptoms of overdose include blurred vision, urinary retention, tachycardia, and absent bowel sounds. For peripheral adverse effects, a quaternary ammonium anticholinesterase, such as neostigmine methylsulfate, may be given I.V. in increments of 0.25 mg in adults; may repeat every 5-10 minutes (up to a maximum of 2.5 mg) based upon decrease in heart rate and return of bowel sounds. For overdose exhibiting CNS symptoms (eg, excitement, restlessness, convulsions, psychotic behavior), physostigmine 0.5-2 mg I.V. slowly, may be given and repeated as necessary, up to 5 mg. Proportionally smaller doses should be used for pediatric patients. Artificial respiration should be given to individuals experiencing a neuromuscular or curare-like effect which could lead to muscular weakness or possible paralysis. Additional care should be symptomatic and supportive.

Dosing

Adults & Elderly:

Reduction of secretions: I.M.:

Preoperative: I.M.: 4 mcg/kg 30-60 minutes before procedure

Intraoperative: I.V.: 0.1 mg repeated as needed at 2- to 3-minute intervals

Reversal of neuromuscular blockade: I.V.: 0.2 mg for each 1 mg of neostigmine or 5 mg of pyridostigmine administered or 5-15 mcg/kg glycopyrrolate with 25-70 mcg/kg of neostigmine or 0.1-0.3 mg/kg of pyridostigmine (agents usually administered simultaneously, but glycopyrrolate may be administered first if bradycardia is present)

Peptic ulcer:

Oral: 1-2 mg 2-3 times/day

I.M., I.V.: 0.1-0.2 mg 3-4 times/day

Pediatrics:

Reduction of secretions:

Preoperative: I.M.:

<2 years: 4-9 mcg/kg 30-60 minutes before procedure

>2 years: 4 mcg/kg 30-60 minutes before procedure

Intraoperative: I.V.: 4 mcg/kg not to exceed 0.1 mg; repeat at 2- to 3-minute intervals as needed.

Chronic:

Oral: 40-100 mcg/kg/dose 3-4 times/day

I.M., I.V.: 4-10 mcg/kg/dose every 3-4 hours; maximum: 0.2 mg/dose or 0.8 mg/24 hours

Reversal of neuromuscular blockade: Refer to adult dosing.

Available Dosage Forms

Injection, solution (Robinul®): 0.2 mg/mL (1 mL, 2 mL, 5 mL, 20 mL) [contains benzyl alcohol]

Tablet:

Robinul®: 1 mg

Robinul® Forte: 2 mg

Nursing Guidelines

Assessment: Assess potential for interactions with other prescriptions, OTC medications, or herbal products patient may be taking (eg, anything that may add to anticholinergic effects). Assess therapeutic effectiveness and adverse response (eg, excessive dryness of eyes, nose, mouth, throat). Teach patient proper use (self-administered), possible side effects/appropriate interventions, and adverse symptoms to report.

Patient Education: Do not take any new medication during therapy unless approved by prescriber. Take as directed before meals; do not increase dose and do not discontinue without consulting prescriber. Void before taking medication. You may experience dizziness or blurred vision (use caution when driving or engaging in tasks that require alertness until response to drug is known); dry mouth (sucking on lozenges may help); photosensitivity (wear dark glasses in bright sunlight); decreased ability to sweat (use caution in hot weather or hot rooms or engaging in strenuous activity); or impotence (temporary). Report excessive and persistent anticholinergic effects (blurred vision, headache, flushing, tachycardia, nervousness, constipation, dizziness, insomnia, mental confusion or excitement, dry mouth, altered taste perception, dysphagia, palpitations, bradycardia, urinary hesitancy or retention, impotence, decreased sweating). **Breast-feeding precaution:** Consult prescriber if breast-feeding.

Geriatric Considerations: Anticholinergic agents are generally not well tolerated in the elderly and their use should be avoided when possible.

Pregnancy Risk Factor: B

Lactation: Excretion in breast milk unknown/use caution

Breast-Feeding Considerations: May suppress lactation

Administration

I.V.: Administer at a rate of 0.2 mg over 1-2 minutes.

Compatibility: Stable in D_5½NS, D_5W, $D_{10}W$, LR, NS

Compatibility in syringe: Incompatible with chloramphenicol, dexamethasone sodium phosphate, diazepam, dimenhydrinate, methohexital, pentazocine, pentobarbital, secobarbital, sodium bicarbonate, thiopental

Compatibility when admixed: Incompatible with methylprednisolone sodium succinate

Storage: Store at 20°C to 25°C (68°F to 77°F).

- Glycopyrronium Bromide *see* Glycopyrrolate *on page 827*
- Glycosum *see* Dextrose *on page 511*
- Glydiazinamide *see* GlipiZIDE *on page 816*
- Glynase® PresTab® *see* GlyBURIDE *on page 820*
- Gly-Oxide® [OTC] *see* Carbamide Peroxide *on page 311*
- GM-CSF *see* Sargramostim *on page 1509*
- Gonak™ [OTC] *see* Hydroxypropyl Methylcellulose *on page 883*
- Gonioscopic Ophthalmic Solution *see* Hydroxypropyl Methylcellulose *on page 883*
- Goniosoft™ *see* Hydroxypropyl Methylcellulose *on page 883*
- Goniosol® [OTC] [DSC] *see* Hydroxypropyl Methylcellulose *on page 883*

Goserelin (GOE se rel in)

U.S. Brand Names Zoladex®

Synonyms D-Ser(Bu^t)^6,Azgly^{10}-LHRH; Goserelin Acetate; ICI-118630; NSC-606864

Pharmacologic Category Gonadotropin Releasing Hormone Agonist

Use Palliative treatment of advanced breast cancer and carcinoma of the prostate; treatment of endometriosis, including pain relief and reduction of endometriotic lesions; endometrial thinning agent as part of treatment for dysfunctional uterine bleeding

Mechanism of Action Goserelin is a synthetic analog of luteinizing-hormone-releasing hormone (LHRH). Following an initial increase in luteinizing hormone (LH) and follicle stimulating hormone (FSH), chronic administration of goserelin results in a sustained suppression of pituitary gonadotropins. Serum testosterone falls to levels comparable to surgical castration. The exact mechanism of this effect is unknown, but may be related to changes in the control of LH or down-regulation of LH receptors.

Pharmacodynamics/Kinetics Note: Data reported using the 1-month implant.

Absorption: SubQ: Rapid and can be detected in serum in 10 minutes

Distribution: V_d: Male: 44.1 L; Female: 20.3 L

Time to peak, serum: SubQ: Male: 12-15 days, Female: 8-22 days

Half-life elimination: SubQ: Male: ~4 hours, Female: ~2 hours; Renal impairment: Male: 12 hours

Excretion: Urine (90%)

Contraindications Hypersensitivity to goserelin or any component of the formulation; pregnancy (or potential to become pregnant); breast-feeding

(Continued)

Goserelin *(Continued)*

Warnings/Precautions Transient worsening of signs and symptoms (tumor flare) may develop during the first few weeks of treatment. Urinary tract obstruction or spinal cord compression have been reported when used for prostate cancer; closely observe patients for weakness, paresthesias, and urinary tract obstruction in first few weeks of therapy. Decreased bone density has been reported in women and may be irreversible; use caution if other risk factors are present; evaluate and institute preventative treatment if necessary. Rare cases of pituitary apoplexy (frequently secondary to pituitary adenoma) have been observed with leuprolide administration (onset from 1 hour to usually <2 weeks); may present as sudden headache, vomiting, visual or mental status changes, and infrequently cardiovascular collapse; immediate medical attention required. Safety and efficacy have not been established in pediatric patients.

Lab Interactions Serum alkaline phosphatase, serum acid phosphatase, serum testosterone, serum LH and FSH, serum estradiol

Adverse Reactions Percentages reported in males with prostatic carcinoma and females with endometriosis using the 1-month implant:

>10%:

- Central nervous system: Headache (female 75%, male 1% to 5%), emotional lability (female 60%), depression (female 54%, male 1% to 5%), pain (female 17%, male 8%), insomnia (female 11%, male 5%)
- Endocrine & metabolic: Hot flashes (female 96%, male 62%), sexual dysfunction (21%), erections decreased (18%), libido decreased (female 61%), breast enlargement (female 18%)
- Genitourinary: Lower urinary symptoms (male 13%), vaginitis (75%), dyspareunia (female 14%)
- Miscellaneous: Diaphoresis (female 45%, male 6%); infection (female 13%)

1% to 10%:

- Cardiovascular: CHF (male 5%), arrhythmia, cerebrovascular accident, hypertension, MI, peripheral vascular disorder, chest pain, palpitation, tachycardia, edema
- Central nervous system: Lethargy (male 8%), dizziness (female 6%, male 5%), abnormal thinking, anxiety, chills, fever, malaise, migraine, somnolence
- Dermatologic: Rash (female >1%, male 6%), alopecia, bruising, dry skin, skin discoloration
- Endocrine & metabolic: Breast pain (female 7%), breast swelling/tenderness (male 1% to 5%), dysmenorrhea, gout, hyperglycemia
- Gastrointestinal: Anorexia (female >1%, male 5%), nausea (male 5%), constipation, diarrhea, flatulence, dyspepsia, ulcer, vomiting, weight increased, xerostomia
- Genitourinary: Renal insufficiency, urinary frequency, urinary obstruction, urinary tract infection, vaginal hemorrhage
- Hematologic: Anemia, hemorrhage
- Neuromuscular & skeletal: Arthralgia, bone mineral density decreased (female; ~4% decrease in 6 months), joint disorder, paresthesia
- Ocular: Amblyopia, dry eyes
- Respiratory: Upper respiratory tract infection (male 7%), COPD (male 5%), pharyngitis (female 5%), bronchitis, cough, epistaxis, rhinitis, sinusitis
- Miscellaneous: Allergic reaction

Postmarketing and/or case reports: Pituitary apoplexy

Overdosage/Toxicology Symptomatic management

Dosing

Adults & Elderly:

Prostate cancer: SubQ:

Monthly implant: 3.6 mg injected into upper abdomen every 28 days

3-month implant: 10.8 mg injected into the upper abdominal wall every 12 weeks

Breast cancer, endometriosis, endometrial thinning: SubQ: Monthly implant: 3.6 mg injected into upper abdomen every 28 days

Note: For breast cancer, treatment may continue indefinitely; for endometriosis, it is recommended that duration of treatment not exceed 6 months. Only 1-2 doses are recommended for endometrial thinning.

Available Dosage Forms

Injection, solution, 1-month implant [disposable syringe; single-dose]: 3.6 mg [with 16-gauge hypodermic needle]

Injection, solution, 3-month implant [disposable syringe; single-dose]: 10.8 mg [with 14-gauge hypodermic needle]

Nursing Guidelines

Assessment: Assess potential for interactions with other prescriptions, OTC medications, or herbal products patient may be taking. Assess therapeutic effectiveness and adverse response periodically during therapy. Teach patient proper use, possible side effects/appropriate interventions, and adverse symptoms to report. **Pregnancy risk factor X:** Determine that patient is not pregnant before beginning treatment. Do not give to women of childbearing age unless female is capable of complying with contraceptive measures 1 month prior to therapy, during therapy, and at least 12 weeks following therapy. Instruct patient in appropriate contraceptive measures.

Patient Education: Do not take any new medication during therapy unless approved by prescriber. This drug must be implanted under the skin of your abdomen every 28 days; it is important to maintain appointment schedule. Males or females, you may experience systemic hot flashes (layered, cool clothes may help); headache (consult prescriber for approved analgesic); constipation (increased bulk and water in diet or stool softener may help); sexual dysfunction (decreased libido, males: decreased erection, females: vaginal dryness); or bone pain (consult prescriber for approved analgesic). Symptoms may worsen temporarily during first weeks of therapy. Report chest pain, palpitations, or respiratory difficulty; swelling of extremities; unusual persistent nausea, vomiting, or constipation; chest pain or respiratory difficulty; unresolved dizziness; or skin rash. **Pregnancy/breast-feeding precautions:** Inform prescriber if you are pregnant; do not get pregnant 1 month before, during, or for 1 month following therapy. Consult prescriber for instruction on appropriate contraceptive measures. This drug may cause severe fetal defects. Do not donate blood during or for 1 month following therapy (same reason). Do not breast-feed.

Pregnancy Risk Factor: X (endometriosis, endometrial thinning); D (advanced breast cancer)

Pregnancy Issues: Goserelin has been found to be teratogenic and increases pregnancy loss in animal studies. Women of childbearing potential should avoid pregnancy. Pregnancy must be ruled out prior to treatment. Use of nonhormonal contraception should be used during therapy and following discontinuation until the return of menses (or for at least 12 weeks).

Lactation: Enters breast milk/contraindicated

Administration

Storage: Zoladex® should be stored at room temperature not to exceed 25°C (77°F). Protect from light. Should be dispensed in a lightproof bag.

- **Goserelin Acetate** *see* Goserelin *on page 829*
- **GP 47680** *see* Oxcarbazepine *on page 1278*
- **GR38032R** *see* Ondansetron *on page 1268*
- **Gramicidin, Neomycin, and Polymyxin B** *see* Neomycin, Polymyxin B, and Gramicidin *on page 1212*

Granisetron (gra NI se tron)

U.S. Brand Names Kytril®

Synonyms BRL 43694

Pharmacologic Category Antiemetic; Selective 5-HT_3 Receptor Antagonist

Medication Safety Issues

Sound-alike/look-alike issues:

Granisetron may be confused with dolasetron, ondansetron, palonosetron

Use Prophylaxis of nausea and vomiting associated with emetogenic chemotherapy and radiation therapy, (including total body irradiation and fractionated abdominal radiation); prophylaxis and treatment of postoperative nausea and vomiting (PONV)

Generally **not** recommended for treatment of existing chemotherapy-induced emesis (CIE) or for prophylaxis of nausea from agents with a low emetogenic potential.

Mechanism of Action Selective 5-HT_3-receptor antagonist, blocking serotonin, both peripherally on vagal nerve terminals and centrally in the chemoreceptor trigger zone

Pharmacodynamics/Kinetics

Duration: Generally up to 24 hours

Absorption: Tablets and oral solution are bioequivalent

Distribution: V_d: 2-4 L/kg; widely throughout body

Protein binding: 65%

(Continued)

Granisetron *(Continued)*

Metabolism: Hepatic via N-demethylation, oxidation, and conjugation; some metabolites may have 5-HT_3 antagonist activity

Half-life elimination: Terminal: 5-9 hours

Excretion: Urine (12% as unchanged drug, 48% to 49% as metabolites); feces (34% to 38% as metabolites)

Contraindications Previous hypersensitivity to granisetron, other 5-HT_3 receptor antagonists, or any component of the formulation

Warnings/Precautions Chemotherapy-related emesis: **Granisetron should be used on a scheduled basis, not on an "as needed" (PRN) basis**, since data support the use of this drug in the prevention of nausea and vomiting and not in the rescue of nausea and vomiting. Granisetron should be used only in the first 24-48 hours of receiving chemotherapy or radiation. Data do not support any increased efficacy of granisetron in delayed nausea and vomiting. May be prescribed for patients who are refractory to or have severe adverse reactions to standard antiemetic therapy or young patients (ie, <45 years of age who are more likely to develop extrapyramidal symptoms to high-dose metoclopramide) who are to receive highly emetogenic chemotherapeutic agents. Should not be prescribed for chemotherapeutic agents with a low emetogenic potential (eg, bleomycin, busulfan, etoposide, 5-fluorouracil, vinblastine, vincristine).

Routine prophylaxis for PONV is not recommended. In patients where nausea and vomiting must be avoided postoperatively, administer to all patients even when expected incidence of nausea and vomiting is low. Use caution following abdominal surgery or in chemotherapy-induced nausea and vomiting; may mask progressive ileus or gastric distention. Use caution in patients with liver disease or in pregnancy. Safety and efficacy in children <2 years of age have not been established. Injection contains benzyl alcohol (1 mg/mL) and should not be used in neonates.

Drug Interactions Substrate of CYP3A4 (minor)

Apomorphine: Due to reports of profound hypotension during concomitant therapy with other 5-HT3 antagonists, the manufacturer of apomorphine contraindicates its use with granisetron.

Nutritional/Herbal/Ethanol Interactions Herb/Nutraceutical: St John's wort may decrease granisetron levels.

Adverse Reactions

>10%:

- Central nervous system: Headache (9% to 21%)
- Gastrointestinal: Constipation (3% to 18%)
- Neuromuscular & skeletal: Weakness (5% to 18%)

1% to 10%:

- Cardiovascular: Hypertension (1% to 2%)
- Central nervous system: Pain (10%), fever (3% to 9%), dizziness (4% to 5%), insomnia (<2% to 5%), somnolence (1% to 4%), anxiety (2%), agitation (<2%), CNS stimulation (<2%)
- Dermatologic: Rash (1%)
- Gastrointestinal: Diarrhea (3% to 9%), abdominal pain (4% to 6%), dyspepsia (3% to 6%), taste perversion (2%)
- Hepatic: Liver enzymes increased (5% to 6%)
- Renal: Oliguria (2%)
- Respiratory: Cough (2%)
- Miscellaneous: Infection (3%)

<1% (Limited to important or life-threatening): Agitation, allergic reactions; anaphylaxis (including hypotension, dyspnea, urticaria); angina, arrhythmias, atrial fibrillation, extrapyramidal syndrome, hot flashes, hypotension, hypersensitivity, syncope

Overdosage/Toxicology Overdoses of up to 38.5 mg have been reported without symptoms or with only slight headache. In the event of an overdose, treatment should be symptomatic and supportive.

Dosing

Adults & Elderly:

Prophylaxis of chemotherapy-related emesis:

Oral: 2 mg once daily up to 1 hour before chemotherapy or 1 mg twice daily; the first 1 mg dose should be given up to 1 hour before chemotherapy.

I.V.:

Within U.S.: 10 mcg/kg/dose (maximum: 1 mg/dose) given 30 minutes prior to chemotherapy; for some drugs (eg, carboplatin, cyclophosphamide) with a later onset of emetic action, 10 mcg/kg every 12 hours may be necessary.

Outside U.S.: 40 mcg/kg/dose (or 3 mg/dose); maximum: 9 mg/24 hours

Breakthrough: Granisetron has not been shown to be effective in teminating nausea or vomiting once it occurs and should not be used for this purpose.

Prophylaxis of radiation therapy-associated emesis: Oral: 2 mg once daily given 1 hour before radiation therapy.

Postoperative nausea and vomiting (PONV): I.V.:

Prevention: 1 mg given undiluted over 30 seconds; administer before induction of anesthesia or immediately before reversal of anesthesia

Treatment: 1 mg given undiluted over 30 seconds

Pediatrics: Prophylaxis associated with cancer chemotherapy: Children >2 years: Refer to adult dosing.

Renal Impairment: No dosage adjustment required.

Hepatic Impairment: Kinetic studies in patients with hepatic impairment showed that total clearance was approximately halved; however, standard doses were very well tolerated, and dose adjustments are not necessary.

Available Dosage Forms

Injection, solution: 1 mg/mL (1 mL, 4 mL) [contains benzyl alcohol]

Injection, solution [preservative free]: 0.1 mg/mL (1 mL)

Solution, oral: 2 mg/10 mL (30 mL) [contains sodium benzoate; orange flavor]

Tablet: 1 mg

Nursing Guidelines

Assessment: See Contraindications, Warnings/Precautions, Dosing, and Administration for use cautions. Blood pressure and cardiac status should be monitored. Assess therapeutic effectiveness (antiemetic) and adverse response (eg, acute headache - see Adverse Reactions) periodically during therapy. Teach patient possible side effects/appropriate interventions and adverse symptoms to report (see Patient Education). Note breast-feeding caution.

Patient Education: This drug will be administered on days when you receive chemotherapy to reduce nausea and vomiting. If outpatient chemotherapy, you may be given oral medication to take after return home; take as directed. May also be given to prevent or treat nausea and vomiting after surgery; take as directed. You may experience drowsiness (use caution when driving); persistent or acute headache (request analgesic from prescriber); or nausea (frequent mouth care, chewing gum, or sucking on lozenges may help). Report unrelieved headache, fever, diarrhea, or constipation. **Breast-feeding precaution:** Consult prescriber if breast-feeding.

Geriatric Considerations: Clinical trials with patients older than 65 years of age are limited; however, the data indicates that safety and efficacy are similar to that observed in younger adults. No adjustment in dose necessary for elderly.

Pregnancy Risk Factor: B

Pregnancy Issues: There are no adequate or well-controlled studies in pregnant women. Teratogenic effects were not observed in animal studies. Injection (1 mg/mL strength) contains benzyl alcohol which may cross the placenta. Use only if benefit exceeds the risk.

Lactation: Excretion in breast milk unknown/use caution

Administration

Oral: Doses should be given up to 1 hour prior to initiation of chemotherapy/radiation

I.V.: Administer I.V. push over 30 seconds or as a 5-10 minute-infusion

Prevention of PONV: Administer before induction of anesthesia or immediately before reversal of anesthesia.

Treatment of PONV: Administer undiluted over 30 seconds.

Compatibility: Stable in D_5½NS, D_5NS, D_5W, NS, bacteriostatic water

Y-site administration: Incompatible with amphotericin B

Storage:

I.V.: Store at 15°C to 30°C (59°F to 86°F). Protect from light. Do not freeze vials. Stable when mixed in NS or D_5W for 7 days under refrigeration and for 3 days at room temperature.

(Continued)

Granisetron *(Continued)*

Oral: Store tablet or oral solution at 15°C to 30°C (59°F to 86°F). Protect from light.

Related Information

Postoperative Nausea and Vomiting *on page 1807*

♦ Granulocyte Colony Stimulating Factor *see* Filgrastim *on page 726*

♦ Granulocyte Colony Stimulating Factor (PEG Conjugate) *see* Pegfilgrastim *on page 1320*

♦ Granulocyte-Macrophage Colony Stimulating Factor *see* Sargramostim *on page 1509*

♦ Guaifen-C *see* Guaifenesin and Codeine *on page 835*

Guaifenesin (gwye FEN e sin)

U.S. Brand Names Allfen Jr; Diabetic Tussin® EX [OTC]; Ganidin NR; Guiatuss™ [OTC]; Humibid® *e* [OTC]; Iophen NR; Mucinex® [OTC]; Naldecon Senior EX® [OTC] [DSC]; Organ-1 NR; Organidin® NR; Phanasin [OTC]; Phanasin® Diabetic Choice [OTC]; Q-Tussin [OTC]; Robitussin® [OTC]; Scot-Tussin® Expectorant [OTC]; Siltussin DAS [OTC]; Siltussin SA [OTC]; Tussin [OTC]; Vicks® Casero™ [OTC]

Synonyms GG; Glycerol Guaiacolate

Pharmacologic Category Expectorant

Medication Safety Issues

Sound-alike/look-alike issues:

Guaifenesin may be confused with guanfacine
Mucinex® may be confused with Mucomyst®
Naldecon® may be confused with Nalfon®

Use Help loosen phlegm and thin bronchial secretions to make coughs more productive

Mechanism of Action Thought to act as an expectorant by irritating the gastric mucosa and stimulating respiratory tract secretions, thereby increasing respiratory fluid volumes and decreasing mucus viscosity

Pharmacodynamics/Kinetics

Absorption: Well absorbed
Half-life elimination: ~1 hour
Excretion: Urine (as unchanged drug and metabolites)

Contraindications Hypersensitivity to guaifenesin or any component of the formulation

Warnings/Precautions Not for persistent cough such as occurs with smoking, asthma, chronic bronchitis, or emphysema or cough accompanied by excessive secretions. When used for self-medication (OTC), contact healthcare provider if needed for >7 days or for a cough with a fever, rash, or persistent headache.

Lab Interactions Possible color interference with determination of 5-HIAA and VMA; discontinue 48 hours prior to test

Adverse Reactions Frequency not defined.

Central nervous system: Dizziness, drowsiness, headache
Dermatologic: Rash
Endocrine & metabolic: Uric acid levels decreased
Gastrointestinal: Nausea, vomiting, stomach pain

Postmarketing and/or case reports: Kidney stone formation (with consumption of large quantities)

Overdosage/Toxicology Symptoms of overdose include vomiting, lethargy, coma, and respiratory depression. Treatment is supportive.

Dosing

Adults & Elderly:

Cough (expectorant): Oral: 200-400 mg every 4 hours to a maximum of 2.4 g/day

Extended release tablet: 600-1200 mg every 12 hours, not to exceed 2.4 g/day

Pediatrics:

Cough (expectorant): Oral: Children:

6 months to 2 years: 25-50 mg every 4 hours, not to exceed 300 mg/day
2-5 years: 50-100 mg every 4 hours, not to exceed 600 mg/day
6-11 years: 100-200 mg every 4 hours, not to exceed 1.2 g/day
>12 years: Refer to adult dosing.

Available Dosage Forms [DSC] = Discontinued product

Liquid: 100 mg/5 mL (120 mL, 480 mL)
Diabetic Tussin EX®: 100 mg/5 mL (120 mL) [alcohol free, sugar free, dye free; contains phenylalanine 8.4 mg/5 mL]
Ganidin NR: 100 mg/5 mL (480 mL) [raspberry flavor]
Iophen NR: 100 mg/5 mL (480 mL)
Naldecon Senior EX®: 200 mg/5 mL (120 mL) [alcohol free, sugar free; contains sodium benzoate] [DSC]
Organidin® NR: 100 mg/5 mL (480 mL) [contains sodium benzoate; raspberry flavor]
Q-Tussin: 100 mg/5 mL (120 mL, 240 mL, 480 mL, 3840 mL) [alcohol free; cherry flavor]
Siltussin DAS: 100 mg/5 mL (120 mL) [alcohol free, dye free, sugar free; strawberry flavor]
Syrup: 100 mg/5 mL (120 mL, 480 mL)
Guiatuss™: 100 mg/5 mL (120 mL, 480 mL) [alcohol free; fruit-mint flavor]
Phanasin: 100 mg/5 mL (120 mL, 240 mL) [alcohol free, sugar free; mint flavor]
Phanasin® Diabetic Choice: 100 mg/5 mL (120 mL) [alcohol free, sugar free; mint flavor]
Robitussin®: 100 mg/5 mL (5 mL, 10 mL, 15 mL, 30 mL, 120 mL, 240 mL, 480 mL) [alcohol free; contains sodium benzoate]
Scot-Tussin® Expectorant: 100 mg/5 mL (120 mL) [alcohol free, dye free, sugar free; contains benzoic acid; grape flavor]
Siltussin SA: 100 mg/5 mL (120 mL, 240 mL, 480 mL) [alcohol free, sugar free; strawberry flavor]
Tussin: 100 mg/5 mL (120 mL, 240 mL)
Vicks® Casero™: 100 mg/6.25 mL (120 mL, 480 mL) [contains phenylalanine 5.5 mg/12.5 mL, sodium 32 mg/12.5 mL, and sodium benzoate; honey menthol flavor]
Syrup, oral drops (Phanasin®): 50 mg/mL (50 mL) [alcohol free, sugar free; fruit flavor]
Tablet: 200 mg
Allfen Jr: 400 mg [dye free]
Humibid® *e*: 400 mg
Organ-1 NR, Organidin® NR: 200 mg
Tablet, extended release (Mucinex®): 600 mg

Nursing Guidelines

Assessment: Assess effectiveness of therapy and adverse reactions (see Adverse Reactions) at beginning of therapy and periodically with long-term use. Teach patient appropriate use, interventions to reduce side effects, and adverse symptoms to report (see Patient Education). Note breast-feeding caution.

Dietary Considerations:
Diabetic Tussin® EX contains phenylalanine 8.4 mg/5 mL.
Vicks® Casero™ contains phenylalanine 5.5 mg/12.5 mL and sodium 32 mg/12.5 mL.

Patient Education: Inform prescriber of all prescriptions, OTC medications, or herbal products you are taking, and any allergies you have. Do not take any new medication during therapy without consulting prescriber. Take as prescribed; do not exceed prescribed dose or frequency. Do not chew or crush extended release tablet. Maintain adequate hydration (2-3 L/day of fluids) unless instructed to restrict fluid intake. You may experience some drowsiness (use caution when driving or engaging in tasks requiring alertness until response to drug is known). Report excessive drowsiness, respiratory difficulty, or lack of improvement or worsening of condition. **Pregnancy/breast-feeding precautions:** Inform prescriber if you are or intend to become pregnant. Consult prescriber if breast-feeding.

Pregnancy Risk Factor: C

Lactation: Excretion in breast milk unknown/use caution

Administration

Oral: Do not crush, chew, or break extended release tablets. Administer with a full glass of water.

♦ Guaifenesin AC *see* Guaifenesin and Codeine *on page 835*

Guaifenesin and Codeine (gwye FEN e sin & KOE deen)

U.S. Brand Names Brontex®; Cheracol®; Cheratussin AC; Diabetic Tussin C®; Gani-Tuss® NR; Guaifen-C; Guaifenesin AC; Guaituss AC®; Iophen-C NR;
(Continued)

Guaifenesin and Codeine *(Continued)*

Kolephrin® #1; Mytussin® AC; Robafen® AC; Romilar® AC; Tussi-Organidin® NR; Tussi-Organidin® S-NR

Synonyms Codeine and Guaifenesin

Pharmacologic Category Antitussive; Cough Preparation; Expectorant

Medication Safety Issues

Sound-alike/look-alike issues:

Halotussin® may be confused with Halotestin®

Use Temporary control of cough due to minor throat and bronchial irritation

Mechanism of Action

Guaifenesin is thought to act as an expectorant by irritating the gastric mucosa and stimulating respiratory tract secretions, thereby increasing respiratory fluid volumes and decreasing phlegm viscosity

Codeine is an antitussive that controls cough by depressing the medullary cough center

Pharmacodynamics/Kinetics See individual agents.

Contraindications

Based on **guaifenesin** component: Hypersensitivity to guaifenesin or any component of the formulation

Based on **codeine** component: Hypersensitivity to codeine or any component of the formulation

Warnings/Precautions

Based on **guaifenesin** component: Not for persistent cough such as occurs with smoking, asthma, or emphysema or cough accompanied by excessive secretions

Based on **codeine** component: Use with caution in patients with hypersensitivity reactions to other phenanthrene derivative opioid agonists (morphine, hydrocodone, hydromorphone, levorphanol, oxycodone, oxymorphone); respiratory diseases including asthma, emphysema, COPD, or severe liver or renal insufficiency; some preparations contain sulfites which may cause allergic reactions; tolerance or drug dependence may result from extended use

Not recommended for use for cough control in patients with a productive cough; not recommended as an antitussive for children <2 years of age; the elderly may be particularly susceptible to the CNS depressant and confusion as well as constipating effects of narcotics

Drug Interactions Increased toxicity: CNS depressant medications produce additive sedative properties

Nutritional/Herbal/Ethanol Interactions Ethanol: Avoid or limit ethanol (may increase CNS depression). Watch for sedation.

Adverse Reactions See individual agents.

Dosing

Adults & Elderly: Cough (antitussive/expectorant): Oral: 5-10 mL every 4-8 hours not to exceed 60 mL/24 hours

Pediatrics: Cough (antitussive/expectorant): Oral:

2-6 years: 1-1.5 mg/kg codeine/day divided into 4 doses administered every 4-6 hours (maximum: 30 mg/24 hours)

6-12 years: 5 mL every 4 hours, not to exceed 30 mL/24 hours

>12 years: 10 mL every 4 hours, up to 60 mL/24 hours

Available Dosage Forms

Liquid:

Brontex®: Guaifenesin 75 mg and codeine phosphate 2.5 mg per 5 mL (480 mL) [alcohol free; strawberry mint flavor]

Diabetic Tussin C®: Guaifenesin 200 mg and codeine phosphate 10 mg per 5 mL (480 mL) [contains phenylalanine 0.03 mcg/5 mL; cherry vanilla flavor]

Gani-Tuss® NR: Guaifenesin 100 mg and codeine phosphate 10 mg per 5 mL (480 mL) [raspberry flavor]

Guaifen-C: Guaifenesin 75 mg and codeine phosphate 2.5 mg per 5 mL (480 mL) [cherry flavor]

Guaifenesin AC: Guaifenesin 100 mg and codeine phosphate 10 mg per 5 mL (120 mL, 480 mL) [alcohol free, sugar free; raspberry flavor]

Iophen-C NR: Guaifenesin 100 mg and codeine phosphate 10 mg per 5 mL (480 mL) [raspberry flavor]

Kolephrin® #1: Guaifenesin 100 mg and codeine phosphate 10 mg per 5 mL (120 mL) [contains sodium 1.1 mg/5 mL and sodium benzoate]

Tussi-Organidin® NR: Guaifenesin 100 mg and codeine phosphate 10 mg per 5 mL (480 mL) [contains sodium benzoate; raspberry flavor]

Tussi-Organidin® S-NR: Guaifenesin 100 mg and codeine phosphate 10 mg per 5 mL (120 mL) [contains sodium benzoate; raspberry flavor]

Syrup:

Cheracol®: Guaifenesin 100 mg and codeine phosphate 10 mg per 5 mL (120 mL) [contains alcohol 4.75% and benzoic acid]

Cheratussin AC: Guaifenesin 100 mg and codeine phosphate 10 mg per 5 mL (120 mL, 240 mL, 480 mL)

Guaituss AC®: Guaifenesin 100 mg and codeine phosphate 10 mg per 5 mL (120 mL, 480 mL) [contains alcohol; sugar free; fruit-mint flavor]

Mytussin® AC: Guaifenesin 100 mg and codeine phosphate 10 mg per 5 mL (120 mL, 480 mL) [contains alcohol; sugar free; fruit flavor]

Robafen® AC: Guaifenesin 100 mg and codeine phosphate 10 mg per 5 mL (120 mL, 480 mL)

Romilar® AC: Guaifenesin 100 mg and codeine phosphate 10 mg per 5 mL (480 mL) [contains benzoic acid and phenylalanine; alcohol free, sugar free, dye free; grape flavor]

Tablet (Brontex®): Guaifenesin 300 mg and codeine phosphate 10 mg

Nursing Guidelines

Assessment: See individual components listed in Related Information. Note breast-feeding caution.

Dietary Considerations: Romilar® AC contains phenylalanine. Diabetic Tussin C® contains phenylalanine 0.03 mcg/5 mL. Kolephrin® #1 contains sodium 1.1 mg/5 mL.

Patient Education: See individual agents. **Pregnancy/breast-feeding precautions:** Inform prescriber if you are or intend to become pregnant. Consult prescriber if breast-feeding.

Pregnancy Risk Factor: C

Lactation: Excretion in breast milk unknown/use caution

Related Information

Codeine *on page 443*

Guaifenesin *on page 834*

- Guaituss AC® *see* Guaifenesin and Codeine *on page 835*
- Guiatuss™ [OTC] *see* Guaifenesin *on page 834*
- Gum Benjamin *see* Benzoin *on page 235*
- Gyne-Lotrimin® 3 [OTC] *see* Clotrimazole *on page 439*
- Gynodiol® *see* Estradiol *on page 649*
- Gynovite® Plus [OTC] *see* Vitamins (Multiple/Oral) *on page 1720*
- Habitrol *see* Nicotine *on page 1223*

Haemophilus b Conjugate Vaccine

(he MOF fi lus bee KON joo gate vak SEEN)

U.S. Brand Names ActHIB®; HibTITER®; PedvaxHIB®

Synonyms Diphtheria CRM_{197} Protein Conjugate; Diphtheria Toxoid Conjugate; *Haemophilus* b Oligosaccharide Conjugate Vaccine; *Haemophilus* b Polysaccharide Vaccine; HbCV; HbOC; Hib Polysaccharide Conjugate; PRP-OMP; PRP-T

Pharmacologic Category Vaccine

Use Routine immunization of children 2 months to 5 years of age against invasive disease caused by *H. influenzae*

Unimmunized children ≥5 years of age with a chronic illness known to be associated with increased risk of *Haemophilus influenzae* type b disease, specifically, persons with anatomic or functional asplenia or sickle cell anemia or those who have undergone splenectomy, should receive *Haemophilus influenzae* type b (Hib) vaccine.

Haemophilus b conjugate vaccines are not indicated for prevention of bronchitis or other infections due to *H. influenzae* in adults; adults with specific dysfunction or certain complement deficiencies who are at especially high risk of *H. influenzae* type b infection (HIV-infected adults); patients with Hodgkin's disease (vaccinated at least 2 weeks before the initiation of chemotherapy or 3 months after the end of chemotherapy)

Mechanism of Action Stimulates production of anticapsular antibodies and provides active immunity to *Haemophilus influenzae*

Pharmacodynamics/Kinetics Seroconversion following one dose of Hib vaccine for children 18 months or 24 months of age or older is 75% to 90% respectively.

(Continued)

Haemophilus b Conjugate Vaccine *(Continued)*

Onset of action: Serum antibody response: 1-2 weeks

Duration: Immunity: 1.5 years

Contraindications Hypersensitivity to *Haemophilus* b polysaccharide vaccine or any component of the formulation

Warnings/Precautions If used in persons with malignancies or those receiving immunosuppressive therapy or who are otherwise immunocompromised, the expected immune response may not be obtained; may be used in patients with HIV infection. Patients who develop symptoms suggestive of hypersensitivity after an injection should not receive further injections of the vaccine. The decision to administer or delay vaccination because of current or recent febrile illness depends on the severity of symptoms and the etiology of the disease. Immunization should be delayed during the course of an acute febrile illness. Use caution in children with coagulation disorders (including thrombocytopenia) where intramuscular injections should not be used. Epinephrine 1:1000 should be readily available.

Children in whom DTP or DT vaccination is deferred: The carrier proteins used in HbOC and PRP-T (but not PRP-OMP) are chemically and immunologically related to toxoids contained in DTP vaccine. Earlier or simultaneous vaccination with diphtheria or tetanus toxoids may be required to elicit an optimal anti-PRP antibody response to HbOC. In contrast, the immunogenicity of PRP-OMP is not affected by vaccination with DTP. In infants in whom DTP or DT vaccination is deferred, PRP-OMP may be advantageous for *Haemophilus influenzae* type b vaccination.

Children with immunologic impairment: Children with chronic illness associated with increased risk of *Haemophilus influenzae* type b disease may have impaired anti-PRP antibody responses to conjugate vaccination. Examples include those with HIV infection, immunoglobulin deficiency, anatomic or functional asplenia, and sickle cell disease, as well as recipients of bone marrow transplants and recipients of chemotherapy for malignancy. Some children with immunologic impairment may benefit from more doses of conjugate vaccine than normally indicated.

Drug Interactions Immunosuppressant medications: The effect of the vaccine may be decreased; consider deferring vaccination for 3 months after immunosuppressant therapy is discontinued.

Lab Interactions May interfere with interpretation of antigen detection tests

Adverse Reactions **All serious adverse reactions must be reported to the U.S. Department of Health and Human Services (DHHS) Vaccine Adverse Event Reporting System (VAERS) 1-800-822-7967.** Frequency not defined:

Central nervous system: Crying (unusual, high pitched, prolonged); fever, irritability, pain, sleepiness

Dermatologic: Rash

Gastrointestinal: Anorexia, diarrhea, vomiting

Local: Injection site: Erythema, induration, pain, soreness, swelling

Otic: Otitis media

Respiratory: Upper respiratory tract infection

Postmarketing and/or case reports: Anaphylactoid reactions, angioedema, erythema multiforme, facial edema, febrile seizures, Guillain-Barré syndrome, headache, hypersensitivity, hypotonia, inflammation, injection site abscess

Vaccination Schedule for Haemophilus b Conjugate Vaccines

Age at 1st Dose (mo)	ActHIBHib®, HibTITER®		PedvaxHIB®	
	Primary Series	Booster	Primary Series	Booster
2-6	3 doses, 2 months apart	15 mo[1]	2 doses, 2 months apart	12-15 mo[1]
7-11	2 doses, 2 months apart	15 mo[1]	2 doses, 2 months apart	12-15 mo[1]
12-14	1 dose	15 mo[1]	1 dose	15 mo[1]
15-71	1 dose	—	1 dose	—

[1]At least 2 months after previous dose.

Note: DTaP/Hib combination vaccines should not be used for infants at ages 2, 4, or 6 months, but can be used as boosters following any Hib vaccine.

(sterile), lethargy, lymphadenopathy, malaise, mass, seizure, skin discoloration, urticaria

Dosing

Pediatrics: Immunization: I.M.: 0.5 mL as a single dose should be administered according to one of the following "brand-specific" schedules; do not inject I.V. (see table)

Available Dosage Forms

Injection, powder for reconstitution (ActHIB®) [preservative free]: *Haemophilus* b capsular polysaccharide 10 mcg and tetanus toxoid 24 mcg per dose [may be reconstituted with provided diluent (forms solution; vial stopper contains latex) or TriHIBit® (forms suspension)]

Injection, solution [preservative free] (HibTITER®): *Haemophilus* b saccharide 10 mcg and diphtheria CRM 197 protein 25 mcg per 0.5 mL (0.5 mL) [vial stopper contains latex]

Injection, suspension (PedvaxHIB®): *Haemophilus* b capsular polysaccharide 7.5 mcg and *Neisseria meningitidis* OMPC 125 mcg per 0.5 mL (0.5 mL) [contains aluminum 225 mcg/0.5 mL]

Nursing Guidelines

Patient Education: May use acetaminophen for postdose fever

Pregnancy Risk Factor: C

Administration

I.M.: For patients at risk of hemorrhage following intramuscular injection, the ACIP recommends "it should be administered intramuscularly if, in the opinion of the physician familiar with the patients bleeding risk, the vaccine can be administered with reasonable safety by this route. If the patient receives antihemophilia or other similar therapy, intramuscular vaccination can be scheduled shortly after such therapy is administered. A fine needle (23 gauge or smaller) can be used for the vaccination and firm pressure applied to the site (without rubbing) for at least 2 minutes. The patient should be instructed concerning the risk of hematoma from the injection."

Storage: Store under refrigeration at 2°C to 8°C (36°F to 46°F). Do not freeze.

ActHIB®: Use within 24 hours following reconstitution with saline; use within 30 minutes following reconstitution with Tripedia®

- ♦ ***Haemophilus* b Oligosaccharide Conjugate Vaccine** *see Haemophilus* b Conjugate Vaccine *on page 837*
- ♦ ***Haemophilus* b Polysaccharide Vaccine** *see Haemophilus* b Conjugate Vaccine *on page 837*
- ♦ **Halcion®** *see* Triazolam *on page 1666*
- ♦ **Haldol®** *see* Haloperidol *on page 839*
- ♦ **Haldol® Decanoate** *see* Haloperidol *on page 839*
- ♦ **Halfprin® [OTC]** *see* Aspirin *on page 189*

Haloperidol (ha loe PER i dole)

U.S. Brand Names Haldol®; Haldol® Decanoate

Synonyms Haloperidol Decanoate; Haloperidol Lactate

Pharmacologic Category Antipsychotic Agent, Typical

Medication Safety Issues

Sound-alike/look-alike issues:

Haloperidol may be confused Halotestin®

Haldol® may be confused with Halcion®, Halenol®, Halog®, Halotestin®, Stadol®

Use Management of schizophrenia; control of tics and vocal utterances of Tourette's disorder in children and adults; severe behavioral problems in children

Unlabeled/Investigational Use Treatment of psychosis; may be used for the emergency sedation of severely-agitated or delirious patients; adjunctive treatment of ethanol dependence; antiemetic

Mechanism of Action Haloperidol is a butyrophenone antipsychotic which blocks postsynaptic mesolimbic dopaminergic D_1 and D_2 receptors in the brain; depresses the release of hypothalamic and hypophyseal hormones; believed to depress the reticular activating system thus affecting basal metabolism, body temperature, wakefulness, vasomotor tone, and emesis

Pharmacodynamics/Kinetics

Onset of action: Sedation: I.V.: ~1 hour

Duration: Decanoate: ~3 weeks

Distribution: Crosses placenta; enters breast milk

Protein binding: 90%

Metabolism: Hepatic to inactive compounds

(Continued)

Haloperidol *(Continued)*

Bioavailability: Oral: 60%

Half-life elimination: 20 hours

Time to peak, serum: 20 minutes

Excretion: Urine (33% to 40% as metabolites) within 5 days; feces (15%)

Contraindications Hypersensitivity to haloperidol or any component of the formulation; Parkinson's disease; severe CNS depression; bone marrow suppression; severe cardiac or hepatic disease; coma

Warnings/Precautions Hypotension may occur, particularly with parenteral administration. Decanoate form should never be administered I.V. Avoid in thyrotoxicosis. May be sedating, use with caution in disorders where CNS depression is a feature. Caution in patients with hemodynamic instability, predisposition to seizures, subcortical brain damage, renal or respiratory disease. Esophageal dysmotility and aspiration have been associated with antipsychotic use - use with caution in patients at risk of pneumonia (ie, Alzheimer's disease). Caution in breast cancer or other prolactin-dependent tumors (may elevate prolactin levels). May alter temperature regulation or mask toxicity of other drugs due to antiemetic effects. May alter cardiac conduction - life-threatening arrhythmias have occurred with therapeutic doses of antipsychotics. Adverse effects of decanoate may be prolonged. May cause orthostatic hypotension - use with caution in patients at risk of this effect or those who would tolerate transient hypotensive episodes (cerebrovascular disease, cardiovascular disease, or other medications which may predispose). Some tablets contain tartrazine.

May cause anticholinergic effects (confusion, agitation, constipation, xerostomia, blurred vision, urinary retention). Therefore, they should be used with caution in patients with decreased gastrointestinal motility, urinary retention, BPH, xerostomia, or visual problems. Conditions which also may be exacerbated by cholinergic blockade include narrow-angle glaucoma (screening is recommended) and worsening of myasthenia gravis. Relative to other neuroleptics, haloperidol has a low potency of cholinergic blockade.

May cause extrapyramidal symptoms, including pseudoparkinsonism, acute dystonic reactions, akathisia, and tardive dyskinesia (risk of these reactions is high relative to other neuroleptics). May be associated with neuroleptic malignant syndrome (NMS) or pigmentary retinopathy.

Drug Interactions Substrate of CYP1A2 (minor), 2D6 (major), 3A4 (major); **Inhibits** CYP2D6 (moderate), 3A4 (moderate)

Acetylcholinesterase inhibitors (central): May increase the risk of antipsychotic-related extrapyramidal symptoms; monitor.

Anticholinergics: May inhibit the therapeutic response to haloperidol and excess anticholinergic effects may occur; tardive dyskinesias have also been reported; includes benztropine and trihexyphenidyl

Antihypertensives: Concurrent use of haloperidol with an antihypertensive may produce additive hypotensive effects (particularly orthostasis)

Bromocriptine: Antipsychotics inhibit the ability of bromocriptine to lower serum prolactin concentrations

Chloroquine: Serum concentrations of haloperidol may be increased by chloroquine

CNS depressants: Sedative effects may be additive; monitor for increased effect; includes barbiturates, benzodiazepines, narcotic analgesics, ethanol and other sedative agents

CYP2D6 inhibitors: May increase the levels/effects of haloperidol. Example inhibitors include chlorpromazine, delavirdine, fluoxetine, miconazole, paroxetine, pergolide, quinidine, quinine, ritonavir, and ropinirole.

CYP2D6 substrates: Haloperidol may increase the levels/effects of CYP2D6 substrates. Example substrates include amphetamines, selected beta-blockers, dextromethorphan, fluoxetine, lidocaine, mirtazapine, nefazodone, paroxetine, risperidone, ritonavir, thioridazine, tricyclic antidepressants, and venlafaxine.

CYP2D6 prodrug substrates: Haloperidol may decrease the levels/effects of CYP2D6 prodrug substrates. Example prodrug substrates include codeine, hydrocodone, oxycodone, and tramadol.

CYP3A4 inducers: CYP3A4 inducers may decrease the levels/effects of haloperidol. Example inducers include aminoglutethimide, carbamazepine, nafcillin, nevirapine, phenobarbital, phenytoin, and rifamycins.

CYP3A4 inhibitors: May increase the levels/effects of haloperidol. Example inhibitors include azole antifungals, clarithromycin, diclofenac, doxycycline, erythromycin, imatinib, isoniazid, nefazodone, nicardipine, propofol, protease inhibitors, quinidine, telithromycin, and verapamil.

CYP3A4 substrates: Haloperidol may increase the levels/effects of CYP3A4 substrates. Example substrates include benzodiazepines, calcium channel blockers, cyclosporine, mirtazapine, nateglinide, nefazodone, sildenafil (and other PDE-5 inhibitors), tacrolimus, and venlafaxine. Selected benzodiazepines (midazolam and triazolam), cisapride, ergot alkaloids, selected HMG-CoA reductase inhibitors (lovastatin and simvastatin), and pimozide are generally contraindicated with strong CYP3A4 inhibitors.

Indomethacin: Haloperidol in combination with indomethacin may result in drowsiness, tiredness, and confusion; monitor for adverse effects

Inhalation anesthetics: Haloperidol in combination with certain forms of induction anesthesia may produce peripheral vasodilitation and hypotension

Levodopa: Haloperidol may inhibit the antiparkinsonian effect of levodopa; avoid this combination

Lithium: Haloperidol may produce neurotoxicity with lithium; this is a rare effect

Methyldopa: Effect of haloperidol may be altered; enhanced effects, as well as reduced efficacy have been reported

Metoclopramide: May increase extrapyramidal symptoms (EPS) or risk.

Nefazodone: Haloperidol and nefazodone may produce additive CNS toxicity, including sedation

Propranolol: Serum concentrations of haloperidol may be increased

Quinidine: May increase haloperidol concentrations; monitor for EPS and/or QT_c prolongation

SSRIs: Fluoxetine, fluvoxamine, and paroxetine may inhibit the metabolism of haloperidol resulting in EPS; monitor for EPS

Sulfadoxine-pyrimethamine: May increase fluphenazine concentrations

Tricyclic antidepressants: Concurrent use may produce increased toxicity or altered therapeutic response

Trazodone: Haloperidol and trazodone may produce additive hypotensive effects

Nutritional/Herbal/Ethanol Interactions

Ethanol: Avoid ethanol (may increase CNS depression).

Herb/Nutraceutical: Avoid valerian, St John's wort, kava kava, gotu kola (may increase CNS depression).

Lab Interactions decreased cholesterol (S)

Adverse Reactions Frequency not defined.

Cardiovascular: Hyper-/hypotension, tachycardia, arrhythmia, abnormal T waves with prolonged ventricular repolarization, torsade de pointes (case-control study ~4%)

Central nervous system: Restlessness, anxiety, extrapyramidal reactions, dystonic reactions, pseudoparkinsonian signs and symptoms, tardive dyskinesia, neuroleptic malignant syndrome (NMS), altered central temperature regulation, akathisia, tardive dystonia, insomnia, euphoria, agitation, drowsiness, depression, lethargy, headache, confusion, vertigo, seizure

Dermatologic: Hyperpigmentation, pruritus, rash, contact dermatitis, alopecia, photosensitivity (rare)

Endocrine & metabolic: Amenorrhea, galactorrhea, gynecomastia, sexual dysfunction, lactation, breast engorgement, mastalgia, menstrual irregularities, hyperglycemia, hypoglycemia, hyponatremia

Gastrointestinal: Nausea, vomiting, anorexia, constipation, diarrhea, hypersalivation, dyspepsia, xerostomia

Genitourinary: Urinary retention, priapism

Hematologic: Cholestatic jaundice, obstructive jaundice

Ocular: Blurred vision

Respiratory: Laryngospasm, bronchospasm

Miscellaneous: Heat stroke, diaphoresis

Overdosage/Toxicology Symptoms of overdose include deep sleep, dystonia, agitation, dysrhythmias, and extrapyramidal symptoms. Treatment is supportive and symptomatic.

Dosing

Adults:

Psychosis:

Oral: 0.5-5 mg 2-3 times/day; usual maximum: 30 mg/day

I.M. (as lactate): 2-5 mg every 4-8 hours as needed

(Continued)

Haloperidol *(Continued)*

I.M. (as decanoate): Initial: 10-20 times the daily oral dose administered at 4-week intervals. Maintenance dose: 10-15 times initial oral dose; used to stabilize psychiatric symptoms

Delirium in the intensive care unit (unlabeled use, unlabeled route):

I.V.: 2-10 mg; may repeat bolus doses every 20-30 minutes until calm achieved then administer 25% of the maximum dose every 6 hours; monitor ECG and QT_c interval

Intermittent I.V.: 0.03-0.15 mg/kg every 30 minutes to 6 hours

Oral: Agitation: 5-10 mg

Continuous I.V. infusion (100 mg/100 mL D_5W): Rates of 3-25 mg/hour have been used

Rapid tranquilization of severely-agitated patient (unlabeled use; administer every 30-60 minutes):

Oral: 5-10 mg

I.M.: 5 mg

Average total dose (oral or I.M.) for tranquilization: 10-20 mg

Elderly: Nonpsychotic patients, dementia behavior: Initial: Oral: 0.25-0.5 mg 1-2 times/day; increase dose at 4- to 7-day intervals by 0.25-0.5 mg/day. Increase dosing intervals (twice daily, 3 times/day, etc) as necessary to control response or side effects.

Pediatrics:

Sedation/psychotic disorders: Oral:

Children: 3-12 years (15-40 kg): Initial: 0.05 mg/kg/day or 0.25-0.5 mg/day given in 2-3 divided doses; increase by 0.25-0.5 mg every 5-7 days; maximum: 0.15 mg/kg/day

Usual maintenance:

Agitation or hyperkinesia: 0.01-0.03 mg/kg/day once daily

Nonpsychotic disorders: 0.05-0.075 mg/kg/day in 2-3 divided doses

Psychotic disorders: 0.05-0.15 mg/kg/day in 2-3 divided doses

Children 6-12 years: Sedation/psychotic disorders: I.M. (as lactate): 1-3 mg/dose every 4-8 hours to a maximum of 0.15 mg/kg/day; change over to oral therapy as soon as able.

Renal Impairment: Hemodialysis/peritoneal dialysis: Supplemental dose is not necessary.

Available Dosage Forms [DSC] = Discontinued product. **Note:** Strength expressed as base.

Injection, oil, as decanoate (Haldol® Decanoate): 50 mg/mL (1 mL, 5 mL); 100 mg/mL (1 mL, 5 mL) [contains benzyl alcohol, sesame oil]

Injection, solution, as lactate: 5 mg/mL (1 mL, 10 mL)

Haldol®: 5 mg/mL (1 mL; 10 mL [DSC])

Solution, oral concentrate, as lactate: 2 mg/mL (15 mL, 120 mL)

Tablet: 0.5 mg, 1 mg, 2 mg, 5 mg, 10 mg, 20 mg

Nursing Guidelines

Assessment: Assess other medications patient is taking for effectiveness and interactions (especially drugs metabolized by P450 enzymes). Review ophthalmic screening. Monitor therapeutic effectiveness and adverse reactions at beginning of therapy and periodically with long-term use. With I.M. or I.V. use, monitor for hypotension. Initiate at lower doses and taper dosage slowly when discontinuing. Assess knowledge/teach patient appropriate use, interventions to reduce side effects, and adverse symptoms to report.

Monitoring Laboratory Tests: Lipid profile, fasting blood glucose/Hgb A_{1c}; BMI

Patient Education: Use exactly as directed; do not increase dose or frequency. It may take 2-3 weeks to achieve desired results; do not discontinue without consulting prescriber. Dilute oral concentration with water or juice. Do not take within 2 hours of any antacid. Store away from light. Avoid alcohol or caffeine and other prescription or OTC medications not approved by prescriber. Maintain adequate hydration (2-3 L/day of fluids) unless instructed to restrict fluid intake. Avoid skin contact with medication; may cause contact dermatitis (wash immediately with warm, soapy water). You may experience excess drowsiness, restlessness, dizziness, or blurred vision (use caution driving or when engaging in tasks requiring alertness until response to drug is known); nausea or vomiting (small frequent meals, frequent mouth care, chewing gum, or sucking lozenges may help); constipation (increased exercise, fluids, fruit, or fiber may help); postural hypotension (use caution climbing stairs or when changing position from lying or sitting to standing); urinary retention (void before taking medication); or decreased perspiration (avoid strenuous exercise in hot environments). Report persistent CNS effects (eg, trembling fingers, altered gait or balance, excessive sedation, seizures, unusual movements, anxiety, abnormal thoughts, confusion, personality changes); chest pain, palpitations, rapid heartbeat, severe dizziness; unresolved urinary retention or changes in urinary pattern; vision changes; skin rash or yellowing of skin; respiratory difficulty; or worsening of condition. **Pregnancy/breast-feeding precautions:** Inform prescriber if you are or intend to become pregnant. Breast-feeding is not recommended.

Geriatric Considerations: (See Warnings/Precautions, Adverse Reactions, and Overdose/Toxicology.) Elderly patients have an increased risk of adverse response to side effects or adverse reactions to antipsychotics.

Pregnancy Risk Factor: C

Lactation: Enters breast milk/not recommended (AAP rates "of concern")

Breast-Feeding Considerations: Decline in developmental scores may be seen in nursing infants.

Perioperative/Anesthesia/Other Concerns:

Delirium in the ICU Patient: Set goals for control of delirium. Haloperidol has not been studied in well-controlled trials enrolling ICU patients with acute delirium or agitation. Avoid use in patients with underlying QT prolongation, in those taking medicines that prolong the QT interval, or cause polymorphic ventricular tachycardia. Even when used at recommended doses, cardiac arrhythmias have occurred. Monitor ECG closely for dose-related QT effects. Once the patient has been stable for a few days, taper the dose and reassess the patient. Haloperidol may cause extrapyramidal symptoms. It is the most frequently implicated antipsychotic associated with neuroleptic malignant syndrome.

Administration

Oral: Dilute the oral concentrate with water or juice before administration. **Note:** Avoid skin contact with oral medication; may cause contact dermatitis.

I.M.: The decanoate injectable formulation should be administered I.M. only; **do not give decanoate I.V.**

I.V.:

Decanoate: Do **not** administer I.V.

Lactate: Although not an FDA-approved route of administration, Haldol® has been administered by this route in many acute care settings.

Reconstitution: Haloperidol lactate may be administered IVPB or I.V. infusion in D_5W solutions. NS solutions should not be used due to reports of decreased stability and incompatibility.

Standardized dose: 0.5-100 mg/50-100 mL D_5W

Stability of standardized solutions is 38 days at room temperature (24°C).

Compatibility: Stable in D_5W

Y-site administration: Incompatible with allopurinol, amphotericin B cholesteryl sulfate complex, cefepime, fluconazole, foscarnet, heparin, piperacillin/tazobactam, sargramostim

Compatibility in syringe: Incompatible with diphenhydramine, heparin, hydroxyzine, ketorolac

Storage: Protect oral dosage forms from light. Haloperidol lactate injection should be stored at controlled room temperature and protected from light, freezing, and temperatures >40°C. Exposure to light may cause discoloration and the development of a grayish-red precipitate over several weeks.

- Haloperidol Decanoate *see* Haloperidol *on page 839*
- Haloperidol Lactate *see* Haloperidol *on page 839*

Halothane (HA loe thane)

Pharmacologic Category General Anesthetic, Inhalation

Medication Safety Issues

Sound-alike/look-alike issues:

Halothane may be confused with Halotestin®

Use Induction and maintenance of general anesthesia

Pharmacodynamics/Kinetics

Onset of action: 1.5-3 minutes

Duration: Emergence time: Depends on blood concentration when halothane is discontinued

Metabolism: Hepatic (20% to 50%) via CYP, both oxidatively and reductively

Excretion: Exhaled gases within 24 hours

(Continued)

Halothane *(Continued)*

Contraindications Hypersensitivity to halothane or any component of the formulation; known or suspected history of malignant hyperthermia; history of hepatitis after a previous anesthetic

Warnings/Precautions Decrease in blood pressure is dose dependent, due to myocardial depression and blunting of the baroreceptor mediated tachycardic response to hypotension. Sinus bradycardia, wandering pacemaker, and junctional rhythm are not uncommon. Respiration is depressed (increase $PaCO_2$ at 1 MAC to 45 mm Hg with spontaneous ventilation). Hypoxic pulmonary vasoconstriction is depressed which may lead to increased pulmonary shunt. Hypoxemia-induced increase in ventilation is abolished at low halothane concentration. Halothane dilates the cerebral vasculature and may, in certain conditions, increase intracranial pressure. Renal, splenic, and hepatic blood flow are reduced. Halothane induces hepatic microsomal enzymes function. Incidence of halothane-induced hepatitis is 1/10,000 to 1/30,000 anesthetics (less in children); it most often occurs following repeat administration (etiology is likely immune-mediated, mortality is 50%). Halothane is a trigger of malignant hyperthermia. Halothane can produce elevated carbon monoxide levels in the presence of a dry carbon dioxide absorbent within the circle breathing system of an anesthetic machine.

Drug Interactions Substrate of CYP2A6 (minor), 2B6 (minor), 2C8/9 (minor), 2D6 (minor), 2E1 (major), 3A4 (minor)

Aminophylline: Increased risk of arrhythmias with combined use.

Antihypertensives: Excessive hypotension may occur with combined use.

Benzodiazepines, opioids: Concurrent use of opioids and/or benzodiazepines decreases the MAC of halothane.

CYP2E1 inhibitors: May increase the levels/effects of halothane. Example inhibitors include disulfiram, isoniazid, and miconazole.

Epinephrine: Increased risk of arrhythmias with combined use. Do not exceed 0.1 mg in 10 minutes or 0.3 mg in 1 hour. Avoid concurrent use.

Isoniazid: Increased risk of hepatotoxicity with combined use.

Neuromuscular-blocking agents (nondepolarizing): Halothane may potentiate the action of nondepolarizing, neuromuscular-blocking agents.

Rifampin: Increased risk of hepatotoxicity with combined use.

Adverse Reactions Frequency not defined.

Cardiovascular: Myocardial depression, hypotension, bradycardia, reflex tachycardia, ventricular or supraventricular arrhythmias

Central nervous system: Agitation, restlessness

Gastrointestinal: Nausea, vomiting

Respiratory: Respiratory depression/arrest, hypoxemia

Miscellaneous: Shivering

Dosing

Adults: Anesthesia: Inhalation: Minimum alveolar concentration (MAC), the concentration at which 50% of patients do not respond to surgical incision, is 0.74% for halothane. The concentration at which amnesia and loss of awareness occur (MAC - awake) is 0.41%. Surgical levels of anesthesia are maintained with concentrations between 0.5% to 2%; inspired concentrations of up to 3% required for induction of anesthesia. MAC is reduced in the elderly.

Elderly: MAC is reduced in the elderly.

Available Dosage Forms Liquid: 125 mL, 250 mL

Nursing Guidelines

Pregnancy Risk Factor: C

Administration

Storage: Halothane mixed with oxygen or air is not flammable or explosive.

Related Information

Inhalational Anesthetics *on page 1850*

- **HandClens® [OTC]** *see* Benzalkonium Chloride *on page 231*
- **Havrix®** *see* Hepatitis A Vaccine *on page 850*
- **HbCV** *see Haemophilus* b Conjugate Vaccine *on page 837*
- **hBNP** *see* Nesiritide *on page 1216*
- **HbOC** *see Haemophilus* b Conjugate Vaccine *on page 837*
- **hCG** *see* Chorionic Gonadotropin (Human) *on page 387*
- **HCTZ (error-prone abbreviation)** *see* Hydrochlorothiazide *on page 862*
- **HDA® Toothache [OTC]** *see* Benzocaine *on page 232*
- **Healon®** *see* Hyaluronate and Derivatives *on page 856*

- ♦ **Healon®5** *see* Hyaluronate and Derivatives *on page 856*
- ♦ **Healon GV®** *see* Hyaluronate and Derivatives *on page 856*
- ♦ **Helistat®** *see* Collagen Hemostat *on page 449*
- ♦ **Helitene®** *see* Collagen Hemostat *on page 449*
- ♦ **Helixate® FS** *see* Antihemophilic Factor (Recombinant) *on page 170*
- ♦ **Hemabate®** *see* Carboprost Tromethamine *on page 315*
- ♦ **Hemocyte Plus®** *see* Vitamins (Multiple/Oral) *on page 1720*
- ♦ **Hemorrhoidal HC** *see* Hydrocortisone *on page 873*
- ♦ **Hemril®-30** *see* Hydrocortisone *on page 873*

Heparin (HEP a rin)

U.S. Brand Names HepFlush®-10; Hep-Lock®

Synonyms Heparin Calcium; Heparin Lock Flush; Heparin Sodium

Pharmacologic Category Anticoagulant

Medication Safety Issues

Sound-alike/look-alike issues:

Heparin may be confused with Hespan®

High alert medication: The Institute for Safe Medication Practices (ISMP) includes this medication among its list of drugs which have a heightened risk of causing significant patient harm when used in error.

Heparin lock flush solution is intended only to maintain patency of I.V. devices and is **not** to be used for anticoagulant therapy.

Note: The 100 unit/mL concentration should not be used in neonates or infants <10 kg, The 10 unit/mL concentration may cause systemic anticoagulation in infants <1 kg who receive frequent flushes.

Use Prophylaxis and treatment of thromboembolic disorders

Note: Heparin lock flush solution is intended only to maintain patency of I.V. devices and is **not** to be used for anticoagulant therapy.

Unlabeled/Investigational Use Acute MI — combination regimen of heparin (unlabeled dose), tenecteplase (half dose), and abciximab (full dose)

Mechanism of Action Potentiates the action of antithrombin III and thereby inactivates thrombin (as well as activated coagulation factors IX, X, XI, XII, and plasmin) and prevents the conversion of fibrinogen to fibrin; heparin also stimulates release of lipoprotein lipase (lipoprotein lipase hydrolyzes triglycerides to glycerol and free fatty acids)

Pharmacodynamics/Kinetics

Onset of action: Anticoagulation: I.V.: Immediate; SubQ: ~20-30 minutes

Absorption: Oral, rectal, I.M.: Erratic at best from all these routes of administration; SubQ absorption is also erratic, but considered acceptable for prophylactic use

Distribution: Does not cross placenta; does not enter breast milk

Metabolism: Hepatic; may be partially metabolized in the reticuloendothelial system

Half-life elimination: Mean: 1.5 hours; Range: 1-2 hours; affected by obesity, renal function, hepatic function, malignancy, presence of pulmonary embolism, and infections

Excretion: Urine (small amounts as unchanged drug)

Contraindications Hypersensitivity to heparin or any component of the formulation; severe thrombocytopenia; uncontrolled active bleeding except when due to DIC; suspected intracranial hemorrhage; not for I.M. use; not for use when appropriate monitoring parameters cannot be obtained

Warnings/Precautions Use cautiously in patients with a documented hypersensitivity reaction and only in life-threatening situations. Hemorrhage is the most common complication. Monitor for signs and symptoms of bleeding. Certain patients are at increased risk of bleeding. Risk factors include bacterial endocarditis; congenital or acquired bleeding disorders; active ulcerative or angiodysplastic GI diseases; severe uncontrolled hypertension; hemorrhagic stroke; or use shortly after brain, spinal, or ophthalmology surgery; patient treated concomitantly with platelet inhibitors; conditions associated with increased bleeding tendencies (hemophilia, vascular purpura); recent GI bleeding; thrombocytopenia or platelet defects; severe liver disease; hypertensive or diabetic retinopathy; or in patients undergoing invasive procedures. A higher incidence of bleeding has been reported in patients >60 years of age, particularly women. They are also more sensitive to the dose.

(Continued)

Heparin *(Continued)*

Patients who develop thrombocytopenia on heparin may be at risk of developing a new thrombus ("White-clot syndrome"). Hypersensitivity reactions can occur. Osteoporosis can occur following long-term use (>6 months). Monitor for hyperkalemia. Discontinue therapy and consider alternatives if platelets are <100,000/ mm^3. Patients >60 years of age may require lower doses of heparin.

Some preparations contain benzyl alcohol as a preservative. In neonates, large amounts of benzyl alcohol (>100 mg/kg/day) have been associated with fatal toxicity (gasping syndrome). The use of preservative-free heparin is, therefore, recommended in neonates. Some preparations contain sulfite which may cause allergic reactions.

Heparin does not possess fibrinolytic activity and, therefore, cannot lyse established thrombi; discontinue heparin if hemorrhage occurs; severe hemorrhage or overdosage may require protamine

Drug Interactions

Cephalosporins which contain the MTT side chain may increase the risk of hemorrhage.

Drugs which affect platelet function (eg, aspirin, NSAIDs, dipyridamole, ticlopidine, clopidogrel, IIb/IIIa antagonists) may potentiate the risk of hemorrhage.

Nitroglycerin (I.V.) may decrease heparin's anticoagulant effect. This interaction has not been validated in some studies, and may only occur at high nitroglycerin dosages.

Penicillins (parenteral) may prolong bleeding time via inhibition of platelet aggregation, potentially increasing the risk of hemorrhage.

Thrombolytic agents increase the risk of hemorrhage.

Warfarin: Risk of bleeding may be increased during concurrent therapy. Heparin is commonly continued during the initiation of warfarin therapy to assure anticoagulation and to protect against possible transient hypercoagulability.

Other drugs reported to increase heparin's anticoagulant effect include antihistamines, tetracycline, quinine, nicotine, and cardiac glycosides (digoxin).

Nutritional/Herbal/Ethanol Interactions

Food: When taking for >6 months, may interfere with calcium absorption.

Herb/Nutraceutical: Avoid cat's claw, dong quai, evening primrose, feverfew, red clover, horse chestnut, garlic, green tea, ginseng, ginkgo (all have additional antiplatelet activity).

Lab Interactions Increased thyroxine (S) (competitive protein binding methods), PT, PTT, bleeding time. A volume of at least 10 mL of blood should be removed and discarded from a heparinized line before blood samples are sent for coagulation testing.

Adverse Reactions

Cardiovascular: Chest pain, vasospasm (possibly related to thrombosis), hemorrhagic shock

Central nervous system: Fever, headache, chills

Dermatologic: Unexplained bruising, urticaria, alopecia, dysesthesia pedis, purpura, eczema, cutaneous necrosis (following deep SubQ injection), erythematous plaques (case reports)

Endocrine & metabolic: Hyperkalemia (supression of aldosterone), rebound hyperlipidemia on discontinuation

Gastrointestinal: Nausea, vomiting, constipation, hematemesis

Genitourinary: Frequent or persistent erection

Hematologic: Hemorrhage, blood in urine, bleeding from gums, epistaxis, adrenal hemorrhage, ovarian hemorrhage, retroperitoneal hemorrhage, thrombocytopenia (see note)

Hepatic: Elevated liver enzymes (AST/ALT)

Local: Irritation, ulceration, cutaneous necrosis have been rarely reported with deep SubQ injections; I.M. injection (not recommended) is associated with a high incidence of these effects

Neuromuscular & skeletal: Peripheral neuropathy, osteoporosis (chronic therapy effect)

Ocular: Conjunctivitis (allergic reaction)

Respiratory: Hemoptysis, pulmonary hemorrhage, asthma, rhinitis, bronchospasm (case reports)

Miscellaneous: Allergic reactions, anaphylactoid reactions

Note: Thrombocytopenia has been reported to occur at an incidence between 0% and 30%. It is often of no clinical significance. However, immunologically mediated heparin-induced thrombocytopenia has been estimated to occur in 1% to 2% of patients, and is marked by a progressive fall in platelet counts and, in some cases, thromboembolic complications (skin necrosis, pulmonary embolism, gangrene of the extremities, stroke or MI). For recommendations regarding platelet monitoring during heparin therapy, consult "Seventh ACCP Consensus Conference on Antithrombotic and Thrombolytic Therapy."

Overdosage/Toxicology The primary symptom of overdose is bleeding. Antidote is protamine; dose 1 mg neutralizes 1 mg (100 units) of heparin. Discontinue all heparin if evidence of progressive immune thrombocytopenia occurs.

Dosing

Adults:

DVT Prophylaxis (low-dose heparin): SubQ: 5000 units every 8-12 hours

Systemic anticoagulation: I.V. infusion (weight-based dosing per institutional nomogram recommended):

Acute coronary syndromes or MI: Fibrinolytic therapy: I.V. infusion:

Full-dose alteplase, reteplase, or tenecteplase with dosing as follows: Concurrent bolus of 60 units/kg (maximum: 4000 units), then 12 units/kg/hour (maximum: 1000 units/hour) as continuous infusion. Check aPTT every 4-6 hours; adjust to target of 1.5-2 times the upper limit of control (50-70 seconds in clinical trials); usual range 10-30 units/kg/hour. Duration of heparin therapy depends on concurrent therapy and the specific patient risks for systemic or venous thromboembolism.

Combination regimen (unlabeled): Half-dose tenecteplase (15-25 mg based on weight) and abciximab 0.25 mg/kg bolus then 0.125 mcg/kg/minute (maximum 10 mcg/minute) for 12 hours with heparin dosing as follows: Concurrent bolus of 40 units/kg (maximum 3000 units), then 7 units/kg/hour (maximum: 800 units/hour) as continuous infusion. Adjust to a aPTT target of 50-70 seconds.

Streptokinase: Heparin use optional depending on concurrent therapy and specific patient risks for systemic or venous thromboembolism (anterior MI, CHF, previous embolus, atrial fibrillation, LV thrombus): If heparin is administered, start when aPTT <2 times the upper limit of control; do not use a bolus, but initiate infusion adjusted to a target aPTT of 1.5-2 times the upper limit of control (50-70 seconds in clinical trials). If heparin is not administered by infusion, 7500-12,500 units SubQ every 12 hours (when aPTT <2 times the upper limit of control) is recommended.

Percutaneous coronary intervention: Heparin bolus and infusion may be administered to an activated clotting time (ACT) of 300-350 seconds if no concurrent GPIIb/IIIa receptor antagonist is administered or 200-250 seconds if a GPIIb/IIIa receptor antagonist is administered.

Unstable angina (high-risk and some intermediate-risk patients): Initial bolus of 60-70 units/kg (maximum: 5000 units), followed by an initial infusion of 12-15 units/kg/hour (maximum: 1000 units/hour). The American College of Chest Physicians consensus conference has recommended dosage adjustments to correspond to a therapeutic range equivalent to heparin levels of 0.3-0.7 units/mL by antifactor Xa determinations.

Venous thromboembolism :

DVT/PE: I.V. push: 80 units/kg followed by continuous infusion of 18 units/kg/hour

DVT: SubQ: 17,500 units every 12 hours

Intermittent I.V. Anticoagulation: Intermittent I.V.: Initial: 10,000 units, then 50-70 units/kg (5000-10,000 units) every 4-6 hours

Maintenance of line patency (line flushing): When using daily flushes of heparin to maintain patency of single and double lumen central catheters, 10 units/mL is commonly used for younger infants (eg, <10 kg) while 100 units/mL is used for older infants, children, and adults. Capped PVC catheters and peripheral heparin locks require flushing more frequently (eg, every 6-8 hours). Volume of heparin flush is usually similar to volume of catheter (or slightly greater). Additional flushes should be given when stagnant blood is observed in catheter, after catheter is used for drug or blood administration, and after blood withdrawal from catheter.

Parenteral nutrition: Addition of heparin (0.5-3 unit/mL) to peripheral and central parenteral nutrition has not been shown to decrease catheter-related thrombosis. The final concentration of heparin used for TPN solutions may need to be decreased to 0.5 units/mL in small infants receiving larger

(Continued)

Heparin *(Continued)*

amounts of volume in order to avoid approaching therapeutic amounts. Arterial lines are heparinized with a final concentration of 1 unit/mL.

Elderly: Patients >60 years of age may have higher serum levels and clinical response (longer aPTTs) as compared to younger patients receiving similar dosages. Lower dosages may be required.

Pediatrics:

Anticoagulation: Intermittent I.V.: Initial: 50-100 units/kg, then 50-100 units/kg every 4 hours

Anticoagulation: I.V. infusion: Initial: 50 units/kg, then 15-25 units/kg/hour; increase dose by 2-4 units/kg/hour every 6-8 hours as required

Note: Refer to adult dosing for notes on line flushing and TPN.

Available Dosage Forms [DSC] = Discontinued product

Infusion, as sodium [premixed in NaCl 0.45%; porcine intestinal mucosa source]: 12,500 units (250 mL); 25,000 units (250 mL, 500 mL)

Infusion, as sodium [preservative free; premixed in D_5W; porcine intestinal mucosa source]: 10,000 units (100 mL) [contains sodium metabisulfite]; 12,500 units (250 mL) [contains sodium metabisulfite]; 20,000 units (500 mL) [contains sodium metabisulfite]; 25,000 units (250 mL, 500 mL) [contains sodium metabisulfite]

Infusion, as sodium [preservative free; premixed in NaCl 0.9%; porcine intestinal mucosa source]: 1000 units (500 mL); 2000 units (1000 mL)

Injection, solution, as sodium [beef lung source; multidose vial]: 1000 units/mL (10 mL, 30 mL); 5000 units/mL (10 mL), 10,000 units/mL (1 mL, 4 mL) [contains benzyl alcohol] [DSC]

Injection, solution, as sodium [lock flush preparation; porcine intestinal mucosa source; multidose vial]: 10 units/mL (1 mL, 10 mL, 30 mL) [contains parabens]; 100 units/mL (1 mL, 5 mL) [contains parabens]

Injection, solution, as sodium [lock flush preparation; porcine intestinal mucosa source; multidose vial]: 10 units/mL (10 mL, 30 mL); 100 units/mL (10 mL, 30 mL) [contains benzyl alcohol]

Hep-Lock®: 10 units/mL (1 mL, 2 mL, 10 mL, 30 mL); 100 units/mL (1 mL, 2 mL, 10 mL, 30 mL) [contains benzyl alcohol]

Injection, solution, as sodium [lock flush preparation; porcine intestinal mucosa source; prefilled syringe]: 10 units/mL (1 mL, 2 mL, 3 mL, 5 mL); 100 units/mL (1 mL, 2 mL, 3 mL, 5 mL) [contains benzyl alcohol]

Injection, solution, as sodium [preservative free; lock flush preparation; porcine intestinal mucosa source; prefilled syringe]: 100 units/mL (5 mL)

Injection, solution, as sodium [preservative free; lock flush preparation; porcine intestinal mucosa source; vial] (HepFlush®-10): 10 units/mL (10 mL)

Injection, solution, as sodium [porcine intestinal mucosa source; multidose vial]: 1000 units/mL (1 mL, 10 mL, 30 mL) [contains benzyl alcohol]; 1000 units/mL (1 mL, 10 mL, 30 mL) [contains methylparabens]; 5000 units/mL (1 mL, 10 mL) [contains benzyl alcohol]; 5000 units/mL (1 mL) [contains methylparabens]; 10,000 units/mL (1 mL, 4 mL) [contains benzyl alcohol]; 10,000 units/mL (1 mL, 5 mL) [contains methylparabens]; 20,000 units/mL (1 mL) [contains methylparabens]

Injection, solution, as sodium [porcine intestinal mucosa source; prefilled syringe]: 5000 units/mL (1 mL) [contains benzyl alcohol]

Injection, solution, as sodium [preservative free; porcine intestinal mucosa source; prefilled syringe]: 10,000 units/mL (0.5 mL)

Injection, solution, as sodium [preservative free; porcine intestinal mucosa source; vial]: 1000 units/mL (2 mL); 2000 units/mL (5 mL); 2500 units/mL (10 mL)

Nursing Guidelines

Assessment: Assess for risk factors for increased bleeding prior to starting therapy. Assess potential for interactions with other pharmacological agents or herbal products patient may be taking (especially anything that will affect coagulation or platelet function). Note specific infusion directions in Administration. Bleeding precautions should be observed at all times during heparin therapy. Assess results of laboratory tests regularly for necessary dosing adjustments and therapeutic effectiveness. Patient response should be assessed regularly during therapy (eg, hypersensitivity reaction, bleeding, chest pain, hyperkalemia, peripheral neuropathy). Teach possible side effects/appropriate interventions (eg, bleeding precautions) and adverse symptoms to report.

Monitoring Laboratory Tests: Platelet counts, hemoglobin, hematocrit, signs of bleeding; aPTT or ACT depending upon indication. For intermittent I.V.

injections, PTT is measured 3.5-4 hours after I.V. injection. **Note:** Continuous I.V. infusion is preferred vs I.V. intermittent injections. For full-dose heparin (ie, nonlow-dose), the dose should be titrated according to PTT results. For anticoagulation, an aPTT 1.5-2.5 times normal is usually desired; aPTT is usually measured prior to heparin therapy, 6-8 hours after initiation of a continuous infusion (following a loading dose), and 6-8 hours after changes in the infusion rate; increase or decrease infusion by 2-4 units/kg/hour dependent on PTT.

Heparin infusion dose adjustment:

aPTT >3x control: Decrease infusion rate 50%.

aPTT 2-3x control: Decrease infusion rate 25%.

aPTT 1.5-2x control: No change.

aPTT <1.5x control: Increase rate of infusion 25%; max 2500 units/hour.

Patient Education: Do not take any new medication, including over-the-counter and biological products, during therapy unless approved by prescriber. This drug can only be administered by infusion or injection. You may have a tendency to bleed easily while taking this drug (brush teeth with soft brush, floss with waxed floss, use electric razor, avoid scissors or sharp knives, and potentially harmful activities). Report immediately any chest pain; difficulty breathing or unusual cough; bleeding or bruising (bleeding gums, nosebleed, blood in urine, dark stool); pain in joints or back; CNS changes (fever, confusion); unusual fever; persistent nausea or GI upset; change in vision, or swelling, pain, or redness at injection site. **Pregnancy precaution:** Inform prescriber if you are pregnant.

Geriatric Considerations: At similar dosages, heparin levels tend to be higher in elderly patients (>60 years of age). In the clinical setting, age has not been shown to be a reliable predictor of a patient's anticoagulant response to heparin. However, it is common for older patients to have a "standard" response for the first 24-48 hours after a loading dose (5000 units) and a maintenance infusion of 800-1000 units/hour. After this period, they then have an exaggerated response (eg, elevated PTT), requiring a lower infusion rate. Hence, monitor closely during this period of therapy. Older women (>60 years of age) are more likely to have bleeding complications and osteoporosis may be a problem when used >3 months or total daily dose exceeds 30,000 units.

Pregnancy Risk Factor: C

Lactation: Does not enter breast milk/compatible

Perioperative/Anesthesia/Other Concerns: In the treatment of unstable angina/non-ST-segment elevation MI, parenteral anticoagulation with unfractionated heparin or low molecular weight heparin is recommended.

Thrombocytopenia: Heparin-associated thrombocytopenia (HAT) commonly occurs within 48-72 hours of initiation. Platelet counts usually fall below 100,000 cells/mm^3 and return to normal within 4 days with continued heparin therapy. Heparin-induced thrombocytopenia (HIT) is a serious, immunoglobulin-mediated reaction with a high risk for thromboembolic events. In HIT, thrombocytopenia usually begins 5-10 days following heparin initiation; HIT can begin within ~10 hours in patients who have received heparin within the previous 100 days (Warkentin T, 2001). Thrombocytopenia can be severe; heparin of all forms must be stopped including flushes and heparin-coated indwelling catheters.

The addition of heparin to parenteral nutrition solutions does not significantly decrease the risk of catheter-related thrombosis (Klerk C, 2003).

Administration

I.M.: Do not administer I.M. due to pain, irritation, and hematoma formation.

I.V.:

Continuous infusion: Infuse via infusion pump.

Heparin lock: Inject via injection cap using positive pressure flushing technique. Heparin lock flush solution is intended only to maintain patency of I.V. devices and is **not** to be used for anticoagulant therapy.

Reconstitution: Stability at room temperature and refrigeration:

Prepared bag: 24 hours

Premixed bag: After seal is broken 4 days

Out of overwrap stability: 30 days

Standard diluent: 25,000 units/500 mL D_5W (premixed)

Minimum volume: 250 mL D_5W

Compatibility: Stable in dextran 6% in dextrose, dextran 6% in NS, D_5LR, $D_5\frac{1}{4}NS$, $D_5\frac{1}{2}NS$, $D_{25}W$, fat emulsion 10%, $\frac{1}{2}NS$, NS

(Continued)

Heparin *(Continued)*

Y-site administration: Incompatible with alatrofloxacin, alteplase, amiodarone, amphotericin B cholesteryl sulfate complex, amsacrine, ciprofloxacin, clarithromycin, diazepam, doxycycline, ergotamine, filgrastim, gatifloxacin, gentamicin, haloperidol, idarubicin, isosorbide dinitrate, levofloxacin, methotrimeprazine, nicardipine, phenytoin, tobramycin, triflupromazine, vancomycin

Compatibility in syringe: Incompatible with amikacin, amiodarone, chlorpromazine, diazepam, doxorubicin, droperidol, droperidol and fentanyl, erythromycin, erythromycin lactobionate, gentamicin, haloperidol, kanamycin, meperidine, methotrimeprazine, pentazocine, promethazine, streptomycin, tobramycin, triflupromazine, vancomycin, warfarin

Compatibility when admixed: Incompatible with alteplase, amikacin, atracurium, ciprofloxacin, cytarabine, daunorubicin, erythromycin lactobionate, gentamicin, hyaluronidase, kanamycin, levorphanol, meperidine, morphine, polymyxin B sulfate, promethazine, streptomycin

Storage: Heparin solutions are colorless to slightly yellow. Minor color variations do not affect therapeutic efficacy. Heparin should be stored at controlled room temperature and protected from freezing and temperatures >40°C.

- **Heparin Calcium** *see* Heparin *on page 845*
- **Heparin Cofactor I** *see* Antithrombin III *on page 173*
- **Heparin Lock Flush** *see* Heparin *on page 845*
- **Heparin Sodium** *see* Heparin *on page 845*

Hepatitis A Vaccine (hep a TYE tis aye vak SEEN)

U.S. Brand Names Havrix®; VAQTA®

Pharmacologic Category Vaccine

Use

Active immunization against disease caused by hepatitis A virus in populations desiring protection against or at high risk of exposure

Populations at high risk of exposure to hepatitis A virus may include children and adolescents in selected states and regions, travelers to developing countries, household and sexual contacts of persons infected with hepatitis A, child day care employees, patients with chronic liver disease, illicit drug users, male homosexuals, institutional workers (eg, institutions for the mentally and physically handicapped persons, prisons), and healthcare workers who may be exposed to hepatitis A virus (eg, laboratory employees)

Mechanism of Action As an inactivated virus vaccine, hepatitis A vaccine offers active immunization against hepatitis A virus infection at an effective immune response rate in up to 99% of subjects

Pharmacodynamics/Kinetics

Onset of action (protection): 4 weeks after a single dose

Duration: Neutralizing antibodies have persisted for up to 8 years; based on kinetic models, antibodies may be present >20 years

Contraindications Hypersensitivity to hepatitis A vaccine or any component of the formulation

Warnings/Precautions Use caution in patients on anticoagulants, with thrombocytopenia, or bleeding disorders (bleeding may occur following intramuscular injection). Treatment for anaphylactic reactions should be immediately available. Postpone vaccination with acute infection or febrile illness. May not prevent infection if adequate antibody titers are not achieved (including immunosuppressed patients, patients on immunosuppressant therapy).

Drug Interactions

Immune globulin: May be administered concomitantly (using separate sites and syringes)

Vaccines: May be administered concomitantly with cholera, diphtheria, MMR II, Japanese encephalitis, poliovirus, rabies, tetanus, typhoid or yellow fever vaccines using separate sites and syringes. May be administered simultaneously with hepatitis B vaccine.

Adverse Reactions All serious adverse reactions must be reported to the U.S. Department of Health and Human Services (DHHS) Vaccine Adverse Event Reporting System (VAERS) 1-800-822-7967.

Frequency dependant upon age, product used, and concomitant vaccine administration. In general, injection site reactions were less common in younger children.

>10%:

Central nervous system: Irritability (11% to 36%), drowsiness (15% to 17%), headache (2% to 16%), fever ≥100.4°F (9% to 11%)

Gastrointestinal: Anorexia (1% to 19%)

Local: Injection site: Pain, soreness, tenderness (3% to 56%), erythema (1% to 22%), warmth (<1% to 17%), swelling (1% to 14%)

1% to 10%:

Central nervous system: Fever ≥102°F (3% to 4%)

Dermatologic: Rash (≤1% to 5%)

Endocrine & metabolic: Menstrual disorder (1%)

Gastrointestinal: Diarrhea (<1% to 6%), vomiting (<1% to 4%), nausea (2%), abdominal pain (<1% to 2%), anorexia (1%)

Local: Injection site bruising (1% to 2%)

Neuromuscular & skeletal: Weakness/fatigue (4%), myalgia (<1% to 2%), arm pain (1%), back pain (1%), stiffness (1%)

Ocular: Conjunctivitis (1%)

Otic: Otitis media (8%), otitis (2%)

Respiratory: Upper respiratory tract infection (<1% to 10%), rhinorrhea (6%), cough (1% to 5%), pharnyngitis (<1% to 3%), respiratory congestion (2%), nasal congestion (1%), laryngotracheobronchitis (1%)

Miscellaneous: Crying (2%), viral exanthema (1%)

<1% (Limited to importantor life threatening): Allergic reaction, anaphylaxis, angioedema, arthralgia, asthma, bronchial constriction, cerebellar ataxia, CK increased, dermatitis, dizziness, dyspnea, encephalitis, erythema multiforme, eosinophilia, Guillain-Barre syndrome, hepatitis, hyperhydrosis, hypertonic episode, injection site hematoma, injection site itching, injection site rash, insomnia, jaundice, liver function tests increased, lymphadenopathy, multiple sclerosis, myelitis, neuropathy, paresthesia, photophobia, pruritus, seizure, somnolence, syncope, taste disturbance, thrombocytopenia, urine protein increased, vertigo, wheezing

Dosing

Adults & Elderly: Immunization: I.M.:

Havrix®:

1440 ELISA units (1 mL) with a booster 6-12 months following primary immunization

VAQTA®:

50 units (1 mL) with 50 units (1 mL) booster to be given 6-18 months after primary immunization (6-12 months if initial dose was with Havrix®)

Pediatrics: Immunization: I.M.:

Havrix®: Children 12 months to 18 years: 720 ELISA units (0.5 mL) with a booster dose of 720 ELISA units 6-12 months following primary immunization

VAQTA®: Children 12 months to 18 years: 25 units (0.5 mL) with 25 units (0.5 mL) booster to be given 6-18 months after primary immunization (6-12 months if initial dose was with Havrix®)

Available Dosage Forms

Injection, suspension, adult:

Havrix®: Viral antigen 1440 ELISA units/mL (1 mL) [contains trace amounts of neomycin; syringe plunger contains latex rubber; available in prefilled syringe or single-dose vial]

VAQTA®: HAV antigen 50 units/mL (1 mL) [vial stopper and syringe plunger contain latex rubber; available in prefilled syringe or single-dose vial]

Injection, suspension, pediatric (Havrix®): Viral antigen 720 ELISA units/0.5 mL (0.5 mL) [contains trace amounts of neomycin; syringe plunger contains latex rubber; available in prefilled syringe or single-dose vial]

Injection, suspension, pediatric/adolescent (VAQTA®): HAV antigen 25 units/0.5 mL (0.5 mL) [vial stopper and syringe plunger contain latex rubber; available in prefilled syringe or single-dose vial]

Nursing Guidelines

Patient Education: Inform patients of side effects; explain need for booster; patients should report side effects lasting longer than 24 hours

Pregnancy Risk Factor: C

Lactation: Excretion in breast milk unknown/use caution

Administration

I.M.: The deltoid muscle is the preferred site for injection. Shake well prior to use. For optimal protection, travelers should receive 1st dose at least 4 weeks prior to departure. For patients at risk of hemorrhage following intramuscular injection, the ACIP recommends "it should be administered intramuscularly if, in the

(Continued)

Hepatitis A Vaccine *(Continued)*

opinion of the physician familiar with the patients bleeding risk, the vaccine can be administered with reasonable safety by this route. If the patient receives antihemophilia or other similar therapy, intramuscular vaccination can be scheduled shortly after such therapy is administered. A fine needle (23 gauge or smaller) can be used for the vaccination and firm pressure applied to the site (without rubbing) for at least 2 minutes. The patient should be instructed concerning the risk of hematoma from the injection."

Storage: Store under refrigeration at 2°C to 8°C (36°F to 46°F). Do not freeze.

♦ **HepFlush®-10** *see* Heparin *on page 845*

♦ **Hep-Lock®** *see* Heparin *on page 845*

♦ **Herceptin®** *see* Trastuzumab *on page 1655*

♦ **HES** *see* Hetastarch *on page 852*

♦ **Hespan®** *see* Hetastarch *on page 852*

Hetastarch (HET a starch)

U.S. Brand Names Hespan®; Hextend®

Synonyms HES; Hydroxyethyl Starch

Pharmacologic Category Plasma Volume Expander, Colloid

Medication Safety Issues

Sound-alike/look-alike issues:

Hespan® may be confused with heparin

Use Blood volume expander used in treatment of hypovolemia

Hespan®: Adjunct in leukapheresis to improve harvesting and increasing the yield of granulocytes by centrifugal means

Unlabeled/Investigational Use Hextend®: Priming fluid in pump oxygenators during cardiopulmonary bypass, and as a plasma volume expander during cardiopulmonary bypass

Mechanism of Action Produces plasma volume expansion by virtue of its highly colloidal starch structure, similar to albumin

Pharmacodynamics/Kinetics

Onset of action: Volume expansion: I.V.: ~30 minutes

Duration: 24-36 hours

Metabolism: Molecules >50,000 daltons require enzymatic degradation by the reticuloendothelial system or amylases in the blood

Excretion: Urine (~40%) within 24 hours; smaller molecular weight molecules readily excreted

Contraindications Hypersensitivity to hydroxyethyl starch or any component of the formulation; severe bleeding disorders, renal failure with oliguria or anuria, or severe congestive heart failure; per the manufacturer, Hextend® is also contraindicated in the treatment of lactic acidosis and in leukapheresis

Warnings/Precautions Anaphylactoid reactions have occurred; use caution in patients allergic to corn (may have cross allergy to hetastarch); use with caution in patients with thrombocytopenia (may interfere with platelet function); large volume may cause drops in hemoglobin concentrations; use with caution in patients at risk from overexpansion of blood volume, including the very young or aged patients, those with CHF or pulmonary edema; volumes >1500 mL may interfere with platelet function and prolong PT and PTT times; use with caution in patients with history of liver disease; note electrolyte content of Hextend® including calcium, lactate, and potassium; use caution in situations where electrolyte and/or acid-base disturbances may be exacerbated (renal impairment, respiratory alkalosis). Safety and efficacy in pediatric patients have not been established, but limited data available.

Adverse Reactions Frequency not defined.

Cardiovascular: Circulatory overload, heart failure, peripheral edema

Central nervous system: Chills, fever, headache, intracranial bleeding

Dermatologic: Itching, pruritus, rash

Endocrine & metabolic: Amylase levels increased, parotid gland enlargement, indirect bilirubin increased, metabolic acidosis

Gastrointestinal: Vomiting

Hematologic: Bleeding, factor VIII:C plasma levels decreased, decreased plasma aggregation decreased, von Willebrand factor decreased, dilutional coagulopathy; prolongation of PT, PTT, clotting time, and bleeding time; thrombocytopenia, anemia, disseminated intravascular coagulopathy (rare), hemolysis (rare)

Neuromuscular & skeletal: Myalgia

Miscellaneous: Anaphylactoid reactions, hypersensitivity, flu-like symptoms (mild)

Overdosage/Toxicology Symptoms of overdose include heart failure, nausea, vomiting, circulatory overload, and bleeding. Treatment is supportive. Hetastarch is not eliminated by hemodialysis.

Dosing

Adults & Elderly:

Volume expansion: 500-1000 mL (up to 1500 mL/day) or 20 mL/kg/day (up to 1500 mL/day); larger volumes (15,000 mL/24 hours) have been used safely in small numbers of patients

Leukapheresis: 250-700 mL; **Note:** Citrate anticoagulant is added before use.

Pediatrics: Safety and efficacy have not been established.

Renal Impairment: Cl_{cr} <10 mL/minute: Initial dose is the same but subsequent doses should be reduced by 20% to 50% of normal.

Available Dosage Forms

Infusion [premixed in lactated electrolyte injection] (Hextend®): 6% (500 mL)

Infusion, solution [premixed in NaCl 0.9%] (Hespan®): 6% (500 mL)

Nursing Guidelines

Assessment: See Use, Contraindications, Warnings/Precautions, and Dosing for use cautions. See Administration specifics. Patient must be monitored closely for hypersensitivity (anaphylactic reaction) and other major adverse reactions (see Adverse Reactions and Overdose/Toxicology). Blood pressure, pulse, central venous pressure, and urine output should be monitored every 5-15 minutes for the first hour and closely thereafter (see below). Patient teaching should be appropriate to patient condition (see Patient Education). Note breast-feeding caution.

Monitoring Laboratory Tests: Hemoglobin, hematocrit

Leukapheresis: CBC, total leukocyte and platelet counts, leukocyte differential count, hemoglobin, hematocrit, PT, PTT

Patient Education: Report immediately any respiratory difficulty, acute headache, muscle pain, or abdominal cramping. **Pregnancy/breast-feeding precautions:** Inform prescriber if you are pregnant. Consult prescriber if breast-feeding.

Pregnancy Risk Factor: C

Lactation: Excretion in breast milk unknown/use caution

Perioperative/Anesthesia/Other Concerns: Hetastarch is a synthetic polymer derived from a waxy starch composed of amylopectin.

Hespan®: 6% hetastarch in 0.9% sodium chloride

Molecular weight: 450,000
Sodium: 154 mEq/L
Chloride: 154 mEq/L

Hextend®: 6% hetastarch in lactated electrolyte injection

Molecular weight: 670,000
Sodium: 143 mEq/L
Chloride: 124 mEq/L
Calcium: 5 mEq/L
Potassium: 3 mEq/L
Magnesium: 0.9 mEq/L
Lactate: 28 mEq/L
Dextrose: 0.99 g/L

Both Hextend® and Hespan® will expand the intravascular volume the same as an equal volume of 5% albumin. Hetastarch will increase the intravascular volume up to 24-36 hours. Hetastarch does not have oxygen-carrying capacity and is not a substitute for blood or plasma. Large volumes of Hespan® or Hextend® may interfere with platelet function, prolong PT and PTT times and cause hemodilution, however, clinically Hextend® has not been associated with coagulation abnormalities in doses >20 mL/kg up to a total of 5000 mL.

Hextend®: Formulated with near physiologic levels of sodium, chloride, calcium, potassium, magnesium; may be associated with less electrolyte abnormalities than Hespan®; not to be used for the treatment of lactic acidosis; should not be administered through the same line as blood products; use with caution in patients with congestive heart failure.

Hespan®: Intraoperative use in patients undergoing cardiac surgery with cardiopulmonary bypass may increase bleeding; each 500 mL provides 77 mEq sodium chloride and may cause hyperchloremic metabolic acidosis in large volumes; critically-ill patients receiving hetastarch infusions (goal: PCWP 12-18 mm Hg) had an increase in cardiac index, oxygen delivery and consumption.

(Continued)

Hetastarch *(Continued)*

Hextend® and Hespan®: May increase serum amylase temporarily without an association with pancreatitis; not eliminated by hemodialysis.

Administration

I.V.: Administer I.V. only; infusion pump is required. May administer up to 1.2 g/kg/hour (20 mL/kg/hour). Change I.V. tubing or flush copiously with normal saline before administering blood through the same line. Change I.V. tubing at least every 24 hours. Do not administer Hextend® with blood through the same administration set. Anaphylactoid reactions can occur, have epinephrine and resuscitative equipment available.

Reconstitution: Do not use if crystalline precipitate forms or is turbid deep brown.

Compatibility: Stable in NS

Y-site administration: Incompatible with amikacin, cefamandole, cefoperazone, cefotaxime, cefoxitin, gentamicin, ranitidine, theophylline, tobramycin

Storage: Store at room temperature; do not freeze. In leukapheresis, admixtures of 500-560 mL of Hespan® with citrate concentrations up to 2.5% are compatible for 24 hours.

Hexachlorophene (heks a KLOR oh feen)

U.S. Brand Names pHisoHex®

Pharmacologic Category Antibiotic, Topical

Medication Safety Issues

Sound-alike/look-alike issues:

pHisoHex® may be confused with Fostex®, pHisoDerm®

Use Surgical scrub and as a bacteriostatic skin cleanser; control an outbreak of gram-positive infection when other procedures have been unsuccessful

Mechanism of Action Bacteriostatic polychlorinated biphenyl which inhibits membrane-bound enzymes and disrupts the cell membrane

Pharmacodynamics/Kinetics

Absorption: Percutaneously through inflamed, excoriated, and intact skin

Distribution: Crosses placenta

Half-life elimination: Infants: 6.1-44.2 hours

Contraindications Hypersensitivity to halogenated phenol derivatives or hexachlorophene; use in premature infants; use on burned or denuded skin; occlusive dressing; application to mucous membranes

Warnings/Precautions Discontinue use if signs of cerebral irritability occur; exposure of preterm infants or patients with extensive burns has been associated with apnea, convulsions, agitation and coma; do not use for bathing infants, premature infants are particularly susceptible to hexachlorophene topical absorption

Drug Interactions No data reported

Adverse Reactions <1%: CNS injury, seizure, irritability, photosensitivity, dermatitis, redness, dry skin

Overdosage/Toxicology

Symptoms of overdose include anorexia, vomiting, abdominal cramps, diarrhea, dehydration, seizures, hypotension, shock

Treatment is supportive

Dosing

Adults & Elderly: Antiseptic (Children and Adults): Topical: Apply 5 mL cleanser and water to area to be cleansed; lather and rinse thoroughly under running water

Pediatrics: Refer to adult dosing.

Available Dosage Forms Liquid, topical: 3% (150 mL, 500 mL, 3840 mL)

Nursing Guidelines

Patient Education: Do not leave on skin for prolonged contact; for external use only; discontinue product if condition persists or worsens and call physician; if suds enter eye, rinse out thoroughly with water

Pregnancy Risk Factor: C

♦ **Hextend®** *see* Hetastarch *on page 852*

♦ **Hibiclens® [OTC]** *see* Chlorhexidine Gluconate *on page 373*

♦ **Hibistat® [OTC]** *see* Chlorhexidine Gluconate *on page 373*

♦ **Hib Polysaccharide Conjugate** *see Haemophilus* b Conjugate Vaccine *on page 837*

♦ **HibTITER®** *see Haemophilus* b Conjugate Vaccine *on page 837*

- **High Gamma Vitamin E Complete™ [OTC]** *see* Vitamin E *on page 1716*
- **Hi-Kovite [OTC** *see* Vitamins (Multiple/Oral) *on page 1720*
- **Hirulog** *see* Bivalirudin *on page 246*

Homatropine (hoe MA troe peen)

U.S. Brand Names Isopto® Homatropine

Synonyms Homatropine Hydrobromide

Pharmacologic Category Anticholinergic Agent, Ophthalmic; Ophthalmic Agent, Mydriatic

Use Producing cycloplegia and mydriasis for refraction; treatment of acute inflammatory conditions of the uveal tract

Mechanism of Action Blocks response of iris sphincter muscle and the accommodative muscle of the ciliary body to cholinergic stimulation resulting in dilation and loss of accommodation

Pharmacodynamics/Kinetics

Onset of action: Accommodation and pupil effect: Ophthalmic:
- Maximum mydriatic effect: Within 10-30 minutes
- Maximum cycloplegic effect: Within 30-90 minutes

Duration:
- Mydriasis: 6 hours to 4 days
- Cycloplegia: 10-48 hours

Contraindications Hypersensitivity to the drug or any component of the formulation; narrow-angle glaucoma, acute hemorrhage

Warnings/Precautions Use with caution in patients with hypertension, cardiac disease, or increased intraocular pressure; safety and efficacy not established in infants and young children, therefore, use with extreme caution due to susceptibility of systemic effects; use with caution in obstructive uropathy, paralytic ileus, ulcerative colitis, unstable cardiovascular status in acute hemorrhage

Adverse Reactions

>10%: Ocular: Blurred vision, photophobia

1% to 10%:
- Local: Irritation
- Ocular: Increased intraocular pressure
- Respiratory: Congestion

<1% (Limited to important or life-threatening): Eczematoid dermatitis, edema, exudate, follicular conjunctivitis, somnolence, vascular congestion

Overdosage/Toxicology

Symptoms of overdose include blurred vision, urinary retention, tachycardia

Anticholinergic toxicity is caused by strong binding of the drug to cholinergic receptors. For anticholinergic overdose with severe life-threatening symptoms, physostigmine 1-2 mg (0.5 mg or 0.02 mg/kg for children) SubQ or I.V., slowly may be given to reverse these effects.

Dosing

Adults & Elderly:

Mydriasis and cycloplegia for refraction: Ophthalmic: Instill 1-2 drops of 2% solution or 1 drop of 5% solution before the procedure; repeat at 5- to 10-minute intervals as needed; maximum of 3 doses for refraction

Uveitis: Ophthalmic: Instill 1-2 drops of 2% or 5% 2-3 times/day up to every 3-4 hours as needed

Pediatrics:

Mydriasis and cycloplegia for refraction: Ophthalmic: Instill 1 drop of 2% solution immediately before the procedure; repeat at 10-minute intervals as needed

Uveitis: Ophthalmic: Instill 1 drop of 2% solution 2-3 times/day

Available Dosage Forms Solution, ophthalmic, as hydrobromide: 2% (5 mL); 5% (5 mL, 15 mL) [contains benzalkonium chloride]

Nursing Guidelines

Patient Education: May cause blurred vision; if irritation persists or increases, discontinue use

Pregnancy Risk Factor: C

- **Homatropine Hydrobromide** *see* Homatropine *on page 855*
- **Horse Antihuman Thymocyte Gamma Globulin** *see* Antithymocyte Globulin (Equine) *on page 174*
- **H.P. Acthar® Gel** *see* Corticotropin *on page 450*
- **Humalog®** *see* Insulin Lispro *on page 923*

- Humalog® Mix 75/25™ *see* Insulin Lispro Protamine and Insulin Lispro *on page 925*
- Human Growth Hormone *see* Somatropin *on page 1555*
- Humanized IgG1 Anti-CD52 Monoclonal Antibody *see* Alemtuzumab *on page 102*
- Humatrope® *see* Somatropin *on page 1555*
- Humibid® *e* [OTC] *see* Guaifenesin *on page 834*
- Humulin® 50/50 *see* Insulin NPH and Insulin Regular *on page 927*
- Humulin® 70/30 *see* Insulin NPH and Insulin Regular *on page 927*
- Humulin® N *see* Insulin NPH *on page 926*
- Humulin® R *see* Insulin Regular *on page 928*
- Humulin® R (Concentrated) U-500 *see* Insulin Regular *on page 928*
- Hurricaine® [OTC] *see* Benzocaine *on page 232*
- Hyalgan® *see* Hyaluronate and Derivatives *on page 856*
- Hyaluronan *see* Hyaluronate and Derivatives *on page 856*

Hyaluronate and Derivatives

(hye al yoor ON ate & dah RIV ah tives)

U.S. Brand Names Biolon™; Euflexxa™; Healon®; Healon®5; Healon GV®; Hyalgan®; Hylaform®; Hylaform® Plus; IPM Wound Gel™ [OTC]; Orthovisc®; Provisc®; Restylane®; Supartz™; Synvisc®; Vitrax®

Synonyms Hyaluronan; Hyaluronic Acid; Hylan Polymers; Sodium Hyaluronate

Pharmacologic Category Antirheumatic Miscellaneous; Ophthalmic Agent, Viscoelastic; Skin and Mucous Membrane Agent, Miscellaneous

Medication Safety Issues

Sound-alike/look-alike issues:

Synvisc® may be confused with Synagis®

Use

Intra-articular injection: Treatment of pain in osteoarthritis in knee in patients who have failed nonpharmacologic treatment and simple analgesics

Intradermal: Correction of moderate-to-severe facial wrinkles or folds

Ophthalmic: Surgical aid in cataract extraction, intraocular implantation, corneal transplant, glaucoma filtration, and retinal attachment surgery

Topical: Management of skin ulcers and wounds

Mechanism of Action Sodium hyaluronate is a polysaccharide which is distributed widely in the extracellular matrix of connective tissue in man (vitreous and aqueous humor of the eye, synovial fluid, skin, and umbilical cord). Sodium hyaluronate and its derivatives form a viscoelastic solution in water (at physiological pH and ionic strength) which makes it suitable for aqueous and vitreous humor in ophthalmic surgery, and functions as a tissue and/or joint lubricant which plays an important role in modulating the interactions between adjacent tissues. Intradermal injection may decrease the depth of facial wrinkles.

Pharmacodynamics/Kinetics

Distribution: Intravitreous injection: Diffusion occurs slowly

Excretion: Ophthalmic: Via Canal of Schlemm

Contraindications Hypersensitivity to hyaluronate or any component of the formulation

Hylaform® (intradermal), Hylaform® Plus (intradermal), Orthovisc® (intra-articular): Additional contraindications include hypersensitivity to avian proteins (egg products, feathers)

Restylane® (intradermal): Additional contraindications include history of or presence of multiple severe allergies; known susceptibility to keloid formation or recurrence; sensitivity to gram-positive bacterial proteins

Intra-articular: Knee joint infections, infections or skin diseases at the site of injection

Warnings/Precautions Not for I.V. injection. Do not inject into blood vessels; may cause occlusion, infarction, embolism, or other systemic adverse events.

Intra-articular: Not for use in infected joints; do not use disinfectants containing quaternary salts for skin preparation (may cause precipitation of hyaluronate). Remove effusion, if present, prior to injection. Use with caution if venous or lymphatic stasis is present in the leg. Avoid strenuous activities for 48 hours after injection. Safety and efficacy have not been established in children.

Intradermal: Do not inject into site of active inflammation or infection. Avoid use in patients susceptible to keloid formation, hypertrophic scarring, or pigmentation disorders. Supplemental "touch up" treatments may be required. Use caution with immunosuppressive treatment. Patient must avoid exposure to ultraviolet rays (sun and UV lamp) or severe cold until swelling and redness is resolved. Laser treatment or chemical peeling may cause acute inflammatory reaction. Use in lip augmentation has not been established.

Ophthalmic: Do not overfill the anterior chamber; carefully monitor intraocular pressure

Topical: Cleansing agents other than normal saline are not recommended

Drug Interactions

Anticoagulants or antiplatelet agents: May increase the risk of injection site bleeding or hematoma.

Adverse Reactions Not all frequencies are defined. Frequencies and/or type of local reaction may vary by formulation and site of application/injection.

Cardiovascular: Blood pressure increased (2% to 4%), edema, flushing, hypotension, tachycardia

Central nervous system: Dizziness, fatigue (1%), headache

Dermatologic: Itching, rash

Gastrointestinal: Nausea (≤2%)

Local: Injection site: Arthralgia, bruising, desquamation, erythema, pain, rash, swelling; nodule, pruritus, skin discoloration

Neuromuscular & skeletal: Back pain (<1% to 6%), tendonitis (2%), parasthesia (1%), hypokinesia (knee)

Ocular (with ophthalmic formulation): Postoperative inflammatory reactions (iritis, hypopyon), corneal edema, corneal decompensation, transient postoperative increase in IOP

Respiratory: Infection (12%), rhinitis (3%)

Miscellaneous: Abscess formation, allergic reactions, anaphylaxis, respiratory difficulties

Dosing

Adults & Elderly:

Surgical aid: Ophthalmic (Biolon™, Healon®, Provisc®, Vitrax®): Depends upon procedure (slowly introduce a sufficient quantity into eye)

Osteoarthritis of the knee: Intra-articular:

Eulexxa™: Inject 20 mg (2 mL) once weekly for 3 weeks

Hyalgan®: Inject 20 mg (2 mL) once weekly for 5 weeks; some patients may benefit with a total of 3 injections

Orthovisc®: Inject 30 mg (2 mL) once weekly for 3-4 weeks

Supartz™: Inject 25 mg (2.5 mL) once weekly for 5 weeks

Synvisc®: Inject 16 mg (2 mL) once weekly for 3 weeks (total of 3 injections)

Facial wrinkles: Intradermal: (Hylaform®, Hylaform® Plus, Restylane®): Inject as required for cosmetic result; typical treatment regimen requires <2 mL; limit injection to ≤1.5 mL per injection site. Hylaform®, Hylaform® Plus: Maximum: 20 mL/60 kg/year

Skin ulcers and wounds: Topical (IPM Wound Gel™): Apply to clean dry ulcer or wound, and cover with nonstick dressing; repeat daily. Discontinue if wound size increase after 3-4 applications.

Available Dosage Forms

Hylan B: Injection, gel:

Hylaform® [500 micron particle]: 5.5 mg/mL (0.75 mL) [prefilled syringe; derived from avian source]

Hylaform® Plus [700 micron particle]: 5.5 mg/mL (0.75 mL) [prefilled syringe; derived from avian source]

Hylan polymers A and B (Hylan G-F 20): Injection, solution, intra-articular (Synvisc®): 8 mg/mL (2 mL) [prefilled syringe; contains trace amounts of *Streptococcus*]

Sodium Hyaluronate:

Gel, topical (IPM Wound Gel™): 2.5% (10 g)

Injection, gel, intradermal (Restylane®): 20 mg/mL [prefilled syringe]

Injection, solution, intra-articular:

Euflexxa™: 10 mg/mL (2 mL) [prefilled syringe; syringe contains latex]

Hyalgan®: 10 mg/mL (2 mL)

Orthovisc®: 15 mg/mL (2 mL) [prefilled syringe; derived from avian source]

Supartz™: 10 mg/mL (2.5 mL) [derived from avian source]

Synvisc®: 8 mg/mL (2 mL) [prefilled syringe; derived from avian source]

Injection, solution, intraocular:

Biolon™: 10 mg/mL (0.5 mL, 1 mL)

Healon®: 10 mg/mL (0.4 mL, 0.55 mL, 0.85 mL, 2 mL)

Healon®5: 23 mg/mL

Healon GV®: 14 mg/mL (0.55 mL, 0.85 mL)

(Continued)

Hyaluronate and Derivatives *(Continued)*

Provisc®: 10 mg/mL (0.4 mL, 0.55 mL, 0.8 mL) [prefilled syringe; contains lactose]

Vitrax®: 30 mg/mL (0.65 mL)

Nursing Guidelines

Pregnancy Risk Factor: C

Lactation: Excretion in breast milk unknown/not recommended

Administration

Compatibility: Incompatible (solution): Disinfectants containing quaternary ammonium salts may precipitate hyaluronic acid. Detergents and benzalkonium chloride may cause solution to have a milky appearance.

Storage:

Euflexxa™: Store under refrigeration at 2°C to 8°C (36°F to 46°F). Do not freeze. Protect from light. Remove from refrigeration at least 20-30 minutes before use.

Healon® products, Provisc®: Store under refrigeration at 2°C to 8°C (36°F to 46°F). Do not freeze. Protect from light.

Hylaform®, Hylaform® Plus: Store at room temperature of 2°C to 30°C. Do not freeze. Do not use if gel separates or becomes cloudy.

Hyalgan®, Orthovisc®: Store below 25°C (77°F). Do not freeze.

IPM Wound Gel™: Store below 35°C (95°F). Do not freeze.

Restylane®: Store at up to 25°C (77°F). Do not freeze. Protect from light. Do not use if gel separates or becomes cloudy.

Synvisc®: Store at room temperature below 30°C (86°F). Do not freeze. Protect from light.

♦ **Hyaluronic Acid** *see* Hyaluronate and Derivatives *on page 856*

Hyaluronidase (hye al yoor ON i dase)

U.S. Brand Names Amphadase™; Hylenex™; Vitrase®

Pharmacologic Category Enzyme

Medication Safety Issues

Sound-alike/look-alike issues:

Wydase may be confused with Lidex®, Wyamine®

Use Increase the dispersion and absorption of other drugs; increase rate of absorption of parenteral fluids given by hypodermoclysis; adjunct in subcutaneous urography for improving resorption of radiopaque agents

Unlabeled/Investigational Use Management of drug extravasations

Mechanism of Action Modifies the permeability of connective tissue through hydrolysis of hyaluronic acid, one of the chief ingredients of tissue cement which offers resistance to diffusion of liquids through tissues; hyaluronidase increases both the distribution and absorption of locally injected substances.

Pharmacodynamics/Kinetics

Onset of action: SubQ: Immediate

Duration: 24-48 hours

Contraindications Hypersensitivity to hyaluronidase or any component of the formulation

Warnings/Precautions Do not inject in or around infected or inflamed areas; may spread localized infection. Should not be used for extravasation management of dopamine or alpha agonists or to reduce swelling of bites or stings. Do not administer intravenously. Do not apply directly to the cornea.

Drug Interactions

Local anesthetics: Hyaluronidase may increase absorption and toxicity of local anesthetics.

Adverse Reactions

Frequency not defined:

Cardiovascular: Edema

Local: Injection site reactions

<1%: Allergic reactions, anaphylactic-like reactions (retrobulbar block or I.V. injections), angioedema, urticaria

Overdosage/Toxicology Symptoms of overdose include local edema, urticaria, erythema, chills, nausea, vomiting, dizziness, tachycardia, and hypotension. Treatment is symptom-directed and supportive.

Dosing

Adults: Note: A preliminary skin test for hypersensitivity can be performed. ACTH, antihistamines, corticosteroids, estrogens, and salicylates, when used in large doses, may cause tissues to be partly resistant to hyaluronidase. May require larger doses of hyaluronidase for the same effect.

Skin test: Intradermal: 0.02 mL (3 units) of a 150 units/mL solution. Positive reaction consists of a wheal with pseudopods appearing within 5 minutes and persisting for 20-30 minutes with localized itching.

Hypodermoclysis: SubQ: 15 units is added to each 100 mL of I.V. fluid to be administered; 150 units facilitates absorption of >1000 mL of solution; rate and volume of a single clysis should not exceed those used for infusion of I.V. fluids

Urography: SubQ: 75 units over each scapula followed by injection of contrast medium at the same site; patient should be in the prone position.

Extravasation (unlabeled use): SubQ: Inject 1 mL of a 150 unit/mL solution (as 5-10 injections of 0.1-0.2 mL) into affected area; doses of 15-250 units have been reported.

Elderly: Refer to adult dosing. Adjust dose carefully to individual patient.

Pediatrics:

Skin test: See "Note" in adult dosing: Intradermal: 0.02 mL (3 units) of a 150 units/mL solution. Positive reaction consists of a wheal with pseudopods appearing within 5 minutes and persisting for 20-30 minutes with localized itching.

Hypodermoclysis: SubQ: 15 units is added to each 100 mL of I.V. fluid to be administered; 150 units facilitates absorption of >1000 mL of solution

Premature Infants and Neonates: Volume of a single clysis should not exceed 25 mL/kg and the rate of administration should not exceed 2 mL/minute

Children <3 years: Volume of a single clysis should not exceed 200 mL

Children ≥3 years: Refer to adult dosing.

Urography: Refer to adult dosing.

Available Dosage Forms

Injection, powder for reconstitution (Vitrase®): 6200 units [ovine derived; contains lactose]

Injection, solution (Amphadase™): 150 units/mL (2 mL) [bovine derived; contains edetate disodium 1 mg, thimerosal ≤0.1 mg]

Injection, solution [preservative free] (Hylenex™): 150 units/mL (1 mL, 2 mL) [recombinant; contains human albumin and edetate disodium]

Injection, solution [preservative free] (Vitrase®): 200 units/mL (2 mL) [ovine derived; contains lactulose]

Nursing Guidelines

Assessment: Results of skin test should be assessed prior to administering. Should not be administered in or around infected or inflamed areas (see Warnings/Precautions). Teach patient possible side effects/interventions, and adverse symptoms to report (see Patient Education). Note breast-feeding caution.

Patient Education: Inform prescriber of any allergies you may have. This drug can only be administered by injection. Report immediately any unusual skin rash, pain, redness, or swelling at or around injection site, swelling of mouth or lips, difficulty breathing, or onset of sudden dizziness. **Pregnancy/breast-feeding precautions:** Inform prescriber if you are or intend to become pregnant. Consult prescriber if breast-feeding.

Geriatric Considerations: The most common use of hyaluronidase in the elderly is in hypodermoclysis. Hypodermoclysis is very useful in dehydrated patients in whom oral intake is minimal and I.V. access is a problem.

Pregnancy Risk Factor: C

Lactation: Excretion in breast milk unknown/use caution

Administration

I.V.: Do **not** administer I.V.

Reconstitution: Vitrase®: Add 6.2 mL of NaCl to vial (1000 units/mL). Further dilute with NaCl before administration.

For 50 units/mL, draw up 0.05 mL of hyaluronidase reconstituted solution (1000 units/mL) and add 0.95 mL of NaCl.

For 75 units/mL, draw up 0.075 mL of hyaluronidase reconstituted solution and add 0.925 mL of NaCl.

For 150 units/mL, draw up 0.15 mL of hyaluronidase reconstituted solution and add 0.85 mL of NaCl.

For 300 units/mL, draw up 0.3 mL of hyaluronidase reconstituted solution and add 0.7 mL of NaCl.

Compatibility:

Incompatible with furosemide, benzodiazepines, phenytoin

(Continued)

Hyaluronidase *(Continued)*

Storage:

Amphadase™, Hylenex™: Store in refrigerator at 2°C to 8°C (35°F to 46°F). Do not freeze.

Vitrase®: Store unopened vial in refrigerator at 2°C to 8°C (35°F to 46°F). After reconstitution, store at 20°C to 25°C (68°F to 77°F) and use within 6 hours.

♦ hycet™ *see* Hydrocodone and Acetaminophen *on page 867*

HydrALAZINE (hye DRAL a zeen)

Synonyms Apresoline [DSC]; Hydralazine Hydrochloride

Pharmacologic Category Vasodilator

Medication Safety Issues

Sound-alike/look-alike issues:

HydrALAZINE may be confused with hydrOXYzine

Use Management of moderate to severe hypertension, congestive heart failure, hypertension secondary to pre-eclampsia/eclampsia; treatment of primary pulmonary hypertension

Mechanism of Action Direct vasodilation of arterioles (with little effect on veins) with decreased systemic resistance

Pharmacodynamics/Kinetics

Onset of action: Oral: 20-30 minutes; I.V.: 5-20 minutes

Duration: Oral: Up to 8 hours; I.V.: 1-4 hours; **Note:** May vary depending on acetylator status of patient

Distribution: Crosses placenta; enters breast milk

Protein binding: 85% to 90%

Metabolism: Hepatically acetylated; extensive first-pass effect (oral)

Bioavailability: 30% to 50%; increased with food

Half-life elimination: Normal renal function: 2-8 hours; End-stage renal disease: 7-16 hours

Excretion: Urine (14% as unchanged drug)

Contraindications Hypersensitivity to hydralazine or any component of the formulation; mitral valve rheumatic heart disease

Warnings/Precautions May cause a drug-induced lupus-like syndrome (more likely on larger doses, longer duration). Adjust dose in severe renal dysfunction. Use with caution in CAD (increase in tachycardia may increase myocardial oxygen demand). Use with caution in pulmonary hypertension (may cause hypotension). Patients may be poorly compliant because of frequent dosing.

Monitor blood pressure closely following I.V. administration. Response may be delayed and unpredictable in some patients. Titrate cautiously to response. Hydralazine-induced fluid and sodium retention may require addition or increased dosage of a diuretics.

Drug Interactions Inhibits CYP3A4 (weak)

Beta-blockers (metoprolol, propranolol) serum concentrations and pharmacologic effects may be increased. Monitor cardiovascular status.

Propranolol increases hydralazine's serum concentrations. Acebutolol, atenolol, and nadolol (low hepatic clearance or no first-pass metabolism) are unlikely to be affected.

NSAIDs may decrease the hemodynamic effects of hydralazine; avoid use if possible or closely monitor cardiovascular status.

Nutritional/Herbal/Ethanol Interactions

Ethanol: Avoid ethanol (may increase CNS depression).

Food: Food enhances bioavailability of hydralazine.

Herb/Nutraceutical: Avoid dong quai if using for hypertension (has estrogenic activity). Avoid ephedra, yohimbe, ginseng (may worsen hypertension). Avoid garlic (may have increased antihypertensive effect).

Adverse Reactions Frequency not defined.

Cardiovascular: Tachycardia, angina pectoris, orthostatic hypotension (rare), dizziness (rare), paradoxical hypertension, peripheral edema, vascular collapse (rare), flushing

Central nervous system: Increased intracranial pressure (I.V., in patient with pre-existing increased intracranial pressure), fever (rare), chills (rare), anxiety*, disorientation*, depression*, coma*

Dermatologic: Rash (rare), urticaria (rare), pruritus (rare)

Gastrointestinal: Anorexia, nausea, vomiting, diarrhea, constipation, adynamic ileus

Genitourinary: Difficulty in micturition, impotence

Hematologic: Hemolytic anemia (rare), eosinophilia (rare), decreased hemoglobin concentration (rare), reduced erythrocyte count (rare), leukopenia (rare), agranulocytosis (rare), thrombocytopenia (rare)

Neuromuscular & skeletal: Rheumatoid arthritis, muscle cramps, weakness, tremor, peripheral neuritis (rare)

Ocular: Lacrimation, conjunctivitis

Respiratory: Nasal congestion, dyspnea

Miscellaneous: Drug-induced lupus-like syndrome (dose related; fever, arthralgia, splenomegaly, lymphadenopathy, asthenia, myalgia, malaise, pleuritic chest pain, edema, positive ANA, positive LE cells, maculopapular facial rash, positive direct Coombs' test, pericarditis, pericardial tamponade), diaphoresis

*Seen in uremic patients and severe hypertension where rapidly escalating doses may have caused hypotension leading to these effects.

Overdosage/Toxicology Symptoms of overdose include hypotension, tachycardia, and shock. Treatment is supportive and symptomatic.

Dosing

Adults:

Hypertension: Oral:

Initial: 10 mg 4 times/day; increase by 10-25 mg/dose every 2-5 days (maximum: 300 mg/day); usual dose range (JNC 7): 25-100 mg/day in 2 divided doses

Acute hypertension: I.M., I.V.: Initial: 10-20 mg/dose every 4-6 hours as needed, may increase to 40 mg/dose; change to oral therapy as soon as possible.

Pre-eclampsia/eclampsia: I.M., I.V.: 5 mg/dose then 5-10 mg every 20-30 minutes as needed

Congestive heart failure: Oral:

Initial dose: 10-25 mg 3-4 times/day

Adjustment: Dosage must be adjusted based on individual response

Target dose: 225-300 mg/day; use in combination with isosorbide dinitrate

Elderly: Oral: Initial: 10 mg 2-3 times/day; increase by 10-25 mg/day every 2-5 days.

Pediatrics:

Hypertension: Oral: Initial: 0.75-1 mg/kg/day in 2-4 divided doses; increase over 3-4 weeks to maximum of 7.5 mg/kg/day in 2-4 divided doses; maximum daily dose: 200 mg/day

Acute hypertension: I.M., I.V.: 0.1-0.2 mg/kg/dose (not to exceed 20 mg) every 4-6 hours as needed, up to 1.7-3.5 mg/kg/day in 4-6 divided doses

Renal Impairment:

Cl_{cr} 10-50 mL/minute: Administer every 8 hours.

Cl_{cr} <10 mL/minute: Administer every 8-16 hours in fast acetylators and every 12-24 hours in slow acetylators.

Hemodialysis effects: Supplemental dose is not necessary.

Peritoneal dialysis effects: Supplemental dose is not necessary.

Available Dosage Forms

Injection, solution, as hydrochloride: 20 mg/mL (1 mL)

Tablet, as hydrochloride: 10 mg, 25 mg, 50 mg, 100 mg

Nursing Guidelines

Assessment: See Contraindications, Warnings/Precautions, and Dosing for use cautions. Assess potential for interactions with other prescriptions, OTC medications, or herbal products patient may be taking (see Drug Interactions). **I.V.:** See Administration specifics. Orthostatic precautions should be observed and patient monitored closely during and following infusion. Assess results of laboratory tests, therapeutic effectiveness (decreased blood pressure), and adverse response (eg, hypotension, fluid retention - see Adverse Reactions and Overdose/Toxicology) periodically during therapy. Teach patient proper use, possible side effects/appropriate interventions, and adverse symptoms to report (see Patient Education).

Monitoring Laboratory Tests: ANA titer

Dietary Considerations: Administer with meals.

Patient Education: Inform prescriber of all prescriptions, OTC medications, or herbal products you are taking, and any allergies you have. Do not take any new medication during therapy unless approved by prescriber. Take as directed, with meals. Avoid alcohol. This medication does not replace other antihypertensive interventions; follow prescriber's instructions for diet and lifestyle changes. Weigh daily at the same time, in the same clothes for the first 2

(Continued)

HydrALAZINE *(Continued)*

weeks and weekly thereafter. Report weight gain >5 lb/week, swelling of feet or ankles. May cause dizziness or weakness (change position slowly when rising from sitting or lying position, climbing stairs, and avoid driving or activities requiring alertness until response to drug is known); nausea or vomiting (small, frequent meals, frequent mouth care, chewing gum, or sucking lozenges may help); impotence (reversible); diarrhea (boiled milk, buttermilk, or yogurt may help); or constipation (increased exercise, fluids, fruit, or fiber may help). Report chest pain, rapid heartbeat, or palpitations; flu-like symptoms; respiratory difficulty; skin rash; numbness and tingling of extremities; muscle cramps, weakness, or tremors; or unresolved GI problems. **Pregnancy precaution:** Inform prescriber if you are or intend to become pregnant

Pregnancy Risk Factor: C

Pregnancy Issues: Crosses the placenta. One report of fetal arrhythmia; transient neonatal thrombocytopenia and fetal distress reported following late 3rd trimester use. A large amount of clinical experience with the use of this drug for management of hypertension during pregnancy is available.

Lactation: Enters breast milk/compatible

Breast-Feeding Considerations: Crosses into breast milk in extremely small amounts. Available evidence suggests safe use during breast-feeding. AAP considers **compatible** with breast-feeding.

Perioperative/Anesthesia/Other Concerns: May be combined with isosorbide dinitrate for the treatment of heart failure. It is considered to be safe for the management of blood pressure during pregnancy.

Administration

I.V.: Inject over 1 minute. Hypotensive effect may be delayed and unpredictable in some patients.

Reconstitution: Hydralazine should be diluted in NS for IVPB administration due to decreased stability in D_5W. Stability of IVPB solution in NS is 4 days at room temperature.

Compatibility: Stable in dextran 6% in dextrose, dextran 6% in NS, D_5LR, $D_5{}^1/_4NS$, $D_5{}^1/_2NS$, D_5NS, $D_{10}W$, LR, $^1/_2NS$, NS; **incompatible** with D_5W

Y-site administration: Incompatible with aminophylline, ampicillin, diazoxide, furosemide

Compatibility when admixed: Incompatible with aminophylline, ampicillin, chlorothiazide, edetate calcium disodium, ethacrynate, hydrocortisone sodium succinate, mephentermine, methohexital, nitroglycerin, phenobarbital, verapamil

Storage: Intact ampuls/vials of hydralazine should not be stored under refrigeration because of possible precipitation or crystallization.

Related Information

Postoperative Hypertension *on page 1815*

♦ **Hydralazine Hydrochloride** *see* HydrALAZINE *on page 860*
♦ **Hydramine® [OTC]** *see* DiphenhydrAMINE *on page 546*
♦ **Hydrated Chloral** *see* Chloral Hydrate *on page 368*

Hydrochlorothiazide (hye droe klor oh THYE a zide)

U.S. Brand Names Microzide™

Synonyms HCTZ (error-prone abbreviation)

Pharmacologic Category Diuretic, Thiazide

Medication Safety Issues

Sound-alike/look-alike issues:

Hydrochlorothiazide may be confused with hydrocortisone, hydroflumethiazide
Esidrix may be confused with Lasix®
HCTZ is an error-prone abbreviation (mistaken as hydrocortisone)

Use Management of mild to moderate hypertension; treatment of edema in congestive heart failure and nephrotic syndrome

Unlabeled/Investigational Use Treatment of lithium-induced diabetes insipidus

Mechanism of Action Inhibits sodium reabsorption in the distal tubules causing increased excretion of sodium and water as well as potassium and hydrogen ions

Pharmacodynamics/Kinetics

Onset of action: Diuresis: ~2 hours
Peak effect: 4-6 hours
Duration: 6-12 hours
Absorption: ~50% to 80%

Distribution: 3.6-7.8 L/kg
Protein binding: 68%
Metabolism: Not metabolized
Bioavailability: 50% to 80%
Half-life elimination: 5.6-14.8 hours
Time to peak: 1-2.5 hours
Excretion: Urine (as unchanged drug)

Contraindications Hypersensitivity to hydrochlorothiazide or any component of the formulation, thiazides, or sulfonamide-derived drugs; anuria; renal decompensation; pregnancy

Warnings/Precautions Avoid in severe renal disease (ineffective). Electrolyte disturbances (hypokalemia, hypochloremic alkalosis, hyponatremia) can occur. Use with caution in severe hepatic dysfunction; hepatic encephalopathy can be caused by electrolyte disturbances. Gout can be precipitate in certain patients with a history of gout, a familial predisposition to gout, or chronic renal failure. Cautious use in diabetics; may see a change in glucose control. Hypersensitivity reactions can occur. Can cause SLE exacerbation or activation. Use with caution in patients with moderate or high cholesterol concentrations. Photosensitization may occur. Correct hypokalemia before initiating therapy.

Chemical similarities are present among sulfonamides, sulfonylureas, carbonic anhydrase inhibitors, thiazides, and loop diuretics (except ethacrynic acid). Use in patients with sulfonamide allergy is specifically contraindicated in product labeling, however, a risk of cross-reaction exists in patients with allergy to any of these compounds; avoid use when previous reaction has been severe.

Drug Interactions

ACE inhibitors: Increased hypotension if aggressively diuresed with a thiazide diuretic.

Beta-blockers increase hyperglycemic effects in type 2 diabetes mellitus (noninsulin dependent, NIDDM)

Cholestyramine: Hydrochlorothiazide absorption may be decreased.

Colestipol: Hydrochlorothiazide absorption may be decreased.

Cyclosporine and thiazides can increase the risk of gout or renal toxicity; avoid concurrent use.

Digoxin toxicity can be exacerbated if a thiazide induces hypokalemia or hypomagnesemia.

Lithium toxicity can occur by reducing renal excretion of lithium; monitor lithium concentration and adjust as needed.

Neuromuscular blocking agents can prolong blockade; monitor serum potassium and neuromuscular status.

NSAIDs can decrease the efficacy of thiazides reducing the diuretic and antihypertensive effects.

Nutritional/Herbal/Ethanol Interactions

Food: Hydrochlorothiazide peak serum levels may be decreased if taken with food. This product may deplete potassium, sodium, and magnesium.

Herb/Nutraceutical: Avoid dong quai if using for hypertension (has estrogenic activity). Dong quai may also cause photosensitization. Avoid ephedra, ginseng, yohimbe (may worsen hypertension). Avoid garlic (may have increased antihypertensive effect).

Lab Interactions Increased creatine phosphokinase [CPK] (S), ammonia (B), amylase (S), calcium (S), chloride (S), cholesterol (S), glucose, acid (S); decreased chloride (S), magnesium, potassium (S), sodium (S); tyramine and phentolamine tests; histamine tests for pheochromocytoma

Adverse Reactions

1% to 10%:

Cardiovascular: Orthostatic hypotension, hypotension
Dermatologic: Photosensitivity
Endocrine & metabolic: Hypokalemia
Gastrointestinal: Anorexia, epigastric distress

<1% (Limited to important or life-threatening): Agranulocytosis, allergic myocarditis, allergic reactions (possibly with life-threatening anaphylactic shock), alopecia, aplastic anemia, eosinophilic pneumonitis, erythema multiforme, exfoliative dermatitis, hemolytic anemia, hepatic function impairment, hypercalcemia, interstitial nephritis, leukopenia, pancreatitis, renal failure, respiratory distress, Stevens-Johnson syndrome, thrombocytopenia, toxic epidermal necrolysis

Overdosage/Toxicology Symptoms of overdose include hypermotility, diuresis, lethargy, confusion, and muscle weakness. Treatment is supportive.

(Continued)

Hydrochlorothiazide *(Continued)*

Dosing

Adults:

Edema (diuresis): Oral: 25-100 mg/day in 1-2 doses; maximum: 200 mg/day

Hypertension: Oral: 12.5-50 mg/day; minimal increase in response and more electrolyte disturbances are seen with doses >50 mg/day

Elderly: Oral: 12.5-25 mg once daily; minimal increase in response and more electrolyte disturbances are seen with doses >50 mg/day (see Geriatric Considerations).

Pediatrics: Hypertension, edema (diuretic): Oral (effect of drug may be decreased when used every day):

Children <6 months: 2-3 mg/kg/day in 2 divided doses

Children >6 months: 2 mg/kg/day in 2 divided doses

Note: In pediatric patients, chlorothiazide may be preferred over hydrochlorothiazide as there are more dosage formulations (eg, suspension) available.

Renal Impairment: Cl_{cr} <10 mL/minute: Avoid use. Usually ineffective with GFR <30 mL/minute. Effective at lower GFR in combination with a loop diuretic.

Available Dosage Forms

Capsule (Microzide™): 12.5 mg

Tablet: 25 mg, 50 mg

Nursing Guidelines

Assessment: Assess allergy history prior to beginning therapy. See Contraindications, Warnings/Precautions, and Dosing for use cautions. Assess potential for interactions with other prescriptions, OTC medications, or herbal products patient may be taking (see Drug Interactions). Assess results of laboratory tests (see below), therapeutic effectiveness (according to purpose for use), and adverse response (see Adverse Reactions and Overdose/Toxicology) regularly during therapy. Caution patients with diabetes to monitor glucose levels closely; may alter glucose control. Teach proper use, possible side effects/appropriate interventions, and adverse symptoms to report (see Patient Education). **Pregnancy risk factor B/D** - see Pregnancy Risk Factor for use cautions. Note breast-feeding caution.

Monitoring Laboratory Tests: Serum electrolytes, BUN, creatinine

Patient Education: Inform prescriber of all prescriptions, OTC medications, or herbal products you are taking, and any allergies you have. Do not take any new medication during therapy unless approved by prescriber. This medication does not replace other antihypertensive interventions; follow prescriber's instructions for diet and lifestyle changes. Take as directed, with meals, early in the day to avoid nocturia. Your prescriber may prescribe a potassium supplement or recommend that you eat foods high in potassium (include bananas and/or orange juice in daily diet). Do not change your diet on your own while taking this medication, especially if you are taking potassium supplements or medications to reduce potassium loss; too much potassium can be as harmful as too little. If you have diabetes, monitor serum glucose closely; this medication may increase serum glucose levels. May cause dizziness or postural hypotension (use caution when rising from sitting or lying position, when driving, climbing stairs, or engaging in tasks that require alertness until response to drug is known); nausea or vomiting (small, frequent meals, frequent mouth care, sucking lozenges, or chewing gum may help); impotence (reversible); constipation (increased exercise, fluids, fruit, or fiber may help); or photosensitivity (use sunscreen, wear protective clothing and eyewear, and avoid direct sunlight). Report persistent flu-like symptoms, chest pain, palpitations, muscle cramping, respiratory difficulty, skin rash or itching, unusual bruising or easy bleeding, or excessive fatigue. **Pregnancy/breast-feeding precautions:** Inform prescriber if you are pregnant. Consult prescriber if breast-feeding.

Geriatric Considerations: Hydrochlorothiazide is not effective in patients with a Cl_{cr} <30 mL/minute, therefore, it may not be a useful agent in many elderly patients.

Pregnancy Risk Factor: B (manufacturer); D (expert analysis)

Pregnancy Issues: Although there are no adequate and well-controlled studies using hydrochlorothiazide in pregnancy, thiazide diuretics may cause an increased risk of congenital defects. Hypoglycemia, hypokalemia, hyponatremia, jaundice, and thrombocytopenia are also reported as possible complications to the fetus or newborn.

Lactation: Enters breast milk/use caution (AAP rates "compatible")

Perioperative/Anesthesia/Other Concerns: If given the morning of surgery it may render the patient volume depleted and blood pressure may be labile during general anesthesia.

Thiazide diuretics are effective first-line therapeutic agents in the management of hypertension and have proven to be of benefit in terms of cardiovascular outcome. They may act synergistically to lower blood pressure when combined with an ACE inhibitor or beta-blocker.

Administration

Oral: May be taken with food or milk. Take early in day to avoid nocturia. Take the last dose of multiple doses no later than 6 PM unless instructed otherwise.

◆ Hydrochlorothiazide and Lisinopril *see* Lisinopril and Hydrochlorothiazide *on page 1051*

◆ Hydrochlorothiazide and Losartan *see* Losartan and Hydrochlorothiazide *on page 1069*

◆ Hydrochlorothiazide and Metoprolol *see* Metoprolol and Hydrochlorothiazide *on page 1153*

◆ Hydrochlorothiazide and Metoprolol Tartrate *see* Metoprolol and Hydrochlorothiazide *on page 1153*

Hydrochlorothiazide and Spironolactone

(hye droe klor oh THYE a zide & speer on oh LAK tone)

U.S. Brand Names Aldactazide®

Synonyms Spironolactone and Hydrochlorothiazide

Pharmacologic Category Antihypertensive Agent, Combination

Medication Safety Issues

Sound-alike/look-alike issues:

Aldactazide® may be confused with Aldactone®

Use Management of mild to moderate hypertension; treatment of edema in congestive heart failure and nephrotic syndrome, and cirrhosis of the liver accompanied by edema and/or ascites

Pharmacodynamics/Kinetics See individual agents.

Contraindications Hypersensitivity to spironolactone, hydrochlorothiazide or any component of the formulation, thiazides, or sulfonamide-derived drugs; anuria; renal decompensation; hyperkalemia

Warnings/Precautions

Based on **hydrochlorothiazide** component: Avoid in severe renal disease (ineffective). Electrolyte disturbances (hypokalemia, hypochloremic alkalosis, hyponatremia) can occur. Use with caution in severe hepatic dysfunction; hepatic encephalopathy can be caused by electrolyte disturbances. Gout can be precipitate in certain patients with a history of gout, a familial predisposition to gout, or chronic renal failure. Cautious use in diabetics; may see a change in glucose control. Hypersensitivity reactions can occur. Can cause SLE exacerbation or activation. Use with caution in patients with moderate or high cholesterol concentrations. Photosensitization may occur. Correct hypokalemia before initiating therapy.

Chemical similarities are present among sulfonamides, sulfonylureas, carbonic anhydrase inhibitors, thiazides, and loop diuretics (except ethacrynic acid). Use in patients with sulfonamide allergy is specifically contraindicated in product labeling, however, a risk of cross-reaction exists in patients with allergy to any of these compounds; avoid use when previous reaction has been severe.

Based on **spironolactone** component: Avoid potassium supplements, potassium-containing salt substitutes, a diet rich in potassium, or other drugs that can cause hyperkalemia. Monitor for fluid and electrolyte imbalances. Gynecomastia is related to dose and duration of therapy. Diuretic therapy should be carefully used in severe hepatic dysfunction; electrolyte and fluid shifts can cause or exacerbate encephalopathy.

Drug Interactions See individual agents.

Nutritional/Herbal/Ethanol Interactions

Food: Avoid food with high potassium content and potassium-containing salt substitutes.

Herb/Nutraceutical: Avoid natural licorice (causes sodium and water retention and increases potassium loss).

Adverse Reactions See individual agents.

(Continued)

Hydrochlorothiazide and Spironolactone *(Continued)*

Dosing

Adults: Hypertension, edema: Oral:

Hydrochlorothiazide 25 mg and spironolactone 25 mg: ½-8 tablets daily

Hydrochlorothiazide 50 mg and spironolactone 50 mg: ½-4 tablets daily in 1-2 doses

Elderly: Oral: Initial: 1 tablet/day; increase as necessary.

Renal Impairment: Efficacy of hydrochlorothiazide is limited in patients with Cl_{cr} <30 mL/minute.

Available Dosage Forms

Tablet: Hydrochlorothiazide 25 mg and spironolactone 25 mg

Aldactazide®:

25/25: Hydrochlorothiazide 25 mg and spironolactone 25 mg

50/50: Hydrochlorothiazide 50 mg and spironolactone 50 mg

Nursing Guidelines

Assessment: See individual components listed in Related Information. Note breast-feeding caution.

Patient Education: See individual agents. **Pregnancy/breast-feeding precautions:** Inform prescriber if you are or intend to become pregnant. Consult prescriber if breast-feeding.

Pregnancy Risk Factor: C

Lactation: Enters breast milk/use caution

Related Information

Hydrochlorothiazide *on page 862*
Spironolactone *on page 1566*

Hydrochlorothiazide and Triamterene

(hye droe klor oh THYE a zide & trye AM ter een)

U.S. Brand Names Dyazide®; Maxzide®; Maxzide®-25

Synonyms Triamterene and Hydrochlorothiazide

Pharmacologic Category Antihypertensive Agent, Combination; Diuretic, Potassium-Sparing; Diuretic, Thiazide

Medication Safety Issues

Sound-alike/look-alike issues:

Dyazide® may be confused with diazoxide, Dynacin®

Maxzide® may be confused with Maxidex®

Use Management of mild to moderate hypertension; treatment of edema in congestive heart failure and nephrotic syndrome

Mechanism of Action

Based on **triamterene** component: Competes with aldosterone for receptor sites in the distal renal tubules, increasing sodium, chloride, and water excretion while conserving potassium and hydrogen ions; may block the effect of aldosterone on arteriolar smooth muscle as well

Based on **hydrochlorothiazide** component: Inhibits sodium reabsorption in the distal tubules causing increased excretion of sodium and water as well as potassium and hydrogen ions

Pharmacodynamics/Kinetics See individual agents.

Contraindications

Based on **hydrochlorothiazide** component: Hypersensitivity to hydrochlorothiazide or any component of the formulation, thiazides, or sulfonamide-derived drugs; anuria; renal decompensation; pregnancy

Based on **triamterene** component: Hypersensitivity to triamterene or any component of the formulation; patients receiving other potassium-sparing diuretics; anuria; severe hepatic disease; hyperkalemia or history of hyperkalemia; severe or progressive renal disease

Warnings/Precautions

Based on **hydrochlorothiazide** component: Avoid in severe renal disease (ineffective). Electrolyte disturbances (hypokalemia, hypochloremic alkalosis, hyponatremia) can occur. Use with caution in severe hepatic dysfunction; hepatic encephalopathy can be caused by electrolyte disturbances. Gout can be precipitate in certain patients with a history of gout, a familial predisposition to gout, or chronic renal failure. Cautious use in diabetics; may see a change in glucose control. Hypersensitivity reactions can occur. Can cause SLE exacerbation or activation. Use with caution in patients with moderate or high cholesterol concentrations. Photosensitization may occur. Correct hypokalemia before initiating therapy.

Chemical similarities are present among sulfonamides, sulfonylureas, carbonic anhydrase inhibitors, thiazides, and loop diuretics (except ethacrynic acid). Use in patients with sulfonamide allergy is specifically contraindicated in product labeling, however, a risk of cross-reaction exists in patients with allergy to any of these compounds; avoid use when previous reaction has been severe.

Based on **triamterene** component: Avoid potassium supplements, potassium-containing salt substitutes, a diet rich in potassium, or other drugs that can cause hyperkalemia. Monitor for fluid and electrolyte imbalances. Diuretic therapy should be carefully used in severe hepatic dysfunction; electrolyte and fluid shifts can cause or exacerbate encephalopathy. Use cautiously in patients with history of kidney stones and diabetes. Can cause photosensitivity.

Safety and efficacy have not been established in pediatric patients.

Drug Interactions See individual agents.

Nutritional/Herbal/Ethanol Interactions Food: Avoid food with high potassium content and potassium-containing salt substitutes.

Adverse Reactions See individual agents.

Dosing

Adults & Elderly: Hypertension, edema: Oral:

Triamterene 37.5 mg and hydrochlorothiazide 25 mg: 1-2 tablets/capsules once daily

Triamterene 75 mg and hydrochlorothiazide 50 mg: $^1/_2$-1 tablet daily

Available Dosage Forms

Capsule (Dyazide®): Hydrochlorothiazide 25 mg and triamterene 37.5 mg

Tablet:

Maxzide®: Hydrochlorothiazide 50 mg and triamterene 75 mg

Maxzide®-25: Hydrochlorothiazide 25 mg and triamterene 37.5 mg

Nursing Guidelines

Assessment: See individual components listed in Related Information. Note breast-feeding caution.

Dietary Considerations: Should be taken after meals.

Patient Education: See individual agents. **Pregnancy/breast-feeding precautions:** Inform prescriber if you are or intend to become pregnant. Consult prescriber if breast-feeding.

Pregnancy Risk Factor: C (per manufacturer)

Lactation: Excretion in breast milk unknown/use caution

Related Information

Hydrochlorothiazide *on page 862*

♦ Hydrochlorothiazide and Valsartan *see* Valsartan and Hydrochlorothiazide *on page 1687*

♦ Hydrocil® Instant [OTC] *see* Psyllium *on page 1438*

Hydrocodone and Acetaminophen

(hye droe KOE done & a seet a MIN oh fen)

U.S. Brand Names Anexsia®; Bancap HC®; Ceta-Plus®; Co-Gesic®; hycet™; Lorcet® 10/650; Lorcet®-HD [DSC]; Lorcet® Plus; Lortab®; Margesic® H; Maxidone™; Norco®; Stagesic®; Vicodin®; Vicodin® ES; Vicodin® HP; Zydone®

Synonyms Acetaminophen and Hydrocodone

Pharmacologic Category Analgesic Combination (Narcotic)

Medication Safety Issues

Sound-alike/look-alike issues:

Lorcet® may be confused with Fioricet®

Lortab® may be confused with Cortef®, Lorabid®, Luride®

Vicodin® may be confused with Hycodan®, Hycomine®, Indocin®, Uridon®

Zydone® may be confused with Vytone®

Use Relief of moderate to severe pain

Mechanism of Action Hydrocodone, as with other narcotic (opiate) analgesics, blocks pain perception in the cerebral cortex by binding to specific receptor molecules (opiate receptors) within the neuronal membranes of synapses. This binding results in a decreased synaptic chemical transmission throughout the CNS thus inhibiting the flow of pain sensations into the higher centers. Mu and (Continued)

Hydrocodone and Acetaminophen *(Continued)*

kappa are the two subtypes of the opiate receptor which hydrocodone binds to cause analgesia.

Acetaminophen inhibits the synthesis of prostaglandins in the CNS and peripherally blocks pain impulse generation; produces antipyresis from inhibition of hypothalamic heat-regulating center.

Pharmacodynamics/Kinetics

Acetaminophen: See Acetaminophen monograph.

Hydrocodone:

Onset of action: Narcotic analgesic: 10-20 minutes

Duration: 4-8 hours

Distribution: Crosses placenta

Metabolism: Hepatic; O-demethylation; N-demethylation and 6-ketosteroid reduction

Half-life elimination: 3.3-4.4 hours

Excretion: Urine

Contraindications Hypersensitivity to hydrocodone, acetaminophen, or any component of the formulation; CNS depression; severe respiratory depression

Warnings/Precautions Use with caution in patients with hypersensitivity reactions to other phenanthrene derivative opioid agonists (morphine, hydromorphone, levorphanol, oxycodone, oxymorphone); tolerance or drug dependence may result from extended use.

Respiratory depressant effects may be increased with head injuries. Use caution with acute abdominal conditions; clinical course may be obscured. Use caution with thyroid dysfunction, prostatic hyperplasia, hepatic or renal disease, and in the elderly. Causes sedation; caution must be used in performing tasks which require alertness (eg, operating machinery or driving).

Limit acetaminophen to <4 g/day. May cause severe hepatic toxicity in acute overdose; in addition, chronic daily dosing in adults has resulted in liver damage in some patients. Use with caution in patients with alcoholic liver disease; consuming ≥3 alcoholic drinks/day may increase the risk of liver damage. Use caution in patients with known G6PD deficiency.

Drug Interactions

Hydrocodone: **Substrate** of CYP2D6 (major)

Acetaminophen: **Substrate** (minor) of CYP1A2, 2A6, 2C8/9, 2D6, 2E1, 3A4; **Inhibits** CYP3A4 (weak)

Acetaminophen component: Refer to Acetaminophen monograph.

Hydrocodone component:

CYP2D6 inhibitors may decrease the effects of hydrocodone. Example inhibitors include chlorpromazine, delavirdine, fluoxetine, miconazole, paroxetine, pergolide, quinidine, quinine, ritonavir, and ropinirole.

CNS depressants (including antianxiety agents, antihistamines, antipsychotics, narcotics): CNS depression is additive; dose adjustment may be needed

MAO inhibitors: May see increased effects of MAO inhibitor and hydrocodone.

Tricyclic antidepressants (TCAs): May see increased effects of TCA and hydrocodone.

Nutritional/Herbal/Ethanol Interactions

Ethanol: Avoid ethanol (may increase CNS depression); consuming ≥3 alcoholic drinks/day may increase the risk of liver damage

Herb/Nutraceutical: Avoid valerian, St John's wort, SAMe, kava kava (may increase risk of excessive sedation).

Adverse Reactions Frequency not defined.

Cardiovascular: Bradycardia, cardiac arrest, circulatory collapse, coma, hypotension

Central nervous system: Anxiety, dizziness, drowsiness, dysphoria, euphoria, fear, lethargy, lightheadedness, malaise, mental clouding, mental impairment, mood changes, physiological dependence, sedation, somnolence, stupor

Dermatologic: Pruritus, rash

Endocrine & metabolic: Hypoglycemic coma

Gastrointestinal: Abdominal pain, constipation, gastric distress, heartburn, nausea, peptic ulcer, vomiting

Genitourinary: Ureteral spasm, urinary retention, vesical sphincter spasm

Hematologic: Agranulocytosis, bleeding time prolonged, hemolytic anemia, iron deficiency anemia, occult blood loss, thrombocytopenia

Hepatic: Hepatic necrosis, hepatitis

Neuromuscular & skeletal: Skeletal muscle rigidity

Otic: Hearing impairment or loss (chronic overdose)
Renal: Renal toxicity, renal tubular necrosis
Respiratory: Acute airway obstruction, apnea, dyspnea, respiratory depression (dose related)
Miscellaneous: Allergic reactions, clamminess, diaphoresis

Overdosage/Toxicology Symptoms of overdose include hepatic necrosis, blood dyscrasias, and respiratory depression. Treatment consists of acetylcysteine 140 mg/kg orally (loading) followed by 70 mg/kg every 4 hours for 17 doses; therapy should be initiated based upon laboratory analysis suggesting a high probability for hepatotoxic potential. Naloxone, 2 mg I.V. with repeat administration as necessary up to a total of 10 mg, can also be used to reverse toxic effects of the opiate. Activated charcoal is effective at binding certain chemicals, and this is especially true for acetaminophen.

Dosing

Adults:

Pain management (analgesic): Oral (doses should be titrated to appropriate analgesic effect): Average starting dose in opioid naive patients: Hydrocodone 5-10 mg 4 times/day; the dosage of acetaminophen should be limited to ≤4 g/day (and possibly less in patients with hepatic impairment or ethanol use).

Dosage ranges (based on specific product labeling): Hydrocodone 2.5-10 mg every 4-6 hours; maximum: 60 mg hydrocodone/day (maximum dose of hydrocodone may be limited by the acetaminophen content of specific product)

Elderly: Doses should be titrated to appropriate analgesic effect; 2.5-5 mg of the hydrocodone component every 4-6 hours. Do not exceed 4 g/day of acetaminophen.

Pediatrics:

Pain management (analgesic): Oral (doses should be titrated to appropriate analgesic effect):

Children 2-13 years or <50 kg: Hydrocodone 0.135 mg/kg/dose every 4-6 hours; do not exceed 6 doses/day or the maximum recommended dose of acetaminophen
Children ≥50 kg: Refer to adult dosing.

Hepatic Impairment: Use with caution. Limited, low-dose therapy usually well tolerated in hepatic disease/cirrhosis; however, cases of hepatotoxicity at daily acetaminophen dosages <4 g/day have been reported. Avoid chronic use in hepatic impairment.

Available Dosage Forms

Capsule (Bancap HC®, Ceta-Plus®, Margesic® H, Stagesic®): Hydrocodone bitartrate 5 mg and acetaminophen 500 mg
Elixir: Hydrocodone bitartrate 7.5 mg and acetaminophen 500 mg per 15 mL (480 mL)
 Lortab®: Hydrocodone bitartrate 7.5 mg and acetaminophen 500 mg per 15 mL (480 mL) [contains alcohol 7%; tropical fruit punch flavor]
Solution, oral (hycet™): Hydrocodone bitartrate 7.5 mg and acetaminophen 325 mg per 15 mL (480 mL) [contains alcohol 7%; tropical fruit punch flavor]
Tablet:
 Hydrocodone bitartrate 2.5 mg and acetaminophen 500 mg
 Hydrocodone bitartrate 5 mg and acetaminophen 325 mg
 Hydrocodone bitartrate 5 mg and acetaminophen 500 mg
 Hydrocodone bitartrate 7.5 mg and acetaminophen 325 mg
 Hydrocodone bitartrate 7.5 mg and acetaminophen 500 mg
 Hydrocodone bitartrate 7.5 mg and acetaminophen 650 mg
 Hydrocodone bitartrate 7.5 mg and acetaminophen 750 mg
 Hydrocodone bitartrate 10 mg and acetaminophen 325 mg
 Hydrocodone bitartrate 10 mg and acetaminophen 500 mg
 Hydrocodone bitartrate 10 mg and acetaminophen 650 mg
 Hydrocodone bitartrate 10 mg and acetaminophen 660 mg
 Anexsia®:
  5/500: Hydrocodone bitartrate 5 mg and acetaminophen 500 mg
  7.5/650: Hydrocodone bitartrate 7.5 mg and acetaminophen 650 mg
 Co-Gesic® 5/500: Hydrocodone bitartrate 5 mg and acetaminophen 500 mg
 Lorcet® 10/650: Hydrocodone bitartrate 10 mg and acetaminophen 650 mg
 Lorcet® Plus: Hydrocodone bitartrate 7.5 mg and acetaminophen 650 mg
 Lortab®:
  2.5/500: Hydrocodone bitartrate 2.5 mg and acetaminophen 500 mg
  5/500: Hydrocodone bitartrate 5 mg and acetaminophen 500 mg

(Continued)

Hydrocodone and Acetaminophen *(Continued)*

7.5/500: Hydrocodone bitartrate 7.5 mg and acetaminophen 500 mg
10/500: Hydrocodone bitartrate 10 mg and acetaminophen 500 mg
Maxidone™: Hydrocodone bitartrate 10 mg and acetaminophen 750 mg
Norco®:
Hydrocodone bitartrate 5 mg and acetaminophen 325 mg
Hydrocodone bitartrate 7.5 mg and acetaminophen 325 mg
Hydrocodone bitartrate 10 mg and acetaminophen 325 mg
Vicodin®: Hydrocodone bitartrate 5 mg and acetaminophen 500 mg
Vicodin® ES: Hydrocodone bitartrate 7.5 mg and acetaminophen 750 mg
Vicodin® HP: Hydrocodone bitartrate 10 mg and acetaminophen 660 mg
Zydone®:
Hydrocodone bitartrate 5 mg and acetaminophen 400 mg
Hydrocodone bitartrate 7.5 mg and acetaminophen 400 mg
Hydrocodone bitartrate 10 mg and acetaminophen 400 mg

Nursing Guidelines

Assessment: Assess patient for history of liver disease or ethanol abuse (acetaminophen and excessive ethanol may have adverse liver effects). Assess other medications patient may be taking for additive or adverse interactions. Monitor therapeutic effectiveness and signs of adverse reactions at beginning of therapy and at regular intervals with long-term use. Order safety precautions for inpatient use. May cause physical and/or psychological dependence. Discontinue slowly after long-term use. Assess knowledge/teach patient appropriate use, adverse reactions to report, and appropriate interventions to reduce side effects.

Patient Education: If self-administered, use exactly as directed; do not increase dose or frequency. Drug may cause physical and/or psychological dependence. Take with food or milk. While using this medication, do not use alcohol and other prescription or OTC medications (especially sedatives, tranquilizers, antihistamines, or pain medications) without consulting prescriber. Maintain adequate hydration (2-3 L/day of fluids) unless instructed to restrict fluid intake. May cause dizziness, lightheadedness, confusion, or drowsiness (use caution when driving, climbing stairs, or changing position - rising from sitting or lying to standing, or when engaging in tasks requiring alertness until response to drug is known); or nausea or vomiting (frequent mouth care, frequent sips of fluids, chewing gum, or sucking lozenges may help). Report chest pain or palpitations; persistent dizziness, shortness of breath, or respiratory difficulty; unusual bleeding or bruising; or unusual fatigue and weakness. **Pregnancy/breast-feeding precautions:** Inform prescriber if you are or intend to become pregnant. Do not breast-feed.

Geriatric Considerations: The elderly may be particularly susceptible to the CNS depressant action (sedation, confusion) and constipating effects of narcotics. If 1 tablet/dose is used, it may be useful to add an additional 325 mg of acetaminophen to maximize analgesic effect and minimize additional risk of narcotic related adverse effects.

Pregnancy Risk Factor: C/D (prolonged use or high doses near term)

Pregnancy Issues: Animal reproduction studies have not been conducted with this combination product. Opioid analgesics are considered FDA risk category D if used for prolonged periods or in large doses near term. Withdrawal symptoms may be observed in babies born to mothers taking opioids regularly during pregnancy. Respiratory depression may be observed in the newborn if opioids are given close to delivery.

Lactation: Excretion in breast milk unknown/contraindicated

Breast-Feeding Considerations: Acetaminophen is excreted in breast milk. The AAP considers it to be "compatible" with breast-feeding. Information is not available for hydrocodone; codeine and other opioids are excreted in breast milk and the AAP considers codeine to be "compatible" with breast-feeding. The manufacturers recommend discontinuing the medication or to discontinue nursing during therapy.

Perioperative/Anesthesia/Other Concerns: Doses of agent must be individualized according to degree of pain; commonly used in place of Tylenol® with Codeine; patients on this drug chronically should have liver function monitored secondary to acetaminophen in the product. Keep acetaminophen dose ≤4 g/day. Patients with chronic alcoholism, liver disease, or those who are fasting can develop severe hepatic disease even at therapeutic doses.

Hydrocodone and Aspirin (hye droe KOE done & AS pir in)

U.S. Brand Names Damason-P®

Synonyms Aspirin and Hydrocodone

Pharmacologic Category Analgesic Combination (Narcotic)

Use Relief of moderate to moderately severe pain

Mechanism of Action

Based on **hydrocodone** component: Binds to opiate receptors in the CNS, altering the perception of and response to pain; suppresses cough in medullary center; produces generalized CNS depression

Based on **aspirin** component: Inhibits prostaglandin synthesis, acts on the hypothalamus heat-regulating center to reduce fever, blocks prostaglandin synthetase action which prevents formation of the platelet-aggregating substance thromboxane A_2

Pharmacodynamics/Kinetics

Aspirin: See Aspirin monograph.

Hydrocodone:

Onset of action: Narcotic analgesic: 10-20 minutes

Duration: 4-8 hours

Distribution: Crosses placenta

Metabolism: Hepatic; O-demethylation; N-demethylation and 6-ketosteroid reduction

Half-life elimination: 3.3-4.4 hours

Excretion: Urine

Contraindications

Based on **hydrocodone** component: Hypersensitivity to hydrocodone or any component of the formulation

Based on **aspirin** component: Hypersensitivity to salicylates, other NSAIDs, or any component of the formulation; asthma; rhinitis; nasal polyps; inherited or acquired bleeding disorders (including factor VII and factor IX deficiency); pregnancy (in 3rd trimester especially); do not use in children (<16 years) for viral infections (chickenpox or flu symptoms), with or without fever, due to a potential association with Reye's syndrome

Warnings/Precautions Use with caution in patients with impaired renal function, erosive gastritis, or peptic ulcer disease; children and teenagers should not use for chickenpox or flu symptoms before a physician is consulted about Reye's syndrome; tolerance or drug dependence may result from extended use

Based on **hydrocodone** component: Use with caution in patients with hypersensitivity reactions to other phenanthrene-derivative opioid agonists (morphine, codeine, hydromorphone, levorphanol, oxycodone, oxymorphone); should be used with caution in elderly or debilitated patients, and those with severe impairment of hepatic or renal function, prostatic hyperplasia, or urethral stricture. Also use caution in patients with head injury, increased intracranial pressure, acute abdomen, or impaired thyroid function. Hydrocodone suppresses the cough reflex; caution should be exercised when this agent is used postoperatively and in patients with pulmonary diseases (including asthma, emphysema, COPD)

Based on **aspirin** component: Use with caution in patients with platelet and bleeding disorders, renal dysfunction, dehydration, erosive gastritis, or peptic ulcer disease. Heavy ethanol use (>3 drinks/day) can increase bleeding risks. Avoid use in severe renal failure or in severe hepatic failure. Discontinue use if tinnitus or impaired hearing occurs. Caution in mild-moderate renal failure (only at high dosages). Patients with sensitivity to tartrazine dyes, nasal polyps and asthma may have an increased risk of salicylate sensitivity. Surgical patients should avoid ASA if possible, for 1-2 weeks prior to surgery, to reduce the risk of excessive bleeding.

Drug Interactions

Based on **hydrocodone** component: **Substrate** of CYP2D6 (major)

CNS depressants, MAO inhibitors, general anesthetics, and tricyclic antidepressants: May potentiate the effects of opiate agonists; dextroamphetamine may enhance the analgesic effect of opiate agonists.

CYP2D6 inhibitors: May decrease the effects of hydrocodone. Example inhibitors include chlorpromazine, delavirdine, fluoxetine, miconazole, paroxetine, pergolide, quinidine, quinine, ritonavir, and ropinirole.

Based on **aspirin** component: **Substrate** of CYP2C8/9 (minor)

ACE inhibitors: The effects of ACE inhibitors may be blunted by aspirin administration, particularly at higher dosages.

Buspirone increases aspirin's free % *in vitro*.

(Continued)

Hydrocodone and Aspirin *(Continued)*

Carbonic anhydrase inhibitors and corticosteroids have been associated with alteration in salicylate serum concentrations.

Heparin and low molecular weight heparins: Concurrent use may increase the risk of bleeding

Methotrexate serum levels may be increased; consider discontinuing aspirin 2-3 days before high-dose methotrexate treatment or avoid concurrent use.

NSAIDs may increase the risk of gastrointestinal adverse effects and bleeding. Serum concentrations of some NSAIDs may be decreased by aspirin.

Platelet inhibitors (IIb/IIIa antagonists): Risk of bleeding may be increased.

Probenecid effects may be antagonized by aspirin.

Sulfonylureas: The effects of older sulfonylurea agents (tolazamide, tolbutamide) may be potentiated due to displacement from plasma proteins. This effect does not appear to be clinically significant for newer sulfonylurea agents (glyburide, glipizide, glimepiride).

Valproic acid may be displaced from its binding sites which can result in toxicity.

Verapamil may potentiate the prolongation of bleeding time associated with aspirin.

Warfarin and oral anticoagulants may increase the risk of bleeding.

Nutritional/Herbal/Ethanol Interactions

Based on **hydrocodone** component: Ethanol: Avoid or limit ethanol (may increase CNS depression). Watch for sedation.

Based on **aspirin** component:

Ethanol: Avoid ethanol (may enhance gastric mucosal damage).

Food: Food may decrease the rate but not the extent of oral absorption. Take with food or large volume of water or milk to minimize GI upset.

Herb/Nutraceutical: Avoid cat's claw, dong quai, evening primrose, feverfew, garlic, ginger, ginkgo, red clover, horse chestnut, green tea, ginseng (all have additional antiplatelet activity).

Lab Interactions Urine glucose, urinary 5-HIAA, serum uric acid

Adverse Reactions

>10%:

Cardiovascular: Hypotension

Central nervous system: Lightheadedness, dizziness, sedation, drowsiness, fatigue

Gastrointestinal: Nausea, heartburn, stomach pain, heartburn, epigastric discomfort

Neuromuscular & skeletal: Weakness

1% to 10%:

Cardiovascular: Bradycardia

Central nervous system: Confusion

Dermatologic: Rash

Gastrointestinal: Vomiting, gastrointestinal ulceration

Genitourinary: Decreased urination

Hematologic: Hemolytic anemia

Respiratory: Dyspnea

Miscellaneous: Anaphylactic shock

<1% (Limited to important or life-threatening): Biliary tract spasm, bronchospasm, hallucinations, hepatotoxicity, histamine release, leukopenia, occult bleeding, physical and psychological dependence with prolonged use, prolongated bleeding time, thrombocytopenia, urinary tract spasm

Overdosage/Toxicology Naloxone is the antidote for hydrocodone. Naloxone, 2 mg I.V. with repeat administration as necessary up to a total of 10 mg, can also be used to reverse toxic effects of the opiate. Nomograms, such as the "Done" nomogram, can be very helpful for estimating the severity of aspirin poisoning and for directing treatment using serum salicylate levels. Treatment can also be based upon symptomatology; symptoms of aspirin overdose include tinnitus, headache, dizziness, confusion, metabolic acidosis, hyperpyrexia, hypoglycemia, and coma.

Dosing

Adults: Pain management (analgesic): Oral: 1-2 tablets every 4-6 hours as needed for pain

Elderly: Refer to dosing in individual monographs.

Available Dosage Forms Tablet: Hydrocodone bitartrate 5 mg and aspirin 500 mg

Nursing Guidelines

Assessment: Do not use for persons with allergic reaction to aspirin or aspirin-containing medications. Assess other medications patient may be taking for additive or adverse interactions. Monitor therapeutic effectiveness and adverse reactions at beginning of therapy and at regular intervals with long-term use. May cause physical and/or psychological dependence. Discontinue slowly after long-term use. Assess knowledge/teach patient appropriate use if self-administered. Teach patient to monitor for adverse reactions, adverse reactions to report, and appropriate interventions to reduce side effects.

Patient Education: If self-administered, use exactly as directed; do not increase dose or frequency. Drug may cause physical and/or psychological dependence. Take with food or milk. While using this medication, do not use alcohol, excessive amounts of vitamin C, or salicylate-containing foods (curry powder, prunes, raisins, tea, or licorice), other aspirin- or salicylate-containing medications, and other prescription or OTC medications (especially sedatives, tranquilizers, antihistamines, or pain medications) without consulting prescriber. Maintain adequate hydration (2-3 L/day of fluids) unless instructed to restrict fluid intake. May cause hypotension, dizziness, drowsiness, impaired coordination, or blurred vision (use caution when driving, climbing stairs, or changing position - rising from sitting or lying to standing, or when engaging in tasks requiring alertness until response to drug is known); nausea, vomiting, or dry mouth (frequent mouth care, small frequent meals, chewing gum, or sucking lozenges may help); or constipation (increased exercise, fluids, fruit, or fiber may help; if unresolved, consult prescriber about use of stool softeners). Report ringing in ears; persistent stomach pain; unresolved nausea or vomiting; respiratory difficulty or shortness of breath; yellowing of skin or eyes; changes in color of stool or urine; or unusual bruising or bleeding. **Pregnancy/breast-feeding precautions:** Use appropriate contraceptive measures; do not get pregnant while taking this drug. Do not breast-feed.

Pregnancy Risk Factor: D

Lactation: Enters breast milk/contraindicated

Breast-Feeding Considerations:

Hydrocodone: No data reported.

Aspirin: Cautious use due to potential adverse effects in nursing infants.

Administration

Oral: Administer with food or a full glass of water to minimize GI distress.

Hydrocortisone (hye droe KOR ti sone)

U.S. Brand Names Anucort-HC®; Anusol-HC®; Anusol® HC-1 [OTC]; Aquanil™ HC [OTC]; Beta-HC®; Caldecort® [OTC]; Cetacort®; Colocort®; Cortaid® Intensive Therapy [OTC]; Cortaid® Maximum Strength [OTC]; Cortaid® Sensitive Skin [OTC]; Cortef®; Corticool® [OTC]; Cortifoam®; Cortizone®-10 Maximum Strength [OTC]; Cortizone®-10 Plus Maximum Strength [OTC]; Cortizone®-10 Quick Shot [OTC]; Dermarest Dricort® [OTC]; Dermtex® HC [OTC]; EarSol® HC; Hemril®-30; HydroZone Plus [OTC]; Hytone®; IvySoothe® [OTC]; Locoid®; Locoid Lipocream®; Nupercainal® Hydrocortisone Cream [OTC]; Nutracort®; Pandel®; Post Peel Healing Balm [OTC]; Preparation H® Hydrocortisone [OTC]; Proctocort®; ProctoCream® HC; Procto-Kit™; Procto-Pak™; Proctosert; Proctosol-HC®; Proctozone-HC™; Sarnol®-HC [OTC]; Solu-Cortef®; Summer's Eve® SpecialCare™ Medicated Anti-Itch Cream [OTC]; Texacort®; Tucks® Anti-Itch [OTC]; Westcort®

Synonyms A-hydroCort; Compound F; Cortisol; Hemorrhoidal HC; Hydrocortisone Acetate; Hydrocortisone Butyrate; Hydrocortisone Probutate; Hydrocortisone Sodium Succinate; Hydrocortisone Valerate

Pharmacologic Category Corticosteroid, Rectal; Corticosteroid, Systemic; Corticosteroid, Topical

Medication Safety Issues

Sound-alike/look-alike issues:

- Hydrocortisone may be confused with hydrocodone, hydroxychloroquine, hydrochlorothiazide
- Anusol® may be confused with Anusol-HC®, Aplisol®, Aquasol®
- Anusol-HC® may be confused with Anusol®
- Cortef® may be confused with Lortab®
- Cortizone® may be confused with cortisone
- HCT (occasional abbreviation for hydrocortisone) is an error-prone abbreviation (mistaken as hydrochlorothiazide)
- Hytone® may be confused with Vytone®
- Proctocort® may be confused with ProctoCream®
- ProctoCream® may be confused with Proctocort®

(Continued)

Hydrocortisone *(Continued)*

Use Management of adrenocortical insufficiency; relief of inflammation of corticosteroid-responsive dermatoses (low and medium potency topical corticosteroid); adjunctive treatment of ulcerative colitis

Mechanism of Action Decreases inflammation by suppression of migration of polymorphonuclear leukocytes and reversal of increased capillary permeability

Pharmacodynamics/Kinetics

Onset of action:

Hydrocortisone acetate: Slow

Hydrocortisone sodium succinate (water soluble): Rapid

Duration: Hydrocortisone acetate: Long

Absorption: Rapid by all routes, except rectally

Metabolism: Hepatic

Half-life elimination: Biologic: 8-12 hours

Excretion: Urine (primarily as 17-hydroxysteroids and 17-ketosteroids)

Contraindications Hypersensitivity to hydrocortisone or any component of the formulation; serious infections, except septic shock or tuberculous meningitis; viral, fungal, or tubercular skin lesions

Warnings/Precautions

Use with caution in patients with hyperthyroidism, cirrhosis, nonspecific ulcerative colitis, hypertension, osteoporosis, thromboembolic tendencies, CHF, convulsive disorders, myasthenia gravis, thrombophlebitis, peptic ulcer, diabetes, glaucoma, cataracts, or tuberculosis. Use caution in hepatic impairment.

May cause HPA axis suppression. Acute adrenal insufficiency may occur with abrupt withdrawal after long-term therapy or with stress; young pediatric patients may be more susceptible to adrenal axis suppression from topical therapy. Avoid use of topical preparations with occlusive dressings or on weeping or exudative lesions.

Because of the risk of adverse effects, systemic corticosteroids should be used cautiously in the elderly, in the smallest possible dose, and for the shortest possible time

Drug Interactions **Substrate** of CYP3A4 (minor); **Induces** CYP3A4 (weak)

Decreased effect:

Insulin decreases hypoglycemic effect

Phenytoin, phenobarbital, ephedrine, and rifampin increase metabolism of hydrocortisone and decrease steroid blood level

Increased toxicity:

Oral anticoagulants change prothrombin time

Potassium-depleting diuretics increase risk of hypokalemia

Cardiac glucosides increase risk of arrhythmias or digitalis toxicity secondary to hypokalemia

Nutritional/Herbal/Ethanol Interactions

Ethanol: Avoid ethanol (may enhance gastric mucosal irritation).

Food: Hydrocortisone interferes with calcium absorption.

Herb/Nutraceutical: St John's wort may decrease hydrocortisone levels. Avoid cat's claw, echinacea (have immunostimulant properties).

Adverse Reactions

Systemic:

>10%:

Central nervous system: Insomnia, nervousness

Gastrointestinal: Increased appetite, indigestion

1% to 10%:

Dermatologic: Hirsutism

Endocrine & metabolic: Diabetes mellitus

Neuromuscular & skeletal: Arthralgia

Ocular: Cataracts

Respiratory: Epistaxis

<1% (Limited to important or life-threatening): Hypertension, edema, euphoria, headache, delirium, hallucinations, seizure, mood swings, acne, dermatitis, skin atrophy, bruising, hyperpigmentation, hypokalemia, hyperglycemia, Cushing's syndrome, sodium and water retention, bone growth suppression, amenorrhea, peptic ulcer, abdominal distention, ulcerative esophagitis, pancreatitis, muscle wasting, hypersensitivity reactions, immunosuppression

Topical:

>10%: Dermatologic: Eczema (12.5%)

1% to 10%: Dermatologic: Pruritus (6%), stinging (2%), dry skin (2%)

<1% (Limited to important or life-threatening): Allergic contact dermatitis, burning, dermal atrophy, folliculitis, HPA axis suppression, hypopigmentation; metabolic effects (hyperglycemia, hypokalemia); striae

Overdosage/Toxicology When consumed in high doses for prolonged periods, systemic hypercorticism and adrenal suppression may occur. In those cases, discontinuation of the corticosteroid should be done judiciously.

Dosing

Adults & Elderly: Dose should be based on severity of disease and patient response.

Acute adrenal insufficiency: I.M., I.V.: Succinate: 100 mg I.V. bolus, then 300 mg/day in divided doses every 8 hours or as a continuous infusion for 48 hours. Once patient is stable change to oral, 50 mg every 8 hours for 6 doses, then taper to 30-50 mg/day in divided doses.

Chronic adrenal corticoid insufficiency/physiologic replacement: Oral: 20-30 mg/day

Anti-inflammatory or immunosuppressive: Oral, I.M., I.V.: Succinate: 15-240 mg every 12 hours

Congenital adrenal hyperplasia: Oral: Initial: 10-20 mg/m^2/day in 3 divided doses; a variety of dosing schedules have been used. **Note:** Inconsistencies have occurred with liquid formulations; tablets may provide more reliable levels. Doses must be individualized by monitoring growth, bone age, and hormonal levels. Mineralocorticoid and sodium supplementation may be required based upon electrolyte regulation and plasma renin activity.

Shock: I.M., I.V.: Succinate: 500 mg to 2 g every 2-6 hours

Status asthmaticus: I.V.: Succinate: 1-2 mg/kg/dose every 6 hours for 24 hours, then maintenance of 0.5-1 mg/kg every 6 hours

Stress dosing (surgery) in patients known to be adrenally-suppressed or on chronic systemic steroids: I.V.:

Minor stress (ie, inguinal herniorrhaphy): 25 mg/day for 1 day

Moderate stress (ie, joint replacement, cholecystectomy): 50-75 mg/day (25 mg every 8-12 hours) for 1-2 days

Major stress (pancreatoduodenectomy, esophagogastrectomy, cardiac surgery): 100-150 mg/day (50 mg every 8-12 hours) for 2-3 days

Rheumatic diseases:

Intralesional, intra-articular, soft tissue injection: Acetate:

Large joints: 25 mg (up to 37.5 mg)

Small joints: 10-25 mg

Tendon sheaths: 5-12.5 mg

Soft tissue infiltration: 25-50 mg (up to 75 mg)

Bursae: 25-37.5 mg

Ganglia: 12.5-25 mg

Dermatosis: Topical: Apply to affected area 2-4 times/day.

Ulcerative colitis: Rectal: 10-100 mg 1-2 times/day for 2-3 weeks

Pediatrics: Dose should be based on severity of disease and patient response.

Acute adrenal insufficiency: I.M., I.V.:

Infants and young Children: Succinate: 1-2 mg/kg/dose bolus, then 25-150 mg/day in divided doses every 6-8 hours

Older Children: Succinate: 1-2 mg/kg bolus then 150-250 mg/day in divided doses every 6-8 hours

Anti-inflammatory or immunosuppressive:

Infants and Children:

Oral: 2.5-10 mg/kg/day **or** 75-300 mg/m^2/day every 6-8 hours

I.M., I.V.: Succinate: 1-5 mg/kg/day **or** 30-150 mg/m^2/day divided every 12-24 hours

Adolescents: Oral, I.M., I.V.: Succinate: 15-240 mg every 12 hours

Congenital adrenal hyperplasia: Oral: Initial: 10-20 mg/m^2/day in 3 divided doses; a variety of dosing schedules have been used. **Note:** Inconsistencies have occurred with liquid formulations; tablets may provide more reliable levels. Doses must be individualized by monitoring growth, bone age, and hormonal levels. Mineralocorticoid and sodium supplementation may be required based upon electrolyte regulation and plasma renin activity

Physiologic replacement: Children:

Oral: 0.5-0.75 mg/kg/day **or** 20-25 mg/m^2/day every 8 hours

I.M.: Succinate: 0.25-0.35 mg/kg/day **or** 12-15 mg/m^2/day once daily

Shock: I.M., I.V.: Succinate:

Children: Initial: 50 mg/kg, then repeated in 4 hours and/or every 24 hours as needed

Adolescents: 500 mg to 2 g every 2-6 hours

(Continued)

Hydrocortisone *(Continued)*

Status asthmaticus: Children: I.V.: Succinate: 1-2 mg/kg/dose every 6 hours for 24 hours, then maintenance of 0.5-1 mg/kg every 6 hours.

Dermatosis: Topical: Children >2 years: Apply to affected area 2-4 times/day (Buteprate: Apply once or twice daily).

Available Dosage Forms [DSC] = Discontinued product

Aerosol, rectal, as acetate (Cortifoam®): 10% (15 g) [90 mg/applicator]
Cream, rectal, as acetate (Nupercainal® Hydrocortisone Cream): 1% (30 g) [strength expressed as base]
Cream, rectal, as base:
  Cortizone®-10: 1% (30 g) [contains aloe]
  Preparation H® Hydrocortisone: 1% (27 g)
Cream, topical, as acetate: 0.5% (9 g, 30 g, 60 g) [available with aloe]; 1% (30 g, 454 g) [available with aloe]
Cream, topical, as base: 0.5% (30 g); 1% (1.5 g, 30 g, 114 g, 454 g); 2.5% (20 g, 30 g, 454 g)
  Anusol-HC®: 2.5% (30 g) [contains benzyl alcohol]
  Caldecort®: 1% (30 g) [contains aloe vera gel]
  Cortaid® Intensive Therapy: 1% (60 g)
  Cortaid® Maximum Strength: 1% (15 g, 30 g, 40 g, 60 g) [contains aloe vera gel and benzyl alcohol]
  Cortaid® Sensitive Skin: 0.5% (15 g) [contains aloe vera gel]
  Cortizone®-10 Maximum Strength: 1% (15 g, 30 g, 60 g) [contains aloe]
  Cortizone®-10 Plus Maximum Strength: 1% (30 g, 60 g) [contains vitamins A, D, E and aloe]
  Dermarest® Dricort®: 1% (15 g, 30 g)
  HydroZone Plus, Proctocort®, Procto-Pak™: 1% (30 g)
  Hytone®: 2.5% (30 g, 60 g)
  IvySoothe®: 1% (30 g) [contains aloe]
  Post Peel Healing Balm: 1% (23 g)
  ProctoCream® HC: 2.5% (30 g) [contains benzyl alcohol]
  Procto-Kit™: 1% (30 g) [packaged with applicator tips and finger cots]; 2.5% (30 g) [packaged with applicator tips and finger cots]
  Proctosol-HC®, Proctozone-HC™: 2.5% (30 g)
  Summer's Eve® SpecialCare™ Medicated Anti-Itch Cream: 1% (30 g)
Cream, topical, as butyrate (Locoid®, Locoid Lipocream®): 0.1% (15 g, 45 g)
Cream, topical, as probutate (Pandel®): 0.1% (15 g, 45 g, 80 g)
Cream, topical, as valerate (Westcort®): 0.2% (15 g, 45 g, 60 g)
Gel, topical, as base (Corticool®): 1% (45 g)
Injection, powder for reconstitution, as sodium succinate (Solu-Cortef®): 100 mg, 250 mg, 500 mg, 1 g [diluent contains benzyl alcohol; strength expressed as base]
Lotion, topical, as base: 1% (120 mL); 2.5% (60 mL)
  Aquanil™ HC: 1% (120 mL)
  Beta-HC®, Cetacort®, Sarnol®-HC: 1% (60 mL)
  HydroZone Plus: 1% (120 mL)
  Hytone®: 2.5% (60 mL)
  Nutracort®: 1% (60 mL, 120 mL); 2.5% (60 mL, 120 mL)
Ointment, topical, as acetate: 1% (30 g) [strength expressed as base; available with aloe]
  Anusol® HC-1: 1% (21 g) [strength expressed as base]
  Cortaid® Maximum Strength: 1% (15 g, 30 g) [strength expressed as base]
Ointment, topical, as base: 0.5% (30 g); 1% (30 g, 454 g); 2.5% (20 g, 30 g, 454 g)
  Cortizone®-10 Maximum Strength: 1% (30 g, 60 g)
  Hytone®: 2.5% (30 g) [DSC]
Ointment, topical, as butyrate (Locoid®): 0.1% (15 g, 45 g)
Ointment, topical, as valerate (Westcort®): 0.2% (15 g, 45 g, 60 g)
Solution, otic, as base (EarSol® HC): 1% (30 mL) [contains alcohol 44%, benzyl benzoate, yerba santa]
Solution, topical, as base (Texacort®): 2.5% (30 mL) [contains alcohol]
Solution, topical, as butyrate (Locoid®): 0.1% (20 mL, 60 mL) [contains alcohol 50%]
Solution, topical spray, as base:
  Cortaid® Intensive Therapy: 1% (60 mL) [contains alcohol]
  Cortizone®-10 Quick Shot: 1% (44 mL) [contains benzyl alcohol]
  Dermtex® HC: 1% (52 mL) [contains menthol 1%]

Suppository, rectal, as acetate: 25 mg (12s, 24s, 100s)
  Anucort-HC®, Tucks® Anti-Itch: 25 mg (12s, 24s, 100s) [strength expressed as base; Anucort-HC® *renamed* Tucks® Anti-Itch]
  Anusol-HC®, Proctosol-HC®: 25 mg (12s, 24s)
  Encort™: 30 mg (12s)
  Hemril®-30, Proctocort®, Proctosert: 30 mg (12s, 24s)
Suspension, rectal, as base: 100 mg/60 mL (7s)
  Colocort®: 100 mg/60 mL (1s, 7s)
Tablet, as base: 20 mg
  Cortef®: 5 mg, 10 mg, 20 mg

Nursing Guidelines

Assessment: Monitor laboratory results, effects and interactions of other medications patient may be taking, response to therapy and adverse effects according to diagnosis, formulation of hydrocortisone, dosage, and extent of time used. Systemic administration and long-term use will require close and frequent monitoring, especially for Cushing's syndrome. Assess for signs of fluid retention. Taper dosage when discontinuing. Assess/teach patient appropriate use, interventions for possible adverse reactions, and symptoms to report. Topical absorption may be minimal.

Monitoring Laboratory Tests: Serum glucose, electrolytes

Dietary Considerations: Systemic use of corticosteroids may require a diet with increased potassium, vitamins A, B_6, C, D, folate, calcium, zinc, phosphorus, and decreased sodium. Sodium content of 1 g (sodium succinate injection): 47.5 mg (2.07 mEq)

Patient Education: Systemic: Take as directed; do not increase doses and do not stop abruptly without consulting prescribed. Dosage of systemic hydrocortisone is usually tapered off gradually. Take oral dose with food to reduce GI upset. Avoid alcohol. Hydrocortisone may cause immunosuppression and mask symptoms of infection; avoid exposure to contagion and notify prescriber of any signs of infection (eg, fever, chills, sore throat, injury) and notify dentist or surgeon (if necessary) that you are taking this medication. You may experience increased appetite, indigestion, or increased nervousness. Report any sudden weight gain (>5 lb/week), swelling of extremities or respiratory difficulty, abdominal pain, severe vomiting, black or tarry stools, fatigue, anorexia, weakness, or unusual mood swings. **Pregnancy/breast-feeding precautions:** Inform prescriber if you are or intend to become pregnant. Consult prescriber if breast-feeding.

Topical: Before applying, wash area gently and thoroughly. Apply a thin film to cleansed area and rub in gently until medication vanishes. Avoid use of occlusive dressings over topical application unless directed by a physician. Avoid use on weeping or exudative lesions. Avoid exposing affected area to sunlight; you will be more sensitive and severe sunburn may occur. Consult prescriber if breast-feeding.

Rectal: Gently insert suppository as high as possible with gloved finger while lying down. Avoid injury with long or sharp fingernails. Remain in resting position for 10 minutes after insertion.

Pregnancy Risk Factor: C

Pregnancy Issues: There are no adequate and well-controlled studies in pregnant women. Corticosteroid use has been associated with cleft palate, neonatal adrenal suppression, low birth weight, and cataracts in the infant; including cases associated with topical administration. Use only if potential benefit to the mother exceeds the potential risk to the fetus. Avoid high doses or prolonged use.

Lactation: Excretion in breast milk unknown/use caution

Breast-Feeding Considerations: It is not known if hydrocortisone is excreted in breast milk, however, other corticosteroids are excreted. Prednisone and prednisolone are excreted in breast milk; the AAP considers them to be "usually compatible" with breast-feeding. Hypertension was reported in a nursing infant when a topical corticosteroid was applied to the nipples of the mother.

Perioperative/Anesthesia/Other Concerns: Hydrocortisone is a long-acting corticosteroid with minimal sodium-retaining potential.

Neuromuscular Effects: ICU-acquired paresis was recently studied in 5 ICUs (3 medical and 2 surgical ICUs) at 4 French hospitals. All ICU patients without pre-existing neuromuscular disease admitted from March 1999 through June 2000 were evaluated (De Jonghe B, 2002). Each patient had to be mechanically ventilated for ≥7 days and was screened daily for awakening. The first day

(Continued)

Hydrocortisone *(Continued)*

the patient was considered awake was Study Day 1. Patients with severe muscle weakness on Study Day 7 were considered to have ICU-acquired paresis. Among the 95 patients who were evaluable, about 25% developed ICU-acquired paresis. Independent predictors included: female gender, the number of days with ≥2 organ dysfunction, and administration of corticosteroids. Further studies may be required to verify and characterize the association between the development of ICU-acquired paresis and use of corticosteroids. Concurrent use of a corticosteroid and muscle relaxant appear to increase the risk of certain ICU myopathies; avoid or administer the corticosteroid at the lowest dose possible.

Adrenal Insufficiency: Patients will often have steroid-induced adverse effects on glucose tolerance and lipid profiles. When discontinuing steroid therapy in patients on long-term steroid supplementation, it is important that the steroid therapy be discontinued gradually. Abrupt withdrawal may result in adrenal insufficiency with hypotension and hyperkalemia. Patients on long-term steroid supplementation will require higher corticosteroid doses when subject to stress (ie, trauma, surgery, severe infection). Guidelines for glucocorticoid replacement during various surgical procedures has been published (Salem M, 1994, Coursin DB, 2002).

Septic Shock: A recent randomized, double-blind, placebo controlled trial assessed whether low dose corticosteroid administration could improve 28-day survival in patients with septic shock and relative adrenal insufficiency. Relative adrenal insufficiency was defined as an inappropriate response to corticotropin administration (increase of serum cortisol of ≤9 mcg/dL from baseline). Cortisol levels were drawn immediately before corticotropin administration and 30 to 60 minutes afterwards. Three hundred adult septic shock patients requiring mechanical ventilation and vasopressor support were randomized to either hydrocortisone (50 mg IVP every 6 hours) and fludrocortisone (50 mcg tablet daily via nasogastric tube) or matching placebos for 7 days. In patients who did not appropriately respond to corticotropin (nonresponders), there were significantly fewer deaths in the active treatment group. Vasopressor therapy was withdrawn more frequently in this subset of the active treatment group. Adverse events were similar in both groups. Patients who lack adrenal reserve and thus have relative adrenal insufficiency during the stress of septic shock may benefit from physiologic steroid replacement. However, there was a trend for increased mortality in patients who responded to the corticotropin test (increase serum cortisol >9 mcg/dL from baseline). These patients may not benefit from physiologic steroid replacement. Further study is required to better characterize the patient populations who may benefit.

Administration

Oral: Administer with food or milk to decrease GI upset.

I.V.:

Parenteral: Hydrocortisone sodium succinate may be administered by I.M. or I.V. routes.

I.V. bolus: Dilute to 50 mg/mL and give over 30 seconds to several minutes (depending on the dose).

I.V. intermittent infusion: Dilute to 1 mg/mL and give over 20-30 minutes.

Note: Should be administered in a 0.1-1 mg/mL concentration due to stability problems.

Reconstitution:

Sodium succinate: Reconstitute 100 mg vials with bacteriostatic water (not >2 mL). Act-O-Vial (self-contained powder for injection plus diluent) may be reconstituted by pressing the activator to force diluent into the powder compartment. Following gentle agitation, solution may be withdrawn via syringe through a needle inserted into the center of the stopper. May be administered (I.V. or I.M.) without further dilution.

Solutions for I.V. infusion: Reconstituted solutions may be added to an appropriate volume of compatible solution for infusion. Concentration should generally not exceed 1 mg/mL. However, in cases where administration of a small volume of fluid is desirable, 100-3000 mg may be added to 50 mL of D_5W or NS (stability limited to 4 hours).

Compatibility:

Hydrocortisone sodium phosphate: Stable in D_5W, NS, fat emulsion 10%

Y-site administration: Incompatible with sargramostim

Compatibility in syringe: Incompatible with doxapram

Hydrocortisone sodium succinate: Stable in dextran 6% in dextrose, dextran 6% in NS, D_5LR, $D_5{}^1/_4NS$, $D_5{}^1/_2NS$, D_5NS, D_5W, $D_{10}W$, $D_{20}W$, LR, $^1/_2NS$, NS, fat emulsion 10%

Y-site administration: Incompatible with ciprofloxacin, diazepam, ergotamine, idarubicin, midazolam, phenytoin, sargramostim

Compatibility in syringe: Incompatible with doxapram

Compatibility when admixed: Incompatible with aminophylline with cephalothin, bleomycin, colistimethate, ephedrine, hydralazine, nafcillin, pentobarbital, phenobarbital, prochlorperazine edisylate, promethazine

Storage: Store at controlled room temperature 20°C to 25°C (59°F to 86°F). Hydrocortisone sodium phosphate and hydrocortisone sodium succinate are clear, light yellow solutions which are heat labile.

Sodium succinate: After initial reconstitution, hydrocortisone sodium succinate solutions are stable for 3 days at room temperature or under refrigeration when protected from light. Stability of parenteral admixture (Solu-Cortef®) at room temperature (25°C) and at refrigeration temperature (4°C) is concentration-dependent:

Stability of concentration 1 mg/mL: 24 hours

Stability of concentration 2 mg/mL to 60 mg/mL: At least 4 hours

Solutions for I.V. infusion: Reconstituted solutions may be added to an appropriate volume of compatible solution for infusion. Concentration should generally not exceed 1 mg/mL. However, in cases where administration of a small volume of fluid is desirable, 100-3000 mg may be added to 50 mL of D_5W or NS (stability limited to 4 hours).

♦ **Hydrocortisone Acetate** *see* Hydrocortisone *on page 873*

♦ **Hydrocortisone, Acetic Acid, and Propylene Glycol Diacetate** *see* Acetic Acid, Propylene Glycol Diacetate, and Hydrocortisone *on page 78*

♦ **Hydrocortisone, Bacitracin, Neomycin, and Polymyxin B** *see* Bacitracin, Neomycin, Polymyxin B, and Hydrocortisone *on page 221*

♦ **Hydrocortisone Butyrate** *see* Hydrocortisone *on page 873*

♦ **Hydrocortisone, Neomycin, and Polymyxin B** *see* Neomycin, Polymyxin B, and Hydrocortisone *on page 1212*

♦ **Hydrocortisone, Neomycin, Colistin, and Thonzonium** *see* Neomycin, Colistin, Hydrocortisone, and Thonzonium *on page 1210*

♦ **Hydrocortisone Probutate** *see* Hydrocortisone *on page 873*

♦ **Hydrocortisone, Propylene Glycol Diacetate, and Acetic Acid** *see* Acetic Acid, Propylene Glycol Diacetate, and Hydrocortisone *on page 78*

♦ **Hydrocortisone Sodium Succinate** *see* Hydrocortisone *on page 873*

♦ **Hydrocortisone Valerate** *see* Hydrocortisone *on page 873*

Hydromorphone (hye droe MOR fone)

U.S. Brand Names Dilaudid®; Dilaudid-HP®; Palladone™ *[Withdrawn]*

Synonyms Dihydromorphinone; Hydromorphone Hydrochloride

Pharmacologic Category Analgesic, Narcotic

Medication Safety Issues

Sound-alike/look-alike issues:

Dilaudid® may be confused with Demerol®, Dilantin®

Hydromorphone may be confused with morphine; significant overdoses have occurred when hydromorphone products have been inadvertently administered instead of morphine sulfate. Commercially available prefilled syringes of both products looks similar and are often stored in close proximity to each other. **Note:** Hydromorphone 1 mg oral is approximately equal to morphine 4 mg oral; hydromorphone 1 mg I.V. is approximately equal to morphine 5 mg I.V.

Dilaudid®, Dilaudid-HP®: Extreme caution should be taken to avoid confusing the highly-concentrated (Dilaudid-HP®) injection with the less-concentrated (Dilaudid®) injectable product.

Use Management of moderate-to-severe pain

Unlabeled/Investigational Use Antitussive

Mechanism of Action Binds to opiate receptors in the CNS, causing inhibition of ascending pain pathways, altering the perception of and response to pain; causes cough supression by direct central action in the medulla; produces generalized CNS depression

Pharmacodynamics/Kinetics

Onset of action: Analgesic: Immediate release formulations:

Oral: 15-30 minutes

(Continued)

Hydromorphone *(Continued)*

Peak effect: Oral: 30-60 minutes

Duration: Immediate release formulations: 4-5 hours

Absorption: I.M.: Variable and delayed; Palladone™: Biphasic

Distribution: V_d: 4 L/kg

Protein binding: ~20%

Metabolism: Hepatic; to inactive metabolites

Bioavailability: 62%

Half-life elimination:

Immediate release formulations: 1-3 hours

Palladone™: 18.6 hours

Excretion: Urine (primarily as glucuronide conjugates)

Contraindications Hypersensitivity to hydromorphone, any component of the formulation, or other phenanthrene derivative; increased intracranial pressure; acute or severe asthma, severe respiratory depression (in absence of resuscitative equipment or ventilatory support); severe CNS depression; pregnancy (prolonged use or high doses at term)

Palladone™ is also contraindicated with known or suspected paralytic ileus.

Warnings/Precautions Controlled release capsules should only be used when continuous analgesia is required over an extended period of time. Palladone™ should only be used in opioid tolerant patients requiring doses of hydromorphone >12 mg/day (or equianalgesic dose of another opioid) and who have been at that dose for >7 days. Controlled release products are not to be used on an as needed basis. Hydromorphone shares toxic potential of opiate agonists, and precaution of opiate agonist therapy should be observed; use with caution in patients with hypersensitivity to other phenanthrene opiates, respiratory disease, biliary tract disease, acute pancreatitis, or severe liver or renal failure; tolerance or drug dependence may result from extended use. Those at risk for opioid abuse include patients with a history of substance abuse or mental illness.

An opioid-containing analgesic regimen should be tailored to each patient's needs and based upon the type of pain being treated (acute versus chronic), the route of administration, degree of tolerance for opioids (naive versus chronic user), age, weight, and medical condition. The optimal analgesic dose varies widely among patients. Doses should be titrated to pain relief/prevention. I.M. use may result in variable absorption and a lag time to peak effect.

Some dosage forms contain trace amounts of sodium bisulfite which may cause allergic reactions in susceptible individuals.

Drug Interactions

CNS depressants: Effects with hydromorphone may be additive.

Pegvisomant: Analgesics (narcotic) may diminish the therapeutic effect of pegvisomant; increased pegvisomant doses may be needed.

Phenothiazines: May enhance the hypotensive and CNS depressant effects of hydromorphone.

Selective serotonin reuptake inhibitors (SSRIs): Serotonergic effects may be additive, leading to serotonin syndrome.

Nutritional/Herbal/Ethanol Interactions

Ethanol: Avoid ethanol (may increase CNS depression).

Herb/Nutraceutical: Avoid valerian, St John's wort, kava kava, gotu kola (may increase CNS depression).

Lab Interactions Increased aminotransferase [ALT (SGPT)/AST (SGOT)] (S)

Adverse Reactions Frequency not defined.

Cardiovascular: Palpitations, hypotension, peripheral vasodilation, tachycardia, bradycardia, flushing of face

Central nervous system: CNS depression, increased intracranial pressure, fatigue, headache, nervousness, restlessness, dizziness, lightheadedness, drowsiness, hallucinations, mental depression, seizure

Dermatologic: Pruritus, rash, urticaria

Endocrine & metabolic: Antidiuretic hormone release

Gastrointestinal: Nausea, vomiting, constipation, stomach cramps, xerostomia, anorexia, biliary tract spasm, paralytic ileus

Genitourinary: Decreased urination, ureteral spasm, urinary tract spasm

Hepatic: LFTs increased, AST increased, ALT increased

Local: Pain at injection site (I.M.)

Neuromuscular & skeletal: Trembling, weakness, myoclonus

Ocular: Miosis

Respiratory: Respiratory depression, dyspnea

Miscellaneous: Histamine release, physical and psychological dependence

Overdosage/Toxicology Symptoms of overdose include CNS depression, respiratory depression, miosis, apnea, pulmonary edema, and convulsions. Along with supportive measures, naloxone, 2 mg I.V. with repeat administration as necessary up to a total of 10 mg, can also be used to reverse toxic effects of the opiate.

Dosing

Adults:

Antitussive (unlabeled use): Oral: 1 mg every 3-4 hours as needed

Acute pain (moderate to severe): Note: These are guidelines and do not represent the maximum doses that may be required in all patients. Doses should be titrated to pain relief/prevention. Doses should be titrated to appropriate analgesic effects; when changing routes of administration, note that oral doses are <50% as effective as parenteral doses (may be only one-fifth as effective).

Oral:

Initial: Opiate-naive: 2-4 mg every 3-4 hours as needed; patients with prior opiate exposure may require higher initial doses

Usual dosage range: 2-8 mg every 3-4 hours as needed

I.V.: Initial: Opiate-naive: 0.2-0.6 mg every 2-3 hours as needed; patients with prior opiate exposure may tolerate higher initial doses

Note: More frequent dosing may be needed.

Mechanically-ventilated patients (based on 70 kg patient): 0.7-2 mg every 1-2 hours as needed; infusion (based on 70 kg patient): 0.5-1 mg/hour

Patient-controlled analgesia (PCA): (Opiate-naive: Consider lower end of dosing range)

Usual concentration: 0.2 mg/mL

Demand dose: Usual: 0.1-0.2 mg; range: 0.05-0.5 mg

Lockout interval: 5-15 minutes

4-hour limit: 4-6 mg

Epidural:

Bolus dose: 1-1.5 mg

Infusion concentration: 0.05-0.075 mg/mL

Infusion rate: 0.04-0.4 mg/hour

Demand dose: 0.15 mg

Lockout interval: 30 minutes

I.M., SubQ: **Note:** I.M. use may result in variable absorption and a lag time to peak effect.

Initial: Opiate-naive: 0.8-1 mg every 4-6 hours as needed; patients with prior opiate exposure may require higher initial doses

Usual dosage range: 1-2 mg every 3-6 hours as needed

Rectal: 3 mg every 4-8 hours as needed

Chronic pain: Note: Patients taking opioids chronically may become tolerant and require doses higher than the usual dosage range to maintain the desired effect. Tolerance can be managed by appropriate dose titration. There is no optimal or maximal dose for hydromorphone in chronic pain. The appropriate dose is one that relieves pain throughout its dosing interval without causing unmanageable side effects.

Controlled release formulation (Hydromorph Contin®, not available in U.S.): Oral: 3-30 mg every 12 hours. **Note:** A patient's hydromorphone requirement should be established using prompt release formulations; conversion to long acting products may be considered when chronic, continuous treatment is required. Higher dosages should be reserved for use only in opioid-tolerant patients.

Extended release formulation (Palladone™): Oral: For use only in opioid-tolerant patients requiring extended treatment of pain. Initial Palladone™ dose should be calculated using standard conversion estimates based on previous total daily opioid dose, rounding off to the most appropriate strength available. Doses should be administered once every 24 hours. Discontinue all previous around-the-clock opioids when treatment is initiated. Dose may be adjusted every 2 days as needed.

Conversion from transdermal fentanyl to oral Palladone™ (limited clinical experience): Initiate Palladone™ 18 hours after removal of patch; substitute Palladone™ 12 mg/day for each fentanyl 50 mcg/hour patch; monitor closely

Conversion from opioid combination drugs: Initial dose: Palladone™ 12 mg/day in patients receiving around-the-clock fixed combination-opioid analgesics with a total dose greater than or equal to oxycodone 45 mg/day, hydrocodone 45 mg/day, or codeine 300 mg/day

(Continued)

Hydromorphone *(Continued)*

Elderly: Doses should be titrated to appropriate analgesic effects. When changing routes of administration, note that oral doses are less than half as effective as parenteral doses (may be only 20% as effective).

Pain: Oral: 1-2 mg every 4-6 hours
Antitussive: Refer to adult dosing.

Pediatrics:

Acute pain (moderate to severe): Note: These are guidelines and do not represent the maximum doses that may be required in all patients. Doses should be titrated to pain relief/prevention.

Young Children ≥6 months and <50 kg:
Oral: 0.03-0.08 mg/kg/dose every 3-4 hours as needed
I.V.: 0.015 mg/kg/dose every 3-6 hours as needed
Older Children >50 kg: Refer to adult dosing.

Antitussive: Oral:
Children 6-12 years: 0.5 mg every 3-4 hours as needed
Children >12 years: 1 mg every 3-4 hours as needed

Hepatic Impairment: Dose adjustment should be considered.

Available Dosage Forms [CAN] = Canadian brand name

Capsule, controlled release (Hydromorph Contin®) [CAN]: 3 mg, 6 mg, 12 mg, 18 mg, 24 mg, 30 mg [not available in U.S.]
Capsule, extended release, as hydrochloride (Palladone™): 12 mg, 16 mg, 24 mg, 32 mg *[withdrawn from market]*
Injection, powder for reconstitution, as hydrochloride (Dilaudid-HP®): 250 mg
Injection, solution, as hydrochloride: 1 mg/mL (1 mL); 2 mg/mL (1 mL, 20 mL); 4 mg/mL (1 mL); 10 mg/mL (1 mL, 5 mL, 10 mL)
Dilaudid®: 1 mg/mL (1 mL); 2 mg/mL (1 mL, 20 mL) [20 mL size contains edetate sodium; vial stopper contains latex]; 4 mg/mL (1 mL)
Dilaudid-HP®: 10 mg/mL (1 mL, 5 mL, 50 mL)
Liquid, oral, as hydrochloride (Dilaudid®): 1 mg/mL (480 mL) [may contain trace amounts of sodium bisulfite]
Suppository, rectal, as hydrochloride (Dilaudid®): 3 mg (6s)
Tablet, as hydrochloride (Dilaudid®): 2 mg, 4 mg, 8 mg (8 mg tablets may contain trace amounts of sodium bisulfite)

Nursing Guidelines

Assessment: Assess other medications patient may be taking for additive or adverse interactions. Monitor for effectiveness of pain relief, adverse reactions, and signs of overdose at beginning of therapy and periodically during long-term use. May cause physical and/or psychological dependence. Monitor blood pressure, CNS and respiratory status, and degree of sedation at beginning of therapy and at regular intervals with long-term use. For inpatients, implement safety measures. Assess knowledge/teach patient appropriate use (if self-administered). Teach patient to monitor for adverse reactions, adverse reactions to report, and appropriate interventions to reduce side effects. Discontinue slowly after prolonged use.

Patient Education: If self-administered, use exactly as directed; do not increase dose or frequency. Drug may cause physical and/or psychological dependence. Palladone™ must be swallowed whole. While using this medication, do not use alcohol and other prescription or OTC medications (especially sedatives, tranquilizers, antihistamines, or pain medications) without consulting prescriber. Maintain adequate hydration (2-3 L/day of fluids) unless instructed to restrict fluid intake. May cause dizziness, drowsiness, impaired coordination, or blurred vision (use caution when driving, climbing stairs, or changing position - rising from sitting or lying to standing, or when engaging in tasks requiring alertness until response to drug is known); loss of appetite, nausea, or vomiting (frequent mouth care, small frequent meals, chewing gum, or sucking lozenges may help); or constipation (increased exercise, fluids, fruit, or fiber may help; if unresolved, consult prescriber about use of stool softeners). Report chest pain, slow or rapid heartbeat, acute dizziness, or persistent headache; swelling of extremities or unusual weight gain; changes in urinary elimination; acute headache; back or flank pain or spasms; or other adverse reactions. **Pregnancy/breast-feeding precautions:** Inform prescriber if you are or intend to become pregnant. Breast-feeding is not recommended.

Geriatric Considerations: Elderly may be particularly susceptible to the CNS depressant and constipating effects of narcotics.

Pregnancy Risk Factor: C/D (prolonged use or high doses at term)

Pregnancy Issues: Hydromorphone was teratogenic in some, but not all, animal studies; however, maternal toxicity was also reported. Hydromorphone crosses the placenta. Chronic opioid use during pregnancy may lead to a withdrawal syndrome in the neonate. Symptoms include irritability, hyperactivity, loss of sleep pattern, abnormal crying, tremor, vomiting, diarrhea, weight loss, or failure to gain weight.

Lactation: Excretion in breast milk unknown/not recommended

Breast-Feeding Considerations: Other opioid analgesics can be found in breast milk; specific data for hydromorphone is not available. The possibility of sedation or respiratory depression in the nursing infant should be considered.

Perioperative/Anesthesia/Other Concerns: When developing a therapeutic plan for pain control, scheduled, intermittent opioid dosing or continuous infusion is preferred over the "as needed" regimen. The 2002 ACCM/SCCM guidelines for analgesia (critically-ill adult) recommend fentanyl in patients who need immediate pain relief because of its rapid onset of action; fentanyl or hydromorphone is preferred in patients who are hypotensive or have renal dysfunction. Morphine or hydromorphone is recommended for intermittent, scheduled therapy. Both have a longer duration of action requiring less frequent administration. Hydromorphone does not have any active metabolites, has less protein binding than other opiates and does not cause histamine release. If the patient has required high-dose analgesia or has used for a prolonged period (~7 days), taper dose to prevent withdrawal; monitor for signs and symptoms of withdrawal.

Equianalgesic doses: Morphine 10 mg I.M. = hydromorphone 1.5 mg I.M.

Administration

Oral:

Hydromorph Contin®: Capsule should be swallowed whole; do not crush or chew; contents may be sprinkled on soft food and swallowed

Palladone™: Capsule must be swallowed whole; do not break open, crush, chew, dissolve, or sprinkle on food.

I.M.: May be given SubQ or I.M.; vial stopper contains latex

I.V.: For IVP, must be given slowly over 2-3 minutes (rapid IVP has been associated with an increase in side effects, especially respiratory depression and hypotension)

Compatibility: Stable in D_5LR, D_5W, $D_5{}^1\!/_2NS$, D_5NS, LR, $^1\!/_2NS$, NS

Y-site administration: Incompatible with amphotericin B cholesteryl sulfate complex, diazepam, minocycline, phenobarbital, phenytoin, sargramostim, tetracycline, thiopental

Compatibility in syringe: Incompatible with ampicillin, diazepam, hyaluronidase, phenobarbital, phenytoin

Compatibility when admixed: Incompatible with sodium bicarbonate, thiopental

Storage: Store injection and oral dosage forms at 25°C (77°F). Protect tablets from light. A slightly yellowish discoloration has not been associated with a loss of potency.

Related Information

Acute Postoperative Pain *on page 1742*

Narcotic / Opioid Analgesics *on page 1880*

- **Hydromorphone Hydrochloride** *see* Hydromorphone *on page 879*
- **Hydroxydaunomycin Hydrochloride** *see* DOXOrubicin *on page 576*
- **Hydroxyethylcellulose** *see* Artificial Tears *on page 187*
- **Hydroxyethyl Starch** *see* Hetastarch *on page 852*
- **Hydroxyldaunorubicin Hydrochloride** *see* DOXOrubicin *on page 576*

Hydroxypropyl Methylcellulose

(hye droks ee PROE pil meth il SEL yoo lose)

U.S. Brand Names Cellugel®; GenTeal® [OTC]; GenTeal® Mild [OTC]; Gonak™ [OTC]; Goniosoft™; Goniosol® [OTC] [DSC]; Isopto® Tears [OTC]; Tearisol® [OTC]; Tears Again® MC [OTC]

Synonyms Gonioscopic Ophthalmic Solution; Hypromellose

Pharmacologic Category Diagnostic Agent, Ophthalmic; Lubricant, Ocular

Medication Safety Issues

Sound-alike/look-alike issues:

Isopto® Tears may be confused with Isoptin®

(Continued)

Hydroxypropyl Methylcellulose *(Continued)*

Use Relief of burning and minor irritation due to dry eyes; diagnostic agent in gonioscopic examination

Contraindications Hypersensitivity to hydroxypropyl methylcellulose or any component of the formulation

Warnings/Precautions Remove contact lenses prior to use. Not labeled for OTC use for >72 hours. Do not use if solution changes color or becomes cloudy.

Dosing

Adults & Elderly: Dry eyes: Ophthalmic: Instill 1-2 drops in affected eye(s) as needed

Available Dosage Forms [DSC] = Discontinued product

Gel, ophthalmic (GenTeal®): 0.3% (10 mL)

Solution, ophthalmic: 0.4% (15 mL)

GenTeal®: 0.3% (15 mL, 25 mL)

GenTeal® Mild: 0.2% (15 mL, 25 mL)

Gonak™: 2.5% (15 mL)

Goniosoft™: 2.5% (15 mL)

Goniosol®: 2.5% (15 mL) [contains benzalkonium chloride] [DSC]

Isopto® Tears: 0.5% (15 mL) [contains benzalkonium chloride]

Tearisol®: 0.5% (15 mL) [contains benzalkonium chloride]

Tears Again® MC: 0.3% (15 mL)

Solution, ophthalmic [for injection] (Cellugel®): 2% (1 mL)

Nursing Guidelines

Patient Education: If you experience eye pain, vision changes, continued redness or irritation of the eye, or if the condition worsens or persists for more than 72 hours, discontinue use and consult a physician

Pregnancy Risk Factor: C

HydrOXYzine (hye DROKS i zeen)

U.S. Brand Names Atarax®; Vistaril®

Synonyms Hydroxyzine Hydrochloride; Hydroxyzine Pamoate

Pharmacologic Category Antiemetic; Antihistamine

Medication Safety Issues

Sound-alike/look-alike issues:

HydrOXYzine may be confused with hydrALAZINE, hydroxyurea

Atarax® may be confused with amoxicillin, Ativan®

Vistaril® may be confused with Restoril®, Versed, Zestril®

Use Treatment of anxiety; preoperative sedative; antipruritic

Unlabeled/Investigational Use Antiemetic; ethanol withdrawal symptoms

Mechanism of Action Competes with histamine for H_1-receptor sites on effector cells in the gastrointestinal tract, blood vessels, and respiratory tract. Possesses skeletal muscle relaxing, bronchodilator, antihistamine, antiemetic, and analgesic properties.

Pharmacodynamics/Kinetics

Onset of action: 15-30 minutes

Duration: 4-6 hours

Absorption: Oral: Rapid

Metabolism: Exact fate unknown

Half-life elimination: 3-7 hours

Time to peak: ~2 hours

Contraindications Hypersensitivity to hydroxyzine or any component of the formulation; early pregnancy

Warnings/Precautions Causes sedation, caution must be used in performing tasks which require alertness (eg, operating machinery or driving). Sedative effects of CNS depressants or ethanol are potentiated. SubQ and intra-arterial administration are not recommended since thrombosis and digital gangrene can occur; should be used with caution in patients with narrow-angle glaucoma, prostatic hyperplasia, and bladder neck obstruction; should also be used with caution in patients with asthma or COPD.

Anticholinergic effects are not well tolerated in the elderly. Hydroxyzine may be useful as a short-term antipruritic, but it is not recommended for use as a sedative or anxiolytic in the elderly.

Drug Interactions **Inhibits** CYP2D6 (weak)

Amantadine, rimantadine: Central and/or peripheral anticholinergic syndrome can occur when administered with amantadine or rimantadine

Anticholinergic agents: Central and/or peripheral anticholinergic syndrome can occur when administered with narcotic analgesics, phenothiazines and other antipsychotics (especially with high anticholinergic activity), tricyclic antidepressants, quinidine and some other antiarrhythmics, and antihistamines

Antipsychotics: Hydroxyzine may antagonize the therapeutic effects of antipsychotics

CNS depressants: Sedative effects of hydroxyzine may be additive with CNS depressants; includes ethanol, benzodiazepines, barbiturates, narcotic analgesics, and other sedative agents; monitor for increased effect

Nutritional/Herbal/Ethanol Interactions

Ethanol: Avoid ethanol (may increase CNS depression).

Herb/Nutraceutical: Avoid valerian, St John's wort, kava kava, gotu kola (may increase CNS depression).

Adverse Reactions Frequency not defined.

Central nervous system: Drowsiness, headache, fatigue, nervousness, dizziness, hallucination

Dermatologic: Pruritus, rash, urticaria

Gastrointestinal: Xerostomia

Neuromuscular & skeletal: Tremor, paresthesia, seizure, involuntary movements

Ocular: Blurred vision

Respiratory: Thickening of bronchial secretions

Miscellaneous: Allergic reaction

Overdosage/Toxicology Symptoms of overdose include seizures, sedation, and hypotension. There is no specific treatment for antihistamine overdose. Clinical toxicity is due to blockade of cholinergic receptors. For anticholinergic overdose with severe life-threatening symptoms, physostigmine 1-2 mg I.V. slowly, may be given to reverse these effects.

Dosing

Adults:

Antiemetic: I.M.: 25-100 mg/dose every 4-6 hours as needed

Anxiety: Oral: 25-100 mg 4 times/day; maximum: 600 mg/day

Preoperative sedation:

Oral: 50-100 mg

I.M.: 25-100 mg

Management of pruritus: Oral: 25 mg 3-4 times/day

Elderly: Management of pruritus: 10 mg 3-4 times/day; increase to 25 mg 3-4 times/day if necessary.

Pediatrics:

Preoperative sedation:

Oral: 0.6 mg/kg/dose every 6 hours

I.M.: 0.5-1.1 mg/kg/dose every 4-6 hours as needed

Pruritus, anxiety: Manufacturer labeling:

<6 years: 50 mg daily in divided doses

≥6 years: 50-100 mg daily in divided doses

Hepatic Impairment: Change dosing interval to every 24 hours in patients with primary biliary cirrhosis.

Available Dosage Forms [DSC] = Discontinued product

Capsule, as pamoate (Vistaril®): 25 mg, 50 mg, 100 mg

Injection, solution, as hydrochloride: 25 mg/mL (1 mL); 50 mg/mL (1 mL, 2 mL, 10 mL)

Suspension, oral, as pamoate (Vistaril®): 25 mg/5 mL (120 mL, 480 mL) [lemon flavor]

Syrup, as hydrochloride: 10 mg/5 mL (120 mL, 480 mL)

Atarax®: 10 mg/5 mL (480 mL) [contains alcohol, sodium benzoate; mint flavor] [DSC]

Tablet, as hydrochloride: 10 mg, 25 mg, 50 mg

Atarax®: 10 mg, 25 mg, 50 mg, 100 mg [DSC]

Nursing Guidelines

Assessment: Assess other medications patient may be taking for effectiveness and possible interactions. **Systemic:** Monitor therapeutic effectiveness and adverse reactions; ensure patient safety (institute safety precautions), have patient void prior to administration; and ensure adequate hydration and environmental temperature control. **Oral:** Monitor therapeutic effectiveness according to purpose for use and adverse reactions. Assess knowledge/teach patient appropriate use, interventions to reduce side effects, and adverse symptoms to report.

(Continued)

HydrOXYzine *(Continued)*

Patient Education: Will cause drowsiness. While using this medication, do not use alcohol and other prescription or OTC medications (especially sedatives, tranquilizers, antihistamines, or pain medications) without consulting prescriber. Use caution when driving or engaging in activities requiring alertness until response to drug is known. **Pregnancy/breast-feeding precautions:** Inform prescriber if you are or intend to become pregnant. Breast-feeding is contraindicated.

Geriatric Considerations: Anticholinergic effects are not well tolerated in the elderly. Hydroxyzine may be useful as a short-term antipruritic, but it is not recommended for use as a sedative or anxiolytic in the elderly.

Pregnancy Risk Factor: C

Pregnancy Issues: Hydroxyzine-induced fetal abnormalities at high dosages in animal studies. Use in early pregnancy is contraindicated by the manufacturer.

Lactation: Enters breast milk/contraindicated

Administration

I.M.: Do not administer SubQ or intra-arterially. Administer I.M. deep in large muscle.

I.V.: Irritant. Use caution when administering I.V. Not generally recommended. May be given as a short (30-60 minute) infusion.

Reconstitution: For I.V. infusion, diilute in 50-250 mL NS or D_5W.

Compatibility:

Y-site administration: Incompatible with allopurinol, amifostine, amphotericin B cholesteryl sulfate complex, cefepime, doxorubicin liposome, fluconazole, fludarabine, paclitaxel, piperacillin/tazobactam, sargramostim

Compatibility in syringe: Incompatible with dimenhydrinate, haloperidol, ketorolac, pentobarbital, ranitidine

Compatibility when admixed: Incompatible with aminophylline, amobarbital, chloramphenicol, penicillin G potassium, penicillin G sodium, pentobarbital, phenobarbital

Storage: Protect from light. Store at 15°C to 30°C.

- **Hydroxyzine Hydrochloride** *see* HydrOXYzine *on page 884*
- **Hydroxyzine Pamoate** *see* HydrOXYzine *on page 884*
- **HydroZone Plus [OTC]** *see* Hydrocortisone *on page 873*
- **Hygroton** *see* Chlorthalidone *on page 383*
- **Hylaform®** *see* Hyaluronate and Derivatives *on page 856*
- **Hylaform® Plus** *see* Hyaluronate and Derivatives *on page 856*
- **Hylan Polymers** *see* Hyaluronate and Derivatives *on page 856*
- **Hylenex™** *see* Hyaluronidase *on page 858*
- **Hyoscine Butylbromide** *see* Scopolamine *on page 1513*
- **Hyoscine Hydrobromide** *see* Scopolamine *on page 1513*

Hyoscyamine (hye oh SYE a meen)

U.S. Brand Names Anaspaz®; Cystospaz®; Cystospaz-M® [DSC]; Hyosine; Levbid®; Levsin®; Levsinex®; Levsin/SL®; NuLev™; Spacol [DSC]; Spacol T/S [DSC]; Symax SL; Symax SR

Synonyms Hyoscyamine Sulfate; *l*-Hyoscyamine Sulfate

Pharmacologic Category Anticholinergic Agent

Medication Safety Issues

Sound-alike/look-alike issues:

Anaspaz® may be confused with Anaprox®, Antispas®
Levbid® may be confused with Lithobid®, Lopid®, Lorabid®
Levsinex® may be confused with Lanoxin®

Use

Oral: Adjunctive therapy for peptic ulcers, irritable bowel, neurogenic bladder/bowel; treatment of infant colic, GI tract disorders caused by spasm; to reduce rigidity, tremors, sialorrhea, and hyperhidrosis associated with parkinsonism; as a drying agent in acute rhinitis

Injection: Preoperative antimuscarinic to reduce secretions and block cardiac vagal inhibitory reflexes; to improve radiologic visibility of the kidneys; symptomatic relief of biliary and renal colic; reduce GI motility to facilitate diagnostic procedures (ie, endoscopy, hypotonic duodenography); reduce pain and hypersecretion in pancreatitis, certain cases of partial heart block associated with vagal activity; reversal of neuromuscular blockade

Mechanism of Action Blocks the action of acetylcholine at parasympathetic sites in smooth muscle, secretory glands and the CNS; increases cardiac output, dries secretions, antagonizes histamine and serotonin

Pharmacodynamics/Kinetics

Onset of action: 2-3 minutes
Duration: 4-6 hours
Absorption: Well absorbed
Distribution: Crosses placenta; small amounts enter breast milk
Protein binding: 50%
Metabolism: Hepatic
Half-life elimination: 3-5 hours
Excretion: Urine

Contraindications Hypersensitivity to belladonna alkaloids or any component of the formulation; glaucoma; obstructive uropathy; myasthenia gravis; obstructive GI tract disease, paralytic ileus, intestinal atony of elderly or debilitated patients, severe ulcerative colitis, toxic megacolon complicating ulcerative colitis; unstable cardiovascular status in acute hemorrhage, myocardial ischemia

Warnings/Precautions Heat prostration may occur in hot weather. Diarrhea may be a sign of incomplete intestinal obstruction, treatment should be discontinued if this occurs. May produce side effects as seen with other anticholinergic medications including drowsiness, dizziness, blurred vision, or psychosis. Children and the elderly may be more susceptible to these effects. Use with caution in children with spastic paralysis. Use with caution in patients with autonomic neuropathy, coronary heart disease, CHF, cardiac arrhythmias, prostatic hyperplasia, hyperthyroidism, hypertension, chronic lung disease, renal disease, and hiatal hernia associated with reflux esophagitis. Use with caution in the elderly, may precipitate undiagnosed glaucoma and/or severely impair memory function (especially in those patients with previous memory problems).

NuLev™: Contains phenylalanine

Drug Interactions

Amantadine: Additive adverse effects may occur due to cholinergic blockade.
Antacids: Antacids may decrease absorption of hyoscyamine; administer hyoscyamine before meals and give antacids after meals.
Antihistamines: Additive adverse effects may occur with some antihistamines due to cholinergic blockade.
Antimuscarinics: Additive adverse effects may occur due to cholinergic blockade.
Haloperidol: Additive adverse effects may occur due to cholinergic blockade.
MAO inhibitors: Additive adverse effects may occur due to cholinergic blockade.
Phenothiazines: Additive adverse effects may occur due to cholinergic blockade.
Tricyclic antidepressants: Additive adverse effects may occur due to cholinergic blockade.

Adverse Reactions Frequency not defined.

Cardiovascular: Palpitations, tachycardia
Central nervous system: Ataxia, dizziness, drowsiness, headache, insomnia, mental confusion/excitement, nervousness, speech disorder
Dermatologic: Urticaria
Endocrine & metabolic: Lactation suppression
Gastrointestinal: Bloating, constipation, dry mouth, loss of taste, nausea, vomiting
Genitourinary: Impotence, urinary hesitancy, urinary retention
Neuromuscular & skeletal: Weakness
Ocular: Blurred vision, cycloplegia, increased ocular tension, mydriasis
Miscellaneous: Allergic reactions, sweating decreased

Overdosage/Toxicology Symptoms of overdose include dilated, unreactive pupils; blurred vision; hot, dry flushed skin; CNS stimulation; dryness of mucous membranes; difficulty swallowing; foul breath; diminished or absent bowel sounds; urinary retention; tachycardia; hyperthermia; hypertension; and increased respiratory rate. For anticholinergic overdose with severe life-threatening symptoms, physostigmine 0.5-2 mg SubQ or I.V. slowly, may be given to reverse these effects; may repeat as necessary to reverse the effects, up to total of 5 mg. Hyoscyamine sulfate is dialyzable.

Dosing

Adults & Elderly:

Gastrointestinal spasms:

Oral or S.L.: 0.125-0.25 mg every 4 hours or as needed (before meals or food); maximum: 1.5 mg/24 hours

Product-specific dosing: Cystospaz®: 0.15-0.3 mg up to 4 times/day

(Continued)

Hyoscyamine *(Continued)*

Oral, timed release: 0.375-0.75 mg every 12 hours; maximum: 1.5 mg/24 hours

I.M., I.V., SubQ: 0.25-0.5 mg; may repeat as needed up to 4 times/day, at 4-hour intervals

Diagnostic procedures: I.V.: 0.25-0.5 mg given 5-10 minutes prior to procedure

Preanesthesia: I.V.: 5 mcg/kg given 30-60 minutes prior to induction of anesthesia or at the time preoperative narcotics or sedatives are administered

To reduce drug-induced bradycardia during surgery: I.V.: 0.125 mg; repeat as needed

Reverse neuromuscular blockade: I.V.: 0.2 mg for every 1 mg neostigmine (or the physostigmine/pyridostigmine equivalent)

Pediatrics:

Gastrointestinal disorders:

Children <2 years: Oral: Dose as listed, based on age and weight (kg) using the 0.125 mg/mL drops. Repeat dose every 4 hours as needed:

3.4 kg: 4 drops; maximum: 24 drops/24 hours
5 kg: 5 drops; maximum: 30 drops/24 hours
7 kg: 6 drops; maximum: 36 drops/24 hours
10 kg: 8 drops; maximum: 48 drops/24 hours

Children 2-12 years: Oral or S.L.: Dose as listed, based on age and weight (kg); repeat dose every 4 hours as needed:

10 kg: 0.031-0.033 mg; maximum: 0.75 mg/24 hours
20 kg: 0.0625 mg; maximum: 0.75 mg/24 hours
40 kg: 0.0938 mg; maximum: 0.75 mg/24 hours
50 kg: 0.125 mg; maximum: 0.75 mg/24 hours

Preanesthesia: Children >2 years: I.V.: Refer to adult dosing.

Available Dosage Forms [DSC] = Discontinued product

Capsule, timed release, as sulfate (Cystospaz-M® [DSC], Levsinex®): 0.375 mg

Elixir, as sulfate: 0.125 mg/5 mL (480 mL)

Hyosine: 0.125 mg/5 mL (480 mL) [contains alcohol 20% and sodium benzoate; orange flavor]

Levsin®: 0.125 mg/5 mL (480 mL) [contains alcohol 20%; orange flavor]

Injection, solution, as sulfate (Levsin®): 0.5 mg/mL (1 mL)

Liquid, as sulfate (Spacol [DSC]): 0.125 mg/5 mL (120 mL) [sugar free, alcohol free, simethicone based, bubble gum flavor]

Solution, oral drops, as sulfate: 0.125 mg/mL (15 mL)

Hyosine: 0.125 mg/mL (15 mL) [contains alcohol 5% and sodium benzoate; orange flavor]

Levsin®: 0.125 mg/mL (15 mL) [contains alcohol 5%; orange flavor]

Tablet (Cystospaz®): 0.15 mg

Tablet, as sulfate (Anaspaz®, Levsin®, Spacol [DSC]): 0.125 mg

Tablet, extended release, as sulfate (Levbid®, Symax SR, Spacol T/S [DSC]): 0.375 mg

Tablet, orally-disintegrating, as sulfate (NuLev™): 0.125 mg [contains phenylalanine 1.7 mg/tablet, mint flavor]

Tablet, sublingual, as sulfate: 0.125 mg

Levsin/SL®: 0.125 mg [peppermint flavor]

Symax SL: 0.125 mg

Nursing Guidelines

Assessment: Assess potential for interactions with other prescriptions, OTC medications, or herbal products patient may be taking (eg, anything that may add to anticholinergic effects). **I.V./I.M.:** Have patient void before administration. Assess therapeutic effectiveness and adverse response (eg, excessive dryness of eyes, nose, mouth, or throat). Teach patient proper use (according to formulations prescribed), possible side effects/appropriate interventions, and adverse symptoms to report.

Dietary Considerations: Should be taken before meals or food; NuLev™ contains phenylalanine

Patient Education: Do not take any new medication during therapy unless approved by prescriber. Take as directed before meals; do not increase dose and do not discontinue without consulting prescriber. Void immediately before taking medication. Do not crush or chew (swallow whole) extended release form. Levbid® and Levsinex® may not completely disintegrate and may be excreted. You may experience dizziness or blurred vision (use caution when driving or engaging in tasks that require alertness until response to drug is known); dry mouth (sucking on lozenges may help); photosensitivity (wear dark glasses in bright sunlight); decreased ability to sweat (use caution in hot weather or hot rooms or when engaging in strenuous activity); or impotence (temporary). Report excessive and persistent anticholinergic effects (blurred vision, headache, flushing, tachycardia, nervousness, constipation, dizziness, insomnia, mental confusion or excitement, dry mouth, altered taste perception, dysphagia, palpitations, bradycardia, urinary hesitancy or retention, impotence, decreased sweating). **Pregnancy/breast-feeding precautions:** Inform prescriber if you are or intend to become pregnant. Breast-feeding is not recommended.

Sublingual tablets: Place tablet under tongue and allow to dissolve.

Orally-disintegrating tablet: Place tablet on tongue and allow to disintegrate before swallowing. Take with or without food.

Geriatric Considerations: Avoid long-term use. The potential for toxic reactions is higher than the potential benefit, elderly are particularly prone to CNS side effects of anticholinergics (eg, confusion, delirium, hallucinations). Side effects often occur before clinical response is obtained. Generally not recommended because of the side effects.

Pregnancy Risk Factor: C

Lactation: Enters breast milk/not recommended

Breast-Feeding Considerations: Excreted in breast milk in trace amounts. May also suppress lactation. Breast-feeding is not recommended.

Administration

Oral: Oral: Tablets should be administered before meals or food.

Levbid®: Tablets are scored and may be broken in half for dose titration; do not crush or chew.

Levsin/SL®: Tablets may be used sublingually, chewed, or swallowed whole.

NuLev™: Tablet is placed on tongue and allowed to disintegrate before swallowing; may take with or without water.

Symax SL: Tablets may be used sublingually or swallowed whole.

I.M.: May be administered without dilution.

I.V.: Inject over at least 1 minute. May be administered without dilution.

Storage: Store at controlled room temperature. Protect NuLev™ from moisture.

- **Hyoscyamine Sulfate** *see* Hyoscyamine *on page 886*
- **Hyosine** *see* Hyoscyamine *on page 886*
- **Hypaque™-76** *see* Diatrizoate Meglumine and Diatrizoate Sodium *on page 514*
- **Hypaque-Cysto™** *see* Diatrizoate Meglumine *on page 513*
- **Hypaque™ Meglumine** *see* Diatrizoate Meglumine *on page 513*
- **Hyperal** *see* Total Parenteral Nutrition *on page 1650*
- **Hyperalimentation** *see* Total Parenteral Nutrition *on page 1650*
- **HypoTears [OTC]** *see* Artificial Tears *on page 187*
- **HypoTears PF [OTC]** *see* Artificial Tears *on page 187*
- **Hypromellose** *see* Hydroxypropyl Methylcellulose *on page 883*
- **Hytone®** *see* Hydrocortisone *on page 873*
- **Hytrin®** *see* Terazosin *on page 1603*
- **Hyzaar®** *see* Losartan and Hydrochlorothiazide *on page 1069*
- **Iberet® [OTC]** *see* Vitamins (Multiple/Oral) *on page 1720*
- **Iberet®-500 [OTC]** *see* Vitamins (Multiple/Oral) *on page 1720*
- **Ibidomide Hydrochloride** *see* Labetalol *on page 996*
- **Ibu-200 [OTC]** *see* Ibuprofen *on page 889*

Ibuprofen (eye byoo PROE fen)

U.S. Brand Names Advil® [OTC]; Advil® Children's [OTC]; Advil® Infants' [OTC]; Advil® Junior [OTC]; Advil® Migraine [OTC]; ElixSure™ IB [OTC]; Genpril® [OTC]; Ibu-200 [OTC]; I-Prin [OTC]; Menadol® [OTC] [DSC]; Midol® Cramp and Body Aches [OTC]; Motrin®; Motrin® Children's [OTC]; Motrin® IB [OTC]; Motrin® Infants' [OTC]; Motrin® Junior Strength [OTC]; Proprinal [OTC]; Ultraprin [OTC]

Synonyms *p*-Isobutylhydratropic Acid

Pharmacologic Category Nonsteroidal Anti-inflammatory Drug (NSAID), Oral

Medication Safety Issues

Sound-alike/look-alike issues:

Haltran® may be confused with Halfprin®

Use Inflammatory diseases and rheumatoid disorders including juvenile rheumatoid arthritis, mild to moderate pain, fever, dysmenorrhea

(Continued)

Ibuprofen *(Continued)*

Unlabeled/Investigational Use Cystic fibrosis, gout, ankylosing spondylitis, acute migraine headache

Mechanism of Action Inhibits prostaglandin synthesis by decreasing the activity of the enzyme, cyclooxygenase, which results in decreased formation of prostaglandin precursors

Pharmacodynamics/Kinetics

Onset of action: Analgesic: 30-60 minutes; Anti-inflammatory: ≤7 days

Peak effect: 1-2 weeks

Duration: 4-6 hours

Absorption: Oral: Rapid (85%)

Protein binding: 90% to 99%

Metabolism: Hepatic via oxidation

Half-life elimination: 2-4 hours; End-stage renal disease: Unchanged

Time to peak: ~1-2 hours

Excretion: Urine (1% as free drug); some feces

Contraindications Hypersensitivity to ibuprofen, aspirin, other NSAIDs, or any component of the formulation; perioperative pain in the setting of coronary artery bypass surgery (CABG); pregnancy (3rd trimester)

Warnings/Precautions NSAIDs are associated with an increased risk of adverse cardiovascular events, including MI, stroke, and new onset or worsening of pre-existing hypertension. Risk may be increased with duration of use or pre-existing cardiovascular risk-factors or disease. Carefully evaluate individual cardiovascular risk profiles prior to prescribing. Use caution with fluid retention, CHF or hypertension.

Use of NSAIDs can compromise existing renal function. Renal toxicity can occur in patient with impaired renal function, dehydration, heart failure, liver dysfunction, those taking diuretics and ACEI and the elderly. Rehydrate patient before starting therapy. Monitor renal function closely. Ibuprofen is not recommended for patients with advanced renal disease.

NSAIDs may increase risk of gastrointestinal irritation, ulceration, bleeding, and perforation. These events may occur at any time during therapy and without warning. Use caution with a history of GI disease (bleeding or ulcers), concurrent therapy with aspirin, anticoagulants and/or corticosteroids, smoking, use of alcohol, the elderly or debilitated patients.

Use the lowest effective dose for the shortest duration of time, consistent with individual patient goals, to reduce risk of cardiovascular or GI adverse events. Alternate therapies should be considered for patients at high risk.

NSAIDs may cause serious skin adverse events including exfoliative dermatitis, Stevens-Johnson syndrome (SJS) and toxic epidermal necrolysis (TEN). Anaphylactoid reactions may occur, even without prior exposure; patients with "aspirin triad" (bronchial asthma, aspirin intolerance, rhinitis) may be at increased risk. Do not use in patients who experience bronchospasm, asthma, rhinitis, or urticaria with NSAID or aspirin therapy.

Use with caution in patients with decreased hepatic function. Closely monitor patients with any abnormal LFT. Severe hepatic reactions (eg, fulminant hepatitis, liver failure) have occurred with NSAID use, rarely; discontinue if signs or symptoms of liver disease develop, or if systemic manifestations occur.

The elderly are at increased risk for adverse effects (especially peptic ulceration, CNS effects, renal toxicity) from NSAIDs even at low doses.

Withhold for at least 4-6 half-lives prior to surgical or dental procedures.

OTC labeling: Prior to self-medication, patients should contact health care provider if they have had recurring stomach pain or upset, ulcers, bleeding problems, high blood pressure, heart or kidney disease, other serious medical problems, are currently taking a diuretic, or are ≥60 years of age. Recommended dosages should not be exceeded, due to an increased risk of GI bleeding. Consuming ≥3 alcoholic beverages/day or taking longer than recommended may increase the risk of GI bleeding. When used for self-medication, patients should contact healthcare provider if used for fever lasting >3 days or for pain lasting >10 days in adults or >3 days in children. In children with a sore throat, do not use for >2 days or administer to children <3 years of age unless instructed by healthcare provider. Consult healthcare provider when sore throat pain is severe, persistent, or accompanied by fever, headache, nausea, and/or vomiting.

Drug Interactions **Substrate** (minor) of CYP2C8/9, 2C19; **Inhibits** CYP2C8/9 (strong)

ACE inhibitors: Antihypertensive effects may be decreased by concurrent therapy with NSAIDs; monitor blood pressure.

Angiotensin II antagonists: Antihypertensive effects may be decreased by concurrent therapy with NSAIDs; monitor blood pressure.

Anticoagulants (warfarin, heparin, LMWHs) in combination with NSAIDs can cause increased risk of bleeding.

Antiplatelet drugs (ticlopidine, clopidogrel, aspirin, abciximab, dipyridamole, eptifibatide, tirofiban) can cause an increased risk of bleeding.

Aspirin: Ibuprofen and other COX-1 inhibitors may reduce the cardioprotective effects of aspirin. Avoid giving prior to aspirin therapy or on a regular basis in patients with CAD.

Corticosteroids: May increase the risk of GI ulceration; avoid concurrent use

Cyclosporine: NSAIDs may increase serum creatinine, potassium, blood pressure, and cyclosporine levels; monitor cyclosporine levels and renal function carefully.

CYP2C8/9 substrates: Ibuprofen may increase the levels/effects of CYP2C8/9 substrates. Example substrates include amiodarone, fluoxetine, glimepiride, glipizide, nateglinide, phenytoin, pioglitazone, rosiglitazone, sertraline, and warfarin.

Hydralazine's antihypertensive effect is decreased; avoid concurrent use

Lithium levels can be increased; avoid concurrent use if possible or monitor lithium levels and adjust dose. Sulindac may have the least effect. When NSAID is stopped, lithium will need adjustment again.

Loop diuretics efficacy (diuretic and antihypertensive effect) is reduced. Indomethacin reduces this efficacy, however, it may be anticipated with any NSAID.

Methotrexate: Severe bone marrow suppression, aplastic anemia, and GI toxicity have been reported with concomitant NSAID therapy. Avoid use during moderate or high-dose methotrexate (increased and prolonged methotrexate levels). NSAID use during low-dose treatment of rheumatoid arthritis has not been fully evaluated; extreme caution is warranted.

Warfarin's INRs may be increased by piroxicam. Other NSAIDs may have the same effect depending on dose and duration. Monitor INR closely. Use the lowest dose of NSAIDs possible and for the briefest duration. May alter the anticoagulant effects of warfarin; concurrent use with other antiplatelet agents or anticoagulants may increase risk of bleeding.

Nutritional/Herbal/Ethanol Interactions

Ethanol: Avoid ethanol (may enhance gastric mucosal irritation).

Food: Ibuprofen peak serum levels may be decreased if taken with food.

Herb/Nutraceutical: Avoid alfalfa, anise, bilberry, bladderwrack, bromelain, cat's claw, celery, coleus, cordyceps, dong quai, evening primrose, feverfew, fenugreek, garlic, ginger, ginkgo biloba, red clover, horse chestnut, grapeseed, green tea, ginseng, guggul, horse chestnut seed, horseradish, licorice, prickly ash, red clover, reishi, SAMe, sweet clover, turmeric, white willow (all have additional antiplatelet activity).

Lab Interactions Increased chloride (S), sodium (S), bleeding time

Adverse Reactions

1% to 10%:

Cardiovascular: Edema (1% to 3%)

Central nervous system: Dizziness (3% to 9%), headache (1% to 3%), nervousness (1% to 3%)

Dermatologic: Itching (1% to 3%), rash (3% to 9%)

Endocrine & metabolic: Fluid retention (1% to 3%)

Gastrointestinal: Dyspepsia (1% to 3%), vomiting (1% to 3%), abdominal pain/cramps/distress (1% to 3%), heartburn (3% to 9%), nausea (3% to 9%), diarrhea (1% to 3%), constipation (1% to 3%), flatulence (1% to 3%), epigastric pain (3% to 9%), appetite decreased (1% to 3%)

Otic: Tinnitus (3% to 9%)

<1% (Limited to important or life-threatening): Acute renal failure, agranulocytosis, anaphylaxis, aplastic anemia, azotemia, blurred vision, bone marrow suppression, confusion, creatinine clearance decreased, duodenal ulcer, edema, eosinophilia, epistaxis, erythema multiforme, gastric ulcer, GI bleed, GI hemorrhage, GI ulceration, hallucinations, hearing decreased, hematuria, hematocrit decreased, hemoglobin decreased, hemolytic anemia, hepatitis, hypertension, inhibition of platelet aggregation, jaundice, liver function tests abnormal, leukopenia, melena, neutropenia, pancreatitis, photosensitivity,

(Continued)

Ibuprofen *(Continued)*

Stevens-Johnson syndrome, thrombocytopenia, toxic amblyopia, toxic epidermal necrolysis, urticaria, vesiculobullous eruptions, vision changes

Overdosage/Toxicology Symptoms of overdose include apnea, metabolic acidosis, coma, nystagmus, seizures, leukocytosis, and renal failure. Management of NSAID intoxication is supportive and symptomatic. Since many NSAIDs undergo enterohepatic cycling, multiple doses of charcoal may be needed to reduce the potential for delayed toxicities.

Dosing

Adults & Elderly:

Inflammatory disease: Oral: 400-800 mg/dose 3-4 times/day (maximum: 3.2 g/day)

Analgesia/pain/fever/dysmenorrhea: Oral: 200-400 mg/dose every 4-6 hours (maximum daily dose: 1.2 g, unless directed by physician)

OTC labeling (analgesic, antipyretic): Oral: 200 mg every 4-6 hours as needed (maximum: 1200 mg/24 hours)

Pediatrics:

Antipyretic: Oral: 6 months to 12 years: Temperature <102.5°F (39°C): 5 mg/kg/dose; temperature >102.5°F: 10 mg/kg/dose given every 6-8 hours; maximum daily dose: 40 mg/kg/day

Juvenile rheumatoid arthritis: Oral: 30-50 mg/kg/24 hours divided every 8 hours; start at lower end of dosing range and titrate upward (maximum: 2.4 g/day)

Analgesic: Oral: 4-10 mg/kg/dose every 6-8 hours

Cystic fibrosis (unlabeled use): Oral: Chronic (>4 years) twice daily dosing adjusted to maintain serum levels of 50-100 mcg/mL has been associated with slowing of disease progression in younger patients with mild lung disease

OTC labeling (analgesic, antipyretic): Oral:

Children 6 months to 11 years: See table; use of weight to select dose is preferred; doses may be repeated every 6-8 hours (maximum: 4 doses/day)

Children ≥12 years: Refer to adult dosing.

Ibuprofen Dosing

Weight (lb)	Age	Dosage (mg)
12-17	6-11 mo	50
18-23	12-23 mo	75
24-35	2-3 y	100
35-47	4-5 y	150
48-59	6-8 y	200
60-71	9-10 y	250
72-95	11 y	300

Hepatic Impairment: Avoid use in severe hepatic impairment.

Available Dosage Forms [DSC] = Discontinued product

Caplet: 200 mg [OTC]
- Advil®: 200 mg [contains sodium benzoate]
- Ibu-200, Motrin® IB: 200 mg
- Motrin® Junior Strength: 100 mg

Capsule, liqui-gel:
- Advil®: 200 mg
- Advil® Migraine: 200 mg [solubilized ibuprofen; contains potassium 20 mg]

Gelcap:
- Advil®: 200 mg [contains coconut oil]
- Motrin® IB: 200 mg [contains benzyl alcohol] [DSC]

Suspension, oral: 100 mg/5 mL (5 mL, 120 mL, 480 mL)
- Advil® Children's: 100 mg/5 mL (60 mL, 120 mL) [contains sodium benzoate; blue raspberry, fruit, and grape flavors]
- ElixSure™ IB: 100 mg/5 mL (120 mL) [berry flavor]
- Motrin® Children's: 100 mg/5 mL (60 mL, 120 mL) [contains sodium benzoate; berry, dye free berry, bubble gum, and grape flavors]

Suspension, oral drops: 40 mg/mL (15 mL)

Advil® Infants': 40 mg/mL (15 mL) [contains sodium benzoate; fruit and grape flavors]

Motrin® Infants': 40 mg/mL (15 mL, 30 mL) [contains sodium benzoate; berry and dye-free berry flavors]

Tablet: 200 mg [OTC], 400 mg, 600 mg, 800 mg

Advil®: 200 mg [contains sodium benzoate]

Advil® Junior: 100 mg [contains sodium benzoate; coated tablets]

Genpril®, I-Prin, Midol® Cramp and Body Aches, Motrin® IB, Proprinal, Ultraprin: 200 mg

Motrin®: 400 mg, 600 mg, 800 mg

Tablet, chewable:

Advil® Children's: 50 mg [contains phenylalanine 2.1 mg; grape flavors]

Advil® Junior: 100 mg [contains phenylalanine 4.2 mg; grape flavors]

Motrin® Children's: 50 mg [contains phenylalanine 1.4 mg; grape and orange flavor]

Motrin® Junior Strength: 100 mg [contains phenylalanine 2.1 mg; grape and orange flavors]

Nursing Guidelines

Assessment: Evaluate cardiac risk and potential for GI bleeding prior to prescribing this medication. Assess patient for allergic reaction to salicylates or other NSAIDs. Assess other medications patient may be taking for additive or adverse interactions. Monitor blood pressure at the beginning of therapy and periodically during use. Monitor therapeutic effectiveness and signs of adverse reactions or overdose at beginning of therapy and periodically during long-term therapy. With long-term therapy, periodic ophthalmic exams are recommended. Assess knowledge/teach patient appropriate use. Teach patient to monitor for adverse reactions, adverse reactions to report, and appropriate interventions to reduce side effects.

Monitoring Laboratory Tests: CBC, periodic liver function, renal function (serum BUN and creatinine)

Dietary Considerations: Should be taken with food. Chewable tablets may contain phenylalanine; amount varies by product, consult manufacturers labeling.

Patient Education: If self-administered, use exactly as directed; do not increase dose or frequency. Adverse reactions can occur with overuse. Consult your prescriber before use if you have hypertension or heart failure. Do not take longer than 3 days for fever, or 10 days for pain without consulting medical advisor. Take with food or milk. While using this medication, do not use alcohol, excessive amounts of vitamin C, or salicylate-containing foods (curry powder, prunes, raisins, tea, or licorice), other prescription or OTC medications containing aspirin or salicylate, or other NSAIDs without consulting prescriber. Maintain adequate hydration (2-3 L/day of fluids) unless instructed to restrict fluid intake. You may experience nausea, vomiting, gastric discomfort (frequent mouth care, small frequent meals, chewing gum, sucking lozenges may help). GI bleeding, ulceration, or perforation can occur with or without pain. Stop taking medication and report ringing in ears; persistent cramping or stomach pain; unresolved nausea or vomiting; respiratory difficulty or shortness of breath; unusual bruising or bleeding (mouth, urine, stool); skin rash; unusual swelling of extremities; chest pain; or palpitations. **Pregnancy/breast-feeding precautions:** Inform prescriber if you are or intend to become pregnant. This drug should not be used in the 3rd trimester of pregnancy. Consult prescriber if breast-feeding.

Geriatric Considerations: Elderly are at a high risk for adverse effects from NSAIDs. As much as 60% of elderly can develop peptic ulceration and/or hemorrhage asymptomatically. The concomitant use of H_2 blockers, omeprazole, and sucralfate is not effective as prophylaxis with the exception of NSAID-induced duodenal ulcers which may be prevented by the use of ranitidine. Misoprostol is the only prophylactic agent proven effective. Also, concomitant disease and drug use contribute to the risk for GI adverse effects. Use lowest effective dose for shortest period possible. Consider renal function decline with age. Use of NSAIDs can compromise existing renal function especially when Cl_{cr} is $\leq$30 mL/minute. Tinnitus may be a difficult and unreliable indication of toxicity due to age-related hearing loss or eighth cranial nerve damage. CNS adverse effects such as confusion, agitation, and hallucination are generally seen in overdose or high-dose situations, but elderly may demonstrate these adverse effects at lower doses than younger adults.

(Continued)

Ibuprofen *(Continued)*

Pregnancy Risk Factor: C/D (3rd trimester)

Lactation: Enters breast milk/use caution (AAP rates "compatible")

Breast-Feeding Considerations: Limited data suggests minimal excretion in breast milk.

Perioperative/Anesthesia/Other Concerns: The 2002 ACCM/SCCM guidelines for analgesia (critically-ill adult) suggest that NSAIDs may be used in combination with opioids in select patients for pain management. Concern about adverse events (increased risk of renal dysfunction, altered platelet function and gastrointestinal irritation) limits its use in patients who have other underlying risks for these events.

In short-term use, NSAIDs vary considerably in their effect on blood pressure. When NSAIDs are used in patients with hypertension, appropriate monitoring of blood pressure responses should be completed and the duration of therapy, when possible, kept short. The use of NSAIDs in the treatment of patients with congestive heart failure may be associated with an increased risk for fluid accumulation and edema. May precipitate renal failure in dehydrated patients.

Administration

Oral: Administer with food.

Related Information

Acute Postoperative Pain *on page 1742*

- IC-Green® *see* Indocyanine Green *on page 905*
- ICI-204,219 *see* Zafirlukast *on page 1730*
- ICI-118630 *see* Goserelin *on page 829*
- ICI-D1033 *see* Anastrozole *on page 168*
- IDEC-C2B8 *see* Rituximab *on page 1484*
- IFLrA *see* Interferon Alfa-2a *on page 933*
- IG *see* Immune Globulin (Intramuscular) *on page 898*
- IGIM *see* Immune Globulin (Intramuscular) *on page 898*
- Imdur® *see* Isosorbide Mononitrate *on page 979*
- Imipemide *see* Imipenem and Cilastatin *on page 894*

Imipenem and Cilastatin (i mi PEN em & sye la STAT in)

U.S. Brand Names Primaxin®

Synonyms Imipemide

Pharmacologic Category Antibiotic, Carbapenem

Medication Safety Issues

Sound-alike/look-alike issues:

Primaxin® may be confused with Premarin®, Primacor®

Use Treatment of respiratory tract, urinary tract, intra-abdominal, gynecologic, bone and joint, skin structure, and polymicrobic infections as well as bacterial septicemia and endocarditis. Antibacterial activity includes resistant gram-negative bacilli (*Pseudomonas aeruginosa* and *Enterobacter* sp), gram-positive bacteria (methicillin-sensitive *Staphylococcus aureus* and *Streptococcus* sp) and anaerobes.

Note: I.M. administration is not intended for severe or life-threatening infections (eg, septicemia, endocarditis, shock)

Mechanism of Action Inhibits bacterial cell wall synthesis by binding to one or more of the penicillin binding proteins (PBPs); which in turn inhibits the final transpeptidation step of peptidoglycan synthesis in bacterial cell walls, thus inhibiting cell wall biosynthesis. Bacteria eventually lyse due to ongoing activity of cell wall autolytic enzymes (autolysins and murein hydrolases) while cell wall assembly is arrested. Cilastatin prevents renal metabolism of imipenem by competitive inhibition of dehydropeptidase along the brush border of the renal tubules.

Pharmacodynamics/Kinetics

Absorption: I.M.: Imipenem: 60% to 75%; cilastatin: 95% to 100%

Distribution: Rapidly and widely to most tissues and fluids including sputum, pleural fluid, peritoneal fluid, interstitial fluid, bile, aqueous humor, reproductive organs, and bone; highest concentrations in pleural fluid, interstitial fluid, peritoneal fluid, and reproductive organs; low concentrations in CSF; crosses placenta; enters breast milk

Metabolism: Renally by dehydropeptidase; activity is blocked by cilastatin; cilastatin is partially metabolized renally

Half-life elimination: Both drugs: 60 minutes; prolonged with renal impairment

Excretion: Both drugs: Urine (~70% as unchanged drug)

Contraindications Hypersensitivity to imipenem/cilastatin or any component of the formulation; consult information on Lidocaine for contraindications associated with I.M. dosing

Warnings/Precautions Dosage adjustment required in patients with impaired renal function; prolonged use may result in superinfection; has been associated with CNS adverse effects, including confusional states and seizures; use with caution in patients with a history of seizures or hypersensitivity to beta-lactams (including penicillins and cephalosporins); serious hypersensitivity reactions, including anaphylaxis, have been reported (some without a history of previous allergic reactions to beta-lactams); elderly patients often require lower doses (adjust carefully to renal function); not recommended in pediatric CNS infections. Doses for I.M. administration are mixed with lidocaine, consult information on lidocaine for associated warnings/precautions. Two different imipenem/cilastin products are available; due to differences in formulation, the I.V. and I.M. preparations **cannot** be interchanged.

Drug Interactions Valproic acid: Imipenem may decrease valproic acid concentrations to subtherapeutic levels; monitor.

Lab Interactions Interferes with urinary glucose determination using Clinitest®

Adverse Reactions

1% to 10%:

Gastrointestinal: Nausea/diarrhea/vomiting (1% to 2%)

Local: Phlebitis (3%), pain at I.M. injection site (1%)

<1% (Limited to important or life-threatening): Anaphylaxis, angioneurotic edema, confusion (acute), drug fever, dyspnea, emergence of resistant strains of *P. aeruginosa*, encephalopathy, eosinophilia, erythema multiforme, hallucinations, hemolytic anemia, hemorrhagic colitis, hepatitis, hypersensitivity, hypotension, increased PT, jaundice, leukopenia, neutropenia (including agranulocytosis), pancytopenia, paresthesia, positive Coombs' test, pruritus, pseudomembranous colitis, psychic disturbances, rash, renal failure (acute), seizure, somnolence, Stevens-Johnson syndrome, thrombocytopenia, toxic epidermal necrolysis, urticaria, vertigo

Overdosage/Toxicology Symptoms of overdose include neuromuscular hypersensitivity and seizures. Hemodialysis may be helpful to aid in removal of the drug from blood; otherwise, treatment is supportive or symptom-directed.

Dosing

Adults & Elderly: Dosage based on **imipenem** content: **Note:** For adults weighing <70 kg, refer to Dosing Adjustment in Renal Impairment:

Moderate infections:

I.M.: 750 mg every 12 hours

I.V.:

Fully-susceptible organisms: 500 mg every 6-8 hours (1.5-2 g/day)

Moderately-susceptible organisms: 500 mg every 6 hours or 1 g every 8 hours (2-3 g/day)

Severe infections: I.V.: **Note:** I.M. administration is not intended for severe or life-threatening infections (eg, septicemia, endocarditis, shock):

Fully-susceptible organisms: 500 mg every 6 hours (2 g/day)

Moderately-susceptible organisms: 1 g every 6-8 hours (3-4 g/day)

Maximum daily dose should not exceed 50 mg/kg or 4 g/day, whichever is lower

Urinary tract infection, uncomplicated: I.V.: 250 mg every 6 hours (1 g/day)

Urinary tract infection, complicated: I.V.: 500 mg every 6 hours (2 g/day)

Mild infections: Note: Rarely a suitable option in mild infections; normally reserved for moderate-severe cases:

I.M.: 500 mg every 12 hours; intra-abdominal infections: 750 mg every 12 hours

I.V.:

Fully-susceptible organisms: 250 mg every 6 hours (1g/day)

Moderately-susceptible organisms: 500 mg every 6 hours (2 g/day)

Pediatrics: Dosage based on **imipenem** content:

Non-CNS infections: I.V.:

Neonates:

<1 week: 25 mg/kg every 12 hours

1-4 weeks: 25 mg/kg every 8 hours

4 weeks to 3 months: 25 mg/kg every 6 hours

Children: >3 months: 15-25 mg/kg every 6 hours

(Continued)

Imipenem and Cilastatin *(Continued)*

Maximum dosage: Susceptible infections: 2 g/day; moderately susceptible organisms: 4 g/day

Cystic fibrosis: I.V.: Children: Doses up to 90 mg/kg/day have been used

Renal Impairment: I.V.: **Note:** Adjustments have not been established for I.M. dosing:

Patients with a Cl_{cr} <5 mL/minute/1.73 m^2 should not receive imipenem/cilastatin unless hemodialysis is instituted within 48 hours.

Patients weighing <30 kg with impaired renal function should not receive imipenem/cilastatin.

Hemodialysis: Use the dosing recommendation for patients with a Cl_{cr} 6-20 mL/minute.

Peritoneal dialysis: Dose as for Cl_{cr} <10 mL/minute.

Continuous arteriovenous or venovenous hemofiltration: Dose as for Cl_{cr} 20-30 mL/minute; monitor for seizure activity. Imipenem is well removed by CAVH but cilastatin is not; removes 20 mg of imipenem per liter of filtrate per day. See table.

Imipenem and Cilastatin Dosage in Renal Impairment

Reduced I.V. Dosage Regimen Based on Creatinine Clearance (mL/minute/1.73 m^2) and/or Body Weight <70 kg					
	Body Weight (kg)				
	≥70	60	50	40	30
Total daily dose for normal renal function: 1 g/day					
Cl_{cr} ≥71	250 mg q6h	250 mg q8h	125 mg q6h	125 mg q6h	125 mg q8h
Cl_{cr} 41-70	250 mg q8h	125 mg q6h	125 mg q6h	125 mg q8h	125 mg q8h
Cl_{cr} 21-40	250 mg q12h	250 mg q12h	125 mg q8h	125 mg q12h	125 mg q12h
Cl_{cr} 6-20	250 mg q12h	125 mg q12h	125 mg q12h	125 mg q12h	125 mg q12h
Total daily dose for normal renal function: 1.5 g/day					
Cl_{cr} ≥71	500 mg q8h	250 mg q6h	250 mg q6h	250 mg q8h	125 mg q6h
Cl_{cr} 41-70	250 mg q6h	250 mg q8h	250 mg q8h	125 mg q6h	125 mg q8h
Cl_{cr} 21-40	250 mg q8h	250 mg q8h	250 mg q12h	125 mg q8h	125 mg q8h
Cl_{cr} 6-20	250 mg q12h	250 mg q12h	250 mg q12h	125 mg q12h	125 mg q12h
Total daily dose for normal renal function: 2 g/day					
Cl_{cr} ≥71	500 mg q6h	500 mg q8h	250 mg q6h	250 mg q6h	250 mg q8h
Cl_{cr} 41-70	500 mg q8h	250 mg q6h	250 mg q6h	250 mg q8h	125 mg q6h
Cl_{cr} 21-40	250 mg q6h	250 mg q8h	250 mg q8h	250 mg q12h	125 mg q8h
Cl_{cr} 6-20	250 mg q12h	250 mg q12h	250 mg q12h	250 mg q12h	125 mg q12h
Total daily dose for normal renal function: 3 g/day					
Cl_{cr} ≥71	1000 mg q8h	750 mg q8h	500 mg q6h	500 mg q8h	250 mg q6h
Cl_{cr} 41-70	500 mg q6h	500 mg q8h	500 mg q8h	250 mg q6h	250 mg q8h
Cl_{cr} 21-40	500 mg q8h	500 mg q8h	250 mg q6h	250 mg q8h	250 mg q8h
Cl_{cr} 6-20	500 mg q12h	500 mg q12h	250 mg q12h	250 mg q12h	250 mg q12h
Total daily dose for normal renal function: 4 g/day					
Cl_{cr} ≥71	1000 mg q6h	1000 mg q8h	750 mg q8h	500 mg q6h	500 mg q8h
Cl_{cr} 41-70	750 mg q8h	750 mg q8h	500 mg q6h	500 mg q8h	250 mg q6h
Cl_{cr} 21-40	500 mg q6h	500 mg q8h	500 mg q8h	250 mg q6h	250 mg q8h
Cl_{cr} 6-20	500 mg q12h	500 mg q12h	500 mg q12h	250 mg q12h	250 mg q12h

Available Dosage Forms

Injection, powder for reconstitution [I.M.]: Imipenem 500 mg and cilastatin 500 mg [contains sodium 32 mg (1.4 mEq)]

Injection, powder for reconstitution [I.V.]: Imipenem 250 mg and cilastatin 250 mg [contains sodium 18.8 mg (0.8 mEq)]; imipenem 500 mg and cilastatin 500 mg [contains sodium 37.5 mg (1.6 mEq)]

Nursing Guidelines

Assessment: See Contraindications, Warnings/Precautions, and Dosing for use cautions. See Administration and Reconstitution. Patient should be monitored for renal, hepatic, hematologic and CNS status. Assess results of laboratory tests (see below), therapeutic effectiveness, and adverse response (see Adverse Reactions and Overdose/Toxicology) periodically during therapy. Advise patients with diabetes about use of Clinitest®. Teach patient possible side effects/appropriate interventions and adverse symptoms to report (see Patient Education). Note breast-feeding caution.

Monitoring Laboratory Tests: Perform culture and sensitivity studies prior to initiating therapy. Periodically monitor renal, hepatic, and hematologic function.

Dietary Considerations: Sodium content of 500 mg injection:

I.M.: 32 mg (1.4 mEq)

I.V.: 37.5 mg (1.6 mEq)

Patient Education: Inform prescriber of all prescriptions, OTC medications, or herbal products you are taking, and any allergies you have. Do not take any new medication during therapy unless approved by prescriber. This medication can only be administered by injection or infusion. Report immediately any warmth, swelling, pain, or redness at infusion or injection site. Maintain adequate hydration (2-3 L/day of fluids) unless instructed to restrict fluid intake, and nutrition (small, frequent meals). May cause false test results with Clinitest®; use of another type of glucose testing is preferable. Report immediately any CNS changes (dizziness, hallucinations, anxiety, visual disturbances); swelling of throat, tongue, lips, or face; chills or fever; or unusual discharge or foul-smelling urine. **Pregnancy/breast-feeding precautions:** Inform prescriber if you are or intend to become pregnant. Consult prescriber if breast-feeding.

Geriatric Considerations: Many of the seizures attributed to imipenem/cilastatin were in elderly patients. Dose must be carefully adjusted for creatinine clearance.

Pregnancy Risk Factor: C

Lactation: Enters breast milk (small amounts)/use caution

Administration

I.M.:

I.M.: Administer by deep injection into a large muscle (gluteal or lateral thigh). Aspiration is necessary to avoid inadvertent injection into a blood vessel. **Only the I.M. formulation can be used for I.M. administration.**

I.V.:

I.V.: Do not administer I.V. push. Infuse doses ≤500 mg over 20-30 minutes; infuse doses ≥750 mg over 40-60 minutes. **Only the I.V. formulation can be used for I.V. administration.**

Reconstitution:

I.M.: Prepare 500 mg vial with 2 mL 1% lidocaine (do not use lidocaine with epinephrine). The I.V. formulation does not form a stable suspension in lidocaine and cannot be used to prepare an I.M dose.

I.V.: Prior to use, dilute dose into 100 mL of an appropriate solution. Imipenem is inactivated at acidic or alkaline pH. Final concentration should not exceed 5 mg/mL. The I.M. formulation is not buffered and cannot be used to prepare I.V. solutions.

Compatibility: Y-site administration: Incompatible with allopurinol, amphotericin B cholesteryl sulfate complex, etoposide phosphate, fluconazole, gemcitabine, lorazepam, meperidine, midazolam, sargramostim, sodium bicarbonate

Storage:

Imipenem/cilastatin powder for injection should be stored at <25°C (77°F).

I.M.: The I.M. suspension should be used within 1 hour of reconstitution.

I.V.: Reconstituted I.V. solutions are stable for 4 hours at room temperature and 24 hours when refrigerated.

♦ **Imitrex®** *see* Sumatriptan *on page 1589*

Immune Globulin (Intramuscular)

(i MYUN GLOB yoo lin, IN tra MUS kyoo ler)

U.S. Brand Names BayGam®

Synonyms Gamma Globulin; IG; IGIM; Immune Serum Globulin; ISG

Pharmacologic Category Immune Globulin

Use Household and sexual contacts of persons with hepatitis A, measles, varicella, and possibly rubella; travelers to high-risk areas outside tourist routes; staff, attendees, and parents of diapered attendees in day-care center outbreaks

For travelers, IG is not an alternative to careful selection of foods and water; immune globulin can interfere with the antibody response to parenterally administered live virus vaccines. Frequent travelers should be tested for hepatitis A antibody, immune hemolytic anemia, and neutropenia (with ITP, I.V. route is usually used).

Mechanism of Action Provides passive immunity by increasing the antibody titer and antigen-antibody reaction potential

Pharmacodynamics/Kinetics

Duration: Immune effect: Usually 3-4 weeks

Half-life elimination: 23 days

Time to peak, serum: I.M.: ~24-48 hours

Contraindications Hypersensitivity to immune globulin, thimerosal, or any component of the formulation; IgA deficiency; I.M. injections in patients with thrombocytopenia or coagulation disorders

Warnings/Precautions Skin testing should not be performed as local irritation can occur and be misinterpreted as a positive reaction; IG should **not** be used to control outbreaks of measles. As a product of human plasma, this product may potentially transmit disease; screening of donors, as well as testing and/or inactivation of certain viruses reduces this risk. Epidemiologic and laboratory data indicate current IMIG products do not have a discernible risk of transmitting HIV. Use caution in patients with thrombocytopenia or coagulation disorders (I.M. injections may be contraindicated). Not for I.V. administration.

Drug Interactions Increased toxicity: Live virus, vaccines (measles, mumps, rubella); do not administer within 3 months after administration of these vaccines

Lab Interactions Skin tests should **not** be done

Adverse Reactions Frequency not defined.

Cardiovascular: Flushing, angioedema

Central nervous system: Chills, lethargy, fever

Dermatologic: Urticaria, erythema

Gastrointestinal: Nausea, vomiting

Local: Pain, tenderness, muscle stiffness at I.M. site

Neuromuscular & skeletal: Myalgia

Miscellaneous: Hypersensitivity reactions

Dosing

Adults & Elderly:

Hepatitis A:

Pre-exposure prophylaxis upon travel into endemic areas (hepatitis A vaccine preferred): I.M.:

0.02 mL/kg for anticipated risk 1-3 months

0.06 mL/kg for anticipated risk >3 months

Repeat approximate dose every 4-6 months if exposure continues

Postexposure prophylaxis: I.M.: 0.02 mL/kg given within 7 days of exposure

Measles:

Prophylaxis: I.M.: 0.25 mL/kg/dose (maximum dose: 15 mL) given within 6 days of exposure followed by live attenuated measles vaccine in 3 months or at 15 months of age (whichever is later)

For patients with leukemia, lymphoma, immunodeficiency disorders, generalized malignancy, or receiving immunosuppressive therapy: I.M.: 0.5 mL/kg (maximum dose: 15 mL)

Hepatitis B (Prophylaxis): I.M.: 0.06 mL/kg/dose (HBIG preferred)

IgG deficiency: I.M.: 1.3 mL/kg, then 0.66 mL/kg in 3-4 weeks

Poliomyelitis (Prophylaxis): I.M.: 0.3 mL/kg/dose as a single dose

Rubella (Prophylaxis): I.M.: 0.55 mL/kg/dose within 72 hours of exposure

Varicella (Prophylaxis): I.M.: 0.6-1.2 mL/kg (varicella zoster immune globulin preferred) within 72 hours of exposure

Available Dosage Forms Injection, solution [preservative free]: 15% to 18% (2 mL, 10 mL)

Nursing Guidelines

Pregnancy Risk Factor: C

Immune Globulin (Intravenous)

(i MYUN GLOB yoo lin, IN tra VEE nus)

U.S. Brand Names Carimune™ NF; Gammagard® Liquid; Gammagard® S/D; Gammar®-P I.V.; Gamunex®; Iveegam EN; Octagam®; Panglobulin® NF; Polygam® S/D

Synonyms IVIG

Pharmacologic Category Immune Globulin

Medication Safety Issues

Sound-alike/look-alike issues:

Gamimune® N may be confused with CytoGam®

Use

Treatment of primary immunodeficiency syndromes (congenital agammaglobulinemia, severe combined immunodeficiency syndromes [SCIDS], common variable immunodeficiency, X-linked immunodeficiency, Wiskott-Aldrich syndrome); idiopathic thrombocytopenic purpura (ITP); Kawasaki disease (in combination with aspirin)

Prevention of bacterial infection in B-cell chronic lymphocytic leukemia (CLL); pediatric HIV infection; bone marrow transplant (BMT)

Unlabeled/Investigational Use Autoimmune diseases (myasthenia gravis, SLE, bullous pemphigoid, severe rheumatoid arthritis), Guillain-Barré syndrome; used in conjunction with appropriate anti-infective therapy to prevent or modify acute bacterial or viral infections in patients with iatrogenically-induced or disease-associated immunodepression; autoimmune hemolytic anemia or neutropenia, refractory dermatomyositis/polymyositis

Mechanism of Action Replacement therapy for primary and secondary immunodeficiencies; interference with F_c receptors on the cells of the reticuloendothelial system for autoimmune cytopenias and ITP; possible role of contained antiviral-type antibodies

Pharmacodynamics/Kinetics

Onset of action: I.V.: Provides immediate antibody levels

Duration: Immune effect: 3-4 weeks (variable)

Distribution: V_d: 0.09-0.13 L/kg

Intravascular portion (primarily): Healthy subjects: 41% to 57%; Patients with congenital humoral immunodeficiencies: ~70%

Half-life elimination: IgG (variable among patients): Healthy subjects: 14-24 days; Patients with congenital humoral immunodeficiencies: 26-40 days; hypermetabolism associated with fever and infection have coincided with a shortened half-life

Contraindications Hypersensitivity to immune globulin or any component of the formulation; selective IgA deficiency

Warnings/Precautions Anaphylactic hypersensitivity reactions can occur, especially in IgA-deficient patients; studies indicate that the currently available products have no discernible risk of transmitting HIV or hepatitis B; aseptic meningitis may occur with high doses (≥2 g/kg). Use with caution in the elderly, patients with renal disease, diabetes mellitus, volume depletion, sepsis, paraproteinemia, and nephrotoxic medications due to risk of renal dysfunction. Patients should be adequately hydrated prior to therapy. Acute renal dysfunction (increased serum creatinine, oliguria, acute renal failure) can rarely occur; usually within 7 days of use (more likely with products stabilized with sucrose). Use caution in patients with a history of thrombotic events or cardiovascular disease; there is clinical evidence of a possible association between thrombotic events and administration of intravenous immune globulin. For intravenous administration only.

Drug Interactions Live virus, vaccines (eg, measles, mumps, rubella): May have impaired response to vaccines; separate administration by at least 3 months.

Lab Interactions Octagam® contains maltose. Falsely-elevated blood glucose levels may occur when glucose monitoring devices and test strips utilizing the glucose dehydrogenase pyrroloquinolinequinone (GDH-PQQ) based methods are used. Glucose monitoring devices and test strips which utilize the glucose-specific method are recommended.

Adverse Reactions Frequency not defined.

Cardiovascular: Flushing of the face, tachycardia, hyper-/hypotension, chest tightness, angioedema, lightheadedness, chest pain, MI, CHF, pulmonary embolism

Central nervous system: Anxiety, chills, dizziness, drowsiness, fatigue, fever, headache, irritability, lethargy, malaise, aseptic meningitis syndrome

(Continued)

Immune Globulin (Intravenous) *(Continued)*

Dermatologic: Pruritus, rash, urticaria
Gastrointestinal: Abdominal cramps, diarrhea, nausea, sore throat, vomiting
Hematologic: Autoimmune hemolytic anemia, hematocrit decreased, leukopenia, mild hemolysis
Hepatic: Liver function test increased
Local: Pain or irritation at the infusion site
Neuromuscular & skeletal: Arthralgia, back or hip pain, myalgia, nuchal rigidity
Ocular: Photophobia, painful eye movements
Renal: Acute renal failure, acute tubular necrosis, anuria, BUN increased, creatinine increased, nephrotic syndrome, oliguria, proximal tubular nephropathy, osmotic nephrosis
Respiratory: Cough, dyspnea, wheezing, nasal congestion, pharyngeal pain, rhinorrhea, sinusitis
Miscellaneous: Diaphoresis, hypersensitivity reactions, anaphylaxis
Postmarketing and/or case reports: Abdominal pain, apnea, ARDS, bronchospasm, bullous dermatitis, cardiac arrest, Coombs' test positive, cyanosis, epidermolysis, erythema multiforme, hepatic dysfunction, hypoxemia, leukopenia, loss of consciousness, pancytopenia, pulmonary edema, rigors, seizure, Stevens-Johnson syndrome, thromboembolism, transfusion-related acute lung injury (TRALI), tremor, vascular collapse

Dosing

Adults & Elderly: Approved doses and regimens may vary between brands; check manufacturer guidelines. **Note:** Some clinicians dose IVIG on ideal body weight or an adjusted ideal body weight in morbidly obese patients.

Primary immunodeficiency disorders: I.V.: 200-400 mg/kg every 4 weeks or as per monitored serum IgG concentrations

Gammagard® Liquid, Gamunex®, Octagam®: 300-600 mg/kg every 3-4 weeks; adjusted based on dosage and interval in conjunction with monitored serum IgG concentrations.

B-cell chronic lymphocytic leukemia (CLL): I.V.: 400 mg/kg/dose every 3 weeks

Idiopathic thrombocytopenic purpura (ITP): I.V.:

Acute: 400 mg/kg/day for 5 days or 1000 mg/kg/day for 1-2 days

Chronic: 400 mg/kg as needed to maintain platelet count >30,000/mm^3; may increase dose to 800 mg/kg (1000 mg/kg if needed)

Kawasaki disease: Initiate therapy within 10 days of disease onset: I.V.: 2 g/kg as a single dose administered over 10 hours, or 400 mg/kg/day for 4 days. **Note:** Must be used in combination with aspirin: 80-100 mg/kg/day in 4 divided doses for 14 days; when fever subsides, dose aspirin at 3-5 mg/kg once daily for ≥6-8 weeks

Acquired immunodeficiency syndrome (patients must be symptomatic) (unlabeled use): I.V.: Various regimens have been used, including:

200-250 mg/kg/dose every 2 weeks

or

400-500 mg/kg/dose every month or every 4 weeks

Autoimmune hemolytic anemia and neutropenia (unlabeled use): I.V.: 1000 mg/kg/dose for 2-3 days

Autoimmune diseases (unlabeled use): I.V.: 400 mg/kg/day for 4 days

Bone marrow transplant: I.V.: 500 mg/kg beginning on days 7 and 2 pretransplant, then 500 mg/kg/week for 90 days post-transplant

Adjuvant to severe cytomegalovirus infections (unlabeled use): I.V.: 500 mg/kg/dose every other day for 7 doses

Guillain-Barré syndrome (unlabeled use): I.V.: Various regimens have been used, including:

400 mg/kg/day for 4 days

or

1000 mg/kg/day for 2 days

or

2000 mg/kg/day for one day

Refractory dermatomyositis (unlabeled use): I.V.: 2 g/kg/dose every month x 3-4 doses

Refractory polymyositis (unlabeled use): I.V.: 1 g/kg/day x 2 days every month x 4 doses

Chronic inflammatory demyelinating polyneuropathy (unlabeled use): I.V.: Various regimens have been used, including:

400 mg/kg/day for 5 doses once each month

or

800 mg/kg/day for 3 doses once each month

or

1000 mg/kg/day for 2 days once each month

Pediatrics: Approved doses and regimens may vary between brands; check manufacturer guidelines. **Note:** Some clinicians dose IVIG on ideal body weight or an adjusted ideal body weight in morbidly obese patients.

Pediatric HIV: I.V.: 400 mg/kg every 28 days

Severe systemic viral and bacterial infections: Children: I.V.: 500-1000 mg/kg/week

Prevention of gastroenteritis: Infants and Children: Oral: 50 mg/kg/day divided every 6 hours

For additional indications, refer to adult dosing.

Renal Impairment: Cl_{cr} <10 mL/minute: Avoid use; in patients at risk of renal dysfunction, consider infusion at a rate less than maximum.

Available Dosage Forms

Injection, powder for reconstitution [preservative free]:
- Gammar®-P I.V.: 5 g, 10 g [stabilized with human albumin and sucrose]
- Iveegam EN: 5 g [stabilized with glucose]

Injection, powder for reconstitution [preservative free, nanofiltered]:
- Carimune™ NF: 3 g, 6 g, 12 g [contains sucrose]
- Panglobulin® NF: 6 g, 12 g [contains sucrose]

Injection, powder for reconstitution [preservative free, solvent detergent treated]
- Gammagard® S/D: 2.5 g, 5 g, 10 g [stabilized with human albumin, glycine, glucose, and polyethylene glycol]
- Polygam® S/D: 5 g, 10 g [stabilized with human albumin, glycine, glucose, and polyethylene glycol]

Injection, solution [preservative free; solvent detergent-treated]:
- Gammagard® Liquid: 10% [100 mg/mL] (10 mL, 25 mL, 50 mL, 100 mL, 200 mL) [latex free, sucrose free; stabilized with glycine]
- Octagam®: 5% [50 mg/mL] (20 mL, 50 mL, 100 mL, 200 mL) [sucrose free; contains sodium 30 mmol/L and maltose]

Injection, solution [preservative free] (Gamunex®): 10% (10 mL, 25 mL, 50 mL, 100 mL, 200 mL) [caprylate/chromatography purified]

Nursing Guidelines

Assessment: Assess for history of previous allergic reactions. Patient should be monitored during infusion for vital sign changes and adverse or allergic reactions. Teach patient adverse symptoms to report.

Dietary Considerations: Octagam® contains sodium 30 mmol/L

Patient Education: This medication can only be administered by infusion. You will be monitored closely during the infusion. If you experience nausea ask for assistance, do not get up alone. Do not have any vaccinations for the next 3 months without consulting prescriber. Immediately report chills; chest pain, tightness, or rapid heartbeat; acute back pain; or respiratory difficulty. **Pregnancy/breast-feeding precautions:** Inform prescriber if you are or intend to become pregnant. Consult prescriber if breast-feeding.

Pregnancy Risk Factor: C

Lactation: Excretion in breast milk unknown

Administration

I.V.: For I.V. use only; for initial treatment, a lower concentration and/or a slower rate of infusion should be used. Refrigerated product should be warmed to room temperature prior to infusion.

Reconstitution: Dilution is dependent upon the manufacturer and brand; do not shake, avoid foaming; discard unused portion:

Carimune™ NF, Panglobulin® NF: Reconstitute with NS, D_5W, or SWFI.
Iveegam EN: Reconstitute with SWFI; use immediately after reconstitution
Gammagard® Liquid: May dilute in D_5W only.
Gammagard® S/D, Polygam® S/D: Reconstitute with sterile water for injection.
Gammar®-P I.V.: Reconstitute with SWFI.
Gamunex®: Dilute in D_5W only.

Compatibility: Stable in D_5W, $D_{15}W$, $D_5{}^1/_4NS$

Storage: Stability and dilution is dependent upon the manufacturer and brand; do not freeze:

Carimune™ NF, Panglobulin® NF: Prior to reconstitution, store at or below 30°C (86°F). Following reconstitution, store under refrigeration; use within 24 hours. Do not freeze.

(Continued)

Immune Globulin (Intravenous) *(Continued)*

Gammagard® Liquid: May be stored for up to 9 months at room temperature of 25°C (77°F) within 24 months of manufacture date. May be stored for up to 36 months under refrigeration at 2°C to 8°C (36°F to 46°F). Do not freeze.

Gammar®-P I.V., Gammagard® S/D, Polygam® S/D, Venoglobulin®-S: Store below 25°C (77°F).

Gammagard® S/D, Polygam® S/D: May store diluted solution under refrigeration for up to 24 hours.

Gamunex®: May be stored for up to 5 months at room temperature up to 25°C (up to 77°F) within 18 months of manufacture date.

Iveegam EN: Store at 2°C to 8°C (36°F to 46°F).

Octagam®: Store at 2°C to 8°C (36°F to 46°F) for 24 months or ≤25°C (77°F) for 18 months.

Polygam® S/D: Store at room temperature at or below 25°C (77°F); do not freeze.

♦ Immune Serum Globulin *see* Immune Globulin (Intramuscular) *on page 898*
♦ Imodium® A-D [OTC] *see* Loperamide *on page 1056*
♦ Imuran® *see* Azathioprine *on page 207*

Inamrinone (eye NAM ri none)

Synonyms Amrinone Lactate

Pharmacologic Category Phosphodiesterase Enzyme Inhibitor

Medication Safety Issues

Sound-alike/look-alike issues:

Amrinone may be confused with amiloride, amiodarone

Use Infrequently used as a last resort, short-term therapy in patients with intractable heart failure

Mechanism of Action Inhibits myocardial cyclic adenosine monophosphate (cAMP) phosphodiesterase activity and increases cellular levels of cAMP resulting in a positive inotropic effect and increased cardiac output; also possesses systemic and pulmonary vasodilator effects resulting in pre- and afterload reduction; slightly increases atrioventricular conduction

Pharmacodynamics/Kinetics

Onset of action: I.V.: 2-5 minutes

Peak effect: ~10 minutes

Duration (dose dependent): Low dose: ~30 minutes; Higher doses: ~2 hours

Half-life elimination, serum: Adults: Healthy volunteers: 3.6 hours, Congestive heart failure: 5.8 hours

Contraindications Hypersensitivity to inamrinone, any component of the formulation, or bisulfites (contains sodium metabisulfite); patients with severe aortic or pulmonic valvular disease

Warnings/Precautions Due to a slight effect on AV conduction, may increase ventricular response rate in atrial fibrillation/atrial flutter; prior treatment with digoxin is recommended. Monitor liver function. Discontinue therapy if alteration in LFTs and clinical symptoms of hepatotoxicity occur. Observe for arrhythmias in this very high-risk patient population. Not recommended in acute MI treatment. Monitor fluid status closely; patients may require adjustment of diuretic and electrolyte replacement therapy. Can cause thrombocytopenia (dose dependent). Correct hypokalemia before initiating therapy. Increase risk of hospitalization and death with long-term therapy.

Drug Interactions

Furosemide: A precipitate forms on admixture with inamrinone.

Diuretics may cause significant hypovolemia and decrease filling pressure.

Digitalis: Inotropic effects are additive.

Adverse Reactions

1% to 10%:

Cardiovascular: Arrhythmias (3%, especially in high-risk patients), hypotension (1% to 2%) (may be infusion rate-related)

Gastrointestinal: Nausea (1% to 2%)

Hematologic: Thrombocytopenia (may be dose related)

<1% (Limited to important or life-threatening): Chest pain, fever, hepatotoxicity, hypersensitivity (especially with prolonged therapy), vomiting; contains sulfites resulting in allergic reactions in susceptible people

Dosing

Adults & Elderly: Dosage is based on clinical response (**Note:** Dose should not exceed 10 mg/kg/24 hours).

Heart failure: 0.75 mg/kg I.V. bolus over 2-3 minutes followed by maintenance infusion of 5-10 mcg/kg/minute; I.V. bolus may need to be repeated in 30 minutes.

Pediatrics: Heart failure: Infants and Children: Refer to adult dosing.

Renal Impairment: Cl_{cr} <10 mL/minute: Administer 50% to 75% of dose.

Available Dosage Forms Injection, solution, as lactate: 5 mg/mL (20 mL) [contains sodium metabisulfite]

Nursing Guidelines

Patient Education: Make position changes slowly because of postural hypotension

Pregnancy Risk Factor: C

Perioperative/Anesthesia/Other Concerns: To avoid confusion with similarly sounding medication names, the generic name "amrinone" changed to "inamrinone" in July, 2000.

Preliminary pharmacokinetic studies estimate total initial bolus doses of 3-4.5 mg/kg given in divided doses in neonates and infants to obtain serum concentrations similar to therapeutic adult levels; the actual use of these higher doses has been reported in a very small number of infants (n=7). Further studies are needed to define pediatric dosing guidelines.

Although the phosphodiesterase inhibitor drugs may induce short-term improvement in clinical status in patients with intractable heart failure, longer-term studies of these drugs in heart failure have suggested that there is a net increase in mortality.

Administration

Compatibility: Stable in NS, ½NS; **incompatible** with D_5W

Y-site administration: Incompatible with sodium bicarbonate

Compatibility when admixed: Incompatible with furosemide

♦ Inapsine® *see* Droperidol *on page 590*

Indapamide (in DAP a mide)

U.S. Brand Names Lozol®

Pharmacologic Category Diuretic, Thiazide-Related

Medication Safety Issues

Sound-alike/look-alike issues:

Indapamide may be confused with Iopidine®

Use Management of mild to moderate hypertension; treatment of edema in congestive heart failure and nephrotic syndrome

Mechanism of Action Diuretic effect is localized at the proximal segment of the distal tubule of the nephron; it does not appear to have significant effect on glomerular filtration rate nor renal blood flow; like other diuretics, it enhances sodium, chloride, and water excretion by interfering with the transport of sodium ions across the renal tubular epithelium

Pharmacodynamics/Kinetics

Onset of action: 1-2 hours

Duration: ≤36 hours

Absorption: Complete

Protein binding, plasma: 71% to 79%

Metabolism: Extensively hepatic

Half-life elimination: 14-18 hours

Time to peak: 2-2.5 hours

Excretion: Urine (~60%) within 48 hours; feces (~16% to 23%)

Contraindications Hypersensitivity to indapamide or any component of the formulation, thiazides, or sulfonamide-derived drugs; anuria; renal decompensation; pregnancy (based on expert analysis)

Warnings/Precautions Use with caution in severe renal disease. Electrolyte disturbances (hypokalemia, hypochloremic alkalosis, hyponatremia) can occur. Use with caution in severe hepatic dysfunction; hepatic encephalopathy can be caused by electrolyte disturbances. Gout can be precipitate in certain patients with a history of gout, a familial predisposition to gout, or chronic renal failure. Cautious use in diabetics; may see a change in glucose control. I.V. use is generally not recommended (but is available). Hypersensitivity reactions can occur. Can cause SLE exacerbation or activation. Use with caution in patients with moderate or high cholesterol concentrations. Photosensitization may occur. Correct hypokalemia before initiating therapy.

(Continued)

Indapamide *(Continued)*

Chemical similarities are present among sulfonamides, sulfonylureas, carbonic anhydrase inhibitors, thiazides, and loop diuretics (except ethacrynic acid). Use in patients with thiazide or sulfonamide allergy is specifically contraindicated in product labeling, however, a risk of cross-reaction exists in patients with allergy to any of these compounds; avoid use when previous reaction has been severe.

Drug Interactions

ACE inhibitors: Increased hypotension if aggressively diuresed with a thiazide diuretic.

Beta-blockers increase hyperglycemic effects in type 2 diabetes mellitus (noninsulin dependent, NIDDM)

Cyclosporine and thiazides can increase the risk of gout or renal toxicity; avoid concurrent use.

Digoxin toxicity can be exacerbated if a thiazide induces hypokalemia or hypomagnesemia.

Lithium toxicity can occur by reducing renal excretion of lithium; monitor lithium concentration and adjust as needed.

Neuromuscular blocking agents can prolong blockade; monitor serum potassium and neuromuscular status.

NSAIDs can decrease the efficacy of thiazides reducing the diuretic and antihypertensive effects.

Nutritional/Herbal/Ethanol Interactions Herb/Nutraceutical: Avoid dong quai if using for hypertension (has estrogenic activity). Avoid ephedra, yohimbe, ginseng (may worsen hypertension). Avoid garlic (may have increased antihypertensive effect).

Adverse Reactions

1% to 10%:

Cardiovascular: Orthostatic hypotension, palpitation, flushing

Central nervous system: Dizziness, lightheadedness, vertigo, headache, weakness, restlessness, drowsiness, fatigue, lethargy, malaise, lassitude, anxiety, agitation, depression, nervousness

Gastrointestinal: Anorexia, gastric irritation, nausea, vomiting, abdominal pain, cramping, bloating, diarrhea, constipation, dry mouth, weight loss

Genitourinary: Nocturia, frequent urination, polyuria

Neuromuscular & skeletal: Muscle cramps, spasm

Ocular: Blurred vision

Respiratory: Rhinorrhea

<1% (Limited to important or life-threatening): Cutaneous vasculitis, glycosuria, hypercalcemia, hyperglycemia, hyperuricemia, impotency, necrotizing angiitis, pancreatitis, purpura, reduced libido, vasculitis

Overdosage/Toxicology Symptoms of overdose include lethargy, diuresis, hypermotility, confusion, and muscle weakness. Treatment is supportive.

Dosing

Adults & Elderly:

Edema (diuretic): Oral: 2.5-5 mg/day. **Note:** There is little therapeutic benefit to increasing the dose >5 mg/day; there is, however, an increased risk of electrolyte disturbances.

Hypertension: Oral: 1.25 mg in the morning, may increase to 5 mg/day by increments of 1.25-2.5 mg; consider adding another antihypertensive and decreasing the dose if response is not adequate.

Available Dosage Forms

Tablet: 1.25 mg, 2.5 mg

Lozol®: 1.25 mg

Nursing Guidelines

Assessment: Assess allergy history prior to beginning therapy. See Contraindications, Warnings/Precautions, and Dosing for use cautions. Assess potential for interactions with other prescriptions, OTC medications, or herbal products patient may be taking (see Drug Interactions). Assess results of laboratory tests (see Monitoring Lab Tests), therapeutic effectiveness, and adverse response (see Adverse Reactions and Overdose/Toxicology) at regular intervals during therapy. Instruct patients with diabetes to monitor glucose levels closely; may interfere with oral hypoglycemic medications. Teach patient proper use, possible side effects (eg, orthostatic hypotension, electrolyte imbalance) and appropriate interventions, and adverse symptoms to report (see Patient Education). **Pregnancy risk factor B/D** - see Pregnancy Risk Factor for use cautions; benefits of use should outweigh possible risks. Note breast-feeding caution.

Monitoring Laboratory Tests: Serum electrolytes, renal function

Dietary Considerations: May be taken with food or milk to decrease GI adverse effects.

Patient Education: Inform prescriber of all prescriptions, OTC medications, or herbal products you are taking, and any allergies you have. Do not take any new medication during therapy unless approved by prescriber. Take as directed, early in the day. Do not exceed recommended dosage. This medication does not replace other antihypertensive interventions; follow prescriber's instructions for diet and lifestyle changes. If you have diabetes, monitor serum glucose closely (medication may decrease effect of oral hypoglycemics). Monitor weight on a regular basis. Report sudden or excessive weight gain (>5 lb/week), swelling of ankles or hands, or respiratory difficulty. You may experience dizziness, weakness, or drowsiness (use caution when rising from sitting or lying position, when climbing stairs and when driving or engaging in tasks that require alertness until response to drug is known); sensitivity to sunlight (use sunblock, wear protective clothing or sunglasses); impotence (reversible); or dry mouth or thirst (frequent mouth care, chewing gum, or sucking lozenges may help). Report any changes in visual acuity; unusual bleeding; chest pain or palpitations; or numbness, tingling, cramping of muscles. **Pregnancy/breast-feeding precaution:** Inform prescriber if you are pregnant. Consult prescriber if breast-feeding.

Geriatric Considerations: Thiazide diuretics lose efficacy when Cl_{cr} is <30-35 mL/minute. Many elderly may have Cl_{cr} below this limit. Calculate Cl_{cr} for elderly before initiating therapy. Indapamide has the advantage over thiazide diuretics in that it is effective when Cl_{cr} is <30 mL/minute.

Pregnancy Risk Factor: B (manufacturer); D (expert analysis)

Lactation: Excretion in breast milk unknown

Administration

Oral: May be taken with food or milk. Take early in day to avoid nocturia. Take the last dose of multiple doses no later than 6 PM unless instructed otherwise.

♦ Inderal® *see* Propranolol *on page 1429*

♦ Inderal® LA *see* Propranolol *on page 1429*

♦ Indocin® *see* Indomethacin *on page 906*

♦ Indocin® I.V. *see* Indomethacin *on page 906*

♦ Indocin® SR *see* Indomethacin *on page 906*

Indocyanine Green (in doe SYE a neen green)

U.S. Brand Names IC-Green®

Pharmacologic Category Diagnostic Agent

Use Determining hepatic function, cardiac output and liver blood flow and for ophthalmic angiography

Adverse Reactions 1% to 10%:

Central nervous system: Headache

Dermatologic: Pruritus, skin discoloration

Miscellaneous: Diaphoresis, anaphylactoid reactions

Dosing

Adults & Elderly:

Angiography: Use 40 mg of dye in 2 mL of aqueous solvent, in some patients, half the volume (1 mL) has been found to produce angiograms of comparable resolution; immediately following the bolus dose of dye, a bolus of sodium chloride 0.9% is given; this regimen will deliver a spatially limited dye bolus of optimal concentration to the choroidal vasculature following I.V. injection

Determination of cardiac output: Dye is injected as rapidly as possible into the right atrium, right ventricle, or pulmonary artery through a cardiac catheter; the usual dose is 1.25 mg for infants, 2.5 mg for children, and 5 mg for adults; total dose should not exceed 2 mg/kg; the dye is diluted with sterile water for injection or sodium chloride 0.9% to make a final volume of 1 mL; doses are repeated periodically to obtain several dilution curves; the dye should be flushed from the catheter with sodium chloride 0.9% to prevent hemolysis

Available Dosage Forms Injection, powder for reconstitution: 25 mg [supplied with diluent]

Nursing Guidelines

Pregnancy Risk Factor: C

Administration

Reconstitution: Reconstitute only with sterile water for injection supplied by manufacturer.

♦ **Indometacin** *see* Indomethacin *on page 906*

Indomethacin (in doe METH a sin)

U.S. Brand Names Indocin®; Indocin® I.V.; Indocin® SR

Synonyms Indometacin; Indomethacin Sodium Trihydrate

Pharmacologic Category Nonsteroidal Anti-inflammatory Drug (NSAID), Oral; Nonsteroidal Anti-inflammatory Drug (NSAID), Parenteral

Medication Safety Issues

Sound-alike/look-alike issues:

Indocin® may be confused with Imodium®, Lincocin®, Minocin®, Vicodin®

Use Acute gouty arthritis, acute bursitis/tendonitis, moderate to severe osteoarthritis, rheumatoid arthritis, ankylosing spondylitis; I.V. form used as alternative to surgery for closure of patent ductus arteriosus in neonates

Mechanism of Action Inhibits prostaglandin synthesis by decreasing the activity of the enzyme, cyclooxygenase, which results in decreased formation of prostaglandin precursors

Pharmacodynamics/Kinetics

Onset of action: ~30 minutes

Duration: 4-6 hours

Absorption: Prompt and extensive

Distribution: V_d: 0.34-1.57 L/kg; crosses blood brain barrier and placenta; enters breast milk

Protein binding: 99%

Metabolism: Hepatic; significant enterohepatic recirculation

Bioavailability: 100%

Half-life elimination: 4.5 hours; prolonged in neonates

Time to peak: Oral: 2 hours

Excretion: Urine (60%, primarily as glucuronide conjugates); feces (33%, primarily as metabolites)

Contraindications Hypersensitivity to indomethacin, aspirin, other NSAIDs, or any component of the formulation; perioperative pain in the setting of coronary artery bypass surgery (CABG); pregnancy (3rd trimester)

Neonates: Necrotizing enterocolitis, impaired renal function, active bleeding, thrombocytopenia, coagulation defects, untreated infection

Warnings/Precautions NSAIDs are associated with an increased risk of adverse cardiovascular events, including MI, stroke, and new onset or worsening of pre-existing hypertension. Risk may be increased with duration of use or pre-existing cardiovascular risk-factors or disease. Carefully evaluate individual cardiovascular risk profiles prior to prescribing. Use caution with fluid retention, CHF or hypertension.

Use of NSAIDs can compromise existing renal function. Renal toxicity can occur in patient with impaired renal function, dehydration, heart failure, liver dysfunction, those taking diuretics and ACEI and the elderly. Rehydrate patient before starting therapy. Monitor renal function closely. Indomethacin is not recommended for patients with advanced renal disease.

NSAIDs may increase risk of gastrointestinal irritation, ulceration, bleeding, and perforation. These events may occur at any time during therapy and without warning. Use caution with a history of GI disease (bleeding or ulcers), concurrent therapy with aspirin, anticoagulants and/or corticosteroids, smoking, use of alcohol, the elderly or debilitated patients.

Use the lowest effective dose for the shortest duration of time, consistent with individual patient goals, to reduce risk of cardiovascular or GI adverse events. Alternate therapies should be considered for patients at high risk.

NSAIDs may cause serious skin adverse events including exfoliative dermatitis, Stevens-Johnson syndrome (SJS) and toxic epidermal necrolysis (TEN). Anaphylactoid reactions may occur, even without prior exposure; patients with "aspirin triad" (bronchial asthma, aspirin intolerance, rhinitis) may be at increased risk. Do not use in patients who experience bronchospasm, asthma, rhinitis, or urticaria with NSAID or aspirin therapy.

Use with caution in patients with decreased hepatic function. Closely monitor patients with any abnormal LFT. Severe hepatic reactions (eg, fulminant hepatitis, liver failure) have occurred with NSAID use, rarely; discontinue if signs or symptoms of liver disease develop, or if systemic manifestations occur.

Withhold for at least 4-6 half-lives prior to surgical or dental procedures.

Drug Interactions **Substrate** (minor) of CYP2C8/9, 2C19; **Inhibits** CYP2C8/9 (strong), 2C19 (weak)

ACE inhibitors: Antihypertensive effects may be decreased by concurrent therapy with NSAIDs; monitor blood pressure.

Aminoglycosides: NSAIDs may decrease the excretion of aminoglycosides.

Angiotensin II antagonists: Antihypertensive effects may be decreased by concurrent therapy with NSAIDs; monitor blood pressure.

Anticoagulants (warfarin, heparin, LMWHs) in combination with NSAIDs can cause increased risk of bleeding.

Antiplatelet drugs (ticlopidine, clopidogrel, aspirin, abciximab, dipyridamole, eptifibatide, tirofiban) can cause an increased risk of bleeding.

Beta-blockers: NSAIDs may diminish the antihypertensive effects of beta blockers.

Bisphosphonates: NSAIDs may increase the risk of gastrointestinal ulceration.

Cholestyramine and colestipol reduce the bioavailability of some NSAIDs; separate administration times.

Corticosteroids may increase the risk of GI ulceration; avoid concurrent use.

Cyclosporine: NSAIDs may increase serum creatinine, potassium, blood pressure, and cyclosporine levels; monitor cyclosporine levels and renal function carefully.

CYP2C8/9 substrates: Indomethacin, a strong CYP2C8/9 inhibitor, may increase the levels/effects of CYP2C8/9 substrates. Example substrates include amiodarone, fluoxetine, glimepiride, glipizide, nateglinide, phenytoin, pioglitazone, rosiglitazone, sertraline, and warfarin.

Gentamicin and amikacin serum concentrations are increased by indomethacin in premature infants. Results may apply to other aminoglycosides and NSAIDs.

Hydralazine's antihypertensive effect is decreased; avoid concurrent use.

Lithium levels can be increased; avoid concurrent use if possible or monitor lithium levels and adjust dose. Sulindac may have the least effect. When NSAID is stopped, lithium will need adjustment again.

Loop diuretics efficacy (diuretic and antihypertensive effect) is reduced. Indomethacin reduces this efficacy, however, it may be anticipated with any NSAID.

Methotrexate: Severe bone marrow suppression, aplastic anemia, and GI toxicity have been reported with concomitant NSAID therapy. Avoid use during moderate or high-dose methotrexate (increased and prolonged methotrexate levels). NSAID use during low-dose treatment of rheumatoid arthritis has not been fully evaluated; extreme caution is warranted.

Pemetrexed: NSAIDs may decrease the excretion of pemetrexed. Patients with Cl_{cr} 45-79 mL/minute should avoid short acting NSAIDs for 2 days before and 2 days after pemetrexed treatment.

Thiazides antihypertensive effects are decreased; avoid concurrent use.

Tiludronate: Indomethacin may increase serum concentration of tiludronate.

Treprostinil: May enhance the risk of bleeding with concurrent use.

Vancomycin: NSAIDs may decrease the excretion of vancomycin.

Nutritional/Herbal/Ethanol Interactions

Ethanol: Avoid ethanol (may enhance gastric mucosal irritation).

Food: Food may decrease the rate but not the extent of absorption. Indomethacin peak serum levels may be delayed if taken with food.

Herb/Nutraceutical: Avoid alfalfa, anise, bilberry, bladderwrack, bromelain, cat's claw, celery, coleus, cordyceps, dong quai, evening primrose, feverfew, fenugreek, garlic, ginger, ginkgo biloba, red clover, horse chestnut, grapeseed, green tea, ginseng, guggul, horse chestnut seed, horseradish, licorice, prickly ash, red clover, reishi, SAMe, sweet clover, turmeric, white willow (all have additional antiplatelet activity).

Lab Interactions False-negative dexamethasone suppression test

Adverse Reactions

>10%: Central nervous system: Headache (12%)

1% to 10%:

Central nervous system: Dizziness (3% to 9%), drowsiness (<1%), fatigue (<3%), vertigo (<3%), depression (<3%), malaise (<3%), somnolence (<3%)

Gastrointestinal: Nausea (3% to 9%), epigastric pain (3% to 9%), abdominal pain/cramps/distress (<3%), heartburn (3% to 9%), indigestion (3% to 9%), constipation (<3%), diarrhea (<3%), dyspepsia (3% to 9%), vomiting

Otic: Tinnitus (<3%)

<1% (Limited to important or life-threatening): Acute respiratory distress, agranulocytosis, allergic rhinitis, anaphylaxis, anemia, angioedema, aplastic anemia,

(Continued)

Indomethacin *(Continued)*

arrhythmia, aseptic meningitis, asthma, bone marrow suppression, bronchospasm, chest pain, cholestatic jaundice, coma, confusion, CHF, cystitis, depersonalization, depression, dilutional hyponatremia (I.V.), diplopia, disseminated intravascular coagulation, dysarthria, dyspnea, ecchymosis, edema, epistaxis, erythema multiforme, erythema nodosum, exfoliative dermatitis, fluid retention, flushing, hair loss, gastritis, GI bleeding, GI ulceration, gynecomastia, hearing decreased, hematuria, hemolytic anemia, hepatitis (including fatal cases), hot flashes, hyperkalemia, hypersensitivity reactions, hypertension, hypoglycemia (I.V.), interstitial nephritis, involuntary muscle movements, leukopenia, necrotizing fasciitis, nephrotic syndrome, oliguria, paresthesias, parkinson's exacerbation, peptic ulcer, peripheral neuropathy, proctitis, psychosis, pulmonary edema, purpura, syncope, renal insufficiency, renal failure, retinal/macular disturbances, seizure exacerbation, shock, somnolence, Stevens-Johnson syndrome, stomatitis, thrombocytopenia, thrombocytopenic purpura, thrombophlebitis, toxic amblyopia, toxic epidermal necrolysis

Overdosage/Toxicology Symptoms of overdose include drowsiness, lethargy, nausea, vomiting, seizures, paresthesia, headache, dizziness, GI bleeding, cerebral edema, tinnitus, leukocytosis, and renal failure. Management of NSAID intoxication is supportive and symptomatic.

Dosing

Adults & Elderly:

Inflammatory/rheumatoid disorders (use lowest effective dose): Oral: 25-50 mg/dose 2-3 times/day; maximum dose: 200 mg/day; extended release capsule should be given on a 1-2 times/day schedule; maximum dose for sustained release is 150 mg/day. In patients with arthritis and persistent night pain and/or morning stiffness may give the larger portion (up to 100 mg) of the total daily dose at bedtime.

Bursitis/tendonitis: Oral: Initial dose: 75-150 mg/day in 3-4 divided doses; usual treatment is 7-14 days

Acute gouty arthritis: Oral: 50 mg 3 times daily until pain is tolerable then reduce dose; usual treatment <3-5 days

Pediatrics:

Patent ductus arteriosus:

Neonates: I.V.: Initial: 0.2 mg/kg, followed by 2 doses depending on postnatal age (PNA):

PNA at time of FIRST dose <48 hours: 0.1 mg/kg at 12- to 24-hour intervals

PNA at time of FIRST dose 2-7 days: 0.2 mg/kg at 12- to 24-hour intervals

PNA at time of FIRST dose >7 days: 0.25 mg/kg at 12- to 24-hour intervals

Note: In general, may use 12-hour dosing interval if urine output >1 mL/kg/hour after prior dose; use 24-hour dosing interval if urine output is <1 mL/kg/hour but >0.6 mL/kg/hour; doses should be withheld if patient has oliguria (urine output <0.6 mL/kg/hour) or anuria

Inflammatory/rheumatoid disorders: Children: Oral: 1-2 mg/kg/day in 2-4 divided doses; maximum dose: 4 mg/kg/day; not to exceed 150-200 mg/day

Available Dosage Forms

Capsule (Indocin®): 25 mg, 50 mg

Capsule, sustained release (Indocin® SR): 75 mg

Injection, powder for reconstitution, as sodium trihydrate (Indocin® I.V.): 1 mg

Suspension, oral (Indocin®): 25 mg/5 mL (237 mL) [contains alcohol 1%; pineapple-coconut-mint flavor]

Nursing Guidelines

Assessment: Evaluate cardiac risk and potential for GI bleeding prior to prescribing this medication. Assess potential for interactions with other prescriptions, OTC medications, or herbal products patient may be taking. Monitor blood pressure at the beginning of therapy and periodically during use. Assess results of laboratory tests, therapeutic effectiveness (according to rationale for use), and adverse response when beginning therapy and at regular intervals during treatment. Teach patient proper use, side effects/appropriate interventions (regular ophthalmic evaluations with long-term use), and adverse symptoms to report.

Monitoring Laboratory Tests: Renal function (serum creatinine and BUN), CBC, liver function

Dietary Considerations: May cause GI upset; take with food or milk to minimize

Patient Education: Do not take any new medication during therapy without consulting prescriber. Use exactly as directed; do not increase dose without consulting prescriber. Do not crush, break, or chew capsules. Take with food or milk to reduce GI distress. Maintain adequate hydration (2-3 L/day of fluids) unless instructed to restrict fluid intake. May cause drowsiness, dizziness, nervousness, or headache (use caution when driving or engaging in tasks that require alertness until response to drug is known); anorexia, nausea, vomiting, or heartburn (small frequent meals, frequent mouth care, chewing gum, or sucking lozenges may help): fluid retention (weigh yourself weekly and report unusually weight gain >3-5 lb/week); or may turn urine green (normal). GI bleeding, ulceration, or perforation can occur with or without pain; discontinue medication and contact prescriber if persistent abdominal pain or cramping or blood in stool occurs. Report difficult breathing or unusual cough; chest pain, rapid heartbeat, or palpitations; unusual bruising or bleeding; blood in urine, gums, or vomitus; swollen extremities; skin rash, irritation, or itching; acute persistent fatigue; or vision changes or ringing in ears. **Pregnancy/ breast-feeding precautions:** Inform prescriber if you are or intend to become pregnant. This drug should not be used in the 3rd trimester of pregnancy. Consult prescriber if breast-feeding.

Geriatric Considerations: Elderly are at high risk for adverse effects from NSAIDs. As much as 60% of elderly can develop peptic ulceration and/or hemorrhage asymptomatically. The concomitant use of H_2 blockers, omeprazole, and sucralfate is not effective as prophylaxis with the exception of NSAID-induced duodenal ulcers which may be prevented by the use of ranitidine. Misoprostol is the only prophylactic agent proven effective. Also, concomitant disease and drug use contribute to the risk for GI adverse effects. Use lowest effective dose for shortest period possible. Consider renal function decline with age. Use of NSAIDs can compromise existing renal function especially when Cl_{cr} is ≤30 mL/minute. Tinnitus may be a difficult and unreliable indication of toxicity due to age-related hearing loss or eighth cranial nerve damage. CNS adverse effects such as confusion, agitation, and hallucination are generally seen in overdose or high-dose situations, but elderly may demonstrate these adverse effects at lower doses than younger adults. Indomethacin frequently causes confusion at recommended doses in the elderly.

Pregnancy Risk Factor: C/D (3rd trimester)

Lactation: Enters breast milk/use caution (AAP rates "compatible")

Perioperative/Anesthesia/Other Concerns: The 2002 ACCM/SCCM guidelines for analgesia (critically-ill adult) suggest that NSAIDs may be used in combination with opioids in select patients for pain management. Concern about adverse events (increased risk of renal dysfunction, altered platelet function and gastrointestinal irritation) limits its use in patients who have other underlying risks for these events.

In short-term use, NSAIDs vary considerably in their effect on blood pressure. When NSAIDs are used in patients with hypertension, appropriate monitoring of blood pressure responses should be completed and the duration of therapy, when possible, kept short. The use of NSAIDs in the treatment of patients with congestive heart failure may be associated with an increased risk for fluid accumulation and edema; may precipitate renal failure in dehydrated patients.

Administration

Oral: Administer with food, milk, or antacids to decrease GI adverse effects. Extended release capsules must be swallowed whole, do not crush.

I.V.: Administer over 20-30 minutes at a concentration of 0.5-1 mg/mL in preservative-free sterile water for injection or normal saline. Reconstitute I.V. formulation just prior to administration; discard any unused portion; avoid I.V. bolus administration or infusion via an umbilical catheter into vessels near the superior mesenteric artery as these may cause vasoconstriction and can compromise blood flow to the intestines. Do not administer intra-arterially.

Reconstitution: Reconstitute just prior to administration; discard any unused portion. Do not use preservative-containing diluents for reconstitution.

Compatibility: Stable in NS

Y-site administration: Incompatible with amino acid injection, calcium gluconate, cimetidine, dobutamine, dopamine, gentamicin, levofloxacin, tobramycin, tolazoline

Storage: I.V.: Store below 30°C (86°F). Protect from light.

◆ **Indomethacin Sodium Trihydrate** *see* Indomethacin *on page 906*

◆ **INF-alpha 2** *see* Interferon Alfa-2b *on page 936*

◆ **Infantaire Gas Drops [OTC]** *see* Simethicone *on page 1533*

♦ **Infants' Tylenol® Cold Plus Cough Concentrated Drops [OTC]** *see* Acetaminophen, Dextromethorphan, and Pseudoephedrine *on page 73*
♦ **INFeD®** *see* Iron Dextran Complex *on page 966*
♦ **Infergen®** *see* Interferon Alfacon-1 *on page 944*

Infliximab (in FLIKS e mab)

U.S. Brand Names Remicade®

Synonyms Infliximab, Recombinant

Pharmacologic Category Antirheumatic, Disease Modifying; Gastrointestinal Agent, Miscellaneous; Monoclonal Antibody; Tumor Necrosis Factor (TNF) Blocking Agent

Medication Safety Issues

Sound-alike/look-alike issues:

Remicade® may be confused with Renacidin®, Rituxan®

Use

Ankylosing spondylitis: Improving signs and symptoms of disease

Crohn's disease: Induction and maintenance of remission in patients with moderate to severe disease who have an inadequate response to conventional therapy; to reduce the number of draining enterocutaneous and rectovaginal fistulas and to maintain fistula closure

Psoriatic arthritis: Improving signs and symptoms of active arthritis in patients with psoriatic arthritis

Rheumatoid arthritis: Inhibits the progression of structural damage and improves physical function in patients with moderate to severe disease; used with methotrexate

Ulcerative colitis (UC): To reduce signs and symptoms, achieve clinical remission and mucosal healing and eliminate corticosteroid use in moderately to severely active UC inadequately responsive to conventional therapy

Mechanism of Action Infliximab is a chimeric monoclonal antibody that binds to human tumor necrosis factor alpha (TNFα), thereby interfering with endogenous TNFα activity. Biological activities of TNFα include the induction of proinflammatory cytokines (interleukins), enhancement of leukocyte migration, activation of neutrophils and eosinophils, and the induction of acute phase reactants and tissue degrading enzymes. Animal models have shown TNFα expression causes polyarthritis, and infliximab can prevent disease as well as allow diseased joints to heal.

Pharmacodynamics/Kinetics

Onset of action: Crohn's disease: ~2 weeks

Half-life elimination: 8-9.5 days

Contraindications Hypersensitivity to murine proteins or any component of the formulation; doses >5 mg/kg in patients with moderate or severe congestive heart failure (NYHA Class III/IV)

Warnings/Precautions Serious infections (including sepsis, pneumonia, and fatal infections) have been reported in patients receiving TNF-blocking agents. Many of the serious infections in patients treated with infliximab have occurred in patients on concomitant immunosuppressive therapy. Caution should be exercised when considering the use of infliximab in patients with a chronic infection or history of recurrent infection. Infliximab should not be given to patients with a clinically important, active infection. Patients who develop a new infection while undergoing treatment with infliximab should be monitored closely. If a patient develops a serious infection or sepsis, infliximab should be discontinued. Rare reactivation of hepatitis B has occurred in chronic virus carriers; evaluate prior to initiation and during treatment. Patients should be evaluated for latent tuberculosis infection with a tuberculin skin test prior to infliximab therapy. Treatment of latent tuberculosis should be initiated before infliximab is used. Tuberculosis (may be disseminated or extrapulmonary) has been reactivated in patients previously exposed to TB while on infliximab. Most cases have been reported within the first 3-6 months of treatment. Other opportunistic infections (eg, invasive fungal infections, listeriosis, *Pneumocystis*) have occurred during therapy. The risk/benefit ratio should be weighed in patients who have resided in regions where histoplasmosis is endemic.

Impact on the development and course of malignancies is not fully defined. As compared to the general population, an increased risk of lymphoma has been noted in clinical trials; however, rheumatoid arthritis has been previously associated with an increased rate of lymphoma.

Severe hepatic reactions have been reported during treatment. Use caution with CHF; if a decision is made to use with CHF, monitor closely and discontinue if exacerbated or new symptoms occur. Use caution with history of hematologic abnormalities; hematologic toxicities (eg, leukopenia, neutropenia, thrombocytopenia, pancytopenia) have been reported; discontinue if significant abnormalities occur. Autoimmune antibodies and a lupus-like syndrome have been reported. If antibodies to double-stranded DNA are confirmed in a patient with lupus-like symptoms, infliximab should be discontinued. Rare cases of optic neuritis and demyelinating disease have been reported; use with caution in patients with pre-existing or recent onset CNS demyelinating disorders, or seizures; discontinue if significant CNS adverse reactions develop.

Medications for the treatment of hypersensitivity reactions should be available for immediate use. Safety and efficacy for use in juvenile rheumatoid arthritis and in pediatric patients with Crohn's disease have not been established.

Drug Interactions Specific drug interaction studies have not been conducted

Abciximab: May increase potential for hypersensitivity reaction to infliximab, and may increase risk of thrombocytopenia and/or reduced therapeutic efficacy of infliximab.

Anakinra: Anti-TNF agents may increase the risk of serious infection when used in combination with anakinra. This effect has been observed with etanercept.

Vaccines, live: Concomitant use has not be studied; currently recommended not to administer live vaccines during infliximab therapy

Adverse Reactions Note: Although profile is similar, frequency of adverse effects may vary with disease state. Except where noted, percentages reported with rheumatoid arthritis:

>10%:

- Central nervous system: Headache (18%)
- Dermatologic: Rash (10%)
- Gastrointestinal: Nausea (21%), diarrhea (12%), abdominal pain (12%, Crohn's 26%)
- Genitourinary: Urinary tract infection (8%)
- Hepatic: ALT increased (risk increased with concomitant methotrexate)
- Local: Infusion reactions (20%)
- Neuromuscular & skeletal: Arthralgia (8%), back pain (8%)
- Respiratory: Upper respiratory tract infection (32%), cough (12%), sinusitis (14%), pharyngitis (12%)
- Miscellaneous: Development of antinuclear antibodies (~50%), infection (36%), development of antibodies to double-stranded DNA (17%); Crohn's patients with fistulizing disease: Development of new abscess (15%)

5% to 10%:

- Cardiovascular: Hypertension (7%)
- Central nervous system: Pain (8%), fatigue (9%), fever (7%)
- Dermatologic: Pruritus (7%)
- Gastrointestinal: Dyspepsia (10%)
- Respiratory: Bronchitis (10%), dyspnea (6%), rhinitis (8%)
- Miscellaneous: Moniliasis (5%)

<5% (Limited to important or life-threatening): Abscess, adult respiratory distress syndrome, allergic reaction, anaphylactic reactions, anemia, angioedema, arrhythmia, basal cell carcinoma, biliary pain, bradycardia, brain infarction, breast cancer, cardiac arrest, cellulitis, cholecystitis, cholelithiasis, circulatory failure, confusion, constipation, dehydration; demyelinating disorders (eg, multiple sclerosis, optic neuritis); diaphoresis increased, dizziness, drug-induced lupus-like syndrome, edema, gastrointestinal hemorrhage, Guillain-Barré syndrome, heart failure, hemolytic anemia, hepatitis, hepatitis B reactivation, hypersensitivity reactions, hypotension, ileus, interstitial fibrosis, interstitial pneumonitis, intervertebral disk herniation, intestinal obstruction, intestinal perforation, intestinal stenosis, jaundice, latent tuberculosis reactivation, leukopenia, liver failure, liver function tests increased, lymphadenopathy, lymphoma, meningitis, menstrual irregularity, metallic taste, MI, neuritis, neuropathy, neutropenia, pancreatitis, pancytopenia, pericardial effusion, peripheral neuropathy, peritonitis pleural effusion, pleurisy, pneumonia, proctalgia, pulmonary edema, pulmonary embolism, renal failure, respiratory insufficiency, seizure, sepsis, serum sickness, suicide attempt, syncope, tachycardia, tendon disorder, thrombocytopenia, thrombophlebitis (deep), ulceration, urticaria, vasculitis (systemic and cutaneous), worsening CHF

Overdosage/Toxicology Doses of up to 20 mg/kg have been given without toxic effects. In case of overdose, treatment should be symptom-directed and supportive.

(Continued)

Infliximab *(Continued)*

Dosing

Adults & Elderly:

Crohn's disease: I.V.:

Induction regimen: 5 mg/kg at 0, 2, and 6 weeks, followed by 5 mg/kg every 8 weeks; dose may be increased to 10 mg/kg in patients who respond but then lose their response. If no response by week 14, consider discontinuing therapy.

Psoriatic arthritis (with or without methotrexate): 5 mg/kg at 0,2, and 6 weeks, then every 8 weeks

Rheumatoid arthritis: I.V. (in combination with methotrexate therapy): 3 mg/kg at 0, 2, and 6 weeks then every 8 weeks thereafter; doses have ranged from 3-10 mg/kg intravenous infusion repeated at 4- to 8-week intervals

Ankylosing spondylitis: I.V.: 5 mg/kg at 0, 2, and 6 weeks, followed by 5 mg/kg every 6 weeks thereafter

Ulcerative colitis: I.V.: 5 mg/kg at 0, 2, and 6 weeks, followed by 5 mg/kg every 8 weeks thereafter

Dosage adjustment with CHF: Weigh risk versus benefits for individual patient:

NYHA Class III or IV: ≤5 mg/kg

Pediatrics: Safety and efficacy have not been established

Renal Impairment: No adjustment is recommended.

Hepatic Impairment: No adjustment necessary.

Available Dosage Forms Injection, powder for reconstitution [preservative free]: 100 mg

Nursing Guidelines

Assessment: Monitor therapeutic effectiveness and adverse reactions. Place and read PPD before initiation. Treatment of latent TB infection should be initiated prior to treatment with infliximab. Monitor for signs or symptoms of infection. Assess for signs of liver dysfunction (eg, unusual fatigue, easy bruising or bleeding, jaundice). Teach patient appropriate interventions to reduce side effects and adverse symptoms to report.

Patient Education: This drug can only be administered by infusion. Avoid receiving immunizations unless approved by prescriber. You will be more prone to infection. Avoid crowds and wash your hands frequently. Report headache or unusual fatigue; increased nausea or abdominal pain; bruising or bleeding easily; cough, runny nose, respiratory difficulty; chest pain or persistent dizziness; fatigue, muscle pain or weakness, back pain; fever or chills; mouth sores; vaginal itching or discharge; sore throat; unhealed sores; or frequent infections. **Breast-feeding precaution:** Breast-feeding is not recommended.

Pregnancy Risk Factor: B (manufacturer)

Pregnancy Issues: Reproduction studies have not been conducted. Use during pregnancy only if clearly needed. A Rheumatoid Arthritis and Pregnancy Registry has been established for women exposed to infliximab during pregnancy (Organization of Teratology Information Services, 877-311-8972).

Lactation: Excretion in breast milk unknown/not recommended

Breast-Feeding Considerations: It is not known whether infliximab is secreted in human milk. Because many immunoglobulins are secreted in milk and the potential for serious adverse reactions exists, a decision should be made whether to discontinue nursing or discontinue the drug, taking into account the importance of the drug to the mother.

Administration

I.V.: Infuse over at least 2 hours.

Reconstitution: Reconstitute vials with 10 mL sterile water for injection; swirl vial gently to dissolve powder, do not shake, allow solution to stand for 5 minutes; total dose of reconstituted product should be further diluted to 250 mL of 0.9% sodium chloride injection; infusion of dose should begin within 3 hours of preparation

Compatibility: Do not infuse with other agents.

Storage: Store vials at 2°C to 8°C (36°F to 46°F). Do not freeze.

♦ **Infliximab, Recombinant** *see* Infliximab *on page 910*

Influenza Virus Vaccine (in floo EN za VYE rus vak SEEN)

U.S. Brand Names Fluarix™; fluMist®; Fluvirin®; Fluzone®

Synonyms Influenza Virus Vaccine (Purified Surface Antigen); Influenza Virus Vaccine (Split-Virus); Influenza Virus Vaccine (Trivalent, Live); Live Attenuated Influenza Vaccine (LAIV); Trivalent Inactivated Influenza Vaccine (TIV)

Pharmacologic Category Vaccine

Medication Safety Issues

Sound-alike/look-alike issues:

Influenza virus vaccine may be confused with tetanus toxoid and tuberculin products. Medication errors have occurred when tuberculin skin tests (PPD) have been inadvertently administered instead of tetanus toxoid products and influenza virus vaccine. These products are refrigerated and often stored in close proximity to each other.

Use Provide active immunity to influenza virus strains contained in the vaccine

Groups at Increased Risk for Influenza-Related Complications: Recommendations for vaccination:

- Persons ≥65 years of age
- Residents of nursing homes and other chronic-care facilities that house persons of any age with chronic medical conditions
- Adults and children with chronic disorders of the pulmonary or cardiovascular systems, including children with asthma
- Adults and children who have required regular medical follow-up or hospitalization during the preceding year because of chronic metabolic diseases (including diabetes mellitus), renal dysfunction, hemoglobinopathies, or immunosuppression (including immunosuppression caused by medications or HIV)
- Adults and children with conditions which may compromise respiratory function, the handling of respiratory secretions, or that can increase the risk of aspiration (eg, cognitive dysfunction, spinal; cord injuries, seizure disorders, other neuromuscular disorders)
- Children and adolescents (6 months to 18 years of age) who are receiving long-term aspirin therapy and therefore, may be at risk for developing Reye's syndrome after influenza
- Women who will be pregnant during the influenza season
- Children 6-23 months of age

Vaccination is also recommended for persons 50-64 years of age, close contacts of children 0-23 months of age, healthy persons who may transmit influenza to those at risk, all healthcare workers, and persons who smoke.

Mechanism of Action Promotes immunity to influenza virus by inducing specific antibody production. Each year the formulation is standardized according to the U.S. Public Health Service. Preparations from previous seasons must not be used.

Pharmacodynamics/Kinetics

Onset: Protective antibody levels achieved ~2 weeks after vaccination

Duration: Protective antibody levels persist approximately ≥6 months

Contraindications Hypersensitivity to influenza virus vaccine, or any component of the formulation; presence of acute respiratory disease or other active infections or illnesses; active neurological disorder (immunization should be delayed)

In addition, for nasal spray: Patients at increased risk for influenza-related complications (see Use); history of Guillain-Barré syndrome; history of asthma or reactive airway disease; children 5-17 years of age receiving aspirin therapy; underlying medical conditions such as diabetes, renal dysfunction, cardiovascular disease, hemoglobinopathies; immunosuppressed or concomitant immunosuppressant therapy; pregnancy

Warnings/Precautions Antigenic response may not be as great as expected in patients requiring immunosuppressive drug or HIV-infected persons with <100 CD4 cells and with >30,000 viral copies of HIV type 1/mL; some products contain thimerosal, latex, or are manufactured with eggs and/or gentamicin; hypersensitivity reactions (presumably to egg proteins) may occur; because of potential for febrile reactions, risks and benefits must carefully be considered in patients with history of febrile convulsions; influenza vaccines from previous seasons must not be used. Inactivated vaccine is preferred over live virus vaccine for household members, healthcare workers and others coming in close contact with severely-immunosuppressed persons requiring care in a protected environment. Treatment for anaphylactic reactions (including epinephrine) should be readily available.

(Continued)

Influenza Virus Vaccine *(Continued)*

Injection: For I.M. use only; use caution with thrombocytopenia or any coagulation disorder. Safety and efficacy for use in children <6 months of age have not been established. Use caution with history of Guillain-Barré syndrome (GBS).

Nasal spray: For intranasal use only. **Avoid contact with severely immunocompromised individuals for at least 7 days following vaccination.** For use in healthy children and adults 5-49 years of age only; safety and efficacy for use in children <5 years or adults ≥50 years of age have not been established. Defer immunization if nasal congestion is present which may impede delivery of vaccine.

Drug Interactions

Aspirin: Concomitant use of aspirin and the nasal spray formulation may increase the risk of Reye syndrome in patients 5-17 years due to the presence of wild-type influenza in the preparation; concomitant use in this age group is contraindicated.

Immunosuppressive agents: Decreased effect of vaccine may occur.

Influenza antiviral agents (amantadine, oseltamivir, ribavirin, rimantadine, zanamivir): Safety and efficacy for use with influenza virus vaccine nasal spray have not been established. Do not administer nasal spray until 48 hours after stopping antiviral; do not administer antiviral for 2 weeks after receiving influenza virus vaccine nasal spray.

Vaccines: Some manufacturers and clinicians recommend that the flu vaccine not be administered concomitantly with DTP due to the potential for increased febrile reactions (specifically whole-cell pertussis) and that one should wait at least 3 days. However, ACIP recommends that children at high risk for influenza may get the vaccine concomitantly with DTP. Safety and efficacy of nasal spray with other vaccines have not been established; do not give within 1 month of other live virus vaccines or within 2 weeks of inactivated or subunit vaccines.

Adverse Reactions **All serious adverse reactions must be reported to the U.S. Department of Health and Human Services (DHHS) Vaccine Adverse Event Reporting System (VAERS) 1-800-822-7967.**

Injection: Frequency not defined:

- Central nervous system: Fever and malaise (may start within 6-12 hours and last 1-2 days; incidence equal to placebo in adults; occurs more frequently than placebo in children); GBS (previously reported with older vaccine formulations; relationship to current formulations not known, however, patients with history of GBS have a greater likelihood of developing GBS than those without)
- Dermatologic: Angioedema, urticaria
- Local: Tenderness, redness, or induration at the site of injection (10% to 64%; may last up to 2 days); injection site pain
- Neuromuscular & skeletal: Myalgia (may start within 6-12 hours and last 1-2 days; incidence equal to placebo in adults; occurs more frequently than placebo in children)
- Miscellaneous: Allergic or anaphylactoid reactions (most likely to residual egg protein; includes allergic asthma, angioedema, hives, systemic anaphylaxis)

Nasal spray: **Note:** Frequency of events reported within 10 days

>10%:

- Central nervous system: Headache (children 18% after first dose, < placebo after second dose; adults 40%) irritability (children 10% to 19%)
- Neuromuscular & skeletal: Tiredness/weakness (adults 26%), muscle aches (children 5% to 6%; adults 17%)
- Respiratory: Cough, nasal congestion/runny nose (children 46% to 48%; adults 9% to 45%), sore throat (children < placebo; adults 28%)
- Miscellaneous: Activity decreased (children 14% after first dose, < placebo after second dose)

1% to 10%:

- Central nervous system: Chills,
- Gastrointestinal: Abdominal pain, diarrhea, vomiting
- Otic: Otitis media

Dosing

Adults & Elderly: Optimal time to receive vaccine is October-November, prior to exposure to influenza; however, vaccination can continue into December and later as long as vaccine is available.

Immunization:

Fluarix™: I.M.: 0.5 mL/dose (1 dose per season)

Fluzone®, Fluvirin®: I.M.: 0.5 mL/dose (1 dose per season)

FluMist®: Intranasal: Adults ≤49 years: 0.5 mL/dose (1 dose per season)

Pediatrics: Optimal time to receive vaccine is October-November, prior to exposure to influenza; however, vaccination can continue into December and later as long as vaccine is available.

Immunization:

Fluzone®: I.M.:

Children 6-35 months: 0.25 mL/dose (1 or 2 doses per season; see **Note**)

Children 3-8 years: 0.5 mL/dose (1 or 2 doses per season; see **Note**)

Children ≥9 years: Refer to adult dosing.

Fluvirin®: I.M.:

Children 4-8 years: 0.5 mL/dose (1 or 2 doses per season; see **Note**)

Children ≥9 years: Refer to adult dosing.

Note: Previously unvaccinated children <9 years should receive 2 doses, given >1 month apart in order to achieve satisfactory antibody response.

fluMist®: Intranasal:

Children 5-8 years, previously **not vaccinated** with influenza vaccine: Initial season: Two 0.5 mL doses separated by 6-10 weeks

Children 5-8 years, previously **vaccinated** with influenza vaccine: 0.5 mL/dose (1 dose per season)

Children ≥9 years: Refer to adult dosing.

Available Dosage Forms

Injection, solution, purified split-virus surface antigen [preservative free] (Fluvirin®): (0.5 mL) [prefilled syringe; contains thimerosal (trace amounts); manufactured using neomycin and polymyxin]; (5 mL) [multidose vial; contains thimerosal; manufactured using neomycin and polymyxin]

Injection, suspension, purified split-virus [produced in chick embryo cell culture]:

Fluarix™ [preservative free]: (0.5 mL) [prefilled syringe; syringe cap and rubber plunger contain natural latex rubber; may contain residual amounts of thimerosal, hydrocortisone, gentamicin, and ovalbumin]

Fluzone®: (5 mL) [vial; contains thimerosal]

Fluzone® [preservative free]: (0.25 mL) [prefilled syringe]; (0.5 mL) [vial]

Solution, nasal spray, trivalent, live virus [preservative free] (fluMist®): (0.5 mL) [manufactured using eggs and gentamicin]

Nursing Guidelines

Patient Education: You may experience the following: Soreness or swelling at injection site, fever, or achiness; some effects may last 1-2 days. Notify your prescriber immediately if these persist or become severe, or if you develop a high fever, allergic reaction (respiratory difficulty, hives, weakness, dizziness, fast heart beat), or have seizures. Prior to vaccination, notify prescriber if you are allergic to eggs (hives, swelling of lip and/or tongue, respiratory difficulty after eating eggs).

Pregnancy Risk Factor: C

Pregnancy Issues: Reproduction studies have not been conducted. Case reports and limited studies suggest pregnancy may increase the risk of serious medical complications from influenza infection. Vaccination is recommended regardless of stage of pregnancy.

Breast-Feeding Considerations: Use of influenza vaccine has not been shown to affect the safety of breast-feeding mothers or their infants. The use of the nasal spray (live virus vaccine) should be used with caution due to the possibility of viral shedding from mother to infant.

Administration

I.M.: For I.M. administration only. Inspect for particulate matter and discoloration prior to administration. Adults and older children should be vaccinated in the deltoid muscle. Infants and young children should be vaccinated in the anterolateral aspect of the thigh. Suspensions should be shaken well prior to use.

For patients at risk of hemorrhage following intramuscular injection, the ACIP recommends "it should be administered intramuscularly if, in the opinion of the physician familiar with the patients bleeding risk, the vaccine can be administered with reasonable safety by this route. If the patient receives antihemophilia or other similar therapy, intramuscular vaccination can be scheduled shortly after such therapy is administered. A fine needle (23 gauge or smaller) can be used for the vaccination and firm pressure applied to the site (without rubbing) for at least 2 minutes. The patient should be instructed concerning the risk of hematoma from the injection."

(Continued)

Influenza Virus Vaccine *(Continued)*

Storage:

Injection: Store between 2°C to 8°C (36°F to 46°F). Potency is destroyed by freezing; do not use if product has been frozen.

Fluarix™: Protect from light.

Nasal spray: Store in a freezer at or below -15°C (5°F); may thaw in refrigerator and store at 2°C to 8°C (36°F to 46°F) ≤60 hours; must be used within 24 hours after removal from the freezer; do not refreeze after thawing.

- ♦ **Influenza Virus Vaccine (Purified Surface Antigen)** *see* Influenza Virus Vaccine *on page 913*
- ♦ **Influenza Virus Vaccine (Split-Virus)** *see* Influenza Virus Vaccine *on page 913*
- ♦ **Influenza Virus Vaccine (Trivalent, Live)** *see* Influenza Virus Vaccine *on page 913*
- ♦ **Infumorph®** *see* Morphine Sulfate *on page 1177*
- ♦ **Infuvite® Adult** *see* Vitamins (Multiple/Injectable) *on page 1719*
- ♦ **Infuvite® Pediatric** *see* Vitamins (Multiple/Injectable) *on page 1719*
- ♦ **INH** *see* Isoniazid *on page 972*
- ♦ **Innohep®** *see* Tinzaparin *on page 1636*
- ♦ **InnoPran XL™** *see* Propranolol *on page 1429*
- ♦ **Insta-Glucose® [OTC]** *see* Dextrose *on page 511*
- ♦ **Instat™** *see* Collagen Hemostat *on page 449*
- ♦ **Instat™ MCH** *see* Collagen Hemostat *on page 449*

Insulin Aspart (IN soo lin AS part)

U.S. Brand Names NovoLog®

Synonyms Aspart Insulin

Pharmacologic Category Antidiabetic Agent, Insulin

Medication Safety Issues

Sound-alike/look-alike issues:

NovoLog® may be confused with Novolin®

NovoLog® Mix 70/30 may be confused with NovoLog®

High alert medication: The Institute for Safe Medication Practices (ISMP) includes this medication among its list of drugs which have a heightened risk of causing significant patient harm when used in error. ***Due to the number of insulin preparations, it is essential to identify/clarify the type of insulin to be used.***

Use Treatment of type 1 diabetes mellitus (insulin dependent, IDDM); type 2 diabetes mellitus (noninsulin dependent, NIDDM) to control hyperglycemia

Mechanism of Action Refer to Insulin Regular monograph *on page 928.* Insulin aspart is a rapid-acting insulin analog.

Pharmacodynamics/Kinetics

Onset of action: 0.2-0.5 hours

Duration: 3-5 hours

Time to peak: 1-3 hours

Excretion: Urine

Contraindications Hypersensitivity to any component of the formulation

Warnings/Precautions Refer to Insulin Regular *on page 928.*

In type 1 diabetes mellitus (insulin dependent, IDDM), insulin lispro (Humalog®) and insulin glulisine (Apidra™) should be used in combination with a long-acting insulin. However, in type 2 diabetes mellitus (noninsulin dependent, NIDDM), insulin lispro (Humalog®) may be used without a long-acting insulin when used in combination with a sulfonylurea.

Drug Interactions Refer to Insulin Regular *on page 928.*

Nutritional/Herbal/Ethanol Interactions Refer to Insulin Regular *on page 928.*

Adverse Reactions Refer to Insulin Regular *on page 928.*

Overdosage/Toxicology Refer to Insulin Regular *on page 928.*

Dosing

Adults & Elderly: Refer to Insulin Regular *on page 928.* Insulin aspart is a rapid-acting insulin analog which is normally administered as a a premeal component of the insulin regimen. It is normally used along with a long-acting (basal) form of insulin.

Pediatrics: Refer to Insulin Regular *on page 928*.

Renal Impairment: Insulin requirements are reduced due to changes in insulin clearance or metabolism.

Available Dosage Forms Injection, solution (NovoLog®): 100 units/mL (3 mL) [FlexPen® prefilled syringe or PenFill® prefilled cartridge]; (10 mL) [vial]

Nursing Guidelines

Assessment: Assess potential for interactions with other prescriptions, OTC medications, or herbal products patient may be taking. Assess results of laboratory tests, therapeutic effectiveness, and adverse response (eg, hypoglycemia) at regular intervals during therapy. Teach patient proper use, including appropriate injection technique and syringe/needle disposal and monitoring requirements (or refer to diabetic educator), possible side effects/appropriate interventions, and adverse symptoms to report.

Monitoring Laboratory Tests: Urine sugar and acetone, serum glucose, electrolytes, Hb A_{1c}, lipid profile; when used intravenously, close monitoring of serum glucose and potassium are required to avoid hypoglycemia and/or hypokalemia

Dietary Considerations: Dietary modification based on ADA recommendations is a key component of therapy.

Patient Education: Do not take any new medication during therapy unless approved by prescriber. This medication is used to control diabetes; it is not a cure. It is imperative to follow other components of prescribed treatment (eg, diet and exercise regimen). Take exactly as directed. Do not change dose or discontinue unless advised by prescriber. With insulin aspart (NovoLog®), you must start eating within 5-10 minutes after injection. If you experience hypoglycemic reaction, contact prescriber immediately. Always carry quick source of sugar with you. Monitor glucose levels as directed by prescriber. Report adverse side effects, including chest pain or palpitations; persistent fatigue, confusion, headache; skin rash or redness; numbness of mouth, lips, or tongue; muscle weakness or tremors; vision changes; respiratory difficulty; or nausea, vomiting, or flu-like symptoms. **Pregnancy precaution:** Inform prescriber if you are or intend to become pregnant.

Geriatric Considerations: How "tightly" a geriatric patient's blood glucose should be controlled is controversial; however, a fasting blood sugar <150 mg/dL is now an acceptable end point. Such a decision should be based on the patient's functional and cognitive status, how well he/she recognizes hypoglycemic or hyperglycemic symptoms, and how to respond to them and any other disease states. Patients who are unable to accurately draw up their dose will need assistance such as prefilled syringes. Initial doses may require considerations for renal function in the elderly with dosing adjusted subsequently based on blood glucose monitoring.

Pregnancy Risk Factor: C

Pregnancy Issues: Does not cross the placenta. Insulin is the drug of choice for control of diabetes mellitus during pregnancy.

Lactation: Excretion in breast milk unknown/compatible

Breast-Feeding Considerations: Endogenous insulin has been detected in breast milk. The gastrointestinal tract destroys insulin when administered orally; therefore, would not be expected to be absorbed intact by the breast-feeding infant.

Administration

I.V.: Insulin aspart may be administered I.V. in selected clinical situations to control hyperglycemia. Appropriate medical supervision is required. May be diluted to a concentration between 0.05 and 1 unit/mL with NS, D_5W, or $D_{10}W$ with 40 mmol/L potassium chloride.

Storage: Insulin aspart (NovoLog®): Store unopened container in refrigerator; do not use if it has been frozen. If not refrigerated, use within 28 days and protect from heat and light. Once opened (in use), vials may be stored in refrigerator or for up to 28 days at room temperature. Cartridges that are in use should be stored at room temperature and used within 28 days; do not refrigerate. Insulin in reservoir should be replaced every 48 hours. Discard if exposed to temperatures ≥37°C (98.6°F).

Related Information

Insulin Regular *on page 928*

♦ **Insulin Aspart and Insulin Aspart Protamine** *see* Insulin Aspart Protamine and Insulin Aspart *on page 918*

Insulin Aspart Protamine and Insulin Aspart

(IN soo lin AS part PROE ta meen & IN soo lin AS part)

U.S. Brand Names NovoLog® Mix 70/30

Synonyms Insulin Aspart and Insulin Aspart Protamine

Pharmacologic Category Antidiabetic Agent, Insulin

Medication Safety Issues

Sound-alike/look-alike issues:

NovoLog® Mix 70/30 may be confused with Novolin® 70/30

High alert medication: The Institute for Safe Medication Practices (ISMP) includes this medication among its list of drugs which have a heightened risk of causing significant patient harm when used in error. ***Due to the number of insulin preparations, it is essential to identify/clarify the type of insulin to be used.***

Use Treatment of type 1 diabetes mellitus (insulin dependent, IDDM); type 2 diabetes mellitus (noninsulin dependent, NIDDM) to control hyperglycemia

Mechanism of Action Refer to Insulin Regular *on page 928*. Insulin aspart protamine and insulin aspart is a combination insulin product with intermediate-acting characteristics. Normally administered twice daily.

Pharmacodynamics/Kinetics

Onset of action: 0.2 hours

Duration: 18-24 hours

Half-life: 8-9 hours

Time to peak: 1-4 hours

Excretion: Urine

Contraindications Hypersensitivity to any component of the formulation; during episodes of hypoglycemia

Warnings/Precautions Refer to Insulin Regular *on page 928*. Safety and efficacy of this insulin product have not been established in pediatric patients.

In type 1 diabetes mellitus (insulin dependent, IDDM), insulin lispro (Humalog®) and insulin glulisine (Apidra™) should be used in combination with a long-acting insulin. However, in type 2 diabetes mellitus (noninsulin dependent, NIDDM), insulin lispro (Humalog®) may be used without a long-acting insulin when used in combination with a sulfonylurea.

Adverse Reactions Refer to Insulin Regular *on page 928*.

Dosing

Adults & Elderly: Refer to Insulin Regular *on page 928*. Fixed insulins (such as insulin aspart protamine and insulin aspart combination) are normally administered in 2 daily doses.

Renal Impairment: Insulin requirements are reduced due to changes in insulin clearance or metabolism.

Available Dosage Forms Injection, suspension (NovoLog® Mix 70/30): Insulin aspart protamine suspension 70% [intermediate acting] and insulin aspart solution 30% [rapid acting]: 100 units/mL (3 mL) [PenFill® prefilled cartridge or FlexPen® prefilled syringe]; (10 mL) [vial]

Nursing Guidelines

Geriatric Considerations: How "tightly" a geriatric patient's blood glucose should be controlled is controversial; however, a fasting blood sugar <150 mg/dL is now an acceptable end point. Such a decision should be based on the patient's functional and cognitive status, how well he/she recognizes hypoglycemic or hyperglycemic symptoms, and how to respond to them and any other disease states. Patients who are unable to accurately draw up their dose will need assistance such as prefilled syringes. Initial doses may require considerations for renal function in the elderly with dosing adjusted subsequently based on blood glucose monitoring.

Pregnancy Risk Factor: C

Pregnancy Issues: Reproduction studies have not been conducted with this combination. Does not cross the placenta. Insulin is the drug of choice for control of diabetes mellitus during pregnancy.

Lactation: Excretion in breast milk unknown/compatible

Breast-Feeding Considerations: Endogenous insulin has been detected in breast milk. The gastrointestinal tract destroys insulin when administered orally; therefore, would not be expected to be absorbed intact by the breast-feeding infant.

Administration

Storage: NovoLog® Mix 70/30: Store unopened container in refrigerator. Do not use if frozen. If refrigeration is not possible, vial (in use) may be stored at room temperature for up to 28 days. The pen in use should **not** be refrigerated, store below 30°C (86°F) away from direct heat or light; discard after 14 days. If refrigeration is not available, opened vials may be stored unrefrigerated in cool place away from heat and sunlight.

Related Information

Insulin Regular *on page 928*

Insulin Detemir (IN soo lin DE te mir)

U.S. Brand Names Levemir®

Synonyms Detemir Insulin

Pharmacologic Category Antidiabetic Agent, Insulin

Medication Safety Issues

High alert medication: The Institute for Safe Medication Practices (ISMP) includes this medication among its list of drugs which have a heightened risk of causing significant patient harm when used in error. ***Due to the number of insulin preparations, it is essential to identify/clarify the type of insulin to be used.***

Use Treatment of type 1 diabetes mellitus (insulin dependent, IDDM); type 2 diabetes mellitus (noninsulin dependent, NIDDM) to control hyperglycemia

Mechanism of Action Refer to Insulin Regular *on page 928*. Insulin detemir is an intermediate-acting insulin analog.

Pharmacodynamics/Kinetics

Onset of action: 3-4 hours

Duration: 6-23 hours

Bioavailability: 60%

Time to peak: 6-8 hours

Excretion: Urine

Contraindications Hypersensitivity to any component of the formulation

Warnings/Precautions Refer to Insulin Regular *on page 928*. Safety and efficacy not established in children <6 years of age.

In type 1 diabetes mellitus (insulin dependent, IDDM), insulin lispro (Humalog®) and insulin glulisine (Apidra™) should be used in combination with a long-acting insulin. However, in type 2 diabetes mellitus (noninsulin dependent, NIDDM), insulin lispro (Humalog®) may be used without a long-acting insulin when used in combination with a sulfonylurea.

Drug Interactions Refer to Insulin Regular *on page 928*.

Nutritional/Herbal/Ethanol Interactions Refer to Insulin Regular *on page 928*.

Adverse Reactions Refer to Insulin Regular *on page 928*.

Overdosage/Toxicology Refer to Insulin Regular *on page 928*.

Dosing

Adults & Elderly: Also refer to Insulin Regular *on page 928*.

Type 1 or type 2 diabetes:

Basal insulin or basal-bolus: May be substituted on a unit-per-unit basis

Insulin-naive patients (type 2 diabetes only): 0.1-0.2 units/kg once daily in the evening or 10 units once or twice daily. Adjust dose to achieve glycemic targets.

Renal Impairment: Insulin requirements are reduced due to changes in insulin clearance or metabolism.

Available Dosage Forms Injection, solution (Levemir®): 100 units/mL (3 mL) [Innolet® prefilled syringe, Penfill® prefilled cartridge, or FlexPen® prefilled syringe]; (10 mL) [vial]

Nursing Guidelines

Assessment: Assess potential for interactions with other prescriptions, OTC medications, or herbal products patient may be taking. Assess results of laboratory tests, therapeutic effectiveness, and adverse response (eg, hypoglycemia) at regular intervals during therapy. Teach patient proper use, including appropriate injection technique and syringe/needle disposal and monitoring requirements (or refer to diabetic educator), possible side effects/appropriate interventions, and adverse symptoms to report.

Monitoring Laboratory Tests: Urine sugar and acetone, serum glucose, electrolytes, Hb A_{1c}, lipid profile

Dietary Considerations: Dietary modification based on ADA recommendations is a key component of therapy.

(Continued)

Insulin Detemir *(Continued)*

Patient Education: Do not take any new medication during therapy unless approved by prescriber. This medication is used to control diabetes; it is not a cure. It is imperative to follow other components of prescribed treatment (eg, diet and exercise regimen). Take exactly as directed. Do not change dose or discontinue unless advised by prescriber. If you experience hypoglycemic reaction, contact prescriber immediately. Always carry quick source of sugar with you. Monitor glucose levels as directed by prescriber. Report adverse side effects, including chest pain or palpitations; persistent fatigue, confusion, headache; skin rash or redness; numbness of mouth, lips, or tongue; muscle weakness or tremors; vision changes; respiratory difficulty; or nausea, vomiting, or flu-like symptoms. **Pregnancy precaution:** Inform prescriber if you are or intend to become pregnant.

Geriatric Considerations: How "tightly" a geriatric patient's blood glucose should be controlled is controversial; however, a fasting blood sugar <150 mg/dL is now an acceptable end point. Such a decision should be based on the patient's functional and cognitive status, how well he/she recognizes hypoglycemic or hyperglycemic symptoms, and how to respond to them and any other disease states. Patients who are unable to accurately draw up their dose will need assistance such as prefilled syringes. Initial doses may require considerations for renal function in the elderly with dosing adjusted subsequently based on blood glucose monitoring.

Pregnancy Risk Factor: C

Pregnancy Issues: Does not cross the placenta. Insulin is the drug of choice for control of diabetes mellitus during pregnancy.

Lactation: Excretion in breast milk unknown/compatible

Breast-Feeding Considerations: Endogenous insulin may be excreted in breast milk. The gastrointestinal tract destroys insulin when administered orally; therefore, would not be expected to be absorbed intact by the breast-feeding infant.

Administration

Storage: Insulin detemir (Levemir®): Store unopened container in refrigerator; do not use if it has been frozen. Once opened (in use), vials may be stored in refrigerator or for up to 42 days at room temperature (below 30°C). Cartridges and prefilled syringes that are in use should be stored at room temperature and used within 42 days; do not refrigerate. Do not store with needle in place. All opened (in-use) vials should be stored away from direct heat and sunlight.

Related Information

Insulin Regular *on page 928*

Insulin Glargine (IN soo lin GLAR jeen)

U.S. Brand Names Lantus®

Synonyms Glargine Insulin

Pharmacologic Category Antidiabetic Agent, Insulin

Medication Safety Issues

Sound-alike/look-alike issues:

Lantus® may be confused with Lente®

Lente® may be confused with Lantus®

High alert medication: The Institute for Safe Medication Practices (ISMP) includes this medication among its list of drugs which have a heightened risk of causing significant patient harm when used in error. ***Due to the number of insulin preparations, it is essential to identify/clarify the type of insulin to be used.***

Use Treatment of type 1 diabetes mellitus (insulin dependent, IDDM); type 2 diabetes mellitus (noninsulin dependent, NIDDM) requiring basal (long-acting) insulin to control hyperglycemia

Mechanism of Action Refer to Insulin Regular *on page 928*. Insulin glargine is a long-acting insulin analog.

Pharmacodynamics/Kinetics

Onset of action: 3-4 hours

Duration: 24 hours

Absorption: Slow; forms microprecipitates which allow small amounts to release over time

Metabolism: Partially metabolized in the skin to form teo active metabolites

Time to peak: No pronounced peak

Excretion: Urine

Contraindications Hypersensitivity to any component of the formulation

Warnings/Precautions Refer to Insulin Regular *on page 928*. Safety and efficacy not established in children <6 years of age.

In type 1 diabetes mellitus (insulin dependent, IDDM), insulin lispro (Humalog®) and insulin glulisine (Apidra™) should be used in combination with a long-acting insulin. However, in type 2 diabetes mellitus (noninsulin dependent, NIDDM), insulin lispro (Humalog®) may be used without a long-acting insulin when used in combination with a sulfonylurea.

Drug Interactions Refer to Insulin Regular *on page 928*.

Nutritional/Herbal/Ethanol Interactions Refer to Insulin Regular *on page 928*.

Adverse Reactions Refer to Insulin Regular *on page 928*.

Overdosage/Toxicology Refer to Insulin Regular *on page 928*.

Dosing

Adults & Elderly: SubQ:

Type 1 diabetes: Refer to Insulin Regular *on page 928*.

Type 2 diabetes:

Patient not already on insulin: 10 units once daily, adjusted according to patient response (range in clinical study: 2-100 units/day)

Patient already receiving insulin: In clinical studies, when changing to insulin glargine from once-daily NPH or Ultralente® insulin, the initial dose was not changed; when changing from twice-daily NPH to once-daily insulin glargine, the total daily dose was reduced by 20% and adjusted according to patient response

Pediatrics: Refer to adult dosing.

Renal Impairment: Insulin requirements are reduced due to changes in insulin clearance or metabolism.

Available Dosage Forms Injection, solution (Lantus®): 100 units/mL (3 mL) [cartridge]; (10 mL) [vial]

Nursing Guidelines

Assessment: Assess potential for interactions with other prescriptions, OTC medications, or herbal products patient may be taking. Assess results of laboratory tests, therapeutic effectiveness, and adverse reactions (eg, hypoglycemia) at regular intervals during therapy. Teach patient proper use, including appropriate injection technique and syringe/needle disposal and monitoring requirements (or refer to diabetic educator), possible side effects/appropriate interventions, and adverse symptoms to report.

Monitoring Laboratory Tests: Urine sugar and acetone, serum glucose, electrolytes, Hb A_{1c}, lipid profile

Patient Education: Do not take any new medication during therapy unless approved by prescriber. This medication is used to control diabetes; it is not a cure. It is imperative to follow other components of prescribed treatment (eg, diet and exercise regimen). Take exactly as directed. Do not change dose or discontinue unless advised by prescriber. If you experience hypoglycemic reaction, contact prescriber immediately. Always carry quick source of sugar with you. Monitor glucose levels as directed by prescriber. Report adverse side effects, including chest pain or palpitations; persistent fatigue, confusion, headache; skin rash or redness; numbness of mouth, lips, or tongue; muscle weakness or tremors; vision changes; respiratory difficulty; or nausea, vomiting, or flu-like symptoms. **Pregnancy precaution:** Inform prescriber if you are or intend to become pregnant.

Pregnancy Risk Factor: C

Pregnancy Issues: Does not cross the placenta. Insulin is the drug of choice for control of diabetes mellitus during pregnancy.

Lactation: Excretion in breast milk unknown/compatible

Breast-Feeding Considerations: Endogenous insulin may be found in breast milk. The gastrointestinal tract destroys insulin when administered orally; therefore, would not be expected to be absorbed intact by the breast-feeding infant.

Administration

Storage: Insulin glargine (Lantus®): Store unopened container in refrigerator; do not use if it has been frozen. If not refrigerated, use within 28 days and protect from heat and light. Once opened (in use), vials may be stored in refrigerator or for up to 28 days at room temperature. Cartridges in use should be stored at room temperature and used within 28 days.

Related Information

Insulin Regular *on page 928*

Insulin Glulisine (IN soo lin gloo LIS een)

U.S. Brand Names Apidra™

Synonyms Glulisine Insulin

Pharmacologic Category Antidiabetic Agent, Insulin

Medication Safety Issues

High alert medication: The Institute for Safe Medication Practices (ISMP) includes this medication among its list of drugs which have a heightened risk of causing significant patient harm when used in error. ***Due to the number of insulin preparations, it is essential to identify/clarify the type of insulin to be used.***

Use Treatment of type 1 diabetes mellitus (insulin dependent, IDDM); type 2 diabetes mellitus (noninsulin dependent, NIDDM) to control hyperglycemia

Mechanism of Action Refer to Insulin Regular *on page 928*. Insulin glulisine is a rapid-acting insulin analog.

Pharmacodynamics/Kinetics

Onset of action: 0.2-0.5 hours

Duration: 3-4 hours

Time to Peak: 30-90 minutes

Excretion: Urine

Contraindications Hypersensitivity to any component of the formulation

Warnings/Precautions Refer to Insulin Regular *on page 928*.

In type 1 diabetes mellitus (insulin dependent, IDDM), insulin lispro (Humalog®) and insulin glulisine (Apidra™) should be used in combination with a long-acting insulin. However, in type 2 diabetes mellitus (noninsulin dependent, NIDDM), insulin lispro (Humalog®) may be used without a long-acting insulin when used in combination with a sulfonylurea.

Drug Interactions Refer to Insulin Regular *on page 928*.

Nutritional/Herbal/Ethanol Interactions Refer to Insulin Regular *on page 928*.

Adverse Reactions Refer to Insulin Regular *on page 928*.

Overdosage/Toxicology Refer to Insulin Regular *on page 928*.

Dosing

Adults & Elderly: Refer to Insulin Regular *on page 928*.

Pediatrics: Refer to Insulin Regular *on page 928*.

Renal Impairment: Insulin requirements are reduced due to changes in insulin clearance or metabolism.

Available Dosage Forms Injection, solution (Apidra™): 100 units/mL (10 mL) [vial]

Nursing Guidelines

Assessment: Assess potential for interactions with other prescriptions, OTC medications, or herbal products patient may be taking. Assess results of laboratory tests, therapeutic effectiveness, and adverse reactions (eg, hypoglycemia) at regular intervals during therapy. Teach patient proper use, including appropriate injection technique and syringe/needle disposal and monitoring requirements (or refer to diabetic educator), possible side effects/appropriate interventions, and adverse symptoms to report.

Monitoring Laboratory Tests: Urine sugar and acetone, serum glucose, electrolytes, Hb A_{1c}, lipid profile

Patient Education: Do not take any new medication during therapy unless approved by prescriber. This medication is used to control diabetes; it is not a cure. It is imperative to follow other components of prescribed treatment (eg, diet and exercise regimen). Take exactly as directed. Do not change dose or discontinue unless advised by prescriber. Insulin glulisine (Apidra™) should be administered within 15 minutes before or within 20 minutes after start of a meal. If you experience hypoglycemic reaction, contact prescriber immediately. Always carry quick source of sugar with you. Monitor glucose levels as directed by prescriber. Report adverse side effects, including chest pain or palpitations; persistent fatigue, confusion, headache; skin rash or redness; numbness of mouth, lips, or tongue; muscle weakness or tremors; vision changes; respiratory difficulty; or nausea, vomiting, or flu-like symptoms. **Pregnancy precaution:** Inform prescriber if you are or intend to become pregnant.

Geriatric Considerations: How "tightly" a geriatric patient's blood glucose should be controlled is controversial; however, a fasting blood sugar <150 mg/dL is now an acceptable end point. Such a decision should be based on the patient's functional and cognitive status, how well he/she recognizes hypoglycemic or hyperglycemic symptoms, and how to respond to them and any other disease states. Patients who are unable to accurately draw up their dose will need assistance such as prefilled syringes. Initial doses may require considerations for renal function in the elderly with dosing adjusted subsequently based on blood glucose monitoring.

Pregnancy Risk Factor: C

Pregnancy Issues: Does not cross the placenta. Insulin is the drug of choice for control of diabetes mellitus during pregnancy.

Lactation: Excretion in breast milk unknown/compatible

Breast-Feeding Considerations: Endogenous insulin has been detected in breast milk. The gastrointestinal tract destroys insulin when administered orally; therefore, would not be expected to be absorbed intact by the breast-feeding infant.

Administration

Storage: Insulin glulisine (Apidra™): Store unopened vials in refrigerator at 2°C to 8°C (36°F to 46°F); do not freeze. Once opened, may store under refrigeration or at room temperature ≤25°C (77°F); use within 28 days. Stable in infusion pump for up to 48 hours. Discard if exposed to temperatures >37°C (98.6°F).

Related Information

Insulin Regular *on page 928*

Insulin Lispro (IN soo lin LYE sproe)

U.S. Brand Names Humalog®

Synonyms Lispro Insulin

Pharmacologic Category Antidiabetic Agent, Insulin

Medication Safety Issues

Sound-alike/look-alike issues:

Humalog® may be confused with Humulin®, Humira®

High alert medication: The Institute for Safe Medication Practices (ISMP) includes this medication among its list of drugs which have a heightened risk of causing significant patient harm when used in error. ***Due to the number of insulin preparations, it is essential to identify/clarify the type of insulin to be used.***

Use Treatment of type 1 diabetes mellitus (insulin dependent, IDDM); type 2 diabetes mellitus (noninsulin dependent, NIDDM) to control hyperglycemia

Note: In type 1 diabetes mellitus (insulin dependent, IDDM), insulin lispro (Humalog®) should be used in combination with a long-acting insulin. However, in type 2 diabetes mellitus (noninsulin dependent, NIDDM), insulin lispro (Humalog®) may be used without a long-acting insulin when used in combination with a sulfonylurea.

Mechanism of Action Refer to Insulin Regular *on page 928*. Insulin lispro is a rapid-acting form of insulin.

Pharmacodynamics/Kinetics

Onset of action: 0.2-0.5 hours

Duration: 3-4 hours

Distribution: 0.26-0.36 L/kg

Bioavailability: 55% to 77%

Time to peak: 30-90 minutes

Excretion: Urine

Contraindications Hypersensitivity to any component of the formulation

Warnings/Precautions Refer to Insulin Regular *on page 928*.

In type 1 diabetes mellitus (insulin dependent, IDDM), insulin lispro (Humalog®) and insulin glulisine (Apidra™) should be used in combination with a long-acting insulin. However, in type 2 diabetes mellitus (noninsulin dependent, NIDDM), insulin lispro (Humalog®) may be used without a long-acting insulin when used in combination with a sulfonylurea.

Drug Interactions Refer to Insulin Regular *on page 928*.

Nutritional/Herbal/Ethanol Interactions Refer to Insulin Regular *on page 928*.

Adverse Reactions Refer to Insulin Regular *on page 928*.

Overdosage/Toxicology Refer to Insulin Regular *on page 928*.

Dosing

Adults & Elderly: Refer to Insulin Regular *on page 928*. Insulin lispro is equipotent to insulin regular, but has a more rapid onset.

Pediatrics: Refer to Insulin Regular *on page 928*. Insulin lispro is equipotent to insulin regular, but has a more rapid onset.

(Continued)

Insulin Lispro *(Continued)*

Renal Impairment: Insulin requirements are reduced due to changes in insulin clearance or metabolism.

Available Dosage Forms Injection, solution (Humalog®): 100 units/mL (3 mL) [prefilled cartridge or prefilled disposable pen]; (10 mL) [vial]

Nursing Guidelines

Assessment: Assess potential for interactions with other prescriptions, OTC medications, or herbal products patient may be taking. Assess results of laboratory tests, therapeutic effectiveness, and adverse reactions (eg, hypoglycemia) at regular intervals during therapy. Teach patient proper use, including appropriate injection technique and syringe/needle disposal and monitoring requirements (or refer to diabetic educator), possible side effects/appropriate interventions, and adverse symptoms to report.

Monitoring Laboratory Tests: Urine sugar and acetone, serum glucose, electrolytes, Hb A_{1c}, lipid profile

Dietary Considerations: Dietary modification based on ADA recommendations is a key component of therapy.

Patient Education: Do not take any new medication during therapy unless approved by prescriber. This medication is used to control diabetes; it is not a cure. It is imperative to follow other components of prescribed treatment (eg, diet and exercise regimen). Take exactly as directed. Do not change dose or discontinue unless advised by prescriber. If you experience hypoglycemic reaction, contact prescriber immediately. Always carry quick source of sugar with you. Monitor glucose levels as directed by prescriber. Report adverse side effects, including chest pain or palpitations; persistent fatigue, confusion, headache; skin rash or redness; numbness of mouth, lips, or tongue; muscle weakness or tremors; vision changes; respiratory difficulty; or nausea, vomiting, or flu-like symptoms. **Pregnancy precaution:** Inform prescriber if you are or intend to become pregnant.

Geriatric Considerations: How "tightly" a geriatric patient's blood glucose should be controlled is controversial; however, a fasting blood sugar <150 mg/dL is now an acceptable end point. Such a decision should be based on the patient's functional and cognitive status, how well he/she recognizes hypoglycemic or hyperglycemic symptoms, and how to respond to them and any other disease states. Patients who are unable to accurately draw up their dose will need assistance such as prefilled syringes. Initial doses may require considerations for renal function in the elderly with dosing adjusted subsequently based on blood glucose monitoring.

Pregnancy Risk Factor: B

Pregnancy Issues: Does not cross the placenta. Insulin is the drug of choice for control of diabetes mellitus during pregnancy.

Lactation: Excretion in breast milk unknown/compatible

Breast-Feeding Considerations: Endogenous insulin can be found in breast milk. The gastrointestinal tract destroys insulin when administered orally; therefore, would not be expected to be absorbed intact by the breast-feeding infant.

Administration

Storage: Insulin lispro (Humalog®): Store unopened container in refrigerator; do not use if it has been frozen. If not refrigerated, use within 28 days and protect from heat and light. Once opened (in use), vials may be stored in refrigerator or for up to 28 days at room temperature. Cartridges/pens should be stored at room temperature and used within 28 days. When used in an external pump, replace insulin in reservoir within 48 hours and cartridges within 7 days; do not expose to temperatures >37°C (98.6°F). If diluted with sterile diluent (available from manufacturer), 1:10 dilutions are stable for 28 days stored at 5°C (41°F) or 14 days stored at 30°C (86°F).

Related Information

Insulin Regular *on page 928*

♦ **Insulin Lispro and Insulin Lispro Protamine** *see* Insulin Lispro Protamine and Insulin Lispro *on page 925*

Insulin Lispro Protamine and Insulin Lispro

(IN soo lin LYE sproe PROE ta meen & IN soo lin LYE sproe)

U.S. Brand Names Humalog® Mix 75/25™

Synonyms Insulin Lispro and Insulin Lispro Protamine

Pharmacologic Category Antidiabetic Agent, Insulin

Medication Safety Issues

Sound-alike/look-alike issues:

Humalog® Mix 75/25™ may be confused with Humulin® 70/30.

High alert medication: The Institute for Safe Medication Practices (ISMP) includes this medication among its list of drugs which have a heightened risk of causing significant patient harm when used in error. ***Due to the number of insulin preparations, it is essential to identify/clarify the type of insulin to be used.***

Use Treatment of type 1 diabetes mellitus (insulin dependent, IDDM); type 2 diabetes mellitus (noninsulin dependent, NIDDM) to control hyperglycemia

Mechanism of Action Refer to Insulin Regular *on page 928*. Insulin lispro protamine and insulin lispro is a combination product with a rapid onset, and a duration of action which is similar to intermediate-acting insulin products.

Pharmacodynamics/Kinetics

Onset of action: 0.2-0.5 hours

Duration: 18-24 hours

Time to peak: 2-12 hours

Excretion: Urine

Contraindications Hypersensitivity to any component of the formulation; during episodes of hypoglycemia

Warnings/Precautions Refer to Insulin Regular *on page 928*. Safety and efficacy in children <18 years of age have not been established.

In type 1 diabetes mellitus (insulin dependent, IDDM), insulin lispro (Humalog®) and insulin glulisine (Apidra™) should be used in combination with a long-acting insulin. However, in type 2 diabetes mellitus (noninsulin dependent, NIDDM), insulin lispro (Humalog®) may be used without a long-acting insulin when used in combination with a sulfonylurea.

Drug Interactions Refer to Insulin Regular *on page 928*.

Nutritional/Herbal/Ethanol Interactions Refer to Insulin Regular *on page 928*.

Adverse Reactions Refer to Insulin Regular *on page 928*.

Dosing

Adults: Refer to Insulin Regular *on page 928*. Fixed ratio insulins (such as insulin lispro protamine and insulin lispro) are normally administered in 2 daily doses.

Renal Impairment: Insulin requirements are reduced due to changes in insulin clearance or metabolism.

Available Dosage Forms Injection, suspension (Humalog® Mix 75/25™): Insulin lispro protamine suspension 75% [intermediate acting] and insulin lispro solution 25% [rapid acting]: 100 units/mL (3 mL) [disposable pen]; (10 mL) [vial]

Nursing Guidelines

Dietary Considerations: Dietary modification based on ADA recommendations is a key component of therapy.

Pregnancy Risk Factor: B

Pregnancy Issues: Insulin is the drug of choice for the control of diabetes mellitus in pregnancy.

Lactation: Excretion in breast milk unknown/compatible

Breast-Feeding Considerations: Endogenous insulin has been found in breast milk. The gastrointestinal tract destroys insulin when administered orally; therefore, would not be expected to be absorbed intact by the breast-feeding infant.

Administration

Storage: Insulin lispro protamine and insulin lispro (Humalog® Mix): Store unopened container in refrigerator; do not use if it has been frozen. Once opened (in use), vials may be stored in refrigerator or for up to 28 days at room temperature. Pens should be stored at room temperature and used within 10 days. Do not expose to temperatures >37°C (98.6°F).

Related Information

Insulin Regular *on page 928*

Insulin NPH (IN soo lin N P H)

U.S. Brand Names Humulin® N; Novolin® N

Synonyms Isophane Insulin; NPH Insulin

Pharmacologic Category Antidiabetic Agent, Insulin

Medication Safety Issues

Sound-alike/look-alike issues:

Humulin® may be confused with Humalog®, Humira®

Novolin® may be confused with NovoLog®

High alert medication: The Institute for Safe Medication Practices (ISMP) includes this medication among its list of drugs which have a heightened risk of causing significant patient harm when used in error. ***Due to the number of insulin preparations, it is essential to identify/clarify the type of insulin to be used.***

Use Treatment of type 1 diabetes mellitus (insulin dependent, IDDM); type 2 diabetes mellitus (noninsulin dependent, NIDDM) to control hyperglycemia

Mechanism of Action Refer to Insulin Regular *on page 928*. Insulin NPH is an intermediate-acting form of insulin.

Pharmacodynamics/Kinetics

Onset of action: 1-2 hours

Duration: 18-24 hours

Time to peak: 6-12 hours

Excretion: Urine

Contraindications Hypersensitivity to any component of the formulation

Warnings/Precautions Refer to Insulin Regular *on page 928*.

In type 1 diabetes mellitus (insulin dependent, IDDM), insulin lispro (Humalog®) and insulin glulisine (Apidra™) should be used in combination with a long-acting insulin. However, in type 2 diabetes mellitus (noninsulin dependent, NIDDM), insulin lispro (Humalog®) may be used without a long-acting insulin when used in combination with a sulfonylurea.

Drug Interactions Refer to Insulin Regular *on page 928*.

Nutritional/Herbal/Ethanol Interactions Refer to Insulin Regular *on page 928*.

Adverse Reactions Refer to Insulin Regular *on page 928*.

Overdosage/Toxicology Refer to Insulin Regular *on page 928*.

Dosing

Adults & Elderly: Refer to Insulin Regular *on page 928*. Insulin NPH is usually administered 1-2 times daily.

Pediatrics: Refer to Insulin Regular *on page 928*. Insulin NPH is usually administered 1-2 times daily.

Renal Impairment: Insulin requirements are reduced due to changes in insulin clearance or metabolism.

Available Dosage Forms [CAN] = Canadian brand name

Injection, suspension:

Humulin® N: 100 units/mL (3 mL) [disposable pen]; (10 mL) [vial]

Novolin® ge NPH [CAN]: 100 units/mL (3 mL) [NovolinSet® prefilled syringe or PenFill® prefilled cartridge]; 10 mL [vial]

Novolin® N: 100 units/mL (3 mL) [InnoLet® prefilled syringe or PenFill® prefilled cartridge]; (10 mL) [vial]

Nursing Guidelines

Assessment: Assess potential for interactions with other prescriptions, OTC medications, or herbal products patient may be taking. Assess results of laboratory tests, therapeutic effectiveness, and adverse response (eg, hypoglycemia) at regular intervals during therapy. Teach patient proper use, including appropriate injection technique and syringe/needle disposal and monitoring requirements (or refer to diabetic educator), possible side effects/appropriate interventions, and adverse symptoms to report.

Monitoring Laboratory Tests: Urine sugar and acetone, serum glucose, electrolytes, Hb A_{1c}, lipid profile

Dietary Considerations: Dietary modification based on ADA recommendations is a key component of therapy.

Patient Education: Do not take any new medication during therapy unless approved by prescriber. This medication is used to control diabetes; it is not a cure. It is imperative to follow other components of prescribed treatment (eg, diet and exercise regimen). Take exactly as directed. Do not change dose or discontinue unless advised by prescriber. If you experience hypoglycemic reaction, contact prescriber immediately. Always carry quick source of sugar with you. Monitor glucose levels as directed by prescriber. Report adverse side effects, including chest pain or palpitations; persistent fatigue, confusion, headache; skin rash or redness; numbness of mouth, lips, or tongue; muscle weakness or tremors; vision changes; respiratory difficulty; or nausea, vomiting, or flu-like symptoms. **Pregnancy precaution:** Inform prescriber if you are or intend to become pregnant.

Geriatric Considerations: How "tightly" a geriatric patient's blood glucose should be controlled is controversial; however, a fasting blood sugar <150 mg/dL is now an acceptable end point. Such a decision should be based on the patient's functional and cognitive status, how well he/she recognizes hypoglycemic or hyperglycemic symptoms, and how to respond to them and any other disease states. Patients who are unable to accurately draw up their dose will need assistance such as prefilled syringes. Initial doses may require considerations for renal function in the elderly with dosing adjusted subsequently based on blood glucose monitoring.

Pregnancy Risk Factor: B

Pregnancy Issues: Insulin is the drug of choice for the control of diabetes mellitus during pregnancy.

Lactation: Excretion in breast milk unknown/compatible

Breast-Feeding Considerations: Endogenous insulin can be found in breast milk. The gastrointestinal tract destroys insulin when administered orally; therefore, would not be expected to be absorbed intact by the breast-feeding infant.

Administration

Storage: Insulin NPH (Humulin® N, Novolin® N): Store unopened container in refrigerator at 2°C to 8°C (36°F to 46°F); do not freeze. Vial in use may be stored under refrigeration or at room temperature. Humulin® N Pen in use should not be refrigerated; store below 30°C (86°F) away from direct heat or light. Discard after 2 weeks.

Related Information

Insulin Regular *on page 928*

Insulin NPH and Insulin Regular

(IN soo lin N P H & IN soo lin REG yoo ler)

U.S. Brand Names Humulin® 50/50; Humulin® 70/30; Novolin® 70/30

Synonyms Insulin Regular and Insulin NPH; Isophane Insulin and Regular Insulin; NPH Insulin and Regular Insulin

Pharmacologic Category Antidiabetic Agent, Insulin

Medication Safety Issues

Sound-alike/look-alike issues:

Humulin® 70/30 may be confused with Humalog® Mix 75/25

Novolin® 70/30 may be confused with NovoLog® Mix 70/30

High alert medication: The Institute for Safe Medication Practices (ISMP) includes this medication among its list of drugs which have a heightened risk of causing significant patient harm when used in error. ***Due to the number of insulin preparations, it is essential to identify/clarify the type of insulin to be used.***

Use Treatment of type 1 diabetes mellitus (insulin dependent, IDDM); type 2 diabetes mellitus (noninsulin dependent, NIDDM) to control hyperglycemia

Mechanism of Action Refer to Insulin Regular *on page 928*. Insulin NPH and insulin regular is a combination insulin product with intermediate-acting characteristics. It may be administered once or twice daily.

Pharmacodynamics/Kinetics

Onset of action: 0.5 hours

Duration: 18-24 hours

Time to peak: 2-12 hours

Excretion: Urine

Contraindications Hypersensitivity to any component of the formulation; during episodes of hypoglycemia

Warnings/Precautions Refer to Insulin Regular *on page 928*.

In type 1 diabetes mellitus (insulin dependent, IDDM), insulin lispro (Humalog®) and insulin glulisine (Apidra™) should be used in combination with a long-acting insulin. However, in type 2 diabetes mellitus (noninsulin dependent, NIDDM), insulin lispro (Humalog®) may be used without a long-acting insulin when used in combination with a sulfonylurea.

(Continued)

Insulin NPH and Insulin Regular *(Continued)*

Dosing

Adults & Elderly:

Refer to Insulin Regular *on page 928*. Fixed ratio insulins are normally administered in 1-2 daily doses.

Pediatrics:

Refer to Insulin Regular *on page 928*. Fixed ratio insulins are normally administered in 1-2 daily doses.

Available Dosage Forms

Injection, suspension:

Humulin® 50/50: Insulin NPH suspension 50% [intermediate acting] and insulin regular solution 50% [short acting]: 100 units/mL (10 mL) [vial]

Humulin® 70/30: Insulin NPH suspension 70% [intermediate acting] and insulin regular solution 30% [short acting]: 100 units/mL (3 mL) [disposable pen]; (10 mL) [vial]

Novolin® 70/30: Insulin NPH suspension 70% [intermediate acting] and insulin regular solution 30% [short acting]: 100 units/mL (3 mL) [InnoLet® prefilled syringe or PenFill® prefilled cartridge]; (10 mL) [vial]

Additional formulations available in Canada: Injection, suspension:

Humulin® 20/80: Insulin regular solution 20% [short acting] and insulin NPH suspension 80% [intermediate acting]: 100 units/mL (3 mL) [PenFill® prefilled cartridge]

Novolin® ge 10/90: Insulin regular solution 10% [short acting] and insulin NPH suspension 90% [intermediate acting]: 100 units/mL (3 mL) [PenFill® prefilled cartridge]

Novolin® ge 20/80: Insulin regular solution 20% [short acting] and insulin NPH suspension 80% [intermediate acting]: 100 units/mL (3 mL) [PenFill® prefilled cartridge]

Novolin® ge 30/70: Insulin regular solution 30% [short acting] and insulin NPH suspension 70% [intermediate acting]: 100 units/mL (3 mL) [prefilled syringe or PenFill® prefilled cartridge]; (10 mL) [vial]

Novolin® ge 40/60: Insulin regular solution 40% [short acting] and insulin NPH suspension 60% [intermediate acting]: 100 units/mL (3 mL) [PenFill® prefilled cartridge]

Novolin® ge 50/50: Insulin regular solution 50% [short acting] and insulin NPH suspension 50% [intermediate acting]: 100 units/mL (3 mL) [PenFill® prefilled cartridge]

Nursing Guidelines

Pregnancy Risk Factor: C

Pregnancy Issues: Reproduction studies have not been conducted with this combination. Does not cross the placenta. Insulin is the drug of choice for control of diabetes mellitus during pregnancy.

Breast-Feeding Considerations: Endogenous insulin has been detected in breast milk. The gastrointestinal tract destroys insulin when administered orally; therefore, would not be expected to be absorbed intact by the breast-feeding infant.

Administration

Storage: Store unopened container in refrigerator. Do not use if it has been frozen. The pen in use should not be refrigerated; store below 30°C (86°F) away from direct heat or light; discard after 10 days. If refrigeration is not available, opened vials may be stored unrefrigerated in cool place away from heat and sunlight.

Related Information

Insulin Regular *on page 928*

Insulin Regular (IN soo lin REG yoo ler)

U.S. Brand Names Humulin® R; Humulin® R (Concentrated) U-500; Novolin® R

Synonyms Regular Insulin

Pharmacologic Category Antidiabetic Agent, Insulin; Antidote

Medication Safety Issues

Sound-alike/look-alike issues:

Humulin® may be confused with Humalog®, Humira®

Novolin® may be confused with NovoLog®

High alert medication: The Institute for Safe Medication Practices (ISMP) includes this medication among its list of drugs which have a heightened risk of causing significant patient harm when used in error. ***Due to the number of***

insulin preparations, it is essential to identify/clarify the type of insulin to be used.

Concentrated solutions (eg, U-500) should not be available in patient care areas.

Use Treatment of type 1 diabetes mellitus (insulin dependent, IDDM); type 2 diabetes mellitus (noninsulin dependent, NIDDM) unresponsive to treatment with diet and/or oral hypoglycemics, to control hyperglycemia; adjunct to parenteral nutrition; diabetic ketoacidosis (DKA)

Unlabeled/Investigational Use Hyperkalemia (regular insulin only; use with glucose to shift potassium into cells to lower serum potassium levels)

Mechanism of Action Insulin acts via specific membrane-bound receptors on target tissues to regulate metabolism of carbohydrate, protein, and fats. Insulin facilitates entry of glucose into muscle, adipose, and other tissues via hexose transporters, including GLUT4. Insulin stimulates the cellular uptake of amino acids and increases cellular permeability to several ions, including potassium, magnesium, and phosphate. By activating sodium-potassium ATPases, insulin promotes the intracellular movement of potassium.

Target organs for insulin include the liver, skeletal muscle, and adipose tissue. Within the liver, insulin stimulates hepatic glycogen synthesis through the activation of the enzymes hexokinase, phosphofructokinase, and glycogen synthase as well as the inhibition of glucose-6 phosphatase. Insulin promotes hepatic synthesis of fatty acids, which are released into the circulation as lipoproteins. Skeletal muscle effects of insulin include increased protein synthesis and increased glycogen synthesis. Within adipose tissue, insulin stimulates the processing of circulating lipoproteins to provide free fatty acids, facilitating triglyceride synthesis and storage by adipocytes. Insulin also directly inhibits the hydrolysis of triglycerides.

Normally secreted by the pancreas, insulin products are manufactured for pharmacologic use through recombinant DNA technology using either *E. coli* or *Saccharomyces cerevisiae*. Insulins are categorized based on promptness and duration of effect, including rapid-, short-, intermediate-, and long-acting insulins.

Pharmacodynamics/Kinetics

Onset of action: 0.5 hours

Duration: 6-8 hours (may increase with dose)

Time to peak: 2-4 hours

Excretion: Urine

Contraindications Hypersensitivity to any component of the formulation

Warnings/Precautions Hypoglycemia is the most common adverse effect of insulin. The timing of hypoglycemia differs among various insulin formulations. Any change of insulin should be made cautiously; changing manufacturers, type, and/or method of manufacture may result in the need for a change of dosage. Human insulin differs from animal-source insulin. Regular insulin is the only insulin to be used I.V. Hypoglycemia may result from increased work or exercise without eating; use of long-acting insulin preparations (insulin glargine, Ultralente®, insulin U) may delay recovery from hypoglycemia. Use with caution in renal or hepatic impairment.

The general objective of insulin replacement therapy is to approximate the physiologic pattern of insulin secretion. This requires a basal level of insulin throughout the day, supplemented by additional insulin at mealtimes. Since combinations of agents are frequently used, dosage adjustment must address the individual component of the insulin regimen which most directly influences the blood glucose value in question, based on the known onset and duration of the insulin component. The frequency of doses and monitoring must be individualized in consideration of the patient's ability to manage therapy. Diabetic education and nutritional counseling are essential to maximize the effectiveness of therapy.

In type 1 diabetes mellitus (insulin dependent, IDDM), insulin lispro (Humalog®) and insulin glulisine (Apidra™) should be used in combination with a long-acting insulin. However, in type 2 diabetes mellitus (noninsulin dependent, NIDDM), insulin lispro (Humalog®) may be used without a long-acting insulin when used in combination with a sulfonylurea.

Drug Interactions **Induces** CYP1A2 (weak)

Drugs which **DECREASE** hypoglycemic effect of insulin:

Contraceptives (oral), corticosteroids, dextrothyroxine, diltiazem, dobutamine, epinephrine, niacin, smoking, thiazide diuretics, thyroid hormone

(Continued)

Insulin Regular *(Continued)*

Drugs which **INCREASE** hypoglycemic effect of insulin:

Alcohol, alpha-blockers, anabolic steroids, beta-blockers (see 'Note', clofibrate, guanethidine, MAO inhibitors, pentamidine, phenylbutazone, salicylates, sulfinpyrazone, tetracyclines. **Note:** Nonselective beta-blockers may delay recovery from hypoglycemic episodes and mask signs/symptoms of hypoglycemia. Cardioselective agents may be alternatives.

Insulin increases the risk of hypoglycemia associated with oral hypoglycemic agents (including sulfonylureas, metformin, pioglitazone, rosiglitazone, and troglitazone).

Nutritional/Herbal/Ethanol Interactions

Ethanol: Caution with ethanol (may increase hypoglycemia).

Food: Insulin shifts potassium from extracellular to intracellular space. Decreases potassium serum concentration.

Herb/Nutraceutical: Use caution with chromium, garlic, gymnema (may increase hypoglycemia).

Adverse Reactions Frequency not defined.

Cardiovascular: Palpitation, pallor, tachycardia

Central nervous system: Fatigue, headache, hypothermia, loss of consciousness, mental confusion

Dermatologic: Urticaria, redness

Endocrine & metabolic: Hypoglycemia

Gastrointestinal: Hunger, nausea, numbness of mouth

Local: Atrophy or hypertrophy of SubQ fat tissue; edema, itching, pain or warmth at injection site; stinging

Neuromuscular & skeletal: Muscle weakness, paresthesia, tremor

Ocular: Transient presbyopia or blurred vision

Miscellaneous: Anaphylaxis, diaphoresis, local allergy, systemic allergic symptoms

Overdosage/Toxicology Symptoms of overdose include tachycardia, anxiety, hunger, tremor, pallor, headache, motor dysfunction, speech disturbances, sweating, palpitations, coma, and death. Antidote is glucose and glucagon, if necessary.

Dosing

Adults & Elderly: SubQ (regular insulin may also be administered I.V.): The number and size of daily doses, time of administration, and diet and exercise require continuous medical supervision. In addition, specific formulations may require distinct administration procedures (see Administration).

Type 1 Diabetes Mellitus: Note: Multiple daily doses guided by blood glucose monitoring are the standard of diabetes care. Combinations of insulin are commonly used.

Initial dose: 0.2-0.6 unit /kg/day in divided doses. Conservative initial doses of 0.2-0.4 units/kg/day are often recommended to avoid the potential for hypoglycemia.

Division of daily insulin requirement: Generally, 50% to 75% of the daily insulin dose is given as an intermediate- or long-acting form of insulin (in 1-2 daily injections). The remaining portion of the 24-hour insulin requirement is divided and administered as a rapid-acting or short-acting form of insulin. These may be given with meals (before or at the time of meals depending on the form of insulin) or at the same time as injections of intermediate forms (some premixed combinations are intended for this purpose).

Adjustment of dose: Dosage must be titrated to achieve glucose control and avoid hypoglycemia. Adjust dose to maintain premeal and bedtime glucose of 80-140 mg/dL (children <5 years: 100-200 mg/dL). Since combinations of agents are frequently used, dosage adjustment must address the individual component of the insulin regimen which most directly influences the blood glucose value in question, based on the known onset and duration of the insulin component.

Usual maintenance range: 0.5-1.2 units/kg/day in divided doses. An estimate of anticipated needs may be based on body weight and/or activity factors as follows:

Adolescents: May require ≤1.5 units/kg/day during growth spurts

Nonobese: 0.4-0.6 units/kg/day

Obese: 0.8-1.2 units/kg/day

Renal failure: Due to alterations in pharmacokinetics of insulin, may require <0.2 units/kg/day

Type 2 Diabetes Mellitus:

Augmentation therapy: Initial dosage of 0.15 (insulin glargine, corresponding to ~10 units) to 0.2 units/kg/day (insulins other than glargine) have been recommended. Dosage must be carefully adjusted.

Note: Administered when residual beta-cell function is present, as a supplemental agent when oral hypoglycemics have not achieved goal glucose control. Twice daily NPH, or an evening dose of NPH, lente, or glargine insulin may be added to oral therapy with metformin or a sulfonylurea. Augmentation to control postprandial glucose may be accomplished with regular, glulisine, aspart, or lispro insulin.

Monotherapy: Initial dose: Highly variable: See Augmentation therapy dosing.

Note: An empirically-defined scheme for dosage estimation based on fasting plasma glucose and degree of obesity has been published with recommended doses ranging from 6-77 units/day (Holman, 1995). In the setting of glucose toxicity (loss of beta-cell sensitivity to glucose concentrations), insulin therapy may be used for short-term management to restore sensitivity of beta-cells; in these cases, the dose may need to be rapidly reduced/withdrawn when sensitivity is re-established.

Hyperkalemia (unlabeled use): I.V.: Administer dextrose at 0.5-1 mL/kg and regular insulin 1 unit for every 4-5 g dextrose given

Diabetic ketoacidosis:

I.V.: Regular insulin 0.15 units/kg initially followed by an infusion of 0.1 units/kg/hour

SubQ, I.M.: Regular insulin 0.4 units/kg given half as I.V. bolus and half as SubQ or I.M., followed by 0.1 units/kg/hour SubQ or I.M.

If serum glucose does not fall by 50-70 mg/dL in the first hour, double insulin dose hourly until glucose falls at an hourly rate of 50-70 mg/dL. Decrease dose to 0.05-0.1 units/kg/hour once serum glucose reaches 250 mg/dL.

Note: Newly-diagnosed patients with IDDM presenting in DKA and patients with blood sugars <800 mg/dL may be relatively "sensitive" to insulin and should receive loading and initial maintenance doses ~50% of those indicated.

Infusion should continue until reversal of acid-base derangement/ketonemia. Serum glucose is not a direct indicator of these abnormalities, and may decrease more rapidly than correction of the range of metabolic abnormalities.

Pediatrics: Diabetes mellitus: Refer to adult dosing. Adolescents (growth spurts): ≤1.5 units/kg/day in divided doses.

Diabetic ketoacidosis: Children <20 years:

I.V.: Regular insulin infused at 0.1 units/kg/hour; continue until acidosis clears, then decrease to 0.05 units/kg/hour until SubQ replacement dosing can be initiated

SubQ, I.M.: If no I.V. infusion access, regular insulin 0.1 units/kg I.M. bolus followed by 0.1 units/kg/hour SubQ or I.M.; continue until acidosis clears, then decrease to 0.05 units/kg/hour until SubQ replacement dosing can be initiated

If serum glucose does not fall by 50-70 mg/dL in the first hour, double insulin dose hourly until glucose falls at an hourly rate of 50-70 mg/dL. Decrease dose to 0.05-0.1 units/kg/hour once serum glucose reaches 250 mg/dL.

Note: Newly-diagnosed patients with IDDM presenting in DKA and patients with blood sugars <800 mg/dL may be relatively "sensitive" to insulin and should receive loading and initial maintenance doses ~50% of those indicated.

Hyperkalemia (unlabeled use): Refer to adult dosing.

Renal Impairment: Insulin requirements are reduced due to changes in insulin clearance or metabolism.

Cl_{cr} 10-50 mL/minute: Administer 75% of normal dose.

Cl_{cr} <10 mL/minute: Administer 25% to 50% of normal dose and monitor glucose closely.

Hemodialysis: Because of a large molecular weight (6000 daltons), insulin is not significantly removed by either peritoneal or hemodialysis.

Supplemental dose is not necessary.

Peritoneal dialysis: Supplemental dose is not necessary.

Continuous arteriovenous or venovenous hemofiltration effects: Supplemental dose is not necessary.

(Continued)

Insulin Regular *(Continued)*

Available Dosage Forms

Injection, solution:

Humulin® R: 100 units/mL (10 mL) [vial]

Novolin® R: 100 units/mL (3 mL) [InnoLet® prefilled syringe or PenFill® prefilled cartridge]; (10 mL) [vial]

Injection, solution, [concentrate] (Humulin® R U-500): 500 units/mL (20 mL vial)

Nursing Guidelines

Assessment: Assess potential for interactions with other prescriptions, OTC medications, or herbal products patient may be taking. Assess results of laboratory tests, therapeutic effectiveness, and adverse response (eg, hypoglycemia) at regular intervals during therapy. Teach patient proper use, including appropriate injection technique and syringe/needle disposal and monitoring requirements (or refer to diabetic educator), possible side effects/appropriate interventions, and adverse symptoms to report.

Monitoring Laboratory Tests: Urine sugar and acetone, serum glucose, electrolytes, Hb A_{1c}, lipid profile

DKA: Arterial blood gases, CBC with differential, urinalysis, serum glucose (baseline and every hour until reaches 250 mg/dL), BUN, creatinine, electrolytes, anion gap

Hyperkalemia: Serum potassium and glucose must be closely monitored to avoid hypoglycemia and/or hypokalemia.

Dietary Considerations: Dietary modification based on ADA recommendations is a part of therapy.

Patient Education: Do not take any new medication during therapy unless approved by prescriber. This medication is used to control diabetes; it is not a cure. It is imperative to follow other components of prescribed treatment (eg, diet and exercise regimen). Take exactly as directed. Do not change dose or discontinue unless advised by prescriber. With insulin aspart (NovoLog®), you must start eating within 5-10 minutes after injection. Insulin glulisine (Apidra™) should be administered within 15 minutes before or within 20 minutes after start of meal. If you experience hypoglycemic reaction, contact prescriber immediately. Always carry quick source of sugar with you. Monitor glucose levels as directed by prescriber. Report adverse side effects, including chest pain or palpitations; persistent fatigue, confusion, headache; skin rash or redness; numbness of mouth, lips, or tongue; muscle weakness or tremors; vision changes; respiratory difficulty; or nausea, vomiting, or flu-like symptoms. **Pregnancy precaution:** Inform prescriber if you are or intend to become pregnant.

Geriatric Considerations: How "tightly" a geriatric patient's blood glucose should be controlled is controversial; however, a fasting blood sugar <150 mg/dL is now an acceptable end point. Such a decision should be based on the patient's functional and cognitive status, how well he/she recognizes hypoglycemic or hyperglycemic symptoms, and how to respond to them and any other disease states. Patients who are unable to accurately draw up their dose will need assistance such as prefilled syringes. Initial doses may require considerations for renal function in the elderly with dosing adjusted subsequently based on blood glucose monitoring.

Pregnancy Risk Factor: B

Pregnancy Issues: Insulin is the drug of choice for the control of diabetes mellitus during pregnancy.

Lactation: Excretion in breast milk unknown/compatible

Breast-Feeding Considerations: Endogenous insulin can be found in breast milk. The gastrointestinal tract destroys insulin when administered orally; therefore, would not be expected to be absorbed intact by the breast-feeding infant.

Perioperative/Anesthesia/Other Concerns: Intensive insulin therapy in critically-ill patients may have beneficial effects on mortality and morbidity. Van den Berghe and colleagues performed a single center, prospective, randomized, controlled study in 1548 surgical intensive care patients. Authors compared "conventional" control of blood glucose (180-200 mg/dL) versus "intensive" control of blood glucose (80-110 mg/dL). Primary outcome was ICU mortality. The authors showed an absolute mortality reduction of 3.4% (8.0% vs 4.6%; p: <0.04). Intensive insulin therapy also reduced bloodstream infections (7.8% vs 4.2%; p: 0.003), acute renal failure requiring hemodialysis (8.2 vs 4.8%; p: 0.007), and critical-illness polyneuropathy (51.9% vs 28.7%; p: <0.001). Greatest mortality reduction appeared in patients with an ICU stay >5 days, reducing mortality by 9.6% (20.2% vs 10.6%; p: 0.005). Other authors have shown intensive insulin therapy to reduce morbidity and mortality after myocardial infarction and coronary bypass.

Administration

I.V.: Regular insulin may be administered by SubQ, I.M., or I.V. routes.

I.V. administration (requires use of an infusion pump): **Only regular insulin** may be administered I.V.

Reconstitution: Standard diluent for regular insulin: 100 units/100 mL NS; **Note:** All bags should be prepared fresh; tubing should be flushed 30 minutes prior to administration to allow adsorption as time permits. Can be given as a more diluted solution (eg, 100 units/250 mL 0.45% NS).

Compatibility:

Y-site administration: Incompatible with dopamine, nafcillin, norepinephrine, ranitidine

Compatibility when admixed: Incompatible with aminophylline, amobarbital, chlorothiazide, cytarabine, dobutamine, methylprednisolone sodium succinate, octreotide, pentobarbital, phenobarbital, phenytoin, thiopental

Storage: Insulin, regular (Humulin® R, Novolin® R): Store unopened containers in refrigerator at 2°C to 8°C (36°F to 46°F); do not freeze. Vial in use may be stored under refrigeration or at room temperature; store below 30°C (86°F) away from direct heat or light. Regular insulin should only be used if clear.

Related Information

Perioperative Management of the Diabetic Patient *on page 1794*

♦ **Insulin Regular and Insulin NPH** *see* Insulin NPH and Insulin Regular *on page 927*

♦ **Intal®** *see* Cromolyn *on page 453*

♦ **Integrilin®** *see* Eptifibatide *on page 625*

♦ **α-2-interferon** *see* Interferon Alfa-2b *on page 936*

Interferon Alfa-2a (in ter FEER on AL fa too aye)

U.S. Brand Names Roferon-A®

Synonyms IFLrA; rIFN-A

Pharmacologic Category Interferon

Medication Safety Issues

Sound-alike/look-alike issues:

Interferon alfa-2a may be confused with interferon alfa-2b

Roferon-A® may be confused with Rocephin®

Use

Patients >18 years of age: Hairy cell leukemia, AIDS-related Kaposi's sarcoma, chronic hepatitis C

Children and Adults: Chronic myelogenous leukemia (CML), Philadelphia chromosome positive, within 1 year of diagnosis (limited experience in children)

Unlabeled/Investigational Use Adjuvant therapy for malignant melanoma, AIDS-related thrombocytopenia, cutaneous ulcerations of Behçet's disease, brain tumors, metastatic ileal carcinoid tumors, cervical and colorectal cancers, genital warts, idiopathic mixed cryoglobulinemia, hemangioma, hepatitis D, hepatocellular carcinoma, idiopathic hypereosinophilic syndrome, mycosis fungoides, Sézary syndrome, low-grade non-Hodgkin's lymphoma, macular degeneration, multiple myeloma, renal cell carcinoma, basal and squamous cell skin cancer, essential thrombocythemia, cutaneous T-cell lymphoma

Mechanism of Action Following activation, multiple effects can be detected including induction of gene transcription. Inhibits cellular growth, alters the state of cellular differentiation, interferes with oncogene expression, alters cell surface antigen expression, increases phagocytic activity of macrophages, and augments cytotoxicity of lymphocytes for target cells

Pharmacodynamics/Kinetics

Absorption: Filtered and absorbed at the renal tubule

Distribution: V_d: 0.223-0.748 L/kg

Metabolism: Primarily renal; filtered through glomeruli and undergoes rapid proteolytic degradation during tubular reabsorption

Bioavailability: I.M.: 83%; SubQ: 90%

Half-life elimination: I.V.: 3.7-8.5 hours (mean ~5 hours)

Time to peak, serum: I.M., SubQ: ~6-8 hours

Contraindications Hypersensitivity to alfa interferon, benzyl alcohol, or any component of the formulation; autoimmune hepatitis; hepatic decompensation (Child-Pugh class B or C)

(Continued)

Interferon Alfa-2a *(Continued)*

Warnings/Precautions Use caution in patients with a history of depression. May cause severe psychiatric adverse events (psychosis, mania, depression, suicidal behavior/ideation) in patients with and without previous psychiatric symptoms; careful neuropsychiatric monitoring is required during therapy. Use with caution in patients with seizure disorders, brain metastases, or compromised CNS function. Higher doses in the elderly or in malignancies other than hairy cell leukemia may result in severe obtundation.

Use caution in patients with autoimmune diseases; development or exacerbation of autoimmune diseases has been reported. Use caution in patients with pre-existing cardiac disease (ischemic or thromboembolic), arrhythmias, renal impairment (Cl_{cr} <50 mL/minute), mild hepatic impairment, or myelosuppression. Also use caution in patients receiving therapeutic immunosuppression. May cause thyroid dysfunction or hyperglycemia, use caution in patients with diabetes or pre-existing thyroid disease. Pulmonary dysfunction may be induced or aggravated by interferon alpha; discontinue if persistent unexplained pulmonary infiltrates are noted. Gastrointestinal ischemia, ulcerative colitis and hemorrhage have been associated rarely with alpha interferons; some cases are severe and life-threatening. Ophthalmologic disorders (including retinal hemorrhages, cotton wool spots, and retinal artery or vein obstruction) have occurred in patients receiving alpha interferons; close monitoring is warranted.

Treatment should be discontinued in patients with worsening or persistently severe signs/symptoms of autoimmune, infectious, ischemic, or neuropsychiatric disorders (including depression and/or suicidal thoughts/behavior). Discontinue treatment if neutrophils $<0.5 \times 10^9$/L or platelets $<25 \times 10^9$/L. **Due to differences in dosage, patients should not change brands of interferons.** Injection solution contains benzyl alcohol; do not use in neonates or infants. Safety and efficacy in children <18 years of age have not been established.

Drug Interactions **Inhibits** CYP1A2 (weak)

Note: May exacerbate the toxicity of other agents with respect to CNS, myelotoxicity, or cardiotoxicity.

ACE inhibitors: Interferons may increase the adverse/toxic effects of ACE inhibitors, specifically the development of granulocytopenia. Risk: Monitor

Clozapine: A case report of agranulocytosis with concurrent use.

Erythropoietin: Case reports of decreased hematopoietic effect

Melphalan: Interferon alpha may decrease the serum concentrations of melphalan; this may or may not decrease the potential toxicity of melphalan. Risk: Monitor

Prednisone: Prednisone may decrease the therapeutic effects of interferon alpha. Risk: Moderate

Ribavirin: Concurrent therapy may increase the risk of hemolytic anemia.

Theophylline: Interferon alpha may decrease the P450 isoenzyme metabolism of theophylline. Risk: Moderate

Warfarin: Interferons may increase the anticoagulant effects of warfarin. Risk: Monitor

Zidovudine: Interferons may decrease the metabolism of zidovudine. Risk: Monitor

Adverse Reactions Flu-like symptoms are common (up to 92%).

>10%:

Cardiovascular: Chest pain (4% to 11%), edema (11%), hypertension (11%)

Central nervous system: Psychiatric disturbances (including depression and suicidal behavior/ideation; reported incidence highly variable, generally >15%), fatigue (90%), headache (52%), dizziness (21%), irritability (15%), insomnia (14%), somnolence, lethargy, confusion, mental impairment, and motor weakness (most frequently seen at high doses [>100 million units], usually reverses within a few days); vertigo (19%); mental status changes (12%)

Dermatologic: Rash (usually maculopapular) on the trunk and extremities (7% to 18%), alopecia (19% to 22%), pruritus (13%), dry skin

Endocrine & metabolic: Hypocalcemia (10% to 51%), hyperglycemia (33% to 39%), transaminases increased (25% to 30%), alkaline phosphatase increased (48%)

Gastrointestinal: Loss of taste, anorexia (30% to 70%), nausea (28% to 53%), vomiting (10% to 30%, usually mild), diarrhea (22% to 34%, may be severe), taste change (13%), dry throat, xerostomia, abdominal cramps, abdominal pain

Hematologic (often due to underlying disease): Myelosuppression; neutropenia (32% to 70%); thrombocytopenia (22% to 70%); anemia (24% to 65%, may be dose-limiting, usually seen only during the first 6 months of therapy)
Onset: 7-10 days
Nadir: 14 days, may be delayed 20-40 days in hairy cell leukemia
Recovery: 21 days
Hepatic: Elevation of AST (SGOT) (77% to 80%), LDH (47%), bilirubin (31%)
Local: Injection site reaction (29%)
Neuromuscular & skeletal: Weakness (may be severe at doses >20,000,000 units/day); arthralgia and myalgia (5% to 73%, usually during the first 72 hours of treatment); rigors
Renal: Proteinuria (15% to 25%)
Respiratory: Cough (27%), irritation of oropharynx (14%)
Miscellaneous: Flu-like syndrome (up to 92% of patients), diaphoresis (15%)

1% to 10%:
Cardiovascular: Hypotension (6%), supraventricular tachyarrhythmia, palpitation (<3%), acute MI (<1% to 1%)
Central nervous system: Confusion (10%), delirium
Dermatologic: Erythema (diffuse), urticaria
Endocrine & metabolic: Hyperphosphatemia (2%)
Gastrointestinal: Stomatitis, pancreatitis (<5%), flatulence, liver pain
Genitourinary: Impotence (6%), menstrual irregularities
Neuromuscular & skeletal: Leg cramps; peripheral neuropathy, paresthesia (7%), and numbness (4%) are more common in patients previously treated with vinca alkaloids or receiving concurrent vinblastine
Ocular: Conjunctivitis (4%)
Respiratory: Dyspnea (7.5%), epistaxis (4%), rhinitis (3%)
Miscellaneous: Antibody production to interferon (10%)

<1% (Limited to important or life-threatening): Angioedema, aplastic anemia, ascites, autoimmune reaction with worsening of liver disease, bronchospasm, bronchiolitis obliterans, cardiomyopathy, coagulopathy, coma, CHF, cutaneous eruptions, diffuse encephalopathy, hallucinations, hemolytic anemia, hyper-/hypothyroidism, hypertriglyceridemia, hyponatremia (SIADH), mania, gastrointestinal hemorrhage, hepatic failure, idiopathic thrombocytopenia purpura, interstitial nephritis, interstitial pneumonitis, ischemic colitis, lupus erythematosus syndrome, myositis, nephrotic syndrome, optic neuritis, pneumonia, pneumonitis, proteinuria, psychotic episodes, Raynaud's phenomenon, renal failure (acute), rhabdomyolysis, sarcoidosis, seizure, stroke, syncope, ulcerative colitis, urticaria, vasculitis, visual acuity decreased

Overdosage/Toxicology Symptoms of overdose include CNS depression, obtundation, flu-like symptoms, and myelosuppression. Treatment is supportive.

Dosing

Adults & Elderly: Refer to individual protocols.

Hairy cell leukemia: SubQ, I.M.: 3 million units/day for 16-24 weeks, then 3 million units 3 times/week for up to 6-24 months

Chronic myelogenous leukemia (CML): SubQ, I.M.: 9 million units/day, continue treatment until disease progression

AIDS-related Kaposi's sarcoma: SubQ, I.M.: 36 million units/day for 10-12 weeks, then 36 million units 3 times/week; to minimize adverse reactions, can use escalating dose (3-, 9-, then 18 million units each day for 3 days, then 36 million units daily thereafter).

Hepatitis C: SubQ, I.M.: 3 million units 3 times/week for 12 months

Pediatrics: Refer to individual protocols. Children (limited data):

Chronic myelogenous leukemia (CML): I.M.: 2.5-5 million units/m^2/day. **Note:** In juveniles, higher dosages (30 million units/m^2/day) have been associated with severe adverse events, including death.

Renal Impairment: Not removed by hemodialysis

Available Dosage Forms Injection, solution, [single-dose prefilled syringe; SubQ use only]: 3 million units/0.5 mL (0.5 mL); 6 million units/0.5 mL (0.5 mL); 9 million units/0.5 mL (0.5 mL) [contains benzyl alcohol]

Nursing Guidelines

Assessment: Assess laboratory results on a regular basis. Monitor for effectiveness of therapy and possible adverse reactions. Monitor for neuropsychiatric changes. Monitor for signs of depression or suicidal ideation. Perform eye exam prior to initiating therapy and periodically during treatment. Monitor weight periodically. Patients with pre-existing cardiac abnormalities or advanced stages of cancer should have ECG before and during treatment. Assess knowledge/

(Continued)

Interferon Alfa-2a *(Continued)*

instruct patient/caregiver on appropriate reconstitution, injection and needle disposal, possible side effects, and symptoms to report.

Monitoring Laboratory Tests: Baseline chest x-ray, ECG, CBC with differential, liver function, electrolytes, platelets

Patient Education: Use as directed; do not change dosage, brand, or schedule of administration without consulting prescriber. Maintain adequate hydration (2-3 L/day of fluids) unless instructed to restrict fluid intake. You may experience flu-like syndrome (acetaminophen may help); nausea, vomiting, dry mouth, or metallic taste (small frequent meals, frequent mouth care, sucking lozenges, or chewing gum may help); or drowsiness, dizziness, agitation, abnormal thinking (use caution when driving or engaging in tasks requiring alertness until response to drug is known). Inform prescriber **immediately** if you feel depressed or have any thoughts of suicide. Report unusual bruising or bleeding; persistent abdominal disturbances; unusual fatigue; muscle pain or tremors; chest pain or palpitation; swelling of extremities or unusual weight gain; respiratory difficulty; pain, swelling, or redness at injection site; change in vision; or other unusual symptoms. **Pregnancy/breast-feeding precautions:** Inform prescriber if you are or intend to become pregnant. Consult prescriber if breast-feeding.

Geriatric Considerations: No specific data is available for the elderly; however, pay close attention to Warnings/Precautions since the elderly often have reduced Cl_{cr} (<50 mL/minute), diabetes, and hyper-/hypothyroidism.

Pregnancy Risk Factor: C

Pregnancy Issues: Safety and efficacy for use during pregnancy have not been established. Interferon alpha has been shown to decrease serum estradiol and progesterone levels in humans. Menstrual irregularities and abortion have been reported in animals. Effective contraception is recommended during treatment.

Lactation: Enters breast milk/contraindicated (AAP rates "compatible")

Breast-Feeding Considerations: Women with hepatitis C should be instructed that there is a theoretical risk the virus may be transmitted in breast milk. HIV-infected mothers are discouraged from breast-feeding to decrease potential transmission of HIV.

Perioperative/Anesthesia/Other Concerns: Indications and dosage regimens are specific for a particular brand of interferon; other brands have different indications and dosage guidelines.

Administration

I.M.: Reconstitute with recommended amount of bacteriostatic water and agitate gently; do not shake. **Note:** Different vial strengths require different amounts of diluent.

Reconstitution: Reconstitute vial with the diluent provided, or SWFI, NS, or D_5W; concentrations ≥3 x 10^6 units/mL are hypertonic.

Storage: Refrigerate (2°C to 8°C/36°F to 46°F); do not freeze; do not shake. After reconstitution, the solution is stable for 24 hours at room temperature and for 1 month when refrigerated.

♦ Interferon Alfa-2a (PEG Conjugate) *see* Peginterferon Alfa-2a *on page 1321*

Interferon Alfa-2b (in ter FEER on AL fa too bee)

U.S. Brand Names Intron® A

Synonyms α-2-interferon; INF-alpha 2; rLFN-α2

Pharmacologic Category Interferon

Medication Safety Issues

Sound-alike/look-alike issues:

Interferon alfa-2b may be confused with interferon alfa-2a

Use

Patients ≥1 year of age: Chronic hepatitis B

Patients ≥18 years of age: Condyloma acuminata, chronic hepatitis C, hairy cell leukemia, malignant melanoma, AIDS-related Kaposi's sarcoma, follicular non-Hodgkin's lymphoma

Unlabeled/Investigational Use AIDS-related thrombocytopenia, cutaneous ulcerations of Behçet's disease, carcinoid syndrome, cervical cancer, lymphomatoid granulomatosis, genital herpes, hepatitis D, chronic myelogenous leukemia (CML), non-Hodgkin's lymphomas (other than follicular lymphoma, see approved use), polycythemia vera, medullary thyroid carcinoma, multiple myeloma, renal cell carcinoma, basal and squamous cell skin cancers, essential thrombocytopenia, thrombocytopenic purpura

Investigational: West Nile virus

Mechanism of Action Following activation, multiple effects can be detected including induction of gene transcription. Inhibits cellular growth, alters the state of cellular differentiation, interferes with oncogene expression, alters cell surface antigen expression, increases phagocytic activity of macrophages, and augments cytotoxicity of lymphocytes for target cells

Pharmacodynamics/Kinetics

Distribution: V_d: 31 L; but has been noted to be much greater (370-720 L) in leukemia patients receiving continuous infusion IFN; IFN does not penetrate the CSF

Metabolism: Primarily renal

Bioavailability: I.M.: 83%; SubQ: 90%

Half-life elimination: I.M., I.V.: 2 hours; SubQ: 3 hours

Time to peak, serum: I.M., SubQ: ~3-12 hours

Contraindications Hypersensitivity to interferon alfa or any component of the formulation; decompensated liver disease; autoimmune hepatitis; history of autoimmune disease; immunosuppressed transplant patients

Warnings/Precautions Suicidal ideation or attempts may occur more frequently in pediatric patients when compared to adults. May cause severe psychiatric adverse events (psychosis, mania, depression, suicidal behavior/ideation) in patients with and without previous psychiatric symptoms, avoid use in severe psychiatric disorders or in patients with a history of depression; careful neuropsychiatric monitoring is required during therapy. Use with caution in patients with a history of seizures, brain metastases, multiple sclerosis, cardiac disease (ischemic or thromboembolic), arrhythmias, myelosuppression, hepatic impairment, or renal dysfunction (use is not recommended if Cl_{cr}<50 mL/minute). Use caution in patients with a history of pulmonary disease, coagulopathy, thyroid disease (monitor thyroid function), hypertension, or diabetes mellitus (particularly if prone to DKA). Caution in patients receiving drugs that may cause lactic acidosis (eg, nucleoside analogues).

Avoid use in patients with autoimmune disorders; worsening of psoriasis and/or development of autoimmune disorders has been associated with alpha interferons. Higher doses in elderly patients, or diseases other than hairy cell leukemia, may result in increased CNS toxicity. Treatment should be discontinued in patients who develop severe pulmonary symptoms with chest x-ray changes, autoimmune disorders, worsening of hepatic function, psychiatric symptoms (including depression and/or suicidal thoughts/behaviors), ischemic and/or infectious disorders. Ophthalmologic disorders (including retinal hemorrhages, cotton wool spots and retinal artery or vein obstruction) have occurred in patients receiving alpha interferons. Hypertriglyceridemia has been reported (discontinue if severe).

Safety and efficacy in children <1 year of age have not been established. Do not treat patients with visceral AIDS-related Kaposi's sarcoma associated with rapidly-progressing or life-threatening disease. A transient increase in SGOT (>2x baseline) is common in patients treated with interferon alfa-2b for chronic hepatitis. Therapy generally may continue, however, functional indicators (albumin, prothrombin time, bilirubin) should be monitored at 2-week intervals. **Due to differences in dosage, patients should not change brands of interferons without the prescribers knowledge.**

Intron® A may cause bone marrow suppression, including very rarely, aplastic anemia. Hemolytic anemia (hemoglobin <10 g/dL) was observed in up to 10% of treated patients in clinical trials when combined with ribavirin; anemia occurred within 1-2 weeks of initiation of therapy.

Drug Interactions Inhibits CYP1A2 (weak)

ACE inhibitors: Interferons may increase the adverse/toxic effects of ACE inhibitors, specifically the development of granulocytopenia; monitor.

Clozapine: A case report of agranulocytosis with concurrent use.

Erythropoietin: Case reports of decreased hematopoietic effect.

Melphalan: Interferon alfa may decrease the serum concentrations of melphalan; this may or may not decrease the potential toxicity of melphalan; monitor.

Prednisone: Prednisone may decrease the therapeutic effects of interferon alfa. Risk: Moderate

Ribavirin: Concurrent therapy may increase the risk of hemolytic anemia.

Theophylline: Interferon alfa may decrease the P450 isoenzyme metabolism of theophylline. Risk: Moderate

Warfarin: Interferons may increase the anticoagulant effects of warfarin; monitor.

Zidovudine: Interferons may decrease the metabolism of zidovudine; monitor.

(Continued)

Interferon Alfa-2b *(Continued)*

Adverse Reactions Flu-like symptoms are common (up to 79%)

>10%:

Cardiovascular: Chest pain (2% to 28%)

Central nervous system: Fatigue (8% to 96%), headache (21% to 62%), fever (34% to 94%), depression (4% to 40%), somnolence (1% to 33%), irritability (1% to 22%), paresthesia (1% to 21%, more common in patients previously treated with vinca alkaloids or receiving concurrent vinblastine), dizziness (7% to 23%), confusion (1% to 12%), malaise (3% to 14%), pain (3% to 15%), insomnia (1% to 12%), impaired concentration (1% to 14%, usually reverses within a few days), amnesia (1% to 14%), chills (45% to 54%)

Dermatologic: Alopecia (8% to 38%), rash (usually maculopapular) on the trunk and extremities (1% to 25%), pruritus (3% to 11%), dry skin (1% to 10%)

Endocrine & metabolic: Hypocalcemia (10% to 51%), hyperglycemia (33% to 39%), amenorrhea (up to 12% in lymphoma), alkaline phosphatase increased (48%)

Gastrointestinal: Anorexia (1% to 69%), nausea (19% to 66%), vomiting (2% to 32%, usually mild), diarrhea (2% to 45%, may be severe), taste change (2% to 24%), xerostomia (1% to 28%), abdominal pain (2% to 23%), gingivitis (2% to 14%), constipation (1% to 14%)

Hematologic: Myelosuppression; neutropenia (30% to 66%); thrombocytopenia (5% to 15%); anemia (15% to 32%, may be dose-limiting, usually seen only during the first 6 months of therapy)

Onset: 7-10 days

Nadir: 14 days, may be delayed 20-40 days in hairy cell leukemia

Recovery: 21 days

Hepatic: Right upper quadrant pain (15% in hepatitis C), transaminases increased (increased SGOT in up to 63%)

Local: Injection site reaction (1% to 20%)

Neuromuscular & skeletal: Weakness (5% to 63%) may be severe at doses >20,000,000 units/day; mild arthralgia and myalgia (5% to 75% - usually during the first 72 hours of treatment), rigors (2% to 42%), back pain (1% to 19%), musculoskeletal pain (1% to 21%), paresthesia (1% to 21%)

Renal: Urinary tract infection (up to 5% in hepatitis C)

Respiratory: Dyspnea (1% to 34%), cough (1% to 31%), pharyngitis (1% to 31%),

Miscellaneous: Loss of smell, flu-like symptoms (5% to 79%), diaphoresis (2% to 21%)

5% to 10%:

Cardiovascular: Hypertension (9% in hepatitis C)

Central nervous system: Anxiety (1% to 9%), nervousness (1% to 3%), vertigo (up to 8% in lymphoma)

Dermatologic: Dermatitis (1% to 8%)

Endocrine & metabolic: Decreased libido (1% to 5%)

Gastrointestinal: Loose stools (1% to 21%), dyspepsia (2% to 8%)

Neuromuscular & skeletal: Hypoesthesia (1% to 10%)

Respiratory: Nasal congestion (1% to 10%)

<5% (Limited to important or life-threatening): Acute hypersensitivity reactions, allergic reactions, angina, aphasia, arrhythmia, ataxia, atrial fibrillation, Bell's palsy, bronchospasm, cardiomyopathy, CHF, coma, depression, epidermal necrolysis, extrapyramidal disorder, gastrointestinal hemorrhage, gingival hyperplasia, granulocytopenia, hallucinations, hemolytic anemia, hemoptysis, hepatic encephalopathy (rare), hepatic failure (rare), hepatotoxic reaction, hypoventilation, jaundice, lupus erythematosus, mania, MI, nephrotic syndrome, pancreatitis, polyarteritis nodosa, psychosis, pulmonary embolism, pulmonary fibrosis, Raynaud's phenomenon, renal failure, seizure, stroke, suicidal ideation, suicide attempt, syncope, tendonitis, thrombocytopenic purpura, thrombosis, vasculitis

Overdosage/Toxicology Symptoms of overdose include CNS depression, obtundation, flu-like symptoms, and myelosuppression. Treatment is supportive.

Dosing

Adults & Elderly: Refer to individual protocols.

Hairy cell leukemia: I.M., SubQ: 2 million units/m^2 3 times/week for 2-6 months

Lymphoma (follicular): SubQ: 5 million units 3 times/week for up to 18 months

Malignant melanoma: 20 million units/m^2 I.V. for 5 consecutive days per week for 4 weeks, then 10 million units/m^2 SubQ 3 times/week for 48 weeks

AIDS-related Kaposi's sarcoma: I.M., SubQ: 30 million units/m^2 3 times/week

Chronic hepatitis B: I.M., SubQ: 5 million units/day or 10 million units 3 times/week for 16 weeks

Chronic hepatitis C: I.M., SubQ: 3 million units 3 times/week for 16 weeks. In patients with normalization of ALT at 16 weeks, continue treatment for 18-24 months; consider discontinuation if normalization does not occur at 16 weeks. **Note:** May be used in combination therapy with ribavirin in previously untreated patients or in patients who relapse following alpha interferon therapy; refer to Interferon Alfa-2b and Ribavirin Combination Pack monograph.

Condyloma acuminata: Intralesionally: 1 million units/lesion (maximum: 5 lesions/treatment) 3 times/week (on alternate days) for 3 weeks. May administer a second course at 12-16 weeks.

Pediatrics: Refer to individual protocols.

Chronic hepatitis B: SubQ: Children 1-17 years: 3 million units/m^2 3 times/week for 1 week; then 6 million units/m^2 3 times/week; maximum: 10 million units 3 times/week; total duration of therapy 16-24 weeks

Renal Impairment:
Combination therapy with ribavirin (hepatitis C) should not be used in patients with reduced renal function (Cl_{cr} <50 mL/minute).

Available Dosage Forms

Injection, powder for reconstitution: 10 million units; 18 million units; 50 million units [contains human albumin]

Injection, solution [multidose prefilled pen]:
- Delivers 3 million units/0.2 mL (1.5 mL) [delivers 6 doses; 18 million units]
- Delivers 5 million units/0.2 mL (1.5 mL) [delivers 6 doses; 30 million units]
- Delivers 10 million units/0.2 mL (1.5 mL) [delivers 6 doses; 60 million units]

Injection, solution [multidose vial]: 6 million units/mL (3 mL); 10 million units/mL (2.5 mL)

Injection, solution [single-dose vial]: 10 million units/ mL (1 mL)

See also Interferon Alfa-2b and Ribavirin Combination Pack monograph.

Nursing Guidelines

Assessment: Assess results of laboratory tests on a regular basis, therapeutic effectiveness, and adverse reactions. Patients with pre-existing cardiac abnormalities, or in advanced stages of cancer should have ECGs taken before and during treatment. Monitor for neuropsychiatric changes. Assess knowledge/instruct patient/caregiver on appropriate reconstitution, injection and needle disposal, possible side effects, and symptoms to report.

Monitoring Laboratory Tests: Baseline chest x-ray, ECG, CBC with differential, liver function, electrolytes, platelets

Patient Education: Use as directed; do not change dosage or schedule of administration without consulting prescriber. Maintain adequate hydration (2-3 L/day of fluids) unless instructed to restrict fluid intake. You may experience flu-like syndrome (acetaminophen may help); nausea, vomiting, dry mouth, or metallic taste (small frequent meals, frequent mouth care, sucking lozenges, or chewing gum may help); fatigue, drowsiness, insomnia, dizziness, agitation, abnormal thinking (use caution when driving or engaging in tasks requiring alertness until response to drug is known). Inform prescriber **immediately** if you feel depressed or have any thoughts of suicide. Report unusual bruising or bleeding; persistent abdominal disturbances; unusual fatigue; muscle pain or tremors; chest pain or palpitation; swelling of extremities or unusual weight gain; respiratory difficulty; pain, swelling, or redness at injection site; or other unusual symptoms. **Pregnancy/breast-feeding precautions:** Inform prescriber if you are or intend to become pregnant. Consult prescriber if breast-feeding.

Pregnancy Risk Factor: C

Pregnancy Issues: Safety and efficacy for use during pregnancy have not been established. Interferon alpha has been shown to decrease serum estradiol and progesterone levels in humans. Menstrual irregularities and abortion have been reported in animals. Effective contraception is recommended during treatment.

Lactation: Enters breast milk/not recommended (AAP rates "compatible")

Breast-Feeding Considerations: Women with hepatitis C should be instructed that there is a theoretical risk the virus may be transmitted in breast milk. HIV-infected mothers are discouraged from breast-feeding to decrease potential transmission of HIV.

Perioperative/Anesthesia/Other Concerns: Indications and dosage regimens are specific for a particular brand of interferon; other brands have different indications and dosage guidelines.

(Continued)

Interferon Alfa-2b *(Continued)*

Administration

Reconstitution: The manufacturer recommends reconstituting vial with the diluent provided (SWFI). To prepare solution for infusion, further dilute appropriate dose in NS 100 mL. Final concentration should not be <10 million units/ 100 mL.

Compatibility: Stable in LR, NS; **incompatible** with D_5W

Storage: Store powder and solution for injection (vials and pens) under refrigeration (2°C to 8°C).

Powder for injection: Following reconstitution, should be used immediately, but may be stored under refrigeration for up to 24 hours.

Prefilled pens: After first use, discard unused portion after 1 month.

Interferon Alfa-2b and Ribavirin

(in ter FEER on AL fa too bee & rye ba VYE rin)

U.S. Brand Names Rebetron®

Synonyms Interferon Alfa-2b and Ribavirin Combination Pack; Ribavirin and Interferon Alfa-2b Combination Pack

Pharmacologic Category Antiviral Agent; Interferon

Use Combination therapy for the treatment of chronic hepatitis C in patients with compensated liver disease previously untreated with alpha interferon or who have relapsed after alpha interferon therapy

Mechanism of Action

Interferon Alfa-2b: Alpha interferons are a family of proteins, produced by nucleated cells, that have antiviral, antiproliferative, and immune-regulating activity. There are 16 known subtypes of alpha interferons. Interferons interact with cells through high affinity cell surface receptors. Following activation, multiple effects can be detected including induction of gene transcription. Inhibits cellular growth, alters the state of cellular differentiation, interferes with oncogene expression, alters cell surface antigen expression, increases phagocytic activity of macrophages, and augments cytotoxicity of lymphocytes for target cells

Ribavirin: Inhibits replication of RNA and DNA viruses; inhibits influenza virus RNA polymerase activity and inhibits the initiation and elongation of RNA fragments resulting in inhibition of viral protein synthesis

Pharmacodynamics/Kinetics See individual agents.

Contraindications Hypersensitivity to interferon alfa-2b, ribavirin, or any component of the formulation; autoimmune hepatitis; males with a pregnant female partner; pregnancy

Warnings/Precautions

Interferon alfa-2b: Suicidal ideation or attempts may occur more frequently in pediatric patients when compared to adults. May cause severe psychiatric adverse events (psychosis, mania, depression, suicidal behavior/ideation) in patients with and without previous psychiatric symptoms, avoid use in severe psychiatric disorders or in patients with a history of depression; careful neuropsychiatric monitoring is required during therapy. Use with caution in patients with a history of seizures, brain metastases, multiple sclerosis, cardiac disease (ischemic or thromboembolic), arrhythmias, myelosuppression, hepatic impairment, or renal dysfunction (use is not recommended if Cl_{cr}<50 mL/minute). Use caution in patients with a history of pulmonary disease, coagulopathy, thyroid disease (monitor thyroid function), hypertension, or diabetes mellitus (particularly if prone to DKA). Caution in patients receiving drugs that may cause lactic acidosis (eg, nucleoside analogues). Avoid use in patients with autoimmune disorders; worsening of psoriasis and/or development of autoimmune disorders has been associated with alpha interferons. Higher doses in elderly patients, or diseases other than hairy cell leukemia, may result in increased CNS toxicity. Treatment should be discontinued in patients who develop severe pulmonary symptoms with chest x-ray changes, autoimmune disorders, worsening of hepatic function, psychiatric symptoms (including depression and/or suicidal thoughts/ behaviors), ischemic and/or infectious disorders. Ophthalmologic disorders (including retinal hemorrhages, cotton wool spots and retinal artery or vein obstruction) have occurred in patients receiving alpha interferons. Hypertriglyceridemia has been reported (discontinue if severe).

Safety and efficacy in children <3 years of age have not been established. Do not treat patients with visceral AIDS-related Kaposi's sarcoma associated with rapidly-progressing or life-threatening disease. A transient increase in SGOT (>2x baseline) is common in patients treated with interferon alfa-2b for chronic hepatitis. Therapy generally may continue, however, functional indicators (albumin, prothrombin time, bilirubin) should be monitored at 2-week intervals. **Due to differences in dosage, patients should not change brands of interferons.**

Intron® A may cause bone marrow suppression, including very rarely, aplastic anemia. Hemolytic anemia (hemoglobin <10 g/dL) was observed in up to 10% of treated patients in clinical trials when combined with ribavirin; anemia occurred within 1-2 weeks of initiation of therapy.

Ribavirin: Oral: Anemia has been observed in patients receiving the interferon/ribavirin combination. Severe psychiatric events have also occurred including depression and suicidal behavior during combination therapy; avoid use in patients with a psychiatric history. Hemolytic anemia is a significant toxicity; usually occurring within 1-2 weeks. Assess cardiac disease before initiation. Anemia may worsen underlying cardiac disease; use caution. If any deterioration in cardiovascular status occurs, discontinue therapy. Use caution in pulmonary disease; pulmonary symptoms have been associated with administration. Use caution in patients with sarcoidosis (exacerbation reported). Negative pregnancy test is required before initiation and monthly thereafter. Avoid pregnancy in female patients and female partners of patients during therapy. Discontinue therapy in suspected/confirmed pancreatitis. Use caution in elderly patients; higher frequency of anemia; take renal function into consideration before initiating. Safety and efficacy have not been established in organ transplant patients, decompensated liver disease, concurrent hepatitis B virus or HIV exposure, or pediatric patients <3 years of age. Use caution in patients receiving concurrent medications which may cause lactic acidosis (eg, nucleoside analogues).

Drug Interactions Interferon Alfa-2b: **Inhibits** CYP1A2 (weak)

ACE inhibitors: Interferons may increase the adverse/toxic effects of ACE inhibitors, specifically the development of granulocytopenia. Risk: Monitor

Antiretroviral (nucleoside): Concomitant use of ribavirin and nucleoside analogues may increase the risk of developing lactic acidosis (includes adefovir, didanosine, lamivudine, stavudine, zalcitabine, zidovudine).

Clozapine: A case report of agranulocytosis with concurrent use.

Erythropoietin: Case reports of decreased hematopoietic effect

Fluorouracil: Possible toxicity with doubling of concentrations in patients with gastrointestinal carcinoma. Monitor and adjust fluorouracil dose if necessary.

Interferon (alfa) and ribavirin: Concomitant therapy may increase the risk of hemolytic anemia.

Melphalan: Interferon alpha may decrease the serum concentrations of melphalan; this may or may not decrease the potential toxicity of melphalan. Risk: Monitor

Prednisone: Prednisone may decrease the therapeutic effects of Interferon alpha. Risk: Moderate

Ribavirin: Concurrent therapy may increase the risk of hemolytic anemia.

Stavudine: Ribavirin may decrease the activity of stavudine; avoid concurrent use.

Theophylline: Interferon alpha may decrease the P450 isoenzyme metabolism of theophylline. Risk: Moderate

Thyroid hormone: Thyroid dysfunction has been reported with interferon/ribavirin therapy; monitor.

Warfarin: Interferons may increase the anticoagulant effects of warfarin. Risk: Monitor

Zidovudine: Interferons may decrease the metabolism of zidovudine. Ribavirin may decrease the activity of zidovudine. Avoid concurrent use.

Adverse Reactions Note: Adverse reactions listed are specific to combination regimen in previously untreated hepatitis patients. See individual agents for additional adverse reactions reported with each agent during therapy for other diseases.

>10%:

Central nervous system: Fatigue (children 61%; adults 68%), headache (63%), insomnia (children 14%; adults 39%), fever (children 61%; adults 37%), depression (children 13%; adults 32% to 36%), irritability (children 10%; adults 23% to 32%), dizziness (17% to 23%), emotional lability (children 16%; adults 7% to 11%), impaired concentration (5% to 14%)

Dermatologic: Alopecia (23% to 32%), pruritus (children 12%; adults 19% to 21%), rash (17% to 28%)

Gastrointestinal: Nausea (33% to 46%), anorexia (children 51%; adults 25% to 27%), dyspepsia (children <1%; adults 14% to 16%), vomiting (children 42%; adults 9% to 11%)

(Continued)

Interferon Alfa-2b and Ribavirin *(Continued)*

Hematologic: Leukopenia, neutropenia (usually recovers within 4 weeks of treatment discontinuation), anemia

Hepatic: Hyperbilirubinemia (27%; only 0.9% to 2% >3.0-6 mg/dL)

Local: Injection site inflammation (13%)

Neuromuscular & skeletal: Myalgia (children 32%; adults 61% to 64%), rigors (40%), arthralgia (children 15%; adults 30% to 33%), musculoskeletal pain (20% to 28%)

Respiratory: Dyspnea (children 5%; adults 18% to 19%)

Miscellaneous: Flu-like syndrome (children 31%; adults 14% to 18%)

1% to 10%:

Cardiovascular: Chest pain (5% to 9%)

Central nervous system: Nervousness (3% to 4%)

Endocrine & metabolic: Thyroid abnormalities (hyper- or hypothyroidism), serum uric acid increased, hyperglycemia

Gastrointestinal: Taste perversion (children <1%; adults 7% to 8%)

Hematologic: Hemolytic anemia (10%), thrombocytopenia

Local: Injection site reaction (7%)

Neuromuscular & skeletal: Weakness (5% to 9%)

Respiratory: Sinusitis (children <1%; adults 9% to 10%)

<1% (Limited to important and life-threatening): Acute hypersensitivity reactions, anaphylaxis, angioedema, aplastic anemia (very rare), arrhythmia, bronchoconstriction, cardiomyopathy, cotton wool spots, diabetes, hallucinations, hearing loss, hepatotoxic reactions, hypertriglyceridemia, hypotension, MI, nephrotic syndrome, pancreatitis, pneumonia, pneumonitis, renal failure, retinal hemorrhages, retinal artery or vein obstruction, sarcoidosis (including exacerbations of sarcoidosis), severe psychiatric reactions, suicidal behavior, suicidal ideation, tinnitus, urticaria; rare cases of autoimmune diseases including vasculitis, polyarteritis reaction, rheumatoid arthritis, lupus erythematosus, and Raynaud's phenomenon

Overdosage/Toxicology Interferon Alfa-2b: Signs and symptoms of overdose include CNS depression, obtundation, flu-like symptoms, myelosuppression; treatment is supportive.

Dosing

Adults & Elderly:

Chronic hepatitis C: Recommended dosage of combination therapy:

Intron® A: SubQ: 3 million int. units 3 times/week **and**

Rebetol® capsule: Oral:

≤75 kg (165 pounds): 1000 mg/day (two 200 mg capsules in the morning and three 200 mg capsules in the evening)

>75 kg: 1200 mg/day (three 200 mg capsules in the morning and three 200 mg capsules in the evening)

Pediatrics: Chronic hepatitis C:

Children ≥3 years: **Note:** Duration of therapy: genotype 1: 48 weeks; genotype 2 or 3: 24 weeks. Discontinue treatment in any patient if HCV-RNA is not below the limits of detection of the assay after 24 weeks of therapy. Combination therapy:

Intron® A: SubQ:

25-61 kg: 3 million int. units/m^2 3 times/week

>61 kg: Refer to Adults dosing

Rebetol®: Oral: **Note:** Oral solution should be used in children 3-5 years of age, children ≤25 kg, or those unable to swallow capsules.

Capsule/solution: 15 mg/kg/day in 2 divided doses (morning and evening)

Capsule dosing recommendations:

25-36 kg: 400 mg/day (200 mg morning and evening)

37-49 kg: 600 mg/day (200 mg in the morning and two 200 mg capsules in the evening)

50-61 kg: 800 mg/day (two 200 mg capsules morning and evening)

>61 kg: Refer to adult dosing.

Renal Impairment: Patients with Cl_{cr} <50 mL/minutes should not receive ribavirin.

Available Dosage Forms Combination package:

For patients ≤75 kg [contains single-dose vials]:

Injection, solution: Interferon alfa-2b (Intron® A): 3 million int. units/0.5 mL (0.5 mL) [6 vials (3 million int. units/vial), 6 syringes, and alcohol swabs]

Capsule: Ribavirin (Rebetol®): 200 mg (70s)

For patients ≤75 kg [contains multidose vials]:

Injection, solution: Interferon alfa-2b (Intron® A): 3 million int. units/0.5 mL (3.8 mL) [1 multidose vial (18 million int. units/vial), 6 syringes, and alcohol swabs]

Capsule: Ribavirin (Rebetol®): 200 mg (70s)

For patients ≤75 kg [contains multidose pen]:

Injection, solution: Interferon alfa-2b (Intron® A): 3 million int. units/0.2 mL (1.5 mL) [1 multidose pen (18 million int. units/pen), 6 needles, and alcohol swabs]

Capsule: Ribavirin (Rebetol®): 200 mg (70s)

For patients >75 kg [contains single-dose vials]:

Injection, solution: Interferon alfa-2b (Intron® A): 3 million int. units/0.5 mL (0.5 mL) [6 vials (3 million int. units/vial), 6 syringes, and alcohol swabs]

Capsule: Ribavirin (Rebetol®): 200 mg (84s)

For patients >75 kg [contains multidose vials]:

Injection, solution: Interferon alfa-2b (Intron® A): 3 million int. units/0.5 mL (3.8 mL) [1 multidose vial (18 million int. units/vial), 6 syringes, and alcohol swabs]

Capsule: Ribavirin (Rebetol®): 200 mg (84s)

For patients >75 kg [contains multidose pen]:

Injection, solution: Interferon alfa-2b (Intron® A): 3 million int. units/0.2 mL (1.5 mL) [1 multidose pen (18 million int. units/pen), 6 needles, and alcohol swabs]

Capsule: Ribavirin (Rebetol®): 200 mg (84s)

For Rebetol® dose reduction [contains single-dose vials]:

Injection, solution: Interferon alfa-2b (Intron® A): 3 million int. units/0.5 mL (0.5 mL) [6 vials (3 million int. units/vial), 6 syringes, and alcohol swabs]

Capsule: Ribavirin (Rebetol®): 200 mg (42s)

For Rebetol® dose reduction [contains multidose vials]:

Injection, solution: Interferon alfa-2b (Intron® A): 3 million int. units/0.5 mL (3.8 mL) [1 multidose vial (18 million int. units/vial), 6 syringes, and alcohol swabs]

Capsule: Ribavirin (Rebetol®): 200 mg (42s)

For Rebetol® dose reduction [contains multidose pen]:

Injection, solution: Interferon alfa-2b (Intron® A): 3 million int. units/0.2 mL (1.5 mL) [1 multidose pen (18 million int. units/pen), 6 needles, and alcohol swabs]

Capsule: Ribavirin (Rebetol®): 200 mg (42s)

Nursing Guidelines

Assessment: Assess other medications patient may be taking for increased risk of drug/drug interactions. Baseline chest x-rays and ECGs are recommended. Patients with pre-existing cardiac abnormalities, or in advanced stages of cancer should have ECGs taken before and during treatment. Monitor for neuropsychiatric changes. Monitor laboratory results and adverse reactions on a frequent and regular basis during therapy (see monographs for Interferon Alfa-2b and Ribavirin). Assess knowledge/teach patient appropriate use (including appropriate injection technique and needle disposal), interventions to reduce side effects, and adverse symptoms to report. **Pregnancy risk factor X:** Determine that patient is not pregnant before beginning treatment and do not give to women of childbearing age or to males who may have intercourse with women of childbearing ages unless both male and female are capable of complying with contraceptive measures for 6 months prior to therapy and for 1 month following therapy.

Monitoring Laboratory Tests: Obtain pretreatment CBC, liver function tests, TSH, and electrolytes and monitor routinely throughout therapy (at 2 weeks and 4 weeks, more frequently if indicated); discontinue if WBC <1.0 x 10^9/L, neutrophils <0.5 x 10^9/L, platelets <25 x 10^9/L, or if hemoglobin <8.5 g/dL (in cardiac patients, discontinue if hemoglobin <12 g/dL after 4 weeks of dosage reduction). Pretreatment and monthly pregnancy test for women of childbearing age. Reticulocyte count, serum HCV RNA levels

Dietary Considerations: Take oral formulation without regard to food, but always in a consistent manner with respect to food intake (ie, always take with food or always take on an empty stomach).

Patient Education: This a combination therapy. Both the injections and the oral capsules are necessary for effective therapy. Follow administration directions exactly and dispose of needles as instructed. Do not discontinue, alter dose or frequency without consulting prescriber. Do not crush, chew, or open capsules. Take at the same times each day. Maintain adequate hydration (2-3 L/day of fluids) unless instructed to restrict fluid intake. You may experience flu-like symptoms (consult prescriber for relief); nausea, vomiting, or GI upset (small frequent meals, frequent mouth care, sucking lozenges, or chewing gum may help); or insomnia, drowsiness, lethargy, fatigue, dizziness, abnormal thinking (use caution when driving or engaging in tasks that require alertness until response to drug is known). Report unusual bruising or bleeding, inflammation

(Continued)

Interferon Alfa-2b and Ribavirin *(Continued)*

or pain at injection site, persistent GI disturbances, muscle pain or tremors, chest pain or palpitations, swelling of extremities, unusual weight gain, or rash. Contact prescriber immediately if you experience unusual agitation, nervousness, feelings of depression, or have thoughts of suicide. **Pregnancy/breast-feeding precautions:** This drug will cause severe fetal defects. Inform prescriber if you are pregnant. Females must not get pregnant or males must not cause a pregnancy during therapy, and for 6 months after therapy is completed. Pregnancy tests are required for females. Consult prescriber for instruction on appropriate contraceptive measures. Breast-feeding is not recommended.

Pregnancy Risk Factor: X

Pregnancy Issues: Abortifacient and teratogenic effects have been reported. Women of childbearing potential should not be treated unless 2 reliable forms of contraception are used. In addition, male patients and their female partners must also use 2 reliable forms of contraception. Pregnancy must be avoided for 6 months following therapy.

Lactation: Excretion in breast milk unknown/not recommended

Breast-Feeding Considerations: Women with hepatitis C should be instructed that there is a theoretical risk the virus may be transmitted in breast milk.

Administration

Oral: Capsule should not be opened, crushed, chewed, or broken. Capsules are not for use in children <5 years of age. Use oral solution for children 3-5 years, those ≤25 kg, or those who cannot swallow capsules.

Storage: Store the Rebetol® capsules plus Intron® A injection combination package refrigerated between 2°C and 8°C (36°F and 46°F)

When separated, the individual carton of Rebetol® capsules should be stored refrigerated between 2°C and 8°C (36°F and 46°F) or at 25°C (77°F); excursions are permitted between 15°C and 30°C (59°F and 86°F)

When separated, the individual carton or vial of Intron® A injection and the Intron® A multidose pen should be stored refrigerated between 2°C and 8°C (36°F and 46°F)

♦ **Interferon Alfa-2b and Ribavirin Combination Pack** *see* Interferon Alfa-2b and Ribavirin *on page 940*

♦ **Interferon Alfa-2b (PEG Conjugate)** *see* Peginterferon Alfa-2b *on page 1325*

Interferon Alfacon-1 (in ter FEER on AL fa con one)

U.S. Brand Names Infergen®

Pharmacologic Category Interferon

Use Treatment of chronic hepatitis C virus (HCV) infection in patients ≥18 years of age with compensated liver disease and anti-HCV serum antibodies or HCV RNA.

Mechanism of Action Alpha interferons are a family of proteins, produced by nucleated cells, that have antiviral, antiproliferative, and immune-regulating activity. There are at least 25 alpha interferons identified. Interferons interact with cells through high affinity cell surface receptors. Following activation, multiple effects can be detected. Interferons induce gene transcription, inhibit cellular growth, alter the state of cellular differentiation, interfere with oncogene expression, alter cell surface antigen expression, increase phagocytic activity of macrophages, and augment cytotoxicity of lymphocytes for target cells. Although all alpha interferons share similar properties, the actual biological effects vary between subtypes.

Pharmacodynamics/Kinetics Pharmacokinetic studies have not been conducted on patients with chronic hepatitis C.

Time to peak: Healthy volunteers: 24-36 hours

Contraindications Hypersensitivity to interferon alfacon-1 or any component of the formulation, other alpha interferons, or *E. coli*-derived products

Warnings/Precautions Severe psychiatric adverse effects, including depression, suicidal ideation, and suicide attempt, may occur. Avoid use in severe psychiatric disorders. Use with caution in patients with a history of depression. Use with caution in patients with prior cardiac disease (ischemic or thromboembolic), arrhythmias, patients who are chronically immunosuppressed, and patients with endocrine disorders. Do not use in patients with hepatic decompensation. Ophthalmologic disorders (including retinal hemorrhages, cotton wool spots and retinal artery or vein obstruction) have occurred in patients using other alpha interferons. Prior to start of therapy, visual exams are recommended for patients with diabetes mellitus or hypertension. Treatment should be discontinued in patients with worsening or persistently severe signs/symptoms of autoimmune, infectious, ischemic (including radiographic changes or worsening hepatic function), or neuropsychiatric disorders (including depression and/or suicidal thoughts/behavior). Use caution in patients with autoimmune disorders; type-1 interferon therapy has been reported to exacerbate autoimmune diseases. Do not use interferon alfacon-1 in patients with autoimmune hepatitis. Use caution in patients with low peripheral blood counts or myelosuppression, including concurrent use of myelosuppressive therapy. Safety and efficacy have not been determined for patients <18 years of age.

Drug Interactions

ACE inhibitors: Interferons may increase the adverse/toxic effects of ACE inhibitors, specifically the development of granulocytopenia. Risk: Monitor

Clozapine: A case report of agranulocytosis with concurrent use.

Erythropoietin: Case reports of decreased hematopoietic effect

Melphalan: Interferon alpha may decrease the serum concentrations of melphalan; this may or may not decrease the potential toxicity of melphalan. Risk: Monitor

Prednisone: Prednisone may decrease the therapeutic effects of Interferon alpha. Risk: Moderate

Theophylline: Interferon alpha may decrease the P450 isoenzyme metabolism of theophylline. Risk: Moderate

Warfarin: Interferons may increase the anticoagulant effects of warfarin. Risk: Monitor

Zidovudine: Interferons may decrease the metabolism of zidovudine. Risk: Monitor

Adverse Reactions Adverse reactions reported using 9 mcg/dose interferon alfacon-1 3 times/week. Reactions listed were reported in ≥5% of patients treated.

>10%:

- Central nervous system: Headache (82%), fatigue (69%), fever (61%), insomnia (39%), nervousness (31%), depression (26%), dizziness (22%), anxiety (19%), noncardiac chest pain (13%), emotional lability (12%), malaise (11%)
- Dermatologic: Alopecia (14%), pruritus (14%), rash (13%)
- Endocrine & metabolic: Hot flashes (13%)
- Gastrointestinal: Abdominal pain (41%), nausea (40%), diarrhea (29%), anorexia (24%), dyspepsia (21%), vomiting (12%)
- Hematologic: Granulocytopenia (23%), thrombocytopenia (19%), leukopenia (15%)
- Local: Injection site erythema (23%)
- Neuromuscular & skeletal: Myalgia (58%), body pain (54%), arthralgia (51%), back pain (42%), limb pain (26%), neck pain (14%), skeletal pain (14%), paresthesia (13%)
- Respiratory: Pharyngitis (34%), upper respiratory tract infection (31%), cough (22%), sinusitis (17%), rhinitis (13%), respiratory tract congestion (12%)
- Miscellaneous: Flu-like syndrome (15%), diaphoresis increased (12%)

1% to 10%:

- Cardiovascular: Peripheral edema (9%), hypertension (5%), tachycardia (4%), palpitation (3%)
- Central nervous system: Amnesia (10%), hypoesthesia (10%), abnormal thinking (8%), agitation (6%), confusion (4%), somnolence (4%)
- Dermatologic: Bruising (6%), erythema (6%), dry skin (6%), wound (4%)
- Endocrine & metabolic: Thyroid test abnormalities (9%), dysmenorrhea (9%), increased triglycerides (6%), menstrual disorder (6%), decreased libido (5%), hypothyroidism (4%)
- Gastrointestinal: Constipation (9%), flatulence (8%), toothache (7%), decreased salivation (6%), hemorrhoids (6%), weight loss (5%), taste perversion (3%)
- Genitourinary: Vaginitis (8%), genital moniliasis (2%)
- Hepatic: Hepatomegaly (5%), liver tenderness (5%), increased prothrombin time (3%)
- Local: Injection site pain (9%), access pain (8%), injection site bruising (6%)
- Neuromuscular & skeletal: Weakness (9%), hypertonia (7%), musculoskeletal disorder (4%)
- Ocular: Conjunctivitis (8%), eye pain (5%), vision abnormalities (3%)
- Otic: Tinnitus (6%), earache (5%), otitis (2%)

(Continued)

Interferon Alfacon-1 *(Continued)*

Respiratory: Upper respiratory tract congestion (10%), epistaxis (8%), dyspnea (7%), bronchitis (6%)

Miscellaneous: Allergic reaction (7%), lymphadenopathy (6%), lymphocytosis (5%), infection (3%)

Flu-like symptoms (which included headache, fatigue, fever, myalgia, rigors, arthralgia, and increased diaphoresis) were the most commonly reported adverse reaction. This was reported separately from flu-like syndrome. Most patients were treated symptomatically.

Other adverse reactions associated with interferon therapy include arrhythmia, autoimmune disorders, chest pain, hepatotoxic reactions, lupus erythematosus, MI, neuropsychiatric disorders (including suicidal thoughts/behavior), pneumonia, pneumonitis, severe hypersensitivity reactions (rare), vasculitis

Overdosage/Toxicology One overdose has been reported. A patient received ten times the prescribed dose (150 mcg) for 3 days. In addition to an increase in anorexia, chills, fever, and myalgia, there was also an increase in ALT, AST, and LDH. Laboratory values reportedly returned to baseline within 30 days.

Dosing

Adults & Elderly: Chronic HCV infection: SubQ: 9 mcg 3 times/week for 24 weeks; allow 48 hours between doses.

Patients who have previously tolerated interferon therapy but did not respond or relapsed: SubQ: 15 mcg 3 times/week for 6 months

Pediatrics: Not indicated for patients <18 years of age.

Hepatic Impairment: Avoid use in decompensated hepatic disease.

Available Dosage Forms Injection, solution [preservative free]: 30 mcg/mL (0.3 mL, 0.5 mL)

Nursing Guidelines

Assessment: Assess other medications patient may be taking for effectiveness and interactions. Monitor for signs of depression and suicidal ideation. Assess results of laboratory tests on a regular basis during therapy. Patient with pre-existing diabetes mellitus or hypertension should have an ophthalmic exam prior to beginning treatment. Patient must be monitored closely for adverse reactions. If self-administered, instruct patient in appropriate storage, injection technique, and syringe disposal. Assess knowledge/teach patient purpose for use, adverse reactions and interventions, and adverse reactions to report.

Monitoring Laboratory Tests: Hemoglobin and hematocrit, white blood cell count, platelets, triglycerides, and thyroid function. Laboratory tests should be taken 2 weeks prior to therapy, after therapy has begun, and periodically during treatment. HCV RNA, and ALT to determine success/response to therapy.

The following guidelines were used during the clinical studies as acceptable baseline values:

- Platelet count ≥75 x 10^9/L
- Hemoglobin ≥100 g/L
- ANC ≥1500 x 10^6/L
- S_{cr} <180 µmol/L (<2 mg/dL) or Cl_{cr} >0.83 mL/second (>50 mL/minute)
- Serum albumin ≥25 g/L
- Bilirubin WNL
- TSH and T_4 WNL

Patient Education: Use exactly as directed (if self-administered, follow exact instructions for injection and syringe disposal). Do not alter dosage or brand of medication without consulting prescriber. You will need frequent laboratory tests during course of therapy. If you have diabetes or hypertension you should have ophthalmic exam prior to beginning therapy. You may experience headache, dizziness, nervousness, anxiety (use caution when driving or engaging in dangerous tasks until response to medication is known); nausea, vomiting, diarrhea, or loss of appetite (small frequent meals, frequent mouth care, sucking hard candy or chewing gum may help); flu-like symptoms such as headache, fatigue, muscle or joint pain, increased perspiration (mild non-narcotic analgesic may help); or hair loss (will probably grow back when treatment is completed). Promptly report any persistent GI upset; insomnia, depression, anxiety, nervousness; chest pain or palpitations; muscle, bone, or joint pain; respiratory difficulties or congestion; vision changes; or other persistent adverse effects. **Pregnancy/breast-feeding precautions:** Inform prescriber if you are or intend to become pregnant. Consult prescriber if breast-feeding.

Pregnancy Risk Factor: C

Pregnancy Issues: There have been no well-controlled studies in pregnant women. Animal studies have shown embryolethal or abortifacient effects. Males and females who are being treated with interferon alfacon-1 should use effective contraception.

Lactation: Excretion in breast milk unknown/use caution (AAP rates "compatible")

Breast-Feeding Considerations: Women with hepatitis C should be instructed that there is a theoretical risk the virus may be transmitted in breast milk.

Perioperative/Anesthesia/Other Concerns: Indications and dosage regimens are specific for a particular brand of interferon; other brands have different indications and dosage guidelines.

Administration

I.V.: Interferon alfacon-1 is given by SubQ injection, 3 times/week, with at least 48 hours between doses.

Storage: Store in refrigerator 2°C to 8°C (36°F to 46°F). Do not freeze. Avoid exposure to direct sunlight. Do not shake vigorously.

Interferon Beta-1a (in ter FEER on BAY ta won aye)

U.S. Brand Names Avonex®; Rebif®

Synonyms rIFN beta-1a

Pharmacologic Category Interferon

Medication Safety Issues

Sound-alike/look-alike issues:

Avonex® may be confused with Avelox®

Use Treatment of relapsing forms of multiple sclerosis (MS)

Mechanism of Action Interferon beta differs from naturally occurring human protein by a single amino acid substitution and the lack of carbohydrate side chains; alters the expression and response to surface antigens and can enhance immune cell activities. Properties of interferon beta that modify biologic responses are mediated by cell surface receptor interactions; mechanism in the treatment of MS is unknown.

Pharmacodynamics/Kinetics Limited data due to small doses used

Half-life elimination: Avonex®: 10 hours; Rebif®: 69 hours

Time to peak, serum: Avonex® (I.M.): 3-15 hours; Rebif® (SubQ): 16 hours

Contraindications Hypersensitivity to natural or recombinant interferons, human albumin, or any other component of the formulation

Warnings/Precautions Interferons have been associated with severe psychiatric adverse events (psychosis, mania, depression, suicidal behavior/ideation) in patients with and without previous psychiatric symptoms, avoid use in severe psychiatric disorders and use caution in patients with a history of depression; patients exhibiting depressive symptoms should be closely monitored and discontinuation of therapy should be considered.

Allergic reactions, including anaphylaxis, have been reported. Caution should be used in patients with hepatic impairment or in those who abuse alcohol. Rare cases of severe hepatic injury, including hepatic failure, have been reported in patients receiving interferon beta-1a; risk may be increased by ethanol use or concurrent therapy with hepatotoxic drugs. Treatment should be suspended if jaundice or symptoms of hepatic dysfunction occur. Some reports indicate symptoms began after 1-6 months of treatment. Hematologic effects, including pancytopenia (rare) and thrombocytopenia, have been reported. Associated with a high incidence of flu-like adverse effects; use of analgesics and/or antipyretics on treatment days may be helpful. Use caution in patients with pre-existing cardiovascular disease, pulmonary disease, seizure disorders, myelosuppression, or renal impairment. Some formulations contain albumin, which may carry a remote risk of transmitting Creutzfeldt-Jakob or other viral diseases. Safety and efficacy in patients <18 years of age have not been established.

Drug Interactions

ACE inhibitors: Interferons may increase the adverse/toxic effects of ACE inhibitors, specifically the development of granulocytopenia; monitor.

Hepatotoxic drugs: May increase the risk of hepatic injury in patients receiving interferon beta-1a.

Warfarin: Interferons may increase the anticoagulant effects of warfarin; monitor.

Zidovudine: Interferons may decrease the metabolism of zidovudine; monitor.

(Continued)

Interferon Beta-1a *(Continued)*

Adverse Reactions

>10%:

Central nervous system: Headache (Avonex® 58%; Rebif® 65% to 70%), fatigue (Rebif® 33% to 41%), fever (Avonex® 20%; Rebif® 25% to 28%), pain (Avonex® 23%), chills (Avonex® 19%), depression (Avonex® 18%), dizziness (Avonex® 14%)

Gastrointestinal: Nausea (Avonex® 23%), abdominal pain (Avonex® 8%; Rebif® 20% to 22%)

Genitourinary: Urinary tract infection (Avonex® 17%)

Hematologic: Leukopenia (Rebif® 28% to 36%)

Hepatic: ALT increased (Rebif® 20% to 27%), AST increased (Rebif® 10% to 17%)

Local: Injection site reaction (Avonex® 3%; Rebif® 89% to 92%)

Neuromuscular & skeletal: Myalgia (Avonex® 29%; Rebif® 25%), back pain (Rebif® 23% to 25%), weakness (Avonex® 24%), skeletal pain (Rebif® 10% to 15%), rigors (Rebif® 6% to 13%)

Ocular: Vision abnormal (Rebif® 7% to 13%)

Respiratory: Sinusitis (Avonex® 14%), upper respiratory tract infection (Avonex® 14%)

Miscellaneous: Flu-like symptoms (Avonex® 49%; Rebif® 56% to 59%), neutralizing antibodies (significance not known; Avonex® 5%; Rebif® 24%), lymphadenopathy (Rebif® 11% to 12%)

1% to 10% (reported with one or both products):

Cardiovascular: Chest pain, vasodilation

Central nervous system: Convulsions, malaise, migraine, somnolence

Dermatologic: Alopecia, erythematous rash, maculopapular rash, urticaria

Endocrine & metabolic: Thyroid disorder

Gastrointestinal: Toothache, xerostomia

Genitourinary: Micturition frequency, urinary incontinence

Hematologic: Anemia, thrombocytopenia

Hepatic: Bilirubinemia, hepatic function abnormal

Local: Injection site bruising, injection site inflammation, injection site necrosis, injection site pain

Neuromuscular & skeletal: Arthralgia, coordination abnormal, hypertonia

Ocular: Eye disorder, xerophthalmia

Respiratory: Bronchitis

Miscellaneous: Infection

<1% (Limited to important and life-threatening): Anaphylaxis, autoimmune hepatitis, cardiomyopathy, CHF, hepatic failure, hepatitis, idiopathic thrombocytopenia, menorrhagia, metrorrhagia, pancytopenia, psychiatric disorders (new or worsening), transaminases increased

Overdosage/Toxicology Symptoms of overdose include CNS depression, obtundation, flu-like symptoms, myelosuppression. Treatment is supportive.

Dosing

Adults & Elderly: Multiple sclerosis: **Note:** Analgesics and/or antipyretics may help decrease flu-like symptoms on treatment days:

I.M. (Avonex®): 30 mcg once weekly

SubQ (Rebif®): Doses should be separated by at least 48 hours:

Target dose 44 mcg 3 times/week: 11

Initial: 8.8 mcg (20 % of final dose) 3 times/week for 8 weeks

Titration: 22 mcg (50% of final dose) 3 times/week for 8 weeks

Final dose: 44 mcg 3 times/week

Target dose 22 mcg 3 times/week:

Initial: 4.4 mcg (20 % of final dose) 3 times/week for 8 weeks

Titration: 11 mcg (50% of final dose) 3 times/week for 8 weeks

Final dose: 22 mcg 3 times/week

Hepatic Impairment: Rebif®: If liver function tests increase or in case of leukopenia: Decrease dose 20% to 50% until toxicity resolves

Available Dosage Forms

Combination package [preservative free] (Rebif® Titration Pack):

Injection, solution: 8.8 mcg/0.2 mL (0.2 mL) [6 prefilled syringes; contains albumin]

Injection, solution: 22 mcg/0.5 mL (0.5 mL) [6 prefilled syringes; contains albumin]

Injection, powder for reconstitution (Avonex®): 33 mcg [6.6 million units; provides 30 mcg/mL following reconstitution] [contains albumin; packaged with SWFI, alcohol wipes, and access pin and needle]

Injection, solution (Avonex®): 30 mcg/0.5 mL (0.5 mL) [albumin free; prefilled syringe; syringe cap contains latex; packaged with alcohol wipes, gauze pad, and adhesive bandages]

Injection, solution [preservative free] (Rebif®): 22 mcg/0.5 mL (0.5 mL) [prefilled syringe; contains albumin]; 44 mcg/0.5 mL (0.5 mL) [prefilled syringe; contains albumin]

Nursing Guidelines

Assessment: Assess results of laboratory tests on a regular a basis, therapeutic effectiveness, and adverse reactions. Monitor for signs of depression and suicidal ideation. Assess knowledge/instruct patient/caregiver on appropriate reconstitution, injection and needle disposal, possible side effects, and symptoms to report.

Monitoring Laboratory Tests: Liver function, blood chemistries, CBC and differential, BUN, creatinine

Avonex®: Frequency of monitoring has not been specifically defined; in clinical trials, monitoring was at 6-month intervals.

Rebif®: CBC and liver function testing at 1-, 3-, and 6 months, then periodically thereafter; thyroid function every 6 months (in patients with pre-existing abnormalities and/or clinical indications)

Patient Education: This is not a cure for MS; you will continue to receive regular treatment and follow-up for MS. Use as directed; do not change dosage or schedule of administration without consulting prescriber. If self-injecting and you miss a dose, take it as soon as you remember, but two injections should not be given within 48 hours of each other. Maintain adequate hydration (2-3 L/day of fluids) unless instructed to restrict fluid intake. You may experience flu-like syndrome (analgesics and/or antipyretics may help); nausea, vomiting, or loss of appetite (small frequent meals, frequent mouth care, sucking lozenges, or chewing gum may help); or drowsiness, sleep disturbances, dizziness, agitation, or abnormal thinking (use caution when driving or engaging in tasks requiring alertness until response to drug is known). Inform prescriber **immediately** if you feel depressed or have any thoughts of suicide. Report unusual bruising or bleeding; persistent abdominal disturbances; unusual fatigue; muscle pain or tremors; chest pain or palpitations; swelling of extremities; visual disturbances; pain, swelling, or redness at injection site; or other unusual symptoms. **Pregnancy/breast-feeding precautions:** Inform prescriber if you are or intend to become pregnant. Breast-feeding is not recommended.

Pregnancy Risk Factor: C

Pregnancy Issues: Safety and efficacy in pregnant women have not been established. Treatment should be discontinued if a woman becomes pregnant, or plans to become pregnant during therapy. A dose-related abortifacient activity was reported in Rhesus monkeys.

Lactation: Excretion in breast milk unknown/not recommended

Breast-Feeding Considerations: Potential for serious adverse reactions. Because its use has not been evaluated during lactation, a decision should be made to either discontinue breast-feeding or discontinue the drug.

Administration

I.M.: Avonex®: Must be given by I.M. injection.

Reconstitution: Avonex®: Reconstitute with 1.1 mL of diluent and swirl gently to dissolve. Do not shake. The reconstituted product contains no preservative and is for single-use only; discard unused portion.

Storage:

Avonex®:

Prefilled syringe: Store at 2°C to 8°C (36°F to 46°F); do not freeze, protect from light. Allow to warm to room temperature prior to use. Use within 12 hours after removing from refrigerator.

Vial: Store unreconstituted vial at 2°C to 8°C (36°F to 46°F). If refrigeration is not available, may be stored at 25°C (77°F) for up to 30 days. Do not freeze, protect from light. Following reconstitution, use immediately, but may be stored up to 6 hours at 2°C to 8°C (36°F to 46°F); do not freeze.

Rebif®: Store at 2°C to 8°C (36°F to 46°F). Do not freeze, protect from light. May also be stored ≤25°C (77°F) for up to 30 days if protected from heat and light.

Interferon Beta-1b (in ter FEER on BAY ta won bee)

U.S. Brand Names Betaseron®

Synonyms rIFN beta-1b

Pharmacologic Category Interferon

Use Treatment of relapsing forms of multiple sclerosis (MS)

Mechanism of Action Interferon beta-1b differs from naturally occurring human protein by a single amino acid substitution and the lack of carbohydrate side chains; mechanism in the treatment of MS is unknown; however, immunomodulatory effects attributed to interferon beta-1b include enhancement of suppressor T cell activity, reduction of proinflammatory cytokines, down-regulation of antigen presentation, and reduced trafficking of lymphocytes into the central nervous system.

Pharmacodynamics/Kinetics Limited data due to small doses used

Half-life elimination: 8 minutes to 4.3 hours

Time to peak, serum: 1-8 hours

Contraindications Hypersensitivity to *E. coli*-derived products, natural or recombinant interferon beta, albumin human or any other component of the formulation

Warnings/Precautions Hepatotoxicity has been reported with all beta interferons, including rare reports of hepatitis (autoimmune) and hepatic failure requiring transplant. Interferons have been associated with severe psychiatric adverse events (psychosis, mania, depression, suicidal behavior/ideation) in patients with and without previous psychiatric symptoms, avoid use in severe psychiatric disorders and use caution in patients with a history of depression; patients exhibiting symptoms of depression should be closely monitored and discontinuation of therapy should be considered. Due to high incidence of flu-like adverse effects, use caution in patients with pre-existing cardiovascular disease, pulmonary disease, seizure disorders, myelosuppression, renal impairment or hepatic impairment. Severe injection site reactions (necrosis) may occur, which may or may not heal with continued therapy; patient and/or caregiver competency in injection technique should be confirmed and periodically re-evaluated. Safety and efficacy in patients <18 years of age have not been established.

Drug Interactions

ACE inhibitors: Interferons may increase the adverse/toxic effects of ACE inhibitors, specifically the development of granulocytopenia. Risk: Monitor

Warfarin: Interferons may increase the anticoagulant effects of warfarin. Risk: Monitor

Zidovudine: Interferons may decrease the metabolism of zidovudine. Risk: Monitor

Adverse Reactions **Note:** Flu-like symptoms (including at least two of the following - headache, fever, chills, malaise, diaphoresis, and myalgia) are reported in the majority of patients (60%) and decrease over time (average duration ~1 week).

>10%:

Cardiovascular: Peripheral edema (15%), chest pain (11%)

Central nervous system: Headache (57%), fever (36%), pain (51%), chills (25%), dizziness (24%), insomnia (24%)

Dermatologic: Rash (24%), skin disorder (12%)

Endocrine & metabolic: Metrorrhagia (11%)

Gastrointestinal: Nausea (27%), diarrhea (19%), abdominal pain (19%), constipation (20%), dyspepsia (14%)

Genitourinary: Urinary urgency (13%)

Hematologic: Lymphopenia (88%), neutropenia (14%), leukopenia (14%)

Local: Injection site reaction (85%), inflammation (53%), pain (18%)

Neuromuscular & skeletal: Weakness (61%), myalgia (27%), hypertonia (50%), myasthenia (46%), arthralgia (31%), incoordination (21%)

Miscellaneous: Flu-like symptoms (60%)

1% to 10%:

Cardiovascular: Palpitation (4%), vasodilation (8%), hypertension (7%), tachycardia (4%), peripheral vascular disorder (6%)

Central nervous system: Anxiety (10%), malaise (8%), nervousness (7%)

Dermatologic: Alopecia (4%)

Endocrine & metabolic: Menorrhagia (8%), dysmenorrhea (7%)

Gastrointestinal: Weight gain (7%)

Genitourinary: Impotence (9%), pelvic pain (6%), cystitis (8%), urinary frequency (7%), prostatic disorder (3%)

Hematologic: Lymphadenopathy (8%)

Hepatic: SGPT increased >5x baseline (10%), SGOT increased >5x baseline (3%)

Local: Injection site necrosis (5%), edema (3%), mass (2%)

Neuromuscular & skeletal: Leg cramps (4%)

Respiratory: Dyspnea (7%)

Miscellaneous: Diaphoresis (8%), hypersensitivity (3%)

<1% (Limited to important or life-threatening): Apnea, arrhythmia, ataxia, bronchospasm, capillary leak syndrome (fatal), cardiac arrest, cardiomegaly, cardiomyopathy, cerebral hemorrhage, coma, confusion, convulsion, delirium, depersonalization, depression, DVT, emotional lability, erythema nodosum, ethanol intolerance, exfoliative dermatitis, gamma GT increase, GI hemorrhage, hallucinations, heart failure, hematemesis, hepatic failure, hepatitis, hyperthyroidism, hyperuricemia, hypocalcemia, mania, MI, paresthesia, pericardial effusion, photosensitivity, pneumonia, pruritus, psychosis, pulmonary embolism, rash, sepsis, shock, SIADH, skin discoloration, skin necrosis, suicidal ideation, syncope, thrombocytopenia, thyroid dysfunction, triglyceride increased, urinary tract infection, urosepsis, urticaria, vaginal hemorrhage, vomiting

Overdosage/Toxicology Symptoms of overdose include CNS depression, obtundation, flu-like symptoms, and myelosuppression. Treatment is supportive.

Dosing

Adults & Elderly: Multiple sclerosis (relapsing-remitting): SubQ: 0.25 mg (8 million units) every other day

Pediatrics: Not recommended in children <18 years of age

Available Dosage Forms Injection, powder for reconstitution [preservative free]: 0.3 mg [9.6 million units] [contains albumin; packaged with prefilled syringe containing diluent]

Nursing Guidelines

Assessment: Monitor laboratory results. Monitor closely for adverse reactions, especially patients with psychiatric or suicidal histories. Assess patient/caregiver knowledge and teach proper administration for SubQ injections and disposal of needles if appropriate. Teach the need for adequate hydration. Monitor for opportunistic infection.

Monitoring Laboratory Tests: Hemoglobin, liver function, blood chemistries

Patient Education: This is not a cure for MS; you will continue to receive regular treatment and follow-up for MS. Use as directed; do not change dosage or schedule of administration without consulting prescriber. Maintain adequate hydration (2-3 L/day of fluids) unless instructed to restrict fluid intake. You may experience flu-like syndrome (acetaminophen may help); nausea, vomiting, or loss of appetite (small frequent meals, frequent mouth care, sucking lozenges, or chewing gum may help); or drowsiness, sleep disturbances, dizziness, agitation, or abnormal thinking (use caution when driving or engaging in tasks requiring alertness until response to drug is known). Inform prescriber **immediately** if you feel depressed or have any thoughts of suicide. Report any broken skin or black-blue discoloration around the injection site. Report unusual bruising or bleeding; persistent abdominal disturbances; unusual fatigue; muscle pain or tremors; chest pain or palpitations, swelling of extremities; visual disturbances; pain, swelling, or redness at injection site; or other unusual symptoms. **Pregnancy/breast-feeding precautions:** Inform prescriber if you are or intend to become pregnant. Do not breast-feed.

Pregnancy Risk Factor: C

Pregnancy Issues: There are no adequate and well-controlled studies in pregnant women. Treatment should be discontinued if a woman becomes pregnant, or plans to become pregnant during therapy.

Lactation: Excretion in breast milk unknown/contraindicated

Breast-Feeding Considerations: Because its use has not been evaluated during lactation, breast-feeding is not recommended

Perioperative/Anesthesia/Other Concerns: Indications and dosage regimens are specific for a particular brand of interferon; other brands have different indications and dosage guidelines.

Administration

Reconstitution: To reconstitute solution, inject 1.2 mL of diluent (provided); gently swirl to dissolve, do not shake. Reconstituted solution provides 0.25 mg/mL. Use product within 3 hours of reconstitution.

Storage: Store at room temperature of 25°C (77°F); excursions permitted to 15°C to 30°C (59°F to 86°F). If not used immediately following reconstitution,

(Continued)

Interferon Beta-1b *(Continued)*

refrigerate solution at 2°C to 8°C (36°F to 46°F); do not freeze or shake solution.

Interferon Gamma-1b (in ter FEER on GAM ah won bee)

U.S. Brand Names Actimmune®

Pharmacologic Category Interferon

Use Reduce frequency and severity of serious infections associated with chronic granulomatous disease; delay time to disease progression in patients with severe, malignant osteopetrosis

Pharmacodynamics/Kinetics

Absorption: I.M., SubQ: Slowly

Half-life elimination: I.V.: 38 minutes; I.M., SubQ: 3-6 hours

Time to peak, plasma: I.M.: 4 hours (1.5 ng/mL); SubQ: 7 hours (0.6 ng/mL)

Contraindications Hypersensitivity to interferon gamma, *E. coli* derived proteins, or any component of the formulation

Warnings/Precautions Patients with pre-existing cardiac disease, seizure disorders, CNS disturbances, or myelosuppression should be carefully monitored; long-term effects on growth and development are unknown; safety and efficacy in children <1 year of age have not been established.

Drug Interactions Inhibits CYP1A2 (weak), 2E1 (weak)

Nutritional/Herbal/Ethanol Interactions Herb/Nutraceutical: Dietary supplements containing aristolochic acid (found most often in Chinese medicines/herbal therapies); cases of nephropathy and ESRD associated with their use.

Adverse Reactions Based on 50 mcg/m^2 dose administered 3 times weekly for chronic granulomatous disease

>10%:

Central nervous system: Fever (52%), headache (33%), chills (14%), fatigue (14%)

Dermatologic: Rash (17%)

Gastrointestinal: Diarrhea (14%), vomiting (13%)

Local: Injection site erythema or tenderness (14%)

1% to 10%:

Central nervous system: Depression (3%)

Gastrointestinal: Nausea (10%), abdominal pain (8%)

Neuromuscular & skeletal: Myalgia (6%), arthralgia (2%), back pain (2%)

Dosing

Adults & Elderly: If severe reactions occur, modify dose (50% reduction) or therapy should be discontinued until adverse reactions abate.

Chronic granulomatous disease: SubQ:

BSA ≤0.5 m^2: 1.5 mcg/kg/dose 3 times/week

BSA >0.5 m^2: 50 mcg/m^2 (1 million int. units/m^2) 3 times/week

Severe, malignant osteopetrosis: Children >1 year: SubQ:

BSA ≤0.5 m^2: 1.5 mcg/kg/dose 3 times/week

BSA >0.5 m^2: 50 mcg/m^2 (1 million int. units/m^2) 3 times/week

Note: Previously expressed as 1.5 million units/m^2; 50 mcg is equivalent to 1 million int. units/m^2.

Pediatrics: Children >1 year: Refer to adult dosing.

Available Dosage Forms Injection, solution [preservative free]: 100 mcg [2 million int. units] (0.5 mL)

Previously, 100 mcg was expressed as 3 million units. This is equivalent to 2 million int. units.

Nursing Guidelines

Assessment: Monitor closely for effectiveness and/or interactions. Assess results of laboratory tests on a regular basis, therapeutic effectiveness, and adverse reactions. Assess knowledge and instruct patient/caregiver on appropriate reconstitution, injection and needle disposal, possible side effects, and symptoms to report.

Monitoring Laboratory Tests: CBC, platelet counts, renal and liver function, urinalysis (at 3-month intervals during treatment)

Patient Education: This is not a cure for MS; you will continue to receive regular treatment and follow-up for MS. Use as directed; do not change the dosage or schedule of administration without consulting prescriber. Maintain adequate hydration (2-3 L/day of fluids) unless instructed to restrict fluid intake. You may experience flu-like syndrome (acetaminophen may help); nausea, vomiting, or loss of appetite (small frequent meals, frequent mouth care, sucking lozenges, or chewing gum may help); or drowsiness, dizziness, agitation, or abnormal thinking (use caution when driving or engaging in tasks requiring alertness until response to drug is known). Report unusual bruising or bleeding; persistent abdominal disturbances; unusual fatigue; muscle pain or tremors; chest pain or palpitations; swelling of extremities; visual disturbances; pain, swelling, or redness at injection site; or other unusual symptoms. **Pregnancy/breast-feeding precautions:** Inform prescriber if you are or intend to become pregnant. Do not breast-feed.

Pregnancy Risk Factor: C

Pregnancy Issues: Safety and efficacy in pregnant women has not been established. Treatment should be discontinued if a woman becomes pregnant, or plans to become pregnant during therapy. A dose-related abortifacient activity was reported in Rhesus monkeys.

Lactation: Excretion in breast milk unknown/contraindicated

Breast-Feeding Considerations: Potential for serious adverse reactions. Because its use has not been evaluated during lactation, breast-feeding is not recommended

Perioperative/Anesthesia/Other Concerns: Indications and dosage regimens are specific for a particular brand of interferon; other brands have different indications and dosage guidelines.

Administration

Storage: Store in refrigerator. Do not freeze. Do not shake. Discard if left unrefrigerated for >12 hours.

- ♦ **Intralipid®** *see* Fat Emulsion *on page 705*
- ♦ **Intravenous Fat Emulsion** *see* Fat Emulsion *on page 705*
- ♦ **Intrifiban** *see* Eptifibatide *on page 625*
- ♦ **Intron® A** *see* Interferon Alfa-2b *on page 936*
- ♦ **Intropin** *see* DOPamine *on page 565*
- ♦ **Invanz®** *see* Ertapenem *on page 631*

Iodixanol (EYE oh dix an ole)

U.S. Brand Names Visipaque™

Pharmacologic Category Iodinated Contrast Media; Radiological/Contrast Media, Nonionic

Medication Safety Issues

Not for intrathecal use

Use

Intra-arterial: Digital subtraction angiography, angiocardiography, peripheral arteriography, visceral arteriography, cerebral arteriography

Intravenous: Contrast enhanced computed tomography imaging, excretory urography, and peripheral venography

Mechanism of Action Opacifies vessels in the path of flow permitting radiographic imaging of internal structures.

Pharmacodynamics/Kinetics

Distribution: V_d: 0.26 L/kg

Protein binding: No

Half-life elimination: Children: 2-4 hours; Adults: 2 hours

Time to peak, plasma: Immediate; peak enhancement at 15-120 seconds; optimum renal contrast at 5-15 minutes; brain contrast at up to 1 hour

Excretion: Urine (97% within 24 hours); feces (<2%)

Contraindications Hypersensitivity to iodixanol or any component of the formulation; not intended for intrathecal use

In pediatric population: Prolonged fasting or laxative administration prior to iodixanol administration

Refer to product labeling for procedure-specific contraindications.

Warnings/Precautions For I.V. or intra-arterial use only; **may be fatal if given intrathecally.** May cause serious thromboembolic events including MI and stroke. Use caution with renal or hepatic dysfunction or cardiovascular disease. May worsen renal insufficiency in multiple myeloma patients. Use caution with thyroid disease; thyroid storm has been reported in patients with history of hyperthyroidism. Minimize exposure of iodixanol and monitor blood pressure closely in patients with pheochromocytoma. May promote sickling in patients with sickle cell disease. Use caution with iodine or contrast dye allergy; may cause serious and potentially fatal anaphylactoid reactions or cardiovascular reactions. Pediatric patients with history of asthma, medication allergies, heart disease, CHF or

(Continued)

Iodixanol *(Continued)*

serum creatinine >1.5 mg/dL are at higher risk for reactions. May cause delayed reaction; monitor for 30-60 minutes after injection. Avoid extravasation.

Drug Interactions Oral cholecystographic agents: May potentiate the renal toxicity of iodixanol.

Lab Interactions Thyroid function tests (protein bound and radioactive iodine uptake studies) may be inaccurate for up to 16 days after administration; may cause false positive urine protein test using Multistix®; may affect urine specific gravity

Adverse Reactions

>10%: Local: Injection site reactions (discomfort/pain/warmth 30%)

1% to 10%:

Cardiovascular: Angina/chest pain (2%)

Central nervous system: Headache/migraine (3%), vertigo (2%)

Dermatologic: Nonurticarial rash/erythema (2%), pruritus (2%)

Gastrointestinal: Taste perversion (4%), nausea (3%)

Neuromuscular & skeletal: Paresthesia (1%)

Respiratory: Parosoma (1%)

<1% (Limited to important or life-threatening): Acute renal failure, anaphylactoid reaction, anaphylaxis, apnea (children only), arrhythmia (children only), asthma, AV block (children only), back pain, bundle branch block (children only), cardiac arrest, cardiac failure (children only), cerebral vascular disorder, disseminated intravascular coagulation (children only), hematoma, hemorrhage, hypersensitivity, hypertension, hypoglycemia, hypotensive collapse, peripheral ischemia, pharyngeal edema, pulmonary edema, pulmonary embolism, respiratory depression, seizure, shock

Overdosage/Toxicology Treatment of overdose should be symptom-directed and supportive. Iodixanol may be dialyzed.

Dosing

Adults & Elderly: Note: Maximum recommended total dose of iodine: 80 g

Intra-arterial: Iodixanol 320 mg iodine/mL: Dose individualized based on injection site and study type; refer to product labeling

I.V.: Iodixanol 270 mg and 320 mg iodine /mL: concentration and dose vary based on study type; refer to product labeling.

Pediatrics: Note: Maximum recommended total dose of iodine: Not been established

Cerebral, cardiac chambers, and related major arteries and visceral studies: Intra-arterial: Children >1 year: Iodixanol 320 mg iodine/mL: 1-2 mL/kg; maximum dose: 4 mL/kg

Contrast-enhanced computer tomography or excretory urography: I.V.: Children >1 year: Iodixanol 270 mg iodine /mL: 1-2 mL/kg; maximum dose: 2 mL/kg

Children >12 years: Refer to adult dosing.

Renal Impairment: Not studied; use caution.

Available Dosage Forms Injection, solution [preservative free]:

270: 550 mg/mL (50 mL, 100 mL, 125 mL, 150 mL, 200 mL) [provides organically-bound iodine 270 mg/mL; contains tromethamine 1.2 mg/mL, edetate calcium disodium]

320: 652 mg/mL (50 mL, 100 mL, 125 mL, 150 mL, 200 mL) [provides organically-bound iodine 320 mg/mL; contains tromethamine 1.2 mg/mL, edetate calcium disodium]

Nursing Guidelines

Pregnancy Risk Factor: B

Lactation: Excretion in breast milk unknown/not recommended

Breast-Feeding Considerations: Due to the potential for adverse reactions, temporary discontinuation of breast-feeding should be considered.

Administration

I.V.: Patients should be adequately hydrated prior to and following administration.

Storage: Store in protective foil at room temperature of 15°C to 30°C (59°F to 86°F); protect from light. Do not freeze; do not use if inadvertently frozen. Vials, glass and polymer bottles (**not** flexible containers) may be stored for up to 1 month at 37°C (98.6°F) in contrast agent warmer.

Iohexol (eye oh HEX ole)

U.S. Brand Names Omnipaque™

Pharmacologic Category Polypeptide Hormone; Radiological/Contrast Media, Nonionic

Use

Intrathecal: Myelography; contrast enhancement for computerized tomography

Intravascular: Angiocardiography, aortography, digital subtraction angiography, peripheral arteriography, excretory urography; contrast enhancement for computed tomographic imaging

Oral/body cavity: Arthrography, GI tract examination, hysterosalpingography, pancreatography, cholangiopancreatography, herniography, cystourethrography; enhanced computed tomography of the abdomen

Contraindications Hypersensitivity to iohexol or any component of the formulation

Refer to product labeling for procedure-specific contraindications

Available Dosage Forms Solution, injection [preservative free]:

140: 302 mg/mL (50 mL) [provides organic iodine 140 mg/mL; contains tromethamine 1.21 mg/mL, edetate calcium disodium]

180: 388 mg/mL (10 mL, 20 mL) [provides organic iodine 180 mg/mL; contains tromethamine 1.21 mg/mL, edetate calcium disodium]

240: 518 mg/mL (10 mL, 20 mL, 50 mL, 100 mL, 150 mL, 200 mL) [provides organic iodine 240 mg/mL; contains tromethamine 1.21 mg/mL, edetate calcium disodium]

300: 647 mg/mL (10 mL, 30 mL, 50 mL, 75 mL, 100 mL, 125 mL, 150 mL, 200 mL) [provides organic iodine 300 mg/mL; contains tromethamine 1.21 mg/mL, edetate calcium disodium]

350: 755 mg/mL (50 mL, 75 mL, 100 mL, 125 mL, 150 mL, 200 mL, 250 mL) [provides organic iodine 350 mg/mL; contains tromethamine 1.21 mg/mL, edetate calcium disodium]

Nursing Guidelines

Pregnancy Risk Factor: B

Lactation: Excretion in breast milk unknown/not recommended

Breast-Feeding Considerations: Bottle feedings are recommended for 24 hours after administration.

Administration

Storage: Solution for injection: Store at room temperature of 20°C to 25°C (68°F to 77°F). Protect from light.

Iopamidol (eye oh PA mi dole)

U.S. Brand Names Isovue®; Isovue-M®; Isovue Multipack®

Pharmacologic Category Iodinated Contrast Media; Radiological/Contrast Media, Nonionic

Use

Intrathecal (Isovue-M®): Neuroradiology; contrast enhancement of computed tomographic cisternography and ventriculography; thoraco-lumbar myelography

Intravascular (Isovue®, Isovue Multipack®): Angiography, excretory urography; contrast enhancement of computed tomographic imaging; evaluation of certain malignancies; image enhancement of non-neoplastic lesions

Contraindications Hypersensitivity to iopamidol or any component of the formulation

Refer to product labeling for product- and procedure-specific contraindications

Available Dosage Forms Injection, solution:

Isovue®:

200: 41% (50 mL, 100 mL, 200 mL) [provides organically-bound iodine 200 mg/mL; contains sodium 0.029 mg (0.001 mEq)/mL, tromethamine 1 mg/mL, edetate calcium disodium]

250: 51% (50 mL, 100 mL, 150 mL, 200 mL) [provides organically-bound iodine 250 mg/mL; contains sodium 0.036 mg (0.002 mEq)/mL, tromethamine 1 mg/mL, edetate calcium disodium]

300: 61% (30 mL, 50 mL, 75 mL, 100 mL, 125 mL, 150 mL, 175 mL) [provides organically-bound iodine 300 mg/mL; contains sodium 0.043 mg (0.002 mEq)/mL, tromethamine 1 mg/mL, edetate calcium disodium]

370: 76% (20 mL, 30 mL, 50 mL, 75 mL, 100 mL, 125 mL, 150 mL, 175 mL, 200 mL) [provides organically-bound iodine 370 mg/mL; contains sodium 0.053 mg (0.002 mEq)/mL, tromethamine 1 mg/mL, edetate calcium disodium]

(Continued)

Iopamidol (Continued)

Isovue-M®:

200: 41% (10 mL, 20 mL) [provides organically-bound iodine 200 mg/mL; contains sodium 0.029 mg (0.001 mEq)/mL, tromethamine 1 mg/mL, edetate calcium disodium]

300: 61% (15 mL) [provides organically-bound iodine 300 mg/mL; contains sodium 0.043 mg (0.002 mEq)/mL, tromethamine 1 mg/mL, edetate calcium disodium]

Isovue Multipack® [pharmacy bulk package]:

250: 51% (200 mL) [provides organically-bound iodine 250 mg/mL; contains sodium 0.036 mg (0.002 mEq)/mL, tromethamine 1 mg/mL, edetate calcium disodium]

300: 61% (200 mL, 500 mL) [provides organically-bound iodine 300 mg/mL; contains sodium 0.043 mg (0.002 mEq)/mL, tromethamine 1 mg/mL, edetate calcium disodium]

370: 76% (200 mL, 500 mL) [provides organically-bound iodine 370 mg/mL; contains sodium 0.053 mg (0.002 mEq)/mL, tromethamine 1 mg/mL, edetate calcium disodium]

Nursing Guidelines

Pregnancy Risk Factor: B

Lactation: Excretion in breast milk unknown/use caution

Administration

Storage: Store at 20°C to 25°C (68°F to 77°F). Protect from light.

♦ **Iophen-C NR** *see* Guaifenesin and Codeine *on page 835*

♦ **Iophen NR** *see* Guaifenesin *on page 834*

♦ **Iopidine®** *see* Apraclonidine *on page 178*

Iothalamate Meglumine (eye oh thal A mate MEG loo meen)

U.S. Brand Names Conray®; Conray® 30; Conray® 43; Cysto-Conray® II

Pharmacologic Category Iodinated Contrast Media; Radiological/Contrast Media, Ionic

Use

Solution for injection: Arthrography, cerebral angiography, cranial computerized angiotomography, digital subtraction angiography, direct cholangiography, endoscopic retrograde cholangiopancreatography, excretory urography, peripheral arteriography, urography, venography; contrast enhancement of computed tomographic images

Solution for instillation: Retrograde cystography and cystourethrography

Contraindications Hypersensitivity to any component of the formulation; intrathecal administration; solution for instillation should not be used intravascularly

Refer to product labeling for product and procedure specific contraindications

Available Dosage Forms

Injection, solution:

Conray®: 60% (30 mL, 50 mL, 100 mL, 150 mL) [provides organically-bound iodine 282 mg/mL; contains edetate calcium disodium]

Conray® 30: 30% (50 mL, 150 mL) [provides organically-bound iodine 141 mg/mL; contains edetate calcium disodium]

Conray® 43: 43% (50 mL, 100 mL, 200 mL, 250 mL) [provides organically-bound iodine 202 mg/mL; contains edetate calcium disodium]

Injection, solution for instillation (Cysto-Conray® II): 17.2% (250 mL, 500 mL) [provides organically-bound iodine 81 mg/mL; contains edetate calcium disodium]

Nursing Guidelines

Pregnancy Risk Factor: B/C (product dependent)

Lactation: Enters breast milk/use caution

Breast-Feeding Considerations: Bottle feedings are recommended for 24 hours after administration.

Administration

Storage: Store below 30°C (86°F). Protect from strong daylight or direct exposure to the sun

Ioversol (EYE oh ver sole)

U.S. Brand Names Optiray®

Pharmacologic Category Iodinated Contrast Media; Radiological/Contrast Media, Nonionic

Use Arteriography, angiography, angiocardiography, ventriculography, excretory urography, and venography procedures; contrast enhanced tomographic imaging

Contraindications Hypersensitivity to any component of the formulation; not intended for intrathecal use

Available Dosage Forms Injection, solution [preservative free]:

160: 34% (50 mL) [provides organically-bound iodine 160 mg/mL; contains tromethamine 3.6 mg/mL, edetate calcium disodium]

240: 51% (50 mL, 100 mL, 125 mL, 200 mL, 500 mL) [provides organically-bound iodine 240 mg/mL; contains tromethamine 3.6 mg/mL, edetate calcium disodium]

300: 64% (50 mL, 100 mL, 150 mL, 200 mL) [provides organically-bound iodine 300 mg/mL; contains tromethamine 3.6 mg/mL, edetate calcium disodium]

320: 68% (20 mL, 30 mL, 50 mL, 75 mL, 100 mL, 125 mL, 150 mL, 200 mL, 250 mL) [provides organically-bound iodine 320 mg/mL; contains tromethamine 3.6 mg/mL, edetate calcium disodium]

350: 74% (50 mL, 75 mL, 100 mL, 150 mL, 200 mL, 250 mL, 500 mL) [provides organically-bound iodine 350 mg/mL; contains tromethamine 3.6 mg/mL, edetate calcium disodium]

Nursing Guidelines

Pregnancy Risk Factor: B

Lactation: Excretion in breast milk unknown/use caution

Breast-Feeding Considerations: Temporary discontinuation of nursing should be considered.

Administration

Storage: Store at room temperature of 15°C to 30°C (59°F to 86°F). Protect from strong light or direct sunlight.

♦ **IPM Wound Gel™ [OTC]** *see* Hyaluronate and Derivatives *on page 856*

Ipratropium (i pra TROE pee um)

U.S. Brand Names Atrovent®; Atrovent® HFA

Synonyms Ipratropium Bromide

Pharmacologic Category Anticholinergic Agent

Medication Safety Issues

Sound-alike/look-alike issues:

Atrovent® may be confused with Alupent®

Use Anticholinergic bronchodilator used in bronchospasm associated with COPD, bronchitis, and emphysema; symptomatic relief of rhinorrhea associated with the common cold and allergic and nonallergic rhinitis

Mechanism of Action Blocks the action of acetylcholine at parasympathetic sites in bronchial smooth muscle causing bronchodilation

Pharmacodynamics/Kinetics

Onset of action: Bronchodilation: 1-3 minutes

Peak effect: 1.5-2 hours

Duration: ≤4 hours

Absorption: Negligible

Distribution: Inhalation: 15% of dose reaches lower airways

Contraindications Hypersensitivity to ipratropium, atropine, its derivatives, or any component of the formulation

In addition, Atrovent® inhalation aerosol is contraindicated in patients with hypersensitivity to soya lecithin or related food products (eg, soybean and peanut). **Note:** Other formulations may include these components; refer to product-specific labeling.

Warnings/Precautions Not indicated for the initial treatment of acute episodes of bronchospasm; use with caution in patients with myasthenia gravis, narrow-angle glaucoma, benign prostatic hyperplasia (BPH), or bladder neck obstruction

Drug Interactions Anticholinergics: Concurrent use with ipratropium may increase risk of adverse events.

Adverse Reactions

Inhalation aerosol and inhalation solution:

>10%: Bronchitis (10% to 23%), upper respiratory tract infection (13%)

1% to 10%:

Cardiovascular: Palpitation

Central nervous system: Dizziness (2% to 3%)

Dermatologic: Rash (1%)

Gastrointestinal: Nausea, xerostomia, stomach upset, dry mucous membranes

Renal: Urinary tract infection

(Continued)

Ipratropium *(Continued)*

Respiratory: Nasal congestion, dyspnea (10%), sputum increased (1%), bronchospasm (2%), pharyngitis (3%), rhinitis (2%), sinusitis (5%)

Miscellaneous: Flu-like syndrome

<1% (Limited to important or life-threatening): Anaphylactic reaction, angioedema, atrial fibrillation, blurred vision, hypersensitivity reactions, laryngospasm, supraventricular tachycardia urinary retention, urticaria

Nasal spray: Respiratory: Epistaxis (8%), nasal dryness (5%), nausea (2%)

Overdosage/Toxicology Symptoms of overdose include dry mouth, drying of respiratory secretions, cough, nausea, GI distress, blurred vision or impaired visual accommodation, headache, and nervousness. Acute overdose with ipratropium by inhalation is unlikely since it is so poorly absorbed. However, if poisoning occurs, it can be treated like any other anticholinergic toxicity. An anticholinergic overdose with severe life-threatening symptoms may be treated with physostigmine 1-2 mg SubQ or I.V. slowly.

Dosing

Adults & Elderly:

Bronchospasm:

Nebulization: 500 mcg (one unit-dose vial) 3-4 times/day with doses 6-8 hours apart

Metered dose inhaler: 2 inhalations 4 times/day, up to 12 inhalations/24 hours

Colds (symptomatic relief of rhinorrhea): Safety and efficacy of use beyond 4 days not established: Nasal spray (0.06%): 2 sprays in each nostril 3-4 times/day

Allergic/nonallergic rhinitis: Nasal spray (0.03%): 2 sprays in each nostril 2-3 times/day

Pediatrics:

Bronchospasm:

Nebulization:

Infants and Children ≤12 years: 125-250 mcg 3 times/day

Children >12 years: Refer to adult dosing.

Metered dose inhaler:

Children 3-12 years: 1-2 inhalations 3 times/day, up to 6 inhalations/24 hours

Children >12 years: Refer to adult dosing.

Colds (symptomatic relief of rhinorrhea): Intranasal: Safety and efficacy of use beyond 4 days in patients with the common cold have not been established:

Children 5-11 years: 0.06%: 2 sprays in each nostril 3 times/day

Children ≥5 years and Adults: 0.06%: 2 sprays in each nostril 3-4 times/day

Allergic/nonallergic rhinitis: Intranasal: Children ≥6 years: Refer to adult dosing.

Available Dosage Forms [DSC] = Discontinued product

Solution for nebulization, as bromide: 0.02% (2.5 mL)

Solution for oral inhalation, as bromide (Atrovent®): 18 mcg/actuation (14 g) [contains soya lecithin and chlorofluorocarbons] [DSC]

Solution for oral inhalation, as bromide (Atrovent® HFA): 17 mcg/actuation (12.9 g)

Solution, intranasal spray, as bromide (Atrovent®): 0.03% (30 mL); 0.06% (15 mL)

Nursing Guidelines

Assessment: Assess potential for interactions with other prescriptions, OTC medications, or herbal products patient may be taking (especially anything that may have anticholinergic properties). Assess patient response on a regular basis throughout therapy. Teach patient proper use, possible side effects/appropriate interventions (eg, importance of adequate hydration), and adverse symptoms to report.

Dietary Considerations: Some dosage forms may contain soya lecithin. Do not use in patients allergic to soya lecithin or related food products such as soybean and peanut.

Patient Education: Do not take any new medication during therapy without consulting prescriber. Use exactly as directed (see below). Do not use more often than recommended. Store solution away from light. Maintain adequate hydration (2-3 L/day of fluids) unless instructed to restrict fluid intake. May cause sensitivity to heat (avoid extremes in temperature); nervousness, dizziness, or fatigue (use caution when driving or engaging in tasks requiring alertness until response to drug is known); dry mouth, unpleasant taste, stomach upset (small frequent meals, frequent mouth care, chewing gum, or sucking hard candy may help); or difficulty urinating (always void before treatment). Report unresolved GI upset, dizziness or fatigue, vision changes, palpitations, persistent inability to void, nervousness, or insomnia. **Breast-feeding precaution:** Consult prescriber if breast-feeding

Inhaler: Follow instructions for use accompanying the product. Close eyes when administering ipratropium; blurred vision may result if sprayed into eyes. Effects are enhanced by holding breath 10 seconds after inhalation; wait at least 1 full minute between inhalations.

Nebulizer: Wash hands before and after treatment. Wash and dry nebulizer after each treatment. Twist open the top of one unit dose vial and squeeze the contents into the nebulizer reservoir. Connect the nebulizer reservoir to the mouthpiece or face mask. Connect nebulizer to compressor. Sit in a comfortable, upright position. Place mouthpiece in your mouth or put on the face mask and turn on the compressor. If a face mask is used, avoid leakage around the mask (temporary blurring of vision, worsening of narrow-angle glaucoma, or eye pain may occur if mist gets into eyes). Breathe calmly and deeply until no more mist is formed in the nebulizer (about 5 minutes). At this point, treatment is finished.

Geriatric Considerations: Older patients may find it difficult to use the metered dose inhaler. A spacer device may be useful. Ipratropium has not been specifically studied in the elderly, but it is poorly absorbed from the airways and appears to be safe in this population.

Pregnancy Risk Factor: B

Lactation: Excretion in breast milk unknown/use caution

Administration

Compatibility: Compatible for 1 hour when mixed with albuterol in a nebulizer

Storage: Store at 15°C to 30°C (59°F to 86°F). Do not store near heat or open flame.

Ipratropium and Albuterol (i pra TROE pee um & al BYOO ter ole)

U.S. Brand Names Combivent®; DuoNeb™

Synonyms Albuterol and Ipratropium

Pharmacologic Category Bronchodilator

Medication Safety Issues

Sound-alike/look-alike issues:

Combivent® may be confused with Combivir®

Use Treatment of COPD in those patients that are currently on a regular bronchodilator who continue to have bronchospasms and require a second bronchodilator

Mechanism of Action See individual agents.

Pharmacodynamics/Kinetics See individual agents.

Contraindications

Based on **ipratropium** component: Hypersensitivity to atropine, its derivatives, or any component of the formulation

In addition, Combivent® inhalation aerosol is contraindicated in patients with hypersensitivity to soya lecithin or related food products (eg, soybean and peanut). **Note:** Other formulations may include these components; refer to product-specific labeling.

Based on **albuterol** component: Hypersensitivity to albuterol, adrenergic amines, or any component of the formulation

Warnings/Precautions

Based on **ipratropium** component: Not indicated for the initial treatment of acute episodes of bronchospasm; use with caution in patients with narrow-angle glaucoma, prostatic hyperplasia, or bladder neck obstruction; ipratropium has not been specifically studied in the elderly, but it is poorly absorbed from the airways and appears to be safe in this population.

Based on **albuterol** component: Use with caution in patients with hyperthyroidism, diabetes mellitus, or sensitivity to sympathomimetic amines; cardiovascular disorders including coronary insufficiency or hypertension; excessive use may result in tolerance. Some adverse reactions may occur more frequently in children 2-5 years of age than in adults and older children. Because of its minimal effect on $beta_1$-receptors and its relatively long duration of action, albuterol is a rational choice in the elderly when a beta agonist is indicated. All patients should utilize a spacer device when using a metered dose inhaler. Oral use should be avoided in the elderly due to adverse effects.

(Continued)

Ipratropium and Albuterol *(Continued)*

Drug Interactions Albuterol: **Substrate** of CYP3A4 (major)

Also see individual agents.

Adverse Reactions See individual agents.

Dosing

Adults & Elderly:

COPD:

Inhalation: 2 metered-dose inhalations 4 times/day; may receive additional doses as necessary, but total number of doses in 24 hours should not exceed 12 inhalations.

Inhalation via nebulization: Initial: 3 mL every 6 hours (maximum: 3 mL every 4 hours)

Available Dosage Forms

Aerosol for oral inhalation (Combivent®): Ipratropium bromide 18 mcg and albuterol sulfate 103 mcg per actuation [200 doses] (14.7 g) [contains soya lecithin]

Solution for oral inhalation (DuoNeb™): Ipratropium bromide 0.5 mg [0.017%] and albuterol base 2.5 mg [0.083%] per 3 mL vial (30s, 60s)

Nursing Guidelines

Assessment: See individual components listed in Related Information. Note breast-feeding caution.

Dietary Considerations: Some dosage forms may contain soya lecithin. Do not use in patients allergic to soya lecithin or related food products such as soybean and peanut.

Patient Education: See individual agents. **Pregnancy/breast-feeding precautions:** Inform prescriber if you are or intend to become pregnant. Consult prescriber if breast-feeding.

Pregnancy Risk Factor: C

Lactation: Excretion in breast milk unknown

Administration

Storage: DuoNeb™: Store at 2°C to 25°C (36°F to 77°F). Protect from light.

Related Information

Albuterol *on page 96*
Ipratropium *on page 957*

♦ **Ipratropium Bromide** *see* Ipratropium *on page 957*
♦ **I-Prin [OTC]** *see* Ibuprofen *on page 889*
♦ **Iproveratril Hydrochloride** *see* Verapamil *on page 1702*
♦ **Iquix®** *see* Levofloxacin *on page 1025*

Irbesartan (ir be SAR tan)

U.S. Brand Names Avapro®

Pharmacologic Category Angiotensin II Receptor Blocker

Medication Safety Issues

Sound-alike/look-alike issues:

Avapro® may be confused with Anaprox®

Use Treatment of hypertension alone or in combination with other antihypertensives; treatment of diabetic nephropathy in patients with type 2 diabetes mellitus (noninsulin dependent, NIDDM) and hypertension

Mechanism of Action Irbesartan is an angiotensin receptor antagonist. Angiotensin II acts as a vasoconstrictor. In addition to causing direct vasoconstriction, angiotensin II also stimulates the release of aldosterone. Once aldosterone is released, sodium as well as water are reabsorbed. The end result is an elevation in blood pressure. Irbesartan binds to the AT1 angiotensin II receptor. This binding prevents angiotensin II from binding to the receptor thereby blocking the vasoconstriction and the aldosterone secreting effects of angiotensin II.

Pharmacodynamics/Kinetics

Onset of action: Peak effect: 1-2 hours
Duration: >24 hours
Distribution: V_d: 53-93 L
Protein binding, plasma: 90%
Metabolism: Hepatic, primarily CYP2C9
Bioavailability: 60% to 80%
Half-life elimination: Terminal: 11-15 hours
Time to peak, serum: 1.5-2 hours
Excretion: Feces (80%); urine (20%)

Contraindications Hypersensitivity to irbesartan or any component of the formulation; hypersensitivity to other A-II receptor antagonists; bilateral renal artery stenosis; pregnancy (2nd and 3rd trimesters)

Warnings/Precautions Avoid use or use smaller doses in patients who are volume depleted; correct depletion first. Deterioration in renal function can occur with initiation. Use with caution in unilateral renal artery stenosis and pre-existing renal insufficiency; significant aortic/mitral stenosis. Safety and efficacy have not been established in pediatric patients <6 years of age.

Drug Interactions **Substrate** of CYP2C8/9 (minor); **Inhibits** CYP2C8/9 (moderate), 2D6 (weak), 3A4 (weak)

CYP2C8/9 substrates: Irbesartan may increase the levels/effects of CYP2C8/9 substrates. Example substrates include amiodarone, fluoxetine, glimepiride, glipizide, nateglinide, phenytoin, pioglitazone, rosiglitazone, sertraline, and warfarin.

Lithium: Risk of toxicity may be increased by irbesartan; monitor lithium levels.

NSAIDs: May decrease angiotensin II antagonist efficacy; effect has been seen with losartan, but may occur with other medications in this class; monitor blood pressure

Potassium-sparing diuretics (amiloride, potassium, spironolactone, triamterene): Increased risk of hyperkalemia.

Potassium supplements may increase the risk of hyperkalemia.

Trimethoprim (high dose) may increase the risk of hyperkalemia.

Nutritional/Herbal/Ethanol Interactions Herb/Nutraceutical: Avoid dong quai if using for hypertension (has estrogenic activity). Avoid ephedra, yohimbe, ginseng (may worsen hypertension). Avoid garlic (may have increased antihypertensive effect).

Adverse Reactions Unless otherwise indicated, percentage of incidence is reported for patients with hypertension.

>10%: Endocrine & metabolic: Hyperkalemia (19%, diabetic nephropathy)

1% to 10%:

Cardiovascular: Orthostatic hypotension (5%, diabetic nephropathy)

Central nervous system: Fatigue (4%), dizziness (10%, diabetic nephropathy)

Gastrointestinal: Diarrhea (3%), dyspepsia (2%)

Respiratory: Upper respiratory infection (9%), cough (2.8% versus 2.7% in placebo)

<1% (Limited to important or life-threatening): Angina, angioedema, arrhythmia, cardiopulmonary arrest, conjunctivitis, depression, dyspnea, ecchymosis, edema, epistaxis, gout, heart failure, hyperkalemia, hypotension, jaundice, libido decreased, MI, orthostatic hypotension, paresthesia, sexual dysfunction, stroke, transaminases increased, urticaria. May be associated with worsening of renal function in patients dependent on renin-angiotensin-aldosterone system.

Overdosage/Toxicology Likely manifestations of overdose include hypotension and tachycardia. Treatment is supportive. Not removed by hemodialysis.

Dosing

Adults & Elderly:

Hypertension: Oral: 150 mg once daily; patients may be titrated to 300 mg once daily. **Note:** Starting dose in volume-depleted patients should be 75 mg.

Nephropathy in patients with type 2 diabetes and hypertension: Oral: Target dose: 300 mg once daily

Pediatrics: Hypertension: Oral:

<6 years: Safety and efficacy have not been established.

≥6-12 years: Initial: 75 mg once daily; may be titrated to a maximum of 150 mg once daily

13-16 years: Refer to adult dosing.

Renal Impairment: No dosage adjustment necessary with mild to severe impairment unless the patient is also volume depleted.

Available Dosage Forms Tablet: 75 mg, 150 mg, 300 mg

Nursing Guidelines

Assessment: See Contraindications, Warnings/Precautions, and Dosing for use cautions. Assess potential for interactions with other prescriptions, OTC medications, or herbal products patient may be taking (see Drug Interactions). Assess results of laboratory tests (see below), therapeutic effectiveness, and adverse response (see Adverse Reactions and Overdose/Toxicology) at regular intervals during therapy. Teach patient proper use, possible side effects/appropriate interventions, and adverse symptoms to report (see Patient Education). **Pregnancy risk factor C/D** - see Pregnancy Risk Factor for use

(Continued)

Irbesartan *(Continued)*

cautions; benefits of use should outweigh possible risks. Instruct patients of childbearing age about appropriate contraceptive measures. Breast-feeding is contraindicated.

Monitoring Laboratory Tests: Electrolytes, serum creatinine, BUN, urinalysis

Dietary Considerations: May be taken with or without food.

Patient Education: Inform prescriber of all prescriptions, OTC medications, or herbal products you are taking, and any allergies you have. Do not take any new medication during therapy unless approved by prescriber. Take exactly as directed; do not discontinue without consulting prescriber. May be taken with or without food. Take first dose at bedtime. This medication does not replace other antihypertensive interventions; follow prescriber's instructions for diet and lifestyle changes. May cause dizziness, fainting, or lightheadedness (use caution when driving or engaging in tasks that require alertness until response to drug is known); nausea, vomiting, or abdominal pain (small, frequent meals, frequent mouth care, sucking lozenges, or chewing gum may help); or diarrhea (buttermilk, boiled milk, yogurt may help). Report chest pain or palpitations, skin rash, fluid retention (swelling of extremities), respiratory difficulty or unusual cough, or other persistent adverse reactions. **Pregnancy/breast-feeding precautions:** Inform prescriber if you are or intend to become pregnant. This drug should not be used in the 2nd or 3rd trimester of pregnancy. Consult prescriber for appropriate contraceptive measures if necessary. Do not breast-feed.

Pregnancy Risk Factor: C/D (2nd and 3rd trimesters)

Pregnancy Issues: The drug should be discontinued as soon as possible after detection of pregnancy. Drugs which act directly on the renin-angiotensin system can cause fetal and neonatal morbidity and death.

Lactation: Excretion in breast milk unknown/contraindicated

Perioperative/Anesthesia/Other Concerns: The angiotensin II receptor antagonists appear to have similar indications as the ACE inhibitors. In heart failure, the angiotensin II antagonists are especially useful in providing an alternative therapy in those patients who have intractable cough in response to ACE inhibitor therapy. Candesartan has been studied as an alternative therapy in chronic heart failure patients who cannot tolerate an ACE-I (CHARM-Alternative) and as an added therapy in heart failure patients who are maintained on an ACE-I (CHARM-Added). In both studies the combined endpoint of cardiovascular death or heart failure hospitalizations was significantly improved over the placebo treated group. Similar to ACE inhibitors, pre-existing volume depletion caused by diuretic therapy may potentiate hypotension in response to angiotensin II antagonists. Concomitant NSAID therapy may attenuate blood pressure control; use of NSAIDs should be avoided or limited, with monitoring of blood pressure control. In the setting of heart failure, NSAID use may be associated with an increased risk for fluid accumulation and edema.

Administration

Storage: Store at room temperature of 15°C to 30°C (59°F to 86°F).

Irinotecan (eye rye no TEE kan)

U.S. Brand Names Camptosar®

Synonyms Camptothecin-11; CPT-11; NSC-616348

Pharmacologic Category Antineoplastic Agent, Natural Source (Plant) Derivative

Use Treatment of metastatic carcinoma of the colon or rectum

Unlabeled/Investigational Use Lung cancer (small cell and nonsmall cell), cervical cancer, gastric cancer, pancreatic cancer, leukemia, lymphoma, breast cancer

Mechanism of Action Irinotecan and its active metabolite (SN-38) bind reversibly to topoisomerase I and stabilize the cleavable complex so that religation of the cleaved DNA strand cannot occur. This results in the accumulation of cleavable complexes and single-strand DNA breaks. This interaction results in single-stranded DNA breaks and cell death consistent with S-phase cell cycle specificity.

Pharmacodynamics/Kinetics

Distribution: V_d: 33-150 L/m^2

Protein binding, plasma: Predominantly albumin; Parent drug: 30% to 68%, SN-38 (active drug): ~95%

Metabolism: Primarily hepatic to SN-38 (active metabolite) by carboxylesterase enzymes; SN-38 undergoes conjugation by UDP- glucuronosyl transferase 1A1 (UGT1A1) to form a glucuronide metabolite. SN-38 is increased by UGT1A1*28 polymorphism (10% of North Americans are homozygous for UGT1A1*28 allele). The lactones of both irinotecan and SN-38 undergo hydrolysis to inactive hydroxy acid forms.

Half-life elimination: SN-38: Mean terminal: 10-20 hours

Time to peak: SN-38: Following 90-minute infusion: ~1 hour

Excretion: Within 24 hours: Urine: Irinotecan (11% to 20%), metabolites (SN-38 <1%, SN-38 glucuronide, 3%)

Contraindications Hypersensitivity to irinotecan or any component of the formulation; concurrent use of atazanavir, ketoconazole, St John's wort; pregnancy

Warnings/Precautions Hazardous agent — use appropriate precautions for handling and disposal. Severe hypersensitivity reactions have occurred.

Deaths due to sepsis following severe myelosuppression have been reported. Therapy should be temporarily discontinued if neutropenic fever occurs or if the absolute neutrophil count is <1000/mm^3. The dose of irinotecan should be reduced if there is a clinically significant decrease in the total WBC (<200/mm^3), neutrophil count (<1500/mm^3), hemoglobin (<8 g/dL), or platelet count (<100,000/mm^3). Routine administration of a colony-stimulating factor is generally not necessary, but may be considered for patients experiencing significant neutropenia.

Patients homozygous for the UGT1A1*28 allele are at increased risk of neutropenia; initial one-level dose reduction should be considered for both single-agent and combination regimens. Heterozygous carriers of the UGT1A1*28 allele may also be at increased risk; however, most patients have tolerated normal starting doses.

Patients with even modest elevations in total serum bilirubin levels (1.0-2.0 mg/dL) have a significantly greater likelihood of experiencing first-course grade 3 or 4 neutropenia than those with bilirubin levels that were <1.0 mg/dL. Patients with abnormal glucuronidation of bilirubin, such as those with Gilbert's syndrome, may also be at greater risk of myelosuppression when receiving therapy with irinotecan. Use caution when treating patients with known hepatic dysfunction or hyperbilirubinemia. Dosage adjustments should be considered.

Patients with diarrhea should be carefully monitored and treated promptly. Severe diarrhea may be dose-limiting and potentially fatal; two severe (life-threatening) forms of diarrhea may occur. Early diarrhea occurs during or within 24 hours of receiving irinotecan and is characterized by cholinergic symptoms (eg, increased salivation, diaphoresis, abdominal cramping); it is usually responsive to atropine. Late diarrhea occurs more than 24 hours after treatment which may lead to dehydration, electrolyte imbalance, or sepsis; it should be promptly treated with loperamide.

Patients should receive fluid and electrolyte replacement as indicated, or antibiotics if ileus, fever, or neutropenia develop. Hold diuretics during dosing due to potential risk of dehydration secondary to vomiting and/or diarrhea induced by irinotecan.

Use caution in patients who previously received pelvic/abdominal radiation, elderly patients with comorbid conditions, or baseline performance status of 2; close monitoring and dosage adjustments are recommended.

Drug Interactions Substrate (major) of CYP2B6, 3A4

Anticonvulsants (carbamazepine, phenobarbital, phenytoin): Decreases the therapeutic effect of irinotecan. Consider replacement of anticonvulsant with a nonenzyme-inducing agent ≥2 weeks prior to irinotecan therapy.

Bevacizumab: May increase the adverse effects of irinotecan (eg, diarrhea, neutropenia).

CYP2B6 inducers: May decrease the levels/effects of irinotecan. Example inducers include carbamazepine, nevirapine, phenobarbital, phenytoin, and rifampin.

CYP2B6 inhibitors: May increase the levels/effects of irinotecan. Example inhibitors include desipramine, paroxetine, and sertraline.

CYP3A4 inducers: CYP3A4 inducers may decrease the levels/effects of irinotecan. Example inducers include aminoglutethimide, carbamazepine, nafcillin, nevirapine, phenobarbital, phenytoin, and rifamycins.

(Continued)

Irinotecan *(Continued)*

CYP3A4 inhibitors: May increase the levels/effects of irinotecan. Example inhibitors include azole antifungals, clarithromycin, diclofenac, doxycycline, erythromycin, imatinib, isoniazid, nefazodone, nicardipine, propofol, protease inhibitors, quinidine, telithromycin, and verapamil.

Ketoconazole: Increases the levels/effects of irinotecan and active metabolite. Discontinue ketoconazole 1 week prior to irinotecan therapy; **concurrent use is contraindicated.**

St John's wort: Decreases the therapeutic effect of irinotecan. Discontinue St John's wort ≥2 weeks prior to irinotecan therapy; **concurrent use is contraindicated.**

Nutritional/Herbal/Ethanol Interactions Herb/Nutraceutical: St John's wort decreases the efficacy of irinotecan.

Adverse Reactions Frequency of adverse reactions reported for single-agent use of irinotecan only. Frequencies vary with alternative dosage regimens or combination therapy.

>10%:

Cardiovascular: Vasodilatation (9% to 11%)

Central nervous system: Pain (23% to 62%), fever (26% to 45%; neutropenic grade 3/4: <1% to 6%), dizziness (15% to 21%), headache (17%), chills (14%), insomnia (19%)

Dermatologic: Rash (13% to 14%), alopecia (17% to 60%, grade 2), hand/foot syndrome (13%), cutaneous reactions (20%)

Gastrointestinal: Gastrointestinal: Diarrhea, early (43% to 51%; grade 3/4: 7% to 22%), diarrhea, late (45% to 88%; grade 3/4: 6% to 31%), nausea (55% to 86%), abdominal pain (17% to 68%), vomiting (32% to 67%), anorexia (19% to 55%), constipation (25% to 32%), mucositis (29% to 30%), flatulence (12%), stomatitis (12%), dyspepsia (10%), abdominal cramping (57%), weight loss (30%), dehydration (15%)

Hepatic: Bilirubin increased (36% to 84%), alkaline phosphatase increased (13%)

Neuromuscular & skeletal: Weakness (48% to 76%), back pain (14%)

Respiratory: Dyspnea (5% to 22%), cough (17% to 20%), rhinitis (16%)

Miscellaneous: Infection (14% to 34%), diaphoresis (16%)

1% to 10%:

Cardiovascular: Hypotension (<1% to 6%), thromboembolic events (5% to 6%), edema (10%)

Central nervous system: Somnolence (9%), confusion (3%)

Gastrointestinal: Abdominal enlargement (10%)

Hepatic: SGOT increased (10%), ascites and/or jaundice (9%)

Respiratory: Pneumonia (4%)

<1%, postmarketing, and/or case reports: Anaphylactoid reaction, anaphylaxis, bleeding, colitis, ileus, pancreatitis, pulmonary toxicity (dyspnea, fever, reticulonodular infiltrates on chest x-ray), renal failure (acute), renal impairment, ulceration

Note: In limited pediatric experience, dehydration (often associated with severe hypokalemia and hyponatremia) was among the most significant grade 3/4 adverse events, with a frequency up to 29%. In addition, grade 3/4 infection was reported in 24%.

Overdosage/Toxicology Symptoms of overdose include bone marrow suppression, leukopenia, thrombocytopenia, nausea, and vomiting. Treatment is supportive.

Dosing

Adults & Elderly: Refer to individual protocols. **Note:** A reduction in the starting dose by one dose level should be considered for patients ≥65 years of age, prior pelvic/abdominal radiotherapy, performance status of 2, homozygosity for UGT1A1*28 allele, or increased bilirubin (dosing for patients with a bilirubin >2 mg/dL cannot be recommended based on lack of data per manufacturer).

Single-agent therapy:

I.V.: Weekly regimen: 125 mg/m² over 90 minutes on days 1, 8, 15, and 22, followed by a 2-week rest

Adjusted dose level -1: 100 mg/m²

Adjusted dose level -2: 75 mg/m²

I.V.: Once-every-3-week regimen: 350 mg/m² over 90 minutes, once every 3 weeks

Adjusted dose level -1: 300 mg/m²

Adjusted dose level -2: 250 mg/m^2

Depending on the patient's ability to tolerate therapy, doses should be adjusted in increments of 25-50 mg/m^2. Irinotecan doses may range from 50-150 mg/m^2 for the weekly regimen. Patients may be dosed as low as 200 mg/m^2 (in 50 mg/m^2 decrements) for the once-every-3-week regimen.

Combination therapy with fluorouracil and leucovorin: Six-week (42-day) cycle:

Regimen 1: I.V.: 125 mg/m^2 over 90 minutes on days 1, 8, 15, and 22; to be given in combination with bolus leucovorin and fluorouracil (leucovorin administered immediately following irinotecan; fluorouracil immediately following leucovorin)

Adjusted dose level -1: 100 mg/m^2

Adjusted dose level -2: 75 mg/m^2

Regimen 2: 180 mg/m^2 over 90 minutes on days 1, 15, and 29; to be given in combination with infusional leucovorin and bolus/infusion fluorouracil (leucovorin administered immediately following irinotecan; fluorouracil immediately following leucovorin)

Adjusted dose level -1: 150 mg/m^2

Adjusted dose level -2: 120 mg/m^2

Note: For all regimens: It is recommended that new courses begin only after the granulocyte count recovers to ≥1500/mm^3, the platelet count recovers to ≥100,000/mm^3, and treatment-related diarrhea has fully resolved. Treatment should be delayed 1-2 weeks to allow for recovery from treatment-related toxicities. If the patient has not recovered after a 2-week delay, consideration should be given to discontinuing irinotecan.

Hepatic Impairment: The manufacturer recommends that no change in dosage or administration be made for patients with liver metastases and normal hepatic function. Consideration may be given to starting irinotecan at a lower dose (eg, 100 mg/m^2) if bilirubin is 1-2 mg/dL; for total serum bilirubin elevations >2.0 mg/dL, specific recommendations are not available.

Available Dosage Forms Injection, solution, as hydrochloride: 20 mg/mL (2 mL, 5 mL)

Nursing Guidelines

Assessment: Use caution and closely monitor use for patients with increased risk of neutropenia, previous pelvic or abdominal radiation, elderly patients with comorbid conditions. Assess potential for interactions with other pharmacological agents prescriptions or herbal products patient may be taking (eg, potential for increased or decreased levels/effects of irinotecan). Premedicate with antiemetic (emetic potential moderately high). Infusion site must be monitored to prevent extravasation. Assess results of laboratory tests (CBC with differential and platelet count), therapeutic effectiveness, and adverse response before each infusion and at regular intervals during therapy (eg, neutropenia, acute diarrhea, sepsis, mucositis and/or stomatitis). Teach patient possible side effects/appropriate interventions, and adverse symptoms to report

Monitoring Laboratory Tests: CBC with differential and platelet count

Patient Education: Do not take any new medication during therapy unless approved by prescriber. This drug can only be administered by infusion. Report immediately any burning, pain, redness, or swelling at infusion site. Maintain adequate hydration (3-4 L/day of fluids) unless instructed to restrict fluid intake during therapy. May cause severe diarrhea; follow instructions for taking antidiarrheal medication. Report immediately if diarrhea persists or you experience signs of dehydration (eg, fainting, dizziness, lightheadedness). You may be more susceptible to infection (avoid crowds and exposure to infection and do not have any vaccinations without consulting prescriber). You may experience nausea or vomiting (small, frequent meals, frequent mouth care, sucking lozenges, or chewing gum may help); hair loss (will regrow after treatment is completed). Report unresolved nausea, or vomiting, alterations in urinary pattern (increased or decreased); opportunistic infection (fever, chills, unusual bruising or bleeding, fatigue, purulent vaginal discharge, unhealed mouth sores), chest pain or respiratory difficulty. **Pregnancy/breast-feeding precautions:** Inform prescriber if you are pregnant. Do not get pregnant or cause a pregnancy (males) while taking this medication. Consult prescriber for use appropriate contraceptive measures (may cause severe fetal defects). Do not breast-feed.

(Continued)

Irinotecan *(Continued)*

Pregnancy Risk Factor: D

Pregnancy Issues: Has shown to be teratogenic in animals. Teratogenic effects include a variety of external, visceral, and skeletal abnormalities. The patient should be warned of potential hazards to the fetus.

Lactation: Excretion in breast milk unknown/not recommended

Administration

I.V.: I.V. infusion, usually over 90 minutes.

Reconstitution: Dilute in 250-500 mL D_5W or NS to a final concentration of 0.12-2.8 mg/mL. Due to the relatively acidic pH, irinotecan appears to be more stable in D_5W than NS.

Compatibility: Stable in D_5W, NS

Y-site administration: Incompatible with gemcitabine

Compatibility when admixed: Incompatible with methylprednisolone sodium succinate

Storage: Store intact vials of injection at room temperature of 15°C to 30°C (59°F to 86°F); protect from light. Solutions diluted in NS may precipitate if refrigerated. Solutions diluted in D_5W are stable for 24 hours at room temperature or 48 hours under refrigeration at 2°C to 8°C.

Iron Dextran Complex (EYE ern DEKS tran KOM pleks)

U.S. Brand Names Dexferrum®; INFeD®

Pharmacologic Category Iron Salt

Medication Safety Issues

Sound-alike/look-alike issues:

Dexferrum® may be confused with Desferal®

Use Treatment of microcytic hypochromic anemia resulting from iron deficiency in patients in whom oral administration is infeasible or ineffective

Mechanism of Action The released iron, from the plasma, eventually replenishes the depleted iron stores in the bone marrow where it is incorporated into hemoglobin

Pharmacodynamics/Kinetics

Absorption:

I.M.: 50% to 90% is promptly absorbed, balance is slowly absorbed over month

I.V.: Uptake of iron by the reticuloendothelial system appears to be constant at about 10-20 mg/hour

Excretion: Urine and feces via reticuloendothelial system

Contraindications Hypersensitivity to iron dextran or any component of the formulation; all anemias that are not involved with iron deficiency; hemochromatosis; hemolytic anemia

Warnings/Precautions Use with caution in patients with history of asthma, hepatic impairment, rheumatoid arthritis; not recommended in children <4 months of age; deaths associated with parenteral administration following anaphylactic-type reactions have been reported (use only where resuscitative equipment and personnel are available); use only in patients where the iron deficient state is not amenable to oral iron therapy. A test dose of 0.5 mL I.V. or I.M. should be given to observe for adverse reactions. Anemia in the elderly is often caused by "anemia of chronic disease" or associated with inflammation rather than blood loss. Iron stores are usually normal or increased, with a serum ferritin >50 ng/mL and a decreased total iron binding capacity. I.V. administration of iron dextran is often preferred over I.M. in the elderly secondary to a decreased muscle mass and the need for daily injections.

Drug Interactions Decreased effect with chloramphenicol

Nutritional/Herbal/Ethanol Interactions Food: Iron bioavailability may be decreased if taken with dairy products.

Lab Interactions May cause falsely elevated values of serum bilirubin and falsely decreased values of serum calcium.

Adverse Reactions

>10%:

Cardiovascular: Flushing

Central nervous system: Dizziness, fever, headache, pain

Gastrointestinal: Nausea, vomiting, metallic taste

Local: Staining of skin at the site of I.M. injection

Miscellaneous: Diaphoresis

1% to 10%:

Cardiovascular: Hypotension (1% to 2%)

Dermatologic: Urticaria (1% to 2%), phlebitis (1% to 2%)
Gastrointestinal: Diarrhea
Genitourinary: Discoloration of urine

<1% (Limited to important or life-threatening): Anaphylactoid reaction, anaphylaxis, shock (cardiovascular collapse, respiratory difficulty; most frequently within minutes of administration)

Note: Diaphoresis, urticaria, arthralgia, fever, chills, dizziness, headache, and nausea may be delayed 24-48 hours after I.V. administration or 3-4 days after I.M. administration.

Overdosage/Toxicology Symptoms of overdose include erosion of GI mucosa, pulmonary edema, hyperthermia, convulsions, tachycardia, hepatic and renal impairment, coma, hematemesis, lethargy, tachycardia, and acidosis. Serum iron level >300 mcg/mL requires treatment of overdose due to severe toxicity. If severe iron overdose (when the serum iron concentration exceeds the total iron-binding capacity) occurs, it may be treated with deferoxamine. Deferoxamine may be administered I.V. (80 mg/kg over 24 hours) or I.M. (40-90 mg/kg every 8 hours).

Dosing

Adults & Elderly:

Note: A 0.5 mL test dose should be given prior to starting iron dextran therapy.

Iron-deficiency anemia: I.M., I.V.:

Dose (mL) = 0.0442 (desired Hgb - observed Hgb) x LBW + (0.26 x LBW)

Desired hemoglobin: Usually 14.8 g/dL

LBW = Lean body weight in kg

Milliliters of Iron Dextran (50 mg/mL) Required for Hemoglobin Restoration and Replacement of Iron Stores

Patient's IBW (kg)	Observed Hemoglobin							
	3 g/dL	4 g/dL	5 g/dL	6 g/dL	7 g/dL	8 g/dL	9 g/dL	10 g/dL
5	3	3	3	3	2	2	2	2
10	7	6	6	5	5	4	4	3
15	10	9	9	8	7	7	6	5
20	16	15	14	13	12	11	10	9
25	20	18	17	16	15	14	13	12
30	23	22	21	19	18	17	15	14
35	27	26	24	23	21	20	18	17
40	31	29	28	26	24	22	21	19
45	35	33	31	29	27	25	23	21
50	39	37	35	32	30	28	26	24
55	43	41	38	36	33	31	28	26
60	47	44	42	39	36	34	31	28
65	51	48	45	42	39	36	34	31
70	55	52	49	45	42	39	36	33
75	59	55	52	49	45	42	39	35
80	63	59	55	52	48	45	41	38
85	66	63	59	55	51	48	44	40
90	70	66	62	58	54	50	46	42
95	74	70	66	62	57	53	49	45
100	78	74	69	65	60	56	52	47

Iron dextran doses calculated for normal adult hemoglobin of 14.8 g/dL for IBW >15 kg, and normal hemoglobin of 12.0 g/dL for IBW ≤15 kg.

IBW (male) = 50 kg + (2.3 kg x inches over 60")

IBW (female) = 45.5 kg + (2.3 kg x inches over 60")

Iron replacement therapy for blood loss: I.M., I.V.: Replacement iron (mg) = blood loss (mL) x Hct

Maximum daily dosage:

Manufacturer's labeling: **Note:** Replacement of larger estimated iron deficits may be achieved by serial administration of smaller incremental dosages. Daily dosages should be limited to: Adults >50 kg: 100 mg iron (2 mL)

Total dose infusion (unlabeled): The entire dose (estimated iron deficit) may be diluted and administered as a one-time I.V. infusion.

Pediatrics: Note: A 0.5 mL test dose (0.25 mL in infants) should be given prior to starting iron dextran therapy.

(Continued)

Iron Dextran Complex *(Continued)*

Iron-deficiency anemia: I.M., I.V.:

Children 5-15 kg: Should not normally be given in the first 4 months of life:

Dose (mL) = 0.0442 (desired Hgb - observed Hgb) x W + (0.26 x W)

Desired hemoglobin: Usually 12 g/dL

W = Weight in kg

Children >15 kg: Refer to adult dosing.

Iron replacement therapy for blood loss: Refer to adult dosing.

Maximum daily dose:

5-10 kg: 50 mg iron (1 mL)

10-50 kg: 100 mg iron (2 mL)

Available Dosage Forms Note: Strength expressed as elemental iron

Injection, solution:

Dexferrum®: 50 mg/mL (1 mL, 2 mL)

INFeD®: 50 mg/mL (2 mL)

Nursing Guidelines

Assessment: Assess results of laboratory tests regularly and patient for adverse reactions. Note that adverse response may occur some time (1-4 days) after administration. Assess patients with rheumatoid arthritis for exacerbated swelling and joint pain; adjust medications as needed.

Monitoring Laboratory Tests: Hemoglobin, hematocrit, reticulocyte count, serum ferritin

Patient Education: You will need frequent blood tests while on this therapy. If you have rheumatoid arthritis, you may experience increased swelling or joint pain; consult prescriber for medication adjustment. If you experience dizziness or severe headache, use caution when driving or engaging in tasks that require alertness until response to drug is known. Small frequent meals, frequent mouth care, sucking lozenges, or chewing gum may relieve nausea and metallic taste. You may experience increased sweating. Report acute GI problems, fever, respiratory difficulty, rapid heartbeat, yellowing of skin or eyes, or swelling of hands and feet. **Pregnancy/breast-feeding precautions:** Inform prescriber if you are or intend to become pregnant. Do not breast-feed.

Geriatric Considerations: Anemia in the elderly is most often caused by "anemia of chronic disease", a result of aging effect in bone marrow, or associated with inflammation rather than blood loss. Iron stores are usually normal or increased, with a serum ferritin >50 ng/mL and a decreased total iron binding capacity. Hence, the anemia is not secondary to iron deficiency but the inability of the reticuloendothelial system to use available iron stores. I.V. administration of iron dextran is often preferred over I.M. in the elderly secondary to a decreased muscle mass and the need for daily injections.

Pregnancy Risk Factor: C

Lactation: Enters breast milk/contraindicated

Administration

I.M.: Note: Test dose: A test dose should be given on the first day of therapy; patient should be observed for 1 hour for hypersensitivity reaction, then the remaining dose (dose minus test dose) should be given. Epinephrine should be available.

I.M.: Use Z-track technique (displacement of the skin laterally prior to injection); injection should be deep into the upper outer quadrant of buttock; subsequent injections should be given into alternate buttock.

I.V.: A test dose should be given on the first day of therapy and administer gradually over at least 5 minutes. Subsequent dose(s) may be administered by I.V. bolus at rate of ≤50 mg/minute or diluted in 250-1000 mL NS and infused over 1-6 hours (initial 25 mL should be given slowly and patient should be observed for allergic reactions); avoid dilutions with dextrose (increased incidence of local pain and phlebitis)

Reconstitution: Stability of parenteral admixture at room temperature (25°C) is 3 months.

Standard diluent: Dose/250-1000 mL NS

Minimum volume: 250 mL NS

Compatibility: Stable in D_5W, NS

Storage: Store at room temperature.

♦ **Iron Gluconate** *see* Ferrous Gluconate *on page 720*

Iron Sucrose (EYE ern SOO krose)

U.S. Brand Names Venofer®

Pharmacologic Category Iron Salt

Use Treatment of iron-deficiency anemia in chronic renal failure, including nondialysis-dependent patients (with or without erythropoietin therapy) and dialysis-dependent patients receiving erythropoietin therapy

Mechanism of Action Iron sucrose is dissociated by the reticuloendothelial system into iron and sucrose. The released iron increases serum iron concentrations and is incorporated into hemoglobin.

Pharmacodynamics/Kinetics

Distribution: V_{dss}: Healthy adults: 7.9 L

Metabolism: Dissociated into iron and sucrose by the reticuloendothelial system

Half-life elimination: Healthy adults: 6 hours

Excretion: Healthy adults: Urine (5%) within 24 hours

Contraindications Hypersensitivity to iron sucrose or any component of the formulation; evidence of iron overload; anemia not caused by iron deficiency

Warnings/Precautions Rare anaphylactic and anaphylactoid reactions, including serious or life-threatening reactions, have been reported. Facilities (equipment and personnel) for cardiopulmonary resuscitation should be available during initial administration until response/tolerance has been established. Hypotension has been reported frequently in hemodialysis dependent patients. The incidence of hypotension in nondialysis patients is substantially lower. Hypotension may be related to total dose or rate of administration (avoid rapid I.V. injection), follow recommended guidelines. Withhold iron in the presence of tissue iron overload; periodic monitoring of hemoglobin, hematocrit, serum ferritin, and transferrin saturation is recommended. Safety and efficacy in children have not been established.

Drug Interactions

ACE inhibitors: Ace Inhibitors may enhance the adverse/toxic effects (erythema, abdominal cramps, nausea, vomiting, hypotension) of iron sucrose.

Iron preparations, oral: Iron sucrose injection may reduce the absorption of oral iron preparations.

Adverse Reactions

>10%:

Cardiovascular: Hypotension (1% to 7%; 39% in hemodialysis patients; may be related to total dose or rate of administration), peripheral edema (2% to 13%)

Central nervous system: Headache (3% to 13%)

Gastrointestinal: Nausea (1% to 15%)

Neuromuscular & skeletal: Muscle cramps (1% to 3%; 29% in hemodialysis patients)

1% to 10%:

Cardiovascular: Hypertension (6% to 8%), edema (1% to 7%), chest pain (1% to 6%), murmur (<1% to 3%), CHF

Central nervous system: Dizziness (1% to 10%), fatigue (2% to 5%), fever (1% to 3%), anxiety

Dermatologic: Pruritus (1% to 7%), rash (<1% to 2%)

Endocrine & metabolic: Gout (2% to 7%), hypoglycemia (<1% to 4%), hyperglycemia (3% to 4%), fluid overload (1% to 3%)

Gastrointestinal: Diarrhea (1% to 10%), vomiting (5% to 9%), taste perversion (1% to 9%), peritoneal infection (8%), constipation (1% to 7%), abdominal pain (1% to 4%), positive fecal occult blood (1% to 3%)

Genitourinary: Urinary tract infection (≤1%)

Local: Injection site reaction (2% to 4%), catheter site infection (4%)

Neuromuscular & skeletal: Muscle pain (1% to 7%), extremity pain (3% to 6%), arthralgia (1% to 4%), weakness (1% to 3%), back pain (1% to 3%)

Ocular: Conjunctivitis (<1% to 3%)

Otic: Ear pain (1% to 7%)

Respiratory: Dyspnea (1% to 10%), pharyngitis (<1% to 7%), cough (1% to 7%), sinusitis (1% to 4%), rhinitis (1% to 3%), upper respiratory infection (1% to 3%), nasal congestion (1%)

Miscellaneous: Graft complication (1% to 10%), hypersensitivity, sepsis

<1% (Limited to important or life-threatening): Anaphylactoid reactions, anaphylactic shock, bronchospasm (with dyspnea), collapse, facial rash, loss of consciousness, hypoesthesia, necrotizing enterocolitis (reported in premature infants, no causal relationship established), seizure, urticaria

(Continued)

Iron Sucrose *(Continued)*

Overdosage/Toxicology Symptoms associated with overdose or rapid infusion include hypotension, headache, vomiting, nausea, dizziness, joint aches, paresthesia, abdominal and muscle pain, edema, and cardiovascular collapse. Reducing rate of infusion can alleviate some symptoms. Most symptoms can be treated with I.V. fluids, hydrocortisone, and/or antihistamines.

For severe iron overdose (serum iron concentration exceeds TIBC), deferoxamine may be administered intravenously.

Dosing

Adults: Doses expressed in mg of **elemental** iron. **Note:** Test dose: Product labeling does not indicate need for a test dose in product-naive patients; test doses were administered in some clinical trials as 50 mg (2.5 mL) in 50 mL 0.9% NaCl administered over 3-10 minutes.

Iron-deficiency anemia in chronic renal disease: I.V.:

Hemodialysis-dependent patient: 100 mg (5 mL of iron sucrose injection) administered 1-3 times/week during dialysis; administer no more than 3 times/week to a cumulative total dose of 1000 mg (10 doses); may continue to administer at lowest dose necessary to maintain target hemoglobin, hematocrit, and iron storage parameters

Peritoneal dialysis-dependent patient: Slow intravenous infusion at the following schedule: Two infusions of 300 mg each over $1^1/_2$ hours 14 days apart followed by a single 400 mg infusion over $2^1/_2$ hours 14 days later (total cumulative dose of 1000 mg in 3 divided doses)

Nondialysis-dependent patient: 200 mg slow injection (over 2-5 minutes) on 5 different occasions within a 14-day period. Total cumulative dose: 1000 mg in 14-day period. **Note:** Dosage has also been administered as two infusions of 500 mg in a maximum of 250 mL 0.9% NaCl infused over 3.5-4 hours on day 1 and day 14 (limited experience)

Elderly: Insufficient data to identify differences between elderly and other adults; use caution.

Available Dosage Forms Injection, solution [preservative free]: 20 mg of elemental iron/mL (5 mL)

Nursing Guidelines

Assessment: Assess other medications patient may be taking for effectiveness and interactions. Facilities for cardiopulmonary resuscitation must be available during administration. Monitor blood pressure closely during infusion. Assess results of laboratory tests, therapeutic effectiveness, and adverse reactions at beginning of therapy and periodically throughout therapy. Assess knowledge/teach patient appropriate use according to product and purpose (dangers of iron overdosing), interventions to reduce side effects, and adverse symptoms to report.

Monitoring Laboratory Tests: Hematocrit, hemoglobin, serum ferritin, transferrin, percent transferrin saturation, TIBC; takes about 4 weeks of treatment to see increased serum iron and ferritin, and decreased TIBC. Serum iron concentrations should be drawn 48 hours after last dose.

Patient Education: You will be watched closely during infusion. You will need frequent blood tests while on this therapy. You may experience hypotension (use caution when driving or climbing stairs or engaging in tasks requiring alertness until response to drug is known); black tarry stools (normal), nausea, vomiting (taking with meals will reduce this), constipation (adequate fluids and exercise may help, may need a stool softener); or diarrhea (buttermilk, boiled milk, or yogurt may help). Report immediately severe unresolved GI irritation (cramping, nausea, vomiting, diarrhea, constipation); headache, lethargy, fatigue, dizziness, or other CNS changes; rapid respiration; leg cramps; chest pain or palpations; vision changes; choking sensation; loss of consciousness; or convulsions. **Breast-feeding precaution:** Consult prescriber if breast-feeding.

Pregnancy Risk Factor: B

Lactation: Excretion in breast milk unknown/use caution

Administration

I.V.: Not for rapid (bolus) I.V. injection; can be administered through dialysis line. Do not mix with other medications or parenteral nutrient solutions.

Slow I.V. injection: 1 mL (20 mg iron) of undiluted solution per minute (100 mg over 2-5 minutes)

Infusion: Dilute 1 vial (100 mg/5 mL) in maximum of 100 mL 0.9% NaCl; infuse over at least 15 minutes; 300 mg/250 mL should be infused over at least $1^1/_2$

hours; 400 mg/250 mL should be infused over at least 2½ hours; 500 mg/250 mL should be infused over at least 3½ hours.

Reconstitution: May be administered via the dialysis line as an undiluted solution or by diluting 100 mg (5 mL) in 100 mL normal saline. Doses ≥200mg should be diluted in a maximum of 250 mL normal saline. Do not mix with other medications.

Storage: Store vials at room temperature of 15°C to 30°C (59°F to 86°F); do not freeze. Following dilution, solutions are stable for 48 hours at room temperature or under refrigeration.

♦ Iron Sulfate *see* Ferrous Sulfate *on page 721*
♦ ISD *see* Isosorbide Dinitrate *on page 976*
♦ ISDN *see* Isosorbide Dinitrate *on page 976*
♦ ISG *see* Immune Globulin (Intramuscular) *on page 898*
♦ ISMN *see* Isosorbide Mononitrate *on page 979*
♦ Ismo® *see* Isosorbide Mononitrate *on page 979*
♦ Isoamyl Nitrite *see* Amyl Nitrite *on page 165*
♦ Isobamate *see* Carisoprodol *on page 316*
♦ Isochron™ *see* Isosorbide Dinitrate *on page 976*

Isoflurane (eye soe FLURE ane)

U.S. Brand Names Forane®

Pharmacologic Category General Anesthetic, Inhalation

Medication Safety Issues

Sound-alike/look-alike issues:

Isoflurane may be confused with enflurane, isoflurophate

Use Maintenance of general anesthesia

Pharmacodynamics/Kinetics

Onset of action: 7-10 minutes (pungent odor limits inhalation rate)

Duration: Emergence time: Depends on blood concentration when discontinued

Metabolism: Hepatic (0.2%)

Excretion: Exhaled gases

Contraindications Hypersensitivity to isoflurane or any component of the formulation; known or suspected history of malignant hyperthermia

Warnings/Precautions Decrease in blood pressure is dose dependent due to peripheral vasodilation primarily in skin and muscle; cardiac output is maintained. Isoflurane may produce cardiac steal (due to coronary vasodilation) in patients with hypertension under certain conditions (eg, unusual coronary artery anatomy). Isoflurane may produce reflex tachycardia, but does not alter atrioventricular conduction or sensitize the myocardium to epinephrine-induced arrhythmias. Respiration is depressed as is the normal hyperventilatory response to hypoxia. Hypoxic pulmonary vasoconstriction is depressed which may lead to pulmonary shunt. Isoflurane dilates the cerebral vasculature and may, in certain conditions, increase intracranial pressure. Renal, splenic, and hepatic blood flow are reduced. Isoflurane is a trigger of malignant hyperthermia. Hypoxemia-induced increase in ventilation is abolished at low isoflurane concentration. Isoflurane can produce elevated carbon monoxide levels in the presence of a dry carbon dioxide absorbent within the circle breathing system of an anesthetic machine.

Drug Interactions **Substrate** of CYP2E1 (major); **Inhibits** CYP2B6 (weak)

Antihypertensives: Excessive hypotension may occur with combined use.

Benzodiazepines, opioids: Concurrent use of opioids and/or benzodiazepines decreases the MAC of isoflurane.

CYP2E1 inhibitors: May increase the levels/effects of isoflurane. Example inhibitors include disulfiram, isoniazid, and miconazole.

Isoniazid: Increased risk of hepatotoxicity with combined use.

Neuromuscular-blocking agents (nondepolarizing): Isoflurane may potentiate the action of nondepolarizing, neuromuscular-blocking agents.

Adverse Reactions Frequency not defined.

Cardiovascular: Hypotension, myocardial depression

Respiratory: Respiratory depression/arrest

Gastrointestinal: Nausea, vomiting

Miscellaneous: Shivering

Dosing

Adults: Anesthesia: Inhalation: Minimum alveolar concentration (MAC), the concentration at which 50% of patients do not respond to surgical incision, is 1.2% for isoflurane. The concentration at which amnesia and loss of awareness

(Continued)

Isoflurane *(Continued)*

occur (MAC - awake) is 0.4%. Surgical levels of anesthesia are achieved with concentrations between 1% to 2.5%.

Elderly: MAC is reduced in the elderly.

Pediatrics: Refer to adult dosing.

Available Dosage Forms Solution: 100 mL, 250 mL

Nursing Guidelines

Pregnancy Risk Factor: C

Perioperative/Anesthesia/Other Concerns: Use of isoflurane for induction of anesthesia is limited by its pungent odor which may cause breath holding or coughing.

Isoniazid (eye soe NYE a zid)

U.S. Brand Names Nydrazid® [DSC]

Synonyms INH; Isonicotinic Acid Hydrazide

Pharmacologic Category Antitubercular Agent

Use Treatment of susceptible tuberculosis infections; treatment of latent tuberculosis infection (LTBI)

Mechanism of Action Unknown, but may include the inhibition of myocolic acid synthesis resulting in disruption of the bacterial cell wall

Pharmacodynamics/Kinetics

Absorption: Rapid and complete; rate can be slowed with food

Distribution: All body tissues and fluids including CSF; crosses placenta; enters breast milk

Protein binding: 10% to 15%

Metabolism: Hepatic with decay rate determined genetically by acetylation phenotype

Half-life elimination: Fast acetylators: 30-100 minutes; Slow acetylators: 2-5 hours; may be prolonged with hepatic or severe renal impairment

Time to peak, serum: 1-2 hours

Excretion: Urine (75% to 95%); feces; saliva

Contraindications Hypersensitivity to isoniazid or any component of the formulation; acute liver disease; previous history of hepatic damage during isoniazid therapy

Warnings/Precautions Use with caution in patients with renal impairment and chronic liver disease. Severe and sometimes fatal hepatitis may occur or develop even after many months of treatment; patients must report any prodromal symptoms of hepatitis, such as fatigue, weakness, malaise, anorexia, nausea, or vomiting. Malnourished patients should receive concomitant pyridoxine therapy. Periodic ophthalmic examinations are recommended even when usual symptoms do not occur; pyridoxine (10-50 mg/day) is recommended in individuals likely to develop peripheral neuropathies.

Drug Interactions Substrate of CYP2E1 (major); **Inhibits** CYP1A2 (weak), 2A6 (moderate), 2C8/9 (moderate), 2C19 (strong), 2D6 (moderate), 2E1 (moderate), 3A4 (strong); **Induces** CYP2E1 (after discontinuation) (weak)

Acetaminophen: Isoniazid may enhance the adverse/toxic effect of acetaminophen.

Antacids: Antacids may decrease the absorption of isoniazid.

Benzodiazepines (metabolized by oxidation): Isoniazid may decrease the metabolism, via CYP isoenzymes, of benzodiazepines (metabolized by oxidation).

Carbamazepine: Isoniazid may decrease the metabolism of carbamazepine.

Cycloserine: Cycloserine may enhance the CNS depressant effect of isoniazid.

CYP2A6 substrates: Isoniazid may increase the levels/effects of CYP2A6 substrates. Example substrates include dexmedetomidine and ifosfamide.

CYP2C8/9 substrates: Isoniazid may increase the levels/effects of CYP2C8/9 substrates. Example substrates include amiodarone, fluoxetine, glimepiride, glipizide, nateglinide, phenytoin, pioglitazone, rosiglitazone, sertraline, and warfarin.

CYP2C19 substrates: Isoniazid may increase the levels/effects of CYP2C19 substrates. Example substrates include citalopram, diazepam, methsuximide, phenytoin, propranolol, and sertraline.

CYP2D6 substrates: Isoniazid may increase the levels/effects of CYP2D6 substrates. Example substrates include amphetamines, selected beta-blockers, dextromethorphan, fluoxetine, lidocaine, mirtazapine, nefazodone, paroxetine, risperidone, ritonavir, thioridazine, tricyclic antidepressants, and venlafaxine.

CYP2D6 prodrug substrates: Isoniazid may decrease the levels/effects of CYP2D6 prodrug substrates. Example prodrug substrates include codeine, hydrocodone, oxycodone, and tramadol.

CYP2E1 substrates: Isoniazid may increase the levels/effects of CYP2E1 substrates. Example substrates include inhalational anesthetics, theophylline, and trimethadione.

CYP3A4 substrates: Isoniazid may increase the levels/effects of CYP3A4 substrates. Example substrates include benzodiazepines, calcium channel blockers, mirtazapine, nateglinide, nefazodone, tacrolimus, and venlafaxine. Selected benzodiazepines (midazolam and triazolam), cisapride, ergot alkaloids, selected HMG-CoA reductase inhibitors (lovastatin and simvastatin), and pimozide are generally contraindicated with strong CYP3A4 inhibitors.

Disulfiram: Isoniazid may enhance the adverse/toxic effect of disulfiram.

Phenytoin: Isoniazid may decrease the metabolism, via CYP isoenzymes, of phenytoin.

Theophylline: Isoniazid may decrease the metabolism, via CYP isoenzymes, of theophylline derivatives.

Valproic Acid: Isoniazid may increase the serum concentration of valproic acid.

Nutritional/Herbal/Ethanol Interactions

Ethanol: Avoid ethanol (increases the risk of hepatitis).

Food: Isoniazid serum levels may be decreased if taken with food. Has some ability to inhibit tyramine metabolism; several case reports of mild reactions (flushing, palpitations) after ingestion of cheese with or without wine. Isoniazid decreases folic acid absorption. Isoniazid alters pyridoxine metabolism.

Lab Interactions False-positive urinary glucose with Clinitest®

Adverse Reactions Frequency not defined.

Cardiovascular: Hypertension, palpitation, tachycardia, vasculitis

Central nervous system: Dizziness, encephalopathy, memory impairment, slurred speech, lethargy, fever, depression, psychosis, seizure

Dermatologic: Rash (morbilliform, maculopapular, pruritic, or exfoliative), flushing

Endocrine & metabolic: Hyperglycemia, metabolic acidosis, gynecomastia, pellagra, pyridoxine deficiency

Gastrointestinal: Anorexia, nausea, vomiting, stomach pain

Hematologic: Agranulocytosis, anemia (sideroblastic, hemolytic, or aplastic), thrombocytopenia, eosinophilia, lymphadenopathy

Hepatic: LFTs mildly increased (10% to 20%); hyperbilirubinemia, jaundice, hepatitis (may involve progressive liver damage; risk increases with age; 2.3% in patients >50 years)

Neuromuscular & skeletal: Weakness, peripheral neuropathy (dose-related incidence, 10% to 20% incidence with 10 mg/kg/day), hyper-reflexia, arthralgia, lupus-like syndrome

Ocular: Blurred vision, loss of vision, optic neuritis and atrophy

Overdosage/Toxicology Symptoms of overdose generally occur within 30 minutes to 3 hours, and may include nausea, vomiting, slurred speech, dizziness, blurred vision, metabolic acidosis, hallucinations, stupor, coma, and intractable seizures. Because of high morbidity and mortality rates with isoniazid overdose, patients who are asymptomatic after an overdose should be monitored for 4-6 hours. Pyridoxine has been shown to be effective in the treatment of intoxication, especially when seizures occur. Pyridoxine I.V. is administered on a milligram to milligram dose. If the amount of isoniazid ingested is unknown, 5 g of pyridoxine should be given over 3-5 minutes and may be followed by an additional 5 g in 30 minutes. Treatment is supportive. Forced diuresis and hemodialysis can result in more rapid removal.

Dosing

Adults & Elderly: Recommendations often change due to resistant strains and newly-developed information; consult *MMWR* for current CDC recommendations. Intramuscular is available in patients who are unable to either take or absorb oral therapy.

Treatment of latent tuberculosis infection (LTBI): 300 mg/day or 900 mg twice weekly for 6-9 months in patients who do not have HIV infection (9 months is optimal, 6 months may be considered to reduce costs of therapy) and 9 months in patients who have HIV infection. Extend to 12 months of therapy if interruptions in treatment occur.

Treatment of active TB infection (drug susceptible):

Daily therapy: 5 mg/kg/day given daily (usual dose: 300 mg/day); 10 mg/kg/day in 1-2 divided doses in patients with disseminated disease

Twice weekly directly observed therapy (DOT): 15 mg/kg (maximum: 900 mg); 3 times/week therapy: 15 mg/kg (maximum: 900 mg)

(Continued)

Isoniazid *(Continued)*

Note: Treatment may be defined by the number of doses administered (eg, "six-month" therapy involves 192 doses of INH and rifampin, and 56 doses of pyrazinamide). Six months is the shortest interval of time over which these doses may be administered, assuming no interruption of therapy.

Note: Concomitant administration of 6-50 mg/day pyridoxine is recommended in malnourished patients or those prone to neuropathy (eg, alcoholics, diabetics)

Pediatrics: Recommendations often change due to resistant strains and newly-developed information; consult *MMWR* for current CDC recommendations. Intramuscular is available in patients who are unable to either take or absorb oral therapy.

Treatment of latent TB infection (LTBI): Infants and Children: Oral: 10-20 mg/kg/day in 1-2 divided doses (maximum: 300 mg/day) or 20-40 mg/kg (maximum: 900 mg/dose) twice weekly for 9 months

Treatment of active TB infection: Infants and Children: Oral:

Daily therapy: 10-15 mg/kg/day in 1-2 divided doses (maximum: 300 mg/day)

Twice weekly directly observed therapy (DOT): 20-30 mg/kg (maximum: 900 mg)

Renal Impairment:

Cl_{cr} <10 mL/minute: Administer 50% of normal dose

Hemodialysis: Dialyzable (50% to 100%)

Administer dose postdialysis

Peritoneal dialysis, continuous arteriovenous or venovenous hemofiltration: Dose for Cl_{cr} <10 mL/minute

Hepatic Impairment: Dose should be reduced in severe hepatic disease.

Available Dosage Forms

Injection, solution (Nydrazid®): 100 mg/mL (10 mL) [DSC]

Syrup: 50 mg/5 mL (473 mL) [orange flavor]

Tablet: 100 mg, 300 mg

Nursing Guidelines

Assessment: See Contraindications and Warnings/Precautions for use cautions. Assess potential for interactions with other prescriptions, OTC medications, or herbal products patient may be taking (see Drug Interactions). Assess results of laboratory tests (see below), therapeutic effectiveness, and adverse response (see Adverse Reactions and Overdose/Toxicology) at regular intervals during therapy. Advise patients with diabetes about use of Clinitest®. Teach patient proper use, possible side effects/appropriate interventions (eg, diet and ophthalmic examinations), and adverse symptoms to report (see Patient Education).

Monitoring Laboratory Tests: Transaminase levels at baseline 1, 3, 6, and 9 months

Dietary Considerations: Should be taken 1 hour before or 2 hours after meals on an empty stomach; increase dietary intake of folate, niacin, magnesium. No need to restrict tyramine-containing foods.

Patient Education: Inform prescriber of all prescriptions, OTC medications, or herbal products you are taking, and any allergies you have. Do not take any new medication during therapy unless approved by prescriber. Best if taken on an empty stomach, 1 hour before or 2 hours after meals. Avoid missing any dose and do not discontinue without notifying prescriber. Avoid alcohol and tyramine-containing foods (eg, aged cheese, broad beans, dry sausage, preserved meats or sausages, liver pate, fish, soy bean, protein supplements, wine) and increase dietary intake of folate, niacin, magnesium. May cause false test results with Clinitest®; use of another type of glucose testing is preferable. You will need to have frequent ophthalmic exams and periodic medical check-ups to evaluate drug effects. You may experience nausea or vomiting (small, frequent meals, frequent mouth care, chewing gum, or sucking lozenges may help). Report tingling or numbness in hands or feet, loss of sensation, unusual weakness, fatigue, nausea or vomiting, dark colored urine, change in urinary pattern, yellowing skin or eyes, or change in color of stool. **Pregnancy precaution:** Inform prescriber if you are or intend to become pregnant.

Geriatric Considerations: Age has not been shown to affect the pharmacokinetics of INH since acetylation phenotype determines clearance and half-life, acetylation rate does not change significantly with age. Most strains of *M. tuberculosis* found the elderly should be susceptible to INH since most acquired their initial infection prior to INH's introduction.

Pregnancy Risk Factor: C

Lactation: Enters breast milk/compatible

Breast-Feeding Considerations: Small amounts of isoniazid are excreted in breast milk. However, women with tuberculosis should not be discouraged from breast-feeding. Pyridoxine supplementation is recommended for the mother and infant.

Administration

Oral: Should be administered 1 hour before or 2 hours after meals on an empty stomach.

Storage: Protect oral dosage forms from light.

- **Isonicotinic Acid Hydrazide** *see* Isoniazid *on page 972*
- **Isonipecaine Hydrochloride** *see* Meperidine *on page 1097*
- **Isophane Insulin** *see* Insulin NPH *on page 926*
- **Isophane Insulin and Regular Insulin** *see* Insulin NPH and Insulin Regular *on page 927*

Isoproterenol (eye soe proe TER e nole)

U.S. Brand Names Isuprel®

Synonyms Isoproterenol Hydrochloride

Pharmacologic Category Beta$_1$- & Beta$_2$-Adrenergic Agonist Agent

Medication Safety Issues

Sound-alike/look-alike issues:

Isuprel® may be confused with Disophrol®, Ismelin®, Isordil®

Use Ventricular arrhythmias due to AV nodal block; hemodynamically compromised bradyarrhythmias or atropine- and dopamine-resistant bradyarrhythmias (when transcutaneous/venous pacing is not available); temporary use in third-degree AV block until pacemaker insertion

Unlabeled/Investigational Use Temporizing measure before transvenous pacing for torsade de pointes; diagnostic aid (vasovagal syncope)

Mechanism of Action Stimulates beta$_1$- and beta$_2$-receptors resulting in relaxation of bronchial, GI, and uterine smooth muscle, increased heart rate and contractility, vasodilation of peripheral vasculature

Pharmacodynamics/Kinetics

Onset of action: Bronchodilation: I.V.: Immediate

Duration: I.V.: 10-15 minutes

Metabolism: Via conjugation in many tissues including hepatic and pulmonary

Half-life elimination: 2.5-5 minutes

Excretion: Urine (primarily as sulfate conjugates)

Contraindications Hypersensitivity to sulfites or isoproterenol, any component of the formulation, or other sympathomimetic amines; angina, pre-existing cardiac arrhythmias (ventricular); tachycardia or AV block caused by cardiac glycoside intoxication

Warnings/Precautions Use with extreme caution; not currently a treatment of choice; use with caution in elderly patients, diabetics, renal or cardiovascular disease, seizure disorder, or hyperthyroidism; excessive or prolonged use may result in decreased effectiveness.

Drug Interactions Increased toxicity: Sympathomimetic agents may cause headaches and elevate blood pressure; general anesthetics may cause arrhythmias

Nutritional/Herbal/Ethanol Interactions Herb/Nutraceutical: Avoid ephedra, yohimbe (may cause CNS stimulation).

Adverse Reactions Frequency not defined.

Cardiovascular: Premature ventricular beats, bradycardia, hyper-/hypotension, chest pain, palpitation, tachycardia, ventricular arrhythmia, MI size increased

Central nervous system: Headache, nervousness or restlessness

Endocrine & metabolic: Serum glucose increased, serum potassium decreased, hypokalemia

Gastrointestinal: Nausea, vomiting

Respiratory: Dyspnea

Overdosage/Toxicology Symptoms of overdose include tachycardia, tremor, hypertension or hypotension, angina, and seizures. Hypokalemia also may occur. Cardiac arrest and death may be associated with abuse of beta-agonist bronchodilators. Treatment includes immediate discontinuation and symptomatic and supportive therapies. Cautious use of beta-adrenergic blocking agents may be considered in severe cases.

(Continued)

Isoproterenol *(Continued)*

Dosing

Adults & Elderly: Cardiac arrhythmias: I.V.: Initial: 2 mcg/minute; titrate to patient response (2-10 mcg/minute)

Pediatrics: Cardiac arrhythmias: I.V.: Start 0.1 mcg/kg/minute (usual effective dose 0.2-2 mcg/kg/minute)

Available Dosage Forms Injection, solution, as hydrochloride: 0.02 mg/mL (10 mL); 0.2 mg/mL (1:5000) (1 mL, 5 mL) [contains sodium metabisulfite]

Nursing Guidelines

Assessment: Assess results of laboratory tests, cardiac, respiratory, and hemodynamic status when used in acute or emergency situations. Assess knowledge/teach patient appropriate use and administration procedures and adverse reactions to report.

Monitoring Laboratory Tests: ECG, arterial blood gas, serum magnesium, serum potassium, serum glucose (in selected patients)

Patient Education: You may experience nervousness, dizziness, or fatigue (use caution when driving or engaging in tasks requiring alertness until response to drug is known); or dry mouth, nausea, or vomiting (small frequent meals may reduce the incidence of nausea or vomiting). If you have diabetes, check blood sugar; blood glucose level may be increased. Report chest pain, rapid heartbeat or palpitations, unresolved/persistent GI upset, dizziness, fatigue, trembling, increased anxiety, sleeplessness, or respiratory difficulty. **Pregnancy/breast-feeding precautions:** Inform prescriber if you are pregnant. Consult prescriber if breast-feeding.

Pregnancy Risk Factor: C

Lactation: Excretion in breast milk unknown

Perioperative/Anesthesia/Other Concerns: An important use for isoproterenol is in the intensive care setting in the treatment of torsade de pointes. In patients with recurrent torsade de pointes, treatment consists of correcting underlying cause (eg, electrolyte abnormalities or drug ingestion). Supportive therapy consists of increasing heart rate so as to decrease the QT interval.

Administration

I.V.: I.V. infusion administration requires the use of an infusion pump. To prepare for infusion: 1 mg isoproterenol to 500 mL D_5W, final concentration 2 mcg/mL

Reconstitution: Stability of parenteral admixture at room temperature (25°C) or at refrigeration (4°C) is 24 hours.

Standard diluent: 2 mg/500 mL D_5W; 4 mg/500 mL D_5W
Minimum volume: 1 mg/100 mL D_5W

Compatibility: Stable in dextran 6% in dextrose, dextran 6% in NS, D_5LR, D_5¼ NS, D_5½NS, D_5NS, D_5W, $D_{10}W$, LR, ½NS, NS; **incompatible** with sodium bicarbonate 5%, and alkaline solutions

Compatibility when admixed: Incompatible with aminophylline, furosemide, sodium bicarbonate

Storage: Isoproterenol solution should be stored at room temperature. It should not be used if a color or precipitate is present. Exposure to air, light, or increased temperature may cause a pink to brownish pink color to develop.

◆ **Isoproterenol Hydrochloride** *see* Isoproterenol *on page 975*
◆ **Isoptin® SR** *see* Verapamil *on page 1702*
◆ **Isopto® Atropine** *see* Atropine *on page 203*
◆ **Isopto® Carbachol** *see* Carbachol *on page 305*
◆ **Isopto® Carpine** *see* Pilocarpine *on page 1365*
◆ **Isopto® Homatropine** *see* Homatropine *on page 855*
◆ **Isopto® Hyoscine** *see* Scopolamine *on page 1513*
◆ **Isopto® Tears [OTC]** *see* Hydroxypropyl Methylcellulose *on page 883*
◆ **Isordil®** *see* Isosorbide Dinitrate *on page 976*

Isosorbide Dinitrate (eye soe SOR bide dye NYE trate)

U.S. Brand Names Dilatrate®-SR; Isochron™; Isordil®

Synonyms ISD; ISDN

Pharmacologic Category Vasodilator

Medication Safety Issues

Sound-alike/look-alike issues:
Isordil® may be confused with Inderal®, Isuprel®

Use Prevention and treatment of angina pectoris; for congestive heart failure; to relieve pain, dysphagia, and spasm in esophageal spasm with GE reflux

Unlabeled/Investigational Use Esophageal spastic disorders

Mechanism of Action Stimulation of intracellular cyclic-GMP results in vascular smooth muscle relaxation of both arterial and venous vasculature. Increased venous pooling decreases left ventricular pressure (preload) and arterial dilatation decreases arterial resistance (afterload). Therefore, this reduces cardiac oxygen demand by decreasing left ventricular pressure and systemic vascular resistance by dilating arteries. Additionally, coronary artery dilation improves collateral flow to ischemic regions; esophageal smooth muscle is relaxed via the same mechanism.

Pharmacodynamics/Kinetics

Onset of action: Sublingual tablet: 2-10 minutes; Chewable tablet: 3 minutes; Oral tablet: 45-60 minutes

Duration: Sublingual tablet: 1-2 hours; Chewable tablet: 0.5-2 hours; Oral tablet: 4-6 hours

Metabolism: Extensively hepatic to conjugated metabolites, including isosorbide 5-mononitrate (active) and 2-mononitrate (active)

Half-life elimination: Parent drug: 1-4 hours; Metabolite (5-mononitrate): 4 hours

Excretion: Urine and feces

Contraindications Hypersensitivity to isosorbide dinitrate or any component of the formulation; hypersensitivity to organic nitrates; concurrent use with phosphodiesterase-5 (PDE-5) inhibitors (sildenafil, tadalafil, or vardenafil); angle-closure glaucoma (intraocular pressure may be increased); head trauma or cerebral hemorrhage (increase intracranial pressure); severe anemia

Warnings/Precautions Severe hypotension can occur. Use with caution in volume depletion, hypotension, and right ventricular infarctions. Paradoxical bradycardia and increased angina pectoris can accompany hypotension. Postural hypotension can also occur. Tolerance does develop to nitrates and appropriate dosing is needed to minimize this. Safety and efficacy have not been established in pediatric patients. Nitrate may aggravate angina caused by hypertrophic cardiomyopathy. Avoid concurrent use with sildenafil.

Drug Interactions Substrate of CYP3A4 (major)

CYP3A4 inducers: CYP3A4 inducers may decrease the levels/effects of isosorbide dinitrate. Example inducers include aminoglutethimide, carbamazepine, nafcillin, nevirapine, phenobarbital, phenytoin, and rifamycins.

CYP3A4 inhibitors: May increase the levels/effects of isosorbide dinitrate. Example inhibitors include azole antifungals, clarithromycin, diclofenac, doxycycline, erythromycin, imatinib, isoniazid, nefazodone, nicardipine, propofol, protease inhibitors, quinidine, telithromycin, and verapamil.

Sildenafil, tadalafil, vardenafil: Significant reduction of systolic and diastolic blood pressure with concurrent use (contraindicated). Do not administer sildenafil, tadalafil, or vardenafil within 24 hours of a nitrate preparation.

Nutritional/Herbal/Ethanol Interactions Ethanol: Caution with ethanol (may increase risk of hypotension).

Lab Interactions Decreased cholesterol (S)

Adverse Reactions Frequency not defined.

Cardiovascular: Hypotension (infrequent), postural hypotension, crescendo angina (uncommon), rebound hypertension (uncommon), pallor, cardiovascular collapse, tachycardia, shock, flushing, peripheral edema, syncope (uncommon)

Central nervous system: Headache (most common), lightheadedness (related to blood pressure changes), dizziness, restlessness

Gastrointestinal: Nausea, vomiting, bowel incontinence, xerostomia

Genitourinary: Urinary incontinence

Hematologic: Methemoglobinemia (rare, overdose)

Neuromuscular & skeletal: Weakness

Ocular: Blurred vision

Miscellaneous: Cold sweat

The incidence of hypotension and adverse cardiovascular events may be increased when used in combination with sildenafil (Viagra®).

Overdosage/Toxicology Symptoms of overdose include hypotension, throbbing headache, palpitations, visual disturbances, tachycardia, methemoglobinemia, flushing, diaphoresis, metabolic acidosis, and coma. High levels or methemoglobinemia can cause signs or symptoms of hypoxemia. Treat symptomatically.

(Continued)

Isosorbide Dinitrate *(Continued)*

Dosing

Adults:

Angina:

Oral: 5-40 mg 4 times/day or 40 mg every 8-12 hours in sustained released dosage form

Sublingual: 2.5-5 mg every 5-10 minutes for maximum of 3 doses in 15-30 minutes; may also use prophylactically 15 minutes prior to activities which may provoke an attack

Congestive heart failure:

Initial dose: 20 mg 3-4 times/day

Target dose: 120-160 mg/day in divided doses; use in combination with hydralazine

Esophageal spastic disorders (unlabeled use):

Oral: 5-10 mg before meals

Sublingual: 2.5 mg after meals

Note: Tolerance to nitrate effects develops with chronic exposure. Dose escalation does not overcome this effect. Tolerance can only be overcome by short periods of nitrate absence from the body. Short periods (10-12 hours) of nitrate withdrawal help minimize tolerance. General recommendations are to take the last dose of short-acting agents no later than 7 PM; administer 2-3 times/day rather than 4 times/day. Sustained release preparations could be administered at times to allow a 15- to 17-hour interval between first and last daily dose. Example: Administer sustained release at 8 AM and 2 PM for a twice daily regimen.

Elderly: Elderly patients should be given lowest recommended adult daily doses initially and titrate upward.

Renal Impairment: Hemodialysis: During hemodialysis, administer dose postdialysis or administer supplemental 10-20 mg dose. During peritoneal dialysis, supplemental dose is not necessary.

Available Dosage Forms [DSC] = Discontinued product

Capsule, sustained release (Dilatrate®-SR): 40 mg

Tablet: 5 mg, 10 mg, 20 mg, 30 mg,

Isordil®: 5 mg, 10 mg [DSC], 20 mg [DSC], 30 mg [DSC], 40 mg

Tablet, extended release (Isochron™): 40 mg

Tablet, sublingual: 2.5 mg, 5 mg

Isordil®: 2.5 mg, 5 mg, 10 mg [DSC]

Nursing Guidelines

Assessment: See Contraindications, Warnings/Precautions, and Drug Interactions for use cautions. Assess potential for interactions with other prescriptions, OTC medications, or herbal products patient may be taking (see Drug Interactions). See Administration warning. Assess results of laboratory tests (see below), therapeutic effectiveness, and adverse response (eg, hypotension - see Adverse Reactions and Overdose/Toxicology) at regular intervals during therapy. When discontinuing, reduce dosage gradually. Teach patient proper use, possible side effects/appropriate interventions, and adverse symptoms to report (see Patient Education). Note breast-feeding caution.

Patient Education: Inform prescriber of all prescriptions, OTC medications, or herbal products you are taking, and any allergies you have. Do not take any new medication during therapy unless approved by prescriber. Take as directed, at the same time each day. Do not chew or swallow sublingual tablets; allow them to dissolve under your tongue. Do not crush or chew sustained release capsules, swallow whole with 8 oz water. Do not change brands without consulting prescriber. Do not discontinue abruptly. Keep medication in original container, tightly closed. Avoid alcohol; combination may cause severe hypotension. May cause postural hypotension (take medication while sitting down and use caution when rising from sitting or lying position or climbing stairs); dizziness, weakness, or blurred vision (use caution when driving or engaging in hazardous activities until response to drug is known); or nausea or vomiting (small, frequent meals, frequent mouth care, chewing gum, or sucking lozenges may help). If chest pain occurs, seek emergency medical help at once. Report acute headache, rapid heartbeat, unusual restlessness or dizziness, muscular weakness, or blurring vision. **Pregnancy/breast-feeding precautions:** Inform prescriber if you are or intend to become pregnant. Consult prescriber if breast-feeding.

Pregnancy Risk Factor: C

Lactation: Excretion in breast milk unknown

Perioperative/Anesthesia/Other Concerns: Nitrates used in right ventricular infarction may induce acute hypotension. Nitrate use in severe pericardial effusion may reduce cardiac filling pressure and precipitate cardiac tamponade. In the management of heart failure, the combination of isosorbide dinitrate and hydralazine confers beneficial effects on disease progression and cardiac outcomes.

Administration

Oral: Do not administer around-the-clock; the first dose of nitrates should be administered in a physician's office to observe for maximal cardiovascular dynamic effects and adverse effects (orthostatic blood pressure drop, headache); when immediate release products are prescribed twice daily (recommend 7 AM and noon); for 3 times/day dosing (recommend 7 AM, noon, and 5 PM); when sustained-release products are indicated, suggest once a day in morning or via twice daily dosing at 8 AM and 2 PM. Do not crush sublingual tablets.

Isosorbide Mononitrate (eye soe SOR bide mon oh NYE trate)

U.S. Brand Names Imdur®; Ismo®; Monoket®

Synonyms ISMN

Pharmacologic Category Vasodilator

Medication Safety Issues

Sound-alike/look-alike issues:

Imdur® may be confused with Imuran®, Inderal LA®, K-Dur®

Monoket® may be confused with Monopril®

Use Long-acting metabolite of the vasodilator isosorbide dinitrate used for the prophylactic treatment of angina pectoris

Mechanism of Action Prevailing mechanism of action for nitroglycerin (and other nitrates) is systemic venodilation, decreasing preload as measured by pulmonary capillary wedge pressure and left ventricular end diastolic volume and pressure; the average reduction in left ventricular end diastolic volume is 25% at rest, with a corresponding increase in ejection fractions of 50% to 60%. This effect improves congestive symptoms in heart failure and improves the myocardial perfusion gradient in patients with coronary artery disease.

Pharmacodynamics/Kinetics

Onset of action: 30-60 minutes

Absorption: Nearly complete and low intersubject variability in its pharmacokinetic parameters and plasma concentrations

Metabolism: Hepatic

Half-life elimination: Mononitrate: ~4 hours

Excretion: Urine and feces

Contraindications Hypersensitivity to isosorbide or any component of the formulation; hypersensitivity to organic nitrates; concurrent use with phosphodiesterase-5 (PDE-5) inhibitors (sildenafil, tadalafil, or vardenafil); angle-closure glaucoma (intraocular pressure may be increased); head trauma or cerebral hemorrhage (increase intracranial pressure); severe anemia

Warnings/Precautions Severe hypotension can occur. Use with caution in volume depletion, hypotension, and right ventricular infarctions. Paradoxical bradycardia and increased angina pectoris can accompany hypotension. Orthostatic hypotension can also occur. Ethanol can accentuate this. Tolerance does develop to nitrates and appropriate dosing is needed to minimize this (drug-free interval). Safety and efficacy have not been established in pediatric patients. Nitrates may aggravate angina caused by hypertrophic cardiomyopathy. Avoid concurrent use with sildenafil.

Drug Interactions **Substrate** of CYP3A4 (major)

CYP3A4 inducers: CYP3A4 inducers may decrease the levels/effects of isosorbide mononitrate. Example inducers include aminoglutethimide, carbamazepine, nafcillin, nevirapine, phenobarbital, phenytoin, and rifamycins.

CYP3A4 inhibitors: May increase the levels/effects of isosorbide mononitrate. Example inhibitors include azole antifungals, clarithromycin, diclofenac, doxycycline, erythromycin, imatinib, isoniazid, nefazodone, nicardipine, propofol, protease inhibitors, quinidine, telithromycin, and verapamil.

Sildenafil, tadalafil, vardenafil: Significant reduction of systolic and diastolic blood pressure with concurrent use (contraindicated). Do not administer sildenafil, tadalafil, or vardenafil within 24 hours of a nitrate preparation.

(Continued)

Isosorbide Mononitrate *(Continued)*

Nutritional/Herbal/Ethanol Interactions Ethanol: Caution with ethanol (may increase risk of hypotension).

Adverse Reactions

>10%: Central nervous system: Headache (19% to 38%)

1% to 10%:

Central nervous system: Dizziness (3% to 5%)

Gastrointestinal: Nausea/vomiting (2% to 4%)

<1% (Limited to important or life-threatening): Angina pectoris, arrhythmia, atrial fibrillation, impotence, methemoglobinemia (rare), pruritus, rash, supraventricular tachycardia, syncope, vomiting

The incidence of hypotension and adverse cardiovascular events may be increased when used in combination with sildenafil (Viagra®).

Overdosage/Toxicology Symptoms of overdose include hypotension, throbbing headache, palpitations, visual disturbances, tachycardia, methemoglobinemia, flushing, diaphoresis, metabolic acidosis, and coma. High levels or methemoglobinemia can cause signs or symptoms of hypoxemia. Treat symptomatically.

Dosing

Adults:

Angina: Oral:

Regular tablet: 5-10 mg twice daily with the two doses given 7 hours apart (eg, 8 AM and 3 PM) to decrease tolerance development; then titrate to 10 mg twice daily in first 2-3 days.

Extended release tablet: Initial: 30-60 mg given in morning as a single dose; titrate upward as needed, giving at least 3 days between increases; maximum daily single dose: 240 mg

Note: Tolerance to nitrate effects develops with chronic exposure. Dose escalation does not overcome this effect. Tolerance can only be overcome by short periods of nitrate absence from the body. Short periods (10-12 hours) of nitrate withdrawal help minimize tolerance. Recommended dosage regimens incorporate this interval. General recommendations are to take the last dose of short-acting agents no later than 7 PM; administer 2 times/day rather than 4 times/day. Administer sustained release tablet once daily in the morning.

Elderly: Start with lowest recommended adult dose.

Renal Impairment: Not necessary for elderly or patients with altered renal or hepatic function. Tolerance to nitrate effects develops with chronic exposure.

Available Dosage Forms

Tablet: 10 mg, 20 mg

Ismo®: 20 mg

Monoket®: 10 mg, 20 mg

Tablet, extended release (Imdur®): 30 mg, 60 mg, 120 mg

Nursing Guidelines

Assessment: See Contraindications, Warnings/Precautions, and Dosing for use cautions. Assess potential for interactions with other prescriptions, OTC medications, or herbal products patient may be taking (see Drug Interactions). See specific Administration directions. Assess results of laboratory tests (see below), therapeutic effectiveness, and adverse response (see Adverse Reactions and Overdose/Toxicology) at regular intervals during therapy. When discontinuing, reduce dosage gradually. Teach patient proper use, possible side effects/appropriate interventions, and adverse symptoms to report (see Patient Education). Note breast-feeding caution.

Monitoring Laboratory Tests: Orthostasis

Patient Education: Inform prescriber of all prescriptions, OTC medications, or herbal products you are taking, and any allergies you have. Do not take any new medication during therapy unless approved by prescriber. Take exactly as directed, at the same time each day. Take last dose in early evening. Do not chew or crush extended forms; swallow whole with 8 oz of water. Do not change brands without consulting prescriber. Do not discontinue abruptly. Keep medication in original container, tightly closed. Avoid alcohol; combination may cause severe hypotension. May cause postural hypotension (take medication while sitting down and use caution when rising from sitting or lying position or climbing stairs); dizziness, weakness, or blurred vision (use caution when driving or engaging in hazardous activities until response to drug is known); or nausea or vomiting (small, frequent meals, frequent mouth care, chewing gum, or sucking lozenges may help). If chest pain occurs, seek emergency medical help at once. Report acute headache, rapid heartbeat, unusual restlessness or dizziness, muscular weakness, or blurring vision. **Pregnancy/breast-feeding precautions:** Inform prescriber if you are or intend to become pregnant. Consult prescriber if breast-feeding.

Geriatric Considerations: The first dose of nitrates (sublingual, chewable, oral) should be taken in a physician's office to observe for maximal cardiovascular dynamic effects and adverse effects (orthostatic blood pressure drop, headache). The use of nitrates for angina may occasionally promote reflux esophagitis. This may require dose adjustments or changing therapeutic agents to correct this adverse effect.

Pregnancy Risk Factor: C

Lactation: Excretion in breast milk unknown

Perioperative/Anesthesia/Other Concerns: Nitrates used in right ventricular infarction may induce acute hypotension. Nitrate use in severe pericardial effusion may reduce cardiac filling pressure and precipitate cardiac tamponade.

Administration

Oral: Do not administer around-the-clock; Monoket® and Ismo® should be scheduled twice daily with doses 7 hours apart (8 AM and 3 PM); Imdur® may be administered once daily. Extended release tablets should not be chewed or crushed. Should be swallowed with a half-glassful of fluid.

Storage: Tablets should be stored in a tight container at room temperature of 15°C to 30°C (59°F to 86°F).

Isotretinoin (eye soe TRET i noyn)

U.S. Brand Names Accutane®; Amnesteem™; Claravis™; Sotret®

Synonyms 13-*cis*-Retinoic Acid

Pharmacologic Category Acne Products; Retinoic Acid Derivative

Medication Safety Issues

Sound-alike/look-alike issues:

Accutane® may be confused with Accolate®, Accupril®

Use Treatment of severe recalcitrant nodular acne unresponsive to conventional therapy

Unlabeled/Investigational Use Investigational: Treatment of children with metastatic neuroblastoma or leukemia that does not respond to conventional therapy

Mechanism of Action Reduces sebaceous gland size and reduces sebum production; regulates cell proliferation and differentiation

Pharmacodynamics/Kinetics

Distribution: Crosses placenta

Protein binding: 99% to 100%; primarily albumin

Metabolism: Hepatic via CYP2B6, 2C8, 2C9, 2D6, 3A4; forms metabolites; major metabolite: 4-oxo-isotretinoin (active)

Half-life elimination: Terminal: Parent drug: 21 hours; Metabolite: 21-24 hours

Time to peak, serum: 3-5 hours

Excretion: Urine and feces (equal amounts)

Contraindications Hypersensitivity to isotretinoin or any component of the formulation; sensitivity to parabens, vitamin A, or other retinoids; pregnancy

Warnings/Precautions This medication should only be prescribed by prescribers competent in treating severe recalcitrant nodular acne, are experienced in the use of systemic retinoids, and are participating in the pregnancy prevention programs authorized by the FDA and product manufacturer. Use with caution in patients with diabetes mellitus, hypertriglyceridemia; acute pancreatitis and fatal hemorrhagic pancreatitis (rare) have been reported. Not to be used in women of childbearing potential unless woman is capable of complying with effective contraceptive measures. Patients must select and commit to two forms of contraception. Therapy is begun after two negative pregnancy tests; effective contraception must be used for at least 1 month before beginning therapy, during therapy, and for 1 month after discontinuation of therapy. Prescriptions should be written for no more than a 1-month supply, and pregnancy testing and counseling should be repeated monthly. Because of the high likelihood of teratogenic effects (~20%), do not prescribe isotretinoin for women who are or who are likely to become pregnant while using the drug. Male and female patients must be enrolled in the manufacturer-sponsored and FDA-approved monitoring programs.

Depression, psychosis, aggressive or violent behavior, and changes in mood. Rarely, suicidal thoughts and actions have been reported during isotretinoin usage. All patients should be observed closely for symptoms of depression or suicidal thoughts. Discontinuation of treatment alone may not be sufficient, further

(Continued)

Isotretinoin *(Continued)*

evaluation may be necessary. Cases of pseudotumor cerebri (benign intracranial hypertension) have been reported, some with concomitant use of tetracycline (avoid using together). Patients with papilledema, headache, nausea, vomiting, and visual disturbances should be referred to a neurologist and treatment with isotretinoin discontinued. Hearing impairment, which can continue after therapy is discontinued, may occur. Clinical hepatitis, elevated liver enzymes, inflammatory bowel disease, skeletal hyperostosis, premature epiphyseal closure, vision impairment, corneal opacities, and decreased night vision have also been reported with the use of isotretinoin. Bone mineral density may decrease; use caution in patients with a genetic predisposition to bone disorders (ie osteoporosis, osteomalacia) and with disease states or concomitant medications that can induce bone disorders. Patients may be at risk when participating in activities with repetitive impact (such as sports). Safety of long-term use is not established and is not recommended.

Drug Interactions

Carbamazepine: Clearance of carbamazepine may be increased, leading to decreased levels.

Corticosteroids: Corticosteroids may cause osteoporosis. Interactive effect with isotretinoin unknown; use with caution.

Oral contraceptives: Retinoic acid derivatives may diminish the therapeutic effect of oral contraceptives. Two forms of contraception are recommended in females of childbearing potential during retinoic acid therapy.

Phenytoin: Phenytoin may cause osteomalacia. Interactive effect with isotretinoin unknown; use with caution.

Tetracycline: Cases of pseudotumor cerebri have been reported with concurrent use; avoid combination.

Nutritional/Herbal/Ethanol Interactions

Ethanol: Avoid or limit ethanol (may increase triglyceride levels if taken in excess).

Food: Isotretinoin bioavailability increased if taken with food or milk.

Herb/Nutraceutical: Avoid dong quai, St John's wort (may also cause photosensitization and may decrease the effectiveness of oral contraceptives). Additional vitamin A supplements may lead to vitamin A toxicity (dry skin, irritation, arthralgias, myalgias, abdominal pain, hepatic changes); avoid use.

Adverse Reactions Frequency not defined.

Cardiovascular: Palpitation, tachycardia, vascular thrombotic disease, stroke, chest pain, syncope, flushing

Central nervous system: Edema, fatigue, pseudotumor cerebri, dizziness, drowsiness, headache, insomnia, lethargy, malaise, nervousness, paresthesia, seizure, stroke, suicidal ideation, suicide attempts, suicide, depression, psychosis, aggressive or violent behavior, emotional instability

Dermatologic: Cutaneous allergic reactions, purpura, acne fulminans, alopecia, bruising, cheilitis, dry mouth, dry nose, dry skin, epistaxis, eruptive xanthomas, fragility of skin, hair abnormalities, hirsutism, hyperpigmentation, hypopigmentation, peeling of palms, peeling of soles, photoallergic reactions, photosensitizing reactions, pruritus, rash, dystrophy, paronychia, facial erythema, seborrhea, eczema, increased sunburn susceptibility, diaphoresis, urticaria, abnormal wound healing

Endocrine & metabolic: Increased triglycerides (25%), elevated blood glucose, increased HDL, increased cholesterol, abnormal menses

Gastrointestinal: Weight loss, inflammatory bowel disease, regional ileitis, pancreatitis, bleeding and inflammation of the gums, colitis, nausea, nonspecific gastrointestinal symptoms

Genitourinary: Nonspecific urogenital findings

Hematologic: Anemia, thrombocytopenia, neutropenia, agranulocytosis, pyogenic granuloma

Hepatic: Hepatitis

Neuromuscular & skeletal: Skeletal hyperostosis, calcification of tendons and ligaments, premature epiphyseal closure, arthralgia, CPK elevations, arthritis, tendonitis, bone abnormalities, weakness, back pain (29% in pediatric patients), rhabdomyolysis (rare), bone mineral density decreased

Ocular: Corneal opacities, decreased night vision, cataracts, color vision disorder, conjunctivitis, dry eyes, eyelid inflammation, keratitis, optic neuritis, photophobia, visual disturbances

Otic: Hearing impairment, tinnitus

Renal: Vasculitis, glomerulonephritis

Respiratory: Bronchospasms, respiratory infection, voice alteration, Wegener's granulomatosis

Miscellaneous: Allergic reactions, anaphylactic reactions, lymphadenopathy, infection, disseminated herpes simplex, diaphoresis

Overdosage/Toxicology Symptoms of overdose include headache, vomiting, flushing, abdominal pain, cheilosis, dizziness, and ataxia. All signs or symptoms have been transient. Patients should not donate blood for at least 30 days following overdose. Male patients should use a condom or avoid sexual activity for 30 days following overdose.

Dosing

Adults & Elderly: Severe recalcitrant nodular acne: Oral: 0.5-2 mg/kg/day in 2 divided doses (dosages as low as 0.05 mg/kg/day have been reported to be beneficial) for 15-20 weeks or until the total cyst count decreases by 70%, whichever is sooner. A second course of therapy may be initiated after a period of ≥2 months off therapy.

Pediatrics:

Neuroblastoma (investigational): Oral: Children: Maintenance therapy for neuroblastoma: 100-250 mg/m^2/day in 2 divided doses

Acne (severe recalcitrant nodular): Children: Refer to adult dosing.

Hepatic Impairment: Empiric dose reductions are recommended in patient with hepatitis.

Available Dosage Forms Capsule:

Accutane®: 10 mg, 20 mg, 40 mg [contains soybean oil and parabens]

Amnesteem™: 10 mg, 20 mg, 40 mg [contains soybean oil]

Claravis™: 10 mg, 20 mg, 40 mg

Sotret®: 10 mg, 20 mg, 30 mg, 40 mg [contains soybean oil]

Nursing Guidelines

Assessment: Assess effectiveness and interactions of other medications patient may be taking. Assess results of laboratory tests, therapeutic effectiveness, and adverse reactions at beginning of therapy and regularly with long-term use. Monitor patients with diabetes closely. Observe for depression or suicidal thoughts. Assess knowledge/teach patient appropriate use, possible side effects/interventions, and adverse symptoms to report. **Pregnancy risk factor X:** Determine that patient is not pregnant before beginning treatment and do not give to women of childbearing age unless female is capable of complying with two contraceptive measures 1 month prior to therapy, during therapy, and 1 month following therapy.

Monitoring Laboratory Tests: Must have two negative pregnancy tests prior to beginning therapy, CBC with differential and platelet count, baseline sedimentation rate, serum triglycerides, liver enzymes

Dietary Considerations: Should be taken with food. Limit intake of vitamin A; avoid use of other vitamin A products. Some formulations may contain soybean oil.

Patient Education: A patient information/consent form must be signed before this medication is prescribed. Do not sign (and do not take this medication) if you do not understand any information on the form. Use exactly as directed; do not take more than recommended. Prescriptions will be written for a 1-month supply and must be filled within 7 days; they will not be honored if filled after that time or if they do not have the appropriate yellow qualification sticker attached. Capsule can be chewed and swallowed, swallowed, or opened with a large needle and contents sprinkled on applesauce or ice cream. Whole capsules should be swallowed with a full glass of liquid. Do not take any other vitamin A products, limit vitamin A intake, and increase exercise during therapy. Limit or avoid alcohol intake. Exacerbations of acne may occur during first weeks of therapy. You may experience headache, loss of night vision, lethargy, or visual disturbances (use caution when driving or engaging in tasks requiring alertness until response to drug is known); photosensitivity (use sunscreen, wear protective clothing and eyewear, and avoid direct sunlight); dry mouth or nausea (small frequent meals, sucking hard candy, or chewing gum may may help); or dryness, redness, or itching of skin, eye irritation, or increased sensitivity to contact lenses (wear regular glasses). Report depression or suicidal thoughts. Discontinue therapy and report acute vision changes, ringing in the ears or changes in hearing, rectal bleeding, abdominal cramping, or unresolved diarrhea. **Pregnancy/breast-feeding precautions:** Inform prescriber if you are pregnant. Do not get pregnant 1 month before, during, or for 1 month following therapy. This drug may cause severe fetal defects. Two forms of contraception and monthly tests to rule out pregnancy are required during therapy. It is

(Continued)

Isotretinoin *(Continued)*

important to note that any type of contraception may fail, it is the responsibility of the patient to be compliant with contraceptive therapy. Do not donate blood during or for 1 month following therapy (same reason). Do not breast-feed.

Pregnancy Risk Factor: X

Pregnancy Issues: Major fetal abnormalities (both internal and external), spontaneous abortion, premature births and low IQ scores in surviving infants have been reported. This medication is contraindicated in females of childbearing potential unless they are able to comply with the guidelines of pregnancy prevention programs put in place by the FDA and the manufacturer of Accutane®.

Lactation: Excretion in breast milk unknown/contraindicated

Administration

Oral: Administer with food. Capsules can be swallowed, or chewed and swallowed. The capsule may be opened with a large needle and the contents placed on applesauce or ice cream for patients unable to swallow the capsule. Whole capsules should be swallowed with a full glass of liquid.

Storage: Store at room temperature and protect from light.

♦ **Isovue®** *see* Iopamidol *on page 955*

♦ **Isovue-M®** *see* Iopamidol *on page 955*

♦ **Isovue Multipack®** *see* Iopamidol *on page 955*

Isradipine (iz RA di peen)

U.S. Brand Names DynaCirc® [DSC]; DynaCirc® CR

Pharmacologic Category Calcium Channel Blocker

Medication Safety Issues

Sound-alike/look-alike issues:

DynaCirc® may be confused with Dynabac®, Dynacin®

Use Treatment of hypertension

Mechanism of Action Inhibits calcium ion from entering the "slow channels" or select voltage-sensitive areas of vascular smooth muscle and myocardium during depolarization, producing a relaxation of coronary vascular smooth muscle and coronary vasodilation; increases myocardial oxygen delivery in patients with vasospastic angina

Pharmacodynamics/Kinetics

Onset of action: Immediate release: 20 minutes
Duration: Immediate release: >12 hours
Absorption: 90% to 95%
Distribution: V_d: 3 L/kg
Protein binding: 95%
Metabolism: Hepatic; CYP3A4 substrate (major); extensive first-pass effect
Bioavailability: 15% to 24%
Half-life elimination: 8 hours
Time to peak, serum: 1-1.5 hours
Excretion: Urine (as metabolites)

Contraindications Hypersensitivity to isradipine or any component of the formulation; hypotension (<90 mm Hg systolic)

Warnings/Precautions Use cautiously in CHF, hypertrophic cardiomyopathy (IHSS), and in hepatic dysfunction. Safety and efficacy have not been established in pediatric patients. Adjust doses at 2- to 4-week intervals.

Drug Interactions Substrate of CYP3A4 (major); **Inhibits** CYP3A4 (weak)

Azole antifungals may inhibit the calcium channel blocker's metabolism; avoid this combination. Try an antifungal like terbinafine (if appropriate) or monitor closely for altered effect of the calcium channel blocker.

Beta-blockers may have increased pharmacokinetic or pharmacodynamic interactions with isradipine.

Calcium may reduce the effect of calcium channel blockers, particularly hypotension.

CYP3A4 inducers: CYP3A4 inducers may decrease the levels/effects of isradipine. Example inducers include aminoglutethimide, carbamazepine, nafcillin, nevirapine, phenobarbital, phenytoin, and rifamycins.

CYP3A4 inhibitors: May increase the levels/effects of isradipine. Example inhibitors include azole antifungals, clarithromycin, diclofenac, doxycycline, erythromycin, imatinib, isoniazid, nefazodone, nicardipine, propofol, protease inhibitors, quinidine, telithromycin, and verapamil.

Rifampin increases the metabolism of the calcium channel blocker; adjust the dose of the calcium channel blocker to maintain efficacy.

Sildenafil, tadalafil, vardenafil: Blood pressure-lowering effects may be additive; use caution.

Nutritional/Herbal/Ethanol Interactions

Food: Administration with food delays absorption, but does not affect availability

Herb/Nutraceutical: St John's wort may decrease isradipine levels. Avoid dong quai if using for hypertension (has estrogenic activity). Avoid ephedra, yohimbe, ginseng (may worsen hypertension). Avoid garlic (may have increased antihypertensive effect).

Adverse Reactions

>10%: Central nervous system: Headache (dose related 1.9% to 22%)

1% to 10%:

Cardiovascular: Edema (dose related 1.2% to 8.7%), palpitation (dose related 0.8% to 5.1%), flushing (dose related 0.8% to 5.1%), tachycardia (1% to 3.4%), chest pain (1.7% to 2.7%)

Central nervous system: Dizziness (1.6% to 8%), fatigue (dose related 0.4% to 8.5%), flushing (9%)

Dermatologic: Rash (1.5% to 2%)

Gastrointestinal: Nausea (1% to 5.1%), abdominal discomfort (0% to 3.3%), vomiting (0% to 1.3%), diarrhea (0% to 3.4%)

Renal: Urinary frequency (1.3% to 3.4%)

Respiratory: Dyspnea (0.5% to 3.4%)

0.5% to 1% (Limited to important or life-threatening): Angioedema, atrial fibrillation, cough, cramps of legs and feet, depression, dyspnea, gingival hyperplasia (incidence unknown), heart failure, hypotension, impotence, insomnia, lethargy, leukopenia, MI, paresthesia, pruritus, stroke, syncope, urticaria, ventricular fibrillation

Overdosage/Toxicology Primary cardiac symptoms of calcium blocker overdose include hypotension and bradycardia. Hypotension is caused by peripheral vasodilation, myocardial depression, and bradycardia. Bradycardia results from sinus bradycardia, second- or third-degree atrioventricular block, or sinus arrest with junctional rhythm. Intraventricular conduction is usually not affected so QRS duration is normal (verapamil does prolong the PR interval and bepridil prolongs the QT interval and may cause ventricular arrhythmias, including torsade de pointes).

Noncardiac symptoms include confusion, stupor, nausea, vomiting, metabolic acidosis and hyperglycemia. Repeated calcium administration may promptly reverse the depressed cardiac contractility (but not sinus node depression or peripheral vasodilation).

Dosing

Adults & Elderly: Hypertension: Oral: 2.5 mg twice daily; antihypertensive response is seen in 2-3 hours; maximal response in 2-4 weeks; increase dose at 2- to 4-week intervals at 2.5-5 mg increments; usual dose range (JNC 7): 2.5-10 mg/day in 2 divided doses. **Note:** Most patients show no improvement with doses >10 mg/day except adverse reaction rate increases. Therefore, maximal dose in older adults should be 10 mg/day.

Available Dosage Forms

Capsule (DynaCirc®): 2.5 mg, 5 mg [DSC]

Tablet, controlled release (DynaCirc® CR): 5 mg, 10 mg

Nursing Guidelines

Assessment: See Contraindications, Warnings/Precautions, and Dosing for use cautions. Assess potential for interactions with other prescriptions, OTC medications, or herbal products patient may be taking (see Drug Interactions). Assess results of laboratory tests (see below), therapeutic effectiveness, and adverse response (eg, cardiac status, blood pressure, fluid balance - see Adverse Reactions and Overdose/Toxicology) at regular intervals during therapy. Teach patient proper use, possible side effects/appropriate interventions, and adverse symptoms to report (see Patient Education). Breastfeeding is not recommended.

Dietary Considerations: May be taken without regard to meals.

Patient Education: Inform prescriber of all prescriptions, OTC medications, or herbal products you are taking, and any allergies you have. Do not take any new medication during therapy unless approved by prescriber. Take as prescribed, with or without food. Do not stop abruptly without consulting prescriber. Do not crush extended release tablets. This medication does not

(Continued)

Isradipine *(Continued)*

replace other antihypertensive interventions; follow prescriber's instructions for diet and lifestyle changes. You may experience headache (if unrelieved, consult prescriber for approved analgesic); nausea or vomiting (small, frequent meals, frequent mouth care, chewing gum, or sucking lozenges may help); constipation (increased dietary bulk and fluids may help); or dizziness, fatigue, confusion (use caution when driving or engaging in potentially hazardous tasks until response to drug is known). Report unrelieved headache, vomiting, or constipation; chest pain, palpitations, or rapid heartbeat; swelling of hands or feet or sudden weight gain (>5 lb/week); or unusual cramps in legs or feet. **Pregnancy/breast-feeding precautions:** Inform prescriber if you are or intend to become pregnant. Breast-feeding is not recommended.

Geriatric Considerations: Elderly may experience a greater hypotensive response. Constipation may be more of a problem in the elderly.

Pregnancy Risk Factor: C

Lactation: Excretion in breast milk unknown/not recommended

Administration

Oral: May open capsule; avoid crushing contents

♦ Istalol™ *see* Timolol *on page 1633*

♦ Isuprel® *see* Isoproterenol *on page 975*

♦ Iveegam EN *see* Immune Globulin (Intravenous) *on page 899*

♦ IVIG *see* Immune Globulin (Intravenous) *on page 899*

♦ Ivy-Rid® [OTC] *see* Benzocaine *on page 232*

♦ IvySoothe® [OTC] *see* Hydrocortisone *on page 873*

♦ Jantoven™ *see* Warfarin *on page 1723*

♦ Kadian® *see* Morphine Sulfate *on page 1177*

Kanamycin (kan a MYE sin)

U.S. Brand Names Kantrex®

Synonyms Kanamycin Sulfate

Pharmacologic Category Antibiotic, Aminoglycoside

Medication Safety Issues

Sound-alike/look-alike issues:

Kanamycin may be confused with Garamycin®, gentamicin

Use Treatment of serious infections caused by susceptible strains of *E. coli*, *Proteus* species, *Enterobacter aerogenes*, *Klebsiella pneumoniae*, *Serratia marcescens*, and *Acinetobacter* species; second-line treatment of *Mycobacterium tuberculosis*

Mechanism of Action Interferes with protein synthesis in bacterial cell by binding to ribosomal subunit

Pharmacodynamics/Kinetics

Distribution:

Relative diffusion from blood into CSF: Good only with inflammation (exceeds usual MICs)

CSF:blood level ratio: Normal meninges: Nil; Inflamed meninges: 43%

Half-life elimination: 2-4 hours; Anuria: 80 hours; End-stage renal disease: 40-96 hours

Time to peak, serum: I.M.: 1-2 hours (decreased in burn patients)

Excretion: Urine (entire amount)

Contraindications Hypersensitivity to kanamycin, any component of the formulation, or other aminoglycosides; pregnancy

Warnings/Precautions Use with caution in patients with pre-existing renal insufficiency, vestibular or cochlear impairment, myasthenia gravis, conditions which depress neuromuscular transmission. Parenteral aminoglycosides are associated with nephrotoxicity or ototoxicity; the ototoxicity may be proportional to the amount of drug given and the duration of treatment; tinnitus or vertigo are indications of vestibular injury and impending hearing loss; renal damage is usually reversible.

Drug Interactions

Amphotericin B: Concomitant use may lead to nephrotoxicity (reported with gentamicin).

Bisphosphonate derivatives: Concomitant use may lead to hypocalcemia (reported with amikacin and clodronate).

Cisplatin: Concomitant use may lead to increased nephrotoxicity.

Loop diuretics: May increase risk of ototoxicity (reported with ethacrynic acid) and nephrotoxicity.

Neuromuscular-blocking agents: Increase risk of neuromuscular blockade

Lab Interactions Some penicillin derivatives may accelerate the degradation of aminoglycosides *in vitro*, leading to a potential underestimation of aminoglycoside serum concentration.

Adverse Reactions Frequency not defined.

Cardiovascular: Edema

Central nervous system: Neurotoxicity, drowsiness, headache, pseudomotor cerebri

Dermatologic: Skin itching, redness, rash, photosensitivity, erythema

Gastrointestinal: Nausea, vomiting, diarrhea, malabsorption syndrome (with prolonged and high-dose therapy of hepatic coma), anorexia, weight loss, salivation increased, enterocolitis

Hematologic: Granulocytopenia, agranulocytosis, thrombocytopenia

Local: Burning, stinging

Neuromuscular & skeletal: Weakness, tremor, muscle cramps

Otic: Ototoxicity (auditory), ototoxicity (vestibular)

Renal: Nephrotoxicity

Respiratory: Dyspnea

Overdosage/Toxicology Symptoms of overdose include ototoxicity, nephrotoxicity, and neuromuscular toxicity. The treatment of choice following a single acute overdose appears to be the maintenance of good urine output of at least 3 mL/kg/hour. Hemodialysis or peritoneal dialysis may enhance kanamycin elimination; exchange transfusion may also be considered in the newborn infant.

Dosing

Adults: Note: Dosing should be based on ideal body weight

Susceptible systemic infections: I.M., I.V.: 5-7.5 mg/kg/dose in divided doses every 8-12 hours (<15 mg/kg/day)

Following surgical contamination, peritonitis: Intraperitoneal: 500 mg

Irrigating solution: 0.25%; maximum 1.5 g/day (via all administration routes)

Aerosol: 250 mg 2-4 times/day

Elderly: I.M., I.V.: Initial dose should be 5-7.5 mg/kg based on ideal body weight (except in obese patients); maintenance dose and interval should be adjusted for estimated renal function; dosing interval in most older patients is every 12-24 hours (see Dosing in Renal Impairment).

Pediatrics: Infections: I.M., I.V.: 15 mg/kg/day in divided doses every 8-12 hours

Note: Dosing should be based on ideal body weight

Renal Impairment:

Cl_{cr} 50-80 mL/minute: Administer 60% to 90% of dose or administer every 8-12 hours.

Cl_{cr} 10-50 mL/minute: Administer 30% to 70% of dose or administer every 12 hours.

Cl_{cr} <10 mL/minute: Administer 20% to 30% of dose or administer every 24-48 hours.

Available Dosage Forms Injection, solution, as sulfate: 1 g/3 mL (3 mL) [contains sodium bisulfate]

Nursing Guidelines

Monitoring Laboratory Tests: Serum creatinine and BUN every 2-3 days; peak and trough concentrations

Patient Education: It is important to maintain adequate hydration (2-3 L/day of fluids) unless instructed to restrict fluid intake. Report change in hearing acuity, ringing or roaring in ears, alteration in balance, vertigo, feeling of fullness in head; pain, tingling, or numbness of any body part; change in urinary pattern or decrease in urine; signs of opportunistic infection (eg, white plaques in mouth, vaginal discharge, unhealed sores, sore throat, unusual fever, chills); pain, redness, or swelling at injection site; skin rash; or other adverse reactions. **Pregnancy/breast-feeding precautions:** Do not get pregnant during therapy with this medication; use appropriate contraceptive measures. Breast-feeding is not recommended.

Pregnancy Risk Factor: D

Lactation: Enters breast milk/not recommended (AAP rates "compatible")

Breast-Feeding Considerations: Due to poor oral absorption, ototoxicity would not be expected in the nursing infant; changes in intestinal flora are possible

(Continued)

Kanamycin *(Continued)*

Administration

I.M.: Administer deeply in upper outer quadrant of the gluteal muscle.

I.V.: Infuse over 30-60 minutes.

Some penicillins (eg, carbenicillin, ticarcillin and piperacillin) have been shown to inactivate aminglycosides *in vitro*. This has been observed to a greater extent with tobramycin and gentamicin, while amikacin has shown greater stability against inactivation. Concurrent use of these agents may pose a risk of reduced antibacterial efficacy *in vivo*, particularly in the setting of profound renal impairment. However, definitive clinical evidence is lacking. If combination penicillin/aminoglycoside therapy is desired in a patient with renal dysfunction, separation of doses (if feasible), and routine monitoring of aminoglycoside levels, CBC, and clinical response should be considered.

Reconstitution:

I.V.: Must be further diluted prior to I.V. infusion. For adults, dilute 500 mg in 100-200 mL of appropriate solution or 1 g in 200-400 mL; for pediatric patients, use sufficient amount to infuse solution over 30-60 minutes.

Intraperitoneal: Dilute dose in 20 mL sterile distilled water.

Aerosol: Dilute 250 mg in 3 mL normal saline.

Compatibility: Stable in D_5NS, D_5W, $D_{10}W$, LR, NS

Compatibility in syringe: Incompatible with ampicillin, heparin, piperacillin

Compatibility when admixed: Incompatible with amphotericin B, cefazolin, cefotaxime, cefotetan, chlorpheniramine, colistimethate, heparin, lincomycin, methohexital, phenobarbital, phenytoin, piperacillin

Storage: Store vial at controlled room temperature. Darkening of vials does not indicate loss of potency.

- **Kanamycin Sulfate** *see* Kanamycin *on page 986*
- **Kanka® Soft Brush™ [OTC]** *see* Benzocaine *on page 232*
- **Kantrex®** *see* Kanamycin *on page 986*
- **Kaon-Cl-10®** *see* Potassium Chloride *on page 1385*
- **Kaon-Cl® 20** *see* Potassium Chloride *on page 1385*
- **Kao-Paverin® [OTC]** *see* Loperamide *on page 1056*
- **Kariva™** *see* Ethinyl Estradiol and Desogestrel *on page 675*
- **Kay Ciel®** *see* Potassium Chloride *on page 1385*
- **Kayexalate®** *see* Sodium Polystyrene Sulfonate *on page 1553*
- **KCl** *see* Potassium Chloride *on page 1385*
- **K-Dur® 10** *see* Potassium Chloride *on page 1385*
- **K-Dur® 20** *see* Potassium Chloride *on page 1385*
- **Keflex®** *see* Cephalexin *on page 364*
- **Kenalog®** *see* Triamcinolone *on page 1660*
- **Kenalog-10®** *see* Triamcinolone *on page 1660*
- **Kenalog-40®** *see* Triamcinolone *on page 1660*
- **Keppra®** *see* Levetiracetam *on page 1021*
- **Kerlone®** *see* Betaxolol *on page 241*
- **Ketalar®** *see* Ketamine *on page 988*

Ketamine (KEET a meen)

U.S. Brand Names Ketalar®

Synonyms Ketamine Hydrochloride

Pharmacologic Category General Anesthetic

Medication Safety Issues

Sound-alike/look-alike issues:

Ketalar® may be confused with Kenalog®

Use Induction and maintenance of general anesthesia, especially when cardiovascular depression must be avoided (ie, hypotension, hypovolemia, cardiomyopathy, constrictive pericarditis); sedation; analgesia

Mechanism of Action Produces a cataleptic-like state in which the patient is dissociated from the surrounding environment by direct action on the cortex and limbic system. Releases endogenous catecholamines (epinephrine, norepinephrine) which maintain blood pressure and heart rate. Reduces polysynaptic spinal reflexes.

Pharmacodynamics/Kinetics

Onset of action:

I.V.: General anesthesia: 1-2 minutes; Sedation: 1-2 minutes

I.M.: General anesthesia: 3-8 minutes
Duration: I.V.: 5-15 minutes; I.M.: 12-25 minutes
Metabolism: Hepatic via hydroxylation and N-demethylation; the metabolite norketamine is 25% as potent as parent compound
Half-life elimination: 11-17 minutes; Elimination: 2.5-3.1 hours
Excretion: Clearance: 18 mL/kg/minute

Contraindications Hypersensitivity to ketamine or any component of the formulation; elevated intracranial pressure; hypertension, aneurysms, thyrotoxicosis, congestive heart failure, angina, psychotic disorders; pregnancy

Warnings/Precautions Use with caution in patients with coronary artery disease, catecholamine depletion, and tachycardia. Postanesthetic emergence reactions which can manifest as vivid dreams, hallucinations and/or frank delirium occur in 12% of patients; these reactions are less common in patients >65 and when given I.M.; emergence reactions, confusion, or irrational behavior may occur up to 24 hours postoperatively and may be reduced by pretreatment with a benzodiazepine. May cause dependence (withdrawal symptoms on discontinuation) and tolerance with prolonged use.

Drug Interactions **Substrate** (major) of CYP2B6, 2C8/9, 3A4

CYP2B6 inhibitors: May increase the levels/effects of ketamine. Example inhibitors include desipramine, paroxetine, and sertraline.
CYP2C8/9 inhibitors: May increase the levels/effects of ketamine. Example inhibitors include delavirdine, fluconazole, gemfibrozil, ketoconazole, nicardipine, NSAIDs, pioglitazone, and sulfonamides.
CYP3A4 inhibitors: May increase the levels/effects of ketamine. Example inhibitors include azole antifungals, clarithromycin, diclofenac, doxycycline, erythromycin, imatinib, isoniazid, nefazodone, nicardipine, propofol, protease inhibitors, quinidine, telithromycin, and verapamil.
Increased effect: Barbiturates, narcotics, hydroxyzine increase prolonged recovery; nondepolarizing may increase effects
Increased toxicity: Muscle relaxants, thyroid hormones may increase blood pressure and heart rate; halothane may decrease BP

Adverse Reactions

>10%:
- Cardiovascular: Hypertension, increased cardiac output, paradoxical direct myocardial depression, tachycardia
- Central nervous system: Increased intracranial pressure, visual hallucinations, vivid dreams
- Neuromuscular & skeletal: Tonic-clonic movements, tremor
- Miscellaneous: Emergence reactions, vocalization

1% to 10%:
- Cardiovascular: Bradycardia, hypotension
- Dermatologic: Pain at injection site, skin rash
- Gastrointestinal: Anorexia, nausea, vomiting
- Ocular: Diplopia, nystagmus
- Respiratory: Respiratory depression

<1% (Limited to important or life-threatening): Anaphylaxis, cardiac arrhythmia, cough reflex may be depressed, decreased bronchospasm, fasciculations, hypersalivation, increased airway resistance, increased intraocular pressure, increased metabolic rate, increased skeletal muscle tone, laryngospasm, myocardial depression, respiratory depression or apnea with large doses or rapid infusions

Overdosage/Toxicology

Symptoms of overdose include respiratory depression with excessive dosing or too rapid administration
Supportive care is the treatment of choice; mechanical support of respiration is preferred

Dosing

Adults & Elderly: Used in combination with anticholinergic agents to decrease hypersalivation

Anesthesia (sedation, analgesia):
I.M.: 3-8 mg/kg
I.V.: Range: 1-4.5 mg/kg; usual induction dosage: 1-2 mg/kg
Maintenance: Supplemental doses of $^{1}/_{3}$ to $^{1}/_{2}$ of initial dose

Pediatrics: Used in combination with anticholinergic agents to decrease hypersalivation

Anesthesia (sedation, analgesia):
Oral: 6-10 mg/kg for 1 dose (mixed in 0.2-0.3 mL/kg of cola or other beverage) given 30 minutes before the procedure

(Continued)

Ketamine *(Continued)*

I.M.: 3-7 mg/kg

I.V.: Range: 0.5-2 mg/kg, use smaller doses (0.5-1 mg/kg) for sedation for minor procedures; usual induction dosage: 1-2 mg/kg. Maintenance: Supplemental doses of 1/3 to 1/2 of initial dose

Continuous I.V. infusion: 5-20 mcg/kg/minute

Available Dosage Forms

Injection, solution: 50 mg/mL (10 mL); 100 mg/mL (5 mL)

Ketalar®: 10 mg/mL (20 mL); 50 mg/mL (10 mL); 100 mg/mL (5 mL)

Nursing Guidelines

Pregnancy Risk Factor: D

Perioperative/Anesthesia/Other Concerns: Produces emergence psychosis including auditory and visual hallucinations, restlessness, disorientation, vivid dreams, and irrational behavior in 15% to 30% of patients; pretreatment with a benzodiazepine reduces incidence of psychosis by >50%. Spontaneous involuntary movements, nystagmus, hypertonus, and vocalizations are also commonly seen.

The analgesia outlasts the general anesthetic component. Bronchodilation is beneficial in asthmatic or COPD patients. Laryngeal reflexes may remain intact or may be obtunded. The direct myocardial depressant action of ketamine can be seen in stressed, catecholamine-deficient patients. Ketamine increases cerebral metabolism and cerebral blood flow while producing a noncompetitive block of the neuronal postsynaptic NMDA receptor. It lowers seizure threshold and stimulates salivary secretions (atropine/scopolamine treatment is recommended).

Ketamine increases myocardial oxygen demand secondary to catecholamine release.

Administration

Oral: Use 100 mg/mL I.V. solution and mix the appropriate dose in 0.2-0.3 mL/kg of cola or other beverage

I.V.: Do not exceed 0.5 mg/kg/minute or administer faster than 60 seconds; do not exceed final concentration of 2 mg/mL; dilute for I.V. administration with normal saline, sterile water, or D_5W

Compatibility: Stable in D_5W, NS

Compatibility in syringe: Incompatible with amobarbital, diazepam, doxapram, methohexital, pentobarbital, phenobarbital, secobarbital, thiopental

Storage: Do not mix with barbiturates or diazepam (precipitation may occur).

Related Information

Intravenous Anesthetic Agents *on page 1853*

♦ **Ketamine Hydrochloride** *see* Ketamine *on page 988*

Ketorolac (KEE toe role ak)

U.S. Brand Names Acular®; Acular LS™; Acular® PF; Toradol®

Synonyms Ketorolac Tromethamine

Pharmacologic Category Nonsteroidal Anti-inflammatory Drug (NSAID), Ophthalmic; Nonsteroidal Anti-inflammatory Drug (NSAID), Oral; Nonsteroidal Anti-inflammatory Drug (NSAID), Parenteral

Medication Safety Issues

Sound-alike/look-alike issues:

Acular® may be confused with Acthar®, Ocular®

Toradol® may be confused with Foradil®, Inderal®, Tegretol®, Torecan®, tramadol

Use

Oral, injection: Short-term (≤5 days) management of moderately-severe acute pain requiring analgesia at the opioid level

Ophthalmic: Temporary relief of ocular itching due to seasonal allergic conjunctivitis; postoperative inflammation following cataract extraction; reduction of ocular pain and photophobia following incisional refractive surgery, reduction of ocular pain, burning and stinging following corneal refractive surgery

Mechanism of Action Inhibits prostaglandin synthesis by decreasing the activity of the enzyme, cyclooxygenase, which results in decreased formation of prostaglandin precursors

Pharmacodynamics/Kinetics

Onset of action: Analgesic: I.M.: ~10 minutes

Peak effect: Analgesic: 2-3 hours

Duration: Analgesic: 6-8 hours
Absorption: Oral: Well absorbed
Distribution: Poor penetration into CSF; crosses placenta; enters breast milk
Protein binding: 99%
Metabolism: Hepatic
Half-life elimination: 2-8 hours; prolonged 30% to 50% in elderly
Time to peak, serum: I.M.: 30-60 minutes
Excretion: Urine (61% as unchanged drug)

Contraindications Hypersensitivity to ketorolac, aspirin, other NSAIDs, or any component of the formulation; active or history of peptic ulcer disease; recent or history of GI bleeding or perforation; patients with advanced renal disease or risk of renal failure; labor and delivery; nursing mothers; prophylaxis before major surgery; suspected or confirmed cerebrovascular bleeding; hemorrhagic diathesis; concurrent ASA or other NSAIDs; epidural or intrathecal administration; concomitant probenecid; perioperative pain in the setting of coronary artery bypass surgery (CABG); pregnancy (3rd trimester)

Warnings/Precautions

Systemic: Treatment should be started with I.V./I.M. administration then changed to oral only as a continuation of treatment. Total therapy is not to exceed 5 days. Should not be used for minor or chronic pain.

May prolong bleeding time; do not use when hemostasis is critical. Patients should be euvolemic prior to treatment. Low doses of narcotics may be needed for breakthrough pain.

NSAIDs are associated with an increased risk of adverse cardiovascular events, including MI, stroke, and new onset or worsening of pre-existing hypertension. Risk may be increased with duration of use or pre-existing cardiovascular risk-factors or disease. Carefully evaluate individual cardiovascular risk profiles prior to prescribing. Use caution with fluid retention, CHF or hypertension.

Use of NSAIDs can compromise existing renal function. Renal toxicity can occur in patient with impaired renal function, dehydration, heart failure, liver dysfunction, those taking diuretics and ACEI and the elderly. Rehydrate patient before starting therapy. Monitor renal function closely. Ketorolac is not recommended for patients with advanced renal disease.

NSAIDs may increase risk of gastrointestinal irritation, ulceration, bleeding, and perforation. These events may occur at any time during therapy and without warning. Use caution with a history of GI disease (bleeding or ulcers), concurrent therapy with aspirin, anticoagulants and/or corticosteroids, smoking, use of alcohol, the elderly or debilitated patients.

Use the lowest effective dose for the shortest duration of time, consistent with individual patient goals, to reduce risk of cardiovascular or GI adverse events. Alternate therapies should be considered for patients at high risk.

NSAIDs may cause serious skin adverse events including exfoliative dermatitis, Stevens-Johnson syndrome (SJS) and toxic epidermal necrolysis (TEN). Anaphylactoid reactions may occur, even without prior exposure; patients with "aspirin triad" (bronchial asthma, aspirin intolerance, rhinitis) may be at increased risk. Do not use in patients who experience bronchospasm, asthma, rhinitis, or urticaria with NSAID or aspirin therapy.

Use with caution in patients with decreased hepatic function. Closely monitor patients with any abnormal LFT. Severe hepatic reactions (eg, fulminant hepatitis, liver failure) have occurred with NSAID use, rarely; discontinue if signs or symptoms of liver disease develop, or if systemic manifestations occur.

The elderly are at increased risk for adverse effects (especially peptic ulceration, CNS effects, renal toxicity) from NSAIDs even at low doses.

Withhold for at least 4-6 half-lives prior to surgical or dental procedures.

Ophthalmic: May increase bleeding time associated with ocular surgery. Use with caution in patients with known bleeding tendencies or those receiving anticoagulants. Healing time may be slowed or delayed. Corneal thinning, erosion, or ulceration have been reported with topical NSAIDs; discontinue if corneal epithelial breakdown occurs. Use caution with complicated ocular surgery, corneal denervation, corneal epithelial defects, diabetes, rheumatoid arthritis, ocular surface disease, or ocular surgeries repeated within short periods of time; risk of corneal epithelial breakdown may be increased. Use for >24 hours prior to or for >14 days following surgery also increases risk of corneal adverse effects. Do not

(Continued)

Ketorolac *(Continued)*

administer while wearing soft contact lenses. Safety and efficacy in pediatric patients <3 years of age have not been established.

Drug Interactions

ACE inhibitors: Antihypertensive effects may be decreased by concurrent therapy with NSAIDs; monitor blood pressure.

Angiotensin II antagonists: Antihypertensive effects may be decreased by concurrent therapy with NSAIDs; monitor blood pressure.

Anticoagulants: Increased risk of bleeding complications with concomitant use; monitor closely.

Antiepileptic drugs (carbamazepine, phenytoin): Sporadic cases of seizures have been reported with concomitant use.

Diuretics: May see decreased effect of diuretics.

Lithium: May increase lithium levels; monitor.

Methotrexate: Severe bone marrow suppression, aplastic anemia, and GI toxicity have been reported with concomitant NSAID therapy. Avoid use during moderate or high-dose methotrexate (increased and prolonged methotrexate levels). NSAID use during low-dose treatment of rheumatoid arthritis has not been fully evaluated; extreme caution is warranted.

Nondepolarizing muscle relaxants: Concomitant use has resulted in apnea.

NSAIDs, salicylates: Concomitant use increases NSAID-induced adverse effects; contraindicated.

Probenecid: Probenecid significantly decreases ketorolac clearance, increases ketorolac plasma levels, and doubles the half-life of ketorolac; concomitant use is contraindicated.

Psychoactive drugs (alprazolam, fluoxetine, thiothixene): Hallucinations have been reported with concomitant use.

Nutritional/Herbal/Ethanol Interactions

Ethanol: Avoid ethanol (may enhance gastric mucosal irritation).

Food: Oral: High-fat meals may delay time to peak (by ~1 hour) and decrease peak concentrations.

Herb/Neutraceuticals: Avoid alfalfa, anise, bilberry, bladderwrack, bromelain, cat's claw, celery, coleus, cordyceps, dong quai, evening primrose, feverfew, fenugreek, garlic, ginger, ginkgo biloboa, red clover, horse chestnut, grapeseed, green tea, ginseng, guggul, horse chestnut seed, horseradish, licorice, prickly ash, red clover, reishi, SAMe, sweet clover, turmeric, white willow (all have additional antiplatelet activity).

Lab Interactions Increased chloride (S), sodium (S), bleeding time

Adverse Reactions

Systemic:

>10%:

Central nervous system: Headache (17%)

Gastrointestinal: Gastrointestinal pain (13%), dyspepsia (12%), nausea (12%)

>1% to 10%:

Cardiovascular: Edema (4%), hypertension

Central nervous system: Dizziness (7%), drowsiness (6%)

Dermatologic: Pruritus, purpura, rash

Gastrointestinal: Diarrhea (7%), constipation, flatulence, gastrointestinal fullness, vomiting, stomatitis

Local: Injection site pain (2%)

Miscellaneous: Diaphoresis

≤1% (Limited to important or life-threatening): Abnormal vision, acute renal failure, anaphylactoid reaction, anaphylaxis, asthma, azotemia, bronchospasm, cholestatic jaundice, convulsions, eosinophilia, epistaxis, esophagitis, extrapyramidal symptoms, GI hemorrhage, GI perforation, hallucinations, hearing loss, hematemesis, hematuria, hepatitis, hypersensitivity reactions, liver failure, Lyell's syndrome, maculopapular rash, nephritis, peptic ulceration, Stevens-Johnson syndrome, tinnitus, toxic epidermal necrolysis, urticaria, vertigo, wound hemorrhage (postoperative)

Ophthalmic solution:

>10%: Ocular: Transient burning/stinging (Acular®: 40%; Acular® PF: 20%)

>1% to 10%:

Central nervous system: Headache

Ocular: Conjunctival hyperemia, corneal infiltrates, iritis, ocular edema, ocular inflammation, ocular irritation, ocular pain, superficial keratitis, superficial ocular infection

Miscellaneous: Allergic reactions

≤1% (Limited to important or life-threatening): Blurred vision corneal ulcer, corneal erosion, corneal perforation, corneal thinning, dry eyes, epithelial breakdown

Overdosage/Toxicology Symptoms of overdose include abdominal pain, peptic ulcers, and metabolic acidosis. Management of NSAID intoxication is supportive and symptomatic. Dialysis is not effective.

Dosing

Adults:

Pain management (acute; moderately-severe): Children ≥16 years and Adults:

Note: The maximum combined duration of treatment (for parenteral and oral) is 5 days; do not increase dose or frequency; supplement with low dose opioids if needed for breakthrough pain. For patients <50 kg and/or ≥65 years of age, see Elderly dosing.

I.M.: 60 mg as a single dose or 30 mg every 6 hours (maximum daily dose: 120 mg)

I.V.: 30 mg as a single dose or 30 mg every 6 hours (maximum daily dose: 120 mg)

Oral: 20 mg, followed by 10 mg every 4-6 hours; do not exceed 40 mg/day; oral dosing is intended to be a continuation of I.M. or I.V. therapy only

Ophthalmic uses:

Seasonal allergic conjunctivitis (relief of ocular itching) (Acular®): Ophthalmic: Instill 1 drop (0.25 mg) 4 times/day for seasonal allergic conjunctivitis

Inflammation following cataract extraction (Acular®): Ophthalmic: Instill 1 drop (0.25 mg) to affected eye(s) 4 times/day beginning 24 hours after surgery; continue for 2 weeks

Pain and photophobia following incisional refractive surgery (Acular® PF): Ophthalmic: Instill 1 drop (0.25 mg) 4 times/day to affected eye for up to 3 days

Pain following corneal refractive surgery (Acular LS™): Ophthalmic: Instill 1 drop 4 times/day as needed to affected eye for up to 4 days

Elderly: Elderly >65 years: Renal insufficiency or weight <50 kg: **Note:** Ketorolac has decreased clearance and increased half-life in the elderly. In addition, the elderly have reported increased incidence of GI bleeding, ulceration, and perforation. The maximum combined duration of treatment (for parenteral and oral) is 5 days.

I.M.: 30 mg as a single dose or 15 mg every 6 hours (maximum daily dose: 60 mg)

I.V.: 15 mg as a single dose or 15 mg every 6 hours (maximum daily dose: 60 mg)

Oral: 10 mg every 4-6 hours; do not exceed 40 mg/day; oral dosing is intended to be a continuation of I.M. or I.V. therapy only

Pediatrics: Note: Do not exceed adult doses.

Anti-inflammatory, single-dose treatment: Children 2-16 years:

I.M.: 1 mg/kg (maximum: 30 mg)

I.V.: 0.5 mg/kg (maximum: 15 mg)

Oral (unlabeled): 1 mg/kg as a single dose reported in one study

Anti-inflammatory, multiple-dose treatment (unlabeled): Children 2-16 years: Limited pediatric studies. The maximum combined duration of treatment (for parenteral and oral) is 5 days.

I.V.: Initial dose: 0.5 mg/kg followed by 0.25-1 mg/kg every 6 hours for up to 48 hours; maximum daily dose: 90 mg

Oral: 0.25 mg/kg every 6 hours

Ophthalmic uses: Children ≥3 years: Refer to adult dosing.

Renal Impairment: Do not use in patients with advanced renal impairment. Patients with moderately-elevated serum creatinine should use half the recommended dose, not to exceed 60 mg/day I.M./I.V.

Hepatic Impairment: Use with caution, may cause elevation of liver enzymes

Available Dosage Forms [DSC] = Discontinued product

Injection, solution, as tromethamine: 15 mg/mL (1 mL); 30 mg/mL (1 mL, 2 mL, 10 mL) [contains alcohol]

Solution, ophthalmic, as tromethamine:

Acular®: 0.5% (3 mL, 5 mL, 10 mL) [contains benzalkonium chloride]

Acular LS™: 0.4% (5 mL) [contains benzalkonium chloride]

Acular® P.F. [preservative free]: 0.5% (0.4 mL)

Tablet, as tromethamine: 10 mg

Toradol®: 10 mg [DSC]

(Continued)

Ketorolac *(Continued)*

Nursing Guidelines

Assessment: Evaluate cardiac risk and potential for GI bleeding prior to prescribing this medication. Assess allergy history prior to beginning therapy. Assess potential for interactions with other prescriptions, OTC medications, or herbal products patient may be taking. **I.V./I.M.:** Vital signs should be monitored on a regular basis during infusion or following injection. Monitor blood pressure at the beginning of therapy and periodically during use. Assess results of laboratory tests, therapeutic effectiveness, and adverse response on a regular basis throughout therapy. Teach patient proper use, possible side effects/ appropriate interventions (eg, importance of adequate hydration), and adverse symptoms to report.

Monitoring Laboratory Tests: CBC, liver function, platelets; renal function (serum creatinine, BUN, urine output)

Dietary Considerations: Administer tablet with food or milk to decrease gastrointestinal distress.

Patient Education: Do not take any new medication during therapy without consulting prescriber (especially aspirin-containing products or other NSAIDs or any other NSAIDs). Use exactly as directed; do not increase dose or frequency. Adverse reactions can occur with overuse. Oral doses may be taken with food or milk. Avoid alcohol. Maintain adequate hydration (2-3 L/day of fluids) unless instructed to restrict fluid intake. May cause nausea or vomiting (frequent mouth care, small frequent meals, chewing gum, or sucking lozenges may help). Report GI bleeding, ulceration or perforation with or without pain (stop medication and report abdominal pain or blood in urine or stool); ringing in ears; unresolved nausea or vomiting; respiratory difficulty or shortness of breath; skin rash; unusual swelling of extremities; chest pain; or palpitations. **Pregnancy/ breast-feeding precautions:** Inform prescriber if you are or intend to become pregnant. This drug should not be used in the 2nd or 3rd trimester of pregnancy. Consult prescriber for appropriate contraceptive measures if necessary. Consult prescriber if breast-feeding.

Ophthalmic: Instill drops as often as recommended. Wash hands before instilling. Sit or lie down to instill. Open eye, look at ceiling, and instill prescribed amount of solution. Close eye and roll eye in all directions. Apply gentle pressure to inner corner of eye for 1-2 minutes after instillation. Do not let tip of applicator touch eye; do not contaminate tip of applicator (may cause eye infection, eye damage, or vision loss). Temporary stinging or blurred vision may occur. Do not wear soft contact lenses. Report persistent pain, burning, double vision, swelling, itching, or worsening of condition.

Geriatric Considerations: Ketorolac is eliminated more slowly in the elderly. It is recommended to use lower doses in the elderly. The elderly are at high risk for adverse effects from NSAIDs. As much as 60% of elderly can develop peptic ulceration and/or hemorrhage asymptomatically. The concomitant use of H_2 blockers, omeprazole, and sucralfate is not effective as prophylaxis with the exception of NSAID-induced duodenal ulcers which may be prevented by the use of ranitidine. Misoprostol is the only prophylactic agent proven effective. Also, concomitant disease and drug use contribute to the risk for GI adverse effects. Use lowest effective dose for shortest period possible. Consider renal function decline with age. Use of NSAIDs can compromise existing renal function especially when Cl_{cr} is ≤30 mL/minute. Tinnitus may be a difficult and unreliable indication of toxicity due to age-related hearing loss or eighth cranial nerve damage. CNS adverse effects such as confusion, agitation, and hallucination are generally seen in overdose or high-dose situations, but elderly may demonstrate these adverse effects at lower doses than younger adults.

Pregnancy Risk Factor: C/D (3rd trimester)

Pregnancy Issues: Ketorolac is contraindicated during labor and delivery (may inhibit uterine contractions and adversely affect fetal circulation). Avoid use of ketorolac ophthalmic solution during late pregnancy.

Lactation: Enters breast milk/contraindicated (AAP rates "compatible")

Perioperative/Anesthesia/Other Concerns: The 2002 ACCM/SCCM guidelines for analgesia (critically-ill adult) recommend that ketorolac therapy be limited to a maximum of 5 days with close attention to gastrointestinal and renal function. The risk of developing renal dysfunction or gastrointestinal bleeding further increases as treatment extends beyond 5 days.

In short-term use, NSAIDs vary considerably in their effect on blood pressure. When NSAIDs are used in patients with hypertension, appropriate monitoring of blood pressure responses should be completed and the duration of therapy, when possible, kept short. The use of NSAIDs in the treatment of patients with congestive heart failure may be associated with an increased risk for fluid accumulation and edema; may precipitate renal failure in dehydrated patients.

Ketorolac is contraindicated during labor and delivery (may inhibit uterine contractions and adversely affect fetal circulation). Avoid use of ketorolac ophthalmic solution during late pregnancy.

Equivalent dosing: 30 mg provides the analgesia comparable to morphine 12 mg or meperidine 100 mg.

Administration

Oral: May take with food to reduce GI upset.

I.M.: Administer slowly and deeply into the muscle. Analgesia begins in 30 minutes and maximum effect within 2 hours.

I.V.: Administer I.V. bolus over a minimum of 15 seconds; onset within 30 minutes; peak analgesia within 2 hours.

Compatibility: Stable in D_5NS, D_5W, LR, NS

Compatibility when admixed: Incompatible with hydroxyzine, meperidine, morphine, promethazine

Storage: Ketorolac injection and ophthalmic solution should be stored at controlled room temperature and protected from light. Injection is clear and has a slight yellow color. Precipitation may occur at relatively low pH values. Store tablets at controlled room temperature.

Related Information

Acute Postoperative Pain *on page 1742*

Labetalol (la BET a lole)

U.S. Brand Names Trandate®

Synonyms Ibidomide Hydrochloride; Labetalol Hydrochloride

Pharmacologic Category Beta Blocker With Alpha-Blocking Activity

Medication Safety Issues

Sound-alike/look-alike issues:

Labetalol may be confused with betaxolol, Hexadrol®, lamotrigine

Trandate® may be confused with tramadol, Trendar®, Trental®, Tridrate®

Use Treatment of mild to severe hypertension; I.V. for hypertensive emergencies

Mechanism of Action Blocks alpha-, $beta_1$-, and $beta_2$-adrenergic receptor sites; elevated renins are reduced

Pharmacodynamics/Kinetics

Onset of action: Oral: 20 minutes to 2 hours; I.V.: 2-5 minutes

Peak effect: Oral: 1-4 hours; I.V.: 5-15 minutes

Duration: Oral: 8-24 hours (dose dependent); I.V.: 2-4 hours

Distribution: V_d: Adults: 3-16 L/kg; mean: <9.4 L/kg; moderately lipid soluble, therefore, can enter CNS; crosses placenta; small amounts enter breast milk

Protein binding: 50%

Metabolism: Hepatic, primarily via glucuronide conjugation; extensive first-pass effect

Bioavailability: Oral: 25%; increased with liver disease, elderly, and concurrent cimetidine

Half-life elimination: Normal renal function: 2.5-8 hours

Excretion: Urine (<5% as unchanged drug)

Clearance: Possibly decreased in neonates/infants

Contraindications Hypersensitivity to labetalol or any component of the formulation; sinus bradycardia; heart block greater than first degree (except in patients with a functioning artificial pacemaker); cardiogenic shock; bronchial asthma; uncompensated cardiac failure; pregnancy (2nd and 3rd trimesters)

Warnings/Precautions Use only with extreme caution in compensated heart failure and monitor for a worsening of the condition. Avoid abrupt discontinuation in patients with a history of CAD; slowly wean while monitoring for signs and symptoms of ischemia. Use caution with concurrent use of beta-blockers and either verapamil or diltiazem; bradycardia or heart block can occur. Avoid concurrent I.V. use of both agents. Patients with bronchospastic disease should not receive beta-blockers. Labetalol may be used with caution in patients with nonallergic bronchospasm (chronic bronchitis, emphysema). Use cautiously in diabetics because it can mask prominent hypoglycemic symptoms. Can mask signs of thyrotoxicosis. Can cause fetal harm when administered in pregnancy. Use cautiously in the hepatically impaired. Use caution when using I.V. labetalol and inhalational anesthetics concurrently (significant myocardial depression).

Drug Interactions **Substrate** of CYP2D6 (major); **Inhibits** CYP2D6 (weak)

Alpha-blockers (prazosin, terazosin): Concurrent use of beta-blockers may increase risk of orthostasis.

Cimetidine increases the bioavailability of labetalol.

CYP2D6 inhibitors: May increase the levels/effects of labetalol. Example inhibitors include chlorpromazine, delavirdine, fluoxetine, miconazole, paroxetine, pergolide, quinidine, quinine, ritonavir, and ropinirole.

Halothane, isoflurane, enflurane (possibly other inhalational anesthetics): Excessive hypotension may occur.

NSAIDs may reduce antihypertensive efficacy of labetalol.

Salicylates may reduce the antihypertensive effects of beta-blockers.

Sulfonylureas: Effects may be decreased by beta-blockers.

Verapamil or diltiazem may have synergistic or additive pharmacological effects when taken concurrently with beta-blockers; avoid concurrent I.V. use.

Nutritional/Herbal/Ethanol Interactions

Food: Labetalol serum concentrations may be increased if taken with food.

Herb/Nutraceutical: Avoid dong quai if using for hypertension (has estrogenic activity). Avoid ephedra, yohimbe, ginseng (may worsen hypertension). Avoid natural licorice (causes sodium and water retention and increases potassium loss). Avoid garlic (may have increased antihypertensive effect).

Lab Interactions False-positive urine catecholamines, VMA if measured by fluorometric or photometric methods; use HPLC or specific catecholamine radioenzymatic technique

Adverse Reactions

>10%:

Central nervous system: Dizziness (1% to 16%)

Gastrointestinal: Nausea (0% to 19%)

1% to 10%:

Cardiovascular: Edema (0% to 2%), hypotension (1% to 5%); with IV use, hypotension may occur in up to 58%

Central nervous system: Fatigue (1% to 10%), paresthesia (1% to 5%), headache (2%), vertigo (2%)

Dermatologic: Rash (1%), scalp tingling (1% to 5%)

Gastrointestinal: Vomiting (<1% to 3%), dyspepsia (1% to 4%)

Genitourinary: Ejaculatory failure (0% to 5%), impotence (1% to 4%)

Hepatic: Transaminases increased (4%)

Neuromuscular & skeletal: Weakness (1%)

Respiratory: Nasal congestion (1% to 6%), dyspnea (2%)

Miscellaneous: Taste disorder (1%), abnormal vision (1%)

<1% (Limited to important or life-threatening): Alopecia (reversible), anaphylactoid reaction, angioedema, bradycardia, bronchospasm, cholestatic jaundice, CHF, diabetes insipidus, heart block, hepatic necrosis, hepatitis, hypersensitivity, hypotension, Peyronie's disease, positive ANA, pruritus, Raynaud's syndrome, syncope, systemic lupus erythematosus, toxic myopathy, urinary retention, urticaria, ventricular arrhythmia (I.V.)

Other adverse reactions noted with beta-adrenergic blocking agents include mental depression, catatonia, short-term memory loss, emotional lability, intensification of pre-existing AV block, laryngospasm, respiratory distress, agranulocytosis, thrombocytopenic purpura, nonthrombocytopenic purpura, mesenteric artery thrombosis, and ischemic colitis.

Overdosage/Toxicology Symptoms of intoxication include cardiac disturbances, CNS toxicity, bronchospasm, hypoglycemia, and hyperkalemia. The most common cardiac symptoms include hypotension and bradycardia. Atrioventricular block, intraventricular conduction disturbances, cardiogenic shock, and asystole may occur with severe overdose, especially with membrane-depressant drugs (eg, propranolol). CNS effects include convulsions, coma, and respiratory arrest and are commonly seen with propranolol and other membrane-depressant and lipid-soluble drugs. Treatment is symptomatic. Glucagon may be administered to improve cardiac function.

Dosing

Adults:

Hypertension: Oral: Initial: 100 mg twice daily, may increase as needed every 2-3 days by 100 mg until desired response is obtained; usual dose: 200-400 mg twice daily; not to exceed 2.4 g/day

Usual dose range (JNC 7): 200-800 mg/day in 2 divided doses

Acute hypertension (hypertensive urgency/emergency):

I.V. bolus: 20 mg or 1-2 mg/kg whichever is lower, IVP over 2 minutes, may give 40-80 mg at 10-minute intervals, up to 300 mg total dose

I.V. infusion: Initial: 2 mg/minute; titrate to response up to 300 mg total dose. Administration requires the use of an infusion pump.

Note: Continuous infusion at low rates (2-4 mg/hour) have been used in some settings for patients unable to transition rapidly to oral medication.

Elderly: Oral: Initial: 100 mg 1-2 times/day increasing as needed

Pediatrics: Note: Due to limited documentation of its use, labetalol should be initiated cautiously in pediatric patients with careful dosage adjustment and blood pressure monitoring.

Hypertension:

Oral: Limited information regarding labetalol use in pediatric patients is currently available in literature. Some centers recommend initial oral doses of 4 mg/kg/day in 2 divided doses. Reported oral doses have started at 3 mg/kg/day and 20 mg/kg/day and have increased up to 40 mg/kg/day.

I.V.: Intermittent bolus doses of 0.3-1 mg/kg/dose have been reported.

Pediatric hypertensive emergencies: Initial continuous infusions of 0.4-1 mg/kg/hour with a maximum of 3 mg/kg/hour have been used; administration requires the use of an infusion pump.

Renal Impairment: Not removed by hemo- or peritoneal dialysis; supplemental dose is not necessary.

Hepatic Impairment: Dosage reduction may be necessary.

Available Dosage Forms

Injection, solution, as hydrochloride: 5 mg/mL (4 mL, 20 mL, 40 mL)

Trandate®: 5 mg/mL (20 mL, 40 mL)

Tablet, as hydrochloride: 100 mg, 200 mg, 300 mg

Trandate®: 100 mg, 200 mg [contains sodium benzoate], 300 mg

(Continued)

Labetalol *(Continued)*

Nursing Guidelines

Assessment: Assess potential for interactions with other prescriptions, OTC medications, or herbal products patient may be taking (especially anything that will effect blood pressure). Blood pressure and heart rate should be assessed prior to and following first dose and any change in dosage. Caution patients with diabetes to monitor glucose levels closely; beta-blockers may alter glucose tolerance. Assess results of laboratory tests, therapeutic effectiveness, and adverse response (eg, CHF). Teach patient proper use, possible side effects/ appropriate interventions, and adverse symptoms to report.

Patient Education: Do not take any new medication during therapy unless approved by prescriber. Take as directed, with meals. Do not skip dose or discontinue without consulting prescriber. This medication does not replace other antihypertensive interventions; follow prescriber's instructions for diet and lifestyle changes. If you have diabetes, monitor serum glucose closely and notify prescriber of changes (this medication can alter hypoglycemic requirements). You may experience drowsiness, dizziness, or impaired judgment (use caution when driving or engaging in tasks that require alertness until response to drug is known); postural hypotension (use caution when rising from sitting or lying position or when climbing stairs); dry mouth, nausea, or loss of appetite (frequent mouth care or sucking lozenges may help); or sexual dysfunction (reversible, may resolve with continued use). Report altered CNS status (eg, fatigue, depression, numbness or tingling of fingers, toes, or skin); palpitations or slowed heartbeat; respiratory difficulty; edema or cold extremities; or other persistent side effects. **Pregnancy/breast-feeding precautions:** Inform prescriber if you are or intend to become pregnant. Consult prescriber if breast-feeding.

Geriatric Considerations: Due to alterations in the beta-adrenergic autonomic nervous system, beta-adrenergic blockade may result in less hemodynamic response than seen in younger adults.

Pregnancy Risk Factor: C (manufacturer); D (2nd and 3rd trimesters - expert analysis)

Pregnancy Issues: Labetalol crosses the placenta. Beta-blockers have been associated with persistent bradycardia, hypotension, and IUGR; IUGR is probably related to maternal hypertension. Available evidence suggests beta-blockers are generally safe during pregnancy (JNC 7). Cases of neonatal hypoglycemia have been reported following maternal use of beta-blockers at parturition or during breast-feeding. Monitor breast-fed infant for symptoms of beta-blockade.

Lactation: Enters breast milk/use caution (AAP rates "compatible")

Breast-Feeding Considerations: Available evidence suggests safe use during breast-feeding. Monitor breast-fed infant for symptoms of beta-blockade.

Perioperative/Anesthesia/Other Concerns: Due to alterations in the beta-adrenergic autonomic nervous system, beta-adrenergic blockade may result in less hemodynamic response in the elderly than seen in younger adults. Despite decreased sensitivity to the chronotropic effects of beta blockade with age, there appears to be an increased myocardial sensitivity to the negative inotropic effect during stress (eg, exercise).

Administration

I.V.: Bolus administered over 2 minutes.

Reconstitution: Stability of parenteral admixture at room temperature (25°C) and refrigeration temperature (4°C) is 3 days.

Standard diluent: 500 mg/250 mL D_5W

Minimum volume: 250 mL D_5W

Compatibility: Stable in D_5LR, $D_5{}^1/_4NS$, $D_5{}^1/_3NS$, D_5NS, D_5W, LR, NS; most stable at pH of 2-4. **Incompatible** with sodium bicarbonate 5% and alkaline solutions.

Y-site administration: Incompatible with amphotericin B cholesteryl sulfate complex, cefoperazone, ceftriaxone, nafcillin, thiopental, warfarin

Compatibility when admixed: Incompatible with sodium bicarbonate

Storage: Labetalol should be stored at room temperature or under refrigeration and should be protected from light and freezing. The solution is clear to slightly yellow.

Related Information

Postoperative Hypertension *on page 1815*

♦ **Labetalol Hydrochloride** *see* Labetalol *on page 996*

♦ **L-AmB** *see* Amphotericin B (Liposomal) *on page 157*
♦ **Lamictal®** *see* Lamotrigine *on page 1002*

Lamivudine (la MI vyoo deen)

U.S. Brand Names Epivir®; Epivir-HBV®

Synonyms 3TC

Pharmacologic Category Antiretroviral Agent, Reverse Transcriptase Inhibitor (Nucleoside)

Medication Safety Issues

Sound-alike/look-alike issues:

Lamivudine may be confused with lamotrigine

Epivir® may be confused with Combivir®

Use

Epivir®: Treatment of HIV infection when antiretroviral therapy is warranted; should always be used as part of a multidrug regimen (at least three antiretroviral agents)

Epivir-HBV®: Treatment of chronic hepatitis B associated with evidence of hepatitis B viral replication and active liver inflammation

Unlabeled/Investigational Use Prevention of HIV following needlesticks (with or without protease inhibitor)

Mechanism of Action Lamivudine is a cytosine analog. After lamivudine is triphosphorylated, the principle mode of action is inhibition of HIV reverse transcription via viral DNA chain termination; inhibits RNA- and DNA-dependent DNA polymerase activities of reverse transcriptase. The monophosphate form of lamivudine is incorporated into the viral DNA by hepatitis B virus polymerase, resulting in DNA chain termination.

Pharmacodynamics/Kinetics

Absorption: Rapid

Distribution: V_d: 1.3 L/kg

Protein binding, plasma: <36%

Metabolism: 5.6% to trans-sulfoxide metabolite

Bioavailability: Absolute; Cp_{max} decreased with food although AUC not significantly affected

Children: 66%

Adults: 87%

Half-life elimination: Children: 2 hours; Adults: 5-7 hours

Excretion: Primarily urine (as unchanged drug)

Contraindications Hypersensitivity to lamivudine or any component of the formulation

Warnings/Precautions A decreased dosage is recommended in patients with renal dysfunction since AUC, C_{max}, and half-life increased with diminishing renal function; use with extreme caution in children with history of pancreatitis or risk factors for development of pancreatitis. Do not use as monotherapy in treatment of HIV. Treatment of HBV in patients with unrecognized/untreated HIV may lead to rapid HIV resistance. In addition, treatment of HIV in patients with unrecognized/untreated HBV may lead to rapid HBV resistance. Patients with HIV infection should receive only dosage forms appropriate for treatment of HIV.

Lactic acidosis and severe hepatomegaly with steatosis have been reported, including fatal cases. Use caution in hepatic impairment. Pregnancy, obesity, and/or prolonged therapy may increase the risk of lactic acidosis and liver damage.

Monitor patients closely for several months following discontinuation of therapy for chronic hepatitis B; clinical exacerbations may occur.

Drug Interactions

Ribavirin: Concomitant use of ribavirin and nucleoside analogues may increase the risk of developing lactic acidosis (includes adefovir, didanosine, lamivudine, stavudine, zalcitabine, zidovudine).

Sulfamethoxazole/trimethoprim: Increased AUC and decreased clearance of lamivudine with concomitant use

Trimethoprim (and other drugs excreted by organic cation transport): May increase serum levels/effects of lamivudine.

Zalcitabine: Intracellular phosphorylation of lamivudine and zalcitabine may be inhibited if used together; concomitant use should be avoided.

Zidovudine: Plasma levels of zidovudine are increased by ~39% with concomitant use.

(Continued)

Lamivudine *(Continued)*

Nutritional/Herbal/Ethanol Interactions Food: Food decreases the rate of absorption and C_{max}; however, there is no change in the systemic AUC. Therefore, may be taken with or without food.

Adverse Reactions (As reported in adults treated for HIV infection)

>10%:

Central nervous system: Headache, fatigue

Gastrointestinal: Nausea, diarrhea, vomiting, pancreatitis (range: 0.5% to 18%; higher percentage in pediatric patients)

Neuromuscular & skeletal: Peripheral neuropathy, paresthesia, musculoskeletal pain

1% to 10%:

Central nervous system: Dizziness, depression, fever, chills, insomnia

Dermatologic: Rash

Gastrointestinal: Anorexia, abdominal pain, heartburn, elevated amylase

Hematologic: Neutropenia

Hepatic: Elevated AST, ALT

Neuromuscular & skeletal: Myalgia, arthralgia

Respiratory: Nasal signs and symptoms, cough

<1% (Limited to important or life-threatening): Alopecia, anaphylaxis, anemia, hepatomegaly, hyperbilirubinemia, hyperglycemia, increased CPK, lactic acidosis, lymphadenopathy, peripheral neuropathy, pruritus, red cell aplasia, rhabdomyolysis, splenomegaly, steatosis, stomatitis, thrombocytopenia, urticaria, weakness

Overdosage/Toxicology Limited information is available, although there have been no clinical signs or symptoms noted, and hematologic tests remained normal in overdose. No antidote is available. Limited (negligible) removal following 4-hour hemodialysis. It is not known if continuous 24-hour hemodialysis would be effective.

Dosing

Adults & Elderly: Note: The formulation and dosage of Epivir-HBV® are not appropriate for patients infected with both HBV and HIV.

HIV: Oral (use with at least two other antiretroviral agents): 150 mg twice daily **or** 300 mg once daily

<50 kg: 4 mg/kg twice daily (maximum: 150 mg twice daily)

Prevention of HIV following needlesticks (unlabeled use): Oral: 150 mg twice daily (with zidovudine with or without a protease inhibitor, depending on risk)

Treatment of hepatitis B (Epivir-HBV®): Oral: 100 mg/day

Pediatrics: Note: The formulation and dosage of Epivir-HBV® are not appropriate for patients infected with both HBV and HIV.

HIV: Oral (use with at least two other antiretroviral agents)

3 months to 16 years: 4 mg/kg twice daily (maximum: 150 mg twice daily)

>16 years: Refer to adult dosing.

Treatment of hepatitis B: Oral: Children 2-17 years: 3 mg/kg once daily (maximum: 100 mg/day)

Renal Impairment: Oral:

Pediatric patients: Insufficient data; however, dose reduction should be considered.

Treatment of HIV patients >16 years:

Cl_{cr} 30-49 mL/minute: Administer 150 mg once daily.

Cl_{cr} 15-29 mL/minute: Administer 150 mg first dose, then 100 mg once daily.

Cl_{cr} 5-14 mL/minute: Administer 150 mg first dose, then 50 mg once daily.

Cl_{cr} <5 mL/minute: Administer 50 mg first dose, then 25 mg once daily.

Dialysis: No data available.

Treatment of hepatitis B patients: Adults:

Cl_{cr} 30-49 mL/minute: Administer 100 mg first dose, then 50 mg once daily.

Cl_{cr} 15-29 mL/minute: Administer 100 mg first dose, then 25 mg once daily.

Cl_{cr} 5-14 mL/minute: Administer 35 mg first dose, then 15 mg once daily.

Cl_{cr} <5 mL/minute: Administer 35 mg first dose, then 10 mg once daily.

Dialysis: Negligible amounts are removed by 4-hour hemodialysis or peritoneal dialysis. Supplemental dosing is not required.

Available Dosage Forms

Solution, oral:

Epivir®: 10 mg/mL (240 mL) [strawberry-banana flavor]

Epivir-HBV®: 5 mg/mL (240 mL) [strawberry-banana flavor]

Tablet:

Epivir®: 150 mg, 300 mg

Epivir-HBV®: 100 mg

Nursing Guidelines

Assessment: Use caution in presence of impaired hepatic or renal function (see Warnings/Precautions for specific use cautions). Assess potential for interactions with other pharmacological agents patient may be taking (eg, increased risk of toxicity; see Drug Interactions). Assess results of laboratory tests, therapeutic effectiveness, and adverse reactions on a regular basis throughout therapy (eg, nausea/vomiting [dehydration], peripheral neuropathy, hepatitis B [jaundice, fatigue, anorexia]; see Adverse Reactions) Monitor patients closely for several months following discontinuation of therapy for chronic hepatitis B and clinical exacerbations. Teach patient proper use (importance of adhering to full treatment regimen), possible side effects/appropriate interventions, and adverse symptoms to report (see Patient Education).

Monitoring Laboratory Tests: Amylase, bilirubin, liver enzymes, CBC

Dietary Considerations: May be taken with or without food. Each 5 mL of oral solution contains 1 g of sucrose.

Patient Education: Do not take any new medication during therapy unless approved by prescriber. Lamivudine is not a cure for HIV or hepatitis B, nor has it been found to reduce transmission. You will need frequent blood tests to adjust dosage for maximum therapeutic effect. Take as directed for full course of therapy; do not discontinue (even if feeling better). Take with or without food. Do not take antacids within 1 hour of lamivudine. Mix four tablets in 3-5 oz water, allow to stand a few minutes, stir, and drink immediately. This may be prescribed as part of a multidrug regimen; it is vital that you maintain that regimen and time medications as instructed. May cause loss of appetite or change in taste (sucking on lozenges, chewing gum, or small frequent meals may help); dizziness or numbness (use caution when driving or engaging in tasks that require alertness until response to drug is known); or headache, fever, or muscle pain (an analgesic may be recommended). Report persistent lethargy or unusual fatigue, yellowing of eyes, pale stool and dark urine; acute headache, severe nausea or vomiting, respiratory difficulty, loss of sensation, rash; or other persistent adverse effects. **Pregnancy/breast-feeding precautions:** Inform prescriber if you are or intend to become pregnant. Do not breast-feed.

Pregnancy Risk Factor: C

Pregnancy Issues: Lamivudine crosses the placenta. The pharmacokinetics of lamivudine during pregnancy are not significantly altered and dosage adjustment is not required. The Perinatal HIV Guidelines Working Group recommends lamivudine for use during pregnancy; the combination of lamivudine with zidovudine is the recommended dual combination NRTI in pregnancy. It may also be used in combination with zidovudine in HIV-infected women who are in labor, but have had no prior antiretroviral therapy, in order to reduce the maternal-fetal transmission of HIV. Cases of lactic acidosis/hepatic steatosis syndrome have been reported in pregnant women receiving nucleoside analogues. It is not known if pregnancy itself potentiates this known side effect; however, pregnant women may be at increased risk of lactic acidosis and liver damage. Hepatic enzymes and electrolytes should be monitored frequently during the 3rd trimester of pregnancy in women receiving nucleoside analogues. Health professionals are encouraged to contact the antiretroviral pregnancy registry to monitor outcomes of pregnant women exposed to antiretroviral medications (1-800-258-4263 or www.APRegistry.com).

Lactation: Enters breast milk/contraindicated

Breast-Feeding Considerations: HIV-infected mothers are discouraged from breast-feeding to decrease potential transmission of HIV.

Administration

Oral: May be taken with or without food. Adjust dosage in renal failure.

Storage: Store at 2°C to 25°C (68°F to 77°F) tightly closed.

◆ **Lamivudine, Abacavir, and Zidovudine** *see* Abacavir, Lamivudine, and Zidovudine *on page 58*

Lamotrigine (la MOE tri jeen)

U.S. Brand Names Lamictal®

Synonyms BW-430C; LTG

Pharmacologic Category Anticonvulsant, Miscellaneous

Medication Safety Issues

Sound-alike/look-alike issues:

Lamotrigine may be confused with labetalol, Lamisil®, lamivudine, Lomotil®, ludiomil

Lamictal® may be confused with Lamisil®, Lomotil®, ludiomil

Use Adjunctive therapy in the treatment of generalized seizures of Lennox-Gastaut syndrome and partial seizures in adults and children ≥2 years of age; conversion to monotherapy in adults with partial seizures who are receiving treatment with valproate or a single enzyme-inducing antiepileptic drug; maintenance treatment of bipolar disorder

Mechanism of Action A triazine derivative which inhibits release of glutamate (an excitatory amino acid) and inhibits voltage-sensitive sodium channels, which stabilizes neuronal membranes. Lamotrigine has weak inhibitory effect on the 5-HT_3 receptor; *in vitro* inhibits dihydrofolate reductase.

Pharmacodynamics/Kinetics

Distribution: V_d: 1.1 L/kg

Protein binding: 55%

Metabolism: Hepatic and renal; metabolized by glucuronic acid conjugation to inactive metabolites

Bioavailability: 98%

Half-life elimination: Adults: 25-33 hours; Concomitant valproic acid therapy: 59-70 hours; Concomitant phenytoin or carbamazepine therapy: 13-14 hours

Time to peak, plasma: 1-4 hours

Excretion: Urine (94%, ~90% as glucuronide conjugates and ~10% unchanged); feces (2%)

Contraindications Hypersensitivity to lamotrigine or any component of the formulation

Warnings/Precautions Severe and potentially life-threatening skin rashes requiring hospitalization have been reported (children 0.8%, adults 0.3%); risk may be increased by coadministration with valproic acid, higher than recommended starting doses, and rapid dose titration. The majority of cases occur in the first 8 weeks; however, isolated cases may occur after prolonged treatment. Discontinue at first sign of rash unless rash is clearly not drug related. Use caution in patients with impaired renal, hepatic, or cardiac function. Avoid abrupt cessation, taper over at least 2 weeks if possible. May cause CNS depression, which may impair physical or mental abilities. Patients must be cautioned about performing tasks which require mental alertness (eg, operating machinery or driving). Effects with other sedative drugs or ethanol may be potentiated. Binds to melanin and may accumulate in the eye and other melanin-rich tissues; the clinical significance of this is not known. Safety and efficacy has not been established for use as initial monotherapy, conversion to monotherapy from nonenzyme-inducing antiepileptic drugs (AED) except valproate, or conversion to monotherapy from two or more AEDs. **Use caution in writing and/or interpreting prescriptions/orders; medication dispensing errors have occurred with similar-sounding medications (Lamisil®, ludiomil, lamivudine, labetalol, and Lomotil®).**

Drug Interactions

Acetaminophen: May reduce serum concentrations of lamotrigine; mechanism not defined; of clinical concern only with chronic acetaminophen dosing (not single doses).

Carbamazepine: Lamotrigine may increase the epoxide metabolite of carbamazepine resulting in toxicity. Carbamazepine may decrease plasma levels of lamotrigine. Dosage adjustments may be needed when adding or withdrawing agents; monitor.

Oral contraceptives (estrogens): Oral contraceptives may decrease the serum concentration of lamotrigine; monitor. Dosage adjustment of lamotrigine may be required when starting/stopping oral contraceptives.

Phenytoin: May decrease plasma levels of lamotrigine. Dosage adjustments may be needed when adding or withdrawing agents; monitor.

Phenobarbital (barbiturates): May increase the metabolism of lamotrigine. Dosage adjustment may be needed when adding or withdrawing agent; monitor.

SSRIs (sertraline): Toxicity has been reported following the addition of sertraline; limited documentation; monitor.

Valproic acid: Inhibits the clearance of lamotrigine, dosage adjustment required when adding or withdrawing valproic acid. Inhibition appears maximal at valproic acid 250-500 mg/day. The incidence of serious rash may be increased by valproic acid.

Nutritional/Herbal/Ethanol Interactions

Ethanol: Avoid ethanol (may increase CNS depression).

Food: Has no effect on absorption.

Herb/Nutraceutical: Avoid evening primrose (seizure threshold decreased).

Adverse Reactions Percentages reported in adults receiving adjunctive therapy:

>10%:

Central nervous system: Headache (29%), dizziness (38%), ataxia (22%), somnolence (14%)

Gastrointestinal: Nausea (19%)

Ocular: Diplopia (28%), blurred vision (16%)

Respiratory: Rhinitis (14%)

1% to 10%:

Cardiovascular: Peripheral edema

Central nervous system: Depression (4%), anxiety (4%), irritability (3%), confusion, speech disorder (3%), difficulty concentrating (2%), malaise, seizure (includes exacerbations) (2% to 3%), incoordination (6%), insomnia (6%), pain, amnesia, hostility, memory decreased, nervousness, vertigo

Dermatologic: Hypersensitivity rash (10%; serious rash requiring hospitalization - adults 0.3%, children 0.8%), pruritus (3%)

Gastrointestinal: Abdominal pain (5%), vomiting (9%), diarrhea (6%), dyspepsia (5%), xerostomia, constipation (4%), anorexia (2%), tooth disorder (3%)

Genitourinary: Vaginitis (4%), dysmenorrhea (7%), amenorrhea (2%)

Neuromuscular & skeletal: Tremor (4%), arthralgia (2%), neck pain (2%)

Ocular: Nystagmus (2%), visual abnormality

Respiratory: Epistaxis, bronchitis, dyspnea

Miscellaneous: Flu syndrome (7%), fever (6%)

<1% (Limited to important or life-threatening): Acne, acute renal failure, agranulocytosis, allergic reactions, alopecia, anemia, angina, angioedema, aplastic anemia, apnea, atrial fibrillation, back pain, bronchospasm, bruising, chills, depersonalization, disseminated intravascular coagulation (DIC), dysarthria, dysphagia, eosinophilia, erythema multiforme, esophagitis, facial edema, GI hemorrhage, gingival hyperplasia, halitosis, hemolytic anemia, hemorrhage, hepatitis, hot flashes, hypersensitivity reactions (including rhabdomyolysis), hypertension, immunosuppression (progressive), impotence, leukopenia, lupus-like reaction, maculopapular rash, malaise, mania, migraine, movement disorder, multiorgan failure, neutropenia, palpitation, pancreatitis, pancytopenia, paralysis, Parkinson's disease exacerbation, photosensitivity (rare), postural hypotension, rash, red cell aplasia, Stevens-Johnson syndrome, stroke, suicidal ideation, thrombocytopenia, tics, toxic epidermal necrolysis, urticaria, vasculitis, vesiculobullous rash

Overdosage/Toxicology Symptoms of overdose include QRS prolongation, AV block, dizziness, drowsiness, sedation, and ataxia. Enhancement of elimination: Multiple dosing of activated charcoal may be useful.

Dosing

Adults & Elderly: Note: Only whole tablets should be used for dosing, round calculated dose down to the nearest whole tablet:

Lennox-Gastaut (adjunctive) or treatment of partial seizures (adjunctive):

Oral:

Patients receiving AED regimens containing valproic acid: Initial dose: 25 mg every other day for 2 weeks, then 25 mg every day for 2 weeks; dose may be increased by 25-50 mg every day for 1-2 weeks in order to achieve maintenance dose. Maintenance dose: 100-400 mg/day in 1-2 divided doses (usual range 100-200 mg/day).

Patients receiving enzyme-inducing AED regimens without valproic acid: Initial dose: 50 mg/day for 2 weeks, then 100 mg in 2 doses for 2 weeks; thereafter, daily dose can be increased by 100 mg every 1-2 weeks to be given in 2 divided doses. Usual maintenance dose: 300-500 mg/day in 2 divided doses; doses as high as 700 mg/day have been reported

Conversion to monotherapy (partial seizures in patients ≥16 years of age):

Adjunctive therapy with valproate: Initiate and titrate as per recommendations to a lamotrigine dose of 200 mg/day. Then taper valproate dose in decrements of not more than 500 mg/day at intervals of one week (or

(Continued)

Lamotrigine *(Continued)*

longer) to a valproate dosage of 500 mg/day; this dosage should be maintained for one week. The lamotrigine dosage should then be increased to 300 mg/day while valproate is decreased to 250 mg/day; this dosage should be maintained for one week. Valproate may then be discontinued, while the lamotrigine dose is increased by 100 mg/day at weekly intervals to achieve a lamotrigine maintenance dose of 500 mg/day.

Adjunctive therapy with enzyme-inducing AED: Initiate and titrate as per recommendations to a lamotrigine dose of 500 mg/day. Concomitant enzyme-inducing AED should then be withdrawn by 20% decrements each week over a 4-week period. Patients should be monitored for rash.

Adjunctive therapy with nonenzyme-inducing AED: No specific guidelines available

Bipolar disorder: 25 mg/day for 2 weeks, followed by 50 mg/day for 2 weeks, followed by 100 mg/day for 1 week; thereafter, daily dosage may be increased to 200 mg/day

Patients receiving valproic acid: Initial: 25 mg every other day for 2 weeks, followed by 25 mg/day for 2 weeks, followed by 50 mg/day for 1 week, followed by 100 mg/day (target dose) thereafter. **Note:** If valproate is discontinued, increase daily lamotrigine dose in 50 mg increments at weekly intervals until daily dosage of 200 mg is attained.

Patients receiving enzyme-inducing drugs (eg, carbamazepine): Initial: 50 mg/day for 2 weeks, followed by 100 mg/day (in divided doses) for 2 weeks, followed by 200 mg/day (in divided doses) for 1 week, followed by 300 mg/day (in divided doses) for 1 week. May increase to 400 mg/day (in divided doses) during week 7 and thereafter. **Note:** If carbamazepine (or other enzyme-inducing drug) is discontinued, decrease daily lamotrigine dose in 100 mg increments at weekly intervals until daily dosage of 200 mg is attained.

Discontinuing therapy: Decrease dose by ~50% per week, over at least 2 weeks unless safety concerns require a more rapid withdrawal.

Restarting therapy after discontinuation: If lamotrigine has been withheld for >5 half-lives, consider restarting according to initial dosing recommendations.

Pediatrics: Note: Only whole tablets should be used for dosing, rounded down to the nearest whole tablet.

Lennox-Gastaut (adjunctive) or partial seizures (adjunctive): Oral:

Children 2-12 years: **Note:** Children 2-6 years will likely require maintenance doses at the higher end of recommended range

Patients receiving AED regimens containing valproic acid:

Weeks 1 and 2: 0.15 mg/kg/day in 1-2 divided doses; round dose down to the nearest whole tablet. For patients >6.7 kg and <14 kg, dosing should be 2 mg every other day.

Weeks 3 and 4: 0.3 mg/kg/day in 1-2 divided doses; round dose down to the nearest whole tablet

Maintenance dose: Titrate dose to effect; after week 4, increase dose every 1-2 weeks by a calculated increment; calculate increment as 0.3 mg/kg/day rounded down to the nearest whole tablet; add this amount to the previously administered daily dose; usual maintenance: 1-5 mg/kg/day in 1-2 divided doses; maximum: 200 mg/day

Patients receiving enzyme-inducing AED regimens without valproic acid:

Weeks 1 and 2: 0.6 mg/kg/day in 2 divided doses; round dose down to the nearest whole tablet

Weeks 3 and 4: 1.2 mg/kg/day in 2 divided doses; round dose down to the nearest whole tablet

Maintenance dose: Titrate dose to effect; after week 4, increase dose every 1-2 weeks by a calculated increment; calculate increment as 1.2 mg/kg/day rounded down to the nearest whole tablet; add this amount to the previously administered daily dose; usual maintenance: 5-15 mg/kg/day in 2 divided doses; maximum: 400 mg/day

Children >12 years: Refer to adult dosing.

Conversion from single enzyme-inducing AED regimen to monotherapy: Children ≥16 years: Refer to adult dosing.

Discontinuing therapy: Decrease dose by ~50% per week, over at least 2 weeks unless safety concerns require a more rapid withdrawal.

Restarting therapy after discontinuation: If lamotrigine has been withheld for >5 half-lives, consider restarting according to initial dosing recommendations.

Renal Impairment: Decreased dosage may be effective in patients with significant renal impairment; use with caution.

Hepatic Impairment:

Child-Pugh Grade B: Reduce initial, escalation, and maintenance doses by 50%.

Child-Pugh Grade C: Reduce initial, escalation, and maintenance doses by 75%.

Available Dosage Forms

Tablet: 25 mg, 100 mg, 150 mg, 200 mg [contains lactose]

Tablet, combination package [each unit-dose starter kit contains]:

Lamictal® (blue kit; for patients taking valproate):

Tablet: Lamotrigine 25 mg (35s)

Lamictal® (green kit; for patients taking carbamazepine, phenytoin, phenobarbital, primidone or rifampin and **not** taking valproate):

Tablet: Lamotrigine 25 mg (84s)

Tablet: Lamotrigine 100 mg (14s)

Lamictal® (orange kit; for patients **not** taking carbamazepine, phenytoin, phenobarbital, primidone, rifampin, or valproate; for use in bipolar patients only):

Tablet: Lamotrigine 25 mg (42s)

Tablet: Lamotrigine 100 mg (7s)

Tablet, dispersible/chewable: 2 mg, 5 mg, 25 mg [black currant flavor]

Nursing Guidelines

Assessment: Assess effectiveness and interactions of other medications patient may be taking. Monitor therapeutic effectiveness, laboratory values, and adverse reactions at beginning of therapy and periodically with long-term use. Taper dosage slowly when discontinuing. Observe and teach seizure/safety precautions. Use caution in writing and/or interpreting prescriptions/orders. Confusion between Lamictal® (lamotrigine) and Lamisil® (terbinafine) has occurred. Assess knowledge/teach patient appropriate use, interventions to reduce side effects, and adverse symptoms to report.

Monitoring Laboratory Tests: Serum levels of concurrent anticonvulsants, LFTs, renal function

Dietary Considerations: Take without regard to meals; drug may cause GI upset.

Patient Education: Take exactly as directed; do not increase dose or frequency or discontinue without consulting prescriber. Only whole tablets should be used for dosing, rounded down to the nearest whole tablet. When having the prescription refilled, contact the prescriber if the medicine looks different or the label name has changed. While using this medication, do not use alcohol and other prescription or OTC medications (especially pain medications, sedatives, antihistamines, or hypnotics) without consulting prescriber. Maintain adequate hydration (2-3 L/day of fluids) unless instructed to restrict fluid intake. You may experience drowsiness, dizziness, or blurred vision (use caution when driving or engaging in tasks requiring alertness until response to drug is known); or nausea, vomiting, loss of appetite, heartburn, or dry mouth (small frequent meals, frequent mouth care, chewing gum, or sucking lozenges may help). Wear identification of epileptic status and medications. Report CNS changes, mentation changes, or changes in cognition; persistent GI symptoms (cramping, constipation, vomiting, anorexia); skin rash; swelling of face, lips, or tongue; easy bruising or bleeding (mouth, urine, stool); vision changes; worsening of seizure activity, or loss of seizure control. **Pregnancy/breast-feeding precautions:** Inform prescriber if you are or intend to become pregnant. Breast-feeding is not recommended.

Geriatric Considerations: Use with caution in the elderly with significant renal impairment.

Pregnancy Risk Factor: C

Pregnancy Issues: Safety and efficacy in pregnant women have not been established. Healthcare providers may enroll patients in the Lamotrigine Pregnancy Registry by calling (800) 336-2176. Patients may enroll themselves in the North American Antiepileptic Drug Pregnancy Registry by calling (888) 233-2334. Dose of lamotrigine may need adjustment during pregnancy to maintain clinical response; lamotrigine serum levels may decrease during pregnancy and return to prepartum levels following delivery.

Lactation: Enters breast milk/not recommended (AAP rates "of concern")

Perioperative/Anesthesia/Other Concerns: Low water solubility; less sedating than other antiepileptic drugs. Use gastric lavage with activated charcoal and a cathartic for overdose. Worsens myoclonic seizure activity.

(Continued)

Lamotrigine *(Continued)*

Administration

Oral: Doses should be rounded down to the nearest whole tablet. Dispersible tablets may be chewed, dispersed in water, or swallowed whole. To disperse tablets, add to a small amount of liquid (just enough to cover tablet); let sit ~1 minute until dispersed; swirl solution and consume immediately. Do not administer partial amounts of liquid. If tablets are chewed, a small amount of water or diluted fruit juice should be used to aid in swallowing.

Storage: Store at 25°C (77°F). Excursions are permitted to 15°C to 30°C (59°F to 86°F). Protect from light.

Related Information

Perioperative Management of Patients on Antiseizure Medication *on page 1801*

- **Lanacane® [OTC]** *see* Benzocaine *on page 232*
- **Lanacane® Maximum Strength [OTC]** *see* Benzocaine *on page 232*
- **Lanoxicaps®** *see* Digoxin *on page 532*
- **Lanoxin®** *see* Digoxin *on page 532*

Lansoprazole (lan SOE pra zole)

U.S. Brand Names Prevacid®; Prevacid® SoluTab™

Pharmacologic Category Proton Pump Inhibitor; Substituted Benzimidazole

Medication Safety Issues

Sound-alike/look-alike issues:

Prevacid® may be confused with Pravachol®, Prevpac®, Prilosec®, Prinivil®

Use

Oral: Short-term treatment of active duodenal ulcers; maintenance treatment of healed duodenal ulcers; as part of a multidrug regimen for *H. pylori* eradication to reduce the risk of duodenal ulcer recurrence; short-term treatment of active benign gastric ulcer; treatment of NSAID-associated gastric ulcer; to reduce the risk of NSAID-associated gastric ulcer in patients with a history of gastric ulcer who require an NSAID; short-term treatment of symptomatic GERD; short-term treatment for all grades of erosive esophagitis; to maintain healing of erosive esophagitis; long-term treatment of pathological hypersecretory conditions, including Zollinger-Ellison syndrome

I.V.: Short-term treatment (≤7 days) of erosive esophagitis in adults unable to take oral medications

Unlabeled/Investigational Use Active ulcer bleeding (parenteral formulation)

Mechanism of Action A proton pump inhibitor which decreases acid secretion in gastric parietal cells

Pharmacodynamics/Kinetics

Duration: >1 day

Absorption: Rapid

Protein binding: 97%

Metabolism: Hepatic via CYP2C19 and 3A4, and in parietal cells to two inactive metabolites

Bioavailability: 80%; decreased 50% to 70% if given 30 minutes after food

Half-life elimination: 2 hours; Elderly: 2-3 hours; Hepatic impairment: ≤7 hours

Time to peak, plasma: 1.7 hours

Excretion: Feces (67%); urine (33%)

Contraindications Hypersensitivity to lansoprazole, substituted benzimidazoles (ie, esomeprazole, omeprazole, pantoprazole, rabeprazole), or any component of the formulation

Warnings/Precautions Severe liver dysfunction may require dosage reductions. Symptomatic response does not exclude malignancy. Safety and efficacy have not been established in children <1 year of age.

Drug Interactions Substrate of CYP2C8/9 (minor), 2C19 (major), 3A4 (major); **Inhibits** CYP2C8/9 (weak), 2C19 (moderate), 2D6 (weak), 3A4 (weak); **Induces** CYP1A2 (weak)

CYP2C19 inducers: May decrease the levels/effects of lansoprazole. Example inducers include aminoglutethimide, carbamazepine, phenytoin, and rifampin.

CYP2C19 substrates: Lansoprazole may increase the levels/effects of CYP2C19 substrates. Example substrates include citalopram, diazepam, methsuximide, phenytoin, propranolol, and sertraline.

CYP3A4 inducers: CYP3A4 inducers may decrease the levels/effects of lansoprazole. Example inducers include aminoglutethimide, carbamazepine, nafcillin, nevirapine, phenobarbital, phenytoin, and rifamycins.

Itraconazole and ketoconazole: Proton pump inhibitors may decrease the absorption of itraconazole and ketoconazole.

Protease inhibitors: Proton pump inhibitors may decrease absorption of some protease inhibitors (atazanavir and indinavir).

Nutritional/Herbal/Ethanol Interactions

Ethanol: Avoid ethanol (may cause gastric mucosal irritation).

Food: Lansoprazole serum concentrations may be decreased if taken with food.

Adverse Reactions

1% to 10%:

Central nervous system: Headache (children 1-11 years 3%, 12-17 years 7%)

Gastrointestinal: Abdominal pain (children 12-17 years 5%; adults 2%), constipation (children 1-11 years 5%; adults 1%), diarrhea (4%; 4% to 7% at doses of 30-60 mg/day), nausea (children 12-17 years 3%; adults 1%)

<1% (Limited to important or life-threatening): Abnormal vision, agitation, allergic reaction, ALT increased, anaphylactoid reaction, anemia, angina, anxiety, aplastic anemia, arrhythmia, AST increased, chest pain, convulsion, depression, dizziness, dry eyes, dry mouth, erythema multiforme, esophagitis, gastrin levels increased, gastrointestinal disorder, glucocorticoids increased, globulins increased, hemolysis, hemolytic anemia, hepatotoxicity, hyperglycemia, LDH increased, maculopapular rash, pancreatitis, photophobia, rash, RBC abnormal, taste perversion, Stevens-Johnson syndrome, thrombocytopenia, tinnitus, toxic epidermal necrolysis (some fatal), tremor, vertigo, visual field defect, vomiting, WBC abnormal

Overdosage/Toxicology No symptoms of toxicity were observed in animal studies; limited human experience in overdose. Treatment is symptomatic and supportive. Lansoprazole is not removed by hemodialysis.

Dosing

Adults & Elderly:

Symptomatic GERD: Oral: Short-term treatment: 15 mg once daily for up to 8 weeks

Erosive esophagitis:

Oral: Short-term treatment: 30 mg once daily for up to 8 weeks; continued treatment for an additional 8 weeks may be considered for recurrence or for patients that do not heal after the first 8 weeks of therapy; maintenance therapy: 15 mg once daily

I.V.: 30 mg once daily for up to 7 days; patients should be switched to an oral formulation as soon as they can take oral medications.

Hypersecretory conditions: Oral: Initial: 60 mg once daily; adjust dose based upon patient response and to reduce acid secretion to <10 mEq/hour (5 mEq/hour in patients with prior gastric surgery); doses of 90 mg twice daily have been used; administer doses >120 mg/day in divided doses

Duodenal ulcer: Oral: Short-term treatment: 15 mg once daily for 4 weeks; maintenance therapy: 15 mg once daily

Peptic ulcer disease: Eradication of *Helicobacter pylori*: Currently accepted recommendations (may differ from product labeling): Oral: Dose varies with regimen: 30 mg once daily or 60 mg/day in 2 divided doses; requires combination therapy with antibiotics

Gastric ulcer: Oral: Short-term treatment: 30 mg once daily for up to 8 weeks

NSAID-associated gastric ulcer (healing): Oral: 30 mg once daily for 8 weeks; controlled studies did not extend past 8 weeks

NSAID-associated gastric ulcer (to reduce risk): Oral: 15 mg once daily for up to 12 weeks; controlled studies did not extend past 12 weeks

Prevention of rebleeding in peptic ulcer bleed (unlabeled use): I.V.: 60 mg, followed by 6 mg/hour infusion for 72 hours

Pediatrics:

GERD, erosive esophagitis: Oral: Children 1-11 years:

≤30 kg: 15 mg once daily

>30 kg: 30 mg once daily

Note: Doses were increased in some pediatric patients if still symptomatic after 2 or more weeks of treatment (maximum dose: 30 mg twice daily)

Erosive esophagitis: Children 12-17 years: Oral: 30 mg once daily for up to 8 weeks

Nonerosive GERD: Children 12-17 years: Oral: 15 mg once daily for up to 8 weeks

(Continued)

Lansoprazole *(Continued)*

Renal Impairment: No adjustment is necessary.

Hepatic Impairment: May require a dose reduction.

Available Dosage Forms

Capsule, delayed release (Prevacid®): 15 mg, 30 mg

Granules, for oral suspension, delayed release (Prevacid®): 15 mg/packet (30s), 30 mg/packet (30s) [strawberry flavor]

Injection, powder for reconstitution (Prevacid®): 30 mg

Tablet, orally-disintegrating (Prevacid® SoluTab™): 15 mg [contains phenylalanine 2.5 mg; strawberry flavor]; 30 mg [contains phenylalanine 5.1 mg; strawberry flavor]

Nursing Guidelines

Assessment: Assess periodic laboratory results and assess effectiveness of medications that require an acid medium for absorption (eg, ketoconazole, itraconazole). Monitor effectiveness of ulcer symptom relief.

Monitoring Laboratory Tests: CBC, liver function, renal function, and serum gastrin levels. Patients with Zollinger-Ellison syndrome should be monitored for gastric acid output, which should be maintained at ≤10 mEq/hour during the last hour before the next lansoprazole dose.

Dietary Considerations: Should be taken before eating; best if taken before breakfast. Prevacid® SoluTab™ contains phenylalanine 2.5 mg per 15 mg tablet; phenylalanine 5.1 mg per 30 mg tablet.

Patient Education: Take as directed, before eating. Do not crush or chew granules. Patients who may have difficulty swallowing capsules may open the delayed-release capsules and sprinkle the contents on applesauce, pudding, cottage cheese, or yogurt. Avoid alcohol. Report unresolved diarrhea. **Breast-feeding precaution:** Breast-feeding is not recommended.

Geriatric Considerations: The clearance of lansoprazole is decreased in the elderly; however, the half-life is only increased by 50% to 100%. This still results in a short half-life and no accumulation is seen in the elderly. The rate of healing and side effects is similar to younger adults; no dosage adjustment is necessary.

Pregnancy Risk Factor: B

Lactation: Excretion in breast milk unknown/not recommended

Perioperative/Anesthesia/Other Concerns: Intravenous omeprazole has been studied in prevention of rebleeding in ulcer patients who are at high risk for rebleeding (endoscopic findings of active bleeding or nonbleeding visible vessel) after successful hemostasis (Lin HJ, 1998; Lau JY, 2000). Lin and his group treated 100 ulcer patients (actively bleeding ulcers or ulcers with nonbleeding visible vessels) endoscopically and then randomized them to cimetidine (300 mg bolus followed by 50 mg/hour infusion) or omeprazole (40 mg bolus, ~7 mg/hour infusion) for 72 hours. Patients were discharged on the oral form of the drug arm they were assigned to. The omeprazole group maintained an intragastric pH >6 for about 84% of the infusion duration, while the cimetidine group maintained their pH >6 only about 50% of the time. Rebleeding occurred significantly more often in the cimetidine group. Lau and his colleagues treated patients with actively bleeding ulcers or ulcers with nonbleeding visible vessels with an epinephrine infusion followed by thermocoagulation. They were then randomized to omeprazole (80 mg bolus followed by a continuous infusion of 8 mg/hour for 72 hours) or placebo. All patients were discharged on oral omeprazole (20 mg/day) for 8 weeks and received *H. pylori* treatment if indicated. The primary goal was to evaluate the rate of rebleeding during the first 30 days after endoscopy. Two hundred and forty patients were enrolled with randomization of 120 into each group. Bleeding recurred in significantly more patients receiving placebo than omeprazole infusion. The authors concluded that after endoscopic therapy, omeprazole reduces the risk of rebleeding in patients with actively bleeding ulcers or ulcers with nonbleeding visible vessels.

Administration

Oral: Administer before food; best if taken before breakfast. The intact granules should not be chewed or crushed; however, in addition to oral suspension, several options are available for those patients unable to swallow capsules:

Capsules may be opened and the intact granules sprinkled on 1 tablespoon of applesauce, Ensure® pudding, cottage cheese, yogurt, or strained pears. The granules should then be swallowed immediately.

Capsules may be opened and emptied into ~60 mL orange juice, apple juice, or tomato juice; mix and swallow immediately. Rinse the glass with additional juice and swallow to assure complete delivery of the dose.

Capsule granules may be mixed with apple, cranberry, grape, orange, pineapple, prune, tomato and V-8® juice and stored for up to 30 minutes.

Delayed release oral suspension granules should be mixed with 2 tablespoonfuls (30 mL) of water; no other liquid should be used. Stir well and drink immediately. Should not be administered through enteral administration tubes.

Orally-disintegrating tablets: Should not be swallowed whole or chewed. Place tablet on tongue; allow to dissolve (with or without water) until particles can be swallowed. Orally-disintegrating tablets may also be administered via an oral syringe: Place the 15 mg tablet in an oral syringe and draw up ~4 mL water, or place the 30 mg tablet in an oral syringe and draw up ~10 mL water. After tablet has dispersed, administer within 15 minutes. Refill the syringe with water (2 mL for the 15 mg tablet; 4 mL for the 30 mg tablet), shake gently, then administer any remaining contents.

I.V.: Administer over 30 minutes. Use of an in-line filter is required. Before and after administration, flush I.V. line with NS, LR, or D_5W. Do not administer with other medications.

Reconstitution:

Oral suspension: Empty packet into container with 2 tablespoons of water. Do **not** mix with other liquids or food. Stir well and drink immediately.

Powder for injection: Reconstitute with sterile water 5 mL; mix gently until dissolved. Prior to administration, further dilute with 50 mL of NS, LR, or D_5W.

Storage: Store at 15°C to 30°C (59°F to 86°F); protect from light and moisture.

Powder for injection: After reconstitution, the solution may be stored for up to 1 hour at room temperature prior to final dilution. Following final dilution, solutions mixed with NS or LR are stable at room temperature for 24 hours; solutions mixed with D_5W are stable for 12 hours

- ♦ **Lantus®** *see* Insulin Glargine *on page 920*
- ♦ **Lapase** *see* Pancrelipase *on page 1301*
- ♦ **Lariam®** *see* Mefloquine *on page 1088*
- ♦ **Lasix®** *see* Furosemide *on page 786*

Latanoprost (la TA noe prost)

U.S. Brand Names Xalatan®

Pharmacologic Category Ophthalmic Agent, Antiglaucoma; Prostaglandin, Ophthalmic

Medication Safety Issues

Sound-alike/look-alike issues:

Xalatan® may be confused with Travatan®, Zarontin®

Use Reduction of elevated intraocular pressure in patients with open-angle glaucoma or ocular hypertension

Mechanism of Action Latanoprost is a prostaglandin F_2-alpha analog believed to reduce intraocular pressure by increasing the outflow of the aqueous humor

Pharmacodynamics/Kinetics

Onset of action: 3-4 hours

Peak effect: Maximum: 8-12 hours

Absorption: Through the cornea where the isopropyl ester prodrug is hydrolyzed by esterases to the biologically active acid. Peak concentration is reached in 2 hours after topical administration in the aqueous humor.

Distribution: V_d: 0.16 L/kg

Metabolism: Primarily hepatic via fatty acid beta-oxidation

Half-life elimination: 17 minutes

Excretion: Urine (as metabolites)

Contraindications Hypersensitivity to latanoprost or any component of the formulation

Warnings/Precautions Latanoprost may gradually change eye color, increasing the amount of brown pigment in the iris by increasing the number of melanosome in melanocytes. The long-term effects on the melanocytes and the consequences of potential injury to the melanocytes or deposition of pigment granules to other areas of the eye is currently unknown. Patients should be examined regularly, and depending on the clinical situation, treatment may be stopped if increased pigmentation ensues.

(Continued)

Latanoprost *(Continued)*

There have been reports of bacterial keratitis associated with the use of multiple-dose containers of topical ophthalmic products. Do not administer while wearing contact lenses.

Drug Interactions

May be used concomitantly with other topical ophthalmic drugs if administration is separated by at least 5 minutes.

Bimatoprost: Combination therapy may result in higher IOP than either agent alone.

Thimerosal-containing eye drops: Precipitation occurs when eye drops containing thimerosal are mixed with latanoprost. If such drugs are used, administer with an interval of at least 5 minutes between applications.

Adverse Reactions

>10%: Ocular: Blurred vision, burning and stinging, conjunctival hyperemia, foreign body sensation, itching, increased pigmentation of the iris, and punctate epithelial keratopathy

1% to 10%:

Cardiovascular: Chest pain, angina pectoris

Dermatologic: Rash, allergic skin reaction

Neuromuscular & skeletal: Myalgia, arthralgia, back pain

Ocular: Dry eye, excessive tearing, eye pain, lid crusting, lid edema, lid erythema, lid discomfort/pain, photophobia

Respiratory: Upper respiratory tract infection, cold, flu

<1% (Limited to important or life-threatening): Asthma, conjunctivitis, corneal edema, corneal erosion, diplopia, discharge from the eye, dyspnea, eyelash change, eyelid skin darkening, herpes keratitis, iritis, keratitis, macular edema, retinal artery embolus, retinal detachment, toxic epidermal necrolysis, uveitis, vitreous hemorrhage from diabetic retinopathy

Overdosage/Toxicology

Symptoms include ocular irritation and conjunctival or episcleral hyperemia

Treatment should be symptomatic

Dosing

Adults & Elderly: Glaucoma: Ophthalmic: 1 drop (1.5 mcg) in the affected eye(s) once daily in the evening; do not exceed the once daily dosage because it has been shown that more frequent administration may decrease the IOP lowering effect

Note: A medication delivery device (Xal-Ease™) is available for use with Xalatan®.

Available Dosage Forms Solution, ophthalmic: 0.005% (2.5 mL) [contains benzalkonium chloride]

Nursing Guidelines

Assessment: Assess potential for interactions with other prescriptions, OTC medications, or herbal products patient may be taking. Assess therapeutic response and adverse effects (eg, blurred vision, burning and stinging, conjunctival hyperemia, foreign body sensation, itching, increased pigmentation of the iris, and punctate epithelial keratopathy). Teach patient proper use, side effects/appropriate interventions, and symptoms to report.

Patient Education: For use in eyes only. Iris color may change because of an increase of the brown pigment (cosmetically different eye coloration that may occur). Iris pigmentation changes may be more noticeable in patients with green-brown, blue/gray-brown, or yellow-brown irides. If any ocular reaction develops, particularly conjunctivitis and lid reactions, immediately notify prescriber. If more than one topical ophthalmic drug is being used, administer the drugs at least 5 minutes apart. Latanoprost contains benzalkonium chloride, which may be absorbed by contact lenses. Remove contact lenses prior to administration; lenses may be reinserted after 15 minutes. Do not let tip of applicator touch eye; do not contaminate tip of applicator (may cause eye infection, eye damage, or vision loss). Serious damage to the eye and subsequent loss of vision may result from using contaminated solutions. A delivery aid, Xal-Ease™, is available for administering Xalatan®. **Pregnancy precaution:** Inform prescriber if you are pregnant.

Pregnancy Risk Factor: C

Administration

Storage: Protect from light; store intact bottles under refrigeration (2°C to 8°C/36°F to 46°F). Once opened, the container may be stored at room temperature up to 25°C (77°F) for 6 weeks.

♦ **Lavacol® [OTC]** *see* Alcohol (Ethyl) *on page 100*
♦ **LCR** *see* VinCRIStine *on page 1710*
♦ **L-Deprenyl** *see* Selegiline *on page 1517*
♦ **LDP-341** *see* Bortezomib *on page 251*

Lepirudin (leh puh ROO din)

U.S. Brand Names Refludan®

Synonyms Lepirudin (rDNA); Recombinant Hirudin

Pharmacologic Category Anticoagulant, Thrombin Inhibitor

Use Indicated for anticoagulation in patients with heparin-induced thrombocytopenia (HIT) and associated thromboembolic disease in order to prevent further thromboembolic complications

Unlabeled/Investigational Use Investigational: Prevention or reduction of ischemic complications associated with unstable angina

Mechanism of Action Lepirudin is a highly specific direct inhibitor of thrombin; lepirudin is a recombinant hirudin derived from yeast cells

Pharmacodynamics/Kinetics

Distribution: Two-compartment model; confined to extracellular fluids.

Metabolism: Via release of amino acids via catabolic hydrolysis of parent drug

Half-life elimination: Initial: ~10 minutes: Terminal: Healthy volunteers: 1.3 hours; Marked renal impairment (Cl_{cr} <15 mL/minute and on hemodialysis): ≤2 days

Excretion: Urine (~48%, 35% as unchanged drug and unchanged drug fragments of parent drug); systemic clearance is proportional to glomerular filtration rate or creatinine clearance

Contraindications Hypersensitivity to hirudins or any component of the formulation

Warnings/Precautions Cautiously administer after a thrombolytic episode; risk of intracranial bleeding. Hemorrhage is the most common complication. Monitor for signs and symptoms of bleeding. Certain patients are at increased risk of bleeding. Risk factors include bacterial endocarditis; congenital or acquired bleeding disorders; recent puncture of large vessels or organ biopsy; recent CVA, stroke, intracerebral surgery, or other neuraxial procedure; severe uncontrolled hypertension; renal impairment; recent major surgery; recent major bleeding (intracranial, GI, intraocular, or pulmonary). With renal impairment, relative overdose might occur even with standard dosage regimen. The bolus dose and rate of infusion must be reduced in patients with known or suspected renal insufficiency. Strict monitoring of aPTT is required; formation of antihirudin antibodies can increase the anticoagulant effect of lepirudin. Use cautiously in cirrhosis. Allergic reactions may occur frequently in patients treated concomitantly with streptokinase. Be cautious in re-exposing patients (anaphylaxis has been reported).

Drug Interactions

Cephalosporins which contain the MTT side chain may increase the risk of hemorrhage.

Drugs which affect platelet function (eg, aspirin, NSAIDs, dipyridamole, ticlopidine, clopidogrel) may potentiate the risk of hemorrhage.

Penicillins (parenteral) may prolong bleeding time via inhibition of platelet aggregation, potentially increasing the risk of hemorrhage.

Thrombolytic agents increase the risk of hemorrhage.

Warfarin: Risk of bleeding may be increased during concurrent therapy. During the initiation of warfarin therapy, heparin is commonly continued to assure anticoagulation and to protect against possible transient hypercoagulability. It is probable that a similar approach would be used in situations where lepirudin is required.

Nutritional/Herbal/Ethanol Interactions Herb/Nutraceutical: Avoid cat's claw, dong quai, evening primrose, feverfew, garlic, ginger, ginkgo, red clover, horse chestnut, green tea, ginseng (all have additional antiplatelet activity)

Adverse Reactions As with all anticoagulants, bleeding is the most common adverse event associated with lepirudin. Hemorrhage may occur at virtually any site. Risk is dependent on multiple variables.

HIT patients:

>10%: Hematologic: Anemia (12%), bleeding from puncture sites (11%), hematoma (11%)

1% to 10%:

Cardiovascular: Heart failure (3%), pericardial effusion (1%), ventricular fibrillation (1%)

Central nervous system: Fever (7%)

Dermatologic: Eczema (3%), maculopapular rash (4%)

(Continued)

Lepirudin *(Continued)*

Gastrointestinal: GI bleeding/rectal bleeding (5%)
Genitourinary: Vaginal bleeding (2%)
Hepatic: Transaminases increased (6%)
Renal: Hematuria (4%)
Respiratory: Epistaxis (4%)

<1% (Limited to important or life-threatening): Allergic reactions, anaphylaxis, hemoperitoneum, hemoptysis, injection site reactions, intracranial bleeding, liver bleeding, mouth bleeding, pruritus, pulmonary bleeding, retroperitoneal bleeding, thrombocytopenia, urticaria

Non-HIT populations (including those receiving thrombolytics and/or contrast media):

1% to 10%: Respiratory: Bronchospasm/stridor/dyspnea/cough

<1% (Limited to important or life-threatening): Allergic reactions (unspecified), anaphylactoid reactions, anaphylaxis, angioedema, intracranial bleeding (0.6%), laryngeal edema, thrombocytopenia, tongue edema

Overdosage/Toxicology Risk of bleeding is increased, and therefore management is directed towards control of bleeding.

Dosing

Adults & Elderly: Note: Maximum dose: Do not exceed 0.21 mg/kg/hour unless an evaluation of coagulation abnormalities limiting response has been completed. **Dosing is weight-based, however, patients weighing >110 kg should not receive doses greater than the recommended dose for a patient weighing 110 kg (44 mg bolus and initial maximal infusion rate of 16.5 mg/hour).**

Heparin-induced thrombocytopenia: I.V.: Bolus dose: 0.4 mg/kg IVP (over 15-20 seconds), followed by continuous infusion at 0.15 mg/kg/hour; bolus and infusion must be reduced in renal insufficiency

Concomitant use with thrombolytic therapy: I.V.: Bolus dose: 0.2 mg/kg IVP (over 15-20 seconds), followed by continuous infusion at 0.1 mg/kg/hour

Dosing adjustments during infusions: Monitor first aPTT 4 hours after the start of the infusion. Subsequent determinations of aPTT should be obtained at least once daily during treatment. More frequent monitoring is recommended in renally impaired patients. Any aPTT ratio measurement out of range (1.5-2.5) should be confirmed prior to adjusting dose, unless a clinical need for immediate reaction exists. If the aPTT is below target range, increase infusion by 20%. If the aPTT is in excess of the target range, decrease infusion rate by 50%. A repeat aPTT should be obtained 4 hours after any dosing change.

Transition to oral anticoagulants: Reduce lepirudin dose gradually to reach aPTT ratio just above 1.5 before starting warfarin therapy; as soon as INR reaches 2.0, lepirudin therapy should be discontinued.

Renal Impairment: All patients with Cl_{cr} <60 or serum creatinine >1.5 mg/dL require dosage reduction.

Initial: Bolus dose: 0.2 mg/kg IVP (over 15-20 seconds); see table. Additional bolus doses of 0.1 mg/kg may be administered every other day (only if aPTT falls below lower therapeutic limit).

Lepirudin Infusion Rates in Patients With Renal Impairment

Creatinine Clearance (mL/min)	Serum Creatinine (mg/dL)	Adjusted Infusion Rate	
		% of Standard Initial Infusion Rate	mg/kg/h
45-60	1.6-2.0	50%	0.075
30-44	2.1-3.0	30%	0.045
15-29	3.1-6.0	15%	0.0225
<15	>6.0	Avoid or STOP infusion	

Available Dosage Forms Injection, powder for reconstitution: 50 mg

Nursing Guidelines

Assessment: See Contraindications, Warnings/Precautions, and Dosing for use cautions. Assess potential for interactions with other prescriptions, OTC medications, or herbal products patient may be taking (especially anything that will affect coagulation or platelet function - see Drug Interactions). See Administration specifics. Bleeding precautions should be observed. Assess results of laboratory tests (see below), therapeutic effectiveness, and adverse response (see Adverse Reactions and Overdose/Toxicology) regularly during therapy. Teach possible side effects/appropriate interventions (eg, bleeding precautions) and adverse symptoms to report (see Patient Education). Note breast-feeding caution.

Monitoring Laboratory Tests: The aPTT ratio should be maintained between 1.5 and 2.5.

Patient Education: Inform prescriber of all prescriptions, OTC medications, or herbal products you are taking, and any allergies you have. Do not take any new medication during therapy unless approved by prescriber. This drug can only be administered by infusion. Report immediately any pain, swelling, burning, or bleeding at infusion site. You may have a tendency to bleed easily while taking this drug (brush teeth with soft brush, floss with waxed floss, use electric razor, avoid scissors or sharp knives, and avoid potentially harmful activities). Report unusual bleeding or bruising (bleeding gums, nosebleed, blood in urine, dark stool); pain in joints or back; CNS changes (fever, confusion); unusual fever; persistent nausea or GI upset; or swelling or pain at injection site. **Breast-feeding precaution:** Consult prescriber if breast-feeding.

Pregnancy Risk Factor: B

Lactation: Enters breast milk/consult prescriber

Perioperative/Anesthesia/Other Concerns: Heparin-Induced Thrombocytopenia (HIT): In a case series of 9 patients with HIT, the combination of lepirudin and a GP IIb/IIIa inhibitor was safe and effective during PCI (Pinto DS, 2003). Another case report describes use in patients with HIT during cardiopulmonary bypass (Liu H, 2002). During prolonged treatment (>5 days) in HIT patients, anticoagulant activity should be monitored daily (Eichler P, 2000). Antihirudin antibodies develop frequently and may enhance lepirudin's activity. In this trial, about half of the patients who developed antihirudin antibodies required a 45% (range: 17% to 90%) decrease in dose.

Administration

Oral: Administer **only** intravenously

I.V.: I.V. bolus: Inject slowly for continuous infusion; solutions with 0.2 or 0.4 mg/mL may be used.

Reconstitution: Reconstitute 50 mg vials with 1 mL water for injection or 0.9% sodium chloride injection. Bolus dose: Prepare 5 mg/mL solution by transferring contents of 1 reconstituted vial to single use, sterile syringe. Dilute to total volume of 10 mL with 0.9 sodium chloride or 5% dextrose injection. To prepare continuous infusion solutions, either 0.9% sodium chloride or 5% dextrose may be used. Add contents of two reconstituted vials to either 250 mL (to prepare 0.4 mg/mL solution) or 500 mL (to prepare 0.2 mg/mL solution). Once reconstituted, use immediately. Reconstituted solutions remain stable for 24 hours (duration of infusion).

♦ **Lepirudin (rDNA)** *see* Lepirudin *on page 1011*

Leucovorin (loo koe VOR in)

Synonyms Calcium Leucovorin; Citrovorum Factor; Folinic Acid; 5-Formyl Tetrahydrofolate; Leucovorin Calcium

Pharmacologic Category Antidote; Vitamin, Water Soluble

Medication Safety Issues

Sound-alike/look-alike issues:

Leucovorin may be confused with Leukeran®, Leukine®

Folinic acid may be confused with folic acid

Use Antidote for folic acid antagonists (methotrexate, trimethoprim, pyrimethamine); treatment of megaloblastic anemias when folate is deficient as in infancy, sprue, pregnancy, and nutritional deficiency when oral folate therapy is not possible; in combination with fluorouracil in the treatment of colon cancer

Mechanism of Action A reduced form of folic acid, leucovorin supplies the necessary cofactor blocked by methotrexate, enters the cells via the same active transport system as methotrexate. Stabilizes the binding of 5-dUMP and thymidylate synthetase, enhancing the activity of fluorouracil.

Pharmacodynamics/Kinetics

Onset of action: Oral: ~30 minutes; I.V.: ~5 minutes

Absorption: Oral, I.M.: Rapid and well absorbed

Metabolism: Intestinal mucosa and hepatically to 5-methyl-tetrahydrofolate (5MTHF; active)

(Continued)

Leucovorin *(Continued)*

Bioavailability: 31% following 200 mg dose; 98% following doses ≤25 mg
Half-life elimination: Leucovorin: 15 minutes; 5MTHF: 33-35 minutes
Excretion: Urine (80% to 90%); feces (5% to 8%)

Contraindications Hypersensitivity to leucovorin or any component of the formulation; pernicious anemia or vitamin B_{12}-deficient megaloblastic anemias

Drug Interactions May decrease efficacy of co-trimoxazole against *Pneumocystis carinii* pneumonitis

Adverse Reactions Frequency not defined.
Dermatologic: Rash, pruritus, erythema, urticaria
Hematologic: Thrombocytosis
Respiratory: Wheezing
Miscellaneous: Anaphylactoid reactions

Dosing

Adults & Elderly:

Treatment of folic acid antagonist overdosage: Oral: 2-15 mg/day for 3 days or until blood counts are normal, **or** 5 mg every 3 days; doses of 6 mg/day are needed for patients with platelet counts <100,000/mm^3.

Folate-deficient megaloblastic anemia: I.M.: 1 mg/day

Megaloblastic anemia secondary to congenital deficiency of dihydrofolate reductase: I.M.: 3-6 mg/day

Rescue dose: Initial: I.V.: 10 mg/m^2, then:

Oral, I.M., I.V., SubQ: 10-15 mg/m^2 every 6 hours until methotrexate level <0.05 micromole/L; if methotrexate level remains >5 micromole/L at 48-72 hours after the end of the methotrexate infusion, increase to 20-100 mg/m^2 every 6 hours until methotrexate level <0.05 micromole/L

Investigational: Post I.T. methotrexate: Oral, I.V.: 12 mg/m^2 as a single dose

Pediatrics: Refer to adult dosing.

Available Dosage Forms

Injection, powder for reconstitution, as calcium: 50 mg, 100 mg, 200 mg, 350 mg, 500 mg
Injection, solution, as calcium: 10 mg/mL (50 mL)
Tablet, as calcium: 5 mg, 10 mg, 15 mg, 25 mg

Nursing Guidelines

Assessment: Monitor for adverse reactions.

Monitoring Laboratory Tests: Plasma methotrexate concentration as a therapeutic guide to high-dose methotrexate therapy with leucovorin factor rescue. Leucovorin is continued until the plasma methotrexate level is <0.05 micromole/L. Each dose of leucovorin is increased if the plasma methotrexate concentration is excessively high. With 4- to 6-hour high-dose methotrexate infusions, plasma drug values in excess of 50 and 1 micromole/L at 24 and 48 hours after starting the infusion, respectively, are often predictive of delayed methotrexate clearance.

Patient Education: Take as directed, at evenly spaced intervals around-the-clock. Maintain hydration (2-3 L of water/day while taking for rescue therapy). For folic acid deficiency, eat foods high in folic acid (eg, meat proteins, bran, dried beans, asparagus, green leafy vegetables). Report respiratory difficulty, lethargy, or rash or itching. **Pregnancy precaution:** Inform prescriber if you are or intend to become pregnant.

Pregnancy Risk Factor: C

Lactation: Enters breast milk/compatible

Administration

Oral: Doses >25 mg should be administered parenterally.

I.V.: Refer to individual protocols. Leucovorin calcium should be administered I.M. or I.V. Leucovorin should not be administered concurrently with methotrexate. It is commonly initiated 24 hours after the start of methotrexate. Toxicity to normal tissues may be irreversible if leucovorin is not initiated by ~40 hours after the start of methotrexate. **Note:** The manufacturer states that leucovorin should not be given intrathecally/intraventricularly; however, it has been given by these routes.

As a rescue after folate antagonists: Leucovorin may be administered by I.V. bolus injection, I.M. injection, or orally. Doses >25 mg should be administered parenterally.

In combination with fluorouracil: When leucovorin is used to modulate fluorouracil activity, the fluorouracil is usually given after, or at the midpoint, of the leucovorin infusion. Leucovorin is usually administered by I.V. bolus injection or short (10-15 minutes) I.V. infusion. Other administration schedules have been used; refer to individual protocols.

Reconstitution: Reconstitute with SWFI, bacteriostatic NS, BWFI, NS, or D_5W; dilute in 100-1000 mL NS, D_5W for infusion

Compatibility: Stable in $D_{10}NS$, D_5W, $D_{10}W$, LR, SWFI, bacteriostatic water, NS, bacteriostatic NS

Y-site administration: Incompatible with amphotericin B cholesteryl sulfate complex, droperidol, foscarnet, sodium bicarbonate

Compatibility in syringe: Incompatible with droperidol

Compatibility when admixed: Incompatible with concentrations >2 mg/mL of leucovorin and >25 mg/mL of fluorouracil

Storage: Store at room temperature; protect from light. Reconstituted solution is chemically stable for 7 days; reconstitutions with bacteriostatic water for injection, U.S.P., must be used within 7 days. Parenteral admixture is stable for 24 hours stored at room temperature (25°C) and for 4 days when stored under refrigeration (4°C).

◆ **Leucovorin Calcium** *see* Leucovorin *on page 1013*

◆ **Leukine®** *see* Sargramostim *on page 1509*

Leuprolide (loo PROE lide)

U.S. Brand Names Eligard®; Lupron®; Lupron Depot®; Lupron Depot-Ped®; Viadur®

Synonyms Abbott-43818; Leuprolide Acetate; Leuprorelin Acetate; NSC-377526; TAP-144

Pharmacologic Category Gonadotropin Releasing Hormone Agonist

Medication Safety Issues

Sound-alike/look-alike issues:

Lupron® may be confused with Nuprin®

Use Palliative treatment of advanced prostate carcinoma; management of endometriosis as initial treatment and/or treatment of recurrent symptoms; preoperative treatment of anemia caused by uterine leiomyomata (fibroids); central precocious puberty

Unlabeled/Investigational Use Treatment of breast, ovarian, and endometrial cancer; infertility; prostatic hyperplasia

Mechanism of Action Potent inhibitor of gonadotropin secretion; continuous daily administration results in suppression of ovarian and testicular steroidogenesis due to decreased levels of LH and FSH with subsequent decrease in testosterone (male) and estrogen (female) levels. Leuprolide may also have a direct inhibitory effect on the testes, and act by a different mechanism not directly related to reduction in serum testosterone.

Pharmacodynamics/Kinetics

Onset of action: Following transient increase, testosterone suppression occurs in ~2-4 weeks of continued therapy

Distribution: Males: V_d: 27 L

Protein binding: 43% to 49%

Metabolism: Major metabolite, pentapeptide (M-1)

Bioavailability: Oral: None; SubQ: 94%

Half-life elimination: 3 hours

Excretion: Urine (<5% as parent and major metabolite)

Contraindications Hypersensitivity to leuprolide, GnRH, GnRH-agonist analogs, or any component of the formulation; spinal cord compression (orchiectomy suggested); undiagnosed abnormal vaginal bleeding; pregnancy; breast-feeding

Warnings/Precautions Transient increases in testosterone serum levels occur at the start of treatment. Tumor flare, bone pain, neuropathy, urinary tract obstruction, and spinal cord compression have been reported when used for prostate cancer; closely observe patients for weakness, paresthesias, hematuria, and urinary tract obstruction in first few weeks of therapy. Observe patients with metastatic vertebral lesions or urinary obstruction closely. Exacerbation of endometriosis or uterine leiomyomata may occur initially. Decreased bone density has been reported when used for ≥6 months. Use caution in patients with a history of psychiatric illness; alteration in mood, memory impairment, and depression have been associated with use. Rare cases of pituitary apoplexy (frequently secondary to pituitary adenoma) have been observed with leuprolide administration (onset from 1 hour to usually <2 weeks); may present as sudden headache, vomiting, visual or mental status changes, and infrequently cardiovascular collapse; immediate medical attention required.

(Continued)

Leuprolide *(Continued)*

Lab Interactions Interferes with pituitary gonadotropic and gonadal function tests during and up to 3 months after therapy. Viadur®: Efficacy and stability of product not affected by MRI or radiographic exposure, although device will be visualized during these diagnostic procedures.

Adverse Reactions

Children:

1% to 10%:

Central nervous system: Pain (2%)
Dermatologic: Acne (2%), rash (2%), seborrhea (2%)
Genitourinary: Vaginitis (2%), vaginal bleeding (2%), vaginal discharge (2%)
Local: Injection site reaction (5%)

<1%: Alopecia, cervix disorder, dysphagia, emotional lability, epistaxis, fever, gingivitis, gynecomastia, headache, nausea, nervousness, peripheral edema, personality disorder, sexual maturity accelerated, skin striae, somnolence, syncope, urinary incontinence, vasodilation, vomiting, weight gain

Adults (frequency dependent upon formulation and indication):

Cardiovascular: Angina, atrial fibrillation, CHF, deep vein thrombosis, edema, hot flashes, hypertension, MI, peripheral edema, syncope, tachycardia
Central nervous system: Abnormal thinking, agitation, amnesia, anxiety, chills, confusion, convulsion, dementia, depression, dizziness, fatigue, fever, headache, insomnia, malaise, pain, vertigo
Dermatologic: Alopecia, bruising, burning, cellulitis, pruritus
Endocrine & metabolic: Bone density decreased, breast enlargement, breast tenderness, dehydration, hirsutism, hyperglycemia, hyperlipidemia, hyperphosphatemia, libido decreased, menstrual disorders, potassium decreased
Gastrointestinal: Anorexia, appetite increased, constipation, diarrhea, dry mucous membranes, dysphagia, eructation, GI hemorrhage, gingivitis, gum hemorrhage, intestinal obstruction, nausea, peptic ulcer, vomiting, weight gain/loss
Genitourinary: Balanitis, impotence, nocturia, penile shrinkage, testicular atrophy; urinary disorder (eg, urgency, incontinence, retention); UTI, vaginitis
Hematologic: Anemia, platelets decreased, PT prolonged, WBC increased
Hepatic: Hepatomegaly, liver function tests abnormal
Local: Abscess, injection site reaction
Neuromuscular & skeletal: Arthritis, bone pain, leg cramps, myalgia, paresthesia, tremor, weakness
Renal: BUN increased
Respiratory: Allergic reaction, dyspnea, emphysema, hemoptysis, hypoxia, lung edema, pulmonary embolism
Miscellaneous: Body odor, diaphoresis, flu-like syndrome, neoplasm, night sweats, voice alteration

Children and Adults: Postmarketing/case reports: Anaphylactic reactions, asthmatic reactions, bone density decreased; fibromyalgia-like symptoms (arthralgia/myalgia, headaches, GI distress); hypotension, induration at the injection site, peripheral neuropathy, photosensitivity, pituitary apoplexy, prostate pain, rash, spinal fracture/paralysis, tenosynovitis-like symptoms, urticaria, WBC decreased

Overdosage/Toxicology Treatment is supportive.

Dosing

Adults & Elderly:

Advanced prostatic carcinoma:

SubQ:

Eligard®: 7.5 mg monthly **or** 22.5 mg every 3 months **or** 30 mg every 4 months **or** 45 mg every 6 months
Lupron®: 1 mg/day
Viadur®: 65 mg implanted subcutaneously every 12 months

I.M.:

Lupron Depot®: 7.5 mg/dose given monthly (every 28-33 days) **or**
Lupron Depot-3®: 22.5 mg every 3 months **or**
Lupron Depot-4®: 30 mg every 4 months

Endometriosis: I.M.: Initial therapy may be with leuprolide alone or in combination with norethindrone; if retreatment for an additional 6 months is necessary, norethindrone should be used. Retreatment is not recommended for longer than one additional 6-month course.

Lupron Depot®: 3.75 mg/month for up to 6 months **or**

Lupron Depot-3®: 11.25 mg every 3 months for up to 2 doses (6 months total duration of treatment)

Uterine leiomyomata (fibroids): I.M. (in combination with iron):

Lupron Depot®: 3.75 mg/month for up to 3 months **or**

Lupron Depot-3®: 11.25 mg as a single injection

Pediatrics:

Precocious puberty (consider discontinuing by age 11 for females and by age 12 for males):

SubQ (Lupron®): 20-45 mcg/kg/day; titrate dose upward by 10 mcg/kg/day if down-regulation is not achieved

I.M. (Lupron Depot-Ped®): 0.3 mg/kg/dose given every 28 days (minimum dose: 7.5 mg)

≤25 kg: 7.5 mg

>25-37.5 kg: 11.25 mg

>37.5 kg: 15 mg

Titrate dose upward in 3.75 mg every 4 weeks if down-regulation is not achieved.

Available Dosage Forms

Implant (Viadur®): 65 mg [released over 12 months; packaged with administration kit]

Injection, solution, as acetate (Lupron®): 5 mg/mL (2.8 mL) [contains benzyl alcohol; packaged with syringes and alcohol swabs]

Injection, powder for reconstitution, as acetate [depot formulation; prefilled syringe]:

Eligard®:

7.5 mg [released over 1 month]

22.5 mg [released over 3 months]

30 mg [released over 4 months]

45 mg [released over 6 months]

Lupron Depot®: 3.75 mg, 7.5 mg [released over 1 month; contains polysorbate 80]

Lupron Depot®-3 Month: 11.25 mg, 22.5 mg [released over 3 months; contains polysorbate 80]

Lupron Depot®-4 Month: 30 mg [released over 4 months; contains polysorbate 80]

Lupron Depot-Ped®: 7.5 mg, 11.25 mg, 15 mg [released over 1 month; contains polysorbate 80]

Nursing Guidelines

Assessment: Assess results of laboratory tests, therapeutic effectiveness, and adverse reactions (eg, urinary tract obstruction, weakness, paresthesias, and urinary tract obstruction in first few weeks of therapy) on a regular basis throughout therapy. Teach patient (or caregiver) proper use (eg, storage, injection technique, syringe/needle disposal), possible side effects/appropriate interventions, and adverse symptoms to report. **Pregnancy risk factor X:** Determine that patient is not pregnant before beginning treatment and do not give to females of childbearing age unless capable of complying with contraceptive measures 1 month prior to therapy, during therapy, and 1 month following therapy. Instruct patient in appropriate contraceptive measures.

Monitoring Laboratory Tests: Precocious puberty: GnRH testing (blood LH and FSH levels), testosterone in males and estradiol in females

Patient Education: Use as directed. Do not discontinue without consulting prescriber. You may experience disease flare (increased bone pain) and urinary retention during early treatment (usually resolves); dizziness, headache, lethargy, or faintness (use caution when driving or engaging in tasks that require alertness until response to drug is known); nausea or vomiting (small frequent meals or analgesics may help); hot flashes, flushing, or redness (cold cloth and cool environment may help); breast swelling or tenderness; or decreased libido. Report irregular or rapid heartbeat, palpitations, chest pain; inability to void or changes in urinary pattern; unresolved nausea or vomiting; numbness of extremities; breast swelling or pain, respiratory difficulty, or redness, swelling or pain at injection sites. **Pregnancy/breast-feeding precautions:** Inform prescriber if you are pregnant. Do not get pregnant. Consult prescriber for appropriate contraceptive use during and for a time following therapy. Do not breast-feed.

Geriatric Considerations: Leuprolide has the advantage of not increasing risk of atherosclerotic vascular disease, causing swelling of breasts, fluid retention, and thromboembolism as compared to estrogen therapy.

(Continued)

Leuprolide *(Continued)*

Pregnancy Risk Factor: X

Pregnancy Issues: Pregnancy must be excluded prior to the start of treatment. Although leuprolide usually inhibits ovulation and stops menstruation, contraception is not ensured and a nonhormonal contraceptive should be used. May cause fetal harm if administered to a pregnant woman.

Lactation: Excretion in breast milk unknown/contraindicated

Perioperative/Anesthesia/Other Concerns:

Eligard® is a nongelatin-based, biodegradable, polymer matrix.

Viadur® is a leuprolide acetate implant containing 72 mg of leuprolide acetate, equivalent to 65 mg leuprolide free base. One Viadur® implant delivers 120 mcg of leuprolide/day over 12 months.

Administration

I.M.:

Eligard®: Packaged in two syringes; one contains the Atrigel® polymer system, and the second contains leuprolide acetate powder; follow instructions for mixing; must be administered within 30 minutes of mixing

Lupron Depot®: Do not use needles smaller than 22 gauge; reconstitute only with diluent provided

Storage:

Lupron®: Store unopened vials of injection in refrigerator, vial in use can be kept at room temperature of ≤30°C (86°F) for several months with minimal loss of potency. Protect from light and store vial in carton until use. Do not freeze.

Eligard®: Store at 2°C to 8°C (36°F to 46°C). Allow to reach room temperature prior to using; once mixed, must be administered within 30 minutes.

Lupron Depot® may be stored at room temperature of 25°C, excursions permitted to 15°C to 30°C (59°F to 86°F). Upon reconstitution, the suspension does not contain a preservative and should be used immediately.

Viadur® may be stored at room temperature of 15°C to 30°C (59°F and 86°F).

◆ **Leuprolide Acetate** *see* Leuprolide *on page 1015*
◆ **Leuprorelin Acetate** *see* Leuprolide *on page 1015*
◆ **Leurocristine Sulfate** *see* VinCRIStine *on page 1710*
◆ **Leustatin®** *see* Cladribine *on page 420*

Levalbuterol (leve al BYOO ter ole)

U.S. Brand Names Xopenex®; Xopenex HFA™

Synonyms Levalbuterol Hydrochloride; Levalbuterol Tartrate; R-albuterol

Pharmacologic Category $Beta_2$-Adrenergic Agonist

Medication Safety Issues

Sound-alike/look-alike issues:

Xopenex® may be confused with Xanax®

Use Treatment or prevention of bronchospasm in children and adults with reversible obstructive airway disease

Mechanism of Action Relaxes bronchial smooth muscle by action on beta-2 receptors with little effect on heart rate

Pharmacodynamics/Kinetics

Onset of action:
- Aerosol: 5.5-10.2 minutes
  - Peak effect: ~77 minutes
- Nebulization: 10-17 minutes (measured as a 15% increase in FEV_1)
  - Peak effect: 1.5 hours

Duration:
- Aerosol: 3-4 hours (up to 6 hours in some patients)
- Nebulization: 5-6 hours (up to 8 hours in some patients)

Absorption: A portion of inhaled dose is absorbed to systemic circulation

Half-life elimination: 3.3-4 hours

Time to peak, serum:
- Aerosol: 0.5 hours
- Nebulization: 0.2 hours

Contraindications Hypersensitivity to levalbuterol, albuterol, or any component of the formulation

Warnings/Precautions Optimize anti-inflammatory treatment before initiating maintenance treatment with levalbuterol. Do not use as a component of chronic therapy without an anti-inflammatory agent. Only the mildest form of asthma (Step 1 and/or exercise-induced) would not require concurrent use based upon asthma guidelines. Patient must be instructed to seek medical attention in cases where acute symptoms are not relieved or a previous level of response is diminished. The need to increase frequency of use may indicate deterioration of asthma, and treatment must not be delayed.

Use caution in patients with cardiovascular disease (arrhythmia or hypertension or CHF), convulsive disorders, diabetes, glaucoma, hyperthyroidism, or hypokalemia. Beta agonists may cause elevation in blood pressure, heart rate, and result in CNS stimulation/excitation. $Beta_2$ agonists may increase risk of arrhythmia, increase serum glucose, or decrease serum potassium.

Do not exceed recommended dose; serious adverse events including fatalities, have been associated with excessive use of inhaled sympathomimetics. Rarely, paradoxical bronchospasm may occur with use of inhaled bronchodilating agents; this should be distinguished from inadequate response. Use with caution during labor and delivery. Safety and efficacy have not been established in patients <4 years of age.

Drug Interactions

Anesthetics (inhaled): Cardiac effects of levalbuterol may be potentiated; use with caution.

Beta-blockers (particularly nonselective agents): May block the effect of levalbuterol and also produce severe bronchospasm.

Diuretics (nonpotassium-sparing): ECG changes and/or hypokalemia may result from concomitant use; use caution.

Digoxin: Plasma levels of digoxin may be decreased by 16% to 22%; monitor.

MAO inhibitors: Cardiac effects of levalbuterol may be potentiated; use with extreme caution or within 2 weeks of discontinuing MAO inhibitor.

Sympathomimetics (including amphetamine, dobutamine): Cardiac effects of levalbuterol may be potentiated; use with caution.

Tricyclic antidepressants (TCAs): Cardiac effects of levalbuterol may be potentiated; use with extreme caution or within 2 weeks of discontinuing TCAs

Adverse Reactions Immediate hypersensitivity reactions have occurred, including angioedema, oropharyngeal edema, urticaria, rash, and anaphylaxis.

>10%:

Endocrine & metabolic: Serum glucose increased, serum potassium decreased

Respiratory: Viral infection (7% to 12%), rhinitis (3% to 11%)

>2% to <10%:

Central nervous system: Nervousness (3% to 10%), tremor (≤7%), anxiety (3%), dizziness (1% to 3%), migraine (≤3%), pain (1% to 3%)

Cardiovascular: Tachycardia (~3%)

Gastrointestinal: Dyspepsia (1% to 3%)

Neuromuscular & skeletal: Leg cramps (≤3%)

Respiratory: Asthma (9%), pharyngitis (8%), cough (1% to 4%), nasal edema (1% to 3%), sinusitis (1% to 4%)

Miscellaneous: Flu-like syndrome (1% to 4%), accidental injury (≤3%)

<2% (Limited to important or life-threatening): Angina, arrhythmia, atrial fibrillation, extrasystole, headache, hematuria, hyper-/hypotension, hypokalemia, insomnia, oropharyngeal dryness, paresthesia, supraventricular arrhythmia, syncope, tremor, vertigo; immediate hypersensitivity reactions have occurred (including angioedema, oropharyngeal edema, urticaria, rash, and anaphylaxis)

Overdosage/Toxicology Symptoms of overdose include tachycardia, tremor, hypertension, angina, and seizures. Hypokalemia also may occur. Cardiac arrest and death may be associated with abuse of beta-agonist bronchodilators. Treatment includes immediate discontinuation and symptomatic and supportive therapies. Cautious use of beta-adrenergic blocking agents may be considered in severe cases.

Dosing

Adults: Bronchospasm:

Metered-dose inhalation: Aerosol: 1-2 puffs every 4-6 hours

Nebulization: 0.63 mg 3 times/day at intervals of 6-8 hours; dosage may be increased to 1.25 mg 3 times/day with close monitoring for adverse effects. Most patients gain optimal benefit from regular use

Elderly: Only a small number of patients have been studied. Although greater sensitivity of some elderly patients cannot be ruled out, no overall differences in safety or effectiveness were observed. An initial dose of 0.63 mg should be used in all patients >65 years of age.

Pediatrics: Bronchospasm:

Metered-dose inhalation: Aerosol: Children ≥4 years: Refer to adult dosing.

(Continued)

Levalbuterol *(Continued)*

Nebulization:

Children 6-11 years: 0.31 mg 3 times/day (maximum dose: 0.63 mg 3 times/day)

Children >12 years: Refer to adult dosing.

Available Dosage Forms Note: Strength expressed as base.

Aerosol, oral, as tartrate: 45 mcg/actuation (15 g) [200 doses; chlorofluorocarbon free]

Solution for nebulization, as hydrochloride: 0.31 mg/3 mL (24s); 0.63 mg/3 mL (24s); 1.25 mg/3 mL (24s)

Solution for nebulization, concentrate, as hydrochloride: 1.25 mg/0.5 mL (30s)

Nursing Guidelines

Assessment: Assess effectiveness and interactions of other medications patient may be taking. Monitor therapeutic effectiveness (patient response and laboratory values), adverse reactions (eg, anaphylaxis or hypertension, first dose administered under supervision), or overdose. Patients with diabetes should monitor serum glucose on a regular basis (possibility of hyperglycemia). Assess knowledge/teach patient appropriate use (safe use of nebulizer), interventions to reduce side effects, and adverse reactions to report.

Monitoring Laboratory Tests: FEV_1 and/or peak expiratory flow rate, arterial blood gases (if condition warrants); serum potassium, serum glucose (in selected patients)

Patient Education: Use only when necessary or as prescribed; tolerance may develop with overuse. Do not administer more frequently than prescribed. First dose should not be used when you are alone. Avoid OTC medications without consulting prescriber. Maintain adequate hydration (2-3 L/day of fluids) unless instructed to restrict fluid intake. Stress or excessive exercising may exacerbate wheezing or bronchospasm (controlled breathing or relaxation techniques may help). If you have diabetes, you will need to monitor serum glucose levels closely until response is known; notify diabetic advisor if hyperglycemia occurs. You may experience tremor, anxiety, dizziness (use caution when driving or engaging in hazardous activities until response to drug is known); or temporarily upset stomach, nausea, or vomiting (small frequent meals, frequent mouth care, chewing gum, or sucking hard candy may help). Paradoxical bronchospasm can occur. Stop drug immediately and notify prescriber if any of the following occur: chest pain, tightness, palpitations; severe headache; respiratory difficulty; increased nervousness, restlessness, or trembling; muscle cramps or weakness; or seizures. Report unusual signs of flu or infection, leg or muscle cramps, unusual cough, persistent GI problems, vision changes, or other adverse effects. **Pregnancy/breast-feeding precautions:** Inform prescriber if you are or intend to become pregnant. Consult prescriber if breast-feeding.

Geriatric Considerations: For aerosol formulation, start with low end of dosage range. Refer to dosing information for nebulization dosing specifics.

Pregnancy Risk Factor: C

Pregnancy Issues: Teratogenic effects were not observed in animal studies; however, racemic albuterol was teratogenic in some species. There are no adequate and well-controlled studies in pregnant women. This drug should be used during pregnancy only if benefit exceeds risk. Use caution if needed for bronchospasm during labor and delivery; has potential to interfere with uterine contractions.

Lactation: Excretion in breast milk unknown/use caution

Breast-Feeding Considerations: It is not known whether levalbuterol is excreted in human milk. Plasma levels following oral inhalation are low. Racemic albuterol was shown to be tumorigenic in animal studies.

Administration

Reconstitution: Concentrated solution should be diluted with 2.5 mL NS prior to use.

Storage: Aerosol: Store at room temperature of 20°C to 25°C (68°F to 77°F); protect from freezing and direct sunlight. Store with mouthpiece up. Discard after 200 actuations.

Solution for nebulization: Store in protective foil pouch at room temperature of 20°C to 25°C (68°F to 77°F). Protect from light and excessive heat. Vials should be used within 2 weeks after opening protective pouch. Use within 1 week and protect from light if removed from pouch. Vials of concentrated solution should be used immediately after removing from protective pouch.

♦ **Levalbuterol Hydrochloride** *see* Levalbuterol *on page 1018*
♦ **Levalbuterol Tartrate** *see* Levalbuterol *on page 1018*
♦ **Levaquin®** *see* Levofloxacin *on page 1025*
♦ **Levarterenol Bitartrate** *see* Norepinephrine *on page 1242*
♦ **Levbid®** *see* Hyoscyamine *on page 886*
♦ **Levemir®** *see* Insulin Detemir *on page 919*

Levetiracetam (lee va tye RA se tam)

U.S. Brand Names Keppra®

Pharmacologic Category Anticonvulsant, Miscellaneous

Medication Safety Issues

Sound-alike/look-alike issues:

Potential for dispensing errors between Keppra® and Kaletra™ (lopinavir/ritonavir)

Use Adjunctive therapy in the treatment of partial onset seizures

Unlabeled/Investigational Use Bipolar disorder

Mechanism of Action The precise mechanism by which levetiracetam exerts its antiepileptic effect is unknown. However, several studies have suggested the mechanism may involve one or more of the following central pharmacologic effects: inhibition of voltage-dependent N-type calcium channels; blockade of GABA-ergic inhibitory transmission through displacement of negative modulators; reduction of delayed rectifier potassium current; and/or binding to synaptic proteins which modulate neurotransmitter release.

Pharmacodynamics/Kinetics

Onset of action: Peak effect: 1 hour

Absorption: Rapid and complete

Protein binding: <10%

Metabolism: Not extensive; primarily by enzymatic hydrolysis; forms metabolites (inactive)

Bioavailability: 100%

Half-life elimination: 6-8 hours

Excretion: Urine (66% as unchanged drug)

Contraindications Hypersensitivity to levetiracetam or any component of the formulation

Warnings/Precautions Psychotic symptoms (psychosis, hallucinations) and behavioral symptoms (including aggression, anger, anxiety, depersonalization, depression, personality disorder) may occur; incidence may be increased in children. Dose reduction may be required. Levetiracetam should be withdrawn gradually to minimize the potential of increased seizure frequency. There is a potential for dispensing errors between Keppra® and Kaletra™ (lopinavir/ritonavir); use caution when prescribing, dispensing, or administering. Use caution with renal impairment (dosage adjustment may be necessary).

Drug Interactions No interaction was observed in pharmacokinetic trials with other anticonvulsants, including phenytoin, carbamazepine, valproic acid, phenobarbital, lamotrigine, gabapentin, and primidone.

Nutritional/Herbal/Ethanol Interactions

Ethanol: Avoid ethanol (may increase CNS depression).

Food: Food may delay, but does not affect the extent of absorption.

Adverse Reactions

>10%:

Central nervous system: Behavioral symptoms (agitation, aggression, anger, anxiety, apathy, depersonalization, depression, emotional lability, hostility, hyperkinesias, irritability, nervousness, neurosis and personality disorder: adults 13%; children 38%), somnolence (15% to 23%), headache (14%), hostility (2% to 12%)

Gastrointestinal: Vomiting (15%), anorexia (13%)

Neuromuscular & skeletal: Weakness (9% to 15%)

Respiratory: Rhinitis (4% to 13%), cough (2% to 11%)

Miscellaneous: Accidental injury (17%), infection (2% to 13%)

1% to 10%:

Cardiovascular: Facial edema (2%)

Central nervous system: Nervousness (4% to 10%), dizziness (7% to 9%), personality disorder (8%), pain (6% to 7%), agitation (6%), emotional lability (2% to 6%), depression (3% to 4%), ataxia (3%), vertigo (3%), amnesia (2%), anxiety (2%), confusion (2%), psychotic symptoms (1%)

Dermatologic: Bruising (4%), pruritus (2%), rash (2%), skin discoloration (2%)

(Continued)

Levetiracetam *(Continued)*

Gastrointestinal: Diarrhea (8%), gastroenteritis (4%), anorexia (3%), constipation (3%), dehydration (2%)
Hematologic: Decreased leukocytes (2% to 3%)
Neuromuscular & skeletal: Neck pain (2%), paresthesia (2%), reflexes increased (2%)
Ocular: Conjunctivitis (3%), diplopia (2%), amblyopia (2%)
Otic: Ear pain (2%)
Renal: Albuminuria (4%), urine abnormality (2%)
Respiratory: Pharyngitis (6% to 10%), asthma (2%), sinusitis (2%)
Miscellaneous: Flu-like symptoms (3%), viral infection (2%)

<1% (Limited to important or life-threatening): Alopecia, attempted suicide, leukopenia, neutropenia, pancreatitis, pancytopenia, suicidal ideation, thrombocytopenia

Overdosage/Toxicology Limited experience. Symptoms would be expected to include drowsiness, somnolence and ataxia. Treatment is symptomatic and supportive. Hemodialysis may be effective (estimated clearance of ~50% in 4 hours).

Dosing

Adults & Elderly:

Partial onset seizures (adjunctive): Oral: Initial: 500 mg twice daily; may increase every 2 weeks by 500 mg/dose to a maximum of 1500 mg twice daily. Doses >3000 mg/day have been used in trials; however, there is no evidence of increased benefit.

Bipolar disorder (unlabeled use): Initial: 500 mg twice daily; if tolerated, increase to 500 mg twice daily; dose may be increased every 3 days until target dose of 3000 mg/day is reached; maximum: 4000 mg/day

Pediatrics:

Partial onset seizures: Oral:

Children 4-15 years: Partial onset seizures: 10 mg/kg/dose given twice daily; may increase every 2 weeks by 10 mg/kg/dose to a maximum of 30 mg/kg/dose twice daily

Children ≥16 years: Refer to adult dosing.

Bipolar disorder (unlabeled use): Oral: Children ≥16 years: Refer to adult dosing.

Renal Impairment: Adults:

Cl_{cr} >80 mL/minute: 500-1500 mg every 12 hours
Cl_{cr} 50-80 mL/minute: 500-1000 mg every 12 hours
Cl_{cr} 30-50 mL/minute: 250-750 mg every 12 hours
Cl_{cr} <30 mL/minute: 250-500 mg every 12 hours
End-stage renal disease patients using dialysis: 500-1000 mg every 24 hours; a supplemental dose of 250-500 mg following dialysis is recommended

Hepatic Impairment: No adjustment necessary.

Available Dosage Forms

Solution, oral: 100 mg/mL (480 mL) [dye free; grape flavor]
Tablet: 250 mg, 500 mg, 750 mg

Nursing Guidelines

Assessment: Assess effectiveness and interactions of other medications patient may be taking. Monitor therapeutic effectiveness, laboratory values, and adverse reactions at beginning of therapy and periodically with long-term use. Monitor for CNS depression (somnolence and fatigue), behavioral abnormalities (psychosis, hallucinations, psychotic depression), and other behavioral symptoms (agitation, anger, aggression, irritability, hostility, anxiety, apathy, emotional lability, depersonalization, and depression). Taper dosage slowly when discontinuing. Observe and teach seizure/safety precautions. Assess knowledge/teach patient appropriate use, interventions to reduce side effects, and adverse symptoms to report.

Dietary Considerations: May be taken with or without food.

Patient Education: Take exactly as directed; do not increase dose or frequency or discontinue without consulting prescriber. While using this medication, do not use alcohol and other prescription or OTC medications (especially pain medications, sedatives, antihistamines, or hypnotics) without consulting prescriber. Maintain adequate hydration (2-3 L/day of fluids) unless instructed to restrict fluid intake. You may experience drowsiness, dizziness, or blurred vision (use caution when driving or engaging in tasks requiring alertness until response to drug is known); or nausea, vomiting, loss of appetite, or dry mouth (small frequent meals, frequent mouth care, chewing gum, or sucking lozenges may help). Wear identification of epileptic status and medications. Report CNS changes, mentation changes, or changes in cognition; muscle cramping, weakness, tremors, changes in gait; persistent GI symptoms (cramping, constipation, vomiting, anorexia); rash or skin irritations; unusual bruising or bleeding (mouth, urine, stool); or worsening of seizure activity or loss of seizure control. **Pregnancy/breast-feeding precautions:** Inform prescriber if you are or intend to become pregnant. Breast-feeding is not recommended.

Pregnancy Risk Factor: C

Pregnancy Issues: Developmental toxicities were observed in animal studies. There are no adequate and well-controlled studies in pregnant women. Two registries are available for women exposed to levetiracetam during pregnancy:

Antiepileptic Drug Pregnancy Registry (888-233-2334 or http://www.mgh.harvard.edu/aed/)

Keppra® pregnancy registry (888-537-7734 or http://www.keppra.com)

Lactation: Enters breast milk/not recommended

Administration

Oral: Tablets may be crushed and placed in food if unable to swallow whole (bitter taste may be expected).

Storage: Store at 25°C (77°F).

Levobupivacaine (LEE voe byoo PIV a kane)

U.S. Brand Names Chirocaine® [DSC]

Pharmacologic Category Local Anesthetic

Use Production of local or regional anesthesia for surgery and obstetrics, and for postoperative pain management

Mechanism of Action Levobupivacaine is the S-enantiomer of bupivacaine. It blocks both the initiation and transmission of nerve impulses by decreasing the neuronal membrane's permeability to sodium ions, which results in inhibition of depolarization with resultant blockade of conduction. Local anesthetics reversibly prevent generation and conduction of electrical impulses in neurons by decreasing the transient increase in permeability to sodium. The differential sensitivity generally depends on the size of the fiber; small fibers are more sensitive than larger fibers and require a longer period for recovery. Sensory pain fibers are usually blocked first, followed by fibers that transmit sensations of temperature, touch, and deep pressure. High concentrations block sympathetic somatic sensory and somatic motor fibers. The spread of anesthesia depends upon the distribution of the solution. This is primarily dependent on the site of administration and volume of drug injected.

Pharmacodynamics/Kinetics

Onset of action: Epidural: 10-14 minutes

Duration (dose dependent): 1-8 hours

Absorption: Dependent on route of administration and dose

Distribution: 67 L

Protein binding, plasma: >97%

Metabolism: Extensively hepatic via CYP3A4 and CYP1A2

Half-life elimination: 1.3 hours

Time to peak: Epidural: 30 minutes

Excretion: Urine (71%) and feces (24%) as metabolites

Contraindications Hypersensitivity to levobupivacaine, any component of the formulation, bupivacaine, or any local anesthetic of the amide type

Warnings/Precautions Unintended intravenous injection may result in cardiac arrest. Use caution when the higher concentration formulations of levobupivacaine are used. Volumes of the high concentration are more likely to produce cardiac toxicity. The 0.75% solution should not be used in obstetrical patients. Use with caution in patients with hypotension, hypovolemia, heart block, hepatic or cardiac impairment.

Local anesthetics should be administered by clinicians familiar with the use of local anesthetic agents and performance of anesthetic procedures, as well as the management of drug-related toxicity and other acute emergencies. Resuscitative equipment and medications should be readily available. Not for use in intravenous regional anesthesia (Bier block) or to produce obstetrical paracervical block anesthesia. Use with caution in patients receiving other local anesthetics or structurally related agents.

Drug Interactions Substrate (minor) of CYP1A2, 3A4

Nutritional/Herbal/Ethanol Interactions Herb/Nutraceutical: St John's wort may decrease levobupivacaine levels.

(Continued)

Levobupivacaine *(Continued)*

Adverse Reactions

>10%:

Cardiovascular: Hypotension (20% to 31%)
Central nervous system: Pain (postoperative) (7% to 18%), fever (7% to 17%)
Gastrointestinal: Nausea (12% to 21%), vomiting (8% to 14%)
Hematologic: Anemia (10% to 12%)

1% to 10%:

Central nervous system: Pain (4% to 8%), headache (5% to 7%), dizziness (5% to 6%), hypoesthesia (3%), somnolence (1%), anxiety (1%), hypothermia (2%)
Cardiovascular: Abnormal ECG (3%), bradycardia (2%), tachycardia (2%), hypertension (1%)
Dermatologic: Pruritus (4% to 9%), purpura (1%)
Endocrine & metabolic: Breast pain - female (1%)
Gastrointestinal: Constipation (3% to 7%), enlarged abdomen (3%), flatulence (2%), abdominal pain (2%), dyspepsia (2%), diarrhea (1%)
Genitourinary: Urinary incontinence (1%), urine flow decreased (1%), urinary tract infection (1%)
Hematologic: Leukocytosis (1%)
Local: Anesthesia (1%)
Neuromuscular & skeletal: Back pain (6%), rigors (3%), paresthesia (2%)
Ocular: Diplopia (3%)
Renal: Albuminuria (3%), hematuria (2%)
Respiratory: Cough (1%)
Miscellaneous: Fetal distress (5% to 10%), delayed delivery (6%), hemorrhage in pregnancy (2%), uterine abnormality (2%), increased wound drainage (1%)

<1% (Limited to important or life-threatening): Apnea, arrhythmia, atrial fibrillation, bronchospasm, cardiac arrest, confusion, dyspnea, generalized spasm, ileus, involuntary muscle contraction, pulmonary edema, skin discoloration, syncope

Overdosage/Toxicology Related to local concentration or due to unintended intrathecal or intravenous injection. Symptoms may include restlessness, anxiety, incoherent speech, lightheadedness, numbness and tingling of the mouth and lips, metallic taste, tinnitus, dizziness, blurred vision, tremors, respiratory arrest, twitching, depression or drowsiness. In addition, cardiac toxicity, including AV block, bradycardia, arrhythmia, and hypotension may occur. Treatment is symptomatic.

Dosing

Adults & Elderly: Note: Rapid injection of a large volume of local anesthetic solution should be avoided. Fractional (incremental) doses are recommended.
Guidelines (individual response varies): See table.

	Concentration	Volume	Dose	Motor Block
Surgical Anesthesia				
Epidural for surgery	0.5%-0.75%	10-20 mL	50-150 mg	Moderate to complete
Epidural for C-section	0.5%	20-30 mL	100-150 mg	Moderate to complete
Peripheral nerve	0.25%-0.5%	0.4 mL/kg (30 mL)	1-2 mg/kg (75-150 mg)	Moderate to complete
Ophthalmic	0.75%	5-15 mL	37.5-112.5 mg	Moderate to complete
Local infiltration	0.25%	60 mL	150 mg	Not applicable
Pain Management				
Levobupivacaine can be used epidurally with fentanyl or clonidine; dilutions for epidural administration should be made with preservative free 0.9% saline according to standard hospital procedures for sterility				
Labor analgesia (epidural bolus)	0.25%	10-20 mL	25-50 mg	Minimal to moderate
Postoperative pain (epidural infusion)	0.125%[1]-0.25%	4-10 mL/h	5-25 mg/h	Minimal to moderate

[1]0.125%: Adjunct therapy with fentanyl or clonidine.

Maximum dosage: Epidural doses up to 375 mg have been administered incrementally to patients during a surgical procedure.
Intraoperative block and postoperative pain: 695 mg in 24 hours
Postoperative epidural infusion over 24 hours: 570 mg
Single-fractionated injection for brachial plexus block: 300 mg

Available Dosage Forms [DSC] = Discontinued product

Injection, solution [preservative free]: 2.5 mg/mL (10 mL, 30 mL); 5 mg/mL (10 mL, 30 mL); 7.5 mg/mL (10 mL, 30 mL) [DSC]

Nursing Guidelines

Assessment: Monitor for effectiveness of anesthesia according to purpose for use. Monitor closely during and after injection for symptoms of CNS, cardiac toxicity, or hypotension. Monitor for return of sensation. Use appropriate patient safety measures until full return of sensation. Teach patient adverse symptoms to report.

Patient Education: This medication is given to reduce sensation and pain. You will experience decreased sensation to pain, heat, or cold in the area and/or decreased muscle strength (depending on area of application). Until sensation returns, use caution to prevent injury (eg, avoid extremes of heat or cold to area, do not use sharp objects, avoid driving, climbing stairs, or sudden moves if muscle strength is affected). Immediately report chest pain or palpitations; increased restlessness, anxiety, dizziness or lightheadedness; sensation of sudden muscle weakness; swelling or tingling of mouth or lips; metallic taste; vision changes or hearing. **Breast-feeding precaution:** Consult prescriber if breast-feeding.

Pregnancy Risk Factor: B

Pregnancy Issues: Local anesthetics rapidly cross the placenta and may cause varying degrees of maternal, fetal, and neonatal toxicity. Close maternal and fetal monitoring (heart rate and electronic fetal monitoring advised) are required during obstetrical use.

Lactation: Excretion in breast milk unknown/use caution

Administration

Compatibility: Stable in 0.9% NS USP. Stable for 24 hours in PVC bags at room temperature when diluted to 0.625-2.5 mg levobupivacaine per mL.

Incompatible with alkaline pH solutions (pH >8.5)

Storage: Store at room temperature (20°C to 25°C/68°F to 77°F). Disinfectants containing heavy metals should not be used for mucous membrane disinfection since they have been related to incidents of swelling and edema. Isopropyl or ethyl alcohol is recommended. Stability of solution in vial has been demonstrated following an autoclave cycle at 121°C for 15 minutes.

Levofloxacin (lee voe FLOKS a sin)

U.S. Brand Names Iquix®; Levaquin®; Quixin™

Pharmacologic Category Antibiotic, Quinolone

Use

Systemic: Treatment of mild, moderate, or severe infections caused by susceptible organisms. Includes the treatment of community-acquired pneumonia, including multidrug resistant strains of *S. pneumoniae* (MDRSP); nosocomial pneumonia; chronic bronchitis (acute bacterial exacerbation); acute bacterial sinusitis; urinary tract infection (uncomplicated or complicated), including acute pyelonephritis caused by *E. coli*; prostatitis (chronic bacterial); skin or skin structure infections (uncomplicated or complicated); prevention of inhalational anthrax (postexposure)

Ophthalmic: Treatment of bacterial conjunctivitis caused by susceptible organisms (Quixin™ 0.5% ophthalmic solution); treatment of corneal ulcer caused by susceptible organisms (Iquix® 1.5% ophthalmic solution)

Mechanism of Action As the S (-) enantiomer of the fluoroquinolone, ofloxacin, levofloxacin, inhibits DNA-gyrase in susceptible organisms thereby inhibits relaxation of supercoiled DNA and promotes breakage of DNA strands. DNA gyrase (topoisomerase II), is an essential bacterial enzyme that maintains the superhelical structure of DNA and is required for DNA replication and transcription, DNA repair, recombination, and transposition.

Pharmacodynamics/Kinetics

Absorption: Rapid and complete

Distribution: V_d: 1.25 L/kg; CSF concentrations ~15% of serum levels; high concentrations are achieved in prostate, lung, and gynecological tissues, sinus, saliva

Protein binding: 50%

Metabolism: Minimally hepatic

Bioavailability: 99%

Half-life elimination: 6-8 hours

Time to peak, serum: 1-2 hours

Excretion: Primarily urine (as unchanged drug)

(Continued)

Levofloxacin *(Continued)*

Contraindications Hypersensitivity to levofloxacin, any component of the formulation, or other quinolones

Warnings/Precautions

Systemic: Not recommended in children <18 years of age; CNS stimulation may occur (tremor, restlessness, confusion, and very rarely hallucinations or seizures); use with caution in patients with known or suspected CNS disorders or renal dysfunction; use caution to avoid possible photosensitivity reactions during and for several days following fluoroquinolone therapy

Rare cases of torsade de pointes have been reported in patients receiving levofloxacin. Risk may be minimized by avoiding use in patients with known prolongation of QT interval, bradycardia, hypokalemia, hypomagnesemia, cardiomyopathy, or in those receiving concurrent therapy with Class Ia or Class III antiarrhythmics.

Severe hypersensitivity reactions, including anaphylaxis, have occurred with quinolone therapy. If an allergic reaction occurs (itching, urticaria, dyspnea or facial edema, loss of consciousness, tingling, cardiovascular collapse), discontinue drug immediately. Prolonged use may result in superinfection; pseudomembranous colitis may occur and should be considered in all patients who present with diarrhea. Tendon inflammation and/or rupture has been reported; risk may be increased with concurrent corticosteroids, particularly in the elderly. Discontinue at first sign of tendon inflammation or pain. Peripheral neuropathies have been linked to levofloxacin use; discontinue if numbness, tingling, or weakness develops. Quinolones may exacerbate myasthenia gravis; use with caution (rare, potentially life-threatening weakness of respiratory muscles may occur).

Ophthalmic solution: For topical use only. Do not inject subconjunctivally or introduce into anterior chamber of the eye. Contact lenses should not be worn during treatment for bacterial conjunctivitis. Safety and efficacy in children <1 year of age (Quixin™) or <6 years of age (Iquix®) have not been established. **Note:** Indications for ophthalmic solutions are product concentration-specific and should not be used interchangeably.

Drug Interactions

Corticosteroids: Concurrent use may increase the risk of tendon rupture, particularly in elderly patients (overall incidence rare).

Glyburide: Quinolones may increase the effect of glyburide; monitor

Metal cations (aluminum, calcium, iron, magnesium, and zinc) bind quinolones in the gastrointestinal tract and inhibit absorption. Concurrent administration of most antacids, oral electrolyte supplements, quinapril, sucralfate, some didanosine formulations (chewable/buffered tablets and pediatric powder for oral suspension), and other highly-buffered oral drugs, should be avoided. Levofloxacin should be administered 2 hours before or 2 hours after these agents.

Probenecid: May decrease renal secretion of levofloxacin.

QT_c-prolonging agents: Effects may be additive with levofloxacin. Avoid concurrent use with Class Ia and Class III antiarrhythmics, erythromycin, cisapride, antipsychotics, and cyclic antidepressants.

Warfarin: The hypoprothrombinemic effect of warfarin may be enhanced by some quinolone antibiotics; monitor INR.

Adverse Reactions

1% to 10%:

Cardiovascular: Chest pain (1%)

Central nervous system: Headache (6%), insomnia (5%), dizziness (2%), fatigue (1%), pain (1%), fever

Dermatologic: Pruritus (1%), rash (1%)

Gastrointestinal: Nausea (7%), diarrhea (5%), abdominal pain (3%), constipation (3%), dyspepsia (2%), vomiting (2%), flatulence (1%)

Genitourinary: Vaginitis (1%)

Hematologic: Lymphopenia (2%)

Ocular (with ophthalmic solution use): Decreased vision (transient), foreign body sensation, transient ocular burning, ocular pain or discomfort, photophobia

Respiratory: Pharyngitis (4%), dyspnea (1%), rhinitis (1%), sinusitis (1%)

<1% (Limited to important or life-threatening):

Systemic: Acute renal failure; allergic reaction (including pneumonitis rash, pneumonitis, and anaphylaxis); agranulocytosis, anaphylactoid reaction, anorexia, anxiety, arrhythmia (including atrial/ventricular tachycardia/fibrillation and torsade de pointes), arthralgia, ascites, bradycardia, bronchospasm, carcinoma, cardiac failure, cerebrovascular disorder, cholecystitis, cholelithiasis, confusion, cnjunctivitis, dehydration, depression, ear disorder, edema, EEG abnormalities, electrolyte abnormality, encephalopathy, eosinophilia, erythema multiforme, gangrene, GI hemorrhage, granulocytopenia, hallucination, heart block, hematoma, hemolytic anemia, hemoptysis, hepatic failure, hyper-/hypotension, infection, INR increased, intestinal obstruction, intracranial hypertension, involuntary muscle contractions, jaundice, leukocytosis, leukopenia, leukorrhea, lymphadenopathy, MI, migraine, multiple organ failure, pancreatitis, paralysis, paresthesia, peripheral neuropathy, phlebitis, photosensitivity (<0.1%), pleural effusion, postural hypotension, prothrombin time increased/decreased, pseudomembraneous colitis, pulmonary edema,pulmonary embolism, purpura, QT_c prolongation, respiratory depression, respiratory disorder, rhabdomyolysis, seizure, skin disorder, somnolence,speech disorder, Stevens-Johnson syndrome, stupor, syncope, taste perversion, tendon rupture, tongue edema, transaminases increased, thrombocythemia, thrombocytopenia, tremor, WBC abnormality

Overdosage/Toxicology

Symptoms of overdose include acute renal failure, seizures

Treatment should include GI decontamination and supportive care; not removed by peritoneal or hemodialysis

Dosing

Adults & Elderly: Note: Sequential therapy (intravenous to oral) may be instituted based on prescriber's discretion.

Bacterial sinusitis (acute): Oral, I.V.: 500 mg every 24 hours for 10-14 days or 750 mg every 24 hours for 5 days

Chronic bronchitis (acute bacterial exacerbation): Oral, I.V.: 500 mg every 24 hours for at least 7 days

Inhalational anthrax: 500 mg every 24 hours for 60 days, beginning as soon as possible after exposure

Pneumonia: Oral, I.V.:

Community-acquired: 500 mg every 24 hours for 7-14 days or 750 mg every 24 hours for 5 days (efficacy of 5-day regimen for MDRSP not established)

Nosocomial: 750 mg every 24 hours for 7-14 days

Prostatitis (chronic bacterial): Oral, I.V.: 500 mg every 24 hours for 28 days

Skin infections: Oral, I.V.:

Uncomplicated: 500 mg every 24 hours for 7-10 days

Complicated: 750 mg every 24 hours for 7-14 days

Urinary tract infections: Oral, I.V.:

Uncomplicated: 250 mg once daily for 3 days

Complicated, including acute pyelonephritis: 250 mg every 24 hours for 10 days

Bacterial conjunctivitis: Ophthalmic (0.5% ophthalmic solution):

Treatment day 1 and day 2: Instill 1-2 drops into affected eye(s) every 2 hours while awake, up to 8 times/day

Treatment day 3 through day 7: Instill 1-2 drops into affected eye(s) every 4 hours while awake, up to 4 times/day

Corneal ulceration: Ophthalmic (1.5% ophthalmic solution):

Treatment day 1 through day 3: Instill 1-2 drops into affected eye(s) every 30 minutes to 2 hours while awake and ~4-6 hours after retiring.

Treatment day 4 to treatment completion: Instill 1-2 drops into affected eye(s) every 1-4 hours while awake.

Pediatrics: Not approved for systemic use in children.

Conjunctivitis (bacterial): Ophthalmic: Children ≥1 year: Refer to adult dosing.

Corneal ulceration: Ophthalmic: Children ≥6 years: Refer to adult dosing.

Renal Impairment:

Chronic bronchitis, acute bacterial sinusitis, uncomplicated skin infection, community-acquired pneumonia, chronic bacterial prostatitis, or inhalational anthrax: Initial: 500 mg, then as follows:

Cl_{cr} 20-49 mL/minute: 250 mg every 24 hours

Cl_{cr} 10-19 mL/minute: 250 mg every 48 hours

Hemodialysis/CAPD: 250 mg every 48 hours

Uncomplicated UTI: No dosage adjustment required

Complicated UTI, acute pyelonephritis: Cl_{cr} 10-19 mL/minute: 250 mg every 48 hours

Complicated skin infection, acute bacterial sinusitis, community-acquired pneumonia, or nosocomial pneumonia: Initial: 750 mg, then as follows:

Cl_{cr} 20-49 mL/minute: 750 mg every 48 hours

(Continued)

Levofloxacin *(Continued)*

Cl_{cr} 10-19 mL/minute: 500 mg every 48 hours

Hemodialysis/CAPD: 500 mg every 48 hours

Available Dosage Forms

Infusion [premixed in D_5W] (Levaquin®): 250 mg (50 mL); 500 mg (100 mL); 750 mg (150 mL)

Injection, solution [preservative free] (Levaquin®): 25 mg/mL (20 mL, 30 mL)

Solution, ophthalmic:

Iquix®: 1.5% (5 mL)

Quixin™: 0.5% (5 mL) [contains benzalkonium chloride]

Solution, oral (Levaquin®): 25 mg/mL (480 mL) [contains benzyl alcohol]

Tablet (Levaquin®): 250 mg, 500 mg, 750 mg

Levaquin® Leva-Pak: 750 mg (5s)

Nursing Guidelines

Assessment: Assess results of culture and sensitivity tests and patient's allergy history before initiating therapy. Use caution with known CNS disorders or renal impairment. Assess potential for interactions with other prescriptions, OTC medications, or herbal products patient may be taking (eg, increased risk of tendon rupture or arrhythmias). See Administration for infusion specifics; if an allergic reaction occurs (itching, urticaria, dyspnea or facial edema, loss of consciousness, tingling, cardiovascular collapse), drug should be discontinued immediately and prescriber notified. Assess results of laboratory tests, therapeutic effectiveness (resolution of infection), and adverse reactions regularly during therapy (eg, hypersensitivity reactions, diarrhea, opportunistic infection, tendon rupture). Teach patient proper use (according to formulation), possible side effects/appropriate interventions, and adverse symptoms to report.

Monitoring Laboratory Tests: Perform culture and sensitivity studies prior to initiating drug therapy. Monitor CBC periodically during therapy. Monitor renal or hepatic function if therapy is prolonged.

Dietary Considerations: Tablets may be taken without regard to meals. Oral solution should be administered on an empty stomach (1 hour before or 2 hours after a meal).

Patient Education: Do not take any new medication during therapy unless approved by prescriber. If administered by infusion, report immediately any chest or back pain, tightness in chest, difficulty swallowing, swelling of face or mouth, or redness, swelling or pain at infusion site. **Pregnancy/breast-feeding precautions:** Inform prescriber if you are or intend to become pregnant. Breast-feeding is not recommended.

Oral: Take exactly as directed; at least 1 hour before or 2 hours after antacids or other drug products containing calcium, iron, or zinc. Take entire prescription even if feeling better. Maintain adequate hydration (2-3 L/day of fluids) unless advised by prescriber to restrict fluid intake. May cause dizziness, lightheadedness, or confusion (use caution when driving or engaging in tasks that require alertness until response to drug is known); nausea or vomiting (small frequent meals, frequent mouth care, sucking lozenges, or chewing gum may help); or photosensitivity (use sunscreen, wear protective clothing and eyewear, and avoid direct sunlight). Discontinue use immediately and report to prescriber if inflammation, tendon pain, or allergic reaction occurs (itching urticaria, respiratory difficulty, facial edema, difficulty swallowing, loss of consciousness, tingling, chest pain, palpitations). Report persistent diarrhea or constipation; signs of infection (unusual fever or chills); vaginal itching or foul-smelling vaginal discharge; or easy bruising or bleeding.

Ophthalmic: Wash hands before instilling solution. Sit or lie down to instill. Open eye, look at ceiling, and instill prescribed amount of solution. Close eye and roll eye in all directions, and apply gentle pressure to inner corner of eye. Do not let tip of applicator touch eye; do not contaminate tip of applicator (may cause eye infection, eye damage, or vision loss). Temporary stinging or blurred vision may occur. Report persistent pain, burning, vision changes, swelling, itching, or worsening of condition. Discontinue medication and contact prescriber immediately if you develop a rash or allergic reaction. Do not wear contact lenses.

Geriatric Considerations: The risk of torsade de pointes and tendon inflammation and/or rupture associated with the concomitant use of corticosteroids and quinolones is increased in the elderly population. Adjust dose for renal function.

Pregnancy Risk Factor: C

Pregnancy Issues: Reports of arthropathy (observed in immature animals and reported rarely in humans) have limited the use of fluoroquinolones in pregnancy. Teratogenic effects were not observed with levofloxacin in animal studies; however, decreased body weight and increased fetal mortality were reported. Based on limited data, quinolones are not expected to be a major human teratogen. Although quinolone antibiotics should not be used as first-line agents during pregnancy, when considering treatment for life-threatening infection and/or prolonged duration of therapy, the potential risk to the fetus must be balanced against the severity of the potential illness.

Lactation: Excretion in breast milk unknown/not recommended

Breast-Feeding Considerations: Other quinolones are known to be excreted in breast milk. Based on data from ofloxacin, excretion of levofloxacin would be expected. The manufacturer recommends to discontinue nursing or to discontinue levofloxacin.

Administration

Oral: Tablets may be administered without regard to meals. Oral solution should be administered 1 hour before or 2 hours after meals.

I.V.: Infuse 250-500 mg I.V. solution over 60 minutes; infuse 750 mg I.V. solution over 90 minutes. Too rapid of infusion can lead to hypotension. Avoid administration through an intravenous line with a solution containing multivalent cations (eg, magnesium, calcium).

Reconstitution: Solution for injection: Single-use vials must be further diluted in compatible solution to a final concentration of 5 mg/mL prior to infusion.

Compatibility: Stable in D_5LR, D_5NS, $D_5{}^1/_2NS$ with 0.15% KCl, D_5W, NS, Plasma-Lyte® 56/5% dextrose, sodium lactate (M/6); **incompatible** with mannitol 20%, sodium bicarbonate 5%

Y-site administration: Incompatible with acyclovir, alprostadil, furosemide, heparin, indomethacin, nitroglycerin, sodium nitroprusside

Storage:

Solution for injection:

Vial: Store at room temperature; protect from light. Diluted solution is stable for 72 hours when stored at room temperature; stable for 14 days when stored under refrigeration. When frozen, stable for 6 months; do not refreeze. Do not thaw in microwave or by bath immersion.

Premixed: Store at ≤25°C (77°F); brief exposure to 40°C (104°F) does not affect product; protect from freezing and light.

Tablet, oral solution: Store at 25°C (77°F); excursions permitted to 15°C to 25°C (59°F to 77°F).

Ophthalmic solution: Store at 15°C to 25°C (59°F to 77°F).

Related Information

Prevention of Wound Infection and Sepsis in Surgical Patients *on page 1830*

♦ Levophed® *see* Norepinephrine *on page 1242*

♦ Levothroid® *see* Levothyroxine *on page 1029*

Levothyroxine (lee voe thye ROKS een)

U.S. Brand Names Levothroid®; Levoxyl®; Synthroid®; Unithroid®

Synonyms Levothyroxine Sodium; *L*-Thyroxine Sodium; T_4

Pharmacologic Category Thyroid Product

Medication Safety Issues

Sound-alike/look-alike issues:

Levothyroxine may be confused with liothyronine
Levoxyl® may be confused with Lanoxin®, Luvox®
Synthroid® may be confused with Symmetrel®

To avoid errors due to misinterpretation of a decimal point, always express dosage in mcg (**not** mg).

Use Replacement or supplemental therapy in hypothyroidism; pituitary TSH suppression

Mechanism of Action Exact mechanism of action is unknown; however, it is believed the thyroid hormone exerts its many metabolic effects through control of DNA transcription and protein synthesis; involved in normal metabolism, growth, and development; promotes gluconeogenesis, increases utilization and mobilization of glycogen stores, and stimulates protein synthesis, increases basal metabolic rate

Pharmacodynamics/Kinetics

Onset of action: Therapeutic: Oral: 3-5 days; I.V. 6-8 hours

(Continued)

Levothyroxine *(Continued)*

Peak effect: I.V.: ~24 hours

Absorption: Oral: Erratic (40% to 80%); decreases with age

Protein binding: >99%

Metabolism: Hepatic to triiodothyronine (active)

Time to peak, serum: 2-4 hours

Half-life elimination: Euthyroid: 6-7 days; Hypothyroid: 9-10 days; Hyperthyroid: 3-4 days

Excretion: Urine and feces; decreases with age

Contraindications Hypersensitivity to levothyroxine sodium or any component of the formulation; recent MI or thyrotoxicosis; uncorrected adrenal insufficiency

Warnings/Precautions Ineffective and potentially toxic for weight reduction; high doses may produce serious or even life-threatening toxic effects particularly when used with some anorectic drugs. Use with caution and reduce dosage in patients with angina pectoris or other cardiovascular disease; use cautiously in elderly since they may be more likely to have compromised cardiovascular functions. Patients with adrenal insufficiency, myxedema, diabetes mellitus and insipidus may have symptoms exaggerated or aggravated; thyroid replacement requires periodic assessment of thyroid status. Chronic hypothyroidism predisposes patients to coronary artery disease. Levoxyl® may rapidly swell and disintegrate causing choking or gagging (should be administered with a full glass of water); use caution in patients with dysphagia or other swallowing disorders.

Drug Interactions

Aluminum- and magnesium-containing antacids, calcium carbonate, simethicone, or sucralfate: May decrease T_4 absorption; separate dose from levothyroxine by at least 4 hours.

Antidiabetic agents (biguanides, meglitinides, sulfonylureas, thiazolidinediones, insulin): Changes in thyroid function may alter requirements of antidiabetic agent. Monitor closely at initiation of therapy, or when dose is changed or discontinued.

Cholestyramine and colestipol: Decrease T_4 absorption; separate dose from levothyroxine by at least 2 hours.

Digoxin: Digoxin levels may be reduced in hyperthyroidism; therapeutic effect may be reduced. Impact of thyroid replacement should be monitored.

Estrogens: May decrease serum free thyroxine concentrations.

Imatinib: May decrease the effects of thyroid replacement therapy; monitor.

Iron: Decreases T_4 absorption; separate dose from levothyroxine by at least 4 hours.

Kayexalate®: Decreases T_4 absorption; separate dose from levothyroxine by at least 4 hours.

Ketamine: May cause marked hypertension and tachycardia; monitor.

Theophylline, caffeine: Decreased theophylline clearance in hypothyroid patients; monitor during thyroid replacement.

Tricyclic and tetracyclic antidepressants: Therapeutic and toxic effects of levothyroxine and the antidepressant are increased.

Warfarin (and other oral anticoagulants): The hypoprothrombinemic response to warfarin may be altered by a change in thyroid function or replacement. Replacement may dramatically increase response to warfarin. However, initiation of warfarin in a patient stabilized on a dose of levothyroxine does not appear to require a significantly different approach.

Nutritional/Herbal/Ethanol Interactions Food: Taking levothyroxine with enteral nutrition may cause reduced bioavailability and may lower serum thyroxine levels leading to signs or symptoms of hypothyroidism. Limit intake of goitrogenic foods (eg, asparagus, cabbage, peas, turnip greens, broccoli, spinach, Brussels sprouts, lettuce, soybeans). Soybean flour (infant formula), cottonseed meal, walnuts, and dietary fiber may decrease absorption of levothyroxine from the GI tract.

Lab Interactions Many drugs may have effects on thyroid function tests: para-aminosalicylic acid, aminoglutethimide, amiodarone, barbiturates, carbamazepine, chloral hydrate, clofibrate, colestipol, corticosteroids, danazol, diazepam, estrogens, ethionamide, fluorouracil, I.V. heparin, insulin, lithium, methadone, methimazole, mitotane, nitroprusside, oxyphenbutazone, phenylbutazone, PTU, perphenazine, phenytoin, propranolol, salicylates, sulfonylureas, and thiazides.

Adverse Reactions Frequency not defined.

Cardiovascular: Angina, arrhythmia, blood pressure increased, cardiac arrest, flushing, heart failure, MI, palpitation, pulse increased, tachycardia

Central nervous system: Anxiety, emotional lability, fatigue, fever, headache, hyperactivity, insomnia, irritability, nervousness, pseudotumor cerebri (children), seizure (rare)

Dermatologic: Alopecia

Endocrine & metabolic: Fertility impaired, menstrual irregularities

Gastrointestinal: Abdominal cramps, appetite increased, diarrhea, vomiting, weight loss

Hepatic: Liver function tests increased

Neuromuscular & skeletal: Bone mineral density decreased, muscle weakness, tremor, slipped capital femoral epiphysis (children)

Respiratory: Dyspnea

Miscellaneous: Diaphoresis, heat intolerance, hypersensitivity (to inactive ingredients, symptoms include urticaria, pruritus, rash, flushing, angioedema, GI symptoms, fever, arthralgia, serum sickness, wheezing)

Levoxyl®: Choking, dysphagia, gagging

Overdosage/Toxicology

Chronic: Chronic overdose may cause hyperthyroidism, weight loss, nervousness, sweating, tachycardia, insomnia, heat intolerance, menstrual irregularities, palpitations, psychosis, and fever. Overtreatment of children may result in premature closure of epiphyses or craniosynostosis (infants). Reduce dose or temporarily discontinue therapy. Hypothalamic-pituitary-thyroid axis will return to normal in 6-8 weeks. Serum T_4 levels do not correlate well with toxicity. Provide general supportive care

Acute: Acute overdose may cause fever, hypoglycemia, CHF, and unrecognized adrenal insufficiency. Acute massive overdose may be life-threatening; treatment should be symptomatic and supportive. Massive overdose may be a require beta-blockers for increased sympathomimetic activity.

Dosing

Adults: Doses should be adjusted based on clinical response and laboratory parameters.

Hypothyroidism:

Oral: 1.7 mcg/kg/day in otherwise healthy adults <50 years old, children in whom growth and puberty are complete, and older adults who have been recently treated for hyperthyroidism or who have been hypothyroid for only a few months. Titrate dose every 6 weeks. Average starting dose ~100 mcg; usual doses are ≤200 mcg/day; doses ≥300 mcg/day are rare (consider poor compliance, malabsorption, and/or drug interactions). **Note:** For patients >50 years or patients with cardiac disease, refer to elderly dosing.

I.M., I.V.: 50% of the oral dose

Severe hypothyroidism: Oral: Initial: 12.5-25 mcg/day; adjust dose by 25 mcg/day every 2-4 weeks as appropriate

Subclinical hypothyroidism (if treated): Oral: 1 mcg/kg/day

TSH suppression: Oral:

Well-differentiated thyroid cancer: Highly individualized; Doses >2 mcg/kg/day may be needed to suppress TSH to <0.1 mU/L.

Benign nodules and nontoxic multinodular goiter: Goal TSH suppression: 0.1-0.3 mU/L

Myxedema coma or stupor: I.V.: 200-500 mcg, then 100-300 mcg the next day if necessary; smaller doses should be considered in patients with cardiovascular disease

Elderly: Doses should be adjusted based on clinical response and laboratory parameters.

Hypothyroidism:

Oral:

>50 years without cardiac disease **or** <50 years with cardiac disease: Initial: 25-50 mcg/day; adjust dose at 6- to 8-week intervals as needed

>50 years with cardiac disease: Initial: 12.5-25 mcg/day; adjust dose by 12.5-25 mcg increments at 4- to 6-week intervals. (**Note:** Many clinicians prefer to adjust at 6- to 8-week intervals.)

Note: Elderly patients may require <1 mcg/kg/day

I.M., I.V.: 50% of the oral dose

Myxedema coma: I.V.: Refer to adult dosing; lower doses may be needed

Pediatrics: Doses should be adjusted based on clinical response and laboratory parameters.

(Continued)

Levothyroxine *(Continued)*

Hypothyroidism:

Oral:

Newborns: Initial: 10-15 mcg/kg/day. Lower doses of 25 mcg/day should be considered in newborns at risk for cardiac failure. Newborns with T_4 levels <5 mcg/dL should be started at 50 mcg/day. Adjust dose at 4- to 6-week intervals.

Infants and Children: Dose based on body weight and age as listed below. Children with severe or chronic hypothyroidism should be started at 25 mcg/day; adjust dose by 25 mcg every 2-4 weeks. In older children, hyperactivity may be decreased by starting with 1/4 of the recommended dose and increasing by 1/4 dose each week until the full replacement dose is reached. Refer to adult dosing once growth and puberty are complete.

0-3 months: 10-15 mcg/kg/day
3-6 months: 8-10 mcg/kg/day
6-12 months: 6-8 mcg/kg/day
1-5 years: 5-6 mcg/kg/day
6-12 years: 4-5 mcg/kg/day
12 years: 2-3 mcg/kg/day

I.M., I.V.: 50% of the oral dose

Available Dosage Forms

Injection, powder for reconstitution, as sodium: 0.2 mg, 0.5 mg

Tablet, as sodium: 25 mcg, 50 mcg, 75 mcg, 88 mcg, 100 mcg, 112 mcg, 125 mcg, 150 mcg, 175 mcg, 200 mcg, 300 mcg

Levothroid®: 25 mcg, 50 mcg, 75 mcg, 88 mcg, 100 mcg, 112 mcg, 125 mcg, 150 mcg, 175 mcg, 200 mcg, 300 mcg

Levoxyl®, Synthroid®: 25 mcg, 50 mcg, 75 mcg, 88 mcg, 100 mcg, 112 mcg, 125 mcg, 137 mcg, 150 mcg, 175 mcg, 200 mcg, 300 mcg

Unithroid®: 25 mcg, 50 mcg, 75 mcg, 88 mcg, 100 mcg, 112 mcg, 125 mcg, 150 mcg, 175 mcg, 200 mcg, 300 mcg

Nursing Guidelines

Assessment: Use with caution in presence of cardiovascular disease, adrenal insufficiency, or diabetes mellitus (see Warnings/Precautions for specific use cautions). Assess potential for interactions with other pharmacological agents patient may be taking (eg, toxic effects with some anorectic drugs, decreased effect of oral hypoglycemics, decreased or increased effect of levothyroxine; see Drug Interactions). See Administration for I.V. specifics. Assess results of laboratory tests, therapeutic benefits, and adverse effects on a regular basis during therapy (eg, hypo- or hyperthyroidism; see Adverse Reactions). **Important:** Many drugs may have effects on thyroid function tests. Teach patient proper use, possible side effects/appropriate interventions (eg, goitrogenic foods), and adverse symptoms to report (see Patient Education).

Monitoring Laboratory Tests: Thyroid function (serum thyroxine, thyrotropin concentrations), resin triiodothyronine uptake (rT_3U), free thyroxine index (FTI), T_4, TSH, TSH may be elevated during the first few months of thyroid replacement despite patients being clinically euthyroid. In cases where T_4 remains low and TSH is within normal limits, an evaluation of "free" (unbound) T_4 is needed to evaluate further increase in dosage.

Dietary Considerations: Should be taken on an empty stomach, at least 30 minutes before food.

Patient Education: Consult prescriber before taking new medication or herbal products during therapy; some other medications or herbals may cause adverse effects with levothyroxine. Thyroid replacement therapy is generally for life. Take as directed, in the morning 30 minutes before breakfast. Do not take antacids or iron preparations within 8 hours of thyroid medication. Do not change brands and do not discontinue without consulting prescriber. Do not eat excessive amounts of goitrogenic foods (eg, asparagus, cabbage, peas, turnip greens, broccoli, spinach, brussel sprouts, lettuce, soybeans). Report chest pain, rapid heart rate, palpitations, heat intolerance, excessive sweating, increased nervousness, agitation, or lethargy.

Geriatric Considerations: The elderly do not have a change in serum thyroxine (T_4) associated with aging; however, plasma T_3 concentrations are decreased 25% to 40% in the elderly. There is not a compensatory rise in thyrotropin suggesting that lower T_3 is not reacted upon as a deficiency by the pituitary. This indicates a slightly lower than normal dosage of thyroid hormone replacement is usually sufficient in older patients than in younger adult patients. TSH must be monitored since insufficient thyroid replacement (elevated TSH) is a risk for coronary artery disease and excessive replacement (low TSH) may cause signs of hyperthyroidism and excessive bone loss. Some clinicians suggest levothyroxine is the drug of choice for replacement therapy.

Pregnancy Risk Factor: A

Pregnancy Issues: Untreated maternal hypothyroidism may have adverse effects on fetal growth and development and is associated with higher rate of complications (spontaneous abortion, pre-eclampsia, stillbirth, premature delivery). Treatment should not be discontinued during pregnancy. TSH levels should be monitored during each trimester and 6-8 weeks postpartum. Increased doses may be needed during pregnancy.

Lactation: Enters breast milk/compatible

Breast-Feeding Considerations: Minimally excreted in human milk; adequate levels are needed to maintain normal lactation

Perioperative/Anesthesia/Other Concerns: Equivalent dosing: Thyroid USP 60 mg ~ levothyroxine 0.05-0.06 mg ~ liothyronine 0.015-0.0375 mg

50-60 mg thyroid ~ 50-60 mcg levothyroxine and 12.5-15 mcg liothyronine

Note: Several medications have effects on thyroid production or conversion. The impact in thyroid replacement has not been specifically evaluated, but patient response should be monitored:

- Methimazole: Decreases thyroid hormone secretion, while propylthiouracil decrease thyroid hormone secretion and decreases conversion of T_4 to T_3.
- Beta-adrenergic antagonists: Decrease conversion of T_4 to T_3 (dose related, propranolol ≥160 mg/day); patients may be clinically euthyroid.
- Iodide, iodine-containing radiographic contrast agents may decrease thyroid hormone secretion; may also increase thyroid hormone secretion, especially in patients with Graves' disease.

Other agents reported to impact on thyroid production/conversion include aminoglutethimide, amiodarone, chloral hydrate, diazepam, ethionamide, interferon-alpha, interleukin-2, lithium, lovastatin (case report), glucocorticoids (dose-related), mercaptopurine, sulfonamides, thiazide diuretics, and tolbutamide.

In addition, a number of medications have been noted to cause transient depression in TSH secretion, which may complicate interpretation of monitoring tests for levothyroxine, including corticosteroids, octreotide, and dopamine. Metoclopramide may increase TSH secretion

Soy protein may interfere with absorption of levothyroxine sodium. An enteral formula without soy protein should be selected and thyroid function monitored during tube feeding.

Administration

Oral: Administer in the morning on an empty stomach, at least 30 minutes before food. Tablets may be crushed and suspended in 1-2 teaspoonfuls of water; suspension should be used immediately. Levoxyl® should be administered with a full glass of water to prevent gagging (due to tablet swelling).

I.V.: Dilute vial with 5 mL normal saline; use immediately after reconstitution; do not mix with other IV fluids

Reconstitution: Dilute vial with 5 mL normal saline. Shake well and use immediately after reconstitution; discard any unused portions.

Compatibility: Do not mix I.V. solution with other I.V. infusion solutions.

Storage: Store tablets and injection at room temperature of 15°C to 30°C (59°F to 86°F). Protect tablets from light and moisture.

- **Levothyroxine Sodium** *see* Levothyroxine *on page 1029*
- **Levoxyl®** *see* Levothyroxine *on page 1029*
- **Levsin®** *see* Hyoscyamine *on page 886*
- **Levsinex®** *see* Hyoscyamine *on page 886*
- **Levsin/SL®** *see* Hyoscyamine *on page 886*
- **Lexapro®** *see* Escitalopram *on page 639*
- ***l*-Hyoscyamine Sulfate** *see* Hyoscyamine *on page 886*
- **LidaMantle®** *see* Lidocaine *on page 1033*
- **Lidex®** *see* Fluocinonide *on page 741*
- **Lidex-E®** *see* Fluocinonide *on page 741*

Lidocaine (LYE doe kane)

U.S. Brand Names Anestacon®; Band-Aid® Hurt-Free™ Antiseptic Wash [OTC]; Burnamycin [OTC]; Burn Jel [OTC]; Burn-O-Jel [OTC]; LidaMantle®; Lidoderm®;

(Continued)

Lidocaine *(Continued)*

L-M-X™ 4 [OTC]; L-M-X™ 5 [OTC]; LTA® 360; Premjact® [OTC]; Solarcaine® Aloe Extra Burn Relief [OTC]; Topicaine® [OTC]; Xylocaine®; Xylocaine® MPF; Xylocaine® Viscous; Zilactin-L® [OTC]

Synonyms Lidocaine Hydrochloride; Lignocaine Hydrochloride

Pharmacologic Category Analgesic, Topical; Antiarrhythmic Agent, Class Ib; Local Anesthetic

Medication Safety Issues

High alert medication: The Institute for Safe Medication Practices (ISMP) includes this medication (I.V. formulation) among its list of drugs which have a heightened risk of causing significant patient harm when used in error.

Transdermal patch may contain conducting metal (eg, aluminum); remove patch prior to MRI.

Use Local anesthetic and acute treatment of ventricular arrhythmias from myocardial infarction, cardiac manipulation, digitalis intoxication; drug of choice for ventricular ectopy, ventricular tachycardia (VT), ventricular fibrillation (VF); for pulseless VT or VF preferably administer **after** defibrillation and epinephrine; control of premature ventricular contractions, wide-complex paroxysmal supraventricular tachycardia (PSVT); control of hemodynamically compromising PVCs; hemodynamically stable VT

Rectal: Temporary relief of pain and itching due to anorectal disorders

Topical: Local anesthetic for use in laser, cosmetic, and outpatient surgeries; minor burns, cuts, and abrasions of the skin

Orphan drug: Lidoderm® Patch: Relief of allodynia (painful hypersensitivity) and chronic pain in postherpetic neuralgia

Mechanism of Action Class Ib antiarrhythmic; suppresses automaticity of conduction tissue, by increasing electrical stimulation threshold of ventricle, His-Purkinje system, and spontaneous depolarization of the ventricles during diastole by a direct action on the tissues; blocks both the initiation and conduction of nerve impulses by decreasing the neuronal membrane's permeability to sodium ions, which results in inhibition of depolarization with resultant blockade of conduction

Pharmacodynamics/Kinetics

Onset of action: Single bolus dose: 45-90 seconds

Duration: 10-20 minutes

Distribution: V_d: 1.1-2.1 L/kg; alterable by many patient factors; decreased in CHF and liver disease; crosses blood-brain barrier

Protein binding: 60% to 80% to $alpha_1$ acid glycoprotein

Metabolism: 90% hepatic; active metabolites monoethylglycinexylidide (MEGX) and glycinexylidide (GX) can accumulate and may cause CNS toxicity

Half-life elimination: Biphasic: Prolonged with congestive heart failure, liver disease, shock, severe renal disease; Initial: 7-30 minutes; Terminal: Infants, premature: 3.2 hours, Adults: 1.5-2 hours

Contraindications Hypersensitivity to lidocaine or any component of the formulation; hypersensitivity to another local anesthetic of the amide type; Adam-Stokes syndrome; severe degrees of SA, AV, or intraventricular heart block (except in patients with a functioning artificial pacemaker); premixed injection may contain corn-derived dextrose and its use is contraindicated in patients with allergy to corn-related products

Warnings/Precautions

Intravenous: Constant ECG monitoring is necessary during I.V. administration. Use cautiously in hepatic impairment, any degree of heart block, Wolff-Parkinson-White syndrome, CHF, marked hypoxia, severe respiratory depression, hypovolemia, history of malignant hyperthermia, or shock. Increased ventricular rate may be seen when administered to a patient with atrial fibrillation. Correct any underlying causes of ventricular arrhythmias. Monitor closely for signs and symptoms of CNS toxicity. The elderly may be prone to increased CNS and cardiovascular side effects. Reduce dose in hepatic dysfunction and CHF.

Injectable anesthetic: Follow appropriate administration techniques so as not to administer any intravascularly. Solutions containing antimicrobial preservatives should not be used for epidural or spinal anesthesia. Some solutions contain a bisulfite; avoid in patients who are allergic to bisulfite. Resuscitative equipment, medicine and oxygen should be available in case of emergency. Use products containing epinephrine cautiously in patients with significant vascular disease, compromised blood flow, or during or following general anesthesia (increased risk of arrhythmias). Adjust the dose for the elderly, pediatric, acutely ill, and debilitated patients.

Topical: L-M-X™ 4 cream: Do not leave on large body areas for >2 hours. Observe young children closely to prevent accidental ingestion. Not for use ophthalmic use or for use on mucous membranes.

Transdermal patch: May contain conducting metal (eg, aluminum); remove patch prior to MRI.

Drug Interactions **Substrate** of CYP1A2 (minor), 2A6 (minor), 2B6 (minor), 2C8/9 (minor), 2D6 (major), 3A4 (major); **Inhibits** CYP1A2 (strong), 2D6 (moderate), 3A4 (moderate)

Cimetidine increases lidocaine blood levels; monitor levels or use an alternative H_2 antagonist.

CYP1A2 substrates: Lidocaine may increase the levels/effects of CYP1A2 substrates. Example substrates include aminophylline, fluvoxamine, mexiletine, mirtazapine, ropinirole, theophylline, and trifluoperazine.

CYP2D6 inhibitors: May increase the levels/effects of lidocaine. Example inhibitors include chlorpromazine, delavirdine, fluoxetine, miconazole, paroxetine, pergolide, quinidine, quinine, ritonavir, and ropinirole.

CYP2D6 substrates: Lidocaine may increase the levels/effects of CYP2D6 substrates. Example substrates include amphetamines, selected beta-blockers, dextromethorphan, fluoxetine, mirtazapine, nefazodone, paroxetine, risperidone, ritonavir, thioridazine, tricyclic antidepressants, and venlafaxine.

CYP2D6 prodrug substrates: Lidocaine may decrease the levels/effects of CYP2D6 prodrug substrates. Example prodrug substrates include codeine, hydrocodone, oxycodone, and tramadol.

CYP3A4 inducers: CYP3A4 inducers may decrease the levels/effects of lidocaine. Example inducers include aminoglutethimide, carbamazepine, nafcillin, nevirapine, phenobarbital, phenytoin, and rifamycins.

CYP3A4 inhibitors: May increase the levels/effects of lidocaine. Example inhibitors include amiodarone (doses >400 mg/day), azole antifungals, clarithromycin, diclofenac, doxycycline, erythromycin, imatinib, isoniazid, nefazodone, nicardipine, propofol, protease inhibitors, quinidine, telithromycin, and verapamil.

CYP3A4 substrates: Lidocaine may increase the levels/effects of CYP3A4 substrates. Example substrates include benzodiazepines, calcium channel blockers, cyclosporine, mirtazapine, nateglinide, nefazodone, sildenafil (and other PDE-5 inhibitors), tacrolimus, and venlafaxine. Selected benzodiazepines (midazolam and triazolam), cisapride, ergot alkaloids, selected HMG-CoA reductase inhibitors (lovastatin and simvastatin), and pimozide are generally contraindicated with strong CYP3A4 inhibitors.

Propranolol: Increases lidocaine blood levels.

Protease inhibitors (eg, amprenavir, ritonavir): May increase lidocaine blood levels.

Nutritional/Herbal/Ethanol Interactions Herb/Nutraceutical: St John's wort may decrease lidocaine levels; avoid concurrent use.

Adverse Reactions Effects vary with route of administration. Many effects are dose related.

Frequency not defined:

Cardiovascular: Bradycardia, hypotension, heart block, arrhythmia, cardiovascular collapse, sinus node supression, increase defibrillator threshold, vascular insufficiency (periarticular injections), arterial spasms

Central nervous system: Agitation, anxiety, coma, dizziness, drowsiness, euphoria, hallucinations, lethargy, lightheadedness, paresthesia, psychosis, seizure, slurred speech

Dermatologic: Angioedema, itching, rash, edema of the skin, contact dermatitis

Gastrointestinal: Nausea, vomiting, taste disorder

Local: Thrombophlebitis

Neuromuscular & skeletal: Transient radicular pain (subarachnoid administration; up to 1.9%), tremor, twitching

Ocular: Diplopia, visual changes

Otic: Tinnitus

Respiratory: Dyspnea, respiratory depression or arrest, bronchospasm

Miscellaneous: Allergic reactions, urticaria, edema, anaphylactoid reaction

Following spinal anesthesia positional headache (3%), shivering (2%) nausea, peripheral nerve symptoms, respiratory inadequacy and double vision (<1%), hypotension, cauda equina syndrome

(Continued)

Lidocaine *(Continued)*

Postmarketing and/or case reports: ARDS (inhalation), asystole, confusion, disorientation, flushing, headache, hyper-/hypoesthesia, hypersensitivity, methemoglobinemia, nervousness, skin reaction, weakness

Overdosage/Toxicology Lidocaine has a narrow therapeutic index. Severe toxicity may occur at doses slightly above the therapeutic range, especially in conjunction with other antiarrhythmic drugs. Symptoms of overdose include sedation, confusion, coma, seizures, respiratory arrest, and cardiac toxicity (sinus arrest, AV block, asystole, and hypotension). QRS and QT intervals are usually normal, although they may be prolonged after massive overdose. Other effects include dizziness, paresthesia, tremor, ataxia, and GI disturbance. Treatment is supportive.

Dosing

Adults & Elderly:

Antiarrhythmic:

I.V.: 1-1.5 mg/kg bolus over 2-3 minutes; may repeat doses of 0.5-0.75 mg/kg in 5-10 minutes up to a total of 3 mg/kg; continuous infusion: 1-4 mg/minute

Infusion rates: 2 g/250 mL D_5W (infusion pump should be used):

1 mg/minute: 7 mL/hour
2 mg/minute: 15 mL/hour
3 mg/minute: 21 mL/hour
4 mg/minute: 30 mL/hour

Ventricular fibrillation (after defibrillation and epinephrine):

I.V.: Initial: 1.5 mg/kg, may repeat boluses as above; follow with continuous infusion after return of perfusion.

Intratracheal: 2-2.5 times the recommended I.V. dose; dilute in 10 mL NS or distilled water. **Note:** Absorption is greater with distilled water, but causes more adverse effects on PaO_2.

Prevention of ventricular fibrillation: Initial bolus: 0.5 mg/kg; repeat every 5-10 minutes to a total dose of 2 mg/kg

Refractory ventricular fibrillation: Repeat 1.5 mg/kg bolus may be given 3-5 minutes after initial dose.

E.T. (loading dose only): 2-2.5 times the I.V. dose

Note: Decrease dose in patients with CHF, shock, or hepatic disease.

Anesthetic, topical:

Cream:

LidaMantle®: Skin irritation: Apply to affected area 2-3 times/day as needed

L-M-X™ 4: Apply ¼ inch thick layer to intact skin. Leave on until adequate anesthetic effect is obtained. Remove cream and cleanse area before beginning procedure.

L-M-X™ 5: Relief of anorectal pain and itching: Rectal: Apply topically to clean, dry area **or** using applicator, insert rectally, up to 6 times/day

Gel, ointment, solution: Apply to affected area ≤3 times/day as needed (maximum dose: 4.5 mg/kg, not to exceed 300 mg)

Jelly: Maximum dose: 30 mL (600 mg) in any 12-hour period:

Anesthesia of male urethra: 5-30 mL (100-600 mg)
Anesthesia of female urethra: 3-5 mL (60-100 mg)
Lubrication of endotracheal tube: Apply a moderate amount to external surface only

Liquid: Cold sores and fever blisters: Apply to affected area every 6 hours as needed

Patch: Postherpetic neuralgia: Apply patch to most painful area. Up to 3 patches may be applied in a single application. Patch may remain in place for up to 12 hours in any 24-hour period.

Anesthetic, local injectable: Varies with procedure, degree of anesthesia needed, vascularity of tissue, duration of anesthesia required, and physical condition of patient; maximum: 4.5 mg/kg/dose; do not repeat within 2 hours.

Pediatrics:

Antiarrhythmic:

I.V., I.O.: (**Note:** For use in pulseless VT or VF, give after defibrillation and epinephrine): Loading dose: 1 mg/kg; follow with continuous infusion; may administer second bolus of 0.5-1 mg/kg if delay between bolus and start of infusion is >15 minutes; continuous infusion: 20-50 mcg/kg/minute. Use 20 mcg/kg/minute in patients with shock, hepatic disease, cardiac arrest, mild CHF; moderate to severe CHF may require ½ loading dose and lower infusion rates to avoid toxicity.

E.T. (loading dose only): 2-10 times the I.V. bolus dose

Anesthetic, topical:

Cream:

LidaMantle®: Skin irritation: Refer to adult dosing.

L-M-X™ 4: Children ≥2 years: Refer to adult dosing.

L-M-X™ 5: Relief of anorectal pain and itching: Rectal: Children ≥12 years: Refer to adult dosing.

Jelly: Children ≥10 years: Dose varies with age and weight (maximum dose: 4.5 mg/kg)

Liquid: Cold sores and fever blisters: Children ≥5 years: Refer to adult dosing.

Injectable local anesthetic: Refer to adult dosing.

Renal Impairment: Not dialyzable (0% to 5%) by hemo- or peritoneal dialysis; supplemental dose is not necessary.

Hepatic Impairment: Reduce dose in acute hepatitis and decompensated cirrhosis by 50%.

Available Dosage Forms [DSC] = Discontinued product

Cream, rectal (L-M-X™ 5): 5% (15 g) [contains benzyl alcohol; packaged with applicator]; (30 g) [contains benzyl alcohol]

Cream, topical (L-M-X™ 4): 4% (5 g) [contains benzyl alcohol; packaged with Tegaderm™ dressing]; (15 g, 30 g) [contains benzyl alcohol]

Cream, topical, as hydrochloride: 3% (30 g)

LidaMantle®: 3% (30 g, 85 g)

Gel, topical:

Burn-O-Jel: 0.5% (90 g)

Topicaine®: 4% (10 g, 30 g, 113 g) [contains alcohol 35%, benzyl alcohol, aloe vera, and jojoba]

Gel, topical, as hydrochloride:

Burn Jel: 2% (3.5 g, 120 g)

Solarcaine® Aloe Extra Burn Relief: 0.5% (113 g, 226 g) [contains aloe vera gel and tartrazine]

Infusion, as hydrochloride [premixed in D_5W]: 0.4% [4 mg/mL] (250 mL, 500 mL); 0.8% [8 mg/mL] (250 mL, 500 mL)

Injection, solution, as hydrochloride: 0.5% [5 mg/mL] (50 mL); 1% [10 mg/mL] (2 mL, 10 mL, 20 mL, 30 mL, 50 mL); 2% [20 mg/mL] (2 mL, 5 mL, 20 mL, 50 mL)

Xylocaine®: 0.5% [5 mg/mL] (50 mL); 1% [10 mg/mL] (10 mL, 20 mL, 50 mL); 2% [20 mg/mL] (1.8 mL, 10 mL, 20 mL, 50 mL)

Injection, solution, as hydrochloride [preservative free]: 0.5% [5 mg/mL] (50 mL); 1% [10 mg/mL] (2 mL, 5 mL, 30 mL); 1.5% [15 mg/mL] (20 mL); 2% [20 mg/mL] (2 mL, 5 mL, 10 mL); 4% [40 mg/mL] (5 mL)

Xylocaine®: 10% [100 mg/mL] (5 mL) [for ventricular arrhythmias]

Xylocaine® MPF: 0.5% [5 mg/mL] (50 mL); 1% [10 mg/mL] (2 mL, 5 mL, 10 mL, 30 mL); 1.5% [15 mg/mL] (10 mL, 20 mL); 2% [20 mg/mL] (2 mL, 5 mL, 10 mL); 4% [40 mg/mL] (5 mL)

Injection, solution, as hydrochloride [premixed in $D_{7.5}W$, preservative free]: 5% (2 mL)

Xylocaine® MPF: 1.5% (2 mL) [DSC]

Jelly, topical, as hydrochloride: 2% (5 mL, 30 mL)

Anestacon®: 2% (15 mL) [contains benzalkonium chloride]

Xylocaine®: 2% (5 mL, 30 mL)

Liquid, topical (Zilactin®-L): 2.5% (7.5 mL)

Lotion, topical, as hydrochloride (LidaMantle®): 3% (177 mL)

Ointment, topical: 5% (37 g, 50 g)

Solution, topical, as hydrochloride: 4% [40 mg/mL] (50 mL)

Band-Aid® Hurt-Free™ Antiseptic Wash: 2% (180 mL)

LTA® 360: 4% [40 mg/mL] (4 mL) [packaged with cannula for laryngotracheal administration

Xylocaine®: 4% [40 mg/mL] (50 mL)

Solution, viscous, as hydrochloride: 2% [20 mg/mL] (20 mL, 100 mL)

Xylocaine® Viscous: 2% [20 mg/mL] (100 mL, 450 mL)

Spray, topical:

Burnamycin: 0.5% (60 mL) [contains aloe vera gel and menthol]

Premjact®: 9.6% (13 mL)

Solarcaine® Aloe Extra Burn Relief: 0.5% (127 g) [contains aloe vera]

Transdermal system, topical (Lidoderm®): 5% (30s)

Nursing Guidelines

Assessment: Assess other medications patient may be taking for adverse interactions. **Local anesthetic:** Monitor for effectiveness of anesthesia and adverse reactions. **Dental/local anesthetic:** Use caution to prevent gagging or

(Continued)

Lidocaine *(Continued)*

choking. Avoid food or drink for 1 hour. Teach patient adverse reactions to report; use and teach appropriate interventions to promote safety. **Antiarrhythmic: I.V.:** ECG and vital signs must be closely and continually monitored. Keep patient supine to reduce hypotensive effects. Assess frequently for adverse reactions or signs of CNS toxicity. Teach patient adverse reactions to report and appropriate interventions to promote safety.

Monitoring Laboratory Tests: I.V.: Serum lidocaine levels. Therapeutic levels range from 1.5-5 mcg/mL; >6 mcg/mL is associated with toxicity.

Dietary Considerations: Premixed injection may contain corn-derived dextrose and its use is contraindicated in patients with allergy to corn-related products.

Patient Education: I.V.: You will be monitored during infusion. Do not get up without assistance. Report dizziness, numbness, double vision, nausea, pain or burning at infusion site, nightmares, hearing strange noises, seeing unusual visions, or respiratory difficulty.

Dermatologic: You will experience decreased sensation to pain, heat, or cold in the area and/or decreased muscle strength (depending on area of application) until effects wear off; use necessary caution to reduce incidence of possible injury until full sensation returns. Report irritation, pain, persistent numbness, tingling, swelling; restlessness, dizziness, acute weakness; blurred vision; ringing in ears; or respiratory difficulty.

Dental/local anesthetic: Lidocaine can cause numbness of tongue, cheeks, and throat. Do not eat or drink for 1 hour after use. Take small sips of water at first to ensure that you can swallow without difficulty. Your tongue and mouth may be numb; use caution avoid biting yourself. Immediately report swelling of face, lips, or tongue

Transdermal patch: Patch may be cut to appropriate size. Apply patch to most painful area. Up to 3 patches may be applied in a single application. Patch may remain in place for up to 12 hours in any 24-hour period. Remove immediately if burning sensation occurs. Wash hands after application.

Pregnancy precaution: Inform prescriber if you are pregnant.

Geriatric Considerations: Due to decreases in Phase I metabolism and possibly decrease in splanchnic perfusion with age, there may be a decreased clearance or increased half-life in the elderly and increased risk for CNS side effects and cardiac effects.

Pregnancy Risk Factor: B

Lactation: Enters breast milk (small amounts)/use caution (AAP rates "compatible")

Perioperative/Anesthesia/Other Concerns:

Cardiac Arrest: Amiodarone was recently compared to lidocaine (ALIVE trial) in out-of-hospital cardiac arrest victims whose ventricular fibrillation was resistant to 3 defibrillation attempts in addition to epinephrine and a fourth defibrillation attempt (Dorian, 2002). Other inclusion criteria included ventricular fibrillation unrelated to trauma (or with other arrhythmias that converted to ventricular fibrillation) and recurrent ventricular fibrillation after successful initial defibrillation. This was a randomized, double-blind comparison. The primary endpoint was the number of patients who were admitted to the hospital intensive care unit alive. Three hundred and forty-seven patients were enrolled. The initial amiodarone dose was 5 mg/kg and the lidocaine dose was 1.5 mg/kg. If ventricular fibrillation persisted after another shock, then the study drug could be administered again (amiodarone 2.5 mg/kg, lidocaine 1.5 mg/kg). Significantly more amiodarone patients (~23%) were admitted to the hospital alive than lidocaine patients (12%). The majority (>90%) of patients in the ALIVE trial had ventricular fibrillation as the initial arrhythmia. The authors concluded that intravenous amiodarone is superior to lidocaine in the treatment of shock-resistant, out-of-hospital ventricular fibrillation. Lidocaine is not as effective as amiodarone for improving intermediate outcomes, but neither has improved survival until hospital discharge among patients with VF cardiac arrest.

Monitoring: Great care is needed in administration of lidocaine in the elderly and in patients with heart failure, shock, or hepatic disease, as toxic effects of lidocaine may become evident earlier in these patients. The half-life of lidocaine increases after 24-48 hours as the drug inhibits its own hepatic metabolism.

The dose should be reduced after 24 hours or blood levels should be monitored. While lidocaine toxicity may elicit seizures, lidocaine may also cause respiratory arrest and cardiac toxicity (eg, sinus arrest, AV block, asystole, and hypotension).

Administration

I.V.: Use microdrip (60 drops/mL) or infusion pump to administer an accurate dose.

Reconstitution: Standard diluent: 2 g/250 mL D_5W

Compatibility: Stable in D_5LR, D_5½NS, D_5NS, D_5W, LR, ¼NS, NS

Y-site administration: Incompatible with amphotericin B cholesteryl sulfate complex, thiopental

Compatibility in syringe: Incompatible with cefazolin

Compatibility when admixed: Incompatible with amphotericin B, dacarbazine, methohexital, phenytoin

Storage: Lidocaine injection is stable at room temperature. Stability of parenteral admixture at room temperature (25°C) is the expiration date on premixed bag; out of overwrap stability is 30 days.

Related Information

Acute Postoperative Pain *on page 1742*
Local Anesthetics *on page 1854*
Management of Postoperative Arrhythmias *on page 1787*

Lidocaine and Epinephrine (LYE doe kane & ep i NEF rin)

U.S. Brand Names LidoSite™; Xylocaine® MPF With Epinephrine; Xylocaine® With Epinephrine

Synonyms Epinephrine and Lidocaine

Pharmacologic Category Local Anesthetic

Medication Safety Issues

Transdermal patch may contain conducting metal (eg, aluminum); remove patch prior to MRI.

Use Local infiltration anesthesia; AVS for nerve block; topical local analgesia for superficial dermatologic procedures

Mechanism of Action Lidocaine blocks both the initiation and conduction of nerve impulses via decreased permeability of sodium ions; epinephrine increases the duration of action of lidocaine by causing vasoconstriction (via alpha effects) which slows the vascular absorption of lidocaine

Pharmacodynamics/Kinetics

Onset of action: Peak effect: ~5 minutes

Duration: ~2 hours; dose and anesthetic procedure dependent

Absorption: Topical: Lidocaine: Minimal; Epinephrine: Minimal

See individual agents.

Contraindications Hypersensitivity to lidocaine, epinephrine, or any component of the formulation; hypersensitivity to other local anesthetics of the amide type; myasthenia gravis; shock; cardiac conduction disease; angle-closure glaucoma

LidoSite™: Hypersensitivity to lidocaine, epinephrine, other local anesthetics of the amide type, or any component of the formulation; patients with electrically-sensitive devices (eg, pacemakers, implantable defibrillators)

Warnings/Precautions Aspirate the syringe (injection solution for infiltration formulation) after tissue penetration and before injection to minimize chance of direct vascular injection. Use caution in endocrine, hepatic, or thyroid disease. Avoid use in presence of flammable anesthetics. Avoid in patients with uncontrolled hyperthyroidism. Use minimal amounts in patients with significant cardiovascular problems (because of epinephrine component). May contain sodium metabisulfite; use caution in patients with a sulfite allergy. Avoid application of topical formulation to distal portions of body (eg, digits, nose, ears, penis). Transdermal patch may contain conducting metal (eg, aluminum); remove patch prior to MRI.

LidoSite™: Do not use near flammable anesthetics. Use with caution in patients with peripheral vascular disease; may have exaggerated vasoconstriction. Use with caution in patients with severe coronary artery disease, hypertension, cardiac dysrhythmias, or patients taking MAO inhibitors or tricyclic antidepressants. Use caution in patients with skin susceptible to injury.

Drug Interactions Lidocaine: **Substrate** of CYP1A2 (minor), 2A6 (minor), 2B6 (minor), 2C8/9 (minor), 2D6 (major), 3A4 (major); **Inhibits** CYP1A2 (strong), 2D6 (strong), 3A4 (moderate)

Also see individual agents. **Note:** Significance of interaction may depend on route of drug delivery and systemic exposure.

(Continued)

Lidocaine and Epinephrine *(Continued)*

Beta-blockers, nonselective: Combination treatment may increase blood pressure.

Epinephrine (and other direct alpha-agonists): Pressor response to I.V. epinephrine, norepinephrine, and phenylephrine may be enhanced in patients receiving TCAs (**Note:** Effect is unlikely with epinephrine or levonordefrin dosages typically administered as infiltration in combination with local anesthetics)

General Anesthetics: May increase sensitivity of myocardium to dysrhythmic effects of epinephrine.

Tricyclic Antidepressants: Combination treatment may increase blood pressure.

Adverse Reactions Degree of adverse effects in the central nervous system and cardiovascular system are directly related to the blood levels of lidocaine. The effects below are more likely to occur after systemic administration rather than infiltration.

Cardiovascular: Myocardial effects include a decrease in contraction force as well as a decrease in electrical excitability and myocardial conduction rate resulting in bradycardia and reduction in cardiac output.

Central nervous system: High blood levels result in anxiety, restlessness, disorientation, confusion, dizziness, tremor, and seizure. This is followed by depression of CNS resulting in somnolence, unconsciousness and possible respiratory arrest. In some cases, symptoms of CNS stimulation may be absent and the primary CNS effects are somnolence and unconsciousness.

Gastrointestinal: Nausea and vomiting may occur

Hypersensitivity reactions: Extremely rare, but may be manifest as dermatologic reactions and edema at injection site. Asthmatic syndromes have occurred. Patients may exhibit hypersensitivity to bisulfites contained in local anesthetic solution to prevent oxidation of epinephrine. In general, patients reacting to bisulfites have a history of asthma and their airways are hyper-reactive to asthmatic syndrome.

Psychogenic reactions: It is common to misinterpret psychogenic responses to local anesthetic injection as an allergic reaction. Intraoral injections are perceived by many patients as a stressful procedure in dentistry. Common symptoms to this stress are diaphoresis, palpitation, hyperventilation, generalized pallor and a fainting feeling

Topical formulation:

>10%: Dermatologic: Papules (up to 12%)

1% to 10%: Dermatologic: Burns (up to 8%), rash (5%), skin irritation, burning sensation, blanching

<1% (Limited to important or life-threatening): Erythema, hematoma, urticaria

Overdosage/Toxicology

Based on **lidocaine** component: Lidocaine has a narrow therapeutic index. Severe toxicity may occur at doses slightly above the therapeutic range, especially in conjunction with other antiarrhythmic drugs. Symptoms of overdose include sedation, confusion, coma, seizures, respiratory arrest, and cardiac toxicity (sinus arrest, AV block, asystole, and hypotension). QRS and QT intervals are usually normal, although they may be prolonged after massive overdose. Other effects include dizziness, paresthesia, tremor, ataxia, and GI disturbance. Treatment is supportive.

Based on **epinephrine** component: Symptoms of overdose include hypertension, which may result in subarachnoid hemorrhage and hemiplegia; arrhythmias; unusually large pupils; pulmonary edema; renal failure; and metabolic acidosis. There is no specific antidote for epinephrine intoxication and treatment is primarily supportive.

Dosing

Adults & Elderly: Dosage varies with the anesthetic procedure, degree of anesthesia needed, vascularity of tissue, duration of anesthesia required, and physical condition of patient.

Dental anesthesia, infiltration, or conduction block:

Children <10 years: 20-30 mg (1-1.5 mL) of lidocaine hydrochloride as a 2% solution with epinephrine 1:100,000; maximum: 4-5 mg of lidocaine hydrochloride/kg of body weight or 100-150 mg as a single dose

Children >10 years and Adults: Do not exceed 6.6 mg/kg body weight or 300 mg of lidocaine hydrochloride and 3 mcg (0.003 mg) of epinephrine/kg of body weight or 0.2 mg epinephrine per dental appointment. The effective anesthetic dose varies with procedure, intensity of anesthesia needed, duration of anesthesia required, and physical condition of the patient. Always use the lowest effective dose along with careful aspiration.

The following numbers of dental carpules (1.8 mL) provide the indicated amounts of lidocaine hydrochloride 2% and epinephrine 1:100,000 (see table):

# of Cartridges (1.8 mL)	Lidocaine HCl (2%) (mg)	Epinephrine 1:100,000 (mg)
1	36	0.018
2	72	0.036
3	108	0.054
4	144	0.072
5	180	0.090
6	216	0.108
7	252	0.126
8	288	0.144
9	324	0.162
10	360	0.180

For most routine dental procedures, lidocaine hydrochloride 2% with epinephrine 1:100,000 is preferred. When a more pronounced hemostasis is required, a 1:50,000 epinephrine concentration should be used. The following numbers of dental carpules (1.8 mL) provide the indicated amounts of lidocaine hydrochloride 2% and epinephrine 1:50,000 (see table):

# of Cartridges (1.8 mL)	Lidocaine HCl (2%) (mg)	Epinephrine 1:50,000 (mg)
1	36	0.036
2	72	0.072
3	108	0.108
4	144	0.144
5	180	0.180
6	216	0.216

Dermatologic procedure: Topical: Place 1 transdermal patch over area requiring analgesia; attach patch to iontophoretic controller and leave on for 10 minutes. Remove patch and perform procedure within 10-20 minutes of patch removal. Do not use another patch for 30 minutes.

Pediatrics: Local anesthetic:

Infiltration: Use lidocaine concentrations of 0.5% to 1% (or even more diluted) to decrease possibility of toxicity. Lidocaine dose should not exceed 7 mg/kg/dose; do not repeat within 2 hours.

Dermatologic procedure: Topical: Children ≥5 years: Refer to adult dosing.

Available Dosage Forms

Injection, solution:

0.5% / 1:200,000: Lidocaine hydrochloride 0.5% and epinephrine 1:200,000 (50 mL)

1% / 1:100,000: Lidocaine hydrochloride 1% and epinephrine 1:100,000 (20 mL, 30 mL, 50 mL)

1% / 1:200,000: Lidocaine hydrochloride 1% and epinephrine 1:200,000 (30 mL)

1.5% / 1:200,000: Lidocaine hydrochloride 1.5% and epinephrine 1:200,000 (30 mL)

2% / 1:50,000: Lidocaine hydrochloride 2% and epinephrine 1:50,000 (1.8 mL)

2% / 1:100,000: Lidocaine hydrochloride 2% and epinephrine 1:100,000 (1.8 mL, 30 mL, 50 mL)

2% / 1:200,000: Lidocaine hydrochloride 2% and epinephrine 1:200,000 (20 mL)

Xylocaine® with Epinephrine:

0.5% / 1:200,000: Lidocaine hydrochloride 0.5% and epinephrine 1:200,000 (50 mL) [contains methylparaben]

1% / 1:100,000: Lidocaine hydrochloride 1% and epinephrine 1:100,000 (10 mL, 20 mL, 50 mL) [contains methylparaben]

(Continued)

Lidocaine and Epinephrine *(Continued)*

2% / 1:50,000: Lidocaine hydrochloride 2% and epinephrine 1:50,000 (1.8 mL) [contains sodium metabisulfite]

2% / 1:100,000: Lidocaine hydrochloride 2% and epinephrine 1:100,000 (1.8 mL) [contains sodium metabisulfite]; (10 mL, 20 mL, 50 mL) [contains methylparaben]

Xylocaine®-MPF with Epinephrine:

1% / 1:200,000: Lidocaine hydrochloride 1% and epinephrine 1:200,000 (5 mL, 10 mL, 30 mL) [contains sodium metabisulfite]

1.5% / 1:200,000: Lidocaine hydrochloride 1.5% and epinephrine 1:200,000 (5 mL, 10 mL, 30 mL) [contains sodium metabisulfite]

2% / 1:200,000: Lidocaine hydrochloride 2% and epinephrine 1:200,000 (5 mL, 10 mL, 20 mL) [contains sodium metabisulfite]

Transdermal system (LidoSite™): Lidocaine hydrochloride 10% and epinephrine 0.1% (25s) [contains sodium metabisulfite; for use only with LidoSite™ controller]

Nursing Guidelines

Assessment: See individual agents.

Patient Education: See individual agents.

Pregnancy Risk Factor: B

Lactation: Enters breast milk/compatible

Breast-Feeding Considerations: Usual infiltration doses of lidocaine with epinephrine given to nursing mothers has not been shown to affect the health of the nursing infant.

Administration

Storage: Solutions with epinephrine should be protected from light. Transdermal system (LidoSite™) should be stored at 20°C to 25°C (68°F to 77°F); avoid freezing.

Related Information

Epinephrine *on page 611*
Lidocaine *on page 1033*

Lidocaine and Prilocaine (LYE doe kane & PRIL oh kane)

U.S. Brand Names EMLA®

Synonyms Prilocaine and Lidocaine

Pharmacologic Category Local Anesthetic

Use Topical anesthetic for use on normal intact skin to provide local analgesia for minor procedures such as I.V. cannulation or venipuncture; has also been used for painful procedures such as lumbar puncture and skin graft harvesting; for superficial minor surgery of genital mucous membranes and as an adjunct for local infiltration anesthesia in genital mucous membranes.

Mechanism of Action Local anesthetic action occurs by stabilization of neuronal membranes and inhibiting the ionic fluxes required for the initiation and conduction of impulses

Pharmacodynamics/Kinetics

EMLA®:

Onset of action: 1 hour

Peak effect: 2-3 hours

Duration: 1-2 hours after removal

Absorption: Related to duration of application and area where applied

3-hour application: 3.6% lidocaine and 6.1% prilocaine

24-hour application: 16.2% lidocaine and 33.5% prilocaine

See individual agents.

Contraindications

Hypersensitivity to amide type anesthetic agents [ie, lidocaine, prilocaine, dibucaine, mepivacaine, bupivacaine, etidocaine]; hypersensitivity to any component of the formulation selected; application on mucous membranes or broken or inflamed skin; infants <1 month of age if gestational age is <37 weeks; infants <12 months of age receiving therapy with methemoglobin-inducing agents; children with congenital or idiopathic methemoglobinemia, or in children who are receiving medications associated with drug-induced methemoglobinemia [ie, acetaminophen (overdosage), benzocaine, chloroquine, dapsone, nitrofurantoin, nitroglycerin, nitroprusside, phenazopyridine, phenelzine, phenobarbital, phenytoin, quinine, sulfonamides]

Warnings/Precautions Use with caution in patients receiving class I antiarrhythmic drugs, since systemic absorption occurs and synergistic toxicity is possible. Although the incidence of systemic adverse reactions with EMLA® is very low, caution should be exercised, particularly when applying over large areas and leaving on for longer than 2 hours.

Drug Interactions Lidocaine: **Substrate** of CYP1A2 (minor), 2A6 (minor), 2B6 (minor), 2C8/9 (minor), 2D6 (major), 3A4 (major); **Inhibits** CYP1A2 (strong), 2D6 (strong), 3A4 (moderate)

Also see individual agents.

Increased toxicity:

Class I antiarrhythmic drugs (tocainide, mexiletine): Effects are additive and potentially synergistic

Drugs known to induce methemoglobinemia

Adverse Reactions Frequency not defined.

Cardiovascular: Hypotension, angioedema

Central nervous system: Shock

Dermatologic: Hyperpigmentation, erythema, itching, rash, burning, urticaria

Genitourinary: Blistering of foreskin (rare)

Local: Burning, stinging, edema

Respiratory: Bronchospasm

Miscellaneous: Alteration in temperature sensation, hypersensitivity reactions

Dosing

Adults & Elderly:

Anesthetic: Topical:

EMLA® cream and EMLA® anesthetic disc: A thick layer of EMLA® cream is applied to intact skin and covered with an occlusive dressing, or alternatively, an EMLA® anesthetic disc is applied to intact skin

Note: Dermal analgesia can be expected to increase for up to 3 hours under occlusive dressing and persist for 1-2 hours after removal of the cream

Minor dermal procedures (eg, I.V. cannulation or venipuncture): Topical: Apply 2.5 g of cream (1/2 of the 5 g tube) over 20-25 cm of skin surface area, or 1 anesthetic disc (1 g over 10 cm^2) for at least 1 hour. **Note:** In clinical trials, 2 sites were usually prepared in case there was a technical problem with cannulation or venipuncture at the first site.

Major dermal procedures (eg, more painful dermatological procedures involving a larger skin area such as split thickness skin graft harvesting): Topical: Apply 2 g of cream per 10 cm^2 of skin and allow to remain in contact with the skin for at least 2 hours.

Adult male genital skin (eg, pretreatment prior to local anesthetic infiltration): Apply a thick layer of cream (1 g/10 cm^2) to the skin surface for 15 minutes. Local anesthetic infiltration should be performed immediately after removal of EMLA® cream.

Adult female genital mucous membranes: Minor procedures (eg, removal of condylomata acuminata, pretreatment for local anesthetic infiltration): Apply 5-10 g (thick layer) of cream for 5-10 minutes

Pediatrics: Note:EMLA® should **not** be used in neonates with a gestational age <37 weeks nor in infants <12 months of age who are receiving treatment with methemoglobin-inducing agents

Local anesthetic (procedures): Topical: Children (intact skin):

Note: Dosing is based on child's age and weight: Although the incidence of systemic adverse effects with EMLA® is very low, caution should be exercised, particularly when applying over large areas and leaving on for >2 hours

Age 0-3 months or <5 kg: Apply a maximum of 1 g over no more than 10 cm^2 of skin; leave on for no longer than 1 hour.

Age 3 months to 12 months and >5 kg: Apply no more than a maximum 2 g total over no more than 20 cm^2 of skin; leave on for no longer than 4 hours.

Age 1-6 years and >10 kg: Apply no more than a maximum of 10 g total over no more than 100 cm^2 of skin; leave on for no longer than 4 hours.

Age 7-12 years and >20 kg: Apply no more than a maximum 20 g total over no more than 200 cm^2 of skin; leave on for no longer than 4 hours.

Note: If a patient greater than 3 months old does not meet the minimum weight requirement, the maximum total dose should be restricted to the corresponding maximum based on patient weight.

Renal Impairment: Smaller areas of treatment are recommended for patients with renal dysfunction.

Hepatic Impairment: Smaller areas of treatment are recommended for patients with hepatic dysfunction.

Available Dosage Forms

Cream, topical: Lidocaine 2.5% and prilocaine 2.5% (5 g, 30 g)

(Continued)

Lidocaine and Prilocaine *(Continued)*

EMLA®: Lidocaine 2.5% and prilocaine 2.5% (5 g, 30 g) [each packaged with Tegaderm® dressings]

Disc, topical: Lidocaine 2.5% and prilocaine 2.5% per disc (2s, 10s) [each 1 g disc is 10 cm^2]

Nursing Guidelines

Assessment: Use on intact skin only. Monitor for effectiveness of anesthesia and adverse reactions. Monitor for return of sensation.

Patient Education: This drug will block sensation to the applied area. Report irritation, pain, burning at application site.

Pregnancy Risk Factor: B

Lactation: Enters breast milk/compatible

Breast-Feeding Considerations: Usual infiltration doses of lidocaine and prilocaine given to nursing mothers has not been shown to affect the health of the nursing infant.

Administration

Storage: Store at room temperature.

◆ **Lidocaine Hydrochloride** *see* Lidocaine *on page 1033*
◆ **Lidoderm®** *see* Lidocaine *on page 1033*
◆ **LidoSite™** *see* Lidocaine and Epinephrine *on page 1039*
◆ **Lignocaine Hydrochloride** *see* Lidocaine *on page 1033*

Linezolid (li NE zoh lid)

U.S. Brand Names Zyvox™

Pharmacologic Category Antibiotic, Oxazolidinone

Medication Safety Issues

Sound-alike/look-alike issues:

Zyvox™ may be confused with Vioxx®, Ziox™, Zosyn®, Zovirax®

Use Treatment of vancomycin-resistant *Enterococcus faecium* (VRE) infections, nosocomial pneumonia caused by *Staphylococcus aureus* including MRSA or *Streptococcus pneumoniae* (including multidrug-resistant strains [MDRSP]), complicated and uncomplicated skin and skin structure infections (including diabetic foot infections without concomitant osteomyelitis), and community-acquired pneumonia caused by susceptible gram-positive organisms

Mechanism of Action Inhibits bacterial protein synthesis by binding to bacterial 23S ribosomal RNA of the 50S subunit. This prevents the formation of a functional 70S initiation complex that is essential for the bacterial translation process. Linezolid is bacteriostatic against enterococci and staphylococci and bactericidal against most strains of streptococci.

Pharmacodynamics/Kinetics

Absorption: Rapid and extensive

Distribution: V_{dss}: Adults: 40-50 L

Protein binding: Adults: 31%

Metabolism: Hepatic via oxidation of the morpholine ring, resulting in two inactive metabolites (aminoethoxyacetic acid, hydroxyethyl glycine); does not involve CYP

Bioavailability: 100%

Half-life elimination: Children ≥1 week (full-term) to 11 years: 1.5-3 hours; Adults: 4-5 hours

Time to peak: Adults: Oral: 1-2 hours

Excretion: Urine (30% as parent drug, 50% as metabolites); feces (9% as metabolites)

Nonrenal clearance: 65%; increased in children ≥1 week to 11 years

Contraindications Hypersensitivity to linezolid or any other component of the formulation

Warnings/Precautions Myelosuppression has been reported and may be dependent on duration of therapy (generally >2 weeks of treatment); use with caution in patients with pre-existing myelosuppression, in patients receiving other drugs which may cause bone marrow suppression, or in chronic infection (previous or concurrent antibiotic therapy). Weekly CBC monitoring is recommended. Discontinue linezolid in patients developing myelosuppression (or in whom myelosuppression worsens during treatment).

Lactic acidosis has been reported with use. Patients who develop recurrent nausea and vomiting, unexplained acidosis, or low bicarbonate levels need immediate evaluation.

Linezolid exhibits mild MAO inhibitor properties and has the potential to have the same interactions as other MAO inhibitors; use with caution in uncontrolled hypertension, pheochromocytoma, carcinoid syndrome, or untreated hyperthyroidism; avoid use with serotonergic agents such as TCAs, venlafaxine, trazodone, sibutramine, meperidine, dextromethorphan, and SSRIs; concomitant use has been associated with the development of serotonin syndrome. Unnecessary use may lead to the development of resistance to linezolid; consider alternatives before initiating outpatient treatment,

Peripheral and optic neuropathy (with vision loss) has been reported and may occur primarily with extended courses of therapy >28 days; any symptoms of visual change or impairment warrant immediate ophthalmic evaluation and possible discontinuation of therapy.

Drug Interactions

Adrenergic agents (eg, phenylpropanolamine, pseudoephedrine, sympathomimetic agents, vasopressor or dopaminergic agents) may cause hypertension.

Myelosuppressive medications: Concurrent use may increase risk of myelosuppression with linezolid.

Serotonergic agents (eg, TCAs, venlafaxine, trazodone, sibutramine, meperidine, dextromethorphan, and SSRIs) may cause a serotonin syndrome (eg, hyperpyrexia, cognitive dysfunction) when used concomitantly.

Tramadol: Concurrent use may increase risk of seizures.

Nutritional/Herbal/Ethanol Interactions

Ethanol: Avoid ethanol (may contain tyramine, hypertensive crisis may result).

Food: Avoid foods (eg, cheese) and beverages containing tyramine in patients receiving linezolid (hypertensive crisis may result).

Adverse Reactions Percentages as reported in adults; frequency similar in pediatric patients

>10%:

Central nervous system: Headache (<1% to 11%)

Gastrointestinal: Diarrhea (3% to 11%)

1% to 10%:

Central nervous system: Insomnia (3%), dizziness (0.4% to 2%), fever (2%)

Dermatologic: Rash (2%)

Gastrointestinal: Nausea (3% to 10%), vomiting (1% to 4%), pancreatic enzymes increased (<1% to 4%), constipation (2%), taste alteration (1% to 2%), tongue discoloration (0.2% to 1%), oral moniliasis (0.4% to 1%), pancreatitis

Genitourinary: Vaginal moniliasis (1% to 2%)

Hematologic: Thrombocytopenia (0.3% to 10%), hemoglobin decreased (0.9% to 7%), anemia, leukopenia, neutropenia; **Note:** Myelosuppression (including anemia, leukopenia, pancytopenia, and thrombocytopenia; may be more common in patients receiving linezolid for >2 weeks)

Hepatic: Abnormal LFTs (0.4% to 1%)

Renal: BUN increased (<1% to 2%)

Miscellaneous: Fungal infection (0.1% to 2%), lactate dehydrogenase increased (<1% to 2%)

<1% or frequency not defined (limited to important or life-threatening): Blurred vision, *C. difficile*-related complications, creatinine increased, dyspepsia, hypertension, localized abdominal pain, pruritus, lactic acidosis, peripheral neuropathy, optic neuropathy, serotonin syndrome (with concurrent use of other serotonergic agents)

Overdosage/Toxicology Treatment includes supportive care. Hemodialysis may improve elimination (30% of a dose is removed during a 3-hour hemodialysis session).

Dosing

Adults & Elderly:

VRE infections: Oral, I.V.: 600 mg every 12 hours for 14-28 days

Nosocomial pneumonia, complicated skin and skin structure infections, community-acquired pneumonia including concurrent bacteremia: Oral, I.V.: 600 mg every 12 hours for 10-14 days

Uncomplicated skin and skin structure infections: Oral: 400 mg every 12 hours for 10-14 days

Pediatrics:

VRE infections: Oral, I.V.:

Preterm neonates (<34 weeks gestational age): 10 mg/kg every 12 hours; neonates with a suboptimal clinical response can be advanced to 10 mg/kg

(Continued)

Linezolid *(Continued)*

every 8 hours. By day 7 of life, all neonates should receive 10 mg/kg every 8 hours.

Infants (excluding preterm neonates <1 week) and Children ≤11 years: 10 mg/kg every 8 hours for 14-28 days

Children ≥12 years: Refer to adult dosing.

Nosocomial pneumonia, complicated skin and skin structure infections, community acquired pneumonia including concurrent bacteremia: Oral, I.V.:

Infants (excluding preterm neonates <1 week) and Children ≤11 years: 10 mg/kg every 8 hours for 10-14 days

Children ≥12 years: Refer to adult dosing.

Uncomplicated skin and skin structure infections: Oral:

Infants (excluding preterm neonates <1 week) and Children <5 years: 10 mg/kg every 8 hours for 10-14 days

Children 5-11 years: 10 mg/kg every 12 hours for 10-14 days

Children ≥12-18 years: 600 mg every 12 hours for 10-14 days

Renal Impairment: No adjustment is recommended. The two primary metabolites may accumulate in patients with renal impairment but the clinical significance is unknown. Weigh the risk of accumulation of metabolites versus the benefit of therapy. Both linezolid and the two metabolites are eliminated by dialysis. Linezolid should be given after hemodialysis.

Hepatic Impairment: No dosage adjustment required for mild to moderate hepatic insufficiency (Child-Pugh class A or B). Use in severe hepatic insufficiency has not been adequately evaluated.

Available Dosage Forms

Infusion [premixed]: 200 mg (100 mL) [contains sodium 1.7 mEq]; 400 mg (200 mL) [contains sodium 3.3 mEq]; 600 mg (300 mL) [contains sodium 5 mEq]

Powder for oral suspension: 20 mg/mL (150 mL) [contains phenylalanine 20 mg/5 mL, sodium benzoate, and sodium 0.4 mEq/5 mL; orange flavor]

Tablet: 600 mg [contains sodium 0.1 mEq/tablet]

Nursing Guidelines

Assessment: Assess for previous drug allergies before administering first dose. See Contraindications and Warnings/Precautions for use cautions. Assess other medications patient may be taking for effectiveness and interactions (see Drug Interactions). Assess results of laboratory tests (see below), therapeutic effectiveness, and adverse reactions (see Adverse Reactions and Overdose/Toxicology) on a regular basis during therapy. Assess knowledge/teach patient appropriate use of oral medication. **Oral/I.V.:** Assess knowledge/teach patient interventions to reduce side effects (including tyramine-free diet) and adverse reactions to report (see Patient Education). Note breast-feeding caution.

Monitoring Laboratory Tests: Weekly CBC and platelet counts, particularly in patients at increased risk of bleeding, with pre-existing myelosuppression, on concomitant medications that cause bone marrow suppression, in those who require >2 weeks of therapy, or in those with chronic infection who have received previous or concomitant antibiotic therapy.

Dietary Considerations: Take with or without food. Avoid foods with high tyramine content (eg, pickled or fermented foods, cheese, beer and wine). Suspension contains 20 mg phenylalanine per teaspoonful. Sodium content: 0.1 mEq/tablet; 0.4 mEq/5 mL; 1.7 mEq/100 mL infusion; 3.3 mEq/200 mL infusion; 5 mEq/300 mL infusion

Patient Education: Oral: Take exactly as directed. Do not alter dosage without consulting prescriber. Complete full course of therapy even if condition appears controlled. Maintain adequate hydration (2-3 L/day of fluids) unless instructed to restrict fluid intake. Avoid alcohol. Avoid tyramine-containing foods (eg, pickles, aged cheese, wine).

Oral/I.V.: You may experience GI discomfort, nausea, vomiting, taste alteration (small, frequent meals, frequent mouth care, sucking lozenges, or chewing gum may help); mild headache (analgesic may help); or constipation (increase exercise, fluids, fruit, or fiber may help). Report immediately unresolved, liquid diarrhea; white plaques in mouth; skin rash or irritation; acute headache, dizziness, blurred vision; or other persistent adverse reactions. **Pregnancy/breast-feeding precautions:** Inform prescriber if you are or intend to become pregnant. Consult prescriber if breast-feeding.

Pregnancy Risk Factor: C

Lactation: Excretion in breast milk unknown/use caution

Perioperative/Anesthesia/Other Concerns: Linezolid has mild MAO inhibitor properties and should be used with caution in patients with cardiovascular disease, particularly those with hypertension. Avoid use with sympathomimetic and dopaminergic agents.

Administration

Oral: Oral suspension: Invert gently to mix prior to administration, do not shake

I.V.: Administer intravenous infusion over 30-120 minutes. Do not mix or infuse with other medications. When the same intravenous line is used for sequential infusion of other medications, flush line with D_5W, NS, or LR before and after infusing linezolid. The yellow color of the injection may intensify over time without affecting potency.

Compatibility:

Y-site administration: Incompatible with amphotericin B, chlorpromazine, diazepam, erythromycin, pentamidine, phenytoin, sulfamethoxazole/trimethoprim

Compatibility when admixed: Incompatible with ceftriaxone

Storage:

Infusion: Store at 25°C (77°F). Protect from light. Keep infusion bags in overwrap until ready for use. Protect infusion bags from freezing.

Oral suspension: Following reconstitution, store at room temperature; use reconstituted suspension within 21 days

- **Lioresal®** *see* Baclofen *on page 222*
- **Lipancreatin** *see* Pancrelipase *on page 1301*
- **Lipitor®** *see* Atorvastatin *on page 198*
- **Liposyn® III** *see* Fat Emulsion *on page 705*
- **Lipram 4500** *see* Pancrelipase *on page 1301*
- **Lipram-CR** *see* Pancrelipase *on page 1301*
- **Lipram-PN** *see* Pancrelipase *on page 1301*
- **Lipram-UL** *see* Pancrelipase *on page 1301*
- **Liquifilm® Tears [OTC]** *see* Artificial Tears *on page 187*

Lisinopril (lyse IN oh pril)

U.S. Brand Names Prinivil®; Zestril®

Pharmacologic Category Angiotensin-Converting Enzyme (ACE) Inhibitor

Medication Safety Issues

Sound-alike/look-alike issues:

Lisinopril may be confused with fosinopril, Lioresal®, Risperdal®

Prinivil® may be confused with Plendil®, Pravachol®, Prevacid®, Prilosec®, Proventil®

Zestril® may be confused with Desyrel®, Restoril®, Vistaril®, Zetia™, Zostrix®

Use Treatment of hypertension, either alone or in combination with other antihypertensive agents; adjunctive therapy in treatment of CHF (afterload reduction); treatment of acute myocardial infarction within 24 hours in hemodynamically-stable patients to improve survival; treatment of left ventricular dysfunction after myocardial infarction

Mechanism of Action Competitive inhibitor of angiotensin-converting enzyme (ACE); prevents conversion of angiotensin I to angiotensin II, a potent vasoconstrictor; results in lower levels of angiotensin II which causes an increase in plasma renin activity and a reduction in aldosterone secretion; a CNS mechanism may also be involved in hypotensive effect as angiotensin II increases adrenergic outflow from CNS; vasoactive kallikreins may be decreased in conversion to active hormones by ACE inhibitors, thus reducing blood pressure

Pharmacodynamics/Kinetics

Onset of action: 1 hour

Peak effect: Hypotensive: Oral: ~6 hours

Duration: 24 hours

Absorption: Well absorbed; unaffected by food

Protein binding: 25%

Half-life elimination: 11-12 hours

Excretion: Primarily urine (as unchanged drug)

Contraindications Hypersensitivity to lisinopril or any component of the formulation; angioedema related to previous treatment with an ACE inhibitor; bilateral renal artery stenosis; pregnancy (2nd and 3rd trimesters)

(Continued)

Lisinopril *(Continued)*

Warnings/Precautions Anaphylactic reactions can occur. Angioedema can occur at any time during treatment (especially following first dose). Angioedema may involve head and neck (potentially affecting the airway) or the intestine (presenting with abdominal pain). Prolonged monitoring may be required as treatment for angioedema may be insufficient. Careful blood pressure monitoring with first dose (hypotension can occur especially in volume-depleted patients). Dosage adjustment needed in renal impairment. Use with caution in hypovolemia; collagen vascular diseases; valvular stenosis (particularly aortic stenosis); hyperkalemia; or before, during, or immediately after anesthesia. Avoid rapid dosage escalation, which may lead to renal insufficiency. Rare toxicities associated with ACE inhibitors include cholestatic jaundice (which may progress to hepatic necrosis) and neutropenia/agranulocytosis with myeloid hyperplasia. If patient has renal impairment then a baseline WBC with differential and serum creatinine should be evaluated and monitored closely during the first 3 months of therapy. Hypersensitivity reactions may be seen during hemodialysis with high-flux dialysis membranes (eg, AN69). Deterioration in renal function can occur with initiation. Use with caution in unilateral renal artery stenosis and pre-existing renal insufficiency. Safety and efficacy have not been established in children <6 years of age.

Drug Interactions

Allopurinol: Case reports (rare) indicate a possible increased risk of hypersensitivity reactions when combined with lisinopril.

$Alpha_1$ blockers: Hypotensive effect increased.

Aspirin: The effects of ACE inhibitors may be blunted by aspirin administration, particularly at higher dosages (see Cardiovascular Considerations) and/or increase adverse renal effects.

Diuretics: Hypovolemia due to diuretics may precipitate acute hypotensive events or acute renal failure.

Insulin: Risk of hypoglycemia may be increased.

Lithium: Risk of lithium toxicity may be increased; monitor lithium levels, especially the first 4 weeks of therapy.

Mercaptopurine: Risk of neutropenia may be increased.

NSAIDs: May attenuate hypertensive efficacy; effect has been seen with captopril and may occur with other ACE inhibitors; monitor blood pressure. May increase adverse renal effects.

Potassium-sparing diuretics (amiloride, spironolactone, triamterene): Increased risk of hyperkalemia.

Potassium supplements may increase the risk of hyperkalemia.

Trimethoprim (high dose) may increase the risk of hyperkalemia.

Nutritional/Herbal/Ethanol Interactions Herb/Nutraceutical: Avoid dong quai if using for hypertension (has estrogenic activity). Avoid ephedra, yohimbe, ginseng (may worsen hypertension). Avoid garlic (may have increased antihypertensive effect).

Lab Interactions May cause false-positive results in urine acetone determinations using sodium nitroprusside reagent; increased potassium (S), serum creatinine/BUN

Adverse Reactions Note: Frequency ranges include data from hypertension and heart failure trials. Higher rates of adverse reactions have generally been noted in patients with CHF. However, the frequency of adverse effects associated with placebo is also increased in this population.

1% to 10%:

- Cardiovascular: Orthostatic effects (1%), hypotension (1% to 4%)
- Central nervous system: Headache (4% to 6%), dizziness (5% to 12%), fatigue (3%)
- Dermatologic: Rash (1% to 2%)
- Endocrine & metabolic: Hyperkalemia (2% to 5%)
- Gastrointestinal: Diarrhea (3% to 4%), nausea (2%), vomiting (1%), abdominal pain (2%)
- Genitourinary: Impotence (1%)
- Hematologic: Decreased hemoglobin (small)
- Neuromuscular & skeletal: Chest pain (3%), weakness (1%)
- Renal: BUN increased (2%); deterioration in renal function (in patients with bilateral renal artery stenosis or hypovolemia); serum creatinine increased (often transient)
- Respiratory: Cough (4% to 9%), upper respiratory infection (2% to 2%)

<1% (Limited to important or life-threatening): Acute renal failure, alopecia, anaphylactoid reactions, angioedema, anuria, arrhythmia, arthralgia, asthma,

ataxia, azotemia, bone marrow suppression, bronchospasm, cardiac arrest, decreased libido, gout, hepatic necrosis, hepatitis, hyperkalemia, hyponatremia, increased bilirubin, transaminases increased, infiltrates, jaundice (cholestatic), MI, neutropenia, oliguria, orthostatic hypotension, pancreatitis, paresthesia, pemphigus, peripheral neuropathy, photosensitivity, pleural effusion, pulmonary embolism, Stevens-Johnson syndrome, stroke, systemic lupus erythematosus, thrombocytopenia, TIA, toxic epidermal necrolysis, tremor, urticaria, vasculitis, vertigo, vision loss. In addition, a syndrome which may include fever, myalgia, arthralgia, interstitial nephritis, vasculitis, rash, eosinophilia and positive ANA, and elevated ESR has been reported with ACE inhibitors.

Overdosage/Toxicology Mild hypotension has been the primary toxic effect seen with acute overdose. Bradycardia may also occur; hyperkalemia occurs even with therapeutic doses, especially in patients with renal insufficiency and those taking NSAIDs. Treatment and is symptomatic and supportive.

Dosing

Adults:

Hypertension: Oral: Usual dosage range (JNC 7): 10-40 mg/day

Not maintained on diuretic: Initial: 10 mg/day

Maintained on diuretic: Initial: 5 mg/day

Note: Antihypertensive effect may diminish toward the end of the dosing interval especially with doses of 10 mg/day. An increased dose may aid in extending the duration of antihypertensive effect. Doses up to 80 mg/day have been used, but do not appear to give greater effect (Zesteril® Product Information, 12/04).

Patients taking diuretics should have them discontinued 2-3 days prior to initiating lisinopril if possible. Restart diuretic after blood pressure is stable if needed. If diuretic cannot be discontinued prior to therapy, begin with 5 mg with close supervision until stable blood pressure. In patients with hyponatremia (<130 mEq/L), start dose at 2.5 mg/day.

Congestive heart failure: Oral: Initial: 2.5-5 mg once daily; then increase by no more than 10 mg increments at intervals no less than 2 weeks to a maximum daily dose of 40 mg. Usual maintenance: 5-40 mg/day as a single dose. Target dose: 20-40 mg once daily (ACC/AHA 2005 Heart Failure Guidelines)

Note: If patient has hyponatremia (serum sodium <130 meq/L) or renal impairment (Cl_{cr} <30 mL/minute or creatinine >3 mg/dL), then initial dose should be 2.5 mg/day

Acute myocardial infarction (within 24 hours in hemodynamically stable patients): Oral: 5 mg immediately, then 5 mg at 24 hours, 10 mg at 48 hours, and 10 mg every day thereafter for 6 weeks. Patients should continue to receive standard treatments such as thrombolytics, aspirin, and beta-blockers.

Elderly: Oral:

Initial: 2.5-5 mg/day; increase doses 2.5-5 mg/day at 1- to 2-week intervals; maximum daily dose: 40 mg

Patients taking diuretics should have them discontinued 2-3 days prior to initiating lisinopril if possible. Restart diuretic after blood pressure is stable if needed. In patients with hyponatremia (<130 mEq/L), start dose at 2.5 mg/day (see Renal Impairment).

Pediatrics:

Hypertension: Children ≥6 years: Oral: Initial: 0.07 mg/kg once daily (up to 5 mg); increase dose at 1- to 2-week intervals; doses >0.61 mg/kg or >40 mg have not been evaluated.

Renal Impairment:

Hypertension:

Adults: Initial doses should be modified and upward titration should be cautious, based on response (maximum: 40 mg/day)

Cl_{cr} >30 mL/minute: Initial: 10 mg/day

Cl_{cr} 10-30 mL/minute: Initial: 5 mg/day

Hemodialysis: Initial: 2.5 mg/day; dialyzable (50%)

Children: Use in not recommended in pediatric patients with GFR <30 mL/minute/1.73 m^2

Congestive heart failure: Adults: Cl_{cr} <30 mL/minute or creatinine >3 mg/dL): Initial: 2.5 mg/day

Available Dosage Forms [DSC] = Discontinued product

Tablet: 2.5 mg, 5 mg, 10 mg, 20 mg, 30 mg, 40 mg

Prinivil®: 2.5 mg [DSC], 5 mg, 10 mg, 20 mg, 30 mg, 40 mg

Zestril®: 2.5 mg, 5 mg, 10 mg, 20 mg, 30 mg, 40 mg

(Continued)

Lisinopril *(Continued)*

Nursing Guidelines

Assessment: Use caution in presence of renal impairment; hypovolemia; collagen vascular diseases; valvular stenosis; hyperkalemia; or before, during, or immediately after anesthesia. Assess potential for interactions with other pharmacological agents or herbal products patient is taking that may impact fluid balance or cardiac status. Patient should be monitored for adverse reactions following first dose, following any increase in dose and regularly during therapy (eg, hypovolemia, postural hypotension, anaphylactic reaction, or angioedema [may effect airway and/or intestine]). Monitor results of laboratory tests and therapeutic effectiveness on a regular basis. Teach patient proper use, possible side effects/appropriate interventions, and adverse symptoms to report (refer to Patient Education).

Monitoring Laboratory Tests: CBC, renal function tests, electrolytes. If patient has renal impairment, a baseline WBC with differential and serum creatinine should be evaluated and monitored closely during the first 3 months of therapy.

Patient Education: Do not take any new medication during therapy unless approved by prescriber. Do not use potassium supplement or salt substitutes without consulting prescriber. Take exactly as directed; do not discontinue without consulting prescriber. Take first dose at bedtime. This drug does not eliminate need for diet or exercise regimen as recommended by prescriber. May cause dizziness, fainting, or lightheadedness (use caution when driving or engaging in tasks that require alertness until response to drug is known); postural hypotension (use caution when rising from lying or sitting position or climbing stairs); or nausea, vomiting, abdominal pain, dry mouth, or transient loss of appetite (small frequent meals, frequent mouth care, sucking lozenges, or chewing gum may help), report if these persist. Report chest pain or palpitations; mouth sores; fever or chills; swelling of extremities, face, mouth, or tongue; skin rash; numbness, tingling, or pain in muscles; respiratory difficulty or unusual cough; other persistent adverse reactions. **Pregnancy/breast-feeding precautions:** Inform prescriber if you are or intend to become pregnant. This drug should not be used in the 2nd or 3rd trimester of pregnancy. Consult prescriber for appropriate contraceptive measures. Breast-feeding is not recommended.

Geriatric Considerations: Due to frequent decreases in glomerular filtration (also creatinine clearance) with aging, elderly patients may have exaggerated responses to ACE inhibitors. Differences in clinical response due to hepatic changes are not observed. ACE inhibitors may be preferred agents in elderly patients with congestive heart failure and diabetes mellitus. Diabetic proteinuria is reduced and insulin sensitivity is enhanced. In general, the side effect profile is favorable in the elderly and causes little or no CNS confusion. Use lowest dose recommendations initially.

Pregnancy Risk Factor: C (1st trimester)/D (2nd and 3rd trimesters)

Pregnancy Issues: ACE inhibitors can cause fetal injury or death if taken during the 2nd or 3rd trimester. Discontinue ACE inhibitors as soon as pregnancy is detected.

Lactation: Excretion in breast milk unknown/not recommended

Breast-Feeding Considerations: Lisinopril is not recommended (per manufacturer) in breast-feeding women. A similar drug, captopril, has been rated as compatible.

Perioperative/Anesthesia/Other Concerns: Due to decreases in glomerular filtration (also creatinine clearance) with aging, severe congestive heart failure and renal failure, these patients may experience renal dysfunction with ACE inhibitor administration.

ACE inhibitor therapy may elicit rapid increases in potassium and creatinine, especially when used in patients with bilateral renal artery stenosis. When ACE inhibition is introduced in patients with pre-existing diuretic therapy who are hypovolemic, the ACE inhibitor may induce acute hypotension. Concomitant NSAID therapy may attenuate blood pressure control. Because of the potent teratogenic effects of ACE inhibitors, these drugs should be avoided, if possible, when treating women of childbearing potential not on effective birth control measures.

Administration

Oral: Watch for hypotensive effects within 1-3 hours of first dose or new higher dose.

Lisinopril and Hydrochlorothiazide

(lyse IN oh pril & hye droe klor oh THYE a zide)

U.S. Brand Names Prinzide®; Zestoretic®

Synonyms Hydrochlorothiazide and Lisinopril

Pharmacologic Category Antihypertensive Agent, Combination

Use Treatment of hypertension

Pharmacodynamics/Kinetics See individual agents.

Contraindications

Based on **lisinopril** component: Hypersensitivity to lisinopril or any component of the formulation; angioedema related to previous treatment with an ACE inhibitor; hereditary or idiopathic angioedema; bilateral renal artery stenosis; pregnancy (2nd and 3rd trimesters)

Based on **hydrochlorothiazide** component: Hypersensitivity to hydrochlorothiazide, thiazides, sulfonamide-derived drugs, or any component of the formulation; anuria; renal decompensation; pregnancy (2nd and 3rd trimesters)

Warnings/Precautions

Based on **lisinopril** component: Anaphylactic reactions can occur. Angioedema can occur at any time during treatment (especially following first dose). Angioedema may involve head and neck (potentially affecting the airway) or the intestine (presenting with abdominal pain). Prolonged monitoring may be required as treatment for angioedema may be insufficient. Careful blood pressure monitoring with first dose (hypotension can occur especially in volume-depleted patients). Dosage adjustment needed in renal impairment. Use with caution in hypovolemia; collagen vascular diseases; valvular stenosis (particularly aortic stenosis); hyperkalemia; or before, during, or immediately after anesthesia. Avoid rapid dosage escalation, which may lead to renal insufficiency. Rare toxicities associated with ACE inhibitors include cholestatic jaundice (which may progress to hepatic necrosis) and neutropenia/agranulocytosis with myeloid hyperplasia. If patient has renal impairment then a baseline WBC with differential and serum creatinine should be evaluated and monitored closely during the first 3 months of therapy. Hypersensitivity reactions may be seen during hemodialysis with high-flux dialysis membranes (eg, AN69). Deterioration in renal function can occur with initiation. Use with caution in unilateral renal artery stenosis and pre-existing renal insufficiency. Safety and efficacy have not been established in children <6 years of age.

Based on **hydrochlorothiazide** component: Avoid in severe renal disease (ineffective). Electrolyte disturbances (hypokalemia, hypochloremic alkalosis, hyponatremia) can occur. Use with caution in severe hepatic dysfunction; hepatic encephalopathy can be caused by electrolyte disturbances. Gout can be precipitate in certain patients with a history of gout, a familial predisposition to gout, or chronic renal failure. Cautious use in diabetics; may see a change in glucose control. Hypersensitivity reactions can occur. Can cause SLE exacerbation or activation. Use with caution in patients with moderate or high cholesterol concentrations. Photosensitization may occur. Correct hypokalemia before initiating therapy.

Chemical similarities are present among sulfonamides, sulfonylureas, carbonic anhydrase inhibitors, thiazides, and loop diuretics (except ethacrynic acid). Use in patients with sulfonamide allergy is specifically contraindicated in product labeling, however, a risk of cross-reaction exists in patients with allergy to any of these compounds; avoid use when previous reaction has been severe.

Drug Interactions See individual agents.

Adverse Reactions See individual agents.

Dosing

Adults & Elderly: Hypertension: Oral: Initial: Lisinopril 10 mg/hydrochlorothiazide 12.5 mg or lisinopril 20 mg/hydrochlorothiazide 12.5 mg with further increases of either or both components could depend on clinical response. Doses >80 mg/day lisinopril or >50 mg/day hydrochlorothiazide are not recommended.

Renal Impairment: Dosage adjustments should be made with caution. Usual regimens of therapy need not be adjusted as long as patient's Cl_{cr} >30 mL/minute. In patients with more severe renal impairment, loop diuretics are preferred.

Available Dosage Forms Tablet:

Lisinopril 10 mg and hydrochlorothiazide 12.5 mg
Lisinopril 20 mg and hydrochlorothiazide 12.5 mg
Lisinopril 20 mg and hydrochlorothiazide 25 mg

(Continued)

Lisinopril and Hydrochlorothiazide *(Continued)*

Nursing Guidelines

Assessment: See individual components listed in Related Information. **Pregnancy risk factor C/D** - see Pregnancy Risk Factor for use cautions. Assess knowledge/instruct patient on need to use appropriate contraceptive measures and the need to avoid pregnancy. Note breast-feeding caution.

Patient Education: See individual agents. **Pregnancy/breast-feeding precautions:** Inform prescriber if you are or intend to become pregnant. Consult prescriber if breast-feeding.

Pregnancy Risk Factor: C/D (2nd and 3rd trimesters)

Lactation:

Hydrochlorothiazide: Compatible

Lisinopril: Excretion in breast milk unknown

Breast-Feeding Considerations: See individual monographs.

Related Information

Hydrochlorothiazide *on page 862*

Lisinopril *on page 1047*

♦ **Lispro Insulin** *see* Insulin Lispro *on page 923*

Lithium (LITH ee um)

U.S. Brand Names Eskalith® [DSC]; Eskalith CR®; Lithobid®

Synonyms Lithium Carbonate; Lithium Citrate

Pharmacologic Category Lithium

Medication Safety Issues

Sound-alike/look-alike issues:

Eskalith® may be confused with Estratest®

Lithobid® may be confused with Levbid®, Lithostat®

Use Management of bipolar disorders; treatment of mania in individuals with bipolar disorder (maintenance treatment prevents or diminishes intensity of subsequent episodes)

Unlabeled/Investigational Use Potential augmenting agent for antidepressants; aggression, post-traumatic stress disorder, conduct disorder in children

Mechanism of Action Alters cation transport across cell membrane in nerve and muscle cells and influences reuptake of serotonin and/or norepinephrine; second messenger systems involving the phosphatidylinositol cycle are inhibited; postsynaptic D2 receptor supersensitivity is inhibited

Pharmacodynamics/Kinetics

Absorption: Rapid and complete

Distribution: V_d: Initial: 0.3-0.4 L/kg; V_{dss}: 0.7-1 L/kg; crosses placenta; enters breast milk at 35% to 50% the concentrations in serum; distribution is complete in 6-10 hours

CSF, liver concentrations: 1/3 to 1/2 of serum concentration

Erythrocyte concentration: ~1/2 of serum concentration

Heart, lung, kidney, muscle concentrations: Equivalent to serum concentration

Saliva concentration: 2-3 times serum concentration

Thyroid, bone, brain tissue concentrations: Increase 50% over serum concentrations

Protein binding: Not protein bound

Metabolism: Not metabolized

Bioavailability: Not affected by food; Capsule, immediate release tablet: 95% to 100%; Extended release tablet: 60% to 90%; Syrup: 100%

Half-life elimination: 18-24 hours; can increase to more than 36 hours in elderly or with renal impairment

Time to peak, serum: Nonsustained release: ~0.5-2 hours; slow release: 4-12 hours; syrup: 15-60 minutes

Excretion: Urine (90% to 98% as unchanged drug); sweat (4% to 5%); feces (1%)

Clearance: 80% of filtered lithium is reabsorbed in the proximal convoluted tubules; therefore, clearance approximates 20% of GFR or 20-40 mL/minute

Contraindications Hypersensitivity to lithium or any component of the formulation; avoid use in patients with severe cardiovascular or renal disease, or with severe debilitation, dehydration, or sodium depletion; pregnancy

Warnings/Precautions Lithium toxicity is closely related to serum levels and can occur at therapeutic doses; serum lithium determinations are required to monitor therapy. Use with caution in patients with thyroid disease, mild-moderate renal impairment, or mild-moderate cardiovascular disease. Use caution in patients receiving medications which alter sodium excretion (eg, diuretics, ACE inhibitors,

NSAIDs), or in patients with significant fluid loss (protracted sweating, diarrhea, or prolonged fever); temporary reduction or cessation of therapy may be warranted. Some elderly patients may be extremely sensitive to the effects of lithium, see Dosage. Chronic therapy results in diminished renal concentrating ability (nephrogenic DI); this is usually reversible when lithium is discontinued. Changes in renal function should be monitored, and re-evaluation of treatment may be necessary. Use caution in patients at risk of suicide (suicidal thoughts or behavior).

Morphologic changes with glomerular and interstitial fibrosis and nephron atrophy have been reported in patients on chronic lithium therapy; morphologic changes have also been reported in manic-depressive patients never exposed to lithium. The relationship between morphologic changes and renal function, and the association with lithium therapy, have not been established.

Use with caution in patients receiving neuroleptic medications - a syndrome resembling NMS has been associated with concurrent therapy. Lithium may impair the patient's alertness, affecting the ability to operate machinery or driving a vehicle. Neuromuscular-blocking agents should be administered with caution; the response may be prolonged.

Higher serum concentrations may be required and tolerated during an acute manic phase; however, the tolerance decreases when symptoms subside. Normal fluid and salt intake must be maintained during therapy.

Safety and efficacy have not been established in children <12 years of age.

Drug Interactions

ACE inhibitors: May increase the risk of lithium toxicity via sodium depletion; monitor

Angiotensin receptor antagonists (losartan): May reduce the renal clearance of lithium; monitor

Caffeine (xanthine derivatives): May lower lithium serum concentrations by increasing urinary lithium excretion; monitor.

Carbamazepine: Concurrent use of lithium with carbamazepine may increase the risk for neurotoxicity; monitor

Carbonic anhydrase inhibitors: May decrease lithium levels; includes acetazolamide; monitor

Calcium channel blockers (diltiazem and verapamil): May increase the risk for neurotoxicity (ataxia, tremors, nausea, vomiting, diarrhea, and/or tinnitus); monitor; does not appear to involve dihydropyridine class

Chlorpromazine: May lower serum concentrations of both drugs; monitor

COX-2 inhibitors (celecoxib): May increase lithium plasma concentrations (similar to NSAIDs); monitor.

Haloperidol: May increase the risk for neurotoxicity and encephalopathy; a rare encephalopathic syndrome resulting in irreversible brain damage has been reported in a few patients (causal relationship not established); monitor

Iodine salts: May enhance the hypothyroid effects of lithium; monitor

Loop diuretics: May decrease the renal excretion of lithium, leading to toxicity; monitor

MAO inhibitors: Should generally be avoided due to use reports of fatal malignant hyperpyrexia when combined with lithium

Methyldopa: May increase the risk for neurotoxicity; monitor

Metronidazole: May increase lithium toxicity (rare); monitor

Neuromuscular-blocking agents: Lithium may potentiate the response to neuromuscular blockade, resulting in prolonged blockade and possible delayed recovery

NSAIDs: Renal lithium excretion may be decreased leading to increased serum lithium concentrations; sulindac and aspirin may be the exceptions; monitor

Phenothiazines: May increase the risk for neurotoxicity; monitor

Phenytoin: May enhance lithium toxicity; monitor

Selegiline: Risk of severe reactions when combined with MAO inhibitors may be decreased when administered with selective MAO type B inhibitor, particularly at selegiline doses <10 mg/day; however, theoretical risk is still present

SSRIs: May increase the risk for neurotoxicity; monitor; effect noted with fluoxetine, fluvoxamine

Sibutramine: Combined use of lithium with sibutramine may increase the risk of serotonin syndrome; this combination is best avoided

Sodium-containing products: Bicarbonate and/or high sodium intake may reduce serum lithium concentrations via enhanced excretion; monitor. **Note:** Reabsorption of lithium in the proximal convoluted tubule occurs against electrical

(Continued)

Lithium *(Continued)*

and concentration gradients that do not distinguish between lithium and sodium. Therefore, lithium clearance may increase or decrease 30% to 50% with sodium load or depletion, respectively. Sodium depletion usually has the greater effect.

Sympathomimetics: Lithium may blunt the pressor response to sympathomimetics (epinephrine, phenylephrine, norepinephrine)

Tetracyclines: May increase lithium levels; monitor

Theophylline: May increase real clearance of lithium, resulting in a decrease in serum lithium concentrations; monitor

Thiazide diuretics: May increase serum lithium concentration via sodium depletion and decreased lithium clearance; a lithium dose reduction of 50% is commonly recommended

Tricyclic antidepressants: May increase the risk for neurotoxicity; monitor

Urea: May lower lithium serum concentrations by increasing urinary excretion; monitor.

Nutritional/Herbal/Ethanol Interactions Food: Lithium serum concentrations may be increased if taken with food. Limit caffeine.

Lab Interactions Increased calcium (S), glucose, magnesium, potassium (S); decreased thyroxine (S)

Adverse Reactions Frequency not defined.

Cardiovascular: Cardiac arrhythmia, hypotension, sinus node dysfunction, flattened or inverted T waves (reversible), edema, bradycardia, syncope

Central nervous system: Dizziness, vertigo, slurred speech, blackout spells, seizure, sedation, restlessness, confusion, psychomotor retardation, stupor, coma, dystonia, fatigue, lethargy, headache, pseudotumor cerebri, slowed intellectual functioning, tics

Dermatologic: Dry or thinning of hair, folliculitis, alopecia, exacerbation of psoriasis, rash

Endocrine & metabolic: Euthyroid goiter and/or hypothyroidism, hyperthyroidism, hyperglycemia, diabetes insipidus

Gastrointestinal: Polydipsia, anorexia, nausea, vomiting, diarrhea, xerostomia, metallic taste, weight gain, salivary gland swelling, excessive salivation

Genitourinary: Incontinence, polyuria, glycosuria, oliguria, albuminuria

Hematologic: Leukocytosis

Neuromuscular & skeletal: Tremor, muscle hyperirritability, ataxia, choreoathetoid movements, hyperactive deep tendon reflexes, myasthenia gravis (rare)

Ocular: Nystagmus, blurred vision, transient scotoma

Miscellaneous: Coldness and painful discoloration of fingers and toes

Overdosage/Toxicology Symptoms include sedation, confusion, tremors, joint pain, visual changes, seizures, and coma. There is no specific antidote for lithium poisoning. For acute ingestion, following initiation of essential overdose management, discontinue lithium and remove any unabsorbed lithium via gastric lavage (activated charcoal is ineffective as it does not bind lithium). Correct fluid and electrolyte imbalances, provide supportive care. In severe cases, patient should be dialyzed. Hemodialysis is preferred (and more effective) than peritoneal dialysis. The goal is to decrease serum lithium level to <1 mEq/L on a serum sample drawn 6-8 hours after completion of dialysis. Agents that increase the excretion of lithium are of questionable value.

Dosing

Adults:

Bipolar disorders: Oral: 900-2400 mg/day in 3-4 divided doses or 900-1800 mg/day in two divided doses of sustained release

Note: Monitor serum concentrations and clinical response (efficacy and toxicity) to determine proper dose

Elderly: Bipolar disorders: Oral: Initial: 300 mg twice daily; increase weekly in increments of 300 mg/day, monitoring levels; rarely need to go >900-1200 mg/day.

Pediatrics:

Bipolar disorders: Oral: Children 6-12 years: 15-60 mg/kg/day in 3-4 divided doses; dose not to exceed usual adult dosage. **Note:** Monitor serum concentrations and clinical response (efficacy and toxicity) to determine proper dose.

Conduct disorder (unlabeled use): Oral: Children 6-12 years: 15-30 mg/kg/day in 3-4 divided doses; dose not to exceed usual adult dosage

Renal Impairment:

Cl_{cr} 10-50 mL/minute: Administer 50% to 75% of normal dose.

Cl_{cr} <10 mL/minute: Administer 25% to 50% of normal dose.

Dialyzable (50% to 100%); 4-7 times more efficient than peritoneal dialysis

Available Dosage Forms

[DSC] = Discontinued product

Capsule, as carbonate: 150 mg, 300 mg, 600 mg

Eskalith®: 300 mg [contains benzyl alcohol] [DSC]

Syrup, as citrate: 300 mg/5 mL (5 mL, 10 mL, 480 mL) [contains alcohol]

Tablet, as carbonate: 300 mg

Tablet, controlled release, as carbonate (Eskalith CR®): 450 mg

Tablet, slow release, as carbonate (Lithobid®): 300 mg

Nursing Guidelines

Assessment: Assess effectiveness and interactions of other medications patient may be taking. Monitor cardiovascular status; assess for fluid retention. Monitor laboratory results at beginning of therapy, when adjusting dose, and periodically thereafter. Monitor effectiveness of therapy and adverse reactions at beginning of therapy and periodically with long-term use. **Note:** Lithium has a very small window of safety (TI). Assess knowledge/teach patient appropriate use, interventions to reduce side effects, and importance of reporting adverse symptoms promptly.

Monitoring Laboratory Tests: Serum lithium every 4-5 days during initial therapy. Monitor renal and thyroid; serum electrolytes; CBC with differential, urinalysis.

Levels should be obtained twice weekly until both patient's clinical status and levels are stable then levels may be obtained every 1-3 months.

Timing of serum samples: Draw trough just before next dose (8-12 hours after previous dose).

Therapeutic levels:

Acute mania: 0.6-1.2 mEq/L (SI: 0.6-1.2 mmol/L)

Protection against future episodes in most patients with bipolar disorder: 0.8-1 mEq/L (SI: 0.8-1.0 mmol/L); a higher rate of relapse is described in subjects who are maintained at <0.4 mEq/L (SI: 0.4 mmol/L).

Elderly patients can usually be maintained at lower end of therapeutic range (0.6-0.8 mEq/L).

Toxic concentration: >1.5 mEq/L (SI: >2 mmol/L)

Adverse effect levels:

GI complaints/tremor: 1.5-2 mEq/L

Confusion/somnolence: 2-2.5 mEq/L

Seizures/death: >2.5 mEq/L

Dietary Considerations: May be taken with meals to avoid GI upset; have patient drink 2-3 L of water daily.

Patient Education: Take exactly as directed; do not change dosage without consulting prescriber. Do not crush or chew extended or slow release tablets or capsules. Maintain adequate hydration (2-3 L/day of fluids) unless instructed to restrict fluid intake (especially in summer). Avoid changes in sodium content (eg, low sodium diets); reduction of sodium can increase lithium toxicity. Limit caffeine intake (diuresis can increase lithium toxicity). Frequent blood test and monitoring will be necessary. You may experience decreased appetite or altered taste sensation (small frequent meals may help maintain nutrition); or drowsiness or dizziness, especially during early therapy (use caution when driving or engaging in tasks requiring alertness until response to drug is known). Immediately report unresolved diarrhea, abrupt changes in weight, muscular tremors or lack of coordination, fever, or changes in urinary volume. **Pregnancy/breast-feeding precautions:** Do not get pregnant while taking this medication; use appropriate contraceptive measures. Do not breast-feed.

Geriatric Considerations: Some elderly patients may be extremely sensitive to the effects of lithium. Initial doses need to be adjusted for renal function in the elderly; thereafter, adjust doses based upon serum concentrations and response.

Pregnancy Risk Factor: D

Pregnancy Issues: Cardiac malformations in the infant, including Ebstein's anomaly, are associated with use of lithium during the first trimester of pregnancy. Nontoxic effects to the newborn include shallow respiration, hypotonia,

(Continued)

Lithium *(Continued)*

lethargy, cyanosis, diabetes insipidus, thyroid depression, and nontoxic goiter when lithium is used near term. Efforts should be made to avoid lithium use during the first trimester; if an alternative therapy is not appropriate, the lowest possible dose of lithium should be used throughout the pregnancy. Fetal echocardiography and ultrasound to screen for anomalies should be conducted between 16-20 weeks of gestation. Lithium levels should be monitored in the mother and may need adjusted following delivery.

Lactation: Enters breast milk/contraindicated

Administration

Oral: Administer with meals to decrease GI upset. Slow release tablets must be swallowed whole; do not crush or chew.

- ♦ **Lithium Carbonate** *see* Lithium *on page 1052*
- ♦ **Lithium Citrate** *see* Lithium *on page 1052*
- ♦ **Lithobid®** *see* Lithium *on page 1052*
- ♦ **Live Attenuated Influenza Vaccine (LAIV)** *see* Influenza Virus Vaccine *on page 913*
- ♦ **LMD®** *see* Dextran *on page 503*
- ♦ **Locoid®** *see* Hydrocortisone *on page 873*
- ♦ **Locoid Lipocream®** *see* Hydrocortisone *on page 873*
- ♦ **Lofibra™** *see* Fenofibrate *on page 708*
- ♦ **L-OHP** *see* Oxaliplatin *on page 1275*
- ♦ **Loniten®** *see* Minoxidil *on page 1165*

Loperamide (loe PER a mide)

U.S. Brand Names Diamode [OTC]; Imodium® A-D [OTC]; Kao-Paverin® [OTC]; K-Pek II [OTC]

Synonyms Loperamide Hydrochloride

Pharmacologic Category Antidiarrheal

Medication Safety Issues

Sound-alike/look-alike issues:

Imodium® A-D may be confused with Indocin®, Ionamin®

Use Treatment of chronic diarrhea associated with inflammatory bowel disease; acute nonspecific diarrhea; increased volume of ileostomy discharge

OTC labeling: Control of symptoms of diarrhea, including Traveler's diarrhea

Unlabeled/Investigational Use Cancer treatment-induced diarrhea (eg, irinotecan induced); chronic diarrhea caused by bowel resection

Mechanism of Action Acts directly on circular and longitudinal intestinal muscles, through the opioid receptor, to inhibit peristalsis and prolong transit time; reduces fecal volume, increases viscosity, and diminishes fluid and electrolyte loss; demonstrates antisecretory activity. Loperamide increases tone on the anal sphincter

Pharmacodynamics/Kinetics

Absorption: Poor

Distribution: Poor penetration into brain; low amounts enter breast milk

Metabolism: Hepatic via oxidative N-demethylation

Half-life elimination: 7-14 hours

Time to peak, plasma: Liquid: 2.5 hours; Capsule: 5 hours

Excretion: Urine and feces (1% as metabolites, 30% to 40% as unchanged drug)

Contraindications Hypersensitivity to loperamide or any component of the formulation; abdominal pain without diarrhea; children <2 years

Avoid use as primary therapy in acute dysentery, acute ulcerative colitis, bacterial enterocolitis, pseudomembranous colitis

Warnings/Precautions Should not be used if diarrhea is accompanied by high fever or blood in stool. Use caution in young children as response may be variable because of dehydration. Concurrent fluid and electrolyte replacement is often necessary in all age groups depending upon severity of diarrhea. Should not be used when inhibition of peristalsis is undesirable or dangerous. Discontinue if constipation, abdominal pain, or ileus develop. Use caution in patients with hepatic impairment because of reduced first pass metabolism. Use caution in treatment of AIDS patients; stop therapy at the sign of abdominal distention. Cases of toxic megacolon have occurred in this population. Loperamide is a symptom-directed treatment; if an underlying diagnosis is made, other disease-specific treatment may be indicated. Use caution in patients with hepatic impairment because of reduced first-pass metabolism; monitor for signs of CNS toxicity.

OTC labeling: If diarrhea lasts longer than 2 days, patient should stop taking loperamide and consult healthcare provider.

Drug Interactions Substrate (minor) of CYP2B6

P-glycoprotein inhibitors: May increase CNS depressant effects of loperamide. Examples of inhibitors include cyclosporine, ketoconazole, quinidine, quinine, and ritonavir. Monitor.

Saquinavir: Loperamide may decrease levels/effects of saquinavir.

Adverse Reactions 1% to 10%:

Central nervous system: Dizziness (1%)

Gastrointestinal: Constipation (2% to 5%), abdominal cramping (<1% to 3%), nausea (<1% to 3%)

Postmarketing and/or case reports: Abdominal distention, abdominal pain, allergic reactions, anaphylactic shock, anaphylactoid reactions, angioedema, bullous eruption (rare), drowsiness, dry mouth, dyspepsia, erythema multiforme (rare), fatigue, flatulence, paralytic ileus, megacolon, pruritus, rash, Stevens-Johnson syndrome, toxic epidermal necrolysis, toxic megacolon, urinary retention, urticaria, vomiting

Overdosage/Toxicology Symptoms of overdose include CNS depression, urinary retention, and paralytic ileus. Treatment of overdose includes gastric lavage followed by 100 g activated charcoal through a nasogastric tube. Naloxone can be given as an antidote. The prolonged action of loperamide may necessitate naloxone's repeated administration and close patient monitoring for recurrent CNS depression.

Dosing

Adults & Elderly:

Acute diarrhea: Oral: Initial: 4 mg, followed by 2 mg after each loose stool, up to 16 mg/day

Chronic diarrhea: Oral: Initial: Follow acute diarrhea; maintenance dose should be slowly titrated downward to minimum required to control symptoms (typically, 4-8 mg/day in divided doses)

Traveler's diarrhea: Oral: Initial: 4 mg after first loose stool, followed by 2 mg after each subsequent stool (maximum dose: 8 mg/day)

Irinotecan-induced diarrhea (unlabeled use): Oral: 4 mg after first loose or frequent bowel movement, then 2 mg every 2 hours until 12 hours have passed without a bowel movement. If diarrhea recurs, then repeat administration

Pediatrics:

Acute diarrhea: Initial doses (in first 24 hours):

2-5 years (13--20 kg): 1 mg 3 times/day

6-8 years (20-30 kg): 2 mg twice daily

8-12 years (>30 kg): 2 mg 3 times/day

Maintenance: After initial dosing, 0.1 mg/kg doses after each loose stool, but not exceeding initial dosage

Traveler's diarrhea:

6-8 years: 2 mg after first loose stool, followed by 1 mg after each subsequent stool (maximum dose: 4 mg/day)

9-11 years: 2 mg after first loose stool, followed by 1 mg after each subsequent stool (maximum dose: 6 mg/day)

≥12 years: Refer to adult dosing.

Hepatic Impairment: No specific guidelines available.

Available Dosage Forms

Caplet, as hydrochloride: 2 mg

Diamode, Imodium® A-D, Kao-Paverin®: 2 mg

Capsule, as hydrochloride: 2 mg

Liquid, oral, as hydrochloride: 1 mg/5 mL (5 mL, 10 mL, 120 mL)

Imodium® A-D: 1 mg/5 mL (60 mL, 120 mL) [contains alcohol, sodium benzoate, benzoic acid; cherry mint flavor]

Imodium® A-D [new formulation]: 1 mg/7.5 mL (60 mL, 120 mL, 360 mL) [contains sodium 10 mg/30 mL, sodium benzoate; creamy mint flavor]

Tablet, as hydrochloride: 2 mg

K-Pek II: 2 mg

Nursing Guidelines

Assessment: Assess for cause of diarrhea before administering first dose. See Contraindications, Warnings/Precautions, and Drug Interactions for use

(Continued)

Loperamide *(Continued)*

cautions. Teach patient proper use, possible side effects/appropriate interventions, and adverse symptoms to report (see Patient Education).

Dietary Considerations:

Imodium® A-D [new formulation] contains sodium 10 mg/30 mL.

Patient Education: Adults should not take more than 8 capsules or 80 mL in 24 hours. May cause drowsiness; use caution. Increased exercise, identifying and avoiding foods that cause diarrhea, safe food preparation and storage, use of buttermilk, yogurt, or boiled milk may help reduce diarrhea. If acute diarrhea lasts longer than 48 hours, consult prescriber. Do not take if diarrhea is bloody.

Geriatric Considerations: Elderly are particularly sensitive to fluid and electrolyte loss. This generally results in lethargy, weakness, and confusion. Repletion and maintenance of electrolytes and water are essential in the treatment of diarrhea. Drug therapy must be limited in order to avoid toxicity with this agent.

Pregnancy Risk Factor: C

Lactation: Enters breast milk/not recommended.

Administration

Storage: Store at 15°C to 25°C (59°F to 77°F).

- Loperamide Hydrochloride *see* Loperamide *on page 1056*
- Lopid® *see* Gemfibrozil *on page 804*
- Lopressor® *see* Metoprolol *on page 1150*
- Lopressor HCT® *see* Metoprolol and Hydrochlorothiazide *on page 1153*
- Loprox® *see* Ciclopirox *on page 390*

Loratadine (lor AT a deen)

U.S. Brand Names Alavert™ [OTC]; Claritin® [OTC]; Claritin® Hives Relief [OTC]; Dimetapp® Children's ND [OTC] [DSC]; Tavist® ND [OTC]; Triaminic® Allerchews™[OTC]

Pharmacologic Category Antihistamine, Nonsedating

Medication Safety Issues

Sound-alike/look-alike issues:

Dimetapp® may be confused with Dermatop®, Dimetabs®, Dimetane®

Use Relief of nasal and non-nasal symptoms of seasonal allergic rhinitis; treatment of chronic idiopathic urticaria

Mechanism of Action Long-acting tricyclic antihistamine with selective peripheral histamine H_1-receptor antagonistic properties

Pharmacodynamics/Kinetics

Onset of action: 1-3 hours

Peak effect: 8-12 hours

Duration: >24 hours

Absorption: Rapid

Distribution: Significant amounts enter breast milk

Metabolism: Extensively hepatic via CYP2D6 and 3A4 to active metabolite

Half-life elimination: 12-15 hours

Excretion: Urine (40%) and feces (40%) as metabolites

Contraindications Hypersensitivity to loratadine or any component of the formulation

Warnings/Precautions Use with caution and modify dose in patients with liver or renal impairment; safety and efficacy in children <2 years of age have not been established

Drug Interactions **Substrate** (minor) of CYP2D6, 3A4; **Inhibits** CYP2C19 (moderate), 2D6 (weak)

CYP2C19 substrates: Loratadine may increase the levels/effects of CYP2C19 substrates. Example substrates include citalopram, diazepam, methsuximide, phenytoin, propranolol, and sertraline.

Protease inhibitors (amprenavir, ritonavir, nelfinavir) may increase the serum levels of loratadine

Increased toxicity: Other antihistamines

Nutritional/Herbal/Ethanol Interactions

Ethanol: Avoid ethanol (although sedation is limited with loratadine, may increase risk of CNS depression).

Food: Increases bioavailability and delays peak.

Herb/Nutraceutical: St John's wort may decrease loratadine levels.

Adverse Reactions

Adults:

Central nervous system: Headache (12%), somnolence (8%), fatigue (4%)
Gastrointestinal: Xerostomia (3%)

Children:

Central nervous system: Nervousness (4% ages 6-12 years), fatigue (3% ages 6-12 years, 2% to 3% ages 2-5 years), malaise (2% ages 6-12 years)
Dermatologic: Rash (2% to 3% ages 2-5 years)
Gastrointestinal: Abdominal pain (2% ages 6-12 years), stomatitis (2% to 3% ages 2-5 years)
Neuromuscular & skeletal: Hyperkinesia (3% ages 6-12 years)
Ocular: Conjunctivitis (2% ages 6-12 years)
Respiratory: Wheezing (4% ages 6-12 years), dysphonia (2% ages 6-12 years), upper respiratory infection (2% ages 6-12 years), epistaxis (2% to 3% ages 2-5 years), pharyngitis (2% to 3% ages 2-5 years), flu-like symptoms (2% to 3% ages 2-5 years)
Miscellaneous: Viral infection (2% to 3% ages 2-5 years)

Adults and Children: <2% (Limited to important or life-threatening): Abnormal hepatic function, agitation, alopecia, altered lacrimation, altered micturition, altered salivation, altered taste, amnesia, anaphylaxis, angioneurotic edema, anorexia, arthralgia, back pain, blepharospasm, blurred vision, breast enlargement, breast pain, bronchospasm, chest pain, confusion, depression, dizziness, dysmenorrhea, dyspnea, erythema multiforme, hemoptysis, hepatic necrosis, hepatitis, hypotension, impaired concentration, impotence, insomnia, irritability, jaundice, menorrhagia, migraine, nausea, palpitation, paresthesia, paroniria, peripheral edema, photosensitivity, pruritus, purpura, rigors, seizure, supraventricular tachyarrhythmia, syncope, tachycardia, tremor, urinary discoloration, urticaria, thrombocytopenia, vaginitis, vertigo, vomiting, weight gain

Overdosage/Toxicology Symptoms of overdose include somnolence, tachycardia, and headache. No specific antidote is available. Treatment is symptomatic and supportive. Loratadine is not eliminated by dialysis.

Dosing

Adults & Elderly: Seasonal allergic rhinitis, chronic idiopathic urticaria: Oral: 10 mg/day

Pediatrics:

Children 2-5 years: Seasonal allergic rhinitis, chronic idiopathic urticaria: Oral: 5 mg once daily
Children ≥6 years: Refer to adult dosing.

Renal Impairment:

Cl_{cr} ≤30 mL/minute:
Children 2-5 years: 5 mg every other day
Children ≥6 years and Adults: 10 mg every other day

Hepatic Impairment:

Elimination half-life increases with severity of disease.
Children 2-5 years: 5 mg every other day
Children ≥6 years and Adults: 10 mg every other day

Available Dosage Forms

Syrup: 5 mg/mL (120 mL)
Claritin®: 1 mg/mL (120 mL) [contains sodium benzoate; fruit flavor]; (60 mL, 120 mL) [alcohol free, dye free, sugar free; contains sodium 6 mg/5mL and sodium benzoate; grape flavor]
Tablet (Alavert™, Claritin®, Claritin® Hives Relief; Tavist® ND): 10 mg
Tablet, rapidly-disintegrating: 10 mg
Alavert™: 10 mg [contains phenylalanine 8.4 mg/tablet]
Claritin® RediTabs®: 10 mg [mint flavor]
Dimetapp® Children's ND: 10 mg [contains phenylalanine 8.4 mg/tablet] [DSC]
Triaminic® Allerchews™: 10 mg

Nursing Guidelines

Assessment: Assess effectiveness and interactions of other medications patient may be taking. Monitor effectiveness of therapy and adverse reactions at beginning of therapy and periodically with long-term use. Assess knowledge/teach patient appropriate use, interventions to reduce side effects, and adverse symptoms to report.

Dietary Considerations: Take on an empty stomach. Alavert™ and Dimetapp® Children's ND contain phenylalanine 8.4 mg per 10 mg tablet.

Patient Education: Take as directed; do not exceed recommended dose. Avoid use of other depressants, alcohol, or sleep-inducing medications unless

(Continued)

Loratadine *(Continued)*

approved by prescriber. You may experience drowsiness or dizziness (use caution when driving or engaging in tasks requiring alertness until response to drug is known); or dry mouth or nausea (small frequent meals, frequent mouth care, chewing gum, or sucking hard candy may help). Report persistent dizziness, sedation, or seizures; chest pain, rapid heartbeat, or palpitations; swelling of face, mouth, lips, or tongue; respiratory difficulty; changes in urinary pattern; yellowing of skin or eyes; dark urine or pale stool; or lack of improvement or worsening or condition. **Breast-feeding precaution:** Consult prescriber if breast-feeding.

Rapidly-disintegrating tablets: Place tablet on tongue; it dissolves rapidly. May be used with or without water. Use within 6 months of opening foil pouch, and immediately after opening individual tablet blister.

Geriatric Considerations: Loratadine is one of the newer, nonsedating antihistamines. Because of its low incidence of side effects, it seems to be a good choice in the elderly. However, there is a wide variation in loratadine half-life reported in the elderly and this should be kept in mind when initiating dosing.

Pregnancy Risk Factor: B

Lactation: Enters breast milk/not recommended (AAP rates "compatible")

Administration

Oral: Take on an empty stomach.

Storage: Store at 2°C to 25°C (36°F to 77°F).

Rapidly-disintegrating tablets: Use within 6 months of opening foil pouch, and immediately after opening individual tablet blister. Store in a dry place.

Loratadine and Pseudoephedrine

(lor AT a deen & soo doe e FED rin)

U.S. Brand Names Alavert™ Allergy and Sinus [OTC]; Claritin-D® 12-Hour [OTC]; Claritin-D® 24-Hour [OTC]

Synonyms Pseudoephedrine and Loratadine

Pharmacologic Category Antihistamine/Decongestant Combination

Use Temporary relief of symptoms of seasonal allergic rhinitis, other upper respiratory allergies, or the common cold

Pharmacodynamics/Kinetics See individual agents.

Contraindications Hypersensitivity to loratadine, pseudoephedrine, or any component of the formulation; use with or within 14 days of MAO inhibitors

Warnings/Precautions Use with caution in hypertension, diabetes mellitus, ischemic heart disease, increased intraocular pressure, hyperthyroidism, and prostatic hyperplasia. Patients with swallowing difficulties (eg, upper GI narrowing or abnormal esophageal peristalsis) should not use Claritin-D® 24-Hour. Use caution with hepatic or renal impairment; dose adjustment may be required. Safety and efficacy have not been established in children <12 years of age. When used for self medication (OTC use) patients should contact health care provider if fever present or if needed for >7 days.

Drug Interactions Loratadine: **Substrate** (minor) of CYP2D6, 3A4; **Inhibits** CYP2C19 (moderate), 2D6 (weak)

Also see individual agents.

Adverse Reactions See individual agents.

Dosing

Adults & Elderly: Seasonal allergic rhinitis/nasal congestion:

Oral: 1 tablet every 12 hours

Extended release: 1 tablet daily

Pediatrics: Seasonal allergic rhinitis/nasal congestion: Children ≥12 years: Refer to adult dosing.

Renal Impairment: Cl_{cr} <30 mL/minute:

Claritin-D® 12-Hour: 1 tablet daily

Claritin-D® 24-Hour: 1 tablet every other day

Hepatic Impairment: Should be avoided.

Available Dosage Forms

Tablet, extended release: Loratadine 10 mg and pseudoephedrine sulfate 240 mg

Alavert™ Allergy and Sinus, Claritin-D® 12-hour: Loratadine 5 mg and pseudoephedrine sulfate 120 mg

Claritin-D® 24-hour: Loratadine 10 mg and pseudoephedrine sulfate 240 mg

Nursing Guidelines

Assessment: See individual components listed in Related Information. Breast-feeding is not recommended.

Patient Education: See individual agents. Do not crush, break, or chew tablet. Take with a full glass of water. **Breast-feeding precaution:** Breast-feeding is not recommended.

Pregnancy Risk Factor: B

Lactation: Enters breast milk/not recommended

Related Information

Loratadine *on page 1058*
Pseudoephedrine *on page 1436*

Lorazepam (lor A ze pam)

U.S. Brand Names Ativan®; Lorazepam Intensol®

Pharmacologic Category Benzodiazepine

Medication Safety Issues

Sound-alike/look-alike issues:

Lorazepam may be confused with alprazolam, clonazepam, diazepam, temazepam

Ativan® may be confused with Atarax®, Atgam®, Avitene®

Use

Oral: Management of anxiety disorders or short-term relief of the symptoms of anxiety or anxiety associated with depressive symptoms

I.V.: Status epilepticus, preanesthesia for desired amnesia, antiemetic adjunct

Unlabeled/Investigational Use Ethanol detoxification; insomnia; psychogenic catatonia; partial complex seizures; agitation (I.V.)

Mechanism of Action Binds to stereospecific benzodiazepine receptors on the postsynaptic GABA neuron at several sites within the central nervous system, including the limbic system, reticular formation. Enhancement of the inhibitory effect of GABA on neuronal excitability results by increased neuronal membrane permeability to chloride ions. This shift in chloride ions results in hyperpolarization (a less excitable state) and stabilization.

Pharmacodynamics/Kinetics

Onset of action:

Hypnosis: I.M.: 20-30 minutes

Sedation: I.V.: 5-20 minutes

Anticonvulsant: I.V.: 5 minutes, oral: 30-60 minutes

Duration: 6-8 hours

Absorption: Oral, I.M.: Prompt

Distribution:

V_d: Neonates: 0.76 L/kg, Adults: 1.3 L/kg; crosses placenta; enters breast milk

Protein binding: 85%; free fraction may be significantly higher in elderly

Metabolism: Hepatic to inactive compounds

Half-life elimination: Neonates: 40.2 hours; Older children: 10.5 hours; Adults: 12.9 hours; Elderly: 15.9 hours; End-stage renal disease: 32-70 hours

Excretion: Urine; feces (minimal)

Contraindications Hypersensitivity to lorazepam or any component of the formulation (cross-sensitivity with other benzodiazepines may exist); acute narrow-angle glaucoma; sleep apnea (parenteral); intra-arterial injection of parenteral formulation; severe respiratory insufficiency (except during mechanical ventilation); pregnancy

Warnings/Precautions Use with caution in elderly or debilitated patients, patients with hepatic disease (including alcoholics) or renal impairment. Use with caution in patients with respiratory disease or impaired gag reflex. Initial doses in elderly or debilitated patients should not exceed 2 mg. Prolonged lorazepam use may have a possible relationship to GI disease, including esophageal dilation.

The parenteral formulation of lorazepam contains polyethylene glycol and propylene glycol. Also contains benzyl alcohol - avoid in neonates. Concurrent administration with scopolamine results in an increased risk of hallucinations, sedation, and irrational behavior.

Causes CNS depression (dose-related) resulting in sedation, dizziness, confusion, or ataxia which may impair physical and mental capabilities. Patients must be cautioned about performing tasks which require mental alertness (eg, operating machinery or driving). Use with caution in patients receiving other CNS depressants or psychoactive agents. Effects with other sedative drugs or ethanol

(Continued)

Lorazepam *(Continued)*

may be potentiated. Benzodiazepines have been associated with falls and traumatic injury and should be used with extreme caution in patients who are at risk of these events (especially the elderly).

Lorazepam may cause anterograde amnesia. Paradoxical reactions, including hyperactive or aggressive behavior have been reported with benzodiazepines, particularly in adolescent/pediatric or psychiatric patients. Does not have analgesic, antidepressant, or antipsychotic properties.

Use caution in patients with depression, particularly if suicidal risk may be present. Use with caution in patients with a history of drug dependence. Benzodiazepines have been associated with dependence and acute withdrawal symptoms on discontinuation or reduction in dose. Acute withdrawal, including seizures, may be precipitated after administration of flumazenil to patients receiving long-term benzodiazepine therapy.

As a hypnotic agent, should be used only after evaluation of potential causes of sleep disturbance. Failure of sleep disturbance to resolve after 7-10 days may indicate psychiatric or medical illness. A worsening of insomnia or the emergence of new abnormalities of thought or behavior may represent unrecognized psychiatric or medical illness and requires immediate and careful evaluation.

Drug Interactions

CNS depressants: Sedative effects and/or respiratory depression may be additive with CNS depressants; includes ethanol, barbiturates, narcotic analgesics, and other sedative agents; monitor for increased effect

Levodopa: Lorazepam may decrease the antiparkinsonian efficacy of levodopa (limited documentation); monitor

Loxapine: There are rare reports of significant respiratory depression, stupor, and/or hypotension with concomitant use of loxapine and lorazepam; use caution if concomitant administration of loxapine and CNS drugs is required

Scopolamine: May increase the incidence of sedation, hallucinations, and irrational behavior; reported only with parenteral lorazepam

Theophylline: May partially antagonize some of the effects of benzodiazepines; monitor for decreased response; may require higher doses for sedation

Nutritional/Herbal/Ethanol Interactions

Ethanol: Avoid or limit ethanol (may increase CNS depression).

Herb/Nutraceutical: Avoid valerian, St John's wort, kava kava, gotu kola (may increase CNS depression).

Lab Interactions May result in elevated liver function tests

Adverse Reactions

>10%:

- Central nervous system: Sedation
- Respiratory: Respiratory depression

1% to 10%:

- Cardiovascular: Hypotension
- Central nervous system: Confusion, dizziness, akathisia, unsteadiness, headache, depression, disorientation, amnesia
- Dermatologic: Dermatitis, rash
- Gastrointestinal: Weight gain/loss, nausea, changes in appetite
- Neuromuscular & skeletal: Weakness
- Respiratory: Nasal congestion, hyperventilation, apnea

<1% (Limited to important or life-threatening): Menstrual irregularities, increased salivation, blood dyscrasias, reflex slowing, physical and psychological dependence with prolonged use, polyethylene glycol or propylene glycol poisoning (prolonged I.V. infusion)

Overdosage/Toxicology Symptoms of overdose include confusion, coma, hypoactive reflexes, dyspnea, labored breathing. **Note:** Prolonged infusions have been associated with toxicity from propylene glycol and/or polyethylene glycol. Treatment for benzodiazepine overdose is supportive. Flumazenil has been shown to selectively block the binding of benzodiazepines to CNS receptors, resulting in a reversal of benzodiazepine-induced CNS depression but not respiratory depression

Dosing

Adults:

Antiemetic: Oral, I.V. (**Note:** May be administered sublingually; not a labeled route): 0.5-2 mg every 4-6 hours as needed

Anxiety and sedation: Oral: 1-10 mg/day in 2-3 divided doses; usual dose: 2-6 mg/day in divided doses; initial dose should not exceed 2 mg in debilitated patients

Insomnia: Oral: 2-4 mg at bedtime

Preoperative:

I.M.: 0.05 mg/kg administered 2 hours before surgery; maximum: 4 mg/dose

I.V.: 0.044 mg/kg 15-20 minutes before surgery; usual maximum: 2 mg/dose

Operative amnesia: I.V.: Up to 0.05 mg/kg; maximum: 4 mg/dose

Status epilepticus: I.V.: 4 mg/dose given slowly over 2-5 minutes; may repeat in 10-15 minutes; usual maximum dose: 8 mg

Rapid tranquilization of agitated patient (administer every 30-60 minutes):

Oral: 1-2 mg

I.M.: 0.5-1 mg

Average total dose for tranquilization: 4-8 mg

Agitation in the ICU patient (unlabeled):

I.V.: 0.02-0.06 mg/kg every 2-6 hours

I.V. infusion: 0.01-0.1 mg/kg/hour

Elderly: Anxiety and sedation: Oral, I.V.: 0.5-4 mg/day; refer to adult dosing for other indications. Dose selection should generally be on the low end of the dosage range (ie, initial dose not to exceed 2 mg)

Pediatrics:

Antiemetic: Children 2-15 years: I.V.: 0.05 mg/kg (up to 2 mg/dose) prior to chemotherapy

Anxiety and sedation: Infants and Children: Oral, I.V.: Usual: 0.05 mg/kg/dose (range: 0.02-0.09 mg/kg) every 4-8 hours

Sedation (preprocedure): Infants and Children:

Oral, I.M., I.V.: Usual: 0.05 mg/kg; range: 0.02-0.09 mg/kg

I.V.: May use smaller doses (eg, 0.01-0.03 mg/kg) and repeat every 20 minutes, as needed to titrate to effect

Status epilepticus: I.V.:

Infants and Children: 0.1 mg/kg slow I.V. over 2-5 minutes, do not exceed 4 mg/single dose; may repeat second dose of 0.05 mg/kg slow I.V. in 10-15 minutes if needed

Adolescents: 0.07 mg/kg slow I.V. over 2-5 minutes; maximum: 4 mg/dose; may repeat in 10-15 minutes

Available Dosage Forms

Injection, solution (Ativan®): 2 mg/mL (1 mL, 10 mL); 4 mg/mL (1 mL, 10 mL) [contains benzyl alcohol]

Solution, oral concentrate (Lorazepam Intensol®): 2 mg/mL (30 mL) [alcohol free, dye free]

Tablet (Ativan®): 0.5 mg, 1 mg, 2 mg

Nursing Guidelines

Assessment: Assess other medications the patient may be taking for effectiveness and interactions. **Oral:** Assess for history of addiction; long-term use can result in dependence, abuse, or tolerance; periodically evaluate need for continued use. For inpatient use, institute safety measures and monitor effectiveness and adverse reactions. For outpatients, monitor therapeutic effectiveness and adverse reactions at beginning of therapy and periodically with long-term use. Taper dosage slowly when discontinuing. Assess knowledge/ teach patient appropriate use, interventions to reduce side effects, and adverse symptoms to report. **I.V./I.M.:** Monitor vital signs and CNS status (possible retrograde amnesia with I.V.), and ability to void. Maintain bedrest for 2-3 hours, and observe when up.

Patient Education: Oral: Take exactly as directed; do not increase dose or frequency. Drug may cause physical and/or psychological dependence. Do not use alcohol or other prescription or OTC medications (especially pain medications, sedatives, antihistamines, or hypnotics) without consulting prescriber. Maintain adequate hydration (2-3 L/day of fluids) unless instructed to restrict fluid intake. You may experience drowsiness, lightheadedness, impaired coordination, dizziness, or blurred vision (use caution when driving or engaging in tasks requiring alertness until response to drug is known); nausea, vomiting, or dry mouth (small frequent meals, frequent mouth care, chewing gum, or sucking lozenges may help); constipation (increased exercise, fluids, fruit, or fiber may help); altered sexual drive or ability (reversible); or photosensitivity (use sunscreen, wear protective clothing and eyewear, and avoid direct sunlight). Report persistent CNS effects (eg, confusion, depression, increased sedation, excitation, headache, agitation, insomnia or nightmares, dizziness, fatigue, impaired coordination, changes in personality, or changes in cognition);

(Continued)

Lorazepam *(Continued)*

changes in urinary pattern; chest pain, palpitations, or rapid heartbeat; muscle cramping, weakness, tremors, or rigidity; ringing in ears or visual disturbances; excessive perspiration; excessive GI symptoms (cramping, constipation, vomiting, anorexia); or worsening of condition. **Pregnancy/breast-feeding precautions:** Do not get pregnant while taking this medication; use appropriate contraceptive measures. Do not breast-feed.

Geriatric Considerations: Because lorazepam is relatively short-acting with an inactive metabolite, it is a preferred agent to use in elderly patients when a benzodiazepine is indicated. Use with caution since elderly patients have decreased pulmonary reserve and are more prone to hypoxia.

Pregnancy Risk Factor: D

Pregnancy Issues: Benzodiazepines cross the placenta. The association between benzodiazepine exposure and malformations remains controversial. A number of types of malformation have been reported (oral cleft, inguinal hernia, cardiac defects, spina bifida, dysmorphic facial features, skeletal defects); however, confounding factors make a clear association difficult. Overall, the risk to the fetus may be low. Nonteratogenic effects (including neonatal flaccidity, respiratory and feeding problems, and withdrawal symptoms) during the postnatal period have also been reported with benzodiazepine use.

Lactation: Enters breast milk/contraindicated (AAP rates "of concern")

Breast-Feeding Considerations: Crosses into breast milk and no data on clinical effects on the infant. AAP states MAY BE OF CONCERN.

Perioperative/Anesthesia/Other Concerns: Lorazepam 2 mg/mL and 4 mg/mL each contains propylene glycol 830 mg/mL (80% v/v).

Agitation in the ICU Patient: Lorazepam has a slower onset of action than midazolam or diazepam, making it less useful for treatment of acute agitation. The polyethylene glycol and propylene glycol solvents in lorazepam injection can accumulate and lead to reversible acute tubular necrosis, lactic acidosis and hyperosmolar states with prolonged, high-dose infusions. Yaucher (2003) and colleagues recently performed a retrospective review of patients who received lorazepam infusions and developed increases in serum creatinine. Eight patients from the medical-surgical intensive care unit or burn unit were evaluated. Lorazepam infusions ranged from 2-28 mg/hour. The mean cumulative dose of lorazepam was 4305 mg and the mean propylene glycol level determined at the time of peak serum creatinine concentration was 1103 mcg/mL. The duration of lorazepam infusion and magnitude of serum creatinine concentration rise correlated (r: 0.60). Propylene glycol levels strongly correlated with both serum osmolality and osmol gap. These authors suggest that serum osmolality and osmol gap may be useful markers of propylene glycol toxicity. A recent case report described a critically-ill man who developed acute tubular necrosis while receiving a lorazepam infusion and sulfamethoxazole-trimethoprim (Hayman, 2003). The addition of sulfamethoxazole-trimethoprim contributed to the development of propylene glycol toxicity. More recently, a prospective, observational study was performed in a medical intensive care unit evaluating patients receiving high-dose lorazepam (≥10 mg/hour) infusions (Arroliga, 2004). The primary objective was to evaluate the relationship between high-dose lorazepam and serum propylene glycol concentrations. Nine patients met the criteria for entry. Baseline creatinine clearances were between 50-100 mL/minute. Propylene glycol accumulation was observed in these patients receiving high-dose lorazepam infusions for ≥48 hours. A significant correlation between high-dose lorazepam infusion rate and serum propylene glycol concentrations was observed. However, osmol gap was the strongest predictor (r^2: 0.80) of serum propylene glycol concentrations. Study findings suggest that in critically-ill adults with normal renal function, serum propylene glycol concentrations may be predicted by the osmol gap. Based on these findings, propylene glycol accumulation may occur as early as 48 hours when using high-dose lorazepam infusions.

More recently, a prospective, observational study was performed in a medical intensive care unit evaluating patients receiving high-dose lorazepam (≥10 mg/hour) infusions (Arroliga, 2004). The primary objective was to evaluate the relationship between high-dose lorazepam and serum propylene glycol concentrations. Nine patients met the criteria for entry. Baseline creatinine clearances were 50-100 mL/minute. Propylene glycol accumulation was observed in these patients receiving high-dose lorazepam infusions for ≥48 hours. A significant correlation between high-dose lorazepam infusion rate and serum propylene glycol concentrations was observed. However, osmol gap was the strongest predictor (R^2 = 0.80) of serum propylene glycol concentrations. Study findings suggest that in critically ill adults with normal renal function, serum propylene glycol concentrations may be predicted by the osmol gap. Based on these findings, propylene glycol accumulation may occur as early as 48 hours when using high-dose lorazepam infusions.

To calculate osmolarity: [2 x sodium (mEq/L)] + [glucose (mg/dL)/18] + [BUN (mg/dL)/2.8]

To calculate osmol gap (normal range: 0-5): (measured osmolality minus calculated osmolarity)

Lorazepam is recommended for the sedation of most patients. Use a defined endpoint in titration of the dose. Use a system to minimize prolonged sedative effects. If patient has received high-dose or >7 days of continuous therapy, consider tapering infusion to prevent withdrawal symptoms.

Status Epilepticus: A randomized, double-blind trial (Treiman, 1998) evaluated the efficacy of four treatments in overt status epilepticus. Treatment arms were designed based upon accepted practices of North American neurologists. The treatments were: 1) lorazepam 0.1 mg/kg, 2) diazepam 0.15 mg/kg followed by phenytoin 18 mg/kg, 3) phenytoin 18 mg/kg alone, and 4) phenobarbital 15 mg/kg. Treatment was considered successful if the seizures were terminated (clinically and by EEG) within 20 minutes of start of therapy without seizure recurrence within 60 minutes from the start of therapy. Patients who failed the first treatment received a second and a third, if necessary. Patients did not receive randomized treatments after the first one, but the treating physician remained blinded. Treatment success: Lorazepam 64.9%, phenobarbital 58.2%, diazepam/phenytoin 55.8%, and phenytoin alone 43.6%. Using an "intention-to-treat" analysis, there was no statistical difference between the groups. Results of subsequent treatments in patients who failed the first therapy indicated that response rate significantly dropped regardless of treatment. Aggregate response rate to the second treatment was 7.0% and third treatment 2.3%.

Administration

I.M.: Should be administered deep into the muscle mass.

I.V.: Continuous infusion solutions should have an in-line filter and the solution should be checked frequently for possible precipitation.

Reconstitution:

I.V.: Dilute with equal volume of compatible diluent (D_5W, NS, SWI).

Infusion: Use 2 mg/mL injectable solution to prepare; dilute ≤1 mg/mL and mix in glass bottle; precipitation may develop; can also be administered undiluted via infusion.

Compatibility:

Y-site administration: Incompatible with aldesleukin, aztreonam, floxacillin, foscarnet, idarubicin, imipenem/cilastatin, omeprazole, ondansetron, sargramostim, sufentanil

Compatibility in syringe: Incompatible with sufentanil

Compatibility when admixed: Incompatible with buprenorphine, dexamethasone sodium phosphate with diphenhydramine and metoclopramide

Storage:

I.V.: Intact vials should be refrigerated, protected from light; do not use discolored or precipitate-containing solutions. May be stored at room temperature for up to 60 days. Parenteral admixture is stable at room temperature (25°C) for 24 hours.

Tablet: Store at room temperature.

Related Information

Conscious Sedation *on page 1779*
Intravenous Anesthetic Agents *on page 1853*

◆ **Lorazepam Intensol®** *see* Lorazepam *on page 1061*

◆ **Lorcet® 10/650** *see* Hydrocodone and Acetaminophen *on page 867*

◆ **Lorcet®-HD [DSC]** *see* Hydrocodone and Acetaminophen *on page 867*

◆ **Lorcet® Plus** *see* Hydrocodone and Acetaminophen *on page 867*

◆ **Lortab®** *see* Hydrocodone and Acetaminophen *on page 867*

Losartan (loe SAR tan)

U.S. Brand Names Cozaar®

Synonyms DuP 753; Losartan Potassium; MK594

Pharmacologic Category Angiotensin II Receptor Blocker

Medication Safety Issues

Sound-alike/look-alike issues:

Losartan may be confused with valsartan

Cozaar® may be confused with Hyzaar®, Zocor®

Use Treatment of hypertension (HTN); treatment of diabetic nephropathy in patients with type 2 diabetes mellitus (noninsulin dependent, NIDDM) and a history of hypertension; stroke risk reduction in patients with HTN and left ventricular hypertrophy (LVH)

Mechanism of Action As a selective and competitive, nonpeptide angiotensin II receptor antagonist, losartan blocks the vasoconstrictor and aldosterone-secreting effects of angiotensin II; losartan interacts reversibly at the AT1 and AT2 receptors of many tissues and has slow dissociation kinetics; its affinity for the AT1 receptor is 1000 times greater than the AT2 receptor. Angiotensin II receptor antagonists may induce a more complete inhibition of the renin-angiotensin system than ACE inhibitors, they do not affect the response to bradykinin, and are less likely to be associated with nonrenin-angiotensin effects (eg, cough and angioedema). Losartan increases urinary flow rate and in addition to being natriuretic and kaliuretic, increases excretion of chloride, magnesium, uric acid, calcium, and phosphate.

Pharmacodynamics/Kinetics

Onset of action: 6 hours

Distribution: V_d: Losartan: 34 L; E-3174: 12 L; does not cross blood brain barrier

Protein binding, plasma: High

Metabolism: Hepatic (14%) via CYP2C9 and 3A4 to active metabolite, E-3174 (40 times more potent than losartan); extensive first-pass effect

Bioavailability: 25% to 33%; AUC of E-3174 is four times greater than that of losartan

Half-life elimination: Losartan: 1.5-2 hours; E-3174: 6-9 hours

Time to peak, serum: Losartan: 1 hour; E-3174: 3-4 hours

Excretion: Urine (4% as unchanged drug, 6% as active metabolite)

Clearance: Plasma: Losartan: 600 mL/minute; Active metabolite: 50 mL/minute

Contraindications Hypersensitivity to losartan or any component of the formulation; hypersensitivity to other A-II receptor antagonists; bilateral renal artery stenosis; pregnancy (2nd and 3rd trimesters)

Warnings/Precautions Avoid use or use a smaller dose in patients who are volume depleted; correct depletion first. Deterioration in renal function can occur with initiation. May cause hyperkalemia; avoid potassium supplementation unless specifically required by healthcare provider. Use with caution in unilateral renal artery stenosis and pre-existing renal insufficiency; significant aortic/mitral stenosis. When used to reduce the risk of stroke in patients with HTN and LVH, may not be effective in the African-American population. Use caution with hepatic dysfunction, dose adjustment may be needed. Safety and efficacy in children <6 years of age have not been established.

Drug Interactions **Substrate** (major) of CYP2C8/9, 3A4; **Inhibits** CYP1A2 (weak), 2C8/9 (moderate), 2C19 (weak), 3A4 (weak)

CYP2C8/9 inducers: May decrease the levels/effects of losartan. Example inducers include carbamazepine, phenobarbital, phenytoin, rifampin, rifapentine, and secobarbital.

CYP2C8/9 substrates: Losartan may increase the levels/effects of CYP2C8/9 substrates. Example substrates include amiodarone, fluoxetine, glimepiride, glipizide, nateglinide, phenytoin, pioglitazone, rosiglitazone, sertraline, and warfarin.

CYP3A4 inducers: CYP3A4 inducers may decrease the levels/effects of losartan. Example inducers include aminoglutethimide, carbamazepine, nafcillin, nevirapine, phenobarbital, phenytoin, and rifamycins.

Fluconazole: Increases plasma levels of losartan via 2C8/9 inhibition (decreases the plasma levels of the active metabolite). Monitor for increased losartan efficacy.

Lithium: Risk of toxicity may be increased by losartan; monitor lithium levels.

NSAIDs: May decrease angiotensin II antagonist efficacy; effect has been seen with losartan, but may occur with other medications in this class; monitor blood pressure

Potassium-sparing diuretics (amiloride, potassium, spironolactone, triamterene): Increased risk of hyperkalemia.

Potassium supplements may increase the risk of hyperkalemia.

Rifampin may reduce antihypertensive efficacy of losartan.

Trimethoprim (high dose) may increase the risk of hyperkalemia.

Nutritional/Herbal/Ethanol Interactions Herb/Nutraceutical: St John's wort may decrease levels. Avoid dong quai if using for hypertension (has estrogenic activity). Avoid ephedra, yohimbe, ginseng (may worsen hypertension). Avoid garlic (may have increased antihypertensive effect).

Adverse Reactions

>10%:

Cardiovascular: Chest pain (12% diabetic nephropathy)

Central nervous system: Fatigue (14% diabetic nephropathy)

Endocrine: Hypoglycemia (14% diabetic nephropathy)

Gastrointestinal: Diarrhea (2% hypertension to 15% diabetic nephropathy)

Genitourinary: Urinary tract infection (13% diabetic nephropathy)

Hematologic: Anemia (14% diabetic nephropathy)

Neuromuscular & skeletal: Weakness (14% diabetic nephropathy), back pain (2% hypertension to 12% diabetic nephropathy)

Respiratory: Cough (≤3% to 11%; similar to placebo; incidence higher in patients with previous cough related to ACE inhibitor therapy)

1% to 10%:

Cardiovascular: Hypotension (7% diabetic nephropathy), orthostatic hypotension (4% hypertension to 4% diabetic nephropathy), first-dose hypotension (dose related: <1% with 50 mg, 2% with 100 mg)

Central nervous system: Dizziness (4%), hypoesthesia (5% diabetic nephropathy), fever (4% diabetic nephropathy), insomnia (1%)

Dermatology: Cellulitis (7% diabetic nephropathy)

Endocrine: Hyperkalemia (<1% hypertension to 7% diabetic nephropathy)

Gastrointestinal: Gastritis (5% diabetic nephropathy), weight gain (4% diabetic nephropathy), dyspepsia (1% to 4%), abdominal pain (2%), nausea (2%)

Neuromuscular & skeletal: Muscular weakness (7% diabetic nephropathy), knee pain (5% diabetic nephropathy), leg pain (1% to 5%), muscle cramps (1%), myalgia (1%)

Respiratory: Bronchitis (10% diabetic nephropathy), upper respiratory infection (8%), nasal congestion (2%), sinusitis (1% hypertension to 6% diabetic nephropathy)

Miscellaneous: Infection (5% diabetic nephropathy), flu-like syndrome (10% diabetic nephropathy)

>1% but frequency ≤ placebo: Edema, abdominal pain, nausea, headache, pharyngitis

<1% (Limited to important or life-threatening): Acute psychosis with paranoid delusions, ageusia, alopecia, anemia, angina, angioedema, arrhythmia, AV block (second degree), depression, dysgeusia, dyspnea, gout, Henoch-Schönlein purpura, hepatitis, hyperkalemia, hyponatremia, impotence, maculopapular rash, MI, panic disorder, pancreatitis, paresthesia, peripheral neuropathy, photosensitivity, renal impairment (patients dependent on renin-angiotensin-aldosterone system), rhabdomyolysis (rare), stroke, syncope, thrombocytopenia (rare), urticaria, vasculitis, vertigo

Overdosage/Toxicology Hypotension and tachycardia may occur with significant overdose. Treatment should be supportive. Not removed via hemodialysis.

Dosing

Adults & Elderly:

Hypertension: Oral: Initial: 25-50 mg once daily; can be administered once or twice daily with total daily doses ranging from 25-100 mg

Usual initial doses in patients receiving diuretics or those with intravascular volume depletion: 25 mg

Nephropathy in patients with type 2 diabetes and hypertension: Oral: Initial: 50 mg once daily; can be increased to 100 mg once daily based on blood pressure response

Stroke reduction (HTN with LVH): Oral: 50 mg once daily (maximum daily dose: 100 mg); may be used in combination with a thiazide diuretic

Pediatrics:

Hypertension: Oral: Children 6-16 years: 0.7 mg/kg once daily (maximum: 50 mg/day); adjust dose based on response; doses >1.4 mg/kg (maximum: 100 mg) have not been studied.

Renal Impairment:

Children: Use is not recommended if Cl_{cr} <30 mL/minute.

(Continued)

Losartan *(Continued)*

Adults: No adjustment necessary.

Hepatic Impairment: Reduce the initial dose to 25 mg/day; divide dosage intervals into two.

Available Dosage Forms Tablet [film coated], as potassium: 25 mg, 50 mg, 100 mg

Nursing Guidelines

Assessment: See Contraindications, Warnings/Precautions, and Dosing for use cautions. Assess potential for interactions with other prescriptions, OTC medications, or herbal products patient may be taking (see Drug Interactions). Assess results of laboratory tests (see below), therapeutic effectiveness, and adverse response (eg, hypotension - see Adverse Reactions and Overdose/Toxicology) on a regular basis during therapy. Teach patient proper use, possible side effects/appropriate interventions, and adverse symptoms to report (see Patient Education). **Pregnancy risk factor C/D** - see Pregnancy Risk Factor for use cautions. Instruct patients of childbearing age about appropriate use of contraceptives (see Pregnancy Issues). Breast-feeding is not recommended.

Monitoring Laboratory Tests: Electrolytes, serum creatinine, BUN, urinalysis, CBC

Dietary Considerations: May be taken with or without food.

Patient Education: Inform prescriber of all prescriptions, OTC medications, or herbal products you are taking, and any allergies you have. Do not take any new medication during therapy unless approved by prescriber. Do not use potassium supplement or salt substitutes without consulting prescriber. Take exactly as directed and do not discontinue without consulting prescriber. This drug does not eliminate need for diet or exercise regimen as recommended by prescriber. May cause dizziness, fainting, or lightheadedness (use caution when driving or engaging in tasks that require alertness until response to drug is known); postural hypotension (use caution when rising from lying or sitting position or climbing stairs); diarrhea (boiled milk, buttermilk, or yogurt may help). Report chest pain or palpitations; unrelenting headache; back or muscle pain or weakness, CNS changes (delusions or depression); swelling of face mouth, tongue or throat; or other persistent adverse reactions. **Pregnancy/breast-feeding precautions:** Inform prescriber if you are or intend to become pregnant. This drug should not be used in the 2nd or 3rd trimester of pregnancy. Consult prescriber for appropriate contraceptive measures. Breast-feeding is not recommended.

Geriatric Considerations: Serum concentrations of losartan and its metabolites are not significantly different in the elderly patient and no initial dose adjustment is necessary even in low creatinine clearance states (<30 mL/minute).

Pregnancy Risk Factor: C/D (2nd and 3rd trimesters)

Pregnancy Issues: Discontinue as soon as possible when pregnancy is detected. Drugs which act directly on renin-angiotensin can cause fetal and neonatal morbidity and death.

Lactation: Excretion in breast milk unknown/not recommended

Breast-Feeding Considerations: Avoid use in the nursing mother, if possible, since it is postulated that losartan is excreted in breast milk. Recommend discontinuing drug or discontinuing nursing based on the importance of the drug to the mother.

Perioperative/Anesthesia/Other Concerns: The angiotensin II receptor antagonists appear to have similar indications as the ACE inhibitors. In heart failure, the angiotensin II antagonists are especially useful in providing an alternative therapy in those patients who have intractable cough in response to ACE inhibitor therapy. Candesartan has been studied as an alternative therapy in chronic heart failure patients who cannot tolerate an ACE-I (CHARM-Alternative) and as an added therapy in heart failure patients who are maintained on an ACE-I (CHARM-Added). In both studies the combined endpoint of cardiovascular death or heart failure hospitalizations was significantly improved over the placebo treated group. Similar to ACE inhibitors, pre-existing volume depletion caused by diuretic therapy may potentiate hypotension in response to angiotensin II antagonists. Concomitant NSAID therapy may attenuate blood pressure control; use of NSAIDs should be avoided or limited, with monitoring of blood pressure control. In the setting of heart failure, NSAID use may be associated with an increased risk for fluid accumulation and edema.

Administration

Oral: May be administered with or without food.

Storage: Store at 15°C to 30°C (59°F to 86°F). Protect from light.

Losartan and Hydrochlorothiazide

(loe SAR tan & hye droe klor oh THYE a zide)

U.S. Brand Names Hyzaar®

Synonyms Hydrochlorothiazide and Losartan

Pharmacologic Category Angiotensin II Receptor Blocker Combination; Antihypertensive Agent, Combination; Diuretic, Thiazide

Medication Safety Issues

Sound-alike/look-alike issues:

Hyzaar® may be confused with Cozaar®

Use Treatment of hypertension; stroke risk reduction in patients with HTN and left ventricular hypertrophy (LVH)

Pharmacodynamics/Kinetics See individual agents.

Contraindications

Hypersensitivity to hydrochlorothiazide, thiazides, sulfonamide-derived drugs, losartan,or any component of the formulation; hypersensitivity to other A-II receptor antagonists; bilateral renal artery stenosis, anuria, renal decompensation; pregnancy (2nd and 3rd trimesters)

Warnings/Precautions

Avoid use or use a smaller dose in patients who are volume depleted; correct depletion first. Deterioration in renal function can occur with initiation. May cause hyperkalemia; monitor. Use with caution in unilateral renal artery stenosis and pre-existing renal insufficiency; significant aortic/mitral stenosis. Avoid in severe renal disease (ineffective). Electrolyte disturbances (hypokalemia, hypochloremic alkalosis, hyponatremia) can occur. Use with caution in severe hepatic dysfunction; hepatic encephalopathy can be caused by electrolyte disturbances. Gout can be precipitate in certain patients with a history of gout, a familial predisposition to gout, or chronic renal failure. Cautious use in diabetics; may see a change in glucose control. Hypersensitivity reactions can occur. Can cause SLE exacerbation or activation. Use with caution in patients with moderate or high cholesterol concentrations. Photosensitization may occur. Correct hypokalemia before initiating therapy.

Chemical similarities are present among sulfonamides, sulfonylureas, carbonic anhydrase inhibitors, thiazides, and loop diuretics (except ethacrynic acid). Use in patients with sulfonamide allergy is specifically contraindicated in product labeling, however, a risk of cross-reaction exists in patients with allergy to any of these compounds; avoid use when previous reaction has been severe. Safety and efficacy in children have not been established.

Drug Interactions Losartan: **Substrate** (major) of CYP2C8/9, 3A4; **Inhibits** CYP1A2 (weak), 2C8/9 (moderate), 2C19 (weak), 3A4 (weak)

Also see individual agents.

Adverse Reactions Based on clinical trials of the combination product in patients with essential hypertension. Also see individual agents.

1% to 10%:

Cardiovascular: Edema (1%), palpitation (1%)

Central nervous system: Dizziness (6%)

Dermatologic: Skin rash (1%)

Gastrointestinal: Abdominal pain (1%)

Neuromuscular & skeletal: Back pain (2%)

Respiratory: Upper respiratory infection (6%), cough (3%), sinusitis (1%)

<1% (Limited to important or life-threatening) or frequency not defined (some reactions attributed to single component): Bilirubin increased (serum), BUN increased, hematocrit decreased, hemoglobin decreased, hyper-/hypotension, hyponatremia, liver enzymes increased, rhabdomyolysis, serum creatinine increased, thrombocytopenia

Dosing

Adults: Hypertension (dosage must be individualized): Oral: 1 tablet/day

Elderly: Refer to dosing in individual monographs.

Renal Impairment: Cl_{cr} ≤30 mL/minute: Use of combination formulation is not recommended.

Hepatic Impairment: Use is not recommended.

Available Dosage Forms Tablet [film coated]:

50-12.5: Losartan potassium 50 mg and hydrochlorothiazide 12.5 mg

100-12.5: Losartan potassium 100 mg and hydrochlorothiazide 12.5 mg

(Continued)

Losartan and Hydrochlorothiazide *(Continued)*

100-25: Losartan potassium 100 mg and hydrochlorothiazide 25 mg

Nursing Guidelines

Assessment: See individual components listed in Related Information. **Pregnancy risk factor C/D** - see Pregnancy Risk Factor for use cautions. Assess knowledge/instruct patient on need to use appropriate contraceptive measures and the need to avoid pregnancy. Breast-feeding is contraindicated.

Patient Education: See individual agents. **Pregnancy/breast-feeding precautions:** Inform prescriber if you are or intend to become pregnant. Do not breast-feed.

Pregnancy Risk Factor: C/D (2nd and 3rd trimesters)

Lactation: Enters breast milk/contraindicated

Related Information

Hydrochlorothiazide *on page 862*
Losartan *on page 1066*

- **Losartan Potassium** *see* Losartan *on page 1066*
- **Lotensin®** *see* Benazepril *on page 228*
- **Lotrel®** *see* Amlodipine and Benazepril *on page 142*
- **Lotrimin® AF Athlete's Foot Cream [OTC]** *see* Clotrimazole *on page 439*
- **Lotrimin® AF Athlete's Foot Solution [OTC]** *see* Clotrimazole *on page 439*
- **Lotrimin® AF Jock Itch Cream [OTC]** *see* Clotrimazole *on page 439*

Lovastatin (LOE va sta tin)

U.S. Brand Names Altoprev™; Mevacor®

Synonyms Mevinolin; Monacolin K

Pharmacologic Category Antilipemic Agent, HMG-CoA Reductase Inhibitor

Medication Safety Issues

Sound-alike/look-alike issues:

Lovastatin may be confused with Leustatin®, Livostin®, Lotensin®

Mevacor® may be confused with Mivacron®

Use

Adjunct to dietary therapy to decrease elevated serum total and LDL-cholesterol concentrations in primary hypercholesterolemia

Primary prevention of coronary artery disease (patients without symptomatic disease with average to moderately elevated total and LDL-cholesterol and below average HDL-cholesterol); slow progression of coronary atherosclerosis in patients with coronary heart disease

Adjunct to dietary therapy in adolescent patients (10-17 years of age, females >1 year postmenarche) with heterozygous familial hypercholesterolemia having LDL >189 mg/dL, **or** LDL >160 mg/dL with positive family history of premature cardiovascular disease (CVD), **or** LDL >160 mg/dL with the presence of at least two other CVD risk factors

Mechanism of Action Lovastatin acts by competitively inhibiting 3-hydroxyl-3-methylglutaryl-coenzyme A (HMG-CoA) reductase, the enzyme that catalyzes the rate-limiting step in cholesterol biosynthesis

Pharmacodynamics/Kinetics

Onset of action: LDL-cholesterol reductions: 3 days

Absorption: 30%; increased with extended release tablets when taken in the fasting state

Protein binding: 95%

Metabolism: Hepatic; extensive first-pass effect; hydrolyzed to B-hydroxy acid (active)

Bioavailability: Increased with extended release tablets

Half-life elimination: 1.1-1.7 hours

Time to peak, serum: 2-4 hours

Excretion: Feces (~80% to 85%); urine (10%)

Contraindications Hypersensitivity to lovastatin or any component of the formulation; active liver disease; unexplained persistent elevations of serum transaminases; pregnancy; breast-feeding

Warnings/Precautions Liver function tests should be assessed before initiation of therapy in patients with a history of liver disease, prior to upwards dosage adjustment to ≥40 mg daily or when otherwise indicated; enzyme levels should be followed periodically thereafter as clinically warranted. Rhabdomyolysis with or without acute renal failure has occurred. Risk is dose-related and is increased with concurrent use of lipid-lowering agents which may cause rhabdomyolysis (gemfibrozil, fibric acid derivatives, or niacin at doses ≥1 g/day) or during concurrent use with potent CYP3A4 inhibitors. Avoid concurrent use of azole antifungals, macrolide antibiotics, and protease inhibitors. Use caution/limit dose with amiodarone, cyclosporine, danazol, gemfibrozil (or other fibrates), lipid-lowering doses of niacin, or verapamil. Patients should be instructed to report unexplained muscle pain or weakness; lovastatin should be discontinued if myopathy is suspected/confirmed. Temporarily discontinue in any patient experiencing an acute or serious condition predisposing to renal failure secondary to rhabdomyolysis. Use with caution in patients who consume large amounts of ethanol or have a history of liver disease. Safety and efficacy of the immediate release tablet have not been evaluated in prepubertal patients, patients <10 years of age, or doses >40 mg/day in appropriately-selected adolescents; extended release tablets have not been studied in patients <20 years of age.

Drug Interactions **Substrate** of CYP3A4 (major); **Inhibits** CYP2C8/9 (weak), 2D6 (weak), 3A4 (weak)

Amiodarone: Inhibits metabolism of lovastatin and may increase lovastatin-induced myopathy and rhabdomyolysis. Concurrent use is not recommended, but if unavoidable, dose of lovastatin should be limited.

Antacids: Plasma concentrations may be decreased when given with magnesium-aluminum hydroxide containing antacids (reported with atorvastatin and pravastatin). Clinical efficacy is not altered, no dosage adjustment is necessary

Azole antifungals: May decrease the metabolism, via CYP isoenzymes, of HMG-CoA reductase inhibitors and may increase risk of lovastatin-induced myopathy and rhabdomyolysis. Avoid concurrent use.

Cholestyramine reduces absorption of several HMG-CoA reductase inhibitors. Separate administration times by at least 4 hours.

Cholestyramine and colestipol (bile acid sequestrants): Cholesterol-lowering effects are additive.

Clofibrate and fenofibrate may increase the risk of myopathy and rhabdomyolysis; limit dose of lovastatin

Cyclosporine: Concurrent use may increase risk of myopathy; limit dose of lovastatin

CYP3A4 inhibitors: May increase the levels/effects of lovastatin. Example inhibitors include azole antifungals, clarithromycin, diclofenac, doxycycline, erythromycin, imatinib, isoniazid, nefazodone, nicardipine, propofol, protease inhibitors, quinidine, telithromycin, and verapamil. Avoid concurrrent use.

Danazol: Concurrent use may increase risk of myopathy; limit dose of lovastatin.

Gemfibrozil: Increased risk of myopathy and rhabdomyolysis; limit dose of lovastatin

Grapefruit juice may inhibit metabolism of lovastatin via CYP3A4; avoid high dietary intakes of grapefruit juice.

Isradipine may decrease lovastatin blood levels.

Macrolide antibiotics: May decrease the metabolism, via CYP isoenzymes, of HMG-CoA reductase inhibitors and may increase risk of lovastatin-induced myopathy and rhabdomyolysis. Avoid concurrent use.

Nefazodone: May decrease the metabolism, via CYP isoenzymes, of HMG-CoA reductase inhibitors and may increase risk of lovastatin-induced myopathy and rhabdomyolysis. Avoid concurrent use.

Niacin (at higher dosages ≥1 g/day) may increase risk of myopathy and rhabdomyolysis; limit dose of lovastatin

Protease inhibitors: Concurrent use increases the risk of myopathy and rhabdomyolysis; concurrent use should be avoided.

Verapamil: Inhibits metabolism of lovastatin and may increase lovastatin-induced myopathy and rhabdomyolysis. Concurrent use is not recommended, but if unavoidable, dose of lovastatin should be limited.

Warfarin effect (hypoprothrombinemic response) may be increased; monitor INR closely when lovastatin is initiated or discontinued.

Nutritional/Herbal/Ethanol Interactions

Ethanol: Avoid excessive ethanol consumption (due to potential hepatic effects).

Food: Food **decreases** the bioavailability of lovastatin extended release tablets and **increases** the bioavailability of lovastatin immediate release tablets. Lovastatin serum concentrations may be increased if taken with grapefruit juice; avoid concurrent intake of large quantities (>1 quart/day). Red yeast rice contains an estimated 2.4 mg lovastatin per 600 mg rice.

Herb/Nutraceutical: St John's wort may decrease lovastatin levels.

Lab Interactions Altered thyroid function tests

Adverse Reactions Percentages as reported with immediate release tablets; similar adverse reactions seen with extended release tablets.

(Continued)

Lovastatin *(Continued)*

>10%: Neuromuscular & skeletal: Increased CPK (>2x normal) (11%)

1% to 10%:

Central nervous system: Headache (2% to 3%), dizziness (0.5% to 1%)

Dermatologic: Rash (0.8% to 1%)

Gastrointestinal: Abdominal pain (2% to 3%), constipation (2% to 4%), diarrhea (2% to 3%), dyspepsia (1% to 2%), flatulence (4% to 5%), nausea (2% to 3%)

Neuromuscular & skeletal: Myalgia (2% to 3%), weakness (1% to 2%), muscle cramps (0.6% to 1%)

Ocular: Blurred vision (0.8% to 1%)

<1% (Limited to important or life-threatening): Acid regurgitation, alopecia, arthralgia, chest pain, dermatomyositis, eye irritation, insomnia, leg pain, paresthesia, pruritus, vomiting, xerostomia

Additional class-related events or case reports (not necessarily reported with lovastatin therapy): Alkaline phosphatase increased, alopecia, alteration in taste, anaphylaxis, angioedema, anorexia, anxiety, arthritis, cataracts, chills, cholestatic jaundice, cirrhosis, CPK increased (>10x normal), depression, dryness of skin/mucous membranes, dyspnea, eosinophilia, erectile dysfunction, erythema multiforme, ESR increased, facial paresis, fatty liver, fever, flushing, fulminant hepatic necrosis, GGT increased, gynecomastia, hemolytic anemia, hepatitis, hepatoma, hyperbilirubinemia, hypersensitivity reaction, impaired extraocular muscle movement, impotence, leukopenia, libido decreased, malaise, memory loss, myopathy, nail changes, nodules, ophthalmoplegia, pancreatitis, paresthesia, peripheral nerve palsy, peripheral neuropathy, photosensitivity, polymyalgia rheumatica, positive ANA, pruritus, psychic disturbance, purpura, rash, renal failure (secondary to rhabdomyolysis), rhabdomyolysis, skin discoloration, Stevens-Johnson syndrome, systemic lupus erythematosus-like syndrome, thrombocytopenia, thyroid dysfunction, toxic epidermal necrolysis, transaminases increased, tremor, urticaria, vasculitis, vertigo, vomiting

Overdosage/Toxicology Few adverse events have been reported. Treatment is symptomatic.

Dosing

Adults & Elderly:

Dyslipidemia and primary prevention of CAD: Oral: Initial: 20 mg with evening meal, then adjust at 4-week intervals; maximum: 80 mg/day immediate release tablet **or** 60 mg/day extended release tablet.

Dosage modification/limits based on concurrent therapy:

Cyclosporine and other immunosuppressant drugs: Initial dose: 10 mg/day with a maximum recommended dose of 20 mg/day

Concurrent therapy with fibrates, danazol, and/or lipid-lowering doses of niacin (>1 g/day): Maximum recommended dose: 20 mg/day. Concurrent use with fibrates should be avoided unless risk to benefit favors use.

Concurrent therapy with amiodarone or verapamil: Maximum recommended dose: 40 mg/day of regular release or 20 mg/day with extended release.

Dosage adjustment in renal impairment: Cl_{cr} <30 mL/minute: Use doses >20 mg/day with caution.

Pediatrics:

Heterozygous familial hypercholesterolemia: Oral (immediate release tablet): Adolescents 10-17 years:

LDL reduction <20%: Initial: 10 mg/day with evening meal

LDL reduction ≥20%: Initial: 20 mg/day with evening meal

Usual range: 10-40 mg with evening meal, then adjust dose at 4-week intervals

Renal Impairment: Cl_{cr} <30 mL/minute: Use with caution and carefully consider doses >20 mg/day.

Available Dosage Forms

Tablet: 10 mg, 20 mg, 40 mg

Mevacor®: 20 mg, 40 mg

Tablet, extended release (Altoprev™): 10 mg, 20 mg, 40 mg, 60 mg

Nursing Guidelines

Assessment: See Contraindications, Warnings/Precautions, and Dosing for use cautions. Assess potential for interactions with other prescriptions, OTC medications, or herbal products patient may be taking (see Drug Interactions). Assess results of laboratory tests (see below) and patient response (see Adverse Reactions and Overdose/Toxicology) on a regular basis throughout therapy. Teach patient proper use, possible side effects/appropriate interventions, and adverse symptoms to report (see Patient Education). **Pregnancy risk factor X** - determine that patient is not pregnant before starting therapy. Do not give to women of childbearing age unless they are capable of complying with effective contraceptive use. Instruct patient in appropriate contraceptive measures. Breast-feeding is contraindicated.

Monitoring Laboratory Tests: Obtain baseline LFTs and total cholesterol profile. LFTs should be performed before initiation of therapy, at 6 and 12 weeks after initiation or first dose, and periodically thereafter.

Dietary Considerations: Before initiation of therapy, patients should be placed on a standard cholesterol-lowering diet for 6 weeks and the diet should be continued during drug therapy. Avoid intake of large quantities of grapefruit juice (≥1 quart/day); may increase toxicity. Red yeast rice contains an estimated 2.4 mg lovastatin per 600 mg rice.

Patient Education: Inform prescriber of all prescriptions, OTC medications, or herbal products you are taking, and any allergies you have. Do not take any new medication during therapy unless approved by prescriber. Take as directed, with food at evening meal. Follow diet and exercise regimen as prescribed. You will have periodic blood tests to assess effectiveness. You may experience nausea or dyspepsia (small, frequent meals, frequent mouth care, chewing gum, or sucking lozenges may help); diarrhea (buttermilk, boiled milk, or yogurt may help); or headache (see prescriber for analgesic). Report muscle pain or cramping; tremor; CNS changes (eg, memory loss, depression, personality changes; numbness, weakness, tingling or pain in extremities). **Pregnancy/breast-feeding precautions:** Inform prescriber if you are pregnant. Consult prescriber for appropriate barrier contraceptive measures to use during and for 1 month following therapy. This drug may cause severe fetal defects. Do not donate blood during or for 1 month following therapy. Do not breast-feed.

Geriatric Considerations: The definition of and, therefore, when to treat hyperlipidemia in the elderly is a controversial issue. The National Cholesterol Education Program recommends that all adults maintain a plasma cholesterol <160 mg/dL. In elderly patients with one additional risk factor, goal LDL would decrease to <130 mg/dL. Pharmacologic treatment should be reserved for those who are unable to obtain a desirable plasma cholesterol concentration by diet alone and for whom the benefits of treatment are believed to outweigh the potential adverse effects, drug interactions, and cost of treatment.

Pregnancy Risk Factor: X

Pregnancy Issues: Cholesterol biosynthesis may be important in fetal development. Contraindicated in pregnancy. Administer to women of childbearing potential only when conception is highly unlikely and patients have been informed of potential hazards.

Lactation: Excretion unknown/contraindicated

Perioperative/Anesthesia/Other Concerns: Myopathy: Currently-marketed HMG-CoA reductase inhibitors appear to have a similar potential for causing myopathy. Incidence of severe myopathy is about 0.08% to 0.09%. The factors that increase risk include advanced age (especially >80 years), gender (occurs in women more frequently than men), small body frame, frailty, multisystem disease (eg, chronic renal insufficiency especially due to diabetes), multiple medications, **perioperative periods (higher risk when continued during hospitalization for major surgery)**, and drug interactions (use with caution or avoid).

Administration

Oral: Administer immediate release tablet with meals. Administer extended release tablet at bedtime; do not crush or chew.

Storage:

Tablet, immediate release: Store between 5°C to 30°C (41°F to 86°F). Protect from light.

Tablet, extended release: Store between 20°C to 25°C (68°F to 77°F). Avoid excessive heat and humidity.

- Lovenox® *see* Enoxaparin *on page 605*
- Lozol® *see* Indapamide *on page 903*
- LTA® 360 *see* Lidocaine *on page 1033*
- LTG *see* Lamotrigine *on page 1002*
- Lu-26-054 *see* Escitalopram *on page 639*
- Lucidex [OTC] *see* Caffeine *on page 284*

- **Lugol's Solution; Strong Iodine Solution** *see* Potassium Iodide and Iodine *on page 1387*
- **Lumigan®** *see* Bimatoprost *on page 244*
- **Luminal® Sodium** *see* Phenobarbital *on page 1343*
- **Lupron®** *see* Leuprolide *on page 1015*
- **Lupron Depot®** *see* Leuprolide *on page 1015*
- **Lupron Depot-Ped®** *see* Leuprolide *on page 1015*
- **Luxiq®** *see* Betamethasone *on page 237*
- **LY170053** *see* Olanzapine *on page 1259*
- **Lymphocyte Immune Globulin** *see* Antithymocyte Globulin (Equine) *on page 174*
- **M-M-R® II** *see* Measles, Mumps, and Rubella Vaccines (Combined) *on page 1082*
- **Maalox® [OTC]** *see* Aluminum Hydroxide, Magnesium Hydroxide, and Simethicone *on page 122*
- **Maalox® Max [OTC]** *see* Aluminum Hydroxide, Magnesium Hydroxide, and Simethicone *on page 122*
- **Maalox® TC (Therapeutic Concentrate) [OTC] [DSC]** *see* Aluminum Hydroxide and Magnesium Hydroxide *on page 122*
- **Macrobid®** *see* Nitrofurantoin *on page 1232*
- **Macrodantin®** *see* Nitrofurantoin *on page 1232*
- **Mag Delay® [OTC]** *see* Magnesium Chloride *on page 1074*
- **Magnesia Magma** *see* Magnesium Hydroxide *on page 1076*
- **Magnesium Carbonate and Aluminum Hydroxide** *see* Aluminum Hydroxide and Magnesium Carbonate *on page 121*

Magnesium Chloride (mag NEE zhum KLOR ide)

U.S. Brand Names Chloromag®; Mag Delay® [OTC]; Mag-SR® [OTC]; Slow-Mag® [OTC]

Pharmacologic Category Magnesium Salt

Use Correction or prevention of hypomagnesemia

Adverse Reactions 1% to 10%:

Cardiovascular: Flushing

Central nervous system: Depressed CNS, somnolence

Gastrointestinal: Diarrhea

Neuromuscular & skeletal: Blocked peripheral neuromuscular transmission, deep tendon reflexes

Respiratory: Respiratory paralysis

Overdosage/Toxicology

Serious, potentially life-threatening electrolyte disturbances may occur with long-term use or overdosage due to diarrhea; hypermagnesemia may occur. CNS depression, confusion, hypotension, muscle weakness, blockage of peripheral neuromuscular transmission.

Serum level >4 mEq/L (4.8 mg/dL): Deep tendon reflexes may be depressed

Serum level ≥10 mEq/L (12 mg/dL): Deep tendon reflexes may disappear, respiratory paralysis may occur, heart block may occur

I.V. calcium (5-10 mEq) will reverse respiratory depression or heart block; in extreme cases, peritoneal dialysis or hemodialysis may be required.

Serum level >12 mEq/L may be fatal, serum level ≥10 mEq/L may cause complete heart block

Dosing

Adults & Elderly: Dietary supplement: Oral: Dietary supplement: 54-283 mg/day in divided doses

In TPN: I.V.: 8-24 mEq/day

Pediatrics:

In TPN: I.V.: Children: 2-10 mEq/day

Note: The usual recommended pediatric maintenance intake of magnesium ranges from 0.2-0.6 mEq/kg/day. The dose of magnesium may also be based on the caloric intake; on that basis, 3-10 mEq/day of magnesium are needed; maximum maintenance dose: 8-16 mEq/day

Renal Impairment: Patients in severe renal failure should not receive magnesium due to toxicity from accumulation. Patients with a Cl_{cr} <25 mL/minute should be monitored by serum magnesium levels.

Available Dosage Forms

Injection, solution (Chloromag®): 200 mg/mL [1.97 mEq/mL] (50 mL)

Tablet [enteric coated] (Slow-Mag®): Elemental magnesium 64 mg [contains elemental calcium 106 mg]

Tablet, extended release (Mag Delay®, Mag-SR®): Magnesium chloride hexahydrate 535 mg [equivalent to elemental magnesium 64 mg]

Nursing Guidelines

Pregnancy Risk Factor: D

Magnesium Citrate (mag NEE zhum SIT rate)

Synonyms Citrate of Magnesia

Pharmacologic Category Laxative, Saline; Magnesium Salt

Use Evacuation of bowel prior to certain surgical and diagnostic procedures or overdose situations

Mechanism of Action Promotes bowel evacuation by causing osmotic retention of fluid which distends the colon with increased peristaltic activity

Pharmacodynamics/Kinetics

Absorption: Oral: 15% to 30%

Excretion: Urine

Contraindications Renal failure, appendicitis, abdominal pain, intestinal impaction, obstruction or perforation, diabetes mellitus, complications in gastrointestinal tract, patients with colostomy or ileostomy, ulcerative colitis or diverticulitis

Warnings/Precautions Use with caution in patients with impaired renal function, especially if Cl_{cr} <30 mL/minute (accumulation of magnesium which may lead to magnesium intoxication); use with caution in digitalized patients (may alter cardiac conduction leading to heart block); use with caution in patients with lithium administration; use with caution with neuromuscular blocking agents, CNS depressants

Lab Interactions Increased magnesium; decreased protein, decreased calcium (S), decreased potassium (S)

Adverse Reactions 1% to 10%:

Cardiovascular: Hypotension

Endocrine & metabolic: Hypermagnesemia

Gastrointestinal: Abdominal cramps, diarrhea, gas formation

Respiratory: Respiratory depression

Overdosage/Toxicology

Serious, potentially life-threatening electrolyte disturbances may occur with long-term use or overdosage due to diarrhea; hypermagnesemia may occur. CNS depression, confusion, hypotension, muscle weakness, blockage of peripheral neuromuscular transmission.

Serum level >4 mEq/L (4.8 mg/dL): Deep tendon reflexes may be depressed

Serum level ≥10 mEq/L (12 mg/dL): Deep tendon reflexes may disappear, respiratory paralysis may occur, heart block may occur

I.V. calcium (5-10 mEq) will reverse respiratory depression or heart block; in extreme cases, peritoneal dialysis or hemodialysis may be required.

Serum level >12 mEq/L may be fatal, serum level ≥10 mEq/L may cause complete heart block

Dosing

Adults & Elderly: Cathartic: Oral: Adults: ½ to 1 full bottle (120-300 mL)

Pediatrics: Cathartic: Oral: Children:

<6 years: 0.5 mL/kg up to a maximum of 200 mL repeated every 4-6 hours until stools are clear

6-12 years: 100-150 mL

≥12 years: Refer to adult dosing.

Renal Impairment: Patients in severe renal failure should not receive magnesium due to toxicity from accumulation. Patients with a Cl_{cr} <25 mL/minute should be monitored by serum magnesium levels.

Available Dosage Forms

Solution, oral: 290 mg/5 mL (300 mL) [cherry and lemon flavors]

Tablet: 100 mg [as elemental magnesium]

Nursing Guidelines

Assessment: Assess therapeutic response and adverse effects.

Dietary Considerations: Magnesium content of 5 mL: 3.85-4.71 mEq

Patient Education: Take with a glass of water, fruit juice, or citrus-flavored carbonated beverage to improve taste. Chill before using. Report severe abdominal pain to physician.

(Continued)

Magnesium Citrate *(Continued)*

Pregnancy Risk Factor: B

Administration

Oral: To increase palatability, chill the solution prior to administration.

Magnesium Hydroxide (mag NEE zhum hye DROKS ide)

U.S. Brand Names Dulcolax® Milk of Magnesia [OTC]; Phillips'® Milk of Magnesia [OTC]

Synonyms Magnesia Magma; Milk of Magnesia; MOM

Pharmacologic Category Antacid; Magnesium Salt

Use Short-term treatment of occasional constipation and symptoms of hyperacidity, magnesium replacement therapy

Mechanism of Action Promotes bowel evacuation by causing osmotic retention of fluid which distends the colon with increased peristaltic activity; reacts with hydrochloric acid in stomach to form magnesium chloride

Pharmacodynamics/Kinetics

Onset of action: Laxative: 4-8 hours

Excretion: Urine (up to 30% as absorbed magnesium ions); feces (as unabsorbed drug)

Contraindications Hypersensitivity to any component of the formulation; patients with colostomy or an ileostomy, intestinal obstruction, fecal impaction, renal failure, appendicitis

Warnings/Precautions Use with caution in patients with severe renal impairment (especially when doses are >50 mEq magnesium/day); hypermagnesemia and toxicity may occur due to decreased renal clearance of absorbed magnesium. Decreased renal function (Cl_{cr} <30 mL/minute) may result in toxicity; monitor for toxicity.

Drug Interactions Decreased effect: Decreased absorption of tetracyclines, digoxin, indomethacin, or iron salts

Lab Interactions Increased magnesium; decreased protein, calcium (S), decreased potassium (S)

Adverse Reactions Frequency not defined.

Cardiovascular: Hypotension

Endocrine & metabolic: Hypermagnesemia

Gastrointestinal: Diarrhea, abdominal cramps

Neuromuscular & skeletal: Muscle weakness

Respiratory: Respiratory depression

Overdosage/Toxicology

Magnesium antacids are also laxative and may cause diarrhea and hypokalemia; in patients with renal failure, magnesium may accumulate to toxic levels.

I.V. calcium (5-10 mEq) will reverse respiratory depression or heart block; in extreme cases, peritoneal dialysis or hemodialysis may be required.

Dosing

Adults & Elderly:

Laxative: Oral: ≥12 years: 30-60 mL/day or in divided doses

Antacid: Oral: 5-15 mL up to 4 times/day as needed

Pediatrics:

Laxative: Oral:

<2 years: 0.5 mL/kg/dose

2-5 years: 5-15 mL/day or in divided doses

6-12 years: 15-30 mL/day or in divided doses

≥12 years: 30-60 mL/day or in divided doses

Antacid: Oral:

Children: 2.5-5 mL as needed up to 4 times/day

Renal Impairment: Patients in severe renal failure should not receive magnesium due to toxicity from accumulation. Patients with a Cl_{cr} <25 mL/minute should be monitored by serum magnesium levels.

Available Dosage Forms

Liquid, oral: 400 mg/5 mL (360 mL, 480 mL, 960 mL, 3780 mL)

Dulcolax® Milk of Magnesia: 400 mg/5 mL (360 mL, 780 mL) [regular and mint flavors]

Phillips'® Milk of Magnesia: 400 mg/5 mL (120 mL, 360 mL, 780 mL) [original, French vanilla, cherry, and mint flavors]

Liquid, oral concentrate: 800 mg/5 mL (100 mL, 400 mL)

Phillips'® Milk of Magnesia [concentrate]: 800 mg/5 mL (240 mL) [strawberry créme flavor]

Tablet, chewable (Phillips'® Milk of Magnesia): 311 mg [mint flavor]

Nursing Guidelines

Pregnancy Risk Factor: B

Administration

Oral: Liquid doses may be diluted with a small amount of water prior to administration. All doses should be followed by 8 ounces of water.

- **Magnesium Hydroxide, Aluminum Hydroxide, and Simethicone** *see* Aluminum Hydroxide, Magnesium Hydroxide, and Simethicone *on page 122*
- **Magnesium Hydroxide and Aluminum Hydroxide** *see* Aluminum Hydroxide and Magnesium Hydroxide *on page 122*
- **Magnesium Hydroxide and Calcium Carbonate** *see* Calcium Carbonate and Magnesium Hydroxide *on page 294*

Magnesium Sulfate (mag NEE zhum SUL fate)

Synonyms Epsom Salts; $MgSO_4$ (error-prone abbreviation)

Pharmacologic Category Antacid; Anticonvulsant, Miscellaneous; Electrolyte Supplement, Parenteral; Laxative, Saline; Magnesium Salt

Medication Safety Issues

Sound-alike/look-alike issues:

Magnesium sulfate may be confused with manganese sulfate, morphine sulfate

$MgSO_4$ is an error-prone abbreviation (mistaken as morphine sulfate)

High alert medication: The Institute for Safe Medication Practices (ISMP) includes this medication (I.V. formulation) among its list of drugs which have a heightened risk of causing significant patient harm when used in error.

Use Treatment and prevention of hypomagnesemia; seizure prevention in severe pre-eclampsia or eclampsia, pediatric acute nephritis; short-term treatment torsade de pointes; treatment of cardiac arrhythmias (VT/VF) caused by hypomagnesemia; short-term treatment of constipation or soaking aid

Mechanism of Action When taken orally, magnesium promotes bowel evacuation by causing osmotic retention of fluid which distends the colon with increased peristaltic activity; parenterally, magnesium decreases acetylcholine in motor nerve terminals and acts on myocardium by slowing rate of S-A node impulse formation and prolonging conduction time

Pharmacodynamics/Kinetics

Onset of action: Oral: Cathartic: 1-2 hours; I.M.: 1 hour; I.V.: Immediate

Duration: I.M.: 3-4 hours; I.V.: 30 minutes

Excretion: Urine (as magnesium)

Contraindications Heart block, serious renal impairment, myocardial damage, hepatitis, Addison's disease

Warnings/Precautions Use with caution in patients with impaired renal function (accumulation of magnesium which may lead to magnesium intoxication); use with caution in digitalized patients (may alter cardiac conduction leading to heart block); monitor serum magnesium level, respiratory rate, deep tendon reflex, renal function when magnesium sulfate is administered parenterally. Use with extreme caution in patients with myasthenia gravis or other neuromuscular disease.

Drug Interactions

Increased effect: Nifedipine decreased blood pressure and increased neuromuscular blockade

Increased toxicity: Aminoglycosides increased neuromuscular blockade; CNS depressants increased CNS depression; neuromuscular antagonists, betamethasone (pulmonary edema), ritodrine increased cardiotoxicity

Lab Interactions Increased magnesium; decreased protein, calcium (S), decreased potassium (S)

Adverse Reactions Hypotension and asystole may occur with rapid administration. Adverse effects on neuromuscular function may occur at lower levels in patients with neuromuscular disease (eg, myasthenia gravis).

Serum magnesium levels >3 mg/dL:

Central nervous system: Depressed CNS

Gastrointestinal: Diarrhea

Neuromuscular & skeletal: Depressed neuromuscular transmission and deep tendon reflexes

Serum magnesium levels >5 mg/dL:

Cardiovascular: Flushing

Central nervous system: Somnolence

(Continued)

Magnesium Sulfate *(Continued)*

Serum magnesium levels >12.5 mg/dL:
- Cardiovascular: Complete heart block
- Respiratory: Respiratory depression

Overdosage/Toxicology

Symptoms of overdose usually present with serum level >4 mEq/L
- Serum magnesium >4: Deep tendon reflexes may be depressed
- Serum magnesium ≥10: Deep tendon reflexes may disappear, respiratory paralysis may occur, heart block may occur
- Serum level >12 mEq/L may be fatal, serum level ≥10 mEq/L may cause complete heart block

I.V. calcium (5-10 mEq) 1-2 g calcium gluconate will reverse respiratory depression or heart block; in extreme cases, peritoneal dialysis or hemodialysis may be required

Dosing

Adults & Elderly:

Daily allowance: The recommended dietary allowance (RDA) of magnesium is 4.5 mg/kg which is a total daily allowance of 350-400 mg for adult men and 280-300 mg for adult women. During pregnancy the RDA is 300 mg and during lactation the RDA is 355 mg. Average daily intakes of dietary magnesium have declined in recent years due to processing of food. The latest estimate of the average American dietary intake was 349 mg/day. Dose represented as magnesium sulfate unless stated otherwise.

Note: Serum magnesium is poor reflection of repletional status as the majority of magnesium is intracellular; serum levels may be transiently normal for a few hours after a dose is given, therefore, aim for consistently high normal serum levels in patients with normal renal function for most efficient repletion

Hypomagnesemia:
- Oral: 3 g every 6 hours for 4 doses as needed
- I.M., I.V.: 1 g every 6 hours for 4 doses; for severe hypomagnesemia: 8-12 g magnesium sulfate/day in divided doses has been used

Eclampsia, pre-eclampsia:
- I.M.: 1-4 g every 4 hours
- I.V.: Initial: 4 g, then switch to I.M. or 1-4 g/hour by continuous infusion
- **Note:** Maximum dose not to exceed 30-40 g/day; maximum rate of infusion: 1-2 g/hour

Life-threatening arrhythmia: I.V.: 1-2 g (8-16 mEq) in 100 mL D_5W, administered over 5-60 minutes followed by an infusion of 0.5-1 g/hour, **or**
1-6 g administered over several minutes, followed by (in some cases) I.V. infusion of 3-20 mg/minute for 5-48 hours (depending on patient response and serum magnesium levels)

Maintenance electrolyte requirements:
- Daily requirements: 0.2-0.5 mEq/kg/24 hours or 3-10 mEq/1000 kcal/24 hours
- Maximum: 8-16 mEq/24 hours

Cathartic: Oral: 10-30 g/day in a single or divided doses

Soaking aid: Topical: Dissolve 2 capfuls of powder per gallon of warm water

Pediatrics:

Note: Serum magnesium is poor reflection of repletional status as the majority of magnesium is intracellular; serum levels may be transiently normal for a few hours after a dose is given, therefore, aim for consistently high normal serum levels in patients with normal renal function for most efficient repletion

Hypomagnesemia:
- Children: I.M., I.V.: 25-50 mg/kg/dose (0.2-0.4 mEq/kg/dose) every 4-6 hours for 3-4 doses, maximum single dose: 2000 mg (16 mEq), may repeat if hypomagnesemia persists (higher dosage up to 100 mg/kg/dose magnesium sulfate I.V. has been used)
  - *Maintenance:* I.V.: 30-60 mg/kg/day (0.25-0.5 mEq/kg/day)

Management of seizures and hypertension: I.M., I.V.: 20-100 mg/kg/dose every 4-6 hours as needed; in severe cases doses as high as 200 mg/kg/dose have been used

Cathartic: Oral: Children:
- 2-5 years: 2.5-5 g/kg/day in a single or divided doses
- 6-11 years: 5-10 g/day in a single or divided doses
- ≥12 years: Refer to adult dosing.

Renal Impairment: Patients in severe renal failure should not receive magnesium due to toxicity from accumulation. Patients with a Cl_{cr} <25 mL/minute should be monitored by serum magnesium levels.

Available Dosage Forms

Infusion [premixed in D_5W]: 10 mg/mL (100 mL); 20 mg/mL (500 mL, 1000 mL)

Infusion [premixed in water for injection]: 40 mg/mL (100 mL, 500 mL, 1000 mL); 80 mg/mL (50 mL)

Injection, solution: 125 mg/mL (8 mL); 500 mg/mL (2 mL, 5 mL, 10 mL, 20 mL, 50 mL)

Powder: Magnesium sulfate USP (480 g, 1810 g, 1920 g)

Nursing Guidelines

Dietary Considerations: Magnesium sulfate oral solution: Mix with water and administer on an empty stomach.

10% elemental magnesium; 8.1 mEq magnesium/g; 4 mmol magnesium/g

500 mg magnesium sulfate = 4.06 mEq magnesium = 49.3 mg elemental magnesium

Patient Education: Take in divided doses. Report diarrhea (>5 stools/day) or changes in mental function to prescriber.

Pregnancy Risk Factor: B

Perioperative/Anesthesia/Other Concerns: Hypomagnesemia can hinder the replenishment of intracellular potassium and should be corrected in order to correct hypokalemia.

Administration

I.M.: A 25% or 50% concentration may be used for adults and a 20% solution is recommended for children

I.V.: Magnesium may be administered IVP, IVPB or I.V. infusion in an auxiliary medication infusion solution (eg, TPN); when giving I.V. push, must dilute first and should not be given any faster than 150 mg/minute

Maximal rate of infusion: 2 g/hour to avoid hypotension; doses of 4 g/hour have been given in emergencies (eclampsia, seizures); optimally, should add magnesium to I.V. fluids or to IVH, but bolus doses are also effective

For I.V., a concentration <20% (200 mg/mL) should be used and the rate of injection should not exceed 1.5 mL of a 10% solution (or equivalent) per minute (150 mg/minute)

Compatibility: Stable in D_5W, LR, NS; **incompatible** with fat emulsion 10%

Y-site administration: Incompatible with alatrofloxacin, amphotericin B cholesteryl sulfate complex, cefepime

Compatibility in syringe: Incompatible with hydrocortisone sodium succinate

Compatibility when admixed: Incompatible with amphotericin B, clindamycin, cyclosporine, dobutamine, polymyxin B sulfate, procaine, sodium bicarbonate

Storage: Refrigeration of intact ampuls may result in precipitation or crystallization. Parenteral admixture is stable at room temperature (25°C) for 60 days.

I.V. is **incompatible** when mixed with fat emulsion (flocculation), calcium gluceptate, clindamycin, dobutamine, hydrocortisone (same syringe), nafcillin, polymyxin B, procaine hydrochloride, tetracyclines, thiopental.

♦ Mag-SR® [OTC] *see* Magnesium Chloride *on page 1074*

Mannitol (MAN i tole)

U.S. Brand Names Osmitrol®; Resectisol®

Synonyms *D*-Mannitol

Pharmacologic Category Diuretic, Osmotic

Medication Safety Issues

Sound-alike/look-alike issues:

Osmitrol® may be confused with esmolol

Use Reduction of increased intracranial pressure associated with cerebral edema; promotion of diuresis in the prevention and/or treatment of oliguria or anuria due to acute renal failure; reduction of increased intraocular pressure; promoting urinary excretion of toxic substances; genitourinary irrigant in transurethral prostatic resection or other transurethral surgical procedures

Mechanism of Action Increases the osmotic pressure of glomerular filtrate, which inhibits tubular reabsorption of water and electrolytes and increases urinary output

Pharmacodynamics/Kinetics

Onset of action: Diuresis: Injection: 1-3 hours; Reduction in intracranial pressure: ~15-30 minutes

Duration: Reduction in intracranial pressure: 1.5-6 hours

(Continued)

Mannitol *(Continued)*

Distribution: Remains confined to extracellular space (except in extreme concentrations); does not penetrate the blood-brain barrier (generally, penetration is low)

Metabolism: Minimally hepatic to glycogen

Half-life elimination: 1.1-1.6 hours

Excretion: Primarily urine (as unchanged drug)

Contraindications Hypersensitivity to mannitol or any component or the formulation; severe renal disease (anuria); severe dehydration; active intracranial bleeding except during craniotomy; progressive heart failure, pulmonary congestion, or renal dysfunction after mannitol administration; severe pulmonary edema or congestion

Warnings/Precautions Should not be administered until adequacy of renal function and urine flow is established;use 1-2 test doses to assess renal response. Diuretic effects may mask and intensify underlying dehydration; excessive loss of water and electrolytes may lead to imbalances and aggravate preexisting hyponatremia. May cause renal dysfunction especially with high doses; use caution in patients taking other nephrotoxic agents, with sepsis or preexisting renal disease. To minimize adverse renal effects, adjust to keep serum osmolality less than 320 mOsm/L. Discontinue if evidence of acute tubular necrosis.

In patients being treated for cerebral edema, mannitol may accumulate in the brain (causing rebound increases in intracranial pressure) if circulating for long periods of time as with continuous infusion; intermittent boluses preferred. Cardiovascular status should also be evaluated; do not administer electrolyte-free mannitol solutions with blood. If hypotension occurs monitor cerebral perfusion pressure to insure adequate.

Drug Interactions Lithium toxicity (with diuretic-induced hyponatremia)

Adverse Reactions Frequency not defined.

Cardiovascular: Chest pain, CHF, circulatory overload, hyper-/hypotension, tachycardia

Central nervous system: Chills, convulsions, dizziness, headache

Dermatologic: Rash, urticaria

Endocrine & metabolic: Fluid and electrolyte imbalance, dehydration and hypovolemia secondary to rapid diuresis, hyperglycemia, hypernatremia, hyponatremia (dilutional), hyperosmolality-induced hyperkalemia, metabolic acidosis (dilutional), osmolar gap increased, water intoxication

Gastrointestinal: Nausea, vomiting, xerostomia

Genitourinary: Dysuria, polyuria

Local: Pain, thrombophlebitis, tissue necrosis

Ocular: Blurred vision

Renal: Acute renal failure, acute tubular necrosis (>200 g/day; serum osmolality >320 mOsm/L)

Respiratory: Pulmonary edema, rhinitis

Miscellaneous: Allergic reactions

Overdosage/Toxicology Symptoms of overdose include acute renal failure, polyuria, hypotension, cardiovascular collapse, pulmonary edema, hyponatremia, hypokalemia, oliguria, and seizures. Increased electrolyte excretion and fluid overload can occur. Hemodialysis will clear mannitol and reduce osmolality.

Dosing

Adults:

Test dose (to assess adequate renal function): I.V.: 12.5 g (200 mg/kg) over 3-5 minutes to produce a urine flow of at least 30-50 mL of urine per hour. If urine flow does not increase, a second test dose may be given. If test dose does not produce an acceptable urine output, then need to reassess management.

Initial: 0.5-1 g/kg

Maintenance: 0.25-0.5 g/kg every 4-6 hours; usual daily dose: 20-200 g/24 hours

Edema (osmotic diuretic): Initial: 0.5-1 g/kg; Maintenance: 0.25-0.5 g/kg every 4-6 hours; usual adult dose: 20-200 g/24 hours

Intracranial pressure/Cerebral edema: I.V.: 0.25-1.5 g/kg/dose I.V. as a 15% to 20% solution over ≥30 minutes; maintain serum osmolality 310 to <320 mOsm/kg.

Prevention of acute renal failure (oliguria): 50-100 g dose

Treatment of oliguria: 100 g dose

Preoperative for neurosurgery: I.V.: 1.5-2 g/kg administered 1-1.5 hours prior to surgery.

Transurethral: Irrigation: Use urogenital solution as required for irrigation.

Elderly: Refer to adult dosing. Consider initiation at lower end of dosing range.

Pediatrics:

Test dose (to assess adequate renal function): I.V.: Children: 200 mg/kg over 3-5 minutes to produce a urine flow of at least 1 mL/kg for 1-3 hours

Edema (osmotic diuretic): I.V.: Children: Initial: 0.5-1 g/kg; Maintenance: 0.25-0.5 g/kg given every 4-6 hours

Renal Impairment:

Contraindicated in severe renal impairment. If test dose does not produce adequate urine output reassess options. Use caution in patients with underlying renal disease.

Hepatic Impairment:

No adjustment required.

Available Dosage Forms

Injection, solution: 5% [50 mg/mL] (1000 mL); 10% [100 mg/mL] (500 mL, 1000 mL); 15% [150 mg/mL] (500 mL); 20% [200 mg/mL] (150 mL, 250 mL, 500 mL); 25% [250 mg/mL] (50 mL)

Osmitrol®: 5% [50 mg/mL] (1000 mL); 10% [100 mg/mL] (500 mL, 1000 mL); 15% [150 mg/mL] (500 mL); 20% [200 mg/mL] (250 mL, 500 mL)

Solution, urogenital (Resectisol®): 5% [50 mg/mL] (2000 mL, 4000 mL)

Nursing Guidelines

Assessment: Assess for adequate renal function and urine flow prior to administration. Lithium toxicity is increased with concurrent use, and concurrent use of other nephrotic agents may increase potential for renal dysfunction. Infusion site must be closely monitored for extravasation; this is a vesicant. Renal and cardiovascular status should be monitored during infusion. Assess results of laboratory tests, therapeutic effectiveness (according to purpose for use), and adverse response (eg, circulatory overload, CHF, rash, water intoxication). Patient teaching should be appropriate to patient condition.

Monitoring Laboratory Tests: Renal function, serum electrolytes, serum and urine osmolality. For treatment of elevated intracranial pressure, maintain serum osmolality 310-320 mOsm/kg

Patient Education: This medication can only be given by infusion. Report immediately any muscle weakness, numbness, tingling, acute headache, nausea, dizziness, blurred vision, eye pain, respiratory difficulty, chest pain, or pain at infusion site. **Pregnancy/breast-feeding precautions:** Inform prescriber if you are pregnant. Consult prescriber if breast-feeding.

Pregnancy Risk Factor: C

Lactation: Excretion in breast milk unknown/use caution

Perioperative/Anesthesia/Other Concerns: Mannitol may autoclave or heat to redissolve crystals.

Mannitol 20% has an approximate osmolarity of 1100 mOsm/L.

Mannitol 25% has an approximate osmolarity of 1375 mOsm/L.

Administration

I.V.: Vesicant. Do not administer with blood. Crenation and agglutination of red blood cells may occur if administered with whole blood. Inspect for crystals prior to administration. If crystals present redissolve by warming solution. Use filter-type administration set.

Compatibility:

Y-site administration: Incompatible with cefepime, doxorubicin liposome, filgrastim

Compatibility when admixed: Incompatible with imipenem/cilastatin, meropenem

Storage: Should be stored at room temperature (15°C to 30°C) and protected from freezing. Crystallization may occur at low temperatures. Do not use solutions that contain crystals, heating in a hot water bath and vigorous shaking may be utilized for resolubilization. Cool solutions to body temperature before using.

◆ **Mantoux** *see* Tuberculin Tests *on page 1673*

◆ **Mapap® [OTC]** *see* Acetaminophen *on page 65*

◆ **Mapap® Arthritis [OTC]** *see* Acetaminophen *on page 65*

◆ **Mapap® Children's [OTC]** *see* Acetaminophen *on page 65*

◆ **Mapap® Extra Strength [OTC]** *see* Acetaminophen *on page 65*

◆ **Mapap® Infants [OTC]** *see* Acetaminophen *on page 65*

◆ **Marcaine®** *see* Bupivacaine *on page 266*

- ♦ **Marcaine® Spinal** *see* Bupivacaine *on page 266*
- ♦ **Marcaine® with Epinephrine** *see* Bupivacaine and Epinephrine *on page 268*
- ♦ **Margesic® H** *see* Hydrocodone and Acetaminophen *on page 867*
- ♦ **Marinol®** *see* Dronabinol *on page 588*
- ♦ **3M™ Avagard™ [OTC]** *see* Chlorhexidine Gluconate *on page 373*
- ♦ **Maxair™ Autohaler™** *see* Pirbuterol *on page 1373*
- ♦ **Maxidex®** *see* Dexamethasone *on page 495*
- ♦ **Maxidone™** *see* Hydrocodone and Acetaminophen *on page 867*
- ♦ **Maxipime®** *see* Cefepime *on page 337*
- ♦ **Maxitrol®** *see* Neomycin, Polymyxin B, and Dexamethasone *on page 1211*
- ♦ **Maxivate®** *see* Betamethasone *on page 237*
- ♦ **Maxzide®** *see* Hydrochlorothiazide and Triamterene *on page 866*
- ♦ **Maxzide®-25** *see* Hydrochlorothiazide and Triamterene *on page 866*
- ♦ **3M™ Cavilon™ Skin Cleanser [OTC]** *see* Benzalkonium Chloride *on page 231*
- ♦ **MCH** *see* Collagen Hemostat *on page 449*
- ♦ **MD-76®R** *see* Diatrizoate Meglumine and Diatrizoate Sodium *on page 514*
- ♦ **MD-Gastroview®** *see* Diatrizoate Meglumine and Diatrizoate Sodium *on page 514*
- ♦ **MDL 73,147EF** *see* Dolasetron *on page 563*

Measles, Mumps, and Rubella Vaccines (Combined)

(MEE zels, mumpz & roo BEL a vak SEENS, kom BINED)

U.S. Brand Names M-M-R® II

Synonyms MMR; Mumps, Measles and Rubella Vaccines, Combined; Rubella, Measles and Mumps Vaccines, Combined

Pharmacologic Category Vaccine, Live Virus

Use Measles, mumps, and rubella prophylaxis

Mechanism of Action As a live, attenuated vaccine, MMR vaccine offers active immunity to disease caused by the measles, mumps, and rubella viruses.

Contraindications Hypersensitivity to measles, mumps, and rubella vaccine or any component of the formulation; hypersensitivity to neomycin or gelatin; current febrile respiratory illness or other febrile infection; severely-immunocompromised persons; blood dyscrasias, cancers affecting the bone marrow or lymphatic systems; children with active untreated tuberculosis

Warnings/Precautions

Females should not become pregnant within 28 days of vaccination.

MMR vaccine should not be given within 3 months of immune globulin or whole blood.

Immediate treatment for anaphylactic/anaphylactoid reaction should be available during vaccine use. Use extreme caution in patients with immediate-type hypersensitivity reactions to eggs.

MMR vaccine should not be administered to severely immunocompromised persons with the exception of asymptomatic children with HIV (ACIP and AAP recommendation).

Severely immunocompromised patients and symptomatic HIV-infected patients who are exposed to measles should receive immune globulin, regardless of prior vaccination status.

The immunogenicity of measles virus vaccine is decreased if vaccine is administered <6 months after immune globulin.

Patients with minor illnesses (diarrhea, mild upper respiratory tract infection with or without low grade fever or other illnesses with low-grade fever) may receive vaccine. Leukemia patients who are in remission and who have not received chemotherapy for at least 3 months may be vaccinated.

Use caution with history of cerebral injury, convulsions, or other conditions where stress due to fever should be avoided. Use caution in patients with thrombocytopenia and those who develop thrombocytopenia after first dose; thrombocytopenia may worsen.

Drug Interactions

Corticosteroids: In patients receiving high doses of systemic corticosteroids for ≥14 days, wait at least 1 month between discontinuing steroid therapy and administering immunization.

Immune globulin, whole blood, plasma: Do not administer together; immune response may be compromised. Defer vaccine administration for ≥3 months.

Immunosuppressant medications: The effect of the vaccine may be decreased.

Lab Interactions Temporary suppression of TB skin test reactivity with onset approximately 3 days after administration

Adverse Reactions All serious adverse reactions must be reported to the U.S. Department of Health and Human Services (DHHS) Vaccine Adverse Event Reporting System (VAERS) 1-800-822-7967.

Frequency not defined:

Cardiovascular: Syncope, vasculitis

Central nervous system: Ataxia, dizziness, febrile convulsions, fever, encephalitis, encephalopathy, Guillain-Barré syndrome, headache, irritability, malaise, measles inclusion body encephalitis, polyneuritis, polyneuropathy, seizure, subacute sclerosing panencephalitis,

Dermatologic: Angioneurotic edema, erythema multiforme, purpura, rash, Stevens-Johnson syndrome, urticaria

Endocrine & metabolic: Diabetes mellitus, parotitis

Gastrointestinal: Diarrhea, nausea, pancreatitis, sore throat, vomiting

Genitourinary: Orchitis

Hematologic: Leukocytosis, thrombocytopenia

Local: Injection site reactions which include burning, induration, redness, stinging, swelling, tenderness, wheal and flare, vesiculation

Neuromuscular & skeletal: Arthralgia/arthritis (variable; highest rates in women, 12% to 26% versus children, up to 3%), myalgia, paresthesia

Ocular: Ocular palsies

Otic: Otitis media

Renal: Conjunctivitis, retinitis, optic neuritis, papillitis, retrobulbar neuritis

Respiratory: Bronchospasm, cough, pneumonitis, rhinitis

Miscellaneous: Anaphylactoid reactions, anaphylaxis, atypical measles, panniculitis, regional lymphadenopathy

Dosing

Pediatrics:

Immunization;

Infants <12 months of age: SubQ: If there is risk of exposure to measles, single-antigen measles vaccine should be administered at 6-11 months of age with a second dose (of MMR) at >12 months.

Children ≥12 months of age: SubQ: 0.5 mL at 12 months and then repeated at 4-6 years of age. If the second dose was not received, the schedule should be completed by the 11- to 12-year old visit. Administer in outer aspect of the upper arm. Recommended age of primary immunization is 12-15 months; revaccination is recommended prior to elementary school.

Available Dosage Forms Injection, powder for reconstitution [preservative free]: Measles virus 1000 $TCID_{50}$, rubella virus 1000 $TCID_{50}$, and mumps virus 20,000 $TCID_{50}$ [contains neomycin 25 mcg, gelatin, human albumin, and bovine serum; produced in chick embryo cell culture]

Nursing Guidelines

Patient Education: This medication is only given by injection. You may experience the following- soreness or swelling in the area where the shot is given, fever, mild rash, swelling in the glands of the cheeks or neck, temporary pain or stiffness in the joints. Some effects may not occur until 1-2 weeks after the injection. Notify your prescriber immediately if these effects continue or are severe, or for a high fever, seizures or allergic reaction (respiratory difficulty, hives, weakness, dizziness, fast heartbeat). **Pregnancy/breast-feeding precautions:** Not to be used during pregnancy; do not get pregnant for 28 days after getting the vaccine. Pregnant women should wait until after giving birth to get the vaccine. Notify prescriber if breast-feeding.

Pregnancy Risk Factor: C

Pregnancy Issues: Animal reproduction studies have not been conducted. It is not known whether the drug can cause fetal harm or affect reproduction capacity (contracting natural measles during pregnancy can increase fetal risk). Do not administer to pregnant females, and avoid pregnancy for 28 days following vaccination.

Lactation:

Measles/mumps: Excretion in breast milk unknown/use caution

Rubella: Enters breast milk/use caution

Breast-Feeding Considerations: Evidence of rubella infection has occurred in breast-fed infants following immunization, most without severe disease.

(Continued)

Measles, Mumps, and Rubella Vaccines (Combined) *(Continued)*

Administration

I.V.: Not for I.V. administration.

Reconstitution: Use entire contents of the provided diluent to reconstitute vaccine. Gently agitate to mix thoroughly. Discard if powder does not dissolve. Use as soon as possible following reconstitution (may be stored at 2°C to 8°C/ 36°F to 46°F; protect from light); discard if not used within 8 hours.

Storage: Prior to reconstitution, store the powder at 2°C to 8°C (36°F to 46°F) or colder (freezing does not affect potency). Protect from light. Diluent may be stored with powder or at room temperature.

Meclizine (MEK li zeen)

U.S. Brand Names Antivert®; Bonine® [OTC]; Dramamine® Less Drowsy Formula [OTC]

Synonyms Meclizine Hydrochloride; Meclozine Hydrochloride

Pharmacologic Category Antiemetic; Antihistamine

Medication Safety Issues

Sound-alike/look-alike issues:

Antivert® may be confused with Axert™

Use Prevention and treatment of symptoms of motion sickness; management of vertigo with diseases affecting the vestibular system

Mechanism of Action Has central anticholinergic action by blocking chemoreceptor trigger zone; decreases excitability of the middle ear labyrinth and blocks conduction in the middle ear vestibular-cerebellar pathways

Pharmacodynamics/Kinetics

Onset of action: ~1 hour

Duration: 8-24 hours

Metabolism: Hepatic

Half-life elimination: 6 hours

Excretion: Urine (as metabolites); feces (as unchanged drug)

Contraindications Hypersensitivity to meclizine or any component of the formulation

Warnings/Precautions Use with caution in patients with angle-closure glaucoma, prostatic hyperplasia, pyloric or duodenal obstruction, or bladder neck obstruction; use with caution in hot weather, and during exercise; elderly may be at risk for anticholinergic side effects such as glaucoma, prostatic hyperplasia, constipation, gastrointestinal obstructive disease; if vertigo does not respond in 1-2 weeks, it is advised to discontinue use

Drug Interactions Increased toxicity: CNS depressants, neuroleptics, anticholinergics

Nutritional/Herbal/Ethanol Interactions Ethanol: Avoid ethanol (may increase CNS depression).

Adverse Reactions

>10%:

- Central nervous system: Slight to moderate drowsiness
- Respiratory: Thickening of bronchial secretions

1% to 10%:

- Central nervous system: Headache, fatigue, nervousness, dizziness
- Gastrointestinal: Appetite increase, weight gain, nausea, diarrhea, abdominal pain, dry mouth
- Neuromuscular & skeletal: Arthralgia
- Respiratory: Pharyngitis

<1% (Limited to important or life-threatening): Bronchospasm, hepatitis, hypotension, palpitation

Overdosage/Toxicology Symptoms of overdose include CNS depression, confusion, nervousness, hallucinations, dizziness, blurred vision, nausea, vomiting, and hyperthermia. There is no specific treatment for antihistamine overdose. Clinical toxicity is due to blockade of cholinergic receptors. For anticholinergic overdose with severe life-threatening symptoms, physostigmine 1-2 mg I.V. slowly, may be given to reverse these effects.

Dosing

Adults & Elderly:

Motion sickness: Oral: 12.5-25 mg 1 hour before travel, repeat dose every 12-24 hours if needed; doses up to 50 mg may be needed

Vertigo: Oral: 25-100 mg/day in divided doses

Pediatrics: Children >12 years: Refer to adult dosing.

Available Dosage Forms

Tablet, as hydrochloride: 12.5 mg, 25 mg

Antivert®: 12.5 mg, 25 mg, 50 mg

Dramamine® Less Drowsy Formula: 25 mg

Tablet, chewable, as hydrochloride (Bonine®): 25 mg

Nursing Guidelines

Assessment: Determine cause of vomiting before beginning therapy. Assess effectiveness and interactions of other medications patient may be taking. Monitor effectiveness of therapy and adverse response. Assess knowledge/teach patient possible side effects/appropriate interventions and adverse symptoms to report.

Patient Education: Take exactly as prescribed; do not increase dose. Avoid alcohol, other CNS depressants, sleeping aids without consulting prescriber. You may experience dizziness, drowsiness, or blurred vision (use caution when driving or engaging in tasks that require alertness until response to drug is known); dry mouth (frequent mouth care, sucking lozenges, or chewing gum may help); constipation (increased exercise, fluids, fruit, or may help); or heat intolerance (avoid excessive exercise, hot environments, maintain adequate hydration). Report CNS change (hallucination, confusion, nervousness); sudden or unusual weight gain; unresolved nausea or diarrhea; chest pain or palpitations; muscle pain; or changes in urinary pattern. **Breast-feeding precaution:** Breast-feeding is not recommended.

Geriatric Considerations: Due to anticholinergic action, use lowest dose in divided doses to avoid side effects and their inconvenience. Limit use if possible. May cause confusion or aggravate symptoms of confusion in those with dementia.

Pregnancy Risk Factor: B

Lactation: Excretion in breast milk unknown/not recommended

- **Meclizine Hydrochloride** *see* Meclizine *on page 1084*
- **Meclozine Hydrochloride** *see* Meclizine *on page 1084*
- **Medicone® [OTC]** *see* Phenylephrine *on page 1350*
- **Medigesic®** *see* Butalbital, Acetaminophen, and Caffeine *on page 280*
- **Medrol®** *see* MethylPREDNISolone *on page 1140*

MedroxyPROGESTERone (me DROKS ee proe JES te rone)

U.S. Brand Names Depo-Provera®; Depo-Provera® Contraceptive; depo-subQ provera 104™; Provera®

Synonyms Acetoxymethylprogesterone; Medroxyprogesterone Acetate; Methylacetoxyprogesterone; MPA

Pharmacologic Category Contraceptive; Progestin

Medication Safety Issues

Sound-alike/look-alike issues:

MedroxyPROGESTERone may be confused with hydroxyprogesterone, methylPREDNISolone, methylTESTOSTERone

Provera® may be confused with Covera®, Parlodel®, Premarin®

Use Endometrial carcinoma or renal carcinoma; secondary amenorrhea or abnormal uterine bleeding due to hormonal imbalance; reduction of endometrial hyperplasia in nonhysterectomized postmenopausal women receiving conjugated estrogens; prevention of pregnancy; management of endometriosis-associated pain

Mechanism of Action Inhibits secretion of pituitary gonadotropins, which prevents follicular maturation and ovulation; causes endometrial thinning

Pharmacodynamics/Kinetics

Absorption: Oral: Well absorbed; I.M.: Slow

Protein binding: 86% to 90% primarily to albumin; does not bind to sex hormone-binding globulin

Metabolism: Extensively hepatic via hydroxylation and conjugation; forms metabolites

Time to peak: Oral: 2-4 hours

Half-life elimination: Oral: 12-17 hours; I.M. (Depo-Provera® Contraceptive): 50 days; SubQ: ~40 days

Excretion: Urine

Contraindications Hypersensitivity to medroxyprogesterone or any component of the formulation; history of or current thrombophlebitis or venous thromboembolic disorders (including DVT, PE); cerebral vascular disease; severe hepatic

(Continued)

MedroxyPROGESTERone *(Continued)*

dysfunction or disease; carcinoma of the breast or genital organs, undiagnosed vaginal bleeding; missed abortion, diagnostic test for pregnancy, pregnancy

Warnings/Precautions Prolonged use of medroxyprogesterone contraceptive injection may result in a loss of bone mineral density (BMD). Loss is related to the duration of use, and may not be completely reversible on discontinuation of the drug. The impact on peak bone mass in adolescents should be considered in treatment decisions. Long-term use (ie, >2 years) should be limited to situations where other birth control methods are inadequate. Consider other methods of birth control in women with (or at risk for) osteoporosis.

Use caution with cardiovascular disease or dysfunction. MPA used in combination with estrogen may increase the risks of hypertension, myocardial infarction (MI), stroke, pulmonary emboli (PE), and deep vein thrombosis; incidence of these effects was shown to be significantly increased in postmenopausal women using conjugated equine estrogens (CEE) in combination with MPA. MPA in combination with estrogens should not be used to prevent coronary heart disease.

The risk of dementia may be increased in postmenopausal women; increased incidence was observed in women ≥65 years of age taking MPA in combination with CEE. An increased risk of invasive breast cancer was observed in postmenopausal women using MPA in combination with CEE. An increase in abnormal mammograms has also been reported with estrogen and progestin therapy.

Discontinue pending examination in cases of sudden partial or complete vision loss, sudden onset of proptosis, diplopia, or migraine; discontinue permanently if papilledema or retinal vascular lesions are observed on examination. Use with caution in patients with diseases that may be exacerbated by fluid retention (including asthma, epilepsy, migraine, diabetes, or renal dysfunction). Use caution with history of depression. Whenever possible, progestins in combination with estrogens should be discontinued at least 4-6 weeks prior to surgeries associated with an increased risk of thromboembolism or during periods of prolonged immobilization. Progestins used in combination with estrogen should be used for shortest duration possible consistent with treatment goals. Conduct periodic risk:benefit assessments.

Drug Interactions Substrate of CYP3A4 (major); **Induces** CYP3A4 (weak)

Acitretin: May diminish the therapeutic effect of progestin contraceptives; contraceptive failure is possible.

CYP3A4 inducers: CYP3A4 inducers may decrease the levels/effects of medroxyprogesterone. Example inducers include aminoglutethimide, carbamazepine, nafcillin, nevirapine, phenobarbital, phenytoin, and rifamycins.

Griseofulvin: May diminish the therapeutic effect of progestin contraceptives; contraceptive failure is possible.

Warfarin: Progestins may diminish the anticoagulant effect of coumarin derivatives. In contrast, enhanced anticoagulant effects have also been noted with some products.

Nutritional/Herbal/Ethanol Interactions

Ethanol: Avoid ethanol (may increase risk of osteoporosis).

Food: Bioavailability of the oral tablet is increased when taken with food; half-life is unchanged.

Herb/Nutraceutical: St John's wort may diminish the therapeutic effect of progestin contraceptives (contraceptive failure is possible).

Lab Interactions

The following tests may be decreased: Steroid levels (plasma and urinary), gonadotropin levels, SHBG concentration, T_3 uptake

The following tests may be increased: Protein-bound iodine, butanol extractable protein-bound iodine, Factors II, VII, VIII, IX, X

Pathologist should be advised of estrogen/progesterone therapy when specimens are submitted.

Adverse Reactions Adverse effects as reported with any dosage form; percent ranges presented are noted with the MPA contraceptive injection:

>5%:

- Central nervous system: Dizziness, headache, nervousness
- Endocrine & metabolic: Libido decreased, menstrual irregularities (includes bleeding, amenorrhea, or both)
- Gastrointestinal: Abdominal pain/discomfort, weight changes (average 3-5 pounds after 1 year, 8 pounds after 2 years)
- Neuromuscular & skeletal: Weakness

1% to 5%:
- Cardiovascular: Edema
- Central nervous system: Depression, fatigue, insomnia, irritability, pain
- Dermatologic: Acne, alopecia, rash
- Endocrine & metabolic: Anorgasmia, breast pain, hot flashes
- Gastrointestinal: Bloating, nausea
- Genitourinary: Cervical smear abnormal, leukorrhea, menometrorrhagia, menorrhagia, pelvic pain, urinary tract infection, vaginitis, vaginal infection, vaginal hemorrhage
- Local: Injection site atrophy, injection site reaction, injection site pain
- Neuromuscular & skeletal: Arthralgia, backache, leg cramp
- Respiratory: Respiratory tract infections

<1% (Limited to important or life-threatening): Allergic reaction, anaphylaxis, anaphylactoid reactions, anemia, angioedema, appetite changes, asthma, axillary swelling, blood dyscrasia, body odor, bone mineral density decreased, breast cancer, breast changes, cervical cancer, chest pain, chills, chloasma, convulsions, deep vein thrombosis, diaphoresis, drowsiness, dry skin, dysmenorrhea, dyspareunia, dyspnea, facial palsy, fever, galactorrhea, genitourinary infections, glucose tolerance decreased, hirsutism, hoarseness, jaundice, lack of return to fertility, lactation decreased, libido increased, melasma, nipple bleeding, osteoporosis, osteoporotic fractures, paralysis, paresthesia, pruritus, pulmonary embolus, rectal bleeding, scleroderma, sensation of pregnancy, somnolence, syncope, tachycardia, thirst, thrombophlebitis, uterine hyperplasia, vaginal cysts, varicose veins; residual lump, sterile abscess, or skin discoloration at the injection site

Overdosage/Toxicology Toxicity is unlikely following single exposure of excessive doses. Supportive treatment is adequate in most cases.

Dosing

Adults & Elderly:

Amenorrhea: Oral: 5-10 mg/day for 5-10 days

Abnormal uterine bleeding: Oral: 5-10 mg for 5-10 days starting on day 16 or 21 of cycle

Contraception:

Depo-Provera® Contraceptive: I.M.: 150 mg every 3 months

depo-subQ provera 104™: SubQ: 104 mg every 3 months (every 12-14 weeks)

Endometriosis: depo-subQ provera 104™: SubQ: 104 mg every 3 months (every 12-14 weeks)

Endometrial or renal carcinoma (Depo-Provera®): I.M.: 400-1000 mg/week

Accompanying cyclic estrogen therapy, postmenopausal: Oral: 5-10 mg for 12-14 consecutive days each month, starting on day 1 or day 16 of the cycle; lower doses may be used if given with estrogen continuously throughout the cycle

Pediatrics: Adolescents:

Amenorrhea: Refer to adult dosing.

Abnormal uterine bleeding: Refer to adult dosing.

Contraception: Refer to adult dosing.

Endometriosis: Refer to adult dosing.

Hepatic Impairment: Use is contraindicated with severe impairment. Consider lower dose or less frequent administration with mild-to-moderate impairment. Use of the contraceptive injection has not been studied in patients with hepatic impairment; consideration should be given to not readminister if jaundice develops

Available Dosage Forms

Injection, suspension, as acetate: 150 mg/mL (1 mL)

Depo-Provera®: 400 mg/mL (2.5 mL)

Depo-Provera® Contraceptive: 150 mg/mL (1 mL) [prefilled syringe or vial]

depo-subQ provera 104™: 104 mg/0.65 mL (0.65 mL) [prefilled syringe]

Tablet, as acetate (Provera®): 2.5 mg, 5 mg, 10 mg

Nursing Guidelines

Assessment: Monitor for effectiveness of therapy and adverse effects. Instruct patient on appropriate dose scheduling (according to purpose of therapy), possible side effects, and symptoms to report. **Pregnancy risk factor X:** Determine that patient is not pregnant before starting therapy. Do not give to sexually-active female patients unless capable of complying with contraceptive use.

Monitoring Laboratory Tests: Must have pregnancy test prior to beginning therapy.

(Continued)

MedroxyPROGESTERone *(Continued)*

Dietary Considerations: Ensure adequate calcium and vitamin D intake when used for the prevention of pregnancy

Patient Education: Follow dosage schedule and do not take more than prescribed. You may experience sensitivity to sunlight (use sunblock, wear protective clothing and eyewear, and avoid extensive exposure to direct sunlight); dizziness, anxiety, depression (use caution when driving or engaging in tasks that require alertness until response to drug is known); changes in appetite; maintain adequate hydration (2-3 L/day of fluids) unless instructed to restrict fluid intake and diet; decreased libido or increased body hair (reversible when drug is discontinued); hot flashes (cool clothes and environment may help). May cause discoloration of stool (green). Report swelling of face, lips, or mouth; absence or altered menses; abdominal pain; vaginal itching, irritation, or discharge; heat, warmth, redness, or swelling of extremities; or sudden onset change in vision. **Pregnancy precaution:** Inform prescriber if you are pregnant. Consult prescriber for instruction on appropriate contraceptive measures.

Injection for contraception: This product does not protect against HIV or other sexually-transmitted diseases.

Geriatric Considerations: No specific recommendations for dosage adjustments. Monitor closely for adverse effects when starting therapy.

Pregnancy Risk Factor: X

Pregnancy Issues: There is an increased risk of minor birth defects in children whose mothers take progesterones during the first 4 months of pregnancy. Hypospadias has been reported in male and mild masculinization of the external genitalia has been reported in female babies exposed during the first trimester. High doses are used to impair fertility. Low birth weight has been reported in neonates from unexpected pregnancies which occurred 1-2 months following injection of medroxyprogesterone (MPA) contraceptive. Ectopic pregnancies have been reported with use of the MPA contraceptive injection. When therapy is discontinued, fertility returns sooner in women of lower body weight. Median time to conception/return to ovulation following discontinuation of MPA contraceptive injection is 10 months following the last injection.

Lactation: Enters breast milk/compatible

Breast-Feeding Considerations: Composition, quality and quantity of breast milk are not affected; adverse developmental and behavioral effects have not been noted following exposure of infant to MPA while breast-feeding.

Administration

I.M.: Depo-Provera® Contraceptive: Administer first dose during the first 5 days of menstrual period, or within the first 5 days postpartum if not breast-feeding, or at the sixth week postpartum if breast feeding exclusively. Shake vigorously prior to administration. Administer by deep I.M. injection in the gluteal or deltoid muscle.

Storage: Store at controlled room temperature.

♦ **Medroxyprogesterone Acetate** *see* MedroxyPROGESTERone *on page 1085*

♦ **Medroxyprogesterone and Estrogens (Conjugated)** *see* Estrogens (Conjugated/Equine) and Medroxyprogesterone *on page 665*

Mefloquine (ME floe kwin)

U.S. Brand Names Lariam®

Synonyms Mefloquine Hydrochloride

Pharmacologic Category Antimalarial Agent

Use Treatment of acute malarial infections and prevention of malaria

Mechanism of Action Mefloquine is a quinoline-methanol compound structurally similar to quinine; mefloquine's effectiveness in the treatment and prophylaxis of malaria is due to the destruction of the asexual blood forms of the malarial pathogens that affect humans, *Plasmodium falciparum*, *P. vivax*, *P. malariae*, *P. ovale*

Pharmacodynamics/Kinetics

Absorption: Well absorbed

Distribution: V_d: 19 L/kg; blood, urine, CSF, tissues; enters breast milk

Protein binding: 98%

Metabolism: Extensively hepatic; main metabolite is inactive

Bioavailability: Increased by food

Half-life elimination: 21-22 days

Time to peak, plasma: 6-24 hours (median: ~17 hours)

Excretion: Primarily bile and feces; urine (9% as unchanged drug, 4% as primary metabolite)

Contraindications Hypersensitivity mefloquine, related compounds (such as quinine and quinidine), or any component of the formulation; history of convulsions; cardiac conduction abnormalities; severe psychiatric disorder (including active or recent history of depression, generalized anxiety disorder, psychosis, or schizophrenia); use with halofantrine

Warnings/Precautions Use with caution in patients with a previous history of depression (see Contraindications regarding severe psychiatric illness, including active/recent depression). May cause a range of psychiatric symptoms (anxiety, paranoia, depression, hallucinations and psychosis). Occasionally, symptoms have been reported to persist long after mefloquine has been discontinued. Rare cases of suicidal ideation and suicide have been reported (no causal relationship established). The appearance of psychiatric symptoms such as acute anxiety, depression, restlessness or confusion may be considered a prodrome to more serious events. When used as prophylaxis, substitute an alternative medication. Discontinue if unexplained neuropsychiatric disturbances occur. Use caution in patients with significant cardiac disease. If mefloquine is to be used for a prolonged period, periodic evaluations including liver function tests and ophthalmic examinations should be performed. (Retinal abnormalities have not been observed with mefloquine in humans; however, it has with long-term administration to rats.) In cases of life-threatening, serious, or overwhelming malaria infections due to *Plasmodium falciparum*, patients should be treated with intravenous antimalarial drug. Mefloquine may be given orally to complete the course. Dizziness, loss of balance, and other CNS disorders have been reported; due to long half-life, effects may persist after mefloquine is discontinued. Use caution in activities requiring alertness and fine motor coordination (driving, piloting planes, operating machinery, deep sea diving, etc).

Drug Interactions **Substrate** of CYP3A4 (major); **Inhibits** CYP2D6 (weak), 3A4 (weak)

Anticonvulsants: Decreased effect of valproic acid, carbamazepine, phenobarbital, or phenytoin.

Antiarrhythmics: Chloroquine and quinidine may produce electrocardiographic changes and increase risk of convulsions. When used as initial treatment of severe malaria, delay mefloquine for 12 hours after the last dose. Use caution with other medications known to alter conduction.

CYP3A4 inducers: CYP3A4 inducers may decrease the levels/effects of mefloquine. Example inducers include aminoglutethimide, carbamazepine, nafcillin, nevirapine, phenobarbital, phenytoin, and rifamycins.

CYP3A4 inhibitors: May increase the levels/effects of mefloquine. Example inhibitors include azole antifungals, clarithromycin, diclofenac, doxycycline, erythromycin, imatinib, isoniazid, nefazodone, nicardipine, propofol, protease inhibitors, quinidine, telithromycin, and verapamil.

Halofantrine: Fatal prolongation of the QT_c interval reported; concomitant use is contraindicated.

Quinine: May produce electrocardiographic changes and increase risk of convulsions. When used as initial treatment of severe malaria, delay mefloquine for 12 hours after the last dose.

Vaccines: Vaccinations with attenuated live bacteria should be completed at least 3 days prior to first dose of mefloquine. Vaccination with oral live attenuated Ty21a vaccine should be delayed for at least 24 hours after the administration of mefloquine.

Nutritional/Herbal/Ethanol Interactions Food: Food increases bioavailability by ~40%.

Adverse Reactions

Frequency not defined: Neuropsychiatric events

1% to 10%:

- Central nervous system: Headache, fever, chills, fatigue
- Dermatologic: Rash
- Gastrointestinal: Vomiting (3%), diarrhea, stomach pain, nausea, appetite decreased
- Neuromuscular & skeletal: Myalgia
- Otic: Tinnitus

<1% (Limited to important or life-threatening): Abnormal dreams, alopecia, ataxia, aggressive behavior, agitation, anaphylaxis, anxiety, arthralgia, AV block, bradycardia, chest pain, conduction abnormalities (transient), confusion, convulsions, depression, diaphoresis (increased), dizziness, dyspepsia, dyspnea, edema, emotional lability, encephalopathy, erythema multiforme, exanthema,

(Continued)

Mefloquine *(Continued)*

extrasystoles, hallucinations, hearing impairment, hypotension, insomnia, leukocytosis, malaise, mood changes, muscle cramps/weakness, palpitation, panic attacks, paranoia, paresthesia, psychosis, pruritus, seizure, somnolence, Stevens-Johnson syndrome, suicidal ideation and behavior (causal relationship not established), syncope, tachycardia, thrombocytopenia, tremor, urticaria, vertigo, visual disturbances, weakness

Overdosage/Toxicology Treatment is supportive. Monitor cardiac function and psychiatric status for at least 24 hours.

Dosing

Adults & Elderly: Dose expressed as mg of mefloquine hydrochloride:

Malaria treatment (mild to moderate infection): Oral: 5 tablets (1250 mg) as a single dose. Take with food and at least 8 oz of water. If clinical improvement is not seen within 48-72 hours, an alternative therapy should be used for retreatment.

Malaria prophylaxis: Oral: 1 tablet (250 mg) weekly starting 1 week before, arrival in endemic area, continuing weekly during travel and for 4 weeks after leaving endemic area. Take with food and at least 8 oz of water.

Pediatrics: Dose expressed as mg of mefloquine hydrochloride: Children ≥6 months and >5 kg:

Malaria treatment: Oral: 20-25 mg/kg in 2 divided doses, taken 6-8 hours apart (maximum: 1250 mg) Take with food and an ample amount of water. If clinical improvement is not seen within 48-72 hours, an alternative therapy should be used for retreatment.

Malaria prophylaxis: Oral: 5 mg/kg/once weekly (maximum dose: 250 mg) starting 1 week before, arrival in endemic area, continuing weekly during travel and for 4 weeks after leaving endemic area. Take with food and an ample amount of water.

Renal Impairment: No dosage adjustment needed in patients with renal impairment or on dialysis.

Hepatic Impairment: Half-life may be prolonged and plasma levels may be higher.

Available Dosage Forms Tablet, as hydrochloride: 250 mg [equivalent to 228 mg base]

Nursing Guidelines

Assessment: See Contraindications, Warnings/Precautions, and Dosing (eg, treatment vs prophylaxis) for use cautions. Assess potential for interactions with other prescriptions, OTC medications, or herbal products patient may be taking (see Drug Interactions). Assess results of laboratory tests (see below), therapeutic effectiveness, and adverse response (eg, CNS changes - see Adverse Reactions and Overdose/Toxicology). Teach patient proper use, possible side effects/interventions (eg, need for ophthalmic exams), and adverse symptoms to report (see Patient Education). Breast-feeding is not recommended.

Monitoring Laboratory Tests: When use is prolonged, periodically monitor liver function tests.

Dietary Considerations: Take with food and with at least 8 oz of water.

Patient Education: Inform prescriber of all prescriptions, OTC medications, or herbal products you are taking, and any allergies you have. Do not take any new medication during therapy unless approved by prescriber. Take as directed; full course of treatment may take several months. For prophylaxis, begin 1 week before traveling to endemic areas, continue during travel period and for 4 weeks following return. Take with 8 oz of water. Avoid alcohol. You should have regular ophthalmic exams (every 4-6 months) if using this medication over extended periods. May cause dizziness, changes in mentation, insomnia, headache, visual disturbances, disturbed sense of balance (use caution when driving or engaging in tasks requiring alertness until response to drug is known); or nausea, vomiting, loss of appetite (small, frequent meals, frequent mouth care, sucking lozenges, or chewing gum may help). Report vision changes, persistent GI disturbances, change in hearing acuity or ringing in the ears, CNS changes, unusual fatigue, or any other persistent adverse reactions. If you are taking this for prophylaxis of malaria and experience symptoms of anxiety, confusion, depression, nervousness, or restlessness, report these symptoms **immediately** to the prescriber (symptoms may worsen) and stop taking this medication. **Pregnancy/breast-feeding precautions:** Inform prescriber if you are pregnant. Use reliable contraception during and for 3 months following treatment. Breast-feeding is not recommended.

Pregnancy Risk Factor: C

Lactation: Enters breast milk/not recommended

Breast-Feeding Considerations: Excreted in small quantities; effect to nursing infant is unknown. Breast-feeding is not recommended during therapy and the long half-life of mefloquine should also be considered once therapy is complete.

Administration

Oral: Administer with food and with at least 8 oz of water. When used for malaria prophylaxis, dose should be taken once weekly on the same day each week. If vomiting occurs within 30-60 minutes after dose, an additional half-dose should be given. Tablets may be crushed and suspended in a small amount of water, milk, or another beverage for persons unable to swallow tablets.

Storage: Store at 25°C (77°F); excursions permitted to 15°C to 30°C (59°F to 86°F)

- ♦ **Mefloquine Hydrochloride** *see* Mefloquine *on page 1088*
- ♦ **Mefoxin®** *see* Cefoxitin *on page 344*

Meloxicam (mel OKS i kam)

U.S. Brand Names Mobic®

Pharmacologic Category Nonsteroidal Anti-inflammatory Drug (NSAID), Oral

Use Relief of signs and symptoms of osteoarthritis, rheumatoid arthritis, and juvenile rheumatoid arthritis (JRA)

Mechanism of Action Inhibits prostaglandin synthesis by decreasing the activity of the enzyme, cyclooxygenase, which results in decreased formation of prostaglandin precursors

Pharmacodynamics/Kinetics

Distribution: 10 L

Protein binding: 99.4%

Metabolism: Hepatic via CYP2C9 and CYP3A4 (minor); forms 4 metabolites (inactive)

Bioavailability: 89%

Half-life elimination: Adults: 15-20 hours

Time to peak: Initial: 5-10 hours; Secondary: 12-14 hours

Excretion: Urine and feces (as inactive metabolites)

Contraindications Hypersensitivity to meloxicam, aspirin, other NSAIDs, or any component of the formulation; perioperative pain in the setting of coronary artery bypass surgery (CABG); pregnancy (3rd trimester)

Warnings/Precautions NSAIDs are associated with an increased risk of adverse cardiovascular events, including MI, stroke, and new onset or worsening of pre-existing hypertension. Risk may be increased with duration of use or pre-existing cardiovascular risk-factors or disease. Carefully evaluate individual cardiovascular risk profiles prior to prescribing. Use caution with fluid retention, CHF or hypertension.

Use of NSAIDs can compromise existing renal function. Renal toxicity can occur in patient with impaired renal function, dehydration, heart failure, liver dysfunction, those taking diuretics and ACEI and the elderly. Rehydrate patient before starting therapy. Monitor renal function closely. Meloxicam is not recommended for patients with advanced renal disease

NSAIDs may increase risk of gastrointestinal irritation, ulceration, bleeding, and perforation. These events may occur at any time during therapy and without warning. Use caution with a history of GI disease (bleeding or ulcers), concurrent therapy with aspirin, anticoagulants and/or corticosteroids, smoking, use of alcohol, the elderly or debilitated patients.

Use the lowest effective dose for the shortest duration of time, consistent with individual patient goals, to reduce risk of cardiovascular or GI adverse events. Alternate therapies should be considered for patients at high risk.

NSAIDs may cause serious skin adverse events including exfoliative dermatitis, Stevens-Johnson syndrome (SJS) and toxic epidermal necrolysis (TEN). Anaphylactoid reactions may occur, even without prior exposure; patients with "aspirin triad" (bronchial asthma, aspirin intolerance, rhinitis) may be at increased risk. Do not use in patients who experience bronchospasm, asthma, rhinitis, or urticaria with NSAID or aspirin therapy.

Use with caution in patients with decreased hepatic function. Closely monitor patients with any abnormal LFT. Severe hepatic reactions (eg, fulminant hepatitis,

(Continued)

Meloxicam *(Continued)*

liver failure) have occurred with NSAID use, rarely; discontinue if signs or symptoms of liver disease develop, or if systemic manifestations occur.

The elderly are at increased risk for adverse effects (especially peptic ulceration, CNS effects, renal toxicity) from NSAIDs even at low doses.

Withhold for at least 4-6 half-lives prior to surgical or dental procedures. Safety and efficacy have not been established in pediatric patients <2 years of age.

Drug Interactions Substrate (minor) of CYP2C8/9, 3A4; **Inhibits** CYP2C8/9 (weak)

ACE inhibitors: Antihypertensive effects may be decreased by concurrent therapy with NSAIDs; monitor blood pressure

Angiotensin II antagonists: Antihypertensive effects may be decreased by concurrent therapy with NSAIDs; monitor blood pressure

Anticoagulants (warfarin, heparin, LMWHs) in combination with NSAIDs can cause increased risk of bleeding.

Antiplatelet drugs (ticlopidine, clopidogrel, aspirin, abciximab, dipyridamole, eptifibatide, tirofiban) can cause an increased risk of bleeding.

Aspirin increases serum concentrations (AUC) of meloxicam (in addition to potential for additive adverse effects); concurrent use is not recommended.

Cholestyramine (and possibly colestipol) increases the clearance of meloxicam.

Corticosteroids may increase the risk of GI ulceration; avoid concurrent use.

Cyclosporine: NSAIDs may increase serum creatinine, potassium, blood pressure, and cyclosporine levels; monitor cyclosporine levels and renal function carefully.

Hydralazine's antihypertensive effect is decreased; avoid concurrent use.

Lithium levels can be increased; avoid concurrent use if possible or monitor lithium levels and adjust dose. When NSAID is stopped, lithium will need adjustment again.

Loop diuretic's efficacy (diuretic and antihypertensive effect) may be reduced by NSAIDs.

Methotrexate: Severe bone marrow suppression, aplastic anemia, and GI toxicity have been reported with concomitant NSAID therapy. Avoid use during moderate or high-dose methotrexate (increased and prolonged methotrexate levels). NSAID use during low-dose treatment of rheumatoid arthritis has not been fully evaluated; extreme caution is warranted.

Thiazide diuretics: Antihypertensive effects of thiazide diuretics are decreased; avoid concurrent use.

Warfarin INRs may be increased by meloxicam. Monitor INR closely, particularly during initiation or change in dose. May increase risk of bleeding. Use lowest possible dose for shortest duration possible.

Nutritional/Herbal/Ethanol Interactions

Ethanol: Avoid ethanol (may enhance gastric mucosal irritation).

Herb/Nutraceutical: Avoid alfalfa, anise, bilberry, bladderwrack, bromelain, cat's claw, celery, coleus, cordyceps, dong quai, evening primrose, feverfew, fenugreek, garlic, ginger, ginkgo biloboa, red clover, horse chestnut, grapeseed, green tea, ginseng, guggul, horse chestnut seed, horseradish, licorice, prickly ash, red clover, reishi, SAMe, sweet clover, turmeric, white willow (all have additional antiplatelet activity).

Adverse Reactions Percentages reported in adult patients; abdominal pain, diarrhea, headache, pyrexia, and vomiting were reported more commonly in pediatric patients

2% to 10%:

Cardiovascular: Edema (<1% to 4%)

Central nervous system: Headache (2% to 8%), dizziness (<1% to 4%), insomnia (<1% to 4%)

Dermatologic: Pruritus (<1% to 2%), rash (<1% to 3%)

Gastrointestinal: Diarrhea (3% to 8%), dyspepsia (4% to 9%), nausea (2% to 7%), abdominal pain (2% to 5%), constipation (<1% to 3%), flatulence (<1% to 3%), vomiting (<1% to 3%)

Hematologic: Anemia (<1% to 4%)

Neuromuscular & skeletal: Arthralgia (<1% to 5%), back pain (<1% to 3%)

Respiratory: Upper respiratory infection (2% to 8%), cough (<1% to 2%), pharyngitis (<1% to 3%)

Miscellaneous: Flu-like symptoms (2% to 6%), falls (3%)

<2% (Limited to important or life-threatening): Agranulocytosis, allergic reaction, anaphylactic reaction, anaphylactoid reaction, angina, angioedema, arrhythmia,

bronchospasm, bullous eruption, cardiac failure, colitis, depression, duodenal perforation, duodenal ulcer, erythema multiforme, gastric perforation, gastric ulcer, gastroesophageal reflux, gastrointestinal hemorrhage, hepatic failure, hepatitis, hyper-/hypotension, interstitial nephritis, intestinal perforation, jaundice, MI, pancreatitis, paresthesia, photosensitivity reaction, renal failure, seizure, shock, somnolence, Stevens-Johnson syndrome, syncope, thrombocytopenia, tinnitus, toxic epidermal necrolysis, tremor, ulcerative stomatitis, urticaria, vasculitis, vertigo

Overdosage/Toxicology Symptoms of overdose include lethargy, drowsiness, nausea, vomiting, and epigastric pain. Rarely, severe symptoms have been associated with NSAID overdose including apnea, metabolic acidosis, coma, nystagmus, seizures, leukocytosis, and renal failure. Management of NSAID intoxication is supportive and symptomatic. Since meloxicam undergoes enterohepatic cycling, multiple doses of charcoal may be needed to reduce the potential for delayed toxicities. Cholestyramine has been shown to increase meloxicam clearance. Meloxicam is not dialyzable.

Dosing

Adults & Elderly: Osteoarthritis, rheumatoid arthritis: Oral: Initial: 7.5 mg once daily; some patients may receive additional benefit from an increased dose of 15 mg once daily.

Pediatrics: JRA: Oral: Children ≥2 years: 0.125 mg/kg/day; maximum dose: 7.5 mg/day

Renal Impairment:

Mild to moderate impairment: No specific dosage recommendations

Significant impairment (Cl_{cr} ≤15 mL/minute): Avoid use

Hemodialysis: Supplemental dose after dialysis not necessary.

Hepatic Impairment:

Mild (Child-Pugh class A) to moderate (Child-Pugh class B) hepatic dysfunction: No dosage adjustment is necessary

Severe hepatic impairment: Patients with severe hepatic impairment have not been adequately studied

Available Dosage Forms

Suspension: 7.5 mg/5 mL (100 mL) [contains sodium benzoate; raspberry flavor]

Tablet: 7.5 mg, 15 mg

Nursing Guidelines

Assessment: Evaluate cardiac risk and potential for GI bleeding prior to prescribing this medication. Assess effectiveness and interactions of other medications patient may be taking. Monitor blood pressure at the beginning of therapy and periodically during use. Assess results of laboratory tests, therapeutic effectiveness, and adverse reactions at beginning of therapy and periodically throughout therapy. Assess knowledge/teach patient appropriate use, interventions to reduce side effects, and adverse symptoms to report.

Monitoring Laboratory Tests: CBC, periodic liver function, renal function (serum BUN, and creatinine)

Dietary Considerations: Should be taken with food or milk to minimize gastrointestinal irritation.

Patient Education: Take this medication exactly as directed; do not increase dose without consulting prescriber. Take with food or milk to reduce GI distress. Maintain adequate hydration (2-3 L/day of fluids) unless instructed to restrict fluid intake. Avoid alcohol, excessive vitamin C intake, or salicylate-containing foods (eg, curry powder, prunes, raisins, tea, or licorice). Do not use aspirin or aspirin-containing medication, or any other anti-inflammatory medications without consulting prescriber. You may experience anorexia, nausea, vomiting, or heartburn (small frequent meals, frequent mouth care, sucking lozenges, or chewing gum may help); drowsiness, dizziness, nervousness, or headache (use caution when driving or engaging in tasks requiring alertness until response to drug is known); or fluid retention (weigh yourself weekly and report unusual (3-5 lb/week) weight gain). GI bleeding, ulceration, or perforation can occur with or without pain; discontinue medication and contact prescriber if persistent abdominal pain or cramping, or blood in stool occurs. Report breathlessness, respiratory difficulty, or unusual cough; chest pain, rapid heartbeat, palpitations; slurring of speech; unusual bruising/bleeding; blood in urine, stool, mouth, or vomitus; swollen extremities; skin blisters, rash, or itching; acute fatigue, jaundice, flu-like symptoms, hearing changes (ringing in ears); or other adverse reactions. **Pregnancy/breast-feeding precautions:** Inform prescriber if you are or intend to become pregnant. This drug should not be used in the 3rd trimester of pregnancy. Do not breast-feed.

(Continued)

Meloxicam *(Continued)*

Geriatric Considerations:

The elderly are at increased risk for adverse effects from NSAIDs. As many as 60% of elderly can develop peptic ulceration and/or hemorrhage asymptomatically. CNS adverse effects such as confusion, agitation, and hallucination are generally seen in overdose or high-dose situations; however, elderly patients may demonstrate these adverse effects at lower doses than younger adults. The elderly are also at increased risk of renal toxicity.

Pregnancy Risk Factor: C/D (3rd trimester)

Pregnancy Issues: May cause premature closure of the ductus arteriosus in the 3rd trimester of pregnancy.

Lactation: Excretion in breast milk unknown/not recommended

Breast-Feeding Considerations: It is not known whether meloxicam is excreted in human milk. Due to a potential for serious adverse reactions, the manufacturer recommends that a decision be made whether to discontinue nursing or discontinue the drug, taking into account the importance of the drug to the mother.

Perioperative/Anesthesia/Other Concerns: The 2002 ACCM/SCCM guidelines for analgesia (critically-ill adult) suggest that NSAIDs may be used in combination with opioids in select patients for pain management. Concern about adverse events (increased risk of renal dysfunction, altered platelet function and gastrointestinal irritation) limits its use in patients who have other underlying risks for these events.

In short-term use, NSAIDs vary considerably in their effect on blood pressure. When NSAIDs are used in patients with hypertension, appropriate monitoring of blood pressure responses should be completed and the duration of therapy, when possible, kept short. The use of NSAIDs in the treatment of patients with congestive heart failure may be associated with an increased risk for fluid accumulation and edema; may precipitate renal failure in dehydrated patients.

Administration

Storage: Store at 25°C (77°F).

Memantine (me MAN teen)

U.S. Brand Names Namenda™

Synonyms Memantine Hydrochloride

Pharmacologic Category N-Methyl-D-Aspartate Receptor Antagonist

Use Treatment of moderate-to-severe dementia of the Alzheimer's type

Unlabeled/Investigational Use Treatment of mild-to-moderate vascular dementia

Mechanism of Action Glutamate, the primary excitatory amino acid in the CNS, may contribute to the pathogenesis of Alzheimer's disease (AD) by overstimulating various glutamate receptors leading to excitotoxicity and neuronal cell death. Memantine is an uncompetitive antagonist of the N-methyl-D-aspartate (NMDA) type of glutamate receptors, located ubiquitously throughout the brain. Under normal physiologic conditions, the (unstimulated) NMDA receptor ion channel is blocked by magnesium ions, which are displaced after agonist-induced depolarization. Pathologic or excessive receptor activation, as postulated to occur during AD, prevents magnesium from reentering and blocking the channel pore resulting in a chronically open state and excessive calcium influx. Memantine binds to the intra-pore magnesium site, but with longer dwell time, and thus functions as an effective receptor blocker only under conditions of excessive stimulation; memantine does not affect normal neurotransmission.

Pharmacodynamics/Kinetics

Distribution: 9-11 L/kg

Protein binding: 45%

Metabolism: Forms 3 metabolites (minimal activity)

Half-life elimination: Terminal: 60-80 hours; severe renal impairment (Cl_{cr} 5-29 mL/minute): 117-156 hours

Time to peak, serum: 3-7 hours

Excretion: Urine (57% to 82% unchanged); excretion reduced by alkaline urine pH

Contraindications Hypersensitivity to memantine or any component of the formulation

Warnings/Precautions Use caution with seizure disorders or hepatic impairment. Caution with use in severe renal impairment; dose adjustment recommended. Clearance is significantly reduced by alkaline urine; use caution with medications, dietary changes, or patient conditions which may alter urine pH.

Drug Interactions

Carbonic anhydrase inhibitors: Carbonic anhydrase inhibitors may alkalinize the urine; clearance of memantine is decreased 80% at urinary pH 8.

Sodium bicarbonate: Sodium bicarbonate may alkalinize the urine; clearance of memantine is decreased 80% at urinary pH 8.

Adverse Reactions

1% to 10%:

Cardiovascular: Hypertension (4%), cardiac failure, syncope, cerebrovascular accident, transient ischemic attack

Central nervous system: Dizziness (7%), confusion (6%), headache (6%), hallucinations (3%), pain (3%), somnolence (3%), fatigue (2%), aggressive reaction, ataxia, vertigo

Dermatologic: Rash

Gastrointestinal: Constipation (5%), vomiting (3%), weight loss

Genitourinary: Micturition

Hematologic: Anemia

Hepatic: Alkaline phosphatase increased

Neuromuscular & skeletal: Back pain (3%), hypokinesia

Ocular: Cataract, conjunctivitis

Respiratory: Cough (4%), dyspnea (2%), pneumonia

<1% (Limited to important or life-threatening): Allergic reaction

Overdosage/Toxicology Loss of consciousness, psychosis, restlessness, somnolence, stupor, and visual hallucinations were reported following ingestion of memantine 400 mg. In case of overdose, treatment should be symptomatic and supportive. Elimination may be increased by acidifying the urine.

Dosing

Adults & Elderly:

Alzheimer's disease: Oral: Initial: 5 mg/day; increase dose by 5 mg/day to a target dose of 20 mg/day; wait at least 1 week between dosage changes. Doses >5 mg/day should be given in 2 divided doses.

Suggested titration: 5 mg/day for ≥1 week; 5 mg twice daily for ≥1 week; 15 mg/day given in 5 mg and 10 mg separated doses for ≥1 week; then 10 mg twice daily.

Mild-to-moderate vascular dementia (unlabeled use): Oral: 10 mg twice daily

Renal Impairment:

Mild-to-moderate impairment: No adjustment required.

Severe impairment: Cl_{cr} 5-29 mL/minute): 5 mg twice daily

Available Dosage Forms

Solution, oral: 2 mg/mL (360 mL) [alcohol free, dye free, sugar free; peppermint flavor]

Tablet, as hydrochloride: 5 mg, 10 mg

Combination package [titration pack contains two separate tablet formulations]: Memantine hydrochloride 5 mg (28s) and memantine hydrochloride 10 mg (21s)

Nursing Guidelines

Assessment: Use with caution and monitor closely in presence of seizure disorders, hepatic or renal impairment, and anything that causes alkaline urine. Assess therapeutic effectiveness and adverse reactions on a regular basis throughout therapy (eg, hypertension, CNS changes, rash, constipation). Teach patient possible side effects/appropriate interventions and adverse symptoms to report.

Dietary Considerations: May be taken with or without food.

Patient Education: Take as directed with or without food. May cause hypertension (monitor if recommended); headache (consult prescriber for analgesic). Report increase or changes in CNS symptoms (confusion, hallucinations, fatigue, aggressive reaction); chest pain or palpitations, dizziness or fainting; difficulty breathing of tightness in chest; rash; alteration in elimination patterns, or other persistent adverse reactions. **Breast-feeding precaution:** Consult prescriber if breast-feeding.

Geriatric Considerations: In clinical trials, patients on memantine had less of a decline in cognitive function and activities of daily living (ADL) as compared to

(Continued)

Memantine *(Continued)*

placebo. This was true for monotherapy with memantine, as well as combination therapy with donepezil, an acetylcholinesterase inhibitor.

Pregnancy Risk Factor: B

Lactation: Excretion in breast milk unknown/use caution

Administration

Storage: Store at controlled room temperature of 15°C to 30°C (59°F to 86°F).

- Memantine Hydrochloride *see* Memantine *on page 1094*
- Menadol® [OTC] [DSC] *see* Ibuprofen *on page 889*
- Menest® *see* Estrogens (Esterified) *on page 669*

Meningococcal Polysaccharide Vaccine (Groups A / C / Y and W-135)

(me NIN joe kok al pol i SAK a ride vak SEEN groops aye, see, why & dubl yoo won thur tee fyve)

U.S. Brand Names Menomune®-A/C/Y/W-135

Synonyms MPSV4

Pharmacologic Category Vaccine

Use Provide active immunity to meningococcal serogroups contained in the vaccine

The ACIP recommends routine vaccination for persons at increased risk for meningococcal disease. (Use of MPSV4 is recommended in children 2-10 years and adults > 55 years. MCV4 is preferred for persons aged 11-55 years; MPSV4 may be used if MCV4 is not available). Persons at increased risk include:

College freshmen living in dormitories

Microbiologists routinely exposed to isolates of *N. meningitides*

Military recruits

Persons traveling to or who reside in countries where *N. meningitides* is hyperendemic or epidemic, particularly if contact with local population will be prolonged

Persons with terminal complement component deficiencies

Persons with anatomic or functional asplenia

Use is also recommended during meningococcal outbreaks caused by vaccine preventable serogroups.

Mechanism of Action Induces the formation of bactericidal antibodies to meningococcal antigens; the presence of these antibodies is strongly correlated with immunity to meningococcal disease caused by *Neisseria meningitidis* groups A, C, Y and W-135.

Pharmacodynamics/Kinetics

Onset of action: Antibody levels: 7-10 days

Duration: Antibodies against group A and C polysaccharides decline markedly (to prevaccination levels) over the first 3 years following a single dose of vaccine, especially in children <4 years of age

Contraindications Hypersensitivity to any component of the formulation; defer immunization during acute illness

Warnings/Precautions Patients who undergo splenectomy secondary to trauma or nonlymphoid tumors respond well; however, those asplenic patients with lymphoid tumors who receive either chemotherapy or irradiation respond poorly. Response may not be as great as desired in immunosuppressed patients. Use in pediatric patients <2 years of age is usually not recommended. Use with caution in patients with latex sensitivity; the stopper to the vial contains dry, natural latex rubber. Some dosage forms contain thimerosal.

Drug Interactions

Immunoglobulin: Decreased effect with administration of immunoglobulin within 1 month.

Vaccines: Should not be administered with whole-cell pertussis or whole-cell typhoid vaccines due to combined endotoxin content.

Adverse Reactions All serious adverse reactions must be reported to the U.S. Department of Health and Human Services (DHHS) Vaccine Adverse Event Reporting System (VAERS) 1-800-822-7967. Percentages reported in adults; incidence of erythema, swelling, or tenderness may be higher in children

>10%: Local: Tenderness (9% to 36%)

1% to 10%:

Central nervous system: Headache (2% to 5%), malaise (2%), fever (100°F to 106°F: 3%), chills (2%)

Local: Pain at injection site (2% to 3%), erythema (1% to 4%), induration (1% to 4%)

Dosing

Adults & Elderly: Immunization: SubQ: 0.5 mL

Note: Revaccination: Not determined, consider revaccination after 3-5 years. May be indicated in patients previously vaccinated with MPSV4 who remain at increased risk for infection. The ACIP recommends the use of MCV4 for revaccination in patients 11-55 years, however use of MPSV4 is also acceptable.

Pediatrics:

Immunization: SubQ:

Children <2 years: Not usually recommended. Two doses (0.5 mL/dose), 3 months apart, may be considered in children 3-18 months to elicit short-term protection against serogroup A disease. A single dose may be considered in children 19-23 months.

Children ≥2 years: Refer to adult dosing.

Revaccination: See **Note** in adult dosing. Children first vaccinated at <4 years: Revaccinate after 2-3 years.

Available Dosage Forms Injection, powder for reconstitution: 50 mcg each of polysaccharide antigen groups A, C, Y, and W-135 [contains lactose; packaged with 0.78 mL preservative free diluent or 6 mL diluent containing thimerosal; vial stoppers contain dry, natural latex rubber]

Nursing Guidelines

Patient Education: Inform patients about common side effects; patients should report serious and unusual effects to physician

Pregnancy Risk Factor: C

Lactation: Excretion in breast milk unknown/use caution

Administration

Reconstitution: Reconstitute using provided diluent; shake well. Use single-dose vial within 30 minutes of reconstitution. Use multidose vial within 35 days of reconstitution.

Storage: Prior to and following reconstitution, store at 2°C to 8°C (35°F to 46°F).

◆ **Menomune®-A/C/Y/W-135** *see* Meningococcal Polysaccharide Vaccine (Groups A / C / Y and W-135) *on page 1096*

◆ **Menostar™** *see* Estradiol *on page 649*

Meperidine (me PER i deen)

U.S. Brand Names Demerol®; Meperitab®

Synonyms Isonipecaine Hydrochloride; Meperidine Hydrochloride; Pethidine Hydrochloride

Pharmacologic Category Analgesic, Narcotic

Medication Safety Issues

Sound-alike/look-alike issues:

Meperidine may be confused with meprobamate

Demerol® may be confused with Demulen®, Desyrel®, dicumarol, Dilaudid®, Dymelor®, Pamelor®

Use Management of moderate to severe pain; adjunct to anesthesia and preoperative sedation

Unlabeled/Investigational Use

Reduce postoperative shivering; reduce rigors from amphotericin

Mechanism of Action Binds to opiate receptors in the CNS, causing inhibition of ascending pain pathways, altering the perception of and response to pain; produces generalized CNS depression

Pharmacodynamics/Kinetics

Onset of action: Analgesic: Oral, SubQ: 10-15 minutes; I.V.: ~5 minutes

Peak effect: SubQ.: ~1 hour; Oral: 2 hours

Duration: Oral, SubQ.: 2-4 hours

Absorption: I.M.: Erratic and highly variable

Distribution: Crosses placenta; enters breast milk

Protein binding: 65% to 75%

Metabolism: Hepatic; hydrolyzed to meperidinic acid (inactive) or undergoes N-demethylation to normeperidine (active; has ½ the analgesic effect and 2-3 times the CNS effects of meperidine)

(Continued)

Meperidine *(Continued)*

Bioavailability: ~50% to 60%; increased with liver disease

Half-life elimination:

Parent drug: Terminal phase: Adults: 2.5-4 hours, Liver disease: 7-11 hours

Normeperidine (active metabolite): 15-30 hours; can accumulate with high doses or with decreased renal function

Excretion: Urine (as metabolites)

Contraindications Hypersensitivity to meperidine or any component of the formulation; use with or within 14 days of MAO inhibitors; pregnancy (prolonged use or high doses near term)

Warnings/Precautions Meperidine is not recommended for the management of chronic pain. When used for acute pain (in patients without renal or CNS disease), treatment should be limited to 48 hours and doses should not exceed 600 mg/24 hours. Oral meperidine is not recommended for acute pain management. Normeperidine (an active metabolite and CNS stimulant) may accumulate and precipitate anxiety, tremors, or seizures; risk increases with renal dysfunction and cumulative dose.

Use only with extreme caution (if at all) in patients with head injury or increased intracranial pressure (ICP); potential to elevate ICP may be greatly exaggerated in these patients. Use caution with pulmonary, hepatic, or renal disorders, supraventricular tachycardias, acute abdominal conditions, hypothyroidism, Addison's disease, BPH, or urethral stricture.

An opioid-containing analgesic regimen should be tailored to each patient's needs and based upon the type of pain being treated (acute versus chronic), the route of administration, degree of tolerance for opioids (naive versus chronic user), age, weight, and medical condition. The optimal analgesic dose varies widely among patients. Doses should be titrated to pain relief/prevention.

Some preparations contain sulfites which may cause allergic reaction. Tolerance or drug dependence may result from extended use.

Drug Interactions

Substrate (minor) of CYP2B6, 2C19, 3A4

Acyclovir: May increase meperidine metabolite concentrations. Use caution.

Barbiturates: May decrease analgesic efficacy and increase sedative and/or respiratory depressive effects of meperidine.

Cimetidine: May increase meperidine metabolite concentrations; use caution.

CNS depressants (including benzodiazepines): May potentiate the sedative and/or respiratory depressive effects of meperidine.

MAO inhibitors: May enhance the serotonergic effect of meperidine, which may cause serotonin syndrome. Concurrent use with or within 14 days of an MAO inhibitor is contraindicated.

Phenothiazines: May potentiate the sedative and/or respiratory depressive effects of meperidine; may increase the incidence of hypotension.

Phenytoin: May decrease the analgesic effects of meperidine

Ritonavir: May increase meperidine metabolite concentrations; use caution.

Serotonin agonists: Serotonin agonists and meperidine may enhance serotonin levels in the brain. Serotonin syndrome may occur.

Serotonin reuptake inhibitors: May potentiate the effects of meperidine, increasing serotonin levels in the brain. Serotonin syndrome may occur.

Sibutramine: May enhance the serotonergic effect of meperidine. Serotonin syndrome may occur.

Tricyclic antidepressants: May potentiate the sedative and/or respiratory depressive effects of meperidine. In addition, potentially may increase the risk of serotonin syndrome.

Nutritional/Herbal/Ethanol Interactions

Ethanol: Avoid or limit ethanol (may increase CNS depression). Watch for sedation.

Herb/Nutraceutical: Avoid valerian, St John's wort, kava kava, gotu kola (may increase CNS depression).

Lab Interactions Increased amylase (S), BSP retention, CPK (I.M. injections)

Adverse Reactions Frequency not defined.

Cardiovascular: Hypotension

Central nervous system: Fatigue, drowsiness, dizziness, nervousness, headache, restlessness, malaise, confusion, mental depression, hallucinations, paradoxical CNS stimulation, increased intracranial pressure, seizure (associated with metabolite accumulation), serotonin syndrome

Dermatologic: Rash, urticaria

Gastrointestinal: Nausea, vomiting, constipation, anorexia, stomach cramps, xerostomia, biliary spasm, paralytic ileus, sphincter of Oddi spasm
Genitourinary: Ureteral spasms, decreased urination
Local: Pain at injection site
Neuromuscular & skeletal: Weakness
Respiratory: Dyspnea
Miscellaneous: Histamine release, physical and psychological dependence

Overdosage/Toxicology Symptoms of overdose include CNS depression, respiratory depression, mydriasis, bradycardia, pulmonary edema, chronic tremor, CNS excitability, and seizures. Treatment is symptomatic. Naloxone, 2 mg I.V. with repeat administration as necessary up to a total dose of 10 mg, can be used to reverse opiate effects. Naloxone should not be used to treat meperidine-induced seizures. Naloxone does not reverse the adverse effects of normeperidine.

Dosing

Adults: Note: Doses should be titrated to necessary analgesic effect. When changing route of administration, note that oral doses are about half as effective as parenteral dose. Not recommended for chronic pain. These are guidelines and do not represent the maximum doses that may be required in all patients. In patients with normal renal function, doses of ≤600 mg/24 hours and use for ≤48 hours are recommended (American Pain Society, 1999).

Pain (analgesic):

Oral: Initial: Opiate-naive: 50 mg every 3-4 hours as needed; usual dosage range: 50-150 mg every 2-4 hours as needed (manufacturers recommendation; oral route is not recommended for acute pain)

I.M., SubQ: Initial: Opiate-naive: 50-75 mg every 3-4 hours as needed; patients with prior opiate exposure may require higher initial doses.

Preoperatively: 50-100 mg given 30-90 minutes before the beginning of anesthesia

Slow I.V.: Initial: 5-10 mg every 5 minutes as needed

Patient-controlled analgesia (PCA): Usual concentration: 10 mg/mL

Initial dose: 10 mg

Demand dose: 1-5 mg (manufacturer recommendations); range 5-25 mg (American Pain Society, 1999).

Lockout interval: 5-10 minutes

Elderly: Note: Doses should be titrated to necessary analgesic effect. When changing route of administration, note that oral doses are about half as effective as parenteral dose. Oral route not recommended for chronic pain. These are guidelines and do not represent the maximum doses that may be required in all patients.

Oral: 50 mg every 4 hours
I.M.: 25 mg every 4 hours

Pediatrics: Pain (analgesic): Refer to 'Note' in adult dosing.

Oral, I.M., I.V., SubQ: Children: 1-1.5 mg/kg/dose every 3-4 hours as needed; 1-2 mg/kg as a single dose preoperative medication may be used; maximum 100 mg/dose. (Oral route is not recommended for acute pain.)

Renal Impairment:

Cl_{cr} 10-50 mL/minute: Administer 75% of normal dose.
Cl_{cr} <10 mL/minute: Administer 50% of normal dose.

Note: Repeated use in renal impairment **should be avoided** due to potential accumulation of neuroexcitatory metabolite.

Hepatic Impairment: Increased narcotic effect in cirrhosis; reduction in dose is more important for oral than I.V. route.

Available Dosage Forms

Injection, solution, as hydrochloride [ampul]: 25 mg/0.5 mL (0.5 mL); 25 mg/mL (1 mL); 50 mg/mL (1 mL, 1.5 mL, 2 mL); 75 mg/mL (1 mL); 100 mg/mL (1 mL)
Injection, solution, as hydrochloride [prefilled syringe]: 25 mg/mL (1 mL); 50 mg/mL (1 mL); 75 mg/mL (1 mL); 100 mg/mL (1 mL)
Injection, solution, as hydrochloride [for PCA pump]: 10 mg/mL (30 mL, 50 mL, 60 mL)
Injection, solution, as hydrochloride [vial]: 25 mg/mL (1 mL); 50 mg/mL (1 mL, 30 mL); 75 mg/mL (1 mL); 100 mg/mL (1 mL, 20 mL) [may contain sodium metabisulfite]
Syrup, as hydrochloride: 50 mg/5 mL (500 mL) [contains sodium benzoate]
Demerol®: 50 mg/5 mL (480 mL) [contains benzoic acid; banana flavor]
Tablet, as hydrochloride (Demerol®, Meperitab®): 50 mg, 100 mg

(Continued)

Meperidine *(Continued)*

Nursing Guidelines

Assessment: Assess other medications patient may be taking for additive or adverse interactions. Monitor therapeutic effectiveness and adverse reactions or overdose at beginning of therapy and at regular intervals with long-term use. Monitor frequently for need, may cause physical and/or psychological dependence. For inpatients, implement safety measures. Assess knowledge/teach patient appropriate use (if self-administered), adverse reactions to report, and appropriate interventions to reduce side effects. Discontinue slowly after prolonged use.

Patient Education: If self-administered, use exactly as directed; do not increase dose or frequency. Drug may cause physical and/or psychological dependence. While using this medication, do not use alcohol and other prescription or OTC medications (especially sedatives, tranquilizers, antihistamines, or pain medications) without consulting prescriber. Maintain adequate hydration (2-3 L/day of fluids) unless instructed to restrict fluid intake. May cause hypotension, dizziness, drowsiness, impaired coordination, or blurred vision (use caution when driving, climbing stairs, or changing position - rising from sitting or lying to standing, or when engaging in tasks requiring alertness until response to drug is known); loss of appetite, nausea, or vomiting (frequent mouth care, small frequent meals, chewing gum, or sucking lozenges may help); or constipation (increased exercise, fluids, fruit, or fiber may help; if unresolved, consult prescriber about use of stool softeners). Report chest pain, slow or rapid heartbeat, acute dizziness or persistent headache; changes in mental status; seizures; swelling of extremities or unusual weight gain; changes in urinary elimination; acute headache; back or flank pain or muscle spasms; blurred vision; skin rash; or shortness of breath. **Pregnancy/breast-feeding precautions:** Inform prescriber if you are or intend to become pregnant. Consult prescriber if breast-feeding.

Geriatric Considerations: Meperidine is not recommended as a drug of first choice for the treatment of chronic pain in the elderly due to the accumulation of its metabolite, normeperidine, which leads to serious CNS side effects (eg, tremor, seizures). For acute pain, its use should be limited to 1-2 doses.

Pregnancy Risk Factor: C/D (prolonged use or high doses at term)

Pregnancy Issues: Meperidine is known to cross the placenta, which may result in respiratory or CNS depression in the newborn.

Lactation: Enters breast milk/contraindicated (AAP rates "compatible")

Breast-Feeding Considerations: Meperidine is excreted in breast milk and may cause CNS and/or respiratory depression in the nursing infant.

Perioperative/Anesthesia/Other Concerns: The 2002 ACCM/SCCM guidelines for analgesia (critically-ill adult) recommend against using meperidine repetitively. The guidelines recommend fentanyl in patients who need immediate pain relief because of its rapid onset of action; fentanyl or hydromorphone is preferred in patients who are hypotensive or have renal dysfunction. Morphine or hydromorphone is recommended for intermittent, scheduled therapy. Both have a longer duration of action requiring less frequent administration.

Administration

Oral: Administer syrup diluted in ½ glass of water; undiluted syrup may exert topical anesthetic effect on mucous membranes

I.V.: Meperidine may be administered I.M., SubQ, or I.V. IVP should be given slowly, use of a 10 mg/mL concentration has been recommended. For continuous I.V. infusions, a more dilute solution (eg, 1 mg/mL) should be used.

Compatibility: Stable in dextran 6% in dextrose, dextran 6% in NS, D_5LR, D_5¼NS, D_5½NS, D_5NS, D_5W, $D_{10}W$, LR, ½NS, NS

Y-site administration: Incompatible with allopurinol, amphotericin B cholesteryl sulfate complex, cefepime, cefoperazone, doxorubicin liposome, idarubicin, imipenem/cilastatin, minocycline

Compatibility in syringe: Incompatible with heparin, morphine, pentobarbital

Compatibility when admixed: Incompatible with aminophylline, amobarbital, floxacillin, furosemide, heparin, morphine, phenobarbital, phenytoin, thiopental

Storage: Meperidine injection should be stored at room temperature and protected from light and freezing. Protect oral dosage forms from light.

Related Information

Conscious Sedation *on page 1779*
Narcotic / Opioid Analgesics *on page 1880*

◆ **Meperidine Hydrochloride** *see* Meperidine *on page 1097*
◆ **Meperitab®** *see* Meperidine *on page 1097*
◆ **Mephyton®** *see* Phytonadione *on page 1363*

Mepivacaine (me PIV a kane)

U.S. Brand Names Carbocaine®; Polocaine®; Polocaine® Dental; Polocaine® MPF

Synonyms Mepivacaine Hydrochloride

Pharmacologic Category Local Anesthetic

Medication Safety Issues

Sound-alike/look-alike issues:

Mepivacaine may be confused with bupivacaine
Polocaine® may be confused with prilocaine

Use Local or regional analgesia; anesthesia by local infiltration, peripheral and central neural techniques including epidural and caudal blocks; **not** for use in spinal anesthesia

Mechanism of Action Mepivacaine is an amide local anesthetic similar to lidocaine; like all local anesthetics, mepivacaine acts by preventing the generation and conduction of nerve impulses

Pharmacodynamics/Kinetics

Onset of action (route and dose dependent): Range: 3-20 minutes
Duration (route and dose dependent): 2-2.5 hours
Protein binding: ~75%
Metabolism: Primarily hepatic via N-demethylation, hydroxylation, and glucuronidation
Half-life elimination: Neonates: 8.7-9 hours; Adults: 1.9-3 hours
Excretion: Urine (95% as metabolites)

Contraindications Hypersensitivity to mepivacaine, other amide-type local anesthetics, or any component of the formulation

Warnings/Precautions Use with caution in patients with cardiac disease, hepatic or renal disease, or hyperthyroidism. Local anesthetics have been associated with rare occurrences of sudden respiratory arrest; convulsions due to systemic toxicity leading to cardiac arrest have been reported presumably due to intravascular injection. A test dose is recommended prior to epidural administration and all reinforcing doses with continuous catheter technique. Do not use solutions containing preservatives for caudal or epidural block. Use caution in debilitated, elderly, or acutely-ill patients; dose reduction may be required.

Adverse Reactions Degree of adverse effects in the CNS and cardiovascular system is directly related to the blood levels of mepivacaine, route of administration, and physical status of the patient. The effects below are more likely to occur after systemic administration rather than infiltration.

Cardiovascular: Bradycardia, cardiac arrest, cardiac output decreased, heart block, hyper-/hypotension, myocardial depression, syncope, tachycardia, ventricular arrhythmias
Central nervous system: Anxiety, chills, convulsions, depression, dizziness, excitation, restlessness, tremors
Dermatologic: Angioneurotic edema, diaphoresis, erythema, pruritus, urticaria
Gastrointestinal: Fecal incontinence, nausea, vomiting
Genitourinary: Incontinence, urinary retention
Neuromuscular & skeletal: Paralysis
Ocular: Blurred vision, pupil constriction
Otic: Tinnitus
Respiratory: Apnea, hypoventilation, sneezing
Miscellaneous: Allergic reaction, anaphylactoid reaction

Overdosage/Toxicology Symptoms of overdose include dizziness, cyanosis, tremor, and bronchial spasm. Treatment is symptomatic and supportive. Termination of anesthesia by pneumatic tourniquet inflation should be attempted when mepivacaine is administered by infiltration or regional injection.

Dosing

Adults & Elderly:

Injectable local anesthetic: Dose varies with procedure, degree of anesthesia needed, vascularity of tissue, duration of anesthesia required, and physical condition of patient. The smallest dose and concentration required to produce the desired effect should be used.

Maximum dose: 400 mg; do not exceed 1000 mg/24 hours

(Continued)

Mepivacaine *(Continued)*

Cervical, brachial, intercostal, pudenal nerve block: 5-40 mL of a 1% solution (maximum: 400 mg) **or** 5-20 mL of a 2% solution (maximum: 400 mg). For pudenal block, inject 1/2 the total dose each side.

Transvaginal block (paracervical plus pudenal): Up to 30 mL (both sides) of a 1% solution (maximum: 300 mg). Inject 1/2 the total dose each side.

Paracervical block: Up to 20 mL (both sides) of a 1% solution (maximum: 200 mg). Inject 1/2 the total dose to each side. This is the maximum recommended dose per 90-minute procedure; inject slowly with 5 minutes between sides.

Caudal and epidural block (preservative free solutions only): 15-30 mL of a 1% solution (maximum: 300 mg) **or** 10-25 mL of a 1.5% solution (maximum: 375 mg) **or** 10-20 mL of a 2% solution (maximum: 400 mg)

Infiltration: Up to 40 mL of a 1% solution (maximum: 400 mg)

Therapeutic block (pain management): 1-5 mL of a 1% solution (maximum: 50 mg) **or** 1-5 mL of a 2% solution (maximum: 100 mg)

Dental anesthesia:

Single site in upper or lower jaw: 54 mg (1.8 mL) as a 3% solution

Infiltration and nerve block of entire oral cavity: 270 mg (9 mL) as a 3% solution. Manufacturer's maximum recommended dose is not more than 400 mg to normal healthy adults.

Pediatrics: Injectable local anesthetic: Dose varies with procedure, degree of anesthesia needed, vascularity of tissue, duration of anesthesia required, and physical condition of patient. The smallest dose and concentration required to produce the desired effect should be used.

Maximum dose: 5-6 mg/kg; only concentrations <2% should be used in children <3 years or <14 kg (30 lbs)

Available Dosage Forms

Injection, solution, as hydrochloride [contains methylparabens]:

Carbocaine®: 1% (50 mL); 2% (50 mL)

Polocaine®: 1% (50 mL); 2% (50 mL)

Injection, solution, as hydrochloride [preservative free]:

Carbocaine®: 1% (30 mL); 1.5% (30 mL); 2% (20 mL); 3% (1.8 mL) [dental cartridge]

Polocaine® Dental: 3% (1.8 ml) [dental cartridge]

Polocaine® MPF: 1% (30 mL); 1.5% (30 mL); 2% (20 mL)

Nursing Guidelines

Assessment: Monitor for effectiveness of anesthesia and adverse reactions. Monitor for return of sensation. **Oral:** Use caution to prevent gagging or choking and avoid food or drink for 1 hour. Teach patient adverse reactions to report; use and teach appropriate interventions to promote safety.

Patient Education: You will experience decreased sensation to pain, heat, or cold in the area and/or decreased muscle strength (depending on area of application) until effects wear off; use necessary caution to reduce incidence of possible injury until full sensation returns. Report irritation, pain, burning at injection site; chest pain or palpitations; or respiratory difficulty.

Oral injection: This will cause numbness of your mouth. Do not eat or drink for 1 hour after use. Take small sips of water at first to ensure that you can swallow without difficulty. Your tongue and/or mouth may be numb, use caution to avoid biting yourself. Report irritation, pain, burning at injection site; chest pain or palpitations; or respiratory difficulty.

Pregnancy precaution: Inform prescriber if you are pregnant.

Pregnancy Risk Factor: C

Pregnancy Issues: Mepivacaine has been used in obstetrical analgesia.

Lactation: Excretion in breast milk unknown/use caution

Perioperative/Anesthesia/Other Concerns:

Peripheral nerve block, caudal/epidural, therapeutic block: 1% or 2% solution

Transvaginal, paracervical block: 1% solution

Infiltration: 0.5% to 1% solution

Dental procedures: Mepivacaine 3% or mepivacaine 2% solution with levonordefrin

Administration

Storage: Store at controlled room temperature of 15°C to 30°C (59°F to 86°F); brief exposure up to 40°C (104°F) does not adversely affect the product. Solutions may be sterilized. Dental solutions should be protected from light.

Related Information

Acute Postoperative Pain *on page 1742*
Local Anesthetics *on page 1854*

♦ **Mepivacaine Hydrochloride** *see* Mepivacaine *on page 1101*
♦ **Mercapturic Acid** *see* Acetylcysteine *on page 80*
♦ **Meridia®** *see* Sibutramine *on page 1529*

Meropenem (mer oh PEN em)

U.S. Brand Names Merrem® I.V.

Pharmacologic Category Antibiotic, Carbapenem

Use Treatment of intra-abdominal infections (complicated appendicitis and peritonitis); treatment of bacterial meningitis in pediatric patients ≥3 months of age caused by *S. pneumoniae*, *H. influenzae*, and *N. meningitidis*; treatment of complicated skin and skin structure infections caused by susceptible organisms

Unlabeled/Investigational Use

Febrile neutropenia, urinary tract infections

Mechanism of Action Inhibits bacterial cell wall synthesis by binding to several of the penicillin-binding proteins, which in turn inhibit the final transpeptidation step of peptidoglycan synthesis in bacterial cell walls, thus inhibiting cell wall biosynthesis; bacteria eventually lyse due to ongoing activity of cell wall autolytic enzymes (autolysins and murein hydrolases) while cell wall assembly is arrested

Pharmacodynamics/Kinetics

Distribution: V_d: Adults: ~0.3 L/kg, Children: 0.4-0.5 L/kg; penetrates well into most body fluids and tissues; CSF concentrations approximate those of the plasma
Protein binding: 2%
Metabolism: Hepatic; metabolized to open beta-lactam form (inactive)
Half-life elimination:
- Normal renal function: 1-1.5 hours
- Cl_{cr} 30-80 mL/minute: 1.9-3.3 hours
- Cl_{cr} 2-30 mL/minute: 3.82-5.7 hours

Time to peak, tissue: 1 hour following infusion
Excretion: Urine (~25% as inactive metabolites)

Contraindications Hypersensitivity to meropenem, any component of the formulation, or other carbapenems (eg, imipenem); patients who have experienced anaphylactic reactions to other beta-lactams

Warnings/Precautions

Hypersensitivity reactions, including anaphylaxis, have occurred and often require immediate drug discontinuation. Seizures and other CNS adverse reactions have occurred, most commonly in patients with renal impairment and/or underlying neurologic disorders (less frequent than with Primaxin®). Use with caution in renal impairment; dose adjustment is necessary. Thrombocytopenia has been reported in patients with significant renal dysfunction. Pseudomembranous colitis has been associated with meropenem use. Superinfection is possible with long courses of therapy. Safety and efficacy have not been established for children <3 months of age

Drug Interactions

Probenecid: May increase meropenem serum concentrations; use caution.
Valproic acid: Meropenem may decrease valproic acid serum concentrations to subtherapeutic levels; monitor.

Lab Interactions Increased SGPT, SGOT, alkaline phosphatase, LDH, bilirubin, platelets, eosinophils, BUN, creatinine; decreased platelets, hemoglobin/hematocrit, WBC; prolonged or shortened PT; prolonged PTT; positive direct or indirect Coombs' test; presence of urine red blood cells

Adverse Reactions

1% to 10%:
- Cardiovascular: Peripheral vascular disorder (<1%)
- Central nervous system: Headache (2% to 8%), pain (5%)
- Dermatologic: Rash (2% to 3%, includes diaper-area moniliasis in pediatrics), pruritus (1%)
- Gastrointestinal: Diarrhea (4% to 5%), nausea/vomiting (1% to 8%), constipation (1% to 7%), oral moniliasis (up to 2% in pediatric patients), glossitis
- Hematologic: Anemia (up to 6%)
- Local: Inflammation at the injection site (2%), phlebitis/thrombophlebitis (1%), injection site reaction (1%)
- Respiratory: Apnea (1%)
- Miscellaneous: Sepsis (2%), septic shock (1%)

(Continued)

Meropenem *(Continued)*

<1% (Limited to important or life-threatening): Agitation/delirium, agranulocytosis, angioedema, arrhythmia, bilirubin increased, bradycardia, BUN increased, cholestatic creatinine increased, jaundice/jaundice, decreased prothrombin time, dyspepsia, dyspnea, eosinophilia, epistaxis, erythema multiforme, gastrointestinal hemorrhage, hallucinations, hearing loss, heart failure, hemoperitoneum, hepatic failure, hyper-/hypotension, ileus, leukopenia, melena, MI, neutropenia, paresthesia, pleural effusion, pulmonary edema, pulmonary embolism, renal failure, seizure, Stevens-Johnson syndrome, syncope, thrombocytopenia, toxic epidermal necrolysis, urticaria, vaginal moniliasis

Overdosage/Toxicology No cases of acute overdosage are reported which have resulted in symptoms. Accidental overdose is possible with the use of large doses in patients with renal impairment. Supportive therapy is recommended. Meropenem and its metabolite are removable by dialysis.

Dosing

Adults & Elderly:

Complicated skin and skin structure infections: I.V.: 500 mg every 8 hours

Intra-abdominal infections: I.V.: 1 g every 8 hours

Meningitis: I.V.: 2 g every 8 hours

Febrile neutropenia, pneumonia, other severe infections (unlabeled use): I.V.: 1 g every 8 hours

Urinary tract infections, complicated (unlabeled use): I.V.: 500 mg to 1 g every 8 hours

Pediatrics:

Complicated skin and skin structure infections:I.V.:

Children >3 months (<50 kg): 10 mg/kg every 8 hours (maximum dose: 500 mg every 8 hours)

Children >50 kg: Refer to adult dosing.

Intra-abdominal infections: I.V.:

Children >3 months (<50 kg): 20 mg/kg every 8 hours (maximum dose: 1 g every 8 hours)

Children >50 kg: 1 g every 8 hours

Meningitis: I.V.:

Children >3 months (<50 kg): 40 mg/kg every 8 hours (maximum dose: 2 g every 8 hours)

Children >50 kg: 2 g every 8 hours

Febrile neutropenia (unlabeled use): I.V.:

Children >3 months (<50 kg): 20 mg/kg every 8 hours (maximum dose: 1 g every 8 hours)

Children >50 kg: Refer to adult dosing.

Renal Impairment:

Cl_{cr} 26-50 mL/minute: Administer recommended dose based on indication every 12 hours

Cl_{cr} 10-25 mL/minute: Administer one-half recommended dose every 12 hours

Cl_{cr} <10 mL/minute: Administer one-half recommended dose every 24 hours

Dialysis: Meropenem and its metabolites are readily dialyzable

Continuous arteriovenous or venovenous hemodiafiltration effects: Dose as Cl_{cr} 10-50 mL/minute

Available Dosage Forms Injection, powder for reconstitution: 500 mg [contains sodium 45.1 mg as sodium carbonate (1.96 mEq)]; 1 g [contains sodium 90.2 mg as sodium carbonate (3.92 mEq)]

Nursing Guidelines

Assessment: Assess history of allergies prior to beginning treatment. See Contraindications, Warnings/Precautions, Drug Interactions, and Dosing for use cautions. See Administration for I.V. specifics. Infusion site should be monitored closely for phlebitis/thrombophlebitis. Assess results of laboratory tests (see below), therapeutic effectiveness, and adverse reactions (see Adverse Reactions and Overdose/Toxicology). Teach patient proper use (according to formulation), possible side effects/appropriate interventions (eg, importance of adequate hydration), and adverse symptoms to report (see Patient Education). Note breast-feeding caution.

Monitoring Laboratory Tests: Perform culture and sensitivity testing prior to initiating therapy. Monitor renal function, liver function, CBC.

Dietary Considerations: 1 g of meropenem contains 90.2 mg of sodium as sodium carbonate (3.92 mEq)

Patient Education: Inform prescriber of all prescriptions, OTC medications, or herbal products you are taking, and any allergies you have. Do not take any new medication during therapy unless approved by prescriber. This medication can only be given by infusion. Report immediately any burning, pain, swelling, or redness at infusion site. Maintain adequate hydration (2-3 L/day of fluids) unless instructed to restrict fluid intake. May cause nausea or vomiting (small, frequent meals, frequent mouth care, chewing gum, or sucking lozenges may help); diarrhea (boiled milk, buttermilk, or yogurt may help); or headache. Report persistent GI distress, diarrhea, mouth sores, respiratory difficulty, headache, or CNS changes (agitation, delirium). **Breast-feeding precaution:** Consult prescriber if breast-feeding.

Geriatric Considerations: Adjust dose based on renal function.

Pregnancy Risk Factor: B

Lactation: Excretion in breast milk unknown/use caution

Administration

I.V.: Administer I.V. infusion over 15-30 minutes; I.V. bolus injection over 3-5 minutes.

Reconstitution: Meropenem infusion vials may be reconstituted with SWFI or a compatible diluent (eg, NS). The 500 mg vials should be reconstituted with 10 mL, and 1 g vials with 20 mL. May be further diluted with compatible solutions for infusion. Consult detailed reference/product labeling for compatibility.

Compatibility:

Y-site administration: Incompatible with amphotericin B, diazepam, metronidazole

Compatibility when admixed: Incompatible with amphotericin B, metronidazole, multivitamins

Storage: Dry powder should be stored at controlled room temperature 20°C to 25°C (68°F to 77°F).

Injection reconstitution: Stability in vial when constituted (up to 50 mg/mL) with:

SWFI: Stable for up to 2 hours at room temperature and for up to 12 hours under refrigeration

Sodium chloride: Stable for up to 2 hours at room temperature or for up to 18 hours under refrigeration.

Dextrose 5% injection: Stable for 1 hour at room temperature or for 8 hours under refrigeration

Infusion admixture (1-20 mg/mL): Solution stability when diluted in NS is 4 hours at room temperature or 24 hours under refrigeration. Stability in D_5W is 1 hour at room temperature and 4 hours under refrigeration.

♦ Merrem® I.V. *see* Meropenem *on page 1103*

♦ Meruvax® II *see* Rubella Virus Vaccine (Live) *on page 1505*

Mesalamine (me SAL a meen)

U.S. Brand Names Asacol®; Canasa™; Pentasa®; Rowasa®

Synonyms 5-Aminosalicylic Acid; 5-ASA; Fisalamine; Mesalazine

Pharmacologic Category 5-Aminosalicylic Acid Derivative

Medication Safety Issues

Sound-alike/look-alike issues:

Mesalamine may be confused with mecamylamine

Asacol® may be confused with Ansaid®, Os-Cal®

Use

Oral: Treatment and maintenance of remission of mildly to moderately active ulcerative colitis

Rectal: Treatment of active mild to moderate distal ulcerative colitis, proctosigmoiditis, or proctitis

Mechanism of Action Mesalamine (5-aminosalicylic acid) is the active component of sulfasalazine; the specific mechanism of action of mesalamine is unknown; however, it is thought that it modulates local chemical mediators of the inflammatory response, especially leukotrienes, and is also postulated to be a free radical scavenger or an inhibitor of tumor necrosis factor (TNF); action appears topical rather than systemic

Pharmacodynamics/Kinetics

Absorption: Rectal: Variable and dependent upon retention time, underlying GI disease, and colonic pH; Oral: Tablet: ~28%, Capsule: ~20% to 30%

Metabolism: Hepatic and via GI tract to acetyl-5-aminosalicylic acid

Half-life elimination: 5-ASA: 0.5-1.5 hours; acetyl-5-ASA: 5-10 hours

Time to peak, serum: 4-7 hours

Excretion: Urine (as metabolites); feces (<2%)

Contraindications Hypersensitivity to mesalamine, sulfasalazine, salicylates, or any component of the formulation; Canasa™ suppositories contain saturated

(Continued)

Mesalamine *(Continued)*

vegetable fatty acid esters (contraindicated in patients with allergy to these components)

Warnings/Precautions May cause an acute intolerance syndrome (cramping, acute abdominal pain, bloody diarrhea; sometimes fever, headache, rash); discontinue if this occurs. Patients with pyloric stenosis may have prolonged gastric retention of tablets, delaying the release of mesalamine in the colon. Pericarditis should be considered in patients with chest pain; pancreatitis should be considered in patients with new abdominal complaints. Use caution in patients with impaired renal or hepatic function. Renal impairment (including minimal change nephropathy and acute/chronic interstitial nephritis) has been reported; use caution with other medications converted to mesalamine. Postmarketing reports suggest an increased incidence of blood dyscrasias in patients >65 years of age. In addition, elderly may have difficulty administering and retaining rectal suppositories and decreased renal function; use with caution and monitor. Safety and efficacy in pediatric patients have not been established.

Rowasa® enema: Contains potassium metabisulfite; may cause severe hypersensitivity reactions (ie, anaphylaxis) in patients with sulfite allergies.

Drug Interactions

Azathioprine, mercaptopurine, thioguanine: Risk of myelosuppression may be increased by aminosalicylates (due to inhibition of TPMT).

Digoxin: Mesalamine may decrease digoxin bioavailability.

Nutritional/Herbal/Ethanol Interactions Food: Oral: Mesalamine serum levels may be decreased if taken with food.

Adverse Reactions Adverse effects vary depending upon dosage form. Effects as reported with tablets, unless otherwise noted:

>10%:

- Central nervous system: Headache (suppository 14%), pain (14%)
- Gastrointestinal: Abdominal pain (18%; enema 8%)
- Genitourinary: Eructation (16%)
- Respiratory: Pharyngitis (11%)

1% to 10%:

- Cardiovascular: Chest pain (3%), peripheral edema (3%)
- Central nervous system: Chills (3%), dizziness (suppository 3%), fever (enema 3%; suppository 1%), insomnia (2%), malaise (2%)
- Dermatologic: Rash (6%; suppository 1%), pruritus (3%; enema 1%), acne (2%; suppository 1%)
- Gastrointestinal: Abdominal pain (enema 8%; suppository 5%), colitis exacerbation (3%; suppository 1%), constipation (5%), diarrhea (suppository 3%), dyspepsia (6%), flatulence (enema 6%; suppository 5%), hemorrhoids (enema 1%), nausea (capsule/suppository 3%), nausea and vomiting (capsule 1%), rectal pain (enema 1%; suppository 2%), vomiting (5%)
- Local: Pain on insertion of enema tip (enema 1%)
- Neuromuscular & skeletal: Back pain (7%; enema 1%), arthralgia (5%), hypertonia (5%), myalgia (3%), arthritis (2%), leg/joint pain (enema 2%)
- Ocular: Conjunctivitis (2%)
- Respiratory: Flu-like syndrome (3%; enema 5%), cough increased (2%)
- Miscellaneous: Diaphoresis (3%)

<1% (Limited to important or life-threatening): Agranulocytosis, alopecia, aplastic anemia, cholestatic jaundice, cholecystitis, edema, elevated liver enzymes, erythema nodosum, fibrosing alveolitis, gout, Guillain-Barré syndrome, hepatitis, hepatocellular damage, hepatotoxicity, interstitial nephritis, Kawasaki-like syndrome, liver failure, liver necrosis, lupus-like syndrome, minimal change nephrotic syndrome, myocarditis, nephropathy, nephrotoxicity, pancreatitis, pancytopenia, pericarditis, thrombocytopenia, vertigo

Overdosage/Toxicology Symptoms of overdose include decreased motor activity, diarrhea, vomiting, and renal function impairment. Treatment is supportive; emesis, gastric lavage, and follow with activated charcoal slurry.

Dosing

Adults & Elderly:

Treatment of ulcerative colitis: Oral:

- Capsule: 1 g 4 times/day
- Tablet: 800 mg 3 times/day for 6 weeks

Maintenance of remission of ulcerative colitis: Oral:

- Capsule: 1 g 4 times/day
- Tablet: 1.6 g/day in divided doses

Distal ulcerative colitis, proctosigmoiditis, or proctitis: Rectal: Retention enema: 60 mL (4 g) at bedtime, retained overnight, approximately 8 hours

Active ulcerative proctitis: Rectal: Rectal suppository (Canasa™):

500 mg: Insert 1 suppository in rectum twice daily; may increase to 3 times/day if inadequate response is seen after 2 weeks

1000 mg: Insert 1 suppository in rectum daily at bedtime

Note: Suppositories should be retained for at least 1-3 hours to achieve maximum benefit.

Note: Some patients may require rectal and oral therapy concurrently.

Available Dosage Forms

Capsule, controlled release (Pentasa®): 250 mg, 500 mg

Suppository, rectal (Canasa™): 500 mg [DSC], 1000 mg [contains saturated vegetable fatty acid esters]

Suspension, rectal: 4 g/60 mL (7s, 28s) [contains potassium metabisulfite and sodium benzoate]

Rowasa®: 4 g/60 mL (7s, 28s) [contains potassium metabisulfite and sodium benzoate]

Tablet, delayed release [enteric coated] (Asacol®): 400 mg

Nursing Guidelines

Assessment: Assess history of allergies prior to beginning treatment. See Contraindications, Warnings/Precautions, Drug Interactions, and Dosing for use cautions. Assess results of laboratory tests (see below), therapeutic effectiveness, and adverse reactions (see Adverse Reactions and Overdose/Toxicology). Teach patient proper use (according to formulation), possible side effects/appropriate interventions (eg, importance of adequate hydration), and adverse symptoms to report (see Patient Education). Note breast-feeding caution.

Monitoring Laboratory Tests: CBC and renal function, particularly in elderly patients

Dietary Considerations: Canasa™ rectal suppository contains saturated vegetable fatty acid esters.

Patient Education: Inform prescriber of all prescriptions, OTC medications, or herbal products you are taking, and any allergies you have. Do not take any new medication during therapy unless approved by prescriber. Take as directed.

Oral: Do not chew or break tablets or capsules. Notify prescriber if whole or partial tablets are repeatedly found in stool.

Enemas: Shake well before using, retain for 8 hours or as long as possible. May cause staining of clothing, undergarments.

Suppository: Do not refrigerate. After removing foil wrapper, insert high in rectum without excessive handling (warmth will melt suppository). Retain suppositories for at least 1-3 hours to achieve maximum benefit. Report severe abdominal pain, unresolved diarrhea, jaundice, severe headache, any unusual pain (back, joint, muscle, swelling of extremities, or chest pain). May cause staining of clothing, undergarments; lubricating gel may be used if needed to assist insertion.

Enema and suppository: May cause staining of clothing, undergarments; lubricating gel may be used if needed to assist insertion.

Breast-feeding precaution: Consult prescriber if breast-feeding.

Geriatric Considerations: Elderly may have difficulty administering and retaining rectal suppositories. Given renal function decline with aging, monitor serum creatinine often during therapy.

Pregnancy Risk Factor: B

Lactation: Excretion in breast milk unknown/use caution

Breast-Feeding Considerations: Adverse effects (diarrhea) in a nursing infant have been reported while the mother received rectal administration of mesalamine within 12 hours after the first dose. The AAP recommends to monitor the infant stool for consistency and to use with caution.

Administration

Oral: Swallow capsules or tablets whole, do not chew or crush.

Storage:

Enema: Store at controlled room temperature. Use promptly once foil wrap is removed; contents may darken with time (do not use if dark brown)

Suppository: Store at controlled room temperature away from direct heat, light, and humidity; do not refrigerate

(Continued)

Mesalamine *(Continued)*

Tablet: Store at controlled room temperature

♦ **Mesalazine** *see* Mesalamine *on page 1105*

Mesna (MES na)

U.S. Brand Names Mesnex®

Synonyms Sodium 2-Mercaptoethane Sulfonate

Pharmacologic Category Antidote

Use Orphan drug: Prevention of hemorrhagic cystitis induced by ifosfamide

Unlabeled/Investigational Use Prevention of hemorrhagic cystitis induced by cyclophosphamide

Mechanism of Action In blood, mesna is oxidized to dimesna which in turn is reduced in the kidney back to mesna, supplying a free thiol group which binds to and inactivates acrolein, the urotoxic metabolite of ifosfamide and cyclophosphamide

Pharmacodynamics/Kinetics

Distribution: No tissue penetration

Protein binding: 69% to 75%

Metabolism: Rapidly oxidized intravascularly to mesna disulfide; mesna disulfide is reduced in renal tubules back to mesna following glomerular filtration.

Bioavailability: Oral: 45% to 79%

Half-life elimination: Parent drug: 24 minutes; Mesna disulfide: 72 minutes

Time to peak, plasma: 2-3 hours

Excretion: Urine; as unchanged drug (18% to 26%) and metabolites

Contraindications Hypersensitivity to mesna or other thiol compounds, or any component of the formulation

Warnings/Precautions Examine morning urine specimen for hematuria prior to ifosfamide or cyclophosphamide treatment; if hematuria (>50 RBC/HPF) develops, reduce the ifosfamide/cyclophosphamide dose or discontinue the drug; will not prevent or alleviate other toxicities associated with ifosfamide or cyclophosphamide and will not prevent hemorrhagic cystitis in all patients. Allergic reactions have been reported; patients with autoimmune disorders may be at increased risk. Symptoms ranged from mild hypersensitivity to systemic anaphylactic reactions. I.V. formulation contains benzyl alcohol; do not use in neonates or infants.

Drug Interactions Decreased effect: Warfarin: Questionable alterations in coagulation control

Lab Interactions False-positive urinary ketones with Multistix® or Labstix®

Adverse Reactions It is difficult to distinguish reactions from those caused by concomitant chemotherapy.

>10%: Gastrointestinal: Bad taste in mouth with oral administration (100%), vomiting (secondary to the bad taste after oral administration, or with high I.V. doses)

<1% (Limited to important or life-threatening): Anaphylaxis, hypersensitivity, hypertonia, injection site reaction, limb pain, myalgia, platelet count decreased, tachycardia, tachypnea

Dosing

Adults & Elderly: Prevention of toxicity: Refer to individual protocols.

I.V.: Recommended dose is 60% of the ifosfamide dose given in 3 divided doses (0, 4, and 8 hours after the start of ifosfamide)

Note: Alternative I.V. regimens include 80% of the ifosfamide dose given in 4 divided doses (0, 3, 6, and 9 hours after the start of ifosfamide) and continuous infusions

I.V./Oral: Recommended dose is 100% of the ifosfamide dose, given as 20% of the ifosfamide dose I.V. at hour 0, followed by 40% of the ifosfamide dose given orally 2 and 6 hours after start of ifosfamide

Pediatrics: Refer to adult dosing.

Available Dosage Forms

Injection, solution: 100 mg/mL (10 mL) [contains benzyl alcohol]

Tablet: 400 mg

Nursing Guidelines

Assessment: Monitor laboratory results and assess frequently for hematuria/bladder hemorrhage.

Monitoring Laboratory Tests: Urinalysis

Patient Education: This drug is given to help prevent side effects of other chemotherapeutic agents you are taking. Report blood in urine. **Breast-feeding precaution:** Do not breast-feed.

Pregnancy Risk Factor: B

Lactation: Excretion in breast milk unknown/not recommended

Administration

Oral: Administer orally in tablet formulation or parenteral solution diluted in water, milk, juice, or carbonated beverages; patients who vomit within 2 hours of taking oral mesna should repeat the dose or receive I.V. mesna

I.V.: Administer by short (15-30 minutes) infusion or continuous (24 hour) infusion

Reconstitution: Dilute in 50-1000 mL NS, D_5W, or lactated Ringer's.

Compatibility: Stable in $D_5{}^1/_4$NS, $D_5{}^1/_3$NS, $D_5{}^1/_2$NS, D_5W, LR, NS

Y-site administration: Incompatible with amphotericin B cholesteryl sulfate complex

Compatibility in syringe: Incompatible with ifosfamide/epirubicin

Compatibility when admixed: Incompatible with carboplatin, cisplatin, ifosfamide/epirubicin

Storage: Store intact vials and tablets at controlled room temperature of 20°C to 25°C (68°F to 77°F). Opened multidose vials may be stored and used for use to 8 days after opening. Infusion solutions diluted in D_5W or lactated Ringer's are stable for at least 48 hours at room temperature. Solutions in NS are stable for at least 24 hours at room temperature. Solutions in plastic syringes are stable for 9 days under refrigeration, or at room or body temperature. Solutions of mesna and ifosfamide in lactated Ringer's are stable for 7 days in a PVC ambulatory infusion pump reservoir. Mesna injection is stable for at least 7 days when diluted 1:2 or 1:5 with grape- and orange-flavored syrups or 11:1 to 1:100 in carbonated beverages for oral administration.

♦ Mesnex® *see* Mesna *on page 1108*

♦ Mestinon® *see* Pyridostigmine *on page 1440*

♦ Mestinon® Timespan® *see* Pyridostigmine *on page 1440*

♦ Metacortandralone *see* PrednisoLONE *on page 1399*

♦ Metadate® CD *see* Methylphenidate *on page 1137*

♦ Metadate® ER *see* Methylphenidate *on page 1137*

♦ Metamucil® [OTC] *see* Psyllium *on page 1438*

♦ Metamucil® Plus Calcium [OTC] *see* Psyllium *on page 1438*

♦ Metamucil® Smooth Texture [OTC] *see* Psyllium *on page 1438*

Metaproterenol (met a proe TER e nol)

U.S. Brand Names Alupent®

Synonyms Metaproterenol Sulfate; Orciprenaline Sulfate

Pharmacologic Category $Beta_2$-Adrenergic Agonist

Medication Safety Issues

Sound-alike/look-alike issues:

Metaproterenol may be confused with metipranolol, metoprolol

Alupent® may be confused with Atrovent®

Use Bronchodilator in reversible airway obstruction due to asthma or COPD; because of its delayed onset of action (1 hour) and prolonged effect (4 or more hours), this may not be the drug of choice for assessing response to a bronchodilator

Mechanism of Action Relaxes bronchial smooth muscle by action on $beta_2$-receptors with very little effect on heart rate

Pharmacodynamics/Kinetics

Onset of action: Bronchodilation: Oral: ~15 minutes; Inhalation: ~60 seconds

Peak effect: Oral: ~1 hour

Duration: ~1-5 hours

Contraindications Hypersensitivity to metaproterenol or any component of the formulation; pre-existing cardiac arrhythmias associated with tachycardia

Warnings/Precautions Optimize anti-inflammatory treatment before initiating maintenance treatment with metaproterenol. Do not use as a component of chronic therapy without an anti-inflammatory agent. Only the mildest form of asthma (Step 1 and/or exercise-induced) would not require concurrent use based upon asthma guidelines. Patient must be instructed to seek medical attention in cases where acute symptoms are not relieved or a previous level of response is

(Continued)

Metaproterenol *(Continued)*

diminished. The need to increase frequency of use may indicate deterioration of asthma, and treatment must not be delayed.

Use caution in patients with cardiovascular disease (arrhythmia or hypertension or CHF), convulsive disorders, diabetes, glaucoma, hyperthyroidism, or hypokalemia. Beta agonists may cause elevation in blood pressure, heart rate, and result in CNS stimulation/excitation. Beta$_2$ agonists may increase risk of arrhythmia, increase serum glucose, or decrease serum potassium.

Do not exceed recommended dose; serious adverse events including fatalities, have been associated with excessive use of inhaled sympathomimetics. Rarely, paradoxical bronchospasm may occur with use of inhaled bronchodilating agents; this should be distinguished from inadequate response. All patients should utilize a spacer device when using a metered-dose inhaler; additionally, a face mask should be used in children <4 years of age.

Metaproterenol has more beta$_1$ activity than beta$_2$-selective agents such as albuterol and, therefore, may no longer be the beta agonist of first choice. Oral use should be avoided due to the increased incidence of adverse effects.

Drug Interactions

Beta-adrenergic blockers (eg, propranolol) antagonize metaproterenol's effects; avoid concurrent use.
Inhaled ipratropium may increase duration of bronchodilation.
MAO inhibitors may increase side effects; monitor heart rate and blood pressure.
TCAs may increase side effects; monitor heart rate and blood pressure.
Sympathomimetics may increase side effects; monitor heart rate and blood pressure.
Halothane may increase risk of malignant arrhythmias; avoid concurrent use.

Lab Interactions Increased potassium (S)

Adverse Reactions

>10%:
- Cardiovascular: Tachycardia (<17%)
- Central nervous system: Nervousness (3% to 14%)
- Endocrine & metabolic: Serum glucose increased, serum potassium decreased
- Neuromuscular & skeletal: Tremor (1% to 33%)

1% to 10%:
- Cardiovascular: Palpitations (<4%)
- Central nervous system: Headache (<4%), dizziness (1% to 4%), insomnia (2%)
- Gastrointestinal: Nausea, vomiting, bad taste, heartburn (≥4%), xerostomia
- Neuromuscular & skeletal: Trembling, muscle cramps, weakness (1%)
- Respiratory: Coughing, pharyngitis (≤4%)
- Miscellaneous: Diaphoresis (increased) (≤4%)

<1% (Limited to important or life-threatening): Angina, chest pain, diarrhea, drowsiness, hypertension, hypokalemia, paradoxical bronchospasm, taste change

Overdosage/Toxicology Symptoms of overdose include tachycardia, tremor, hypertension, angina, and seizures. Hypokalemia also may occur. Cardiac arrest and death may be associated with abuse of beta-agonist bronchodilators. Treatment includes immediate discontinuation and symptomatic and supportive therapies. Cautious use of beta-adrenergic blocking agents may be considered in severe cases.

Dosing

Adults:

Bronchoconstriction (Asthma, COPD):

Oral: 20 mg 3-4 times/day

Inhalation: 2-3 inhalations every 3-4 hours, up to 12 inhalations in 24 hours

Nebulizer: 5-20 breaths of full strength 5% metaproterenol **or** 0.2 to 0.3 mL 5% metaproterenol in 2.5-3 mL normal saline until nebulized every 4-6 hours (can be given more frequently according to need)

Elderly: Oral: Initial: 10 mg 3-4 times/day; increase as necessary up to 20 mg 3-4 times/day.

Pediatrics:

Bronchoconstriction (asthma):

Oral:

<2 years: 0.4 mg/kg/dose given 3-4 times/day; in infants, the dose can be given every 8-12 hours

2-6 years: 1-2.6 mg/kg/day divided every 6 hours

6-9 years: 10 mg/dose 3-4 times/day

>9 years: 20 mg 3-4 times/day

Inhalation: >12 years: Refer to adult dosing.

Nebulizer:

Infants and Children: 0.01-0.02 mL/kg of 5% solution; minimum dose: 0.1 mL; maximum dose: 0.3 mL diluted in 2-3 mL normal saline every 4-6 hours (may be given more frequently according to need)

Adolescents: Refer to adult dosing.

Available Dosage Forms

Aerosol for oral inhalation, as sulfate (Alupent®): 0.65 mg/inhalation (14 g) [200 doses]

Solution for oral inhalation, as sulfate [preservative free]: 0.4% [4 mg/mL] (2.5 mL); 0.6% [6 mg/mL] (2.5 mL)

Syrup, as sulfate: 10 mg/5 mL (480 mL) [may contain sodium benzoate]

Tablet, as sulfate: 10 mg, 20 mg

Nursing Guidelines

Assessment: Assess effectiveness and interactions of other medications patient may be taking. Monitor effectiveness of therapy (relief of airway obstruction) and adverse reactions at beginning of therapy and periodically with long-term use. For inpatient care, vital signs and lung sounds should be monitored prior to and periodically during therapy. Assess knowledge/teach patient appropriate use, interventions to reduce side effects, and adverse symptoms to report.

Monitoring Laboratory Tests: FEV_1, peak flow, and/or other pulmonary function tests; serum potassium, serum glucose (in selected patients)

Patient Education: Use exactly as directed (see following administration information). Do not use more often than recommended. Maintain adequate hydration (2-3 L/day of fluids) unless instructed to restrict fluid intake. You may experience nervousness, dizziness, or fatigue (use caution when driving or engaging in tasks requiring alertness until response to drug is known); dry mouth, unpleasant aftertaste, stomach upset (small frequent meals, frequent mouth care, chewing gum, or sucking hard candy may help); or increased perspiration. If you have diabetes, check blood sugar; blood glucose level may be increased. Report unresolved GI upset; dizziness or fatigue; vision changes; chest pain, rapid heartbeat, or palpitations; nervousness or insomnia; muscle cramping or tremor; or unusual cough. **Pregnancy/breast-feeding precautions:** Inform prescriber if you are or intend to become pregnant. Consult prescriber if breast-feeding.

Self-administered inhalation: Store canister upside down; do not freeze. Shake canister before using. Sit when using medication. Close eyes when administering metaproterenol to avoid spray getting into eyes. Exhale slowly and completely through nose; inhale deeply through mouth while administering aerosol. Hold breath for 5-10 seconds after inhalation. Wait at least 1 full minute between inhalations. Wash mouthpiece between use. If more than one inhalation medication is used, use bronchodilator first and wait 5 minutes between medications.

Self-administered nebulizer: Wash hands before and after treatment. Wash and dry nebulizer after each treatment. Twist open the top of one unit dose vial and squeeze contents into nebulizer reservoir. Connect nebulizer reservoir to the mouthpiece or face mask. Connect nebulizer to compressor. Sit in comfortable, upright position. Place mouthpiece in your mouth or put on face mask and turn on compressor. If face mask is used, avoid leakage around the mask to avoid mist getting into eyes which may cause vision problems. Breathe calmly and deeply until no more mist is formed in nebulizer (about 5 minutes). At this point treatment is finished.

Geriatric Considerations: Metaproterenol has more $beta_1$ activity than other sympathomimetics such as albuterol and, therefore, may no longer be the beta agonist of first choice. The elderly may find it beneficial to utilize a spacer device when using a metered dose inhaler. Oral use should be avoided due to the increased incidence of adverse effects.

Pregnancy Risk Factor: C

Lactation: Excretion in breast milk unknown

Breast-Feeding Considerations: No data on crossing into breast milk or clinical effects on the infant.

(Continued)

Metaproterenol *(Continued)*

Perioperative/Anesthesia/Other Concerns: Hypertension and tachycardia are increased with exogenous sympathomimetics. During endotracheal intubation, $beta_2$-specific agent is more appropriate for perioperative use. Use with caution perioperatively due to $beta_1$ effect of agent.

Administration

Oral: Administer around-the-clock to promote less variation in peak and trough serum levels.

Storage: Store in a tight, light-resistant container. Do not use if brown solution or contains a precipitate.

♦ Metaproterenol Sulfate *see* Metaproterenol *on page 1109*

Metformin (met FOR min)

U.S. Brand Names Fortamet™; Glucophage®; Glucophage® XR; Riomet™

Synonyms Metformin Hydrochloride

Pharmacologic Category Antidiabetic Agent, Biguanide

Medication Safety Issues

Sound-alike/look-alike issues:

Metformin may be confused with metronidazole

Glucophage® may be confused with Glucotrol®, Glutofac®

Use Management of type 2 diabetes mellitus (noninsulin dependent, NIDDM) as monotherapy when hyperglycemia cannot be managed on diet alone. May be used concomitantly with a sulfonylurea or insulin to improve glycemic control.

Unlabeled/Investigational Use Treatment of HIV lipodystrophy syndrome

Mechanism of Action Decreases hepatic glucose production, decreasing intestinal absorption of glucose and improves insulin sensitivity (increases peripheral glucose uptake and utilization)

Pharmacodynamics/Kinetics

Onset of action: Within days; maximum effects up to 2 weeks

Distribution: V_d: 654 ± 358 L

Protein binding: Negligible

Bioavailability: Absolute: Fasting: 50% to 60%

Half-life elimination, plasma: 6.2 hours

Excretion: Urine (90% as unchanged drug)

Contraindications Hypersensitivity to metformin or any component of the formulation; renal disease or renal dysfunction (serum creatinine ≥1.5 mg/dL in males or ≥1.4 mg/dL in females or abnormal creatinine clearance from any cause, including shock, acute myocardial infarction, or septicemia); congestive heart failure requiring pharmacological management; acute or chronic metabolic acidosis with or without coma (including diabetic ketoacidosis)

Note: Temporarily discontinue in patients undergoing radiologic studies in which intravascular iodinated contrast materials are utilized.

Warnings/Precautions Lactic acidosis is a rare, but potentially severe consequence of therapy with metformin. Lactic acidosis should be suspected in any diabetic patient receiving metformin who has evidence of acidosis when evidence of ketoacidosis is lacking. Discontinue metformin in clinical situations predisposing to hypoxemia, including conditions such as cardiovascular collapse, respiratory failure, acute myocardial infarction, acute congestive heart failure, and septicemia.

Metformin is substantially excreted by the kidney. The risk of accumulation and lactic acidosis increases with the degree of impairment of renal function. Patients with renal function below the limit of normal for their age should not receive metformin. In elderly patients, renal function should be monitored regularly; should not be used in any patient ≥80 years of age unless measurement of creatinine clearance verifies normal renal function. Use of concomitant medications that may affect renal function (ie, affect tubular secretion) may also affect metformin disposition. Metformin should be suspended in patients with dehydration and/or prerenal azotemia. Therapy should be suspended for any surgical procedures (resume only after normal intake resumed and normal renal function is verified). Metformin should also be temporarily discontinued for 48 hours in patients undergoing radiologic studies involving the intravascular administration of iodinated contrast materials (potential for acute alteration in renal function).

Avoid use in patients with impaired liver function. Patient must be instructed to avoid excessive acute or chronic ethanol use. Administration of oral antidiabetic drugs has been reported to be associated with increased cardiovascular mortality;

metformin does not appear to share this risk. Safety and efficacy of metformin have been established for use in children ≥10 years of age; the extended release preparation is for use in patients ≥17 years of age.

Drug Interactions

Drugs which tend to produce hyperglycemia (eg, diuretics, corticosteroids, phenothiazines, thyroid products, estrogens, oral contraceptives, phenytoin, nicotinic acid, sympathomimetics, calcium channel blocking drugs, isoniazid) may lead to a loss of glycemic control

Cationic drugs (eg, amiloride, digoxin, morphine, procainamide, quinidine, quinine, ranitidine, triamterene, trimethoprim, and vancomycin) which are eliminated by renal tubular secretion could have the potential for interaction with metformin by competing for common renal tubular transport systems

Cimetidine increases (by 60%) peak metformin plasma and whole blood concentrations

Contrast agents: May increase the risk of metformin-induced lactic acidosis. Discontinue metformin prior to exposure and withhold for 48 hours.

Furosemide increased the metformin plasma and blood C_{max} without altering metformin renal clearance in a single dose study

Nutritional/Herbal/Ethanol Interactions

Ethanol: Avoid or limit ethanol (incidence of lactic acidosis may be increased; may cause hypoglycemia).

Food: Food decreases the extent and slightly delays the absorption. May decrease absorption of vitamin B_{12} and/or folic acid.

Herb/Nutraceutical: Caution with chromium, garlic, gymnema (may cause hypoglycemia).

Adverse Reactions

>10%:

Gastrointestinal: Nausea/vomiting (6% to 25%), diarrhea (10% to 53%), flatulence (12%)

Neuromuscular & skeletal: Weakness (9%)

1% to 10%:

Cardiovascular: Chest discomfort, flushing, palpitation

Central nervous system: Headache (6%), chills, dizziness, lightheadedness

Dermatologic: Rash

Endocrine & metabolic: Hypoglycemia

Gastrointestinal: Indigestion (7%), abdominal discomfort (6%), abdominal distention, abnormal stools, constipation, dyspepsia/ heartburn, taste disorder

Neuromuscular & skeletal: Myalgia

Respiratory: Dyspnea, upper respiratory tract infection

Miscellaneous: Decreased vitamin B_{12} levels (7%), increased diaphoresis, flu-like syndrome, nail disorder

<1% (Limited to important or life-threatening): Lactic acidosis, megaloblastic anemia

Overdosage/Toxicology Hypoglycemia (10% of cases) or lactic acidosis (~32% of cases) may occur. Metformin is dialyzable with a clearance of up to 170 mL/minute. Hemodialysis may be useful for removal of accumulated drug from patients in whom metformin overdose is suspected. Treatment is supportive.

Dosing

Adults: Note: Oral (allow 1-2 weeks between dose titrations): Generally, clinically significant responses are not seen at doses <1500 mg daily; however, a lower recommended starting dose and gradual increased dosage is recommended to minimize gastrointestinal symptoms

Management of type 2 diabetes mellitus: Oral:

Immediate release tablet or oral solution: Initial: 500 mg twice daily (give with the morning and evening meals) **or** 850 mg once daily; increase dosage incrementally.

Adjustment: Incremental dosing recommendations are based on dosage form:

500 mg tablet: One tablet/day at weekly intervals

850 mg tablet: One tablet/day every other week

Oral solution: 500 mg twice daily every other week

Note: Doses of up to 2000 mg/day may be given twice daily. If a dose >2000 mg/day is required, it may be better tolerated in three divided doses. Maximum recommended dose 2550 mg/day.

Extended release tablet: Initial: 500 mg once daily (with the evening meal); dosage may be increased by 500 mg weekly; maximum dose: 2000 mg once daily. If glycemic control is not achieved at maximum dose, may divide

(Continued)

Metformin *(Continued)*

dose to 1000 mg twice daily. If doses >2000 mg/day are needed, switch to regular release tablets and titrate to maximum dose of 2550 mg/day.

Transfer from other antidiabetic agents: No transition period is generally necessary except when transferring from chlorpropamide. When transferring from chlorpropamide, care should be exercised during the first 2 weeks because of the prolonged retention of chlorpropamide in the body, leading to overlapping drug effects and possible hypoglycemia.

Concomitant metformin and oral sulfonylurea therapy: If patients have not responded to 4 weeks of the maximum dose of metformin monotherapy, consider a gradual addition of an oral sulfonylurea, even if prior primary or secondary failure to a sulfonylurea has occurred. Continue metformin at the maximum dose.

Failed sulfonylurea therapy: Patients with prior failure on glyburide may be treated by gradual addition of metformin. Initiate with glyburide 20 mg and metformin 500 mg daily. Metformin dosage may be increased by 500 mg/day at weekly intervals, up to a maximum of 2500 mg/day (dosage of glyburide maintained at 20 mg/day).

Concomitant metformin and insulin therapy:

Initial: 500 mg metformin once daily, continue current insulin dose; increase by 500 mg metformin weekly until adequate glycemic control is achieved

Maximum dose: 2500 mg metformin; 2000 mg metformin extended release

Note: Decrease insulin dose 10% to 25% when FPG <120 mg/dL; monitor and make further adjustments as needed

Elderly: The initial and maintenance dosing should be conservative, due to the potential for decreased renal function. Generally, elderly patients should **not** be titrated to the maximum dose of metformin. See Geriatric Considerations.

Pediatrics: Note: Allow 1-2 weeks between dose titrations: Generally, clinically significant responses are not seen at doses <1500 mg daily; however, a lower recommended starting dose and gradual increased dosage is recommended to minimize gastrointestinal symptoms

Management of type 2 diabetes mellitus: Children 10-16 years: Oral (500 mg tablet or oral solution): Initial: 500 mg twice daily (given with the morning and evening meals); increases in daily dosage should be made in increments of 500 mg at weekly intervals, given in divided doses, up to a maximum of 2000 mg/day

Renal Impairment: The plasma and blood half-life of metformin is prolonged and the renal clearance is decreased in proportion to the decrease in creatinine clearance. Per the manufacturer, metformin is contraindicated in the presence of renal dysfunction defined as a serum creatinine >1.5 mg/dL in males, or >1.4 mg/dL in females and in patients with abnormal clearance. Clinically, it has been recommended that metformin be avoided in patients with Cl_{cr} <60-70 mL/minute (DeFronzo, 1999).

Hepatic Impairment: Avoid metformin; liver disease is a risk factor for the development of lactic acidosis during metformin therapy.

Available Dosage Forms

Solution, oral, as hydrochloride (Riomet™): 100 mg/mL (118 mL, 473 mL) [contains saccharin; cherry flavor]

Tablet, as hydrochloride (Glucophage®): 500 mg, 850 mg, 1000 mg

Tablet, extended release, as hydrochloride: 500 mg

Fortamet™: 500 mg, 1000 mg

Glucophage® XR: 500 mg, 750 mg

Nursing Guidelines

Assessment: Assess potential for interactions with other prescriptions, OTC medications, or herbal products patient may be taking (eg, anything that may effect glucose levels). Assess results of laboratory tests, therapeutic effectiveness, and adverse response (eg, assess for signs and symptoms of vitamin B_{12} and/or folic acid deficiency; supplementation may be required) during therapy. Teach patient (or refer patient to diabetic educator for instruction) in appropriate use, possible side effects/appropriate interventions, and adverse symptoms to report.

Monitoring Laboratory Tests: Urine for glucose and ketones, fasting blood glucose, hemoglobin A_{1c}, and fructosamine. Initial and periodic monitoring of hematologic parameters (eg, hemoglobin/hematocrit and red blood cell indices) and renal function should be performed, at least annually. While megaloblastic anemia has been rarely seen with metformin, if suspected, vitamin B_{12} deficiency should be excluded.

Dietary Considerations: Drug may cause GI upset; take with food (to decrease GI upset). Take at the same time each day. Dietary modification based on ADA recommendations is a part of therapy. Monitor for signs and symptoms of vitamin B_{12} and/or folic acid deficiency; supplementation may be required.

Patient Education: Do not take any new medication during therapy unless approved by prescriber. Take as directed (may take with food to decrease GI upset). Do not chew or crush tablets. Parts of extended-release tablets may be excreted in the stool (normal). Do not change dosage or discontinue without consulting prescriber. Avoid overuse of alcohol (could cause severe reaction). It is important to follow dietary and lifestyle recommendations of prescriber. You will be instructed in signs of hypo- or hyperglycemia by prescriber or diabetic educator. May cause drowsiness or dizziness (use caution driving or engaging in potentially hazardous tasks until response to drug is known); nausea or vomiting (taking with meals, eating small frequent meals, frequent mouth care, or sucking lozenges may help); or abdominal distention, flatulence, diarrhea, constipation, or heartburn (if these persist consult prescriber for approved medication). Report immediately unusual weakness or fatigue; unusual muscle pain; persistent GI discomfort; dizziness or lightheadedness; sudden respiratory difficulty, chest discomfort, slow or irregular heartbeat; or other adverse reactions. **Breast-feeding precaution:** Breast-feeding is not recommended.

Geriatric Considerations: Limited data suggests that metformin's total body clearance may be decreased and AUC and half-life increased in older patients; presumably due to decreased renal clearance. Metformin has been well tolerated by the elderly but lower doses and frequent monitoring are recommended.

Pregnancy Risk Factor: B

Pregnancy Issues: Abnormal blood glucose levels are associated with a higher incidence of congenital abnormalities. Insulin is the drug of choice for the control of diabetes mellitus during pregnancy.

Lactation: Excretion in breast milk unknown/not recommended

Breast-Feeding Considerations: It is not known if metformin is excreted in human breast milk (excretion occurs in animal models); insulin therapy should be considered in breast-feeding women.

Perioperative/Anesthesia/Other Concerns: While megaloblastic anemia has been rarely seen with metformin, if suspected, vitamin B_{12} deficiency should be excluded. Metformin has a large volume of distribution in liver, kidney, and GI tract where concentration is much larger than in the plasma.

Lactic acidosis is an uncommon side effect in patients without renal or respiratory insufficiency, hepatic failure, or conditions that predispose to hypoxemia. Metformin should be avoided in diabetic patients with heart failure.

Administration

Oral: Extended release dosage form should be swallowed whole; do not crush, break, or chew. Patients who are anorexic or NPO may need to have their dose held to avoid hypoglycemia.

Storage: Store tablets and oral solution at 20°C to 25°C (68°F to 77°F).

Related Information

Perioperative Management of the Diabetic Patient *on page 1794*

- **Metformin and Glyburide** *see* Glyburide and Metformin *on page 823*
- **Metformin and Rosiglitazone** *see* Rosiglitazone and Metformin *on page 1502*
- **Metformin Hydrochloride** *see* Metformin *on page 1112*
- **Metformin Hydrochloride and Rosiglitazone Maleate** *see* Rosiglitazone and Metformin *on page 1502*
- **Methadex** *see* Neomycin, Polymyxin B, and Dexamethasone *on page 1211*

Methadone (METH a done)

U.S. Brand Names Dolophine®; Methadone Diskets®; Methadone Intensol™; Methadose®

Synonyms Methadone Hydrochloride

Pharmacologic Category Analgesic, Narcotic

Medication Safety Issues

Sound-alike/look-alike issues:

Methadone may be confused with Mephyton®, methylphenidate

(Continued)

Methadone *(Continued)*

Use Management of severe pain; detoxification and maintenance treatment of narcotic addiction (if used for detoxification and maintenance treatment of narcotic addiction, it must be part of an FDA-approved program)

Mechanism of Action Binds to opiate receptors in the CNS, causing inhibition of ascending pain pathways, altering the perception of and response to pain; produces generalized CNS depression

Pharmacodynamics/Kinetics

Onset of action: Oral: Analgesic: 0.5-1 hour; Parenteral: 10-20 minutes

Peak effect: Parenteral: 1-2 hours

Duration: Oral: 4-8 hours, increases to 22-48 hours with repeated doses

Distribution: V_{dss}: 1-8 L/kg

Protein binding: 85% to 90%

Metabolism: Hepatic; N-demethylation primarily via CYP3A4, CYP2B6, and CYP2C19 to inactive metabolites

Bioavailability: Oral: 36% to 100%

Half-life elimination: 7-59 hours; may be prolonged with alkaline pH, decreased during pregnancy

Excretion: Urine (<10% as unchanged drug); increased with urine pH <6

Contraindications Hypersensitivity to methadone or any component of the formulation; respiratory depression (in the absence of resuscitative equipment or in an unmonitored setting); acute bronchial asthma or hypercarbia; pregnancy (prolonged use or high doses near term)

Warnings/Precautions An opioid-containing analgesic regimen should be tailored to each patient's needs and based upon the type of pain being treated (acute versus chronic), the route of administration, degree of tolerance for opioids (naive versus chronic user), age, weight, and medical condition. The optimal analgesic dose varies widely among patients. Doses should be titrated to pain relief/prevention. Patients maintained on stable doses of methadone may need higher and/or more frequent doses in case of acute pain (eg, postoperative pain, physical trauma). Methadone is ineffective for the relief of anxiety.

May prolong the QT interval; use caution in patients at risk for QT prolongation, with medications known to prolong the QT interval, or history of conduction abnormalities. QT interval prolongation and torsade de pointes may be associated with doses >200 mg/day, but have also been observed with lower doses. May cause severe hypotension; use caution with severe volume depletion or other conditions which may compromise maintenance of normal blood pressure. Use caution with cardiovascular disease or patients predisposed to dysrhythmias.

May cause respiratory depression. Use caution in patients with respiratory disease or pre-existing respiratory conditions (eg, severe obesity, asthma, COPD, sleep apnea, CNS depression). Because the respiratory effects last longer than the analgesic effects, slow titration is required. Abrupt cessation may precipitate withdrawal symptoms.

May cause CNS depression, which may impair physical or mental abilities. Patients must be cautioned about performing tasks which require mental alertness (eg, operating machinery or driving). Effects with other sedative drugs or ethanol may be potentiated. Use with caution in patients with depression or suicidal tendencies, or in patients with a history of drug abuse. Tolerance or psychological and physical dependence may occur with prolonged use.

Use with caution in patients with head injury or increased intracranial pressure. May obscure diagnosis or clinical course of patients with acute abdominal conditions. Elderly may be more susceptible to adverse effects (eg, CNS, respiratory, gastrointestinal). Decrease initial dose and use caution in the elderly or debilitated; with hyper/hypothyroidism, prostatic hypertrophy, or urethral stricture; or with severe renal or hepatic failure. Safety and efficacy have not been established in patients <18 years of age. Tablets contain excipients to deter use by injection.

Drug Interactions **Substrate** of CYP2C8/9 (minor), 2C19 (minor), 2D6 (minor), 3A4 (major); **Inhibits** CYP2D6 (moderate), 3A4 (weak)

Agonist/antagonist analgesics (buprenorphine, butorphanol, nalbuphine, pentazocine): May decrease analgesic effect of methadone and precipitate withdrawal symptoms; use is not recommended.

Antiretroviral agents, NNRTI: May decrease levels of methadone, opioid withdrawal syndrome has been reported. Effect reported with efavirenz and nevirapine.

Antiretroviral agents, NRTI: Methadone may increase bioavailability and toxic effects of zidovudine. Methadone may decrease bioavailability of didanosine and stavudine.

Antiretroviral agent, PI: Ritonavir (and combinations) may decrease levels of methadone; withdrawal symptoms have inconsistently been observed, monitor.

CNS depressants (including but not limited to opioid analgesics, general anesthetics, sedatives, hypnotics, ethanol): May cause respiratory depression, hypotension, profound sedation, or coma.

CYP2D6 substrates: Methadone may increase the levels/effects of CYP2D6 substrates. Example substrates include amphetamines, selected beta-blockers, dextromethorphan, fluoxetine, lidocaine, mirtazapine, nefazodone, paroxetine, risperidone, ritonavir, thioridazine, tricyclic antidepressants, and venlafaxine.

CYP2D6 prodrug substrates: Methadone may decrease the levels/effects of CYP2D6 prodrug substrates. Example prodrug substrates include codeine, hydrocodone, oxycodone, and tramadol.

CYP3A4 inducers: CYP3A4 inducers may decrease the levels/effects of methadone. Example inducers include aminoglutethimide, carbamazepine, nafcillin, nevirapine, phenobarbital, phenytoin, and rifamycins.

CYP3A4 inhibitors: May increase the levels/effects of methadone. Example inhibitors include azole antifungals, clarithromycin, diclofenac, doxycycline, erythromycin, imatinib, isoniazid, nefazodone, nicardipine, propofol, protease inhibitors, quinidine, telithromycin, and verapamil.

Desipramine: Levels of desipramine may be increased by methadone.

QT_c interval-prolonging agents (including but may not be limited to amitriptyline, astemizole, bepridil, disopyramide, erythromycin, haloperidol, imipramine, quinidine, pimozide, procainamide, sotalol, and thioridazine): Effect/toxicity increased; use with caution.

Ritonavir: May increase levels/effects of methadone shortly after initiation. May decrease levels/effects of methadone with continued dosing.

Somatostatin: Therapeutic effect of methadone may be decreased; limited documentation; monitor

Zidovudine: serum concentrations may be increased by methadone; monitor

Nutritional/Herbal/Ethanol Interactions

Ethanol: Avoid ethanol (may increase CNS effects). Watch for sedation.

Herb/Nutraceutical: Avoid St John's wort (may decrease methadone levels; may increase CNS depression). Avoid valerian, kava kava, gotu kola (may increase CNS depression). Methadone is metabolized by CYP3A4 in the intestines; avoid concurrent use of grapefruit juice.

Lab Interactions Increased thyroxine (S), aminotransferase [ALT (SGPT)/AST (SGOT)] (S)

Adverse Reactions Frequency not defined. During prolonged administration, adverse effects may decrease over several weeks; however, constipation and sweating may persist.

Cardiovascular: Bradycardia, peripheral vasodilation, cardiac arrest, syncope, faintness, shock, hypotension, edema, arrhythmia, bigeminal rhythms, extrasystoles, tachycardia, torsade de pointes, ventricular fibrillation, ventricular tachycardia, ECG changes, QT interval prolonged, T-wave inversion, cardiomyopathy, flushing, heart failure, palpitation, phlebitis, orthostatic hypotension

Central nervous system: Euphoria, dysphoria, headache, insomnia, agitation, disorientation, drowsiness, dizziness, lightheadedness, sedation, confusion, seizure

Dermatologic: Pruritus, urticaria, rash, hemorrhagic urticaria

Endocrine & metabolic: Libido decreased, hypokalemia, hypomagnesemia, antidiuretic effect, amenorrhea

Gastrointestinal: Nausea, vomiting, constipation, anorexia, stomach cramps, xerostomia, biliary tract spasm, abdominal pain, glossitis, weight gain

Genitourinary: Urinary retention or hesitancy, impotence

Hematologic: Thrombocytopenia (reversible, reported in patients with chronic hepatitis)

Neuromuscular & skeletal: Weakness

Local: I.M./SubQ injection: Pain, erythema, swelling; I.V. injection: pruritus, urticaria, rash, hemorrhagic urticaria (rare)

Ocular: Miosis, visual disturbances

Respiratory: Respiratory depression, respiratory arrest, pulmonary edema

Miscellaneous: Physical and psychological dependence, death, diaphoresis

(Continued)

Methadone *(Continued)*

Overdosage/Toxicology Symptoms include respiratory depression, CNS depression, miosis, hypothermia, circulatory collapse, and convulsions. Treatment includes naloxone 2 mg I.V. (0.01 mg/kg for children), with repeat administration as necessary, up to a total of 10 mg, or as a continuous infusion. Nalmefene may also be used to reverse signs of intoxication. Patient should be monitored for depressant effects of methadone for 36-48 hours and other supportive measures should be employed as needed. Forced diuresis, peritoneal dialysis, hemodialysis, or charcoal hemoperfusion have not been established as beneficial for increasing methadone or metabolite elimination.

Dosing

Adults: Regulations regarding methadone use may vary by state and/or country. Obtain advice from appropriate regulatory agencies and/or consult with pain management/palliative care specialists. **Note:** These are guidelines and do not represent the maximum doses that may be required in all patients. Methadone accumulates with repeated doses and dosage may need reduction after 3-5 days to prevent CNS depressant effects. Some patients may benefit from every 8-12 hour dosing interval for chronic pain management. Doses should be titrated to appropriate effects.

Pain (analgesia):

Oral: Initial: 5-10 mg; dosing interval may range from 4-12 hours during initial therapy; decrease in dose or frequency may be required (~days 2-5) due to accumulation with repeated doses

Manufacturer's labeling: 2.5-10 mg every 3-4 hours as needed

I.V.: Manufacturers labeling: Initial: 2.5-10 mg every 8-12 hours in opioid-naive patients; titrate slowly to effect; may also be administered by SubQ or I.M. injection

Note: Conversion from oral to parenteral dose: Initial dose: Oral: parenteral: 2:1 ratio

Detoxification: *Oral:*

Initial: Should not exceed 30 mg; lower doses should be considered in patients with low tolerance at initiation (eg, absence of opioids ≥5 days); an additional 5-10 mg of methadone may be provided if withdrawal symptoms have not been suppressed or if symptoms reappear after 2-4 hours; total daily dose on the first day should not exceed 40 mg, unless the program physician documents in the patient's record that 40 mg did not control opiate abstinence symptoms.

Maintenance: Usual range: 80-120 mg/day (titration should occur cautiously)

Withdrawal: Dose reductions should be <10% of the maintenance dose, every 10-14 days

Detoxification (short-term): *Oral:*

Initial: Titrate to 40 mg/day in 2 divided doses

Maintenance: Continue 40 mg dose for 2-3 days

Withdrawal: Decrease daily or every other day, keeping withdrawal symptoms tolerable; hospitalized patients may tolerate a 20% reduction/day; ambulatory patients may require a slower reduction

Dosage adjustment during pregnancy: Methadone dose may need to be increased, or the dosing interval decreased; see Pregnancy Implications — use should be reserved for cases where the benefits clearly outweigh the risks

Elderly: Oral, I.M.: 2.5 mg every 8-12 hours; refer to adult dosing.

Pediatrics: Regulations regarding methadone use may vary by state and/or country. Obtain advice from appropriate regulatory agencies and/or consult with pain management/palliative care specialists. **Note:** These are guidelines and do not represent the maximum doses that may be required in all patients. Methadone accumulates with repeated doses and dosage may need reduction after 3-5 days to prevent CNS depressant effects. Some patients may benefit from every 8-12 hour dosing interval for chronic pain management. Doses should be titrated to appropriate effects.

Pain (analgesia):

Oral (unlabeled use): Initial: 0.1-0.2 mg/kg 4-8 hours initially for 2-3 doses, then every 6-12 hours as needed. Dosing interval may range from 4-12 hours during initial therapy; decrease in dose or frequency may be required (~ days 2-5) due to accumulation with repeated doses (maximum dose: 5-10 mg)

I.V. (unlabeled use): 0.1 mg/kg every 4-8 hours initially for 2-3 doses, then every 6-12 hours as needed. Dosing interval may range from 4-12 hours during initial therapy; decrease in dose or frequency may be required (~ days 2-5) due to accumulation with repeated doses (maximum dose: 5-8 mg)

Iatrogenic narcotic dependency (unlabeled): Oral: General guidelines: Initial: 0.05-0.1 mg/kg/dose every 6 hours; increase by 0.05 mg/kg/dose until withdrawal symptoms are controlled; after 24-48 hours, the dosing interval can be lengthened to every 12-24 hours; to taper dose, wean by 0.05 mg/kg/ day; if withdrawal symptoms recur, taper at a slower rate

Renal Impairment: Cl_{cr} <10 mL/minute: Administer 50% to 75% of normal dose.

Hepatic Impairment: Avoid in severe liver disease.

Available Dosage Forms

Injection, solution, as hydrochloride: 10 mg/mL (20 mL)

Solution, oral, as hydrochloride: 5 mg/5 mL (500 mL); 10 mg/5 mL (500 mL) [contains alcohol 8%; citrus flavor]

Solution, oral concentrate, as hydrochloride: 10 mg/mL (946 mL)

Methadone Intensol™: 10 mg/mL (30 mL)

Methadose®: 10 mg/mL (1000 mL) [cherry flavor]

Methadose®: 10 mg/mL (1000 mL) [dye free, sugar free, unflavored]

Tablet, as hydrochloride (Dolophine®, Methadose®): 5 mg, 10 mg

Tablet, dispersible, as hydrochloride:

Methadose®: 40 mg

Methadone Diskets®: 40 mg [orange-pineapple flavor]

Nursing Guidelines

Assessment: Assess other medications patient may be taking for additive or adverse interactions. Monitor therapeutic effectiveness and adverse reactions of overdose at beginning of therapy and at regular intervals with long-term use. May cause physical and/or psychological dependence. Monitor blood pressure, respiratory and CNS status (degree of sedation). For inpatients, implement safety measures. Assess knowledge/teach patient appropriate use (if self-administered) adverse reactions to report, and appropriate interventions to reduce side effects. Discontinue slowly after prolonged use.

Patient Education: If self-administered, use exactly as directed; do not increase dose or frequency. Drug may cause physical and/or psychological dependence. While using this medication, do not use alcohol and other prescription or OTC medications (especially sedatives, tranquilizers, antihistamines, or pain medications) without consulting prescriber. Maintain adequate hydration (2-3 L/day of fluids) unless instructed to restrict fluid intake. May cause hypotension, dizziness, drowsiness, impaired coordination, or blurred vision (use caution when driving, climbing stairs, or changing position - rising from sitting or lying to standing, or when engaging in tasks requiring alertness until response to drug is known); loss of appetite, nausea, or vomiting (frequent mouth care, small frequent meals, chewing gum, or sucking lozenges may help); or constipation (increased exercise, fluids, fruit, or fiber may help; if unresolved, consult prescriber about use of stool softeners). Report chest pain, slow or rapid heartbeat, acute dizziness or persistent headache; changes in mental status; swelling of extremities or unusual weight gain; changes in urinary elimination; acute headache; back or flank pain or muscle spasms; blurred vision; skin rash; or shortness of breath. **Pregnancy/breast-feeding precautions:** Inform prescriber if you are or intend to become pregnant. If you are breast-feeding, take medication immediately after breast-feeding or 3-4 hours prior to next feeding.

Geriatric Considerations: Because of its long half-life and risk of accumulation, methadone is not considered a drug of first choice in the elderly. The elderly may be particularly susceptible to the CNS depressant and constipating effects of narcotics. Adjust dose for renal function.

Pregnancy Risk Factor: C/D (prolonged use or high doses at term)

Pregnancy Issues: Teratogenic effects have been observed in some, but not all, animal studies. Data collected by the Teratogen Information System are complicated by maternal use of illicit drugs, nutrition, infection, and psychosocial circumstances. However, pregnant women in methadone treatment programs are reported to have improved fetal outcomes compared to pregnant women using illicit drugs. Methadone can be detected in the amniotic fluid, cord plasma, and newborn urine. Fetal growth, birth weight, length, and/or head circumference may be decreased in infants born to narcotic-addicted mothers treated with methadone during pregnancy. Growth deficits do not appear to

(Continued)

Methadone *(Continued)*

persist; however, decreased performance on psychometric and behavioral tests has been found to continue into childhood. Abnormal fetal nonstress tests have also been reported. Withdrawal symptoms in the neonate may be observed up to 2-4 weeks after delivery. The manufacturer states that methadone should be used during pregnancy only if clearly needed. Because methadone clearance in pregnant women is increased and half-life is decreased during the 2nd and 3rd trimesters of pregnancy, withdrawal symptoms may be observed in the mother; dosage of methadone may need increased or dosing interval decreased during pregnancy.

Lactation: Enters breast milk/not recommended (AAP rates "compatible")

Breast-Feeding Considerations: Peak methadone levels appear in breast milk 4-5 hours after an oral dose. Methadone has been detected in the plasma of some breast-fed infants whose mothers are taking methadone. Use during breast-feeding is not recommended, and the manufacturer recommends that women on high dose methadone maintenance who already are breast-feeding be instructed to wean breast-feeding gradually to avoid neonatal abstinence syndrome. Unless otherwise contraindicated (concurrent medical conditions, other medications of abuse), the AAP rates methadone "compatible" with breast-feeding.

Perioperative/Anesthesia/Other Concerns: Methadone accumulates with repeated doses and dosage may need to be adjusted downward after 3-5 days to prevent toxic effects. Some patients may benefit from every 8- to 12-hour dosing interval (pain control). Oral dose for detoxification and maintenance may be administered in fruit juice or water.

Administration

Oral: Oral dose for detoxification and maintenance may be administered in fruit juice or water.

Compatibility: Stable in NS

Storage:

Injection: Store at controlled room temperature of 15°C to 30°C (59°F to 86°F). Protect from light.

Oral concentrate, oral solution, tablet: Store at controlled room temperature of 15°C to 30°C (59°F to 86°F).

Related Information

Narcotic / Opioid Analgesics *on page 1880*

- **Methadone Diskets®** *see* Methadone *on page 1115*
- **Methadone Hydrochloride** *see* Methadone *on page 1115*
- **Methadone Intensol™** *see* Methadone *on page 1115*
- **Methadose®** *see* Methadone *on page 1115*

Methazolamide (meth a ZOE la mide)

Pharmacologic Category Carbonic Anhydrase Inhibitor; Diuretic, Carbonic Anhydrase Inhibitor; Ophthalmic Agent, Antiglaucoma

Medication Safety Issues

Sound-alike/look-alike issues:

Methazolamide may be confused with methenamine, metolazone

Neptazane® may be confused with Nesacaine®

Use Adjunctive treatment of open-angle or secondary glaucoma; short-term therapy of narrow-angle glaucoma when delay of surgery is desired

Mechanism of Action Noncompetitive inhibition of the enzyme carbonic anhydrase; thought that carbonic anhydrase is located at the luminal border of cells of the proximal tubule. When the enzyme is inhibited, there is an increase in urine volume and a change to an alkaline pH with a subsequent decrease in the excretion of titratable acid and ammonia.

Pharmacodynamics/Kinetics

Onset of action: Slow in comparison with acetazolamide (2-4 hours)

Peak effect: 6-8 hours

Duration: 10-18 hours

Absorption: Slow

Distribution: Well into tissue

Protein binding: ~55%

Metabolism: Slowly from GI tract

Half-life elimination: ~14 hours

Excretion: Urine (~25% as unchanged drug)

Contraindications Hypersensitivity to methazolamide or any component of the formulation; marked kidney or liver dysfunction; severe pulmonary obstruction

Warnings/Precautions Sulfonamide-type reactions can occur. Chemical similarities are present among sulfonamides, sulfonylureas, carbonic anhydrase inhibitors, thiazides, and loop diuretics (except ethacrynic acid). In patients with allergy to one of these compounds, a risk of cross-reaction exists; avoid use when previous reaction has been severe. Use with caution in patients with respiratory acidosis and diabetes mellitus; impairment of mental alertness and/or physical coordination. Malaise and complaints of tiredness and myalgia are signs of excessive dosing and acidosis in the elderly.

Drug Interactions

Increased toxicity:

May induce hypokalemia which would sensitize a patient to digitalis toxicity

May increase the potential for salicylate toxicity

Hypokalemia may be compounded with concurrent diuretic use or steroids

Primidone absorption may be delayed

Decreased effect: Increased lithium excretion and altered excretion of other drugs by alkalinization of the urine, such as amphetamines, quinidine, procainamide, methenamine, phenobarbital, salicylates

Adverse Reactions Frequency not defined.

Central nervous system: Malaise, fever, mental depression, drowsiness, dizziness, nervousness, headache, confusion, seizure, fatigue, trembling, unsteadiness

Dermatologic: Urticaria, pruritus, photosensitivity, rash, Stevens-Johnson syndrome

Endocrine & metabolic: Hyperchloremic metabolic acidosis, hypokalemia, hyperglycemia

Gastrointestinal: Metallic taste, anorexia, nausea, vomiting, diarrhea, constipation, weight loss, GI irritation, xerostomia, black tarry stools

Genitourinary: Polyuria, crystalluria, hematuria, renal calculi, impotence

Hematologic: Bone marrow depression, thrombocytopenia, thrombocytopenic purpura, hemolytic anemia, leukopenia, pancytopenia, agranulocytosis

Hepatic: Hepatic insufficiency

Neuromuscular & skeletal: Weakness, ataxia, paresthesia

Miscellaneous: Hypersensitivity

Dosing

Adults & Elderly: Glaucoma: Oral: 50-100 mg 2-3 times/day

Available Dosage Forms Tablet: 25 mg, 50 mg

Nursing Guidelines

Assessment: Assess allergy history. Monitor blood pressure prior to beginning therapy and after first few doses, especially patients on another concomitant diuretic therapy. If diabetic, blood glucose levels may be elevated. Monitor blood sugars closely. Monitor for and/or teach patient to monitor and report adverse reactions. Use and teach patient postural hypotension precautions.

Patient Education: Take with food; swallow whole, do not chew or crush. You may experience GI upset and loss of appetite; small frequent meals are advised to reduce these effects and the metallic taste that sometimes occurs with this medication. You may experience lightheadedness, depression, dizziness, or weakness for a few days; use caution when driving or engaging in tasks that require alertness until response to drug is known. Report excessive tiredness; loss of appetite; cramping, pain, or weakness in muscles; acute GI symptoms; CNS changes (depression, drowsiness); difficulty or pain on urination; visual changes; or skin rash. **Pregnancy/breast-feeding precautions:** Inform prescriber if you are or intend to become pregnant. Consult prescriber if breast-feeding.

Geriatric Considerations: Malaise and complaints of tiredness and myalgia are signs of excessive dosing and acidosis in the elderly.

Pregnancy Risk Factor: C

Lactation: Excretion in breast milk unknown

◆ **Methergine®** *see* Methylergonovine *on page 1135*

Methimazole (meth IM a zole)

U.S. Brand Names Tapazole®

Synonyms Thiamazole

Pharmacologic Category Antithyroid Agent

Medication Safety Issues

Sound-alike/look-alike issues:

Methimazole may be confused with metolazone

Use Palliative treatment of hyperthyroidism, return the hyperthyroid patient to a normal metabolic state prior to thyroidectomy, and to control thyrotoxic crisis that may accompany thyroidectomy. The use of antithyroid thioamides is as effective in elderly as they are in younger adults; however, the expense, potential adverse effects, and inconvenience (compliance, monitoring) make them undesirable. The use of radioiodine due to ease of administration and less concern for long-term side effects and reproduction problems (some older males) makes it a more appropriate therapy.

Mechanism of Action Inhibits the synthesis of thyroid hormones by blocking the oxidation of iodine in the thyroid gland, blocking iodine's ability to combine with tyrosine to form thyroxine and triiodothyronine (T_3), does not inactivate circulating T_4 and T_3

Pharmacodynamics/Kinetics

Onset of action: Antithyroid: Oral: 12-18 hours

Duration: 36-72 hours

Distribution: Concentrated in thyroid gland; crosses placenta; enters breast milk (1:1)

Protein binding, plasma: None

Metabolism: Hepatic

Bioavailability: 80% to 95%

Half-life elimination: 4-13 hours

Excretion: Urine (80%)

Contraindications Hypersensitivity to methimazole or any component of the formulation; nursing mothers (per manufacturer; however, expert analysis and the AAP state this drug may be used with caution in nursing mothers); pregnancy

Warnings/Precautions Use with extreme caution in patients receiving other drugs known to cause myelosuppression particularly agranulocytosis, patients >40 years of age; avoid doses >40 mg/day (increased myelosuppression); may cause acneiform eruptions or worsen the condition of the thyroid

Drug Interactions **Inhibits** CYP1A2 (weak), 2A6 (weak), 2B6 (weak), 2C8/9 (weak), 2C19 (weak), 2D6 (moderate), 2E1 (weak), 3A4 (weak)

Beta-blockers: Methimazole may decrease beta-blocker clearance due to changes in thyroid function.

Digoxin: Methimazole may increase digoxin levels due to changes in thyroid function.

CYP2D6 substrates: Methimazole may increase the levels/effects of CYP2D6 substrates. Example substrates include amphetamines, selected beta-blockers, dextromethorphan, fluoxetine, lidocaine, mirtazapine, nefazodone, paroxetine, risperidone, ritonavir, thioridazine, tricyclic antidepressants, and venlafaxine.

CYP2D6 prodrug substrates: Methimazole may decrease the levels/effects of CYP2D6 prodrug substrates. Example prodrug substrates include codeine, hydrocodone, oxycodone, and tramadol.

Theophylline: Methimazole may decrease theophylline clearance due to changes in thyroid function.

Warfarin: Anticoagulant effect of warfarin may be decreased.

Adverse Reactions Frequency not defined.

Cardiovascular: Edema

Central nervous system: Headache, vertigo, drowsiness, CNS stimulation, depression

Dermatologic: Skin rash, urticaria, pruritus, erythema nodosum, skin pigmentation, exfoliative dermatitis, alopecia

Endocrine & metabolic: Goiter

Gastrointestinal: Nausea, vomiting, stomach pain, abnormal taste, constipation, weight gain, salivary gland swelling

Hematologic: Leukopenia, agranulocytosis, granulocytopenia, thrombocytopenia, aplastic anemia, hypoprothrombinemia

Hepatic: Cholestatic jaundice, jaundice, hepatitis

Neuromuscular & skeletal: Arthralgia, paresthesia

Renal: Nephrotic syndrome

Miscellaneous: SLE-like syndrome

Overdosage/Toxicology Symptoms of overdose include nausea, vomiting, epigastric distress, headache, fever, arthralgia, pruritus, edema, pancytopenia, and signs of hypothyroidism. Management of overdose is supportive.

Dosing

Adults & Elderly:

Hyperthyroidism: Oral: Administer in 3 equally divided doses at approximately 8-hour intervals

Initial: 15 mg/day for mild hyperthyroidism; 30-40 mg/day in moderately severe hyperthyroidism; 60 mg/day in severe hyperthyroidism; maintenance: 5-15 mg/day

Adjustment: Adjust dosage as required to achieve and maintain serum T_3, T_4, and TSH levels in the normal range. An elevated T_3 may be the sole indicator of inadequate treatment. An elevated TSH indicates excessive antithyroid treatment.

Pediatrics: Note: Administer in 3 equally divided doses at ~8-hour intervals.

Hyperthyroidism: Oral:

Initial: 0.4 mg/kg/day in 3 divided doses; maintenance: 0.2 mg/kg/day in 3 divided doses up to 30 mg/24 hours maximum

Alternatively: Initial: 0.5-0.7 mg/kg/day **or** 15-20 mg/m^2/day in 3 divided doses

Maintenance: $^1/_3$ to $^2/_3$ of the initial dose beginning when the patient is euthyroid

Maximum: 30 mg/24 hours

Available Dosage Forms

Tablet: 5 mg, 10 mg, 20 mg

Tapazole® 5 mg, 10 mg

Nursing Guidelines

Assessment: See Contraindications, Warnings/Precautions, and Dosing for use cautions. Assess potential for interactions with other prescriptions, OTC medications, or herbal products patient may be taking (see Drug Interactions). Assess results of laboratory tests (see below), therapeutic effectiveness, and adverse reactions (eg, hyper-/hypothyroidism - see Adverse Reactions and Overdose/Toxicology) during therapy. Teach patient proper use, possible side effects/appropriate interventions, and adverse symptoms to report (see Patient Education). **Pregnancy risk factor D** - determine that patient is not pregnant before beginning treatment. Instruct patient in appropriate use of contraceptive measures during therapy. See Lactation for breast-feeding considerations.

Monitoring Laboratory Tests: T_4, T_3, CBC with differential, liver function (baseline and as needed), serum thyroxine, free thyroxine index

Dietary Considerations: Should be taken consistently in relation to meals every day.

Patient Education: Inform prescriber of all prescriptions, OTC medications, or herbal products you are taking, and any allergies you have. Do not take any new medication during therapy unless approved by prescriber. Take as directed, at the same time each day, around-the-clock (eg, every 8 hours). Do not miss doses or make up missed doses. This drug will need to be taken for an extended period of time to achieve appropriate results. May cause nausea or vomiting (small, frequent meals may help); or dizziness or drowsiness (use caution when driving or engaging in tasks that require alertness until response to drug is known). Report rash, fever, unusual bleeding or bruising, unresolved headache, yellowing of eyes or skin, changes in color of urine or feces, or unresolved malaise. **Pregnancy/breast-feeding precautions:** Inform prescriber if you are pregnant and do not get pregnant while taking this medicine. Consult prescriber for appropriate contraceptive measures. Consult prescriber if breast-feeding.

Geriatric Considerations: The use of antithyroid thioamides is as effective in the elderly as in younger adults; however, the expense, potential adverse effects, and inconvenience (compliance, monitoring) make them undesirable.

Pregnancy Risk Factor: D

Pregnancy Issues: Hypothyroidism and congenital defects (rare) may occur.

Lactation: Enters breast milk/contraindicated (AAP rates "compatible")

Breast-Feeding Considerations: Use with caution; consider monitoring thyroid function in the infant (weekly or biweekly)

Perioperative/Anesthesia/Other Concerns: Hypothyroidism and congenital defects (rare) may occur. Agranulocytosis, when it occurs, is usually seen during the first several months of therapy and with maintenance doses >40 mg/day.

(Continued)

Methimazole *(Continued)*

Administration

Storage: Protect from light.

Methocarbamol (meth oh KAR ba mole)

U.S. Brand Names Robaxin®

Pharmacologic Category Skeletal Muscle Relaxant

Medication Safety Issues

Sound-alike/look-alike issues:

Methocarbamol may be confused with mephobarbital

Robaxin® may be confused with Rubex®

Use Treatment of muscle spasm associated with acute painful musculoskeletal conditions; supportive therapy in tetanus

Mechanism of Action Causes skeletal muscle relaxation by general CNS depression

Pharmacodynamics/Kinetics

Onset of action: Muscle relaxation: Oral: ~30 minutes

Protein binding: 46% to 50%

Metabolism: Hepatic via dealkylation and hydroxylation

Half-life elimination: 1-2 hours

Time to peak, serum: ~2 hours

Excretion: Urine (as metabolites)

Contraindications Hypersensitivity to methocarbamol or any component of the formulation; renal impairment (injection formulation)

Warnings/Precautions

Oral: Use caution with renal or hepatic impairment.

Injection: Rate of injection should not exceed 3 mL/minute; solution is hypertonic; avoid extravasation. Use with caution in patients with a history of seizures. Use caution with hepatic impairment.

Drug Interactions Increased effect/toxicity with CNS depressants; pyridostigmine (a single case of worsening myasthenia has been reported following methocarbamol administration)

Nutritional/Herbal/Ethanol Interactions

Ethanol: Avoid ethanol (may increase CNS depression).

Herb/Nutraceutical: Avoid valerian, St John's wort, kava kava, gotu kola (may increase CNS depression).

Lab Interactions May cause color interference in certain screening tests for 5-HIAA using nitrosonaphthol reagent and in screening tests for urinary VMA using the Gitlow method.

Adverse Reactions Frequency not defined.

Cardiovascular: Flushing of face, bradycardia, hypotension, syncope

Central nervous system: Drowsiness, dizziness, lightheadedness, convulsion, vertigo, headache, fever, amnesia, confusion, insomnia, sedation, coordination impaired (mild)

Dermatologic: Allergic dermatitis, urticaria, pruritus, rash, angioneurotic edema

Gastrointestinal: Nausea, vomiting, metallic taste, dyspepsia

Hematologic: Leukopenia

Hepatic: Jaundice

Local: Pain at injection site, thrombophlebitis

Ocular: Nystagmus, blurred vision, diplopia, conjunctivitis

Renal: Renal impairment

Respiratory: Nasal congestion

Miscellaneous: Allergic manifestations, anaphylactic reaction

Overdosage/Toxicology Symptoms of overdose include cardiac arrhythmias, nausea, vomiting, drowsiness, and coma. Treatment is supportive.

Dosing

Adults:

Muscle spasm:

Oral: 1.5 g 4 times/day for 2-3 days (up to 8 g/day may be given in severe conditions), then decrease to 4-4.5 g/day in 3-6 divided doses

I.M., I.V.: 1 g every 8 hours if oral not possible; injection should not be used for more than 3 consecutive days. If condition persists, may repeat course of therapy after a drug-free interval of 48 hours.

Tetanus: I.V.: Initial dose: 1-3 g; may repeat dose every 6 hours until oral dosing is possible; injection should not be used for more than 3 consecutive days

Elderly: Muscle spasm: Oral: Initial: 500 mg 4 times/day; titrate to response

Pediatrics:

Tetanus (recommended **only** for use in tetanus): I.V.: 15 mg/kg/dose or 500 mg/m²/dose, may repeat every 6 hours if needed; maximum dose: 1.8 g/m²/day for 3 days only

Muscle spasm: Children ≥16 years: Refer to adult dosing.

Renal Impairment: Do not administer parenteral formulation to patients with renal dysfunction.

Hepatic Impairment: Specific dosing guidelines are not available. Plasma protein binding and clearance are decreased; half-life is increased.

Available Dosage Forms

Injection, solution: 100 mg/mL (10 mL) [in polyethylene glycol; vial stopper contains latex]

Tablet: 500 mg, 750 mg

Nursing Guidelines

Assessment: Assess other medications for excess CNS depression. Monitor effectiveness of therapy (according to rationale for therapy) and adverse reactions at beginning and periodically during therapy. Monitor I.V. site closely to prevent extravasation. Assess knowledge/teach patient appropriate use, interventions to reduce side effects, and adverse symptoms to report.

Patient Education: Take exactly as directed. Do not increase dose or discontinue without consulting prescriber. Do not use alcohol, prescriptive or OTC antidepressants, sedatives, or pain medications without consulting prescriber. You may experience drowsiness, dizziness, lightheadedness (avoid driving or engaging in tasks requiring alertness until response to drug is known); or nausea or vomiting (small frequent meals, frequent mouth care, or sucking hard candy may help). Report excessive drowsiness or mental agitation, chest pain, skin rash, swelling of mouth/face, difficulty speaking, or vision changes. **Pregnancy/breast-feeding precautions:** Inform prescriber if you are or intend to become pregnant. Consult prescriber if breast-feeding.

Geriatric Considerations: There is no specific information on the use of skeletal muscle relaxants in the elderly. Methocarbamol has a short half-life, so it may be considered one of the safer agents in this class.

Pregnancy Risk Factor: C

Lactation: Excretion in breast milk unknown/use caution

Administration

Oral: Tablets may be crushed and mixed with food or liquid if needed. Avoid alcohol.

I.M.: A maximum of 5 mL can be administered into each gluteal region.

I.V.: Maximum rate: 3 mL/minute; injection should not be used for more than 3 consecutive days; may be administered undiluted

Reconstitution: Injection may be diluted to 4 mg/mL in sterile water, 5% dextrose, or 0.9% saline.

Storage:

Injection: Prior to dilution, store at controlled room temperature of 20°C to 25°C (68°F to 77°F). Injection when diluted to 4 mg/mL in sterile water, 5% dextrose, or 0.9% saline is stable for 6 days at room temperature; do **not** refrigerate after dilution

Tablet: Store at controlled room temperature of 20°C to 25°C (68°F to 77°F).

Methohexital (meth oh HEKS i tal)

U.S. Brand Names Brevital® Sodium

Synonyms Methohexital Sodium

Pharmacologic Category Barbiturate

Medication Safety Issues

Sound-alike/look-alike issues:

Brevital® may be confused with Brevibloc®

Use Induction and maintenance of general anesthesia for short procedures

Can be used in pediatric patients ≥1 month of age as follows: For rectal or intramuscular induction of anesthesia prior to the use of other general anesthetic agents, as an adjunct to subpotent inhalational anesthetic agents for short surgical procedures, or for short surgical, diagnostic, or therapeutic procedures associated with minimal painful stimuli

Unlabeled/Investigational Use Wada test

Mechanism of Action Ultra short-acting I.V. barbiturate anesthetic

Pharmacodynamics/Kinetics

Onset of action: I.V.: Immediately

(Continued)

Methohexital *(Continued)*

Duration: Single dose: 10-20 minutes

Contraindications Hypersensitivity to methohexital or any component of the formulation; porphyria

Warnings/Precautions Use with extreme caution in patients with liver impairment, asthma, cardiovascular instability

Drug Interactions

Acetaminophen: Barbiturates may enhance the hepatotoxic potential of acetaminophen overdoses

Antiarrhythmics: Barbiturates may increase the metabolism of antiarrhythmics, decreasing their clinical effect; includes disopyramide, propafenone, and quinidine

Anticonvulsants: Barbiturates may increase the metabolism of anticonvulsants; includes ethosuximide, felbamate (possibly), lamotrigine, phenytoin, tiagabine, topiramate, and zonisamide; does not appear to affect gabapentin or levetiracetam

Antineoplastics: Limited evidence suggests that enzyme-inducing anticonvulsant therapy may reduce the effectiveness of some chemotherapy regimens (specifically in ALL); teniposide and methotrexate may be cleared more rapidly in these patients

Antipsychotics: Barbiturates may enhance the metabolism (decrease the efficacy) of antipsychotics; monitor for altered response; dose adjustment may be needed

Beta-blockers: Metabolism of beta-blockers may be increased and clinical effect decreased; atenolol and nadolol are unlikely to interact given their renal elimination

Calcium channel blockers: Barbiturates may enhance the metabolism of calcium channel blockers, decreasing their clinical effect

Chloramphenicol: Barbiturates may increase the metabolism of chloramphenicol and chloramphenicol may inhibit barbiturate metabolism; monitor for altered response

Cimetidine: Barbiturates may enhance the metabolism of cimetidine, decreasing its clinical effect

CNS depressants: Sedative effects and/or respiratory depression with barbiturates may be additive with other CNS depressants; monitor for increased effect; includes ethanol, sedatives, antidepressants, narcotic analgesics, and benzodiazepines

Corticosteroids: Barbiturates may enhance the metabolism of corticosteroids, decreasing their clinical effect

Cyclosporine: Levels may be decreased by barbiturates; monitor

Doxycycline: Barbiturates may enhance the metabolism of doxycycline, decreasing its clinical effect; higher dosages may be required

Estrogens: Barbiturates may increase the metabolism of estrogens and reduce their efficacy

Felbamate may inhibit the metabolism of barbiturates and barbiturates may increase the metabolism of felbamate

Griseofulvin: Barbiturates may impair the absorption of griseofulvin, and griseofulvin metabolism may be increased by barbiturates, decreasing clinical effect

Guanfacine: Effect may be decreased by barbiturates

Immunosuppressants: Barbiturates may enhance the metabolism of immunosuppressants, decreasing its clinical effect; includes both cyclosporine and tacrolimus

Loop diuretics: Metabolism may be increased and clinical effects decreased; established for furosemide, effect with other loop diuretics not established

MAO inhibitors: Metabolism of barbiturates may be inhibited, increasing clinical effect or toxicity of the barbiturates

Methadone: Barbiturates may enhance the metabolism of methadone resulting in methadone withdrawal

Methoxyflurane: Barbiturates may enhance the nephrotoxic effects of methoxyflurane

Oral contraceptives: Barbiturates may enhance the metabolism of oral contraceptives, decreasing their clinical effect; an alternative method of contraception should be considered

Theophylline: Barbiturates may increase metabolism of theophylline derivatives and decrease their clinical effect

Tricyclic antidepressants: Barbiturates may increase metabolism of tricyclic antidepressants and decrease their clinical effect; sedative effects may be additive

Valproic acid: Metabolism of barbiturates may be inhibited by valproic acid; monitor for excessive sedation; a dose reduction may be needed

Warfarin: Barbiturates inhibit the hypoprothrombinemic effects of oral anticoagulants via increased metabolism; this combination should generally be avoided

Adverse Reactions Frequency not defined.

Cardiovascular: Hypotension, peripheral vascular collapse

Central nervous system: Seizures, headache

Gastrointestinal: Cramping, diarrhea, rectal bleeding, nausea, vomiting, abdominal pain

Hematologic: Hemolytic anemia, thrombophlebitis

Hepatic: Transaminases increased

Local: Pain on I.M. injection

Neuromuscular & skeletal: Tremor, twitching, rigidity, involuntary muscle movement, radial nerve palsy

Respiratory: Apnea, respiratory depression, laryngospasm, cough, hiccups

Overdosage/Toxicology

Symptoms of overdose include apnea, tachycardia, hypotension

Treatment is primarily supportive with mechanical ventilation if needed

Dosing

Adults & Elderly:

Anesthesia (doses must be titrated to effect): I.V.: Induction: 50-120 mg to start; 20-40 mg every 4-7 minutes

Wada test (unlabeled): I.V.: 3-4 mg over 3 second; following signs of recovery, administer a second dose of 2 mg over 2 seconds

Pediatrics: Anesthesia: Doses must be titrated to effect

Manufacturer's recommendations:

Infants <1 month: Safety and efficacy not established

Infants ≥ 1 month and Children:

I.M.: Induction: 6.6-10 mg/kg of a 5% solution

Rectal: Induction: Usual: 25 mg/kg of a 1% solution

Alternative pediatric dosing:

Children 3-12 years:

I.M.: Preoperative: 5-10 mg/kg/dose

I.V.: Induction: 1-2 mg/kg/dose

Rectal: Preoperative/induction: 20-35 mg/kg/dose; usual: 25 mg/kg/dose; maximum dose: 500 mg/dose; give as 10% aqueous solution

Hepatic Impairment: Lower dosage and monitor closely.

Available Dosage Forms Injection, powder for reconstitution, as sodium: 500 mg, 2.5 g, 5 g

Nursing Guidelines

Dietary Considerations: Should not be given to patients with food in stomach because of danger of vomiting during anesthesia.

Patient Education: May cause drowsiness

Pregnancy Risk Factor: C

Perioperative/Anesthesia/Other Concerns: Methohexital does not possess analgesic properties.

Administration

I.V.: Dilute to a maximum concentration of 1% for I.V. use; for Wada testing, a dilution of 1 mg/mL has been reported

Compatibility: Stable in D_5LR, D_5NS, D_5W, LR, NS

Compatibility in syringe: Incompatible with glycopyrrolate

Compatibility when admixed: Incompatible with atracurium, atropine, chlorpromazine, cimetidine, clindamycin, droperidol, fentanyl, hydralazine, kanamycin, lidocaine, mechlorethamine, methyldopate, metocurine, pancuronium, pentazocine, prochlorperazine mesylate, promazine, promethazine, propiomazine, scopolamine, streptomycin, succinylcholine, thiamine, tubocurarine

Related Information

Conscious Sedation *on page 1779*

Intravenous Anesthetic Agents *on page 1853*

♦ **Methohexital Sodium** *see* Methohexital *on page 1125*

Methotrexate (meth oh TREKS ate)

U.S. Brand Names Rheumatrex®; Trexall™

Synonyms Amethopterin; Methotrexate Sodium; MTX (error-prone abbreviation); NSC-740

(Continued)

Methotrexate *(Continued)*

Pharmacologic Category Antineoplastic Agent, Antimetabolite (Antifolate)

Medication Safety Issues

Sound-alike/look-alike issues:

Methotrexate may be confused with metolazone, mitoxantrone

MTX is an error-prone abbreviation (mistaken as mitoxantrone)

High alert medication: The Institute for Safe Medication Practices (ISMP) includes this medication among its list of drugs which have a heightened risk of causing significant patient harm when used in error.

Errors have occurred (resulting in death) when oral methotrexate was administered as "daily" dose instead of the recommended "weekly" dose.

Use Treatment of trophoblastic neoplasms; leukemias; psoriasis; rheumatoid arthritis (RA), including polyarticular-course juvenile rheumatoid arthritis (JRA); breast, head and neck, and lung carcinomas; osteosarcoma; soft-tissue sarcomas; carcinoma of gastrointestinal tract, esophagus, testes; lymphomas

Unlabeled/Investigational Use

Treatment and maintenance of remission in Crohn's disease

Mechanism of Action Methotrexate is a folate antimetabolite that inhibits DNA synthesis. Methotrexate irreversibly binds to dihydrofolate reductase, inhibiting the formation of reduced folates, and thymidylate synthetase, resulting in inhibition of purine and thymidylic acid synthesis. Methotrexate is cell cycle specific for the S phase of the cycle.

The MOA in the treatment of rheumatoid arthritis is unknown, but may affect immune function. In psoriasis, methotrexate is thought to target rapidly proliferating epithelial cells in the skin.

In Crohn's disease, it may have immune modulator and anti-inflammatory activity

Pharmacodynamics/Kinetics

Onset of action: Antirheumatic: 3-6 weeks; additional improvement may continue longer than 12 weeks

Absorption: Oral: Rapid; well absorbed at low doses (<30 mg/m^2), incomplete after large doses; I.M.: Complete

Distribution: Penetrates slowly into 3rd space fluids (eg, pleural effusions, ascites), exits slowly from these compartments (slower than from plasma); crosses placenta; small amounts enter breast milk; sustained concentrations retained in kidney and liver

Protein binding: 50%

Metabolism: <10%; degraded by intestinal flora to DAMPA by carboxypeptidase; hepatic aldehyde oxidase converts methotrexate to 7-OH methotrexate; polyglutamates are produced intracellularly and are just as potent as methotrexate; their production is dose- and duration-dependent and they are slowly eliminated by the cell once formed

Half-life elimination: Low dose: 3-10 hours; High dose: 8-12 hours

Time to peak, serum: Oral: 1-2 hours; I.M.: 30-60 minutes

Excretion: Urine (44% to 100%); feces (small amounts)

Contraindications Hypersensitivity to methotrexate or any component of the formulation; severe renal or hepatic impairment; pre-existing profound bone marrow suppression in patients with psoriasis or rheumatoid arthritis, alcoholic liver disease, AIDS, pre-existing blood dyscrasias; pregnancy (in patients with psoriasis or rheumatoid arthritis); breast-feeding

Warnings/Precautions Hazardous agent - use appropriate precautions for handling and disposal. May cause potentially life-threatening pneumonitis (may occur at any time during therapy and at any dosage); monitor closely for pulmonary symptoms, particularly dry, nonproductive cough. Methotrexate may cause photosensitivity and/or severe dermatologic reactions which are not dose-related. Methotrexate has been associated with acute and chronic hepatotoxicity, fibrosis, and cirrhosis. Risk is related to cumulative dose and prolonged exposure. Ethanol abuse, obesity, advanced age, and diabetes may increase the risk of hepatotoxic reactions.

Methotrexate may cause renal failure, gastrointestinal toxicity, or bone marrow depression. Use with caution in patients with renal impairment, peptic ulcer disease, ulcerative colitis, or pre-existing bone marrow suppression. Diarrhea and ulcerative stomatitis may require interruption of therapy; death from hemorrhagic enteritis or intestinal perforation has been reported. Methotrexate penetrates slowly into 3rd space fluids, such as pleural effusions or ascites, and exits slowly from these compartments (slower than from plasma). Dosage reduction may be necessary in patients with renal or hepatic impairment, ascites, and pleural effusion. Toxicity from methotrexate or any immunosuppressive is increased in the elderly.

Severe bone marrow suppression, aplastic anemia, and GI toxicity have occurred during concomitant administration with NSAIDs. Use caution when used with other hepatotoxic agents (azathioprine, retinoids, sulfasalazine). Methotrexate given concomitantly with radiotherapy may increase the risk of soft tissue necrosis and osteonecrosis. Immune suppression may lead to opportunistic infections.

For rheumatoid arthritis and psoriasis, immunosuppressive therapy should only be used when disease is active and less toxic; traditional therapy is ineffective. Discontinue therapy in RA or psoriasis if a significant decrease in hematologic components is noted. Methotrexate formulations and/or diluents containing preservatives should not be used for intrathecal or high-dose therapy. Methotrexate injection may contain benzyl alcohol and should not be used in neonates.

Drug Interactions

Acitretin: May enhance the hepatotoxic effect of methotrexate. Avoid concurrent use.

Cholestyramine: May decrease levels of methotrexate.

Corticosteroids: May decrease uptake of methotrexate into leukemia cells. Administration of these drugs should be separated by 12 hours. Dexamethasone has been reported to not affect methotrexate influx into cells.

Cyclosporine: Concomitant administration with methotrexate may increase levels and toxicity of each.

Cytarabine: Methotrexate, when administered prior to cytarabine, may enhance the efficacy and toxicity of cytarabine. Some combination treatment regimens (eg, hyper-CVAD) have been designed to take advantage of this interaction.

Hepatotoxic agents (azathioprine, retinoids, sulfasalazine) may increase the risk of hepatotoxic reactions

Mercaptopurine: Methotrexate may increase mercaptopurine levels. Dosage adjustment may be required.

NSAIDs: Severe bone marrow suppression, aplastic anemia, and GI toxicity have been reported with concomitant therapy. Should not be used during moderate or high-dose methotrexate due to increased and prolonged methotrexate levels (may increase toxicity); NSAID use during treatment of rheumatoid arthritis has not been fully explored, but continuation of prior regimen has been allowed in some circumstances, with cautious monitoring

Penicillins: May increase methotrexate concentrations (due to a reduction in renal tubular secretion). Primarily a concern with high doses of penicillins and higher dosages of methotrexate.

Probenecid: May increase methotrexate concentrations (due to a reduction in renal tubular secretion). Primarily a concern with higher dosages of methotrexate.

Salicylates: May increase the serum concentration of Methotrexate. Salicylate doses used for prophylaxis of cardiovascular events are not likely to be of concern.

Sulfonamides: May increase methotrexate concentrations (due to a reduction in renal tubular secretion). In addition, sulfonamides may reduce folate levels, increasing the risk/severity of bone marrow suppression. Particularly a concern with higher dosages of methotrexate.

Tetracyclines: May increase methotrexate toxicity; monitor

Theophylline: Methotrexate may increase theophylline levels.

Vaccines (live virus): Concurrent use with methotrexate may result in vaccinia infections.

Nutritional/Herbal/Ethanol Interactions

Ethanol: Avoid ethanol (may be associated with increased liver injury).

Food: Methotrexate peak serum levels may be decreased if taken with food. Milk-rich foods may decrease methotrexate absorption. Folate may decrease drug response.

Herb/Nutraceutical: Avoid echinacea (has immunostimulant properties).

Adverse Reactions Note: Adverse reactions vary by route and dosage. Hematologic and/or gastrointestinal toxicities may be common at dosages used in chemotherapy; these reactions are much less frequent when used at typical dosages for rheumatic diseases.

(Continued)

Methotrexate *(Continued)*

>10%:

Central nervous system (with I.T. administration or very high-dose therapy):

Arachnoiditis: Acute reaction manifested as severe headache, nuchal rigidity, vomiting, and fever; may be alleviated by reducing the dose

Subacute toxicity: 10% of patients treated with 12-15 mg/m^2 of I.T. methotrexate may develop this in the second or third week of therapy; consists of motor paralysis of extremities, cranial nerve palsy, seizure, or coma. This has also been seen in pediatric cases receiving very high-dose I.V. methotrexate.

Demyelinating encephalopathy: Seen months or years after receiving methotrexate; usually in association with cranial irradiation or other systemic chemotherapy

Dermatologic: Reddening of skin

Endocrine & metabolic: Hyperuricemia, defective oogenesis or spermatogenesis

Gastrointestinal: Ulcerative stomatitis, glossitis, gingivitis, nausea, vomiting, diarrhea, anorexia, intestinal perforation, mucositis (dose dependent; appears in 3-7 days after therapy, resolving within 2 weeks)

Hematologic: Leukopenia, thrombocytopenia

Renal: Renal failure, azotemia, nephropathy

Respiratory: Pharyngitis

1% to 10%:

Cardiovascular: Vasculitis

Central nervous system: Dizziness, malaise, encephalopathy, seizure, fever, chills

Dermatologic: Alopecia, rash, photosensitivity, depigmentation or hyperpigmentation of skin

Endocrine & metabolic: Diabetes

Genitourinary: Cystitis

Hematologic: Hemorrhage

Myelosuppressive: This is the primary dose-limiting factor (along with mucositis) of methotrexate; occurs about 5-7 days after methotrexate therapy, and should resolve within 2 weeks

WBC: Mild

Platelets: Moderate

Onset: 7 days

Nadir: 10 days

Recovery: 21 days

Hepatic: Cirrhosis and portal fibrosis have been associated with chronic methotrexate therapy; acute elevation of liver enzymes are common after high-dose methotrexate, and usually resolve within 10 days.

Neuromuscular & skeletal: Arthralgia

Ocular: Blurred vision

Renal: Renal dysfunction: Manifested by an abrupt rise in serum creatinine and BUN and a fall in urine output; more common with high-dose methotrexate, and may be due to precipitation of the drug.

Respiratory: Pneumonitis: Associated with fever, cough, and interstitial pulmonary infiltrates; treatment is to withhold methotrexate during the acute reaction; interstitial pneumonitis has been reported to occur with an incidence of 1% in patients with RA (dose 7.5-15 mg/week)

<1% (Limited to important or life-threatening): Acute neurologic syndrome (at high dosages - symptoms include confusion, hemiparesis, transient blindness, and coma); anaphylaxis, alveolitis, cognitive dysfunction (has been reported at low dosage), decreased resistance to infection, erythema multiforme, hepatic failure, leukoencephalopathy (especially following craniospinal irradiation or repeated high-dose therapy), lymphoproliferative disorders, osteonecrosis and soft tissue necrosis (with radiotherapy), pericarditis, plaque erosions (psoriasis), seizure (more frequent in pediatric patients with ALL), Stevens-Johnson syndrome, thromboembolism

Overdosage/Toxicology Symptoms of overdose include nausea, vomiting, alopecia, melena, and renal failure. Administer leucovorin (see Dosage).

Hydration and alkalinization may be used to prevent precipitation of methotrexate or methotrexate metabolites in the renal tubules. Severe bone marrow toxicity can result from overdose. Generally, neither peritoneal nor hemodialysis have been shown to increase elimination. However, effective clearance of methotrexate has been reported with acute, intermittent hemodialysis using a high-flux dialyzer.

Dosing

Adults: Refer to individual protocols.

Note: Doses between 100-500 mg/m^2 **may require** leucovorin rescue. Doses >500 mg/m^2 **require** leucovorin rescue: I.V., I.M., Oral: Leucovorin 10-15 mg/m^2 every 6 hours for 8 or 10 doses, starting 24 hours after the start of methotrexate infusion. Continue until the methotrexate level is ≤0.1 micromolar (10^{-7}M). Some clinicians continue leucovorin until the methotrexate level is <0.05 micromolar (5 x 10^{-8}M) or 0.01 micromolar (10^{-8}M).

If the 48-hour methotrexate level is >1 micromolar (10^{-7}M) or the 72-hour methotrexate level is >0.2 micromolar (2 x 10^{-7}M): I.V., I.M, Oral: Leucovorin 100 mg/m^2 every 6 hours until the methotrexate level is ≤0.1 micromolar (10^{-7}M). Some clinicians continue leucovorin until the methotrexate level is <0.05 micromolar (5 x 10^{-8}M) or 0.01 micromolar (10^{-8}M).

Antineoplastic dosage range: I.V.: Range is wide from 30-40 mg/m^2/week to 100-12,000 mg/m^2 with leucovorin rescue

Trophoblastic neoplasms:
Oral, I.M.: 15-30 mg/day for 5 days; repeat in 7 days for 3-5 courses
I.V.: 11 mg/m^2 days 1 through 5 every 3 weeks

Head and neck cancer: Oral, I.M., I.V.: 25-50 mg/m^2 once weekly

Mycosis fungoides (cutaneous T-cell lymphoma): Oral, I.M.: Initial (early stages):
5-50 mg once weekly **or**
15-37.5 mg twice weekly

Bladder cancer: I.V.:
30 mg/m^2 day 1 and 8 every 3 weeks **or**
30 mg/m^2 day 1, 15, and 22 every 4 weeks

Breast cancer: I.V.: 30-60 mg/m^2 Day 1 and 8 every 3-4 weeks

Gastric cancer: I.V.:1500 mg/m^2 every 4 weeks

Lymphoma, non-Hodgkin's: I.V.:
30 mg/m^2 days 3 and 10 every 3 weeks **or**
120 mg/m^2 day 8 and 15 every 3-4 weeks **or**
200 mg/m^2 day 8 and 15 every 3 weeks **or**
400 mg/m^2 every 4 weeks for 3 cycles **or**
1 g/m^2 every 3 weeks **or**
1.5 g/m^2 every 4 weeks

Sarcoma: I.V.: 8-12 g/m^2 weekly for 2-4 weeks

Rheumatoid arthritis: Oral: 7.5 mg once weekly **or** 2.5 mg every 12 hours for 3 doses/week, not to exceed 20 mg/week

Psoriasis: Oral: 2.5-5 mg/dose every 12 hours for 3 doses given weekly **or** Oral, I.M.: 10-25 mg/dose given once weekly

Ectopic pregnancy: I.M., I.V.: 50 mg/m^2 single-dose

Active Crohn's disease (unlabeled use): Induction of remission: I.M., SubQ: 15-25 mg once weekly; remission maintenance: 15 mg once weekly

Note: Oral dosing has been reported as effective but oral absorption is highly variable. If patient relapses after a switch to oral, may consider returning to injectable.

Elderly: Refer to individual protocols; adjust for renal impairment.

Rheumatoid arthritis/psoriasis: Oral: Initial: 5-7.5 mg/week, not to exceed 20 mg/week

Pediatrics: Refer to individual protocols.

Note: Doses between 100-500 mg/m^2 **may require** leucovorin rescue. Doses >500 mg/m^2 **require** leucovorin rescue: I.V., I.M., Oral: Leucovorin 10-15 mg/m^2 every 6 hours for 8 or 10 doses, starting 24 hours after the start of methotrexate infusion. Continue until the methotrexate level is ≤0.1 micromolar (10^{-7}M). Some clinicians continue leucovorin until the methotrexate level is <0.05 micromolar (5 x 10^{-8}M) or 0.01 micromolar (10^{-8}M).

If the 48-hour methotrexate level is >1 micromolar (10^{-7}M) or the 72-hour methotrexate level is >0.2 micromolar (2 x 10^{-7}M): I.V., I.M, Oral: Leucovorin 100 mg/m^2 every 6 hours until the methotrexate level is ≤0.1 micromolar (10^{-7}M). Some clinicians continue leucovorin until the methotrexate level is <0.05 micromolar (5 x 10^{-8}M) or 0.01 micromolar (10^{-8}M).

Dermatomyositis: Oral: 15-20 mg/m^2/week as a single dose once weekly **or** 0.3-1 mg/kg/dose once weekly

Juvenile rheumatoid arthritis: Oral, I.M.:10 mg/m^2 once weekly, then 5-15 mg/m^2/week as a single dose **or** as 3 divided doses given 12 hours apart

Antineoplastic dosage range:
Oral, I.M.: 7.5-30 mg/m^2/week **or** every 2 weeks

(Continued)

Methotrexate *(Continued)*

I.V.: 10-18,000 mg/m² bolus dosing **or** continuous infusion over 6-42 hours
For dosing schedules, see table.

Methotrexate Dosing Schedules

Dose	Route	Frequency
Conventional		
15-20 mg/m²	P.O.	Twice weekly
30-50 mg/m²	P.O., I.V.	Weekly
15 mg/day for 5 days	P.O., I.M.	Every 2-3 weeks
Intermediate		
50-150 mg/m²*	I.V. push	Every 2-3 weeks
240 mg/m²*	I.V. infusion	Every 4-7 days
0.5-1 g/m²**	I.V. infusion	Every 2-3 weeks
High		
1-25 g/m²*	I.V. infusion	Every 1-3 weeks

*Doses between 100-500 mg/m² may require leucovorin rescue in some patients.

**Followed with leucovorin rescue - refer to Leucovorin monograph for details.

Pediatric solid tumors (high-dose): I.V.:
<12 years: 12-25 g/m²
≥12 years: 8 g/m²

Acute lymphocytic leukemia (intermediate-dose): I.V.: Loading: 100 mg/m² bolus dose, followed by 900 mg/m²/day infusion over 23-41 hours.

Meningeal leukemia: I.T.: 10-15 mg/m² (maximum dose: 15 mg) **or** an age-based dosing regimen; one possible system is:
≤3 months: 3 mg/dose
4-11 months: 6 mg/dose
1 year: 8 mg/dose
2 years: 10 mg/dose
≥3 years: 12 mg/dose

Renal Impairment:
Cl_{cr} 61-80 mL/minute: Reduce dose to 75%.
Cl_{cr} 51-60 mL/minute: Reduce dose to 70%.
Cl_{cr} 10-50 mL/minute: Reduce dose to 30% to 50%.
Cl_{cr} <10 mL/minute: Avoid use.
Hemodialysis effects: Not dialyzable (0% to 5%)
Supplemental dose is not necessary.
Peritoneal dialysis effects: Supplemental dose is not necessary.
CAVH effects: Unknown

Hepatic Impairment:
Bilirubin 3.1-5 mg/dL or AST >180 units: Administer 75% of dose.
Bilirubin >5 mg/dL: Do not use.

Available Dosage Forms

Injection, powder for reconstitution [preservative free]: 20 mg, 1 g
Injection, solution: 25 mg/mL (2 mL, 10 mL) [contains benzyl alcohol]
Injection, solution [preservative free]: 25 mg/mL (2 mL, 4 mL, 8 mL, 10 mL)
Tablet: 2.5 mg
Trexall™: 5 mg, 7.5 mg, 10 mg, 15 mg
Tablet, as sodium [dose pack] (Rheumatrex® Dose Pack): 2.5 mg (4 cards with 2, 3, 4, 5, or 6 tablets each)

Nursing Guidelines

Assessment: Monitor closely if used in presence of preexisting conditions that increase potential for toxicity (eg, renal impairment, peptic ulcer disease, ulcerative colitis, hepatic impairment, bone marrow suppression). Assess potential for interactions with other pharmacological agents and herbal products patient may be using (eg, NSAIDs and salicylates or other hepatotoxic agents, or drugs that may effect the levels/effects of methotrexate). Evaluate results of laboratory tests prior to therapy and at frequent intervals during therapy. Patient should be monitored closely for adverse reactions (eg, hyper- or hypothyroidism, pneumonitis [dry, nonproductive cough], gastrointestinal disturbance [ulcerative stomatitis, pain, intestinal perforation], renal failure [decreased urine output]). Assess effectiveness at regular intervals (according to purpose for use). Teach patient proper use, possible side effects/appropriate interventions, and adverse symptoms to report. **Pregnancy risk factor X:** Determine that patient is not pregnant before beginning treatment. Instruct patient of childbearing age (or males who may have intercourse with women of childbearing age) in appropriate use of contraceptive measures during therapy and for 3 months following treatment of males or 1 ovulatory cycle in females.

Monitoring Laboratory Tests: For prolonged use (especially rheumatoid arthritis, psoriasis) a baseline liver biopsy, repeated at each 1-1.5 g cumulative dose interval, should be performed; WBC and platelet counts every 4 weeks; CBC and creatinine, LFTs every 3-4 months; chest x-ray

Dietary Considerations:

Sodium content of 100 mg injection: 20 mg (0.86 mEq)

Sodium content of 100 mg (low sodium) injection: 15 mg (0.65 mEq)

Patient Education: Do not take any new medication during therapy unless approved by prescriber. **Infusion/injection:** Report immediately any redness, swelling, pain, or burning at infusion/injection site. It is very important to maintain adequate hydration (2-3 L/day of fluids) unless instructed to restrict fluid intake and nutrition (small frequent meals may help). Avoid alcohol to prevent serious side effects. You will be more susceptible to infection (avoid crowds and exposure to infection and do not have any vaccinations without consulting prescriber). May cause sensitivity to sunlight (use sunscreen, wear protective clothing, and eyewear); nausea or vomiting (small frequent meals, frequent mouth care, sucking lozenges, or chewing gum may help; if unresolved, contact prescriber); drowsiness, dizziness, numbness, or blurred vision (use caution when driving or engaging in tasks that require alertness until response to drug is known); loss of hair (may be reversible); color change of skin; permanent sterility; or mouth sores (frequent mouth care with soft toothbrush or cotton swabs and frequent rinses may help). Report immediately any rash, excessive or unusual fatigue, or respiratory difficulty. Report rapid heartbeat or palpitations, black or tarry stools, fever, chills, unusual bleeding or bruising, shortness of breath, persistent GI disturbances, diarrhea, constipation, pain on urination or change in urinary patterns, or any other persistent adverse effects. **Pregnancy/breast-feeding precautions:** Do not get pregnant while taking this medication. Consult prescriber for appropriate contraceptive measures. This drug may cause birth defects. Do not breast-feed.

Geriatric Considerations: Toxicity to methotrexate or any immunosuppressive is increased in the elderly. Must monitor carefully. For rheumatoid arthritis and psoriasis, immunosuppressive therapy should only be used when disease is active and less toxic, traditional therapy is ineffective. Recommended doses should be reduced when initiating therapy in the elderly due to possible decreased metabolism, reduced renal function, and presence of interacting diseases and drugs. Adjust dose as needed for renal function (Cl_{cr}).

Pregnancy Risk Factor: X (psoriasis, rheumatoid arthritis)

Lactation: Enters breast milk/contraindicated

Administration

I.M.: May be administered I.M.

I.V.: May be administered I.V.; I.V. administration may be as slow push, short bolus infusion, or 24- to 42-hour continuous infusion

Specific dosing schemes vary, but high dose should be followed by leucovorin calcium to prevent toxicity; refer to Leucovorin monograph *on page 1013*

Reconstitution: Dilute powder with D_5W or NS to a concentration of ≤25 mg/mL (20 mg and 50 mg vials) and 50 mg/mL (1 g vial). Intrathecal solutions may be reconstituted to 2.5-5 mg/mL with NS, D_5W, lactated Ringer's, or Elliott's B solution. **Use preservative free preparations for intrathecal or high-dose administration.**

Compatibility: Stable in D_5NS, D_5W, NS

Y-site administration: Incompatible with chlorpromazine, gemcitabine, idarubicin, ifosfamide, midazolam, nalbuphine, promethazine, propofol

Compatibility when admixed: Incompatible with bleomycin

Storage: Store tablets and intact vials at room temperature (15°C to 25°C); protect from light. Solution diluted in D_5W or NS is stable for 24 hours at room temperature (21°C to 25°C). Reconstituted solutions with a preservative may be stored under refrigeration for up to 3 months, and up to 4 weeks at room temperature. Intrathecal dilutions are stable at room temperature for 7 days, but it is generally recommended that they be used within 4-8 hours.

♦ **Methotrexate Sodium** *see* Methotrexate *on page 1127*

♦ **Methylacetoxyprogesterone** *see* MedroxyPROGESTERone *on page 1085*

Methylene Blue (METH i leen bloo)

U.S. Brand Names Urolene Blue®

Pharmacologic Category Antidote

Medication Safety Issues Due to potential toxicity (hemolytic anemia), do not use methylene blue to color enteral feedings to detect aspiration.

Use Antidote for cyanide poisoning and drug-induced methemoglobinemia, indicator dye

Unlabeled/Investigational Use Has been used topically (0.1% solutions) in conjunction with polychromatic light to photoinactivate viruses such as herpes simplex; has been used alone or in combination with vitamin C for the management of chronic urolithiasis

Mechanism of Action Weak germicide in low concentrations, hastens the conversion of methemoglobin to hemoglobin; has opposite effect at high concentrations by converting ferrous ion of reduced hemoglobin to ferric ion to form methemoglobin; in cyanide toxicity, it combines with cyanide to form cyanmethemoglobin preventing the interference of cyanide with the cytochrome system

Pharmacodynamics/Kinetics

Absorption: Oral: 53% to 97%

Excretion: Urine and feces

Contraindications Hypersensitivity to methylene blue or any component of the formulation; intraspinal injection; renal insufficiency; pregnancy (injected intra-amniotically)

Warnings/Precautions Do not inject SubQ or intrathecally; use with caution in young patients and in patients with G6PD deficiency; continued use can cause profound anemia

Adverse Reactions Frequency not defined.

Cardiovascular: Hypertension, precordial pain

Central nervous system: Dizziness, mental confusion, headache, fever

Dermatologic: Staining of skin

Gastrointestinal: Fecal discoloration (blue-green), nausea, vomiting, abdominal pain

Genitourinary: Discoloration of urine (blue-green), bladder irritation

Hematologic: Anemia

Miscellaneous: Diaphoresis

Overdosage/Toxicology

Symptoms of overdose include nausea, vomiting, precordial pain, hypertension, methemoglobinemia, cyanosis; overdosage has resulted in methemoglobinemia and cyanosis

Treatment is symptomatic and supportive

Dosing

Adults & Elderly:

Methemoglobinemia: I.V.: 1-2 mg/kg or 25-50 mg/m^2 over several minutes; may be repeated in 1 hour if necessary

Genitourinary antiseptic: Oral: 65-130 mg 3 times/day with a full glass of water (maximum: 390 mg/day)

Pediatrics:

NADPH-methemoglobin reductase deficiency: Oral: Children: 1-1.5 mg/kg/day (maximum: 300 mg/day) given with 5-8 mg/kg/day of ascorbic acid

Methemoglobinemia: Children: Refer to adult dosing.

Available Dosage Forms

Injection, solution: 10 mg/mL (1 mL, 10 mL)

Tablet (Urolene Blue®): 65 mg

Nursing Guidelines

Patient Education: May discolor urine and feces blue-green; take oral formulation after meals with a glass of water; skin stains may be removed using a hypochlorite solution

Pregnancy Risk Factor: C/D (injected intra-amniotically)

Administration

I.V.: Administer undiluted by direct I.V. injection over several minutes.

♦ Methylergometrine Maleate *see* Methylergonovine *on page 1135*

Methylergonovine (meth il er goe NOE veen)

U.S. Brand Names Methergine®

Synonyms Methylergometrine Maleate; Methylergonovine Maleate

Pharmacologic Category Ergot Derivative

Medication Safety Issues

Sound-alike/look-alike issues:

Methylergonovine and terbutaline parenteral dosage forms look similar. Due to their contrasting indications, use care when administering these agents.

Use Prevention and treatment of postpartum and postabortion hemorrhage caused by uterine atony or subinvolution

Mechanism of Action Similar smooth muscle actions as seen with ergotamine; however, it affects primarily uterine smooth muscles producing sustained contractions and thereby shortens the third stage of labor

Pharmacodynamics/Kinetics

Onset of action: Oxytocic: Oral: 5-10 minutes; I.M.: 2-5 minutes; I.V.: Immediately

Duration: Oral: ~3 hours; I.M.: ~3 hours; I.V.: 45 minutes

Absorption: Rapid

Distribution: V_d: 39-73 L

Rapid; primarily to plasma and extracellular fluid following I.V. administration; tissues

Metabolism: Hepatic

Bioavailability: Oral: 60%; I.M.: 78%

Half-life elimination: Biphasic: Initial: 1-5 minutes; Terminal: 0.5-2 hours

Time to peak, serum: Oral: 0.3-2 hours; I.M.: 0.2-0.6 hours

Excretion: Urine and feces

Contraindications Hypersensitivity to methylergonovine or any component of the formulation; ergot alkaloids are contraindicated with potent inhibitors of CYP3A4 (includes protease inhibitors, azole antifungals, and some macrolide antibiotics); hypertension; toxemia; pregnancy

Warnings/Precautions Use caution in patients with sepsis, obliterative vascular disease, hepatic, or renal involvement, or second stage of labor; administer with extreme caution if using intravenously. Pleural and peritoneal fibrosis have been reported with prolonged daily use. Cardiac valvular fibrosis has also been associated with ergot alkaloids.

Drug Interactions Substrate of CYP3A4 (major)

Antifungals, azole derivatives (itraconazole, ketoconazole) increase levels of ergot alkaloids by inhibiting CYP3A4 metabolism, resulting in toxicity; concomitant use is contraindicated.

Antipsychotics: May diminish the effects of methylergonovine (due to dopamine antagonism); these combinations should generally be avoided.

Beta blockers: severe peripheral vasoconstriction has been reported with concomitant use of beta blockers and ergot derivatives. Monitor.

CYP3A4 inhibitors: May increase the levels/effects of methylergonovine. Example inhibitors include azole antifungals, clarithromycin, diclofenac, doxycycline, erythromycin, imatinib, isoniazid, nefazodone, nicardipine, propofol, protease inhibitors, quinidine, telithromycin, and verapamil.

Macrolide antibiotics: Erythromycin, clarithromycin, and troleandomycin may increase levels of ergot alkaloids by inhibiting CYP3A4 metabolism, resulting in toxicity (ischemia, vasospasm); concomitant use is contraindicated.

MAO inhibitors: The serotonergic effects of ergot derivatives may be increased by MAO inhibitors. Monitor for signs and symptoms of serotonin syndrome.

Metoclopramide: May diminish the effects of methylergonovine (due to dopamine antagonism); concurrent therapy should generally be avoided.

Protease inhibitors (ritonavir, amprenavir, atazanavir, indinavir, nelfinavir, and saquinavir) increase blood levels of ergot alkaloids by inhibiting CYP3A4 metabolism, acute ergot toxicity has been reported; concomitant use is contraindicated.

Serotonin agonists: Concurrent use with methylergonovine may increase the risk of serotonin syndrome (includes buspirone, SSRIs, TCAs, nefazodone, sumatriptan, and trazodone).

Sibutramine: May cause serotonin syndrome; concurrent use with ergot alkaloids is contraindicated.

Sumatriptan and other serotonin 5-HT_1 receptor agonists: Prolong vasospastic reactions; do not use sumatriptan or ergot-containing drugs within 24 hours of each other.

Vasoconstrictors: Concomitant use with peripheral vasoconstrictors may cause synergistic elevation of blood pressure; use is contraindicated.

(Continued)

Methylergonovine *(Continued)*

Adverse Reactions Frequency not defined.

Cardiovascular: Acute MI, hypertension, temporary chest pain, palpitation
Central nervous system: Hallucinations, dizziness, seizure, headache
Endocrine & metabolic: Water intoxication
Gastrointestinal: Nausea, vomiting, diarrhea, foul taste
Local: Thrombophlebitis
Neuromuscular & skeletal: Leg cramps
Otic: Tinnitus
Renal: Hematuria
Respiratory: Dyspnea, nasal congestion
Miscellaneous: Diaphoresis

Overdosage/Toxicology Symptoms of overdose include prolonged gangrene, numbness in extremities, acute nausea, vomiting, abdominal pain, respiratory depression, hypotension, and seizures. Treatment is symptomatic and supportive.

Dosing

Adults & Elderly: Prevention of hemorrhage:

Oral: 0.2 mg 3-4 times/day for 2-7 days

I.M., I.V.: 0.2 mg after delivery of anterior shoulder, after delivery of placenta, or during puerperium; may be repeated as required at intervals of 2-4 hours

Available Dosage Forms

Injection, solution, as maleate: 0.2 mg/mL (1 mL)
Tablet, as maleate: 0.2 mg

Nursing Guidelines

Assessment: See Contraindications, Warnings/Precautions, Dosing, and Drug Interactions for use cautions. Blood pressure, CNS status, and vaginal bleeding should be monitored on a regular basis - especially with infusion or injection. Assess therapeutic effectiveness and adverse response (eg, ergotamine toxicity: headache, ringing in ears, nausea and vomiting, diarrhea, numbness or coldness of extremities, confusion, hallucinations, dyspnea, chest pain, convulsions - see Adverse Reactions and Overdose/Toxicology). Teach patient proper use (when self-administered) and possible side effects/appropriate interventions (see Patient Education).

Patient Education: This drug will generally not be needed for more than a week. May cause nausea and vomiting (small, frequent meals may help), dizziness, headache, or ringing in the ears (will reverse when drug is discontinued). Report immediately any chest pain or tightness, jaw, shoulder or midback pain; difficulty breathing; acute headache; numb, cold, or cramping extremities; or severe abdominal cramping. **Breast-feeding precaution:** Consult prescriber if breast-feeding.

Pregnancy Risk Factor: C

Pregnancy Issues: Prolonged constriction of the uterine vessels and/or increased myometrial tone may lead to reduced placental blood flow. This has contributed to fetal growth retardation in animals. Methylergonovine is intended for use after delivery of the infant.

Lactation: Enters breast milk/use caution

Perioperative/Anesthesia/Other Concerns: This drug should be used extremely carefully because of it's potent vasoconstrictor action. I.V. use may induce sudden hypertension and cerebrovascular accidents. As a last resort, give I.V. slowly over several minutes and monitor blood pressure closely.

Administration

I.V.: Administer over ≥60 seconds. Should not be routinely administered I.V. because of possibility of inducing sudden hypertension and cerebrovascular accident.

Compatibility: Stable in NS

Storage:

Ampul: Store under refrigeration at 2°C to 8°C (36°F to 46°F). Protect from light.
Tablet: Store below 25°C (77°F).

- **Methylergonovine Maleate** *see* Methylergonovine *on page 1135*
- **Methylin®** *see* Methylphenidate *on page 1137*
- **Methylin® ER** *see* Methylphenidate *on page 1137*
- **Methylmorphine** *see* Codeine *on page 443*

Methylphenidate (meth il FEN i date)

U.S. Brand Names Concerta®; Metadate® CD; Metadate® ER; Methylin®; Methylin® ER; Ritalin®; Ritalin® LA; Ritalin-SR®

Synonyms Methylphenidate Hydrochloride

Pharmacologic Category Central Nervous System Stimulant

Medication Safety Issues

Sound-alike/look-alike issues:

Methylphenidate may be confused with methadone

Ritalin® may be confused with Ismelin®, Rifadin®

Use Treatment of attention-deficit/hyperactivity disorder (ADHD); symptomatic management of narcolepsy

Unlabeled/Investigational Use Depression (especially elderly or medically ill)

Mechanism of Action Mild CNS stimulant; blocks the reuptake mechanism of dopaminergic neurons; appears to stimulate the cerebral cortex and subcortical structures similar to amphetamines

Pharmacodynamics/Kinetics

Onset of action: Peak effect:

Immediate release tablet: Cerebral stimulation: ~2 hours

Extended release capsule (Metadate® CD): Biphasic; initial peak similar to immediate release product, followed by second rising portion (corresponding to extended release portion)

Sustained release tablet: 4-7 hours

Osmotic release tablet (Concerta®): Initial: 1-2 hours

Duration: Immediate release tablet: 3-6 hours; Sustained release tablet: 8 hours

Absorption: Readily

Metabolism: Hepatic via de-esterification to active metabolite

Half-life elimination: 2-4 hours

Time to peak: C_{max}: 6-8 hours

Excretion: Urine (90% as metabolites and unchanged drug)

Contraindications Hypersensitivity to methylphenidate, any component of the formulation, or idiosyncrasy to sympathomimetic amines; marked anxiety, tension, and agitation; glaucoma; use during or within 14 days following MAO inhibitor therapy; Tourette's syndrome or tics

Warnings/Precautions Has demonstrated value as part of a comprehensive treatment program for ADHD. Safety and efficacy in children <6 years of age not established. Use with caution in patients with bipolar disorder, diabetes mellitus, cardiovascular disease, hyperthyroidism, seizure disorders, insomnia, porphyria, or hypertension. Use caution in patients with history of ethanol or drug abuse. May exacerbate symptoms of behavior and thought disorder in psychotic patients. Do not use to treat severe depression or fatigue states. Potential for drug dependency exists - avoid abrupt discontinuation in patients who have received for prolonged periods. Visual disturbances have been reported (rare). Stimulant use has been associated with growth suppression. Growth should be monitored during treatment. Stimulants may unmask tics in individuals with coexisting Tourette's syndrome. Concerta® should not be used in patients with esophageal motility disorders or pre-existing severe gastrointestinal narrowing (small bowel disease, short gut syndrome, history of peritonitis, cystic fibrosis, chronic intestinal pseudo-obstruction, Meckel's diverticulum).

Drug Interactions Substrate of CYP2D6 (major); **Inhibits** CYP2D6 (weak)

Antihypertensive agents: Effectiveness of antihypertensive agent may be decreased; use with caution

Carbamazepine: Carbamazepine may decrease the serum concentration of methylphenidate.

Clonidine: Severe toxic reactions have been reported in combined use with methylphenidate.

CYP2D6 inhibitors: May increase the levels/effects of methylphenidate. Example inhibitors include chlorpromazine, delavirdine, fluoxetine, miconazole, paroxetine, pergolide, quinidine, quinine, ritonavir, and ropinirole.

Linezolid: Due to MAO inhibition (see note on MAO inhibitors), concurrent use with methylphenidate should generally be avoided.

MAO inhibitors: Severe hypertensive episodes have occurred with amphetamine when used in patients receiving nonselective MAO inhibitors; methylphenidate may be less likely to interact, or reactions may be less severe; use with caution only when warranted; wait 14 days following discontinuation of MAO inhibitor.

Phenobarbital: Serum levels may be increased by methylphenidate (in some patients); monitor

(Continued)

Methylphenidate *(Continued)*

Phenytoin: Serum levels may be increased by methylphenidate (in some patients); monitor

Selegiline: When selegiline is used at low dosages (<10 mg/day), an interaction with methylphenidate is less likely than with nonselective MAO inhibitors (see MAO inhibitor information), but theoretically possible; monitor

Sibutramine: Potential for reactions noted with amphetamines (severe hypertension and tachycardia) appears to be low; use with caution

Tricyclic antidepressants: Methylphenidate may increase serum concentrations of some tricyclic agents; clinical reports of toxicity are limited; dosage reduction of tricyclic antidepressants may be required; monitor

Venlafaxine: NMS has been reported in a patient receiving methylphenidate and venlafaxine.

Warfarin: Methylphenidate may decrease metabolism of coumarin anticoagulants; effect has not been confirmed in all studies; monitor INR

Nutritional/Herbal/Ethanol Interactions

Ethanol: Avoid ethanol (may cause CNS depression).

Food: Food may increase oral absorption; Concerta® formulation is not affected. Food delays early peak and high-fat meals increase C_{max} and AUC of Metadate® CD formulation.

Herb/Nutraceutical: Avoid ephedra (may cause hypertension or arrhythmias) and yohimbe (also has CNS stimulatory activity).

Adverse Reactions Frequency not defined.

Cardiovascular: Angina, cardiac arrhythmia, cerebral arteritis, cerebral occlusion, hyper-/hypotension, palpitation, pulse increase/decrease, tachycardia

Central nervous system: Depression, dizziness, drowsiness, fever, headache, insomnia, nervousness, neuroleptic malignant syndrome (NMS), Tourette's syndrome, toxic psychosis

Dermatologic: Erythema multiforme, exfoliative dermatitis, hair loss, rash, urticaria

Endocrine & metabolic: Growth retardation

Gastrointestinal: Abdominal pain, anorexia, diarrhea, nausea, vomiting, weight loss

Hematologic: Anemia, leukopenia, thrombocytopenic purpura

Hepatic: Liver function tests abnormal, hepatic coma, transaminases increased

Neuromuscular & skeletal: Arthralgia, dyskinesia

Ocular: Blurred vision

Renal: Necrotizing vasculitis

Respiratory: Cough increased, pharyngitis, sinusitis, upper respiratory tract infection

Miscellaneous: Accidental injury. hypersensitivity reactions

Overdosage/Toxicology Symptoms of overdose include vomiting, agitation, tremor, hyperpyrexia, muscle twitching, hallucinations, tachycardia, mydriasis, sweating, and palpitations. There is no specific antidote; treatment is supportive.

Dosing

Adults & Elderly:

Narcolepsy: Oral: 10 mg 2-3 times/day, up to 60 mg/day

Depression: Oral: Initial: 2.5 mg every morning before 9 AM; dosage may be increased by 2.5-5 mg every 2-3 days as tolerated to a maximum of 20 mg/day. May be divided (eg, 7 AM and 12 noon), but should not be given after noon. Do not use sustained release product.

ADHD: Oral: Refer to pediatric dosing.

Note: Discontinue periodically to re-evaluate or if no improvement occurs within 1 month.

Pediatrics: Note: Oral: Discontinue periodically to re-evaluate or if no improvement occurs within 1 month.

ADHD: Oral: Children ≥6 years: Initial: 0.3 mg/kg/dose or 2.5-5 mg/dose given before breakfast and lunch; increase by 0.1 mg/kg/dose or by 5-10 mg/day at weekly intervals; usual dose: 0.5-1 mg/kg/day; maximum dose: 2 mg/kg/day or 90 mg/day

Extended release products:

Metadate® ER, Methylin® ER, Ritalin® SR: Duration of action is 8 hours. May be given in place of regular tablets, once the daily dose is titrated using the regular tablets and the titrated 8-hour dosage corresponds to sustained release tablet size.

Metadate® CD, Ritalin® LA: Initial: 20 mg once daily; may be adjusted in 10-20 mg increments at weekly intervals; maximum: 60 mg/day

Concerta®:

Initial dose:

Children not currently taking methylphenidate: 18 mg once daily in the morning

Children currently taking methylphenidate: **Note:** Dosing based on current regimen and clinical judgment; suggested dosing listed below:

Patients taking methylphenidate 5 mg 2-3 times/day or 20 mg/day sustained release formulation: 18 mg once every morning

Patients taking methylphenidate 10 mg 2-3 times/day or 40 mg/day sustained release formulation: 36 mg once every morning

Patients taking methylphenidate 15 mg 2-3 times/day or 60 mg/day sustained release formulation: 54 mg once every morning

Dose adjustment: May increase dose in increments of 18 mg; dose may be adjusted at weekly intervals. A dosage strength of 27 mg is available for situations in which a dosage between 18-36 mg is desired. Maximum dose should not exceed 2 mg/kg/day **or** 54 mg/day in children 6-12 years or 72 mg/day in children 13-17 years.

Available Dosage Forms

Capsule, extended release, as hydrochloride:

Metadate® CD: 10 mg, 20 mg, 30 mg

Ritalin® LA: 10 mg, 20 mg, 30 mg, 40 mg

Solution, oral, as hydrochloride:

Methylin®: 5 mg/5 mL (500 mL) [grape flavor]; 10 mg/5 mL (500 mL) [grape flavor]

Tablet, as hydrochloride: 5 mg, 10 mg, 20 mg

Methylin®, Ritalin®: 5 mg, 10 mg, 20 mg

Tablet, chewable, as hydrochloride:

Methylin®: 2.5 mg [contains phenylalanine 0.42 mg; grape flavor]; 5 mg [contains phenylalanine 0.84 mg; grape flavor]; 10 mg [contains phenylalanine 1.68 mg; grape flavor]

Tablet, extended release, as hydrochloride: 20 mg

Concerta®: 18 mg, 27 mg, 36 mg, 54 mg [osmotic controlled release]

Metadate® ER, Methylin® ER: 10 mg, 20 mg

Tablet, sustained release, as hydrochloride (Ritalin-SR®): 20 mg

Nursing Guidelines

Assessment: Assess effectiveness and interactions of other medications patient may be taking. Assess for history of addiction; long-term use can result in dependence, abuse, or tolerance. Evaluate periodically for need for continued use. After long-term use, taper dosage slowly when discontinuing. In children, monitor growth pattern. If growth/weight gain is not as expected, may need to discontinue medication. Assess results of laboratory tests, therapeutic effectiveness, and adverse reactions at beginning of therapy and periodically with long-term use. Monitor blood pressure and pulse periodically. Assess knowledge/teach patient appropriate use, interventions to reduce side effects, and importance of reporting adverse symptoms promptly.

Dietary Considerations: Should be taken 30-45 minutes before meals. Concerta® is not affected by food and should be taken with water, milk, or juice. Metadate® CD should be taken before breakfast. Metadate™ ER should be taken before breakfast and lunch.

Patient Education: Take exactly as directed, 30-45 minutes before meals with a full glass of water. Do not change dosage or discontinue without consulting prescriber. Response may take some time. Do not crush or chew sustained release dosage forms. Tablets and sustained release tablets should be taken 30-45 minutes before meals. Concerta® may be taken with or without food, but must be taken with water, milk, or juice. Metadate® CD and Ritalin® LA capsules may be opened and the contents sprinkled onto a small amount (equal to 1 tablespoon) of applesauce. Swallow applesauce without chewing. Do not crush or chew capsule contents. Avoid alcohol, caffeine, or other stimulants. Maintain adequate hydration (2-3 L/day of fluids) unless instructed to restrict fluid intake. You may experience decreased appetite or weight loss (small frequent meals may help maintain adequate nutrition); or restlessness, impaired judgment, or dizziness, especially during early therapy (use caution when driving or engaging in tasks requiring alertness until response to drug is known). Report unresolved rapid heartbeat; excessive agitation, nervousness, insomnia, tremors, or dizziness; change in vision; blackened stool; skin rash or irritation; or altered gait or movement. Concerta® tablet shell may appear intact in stool; this is normal. Pediatrics: Monitor growth. **Pregnancy/breast-feeding**

(Continued)

Methylphenidate *(Continued)*

precautions: Inform prescriber if you are or intend to become pregnant. Consult prescriber if breast-feeding.

Geriatric Considerations: Methylphenidate is often useful in treating elderly patients who are discouraged, withdrawn, apathetic, or disinterested in their activities. In particular, it is useful in patients who are starting a rehabilitation program but have resigned themselves to fail; these patients may not have a major depressive disorder; will not improve memory or cognitive function; use with caution in patients with dementia who may have increased agitation and confusion (see Dosage and Adverse Reactions).

Pregnancy Risk Factor: C

Lactation: Excretion in breast milk unknown/use caution

Administration

Oral: Do not crush or allow patient to chew sustained release dosage form. To effectively avoid insomnia, dosing should be completed by noon.

Concerta®: Administer dose once daily in the morning. May be taken with or without food, but must be taken with water, milk, or juice.

Metadate® CD, Ritalin® LA: Capsules may be opened and the contents sprinkled onto a small amount (equal to 1 tablespoon) of applesauce. Swallow applesauce without chewing. Do not crush or chew capsule contents.

Methylin® chewable tablet: Administer with at least 8 ounces of water or other fluid.

Storage:

Chewable tablet: Store at room temperature of 20°C to 25°C (68°F to 77°F). Protect from moisture.

Extended release capsule: Store in dose pack provided at 25°C (77°F).

Immediate release tablet: Do not store above 30°C (86°F). Protect from light .

Osmotic controlled release tablet (Concerta®): Store at 25°C (77°F). Protect from humidity.

Solution: Store at room temperature of 20°C to 25°C (68°F to 77°F).

Sustained release tablet: Do not store above 30°C (86°F). Protect from moisture.

♦ **Methylphenidate Hydrochloride** *see* Methylphenidate *on page 1137*
♦ **Methylphenyl Isoxazolyl Penicillin** *see* Oxacillin *on page 1274*
♦ **Methylphytyl Napthoquinone** *see* Phytonadione *on page 1363*

MethylPREDNISolone (meth il pred NIS oh lone)

U.S. Brand Names Depo-Medrol®; Medrol®; Solu-Medrol®

Synonyms 6-α-Methylprednisolone; A-Methapred; Methylprednisolone Acetate; Methylprednisolone Sodium Succinate

Pharmacologic Category Corticosteroid, Systemic

Medication Safety Issues

Sound-alike/look-alike issues:

MethylPREDNISolone may be confused with medroxyPROGESTERone, predniSONE

Depo-Medrol® may be confused with Solu-Medrol®

Medrol® may be confused with Mebaral®

Solu-Medrol® may be confused with Depo-Medrol®

Use Primarily as an anti-inflammatory or immunosuppressant agent in the treatment of a variety of diseases including those of hematologic, allergic, inflammatory, neoplastic, and autoimmune origin. Prevention and treatment of graft-versus-host disease following allogeneic bone marrow transplantation.

Unlabeled/Investigational Use Treatment of fibrosing-alveolitis phase of adult respiratory distress syndrome (ARDS)

Mechanism of Action In a tissue-specific manner, corticosteroids regulate gene expression subsequent to binding specific intracellular receptors and translocation into the nucleus. Corticosteroids exert a wide array of physiologic effects including modulation of carbohydrate, protein, and lipid metabolism and maintenance of fluid and electrolyte homeostasis. Moreover cardiovascular, immunologic, musculoskeletal, endocrine, and neurologic physiology are influenced by corticosteroids. Decreases inflammation by suppression of migration of polymorphonuclear leukocytes and reversal of increased capillary permeability.

Pharmacodynamics/Kinetics

Onset of action: Peak effect (route dependent): Oral: 1-2 hours; I.M.: 4-8 days; Intra-articular: 1 week; methylprednisolone sodium succinate is highly soluble and has a rapid effect by I.M. and I.V. routes

Duration (route dependent): Oral: 30-36 hours; I.M.: 1-4 weeks; Intra-articular: 1-5 weeks; methylprednisolone acetate has a low solubility and has a sustained I.M. effect

Distribution: V_d: 0.7-1.5 L/kg

Half-life elimination: 3-3.5 hours; reduced in obese

Excretion: Clearance: Reduced in obese

Contraindications Hypersensitivity to methylprednisolone or any component of the formulation; viral, fungal, or tubercular skin lesions; administration of live virus vaccines; serious infections, except septic shock or tuberculous meningitis. Methylprednisolone formulations containing benzyl alcohol preservative are contraindicated in infants.

Warnings/Precautions Use with caution in patients with hyperthyroidism, cirrhosis, nonspecific ulcerative colitis, hypertension, osteoporosis, thromboembolic tendencies, CHF, convulsive disorders, myasthenia gravis, thrombophlebitis, peptic ulcer, diabetes, glaucoma, cataracts, or tuberculosis. Use caution in hepatic impairment. Because of the risk of adverse effects, systemic corticosteroids should be used cautiously in the elderly, in the smallest possible dose, and for the shortest possible time

Acute adrenal insufficiency may occur with abrupt withdrawal after long-term therapy or with stress; young pediatric patients may be more susceptible to adrenal axis suppression from topical therapy

Drug Interactions **Substrate** of CYP3A4 (minor); **Inhibits** CYP3A4 (weak)

Decreased effect:

Phenytoin, phenobarbital, rifampin increase clearance of methylprednisolone

Potassium depleting diuretics enhance potassium depletion

Increased toxicity:

Skin test antigens, immunizations decrease response and increase potential infections

Methylprednisolone may increase circulating glucose levels and may need adjustments of insulin or oral hypoglycemics

Nutritional/Herbal/Ethanol Interactions

Ethanol: Avoid ethanol (may increase gastric mucosal irritation).

Food: Methylprednisolone interferes with calcium absorption. Limit caffeine.

Herb/Nutraceutical: St John's wort may decrease methylprednisolone levels. Avoid cat's claw, echinacea (have immunostimulant properties).

Lab Interactions Interferes with skin tests

Adverse Reactions Frequency not defined.

Cardiovascular: Edema, hypertension, arrhythmia

Central nervous system: Insomnia, nervousness, vertigo, seizure, psychoses, pseudotumor cerebri, headache, mood swings, delirium, hallucinations, euphoria

Dermatologic: Hirsutism, acne, skin atrophy, bruising, hyperpigmentation

Endocrine & metabolic: Diabetes mellitus, adrenal suppression, hyperlipidemia, Cushing's syndrome, pituitary-adrenal axis suppression, growth suppression, glucose intolerance, hypokalemia, alkalosis, amenorrhea, sodium and water retention, hyperglycemia

Gastrointestinal: Increased appetite, indigestion, peptic ulcer, nausea, vomiting, abdominal distention, ulcerative esophagitis, pancreatitis

Hematologic: Transient leukocytosis

Neuromuscular & skeletal: Arthralgia, muscle weakness, osteoporosis, fractures

Ocular: Cataracts, glaucoma

Miscellaneous: Infections, hypersensitivity reactions, avascular necrosis, secondary malignancy, intractable hiccups

Overdosage/Toxicology When consumed in high doses for prolonged periods, systemic hypercorticism and adrenal suppression may occur. In these cases, discontinuation should be done judiciously. Arrhythmias and cardiovascular collapse are possible with rapid intravenous infusion of high-dose methylprednisolone. May mask signs and symptoms of infection.

Dosing

Adults: Only sodium succinate may be given I.V.; methylprednisolone sodium succinate is highly soluble and has a rapid effect by I.M. and I.V. routes. Methylprednisolone acetate has a low solubility and has a sustained I.M. effect.

Anti-inflammatory or immunosuppressive:

Oral: 2-60 mg/day in 1-4 divided doses to start, followed by gradual reduction in dosage to the lowest possible level consistent with maintaining an adequate clinical response.

I.M. (sodium succinate): 10-80 mg/day once daily

(Continued)

MethylPREDNISolone *(Continued)*

I.M. (acetate): 10-80 mg every 1-2 weeks

I.V. (sodium succinate): 10-40 mg over a period of several minutes and repeated I.V. or I.M. at intervals depending on clinical response; when high dosages are needed, give 30 mg/kg over a period ≥30 minutes and may be repeated every 4-6 hours for 48 hours.

Status asthmaticus: I.V. (sodium succinate): Loading dose: 2 mg/kg/dose, then 0.5-1 mg/kg/dose every 6 hours for up to 5 days

Acute spinal cord injury: I.V. (sodium succinate): 30 mg/kg over 15 minutes, followed in 45 minutes by a continuous infusion of 5.4 mg/kg/hour for 23 hours

Lupus nephritis: High-dose "pulse" therapy: I.V. (sodium succinate): 1 g/day for 3 days

Aplastic anemia: I.V. (sodium succinate): 1 mg/kg/day or 40 mg/day (whichever dose is higher), for 4 days. After 4 days, change to oral and continue until day 10 or until symptoms of serum sickness resolve, then rapidly reduce over approximately 2 weeks.

Pneumonia in AIDS patients due to *Pneumocystis:* I.V.: 40-60 mg every 6 hours for 7-10 days

Arthritis: Intra-articular (acetate): Administer every 1-5 weeks.

Large joints: 20-80 mg

Small joints: 4-10 mg

Intralesional (acetate): 20-60 mg every 1-5 weeks

Elderly: Only sodium succinate salt may be given I.V. Use the lowest effective adult dose.

Pediatrics: Dosing should be based on the lesser of ideal body weight or actual body weight. **Only sodium succinate may be given I.V.;** methylprednisolone sodium succinate is highly soluble and has a rapid effect by I.M. and I.V. routes. Methylprednisolone acetate has a low solubility and has a sustained I.M. effect.

Anti-inflammatory or immunosuppressive: Oral, I.M., I.V. (sodium succinate): Children: 0.5-1.7 mg/kg/day **or** 5-25 mg/m^2/day in divided doses every 6-12 hours; "Pulse" therapy: 15-30 mg/kg/dose over ≥30 minutes given once daily for 3 days

Status asthmaticus: Children: I.V. (sodium succinate): Loading dose: 2 mg/kg/dose, then 0.5-1 mg/kg/dose every 6 hours for up to 5 days

Acute spinal cord injury: I.V. (sodium succinate): 30 mg/kg over 15 minutes, followed in 45 minutes by a continuous infusion of 5.4 mg/kg/hour for 23 hours

Lupus nephritis: I.V. (sodium succinate): 30 mg/kg over ≥30 minutes every other day for 6 doses

Renal Impairment:

Hemodialysis effects: Slightly dialyzable (5% to 20%)

Administer dose posthemodialysis.

Available Dosage Forms

Injection, powder for reconstitution, as sodium succinate: 125 mg [strength expressed as base]

Solu-Medrol®: 40 mg, 125 mg, 500 mg, 1 g, 2 g [packaged with diluent; diluent contains benzyl alcohol; strength expressed as base]

Solu-Medrol®: 500 mg, 1 g

Injection, suspension, as acetate (Depo-Medrol®): 20 mg/mL (5 mL); 40 mg/mL (5 mL); 80 mg/mL (5 mL) [contains benzyl alcohol; strength expressed as base]

Injection, suspension, as acetate [single-dose vial] (Depo-Medrol®): 40 mg/mL (1 mL, 10 mL); 80 mg/mL (1 mL)

Tablet: 4 mg

Medrol®: 2 mg, 4 mg, 8 mg, 16 mg, 32 mg

Tablet, dose-pack: 4 mg (21s)

Medrol® Dosepack™: 4 mg (21s)

Nursing Guidelines

Assessment: Assess effectiveness and interactions of other medications patient may be taking. Monitor for effectiveness of therapy and adverse reactions according to dose, route, and length of therapy (especially with systemic administration). Assess knowledge/teach patient appropriate use, possible side effects/interventions, and adverse symptoms to report (ie, opportunistic infection, adrenal suppression). Instruct patients with diabetes to monitor serum glucose levels closely; corticosteroids can alter glycemic response. Dose may need to be increased if patient is experiencing higher than normal levels of stress. When discontinuing, taper dose and frequency slowly.

Monitoring Laboratory Tests: Blood glucose, electrolytes

Dietary Considerations: Should be taken after meals or with food or milk; need diet rich in pyridoxine, vitamin C, vitamin D, folate, calcium, phosphorus, and protein.

Sodium content of 1 g sodium succinate injection: 2.01 mEq; 53 mg of sodium succinate salt is equivalent to 40 mg of methylprednisolone base

Methylprednisolone acetate: Depo-Medrol®

Methylprednisolone sodium succinate: Solu-Medrol®

Patient Education: Maintain adequate nutritional intake; consult prescriber for possibility of special dietary instructions. If you have diabetes, monitor serum glucose closely and notify prescriber of any changes; this medication can alter glycemic response. Avoid alcohol. Inform prescriber if you are experiencing unusual stress; dosage may need to be adjusted. You will be susceptible to infection (avoid crowds and and exposure to infection). You may experience insomnia or nervousness; use caution when driving or engaging in tasks requiring alertness until response to drug is known. Report increased pain, swelling, or redness in area being treated; excessive or sudden weight gain; swelling of extremities; respiratory difficulty; muscle pain or weakness; change in menstrual pattern; vision changes; signs of hyperglycemia; signs of infection (eg, fever, chills, mouth sores, perianal itching, vaginal discharge); blackened stool; other persistent side effects; or worsening of condition. **Pregnancy/breast-feeding precautions:** Inform prescriber if you are or intend to become pregnant. Consult prescriber if breast-feeding.

Oral: Take as directed, with food or milk. Take once-a-day dose in the morning. Do not take more than prescribed or discontinue without consulting prescriber.

Intra-articular: Refrain from excessive use of joint following therapy, even if pain is gone.

Geriatric Considerations: Because of the risk of adverse effects, systemic corticosteroids should be used cautiously in the elderly, in the smallest possible dose, and for the shortest possible time.

Pregnancy Risk Factor: C

Lactation: Excretion in breast milk unknown

Perioperative/Anesthesia/Other Concerns:

Neuromuscular Effects: ICU-acquired paresis was recently studied in 5 ICUs (3 medical and 2 surgical ICUs) at 4 French hospitals. All ICU patients without pre-existing neuromuscular disease admitted from March 1999 through June 2000 were evaluated (De Jonghe B, 2002). Each patient had to be mechanically ventilated for ≥7 days and was screened daily for awakening. The first day the patient was considered awake was Study Day 1. Patients with severe muscle weakness on Study Day 7 were considered to have ICU-acquired paresis. Among the 95 patients who were evaluable, about 25% developed ICU-acquired paresis. Independent predictors included female gender, the number of days with ≥2 organ dysfunction, and administration of corticosteroids. Further studies may be required to verify and characterize the association between the development of ICU-acquired paresis and use of corticosteroids. Concurrent use of a corticosteroid and muscle relaxant appear to increase the risk of certain ICU myopathies; avoid or administer the corticosteroid at the lowest dose possible.

Adrenal Insufficiency: Patients will often have steroid-induced adverse effects on glucose tolerance and lipid profiles. When discontinuing steroid therapy in patients on long-term steroid supplementation, it is important that the steroid therapy be discontinued gradually. Abrupt withdrawal may result in adrenal insufficiency with hypotension and hyperkalemia. Patients on long-term steroid supplementation will require higher corticosteroid doses when subject to stress (ie, trauma, surgery, severe infection). Guidelines for glucocorticoid replacement during various surgical procedures has been published (Salem M, 1994, Coursin DB, 2002).

Septic Shock: A recent randomized, double-blind, placebo controlled trial assessed whether low dose corticosteroid administration could improve 28-day survival in patients with septic shock and relative adrenal insufficiency. Relative adrenal insufficiency was defined as an inappropriate response to corticotropin administration (increase of serum cortisol of ≤9 mcg/dL from baseline). Cortisol levels were drawn immediately before corticotropin administration and 30 to 60 minutes afterwards. Three hundred adult septic shock patients requiring mechanical ventilation and vasopressor support were randomized to either hydrocortisone (50 mg IVP every 6 hours) and fludrocortisone (50 mcg tablet

(Continued)

MethylPREDNISolone *(Continued)*

daily via nasogastric tube) or matching placebos for 7 days. In patients who did not appropriately respond to corticotropin (nonresponders), there were significantly fewer deaths in the active treatment group. Vasopressor therapy was withdrawn more frequently in this subset of the active treatment group. Adverse events were similar in both groups. Patients who lack adrenal reserve and thus have relative adrenal insufficiency during the stress of septic shock may benefit from physiologic steroid replacement. However, there was a trend for increased mortality in patients who responded to the corticotropin test (increase serum cortisol >9 mcg/dL from baseline). These patients may not benefit from physiologic steroid replacement. Further study is required to better characterize the patient populations who may benefit.

Administration

Oral: Give oral formulation with meals to decrease GI upset. Give daily dose in the morning to mimic normal peak blood levels.

I.V.: Only sodium succinate formulation may be given I.V. Acetate salt should not be given I.V.

Parenteral: Methylprednisolone sodium succinate may be administered I.M. or I.V.; I.V. administration may be IVP over one to several minutes or IVPB or continuous I.V. infusion.

I.V.: Succinate:

Low dose: ≤1.8 mg/kg or ≤125 mg/dose: I.V. push over 3-15 minutes
Moderate dose: ≥2 mg/kg or 250 mg/dose: I.V. over 15-30 minutes
High dose: 15 mg/kg or ≥500 mg/dose: I.V. over ≥30 minutes
Doses >15 mg/kg or ≥1 g: Administer over 1 hour

Do **not** administer high-dose I.V. push; hypotension, cardiac arrhythmia, and sudden death have been reported in patients given high-dose methylprednisolone I.V. push over <20 minutes. Intermittent infusion over 15-60 minutes; maximum concentration: I.V. push 125 mg/mL.

Reconstitution:

Standard diluent (Solu-Medrol®): 40 mg/50 mL D_5W; 125 mg/50 mL D_5W
Minimum volume (Solu-Medrol®): 50 mL D_5W

Compatibility: Incompatible with D_5½NS

Y-site administration: Incompatible with allopurinol, amsacrine, ciprofloxacin, docetaxel, etoposide phosphate, filgrastim, gemcitabine, ondansetron, paclitaxel, propofol, sargramostim, vinorelbine

Compatibility in syringe: Incompatible with doxapram

Compatibility when admixed: Incompatible with calcium gluconate, glycopyrrolate, insulin (regular), metaraminol, nafcillin, penicillin G sodium

Storage: Intact vials of methylprednisolone sodium succinate should be stored at controlled room temperature. Reconstituted solutions of methylprednisolone sodium succinate should be stored at room temperature (15°C to 30°C) and used within 48 hours. Stability of parenteral admixture at room temperature (25°C) and at refrigeration temperature (4°C) is 48 hours.

Related Information

Contrast Media Reactions, Premedication for Prophylaxis *on page 1911*

- **6-α-Methylprednisolone** *see* MethylPREDNISolone *on page 1140*
- **Methylprednisolone Acetate** *see* MethylPREDNISolone *on page 1140*
- **Methylprednisolone Sodium Succinate** *see* MethylPREDNISolone *on page 1140*
- **Methylrosaniline Chloride** *see* Gentian Violet *on page 811*

Metoclopramide (met oh kloe PRA mide)

U.S. Brand Names Reglan®

Pharmacologic Category Antiemetic; Gastrointestinal Agent, Prokinetic

Medication Safety Issues

Sound-alike/look-alike issues:
Metoclopramide may be confused with metolazone
Reglan® may be confused with Megace®, Regonol®, Renagel®

Use

Oral: Symptomatic treatment of diabetic gastric stasis; gastroesophageal reflux

I.V., I.M.: Symptomatic treatment of diabetic gastric stasis; postpyloric placement of enteral feeding tubes; prevention and/or treatment of nausea and vomiting associated with chemotherapy, or postsurgery; to stimulate gastric emptying and intestinal transit of barium during radiological examination

Mechanism of Action Blocks dopamine receptors and (when given in higher doses) also blocks serotonin receptors in chemoreceptor trigger zone of the CNS; enhances the response to acetylcholine of tissue in upper GI tract causing enhanced motility and accelerated gastric emptying without stimulating gastric, biliary, or pancreatic secretions; increases lower esophageal sphincter tone

Pharmacodynamics/Kinetics

Onset of action: Oral: 0.5-1 hour; I.V.: 1-3 minutes; I.M.: 10-15 minutes
Duration: Therapeutic: 1-2 hours, regardless of route
Distribution: V_d: 2-4 L/kg
Protein binding: 30%
Bioavailability: Oral: 65% to 95%
Half-life elimination: Normal renal function: 4-6 hours (may be dose dependent)
Time to peak, serum: Oral: 1-2 hours
Excretion: Urine (~85%)

Contraindications Hypersensitivity to metoclopramide or any component of the formulation; GI obstruction, perforation or hemorrhage; pheochromocytoma; history of seizures

Warnings/Precautions Use caution with a history of mental illness; has been associated with extrapyramidal symptoms (EPS) and depression. The frequency of EPS is higher in pediatric patients and adults <30 years of age; risk is increased at higher dosages. Extrapyramidal reactions typically occur within the initial 24-48 hours of treatment. Use caution with concurrent use of other drugs associated with EPS. Use caution in the elderly and with Parkinson's disease; may have increased risk of tardive dyskinesia. Use caution in patients with a history of seizures; risk of metoclopramide-associated seizures is increased. Neuroleptic malignant syndrome (NMS) has been reported (rarely) with metoclopramide. Use lowest recommended doses initially; may cause transient increase in serum aldosterone; use caution in patients who are at risk of fluid overload (CHF, cirrhosis). Use caution in patients with hypertension or following surgical anastomosis/closure. Patients with NADH-cytochrome b5 reductase deficiency are at increased risk of methemoglobinemia and/or sulfhemoglobinemia. Abrupt discontinuation may (rarely) result in withdrawal symptoms (dizziness, headache, nervousness). Use caution and adjust dose in renal impairment.

Drug Interactions Substrate (minor) of CYP1A2, 2D6; **Inhibits** CYP2D6 (weak)

Anticholinergic agents antagonize metoclopramide's actions
Antipsychotic agents: Metoclopramide may increase extrapyramidal symptoms (EPS) or risk when used concurrently.
Cyclosporine: Metoclopramide may increase cyclosporine levels.
Opiate analgesics may increase CNS depression

Nutritional/Herbal/Ethanol Interactions Ethanol: Avoid ethanol (may increase CNS depression).

Lab Interactions Increased aminotransferase [ALT (SGPT)/AST (SGOT)] (S), amylase (S)

Adverse Reactions Frequency not always defined.

Cardiovascular: AV block, bradycardia, CHF, fluid retention, flushing (following high I.V. doses), hyper-/hypotension, supraventricular tachycardia
Central nervous system: Drowsiness (~10% to 70%; dose related), fatigue (~10%), restlessness (~10%), acute dystonic reactions (<1% to 25%; dose and age related), akathisia, confusion, depression, dizziness, hallucinations (rare), headache, insomnia, neuroleptic malignant syndrome (rare), Parkinsonian-like symptoms, suicidal ideation, seizures, tardive dyskinesia
Dermatologic: Angioneurotic edema (rare), rash, urticaria
Endocrine & metabolic: Amenorrhea, galactorrhea, gynecomastia, impotence
Gastrointestinal: Diarrhea, nausea
Genitourinary: Incontinence, urinary frequency
Hematologic: Agranulocytosis, leukopenia, neutropenia, porphyria
Hepatic: Hepatotoxicity (rare)
Ocular: Visual disturbance
Respiratory: Bronchospasm, laryngeal edema (rare)
Miscellaneous: Allergic reactions, methemoglobinemia, sulfhemoglobinemia

Overdosage/Toxicology Symptoms of overdose include drowsiness, ataxia, extrapyramidal symptoms, seizures, methemoglobinemia (in infants). Disorientation, muscle hypertonia, irritability, and agitation are common. Metoclopramide often causes extrapyramidal symptoms (eg, dystonic reactions) requiring management with diphenhydramine 1-2 mg/kg (adults) up to a maximum of 50-100 mg I.M. or I.V. slow push followed by a maintenance dose (25-50 mg orally every 4-6 hours) for 48-72 hours. When these reactions are unresponsive to diphenhydramine, benztropine mesylate I.V. 1-2 mg (adults) may be effective.
(Continued)

Metoclopramide *(Continued)*

These agents are generally effective within 2-5 minutes. Methylene blue is not recommended in patients with G6PD deficiency who experience methemoglobinemia due to metoclopramide.

Dosing

Adults:

Gastroesophageal reflux: Oral: 10-15 mg/dose up to 4 times/day 30 minutes before meals or food and at bedtime; single doses of 20 mg are occasionally needed for provoking situations. Treatment >12 weeks has not been evaluated.

Diabetic gastric stasis:

Oral: 10 mg 30 minutes before each meal and at bedtime

I.M., I.V. (for severe symptoms): 10 mg over 1-2 minutes; 10 days of I.V. therapy may be necessary for best response

Chemotherapy-induced emesis:

I.V.: 1-2 mg/kg 30 minutes before chemotherapy and repeated every 2 hours for 2 doses, then every 3 hours for 3 doses (manufacturer labeling)

Alternate dosing (with or without diphenhydramine):

Moderate emetic risk chemotherapy: 0.5 mg/kg every 6 hours on days 2-4

Low and minimal risk chemotherapy: 1-2 mg/kg every 3-4 hours

Breakthrough treatment: 1-2 mg/kg every 3-4 hours

Oral (unlabeled use; with or without diphenhydramine):

Moderate emetic risk chemotherapy: 0.5 mg/kg every 6 hours or 20 mg 4 times/day on days 2-4

Low and minimal risk chemotherapy: 20-40 mg every 4-6 hours

Breakthrough treatment: 20-40 mg every 4-6 hours

Postoperative nausea and vomiting: I.M., I.V.: 10-20 mg near end of surgery

Postpyloric feeding tube placement, radiological exam: I.V.: 10 mg

Elderly:

Gastroesophageal reflux: Oral: 5 mg 4 times/day (30 minutes before meals or food and at bedtime); increase dose to 10 mg 4 times/day if no response at lower dose

Gastrointestinal hypomotility:

Oral: Initial: 5 mg 30 minutes before meals and at bedtime; increase if necessary to 10 mg doses

I.V.: Initiate at 5 mg over 1-2 minutes; increase to 10 mg if necessary

Postoperative nausea and vomiting: I.M., I.V.: 5 mg near end of surgery; may repeat dose if necessary

Pediatrics:

Gastroesophageal reflux (unlabeled use): Oral: 0.1-0.2 mg/kg/dose 4 times/day

Chemotherapy-induced emesis (unlabeled use): I.V.: 1-2 mg/kg 30 minutes before chemotherapy and every 2-4 hours

Postpyloric feeding tube placement: I.V.:

<6 years: 0.1 mg/kg

6-14 years: 2.5-5 mg

>14 years: Refer to Adults dosing.

Renal Impairment:

Cl_{cr} <40 mL/minute: Administer 50% of normal dose.

Not dialyzable (0% to 5%); supplemental dose is not necessary.

Available Dosage Forms

Injection, solution (Reglan®): 5 mg/mL (2 mL, 10 mL, 30 mL)

Syrup: 5 mg/5 mL (10 mL, 480 mL)

Tablet (Reglan®): 5 mg, 10 mg

Nursing Guidelines

Assessment: Assess potential for interactions with other pharmacological agents patient may be taking (eg, any antipsychotic agents, opioids, anticholinergics). Vital signs should be monitored during intravenous administration. Inpatients should use safety measures (eg, side rails up, call light within reach) and caution patient to call for assistance with ambulation. Assess results of laboratory tests (periodic renal function tests), therapeutic effectiveness (relief of symptoms), and adverse reactions (eg, extrapyramidal effects, parkinsonian-like reactions, seizures, fluid retention, adverse CNS changes). Teach patient proper use, possible side effects/appropriate interventions, and adverse symptoms to report (eg, CNS restlessness, drowsiness, depression, rash).

Monitoring Laboratory Tests: Periodic renal function

Patient Education: Do not take any new medication during therapy unless approved by prescriber. Oral: Take this drug as prescribed, 30 minutes prior to eating. Do not increase dosage. Avoid alcohol; may increase adverse effects. May cause dizziness, drowsiness, or blurred vision (use caution when driving or engaging in tasks that require alertness until response to drug is known); cause restlessness, anxiety, depression, or insomnia (will reverse when medication is discontinued). Report any CNS changes, spasticity or involuntary movements, unresolved diarrhea, fluid retention (swelling of extremities, weight gain); visual disturbances; palpitations or rapid heart beat; or any other persistent adverse effects. **Breast-feeding precaution:** Breast-feeding is not recommended.

Geriatric Considerations: Elderly are more likely to develop tardive dyskinesia syndrome (especially elderly females) reactions than younger adults. Use lowest recommended doses initially. Must consider renal function (estimate creatinine clearance). It is recommended to do involuntary movement assessments on elderly using this medication at high doses and for long-term therapy.

Pregnancy Risk Factor: B

Pregnancy Issues: Crosses the placenta; available evidence suggests safe use during pregnancy.

Lactation: Enters breast milk/use caution

Breast-Feeding Considerations: Enters breast milk; may increase milk production

Perioperative/Anesthesia/Other Concerns: To prevent extrapyramidal symptoms associated with antiemetic dosages, patients may be pretreated with diphenhydramine.

Administration

I.M.: May be administered I.M.

I.V.: Injection solution may be given I.M., direct I.V. push, short infusion (15-30 minutes), or continuous infusion; lower doses (≤10 mg) of metoclopramide can be given I.V. push undiluted over 1-2 minutes; higher doses to be given IVPB over at least 15 minutes; continuous SubQ infusion and rectal administration have been reported. **Note:** Rapid I.V. administration may be associated with a transient (but intense) feeling of anxiety and restlessness, followed by drowsiness.

Compatibility: Stable in D_5½NS, D_5W, mannitol 20%, LR, NS

Y-site administration: Incompatible with allopurinol, amphotericin B cholesteryl sulfate complex, amsacrine, cefepime, doxorubicin liposome, furosemide, propofol

Compatibility in syringe: Incompatible with ampicillin, calcium gluconate, chloramphenicol, furosemide, penicillin G potassium, sodium bicarbonate

Compatibility when admixed: Incompatible with dexamethasone sodium phosphate with lorazepam and diphenhydramine, erythromycin lactobionate, floxacillin, fluorouracil, furosemide

Storage:

Injection: Store intact vial at controlled room temperature; injection is photosensitive and should be protected from light during storage; parenteral admixtures in D_5W or NS are stable for at least 24 hours, and do not require light protection if used within 24 hours.

Tablet: Store at controlled room temperature.

Related Information

Postoperative Nausea and Vomiting *on page 1807*

Metolazone (me TOLE a zone)

U.S. Brand Names Zaroxolyn®

Pharmacologic Category Diuretic, Thiazide-Related

Medication Safety Issues

Sound-alike/look-alike issues:

Metolazone may be confused with metaxalone, methazolamide, methimazole, methotrexate, metoclopramide, metoprolol, minoxidil

Zaroxolyn® may be confused with Zarontin®

Use Management of mild to moderate hypertension; treatment of edema in congestive heart failure and nephrotic syndrome, impaired renal function

Mechanism of Action Inhibits sodium reabsorption in the distal tubules causing increased excretion of sodium and water, as well as, potassium and hydrogen ions

Pharmacodynamics/Kinetics

Onset of action: Diuresis: ~60 minutes

(Continued)

Metolazone *(Continued)*

Duration: 12-24 hours
Absorption: Incomplete
Distribution: Crosses placenta; enters breast milk
Protein binding: 95%
Metabolism: Undergoes enterohepatic recirculation
Bioavailability: Mykrox® reportedly has highest
Half-life elimination (renal function dependent): 6-20 hours
Excretion: Urine (80% to 95%)

Contraindications Hypersensitivity to metolazone, any component of the formulation, other thiazides, and sulfonamide derivatives; anuria; hepatic coma; pregnancy (expert analysis)

Warnings/Precautions Electrolyte disturbances (hypokalemia, hypochloremic alkalosis, hyponatremia) can occur. Use with caution in severe hepatic dysfunction; hepatic encephalopathy can be caused by electrolyte disturbances. Gout can be precipitate in certain patients with a history of gout, a familial predisposition to gout, or chronic renal failure. Cautious use in diabetics; may see a change in glucose control. Hypersensitivity reactions can occur. Can cause SLE exacerbation or activation. Use caution in severe renal impairment. Orthostatic hypotension may occur (potentiated by alcohol, barbiturates, narcotics, other antihypertensive drugs). Mykrox® tablets are not interchangeable with Zaroxolyn® tablets. Use with caution in patients with moderate or high cholesterol concentrations. Photosensitization may occur.

Chemical similarities are present among sulfonamides, sulfonylureas, carbonic anhydrase inhibitors, thiazides, and loop diuretics (except ethacrynic acid). Use in patients with thiazide or sulfonamide allergy is specifically contraindicated in product labeling, however, a risk of cross-reaction exists in patients with allergy to any of these compounds; avoid use when previous reaction has been severe.

Drug Interactions

ACE inhibitors: Increased hypotension if aggressively diuresed with a thiazide-type diuretic.

Beta-blockers increase hyperglycemic effects in type 2 diabetes mellitus (noninsulin dependent, NIDDM).

Cholestyramine and colestipol may decrease metolazone absorption.

Cyclosporine and thiazide-type compounds can increase the risk of gout or renal toxicity; avoid concurrent use.

Digoxin toxicity can be exacerbated if a diuretic induces hypokalemia or hypomagnesemia.

Lithium toxicity can occur due to a reduced renal excretion of lithium; monitor lithium concentration and adjust as needed.

Loop diuretics (eg, furosemide) may increase the effect of metolazone.

Neuromuscular blocking agents effects may be prolonged; monitor serum potassium and neuromuscular status.

NSAIDs can decrease the efficacy of thiazide-type diuretics.

Nutritional/Herbal/Ethanol Interactions Herb/Nutraceutical: Avoid dong quai if using for hypertension (has estrogenic activity). Avoid dong quai, St John's wort (may also cause photosensitization). Avoid ephedra, yohimbe, ginseng (may worsen hypertension). Avoid natural licorice. Avoid garlic (may have increased antihypertensive effect).

Adverse Reactions

>10%: Central nervous system: Dizziness

1% to 10%:

Cardiovascular: Orthostatic hypotension, palpitation, chest pain, cold extremities (rapidly acting), edema (rapidly acting), venous thrombosis (slow acting), syncope (slow acting)

Central nervous system: Headache, fatigue, lethargy, malaise, lassitude, anxiety, depression, nervousness, "weird" feeling (rapidly acting), chills (slow acting)

Dermatologic: Rash, pruritus, dry skin (rapidly acting)

Endocrine & metabolic: Hypokalemia, impotence, reduced libido, excessive volume depletion (slow acting), hemoconcentration (slow acting), acute gouty attach (slow acting)

Gastrointestinal: Nausea, vomiting, abdominal pain, cramping, bloating, diarrhea or constipation, dry mouth

Genitourinary: Nocturia

Neuromuscular & skeletal: Muscle cramps, spasm, weakness

Ocular: Eye itching (rapidly acting)

Otic: Tinnitus (rapidly acting)

Respiratory: Cough (rapidly acting), epistaxis (rapidly acting), sinus congestion (rapidly acting), sore throat (rapidly acting)

<1% (Limited to important or life-threatening): Agranulocytosis, aplastic anemia, cholestasis, cutaneous vasculitis, glycosuria, hepatitis, hypercalcemia, hyperglycemia, leukopenia, pancreatitis, photosensitivity, pruritus, purpura, Stevens-Johnson syndrome, thrombocytopenia, toxic epidermal necrolysis

Overdosage/Toxicology Symptoms of overdose include orthostatic hypotension, dizziness, drowsiness, syncope, hemoconcentration and hemodynamic changes due to plasma volume depletion. Treatment is symptomatic and supportive.

Dosing

Adults:

Edema: Oral: 2.5-20 mg/dose every 24 hours (ACC/AHA 2005 Heart Failure Guidelines)

Hypertension:

Zaroxolyn®: Oral: 2.5-5 mg/dose every 24 hours

Mykrox®: Oral: 0.5 mg/day; if response is not adequate, increase dose to maximum of 1 mg/day.

Elderly: Oral:

Zaroxolyn®: Initial: 2.5 mg/day or every other day

Mykrox®: 0.5 mg once daily; may increase to 1 mg if response is inadequate; do not use more than 1 mg/day.

Pediatrics: Limited experience in pediatric patients. Doses used have generally ranged from 0.05 to 0.1 mg/kg administered once daily. Prolonged use is not recommended.

Renal Impairment: Not dialyzable (0% to 5%)

Available Dosage Forms Tablet, slow acting: 2.5 mg, 5 mg, 10 mg

Nursing Guidelines

Assessment: Assess allergy history prior to beginning therapy. See Contraindications, Warnings/Precautions, and Dosing for use cautions. Assess potential for interactions with other prescriptions, OTC medications, or herbal products patient may be taking (eg, any substance that will affect blood pressure - see Drug Interactions). Assess results of laboratory tests (see below), therapeutic effectiveness, and adverse reactions (eg, electrolyte imbalance, hypotension - see Adverse Reactions and Overdose/Toxicology). Caution patients with diabetes (may see a change in glucose control). Teach patient proper use, possible side effects/appropriate interventions, and adverse symptoms to report (see Patient Education). **Pregnancy risk factor B/D** - see Pregnancy Risk Factor for use cautions; benefits of use should outweigh possible risks. Note breast-feeding caution.

Monitoring Laboratory Tests: Serum electrolytes (potassium, sodium, chloride, bicarbonate), renal function

Dietary Considerations: Should be taken after breakfast; may require potassium supplementation

Patient Education: Inform prescriber of all prescriptions, OTC medications, or herbal products you are taking, and any allergies you have. Do not take any new medication during therapy unless approved by prescriber. Take exactly as directed, after breakfast. Include bananas or orange juice in daily diet but do not take potassium supplements without advice of prescriber. This medication does not replace other antihypertensive interventions; follow prescriber's instructions for diet and lifestyle changes. Weigh yourself weekly at the same time, in the same clothes. Report weight gain >5 lb/week. May cause dizziness or weakness (change position slowly when rising from sitting or lying, avoid driving or tasks requiring alertness until response to drug is known); nausea or loss of appetite (small, frequent meals, frequent mouth care, chewing gum, or sucking lozenges may help); impotence (reversible); constipation (increased exercise, fluids, fruit, or fiber may help); or photosensitivity (use sunscreen, wear protective clothing and eyewear, and avoid direct sunlight). Report flu-like symptoms, headache, joint soreness or weakness, respiratory difficulty, skin rash, excessive fatigue, swelling of extremities, or respiratory difficulty. **Pregnancy/breast-feeding precautions:** Inform prescriber if you are pregnant. Do not get pregnant while taking this medication. Consult prescriber for appropriate contraceptives. Consult prescriber if breast-feeding.

Geriatric Considerations: When metolazone is used in combination with other diuretics, there is an increased risk of azotemia and electrolyte depletion, particularly in the elderly, monitor closely. May be effective in patients with

(Continued)

Metolazone *(Continued)*

glomerular filtration rate <20 mL/minute. Metolazone is often used in combination with a loop diuretic in patients who are unresponsive to the loop diuretic alone.

Pregnancy Risk Factor: B (manufacturer); D (expert analysis)

Lactation: Enters breast milk/use caution

Perioperative/Anesthesia/Other Concerns: Metolazone 5 mg is approximately equivalent to hydrochlorothiazide 50 mg; taken the day of surgery may cause hypovolemia and the hypertensive patient undergoing general anesthesia to have labile blood pressure; use with caution prior to surgery or perioperatively

Metolazone is a potent diuretic and is often used in patients refractory to thiazide or loop diuretics. It is important that the patient be closely monitored to avoid profound volume depletion. Also watch for hypomagnesemia.

Administration

Oral: May be taken with food or milk. Take early in day to avoid nocturia. Take the last dose of multiple doses no later than 6 PM unless instructed otherwise.

Metoprolol (me toe PROE lole)

U.S. Brand Names Lopressor®; Toprol-XL®

Synonyms Metoprolol Succinate; Metoprolol Tartrate

Pharmacologic Category Beta Blocker, $Beta_1$ Selective

Medication Safety Issues

Sound-alike/look-alike issues:

Metoprolol may be confused with metaproterenol, metolazone, misoprostol

Toprol-XL® may be confused with Tegretol®, Tegretol®-XR, Topamax®

Use Treatment of hypertension and angina pectoris; prevention of myocardial infarction, atrial fibrillation, flutter, symptomatic treatment of hypertrophic subaortic stenosis; to reduce mortality/hospitalization in patients with congestive heart failure (stable NYHA Class II or III) in patients already receiving ACE inhibitors, diuretics, and/or digoxin (sustained-release only)

Unlabeled/Investigational Use Treatment of ventricular arrhythmias, atrial ectopy, migraine prophylaxis, essential tremor, aggressive behavior

Mechanism of Action Selective inhibitor of $beta_1$-adrenergic receptors; competitively blocks $beta_1$-receptors, with little or no effect on $beta_2$-receptors at doses <100 mg; does not exhibit any membrane stabilizing or intrinsic sympathomimetic activity

Pharmacodynamics/Kinetics

Onset of action: Peak effect: Antihypertensive: Oral: 1.5-4 hours

Duration: 10-20 hours

Absorption: 95%

Protein binding: 8%

Metabolism: Extensively hepatic; significant first-pass effect

Bioavailability: Oral: 40% to 50%

Half-life elimination: 3-4 hours; End-stage renal disease: 2.5-4.5 hours

Excretion: Urine (3% to 10% as unchanged drug)

Contraindications Hypersensitivity to metoprolol or any component of the formulation; sinus bradycardia; heart block greater than first degree (except in patients with a functioning artificial pacemaker); cardiogenic shock; uncompensated cardiac failure; pregnancy (2nd and 3rd trimesters)

Warnings/Precautions Must use care in compensated heart failure and monitor closely for a worsening of the condition (efficacy has not been established for metoprolol). Beta-blocker therapy should not be withdrawn abruptly (particularly in patients with CAD), but gradually tapered to avoid acute tachycardia, hypertension, and/or ischemia. Beta-blockers may increase the risk of anaphylaxis (in predisposed patients) and blunt response to epinephrine. Use caution in patients with PVD (can aggravate arterial insufficiency). Use caution with concurrent use of beta-blockers and either verapamil or diltiazem; bradycardia or heart block can occur. Avoid concurrent I.V. use of both agents. In general, beta-blockers should be avoided in patients with bronchospastic disease. Metoprolol, with B1 selectivity, should be used cautiously in bronchospastic disease with close monitoring. Use cautiously in diabetics because it can mask prominent hypoglycemic symptoms. Can mask signs of thyrotoxicosis. Can cause fetal harm when administered in pregnancy. Use cautiously in the hepatically impaired. Use care with anesthetic agents which decrease myocardial function. The extended release formulation consists of drug within a nondeformable matrix; following drug release/absorption, the matrix/shell is expelled in the stool. The use of nondeformable products in patients with known stricture/narrowing of the GI tract has been associated with symptoms of obstruction.

Drug Interactions **Substrate** of CYP2C19 (minor), 2D6 (major); **Inhibits** CYP2D6 (weak)

Alpha-blockers (prazosin, terazosin): Concurrent use of beta-blockers may increase risk of orthostasis.

AV conduction-slowing agents (digoxin): Effects may be additive with beta-blockers.

Clonidine: Hypertensive crisis after or during withdrawal of either agent.

CYP2D6 inhibitors: May increase the levels/effects of metoprolol. Example inhibitors include chlorpromazine, delavirdine, fluoxetine, miconazole, paroxetine, pergolide, quinidine, quinine, ritonavir, and ropinirole.

Fluoxetine may inhibit the metabolism of metoprolol resulting in cardiac toxicity.

Glucagon: Metoprolol may blunt the hyperglycemic action of glucagon.

Hydralazine may enhance the bioavailability of metoprolol.

Insulin and oral hypoglycemics: Metoprolol may mask tachycardia from hypoglycemia.

Metoprolol reduces antipyrine's clearance by 18%.

NSAIDs (ibuprofen, indomethacin, naproxen, piroxicam) may reduce the antihypertensive effects of beta-blockers.

Oral contraceptives may increase the AUC and C_{max} of metoprolol.

Salicylates may reduce the antihypertensive effects of beta-blockers.

Sulfonylureas: Beta-blockers may alter response to hypoglycemic agents.

Verapamil or diltiazem may have synergistic or additive pharmacological effects when taken concurrently with beta-blockers; avoid concurrent I.V. use.

Nutritional/Herbal/Ethanol Interactions

Food: Food increases absorption. Metoprolol serum levels may be increased if taken with food.

Herb/Nutraceutical: Avoid dong quai if using for hypertension (has estrogenic activity). Avoid ephedra, yohimbe, ginseng (may worsen hypertension). Avoid garlic (may have increased antihypertensive effect).

Adverse Reactions

>10%:

Central nervous system: Drowsiness, insomnia

Endocrine & metabolic: Decreased sexual ability

1% to 10%:

Cardiovascular: Bradycardia, palpitation, edema, CHF, reduced peripheral circulation

Central nervous system: Mental depression

Gastrointestinal: Diarrhea or constipation, nausea, stomach discomfort

Respiratory: Bronchospasm

Miscellaneous: Cold extremities

<1% (Limited to important or life-threatening): Arrhythmias, arthralgia, chest pain, confusion (especially in the elderly), depression, dyspnea, hallucinations, headache, heart block (second- and third-degree), hepatic dysfunction, hepatitis, jaundice, leukopenia, nervousness, orthostatic hypotension, paresthesia, photosensitivity, thrombocytopenia, vomiting

Overdosage/Toxicology Symptoms of intoxication include cardiac disturbances, CNS toxicity, bronchospasm, hypoglycemia and hyperkalemia. The most common cardiac symptoms include hypotension and bradycardia. Atrioventricular block, intraventricular conduction disturbances, cardiogenic shock, and asystole may occur with severe overdose, especially with membrane-depressant drugs (eg, propranolol). CNS effects include convulsions, coma, and respiratory arrest. Treatment is symptom-directed and supportive.

Dosing

Adults:

Hypertension: Oral: 100-450 mg/day in 2-3 divided doses, begin with 50 mg twice daily and increase doses at weekly intervals to desired effect; usual dosage range (JNC 7): 50-100 mg/day

Extended release: Initial: 25-100 mg/day (maximum: 400 mg/day)

Angina, SVT, MI prophylaxis: Oral: 100-450 mg/day in 2-3 divided doses, begin with 50 mg twice daily and increase doses at weekly intervals to desired effect

Extended release: Initial: 100 mg/day (maximum: 400 mg/day)

Hypertension/ventricular rate control: I.V. (in patients having nonfunctioning GI tract): Initial: 1.25-5 mg every 6-12 hours; titrate initial dose to response.

(Continued)

Metoprolol *(Continued)*

Initially, low doses may be appropriate to establish response; however, up to 15 mg every 3-6 hours has been employed.

Congestive heart failure: Oral (extended release): Initial: 25 mg once daily (reduce to 12.5 mg once daily in NYHA class higher than class II); may double dosage every 2 weeks as tolerated, up to 200 mg/day

Myocardial infarction (acute): I.V.: 5 mg every 2 minutes for 3 doses in early treatment of myocardial infarction; thereafter give 50 mg orally every 6 hours 15 minutes after last I.V. dose and continue for 48 hours; then administer a maintenance dose of 100 mg twice daily.

Elderly: Oral: Initial: 25 mg/day; usual dose range: 25-300 mg/day; increase at 1- to 2-week intervals.

Extended release: 25-50 mg/day initially as a single dose; increase at 1- to 2-week intervals.

Pediatrics:

Hypertension, arrhythmia: Oral: Children: 1-5 mg/kg/24 hours divided twice daily; allow 3 days between dose adjustments.

Renal Impairment: Hemodialysis: Administer dose posthemodialysis or administer 50 mg supplemental dose. Supplemental dose is not necessary following peritoneal dialysis.

Hepatic Impairment: Reduced dose is probably necessary.

Available Dosage Forms

Injection, solution, as tartrate (Lopressor®): 1 mg/mL (5 mL)

Tablet, as tartrate 25 mg, 50 mg, 100 mg

Lopressor®: 50 mg, 100 mg

Tablet, extended release, as succinate (Toprol-XL®): 25 mg, 50 mg, 100 mg, 200 mg [expressed as mg equivalent to tartrate]

Nursing Guidelines

Assessment: Assess potential for interactions with other prescriptions, OTC medications, or herbal products patient may be taking. **I.V.:** See specifics below and monitor blood pressure and cardiac status. Assess therapeutic effectiveness and adverse reactions (eg, fluid balance, CHF, postural hypotension). Caution patients with diabetes to monitor serum glucose closely; may decrease the effect of sulfonylureas and can mask prominent hypoglycemic symptoms. Teach patient proper use (oral), possible side effects/appropriate interventions, and adverse symptoms to report.

Dietary Considerations: Regular tablets should be taken with food. Extended release tablets may be taken without regard to meals.

Patient Education: I.V. use in emergency situations: Patient information is appropriate to patient condition.

Oral: Do not take any new medication during therapy unless approved by prescriber. Take exactly as directed. Do not change dosage or discontinue without consulting prescriber. Take pulse daily, prior to medication and follow prescriber's instruction about holding medication. Do not take with antacids. If you have diabetes, monitor serum sugar closely (drug may alter glucose tolerance or mask signs of hypoglycemia). May cause fatigue, dizziness, or postural hypotension (use caution when changing position from lying or sitting to standing, when driving, or when climbing stairs until response to medication is known); or alteration in sexual performance (reversible). Report unresolved swelling of extremities, respiratory difficulty or new cough, unresolved fatigue, unusual weight gain, unresolved constipation, or unusual muscle weakness. **Pregnancy/breast-feeding precautions:** Inform prescriber if you are or intend to become pregnant. Consult prescriber if breast-feeding.

Geriatric Considerations: Due to alterations in the beta-adrenergic autonomic nervous system, beta-adrenergic blockade may result in less hemodynamic response than seen in younger adults.

Pregnancy Risk Factor: C (manufacturer); D (2nd and 3rd trimesters - expert analysis)

Pregnancy Issues: Metoprolol crosses the placenta. Beta-blockers have been associated with bradycardia, hypotension, and IUGR; IUGR is probably related to maternal hypertension. Available evidence suggests beta-blockers are generally safe during pregnancy (JNC 7). Cases of neonatal hypoglycemia have been reported following maternal use of beta-blockers at parturition or during breast-feeding. Monitor breast-fed infant for symptoms of beta-blockade.

Lactation: Enters breast milk/use caution (AAP rates "compatible")

Breast-Feeding Considerations: Metoprolol is considered compatible by the AAP. However, monitor the infant for signs of beta-blockade (hypotension, bradycardia, etc) with long-term use.

Perioperative/Anesthesia/Other Concerns: Symptomatic bradycardia may be treated with atropine.

Surgery: Atenolol has also been shown to improve cardiovascular outcomes when used in the perioperative period in patients with underlying cardiovascular disease who are undergoing noncardiac surgery. Bisoprolol in high-risk patients undergoing vascular surgery reduced the perioperative incidence of death from cardiac causes and nonfatal myocardial infarction.

Withdrawal: Beta-blocker therapy should not be withdrawn abruptly, but gradually tapered to avoid acute tachycardia and hypertension.

Administration

Oral: Extended release tablets may be divided in half; do not crush or chew.

I.V.: When administered acutely for cardiac treatment, monitor ECG and blood pressure. May administer by rapid infusion (I.V. push) over 1 minute or by slow infusion (ie, 5-10 mg of metoprolol in 50 mL of fluid) over ~30 minutes. Necessary monitoring for surgical patients who are unable to take oral beta-blockers (prolonged ileus) has not been defined. Some institutions require monitoring of baseline and postinfusion heart rate and blood pressure when a patient's response to beta-blockade has not been characterized (ie, the patient's initial dose or following a change in dose). Consult individual institutional policies and procedures.

Compatibility: Stable in D_5W, NS

Y-site administration: Incompatible with amphotericin B cholesteryl sulfate complex

Storage:

Injection: Do not store above 30°C (86°F). Protect from light.

Tablet: Store between 15°C to 30°C (59°F to 86°F).

Related Information

Management of Postoperative Arrhythmias *on page 1787*

Metoprolol and Hydrochlorothiazide

(me toe PROE lole & hye droe klor oh THYE a zide)

U.S. Brand Names Lopressor HCT®

Synonyms Hydrochlorothiazide and Metoprolol; Hydrochlorothiazide and Metoprolol Tartrate; Metoprolol Tartrate and Hydrochlorothiazide

Pharmacologic Category Beta Blocker, $Beta_1$ Selective; Diuretic, Thiazide

Use Treatment of hypertension

Mechanism of Action See individual agents.

Pharmacodynamics/Kinetics See individual agents.

Contraindications Hypersensitivity to metoprolol, hydrochlorothiazide, sulfonamide-derived drugs or any component of the formulation; sinus bradycardia; heart block greater than first degree; cardiogenic shock; overt cardiac failure; anuria

Warnings/Precautions Used as a replacement for separate dosing of components or combination when response to single agent is suboptimal; the fixed combination is not indicated for initial treatment of hypertension; see individual monographs for additional warnings/precautions. Safety and efficacy not established in pediatric patients.

Drug Interactions Metoprolol: **Substrate** of CYP2C19 (minor), 2D6 (major); Inhibits CYP2D6 (weak)

Also see individual agents.

Nutritional/Herbal/Ethanol Interactions See individual agents.

Lab Interactions See individual agents.

Adverse Reactions Reactions noted here have been reported with the combination product; see individual drug monographs for additional adverse reactions that may be expected from each agent.

1% to 10%:

Cardiovascular: Bradycardia (6%), edema (1%)

Central nervous system: Fatigue (10%), dizziness (10%), drowsiness (10%), headache (10%), vertigo (10%), abnormal dreams (1%)

Dermatologic: Purpura (1%)

Endocrine & metabolic: Hypokalemia, gout (1%)

Gastrointestinal: Anorexia (1%), constipation (1%), diarrhea (1%), nausea (1%), vomiting (1%), xerostomia (1%)

(Continued)

Metoprolol and Hydrochlorothiazide *(Continued)*

Genitourinary: Impotence (1%)
Neuromuscular & skeletal: Myalgia
Ocular: Blurred vision (1%)
Otic: Earache (1%), tinnitus (1%)
Respiratory: Dyspnea (1%)
Miscellaneous: Flu-like syndrome (10%), diaphoresis (1%), exercise tolerance decreased (1%)

Overdosage/Toxicology Symptoms may include hypotension, bradycardia, bronchospasm, or cardiac failure. Nausea, thirst, muscle cramps, or confusion may also occur. Inducement of vomiting, gastric lavage, and activated charcoal are recommended. Treatment is supportive; fluid, electrolyte balance, and renal function should be monitored.

Dosing

Adults & Elderly: Hypertension: Oral: Dosage should be determined by titration of the individual agents and the combination product substituted based upon the daily requirements.

Usual dose: Metoprolol 50-100 mg and hydrochlorothiazide 25-50 mg administered daily as single or divided doses (twice daily)

Note: Hydrochlorothiazide >50 mg/day is not recommended.

Concomitant therapy: It is recommended that if an additional antihypertensive agent is required, gradual titration should occur using 1/2 the usual starting dose of the other agent to avoid hypotension.

Available Dosage Forms Tablet:
50/25: Metoprolol tartrate 50 mg and hydrochlorothiazide 25 mg
100/25: Metoprolol tartrate 100 mg and hydrochlorothiazide 25 mg
100/50: Metoprolol tartrate 100 mg and hydrochlorothiazide 50 mg

Nursing Guidelines

Monitoring Laboratory Tests: Serum electrolytes, BUN, creatinine

Patient Education: See individual agents. **Pregnancy/breast-feeding precautions:** Inform prescriber if you are or intend to become pregnant. Consult prescriber if breast-feeding.

Pregnancy Risk Factor: C/D (expert analysis)

Lactation: Enters breast milk/not recommended

Breast-Feeding Considerations: See individual agents.

Administration

Oral: Administer with or immediately following meals (or as directed). To avoid nocturia, doses should be taken early in the day and last dose of multiple doses should be taken no later than 6 pm.

Storage: Store between 15°C to 30°C (59°F to 86°F). Protect from moisture.

Related Information

Hydrochlorothiazide *on page 862*
Metoprolol *on page 1150*

♦ **Metoprolol Succinate** *see* Metoprolol *on page 1150*
♦ **Metoprolol Tartrate** *see* Metoprolol *on page 1150*
♦ **Metoprolol Tartrate and Hydrochlorothiazide** *see* Metoprolol and Hydrochlorothiazide *on page 1153*
♦ **Metrizamide** *see* Radiological/Contrast Media (Nonionic) *on page 1459*
♦ **MetroCream®** *see* Metronidazole *on page 1154*
♦ **MetroGel®** *see* Metronidazole *on page 1154*
♦ **MetroGel-Vaginal®** *see* Metronidazole *on page 1154*
♦ **MetroLotion®** *see* Metronidazole *on page 1154*

Metronidazole (me troe NI da zole)

U.S. Brand Names Flagyl®; Flagyl ER®; Flagyl® I.V. RTU™; MetroCream®; MetroGel®; MetroGel-Vaginal®; MetroLotion®; Noritate®; Vandazole™

Synonyms Metronidazole Hydrochloride

Pharmacologic Category Amebicide; Antibiotic, Miscellaneous; Antibiotic, Topical; Antiprotozoal, Nitroimidazole

Medication Safety Issues

Sound-alike/look-alike issues:
Metronidazole may be confused with metformin.

Use Treatment of susceptible anaerobic bacterial and protozoal infections in the following conditions: Amebiasis, symptomatic and asymptomatic trichomoniasis; skin and skin structure infections; CNS infections; intra-abdominal infections (as part of combination regimen); systemic anaerobic infections; treatment of antibiotic-associated pseudomembranous colitis (AAPC), bacterial vaginosis; as part of a multidrug regimen for *H. pylori* eradication to reduce the risk of duodenal ulcer recurrence

Topical: Treatment of inflammatory lesions and erythema of rosacea

Unlabeled/Investigational Use Crohn's disease

Mechanism of Action After diffusing into the organism, interacts with DNA to cause a loss of helical DNA structure and strand breakage resulting in inhibition of protein synthesis and cell death in susceptible organisms

Pharmacodynamics/Kinetics

Absorption: Oral: Well absorbed; Topical: Concentrations achieved systemically after application of 1 g topically are 10 times less than those obtained after a 250 mg oral dose

Distribution: To saliva, bile, seminal fluid, breast milk, bone, liver, and liver abscesses, lung and vaginal secretions; crosses placenta and blood-brain barrier

CSF:blood level ratio: Normal meninges: 16% to 43%; Inflamed meninges: 100%

Protein binding: <20%

Metabolism: Hepatic (30% to 60%)

Half-life elimination: Neonates: 25-75 hours; Others: 6-8 hours, prolonged with hepatic impairment; End-stage renal disease: 21 hours

Time to peak, serum: Oral: Immediate release: 1-2 hours

Excretion: Urine (20% to 40% as unchanged drug); feces (6% to 15%)

Contraindications Hypersensitivity to metronidazole, nitroimidazole derivatives, or any component of the formulation; pregnancy (1st trimester - found to be carcinogenic in rats)

Warnings/Precautions Use with caution in patients with liver impairment due to potential accumulation, blood dyscrasias; history of seizures, CHF, or other sodium retaining states; reduce dosage in patients with severe liver impairment, CNS disease, and severe renal failure (Cl_{cr} <10 mL/minute); if *H. pylori* is not eradicated in patients being treated with metronidazole in a regimen, it should be assumed that metronidazole-resistance has occurred and it should not again be used; seizures and neuropathies have been reported especially with increased doses and chronic treatment; if this occurs, discontinue therapy

Drug Interactions Inhibits CYP2C8/9 (weak), 3A4 (moderate)

Cimetidine may increase metronidazole levels.

Cisapride: May inhibit metabolism of cisapride, causing potential arrhythmias; avoid concurrent use

CYP3A4 substrates: Metronidazole may increase the levels/effects of CYP3A4 substrates. Example substrates include benzodiazepines, calcium channel blockers, cyclosporine, mirtazapine, nateglinide, nefazodone, sildenafil (and other PDE-5 inhibitors), tacrolimus, and venlafaxine. Selected benzodiazepines (midazolam and triazolam), cisapride, ergot alkaloids, selected HMG-CoA reductase inhibitors (lovastatin and simvastatin), and pimozide are generally contraindicated with strong CYP3A4 inhibitors.

Ethanol: Ethanol results in disulfiram-like reactions.

Lithium: Metronidazole may increase lithium levels/toxicity; monitor lithium levels.

Phenytoin, phenobarbital may increase metabolism of metronidazole, potentially decreasing its effect.

Warfarin: Metronidazole increases P-T prolongation with warfarin.

Nutritional/Herbal/Ethanol Interactions

Ethanol: The manufacturer recommends to avoid all ethanol or any ethanol-containing drugs (may cause disulfiram-like reaction characterized by flushing, headache, nausea, vomiting, sweating or tachycardia).

Food: Peak antibiotic serum concentration lowered and delayed, but total drug absorbed not affected.

Lab Interactions May cause falsely decreased AST and ALT levels.

Adverse Reactions

Systemic: Frequency not defined:

Cardiovascular: Flattening of the T-wave, flushing

Central nervous system: Ataxia, confusion, coordination impaired, dizziness, fever, headache, insomnia, irritability, seizure, vertigo

Dermatologic: Erythematous rash, urticaria

Endocrine & metabolic: Disulfiram-like reaction, dysmenorrhea, libido decreased

(Continued)

Metronidazole *(Continued)*

Gastrointestinal: Nausea (~12%), anorexia, abdominal cramping, constipation, diarrhea, furry tongue, glossitis, proctitis, stomatitis, unusual/metallic taste, vomiting, xerostomia

Genitourinary: Cystitis, darkened urine (rare), dysuria, incontinence, polyuria, vaginitis

Hematologic: Neutropenia (reversible), thrombocytopenia (reversible, rare)

Neuromuscular & skeletal: Peripheral neuropathy, weakness

Respiratory: Nasal congestion, rhinitis, sinusitis, pharyngitis

Miscellaneous: Flu-like syndrome, moniliasis

Topical: Frequency not defined:

Central nervous system: Headache

Dermatologic: Burning, contact dermatitis, dryness, erythema, irritation, pruritus, rash

Gastrointestinal: Unusual/metallic taste, nausea, constipation

Local: Local allergic reaction

Neuromuscular & skeletal: Tingling/numbness of extremities

Ocular: Eye irritation

Vaginal:

>10%: Genitourinary: Vaginal discharge (12%)

1% to 10%:

Central nervous system: Headache (5%), dizziness (2%)

Gastrointestinal: Gastrointestinal discomfort (7%), nausea and/or vomiting (4%), unusual/metallic taste (2%), diarrhea (1%)

Genitourinary: Vaginitis (10%), vulva/vaginal irritation (9%), pelvic discomfort (3%)

Hematologic: WBC increased (2%)

<1%: Abdominal bloating, abdominal gas, darkened urine, depression, fatigue, itching, rash, thirst, xerostomia

Overdosage/Toxicology Symptoms of overdose include nausea, vomiting, ataxia, seizures, and peripheral neuropathy. Treatment is symptomatic and supportive.

Dosing

Adults:

Anaerobic infections (diverticulitis, intra-abdominal, peritonitis, cholangitis, or abscess): Oral, I.V.: 500 mg every 6-8 hours, not to exceed 4 g/day

Acne rosacea: Topical:

0.75%: Apply and rub a thin film twice daily, morning and evening, to entire affected areas after washing. Significant therapeutic results should be noticed within 3 weeks. Clinical studies have demonstrated continuing improvement through 9 weeks of therapy.

1%: Apply thin film to affected area once daily

Amebiasis: Oral: 500-750 mg every 8 hours for 5-10 days

Antibiotic-associated pseudomembranous colitis: Oral: 250-500 mg 3-4 times/day for 10-14 days

Giardiasis: 500 mg twice daily for 5-7 days

Peptic ulcer disease: *Helicobacter pylori* eradication: Oral: 250-500 mg with meals and at bedtime for 14 days; requires combination therapy with at least one other antibiotic and an acid-suppressing agent (proton pump inhibitor or H_2 blocker)

Bacterial vaginosis or vaginitis due to *Gardnerella, Mobiluncus*:

Oral: 500 mg twice daily (regular release) or 750 mg once daily (extended release tablet) for 7 days

Vaginal: 1 applicatorful (~37.5 mg metronidazole) intravaginally once or twice daily for 5 days; apply once in morning and evening if using twice daily, if daily, use at bedtime

Trichomoniasis: Oral: 250 mg every 8 hours for 7 days **or** 375 mg twice daily for 7 days **or** 2 g as a single dose

Elderly: Use the lower end of the dosing recommendations for adults; do not administer as single dose as efficacy has not been established.

Pediatrics:

Anaerobic infections: Oral, I.V.:

Postnatal age >7 days:

1200-2000 g: 15 mg/kg/day in divided doses every 12 hours

>2000 g: 30 mg/kg/day in divided doses every 12 hours

Infants and Children:

Oral: 15-35 mg/kg/day in divided doses every 8 hours

I.V.: 30 mg/kg/day in divided doses every 6 hours

Colitis due to *Clostridium difficile*: Oral: 20 mg/kg/day divided every 6 hours. Maximum dose: 2 g/day

Amebiasis: Infants and Children: Oral: 35-50 mg/kg/day in divided doses every 8 hours for 10 days

Trichomoniasis: Infants and Children: Oral: 15-30 mg/kg/day in divided doses every 8 hours for 7 days

Renal Impairment:

Cl_{cr} <10 mL/minute: Administer 50% of dose or every 12 hours.

Hemodialysis effects: Extensively removed by hemodialysis and peritoneal dialysis (50% to 100%). Administer dose posthemodialysis. During peritoneal dialysis, dose as for Cl_{cr} <10 mL/minute.

Continuous arteriovenous or venovenous hemofiltration: Dose as for normal renal function

Hepatic Impairment: Unchanged in mild liver disease; reduce dosage in severe liver disease.

Available Dosage Forms

Capsule (Flagyl®): 375 mg

Cream, topical: 0.75% (45 g)

MetroCream®: 0.75% (45 g) [contains benzyl alcohol]

Noritate®: 1% (60 g)

Gel, topical (MetroGel®): 0.75% (45 g), 1% (45 g)

Gel, vaginal (MetroGel-Vaginal®, Vandazole™): 0.75% (70 g)

Infusion (Flagyl® I.V. RTU™) [premixed iso-osmotic sodium chloride solution]: 500 mg (100 mL) [contains sodium 14 mEq]

Lotion, topical (MetroLotion®): 0.75% (60 mL) [contains benzyl alcohol]

Tablet (Flagyl®): 250 mg, 500 mg

Tablet, extended release (Flagyl® ER): 750 mg

Nursing Guidelines

Assessment: Assess effectiveness and interactions of other medications patient may be taking. Assess results of laboratory tests, therapeutic effectiveness, and adverse reactions according to dose, route of administration, and purpose of therapy. Assess knowledge/teach patient appropriate use, interventions to reduce side effects, and adverse symptoms to report.

Dietary Considerations: Take on an empty stomach. Drug may cause GI upset; if GI upset occurs, take with food. Extended release tablets should be taken on an empty stomach (1 hour before or 2 hours after meals). Sodium content of 500 mg (I.V.): 322 mg (14 mEq). The manufacturer recommends that ethanol be avoided during treatment and for 3 days after therapy is complete.

Patient Education: Take exactly as directed. May take with or without food. Take with food if medication causes upset stomach. Avoid alcohol during and for 72 hours after last dose. With alcohol you may experience severe flushing, headache, nausea, vomiting, or chest and abdominal pain. May discolor urine (brown/black/dark) (normal). You may experience 'metallic' taste disturbance or nausea or vomiting (small frequent meals, frequent mouth care, chewing gum, or sucking lozenges may help). Refrain from intercourse or use a contraceptive if being treated for trichomoniasis. Report unresolved or severe fatigue; weakness; fever or chills; mouth or vaginal sores; numbness, tingling, or swelling of extremities; respiratory difficulty; or lack of improvement or worsening of condition. **Pregnancy/breast-feeding precautions:** Inform prescriber if you are pregnant. Breast-feeding is not recommended.

Topical: Wash hands and area before applying. Apply medication thinly. Wash hands after applying. Avoid contact with eyes. Do not cover with occlusive dressing. Report severe skin irritation or if condition does not improve.

Geriatric Considerations: Adjust dose based on renal function.

Pregnancy Risk Factor: B (may be contraindicated in 1st trimester)

Pregnancy Issues: Crosses the placenta; contraindicated for the treatment of trichomoniasis during the first trimester of pregnancy, unless alternative treatment is inadequate. Until safety and efficacy for other indications have been established, use only during pregnancy when the benefit to the mother outweighs the potential risk to the fetus.

Lactation: Enters breast milk/not recommended (AAP rates "of concern")

Breast-Feeding Considerations: It is suggested to stop breast-feeding for 12-24 hours following single dose therapy to allow excretion of dose.

(Continued)

Metronidazole *(Continued)*

Perioperative/Anesthesia/Other Concerns: Metronidazole may have effects similar to that of disulfiram (Antabuse®). If ethanol is taken during and within 24 hours of the last dose of metronidazole, patients may have severe flushing, headache, nausea, vomiting, or chest and abdominal pain.

Administration

Oral: May be taken with food to minimize stomach upset. Extended release tablets should be taken on an empty stomach (1 hour before or 2 hours after meals).

Reconstitution: Standard diluent: 500 mg/100 mL NS

Compatibility: Stable in D_5W, NS

Y-site administration: Incompatible with amphotericin B cholesteryl sulfate complex, aztreonam, filgrastim, meropenem, warfarin

Compatibility when admixed: Incompatible with aztreonam, dopamine, meropenem

Storage: Metronidazole injection should be stored at 15°C to 30°C and protected from light. Product may be refrigerated but crystals may form; crystals redissolve on warming to room temperature. Prolonged exposure to light will cause a darkening of the product. However, short-term exposure to normal room light does not adversely affect metronidazole stability. Direct sunlight should be avoided. Stability of parenteral admixture at room temperature (25°C): Out of overwrap stability: 30 days.

Related Information

Prevention of Wound Infection and Sepsis in Surgical Patients *on page 1830*

- ♦ **Metronidazole Hydrochloride** *see* Metronidazole *on page 1154*
- ♦ **Mevacor®** *see* Lovastatin *on page 1070*
- ♦ **Mevinolin** *see* Lovastatin *on page 1070*
- ♦ **$MgSO_4$ (error-prone abbreviation)** *see* Magnesium Sulfate *on page 1077*
- ♦ **Miacalcin®** *see* Calcitonin *on page 287*
- ♦ **Mi-Acid [OTC]** *see* Aluminum Hydroxide, Magnesium Hydroxide, and Simethicone *on page 122*
- ♦ **Mi-Acid™ Double Strength [OTC]** *see* Calcium Carbonate and Magnesium Hydroxide *on page 294*
- ♦ **Mi-Acid Maximum Strength [OTC]** *see* Aluminum Hydroxide, Magnesium Hydroxide, and Simethicone *on page 122*
- ♦ **MICRhoGAM®** *see* Rh_o(D) Immune Globulin *on page 1471*
- ♦ **Microfibrillar Collagen Hemostat** *see* Collagen Hemostat *on page 449*
- ♦ **microK®** *see* Potassium Chloride *on page 1385*
- ♦ **microK® 10** *see* Potassium Chloride *on page 1385*
- ♦ **Micronase®** *see* GlyBURIDE *on page 820*
- ♦ **microNefrin®** *see* Epinephrine (Racemic/Dental) *on page 615*
- ♦ **Microzide™** *see* Hydrochlorothiazide *on page 862*

Midazolam (MID aye zoe lam)

Synonyms Midazolam Hydrochloride; Versed

Pharmacologic Category Benzodiazepine

Medication Safety Issues

Sound-alike/look-alike issues:

Versed may be confused with VePesid®, Vistaril®

Use Preoperative sedation and provides conscious sedation prior to diagnostic or radiographic procedures; ICU sedation (continuous infusion); intravenous anesthesia (induction); intravenous anesthesia (maintenance)

Unlabeled/Investigational Use Anxiety, status epilepticus

Mechanism of Action Binds to stereospecific benzodiazepine receptors on the postsynaptic GABA neuron at several sites within the central nervous system, including the limbic system, reticular formation. Enhancement of the inhibitory effect of GABA on neuronal excitability results by increased neuronal membrane permeability to chloride ions. This shift in chloride ions results in hyperpolarization (a less excitable state) and stabilization.

Pharmacodynamics/Kinetics

Onset of action: I.M.: Sedation: ~15 minutes; I.V.: 1-5 minutes

Peak effect: I.M.: 0.5-1 hour

Duration: I.M.: Up to 6 hours; Mean: 2 hours

Absorption: Oral: Rapid

Distribution: V_d: 0.8-2.5 L/kg; increased with congestive heart failure (CHF) and chronic renal failure

Protein binding: 95%

Metabolism: Extensively hepatic via CYP3A4

Bioavailability: Mean: 45%

Half-life elimination: 1-4 hours; prolonged with cirrhosis, congestive heart failure, obesity, and elderly

Excretion: Urine (as glucuronide conjugated metabolites); feces (~2% to 10%)

Contraindications Hypersensitivity to midazolam or any component of the formulation, including benzyl alcohol (cross-sensitivity with other benzodiazepines may exist); parenteral form is not for intrathecal or epidural injection; narrow-angle glaucoma; concurrent use of potent inhibitors of CYP3A4 (amprenavir, atazanavir, or ritonavir); pregnancy

Warnings/Precautions May cause severe respiratory depression, respiratory arrest, or apnea. Use with extreme caution, particularly in noncritical care settings. Appropriate resuscitative equipment and qualified personnel must be available for administration and monitoring. Initial dosing must be cautiously titrated and individualized, particularly in elderly or debilitated patients, patients with hepatic impairment (including alcoholics), or in renal impairment, particularly if other CNS depressants (including opiates) are used concurrently. Initial doses in elderly or debilitated patients should not exceed 2.5 mg. Use with caution in patients with respiratory disease or impaired gag reflex. Use during upper airway procedures may increase risk of hypoventilation. Prolonged responses have been noted following extended administration by continuous infusion (possibly due to metabolite accumulation) or in the presence of drugs which inhibit midazolam metabolism.

May cause hypotension - hemodynamic events are more common in pediatric patients or patients with hemodynamic instability. Hypotension and/or respiratory depression may occur more frequently in patients who have received narcotic analgesics. Use with caution in obese patients, chronic renal failure, and CHF. Parenteral form contains benzyl alcohol - avoid rapid injection in neonates or prolonged infusions. Does not protect against increases in heart rate or blood pressure during intubation. Should not be used in shock, coma, or acute alcohol intoxication. Avoid intra-arterial administration or extravasation of parenteral formulation.

Causes CNS depression (dose-related) resulting in sedation, dizziness, confusion, or ataxia which may impair physical and mental capabilities. Patients must be cautioned about performing tasks which require mental alertness (eg, operating machinery or driving). A minimum of 1 day should elapse after midazolam administration before attempting these tasks. Use with caution in patients receiving other CNS depressants or psychoactive agents. Effects with other sedative drugs or ethanol may be potentiated. Benzodiazepines have been associated with falls and traumatic injury and should be used with extreme caution in patients who are at risk of these events (especially the elderly).

Midazolam causes anterograde amnesia. Paradoxical reactions, including hyperactive or aggressive behavior have been reported with benzodiazepines, particularly in adolescent/pediatric or psychiatric patients. Does not have analgesic, antidepressant, or antipsychotic properties.

Benzodiazepines have been associated with dependence and acute withdrawal symptoms on discontinuation or reduction in dose. Acute withdrawal, including seizures, may be precipitated after administration of flumazenil to patients receiving long-term benzodiazepine therapy.

Drug Interactions **Substrate** of CYP2B6 (minor), 3A4 (major); **Inhibits** CYP2C8/9 (weak), 3A4 (weak)

CNS depressants: Sedative effects and/or respiratory depression may be additive with CNS depressants; includes ethanol, barbiturates, narcotic analgesics, and other sedative agents; monitor for increased effect. **If narcotics or other CNS depressants are administered concomitantly, the midazolam dose should be reduced by 30% if <65 years of age, or by at least 50% if >65 years of age.**

CYP3A4 inducers: CYP3A4 inducers may decrease the levels/effects of midazolam. Example inducers include aminoglutethimide, carbamazepine, nafcillin, nevirapine, phenobarbital, phenytoin, and rifamycins.

(Continued)

Midazolam *(Continued)*

CYP3A4 inhibitors: May increase the levels/effects of midazolam. Example inhibitors include azole antifungals, clarithromycin, diclofenac, doxycycline, erythromycin, imatinib, isoniazid, nefazodone, nicardipine, propofol, protease inhibitors, quinidine, telithromycin, and verapamil.

Levodopa: Therapeutic effects may be diminished in some patients following the addition of a benzodiazepine; limited/inconsistent data

Oral contraceptives: May decrease the clearance of some benzodiazepines (those which undergo oxidative metabolism); monitor for increased benzodiazepine effect

Saquinavir: A 56% reduction in clearance and a doubling of midazolam's half-life were seen with concurrent administration with saquinavir.

Theophylline: May partially antagonize some of the effects of benzodiazepines; monitor for decreased response; may require higher doses for sedation

Nutritional/Herbal/Ethanol Interactions

Ethanol: Avoid ethanol (may increase CNS depression).

Food: Grapefruit juice may increase serum concentrations of midazolam; avoid concurrent use with oral form.

Herb/Nutraceutical: Avoid concurrent use with St John's wort (may decrease midazolam levels, may increase CNS depression). Avoid concurrent use with valerian, kava kava, gotu kola (may increase CNS depression).

Adverse Reactions As reported in adults unless otherwise noted:

>10%: Respiratory: Decreased tidal volume and/or respiratory rate decrease, apnea (3% children)

1% to 10%:

- Cardiovascular: Hypotension (3% children)
- Central nervous system: Drowsiness (1%), oversedation, headache (1%), seizure-like activity (1% children)
- Gastrointestinal: Nausea (3%), vomiting (3%)
- Local: Pain and local reactions at injection site (4% I.M., 5% I.V.; severity less than diazepam)
- Ocular: Nystagmus (1% children)
- Respiratory: Cough (1%)
- Miscellaneous: Physical and psychological dependence with prolonged use, hiccups (4%, 1% children), paradoxical reaction (2% children)

<1% (Limited to important or life-threatening): Agitation, amnesia, bigeminy, bronchospasm, emergence delirium, euphoria, hallucinations, laryngospasm, rash

Overdosage/Toxicology Symptoms of overdose include respiratory depression, hypotension, coma, stupor, confusion, and apnea. Treatment for benzodiazepine overdose is supportive. Flumazenil has been shown to selectively block the binding of benzodiazepines to its receptor, resulting in reversal of CNS depression but not always respiratory depression.

Dosing

Adults:

Note: The dose of midazolam needs to be individualized based on the patient's age, underlying diseases, and concurrent medications. Decrease dose (by ~30%) if narcotics or other CNS depressants are administered concomitantly. **Personnel and equipment needed for standard respiratory resuscitation should be immediately available during midazolam administration.**

Preoperative sedation:

I.M.: 0.07-0.08 mg/kg 30-60 minutes prior to surgery/procedure; usual dose: 5 mg; **Note:** Reduce dose in patients with COPD, high-risk patients, patients ≥60 years of age, and patients receiving other narcotics or CNS depressants

I.V.: 0.02-0.04 mg/kg; repeat every 5 minutes as needed to desired effect or up to 0.1-0.2 mg/kg

Intranasal (not an approved route): 0.2 mg/kg (up to 0.4 mg/kg in some studies); administer 30-45 minutes prior to surgery/procedure

Conscious sedation: I.V.: Initial: 0.5-2 mg slow I.V. over at least 2 minutes; slowly titrate to effect by repeating doses every 2-3 minutes if needed; usual total dose: 2.5-5 mg; use decreased doses in elderly.

Healthy Adults <60 years:

Initial: Some patients respond to doses as low as 1 mg; no more than 2.5 mg should be administered over a period of 2 minutes. Additional doses of midazolam may be administered after a 2-minute waiting period and evaluation of sedation after each dose increment. A total dose >5 mg is generally not needed. If narcotics or other CNS depressants are administered concomitantly, the midazolam dose should be reduced by 30%. *Refer to elderly dosing for patients ≥60 years, debilitated, or chronically ill.*

Maintenance: 25% of dose used to reach sedative effect

Anesthesia: I.V.:

Induction:

Unpremedicated patients: 0.3-0.35 mg/kg (up to 0.6 mg/kg in resistant cases)

Premedicated patients: 0.15-0.35 mg/kg

Maintenance: 0.05-0.3 mg/kg as needed, or continuous infusion 0.25-1.5 mcg/kg/minute

Sedation in mechanically-ventilated patients: I.V. continuous infusion: 100 mg in 250 mL D_5W or NS (if patient is fluid-restricted, may concentrate up to a maximum of 0.5 mg/mL); initial dose: 0.02-0.08 mg/kg (~1 mg to 5 mg in 70 kg adult) initially and either repeated at 5-15 minute intervals until adequate sedation is achieved or continuous infusion rates of 0.04-0.2 mg/kg/hour and titrate to reach desired level of sedation

Elderly: The dose of midazolam needs to be individualized based on the patient's age, underlying diseases, and concurrent medications. Decrease dose (by ~30%) if narcotics or other CNS depressants are administered concomitantly. **Personnel and equipment needed for standard respiratory resuscitation should be immediately available during midazolam administration.**

I.V.: Conscious sedation: Initial: 0.5 mg slow I.V.; give no more than 1.5 mg in a 2-minute period. If additional titration is needed, give no more than 1 mg over 2 minutes, waiting another 2 or more minutes to evaluate sedative effect. A total dose >3.5 mg is rarely necessary.

Pediatrics:

Notes: The dose of midazolam needs to be individualized based on the patient's age, underlying diseases, and concurrent medications. Decrease dose (by ~30%) if narcotics or other CNS depressants are administered concomitantly. **Personnel and equipment needed for standard respiratory resuscitation should be immediately available during midazolam administration.** Children <6 years may require higher doses and closer monitoring than older children; calculate dose on ideal body weight

Conscious sedation for procedures or preoperative sedation:

Oral: 0.25-0.5 mg/kg as a single dose preprocedure, up to a maximum of 20 mg; administer 30-40 minutes prior to procedure. Children <6 years, or less cooperative patients may require as much as 1 mg/kg as a single dose; 0.25 mg/kg may suffice for children 6-16 years of age.

Intranasal (not an approved route): 0.2 mg/kg (up to 0.4 mg/kg in some studies), administered 30-45 minutes prior to procedure

I.M.: 0.1-0.15 mg/kg 30-60 minutes before surgery or procedure; range 0.05-0.15 mg/kg; doses up to 0.5 mg/kg have been used in more anxious patients; maximum total dose: 10 mg

I.V.:

Infants <6 months: Limited information is available in nonintubated infants; dosing recommendations not clear; infants <6 months are at higher risk for airway obstruction and hypoventilation; titrate dose in small increments to desired effect; monitor carefully

Infants 6 months to Children 5 years: Initial: 0.05-0.1 mg/kg; titrate dose carefully; total dose of 0.6 mg/kg may be required; usual maximum total dose: 6 mg

Children 6-12 years: Initial: 0.025-0.05 mg/kg; titrate dose carefully; total doses of 0.4 mg/kg may be required; usual maximum total dose: 10 mg

Children 12-16 years: Dose as adults; usual maximum total dose: 10 mg

Conscious sedation during mechanical ventilation: I.V.: Children: Loading dose: 0.05-0.2 mg/kg, followed by initial continuous infusion: 1-2 mcg/kg/minute; titrate to the desired effect; usual range: 0.4-6 mcg/kg/minute

Status epilepticus refractory to standard therapy: I.V.: Infants >2 months and Children: Loading dose: 0.15 mg/kg followed by a continuous infusion of 1 mcg/kg/minute; titrate dose upward every 5 minutes until clinical seizure activity is controlled; mean infusion rate required in 24 children was 2.3 mcg/kg/minute with a range of 1-18 mcg/kg/minute

Renal Impairment:

Hemodialysis: Supplemental dose is not necessary.

(Continued)

Midazolam *(Continued)*

Peritoneal dialysis: Significant drug removal is unlikely based on physicochemical characteristics.

Available Dosage Forms

Injection, solution: 1 mg/mL (2 mL, 5 mL, 10 mL); 5 mg/mL (1 mL, 2 mL, 5 mL, 10 mL) [contains benzyl alcohol 1%]

Injection, solution [preservative free]: 1 mg/mL (2 mL, 5 mL); 5 mg/mL (1 mL, 2 mL)

Syrup: 2 mg/mL (118 mL) [contains sodium benzoate; cherry flavor]

Nursing Guidelines

Assessment: Assess other medications the patient may be taking for effectiveness and interactions. For inpatient use, institute safety measures and monitor effectiveness and adverse reactions. For outpatients, monitor therapeutic effectiveness and adverse reactions at beginning of therapy and periodically with long-term use. **I.V.:** Monitor cardiac and respiratory status continuously. Monitor I.V. infusion site carefully for extravasation. **I.V./I.M.:** Monitor closely following administration. Bedrest and assistance with ambulation necessary for several hours. **Note:** Full recovery usually occurs within 2-3 hours, but may take 6 hours.

Dietary Considerations: Injection: Sodium content of 1 mL: 0.14 mEq

Patient Education: Avoid use of alcohol, prescription or OTC sedatives, or hypnotics for a minimum of 24 hours after administration. Avoid driving or engaging in any tasks that require alertness for 24 hours following administration. You may experience some loss of memory following administration. **Pregnancy/breast-feeding precautions:** Advise prescriber if you are pregnant; this medication is contraindicated for pregnant women. Breast-feeding is not recommended.

Geriatric Considerations: If concomitant CNS depressant medications are used in the elderly, the midazolam dose will be at least 50% less than doses used in healthy, young, unpremedicated patients (see Warnings/Precautions and Pharmacokinetics).

Pregnancy Risk Factor: D

Pregnancy Issues: Benzodiazepines cross the placenta. The association between benzodiazepine exposure and malformations remains controversial. A number of types of malformation have been reported (oral cleft, inguinal hernia, cardiac defects, spina bifida, dysmorphic facial features, skeletal defects); however, confounding factors make a clear association difficult. Overall, the risk to the fetus may be low. Nonteratogenic effects (including neonatal flaccidity, respiratory and feeding problems, and withdrawal symptoms) during the postnatal period have also been reported with benzodiazepine use.

Lactation: Enters breast milk/not recommended (AAP rates "of concern")

Perioperative/Anesthesia/Other Concerns:

Agitation in the ICU Patient: Diazepam or midazolam is recommended for rapid sedation of the acutely-agitated patient. Midazolam may accumulate in obesity, in patients with hypoalbuminemia, or renal failure. Concurrent use of CYP3A4 inhibitors may inhibit midazolam's metabolism and prolong its sedative effects. The ACCM/SCCM task force does not recommend midazolam use for ongoing sedation in the practice guidelines for sustained use of sedatives and analgesics in the critically-ill adult. Midazolam is 3-4 times as potent as diazepam. Paradoxical reactions associated with midazolam use in children (eg, agitation, restlessness, combativeness) have been successfully treated with flumazenil.

Administration

Oral: Do not mix with any liquid (such as grapefruit juice) prior to administration.

I.M.: Give deep I.M. into large muscle.

I.V.: Administer by slow I.V. injection over at least 2-5 minutes at a concentration of 1-5 mg/mL or by I.V. infusion. Continuous infusions should be administered via an infusion pump.

Compatibility: Stable in D_5NS, D_5W, NS; **incompatible** with LR

Y-site administration: Incompatible with albumin, amphotericin B cholesteryl sulfate complex, ampicillin, bumetanide, butorphanol, ceftazidime, cefuroxime, clonidine, dexamethasone sodium succinate, floxacillin, foscarnet, fosphenytoin, furosemide, hydrocortisone sodium succinate, imipenem/cilastatin, methotrexate, nafcillin, omeprazole, sodium bicarbonate, thiopental, trimethoprim/sulfamethoxazole

Compatibility in syringe: Incompatible with dimenhydrinate, pentobarbital, perphenazine, prochlorperazine edisylate, ranitidine

Storage: Stable for 24 hours at room temperature/refrigeration; at a final concentration of 0.5 mg/mL, stable for up to 24 hours when diluted with D_5W or NS, or for up to 4 hours when diluted with lactated Ringer's; admixtures do not require protection from light for short-term storage

Related Information

Conscious Sedation *on page 1779*

Intravenous Anesthetic Agents *on page 1853*

- **Midazolam Hydrochloride** *see* Midazolam *on page 1158*
- **Midol® Cramp and Body Aches [OTC]** *see* Ibuprofen *on page 889*
- **Midol® Extended Relief** *see* Naproxen *on page 1203*
- **Migranal®** *see* Dihydroergotamine *on page 537*
- **Milk of Magnesia** *see* Magnesium Hydroxide *on page 1076*

Milrinone (MIL ri none)

U.S. Brand Names Primacor®

Synonyms Milrinone Lactate

Pharmacologic Category Phosphodiesterase Enzyme Inhibitor

Medication Safety Issues

Sound-alike/look-alike issues:

Primacor® may be confused with Primaxin®

Use Short-term I.V. therapy of congestive heart failure; calcium antagonist intoxication

Mechanism of Action Phosphodiesterase inhibitor resulting in vasodilation

Pharmacodynamics/Kinetics

Onset of action: I.V.: 5-15 minutes

Serum level: I.V.: Following a 125 mcg/kg dose, peak plasma concentrations ~1000 ng/mL were observed at 2 minutes postinjection, decreasing to <100 ng/mL in 2 hours

Drug concentration levels:

Therapeutic:

Serum levels of 166 ng/mL, achieved during I.V. infusions of 0.25-1 mcg/kg/minute, were associated with sustained hemodynamic benefit in severe congestive heart failure patients over a 24-hour period

Maximum beneficial effects on cardiac output and pulmonary capillary wedge pressure following I.V. infusion have been associated with plasma milrinone concentrations of 150-250 ng/mL

Toxic: Serum concentrations >250-300 ng/mL have been associated with marked reductions in mean arterial pressure and tachycardia; however, more studies are required to determine the toxic serum levels for milrinone

Distribution: V_{dss}: 0.32 L/kg; Severe congestive heart failure (CHF): V_d: 0.33-0.47 L/kg; not significantly bound to tissues; excretion in breast milk unknown

Protein binding, plasma: ~70%

Metabolism: Hepatic (12%)

Half-life elimination: I.V.: 136 minutes in patients with CHF; patients with severe CHF have a more prolonged half-life, with values ranging from 1.7-2.7 hours. Patients with CHF have a reduction in the systemic clearance of milrinone, resulting in a prolonged elimination half-life. Alternatively, one study reported that 1 month of therapy with milrinone did not change the pharmacokinetic parameters for patients with CHF despite improvement in cardiac function.

Excretion: I.V.: Urine (85% as unchanged drug) within 24 hours; active tubular secretion is a major elimination pathway for milrinone

Clearance: I.V. bolus: 25.9 ± 5.7 L/hour (0.37 L/hour/kg); Severe congestive heart failure: 0.11-0.13 L/hour/kg. The reduction in clearance may be a result of reduced renal function. Creatinine clearance values were ½ those reported for healthy adults in patients with severe congestive heart failure (52 vs 119 mL/minute).

Contraindications Hypersensitivity to milrinone, inamrinone, or any component of the formulation; concurrent use of inamrinone

Warnings/Precautions Avoid in severe obstructive aortic or pulmonic valvular disease. It may aggravate outflow tract obstruction in hypertrophic subaortic stenosis. Supraventricular and ventricular arrhythmias have developed in high-risk patients. Monitor closely during the infusion. Ensure that ventricular rate controlled in atrial fibrillation/flutter before initiating. Not recommended for use in

(Continued)

Milrinone *(Continued)*

acute MI patients. Monitor and correct fluid and electrolyte problems. Adjust dose in renal dysfunction.

Adverse Reactions

>10%: Cardiovascular: Ventricular arrhythmia (ectopy 9%, NSVT 3%, sustained ventricular tachycardia 1%, ventricular fibrillation <1%); life-threatening arrhythmia are infrequent, often associated with underlying factors (eg, pre-existing arrhythmia, electrolyte disturbances, catheter insertion)

1% to 10%:

Cardiovascular: Supraventricular arrhythmia (4%), hypotension

Central nervous system: Headache

<1% (Limited to important or life-threatening): Anaphylaxis, atrial fibrillation, bronchospasm, chest pain, hypokalemia, liver function abnormalities, MI, rash, thrombocytopenia, torsade de pointes, tremor, ventricular fibrillation

Overdosage/Toxicology Treatment is supportive and symptomatic.

Dosing

Adults & Elderly: CHF/Hemodynamic support: I.V.: Loading dose: 50 mcg/kg administered over 10 minutes followed by a maintenance dose titrated according to the hemodynamic and clinical response, see table.

Maintenance Dosage	Dose Rate (mcg/kg/min)	Total Dose (mg/kg/24 h)
Minimum	0.375	0.59
Standard	0.500	0.77
Maximum	0.750	1.13

Renal Impairment:

Cl_{cr} 50 mL/minute/1.73 m^2: Administer 0.43 mcg/kg/minute.
Cl_{cr} 40 mL/minute/1.73 m^2: Administer 0.38 mcg/kg/minute.
Cl_{cr} 30 mL/minute/1.73 m^2: Administer 0.33 mcg/kg/minute.
Cl_{cr} 20 mL/minute/1.73 m^2: Administer 0.28 mcg/kg/minute.
Cl_{cr} 10 mL/minute/1.73 m^2: Administer 0.23 mcg/kg/minute.
Cl_{cr} 5 mL/minute/1.73 m^2: Administer 0.2 mcg/kg/minute.

Available Dosage Forms [DSC] = Discontinued product

Infusion [premixed in D_5W] (Primacor®): 200 mcg/mL (100 mL, 200 mL)

Injection, solution: 1 mg/mL (10 mL, 20 mL, 50 mL)

Primacor®: 1 mg/mL (10 mL, 20 mL; 50 mL [DSC])

Nursing Guidelines

Assessment: Use infusion pump. Monitor cardiac/hemodynamic status continuously during therapy and serum potassium at regular intervals. Monitor for fluid retention.

Monitoring Laboratory Tests: Serum potassium

Patient Education: This drug can only be given intravenously. If you experience increased voiding call for assistance. Report pain at infusion site, numbness or tingling of extremities, or respiratory difficulty. **Pregnancy/ breast-feeding precautions:** Inform prescriber if you are pregnant. Consult prescriber if breast-feeding.

Pregnancy Risk Factor: C

Lactation: Excretion in breast milk unknown

Perioperative/Anesthesia/Other Concerns: Inotrope of choice for severe congestive heart failure patients taking beta-blockers. Milrinone may be useful for severe CHF patients on beta-blocker who require an intravenous inotrope. If hypotension is a problem, loading doses may be omitted and maintenance infusions initiated. There is some delay in hemodynamic effects, but it is minimal (1-3 hours). Lower maintenance infusions have also been used (0.18-0.25 mcg/kg/minute).

Administration

I.V.: Infuse via infusion pump.

Reconstitution: Stable at 0.2 mg/mL in 0.9% sodium chloride or D_5W for 72 hours at room temperature in normal light.

Standard dilution: For a final concentration of 0.2 mg/mL: Dilute Primacor® 1 mg/mL (20 mL) with 80 mL diluent (final volume: 100 mL); may also dilute 1 mg/mL (10 mL) with 40 mL diluent (final volume: 50 mL)

Compatibility: Stable in D_5W, LR, ½NS, NS

Y-site administration: Incompatible with furosemide, procainamide

Compatibility in syringe: Incompatible with furosemide

Compatibility when admixed: Incompatible with bumetanide, furosemide, procainamide

Storage: Colorless to pale yellow solution. Store at room temperature and protect from light.

♦ **Milrinone Lactate** *see* Milrinone *on page 1163*

♦ **Minidyne® [OTC]** *see* Povidone-Iodine *on page 1392*

♦ **Minitran™** *see* Nitroglycerin *on page 1234*

Minoxidil (mi NOKS i dil)

U.S. Brand Names Loniten®; Rogaine® Extra Strength for Men [OTC]; Rogaine® for Men [OTC]; Rogaine® for Women [OTC]

Pharmacologic Category Topical Skin Product; Vasodilator

Medication Safety Issues

Sound-alike/look-alike issues:

Minoxidil may be confused with metolazone, Monopril®

Loniten® may be confused with clonidine, Lioresal®, Lotensin®

Use Management of severe hypertension (usually in combination with a diuretic and beta-blocker); treatment (topical formulation) of alopecia androgenetica in males and females

Mechanism of Action Produces vasodilation by directly relaxing arteriolar smooth muscle, with little effect on veins; effects may be mediated by cyclic AMP; stimulation of hair growth is secondary to vasodilation, increased cutaneous blood flow and stimulation of resting hair follicles

Pharmacodynamics/Kinetics

Onset of action: Hypotensive: Oral: ~30 minutes

Peak effect: 2-8 hours

Duration: 2-5 days

Protein binding: None

Metabolism: 88%, primarily via glucuronidation

Bioavailability: Oral: 90%

Half-life elimination: Adults: 3.5-4.2 hours

Excretion: Urine (12% as unchanged drug)

Contraindications Hypersensitivity to minoxidil or any component of the formulation; pheochromocytoma; acute MI; dissecting aortic aneurysm

Warnings/Precautions Maximum therapeutic doses of a diuretic and two antihypertensives should be used before this drug is ever added. It can cause pericardial effusion, tamponade, or exacerbate angina pectoris. Monitor patients who are receiving guanethidine concurrently (orthostasis can be problematic). May need to add a diuretic to minimize fluid gain and a beta-blocker (if no contraindications) to treat tachycardia. Rapid control of blood pressure can lead to syncope, CVA, MI, ischemia. Hypersensitivity reactions occur rarely. Avoid use for a month after acute MI. Inform patients of hair growth patterns before initiating therapy. May take 1-6 months for hypertrichosis to reverse itself after discontinuation of the drug. Use with caution in patients with pulmonary hypertension, significant renal failure, CHF, or ischemic disease. Renal failure and dialysis patients may require a smaller dose.

Drug Interactions

Antihypertensives: Effects may be additive.

Guanethidine can cause severe orthostasis; avoid concurrent use - discontinue 1-3 weeks prior to initiating minoxidil.

Nutritional/Herbal/Ethanol Interactions Herb/Nutraceutical: Avoid natural licorice (causes sodium and water retention and increases potassium loss).

Adverse Reactions

>10%:

Cardiovascular: CHF, edema, ECG (transient change in T-wave amplitude and direction), tachycardia

Dermatologic: Hypertrichosis (commonly occurs within 1-2 months of therapy)

1% to 10%: Endocrine & metabolic: Fluid and electrolyte imbalance

<1% (Limited to important or life-threatening): Angina, coarsening facial features, leukopenia, pericardial effusion tamponade, rash, Stevens-Johnson syndrome, thrombocytopenia, weight gain

Overdosage/Toxicology

Symptoms of overdose include hypotension, tachycardia, headache, nausea, dizziness, weakness syncope, warm flushed skin and palpitations; lethargy and ataxia may occur in children

(Continued)

Minoxidil *(Continued)*

Hypotension usually responds to I.V. fluids, Trendelenburg positioning or vasoconstrictor; treatment is primarily supportive and symptomatic

Dosing

Adults:

Hypertension: Oral: Initial: 5 mg once daily, increase gradually every 3 days (maximum: 100 mg/day); usual dose range (JNC 7): 2.5-80 mg/day in 1-2 divided doses

Alopecia: Topical: Apply twice daily; 4 months of therapy may be necessary for hair growth.

Note: Dosage adjustment is needed when added to concomitant therapy.

Elderly: Hypertension: Initial: 2.5 mg once daily; increase gradually.

Pediatrics:

Hypertension: Oral:

Children <12 years: Initial: 0.1-0.2 mg/kg once daily; maximum: 5 mg/day; increase gradually every 3 days; usual dosage: 0.25-1 mg/kg/day in 1-2 divided doses; maximum: 50 mg/day

Children >12 years: Refer to adult dosing.

Renal Impairment: Dialysis: Supplemental dose is not necessary via hemo- or peritoneal dialysis.

Available Dosage Forms [DSC] = Discontinued product

Solution, topical: 2% [20 mg/metered dose] (60 mL); 5% [50 mg/metered dose] (60 mL)

Rogaine® for Men, Rogaine® for Women: 2% [20 mg/metered dose] (60 mL)

Rogaine® Extra Strength for Men: 5% [50 mg/metered dose] (60 mL)

Tablet: 2.5 mg, 10 mg

Loniten®: 2.5 mg [DSC], 10 mg

Nursing Guidelines

Patient Education: Topical product is for external use only. When using the topical product, do not use other topical medications on the scalp. Topical product must be used every day. Hair growth usually takes 4 months. Notify physician if any of the following occur: Heart rate ≥20 beats per minute over normal; rapid weight gain >5 lb (2 kg); unusual swelling of extremities, face, or abdomen; breathing difficulty, especially when lying down; rise slowly from prolonged lying or sitting; new or aggravated angina symptoms (chest, arm, or shoulder pain); severe indigestion; dizziness, lightheadedness, or fainting; nausea or vomiting may occur. Do not make up for missed doses. **Pregnancy precaution:** Inform prescriber if you are or intend to become pregnant.

Pregnancy Risk Factor: C

Perioperative/Anesthesia/Other Concerns: Minoxidil when used in patients with hypertension will not cause regression of left ventricular hypertrophy.

Administration

Storage: Store at controlled room temperature of 20°C to 25°C (68°F to 77°F).

- **Mintox Extra Strength [OTC]** *see* Aluminum Hydroxide, Magnesium Hydroxide, and Simethicone *on page 122*
- **Mintox Plus [OTC]** *see* Aluminum Hydroxide, Magnesium Hydroxide, and Simethicone *on page 122*
- **Miochol-E®** *see* Acetylcholine *on page 79*
- **Miostat®** *see* Carbachol *on page 305*
- **Mirapex®** *see* Pramipexole *on page 1394*
- **Mircette®** *see* Ethinyl Estradiol and Desogestrel *on page 675*

Misoprostol (mye soe PROST ole)

U.S. Brand Names Cytotec®

Pharmacologic Category Prostaglandin

Medication Safety Issues

Sound-alike/look-alike issues:

Misoprostol may be confused with metoprolol

Cytotec® may be confused with Cytoxan®, Sytobex®

Use Prevention of NSAID-induced gastric ulcers; medical termination of pregnancy of ≤49 days (in conjunction with mifepristone)

Unlabeled/Investigational Use Cervical ripening and labor induction; NSAID-induced nephropathy; fat malabsorption in cystic fibrosis

Mechanism of Action Misoprostol is a synthetic prostaglandin E_1 analog that replaces the protective prostaglandins consumed with prostaglandin-inhibiting therapies (eg, NSAIDs); has been shown to induce uterine contractions

Pharmacodynamics/Kinetics

Absorption: Rapid

Metabolism: Hepatic; rapidly de-esterified to misoprostol acid (active)

Half-life elimination: Metabolite: 20-40 minutes

Time to peak, serum: Active metabolite: Fasting: 15-30 minutes

Excretion: Urine (64% to 73%) and feces (15%) within 24 hours

Contraindications Hypersensitivity to misoprostol, prostaglandins, or any component of the formulation; pregnancy (when used to reduce NSAID-induced ulcers)

Warnings/Precautions Safety and efficacy have not been established in children <18 years of age; use with caution in patients with renal impairment and the elderly; not to be used in women of childbearing potential unless woman is capable of complying with effective contraceptive measures; therapy is normally begun on the second or third day of next normal menstrual period. Uterine perforation and/or rupture have been reported in association with intravaginal use to induce labor or with combined oral/intravaginal use to induce abortion. The manufacturer states that Cytotec® should not be used as a cervical-ripening agent for induction of labor. However, The American College of Obstetricians and Gynecologists (ACOG) continues to support this off-label use.

Drug Interactions

Oxytocin: Misoprostol may increase the effect of oxytocin; wait 6-12 hours after misoprostol administration before initiating oxytocin.

Nutritional/Herbal/Ethanol Interactions Food: Misoprostol peak serum concentrations may be decreased if taken with food (not clinically significant).

Adverse Reactions

>10%: Gastrointestinal: Diarrhea, abdominal pain

1% to 10%:

Central nervous system: Headache

Gastrointestinal: Constipation, flatulence, nausea, dyspepsia, vomiting

<1% (Limited to important or life-threatening): Anaphylaxis, anxiety, appetite changes, arrhythmia, arterial thrombosis, bronchospasm, confusion, cramps, depression, drowsiness, edema, fetal or infant death (when used during pregnancy), fever, GI bleeding, GI inflammation, gingivitis, gout, hyper-/hypotension, impotence, loss of libido, MI, neuropathy, neurosis, pulmonary embolism, purpura, rash, reflux, rigors, thrombocytopenia, uterine rupture, weakness, weight changes

Overdosage/Toxicology Symptoms of overdose include sedation, tremor, convulsions, dyspnea, abdominal pain, diarrhea, hypotension, and bradycardia. Treatment is symptom-directed and supportive.

Dosing

Adults:

Prevention of NSAID-induced ulcers: Oral: 200 mcg 4 times/day with food; if not tolerated, may decrease dose to 100 mcg 4 times/day with food or 200 mcg twice daily with food. Last dose of the day should be taken at bedtime.

Labor induction or cervical ripening (unlabeled uses): Intravaginal: 25 mcg (1/4 of 100 mcg tablet); may repeat at intervals no more frequent than every 3-6 hours. Do not use in patients with previous cesarean delivery or prior major uterine surgery.

Medical termination of pregnancy: Oral: Refer to Mifepristone monograph.

Elderly: Oral: 100-200 mcg 4 times/day with food; if 200 mcg 4 times/day not tolerated, reduce to 100 mcg 4 times/day or 200 mcg twice daily with food. **Note:** To avoid the diarrhea potential, doses can be initiated at 100 mcg/day and increased 100 mcg/day at 3-day intervals until desired dose is achieved; also, recommend administering with food to decrease diarrhea incidence.

Pediatrics: Children 8-16 years: Oral: Fat absorption in cystic fibrosis (unlabeled use): 100 mcg 4 times/day

Available Dosage Forms Tablet: 100 mcg, 200 mcg

Nursing Guidelines

Assessment: Assess knowledge/teach appropriate antiulcer diet and lifestyle. Monitor renal function and fluid balance. **Pregnancy risk factor X:** Determine that patient is not pregnant before beginning treatment and do not give to women of childbearing age or to males who may have intercourse with women of childbearing age unless both male and female are capable of complying with contraceptive measures during therapy and for 1 month following therapy.

(Continued)

Misoprostol *(Continued)*

Dietary Considerations: Should be taken with food; incidence of diarrhea may be lessened by having patient take dose right after meals.

Patient Education: Take as directed; continue taking your NSAIDs while taking this medication. Take with meals or after meals to prevent nausea, diarrhea, and flatulence. Avoid using antacids. You may experience increased menstrual pain, or cramping; request analgesics. Report abnormal menstrual periods, spotting (may occur even in postmenstrual women), or severe menstrual bleeding. **Pregnancy/breast-feeding precautions:** When used to prevent NSAID-induced ulcers: Inform prescriber if you are pregnant. Do not get pregnant during or for 1 month following therapy. Male: Do not cause a female to become pregnant. Male/female: Consult prescriber for instruction on appropriate contraceptive measures. This drug may cause severe fetal defects, miscarriage, or abortion; do not share medication with others. Do not breast-feed.

Geriatric Considerations: Elderly, due to extensive use of NSAIDs and the high percentage of asymptomatic hemorrhage and perforation from NSAIDs, are at risk for NSAID-induced ulcers and may be candidates for misoprostol use. However, routine use for prophylaxis is not justified. Patients must be selected upon demonstration that they are at risk for NSAID-induced lesions. Misoprostol should not be used as a first-line therapy for gastric or duodenal ulcers.

Pregnancy Risk Factor: X

Pregnancy Issues: Misoprostol is an abortifacient. During pregnancy, use to prevent NSAID-induced ulcers is contraindicated. Reports of fetal death, congenital anomalies, uterine perforation, and abortion have been received after the use of misoprostol in pregnancy.

Lactation: Excretion in breast milk unknown/contraindicated

Breast-Feeding Considerations: It is not known if misoprostol is excreted in human milk, however, because significant diarrhea may occur in a nursing infant, breast-feeding is contraindicated

Administration

Oral: Incidence of diarrhea may be lessened by having patient take dose right after meals. Therapy is usually begun on the second or third day of the next normal menstrual period.

Storage: Store at or below 25°C (77°F).

Mitomycin (mye toe MYE sin)

U.S. Brand Names Mutamycin®

Synonyms Mitomycin-C; Mitomycin-X; MTC; NSC-26980

Pharmacologic Category Antineoplastic Agent, Antibiotic

Medication Safety Issues

Sound-alike/look-alike issues:

Mitomycin may be confused with mithramycin, mitotane, mitoxantrone, Mutamycin®

Mutamycin® may be confused with mitomycin

Use Treatment of adenocarcinoma of stomach or pancreas, bladder cancer, breast cancer, or colorectal cancer

Unlabeled/Investigational Use Prevention of excess scarring in glaucoma filtration procedures in patients at high risk of bleb failure

Mechanism of Action Acts like an alkylating agent and produces DNA cross-linking (primarily with guanine and cytosine pairs); cell-cycle nonspecific; inhibits DNA and RNA synthesis; degrades preformed DNA, causes nuclear lysis and formation of giant cells. While not phase-specific *per se*, mitomycin has its maximum effect against cells in late G and early S phases.

Pharmacodynamics/Kinetics

Distribution: V_d: 22 L/m^2; high drug concentrations found in kidney, tongue, muscle, heart, and lung tissue; probably not distributed into the CNS

Metabolism: Hepatic

Half-life elimination: 23-78 minutes; Terminal: 50 minutes

Excretion: Urine (<10% as unchanged drug), with elevated serum concentrations

Contraindications Hypersensitivity to mitomycin or any component of the formulation; thrombocytopenia; coagulation disorders, increased bleeding tendency; pregnancy

Warnings/Precautions Hazardous agent - use appropriate precautions for handling and disposal. Use with caution in patients who have received radiation therapy or in the presence of hepatobiliary dysfunction; reduce dosage in patients who are receiving radiation therapy simultaneously. Hemolytic-uremic syndrome, potentially fatal, occurs in some patients receiving long-term therapy. It is correlated with total dose (single doses ≥60 mg or cumulative doses ≥50 mg/m^2) and total duration of therapy (>5-11 months). **Mitomycin is a potent vesicant, may cause ulceration, necrosis, cellulitis, and tissue sloughing if infiltrated.**

Drug Interactions *Vinca* alkaloids or doxorubicin may enhance cardiac toxicity when coadministered with mitomycin.

Nutritional/Herbal/Ethanol Interactions Herb/Nutraceutical: Avoid black cohosh, dong quai in estrogen-dependent tumors.

Adverse Reactions

>10%:

Cardiovascular: CHF (3% to 15%) (doses >30 mg/m^2)

Central nervous system: Fever (14%)

Dermatologic: Alopecia, nail banding/discoloration

Gastrointestinal: Nausea, vomiting and anorexia (14%)

Hematologic: Anemia (19% to 24%); myelosuppression, common, dose-limiting, delayed

Onset: 3 weeks

Nadir: 4-6 weeks

Recovery: 6-8 weeks

1% to 10%:

Dermatologic: Rash

Gastrointestinal: Stomatitis

Neuromuscular: Paresthesias

Renal: Creatinine increase (2%)

Respiratory: Interstitial pneumonitis, infiltrates, dyspnea, cough (7%)

<1% (Limited to important or life-threatening): Extravasation reactions, hemolytic uremic syndrome, malaise, pruritus, renal failure, bladder fibrosis/contraction (intravesical administration)

Overdosage/Toxicology Symptoms of overdose include bone marrow suppression, nausea, vomiting, and alopecia. Treatment is symptom-directed and supportive.

Dosing

Adults & Elderly: Refer to individual protocols:

Single-agent therapy: I.V.: 20 mg/m^2 every 6-8 weeks

Combination therapy: I.V.: 10 mg/m^2 every 6-8 weeks

Bladder carcinoma: Intravesicular instillations (unapproved route): 20-40 mg/dose instilled into the bladder for 3 hours repeated up to 3 times/week for up to 20 procedures per course.

Glaucoma surgery (unlabeled use): Dosages and techniques vary; 0.2-0.5 mg may be applied to a pledget (using a 0.2-0.5 mg/mL solution), and placed in contact with the surgical wound for 2-5 minutes; other protocols have been reported

Pediatrics: Refer to adult dosing.

Renal Impairment: Varying approaches to dosing adjustments have been published; one representative recommendation: Cl_{cr} <10 mL/minute: Administer 75% of normal dose

Note: The manufacturers state that products should not be given to patients with serum creatinine >1.7 mg/dL.

Hemodialysis: Unknown

CAPD effects: Unknown

CAVH effects: Unknown

Hepatic Impairment: Although some mitomycin may be excreted in the bile, no specific guidelines regarding dosage adjustment in hepatic impairment can be made.

Available Dosage Forms Injection, powder for reconstitution: 5 mg, 20 mg, 40 mg

Nursing Guidelines

Assessment: See Contraindications, Warnings/Precautions, and Dosing for use cautions. Assess potential for interactions with other prescriptions, OTC medications, or herbal products patient may be taking (see Drug Interactions). **I.V.:** See Administration for specifics; infusion site must be closely monitored to prevent extravasation (eg, mitomycin is a potent vesicant, may cause ulceration, necrosis, cellulitis, and tissue sloughing if infiltrated - see Extravasation Management). Assess results of laboratory tests (see below), therapeutic effectiveness, and adverse reactions (eg, signs of CHF, hydration, nutritional status,

(Continued)

Mitomycin *(Continued)*

and opportunistic infection - see Adverse Reactions and Overdose/Toxicology) on a regular basis throughout therapy. Teach patient possible side effects/ appropriate interventions and adverse symptoms to report (see Patient Education). **Pregnancy risk factor D** - determine that patient is not pregnant before beginning treatment. Instruct patients of childbearing age about appropriate contraceptive measures. Breast-feeding is contraindicated.

Monitoring Laboratory Tests: Platelet count, CBC with differential, prothrombin time, renal and pulmonary function

Patient Education: Inform prescriber of all prescriptions, OTC medications, or herbal products you are taking, and any allergies you have. Do not take any new medication during therapy unless approved by prescriber. This drug can only be given intravenously. Report immediately any redness, swelling, burning, or pain at infusion site. Maintain adequate hydration (2-3 L/day of fluids) unless instructed to restrict fluid intake, and nutrition. May cause nausea, vomiting, or anorexia (small, frequent meals, frequent mouth care, chewing gum, or sucking lozenges may help); mouth sores (use soft toothbrush, waxed dental floss, and frequent mouth rinses); or loss of hair or discoloration of nails (may be reversible when therapy is discontinued). Report rash or itching, unresolved nausea or diarrhea; respiratory difficulty, swelling of extremities, sudden weight gain, or unusual cough; any numbness, tingling, or loss of sensation; or opportunistic infection (fever, chills, sore throat, burning urination, fatigue). **Pregnancy/ breast-feeding precautions:** Do not get pregnant while taking this medication. Consult prescriber for appropriate contraceptive measures. Do not breast-feed.

Pregnancy Risk Factor: D

Pregnancy Issues: Mitomycin can cause fetal harm in humans. Animal studies show delayed fetal development, fetal external anomalies, and neonatal anomalies.

Lactation: Enters breast milk/contraindicated

Administration

I.V.: Vesicant. Administer slow I.V. push or by slow (15-30 minute) infusion via a freely-running dextrose or saline infusion. Consider using a central venous catheter.

Reconstitution: Dilute powder with SWFI or 0.9% sodium chloride to a concentration of 0.5-1 mg/mL.

Compatibility: Stable in LR

Y-site administration: Incompatible with aztreonam, cefepime, etoposide phosphate, filgrastim, gemcitabine, piperacillin/tazobactam, sargramostim, topotecan, vinorelbine

Compatibility when admixed: Incompatible with bleomycin

Storage: Store intact vials at controlled room temperature. Mitomycin solution is stable for 7 days at room temperature and 14 days when refrigerated if protected from light. Solution of 0.5 mg/mL in a syringe is stable for 7 days at room temperature and 14 days when refrigerated and protected from light.

Further dilution to 20-40 mcg/mL:

In normal saline: Stable for 12 hours at room temperature.

In sodium lactate: Stable for 24 hours at room temperature.

♦ Mitomycin-X *see* Mitomycin *on page 1168*
♦ Mitomycin-C *see* Mitomycin *on page 1168*
♦ Mivacron® *see* Mivacurium *on page 1170*

Mivacurium (mye va KYOO ree um)

U.S. Brand Names Mivacron®

Synonyms Mivacurium Chloride

Pharmacologic Category Neuromuscular Blocker Agent, Nondepolarizing

Medication Safety Issues

Sound-alike/look-alike issues:

Mivacron® may be confused with Mevacor®

Use Adjunct to general anesthesia to facilitate endotracheal intubation and to relax skeletal muscles during surgery; to facilitate mechanical ventilation in ICU patients; does not relieve pain or produce sedation

Mechanism of Action Mivacurium is a short-acting, nondepolarizing, neuromuscular-blocking agent. Like other nondepolarizing drugs, mivacurium antagonizes acetylcholine by competitively binding to cholinergic sites on motor endplates in skeletal muscle. This inhibits contractile activity in skeletal muscle leading to muscle paralysis. This effect is reversible with cholinesterase inhibitors such as edrophonium, neostigmine, and physostigmine.

Pharmacodynamics/Kinetics

Onset of action: Neuromuscular blockade (dose dependent): I.V.: 1.5-3 minutes

Duration: Short due to rapid hydrolysis by plasma cholinesterases; clinically effective block may last for 12-20 minutes; spontaneous recovery may be 95% complete in 25-30 minutes; duration shorter in children and may be slightly longer in elderly

Metabolism: Via plasma cholinesterase, inactive metabolites

Half-life elimination: 2 minutes (more active isomers only)

Excretion: Urine (<10%)

Contraindications Hypersensitivity to mivacurium chloride, any component of the formulation, or other benzylisoquinolinium agents; use of multidose vials in patients with allergy to benzyl alcohol; pre-existing tachycardia

Warnings/Precautions Ventilation must be supported during neuromuscular blockade; does not counteract bradycardia produced by anesthetics/vagal stimulation; prolonged neuromuscular block may be seen in patients with reduced or atypical plasma cholinesterase activity (eg, pregnancy, liver or kidney disease, infections, peptic ulcer, anemia); patients homozygous for the atypical plasma cholinesterase gene are extremely sensitive to the neuromuscular blocking effect of mivacurium (use extreme caution if at all in those patients); duration prolonged in patients with renal and/or hepatic impairment; reduce initial dosage and inject slowly (over 60 seconds) in patients in whom substantial histamine release would be potentially hazardous; certain clinical conditions may result in potentiation or antagonism of neuromuscular blockade:

Potentiation: Electrolyte abnormalities, severe hyponatremia, severe hypocalcemia, severe hypokalemia, hypermagnesemia, neuromuscular diseases, acidosis, acute intermittent porphyria, renal failure, hepatic failure

Antagonism: Alkalosis, hypercalcemia, demyelinating lesions, peripheral neuropathies, diabetes mellitus

Increased sensitivity in patients with myasthenia gravis, Eaton-Lambert syndrome, resistance in burn patients (>30% of body) for period of 5-70 days postinjury; resistance in patients with muscle trauma, denervation, immobilization, infection. Cross-sensitivity with other neuromuscular-blocking agents may occur; use extreme caution in patients with previous anaphylactic reactions.

Drug Interactions Prolonged neuromuscular blockade: Inhaled anesthetics; local anesthetics; calcium channel blockers; antiarrhythmics (eg, quinidine or procainamide); antibiotics (eg, aminoglycosides, tetracyclines, vancomycin, clindamycin); immunosuppressants (eg, cyclosporine)

Adverse Reactions

>10%: Cardiovascular: Flushing of face

1% to 10%: Cardiovascular: Hypotension

<1% (Limited to important or life-threatening): Acute quadriplegic myopathy syndrome (prolonged use), anaphylactoid reaction, anaphylaxis, bradycardia, bronchospasm, cutaneous erythema, dizziness, endogenous histamine release, hypersensitivity reactions, hypoxemia, injection site reaction, muscle spasms, myositis ossificans (prolonged use), rash, tachycardia, wheezing

Dosing

Adults & Elderly: Note: Continuous infusion requires an infusion pump; dose should be based on ideal body weight

Neuromuscular blockade: Initial: I.V.: 0.15-0.25 mg/kg bolus followed by maintenance doses of 0.1 mg/kg at approximately 15-minute intervals; for prolonged neuromuscular block, initial infusion of 9-10 mcg/kg/minute is used upon evidence of spontaneous recovery from initial dose, usual infusion rate of 6-7 mcg/kg/minute (1-15 mcg/kg/minute) under balanced anesthesia; initial dose after succinylcholine for intubation (balanced anesthesia): Adults: 0.1 mg/kg

Pretreatment/priming: 10% of intubating dose given 3-5 minutes before initial dose

Pediatrics: Note: Continuous infusion requires an infusion pump; dose should be based on ideal body weight

Neuromuscular blockade: I.V.: Children 2-12 years (duration of action is shorter and dosage requirements are higher): 0.2 mg/kg followed by average infusion rate of 14 mcg/kg/minute (range: 5-31 mcg/kg/minute) upon evidence of spontaneous recovery from initial dose

(Continued)

Mivacurium *(Continued)*

Renal Impairment: 150 mcg/kg I.V. bolus; duration of action of blockade: 1.5 times longer in ESRD, may decrease infusion rates by as much as 50%, dependent on degree of renal impairment.

Hepatic Impairment: 150 mcg/kg I.V. bolus; duration of blockade: 3 times longer in ESLD, may decrease rate of infusion by as much as 50% in ESLD, dependent on the degree of impairment

Available Dosage Forms

Injection, solution [preservative free]: 2 mg/mL (5 mL, 10 mL)

Injection, solution: 2 mg/mL (20 mL, 50 mL) [with benzyl alcohol]

Nursing Guidelines

Assessment: Only clinicians experienced in the use of neuromuscular blocking agents should administer and/or manage the use of mivacurium. Assess potential for interactions with other prescriptions, OTC medications, or herbal products patient may be taking (eg, other drugs that affect neuromuscular activity may increase/decrease neuromuscular block induced by mivacurium). Ventilatory support must be instituted and maintained until adequate respiratory muscle function and/or airway protection are assured. This drug does not cause anesthesia or analgesia; pain must be treated with appropriate agents. Continuous monitoring of vital signs, cardiac and respiratory status, and neuromuscular block (objective assessment with peripheral external nerve stimulator) are mandatory until full muscle tone has returned. Safety precautions must be maintained until full muscle tone has returned. **Note:** It may take longer for return of muscle tone in elderly persons or patients with myasthenia gravis, myopathy, other neuromuscular diseases, dehydration, electrolyte imbalance, or severe acid/base imbalance. Provide appropriate teaching/support prior to, during, and following administration.

Long-term use: Monitor vital signs and fluid levels regularly during treatment. Every 2- to 3-hour repositioning, and skin, mouth, and eye care is necessary while patient is sedated. Emotional and sensory support (auditory and environmental) should be provided.

Patient Education: Patient education should be appropriate for patient condition. Reassurance of constant monitoring and emotional support should precede and follow administration. Patients should be reminded as muscle tone returns not to attempt to change position or rise from bed without assistance and to report any skin rash, hives, pounding heartbeat, respiratory difficulty, or muscle tremors. **Pregnancy/breast-feeding precaution:** Inform prescriber if you are pregnant. Consult prescriber if breast-feeding.

Pregnancy Risk Factor: C

Lactation: Excretion in breast milk unknown/use caution

Perioperative/Anesthesia/Other Concerns: Mivacurium is classified as a short duration neuromuscular-blocking agent; do not mix with barbiturates in same syringe; does not appear to have a cumulative effect on the duration of blockade.

Critically-Ill Adult Patients: The 2002 ACCM/SCCM/ASHP clinical practice guidelines for sustained neuromuscular blockade in the adult critically-ill patient recommend:

Optimize sedatives and analgesics prior to initiation and monitor and adjust accordingly during course. Neuromuscular blockers do not relieve pain or produce sedation.

Protect patient's eyes from development of keratitis and corneal abrasion by administering ophthalmic ointment and taping eyelids closed or using eye patches. Reposition patient routinely to protect pressure points from breakdown. Address DVT prophylaxis.

Concurrent use of a neuromuscular blocker and corticosteroids appear to increase the risk of certain ICU myopathies; avoid or administer the corticosteroid at the lowest dose possible. Reassess need for neuromuscular blocker daily.

Using daily drug holidays (stopping neuromuscular-blocking agent until patient requires it again) may decrease the incidence of acute quadriplegic myopathy syndrome.

Tachyphylaxis can develop; switch to another neuromuscular blocker (taking into consideration the patient's organ function) if paralysis is still necessary.

Atracurium or cisatracurium is recommended for patients with significant hepatic or renal disease, due to organ-independent Hofmann elimination.

Monitor patients clinically and via "Train of Four" (TOF) testing with a goal of adjusting the degree of blockade to 1-2 twitches or based upon the patient's clinical condition.

Administration

I.V.: Children require higher mivacurium infusion rates than adults; during opioid/nitrous oxide/oxygen anesthesia, the infusion rate required to maintain 89% to 99% neuromuscular block averages 14 mcg/kg/minute (range: 5-31). For adults and children, the amount of infusion solution required per hour depends upon the clinical requirements of the patient, the concentration of mivacurium in the infusion solution, and the patient's weight. The contribution of the infusion solution to the fluid requirements of the patient must be considered.

Compatibility: Stable in D_5LR, D_5NS, D_5W, LR, NS

Storage: Store at room temperature of 15°C to 25°C (59°F to 77°F); protect from direct ultraviolet light.

- **Mivacurium Chloride** *see* Mivacurium *on page 1170*
- **MK594** *see* Losartan *on page 1066*
- **MK0826** *see* Ertapenem *on page 631*
- **MLN341** *see* Bortezomib *on page 251*
- **MMF** *see* Mycophenolate *on page 1188*
- **MMR** *see* Measles, Mumps, and Rubella Vaccines (Combined) *on page 1082*
- **Mobic®** *see* Meloxicam *on page 1091*

Modafinil (moe DAF i nil)

U.S. Brand Names Provigil®

Pharmacologic Category Stimulant

Use Improve wakefulness in patients with excessive daytime sleepiness associated with narcolepsy and shift work sleep disorder (SWSD); adjunctive therapy for obstructive sleep apnea/hypopnea syndrome (OSAHS)

Unlabeled/Investigational Use Attention-deficit/hyperactivity disorder (ADHD); treatment of fatigue in MS and other disorders

Mechanism of Action The exact mechanism of action is unclear, it does not appear to alter the release of dopamine or norepinephrine, it may exert its stimulant effects by decreasing GABA-mediated neurotransmission, although this theory has not yet been fully evaluated; several studies also suggest that an intact central alpha-adrenergic system is required for modafinil's activity; the drug increases high-frequency alpha waves while decreasing both delta and theta wave activity, and these effects are consistent with generalized increases in mental alertness

Pharmacodynamics/Kinetics Modafinil is a racemic compound (10% *d*-isomer and 90% *l*-isomer at steady state) whose enantiomers have different pharmacokinetics

Distribution: V_d: 0.9 L/kg

Protein binding: 60%, primarily to albumin

Metabolism: Hepatic; multiple pathways including CYP3A4

Half-life elimination: Effective half-life: 15 hours; Steady-state: 2-4 days

Time to peak, serum: 2-4 hours

Excretion: Urine (as metabolites, <10% as unchanged drug)

Contraindications Hypersensitivity to modafinil or any component of the formulation

Warnings/Precautions Use is not recommended with a history of angina, cardiac ischemia, recent history of myocardial infarction, left ventricular hypertrophy, or patients with mitral valve prolapse who have developed mitral valve prolapse syndrome with previous CNS stimulant use. Caution should be exercised when modafinil is given to patients with a history of psychosis; caution is warranted when operating machinery or driving, although functional impairment has not been demonstrated with modafinil, all CNS-active agents may alter judgment, thinking and/or motor skills. Stimulants may unmask tics in individuals with coexisting Tourette's syndrome. Use caution with renal or hepatic impairment. Safety and efficacy in children ≤16 years of age have not been established.

Drug Interactions Substrate of CYP3A4 (major); **Inhibits** CYP1A2 (weak), 2A6 (weak), 2C8/9 (weak), 2C19 (strong), 2E1 (weak), 3A4 (weak); **Induces** CYP1A2 (weak), 2B6 (weak), 3A4 (weak)

Cyclosporine: Metabolism of cyclosporine may be increased; monitor serum levels.

(Continued)

Modafinil *(Continued)*

CYP2C19 substrates: Modafinil may increase the levels/effects of CYP2C19 substrates. Example substrates include citalopram, diazepam, methsuximide, phenytoin, propranolol, and sertraline.

CYP3A4 inducers: CYP3A4 inducers may decrease the levels/effects of modafinil. Example inducers include aminoglutethimide, carbamazepine, nafcillin, nevirapine, phenobarbital, phenytoin, and rifamycins.

CYP3A4 inhibitors: May increase the levels/effects of modafinil. Example inhibitors include azole antifungals, clarithromycin, diclofenac, doxycycline, erythromycin, imatinib, isoniazid, nefazodone, nicardipine, propofol, protease inhibitors, quinidine, telithromycin, and verapamil.

Oral contraceptives; Serum concentrations may be reduced (enzyme induction); contraceptive failure may result; alternative contraceptive measures are recommended during therapy and for 1 month after modafinil is discontinued.

Phenytoin: Serum concentrations may be increased by modafinil (enzyme inhibition); modafinil concentrations may be reduced by phenytoin (enzyme induction)

SSRIs: In populations genetically deficient in the CYP2D6 isoenzyme, where CYP2C19 acts as a secondary metabolic pathway, concentrations of selective serotonin reuptake inhibitors may be increased during coadministration

Tricyclic antidepressants: In populations genetically deficient in the CYP2D6 isoenzyme, where CYP2C19 acts as a secondary metabolic pathway, concentrations of tricyclic antidepressants may be increased during coadministration

Warfarin: Serum concentrations/effect may be increased by modafinil

Nutritional/Herbal/Ethanol Interactions

Ethanol: Avoid or limit ethanol.

Food: Delays absorption, but does not affect bioavailability.

Adverse Reactions

>10%:

- Central nervous system: Headache (34%, dose related)
- Gastrointestinal: Nausea (11%)

1% to 10%:

- Cardiovascular: Chest pain (3%), hypertension (3%), palpitation (2%), tachycardia (2%), vasodilation (2%), edema (1%)
- Central nervous system: Nervousness (7%), dizziness (5%), depression (2%), anxiety (5%, dose related), insomnia (5%), somnolence (2%), chills (1%), agitation (1%), confusion (1%), emotional lability (1%), vertigo (1%)
- Gastrointestinal: Diarrhea (6%), dyspepsia (5%), xerostomia (4%), anorexia (4%), constipation (2%), flatulence (1%), mouth ulceration (1%), taste perversion (1%)
- Genitourinary: Abnormal urine (1%), hematuria (1%), pyuria (1%)
- Hematologic: Eosinophilia (1%)
- Hepatic: Abnormal LFTs (2%)
- Neuromuscular & skeletal: Back pain (6%), paresthesia (2%), dyskinesia (1%), hyperkinesia (1%), hypertonia (1%), neck rigidity (1%), tremor (1%)
- Ocular: Amblyopia (1%), abnormal vision (1%), eye pain (1%)
- Respiratory: Pharyngitis (4%), rhinitis (7%), lung disorder (2%), asthma (1%), epistaxis (1%)
- Miscellaneous: Diaphoresis

Postmarketing and/or case reports: Agranulocytosis, mania, psychosis

Overdosage/Toxicology Symptoms of overdose include agitation, irritability, aggressiveness, confusion, nervousness, tremor, insomnia, palpitations, and elevations in hemodynamic parameters. Treatment is symptomatic and supportive. Cardiac monitoring is warranted.

Dosing

Adults:

ADHD (unlabeled use): Oral: 100-300 mg once daily

Narcolepsy, OSAHS: Oral: Initial: 200 mg as a single daily dose in the morning.

SWSD: Oral: Initial: 200 mg as a single dose taken ~1 hour prior to start of work shift.

Note: Doses of 400 mg/day, given as a single dose, have been well tolerated, but there is no consistent evidence that this dose confers additional benefit.

Elderly: Elimination of modafinil and its metabolites may be reduced as a consequence of aging and as a result, lower doses should be considered.

Pediatrics:

ADHD (unlabeled use): Oral: 50-100 mg once daily

Renal Impairment: Inadequate data to determine safety and efficacy in severe renal impairment.

Hepatic Impairment: Dose should be reduced to one-half of that recommended for patients with normal liver function.

Available Dosage Forms Tablet: 100 mg, 200 mg

Nursing Guidelines

Assessment: Assess effectiveness and interactions of other medications, especially those that are metabolized by P450 enzymes. Note that modafinil has potential for abuse; caution patient about inappropriate or overuse. Assess knowledge/teach patient appropriate use, adverse symptoms to report. and interventions to reduce side effects.

Patient Education: Take exactly as prescribed; do not exceed recommended dosage without consulting prescriber. Avoid drinking alcohol. Do not share medication with anyone else. Void before taking medication. You may experience headache, nervousness, confusion, or dizziness (use caution when driving or engaging in tasks requiring alertness until response to drug is known); diarrhea (yogurt or buttermilk may help); or dry mouth or sore mouth, loss of appetite, or vomiting (small frequent meals, frequent mouth care, chewing gum, or sucking lozenges may help). If you have diabetes, monitor glucose levels closely. Report chest pain or palpitations; respiratory difficulty; excessive insomnia, CNS agitation, depression, or memory disturbances; vision changes; changes in urinary pattern or ejaculation disturbances; or persistent joint pain or stiffness. **Pregnancy/breast-feeding precautions:** Inform prescriber if you are or intend to become pregnant. Consult prescriber if breast-feeding.

Pregnancy Risk Factor: C

Pregnancy Issues: Embryotoxic effects have been observed in some, but not all animal studies. There are no adequate and well-controlled studies in pregnant women; use only when the potential risk of drug therapy is outweighed by the drug's benefits. Efficacy of steroidal contraceptives may be decreased; alternate means of contraception should be considered during therapy and for 1 month after modafinil is discontinued.

Lactation: Excretion in breast milk unknown/use caution

- **Modane® Bulk [OTC]** *see* Psyllium *on page 1438*
- **Modane Tablets® [OTC]** *see* Bisacodyl *on page 245*
- **Modified Dakin's Solution** *see* Sodium Hypochlorite Solution *on page 1549*
- **Modified Shohl's Solution** *see* Sodium Citrate and Citric Acid *on page 1548*
- **Moisture® Eyes [OTC]** *see* Artificial Tears *on page 187*
- **Moisture® Eyes PM [OTC]** *see* Artificial Tears *on page 187*
- **MOM** *see* Magnesium Hydroxide *on page 1076*
- **Monacolin K** *see* Lovastatin *on page 1070*
- **Monocaps [OTC]** *see* Vitamins (Multiple/Oral) *on page 1720*
- **Monodox®** *see* Doxycycline *on page 584*
- **Monoket®** *see* Isosorbide Mononitrate *on page 979*
- **MonoNessa™** *see* Ethinyl Estradiol and Norgestimate *on page 689*
- **Monopril®** *see* Fosinopril *on page 778*

Montelukast (mon te LOO kast)

U.S. Brand Names Singulair®

Synonyms Montelukast Sodium

Pharmacologic Category Leukotriene-Receptor Antagonist

Medication Safety Issues

Sound-alike/look-alike issues:

Singulair® may be confused with Sinequan®

Use Prophylaxis and chronic treatment of asthma; relief of symptoms of seasonal allergic rhinitis and perennial allergic rhinitis

Unlabeled/Investigational Use Acute asthma

Mechanism of Action Selective leukotriene receptor antagonist that inhibits the cysteinyl leukotriene receptor. Cysteinyl leukotrienes and leukotriene receptor occupation have been correlated with the pathophysiology of asthma, including airway edema, smooth muscle contraction, and altered cellular activity associated with the inflammatory process, which contribute to the signs and symptoms of asthma.

Pharmacodynamics/Kinetics

Duration: >24 hours

(Continued)

Montelukast *(Continued)*

Absorption: Rapid

Distribution: V_d: 8-11 L

Protein binding, plasma: >99%

Metabolism: Extensively hepatic via CYP3A4 and 2C8/9

Bioavailability: Tablet: 10 mg: Mean: 64%; 5 mg: 63% to 73%

Half-life elimination, plasma: Mean: 2.7-5.5 hours

Time to peak, serum: Tablet: 10 mg: 3-4 hours; 5 mg: 2-2.5 hours; 4 mg: 2 hours

Excretion: Feces (86%); urine (<0.2%)

Contraindications Hypersensitivity to montelukast or any component of the formulation

Warnings/Precautions Montelukast is not FDA approved for use in the reversal of bronchospasm in acute asthma attacks; some clinicians, however, support its use (Cylly, 2003; Camargo, 2003; Ferreira, 2001). Should not be used as monotherapy for the treatment and management of exercise-induced bronchospasm. Advise patients to have appropriate rescue medication available. Appropriate clinical monitoring and caution are recommended when systemic corticosteroid reduction is considered in patients receiving montelukast. Inform phenylketonuric patients that the chewable tablet contains phenylalanine. Safety and efficacy in children <6 months of age have not been established.

In rare cases, patients on therapy with montelukast may present with systemic eosinophilia, sometimes presenting with clinical features of vasculitis consistent with Churg-Strauss syndrome, a condition which is often treated with systemic corticosteroid therapy. Healthcare providers should be alert to eosinophilia, vasculitic rash, worsening pulmonary symptoms, cardiac complications, and/or neuropathy presenting in their patients. A causal association between montelukast and these underlying conditions has not been established.

Drug Interactions Substrate (major) of CYP2C8/9, 3A4; **Inhibits** CYP2C8/9 (weak)

CYP2C8/9 inducers: May decrease the levels/effects of montelukast. Example inducers include carbamazepine, phenobarbital, phenytoin, rifampin, rifapentine, and secobarbital.

CYP3A4 inducers: CYP3A4 inducers may decrease the levels/effects of montelukast. Example inducers include aminoglutethimide, carbamazepine, nafcillin, nevirapine, phenobarbital, phenytoin, and rifamycins.

Nutritional/Herbal/Ethanol Interactions Herb/Nutraceutical: St John's wort may decrease montelukast levels.

Adverse Reactions (As reported in adults)

1% to 10%:

Central nervous system: Dizziness (2%), fatigue (2%), fever (2%)

Dermatologic: Rash (2%)

Gastrointestinal: Abdominal pain (3%), dyspepsia (2%), dental pain (2%), gastroenteritis (2%)

Neuromuscular & skeletal: Weakness (2%)

Respiratory: Cough (3%), nasal congestion (2%), upper respiratory infection (2%)

Miscellaneous: Flu-like symptoms (4%), trauma (1%)

<1% (Limited to important or life-threatening): Agitation, anaphylaxis, angioedema, arthralgia, cholestasis (rare), Churg-Strauss syndrome, eosinophilia, hallucinations, hepatic eosinophilic infiltration (rare); hepatitis (mixed pattern, hepatocellular, and cholestatic); hypoesthesia, insomnia, myalgia, palpitation, pancreatitis, paresthesia, pruritus, seizure, vasculitis

Overdosage/Toxicology No specific antidote

Remove unabsorbed material from the GI tract, employ clinical monitoring and institute supportive therapy if required. Abdominal pain, hyperkinesia, mydriasis, somnolence, and thirst have been reported with acute overdose of ≥150 mg/day.

Dosing

Adults & Elderly:

Asthma, allergic seasonal or perennial rhinitis: Oral: One 10 mg tablet daily in the evening

Asthma, acute (unlabeled use): 10 mg as a single dose administered with first-line therapy

Pediatrics:

Asthma: Oral:

6-11 months (unlabeled use): 4 mg (oral granules) once daily, taken in the evening

12-23 months: 4 mg (oral granules) once daily, taken in the evening

Seasonal or perennial allergic rhinitis: Oral: *6-23 months:* 4 mg (oral granules) once daily

Asthma, seasonal or perennial allergic rhinitis: Oral:

2-5 years: 4 mg (chewable tablet or oral granules) once daily, taken in the evening

6-14 years: Chew one 5 mg chewable tablet/day, taken in the evening

≥15 years: Refer to adult dosing.

Renal Impairment: No adjustment is necessary.

Hepatic Impairment: No adjustment necessary in mild-to-moderate hepatic disease. Patients with severe hepatic disease were **not** studied.

Available Dosage Forms

Granules: 4 mg/packet

Tablet: 10 mg

Tablet, chewable: 4 mg [contains phenylalanine 0.674 mg; cherry flavor]; 5 mg [contains phenylalanine 0.842 mg; cherry flavor]

Nursing Guidelines

Assessment: Not for use in acute asthma attacks, including status asthmaticus. Assess effectiveness and interactions of other medications patient may be taking. Monitor effectiveness of therapy and adverse reactions at beginning of therapy and periodically with long-term use. Assess knowledge/teach patient appropriate use, interventions to reduce side effects, and adverse symptoms to report.

Dietary Considerations: Tablet, chewable: 4 mg strength contains phenylalanine 0.674 mg; 5 mg strength contains phenylalanine 0.842 mg

Patient Education: Do not stop other asthma medication unless advised by prescriber. Chewable tablet contains phenylalanine. Take every evening on a continuous basis; do not discontinue even if feeling better (this medication may help reduce incidence of acute attacks). Granules may be administered directly in the mouth or mixed with applesauce, carrots, rice, or ice cream (do not mix in liquids); administer within 15 minutes of opening packet. You may experience mild headache (mild analgesic may help); or fatigue or dizziness (use caution when driving). Report skin rash or itching, abdominal pain or persistent GI upset, unusual cough or congestion, feeling of numbness in arms or legs, flu-like illness, or worsening of asthmatic condition. **Breast-feeding precaution:** Consult prescriber if breast-feeding.

Pregnancy Risk Factor: B

Lactation: Excretion in breast milk unknown/use caution

Breast-Feeding Considerations: Zafirlukast, another leukotriene receptor antagonist, is excreted in breast milk and use while breast-feeding is not recommended.

Administration

Oral: When treating asthma, administer dose in the evening. Granules may be administered directly in the mouth or mixed with applesauce, carrots, rice, ice cream, baby formula, or breast milk; do not add to any other liquids. Administer within 15 minutes of opening packet.

Storage: Store at room temperature of 15°C to 30°C (59°F to 86°F). Protect from moisture and light.

Granules: Use within 15 minutes of opening packet.

♦ **Montelukast Sodium** *see* Montelukast *on page 1175*

Morphine Sulfate (MOR feen SUL fate)

U.S. Brand Names Astramorph/PF™; Avinza®; DepoDur™; Duramorph®; Infumorph®; Kadian®; MS Contin®; Oramorph SR®; RMS®; Roxanol™; Roxanol 100™; Roxanol™-T [DSC]

Synonyms MSO_4 (error-prone abbreviation and should not be used)

Pharmacologic Category Analgesic, Narcotic

Medication Safety Issues

Sound-alike/look-alike issues:

Morphine may be confused with hydromorphone

Morphine sulfate may be confused with magnesium sulfate

MSO_4 is an error-prone abbreviation (mistaken as magnesium sulfate)

Avinza® may be confused with Evista®, Invanz®

(Continued)

Morphine Sulfate *(Continued)*

Roxanol™ may be confused with OxyFast®, Roxicet™

Use care when prescribing and/or administering morphine solutions. These products are available in different concentrations. Always prescribe dosage in mg; **not** by volume (mL).

Use Relief of moderate to severe acute and chronic pain; relief of pain of myocardial infarction; relief of dyspnea of acute left ventricular failure and pulmonary edema; preanesthetic medication

DepoDur™: Epidural (lumbar) single-dose management of surgical pain

Infumorph®: Used in microinfusion devices for intraspinal administration in treatment of intractable chronic pain

Mechanism of Action Binds to opiate receptors in the CNS, causing inhibition of ascending pain pathways, altering the perception of and response to pain; produces generalized CNS depression

Pharmacodynamics/Kinetics

Onset of action: Oral (immediate release): ~30 minutes; I.V.: 5-10 minutes

Duration: Pain relief:

Immediate release formulations: 4 hours

Extended release epidural injection (DepoDur™): >48 hours

Absorption: Variable

Distribution: V_d: 3-4 L/kg; binds to opioid receptors in the CNS and periphery (eg, GI tract)

Protein binding: 30% to 35%

Metabolism: Hepatic via conjugation with glucuronic acid to morphine-3-glucuronide (inactive), morphine-6-glucuronide (active), and in lesser amounts, morphine-3-6-diglucuronide; other minor metabolites include normorphine (active) and the 3-ethereal sulfate

Bioavailability: Oral: 17% to 33% (first-pass effect limits oral bioavailability; oral:parenteral effectiveness reportedly varies from 1:6 in opioid naive patients to 1:3 with chronic use)

Half-life elimination: Adults: 2-4 hours (immediate release forms)

Time to peak, plasma: Kadian®: ~10 hours

Excretion: Urine (primarily as morphine-3-glucuronide, ~2% to 12% excreted unchanged); feces (~7% to 10%). It has been suggested that accumulation of morphine-6-glucuronide might cause toxicity with renal insufficiency. All of the metabolites (ie, morphine-3-glucuronide, morphine-6-glucuronide, and normorphine) have been suggested as possible causes of neurotoxicity (eg, myoclonus).

Contraindications Hypersensitivity to morphine sulfate or any component of the formulation; increased intracranial pressure; severe respiratory depression; acute or severe asthma; known or suspected paralytic ileus; sustained release products are not recommended with gastrointestinal obstruction or in acute/postoperative pain; pregnancy (prolonged use or high doses at term)

Warnings/Precautions An opioid-containing analgesic regimen should be tailored to each patient's needs and based upon the type of pain being treated (acute versus chronic), the route of administration, degree of tolerance for opioids (naive versus chronic user), age, weight, and medical condition. The optimal analgesic dose varies widely among patients. Doses should be titrated to pain relief/prevention. When used as an epidural injection, monitor for delayed sedation.

May cause respiratory depression; use with caution in patients (particularly elderly or debilitated) with impaired respiratory function or severe hepatic dysfunction and in patients with hypersensitivity reactions to other phenanthrene derivative opioid agonists (codeine, hydrocodone, hydromorphone, levorphanol, oxycodone, oxymorphone). Infants <3 months of age are more susceptible to respiratory depression, use with caution and generally in reduced doses in this age group. May cause hypotension in patients with acute myocardial infarction, volume depletion, or concurrent drug therapy which may exaggerate vasodilation. Tolerance or drug dependence may result from extended use. MS Contin® 200 mg tablets are for use only in opioid-tolerant patients requiring >400 mg/day. Infumorph® solutions are **for use in microinfusion devices only**; not for I.V., I.M., or SubQ administration.

Use caution in CNS depression, toxic psychosis, delirium tremens, or convulsive disorders. Sedation and psychomotor impairment are likely, and are additive with other CNS depressants or ethanol. Use caution in renal impairment, gastrointestinal motility disturbances, biliary tract disease (including acute pancreatitis), prostatic hyperplasia, urethral stricture, thyroid disorders (Addison's disease, myxedema, or hypothyroidism). Extended or sustained release dosage forms should not be crushed or chewed. Do not administer Avinza® with alcoholic beverages or ethanol-containing products, which may disrupt extended-release characteristic of product. Controlled-, extended-, or sustained-release products are not intended for "as needed (PRN)" use. Some preparations contain sulfites which may cause allergic reactions.

Elderly and/or debilitated may be particularly susceptible to the CNS depressant and constipating effects of narcotics. May mask diagnosis or clinical course in patients with acute abdominal conditions.

Drug Interactions Substrate of CYP2D6 (minor)

Antipsychotic agents: May increase hypotensive effects of morphine; monitor.

CNS depressants: May increase the effects/toxicity of morphine; monitor.

MAO inhibitors: May increase the effects/toxicity of morphine; some manufacturers recommend avoiding use within 14 days of MAO inhibitors

Pegvisomant: Therapeutic efficacy may be decreased by concomitant opiates, possibly requiring dosage adjustment of pegvisomant.

Rifamycin derivatives: May decrease levels/effects of morphine; monitor.

Selective serotonin reuptake inhibitors (SSRIs) and meperidine: Serotonergic effects may be additive, leading to serotonin syndrome.

Nutritional/Herbal/Ethanol Interactions

Ethanol: Avoid ethanol (may increase CNS depression).

- Avinza®: Alcoholic beverages or ethanol-containing products may disrupt extended-release formulation resulting in rapid release of entire morphine dose.

Food: Administration of oral morphine solution with food may increase bioavailability (ie, a report of 34% increase in morphine AUC when morphine oral solution followed a high-fat meal). The bioavailability of Oramorph SR® or Kadian® does not appear to be affected by food.

Herb/Nutraceutical: Avoid valerian, St John's wort, kava kava, gotu kola (may increase CNS depression).

Lab Interactions Increased aminotransferase [ALT (SGPT)/AST (SGOT)] (S)

Adverse Reactions Note: Individual patient differences are unpredictable, and percentage may differ in acute pain (surgical) treatment.

Frequency not defined: Flushing, CNS depression, sedation, antidiuretic hormone release, physical and psychological dependence, diaphoresis

>10%:

- Cardiovascular: Palpitations, hypotension, bradycardia
- Central nervous system: Drowsiness (48%, tolerance usually develops to drowsiness with regular dosing for 1-2 weeks); dizziness (20%), confusion, headache (following epidural or intrathecal use)
- Dermatologic: Pruritus (may be secondary to histamine release)
  - **Note:** Pruritus may be dose-related, but not confined to the site of administration.
- Gastrointestinal: Nausea (28%, tolerance usually develops to nausea and vomiting with chronic use); constipation (40%, tolerance develops very slowly if at all); xerostomia (78%)
- Genitourinary: Urinary retention (16%; may be prolonged, up to 20 hours, following epidural or intrathecal use)
- Local: Pain at injection site
- Neuromuscular & skeletal: Weakness
- Miscellaneous: Histamine release

1% to 10%:

- Cardiovascular: Atrial fibrillation (<3%), chest pain (<3%), edema (<3%), syncope (<3%), tachycardia (<3%)
- Central nervous system: Amnesia, anxiety, apathy, ataxia, chills, depression, euphoria, false feeling of well being, fever, headache, hypoesthesia, insomnia, lethargy, malaise, restlessness, seizure, vertigo
- Endocrine & metabolic: Hyponatremia (<3%), gynecomastia (<3%)
- Gastrointestinal: Anorexia, biliary colic, dyspepsia, dysphagia, GERD, GI irritation, paralytic ileus, vomiting (9%)
- Genitourinary: Decreased urination
- Hematologic: Anemia (<3%), leukopenia (<3%), thrombocytopenia (<3%)
- Neuromuscular & skeletal: Arthralgia, back pain, bone pain, paresthesia, trembling

(Continued)

Morphine Sulfate *(Continued)*

Ocular: Vision problems

Respiratory: Asthma, atelectasis, dyspnea, hiccups, hypoxia, noncardiogenic pulmonary edema, respiratory depression, rhinitis

Miscellaneous: Diaphoresis, flu-like syndrome, withdrawal syndrome

<1% (Limited to important or life-threatening): Amenorrhea, anaphylaxis, biliary tract spasm, hallucinations, intestinal obstruction, intracranial pressure increased, liver function tests increased, menstrual irregularities, mental depression, miosis, muscle rigidity, myoclonus, oliguria, paradoxical CNS stimulation, peripheral vasodilation, urinary tract spasm, transaminases increased

Overdosage/Toxicology Symptoms of overdose include respiratory depression, miosis, hypotension, bradycardia, apnea, and pulmonary edema. Treatment is symptomatic. Naloxone, 2 mg I.V. with repeat administration as necessary up to a total dose of 10 mg, can be used to reverse opiate effects.

Dosing

Adults: Note: These are guidelines and do not represent the doses that may be required in all patients. Doses should be titrated to pain relief/prevention.

Acute pain (moderate-to-severe):

Oral: Prompt release formulations: Opiate-naive: Initial: 10 mg every 3 to 4 hours as needed; patients with prior opiate exposure may require higher initial doses: usual dosage range: 10-30 mg every 3-4 hours as needed

I.M., SubQ: **Note:** Repeated SubQ administration causes local tissue irritation, pain, and induration.

Initial: Opiate-naive: 5-10 mg every 3-4 hours as needed; patients with prior opiate exposure may require higher initial doses; usual dosage range: 5-20 mg every 3-4 hours as needed

Rectal: 10-20 mg every 3-4 hours

I.V.: Initial: Opiate-naive: 2.5-5 mg every 3 to 4 hours; patients with prior opiate exposure may require higher initial doses. **Note:** Repeated doses (up to every 5 minutes if needed) in small increments (eg, 1-4 mg) may be preferred to larger and less frequent doses.

I.V., SubQ continuous infusion: 0.8-10 mg/hour; usual range: Up to 80 mg/hour

Mechanically-ventilated patients (based on 70 kg patient): 0.7-10 mg every 1-2 hours as needed; infusion: 5-35 mg/hour

Patient-controlled analgesia (PCA): (Opiate-naive: Consider lower end of dosing range):

Usual concentration: 1 mg/mL

Demand dose: Usual: 1 mg; range: 0.5-2.5 mg

Lockout interval: 5-10 minutes

Intrathecal (I.T.): **Note:** Administer with extreme caution and in reduced dosage to geriatric or debilitated patients.

Opioid-naive: 0.2-0.25 mg/dose (may provide adequate relief for 24 hours); repeat doses are **not** recommended.

Epidural: **Note:** Administer with extreme caution and in reduced dosage to geriatric or debilitated patients. Vigilant monitoring is particularly important in these patients.

Pain management:

Single-dose (Duramorph®): Initial: 3-5 mg

Infusion:

Bolus dose: 1-6 mg

Infusion rate: 0.1-0.2 mg/hour

Maximum dose: 10 mg/24 hours

Surgical anesthesia: Epidural: Single-dose (extended release, Depo-Dur™): Lumbar epidural only; not recommended in patients <18 years of age:

Cesarean section: 10 mg

Lower abdominal/pelvic surgery: 10-15 mg

Major orthopedic surgery of lower extremity: 15 mg

For Depo-Dur™: To minimize the pharmacokinetic interaction resulting in higher peak serum concentrations of morphine, administer the test dose of the local anesthetic at least 15 minutes prior to Depo-Dur™ administration. Use of Depo-Dur™ with epidural local anesthetics has not been studied.

Note: Some patients may benefit from a 20 mg dose, however, the incidence of adverse effects may be increased.

Chronic pain: Note: Patients taking opioids chronically may become tolerant and require doses higher than the usual dosage range to maintain the desired effect. Tolerance can be managed by appropriate dose titration. There is no optimal or maximal dose for morphine in chronic pain. The appropriate dose is one that relieves pain throughout its dosing interval without causing unmanageable side effects.

Oral: Controlled-, extended-, or sustained-release formulations: A patient's morphine requirement should be established using prompt-release formulations. Conversion to long-acting products may be considered when chronic, continuous treatment is required. Higher dosages should be reserved for use only in opioid-tolerant patients.

Capsules, extended release (Avinza™): Daily dose administered once daily (for best results, administer at same time each day)

Capsules, sustained release (Kadian®): Daily dose administered once daily or in 2 divided doses daily (every 12 hours)

Tablets, controlled release (MS Contin®), sustained release (Oramorph SR®), or extended release: Daily dose divided and administered every 8 or every 12 hours

Elderly: Refer to adult dosing. Use with caution; may require reduced dosage in the elderly and debilitated patients.

Pediatrics: Note: These are guidelines and do not represent the doses that may be required in all patients. Doses should be titrated to pain relief/prevention.

Acute pain (moderate-to-severe): Children >6 months and <50 kg:

Oral (prompt release): 0.15-0.3 mg/kg every 3-4 hours as needed

I.M.: 0.1 mg/kg every 3-4 hours as needed

I.V.: 0.05-0.1 mg/kg every 3-4 hours as needed

I.V. infusion: Range: 10-30 mcg/kg/hour

Sedation/analgesia for procedures: Adolescents >12 years: I.V.: 3-4 mg and repeat in 5 minutes if necessary

Renal Impairment:

Cl_{cr} 10-50 mL/minute: Administer 75% of normal dose.

Cl_{cr} <10 mL/minute: Administer 50% of normal dose.

Hepatic Impairment: Unchanged in mild liver disease; substantial extrahepatic metabolism may occur. Excessive sedation may occur in cirrhosis.

Available Dosage Forms

[DSC] = Discontinued product

Capsule, extended release (Avinza®): 30 mg, 60 mg, 90 mg, 120 mg

Capsule, sustained release (Kadian®): 20 mg, 30 mg, 50 mg, 60 mg, 100 mg

Infusion [premixed in D_5W]: 1 mg/mL (100 mL, 250 mL)

Injection, extended release liposomal suspension [lumbar epidural injection, preservative free] (DepoDur™): 10 mg/mL (1 mL, 1.5 mL, 2 mL)

Injection, solution: 2 mg/mL (1 mL); 4 mg/mL (1 mL); 5 mg/mL (1 mL); 8 mg/mL (1 mL); 10 mg/mL (1 mL, 10 mL); 15 mg/mL (1 mL, 20 mL); 25 mg/mL (4 mL, 10 mL, 20 mL, 40 mL, 50 mL, 100 mL, 250 mL); 50 mg/mL (20 mL, 40 mL) [some preparations contain sodium metabisulfite]

Injection, solution [epidural, intrathecal, or I.V. infusion; preservative free]:

Astramorph/PF™: 0.5 mg/mL (2 mL, 10 mL); 1 mg/mL (2 mL, 10 mL)

Duramorph®: 0.5 mg/mL (10 mL); 1 mg/mL (10 mL)

Injection, solution [epidural or intrathecal infusion via microinfusion device; preservative free] (Infumorph®): 10 mg/mL (20 mL); 25 mg/mL (20 mL)

Injection, solution [I.V. infusion via PCA pump]: 0.5 mg/mL (30 mL); 1 mg/mL (30 mL, 50 mL); 2 mg/mL (30 mL); 5 mg/mL (30 mL, 50 mL)

Injection, solution [preservative free]: 0.5 mg/mL (10 mL); 1 mg/mL (10 mL); 25 mg/mL (4 mL, 10 mL, 20 mL)

Solution, oral: 10 mg/5 mL (5 mL, 10 mL, 100 mL, 500 mL); 20 mg/5 mL (100 mL, 500 mL); 20 mg/mL (30 mL, 120 mL, 240 mL)

Roxanol™: 20 mg/mL (30 mL, 120 mL)

Roxanol 100™: 100 mg/5 mL (240 mL) [with calibrated spoon]

Roxanol™-T: 20 mg/mL (30 mL, 120 mL) [tinted, flavored] [DSC]

Suppository, rectal (RMS®): 5 mg (12s), 10 mg (12s), 20 mg (12s), 30 mg (12s)

Tablet: 15 mg, 30 mg

Tablet, controlled release (MS Contin®): 15 mg, 30 mg, 60 mg, 100 mg, 200 mg

Tablet, extended release: 15 mg, 30 mg, 60 mg, 100 mg, 200 mg

Tablet, sustained release (Oramorph SR®): 15 mg, 30 mg, 60 mg, 100 mg

Nursing Guidelines

Assessment: Assess other medications patient may be taking for additive or adverse interactions. Monitor vital signs, respiratory and CNS status, therapeutic effectiveness, and adverse reactions or overdose at regular intervals with long-term use. May cause physical and/or psychological dependence. For

(Continued)

Morphine Sulfate *(Continued)*

inpatients, implement safety measures. Assess knowledge/teach patient appropriate use (if self-administered), adverse reactions to report, and appropriate interventions to reduce side effects. Discontinue slowly after prolonged use.

Dietary Considerations: Morphine may cause GI upset; take with food if GI upset occurs. Be consistent when taking morphine with or without meals.

Patient Education: If self-administered, use exactly as directed; do not increase dose or frequency. Do not crush or chew controlled release tablet or capsule. May cause physical and/or psychological dependence. While using this medication, do not use alcohol and other prescription or OTC medications (especially sedatives, tranquilizers, antihistamines, or pain medications) without consulting prescriber. Maintain adequate hydration (2-3 L/day of fluids) unless instructed to restrict fluid intake. May cause hypotension, dizziness, drowsiness, impaired coordination, or blurred vision (use caution when driving, climbing stairs, or changing position - rising from sitting or lying to standing, or when engaging in tasks requiring alertness until response to drug is known); loss of appetite, nausea, or vomiting (frequent mouth care, small frequent meals, chewing gum, or sucking lozenges may help); or constipation (increased exercise, fluids, fruit, or fiber may help; if unresolved, consult prescriber about use of stool softeners and/or laxatives). Report chest pain, slow or rapid heartbeat, acute dizziness, or persistent headache; changes in mental status; swelling of extremities or unusual weight gain; changes in urinary elimination or pain on urination; acute headache; back or flank pain; muscle spasms; blurred vision; skin rash; or shortness of breath. **Pregnancy/breast-feeding precautions:** Inform prescriber if you are or intend to become pregnant. If you are breast-feeding, take medication immediately after breast-feeding or 3-4 hours (for Depo-Dur™, 48 hours) prior to next feeding.

Geriatric Considerations: The elderly may be particularly susceptible to the CNS depressant and constipating effects of narcotics. For chronic administration of narcotic analgesics, morphine is preferable in the elderly due to its pharmacokinetics and side effect profile as compared to meperidine and methadone.

Pregnancy Risk Factor: C/D (prolonged use or high doses at term)

Pregnancy Issues: Morphine crosses the placenta. The frequency of congenital malformations has not been reported to be greater than expected in children from mothers treated with morphine during pregnancy. Reduced growth and behavioral abnormalities in offspring have been observed in animal studies. Neonates born to mothers receiving chronic opioids during pregnancy should be monitored for neonatal withdrawal syndrome.

DepoDur™ may be used in women undergoing cesarean section following clamping of the umbilical cord; not for use in vaginal labor and delivery.

Lactation: Enters breast milk/use caution (AAP rates "compatible")

Breast-Feeding Considerations: Morphine concentrates in breast milk, with a milk to plasma ratio of 2.5:1. Detectable serum levels of morphine can be found in infants following morphine administration to nursing mothers. Treatment of the mother with single doses of morphine is not expected to cause detrimental effects in nursing infants. Breast-feeding following chronic use or in neonates with hepatic or renal dysfunction may lead to higher levels of morphine in the infant and a risk of adverse effects. Some clinicians recommend administering morphine immediately after breast-feeding or 3-4 hours prior to the next feeding. Breast-feeding should be delayed for 48 hours after DepoDur™ administration.

Perioperative/Anesthesia/Other Concerns: When developing a therapeutic plan for pain control, scheduled, intermittent opioid dosing or continuous infusion is preferred over the "as needed" regimen. The 2002 ACCM/SCCM guidelines for analgesia (critically-ill adult) recommend fentanyl in patients who need immediate pain relief because of its rapid onset of action; fentanyl or hydromorphone is preferred in patients who are hypotensive or have renal dysfunction. Morphine or hydromorphone is recommended for intermittent, scheduled therapy. Both have a longer duration of action requiring less frequent administration. If the patient has required high-dose analgesia or has used for a prolonged period (~7 days), taper dose to prevent withdrawal; monitor for signs and symptoms of withdrawal. Use only preservative-free injections for epidural or intrathecal administration; less adverse effects are associated with epidural compared to intrathecal route of administration.

Administration

Oral: Do not crush controlled release drug product, swallow whole. Kadian® and Avinza® can be opened and sprinkled on applesauce; do not crush or chew the beads. Contents of Kadian® capsules may be opened and sprinkled over 10 mL water and flushed through prewetted 16F gastrostomy tube; do not administer Kadian® through nasogastric tube. Administration of oral morphine solution with food may increase bioavailability (not observed with Oramorph SR®).

I.V.: When giving morphine I.V. push, it is best to first dilute in 4-5 mL of sterile water, and then to administer slowly (eg, 15 mg over 3-5 minutes).

Reconstitution: Usual concentration for continuous I.V. infusion: 0.1-1 mg/mL in D_5W. DepoDur™ may be diluted in preservative-free NS to a volume of 5 mL.

Compatibility: Stable in dextran 6% in dextrose, dextran 6% in NS, D_5LR, $D_5{}^1/_4NS$, $D_5{}^1/_2NS$, D_5NS, D_5W, $D_{10}W$, LR, ½NS, NS

Y-site administration: Incompatible with alatrofloxacin, amphotericin B cholesteryl sulfate complex, cefepime, doxorubicin liposome, minocycline, sargramostim

Compatibility in syringe: Incompatible with meperidine, thiopental

Compatibility when admixed: Incompatible with aminophylline, amobarbital, chlorothiazide, floxacillin, fluorouracil, heparin, meperidine, phenobarbital, phenytoin, sodium bicarbonate, thiopental

DepoDur™: Do not mix with other medications.

Storage:

Capsule, sustained release (Kadian®): Store at controlled room temperature 15°C to 30°C (59°F to 86°F). Protect from light and moisture.

Suppositories: Store at controlled room temperature 25°C (77°F). Protect from light.

Injection: Store at controlled room temperature. Protect from light. Degradation depends on pH and presence of oxygen; relatively stable in pH ≤4; darkening of solutions indicate degradation.

DepoDur™: Store under refrigeration, 2°C to 8°C (36°F to 46°F). Do not freeze. May store at room temperature for up to 7 days. Once vial is opened, use within 4 hours.

Related Information

Acute Postoperative Pain *on page 1742*
Conscious Sedation *on page 1779*
Narcotic / Opioid Analgesics *on page 1880*

♦ Motrin® *see* Ibuprofen *on page 889*
♦ Motrin® Children's [OTC] *see* Ibuprofen *on page 889*
♦ Motrin® IB [OTC] *see* Ibuprofen *on page 889*
♦ Motrin® Infants' [OTC] *see* Ibuprofen *on page 889*
♦ Motrin® Junior Strength [OTC] *see* Ibuprofen *on page 889*

Moxifloxacin (moxs i FLOKS a sin)

U.S. Brand Names Avelox®; Avelox® I.V.; Vigamox™

Synonyms Moxifloxacin Hydrochloride

Pharmacologic Category Antibiotic, Ophthalmic; Antibiotic, Quinolone

Medication Safety Issues

Sound-alike/look-alike issues:

Avelox® may be confused with Avonex®

Use Treatment of mild-to-moderate community-acquired pneumonia, including multidrug-resistant *Streptococcus pneumoniae* (MDRSP); acute bacterial exacerbation of chronic bronchitis; acute bacterial sinusitis; complicated and uncomplicated skin and skin structure infections; complicated intra-abdominal infections; bacterial conjunctivitis (ophthalmic formulation)

Mechanism of Action Moxifloxacin is a DNA gyrase inhibitor, and also inhibits topoisomerase IV. DNA gyrase (topoisomerase II) is an essential bacterial enzyme that maintains the superhelical structure of DNA. DNA gyrase is required for DNA replication and transcription, DNA repair, recombination, and transposition; inhibition is bactericidal.

Pharmacodynamics/Kinetics

Absorption: Well absorbed; not affected by high fat meal or yogurt

Distribution: V_d: 1.7 to 2.7 L/kg; tissue concentrations often exceed plasma concentrations in respiratory tissues, alveolar macrophages, abdominal tissues/fluids, and sinus tissues

Protein binding: 30% to 50%

(Continued)

Moxifloxacin *(Continued)*

Metabolism: Hepatic (52% of dose) via glucuronide (14%) and sulfate (38%) conjugation

Bioavailability: 90%

Half-life elimination: Oral: 12 hours; I.V.: 15 hours

Excretion: Approximately 45% of a dose is excreted in feces (25%) and urine (20%) as unchanged drug

Metabolites: Sulfate conjugates in feces, glucuronide conjugates in urine

Contraindications Hypersensitivity to moxifloxacin, other quinolone antibiotics, or any component of the formulation

Warnings/Precautions Use with caution in patients with significant bradycardia or acute myocardial ischemia. Moxifloxacin causes a concentration-dependent QT prolongation. Do not exceed recommended dose or infusion rate. Avoid use with uncorrected hypokalemia, with other drugs that prolong the QT interval or induce bradycardia, or with class IA or III antiarrhythmic agents. Use with caution in individuals at risk of seizures (CNS disorders or concurrent therapy with medications which may lower seizure threshold). Discontinue in patients who experience significant CNS adverse effects (dizziness, hallucinations, suicidal ideation or actions). Not recommended in patients with moderate to severe hepatic insufficiency. Use with caution in diabetes; glucose regulation may be altered. Tendon inflammation and/or rupture have been reported with quinolone antibiotics. Risk may be increased with concurrent corticosteroids, particularly in the elderly. Discontinue at first signs or symptoms of tendon pain.

Severe hypersensitivity reactions, including anaphylaxis, have occurred with quinolone therapy. If an allergic reaction occurs (itching, urticaria, dyspnea or facial edema, loss of consciousness, tingling, cardiovascular collapse) discontinue drug immediately. May cause photosensitivity. Prolonged use may result in superinfection; pseudomembranous colitis may occur and should be considered in all patients who present with diarrhea. Quinolones may exacerbate myasthenia gravis, use with caution (rare, potentially life-threatening weakness of respiratory muscles may occur). Peripheral neuropathy may rarely occur. Safety and efficacy of systemically administered moxifloxacin (oral, intravenous) in patients <18 years of age have not been established.

Ophthalmic: Eye drops should not be injected subconjunctivally or introduced directly into the anterior chamber of the eye. Contact lenses should not be worn during therapy.

Drug Interactions

Corticosteroids: Concurrent use may increase the risk of tendon rupture, particularly in elderly patients (overall incidence rare).

Glyburide: Quinolones may increase the effect of glyburide; monitor

Metal cations (aluminum, calcium, iron, magnesium, and zinc) bind quinolones in the gastrointestinal tract and inhibit absorption. Concurrent administration of most antacids, oral electrolyte supplements, quinapril, sucralfate, some didanosine formulations (chewable/buffered tablets and pediatric powder for oral suspension), and other higly-buffered oral drugs, should be avoided. Moxifloxacin should be administered 4 hours before or 8 hours after these agents. Calcium products do not appear to significantly affect moxifloxacin absorption.

QT_c-prolonging agents: Effects may be additive with moxifloxacin. Avoid concurrent use with Class Ia and Class III antiarrhythmics, erythromycin, cisapride, antipsychotics, and cyclic antidepressants.

Warfarin: The hypoprothrombinemic effect of warfarin may be enhanced by some quinolone antibiotics; monitor INR.

Nutritional/Herbal/Ethanol Interactions Food: Absorption is not affected by administration with a high-fat meal or yogurt.

Adverse Reactions

Systemic:

3% to 10%: Gastrointestinal: Nausea (6%), diarrhea (5%)

0.1% to 3%:

Central nervous system: Anxiety, chills, dizziness (2%), headache, insomnia, malaise, nervousness, pain, somnolence, tremor, vertigo

Dermatologic: Dry skin, pruritus, rash (maculopapular, purpuric, pustular)

Endocrine & metabolic: Serum chloride increased (≥2%), serum ionized calcium increased (≥2%), serum glucose decreased (≥2%)

Gastrointestinal: Abdominal pain, amylase increased, amylase decreased (≥2%), anorexia, constipation, dry mouth, dyspepsia, flatulence, glossitis, lactic dehydrogenase increased, stomatitis, taste perversion, vomiting

Genitourinary: Vaginal moniliasis, vaginitis
Hematologic: Anemia, eosinophilia, leukopenia, prothrombin time prolonged, increased INR, thrombocythemia
Increased serum levels of the following (≥2%): MCH, neutrophils, WBC
Decreased serum levels of the following (≥2%): Basophils, eosinophils, hemoglobin, RBC, neutrophils
Hepatic: Bilirubin decreased or increased (≥2%), GGTP increased, liver function test abnormal
Local: Injection site reaction
Neuromuscular & skeletal: Arthralgia, myalgia, weakness
Renal: Serum albumin increased (≥2%)
Respiratory: Pharyngitis, pneumonia, rhinitis, sinusitis, pO_2 increased (≥2%)
Miscellaneous: Allergic reaction, infection, diaphoresis, oral moniliasis

Additional reactions with **ophthalmic** preparation: 1% to 6%: Conjunctivitis, dry eye, ocular discomfort, ocular hyperemia, ocular pain, ocular pruritus, subconjunctival hemorrhage, tearing, visual acuity decreased

Overdosage/Toxicology Potential symptoms of overdose may include CNS excitation, seizures, QT prolongation, and arrhythmias (including torsade de pointes). Patients should be monitored by continuous ECG in the event of an overdose. Management is supportive and symptomatic. Hemodialysis only removes ~9% of dose.

Dosing

Adults & Elderly:

Acute bacterial sinusitis: Oral, I.V.: 400 mg every 24 hours for 10 days

Chronic bronchitis, acute bacterial exacerbation: Oral, I.V.: 400 mg every 24 hours for 5 days

Note: Avelox® ABC Pack™ (Avelox® Bronchitis Course) contains five tablets of 400 mg each.

Community-acquired pneumonia (including MDRSP and methcillin-suspectible *Staphylococcus aureus*): 400 mg every 24 hours for 7-14 days

Intra-abdominal infections, complicated: 400 mg every 24 hours for 5-14 days (initiate with I.V.)

Skin and skin structure infections:
Complicated: 400 mg every 24 hours for 7-21 days
Uncomplicated: 400 mg every 24 hours for 7 days

Bacterial conjunctivitis: Ophthalmic: Instill 1 drop into affected eye(s) 3 times/day for 7 days

Pediatrics: Bacterial conjunctivitis: Ophthalmic: Children ≥1 year: Refer to adult dosing.

Renal Impairment: No adjustment is necessary, including patients on hemodialysis or CAPD.

Hepatic Impairment: No dosage adjustment is required in mild to moderate hepatic insufficiency (Child-Pugh Classes A and B). Not recommended in patients with severe hepatic insufficiency.

Available Dosage Forms

Infusion [premixed in sodium chloride 0.8%] (Avelox® I.V.): 400 mg (250 mL)
Solution, ophthalmic (Vigamox™): 0.5% (3 mL)
Tablet [film coated]:
Avelox®: 400 mg
Avelox® ABC Pack [unit-dose pack]: 400 mg (5s)

Nursing Guidelines

Assessment: Assess results of any culture and sensitivity tests and patient's allergy history before initiating therapy. Use caution with known CNS disorders, bradycardia, or hepatic impairment. Assess potential for interactions with other pharmacological agents or herbal products patient is taking that may increase risk of tendon rupture or arrhythmias. See Administration for infusion specifics; if an allergic reaction occurs (itching, urticaria, dyspnea or facial edema, loss of consciousness, tingling, cardiovascular collapse), drug should be discontinued immediately and prescriber notified. Assess results of laboratory tests, therapeutic effectiveness (resolution of infection), and adverse effects. Teach patient proper use, possible side effects/appropriate interventions, and adverse symptoms to report (refer to Patient Education).

Monitoring Laboratory Tests: WBC

Dietary Considerations: May be taken with or without food. Take 4 hours before or 8 hours after multiple vitamins, antacids, or other products containing magnesium, aluminum, iron, or zinc.

(Continued)

Moxifloxacin *(Continued)*

Patient Education: Inform prescriber of all prescriptions, OTC medications, or herbal products you are taking, and any allergies you have. Do not take any new medication during therapy unless approved by prescriber. **Pregnancy/breast-feeding precautions:** Inform prescriber if you are or intend to become pregnant. Breast-feeding is not recommended.

I.V.: Report any redness, swelling, or pain at infusion site; any swelling of mouth, lips, tongue, or throat; chest pain or tightness; respiratory difficulty; back pain; itching; skin rash; tingling; tendon pain; dizziness; abnormal thinking; or anxiety.

Oral: Take exactly as directed with or without food. Do not take antacids 4 hours before or 8 hours after taking this medication. Do not miss a dose (take a missed dose as soon as possible, unless it is almost time for your next dose). Take entire prescription even if feeling better. Maintain adequate hydration (2-3 L/day of fluids) unless instructed to restrict fluid intake. May cause nausea, vomiting, taste perversion (small, frequent meals, good mouth care, chewing gum, or sucking hard candy may help); headache, dizziness, insomnia, anxiety (use caution when driving or engaging in tasks requiring alertness until response to drug is known). Report immediately any swelling of mouth, lips, tongue or throat; chest pain or tightness; respiratory difficulty; back pain; itching; skin rash; tingling; tendon pain; pain or numbness (loss of sensation) in extremities; confusion, dizziness, abnormal thinking, or anxiety; or insomnia. Report changes in voiding pattern; vaginal itching, burning, or discharge; vision changes or hearing; abnormal bruising or bleeding or blood in urine; or other adverse reactions.

Ophthalmic: Wash hands before instilling solution. Sit or lie down to instill. Open eye, look at ceiling, and instill prescribed amount of solution as directed. Do not touch tip of applicator or let tip of applicator touch eye. Do not wear contact lenses during therapy. Temporary stinging or blurred vision, or dry eyes may occur. Report persistent pain, burning, excessive tearing, decreased visual acuity, swelling, itching, or worsening of condition.

Pregnancy Risk Factor: C

Pregnancy Issues: Reports of arthropathy (observed in immature animals and reported rarely in humans) have limited the use of fluoroquinolones during pregnancy. Teratogenic effects were not observed with moxifloxacin in animal studies; however, delayed skeletal development and smaller fetuses were observed in some species. There are no adequate and well-controlled studies in pregnant women. Based on limited data, quinolones are not expected to be a major human teratogen. Although quinolone antibiotics should not be used as first-line agents during pregnancy, when considering treatment for life-threatening infection and/or prolonged duration of therapy, the potential risk to the fetus must be balanced against the severity of the potential illness.

Lactation: Excretion in breast milk unknown/not recommended

Breast-Feeding Considerations: Other quinolones are known to be excreted in breast milk. The manufacturer recommends to discontinue nursing or to discontinue moxifloxacin.

Perioperative/Anesthesia/Other Concerns: Moxifloxacin causes a dose-dependent QT prolongation. Coadministration of moxifloxacin with other drugs that also prolong the QT interval or induce bradycardia (eg, beta-blockers, amiodarone) should be avoided. Careful consideration should be given in the use of moxifloxacin in patients with cardiovascular disease, in those with conduction abnormalities.

Administration

I.V.: I.V.: Infuse over 60 minutes; do not infuse by rapid or bolus intravenous infusion

Compatibility: Stable in NS, D_5W, $D_{10}W$, SWFI, LR

Do not add other medications to intravenous solution

Storage: Store at 15°C to 30°C (59°F to 86°F). Do not refrigerate infusion solution.

Related Information

Prevention of Wound Infection and Sepsis in Surgical Patients *on page 1830*

- **Moxifloxacin Hydrochloride** *see* Moxifloxacin *on page 1183*
- **Moxilin®** *see* Amoxicillin *on page 144*
- **MPA** *see* Mycophenolate *on page 1188*

- **MPA and Estrogens (Conjugated)** *see* Estrogens (Conjugated/Equine) and Medroxyprogesterone *on page 665*
- **MPSV4** *see* Meningococcal Polysaccharide Vaccine (Groups A / C / Y and W-135) *on page 1096*
- **MS Contin®** *see* Morphine Sulfate *on page 1177*
- **MSO_4 (error-prone abbreviation and should not be used)** *see* Morphine Sulfate *on page 1177*
- **MTC** *see* Mitomycin *on page 1168*
- **MTX (error-prone abbreviation)** *see* Methotrexate *on page 1127*
- **Mucinex® [OTC]** *see* Guaifenesin *on page 834*
- **Mucomyst®** *see* Acetylcysteine *on page 80*
- **Multiple Vitamins** *see* Vitamins (Multiple/Oral) *on page 1720*
- **Multiret Folic 500** *see* Vitamins (Multiple/Oral) *on page 1720*
- **Multivitamins/Fluoride** *see* Vitamins (Multiple/Pediatric) *on page 1720*
- **Mumps, Measles and Rubella Vaccines, Combined** *see* Measles, Mumps, and Rubella Vaccines (Combined) *on page 1082*

Mupirocin (myoo PEER oh sin)

U.S. Brand Names Bactroban®; Bactroban® Nasal; Centany™

Synonyms Mupirocin Calcium; Pseudomonic Acid A

Pharmacologic Category Antibiotic, Topical

Medication Safety Issues

Sound-alike/look-alike issues:

Bactroban® may be confused with bacitracin, baclofen

Use

Intranasal: Eradication of nasal colonization with MRSA in adult patients and healthcare workers

Topical treatment of impetigo due to *Staphylococcus aureus*, beta-hemolytic *Streptococcus*, and *S. pyogenes*

Unlabeled/Investigational Use Intranasal: Surgical prophylaxis to prevent wound infections

Mechanism of Action Binds to bacterial isoleucyl transfer-RNA synthetase resulting in the inhibition of protein and RNA synthesis

Pharmacodynamics/Kinetics

Absorption: Topical: Penetrates outer layers of skin; systemic absorption minimal through intact skin

Protein binding: 95%

Metabolism: Skin: 3% to monic acid

Half-life elimination: 17-36 minutes

Excretion: Urine

Contraindications Hypersensitivity to mupirocin, polyethylene glycol, or any component of the formulation

Warnings/Precautions Potentially toxic amounts of polyethylene glycol contained in the vehicle may be absorbed percutaneously in patients with extensive burns or open wounds; prolonged use may result in over growth of nonsusceptible organisms; for external use only; not for treatment of pressure sores

Drug Interactions No data reported

Adverse Reactions Frequency not defined.

Central nervous system: Dizziness, headache

Dermatologic: Pruritus, rash, erythema, dry skin, cellulitis, dermatitis

Gastrointestinal: Nausea, taste perversion

Local: Burning, stinging, tenderness, edema, pain

Respiratory: Rhinitis, upper respiratory tract infection, pharyngitis, cough

Dosing

Adults & Elderly:

Impetigo: Topical: Apply small amount to affected area 2-5 times/day for 5-14 days.

Elimination of MRSA colonization: Nasal: Approximately one-half of the ointment from the single-use tube should be applied into one nostril and the other half into the other nostril twice daily for 5 days.

Pediatrics:

Topical: Children: Refer to adult dosing.

Nasal: ≥12 years: Refer to adult dosing.

Available Dosage Forms

Cream, topical, as calcium (Bactroban®): 2% (15 g, 30 g) [contains benzyl alcohol]

(Continued)

Mupirocin *(Continued)*

Ointment, intranasal, topical, as calcium (Bactroban® Nasal): 2% (1 g) [single-use tube]

Ointment, topical: 2% (0.9 g, 22 g)
Bactroban®: 2% (22 g)
Centany™: 2% (15 g, 30 g)

Nursing Guidelines

Assessment: See Warnings/Precautions and Contraindications for use cautions. Assess for effectiveness of therapy and symptoms of infection. Assess knowledge/teach patient appropriate application and use and adverse symptoms (see Adverse Reactions) to report. Note breast-feeding caution.

Patient Education: For external use only. Wash hands before and after application. Apply thin film over affected areas exactly as directed. Avoid getting in eyes. Report rash, persistent burning, stinging, swelling, itching, or pain. Contact prescriber if no improvement is seen in 3-5 days. **Breast-feeding precaution:** Consult prescriber if breast-feeding.

Pregnancy Risk Factor: B

Lactation: Excretion in breast milk unknown/use caution

Administration

Compatibility: Do not mix with Aquaphor®, coal tar solution, or salicylic acid.

- **Mupirocin Calcium** *see* Mupirocin *on page 1187*
- **Murine® Ear Wax Removal System [OTC]** *see* Carbamide Peroxide *on page 311*
- **Murine® Tears [OTC]** *see* Artificial Tears *on page 187*
- **Muro 128® [OTC]** *see* Sodium Chloride *on page 1545*
- **Murocel® [OTC]** *see* Artificial Tears *on page 187*
- **Muse®** *see* Alprostadil *on page 113*
- **Mutamycin®** *see* Mitomycin *on page 1168*
- **M.V.I.®-12 [DSC]** *see* Vitamins (Multiple/Injectable) *on page 1719*
- **M.V.I. Adult™** *see* Vitamins (Multiple/Injectable) *on page 1719*
- **M.V.I® Pediatric** *see* Vitamins (Multiple/Injectable) *on page 1719*
- **Mycelex®** *see* Clotrimazole *on page 439*
- **Mycelex®-7 [OTC]** *see* Clotrimazole *on page 439*
- **Mycelex® Twin Pack [OTC]** *see* Clotrimazole *on page 439*
- **Mycinaire™ [OTC]** *see* Sodium Chloride *on page 1545*
- **Mycinettes® [OTC]** *see* Benzocaine *on page 232*

Mycophenolate (mye koe FEN oh late)

U.S. Brand Names CellCept®; Myfortic®

Synonyms MMF; MPA; Mycophenolate Mofetil; Mycophenolate Sodium; Mycophenolic Acid

Pharmacologic Category Immunosuppressant Agent

Use Prophylaxis of organ rejection concomitantly with cyclosporine and corticosteroids in patients receiving allogenic renal (CellCept®, Myfortic®), cardiac (CellCept®), or hepatic (CellCept®) transplants

Unlabeled/Investigational Use Treatment of rejection in liver transplant patients unable to tolerate tacrolimus or cyclosporine due to neurotoxicity; mild rejection in heart transplant patients; treatment of moderate-severe psoriasis; treatment of proliferative lupus nephritis

Mechanism of Action MPA exhibits a cytostatic effect on T and B lymphocytes. It is an inhibitor of inosine monophosphate dehydrogenase (IMPDH) which inhibits *de novo* guanosine nucleotide synthesis. T and B lymphocytes are dependent on this pathway for proliferation.

Pharmacodynamics/Kinetics

Onset of action: Peak effect: Correlation of toxicity or efficacy is still being developed, however, one study indicated that 12-hour AUCs >40 mcg/mL/hour were correlated with efficacy and decreased episodes of rejection

T_{max}: Oral: MPA:
CellCept®: 1-1.5 hours
Myfortic®: 1.5-2.5 hours

Absorption: AUC values for MPA are lower in the early post-transplant period versus later (>3 months) post-transplant period. The extent of absorption in pediatrics is similar to that seen in adults, although there was wide variability reported.

Oral: Myfortic®: 93%

Distribution:

CellCept®: MPA: Oral: 4 L/kg; I.V.: 3.6 L/kg

Myfortic®: MPA: Oral: 54 L (at steady state); 112 L (elimination phase)

Protein binding: MPA: 97%, MPAG 82%

Metabolism: Hepatic and via GI tract; CellCept® is completely hydrolyzed in the liver to mycophenolic acid (MPA; active metabolite); enterohepatic recirculation of MPA may occur; MPA is glucuronidated to MPAG (inactive metabolite)

Bioavailability: Oral: CellCept®: 94%; Myfortic®: 72%

Half-life elimination:

CellCept®: MPA: Oral: 18 hours; I.V.: 17 hours

Myfortic®: MPA: Oral: 8-16 hours; MPAG: 13-17 hours

Excretion:

CellCept®: MPA: Urine (<1%), feces (6%); MPAG: Urine (87%)

Myfortic®: MPA: Urine (3%), feces; MPAG: Urine (>60%)

Contraindications Hypersensitivity to mycophenolate mofetil, mycophenolic acid, mycophenolate sodium, or any component of the formulation; intravenous formulation is contraindicated in patients who are allergic to polysorbate 80

Warnings/Precautions Risk for infection and development of lymphoproliferative disorders (particularly of the skin) is increased. Patients should be monitored appropriately, instructed to limit exposure to sunlight/UV light, and given supportive treatment should these conditions occur. Severe neutropenia may occur, requiring interruption of treatment (risk greater from day 31-180 post-transplant). Use caution with active peptic ulcer disease; may be associated with GI bleeding and/or perforation. Use caution in renal impairment as toxicity may be increased; may require dosage adjustment in severe impairment. Patients may be at increased risk of infection.

Because mycophenolate mofetil has demonstrated teratogenic effects in rats and rabbits, tablets should not be crushed, and capsules should not be opened or crushed. Avoid inhalation or direct contact with skin or mucous membranes of the powder contained in the capsules and the powder for oral suspension. Caution should be exercised in the handling and preparation of solutions of intravenous mycophenolate. Avoid skin contact with the intravenous solution and reconstituted suspension. If such contact occurs, wash thoroughly with soap and water, rinse eyes with plain water.

Theoretically, use should be avoided in patients with the rare hereditary deficiency of hypoxanthine-guanine phosphoribosyltransferase (such as Lesch-Nyhan or Kelley-Seegmiller syndrome). Intravenous solutions should be given over at least 2 hours; **never** administer intravenous solution by rapid or bolus injection.

Note: CellCept® and Myfortic® dosage forms should not be used interchangeably due to differences in absorption.

Drug Interactions

Acyclovir and valacyclovir: Levels of both drugs may increase due to competition for tubular secretion; monitor carefully

Antacids (magnesium- and aluminum hydroxide-containing products): Decrease absorption of mycophenolate; do not administer together

Azathioprine: Bone marrow suppression may be caused by both agents; do not administer together

Cholestyramine: Decreases AUC which may lead to decreased efficacy; do not administer together

Ganciclovir and valganciclovir: Levels of both drugs may increase due to competition for tubular secretion; monitor carefully

Oral contraceptives: Progesterone levels are not significantly affected, however, effect on estrogen component varies; although the ovulation-suppression action may not be affected, an additional form of contraception should be used

Probenecid: May increase mycophenolate levels due to inhibition of tubular secretion

Vaccines: Avoid use of live vaccines; vaccinations may be less effective. Influenza vaccine may be of value.

Nutritional/Herbal/Ethanol Interactions

Food: Decreases C_{max} of MPA by 40% following CellCept® administration and 33% following Myfortic® use; the extent of absorption is not changed

Herb/Nutraceutical: Avoid cat's claw, echinacea (have immunostimulant properties)

Adverse Reactions As reported in adults following oral dosing of CellCept® alone in renal, cardiac, and hepatic allograft rejection studies. In general, lower doses

(Continued)

Mycophenolate *(Continued)*

used in renal rejection patients had less adverse effects than higher doses. Rates of adverse effects were similar for each indication, except for those unique to the specific organ involved. The type of adverse effects observed in pediatric patients was similar to those seen in adults; abdominal pain, anemia, diarrhea, fever, hypertension, infection, pharyngitis, respiratory tract infection, sepsis, and vomiting were seen in higher proportion; lymphoproliferative disorder was the only type of malignancy observed. Percentages of adverse reactions were similar in studies comparing CellCept® to Myfortic® in patients following renal transplant.

>20%:

Cardiovascular: Hypertension (28% to 77%), hypotension (up to 33%), peripheral edema (27% to 64%), edema (27% to 28%), tachycardia (20% to 22%)

Central nervous system: Pain (31% to 76%), headache (16% to 54%), insomnia (41% to 52%), fever (21% to 52%), dizziness (up to 29%), anxiety (28%)

Dermatologic: Rash (up to 22%)

Endocrine & metabolic: Hyperglycemia (44% to 47%), hypercholesterolemia (41%), hypokalemia (32% to 37%), hypocalcemia (up to 30%), hypomagnesemia (up to 39%), hyperkalemia (up to 22%)

Gastrointestinal: Abdominal pain (25% to 62%), nausea (20% to 54%), diarrhea (31% to 52%), constipation (18% to 41%), vomiting (33% to 34%), anorexia (up to 25%), dyspepsia (22%)

Genitourinary: Urinary tract infection (37%)

Hematologic: Leukopenia (23% to 46%), leukocytosis (22% to 40%), hypochromic anemia (26% to 43%), thrombocytopenia (24% to 36%)

Hepatic: Liver function tests abnormal (up to 25%), ascites (24%)

Neuromuscular & skeletal: Back pain (35% to 47%), weakness (35% to 43%), tremor (24% to 34%), paresthesia (21%)

Renal: BUN increased (up to 35%), creatinine increased (up to 39%)

Respiratory: Dyspnea (31% to 37%), respiratory tract infection (22% to 37%), cough (31%), lung disorder (22% to 30%)

Miscellaneous: Infection (18% to 27%), *Candida* (11% to 22%), herpes simplex (10% to 21%)

3% to <20%:

Cardiovascular: Angina, arrhythmia, arterial thrombosis, atrial fibrillation, atrial flutter, bradycardia, cardiac arrest, cardiac failure, CHF, extrasystole, facial edema, hypervolemia, pallor, palpitation, pericardial effusion, peripheral vascular disorder, postural hypotension, supraventricular extrasystoles, supraventricular tachycardia, syncope, thrombosis, vasodilation, vasospasm, venous pressure increased, ventricular extrasystole, ventricular tachycardia

Central nervous system: Agitation, chills with fever, confusion, convulsion, delirium, depression, emotional lability, hallucinations, hypoesthesia, malaise, nervousness, psychosis, somnolence, thinking abnormal, vertigo

Dermatologic: Acne, alopecia, bruising, cellulitis, hirsutism, petechia, pruritus, skin carcinoma, skin hypertrophy, skin ulcer, vesiculobullous rash

Endocrine & metabolic: Acidosis, Cushing's syndrome, dehydration, diabetes mellitus, gout, hypercalcemia, hyperlipemia, hyperphosphatemia, hyperuricemia, hypochloremia, hypoglycemia, hyponatremia, hypoproteinemia, hypothyroidism, parathyroid disorder, weight gain/loss

Gastrointestinal: Abdomen enlarged, dry mouth, dysphagia, esophagitis, flatulence, gastritis, gastroenteritis, gastrointestinal hemorrhage, gastrointestinal moniliasis, gingivitis, gum hyperplasia, ileus, melena, mouth ulceration, oral moniliasis, stomach disorder, stomatitis

Genitourinary: Impotence, nocturia, pelvic pain, prostatic disorder, scrotal edema, urinary frequency, urinary incontinence, urinary retention, urinary tract disorder

Hematologic: Coagulation disorder, hemorrhage, neutropenia, pancytopenia, polycythemia, prothrombin time increased, thromboplastin increased

Hepatic: Alkaline phosphatase increased, alkalosis, bilirubinemia, cholangitis, cholestatic jaundice, GGT increased, hepatitis, jaundice, liver damage, transaminases increased

Local: Abscess

Neuromuscular & skeletal: Arthralgia, hypertonia, joint disorder, leg cramps, myalgia, myasthenia, neck pain, neuropathy, osteoporosis

Ocular: Amblyopia, cataract, conjunctivitis, eye hemorrhage, lacrimation disorder, vision abnormal

Otic: Deafness, ear disorder, ear pain, tinnitus

Renal: Albuminuria, creatinine increased, dysuria, hematuria, hydronephrosis, kidney failure, kidney tubular necrosis, oliguria

Respiratory: Apnea, asthma, atelectasis, bronchitis, epistaxis, hemoptysis, hiccup, hyperventilation, hypoxia, respiratory acidosis, lung edema, pharyngitis, pleural effusion, pneumonia, pneumothorax, pulmonary hypertension, respiratory moniliasis, rhinitis, sinusitis, sputum increased, voice alteration

Miscellaneous: *Candida* (mucocutaneous 15% to 18%), CMV viremia/syndrome (12% to 14%), CMV tissue invasive disease (6% to 11%), herpes zoster cutaneous disease (4% to 10%), cyst, diaphoresis, flu-like syndrome, fungal dermatitis, healing abnormal, hernia, ileus infection, lactic dehydrogenase increased, peritonitis, pyelonephritis, thirst

Postmarketing and/or case reports: Atypical mycobacterial infection, colitis, infectious endocarditis, interstitial lung disorder, intestinal villous atrophy, meningitis, pancreatitis, pulmonary fibrosis (fatal), tuberculosis

Overdosage/Toxicology There are no reported overdoses with mycophenolate. At plasma concentrations >100 mcg/mL, small amounts of the inactive metabolite MPAG are removed by hemodialysis. Excretion of the active metabolite, MPA, may be increased by using bile acid sequestrants (cholestyramine).

Dosing

Adults: The initial dose should be given as soon as possible following transplantation; intravenous solution may be given until the oral medication can be tolerated (up to 14 days)

Renal transplant:

CellCept®:

Oral: 1 g twice daily. Although a dose of 1.5 g twice daily was used in clinical trials and shown to be effective, no efficacy advantage was established. Patients receiving 2 g/day demonstrated an overall better safety profile than patients receiving 3 g/day. Doses >2 g/day are not recommended in these patients because of the possibility for enhanced immunosuppression as well as toxicities.

I.V.: 1 g twice daily

Myfortic®: Oral: 720 mg twice daily (1440 mg/day)

Cardiac transplantation:

Oral (CellCept®): 1.5 g twice daily

I.V. (CellCept®): 1.5 g twice daily

Hepatic transplantation:

Oral (CellCept®): 1.5 g twice daily

I.V. (CellCept®): 1 g twice daily

Dosing adjustment for toxicity (neutropenia): ANC <1.3 x $10^3/\mu L$: Dosing should be interrupted or the dose reduced, appropriate diagnostic tests performed and patients managed appropriately

Elderly: Dosage is the same as younger patients, however, dosing should be cautious due to possibility of increased hepatic, renal, or cardiac dysfunction. Elderly patients may be at an increased risk of certain infections, gastrointestinal hemorrhage, and pulmonary edema, as compared to younger patients.

Pediatrics:

Renal transplant: Oral:

CellCept® suspension: 600 mg/m²/dose twice daily; maximum dose: 1 g twice daily

Alternatively, may use solid dosage forms according to BSA as follows:

BSA 1.25-1.5 m^2: 750 mg capsule twice daily

BSA >1.5 m^2: 1 g capsule or tablet twice daily

Myfortic®: 400 mg/m^2/dose twice daily; maximum dose: 720 mg twice daily

BSA <1.19 m^2: Use of this formulation is not recommended

BSA 1.19-1.58 m^2: 540 mg twice daily (maximum: 1080 mg/day)

BSA >1.58 m^2: 720 mg twice daily (maximum: 1440 mg/day)

Renal Impairment:

Renal transplant: GFR <25 mL/minute in patients outside the immediate post-transplant period:

CellCept®: Doses of >1 g administered twice daily should be avoided; patients should also be carefully observed; no dose adjustments are needed in renal transplant patients experiencing delayed graft function postoperatively

Myfortic®: Cl_{cr} <25 mL/minute: Monitor carefully

Cardiac or liver transplant: No data available; mycophenolate may be used in cardiac or hepatic transplant patients with severe chronic renal impairment if the potential benefit outweighs the potential risk.

Hemodialysis: Not removed; supplemental dose is not necessary.

(Continued)

Mycophenolate *(Continued)*

Peritoneal dialysis: Supplemental dose is not necessary.

Hepatic Impairment: No dosage adjustment is recommended for renal patients with severe hepatic parenchymal disease; however, it is not currently known whether dosage adjustments are necessary for hepatic disease with other etiologies.

Available Dosage Forms

Capsule, as mofetil (CellCept®): 250 mg

Injection, powder for reconstitution, as mofetil hydrochloride (CellCept®): 500 mg [contains polysorbate 80]

Powder for oral suspension, as mofetil (CellCept®): 200 mg/mL (225 mL) [provides 175 mL suspension following reconstitution; contains phenylalanine 0.56 mg/mL; mixed fruit flavor]

Tablet, as mofetil [film coated] (CellCept®): 500 mg [may contain ethyl alcohol]

Tablet, delayed release, as mycophenolic acid [film coated] (Myfortic®): 180 mg, 360 mg [formulated as a sodium salt]

Nursing Guidelines

Assessment: Assess other medications patient may be taking for effectiveness and interactions. Assess results of laboratory tests, therapeutic effectiveness, and adverse reactions. Patients with diabetes should monitor glucose levels closely (this medication may alter glucose levels). Monitor/instruct patient on appropriate interventions to reduce side effects, to monitor for signs of opportunistic infection, and adverse reactions to report.

Monitoring Laboratory Tests: Renal and liver function, CBC

Dietary Considerations: Oral dosage formulations should be taken on an empty stomach to avoid variability in MPA absorption. However, in stable renal transplant patients, may be administered with food if necessary. Oral suspension contains 0.56 mg phenylalanine/mL; use caution if administered to patients with phenylketonuria.

Patient Education: Take oral formulations as directed, preferably 1 hour before or 2 hours after meals. Do not take within 1 hour before or 2 hours after antacids or cholestyramine medications. Do not alter dose and do not discontinue without consulting prescriber. Maintain adequate hydration (2-3 L/day of fluids) during entire course of therapy unless instructed to restrict fluid intake. You will be susceptible to infection (avoid crowds and exposure to infection). May be at increased risk for skin cancer, wear protective clothing and use sunscreen with high protective factor to help limit exposure to sunlight and UV light. If you have diabetes, monitor glucose levels closely (drug may alter glucose levels). You may experience dizziness or trembling (use caution until response to medication is known); nausea or vomiting (small frequent meals, frequent mouth care may help); diarrhea (boiled milk, yogurt, or buttermilk may help); sores or white plaques in mouth (frequent rinsing of mouth and frequent mouth care may help); or muscle or back pain (mild analgesics may be recommended). Report chest pain; acute headache or dizziness; symptoms of respiratory infection, cough, or respiratory difficulty; unresolved GI effects; fatigue, chills, fever unhealed sores, white plaques in mouth; irritation in genital area or unusual discharge; unusual bruising or bleeding; or other unusual effects related to this medication. **Pregnancy/breast-feeding precautions:** Inform prescriber if you are or intend to become pregnant. Two reliable forms of contraception should be used prior to, during, and for 6 weeks after therapy. Breast-feeding is not recommended.

Pregnancy Risk Factor: C (manufacturer)

Pregnancy Issues: There are no adequate and well-controlled studies using mycophenolate in pregnant women, however, it may cause fetal harm. Women of childbearing potential should have a negative pregnancy test within 1 week prior to beginning therapy. Two reliable forms of contraception should be used prior to, during, and for 6 weeks after therapy.

Lactation: Excretion in breast milk unknown/not recommended

Breast-Feeding Considerations: It is unknown if mycophenolate is excreted in human milk. Due to potentially serious adverse reactions, the decision to discontinue the drug or discontinue breast-feeding should be considered. Breast-feeding is not recommended during therapy or for 6 weeks after treatment is complete.

Perioperative/Anesthesia/Other Concerns: Avoid inhalation or direct contact with skin or mucous membranes of the powder in CellCept® capsules. If such contact occurs, wash with soap and water; rinse eyes with plain water. Capsules should not be opened or crushed.

Hypertension may accompany the use of mycophenolate in patients post-transplantation. Furthermore, this drug may also induce increases in cholesterol and potassium, and impair glucose tolerance and phosphate and potassium depletion.

Administration

Oral: Oral dosage formulations (tablet, capsule, suspension) should be administered as soon as possible following transplantation. Oral dosage forms should be administered on an empty stomach to avoid variability in MPA absorption. The oral solution may be administered via a nasogastric tube (minimum 8 French, 1.7 mm interior diameter); oral suspension should not be mixed with other medications. Delayed release tablets should not be crushed, cut, or chewed.

I.V.: Intravenous solutions should be given over at least 2 hours. Do not administer intravenous solution by rapid or bolus injection.

Reconstitution:

Oral suspension: Should be constituted by a pharmacist prior to dispensing to the patient and **not** mixed with any other medication. Closed bottle should be tapped to loosen the powder. Add 47 mL of water to the bottle and shake well for ~1 minute. Add another 47 mL of water to the bottle and shake well for an additional minute. Remove child-resistant cap and push bottle adapter into neck of the bottle; close bottle with child-resistant cap tightly to assure proper placement of adapter and status of child-resistant cap. Final concentration is 200 mg/mL of mycophenolate mofetil.

Injection: Does not contain an antibacterial preservative; therefore, reconstitution and dilution of the product must be done under aseptic conditions. Preparation of intravenous formulation should take place in a vertical laminar flow hood with the same precautions as antineoplastic agents. **Note:** Vial is vacuum-sealed; if a lack of vacuum is noted during preparation, the vial should not be used.

I.V. preparation procedure Step 1:

a. Two vials of mycophenolate injection are used for preparing a 1 g dose, whereas 3 vials are needed for each 1.5 g dose. Reconstitute the contents of each vial by injecting 14 mL of 5% dextrose injection.

b. Gently shake the vial to dissolve the drug

c. Inspect the resulting slightly yellow solution for particulate matter and discoloration prior to further dilution. Discard the vial if particulate matter or discoloration is observed.

I.V. preparation procedure Step 2:

a. To prepare a 1 g dose, further dilute the contents of the two reconstituted vials into 140 mL of 5% dextrose in water. To prepare a 1.5 g dose, further dilute the contents of the three reconstituted vials into 210 mL of 5% dextrose in water. The final concentration of both solutions is 6 mg mycophenolate mofetil per mL.

b. Inspect the infusion solution for particulate matter or discoloration. Discard the infusion solution if particulate matter or discoloration is observed.

Storage:

Capsules: Store at room temperature of 15°C to 39°C (59°F to 86°F).

Tablets: Store at room temperature of 15°C to 39°C (59°F to 86°F). Protect from light.

Oral suspension: Store powder for oral suspension at room temperature of 15°C to 39°C (59°F to 86°F). Once reconstituted, the oral solution may be stored at room temperature or under refrigeration. Do not freeze. The mixed suspension is stable for 60 days.

Injection: Store intact vials at room temperature 15°C to 30°C (59°F to 86°F). Stability of the infusion solution: 4 hours from reconstitution and dilution of the product. Store solutions at 15°C to 30°C (59°F to 86°F).

- Mycophenolate Mofetil *see* Mycophenolate *on page 1188*
- Mycophenolate Sodium *see* Mycophenolate *on page 1188*
- Mycophenolic Acid *see* Mycophenolate *on page 1188*
- Mycostatin® *see* Nystatin *on page 1249*
- Mydfrin® *see* Phenylephrine *on page 1350*
- Mydral™ *see* Tropicamide *on page 1672*
- Mydriacyl® *see* Tropicamide *on page 1672*
- My First Flintstones® [OTC] *see* Vitamins (Multiple/Pediatric) *on page 1720*
- Myfortic® *see* Mycophenolate *on page 1188*

- **Mylanta® Children's [OTC]** *see* Calcium Carbonate *on page 291*
- **Mylanta® Gas [OTC]** *see* Simethicone *on page 1533*
- **Mylanta® Gas Maximum Strength [OTC]** *see* Simethicone *on page 1533*
- **Mylanta® Gelcaps® [OTC]** *see* Calcium Carbonate and Magnesium Hydroxide *on page 294*
- **Mylanta® Liquid [OTC]** *see* Aluminum Hydroxide, Magnesium Hydroxide, and Simethicone *on page 122*
- **Mylanta® Maximum Strength Liquid [OTC]** *see* Aluminum Hydroxide, Magnesium Hydroxide, and Simethicone *on page 122*
- **Mylanta® Supreme [OTC]** *see* Calcium Carbonate and Magnesium Hydroxide *on page 294*
- **Mylanta® Ultra [OTC]** *see* Calcium Carbonate and Magnesium Hydroxide *on page 294*
- **Mylicon® Infants [OTC]** *see* Simethicone *on page 1533*
- **Mytussin® AC** *see* Guaifenesin and Codeine *on page 835*
- **NAC** *see* Acetylcysteine *on page 80*
- ***N*-Acetyl-L-cysteine** *see* Acetylcysteine *on page 80*
- ***N*-Acetylcysteine** *see* Acetylcysteine *on page 80*
- **N-Acetyl-P-Aminophenol** *see* Acetaminophen *on page 65*
- **NaCl** *see* Sodium Chloride *on page 1545*

Nafcillin (naf SIL in)

Synonyms Ethoxynaphthamido Penicillin Sodium; Nafcillin Sodium; Nallpen; Sodium Nafcillin

Pharmacologic Category Antibiotic, Penicillin

Use Treatment of infections such as osteomyelitis, septicemia, endocarditis, and CNS infections caused by susceptible strains of staphylococci species

Mechanism of Action Interferes with bacterial cell wall synthesis during active multiplication, causing cell wall death and resultant bactericidal activity against susceptible bacteria

Pharmacodynamics/Kinetics

Distribution: Widely distributed; CSF penetration is poor but enhanced by meningeal inflammation; crosses placenta

Protein binding: 70% to 90%

Metabolism: Primarily hepatic; undergoes enterohepatic recirculation

Half-life elimination:

Neonates: <3 weeks: 2.2-5.5 hours; 4-9 weeks: 1.2-2.3 hours

Children 3 months to 14 years: 0.75-1.9 hours

Adults: 30 minutes to 1.5 hours with normal renal and hepatic function

Time to peak, serum: I.M.: 30-60 minutes

Excretion: Primarily feces; urine (10% to 30% as unchanged drug)

Contraindications Hypersensitivity to nafcillin, or any component of the formulation, or penicillins

Warnings/Precautions Extravasation of I.V. infusions should be avoided; modification of dosage is necessary in patients with both severe renal and hepatic impairment; elimination rate will be slow in neonates; use with caution in patients with cephalosporin hypersensitivity

Drug Interactions **Induces** CYP3A4 (strong)

Chloramphenicol: May decrease efficacy of nafcillin

Cyclosporine: Levels may be decreased by nafcillin

CYP3A4 substrates: Nafcillin may decrease the levels/effects of CYP3A4 substrates. Example substrates include benzodiazepines, calcium channel blockers, clarithromycin, cyclosporine, erythromycin, estrogens, mirtazapine, nateglinide, nefazodone, nevirapine, protease inhibitors, tacrolimus, and venlafaxine

Methotrexate: Penicillins may increase the exposure to methotrexate during concurrent therapy; monitor.

Oral contraceptives: Anecdotal reports suggesting decreased contraceptive efficacy with penicillins have been refuted by more rigorous scientific and clinical data.

Probenecid: May increase levels of penicillins (nafcillin)

Warfarin, oral anticoagulants: Effects of anticoagulants may be decreased

Lab Interactions Positive Coombs' test (direct)

Adverse Reactions Frequency not defined.

Central nervous system: Pain, fever

Dermatologic: Rash

Gastrointestinal: Nausea, diarrhea

Hematologic: Agranulocytosis, bone marrow depression, neutropenia

Local: Pain, swelling, inflammation, phlebitis, skin sloughing, and thrombophlebitis at the injection site; oxacillin (less likely to cause phlebitis) is often preferred in pediatric patients

Renal: Interstitial nephritis (acute)

Miscellaneous: Hypersensitivity reactions

Overdosage/Toxicology Symptoms of penicillin overdose include neuromuscular hypersensitivity (eg, agitation, hallucinations, asterixis, encephalopathy, confusion, and seizures). Electrolyte imbalance may occur if the preparation contains potassium or sodium salts, especially in renal failure. Treatment is supportive or symptom-directed.

Dosing

Adults & Elderly:

Susceptible infections:

I.M.: 500 mg every 4-6 hours

I.V.: 500-2000 mg every 4-6 hours

Pediatrics:

Susceptible infections: Children:

I.M.: 25 mg/kg twice daily

I.V.:

Mild to moderate infections: 50-100 mg/kg/day in divided doses every 6 hours

Severe infections: 100-200 mg/kg/day in divided doses every 4-6 hours

Maximum dose: 12 g/day

Renal Impairment: No adjustment is necessary.

Hemodialysis effects: Not dialyzable (0% to 5%) via hemodialysis. Supplemental dose is not necessary with hemo- or peritoneal dialysis or continuous arteriovenous or venovenous hemofiltration.

Hepatic Impairment: In patients with both hepatic and renal impairment, modification of dosage may be necessary; no data available.

Available Dosage Forms

Infusion [premixed iso-osmotic dextrose solution]: 1 g (50 mL); 2 g (100 mL)

Injection, powder for reconstitution, as sodium: 1 g, 2 g, 10 g

Nursing Guidelines

Assessment: Assess for allergy history prior to starting therapy. See Contraindications and Warnings/Precautions for use cautions. Assess potential for interactions with other prescriptions, OTC medications, or herbal products patient may be taking (see Drug Interactions). Infusion/Injection site must be monitored closely to prevent extravasation (see Administration). Assess for therapeutic effect and adverse reactions (eg, opportunistic infection (eg, fever, chills, unhealed sores, white plaques in mouth or vagina, purulent vaginal discharge, fatigue) - see Adverse Reactions and Overdose/Toxicology). Teach patient possible side effects/appropriate interventions and adverse symptoms to report (see Patient Education). Note breast-feeding caution.

Monitoring Laboratory Tests: Perform culture and sensitivity studies prior to initiating drug therapy. Monitor renal, hepatic, CBC with prolonged therapy.

Dietary Considerations: Sodium content of 1 g: 76.6 mg (3.33 mEq)

Patient Education: Inform prescriber of all prescriptions, OTC medications, or herbal products you are taking, and any allergies you have. Do not take any new medication during therapy unless approved by prescriber. This medication can only be administered by infusion or injection. Report immediately any redness, swelling, burning, or pain at injection/infusion site; respiratory difficulty or swallowing; chest pain; or rash. May cause nausea (small, frequent meals, frequent mouth care, chewing gum, or sucking lozenges may help); or opportunistic infection (eg, fever, chills, sore throat, burning urination, fatigue). Report persistent side effects or if condition does not respond to treatment. **Breast-feeding precaution:** Consult prescriber if breast-feeding.

Geriatric Considerations: Nafcillin has not been studied exclusively in the elderly, however, given its route of elimination, dosage adjustments based upon age and renal function are not necessary. Consider sodium content in patients who may be sensitive to volume expansion (ie, CHF).

(Continued)

Nafcillin *(Continued)*

Pregnancy Risk Factor: B

Lactation: Enters breast milk/use caution

Administration

I.M.: Rotate injection sites.

I.V.: Vesicant. Administer around-the-clock to promote less variation in peak and trough serum levels. Infuse over 30-60 minutes.

Compatibility: Stable in dextran 40 10% in dextrose, D_5LR, $D_5{1/4}NS$, $D_5{1/2}NS$, D_5NS, D_5W, $D_{10}NS$, $D_{10}W$, LR, NS

Y-site administration: Incompatible with droperidol, fentanyl and droperidol, insulin (regular), labetalol, midazolam, nalbuphine, pentazocine, verapamil

Compatibility when admixed: Incompatible with ascorbic acid injection, aztreonam, bleomycin, cytarabine, gentamicin, hydrocortisone sodium succinate, methylprednisolone sodium succinate, promazine

Storage: Reconstituted parenteral solution is stable for 3 days at room temperature, 7 days when refrigerated, or 12 weeks when frozen. For I.V. infusion in NS or D_5W, solution is stable for 24 hours at room temperature and 96 hours when refrigerated.

♦ **Nafcillin Sodium** *see* Nafcillin *on page 1194*
♦ **$NaHCO_3$** *see* Sodium Bicarbonate *on page 1542*

Nalbuphine (NAL byoo feen)

U.S. Brand Names Nubain®

Synonyms Nalbuphine Hydrochloride

Pharmacologic Category Analgesic, Narcotic

Medication Safety Issues

Sound-alike/look-alike issues:

Nubain® may be confused with Navane®, Nebcin®

Use Relief of moderate to severe pain; preoperative analgesia, postoperative and surgical anesthesia, and obstetrical analgesia during labor and delivery

Mechanism of Action Agonist of kappa opiate receptors and partial antagonist of mu opiate receptors in the CNS, causing inhibition of ascending pain pathways, altering the perception of and response to pain; produces generalized CNS depression

Pharmacodynamics/Kinetics

Onset of action: Peak effect: SubQ, I.M.: <15 minutes; I.V.: 2-3 minutes

Metabolism: Hepatic

Half-life elimination: 5 hours

Excretion: Feces; urine (~7% as metabolites)

Contraindications Hypersensitivity to nalbuphine or any component of the formulation

Warnings/Precautions Use caution in CNS depression. Sedation and psychomotor impairment are likely, and are additive with other CNS depressants or ethanol. May cause respiratory depression. Ambulatory patients must be cautioned about performing tasks which require mental alertness (eg, operating machinery or driving). Use with caution in patients with recent myocardial infarction, biliary tract surgery, head trauma, or increased intracranial pressure. Use caution in patients with decreased hepatic or renal function. May result in tolerance and/or drug dependence with chronic use; use with caution in patients with a history of drug dependence. Abrupt discontinuation following prolonged use may lead to withdrawal symptoms. May precipitate withdrawal symptoms in patients following prolonged therapy with mu opiod agonists. Use with caution in pregnancy (close neonatal monitoring required when used in labor and delivery). Safety and efficacy in pediatric patients (<18 years of age) have not been established.

Drug Interactions Increased toxicity: Barbiturate anesthetics may increase CNS depression

Nutritional/Herbal/Ethanol Interactions

Ethanol: Avoid ethanol (may increase CNS depression).

Herb/Nutraceutical: Avoid valerian, St John's wort, kava kava, gotu kola (may increase CNS depression).

Adverse Reactions

>10%: Central nervous system: Sedation (36%)

1% to 10%:

Central nervous system: Dizziness (5%), headache (3%)

Gastrointestinal: Nausea/vomiting (6%), xerostomia (4%)

Miscellaneous: Clamminess (9%)

<1% (Limited to important or life-threatening): Abdominal pain, agitation, allergic reaction, anaphylaxis, anaphylactoid reaction, anxiety, asthma, bitter taste, blurred vision, bradycardia, cardiac arrest, confusion, crying, delusion, depersonalization, depression, diaphoresis, dreams (abnormal), dyspepsia, dysphoria, dyspnea, euphoria, faintness, fever, floating sensation, flushing, gastrointestinal cramps, hallucinations, hostility, hypertension, hypotension, injection site reactions (pain, swelling, redness, burning); laryngeal edema, loss of consciousness, nervousness, numbness, pruritus, pulmonary edema, rash, respiratory depression, respiratory distress, restlessness, seizure, sensation of warmth/burning, somnolence, speech disorder, stridor, tachycardia, tingling, tremor, unreality, urinary urgency, urticaria

Overdosage/Toxicology Symptoms of overdose include CNS depression, respiratory depression, miosis, hypotension, and bradycardia. Treatment is symptomatic. Naloxone, 2 mg I.V. with repeat administration as necessary up to a total dose of 10 mg, can be used to reverse opiate effects.

Dosing

Adults:

Pain management: I.M., I.V., SubQ: 10 mg/70 kg every 3-6 hours; maximum single dose in nonopioid-tolerant patients: 20 mg; maximum daily dose: 160 mg

Surgical anesthesia supplement: I.V.: Induction: 0.3-3 mg/kg over 10-15 minutes; maintenance doses of 0.25-0.5 mg/kg may be given as required

Elderly: Refer to adult dosing; use with caution.

Pediatrics: Pain management (unlabeled use): Children ≥1 year: I.M., I.V., SubQ: 0.1-0.2 mg/kg every 3-4 hours as needed; maximum: 20 mg/dose and/or 160 mg/day

Renal Impairment: Use with caution and reduce dose. Monitor.

Hepatic Impairment: Use with caution and reduce dose.

Available Dosage Forms [DSC] = Discontinued product

Injection, solution, as hydrochloride: 10 mg/mL (10 mL); 20 mg/mL (10 mL)

Nubain®: 10 mg/mL (10 mL) [DSC]; 20 mg/mL (10 mL)

Injection, solution, as hydrochloride [preservative free]: 10 mg/mL (1 mL); 20 mg/mL (1 mL)

Nubain®: 10 mg/mL (1 mL); 20 mg/mL (1 mL)

Nursing Guidelines

Assessment: Assess effectiveness and interactions of other medications patient may be taking. Monitor therapeutic effectiveness (eg, pain relief) and adverse reactions at beginning of therapy and periodically throughout therapy. Monitor blood pressure, CNS and respiratory status, and degree of sedation at beginning of therapy and at regular intervals during use. For inpatients, implement safety measures. Generally used in conjunction with surgical anesthesia or during labor and delivery; however, if self-administered for relief of pain, assess knowledge/teach patient appropriate use, adverse reactions to report, and appropriate interventions to reduce side effects.

Patient Education: If self-administered, use exactly as directed; do not increase dose or frequency. Drug may cause physical and/or psychological dependence. While using this medication, do not use alcohol and other prescription or OTC medications (especially sedatives, tranquilizers, antihistamines, or pain medications) without consulting prescriber. Maintain adequate hydration (2-3 L/day of fluids) unless instructed to restrict fluid intake. May cause hypotension, dizziness, drowsiness, impaired coordination, or blurred vision (use caution when driving, climbing stairs, or changing position - rising from sitting or lying to standing, or when engaging in tasks requiring alertness until response to drug is known); loss of appetite, nausea, or vomiting (frequent mouth care, small frequent meals, chewing gum, or sucking lozenges may help); or constipation (increased exercise, fluids, fruit, or fiber may help; if unresolved, consult prescriber about use of stool softeners). Report chest pain, slow or rapid heartbeat, acute dizziness or persistent headache; changes in mental status; swelling of extremities or unusual weight gain; changes in urinary elimination or pain on urination; acute headache; back or flank pain or muscle spasms; blurred vision; skin rash; or shortness of breath. **Pregnancy/breast-feeding precautions:** Inform prescriber if you are or intend to become pregnant. If you are breast-feeding, take medication immediately after breast-feeding or 3-4 hours prior to next feeding.

Geriatric Considerations: The elderly may be particularly susceptible to CNS effects; monitor closely.

(Continued)

Nalbuphine *(Continued)*

Pregnancy Risk Factor: B/D (prolonged use or high doses at term)

Pregnancy Issues: Severe fetal bradycardia has been reported following use in labor/delivery. Fetal bradycardia may occur when administered earlier in pregnancy (not documented). Use only if clearly needed, with monitoring to detect and manage possible adverse fetal effects. Naloxone has been reported to reverse bradycardia. Newborn should be monitored for respiratory depression or bradycardia following nalbuphine use in labor.

Lactation: Enters breast milk/use caution

Perioperative/Anesthesia/Other Concerns: Abrupt discontinuation after sustained use (generally >10 days) may cause withdrawal symptoms.

Mixed agonist-antagonist: Incidence of psychomimetic effect is lower than with pentazocine; may precipitate withdrawal in narcotic-dependent patients.

Administration

Compatibility: Stable in D_5NS, $D_{10}W$, LR, NS

Y-site administration: Incompatible with allopurinol, amphotericin B cholesteryl sulfate complex, cefepime, docetaxel, ketorolac, methotrexate, nafcillin, piperacillin/tazobactam, sargramostim, sodium bicarbonate

Compatibility in syringe: Incompatible with diazepam, ketorolac, pentobarbital

Storage: Store at room temperature of 15°C to 30°C (59°F to 86°F). Protect from light.

Related Information

Narcotic / Opioid Analgesics *on page 1880*

- **Nalbuphine Hydrochloride** *see* Nalbuphine *on page 1196*
- **Naldecon Senior EX® [OTC] [DSC]** *see* Guaifenesin *on page 834*
- **Nallpen** *see* Nafcillin *on page 1194*
- ***N*-allylnoroxymorphine Hydrochloride** *see* Naloxone *on page 1200*

Nalmefene (NAL me feen)

U.S. Brand Names Revex®

Synonyms Nalmefene Hydrochloride

Pharmacologic Category Antidote

Medication Safety Issues

Sound-alike/look-alike issues:

Revex® may be confused with Nimbex®, ReVia®

Use Complete or partial reversal of opioid drug effects, including respiratory depression induced by natural or synthetic opioids; reversal of postoperative opioid depression; management of known or suspected opioid overdose

Mechanism of Action As a 6-methylene analog of naltrexone, nalmefene acts as a competitive antagonist at opioid receptor sites, preventing or reversing the respiratory depression, sedation, and hypotension induced by opiates; no pharmacologic activity of its own (eg, opioid agonist activity) has been demonstrated

Pharmacodynamics/Kinetics

Onset of action: I.M., SubQ: 5-15 minutes

Distribution: V_d: 8.6 L/kg; rapid

Protein binding: 45%

Metabolism: Hepatic via glucuronide conjugation to metabolites with little or no activity

Bioavailability: I.M., I.V., SubQ: 100%

Half-life elimination: 10.8 hours

Time to peak, serum: I.M.: 2.3 hours; I.V.: <2 minutes; SubQ: 1.5 hours

Excretion: Feces (17%); urine (<5% as unchanged drug)

Clearance: 0.8 L/hour/kg

Contraindications Hypersensitivity to nalmefene, naltrexone, or any component of the formulation

Warnings/Precautions May induce symptoms of acute withdrawal in opioid-dependent patients; recurrence of respiratory depression is possible if the opioid involved is long-acting; observe patients until there is no reasonable risk of recurrent respiratory depression. Safety and efficacy have not been established in children. Avoid abrupt reversal of opioid effects in patients of high cardiovascular risk or who have received potentially cardiotoxic drugs. Pulmonary edema and cardiovascular instability have been reported in association with abrupt reversal with other narcotic antagonists. Animal studies indicate nalmefene may not completely reverse buprenorphine-induced respiratory depression.

Drug Interactions

Flumazenil: May increase the risk of toxicity with flumazenil. An increased risk of seizures has been associated with flumazenil and nalmefene coadministration

Narcotic analgesics: Decreased effect of narcotic analgesics; may precipitate acute withdrawal reaction in physically dependent patients

Adverse Reactions

>10%: Gastrointestinal: Nausea

1% to 10%:

Cardiovascular: Tachycardia, hyper-/hypotension, vasodilation

Central nervous system: Fever, dizziness, headache, chills

Gastrointestinal: Vomiting

Miscellaneous: Postoperative pain

<1% (Limited to important or life-threatening): Agitation, arrhythmia, bradycardia, confusion, depression, diarrhea, myoclonus, nervousness, pharyngitis, pruritus, somnolence, tremor, urinary retention, xerostomia

Overdosage/Toxicology No reported symptoms with significant overdose. Large doses of opioids administered to overcome a full blockade of opioid antagonists, however, have resulted in adverse respiratory and circulatory reactions.

Dosing

Adults & Elderly:

Reversal of postoperative opioid depression: I.V.: Blue labeled product (100 mcg/mL): Titrate to reverse the undesired effects of opioids; initial dose for nonopioid dependent patient: 0.25 mcg/kg followed by 0.25 mcg/kg incremental doses at 2- to 5-minute intervals. After a total dose >1 mcg/kg, further therapeutic response is unlikely.

Management of known/suspected opioid overdose: I.V.: Green labeled product (1000 mcg/mL): Initial: 0.5 mg/70 kg; may repeat with 1 mg/70 kg in 2-5 minutes. Further increase beyond a total dose of 1.5 mg/70 kg will not likely result in improved response and may result in cardiovascular stress and precipitated withdrawal syndrome. (If opioid dependency is suspected, administer a challenge dose of 0.1 mg/70 kg; if no withdrawal symptoms are observed in 2 minutes, the recommended doses can be administered).

Recurrence of respiratory depression: If noted, dose may again be titrated to clinical effect using incremental doses.

Loss of I.V. access: If I.V. access is lost or not readily obtainable, a single SubQ or I.M. dose of 1 mg may be effective in 5-15 minutes.

Renal Impairment: Not necessary with single uses, however, slow administration (over 60 seconds) of incremental doses is recommended to minimize hypertension and dizziness.

Hepatic Impairment: Not necessary with single uses, however, slow administration (over 60 seconds) of incremental doses is recommended to minimize hypertension and dizziness.

Available Dosage Forms Injection, solution: 100 mcg/mL (1 mL) [blue label]; 1000 mcg/mL (2 mL) [green label]

Nursing Guidelines

Assessment: Assess patient for opioid dependency. Monitor vital signs, respiratory, and cardiac status carefully during infusion and for some time thereafter (effects may continue for several days, use nonopioid analgesics for pain).

Patient Education: This drug can only be administered I.V. You may experience drowsiness, dizziness, or blurred vision for several days; use caution when driving or engaging in tasks requiring alertness until response to drug is known. Small frequent meals and good mouth care may reduce any nausea or vomiting. Report yellowing of eyes or skin, unusual bleeding, dark or tarry stools, acute headache, or palpitations. **Breast-feeding precaution:** Consult prescriber if breast-feeding.

Pregnancy Risk Factor: B

Pregnancy Issues: Limited information available

Lactation: Enters breast milk/use caution

Breast-Feeding Considerations: Limited information available; do not use in lactating women if possible.

Perioperative/Anesthesia/Other Concerns: Proper steps should be used to prevent use of the incorrect dosage strength. The goal of treatment in the postoperative setting is to achieve reversal of excessive opioid effects without inducing a complete reversal and acute pain. If opioid dependence is suspected, nalmefene should only be used in opioid overdose if the likelihood of overdose is high, based on history or the clinical presentation of respiratory depression with concurrent pupillary constriction present.

(Continued)

Nalmefene *(Continued)*

Administration

I.M.: If I.V. access is lost or not readily obtainable, a single SubQ or I.M. dose of 1 mg may be effective in 5-15 minutes.

I.V.: Slow administration (over 60 seconds) of incremental doses is recommended to minimize hypertension and dizziness.

Compatibility: Stable in D_5LR, $D_5{}^1/_2NS$, D_5W, LR, sodium bicarbonate 5%, $^1/_2NS$, NS

♦ Nalmefene Hydrochloride *see* Nalmefene *on page 1198*

Naloxone (nal OKS one)

U.S. Brand Names Narcan® [DSC]

Synonyms *N*-allylnoroxymorphine Hydrochloride; Naloxone Hydrochloride

Pharmacologic Category Antidote

Medication Safety Issues

Sound-alike/look-alike issues:

Naloxone may be confused with naltrexone

Narcan® may be confused with Marcaine®, Norcuron®

Use

Complete or partial reversal of opioid depression, including respiratory depression, induced by natural and synthetic opioids, including propoxyphene, methadone, and certain mixed agonist-antagonist analgesics: nalbuphine, pentazocine, and butorphanol

Diagnosis of suspected opioid tolerance or acute opioid overdose

Adjunctive agent to increase blood pressure in the management of septic shock

Unlabeled/Investigational Use PCP and ethanol ingestion

Mechanism of Action Pure opioid antagonist that competes and displaces narcotics at opioid receptor sites

Pharmacodynamics/Kinetics

Onset of action: Endotracheal, I.M., SubQ: 2-5 minutes; I.V.: ~2 minutes

Duration: 20-60 minutes; since shorter than that of most opioids, repeated doses are usually needed

Distribution: Crosses placenta

Metabolism: Primarily hepatic via glucuronidation

Half-life elimination: Neonates: 1.2-3 hours; Adults: 1-1.5 hours

Excretion: Urine (as metabolites)

Contraindications Hypersensitivity to naloxone or any component of the formulation

Warnings/Precautions Due to an association between naloxone and acute pulmonary edema, use with caution in patients with cardiovascular disease or in patients receiving medications with potential adverse cardiovascular effects (eg, hypotension, pulmonary edema or arrhythmias). Excessive dosages should be avoided after use of opiates in surgery. Abrupt postoperative reversal may result in nausea, vomiting, sweating, tachycardia, hypertension, seizures, and other cardiovascular events (including pulmonary edema and arrhythmias). May precipitate withdrawal symptoms in patients addicted to opiates, including pain, hypertension, sweating, agitation, irritability; in neonates: shrill cry, failure to feed. Recurrence of respiratory depression is possible if the opioid involved is long-acting; observe patients until there is no reasonable risk of recurrent respiratory depression.

Drug Interactions Narcotic analgesics: Decreased effect of narcotic analgesics; may precipitate acute withdrawal reaction in physically dependent patients

Adverse Reactions Frequency not defined.

Cardiovascular: Hyper-/hypotension, tachycardia, ventricular arrhythmia, cardiac arrest

Central nervous system: Irritability, anxiety, narcotic withdrawal, restlessness, seizure

Gastrointestinal: Nausea, vomiting, diarrhea

Neuromuscular & skeletal: Tremulousness

Respiratory: Dyspnea, pulmonary edema, runny nose, sneezing

Miscellaneous: Diaphoresis

Overdosage/Toxicology Naloxone is the drug of choice for respiratory depression that is known or suspected to be caused by overdose of an opiate or opioid. **Caution:** Naloxone's effects are due to its action on narcotic reversal, not due to any direct effect upon opiate receptors. Therefore, adverse events occur secondarily to reversal (withdrawal) of narcotic analgesia and sedation, which can cause severe reactions.

Dosing

Adults & Elderly:

Narcotic overdose:

I.V. (preferred), I.M., intratracheal, SubQ: 0.4-2 mg every 2-3 minutes as needed; may need to repeat doses every 20-60 minutes. If no response is observed after 10 mg, question the diagnosis. **Note:** Use 0.1-0.2 mg increments in patients who are opioid dependent and in postoperative patients to avoid large cardiovascular changes.

Continuous infusion: I.V.: If continuous infusion is required, calculate dosage/hour based on effective intermittent dose used and duration of adequate response seen; adult dose typically 0.25-6.25 mg/hour (short-term infusions as high as 2.4 mg/kg/hour have been tolerated in adults during treatment for septic shock); alternatively, continuous infusion utilizes $^2/_3$ of the initial naloxone bolus on an hourly basis; add 10 times this dose to each liter of D_5W and infuse at a rate of 100 mL/hour; $^1/_2$ of the initial bolus dose should be readministered 15 minutes after initiation of the continuous infusion to prevent a drop in naloxone levels; increase infusion rate as needed to assure adequate ventilation

Pediatrics:

Postanesthesia narcotic reversal: I.M., I.V. (preferred), intratracheal, SubQ: Infants and Children: 0.01 mg/kg; may repeat every 2-3 minutes as needed based on response

Narcotic overdose:

I.M., I.V. (preferred), intratracheal, SubQ:

Birth (including premature infants) to 5 years or <20 kg: 0.1 mg/kg; repeat every 2-3 minutes if needed; may need to repeat doses every 20-60 minutes

>5 years or ≥20 kg: 2 mg/dose; if no response, repeat every 2-3 minutes; may need to repeat doses every 20-60 minutes

Continuous infusion: I.V.: Refer to adult dosing.

Available Dosage Forms

Injection, solution, as hydrochloride: 0.4 mg/mL (1 mL, 10 mL)

Narcan®: 0.4 mg/mL (1 mL) [DSC]

Nursing Guidelines

Assessment: Assess patient for opioid dependency. Monitor vital signs and cardiorespiratory status continuously during infusion, maintain patent airway.

Patient Education: This drug can only be administered I.V.; if patient is responsive, instructions are individualized. Report respiratory difficulty, palpitations, or tremors. **Breast-feeding precaution:** Breast-feeding is not recommended.

Geriatric Considerations: In small trials, naloxone has shown temporary improvement in Alzheimer's disease; however, is not recommended for treatment.

Pregnancy Risk Factor: C

Pregnancy Issues: Consider benefit to the mother and the risk to the fetus before administering to a pregnant woman who is known or suspected to be opioid dependent. May precipitate withdrawal in both the mother and fetus.

Lactation: Excretion in breast milk unknown/not recommended

Breast-Feeding Considerations: No data reported. Since naloxone is used for opiate reversal the concern should be on opiate drug levels in a breast-feeding mother and transfer to the infant rather than naloxone exposure. The safest approach would be **not** to breast-feed.

Perioperative/Anesthesia/Other Concerns: Naloxone may contain methyl and propylparabens. Proper steps should be used to prevent use of the incorrect dosage strength. the goal of treatment in the postoperative setting is to achieve reversal of excessive opioid effects without inducing a complete reversal and acute pain.

Administration

I.V.:

I.V. push: Administer over 30 seconds as undiluted preparation

I.V. continuous infusion: Dilute to 4 mcg/mL in D_5W or normal saline

Reconstitution: Stable in 0.9% sodium chloride and D_5W at 4 mcg/mL for 24 hours.

(Continued)

Naloxone *(Continued)*

Compatibility: Stable in D_5W, NS

Y-site administration: Incompatible with amphotericin B cholesteryl sulfate complex

Storage: Store at 25°C (77°F). Protect from light.

Related Information

Conscious Sedation *on page 1779*

♦ **Naloxone Hydrochloride** *see* Naloxone *on page 1200*

Naltrexone (nal TREKS one)

U.S. Brand Names Depade®; ReVia®

Synonyms Naltrexone Hydrochloride

Pharmacologic Category Antidote

Medication Safety Issues

Sound-alike/look-alike issues:

Naltrexone may be confused with naloxone

ReVia® may be confused with Revex®

Use Treatment of ethanol dependence; blockade of the effects of exogenously administered opioids

Mechanism of Action Naltrexone (a pure opioid antagonist) is a cyclopropyl derivative of oxymorphone similar in structure to naloxone and nalorphine (a morphine derivative); it acts as a competitive antagonist at opioid receptor sites

Pharmacodynamics/Kinetics

Duration: 50 mg: 24 hours; 100 mg: 48 hours; 150 mg: 72 hours

Absorption: Almost complete

Distribution: V_d: 19 L/kg; widely throughout the body but considerable interindividual variation exists

Protein binding: 21%

Metabolism: Extensive first-pass effect to 6-β-naltrexol

Half-life elimination: 4 hours; 6-β-naltrexol: 13 hours

Time to peak, serum: ~60 minutes

Excretion: Primarily urine (as metabolites and unchanged drug)

Contraindications Hypersensitivity to naltrexone or any component of the formulation; narcotic dependence or current use of opioid analgesics; acute opioid withdrawal; failure to pass Narcan® challenge or positive urine screen for opioids; acute hepatitis; liver failure

Warnings/Precautions Dose-related hepatocellular injury is possible; the margin of separation between the apparent safe and hepatotoxic doses appear to be only fivefold or less. May precipitate withdrawal symptoms in patients addicted to opiates, including pain, hypertension, sweating, agitation, irritability; in neonates: shrill cry, failure to feed. Use with caution in patients with hepatic or renal impairment.

Patients who had been treated with naltrexone may respond to lower opioid doses than previously used. This could result in potentially life-threatening opioid intoxication. Patients should be aware that they may be more sensitive to lower doses of opioids after naltrexone treatment is discontinued. Use of naltrexone does not eliminate or diminish withdrawal symptoms.

Drug Interactions

Narcotic analgesics: Decreased effect of narcotic analgesics; may precipitate acute withdrawal reaction in physically dependent patients; concurrent use is contraindicated

Thioridazine: Lethargy and somnolence have been reported with the combination of naltrexone and thioridazine

Adverse Reactions

>10%:

Central nervous system: Insomnia, nervousness, headache, low energy

Gastrointestinal: Abdominal cramping, nausea, vomiting

Neuromuscular & skeletal: Arthralgia

1% to 10%:

Central nervous system: Increased energy, feeling down, irritability, dizziness, anxiety, somnolence

Dermatologic: Rash

Endocrine & metabolic: Polydipsia

Gastrointestinal: Diarrhea, constipation

Genitourinary: Delayed ejaculation, impotency

<1% (Limited to important or life-threatening): Depression, disorientation, hallucinations, narcotic withdrawal, paranoia, restlessness, suicide attempts

Overdosage/Toxicology Symptoms of overdose include clonic-tonic convulsions and respiratory failure. Patients receiving up to 800 mg/day for 1 week have shown no toxicity. Seizures and respiratory failure have been seen in animals.

Dosing

Adults & Elderly: Opioid dependence or alcoholism (Do not give until patient is opioid-free for 7-10 days as required by urine analysis): Oral: 25 mg; if no withdrawal signs within 1 hour give another 25 mg; maintenance regimen is flexible, variable and individualized (50 mg/day to 100-150 mg 3 times/week).

Renal Impairment: Use caution.

Hepatic Impairment: Use caution. An increase in naltrexone AUC of approximately five- and 10-fold in patients with compensated or decompensated liver cirrhosis respectively, compared with normal liver function has been reported.

Available Dosage Forms

Tablet, as hydrochloride: 50 mg
- Depade®: 25 mg, 50 mg, 100 mg
- ReVia®: 50 mg

Nursing Guidelines

Assessment: Do not use until patient has been opioid-free for 7-10 days. Assess carefully for several days following start of therapy for narcotic withdrawal symptoms or severe adverse reactions. Use non-narcotic analgesics for pain.

Monitoring Laboratory Tests: Periodic LFTs

Patient Education: This medication will help you achieve abstinence from opiates if taken as directed. Do not increase or change dose. Do not use opiates or any medications not approved by your prescriber during naltrexone therapy. You may experience drowsiness, dizziness, or blurred vision (use caution when driving or engaging in tasks requiring alertness until response to drug is known); abdominal cramping, nausea or vomiting (small frequent meals, frequent mouth care, chewing gum, or sucking lozenges may help); low energy; or decreased sexual function (reversible when drug is discontinued). Report yellowing of skin or eyes, change in color of stool or urine, increased perspiration or chills, acute headache, palpitations, or unusual joint pain. **Pregnancy/breast-feeding precautions:** Inform prescriber if you are or intend to become pregnant. Consult prescriber if breast-feeding.

Pregnancy Risk Factor: C

Lactation: Excretion in breast milk unknown

Perioperative/Anesthesia/Other Concerns: May also be used in detoxification with special guidelines

- ♦ **Naltrexone Hydrochloride** *see* Naltrexone *on page 1202*
- ♦ **Namenda™** *see* Memantine *on page 1094*
- ♦ **Naprelan®** *see* Naproxen *on page 1203*
- ♦ **Naprosyn®** *see* Naproxen *on page 1203*

Naproxen (na PROKS en)

U.S. Brand Names Aleve® [OTC]; Anaprox®; Anaprox® DS; EC-Naprosyn®; Midol® Extended Relief; Naprelan®; Naprosyn®; Pamprin® Maximum Strength All Day Relief [OTC]

Synonyms Naproxen Sodium

Pharmacologic Category Nonsteroidal Anti-inflammatory Drug (NSAID), Oral

Medication Safety Issues

Sound-alike/look-alike issues:
- Naproxen may be confused with Natacyn®, Nebcin®
- Aleve® may be confused with Alesse®
- Anaprox® may be confused with Anaspaz®, Avapro®
- Naprelan® may be confused with Naprosyn®
- Naprosyn® may be confused with Naprelan®, Natacyn®, Nebcin®

Use Management of ankylosing spondylitis, osteoarthritis, and rheumatoid disorders (including juvenile rheumatoid arthritis); acute gout; mild to moderate pain; tendonitis, bursitis; dysmenorrhea; fever, migraine headache

Mechanism of Action Inhibits prostaglandin synthesis by decreasing the activity of the enzyme, cyclooxygenase, which results in decreased formation of prostaglandin precursors

Pharmacodynamics/Kinetics

Onset of action: Analgesic: 1 hour; Anti-inflammatory: ~2 weeks

(Continued)

Naproxen *(Continued)*

Peak effect: Anti-inflammatory: 2-4 weeks

Duration: Analgesic: ≤7 hours; Anti-inflammatory: ≤12 hours

Absorption: Almost 100%

Protein binding: >99%; increased free fraction in elderly

Half-life elimination: Normal renal function: 12-17 hours; End-stage renal disease: No change

Time to peak, serum: 1-4 hours

Excretion: Urine (95%)

Contraindications Hypersensitivity to naproxen, aspirin, other NSAIDs, or any component of the formulation; perioperative pain in the setting of coronary artery bypass surgery (CABG); pregnancy (3rd trimester)

Warnings/Precautions NSAIDs are associated with an increased risk of adverse cardiovascular events, including MI, stroke, and new onset or worsening of pre-existing hypertension. Risk may be increased with duration of use or pre-existing cardiovascular risk-factors or disease. Carefully evaluate individual cardiovascular risk profiles prior to prescribing. Use caution with fluid retention, CHF or hypertension.

Use of NSAIDs can compromise existing renal function. Renal toxicity can occur in patient with impaired renal function, dehydration, heart failure, liver dysfunction, those taking diuretics and ACEI and the elderly. Rehydrate patient before starting therapy. Monitor renal function closely. Naproxen is not recommended for patients with advanced renal disease.

NSAIDs may increase risk of gastrointestinal irritation, ulceration, bleeding, and perforation. These events may occur at any time during therapy and without warning. Use caution with a history of GI disease (bleeding or ulcers), concurrent therapy with aspirin, anticoagulants and/or corticosteroids, smoking, use of alcohol, the elderly or debilitated patients.

Use the lowest effective dose for the shortest duration of time, consistent with individual patient goals, to reduce risk of cardiovascular or GI adverse events. Alternate therapies should be considered for patients at high risk.

NSAIDs may cause serious skin adverse events including exfoliative dermatitis, Stevens-Johnson Syndrome (SJS) and toxic epidermal necrolysis (TEN). Anaphylactoid reactions may occur, even without prior exposure; patients with "aspirin triad" (bronchial asthma, aspirin intolerance, rhinitis) may be at increased risk. Do not use in patients who experience bronchospasm, asthma, rhinitis, or urticaria with NSAID or aspirin therapy.

Use with caution in patients with decreased hepatic function. Closely monitor patients with any abnormal LFT. Severe hepatic reactions (eg, fulminant hepatitis, liver failure) have occurred with NSAID use, rarely; discontinue if signs or symptoms of liver disease develop, or if systemic manifestations occur.

The elderly are at increased risk for adverse effects (especially peptic ulceration, CNS effects, renal toxicity) from NSAIDs even at low doses.

Withhold for at least 4-6 half-lives prior to surgical or dental procedures. Safety and efficacy have not been established in children <2 years of age.

OTC labeling: Prior to self-medication, patients should contact health care provider if they have had recurring stomach pain or upset, ulcers, bleeding problems, high blood pressure, heart or kidney disease, other serious medical problems, are currently taking a diuretic, or are ≥60 years of age. Recommended dosages should not be exceeded, due to an increased risk of GI bleeding. Consuming ≥3 alcoholic beverages/day or taking longer than recommended may increase the risk of GI bleeding. When used for self-medication, patients should be instructed to contact healthcare provider if used for fever lasting >3 days or for pain lasting >10 days in adults or >3 days in children. Not for self-medication (OTC use) in children <12 years of age.

Drug Interactions Substrate (minor) of CYP1A2, 2C8/9

ACE inhibitors: Antihypertensive effects may be decreased by concurrent therapy with NSAIDs; monitor blood pressure.

Angiotensin II antagonists: Antihypertensive effects may be decreased by concurrent therapy with NSAIDs; monitor blood pressure.

Anticoagulants (warfarin, heparin, LMWHs) in combination with NSAIDs can cause increased risk of bleeding.

Antiplatelet drugs (ticlopidine, clopidogrel, aspirin, abciximab, dipyridamole, eptifibatide, tirofiban) can cause an increased risk of bleeding.

Corticosteroids may increase the risk of GI ulceration; avoid concurrent use.

Cyclosporine: NSAIDs may increase serum creatinine, potassium, blood pressure, and cyclosporine levels; monitor cyclosporine levels and renal function carefully.

Hydralazine's antihypertensive effect is decreased; avoid concurrent use.

Lithium levels can be increased; avoid concurrent use if possible or monitor lithium levels and adjust dose. Sulindac may have the least effect. When NSAID is stopped, lithium will need adjustment again.

Loop diuretics efficacy (diuretic and antihypertensive effect) is reduced. Indomethacin reduces this efficacy, however, it may be anticipated with any NSAID.

Methotrexate: Severe bone marrow suppression, aplastic anemia, and GI toxicity have been reported with concomitant NSAID therapy. Avoid use during moderate or high-dose methotrexate (increased and prolonged methotrexate levels). NSAID use during low-dose treatment of rheumatoid arthritis has not been fully evaluated; extreme caution is warranted.

Thiazides antihypertensive effects are decreased; avoid concurrent use.

Warfarin's INRs may be increased by naproxen. Other NSAIDs may have the same effect depending on dose and duration. Monitor INR closely. Use the lowest dose of NSAIDs possible and for the briefest duration.

Nutritional/Herbal/Ethanol Interactions

Ethanol: Avoid ethanol (may enhance gastric mucosal irritation).

Food: Naproxen absorption ratelevels may be decreased if taken with food.

Herb/Nutraceutical: Avoid alfalfa, anise, bilberry, bladderwrack, bromelain, cat's claw, celery, coleus, cordyceps, dong quai, evening primrose, feverfew, fenugreek, garlic, ginger, ginkgo biloboa, red clover, horse chestnut, grapeseed, green tea, ginseng, guggul, horse chestnut seed, horseradish, licorice, prickly ash, red clover, reishi, SAMe, sweet clover, turmeric, white willow (all have additional antiplatelet activity).

Lab Interactions Increased chloride (S), sodium (S), bleeding time

Adverse Reactions

1% to 10%:

Cardiovascular: Edema (3% to 9%), palpitations (<3%)

Central nervous system: Dizziness (3% to 9%), drowsiness (3% to 9%), headache (3% to 9%), lightheadedness (<3%), vertigo (<3%)

Dermatologic: Pruritus (3% to 9%), skin eruption (3% to 9%), rash, ecchymosis (3% to 9%), purpura (<3%)

Endocrine & metabolic: Fluid retention (3% to 9%)

Gastrointestinal: Abdominal pain (3% to 9%), constipation (3% to 9%), nausea (3% to 9%), heartburn (3% to 9%), diarrhea (<3%), dyspepsia (<3%), stomatitis (<3%), heartburn (<3%), flatulence, gross bleeding/perforation, indigestion, ulcers, vomiting

Genitourinary: Abnormal renal function

Hematologic: Hemolysis (3% to 9%), ecchymosis (3% to 9%), anemia, bleeding time increased

Hepatic: LFTS increased

Ocular: Visual disturbances (<3%)

Otic: Tinnitus (3% to 9%), hearing disturbances (<3%)

Respiratory: Dyspnea (3% to 9%)

Miscellaneous: Diaphoresis (<3%), thirst (<3%)

<1% (Limited to important or life-threatening): Agranulocytosis, alopecia, anaphylactic/anaphylactoid reaction, angioneurotic edema, arrhythmia, aseptic meningitis, asthma, blurred vision, cognitive dysfunction, colitis, coma, confusion, CHF, conjunctivitis, cystitis, depression, dream abnormalities, dysuria, eosinophilia, eosinophilic pneumonitis, erythema multiforme, exfoliative dermatitis, glossitis, granulocytopenia, hallucinations, hematemesis, hepatitis, hyper-/hypoglycemia, hyper-/hypotension, infection, interstitial nephritis, melena, jaundice, leukopenia, liver failure, lymphadenopathy, menstrual disorders, malaise, MI, myalgia, muscle weakness, oliguria, pancreatitis, paresthesia,pancytopenia, photosensitivity, pneumonia, polyuria, proteinuria, pyrexia, rectal bleeding, renal failure, renal papillary necrosis, respiratory depression, sepsis, Stevens-Johnson syndrome, tachycardia, seizure, syncope, thrombocytopenia, toxic epidermal necrolysis ulcerative stomatitis, vasculitis

Overdosage/Toxicology Symptoms of overdose include drowsiness, heartburn, vomiting, CNS depression, leukocytosis, and renal failure. Management is supportive and symptomatic. Seizures tend to be very short-lived and often do not require drug treatment.

(Continued)

Naproxen *(Continued)*

Dosing

Adults: Note: Dosage expressed as naproxen base; 200 mg naproxen base is equivalent to 220 mg naproxen sodium.

Acute gout: Oral: Initial: 750 mg, followed by 250 mg every 8 hours until attack subsides; **Note:** EC-Naprosyn® is not recommended

Rheumatoid arthritis, osteoarthritis, and ankylosing spondylitis: 500-1000 mg/day in 2 divided doses; may increase to 1.5 g/day of naproxen base for limited time period

Mild-to-moderate pain, dysmenorrhea, acute tendonitis, bursitis: Oral: Initial: 500 mg, then 250 mg every 6-8 hours; maximum: 1250 mg/day naproxen base

OTC labeling: Pain/fever:

Adults ≤65 years: 200 mg naproxen base every 8-12 hours; if needed, may take 400 mg naproxen base for the initial dose; maximum: 600 mg naproxen base/24 hours

Adults >65 years: Refer to elderly dosing.

Elderly: Refer to adult dosing and Geriatric Considerations.

OTC labeling: Pain/fever: Adults >65 years: 200 mg naproxen base every 12 hours

Pediatrics: Note: Dosage expressed as naproxen base; 200 mg naproxen base is equivalent to 220 mg naproxen sodium.

Fever: Oral: Children >2 years: 2.5-10 mg/kg/dose; maximum: 10 mg/kg/day

Juvenile arthritis: Oral: Children >2 years: 10 mg/kg/day in 2 divided doses

OTC labeling: Pain/fever: Oral: Children ≥12 years: Refer to adult dosing.

Renal Impairment: Cl_{cr} <30 mL/minute: use is not recommended.

Available Dosage Forms

Caplet, as sodium (Aleve®, Midol® Extended Relief, Pamprin® Maximum Strength All Day Relief): 220 mg [equivalent to naproxen 200 mg and sodium 20 mg]

Gelcap, as sodium (Aleve®): 220 mg [equivalent to naproxen 200 mg and sodium 20 mg]

Suspension, oral (Naprosyn®): 125 mg/5 mL (480 mL) [contains sodium 0.3 mEq/mL; orange-pineapple flavor]

Tablet (Naprosyn®): 250 mg, 375 mg, 500 mg

Tablet, as sodium: 220 mg [equivalent to naproxen 200 mg and sodium 20 mg]; 275 mg [equivalent to naproxen 250 mg and sodium 25 mg]; 550 mg [equivalent to naproxen 500 mg and sodium 50 mg]

Aleve®: 220 mg [equivalent to naproxen 200 mg and sodium 20 mg]

Anaprox®: 275 mg [equivalent to naproxen 250 mg and sodium 25 mg]

Anaprox® DS: 550 mg [equivalent to naproxen 500 mg and sodium 50 mg]

Tablet, controlled release, as sodium: 550 mg [equivalent to naproxen 500 mg and sodium 50 mg]

Naprelan®: 421.5 mg [equivalent to naproxen 375 mg and sodium 37.5 mg]; 550 mg [equivalent to naproxen 500 mg and sodium 50 mg]

Tablet, delayed release (EC-Naprosyn®): 375 mg, 500 mg

Nursing Guidelines

Assessment: Evaluate cardiac risk and potential for GI bleeding prior to prescribing this medication. Assess effectiveness and interactions of other medications patient may be taking. Monitor blood pressure at the beginning of therapy and periodically during use. Assess results of laboratory tests, therapeutic effectiveness, and adverse reactions (eg, GI effects, hepatotoxicity, or ototoxicity) at beginning of therapy and periodically throughout therapy. Schedule ophthalmic evaluations for patients who develop eye complaints during long-term NSAID therapy. Assess knowledge/teach patient appropriate use, interventions to reduce side effects, and adverse symptoms to report.

Monitoring Laboratory Tests: Periodic liver function, CBC, BUN, serum creatinine

Dietary Considerations: Drug may cause GI upset, bleeding, ulceration, perforation; take with food or milk to minimize GI upset.

Patient Education: Take this medication exactly as directed; do not increase dose without consulting prescriber. Do not crush tablets. Take with food or milk to reduce GI distress. Maintain adequate hydration (2-3 L/day of fluids) unless instructed to restrict fluid intake. Do not use alcohol, aspirin or aspirin-containing medication, or any other anti-inflammatory medications without consulting prescriber. You may experience drowsiness, dizziness, lightheadedness, or headache (use caution when driving or engaging in tasks requiring alertness until response to drug is known); anorexia, nausea, vomiting, or heartburn (small frequent meals, frequent mouth care, sucking lozenges, or chewing gum may help); or fluid retention (weigh yourself weekly and report unusual [3-5 lb/week] weight gain), GI bleeding, ulceration, or perforation can occur with or without pain; or discontinue medication and contact prescriber if persistent abdominal pain or cramping, or blood in stool occurs. Report breathlessness, respiratory difficulty, or unusual cough; chest pain, rapid heartbeat, palpitations; unusual bruising/bleeding; blood in urine, stool, mouth, or vomitus; swollen extremities; skin rash or itching; acute fatigue; or changes in eyesight (double vision, color changes, blurred vision), hearing, or ringing in ears. **Breast-feeding precautions:** Notify prescriber if you are or intend to become pregnant. Do not take this drug during last trimester of pregnancy.

Geriatric Considerations: Elderly are at high risk for adverse effects from NSAIDs. As much as 60% of elderly can develop peptic ulceration and/or hemorrhage asymptomatically. The concomitant use of H_2 blockers, omeprazole, and sucralfate is not effective as prophylaxis with the exception of NSAID-induced duodenal ulcers which may be prevented by the use of ranitidine. Misoprostol is the only prophylactic agent proven effective. Also, concomitant disease and drug use contribute to the risk for GI adverse effects. Use lowest effective dose for shortest period possible. Consider renal function decline with age. Use of NSAIDs can compromise existing renal function especially when Cl_{cr} is ≤30 mL/minute. Tinnitus may be a difficult and unreliable indication of toxicity due to age-related hearing loss or eighth cranial nerve damage. CNS adverse effects such as confusion, agitation, and hallucination are generally seen in overdose or high-dose situations, but elderly may demonstrate these adverse effects at lower doses than younger adults.

Pregnancy Risk Factor: C/D (3rd trimester)

Lactation: Enters breast milk/not recommended (AAP rates "compatible")

Perioperative/Anesthesia/Other Concerns: The 2002 ACCM/SCCM guidelines for analgesia (critically-ill adult) suggest that NSAIDs may be used in combination with opioids in select patients for pain management. Concern about adverse events (increased risk of renal dysfunction, altered platelet function and gastrointestinal irritation) limits its use in patients who have other underlying risks for these events.

In short-term use, NSAIDs vary considerably in their effect on blood pressure. When NSAIDs are used in patients with hypertension, appropriate monitoring of blood pressure responses should be completed and the duration of therapy, when possible, kept short. The use of NSAIDs in the treatment of patients with congestive heart failure may be associated with an increased risk for fluid accumulation and edema; may precipitate renal failure in dehydrated patients.

Administration

Oral: Administer with food, milk, or antacids to decrease GI adverse effects

Suspension: Shake suspension well before administration.

Tablet, extended release: Swallow tablet whole; do not break, crush, or chew.

Storage: Store oral suspension and tablet at 15°C to 30°C (59°F to 86°F).

Related Information

Acute Postoperative Pain *on page 1742*

- ♦ Naproxen Sodium *see* Naproxen *on page 1203*
- ♦ Narcan® [DSC] *see* Naloxone *on page 1200*
- ♦ Naropin® *see* Ropivacaine *on page 1498*
- ♦ Nasacort® AQ *see* Triamcinolone *on page 1660*
- ♦ Nasacort® HFA *see* Triamcinolone *on page 1660*
- ♦ NaSal™ [OTC] *see* Sodium Chloride *on page 1545*
- ♦ NasalCrom® [OTC] *see* Cromolyn *on page 453*
- ♦ Nasal Moist® [OTC] *see* Sodium Chloride *on page 1545*
- ♦ Nascobal® *see* Cyanocobalamin *on page 457*
- ♦ NataChew™ *see* Vitamins (Multiple/Prenatal) *on page 1721*
- ♦ NataFort® *see* Vitamins (Multiple/Prenatal) *on page 1721*
- ♦ NatalCare® CFe 60 [DSC] *see* Vitamins (Multiple/Prenatal) *on page 1721*
- ♦ NatalCare® GlossTabs™ *see* Vitamins (Multiple/Prenatal) *on page 1721*
- ♦ NatalCare® PIC *see* Vitamins (Multiple/Prenatal) *on page 1721*
- ♦ NatalCare® PIC Forte *see* Vitamins (Multiple/Prenatal) *on page 1721*
- ♦ NatalCare® Plus *see* Vitamins (Multiple/Prenatal) *on page 1721*
- ♦ NatalCare® Rx *see* Vitamins (Multiple/Prenatal) *on page 1721*

♦ **NatalCare® Three** *see* Vitamins (Multiple/Prenatal) *on page 1721*
♦ **NataTab™ CFe** *see* Vitamins (Multiple/Prenatal) *on page 1721*
♦ **NataTab™ FA** *see* Vitamins (Multiple/Prenatal) *on page 1721*
♦ **NataTab™ Rx** *see* Vitamins (Multiple/Prenatal) *on page 1721*
♦ **Natrecor®** *see* Nesiritide *on page 1216*
♦ **Natriuretic Peptide** *see* Nesiritide *on page 1216*
♦ **Natural Fiber Therapy [OTC]** *see* Psyllium *on page 1438*
♦ **Nature's Tears® [OTC]** *see* Artificial Tears *on page 187*
♦ **Navelbine®** *see* Vinorelbine *on page 1713*
♦ **Na-Zone® [OTC]** *see* Sodium Chloride *on page 1545*
♦ **NebuPent®** *see* Pentamidine *on page 1334*
♦ **Nembutal®** *see* Pentobarbital *on page 1336*
♦ **Neo-Fradin™** *see* Neomycin *on page 1208*

Neomycin (nee oh MYE sin)

U.S. Brand Names Neo-Fradin™; Neo-Rx

Synonyms Neomycin Sulfate

Pharmacologic Category Ammonium Detoxicant; Antibiotic, Aminoglycoside; Antibiotic, Topical

Medication Safety Issues

Sound-alike/look-alike issues:

Myciguent may be confused with Mycitracin®

Use Orally to prepare GI tract for surgery; topically to treat minor skin infections; treatment of diarrhea caused by *E. coli*; adjunct in the treatment of hepatic encephalopathy; bladder irrigation; ocular infections

Mechanism of Action Interferes with bacterial protein synthesis by binding to 30S ribosomal subunits

Pharmacodynamics/Kinetics

Absorption: Oral, percutaneous: Poor (3%)

Distribution: V_d: 0.36 L/kg

Metabolism: Slightly hepatic

Half-life elimination (age and renal function dependent): 3 hours

Time to peak, serum: Oral: 1-4 hours

Excretion: Feces (97% of oral dose as unchanged drug); urine (30% to 50% of absorbed drug as unchanged drug)

Contraindications Hypersensitivity to neomycin or any component of the formulation, or other aminoglycosides; intestinal obstruction

Warnings/Precautions Use with caution in patients with renal impairment, pre-existing hearing impairment, neuromuscular disorders; neomycin is more toxic than other aminoglycosides when given parenterally; **do not administer parenterally**; topical neomycin is a contact sensitizer with sensitivity occurring in 5% to 15% of patients treated with the drug; symptoms include itching, reddening, edema, and failure to heal; **do not use as peritoneal lavage** due to significant systemic adsorption of the drug

Drug Interactions

Decreased effect: May decrease GI absorption of digoxin and methotrexate

Increased effect: Synergistic effects with penicillins

Increased toxicity:

Oral neomycin may potentiate the effects of oral anticoagulants

Increased adverse effects with other neurotoxic, ototoxic, or nephrotoxic drugs

Adverse Reactions

Oral:

>10%: Gastrointestinal: Nausea, diarrhea, vomiting, irritation or soreness of the mouth or rectal area

<1% (Limited to important or life-threatening): Dyspnea, eosinophilia, nephrotoxicity, neurotoxicity, ototoxicity (auditory), ototoxicity (vestibular)

Topical: >10%: Dermatologic: Contact dermatitis

Overdosage/Toxicology Symptoms of overdose (rare due to poor oral bioavailability) include ototoxicity, nephrotoxicity, and neuromuscular toxicity. The treatment of choice following a single acute overdose appears to be maintenance of urine output of at least 3 mL/kg/hour during the acute treatment phase. Dialysis is of questionable value in enhancing aminoglycoside elimination. If required, hemodialysis is preferred over peritoneal dialysis in patients with normal renal function. Chelation with penicillin may be of benefit.

Dosing

Adults & Elderly:

Dermatologic infections: Topical: Topical solutions containing 0.1% to 1% neomycin have been used for irrigation

Preoperative intestinal antisepsis: Oral: 1 g each hour for 4 doses then 1 g every 4 hours for 5 doses; or 1 g at 1 PM, 2 PM, and 11 PM on day preceding surgery as an adjunct to mechanical cleansing of the bowel and oral erythromycin; or 6 g/day divided every 4 hours for 2-3 days

Hepatic encephalopathy: Oral: 500-2000 mg every 6-8 hours or 4-12 g/day divided every 4-6 hours for 5-6 days

Chronic hepatic insufficiency: Oral: 4 g/day for an indefinite period

Pediatrics:

Preoperative intestinal antisepsis: Oral: Children: 90 mg/kg/day divided every 4 hours for 2 days; or 25 mg/kg at 1 PM, 2 PM, and 11 PM on the day preceding surgery as an adjunct to mechanical cleansing of the intestine and in combination with erythromycin base

Hepatic encephalopathy: Oral: Children: 50-100 mg/kg/day in divided doses every 6-8 hours or 2.5-7 g/m^2/day divided every 4-6 hours for 5-6 days not to exceed 12 g/day

Dermatologic infections: Topical: Children: Refer to adult dosing.

Available Dosage Forms

Powder, micronized, as sulfate [for prescription compounding] (Neo-Rx): (10 g, 100 g)

Solution, oral, as sulfate (Neo-Fradin™): 125 mg/5 mL (60 mL, 480 mL) [contains benzoic acid; cherry flavor]

Tablet, as sulfate: 500 mg

Nursing Guidelines

Assessment: Assess effectiveness and interactions of other medications patient may be taking. Assess results of laboratory tests, therapeutic effectiveness, and adverse response (eg, ototoxicity, nephrotoxicity, neurotoxicity). Assess knowledge/teach patient appropriate use (application of cream/ointment), possible side effects/interventions, and adverse symptoms to report. Minimal absorption across GI mucosa or skin surfaces; however with ulceration, open or burned surfaces (especially large surfaces), absorption is possible.

Monitoring Laboratory Tests: Renal function; perform culture and sensitivity prior to initiating therapy.

Patient Education: Oral: Take as directed. Maintain adequate hydration (2-3 L/day of fluids) unless instructed to restrict fluid intake. You may experience nausea or vomiting (small frequent meals, frequent mouth care, sucking lozenges, or chewing gum may help); constipation (increased exercise, fluids, fruit, or fiber may help, or consult prescriber); or diarrhea (buttermilk, boiled milk, or yogurt may help). Report immediately any change in hearing; ringing or sense of fullness in ears; persistent diarrhea; changes in voiding patterns; or numbness, tingling, or pain in any extremity. **Pregnancy/breast-feeding precautions:** Inform prescriber if you are or intend to become pregnant. Consult prescriber if breast-feeding.

Pregnancy Risk Factor: D

Lactation: Excretion in breast milk unknown

Related Information

Prevention of Wound Infection and Sepsis in Surgical Patients *on page 1830*

Neomycin and Polymyxin B (nee oh MYE sin & pol i MIKS in bee)

U.S. Brand Names Neosporin® G.U. Irrigant

Synonyms Polymyxin B and Neomycin

Pharmacologic Category Antibiotic, Topical

Use Short-term as a continuous irrigant or rinse in the urinary bladder to prevent bacteriuria and gram-negative rod septicemia associated with the use of indwelling catheters; to help prevent infection in minor cuts, scrapes, and burns

Mechanism of Action See individual agents.

Pharmacodynamics/Kinetics

Absorption: Topical: Not absorbed following application to intact skin; absorbed through denuded or abraded skin, peritoneum, wounds, or ulcers

See individual agents.

Contraindications Hypersensitivity to neomycin, polymyxin B, or any component of the formulation; pregnancy (GU irrigant)

Drug Interactions No data reported

(Continued)

Neomycin and Polymyxin B *(Continued)*

Adverse Reactions Frequency not defined.

Dermatologic: Contact dermatitis, erythema, rash, urticaria
Genitourinary: Bladder irritation
Local: Burning
Neuromuscular & skeletal: Neuromuscular blockade
Otic: Ototoxicity
Renal: Nephrotoxicity

Dosing

Adults & Elderly: Bladder irrigation: **Not for I.V. injection**; add 1 mL irrigant to 1 liter isotonic saline solution and connect container to the inflow of lumen of 3-way catheter. Continuous irrigant or rinse in the urinary bladder for up to a maximum of 10 days with administration rate adjusted to patient's urine output; usually no more than 1 L of irrigant is used per day.

Pediatrics: Refer to adult dosing.

Available Dosage Forms Solution, irrigant: Neomycin 40 mg and polymyxin B sulfate 200,000 units per mL (1 mL, 20 mL)

Nursing Guidelines

Assessment: Pregnancy risk factor C/D - see Pregnancy Risk Factor for use cautions. Assess knowledge/instruct patient on need to use appropriate contraceptive measures and the need to avoid pregnancy. Note breast-feeding caution.

Patient Education:

Pregnancy/breast-feeding precautions: Inform prescriber if you are or intend to become pregnant. Consult prescriber if breast-feeding.

Pregnancy Risk Factor: C/D (for G.U. irrigant)

Lactation: Excretion in breast milk unknown

Administration

Storage: Store irrigation solution in refrigerator; aseptic prepared dilutions (1 mL/1 L) should be stored in the refrigerator and discarded after 48 hours

♦ **Neomycin, Bacitracin, and Polymyxin B** *see* Bacitracin, Neomycin, and Polymyxin B *on page 220*

♦ **Neomycin, Bacitracin, Polymyxin B, and Hydrocortisone** *see* Bacitracin, Neomycin, Polymyxin B, and Hydrocortisone *on page 221*

Neomycin, Colistin, Hydrocortisone, and Thonzonium

(nee oh MYE sin, koe LIS tin, hye droe KOR ti sone, & thon ZOE nee um)

U.S. Brand Names Coly-Mycin® S; Cortisporin®-TC

Synonyms Colistin, Neomycin, Hydrocortisone, and Thonzonium; Hydrocortisone, Neomycin, Colistin, and Thonzonium; Thonzonium, Neomycin, Colistin, and Hydrocortisone

Pharmacologic Category Antibiotic/Corticosteroid, Otic

Use Treatment of superficial and susceptible bacterial infections of the external auditory canal; for treatment of susceptible bacterial infections of mastoidectomy and fenestration cavities

Contraindications Hypersensitivity to any component of the formulation and/or aminoglycosides; herpes simplex, vaccinia, varicella

Warnings/Precautions Prolonged treatment may result in overgrowth of nonsusceptible organisms. Discontinue if irritation occurs. Use caution in longstanding otitis media or tympanic perforation; risk of ototoxicity is increased. Do not use for longer than 10 days.

Drug Interactions Hydrocortisone: **Substrate** of CYP3A4 (minor); **Induces** CYP3A4 (weak)

Adverse Reactions Frequency not defined.

Dermatologic: Hypersensitivity reaction, irritation
Otic: Ototoxicity (rare)

Dosing

Adults & Elderly: Ear inflammation/infection: Otic:

Calibrated dropper: 5 drops in affected ear 3-4 times/day
Dropper bottle: 4 drops in affected ear 3-4 times/day

Note: Alternatively, a cotton wick may be inserted in the ear canal and saturated with suspension every 4 hours; wick should be replaced at least every 24 hours

Pediatrics: Ear inflammation/infection: Otic:

Calibrated dropper: 4 drops in affected ear 3-4 times/day
Dropper bottle: 3 drops in affected ear 3-4 times/day

Note: Alternatively, a cotton wick may be inserted in the ear canal and saturated with suspension every 4 hours; wick should be replaced at least every 24 hours

Available Dosage Forms Suspension, otic [drops]:

Coly-Mycin® S: Neomycin 0.33%, colistin 0.3%, hydrocortisone acetate 1%, and thonzonium bromide 0.05% (5 mL) [contains thimerosal; packaged with dropper]

Cortisporin®-TC: Neomycin 0.33%, colistin 0.3%, hydrocortisone acetate 1%, and thonzonium bromide 0.05% (10 mL) [contains thimerosal; packaged with dropper]

Nursing Guidelines

Assessment: See individual agents.

Patient Education: Shake well before using.

Neomycin, Polymyxin B, and Dexamethasone

(nee oh MYE sin, pol i MIKS in bee, & deks a METH a sone)

U.S. Brand Names AK-Trol®; Dexacidin® [DSC]; Dexacine™ [DSC]; Dexasporin; Maxitrol®; Methadex

Synonyms Dexamethasone, Neomycin, and Polymyxin B; Polymyxin B, Neomycin, and Dexamethasone

Pharmacologic Category Antibiotic/Corticosteroid, Ophthalmic

Medication Safety Issues

Sound-alike/look-alike issues:

AK-Trol® may be confused with AKTob®

Use Steroid-responsive inflammatory ocular conditions in which a corticosteroid is indicated and where bacterial infection or a risk of bacterial infection exists

Mechanism of Action See individual agents.

Pharmacodynamics/Kinetics See individual agents.

Contraindications Hypersensitivity to neomycin, polymyxin B, dexamethasone, or any component of the formulation; viral, fungal, or tuberculosis diseases of the eye

Warnings/Precautions Sensitivity to neomycin may develop; discontinue if sensitivity reaction occurs. Prolonged use of corticosteroids may result in glaucoma; damage to the optic nerve, defects in visual acuity and fields of vision, and posterior subcapsular cataract formation may occur. Prolonged use of corticosteroids may increase the incidence of secondary ocular infection or mask acute infection (including fungal infections); may prolong or exacerbate ocular viral infections; use following cataract surgery may delay healing or increase the incidence of bleb formation. A maximum of 8 g of ointment or 20 mL of suspension should be prescribed initially; patients should be evaluated prior to additional refills. Suspension contains benzalkonium chloride which may be adsorbed by contact lenses; contact lenses should not be worn during treatment of ophthalmic infections.

Drug Interactions Dexamethasone: **Substrate** of CYP3A4 (minor); **Induces** CYP2A6 (weak), 2B6 (weak), 2C8/9 (weak), 3A4 (weak)

Also see individual agents.

Adverse Reactions Frequency not defined: Ocular: Allergic sensitivity, cutaneous sensitization, eye pain, development of glaucoma, cataract, increased intraocular pressure, optic nerve damage, wound healing delayed

Dosing

Adults & Elderly: Ocular inflammation/infection: Ophthalmic:

Ointment: Place a small amount (~1/2") in the affected eye 3-4 times/day or apply at bedtime as an adjunct with drops

Suspension: Instill 1-2 drops into affected eye(s) every 3-4 hours; in severe disease, drops may be used hourly and tapered to discontinuation

Pediatrics: Refer to adult dosing.

Available Dosage Forms [DSC] = Discontinued product

Ointment, ophthalmic (Dexacine™ [DSC], Maxitrol®): Neomycin 3.5 mg, polymyxin B sulfate 10,000 units, and dexamethasone 0.1% per g (3.5 g)

Suspension, ophthalmic (AK-Trol®, Dexacidin® [DSC], Dexasporin, Maxitrol®, Methadex): Neomycin 3.5 mg, polymyxin B sulfate 10,000 units, and dexamethasone 0.1% per mL (5 mL) [contains benzalkonium chloride]

Nursing Guidelines

Patient Education: Notify prescriber if condition worsens or does not improve in 3-4 days

(Continued)

Neomycin, Polymyxin B, and Dexamethasone *(Continued)*

Pregnancy Risk Factor: C

Lactation: Excretion in breast milk unknown/use caution

Breast-Feeding Considerations: It is unknown if topical use results in sufficient absorption to produce detectable quantities in breast milk.

Related Information

Dexamethasone *on page 495*

Neomycin *on page 1208*

Polymyxin B *on page 1380*

Neomycin, Polymyxin B, and Gramicidin

(nee oh MYE sin, pol i MIKS in bee, & gram i SYE din)

U.S. Brand Names Neosporin® Ophthalmic Solution

Synonyms Gramicidin, Neomycin, and Polymyxin B; Polymyxin B, Neomycin, and Gramicidin

Pharmacologic Category Antibiotic, Ophthalmic

Use Treatment of superficial ocular infection

Mechanism of Action Interferes with bacterial protein synthesis by binding to 30S ribosomal subunits; binds to phospholipids, alters permeability, and damages the bacterial cytoplasmic membrane permitting leakage of intracellular constituents

Contraindications Hypersensitivity to neomycin, polymyxin B, gramicidin or any component of the formulation

Warnings/Precautions Symptoms of neomycin sensitization include itching, reddening, edema, failure to heal; prolonged use may result in glaucoma, defects in visual acuity, posterior subcapsular cataract formation, and secondary ocular infections

Drug Interactions No data reported

Adverse Reactions Frequency not defined: Ocular: Transient irritation, burning, stinging, itching, inflammation, angioneurotic edema, urticaria, vesicular and maculopapular dermatitis

Dosing

Adults & Elderly: Children and Adults: Ophthalmic: Instill 1-2 drops 4-6 times/day or more frequently as required for severe infections

Pediatrics: Refer to adult dosing.

Available Dosage Forms Solution, ophthalmic: Neomycin 1.75 mg, polymyxin B 10,000 units, and gramicidin 0.025 mg per mL (10 mL) [contains alcohol 0.5% and thimerosal]

Nursing Guidelines

Patient Education: Tilt head back, place medication in conjunctival sac, and close eyes; apply finger pressure on lacrimal sac for 1 minute following instillation

Pregnancy Risk Factor: C

Related Information

Neomycin *on page 1208*

Polymyxin B *on page 1380*

Prevention of Wound Infection and Sepsis in Surgical Patients *on page 1830*

Neomycin, Polymyxin B, and Hydrocortisone

(nee oh MYE sin, pol i MIKS in bee, & hye droe KOR ti sone)

U.S. Brand Names AntibiOtic® Ear; Cortisporin® Cream; Cortisporin® Ophthalmic; Cortisporin® Otic; PediOtic®

Synonyms Hydrocortisone, Neomycin, and Polymyxin B; Polymyxin B, Neomycin, and Hydrocortisone

Pharmacologic Category Antibiotic/Corticosteroid, Ophthalmic; Antibiotic/Corticosteroid, Otic; Topical Skin Product

Use Steroid-responsive inflammatory condition for which a corticosteroid is indicated and where bacterial infection or a risk of bacterial infection exists

Mechanism of Action See individual agents.

Pharmacodynamics/Kinetics See individual agents.

Contraindications Hypersensitivity to neomycin, polymyxin B, hydrocortisone, or any component of the formulation

Drug Interactions Hydrocortisone: **Substrate** of CYP3A4 (minor); **Induces** CYP3A4 (weak)

Also see individual agents.

Adverse Reactions Frequency not defined.

Dermatologic: Contact dermatitis, erythema, rash, urticaria

Local: Burning, itching, swelling, pain, stinging

Ocular: Intraocular pressure increased, glaucoma, cataracts, conjunctival erythema, transient irritation, burning, stinging, itching, inflammation, angioneurotic edema, urticaria, vesicular and maculopapular dermatitis

Otic: Ototoxicity

Miscellaneous: Hypersensitivity, sensitization to neomycin, secondary infection

Dosing

Adults & Elderly:

Note: Duration of use should be limited to 10 days unless otherwise directed by the physician. Otic solution is used **only** for swimmer's ear (infections of external auditory canal)

Auditory canal inflammation/infection: Otic: Instill 4 drops 3-4 times/day; otic suspension is the preferred otic preparation

Ocular inflammation/infection: Ophthalmic: Instill 1-2 drops 2-4 times/day, or more frequently as required for severe infections; in acute infections, instill 1-2 drops every 15-30 minutes gradually reducing the frequency of administration as the infection is controlled

Dermatologic inflammation/infection: Topical: Apply a thin layer 1-4 times/day. Therapy should be discontinued when control is achieved; if no improvement is seen, reassessment of diagnosis may be necessary.

Pediatrics:

Note: Duration of use should be limited to 10 days unless otherwise directed by the physician. Otic solution is used **only** for swimmer's ear (infections of external auditory canal).

Auditory canal inflammation/infection: Otic: Children: Instill 3 drops into affected ear 3-4 times/day.

Ocular inflammation/infection: Children: Refer to adult dosing.

Dermatologic inflammation/infection: Children: Refer to adult dosing.

Available Dosage Forms

Cream, topical (Cortisporin®): Neomycin 3.5 mg, polymyxin B 10,000 units, and hydrocortisone 5 mg per g (7.5 g)

Solution, otic (AntibiOtic® Ear; Cortisporin®): Neomycin 3.5 mg, polymyxin B 10,000 units, and hydrocortisone 10 mg per mL (10 mL) [contains potassium metabisulfite]

Suspension, ophthalmic (Cortisporin®): Neomycin 3.5 mg, polymyxin B 10,000 units, and hydrocortisone 10 mg per mL (7.5 mL) [contains thimerosal]

Suspension, otic: Neomycin 3.5 mg, polymyxin B 10,000 units, and hydrocortisone 10 mg per mL (10 mL)

AntibiOtic® Ear, Cortisporin®: Neomycin 3.5 mg, polymyxin B 10,000 units, and hydrocortisone 10 mg per mL (10 mL) [contains thimerosal]

PediOtic®: Neomycin 3.5 mg, polymyxin B 10,000 units, and hydrocortisone 10 mg per mL (7.5 mL) [contains thimerosal]

Nursing Guidelines

Assessment: See individual agents.

Patient Education:

Otic: Hold container in hand to warm; if drops are in suspension form, shake well for approximately 10 seconds, lie on your side with affected ear up; for adults hold the ear lobe up and back, for children hold the ear lobe down and back; instill drops in ear without inserting dropper into ear; maintain tilted ear for 2 minutes.

Ophthalmic: May cause sensitivity to bright light; may cause temporary blurring of vision or stinging following administration, but discontinue product and see prescriber if problems persist or increase; to use, tilt head back and place medication in conjunctival sac and close eyes; apply light pressure on lacrimal sac for 1 minute.

Cream: Discontinue product if irritation persists or increases.

Pregnancy Risk Factor: C

Related Information

Hydrocortisone *on page 873*

Neomycin *on page 1208*

Polymyxin B *on page 1380*

- **Neomycin Sulfate** *see* Neomycin *on page 1208*
- **Neoral®** *see* CycloSPORINE *on page 465*
- **Neo-Rx** *see* Neomycin *on page 1208*

- ♦ **Neosporin® G.U. Irrigant** *see* Neomycin and Polymyxin B *on page 1209*
- ♦ **Neosporin® Neo To Go® [OTC]** *see* Bacitracin, Neomycin, and Polymyxin B *on page 220*
- ♦ **Neosporin® Ophthalmic Ointment [DSC]** *see* Bacitracin, Neomycin, and Polymyxin B *on page 220*
- ♦ **Neosporin® Ophthalmic Solution** *see* Neomycin, Polymyxin B, and Gramicidin *on page 1212*
- ♦ **Neosporin® Topical [OTC]** *see* Bacitracin, Neomycin, and Polymyxin B *on page 220*

Neostigmine (nee oh STIG meen)

U.S. Brand Names Prostigmin®

Synonyms Neostigmine Bromide; Neostigmine Methylsulfate

Pharmacologic Category Acetylcholinesterase Inhibitor

Medication Safety Issues

Sound-alike/look-alike issues:

Prostigmin® may be confused with physostigmine

Use Diagnosis and treatment of myasthenia gravis; prevention and treatment of postoperative bladder distention and urinary retention; reversal of the effects of nondepolarizing neuromuscular-blocking agents after surgery

Mechanism of Action Inhibits destruction of acetylcholine by acetylcholinesterase which facilitates transmission of impulses across myoneural junction

Pharmacodynamics/Kinetics

Onset of action: I.M.: 20-30 minutes; I.V.: 1-20 minutes

Duration: I.M.: 2.5-4 hours; I.V.: 1-2 hours

Absorption: Oral: Poor, <2%

Metabolism: Hepatic

Half-life elimination: Normal renal function: 0.5-2.1 hours; End-stage renal disease: Prolonged

Excretion: Urine (50% as unchanged drug)

Contraindications Hypersensitivity to neostigmine, bromides, or any component of the formulation; GI or GU obstruction

Warnings/Precautions Does **not** antagonize and may prolong the phase I block of depolarizing muscle relaxants (eg, succinylcholine); use with caution in patients with epilepsy, asthma, bradycardia, hyperthyroidism, cardiac arrhythmias, or peptic ulcer; adequate facilities should be available for cardiopulmonary resuscitation when testing and adjusting dose for myasthenia gravis; have atropine and epinephrine ready to treat hypersensitivity reactions; overdosage may result in cholinergic crisis, this must be distinguished from myasthenic crisis; anticholinesterase insensitivity can develop for brief or prolonged periods

Drug Interactions

Anticholinergics: Effects may be reduced with cholinesterase inhibitors; atropine antagonizes the muscarinic effects of cholinesterase inhibitors

Beta-blockers without ISA: Activity may increase risk of bradycardia

Calcium channel blockers (diltiazem or verapamil): May increase risk of bradycardia

Cholinergic agonists: Effects may be increased with cholinesterase inhibitors

Corticosteroids: May see increased muscle weakness and decreased response to anticholinesterases shortly after onset of corticosteroid therapy in the treatment of myasthenia gravis. Deterioration in muscle strength, including severe muscular depression, has been documented in patients with myasthenia gravis while receiving corticosteroids and anticholinesterases.

Digoxin: Increased risk of bradycardia with concurrent use

Neuromuscular blockers: Depolarizing neuromuscular blocking agents effects may be increased with cholinesterase inhibitors; nondepolarizing agents are antagonized by cholinesterase inhibitors

Lab Interactions Increased aminotransferase [ALT (SGPT)/AST (SGOT)] (S), amylase (S)

Adverse Reactions Frequency not defined.

Cardiovascular: Arrhythmias (especially bradycardia), hypotension, decreased carbon monoxide, tachycardia, AV block, nodal rhythm, nonspecific ECG changes, cardiac arrest, syncope, flushing

Central nervous system: Convulsions, dysarthria, dysphonia, dizziness, loss of consciousness, drowsiness, headache

Dermatologic: Skin rash, thrombophlebitis (I.V.), urticaria

Gastrointestinal: Hyperperistalsis, nausea, vomiting, salivation, diarrhea, stomach cramps, dysphagia, flatulence

Genitourinary: Urinary urgency
Neuromuscular & skeletal: Weakness, fasciculations, muscle cramps, spasms, arthralgia
Ocular: Small pupils, lacrimation
Respiratory: Increased bronchial secretions, laryngospasm, bronchiolar constriction, respiratory muscle paralysis, dyspnea, respiratory depression, respiratory arrest, bronchospasm
Miscellaneous: Diaphoresis (increased), anaphylaxis, allergic reactions

Overdosage/Toxicology Symptoms of overdose include muscle weakness, blurred vision, excessive sweating, tearing and salivation, nausea, vomiting, diarrhea, hypertension, bradycardia, muscle weakness, and paralysis. Atropine sulfate injection should be readily available as an antagonist for the effects of neostigmine.

Dosing

Adults & Elderly:

Myasthenia gravis, diagnosis: I.M.: 0.02 mg/kg as a single dose

Myasthenia gravis, treatment:

Oral: 15 mg/dose every 3-4 hours up to 375 mg/day maximum

I.M., I.V., SubQ: 0.5-2.5 mg every 1-3 hours up to 10 mg/24 hours maximum

Reversal of nondepolarizing neuromuscular blockade after surgery in conjunction with atropine: I.V.: 0.5-2.5 mg; total dose not to exceed 5 mg; must administer atropine several minutes prior to neostigmine

Bladder atony: I.M., SubQ:

Prevention: 0.25 mg every 4-6 hours for 2-3 days

Treatment: 0.5-1 mg every 3 hours for 5 doses after bladder has emptied

Pediatrics:

Myasthenia gravis, diagnosis: I.M.: Children: 0.04 mg/kg as a single dose

Myasthenia gravis, treatment: Children:

Oral: 2 mg/kg/day divided every 3-4 hours

I.M., I.V., SubQ: 0.01-0.04 mg/kg every 2-4 hours

Reversal of nondepolarizing neuromuscular blockade after surgery in conjunction with atropine (must administer atropine several minutes prior to neostigmine): I.V.:

Infants: 0.025-0.1 mg/kg/dose

Children: 0.025-0.08 mg/kg/dose

Renal Impairment:

Cl_{cr} 10-50 mL/minute: Administer 50% of normal dose.

Cl_{cr} <10 mL/minute: Administer 25% of normal dose.

Available Dosage Forms

Injection, solution, as methylsulfate: 0.5 mg/mL (1 mL, 10 mL); 1 mg/mL (10 mL)
Tablet, as bromide: 15 mg

Nursing Guidelines

Assessment: Used for MG diagnosis by physicians. For bladder atony, assess bladder adequacy prior to administering medication. Monitor therapeutic effectiveness and adverse effects (including cholinergic crisis). Teach patient symptoms to report.

Patient Education: Take this drug exactly as prescribed. You may experience visual difficulty (eg, blurring and dark adaptation, use caution at night) or urinary frequency. Promptly report any muscle weakness, respiratory difficulty, severe or unresolved diarrhea, persistent abdominal cramping or vomiting, sweating, or tearing. **Pregnancy/breast-feeding precautions:** Inform prescriber if you are pregnant. Breast-feeding is not recommended.

Geriatric Considerations: Many elderly will have diseases which may influence the use of neostigmine. Also, many elderly will need doses reduced 50% due to creatinine clearances in the 10-50 mL/minute range (common in the aged). Side effects or concomitant disease may warrant use of pyridostigmine.

Pregnancy Risk Factor: C

Lactation: Excretion in breast milk unknown/not recommended

Administration

I.M.: In the diagnosis of myasthenia gravis, all anticholinesterase medications should be discontinued for at least 8 hours before administering neostigmine.

Compatibility: Stable in NS

♦ **Neostigmine Bromide** *see* Neostigmine *on page 1214*
♦ **Neostigmine Methylsulfate** *see* Neostigmine *on page 1214*
♦ **Neo-Synephrine® 12 Hour [OTC]** *see* Oxymetazoline *on page 1290*

- ♦ **Neo-Synephrine® 12 Hour Extra Moisturizing [OTC]** *see* Oxymetazoline *on page 1290*
- ♦ **Neo-Synephrine® Extra Strength [OTC]** *see* Phenylephrine *on page 1350*
- ♦ **Neo-Synephrine® Mild [OTC]** *see* Phenylephrine *on page 1350*
- ♦ **Neo-Synephrine® Ophthalmic [DSC]** *see* Phenylephrine *on page 1350*
- ♦ **Neo-Synephrine® Regular Strength [OTC]** *see* Phenylephrine *on page 1350*
- ♦ **NephPlex® Rx** *see* Vitamin B Complex Combinations *on page 1716*
- ♦ **Nephro-Calci® [OTC]** *see* Calcium Carbonate *on page 291*
- ♦ **Nephrocaps®** *see* Vitamin B Complex Combinations *on page 1716*
- ♦ **Nephron FA®** *see* Vitamin B Complex Combinations *on page 1716*
- ♦ **Nephro-Vite®** *see* Vitamin B Complex Combinations *on page 1716*
- ♦ **Nephro-Vite® Rx** *see* Vitamin B Complex Combinations *on page 1716*
- ♦ **Nesacaine®** *see* Chloroprocaine *on page 375*
- ♦ **Nesacaine®-MPF** *see* Chloroprocaine *on page 375*

Nesiritide (ni SIR i tide)

U.S. Brand Names Natrecor®

Synonyms B-type Natriuretic Peptide (Human); hBNP; Natriuretic Peptide

Pharmacologic Category Natriuretic Peptide, B-Type, Human; Vasodilator

Medication Safety Issues

High alert medication: The Institute for Safe Medication Practices (ISMP) includes this medication among its list of drugs which have a heightened risk of causing significant patient harm when used in error.

Use Treatment of acutely decompensated congestive heart failure (CHF) in patients with dyspnea at rest or with minimal activity

Mechanism of Action Binds to guanylate cyclase receptor on vascular smooth muscle and endothelial cells, increasing intracellular cyclic GMP, resulting in smooth muscle cell relaxation. Has been shown to produce dose-dependent reductions in pulmonary capillary wedge pressure (PCWP) and systemic arterial pressure.

Pharmacodynamics/Kinetics

Onset of action: 15 minutes (60% of 3-hour effect achieved)

Duration: >60 minutes (up to several hours) for systolic blood pressure; hemodynamic effects persist longer than serum half-life would predict

Distribution: V_{ss}: 0.19 L/kg

Metabolism: Proteolytic cleavage by vascular endopeptidases and proteolysis following receptor binding and cellular internalization

Half-life elimination: Initial (distribution) 2 minutes; Terminal: 18 minutes

Time to peak: 1 hour

Excretion: Urine

Contraindications Hypersensitivity to natriuretic peptide or any component of the formulation; cardiogenic shock (when used as primary therapy); hypotension (systolic blood pressure <90 mm Hg)

Warnings/Precautions May cause hypotension; administer in clinical situations when blood pressure may be closely monitored. Use caution in patients with systolic blood pressure <100 mm Hg (contraindicated if <90 mm Hg); more likely to experience hypotension. Effects may be additive with other agents capable of causing hypotension. Hypotensive effects may last for several hours.

Should not be used in patients with low filling pressures, or in patients with conditions which depend on venous return including significant valvular stenosis, restrictive or obstructive cardiomyopathy, constrictive pericarditis, and pericardial tamponade. May be associated with development of azotemia; use caution in patients with renal impairment or in patients where renal perfusion is dependent on renin-angiotensin-aldosterone system.

Atrial natriuretic peptide (ANP), a related peptide, has been associated with increased vascular permeability and decreased intravascular volume. This has not been observed in clinical trials with nesiritide, however, patients should be monitored for this effect.

Prepared through recombinant technology using *E. coli*; monitor for allergic or anaphylactic reactions. Use caution with prolonged infusions; limited experience for infusions >48 hours. Safety and efficacy in pediatric patients have not been established.

Drug Interactions

ACE inhibitors: An increased frequency of symptomatic hypotension was observed with concurrent administration.

Diuretics: Use caution in patients who may have decreased intravascular volume due to diuretic therapy (risk of hypotension and/or renal impairment may be increased). Nesiritide should be avoided in patients with low filling pressures.

Hypotensive agents: Effects on blood pressure are likely to be additive with nesiritide.

Adverse Reactions Note: Frequencies cited below were recorded in VMAC trial at dosages similar to approved labeling. Higher frequencies have been observed in trials using higher dosages of nesiritide.

>10%:

Cardiovascular: Hypotension (total: 11%; symptomatic: 4% at recommended dose, up to 17% at higher doses)

Renal: Increased serum creatinine (28% with >0.5 mg/dL increase over baseline)

1% to 10%:

Cardiovascular: Ventricular tachycardia (3%)*, ventricular extrasystoles (3%)*, angina (2%)*, bradycardia (1%), tachycardia, atrial fibrillation, AV node conduction abnormalities

Central nervous system: Headache (8%)*, dizziness (3%)*, insomnia (2%), anxiety (3%), fever, confusion, paresthesia, somnolence, tremor

Dermatologic: Pruritus, rash

Gastrointestinal: Nausea (4%)*, abdominal pain (1%)*, vomiting (1%)*

Hematologic: Anemia

Local: Injection site reaction

Neuromuscular & skeletal: Back pain (4%), leg cramps

Ocular: Amblyopia

Respiratory: Cough (increased), hemoptysis, apnea

Miscellaneous: Increased diaphoresis

*Frequency less than or equal to placebo or other standard therapy

Overdosage/Toxicology No data. Symptoms of overdose would be expected to include excessive and/or prolonged hypotension. Treatment is symptomatic and supportive. Drug discontinuation and/or dosage reduction may be required.

Dosing

Adults & Elderly:

Congestive heart failure: I.V.: Initial: 2 mcg/kg (bolus); followed by continuous infusion at 0.01 mcg/kg/minute; **Note:** Should not be initiated at a dosage higher than initial recommended dose. At intervals of ≥3 hours, the dosage may be increased by 0.005 mcg/kg/minute (preceded by a bolus of 1 mcg/kg), up to a maximum of 0.03 mcg/kg/minute. Increases beyond the initial infusion rate should be limited to selected patients and accompanied by hemodynamic monitoring.

Patients experiencing hypotension during the infusion: Infusion should be interrupted. May attempt to restart at a lower dose (reduce initial infusion dose by 30% and omit bolus).

Renal Impairment: No adjustment required

Available Dosage Forms Injection, powder for reconstitution: 1.5 mg

Nursing Guidelines

Assessment: Assess potential for interactions with other prescriptions, OTC medications, or herbal products patient may be taking (eg, other hypotensive agents or diuretics). Blood pressure and cardiac function should be monitored before and at frequent intervals during and for 24 hours following infusion (hemodynamic monitoring with larger doses). Assess results of laboratory tests, renal function, and patient response on a regular basis throughout therapy (eg, hypersensitivity, hypotension). Teach patient possible side effects/appropriate interventions and adverse symptoms to report.

Patient Education: This medication can only be administered by infusion; you will be monitored closely during and following infusion. Report immediately any pain, burning, swelling at infusion site, or any signs of allergic reaction (eg, respiratory or swallowing difficulty, back pain, chest tightness, rash, hives, swelling of lips or mouth). Remain in bed until advised otherwise; call for assistance with turning or changing position. Report any chest pain, respiratory difficulty, confusion, nausea, leg cramps, swelling of extremities, sudden or extensive weight gain, or any other adverse effects. **Pregnancy/breast-feeding precautions:** Inform prescriber if you are or intend to become pregnant. Consult prescriber if breast-feeding.

Geriatric Considerations: No specific data to date; elderly are liable to have hypotension, see Warnings/Precautions for blood pressure criteria. Elderly with reduced renal function should be monitored closely.

(Continued)

Nesiritide *(Continued)*

Pregnancy Risk Factor: C

Lactation: Excretion in breast milk unknown/use caution

Administration

I.V.: Do not administer through a heparin-coated catheter (concurrent administration of heparin via a separate catheter is acceptable, per manufacturer).

Reconstitution: Reconstitute 1.5 mg vial with 5 mL of diluent removed from a premixed plastic I.V. bag (compatible with 5% dextrose, 0.9% sodium chloride, 5% dextrose and 0.45% sodium chloride, or 5% dextrose and 0.2% sodium chloride). Do not shake vial to dissolve (roll gently). Withdraw entire contents of vial and add to 250 mL I.V. bag. Resultant concentration of solution approximately 6 mcg/mL.

Compatibility: Incompatible with heparin, insulin, ethacrynate sodium, bumetanide, enalaprilat, hydralazine, and furosemide. Do not administer through the same catheter. Do not administer with any solution containing sodium metabisulfite. Catheter must be flushed between administration of nesiritide and physically incompatible drugs.

Storage: Vials may be stored at controlled room temperature of 20°C to 25°C (68°F to 77 °F) or under refrigeration at 2°C to 8°C (36°F to 46°F). Following reconstitution, vials are stable under these conditions for up to 24 hours.

- **Nestabs® CBF** *see* Vitamins (Multiple/Prenatal) *on page 1721*
- **Nestabs® FA** *see* Vitamins (Multiple/Prenatal) *on page 1721*
- **Nestabs® RX** *see* Vitamins (Multiple/Prenatal) *on page 1721*
- **Neulasta®** *see* Pegfilgrastim *on page 1320*
- **Neupogen®** *see* Filgrastim *on page 726*
- **Neurontin®** *see* Gabapentin *on page 790*
- **Neut®** *see* Sodium Bicarbonate *on page 1542*
- **Neutra-Phos® [OTC]** *see* Potassium Phosphate and Sodium Phosphate *on page 1391*
- **Neutra-Phos®-K [OTC]** *see* Potassium Phosphate *on page 1389*
- **Nexium®** *see* Esomeprazole *on page 647*

Niacin (NYE a sin)

U.S. Brand Names Niacor®; Niaspan®; Slo-Niacin® [OTC]

Synonyms Nicotinic Acid; Vitamin B_3

Pharmacologic Category Antilipemic Agent, Miscellaneous; Vitamin, Water Soluble

Medication Safety Issues

Sound-alike/look-alike issues:

Niacin may be confused with Minocin®, Niaspan®, Nispan®

Niaspan® may be confused with niacin

Nicobid® may be confused with Nitro-Bid®

Use Adjunctive treatment of dyslipidemias (types IIa and IIb or primary hypercholesterolemia) to lower the risk of recurrent MI and/or slow progression of coronary artery disease, including combination therapy with other antidyslipidemic agents when additional triglyceride-lowering or HDL-increasing effects are desired; treatment of hypertriglyceridemia in patients at risk of pancreatitis; treatment of peripheral vascular disease and circulatory disorders; treatment of pellagra; dietary supplement

Mechanism of Action Component of two coenzymes which is necessary for tissue respiration, lipid metabolism, and glycogenolysis; inhibits the synthesis of very low density lipoproteins

Pharmacodynamics/Kinetics

Absorption: Rapid and extensive (60% to 76%)

Distribution: Mainly to hepatic, renal, and adipose tissue

Metabolism: Extensive first-pass effects; converted to nicotinamide adenine dinucleotide, nicotinuric acid, and other metabolites

Half-life elimination: 45 minutes

Time to peak, serum: Immediate release formulation: ~45 minutes; extended release formulation: 4-5 hours

Excretion: Urine 60% to 88% (unchanged drug and metabolites)

Contraindications Hypersensitivity to niacin, niacinamide, or any component of the formulation; active hepatic disease; active peptic ulcer; arterial hemorrhage

Warnings/Precautions Use caution in heavy ethanol users, unstable angina or MI, diabetes (interferes with glucose control), renal disease, active gallbladder disease (can exacerbate), gout, past history of hepatic disease, or with anticoagulants. Monitor glucose and liver function tests. Rare cases of rhabdomyolysis have occurred during concomitant use with HMG-CoA reductase inhibitors. With concurrent use or if symptoms suggestive of myopathy occur, monitor creatinine phosphokinase (CPK) and potassium. Immediate and extended or sustained release products should not be interchanged. Flushing is common and can be attenuated with a gradual increase in dose, and/or by taking aspirin 30-60 minutes before dosing. Compliance is enhanced with twice daily dosing.

Niaspan®: 500 mg and 750 mg tablets are not interchangeable (eg, three 500 mg tablets are not equivalent to two 750 mg tablets).

Nutritional/Herbal/Ethanol Interactions Ethanol: Avoid heavy use; avoid use around niacin dose.

Lab Interactions False elevations in some fluorometric determinations of urinary catecholamines; false-positive urine glucose (Benedict's reagent)

Adverse Reactions Frequency not defined.

Cardiovascular: Arrhythmias, atrial fibrillation, edema, flushing, hypotension, orthostasis, palpitation, syncope (rare), tachycardia

Central nervous system: Chills, dizziness, insomnia, migraine

Dermatologic: Acanthosis nigricans, dry skin, hyperpigmentation, maculopapular rash, pruritus, rash, urticaria

Endocrine & metabolic: Glucose tolerance decreased, gout, phosphorous levels decreased, uric acid level increased

Gastrointestinal: Abdominal pain, dyspepsia, eructation, flatulence, nausea, peptic ulcers, vomiting

Hematologic: Platelet counts decreased, prothrombin time increased

Hepatic: Hepatic necrosis (rare), jaundice, liver enzymes increased

Neuromuscular & skeletal: Leg cramps, myalgia, myasthenia, myopathy (with concurrent HMG-CoA reductase inhibitor), pain, rhabdomyolysis (with concurrent HMG-CoA reductase inhibitor; rare), weakness

Ocular: Cystoid macular edema, toxic amblyopia

Respiratory: Dyspnea

Miscellaneous: Diaphoresis, hypersensitivity reactions (rare)

Overdosage/Toxicology Symptoms of acute overdose include flushing, GI distress, and pruritus. Chronic excessive use has been associated with hepatitis. Antihistamines may relieve niacin-induced histamine release; otherwise treatment is symptomatic.

Dosing

Adults & Elderly:

Recommended daily allowances:

Male: 25-50 years: 19 mg/day; >51 years: 15 mg/day

Female: 25-50 years: 15 mg/day; >51 years: 13 mg/day

Hyperlipidemia: Oral: Usual target dose: 1.5-6 g/day in 3 divided doses with or after meals using a dosage titration schedule; extended release: 375 mg to 2 g once daily at bedtime

Regular release formulation (Niacor®): Initial: 250 mg once daily (with evening meal); increase frequency and/or dose every 4-7 days to desired response or first-level therapeutic dose (1.5-2 g/day in 2-3 divided doses); after 2 months, may increase at 2- to 4-week intervals to 3 g/day in 3 divided doses

Extended release formulation (Niaspan®): 500 mg at bedtime for 4 weeks, then 1 g at bedtime for 4 weeks; adjust dose to response and tolerance; can increase to a maximum of 2 g/day, but only at 500 mg/day at 4-week intervals

Pellagra: Oral: 50-100 mg 3-4 times/day, maximum: 500 mg/day

Niacin deficiency: Oral: 10-20 mg/day, maximum: 100 mg/day

Pediatrics:

Pellagra: Oral: Children: 50-100 mg/dose 3 times/day

Recommended daily allowances:

0-0.5 years: 5 mg/day

0.5-1 year: 6 mg/day

1-3 years: 9 mg/day

4-6 years: 12 mg/day

7-10 years: 13 mg/day

RDA: Children and Adolescents:

Male:

11-14 years: 17 mg/day

15-18 years: 20 mg/day

(Continued)

Niacin *(Continued)*

19-24 years: 19 mg/day

Female: 11-24 years: 15 mg/day

Renal Impairment: Use with caution.

Hepatic Impairment: Not recommended for use in patients with significant or unexplained hepatic dysfunction.

Available Dosage Forms

Capsule, extended release: 125 mg, 250 mg, 400 mg, 500 mg

Capsule, timed release: 250 mg

Tablet: 50 mg, 100 mg, 250 mg, 500 mg

Niacor®: 500 mg

Tablet, controlled release (Slo-Niacin®): 250 mg, 500 mg, 750 mg

Tablet, extended release (Niaspan®): 500 mg, 750 mg, 1000 mg

Note: 500 mg and 750 mg tablets are not interchangeable (eg, three 500 mg tablets are not equivalent to two 750 mg tablets)

Tablet, timed release: 250 mg, 500 mg, 750 mg, 1000 mg

Nursing Guidelines

Assessment: Assess other medications patient may be taking for increased risk of drug/drug interactions. Teach patient appropriate use, interventions to reduce side effects, and adverse symptoms to report.

Monitoring Laboratory Tests: Blood glucose; liver function tests (dyslipidemia, high dose, prolonged therapy) pretreatment and every 6-12 weeks for first year then periodically; lipid profile

Dietary Considerations: Should be taken with meal; low-fat meal if treating hyperlipidemia. Avoid hot drinks around the time of niacin dose.

Patient Education: Take exactly as directed; do not exceed recommended dosage. Take with food to reduce incidence of GI upset. Do not crush sustained release capsules. You may experience flushing, sensation of heat, or headache; these reactions may be decreased by increasing dose slowly or by taking aspirin (consult prescriber) 30 minutes prior to taking niacin. Avoid alcohol or hot drinks around time of taking medication to minimize flushing. Taking at bedtime is also recommended. You may experience dizziness, lightheadedness (use caution when driving or engaging in tasks requiring alertness until response to drug is known). Report persistent GI disturbance or changes in color of urine or stool. **Pregnancy/breast-feeding precautions:** Inform prescriber if you are pregnant. Consult prescriber if breast-feeding

Pregnancy Risk Factor: A/C (dose exceeding RDA recommendation)

Lactation: Enters breast milk/consult prescriber

Administration

Oral: Administer with food. Administer Niaspan® at bedtime. Niaspan® tablet strengths are not interchangeable. When switching from immediate release tablet, initiate Niaspan® at lower dose and titrate. Long-acting forms should not be crushed, broken, or chewed. Do not substitute long-acting forms for immediate release ones.

♦ **Niacor®** *see* Niacin *on page 1218*
♦ **Niaspan®** *see* Niacin *on page 1218*

NiCARdipine (nye KAR de peen)

U.S. Brand Names Cardene®; Cardene® I.V.; Cardene® SR

Synonyms Nicardipine Hydrochloride

Pharmacologic Category Calcium Channel Blocker

Medication Safety Issues

Sound-alike/look-alike issues:

NiCARdipine may be confused with niacinamide, NIFEdipine, nimodipine

Cardene® may be confused with Cardizem®, Cardura®, codeine

Use Chronic stable angina (immediate-release product only); management of essential hypertension (immediate and sustained release; parenteral only for short time that oral treatment is not feasible)

Unlabeled/Investigational Use Congestive heart failure

Mechanism of Action Inhibits calcium ion from entering the "slow channels" or select voltage-sensitive areas of vascular smooth muscle and myocardium during depolarization, producing a relaxation of coronary vascular smooth muscle and coronary vasodilation; increases myocardial oxygen delivery in patients with vasospastic angina

Pharmacodynamics/Kinetics

Onset of action: Oral: 0.5-2 hours; I.V.: 10 minutes; Hypotension: ~20 minutes

Duration: ≤8 hours
Absorption: Oral: ~100%
Protein binding: >95%
Metabolism: Hepatic; CYP3A4 substrate (major); extensive first-pass effect (saturable)
Bioavailability: 35%
Half-life elimination: 2-4 hours
Time to peak, serum: 30-120 minutes
Excretion: Urine (60% as metabolites); feces (35%)

Contraindications Hypersensitivity to nicardipine or any component of the formulation; advanced aortic stenosis; severe hypotension; cardiogenic shock; ventricular tachycardia

Warnings/Precautions Blood pressure lowering should be done at a rate appropriate for the patient's condition. Rapid drops in blood pressure can lead to arterial insufficiency. Use with caution in CAD (can cause increase in angina), CHF (can worsen heart failure symptoms), and pheochromocytoma (limited clinical experience). Peripheral infusion sites (for I.V. therapy) should be changed ever 12 hours. Titrate I.V. dose cautiously in patients with CHF, renal, or hepatic dysfunction. Use the I.V. form cautiously in patients with portal hypertension (can cause increase in hepatic pressure gradient). Safety and efficacy have not been demonstrated in pediatric patients. Abrupt withdrawal may cause rebound angina in patients with CAD.

Drug Interactions **Substrate** of CYP1A2 (minor), 2C8/9 (minor), 2D6 (minor), 2E1 (minor), 3A4 (major); **Inhibits** CYP2C8/9 (strong), 2C19 (moderate), 2D6 (moderate), 3A4 (strong)

Azole antifungals may inhibit the calcium channel blocker's metabolism; avoid this combination. Try an antifungal like terbinafine (if appropriate) or monitor closely for altered effect of the calcium channel blocker.

Calcium may reduce the calcium channel blocker's effects, particularly hypotension.

Cyclosporine's serum concentrations are increased by nicardipine; avoid this combination. Use another calcium channel blocker or monitor cyclosporine trough levels and renal function closely. Tacrolimus may be affected similarly.

CYP2C8/9 substrates: Nicardipine may increase the levels/effects of CYP2C8/9 substrates. Example substrates include amiodarone, fluoxetine, glimepiride, glipizide, nateglinide, phenytoin, pioglitazone, rosiglitazone, sertraline, and warfarin.

CYP2C19 substrates: Nicardipine may increase the levels/effects of CYP2C19 substrates. Example substrates include citalopram, diazepam, methsuximide, phenytoin, propranolol, and sertraline.

CYP2D6 substrates: Nicardipine may increase the levels/effects of CYP2D6 substrates. Example substrates include amphetamines, selected beta-blockers, dextromethorphan, fluoxetine, lidocaine, mirtazapine, nefazodone, paroxetine, risperidone, ritonavir, thioridazine, tricyclic antidepressants, and venlafaxine.

CYP2D6 prodrug substrates: Nicardipine may decrease the levels/effects of CYP2D6 prodrug substrates. Example prodrug substrates include codeine, hydrocodone, oxycodone, and tramadol.

CYP3A4 inducers: CYP3A4 inducers may decrease the levels/effects of nicardipine. Example inducers include aminoglutethimide, carbamazepine, nafcillin, nevirapine, phenobarbital, phenytoin, and rifamycins.

CYP3A4 inhibitors: May increase the levels/effects of nicardipine. Example inhibitors include azole antifungals, clarithromycin, diclofenac, doxycycline, erythromycin, imatinib, isoniazid, nefazodone, propofol, protease inhibitors, quinidine, telithromycin, and verapamil.

CYP3A4 substrates: Nicardipine may increase the levels/effects of CYP3A4 substrates. Example substrates include benzodiazepines, calcium channel blockers, mirtazapine, nateglinide, nefazodone, tacrolimus, and venlafaxine. Selected benzodiazepines (midazolam and triazolam), cisapride, ergot alkaloids, selected HMG-CoA reductase inhibitors (lovastatin and simvastatin), and pimozide are generally contraindicated with strong CYP3A4 inhibitors.

Metoprolol: Concentration of metoprolol is increased by 25% with concurrent use.

Nafcillin decreases plasma concentration of nicardipine; avoid this combination.

Propranolol: May decrease the metabolism of nicardipine.

Protease inhibitor like amprenavir and ritonavir may increase nicardipine's serum concentration.

Rifampin increases the metabolism of the calcium channel blocker; adjust the dose of the calcium channel blocker to maintain efficacy.

(Continued)

NiCARdipine *(Continued)*

Sildenafil, tadalafil, vardenafil: Blood pressure-lowering effects may be additive; use caution.

Vecuronium: Clearance of vecuronium is decreased by 25% with use of I.V. nicardipine; reduce dose of muscle relaxant.

Nutritional/Herbal/Ethanol Interactions

Ethanol: Avoid ethanol (may increase CNS depression).

Food: Nicardipine average peak concentrations may be decreased if taken with food. Serum concentrations/toxicity of nicardipine may be increased by grapefruit juice; avoid concurrent use.

Herb/Nutraceutical: St John's wort may decrease levels. Avoid dong quai if using for hypertension (has estrogenic activity). Avoid ephedra, yohimbe, ginseng (may worsen hypertension). Avoid garlic (may have increased antihypertensive effect).

Adverse Reactions

1% to 10%:

Cardiovascular: Flushing (6% to 10%), palpitation (3% to 4%), tachycardia (1% to 3%), peripheral edema (dose related 7% to 8%), increased angina (dose related 5.6%)

Central nervous system: Headache (6% to 8%), dizziness (4% to 7%), somnolence (4% to 6%), paresthesia (1%)

Dermatologic: Rash (1%)

Gastrointestinal: Nausea (2% to 5%), dry mouth (1%)

Neuromuscular & skeletal: Weakness (4% to 6%), myalgia (1%)

<1% (Limited to important or life-threatening): Abnormal ECG, dyspnea, gingival hyperplasia, nervousness, parotitis, sustained tachycardia, syncope

Overdosage/Toxicology The primary cardiac symptoms of calcium blocker overdose include hypotension and bradycardia. Noncardiac symptoms include confusion, stupor, nausea, vomiting, metabolic acidosis, and hyperglycemia. Following initial gastric decontamination, if possible, repeated calcium administration may promptly reverse the depressed cardiac contractility (but not sinus node depression or peripheral vasodilation). Glucagon and epinephrine may treat refractory hypotension. Glucagon and epinephrine also increase the heart rate (outside the U.S., 4-aminopyridine may be available as an antidote). Dialysis and hemoperfusion are not effective in enhancing elimination although repeat-dose activated charcoal may serve as an adjunct with sustained-release preparations.

Dosing

Adults & Elderly:

Angina: Immediate release: Oral: 20 mg 3 times/day; usual range: 60-120 mg/day; increase dose at 3-day intervals

Hypertension: Oral:

Immediate release: Initial: 20 mg 3 times/day; usual: 20-40 mg 3 times/day (allow 3 days between dose increases)

Sustained release: Initial: 30 mg twice daily, titrate up to 60 mg twice daily

Note: The total daily dose of immediate-release product may not automatically be equivalent to the daily sustained-release dose; use caution in converting.

Acute hypertension: I.V. (dilute to 0.1 mg/mL): Initial: 5 mg/hour increased by 2.5 mg/hour every 15 minutes to a maximum of 15 mg/hour; consider reduction to 3 mg/hour after response is achieved. Monitor and titrate to lowest dose necessary to maintain stable blood pressure.

Substitution for oral therapy (approximate equivalents):

20 mg every 8 hours oral, equivalent to 0.5 mg/hour I.V. infusion
30 mg every 8 hours oral, equivalent to 1.2 mg/hour I.V. infusion
40 mg every 8 hours oral, equivalent to 2.2 mg/hour I.V. infusion

Renal Impairment: Titrate dose beginning with 20 mg 3 times/day (immediate release) or 30 mg twice daily (sustained release). Specific guidelines for adjustment of I.V. nicardipine are not available, but careful monitoring/adjustment is warranted.

Hepatic Impairment: Starting dose: 20 mg twice daily (immediate release) with titration. Refer to "Note" in adult dosing. Specific guidelines for adjustment of I.V. nicardipine are not available, but careful monitoring/adjustment is warranted.

Available Dosage Forms

Capsule (Cardene®): 20 mg, 30 mg

Capsule, sustained release (Cardene® SR): 30 mg, 45 mg, 60 mg

Injection, solution (Cardene® IV): 2.5 mg/mL (10 mL)

Nursing Guidelines

Assessment: See Contraindications, Warnings/Precautions, and Dosing for use cautions. Assess potential for interactions with other prescriptions, OTC medications, or herbal products patient may be taking (see Drug Interactions). See infusion specifics below; infusion site must be monitored closely to prevent extravasation and peripheral infusion sites (for I.V. therapy) should be changed ever 12 hours. Assess therapeutic effectiveness and adverse response (eg, cardiac status and blood pressure when starting, adjusting dose, or discontinuing - see Adverse Reactions and Overdose/Toxicology). Teach patient proper use, possible side effects/appropriate interventions (eg, orthostatic precautions), and adverse symptoms to report (see Patient Education). Breast-feeding is not recommended.

Patient Education: Inform prescriber of all prescriptions, OTC medications, or herbal products you are taking, and any allergies you have. Do not take any new medication during therapy unless approved by prescriber.

I.V.: Report immediately any swelling, redness, burning, or pain at infusion site.

Oral: Take as directed; do not alter dose or decrease without consulting prescriber. Do not crush or chew sustained release forms; swallow whole. Take with nonfatty food. Avoid caffeine and alcohol. Consult prescriber before increasing exercise routine (decreased angina does not mean it is safe to increase exercise). May cause orthostatic hypotension (change position slowly from sitting or lying to standing, or when climbing stairs); sore mouth (inspect gums for swelling or redness - use soft toothbrush, waxed dental floss, and frequent mouth rinses); dizziness or fatigue (use caution when driving or engaging in tasks that require alertness until response to drug is known); or nausea and dry mouth (small, frequent meals, frequent mouth care, chewing gum, or sucking lozenges may help). Report chest pain, palpitations, rapid heartbeat; swelling of extremities; muscle weakness or pain; respiratory difficulty; or nervousness. **Pregnancy/breast-feeding precautions:** Inform prescriber if you are or intend to become pregnant. Breast-feeding is not recommended.

Geriatric Considerations: Elderly may experience a greater hypotensive response. Constipation may be more of a problem in the elderly.

Pregnancy Risk Factor: C

Lactation: Enters breast milk/not recommended

Perioperative/Anesthesia/Other Concerns: I.V. ampuls must be diluted; dilute each ampul in 240 mL to result in 250 mL of 0.1 mg/mL nicardipine. Nicardipine should be used with caution in patients with heart failure.

Administration

Oral: Do not chew or crush the sustained release formulation, swallow whole. Do not open or cut capsules.

I.V.: Ampuls must be diluted before use. Administer as a slow continuous infusion.

Compatibility: Stable in D_5W with KCl 40 mEq, $D_5{}^1/_2NS$, D_5NS, D_5W, $^1/_2NS$, NS; **incompatible** with sodium bicarbonate 5%, LR

Y-site administration: Incompatible with furosemide, heparin, thiopental

Storage: I.V.: Store at room temperature. Protect from light. Freezing does not affect stability.

Related Information

Postoperative Hypertension *on page 1815*

♦ **Nicardipine Hydrochloride** *see* NiCARdipine *on page 1220*

♦ **NicoDerm® CQ® [OTC]** *see* Nicotine *on page 1223*

♦ **Nicorette® [OTC]** *see* Nicotine *on page 1223*

Nicotine (nik oh TEEN)

U.S. Brand Names Commit™ [OTC]; NicoDerm® CQ® [OTC]; Nicorette® [OTC]; Nicotrol® Inhaler; Nicotrol® NS; Nicotrol® Patch [OTC]

Synonyms Habitrol

Pharmacologic Category Smoking Cessation Aid

Medication Safety Issues

Sound-alike/look-alike issues:

NicoDerm® may be confused with Nitroderm

Nicorette® may be confused with Nordette®

(Continued)

Nicotine *(Continued)*

Transdermal patch may contain conducting metal (eg, aluminum); remove patch prior to MRI.

Use Treatment to aid smoking cessation for the relief of nicotine withdrawal symptoms (including nicotine craving)

Unlabeled/Investigational Use Management of ulcerative colitis (transdermal)

Mechanism of Action Nicotine is one of two naturally-occurring alkaloids which exhibit their primary effects via autonomic ganglia stimulation. The other alkaloid is lobeline which has many actions similar to those of nicotine but is less potent. Nicotine is a potent ganglionic and central nervous system stimulant, the actions of which are mediated via nicotine-specific receptors. Biphasic actions are observed depending upon the dose administered. The main effect of nicotine in small doses is stimulation of all autonomic ganglia; with larger doses, initial stimulation is followed by blockade of transmission. Biphasic effects are also evident in the adrenal medulla; discharge of catecholamines occurs with small doses, whereas prevention of catecholamines release is seen with higher doses as a response to splanchnic nerve stimulation. Stimulation of the central nervous system (CNS) is characterized by tremors and respiratory excitation. However, convulsions may occur with higher doses, along with respiratory failure secondary to both central paralysis and peripheral blockade to respiratory muscles.

Pharmacodynamics/Kinetics

Onset of action: Intranasal: More closely approximate the time course of plasma nicotine levels observed after cigarette smoking than other dosage forms

Duration: Transdermal: 24 hours

Absorption: Transdermal: Slow

Metabolism: Hepatic, primarily to cotinine ($^1/_5$ as active)

Half-life elimination: 4 hours

Time to peak, serum: Transdermal: 8-9 hours

Excretion: Urine

Clearance: Renal: pH dependent

Contraindications Hypersensitivity to nicotine or any component of the formulation; patients who are smoking during the postmyocardial infarction period; patients with life-threatening arrhythmias, or severe or worsening angina pectoris; active temporomandibular joint disease (gum); pregnancy; not for use in nonsmokers

Warnings/Precautions The risk versus the benefits must be weighed for each of these groups: patients with CAD, serious cardiac arrhythmias, vasospastic disease. Use caution in patients with hyperthyroidism, pheochromocytoma, or insulin-dependent diabetes. Use with caution in oropharyngeal inflammation and in patients with history of esophagitis, peptic ulcer, coronary artery disease, vasospastic disease, angina, hypertension, hyperthyroidism, pheochromocytoma, diabetes, severe renal dysfunction, and hepatic dysfunction. The inhaler should be used with caution in patients with bronchospastic disease (other forms of nicotine replacement may be preferred). Transdermal patch may contain conducting metal (eg, aluminum); remove patch prior to MRI. Cautious use of topical nicotine in patients with certain skin diseases. Hypersensitivity to the topical products can occur. Dental problems may be worsened by chewing the gum. Urge patients to stop smoking completely when initiating therapy. Safety and efficacy have not been established in pediatric patients.

Drug Interactions Substrate (minor) of CYP1A2, 2A6, 2B6, 2C8/9, 2C19, 2D6, 2E1, 3A4; **Inhibits** CYP2A6 (weak), 2E1 (weak)

Adenosine: Nicotine increases the hemodynamic and AV blocking effects of adenosine; monitor

Bupropion: Monitor for treatment-emergent hypertension in patients treated with the combination of nicotine patch and bupropion

Cimetidine; May increases nicotine concentrations; therefore, may decrease amount of gum or patches needed

Nutritional/Herbal/Ethanol Interactions Food: Lozenge: Acidic foods/beverages decrease absorption of nicotine.

Adverse Reactions

Chewing gum/lozenge:

>10%:

Cardiovascular: Tachycardia

Central nervous system: Headache (mild)

Gastrointestinal: Nausea, vomiting, indigestion, excessive salivation, belching, increased appetite

Miscellaneous: Mouth or throat soreness, jaw muscle ache, hiccups

1% to 10%:
- Central nervous system: Insomnia, dizziness, nervousness
- Endocrine & metabolic: Dysmenorrhea
- Gastrointestinal: GI distress, eructation
- Neuromuscular & skeletal: Muscle pain
- Respiratory: Hoarseness

<1% (Limited to important or life-threatening): Atrial fibrillation, erythema, hypersensitivity reactions, itching

Transdermal systems:

>10%:
- Central nervous system: Insomnia, abnormal dreams
- Dermatologic: Pruritus, erythema
- Local: Application site reaction
- Respiratory: Rhinitis, cough, pharyngitis, sinusitis

1% to 10%:
- Cardiovascular: Chest pain
- Central nervous system: Dysphoria, anxiety, difficulty concentrating, dizziness, somnolence
- Dermatologic: Rash
- Gastrointestinal: Diarrhea, dyspepsia, nausea, xerostomia, constipation, anorexia, abdominal pain
- Neuromuscular & skeletal: Arthralgia, myalgia

<1% (Limited to important or life-threatening): Atrial fibrillation, hypersensitivity reactions, itching, nervousness, taste perversion, thirst, tremor

Overdosage/Toxicology Symptoms of overdose include nausea, vomiting, abdominal pain, mental confusion, diarrhea, salivation, tachycardia, respiratory and cardiovascular collapse. Treatment is symptomatic and supportive. Remove patch, rinse area with water, and dry. Do not use soap as this may increase absorption.

Dosing

Adults & Elderly:

Tobacco cessation (patients should be advised to completely stop smoking upon initiation of therapy):

Gum: Chew 1 piece of gum when urge to smoke, up to 30 pieces/day; most patients require 10-12 pieces of gum/day

Inhaler: Usually 6 to 16 cartridges per day; best effect was achieved by frequent continuous puffing (20 minutes); recommended duration of treatment is 3 months, after which patients may be weaned from the inhaler by gradual reduction of the daily dose over 6-12 weeks

Lozenge: Patients who smoke their first cigarette within 30 minutes of waking should use the 4 mg strength; otherwise the 2 mg strength is recommended.

Weeks 1-6: One lozenge every 1-2 hours

Weeks 7-9: One lozenge every 2-4 hours

Weeks 10-12: One lozenge every 4-8 hours

Note: Use at least 9 lozenges/day during first 6 weeks to improve chances of quitting; do not use more than one lozenge at a time (maximum: 5 lozenges every 6 hours, 20 lozenges/day)

Spray: 1-2 sprays/hour; do not exceed more than 5 doses (10 sprays) per hour; each dose (2 sprays) contains 1 mg of nicotine. **Warning:** A dose of 40 mg can cause fatalities

Transdermal patch: Apply new patch every 24 hours to nonhairy, clean, dry skin on the upper body or upper outer arm; each patch should be applied to a different site. **Note:** Adjustment may be required during initial treatment (move to higher dose if experiencing withdrawal symptoms; lower dose if side effects are experienced).

Habitrol®, NicoDerm CQ®:

Patients smoking ≥10 cigarettes/day: Begin with step 1 (21 mg/day) for 4-6 weeks, **followed by** step 2 (14 mg/day) for 2 weeks; **finish with** step 3 (7 mg/day) for 2 weeks

Patients smoking <10 cigarettes/day: Begin with step 2 (14 mg/day) for 6 weeks, **followed by** step 3 (7 mg/day) for 2 weeks

Note: Initial starting dose for patients <100 pounds, history of cardiovascular disease: 14 mg/day for 4-6 weeks, **followed by** 7 mg/day for 2-4 weeks

Note: Patients who are receiving >600 mg/day of cimetidine: Decrease to the next lower patch size

Nicotrol®: One patch daily for 6 weeks

(Continued)

Nicotine *(Continued)*

Benefits of use of nicotine transdermal patches beyond 3 months have not been demonstrated

Ulcerative colitis (unlabeled use): Transdermal: Titrated to 22-25 mg/day

Available Dosage Forms

Gum, chewing, as polacrilex: 2 mg (48s, 108s); 4 mg (48s, 108s)

Nicorette®: 2 mg (48s, 50s, 108s, 110s, 168s, 170s, 192s, 200s, 216s); 4 mg (48s, 108s, 168s) [mint, fresh mint, orange, and original flavors]

Lozenge, as polacrilex (Commit™): 2 mg (48s, 72s) [contains phenylalanine 3.4 mg/lozenge; mint flavor]; 4 mg (48s, 72s) [contains phenylalanine 3.4 mg/lozenge; mint flavor]

Oral inhalation system (Nicotrol® Inhaler): 10 mg cartridge [delivering 4 mg nicotine] (168s) [each unit consists of 5 mouthpieces, 28 storage trays each containing 6 cartridges, and 1 storage case]

Patch, transdermal: 7 mg/24 (30s); 14 mg/24 hours (30s); 21 mg/24 hours (30s)

NicoDerm® CQ®: 7 mg/24 hours (14s); 14 mg/24 hours (14s); 21 mg/24 hours (14s) [available in tan or clear patch]

Nicotrol®: 15 mg/16 hours (7s, 14s) [step 1]; 10 mg/16 hours (14s) [step 2]; 5 mg/16 hours (14s) [step 3]

Solution, intranasal spray (Nicotrol® NS): 10 mg/mL (10 mL) [delivers 0.5 mg/spray; 200 sprays]

Nursing Guidelines

Assessment: Monitor cardiac status and vital signs prior to, when beginning, and periodically during therapy. Monitor effectiveness of therapy (according to rationale for therapy), and adverse reactions at beginning and periodically during therapy. Assess knowledge/teach patient appropriate use, interventions to reduce side effects, and adverse symptoms to report for prescribed form of drug. **Pregnancy risk factor D/X:** See Pregnancy Risk Factor for use cautions. Determine that patient is not pregnant before beginning treatment and do not give to women of childbearing age unless female is capable of complying with contraceptive measures.

Dietary Considerations: Each lozenge contains phenylalanine 3.4 mg.

Patient Education: Use exactly as directed; do not use more often than prescribed. Stop smoking completely during therapy. Do not smoke, chew tobacco, use snuff, nicotine gum, or any other form of nicotine. Nicotine overdose could occur.

Gum: Chew slowly for 30 minutes. Discard chewed gum away from access by children.

Lozenge: Allow to dissolve slowly in the mouth. Do not chew or swallow lozenge whole. Avoid food or drink 15 minutes prior to, during, or after lozenge.

Transdermal patch: Follow directions in package for dosing schedule and use. Do not cut patches or wear more than one patch at a time. Remove backing from patch and press immediately on skin. Hold for 10 seconds. Apply to clean, dry skin in different site each day. Do not touch eyes; wash hands after application. You may experience vivid dreams and sleep disturbances, dizziness or lightheadedness (use caution driving or when engaging in tasks requiring alertness until response to drug is known). For nausea, vomiting or GI upset, small frequent meals, chewing gum, and frequent oral care may help. Report persistent vomiting, diarrhea, chills, sweating, chest pain or palpitations, or burning or redness at application site.

Spray: Follow directions in package. Blow nose gently before use. Use 1-2 sprays/hour; do not exceed 5 doses (10 sprays) per hour. Excessive use can result in severe (even life-threatening) reactions. You may experience temporary stinging or burning after spray.

Pregnancy/breast-feeding precautions: Inform prescriber if you are pregnant. Do not get pregnant during or for 1 month following therapy. Consult prescriber for instruction on appropriate contraceptive measures. This drug may cause severe fetal defects. Do not breast-feed.

Geriatric Considerations: Must evaluate benefit in the elderly who may have chronic diseases mentioned (see Warnings/Precautions and Contraindications). The transdermal systems are as effective in the elderly as they are in younger adults; however, complaints of body aches, dizziness, and asthenia were reported more often in the elderly.

Pregnancy Risk Factor: D (transdermal); X (chewing gum)

Lactation: Excretion in breast milk unknown/contraindicated

Administration

Oral:

Gum: Should be chewed slowly to avoid jaw ache and to maximize benefit.

Lozenge: Should not be chewed or swallowed.

Storage: Store inhaler cartridge at room temperature not to exceed 30°C (86°F); protect cartridges from light

♦ **Nicotinic Acid** *see* Niacin *on page 1218*
♦ **Nicotrol® Inhaler** *see* Nicotine *on page 1223*
♦ **Nicotrol® NS** *see* Nicotine *on page 1223*
♦ **Nicotrol® Patch [OTC]** *see* Nicotine *on page 1223*
♦ **Nifediac™ CC** *see* NIFEdipine *on page 1227*
♦ **Nifedical™ XL** *see* NIFEdipine *on page 1227*

NIFEdipine (nye FED i peen)

U.S. Brand Names Adalat® CC; Afeditab™ CR; Nifediac™ CC; Nifedical™ XL; Procardia®; Procardia XL®

Pharmacologic Category Calcium Channel Blocker

Medication Safety Issues

Sound-alike/look-alike issues:

NIFEdipine may be confused with niCARdipine, nimodipine, nisoldipine

Procardia XL® may be confused with Cartia® XT

Use Angina and hypertension (sustained release only), pulmonary hypertension

Mechanism of Action Inhibits calcium ion from entering the "slow channels" or select voltage-sensitive areas of vascular smooth muscle and myocardium during depolarization, producing a relaxation of coronary vascular smooth muscle and coronary vasodilation; increases myocardial oxygen delivery in patients with vasospastic angina

Pharmacodynamics/Kinetics

Onset of action: Immediate release: ~20 minutes

Protein binding (concentration dependent): 92% to 98%

Metabolism: Hepatic to inactive metabolites

Bioavailability: Capsule: 40% to 77%; Sustained release: 65% to 89% relative to immediate release capsules

Half-life elimination: Adults: Healthy: 2-5 hours, Cirrhosis: 7 hours; Elderly: 6.7 hours

Excretion: Urine (as metabolites)

Contraindications Hypersensitivity to nifedipine or any component of the formulation; immediate release preparation for treatment of urgent or emergent hypertension; acute MI

Warnings/Precautions **The use of sublingual short-acting nifedipine in hypertensive emergencies and pseudoemergencies is neither safe nor effective and SHOULD BE ABANDONED!** Serious adverse events (cerebrovascular ischemia, syncope, heart block, stroke, sinus arrest, severe hypotension, acute myocardial infarction, ECG changes, and fetal distress) have been reported in relation to such use.

Blood pressure lowering should be done at a rate appropriate for the patient's condition. Rapid drops in blood pressure can lead to arterial insufficiency. Increased angina and/or MI has occurred with initiation or dosage titration of calcium channel blockers. Severe hypotension may occur in patients taking immediate release nifepine concurrently with beta blockers when undergoing CABG with high dose fentanyl anesthesia. When considering surgery with high dose fentanyl, may consider withdrawing nifedipine (>36 hours) before surgery if possible. Use caution in severe aortic stenosis. Use caution in patients with severe hepatic impairment (may need dosage adjustment). Abrupt withdrawal may cause rebound angina in patients with CAD. Use caution in CHF (may cause worsening of symptoms).

The extended release formulation consists of drug within a nondeformable matrix; following drug release/absorption, the matrix/shell is expelled in the stool. The use of nondeformable products in patients with known stricture/narrowing of the GI tract has been associated with symptoms of obstruction. Avoid grapefruit juice during treatment with nifedipine.

Drug Interactions **Substrate** of CYP2D6 (minor), 3A4 (major); **Inhibits** CYP1A2 (moderate), 2C8/9 (weak), 2D6 (weak), 3A4 (weak)

(Continued)

NIFEdipine *(Continued)*

Alpha 1-blockers: May enhance the effects of calcium channel blockers; monitor blood pressure.

Azole antifungals: May inhibit the calcium channel blocker's metabolism; monitor for the toxic effects of calcium channel blocker and adjust accordingly.

Barbiturates: May increase metabolism of calcium channel blocker. Consider therapy modification.

Calcium may reduce the calcium channel blocker's effects.

Calcium channel blocker (nondihydropyridine): May enhance the hypotensive effects of calcium channel blocker (dihydropyridine).

Carbamazepine: May decrease nifedipine serum concentration.

Cimetidine: May increase nifedipine serum concentrations; monitor for toxic effects of calcium channel blocker or choose an alternative H_2 antagonist.

Cisapride: May increase nifedipine's effects; monitor blood pressure.

Cyclosporine: May decrease metabolism of calcium channel blocker (dihydropyridine); monitor for toxic effects of calcium channel blocker.

CYP1A2 substrates: Nifedipine may increase the levels/effects of CYP1A2 substrates. Example substrates include aminophylline, fluvoxamine, mexiletine, mirtazapine, ropinirole, theophylline, and trifluoperazine.

CYP3A4 inducers: CYP3A4 inducers may decrease the levels/effects of nifedipine. Example inducers include aminoglutethimide, carbamazepine, nafcillin, nevirapine, phenobarbital, phenytoin, and rifamycins.

CYP3A4 inhibitors: May increase the levels/effects of nifedipine. Example inhibitors include azole antifungals, clarithromycin, diclofenac, doxycycline, erythromycin, imatinib, isoniazid, nefazodone, nicardipine, propofol, protease inhibitors, quinidine, telithromycin, and verapamil.

Erythromycin: May increase nifedipine serum concentration; monitor blood pressure and adjust if necessary.

Grapefruit juice increases the bioavailability of nifedipine; avoid grapefruit juice.

Magnesium salts: Concurrent use may enhance the adverse/toxic effects of magnesium and enhance the hypotensive effects of the calcium channel blocker.

Nafcillin decreases plasma concentration of nifedipine; avoid this combination.

Neuromuscular-blocking agent (nondepolarizing): Calcium channel blockers may enhance the neuromuscular blocking effect; monitor.

Phenobarbital reduces the plasma concentration of nifedipine. May require much higher dose of nifedipine.

Phenytoin: May decrease nifedipine serum concentration; monitor and adjust if necessary.

Protease inhibitors like amprenavir and ritonavir may increase nifedipine's serum concentration.

Quinidine's serum concentration is reduced and nifedipine's is increased; adjust doses as needed.

Quinupristin/dalfopristin: May increase nifedipine serum concentration; monitor blood pressure and adjust if necessary.

Rifamycin derivatives: Increase the metabolism of the calcium channel blocker; adjust the dose of the calcium channel blocker to maintain efficacy.

Tacrolimus's serum concentrations are increased by nifedipine; monitor tacrolimus trough levels and renal function closely.

Vincristine's half-life is increased by nifedipine; monitor closely for vincristine dose adjustment.

Nutritional/Herbal/Ethanol Interactions

Ethanol: Avoid ethanol (may increase CNS depression and may increase the effects of nifedipine). Monitor.

Food: Nifedipine serum levels may be decreased if taken with food. Food may decrease the rate but not the extent of absorption of Procardia XL®. Increased therapeutic and vasodilator side effects, including severe hypotension and myocardial ischemia, may occur if nifedipine is taken by patients ingesting grapefruit.

Herb/Nutraceutical: St John's wort may decrease nifedipine levels. Avoid dong quai if using for hypertension (has estrogenic activity). Avoid ephedra, yohimbe, ginseng (may worsen hypertension). Avoid garlic (may have increased antihypertensive effect).

Adverse Reactions

>10%:

Cardiovascular: Flushing (10% to 25%), peripheral edema (dose related 7% to 10%; up to 50%)

Central nervous system: Dizziness/lightheadedness/giddiness (10% to 27%), headache (10% to 23%)
Gastrointestinal: Nausea/heartburn (10% to 11%)
Neuromuscular & skeletal: Weakness (10% to 12%)

≥1% to 10%:
Cardiovascular: Palpitations (≤2% to 7%), transient hypotension (dose related 5%), CHF (2%)
Central nervous system: Nervousness/mood changes (≤2% to 7%), shakiness (≤2%), jitteriness (≤2%), sleep disturbances (≤2%), difficulties in balance (≤2%), fever (≤2%), chills (≤2%)
Dermatologic: Dermatitis (≤2%), pruritus (≤2%), urticaria (≤2%)
Endocrine & metabolic: Sexual difficulties (≤2%)
Gastrointestinal: Diarrhea (≤2%), constipation (≤2%), cramps (≤2%), flatulence (≤2%), gingival hyperplasia (≤10%)
Neuromuscular & skeletal: Muscle cramps/tremor (≤2% to 8%), inflammation (≤2%), joint stiffness (≤2%)
Ocular: Blurred vision (≤2%)
Respiratory: Cough/wheezing (6%), nasal congestion/sore throat (≤2% to 6%), chest congestion (≤2%), dyspnea (≤2%)
Miscellaneous: Diaphoresis (≤2%)

<1% (Limited to important or life-threatening): Agranulocytosis, allergic hepatitis, angina, angioedema, aplastic anemia, arthritis with positive ANA, bezoars (sustained-release preparations), cerebral ischemia, depression, erythema multiforme, erythromelalgia, exfoliative dermatitis, extrapyramidal symptoms, fever, gingival hyperplasia, gynecomastia, leukopenia, memory dysfunction, paranoid syndrome, photosensitivity, purpura, Stevens-Johnson syndrome, syncope, thrombocytopenia, tinnitus, transient blindness

Reported with use of sublingual short-acting nifedipine: Acute MI, cerebrovascular ischemia, ECG changes, fetal distress, heart block, severe hypotension, sinus arrest, stroke, syncope

Overdosage/Toxicology Primary cardiac symptoms of calcium blocker overdose include hypotension and bradycardia. Noncardiac symptoms include confusion, stupor, nausea, vomiting, metabolic acidosis, and hyperglycemia. Following initial gastric decontamination, treat symptomatically.

Dosing

Adults & Elderly:

Hypertension: Oral: Initial: 10 mg 3 times/day as capsules or 30 mg once daily as sustained release

Usual dose: 10-30 mg 3 times/day as capsules or 30-60 mg once daily as sustained release

Maximum: 120-180 mg/day

Note: Adjustment of sustained release formulations should be made at 7- to 14-day intervals

Pediatrics:

Hypertrophic cardiomyopathy (unlabeled use): Oral: Children: 0.6-0.9 mg/kg/24 hours in 3-4 divided doses

Hypertension: Oral: Adolescents: Refer to adult dosing.

Hepatic Impairment: Reduce oral dose by 50% to 60% in patients with cirrhosis.

Available Dosage Forms

Capsule, softgel: 10 mg, 20 mg
Procardia®: 10 mg

Tablet, extended release: 30 mg, 60 mg, 90 mg
Adalat® CC, Procardia XL®: 30 mg, 60 mg, 90 mg
Afeditab™ CR, Nifedical™ XL: 30 mg, 60 mg
Nifediac™ CC: 30 mg, 60 mg, 90 mg [90 mg tablet contains tartrazine]

Nursing Guidelines

Assessment: Use caution in severe aortic stenosis or severe hepatic impairment. Assess potential for interactions with other pharmacological agents or herbal products patient is taking that may increase risk of hypotension and toxicity. Assess therapeutic effectiveness (blood pressure and cardiac status) and adverse reactions (eg, hypotension, peripheral edema, gastrointestinal upset, CNS changes) when starting, adjusting dose, or discontinuing. Teach patient proper use, possible side effects/appropriate interventions (eg, orthostatic precautions), and adverse symptoms to report (refer to Patient Education).

(Continued)

NIFEdipine *(Continued)*

Dietary Considerations: Capsule is rapidly absorbed orally if it is administered without food, but may result in vasodilator side effects; administration with low-fat meals may decrease flushing. Avoid grapefruit juice.

Patient Education: Inform prescriber of all prescriptions, OTC medications, or herbal products you are taking, and any allergies you have. Do not take any new medication during therapy unless approved by prescriber. Take as directed; do not alter dose or decrease without consulting prescriber. Do not crush or chew sustained release forms, swallow whole. Take with nonfatty food. Avoid caffeine, alcohol, and grapefruit juice. Consult prescriber before increasing exercise routine (decreased angina does not mean it is safe to increase exercise). May cause orthostatic hypotension (change position slowly from sitting or lying to standing, or when climbing stairs); sore mouth (inspect gums for swelling or redness - use soft toothbrush, waxed dental floss, and frequent mouth rinses); dizziness, difficulties in balance, or fatigue (use caution when driving or engaging in tasks that require alertness until response to drug is known); or nausea or heartburn (small, frequent meals, frequent mouth care, chewing gum, or sucking lozenges may help). Report chest pain, palpitations, rapid heartbeat; swelling of extremities; muscle weakness or pain; respiratory difficulty; nervousness or mood change, rash; or vision changes. **Pregnancy precaution:** Inform prescriber if you are or intend to become pregnant.

Geriatric Considerations: Elderly may experience a greater hypotensive response. Theoretically, constipation may be more of a problem in elderly patients. The half-life of nifedipine is extended in elderly patients (6.7 hours) as compared to younger subjects (3.8 hours).

Pregnancy Risk Factor: C

Pregnancy Issues: Hypotension, IUGR reported. IUGR probably related to maternal hypertension. May exhibit tocolytic effects.

Lactation: Enters breast milk/compatible

Breast-Feeding Considerations: Crosses into breast milk. Available evidence suggests safe use during breast-feeding. AAP considers **compatible** with breast-feeding.

Perioperative/Anesthesia/Other Concerns: Considerable attention has been directed to potential increases in mortality and morbidity when short-acting nifedipine is used in treating hypertension. The rapid reduction in blood pressure may precipitate adverse cardiovascular events. At this time, there is no indication for the use of short-acting calcium channel blocker therapy for angina and hypertension. Nifedipine also has potent negative inotropic effects and can worsen heart failure.

Administration

Oral: Extended release tablets should be swallowed whole; do not crush or chew.

- ♦ **Niferex®-PN** *see* Vitamins (Multiple/Prenatal) *on page 1721*
- ♦ **Niferex®-PN Forte** *see* Vitamins (Multiple/Prenatal) *on page 1721*
- ♦ **Nimbex®** *see* Cisatracurium *on page 409*
- ♦ **Niravam™** *see* Alprazolam *on page 110*

Nisoldipine (NYE sole di peen)

U.S. Brand Names Sular®

Pharmacologic Category Calcium Channel Blocker

Medication Safety Issues

Sound-alike/look-alike issues:

Nisoldipine may be confused with NIFEdipine

Use Management of hypertension, alone or in combination with other antihypertensive agents

Mechanism of Action As a dihydropyridine calcium channel blocker, structurally similar to nifedipine, nisoldipine impedes the movement of calcium ions into vascular smooth muscle and cardiac muscle. Dihydropyridines are potent vasodilators and are not as likely to suppress cardiac contractility and slow cardiac conduction as other calcium antagonists such as verapamil and diltiazem; nisoldipine is 5-10 times as potent a vasodilator as nifedipine.

Pharmacodynamics/Kinetics

Duration: >24 hours

Absorption: Well absorbed

Protein binding: >99%

Metabolism: Extensively hepatic; 1 active metabolite (10% of parent); first-pass effect

Bioavailability: 5%

Half-life elimination: 7-12 hours

Time to peak: 6-12 hours

Excretion: Urine (as metabolites)

Contraindications Hypersensitivity to nisoldipine, any component of the formulation, or other dihydropyridine calcium channel blockers

Warnings/Precautions Increased angina and/or myocardial infarction in patients with coronary artery disease. Use with caution in patients with hypotension, CHF, and hepatic impairment. Blood pressure lowering must be done at a rate appropriate for the patient's condition.

Drug Interactions **Substrate** of CYP3A4 (major); **Inhibits** CYP1A2 (weak), 3A4 (weak)

Azole antifungals may inhibit the calcium channel blocker's metabolism; avoid this combination. Try an antifungal like terbinafine (if appropriate) or monitor closely for altered effect of the calcium channel blocker.

Beta-blockers may have increased pharmacokinetic or pharmacodynamic interactions with nisoldipine.

Calcium may reduce the calcium channel blocker's effects, particularly hypotension.

CYP3A4 inducers: CYP3A4 inducers may decrease the levels/effects of nisoldipine. Example inducers include aminoglutethimide, carbamazepine, nafcillin, nevirapine, phenobarbital, phenytoin, and rifamycins.

CYP3A4 inhibitors: May increase the levels/effects of nisoldipine. Example inhibitors include azole antifungals, clarithromycin, diclofenac, doxycycline, erythromycin, imatinib, isoniazid, nefazodone, nicardipine, propofol, protease inhibitors, quinidine, telithromycin, and verapamil.

Grapefruit juice increases the bioavailability of nisoldipine; monitor for altered nisoldipine effects.

Phenytoin decreases nisoldipine to undetectable levels. Avoid use of any CYP3A4 inducer with nisoldipine.

Rifampin increases the metabolism of the calcium channel blocker; adjust the dose of the calcium channel blocker to maintain efficacy.

Sildenafil, tadalafil, vardenafil: Blood pressure-lowering effects may be additive; use caution.

Nutritional/Herbal/Ethanol Interactions

Food: Nisoldipine bioavailability may be increased if taken with high-lipid foods or with grapefruit juice. Avoid grapefruit products before and after dosing.

Herb/Nutraceutical: St John's wort may decrease nisoldipine levels. Avoid dong quai if using for hypertension (has estrogenic activity). Avoid ephedra, yohimbe, ginseng (may worsen hypertension). Avoid garlic (may have increased antihypertensive effect).

Adverse Reactions

>10%:

- Cardiovascular: Peripheral edema (dose related 7% to 29%)
- Central nervous system: Headache (22%)

1% to 10%:

- Cardiovascular: Chest pain (2%), palpitation (3%), vasodilation (4%)
- Central nervous system: Dizziness (3% to 10%)
- Dermatologic: Rash (2%)
- Gastrointestinal: Nausea (2%)
- Respiratory: Pharyngitis (5%), sinusitis (3%), dyspnea (3%), cough (5%)

<1% (Limited to important or life-threatening): Alopecia, amblyopia, angina, anxiety, ataxia, atrial fibrillation, cerebral ischemia, cholestatic jaundice, confusion, CHF, depression, dyspnea, exfoliative dermatitis, first-degree AV block, GI hemorrhage, gingival hyperplasia, gout, impotence, leukopenia, migraine, myasthenia, MI, paresthesia, pruritus, pulmonary edema, rash, somnolence, stroke, supraventricular tachycardia, syncope, temporary unilateral loss of vision, tinnitus, T-wave abnormalities on ECG (flattening, inversion, nonspecific changes), urticaria, vaginal hemorrhage, ventricular extrasystoles, vertigo

Overdosage/Toxicology Primary cardiac symptoms of calcium blocker overdose include hypotension and bradycardia. Noncardiac symptoms include confusion, stupor, nausea, vomiting, metabolic acidosis and hyperglycemia. Treat symptomatically.

(Continued)

Nisoldipine *(Continued)*

Dosing

Adults:

Hypertension: Oral: Initial: 20 mg once daily, then increase by 10 mg/week (or longer intervals) to attain adequate control of blood pressure

Usual dose range (JNC 7): 10-40 mg once daily; doses >60 mg once daily are not recommended.

Elderly: Initial dose: 10 mg/day, increase by 10 mg/week (or longer intervals) to attain adequate blood pressure control. Those with hepatic disease should be started with 10 mg/day.

Hepatic Impairment: A starting dose not exceeding 10 mg/day is recommended for patients with hepatic impairment.

Available Dosage Forms Tablet, extended release: 10 mg, 20 mg, 30 mg, 40 mg

Nursing Guidelines

Assessment: See Contraindications, Warnings/Precautions, and Dosing for use cautions. Assess potential for interactions with other prescriptions, OTC medications, or herbal products patient may be taking (eg, other antihypertensives - see Drug Interactions). Assess therapeutic effectiveness and adverse response (eg, cardiac status and blood pressure when starting or adjusting dose and periodically during long-term therapy - see Adverse Reactions and Overdose/Toxicology). Taper dose gradually (over 2 weeks) when discontinuing. Teach patient proper use, possible side effects/appropriate interventions, and adverse symptoms to report (see Patient Education). Note breast-feeding caution.

Patient Education: Inform prescriber of all prescriptions, OTC medications, or herbal products you are taking, and any allergies you have. Do not take any new medication during therapy unless approved by prescriber. Take exactly as directed; do not alter dose or decrease without consulting prescriber. Do not crush or chew capsules; swallow whole. Take with food, but avoid fatty food and grapefruit juice. This drug does not replace diet and other exercise recommendations of prescriber. May cause orthostatic hypotension (change position slowly when rising from sitting or lying, or when climbing stairs); headache (consult prescriber for approved analgesic); dizziness (use caution when driving or engaging in tasks that require alertness until response to drug is known); or nausea (small, frequent meals, frequent mouth care, chewing gum, or sucking lozenges may help). Report chest pain, palpitations, irregular heartbeat; respiratory difficulty; unusual cough; rash; vision changes; anxiety, confusion, depression, or other CNS changes; or other persistent adverse reactions. **Pregnancy/breast-feeding precautions:** Inform prescriber if you are or intend to become pregnant. Consult prescriber if breast-feeding.

Geriatric Considerations: Elderly may experience a greater hypotensive response. Constipation may be more of a problem in the elderly. Calcium channel blockers are no more effective in the elderly than other therapies; however, they do not cause significant CNS effects which is an advantage over some antihypertensive agents.

Pregnancy Risk Factor: C

Lactation: Excretion in breast milk unknown

Administration

Oral: Administer at the same time each day to ensure minimal fluctuation of serum levels. Avoid high-fat diet.

♦ **Nitalapram** *see* Citalopram *on page 416*
♦ **Nitrek®** *see* Nitroglycerin *on page 1234*
♦ **Nitro-Bid®** *see* Nitroglycerin *on page 1234*
♦ **Nitro-Dur®** *see* Nitroglycerin *on page 1234*

Nitrofurantoin (nye troe fyoor AN toyn)

U.S. Brand Names Furadantin®; Macrobid®; Macrodantin®

Pharmacologic Category Antibiotic, Miscellaneous

Use Prevention and treatment of urinary tract infections caused by susceptible gram-negative and some gram-positive organisms; *Pseudomonas*, *Serratia*, and most species of *Proteus* are generally resistant to nitrofurantoin

Mechanism of Action Inhibits several bacterial enzyme systems including acetyl coenzyme A interfering with metabolism and possibly cell wall synthesis

Pharmacodynamics/Kinetics

Absorption: Well absorbed; macrocrystalline form absorbed more slowly due to slower dissolution (causes less GI distress)

Distribution: V_d: 0.8 L/kg; crosses placenta; enters breast milk

Protein binding: 60% to 90%

Metabolism: Body tissues (except plasma) metabolize 60% of drug to inactive metabolites

Bioavailability: Increased with food

Half-life elimination: 20-60 minutes; prolonged with renal impairment

Excretion:

Suspension: Urine (40%) and feces (small amounts) as metabolites and unchanged drug

Macrocrystals: Urine (20% to 25% as unchanged drug)

Contraindications Hypersensitivity to nitrofurantoin or any component of the formulation; renal impairment (anuria, oliguria, significantly elevated serum creatinine, or Cl_{cr}< 60 mL/minute); infants <1 month (due to the possibility of hemolytic anemia); pregnancy at term (38-42 weeks gestation), during labor and delivery, or when the onset of labor is imminent

Warnings/Precautions Use with caution in patients with G6PD deficiency or in patients with anemia. Therapeutic concentrations of nitrofurantoin are not attained in urine of patients with Cl_{cr}<60 mL/minute. Use with caution if prolonged therapy is anticipated due to possible pulmonary toxicity. Acute, subacute, or chronic (usually after 6 months of therapy) pulmonary reactions have been observed in patients treated with nitrofurantoin; if these occur, discontinue therapy immediately; monitor closely for malaise, dyspnea, cough, fever, radiologic evidence of diffuse interstitial pneumonitis or fibrosis. Rare, but severe hepatic reactions have been associated with nitrofurantoin (onset may be insidious); discontinue immediately if hepatitis occurs. Has been associated with peripheral neuropathy (rare); risk may be increased by renal impairment, diabetes, vitamin B deficiency, or electrolyte imbalance; use caution.

Drug Interactions

Decreased effect: Antacids, especially magnesium salts, decrease absorption of nitrofurantoin; nitrofurantoin may antagonize effects of norfloxacin

Increased toxicity: Probenecid (decreases renal excretion of nitrofurantoin); anticholinergic drugs increase absorption of nitrofurantoin

Nutritional/Herbal/Ethanol Interactions

Ethanol: Avoid ethanol (may increase CNS depression).

Food: Nitrofurantoin serum concentrations may be increased if taken with food.

Lab Interactions False-positive urine glucose (Benedict's and Fehling's methods); no false positives with enzymatic tests

Adverse Reactions Frequency not defined.

Cardiovascular: Chest pain, cyanosis, ECG changes (associated with pulmonary toxicity)

Central nervous system: Chills, depression, dizziness, drowsiness, fatigue, fever, headache, pseudotumor cerebri, psychotic reaction

Dermatologic: Alopecia, erythema multiforme, exfoliative dermatitis, pruritus, rash, Stevens-Johnson syndrome

Gastrointestinal: Abdominal pain, *C. difficile*-colitis, constipation, diarrhea, dyspepsia, loss of appetite, nausea (most common), pancreatitis, sore throat, vomiting

Hematologic: Agranulocytosis, aplastic anemia, eosinophilia, hemolytic anemia, methemoglobinemia, thrombocytopenia

Hepatic: Cholestasis, hepatitis, hepatic necrosis, transaminases increased, jaundice (cholestatic)

Neuromuscular & skeletal: Arthralgia, numbness, paresthesia, peripheral neuropathy, weakness

Ocular: Amblyopia, nystagmus, optic neuritis (rare)

Respiratory: Cough, dyspnea, pneumonitis, pulmonary fibrosis

Miscellaneous: Hypersensitivity (including acute pulmonary hypersensitivity), lupus-like syndrome

Overdosage/Toxicology Symptoms of overdose include vomiting. Treatment is supportive.

Dosing

Adults:

Treatment of UTI: Oral: 50-100 mg/dose every 6 hours (not to exceed 400 mg/24 hours)

Prophylaxis of UTI: Oral: 50-100 mg/dose at bedtime

(Continued)

Nitrofurantoin *(Continued)*

Elderly: Refer to adult dosing (see Geriatric Considerations).

Pediatrics:

Treatment of UTI: Oral: Children >1 month: 5-7 mg/kg/day in divided doses every 6 hours; maximum: 400 mg/day

Chronic therapy: Oral: 1-2 mg/kg/day in divided doses every 12-24 hours; maximum: 100 mg/day

Renal Impairment:

Cl_{cr} <60 mL/minute: Contraindicated

Contraindicated in hemo- and peritoneal dialysis and continuous arteriovenous or venovenous hemofiltration.

Available Dosage Forms

Capsule, macrocrystal: 50 mg, 100 mg

Macrodantin®: 25 mg, 50 mg, 100 mg

Capsule, macrocrystal/monohydrate (Macrobid®): 100 mg

Suspension, oral (Furadantin®): 25 mg/5 mL (470 mL)

Nursing Guidelines

Assessment: See Contraindications, Warnings/Precautions, and Drug interactions for use cautions. Assess results of laboratory tests (see below), therapeutic effectiveness, and adverse response (see Adverse Reactions and Overdose/Toxicology). Advise patients with diabetes about use of Clinitest® (may cause false-positive urine glucose). Teach patient proper use, possible side effects/appropriate interventions, and adverse symptoms to report (see Patient Education).

Monitoring Laboratory Tests: CBC, periodic liver function. Perform culture and sensitivity prior to initiating therapy.

Patient Education: Inform prescriber of all prescriptions, OTC medications, or herbal products you are taking, and any allergies you have. Do not take any new medication during therapy unless approved by prescriber. Take entire prescription, even if you are feeling better. Take with food. Maintain adequate hydration (2-3 L/day of fluids) unless instructed to restrict fluid intake. If you have diabetes, drug may cause false test results with Clinitest® urine glucose monitoring; use of another type of glucose monitoring is preferable. May cause nausea or vomiting (small, frequent meals, frequent mouth care, sucking lozenges, or chewing gum may help); or diarrhea (buttermilk, boiled milk, or yogurt may help). Report immediately and rash; swelling of face, tongue, mouth, or throat; or chest tightness. Report if condition being treated worsens or does not improve by the time prescription is completed.

Geriatric Considerations: Because of nitrofurantoin's decreased efficacy in patients with a Cl_{cr} <60 mL/minute and its side effect profile, it is not an antibiotic of choice for acute or prophylactic treatment of urinary tract infections in the elderly. An increased rate of severe hepatic toxicity has been suggested by postmarketing reports.

Pregnancy Risk Factor: B (contraindicated at term)

Pregnancy Issues: Teratogenic effects have not been observed, however may cause hemolytic anemia in infants. Use of nitrofurantoin is contraindicated at term (38-42 weeks gestation), during labor and delivery, or when the onset of labor is imminent.

Lactation: Enters breast milk/not recommended (infants <1 month); AAP rates "compatible"

Breast-Feeding Considerations: Excreted in trace amounts in breast milk; may cause hyperbilirubinemia or hemolytic anemia in infants (<1 month of age). AAP rates "compatible." Use caution in G6PD deficiency.

Administration

Oral: Suspension: Shake well before use. Higher peak serum levels may cause increased GI upset. Give with meals to slow the rate of absorption and decrease adverse effects.

Storage: Store at room temperature 15°C to 30°C (59°F to 86°F).

Nitroglycerin (nye troe GLI ser in)

U.S. Brand Names Minitran™; Nitrek®; Nitro-Bid®; Nitro-Dur®; Nitrolingual®; Nitro-Quick®; Nitrostat®; Nitro-Tab®; NitroTime®

Synonyms Glyceryl Trinitrate; Nitroglycerol; NTG

Pharmacologic Category Vasodilator

Medication Safety Issues

Sound-alike/look-alike issues:

Nitroglycerin may be confused with nitroprusside
Nitro-Bid® may be confused with Nicobid®
Nitroderm may be confused with NicoDerm®
Nitrol® may be confused with Nizoral®
Nitrostat® may be confused with Hyperstat®, Nilstat®, nystatin

Nitroglycerin transdermal patches should be removed prior to defibrillation or MRI study.

Use Treatment of angina pectoris; I.V. for congestive heart failure (especially when associated with acute myocardial infarction); pulmonary hypertension; hypertensive emergencies occurring perioperatively (especially during cardiovascular surgery)

Unlabeled/Investigational Use Esophageal spastic disorders (sublingual)

Mechanism of Action Works by relaxation of smooth muscle, producing a vasodilator effect on the peripheral veins and arteries with more prominent effects on the veins. Primarily reduces cardiac oxygen demand by decreasing preload (left ventricular end-diastolic pressure); may modestly reduce afterload; dilates coronary arteries and improves collateral flow to ischemic regions

Pharmacodynamics/Kinetics

Onset of action: Sublingual tablet: 1-3 minutes; Translingual spray: 2 minutes; Sustained release: 20-45 minutes; Topical: 15-60 minutes; Transdermal: 40-60 minutes; I.V. drip: Immediate

Peak effect: Sublingual tablet: 4-8 minutes; Translingual spray: 4-10 minutes; Sustained release: 45-120 minutes; Topical: 30-120 minutes; Transdermal: 60-180 minutes; I.V. drip: Immediate

Duration: Sublingual tablet: 30-60 minutes; Translingual spray: 30-60 minutes; Sustained release: 4-8 hours; Topical: 2-12 hours; Transdermal: 18-24 hours; I.V. drip: 3-5 minutes

Protein binding: 60%

Metabolism: Extensive first-pass effect

Half-life elimination: 1-4 minutes

Excretion: Urine (as inactive metabolites)

Contraindications Hypersensitivity to organic nitrates; hypersensitivity to isosorbide, nitroglycerin, or any component of the formulation; concurrent use with phosphodiesterase-5 (PDE-5) inhibitors (sildenafil, tadalafil, or vardenafil); angle-closure glaucoma (intraocular pressure may be increased); head trauma or cerebral hemorrhage (increase intracranial pressure); severe anemia; allergy to adhesive (transdermal product)

Additional contraindications for I.V. product: Hypotension; uncorrected hypovolemia; inadequate cerebral circulation; constrictive pericarditis; pericardial tamponade

Warnings/Precautions Severe hypotension can occur. Use with caution in volume depletion, hypotension, and right ventricular infarctions. Paradoxical bradycardia and increased angina pectoris can accompany hypotension. Orthostatic hypotension can also occur. Ethanol can accentuate this. Tolerance does develop to nitrates and appropriate dosing is needed to minimize this (drug-free interval). Safety and efficacy have not been established in pediatric patients. Avoid use of long-acting agents in acute MI or CHF; cannot easily reverse. Nitrate may aggravate angina caused by hypertrophic cardiomyopathy. Nitroglycerin transdermal patches should be removed prior to defibrillation or MRI study.

Drug Interactions

Alteplase (tissue plasminogen activator) has a lesser effect when used with I.V. nitroglycerin; avoid concurrent use.

Ergot alkaloids may cause an increase in blood pressure and decrease in antianginal effects; avoid concurrent use.

Ethanol can cause hypotension when nitrates are taken 1 hour or more after ethanol ingestion.

Heparin's effect may be reduced by I.V. nitroglycerin. May affect only a minority of patients.

Sildenafil, tadalafil, vardenafil: Significant reduction of systolic and diastolic blood pressure with concurrent use (contraindicated). Do not administer sildenafil, tadalafil, or vardenafil within 24 hours of a nitrate preparation.

(Continued)

Nitroglycerin *(Continued)*

Adverse Reactions

Spray or patch:

>10%: Central nervous system: Headache (patch 63%, spray 50%)

1% to 10%:

Cardiovascular: Hypotension (patch 4%), increased angina (patch 2%), syncope (patch 4%)

Central nervous system: Lightheadedness (patch 6%)

<1% (Limited to important or life-threatening): Allergic reactions, application site irritation (patch), collapse, dizziness, exfoliative dermatitis, methemoglobinemia (rare, overdose), pallor, palpitation, perspiration, rash, restlessness, vertigo, weakness

Topical, sublingual, intravenous: Frequency not defined:

Cardiovascular: Hypotension (infrequent), postural hypotension, crescendo angina (uncommon), rebound hypertension (uncommon), pallor, cardiovascular collapse, tachycardia, shock, flushing, peripheral edema

Central nervous system: Headache (most common), lightheadedness (related to blood pressure changes), syncope (uncommon), dizziness, restlessness

Gastrointestinal: Nausea, vomiting, bowel incontinence, xerostomia

Genitourinary: Urinary incontinence

Hematologic: Methemoglobinemia (rare, overdose)

Neuromuscular & skeletal: Weakness

Ocular: Blurred vision

Miscellaneous: Cold sweat

Overdosage/Toxicology Symptoms of overdose include hypotension, throbbing headache, palpitations, bloody diarrhea, bradycardia, cyanosis, tissue hypoxia, metabolic acidosis, clonic convulsions, circulatory collapse, and methemoglobinemia with extremely large overdoses. Treatment is supportive and symptomatic. Methemoglobinemia should be treated with methylene blue (1-2 mg/kg over 5 minutes). Additional doses may be necessary (0.5-1 mg/kg) based on follow-up methemoglobin levels (obtained after 30 minutes).

Dosing

Adults & Elderly: Note: Hemodynamic and antianginal tolerance often develop within 24-48 hours of continuous nitrate administration. Nitrate-free interval (10-12 hours/day) is recommended to avoid tolerance development; gradually decrease dose in patients receiving NTG for prolonged period to avoid withdrawal reaction.

Angina/coronary artery disease:

Oral: 2.5-9 mg 2-4 times/day (up to 26 mg 4 times/day)

I.V.: 5 mcg/minute, increase by 5 mcg/minute every 3-5 minutes to 20 mcg/minute. If no response at 20 mcg/minute increase by 10 mcg/minute every 3-5 minutes, up to 200 mcg/minute.

Topical ointment: Include a nitrate free interval, ~10 to 12 hours; Apply 0.5" to 2" every 6 hours with a nitrate free interval.

Topical patch, transdermal: 0.2-0.4 mg/hour initially and titrate to doses of 0.4-0.8 mg/hour. Tolerance is minimized by using a patch-on period of 12-14 hours and patch-off period of 10-12 hours.

Sublingual: 0.2-0.6 mg every 5 minutes for maximum of 3 doses in 15 minutes; may also use prophylactically 5-10 minutes prior to activities which may provoke an attack.

Esophageal spastic disorders (unlabeled use): 0.3-0.4 mg 5 minutes before meals

Translingual: 1-2 sprays into mouth under tongue every 3-5 minutes for maximum of 3 doses in 15 minutes, may also be used 5-10 minutes prior to activities which may provoke an attack prophylactically.

Pediatrics:

Pulmonary hypertension: I.V. Continuous infusion: Children: Start 0.25-0.5 mcg/kg/minute and titrate by 1 mcg/kg/minute at 20- to 60-minute intervals to desired effect; usual dose: 1-3 mcg/kg/minute; maximum: 5 mcg/kg/minute

Note: Hemodynamic and antianginal tolerance often develop within 24-48 hours of continuous nitrate administration.

Available Dosage Forms

Capsule, extended release (Nitro-Time®): 2.5 mg, 6.5 mg, 9 mg

Infusion [premixed in D_5W]: 25 mg (250 mL) [0.1 mg/mL]; 50 mg (250 mL) [0.2 mg/mL]; 50 mg (500 mL) [0.1 mg/mL]; 100 mg (250 mL) [0.4 mg/mL]; 200 mg (500 mL) [0.4 mg/mL]

Injection, solution: 5 mg/mL (5 mL, 10 mL) [contains alcohol and propylene glycol]

Ointment, topical (Nitro-Bid®): 2% [20 mg/g] (1 g, 30 g, 60 g)

Solution, translingual spray (Nitrolingual®): 0.4 mg/metered spray (4.9 g) [contains alcohol 20%; 60 metered sprays]; (12 g) [contains alcohol 20%; 200 metered sprays]

Tablet, sublingual (NitroQuick®, Nitrostat®, Nitro-Tab®): 0.3 mg, 0.4 mg, 0.6 mg

Transdermal system [once daily patch]: 0.1 mg/hour (30s); 0.2 mg/hour (30s); 0.4 mg/hour (30s); 0.6 mg/hour (30s)

Minitran™: 0.1 mg/hour (30s); 0.2 mg/hour (30s); 0.4 mg/hour (30s); 0.6 mg/hour (30s)

Nitrek®: 0.2 mg/hour (30s); 0.4 mg/hour (30s); 0.6 mg/hour (30s)

Nitro-Dur®: 0.1 mg/hour (30s); 0.2 mg/hour (30s); 0.3 mg/hour (30s); 0.4 mg/hour (30s); 0.6 mg/hour (30s); 0.8 mg/hour (30s)

Nursing Guidelines

Assessment: See Contraindications, Warnings/Precautions, and Dosing for use cautions. Assess potential for interactions with other prescriptions, OTC medications, or herbal products patient may be taking (see Drug Interactions). See Administration specifics for different formulations below. Assess therapeutic effectiveness (cardiac status) and adverse response (eg, hypotension and arrhythmias - see Adverse Reactions and Overdose/Toxicology). Dose should be reduced gradually when discontinuing after long-term therapy. Teach patient proper use (according to purpose and formulation), possible side effects/appropriate interventions (eg, drug-free intervals), and adverse symptoms to report (see Patient Education). Note breast-feeding caution.

Patient Education: Inform prescriber of all prescriptions, OTC medications, or herbal products you are taking, and any allergies you have. Do not take any new medication during therapy unless approved by prescriber. Take as per directions (see below). Do not change brands without consulting prescriber. Do not discontinue abruptly. Keep medication in original container, tightly closed. If anginal chest pain is unresolved in 15 minutes, seek emergency medical help at once. Daily use may cause dizziness or lightheadedness (use caution when driving or engaging in hazardous activities until response to drug is known); headache (consult prescriber for approved analgesic); hypotension (use care when changing position from sitting or lying to standing, when climbing stairs or when engaging in tasks that are potentially hazardous until response to drug is known); GI disturbances (small, frequent meals, frequent mouth care, chewing gum, or sucking lozenges may help). Report acute headache, rapid heartbeat, unusual restlessness or dizziness, muscular weakness, or blurred vision or seeing abnormal colors. **Pregnancy/breast-feeding precautions:** Inform prescriber if you are or intend to become pregnant. Consult prescriber if breast-feeding.

Oral: Take as directed. Do not chew or swallow sublingual tablets; allow to dissolve under tongue. Sit down before using sublingual or buccal tablet or spray form. Do not chew or crush extended release capsules; swallow with 8 oz of water.

Spray: Spray directly on mucous membranes; do not inhale.

Topical: Spread prescribed amount thinly on applicator; rotate application sites.

Transdermal: Use as directed; place on hair-free area of skin, rotate sites (usually, patches will be removed for a period each day)

Geriatric Considerations: Caution should be used when using nitrate therapy in the elderly due to hypotension. Hypotension is enhanced in the elderly due to decreased baroreceptor response, decreased venous tone, and often hypovolemia (dehydration) or other hypotensive drugs. Elderly patients may be at greater risk of falling due to nitroglycerin-associated hypotension/orthostasis.

Pregnancy Risk Factor: C

Lactation: Excretion in breast milk unknown/use caution

Perioperative/Anesthesia/Other Concerns: Nitroglycerin 5 mg/mL contains propylene glycol 518 mg/mL (30% v/v).

In the treatment of unstable angina/non-ST-segment elevation MI, nitroglycerin (sublingual tablet or spray), followed by intravenous administration, is recommended for immediate relief of ischemia and associated symptoms. Note that nitrate use may result in significant hypotension in individuals who are volume depleted.

(Continued)

Nitroglycerin *(Continued)*

Nitrate use in right ventricular infarction may induce acute hypotension. Nitrate use in severe pericardial effusion may reduce cardiac filling pressure and precipitate cardiac tamponade.

Administration

Oral: Do not crush sublingual drug product.

I.V.: I.V. must be prepared in glass bottles and use special sets intended for nitroglycerin. glass I.V. bottles and administration sets provided by manufacturer.

Reconstitution: Doses should be made in glass bottles, Excel® or PAB® containers; adsorption occurs to soft plastic (eg, PVC). Nitroglycerin diluted in D_5W or NS in glass containers is physically and chemically stable for 48 hours at room temperature and 7 days under refrigeration. In D_5W or NS in Excel®/PAB® containers is physically and chemically stable for 24 hours at room temperature and 14 days under refrigeration.

Standard diluent: 50 mg/250 mL D_5W; 50 mg/500 mL D_5W

Minimum volume: 100 mg/250 mL D_5W; concentration should not exceed 400 mcg/mL.

Compatibility: Stable in D_5LR, D_5½NS, D_5NS, LR, ½NS

Y-site administration: Incompatible with alteplase, levofloxacin

Compatibility when admixed: Dose is variable and may require titration, therefore it is not advisable to mix with other agents. **Incompatible** with hydralazine, phenytoin

Storage: Doses should be made in glass bottles, Excel® or PAB® containers. Adsorption occurs to soft plastic (eg, PVC). Premixed bottles are stable according to the manufacturer's expiration dating. Store sublingual tablets and ointment in tightly closed containers at 15°C to 30°C. Store spray and transdermal patch at 25°C, excursions permitted to 15°C to 30°C (59°F to 86°F).

Related Information

Postoperative Hypertension *on page 1815*

♦ **Nitroglycerol** *see* Nitroglycerin *on page 1234*
♦ **Nitrolingual®** *see* Nitroglycerin *on page 1234*
♦ **Nitropress®** *see* Nitroprusside *on page 1238*

Nitroprusside (nye troe PRUS ide)

U.S. Brand Names Nitropress®

Synonyms Nitroprusside Sodium; Sodium Nitroferricyanide; Sodium Nitroprusside

Pharmacologic Category Vasodilator

Medication Safety Issues

Sound-alike/look-alike issues:

Nitroprusside may be confused with nitroglycerin

High alert medication: The Institute for Safe Medication Practices (ISMP) includes this medication among its list of drugs which have a heightened risk of causing significant patient harm when used in error.

Use Management of hypertensive crises; congestive heart failure; used for controlled hypotension to reduce bleeding during surgery

Mechanism of Action Causes peripheral vasodilation by direct action on venous and arteriolar smooth muscle, thus reducing peripheral resistance; will increase cardiac output by decreasing afterload; reduces aortal and left ventricular impedance

Pharmacodynamics/Kinetics

Onset of action: BP reduction <2 minutes

Duration: 1-10 minutes

Metabolism: Nitroprusside is converted to cyanide ions in the bloodstream; decomposes to prussic acid which in the presence of sulfur donor is converted to thiocyanate (hepatic and renal rhodanase systems)

Half-life elimination: Parent drug: <10 minutes; Thiocyanate: 2.7-7 days

Excretion: Urine (as thiocyanate)

Contraindications Hypersensitivity to nitroprusside or any component of the formulation; treatment of compensatory hypertension (aortic coarctation, arteriovenous shunting); high output failure; congenital optic atrophy or tobacco amblyopia

Warnings/Precautions Except when used briefly or at low (<2 mcg/kg/minute) infusion rates, nitroprusside gives rise to large cyanide quantities. Do not use the maximum dose for more than 10 minutes. Use with extreme caution in patients with elevated intracranial pressure. Use extreme caution in patients with hepatic or renal dysfunction. Watch for cyanide toxicity in patients with impaired hepatic function. Use the lowest end of the dosage range with renal impairment. Thiocyanate toxicity occurs in patients with renal impairment or those on prolonged infusions. Continuous blood pressure monitoring is needed.

Drug Interactions None noted

Adverse Reactions 1% to 10%:

Cardiovascular: Excessive hypotensive response, palpitation, substernal distress
Central nervous system: Disorientation, psychosis, headache, restlessness
Endocrine & metabolic: Thyroid suppression
Gastrointestinal: Nausea, vomiting
Neuromuscular & skeletal: Weakness, muscle spasm
Otic: Tinnitus
Respiratory: Hypoxia
Miscellaneous: Diaphoresis, thiocyanate toxicity

Overdosage/Toxicology Symptoms of overdose include hypotension, vomiting, hyperventilation, tachycardia, muscular twitching, hypothyroidism, cyanide or thiocyanate toxicity. Thiocyanate toxicity includes psychosis, hyper-reflexia, confusion, weakness, tinnitus, seizures, and coma; cyanide toxicity includes acidosis (decreased HCO_3, decreased pH, increased lactate), increase in mixed venous blood oxygen tension, tachycardia, altered consciousness, coma, convulsions, and almond smell on breath.

Nitroprusside has been shown to release cyanide *in vivo* with hemoglobin. Cyanide toxicity does not usually occur because of the rapid uptake of cyanide by erythrocytes and its eventual incorporation into thiocyanate in the liver. However, high doses, prolonged administration of nitroprusside, or reduced elimination can lead to cyanide poisoning or thiocyanate intoxication. Anemia and liver impairment pose a risk for cyanide accumulation, while renal impairment predisposes thiocyanate accumulation. If toxicity develops, airway support with oxygen therapy is appropriate, followed closely with antidotal therapy of amyl nitrate perles, sodium nitrate 300 mg I.V. for adults (range based on hemoglobin concentration: 6-12 mg/kg for children) and sodium thiosulfate 12.5 g I.V. for adults (range based on hemoglobin concentration: 0.95-1.95 mL/kg of the 25% solution for children); nitrates should not be administered to neonates and small children. Thiocyanate is dialyzable. May be mixed with sodium thiosulfate in I.V. to prevent cyanide toxicity.

Dosing

Adults & Elderly:

Acute hypertension: I.V.: Initial: 0.3-0.5 mcg/kg/minute; increase in increments of 0.5 mcg/kg/minute, titrating to the desired hemodynamic effect or the appearance of headache or nausea; usual dose: 3 mcg/kg/minute; rarely need >4 mcg/kg/minute; maximum: 10 mcg/kg/minute. When >500 mcg/kg is administered by prolonged infusion of faster than 2 mcg/kg/minute, cyanide is generated faster than an unaided patient can handle.

Note: Administration requires the use of an infusion pump. Average dose: 5 mcg/kg/minute.

Pediatrics:

Pulmonary hypertension: I.V.: Children: Initial: 1 mcg/kg/minute by continuous I.V. infusion; increase in increments of 1 mcg/kg/minute at intervals of 20-60 minutes; titrating to the desired response; usual dose: 3 mcg/kg/minute, rarely need >4 mcg/kg/minute; maximum: 5 mcg/kg/minute.

Note: Administration requires the use of an infusion pump. Average dose: 5 mcg/kg/minute.

Renal Impairment: Limit use; accumulation of thiocyanate may occur.

Hepatic Impairment: Limit use; risk of cyanide toxicity.

Available Dosage Forms Injection, solution, as sodium: 25 mg/mL (2 mL)

Nursing Guidelines

Assessment: See Contraindications, Warnings/Precautions, and Dosing for use cautions. Assess potential for interactions with other prescriptions, OTC medications, or herbal products patient may be taking (see Drug Interactions). See Administration, Storage, and Reconstitution for infusion specifics. Infusion site must be monitored closely to prevent extravasation. Continuous blood pressure monitoring is needed. Assess therapeutic effectiveness and adverse response (see Adverse Reactions and Overdose/Toxicology - eg, acid/base balance, metabolic acidosis is early sign of cyanide toxicity). Provide patient teaching according to patient condition (see Patient Education). Note breast-feeding caution.

(Continued)

Nitroprusside *(Continued)*

Patient Education: Patient condition should indicate extent of education and instruction needed. This drug can only be given I.V. You will be monitored at all times during infusion. Promptly report any chest pain or pain/burning at site of infusion. **Breast-feeding precaution:** Consult prescriber if breast-feeding.

Geriatric Considerations: Elderly patients may have an increased sensitivity to nitroprusside possibly due to a decreased baroreceptor reflex, altered sensitivity to vasodilating effects or a resistance of cardiac adrenergic receptors to stimulation by catecholamines.

Pregnancy Risk Factor: C

Lactation: Excretion in breast milk unknown

Perioperative/Anesthesia/Other Concerns:

Elderly patients may have an increased sensitivity to nitroprusside possibly due to a decreased baroreceptor reflex, altered sensitivity to vasodilating effects or a resistance of cardiac adrenergic receptors to stimulation by catecholamines.

Nitroprusside preparations must be wrapped with aluminum foil to protect from light in order to prevent breakdown of the parent drug to cyanide. A bluish tint to the solution indicates breakdown to cyanide. Thiocyanate levels should be monitored if high doses are used for more than 24 hours. Nitroprusside may also be useful for afterload reduction in patients with severe heart failure. Nitroprusside should be avoided in patients with aortic stenosis or coarctation. Nitroprusside should also be used cautiously in patients with acute myocardial infarction, because of hemodynamic effects and possible coronary steal.

Administration

I.V.: I.V. infusion only, use only as an infusion with 5% dextrose in water. Infusion pump required. Not for direct injection.

Reconstitution: Brownish solution is usable, discard if bluish in color. Nitroprusside sodium should be reconstituted freshly by diluting 50 mg in 250-1000 mL of D_5W. Use only clear solutions; solutions of nitroprusside exhibit a color described as brownish, brown, brownish-pink, light orange, and straw. Solutions are highly sensitive to light. Exposure to light causes decomposition, resulting in a highly colored solution of orange, dark brown or blue. **A blue color indicates almost complete degradation and breakdown to cyanide. Solutions should be wrapped with aluminum foil or other opaque material to protect from light (do as soon as possible)**. Stability of parenteral admixture at room temperature (25°C) and at refrigeration temperature (4°C) is 24 hours.

Compatibility: Stable in LR

Y-site administration: Incompatible with levofloxacin

Compatibility when admixed: Incompatible with atracurium

Storage:

Use only clear solutions; solutions of nitroprusside exhibit a color described as brownish, brown, brownish-pink, light orange, and straw. Solutions are highly sensitive to light. Exposure to light causes decomposition, resulting in a highly colored solution of orange, dark brown or blue. **A blue color indicates almost complete degradation and breakdown to cyanide.**

Solutions should be wrapped with aluminum foil or other opaque material to protect from light (do as soon as possible)

Stability of parenteral admixture at room temperature (25°C) and at refrigeration temperature (4°C): 24 hours

Related Information

Postoperative Hypertension *on page 1815*

- **Nitroprusside Sodium** *see* Nitroprusside *on page 1238*
- **NitroQuick®** *see* Nitroglycerin *on page 1234*
- **Nitrostat®** *see* Nitroglycerin *on page 1234*
- **Nitro-Tab®** *see* Nitroglycerin *on page 1234*
- **NitroTime®** *see* Nitroglycerin *on page 1234*

Nizatidine (ni ZA ti deen)

U.S. Brand Names Axid®; Axid® AR [OTC]

Pharmacologic Category Histamine H_2 Antagonist

Medication Safety Issues

Sound-alike/look-alike issues:

Axid® may be confused with Ansaid®

Use Treatment and maintenance of duodenal ulcer; treatment of benign gastric ulcer; treatment of gastroesophageal reflux disease (GERD); OTC tablet used for the prevention of meal-induced heartburn, acid indigestion, and sour stomach

Unlabeled/Investigational Use Part of a multidrug regimen for *H. pylori* eradication to reduce the risk of duodenal ulcer recurrence

Mechanism of Action Competitive inhibition of histamine at H_2-receptors of the gastric parietal cells resulting in reduced gastric acid secretion, gastric volume and hydrogen ion concentration reduced. In healthy volunteers, nizatidine suppresses gastric acid secretion induced by pentagastrin infusion or food.

Pharmacodynamics/Kinetics

Distribution: V_d: 0.8-1.5 L/kg

Protein binding: 35% to α_1-acid glycoprotein

Metabolism: Partially hepatic; forms metabolites

Bioavailability: >70%

Half-life elimination: 1-2 hours; prolonged with renal impairment

Time to peak, plasma: 0.5-3.0 hours

Excretion: Urine (90%; ~60% as unchanged drug); feces (<6%)

Contraindications Hypersensitivity to nizatidine or any component of the formulation; hypersensitivity to other H_2 antagonists (cross-sensitivity has been observed)

Warnings/Precautions Use with caution in children <12 years of age; use with caution in patients with liver and renal impairment; dosage modification required in patients with renal impairment

Drug Interactions Inhibits 3A4 (weak)

Antifungal agents (imidazole): Nizatidine may decrease the absorption of itraconazole or ketoconazole.

Nutritional/Herbal/Ethanol Interactions

Ethanol: Avoid ethanol (may cause gastric mucosal irritation).

Food: Administration with apple juice may decrease absorption.

Lab Interactions False-positive urine protein using Multistix®, gastric acid secretion test, skin tests allergen extracts, serum creatinine and serum transaminase concentrations, urine protein test

Adverse Reactions

>10%: Central nervous system: Headache (16%)

1% to 10%:

- Central nervous system: Anxiety, dizziness, fever (reported in children), insomnia, irritability (reported in children), somnolence, nervousness
- Dermatologic: Pruritus, rash
- Gastrointestinal: Abdominal pain, anorexia, constipation, diarrhea, dry mouth, flatulence, heartburn, nausea, vomiting
- Respiratory: Reported in children: Cough, nasal congestion, nasopharyngitis

<1% (Limited to important or life-threatening): Alkaline phosphatase increased, anaphylaxis, anemia, AST/ALT increased, bronchospasm, confusion, eosinophilia, exfoliative dermatitis, gynecomastia, hepatitis, jaundice, laryngeal edema, serum-sickness like reactions, thrombocytopenia, thrombocytopenic purpura, vasculitis, ventricular tachycardia

Overdosage/Toxicology Symptoms of overdose include muscular tremor, vomiting, and rapid respiration. LD_{50} ~80 mg/kg. Treatment is symptomatic and supportive.

Dosing

Adults & Elderly:

Duodenal ulcer: Oral:

Treatment of active ulcer: 300 mg at bedtime or 150 mg twice daily

Maintenance of healed ulcer: 150 mg/day at bedtime

Gastric ulcer: Oral: 150 mg twice daily or 300 mg at bedtime

GERD: Oral: 150 mg twice daily

Meal-induced heartburn, acid indigestion, and sour stomach (OTC labeling): Oral: 75 mg tablet [OTC] twice daily, 30-60 minutes prior to consuming food or beverages

Eradication of *Helicobacter pylori* (unlabeled use): Oral: 150 mg twice daily; requires combination therapy

Pediatrics:

GERD (unlabeled use): Oral:

Children <12 years: 10 mg/kg/day in divided doses given twice daily; may not be as effective in children <12 years

Children ≥12 years: Refer to adult dosing.

(Continued)

Nizatidine *(Continued)*

Meal-induced heartburn, acid indigestion and sour stomach: Oral: Children ≥12 years: Refer to adult dosing.

Renal Impairment:

Active treatment:

Cl_{cr} 20-50 mL/minute: 150 mg/day

Cl_{cr} <20 mL/minute: 150 mg every other day

Maintenance treatment:

Cl_{cr} 20-50 mL/minute: 150 mg every other day

Cl_{cr} <20 mL/minute: 150 mg every 3 days

Available Dosage Forms

Capsule (Axid®): 150 mg, 300 mg

Solution, oral (Axid®): 15 mg/mL (120 mL, 480 mL) [bubble gum flavor]

Tablet (Axid® AR): 75 mg

Nursing Guidelines

Assessment: See Contraindications, Warnings/Precautions, Drug Interactions, and Dosing for use cautions. Assess therapeutic effectiveness and adverse response (see Adverse Reactions and Overdose/Toxicology). Teach patient proper use, possible side effects/appropriate interventions, and adverse symptoms to report (see Patient Education). **Pregnancy risk factor B** - benefits of use should outweigh possible risks.

Patient Education: Inform prescriber of all prescriptions, OTC medications, or herbal products you are taking, and any allergies you have. Do not take any new medication during therapy unless approved by prescriber. Take as directed; do not change dose or discontinue without consulting prescriber. Do not take within 1 hour of any antacids. Follow diet instructions of prescriber. May cause drowsiness; use caution when driving or engaging in tasks that require alertness until response to drug is known. Report fever, sore throat, tarry stools, CNS changes, or muscle or joint pain. **Pregnancy precaution:** Inform prescriber if you are or intend to become pregnant.

Geriatric Considerations: H_2 blockers are the preferred drugs for treating peptic ulcer disorder (PUD) in the elderly due to cost and ease of administration. These agents are no less or more effective than any other therapy. The preferred agents (due to side effects and drug interaction profile and pharmacokinetics) are ranitidine, famotidine, and nizatidine. Treatment for PUD in the elderly is recommended for 12 weeks since their lesions are larger, and therefore, take longer to heal. Always adjust dose based upon creatinine clearance.

Pregnancy Risk Factor: B

Lactation: Enters breast milk/may be compatible

Breast-Feeding Considerations: The amount of nizatidine excreted in breast milk is 0.1%.

- **No Doz® Maximum Strength [OTC]** *see* Caffeine *on page 284*
- **Noradrenaline** *see* Norepinephrine *on page 1242*
- **Noradrenaline Acid Tartrate** *see* Norepinephrine *on page 1242*
- **Norco®** *see* Hydrocodone and Acetaminophen *on page 867*
- **Norcuron® [DSC]** *see* Vecuronium *on page 1695*
- **Nordeoxyguanosine** *see* Ganciclovir *on page 794*
- **Norditropin®** *see* Somatropin *on page 1555*
- **Norditropin® NordiFlex®** *see* Somatropin *on page 1555*
- **Norelgestromin and Ethinyl Estradiol** *see* Ethinyl Estradiol and Norelgestromin *on page 684*

Norepinephrine (nor ep i NEF rin)

U.S. Brand Names Levophed®

Synonyms Levarterenol Bitartrate; Noradrenaline; Noradrenaline Acid Tartrate; Norepinephrine Bitartrate

Pharmacologic Category Alpha/Beta Agonist

Use Treatment of shock which persists after adequate fluid volume replacement

Mechanism of Action Stimulates $beta_1$-adrenergic receptors and alpha-adrenergic receptors causing increased contractility and heart rate as well as vasoconstriction, thereby increasing systemic blood pressure and coronary blood flow; clinically alpha effects (vasoconstriction) are greater than beta effects (inotropic and chronotropic effects)

Pharmacodynamics/Kinetics

Onset of action: I.V.: Very rapid-acting

Duration: Limited

Metabolism: Via catechol-o-methyltransferase (COMT) and monoamine oxidase (MAO)

Excretion: Urine (84% to 96% as inactive metabolites)

Contraindications Hypersensitivity to norepinephrine, bisulfites (contains metabisulfite), or any component of the formulation; hypotension from hypovolemia except as an emergency measure to maintain coronary and cerebral perfusion until volume could be replaced; mesenteric or peripheral vascular thrombosis unless it is a lifesaving procedure; during anesthesia with cyclopropane or halothane anesthesia (risk of ventricular arrhythmias)

Warnings/Precautions Assure adequate circulatory volume to minimize need for vasoconstrictors. Avoid hypertension; monitor blood pressure closely and adjust infusion rate. Infuse into a large vein if possible. Avoid infusion into leg veins. Watch I.V. site closely. Avoid extravasation. Never use leg veins for infusion sites.

Drug Interactions

Beta-blockers (nonselective ones) may increase hypertensive effect; avoid concurrent use.

Cocaine may cause malignant arrhythmias; avoid concurrent use.

Guanethidine can increase the pressor response; be aware of the patient's drug regimen.

MAO inhibitors potentiate hypertension and hypertensive crisis; avoid concurrent use.

Methyldopa can increase the pressor response; be aware of patient's drug regimen.

Reserpine increases the pressor response; be aware of patient's drug regimen.

TCAs increase the pressor response; be aware of patient's drug regimen.

Adverse Reactions Frequency not defined.

Cardiovascular: Bradycardia, arrhythmia, peripheral (digital) ischemia

Central nervous system: Headache (transient), anxiety

Local: Skin necrosis (with extravasation)

Respiratory: Dyspnea, respiratory difficulty

Overdosage/Toxicology Symptoms of overdose include hypertension, sweating, cerebral hemorrhage, and convulsions. Infiltrate the area of extravasation with phentolamine 5-10 mg in 10-15 mL of saline solution; inject a small amount of this dilution into extravasated area; blanching should reverse immediately. Monitor site; if blanching should recur, additional injections of phentolamine may be needed.

Dosing

Adults & Elderly: Note: Norepinephrine dosage is stated in terms of norepinephrine base and intravenous formulation is norepinephrine bitartrate.

Norepinephrine bitartrate 2 mg = norepinephrine base 1 mg

Hypotension/shock: Continuous I.V. infusion:

Adults: Initial: 0.5-1 mcg/minute and titrate to desired response; 8-30 mcg/minute is usual range; range used in clinical trials: 0.01-3 mcg/kg/minute;

ACLS dosing range: 0.5-30 mcg/minute

Rate of infusion: 4 mg in 500 mL D_5W

2 mcg/minute = 15 mL/hour

4 mcg/minute = 30 mL/hour

6 mcg/minute = 45 mL/hour

8 mcg/minute = 60 mL/hour

10 mcg/minute = 75 mL/hour

Pediatrics: Administration requires the use of an infusion pump

Note: Norepinephrine dosage is stated in terms of norepinephrine base and intravenous formulation is norepinephrine bitartrate.

Norepinephrine bitartrate 2 mg = Norepinephrine base 1 mg

Hypotension/shock: Continuous I.V. infusion: Children: Initial: 0.05-0.1 mcg/kg/minute; titrate to desired effect; maximum dose: 1-2 mcg/kg/minute

Available Dosage Forms Injection, solution, as bitartrate: 1 mg/mL (4 mL) [contains sodium metabisulfite]

Nursing Guidelines

Assessment: Assess other medications patient may be taking. Monitor blood pressure and cardiac status, CNS status, skin temperature and color during and following infusion. Monitor fluid status. Assess infusion site frequently for extravasation. Blanching along vein pathway is a preliminary sign of extravasation.

(Continued)

Norepinephrine *(Continued)*

Patient Education: This drug is used in emergency situations. Patient information is based on patient condition.

Pregnancy Risk Factor: C

Lactation: Excretion in breast milk unknown

Perioperative/Anesthesia/Other Concerns: Norepinephrine is effective at increasing arterial blood pressure through vasoconstriction with little change in heart rate or cardiac output. Adequate fluid resuscitation is essential to the success of norepinephrine in raising blood pressure; may successfully increase blood pressure without causing a deterioration in cardiac index or organ function in patients with septic shock. It should be used early and not withheld as a last resort. The 1999 ACCM/SCCM Practice Parameters for Hemodynamic Support of Sepsis in Adult Patients recommends either dopamine or norepinephrine as vasopressor therapy. Norepinephrine may be more effective in some patients.

Administration

I.V.: Administer into large vein to avoid the potential for extravasation; potent drug, must be diluted prior to use; do not administer $NaHCO_3$ through an I.V. line containing norepinephrine. Central line administration is required. Do not administer $NaHCO_3$ through an I.V. line containing norepinephrine.

Reconstitution: Dilute with D_5W or D_5NS, but not recommended to dilute in normal saline. Stability of parenteral admixture at room temperature (25°C) is 24 hours.

Compatibility: Stable in D_5NS, D_5W, LR; may dilute with D_5W or D_5NS, but not recommended to dilute in normal saline; not stable in alkaline solutions. Stability of parenteral admixture at room temperature (25°C) is 24 hours.

Y-site administration: Incompatible with insulin (regular), thiopental

Compatibility when admixed: Incompatible with aminophylline, amobarbital, chlorothiazide, chlorpheniramine, pentobarbital, phenobarbital, phenytoin, sodium bicarbonate, streptomycin, thiopental

Storage: Readily oxidized; protect from light. Do not use if brown coloration.

- ♦ **Norepinephrine Bitartrate** *see* Norepinephrine *on page 1242*
- ♦ **Norethindrone and Estradiol** *see* Estradiol and Norethindrone *on page 655*
- ♦ **Norgestimate and Ethinyl Estradiol** *see* Ethinyl Estradiol and Norgestimate *on page 689*
- ♦ **Noritate®** *see* Metronidazole *on page 1154*
- ♦ **Normal Human Serum Albumin** *see* Albumin *on page 94*
- ♦ **Normal Saline** *see* Sodium Chloride *on page 1545*
- ♦ **Normal Serum Albumin (Human)** *see* Albumin *on page 94*
- ♦ **Norpace®** *see* Disopyramide *on page 552*
- ♦ **Norpace® CR** *see* Disopyramide *on page 552*

Nortriptyline (nor TRIP ti leen)

U.S. Brand Names Pamelor®

Synonyms Nortriptyline Hydrochloride

Pharmacologic Category Antidepressant, Tricyclic (Secondary Amine)

Medication Safety Issues

Sound-alike/look-alike issues:

Nortriptyline may be confused with amitriptyline, desipramine, Norpramin®

Aventyl® HCl may be confused with Bentyl®

Pamelor® may be confused with Demerol®, Dymelor®

Use Treatment of symptoms of depression

Unlabeled/Investigational Use Chronic pain, anxiety disorders, enuresis, attention-deficit/hyperactivity disorder (ADHD); adjunctive therapy for smoking cessation

Mechanism of Action Traditionally believed to increase the synaptic concentration of serotonin and/or norepinephrine in the central nervous system by inhibition of their reuptake by the presynaptic neuronal membrane. However, additional receptor effects have been found including desensitization of adenyl cyclase, down regulation of beta-adrenergic receptors, and down regulation of serotonin receptors.

Pharmacodynamics/Kinetics

Onset of action: Therapeutic: 1-3 weeks

Distribution: V_d: 21 L/kg

Protein binding: 93% to 95%

Metabolism: Primarily hepatic; extensive first-pass effect
Half-life elimination: 28-31 hours
Time to peak, serum: 7-8.5 hours
Excretion: Urine (as metabolites and small amounts of unchanged drug); feces (small amounts)

Contraindications Hypersensitivity to nortriptyline and similar chemical class, or any component of the formulation; use of MAO inhibitors within 14 days; use in a patient during the acute recovery phase of MI; pregnancy

Warnings/Precautions Antidepressants increase the risk of suicidal thinking and behavior in children and adolescents with major depressive disorder (MDD) and other depressive disorders; consider risk prior to prescribing. Closely monitor for clinical worsening, suicidality, or unusual changes in behavior; the child's family or caregiver should be instructed to closely observe the patient and communicate condition with healthcare provider. Such observation would generally include at least weekly face-to-face contact with patients or their family members or caregivers during the first 4 weeks of treatment, then every other week visits for the next 4 weeks, then at 12 weeks, and as clinically indicated beyond 12 weeks. Additional contact by telephone may be appropriate between face-to-face visits. Adults treated with antidepressants should be observed similarly for clinical worsening and suicidality, especially during the initial few months of a course of drug therapy, or at times of dose changes, either increases or decreases. A medication guide should be dispensed with each prescription. **Nortriptyline is not FDA approved for use in children.**

The possibility of a suicide attempt is inherent in major depression and may persist until remission occurs. Monitor for worsening of depression or suicidality, especially during initiation of therapy or with dose increases or decreases. Worsening depression and severe abrupt suicidality that are not part of the presenting symptoms may require discontinuation or modification of drug therapy. Use caution in high-risk patients during initiation of therapy. Prescriptions should be written for the smallest quantity consistent with good patient care. The patient's family or caregiver should be alerted to monitor patients for the emergence of suicidality and associated behaviors such as anxiety, agitation, panic attacks, insomnia, irritability, hostility, impulsivity, akathisia, hypomania, and mania; patients should be instructed to notify their healthcare provider if any of these symptoms or worsening depression occur.

May worsen psychosis in some patients or precipitate a shift to mania or hypomania in patients with bipolar disorder. Monotherapy in patients with bipolar disorder should be avoided. Patients presenting with depressive symptoms should be screened for bipolar disorder. **Nortriptyline is not FDA approved for the treatment of bipolar depression.**

May cause sedation, resulting in impaired performance of tasks requiring alertness (eg, operating machinery or driving). Sedative effects may be additive with other CNS depressants and/or ethanol. The degree of sedation is low-moderate relative to other antidepressants. May increase the risks associated with electroconvulsive therapy. Consider discontinuing, when possible, prior to elective surgery. Therapy should not be abruptly discontinued in patients receiving high doses for prolonged periods. May alter glucose regulation - use caution in patients with diabetes.

May cause orthostatic hypotension (risk is low relative to other antidepressants) - use with caution in patients at risk of hypotension or in patients where transient hypotensive episodes would be poorly tolerated (cardiovascular disease or cerebrovascular disease). The degree of anticholinergic blockade produced by this agent is moderate relative to other cyclic antidepressants, however, caution should still be used in patients with urinary retention, benign prostatic hyperplasia, narrow-angle glaucoma, xerostomia, visual problems, constipation, or history of bowel obstruction.

Use with caution in patients with a history of cardiovascular disease (including previous MI, stroke, tachycardia, or conduction abnormalities). The risk conduction abnormalities with this agent is moderate relative to other antidepressants. Use caution in patients with a previous seizure disorder or condition predisposing to seizures such as brain damage, alcoholism, or concurrent therapy with other drugs which lower the seizure threshold. Use with caution in hyperthyroid patients or those receiving thyroid supplementation. Use with caution in patients with hepatic or renal dysfunction and in elderly patients.

Drug Interactions Substrate of CYP1A2 (minor), 2C19 (minor), 2D6 (major), 3A4 (minor); **Inhibits** CYP2D6 (weak), 2E1 (weak)

(Continued)

Nortriptyline *(Continued)*

Altretamine: Concurrent use may cause orthostatic hypertension

Amphetamines: TCAs may enhance the effect of amphetamines; monitor for adverse CV effects

Anticholinergics: Combined use with TCAs may produce additive anticholinergic effects

Antihypertensives: TCAs may inhibit the antihypertensive response tó bethanidine, clonidine, debrisoquin, guanadrel, guanethidine, guanabenz, guanfacine; monitor BP; consider alternate antihypertensive agent

Beta-agonists: When combined with TCAs may predispose patients to cardiac arrhythmias

Bupropion: May increase the levels of tricyclic antidepressants; based on limited information; monitor response

Carbamazepine: Tricyclic antidepressants may increase carbamazepine levels; monitor

Cholestyramine and colestipol: May bind TCAs and reduce their absorption; monitor for altered response

Clonidine: Abrupt discontinuation of clonidine may cause hypertensive crisis, amitriptyline may enhance the response

CNS depressants: Sedative effects may be additive with TCAs; monitor for increased effect; includes benzodiazepines, barbiturates, antipsychotics, ethanol and other sedative medications

CYP2D6 inhibitors: May increase the levels/effects of nortriptyline. Example inhibitors include chlorpromazine, delavirdine, fluoxetine, miconazole, paroxetine, pergolide, quinidine, quinine, ritonavir, and ropinirole.

Epinephrine (and other direct alpha-agonists): Pressor response to I.V. epinephrine, norepinephrine, and phenylephrine may be enhanced in patients receiving TCAs (**Note:** Effect is unlikely with epinephrine or levonordefrin dosages typically administered as infiltration in combination with local anesthetics)

Fenfluramine: May increase tricyclic antidepressant levels/effects

Hypoglycemic agents (including insulin): TCAs may enhance the hypoglycemic effects of tolazamide, chlorpropamide, or insulin; monitor for changes in blood glucose levels; reported with chlorpropamide, tolazamide, and insulin

Levodopa: Tricyclic antidepressants may decrease the absorption (bioavailability) of levodopa; rare hypertensive episodes have also been attributed to this combination

Linezolid: Hyperpyrexia, hypertension, tachycardia, confusion, seizures, and **deaths have been reported** with agents which inhibit MAO (serotonin syndrome); this combination should be avoided

Lithium: Concurrent use with a TCA may increase the risk for neurotoxicity

MAO inhibitors: Hyperpyrexia, hypertension, tachycardia, confusion, seizures, and **deaths have been reported** (serotonin syndrome); this combination should be avoided

Methylphenidate: Metabolism of TCAs may be decreased

Phenothiazines: Serum concentrations of some TCAs may be increased; in addition, TCAs may increase concentration of phenothiazines; monitor for altered clinical response

QT_c-prolonging agents: Concurrent use of tricyclic agents with other drugs which may prolong QT_c interval may increase the risk of potentially fatal arrhythmias; includes type Ia and type III antiarrhythmics agents, selected quinolones (sparfloxacin, gatifloxacin, moxifloxacin, grepafloxacin), cisapride, and other agents

Ritonavir: Combined use of high-dose tricyclic antidepressants with ritonavir may cause serotonin syndrome in HIV-positive patients; monitor

Sucralfate: Absorption of tricyclic antidepressants may be reduced with coadministration

Sympathomimetics, indirect-acting: Tricyclic antidepressants may result in a decreased sensitivity to indirect-acting sympathomimetics; includes dopamine and ephedrine; also see interaction with epinephrine (and direct-acting sympathomimetics)

Tramadol: Tramadol's risk of seizures may be increased with TCAs

Valproic acid: May increase serum concentrations/adverse effects of some tricyclic antidepressants

Warfarin (and other oral anticoagulants): TCAs may increase the anticoagulant effect in patients stabilized on warfarin; monitor INR

Nutritional/Herbal/Ethanol Interactions

Ethanol: Avoid ethanol (may increase CNS depression).

Food: Grapefruit juice may inhibit the metabolism of some TCAs and clinical toxicity may result.

Herb/Nutraceutical: Avoid valerian, St John's wort, SAMe, kava kava (may increase risk of serotonin syndrome and/or excessive sedation).

Lab Interactions Increased glucose

Adverse Reactions Frequency not defined.

Cardiovascular: Postural hypotension, arrhythmia, hypertension, heart block, tachycardia, palpitation, MI

Central nervous system: Confusion, delirium, hallucinations, restlessness, insomnia, disorientation, delusions, anxiety, agitation, panic, nightmares, hypomania, exacerbation of psychosis, incoordination, ataxia, extrapyramidal symptoms, seizure

Dermatologic: Alopecia, photosensitivity, rash, petechiae, urticaria, itching

Endocrine & metabolic: Sexual dysfunction, gynecomastia, breast enlargement, galactorrhea, increase or decrease in libido, increase in blood sugar, SIADH

Gastrointestinal: Xerostomia, constipation, vomiting, anorexia, diarrhea, abdominal cramps, black tongue, nausea, unpleasant taste, weight gain/loss

Genitourinary: Urinary retention, delayed micturition, impotence, testicular edema

Hematologic: Rarely agranulocytosis, eosinophilia, purpura, thrombocytopenia

Hepatic: Increased liver enzymes, cholestatic jaundice

Neuromuscular & skeletal: Tremor, numbness, tingling, paresthesia, peripheral neuropathy

Ocular: Blurred vision, eye pain, disturbances in accommodation, mydriasis

Otic: Tinnitus

Miscellaneous: Diaphoresis (excessive), allergic reactions

Overdosage/Toxicology Symptoms of overdose include agitation, confusion, hallucinations, urinary retention, hypothermia, hypotension, seizures, and ventricular tachycardia. Treatment is symptomatic and supportive. Alkalinization by sodium bicarbonate and/or hyperventilation may limit cardiac toxicity.

Dosing

Adults:

Depression: Oral: 25 mg 3-4 times/day up to 150 mg/day

Chronic urticaria, angioedema, nocturnal pruritus (unlabeled use): Oral: 75 mg/day

Smoking cessation (unlabeled use): Oral: 25-75 mg/day beginning 10-14 days before "quit" day; continue therapy for ≥12 weeks after "quit" day

Elderly: Note: Nortriptyline is one of the best tolerated TCAs in the elderly.

Initial: 10-25 mg at bedtime

Dosage can be increased by 25 mg every 3 days for inpatients and weekly for outpatients if tolerated.

Usual maintenance dose: 75 mg as a single bedtime dose or 2 divided doses; however, lower or higher doses may be required to stay within the therapeutic window.

Pediatrics:

Nocturnal enuresis (unlabeled use): Oral: 10-20 mg/day; titrate to a maximum of 40 mg/day

Depression (unlabeled use): Oral: 1-3 mg/kg/day

Hepatic Impairment: Lower doses and slower titration are recommended dependent on individualization of dosage.

Available Dosage Forms

Capsule, as hydrochloride: 10 mg, 25 mg, 50 mg, 75 mg

Pamelor®: 10 mg, 25 mg, 50 mg, 75 mg [may contain benzyl alcohol; 50 mg may also contain sodium bisulfite]

Solution, as hydrochloride (Pamelor®): 10 mg/5 mL (473 mL) [contains alcohol 4% and benzoic acid]

Nursing Guidelines

Assessment: Assess potential for interactions with other prescriptions, OTC medications, or herbal products patient may be taking. Assess for suicidal tendencies before beginning therapy. May cause physiological or psychological dependence, tolerance, or abuse; periodically evaluate need for continued use. Assess therapeutic effectiveness (mental status, mood, affect) and adverse reactions (eg, suicidal ideation) at beginning of therapy and periodically with long-term use. Taper dosage slowly when discontinuing (allow 3-4 weeks between discontinuing this medication and starting another antidepressant). Caution patients with diabetes to monitor glucose levels closely; may increase or decrease serum glucose levels. Teach patient appropriate use, interventions to reduce side effects, and adverse symptoms to report.

(Continued)

Nortriptyline *(Continued)*

Patient Education: Do not take any new medication during therapy unless approved by prescriber. Take exactly as directed; take once-a-day dose at bedtime. Do not increase dose or frequency; may take 2-3 weeks to achieve desired results. This drug may cause physical and/or psychological dependence. Avoid alcohol and grapefruit juice. Maintain adequate hydration (2-3 L/day of fluids) unless instructed to restrict fluid intake. May cause drowsiness, lightheadedness, impaired coordination, dizziness, or blurred vision (use caution when driving or engaging in tasks requiring alertness until response to drug is known); nausea, vomiting, loss of appetite, or disturbed taste (small frequent meals, good mouth care, chewing gum, or sucking lozenges may help); constipation (increased exercise, fluids, fruit, or fiber may help); urinary retention (void before taking medication); postural hypotension (use caution climbing stairs or when changing position from lying or sitting to standing); altered sexual drive or ability (reversible); or photosensitivity (use sunscreen, wear protective clothing and eyewear, and avoid direct sunlight). Report chest pain, palpitations, or rapid heartbeat; persistent adverse CNS effects (eg, suicidal ideation, nervousness, restlessness, insomnia, anxiety, excitation, headache, agitation, impaired coordination, changes in cognition); muscle cramping, weakness, tremors, or rigidity; blurred vision or eye pain; breast enlargement or swelling; yellowing of skin or eyes; or worsening of condition. **Pregnancy/breast-feeding precautions:** Inform prescriber if you pregnant. Do not get pregnant while taking this medication. Consult prescriber for appropriate contraceptive measures. Do not breast-feed.

Geriatric Considerations: Since nortriptyline is the least likely of the tricyclic antidepressants (TCAs) to cause orthostatic hypotension and one of the least anticholinergic and sedating TCAs, it is a preferred agent when a TCA is indicated. Data from a clinical trial comparing fluoxetine to tricyclics suggests that fluoxetine is significantly less effective than nortriptyline in hospitalized elderly patients with unipolar affective disorder, especially those with melancholia and concurrent cardiovascular disease.

Pregnancy Risk Factor: D

Lactation: Enters breast milk/contraindicated (AAP rates "of concern")

Perioperative/Anesthesia/Other Concerns: Its maximum antidepressant effect may not be seen for ≥2 weeks after initiation of therapy.

Administration

Storage: Protect from light.

- **Nortriptyline Hydrochloride** *see* Nortriptyline *on page 1244*
- **Norvasc®** *see* Amlodipine *on page 140*
- **Novarel™** *see* Chorionic Gonadotropin (Human) *on page 387*
- **Novocain®** *see* Procaine *on page 1411*
- **Novolin® 70/30** *see* Insulin NPH and Insulin Regular *on page 927*
- **Novolin® N** *see* Insulin NPH *on page 926*
- **Novolin® R** *see* Insulin Regular *on page 928*
- **NovoLog®** *see* Insulin Aspart *on page 916*
- **NovoLog® Mix 70/30** *see* Insulin Aspart Protamine and Insulin Aspart *on page 918*
- **NovoSeven®** *see* Factor VIIa (Recombinant) *on page 700*
- **NPH Insulin** *see* Insulin NPH *on page 926*
- **NPH Insulin and Regular Insulin** *see* Insulin NPH and Insulin Regular *on page 927*
- **NRS® [OTC]** *see* Oxymetazoline *on page 1290*
- **NSC-740** *see* Methotrexate *on page 1127*
- **NSC-26271** *see* Cyclophosphamide *on page 462*
- **NSC-26980** *see* Mitomycin *on page 1168*
- **NSC-49842** *see* VinBLAStine *on page 1707*
- **NSC-63878** *see* Cytarabine *on page 477*
- **NSC-67574** *see* VinCRIStine *on page 1710*
- **NSC-123127** *see* DOXOrubicin *on page 576*
- **NSC-125066** *see* Bleomycin *on page 248*
- **NSC-125973** *see* Paclitaxel *on page 1294*
- **NSC-266046** *see* Oxaliplatin *on page 1275*
- **NSC-377526** *see* Leuprolide *on page 1015*
- **NSC-409962** *see* Carmustine *on page 318*

♦ NSC-606864 *see* Goserelin *on page 829*
♦ NSC-616348 *see* Irinotecan *on page 962*
♦ NSC-628503 *see* Docetaxel *on page 557*
♦ NSC-706363 *see* Arsenic Trioxide *on page 184*
♦ NTG *see* Nitroglycerin *on page 1234*
♦ Nubain® *see* Nalbuphine *on page 1196*
♦ NuLev™ *see* Hyoscyamine *on page 886*
♦ Nupercainal® [OTC] *see* Dibucaine *on page 520*
♦ Nupercainal® Hydrocortisone Cream [OTC] *see* Hydrocortisone *on page 873*
♦ Nuromax® *see* Doxacurium *on page 570*
♦ Nu-Tears® [OTC] *see* Artificial Tears *on page 187*
♦ Nu-Tears® II [OTC] *see* Artificial Tears *on page 187*
♦ Nutracort® *see* Hydrocortisone *on page 873*
♦ NutriNate® *see* Vitamins (Multiple/Prenatal) *on page 1721*
♦ Nutropin® *see* Somatropin *on page 1555*
♦ Nutropin AQ® *see* Somatropin *on page 1555*
♦ NVB *see* Vinorelbine *on page 1713*
♦ Nyamyc™ *see* Nystatin *on page 1249*
♦ Nydrazid® [DSC] *see* Isoniazid *on page 972*

Nystatin (nye STAT in)

U.S. Brand Names Bio-Statin®; Mycostatin®; Nyamyc™; Nystat-Rx®; Nystop®; Pedi-Dri®

Pharmacologic Category Antifungal Agent, Oral Nonabsorbed; Antifungal Agent, Topical; Antifungal Agent, Vaginal

Medication Safety Issues

Sound-alike/look-alike issues:

Nystatin may be confused with Nilstat®, Nitrostat®

Nilstat may be confused with Nitrostat®, nystatin

Use Treatment of susceptible cutaneous, mucocutaneous, and oral cavity fungal infections normally caused by the *Candida* species

Mechanism of Action Binds to sterols in fungal cell membrane, changing the cell wall permeability allowing for leakage of cellular contents

Pharmacodynamics/Kinetics

Onset of action: Symptomatic relief from candidiasis: 24-72 hours

Absorption: Topical: None through mucous membranes or intact skin; Oral: Poorly absorbed

Excretion: Feces (as unchanged drug)

Contraindications Hypersensitivity to nystatin or any component of the formulation

Drug Interactions No data reported

Adverse Reactions

Frequency not defined: Dermatologic: Contact dermatitis, Stevens-Johnson syndrome

1% to 10%: Gastrointestinal: Nausea, vomiting, diarrhea, stomach pain

<1% (Limited to important or life-threatening): Hypersensitivity reactions

Overdosage/Toxicology Symptoms of overdose include nausea, vomiting, and diarrhea. Treatment is supportive.

Dosing

Adults & Elderly:

Oral candidiasis: Suspension (swish and swallow orally): 400,000-600,000 units 4 times/day

Mucocutaneous infections: Topical: Apply 2-3 times/day to affected areas; very moist topical lesions are treated best with powder.

Intestinal infections: Oral tablets: 500,000-1,000,000 units every 8 hours

Vaginal infections: Vaginal tablets: Insert 1 tablet/day at bedtime for 2 weeks. (May also be given orally.)

Note: Powder for compounding: $^1/_8$ teaspoon (500,000 units) to equal approximately $^1/_2$ cup of water; give 4 times/day

Pediatrics:

Oral candidiasis:

Suspension (swish and swallow orally):

Premature infants: 100,000 units 4 times/day

Infants: 200,000 units 4 times/day or 100,000 units to each side of mouth 4 times/day

(Continued)

Nystatin *(Continued)*

Children: 400,000-600,000 units 4 times/day

Powder for compounding: Children: Refer to adult dosing.

Mucocutaneous infections: Children: Refer to adult dosing.

Available Dosage Forms

Capsule (Bio-Statin®): 500,000 units, 1 million units

Cream: 100,000 units/g (15 g, 30 g)

Mycostatin®: 100,000 units/g (30 g)

Ointment, topical: 100,000 units/g (15 g, 30 g)

Powder, for prescription compounding: 50 million units (10 g); 150 million units (30 g); 500 million units (100 g); 2 billion units (400 g)

Nystat-Rx®: 50 million units (10 g); 150 million units (30 g); 500 million units (100 g); 1 billion units (190 g); 2 billion units (350 g)

Powder, topical:

Mycostatin®: 100,000 units/g (15 g)

Nyamyc™: 100,000 units/g (15 g, 30 g)

Nystop®: 100,000 units/g (15 g, 30 g, 60 g)

Pedi-Dri®: 100,000 units/g (56.7 g)

Suspension, oral: 100,000 units/mL (5 mL, 60 mL, 480 mL)

Tablet: 500,000 units

Tablet, vaginal: 100,000 units (15s) [packaged with applicator]

Nursing Guidelines

Assessment: Determine that cause of infection is fungal. Avoid skin contact when applying. Monitor therapeutic effectiveness, adverse reactions at beginning of therapy and periodically throughout therapy. Assess knowledge/teach patient appropriate use, interventions to reduce side effects, and adverse symptoms to report.

Patient Education: Take as directed. Maintain adequate hydration (2-3 L/day of fluids) unless instructed to restrict fluid intake. Do not allow medication to come in contact with eyes. Report persistent nausea, vomiting, or diarrhea; or if condition being treated worsens or does not improve. **Pregnancy precaution:** Inform prescriber if you are pregnant.

Oral tablet: Swallow whole; do not crush or chew.

Oral suspension: Shake well before using. Remove dentures, clean mouth (do not replace dentures until after using medications). Swish suspension in mouth for several minutes before swallowing

Oral troche: Remove dentures, clean mouth (do not replace dentures until after using medication). Allow troche to dissolve in mouth; do not chew or swallow whole.

Topical: Wash and dry area before applying (do not reuse towels without washing, apply clean clothing after use). Report unresolved burning, redness, or swelling in treated areas.

Vaginal tablet: Wash hands before using. Lie down to insert high into vagina at bedtime.

Geriatric Considerations: For oral infections, patients who wear dentures must have them removed and cleaned in order to eliminate source of reinfection.

Pregnancy Risk Factor: B/C (oral)

Lactation: Does not enter breast milk/compatible (not absorbed orally)

Administration

Oral: Suspension: Shake well before using. Should be swished about the mouth and retained in the mouth for as long as possible (several minutes) before swallowing.

Storage: Vaginal insert: Store in refrigerator. Protect from temperature extremes, moisture, and light.

Oral tablet, ointment, topical powder, and oral suspension: Store at controlled room temperature 15°C to 25°C (59°F to 77°F).

◆ **Nystat-Rx®** *see* Nystatin *on page 1249*

◆ **Nystop®** *see* Nystatin *on page 1249*

◆ **Nytol® Quick Caps [OTC]** *see* DiphenhydrAMINE *on page 546*

◆ **Nytol® Quick Gels [OTC]** *see* DiphenhydrAMINE *on page 546*

◆ **NāSop™** *see* Phenylephrine *on page 1350*

◆ **Nōstrilla® [OTC]** *see* Oxymetazoline *on page 1290*

- ♦ **OB-20** *see* Vitamins (Multiple/Prenatal) *on page 1721*
- ♦ **Obegyn®** *see* Vitamins (Multiple/Prenatal) *on page 1721*
- ♦ **OCBZ** *see* Oxcarbazepine *on page 1278*
- ♦ **Ocean® [OTC]** *see* Sodium Chloride *on page 1545*
- ♦ **Oceant® for Kids [OTC]** *see* Sodium Chloride *on page 1545*
- ♦ **Octagam®** *see* Immune Globulin (Intravenous) *on page 899*

Octreotide (ok TREE oh tide)

U.S. Brand Names Sandostatin®; Sandostatin LAR®

Synonyms Octreotide Acetate

Pharmacologic Category Antidiarrheal; Somatostatin Analog

Medication Safety Issues

Sound-alike/look-alike issues:

Sandostatin® may be confused with Sandimmune®

Use Control of symptoms in patients with metastatic carcinoid and vasoactive intestinal peptide-secreting tumors (VIPomas); acromegaly

Unlabeled/Investigational Use AIDS-associated secretory diarrhea (including *Cryptosporidiosis*), control of bleeding of esophageal varices, breast cancer, cryptosporidiosis, Cushing's syndrome (ectopic), insulinomas, small bowel fistulas, pancreatic tumors, gastrinoma, postgastrectomy dumping syndrome, chemotherapy-induced diarrhea, graft-versus-host disease (GVHD) induced diarrhea, Zollinger-Ellison syndrome, congenital hyperinsulinism

Mechanism of Action Mimics natural somatostatin by inhibiting serotonin release, and the secretion of gastrin, VIP, insulin, glucagon, secretin, motilin, and pancreatic polypeptide. Decreases growth hormone and IGF-1 in acromegaly.

Pharmacodynamics/Kinetics

Duration: SubQ: 6-12 hours

Absorption: SubQ: Rapid

Distribution: V_d: 14 L (13-30 L in acromegaly)

Protein binding: 65%

Metabolism: Extensively hepatic

Bioavailability: SubQ: 100%

Half-life elimination: 1.7-1.9 hours; up to 3.7 hours with cirrhosis

Time to peak, plasma: SubQ: 0.4 hours (0.7 hours acromegaly)

Excretion: Urine (32%)

Contraindications Hypersensitivity to octreotide or any component of the formulation

Warnings/Precautions May impair gall bladder function; monitor patients for cholelithiasis. Use with caution in patients with renal impairment. Somatostatin analogs may affect glucose regulation; in type I diabetes, severe hypoglycemia may occur; in type II diabetes or nondiabetic patients, hyperglycemia may occur. Insulin and other hypoglycemic medication requirements may change. Bradycardia, conduction abnormalities, and arrhythmia have been observed in acromegalic patients; use caution with CHF or concomitant medications that alter heart rate or rhythm. May alter absorption of dietary fats; monitor for pancreatitis. Chronic treatment has been associated with abnormal Schillings test; monitor vitamin B_{12} levels.

Drug Interactions

Cyclosporine: Case reports of transplant rejection due to reduction of serum cyclosporine levels when cyclosporine was given orally in conjunction with a somatostatin analogue.

Adverse Reactions Adverse reactions vary by route of administration. Frequency of cardiac, endocrine, and gastrointestinal adverse reactions were generally higher in acromegalics.

>16%:

Cardiovascular: Sinus bradycardia (19% to 25%), chest pain (16% to 20%)

Central nervous system: Fatigue (1% to 20%), malaise (16% to 20%), dizziness (5% to 20%), headache (6% to 20%), fever (16% to 20%)

Endocrine & metabolic: Hyperglycemia (2% to 27%)

Gastrointestinal: Diarrhea (5% to 61%), abdominal discomfort (5% to 61%), flatulence (<10% to 38%), constipation (9% to 21%), nausea (5% to 61%), cholelithiasis (27%; length of therapy dependent), biliary duct dilatation (12%), biliary sludge (24%; length of therapy dependent), loose stools (5% to 61%), vomiting (4% to 21%)

Hematologic: Antibodies to octreotide (up to 25%; no efficacy change)

Local: Injection pain (2% to 50%; dose- and formulation-related)

Neuromuscular & skeletal: Backache (1% to 20%), arthropathy (16% to 20%)

(Continued)

Octreotide *(Continued)*

Respiratory: Dyspnea (16% to 20%), upper respiratory infection (16% to 20%)
Miscellaneous: Flu symptoms (1% to 20%)

5% to 15%:

Cardiovascular: Conduction abnormalities (9% to 10%), arrhythmia (3% to 9%), hypertension, palpitations, peripheral edema
Central nervous system: Anxiety, confusion, depression, hypoesthesia, insomnia, vertigo
Dermatologic: Pruritus, rash
Endocrine & metabolic: Hypothyroidism (2% to 12%), goiter (2% to 8%)
Gastrointestinal: Abdominal pain, anorexia, cramping, dehydration, discomfort, hemorrhoids, tenesmus (4% to 6%), dyspepsia (4% to 6%), steatorrhea (4% to 6%), feces discoloration (4% to 6%), weight loss
Genitourinary: UTI
Hematologic: Anemia
Hepatic: Hepatitis
Neuromuscular & skeletal: Arthralgia, leg cramps, myalgia, paresthesia, rigors, weakness
Otic: Ear ache, otitis media
Renal: Renal calculus
Respiratory: Coughing, pharyngitis, rhinitis, sinusitis
Miscellaneous: Allergy, diaphoresis

1% to 4%:

Cardiovascular: Angina, cardiac failure, cerebral vascular disorder, edema, flushing, hematoma, phlebitis, tachycardia
Central nervous system: Abnormal gait, amnesia, dysphonia, hallucinations, nervousness, neuralgia, neuropathy, somnolence, tremor, vertigo
Dermatologic: Acne, alopecia, bruising, cellulitis, urticaria
Endocrine & metabolic: Hypoglycemia (2% to 4%), hypokalemia, hypoproteinemia, gout, cachexia, menstrual irregularities, breast pain, impotence
Gastrointestinal: Colitis, diverticulitis, dysphagia, fat malabsorption, gastritis, gastroenteritis, gingivitis, glossitis, melena, rectal bleeding, stomatitis, taste perversion, xerostomia
Genitourinary: Incontinence
Hematologic: Epistaxis
Hepatic: Ascites, jaundice
Local: Injection hematoma
Neuromuscular & skeletal: Hyperkinesia, hypertonia, joint pain
Ocular: Blurred vision, visual disturbance
Otic: Tinnitus
Renal: Albuminuria, renal abscess
Respiratory: Bronchitis, pleural effusion, pneumonia, pulmonary embolism
Miscellaneous: Bacterial infection, cold symptoms, moniliasis

<1% (Limited to important or life-threatening): Abdomen enlarged, anaphylactic shock, anaphylactoid reaction, aneurysm, aphasia, appendicitis, arthritis, atrial fibrillation, basal cell carcinoma, Bell's palsy, breast carcinoma, burning eyes, cardiac arrest, CHF, CK increased, creatinine increased, deafness, diabetes insipidus, diabetes mellitus, facial edema, fatty liver, galactorrhea, gallbladder polyp, gallstones, GI hemorrhage, glaucoma, gynecomastia, hematuria, hemiparesis, hepatitis, hyperesthesia, hypertensive reaction, hypoadrenalism, intestinal obstruction, intracranial hemorrhage, iron deficiency, ischemia, joint effusion, lactation, leg cramps, LFTs increased, libido decreased, malignant hyperpyrexia, MI, migraine, muscle cramping, nephrolithiasis, orthostatic hypotension, pancreatitis, paranoia, paresis, peptic ulcer, petechiae, pituitary apoplexy, pneumothorax, pulmonary hypertension, pulmonary nodule, Raynaud's syndrome, renal insufficiency, retinal vein thrombosis, rhinorrhea, scotoma, seizure, status asthmaticus, suicide attempt, throat discomfort, thrombocytopenia, thrombophlebitis, thrombosis, vaginitis, visual field defect, wheal/erythema

Overdosage/Toxicology Symptoms of overdose include hypo- or hyperglycemia, blurred vision, dizziness, drowsiness, and loss of motor function. Well tolerated bolus doses up to 1000 mcg have failed to produce adverse effects.

Dosing

Adults & Elderly: SubQ, I.V.: Initial: 50 mcg 2-3 times/day; titrate dose based on response, tolerance, and indication

Carcinoid tumors:

SubQ, I.V.: Initial 2 weeks: 100-600 mcg/day in 2-4 divided doses; usual range 50-1500 mcg/day

I.M. Depot injection: Patients must be stabilized on subcutaneous octreotide for at least 2 weeks before switching to the long-acting depot: Upon switch: 20 mg I.M. intragluteally every 4 weeks for 2-3 months, then the dose may be modified based upon response

Dosage adjustment: See dosing for VIPomas.

VIPomas:

SubQ, I.V.: Initial 2 weeks: 200-300 mcg/day in 2-4 divided doses; titrate dose based on response/tolerance. Range: 150-750 mcg/day (doses >450 mcg/day are rarely required)

I.M. Depot injection: Patients must be stabilized on subcutaneous octreotide for at least 2 weeks before switching to the long-acting depot: Upon switch: 20 mg I.M. intragluteally every 4 weeks for 2-3 months, then the dose may be modified based upon response

Dosage adjustment for carcinoid tumors and VIPomas: After 2 months of depot injections the dosage may be continued or modified as follows:

Increase to 30 mg I.M. every 4 weeks if symptoms are inadequately controlled

Decrease to 10 mg I.M. every 4 weeks, for a trial period, if initially responsive to 20 mg dose

Dosage >30 mg is not recommended

Diarrhea: I.V.: Initial: 50-100 mcg every 8 hours; increase by 100 mcg/dose at 48-hour intervals; maximum dose: 500 mcg every 8 hours

Esophageal varices bleeding (unlabeled use): I.V. bolus: 25-50 mcg followed by continuous I.V. infusion of 25-50 mcg/hour

Acromegaly:

SubQ, I.V.: Initial: 50 mcg 3 times/day; titrate to achieve growth hormone levels <5 ng/mL or IGF-I (somatomedin C) levels <1.9 U/mL in males and <2.2 U/mL in females. Usual effective dose 100 mcg 3 times/day. Range 300-1500 mcg/day. **Note:** Should be withdrawn yearly for a 4 week interval (8 weeks for depot injection) in patients who have received irradiation. Resume if levels increase and signs/symptoms recur.

I.M. Depot injection: Patients must be stabilized on subcutaneous octreotide for at least 2 weeks before switching to the long-acting depot: Upon switch: 20 mg I.M. intragluteally every 4 weeks for 2-3 months, then the dose may be modified based upon response

Dosage adjustment for acromegaly: After 3 months of depot injections the dosage may be continued or modified as follows:

GH ≤1 ng/mL, IGF-1 is normal, symptoms controlled: Reduce octreotide LAR® to 10 mg I.M. every 4 weeks

GH ≤2.5 ng/mL, IGF-1 is normal, symptoms controlled: Maintain octreotide LAR® at 20 mg I.M. every 4 weeks

GH >2.5 ng/mL, IGF-1 is elevated, or symptoms uncontrolled: Increase octreotide LAR® to 30 mg I.M. every 4 weeks

Dosages >40 mg are not recommended

Pediatrics: Infants and Children:

Secretory diarrhea (unlabeled use): I.V., SubQ: Doses of 1-10 mcg/kg every 12 hours have been used in children beginning at the low end of the range and increasing by 0.3 mcg/kg/dose at 3-day intervals. Suppression of growth hormone (animal data) is of concern when used as long-term therapy.

Congenital hyperinsulinism (unlabeled use): SubQ: Doses of 3-40 mcg/kg/day have been used.

Renal Impairment: Half-life may be increased, requiring adjustment of maintenance dose.

Available Dosage Forms

Injection, microspheres for suspension, as acetate [depot formulation] (Sandostatin LAR®): 10 mg, 20 mg, 30 mg [with diluent and syringe]

Injection, solution, as acetate (Sandostatin®): 0.05 mg/mL (1 mL); 0.1 mg/mL (1 mL); 0.2 mg/mL (5 mL); 0.5 mg/mL (1 mL); 1 mg/mL (5 mL)

Nursing Guidelines

Assessment: See Contraindications, Warnings/Precautions, and Dosing for use cautions. Assess potential for interactions with other prescriptions, OTC medications, or herbal products patient may be taking (see extensive list of Drug Interactions). See Administration specifics. Assess results of laboratory tests (see below), therapeutic effectiveness, and adverse effects (see Adverse Reactions and Overdose/Toxicology). Caution patients with diabetes to monitor

(Continued)

Octreotide *(Continued)*

serum glucose closely; may increase the effect of insulin or sulfonylureas, which may result in hypoglycemia. Teach patient proper use if self-administered (appropriate injection technique and syringe/needle disposal), possible side effects/appropriate interventions, and adverse symptoms to report (see Patient Education). Breast-feeding is contraindicated.

Monitoring Laboratory Tests: Blood glucose

Acromegaly: Growth hormone, somatomedin C (IGF-1), heart rate, EKG

Carcinoid: 5-HIAA, plasma serotonin and plasma substance P

VIPomas: Vasoactive intestinal peptide

Chronic therapy: Thyroid function (baseline and periodic), vitamin B_{12} level

Dietary Considerations: Schedule injections between meals to decrease GI effects. May alter absorption of dietary fats.

Patient Education: Inform prescriber of all prescriptions, OTC medications, or herbal products you are taking, and any allergies you have. Do not take any new medication during therapy unless approved by prescriber. If self-administered, follow instructions for injection and syringe/needle disposal. Schedule injections between meals to decrease GI effects. Consult prescriber about appropriate diet. If you have diabetes, monitor serum glucose closely and notify prescriber of significant changes (this drug may increase the effects of insulin or sulfonylureas). May cause skin flushing; nausea or vomiting (small, frequent meals, frequent mouth care, sucking lozenges, or chewing gum may help); or dizziness, fatigue, or drowsiness (use caution when driving or engaging in tasks that require alertness until response to drug is known). Report unusual weight gain, swelling of extremities, or respiratory difficulty; acute or persistent GI distress (eg, diarrhea, vomiting, constipation, abdominal pain); muscle weakness or tremors or loss of motor function; chest pain or palpitations; blurred vision; depression; or redness, swelling, burning, or pain at injection site. **Breast-feeding precaution:** Do not breast-feed.

Pregnancy Risk Factor: B

Lactation: Excretion in breast milk unknown/use caution

Administration

I.M.: Depot formulation: Administer I.M. intragluteal (avoid deltoid administration); do not administer Sandostatin LAR® intravenously or subcutaneously; must be administered immediately after mixing

I.V.: Regular injection only (not suspension): IVP should be administered undiluted over 3 minutes. IVPB should be administered over 15-30 minutes. Continuous I.V. infusion rates have ranged from 25-50 mcg/hour for the treatment of esophageal variceal bleeding.

Compatibility: Stable in D_5W, NS; **incompatible** with fat emulsion 10%.

The manufacturer states that octreotide solution is not compatible in TPN solutions due to the formation of a glycosyl octreotide conjugate which may have decreased activity; other sources give it limited compatibility.

Storage:

Solution: Octreotide is a clear solution and should be stored under refrigeration; may be stored at room temperature for up to 14 days when protected from light. Stability of parenteral admixture is stable in NS for 96 hours at room temperature (25°C) and in D_5W for 24 hours.

Suspension: Prior to dilution, store under refrigeration and protect from light; may be at room temperature for 30-60 minutes prior to use; use suspension immediately after preparation.

♦ **Octreotide Acetate** *see* Octreotide *on page 1251*

♦ **OcuCoat® [OTC]** *see* Artificial Tears *on page 187*

♦ **OcuCoat® PF [OTC]** *see* Artificial Tears *on page 187*

♦ **Ocufen®** *see* Flurbiprofen *on page 757*

♦ **Ocuflox®** *see* Ofloxacin *on page 1255*

♦ **Ocuvite® [OTC]** *see* Vitamins (Multiple/Oral) *on page 1720*

♦ **Ocuvite® Extra® [OTC]** *see* Vitamins (Multiple/Oral) *on page 1720*

♦ **Ocuvite® Lutein [OTC]** *see* Vitamins (Multiple/Oral) *on page 1720*

Ofloxacin (oh FLOKS a sin)

U.S. Brand Names Floxin®; Ocuflox®

Synonyms Floxin Otic Singles

Pharmacologic Category Antibiotic, Quinolone

Medication Safety Issues

Sound-alike/look-alike issues:

Floxin® may be confused with Flexeril®

Ocuflox® may be confused with Ocufen®

Use Quinolone antibiotic for the treatment of acute exacerbations of chronic bronchitis, community-acquired pneumonia, skin and skin structure infections (uncomplicated), urethral and cervical gonorrhea (acute, uncomplicated), urethritis and cervicitis (nongonococcal), mixed infections of the urethra and cervix, pelvic inflammatory disease (acute), cystitis (uncomplicated), urinary tract infections (complicated), prostatitis

Ophthalmic: Treatment of superficial ocular infections involving the conjunctiva or cornea due to strains of susceptible organisms

Otic: Otitis externa, chronic suppurative otitis media, acute otitis media

Unlabeled/Investigational Use Epididymitis (gonorrhea)

Mechanism of Action Ofloxacin is a DNA gyrase inhibitor. DNA gyrase is an essential bacterial enzyme that maintains the superhelical structure of DNA. DNA gyrase is required for DNA replication and transcription, DNA repair, recombination, and transposition; bactericidal

Pharmacodynamics/Kinetics

Absorption: Well absorbed; food causes only minor alterations

Distribution: V_d: 2.4-3.5 L/kg

Protein binding: 20%

Bioavailability: Oral: 98%

Half-life elimination: Biphasic: 5-7.5 hours and 20-25 hours (accounts for <5%); prolonged with renal impairment

Excretion: Primarily urine (as unchanged drug)

Contraindications Hypersensitivity to ofloxacin or other members of the quinolone group such as nalidixic acid, oxolinic acid, cinoxacin, norfloxacin, and ciprofloxacin; hypersensitivity to any component of the formulation

Warnings/Precautions Use with caution in patients with epilepsy or other CNS diseases which could predispose seizures; use with caution in patients with renal or hepatic impairment. Tendon inflammation and/or rupture have been reported with quinolone antibiotics, including ofloxacin. Risk may be increased with concurrent corticosteroids, particularly in the elderly. Discontinue at first sign of tendon inflammation or pain. Peripheral neuropathies have been linked to ofloxacin use; discontinue if numbness, tingling, or weakness develops.

Rare cases of torsade de pointes have been reported in patients receiving ofloxacin and other quinolones. Risk may be minimized by avoiding use in patients with known prolongation of the QT interval, bradycardia, hypokalemia, hypomagnesemia, cardiomyopathy, or in those receiving concurrent therapy with Class Ia or Class III antiarrhythmics.

Severe hypersensitivity reactions, including anaphylaxis, have occurred with quinolone therapy. If an allergic reaction occurs (itching, urticaria, dyspnea, facial edema, loss of consciousness, tingling, cardiovascular collapse), discontinue drug immediately. Prolonged use may result in superinfection; pseudomembranous colitis may occur and should be considered in all patients who present with diarrhea. Quinolones may exacerbate myasthenia gravis, use with caution (rare, potentially life-threatening weakness of respiratory muscles may occur).

Drug Interactions **Inhibits** CYP1A2 (strong)

Corticosteroids: Concurrent use may increase the risk of tendon rupture, particularly in elderly patients (overall incidence rare).

CYP1A2 substrates: Ofloxacin may increase the levels/effects of CYP1A2 substrates. Example substrates include aminophylline, fluvoxamine, mexiletine, mirtazapine, ropinirole, and trifluoperazine.

Glyburide: Quinolones may increase the effect of glyburide; monitor.

Metal cations (aluminum, calcium, iron, magnesium, and zinc) bind quinolones in the gastrointestinal tract and inhibit absorption. Concurrent administration of most antacids, oral electrolyte supplements, quinapril, sucralfate, some didanosine formulations (chewable/buffered tablets and pediatric powder for oral suspension), and other highly-buffered oral drugs, should be avoided. Ofloxacin should be administered 2 hours before or 2 hours after these agents.

Probenecid: May decrease renal secretion of ofloxacin.

(Continued)

Ofloxacin *(Continued)*

QT_c-prolonging agents: Effects may be additive with ofloxacin. Avoid concurrent use with Class Ia and Class III antiarrhythmics; use caution with other drugs known to prolong QT_c, including erythromycin, cisapride, antipsychotics, and cyclic antidepressants.

Theophylline: Ofloxacin may increase plasma levels of theophylline. Monitor.

Warfarin: The hypoprothrombinemic effect of warfarin may be enhanced by some quinolone antibiotics; monitor INR.

Nutritional/Herbal/Ethanol Interactions

Food: Ofloxacin average peak serum concentrations may be decreased by 20% if taken with food.

Herb/Nutraceutical: Avoid dong quai, St John's wort (may also cause photosensitization).

Adverse Reactions

Systemic:

1% to 10%:

Cardiovascular: Chest pain (1% to 3%)

Central nervous system: Headache (1% to 9%), insomnia (3% to 7%), dizziness (1% to 5%), fatigue (1% to 3%), somnolence (1% to 3%), sleep disorders (1% to 3%), nervousness (1% to 3%), pyrexia (1% to 3%)

Dermatologic: Rash/pruritus (1% to 3%)

Gastrointestinal: Diarrhea (1% to 4%), vomiting (1% to 4%), GI distress (1% to 3%), abdominal cramps (1% to 3%), flatulence (1% to 3%), abnormal taste (1% to 3%), xerostomia (1% to 3%), decreased appetite (1% to 3%), nausea (3% to 10%), constipation (1% to 3%)

Genitourinary: Vaginitis (1% to 5%), external genital pruritus in women (1% to 3%)

Ocular: Visual disturbances (1% to 3%)

Respiratory: Pharyngitis (1% to 3%)

Miscellaneous: Trunk pain

<1%, postmarketing, and/or case reports (limited to important or life-threatening): Anaphylaxis reactions, anxiety, blurred vision, chills, cognitive change, cough, depression, dream abnormality, ecchymosis, edema, erythema nodosum, euphoria, extremity pain, hallucinations, hearing acuity decreased, hepatic dysfunction, hepatitis, hyper/hypoglycemia, hypertension, interstitial nephritis, lightheadedness, malaise, myasthenia gravis exacerbation, palpitation, paresthesia, peripheral neuropathy, photophobia, photosensitivity, psychotic reactions, rhabdomyolysis, seizure, Stevens-Johnson syndrome, syncope, tendonitis and tendon rupture, thirst, tinnitus, torsade de pointes, Tourette's syndrome, toxic epidermal necrolysis, vasculitis, vasodilation, vertigo, weakness, weight loss

Ophthalmic: Frequency not defined:

Central nervous system: Dizziness

Gastrointestinal: Nausea

Ocular: Blurred vision, burning, chemical conjunctivitis/keratitis, discomfort, dryness, edema, eye pain, foreign body sensation, itching, photophobia, redness, stinging, tearing

Otic:

>10%: Local: Application site reaction (<1% to 17%)

1% to 10%:

Central nervous system: Dizziness (≤1%), vertigo (≤1%)

Dermatologic: Pruritus (1% to 4%), rash (1%)

Gastrointestinal: Taste perversion (7%)

Neuromuscular & skeletal: Paresthesia (1%)

<1% (Limited to important or life-threatening): Diarrhea, fever, headache, hearing loss (transient), hypertension, nausea, otorrhagia, tinnitus, transient neuropsychiatric disturbances, tremor, vomiting, xerostomia

Overdosage/Toxicology Symptoms of overdose include acute renal failure, seizures, nausea, and vomiting. Treatment includes GI decontamination, if possible, and supportive care. Not removed by peritoneal or hemodialysis.

Dosing

Adults:

Chronic bronchitis (acute exacerbation), community-acquired pneumonia, skin and skin structure infections (uncomplicated): 400 mg every 12 hours for 10 days

Urethral and cervical gonorrhea (acute, uncomplicated): 400 mg as a single dose

Cervicitis/urethritis (nongonococcal) due to *C. trachomatis*, mixed infection of urethra and cervix due to *C. trachomatis* and *N. gonorrhoea*: 300 mg every 12 hours for 7 days

Pelvic inflammatory disease (acute): 400 mg every 12 hours for 10-14 days

Cystitis (uncomplicated):

Due to *E. coli* or *K. pneumoniae*: 200 mg every 12 hours for 3 days

Due to other organisms: 200 mg every 12 hours for 7 days

UTI (complicated): 200 mg every 12 hours for 10 days

Prostatitis: 200 mg every 12 hours for 6 weeks

Epididymitis (gonorrhea; unlabeled use): 300 mg twice daily for 10 days

Conjunctivitis: Ophthalmic: Instill 1-2 drops in affected eye(s) every 2-4 hours for the first 2 days, then use 4 times/day for an additional 5 days.

Corneal ulcer: Ophthalmic: Instill 1-2 drops every 30 minutes while awake and every 4-6 hours after retiring for the first 2 days; beginning on day 3, instill 1-2 drops every hour while awake for 4-6 additional days; thereafter, 1-2 drops 4 times/day until clinical cure.

Chronic suppurative otitis media with perforated tympanic membranes: Otic: Instill 10 drops (or the contents of 2 single-dose containers) into affected ear twice daily for 14 days

Otitis externa: Otic: Instill 10 drops (or the contents of 2 single-dose containers) into affected ear(s) once daily for 7 days

Elderly: Oral: 200-400 mg every 12-24 hours (based on estimated renal function) for 7 days to 6 weeks depending on indication.

Pediatrics: Not for systemic use

Conjunctivitis: Ophthalmic: Children ≥1 year: Refer to adult dosing.

Corneal ulcer: Ophthalmic: Children ≥1 year: Refer to adult dosing.

Chronic suppurative otitis media with perforated tympanic membranes: Otic: Children >12 years: Refer to adult dosing.

Otitis externa: Otic:

Children 6 months to 13 years: Instill 5 drops (or the contents of 1 single-dose container) into affected ear(s) once daily for 7 days

Children ≥13 years: Refer to adult dosing.

Acute otitis media with tympanotomy tubes: Otic: Children 1-12 years: Instill 5 drops (or the contents of 1 single-dose container) into affected ear twice daily for 10 days.

Renal Impairment: Adults: Oral: After a normal initial dose, adjust as follows:

Cl_{cr} 20-50 mL/minute: Administer usual dose every 24 hours

Cl_{cr} <20 mL/minute: Administer half the usual dose every 24 hours

Continuous arteriovenous or venovenous hemodiafiltration effects: Administer 300 mg every 24 hours

Hepatic Impairment: Severe impairment: Maximum dose: 400 mg/day

Available Dosage Forms [DSC] = Discontinued product

Solution, ophthalmic (Ocuflox®): 0.3% (5 mL; 10 mL [DSC]) [contains benzalkonium chloride]

Solution, otic:

Floxin®: 0.3% (5 mL, 10 mL) [contains benzalkonium chloride]

Floxin® Otic Singles™: 0.3% (0.25 mL) [contains benzalkonium chloride; packaged as 2 single-dose containers per pouch, 10 pouches per carton, total net volume 5 mL]

Tablet (Floxin®): 200 mg, 300 mg, 400 mg

Nursing Guidelines

Assessment: Assess allergy history before initiating therapy. See Contraindications, Warnings/Precautions, and Dosing for use cautions. Assess potential for interactions with other prescriptions, OTC medications, or herbal products patient may be taking (see extensive list of Drug Interactions). See administration specifics for different formulations below. Assess results of laboratory tests (see below), therapeutic effectiveness, and adverse effects (see Adverse Reactions and Overdose/Toxicology). Teach patient appropriate use (according to formulation), possible side effects/appropriate interventions, and adverse symptoms to report (see Patient Education). Breast-feeding is not recommended.

Monitoring Laboratory Tests: Perform culture and sensitivity studies before initiating therapy. Monitor CBC, renal and hepatic function periodically if therapy is prolonged.

(Continued)

Ofloxacin *(Continued)*

Patient Education: Inform prescriber of all prescriptions, OTC medications, or herbal products you are taking, and any allergies you have. Do not take any new medication during therapy unless approved by prescriber.

Oral: Take per recommended schedule; complete full course of therapy and do not skip doses. Take on an empty stomach (1 hour before or 2 hours after meals, dairy products, antacids, or other medication). Maintain adequate hydration (2-3 L/day of fluids) unless advised by prescriber to restrict fluids. May cause dizziness, lightheadedness, or headache (use caution when driving or engaging in tasks that require alertness until response to drug is known); nausea, vomiting, or taste perversion (small, frequent meals, frequent mouth care, sucking lozenges, or chewing gum may help); photosensitivity (use sunscreen, wear protective clothing and eyewear, and avoid direct sunlight). If inflammation or tendon pain occurs, discontinue use immediately and report to prescriber. If chest pain, palpitations, rapid heart beat, or unusual dizziness occurs, contact prescriber immediately. If sign of allergic reaction (eg, itching, urticaria, respiratory difficulty, facial edema or difficulty swallowing, loss of consciousness, tingling, chest pain, palpitations) occurs, discontinue use immediately and report to prescriber. Report GI disturbances; CNS changes (eg, excessive sleepiness, agitation, or tremors); skin rash; vision changes; respiratory difficulty; signs of opportunistic infection (eg, sore throat, chills, fever, burning, itching on urination, vaginal discharge, white plaques in mouth); or worsening of condition.

Pregnancy/breast-feeding precautions: Inform prescriber if you are or intend to become pregnant. Breast-feeding is not recommended.

Ophthalmic: Tilt head back, instill 1-2 drops in affected eye as frequently as prescribed. Do not let tip of applicator touch eye; do not contaminate tip of applicator (may cause eye infection, eye damage, or vision loss). May cause some stinging or burning or a bad taste in you mouth after instillation. Report persistent pain, burning, swelling, or visual disturbances.

Otic: Wash hands before and after applying drops. Lie with affected ear up and instill prescribed number of drops into ear. Remain on side with ear up for 5 minutes.

Geriatric Considerations: The risk of torsade de pointes and tendon inflammation and/or rupture associated with the concomitant use of corticosteroids and quinolones is increased in the elderly population. Dosage must be carefully adjusted to renal function. The half-life of ofloxacin may be prolonged, and serum concentrations are elevated in elderly patients even in the absence of overt renal impairment.

Pregnancy Risk Factor: C

Pregnancy Issues: Reports of arthropathy (observed in immature animals and reported rarely in humans) have limited the use of fluoroquinolones in pregnancy. Teratogenic effects were not observed with ofloxacin in animal studies; however, decreased fetal body weight and increased fetal mortality were observed in some species. Ofloxacin crosses the placenta. Although quinolone antibiotics should not be used as first-line agents during pregnancy, when considering treatment for life-threatening infection and/or prolonged duration of therapy, the potential risk to the fetus must be balanced against the severity of the potential illness.

Lactation: Enters breast milk/not recommended (AAP rates "compatible")

Breast-Feeding Considerations: Following oral use, levels of ofloxacin in breast milk are similar to those in plasma. The manufacturer recommends to discontinue nursing or to discontinue ofloxacin.

Administration

Oral: Do not take within 2 hours of food or any antacids which contain zinc, magnesium, or aluminum.

Storage:

Ophthalmic and otic solution: Store between 15°C to 25°C (59°F to 77°F).

Otic Singles™: Store between 15°C to 30°C (59°F to 86°F). Store in pouch to protect from light.

Tablet: Store below 30°C (86°F).

Related Information

Prevention of Wound Infection and Sepsis in Surgical Patients *on page 1830*

Olanzapine (oh LAN za peen)

U.S. Brand Names Zyprexa®; Zyprexa® Zydis®

Synonyms LY170053; Zyprexa Zydis

Pharmacologic Category Antipsychotic Agent, Atypical

Medication Safety Issues

Sound-alike/look-alike issues:

Olanzapine may be confused with olsalazine

Zyprexa® may be confused with Celexa™, Zyrtec®

Use Treatment of the manifestations of schizophrenia; treatment of acute or mixed mania episodes associated with Bipolar I Disorder (as monotherapy or in combination with lithium or valproate); maintenance treatment of bipolar disorder; acute agitation (patients with schizophrenia or bipolar mania)

Unlabeled/Investigational Use Treatment of psychotic symptoms; chronic pain

Mechanism of Action Olanzapine is a thienobenzodiazepine antipsychotic which is a potent selective antagonist of serotonin 5-HT_{2A} and 5-HT_{2C}, dopamine D_{1-4}, muscarinic M_{1-5}, histamine H_1- and alpha$_1$-adrenergic receptors. Olanzapine shows moderate antagonism of 5-HT_3 and muscarinic M_{1-5} receptors, and weak binding to GABA-A, BZD, and beta-adrenergic receptors. Although the precise mechanism of action in schizophrenia and bipolar disorder is not known, the efficacy of olanzapine is thought to be mediated through combined antagonism of dopamine and serotonin type 2 receptor sites.

Pharmacodynamics/Kinetics

Absorption:

I.M.: Rapidly absorbed

Oral: Well absorbed; not affected by food; tablets and orally-disintegrating tablets are bioequivalent

Distribution: V_d: Extensive, 1000 L

Protein binding, plasma: 93% bound to albumin and alpha$_1$-glycoprotein

Metabolism: Highly metabolized via direct glucuronidation and cytochrome P450 mediated oxidation (CYP1A2, CYP2D6)

Bioavailability: >57%

Half-life elimination: 21-54 hours; ~1.5 times greater in elderly

Time to peak, plasma: Maximum plasma concentrations after I.M. administration are 5 times higher than maximum plasma concentrations produced by an oral dose.

I.M.: 15-45 minutes

Oral: ~6 hours

Excretion: 40% removed via first pass metabolism; urine (57%, 7% as unchanged drug); feces (30%)

Clearance: 40% increase in olanzapine clearance in smokers

Contraindications Hypersensitivity to olanzapine or any component of the formulation

Warnings/Precautions Patients with dementia-related behavioral disorders treated with atypical antipsychotics are at an increased risk of death compared to placebo. Olanzapine is not approved for this indication.

Moderate to highly sedating, use with caution in disorders where CNS depression is a feature; patients must be cautioned about performing tasks which require mental alertness (eg, operating machinery or driving). Use with caution in Parkinson's disease; in patients with hemodynamic instability; bone marrow suppression; predisposition to seizures; subcortical brain damage; severe cardiac, hepatic, renal, or respiratory disease. Esophageal dysmotility and aspiration have been associated with antipsychotic use; use with caution in patients at risk of pneumonia (ie, Alzheimer's disease). Caution in breast cancer or other prolactin-dependent tumors (may elevate prolactin levels). May alter temperature regulation or mask toxicity of other drugs due to antiemetic effects. Life-threatening arrhythmias have occurred with therapeutic doses of some neuroleptics. An increased incidence of cerebrovascular adverse events (including fatalities) has been reported in elderly patients with dementia-related psychosis. Significant weight gain may occur.

May cause anticholinergic effects (constipation, xerostomia, blurred vision, urinary retention); therefore, they should be used with caution in patients with decreased gastrointestinal motility, urinary retention, BPH, xerostomia, or visual problems. Conditions which also may be exacerbated by cholinergic blockade include narrow-angle glaucoma (screening is recommended) and worsening of myasthenia gravis. Relative to other neuroleptics, olanzapine has a moderate potency of cholinergic blockade.

(Continued)

Olanzapine *(Continued)*

May cause extrapyramidal symptoms, including pseudoparkinsonism, acute dystonic reactions, akathisia, and tardive dyskinesia (risk of these reactions is very low relative to other neuroleptics). May be associated with neuroleptic malignant syndrome (NMS). May cause hyperglycemia; in some cases may be extreme and associated with ketoacidosis, hyperosmolar coma, or death. Use with caution in patients with diabetes or other disorders of glucose regulation; monitor for worsening of glucose control. Olanzapine levels may be lower in patients who smoke, requiring dosage adjustment.

The possibility of a suicide attempt is inherent in psychotic illness or bipolar disorder; use caution in high-risk patients during initiation of therapy. Prescriptions should be written for the smallest quantity consistent with good patient care.

Drug Interactions Substrate of CYP1A2 (major), 2D6 (minor); **Inhibits** CYP1A2 (weak), 2C8/9 (weak), 2C19 (weak), 2D6 (weak), 3A4 (weak)

Acetylcholinesterase inhibitors (central): May increase the risk of antipsychotic-related extrapyramidal symptoms; monitor.

Anticholinergics: Adverse effects/toxicity may be additive with olanzapine.

Carbamazepine: May decreases olanzapine levels/effects; monitor.

Ciprofloxacin; May increase the levels/effects of olanzapine.

CNS depressants: Sedative effects and may be additive with CNS depressants; includes ethanol, barbiturates, narcotic analgesics, and other sedative agents; monitor for increased effect.

CYP1A2 inhibitors: May increase the levels/effects of olanzapine. Example inhibitors include amiodarone, ciprofloxacin, fluvoxamine, ketoconazole, norfloxacin, ofloxacin, and rofecoxib.

Fluvoxamine: Increases olanzapine levels; consider using a lower dose of olanzapine in patients receiving concomitant treatment with fluvoxamine.

Nutritional/Herbal/Ethanol Interactions

Ethanol: Avoid ethanol (may increase CNS depression).

Herb/Nutraceutical: Avoid dong quai, St John's wort (may also cause photosensitization). Avoid kava kava, gotu kola, valerian, St John's wort (may increase CNS depression).

Adverse Reactions

>10%:

- Central nervous system: Somnolence (6% to 39% dose-dependent), extrapyramidal symptoms (15% to 32% dose-dependent), insomnia (up to 12%), dizziness (4% to 18%)
- Gastrointestinal: Dyspepsia (7% to 11%), constipation (9% to 11%), weight gain (5% to 6%, has been reported as high as 40%), xerostomia (9% to 22% dose-dependent)
- Neuromuscular & skeletal: Weakness (2% to 20% dose-dependent)
- Miscellaneous: Accidental injury (12%)

1% to 10%:

- Cardiovascular: Postural hypotension (1% to 5%), tachycardia (up to 3%), peripheral edema (up to 3%), chest pain (up to 3%), hyper-/hypotension (up to 2%)
- Central nervous system: Personality changes (8%), speech disorder (7%), fever (up to 6%), abnormal dreams, euphoria, amnesia, delusions, emotional lability, mania, schizophrenia
- Dermatologic: Bruising (up to 5%)
- Endocrine & metabolic: Cholesterol increased, prolactin increased
- Gastrointestinal: Nausea (up to 9% dose-dependent), appetite increased (3% to 6%), vomiting (up to 4%), flatulence, salivation increased, thirst
- Genitourinary: Incontinence (up to 2%), UTI (up to 2%), vaginitis
- Local: Injection site pain (I.M. administration)
- Neuromuscular & skeletal: Twitching, hypertonia (up to 3%), tremor (up to 7% dose-dependent), back pain (up to 5%), abnormal gait (6%), joint/extremity pain (up to 5%) akathisia (3% to 5%), articulation impairment (up to 2%), falling (particularly in older patients), joint stiffness
- Ocular: Amblyopia (up to 3%), conjunctivitis
- Respiratory: Rhinitis (up to 7%), cough (up to 6%), pharyngitis (up to 4%), dyspnea
- Miscellaneous: Dental pain, diaphoresis, flu-like symptoms

<1% (Limited to important or life-threatening): Acidosis, akinesia, albuminuria, alkaline phosphatase increased, anaphylactoid reaction, anemia, angioedema, apnea, arteritis, asthma, ataxia, atelectasis, atrial fibrillation, AV block, bilirubinemia, bradycardia, cataract, cerebrovascular accident, CNS stimulation,

coma, confusion, congestive heart failure, creatine phosphokinase increased, cyanosis, deafness, dehydration, diabetes mellitus, diabetic acidosis, dyskinesia, encephalopathy, enteritis, esophageal ulcer, facial paralysis, fecal impaction, glaucoma, heart arrest, heart block, heart failure, hematuria, hemoptysis; hemorrhage (eye, rectal, subarachnoid, vaginal), hepatitis, hyper-/hypoglycemia, hypo-/hyperkalemia, hyperlipemia, hypo-/hypernatremia, hyperuricemia, hyper-/hypoventilation, hypoproteinemia, hypoxia, ileus, ketosis, leukocytosis, leukopenia, liver fatty deposit, lung edema, lymphadenopathy, myasthenia, myopathy, neuroleptic malignant syndrome, neuropathy, normocytic anemia, osteoporosis, palpitation, pancreatitis, paralysis, pulmonary embolus, rhabdomyolysis, rheumatoid arthritis, seizure, stridor, sudden death, suicide attempt, syncope, tardive dyskinesia, thrombocythemia, thrombocytopenia, ventricular extrasystoles, venous thrombotic events, withdrawal syndrome

Overdosage/Toxicology Signs and symptoms of overdose include CNS depression (ranging from drowsiness to coma), extrapyramidal movements, fasciculations, hypotension (possible, though not described), miosis, respiratory depression, rhinitis (10%), slurred speech, tachycardia, trismus. Treatment is symptom-directed and supportive. Activated charcoal (1 g) may reduce the C_{max} and AUC of olanzapine by ~60%.

Dosing

Adults:

Schizophrenia: Initial: 5-10 mg once daily, increase to 10 mg once daily within 5-7 days; thereafter, adjust by 5 mg/day at 1-week intervals, up to a recommended maximum of 20 mg/day. Maintenance: 10-20 mg once daily. **Note:** Doses of 30-50 mg/day have been used; however, safety and efficacy of doses >20 mg/day have not been evaluated.

Acute mania associated with bipolar disorder: Oral:

Monotherapy: Initial: 10-15 mg once daily; increase by 5 mg/day at intervals of not less than 24 hours. Maintenance: 5-20 mg/day; recommended maximum dose: 20 mg/day

Combination therapy (with lithium or valproate): Initial: 10 mg once daily; dosing range: 5-20 mg/day

Agitation (acute, associated with bipolar disorder or schizophrenia): I.M.: Initial dose: 5-10 mg (a lower dose of 2.5 mg may be considered when clinical factors warrant); additional doses (2.5-10 mg) may be considered; however, 2-4 hours should be allowed between doses to evaluate response (maximum total daily dose: 30 mg, per manufacturer's recommendation)

Elderly: Refer to adult dosing. Consider lower starting dose of 2.5-5 mg/day for elderly or debilitated patients; may increase as clinically indicated and tolerated with close monitoring of orthostatic blood pressure.

Pediatrics:

Schizophrenia/bipolar disorder: Oral: Initial: 2.5 mg/day; titrate as necessary to 20 mg/day (0.12-0.29 mg/kg/day)

Renal Impairment: No dosage adjustment required. Not removed by dialysis

Hepatic Impairment: Dosage adjustment may be necessary, however, there are no specific recommendations. Monitor closely.

Available Dosage Forms

Injection, powder for reconstitution (Zyprexa® IntraMuscular): 10 mg [contains lactose 50 mg]

Tablet (Zyprexa®): 2.5 mg, 5 mg, 7.5 mg, 10 mg, 15 mg, 20 mg

Tablet, orally-disintegrating (Zyprexa® Zydis®): 5 mg [contains phenylalanine 0.34 mg/tablet], 10 mg [contains phenylalanine 0.45 mg/tablet], 15 mg [contains phenylalanine 0.67 mg/tablet], 20 mg [contains phenylalanine 0.9 mg/tablet]

Nursing Guidelines

Assessment: Assess potential for interactions with other prescriptions, OTC medications, or herbal products patient may be taking. Initiate at lower doses and taper dosage slowly when discontinuing. Instruct patients with diabetes to monitor blood glucose levels closely (may cause hyperglycemia). Monitor therapeutic effectiveness, and adverse reactions at beginning of therapy and periodically with long-term use. Monitor weight prior to initiating therapy and at least monthly. Consider titrating to a different antipsychotic agent for a weight gain ≥ 5% of initial weight. Teach patient appropriate administration, interventions to reduce side effects, and adverse symptoms to report.

Monitoring Laboratory Tests: Fasting lipid profile and fasting blood glucose/Hgb A_{1c} (prior to treatment, at 3 months, then annually); periodic assessment of hepatic transaminases (in patients with hepatic disease)

(Continued)

Olanzapine *(Continued)*

Dietary Considerations: Tablets may be taken with or without food/meals. Zyprexa® Zydis®: 5 mg tablet contains phenylalanine 0.34 mg; 10 mg tablet contains phenylalanine 0.45 mg; 15 mg tablet contains phenylalanine 0.67 mg; 20 mg tablet contains phenylalanine 0.9 mg

Patient Education: Do not take any new medication during therapy unless approved by prescriber. Use exactly as directed; do not increase dose or frequency. It may take 2-3 weeks to achieve desired results; do not discontinue without consulting prescriber. Avoid alcohol or caffeine and other prescription or OTC medications not approved by prescriber. Maintain adequate hydration (2-3 L/day of fluids) unless instructed to restrict fluid intake. If diabetic, you may experience increased blood sugars. Monitor blood sugars closely. If you have glaucoma periodic ophthalmic exams are recommended. You may experience excess drowsiness, restlessness, dizziness, or blurred vision (use caution driving or when engaging in tasks requiring alertness until response to drug is known); or constipation (increased exercise, fluids, fruit, or fiber may help). Report persistent CNS effects (eg, trembling fingers, altered gait or balance, excessive sedation, seizures, unusual movements, anxiety, abnormal thoughts, confusion, personality changes); unresolved constipation or GI effects; vision changes; respiratory difficulty; unusual cough or flu-like symptoms; or worsening of condition. **Pregnancy/breast-feeding precautions:** Inform prescriber if you are or intend to become pregnant. Breast-feeding is not recommended.

Orally-disintegrating tablet: Remove from foil blister by peeling back (do not push tablet through the foil). Place tablet in mouth immediately upon removal. Tablet dissolves rapidly in saliva and may be swallowed with or without liquid.

Geriatric Considerations: (See Warnings/Precautions and Adverse Reactions). Elderly patients have an increased risk of adverse response to side effects or adverse reactions to antipsychotics. A higher incidence of falls has been reported in elderly patients, particularly in debilitated patients. Olanzapine half-life that was 1.5 times that of younger (<65 years of age) adults; therefore, lower initial doses are recommended.

Pregnancy Risk Factor: C

Lactation: Enters breast milk/not recommended

Administration

Oral:

Tablet: May be administered with or without food/meals.

Orally-disintegrating tablet: Remove from foil blister by peeling back (do not push tablet through the foil). Place tablet in mouth immediately upon removal. Tablet dissolves rapidly in saliva and may be swallowed with or without liquid. May be administered with or without food/meals.

I.M.: Injection: For I.M. administration only; inject slowly, deep into muscle. If dizziness and/or drowsiness are noted, patient should remain recumbent until examination indicates postural hypotension and/or bradycardia are not a problem.

I.V.: Do not administer injection intravenously.

Reconstitution: Injection, powder for reconstitution: Reconstitute 10 mg vial with 2.1 mL SWFI; resulting solution is ~5 mg/mL. Use immediately (within 1 hour) following reconstitution. Discard any unused portion.

Storage:

Tablet and orally-disintegrating tablet: Store at room temperature of 15°C to 25°C (59°F to 86°F). Protect from light and moisture.

Injection, powder for reconstitution: Store at room temperature 15°C to 25°C (59°F to 86°F). Protect from light. Do not freeze.

- ♦ **Olay® Vitamins Complete Women's [OTC]** *see* Vitamins (Multiple/Oral) *on page 1720*
- ♦ **Olay® Vitamins Complete Women's 50+[OTC]** *see* Vitamins (Multiple/Oral) *on page 1720*
- ♦ **Olay® Vitamins Even Complexion [OTC]** *see* Vitamins (Multiple/Oral) *on page 1720*

Olopatadine (oh loe pa TA deen)

U.S. Brand Names Patanol®

Pharmacologic Category Antihistamine; Ophthalmic Agent, Miscellaneous

Medication Safety Issues

Sound-alike/look-alike issues:

Patanol® may be confused with Platinol®

Use Treatment of the signs and symptoms of allergic conjunctivitis

Pharmacodynamics/Kinetics

Absorption: Low systemic absorption following topical administration

Half-life elimination: ~3 hours

Excretion: Urine (60% to 70%)

Contraindications Hypersensitivity to olopatadine hydrochloride or any component of the formulation

Warnings/Precautions Contains benzalkonium chloride which may be absorbed by contact lenses; do not wear contact lenses if eyes are red. Safety and efficacy in children <3 years of age have not been established.

Drug Interactions Studies evaluating drug interactions with olopatadine hydrochloride have not been conducted

Adverse Reactions

>5%: Central nervous system: Headache (7%)

<5%:

- Central nervous system: Cold syndrome
- Gastrointestinal: Nausea, taste perversion
- Neuromuscular & skeletal: Weakness
- Ocular: Blurred vision, burning, stinging, dry eyes, foreign body sensation, hyperemia, keratitis, eyelid edema, itching
- Respiratory: Pharyngitis, rhinitis, sinusitis

Dosing

Adults & Elderly: Allergic conjunctivitis: Ophthalmic: Instill 1 to 2 drops into affected eye(s) twice daily (allowing 6-8 hours between doses); results from an environmental study demonstrated that olopatadine was effective when dosed twice daily for up to 6 weeks

Available Dosage Forms Solution, ophthalmic: 0.1% (5 mL) [contains benzalkonium chloride]

Nursing Guidelines

Assessment: Assess therapeutic response and adverse effects. Teach patient proper use, side effects/appropriate interventions, and symptoms to report.

Patient Education: For use in eyes only. Do not let tip of applicator touch eye; do not contaminate tip of applicator (may cause eye infection, eye damage, or vision loss). **Pregnancy precaution:** Inform prescriber if you are pregnant.

Pregnancy Risk Factor: C

♦ **Omacor®** *see* Omega-3-Acid Ethyl Esters *on page 1263*

Omega-3-Acid Ethyl Esters (oh MEG a three AS id ETH il ES ters)

U.S. Brand Names Omacor®

Synonyms Ethyl Esters of Omega-3 Fatty Acids; Fish Oil

Pharmacologic Category Antilipemic Agent, Miscellaneous

Medication Safety Issues

Sound-alike/look-alike issues:

Omacor® may be confused with Amicar®

Use Omacor®: Treatment of hypertriglyceridemia (≥500 mg/dL)

Note: A number of OTC formulations containing omega-3 fatty acids are marketed as nutritional supplements; these do not have FDA-approved indications.

Unlabeled/Investigational Use Omacor®: Treatment of IgA nephropathy

Mechanism of Action Mechanism has not been completely defined. Possible mechanisms include inhibition of acyl CoA:1,2 diacylglycerol acyltransferase, increased hepatic beta-oxidation, or a reduction in the hepatic synthesis of triglycerides.

Contraindications Hypersensitivity to omega-3-acid ethyl esters or any component of the formulation

Warnings/Precautions Use with caution in patients with known allergy to fish. Should be used as an adjunct to diet and exercise only in those with very high triglyceride levels. Treatment of primary metabolic disorders (eg, diabetes, thyroid disease) and/or evaluation of the patient's medication regimen for possible etiologic agents should be completed prior to a decision to initiate therapy. If triglyceride levels do not adequately respond after 2 months of treatment with omega-3-acid ethyl esters, discontinue treatment. Prolongation of bleeding time has been observed in some clinical studies. Use caution in patients with coagulopathy or in those receiving therapeutic anticoagulation. Safety and efficacy have not been established in children (<18 years of age).

(Continued)

Omega-3-Acid Ethyl Esters *(Continued)*

Drug Interactions

Anticoagulants: Omega-3-acid ethyl esters may prolong bleeding time. The effect of concurrent anticoagulant therapy has not been evaluated.

Antiplatelet agents, salicylates, and nonsteroidal anti-inflammatory agents: Omega-3-acid ethyl esters may prolong bleeding time. The effect of concurrent medications which may alter platelet function has not been evaluated.

Beta-blockers: May decrease the therapeutic effect of omega-3-acid ethyl esters. Omega-3-acid ethyl esters may augment the antihypertensive effect of beta-blockers.

Estrogens: May decrease the therapeutic effect of omega-3-acid ethyl esters.

Thiazide diuretics: May decrease the therapeutic effect of omega-3-acid ethyl esters. Thiazide diuretics may increase serum triglycerides. Omega-3-acid ethyl esters may augment the antihypertensive effect of thiazide diuretics.

Nutritional/Herbal/Ethanol Interactions

Ethanol: Monitor ethanol use (alcohol use may increase triglycerides).

Adverse Reactions

Cardiovascular: Angina (1%)

Central nervous system: Pain (2%)

Dermatologic: Rash (2%)

Gastrointestinal: Eructation (5%), dyspepsia (3%), taste perversion (3%)

Neuromuscular and skeletal: Back pain (2%)

Miscellaneous: Flu-like syndrome (4%), infection (4%)

<1% (Limited to important or life-threatening): Body odor, epistaxis, fecal incontinence, ALT increased, AST increased

Dosing

Adults & Elderly:

Hypertriglyceridemia: Oral: 4 g/day as a single daily dose or in 2 divided doses.

Treatment of IgA nephropathy (unlabeled use): Oral: 4 g/day

Renal Impairment: No dosage adjustment required.

Available Dosage Forms Capsule: 1 g [contains EPA ~465 mg and DHA ~375 mg]

Nursing Guidelines

Assessment: Do not use if allergic to fish. Encourage diet and exercise along with use of this medication.

Monitoring Laboratory Tests: Triglycerides and other lipids (LDL-C) should be monitored at baseline and periodically. Hepatic transaminase levels, particularly ALT, should be monitored periodically.

Dietary Considerations: May be taken with meals. Dietary modification is important in the control of severe hypertriglyceridemia. Maintain dietary restrictions during therapy.

Patient Education: Do not use if allergic to fish. This medication should be used in addition to diet and exercise. Avoid alcohol use. You may experience flu-like syndrome, fever, burping, or an "upset stomach". Report any significant or continued problems to prescriber. **Pregnancy/breast-feeding precautions:** Inform prescriber if you are or intend to become pregnant. Consult prescriber before breast-feeding.

Geriatric Considerations: Specific information about the safety and efficacy of omega-3-acid ethyl esters is limited. The manufacturer states there were no apparent differences between persons <60 and >60 years of age.

Pregnancy Risk Factor: C

Lactation: Excretion in breast milk unknown/use caution

Administration

Oral: May be administered with meals.

Storage: Store at 25°C (77°F); excursions permitted to 15°C to 30°C (59°F to 86°F). Do not freeze.

Omeprazole (oh ME pray zol)

U.S. Brand Names Prilosec®; Prilosec OTC™ [OTC]; Zegerid™

Pharmacologic Category Proton Pump Inhibitor; Substituted Benzimidazole

Medication Safety Issues

Sound-alike/look-alike issues:

Prilosec® may be confused with Plendil®, Prevacid®, predniSONE, prilocaine, Prinivil®, Proventil®, Prozac®

Use Short-term (4-8 weeks) treatment of active duodenal ulcer disease or active benign gastric ulcer; treatment of heartburn and other symptoms associated with gastroesophageal reflux disease (GERD); short-term (4-8 weeks) treatment of endoscopically-diagnosed erosive esophagitis; maintenance healing of erosive esophagitis; long-term treatment of pathological hypersecretory conditions; as part of a multidrug regimen for *H. pylori* eradication to reduce the risk of duodenal ulcer recurrence; reduction of risk of upper gastrointestinal bleeding in critically-ill patients (Zegerid™)

OTC labeling: Short-term treatment of frequent, uncomplicated heartburn occurring ≥2 days/week

Unlabeled/Investigational Use Healing NSAID-induced ulcers; prevention of NSAID-induced ulcers

Mechanism of Action Suppresses gastric basal and stimulated acid secretion by inhibiting the parietal cell H+/K+ ATP pump

Pharmacodynamics/Kinetics

Onset of action: Antisecretory: ~1 hour

Peak effect: 2 hours

Duration: 72 hours

Protein binding: 95%

Metabolism: Extensively hepatic to inactive metabolites

Bioavailability: Oral: 30% to 40%; increased in Asian patients and patients with hepatic dysfunction

Half-life elimination: Delayed release capsule: 0.5-1 hour; Oral suspension: 0.4-3.2 hours

Excretion: Urine (77% as metabolites, very small amount as unchanged drug); feces

Contraindications Hypersensitivity to omeprazole, substituted benzimidazoles (ie, esomeprazole, lansoprazole, pantoprazole, rabeprazole), or any component of the formulation

Warnings/Precautions In long-term (2-year) studies in rats, omeprazole produced a dose-related increase in gastric carcinoid tumors. While available endoscopic evaluations and histologic examinations of biopsy specimens from human stomachs have not detected a risk from short-term exposure to omeprazole, further human data on the effect of sustained hypochlorhydria and hypergastrinemia are needed to rule out the possibility of an increased risk for the development of tumors in humans receiving long-term therapy. Bioavailability may be increased in the elderly, Asian population, and with hepatic dysfunction. Use Zegerid™ with caution in patients with Bartter's syndrome, hypocalcemia, hypokalemia, sodium-restricted diets, and respiratory alkalosis (contains sodium bicarbonate). Safety and efficacy have not been established in children <2 years of age. When used for self-medication (OTC), do not use for >14 days; treatment should not be repeated more often than every 4 months; OTC and oral suspension are not approved for use in children <18 years of age.

Drug Interactions **Substrate** of CYP2A6 (minor), 2C8/9 (minor), 2C19 (major), 2D6 (minor), 3A4 (minor); **Inhibits** CYP1A2 (weak), 2C8/9 (moderate), 2C19 (strong), 2D6 (weak), 3A4 (weak); **Induces** CYP1A2 (weak)

Benzodiazepines metabolized by oxidation (eg, diazepam, midazolam, triazolam): Esomeprazole and omeprazole may increase levels of benzodiazepines metabolized by oxidation.

Carbamazepine: Esomeprazole and omeprazole may increase carbamazepine levels.

CYP2C8/9 substrates: Omeprazole may increase the levels/effects of CYP2C8/9 substrates. Example substrates include amiodarone, fluoxetine, glimepiride, glipizide, nateglinide, phenytoin, pioglitazone, rosiglitazone, sertraline, and warfarin.

CYP2C19 inducers: May decrease the levels/effects of omeprazole. Example inducers include aminoglutethimide, carbamazepine, phenytoin, and rifampin.

CYP2C19 substrates: Omeprazole may increase the levels/effects of CYP2C19 substrates. Example substrates include citalopram, diazepam, methsuximide, phenytoin, propranolol, and sertraline.

Itraconazole and ketoconazole: Proton pump inhibitors may decrease the absorption of itraconazole and ketoconazole.

Phenytoin: Elimination of phenytoin may be prolonged; monitor. Phenytoin may decrease omeprazole levels/effects.

Protease inhibitors: Proton pump inhibitors may decrease absorption of some protease inhibitors (atazanavir and indinavir).

Warfarin: Elimination of warfarin may be prolonged; monitor.

(Continued)

Omeprazole *(Continued)*

Nutritional/Herbal/Ethanol Interactions

Ethanol: Avoid ethanol (may cause gastric mucosal irritation).

Food: Food delays absorption. When Zegerid™ is given 1 hour after a meal, absorption is reduced.

Herb/Nutraceutical: St John's wort may decrease omeprazole levels.

Adverse Reactions

Zegerid™ oral powder for suspension:

>10%:

Central nervous system: Pyrexia (20%)

Endocrine & metabolic: Hypokalemia (12%), hyperglycemia (11%)

Respiratory: Nosocomial pneumonia (11%)

1% to 10%:

Cardiovascular: Hypotension (10%), hypertension (8%), atrial fibrillation (6%), ventricular tachycardia (5%), tachycardia (3%), supraventricular tachycardia (3%), edema (3%)

Central nervous system: Hyperpyrexia (5%), agitation (3%)

Dermatological: Rash (6%), decubitus ulcer (3%)

Endocrine & metabolic: Hypomagnesemia (10%), hypocalcemia (6%), hypophosphatemia (6%), fluid overload (5%), hypoglycemia (3%), hyponatremia (4%), hypernatremia (2%), hyperkalemia (2%)

Gastrointestinal: Constipation (5%), diarrhea (4%), hypomotility (2%)

Genitourinary: Urinary tract infection (2%)

Hematological: Thrombocytopenia (10%), anemia (8%), anemia increased (2%)

Hepatic: LFTs increased (2%)

Respiratory: ARDS (3%), respiratory failure (2%)

Miscellaneous: Sepsis (5%), oral candidiasis (4%), candidal infection (2%)

Capsule and tablet: 1% to 10%:

Central nervous system: Headache (3% to 7%), dizziness (2%)

Dermatologic: Rash (2%)

Gastrointestinal: Diarrhea (3% to 4%), abdominal pain (2% to 5 %), nausea (2% to 4%), vomiting (2% to 3%), flatulence (3%), acid regurgitation (2%), constipation (1% to 2%), taste perversion

Neuromuscular & skeletal: Weakness (1%), back pain (1%)

Respiratory: Upper respiratory infection (2%), cough (1%)

<1% (Limited to important or life-threatening; adverse event occurrence may vary based on formulation): Abdominal swelling, abnormal dreams, aggression, agranulocytosis, allergic reactions, alopecia, anaphylaxis, anemia, angina, angioedema, anorexia, anxiety, apathy, atrophic gastritis, benign gastric polyps, blurred vision, bradycardia, jaundice, confusion, depression, diaphoresis, double vision, dry mouth, dry skin, epistaxis, erythema multiforme, esophageal candidiasis, fatigue, fecal discoloration, fever, flatulence, glycosuria, gynecomastia, hallucinations, hematuria, hemifacial dysesthesia, hemolytic anemia, hepatic encephalopathy, hepatic failure, hepatic necrosis, hypertension, hypoglycemia, hyponatremia, insomnia, interstitial nephritis, irritable colon, joint pain, leg pain, leukocytosis, leukopenia; liver disease (hepatocellular, cholestatic, mixed); liver enzymes increased, malaise, microscopic pyuria, mucosal atrophy (tongue), muscle cramps, muscle weakness, myalgia, nervousness, neutropenia, ocular irritation, pain, palpitation, pancreatitis, pancytopenia, paresthesia, peripheral edema, pharyngeal pain, proteinuria, photosensitivity, pruritus, psychic disturbance, rash, serum alkaline increased, serum creatinine increased, serum transaminases increased, skin inflammation, somnolence, Stevens-Johnson syndrome, stomatitis, tachycardia, testicular pain, thrombocytopenia, tinnitus, toxic epidermal necrolysis, tremor, urinary frequency, urinary tract infection, urticaria, vertigo, weight gain

Overdosage/Toxicology Limited experience with overdose in humans. Symptoms include confusion, drowsiness, blurred vision, tachycardia, nausea, flushing, diaphoresis, headache, dry mouth. Treatment is symptom-directed and supportive.

Zegerid™: Also consider signs and symptoms of sodium bicarbonate overdose. Electrolytes (including sodium, potassium, calcium) may be altered; monitoring may be required.

Dosing

Adults & Elderly:

Active duodenal ulcer: Oral: 20 mg/day for 4-8 weeks

Gastric ulcers: Oral: 40 mg/day for 4-8 weeks

Symptomatic GERD: Oral: 20 mg/day for up to 4 weeks

Erosive esophagitis: Oral: 20 mg/day for 4-8 weeks

Peptic ulcer disease: Eradication of *Helicobacter pylori*: Oral: Dose varies with regimen: 20 mg once daily **or** 40 mg/day as single dose or in 2 divided doses; requires combination therapy with antibiotics

Pathological hypersecretory conditions: Oral: Initial: 60 mg once daily; doses up to 120 mg 3 times/day have been administered; administer daily doses >80 mg in divided doses

Frequent heartburn (OTC labeling): Oral: 20 mg/day for 14 days; treatment may be repeated after 4 months if needed

Risk reduction of upper GI bleeding in critically-ill patients (Zegerid™):

Loading dose: Day 1: 40 mg every 6-8 hours for two doses

Maintenance dose: 40 mg/day for up to 14 days; therapy >14 days has not been evaluated

Pediatrics:

GERD or other acid-related disorders: Oral: Children ≥2 years:

<20 kg: 10 mg once daily

≥20 kg: 20 mg once daily

Renal Impairment: No adjustment is necessary.

Hepatic Impairment: Specific guidelines are not available; bioavailability is increased with chronic liver disease.

Available Dosage Forms

Capsule, delayed release: 10 mg, 20 mg

Prilosec®: 10 mg, 20 mg, 40 mg

Powder for oral suspension [packet] (Zegerid™): 20 mg (30s), 40 mg (30s) [both strengths contain sodium bicarbonate 1680 mg, equivalent to sodium 460 mg per packet]

Tablet, delayed release (Prilosec OTC™): 20 mg

Nursing Guidelines

Assessment: Assess other medications patient may be taking for effectiveness and interactions (especially those dependent on cytochrome P450 metabolism or those dependent on a acid environment for absorption). Monitor effectiveness of therapeutic effectiveness and adverse reactions at beginning of therapy and periodically throughout therapy. Assess knowledge/teach appropriate use of this medication, interventions to reduce side effects, and adverse symptoms to report.

Dietary Considerations:

Should be taken on an empty stomach; best if taken before breakfast.

Zegerid™: Take 1 hour before a meal; each 20 mg or 40 mg packet contains sodium bicarbonate 1680 mg (20 mEq), equivalent to sodium 460 mg (20 mEq) per dose

Patient Education: Take as directed, before eating. Do not crush or chew capsules. Capsule may be opened and contents added to applesauce. Avoid alcohol. You may experience anorexia; small frequent meals may help to maintain adequate nutrition. Report changes in urination or pain on urination, unresolved severe diarrhea, testicular pain, or changes in respiratory status. **Pregnancy/breast-feeding precautions:** Inform prescriber if you are or intend to become pregnant. Breast-feeding is not recommended.

Geriatric Considerations: The incidence of side effects in the elderly is no different than that of younger adults (≤65 years) despite slight decrease in elimination and increase in bioavailability. Bioavailability may be increased in the elderly (≥65 years of age), however, dosage adjustments are not necessary.

Pregnancy Risk Factor: C

Pregnancy Issues: Crosses the placenta; congenital abnormalities have been reported sporadically following omeprazole use during pregnancy. Based on data collected by the Teratogen Information System (TERIS), it was concluded that therapeutic doses used during pregnancy would be unlikely to pose a substantial teratogenic risk (quantity/quality of data: fair). Because the possibility of harm still exists, the manufacturer recommends use during pregnancy only if the potential benefit to the mother outweighs the possible risk to the fetus. Zegerid™ contains sodium bicarbonate; chronic use may lead to systemic alkalosis, edema, and weight gain; metabolic alkalosis and fluid overload may occur in mother and fetus.

(Continued)

Omeprazole *(Continued)*

Lactation: Enters breast milk/not recommended

Perioperative/Anesthesia/Other Concerns: A 2 mg/mL oral omeprazole solution (Simplified Omeprazole Solution) can be prepared with five omeprazole 20 mg capsules and 50 mL 8.4% sodium bicarbonate. Empty capsules into beaker. Add sodium bicarbonate solution. Gently stir (about 15 minutes) until a white suspension is formed. Transfer to amber-colored syringe or bottle. Stable for 14 days at room temperature or for 30 days under refrigeration.

DiGiancinto JL, Olsen KM, Bergman KL, et al, "Stability of Suspension Formulations of Lansoprazole and Omeprazole Stored in Amber-Colored Plastic Oral Syringes," *Ann Pharmacother*, 2000, 34:600-5.

Quercia R, Fan C, Liu X, et al, "Stability of Omeprazole in an Extemporaneously Prepared Oral Liquid," *Am J Health Syst Pharm*, 1997, 54:1833-6.

Sharma V, "Comparison of 24-hour Intragastric pH Using Four Liquid Formulations of Lansoprazole and Omeprazole," *Am J Health Syst Pharm*, 1999, 56(Suppl 4):S18-21.

Administration

Oral:

Capsule: Should be swallowed whole; do not chew, crush, or open. Best if taken before breakfast. May be opened and contents added to applesauce. Administration via NG tube should be in an acidic juice.

Powder for oral suspension (Zegerid™): Administer 1 hour before a meal. Mix with 2 tablespoons of water; stir well and drink immediately. Rinse cup with water and drink.

Tablet: Should be swallowed whole; do not crush or chew.

Storage: Store at 15°C to 30°C (59°F to 86°F).

♦ **Omnicef®** *see* Cefdinir *on page 333*
♦ **Omnipaque™** *see* Iohexol *on page 955*

Ondansetron (on DAN se tron)

U.S. Brand Names Zofran®; Zofran® ODT

Synonyms GR38032R; Ondansetron Hydrochloride

Pharmacologic Category Antiemetic; Selective 5-HT_3 Receptor Antagonist

Medication Safety Issues

Sound-alike/look-alike issues:

Ondansetron may be confused with dolasetron, granisetron, palonosetron
Zofran® may be confused with Zantac®, Zosyn®

Use Prevention of nausea and vomiting associated with moderately- to highly-emetogenic cancer chemotherapy [not recommended for treatment of **existing** chemotherapy-induced emesis (CIE)]; radiotherapy in patients receiving total body irradiation or fractions to the abdomen; prevention of postoperative nausea and vomiting (PONV); treatment of PONV if no prophylactic dose received

Unlabeled/Investigational Use Treatment of early-onset alcoholism; hyperemesis gravidarum

Mechanism of Action Selective 5-HT_3-receptor antagonist, blocking serotonin, both peripherally on vagal nerve terminals and centrally in the chemoreceptor trigger zone

Pharmacodynamics/Kinetics

Onset of action: ~30 minutes

Distribution: V_d: Children: 1.7-3.7 L/kg; Adults: 2.2-2.5 L/kg

Protein binding, plasma: 70% to 76%

Metabolism: Extensively hepatic via hydroxylation, followed by glucuronide or sulfate conjugation; CYP1A2, CYP2D6, and CYP3A4 substrate; some demethylation occurs

Bioavailability: Oral: 56% to 71%; Rectal: 58% to 74%

Half-life elimination: Children <15 years: 2-7 hours; Adults: 3-6 hours
Mild-to-moderate hepatic impairment: Adults: 12 hours
Severe hepatic impairment (Child-Pugh C): Adults: 20 hours

Time to peak: Oral: ~2 hours

Excretion: Urine (44% to 60% as metabolites, 5% to 10% as unchanged drug); feces (~25%)

Contraindications Hypersensitivity to ondansetron, other selective 5-HT_3 antagonists, or any component of the formulation

Warnings/Precautions For chemotherapy, ondansetron should be used on a scheduled basis, not on an "as needed" (PRN) basis, since data support the use of this drug only in the prevention of nausea and vomiting (due to antineoplastic therapy) and not in the rescue of nausea and vomiting. Ondansetron should only be used in the first 24-48 hours of chemotherapy. Data do not support any increased efficacy of ondansetron in delayed nausea and vomiting. Does not stimulate gastric or intestinal peristalsis; may mask progressive ileus and/or gastric distension. Orally-disintegrating tablets contain phenylalanine. Safety and efficacy for children <1 month of age have not been established.

Drug Interactions **Substrate** of CYP1A2 (minor), 2C8/9 (minor), 2D6 (minor), 2E1 (minor), 3A4 (major); **Inhibits** CYP1A2 (weak), 2C8/9 (weak), 2D6 (weak)

Apomorphine: Due to reports of profound hypotension during concomitant therapy, the manufacturer of apomorphine contraindicates its use with ondansetron.

CYP3A4 inducers: CYP3A4 inducers may decrease the levels/effects of ondansetron. Example inducers include aminoglutethimide, carbamazepine, nafcillin, nevirapine, phenobarbital, phenytoin, and rifamycins. The manufacturer does not recommend dosage adjustment in patients receiving CYP3A4 inducers.

Nutritional/Herbal/Ethanol Interactions

Food: Food increases the extent of absorption. The C_{max} and T_{max} do not change much.

Herb/Nutraceutical: St John's wort may decrease ondansetron levels.

Adverse Reactions

Note: Percentages reported in adult patients.

>10%:

Central nervous system: Headache (9% to 27%), malaise/fatigue (9% to 13%)
Gastrointestinal: Constipation (6% to 11%)

1% to 10%:

Central nervous system: Drowsiness (8%), fever (2% to 8%), dizziness (4% to 7%), anxiety (6%), cold sensation (2%)
Dermatologic: Pruritus (2% to 5%), rash (1%)
Gastrointestinal: Diarrhea (2% to 7%)
Genitourinary: Gynecological disorder (7%), urinary retention (5%)
Hepatic: ALT/AST increased (1% to 5%)
Local: Injection site reaction (4%; pain, redness, burning)
Neuromuscular & skeletal: Paresthesia (2%)
Respiratory: Hypoxia (9%)

<1% (Limited to important or life-threatening): Anaphylactoid reactions, anaphylaxis, angina, angioedema, arrhythmia, blindness (transient/following infusion), blurred vision (transient/following infusion), bradycardia, bronchospasm, cardiopulmonary arrest, dyspnea, dystonic reaction, ECG changes, electrocardiographic alterations (second degree heart block and ST-segment depression), extrapyramidal symptoms, flushing, grand mal seizure, hiccups, hypersensitivity reaction, hypokalemia, hypotension, laryngeal edema, laryngospasm, oculogyric crisis, palpitation, premature ventricular contractions (PVC), shock, stridor, supraventricular tachycardia, syncope, tachycardia, urticaria, vascular occlusive events, ventricular arrhythmia

Overdosage/Toxicology Sudden transient blindness, severe constipation, hypotension, and vasovagal episode with transient secondary heart block have been reported in some cases of overdose. I.V. doses of up to 252 mg/day have been inadvertently given without adverse effects. There is no specific antidote. Treatment is symptom-directed and supportive.

Dosing

Adults & Elderly: **Note:** Studies in adults have shown a single daily dose of 8-12 mg I.V. or 8-24 mg orally to be as effective as mg/kg dosing, and should be considered for **all** patients whose mg/kg dose exceeds 8-12 mg I.V.; oral solution and ODT formulations are bioequivalent to corresponding doses of tablet formulation.

Prevention of chemotherapy-induced emesis:

I.V.:

0.15 mg/kg 3 times/day beginning 30 minutes prior to chemotherapy **or**
0.45 mg/kg once daily **or**
8-10 mg 1-2 times/day **or**
24 mg or 32 mg once daily

Highly-emetogenic agents/single-day therapy: Oral: 24 mg given 30 minutes prior to the start of therapy

Moderately-emetogenic agents: Oral: 8 mg every 12 hours beginning 30 minutes before chemotherapy, continuously for 1-2 days after chemotherapy completed

(Continued)

Ondansetron *(Continued)*

Total body irradiation: Oral: 8 mg 1-2 hours before each daily fraction of radiotherapy

Single high-dose fraction radiotherapy to abdomen: Oral: 8 mg 1-2 hours before irradiation, then 8 mg every 8 hours after first dose for 1-2 days after completion of radiotherapy

Daily fractionated radiotherapy to abdomen: 8 mg 1-2 hours before irradiation, then 8 mg 8 hours after first dose for each day of radiotherapy

Postoperative nausea and vomiting (PONV):

Oral: 16 mg given one hour prior to induction of anesthesia

I.M., I.V.: 4 mg as a single dose immediately before induction of anesthesia, or shortly following procedure if vomiting occurs

Note: Repeat doses given in response to inadequate control of nausea/vomiting from preoperative doses are generally ineffective.

Treatment of hyperemesis gravidum (unlabeled use):

Oral: 8 mg every 12 hours

I.V.: 8 mg administered over 15 minutes every 12 hours or 1 mg/hour infused continuously for up to 24 hours

Pediatrics: Note: Studies in adults have shown a single daily dose of 8-12 mg I.V. or 8-24 mg orally to be as effective as mg/kg dosing, and should be considered for **all** patients whose mg/kg dose exceeds 8-12 mg I.V.; oral solution and ODT formulations are bioequivalent to corresponding doses of tablet formulation.

Prevention of chemotherapy-induced emesis:

I.V.: Children 6 months to 18 years: 0.15 mg/kg/dose administered 30 minutes prior to chemotherapy, 4 and 8 hours after the first dose **or** 0.45 mg/kg/day as a single dose

Oral:

4-11 years: 4 mg 30 minutes before chemotherapy; repeat 4 and 8 hours after initial dose, then 4 mg every 8 hours for 1-2 days after chemotherapy completed

≥12 years: Refer to adult dosing.

Prevention of postoperative nausea and vomiting (PONV): I.V.: Children 1 month to 12 years:

≤40 kg: 0.1 mg/kg as a single dose

>40 kg: 4 mg as a single dose

Renal Impairment: No adjustment is necessary.

Hepatic Impairment: Severe liver disease (Child-Pugh C): Maximum daily dose: 8 mg

Available Dosage Forms

Infusion [premixed in D_5W, preservative free] (Zofran®): 32 mg (50 mL)

Injection, solution (Zofran®): 2 mg/mL (2 mL, 20 mL)

Solution, oral (Zofran®): 4 mg/5 mL (50 mL) [contains sodium benzoate; strawberry flavor]

Tablet (Zofran®): 4 mg, 8 mg, 24 mg

Tablet, orally-disintegrating (Zofran® ODT): 4 mg, 8 mg [each strength contains phenylalanine <0.03 mg/tablet; strawberry flavor]

Nursing Guidelines

Assessment: See Contraindications, Warnings/Precautions, and Dosing for use cautions. Assess potential for interactions with other prescriptions, OTC medications, or herbal products patient may be taking (see extensive list of Drug Interactions). See Administration specifics. Assess therapeutic effectiveness and adverse effects (see Adverse Reactions and Overdose/Toxicology). Teach patient appropriate use (according to formulation), possible side effects/appropriate interventions, and adverse symptoms to report (see Patient Education).

Dietary Considerations: Take without regard to meals.

Orally-disintegrating tablet contains <0.03 mg phenylalanine

Patient Education: Inform prescriber of all prescriptions, OTC medications, or herbal products you are taking, and any allergies you have. Do not take any new medication during therapy unless approved by prescriber. If self-administered, take as directed. May cause drowsiness or dizziness (use caution when driving or engaging in tasks that require alertness until response to drug is known): or fatigue, diarrhea, constipation, or headache (request appropriate treatment from prescriber). Do not change position rapidly (rise slowly). Report persistent headache, excessive drowsiness, fever, numbness or tingling, or changes in elimination patterns (constipation or diarrhea); or chest pain or palpitations.

Orally-disintegrating tablets: Do not remove from blister until needed. Peel backing off the blister, do not push tablet through. Using dry hands, place tablet on tongue and allow to dissolve. Swallow with saliva. Contains <0.03 mg phenylalanine/tablet.

Geriatric Considerations: Elderly have a slightly decreased hepatic clearance rate. This does not, however, require a dose adjustment.

Pregnancy Risk Factor: B

Lactation: Excretion in breast milk unknown/use caution

Administration

Oral: Oral dosage forms should be given 30 minutes prior to chemotherapy; 1-2 hours before radiotherapy; 1 hour prior to the induction of anesthesia

Orally-disintegrating tablets: Do not remove from blister until needed. Peel backing off the blister, do not push tablet through. Using dry hands, place tablet on tongue and allow to dissolve. Swallow with saliva.

The I.V. preparation has been successful when administered orally.

I.M.: Should be given undiluted

I.V.: Give first dose 30 minutes prior to beginning chemotherapy; the I.V. preparation has been successful when administered orally

I.V. injection: Single doses for prevention of postoperative nausea and vomiting may be administered I.V. over 2-5 minutes as undiluted solution

IVPB: Dilute in 50 mL D_5W or NS. Infuse over 15-30 minutes; 24-hour continuous infusions have been reported, but are rarely used

Reconstitution: Prior to I.V. infusion, dilute in 50 mL D_5W or NS.

Compatibility: Stable in $D_5{}^1/_2NS$, D_5NS, D_5W, mannitol 10%, LR, NS, NS 3%; do not mix injection with alkaline solutions

Y-site administration: Incompatible with acyclovir, allopurinol, aminophylline, amphotericin B, amphotericin B cholesteryl sulfate complex, ampicillin, ampicillin/sulbactam, amsacrine, cefepime, cefoperazone, furosemide, ganciclovir, lorazepam, methylprednisolone sodium succinate, piperacillin, sargramostim, sodium bicarbonate

Storage:

Oral solution: Store between 15°C and 30°C (59°F and 86°F). Protect from light.

Premixed bag: Store between 2°C and 30°C (36°F and 86°F). Protect from light.

Tablet: Store between 2°C and 30°C (36°F and 86°F)

Vial: Store between 2°C and 30°C (36°F and 86°F). Protect from light. Stable when mixed in D_5W or NS for 48 hours at room temperature.

Related Information

Postoperative Nausea and Vomiting *on page 1807*

- **Ondansetron Hydrochloride** *see* Ondansetron *on page 1268*
- **One-A-Day® 50 Plus Formula [OTC]** *see* Vitamins (Multiple/Oral) *on page 1720*
- **One-A-Day® Active Formula [OTC]** *see* Vitamins (Multiple/Oral) *on page 1720*
- **One-A-Day® Carb Smart [OTC]** *see* Vitamins (Multiple/Oral) *on page 1720*
- **One-A-Day® Cholesterol Plus™ [OTC]** *see* Vitamins (Multiple/Oral) *on page 1720*
- **One-A-Day® Essential Formula [OTC]** *see* Vitamins (Multiple/Oral) *on page 1720*
- **One-A-Day® Kids Bugs Bunny and Friends Complete [OTC]** *see* Vitamins (Multiple/Pediatric) *on page 1720*
- **One-A-Day® Kids Bugs Bunny and Friends Plus Extra C [OTC]** *see* Vitamins (Multiple/Pediatric) *on page 1720*
- **One-A-Day® Kids Extreme Sports [OTC]** *see* Vitamins (Multiple/Pediatric) *on page 1720*
- **One-A-Day® Kids Scooby-Doo! Complete [OTC]** *see* Vitamins (Multiple/Pediatric) *on page 1720*
- **One-A-Day® Kids Scooby-Doo! Fizzy Vites [OTC]** *see* Vitamins (Multiple/Pediatric) *on page 1720*
- **One-A-Day® Kids Scooby-Doo! Plus Calcium [OTC]** *see* Vitamins (Multiple/Pediatric) *on page 1720*
- **One-A-Day® Maximum Formula [OTC]** *see* Vitamins (Multiple/Oral) *on page 1720*
- **One-A-Day® Men's Formula [OTC]** *see* Vitamins (Multiple/Oral) *on page 1720*
- **One-A-Day® Today [OTC]** *see* Vitamins (Multiple/Oral) *on page 1720*
- **One-A-Day® Weight Smart [OTC** *see* Vitamins (Multiple/Oral) *on page 1720*

- ♦ **One-A-Day® Women's Formula [OTC]** *see* Vitamins (Multiple/Oral) *on page 1720*
- ♦ **Onxol™** *see* Paclitaxel *on page 1294*
- ♦ **Ony-Clear [OTC] [DSC]** *see* Benzalkonium Chloride *on page 231*
- ♦ **OPC-13013** *see* Cilostazol *on page 394*
- ♦ **Operand® [OTC]** *see* Povidone-Iodine *on page 1392*
- ♦ **Operand® Chlorhexidine Gluconate [OTC]** *see* Chlorhexidine Gluconate *on page 373*
- ♦ **Ophthetic®** *see* Proparacaine *on page 1420*
- ♦ **Opium and Belladonna** *see* Belladonna and Opium *on page 227*

Opium Tincture (OH pee um TING chur)

Synonyms DTO (error-prone abbreviation); Opium Tincture, Deodorized

Pharmacologic Category Analgesic, Narcotic; Antidiarrheal

Medication Safety Issues

Sound-alike/look-alike issues:

Opium tincture may be confused with camphorated tincture of opium (paregoric)

Use care when prescribing opium tincture; each mL contains the equivalent of morphine 10 mg; paregoric contains the equivalent of morphine 0.4 mg/mL

DTO is an error-prone abbreviation (mistaken as Diluted Tincture of Opium; dose equivalency of paregoric)

Use Treatment of diarrhea or relief of pain

Mechanism of Action Contains many narcotic alkaloids including morphine; its mechanism for gastric motility inhibition is primarily due to this morphine content; it results in a decrease in digestive secretions, an increase in GI muscle tone, and therefore a reduction in GI propulsion

Pharmacodynamics/Kinetics

Duration: 4-5 hours

Absorption: Variable

Metabolism: Hepatic

Excretion: Urine

Contraindications Hypersensitivity to morphine sulfate or any component of the formulation; increased intracranial pressure; severe respiratory depression; severe hepatic or renal insufficiency; pregnancy (prolonged use or high dosages near term)

Warnings/Precautions Opium shares the toxic potential of opiate agonists, and usual precautions of opiate agonist therapy should be observed; some preparations contain sulfites which may cause allergic reactions; infants <3 months of age are more susceptible to respiratory depression, use with caution and generally in reduced doses in this age group; this is **not** paregoric, dose accordingly

Drug Interactions Increased toxicity: CNS depressants, MAO inhibitors, tricyclic antidepressants may potentiate the effects of opiate agonists; dextroamphetamine may enhance the analgesic effect of opiate agonists

Nutritional/Herbal/Ethanol Interactions Ethanol: Avoid ethanol (may increase CNS depression).

Lab Interactions Increased aminotransferase [ALT (SGPT)/AST (SGOT)] (S)

Adverse Reactions Frequency not defined.

Cardiovascular: Palpitations, hypotension, bradycardia, peripheral vasodilation

Central nervous system: Drowsiness, dizziness, restlessness, headache, malaise, CNS depression, increased intracranial pressure, insomnia, mental depression

Gastrointestinal: Nausea, vomiting, constipation, anorexia, stomach cramps, biliary tract spasm

Genitourinary: Decreased urination, urinary tract spasm

Neuromuscular & skeletal: Weakness

Ocular: Miosis

Respiratory: Respiratory depression

Miscellaneous: Histamine release, physical and psychological dependence

Overdosage/Toxicology Primary attention should be directed to ensuring adequate respiratory exchange. Naloxone, 2 mg I.V. with repeat administration as necessary up to a total of 10 mg, can also be used to reverse toxic effects of the opiate.

Dosing

Adults & Elderly:

Diarrhea: Oral: 0.3-1 mL/dose every 2-6 hours to maximum of 6 mL/24 hours

Analgesia: Oral: 0.6-1.5 mL/dose every 3-4 hours

Pediatrics:

Diarrhea: Oral: Children: 0.005-0.01 mL/kg/dose every 3-4 hours for a maximum of 6 doses/24 hours

Analgesia: Oral: Children: 0.01-0.02 mL/kg/dose every 3-4 hours

Available Dosage Forms Liquid: 10% (120 mL, 480 mL) [0.6 mL equivalent to morphine 6 mg; contains alcohol 19%]

Nursing Guidelines

Assessment: Assess other medications patient may be taking for additive or adverse interactions. Monitor vital signs, effectiveness of pain relief, adverse reactions, and signs of overdose at beginning of therapy and at regular intervals with long-term use. May cause physical and/or psychological dependence. For inpatients, implement safety measures. Assess knowledge/teach patient appropriate use (if self-administered). Teach patient to monitor for adverse reactions, adverse reactions to report, and appropriate interventions to reduce side effects. Discontinue slowly after prolonged use.

Patient Education: If self-administered, use exactly as directed; do not increase dose or frequency. Drug may cause physical and/or psychological dependence. While using this medication, do not use alcohol and other prescription or OTC medications (especially sedatives, tranquilizers, antihistamines, or pain medications) without consulting prescriber. Maintain adequate hydration (2-3 L/day of fluids). May cause hypotension, dizziness, drowsiness, impaired coordination, or blurred vision (use caution when driving, climbing stairs, or changing position - rising from sitting or lying to standing, or when engaging in tasks requiring alertness until response to drug is known); or dry mouth (frequent mouth care, small frequent meals, chewing gum, or sucking lozenges may help). Report slow or rapid heartbeat, acute dizziness, or persistent headache; changes in mental status; swelling of extremities or unusual weight gain; changes in urinary elimination or pain on urination; acute headache; trembling or muscle spasms; blurred vision; skin rash; or shortness of breath. **Pregnancy/breast-feeding precautions:** Inform prescriber if you are or intend to become pregnant.

Pregnancy Risk Factor: B/D (prolonged use or high doses at term)

Lactation: Enters breast milk/use caution

Administration

Storage: Protect from light

- **Opium Tincture, Deodorized** *see* Opium Tincture *on page 1272*
- **Opticrom®** *see* Cromolyn *on page 453*
- **Optiray®** *see* Ioversol *on page 956*
- **Optivar®** *see* Azelastine *on page 210*
- **Optivite® P.M.T. [OTC]** *see* Vitamins (Multiple/Oral) *on page 1720*
- **Orabase® with Benzocaine [OTC]** *see* Benzocaine *on page 232*
- **Oracit®** *see* Sodium Citrate and Citric Acid *on page 1548*
- **Orajel® Baby Daytime and Nighttime [OTC]** *see* Benzocaine *on page 232*
- **Orajel® Baby Teething [OTC]** *see* Benzocaine *on page 232*
- **Orajel® Baby Teething Nighttime [OTC]** *see* Benzocaine *on page 232*
- **Orajel® Denture Plus [OTC]** *see* Benzocaine *on page 232*
- **Orajel® Maximum Strength [OTC]** *see* Benzocaine *on page 232*
- **Orajel® Medicated Toothache [OTC]** *see* Benzocaine *on page 232*
- **Orajel® Mouth Sore [OTC]** *see* Benzocaine *on page 232*
- **Orajel® Multi-Action Cold Sore [OTC]** *see* Benzocaine *on page 232*
- **Orajel® Perioseptic® Spot Treatment [OTC]** *see* Carbamide Peroxide *on page 311*
- **Orajel PM® [OTC]** *see* Benzocaine *on page 232*
- **Orajel® Ultra Mouth Sore [OTC]** *see* Benzocaine *on page 232*
- **Oramorph SR®** *see* Morphine Sulfate *on page 1177*
- **Oranyl [OTC]** *see* Pseudoephedrine *on page 1436*
- **Orapred®** *see* PrednisoLONE *on page 1399*
- **Orciprenaline Sulfate** *see* Metaproterenol *on page 1109*
- **ORG 946** *see* Rocuronium *on page 1489*
- **Organ-1 NR** *see* Guaifenesin *on page 834*
- **Organidin® NR** *see* Guaifenesin *on page 834*
- **ORG NC 45** *see* Vecuronium *on page 1695*
- **Ortho-Cept®** *see* Ethinyl Estradiol and Desogestrel *on page 675*

- **Ortho-Cyclen®** *see* Ethinyl Estradiol and Norgestimate *on page 689*
- **Ortho Evra®** *see* Ethinyl Estradiol and Norelgestromin *on page 684*
- **Ortho Tri-Cyclen®** *see* Ethinyl Estradiol and Norgestimate *on page 689*
- **Ortho Tri-Cyclen® Lo** *see* Ethinyl Estradiol and Norgestimate *on page 689*
- **Orthovisc®** *see* Hyaluronate and Derivatives *on page 856*
- **Os-Cal® 500 [OTC]** *see* Calcium Carbonate *on page 291*
- **Osmitrol®** *see* Mannitol *on page 1079*
- **Osmoglyn® [DSC]** *see* Glycerin *on page 826*
- **Oticaine** *see* Benzocaine *on page 232*
- **Otocaine™** *see* Benzocaine *on page 232*
- **Outgro® [OTC]** *see* Benzocaine *on page 232*
- **Ovace™** *see* Sulfacetamide *on page 1579*
- **Ovidrel®** *see* Chorionic Gonadotropin (Recombinant) *on page 389*

Oxacillin (oks a SIL in)

Synonyms Methylphenyl Isoxazolyl Penicillin; Oxacillin Sodium

Pharmacologic Category Antibiotic, Penicillin

Use Treatment of infections such as osteomyelitis, septicemia, endocarditis, and CNS infections caused by susceptible strains of *Staphylococcus*

Mechanism of Action Inhibits bacterial cell wall synthesis by binding to one or more of the penicillin binding proteins (PBPs); which in turn inhibits the final transpeptidation step of peptidoglycan synthesis in bacterial cell walls, thus inhibiting cell wall biosynthesis. Bacteria eventually lyse due to ongoing activity of cell wall autolytic enzymes (autolysins and murein hydrolases) while cell wall assembly is arrested.

Pharmacodynamics/Kinetics

Distribution: Into bile, synovial and pleural fluids, bronchial secretions, peritoneal, and pericardial fluids; crosses placenta; enters breast milk; penetrates the blood-brain barrier only when meninges are inflamed

Protein binding: ~94%

Metabolism: Hepatic to active metabolites

Half-life elimination: Children 1 week to 2 years: 0.9-1.8 hours; Adults: 23-60 minutes; prolonged in neonates and with renal impairment

Time to peak, serum: I.M.: 30-60 minutes

Excretion: Urine and feces (small amounts as unchanged drug and metabolites)

Contraindications Hypersensitivity to oxacillin or other penicillins or any component of the formulation

Warnings/Precautions Elimination rate will be slow in neonates; modify dosage in patients with renal impairment and in the elderly; use with caution in patients with cephalosporin hypersensitivity

Drug Interactions

Methotrexate: Penicillins may increase the exposure to methotrexate during concurrent therapy; monitor.

Oral contraceptives: Anecdotal reports suggesting decreased contraceptive efficacy with penicillins have been refuted by more rigorous scientific and clinical data.

Probenecid, disulfiram: May increase levels of penicillins (oxacillin)

Warfarin: Effects of warfarin may be increased

Lab Interactions May interfere with urinary glucose tests using cupric sulfate (Benedict's solution, Clinitest®); may inactivate aminoglycosides *in vitro*; false-positive urinary and serum proteins

Adverse Reactions Frequency not defined.

Central nervous system: Fever

Dermatologic: Rash

Gastrointestinal: Nausea, diarrhea, vomiting

Hematologic: Eosinophilia, leukopenia, neutropenia, thrombocytopenia, agranulocytosis

Hepatic: Hepatotoxicity, AST increased

Renal: Acute interstitial nephritis, hematuria

Miscellaneous: Serum sickness-like reactions

Overdosage/Toxicology Symptoms of penicillin overdose include neuromuscular hypersensitivity (eg, agitation, hallucinations, asterixis, encephalopathy, confusion, and seizures). Electrolyte imbalance may occur if the preparation contains potassium or sodium salts, especially in renal failure. Hemodialysis may be helpful to aid in removal of the drug from blood; otherwise, treatment is supportive or symptom-directed.

Dosing

Adults & Elderly: Susceptible infections: I.M., I.V.:

Mild-to-moderate infections: 250-500 mg every 4-6 hours

Severe infections: 1-2 g every 4-6 hours

Pediatrics: Susceptible infections: I.M., I.V.: Infants and Children:

Mild-to-moderate infections: 100-150 mg/kg/day in divided doses every 6 hours (maximum: 4 g/day)

Severe infections: 150-200 mg/kg/day in divided doses every 6 hours (maximum: 12 g/day)

Renal Impairment:

Cl_{cr} <10 mL/minute: Clinical practice varies; some clinicians recommend adjustment to the lower range of the usual dosage as based on severity of infection.

Not dialyzable (0% to 5%)

Available Dosage Forms

Infusion [premixed iso-osmotic dextrose solution]: 1 g (50 mL); 2 g (50 mL)

Injection, powder for reconstitution, as sodium: 1 g, 2 g, 10 g

Nursing Guidelines

Assessment: Assess patient reports of allergy or sensitivity before administering. I.V. - monitor infusion site for extravasation. Monitor response to therapy; if no response, therapy should be re-evaluated.

Monitoring Laboratory Tests: Perform culture and sensitivity studies prior to initiating therapy.

Dietary Considerations: Sodium content of 1 g: 92.4 mg (4.02 mEq)

Patient Education: Complete course of treatment as prescribed. You may experience nausea or vomiting; small, frequent meals and good mouth care may help. If you have diabetes, drug may cause false test results with Clinitest® urine glucose monitoring; use of glucose oxidase methods (Clinistix®) or serum glucose monitoring is preferable. Report persistent fever, sore throat, sores in mouth, diarrhea, unusual bleeding or bruising, respiratory difficulty, or skin rash. Notify prescriber if condition does not respond to treatment.

Geriatric Considerations: Oxacillin has not been studied in the elderly. Dosing adjustments are not necessary except in renal failure (eg, Cl_{cr} <10 mL/minute). Consider sodium content in patients who may be sensitive to volume expansion (ie, CHF).

Pregnancy Risk Factor: B

Lactation: Enters breast milk/compatible

Breast-Feeding Considerations: No adverse effects have been reported in the nursing infant. Theoretically, the antibiotic effect of oxacillin may appear in the infant and change the bowel flora or affect culture results.

Administration

I.V.: Administer around-the-clock to promote less variation in peak and trough serum levels. Administer IVP over 10 minutes. Administer IVPB over 30 minutes.

Compatibility: Stable in dextran 70 6% in dextrose, dextran 40 10% in dextrose, D_5LR, $D_{10}W$, hetastarch 6%, LR

Y-site administration: Incompatible with sodium bicarbonate, verapamil

Compatibility when admixed: Incompatible with cytarabine

Storage: Reconstituted parenteral solution is stable for 3 days at room temperature and 7 days when refrigerated. For I.V. infusion in NS or D_5W, solution is stable for 6 hours at room temperature.

♦ **Oxacillin Sodium** *see* Oxacillin *on page 1274*

Oxaliplatin (ox AL i pla tin)

U.S. Brand Names Eloxatin™

Synonyms Diaminocyclohexane Oxalatoplatinum; L-OHP; NSC-266046

Pharmacologic Category Antineoplastic Agent, Alkylating Agent

Medication Safety Issues

Sound-alike/look-alike issues:

Oxaliplatin may be confused with Aloxi™

Use Treatment of advanced colon cancer and advanced rectal carcinoma

Unlabeled/Investigational Use Head and neck cancer, nonsmall cell lung cancer, non-Hodgkin's lymphoma, ovarian cancer

Mechanism of Action Oxaliplatin is an alkylating agent. Following intracellular hydrolysis, the platinum compound binds to DNA, RNA, or proteins. Cytotoxicity is cell-cycle nonspecific.

(Continued)

Oxaliplatin *(Continued)*

Pharmacodynamics/Kinetics

Distribution: V_d: 440 L

Protein binding: >90% primarily albumin and gamma globulin (irreversible binding to platinum)

Metabolism: Nonenzymatic (rapid and extensive), forms active and inactive derivatives

Half-life elimination: 391 hours; Distribution: Alpha phase: 0.4 hours, Beta phase: 16.8 hours

Excretion: Primarily urine

Contraindications Hypersensitivity to oxaliplatin, other platinum-containing compounds, or any component of the formulation; pregnancy

Warnings/Precautions The U.S. Food and Drug Administration (FDA) currently recommends that procedures for proper handling and disposal of antineoplastic agents be considered. Anaphylactic-like reaction may occur within minutes of oxaliplatin administration. Two different types of neuropathy may occur: First, an acute (within first 2 days), reversible (resolves within 14 days), primarily peripheral symptoms that are often exacerbated by cold (may include pharyngolaryngeal dysesthesia); and secondly, a more persistent (>14 days) presentation that often interferes with daily activities (eg, writing, buttoning, swallowing), these symptoms may improve upon discontinuing treatment. May cause pulmonary fibrosis or hepatotoxicity. The presence of hepatic vascular disorders (including veno-occlusive disease) should be considered, especially in individuals developing portal hypertension or who present with increased liver function tests. Caution in renal dysfunction. Safety and efficacy in pediatric patients have not been established.

Drug Interactions

Anticoagulant therapy: Prolonged prothrombin time and increased INR associated with hemorrhage have been reported in patients receiving oxaliplatin/fluorouracil/leucovorin concomitantly with oral anticoagulants; may require monitoring.

Docetaxel, paclitaxel (taxane derivatives): When administered as sequential infusions, taxane derivatives should be administered before platinum derivatives to limit myelosuppression and to enhance efficacy.

Nephrotoxic drugs: May increase risk of toxicity.

Adverse Reactions Based on clinical trial data using oxaliplatin alone. Some adverse effects (eg, thrombocytopenia, hemorrhagic events, neutropenia) may be increased when therapy is combined with fluorouracil/leucovorin.

>10%:

- Central nervous system: Fatigue (61%), fever (25%), pain (14%), headache (13%), insomnia (11%)
- Gastrointestinal: Nausea (64%), diarrhea (46%), vomiting (37%), abdominal pain (31%), constipation (31%), anorexia (20%), stomatitis (14%)
- Hematologic: Anemia (64%), thrombocytopenia (30%), leukopenia (13%)
- Hepatic: SGOT increased (54%), SGPT increased (36%); total bilirubin increased (13%)
- Neuromuscular & skeletal: Neuropathy (may be dose-limiting), peripheral (acute 56%, persistent 48%), back pain (11%)
- Respiratory: Dyspnea (13%), cough (11%)

1% to 10%:

- Cardiovascular: Edema (10%), chest pain (5%), flushing (3%), thrombosis (2% to 6%), thromboembolism (6% to 9%)
- Central nervous system: Rigors (9%), dizziness (7%), hand-foot syndrome (1%)
- Dermatologic: Rash (5%), alopecia (3%)
- Endocrine & metabolic: Dehydration (5%), hypokalemia (3%)
- Gastrointestinal: Dyspepsia (7%), taste perversion (5%), flatulence (3%), mucositis (2%), gastroesophageal reflux (1%), dysphagia (acute 1% to 2%)
- Genitourinary: Dysuria (1%)
- Hematologic: Neutropenia (7%)
- Local: Injection site reaction (9%)
- Neuromuscular & skeletal: Arthralgia (7%)
- Ocular: Abnormal lacrimation (1%)
- Renal: Serum creatinine increased (10%)
- Respiratory: URI (7%), rhinitis (6%), epistaxis (2%), pharyngitis (2%), pharyngolaryngeal dysesthesia (1% to 2%)
- Miscellaneous: Allergic reactions (3%), hiccup (2%)

Postmarketing and/or case reports: Anaphylactic shock, angioedema, colitis, cranial nerve palsies, deep tendon reflex loss, deafness, dysarthria, fasciculations, hemolytic anemia (immuno-allergic), hemolytic uremia syndrome, ileus, interstitial lung diseases, intestinal obstruction, Lhermittes' sign, metabolic acidosis, optic neuritis, pancreatitis, pulmonary fibrosis, thrombocytopenia (immuno-allergic), veno-occlusive disease of the liver, visual acuity decreased, visual field disturbance

Overdosage/Toxicology Overdose symptoms are extensions of known side effects (eg, thrombocytopenia, myelosuppression, nausea, vomiting, neurotoxicity, respiratory symptoms). Treatment should be supportive.

Dosing

Adults:

Colorectal cancer (labeled dosing): Refer to individual protocols. I.V.:

85 mg/m^2 every 2 weeks **or**

20-25 mg/m^2 days 1-5 every 3 weeks **or**

100-130 mg/m^2 every 2-3 weeks

Elderly: No dosing adjustment recommended.

Renal Impairment: Consider omitting dose or changing chemotherapy regimen if Cl_{cr} ≤19 mL/minute.

Available Dosage Forms

Injection, powder for reconstitution: 50 mg, 100 mg [contains lactose]

Injection, solution [preservative free]: 5 mg/mL (10 mL, 20 mL)

Nursing Guidelines

Assessment: See Contraindications, Warnings/Precautions, and Dosing for use cautions. Assess potential for interactions with other prescriptions, OTC medications, or herbal products patient may be taking (see Drug Interactions). See I.V. Administration specifics. Patient must be observed closely for hypersensitivity reaction (which can occur within minutes of administration). Assess results of laboratory tests, therapeutic effectiveness, and adverse reactions (eg, neuropathy - see Adverse Reactions and Overdose/Toxicology) prior to initiating therapy and on a regular basis throughout therapy. Teach patient possible side effects/appropriate interventions and adverse symptoms to report (see Patient Education). **Pregnancy risk factor D** - determine that patient is not pregnant before beginning treatment. Instruct patients of childbearing age about appropriate barrier contraceptive measures during therapy and for 1 month following therapy. Breast-feeding is not recommended.

Patient Education: Inform prescriber of all prescriptions, OTC medications, or herbal products you are taking, and any allergies you have. Do not take any new medication during therapy without consulting prescriber. This medication can only be administered by infusion; you will be monitored closely during and following infusion. Report immediately any pain, burning, swelling at infusion site, or any signs of allergic reaction (eg, respiratory difficulty or swallowing, back pain, chest tightness, rash, hives, swelling of lips or mouth). It is important that you maintain adequate nutrition (small, frequent meals may help) and adequate hydration (2-3 L/day of fluids) unless instructed to restrict fluid intake. You will be susceptible to infection (avoid crowds and exposure to infection and do not have any vaccinations without consulting prescriber). May cause nausea, vomiting, loss of appetite, or taste perversion (small, frequent meals, frequent mouth care, chewing gum, or sucking lozenges may help - if nausea/vomiting is unresolved, consult prescriber for approved antiemetic); mouth sores (use soft toothbrush or cotton swabs for mouth care); diarrhea (boiled milk, buttermilk, or yogurt may help); or loss of hair (reversible). Report any numbness, pain, tingling, or loss of sensation of extremities; chest pain or palpitations; swelling, pain, or hot areas in legs; unusual fatigue; unusual bruising or bleeding; respiratory difficulty; muscle cramps or twitching; change in hearing acuity; or other persistent adverse effects. **Pregnancy/breast-feeding precautions:** Do not get pregnant while taking this medication; use appropriate barrier contraceptive measures. Breast-feeding is not recommended.

Pregnancy Risk Factor: D

Lactation: Excretion in breast milk unknown/not recommended

Administration

I.V.: Administer as I.V. infusion over 2-6 hours. Longer infusion times (eg, those approaching or equal to 6 hours) may mitigate signs/symptoms of acute reactions. Flush infusion line with D_5W prior to administration of any concomitant medication.

(Continued)

Oxaliplatin *(Continued)*

Reconstitution: Do not reconstitute using a chloride-containing solution (eg, NaCl). Further dilution with D_5W (250 or 500 mL) is required prior to administration. Reconstituted solution does not require protection from light.

Compatibility: Incompatible with alkaline solutions (eg, fluorouracil) and chloride-containing solutions. Flush infusion line with D_5W prior to, and following, administration of concomitant medications via same I.V. line.

Storage: Store in original outer carton at room temperature of 15°C to 30°C (59°F to 86°F); do not freeze. Protect from light. Diluted solution is stable up to 6 hours at room temperature of 20°C to 25°C (68°F to 77°F) or up to 24 hours under refrigeration at 2°C to 8°C (36°F to 46°F).

Oxcarbazepine (ox car BAZ e peen)

U.S. Brand Names Trileptal®

Synonyms GP 47680; OCBZ

Pharmacologic Category Anticonvulsant, Miscellaneous

Use Monotherapy or adjunctive therapy in the treatment of partial seizures in adults and children ≥4 years of age with epilepsy; adjunctive therapy in the treatment of partial seizures in children ≥2 years of age with epilepsy.

Unlabeled/Investigational Use Bipolar disorder; treatment of neuropathic pain

Mechanism of Action Pharmacological activity results from both oxcarbazepine and its monohydroxy metabolite (MHD). Precise mechanism of anticonvulsant effect has not been defined. Oxcarbazepine and MHD block voltage sensitive sodium channels, stabilizing hyperexcited neuronal membranes, inhibiting repetitive firing, and decreasing the propagation of synaptic impulses. These actions are believed to prevent the spread of seizures. Oxcarbazepine and MHD also increase potassium conductance and modulate the activity of high-voltage activated calcium channels.

Pharmacodynamics/Kinetics

Absorption: Complete; food has no affect on rate or extent

Distribution: MHD: V_d: 49 L

Protein binding, serum: MHD: 40%

Metabolism: Hepatic to 10-monohydroxy metabolite (MHD; active); MHD is further conjugated to DHD (inactive)

Bioavailability: Decreased in children <8 years; increased in elderly >60 years

Half-life elimination: Parent drug: 2 hours; MHD: 9 hours; renal impairment (Cl_{cr} 30 mL/minute): MHD: 19 hours

Clearance of MHD is increased in younger children (~80% in children 2-4 years of age) and approaches that of adults by ~13 years of age

Time to peak, serum: 4.5 hours (3-13 hours)

Excretion: Urine (95%, <1% as unchanged oxcarbazepine, 27% as unchanged MHD, 49% as MHD glucuronides); feces (<4%)

Contraindications Hypersensitivity to oxcarbazepine or any component of the formulation

Warnings/Precautions Clinically-significant hyponatremia (sodium <125 mmol/L) can develop during oxcarbazepine use; monitor serum sodium, particularly during the first 3 months of therapy or in patients at risk for hyponatremia. Potentially serious, sometimes fatal, dermatologic reactions (eg, Stevens-Johnson, toxic epidermal necrolysis) and multiorgan hypersensitivity reactions have been reported in adults and children; monitor for signs and symptoms of skin reactions and possible disparate manifestations associated with lymphatic, hepatic, renal and/or hematologic organ systems; gradual discontinuation and conversion to alternate therapy may be required. As with all antiepileptic drugs, oxcarbazepine should be withdrawn gradually to minimize the potential of increased seizure frequency. Use of oxcarbazepine has been associated with CNS related adverse events, most significant of these were cognitive symptoms including psychomotor slowing, difficulty with concentration, and speech or language problems, somnolence or fatigue, and coordination abnormalities, including ataxia and gait disturbances. Use caution in patients with previous hypersensitivity to carbamazepine (cross-sensitivity occurs in 25% to 30%). May reduce the efficacy of oral contraceptives (nonhormonal contraceptive measures are recommended).

Drug Interactions Inhibits CYP2C19 (weak); **Induces** CYP3A4 (strong)

Carbamazepine: Oxcarbazepine serum concentrations may be reduced by a mean 40%

CYP3A4 substrates: Oxcarbazepine may decrease the levels/effects of CYP3A4 substrates. Example substrates include benzodiazepines, calcium channel blockers, clarithromycin, cyclosporine, erythromycin, estrogens, mirtazapine, nateglinide, nefazodone, nevirapine, protease inhibitors, tacrolimus, and venlafaxine.

Felodipine: Metabolism is increased due to enzyme induction; similar effects may be anticipated with other dihydropyridine calcium channel blockers

Hormonal contraceptives: Metabolism may be increased due to enzyme induction; use alternative contraceptive measures; oxcarbazepine with oral contraceptives has been shown to decrease plasma concentrations of the two hormonal components, ethinyl estradiol (48% and 52%) and levonorgestrel (32% and 52%).

Phenobarbital: Phenobarbital levels are increased (average of 14%); oxcarbazepine levels are decreased (average of 25%)

Phenytoin: Phenytoin levels may be increased (high dosages) by an average of 40%; oxcarbazepine levels may be decreased (by an average of 30%) during concurrent therapy; monitor phenytoin levels

Valproic acid decreases oxcarbazepine levels by an average of 18%

Verapamil's metabolism may be increased due to enzyme induction; verapamil may reduce blood levels of oxcarbazepine's active metabolite (MHD)

Nutritional/Herbal/Ethanol Interactions

Ethanol: Avoid ethanol (may increase CNS depression).

Herb/Nutraceutical: St John's wort may decrease oxcarbazepine levels. Avoid evening primrose (seizure threshold decreased). Avoid valerian, St John's wort, kava kava, gotu kola.

Lab Interactions Thyroid function tests may depress serum T_4 without affecting T_3 levels or TSH.

Adverse Reactions As reported in adults with doses of up to 2400 mg/day (includes patients on monotherapy, adjunctive therapy, and those not previously on AEDs); incidence in children was similar.

>10%:

Central nervous system: Dizziness (22% to 49%), somnolence (20% to 36%), headache (13% to 32%, placebo 23%), ataxia (5% to 31%), fatigue (12% to 15%), vertigo (6% to 15%)

Gastrointestinal: Vomiting (7% to 36%), nausea (15% to 29%), abdominal pain (10% to 13%)

Neuromuscular & skeletal: Abnormal gait (5% to 17%), tremor (3% to 16%)

Ocular: Diplopia (14% to 40%), nystagmus (7% to 26%), abnormal vision (4% to 14%)

1% to 10%:

Cardiovascular: Hypotension (1% to 2%)

Central nervous system: Nervousness (2% to 5%), amnesia (4%), agitation (1% to 2%)

Dermatologic: Rash (4%)

Endocrine & metabolic: Hyponatremia (1% to 3%)

Gastrointestinal: Diarrhea (5% to 7%), gastritis (1% to 2%)

Neuromuscular & skeletal: Weakness (3% to 6%), back pain (4%), falls (4%), abnormal coordination (1% to 4%), muscle weakness (1% to 2%)

Ocular: Abnormal accommodation (2%)

Respiratory: Upper respiratory tract infection (7%)

<1% (Limited to important or life-threatening): Aggressive reaction, alopecia, angioedema, aphasia, asthma, blood in stool, cardiac failure, cataract, cerebral hemorrhage, cholelithiasis, convulsions aggravated, delirium, duodenal ulcer, dysphagia, dysphonia, dyspnea, dystonia, erythema multiforme, eosinophilia, extrapyramidal disorder, gastric ulcer, genital pruritus, gingival hyperplasia, hematemesis, hematuria, hemianopia, hemiplegia, hypersensitivity reaction, intermenstrual bleeding, laryngismus, leukopenia, maculopapular rash, malaise, manic reaction, menorrhagia, migraine, muscle contractions (involuntary), neuralgia, oculogyric crisis, paralysis, photosensitivity reaction, postural hypotension, priapism, purpura, psychosis, scotoma, sialoadenitis, Stevens-Johnson syndrome, stupor, syncope, systemic lupus erythematosus, tetany, thrombocytopenia, toxic epidermal necrolysis, urticaria

Overdosage/Toxicology Symptoms may include CNS depression (somnolence, ataxia). Treatment is symptomatic and supportive.

Dosing

Adults & Elderly:

Adjunctive therapy, partial seizures (epilepsy): Oral: Initial: 300 mg twice daily; dosage may be increased by 600 mg/day at approximate weekly intervals. Recommended daily dose is 1200 mg/day in 2 divided doses. Although

(Continued)

Oxcarbazepine *(Continued)*

daily doses >1200 mg/day demonstrated greater efficacy, most patients were unable to tolerate 2400 mg/day (due to CNS effects).

Conversion to monotherapy, partial seizures (epilepsy): Oral: Patients receiving concomitant antiepileptic drugs (AEDs): Initial: 300 mg twice daily while simultaneously reducing the dose of concomitant AEDs. Withdraw concomitant AEDs completely over 3-6 weeks, while increasing the oxcarbazine dose in increments of 600 mg/day at weekly intervals, reaching the maximum oxcarbazine dose (2400 mg/day) in about 2-4 weeks (lower doses have been effective in patients in whom monotherapy has been initiated).

Initiation of monotherapy, partial seizures (epilepsy): Oral: Patients not receiving prior AEDs: 300 mg twice daily (total dose 600 mg/day). Increase dose by 300 mg/day every third day to a dose of 1200 mg/day. Higher dosages (2400 mg/day) have been shown to be effective in patients converted to monotherapy from other AEDs.

Pediatrics:

Adjunctive treatment, partial seizures (epilepsy): Oral: Children 2-16 years:

Initial: 8-10 mg/kg/day (not to exceed 600 mg/day) given in a twice daily regimen.

Maintenance: The target maintenance dose should be achieved over 2 weeks, and depends on weight of the child:

<20 kg: 600 mg/day in 2 divided doses; consider initiating dose at 16-20 mg/kg/day; maximum maintenance dose should be achieved over 2-4 weeks and should not exceed 60 mg/kg/day
20-29 kg: 900 mg/day in 2 divided doses
29.1-39 kg: 1200 mg/day in 2 divided doses
>39 kg: 1800 mg/day in 2 divided doses

Conversion to monotherapy: Children 4-16 years: Oxcarbazepine 8-10 mg/kg/day in twice daily divided doses, while simultaneously initiating the reduction of the dose of the concomitant antiepileptic drug; the concomitant drug should be withdrawn over 3-6 weeks. Oxcarbazepine dose may be increased by a maximum of 10 mg/kg/day at weekly intervals. See below for recommended total daily dose by weight.

Initiation of monotherapy: Children 4-16 years: Oxcarbazepine should be initiated at 8-10 mg/kg/day in twice daily divided doses; doses may be titrated by 5 mg/kg/day every third day. See below for recommended total daily dose by weight.

Range of maintenance doses by weight during monotherapy:

20 kg: 600-900 mg/day
25-30 kg: 900-1200 mg/day
35-40 kg: 900-1500 mg/day
45 kg: 1200-1500 mg/day
50-55 kg: 1200-1800 mg/day
60-65 kg: 1200-2100 mg/day
70 kg: 1500-2100 mg/day

Renal Impairment: Cl_{cr} <30 mL/minute: Therapy should be initiated at one-half the usual starting dose (300 mg/day in adults) and increased slowly to achieve the desired clinical response

Hepatic Impairment: No dosage adjustment recommended in mild to moderate hepatic impairment. Patients with severe hepatic impairment have not been evaluated.

Available Dosage Forms

Suspension, oral: 300 mg/5 mL (250 mL) [contains ethanol; packaged with oral syringe]

Tablet [film coated]: 150 mg, 300 mg, 600 mg

Nursing Guidelines

Assessment: Assess complete allergy history (carbamazepine). Assess effectiveness and interactions of other medications. Monitor therapeutic effectiveness (seizure activity, frequency, duration, type), laboratory results, and adverse reactions (eg, sedation, CNS changes, visual changes). Monitor for skin reactions. Dosage should be tapered when discontinuing to reduce risk of increased seizures. Assess knowledge/teach patient appropriate use, interventions to reduce side effects, and adverse reactions to report. **Note:** Oxcarbazepine may reduce the effectiveness of oral contraceptives, nonhormonal contraception is recommended.

Monitoring Laboratory Tests: Serum sodium (particularly during first 3 months of therapy); additional serum sodium monitoring is recommended during maintenance treatment in patients receiving other medications known to decrease sodium levels, in patients with signs/symptoms of hyponatremia, and in patients with an increase in seizure frequency or severity.

Dietary Considerations: May be taken with or without food.

Patient Education: Do not increase dose or frequency or discontinue without consulting prescriber. While using the medication do not use alcohol and other prescription or OTC medications (especially medications to relieve pain, induce sleep, reduce anxiety, treat or prevent cold, coughs, or allergies) unless approved by prescriber. Maintain adequate hydration (2-3 L/day of fluids) unless instructed to restrict fluid intake. You may experience drowsiness, dizziness, or blurred vision (use caution when driving or engaging in tasks requiring alertness until response to drug is known); nausea or vomiting (small frequent meals, good mouth care, chewing gum, or sucking hard candy may help, or contact prescriber). Report CNS changes, increase in seizure frequency or severity, mentation changes, changes in cognition or memory, acute fatigue or weakness, or insomnia; muscle cramping, weakness, or pain; rash or skin irritations; unusual bruising or bleeding (mouth, urine, stool); swelling of extremities; or other adverse response. **Pregnancy/breast-feeding precautions:** Inform prescriber if you are or intend to become pregnant. **Note:** Oxcarbazepine may reduce the effectiveness of oral contraceptives, nonhormonal contraception is recommended. Breast-feeding is not recommended.

Geriatric Considerations: Studies in elderly volunteers (60-82 years of age) with both single dose (300 mg) and multiple doses (600 mg/day) reported maximum plasma concentrations and AUC as being 30% to 60% higher than younger volunteers (18-32 years of age). These results were due to differences in creatinine clearance between the two groups. Since elderly may have Cl_{cr} <30 mL/minute, dose reductions may be needed. See dosing information.

Pregnancy Risk Factor: C

Pregnancy Issues: Although many epidemiological studies of congenital anomalies in infants born to women treated with various anticonvulsants during pregnancy have been reported, none of these investigations includes enough women treated with oxcarbazepine to assess possible teratogenic effects of this drug. Given that teratogenic effects have been observed in animal studies, and that oxcarbazepine is structurally related to carbamazepine (teratogenic in humans), use during pregnancy only if the benefit to the mother outweighs the potential risk to the fetus.

Lactation: Enters breast milk/not recommended

Breast-Feeding Considerations: Oxcarbazepine and its active metabolite (MHD) are excreted in human breast milk. A milk-to-plasma concentration ratio of 0.5 was found for both. Because of the potential for serious adverse reactions to oxcarbazepine in nursing infants, a decision should be made whether to discontinue nursing or to discontinue the drug in nursing women.

Administration

Oral: Suspension: Prior to using for the first time, firmly insert the plastic adapter provided with the bottle. Cover adapter with child-resistant cap when not in use. Shake bottle for at least 10 seconds, remove child-resistant cap and insert the oral dosing syringe provided to withdraw appropriate dose. Dose may be taken directly from oral syringe or may be mixed in a small glass of water immediately prior to swallowing. Rinse syringe with warm water after use and allow to dry thoroughly. Discard any unused portion after 7 weeks of first opening bottle.

Storage: Store tablets and suspension at 25°C (77°F). Use suspension within 7 weeks of first opening container.

- **Oxidized Regenerated Cellulose** *see* Cellulose (Oxidized Regenerated) *on page 362*
- **Oxpentifylline** *see* Pentoxifylline *on page 1340*

Oxybutynin (oks i BYOO ti nin)

U.S. Brand Names Ditropan®; Ditropan® XL; Oxytrol™

Synonyms Oxybutynin Chloride

Pharmacologic Category Antispasmodic Agent, Urinary

Medication Safety Issues

Sound-alike/look-alike issues:

Oxybutynin may be confused with OxyContin®

Ditropan® may be confused with Detrol®, diazepam, Diprivan®, dithranol

(Continued)

Oxybutynin *(Continued)*

Transdermal patch may contain conducting metal (eg, aluminum); remove patch prior to MRI.

Use Antispasmodic for neurogenic bladder (urgency, frequency, urge incontinence) and uninhibited bladder

Mechanism of Action Direct antispasmodic effect on smooth muscle, also inhibits the action of acetylcholine on smooth muscle (exhibits $^1/_5$ the anticholinergic activity of atropine, but is 4-10 times the antispasmodic activity); does not block effects at skeletal muscle or at autonomic ganglia; increases bladder capacity, decreases uninhibited contractions, and delays desire to void; therefore, decreases urgency and frequency

Pharmacodynamics/Kinetics

Onset of action: Oral: 30-60 minutes

Peak effect: 3-6 hours

Duration: 6-10 hours (up to 24 hours for extended release oral formulation)

Absorption: Oral: Rapid and well absorbed; Transdermal: High

Distribution: V_d: 193 L

Metabolism: Hepatic via CYP3A4; Oral: High first-pass metabolism; I.V.: Forms active and inactive metabolites

Half-life elimination: I.V.: ~2 hours (parent drug), 7-8 hours (metabolites)

Time to peak, serum: Oral: ~60 minutes; Transdermal: 24-48 hours

Excretion: Urine (<0.1%)

Contraindications Hypersensitivity to oxybutynin or any component of the formulation; untreated glaucoma; partial or complete GI obstruction; GU obstruction; urinary retention; megacolon; toxic megacolon

Warnings/Precautions Use with caution in patients with urinary tract obstruction, angle-closure glaucoma (treated), hyperthyroidism, reflux esophagitis (including concurrent therapy with oral bisphosphonates or drugs which may increase the risk of esophagitis), heart disease, hepatic or renal disease, prostatic hyperplasia, autonomic neuropathy, ulcerative colitis (may cause ileus and toxic megacolon), hypertension, hiatal hernia, myasthenia gravis, ulcerative colitis, or intestinal atony. The extended release formulation consists of drug within a nondeformable matrix; following drug release/absorption, the matrix/shell is expelled in the stool. Transdermal patch may contain conducting metal (eg, aluminum); remove patch prior to MRI. The use of nondeformable products in patients with known stricture/narrowing of the GI tract has been associated with symptoms of obstruction. Caution should be used in elderly due to anticholinergic activity (eg, confusion, constipation, blurred vision, and tachycardia). May increase the risk of heat prostration.

Drug Interactions **Substrate** of CYP3A4 (minor); **Inhibits** CYP2D6 (weak), 3A4 (weak)

Anticholinergic agents: Additive anticholinergic effects may occur with concurrent antihistamines and anticholinergic agents.

CNS depressants: Additive sedation with CNS depressants and ethanol.

Nutritional/Herbal/Ethanol Interactions Ethanol: Use ethanol with caution (may increase CNS depression and toxicity). Watch for sedation.

Lab Interactions May suppress the wheal and flare reactions to skin test antigens.

Adverse Reactions

Oral:

>10%:

Central nervous system: Dizziness (6% to 16%), somnolence (12% to 13%)

Gastrointestinal: Xerostomia (61% to 71%), constipation (13%)

Genitourinary: Urination impaired (11%)

1% to 10%:

Cardiovascular: Palpitation (2% to <5%), peripheral edema (2% to <5%), hypertension (2% to <5%), vasodilation (2% to <5%)

Central nervous system: Headache (6% to 10%), pain (7%), confusion (2% to <5%), insomnia (2% to <5%), nervousness (2% to <5%)

Dermatologic: Dry skin (2% to <5%), skin rash (2% to <5%)

Gastrointestinal: Nausea (9% to 10%), dyspepsia (7%), abdominal pain (2% to 6%), diarrhea (5% to 9%), flatulence (2% to <5%), gastrointestinal reflux (2% to <5%), taste perversion (2% to <5%)

Genitourinary: Postvoid residuals increased (2% to 9%), urinary tract infection (5%)

Neuromuscular & skeletal: Weakness (2% to 7%)

Ocular: Blurred vision (8% to 9%), dry eyes (2% to 6%)

Respiratory: Rhinitis (6%), dry nasal and sinus membranes (2% to <5%)

Transdermal:
>10%: Local: Application site reaction (17%), pruritus (14%)
1% to 10%:
Gastrointestinal: Xerostomia (4% to 10%), diarrhea (3%), constipation (3%)
Genitourinary: Dysuria (2%)
Local: Erythema (6% to 8%), vesicles (3%), rash (3%)
Ocular: Vision changes (3%)

Postmarketing and/or case reports: Cardiac arrhythmia, cycloplegia, hallucinations, lactation suppressed, myocarditis, impotence, seizure, sweating decreased, tachycardia

Overdosage/Toxicology Symptoms of overdose include hypotension, circulatory failure, psychotic behavior, flushing, respiratory failure, paralysis, tremor, irritability, seizures, delirium, hallucinations, and coma. Treatment is symptomatic and supportive. For anticholinergic overdose with severe life-threatening symptoms, physostigmine 1-2 mg I.V. slowly, may be given to reverse these effects.

Dosing

Adults:

Bladder spasms:

Oral:
Regular release: 5 mg 2-3 times/day up to maximum of 5 mg 4 times/day
Extended release: Initial: 5-10 mg once daily, may increase in 5-10 mg increments; maximum: 30 mg daily

Transdermal: Apply one 3.9 mg/day patch twice weekly (every 3-4 days)

Note: Should be discontinued periodically to determine whether the patient can manage without the drug and to minimize resistance to the drug.

Elderly:
Oral: 2.5-5 mg 2-3 times/day
Transdermal: Refer to adult dosing. **Note:** Should be discontinued periodically to determine whether the patient can manage without the drug and to minimize resistance to the drug.

Pediatrics:

Bladder spasms: Oral: Children:
1-5 years (unlabeled use): 0.2 mg/kg/dose 2-4 times/day
>5 years: 5 mg twice daily, up to 5 mg 3 times/day maximum
>6 years: Extended release: 5 mg once daily; maximum dose: 20 mg/day

Available Dosage Forms
Syrup, as chloride (Ditropan®): 5 mg/5 mL (473 mL)
Tablet, as chloride (Ditropan®): 5 mg
Tablet, extended release, as chloride (Ditropan® XL): 5 mg, 10 mg, 15 mg
Transdermal system (Oxytrol™): 3.9 mg/day (8s) [39 cm^2; total oxybutynin 36 mg]

Nursing Guidelines

Assessment: Assess other prescriptions, OTC medications, or herbal products patient may be taking for interactions. Assess voiding pattern, incontinent episodes, frequency, urgency, distention, and urinary retention prior to beginning therapy and periodically with long-term use. Assess knowledge/teach patient appropriate use, possible side effects, and symptoms to report.

Dietary Considerations: Food causes a slight delay in the absorption of the oral solution and bioavailability is deceased by ~25%. Absorption of the extended release tablet is not affected by food.

Patient Education: Take prescribed oral dose preferably on an empty stomach, 1 hour before or 2 hours after meals. Swallow extended-release tablets whole, do not chew or crush. You may experience dizziness, lightheadedness, or drowsiness (use caution when driving or engaging in tasks requiring alertness until response to drug is known); dry mouth or changes in appetite (small frequent meals, frequent mouth care, sucking lozenges, or chewing gum may help); constipation (increased exercise, fluids, fruit, fiber, or stool softener may help); decreased sexual ability (reversible with discontinuance of drug); or decreased sweating (use caution in hot weather, avoid extreme exercise or activity). Use alcohol with caution; may increase drowsiness. Report rapid heartbeat, palpitations, or chest pain; difficulty voiding; or vision changes.

Geriatric Considerations: Caution should be used in the elderly due to anticholinergic activity (eg, confusion, constipation, blurred vision, and tachycardia). Start with lower doses. Transdermal dosage form may have less potential for these effects. Oxybutynin may cause memory problems in the elderly. A study of 12 healthy volunteers with an average age of 69 showed cognitive decline while taking the drug (*J Am Geriatr Soc*, 1998, L46:8-13).

(Continued)

Oxybutynin *(Continued)*

Pregnancy Risk Factor: B

Lactation: Excretion in breast milk unknown/use caution

Breast-Feeding Considerations: Suppression of lactation has been reported (rarely).

Administration

Oral: Immediate release tablets and solution should be administered on an empty stomach with water. Extended release tablets may be taken with or without food and must be swallowed whole; do not crush, divide, or chew.

Storage: Store at controlled room temperature. Protect syrup from light. Keep transdermal patch in sealed pouch.

♦ **Oxybutynin Chloride** *see* Oxybutynin *on page 1281*

Oxycodone (oks i KOE done)

U.S. Brand Names OxyContin®; Oxydose™; OxyFast®; OxyIR®; Roxicodone™; Roxicodone™ Intensol™

Synonyms Dihydrohydroxycodeinone; Oxycodone Hydrochloride

Pharmacologic Category Analgesic, Narcotic

Medication Safety Issues

Sound-alike/look-alike issues:

Oxycodone may be confused with OxyContin®

OxyContin® may be confused with oxybutynin, oxycodone

OxyFast® may be confused with Roxanol™

Use Management of moderate to severe pain, normally used in combination with non-narcotic analgesics

OxyContin® is indicated for around-the-clock management of moderate to severe pain when an analgesic is needed for an extended period of time. **Note:** OxyContin® is not intended for use as an "as needed" analgesic or for immediately-postoperative pain management (should be used postoperatively only if the patient has received it prior to surgery or if severe, persistent pain is anticipated).

Mechanism of Action Binds to opiate receptors in the CNS, causing inhibition of ascending pain pathways, altering the perception of and response to pain; produces generalized CNS depression

Pharmacodynamics/Kinetics

Onset of action: Pain relief: 10-15 minutes

Peak effect: 0.5-1 hour

Duration: 3-6 hours; Controlled release: ≤12 hours

Metabolism: Hepatic

Half-life elimination: 2-3 hours

Excretion: Urine

Contraindications Hypersensitivity to oxycodone or any component of the formulation; significant respiratory depression; hypercarbia; acute or severe bronchial asthma; OxyContin® is also contraindicated in paralytic ileus (known or suspected); pregnancy (prolonged use or high doses at term)

Warnings/Precautions Use with caution in patients with hypersensitivity reactions to other phenanthrene derivative opioid agonists (morphine, hydrocodone, hydromorphone, levorphanol, oxycodone, oxymorphone), respiratory diseases including asthma, emphysema, or COPD. Use with caution in pancreatitis or biliary tract disease, acute alcoholism (including delirium tremens), adrenocortical insufficiency, CNS depression/coma, kyphoscoliosis (or other skeletal disorder which may alter respiratory function), hypothyroidism (including myxedema), prostatic hyperplasia, urethral stricture, and toxic psychosis.

Use with caution in the elderly, debilitated, severe hepatic or renal function. Hemodynamic effects (hypotension, orthostasis) may be exaggerated in patients with hypovolemia, concurrent vasodilating drugs, or in patients with head injury. Respiratory depressant effects and capacity to elevate CSF pressure may be exaggerated in presence of head injury, other intracranial lesion, or pre-existing intracranial pressure. Tolerance or drug dependence may result from extended use. Healthcare provider should be alert to problems of abuse, misuse, and diversion. Do **not** crush controlled-release tablets. Some preparations contain sulfites which may cause allergic reactions. OxyContin® 80 mg and 160 mg strengths are for use only in opioid-tolerant patients requiring high daily dosages >160 mg (80 mg formulation) or >320 mg (160 mg formulation).

Drug Interactions Substrate of CYP2D6 (major)

CNS depressants, MAO inhibitors, general anesthetics, and tricyclic antidepressants: May potentiate the effects of opiate agonists; dextroamphetamine may enhance the analgesic effect of opiate agonists

CYP2D6 inhibitors: May decrease the effects of oxycodone. Example inhibitors include chlorpromazine, delavirdine, fluoxetine, miconazole, paroxetine, pergolide, quinidine, quinine, ritonavir, and ropinirole.

Nutritional/Herbal/Ethanol Interactions

Ethanol: Avoid ethanol (may increase CNS depression).

Food: When taken with a high-fat meal, peak concentration is 25% greater following a single OxyContin® 160 mg tablet as compared to two 80 mg tablets.

Herb/Nutraceutical: Avoid valerian, St John's wort, kava kava, gotu kola (may increase CNS depression).

Adverse Reactions

>10%:

Central nervous system: Fatigue, drowsiness, dizziness, somnolence

Dermatologic: Pruritus

Gastrointestinal: Nausea, vomiting, constipation

Neuromuscular & skeletal: Weakness

1% to 10%:

Cardiovascular: Postural hypotension

Central nervous system: Nervousness, headache, restlessness, malaise, confusion, anxiety, abnormal dreams, euphoria, thought abnormalities

Dermatologic: Rash

Gastrointestinal: Anorexia, stomach cramps, xerostomia, biliary spasm, abdominal pain, dyspepsia, gastritis

Genitourinary: Ureteral spasms, decreased urination

Local: Pain at injection site

Respiratory: Dyspnea, hiccups

Miscellaneous: Diaphoresis

<1% (Limited to important or life-threatening): Anaphylaxis, anaphylactoid reaction, dysphagia, exfoliative dermatitis, hallucinations, histamine release, hyponatremia, ileus, intracranial pressure increased, mental depression, paradoxical CNS stimulation, paralytic ileus, physical and psychological dependence, SIADH, syncope, urinary retention, urticaria, vasodilation, withdrawal syndrome (may include seizure)

Note: Deaths due to overdose have been reported due to misuse/abuse after crushing the sustained release tablets.

Overdosage/Toxicology Symptoms of toxicity include CNS depression, respiratory depression, and miosis. Naloxone, 2 mg I.V. with repeat administration as necessary up to a total of 10 mg, can also be used to reverse toxic effects of the opiate.

Dosing

Adults & Elderly: Management of pain: Oral:

Regular or immediate release formulations: 2.5-5 mg every 6 hours as needed

Controlled release:

Opioid naive (not currently on opioid): 10 mg every 12 hours

Currently on opioid/ASA or acetaminophen or NSAID combination:

1-5 tablets: 10-20 mg every 12 hours

6-9 tablets: 20-30 mg every 12 hours

10-12 tablets: 30-40 mg every 12 hours

May continue the nonopioid as a separate drug.

Currently on opioids: Use standard conversion chart to convert daily dose to oxycodone equivalent. Divide daily dose in 2 (for every 12-hour dosing) and round down to nearest dosage form.

Note: 80 mg or 160 mg tablets are for use **only** in opioid-tolerant patients. Special safety considerations must be addressed when converting to OxyContin® doses ≥160 mg every 12 hours. Dietary caution must be taken when patients are initially titrated to 160 mg tablets.

Pediatrics: Oral: Regular or immediate release formulations:

6-12 years: 1.25 mg every 6 hours as needed

>12 years: 2.5 mg every 6 hours as needed

Hepatic Impairment: Reduce dosage in patients with severe liver disease.

Available Dosage Forms

Capsule, immediate release, as hydrochloride (OxyIR®): 5 mg

Solution, oral, as hydrochloride: 5 mg/5 mL (500 mL)

Roxicodone™: 5 mg/5 mL (5 mL, 500 mL) [contains alcohol]

Solution, oral concentrate, as hydrochloride: 20 mg/mL (30 mL)

(Continued)

Oxycodone *(Continued)*

Oxydose™: 20 mg/mL (30 mL) [contains sodium benzoate; berry flavor]
OxyFast®, Roxicodone™ Intensol™: 20 mg/mL (30 mL) [contains sodium benzoate]

Tablet, as hydrochloride: 5 mg, 15 mg, 30 mg
Roxicodone™: 5 mg, 15 mg, 30 mg

Tablet, controlled release, as hydrochloride (OxyContin®): 10 mg, 20 mg, 40 mg, 80 mg, 160 mg

Tablet, extended release, as hydrochloride: 10 mg, 20 mg, 40 mg, 80 mg

Nursing Guidelines

Assessment: Assess other medications patient may be taking for additive or adverse interactions. Monitor for effectiveness of pain relief and monitor for signs of overdose. Monitor vital signs, CNS and respiratory status, and degree of sedation at beginning of therapy and at regular intervals with long-term use. May cause physical and/or psychological dependence. For inpatients, implement safety measures. Assess knowledge/teach patient appropriate use (if self-administered). Teach patient to monitor for adverse reactions, adverse reactions to report, and appropriate interventions to reduce side effects.

Dietary Considerations: Instruct patient to avoid high-fat meals when taking OxyContin® 160 mg tablets.

Patient Education: If self-administered, use exactly as directed; do not increase dose or frequency. Drug may cause physical and/or psychological dependence. Do not crush or chew controlled-release tablets. While using this medication, do not use alcohol and other prescription or OTC medications (especially sedatives, tranquilizers, antihistamines, or pain medications) without consulting prescriber. Maintain adequate hydration (2-3 L/day of fluids) unless instructed to restrict fluid intake. May cause hypotension, dizziness, drowsiness, impaired coordination, or blurred vision (use caution when driving, climbing stairs, or changing position - rising from sitting or lying to standing, or when engaging in tasks requiring alertness until response to drug is known); nausea, vomiting, or dry mouth (frequent mouth care, small frequent meals, chewing gum, or sucking lozenges may help); or constipation (increased exercise, fluids, fruit, or fiber may help; if unresolved, consult prescriber about use of stool softeners). Report persistent dizziness or headache; excessive fatigue or sedation; changes in mental status; changes in urinary elimination or pain on urination; weakness or trembling; blurred vision; or shortness of breath. **Pregnancy/breast-feeding precautions:** Inform prescriber if you are or intend to become pregnant. If you are breast-feeding, take medication immediately after breast-feeding or 3-4 hours prior to next feeding.

Geriatric Considerations: The elderly may be particularly susceptible to the CNS depressant and constipating effects of narcotics. Serum levels at a given dose may also be increased relative to concentrations in younger patients.

Pregnancy Risk Factor: B/D (prolonged use or high doses at term)

Pregnancy Issues: Use of narcotics during pregnancy may produce physical dependence in the neonate; respiratory depression may occur in the newborn if narcotics are used prior to delivery (especially high doses).

Lactation: Enters breast milk/use caution

Administration

Oral: Do not crush controlled-release tablets; 80 mg and 160 mg tablets are for use **only** in opioid-tolerant patients. Do not administer OxyContin® 160 mg tablet with a high-fat meal.

Storage: Tablets should be stored at room temperature.

Related Information

Acute Postoperative Pain *on page 1742*
Narcotic / Opioid Analgesics *on page 1880*

Oxycodone and Acetaminophen

(oks i KOE done & a seet a MIN oh fen)

U.S. Brand Names Endocet®; Percocet®; Roxicet™; Roxicet™ 5/500; Tylox®

Synonyms Acetaminophen and Oxycodone

Pharmacologic Category Analgesic, Narcotic

Medication Safety Issues

Sound-alike/look-alike issues:
Percocet® may be confused with Percodan®
Roxicet™ may be confused with Roxanol™
Tylox® may be confused with Trimox®, Tylenol®, Wymox®, Xanax®

Use Management of moderate to severe pain

Mechanism of Action

Oxycodone, as with other narcotic (opiate) analgesics, blocks pain perception in the cerebral cortex by binding to specific receptor molecules (opiate receptors) within the neuronal membranes of synapses. This binding results in a decreased synaptic chemical transmission throughout the CNS thus inhibiting the flow of pain sensations into the higher centers. Mu and kappa are the two subtypes of the opiate receptor to which oxycodone binds to cause analgesia.

Acetaminophen inhibits the synthesis of prostaglandins in the CNS and peripherally blocks pain impulse generation; produces antipyresis from inhibition of hypothalamic heat-regulating center

Pharmacodynamics/Kinetics See individual agents.

Contraindications Hypersensitivity to oxycodone, acetaminophen, or any component of the formulation; severe respiratory depression (in absence of resuscitative equipment or ventilatory support); pregnancy (prolonged periods or high doses at term)

Warnings/Precautions Use with caution in patients with hypersensitivity reactions to other phenanthrene-derivative opioid agonists (morphine, codeine, hydrocodone, hydromorphone, levorphanol, oxymorphone); respiratory diseases including asthma, emphysema, COPD, or severe liver or renal insufficiency, hypothyroidism, Addison's disease, prostatic hypertrophy, or urethral stricture; some preparations contain sulfites which may cause allergic reactions; may be habit-forming

Use with caution in patients with head injury and increased intracranial pressure (respiratory depressant effects increased and may also elevate CSF pressure). May mask diagnosis or clinical course in patients with acute abdominal conditions.

Enhanced analgesia has been seen in elderly patients on therapeutic doses of narcotics; duration of action may be increased in the elderly; the elderly may be particularly susceptible to the CNS depressant and constipating effects of narcotics

Drug Interactions Also see individual agents.

Oxycodone: **Substrate** of CYP2D6 (major)

Acetaminophen: **Substrate** (minor) of CYP1A2, 2A6, 2C8/9, 2D6, 2E1, 3A4

Anesthetics, general: May have additive CNS depression; consider lowering dose of one or both agents

Anticholinergics: Concomitant use may lead to paralytic ileus

CNS depressants: May have additive CNS depression; consider lowering dose of one or both agents

CYP2D6 inhibitors: May decrease the effects of oxycodone. Example inhibitors include chlorpromazine, delavirdine, fluoxetine, miconazole, paroxetine, pergolide, quinidine, quinine, ritonavir, and ropinirole.

Phenothiazines: May have additive CNS depression with phenothiazine and other tranquilizers; consider lowering dose of one or both agents

Sedative hypnotics: May have additive CNS depression; consider lowering dose of one or both agents

Nutritional/Herbal/Ethanol Interactions Ethanol: May have additive CNS depression. In addition, excessive intake of ethanol may increase the risk of acetaminophen-induced hepatotoxicity. Avoid ethanol or limit to <3 drinks/day.

Adverse Reactions Frequency not defined (also see individual agents): Allergic reaction, constipation, dizziness, dysphoria, euphoria, lightheadedness, nausea, pruritus, respiratory depression, sedation, skin rash, vomiting

Overdosage/Toxicology See individual agents.

Dosing

Adults:

Note: Initial dose is based on the **oxycodone** content; however, the maximum daily dose is based on the **acetaminophen** content.

Management of pain: Doses should be given every 4-6 hours as needed and titrated to appropriate analgesic effects.

Maximum daily dose, based on acetaminophen content: Oral: 4 g/day.

Mild to moderate pain: Oral: Initial dose, **based on oxycodone content:** 5 mg

Severe pain: Oral: Initial dose, **based on oxycodone content:** 15-30 mg

Elderly: Doses should be titrated to appropriate analgesic effects: Oral: Initial dose, **based on oxycodone content:** 2.5-5 mg every 6 hours. Do not exceed 4 g/day of acetaminophen.

(Continued)

Oxycodone and Acetaminophen *(Continued)*

Pediatrics:

Note: Initial dose is based on the **oxycodone** content; however, the maximum daily dose is based on the **acetaminophen** content.

Management of pain: Doses should be given every 4-6 hours as needed and titrated to appropriate analgesic effects.

Mild to moderate pain: Oral: Initial dose, **based on oxycodone content:** 0.05-0.1 mg/kg/dose

Severe pain: Oral: Initial dose, **based on oxycodone content:** 0.3 mg/kg/dose

Maximum dose, based on acetaminophen content: Oral: Children <45 kg: 90 mg/kg/day; children >45 kg: 4 g/day

Hepatic Impairment: Dose should be reduced in patients with severe liver disease.

Available Dosage Forms

Caplet (Roxicet™ 5/500): Oxycodone hydrochloride 5 mg and acetaminophen 500 mg

Capsule: Oxycodone hydrochloride 5 mg and acetaminophen 500 mg

Tylox®: Oxycodone hydrochloride 5 mg and acetaminophen 500 mg [contains sodium benzoate and sodium metabisulfite]

Solution, oral (Roxicet™): Oxycodone hydrochloride 5 mg and acetaminophen 325 mg per 5 mL (5 mL, 500 mL) [contains alcohol <0.5%]

Tablet: Oxycodone hydrochloride 5 mg and acetaminophen 325 mg; oxycodone hydrochloride 7.5 mg and acetaminophen 325 mg; oxycodone hydrochloride 7.5 mg and acetaminophen 500 mg; oxycodone hydrochloride 10 mg and acetaminophen 325 mg; oxycodone hydrochloride 10 mg and acetaminophen 650 mg

Endocet® 5/325 [scored]: Oxycodone hydrochloride 5 mg and acetaminophen 325 mg

Endocet® 7.5/325: Oxycodone hydrochloride 7.5 mg and acetaminophen 325 mg

Endocet® 7.5/500: Oxycodone hydrochloride 7.5 mg and acetaminophen 500 mg

Endocet® 10/325: Oxycodone hydrochloride 10 mg and acetaminophen 325 mg

Endocet® 10/650: Oxycodone hydrochloride 10 mg and acetaminophen 650 mg

Percocet® 2.5/325: Oxycodone hydrochloride 2.5 mg and acetaminophen 325 mg

Percocet® 5/325 [scored]: Oxycodone hydrochloride 5 mg and acetaminophen 325 mg

Percocet® 7.5/325: Oxycodone hydrochloride 7.5 mg and acetaminophen 325 mg

Percocet® 7.5/500: Oxycodone hydrochloride 7.5 mg and acetaminophen 500 mg

Percocet® 10/325: Oxycodone hydrochloride 10 mg and acetaminophen 325 mg

Percocet® 10/650: Oxycodone hydrochloride 10 mg and acetaminophen 650 mg

Roxicet™ [scored]: Oxycodone hydrochloride 5 mg and acetaminophen 325 mg

Nursing Guidelines

Assessment: Pregnancy risk factor C/D - see Pregnancy Risk Factor for use cautions; benefits of use should outweigh possible risks. Note breast-feeding caution.

Patient Education: See individual agents. **Pregnancy/breast-feeding precautions:** Inform prescriber if you are or intend to become pregnant. Consult prescriber if breast-feeding.

Pregnancy Risk Factor: C/D (prolonged periods or high doses at term)

Pregnancy Issues: Use of narcotics during pregnancy may produce physical dependence in the neonate; respiratory depression may occur in the newborn if narcotics are used prior to delivery (especially high doses).

Lactation: Enters breast milk/use caution

Breast-Feeding Considerations:

Oxycodone: Excreted in breast milk. If occasional doses are used during breast-feeding, monitor infant for sedation, GI effects and changes in feeding pattern.

Acetaminophen: May be taken while breast-feeding

Administration

Storage: Store at controlled room temperature of 15°C to 30°C (59°F to 86°F). Protect from moisture.

Oxycodone and Aspirin (oks i KOE done & AS pir in)

U.S. Brand Names Endodan®; Percodan®

Synonyms Aspirin and Oxycodone

Pharmacologic Category Analgesic, Narcotic

Medication Safety Issues

Sound-alike/look-alike issues:

Percodan® may be confused with Decadron®, Percocet®, Percogesic®, Periactin®

Use Management of moderate to severe pain

Mechanism of Action

Oxycodone, as with other narcotic (opiate) analgesics, blocks pain perception in the cerebral cortex by binding to specific receptor molecules (opiate receptors) within the neuronal membranes of synapses. This binding results in a decreased synaptic chemical transmission throughout the CNS thus inhibiting the flow of pain sensations into the higher centers. Mu and kappa are the two subtypes of the opiate receptor to which oxycodone binds to cause analgesia.

Aspirin inhibits prostaglandin synthesis by decreasing the activity of the enzyme, cyclooxygenase, which results in decreased formation of prostaglandin precursors, acts on the hypothalamic heat-regulating center to reduce fever, blocks thromboxane synthetase action which prevents formation of the platelet-aggregating substance thromboxane A_2

Pharmacodynamics/Kinetics See individual agents.

Contraindications Hypersensitivity to oxycodone, salicylates, other NSAIDs, or any component of the formulation; patients with the syndrome of asthma, rhinitis, and nasal polyps; inherited or acquired bleeding disorders (including factor VII and factor IX deficiency); do not use in children (<16 years of age) in the presence of viral infections (chickenpox or flu symptoms), with or without fever, due to a potential association with Reye's syndrome; significant respiratory depression; hypercarbia; known or suspected paralytic ileus; acute or severe bronchial asthma; pregnancy (3rd trimester)

Warnings/Precautions Use with caution in patients with hypersensitivity reactions to other phenanthrene derivative opioid agonists (morphine, hydrocodone, hydromorphone, levorphanol, oxycodone, oxymorphone), respiratory diseases including asthma, emphysema, or COPD. Use with caution in pancreatitis or biliary tract disease, acute alcoholism (including delirium tremens), adrenocortical insufficiency, CNS depression/coma, kyphoscoliosis (or other skeletal disorder which may alter respiratory function), hypothyroidism (including myxedema), prostatic hyperplasia, urethral stricture, and toxic psychosis.

Use with caution in the elderly, debilitated, severe hepatic or renal dysfunction. Hemodynamic effects (hypotension, orthostasis) may be exaggerated in patients with dehydration, hypovolemia, concurrent vasodilating drugs, or in patients with head injury. Respiratory depressant effects and capacity to elevate CSF pressure may be exaggerated in presence of head injury, other intracranial lesion, or pre-existing elevation of intracranial pressure. Tolerance or drug dependence may result from extended use. Healthcare provider should be alert to problems of abuse, misuse, and diversion. Taper dose gradually to avoid withdrawal symptoms in physically dependent patients.

Use with caution in patients with platelet and bleeding disorders, erosive gastritis, or peptic ulcer disease. Heavy ethanol use (>3 drinks/day) can increase bleeding risks. Discontinue use if tinnitus or impaired hearing occurs. Patients with sensitivity to tartrazine dyes, nasal polyps and asthma may have an increased risk of salicylate sensitivity. Surgical patients should avoid ASA if possible, for 1-2 weeks prior to surgery, to reduce the risk of excessive bleeding.

Drug Interactions

Oxycodone: **Substrate** of CYP2D6 (major)

Aspirin: **Substrate** of CYP2C8/9 (minor)

Also see individual agents.

CYP2D6 inhibitors: May decrease the effects of oxycodone. Example inhibitors include chlorpromazine, delavirdine, fluoxetine, miconazole, paroxetine, pergolide, quinidine, quinine, ritonavir, and ropinirole.

Increased effect/toxicity with CNS depressants, TCAs, dextroamphetamine

Lab Interactions May cross-react with urine tests for cocaine or marijuana.

(Continued)

Oxycodone and Aspirin *(Continued)*

Adverse Reactions Note: Also refer to individual agents

Common (frequency not defined):

Central nervous system: Dizziness, drowsiness, lightheadedness, sedation
Dermatologic: Pruritus
Gastrointestinal: Nausea, vomiting, constipation

<1%, postmarketing, and/or case reports (limited to important or life-threatening): Allergic reaction, anaphylaxis, anaphylactoid reaction, angioedema, apnea, asthma, bradycardia, bronchospasm, circulatory depression, confusion, duodenal ulcer, dysphoria, dyspnea, ecchymosis, euphoria, gastric ulcer, gastrointestinal bleeding, hallucination, hemorrhage, hepatitis, hepatotoxicity, hypotension, hypoglycemia, hyperglycemia, ileus, interstitial nephritis, intestinal obstruction, laryngeal edema, metabolic acidosis, pancreatitis, papillary necrosis, paresthesia, purpura, pulmonary edema, proteinuria, rash, renal failure, respiratory alkalosis, respiratory depression, Reye syndrome, rhabdomyolysis, seizure, shock, thrombocytopenia, tinnitus

Dosing

Adults & Elderly: Analgesic: Oral (based on oxycodone combined salts): Percodan®: 1 tablet every 6 hours as needed for pain; maximum aspirin dose should not exceed 4 g/day.

Pediatrics: Analgesic: Oral (based on oxycodone combined salts): Maximum oxycodone: 5 mg/dose; maximum aspirin dose should not exceed 4 g/day. Doses should be given every 6 hours as needed.

Mild-to-moderate pain: Initial dose, **based on oxycodone content:** 0.05-0.1 mg/kg/dose

Severe pain: Initial dose, **based on oxycodone content:** 0.3 mg/kg/dose

Hepatic Impairment: Dose should be reduced in patients with severe liver disease.

Available Dosage Forms

Tablet: Oxycodone hydrochloride 4.5 mg, oxycodone terephthalate 0.38 mg, and aspirin 325 mg

Endodan®, Percodan®: Oxycodone hydrochloride 4.5 mg, oxycodone terephthalate 0.38 mg, and aspirin 325 mg

Nursing Guidelines

Assessment: Pregnancy risk factor D - determine that patient is not pregnant before beginning treatment. Instruct patients of childbearing age about appropriate barrier contraceptive measures. Note breast-feeding caution.

Dietary Considerations: May be taken with food or water.

Patient Education: See individual agents. **Pregnancy/breast-feeding precautions:** Inform prescriber if you are or intend to become pregnant. Consult prescriber if breast-feeding.

Pregnancy Risk Factor: D

Lactation: Enters breast milk/use caution

Breast-Feeding Considerations:

Aspirin: Caution is suggested due to potential adverse effects in nursing infants.
Oxycodone: No data reported.

- **Oxycodone Hydrochloride** *see* Oxycodone *on page 1284*
- **OxyContin®** *see* Oxycodone *on page 1284*
- **Oxydose™** *see* Oxycodone *on page 1284*
- **OxyFast®** *see* Oxycodone *on page 1284*
- **OxyIR®** *see* Oxycodone *on page 1284*

Oxymetazoline (oks i met AZ oh leen)

U.S. Brand Names Afrin® Extra Moisturizing [OTC]; Afrin® Original [OTC]; Afrin® Severe Congestion [OTC]; Afrin® Sinus [OTC]; Duramist® Plus [OTC]; Duration® [OTC]; Genasal [OTC]; Neo-Synephrine® 12 Hour [OTC]; Neo-Synephrine® 12 Hour Extra Moisturizing [OTC]; Nōstrilla® [OTC]; NRS® [OTC]; Vicks Sinex® 12 Hour [OTC]; Vicks Sinex® 12 Hour Ultrafine Mist [OTC]; Visine® L.R. [OTC]; 4-Way® 12 Hour [OTC]

Synonyms Oxymetazoline Hydrochloride

Pharmacologic Category Adrenergic Agonist Agent; Vasoconstrictor

Medication Safety Issues

Sound-alike/look-alike issues:

Oxymetazoline may be confused with oxymetholone

Afrin® may be confused with aspirin

Visine® may be confused with Visken®

Use Adjunctive therapy of middle ear infections, associated with acute or chronic rhinitis, the common cold, sinusitis, hay fever, or other allergies

Ophthalmic: Relief of redness of eye due to minor eye irritations

Mechanism of Action Stimulates alpha-adrenergic receptors in the arterioles of the nasal mucosa to produce vasoconstriction

Pharmacodynamics/Kinetics

Onset of action: Intranasal: 5-10 minutes

Duration: 5-6 hours

Contraindications Hypersensitivity to oxymetazoline or any component of the formulation

Warnings/Precautions

Nasal: Rebound congestion may occur with extended use (>3 days). Prior to self-medication (OTC use), contact healthcare provider in the presence of hypertension, diabetes, hyperthyroidism, heart disease, coronary artery disease, cerebral arteriosclerosis, or long-standing bronchial asthma.

Ophthalmic: Prior to OTC use, contact healthcare provider in the presence of glaucoma or if needed for >72 hours.

Drug Interactions Increased toxicity with MAO inhibitors

Adverse Reactions Frequency not defined.

Cardiovascular: Hypertension, palpitation

Local: Transient burning, stinging

Respiratory: Dryness of the nasal mucosa, rebound congestion with prolonged use, sneezing

Dosing

Adults & Elderly:

Nasal congestion: Intranasal (therapy should not exceed 3 days): 0.05% solution: Instill 2-3 sprays into each nostril twice daily

Relief of eye redness: Ophthalmic: 0.025% solution: Instill 1-2 drops in affected eye(s) every 6 hours as needed or as directed by healthcare provider

Pediatrics:

Nasal congestion: Intranasal: Refer to adult dosing.

Relief of eye redness: Ophthalmic: Children >6 years: 0.025% solution: Instill 1-2 drops in affected eye(s) every 6 hours as needed or as directed by healthcare provider

Available Dosage Forms

Solution, intranasal spray, as hydrochloride: 0.05% (15 mL, 30 mL)

Afrin® Extra Moisturizing: 0.05% (15 mL) [contains benzyl alcohol and glycerin; regular or no drip formula]

Afrin® Original: 0.05% (15 mL, 30 mL) [contains benzalkonium chloride]

Afrin® Original: 0.05% (15 mL) [contains benzyl alcohol and benzalkonium chloride; no drip formula]

Afrin® Severe Congestion: 0.05% (15 mL) [contains benzyl alcohol and menthol; regular or no drip formula]

Afrin® Sinus: 0.05% (15 mL) [contains benzyl alcohol, benzalkonium chloride, camphor, phenol; regular or no drip formula]

Duramist® Plus, Neo-Synephrine® 12 Hour, Nōstrilla®, Vicks Sinex® 12 Hour Ultrafine Mist, Vicks Sinex® 12 Hour, 4-Way® 12 Hour: 0.05% (15 mL) [contains benzalkonium chloride]

Duration®: 0.05% (30 mL) [contains benzalkonium chloride]

Genasal, NRS®: 0.05% (15 mL, 30 mL) [contains benzalkonium chloride]

Neo-Synephrine® 12 Hour Extra Moisturizing: 0.05% (15 mL) [contains glycerin]

Solution, ophthalmic, as hydrochloride (Visine® L.R.): 0.025% (15 mL, 30 mL) [contains benzalkonium chloride]

Nursing Guidelines

Patient Education: Should not be used for self-medication for longer than 3 days, if symptoms persist, drug should be discontinued and prescriber consulted; notify prescriber of insomnia, tremor, or irregular heartbeat; burning, stinging, or drying of the nasal mucosa may occur

Administration

Storage: Store at room temperature.

♦ **Oxymetazoline Hydrochloride** *see* Oxymetazoline *on page 1290*

Oxytetracycline (oks i tet ra SYE kleen)

U.S. Brand Names Terramycin® I.M.

Synonyms Oxytetracycline Hydrochloride

Pharmacologic Category Antibiotic, Tetracycline Derivative

Medication Safety Issues

Sound-alike/look-alike issues:

Terramycin® may be confused with Garamycin®

Use Treatment of susceptible bacterial infections; both gram-positive and gram-negative, as well as, *Rickettsia* and *Mycoplasma* organisms

Mechanism of Action Inhibits bacterial protein synthesis by binding with the 30S and possibly the 50S ribosomal subunit(s) of susceptible bacteria, cell wall synthesis is not affected

Pharmacodynamics/Kinetics

Absorption: Poor

Distribution: Crosses placenta

Metabolism: Hepatic (small amounts)

Half-life elimination: 8.5-9.6 hours; prolonged with renal impairment

Excretion: Urine; feces

Contraindications Hypersensitivity to tetracycline or any component of the formulation

Warnings/Precautions Avoid in children ≤8 years of age, pregnant and nursing women; photosensitivity can occur with oxytetracycline

Drug Interactions

Barbiturates, phenytoin, and carbamazepine decrease serum levels of tetracyclines.

Oral contraceptives: Anecdotal reports suggesting decreased contraceptive efficacy with tetracyclines have been refuted by more rigorous scientific and clinical data.

Increased effect of warfarin

Adverse Reactions Frequency not defined; also refer to Tetracycline monograph

Cardiovascular: Pericarditis

Central nervous system: Bulging fontanels (infants), intracranial hypertension (adults)

Dermatologic: Angioneurotic edema, erythematous rash, exfoliative dermatitis (uncommon), maculopapular rash, photosensitivity, urticaria

Gastrointestinal: Anogenital inflammatory lesions, diarrhea, dysphagia, enamel hypoplasia, enterocolitis, glossitis, nausea, tooth discoloration, vomiting

Hematologic: Anemia, eosinophilia, neutropenia, thrombocytopenia

Local: Irritation

Renal: BUN increased

Miscellaneous: Anaphylactoid purpura, anaphylaxis, hypersensitivity reaction, SLE exacerbation

Overdosage/Toxicology Symptoms of overdose include nausea, anorexia, diarrhea. Following GI decontamination, supportive care only.

Dosing

Adults & Elderly: I.M.: Usual dosage: 250 mg every 24 hours or 300 mg/day divided every 8-12 hours

Pediatrics: I.M.: Children >8 years: 15-25 mg/kg/day (maximum: 250 mg/dose) in divided doses every 8-12 hours

Renal Impairment: Cl_{cr} <10 mL/minute: Administer every 24 hours or avoid use if possible

Hepatic Impairment: Avoid use in patients with severe liver disease.

Available Dosage Forms Injection, solution: 5% [50 mg/mL] (10 mL) [contains lidocaine hydrochloride 2%]

Nursing Guidelines

Patient Education: You may be sensitive to sunlight; use sunblock, wear protective clothing, and avoid direct sun. Report rash, respiratory difficulty, yellowing of skin or eyes, change in color of urine or stool, easy bruising or bleeding, fever, chills, perianal itching, purulent vaginal discharge, white plaques in mouth, or persistent diarrhea. **Pregnancy/breast-feeding precautions:** Do not get pregnant while taking this medication. Breast-feeding is not recommended.

Pregnancy Risk Factor: D

Lactation: Enters breast milk/not recommended

Administration

I.M.: Injection for intramuscular use only.

♦ **Oxytetracycline Hydrochloride** *see* Oxytetracycline *on page 1292*

Oxytocin (oks i TOE sin)

U.S. Brand Names Pitocin®

Synonyms Pit

Pharmacologic Category Oxytocic Agent

Medication Safety Issues

Sound-alike/look-alike issues:

Pitocin® may be confused with Pitressin®

Use Induction of labor at term; control of postpartum bleeding; adjunctive therapy in management of abortion

Mechanism of Action Produces the rhythmic uterine contractions characteristic to delivery

Pharmacodynamics/Kinetics

Onset of action: Uterine contractions: I.M.: 3-5 minutes; I.V.: ~1 minute

Duration: I.M.: 2-3 hour; I.V.: 1 hour

Metabolism: Rapidly hepatic and via plasma (by oxytocinase) and to a smaller degree the mammary gland

Half-life elimination: 1-5 minutes

Excretion: Urine

Contraindications Hypersensitivity to oxytocin or any component of the formulation; significant cephalopelvic disproportion; unfavorable fetal positions; fetal distress; hypertonic or hyperactive uterus; contraindicated vaginal delivery (invasive cervical cancer, active genital herpes, prolapse of the cord, cord presentation, total placenta previa, or vasa previa)

Warnings/Precautions To be used for medical rather than elective induction of labor; may produce antidiuretic effect (ie, water intoxication and excess uterine contractions); high doses or hypersensitivity to oxytocin may cause uterine hypertonicity, spasm, tetanic contraction, or rupture of the uterus; severe water intoxication with convulsions, coma, and death is associated with a slow oxytocin infusion over 24 hours

Drug Interactions

Dinoprostone, misoprostol: May increase the effect of oxytocin; wait 6-12 hours after dinoprostone or misoprostol administration before initiating oxytocin.

Adverse Reactions Frequency not defined.

Fetus or neonate:

Cardiovascular: Arrhythmias (including premature ventricular contractions), bradycardia

Central nervous system: Brain or CNS damage (permanent), neonatal seizure

Hepatic: Neonatal jaundice

Ocular: Neonatal retinal hemorrhage

Miscellaneous: Fetal death, low Apgar score (5 minute)

Mother:

Cardiovascular: Arrhythmias, hypertensive episodes, premature ventricular contractions

Gastrointestinal: Nausea, vomiting

Genitourinary: Pelvic hematoma, postpartum hemorrhage, uterine hypertonicity, tetanic contraction of the uterus, uterine rupture, uterine spasm

Hematologic: Afibrinogenemia (fatal)

Miscellaneous: Anaphylactic reaction, subarachnoid hemorrhage

Overdosage/Toxicology Symptoms of overdose include tetanic uterine contractions, impaired uterine blood flow, amniotic fluid embolism, uterine rupture, SIADH, and seizures. Treatment is symptom-directed and supportive.

Dosing

Adults: Note: I.V. administration requires the use of an infusion pump.

Induction of labor: I.V.: 0.5-1 milliunits/minute; gradually increase dose in increments of 1-2 milliunits/minute until desired contraction pattern is established; dose may be decreased after desired frequency of contractions is reached and labor has progressed to 5-6 cm dilation. Infusion rates of 6 milliunits/minute provide oxytocin levels similar to those at spontaneous labor; rates of >9-10 milliunits/minute are rarely required.

Postpartum bleeding:

I.M.: Total dose of 10 units after delivery

(Continued)

Oxytocin *(Continued)*

I.V.: 10-40 units by I.V. infusion in 1000 mL of intravenous fluid at a rate sufficient to control uterine atony

Adjunctive treatment of abortion: I.V.: 10-20 milliunits/minute; maximum total dose: 30 units/12 hours

Available Dosage Forms

Injection, solution: 10 units/mL (1 mL, 10 mL)

Pitocin®: 10 units/mL (1 mL)

Nursing Guidelines

Assessment: Monitor blood pressure, fluid intake and output, and labor closely if using oxytocin for induction; fetal monitoring is strongly recommended. **Pregnancy risk factor X.**

Patient Education: I.V./I.M.: Generally used in emergency situations. Drug teaching should be incorporated in other situational teaching. **Breast-feeding precaution:** Use caution.

Pregnancy Risk Factor: X

Pregnancy Issues: Reproduction studies have not been conducted. When used as indicated, teratogenic effects would not be expected. Nonteratogenic adverse reactions are reported in the neonate as well as the mother.

Lactation: Excretion in breast milk unknown/use caution

Breast-Feeding Considerations: Endogenous levels of oxytocin naturally increase during breast-feeding.

Administration

I.V.: Refer to Reconstitution for dilution information. An infusion pump is required for administration.

Reconstitution: I.V.

Induction or stimulation of labor: Add oxytocin 10 units to NS or LR 1000 mL to yield a solution containing oxytocin 10 milliunits/mL; rotate solution to mix

Postpartum uterine bleeding: Add oxytocin 10-40 units to running I.V. infusion; maximum: 40 units/1000 mL

Adjunctive management of abortion: Add oxytocin 10 units to 500 mL of a physiologic saline solution or D_5W

Compatibility: Stable in dextran 6% in dextrose, dextran 6% in NS, D_5LR, $D_5{}^1/_4NS$, $D_5{}^1/_2NS$, D_5NS, D_5W, $D_{10}W$, LR, $^1/_2NS$, NS

Compatibility when admixed: Incompatible with fibrinolysin (human), norepinephrine, prochlorperazine edisylate, warfarin

Storage: Store oxytocin at 2°C to 8°C (36°F to 46°F); protect from freezing. Pitocin® may also be stored at 15°C to 25°C (59°F to 77°F) for up to 30 days.

- **Oxytrol™** *see* Oxybutynin *on page 1281*
- **Oysco 500 [OTC]** *see* Calcium Carbonate *on page 291*
- **Oyst-Cal 500 [OTC]** *see* Calcium Carbonate *on page 291*
- **P-071** *see* Cetirizine *on page 366*
- **Pacerone®** *see* Amiodarone *on page 130*

Paclitaxel (PAK li taks el)

U.S. Brand Names Onxol™; Taxol®

Synonyms NSC-125973

Pharmacologic Category Antineoplastic Agent, Antimicrotubular; Antineoplastic Agent, Natural Source (Plant) Derivative

Medication Safety Issues

Sound-alike/look-alike issues:

Paclitaxel may be confused with paroxetine, Paxil®

Paclitaxel (conventional) may be confused with paclitaxel (protein-bound)

Taxol® may be confused with Abraxane™, Paxil®, Taxotere®

Use Treatment of breast, lung (small cell and nonsmall cell), and ovarian cancers

Mechanism of Action Paclitaxel promotes microtubule assembly by enhancing the action of tubulin dimers, stabilizing existing microtubules, and inhibiting their disassembly, interfering with the late G_2 mitotic phase, and inhibiting cell replication. In addition, the drug can distort mitotic spindles, resulting in the breakage of chromosomes. Paclitaxel may also suppress cell proliferation and modulate immune response.

Pharmacodynamics/Kinetics

Distribution:

V_d: Widely distributed into body fluids and tissues; affected by dose and duration of infusion

V_{dss}:
1- to 6-hour infusion: 67.1 L/m^2
24-hour infusion: 227-688 L/m^2
Protein binding: 89% to 98%
Metabolism: Hepatic via CYP2C8/9 and 3A4; forms metabolites
Half-life elimination:
1- to 6-hour infusion: Mean (beta): 6.4 hours
3-hour infusion: Mean (terminal): 13.1-20.2 hours
24-hour infusion: Mean (terminal): 15.7-52.7 hours
Excretion: Feces (~70%, 5% as unchanged drug); urine (14%)
Clearance: Mean: Total body: After 1- and 6-hour infusions: 5.8-16.3 L/hour/m^2; After 24-hour infusions: 14.2-17.2 L/hour/m^2

Contraindications Hypersensitivity to paclitaxel, Cremophor® EL (polyoxyethylated castor oil), or any component of the formulation; pregnancy

Warnings/Precautions Hazardous agent - use appropriate precautions for handling and disposal. Severe hypersensitivity reactions have been reported; prolongation of the infusion (to ≥6 hours) plus premedication may minimize this effect. When administered as sequential infusions, taxane derivatives (docetaxel, paclitaxel) should be administered before platinum derivatives (carboplatin, cisplatin) to limit myelosuppression. Elderly patients have an increased risk of toxicity (neutropenia, neuropathy).

Drug Interactions Substrate (major) of CYP2C8/9, 3A4; **Induces** CYP3A4 (weak)

Carboplatin, cisplatin (platinum derivatives): When administered as sequential infusions, taxane derivatives should be administered before platinum derivatives to limit myelosuppression and to enhance efficacy.

CYP2C8/9 inducers: May decrease the levels/effects of paclitaxel. Example inducers include carbamazepine, phenobarbital, phenytoin, rifampin, rifapentine, and secobarbital.

CYP2C8/9 inhibitors: May increase the levels/effects of paclitaxel. Example inhibitors include delavirdine, fluconazole, gemfibrozil, ketoconazole, nicardipine, NSAIDs, pioglitazone, and sulfonamides.

CYP3A4 inducers: CYP3A4 inducers may decrease the levels/effects of paclitaxel. Example inducers include aminoglutethimide, carbamazepine, nafcillin, nevirapine, phenobarbital, phenytoin, and rifamycins.

CYP3A4 inhibitors: May increase the levels/effects of paclitaxel. Example inhibitors include azole antifungals, clarithromycin, diclofenac, doxycycline, erythromycin, imatinib, isoniazid, nefazodone, nicardipine, propofol, protease inhibitors, quinidine, telithromycin, and verapamil.

Doxorubicin: Paclitaxel may increase doxorubicin levels/toxicity.

Nutritional/Herbal/Ethanol Interactions Herb/Nutraceutical: Avoid black cohosh, dong quai in estrogen-dependent tumors. Avoid valerian, St John's wort, kava kava, gotu kola (may increase CNS depression).

Adverse Reactions

>10%:

Allergic: Appear to be primarily nonimmunologically mediated release of histamine and other vasoactive substances; almost always seen within the first hour of an infusion (~75% occur within 10 minutes of starting the infusion); incidence is significantly reduced by premedication

Cardiovascular: Bradycardia (transient, 25%)

Dermatologic: Alopecia (87%), venous erythema, tenderness, discomfort

Hematologic: Myelosuppression, leukopenia, neutropenia (6% to 21%), thrombocytopenia

Hepatic: Mild increases in liver enzymes
Onset: 8-11 days
Nadir: 15-21 days
Recovery: 21 days

Neurotoxicity: Sensory and/or autonomic neuropathy (numbness, tingling, burning pain), myopathy or myopathic effects (25% to 55%), and central nervous system toxicity. May be cumulative and dose-limiting. **Note:** Motor neuropathy is uncommon at doses <250 mg/m^2; sensory neuropathy is almost universal at doses >250 mg/m^2; myopathic effects are common with doses >250 mg/m^2, generally occurring within 2-3 days of treatment, resolving over 5-6 days; pre-existing neuropathy may increase the risk of neuropathy.

Gastrointestinal: Severe, potentially dose-limiting mucositis, stomatitis (15%), most common at doses >390 mg/m^2

Neuromuscular & skeletal: Arthralgia, myalgia

(Continued)

Paclitaxel *(Continued)*

1% to 10%:

Cardiovascular: Myocardial infarction

Dermatologic: Phlebitis (2%)

Gastrointestinal: Mild nausea and vomiting (5% to 6%), diarrhea (5% to 6%)

Hematologic: Anemia

<1% (Limited to important or life-threatening): Ataxia, atrial fibrillation, enterocolitis, hepatic encephalopathy, intestinal obstruction, interstitial pneumonia, necrotic changes and ulceration following extravasation, neuroencephalopathy, ototoxicity (tinnitus and hearing loss), pancreatitis, paralytic ileus, pruritus, pulmonary fibrosis, radiation recall, radiation pneumonitis, rash, seizure, Stevens-Johnson syndrome, toxic epidermal necrolysis, visual disturbances (scintillating scotomata)

Dosing

Adults & Elderly: Note: Premedication with dexamethasone (20 mg orally or I.V. at 12 and 6 hours **or** 14 and 7 hours before the dose), diphenhydramine (50 mg I.V. 30-60 minutes prior to the dose), and cimetidine, famotidine or ranitidine (I.V. 30-60 minutes prior to the dose) is recommended

Ovarian carcinoma: I.V.: 135-175 mg/m^2 over 3 hours every 3 weeks **or**
50-80 mg/m^2 over 1-3 hours weekly **or**
1.4-4 mg/m^2/day continuous infusion for 14 days every 4 weeks

Metastatic breast cancer: 175-250 mg/m^2 over 3 hours every 3 weeks **or**
50-80 mg/m^2 weekly **or**
1.4-4 mg/m^2/day continuous infusion for 14 days every 4 weeks

Nonsmall cell lung carcinoma: 135 mg/m^2 over 24 hours every 3 weeks

AIDS-related Kaposi's sarcoma: 135 mg/m^2 over 3 hours every 3 weeks **or** 100 mg/m^2 over 3 hours every 2 weeks

Hepatic Impairment:

Note: These recommendations are based upon the patient's first course of therapy where the usual dose would be 135 mg/m^2 dose over 24 hours or the 175 mg/m^2 dose over 3 hours in patients with normal hepatic function. Dosage in subsequent courses should be based upon individual tolerance. Adjustments for other regimens are not available.

24-hour infusion:

- If transaminase levels <2 times upper limit of normal (ULN) and bilirubin level ≤1.5 mg/dL: 135 mg/m^2
- If transaminase levels 2-<10 times ULN and bilirubin level ≤1.5 mg/dL: 100 mg/m^2
- If transaminase levels <10 times ULN and bilirubin level 1.6-7.5 mg/dL: 50 mg/m^2
- If transaminase levels ≥10 times ULN and bilirubin level >7.5 mg/dL: Avoid use

3-hour infusion:

- If transaminase levels <10 times ULN and bilirubin level ≤1.25 times ULN: 175 mg/m^2
- If transaminase levels <10 times ULN and bilirubin level 1.26-2 times ULN: 135 mg/m^2
- If transaminase levels <10 times ULN and bilirubin level 2.01-5 times ULN: 90 mg/m^2
- If transaminase levels ≥10 times ULN and bilirubin level >5 times ULN: Avoid use

Available Dosage Forms

Injection, solution: 6 mg/mL (5 mL, 16.7 mL, 50 mL) [contains alcohol and purified Cremophor® EL (polyoxyethylated castor oil)]

Onxol™: 6 mg/mL (5 mL, 25 mL, 50 mL) [contains alcohol] [contains alcohol and purified Cremophor® EL (polyoxyethylated castor oil)]

Taxol®: 6 mg/mL (5 mL, 16.7 mL, 50 mL) [contains alcohol and purified Cremophor® EL (polyoxyethylated castor oil)]

Nursing Guidelines

Assessment: See Contraindications, Warnings/Precautions, and Dosing for use cautions. Assess potential for interactions with other prescriptions, OTC medications, or herbal products patient may be taking (see Drug Interactions). See below for infusion specifics. Premedication prior to infusion is recommended (see Dosing). Infusion site should be monitored to prevent extravasation. Assess results of laboratory tests (see below) prior to and regularly during therapy, therapeutic effectiveness, and adverse response (eg, peripheral neuropathy, myelosuppression, opportunistic infection, and hypersensitivity -

see Adverse Reactions and Overdose/Toxicology). Teach patient possible side effects/appropriate interventions and adverse symptoms to report (see Patient Education). **Pregnancy risk factor D** - determine that patient is not pregnant before beginning treatment. Instruct patients of childbearing age about appropriate barrier contraceptive measures. Breast-feeding is contraindicated.

Monitoring Laboratory Tests: CBC with differential and platelet count, liver and kidney function

Patient Education: Inform prescriber of all prescriptions, OTC medications, or herbal products you are taking, and any allergies you have. Do not take any new medication during therapy unless approved by prescriber. This drug can only be given by infusion. Report immediately any redness, swelling, burning, pain at infusion site or signs of allergic reaction (eg, respiratory difficulty or swallowing, chest tightness, rash, hives, swelling of lips or mouth). Maintain adequate hydration (2-3 L/day of fluids) unless instructed to restrict fluid intake, and nutrition. You will be more susceptible to infection (avoid crowds and exposure to infection and do not have any vaccinations without consulting prescriber). May cause loss of hair (will grow back after therapy); experience nausea or vomiting (consult prescriber for approved antiemetic); feel weak or lethargic (use caution when driving or engaging in tasks that require alertness until response to drug is known); or mouth sores (use good oral care, bush with soft toothbrush and use waxed dental floss). Report numbness or tingling in fingers or toes (use care to prevent injury); signs of opportunistic infection (fever, chills, sore throat, burning urination, fatigue); unusual bleeding (tarry stools, easy bruising, or blood in stool, urine, or mouth); unresolved mouth sores; nausea or vomiting; or skin rash or itching. **Pregnancy/breast-feeding precautions:** Do not get pregnant while taking this medication. Consult prescriber for appropriate barrier contraceptive measures. Do not breast-feed.

Geriatric Considerations: Elderly patients may have a higher incidence of severe neuropathy, severe myelosuppression, or cardiovascular events as compared to younger patients.

Pregnancy Risk Factor: D

Pregnancy Issues: Teratogenic effects have been observed in animal studies; women of childbearing potential should be advised to avoid becoming pregnant.

Lactation: Excretion in breast milk unknown/contraindicated

Breast-Feeding Considerations: Antineoplastic agents are generally contraindicated.

Administration

I.V.: Irritant. Manufacturer recommends administration over 1-24 hours. Other routes are being studied. When administered as sequential infusions, taxane derivatives should be administered before platinum derivatives (cisplatin, carboplatin) to limit myelosuppression and to enhance efficacy.

Premedication with dexamethasone (20 mg orally or I.V. at 12 and 6 hours **or** 14 and 7 hours before the dose), diphenhydramine (50 mg I.V. 30-60 minutes prior to the dose), and cimetidine, famotidine or ranitidine (I.V. 30-60 minutes prior to the dose) is recommended

Administer I.V. infusion over 1-24 hours; use of a 0.22 micron in-line filter and nonsorbing administration set is recommended during the infusion

Nonpolyvinyl (non-PVC) tubing (eg, polyethylene) should be used to minimize leaching. Formulated in a vehicle known as Cremophor® EL (polyoxyethylated castor oil). Cremophor® EL has been found to leach the plasticizer DEHP from polyvinyl chloride infusion bags or administration sets. Contact of the undiluted concentrate with plasticized polyvinyl chloride (PVC) equipment or devices is not recommended. Administer through I.V. tubing containing an in-line (NOT >0.22 μ) filter; administration through IVEX-2® filters (which incorporate short inlet and outlet polyvinyl chloride-coated tubing) has not resulted in significant leaching of DEHP.

Reconstitution: Dilute in 250-1000 mL D_5W, D_5LR, D_5NS, or NS to a concentration of of 0.3-1.2 mg/mL.

Compatibility: Stable in D_5W, D_5NS, D_5LR, NS

Y-site administration: Incompatible with amphotericin B, amphotericin B cholesteryl sulfate complex, chlorpromazine, doxorubicin liposome, hydroxyzine, methylprednisolone sodium succinate, mitoxantrone

Storage: Store intact vials at room temperature of 20°C to 25°C (68°F to 77°F). Protect from light. Per the manufacturer, reconstituted solution is stable for up to 27 hours at room temperature (25°C) and ambient light conditions. Other

(Continued)

Paclitaxel *(Continued)*

sources report that solutions in D_5W and NS are stable for up to 3 days at room temperature (25°C).

Paclitaxel should be dispensed in either glass or Excel™/PAB™ containers. Should also use **nonpolyvinyl** (non-PVC) tubing (eg, polyethylene) to minimize leaching. Formulated in a vehicle known as Cremophor® EL (polyoxyethylated castor oil). Cremophor® EL has been found to leach the plasticizer DEHP from polyvinyl chloride infusion bags or administration sets. Contact of the undiluted concentrate with plasticized polyvinyl chloride (PVC) equipment or devices is not recommended.

♦ Pain-A-Lay® [OTC] *see* Phenol *on page 1347*
♦ Palladone™ *[Withdrawn]* *see* Hydromorphone *on page 879*
♦ Pamelor® *see* Nortriptyline *on page 1244*

Pamidronate (pa mi DROE nate)

U.S. Brand Names Aredia®

Synonyms Pamidronate Disodium

Pharmacologic Category Antidote; Bisphosphonate Derivative

Medication Safety Issues

Sound-alike/look-alike issues:

Aredia® may be confused with Adriamycin

Use Treatment of hypercalcemia associated with malignancy; treatment of osteolytic bone lesions associated with multiple myeloma or metastatic breast cancer; moderate to severe Paget's disease of bone

Unlabeled/Investigational Use Treatment of pediatric osteoporosis, treatment of osteogenesis imperfecta

Mechanism of Action A bisphosphonate which inhibits bone resorption via actions on osteoclasts or on osteoclast precursors. Does not appear to produce any significant effects on renal tubular calcium handling and is poorly absorbed following oral administration (high oral doses have been reported effective); therefore, I.V. therapy is preferred.

Pharmacodynamics/Kinetics

Onset of action: 24-48 hours

Peak effect: Maximum: 5-7 days

Absorption: Poor; pharmacokinetic studies lacking

Metabolism: Not metabolized

Half-life elimination: 21-35 hours

Excretion: Biphasic; urine (~50% as unchanged drug) within 120 hours

Contraindications Hypersensitivity to pamidronate, other bisphosphonates, or any component of the formulation; pregnancy

Warnings/Precautions Bisphosphonate therapy has been associated with osteonecrosis, primarily of the jaw; this has been observed mostly in cancer patients, but also in patients with postmenopausal osteoporosis and other diagnoses. Risk factors include a diagnosis of cancer, with concomitant chemotherapy, radiotherapy or corticosteroids; anemia, coagulopathy, infection or pre-existing dental disease. Symptoms included nonhealing extraction socket or an exposed jawbone. There are no data addressing whether discontinuation of therapy reduces the risk of developing osteonecrosis. However, as a precautionary measure, dental exams and preventative dentistry should be performed prior to placing patients with risk factors on chronic bisphosphonate therapy. Invasive dental procedures should be avoided during treatment.

May cause deterioration in renal function. Use caution in patients with renal impairment and avoid in severe renal impairment. Assess serum creatinine prior to each dose; withhold dose in patients with bone metastases who experience deterioration in renal function. Leukopenia has been observed with oral pamidronate and monitoring of white blood cell counts is suggested. Patients with pre-existing anemia, leukopenia, or thrombocytopenia should be closely monitored during the first 2 weeks of treatment.

Vein irritation and thrombophlebitis may occur with infusions. Monitor serum electrolytes, especially in the elderly.

Severe (and occasionally debilitating) bone, joint, and/or muscle pain have been reported infrequently during bisphosphonate treatment. Onset of pain ranged from a single day to several months, with relief in most cases upon discontinuation of the drug. Patients may experience recurrence when rechallenged with the same drug or another bisphosphonate.

Drug Interactions

Aminoglycosides: Aminoglycosides may lower serum calcium levels with prolonged administration. Concomitant use may have an additive hypocalcemic effect.

Nonsteroidal anti-inflammatory drugs (NSAIDs): May enhance the gastrointestinal adverse/toxic effects (increased incidence of GI ulcers) of pamidronate.

Phosphate supplements: Pamidronate may increase the hypocalcemic effects of phosphate supplements.

Lab Interactions Bisphosphonates may interfere with diagnostic imaging agents such as technetium-99m-diphosphonate in bone scans.

Adverse Reactions Percentage of adverse effect varies upon dose and duration of infusion.

>10%:

Central nervous system: Fatigue (12% to 40%), fever (18% to 39%), headache (24% to 27%), anxiety (8% to 18%), insomnia (1% to 25%), pain (13% to 15%)

Endocrine & metabolic: Hypophosphatemia (9% to 18%), hypokalemia (4% to 18%), hypomagnesemia (4% to 12%), hypocalcemia (1% to 12%)

Gastrointestinal: Nausea (4% to 64%), vomiting (4% to 46%), anorexia (1% to 31%), abdominal pain (1% to 24%), dyspepsia (4% to 23%)

Genitourinary: Urinary tract infection (15% to 20%)

Hematologic: Anemia (6% to 48%), leukopenia (4% to 21%)

Local: Infusion site reaction (4% to 18%)

Neuromuscular & skeletal: Weakness (16% to 26%), myalgia (1% to 26%), arthralgia (11% to 15%)

Renal: Serum creatinine increased (19%)

Respiratory: Dyspnea (22% to 35%), cough (25% to 26%), upper respiratory tract infection (3% to 20%), sinusitis (15% to 16%), pleural effusion (3% to 15%)

1% to 10%:

Cardiovascular: Atrial fibrillation (6%), hypertension (6%), syncope (6%), tachycardia (6%), atrial flutter (1%), cardiac failure (1%), edema (1%)

Central nervous system: Somnolence (1% to 6%), psychosis (4%)

Endocrine & metabolic: Hypothyroidism (6%)

Gastrointestinal: Constipation (4% to 6%), gastrointestinal hemorrhage (6%), diarrhea (1%), stomatitis (1%)

Hematologic: Neutropenia (1%), thrombocytopenia (1%)

Neuromuscular & skeletal: Back pain (5%), bone pain (5%)

Renal: Uremia (4%)

Respiratory: Rales (6%), rhinitis (6%)

Miscellaneous: Moniliasis (6%)

<1% (Limited to important or life-threatening): Allergic reaction, anaphylactic shock, angioedema, episcleritis, hypotension, interstitial pneumonitis, iritis, joint and/or muscle pain, malaise, osteonecrosis (primarily jaws), renal deterioration, scleritis, uveitis

Overdosage/Toxicology Symptoms of overdose include hypocalcemia, hypotension, ECG changes, seizures, bleeding, paresthesia, carpopedal spasm, and fever. Treat with I.V. calcium gluconate, and general supportive care; fever and hypotension can be treated with corticosteroids.

Dosing

Adults: Note: Drug must be diluted properly before administration and infused intravenously slowly. Due to risk of nephrotoxicity, doses should not exceed 90 mg.

Hypercalcemia of malignancy: I.V.:

Moderate cancer-related hypercalcemia (corrected serum calcium: 12-13.5 mg/dL): 60-90 mg, as a single dose

Severe cancer-related hypercalcemia (corrected serum calcium: >13.5 mg/dL): 90 mg, as a single dose

Repeat dosing: A period of 7 days should elapse before the use of second course; repeat infusions every 2-3 weeks have been suggested, however, could be administered every 2-3 months according to the degree and of severity of hypercalcemia and/or the type of malignancy.

Osteolytic bone lesions with multiple myeloma: I.V.: 90 mg monthly

Osteolytic bone lesions with metastatic breast cancer: I.V.: 90 mg repeated every 3-4 weeks

(Continued)

Pamidronate *(Continued)*

Paget's disease: I.V.: 30 mg for 3 consecutive days

Elderly: Refer to adult dosing. Begin at lower end of adult dosing range.

Renal Impairment: Not recommended in severe renal impairment (patients with bone metastases). Safety and efficacy have not been established in patients with serum creatinine >5 mg/dL. Studies are limited in multiple myeloma patients with serum creatinine ≥3 mg/dL.

Dosing adjustment in renal toxicity: In patients with bone metastases, treatment should be withheld in patients who experience deterioration in renal function (increase of serum creatinine ≥0.5 mg/dL in patients with normal baseline or ≥1.0 mg/dL in patients with abnormal baseline). Resumption of therapy may be considered when serum creatinine returns to within 10% of baseline.

Available Dosage Forms

Injection, powder for reconstitution, as disodium (Aredia®): 30 mg, 90 mg

Injection, solution: 3 mg/mL (10 mL); 6 mg/mL (10 mL); 9 mg/mL (10 mL)

Nursing Guidelines

Assessment: Assess results of laboratory tests, therapeutic effectiveness, and adverse reactions. Teach patient lifestyle and dietary changes that will be beneficial, possible side effects, interventions to reduce side effects, and adverse reactions to report.

Monitoring Laboratory Tests: Serum calcium, electrolytes, phosphate, magnesium, CBC with differential; monitor for hypocalcemia for at least 2 weeks after therapy; monitor serum creatinine prior to each dose; patients with pre-existing anemia, leukopenia or thrombocytopenia should be closely monitored during the first 2 weeks of treatment

Patient Education: Do not take any new medication during therapy unless approved by prescriber. This medication can only be administered intravenously; report immediately any difficulty breathing, chest tightness, difficulty swallowing, redness, swelling, or pain at infusion site. You may experience nausea or vomiting (small frequent meals and good mouth care may help); recurrent bone pain (consult prescriber for analgesic); increased fatigue (adequate rest is important); dizziness (use caution when driving or engaged in potentially dangerous tasks until response to drug is known). Report palpitations or rapid heart beat, unusual muscle twitching or spasms, persistent diarrhea/constipation, or acute bone pain, respiratory difficulty, or other persistent adverse effects. **Pregnancy/breast-feeding precautions:** Inform prescriber if you are pregnant. Do not get pregnant while taking this medication. Consult prescriber for appropriate contraceptive measures. Consult prescriber if breast-feeding.

Geriatric Considerations: No overall differences in safety for the elderly were observed in studies. The elderly may be more sensitive to the effects of pamidronate. Consider initiating doses for the elderly at the lower end of the dosing range. Monitor serum electrolytes periodically since elderly are often receiving diuretics which can result in decreases in serum calcium, potassium, and magnesium.

Pregnancy Risk Factor: D

Pregnancy Issues: Pamidronate has been shown to cross the placenta and cause nonteratogenic embryo/fetal effects in animals. There are no adequate and well-controlled studies in pregnant women; manufacturer states pamidronate should not be used in pregnancy. Based on limited case reports, serum calcium levels in the newborn may be altered if pamidronate is administered during pregnancy. Bisphosphonates are incorporated into the bone matrix and gradually released over time. Theoretically, there may be a risk of fetal harm when pregnancy follows the completion of therapy. Women of childbearing potential should be advised to use effective contraception and avoid becoming pregnant during therapy.

Lactation: Excretion in breast milk unknown/use caution

Administration

I.V.: I.V. infusion over 2-24 hours.

Reconstitution: Powder for injection: Reconstitute by adding 10 mL of SWFI to each vial of lyophilized pamidronate disodium powder, the resulting solution will be 30 mg/10 mL or 90 mg/10 mL.

Pamidronate may be further diluted in 250-1000 mL of 0.45% or 0.9% sodium chloride or 5% dextrose.

Compatibility: Incompatible with calcium-containing infusion solutions such as lactated Ringer's

Storage:

Powder for reconstitution: Store below 30°C (86°F). The reconstituted solution is stable for 24 hours stored under refrigeration at 2°C to 8°C (36°F to 46°F).

Solution for injection: Store below 25°C (77°F).

Pamidronate solution for infusion is stable at room temperature for up to 24 hours.

- **Pamidronate Disodium** *see* Pamidronate *on page 1298*
- **p-Aminoclonidine** *see* Apraclonidine *on page 178*
- **Pamprin® Maximum Strength All Day Relief [OTC]** *see* Naproxen *on page 1203*
- **Pan-B Antibody** *see* Rituximab *on page 1484*
- **Pancrease®** *see* Pancrelipase *on page 1301*
- **Pancrease® MT** *see* Pancrelipase *on page 1301*
- **Pancrecarb MS®** *see* Pancrelipase *on page 1301*

Pancrelipase (pan kre LI pase)

U.S. Brand Names Creon®; Dygase; ku-zyme® HP; Lapase; Lipram 4500; Lipram-CR; Lipram-PN; Lipram-UL; Pancrease®; Pancrease® MT; Pancrecarb MS®; Pangestyme™ CN; Pangestyme™ EC; Pangestyme™ MT; Pangestyme™ UL; Panokase®; Panokase® 16; Plaretase® 8000; Ultrase®; Ultrase® MT; Viokase®

Synonyms Lipancreatin

Pharmacologic Category Enzyme

Use Replacement therapy in symptomatic treatment of malabsorption syndrome caused by pancreatic insufficiency

Unlabeled/Investigational Use Treatment of occluded feeding tubes

Mechanism of Action Pancrelipase is a natural product harvested from the hog pancreas. It contains a combination of lipase, amylase, and protease. Products are formulated to dissolve in the more basic pH of the duodenum so that they may act locally to break down fats, protein, and starch.

Pharmacodynamics/Kinetics

Absorption: None; acts locally in GI tract

Excretion: Feces

Contraindications Hypersensitivity to pork protein or any component of the formulation; acute pancreatitis or acute exacerbations of chronic pancreatic disease

Warnings/Precautions Pancrelipase is inactivated by acids; use microencapsulated products whenever possible, since these products permit better dissolution of enzymes in the duodenum and protect the enzyme preparations from acid degradation in the stomach. Fibrotic strictures in the colon, some requiring surgery, have been reported with high doses; use caution, especially in children with cystic fibrosis. Use caution when adjusting doses or changing brands. Avoid inhalation of powder, may cause nasal and respiratory tract irritation.

Nutritional/Herbal/Ethanol Interactions Food: Avoid placing contents of opened capsules on alkaline food (pH >5.5); pancrelipase may impair absorption of oral iron and folic acid.

Adverse Reactions Frequency not defined; occurrence of events may be dose related.

Central nervous system: Pain

Dermatologic: Rash

Endocrine & metabolic: Hyperuricemia

Gastrointestinal: Nausea, cramps, constipation, diarrhea, perianal irritation/inflammation (large doses), irritation of the mouth, abdominal pain, intestinal obstruction, vomiting, flatulence, melena, weight loss, fibrotic strictures, greasy stools

Ocular: Lacrimation

Renal: Hyperuricosuria

Respiratory: Sneezing, dyspnea, bronchospasm

Miscellaneous: Allergic reactions

Overdosage/Toxicology Symptoms of overdose include diarrhea, other transient intestinal upset, hyperuricosuria, and hyperuricemia. Treatment is supportive.

(Continued)

Pancrelipase *(Continued)*

Dosing

Adults & Elderly:

Malabsorption: Oral:

Powder: Actual dose depends on the condition being treated and the digestive requirements of the patient: 0.7 g ($^1/_4$ teaspoonful) with meals

Capsules/tablets: The following dosage recommendations are only an approximation for initial dosages. The actual dosage will depend on the condition being treated and the digestive requirements of the individual patient.

Note: Dosage adjustment: Adjust dose based on body weight and stool fat content. Total daily dose reflects ~3 meals/day and 2-3 snacks/day, with half the mealtime dose given with a snack. Older patients may need less units/kg due to increased weight, but decreased ingestion of fat/kg. Maximum dose: 2500 units of lipase/kg/meal (10,000 units of lipase/kg/day): 4000-48,000 units of lipase with meals and with snacks

Occluded feeding tubes (unlabeled use): One tablet of Viokase® crushed with one 325 mg tablet of sodium bicarbonate (to activate the Viokase®) in 5 mL of water can be instilled into the nasogastric tube and clamped for 5 minutes; then, flushed with 50 mL of tap water

Pediatrics:

Malabsorption: Oral:

Powder: Actual dose depends on the condition being treated and the digestive requirements of the patient: Children <1 year: Start with $^1/_8$ teaspoonful with feedings

Capsules/tablets: Children: Approximate initial dosages; actual dosage will depend on the condition being treated and the digestive requirements of the individual patient.

<1 year: 2000 units of lipase with meals

1-6 years: 4000-8000 units of lipase with meals and 4000 units with snacks

7-12 years: 4000-12,000 units of lipase with meals and snacks

Note: Dosage adjustment: Adjust dose based on body weight and stool fat content. Total daily dose reflects ~3 meals/day and 2-3 snacks/day, with half the mealtime dose given with a snack.

Available Dosage Forms [DSC] = Discontinued product

Capsule:

Dygase: Lipase 2400 units, protease 30,000 units, and amylase 30,000 units

ku-zyme® HP: Lipase 8000 units, protease 30,000 units, and amylase 30,000 units

Lapase: Lipase 1200 units, protease 15,000 units, and amylase 15,000 units [contains tartrazine]

Capsule, delayed release, enteric coated granules:

Pangestyme™ CN-10: Lipase 10,000 units, protease 37,500 units, amylase 33,200 units

Pangestyme™ CN-20: Lipase 20,000 units, protease 75,000 units, amylase 66,400 units

Pangestyme™ EC: Lipase 4500 units, protease 25,000 units, and amylase 20,000 units

Pangestyme™ MT16: Lipase 16,000 units, protease 48,000 units, and amylase 48,000 units

Pangestyme™ UL 12: Lipase 12,000 units, protease 39,000 units, and amylase 39,000 units

Pangestyme™ UL 18: Lipase 18,000 units, protease 58,500 units, and amylase 58,500 units

Pangestyme™ UL 20: Lipase 20,000 units, protease 65,000 units, and amylase 65,000 units

Capsule, delayed release, enteric coated microspheres: Lipase 4,500 units, protease 25,000 units, and amylase 25,000 units

Creon® 5: Lipase 5000 units, protease 18,750 units, and amylase 16,600 units

Creon® 10: Lipase 10,000 units, protease 37,500 units, and amylase 33,200 units

Creon® 20: Lipase 20,000 units, protease 75,000 units, and amylase 66,400 units

Lipram 4500: Lipase 4500 units, protease 25,000 units, and amylase 20,000 units

Lipram-CR5: Lipase 5000 units, protease 18,750 units, and amylase 16,600 units [DSC]

Lipram-CR10: Lipase 10,000 units, protease 37,500 units, and amylase 33,200 units

Lipram-CR20: Lipase 20,000 units, protease 75,000 units, and amylase 66,400 units

Lipram-PN10: Lipase 10,000 units, protease 30,000 units, and amylase 30,000 units

Lipram-PN16: Lipase 16,000 units, protease 48,000 units, and amylase 48,000 units

Lipram-PN20: Lipase 20,000 units, protease 44,000 units, and amylase 56,000 units

Lipram-UL12: Lipase 12,000 units, protease 39,000 units, and amylase 39,000 units

Lipram-UL18: Lipase 18,000 units, protease 58,500 units, and amylase 58,500 units

Lipram-UL20: Lipase 20,000 units, protease 65,000 units, and amylase 65,000 units

Pancrecarb MS-4®: Lipase 4000 units, protease 25,000 units, and amylase 25,000 units [buffered]

Pancrecarb MS-8®: Lipase 8000 units, protease 45,000 units, and amylase 40,000 units [buffered]

Capsule, enteric coated microspheres (Pancrease®, Ultrase®): Lipase 4500 units, protease 25,000 units, and amylase 20,000 units

Capsule, enteric coated microtablets:

Pancrease® MT 4: Lipase 4000 units, protease 12,000 units, and amylase 12,000 units

Pancrease® MT 10: Lipase 10,000 units, protease 30,000 units, and amylase 30,000 units

Pancrease® MT 16: Lipase 16,000 units, protease 48,000 units, and amylase 48,000 units

Pancrease® MT 20: Lipase 20,000 units, protease 44,000 units, and amylase 56,000 units

Capsule, enteric coated minitablets:

Ultrase® MT12: Lipase 12,000 units, protease 39,000 units, and amylase 39,000 units

Ultrase® MT18: Lipase 18,000 units, protease 58,500 units, and amylase 58,500 units

Ultrase® MT20: Lipase 20,000 units, protease 65,000 units, and amylase 65,000 units

Powder (Viokase®): Lipase 16,800 units, protease 70,000 units, and amylase 70,000 units per 0.7 g (227 g)

Tablet: Lipase 8000 units, protease 30,000 units, and amylase 30,000 units

Panokase®: Lipase 8,000 units, protease 30,000 units, and amylase 30,000 units

Panokase® 16: Lipase 16,000 units, protease 60,000 units, and amylase 60,000 units

Plaretase™ 8000: Lipase 8,000 units, protease 30,000 units, and amylase 30,000 units

Viokase® 8: Lipase 8000 units, protease 30,000 units, and amylase 30,000 units

Viokase® 16: Lipase 16,000 units, protease 60,000 units, and amylase 60,000 units

Nursing Guidelines

Assessment: See Contraindications, Warnings/Precautions, Drug Interactions, and Dosing for use cautions. If powder spills on skin, wash off immediately, do not inhale powder when preparing. Assess patient response (see Adverse Reactions and Overdose/Toxicology). Teach patient proper use, possible side effects/appropriate interventions and adverse symptoms to report (see Patient Education). **Pregnancy risk factor B/C** - see Pregnancy Risk Factor for use cautions; benefits of use should outweigh possible risks. Note breast-feeding caution.

Dietary Considerations: Should be used as part of a high-calorie diet, appropriate for age and clinical status. Administer with meals or snacks and swallow whole with a generous amount of liquid. Do not crush or chew. Delayed-release capsules containing enteric coated microspheres or microtablets may also be opened and the contents sprinkled on soft food with a low pH such as applesauce, gelatin; apricot, banana, or sweet potato baby food; baby formula. Dairy products such as milk, custard or ice cream may have a high pH and should be avoided.

(Continued)

Pancrelipase *(Continued)*

Patient Education: Inform prescriber of all prescriptions, OTC medications, or herbal products you are taking, and any allergies you have. Do not take any new medication during therapy unless approved by prescriber. Take right before or with meals. Avoid taking with alkaline food. Do not chew, crush, or dissolve delayed release capsules; swallow whole. If powder spills on skin, wash off immediately, do not inhale powder when preparing. You may experience some gastric discomfort. Report unusual rash, persistent GI upset; or respiratory difficulty. **Pregnancy/breast-feeding precautions:** Inform prescriber if you are or intend to become pregnant. Consult prescriber if breast-feeding.

Geriatric Considerations: No special considerations are necessary since drug is dosed to response; however, drug-induced diarrhea can result in unwanted side effects (confusion, hypotension, lethargy, fluid and electrolyte loss).

Pregnancy Risk Factor: B/C (product specific)

Lactation: Excretion in breast milk unknown/use caution

Breast-Feeding Considerations: Systemic absorption and concentration in the breast milk is unlikely, but unknown.

Administration

Oral: Oral: Administer with meals or snacks and swallow whole with a generous amount of liquid. Do not crush or chew; retention in the mouth before swallowing may cause mucosal irritation and stomatitis. Delayed-release capsules containing enteric-coated microspheres or microtablets may also be opened and the contents sprinkled on soft food with a low pH that does not require chewing, such as applesauce, gelatin; apricot, banana, or sweet potato baby food; baby formula. Dairy products such as milk, custard, or ice cream may have a high pH and should be avoided. Avoid inhalation of powder, may cause nasal and respiratory tract irritation.

Storage: Store between 15°C to 25°C (59°F to 77°F). Keep in a dry place. Do not refrigerate.

Pancuronium (pan kyoo ROE nee um)

Synonyms Pancuronium Bromide; Pavulon [DSC]

Pharmacologic Category Neuromuscular Blocker Agent, Nondepolarizing

Medication Safety Issues

Sound-alike/look-alike issues:

Pancuronium may be confused with pipecuronium

Use Adjunct to general anesthesia to facilitate endotracheal intubation and to relax skeletal muscles during surgery; to facilitate mechanical ventilation in ICU patients; does not relieve pain or produce sedation

Drug of choice for neuromuscular blockade except in patients with renal failure, hepatic failure, or cardiovascular instability or in situations not suited for pancuronium's long duration of action

Mechanism of Action Blocks neural transmission at the myoneural junction by binding with cholinergic receptor sites

Pharmacodynamics/Kinetics

Onset of effect: Peak effect: I.V.: 2-3 minutes

Duration (dose dependent): 60-100 minutes

Metabolism: Hepatic (30% to 45%); active metabolite 3-hydroxypancuronium ($^1/_3$ to $^1/_2$ the activity of parent drug)

Half-life elimination: 110 minutes

Excretion: Urine (55% to 70% as unchanged drug)

Contraindications Hypersensitivity to pancuronium, bromide, or any component of the formulation

Warnings/Precautions Ventilation must be supported during neuromuscular blockade; use with caution in patients with renal and/or hepatic impairment (adjust dose appropriately); certain clinical conditions may result in potentiation or antagonism of neuromuscular blockade:

Potentiation: Electrolyte abnormalities, severe hyponatremia, severe hypocalcemia, severe hypokalemia, hypermagnesemia, neuromuscular diseases, acidosis, acute intermittent porphyria, renal failure, hepatic failure

Antagonism: Alkalosis, hypercalcemia, demyelinating lesions, peripheral neuropathies, diabetes mellitus

Increased sensitivity in patients with myasthenia gravis, Eaton-Lambert syndrome; resistance in burn patients (>30% of body) for period of 5-70 days postinjury; resistance in patients with muscle trauma, denervation, immobilization, infection. Cross-sensitivity with other neuromuscular-blocking agents may occur; use extreme caution in patients with previous anaphylactic reactions.

Drug Interactions See table.

Potential Drug Interactions

Potentiation	Antagonism
Anesthetics	Calcium
Desflurane, sevoflurane, enflurane and isoflurane > halothane > nitrous oxide-narcotics	Carbamazepine
Antibiotics	Phenytoin
Aminoglycosides, polymyxins, clindamycin, vancomycin	Steroids (chronic administration)
Magnesium sulfate	Theophylline
Antiarrhythmics	Anticholinesterases[1]
Quinidine, procainamide, bretylium, and possibly lidocaine	Neostigmine, pyridostigmine, edrophonium, echothiophate ophthalmic solution
Diuretics	Caffeine
Furosemide, mannitol	Azathioprine
Amphotericin B (secondary to hypokalemia)	
Local anesthetics	
Dantrolene (directly depresses skeletal muscle)	
Beta agonists	
Beta blockers	
Calcium channel blockers	
Ketamine	
Lithium	
Succinylcholine (when administered prior to nondepolarizing NMB agent)	

[1]Can prolong the effects of acetylcholine.

Adverse Reactions Frequency not defined.

Cardiovascular: Elevation in pulse rate, elevated blood pressure and cardiac output, tachycardia, edema, skin flushing, circulatory collapse

Dermatologic: Rash, itching, erythema, burning sensation along the vein

Gastrointestinal: Excessive salivation

Neuromuscular & skeletal: Profound muscle weakness

Respiratory: Wheezing, bronchospasm

Miscellaneous: Hypersensitivity reaction

Postmarketing and/or case reports: Acute quadriplegic myopathy syndrome (prolonged use), myositis ossificans (prolonged use)

Overdosage/Toxicology Symptoms of overdose include apnea, respiratory depression, and cardiovascular collapse. Pyridostigmine, neostigmine, or edrophonium in conjunction with atropine will usually antagonize the action of pancuronium.

Dosing

Adults & Elderly: Administer I.V.; dose to effect; doses will vary due to interpatient variability; use ideal body weight for obese patients

Neuromuscular blockade: Initial: 0.06-0.1 mg/kg or 0.05 mg/kg after initial dose of succinylcholine for intubation; maintenance dose: 0.01 mg/kg 60-100 minutes after initial dose and then 0.01 mg/kg every 25-60 minutes

Pretreatment/priming: 10% of intubating dose given 3-5 minutes before initial dose

Neuromuscular blockade in the ICU: 0.05-0.1 mg/kg bolus followed by 0.8-1.7 mcg/kg/minute once initial recovery from bolus observed or 0.1-0.2 mg/kg every 1-3 hours

Pediatrics: Infants >1 month and Children: Refer to adult dosing.

Renal Impairment: Elimination half-life is doubled, plasma clearance is reduced, and rate of recovery is sometimes much slower.

Cl_{cr} 10-50 mL/minute: Administer 50% of normal dose.

(Continued)

Pancuronium *(Continued)*

Cl_{cr} <10 mL/minute: Do not use.

Hepatic Impairment: Elimination half-life is doubled, plasma clearance is doubled, recovery time is prolonged, volume of distribution is increased (50%) and results in a slower onset, higher total dosage, and prolongation of neuromuscular blockade. Patients with liver disease may develop slow resistance to nondepolarizing muscle relaxant. Large doses may be required and problems may arise in antagonism.

Available Dosage Forms Injection, solution, as bromide: 1 mg/mL (10 mL); 2 mg/mL (2 mL, 5 mL) [may contain benzyl alcohol]

Nursing Guidelines

Assessment: Only clinicians experienced in the use of neuromuscular blocking drugs should administer and/or manage the use of pancuronium. Dosage and rate of administration should be individualized and titrated to the desired effect, according to relevant clinical factors, premedication, concomitant medications, age, and general condition of the patient. Ventilatory support must be instituted and maintained until adequate respiratory muscle function and/or airway protection are assured. Assess other medications for effectiveness and safety. Other drugs that affect neuromuscular activity may increase/decrease neuromuscular block induced by pancuronium. This drug does not cause anesthesia or analgesia; pain must be treated with appropriate analgesic agents. Continuous monitoring of vital signs, cardiac status, respiratory status, and degree of neuromuscular block (objective assessment with peripheral external nerve stimulator) is mandatory and until full muscle tone has returned. Muscle tone returns in a predictable pattern, starting with diaphragm, abdomen, chest, limbs, and finally muscles of the neck, face, and eyes. Safety precautions must be maintained until full muscle tone has returned. **Note:** It may take longer for return of muscle tone in obese or elderly patients or patients with renal or hepatic disease, myasthenia gravis, myopathy, other neuromuscular disease, dehydration, electrolyte imbalance, or severe acid/base imbalance. Provide appropriate patient teaching/support prior to and following administration.

Long-term use: Monitor fluid levels (intake and output) during and following infusion. Reposition patient and provide appropriate skin care, mouth care, and care of patient's eyes every 2-3 hours while sedated. Provide appropriate emotional and sensory support (auditory and environmental).

Patient Education: Patient will usually be unconscious prior to administration. Patient education should be appropriate to individual situation. Reassurance of constant monitoring and emotional support to reduce fear and anxiety should precede and follow administration. Following return of muscle tone, do not attempt to change position or rise from bed without assistance. Report immediately any skin rash or hives, pounding heartbeat, respiratory difficulty, or muscle tremors. **Pregnancy/breast-feeding precautions:** Inform prescriber if you are pregnant. Breast-feeding is not recommended.

Pregnancy Risk Factor: C

Lactation: Excretion in breast milk unknown/not recommended

Perioperative/Anesthesia/Other Concerns: Classified as a long duration neuromuscular-blocking agent; neuromuscular blockade will be prolonged in patients with decreased renal function; may produce cumulative effect on duration of blockade; produces tachycardia secondary to vagolytic activity and sympathetic stimulation.

Critically-Ill Adult Patients: The 2002 ACCM/SCCM/ASHP clinical practice guidelines for sustained neuromuscular blockade in the adult critically-ill patient recommend:

Optimize sedatives and analgesics prior to initiation and monitor and adjust accordingly during course. Neuromuscular blockers do not relieve pain or produce sedation.

Protect patient's eyes from development of keratitis and corneal abrasion by administering ophthalmic ointment and taping eyelids closed or using eye patches. Reposition patient routinely to protect pressure points from breakdown. Address DVT prophylaxis.

Concurrent use of a neuromuscular blocker and corticosteroids appear to increase the risk of certain ICU myopathies; avoid or administer the corticosteroid at the lowest dose possible. Reassess need for neuromuscular blocker daily.

Using daily drug holidays (stopping neuromuscular-blocking agent until patient requires it again) may decrease the incidence of acute quadriplegic myopathy syndrome.

Tachyphylaxis can develop; switch to another neuromuscular blocker (taking into consideration the patient's organ function) if paralysis is still necessary.

Atracurium or cisatracurium is recommended for patients with significant hepatic or renal disease, due to organ-independent Hofmann elimination.

Monitor patients clinically and via "Train of Four" (TOF) testing with a goal of adjusting the degree of blockade to 1-2 twitches or based upon the patient's clinical condition.

Administration

I.V.: May be administered undiluted by rapid I.V. injection.

Compatibility: Stable in D_5NS, D_5W, LR, NS

Y-site administration: Incompatible with diazepam, thiopental

Storage: Refrigerate; however, is stable for up to 6 months at room temperature.

- **Pancuronium Bromide** *see* Pancuronium *on page 1304*
- **Pandel®** *see* Hydrocortisone *on page 873*
- **Pangestyme™ CN** *see* Pancrelipase *on page 1301*
- **Pangestyme™ EC** *see* Pancrelipase *on page 1301*
- **Pangestyme™ MT** *see* Pancrelipase *on page 1301*
- **Pangestyme™ UL** *see* Pancrelipase *on page 1301*
- **Panglobulin® NF** *see* Immune Globulin (Intravenous) *on page 899*
- **Panixine DisperDose™** *see* Cephalexin *on page 364*
- **Panokase®** *see* Pancrelipase *on page 1301*
- **Panokase® 16** *see* Pancrelipase *on page 1301*

Pantoprazole (pan TOE pra zole)

U.S. Brand Names Protonix®

Pharmacologic Category Proton Pump Inhibitor; Substituted Benzimidazole

Medication Safety Issues

Sound-alike/look-alike issues:

Protonix® may be confused with Lotronex®, Lovenox®, protamine

Vials containing Protonix® I.V. for injection are not recommended for use with spiked I.V. system adaptors. Nurses and pharmacists have reported breakage of the glass vials during attempts to connect spiked I.V. system adaptors, which may potentially result in injury to healthcare professionals.

Use

Oral: Treatment and maintenance of healing of erosive esophagitis associated with GERD; reduction in relapse rates of daytime and nighttime heartburn symptoms in GERD; hypersecretory disorders associated with Zollinger-Ellison syndrome or other neoplastic disorders

I.V.: Short-term treatment (7-10 days) of patients with gastroesophageal reflux disease (GERD) and a history of erosive esophagitis; hypersecretory disorders associated with Zollinger-Ellison syndrome or other neoplastic disorders

Unlabeled/Investigational Use Peptic ulcer disease, active ulcer bleeding (parenteral formulation); adjunct treatment with antibiotics for *Helicobacter pylori* eradication

Mechanism of Action Suppresses gastric acid secretin by inhibiting the parietal cell H^+/K^+ ATP pump

Pharmacodynamics/Kinetics

Absorption: Well absorbed

Distribution: V_d: 11-24 L

Protein binding: 98%, primarily to albumin

Metabolism: Extensively hepatic; CYP2C19 (demethylation), CYP3A4; no evidence that metabolites have pharmacologic activity

Bioavailability: 77%

Half-life elimination: 1 hour; increased to 3.5-10 hours with CYP2C19 deficiency

Time to peak: Oral: 2.5 hours

Excretion: Urine (71%); feces (18%)

Contraindications Hypersensitivity to pantoprazole, substituted benzamidazoles (ie, esomeprazole, lansoprazole, omeprazole, rabeprazole), or any component of the formulation

Warnings/Precautions Symptomatic response does not preclude gastric malignancy. Not indicated for maintenance therapy; safety and efficacy for use beyond 16 weeks have not been established. Prolonged treatment (typically >3 years)

(Continued)

Pantoprazole *(Continued)*

may lead to vitamin B_{12} malabsorption. Intravenous preparation contains edetate sodium (EDTA); use caution in patients who are risk for zinc deficiency if other EDTA-containing solutions are coadministered. Safety and efficacy in pediatric patients have not been established.

Drug Interactions Substrate of CYP2C19 (major), 3A4 (minor); **Inhibits** 2C8/9 (moderate); **Induces** CYP1A2 (weak), 3A4 (weak)

CYP2C8/9 substrates: Pantoprazole may increase the levels/effects of CYP2C8/9 substrates. Example substrates include amiodarone, fluoxetine, glimepiride, glipizide, nateglinide, phenytoin, pioglitazone, rosiglitazone, sertraline, and warfarin.

CYP2C19 inducers: May decrease the levels/effects of pantoprazole. Example inducers include aminoglutethimide, carbamazepine, phenytoin, and rifampin.

Iron salts: Oral absorption may be reduced by pantoprazole.

Itraconazole and ketoconazole: Proton pump inhibitors may decrease the absorption of itraconazole and ketoconazole.

Protease inhibitors: Proton pump inhibitors may decrease absorption of some protease inhibitors (atazanavir and indinavir).

Warfarin: Increased anticoagulant effects/INR have been reported with concurrent use (postmarketing case reports); monitor INR closely.

Nutritional/Herbal/Ethanol Interactions

Ethanol: Avoid ethanol (may cause gastric mucosal irritation).

Herb/Nutraceutical: Prolonged treatment (typically >3 years) may lead to vitamin B_{12} malabsorption.

Lab Interactions False-positive urine screening tests for tetrahydrocannabinol (THC) have been reported in patients receiving proton pump inhibitors, including pantoprazole.

Adverse Reactions

≥1%:

Cardiovascular: Chest pain

Central nervous system: Headache (5% to 9%), insomnia (<1% to 1%), dizziness, migraine, anxiety

Dermatologic: Rash (<1% to 2%)

Endocrine and metabolic: Hyperglycemia (<1% to 1%), hyperlipidemia

Gastrointestinal: Diarrhea (4% to 6%), flatulence (2% to 4%), abdominal pain (1% to 4%), nausea (≤2%), vomiting (≤2%), eructation (≤1%), constipation, dyspepsia, gastroenteritis, rectal disorder

Genitourinary: Urinary frequency, UTI

Hepatic: Liver function abnormal (up to 2%)

Local: Injection site reaction (includes thrombophlebitis and abscess)

Neuromuscular & skeletal: Arthralgia, back pain, hypertonia, neck pain, weakness

Respiratory: Bronchitis, cough, dyspnea, pharyngitis, rhinitis, sinusitis, upper respiratory tract infection

Miscellaneous: Flu syndrome, infection, pain

<1% (Limited to important or life-threatening): Anaphylaxis, angioedema, anterior ischemic optic neuropathy, albuminuria, alkaline phosphatase increased, allergic reaction, anemia, angina pectoris, aphthous stomatitis, arrhythmia, asthma, atrial fibrillation/flutter, bone pain, breast pain, bursitis, cataract, CHF, cholecystitis, cholelithiasis, CPK increased, colitis, confusion, contact dermatitis, convulsion, creatinine increased, cystitis, deafness, decreased reflexes, dehydration, depression, diabetes mellitus, duodenitis, dysarthria, dysmenorrhea, dysphagia, dysuria, ecchymosis, eczema, ECG abnormality, eosinophilia, epididymitis, erythema multiforme, extraocular palsy, fever, fungal dermatitis, gastrointestinal carcinoma, gastrointestinal hemorrhage, gastrointestinal moniliasis, generalized edema, glaucoma, glycosuria, goiter, gout, hallucinations, hematuria, hemorrhage, hepatic failure, hepatitis, herpes simplex, herpes zoster, hyperkinesia, hyper-/hypotension, hyperuricemia, hypokinesia, impaired urination, impotence, interstitial nephritis, jaundice, kidney calculus, kidney pain, laryngitis, leukocytosis, leukopenia, lichenoid dermatitis, maculopapular rash, mouth ulceration, myalgia, myocardial ischemia, neoplasm, neuralgia, neuritis, optic neuropathy, palpitation, pancreatitis, pancytopenia, paresthesia, pneumonia, pyelonephritis, rhabdomyolysis, rectal hemorrhage, retinal vascular disorder, scrotal edema, skin ulcer, somnolence, Stevens-Johnson syndrome, stomach ulcer, stomatitis, syncope, tachycardia, tenosynovitis, thrombocytopenia, thrombosis, toxic epidermal necrolysis, urethritis, vasodilation, vision abnormal

Overdosage/Toxicology Treatment of an overdose would include appropriate supportive treatment. No adverse events were seen with ingestions of 400 and 600 mg doses. Pantoprazole is not removed by hemodialysis.

Dosing

Adults & Elderly:

Erosive esophagitis associated with GERD:

Oral:

Treatment: 40 mg once daily for up to 8 weeks; an additional 8 weeks may be used in patients who have not healed after an 8-week course

Maintenance of healing: 40 mg once daily

Note: Lower doses (20 mg once daily) have been used successfully in mild GERD treatment and maintenance of healing

I.V.: 40 mg once daily for 7-10 days

Peptic ulcer disease: Eradication of *Helicobacter pylori* (unlabeled use): Oral: Doses up to 40 mg twice daily have been used as part of combination therapy

Hypersecretory disorders (including Zollinger-Ellison):

Oral: Initial: 40 mg twice daily; adjust dose based on patient needs; doses up to 240 mg/day have been administered

I.V.: 80 mg twice daily; adjust dose based on acid output measurements; 160-240 mg/day in divided doses has been used for a limited period (up to 7 days)

Prevention of rebleeding in peptic ulcer bleed (unlabeled use): I.V.: 80 mg, followed by 8 mg/hour infusion for 72 hours. **Note:** A daily infusion of 40 mg does not raise gastric pH sufficiently to enhance coagulation in active GI bleeds.

Renal Impairment: No adjustment is required. Pantoprazole is not removed by hemodialysis.

Hepatic Impairment: No adjustment is required.

Available Dosage Forms [DSC] = Discontinued product; **Note:** Strength expressed as base

Injection, powder for reconstitution, as sodium: 40 mg [original formulation] [DSC]

Injection, powder for reconstitution, as sodium: 40 mg [contains edetate sodium 1 mg]

Tablet, delayed release, as sodium: 20 mg, 40 mg

Nursing Guidelines

Assessment: Assess other medications for effectiveness and interactions (cytochrome P450 enzyme substrate), especially those drugs where absorption is determined by an acidic gastric pH. Monitor therapeutic effectiveness and adverse effects at beginning of therapy and regularly with long-term use. Assess knowledge/teach patient appropriate use, possible side effects/interventions, and adverse symptoms to report.

Dietary Considerations:

Oral: May be taken with or without food; best if taken before breakfast.

I.V.: Due to EDTA in preparation, zinc supplementation may be needed in patients prone to zinc deficiency.

Patient Education: Take as directed; do not alter dosage without consulting prescriber. Take at similar time each day. Swallow tablet whole (do not crush or chew). Avoid alcohol. You may experience dizziness, headache, or anxiety (use caution when driving or engaging in dangerous activities until response to medication is known); vomiting or loss of appetite (small frequent meals, frequent mouth care, sucking lozenges, or chewing gum may help); or diarrhea (boiled milk, yogurt, or buttermilk may help). Report persistent abdominal discomfort; chest pain or palpitations; acute headache; unresolved diarrhea; excessive fatigue; increased muscle, joint, or body pain; shortness of breath or wheezing; cold or flu symptoms; changes in urinary pattern; or other persistent adverse reactions. **Pregnancy/breast-feeding precautions:** Inform prescriber if you are pregnant. Breast-feeding is not recommended.

Pregnancy Risk Factor: B

Lactation: Enters breast milk/not recommended

Breast-Feeding Considerations: Not recommended due to carcinogenicity in animal studies.

Perioperative/Anesthesia/Other Concerns: Intravenous omeprazole has been studied in prevention of rebleeding in ulcer patients who are at high risk for rebleeding (endoscopic findings of active bleeding or nonbleeding visible vessel) after successful hemostasis (Lin HJ, 1998; Lau JYW, 2000). Lin and his group treated 100 ulcer patients (actively bleeding ulcers or ulcers with nonbleeding visible vessels) endoscopically and then randomized them to

(Continued)

Pantoprazole *(Continued)*

cimetidine (300 mg bolus followed by 50 mg/hour infusion) or omeprazole (40 mg bolus, ~7 mg/hour infusion) for 72 hours. Patients were discharged on the oral form of the drug arm they were assigned to. The omeprazole group maintained an intragastric pH >6 for about 84% of the infusion duration, while the cimetidine group maintained their pH >6 only about 50% of the time. Rebleeding occurred significantly more often in the cimetidine group. Lau and his colleagues treated patients with actively bleeding ulcers or ulcers with nonbleeding visible vessels with an epinephrine infusion followed by thermocoagulation. They were then randomized to omeprazole (80 mg bolus followed by a continuous infusion of 8 mg/hour for 72 hours) or placebo. All patients were discharged on oral omeprazole (20 mg/day) for 8 weeks and received *H. pylori* treatment if indicated. The primary goal was to evaluate the rate of rebleeding during the first 30 days after endoscopy. Two hundred and forty patients were enrolled with randomization of 120 into each group. Bleeding recurred in significantly more patients receiving placebo than omeprazole infusion. The authors concluded that after endoscopic therapy, omeprazole reduces the risk of rebleeding in patients with actively bleeding ulcers or ulcers with nonbleeding visible vessels.

Administration

Oral: Tablets should be swallowed whole, do not crush or chew. Best if taken before breakfast.

I.V.: Flush I.V. line before and after administration. Solutions prepared from original formulation must be infused through an inline filter. Solutions prepared from the EDTA-stabilized formulation do not require an in-line filter (per manufacturer).

2-minute infusion: The volume of reconstituted solution (4 mg/mL) to be injected may be administered intravenously over at least 2 minutes.

15-minute infusion: Infuse over 15 minutes at a rate not to exceed 7 mL/minute (3 mg/minute).

Reconstitution: Reconstitute with 10 mL NS (final concentration 4 mg/mL). Reconstituted solution may be given intravenously (over 2 minutes) or may be added to 100 mL D_5W, NS, or LR (for 15-minute infusion).

Compatibility: Y-site administration: Incompatible: Midazolam, zinc

Storage:

Oral: Store tablet at 15°C to 30°C (59°F to 77°F)

I.V.:

EDTA-stabilized formulation: Prior to use: Store at 15°C to 30°C (59°F to 86°F). Protect from light. When reconstituted with 10 mL NS (final concentration 4 mg/mL), solution is stable up to 24 hours at room temperature. Diluted solution is stable at room temperature for up to 24 hours from the time of initial reconstitution; potection from light not required.

Original formulation (discontinued): Store at 2°C to 8°C (36°F to 46°F). Protect from light. When reconstituted with 10 mL NS (final concentration 4 mg/mL), solution is stable up to 2 hours at room temperature; protection from light not required. When diluted in 100 mL D_5W, LR, or NS, may be stored at room temperature for up to 12 hours.

Papaverine (pa PAV er een)

U.S. Brand Names Para-Time SR®

Synonyms Papaverine Hydrochloride; Pavabid [DSC]

Pharmacologic Category Vasodilator

Use Oral: Relief of peripheral and cerebral ischemia associated with arterial spasm and myocardial ischemia complicated by arrhythmias

Unlabeled/Investigational Use Investigational: Parenteral: Various vascular spasms associated with muscle spasms as in myocardial infarction, angina, peripheral and pulmonary embolism, peripheral vascular disease, angiospastic states, and visceral spasm (ureteral, biliary, and GI colic); testing for impotence

Mechanism of Action Smooth muscle spasmolytic producing a generalized smooth muscle relaxation including: vasodilatation, gastrointestinal sphincter relaxation, bronchiolar muscle relaxation, and potentially a depressed myocardium (with large doses); muscle relaxation may occur due to inhibition or cyclic nucleotide phosphodiesterase, increasing cyclic AMP; muscle relaxation is unrelated to nerve innervation; papaverine increases cerebral blood flow in normal subjects; oxygen uptake is unaltered

Pharmacodynamics/Kinetics

Onset of action: Oral: Rapid

Protein binding: 90%
Metabolism: Rapidly hepatic
Half-life elimination: 0.5-1.5 hours
Excretion: Primarily urine (as metabolites)

Contraindications Hypersensitivity to papaverine or any component of the formulation

Warnings/Precautions Use with caution in patients with glaucoma; administer I.V. cautiously since apnea and arrhythmias may result; may, in large doses, depress AV and intraventricular cardiac conduction leading to serious arrhythmias (eg, premature beats, paroxysmal tachycardia); chronic hepatitis noted with jaundice, eosinophilia, and abnormal LFTs

Drug Interactions

Decreased effect: Papaverine decreases the effects of levodopa
Increased toxicity: Additive effects with CNS depressants

Nutritional/Herbal/Ethanol Interactions Ethanol: Avoid ethanol (may increase CNS depression).

Adverse Reactions Frequency not defined.

Cardiovascular: Arrhythmias (with rapid I.V. use), flushing of the face, mild hypertension, tachycardia
Central nervous system: Drowsiness, headache, lethargy, sedation, vertigo
Gastrointestinal: Abdominal distress, anorexia, constipation, diarrhea, nausea
Hepatic: Chronic hepatitis, hepatic hypersensitivity
Respiratory: Apnea (with rapid I.V. use)

Overdosage/Toxicology Symptoms of overdose include nausea, vomiting, weakness, gastric distress, ataxia, hepatic dysfunction, drowsiness, nystagmus, hyperventilation, hypotension, and hypokalemia. Treatment is supportive.

Dosing

Adults & Elderly: Arterial spasm:

Oral, sustained release: 150-300 mg every 12 hours; in difficult cases: 150 mg every 8 hours
I.M., I.V.: 30-65 mg (rarely up to 120 mg); may repeat every 3 hours

Pediatrics: Arterial spasm: I.M., I.V.: 6 mg/kg/day in 4 divided doses

Available Dosage Forms

Capsule, sustained release, as hydrochloride (Para-Time SR®): 150 mg
Injection, solution, as hydrochloride: 30 mg/mL (2 mL, 10 mL)

Nursing Guidelines

Assessment: See Contraindications, Warnings/Precautions, Drug Interactions, and Dosing for use cautions. **I.V., I.M.:** Blood pressure and heart rate should be monitored. **Oral:** Blood pressure and heart rate should be monitored prior to therapy and at frequent intervals thereafter. Assess therapeutic effectiveness and adverse response (see Adverse Reactions and Overdose/Toxicology). Teach patient proper use, possible side effects/appropriate interventions and adverse symptoms to report (see Patient Education). Breast-feeding is not recommended.

Dietary Considerations: May be taken with food.

Patient Education: Inform prescriber of all prescriptions, OTC medications, or herbal products you are taking, and any allergies you have. Do not take any new medication during therapy unless approved by prescriber. Take as directed; do not alter dose or discontinue without consulting prescriber. Swallow extended release capsules whole; do not chew, crush, or dissolve. May cause dizziness, confusion, or blurred vision (avoid driving or engaging in tasks that require alertness until response to drug is known); or constipation (increased exercise, fluids, fruit, or fiber may help). Report rapid heartbeat or palpitations and CNS changes (eg, depression, persistent sedation or lethargy, or acute headache). **Pregnancy/breast-feeding precautions:** Inform prescriber if you are or intend to become pregnant. Breast-feeding is not recommended.

Geriatric Considerations: Vasodilators have been used to treat dementia upon the premise that dementia is secondary to a cerebral blood flow insufficiency. The hypothesis is that if blood flow could be increased, cognitive function would be increased. This hypothesis is no longer valid. The use of vasodilators for cognitive dysfunction is not recommended or proven by appropriate scientific study.

Pregnancy Risk Factor: C

Lactation: Excretion in breast milk unknown/not recommended

Perioperative/Anesthesia/Other Concerns: The use of vasodilators for cognitive dysfunction is **not** recommended.

(Continued)

Papaverine *(Continued)*

Administration

I.V.: Rapid I.V. administration may result in arrhythmias and fatal apnea; administer no faster than over 1-2 minutes.

Reconstitution: Solutions should be clear to pale yellow. Precipitates with lactated Ringer's.

Compatibility: Stable in dextran 6% in dextrose, dextran 6% in NS, D_5LR, $D_5{}^1/_4NS$, $D_5{}^1/_2NS$, D_5NS, D_5W, $D_{10}W$, $^1/_2NS$, NS; **incompatible** with LR

Compatibility in syringe: Incompatible with diatrizoate meglumine 52%, diatrizoate sodium 8%

Compatibility when admixed: Incompatible with aminophylline with trimecaine

Storage: Protect from heat or freezing. Refrigerate injection at 2°C to 8°C (35°F to 46°F).

◆ Papaverine Hydrochloride *see* Papaverine *on page 1310*
◆ Paracetamol *see* Acetaminophen *on page 65*
◆ Paraplatin® *see* Carboplatin *on page 313*
◆ Para-Time SR® *see* Papaverine *on page 1310*

Paregoric (par e GOR ik)

Synonyms Camphorated Tincture of Opium (error-prone synonym)

Pharmacologic Category Analgesic, Narcotic

Medication Safety Issues

Sound-alike/look-alike issues:

Camphorated tincture of opium is an error-prone synonym (mistaken as opium tincture)

Paregoric may be confused with Percogesic®

Use care when prescribing opium tincture; each mL contains the equivalent of morphine 10 mg; paregoric contains the equivalent of morphine 0.4 mg/mL

Use Treatment of diarrhea or relief of pain; neonatal opiate withdrawal

Mechanism of Action Increases smooth muscle tone in GI tract, decreases motility and peristalsis, diminishes digestive secretions

Pharmacodynamics/Kinetics In terms of opium:

Metabolism: Hepatic

Excretion: Urine (primarily as morphine glucuronide conjugates and unchanged drug - morphine, codeine, papaverine, etc)

Contraindications Hypersensitivity to opium or any component of the formulation; diarrhea caused by poisoning until the toxic material has been removed; pregnancy (prolonged use or high doses)

Warnings/Precautions Use with caution in patients with respiratory, hepatic or renal dysfunction, severe prostatic hyperplasia, or history of narcotic abuse; opium shares the toxic potential of opiate agonists, and usual precautions of opiate agonist therapy should be observed; some preparations contain sulfites which may cause allergic reactions; infants <3 months of age are more susceptible to respiratory depression, use with caution and generally in reduced doses in this age group; tolerance or drug dependence may result from extended use

Drug Interactions Increased effect/toxicity with CNS depressants (eg, alcohol, narcotics, benzodiazepines, TCAs, MAO inhibitors, phenothiazine)

Nutritional/Herbal/Ethanol Interactions Ethanol: Avoid ethanol (may increase CNS depression).

Lab Interactions Increased aminotransferase [ALT (SGPT)/AST (SGOT)] (S)

Adverse Reactions Frequency not defined.

Cardiovascular: Hypotension, peripheral vasodilation

Central nervous system: Drowsiness, dizziness, insomnia, CNS depression, mental depression, increased intracranial pressure, restlessness, headache, malaise

Gastrointestinal: Constipation, anorexia, stomach cramps, nausea, vomiting, biliary tract spasm

Genitourinary: Ureteral spasms, decreased urination, urinary tract spasm

Hepatic: Increased liver function tests

Neuromuscular & skeletal: Weakness

Ocular: Miosis

Respiratory: Respiratory depression

Miscellaneous: Physical and psychological dependence, histamine release

Overdosage/Toxicology Symptoms of overdose include hypotension, drowsiness, seizures, and respiratory depression. Naloxone, 2 mg I.V. with repeat administration as necessary up to a total of 10 mg, can be used to reverse opiate effects.

Dosing

Adults & Elderly: Diarrhea: Oral: 5-10 mL 1-4 times/day

Pediatrics:

Neonatal opiate withdrawal: Oral: 3-6 drops every 3-6 hours as needed, or initially 0.2 mL every 3 hours; increase dosage by approximately 0.05 mL every 3 hours until withdrawal symptoms are controlled; it is rare to exceed 0.7 mL/dose. Stabilize withdrawal symptoms for 3-5 days, then gradually decrease dosage over a 2- to 4-week period.

Diarrhea: Oral: Children: 0.25-0.5 mL/kg 1-4 times/day

Available Dosage Forms Liquid, oral: Morphine equivalent 2 mg/5 mL (473 mL) [equivalent to opium 20 mg powder; contains alcohol 45% and benzoic acid]

Nursing Guidelines

Assessment: Monitor for excessive sedation, respiratory depression, or hypotension. Has potential for psychological or physiological dependence

Patient Education: Take exactly as directed; do not increase dosage. May cause dependence with prolonged or excessive use. Avoid alcohol or any other prescription and OTC medications that may cause sedation (sleeping medications, some cough/cold remedies, antihistamines, etc). You may experience drowsiness, dizziness, or impaired judgment (use caution when driving or engaging in tasks that require alertness until response to drug is known) or postural hypotension (use caution when rising from sitting or lying position or when climbing stairs). You may experience nausea or loss of appetite (small frequent meals may help) or constipation (a laxative may be necessary). Report unresolved nausea, vomiting, respiratory difficulty (shortness of breath or decreased respirations), chest pain, or palpitations. **Pregnancy/breast-feeding precautions:** Inform prescriber if you are pregnant. If nursing, take immediately after feeding or 4-6 hour before next feeding.

Pregnancy Risk Factor: B/D (prolonged use or high doses)

Lactation: Enters breast milk/use caution

Breast-Feeding Considerations: Information regarding use while breast-feeding is based on experience with morphine. Probably safe with low doses and by administering dose after breast-feeding to further minimize exposure to the drug. Monitor the infant for possible side effects related to opiates.

Administration

Storage: Store in light-resistant, tightly closed container

♦ **Parenteral Nutrition** *see* Total Parenteral Nutrition *on page 1650*

♦ **Pariprazole** *see* Rabeprazole *on page 1457*

Paroxetine (pa ROKS e teen)

U.S. Brand Names Paxil®; Paxil CR®; Pexeva®

Synonyms Paroxetine Hydrochloride; Paroxetine Mesylate

Pharmacologic Category Antidepressant, Selective Serotonin Reuptake Inhibitor

Medication Safety Issues

Sound-alike/look-alike issues:

Paroxetine may be confused with paclitaxel, pyridoxine

Paxil® may be confused with Doxil®, paclitaxel, Plavix®, Taxol®

Use Treatment of depression in adults; treatment of panic disorder with or without agoraphobia; obsessive-compulsive disorder (OCD) in adults; social anxiety disorder (social phobia); generalized anxiety disorder (GAD); post-traumatic stress disorder (PTSD)

Paxil CR®: Treatment of depression; panic disorder; premenstrual dysphoric disorder (PMDD); social anxiety disorder (social phobia)

Unlabeled/Investigational Use May be useful in eating disorders, impulse control disorders, self-injurious behavior; premenstrual disorders, vasomotor symptoms of menopause; treatment of depression and obsessive-compulsive disorder (OCD) in children

Mechanism of Action Paroxetine is a selective serotonin reuptake inhibitor, chemically unrelated to tricyclic, tetracyclic, or other antidepressants; presumably, the inhibition of serotonin reuptake from brain synapse stimulated serotonin activity in the brain

(Continued)

Paroxetine *(Continued)*

Pharmacodynamics/Kinetics

Absorption: Completely absorbed following oral administration

Distribution: V_d: 8.7 L/kg (3-28 L/kg)

Protein binding: 93% to 95%

Metabolism: Extensively hepatic via CYP enzymes via oxidation and methylation; nonlinear pharmacokinetics may be seen with higher doses and longer duration of therapy. Saturation of CYP2D6 appears to account for the nonlinearity. C_{min} concentrations 70% to 80% greater in the elderly compared to nonelderly patients; clearance is also decreased.

Half-life elimination: 21 hours (3-65 hours)

Time to peak, serum: Immediate release: 5.2 hours; controlled release: 6-10 hours

Excretion: Urine (64%, 2% as unchanged drug); feces (36% primarily via bile)

Contraindications Hypersensitivity to paroxetine or any component of the formulation; use of MAO inhibitors or within 14 days; concurrent use with thioridazine or pimozide

Warnings/Precautions

Major psychiatric warnings:

- Antidepressants increase the risk of suicidal thinking and behavior in children and adolescents with major depressive disorder (MDD) and other depressive disorders; consider risk prior to prescribing.
- Closely monitor for clinical worsening, suicidality, or unusual changes in behavior; the child's family or caregiver should be instructed to closely observe the patient and communicate condition with healthcare provider. **Paroxetine is not FDA approved for use in children.**
- Adults treated with antidepressants should be observed similarly for clinical worsening and suicidality, especially during the initial few months of a course of drug therapy, or at times of dose changes, either increases or decreases. A medication guide should be dispensed with each prescription.
- The possibility of a suicide attempt is inherent in major depression and may persist until remission occurs. Worsening depression and severe abrupt suicidality that are not part of the presenting symptoms may require discontinuation or modification of drug therapy. Use caution in high-risk patients during initiation of therapy.
- Prescriptions should be written for the smallest quantity consistent with good patient care. The patient's family or caregiver should be alerted to monitor patients for the emergence of suicidality and associated behaviors such as anxiety, agitation, panic attacks, insomnia, irritability, hostility, impulsivity, akathisia, hypomania, and mania; patients should be instructed to notify their healthcare provider if any of these symptoms or worsening depression or psychosis occur.
- May worsen psychosis in some patients or precipitate a shift to mania or hypomania in patients with bipolar disorder. Monotherapy in patients with bipolar disorder should be avoided. Patients presenting with depressive symptoms should be screened for bipolar disorder. **Paroxetine is not FDA approved for the treatment of bipolar depression.**

Key adverse effects:

- Anticholinergic effects: Has low potential for sedation and anticholinergic effects relative to cyclic antidepressants; however among the SSRI class these effects are relatively higher.
- CNS depression: Has a low potential to impair cognitive or motor performance; caution operating hazardous machinery or driving.
- SIADH and hyponatremia: Has been associated with the development of SIADH; hyponatremia has been reported rarely, predominately in the elderly

Concurrent disease:

- Cardiovascular disease: Use caution in patients with cardiovascular disease; paroxetine has not been systemically evaluated in patients with a recent history of MI or unstable heart disease.
- Hepatic impairment: Use caution; clearance is decreased and plasma concentrations are increased; a lower dosage may be needed.
- Narrow-angle glaucoma: Associated with an increased risk of mydriasis in patients with controlled narrow angle glaucoma.
- Platelet aggregation: May impair platelet aggregation, resulting in bleeding.
- Renal impairment: Use caution; clearance is decreased and plasma concentrations are increased; a lower dosage may be needed.

- Seizure disorders: Use caution with a previous seizure disorder or condition predisposing to seizures such as brain damage or alcoholism.
- Sexual dysfunction: May cause or exacerbate sexual dysfunction.

Concurrent drug therapy:

- Agents which lower seizure threshold: Concurrent therapy with other drugs which lower the seizure threshold.
- Anticoagulants/Antiplatelets: Use caution with concomitant use of NSAIDs, ASA, or other drugs that affect coagulation; the risk of bleeding is potentiated.
- CNS depressants: Use caution with concomitant therapy.
- MAO inhibitors: Potential for severe reaction when used with MAO inhibitors; autonomic instability, coma, death, delirium, diaphoresis, hyperthermia, mental status changes/agitation, muscular rigidity, myoclonus, neuroleptic malignant syndrome features, and seizures may occur.

Special populations:

- Elderly: Use caution in elderly patients.
- Pregnancy: Avoid use in the first trimester.

Special notes:

- Electroconvulsive therapy: May increase the risks associated with electroconvulsive therapy; consider discontinuing, when possible, prior to ECT treatment.
- Withdrawal syndrome: May cause dysphoric mood, irritability, agitation, dizziness, sensory disturbances, anxiety, confusion, headache, lethargy, emotional lability, insomnia, hypomania, tinnitus, and seizures. Upon discontinuation of venlafaxine therapy, gradually taper dose. If intolerable symptoms occur following a decrease in dosage or upon discontinuation of therapy, then resuming the previous dose with a more gradual taper should be considered.

Drug Interactions **Substrate** of CYP2D6 (major); **Inhibits** CYP1A2 (weak), 2B6 (moderate), 2C8/9 (weak), 2C19 (weak), 2D6 (strong), 3A4 (weak)

Amphetamines: SSRIs may increase the sensitivity to amphetamines, and amphetamines may increase the risk of serotonin syndrome

Aspirin (and other antiplatelet drugs): Concomitant use of paroxetine and NSAIDs, aspirin, or other drugs affecting coagulation has been associated with an increased risk of bleeding; monitor.

Atomoxetine: Paroxetine may increase the levels/effects; dose reduction of atomoxetine may be required.

Buspirone: Combined use with SSRIs may cause serotonin syndrome

Carbamazepine: May increase levels/effects of paroxetine; monitor.

Carvedilol: Serum concentrations may be increased; monitor carefully for increased carvedilol effect (hypotension and bradycardia)

Cimetidine: Cimetidine may reduce the first-pass metabolism of paroxetine resulting in elevated paroxetine serum concentrations; consider an alternative H_2antagonist

Clozapine: May increase serum levels of clozapine; monitor for increased effect/toxicity

CYP2B6 substrates: Paroxetine may increase the levels/effects of CYP2B6 substrates. Example substrates include bupropion, promethazine, propofol, selegiline, and sertraline.

CYP2D6 inhibitors: May increase the levels/effects of paroxetine. Example inhibitors include chlorpromazine, delavirdine, fluoxetine, miconazole, pergolide, quinidine, quinine, ritonavir, and ropinirole.

CYP2D6 substrates: Paroxetine may increase the levels/effects of CYP2D6 substrates. Example substrates include amphetamines, selected beta-blockers, dextromethorphan, fluoxetine, lidocaine, mirtazapine, nefazodone, risperidone, ritonavir, thioridazine, tricyclic antidepressants, and venlafaxine.

CYP2D6 prodrug substrates: Paroxetine may decrease the levels/effects of CYP2D6 prodrug substrates. Example prodrug substrates include codeine, hydrocodone, oxycodone, and tramadol.

Cyproheptadine: May inhibit the effects of serotonin reuptake inhibitors; monitor for altered antidepressant response; cyproheptadine acts as a serotonin agonist

Dextromethorphan: Metabolism of dextromethorphan may be inhibited; visual hallucinations occurred; monitor

Galantamine: Paroxetine may increase levels/effects; monitor.

Haloperidol: Metabolism may be inhibited and cause extrapyramidal symptoms (EPS); monitor patients for EPS if combination is utilized

(Continued)

Paroxetine *(Continued)*

HMG-CoA reductase inhibitors: Metabolism may be inhibited by SSRIs; particularly lovastatin and simvastatin resulting in myositis and rhabdomyolysis; paroxetine appears to have weak interaction with CYP3A4, and therefore, appears to have a low risk of this interaction

Lithium: Patients receiving SSRIs and lithium have developed neurotoxicity; if combination is used; monitor for neurotoxicity

Loop diuretics: SSRIs may cause hyponatremia; additive hyponatremic effects may be seen with combined use of a loop diuretic (bumetanide, furosemide, torsemide); monitor for hyponatremia

MAO inhibitors: SSRIs should not be used with nonselective MAO inhibitors (isocarboxazid, phenelzine); fatal reactions have been reported; this combination should be avoided

Meperidine: Combined use may cause serotonin syndrome; monitor

Nefazodone and trazodone: May increase the risk of serotonin syndrome with SSRIs; monitor.

NSAIDs: Concomitant use of paroxetine and NSAIDs, aspirin, or other drugs affecting coagulation has been associated with an increased risk of bleeding; monitor.

Phenytoin: Metabolism of phenytoin may be inhibited, resulting in phenytoin toxicity; monitor for toxicity (ataxia, confusion, dizziness, nystagmus, involuntary muscle movement).

Pimozide: Paroxetine may increase the levels/effects; concomitant use contraindicated.

Procyclidine: Paroxetine increases AUC of procyclidine by 35%; this may result in increased anticholinergic effects; procyclidine dose reduction may be necessary.

Risperidone: Paroxetine, a potent CYP2D6 inhibitor, inhibits the metabolism of risperidone (CYP2D6 substrate) resulting in elevated plasma risperidone levels. The clinical implications are unclear, but clinicians should monitor for potential extrapyramidal symptoms (EPS).

Ritonavir: Combined use of paroxetine with ritonavir may cause serotonin syndrome; monitor

Selegiline: SSRIs have been reported to cause mania or hypertension when combined with selegiline; this combination is best avoided; concurrent use with SSRIs has also been reported to cause serotonin syndrome; as an MAO type B inhibitor, the risk of serotonin syndrome may be less than with nonselective MAO inhibitors

Serotonergic uptake inhibitors: Combined use with other drugs which inhibit the reuptake may cause serotonin syndrome

Sibutramine: May increase the risk of serotonin syndrome with SSRIs; avoid coadministration

Sumatriptan (and other serotonin agonists): Concurrent use may result in toxicity; weakness, hyper-reflexia, and incoordination have been observed with sumatriptan and SSRIs. In addition, concurrent use may theoretically increase the risk of serotonin syndrome; includes sumatriptan, naratriptan, rizatriptan, and zolmitriptan.

Sympathomimetics: May increase the risk of serotonin syndrome with SSRIs

Theophylline: Paroxetine may elevate serum levels of theophylline; monitor

Thioridazine: Paroxetine may inhibit the metabolism of thioridazine, resulting in increased plasma levels and increasing the risk of QT_c interval prolongation. Concurrent use is contraindicated.

Tramadol: Combined use may cause serotonin syndrome; monitor

Tricyclic antidepressants: The metabolism of tricyclic antidepressants (amitriptyline, desipramine, imipramine, nortriptyline) may be inhibited by SSRIs resulting is elevated serum levels; if combination is warranted, a low dose of TCA (10-25 mg/day) should be utilized.

Tryptophan: May increase serotonergic effects; concomitant use not recommended.

Venlafaxine: Combined use with paroxetine may increase the risk of serotonin syndrome

Warfarin: May alter the hypoprothrombinemic response to warfarin; monitor INR

Zolpidem: At least one case of acute delirium in association with combined therapy has been reported

Nutritional/Herbal/Ethanol Interactions

Ethanol: Avoid ethanol.

Food: Peak concentration is increased, but bioavailability is not significantly altered by food.

Herb/Nutraceutical: Avoid valerian, St John's wort, SAMe, kava kava.

Lab Interactions Increased LFTs

Adverse Reactions Frequency varies by dose and indication. Adverse reactions reported as a composite of all indications.

>10%:

Central nervous system: Somnolence (15% to 24%), insomnia (11% to 24%), headache (17% to 18%), dizziness (6% to 14%)

Endocrine & metabolic: Libido decreased (6% to 15%)

Gastrointestinal: Nausea (19% to 26%), xerostomia (9% to 18%), constipation (5% to 16%), diarrhea (9% to 12%)

Genitourinary: Ejaculatory disturbances (10% to 28%)

Neuromuscular & skeletal: Weakness (12% to 22%), tremor (4% to 11%)

Miscellaneous: Diaphoresis (5% to 14%)

1% to 10%:

Cardiovascular: Vasodilation (2% to 4%), chest pain (3%), palpitations (2% to 3%), hypertension (≥1%), tachycardia (≥1%)

Central nervous system: Nervousness (4% to 9%), anxiety (5%), agitation (3% to 5%), abnormal dreams (3% to 4%), concentration impaired (3% to 4%), yawning (2% to 4%), depersonalization (up to 3%), amnesia (2%), emotional lability (≥1%), vertigo (≥1%), confusion (1%), chills (2%)

Dermatologic: Rash (2% to 3%), pruritus (≥1%)

Endocrine & metabolic: Orgasmic disturbance (2% to 9%), dysmenorrhea (5%)

Gastrointestinal: Anorexia, appetite decreased (5% to 9%), dyspepsia (2% to 5%), flatulence (4%), abdominal pain (4%), appetite increased (2% to 4%), vomiting (2% to 3%), taste perversion (2%), weight gain (≥1%)

Genitourinary: Impotence (2% to 9%), genital disorder (female 2% to 9%), urinary frequency (2% to 3%), urinary tract infection (2%)

Neuromuscular & skeletal: paresthesia (4%), myalgia (2% to 4%), back pain (3%), myoclonus (2% to 3%), myopathy (2%), myasthenia (1%), arthralgia (≥1%)

Ocular: Blurred vision (4%), abnormal vision (2% to 3%)

Otic: Tinnitus (≥1%)

Respiratory: Respiratory disorder (up to 7%), pharyngitis (4%), sinusitis (up to 4%), rhinitis (3%)

Miscellaneous: Infection (5% to 6%)

<1%, postmarketing, and/or case reports (limited to important or life-threatening): Acute renal failure, adrenergic syndrome, akinesia, alkaline phosphatase increased, allergic reaction, anaphylaxis, anemias (various), angina pectoris, angioedema, aphasia, aphthous stomatitis, arrhythmias (atrial and ventricular), arthrosis, asthma, behavioral disturbances (various), bilirubinemia, bleeding time increased, blood dyscrasias, bloody diarrhea, bradycardia, bronchitis, bulimia, BUN increased, bundle branch block, cardiospasm, cataract, cellulitis, cerebral ischemia, cerebrovascular accident, cholelithiasis, colitis, congestive heart failure, creatinine phosphokinase increased, deafness, dehydration, delirium, diabetes mellitus, drug dependence, dyskinesia, dysphagia, dyspnea, dystonia, ecchymosis, eclampsia, electrolyte abnormalities, emphysema, erythema, exfoliative dermatitis, extrapyramidal syndrome, fecal impactions, fungal dermatitis, gamma globulins increased, gastroenteritis, glaucoma, goiter, Guillain-Barré syndrome, hematemesis, hematoma, hemorrhage, hemoptysis, hepatic necrosis, hepatitis, hypercholesteremia, hyper-/hypoglycemia, hyper-/hypothyroidism, hypotension, ileus, jaundice, ketosis, lactic dehydrogenase increased, liver function tests abnormal, low cardiac output, lung fibrosis, lymphadenopathy, meningitis, MI, migraine, myelitis, neuroleptic malignant syndrome, neuropathy, osteoporosis, pancreatitis, peptic ulcer, peritonitis, phlebitis, pneumonia, platelet count abnormalities, pulmonary edema, pulmonary embolus, pulmonary hypertension, seizure, sepsis, serotonin syndrome, syncope, tetany, tongue edema, torsade de pointes, toxic epidermal necrolysis

Overdosage/Toxicology Symptoms of overdose include somnolence, nausea, vomiting, hepatic dysfunction, drowsiness, sinus tachycardia, urinary retention, renal failure (acute), and dilated pupils. Convulsions, status epilepticus, and ventricular arrhythmias (including torsade de pointes) have been reported, as well as serotonin syndrome and manic reaction. There are no specific antidotes, following attempts at decontamination, treatment is supportive and symptom-directed . Forced diuresis, dialysis, and hemoperfusion are unlikely to be beneficial.

(Continued)

Paroxetine *(Continued)*

Dosing

Adults:

Depression: Oral:

Paxil®, Pexeva®: Initial: 20 mg once daily, preferably in the morning; increase if needed by 10 mg/day increments at intervals of at least 1 week; maximum dose: 50 mg/day

Paxil CR®: Initial: 25 mg once daily; increase if needed by 12.5 mg/day increments at intervals of at least 1 week; maximum dose: 62.5 mg/day

GAD (Paxil®): Oral: Initial: 20 mg once daily, preferably in the morning; doses of 20-50 mg/day were used in clinical trials, however, no greater benefit was seen with doses >20 mg. If dose is increased, adjust in increments of 10 mg/day at 1-week intervals.

OCD (Paxil®, Pexeva®): Oral: Initial: 20 mg once daily, preferably in the morning; increase if needed by 10 mg/day increments at intervals of at least 1 week; recommended dose: 40 mg/day; range: 20-60 mg/day; maximum dose: 60 mg/day

Panic disorder: Oral:

Paxil®, Pexeva®: Initial: 10 mg once daily, preferably in the morning; increase if needed by 10 mg/day increments at intervals of at least 1 week; recommended dose: 40 mg/day; range: 10-60 mg/day; maximum dose: 60 mg/day

Paxil CR®: Initial: 12.5 mg once daily; increase if needed by 12.5 mg/day at intervals of at least 1 week; maximum dose: 75 mg/day

PMDD (Paxil CR®): Oral: Initial: 12.5 mg once daily in the morning; may be increased to 25 mg/day; dosing changes should occur at intervals of at least 1 week. May be given daily throughout the menstrual cycle or limited to the luteal phase.

PTSD (Paxil®): Oral: Initial: 20 mg once daily, preferably in the morning; increase if needed by 10 mg/day increments at intervals of at least 1 week; range: 20-50 mg

Social anxiety disorder: Oral:

Paxil®: Initial: 20 mg once daily, preferably in the morning; recommended dose: 20 mg/day; range: 20-60 mg/day; doses >20 mg may not have additional benefit

Paxil CR®: Initial: 12.5 mg once daily, preferably in the morning; may be increased by 12.5 mg/day at intervals of at least 1 week; maximum dose: 37.5 mg/day

Menopause-associated vasomotor symptoms (unlabeled use, Paxil CR®): Oral: 12.5-25 mg/day

Elderly:

Depression, obsessive compulsive disorder, panic attack, social anxiety disorder:

Paxil®, Pexeva®: Oral: Initial: 10 mg/day; increase if needed by 10 mg/day increments at intervals of at least 1 week; maximum dose: 40 mg/day

Paxil CR®: Initial: 12.5 mg/day; increase if needed by 12.5 mg/day increments at intervals of at least 1 week; maximum dose: 50 mg/day

Pediatrics:

Depression (unlabeled use; not recommended by FDA): Oral: Initial: 10 mg/day and adjusted upward on an individual basis to 20 mg/day

OCD (unlabeled use): Oral: Initial: 10 mg/day and titrate up as necessary to 60 mg/day

Self-Injurious behavior (unlabeled use): Oral: 20 mg/day

Social phobia (unlabeled use): Oral: 2.5-15 mg/day

Renal Impairment:

Cl_{cr} <30 mL/minute: Mean plasma concentrations ~4 times that seen in normal function.

Cl_{cr} 30-60 mL/minute: Plasma concentrations 2 times that seen in normal function.

Paxil®, Pexeva®: Adults: Initial: 10 mg/day; increase if needed by 10 mg/day increments at intervals of at least 1 week; maximum dose: 40 mg/day

Paxil CR®; Initial: 12.5 mg/day; increase if needed by 12.5 mg/day increments at intervals of at least 1 week; maximum dose: 50 mg/day

Hepatic Impairment: In hepatic dysfunction, plasma concentration is 2 times that seen in normal function.

Paxil®, Pexeva®: Adults: Initial: 10 mg/day; increase if needed by 10 mg/day increments at intervals of at least 1 week; maximum dose: 40 mg/day

Paxil CR®; Initial: 12.5 mg/day; increase if needed by 12.5 mg/day increments at intervals of at least 1 week; maximum dose: 50 mg/day

Available Dosage Forms Note: Available as paroxetine hydrochloride or mesylate; mg strength refers to paroxetine

Suspension, oral, as hydrochloride (Paxil®): 10 mg/5 mL (250 mL) [orange flavor]

Tablet, as hydrochloride (Paxil®): 10 mg, 20 mg, 30 mg, 40 mg

Tablet, as mesylate (Pexeva®): 10 mg, 20 mg, 30 mg, 40 mg

Tablet, controlled release, as hydrochloride (Paxil CR®): 12.5 mg, 25 mg, 37.5 mg

Nursing Guidelines

Assessment: Assess potential for interactions with other prescription or OTC medications or herbal products patient may be taking. Assess results of laboratory tests. Assess therapeutic effectiveness (according to rationale for prescribing), and adverse reactions at beginning of therapy and frequently with long-term use. Monitor for clinical worsening and suicidal ideation. Taper dosage slowly when discontinuing. Assess knowledge/teach patient appropriate use, interventions to reduce side effects, and adverse symptoms to report

Monitoring Laboratory Tests: Hepatic and renal function

Dietary Considerations: May be taken with or without food.

Patient Education: Take exactly as directed; do not increase dose or frequency or discontinue without consulting prescriber. It may take 2-3 weeks to achieve desired results. Take in the morning to reduce the incidence of insomnia (may be taken with or without food). Do not crush, break, or chew controlled release (Paxil CR®) tablets. Avoid alcohol, caffeine, and other prescription or OTC medications not approved by prescriber. Maintain adequate hydration (2-3 L/day of fluids) unless instructed to restrict fluid intake. You may experience drowsiness, dizziness, or lightheadedness (use caution when driving or engaging in tasks requiring alertness until response to drug is known); nausea, vomiting, anorexia, or dry mouth (small frequent meals, frequent mouth care, chewing gum, or sucking lozenges may help); or orthostatic hypotension (use caution when climbing stairs or changing position from lying or sitting to standing). Report persistent insomnia or excessive daytime sedation; muscle cramping, tremors, weakness, or change in gait; chest pain, palpitations, or rapid heartbeat; vision changes or eye pain; respiratory difficulty or breathlessness; abdominal pain or blood in stool; change in affect or thought processes, unusual agitation, or abnormal dreams; worsening of condition; or suicidal ideation. **Pregnancy/breast-feeding precautions:** Inform prescriber if you are or intend to become pregnant. Consult prescriber if breast-feeding.

Geriatric Considerations: Paroxetine's favorable side effect profile make it a useful alternative to traditional tricyclic antidepressants. Paroxetine is the most sedating of the currently available selective serotonin reuptake inhibitors. Paroxetine's half-life is approximately 21 hours and it has no active metabolites.

Pregnancy Risk Factor: D

Pregnancy Issues: Teratogenic effects were not observed in animal studies. Preliminary results from a retrospective epidemiologic studies in humans show the risk of congenital malformations, specifically atrial or ventricular septal defects, may be increased with paroxetine relative to other antidepressants. Nonteratogenic effects including respiratory distress, cyanosis, apnea, seizures, temperature instability, feeding difficulty, vomiting, hypoglycemia, hypo- or hypertonia, hyper-reflexia, jitteriness, irritability, constant crying, and tremor have been reported in the neonate immediately following delivery after exposure late in the third trimester. Adverse effects may be due to toxic effects of SSRI or drug discontinuation. There are no adequate and well-controlled studies in pregnant women. Use during pregnancy only if the potential benefit to the mother outweighs the possible risk to the fetus. If treatment during pregnancy is required, consider tapering therapy during the third trimester.

Lactation: Enters breast milk/use caution (AAP rates "of concern")

Perioperative/Anesthesia/Other Concerns: Paroxetine has properties similar to fluvoxamine maleate. Buspirone (15-60 mg/day) may be useful in treatment of sexual dysfunction during treatment with a selective serotonin reuptake inhibitor.

Administration

Oral: May be administered with or without food. Do not crush, break, or chew controlled release tablets.

Storage:

Suspension: Store at ≤25°C (≤77°F)

Tablet: Store at 15°C to 30°C (59°F to 86°F)

♦ **Paroxetine Hydrochloride** *see* Paroxetine *on page 1313*

- ♦ **Paroxetine Mesylate** *see* Paroxetine *on page 1313*
- ♦ **Patanol®** *see* Olopatadine *on page 1262*
- ♦ **Pavabid [DSC]** *see* Papaverine *on page 1310*
- ♦ **Pavulon [DSC]** *see* Pancuronium *on page 1304*
- ♦ **Paxil®** *see* Paroxetine *on page 1313*
- ♦ **Paxil CR®** *see* Paroxetine *on page 1313*
- ♦ **PCA (error-prone abbreviation)** *see* Procainamide *on page 1407*
- ♦ **PCE®** *see* Erythromycin *on page 634*
- ♦ **PCV7** *see* Pneumococcal Conjugate Vaccine (7-Valent) *on page 1376*
- ♦ **PediaCare® Decongestant Infants [OTC]** *see* Pseudoephedrine *on page 1436*
- ♦ **Pediapred®** *see* PrednisoLONE *on page 1399*
- ♦ **Pediarix™** *see* Diphtheria, Tetanus Toxoids, Acellular Pertussis, Hepatitis B (Recombinant), and Poliovirus (Inactivated) Vaccine *on page 550*
- ♦ **Pedi-Dri®** *see* Nystatin *on page 1249*
- ♦ **PediOtic®** *see* Neomycin, Polymyxin B, and Hydrocortisone *on page 1212*
- ♦ **PedvaxHIB®** *see* *Haemophilus* b Conjugate Vaccine *on page 837*
- ♦ **Pegasys®** *see* Peginterferon Alfa-2a *on page 1321*

Pegfilgrastim (peg fil GRA stim)

U.S. Brand Names Neulasta®

Synonyms G-CSF (PEG Conjugate); Granulocyte Colony Stimulating Factor (PEG Conjugate)

Pharmacologic Category Colony Stimulating Factor

Use Decrease the incidence of infection, by stimulation of granulocyte production, in patients with nonmyeloid malignancies receiving myelosuppressive therapy associated with a significant risk of febrile neutropenia

Mechanism of Action Stimulates the production, maturation, and activation of neutrophils, pegfilgrastim activates neutrophils to increase both their migration and cytotoxicity. Pegfilgrastim has a prolonged duration of effect relative to filgrastim and a reduced renal clearance.

Pharmacodynamics/Kinetics Half-life elimination: SubQ: 15-80 hours

Contraindications Hypersensitivity to pegfilgrastim, filgrastim, *E. coli*-derived proteins, or any component of the formulation; concurrent myelosuppressive, chemotherapy, or radiation therapy

Warnings/Precautions Complete blood count and platelet count should be obtained prior to chemotherapy. Do not use pegfilgrastim in the period 14 days before to 24 hours after administration of cytotoxic chemotherapy because of the potential sensitivity of rapidly dividing myeloid cells to cytotoxic chemotherapy. Pegfilgrastim can potentially act as a growth factor for any tumor type, particularly myeloid malignancies. Precaution should be exercised in the usage of pegfilgrastim in any malignancy with myeloid characteristics. Tumors of nonhematopoietic origin may have surface receptors for pegfilgrastim. Pegfilgrastim has not been evaluated for peripheral blood progenitor cell (PBPC) mobilization.

Allergic-type reactions have occurred in patients receiving the parent compound, filgrastim (G-CSF) with first or later doses. Reactions tended to occur more frequently with intravenous administration and within 30 minutes of infusion. Rare cases of splenic rupture or adult respiratory distress syndrome have been reported in association with filgrastim; patients must be instructed to report left upper quadrant pain or shoulder tip pain or respiratory distress. Use caution in patients with sickle cell diseases; sickle cell crises have been reported following filgrastim therapy. Safety and efficacy in pediatric patients have not been established. The 6 mg fixed dose should not be used in adolescents weighing <45 kg.

Drug Interactions No formal drug interactions studies have been conducted.

Lithium: May potentiate release of neutrophils from bone marrow.

Adverse Reactions

>10%:

Cardiovascular: Peripheral edema (12%)

Central nervous system: Headache (16%)

Gastrointestinal: Vomiting (13%), constipation (12%)

Neuromuscular & skeletal: Bone pain (57%), myalgia (21%), arthralgia (16%), weakness (13%)

<1% (Limited to important or life-threatening): Leukocytosis, hypoxia. **Note**: Rare adverse reactions reported for filgrastim and pegfilgrastim include adult respiratory distress syndrome, allergic reactions (including urticaria, rash or anaphylaxis), sickle cell crisis, and splenic rupture. Cytopenias resulting from an

antibody response to exogenous growth factors have been reported on rare occasions in patients treated with other recombinant growth factors.

Overdosage/Toxicology No clinical adverse effects have been seen with high doses producing ANC >10,000/mm^3. Duration of leukocytosis has ranged from 6-13 days. Leukapheresis may be considered in symptomatic individuals.

Dosing

Adults & Elderly: Myelosuppressive therapy: SubQ: 6 mg once per chemotherapy cycle; do not administer in the period between 14 days before and 24 hours after administration of cytotoxic chemotherapy

Pediatrics: Adolescents >45 kg: Refer to adult dosing.

Renal Impairment: No adjustment necessary.

Available Dosage Forms Injection, solution [preservative free]: 10 mg/mL (0.6 mL) [prefilled syringe]

Nursing Guidelines

Monitoring Laboratory Tests: Complete blood count and platelet count should be obtained prior to chemotherapy. Leukocytosis (white blood cell counts 100,000/mm^3) has been observed in <1% of patients receiving pegfilgrastim. Monitor platelets and hematocrit regularly.

Patient Education: Follow directions for proper storage and administration of SubQ medication. Never reuse syringes or needles. You may experience bone pain (request analgesic). Report unusual fever or chills; unhealed sores; severe bone pain; pain, redness, or swelling at injection site; pain in the upper abdomen or shoulder tip; unusual swelling of extremities or respiratory difficulty; or chest pain and palpitations. **Pregnancy/breast-feeding precautions:** Inform prescriber if you are or intend to become pregnant. Consult prescriber if breast-feeding.

Pregnancy Risk Factor: C

Lactation: Excretion in breast milk unknown/use caution

Administration

Storage: Store under refrigeration 2°C to 8°C (36°F to 46°F). Protect from light. Allow to reach room temperature prior to injection. May be kept at room temperature for 48 hours. Do not freeze. If inadvertently frozen, allow to thaw in refrigerator; discard if frozen more than one time.

Peginterferon Alfa-2a (peg in ter FEER on AL fa too aye)

U.S. Brand Names Pegasys®

Synonyms Interferon Alfa-2a (PEG Conjugate); Pegylated Interferon Alfa-2a

Pharmacologic Category Interferon

Use Treatment of chronic hepatitis C (CHC), alone or in combination with ribavirin, in patients with compensated liver disease and histological evidence of cirrhosis (Child-Pugh class A) and patients with clinically-stable HIV disease; treatment of patients with HBeAg positive and HBeAg negative chronic hepatitis B with compensated liver disease and evidence of viral replication and liver inflammation

Mechanism of Action Alpha interferons are a family of proteins, produced by nucleated cells, that have antiviral, antiproliferative, and immune-regulating activity. There are 16 known subtypes of alpha interferons. Interferons interact with cells through high affinity cell surface receptors. Following activation, multiple effects can be detected including induction of gene transcription. Inhibits cellular growth, alters the state of cellular differentiation, interferes with oncogene expression, alters cell surface antigen expression, increases phagocytic activity of macrophages, and augments cytotoxicity of lymphocytes for target cells.

Pharmacodynamics/Kinetics

Half-life elimination: Terminal: 50-140 hours; increased with renal dysfunction

Time to peak, serum: 72-96 hours

Contraindications Hypersensitivity to polyethylene glycol (PEG), interferon alfa, or any component of the formulation; autoimmune hepatitis; decompensated liver disease in cirrhotic patients (Child-Pugh score >6); decompensated liver disease (Child-Pugh score ≥6, class B and C) in CHC coinfected with HIV; neonates and infants

Warnings/Precautions Severe acute hypersensitivity reactions have occurred rarely; prompt discontinuation is advised. Use caution with prior cardiovascular disease, endocrine disorders, autoimmune disorders, and pulmonary dysfunction. Discontinue treatment with worsening or persistently severe signs/symptoms of autoimmune, infectious, respiratory, or neuropsychiatric disorders (including depression and/or suicidal thoughts/behavior). Severe psychiatric adverse effects (including depression, suicidal ideation, and suicide attempt) may occur. Avoid use in severe psychiatric disorders; use caution in patients with a history of

(Continued)

Peginterferon Alfa-2a *(Continued)*

depression. Patients who experience dizziness, confusion, somnolence or fatigue should use caution when performing tasks which require mental alertness (eg, operating machinery or driving).

Hepatic decompensation and death have been associated with the use of alpha interferons including Pegasys®, in cirrhotic chronic hepatitis C patients; patients coinfected with HIV and receiving highly active antiretroviral therapy have shown an increased risk. Monitor hepatic function; discontinue if decompensation occurs (Child-Pugh score >6) in monoinfected patients and (Child-Pugh score ≥6, class B and C) in patients coinfected with HIV. In hepatitis B patients, flares (transient and potentially severe increases in serum ALT) may occur during or after treatment; more frequent monitoring of LFTs and a dose reduction are recommended. Discontinue if ALT elevation continues despite dose reduction or if increased bilirubin or hepatic decompensation occur.

May cause myelosuppression (including neutropenia, lymphopenia, aplastic anemia); use caution with renal dysfunction (Cl_{cr} <50 mL/minute). Patients with renal dysfunction should be monitored for signs/symptoms of toxicity (dosage adjustment required if toxicity occurs). Discontinue if new or worsening ophthalmologic disorders occur including retinal hemorrhages, cotton wool spots, and retinal artery or vein obstruction; visual exams are recommended in these instances, at the initiation of therapy, and periodically during therapy.

Use caution with baseline neutrophil count <1500/mm^3, platelet count <90,000/mm^3 or hemoglobin <10 g/dL. Discontinue therapy (at least temporarily) if ANC <500/mm^3 or platelet count <25,000/mm^3, colitis develops, or if known or suspected pancreatitis develops. Use caution in patients with an increased risk for severe anemia (eg, spherocytosis, history of GI bleeding).

Use caution in geriatric patients. Safety and efficacy have not been established in patients who have failed other alpha interferon therapy, received organ transplants, been coinfected with HBV and HCV or HIV; or with HCV and HIV with a $CD4^+$ cell count <100 cells/microL, or been treated for >48 weeks. Due to differences in dosage, patients should not change brands of interferon. Safety and efficacy have not been established in children.

Drug Interactions Inhibits CYP1A2 (weak)

ACE inhibitors: Interferons may increase the risk of neutropenia.

Fluorouracil: Concentrations of fluorouracil doubled in patients with gastrointestinal carcinoma who received interferon alfa-2b.

Melphalan: Interferon alfa may decrease the serum concentrations of melphalan.

Prednisone: Prednisone may decrease the therapeutic effects of interferon alfa.

Ribavirin: Concurrent therapy may increase the risk of hemolytic anemia.

Theophylline: Interferon alfa may decrease the CYP450 metabolism of theophylline.

Warfarin: Interferons may increase the anticoagulant effects of warfarin.

Zidovudine: Interferons may decrease the metabolism of zidovudine.

Nutritional/Herbal/Ethanol Interactions Ethanol: Avoid use in patients with hepatitis C virus.

Adverse Reactions Note: Percentages are reported for peginterferon alfa-2a in chronic hepatitis C (CHC) patients. Other percentages indicated as "with ribavirin" or "in HIV/CHC" are those which significantly exceed incidence reported for peginterferon monotherapy in CHC patients.

>10%:

Central nervous system: Headache (54%), fatigue (50%), pyrexia (37%; 41% with ribavirin; 54% in hepatitis B), insomnia (19%; 30% with ribavirin), depression (18%), dizziness (16%), irritability/anxiety/nervousness (19%; 33% with ribavirin), pain (11%)

Dermatologic: Alopecia (23%; 28% with ribavirin), pruritus (12%; 19% with ribavirin), dermatitis (16% with ribavirin)

Gastrointestinal: Nausea/vomiting (24%), anorexia (17%; 24% with ribavirin), diarrhea (16%), weight loss (16% in HIV/CHC), abdominal pain (15%)

Hematologic: Neutropenia (21%; 27% with ribavirin; 40% in HIV/CHC), lymphopenia (14% with ribavirin), anemia (11% with ribavirin; 14% in HIV/CHC)

Hepatic: ALT increases 5-10 x ULN during treatment (25% to 27% in hepatitis B); ALT increases >10 x ULN during treatment (12% to 18% in hepatitis B); ALT increases 5-10 x ULN after treatment (13% to 16% in hepatitis B); ALT increases >10 x ULN after treatment (7% to 12% in hepatitis B)

Local: Injection site reaction (22%)

Neuromuscular & skeletal: Weakness (56%; 65% with ribavirin), myalgia (37%), rigors (32%; 25% to 27% in hepatitis B), arthralgia (28%)
Respiratory: Dyspnea (13% with ribavirin)

1% to 10%:

Central nervous system: Concentration impaired (8%), memory impaired (5%), mood alteration (3%; 9% in HIV/CHC)
Dermatologic: Dermatitis (8%), rash (5%), dry skin (4%; 10% with ribavirin), eczema (5% with ribavirin)
Endocrine & metabolic: Hypothyroidism (4%), hyperthyroidism (1%)
Gastrointestinal: Xerostomia (6%), dyspepsia (6% with ribavirin), weight loss (4%; 10% with ribavirin)
Hematologic: Thrombocytopenia (5%), platelets decreased <50,000/mm^3 (5%), lymphopenia (3%), anemia (2%)
Hepatic: Hepatic decompensation (2% CHC/HIV patients)
Neuromuscular & skeletal: Back pain (9%)
Ocular: Blurred vision (4%)
Respiratory: Cough (4%; 10 % with ribavirin), dyspnea (4%), exertional dyspnea (4% with ribavirin)
Miscellaneous: Diaphoresis (6%), bacterial infection (3%; 5% in HIV/CHC)

≤1% (Limited to important or life-threatening): Anaphylaxis, angioedema, angina, aggression, arrhythmia, autoimmune disorders, bronchiolitis obliterans, bronchoconstriction, cerebral hemorrhage, chest pain, cholangitis, colitis, coma, corneal ulcer, cotton wool spots, diabetes mellitus, endocarditis, exertional dyspnea, fatty liver, gastrointestinal bleeding, hearing impairment, hearing loss, hemoglobin decreased, hematocrit decreased, hepatic dysfunction, hepatic decompensation, hyper-/hypoglycemia, hypersensitivity reactions, hypertension, influenza, interstitial pneumonitis, MI, myositis, optic neuritis, papilledema, pancreatitis, peptic ulcer, peripheral neuropathy, pneumonia, psychosis, pulmonary embolism, pulmonary infiltrates, retinal hemorrhage, retinopathy, sarcoidosis, substance overdose, suicidal ideation, suicide, supraventricular arrhythmia, thrombotic thrombocytopenic purpura, urticaria, vision decreased/loss

Overdosage/Toxicology Experience with overdosage is limited and no serious reactions have been reported. Dose-limiting toxicities include fatigue, elevated liver enzymes, neutropenia and thrombocytopenia. In case of overdose, treatment should be symptom-directed and supportive. Hemodialysis and peritoneal dialysis are not effective.

Dosing

Adults:

Chronic hepatitis C (monoinfection or coinfection with HIV): SubQ:
Monotherapy: 180 mcg once weekly for 48 weeks
Combination therapy with ribavirin: Recommended dosage: 180 mcg once/week with ribavirin (Copegus®)
Duration of therapy: Monoinfection (based on genotype):
Genotype 1,4: 48 weeks
Genotype 2,3: 24 weeks
Duration of therapy: Coinfection: 48 weeks

Chronic hepatitis B: SubQ: 180 mcg once weekly for 48 weeks

Dose modifications:

For moderate to severe adverse reactions: Initial: 135 mcg/week; may need decreased to 90 mcg/week in some cases
Based on hematologic parameters:
ANC <750/mm^3: 135 mcg/week
ANC <500/mm^3: Suspend therapy until >1000/mm^3, then restart at 90 mcg/week and monitor
Platelet count <50,000/mm^3: 90 mcg/week
Platelet count <25,000/mm^3: Discontinue therapy
Depression (severity based on DSM-IV criteria):
Mild depression: No dosage adjustment required; evaluate once weekly by visit/phone call. If depression remains stable, continue weekly visits. If depression improves, resume normal visit schedule
Moderate depression: Decrease interferon dose to 90-135 mcg once/week; evaluate once weekly with an office visit at least every other week. If depression remains stable, consider psychiatric evaluation and continue with reduced dosing. If symptoms improve and remain stable for 4 weeks, resume normal visit schedule; continue reduced dosing or return to normal dose.

(Continued)

Peginterferon Alfa-2a *(Continued)*

Severe depression: Discontinue interferon permanently. Obtain immediate psychiatric consultation. Discontinue ribavirin if using concurrently.

Renal Impairment:

Cl_{cr} <50 mL/minute: Use caution; monitor for toxicity

End-stage renal disease requiring hemodialysis: 135 mcg/week; monitor for toxicity

Hepatic Impairment:

HCV: ALT progressively rising above baseline: Decrease dose to 135 mcg/week. If ALT continues to rise or is accompanied by increased bilirubin or hepatic decompensation, discontinue therapy immediately.

HBV:

ALT >5 x ULN: Monitor LFTs more frequently; consider decreasing dose to 135 mcg/week or temporarily discontinuing (may resume after ALT flare subsides).

ALT >10 x ULN: Consider discontinuing.

Available Dosage Forms Injection, solution:

180 mcg/0.5 mL (0.5 mL) [prefilled syringe; contains benzyl alcohol; packaged with needles and alcohol swabs]

180 mcg/mL (1 mL) [contains benzyl alcohol]

Nursing Guidelines

Assessment: Assess potential for interactions with other prescriptions, OTC medications, or herbal products patient may be taking. Assess results of laboratory tests prior to and periodically during therapy. Evaluate for depression and other psychiatric symptoms before and during therapy; baseline eye examination and periodically in patients with baseline disorders; baseline echocardiogram in patients with cardiac disease; assess therapeutic effectiveness and adverse response at beginning of and at regular intervals during therapy. Teach patient proper use if self-administered (appropriate injection technique and syringe/needle disposal), possible side effects/appropriate interventions, and adverse symptoms to report.

Monitoring Laboratory Tests: Standard hematological tests should be performed prior to therapy, at week 2, and periodically. Standard biochemical tests should be performed prior to therapy, at week 4, and periodically. Baseline eye examination and periodically in patients with baseline disorders; baseline echocardiogram in patients with cardiac disease; serum HCV RNA levels after 12 weeks of treatment

Clinical studies tested as follows: CBC (including hemoglobin, WBC, and platelets) and chemistries (including liver function tests and uric acid) measured at weeks 1, 2, 4, 6, and 8, and then every 4 weeks; TSH measured every 12 weeks

In addition, the following baseline values were used as entrance criteria:

Platelet count ≥ 90,000/mm^3 (as low as 75,000/mm^3 in patients with cirrhosis or transition to cirrhosis)

ANC ≥ 1500/mm^3

Serum creatinine <1.5 times ULN

TSH and T_4 within normal limits or adequately controlled

Consider discontinuing treatment if virologic tests indicate no response by week 12.

Dietary Considerations: Avoid ethanol use in patients with hepatitis C virus.

Patient Education: Inform prescriber of all prescriptions, OTC medications, or herbal products you are taking, and any allergies you have. Do not take any new medication during therapy without consulting prescriber. This medication must be given by injection; if self-administered, follow exact instructions for injection and syringe/needle disposal. Avoid alcohol. You will need laboratory tests and ophthalmic exams prior to and during therapy. May cause headache, insomnia, dizziness (use caution when driving or engaging in potentially hazardous tasks until response to drug is known); loss of hair (will grow back after therapy); nausea or anorexia (small frequent meals or frequent mouth care may help); diarrhea (boiled milk, buttermilk, or yogurt may help); weakness, fatigue; muscle, skeletal, or joint pain; or increased perspiration. Report any severe or persistent adverse effects, including nausea, vomiting, or abdominal pain; severe depression, anxiety, or suicidal ideation; skin rash; pain, redness, or swelling at injection site; signs of infection, unusual bleeding or bruising, changes in vision, chest pain, palpitations, or respiratory difficulty. **Pregnancy/breast-feeding precautions:** Inform prescriber if you are or intend to become pregnant. Consult prescriber for appropriate contraceptive measures. Breast-feeding is not recommended.

Pregnancy Risk Factor: C; X when used with ribavirin

Pregnancy Issues: Animal teratogenicity studies have not been conducted; very high doses are abortifacient in Rhesus monkeys. Assumed to have abortifacient potential in humans. There are no adequate and well-controlled studies in pregnant women; use during pregnancy only if the potential benefit to the mother outweighs the possible risk to the fetus. Risk of maternal-infant transmission of hepatitis C is <5%. Reliable contraception should be used in women of childbearing potential.

Lactation: Excretion in breast milk unknown/not recommended

Administration

Storage: Store in refrigerator at 2°C to 8°C (36°F to 46°F). Do not freeze or shake; protect from light. Discard unused solution.

Peginterferon Alfa-2b (peg in ter FEER on AL fa too bee)

U.S. Brand Names PEG-Intron®

Synonyms Interferon Alfa-2b (PEG Conjugate); Pegylated Interferon Alfa-2b

Pharmacologic Category Interferon

Use Treatment of chronic hepatitis C (as monotherapy or in combination with ribavirin) in adult patients who have never received interferon alpha and have compensated liver disease

Mechanism of Action Alpha interferons are a family of proteins, produced by nucleated cells, that have antiviral, antiproliferative, and immune-regulating activity. There are 16 known subtypes of alpha interferons. Interferons interact with cells through high affinity cell surface receptors. Following activation, multiple effects can be detected including induction of gene transcription. Inhibits cellular growth, alters the state of cellular differentiation, interferes with oncogene expression, alters cell surface antigen expression, increases phagocytic activity of macrophages, and augments cytotoxicity of lymphocytes for target cells.

Pharmacodynamics/Kinetics

Bioavailability: Increases with chronic dosing

Half-life elimination: 40 hours

Time to peak: 15-44 hours

Excretion: Urine (30%)

Contraindications Hypersensitivity to polyethylene glycol (PEG), interferon alfa, or any component of the formulation; autoimmune hepatitis; decompensated liver disease; previous treatment with interferon; severe psychiatric disorder; pregnancy (in combination with ribavirin)

Warnings/Precautions Severe psychiatric adverse effects, including depression, suicidal ideation, and suicide attempt, may occur; use caution with a history of depression. Avoid use in severe psychiatric disorders and discontinue if worsening or persistently severe signs/symptoms of neuropsychiatric disorders (including depression and/or suicidal thoughts/behavior) occur. Use with caution in patients who are chronically immunosuppressed, with low peripheral blood counts or myelosuppression, including concurrent use of myelosuppressive therapy. Discontinue therapy when significant decreases in neutrophil (<0.5 x 10^9/L) or platelet counts (<50,000/mm^3 occur).

Use with caution in patients with prior cardiovascular disease, endocrine disorders, autoimmune disorders, and pulmonary dysfunction; may cause or aggravate fatal or life-threatening conditions. Discontinue therapy if colitis develops or known or suspected pancreatitis develops. Patients with renal dysfunction should be monitored for signs/symptoms of toxicity (dosage adjustment required if toxicity occurs); avoid use of combination therapy with ribavirin in renal dysfunction (Cl_{cr} <50 mL/minute). Ophthalmologic disorders (including retinal hemorrhages, cotton wool spots, and retinal artery or vein obstruction) have occurred in patients using other alpha interferons. Prior to start of therapy, visual exams are recommended for patients with diabetes mellitus or hypertension. Transient rashes do not necessitate interruption of therapy.

Due to differences in dosages, patients should not change brands. Safety and efficacy have not been established in patients who have failed other alpha interferon (including peginterferon alfa-2b) therapy, received organ transplants, been

(Continued)

Peginterferon Alfa-2b *(Continued)*

infected with HIV or hepatitis B, or received treatment for >48 weeks. Use caution in geriatric patients. Safety and efficacy have not been established in children.

Drug Interactions Inhibits CYP1A2 (weak)

ACE inhibitors: Interferons may increase the risk of neutropenia. Risk: Monitor
Clozapine: A case report of agranulocytosis with concurrent use.
Erythropoietin: Case reports of decreased hematopoietic effect
Fluorouracil: Concentrations of fluorouracil doubled in patients with gastrointestinal carcinoma who received interferon alfa-2b.
Melphalan: Interferon alfa may decrease the serum concentrations of melphalan; monitor.
Prednisone: Prednisone may decrease the therapeutic effects of interferon alfa. Risk: Moderate.
Ribavirin: Concurrent therapy may increase the risk of hemolytic anemia.
Theophylline: Interferon alfa may decrease the P450 isoenzyme metabolism of theophylline. Risk: Moderate.
Warfarin: Interferons may increase the anticoagulant effects of warfarin; monitor.
Zidovudine: Interferons may decrease the metabolism of zidovudine; monitor.

Nutritional/Herbal/Ethanol Interactions Ethanol: Avoid use in patients with hepatitis C virus.

Adverse Reactions

>10%:

Central nervous system: Headache (56%), fatigue (52%), depression (16% to 29%), anxiety/emotional liability/irritability (28%), insomnia (23%), fever (22%), dizziness (12%), impaired concentration (5% to 12%), pain (12%)
Dermatologic: Alopecia (22%), pruritus (12%), dry skin (11%)
Gastrointestinal: Nausea (26%), anorexia (20%), diarrhea (18%), abdominal pain (15%), weight loss (11%)
Local: Injection site inflammation/reaction (47%),
Neuromuscular & skeletal: Musculoskeletal pain (56%), myalgia (38% to 42%), rigors (23% to 45%)
Respiratory: Epistaxis (14%), nasopharyngitis (11%)
Miscellaneous: Flu-like syndrome (46%), viral infection (11%)

>1% to 10%:

Cardiovascular: Flushing (6%)
Central nervous system: Malaise (8%)
Dermatologic: Rash (6%), dermatitis (7%)
Endocrine & metabolic: Hypothyroidism (5%)
Gastrointestinal: Vomiting (7%), dyspepsia (6%), taste perversion
Hematologic: Neutropenia, thrombocytopenia
Hepatic: Hepatomegaly (6%), transaminases increased (10%; transient)
Local: Injection site pain (2%)
Neuromuscular & skeletal: Hypertonia (5%)
Respiratory: Pharyngitis (10%), sinusitis (7%), cough (6%)
Miscellaneous: Diaphoresis (6%)

≤1% (Limited to important or life-threatening): Anaphylaxis, angioedema, aplastic anemia, arrhythmia, autoimmune disorder (eg, thyroiditis, thrombocytopenia, rheumatoid arthritis, interstitial nephritis, systemic lupus erythematosus, psoriasis), diabetes mellitus, dyspnea, facial oculomotor nerve palsy, hallucinations, hemorrhagic colitis, homicidal ideation, hyperthyroidism, hypotension, MI, nerve palsy, neutralizing antibodies, pancreatitis, pneumonia, pneumonitis, psychosis, pulmonary infiltrates, retinal hemorrhage, retinal ischemia, severe depression, severe neutropenia (<0.5 x 10^9/L), severe thrombocytopenia (<50,000/mm^3), suicidal behavior, suicidal ideation, supraventricular arrhythmia, tachycardia, transient ischemic attack, urticaria

Overdosage/Toxicology Limited experience with accidental use of doses >10.5 times the intended dose. No serious side effects noted. Treatment is symptom-directed and supportive.

Dosing

Adults:

Chronic hepatitis C: SubQ: Administer dose once weekly; **Note:** Usual duration is for 1 year; after 24 weeks of treatment, if serum HCV RNA is not below the limit of detection of the assay, consider discontinuation:

Monotherapy: Initial:

≤45 kg: 40 mcg
46-56 kg: 50 mcg
57-72 kg: 64 mcg

73-88 kg: 80 mcg
89-106 kg: 96 mcg
107-136 kg: 120 mcg
137-160 kg: 150 mcg

Combination therapy with ribavirin (400 mg twice daily): Initial: 1.5 mcg/kg/week
<40 kg: 50 mcg
40-50 kg: 64 mcg
51-60 kg: 80 mcg
61-75 kg: 96 mcg
76-85 kg: 120 mcg
>85 kg: 150 mcg

Dose adjustment if serious adverse event occurs: Depression (severity based upon DSM-IV criteria):

Mild depression: No dosage adjustment required; evaluate once weekly by visit/phone call. If depression remains stable, continue weekly visits. If depression improves, resume normal visit schedule.

Moderate depression: Decrease interferon dose by 50%; evaluate once weekly with an office visit at least every other week. If depression remains stable, consider psychiatric evaluation and continue with reduced dosing. If symptoms improve and remain stable for 4 weeks, resume normal visit schedule; continue reduced dosing or return to normal dose.

Severe depression: Discontinue interferon and ribavirin permanently. Obtain immediate psychiatric consultation.

Elderly: May require dosage reduction based upon renal dysfunction, but no established guidelines are available.

Pediatrics: Safety and efficacy have not been established.

Renal Impairment: Monitor for signs and symptoms of toxicity and if toxicity occurs then adjust dose. Do not use in patients with Cl_{cr} <50 mL/minute. Patients were excluded from the clinical trials if serum creatinine >1.5 times the upper limits of normal.

Hepatic Impairment: Contraindicated in decompensated liver disease

Available Dosage Forms

Injection, powder for reconstitution [prefilled syringe] (Redipen™): 50 mcg, 80 mcg, 120 mcg, 150 mcg [packaged with alcohol swabs and needle for injection]

Injection, powder for reconstitution [vial]: 50 mcg, 80 mcg, 120 mcg, 150 mcg [packaged with SWFI, alcohol swabs, and syringes]

Nursing Guidelines

Patient Education: You may be taught to give yourself the injection if you are willing and able to learn. Blood work will be done before the start of this medicine and during its use. Other tests may be needed depending on your medical history. If you have diabetes or have high blood pressure, get an eye examination before starting treatment. Maintain adequate hydration (2-3 L/day of fluids) unless instructed to restrict fluid intake. Avoid alcohol. You may experience flu-like syndrome (giving the medicine at bedtime or using acetaminophen may help), nausea and vomiting (small, frequent meals, frequent mouth care, sucking lozenges, or chewing gum may help), feeling tired (use caution when driving or engaging in tasks requiring alertness until response to drug is known), or headache. Report persistent abdominal pain, bloody diarrhea, and fever; symptoms of depression, suicidal ideas; unusual bruising or bleeding, any signs or symptoms of infection, unusual fatigue, chest pain or palpitations, respiratory difficulty, wheezing, severe nausea or vomiting. **Pregnancy/breast-feeding precautions:** Do not use in pregnancy. Reliable contraception should be used in women of childbearing potential. Breast-feeding is not recommended.

Pregnancy Risk Factor: C (manufacturer) as monotherapy; X in combination with ribavirin

Pregnancy Issues: Very high doses are abortifacient in Rhesus monkeys. Assumed to have abortifacient potential in humans. Case reports of use in pregnant women (usually interferon alfa-2a) did not result in adverse effects in the fetus or newborn. There are no adequate and well-controlled studies in pregnant women. Risk of maternal-infant transmission of hepatitis C is <5%. Reliable contraception should be used in women of childbearing potential. Not recommended for use in pregnancy (per manufacturer).

Lactation: Excretion in breast milk unknown/not recommended

Breast-Feeding Considerations: Case report of interferon alfa-2b: Too large in molecular weight to transfer into human milk in clinically relevant amounts.

(Continued)

Peginterferon Alfa-2b *(Continued)*

Breast-feeding is not linked to the spread of hepatitis C virus; however, if nipples are cracked or bleeding, breast-feeding is not recommended.

Administration

Reconstitution:

Redipen™: Hold cartridge upright and press the two halves together until there is a "click"; gently invert to mix, do not shake.

Vial: Add 0.7 mL of sterile water for injection, USP (supplied diluent) to the vial. Gently swirl. Do not re-enter vial after dose removed. Discard unused portion.

Compatibility: Do not mix with any other medicines.

Storage: Prior to reconstitution, store Redipen™ at 2°C to 8°C (36°F to 46°F) and store vials at 15°C to 30°C (59°F to 86°F). Once reconstituted each product should be used immediately or may be stored for ≤24 hours at 2°C to 8°C (36°F to 46°F). Products do not contain preservative. Do not freeze.

♦ **PEG-Intron®** *see* Peginterferon Alfa-2b *on page 1325*

♦ **Pegylated Interferon Alfa-2a** *see* Peginterferon Alfa-2a *on page 1321*

♦ **Pegylated Interferon Alfa-2b** *see* Peginterferon Alfa-2b *on page 1325*

Penicillin V Potassium (pen i SIL in vee poe TASS ee um)

U.S. Brand Names Veetids®

Synonyms Pen VK; Phenoxymethyl Penicillin

Pharmacologic Category Antibiotic, Penicillin

Medication Safety Issues

Sound-alike/look-alike issues:

Penicillin V procaine may be confused with penicillin G potassium

Use Treatment of infections caused by susceptible organisms involving the respiratory tract, otitis media, sinusitis, skin, and urinary tract; prophylaxis in rheumatic fever

Mechanism of Action Inhibits bacterial cell wall synthesis by binding to one or more of the penicillin binding proteins (PBPs); which in turn inhibits the final transpeptidation step of peptidoglycan synthesis in bacterial cell walls, thus inhibiting cell wall biosynthesis. Bacteria eventually lyse due to ongoing activity of cell wall autolytic enzymes (autolysins and murein hydrolases) while cell wall assembly is arrested.

Pharmacodynamics/Kinetics

Absorption: 60% to 73%

Distribution: Enters breast milk

Protein binding, plasma: 80%

Half-life elimination: 30 minutes; prolonged with renal impairment

Time to peak, serum: 0.5-1 hour

Excretion: Urine (as unchanged drug and metabolites)

Contraindications Hypersensitivity to penicillin or any component of the formulation

Warnings/Precautions Use with caution in patients with severe renal impairment (modify dosage), history of seizures, or hypersensitivity to cephalosporins

Drug Interactions

Aminoglycosides: May be synergistic against selected organisms

Methotrexate: Penicillins may increase the exposure to methotrexate during concurrent therapy; monitor.

Oral contraceptives: Anecdotal reports suggesting decreased contraceptive efficacy with penicillins have been refuted by more rigorous scientific and clinical data.

Probenecid, disulfiram: May increase penicillin levels

Tetracyclines: May decrease penicillin effectiveness

Warfarin: Effects of warfarin may be increased

Nutritional/Herbal/Ethanol Interactions Food: Decreases drug absorption rate; decreases drug serum concentration.

Lab Interactions False-positive or negative urinary glucose determination using Clinitest®; positive Coombs' [direct]; false-positive urinary and/or serum proteins

Adverse Reactions

>10%: Gastrointestinal: Mild diarrhea, vomiting, nausea, oral candidiasis

<1% (Limited to important or life-threatening): Acute interstitial nephritis, convulsions, hemolytic anemia, positive Coombs' reaction

Overdosage/Toxicology Symptoms of penicillin overdose include neuromuscular hypersensitivity (eg, agitation, hallucinations, asterixis, encephalopathy, confusion, and seizures). Electrolyte imbalance may occur if the preparation contains potassium or sodium salts, especially in renal failure. Hemodialysis may be helpful to aid in removal of the drug from blood; otherwise, treatment is supportive or symptom-directed.

Dosing

Adults & Elderly:

Systemic infections: Oral: 125-500 mg every 6-8 hours

Prophylaxis of pneumococcal infections: Oral: 250 mg twice daily

Prophylaxis of recurrent rheumatic fever: Oral: 250 mg twice daily

Pediatrics:

Systemic infections: Oral:

<12 years: 25-50 mg/kg/day in divided doses every 6-8 hours; maximum dose: 3 g/day

≥12 years: 125-500 mg every 6-8 hours

Prophylaxis of pneumococcal infections: Oral:

<5 years: 125 mg twice daily

≥5 years: 250 mg twice daily

Prophylaxis of recurrent rheumatic fever: Oral:

<5 years: 125 mg twice daily

≥5 years: 250 mg twice daily

Renal Impairment:

Cl_{cr} 10-50 mL/minute: Administer every 8-12 hours.

Cl_{cr} <10 mL/minute: Administer every 12-16 hours.

Available Dosage Forms Note: 250 mg = 400,000 units

Powder for oral solution: 125 mg/5 mL (100 mL, 200 mL); 250 mg/5 mL (100 mL, 200 mL)

Tablet: 250 mg, 500 mg

Nursing Guidelines

Assessment: Assess for allergy history prior to starting therapy. See Contraindications and Warnings/Precautions for use cautions. Assess potential for interactions with other prescriptions, OTC medications, or herbal products patient may be taking (see Drug Interactions). Advise patients with diabetes about use of Clinitest®. Assess results of laboratory tests (see below), therapeutic effectiveness, and adverse reactions (see Adverse Reactions and Overdose/Toxicology). Teach patient proper use, possible side effects/appropriate interventions, and adverse symptoms to report (see Patient Education).

Monitoring Laboratory Tests: Periodic renal and hematologic function during prolonged therapy; perform culture and sensitivity before administering first dose

Dietary Considerations: Take on an empty stomach 1 hour before or 2 hours after meals.

Patient Education: Inform prescriber of all prescriptions, OTC medications, or herbal products you are taking, and any allergies you have. Do not take any new medication during therapy unless approved by prescriber. Take as directed at intervals around-the-clock, preferable on an empty stomach (1 hour before or 2 hours after a meal). Take entire prescription; do not skip doses or discontinue without consulting prescriber. Take a missed dose as soon as possible. If almost time for next dose, skip the missed dose and return to your regular schedule. Do not take a double dose. Maintain adequate hydration (2-3 L/day of fluids) unless instructed to restrict fluid intake. If you have diabetes, drug may cause false test results with Clinitest®, consult prescriber for alternative method of glucose monitoring. May cause nausea or vomiting (small, frequent meals, frequent mouth care, chewing gum, or sucking lozenges may help); or diarrhea (buttermilk, boiled milk, or yogurt may help). Report persistent adverse effects; signs of opportunistic infection (eg, fever, chills, unhealed sores, white plaques in mouth or vagina, purulent vaginal discharge, fatigue); or signs of hypersensitivity reaction (rash, hives, itching, swelling of lips, tongue, mouth, or throat).

Pregnancy Risk Factor: B

Lactation: Enters breast milk (other penicillins are compatible with breast-feeding)

Breast-Feeding Considerations: No data reported; however, other penicillins may be taken while breast-feeding.

Administration

Oral: Administer around-the-clock to promote less variation in peak and trough serum levels. Take on an empty stomach 1 hour before or 2 hours after meals, to enhance absorption, take until gone, do not skip doses.

Storage: Refrigerate suspension after reconstitution; discard after 14 days.

(Continued)

Penicillin G Benzathine (pen i SIL in jee BENZ a theen)

U.S. Brand Names Bicillin® L-A

Synonyms Benzathine Benzylpenicillin; Benzathine Penicillin G; Benzylpenicillin Benzathine

Pharmacologic Category Antibiotic, Penicillin

Medication Safety Issues

Sound-alike/look-alike issues:

Penicillin may be confused with penicillamine

Bicillin® may be confused with Wycillin®

Bicillin® C-R (penicillin G benzathine and penicillin G procaine) may be confused with Bicillin® L-A (penicillin G benzathine). Penicillin G benzathine is the only product currently approved for the treatment of syphilis. Administration of penicillin G benzathine and penicillin G procaine combination instead of Bicillin® L-A may result in inadequate treatment response.

Penicillin G benzathine may only be administered by deep intramuscular injection; intravenous administration of penicillin G benzathine has been associated with cardiopulmonary arrest and death.

Use Active against some gram-positive organisms, few gram-negative organisms such as *Neisseria gonorrhoeae*, and some anaerobes and spirochetes; used in the treatment of syphilis; used only for the treatment of mild to moderately severe infections caused by organisms susceptible to low concentrations of penicillin G or for prophylaxis of infections caused by these organisms

Mechanism of Action Interferes with bacterial cell wall synthesis during active multiplication, causing cell wall death and resultant bactericidal activity against susceptible bacteria

Pharmacodynamics/Kinetics

Duration: 1-4 weeks (dose dependent); larger doses result in more sustained levels

Absorption: I.M.: Slow

Time to peak, serum: 12-24 hours

Contraindications Hypersensitivity to penicillin or any component of the formulation

Warnings/Precautions Use with caution in patients with impaired renal function, seizure disorder, or history of hypersensitivity to other beta-lactams; CDC and AAP do not currently recommend the use of penicillin G benzathine to treat congenital syphilis or neurosyphilis due to reported treatment failures and lack of published clinical data on its efficacy

Drug Interactions

Aminoglycosides: May be synergistic against selected organisms

Heparin: Heparin and parenteral penicillins may result in increased bleeding

Methotrexate: Penicillins may increase the exposure to methotrexate during concurrent therapy; monitor.

Oral contraceptives: Anecdotal reports suggesting decreased contraceptive efficacy with penicillins have been refuted by more rigorous scientific and clinical data.

Probenecid, disulfiram: May increase penicillin levels

Tetracyclines: May decrease penicillin effectiveness

Warfarin: Effects of warfarin may be increased

Lab Interactions Positive Coombs' [direct], false-positive urinary and/or serum proteins; false-positive or negative urinary glucose using Clinitest®

Adverse Reactions Frequency not defined.

Central nervous system: Convulsions, confusion, drowsiness, myoclonus, fever

Dermatologic: Rash

Endocrine & metabolic: Electrolyte imbalance

Hematologic: Positive Coombs' reaction, hemolytic anemia

Local: Pain, thrombophlebitis

Renal: Acute interstitial nephritis

Miscellaneous: Anaphylaxis, hypersensitivity reactions, Jarisch-Herxheimer reaction

Overdosage/Toxicology Symptoms of penicillin overdose include neuromuscular hypersensitivity (eg, agitation, hallucinations, asterixis, encephalopathy, confusion, and seizures). Electrolyte imbalance may occur if the preparation contains potassium or sodium salts, especially in renal failure. Hemodialysis may be helpful to aid in removal of the drug from blood; otherwise, treatment is supportive or symptom-directed.

Dosing

Adults & Elderly:

Group A streptococcal upper respiratory infection: I.M.: 1.2 million units as a single dose

Prophylaxis of recurrent rheumatic fever: I.M.: 1.2 million units every 3-4 weeks or 600,000 units twice monthly

Early syphilis: I.M.: 2.4 million units as a single dose in 2 injection sites

Syphilis of more than 1-year duration: I.M.: 2.4 million units in 2 injection sites once weekly for 3 doses

Note: Not indicated as single drug therapy for neurosyphilis, but may be given 1 time/week for 3 weeks following I.V. treatment (refer to Penicillin G monograph for dosing)

Pediatrics:

Asymptomatic congenital syphilis: I.M.: Neonates >1200 g: 50,000 units/kg for 1 dose

Group A streptococcal upper respiratory infection: I.M.: Infants and Children: 25,000-50,000 units/kg as a single dose; maximum: 1.2 million units

Prophylaxis of recurrent rheumatic fever: I.M.: Infants and Children: 25,000-50,000 units/kg every 3-4 weeks; maximum: 1.2 million units/dose

Early syphilis: I.M.: Infants and Children: 50,000 units/kg as a single injection; maximum: 2.4 million units

Syphilis of more than 1-year duration: I.M.: Infants and Children: 50,000 units/kg every week for 3 doses; maximum: 2.4 million units/dose

Available Dosage Forms Injection, suspension [prefilled syringe]: 600,000 units/mL (1 mL, 2 mL, 4 mL)

Nursing Guidelines

Assessment: Assess for allergy history prior to starting therapy. See Contraindications and Warnings/Precautions for use cautions. Assess potential for interactions with other prescriptions, OTC medications, or herbal products patient may be taking (see Drug Interactions). Advise patients with diabetes about use of Clinitest®. Assess for therapeutic effectiveness and adverse reactions (eg, hypersensitivity reactions, opportunistic infection - see Adverse Reactions and Overdose/Toxicology). Teach patient possible side effects/appropriate interventions and adverse symptoms to report (see Patient Education).

Monitoring Laboratory Tests: Perform culture and sensitivity before administering first dose.

Patient Education: Inform prescriber of all prescriptions, OTC medications, or herbal products you are taking, and any allergies you have. Do not take any new medication during therapy unless approved by prescriber. This drug can only be given by injection. Report immediately any redness, swelling, burning, or pain at infusion site or any signs of allergic reaction (eg, respiratory difficulty or swallowing, chest tightness, rash, hives, swelling of lips or mouth). Maintain adequate hydration (2-3 L/day of fluids) unless instructed to restrict fluid intake. If being treated for sexually-transmitted disease, partner will also need to be treated. If you have diabetes, drug may cause false test results with Clinitest®; consult prescriber for alternative method of glucose monitoring. May cause confusion or drowsiness (use caution when driving or engaging in tasks that require alertness until response to drug is known). Report persistent adverse effects or signs of opportunistic infection (eg, fever, chills, unhealed sores, white plaques in mouth or vagina, purulent vaginal discharge, fatigue).

Pregnancy Risk Factor: B

Lactation: Enters breast milk/compatible

Administration

I.M.: Administer by deep I.M. injection in the upper outer quadrant of the buttock. Do **not** give I.V., intra-arterially, or SubQ. When doses are repeated, rotate the injection site.

Storage: Store in refrigerator.

Penicillin G (Parenteral/Aqueous)

(pen i SIL in jee, pa REN ter al, AYE kwee us)

U.S. Brand Names Pfizerpen®

Synonyms Benzylpenicillin Potassium; Benzylpenicillin Sodium; Crystalline Penicillin; Penicillin G Potassium; Penicillin G Sodium

(Continued)

Penicillin G (Parenteral/Aqueous) *(Continued)*

Pharmacologic Category Antibiotic, Penicillin

Medication Safety Issues

Sound-alike/look-alike issues:

Penicillin may be confused with penicillamine

Use Active against some gram-positive organisms, generally not *Staphylococcus aureus*; some gram-negative organisms such as *Neisseria gonorrhoeae*, and some anaerobes and spirochetes

Mechanism of Action Interferes with bacterial cell wall synthesis during active multiplication, causing cell wall death and resultant bactericidal activity against susceptible bacteria

Pharmacodynamics/Kinetics

Distribution: Poor penetration across blood-brain barrier, despite inflamed meninges; crosses placenta; enters breast milk

Relative diffusion from blood into CSF: Good only with inflammation (exceeds usual MICs)

CSF:blood level ratio: Normal meninges: <1%; Inflamed meninges: 3% to 5%

Protein binding: 65%

Metabolism: Hepatic (30%) to penicilloic acid

Half-life elimination:

Neonates: <6 days old: 3.2-3.4 hours; 7-13 days old: 1.2-2.2 hours; >14 days old: 0.9-1.9 hours

Children and Adults: Normal renal function: 20-50 minutes

End-stage renal disease: 3.3-5.1 hours

Time to peak, serum: I.M.: ~30 minutes; I.V. ~1 hour

Excretion: Urine

Contraindications Hypersensitivity to penicillin or any component of the formulation

Warnings/Precautions Avoid intra-arterial administration or injection into or near major peripheral nerves or blood vessels since such injections may cause severe and/or permanent neurovascular damage; use with caution in patients with renal impairment (dosage reduction required), pre-existing seizure disorders, or with a history of hypersensitivity to cephalosporins

Drug Interactions

Aminoglycosides: May be synergistic against selected organisms

Methotrexate: Penicillins may increase the exposure to methotrexate during concurrent therapy; monitor.

Oral contraceptives: Anecdotal reports suggesting decreased contraceptive efficacy with penicillins have been refuted by more rigorous scientific and clinical data.

Probenecid, disulfiram: May increase penicillin levels

Tetracyclines: May decrease penicillin effectiveness

Warfarin: Effects of warfarin may be increased

Lab Interactions False-positive or negative urinary glucose determination using Clinitest®; positive Coombs' [direct]; false-positive urinary and/or serum proteins

Adverse Reactions Frequency not defined.

Central nervous system: Convulsions, confusion, drowsiness, myoclonus, fever

Dermatologic: Rash

Endocrine & metabolic: Electrolyte imbalance

Hematologic: Positive Coombs' reaction, hemolytic anemia

Local: Injection site reaction, thrombophlebitis

Renal: Acute interstitial nephritis

Miscellaneous: Anaphylaxis, hypersensitivity reactions, Jarisch-Herxheimer reaction

Overdosage/Toxicology Symptoms of penicillin overdose include neuromuscular hypersensitivity (eg, agitation, hallucinations, asterixis, encephalopathy, confusion, and seizures). Electrolyte imbalance may occur if the preparation contains potassium or sodium salts, especially in renal failure. Treatment is supportive or symptom-directed.

Dosing

Adults & Elderly:

Susceptible infections: I.M., I.V.: 2-24 million units/day in divided doses every 4 hours depending on sensitivity of the organism and severity of the infection

Neurosyphilis: I.M., I.V.: 18-24 million units/day in divided doses every 4 hours (or by continuous infusion) for 10-14 days

Pediatrics:

Susceptible infections: I.M., I.V.:

Neonates:

<7 days, <2000 g: 25,000-50,000 units/kg every 12 hours
<7 days, >2000 g: 25,000-50,000 units/kg every 8 hours
>7 days, <2000 g: 25,000-50,000 units/kg every 8 hours
>7 days, >2000 g: 25,000-50,000 units/kg every 6 hours

Infants and Children:

Mild-to-moderate infections: 25,000-50,000 units/kg/day in 4 divided doses
Severe infections: 250,000 to 400,000 units/kg/day in divided doses every 4-6 hours; maximum dose: 24 million units/day

Congenital syphilis:

Neonates:

≤7 days: 50,000 units/kg I.V. every 12 hours for a total of 10 days
>7 days: 50,000 units/kg I.V. every 8 hours for a total of 10 days

Infants: 50,000 units/kg every 4-6 hours for 10 days

Renal Impairment: Dosage modification is required in patients with renal insufficiency.

Cl_{cr} >10 mL/minute: Administer full loading dose followed by ½ loading dose given every 4-5 hours

Cl_{cr} <10 mL/minute: Administer full loading dose followed by ½ loading dose given every 8-10 hours

Available Dosage Forms

Infusion, as potassium [premixed iso-osmotic dextrose solution, frozen]: 1 million units (50 mL), 2 million units (50 mL), 3 million units (50 mL) [contains sodium 1.02 mEq and potassium 1.7 mEq per 1 million units]

Injection, powder for reconstitution, as potassium (Pfizerpen®): 5 million units, 20 million units [contains sodium 6.8 mg (0.3 mEq) and potassium 65.6 mg (1.68 mEq) per 1 million units]

Injection, powder for reconstitution, as sodium: 5 million units [contains sodium 1.68 mEq per 1 million units]

Nursing Guidelines

Assessment: Assess results of culture and sensitivity tests and patient's allergy history prior to starting therapy. Use with caution and monitor closely in presence of renal impairment or seizure disorder. Assess potential for interactions with other pharmacological agents (eg, decreased or increased levels/effects of penicillin G). Avoid intravascular or intra-arterial administration or injection into or near major peripheral nerves or blood vessels; may cause severe and/or permanent neurovascular damage. Advise patients with diabetes about use of Clinitest®; may cause false positive or negative. Assess effectiveness (resolution of infections) and adverse reactions (eg, hypersensitivity reactions, opportunistic infection [fever, chills, unhealed sores, white plaques in mouth or vagina, purulent vaginal discharge, fatigue], CNS changes, thrombophlebitis). Teach patient possible side effects/appropriate interventions and adverse symptoms to report.

Monitoring Laboratory Tests: Perform culture and sensitivity before administering first dose.

Dietary Considerations:

Injection powder for reconstitution as potassium contains sodium 6.8 mg (0.3 mEq) and potassium 65.6 mg (1.68 mEq) per 1 million units

Patient Education: This drug can only be given by injection or infusion. Report immediately any redness, swelling, burning, or pain at infusion site or any signs of allergic reaction (eg, respiratory or swallowing difficulty, chest tightness, rash, hives, swelling of lips or mouth). Maintain adequate hydration (2-3 L/day of fluids) unless instructed to restrict fluid intake. If being treated for sexually-transmitted disease, partner will also need to be treated. If you have diabetes, drug may cause false test results with Clinitest®, consult prescriber for alternative method of glucose monitoring. May cause confusion or drowsiness (use caution when driving or engaging in tasks that require alertness until response to drug is known). Report persistent adverse effects or signs of opportunistic infection (eg, fever, chills, unhealed sores, white plaques in mouth or vagina, purulent vaginal discharge, fatigue).

Geriatric Considerations: Despite a reported prolonged half-life, it is usually not necessary to adjust the dose of penicillin G or VK in the elderly to account for renal function changes with age, however, it is advised to calculate an estimated creatinine clearance and adjust dose accordingly. Consider sodium content in patients who may be sensitive to volume expansion (ie, CHF).

(Continued)

Penicillin G (Parenteral/Aqueous) *(Continued)*

Pregnancy Risk Factor: B

Lactation: Enters breast milk/compatible

Perioperative/Anesthesia/Other Concerns: One million units is approximately equal to 625 mg.

Administration

I.M.: Administer I.M. by deep injection in the upper outer quadrant of the buttock. Administer injection around-the-clock to promote less variation in peak and trough levels.

I.V.: While I.M. route is preferred route of administration, large doses should be administered by continuous I.V. infusion. Determine volume and rate of fluid administration required in a 24-hour period. Add appropriate daily dosage to this fluid. Rapid administration or excessive dosage can cause electrolyte imbalance, cardiac arrhythmias, and/or seizures.

Compatibility: Inactivated in acidic or alkaline solutions

Penicillin G potassium: Stable in dextran 6% in dextrose, dextran 6% in NS, D_5LR, $D_5{}^1/_4NS$, $D_5{}^1/_2NS$, D_5NS, D_5W, $D_{10}W$, LR, $^1/_2NS$, NS, hetastarch 6%; **incompatible** with dextran 70 6% in dextrose, dextran 40 10% in dextrose

Compatibility in syringe: Incompatible with metoclopramide

Compatibility when admixed: Incompatible with aminoglycosides, aminophylline, amphotericin B, chlorpromazine, dopamine, floxacillin, hydroxyzine, metaraminol, pentobarbital, phenytoin, prochlorperazine mesylate, promazine, thiopental, vancomycin, vitamin B complex with C with oxytetracycline

Penicillin G sodium: Stable in dextran 40 10%; **incompatible** with fat emulsion 10%

Compatibility when admixed: Incompatible with amphotericin B, bleomycin, chlorpromazine, cytarabine, floxacillin, hydroxyzine, methylprednisolone sodium succinate, prochlorperazine mesylate, promethazine, vancomycin

Storage:

Penicillin G potassium powder for injection should be stored below 86°F (30°C); following reconstitution, solution may be stored for up to 7 days under refrigeration. Premixed bags for infusion should be stored in the freezer (-20°C to -4°F); frozen bags may be thawed at room temperature or in refrigerator. Once thawed, solution is stable for 14 days if stored in refrigerator or for 24 hours when stored at room temperature. Do not re-freeze once thawed.

Penicillin G sodium powder for injection should be stored at controlled room temperature; reconstituted solution may be stored under refrigeration for up to 3 days.

Related Information

Prevention of Wound Infection and Sepsis in Surgical Patients *on page 1830*

- **Penicillin G Potassium** *see* Penicillin G (Parenteral/Aqueous) *on page 1331*
- **Penicillin G Sodium** *see* Penicillin G (Parenteral/Aqueous) *on page 1331*
- **Penlac®** *see* Ciclopirox *on page 390*
- **Pentam-300®** *see* Pentamidine *on page 1334*

Pentamidine (pen TAM i deen)

U.S. Brand Names NebuPent®; Pentam-300®

Synonyms Pentamidine Isethionate

Pharmacologic Category Antibiotic, Miscellaneous

Use Treatment and prevention of pneumonia caused by *Pneumocystis carinii* (PCP)

Unlabeled/Investigational Use Treatment of trypanosomiasis and visceral leishmaniasis

Mechanism of Action Interferes with RNA/DNA, phospholipids and protein synthesis, through inhibition of oxidative phosphorylation and/or interference with incorporation of nucleotides and nucleic acids into RNA and DNA, in protozoa

Pharmacodynamics/Kinetics

Absorption: I.M.: Well absorbed; Inhalation: Limited systemic absorption

Half-life elimination: Terminal: 6.4-9.4 hours; may be prolonged with severe renal impairment

Excretion: Urine (33% to 66% as unchanged drug)

Contraindications Hypersensitivity to pentamidine isethionate or any component of the formulation (inhalation and injection)

Warnings/Precautions Use with caution in patients with diabetes mellitus, renal or hepatic dysfunction, hyper-/hypotension, leukopenia, thrombocytopenia, asthma, or hypo-/hyperglycemia.

Drug Interactions **Substrate** of CYP2C19 (major); **Inhibits** CYP2C8/9 (weak), 2C19 (weak), 2D6 (weak), 3A4 (weak)

CYP2C19 inducers: May decrease the levels/effects of pentamidine. Example inducers include aminoglutethimide, carbamazepine, phenytoin, and rifampin.

CYP2C19 inhibitors: May increase the levels/effects of pentamidine. Example inhibitors include delavirdine, fluconazole, fluvoxamine, gemfibrozil, isoniazid, omeprazole, and ticlopidine.

QT_c-prolonging agents: Pentamidine may potentiate the effect of other drugs which prolong QT interval (cisapride, sparfloxacin, gatifloxacin, moxifloxacin, pimozide, and type Ia and type III antiarrhythmics).

Nutritional/Herbal/Ethanol Interactions Ethanol: Avoid ethanol (may increase CNS depression or aggravate hypoglycemia).

Adverse Reactions

Inhalation:

>10%:

Cardiovascular: Chest pain

Dermatologic: Rash

Respiratory: Wheezing, dyspnea, cough, pharyngitis

1% to 10%: Gastrointestinal: Bitter or metallic taste

<1% (Limited to important or life-threatening): Hypoglycemia, renal insufficiency

Systemic:

>10%:

Cardiovascular: Hypotension

Dermatologic: Rash

Endocrine & metabolic: Hyperglycemia or hypoglycemia

Gastrointestinal: Nausea, vomiting, anorexia, diarrhea

Hematologic: Leukopenia or neutropenia, thrombocytopenia

Hepatic: Elevated LFTs

Renal: Nephrotoxicity

1% to 10%:

Cardiovascular: Cardiac arrhythmia

Gastrointestinal: Pancreatitis, metallic taste

Hematologic: Anemia

Local: Local reactions at injection site

<1% (Limited to important or life-threatening): Arrhythmias

Overdosage/Toxicology Symptoms of overdose include hypotension, hypoglycemia, and cardiac arrhythmias. Treatment is supportive.

Dosing

Adults & Elderly:

Treatment of PCP pneumonia: I.M., I.V. (I.V. preferred): 4 mg/kg/day once daily for 14 days

Prevention of PCP pneumonia: Inhalation: 300 mg every 4 weeks via Respirgard® II nebulizer

Pediatrics:

Treatment of PCP pneumonia: I.M., I.V. (I.V. preferred): Children: 4 mg/kg/day once daily for 10-14 days

Prevention of PCP pneumonia: Children:

I.M., I.V.: 4 mg/kg monthly or every 2 weeks

Inhalation (aerosolized pentamidine in children ≥5 years): 300 mg/dose given every 3-4 weeks via Respirgard® II inhaler (8 mg/kg dose has also been used in children <5 years)

Treatment of trypanosomiasis (unlabeled use): I.V.: 4 mg/kg/day once daily for 10 days

Renal Impairment:

Cl_{cr} 10-50 mL/minute: Administer dose every 24-36 hours.

Cl_{cr} <10 mL/minute: Administer dose every 48 hours.

Not removed by hemo- or peritoneal dialysis or continuous arteriovenous or venovenous hemofiltration. Supplemental dose is not necessary.

Available Dosage Forms

Injection, powder for reconstitution, as isethionate (Pentam-300®): 300 mg

Powder for nebulization, as isethionate (NebuPent®): 300 mg

(Continued)

Pentamidine *(Continued)*

Nursing Guidelines

Assessment: Assess for allergy history prior to starting therapy. See Contraindications and Warnings/Precautions for use cautions. Assess potential for interactions with other prescriptions, OTC medications, or herbal products patient may be taking (see Drug Interactions). **I.V./I.M.:** Patients should be lying down. Blood pressure, cardiac status, and respiratory function should be monitored closely during I.V. administration or following I.M. injection. Assess results of laboratory tests (see below), therapeutic effectiveness, and adverse reactions (see Adverse Reactions and Overdose/Toxicology). Teach patient proper use, possible side effects/appropriate interventions, and adverse symptoms to report (see Patient Education). Breast-feeding is contraindicated.

Monitoring Laboratory Tests: Liver and renal function, blood glucose, serum potassium and calcium, ECG, CBC with platelets

Patient Education: Inform prescriber of all prescriptions, OTC medications, or herbal products you are taking, and any allergies you have. Do not take any new medication during therapy without consulting prescriber. I.V. or I.M. preparations must be given every day. Inhalant drug must be prepared and used with a nebulizer as directed once every 4 weeks. Frequent blood tests and blood pressure checks will be required while using this drug. PCP pneumonia may still occur despite pentamidine use. Maintain adequate hydration (2-3 L/day of fluids) unless instructed to restrict fluid intake. Avoid alcohol. If you have diabetes, monitor glucose levels closely and frequently. May cause hypotension (use caution when rising from sitting or lying position or when climbing stairs); or metallic taste, nausea, vomiting, or anorexia (small, frequent meals, frequent mouth care, chewing gum, or sucking lozenges may help). Report chest pain or irregular heartbeat; unusual confusion or hallucinations; rash; or unusual wheezing, coughing, or respiratory difficulty. **Pregnancy/breast-feeding precautions:** Inform prescriber if you are or intend to become pregnant. Do not breast-feed.

Geriatric Considerations: Ten percent of acquired immunodeficiency syndrome (AIDS) cases are in the elderly and this figure is expected to increase. Pentamidine has not as yet been studied exclusively in this population. Adjust dose for renal function.

Pregnancy Risk Factor: C

Lactation: Excretion in breast milk unknown/contraindicated

Administration

I.M.: Deep I.M.

I.V.: Do not use NS as a diluent. Infuse I.V. slowly over a period of at least 60 minutes or administer deep I.M.

Reconstitution: Powder for inhalation should be reconstituted with sterile water for injection (6 mL per 300 mg vial). Powder for injection may be reconstituted with sterile water for injection or D_5W (SWFI should be used for I.M. injections). **Do not use NS as a diluent.**

Compatibility: Reconstituted vials with SWFI (60-100 mg/mL) are stable for 48 hours at room temperature protected from light. Solutions for injection (1-2.5 mg/mL) in D_5W are stable for at least 24 hours at room temperature.

Y-site administration: Incompatible: Aldesleukin, cefazolin, cefoperazone, cefotaxime, cefoxitin, ceftazidime, ceftriaxone, fluconazole, foscarnet, linezolid

Storage: Store intact vials at controlled room temperature and protect from light. Reconstituted vials with SWFI (60-100 mg/mL) are stable for 48 hours at room temperature and do not require light protection. Diluted solutions in 50-250 mL D_5W for infusion (1-2.5 mg/mL) are stable for at least 24 hours at room temperature.

♦ **Pentamidine Isethionate** *see* Pentamidine *on page 1334*
♦ **Pentasa®** *see* Mesalamine *on page 1105*

Pentobarbital (pen toe BAR bi tal)

U.S. Brand Names Nembutal®

Synonyms Pentobarbital Sodium

Pharmacologic Category Anticonvulsant, Barbiturate; Barbiturate

Medication Safety Issues

Sound-alike/look-alike issues:

Pentobarbital may be confused with phenobarbital

Nembutal® may be confused with Myambutol®

Use Sedative/hypnotic; preanesthetic; high-dose barbiturate coma for treatment of increased intracranial pressure or status epilepticus unresponsive to other therapy

Mechanism of Action Short-acting barbiturate with sedative, hypnotic, and anticonvulsant properties. Barbiturates depress the sensory cortex, decrease motor activity, alter cerebellar function, and produce drowsiness, sedation, and hypnosis. In high doses, barbiturates exhibit anticonvulsant activity; barbiturates produce dose-dependent respiratory depression.

Pharmacodynamics/Kinetics

Onset of action: I.M.: 10-15 minutes; I.V.: ~1 minute

Duration: I.V.: 15 minutes

Distribution: V_d: Children: 0.8 L/kg; Adults: 1 L/kg

Protein binding: 35% to 55%

Metabolism: Extensively hepatic via hydroxylation and oxidation pathways

Half-life elimination: Terminal: Children: 25 hours; Adults: Healthy: 22 hours (range: 15-50 hours)

Excretion: Urine (<1% as unchanged drug)

Contraindications Hypersensitivity to barbiturates or any component of the formulation; marked hepatic impairment; dyspnea or airway obstruction; porphyria; pregnancy

Warnings/Precautions Tolerance to hypnotic effect can occur; do not use for >2 weeks to treat insomnia. Potential for drug dependency exists, abrupt cessation may precipitate withdrawal, including status epilepticus in epileptic patients. Do not administer to patients in acute pain. Use caution in elderly, debilitated, renally impaired, hepatic dysfunction, or pediatric patients. May cause paradoxical responses, including agitation and hyperactivity, particularly in acute pain and pediatric patients. Use with caution in patients with depression or suicidal tendencies, or in patients with a history of drug abuse. Tolerance, psychological and physical dependence may occur with prolonged use.

May cause CNS depression, which may impair physical or mental abilities. Patients must be cautioned about performing tasks which require mental alertness (eg, operating machinery or driving). Effects with other sedative drugs or ethanol may be potentiated. Use of this agent as a hypnotic in the elderly is not recommended due to its long half-life and potential for physical and psychological dependence.

May cause respiratory depression or hypotension, particularly when administered intravenously. Use with caution in hemodynamically unstable patients or patients with respiratory disease. High doses (loading doses of 15-35 mg/kg given over 1-2 hours) have been utilized to induce pentobarbital coma, but these higher doses often cause hypotension requiring vasopressor therapy.

Drug Interactions Induces CYP2A6 (strong), 3A4 (strong)

Acetaminophen: Barbiturates may enhance the hepatotoxic potential of acetaminophen overdoses

Antiarrhythmics: Barbiturates may increase the metabolism of antiarrhythmics, decreasing their clinical effect; includes disopyramide, propafenone, and quinidine

Anticonvulsants: Barbiturates may increase the metabolism of anticonvulsants; includes ethosuximide, felbamate (possibly), lamotrigine, phenytoin, tiagabine, topiramate, and zonisamide; does not appear to affect gabapentin or levetiracetam

Antineoplastics: Limited evidence suggests that enzyme-inducing anticonvulsant therapy may reduce the effectiveness of some chemotherapy regimens (specifically in ALL); teniposide and methotrexate may be cleared more rapidly in these patients

Antipsychotics: Barbiturates may enhance the metabolism (decrease the efficacy) of antipsychotics; monitor for altered response; dose adjustment may be needed

Beta-blockers: Metabolism of beta-blockers may be increased and clinical effect decreased; atenolol and nadolol are unlikely to interact given their renal elimination

Calcium channel blockers: Barbiturates may enhance the metabolism of calcium channel blockers, decreasing their clinical effect

Chloramphenicol: Barbiturates may increase the metabolism of chloramphenicol and chloramphenicol may inhibit barbiturate metabolism; monitor for altered response

(Continued)

Pentobarbital *(Continued)*

Cimetidine: Barbiturates may enhance the metabolism of cimetidine, decreasing its clinical effect

CNS depressants: Sedative effects and/or respiratory depression with barbiturates may be additive with other CNS depressants; monitor for increased effect; includes ethanol, sedatives, antidepressants, narcotic analgesics, and benzodiazepines

Corticosteroids: Barbiturates may enhance the metabolism of corticosteroids, decreasing their clinical effect

Cyclosporine: Levels may be decreased by barbiturates; monitor

CYP2A6 substrates: Pentobarbital may decrease the levels/effects of CYP2A6 substrates. Example substrates include ifosfamide and rifampin.

CYP3A4 substrates: Pentobarbital may decrease the levels/effects of CYP3A4 substrates. Example substrates include benzodiazepines, calcium channel blockers, clarithromycin, cyclosporine, erythromycin, estrogens, mirtazapine, nateglinide, nefazodone, nevirapine, protease inhibitors, tacrolimus, and venlafaxine.

Doxycycline: Barbiturates may enhance the metabolism of doxycycline, decreasing its clinical effect; higher dosages may be required

Estrogens: Barbiturates may increase the metabolism of estrogens and reduce their efficacy

Felbamate may inhibit the metabolism of barbiturates and barbiturates may increase the metabolism of felbamate

Griseofulvin: Barbiturates may impair the absorption of griseofulvin, and griseofulvin metabolism may be increased by barbiturates, decreasing clinical effect

Guanfacine: Effect may be decreased by barbiturates

Immunosuppressants: Barbiturates may enhance the metabolism of immunosuppressants, decreasing its clinical effect; includes both cyclosporine and tacrolimus

Loop diuretics: Metabolism may be increased and clinical effects decreased; established for furosemide, effect with other loop diuretics not established

MAO inhibitors: Metabolism of barbiturates may be inhibited, increasing clinical effect or toxicity of the barbiturates

Methadone: Barbiturates may enhance the metabolism of methadone resulting in methadone withdrawal

Methoxyflurane: Barbiturates may enhance the nephrotoxic effects of methoxyflurane

Oral contraceptives: Barbiturates may enhance the metabolism of oral contraceptives, decreasing their clinical effect; an alternative method of contraception should be considered

Theophylline: Barbiturates may increase metabolism of theophylline derivatives and decrease their clinical effect

Tricyclic antidepressants: Barbiturates may increase metabolism of tricyclic antidepressants and decrease their clinical effect; sedative effects may be additive

Valproic acid: Metabolism of barbiturates may be inhibited by valproic acid; monitor for excessive sedation; a dose reduction may be needed

Warfarin: Barbiturates inhibit the hypoprothrombinemic effects of oral anticoagulants via increased metabolism; this combination should generally be avoided

Nutritional/Herbal/Ethanol Interactions Ethanol: Avoid ethanol (may increase CNS depression).

Lab Interactions Increased ammonia (B); decreased bilirubin (S)

Adverse Reactions Frequency not defined.

Cardiovascular: Bradycardia, hypotension, syncope

Central nervous system: Drowsiness, lethargy, CNS excitation or depression, impaired judgment, "hangover" effect, confusion, somnolence, agitation, hyperkinesia, ataxia, nervousness, headache, insomnia, nightmares, hallucinations, anxiety, dizziness

Dermatologic: Rash, exfoliative dermatitis, Stevens-Johnson syndrome

Gastrointestinal: Nausea, vomiting, constipation

Hematologic: Agranulocytosis, thrombocytopenia, megaloblastic anemia

Local: Pain at injection site, thrombophlebitis with I.V. use

Renal: Oliguria

Respiratory: Laryngospasm, respiratory depression, apnea (especially with rapid I.V. use), hypoventilation

Miscellaneous: Gangrene with inadvertent intra-arterial injection

Overdosage/Toxicology Symptoms of overdose include unsteady gait, slurred speech, confusion, jaundice, hypothermia, hypotension, respiratory depression, and coma. Treat symptomatically. Charcoal hemoperfusion may be beneficial in stage IV coma due to high serum concentration.

Dosing

Adults:

Hypnotic:

I.M.: 150-200 mg

I.V.: Initial: 100 mg, may repeat every 1-3 minutes up to 200-500 mg total dose

Preoperative sedation: I.M.: 150-200 mg

Barbiturate coma in head injury patients or status epilepticus: I.V.: Loading dose: 5-10 mg/kg given slowly over 1-2 hours; monitor blood pressure and respiratory rate; maintenance infusion: initial: 1 mg/kg/hour; may increase to 2-3 mg/kg/hour; maintain burst suppression on EEG

Status epilepticus: I.V.: Loading dose: 2-15 mg/kg given slowly over 1-2 hours; maintenance infusion: 0.5-3 mg/kg/hour. **Note**: Intubation required; monitor hemodynamics

Elderly: Not recommended for use in the elderly (see Geriatric Considerations).

Pediatrics:

Hypnotic: I.M.: 2-6 mg/kg; maximum: 100 mg/dose

Preoperative/preprocedure sedation: ≥6 months:

Note: Limited information is available for infants <6 months of age.

I.M.: 2-6 mg/kg; maximum: 100 mg/dose

I.V.: 1-3 mg/kg to a maximum of 100 mg until asleep

Conscious sedation prior to a procedure: I.V.:

Children 5-12 years: I.V.: 2 mg/kg 5-10 minutes before procedures, may repeat one time

Adolescents: 100 mg prior to a procedure

Barbiturate coma in head injury patients: I.V.: Loading dose: 5-10 mg/kg given slowly over 1-2 hours; monitor blood pressure and respiratory rate; Maintenance infusion: Initial: 1 mg/kg/hour; may increase to 2-3 mg/kg/hour; maintain burst suppression on EEG

Status epilepticus: I.V.: **Note**: Intubation required; monitor hemodynamics: Loading dose: 5-15 mg/kg given slowly over 1-2 hours; maintenance infusion: 0.5-5 mg/kg/hour

Hepatic Impairment: Reduce dosage in patients with severe liver dysfunction.

Available Dosage Forms Injection, solution, as sodium: 50 mg/mL (20 mL, 50 mL) [contains alcohol 10% and propylene glycol 40%]

Nursing Guidelines

Assessment: Assess effectiveness and interactions of other medications patient may be taking. Assess for history of addiction; long-term use can result in dependence, abuse, or tolerance. Periodically evaluate the need for continued use. **I.V.:** Keep patient under observation. Monitor cardio/respiratory status and institute patient safety precautions. Monitor effectiveness of therapy and adverse reactions.

Patient Education: Patient instructions and information are determined by patient condition and therapeutic purpose. Drug may cause physical and/or psychological dependence. While using this medication, do not use alcohol and other prescription or OTC medications (especially pain medications, sedatives, antihistamines, or hypnotics) without consulting prescriber. Maintain adequate hydration (2-3 L/day of fluids) unless instructed to restrict fluid intake. You may experience drowsiness, dizziness, or blurred vision (use caution when driving or engaging in tasks requiring alertness until response to drug is known); nausea, vomiting, or loss of appetite (small frequent meals, frequent mouth care, chewing gum, or sucking lozenges may help); or constipation (increased exercise, fluids, fruit, or fiber may help). Report skin rash or irritation; CNS changes (confusion, depression, increased sedation, excitation, headache, insomnia, or nightmares); respiratory difficulty or shortness of breath; changes in urinary pattern or menstrual pattern; muscle weakness or tremors; or difficulty swallowing or feeling of tightness in throat. **Pregnancy/breast-feeding precautions:** Do not get pregnant; use appropriate contraceptive measures to prevent possible harm to the fetus. Do not breast-feed.

Geriatric Considerations: Use of this agent as a hypnotic in the elderly is not recommended due to its long half-life and addiction potential.

Pregnancy Risk Factor: D

Lactation: Enters breast milk/contraindicated

Perioperative/Anesthesia/Other Concerns: Pentobarbital 50 mg/mL contains propylene glycol 414.4 mg/mL (40% v/v).

(Continued)

Pentobarbital *(Continued)*

Pentobarbital is one of the standard choices for refractory status epilepticus. Most patients will require systemic and pulmonary arterial catheterization with fluid and vasoactive therapy to maintain blood pressure. High-dose pentobarbital generally produces poikilothermia. Maintenance anticonvulsant treatment may be substantial in order to wean pentobarbital. High doses of barbiturates are potentially immunosuppressive; guard against infection.

Administration

I.M.: Pentobarbital may be administered by deep I.M.: No more than 5 mL (250 mg) should be injected at any one site because of possible tissue irritation.

I.V.: Pentobarbital must be administered by slow I.V. injection. I.V. push doses can be given undiluted, but should be administered no faster than 50 mg/minute. Avoid intra-arterial injection. Has many incompatibilities when given I.V.

Compatibility: Stable in dextran 6% in dextrose, dextran 6% in NS, D_5LR, $D_5{}^1/_4NS$, $D_5{}^1/_2NS$, D_5NS, $D_{10}W$, LR, $^1/_2NS$

Y-site administration: Incompatible with amphotericin B cholesteryl sulfate complex

Compatibility in syringe: Incompatible with atropine with cimetidine, butorphanol, chlorpromazine, cimetidine, dimenhydrinate, diphenhydramine, droperidol, fentanyl, glycopyrrolate, hydroxyzine, meperidine, midazolam, nalbuphine, pentazocine, perphenazine, prochlorperazine edisylate, promazine, promethazine, ranitidine

Compatibility when admixed: Incompatible with cefazolin, chlorpheniramine, cimetidine, clindamycin, droperidol, ephedrine, fentanyl, hydrocortisone sodium succinate, hydroxyzine, insulin (regular), levorphanol, norepinephrine, pancuronium, penicillin G potassium, pentazocine, phenytoin, promazine, promethazine, streptomycin, triflupromazine, vancomycin

Storage: Protect from freezing. Aqueous solutions are not stable; a commercially available vehicle (containing propylene glycol) is more stable. When mixed with an acidic solution, precipitate may form. Use only clear solution.

♦ **Pentobarbital Sodium** *see* Pentobarbital *on page 1336*

♦ **Pentothal®** *see* Thiopental *on page 1624*

Pentoxifylline (pen toks I fi leen)

U.S. Brand Names Pentoxil®; Trental®

Synonyms Oxpentifylline

Pharmacologic Category Blood Viscosity Reducer Agent

Medication Safety Issues

Sound-alike/look-alike issues:

Pentoxifylline may be confused with tamoxifen

Trental® may be confused with Bentyl®, Tegretol®, Trandate®

Use Treatment of intermittent claudication on the basis of chronic occlusive arterial disease of the limbs; may improve function and symptoms, but not intended to replace more definitive therapy

Unlabeled/Investigational Use AIDS patients with increased TNF, CVA, cerebrovascular diseases, diabetic atherosclerosis, diabetic neuropathy, gangrene, hemodialysis shunt thrombosis, vascular impotence, cerebral malaria, septic shock, sickle cell syndromes, and vasculitis

Mechanism of Action Reduces blood viscosity via increased leukocyte and erythrocyte deformability and decreased neutrophil adhesion/activation; improves peripheral tissue oxygenation presumably through enhanced blood flow.

Pharmacodynamics/Kinetics

Absorption: Well absorbed

Metabolism: Hepatic and via erythrocytes; extensive first-pass effect

Half-life elimination: Parent drug: 24-48 minutes; Metabolites: 60-96 minutes

Time to peak, serum: 2-4 hours

Excretion: Primarily urine (active metabolites); feces (4%)

Contraindications Hypersensitivity to pentoxifylline, xanthines (eg, caffeine, theophylline), or any component of the formulation; recent cerebral and/or retinal hemorrhage

Warnings/Precautions Use with caution in patients with renal and hepatic impairment; start with lower doses in elderly patients and monitor renal function. Use caution in patients receiving anticoagulant therapy or at risk for bleeding complications; monitor PT/INR, hematocrit, and/or hemoglobin as necessary. May lower blood pressure; monitor with concomitant antihypertensive agent use. Safety and efficacy in pediatric patients have not been established.

Drug Interactions
Theophylline: Increased toxicity

Nutritional/Herbal/Ethanol Interactions Food: Food may decrease rate but not extent of absorption. Pentoxifylline peak serum levels may be decreased if taken with food.

Lab Interactions Decreased calcium (S), magnesium (S); false-positive theophylline levels

Adverse Reactions
1% to 10%: Gastrointestinal: Nausea (2%), vomiting (1%)
<1% (Limited to important or life-threatening): Anaphylactoid reaction, angioedema, angina, anorexia, anxiety, aplastic anemia, arrhythmia, aseptic meningitis, bloating, blurred vision, brittle fingernails, chest pain, cholecystitis, confusion, conjunctivitis, constipation, depression, dyspnea, ear ache, edema, epistaxis, eructation, fibrinogen decreased (serum), flatus, flu-like symptoms, hallucinations, hepatitis, hypotension, jaundice, laryngitis, leukemia, leukopenia, liver enzymes increased, malaise, nasal congestion, pancytopenia, pruritus, purpura, rash, scotoma, seizure, sialism, sore throat, taste perversion, tachycardia, thrombocytopenia, tremor, urticaria, weight change, xerostomia

Overdosage/Toxicology Symptoms of overdose have been reported to occur 4-5 hours postingestion and last approximately 12 hours. Symptoms may include hypotension, flushing, convulsions, deep sleep, agitation, bradycardia, and AV block. Treatment should be symptom-directed and supportive.

Dosing
Adults & Elderly: Peripheral vascular disease: Oral: 400 mg 3 times/day with meals; maximal therapeutic benefit may take 2-4 weeks to develop; recommended to maintain therapy for at least 8 weeks. May reduce to 400 mg twice daily if GI or CNS side effects occur.

Available Dosage Forms Tablet, extended release (Pentoxil®, Trental®): 400 mg

Nursing Guidelines
Assessment: Assess potential for interactions with other prescriptions, OTC medications, or herbal products patient may be taking. Assess therapeutic effectiveness, and adverse reactions at regular intervals during therapy (eg, cardiac status and blood pressure). Teach patient proper use, possible side effects/appropriate interventions, and adverse symptoms to report.

Dietary Considerations: May be taken with meals or food.

Patient Education: Do not take any new medication during therapy unless approved by prescriber. This may relieve pain of claudication, but additional therapy may be recommended. Take as prescribed for full length of prescription. May cause dizziness (use caution when driving or engaging in tasks that are potentially hazardous until response to drug is known); or heartburn, nausea, or vomiting (small frequent meals, frequent mouth care, chewing gum, or sucking lozenges may help). Report chest pain; swelling of lips, mouth, or tongue; persistent headache; respiratory difficulty; rash; or unrelieved nausea or vomiting. **Pregnancy/breast-feeding precautions:** Inform prescriber if you are or intend to become pregnant. Consult prescriber if breast-feeding.

Geriatric Considerations: Pentoxifylline's value in the treatment of intermittent claudication is controversial. Walking distance improved statistically in some clinical trials, but the actual distance was minimal when applied to improving physical activity.

Pregnancy Risk Factor: C

Lactation: Enters breast milk/not recommended

Perioperative/Anesthesia/Other Concerns: Pentoxifylline may be used in the treatment of peripheral vascular disease, however, its efficacy is not fully established. Therapeutic effects may be seen after 2-4 weeks.

Administration
Oral: Tablets should be swallowed whole; do not chew, break, or crush.
Storage:
Store between 15°C to 30°C (59°F to 86°F).

- **Pentoxil®** *see* Pentoxifylline *on page 1340*
- **Pen VK** *see* Penicillin V Potassium *on page 1328*
- **Pepcid®** *see* Famotidine *on page 702*
- **Pepcid® AC [OTC]** *see* Famotidine *on page 702*
- **Percocet®** *see* Oxycodone and Acetaminophen *on page 1286*
- **Percodan®** *see* Oxycodone and Aspirin *on page 1289*
- **Perdiem® Overnight Relief [OTC]** *see* Senna *on page 1520*
- **Periactin** *see* Cyproheptadine *on page 472*

- **Peri-Colace® [DSC] [OTC]** *see* Docusate and Casanthranol *on page 561*
- **Peri-Colace® *(reformulation)* [OTC]** *see* Docusate and Senna *on page 562*
- **Peridex®** *see* Chlorhexidine Gluconate *on page 373*
- **PerioChip®** *see* Chlorhexidine Gluconate *on page 373*
- **PerioGard®** *see* Chlorhexidine Gluconate *on page 373*
- **Periostat®** *see* Doxycycline *on page 584*
- **Pethidine Hydrochloride** *see* Meperidine *on page 1097*
- **Pexeva®** *see* Paroxetine *on page 1313*
- **PFA** *see* Foscarnet *on page 775*
- **Pfizerpen®** *see* Penicillin G (Parenteral/Aqueous) *on page 1331*
- **PGE_1** *see* Alprostadil *on page 113*
- **PGI_2** *see* Epoprostenol *on page 622*
- **PGX** *see* Epoprostenol *on page 622*
- **Phanasin [OTC]** *see* Guaifenesin *on page 834*
- **Phanasin® Diabetic Choice [OTC]** *see* Guaifenesin *on page 834*
- **Phazyme® Quick Dissolve [OTC]** *see* Simethicone *on page 1533*
- **Phazyme® Ultra Strength [OTC]** *see* Simethicone *on page 1533*
- **Phenadoz™** *see* Promethazine *on page 1417*
- **Phenaseptic [OTC]** *see* Phenol *on page 1347*

Phenazopyridine (fen az oh PEER i deen)

U.S. Brand Names AZO-Gesic® [OTC]; AZO-Standard® [OTC]; Baridium® [OTC]; Pyridium®; ReAzo [OTC]; Uristat® [OTC]; UTI Relief® [OTC]

Synonyms Phenazopyridine Hydrochloride; Phenylazo Diamino Pyridine Hydrochloride

Pharmacologic Category Analgesic, Urinary

Medication Safety Issues

Sound-alike/look-alike issues:

Pyridium® may be confused with Dyrenium®, Perdiem®, pyridoxine, pyrithione

Use Symptomatic relief of urinary burning, itching, frequency and urgency in association with urinary tract infection or following urologic procedures

Mechanism of Action An azo dye which exerts local anesthetic or analgesic action on urinary tract mucosa through an unknown mechanism

Pharmacodynamics/Kinetics

Metabolism: Hepatic and via other tissues

Excretion: Urine (65% as unchanged drug)

Contraindications Hypersensitivity to phenazopyridine or any component of the formulation; kidney or liver disease; patients with a Cl_{cr} <50 mL/minute

Warnings/Precautions Does not treat infection, acts only as an analgesic; drug should be discontinued if skin or sclera develop a yellow color; use with caution in patients with renal impairment. Use of this agent in the elderly is limited since accumulation of phenazopyridine can occur in patients with renal insufficiency. Use is contraindicated in patients with a Cl_{cr} <50 mL/minute.

Drug Interactions No data reported

Lab Interactions Phenazopyridine may cause delayed reactions with glucose oxidase reagents (Clinistix®); cupric sulfate tests (Clinitest®) are not affected; interference may also occur with urine ketone tests (Acetest®, Ketostix®) and urinary protein tests; tests for urinary steroids and porphyrins may also occur

Adverse Reactions

1% to 10%:

Central nervous system: Headache, dizziness

Gastrointestinal: Stomach cramps

<1% (Limited to important or life-threatening): Acute renal failure, hemolytic anemia, hepatitis, methemoglobinemia

Overdosage/Toxicology Symptoms of overdose include methemoglobinemia, hemolytic anemia, skin pigmentation, and renal and hepatic impairment. For methemoglobinemia, the antidote is methylene blue 1-2 mg/kg I.V.

Dosing

Adults & Elderly: Urinary analgesic: Oral: 100-200 mg 3 times/day after meals for 2 days when used concomitantly with an antibacterial agent

Pediatrics: Urinary analgesic: Oral: Children: 12 mg/kg/day in 3 divided doses administered after meals for 2 days

Renal Impairment:

Cl_{cr} 50-80 mL/minute: Administer every 8-16 hours.

Cl_{cr} <50 mL/minute: Avoid use.

Available Dosage Forms

Tablet, as hydrochloride: 100 mg, 200 mg

AZO-Gesic®, AZO-Standard®, Uristat®: 95 mg

Baridium®: 97.2 mg

ReAzo: 95 mg

Pyridium®: 100 mg, 200 mg

UTI Relief®: 97.2 mg

Nursing Guidelines

Assessment: Assess therapeutic effectiveness (according to rationale for use). Instruct patients with diabetes to use serum glucose monitoring (phenazopyridine may interfere with certain urine testing reagents). Teach patient appropriate use, side effects/appropriate interventions, and adverse symptoms to report.

Dietary Considerations: Should be taken after meals.

Patient Education: Take exactly as directed. May discolor urine (orange/yellow); this is normal, but will also stain fabric. If you have diabetes, use serum glucose tests; this medication may interfere with accuracy of urine testing. Report persistent headache, dizziness, or stomach cramping. **Breast-feeding precaution:** Consult prescriber if breast-feeding.

Geriatric Considerations: Use of this agent in the elderly is limited since accumulation of phenazopyridine can occur in patients with renal insufficiency. It should not be used in patients with a Cl_{cr} <50 mL/minute.

Pregnancy Risk Factor: B

Lactation: Excretion in breast milk unknown

♦ **Phenazopyridine Hydrochloride** *see* Phenazopyridine *on page 1342*

♦ **Phenergan®** *see* Promethazine *on page 1417*

Phenobarbital (fee noe BAR bi tal)

U.S. Brand Names Luminal® Sodium

Synonyms Phenobarbital Sodium; Phenobarbitone; Phenylethylmalonylurea

Pharmacologic Category Anticonvulsant, Barbiturate; Barbiturate

Medication Safety Issues

Sound-alike/look-alike issues:

Phenobarbital may be confused with pentobarbital

Luminal® may be confused with Tuinal®

Use Management of generalized tonic-clonic (grand mal) and partial seizures; sedative

Unlabeled/Investigational Use Febrile seizures in children; may also be used for prevention and treatment of neonatal hyperbilirubinemia and lowering of bilirubin in chronic cholestasis; neonatal seizures; management of sedative/hypnotic withdrawal

Mechanism of Action Short-acting barbiturate with sedative, hypnotic, and anticonvulsant properties. Barbiturates depress the sensory cortex, decrease motor activity, alter cerebellar function, and produce drowsiness, sedation, and hypnosis. In high doses, barbiturates exhibit anticonvulsant activity; barbiturates produce dose-dependent respiratory depression.

Pharmacodynamics/Kinetics

Onset of action: Oral: Hypnosis: 20-60 minutes; I.V.: ~5 minutes

Peak effect: I.V.: ~30 minutes

Duration: Oral: 6-10 hours; I.V.: 4-10 hours

Absorption: Oral: 70% to 90%

Protein binding: 20% to 45%; decreased in neonates

Metabolism: Hepatic via hydroxylation and glucuronide conjugation

Half-life elimination: Neonates: 45-500 hours; Infants: 20-133 hours; Children: 37-73 hours; Adults: 53-140 hours

Time to peak, serum: Oral: 1-6 hours

Excretion: Urine (20% to 50% as unchanged drug)

Contraindications Hypersensitivity to barbiturates or any component of the formulation; marked hepatic impairment; dyspnea or airway obstruction; porphyria; pregnancy

Warnings/Precautions Potential for drug dependency exists, abrupt cessation may precipitate withdrawal, including status epilepticus in epileptic patients. Do not administer to patients in acute pain. Use caution in elderly, debilitated, renally or hepatic dysfunction, and pediatric patients. May cause paradoxical responses, including agitation and hyperactivity, particularly in acute pain and pediatric patients. Use with caution in patients with depression or suicidal tendencies, or in

(Continued)

Phenobarbital *(Continued)*

patients with a history of drug abuse. Tolerance, psychological and physical dependence may occur with prolonged use. May cause CNS depression, which may impair physical or mental abilities. Patients must cautioned about performing tasks which require mental alertness (eg, operating machinery or driving). Effects with other sedative drugs or ethanol may be potentiated. May cause respiratory depression or hypotension, particularly when administered intravenously. Use with caution in hemodynamically unstable patients (hypovolemic shock, CHF) or patients with respiratory disease. Due to its long half-life and risk of dependence, phenobarbital is not recommended as a sedative in the elderly. Use has been associated with cognitive deficits in children. Use with caution in patients with hypoadrenalism.

Drug Interactions Substrate of CYP2C8/9 (minor), 2C19 (major), 2E1 (minor); **Induces** CYP1A2 (strong), 2A6 (strong), 2B6 (strong), 2C8/9 (strong), 3A4 (strong)

Acetaminophen: Barbiturates may enhance the hepatotoxic potential of acetaminophen overdoses

Antiarrhythmics: Barbiturates may increase the metabolism of antiarrhythmics, decreasing their clinical effect; includes disopyramide, propafenone, and quinidine

Anticonvulsants: Barbiturates may increase the metabolism of anticonvulsants; includes ethosuximide, felbamate (possibly), lamotrigine, phenytoin, tiagabine, topiramate, and zonisamide; does not appear to affect gabapentin or levetiracetam

Antineoplastics: Limited evidence suggests that enzyme-inducing anticonvulsant therapy may reduce the effectiveness of some chemotherapy regimens (specifically in ALL); teniposide and methotrexate may be cleared more rapidly in these patients

Antipsychotics: Barbiturates may enhance the metabolism (decrease the efficacy) of antipsychotics; monitor for altered response; dose adjustment may be needed

Beta-blockers: Metabolism of beta-blockers may be increased and clinical effect decreased; atenolol and nadolol are unlikely to interact given their renal elimination

Calcium channel blockers: Barbiturates may enhance the metabolism of calcium channel blockers, decreasing their clinical effect

Chloramphenicol: Barbiturates may increase the metabolism of chloramphenicol and chloramphenicol may inhibit barbiturate metabolism; monitor for altered response

Cimetidine: Barbiturates may enhance the metabolism of cimetidine, decreasing its clinical effect

CNS depressants: Sedative effects and/or respiratory depression with barbiturates may be additive with other CNS depressants; monitor for increased effect; includes ethanol, sedatives, antidepressants, narcotic analgesics, and benzodiazepines

Corticosteroids: Barbiturates may enhance the metabolism of corticosteroids, decreasing their clinical effect

Cyclosporine: Levels may be decreased by barbiturates; monitor

CYP1A2 substrates: Phenobarbital may decrease the levels/effects of CYP1A2 substrates. Example substrates include aminophylline, estrogens, fluvoxamine, mirtazapine, ropinirole, and theophylline.

CYP2A6 substrates: Phenobarbital may decrease the levels/effects of CYP2A6 substrates. Example substrates include ifosfamide and rifampin.

CYP2B6 substrates: Phenobarbital may decrease the levels/effects of CYP2B6 substrates. Example substrates include bupropion, efavirenz, promethazine, selegiline, and sertraline.

CYP2C8/9 substrates: Phenobarbital may decrease the levels/effects of CYP2C8/9 substrates. Example substrates include amiodarone, fluoxetine, glimepiride, glipizide, losartan, nateglinide, phenytoin, pioglitazone, rosiglitazone, sertraline, sulfonamides, warfarin, and zafirlukast.

CYP2C19 inducers: May decrease the levels/effects of phenobarbital. Example inducers include aminoglutethimide, carbamazepine, phenytoin, and rifampin.

CYP2C19 inhibitors: May increase the levels/effects of phenobarbital. Example inhibitors include delavirdine, fluconazole, fluvoxamine, gemfibrozil, isoniazid, omeprazole, and ticlopidine.

CYP3A4 substrates: Phenobarbital may decrease the levels/effects of CYP3A4 substrates. Example substrates include benzodiazepines, calcium channel blockers, clarithromycin, cyclosporine, erythromycin, estrogens, mirtazapine, nateglinide, nefazodone, nevirapine, protease inhibitors, tacrolimus, and venlafaxine.

Doxycycline: Barbiturates may enhance the metabolism of doxycycline, decreasing its clinical effect; higher dosages may be required

Estrogens: Barbiturates may increase the metabolism of estrogens and reduce their efficacy

Felbamate may inhibit the metabolism of barbiturates and barbiturates may increase the metabolism of felbamate

Griseofulvin: Barbiturates may impair the absorption of griseofulvin, and griseofulvin metabolism may be increased by barbiturates, decreasing clinical effect

Guanfacine: Effect may be decreased by barbiturates

Immunosuppressants: Barbiturates may enhance the metabolism of immunosuppressants, decreasing its clinical effect; includes both cyclosporine and tacrolimus

Loop diuretics: Metabolism may be increased and clinical effects decreased; established for furosemide, effect with other loop diuretics not established

MAO inhibitors: Metabolism of barbiturates may be inhibited, increasing clinical effect or toxicity of the barbiturates

Methadone: Barbiturates may enhance the metabolism of methadone resulting in methadone withdrawal

Methoxyflurane: Barbiturates may enhance the nephrotoxic effects of methoxyflurane

Oral contraceptives: Barbiturates may enhance the metabolism of oral contraceptives, decreasing their clinical effect; an alternative method of contraception should be considered

Theophylline: Barbiturates may increase metabolism of theophylline derivatives and decrease their clinical effect

Tricyclic antidepressants: Barbiturates may increase metabolism of tricyclic antidepressants and decrease their clinical effect; sedative effects may be additive

Valproic acid: Metabolism of barbiturates may be inhibited by valproic acid; monitor for excessive sedation; a dose reduction may be needed

Warfarin: Barbiturates inhibit the hypoprothrombinemic effects of oral anticoagulants via increased metabolism; this combination should generally be avoided

Nutritional/Herbal/Ethanol Interactions

Ethanol: Avoid ethanol (may increase CNS depression).

Food: May cause decrease in vitamin D and calcium.

Herb/Nutraceutical: Avoid evening primrose (seizure threshold decreased). Avoid valerian, St John's wort, kava kava, gotu kola (may increase CNS depression).

Lab Interactions Increased ammonia (B), LFTs, copper (serum); decreased bilirubin (S); assay interference of LDH

Adverse Reactions Frequency not defined.

Cardiovascular: Bradycardia, hypotension, syncope

Central nervous system: Drowsiness, lethargy, CNS excitation or depression, impaired judgment, "hangover" effect, confusion, somnolence, agitation, hyperkinesia, ataxia, nervousness, headache, insomnia, nightmares, hallucinations, anxiety, dizziness

Dermatologic: Rash, exfoliative dermatitis, Stevens-Johnson syndrome

Gastrointestinal: Nausea, vomiting, constipation

Hematologic: Agranulocytosis, thrombocytopenia, megaloblastic anemia

Local: Pain at injection site, thrombophlebitis with I.V. use

Renal: Oliguria

Respiratory: Laryngospasm, respiratory depression, apnea (especially with rapid I.V. use), hypoventilation

Miscellaneous: Gangrene with inadvertent intra-arterial injection

Overdosage/Toxicology Symptoms of overdose include unsteady gait, slurred speech, confusion, jaundice, hypothermia, hypotension, respiratory depression, and coma. In severe overdose, charcoal hemoperfusion may accelerate removal. Treatment is symptom-directed and supportive.

Dosing

Adults:

Sedation: Oral, I.M.: 30-120 mg/day in 2-3 divided doses

Hypnotic: Oral, I.M., I.V., SubQ: 100-320 mg at bedtime

Preoperative sedation: I.M.: 100-200 mg 1-1.5 hours before procedure

Anticonvulsant/status epilepticus:

Loading dose: I.V.: 300-800 mg initially followed by 120-240 mg/dose at 20-minute intervals until seizures are controlled or a total dose of 1-2 g

(Continued)

Phenobarbital *(Continued)*

Maintenance dose: Oral, I.V.: 1-3 mg/kg/day in divided doses or 50-100 mg 2-3 times/day

Sedative/hypnotic withdrawal (unlabeled use): Initial daily requirement is determined by substituting phenobarbital 30 mg for every 100 mg pentobarbital used during tolerance testing; then daily requirement is decreased by 10% of initial dose.

Elderly: Geriatric patients should be started at the lowest recommended dose. Refer to adult dosing.

Pediatrics:

Sedation: Oral: Children: 2 mg/kg 3 times/day

Hypnotic: I.M., I.V., SubQ: Children: 3-5 mg/kg at bedtime

Preoperative sedation: Oral, I.M., I.V.: Children: 1-3 mg/kg 1-1.5 hours before procedure

Anticonvulsant/Status epilepticus (Loading dose): I.V.: Infants and Children: 10-20 mg/kg in a single or divided dose; in select patients may administer additional 5 mg/kg/dose every 15-30 minutes until seizure is controlled or a total dose of 40 mg/kg is reached

Anticonvulsant maintenance dose: Oral, I.V.:

Infants: 5-8 mg/kg/day in 1-2 divided doses

Children:

1-5 years: 6-8 mg/kg/day in 1-2 divided doses

5-12 years: 4-6 mg/kg/day in 1-2 divided doses

>12 years: 1-3 mg/kg/day in divided doses or 50-100 mg 2-3 times/day

Renal Impairment:

Cl_{cr} <10 mL/minute: Administer every 12-16 hours.

Moderately dialyzable (20% to 50%)

Hepatic Impairment: Increased side effects may occur in severe liver disease. Monitor plasma levels and adjust dose accordingly.

Available Dosage Forms

Elixir: 20 mg/5 mL (473 mL) [contains alcohol]

Injection, solution, as sodium: 65 mg/mL (1 mL); 130 mg/mL (1 mL) [contains alcohol and propylene glycol]

Luminal® Sodium: 60 mg/mL (1 mL); 130 mg/mL (1 mL) [contains alcohol 10% and propylene glycol]

Tablet: 15 mg, 30 mg, 32 mg, 60 mg, 65 mg, 100 mg

Nursing Guidelines

Assessment: Assess effectiveness and interactions of other medications patient may be taking. Assess for history of addiction; long-term use can result in dependence, abuse, or tolerance; periodically evaluate need for continued use. Monitor cardio/respiratory and CNS status; use safety precautions. Monitor effectiveness of therapy and adverse reactions. **Oral**: Monitor therapeutic effectiveness and adverse reactions at beginning of therapy and periodically with long-term use. Assess knowledge/teach patient appropriate use, possible side effects, and symptoms to report.

Monitoring Laboratory Tests: Phenobarbital serum concentrations, CBC, LFTs

Dietary Considerations: Vitamin D: Loss in vitamin D due to malabsorption; increase intake of foods rich in vitamin D. Supplementation of vitamin D and/or calcium may be necessary. Sodium content of injection (65 mg, 1 mL): 6 mg (0.3 mEq).

Patient Education: I.M./I.V.: Patient instructions and information are determined by patient condition and therapeutic purpose. If self-administered, use exactly as directed; do not increase dose or frequency. Drug may cause physical and/or psychological dependence. While using this medication, do not use alcohol and other prescription or OTC medications (especially pain medications, sedatives, antihistamines, or hypnotics) without consulting prescriber. Maintain adequate hydration (2-3 L/day of fluids) unless instructed to restrict fluid intake. You may experience drowsiness, dizziness, or blurred vision (use caution when driving or engaging in tasks requiring alertness until response to drug is known); nausea, vomiting, or loss of appetite (small frequent meals, frequent mouth care, chewing gum, or sucking lozenges may help); or constipation (increased exercise, fluids, fruit, or fiber may help). Report skin rash or irritation; CNS changes (confusion, depression, increased sedation, excitation, headache, insomnia, or nightmares); respiratory difficulty or shortness of breath; changes in urinary pattern or menstrual pattern; muscle weakness or tremors; or difficulty swallowing or feeling of tightness in throat. **Pregnancy/**

breast-feeding precautions: Do not get pregnant while taking this medication; use appropriate contraceptive measures. Breast-feeding is not recommended.

Geriatric Considerations: Due to its long half-life and risk of dependence, phenobarbital is not recommended as a sedative or hypnotic in the elderly. Interpretive guidelines from the Health Care Financing Administration discourage the use of this agent as a sedative/hypnotic in long-term care residents.

Pregnancy Risk Factor: D

Pregnancy Issues: Crosses the placenta. Cardiac defect reported; hemorrhagic disease of newborn due to fetal vitamin K depletion may occur; may induce maternal folic acid deficiency; withdrawal symptoms observed in infant following delivery. Epilepsy itself, number of medications, genetic factors, or a combination of these probably influence the teratogenicity of anticonvulsant therapy. Benefit:risk ratio usually favors continued use during pregnancy.

Lactation: Enters breast milk/not recommended (AAP recommends use "with caution")

Breast-Feeding Considerations: Sedation has been reported in nursing infants; infantile spasms may occur after weaning from breast milk. AAP recommends USE WITH CAUTION.

Perioperative/Anesthesia/Other Concerns: Phenobarbital 65 mg/mL and 130 mg/mL each contains propylene glycol 702.4 mg/mL (67.8% v/v).

Status Epilepticus: A randomized, double-blind trial (Treiman D, 1998) evaluated the efficacy of four treatments in overt status epilepticus. Treatment arms were designed based upon accepted practices of North American neurologists. The treatments were: 1) lorazepam 0.1 mg/kg, 2) diazepam 0.15 mg/kg followed by phenytoin 18 mg/kg, 3) phenytoin 18 mg/kg alone, and 4) phenobarbital 15 mg/kg. Treatment was considered successful if the seizures were terminated (clinically and by EEG) within 20 minutes of start of therapy without seizure recurrence within 60 minutes from the start of therapy. Patients who failed the first treatment received a second and a third, if necessary. Patients did not receive randomized treatments after the first one but the treating physician remained blinded. Treatment success: Lorazepam 64.9%, phenobarbital 58.2%, diazepam/phenytoin 55.8%, and phenytoin alone 43.6%. Using an "intention-to-treat" analysis, there was no statistical difference between the groups. Results of subsequent treatments in patients who failed the first therapy indicated that response rate significantly dropped regardless of treatment. Aggregate response rate to the second treatment was 7.0% and third treatment 2.3%.

Administration

I.V.: Avoid rapid I.V. administration >50 mg/minute. Avoid intra-arterial injection.

Compatibility: Stable in dextran 6% in dextrose, dextran 6% in NS, D_5LR, $D_5{}^1/_4NS$, $D_5{}^1/_2NS$, D_5NS, D_5W, $D_{10}W$, LR, $^1/_2NS$, NS

Y-site administration: Incompatible with amphotericin B cholesteryl sulfate complex, hydromorphone

Compatibility in syringe: Incompatible with hydromorphone, pentazocine, ranitidine, sufentanil

Compatibility when admixed: Incompatible with chlorpromazine, cimetidine, clindamycin, dimenhydrinate, diphenhydramine, droperidol, ephedrine, hydralazine, hydrocortisone sodium succinate, hydroxyzine, insulin (regular), kanamycin, levorphanol, meperidine, morphine, norepinephrine, pancuronium, penicillin G, pentazocine, phenytoin, procaine, prochlorperazine edisylate, prochlorperazine mesylate, promazine, promethazine, streptomycin, succinylcholine, vancomycin

Storage: Protect elixir from light. Not stable in aqueous solutions. Use only clear solutions. Do not add to acidic solutions; precipitation may occur.

Related Information

Perioperative Management of Patients on Antiseizure Medication *on page 1801*

♦ **Phenobarbital Sodium** *see* Phenobarbital *on page 1343*

♦ **Phenobarbitone** *see* Phenobarbital *on page 1343*

Phenol (FEE nol)

U.S. Brand Names Castellani Paint Modified [OTC]; Cepastat® [OTC]; Cepastat® Extra Strength [OTC]; Cheracol® [OTC]; Chloraseptic® Gargle [OTC]; Chloraseptic® Mouth Pain [OTC]; Chloraseptic® Rinse [OTC]; Chloraseptic® Spray [OTC]; Chloraseptic® Spray for Kids [OTC]; Pain-A-Lay® [OTC]; Phenaseptic [OTC]; Phenol EZ® [OTC]; Ulcerease® [OTC]

(Continued)

Phenol *(Continued)*

Synonyms Carbolic Acid

Pharmacologic Category Anesthetic, Topical

Medication Safety Issues

Sound-alike/look-alike issues:

Cēpastat® may be confused with Capastat®

Use Relief of sore throat pain, mouth, gum, and throat irritations; antiseptic; topical anesthetic

Warnings/Precautions

When used for self-medication (OTC) for sore throat: Not for use >7 days or if pain, redness, or irritation continues. If sore throat is severe, not for use >2 days or if followed by fever, headache, rash, nausea, or vomiting. Oral gargles and sprays should not be swallowed.

When used for self-medication (OTC) as a topical antiseptic: Do not use in eyes, or apply to large areas of the body, deep or puncture wounds, animal bites or burns. Do not use for >7 days; do not bandage affected area.

Dosing

Adults & Elderly:

Sore throat: Oral:

Cēpastat® Extra Strength, Cēpastat®: Up to 2 lozenges every 2 hours as needed

Cheracol®, Pain-A-Lay® Spray: Spray directly in throat; rinse for 15 seconds then expectorate; may repeat every 2 hours

Chloraseptic®: Five sprays onto throat or affected area; may repeat every 2 hours

Chloraseptic® Gargle, Cēpastat® Mouth Pain, Pain-A-Lay® Gargle, Ulcerease®: Gargle or swish for 15 seconds, then expectorate; may repeat every 2 hours

Antiseptic: Topical: Castellani Paint Modified: Apply small amount to affected area 1-3 times/day

Pediatrics: Sore throat: Oral:

Children 2-12 years:

Chloraseptic®: Three sprays onto throat or affected area; may repeat every 2 hours

Chloraseptic® for Kids: Five sprays onto throat or affected area; may repeat every 2 hours

Children >3 year (Ulcerease®): Refer to adult dosing.

Children 6-12 years:

Cēpastat® Extra Strength: Up to 1 lozenge every 2 hours as needed (maximum: 10 lozenges/24 hours)

Cēpastat®: Up to 1 lozenge every 2 hours as needed (maximum: 18 lozenges/24 hours)

Pain-A-Lay® Gargle: Using gauze pad, apply 10 mL to affected area, or gargle or swish for 15 seconds, then expectorate

Children ≥12 years: Cēpastat® Extra Strength, Cēpastat®,Cheracol®, Pain-A-Lay® (spray/gargle), Chloraseptic® (spray/gargle), Chloraseptic® Mouth Pain: Refer to adult dosing.

Available Dosage Forms

Lozenge, oral:

Cēpastat®: 14.5 mg (18s) [sugar free; contains menthol; cherry flavor]

Cēpastat® Extra Strength: 29 mg (18s) [sugar free; contains menthol; eucalyptus flavor]

Solution, oral: 1.4% (180 mL) [spray]

Cheracol® [spray]: Phenol 1.4% (180 mL) [alcohol and sugar free; contains tartrazine]

Chloraseptic® [gargle]: 1.4% (296 mL) [alcohol and sugar free; cool mint flavor]

Chloraseptic® Mouth Pain [rinse]: 1.4% (240 mL) [cinnamon flavor]

Chloraseptic® [spray]: 1.4% (20 mL, 30 mL) [alcohol and sugar free; cherry flavor]; (180 mL) [alcohol and sugar free; cherry, cool mint, and menthol flavors]

Chloraseptic® for Kids [spray]: 0.5% (177 mL) [grape flavor]

Pain-A-Lay® [gargle]: 1.4% (240 mL, 540 mL) [contains tartrazine]

Pain-A-Lay® [spray]: 1.4% (180 mL) [contains tartrazine]

Phenaseptic [spray]: 1.4% (180 mL) [cherry flavor]

Ulcerease® [gargle]: 0.6% (180 mL) [alcohol, dye, and sugar free; contains glycerin]

Solution, topical:

Castellani Paint Modified: Phenol 1.5% (30 mL) [contains alcohol 13%, acetone, basic fuchsin, resorcinol]

Castellani Paint Modified [colorless]: Phenol 1.5% (30 mL) [contains alcohol 13%, acetone, and resorcinol]

Swabs, topical (Phenol EZ®): 89% (30s) [~0.2 mL]

Nursing Guidelines

Patient Education: Severe or persistent sore throat accompanied by high fever, headache, nausea or vomiting may be serious

Administration

Oral: Allow to lozenge dissolve slowly in mouth. Spray should be allowed to remain in mouth for ~15 seconds, then expectorate.

♦ **Phenol EZ® [OTC]** *see* Phenol *on page 1347*

♦ **Phenoxymethyl Penicillin** *see* Penicillin V Potassium *on page 1328*

Phentolamine (fen TOLE a meen)

Synonyms Phentolamine Mesylate; Regitine [DSC]

Pharmacologic Category $Alpha_1$ Blocker

Medication Safety Issues

Sound-alike/look-alike issues:

Phentolamine may be confused with phentermine, Ventolin®

Use Diagnosis of pheochromocytoma and treatment of hypertension associated with pheochromocytoma or other forms of hypertension caused by excess sympathomimetic amines; as treatment of dermal necrosis after extravasation of drugs with alpha-adrenergic effects (norepinephrine, dopamine, epinephrine)

Unlabeled/Investigational Use Treatment of pralidoxime-induced hypertension

Mechanism of Action Competitively blocks alpha-adrenergic receptors to produce brief antagonism of circulating epinephrine and norepinephrine to reduce hypertension caused by alpha effects of these catecholamines; also has a positive inotropic and chronotropic effect on the heart

Pharmacodynamics/Kinetics

Onset of action: I.M.: 15-20 minutes; I.V.: Immediate

Duration: I.M.: 30-45 minutes; I.V.: 15-30 minutes

Metabolism: Hepatic

Half-life elimination: 19 minutes

Excretion: Urine (10% as unchanged drug)

Contraindications Hypersensitivity to phentolamine or any component of the formulation; renal impairment; coronary or cerebral arteriosclerosis; concurrent use with phosphodiesterase-5 (PDE-5) inhibitors including sildenafil (>25 mg), tadalafil, or vardenafil

Warnings/Precautions Myocardial infarction, cerebrovascular spasm and cerebrovascular occlusion have occurred following administration. Use with caution in patients with gastritis or peptic ulcer, tachycardia, or a history of cardiac arrhythmias.

Drug Interactions

Epinephrine, ephedrine: Effects may be decreased.

Ethanol: Increased toxicity (disulfiram reaction).

Sildenafil, tadalafil, vardenafil: Blood pressure-lowering effects are additive. Use of tadalafil or vardenafil is contraindicated by the manufacturer. Use sildenafil with extreme caution (dose ≤25 mg).

Lab Interactions Increased LFTs rarely

Adverse Reactions Frequency not defined.

Cardiovascular: Hypotension, tachycardia, arrhythmia, flushing, orthostatic hypotension

Central nervous system: Dizziness

Gastrointestinal: Nausea, vomiting, diarrhea

Neuromuscular & skeletal: Weakness

Respiratory: Nasal congestion

Postmarketing and/or case reports: Pulmonary hypertension

Overdosage/Toxicology Symptoms of overdose include tachycardia, shock, vomiting, and dizziness. If fluid replacement is inadequate to treat hypotension, only alpha-adrenergic vasopressors such as norepinephrine should be used. Mixed agents such as epinephrine may cause more hypotension.

(Continued)

Phentolamine *(Continued)*

Dosing

Adults & Elderly:

Treatment of alpha-adrenergic drug extravasation: SubQ:

Infiltrate area with a small amount (eg, 1 mL) of solution (made by diluting 5-10 mg in 10 mL of NS) within 12 hours of extravasation; do not exceed 0.1-0.2 mg/kg or 5 mg total

If dose is effective, normal skin color should return to the blanched area within 1 hour.

Diagnosis of pheochromocytoma: I.M., I.V.: 5 mg

Surgery for pheochromocytoma: Hypertension: I.M., I.V.: 5 mg given 1-2 hours before procedure and repeated as needed every 2-4 hours

Hypertensive crisis: I.V.: 5-20 mg

Treatment of pralidoxime-induced hypertension (unlabeled use): I.V.: 5 mg

Pediatrics:

Treatment of alpha-adrenergic drug extravasation: SubQ: Infiltrate area with a small amount (eg, 1 mL) of solution (made by diluting 5-10 mg in 10 mL of NS) within 12 hours of extravasation; do not exceed 0.1-0.2 mg/kg or 5 mg total

Diagnosis of pheochromocytoma: I.M., I.V.: 0.05-0.1 mg/kg/dose, maximum single dose: 5 mg

Surgery for pheochromocytoma: Hypertension: I.M., I.V.: 0.05-0.1 mg/kg/dose given 1-2 hours before procedure; repeat as needed every 2-4 hours until hypertension is controlled; maximum single dose: 5 mg.

Treatment of pralidoxime-induced hypertension (unlabeled use): I.V.: 1 mg

Available Dosage Forms Injection, powder for reconstitution, as mesylate: 5 mg

Nursing Guidelines

Assessment: See Contraindications, Warnings/Precautions, and Drug Interactions for use cautions. See Dosing and Administration for specifics according to purpose for use. When used to treat dermal necrosis after extravasation of drugs with alpha-adrenergic effects, monitor effectiveness of treatment closely. Assess patient response (eg, Cardiac status - Adverse Reactions and Overdose/Toxicology). Teach patient adverse symptoms to report (see Patient Education). Note breast-feeding caution.

Patient Education: This medication can only be administered by infusion or injection. Report immediately any pain at infusion/injection site. May cause orthostatic hypotension (use caution when changing position or call for assistance). Report dizziness, rapid heartbeat, feelings of weakness, or nausea/vomiting. **Pregnancy/breast-feeding precautions:** Inform prescriber if you are or intend to become pregnant. Consult prescriber if breast-feeding.

Pregnancy Risk Factor: C

Lactation: Excretion in breast milk unknown

Administration

I.V.:

Vasoconstrictor (alpha-adrenergic agonist) extravasation: Infiltrate the area of extravasation with multiple small injections using only 27- or 30-gauge needles and changing the needle between each skin entry. Be careful not to cause so much swelling of the extremity or digit that a compartment syndrome occurs. If infiltration is severe, may also need to consult vascular surgeon.

Pheochromocytoma: Inject each 5 mg over 1 minute.

Reconstitution: Reconstituted solution is stable for 48 hours at room temperature and 1 week when refrigerated.

Compatibility: Stable in NS

♦ **Phentolamine Mesylate** *see* Phentolamine *on page 1349*

♦ **Phenylazo Diamino Pyridine Hydrochloride** *see* Phenazopyridine *on page 1342*

Phenylephrine (fen il EF rin)

U.S. Brand Names AH-chew® D [OTC]; AK-Dilate®; Altafrin; Anu-Med [OTC]; Formulation R™ [OTC]; Medicone® [OTC]; Mydfrin®; NāSop™; Neo-Synephrine® Extra Strength [OTC]; Neo-Synephrine® Mild [OTC]; Neo-Synephrine® Ophthalmic [DSC]; Neo-Synephrine® Regular Strength [OTC]; Rectacaine [OTC]; Relief® [OTC]; Rhinall [OTC]; Sudafed PE™ [OTC]; Tronolane® Suppository [OTC]; Vicks® Sinex® Nasal Spray [OTC]; Vicks® Sinex® UltraFine Mist [OTC]

Synonyms Phenylephrine Hydrochloride; Phenylephrine Tannate

Pharmacologic Category Alpha/Beta Agonist; Ophthalmic Agent, Antiglaucoma; Ophthalmic Agent, Mydriatic

Medication Safety Issues

Sound-alike/look-alike issues:

Mydfrin® may be confused with Midrin®

Use Treatment of hypotension, vascular failure in shock; as a vasoconstrictor in regional analgesia; as a mydriatic in ophthalmic procedures and treatment of wide-angle glaucoma; supraventricular tachycardia

For OTC use as symptomatic relief of nasal and nasopharyngeal mucosal congestion, treatment of hemorrhoids, relief of redness of the eye due to irritation

Mechanism of Action Potent, direct-acting alpha-adrenergic stimulator with weak beta-adrenergic activity; causes vasoconstriction of the arterioles of the nasal mucosa and conjunctiva; activates the dilator muscle of the pupil to cause contraction; produces vasoconstriction of arterioles in the body; produces systemic arterial vasoconstriction

Pharmacodynamics/Kinetics

Onset of action: I.M., SubQ: 10-15 minutes; I.V.: Immediate; Ophthalmic: 10-15 minutes

Duration: I.M.: 0.5-2 hours; I.V.: 15-30 minutes; SubQ: 1 hour; Ophthalmic: Maximal mydriasis: 1 hour, recover time: 3-6 hours

Metabolism: Hepatic, via intestinal monoamine oxidase to phenolic conjugates

Excretion: Urine (90%)

Contraindications Hypersensitivity to phenylephrine or any component of the formulation; hypertension; ventricular tachycardia

Oral: Use with or within 14 days of MAO inhibitor therapy

Ophthalmic: Narrow-angle glaucoma

Warnings/Precautions Some products contain sulfites which may cause allergic reactions in susceptible individuals.

Intravenous: Use with caution in the elderly, patients with hyperthyroidism, bradycardia, partial heart block, myocardial disease, or severe CAD. Not a substitute for volume replacement. Avoid hypertension; monitor blood pressure closely and adjust infusion rate. Infuse into a large vein if possible. Watch I.V. site closely. Avoid extravasation.

Nasal, oral, rectal: Use caution with hyperthyroidism, diabetes mellitus, cardiovascular disease, ischemic heart disease, increased intraocular pressure, prostatic hyperplasia or in the elderly. Rebound congestion may occur when nasal products are discontinued after chronic use. When used for self-medication (OTC), notify healthcare provider if symptoms do not improve within 7 days (oral, rectal) or 3 days (nasal), are accompanied by fever (oral), or if bleeding occurs (rectal).

Ophthalmic: Use caution with or within 21 days of MAO inhibitor therapy. When used for self-medication (OTC), notify healthcare provider in case of vision changes, continued redness, or if symptoms worsen or do not improve within 3 days.

Drug Interactions

Beta-blockers (nonselective) may increase hypertensive effect; avoid concurrent use.

MAO inhibitors: May potentiate hypertension and hypertensive crisis; avoid concurrent use.

Methyldopa can increase the pressor response; be aware of patient's drug regimen.

Tricyclic antidepressants: May enhance the vasopressor effect phenylephrine; avoid concurrent use.

Nutritional/Herbal/Ethanol Interactions Herb/Nutraceutical: Avoid ephedra, yohimbe (may cause CNS stimulation).

Adverse Reactions Frequency not defined.

Cardiovascular: Reflex bradycardia, excitability, restlessness, arrhythmia (rare), precordial pain or discomfort, pallor, hypertension, severe peripheral and visceral vasoconstriction, decreased cardiac output

Central nervous system: Headache, anxiety, dizziness, tremor, paresthesia, restlessness

Endocrine & metabolic: Metabolic acidosis

Local: I.V.: Extravasation which may lead to necrosis and sloughing of surrounding tissue, blanching of skin

Neuromuscular & skeletal: Pilomotor response, weakness

(Continued)

Phenylephrine *(Continued)*

Renal: Decreased renal perfusion, reduced urine output

Respiratory: Respiratory distress

Overdosage/Toxicology Symptoms of overdose include vomiting, hypertension, palpitations, paresthesia, and ventricular extrasystoles. Treatment is supportive. In extreme cases, I.V. phentolamine may be used.

Dosing

Adults:

Hemorrhoids: Rectal:

Cream/ointment: Apply to clean dry area, up to 4 times/day; may be used externally or inserted rectally using applicator.

Suppository: Insert 1 suppository rectally, up to 4 times/day

Hypotension/shock:

I.V. bolus: 0.1-0.5 mg/dose every 10-15 minutes as needed (initial dose should not exceed 0.5 mg)

I.V. infusion: Initial dose: 100-180 mcg/minute; when blood pressure is stabilized, maintenance rate: 40-60 mcg/minute; rates up to 360 mcg/minute have been reported; dosing range: 0.4-9.1 mcg/kg/minute

Nasal congestion:

Intranasal: Instill 1-2 sprays or instill 1-2 drops every 4 hours of 0.25% to 0.5% solution as needed; 1% solution may be used in adult in cases of extreme nasal congestion; do not use nasal solutions more than 3 days

Oral:

Hydrochloride salt: 10-20 mg every 4 hours

Tannate salt (NāSop™ suspension): 7.5-15 mg every 12 hours

Ocular procedures: Ophthalmic: Instill 1 drop of 2.5% or 10% solution, may repeat in 10-60 minutes as needed.

Paroxysmal supraventricular tachycardia: I.V.: 0.25-0.5 mg/dose over 20-30 seconds

Reduction in ocular redness (OTC formulation): Ophthalmic: Instill 1-2 drops 0.12% solution into affected eye, up to 4 times/day; do not use for >72 hours

Elderly:

Nasal decongestant: Administer 2-3 drops or 1-2 sprays every 4 hours of 0.125% to 0.25% solution as needed; do not use more than 3 days.

Ophthalmic preparations for pupil dilation: Instill 1 drop of 2.5% solution, may repeat in 1 hour if necessary.

Refer to adult dosing for other uses and Geriatric Considerations for cautions on I.V. use.

Pediatrics:

Hemorrhoids: Children >12 years: Refer to adult dosing.

Hypotension/shock: Children:

I.V. bolus: 5-20 mcg/kg/dose every 10-15 minutes as needed

I.V. infusion: 0.1-0.5 mcg/kg/minute

Nasal congestion:

2-6 years:

Intranasal: Instill 1 drop every 2-4 hours of 0.125% solution as needed. (**Note:** Therapy should not exceed 3 continuous days.)

Oral: Tannate salt (NāSop™ suspension): 1.87-3.75 mg every 12 hours

6-12 years:

Intranasal: Instill 1-2 sprays or instill 1-2 drops every 4 hours of 0.25% solution as needed. (**Note:** Therapy should not exceed 3 continuous days.)

Oral:

Hydrochloride salt: 10 mg every 4 hours

Tannate salt (NāSop™ suspension): 3.75-7.5 mg every 12 hours

>12 years: Refer to adult dosing.

Ocular procedures: Ophthalmic:

Infants <1 year: Instill 1 drop of 2.5% 15-30 minutes before procedures

Children: Refer to adult dosing.

Paroxysmal supraventricular tachycardia: I.V.: Children: 5-10 mcg/kg/dose over 20-30 seconds

Available Dosage Forms [DSC] = Discontinued product

Cream, rectal, as hydrochloride (Formulation R™): 0.25% (54 g) [contains sodium benzoate]

Injection, solution, as hydrochloride: 1% [10 mg/mL] (1 mL, 5 mL) [may contain sodium metabisulfite]

Neo-Synephrine®: 1% (1 mL) [contains sodium metabisulfite]
Ointment, rectal, as hydrochloride:
Formulation R™: 0.25% (30 g, 60 g) [contains benzoic acid]
Rectacaine: 0.25% (30 g) [contains shark liver oil]
Solution, intranasal drops, as hydrochloride:
Neo-Synephrine® Extra Strength: 1% (15 mL) [contains benzalkonium chloride]
Neo-Synephrine® Regular Strength: 0.5% (15 mL) [contains benzalkonium chloride]
Rhinall: 0.25% (30 mL) [contains benzalkonium chloride and sodium bisulfite]
Solution, intranasal spray, as hydrochloride:
Neo-Synephrine® Extra Strength: 1% (15 mL) [contains benzalkonium chloride]
Neo-Synephrine® Mild: 0.25% (15 mL) [contains benzalkonium chloride]
Neo-Synephrine® Regular Strength: 0.5% (15 mL) [contains benzalkonium chloride]
Rhinall: 0.25% (40 mL) [contains benzalkonium chloride and sodium bisulfite]
Vicks® Sinex®, Vicks® Sinex® UltraFine Mist: 0.5% (15 mL) [contains benzalkonium chloride]
Solution, ophthalmic, as hydrochloride: 2.5% (1 mL, 2 mL, 3 mL, 5 mL, 15 mL) [may contain sodium bisulfite]
AK-Dilate®: 2.5% (2 mL, 15 mL); 10% (5 mL)
Altrafrin: 0.12% (15 mL) [OTC]; 2.5% (5 mL, 15 mL) [RX; contains benzalkonium chloride]; 10% (5 mL) [RX; contains benzalkonium chloride]
Mydfrin®: 2.5% (3 mL, 5 mL) [contains sodium bisulfite]
Neo-Synephrine®: 2.5% (15 mL); 10% (5 mL) [contains benzalkonium chloride] [DSC]
Neo-Synephrine® Viscous: 10% (5 mL) [contains benzalkonium chloride] [DSC]
Suppository, rectal, as hydrochloride: 0.25% (12s)
Anu-Med, Tronolane®: 0.25% (12s)
Medicone®: 0.25% (18s, 24s)
Rectacaine: 0.25% (12s) [contains shark liver oil]
Suspension, oral, as tannate (NāSop™): 7.5 mg/5 mL (120 mL) [orange flavor]
Tablet, as hydrochloride (Sudafed PE™): 10 mg
Tablet, chewable, as hydrochloride (AH-chew® D): 10 mg
Tablet, orally dissolving, as hydrochloride (NāSop™): 10 mg [contains phenylalanine 4 mg/tablet; bubble gum flavor]

Nursing Guidelines

Assessment: Assess other medications patient may be taking for effectiveness and interactions. Monitor therapeutic effectiveness and adverse reactions according to use. **Parenteral:** Monitor arterial blood gases, vital signs, adverse reactions, and infusion site. **Nasal/ophthalmic:** Assess knowledge/teach patient appropriate use, interventions to reduce side effects, and adverse symptoms to report. Systemic absorption from ophthalmic instillation is minimal.

Dietary Considerations: NāSop™ contains phenylalanine 4 mg/tablet.

Patient Education:

Nasal decongestant: Do not use for more than 3 days in a row. Clear nose as much as possible before use. Tilt head back and instill recommended dose of drops or spray. Do not blow nose for 5-10 minutes. You may experience transient stinging or burning.

Ophthalmic: Do not let tip of applicator touch eye; do not contaminate tip of applicator (may cause eye infection, eye damage, or vision loss). Open eye, look at ceiling, and instill prescribed amount of solution. Close eye and roll eye in all directions, and apply gentle pressure to inner corner of eye for 1-2 minutes after instillation. Temporary stinging or blurred vision may occur. Report persistent pain, burning, double vision, severe headache, or if condition worsens.

Pregnancy/breast-feeding precautions: Inform prescriber if you are pregnant. Consult prescriber if breast-feeding.

Geriatric Considerations: Phenylephrine I.V. should be used with extreme caution in the elderly. The 10% ophthalmic solution has caused increased blood pressure in elderly patients and its use should, therefore, be avoided. Since topical decongestants can be obtained OTC, elderly patients should be counseled about their proper use and in what disease states they should be avoided (see Warnings/Precautions).

Pregnancy Risk Factor: C

Lactation: Excretion in breast milk unknown/not recommended

Perioperative/Anesthesia/Other Concerns: Phenylephrine allows for close titration of blood pressure and may be used in patients with hypotension or shock due to peripheral vasodilation; can increase blood pressure in

(Continued)

Phenylephrine *(Continued)*

fluid-resuscitated septic shock patients; does not impair cardiac or renal function. May be a good choice when tachyarrhythmias limit use of other vasopressors, although experience in patients with septic shock is limited. An increase in oxygen delivery and consumption may occur in >15% of patients according to one study (Flancbaum, 1997).

Extravasation Management: Antidote for peripheral ischemia caused by phenylephrine extravasation: To prevent sloughing and necrosis in ischemic areas, the area should be infiltrated as soon as possible with 5-10 mg of Regitine® (phentolamine), an adrenergic blocking agent, diluted in 10-15 mL of saline. A syringe with a fine hypodermic needle should be used, and the solution liberally infiltrated throughout the ischemic area. Sympathetic blockade with phentolamine causes immediate and conspicuous local hyperemic changes if the area is infiltrated within 12 hours. Therefore, phentolamine should be given as soon as possible after the extravasation is noted, as phentolamine may be ineffective if given >12 hours after extravasation.

Administration

Oral: NāSop™: Place tablet on tongue and allow to dissolve

Reconstitution: Solution for injection:

I.V. infusion: May dilute 10 mg in 500 mL NS or D_5W.

I.V. injection: Dilute with SWFI to a concentration of 1 mg/mL.

Compatibility: Stable in dextran 6% in dextrose, dextran 6% in NS, D_5LR, $D_5{}^1/_4NS$, $D_5{}^1/_2NS$, D_5NS, D_5W, $D_{10}W$, LR, $^1/_2NS$, NS, sodium bicarbonate 5%

Y-site administration: Incompatible with thiopental

Storage:

Solution for injection: Store vials at controlled room temperature of 15°C to 30°C (59°F to 86°F). Protect from light. Do not use solution if brown or contains a precipitate.

Ophthalmic solution:

0.12%: Store at controlled room temperature. Protect from light and excessive heat.

2.5% and 10%: Refer to product labeling. Some products are labeled to store at room temperature, others should be stored under refrigeration at 2°C to 8°C (36°F to 46°F); do not use solution if brown or contains a precipitate.

- ♦ **Phenylephrine and Cyclopentolate** *see* Cyclopentolate and Phenylephrine *on page 461*
- ♦ **Phenylephrine Hydrochloride** *see* Phenylephrine *on page 1350*
- ♦ **Phenylephrine Tannate** *see* Phenylephrine *on page 1350*
- ♦ **Phenylethylmalonylurea** *see* Phenobarbital *on page 1343*
- ♦ **Phenytek™** *see* Phenytoin *on page 1354*

Phenytoin (FEN i toyn)

U.S. Brand Names Dilantin®; Phenytek™

Synonyms Diphenylhydantoin; DPH; Phenytoin Sodium; Phenytoin Sodium, Extended; Phenytoin Sodium, Prompt

Pharmacologic Category Antiarrhythmic Agent, Class Ib; Anticonvulsant, Hydantoin

Medication Safety Issues

Sound-alike/look-alike issues:

Phenytoin may be confused with phenelzine, phentermine

Dilantin® may be confused with Dilaudid®, diltiazem, Dipentum®

Use Management of generalized tonic-clonic (grand mal), complex partial seizures; prevention of seizures following head trauma/neurosurgery

Unlabeled/Investigational Use Ventricular arrhythmias, including those associated with digitalis intoxication, prolonged QT interval and surgical repair of congenital heart diseases in children; epidermolysis bullosa

Mechanism of Action Stabilizes neuronal membranes and decreases seizure activity by increasing efflux or decreasing influx of sodium ions across cell membranes in the motor cortex during generation of nerve impulses; prolongs effective refractory period and suppresses ventricular pacemaker automaticity, shortens action potential in the heart

Pharmacodynamics/Kinetics

Onset of action: I.V.: ~0.5-1 hour

Absorption: Oral: Slow

Distribution: V_d:

Neonates: Premature: 1-1.2 L/kg; Full-term: 0.8-0.9 L/kg

Infants: 0.7-0.8 L/kg

Children: 0.7 L/kg

Adults: 0.6-0.7 L/kg

Protein binding:

Neonates: ≥80% (≤20% free)

Infants: ≥85% (≤15% free)

Adults: 90% to 95%

Others: Decreased protein binding

Disease states resulting in a decrease in serum albumin concentration: Burns, hepatic cirrhosis, nephrotic syndrome, pregnancy, cystic fibrosis

Disease states resulting in an apparent decrease in affinity of phenytoin for serum albumin: Renal failure, jaundice (severe), other drugs (displacers), hyperbilirubinemia (total bilirubin >15 mg/dL), Cl_{cr} <25 mL/minute (unbound fraction is increased two- to threefold in uremia)

Metabolism: Follows dose-dependent capacity-limited (Michaelis-Menten) pharmacokinetics with increased V_{max} in infants >6 months of age and children versus adults; major metabolite (via oxidation), HPPA, undergoes enterohepatic recirculation

Bioavailability: Form dependent

Half-life elimination: Oral: 22 hours (range: 7-42 hours)

Time to peak, serum (form dependent): Oral: Extended-release capsule: 4-12 hours; Immediate release preparation: 2-3 hours

Excretion: Urine (<5% as unchanged drug); as glucuronides

Clearance: Highly variable, dependent upon intrinsic hepatic function and dose administered; increased clearance and decreased serum concentrations with febrile illness

Contraindications Hypersensitivity to phenytoin, other hydantoins, or any component of the formulation; pregnancy

Warnings/Precautions May increase frequency of petit mal seizures; I.V. form may cause hypotension, skin necrosis at I.V. site; avoid I.V. administration in small veins; use with caution in patients with porphyria; discontinue if rash or lymphadenopathy occurs; use with caution in patients with hepatic dysfunction, sinus bradycardia, SA block, or AV block; use with caution in elderly or debilitated patients, or in any condition associated with low serum albumin levels, which will increase the free fraction of phenytoin in the serum and, therefore, the pharmacologic response. Sedation, confusional states, or cerebellar dysfunction (loss of motor coordination) may occur at higher total serum concentrations, or at lower total serum concentrations when the free fraction of phenytoin is increased. Abrupt withdrawal may precipitate status epilepticus.

Drug Interactions Substrate of CYP2C8/9 (major), 2C19 (major), 3A4 (minor); **Induces** CYP2B6 (strong), 2C8/9 (strong), 2C19 (strong), 3A4 (strong)

Acetaminophen: Phenytoin may enhance the hepatotoxic potential of acetaminophen overdoses

Acetazolamide: Concurrent use with phenytoin may result in an increased risk of osteomalacia

Acyclovir: May decrease phenytoin serum levels; limited documentation; monitor

Allopurinol: May increase phenytoin serum concentrations; monitor

Antacids: May decrease absorption of phenytoin; separate oral doses by several hours

Antiarrhythmics: Phenytoin may increase the metabolism of antiarrhythmics, decreasing their clinical effect; includes disopyramide, propafenone, and quinidine; amiodarone also may increase phenytoin concentrations (see CYP inhibitors)

Anticonvulsants: Phenytoin may increase the metabolism of anticonvulsants; includes barbiturates, carbamazepine, ethosuximide, felbamate, lamotrigine, tiagabine, topiramate, and zonisamide; does not appear to affect gabapentin or levetiracetam; felbamate and gabapentin may increase phenytoin levels; monitor

Antineoplastics: Several chemotherapeutic agents have been associated with a decrease in serum phenytoin levels; includes cisplatin, bleomycin, carmustine, methotrexate, and vinblastine; monitor phenytoin serum levels. Limited evidence also suggest that enzyme-inducing anticonvulsant therapy may reduce the effectiveness of some chemotherapy regimens (specifically in ALL). Teniposide and methotrexate may be cleared more rapidly in these patients.

(Continued)

Phenytoin *(Continued)*

Antipsychotics: Phenytoin may enhance the metabolism (decrease the efficacy) of antipsychotics; monitor for altered response; dose adjustment may be needed; also see note on clozapine

Benzodiazepines: Phenytoin may decrease the serum concentrations of some benzodiazepines; monitor for decreased benzodiazepine effect

Beta-blockers: Metabolism of beta-blockers may be increased and clinical effect decreased; atenolol and nadolol are unlikely to interact given their renal elimination

Calcium channel blockers: Phenytoin may enhance the metabolism of calcium channel blockers, decreasing their clinical effect; calcium channel blockers (diltiazem, nifedipine) have been reported to increase phenytoin levels (case report); monitor.

Capecitabine: May increase the serum concentrations of phenytoin; monitor

Chloramphenicol: Phenytoin may increase the metabolism of chloramphenicol and chloramphenicol may inhibit phenytoin metabolism; monitor for altered response

Cimetidine: May increase the serum concentrations of phenytoin; monitor.

Ciprofloxacin: May decrease serum phenytoin concentrations; monitor.

Clozapine: Phenytoin may decrease levels/effects of clozapine; monitor.

CNS depressants: Sedative effects may be additive with other CNS depressants; monitor for increased effect; includes ethanol, barbiturates, sedatives, antidepressants, narcotic analgesics, and benzodiazepines

Corticosteroids: Phenytoin may increase the metabolism of corticosteroids, decreasing their clinical effect; also see dexamethasone

Cyclosporine and tacrolimus: Levels may be decreased by phenytoin; monitor

CYP2B6 substrates: Phenytoin may decrease the levels/effects of CYP2B6 substrates. Example substrates include bupropion, efavirenz, promethazine, selegiline, and sertraline.

CYP2C8/9 inducers: May decrease the levels/effects of phenytoin. Example inducers include carbamazepine, phenobarbital, rifampin, rifapentine, and secobarbital.

CYP2C8/9 inhibitors: May increase the levels/effects of phenytoin. Example inhibitors include delavirdine, fluconazole, gemfibrozil, ketoconazole, nicardipine, NSAIDs, pioglitazone, and sulfonamides.

CYP2C8/9 substrates: Phenytoin may decrease the levels/effects of CYP2C8/9 substrates. Example substrates include amiodarone, fluoxetine, glimepiride, glipizide, losartan, nateglinide, pioglitazone, rosiglitazone, sertraline, sulfonamides, warfarin, and zafirlukast.

CYP2C19 inducers: May decrease the levels/effects of phenytoin. Example inducers include aminoglutethimide, carbamazepine, phenytoin, and rifampin.

CYP2C19 inhibitors: May increase the levels/effects of phenytoin. Example inhibitors include delavirdine, fluconazole, fluvoxamine, gemfibrozil, isoniazid, omeprazole, and ticlopidine.

CYP2C19 substrates: Phenytoin may decrease the levels/effects of CYP2C19 substrates. Example substrates include citalopram, diazepam, methsuximide, propranolol, proton pump inhibitors, sertraline, and voriconazole.

CYP3A4 substrates: Phenytoin may decrease the levels/effects of CYP3A4 substrates. Example substrates include benzodiazepines, calcium channel blockers, clarithromycin, cyclosporine, erythromycin, estrogens, mirtazapine, nateglinide, nefazodone, nevirapine, protease inhibitors, tacrolimus, and venlafaxine.

Digoxin: Effects and/or levels of digitalis glycosides may be decreased by phenytoin

Disulfiram: May increase serum phenytoin concentrations; monitor

Dopamine: Phenytoin (I.V.) may increase the effect of dopamine (enhanced hypotension)

Doxycycline: Phenytoin may enhance the metabolism of doxycycline, decreasing its clinical effect; higher dosages may be required

Estrogens: Phenytoin may increase the metabolism of estrogens, decreasing their clinical effect; monitor

Folic acid: Replacement of folic acid has been reported to increase the metabolism of phenytoin, decreasing its serum concentrations and/or increasing seizures

HMG-CoA reductase inhibitors: Phenytoin may increase the metabolism of these agents, reducing their clinical effect; monitor

Itraconazole: Phenytoin may decrease the effect of itraconazole

Levodopa: Phenytoin may inhibit the anti-Parkinson effect of levodopa
Lithium: Concurrent use of phenytoin and lithium has resulted in lithium intoxication
Methadone: Phenytoin may enhance the metabolism of methadone resulting in methadone withdrawal
Methylphenidate: May increase serum phenytoin concentrations; monitor
Metronidazole: May increase the serum concentrations of phenytoin; monitor.
Neuromuscular-blocking agents: Duration of effect may be decreased by phenytoin
Omeprazole: May increase serum phenytoin concentrations; monitor
Oral contraceptives: Phenytoin may enhance the metabolism of oral contraceptives, decreasing their clinical effect; an alternative method of contraception should be considered
Primidone: Phenytoin enhances the conversion of primidone to phenobarbital resulting in elevated phenobarbital serum concentrations
Quetiapine: Serum concentrations may be substantially reduced by phenytoin, potentially resulting in a loss of efficacy; limited documentation; monitor
SSRIs: May increase phenytoin serum concentrations; fluoxetine and fluvoxamine are known to inhibit metabolism via CYP enzymes; sertraline and paroxetine have also been shown to increase concentrations in some patients; monitor
Sucralfate: May reduce the GI absorption of phenytoin; monitor
Theophylline: Phenytoin may increase metabolism of theophylline derivatives and decrease their clinical effect; theophylline may also increase phenytoin concentrations
Thyroid hormones (including levothyroxine): Phenytoin may alter the metabolism of thyroid hormones, reducing its effect; there is limited documentation of this interaction, but monitoring should be considered
Ticlopidine: May increase serum phenytoin concentrations and/or toxicity; monitor
Tricyclic antidepressants: Phenytoin may increase metabolism of tricyclic antidepressants and decrease their clinical effect; sedative effects may be additive; tricyclics may also increase phenytoin concentrations
Topiramate: Phenytoin may decrease serum levels of topiramate; topiramate may increase the effect of phenytoin
Trazodone: Serum levels of phenytoin may be increased; limited documentation; monitor
Trimethoprim: May increase serum phenytoin concentrations; monitor
Valproic acid (and sulfisoxazole): May displace phenytoin from binding sites; valproic acid may increase, decrease, or have no effect on phenytoin serum concentrations
Vigabatrin: May reduce phenytoin serum concentrations; monitor
Warfarin: Phenytoin transiently increased the hypothrombinemia response to warfarin initially; this is followed by an inhibition of the hypoprothrombinemic response

Nutritional/Herbal/Ethanol Interactions

Ethanol:

Acute use: Avoid or limit ethanol (inhibits metabolism of phenytoin). Watch for sedation.

Chronic use: Avoid or limit ethanol (stimulates metabolism of phenytoin).

Food: Phenytoin serum concentrations may be altered if taken with food. If taken with enteral nutrition, phenytoin serum concentrations may be decreased. Tube feedings decrease bioavailability; hold tube feedings 2 hours before and 2 hours after phenytoin administration. May decrease calcium, folic acid, and vitamin D levels.

Herb/Nutraceutical: Avoid evening primrose (seizure threshold decreased). Avoid valerian, St John's wort, kava kava, gotu kola (may increase CNS depression).

Lab Interactions Increased glucose, alkaline phosphatase (S); decreased thyroxine (S), calcium (S)

Adverse Reactions I.V. effects: Hypotension, bradycardia, cardiac arrhythmia, cardiovascular collapse (especially with rapid I.V. use), venous irritation and pain, thrombophlebitis

Effects not related to plasma phenytoin concentrations: Hypertrichosis, gingival hypertrophy, thickening of facial features, carbohydrate intolerance, folic acid deficiency, peripheral neuropathy, vitamin D deficiency, osteomalacia, systemic lupus erythematosus

Concentration-related effects: Nystagmus, blurred vision, diplopia, ataxia, slurred speech, dizziness, drowsiness, lethargy, coma, rash, fever, nausea,

(Continued)

Phenytoin *(Continued)*

vomiting, gum tenderness, confusion, mood changes, folic acid depletion, osteomalacia, hyperglycemia

Related to elevated concentrations:

>20 mcg/mL: Far lateral nystagmus

>30 mcg/mL: 45° lateral gaze nystagmus and ataxia

>40 mcg/mL: Decreased mentation

>100 mcg/mL: Death

Cardiovascular: Hypotension, bradycardia, cardiac arrhythmia, cardiovascular collapse

Central nervous system: Psychiatric changes, slurred speech, dizziness, drowsiness, headache, insomnia

Dermatologic: Rash

Gastrointestinal: Constipation, nausea, vomiting, gingival hyperplasia, enlargement of lips

Hematologic: Leukopenia, thrombocytopenia, agranulocytosis

Hepatic: Hepatitis

Local: Thrombophlebitis

Neuromuscular & skeletal: Tremor, peripheral neuropathy, paresthesia

Ocular: Diplopia, nystagmus, blurred vision

Rarely seen effects: Blood dyscrasias, coarsening of facial features, dyskinesias, hepatitis, hypertrichosis, lymphadenopathy, lymphoma, pseudolymphoma, SLE-like syndrome, Stevens-Johnson syndrome, venous irritation and pain

Overdosage/Toxicology Symptoms of overdose include unsteady gait, slurred speech, confusion, nausea, hypothermia, fever, hypotension, respiratory depression, coma. Treatment is symptomatic.

Dosing

Adults & Elderly:

Status epilepticus: I.V.: Loading dose: Manufacturer recommends 10-15 mg/kg, however, 15-25 mg/kg has been used clinically; maintenance dose: 300 mg/day or 5-6 mg/kg/day in 3 divided doses or 1-2 divided doses using extended release

Anticonvulsant: Oral: Loading dose: 15-20 mg/kg; based on phenytoin serum concentrations and recent dosing history; administer oral loading dose in 3 divided doses given every 2-4 hours to decrease GI adverse effects and to ensure complete oral absorption; maintenance dose: 300 mg/day or 5-6 mg/kg/day in 3 divided doses or 1-2 divided doses using extended release (range 200-1200 mg/day)

Pediatrics:

Status epilepticus: I.V.:

Infants and Children: Loading dose: 15-20 mg/kg in a single or divided dose; maintenance dose: Initial: 5 mg/kg/day in 2 divided doses, usual doses:

6 months to 3 years: 8-10 mg/kg/day

4-6 years: 7.5-9 mg/kg/day

7-9 years: 7-8 mg/kg/day

10-16 years: 6-7 mg/kg/day, some patients may require every 8 hours dosing

Anticonvulsant: Children: Oral: Refer to adult dosing.

Renal Impairment: Phenytoin level in serum may be difficult to interpret in renal failure. Monitoring of free (unbound) concentrations or adjustment to allow interpretation is recommended.

Hepatic Impairment: Safe in usual doses in mild liver disease; clearance may be substantially reduced in cirrhosis and plasma level monitoring with dose adjustment advisable. Free phenytoin levels should be monitored closely.

Available Dosage Forms

Capsule, extended release, as sodium: 100 mg

Dilantin®: 30 mg [contains sodium benzoate], 100 mg

Phenytek™: 200 mg, 300 mg

Capsule, prompt release, as sodium: 100 mg

Injection, solution, as sodium: 50 mg/mL (2 mL, 5 mL) [contains alcohol and propylene glycol]

Suspension, oral (Dilantin®): 125 mg/5 mL (240 mL) [contains alcohol <0.6%, sodium benzoate; banana flavor]

Tablet, chewable (Dilantin®): 50 mg

Nursing Guidelines

Assessment: Assess potential for numerous interactions with other prescriptions, OTC medications, or herbal products patient may be taking (see extensive list of Drug Interactions). Assess results of laboratory tests, therapeutic effectiveness, and adverse response when beginning therapy and at regular intervals during treatment. When discontinuing oral formulation, taper dose gradually; abrupt discontinuance can cause status epilepticus. Teach patient proper use (oral), side effects/appropriate interventions, and adverse symptoms to report. **I.V.:** Monitor blood pressure. Infusion site should be monitored closely (vesicant). Patient should be monitored closely for adverse/toxic results.

Monitoring Laboratory Tests: Plasma phenytoin level, CBC, liver function. **Note:** Serum phenytoin concentrations should be interpreted in terms of the unbound concentration. Adjustment should be made in patients with renal impairment and/or hypoalbuminemia.

Dietary Considerations:

Folic acid: Phenytoin may decrease mucosal uptake of folic acid; to avoid folic acid deficiency and megaloblastic anemia, some clinicians recommend giving patients on anticonvulsants prophylactic doses of folic acid and cyanocobalamin. However, folate supplementation may increase seizures in some patients (dose dependent). Discuss with healthcare provider prior to using any supplements.

Calcium: Hypocalcemia has been reported in patients taking prolonged high-dose therapy with an anticonvulsant. Some clinicians have given an additional 4000 units/week of vitamin D (especially in those receiving poor nutrition and getting no sun exposure) to prevent hypocalcemia.

Vitamin D: Phenytoin interferes with vitamin D metabolism and osteomalacia may result; may need to supplement with vitamin D

Tube feedings: Tube feedings decrease phenytoin absorption. To avoid decreased serum levels with continuous NG feeds, hold feedings for 2 hours prior to and 2 hours after phenytoin administration, if possible. There is a variety of opinions on how to administer phenytoin with enteral feedings. Be **consistent** throughout therapy.

Sodium content of 1 g injection: 88 mg (3.8 mEq)

Patient Education: Do not take any new medication during therapy without consulting prescriber. Take exactly as directed, preferably on an empty stomach. Do not alter dose or discontinue without consulting prescriber. Do not crush, break, or chew extended release capsules. Shake liquid suspension well before using. Follow recommended diet, avoid alcohol, and maintain adequate hydration (2-3 L/day of fluids) unless instructed to restrict fluid intake. May cause gum or mouth soreness (use good oral hygiene and have frequent dental exams); drowsiness, dizziness, nervousness, or headache (use caution when driving or engaging in tasks that require alertness until response to drug is known); or nausea or vomiting (small frequent meals, frequent mouth care, chewing gum, or sucking lozenges may help). Report chest pain, irregular heartbeat, or palpitations; slurred speech, unsteady gait, coordination difficulties, or change in mentation; skin rash; unresolved nausea, vomiting, or constipation; swollen glands; swollen, sore, or bleeding gums; unusual bruising or bleeding; acute persistent fatigue; vision changes; or other persistent adverse effects. **Pregnancy/breast-feeding precautions:** Do not get pregnant; use contraceptive measures to prevent possible harm to the fetus (effectiveness of oral contraceptives may be affected by phenytoin). Consult prescriber if breast-feeding.

Geriatric Considerations: Elderly may have low albumin which will increase free fraction and increase drug response. Monitor closely in those who are hypoalbuminemic. Free fraction measurements advised, also elderly may display a higher incidence of adverse effects (cardiovascular) when using the I.V. loading regimen; therefore, recommended to decrease loading I.V. dose to 25 mg/minute (see Warnings/Precautions).

Pregnancy Risk Factor: D

Pregnancy Issues: Phenytoin crosses the placenta. Congenital malformations (including a pattern of malformations termed the "fetal hydantoin syndrome" or "fetal anticonvulsant syndrome") have been reported in infants. Isolated cases of malignancies (including neuroblastoma) and coagulation defects in the neonate following delivery have also been reported. Epilepsy itself, the number of medications, genetic factors, or a combination of these probably influence the teratogenicity of anticonvulsant therapy.

(Continued)

Phenytoin *(Continued)*

Total plasma concentrations of phenytoin are decreased by 56% in the mother during pregnancy; unbound plasma (free) concentrations are decreased by 31%. Because protein binding is decreased, monitoring of unbound plasma concentrations is recommended. Concentrations should be monitored through the 8th week postpartum. The use of folic acid throughout pregnancy and vitamin K during the last month of pregnancy is recommended.

A pregnancy registry is available for women exposed to antiepileptic drug (including phenytoin) at the Genetics and Teratology Unit Massachusetts General Hospital, 1-888-233-2334.

Lactation: Enters breast milk/not recommended (AAP rates "compatible")

Breast-Feeding Considerations: Phenytoin is excreted in breast milk; however, the amount to which the infant is exposed is considered small. The manufacturers of phenytoin do not recommend breast-feeding during therapy, however, the AAP considers it to be usually compatible. Women should be counseled of the possible risks and benefits associated with breast-feeding while on phenytoin.

Perioperative/Anesthesia/Other Concerns: Because phenytoin induces the metabolism of many drugs, it may alter their effective blood concentration.

The vehicle which contains propylene glycol, ethanol, and sodium hydroxide, may cause hypotension, bradycardia, arrhythmias, or asystole refractory to defibrillation. Phenytoin 50 mg/mL contains propylene glycol 414.4 mg/mL (40% v/v).

Patients on chronic phenytoin therapy require larger and more frequent doses of nondepolarizing muscle relaxants to attain the same degree of muscle relaxation. This is probably due to increased levels of $alpha_1$-acid glycoprotein released by the liver (which bind free phenytoin) during hepatic enzyme induction.

Rapid intravenous administration may cause hypotension. Infuse at a rate no greater than 50 mg/minute in adults and 25 mg/minute in the elderly.

Status Epilepticus: A randomized, double-blind trial (Treiman D, 1998) evaluated the efficacy of four treatments in overt status epilepticus. Treatment arms were designed based upon accepted practices of North American neurologists. The treatments were: 1) lorazepam 0.1 mg/kg, 2) diazepam 0.15 mg/kg followed by phenytoin 18 mg/kg, 3) phenytoin 18 mg/kg alone, and 4) phenobarbital 15 mg/kg. Treatment was considered successful if the seizures were terminated (clinically and by EEG) within 20 minutes of start of therapy without seizure recurrence within 60 minutes from the start of therapy. Patients who failed the first treatment received a second and a third, if necessary. Patients did not receive randomized treatments after the first one but the treating physician remained blinded. Treatment success: Lorazepam 64.9%, phenobarbital 58.2%, diazepam/phenytoin 55.8%, and phenytoin alone 43.6%. Using an intention to treat analysis, there was no statistical difference between the groups. Results of subsequent treatments in patients who failed the first therapy indicated that response rate significantly dropped regardless of treatment. Aggregate response rate to the second treatment was 7.0% and third treatment 2.3%.

Administration

Oral: Suspension: Shake well prior to use. Absorption is impaired when phenytoin suspension is given concurrently to patients who are receiving continuous nasogastric feedings. A method to resolve this interaction is to divide the daily dose of phenytoin and withhold the administration of nutritional supplements for 1-2 hours before and after each phenytoin dose.

I.M.: Although approved for I.M. use, I.M. administration is not recommended due to erratic absorption and pain on injection. Fosphenytoin may be considered.

I.V.: Vesicant. Fosphenytoin may be considered for loading in patients who are in status epilepticus, hemodynamically unstable or develop hypotension/bradycardia with I.V. administration of phenytoin. Phenytoin may be administered by IVP or IVPB administration. The maximum rate of I.V. administration is 50 mg/minute. Highly sensitive patients (eg, elderly, patients with pre-existing cardiovascular conditions) should receive phenytoin more slowly (eg, 20 mg/minute).

Reconstitution: I.V.: Further dilution of the solution for I.V. infusion is controversial and no consensus exists as to the optimal concentration and length of stability. Stability is concentration and pH dependent. Based on limited clinical consensus, NS or LR are recommended diluents; dilutions of 1-10 mg/mL have been used and should be administered as soon as possible after preparation (some recommend to discard if not used within 4 hours). Do not refrigerate.

Compatibility: Incompatible with D_5NS, D_5W, fat emulsion 10%, LR, ½NS

Compatibility in syringe: Incompatible with hydromorphone, sufentanil

Compatibility when admixed: Incompatible with amikacin, aminophylline, bretylium, chloramphenicol, dimenhydrinate, diphenhydramine, dobutamine, hydroxyzine, insulin (regular), kanamycin, levorphanol, lidocaine, lincomycin, meperidine, metaraminol, morphine, nitroglycerin, norepinephrine, penicillin G potassium, pentobarbital, phenobarbital, phenylephrine, phytonadione, procainamide, procaine, prochlorperazine edisylate, promazine, promethazine, streptomycin, vancomycin, vitamin B complex with C

Storage:

Capsule, tablet: Store below 30°C (86°F); protect from light and moisture

Oral suspension: Store at room temperature of 20°C to 25°C (68°F to 77°F); protect from freezing and light.

Solution for injection: Store at room temperature of 15°C to 30°C (59°F to 86°F); use only clear solutions free of precipitate and haziness, slightly yellow solutions may be used. Precipitation may occur if solution is refrigerated and may dissolve at room temperature.

Related Information

Perioperative Management of Patients on Antiseizure Medication *on page 1801*

- **Phenytoin Sodium** *see* Phenytoin *on page 1354*
- **Phenytoin Sodium, Extended** *see* Phenytoin *on page 1354*
- **Phenytoin Sodium, Prompt** *see* Phenytoin *on page 1354*
- **Phillips'® Milk of Magnesia [OTC]** *see* Magnesium Hydroxide *on page 1076*
- **Phillips'® Stool Softener Laxative [OTC]** *see* Docusate *on page 560*
- **pHisoHex®** *see* Hexachlorophene *on page 854*
- **Phos-NaK** *see* Potassium Phosphate and Sodium Phosphate *on page 1391*
- **Phospha 250™ Neutral** *see* Potassium Phosphate and Sodium Phosphate *on page 1391*
- **Phosphate, Potassium** *see* Potassium Phosphate *on page 1389*
- **Phosphonoformate** *see* Foscarnet *on page 775*
- **Phosphonoformic Acid** *see* Foscarnet *on page 775*
- ***p*-Hydroxyampicillin** *see* Amoxicillin *on page 144*
- **Phylloquinone** *see* Phytonadione *on page 1363*

Physostigmine (fye zoe STIG meen)

Synonyms Eserine Salicylate; Physostigmine Salicylate; Physostigmine Sulfate

Pharmacologic Category Acetylcholinesterase Inhibitor

Medication Safety Issues

Sound-alike/look-alike issues:

Physostigmine may be confused with Prostigmin®, pyridostigmine

Use Reverse toxic CNS effects caused by anticholinergic drugs

Mechanism of Action Inhibits destruction of acetylcholine by acetylcholinesterase which facilitates transmission of impulses across myoneural junction and prolongs the central and peripheral effects of acetylcholine

Pharmacodynamics/Kinetics

Onset of action: ~5 minutes

Duration: 0.5-5 hours

Absorption: I.M., SubQ: Readily absorbed

Distribution: Crosses blood-brain barrier readily and reverses both central and peripheral anticholinergic effects

Metabolism: Hepatic and via hydrolysis by cholinesterases

Half-life elimination: 15-40 minutes

Contraindications Hypersensitivity to physostigmine or any component of the formulation; GI or GU obstruction; physostigmine therapy of drug intoxications should be used with extreme caution in patients with asthma, gangrene, severe cardiovascular disease, or mechanical obstruction of the GI tract or urogenital tract. In these patients, physostigmine should be used only to treat life-threatening conditions.

Warnings/Precautions Use with caution in patients with epilepsy, asthma, diabetes, gangrene, cardiovascular disease, bradycardia. Discontinue if excessive salivation or emesis, frequent urination or diarrhea occur. Reduce dosage if excessive sweating or nausea occurs. Administer I.V. slowly or at a controlled rate not faster than 1 mg/minute. Due to the possibility of hypersensitivity or

(Continued)

Physostigmine *(Continued)*

overdose/cholinergic crisis, atropine should be readily available; not intended as a first-line agent for anticholinergic toxicity or Parkinson's disease.

Drug Interactions Increased toxicity: Bethanechol, methacholine, succinylcholine may increase neuromuscular blockade with systemic administration

Lab Interactions Increased aminotransferase [ALT (SGPT)/AST (SGOT)] (S), amylase (S)

Adverse Reactions Frequency not defined.

Cardiovascular: Palpitations, bradycardia
Central nervous system: Restlessness, nervousness, hallucinations, seizure
Gastrointestinal: Nausea, salivation, diarrhea, stomach pain
Genitourinary: Frequent urge to urinate
Neuromuscular & skeletal: Muscle twitching
Ocular: Lacrimation, miosis
Respiratory: Dyspnea, bronchospasm, respiratory paralysis, pulmonary edema
Miscellaneous: Diaphoresis

Overdosage/Toxicology Symptoms of overdose include muscle weakness, blurred vision, excessive sweating, tearing and salivation, nausea, vomiting, bronchospasm, and seizures. If physostigmine is used in excess or in the absence of an anticholinergic overdose, patients may manifest signs of cholinergic toxicity. At this point, an anticholinergic agent (eg, atropine 0.015-0.05 mg/kg) may be necessary.

Dosing

Adults & Elderly:

Anticholinergic drug overdose:

I.M., I.V., SubQ: 0.5-2 mg to start; repeat every 20 minutes until response occurs or adverse effect occurs.

Repeat 1-4 mg every 30-60 minutes as life-threatening signs (arrhythmias, seizures, deep coma) recur; maximum I.V. rate: 1 mg/minute.

Pediatrics: Anticholinergic drug overdose (Reserve for life-threatening situations only): children: I.V.: 0.01-0.03 mg/kg/dose (maximum: 0.5 mg/minute). May repeat after 5-10 minutes to a maximum total dose of 2 mg or until response occurs or adverse cholinergic effects occur,

Available Dosage Forms Injection, solution, as salicylate: 1 mg/mL (2 mL) [contains benzyl alcohol and sodium metabisulfite]

Nursing Guidelines

Assessment: When used to reverse neuromuscular block, patient must be monitored closely until full return of neuromuscular functioning. Assess bladder and sphincter adequacy prior to administering medication. Assess other medications patient may be taking for effectiveness and interactions. Monitor therapeutic effectiveness and adverse reactions (cholinergic crisis). Assess knowledge/teach patient appropriate use of ophthalmic forms, interventions to reduce side effects, and adverse symptoms to report.

Patient Education: Maintain adequate hydration (2-3 L/day of fluids) unless instructed to restrict fluid intake. May cause dizziness, drowsiness, or hypotension (rise slowly from sitting or lying position and use caution when driving or climbing stairs); vomiting or loss of appetite (small frequent meals, frequent mouth care, chewing gum, or sucking lozenges may help); or diarrhea (boiled milk, yogurt, or buttermilk may help). Report persistent abdominal discomfort; significantly increased salivation, sweating, tearing, or urination; flushed skin; chest pain or palpitations; acute headache; unresolved diarrhea; excessive fatigue, insomnia, dizziness, or depression; increased muscle, joint, or body pain; vision changes or blurred vision; or shortness of breath or wheezing. **Pregnancy/breast-feeding precautions:** Inform prescriber if you are or intend to become pregnant. Consult prescriber if breast-feeding.

Geriatric Considerations: Studies on the use of physostigmine in Alzheimer's disease have reported variable results. Doses generally were in the range of 2-4 mg 4 times/day. Limitations to the use of physostigmine include a short half-life requiring frequent dosing, variable absorption from the GI tract, and no commercially available oral product; therefore, not recommended for treatment of Alzheimer's disease.

Pregnancy Risk Factor: C

Lactation: Excretion in breast milk unknown

Perioperative/Anesthesia/Other Concerns: Cholinergic effects of physostigmine include bradycardia and bradydysrhythmias.

Administration

I.V.: Infuse slowly I.V. at a maximum rate of 0.5 mg/minute in children or 1 mg/minute in adults. Too rapid administration (I.V. rate not to exceed 1 mg/minute) can cause bradycardia, hypersalivation leading to respiratory difficulties and seizures.

Compatibility: Stable in dextran 6% in dextrose, dextran 6% in NS, D_5W, $D_{10}W$, D_5LR, $D_5{}^1/_4NS$, $D_5{}^1/_2NS$, D_5NS, fat emulsion 10%, LR, $^1/_2NS$, NS

Y-site administration: Incompatible with dobutamine

Compatibility when admixed: Incompatible with phenytoin, ranitidine

Storage: Do not use solution if cloudy or dark brown.

♦ **Physostigmine Salicylate** *see* Physostigmine *on page 1361*

♦ **Physostigmine Sulfate** *see* Physostigmine *on page 1361*

♦ **Phytomenadione** *see* Phytonadione *on page 1363*

Phytonadione (fye toe na DYE one)

U.S. Brand Names Mephyton®

Synonyms Methylphytyl Napthoquinone; Phylloquinone; Phytomenadione; Vitamin K_1

Pharmacologic Category Vitamin, Fat Soluble

Medication Safety Issues

Sound-alike/look-alike issues:

Mephyton® may be confused with melphalan, methadone

Use Prevention and treatment of hypoprothrombinemia caused by coumarin derivative-induced or other drug-induced vitamin K deficiency, hypoprothrombinemia caused by malabsorption or inability to synthesize vitamin K; hemorrhagic disease of the newborn

Mechanism of Action Promotes liver synthesis of clotting factors (II, VII, IX, X); however, the exact mechanism as to this stimulation is unknown. Menadiol is a water soluble form of vitamin K; phytonadione has a more rapid and prolonged effect than menadione; menadiol sodium diphosphate (K_4) is half as potent as menadione (K_3).

Pharmacodynamics/Kinetics

Onset of action: Increased coagulation factors: Oral: 6-10 hours; I.V.: 1-2 hours

Peak effect: INR values return to normal: Oral: 24-48 hours; I.V.: 12-14 hours

Absorption: Oral: From intestines in presence of bile; SubQ: Variable

Metabolism: Rapidly hepatic

Excretion: Urine and feces

Contraindications Hypersensitivity to phytonadione or any component of the formulation

Warnings/Precautions

Allergic reactions (injectable): Severe reactions resembling hypersensitivity (eg, anaphylaxis) reactions have occurred rarely during or immediately after I.V. administration (even with proper dilution and rate of administration). Allergic reactions have also occurred with I.M. and SubQ injections.

Route: Oral administration is the safest and requires the presence of bile salts for absorption. In obstructive jaundice or with biliary fistulas, concurrent administration of bile salts would be necessary for proper absorption. Manufacturers recommend the SubQ route over other parenteral routes, however, SubQ is less predictable when compared to the oral route, and efficacy may be delayed. The American College of Chest Physicians recommends the I.V. route in patients with serious or life-threatening bleeding secondary to use of vitamin K antagonists such as warfarin. The I.V. route should be restricted to emergency situations only where oral phytonadione cannot be used. Efficacy (eg, control of bleeding, decrease in INR) is delayed regardless of route of administration; patient management may require other treatments in the interim.

Reversing anticoagulant induced hypoprothrombinemia: Administer a dose that will quickly lower the INR into a safe range without causing resistance to warfarin. High phytonadione doses may lead to warfarin resistance for at least one week.

Newborns: Use caution in newborns, especially premature infants; hemolysis, jaundice, and hyperbilirubinemia have been reported with larger than recommended doses. Some dosage forms contain benzyl alcohol which has been associated with "gasping syndrome" in premature infants.

(Continued)

Phytonadione *(Continued)*

Hypoprothrombinemia caused by liver disease: If initial doses do not reverse coagulopathy, then higher doses are unlikely to have any effect. **Note:** Ineffective in hereditary hypoprothrombinemia.

Renal dysfunction: Use caution with renal dysfunction (including premature infants). Injectable products may contain aluminum; may result in toxic levels following prolonged administration.

Drug Interactions

Coumarin derivatives: Phytonadione may diminish the anticoagulant effect; monitor INR.

Orlistat: Phytonadione (oral) may not be properly absorbed when administered concurrently; separate doses by at least 2 hours.

Adverse Reactions Parenteral administration: Frequency not defined.

Cardiovascular: Cyanosis, flushing, hypotension

Central nervous system: Dizziness

Dermatologic: Scleroderma-like lesions

Endocrine & metabolic: Hyperbilirubinemia (newborn; greater than recommended doses)

Gastrointestinal: Abnormal taste

Local: Injection site reactions

Respiratory: Dyspnea

Miscellaneous: Anaphylactoid reactions, diaphoresis, hypersensitivity reactions

Management of Elevated INR

INR	Symptom	Action
Above therapeutic range to <5	No significant bleeding	Lower or hold the next dose and monitor frequently; when INR approaches desired range, may resume dosing with a lower dose if INR was significantly above therapeutic range.
≥5 and <9	No significant bleeding	Omit the next 1or 2 doses; monitor INR and resume with a lower dose when the INR approaches the desired range. Alternatively, if there are other risk factors for bleeding, omit the next dose and give vitamin K_1 orally ≤5 mg; resume with a lower dose when the INR approaches the desired range. If rapid reversal is required for surgery, then given vitamin K_1 orally 2-4 mg and hold warfarin. Expect a response within 24 hours; another 1-2 mg may be given orally if needed.
≥9	No significant bleeding	Hold warfarin, give vitamin K_1 orally 5-10 mg, expect the INR to be reduced within 24-48 hours; monitor INR and administer additional vitamin K if necessary. Resume warfarin at lower doses when INR is in the desired range.
Any INR elevation	Serious bleeding	Hold warfarin, give vitamin K_1 (10 mg by slow I.V. infusion), and supplement with fresh plasma transfusion or prothrombin complex concentrate (Factor X complex); recombinant factor VIIa is an alternative to prothrombin complex concentrate. Vitamin K_1 injection can be repeated every 12 hours.
Any INR elevation	Life-threatening bleeding	Hold warfarin, give prothrombin complex concentrate, supplemented with vitamin K_1 (10 mg by slow I.V. infusion); repeat if necessary. Recombinant factor VIIa is an alternative to prothrombin complex concentrate.

Note: Use of high doses of vitamin K_1 (10-15 mg) may cause resistance to warfarin for up to a week. Heparin or low molecular weight heparin can be given until the patient becomes responsive to warfarin. **Reference:** Ansell J, Hirsh J, Poller L et al. "The Pharmacology and Management of the Vitamin K Antagonists," *Chest*, 2004, 126 (3 Suppl):204-33.

Dosing

Adults & Elderly:

Adequate intake: Males: 120 mcg/day; Females: 90 mcg/day

Hypoprothrombinemia due to drugs (other than coumarin derivatives) or factors limiting absorption or synthesis: Oral, SubQ, I.M., I.V.: Initial: 2.5-25 mg (rarely up to 50 mg)

Vitamin K deficiency secondary to coumarin derivative: See table on previous page:

Pediatrics:

Adequate intake:

1-3 years: 30 mcg/day

4-8 years: 55 mcg/day

9-13 years: 60 mcg/day

14-18 years: 75 mcg/day

Hemorrhagic disease of the newborn:

Prophylaxis: I.M.: 0.5-1 mg within 1 hour of birth

Treatment: I.M., SubQ: 1 mg/dose/day; higher doses may be necessary if mother has been receiving oral anticoagulants

Available Dosage Forms

Injection, aqueous colloidal: 2 mg/mL (0.5 mL); 10 mg/mL (1 mL) [contains benzyl alcohol]

Tablet: 5 mg

Nursing Guidelines

Assessment: Note dosing specifics according to purpose for use. Assess results of laboratory tests and patient response (degree of bleeding). Teach patient proper use, possible side effects/appropriate interventions, and adverse symptoms to report.

Monitoring Laboratory Tests: PT, INR

Patient Education: Do not take any new medication during therapy (especially any aspirin-containing products or NSAIDs) without consulting prescriber. Oral: Take only as directed; do not take more or more often than prescribed. Consult prescriber for recommended diet. Report bleeding gums; blood in urine, stool, or vomitus; unusual bruising or bleeding; or abdominal cramping. **Pregnancy precaution:** Inform prescriber if you are or intend to become pregnant.

Pregnancy Risk Factor: C

Lactation: Enters breast milk/use caution (APP rates "compatible")

Administration

I.V.: Infuse slowly; rate of infusion should not exceed 1 mg/minute. The injectable route should be used only if the oral route is not feasible or there is a greater urgency to reverse anticoagulation.

Reconstitution: Dilute injection solution in preservative-free NS, D_5W, or D_5NS.

Storage:

Injection: Store at 15°C to 30°C (59°F to 86°F). **Note:** Store Hospira product at 20°C to 25°C (68°F to 77°F).

Oral: Store tablets at 15°C to 30°C (59°F to 86°F); protect from light.

♦ **Pidorubicin** *see* Epirubicin *on page 615*

♦ **Pidorubicin Hydrochloride** *see* Epirubicin *on page 615*

Pilocarpine (pye loe KAR peen)

U.S. Brand Names Isopto® Carpine; Pilopine HS®; Salagen®

Synonyms Pilocarpine Hydrochloride

Pharmacologic Category Cholinergic Agonist; Ophthalmic Agent, Antiglaucoma; Ophthalmic Agent, Miotic

Medication Safety Issues

Sound-alike/look-alike issues:

Isopto® Carpine may be confused with Isopto® Carbachol

Salagen® may be confused with Salacid®, selegiline

Use

Ophthalmic: Management of chronic simple glaucoma, chronic and acute angle-closure glaucoma

Oral: Symptomatic treatment of xerostomia caused by salivary gland hypofunction resulting from radiotherapy for cancer of the head and neck or Sjögren's syndrome

Unlabeled/Investigational Use Counter effects of cycloplegics

(Continued)

Pilocarpine *(Continued)*

Mechanism of Action Directly stimulates cholinergic receptors in the eye causing miosis (by contraction of the iris sphincter), loss of accommodation (by constriction of ciliary muscle), and lowering of intraocular pressure (with decreased resistance to aqueous humor outflow)

Pharmacodynamics/Kinetics

Onset of action:

Ophthalmic: Miosis: 10-30 minutes; Intraocular pressure reduction: 1 hour
Oral: 20 minutes

Duration:

Ophthalmic: Miosis: 4-8 hours; Intraocular pressure reduction: 4-12 hours
Oral: 3-5 hours

Half-life elimination: Oral: 0.76-1.35 hours; increased with hepatic impairment

Excretion: Urine

Contraindications Hypersensitivity to pilocarpine or any component of the formulation; acute inflammatory disease of the anterior chamber of the eye; in addition, tablets are also contraindicated in patients with uncontrolled asthma, angle-closure glaucoma, severe hepatic impairment

Warnings/Precautions Use caution with cardiovascular disease; patients may have difficulty compensating for transient changes in hemodynamics or rhythm induced by pilocarpine.

Ophthalmic products: May cause decreased visual acuity, especially at night or with reduced lighting.

Oral tablets: Use caution with controlled asthma, chronic bronchitis or COPD; may increase airway resistance, bronchial smooth muscle tone, and bronchial secretions. Use caution with cholelithiasis, biliary tract disease, nephrolithiasis; adjust dose with moderate hepatic impairment.

Drug Interactions **Inhibits** CYP2A6 (weak), 2E1 (weak), 3A4 (weak)

Concurrent use with beta-blockers may cause conduction disturbances; pilocarpine may antagonize the effects of anticholinergic drugs

Nutritional/Herbal/Ethanol Interactions Food: Avoid administering oral formulation with high-fat meal; fat decreases the rate of absorption, maximum concentration and increases the time it takes to reach maximum concentration.

Adverse Reactions

Ophthalmic: Frequency not defined:

Cardiovascular: Hypertension, tachycardia
Gastrointestinal: Diarrhea, nausea, salivation, vomiting
Ocular: Burning, ciliary spasm, conjunctival vascular congestion, corneal granularity (gel 10%), lacrimation, lens opacity, myopia, retinal detachment, supraorbital or temporal headache, visual acuity decreased
Respiratory: Bronchial spasm, pulmonary edema
Miscellaneous: Diaphoresis

Oral (frequency varies by indication and dose):

>10%:

Cardiovascular: Flushing (8% to 13%)
Central nervous system: Chills (3% to 15%), dizziness (5% to 12%), headache (11%)
Gastrointestinal: Nausea (6% to 15%)
Genitourinary: Urinary frequency (9% to 12%)
Neuromuscular & skeletal: Weakness (2% to 12%)
Respiratory: Rhinitis (5% to 14%)
Miscellaneous: Diaphoresis (29% to 68%)

1% to 10%:

Cardiovascular: Edema (<1% to 5%), facial edema, hypertension (3%), palpitation, tachycardia
Central nervous system: Pain (4%), fever, somnolence
Dermatologic: Pruritus, rash
Gastrointestinal: Diarrhea (4% to 7%), dyspepsia (7%), vomiting (3% to 4%), constipation, flatulence, glossitis, salivation increased, stomatitis, taste perversion
Genitourinary: Vaginitis, urinary incontinence
Neuromuscular & skeletal: Myalgias, tremor
Ocular: Lacrimation (6%), amblyopia (4%), abnormal vision, blurred vision, conjunctivitis
Otic: Tinnitus
Respiratory: Cough increased, dysphagia, epistaxis, sinusitis

Miscellaneous: Allergic reaction, voice alteration

<1% (Limited to important or life-threatening): Abnormal dreams, alopecia, angina pectoris, anorexia, anxiety, arrhythmia, body odor, bone disorder, cholelithiasis, colitis, confusion, dry eyes, dry mouth, ECG abnormality, myasthenia, photosensitivity reaction, nervousness, pancreatitis, paresthesia, salivary gland enlargement, sputum increased, taste loss, tongue disorder, urinary impairment, urinary urgency, yawning

Overdosage/Toxicology Symptoms of overdose include bronchospasm, bradycardia, involuntary urination, vomiting, hypotension, and tremor. Atropine is the treatment of choice for intoxications manifesting with significant muscarinic symptoms. Atropine I.V. 2-4 mg every 3-60 minutes should be repeated to control symptoms and then continued as needed for 1-2 days following acute ingestion. Epinephrine 0.1-1 mg SubQ may be useful for reversing severe cardiovascular or pulmonary sequelae.

Dosing

Adults & Elderly:

Glaucoma: Ophthalmic

Solution: Instill 1-2 drops up to 6 times/day; adjust the concentration and frequency as required to control elevated intraocular pressure.

Gel: Instill 0.5" ribbon into lower conjunctival sac once daily at bedtime.

To counteract the mydriatic effects of sympathomimetic agents (unlabeled use): Ophthalmic solution: Instill 1 drop of a 1% solution in the affected eye.

Xerostomia: Oral:

Following head and neck cancer: 5 mg 3 times/day, titration up to 10 mg 3 times/day may be considered for patients who have not responded adequately; do not exceed 2 tablets/dose

Sjögren's syndrome: 5 mg 4 times/day

Hepatic Impairment: Oral: Patients with moderate impairment: 5 mg 2 times/day regardless of indication; adjust dose based on response and tolerability. Do not use with severe impairment (Child-Pugh score 10-15)

Available Dosage Forms

Gel, ophthalmic, as hydrochloride (Pilopine HS®): 4% (4 g) [contains benzalkonium chloride]

Solution, ophthalmic, as hydrochloride: 0.5% (15 mL); 1% (2 mL, 15 mL); 2% (2 mL, 15 mL); 3% (15 mL); 4% (2 mL, 15 mL); 6% (15 mL) [may contain benzalkonium chloride]

Isopto® Carpine: 1% (15 mL); 2% (15 mL); 4% (15 mL) [contains benzalkonium chloride]

Tablet, as hydrochloride: 5 mg

Salagen®: 5 mg, 7.5 mg

Nursing Guidelines

Assessment: Monitor for adverse effects and response to treatment. Assess results of intraocular pressure testing, fundoscopic exam, and visual field testing on a periodic basis. Teach patient appropriate administration of ophthalmic solution.

Patient Education: Use as often as recommended. Avoid taking oral medication with a high fat meal.

Ophthalmic: Wash hands before using. Do not let tip of applicator touch eye; do not contaminate tip of applicator (may cause eye infection, eye damage, or vision loss). Sit or lie down. Open eye, look at ceiling, and instill prescribed amount of solution. Do not blink for 30 seconds, close eye and roll eye in all directions, and apply gentle pressure to inner corner of eye for 1-2 minutes. Temporary stinging or blurred vision may occur. You may experience altered dark adaptation; use caution when driving at night or in poorly lit environments. Report persistent pain, redness, burning, double vision, or severe headache. **Pregnancy/breast-feeding precautions:** Inform prescriber if you are pregnant. Breast-feeding is not recommended

Geriatric Considerations: Assure the patient or a caregiver can adequately administer ophthalmic medication dosage form.

Pregnancy Risk Factor: C

Lactation: Excretion in breast milk unknown/not recommended

Administration

Oral: Avoid administering with high-fat meal. Fat decreases the rate of absorption, maximum concentration, and increases the time it takes to reach maximum concentration.

(Continued)

Pilocarpine *(Continued)*

Storage:

Gel: Store at room temperature of 2°C to 27°C (36°F to 80°F). Do not freeze; avoid excessive heat.

Tablets: Store at controlled room temperature of 15°C to 30°C (59°F to 86°F).

♦ **Pilocarpine Hydrochloride** *see* Pilocarpine *on page 1365*

♦ **Pilopine HS®** *see* Pilocarpine *on page 1365*

Piperacillin (pi PER a sil in)

Synonyms Piperacillin Sodium

Pharmacologic Category Antibiotic, Penicillin

Use Treatment of susceptible infections such as septicemia, acute and chronic respiratory tract infections, skin and soft tissue infections, and urinary tract infections due to susceptible strains of *Pseudomonas*, *Proteus*, and *Escherichia coli* and *Enterobacter*; active against some streptococci and some anaerobic bacteria; febrile neutropenia (as part of combination regimen)

Mechanism of Action Inhibits bacterial cell wall synthesis by binding to one or more of the penicillin binding proteins (PBPs); which in turn inhibits the final transpeptidation step of peptidoglycan synthesis in bacterial cell walls, thus inhibiting cell wall biosynthesis. Bacteria eventually lyse due to ongoing activity of cell wall autolytic enzymes (autolysins and murein hydrolases) while cell wall assembly is arrested.

Pharmacodynamics/Kinetics

Absorption: I.M.: 70% to 80%

Distribution: Crosses placenta; low concentrations enter breast milk

Protein binding: 22%

Half-life elimination (dose dependent; prolonged with moderately severe renal or hepatic impairment):

Neonates: 1-5 days old: 3.6 hours; >6 days old: 2.1-2.7 hours

Children: 1-6 months: 0.79 hour; 6 months to 12 years: 0.39-0.5 hour

Adults: 36-80 minutes

Time to peak, serum: I.M.: 30-50 minutes

Excretion: Primarily urine; partially feces

Contraindications Hypersensitivity to piperacillin, other beta-lactam antibiotics (penicillins or cephalosporins), or any component of the formulation

Warnings/Precautions Dosage modification required in patients with impaired renal function. Use caution in patients with history of seizure activity. Leukopenia and neutropenia have been reported (during prolonged therapy). An increased frequency of fever and rash has been reported in patients with cystic fibrosis.

Drug Interactions

Aminoglycosides: May be synergistic against selected organisms; physical inactivation of aminoglycosides in the presence of high concentrations of piperacillin and potential toxicity in patients with mild to moderate renal dysfunction

Heparin: Concomitant use with high-dose parenteral penicillins may result in increased risk of bleeding

Methotrexate: Penicillins may increase the exposure to methotrexate during concurrent therapy; monitor.

Neuromuscular blockers: May increase duration of blockade

Oral contraceptives: Anecdotal reports suggesting decreased contraceptive efficacy with penicillins have been refuted by more rigorous scientific and clinical data.

Probenecid: May increase levels of penicillins (piperacillin)

Tetracyclines: May decrease effectiveness of penicillins (piperacillin)

Warfarin: Effects of warfarin may be increased

Lab Interactions May interfere with urinary glucose tests using cupric sulfate (Benedict's solution, Clinitest®); false-positive urinary and serum proteins, positive Coombs' test [direct]. False-positive Platelia® *Aspergillus* EIA test (Bio-Rad Laboratories) has been reported.

Some penicillin derivatives may accelerate the degradation of aminoglycosides *in vitro*, leading to a potential underestimation of aminoglycoside serum concentration.

Adverse Reactions Frequency not defined.

Central nervous system: Confusion, convulsions, drowsiness, fever, Jarisch-Herxheimer reaction

Dermatologic: Rash, toxic epidermal necrolysis, urticaria

Endocrine & metabolic: Electrolyte imbalance, hypokalemia

Hematologic: Abnormal platelet aggregation and prolonged PT (high doses), agranulocytosis, Coombs' reaction (positive), hemolytic anemia, pancytopenia

Local: Thrombophlebitis

Neuromuscular & skeletal: Myoclonus

Renal: Acute interstitial nephritis, acute renal failure

Miscellaneous: Anaphylaxis, hypersensitivity reactions

Overdosage/Toxicology Symptoms of penicillin overdose include neuromuscular hypersensitivity (eg, agitation, hallucinations, asterixis, encephalopathy, confusion, and seizures). Electrolyte imbalance may occur if the preparation contains potassium or sodium salts, especially in renal failure. Hemodialysis may be helpful to aid in removal of the drug from blood; otherwise, treatment is supportive or symptom-directed.

Dosing

Adults: Usual dosage range:

I.M.: 2-3 g/dose every 6-12 hours; maximum: 24 g/24 hours

I.V.: 3-4 g/dose every 4-6 hours; maximum: 24 g/24 hours

Elderly: Adjust dose for renal impairment:

I.M.: 1-2 g every 8-12 hours

I.V.: 2-4 g every 6-8 hours

Pediatrics: Usual dosage range:

Infants and Children: I.M., I.V.: 200-300 mg/kg/day in divided doses every 4-6 hours

Note: In cystic fibrosis, dosages up to 350-500 mg/kg/day in divided doses every 4-6 hours have been used.

Renal Impairment:

Cl_{cr} 10-50 mL/minute: Administer every 6-8 hours.

Cl_{cr} <10 mL/minute: Administer every 8 hours.

Moderately dialyzable (20% to 50%)

Continuous arteriovenous or venovenous hemofiltration: Dose as for Cl_{cr} 10-50 mL/minute.

Available Dosage Forms Injection, powder for reconstitution: 2 g, 3 g, 4 g, 40 g

Nursing Guidelines

Assessment: Assess for allergy history prior to starting therapy. See Contraindications and Warnings/Precautions for use cautions. Assess potential for interactions with other prescriptions, OTC medications, or herbal products patient may be taking (see Drug Interactions). Assess for therapeutic effectiveness and adverse reactions (eg, hypersensitivity reactions, opportunistic infection - see Adverse Reactions and Overdose/Toxicology). Advise patients with diabetes about use of Clinitest®. Teach patient possible side effects/appropriate interventions and adverse symptoms to report (see Patient Education).

Monitoring Laboratory Tests: Perform culture and sensitivity before administering first dose.

Dietary Considerations: Sodium content of 1 g: 1.85 mEq

Patient Education: Inform prescriber of all prescriptions, OTC medications, or herbal products you are taking, and any allergies you have. Do not take any new medication during therapy unless approved by prescriber. This drug can only be given by injection or infusion. Report immediately any redness, swelling, burning, or pain at infusion site or any signs of allergic reaction (eg, respiratory difficulty or swallowing, chest tightness, rash, hives, swelling of lips or mouth). Maintain adequate hydration (2-3 L/day of fluids) unless instructed to restrict fluid intake. If you have diabetes, drug may cause false test results with Clinitest®, consult prescriber for alternative method of glucose monitoring. May cause confusion or drowsiness (use caution when driving or engaging in tasks that require alertness until response to drug is known). Report chest pain, palpitations, or irregular heartbeat; persistent adverse effects.

Geriatric Considerations: Antipseudomonal penicillins should not be used alone and are often combined with an aminoglycoside as empiric therapy for lower respiratory infection and sepsis in which gram-negative (including *Pseudomonas*) and/or anaerobes are of a high probability. Because of piperacillin's lower sodium content, it is preferred over ticarcillin in patients with a history of heart failure and/or renal or hepatic disease. Adjust dose for renal function.

Pregnancy Risk Factor: B

Lactation: Enters breast milk (small amounts - other penicillins are compatible with breast-feeding)

(Continued)

Piperacillin *(Continued)*

Administration

I.M.: Do not administer more than 2 g per injection site.

I.V.: Administer around-the-clock to promote less variation in peak and trough serum levels. Give at least 1 hour apart from aminoglycosides. Rapid administration can lead to seizures. Administer direct I.V. over 3-5 minutes. Intermittently infusion over 30 minutes.

Some penicillins (eg, carbenicillin, ticarcillin and piperacillin) have been shown to inactivate aminglycosides *in vitro*. This has been observed to a greater extent with tobramycin and gentamicin, while amikacin has shown greater stability against inactivation. Concurrent use of these agents may pose a risk of reduced antibacterial efficacy *in vivo*, particularly in the setting of profound renal impairment. However, definitive clinical evidence is lacking. If combination penicillin/aminoglycoside therapy is desired in a patient with renal dysfunction, separation of doses (if feasible), and routine monitoring of aminoglycoside levels, CBC, and clinical response should be considered.

Compatibility: Stable in dextran 6% in NS, D_5NS, D_5W, LR, NS, SWFI, bacteriostatic water

Y-site administration: Incompatible with amphotericin B cholesteryl sulfate complex, filgrastim, fluconazole, gatifloxacin, gemcitabine, ondansetron, sargramostim, vinorelbine

Compatibility when admixed: Incompatible with aminoglycosides

Storage: Reconstituted solution is stable (I.V. infusion) in NS or D_5W for 24 hours at room temperature, 7 days when refrigerated, or 4 weeks when frozen. After freezing, thawed solution is stable for 24 hours at room temperature or 48 hours when refrigerated. 40 g bulk vial should **not** be frozen after reconstitution.

Piperacillin and Tazobactam Sodium

(pi PER a sil in & ta zoe BAK tam SOW dee um)

U.S. Brand Names Zosyn®

Synonyms Piperacillin Sodium and Tazobactam Sodium

Pharmacologic Category Antibiotic, Penicillin

Medication Safety Issues

Sound-alike/look-alike issues:

Zosyn® may be confused with Zofran®, Zyvox™

Use Treatment of moderate-to-severe infections caused by susceptible organisms, including infections of the lower respiratory tract (community-acquired pneumonia, nosocomial pneumonia); urinary tract; uncomplicated and complicated skin and skin structures; gynecologic (endometritis, pelvic inflammatory disease); bone and joint infections; intra-abdominal infections (appendicitis with rupture/abscess, peritonitis); and septicemia. Tazobactam expands activity of piperacillin to include beta-lactamase producing strains of *S. aureus*, *H. influenzae*, *Bacteroides*, and other gram-negative bacteria.

Mechanism of Action Inhibits bacterial cell wall synthesis by binding to one or more of the penicillin binding proteins (PBPs); which in turn inhibits the final transpeptidation step of peptidoglycan synthesis in bacterial cell walls, thus inhibiting cell wall biosynthesis. Bacteria eventually lyse due to ongoing activity of cell wall autolytic enzymes (autolysins and murein hydrolases) while cell wall assembly is arrested. Tazobactam inhibits many beta-lactamases, including staphylococcal penicillinase and Richmond and Sykes types II, III, IV, and V, including extended spectrum enzymes; it has only limited activity against class I beta-lactamases other than class Ic types.

Pharmacodynamics/Kinetics Both AUC and peak concentrations are dose proportional; hepatic impairment does not affect kinetics

Distribution: Well into lungs, intestinal mucosa, skin, muscle, uterus, ovary, prostate, gallbladder, and bile; penetration into CSF is low in subject with noninflamed meninges

Protein binding: Piperacillin and tazobactam: ~30%

Metabolism:

Piperacillin: 6% to 9% to desethyl metabolite (weak activity)

Tazobactam: ~26% to inactive metabolite

Half-life elimination: Piperacillin and tazobactam: 0.7-1.2 hours

Time to peak, plasma: Immediately following infusion of 30 minutes

Excretion: Clearance of both piperacillin and tazobactam are directly proportional to renal function

Piperacillin: Urine (68% as unchanged drug); feces (10% to 20%)

Tazobactam: Urine (80% as inactive metabolite)

Contraindications Hypersensitivity to penicillins, beta-lactamase inhibitors, or any component of the formulation

Warnings/Precautions Bleeding disorders have been observed, particularly in patients with renal impairment; discontinue if thrombocytopenia or bleeding occurs. Due to sodium load and to the adverse effects of high serum concentrations of penicillins, dosage modification is required in patients with impaired or underdeveloped renal function; use with caution in patients with seizures or in patients with history of beta-lactam allergy; associated with an increased incidence of rash and fever in cystic fibrosis patients. Prolonged use may result in superinfection, including pseudomembranous colitis. Safety and efficacy have not been established in children.

Drug Interactions

Aminoglycosides: May be synergistic against selected organisms; physical inactivation of aminoglycosides in the presence of high concentrations of piperacillin and potential toxicity in patients with mild to moderate renal dysfunction

Heparin: Concomitant use with high-dose parenteral penicillins may result in increased risk of bleeding

Methotrexate: Penicillins may increase the exposure to methotrexate during concurrent therapy; monitor.

Neuromuscular blockers: May increase duration of blockade

Oral contraceptives: Anecdotal reports suggesting decreased contraceptive efficacy with penicillins have been refuted by more rigorous scientific and clinical data.

Probenecid: May increase levels of penicillins (piperacillin)

Tetracyclines: May decrease effectiveness of penicillins (piperacillin)

Warfarin: Effects of warfarin may be increased

Lab Interactions Positive Coombs' [direct] test; false positive reaction for urine glucose using copper-reduction method (Clinitest®); may result in false positive results with the Platelia® *Aspergillus* enzyme immunoassay (EIA)

Some penicillin derivatives may accelerate the degradation of aminoglycosides *in vitro*, leading to a potential underestimation of aminoglycoside serum concentration.

Adverse Reactions

>10%: Gastrointestinal: Diarrhea (11%)

>1% to 10%:

Cardiovascular: Hypertension (2%), chest pain, edema

Central nervous system: Insomnia (7%), headache (7% to 8%), agitation (2%), fever (2%), pain (2%), anxiety, dizziness

Dermatologic: Rash (4%), pruritus (3%)

Gastrointestinal: Constipation (7% to 8%), nausea (7%), vomiting (3%), dyspepsia (3%), stool changes (2%), abdominal pain

Hepatic: Transaminases increased

Respiratory: Dyspnea, rhinitis

Miscellaneous: Moniliasis (2%)

≤1%, postmarketing, and/or case reports: Agranulocytosis, anaphylaxis/anaphylactoid reaction, anemia, arrhythmia, arthralgia, atrial fibrillation, back pain, bradycardia, bronchospasm, candidiasis, cardiac arrest, cardiac failure, circulatory failure, cholestatic jaundice, confusion, convulsions, coughing, depression, diaphoresis, dysuria, epistaxis, erythema multiforme, flatulence, flushing, gastritis, genital pruritus, hallucination, hematuria, hemolytic anemia, hemorrhage, hepatitis, hiccough, hypoglycemia, hypotension, ileus, incontinence, injection site reaction, interstitial nephritis, leukorrhea, malaise, melena, mesenteric embolism, myalgia, myocardial infarction, oliguria, pancytopenia, pharyngitis, phlebitis, photophobia, pseudomembranous colitis, pulmonary edema, pulmonary embolism, purpura, renal failure, retention, rigors, seizure, Stevens-Johnson syndrome, syncope, tachycardia (supraventricular and ventricular), taste perversion, thirst, thrombocytosis, tinnitus, toxic epidermal necrolysis, tremor, ulcerative stomatitis, vaginitis, ventricular fibrillation, vertigo

Overdosage/Toxicology Symptoms of penicillin overdose include neuromuscular hypersensitivity (eg, agitation, hallucinations, asterixis, encephalopathy, confusion, and seizures). Electrolyte imbalance may occur if the preparation contains potassium or sodium salts, especially in renal dysfunction. Hemodialysis may be helpful to aid in removal of the drug from blood; otherwise, treatment is supportive or symptom-directed.

(Continued)

Piperacillin and Tazobactam Sodium *(Continued)*

Dosing

Adults & Elderly:

Nosocomial pneumonia: I.V.: 4.5 g every 6 hours for 7-14 days (when used empirically, combination with an aminoglycoside is recommended; consider discontinuation of aminoglycoside if *P. aeruginosa* is not isolated)

Severe infections: I.V.: 4.5 g every 8 hours or 3.375 g every 6 hours for 7-10 days

Moderate infections: I.M.: 2.25 g every 6-8 hours; treatment should be continued for ≥7-10 days depending on severity of disease (**Note:** I.M. route not FDA-approved)

Pediatrics: Children ≥6 months (≤50 kg) (unlabeled use): I.V.: 240 mg of piperacillin component/kg/day in divided doses every 4-6 hours for severe infections

Higher doses have been used for serious pseudomonal infections: 300-450 mg of piperacillin component/kg/day in divided doses every 6-8 hours

Renal Impairment:

Cl_{cr} 20-40 mL/minute: Administer 2.25 g every 6 hours (3.375 g every 6 hours for nosocomial pneumonia)

Cl_{cr} <20 mL/minute: Administer 2.25 g every 8 hours (2.25 g every 6 hours for nosocomial pneumonia)

Hemodialysis/CAPD: Administer 2.25 g every 12 hours (every 8 hours for nosocomial pneumonia) with an additional dose of 0.75 g after each dialysis

Continuous arteriovenous or venovenous hemodiafiltration effects: Dose as for Cl_{cr} 10-50 mL/minute

Hepatic Impairment: Hepatic impairment does not affect the kinetics of piperacillin or tazobactam significantly.

Available Dosage Forms Note: 8:1 ratio of piperacillin sodium/tazobactam sodium

Infusion [premixed iso-osmotic solution, frozen]:

2.25 g: Piperacillin 2 g and tazobactam 0.25 g (50 mL) [contains sodium 5.58 mEq (128 mg)]

3.375 g: Piperacillin 3 g and tazobactam 0.375 g (50 mL) [contains sodium 8.38 mEq (192 mg)]

4.5 g: Piperacillin 4 g and tazobactam 0.5 g (50 mL) [contains sodium 11.17 mEq (256 mg)]

Injection, powder for reconstitution:

2.25 g: Piperacillin 2 g and tazobactam 0.25 g [contains sodium 5.58 mEq (128 mg)]

3.375 g: Piperacillin 3 g and tazobactam 0.375 g [contains sodium 8.38 mEq (192 mg)]

4.5 g: Piperacillin 4 g and tazobactam 0.5 g [contains sodium 11.17 mEq (256 mg)]

40.5 g: Piperacillin 36 g and tazobactam 4.5 g [contains sodium 100.4 mEq (2304 mg); bulk pharmacy vial]

Nursing Guidelines

Assessment: Assess results of culture and sensitivity tests and patient's allergy history prior to starting therapy. Use caution with impaired renal function and history of seizure activity (see Warnings/Precautions). Assess potential for interactions with other pharmacological agents patient may be taking (eg, may increase or decrease levels/effects of penicillin or increase risk of toxicity [aminoglycosides, neuromuscular blockers]; see Drug Interactions). See Administration for infusion specifics. Assess effectiveness (resolution of infection) and adverse reactions (eg, hypersensitivity reactions, opportunistic infection [fever, chills, unhealed sores, white plaques in mouth or vagina, purulent vaginal discharge, fatigue], confusion, convulsions, rash, thrombophlebitis; see Adverse Reactions). Advise patients with diabetes about use of Clinitest®. Teach patient possible side effects/appropriate interventions and adverse symptoms to report (see Patient Education).

Monitoring Laboratory Tests: LFTs, creatinine, BUN, CBC with differential, serum electrolytes, urinalysis, PT, PTT; perform culture and sensitivity before administering first dose.

Dietary Considerations:

Infusion, premixed: 2.25 g contains sodium 5.58 mEq (128 mg); 3.375 g contains sodium 8.38 mEq (192 mg); 4.5 g contains sodium 11.17 mEq (256 mg)

Injection, powder for reconstitution: 2.25 g contains sodium 5.58 mEq (128 mg); 3.375 g contains sodium 8.38 mEq (192 mg); 4.5 g contains sodium 11.17

mEq (256 mg); 40.5 g contains sodium 100.4 mEq (2304 mg, bulk pharmacy vial)

Patient Education: This drug can only be given by injection or infusion; report immediately any redness, swelling, burning, or pain at infusion site or any signs of allergic reaction (eg, respiratory or swallowing difficulty, chest tightness, rash, hives, swelling of lips or mouth). Maintain adequate hydration (2-3 L/day of fluids) unless instructed to restrict fluid intake. If you have diabetes, drug may cause false test results with Clinitest®, consult prescriber for alternative method of glucose monitoring. May cause diarrhea (consult prescriber for approved medication); nausea or vomiting (small frequent meals, frequent mouth care, chewing gum, or sucking lozenges may help); or constipation (increased exercise, fluids, fruit, or fiber may help). Report acute or persistent headache; rash; CNS changes (eg, agitation, confusion, hallucinations, or seizures); persistent abdominal pain, cramping or diarrhea; unusual fever; or other persistent adverse effects. **Breast-feeding precaution:** Consult prescriber if breast-feeding.

Geriatric Considerations: Has not been studied exclusively in the elderly.

Pregnancy Risk Factor: B

Lactation: Enters breast milk/use caution

Breast-Feeding Considerations: Piperacillin is excreted in breast milk.

Administration

I.V.: Administer by I.V. infusion over 30 minutes.

Some penicillins (eg, carbenicillin, ticarcillin and piperacillin) have been shown to inactivate aminglycosides *in vitro*. This has been observed to a greater extent with tobramycin and gentamicin, while amikacin has shown greater stability against inactivation. Concurrent use of these agents may pose a risk of reduced antibacterial efficacy *in vivo*, particularly in the setting of profound renal impairment. However, definitive clinical evidence is lacking. If combination penicillin/aminoglycoside therapy is desired in a patient with renal dysfunction, separation of doses (if feasible), and routine monitoring of aminoglycoside levels, CBC, and clinical response should be considered.

Reconstitution: Use single-dose vials immediately after reconstitution (discard unused portions after 24 hours at room temperature and 48 hours if refrigerated). Reconstitute with 5 mL of diluent per 1 g of piperacillin and then further dilute. Compatible diluents include NS, SW, dextran 6%, D_5W, D_5W with potassium chloride 40 mEq, bacteriostatic saline and water.

Compatibility: Stable in dextran 6% in NS, D_5W, NS, SWFI **incompatible** with LR

Y-site administration: Incompatible with acyclovir, alatrofloxacin, amphotericin B, amphotericin B cholesteryl sulfate complex, chlorpromazine, cisplatin, dacarbazine, daunorubicin, dobutamine, doxorubicin, doxorubicin liposome, doxycycline, droperidol, famotidine, ganciclovir, gatifloxacin, gemcitabine, haloperidol, hydroxyzine, idarubicin, minocycline, mitomycin, mitoxantrone, nalbuphine, prochlorperazine edisylate, promethazine, streptozocin

Compatibility when admixed: Incompatible: Aminoglycosides

Storage:

Vials: Store at controlled room temperature of 20°C to 25°C (68°F to 77°F). Use single-dose vials immediately after reconstitution (discard unused portions after 24 hours at room temperature and 48 hours if refrigerated). After reconstitution, solution is stable in NS or D_5W for 24 hours at room temperature and 7 days when refrigerated.

Premixed solution: Store frozen at -20°C (-4°F). Thawed solution is stable for 24 hours at room temperature or 14 days under refrigeration; do not refreeze.

♦ **Piperacillin Sodium** *see* Piperacillin *on page 1368*

♦ **Piperacillin Sodium and Tazobactam Sodium** *see* Piperacillin and Tazobactam Sodium *on page 1370*

Pirbuterol (peer BYOO ter ole)

U.S. Brand Names Maxair™ Autohaler™

Synonyms Pirbuterol Acetate

Pharmacologic Category Beta$_2$-Adrenergic Agonist

Use Prevention and treatment of reversible bronchospasm including asthma

Mechanism of Action Pirbuterol is a beta$_2$-adrenergic agonist with a similar structure to albuterol, specifically a pyridine ring has been substituted for the benzene ring in albuterol. The increased beta$_2$ selectivity of pirbuterol results from the substitution of a tertiary butyl group on the nitrogen of the side chain, which additionally imparts resistance of pirbuterol to degradation by monoamine (Continued)

Pirbuterol *(Continued)*

oxidase and provides a lengthened duration of action in comparison to the less selective previous beta-agonist agents.

Pharmacodynamics/Kinetics

Onset of action: Peak effect: Therapeutic: Oral: 2-3 hours with peak serum concentration of 6.2-9.8 mcg/L; Inhalation: 0.5-1 hour

Half-life elimination: 2-3 hours

Metabolism: Hepatic

Excretion: Urine (10% as unchanged drug)

Contraindications Hypersensitivity to pirbuterol, albuterol, or any component of the formulation

Warnings/Precautions Optimize anti-inflammatory treatment before initiating maintenance treatment with pirbuterol. Do not use as a component of chronic therapy without an anti-inflammatory agent. Only the mildest form of asthma (Step 1 and/or exercise-induced) would not require concurrent use based upon asthma guidelines. Patient must be instructed to seek medical attention in cases where acute symptoms are not relieved or a previous level of response is diminished. The need to increase frequency of use may indicate deterioration of asthma, and treatment must not be delayed.

Use caution in patients with cardiovascular disease (arrhythmia or hypertension or CHF), convulsive disorders, diabetes, glaucoma, hyperthyroidism, or hypokalemia. Beta agonists may cause elevation in blood pressure, heart rate, and result in CNS stimulation/excitation. $Beta_2$ agonists may increase risk of arrhythmia, increase serum glucose, or decrease serum potassium.

Do not exceed recommended dose; serious adverse events including fatalities, have been associated with excessive use of inhaled sympathomimetics. Rarely, paradoxical bronchospasm may occur with use of inhaled bronchodilating agents; this should be distinguished from inadequate response. All patients should utilize a spacer device when using a metered-dose inhaler. Safety and efficacy have not been established in children <12 years of age.

Drug Interactions

Decreased effect with beta-blockers

Increased toxicity with other beta agonists, MAO inhibitors, TCAs

Adverse Reactions

>10%:

Central nervous system: Nervousness, restlessness

Endocrine & metabolic: Serum glucose increased, serum potassium decreased

Neuromuscular & skeletal: Trembling

1% to 10%:

Cardiovascular: Tachycardia, pounding heartbeat

Central nervous system: Headache, dizziness, lightheadedness

Gastrointestinal: Taste changes, vomiting, nausea

<1% (Limited to important or life-threatening): Arrhythmias, chest pain, hypertension, hypokalemia, insomnia, paradoxical bronchospasm

Overdosage/Toxicology Symptoms of overdose include tachycardia, tremor, hypertension, angina, and seizures. Hypokalemia also may occur. Cardiac arrest and death may be associated with abuse of beta-agonist bronchodilators. Treatment includes immediate discontinuation and symptomatic and supportive therapies. Cautious use of beta-adrenergic blocking agents may be considered in severe cases.

Dosing

Adults & Elderly: Bronchospasm: Inhalation: 2 inhalations every 4-6 hours for prevention; 2 inhalations at an interval of at least 1-3 minutes, followed by a third inhalation in treatment of bronchospasm, not to exceed 12 inhalations/day

Pediatrics: Children ≥12 years: Refer to adult dosing.

Available Dosage Forms Aerosol for oral inhalation, as acetate:

Maxair™ Autohaler™: 14 g [400 inhalations; contains chlorofluorocarbons]

Nursing Guidelines

Assessment: Assess effectiveness and interactions of other medications patient may be taking. Monitor effectiveness of therapy and adverse reactions at beginning of therapy and periodically with long-term use. For inpatient care, monitor vital signs and lung sounds prior to and periodically during therapy. Assess knowledge/teach patient appropriate use, interventions to reduce side effects, and adverse symptoms to report.

Monitoring Laboratory Tests: FEV_1, peak flow, and/or other pulmonary function tests; serum potassium, serum glucose (in selected patients)

Patient Education: Use exactly as directed. Do not use more often than recommended. Maintain adequate hydration (2-3 L/day of fluids) unless instructed to restrict fluid intake. You may experience nervousness, dizziness, or fatigue (use caution when driving or engaging in tasks requiring alertness until response to drug is known); or dry mouth or stomach upset (small frequent meals, frequent mouth care, chewing gum, or sucking hard candy may help). If you have diabetes, check blood sugar; blood glucose levels may be increased. Report unresolved GI upset; dizziness or fatigue; vision changes; chest pain, rapid heartbeat, or palpitations; nervousness or insomnia; muscle cramping or tremor; or unusual cough. **Pregnancy/breast-feeding precautions:** Inform prescriber if you are or intend to become pregnant. Consult prescriber if breast-feeding.

Aerosol: Store canister upside down; do not freeze. Shake canister before using. Sit when using medication. Close eyes when administering pirbuterol to avoid spray getting into eyes. Exhale slowly and completely through nose; inhale deeply through mouth while administering aerosol. Hold breath for 5-10 seconds after inhalation. Wait at least 1 full minute between inhalations. Wash mouthpiece between use. If more than one inhalation medication is used, use bronchodilator first and wait 5 minutes between medications

Maxair™ Autohaler™: Hold upright. Raise lever so that it stays up and snaps into place. Shake well. Exhale. Seal lips tightly around mouthpiece, inhale deeply. A 'click' will be heard and you will feel a soft puff when the medication has been triggered. Continue to take a full, deep breath. Remove inhaler from mouth, hold breath for 10 seconds, then exhale slowly. **Note:** A test-fire slide has been added to the bottom of the Autohaler™ actuator/mouthpiece. The inhaler should be primed prior to using for the first time or if it has not been used in 48 hours. To prime, remove mouthpiece; point mouthpiece away from yourself or others, and push the lever so that it stays up. Push the white test-fire slide located on the bottom of the mouthpiece to release the priming spray. In order to release a second priming spray, push lever to 'down' position, then repeat steps. When two priming sprays have been done, return lever to 'down' position.

Geriatric Considerations: Elderly patients may find it beneficial to utilize a spacer device when using a metered dose inhaler. Difficulty in using the inhaler often limits its effectiveness. The Maxair™ Autohaler™ may be easier for the elderly to use.

Pregnancy Risk Factor: C

Lactation: Excretion in breast milk unknown

Administration

Storage: Store between 15°C and 30°C (59°F and 86°F).

♦ **Pirbuterol Acetate** *see* Pirbuterol *on page 1373*

♦ ***p*-Isobutylhydratropic Acid** *see* Ibuprofen *on page 889*

♦ **Pit** *see* Oxytocin *on page 1293*

♦ **Pitocin®** *see* Oxytocin *on page 1293*

♦ **Pitressin®** *see* Vasopressin *on page 1691*

♦ **Plantago Seed** *see* Psyllium *on page 1438*

♦ **Plantain Seed** *see* Psyllium *on page 1438*

♦ **Plaretase® 8000** *see* Pancrelipase *on page 1301*

♦ **Plasbumin®** *see* Albumin *on page 94*

♦ **Plasmanate®** *see* Plasma Protein Fraction *on page 1375*

Plasma Protein Fraction (PLAS mah PROE teen FRAK shun)

U.S. Brand Names Plasmanate®

Pharmacologic Category Blood Product Derivative

Use Plasma volume expansion and maintenance of cardiac output in the treatment of certain types of shock or impending shock

Dosing

Adults & Elderly: Volume expansion: I.V.: 250-1500 mL/day

Available Dosage Forms Injection, solution [human]: 5% (50 mL, 250 mL) [contains sodium 145 mEq/L]

(Continued)

Plasma Protein Fraction *(Continued)*

Nursing Guidelines

Dietary Considerations: Injection solution contains sodium 145 mEq/L

Pregnancy Risk Factor: C

Administration

I.M.: Administration must be completed within 4 hours after entering the container; rapid infusion may cause vascular overload

- **Platinol®-AQ [DSC]** *see* Cisplatin *on page 412*
- **Plavix®** *see* Clopidogrel *on page 437*
- **Plendil®** *see* Felodipine *on page 706*
- **Pletal®** *see* Cilostazol *on page 394*
- **PN** *see* Total Parenteral Nutrition *on page 1650*
- **Pneumococcal 7-Valent Conjugate Vaccine** *see* Pneumococcal Conjugate Vaccine (7-Valent) *on page 1376*

Pneumococcal Conjugate Vaccine (7-Valent)

(noo moe KOK al KON ju gate vak SEEN, seven vay lent)

U.S. Brand Names Prevnar®

Synonyms Diphtheria CRM_{197} Protein; PCV7; Pneumococcal 7-Valent Conjugate Vaccine

Pharmacologic Category Vaccine

Medication Safety Issues

Sound-alike/look-alike issues:

Prevnar® may be confused with PREVEN®

Use Immunization of infants and toddlers against *Streptococcus pneumoniae* infection caused by serotypes included in the vaccine

Advisory Committee on Immunization Practices (ACIP) guidelines also recommend PCV7 for use in:

All children 2-23 months

Children ≥2-59 months with cochlear implants

Children ages 24-59 months with: Sickle cell disease (including other sickle cell hemoglobinopathies, asplenia, splenic dysfunction), HIV infection, immunocompromising conditions (congenital immunodeficiencies, renal failure, nephrotic syndrome, diseases associated with immunosuppressive or radiation therapy, solid organ transplant), chronic illnesses (cardiac disease, cerebrospinal fluid leaks, diabetes mellitus, pulmonary disease excluding asthma unless on high dose corticosteroids)

Consider use in all children 24-59 months with priority given to:

Children 24-35 months

Children 24-59 months who are of Alaska native, American Indian, or African-American descent

Children 24-59 months who attend group day care centers

Mechanism of Action Promotes active immunization against invasive disease caused by *S. pneumoniae* capsular serotypes 4, 6B, 9V, 18C, 19F, and 23F, all which are individually conjugated to CRM197 protein

Contraindications Hypersensitivity to pneumococcal vaccine or any component of the formulation, including diphtheria toxoid; current or recent severe or moderate febrile illness

Warnings/Precautions Use caution in latex sensitivity. Children with impaired immune responsiveness may have a reduced response to active immunization. The decision to administer or delay vaccination because of current or recent febrile illness depends on the severity of symptoms and the etiology of the disease. Immunization should be delayed during the course of an acute febrile illness. Use caution in children with coagulation disorders (including thrombocytopenia) where intramuscular injections should not be used. Epinephrine 1:1000 should be readily available. Use of pneumococcal conjugate vaccine does not replace use of the 23-valent pneumococcal polysaccharide vaccine in children ≥24 months of age with sickle cell disease, asplenia, HIV infection, chronic illness or if immunocompromised. Safety and efficacy have not been established in children <6 weeks or ≥10 years of age. Not for I.V. use.

Drug Interactions Immunosuppressants: May decrease response to active immunizations

Vaccines: May be administered simultaneously with DTaP, HbOC, IPV, hepatitis B vaccines, MMR, and varicella vaccine, when given in separate sites.

Adverse Reactions All serious adverse reactions must be reported to the U.S. Department of Health and Human Services (DHHS) Vaccine Adverse Event Reporting System (VAERS) 1-800-822-7967.

>10%:

Central nervous system: Fever, irritability, drowsiness, restlessness

Dermatologic: Erythema

Gastrointestinal: Decreased appetite, vomiting, diarrhea

Local: Induration, tenderness, nodule

1% to 10%: Dermatologic: Rash

Postmarketing and/or case reports: Anaphylactic reaction, anaphylactoid reaction, angioneurotic edema, apnea, bronchospasm, dyspnea, erythema multiforme, facial edema, febrile seizure, hypersensitivity reaction, injection site reaction (eg, dermatitis, lymphadenopathy, pruritus, urticaria, shock)

Overdosage/Toxicology

Higher than recommended doses, and doses administered closer than the recommended interval, have been reported. Adverse events were similar to those reported with single doses; most patients were asymptomatic.

Dosing

Adults & Elderly: Dosing established for infants and toddlers

Pediatrics:

Immunization: Infants: 2-6 months: I.M.: 0.5 mL at approximately 2-month intervals for 3 consecutive doses, followed by a fourth dose of 0.5 mL at 12-15 months of age; first dose may be given as young as 6 weeks of age, but is typically given at 2 months of age. In case of a moderate shortage of vaccine, defer the fourth dose until shortage is resolved; in case of a severe shortage of vaccine, defer third and fourth doses until shortage is resolved.

Previously Unvaccinated Older Infants and Children: I.M.:

7-11 months: 0.5 mL for a total of 3 doses; 2 doses at least 4 weeks apart, followed by a third dose after the 1-year birthday (12-15 months), separated from the second dose by at least 2 months. In case of a severe shortage of vaccine, defer the third dose until shortage is resolved.

12-23 months: 0.5 mL for a total of 2 doses, separated by at least 2 months. In case of a severe shortage of vaccine, defer the second dose until shortage is resolved.

24-59 months:

Healthy Children: 0.5 mL as a single dose. In case of a severe shortage of vaccine, defer dosing until shortage is resolved.

Children with sickle cell disease, asplenia, HIV infection, chronic illness or immunocompromising conditions (not including bone marrow transplants - results pending; use PPV23 [pneumococcal polysaccharide vaccine, polyvalent] at 12-and 24-months until studies are complete): 0.5 mL for a total of 2 doses, separated by 2 months

Previously Vaccinated Children with a lapse in vaccine administration: I.M.:

7-11 months: Previously received 1 or 2 doses PCV7: 0.5 mL dose at 7-11 months of age, followed by a second dose ≥2 months later at 12-15 months of age

12-23 months:

Previously received 1 dose before 12 months of age: 0.5 mL dose, followed by a second dose ≥2 months later

Previously received 2 doses before age 12 months: 0.5 mL dose ≥2 months after the most recent dose

24-59 months: Any incomplete schedule: 0.5 mL as a single dose; **Note:** Patients with chronic diseases or immunosuppressing conditions should receive 2 doses ≥2 months apart

Available Dosage Forms Injection, suspension: 2 mcg of each saccharide for serotypes 4, 9V, 14, 18C, 19F, and 23F, and 4 mcg of serotype 6B per 0.5 mL (0.5 mL) [contains 16 mcg total saccharide; also contains diphtheria CRM197 carrier protein ~20 mcg/0.5 mL and aluminum 0.125 mg/0.5 mL (as aluminum phosphate adjuvant); serotypes grown in soy peptone broth; vial stopper contains latex]

Nursing Guidelines

Patient Education: This vaccine is used to prevent bacterial meningitis and ear infections in infants and toddlers. This vaccine will help prevent the disease and stop its spread from person to person. It may be given with other childhood vaccines. Children who are moderately to severely ill should not get this vaccine until they have recovered. This vaccine may be given during a minor

(Continued)

Pneumococcal Conjugate Vaccine (7-Valent) *(Continued)*

illness, such as a cold. Side effects from this vaccine include redness, tenderness, or swelling at the injection site and mild fever. Contact your prescriber immediately for high fever, unusual behavior, or signs of allergic reaction (respiratory difficulty, hoarseness or wheezing, hives, paleness, weakness, fast heartbeat, dizziness, or swelling of the throat).

Pregnancy Risk Factor: C

Lactation:

Excretion in breast milk unknown/not recommended

Administration

I.M.: Shake well prior to use. Do not inject I.V.; avoid intradermal route; administer I.M. (deltoid muscle for toddlers and young children or lateral midthigh in infants).

For patients at risk of hemorrhage following intramuscular injection, the ACIP recommends "it should be administered intramuscularly if, in the opinion of the physician familiar with the patients bleeding risk, the vaccine can be administered with reasonable safety by this route. If the patient receives antihemophilia or other similar therapy, intramuscular vaccination can be scheduled shortly after such therapy is administered. A fine needle (23 gauge or smaller) can be used for the vaccination and firm pressure applied to the site (without rubbing) for at least 2 minutes. The patient should be instructed concerning the risk of hematoma from the injection."

Storage: Store refrigerated at 2°C to 8°C (36°F to 46°F).

Pneumococcal Polysaccharide Vaccine (Polyvalent)

(noo moe KOK al pol i SAK a ride vak SEEN, pol i VAY lent)

U.S. Brand Names Pneumovax® 23

Synonyms PPV23; 23PS; 23-Valent Pneumococcal Polysaccharide Vaccine

Pharmacologic Category Vaccine

Use Children ≥2 years of age and adults who are at increased risk of pneumococcal disease and its complications because of underlying health conditions (including patients with cochlear implants); routine use in older adults >50 years of age, including all those ≥65 years

Current Advisory Committee on Immunization Practices (ACIP) guidelines recommend **pneumococcal 7-valent conjugate vaccine (PCV7)** be used for children 2-23 months of age and, in certain situations, children up to 59 months of age

Mechanism of Action Although there are more than 80 known pneumococcal capsular types, pneumococcal disease is mainly caused by only a few types of pneumococci. Pneumococcal vaccine contains capsular polysaccharides of 23 pneumococcal types of *Streptococcal pneumoniae* which represent at least 85% to 90% of pneumococcal disease isolates in the United States. The pneumococcal vaccine with 23 pneumococcal capsular polysaccharide types became available in 1983. The 23 capsular pneumococcal vaccine contains purified capsular polysaccharides of pneumococcal types 1, 2, 3, 4, 5, 6B, 7F, 8, 9N, 9V, 10A, 11A, 12F, 14, 15B, 17F, 18C, 19F, 19A, 20, 22F, 23F, and 33F. These are the main pneumococcal types associated with serious infections in the United States.

Contraindications Hypersensitivity to pneumococcal vaccine or any component of the formulation

Warnings/Precautions Use caution in patients with severe cardiovascular or pulmonary disease where a systemic reaction may pose a significant risk. Use caution and consider delay of vaccination in any active infection. Use caution in individuals who have had episodes of pneumococcal infection within the preceding 3 years (pre-existing pneumococcal antibodies may result in increased reactions to vaccine); may cause relapse in patients with stable idiopathic thrombocytopenia purpura. Epinephrine injection (1:1000) must be immediately available in the case of anaphylaxis.

Patients who will be receiving immunosuppressive therapy (including Hodgkin's disease, cancer chemotherapy, or transplantation) should be vaccinated at least 2 weeks prior to the initiation of therapy. Immune responses may be impaired for several months following intensive immunosuppressive therapy (up to 2 years in Hodgkin's disease patients). Patients who will undergo splenectomy should also be vaccinated 2 weeks prior to surgery, if possible. Patients with HIV should be vaccinated as soon as possible (following confirmation of the diagnosis). Not recommended in children <2 years of age.

Drug Interactions Immunosuppressant medications: The effect of the vaccine may be decreased.

Vaccines: May be administered at the same time as influenza vaccine, by separate injection and injection site.

Adverse Reactions All serious adverse reactions must be reported to the U.S. Department of Health and Human Services (DHHS) Vaccine Adverse Event Reporting System (VAERS) 1-800-822-7967.

Frequency not defined.
Cardiovascular: Malaise
Central nervous system: Guillain-Barré syndrome, fever ≤102°F*, fever >102°F, headache, radiculoneuropathy
Dermatologic: Angioneurotic edema, cellulitis, rash, urticaria
Gastrointestinal: Nausea, vomiting
Hematologic: Hemolytic anemia (in patients with other hematologic disorders), thrombocytopenia (in patients with stabilized ITP)
Local: Injection site reaction* (erythema, induration, swelling, soreness, warmth)
Neuromuscular & skeletal: Arthralgia, arthritis, myalgia, paresthesia, weakness
Miscellaneous: Anaphylactoid reaction, lymphadenitis, serum sickness
*Reactions most commonly reported in clinical trials.

Dosing

Adults & Elderly: Immunization: I.M., SubQ:

Children ≥2 years and Adults: 0.5 mL

Previously vaccinated with PCV7 vaccine: Children ≥2 years and Adults:

With sickle cell disease, asplenia, immunocompromised or HIV infection: 0.5 mL at ≥2 years of age and ≥2 months after last dose of PCV7; revaccination with PPV23 should be given ≥5 years for children >10 years of age and every 3-5 years for children ≤10 years of age; revaccination should not be administered <3 years after the previous PPV23 dose

With chronic illness: 0.5 mL at ≥2 years of age and ≥2 months after last dose of PCV7; revaccination with PPV23 is not recommended

Following bone marrow transplant (use of PCV7 under study): Administer one dose PPV23 at 12- and 24-months following BMT

Revaccination should be considered:

1. If ≥6 years since initial vaccination has elapsed, or
2. In patients who received 14-valent pneumococcal vaccine and are at highest risk (asplenic) for fatal infection or
3. At ≥6 years in patients with nephrotic syndrome, renal failure, or transplant recipients, or
4. 3-5 years in children with nephrotic syndrome, asplenia, or sickle cell disease

Pediatrics: Children ≥2 years: Refer to adult dosing.

Available Dosage Forms Injection, solution: 25 mcg each of 23 polysaccharide isolates/0.5 mL (0.5 mL, 2.5 mL)

Nursing Guidelines

Patient Education: This vaccine is used to prevent pneumococcal disease which causes bacterial meningitis and pneumonia. It can be used in some children and in adults. Side effects from this vaccine include redness, tenderness, or swelling at the injection site and mild fever. Contact your prescriber immediately for high fever or signs of allergic reaction (respiratory difficulty, hoarseness or wheezing, hives, paleness, weakness, fast heartbeat, dizziness, swelling of the throat). **Pregnancy/breast-feeding precautions:** This vaccine is not usually given during pregnancy. Notify your prescriber if you are pregnant or breast-feeding.

Pregnancy Risk Factor: C

Lactation:

Excretion in breast milk unknown/use caution

Administration

I.M.: Do not inject I.V., avoid intradermal, administer SubQ or I.M. (deltoid muscle or lateral midthigh)

For patients at risk of hemorrhage following intramuscular injection, the ACIP recommends "it should be administered intramuscularly if, in the opinion of the physician familiar with the patients bleeding risk, the vaccine can be administered with reasonable safety by this route. If the patient receives antihemophilia or other similar therapy, intramuscular vaccination can be scheduled shortly after such therapy is administered. A fine needle (23 gauge or smaller) can be used for the vaccination and firm pressure applied to the site (without rubbing)

(Continued)

Pneumococcal Polysaccharide Vaccine (Polyvalent) *(Continued)*

for at least 2 minutes. The patient should be instructed concerning the risk of hematoma from the injection."

Storage: Store under refrigeration at 2°C to 8°C (36°F to 46°F).

- ♦ **Pneumovax® 23** *see* Pneumococcal Polysaccharide Vaccine (Polyvalent) *on page 1378*
- ♦ **Polocaine®** *see* Mepivacaine *on page 1101*
- ♦ **Polocaine® Dental** *see* Mepivacaine *on page 1101*
- ♦ **Polocaine® MPF** *see* Mepivacaine *on page 1101*
- ♦ **Polygam® S/D** *see* Immune Globulin (Intravenous) *on page 899*

Polymyxin B (pol i MIKS in bee)

U.S. Brand Names Poly-Rx

Synonyms Polymyxin B Sulfate

Pharmacologic Category Antibiotic, Irrigation; Antibiotic, Miscellaneous

Use Treatment of acute infections caused by susceptible strains of *Pseudomonas aeruginosa*; used occasionally for gut decontamination; parenteral use of polymyxin B has mainly been replaced by less toxic antibiotics, reserved for life-threatening infections caused by organisms resistant to the preferred drugs (eg, pseudomonal meningitis - intrathecal administration)

Mechanism of Action Binds to phospholipids, alters permeability, and damages the bacterial cytoplasmic membrane permitting leakage of intracellular constituents

Pharmacodynamics/Kinetics

Absorption: Well absorbed from peritoneum; minimal from GI tract (except in neonates) from mucous membranes or intact skin

Distribution: Minimal into CSF; does not cross placenta

Half-life elimination: 4.5-6 hours; prolonged with renal impairment

Time to peak, serum: I.M.: ~2 hours

Excretion: Urine (>60% primarily as unchanged drug)

Contraindications Hypersensitivity to polymyxin B or any component of the formulation; concurrent use of neuromuscular blockers

Warnings/Precautions Use with caution in patients with impaired renal function (modify dosage); polymyxin B-induced nephrotoxicity may be manifested by albuminuria, cellular casts, and azotemia. Discontinue therapy with decreasing urinary output and increasing BUN; neurotoxic reactions are usually associated with high serum levels, often in patients with renal dysfunction. Avoid concurrent or sequential use of other nephrotoxic and neurotoxic drugs (eg, aminoglycosides). The drug's neurotoxicity can result in respiratory paralysis from neuromuscular blockade, especially when the drug is given soon after anesthesia or muscle relaxants. Polymyxin B sulfate is most toxic when given parenterally; avoid parenteral use whenever possible.

Drug Interactions Polymyxin may increase/prolong effect of neuromuscular blocking agents; aminoglycosides may increase polymyxin's risk of respiratory paralysis and renal dysfunction

Adverse Reactions Frequency not defined (limited to important or life-threatening):

Central nervous system: Neurotoxicity (irritability, drowsiness, ataxia, perioral paresthesia, numbness of the extremities, and blurred vision); dizziness

Neuromuscular & skeletal: Neuromuscular blockade

Renal: Nephrotoxicity

Respiratory: Respiratory arrest

Overdosage/Toxicology Symptoms of overdose include respiratory paralysis, ototoxicity, and nephrotoxicity. Supportive care is indicated as treatment.

Dosing

Adults & Elderly:

Ear canal infections (external): Otic (in combination with other drugs): Instill 1-2 drops, 3-4 times/day; should be used sparingly to avoid accumulation of excess debris.

Systemic infections:

I.M.: 25,000-30,000 units/kg/day divided every 4-6 hours

I.V.: 15,000-25,000 units/kg/day divided every 12 hours

Intrathecal: 50,000 units/day for 3-4 days, then every other day for at least 2 weeks

Note: Total daily dose should not exceed 2,000,000 units/day.

Bladder irrigation (in combination with 57 mg neomycin sulfate): Continuous irrigant or rinse in the urinary bladder for up to 10 days using 20 mg (equal to 200,000 units) added to 1 L of normal saline; usually no more than 1 L of irrigant is used per day unless urine flow rate is high; administration rate is adjusted to patient's urine output.

Topical irrigation or topical solution: 500,000 units/L of normal saline; topical irrigation should not exceed 2 million units/day in adults.

Ocular infections: Ophthalmic: A concentration of 0.1% to 0.25% is administered as 1-3 drops every hour, then increasing the interval as response indicates to 1-2 drops 4-6 times/day.

Pediatrics:

Ear canal infections (external): Otic (in combination with other drugs): 1-2 drops, 3-4 times/day; should be used sparingly to avoid accumulation of excess debris

Systemic infections: Infants <2 years:

I.M.: Up to 40,000 units/kg/day divided every 6 hours (not routinely recommended due to pain at injection sites)

I.V.: Up to 40,000 units/kg/day divided every 12 hours

Intrathecal: 20,000 units/day for 3-4 days, then 25,000 units every other day for at least 2 weeks after CSF cultures are negative and CSF (glucose) has returned to within normal limits

Children ≥2 years: Refer to adult dosing.

Renal Impairment:

Cl_{cr} 20-50 mL/minute: Administer 75% to 100% of normal dose every 12 hours.

Cl_{cr} 5-20 mL/minute: Administer 50% of normal dose every 12 hours.

Cl_{cr} <5 mL/minute: Administer 15% of normal dose every 12 hours.

Available Dosage Forms

Injection, powder for reconstitution: 500,000 units

Powder [for prescription compounding] (Poly-Rx): 100 million units (13 g)

Nursing Guidelines

Assessment: Assess for allergy history prior to starting therapy. See Contraindications, Warnings/Precautions, and Dosing for use cautions. Assess potential for interactions with other prescriptions, OTC medications, or herbal products patient may be taking (eg, other nephrotoxic and neurotoxic drugs - see Drug Interactions). See Administration specifics; infusion site must be monitored closely to prevent extravasation. Assess results of laboratory tests (see below), therapeutic effectiveness, and adverse reactions (eg, neurotoxicity - irritability, drowsiness, ataxia, perioral paresthesia, numbness of the extremities, and blurring of vision; neuromuscular blockade - see Adverse Reactions and Overdose/Toxicology). Teach patient possible side effects/appropriate interventions and adverse symptoms to report (see Patient Education). Note breast-feeding caution.

Monitoring Laboratory Tests: Perform culture and sensitivity prior to beginning therapy. Establish baseline renal function prior to initiating therapy. Monitor renal function closely.

Patient Education: Wound irrigation/bladder irrigation/gut sterilization/I.V.: Immediately report numbness or tingling of mouth, tongue, or extremities; constant blurring of vision; increased nervousness or irritability; excessive drowsiness; or respiratory difficulty. For I.V. immediately report swelling, redness, burning, or pain at infusion site.

Ophthalmic: Tilt head back, place medication into eyes (as frequently as prescribed), close eyes, apply light pressure over inside corner of the eye for 1 minute. Do not let tip of applicator touch eye; do not contaminate tip of applicator (may cause eye infection, eye damage, or vision loss). You may experience some stinging or burning or temporary blurring of vision; use caution driving or when engaging in hazardous tasks until vision clears. Report any adverse effects including respiratory difficulty or unusual numbness or tingling of mouth or tongue, increased nervousness or irritability, or excessive drowsiness.

Breast-feeding precaution: Consult prescriber if breast-feeding.

Pregnancy Risk Factor: B (per expert opinion)

Lactation: Excretion in breast milk unknown/use caution

Administration

I.M.: Administer into upper outer quadrant of gluteal muscle; however, I.M. route is not recommended due to severe pain at injection site.

(Continued)

Polymyxin B *(Continued)*

I.V.: Infuse over 60-90 minutes.

Compatibility: Compatibility when admixed: Incompatible with amphotericin B, calcium chloride, calcium gluconate, cefazolin, chloramphenicol, chlorothiazide, heparin, magnesium sulfate

Storage: Prior to reconstitution, store at room temperature of 15°C to 30°C (59°F to 86°F) and protect from light. After reconstitution, store under refrigeration at 2°C to 8°C (36°F to 46°F). Discard any unused solution after 72 hours. **Incompatible** with strong acids/alkalies, calcium, magnesium, cephalothin, cefazolin, chloramphenicol, heparin, penicillins.

- ♦ **Polymyxin B and Bacitracin** *see* Bacitracin and Polymyxin B *on page 219*
- ♦ **Polymyxin B and Neomycin** *see* Neomycin and Polymyxin B *on page 1209*
- ♦ **Polymyxin B and Trimethoprim** *see* Trimethoprim and Polymyxin B *on page 1670*
- ♦ **Polymyxin B, Bacitracin, and Neomycin** *see* Bacitracin, Neomycin, and Polymyxin B *on page 220*
- ♦ **Polymyxin B, Bacitracin, Neomycin, and Hydrocortisone** *see* Bacitracin, Neomycin, Polymyxin B, and Hydrocortisone *on page 221*
- ♦ **Polymyxin B, Neomycin, and Dexamethasone** *see* Neomycin, Polymyxin B, and Dexamethasone *on page 1211*
- ♦ **Polymyxin B, Neomycin, and Gramicidin** *see* Neomycin, Polymyxin B, and Gramicidin *on page 1212*
- ♦ **Polymyxin B, Neomycin, and Hydrocortisone** *see* Neomycin, Polymyxin B, and Hydrocortisone *on page 1212*
- ♦ **Polymyxin B Sulfate** *see* Polymyxin B *on page 1380*
- ♦ **Poly-Rx** *see* Polymyxin B *on page 1380*
- ♦ **Polysporin® Ophthalmic** *see* Bacitracin and Polymyxin B *on page 219*
- ♦ **Polysporin® Topical [OTC]** *see* Bacitracin and Polymyxin B *on page 219*
- ♦ **Polytrim®** *see* Trimethoprim and Polymyxin B *on page 1670*
- ♦ **Poly-Vi-Flor®** *see* Vitamins (Multiple/Pediatric) *on page 1720*
- ♦ **Poly-Vi-Flor® With Iron** *see* Vitamins (Multiple/Pediatric) *on page 1720*
- ♦ **Polyvinyl Alcohol** *see* Artificial Tears *on page 187*
- ♦ **Polyvinylpyrrolidone with Iodine** *see* Povidone-Iodine *on page 1392*
- ♦ **Poly-Vi-Sol® [OTC]** *see* Vitamins (Multiple/Pediatric) *on page 1720*
- ♦ **Poly-Vi-Sol® with Iron [OTC]** *see* Vitamins (Multiple/Pediatric) *on page 1720*
- ♦ **Pontocaine®** *see* Tetracaine *on page 1612*
- ♦ **Pontocaine® Niphanoid®** *see* Tetracaine *on page 1612*
- ♦ **Post Peel Healing Balm [OTC]** *see* Hydrocortisone *on page 873*

Potassium Acetate (poe TASS ee um AS e tate)

Pharmacologic Category Electrolyte Supplement, Parenteral

Medication Safety Issues

Consider special storage requirements for intravenous potassium salts; I.V. potassium salts have been administered IVP in error, leading to fatal outcomes.

Use Potassium deficiency; to avoid chloride when high concentration of potassium is needed, source of bicarbonate

Mechanism of Action Potassium is the major cation of intracellular fluid and is essential for the conduction of nerve impulses in heart, brain, and skeletal muscle; contraction of cardiac, skeletal and smooth muscles; maintenance of normal renal function, acid-base balance, carbohydrate metabolism, and gastric secretion

Pharmacodynamics/Kinetics

Distribution: Enters cells via active transport from extracellular fluid

Excretion: Primarily urine; skin and feces (small amounts); most intestinal potassium reabsorbed

Contraindications Severe renal impairment; hyperkalemia

Warnings/Precautions Use with caution in patients with renal disease, hyperkalemia, cardiac disease, metabolic alkalosis; must be administered in patients with adequate urine flow. Potassium acetate solution for injection contains aluminum; use caution with impaired renal function and in premature infants.

Drug Interactions Increased effect/levels with potassium-sparing diuretics, salt substitutes, ACE inhibitors

Adverse Reactions

1% to 10%:

Cardiovascular: Bradycardia

Endocrine & metabolic: Hyperkalemia

Neuromuscular & skeletal: Weakness

Respiratory: Dyspnea

Local: Local tissue necrosis with extravasation

<1% (Limited to important or life-threatening): Abdominal pain, alkalosis, chest pain, mental confusion, paralysis, paresthesia, phlebitis, throat pain

Overdosage/Toxicology Symptoms of overdose include muscle weakness, paralysis, peaked T waves, flattened P waves, prolongation of chloride. QRS complex, ventricular arrhythmias. Removal of potassium can be accomplished by various means; removal through the GI tract with Kayexalate® administration; by way of the kidney through diuresis, mineralocorticoid administration or increased sodium intake; by hemodialysis or peritoneal dialysis; or by shifting potassium back into the cells by insulin and glucose infusion or administration of sodium bicarbonate; calcium chloride will reverse cardiac effects.

Dosing

Adults & Elderly: I.V. doses should be incorporated into the patient's maintenance I.V. fluids, intermittent I.V. potassium administration should be reserved for severe depletion situations and requires ECG monitoring; doses listed as mEq of potassium

Treatment of hypokalemia: I.V.: 40-100 mEq/day

I.V. intermittent infusion (must be diluted prior to administration):

5-10 mEq/dose (maximum: 40 mEq/dose) to infuse over 2-3 hours (maximum: 40 mEq over 1 hour)

Note: Continuous cardiac monitor recommended for rates >0.5 mEq/hour

Potassium dosage/rate of infusion guidelines:

Serum potassium >2.5 mEq/L: Maximum infusion rate: 10 mEq/hour; maximum concentration: 40 mEq/L; maximum 24-hour dose: 200 mEq

Serum potassium <2.5 mEq/L: Maximum infusion rate: 40 mEq/hour; maximum concentration: 80 mEq/L; maximum 24-hour dose: 400 mEq

Pediatrics: I.V. doses should be incorporated into the patient's maintenance I.V. fluids, intermittent I.V. potassium administration should be reserved for severe depletion situations and requires ECG monitoring; doses listed as mEq of potassium.

Note: Use caution in premature neonates; potassium acetate for injection contains aluminum.

Treatment of hypokalemia: I.V.: 2-5 mEq/kg/day

I.V. intermittent infusion (must be diluted prior to administration): 0.5-1 mEq/kg/dose (maximum: 30 mEq/dose) to infuse at 0.3-0.5 mEq/kg/hour (maximum: 1 mEq/kg/hour)

Note: Continuous cardiac monitor recommended for rates >0.5 mEq/hour

Potassium dosage/rate of infusion guidelines:

Serum potassium >2.5 mEq/L: Maximum infusion rate: 10 mEq/hour; maximum concentration: 40 mEq/L; maximum 24-hour dose: 200 mEq

Serum potassium <2.5 mEq/L: Maximum infusion rate: 40 mEq/hour; maximum concentration: 80 mEq/L; maximum 24-hour dose: 400 mEq

Renal Impairment: Use caution; potassium acetate injection contains aluminum.

Available Dosage Forms Injection, solution: 2 mEq/mL (20 mL, 50 mL, 100 mL); 4 mEq/mL (50 mL) [contains aluminum ≤200 mcg/mL]

Nursing Guidelines

Monitoring Laboratory Tests: Serum potassium

Patient Education: This form of potassium may only be given I.V. Report immediately any burning or pain at infusion site, chest pain, palpitations, unusual weakness in muscles, tarry stools, or easy bruising.

Pregnancy Risk Factor: C

Potassium Bicarbonate (poe TASS ee um bye KAR bun ate)

Pharmacologic Category Electrolyte Supplement, Oral

Use Potassium deficiency, hypokalemia

Warnings/Precautions Use with caution in patients with renal disease, cardiac disease.

Drug Interactions Increased effect/levels with potassium-sparing diuretics, salt substitutes, salicylates, ACE inhibitors

(Continued)

Potassium Bicarbonate *(Continued)*

Dosing

Adults & Elderly: Hypokalemia: Oral: 25 mEq 2-4 times/day

Pediatrics: Hypokalemia: Oral: Children: 1-4 mEq/kg/day

Available Dosage Forms Tablet for oral solution, effervescent: Potassium 25 mEq

Nursing Guidelines

Monitoring Laboratory Tests: Serum potassium, serum bicarbonate

Patient Education: Dissolve completely in 3-8 oz cold water, juice, or other suitable beverage and drink slowly.

Pregnancy Risk Factor: C

Potassium Bicarbonate and Potassium Chloride

(poe TASS ee um bye KAR bun ate & poe TASS ee um KLOR ide)

U.S. Brand Names K-Lyte/Cl®; K-Lyte/Cl® 50

Synonyms Potassium Bicarbonate and Potassium Chloride (Effervescent)

Pharmacologic Category Electrolyte Supplement, Oral

Use Treatment or prevention of hypokalemia

Contraindications Hypersensitivity to any component of the formulation; hyperkalemia

Warnings/Precautions Use with caution in patients with renal disease, cardiac disease.

Drug Interactions See individual agents.

Adverse Reactions Frequency not defined: Gastrointestinal: Abdominal discomfort, diarrhea, nausea, vomiting

Overdosage/Toxicology Signs and symptoms of hyperkalemia include arrhythmias, confusion, anxiety, unexplained numbness or tingling, difficulty breathing, unusual tiredness or weakness.

Dosing

Adults & Elderly: Hypokalemia: Oral:

Prevention: 16-24 mEq/day in 2-4 divided doses

Treatment: 40-100 mEq/day in 2-4 divided doses

Available Dosage Forms Tablet for oral solution, effervescent:

K-Lyte/Cl®: Potassium chloride 25 mEq [potassium chloride 1.5 g and potassium bicarbonate 0.5 g; citrus or fruit punch flavor]

K-Lyte/Cl® 50: Potassium chloride 50 mEq [potassium chloride 2.24 g and potassium bicarbonate 2 g; citrus flavor]

Nursing Guidelines

Assessment: Assess for adequate kidney function, use of ACE inhibitors, or potassium-sparing diuretics prior to starting therapy. Monitor cardiac status and serum potassium levels on a regular basis with long-term therapy. Instruct patient on appropriate diet and administration.

Monitoring Laboratory Tests: Serum potassium, serum bicarbonate

Dietary Considerations: Should be taken with meals.

Patient Education: Take as directed; do not take more than directed. Dissolve tablets in water or juice and stir before drinking. Do not take on an empty stomach; take with or after meals. Consult prescriber about increasing dietary potassium intake (eg, salt substitutes, orange juice, bananas). Report tingling of hands or feet, unresolved nausea or vomiting, chest pain, palpitations, persistent abdominal pain, muscle cramping or weakness, tarry stools, easy bruising, or unusual bleeding. **Pregnancy precaution:** Inform prescriber if you are pregnant.

Pregnancy Risk Factor: C

Lactation: Enters breast milk/compatible

Administration

Oral: Administer with meals; solution should be sipped slowly, over 5-10 minutes

Reconstitution: Tablet for oral solution:

25 mEq: Dissolve in 3-4 ounces of cold water.

50 mEq: Dissolve in 6-8 ounces of cold water.

Storage: Store below 30°C (86°F).

Related Information

Potassium Bicarbonate *on page 1383*

Potassium Chloride *on page 1385*

♦ **Potassium Bicarbonate and Potassium Chloride (Effervescent)** *see* Potassium Bicarbonate and Potassium Chloride *on page 1384*

Potassium Chloride (poe TASS ee um KLOR ide)

U.S. Brand Names Kaon-Cl-10®; Kaon-Cl® 20; Kay Ciel®; K-Dur® 10; K-Dur® 20; K-Lor®; Klor-Con®; Klor-Con® 8; Klor-Con® 10; Klor-Con®/25; Klor-Con® M; K+ Potassium; K-Tab®; microK®; microK® 10; Rum-K®

Synonyms KCl

Pharmacologic Category Electrolyte Supplement, Oral; Electrolyte Supplement, Parenteral

Medication Safety Issues

Sound-alike/look-alike issues:

Kaon-Cl-10® may be confused with kaolin
KCl may be confused with HCl
K-Dur® may be confused with Cardura®, Imdur®
K-Lor® may be confused with Kaochlor®, Klor-Con®
Klor-Con® may be confused with Klaron®, K-Lor®
Klotrix® may be confused with liotrix
microK® may be confused with Micronase®

High alert medication: The Institute for Safe Medication Practices (ISMP) includes this medication (I.V. formulation) among its list of drugs which have a heightened risk of causing significant patient harm when used in error.

Per JCAHO recommendations, concentrated electrolyte solutions should not be available in patient care areas.

Consider special storage requirements for intravenous potassium salts; I.V. potassium salts have been administered IVP in error, leading to fatal outcomes.

Use Treatment or prevention of hypokalemia

Mechanism of Action Potassium is the major cation of intracellular fluid and is essential for the conduction of nerve impulses in heart, brain, and skeletal muscle; contraction of cardiac, skeletal and smooth muscles; maintenance of normal renal function, acid-base balance, carbohydrate metabolism, and gastric secretion

Pharmacodynamics/Kinetics

Absorption: Well absorbed from upper GI tract

Distribution: Enters cells via active transport from extracellular fluid

Excretion: Primarily urine; skin and feces (small amounts); most intestinal potassium reabsorbed

Contraindications Severe renal impairment, untreated Addison's disease, heat cramps, hyperkalemia, severe tissue trauma; solid oral dosage forms are contraindicated in patients in whom there is a structural, pathological, and/or pharmacologic cause for delay or arrest in passage through the GI tract; an oral liquid potassium preparation should be used in patients with esophageal compression or delayed gastric emptying time

Warnings/Precautions Use with caution in patients with cardiac disease, severe renal impairment, hyperkalemia

Drug Interactions Increased effect/levels with potassium-sparing diuretics, salt substitutes, ACE inhibitors

Adverse Reactions

>10%: Gastrointestinal: Diarrhea, nausea, stomach pain, flatulence, vomiting (oral)

1% to 10%:

Cardiovascular: Bradycardia
Endocrine & metabolic: Hyperkalemia
Local: Local tissue necrosis with extravasation, pain at the site of injection
Neuromuscular & skeletal: Weakness
Respiratory: Dyspnea

<1% (Limited to important or life-threatening): Abdominal pain, alkalosis, arrhythmia, chest pain, heart block, hypotension, mental confusion, paralysis, paresthesia, phlebitis, rash, throat pain

Overdosage/Toxicology

Symptoms of overdose include muscle weakness, paralysis, peaked T waves, flattened P waves, prolongation of QRS complex, ventricular arrhythmias

Removal of potassium can be accomplished by various means; removal through the GI tract with Kayexalate® administration; by way of the kidney through diuresis, mineralocorticoid administration or increased sodium intake; by hemodialysis or peritoneal dialysis; or by shifting potassium back into the cells by insulin and glucose infusion or sodium bicarbonate; calcium chloride reverses cardiac effects.

(Continued)

Potassium Chloride *(Continued)*

Dosing

Adults & Elderly: I.V. doses should be incorporated into the patient's maintenance I.V. fluids; intermittent I.V. potassium administration should be reserved for severe depletion situations in patients undergoing ECG monitoring.

Normal daily requirements: Oral, I.V.: 40-80 mEq/day

Prevention of hypokalemia during diuretic therapy: Oral: 20-40 mEq/day in 1-2 divided doses

Treatment of hypokalemia (guidelines):

Potassium >2.5 mEq/L:

Oral: 60-80 mEq/day plus additional amounts if needed

I.V.: 10 mEq over 1 hour with additional doses if needed

Potassium <2.5 mEq/L:

Oral: Up to 40-60 mEq initial dose, followed by further doses based on lab values

I.V.: Up to 40 mEq over 1 hour, with doses based on frequent lab monitoring; deficits at a plasma level of 2 mEq/L may be as high as 400-800 mEq of potassium

Acute hypokalemia:

I.V. intermittent infusion: 5-10 mEq/hour (continuous cardiac monitor recommended for rates >5 mEq/hour), not to exceed 40 mEq/hour; usual adult maximum per 24 hours: 400 mEq/day.

Potassium dosage/rate of infusion guidelines:

Serum potassium >2.5 mEq/L: Maximum infusion rate: 10 mEq/hour; maximum concentration: 40 mEq/L; maximum 24-hour dose: 200 mEq

Serum potassium <2.5 mEq/L: Maximum infusion rate: 40 mEq/hour; maximum concentration: 80 mEq/L; maximum 24-hour dose: 400 mEq

Pediatrics: I.V. doses should be incorporated into the patient's maintenance I.V. fluids; intermittent I.V. potassium administration should be reserved for severe depletion situations in patients undergoing ECG monitoring.

Normal daily requirements: Oral, I.V.:

Premature infants: 2-6 mEq/kg/24 hours

Term infants 0-24 hours: 0-2 mEq/kg/24 hours

Infants >24 hours: 1-2 mEq/kg/24 hours

Children: 2-3 mEq/kg/day

Prevention of hypokalemia during diuretic therapy: Oral: Children: 1-2 mEq/kg/day in 1-2 divided doses

Treatment of hypokalemia: Children:

Oral: 1-2 mEq/kg initially, then as needed based on frequently obtained lab values. If deficits are severe or ongoing losses are great, I.V. route should be considered.

I.V.: 1 mEq/kg over 1-2 hours initially, then repeated as needed based on frequently obtained lab values; severe depletion or ongoing losses may require >200% of normal limit needs

I.V. intermittent infusion: Dose should not exceed 1 mEq/kg/hour, or 40 mEq/hour; if it exceeds 0.5 mEq/kg/hour, physician should be at bedside and patient should have continuous ECG monitoring; usual pediatric maximum: 3 mEq/kg/day or 40 mEq/m^2/day

Available Dosage Forms [DSC] = Discontinued product

Capsule, extended release: 10 mEq [750 mg]

microK® [microencapsulated]: 8 mEq [600 mg]

microK® 10 [microencapsulated]: 10 mEq [750 mg]

Infusion [premixed in D_5W]: 20 mEq (1000 mL); 30 mEq (1000 mL); 40 mEq (1000 mL)

Infusion [premixed in D_5W and LR]: 20 mEq (1000 mL); 30 mEq (1000 mL); 40 mEq (1000 mL)

Infusion [premixed in D_5W and ¼NS]: 10 mEq (500 mL, 1000 mL); 20 mEq (250 mL, 500 mL, 1000 mL); 30 mEq (1000 mL); 40 mEq (1000 mL)

Infusion [premixed in D_5W and ½NS]: 10 mEq (500 mL, 1000 mL); 20 mEq (500 mL, 1000 mL); 30 mEq (1000 mL); 40 mEq (1000 mL)

Infusion [premixed in D_5 and NS]: 20 mEq (1000 mL); 40 mEq (1000 mL)

Infusion [premixed in D_5W and sodium chloride 0.3%]: 10 mEq (500 mL); 20 mEq (1000 mL); 30 mEq (1000 mL); 40 mEq (1000 mL)

Infusion [premixed in $D_{10}W$ and sodium chloride 0.2%]: 20 mEq (250 mL)

Infusion [premixed in NS]: 20 mEq (1000 mL); 40 mEq (1000 mL)

Infusion [premixed in SWFI; concentrate]: 10 mEq (50 mL, 100 mL); 20 mEq (50 mL, 100 mL); 30 mEq (100 mL); 40 mEq (100 mL)
Injection, solution [concentrate]: 2 mEq/mL (5 mL, 10 mL, 15 mL, 20 mL, 30 mL, 250 mL, 500 mL)
Powder, for oral solution: 20 mEq/packet (30s, 100s, 1000s)
K-Lor™: 20 mEq/packet (30s, 100s) [fruit flavor]
K+ Potassium: 20 mEq/packet (30s) [orange flavor]
Kay Ciel® 10%: 20 mEq/packet (30s, 100s) [sugar free]
Klor-Con®: 20 mEq/packet (30s, 100s) [sugar free; fruit flavor]
Klor-Con®/25: 25 mEq/packet (30s, 100s) [sugar free; fruit flavor]
Solution, oral: 20 mEq/15 mL (480 mL, 3840 mL); 40 mEq/15 mL (480 mL)
Kaon-Cl® 20: 40 mEq/15 mL (480 mL) [sugar free; contains alcohol; cherry flavor]
Kay Ciel®: 10%: 20 mEq/15 mL (480 mL) [sugar free; contains alcohol] [DSC]
Rum-K®: 20 mEq/10 mL (480 mL) [alcohol free, sugar free; butter/rum flavor]
Tablet, extended release: 8 mEq [600 mg]; 10 mEq [750 mg]; 20 mEq [1500 mg]
K-Dur® 10 [microencapsulated]: 10 mEq [750 mg]
K-Dur® 20 [microencapsulated]: 20 mEq [1500 mg; scored]
K-Tab®: 10 mEq [750 mg]
Kaon-Cl® 10 [film coated]: 10 mEq [750 mg]
Klor-Con® 8: 8 mEq [600 mg; wax matrix]
Klor-Con® 10: 10 mEq [750 mg; wax matrix]
Klor-Con® M10 [microencapsulated]: 10 mEq [750 mg]
Klor-Con® M15 [microencapsulated]: 15 mEq [1125 mg; scored]
Klor-Con® M20 [microencapsulated]: 20 mEq [1500 mg; scored]

Nursing Guidelines

Assessment: Assess therapeutic response and adverse effects.

Monitoring Laboratory Tests: Serum potassium

Dietary Considerations: Administer with plenty of fluid and/or food because of stomach irritation and discomfort.

Patient Education: Long-acting and wax matrix tablets should be swallowed whole; do not crush or chew. Powder must be dissolved in water before use. Take with food. Liquid can be diluted or dissolved in water or juice.

Pregnancy Risk Factor: A

Administration

Oral: Wax matrix tablets must be swallowed and not allowed to dissolve in mouth.

I.V.: Potassium must be diluted prior to parenteral administration; maximum recommended concentration (peripheral line): 80 mEq/L; maximum recommended concentration (central line): 150 mEq/L or 15 mEq/100 mL; in severely fluid-restricted patients (with central lines): 200 mEq/L or 20 mEq/100 mL has been used; maximum rate of infusion, see Dosage, I.V. intermittent infusion

Compatibility: Stable in dextran 6% in dextrose, dextran 6% in NS, D_5LR, $D_5 1/4NS$, $D_5 1/2NS$, D_5NS, D_5W, $D_{10}W$, $D_{20}W$, LR, 1/2NS, NS, sodium chloride 3%

Y-site administration: Incompatible with amphotericin B cholesteryl sulfate complex, diazepam, ergotamine, phenytoin

Compatibility when admixed: Incompatible with amphotericin B

Storage: Store at room temperature, protect from freezing; use only clear solutions; use admixtures within 24 hours

Potassium Iodide and Iodine

(poe TASS ee um EYE oh dide & EYE oh dine)

Synonyms Lugol's Solution; Strong Iodine Solution

Pharmacologic Category Antithyroid Agent

Medication Safety Issues

Sound-alike/look-alike issues:

Potassium iodide and iodine (Strong Iodide Solution or Lugol's solution) may be confused with potassium iodide products, including saturated solution of potassium iodide (SSKI®)

Use Reduce thyroid vascularity prior to thyroidectomy and management of thyrotoxic crisis; block thyroidal uptake of radioactive isotopes of iodine in a radiation emergency or other exposure to radioactive iodine

Mechanism of Action Inhibits secretion of thyroid hormone, fosters colloid accumulation in thyroid follicles. Following radioactive iodine exposure, potassium iodide blocks uptake of radioiodine by the thyroid, reducing the risk of thyroid cancer.

(Continued)

Potassium Iodide and Iodine *(Continued)*

Pharmacodynamics/Kinetics

Onset of action: Hyperthyroidism: 24-48 hours

Peak effect: 10-15 days after continuous therapy

Contraindications Hypersensitivity to iodine or any component of the formulation; hyperkalemia; pulmonary edema; impaired renal function; hyperthyroidism; iodine-induced goiter; dermatitis herpetiformis; hypocomplementemic vasculitis

Warnings/Precautions Prolonged use can lead to hypothyroidism; cystic fibrosis patients have an exaggerated response; can cause acne flare-ups, can cause dermatitis; use with caution in patients with a history of thyroid disease, Addison's disease, cardiac disease, myotonia congenita, tuberculosis, acute bronchitis

Drug Interactions

ACE inhibitors: Concurrent use may lead to hyperkalemia, cardiac arrhythmias or cardiac arrest.

Diuretics, potassium-sparing: Concurrent use may lead to hyperkalemia, cardiac arrhythmias, or cardiac arrest.

Lithium: May cause additive hypothyroid effects.

Potassium (and potassium-containing products): Concurrent use may lead to hyperkalemia, cardiac arrhythmias, or cardiac arrest.

Lab Interactions May alter thyroid function tests.

Adverse Reactions Frequency not defined.

Cardiovascular: Irregular heart beat

Central nervous system: Confusion, tiredness, fever

Dermatologic: Skin rash

Endocrine & metabolic: Goiter, salivary gland swelling/tenderness, thyroid adenoma, swelling of neck/throat, myxedema, lymph node swelling, hyper-/hypothyroidism

Gastrointestinal: Diarrhea, gastrointestinal bleeding, metallic taste, nausea, stomach pain, stomach upset, vomiting

Neuromuscular & skeletal: Numbness, tingling, weakness, joint pain

Miscellaneous: Chronic iodine poisoning (with prolonged treatment/high doses); iodism, hypersensitivity reactions (angioedema, cutaneous and mucosal hemorrhage, serum sickness-like symptoms)

Overdosage/Toxicology Symptoms of overdose include angioedema, laryngeal edema or cutaneous hemorrhages, muscle weakness, paralysis, peaked T waves, flattened P waves, prolongation of QRS complex, and ventricular arrhythmias.

Symptoms of iodism or chronic iodine poisoning may manifest as burning of mouth or throat, severe headache, metallic taste, sore teeth and gums, head cold symptoms, eye irritation including eyelid swelling, unusual increase in salivation, acneform skin lesions in seborrheic areas, or severe skin eruption (rare).

Removal of potassium can be accomplished by various means: Removal through the GI tract with Kayexalate® administration; by way of the kidney through diuresis, mineralocorticoid administration, or increased sodium intake; by hemodialysis or peritoneal dialysis; or by shifting potassium back into the cells by insulin and glucose infusion or by administration of sodium bicarbonate. Calcium chloride reverses cardiac effects.

Dosing

Adults & Elderly: RDA, Adults: 150 mcg (iodine)

Preoperative thyroidectomy: Oral: 0.1-0.3 mL (3-5 drops) of strong iodine (Lugol's solution) 3 times/day; administer for 10 days before surgery

Thyrotoxic crisis: Oral: 1 mL strong iodine (Lugol's solution) 3 times/day

Pediatrics:

Refer to adult dosing.

Available Dosage Forms Solution, oral (Lugol's solution, strong iodine): Potassium iodide 100 mg/mL and iodine 50 mg/mL (15 mL, 480 mL)

Nursing Guidelines

Assessment: Use caution in presence of history of thyroid disease, Addison's disease, cardiac disease, myotonia congenital, tuberculosis, or acute bronchitis. Assess potential for interactions with other pharmacological agents or herbal products patient is taking that may increase risk of hyperkalemia, hypokalemia., or additive hypothyroid effects. Assess need for laboratory monitoring, therapeutic effects (according to purpose for use), and adverse reactions. Teach patient or caregiver purpose for use, necessity for contraception for sexually active female patients, possible side effects/appropriate interventions, and adverse symptoms to report (refer to Patient Education).

Patient Education: Take this medication exactly as directed; do not exceed recommended dosage. May cause metallic taste, nausea, or vomiting (small frequent meals, frequent mouth care, chewing gum, or sucking lozenges may help); soreness of teeth, gums, or glands (use soft toothbrush and frequent mouth rinses; fever, headache or sore joints (consult prescriber for approved analgesic); confusion or tiredness (use caution when driving or engaged in potential hazardous tasks until response to medication is known). Report immediately any swelling of lips, mouth, or tongue; difficulty swallowing; chest pain or irregular heartbeat; muscle weakness; eye irritation or eyelid swelling; skin rash or other persistent adverse effects. **Pregnancy/breast-feeding precautions:** Inform prescriber if you are pregnant. Do not get pregnant during therapy. Consult prescriber for instruction on appropriate contraceptive measures. This drug may cause fetal defects. Consult prescriber if breast-feeding.

Geriatric Considerations:
Elderly may have reduced renal function and require close monitoring of serum potassium. May be also recommended to check serum magnesium.

Pregnancy Risk Factor: D (potassium iodide)

Lactation: Enters breast milk/use caution (AAP rates "compatible")

Breast-Feeding Considerations: AAP considers this drug 'compatible,' but recommends avoiding breast-feeding following radioactive iodine exposure unless no alternative is available. Skin rash in the nursing infant has been reported with maternal intake of potassium iodide. Refer to Iodine monograph for additional information.

Administration

Storage: Store at controlled room temperature of 25°C (77°F) excursions permitted to 15°C to 30°C (59°F to 86°F). Protect from light and keep container tightly closed.

Potassium Phosphate (poe TASS ee um FOS fate)

U.S. Brand Names Neutra-Phos®-K [OTC]

Synonyms Phosphate, Potassium

Pharmacologic Category Electrolyte Supplement, Oral; Electrolyte Supplement, Parenteral

Medication Safety Issues

Sound-alike/look-alike issues:

Neutra-Phos®-K may be confused with K-Phos Neutral®

High alert medication: The Institute for Safe Medication Practices (ISMP) includes this medication (I.V. formulation) among its list of drugs which have a heightened risk of causing significant patient harm when used in error.

Per JCAHO recommendations, concentrated electrolyte solutions should not be available in patient care areas.

Consider special storage requirements for intravenous potassium salts; I.V. potassium salts have been administered IVP in error, leading to fatal outcomes.

Use Treatment and prevention of hypophosphatemia or hypokalemia

Contraindications Hyperphosphatemia, hyperkalemia, hypocalcemia, hypomagnesemia, renal failure

Warnings/Precautions Use with caution in patients with renal insufficiency, cardiac disease, metabolic alkalosis; admixture of phosphate and calcium in I.V. fluids can result in calcium phosphate precipitation

Drug Interactions

Decreased effect/levels with aluminum and magnesium-containing antacids or sucralfate which can act as phosphate binders

Increased effect/levels with potassium-sparing diuretics, salt substitutes, or ACE inhibitors; increased effect of digitalis

Nutritional/Herbal/Ethanol Interactions Food: Avoid administering with oxalate (berries, nuts, chocolate, beans, celery, tomato) or phytate-containing foods (bran, whole wheat).

Lab Interactions Decreased ammonia (B)

Adverse Reactions

>10%: Gastrointestinal: Diarrhea, nausea, stomach pain, flatulence, vomiting

1% to 10%:

- Cardiovascular: Bradycardia
- Endocrine & metabolic: Hyperkalemia
- Neuromuscular & skeletal: Weakness
- Respiratory: Dyspnea

(Continued)

Potassium Phosphate *(Continued)*

<1% (Limited to important or life-threatening): Acute renal failure, arrhythmia, chest pain, decreased urine output, dyspnea, edema, mental confusion, paralysis, paresthesia, phlebitis, tetany (with large doses of phosphate)

Overdosage/Toxicology

Symptoms of overdose include muscle weakness, paralysis, peaked T waves, flattened P waves, prolongation of QRS complex, ventricular arrhythmias, tetany, calcium-phosphate precipitation

Removal of potassium can be accomplished by various means; removal through the GI tract with Kayexalate® administration; by way of the kidney through diuresis, mineralocorticoid administration or increased sodium intake; by hemodialysis or peritoneal dialysis; or by shifting potassium back into the cells by insulin, glucose infusion, or sodium bicarbonate; calcium chloride reverses cardiac effects.

Dosing

Adults & Elderly: I.V. doses should be incorporated into the patient's maintenance I.V. fluids; intermittent I.V. infusion should be reserved for severe depletion situations in patients undergoing continuous ECG monitoring. It is difficult to determine total body phosphorus deficit; the following dosages are empiric guidelines:

Normal requirements elemental phosphorus: Oral:

Pregnancy lactation: Additional 400 mg/day

Adults: 800 mg

Treatment of hypophosphatemia: It is difficult to provide concrete guidelines for the treatment of severe hypophosphatemia because the extent of total body deficits and response to therapy are difficult to predict. Aggressive doses of phosphate may result in a transient serum elevation followed by redistribution into intracellular compartments or bone tissue. It is recommended that repletion of severe hypophosphatemia (<1 mg/dL in adults) be done I.V. because large doses of oral phosphate may cause diarrhea and intestinal absorption may be unreliable

Adult I.V. phosphate repletion:

Initial dose: 0.08 mmol/kg if recent uncomplicated hypophosphatemia

Initial dose: 0.16 mmol/kg if prolonged hypophosphatemia with presumed total body deficits; increase dose by 25% to 50% if patient symptomatic with severe hypophosphatemia

Do not exceed 0.24 mmol/kg/dose; administer over 6-12 hours by I.V. infusion. Some investigators have used more rapid infusions.

Note: With orders for I.V. phosphate, there is considerable confusion associated with the use of millimoles (mmol) versus milliequivalents (mEq) to express the phosphate requirement. Because inorganic phosphate exists as monobasic and dibasic anions, with the mixture of valences dependent on pH, ordering by mEq amounts is unreliable and may lead to large dosing errors. In addition, I.V. phosphate is available in the sodium and potassium salt; therefore, the content of these cations must be considered when ordering phosphate. The most reliable method of ordering I.V. phosphate is by millimoles, then specifying the potassium or sodium salt. For example, an order for 15 mmol of phosphate as potassium phosphate in one liter of normal saline. The dosing of phosphate should be 0.2-0.3 mmol/kg with a usual daily requirement of 30-60 mmol/day or 15 mmol of phosphate per liter of TPN or 15 mmol phosphate per 1000 calories of dextrose. Would also provide 22 mEq of potassium.

Maintenance:

I.V. solutions: 15-30 mmol/24 hours I.V. or 50-150 mmol/24 hours orally in divided doses

Oral: 1-2 capsules (250-500 mg phosphorus/8-16 mmol) 4 times/day; dilute as instructed

Pediatrics: I.V. doses should be incorporated into the patient's maintenance I.V. fluids; intermittent I.V. infusion should be reserved for severe depletion situations in patients undergoing continuous ECG monitoring. It is difficult to determine total body phosphorus deficit; the following are empiric guidelines

Note: Refer to notes under Adult dosing

Pediatric I.V. phosphate repletion:

Children: 0.25-0.5 mmol/kg **administer over 4-6 hours and repeat if symptomatic hypophosphatemia persists**; to assess the need for further phosphate administration, obtain serum inorganic phosphate after administration of the first dose and base further doses on serum levels and clinical status

Maintenance:

I.V. solutions: Children: 0.5-1.5 mmol/kg/24 hours I.V. or 2-3 mmol/kg/24 hours orally in divided doses

Oral:

Children <4 years: 1 capsule (250 mg phosphorus/8 mmol) 4 times/day; dilute as instructed

Children >4 years: Refer to adult dosing.

Available Dosage Forms

Injection, solution: Phosphate 3 mmol and potassium 4.4 mEq per mL (5 mL, 15 mL, 50 mL) [equivalent to phosphate 285 mg and potassium 170 mg per mL]

Powder for oral solution [packet] (Neutra-Phos®-K): Monobasic potassium phosphate and dibasic potassium phosphate/packet (100s) [equivalent to elemental phosphorus 250 mg and potassium 556 mg (14.2 mEq) per packet; sodium free]

Nursing Guidelines

Assessment: Assess therapeutic response and adverse effects.

Monitoring Laboratory Tests: Serum potassium, phosphate

Patient Education: Empty contents of capsule into 3-4 oz of water; do not swallow the capsule. Take with food to reduce the risk of diarrhea.

Pregnancy Risk Factor: C

Administration

Compatibility: Stable in dextran 6% in dextrose, dextran 6% in NS, D_{10}LR, $D_5$1/4NS, $D_5$1/2NS, D_5NS, D_5W, D_{10}W, 1/2NS, NS; **incompatible** with D_5LR, D_{10}NS, LR

Y-site administration: Incompatible with gatifloxacin

Compatibility when admixed: Incompatible with dobutamine

Potassium Phosphate and Sodium Phosphate

(poe TASS ee um FOS fate & SOW dee um FOS fate)

U.S. Brand Names K-Phos® MF; K-Phos® Neutral; K-Phos® No. 2; Neutra-Phos® [OTC]; Phos-NaK; Phospha 250™ Neutral; Uro-KP-Neutral®

Synonyms Sodium Phosphate and Potassium Phosphate

Pharmacologic Category Electrolyte Supplement, Oral

Medication Safety Issues

Sound-alike/look-alike issues:

K-Phos® Neutral may be confused with Neutra-Phos-K®

Use Treatment of conditions associated with excessive renal phosphate loss or inadequate GI absorption of phosphate; to acidify the urine to lower calcium concentrations; to increase the antibacterial activity of methenamine; reduce odor and rash caused by ammonia in urine

Pharmacodynamics/Kinetics Excretion: Urine

Contraindications Addison's disease, hyperkalemia, hyperphosphatemia, infected urolithiasis or struvite stone formation, patients with severely impaired renal function

Warnings/Precautions Use with caution in patients with renal disease, cardiac disease, metabolic alkalosis, acute dehydration, hepatic impairment, hypernatremia, and hypotension. Products also contain potassium and sodium.

Drug Interactions

Decreased effect/levels with aluminum and magnesium-containing antacids or sucralfate which can act as phosphate binders

Increased effect/levels with potassium-sparing diuretics or ACE inhibitors; salicylates

Adverse Reactions Frequency not defined.

Cardiovascular: Bradycardia, arrhythmia, chest pain, edema, tachycardia

Central nervous system: Mental confusion, tetany (with large doses of phosphate), headache, dizziness, seizure

Endocrine & metabolic: Hyperkalemia, alkalosis

Gastrointestinal: Diarrhea, nausea, stomach pain, flatulence, vomiting, throat pain, weight gain

Genitourinary: Urine output decreased

Local: Phlebitis

Neuromuscular & skeletal: Weakness, arthralgia, bone pain, paralysis, paresthesia, pain/weakness of extremities, muscle cramps

Renal: Acute renal failure

Respiratory: Dyspnea

(Continued)

Potassium Phosphate and Sodium Phosphate *(Continued)*

Miscellaneous: Thirst

Overdosage/Toxicology Symptoms of overdose include muscle weakness, paralysis, peaked T waves, flattened P waves, prolongation of QRS complex, ventricular arrhythmias, tetany, calcium phosphate precipitation. Removal of potassium can be accomplished by various means; removal through the GI tract with Kayexalate® administration; by way of the kidney through diuresis, mineralocorticoid administration or increased sodium intake; by hemodialysis or peritoneal dialysis; or by shifting potassium back into the cells by insulin and glucose infusion; calcium chloride reverses cardiac effects.

Dosing

Adults & Elderly: Note: All dosage forms to be mixed in 6-8 oz of water prior to administration

Phosphate supplement: Oral: Elemental phosphorus 250-500 mg 4 times/day after meals and at bedtime

Pediatrics: Note: All dosage forms to be mixed in 6-8 oz of water prior to administration

Phosphate supplement: Oral: Children ≥4 years: Elemental phosphorus 250 mg 4 times/day after meals and at bedtime

Available Dosage Forms

Powder, for oral solution (Neutra-Phos®, Phos-NaK): Monobasic sodium, dibasic sodium, and potassium phosphate/packet (100s) [equivalent to elemental phosphorus 250 mg, sodium 164 mg (7.1 mEq), and potassium 278 mg (7.1 mEq) per packet]

Tablet:

K-Phos® MF: Potassium acid phosphate 155 mg and sodium acid phosphate 350 mg [equivalent to elemental phosphorus 125.6 mg, sodium 67 mg (2.9 mEq), and potassium 44.5 mg (1.1 mEq)]

K-Phos® Neutral: Dibasic sodium phosphate 852 mg, monobasic potassium phosphate 155 mg, and monobasic sodium phosphate 130 mg [equivalent to elemental phosphorus 250 mg, sodium 298 mg (13 mEq), and potassium 45 mg (1.1 mEq)]

K-Phos® No. 2: Potassium acid phosphate 305 mg and sodium acid phosphate 700 mg [equivalent to elemental phosphorus 250 mg, sodium 134 mg (5.8 mEq), and potassium 88 mg (2.3 mEq)]

Phospha 250™ Neutral: Dibasic sodium phosphate 852 mg, monobasic potassium phosphate 155 mg, and monobasic sodium phosphate 130 mg [equivalent to elemental phosphorus 250 mg, sodium 298 mg (13 mEq), and potassium 45 mg (1.1 mEq)]

Uro-KP-Neutral®: Sodium phosphate monobasic, dipotassium phosphate, and disodium phosphate [equivalent to elemental phosphorus 258 mg, sodium 262.4 mg (10.8 mEq), and potassium 49.4 mg (1.3 mEq)]

Nursing Guidelines

Monitoring Laboratory Tests: Serum potassium, phosphate

Dietary Considerations: Should be taken after meals. In addition to phosphate, products contain potassium and sodium.

Patient Education: Powder packets are to be mixed in 6-8 oz of water; following dilution, solution may be chilled to increase palatability. Tablets should be taken with a full glass of water.

Pregnancy Risk Factor: C

Administration

Oral:

Powder: Following dilution of powder, solution may be chilled to increase palatability.

Tablet: Should be taken with a full glass of water.

♦ **Povidine™ [OTC]** *see* Povidone-Iodine *on page 1392*

Povidone-Iodine (POE vi done EYE oh dyne)

U.S. Brand Names Betadine® [OTC]; Betadine® Ophthalmic; Minidyne® [OTC]; Operand® [OTC]; Povidine™ [OTC]; Summer's Eve® Medicated Douche [OTC]; Vagi-Gard® [OTC]

Synonyms Polyvinylpyrrolidone with Iodine; PVP-I

Pharmacologic Category Antiseptic, Ophthalmic; Antiseptic, Topical; Antiseptic, Vaginal; Topical Skin Product

Medication Safety Issues

Sound-alike/look-alike issues:

Betadine® may be confused with Betagan®, betaine

Use External antiseptic with broad microbicidal spectrum for the prevention or treatment of topical infections associated with surgery, burns, minor cuts/scrapes; relief of minor vaginal irritation

Mechanism of Action Povidone-iodine is known to be a powerful broad spectrum germicidal agent effective against a wide range of bacteria, viruses, fungi, protozoa, and spores.

Pharmacodynamics/Kinetics Absorption: Topical: Absorbed systemically as iodine; amount depends upon concentration, route of administration, characteristics of skin

Contraindications Hypersensitivity to iodine or any component of the formulation

Warnings/Precautions Use caution in patients with thyroid disorders. Toxicity may occur following application of large or prolonged quantities; use caution with renal dysfunction, burns, pediatric patients. When used for self-medication (OTC use) do not apply to deep puncture wounds or serious burns; discontinue in case of redness, swelling, irritation or pain; do not use for longer than 1 week.

Drug Interactions No data reported

Adverse Reactions Frequency not defined.

Local: Edema, irritation, pruritus, rash

Dosing

Adults & Elderly:

Antiseptic: Topical: Apply to affected area as needed. Ophthalmic solution may be used to irrigate the eye or applied to area around the eye such as skin, eyelashes, or lid margins.

Surgical scrub: Topical: Apply solution to wet skin or hands, scrub for ~5 minutes, rinse; refer to product labeling for specific procedure-related instructions.

Vaginal irritation: Douche: Insert 0.3% solution vaginally once daily for 5-7 days

Available Dosage Forms [DSC] = Discontinued product

Gel, topical (Operand®): 10% (120 g)

Liquid, topical: 10% (30 mL)

Ointment, topical: 10% (1 g, 30 g)

Betadine®: 10% (0.9 g, 3.7 g, 30 g) [DSC]

Povidine™: 10% (30 g)

Pad [prep pads]: 10% (200s)

Betadine® SwabAids: 10% (100s)

Scrub brush [solution impregnated]: 7.5% (30s)

Solution, ophthalmic (Betadine®): 5% (50 mL)

Solution, perineal (Operand®): 10% (240 mL) [concentrate]

Solution, topical: 10% (240 mL, 480 mL, 3840 mL)

Betadine®: 10% (15 mL, 120 mL, 240 mL, 480 mL, 960 mL, 3840 mL)

Minidyne®: 10% (15 mL)

Operand®: 10% (60 mL, 120 mL, 240 mL, 480 mL, 960 mL, 3840 mL)

Solution, topical scrub:

Betadine® Surgical Scrub: 7.5% (120 mL, 480 mL, 960 mL, 3840 mL)

Betadine® Skin Cleanser: 7.5% (120 mL)

Operand®: 7.5% (60 mL, 120 mL, 240 mL, 480 mL, 960 mL, 3840 mL)

Solution, topical spray

Betadine®: 5% (90 mL) [CFC free; contains dry natural rubber]

Operand®: 10% (59 mL)

Solution, vaginal douche:

Operand®: 10% (240 mL) [concentrate]

Summer's Eve® Medicated Douche: 0.3% (135 mL)

Vagi-Gard®: 10% (180 mL, 240 mL) [concentrate]

Solution, whirlpool (Operand®): 10% (3840 mL) [concentrate]

Swab [prep-swab ampul]: 10% (0.65 mL)

Swabsticks: 10% (25s, 50s)

Betadine®: 10% (50s, 150s, 200s)

Swabsticks [gel saturated]: 10% (50s)

Swabsticks, topical scrub: 7.5% (25s, 50s)

(Continued)

Povidone-Iodine *(Continued)*

Nursing Guidelines

Patient Education: Do not swallow; avoid contact with eyes

Pregnancy Risk Factor: C (ophthalmic)

Pregnancy Issues: Reproduction studies have not been conducted. Vaginal products should not be used during pregnancy. Absorbed systemically as iodine. Transient hypothyroidism in the newborn has been reported following topical or vaginal use prior to delivery.

Lactation: Enters breast milk/use caution (AAP rates 'compatible')

- ♦ **PPD** *see* Tuberculin Tests *on page 1673*
- ♦ **PPV23** *see* Pneumococcal Polysaccharide Vaccine (Polyvalent) *on page 1378*

Pramipexole (pra mi PEKS ole)

U.S. Brand Names Mirapex®

Pharmacologic Category Anti-Parkinson's Agent, Dopamine Agonist

Medication Safety Issues

Sound-alike/look-alike issues:

Mirapex® may be confused with Mifeprex®, MiraLax™

Use Treatment of the signs and symptoms of idiopathic Parkinson's disease

Unlabeled/Investigational Use Treatment of depression

Mechanism of Action Pramipexole is a nonergot dopamine agonist with specificity for the D_2 subfamily dopamine receptor, and has also been shown to bind to D_3 and D_4 receptors. By binding to these receptors, it is thought that pramipexole can stimulate dopamine activity on the nerves of the striatum and substantia nigra.

Pharmacodynamics/Kinetics

Protein binding: 15%

Bioavailability: 90%

Half-life elimination: ~8 hours; Elderly: 12-14 hours

Time to peak, serum: ~2 hours

Excretion: Urine (90% as unchanged drug)

Contraindications Hypersensitivity to pramipexole or any component of the formulation

Warnings/Precautions Caution should be taken in patients with renal insufficiency and in patients with pre-existing dyskinesias. May cause orthostatic hypotension; Parkinson's disease patients appear to have an impaired capacity to respond to a postural challenge. Use with caution in patients at risk of hypotension (such as those receiving antihypertensive drugs) or where transient hypotensive episodes would be poorly tolerated (cardiovascular disease or cerebrovascular disease). Parkinson's patients being treated with dopaminergic agonists ordinarily require careful monitoring for signs and symptoms of postural hypotension, especially during dose escalation, and should be informed of this risk. May cause hallucinations, particularly in older patients. Pathologic degenerative changes were observed in the retinas of albino rats during studies with this agent, but were not observed in the retinas of pigmented rats or in other species. The significance of these data for humans remains uncertain.

Although not reported for pramipexole, other dopaminergic agents have been associated with a syndrome resembling neuroleptic malignant syndrome on withdrawal or significant dosage reduction after long-term use. Dopaminergic agents from the ergot class have also been associated with fibrotic complications, such as retroperitoneum, lungs, and pleura.

Pramipexole has been associated with somnolence, particularly at higher dosages (>1.5 mg/day). In addition, patients have been reported to fall asleep during activities of daily living, including driving, while taking this medication. Whether these patients exhibited somnolence prior to these events is not clear. Patients should be advised of this issue and factors which may increase risk (sleep disorders, other sedating medications, or concomitant medications which increase pramipexole concentrations) and instructed to report daytime somnolence or sleepiness to the prescriber. Patients should use caution in performing activities which require alertness (driving or operating machinery), and to avoid other medications which may cause CNS depression, including ethanol.

Drug Interactions

Antipsychotics: May decrease the efficiency of pramipexole due to dopamine antagonism

Cationic drugs: Drugs secreted by the cationic transport system (diltiazem, triamterene, verapamil, quinidine, quinine, ranitidine) decrease the clearance of pramipexole by ~20%

Cimetidine: May increase serum concentrations; cimetidine in combination with pramipexole produced a 50% increase in AUC and a 40% increase in half-life

Metoclopramide: May decrease the efficiency of pramipexole due to dopamine antagonism

Nutritional/Herbal/Ethanol Interactions

Ethanol: Avoid ethanol (may increase CNS depression).

Food: Food intake does not affect the extent of drug absorption, although the time to maximal plasma concentration is delayed by 60 minutes when taken with a meal.

Herb/Nutraceutical: Avoid valerian, St John's wort, SAMe, kava kava (may increase risk of serotonin syndrome and/or excessive sedation).

Adverse Reactions

>10%:

Cardiovascular: Postural hypotension

Central nervous system: Asthenia, dizziness, somnolence, insomnia, hallucinations, abnormal dreams

Gastrointestinal: Nausea, constipation

Neuromuscular & skeletal: Weakness, dyskinesia, EPS

1% to 10%:

Cardiovascular: Edema, syncope, tachycardia, chest pain

Central nervous system: Malaise, confusion, amnesia, dystonias, akathisia, thinking abnormalities, myoclonus, hyperesthesia, paranoia, fever

Endocrine & metabolic: Decreased libido

Gastrointestinal: Anorexia, weight loss, xerostomia, dysphagia

Genitourinary: Urinary frequency, impotence, urinary incontinence

Neuromuscular & skeletal: Muscle twitching, leg cramps, arthritis, bursitis, myasthenia, hypertonia, gait abnormalities

Ocular: Vision abnormalities

Respiratory: Dyspnea, rhinitis

<1% (Limited to important or life-threatening): Compulsive gambling, liver transaminases increased, rhabdomyolysis

Frequency not defined, dose related: Falling asleep during activities of daily living

Dosing

Adults & Elderly: Parkinson's disease: Oral: Initial: 0.375 mg/day given in 3 divided doses; increase gradually by 0.125 mg/dose every 5-7 days; range: 1.5-4.5 mg/day.

Renal Impairment:

Cl_{cr} 35-59 mL/minute: Initial: 0.125 mg twice daily (maximum dose: 1.5 mg twice daily)

Cl_{cr} 15-34 mL/minute: Initial: 0.125 mg once daily (maximum dose: 1.5 mg once daily)

Cl_{cr} <15 mL/minute (or hemodialysis patients): Not adequately studied.

Available Dosage Forms Tablet, as dihydrochloride monohydrate: 0.125 mg, 0.25 mg, 0.5 mg, 1 mg, 1.5 mg

Nursing Guidelines

Assessment: Assess potential for interactions with other prescriptions, OTC medications, or herbal products patient may be taking. Monitor blood pressure. Assess degree of somnolence. Assess for therapeutic effectiveness (improvement of symptoms) and adverse response. Teach patient appropriate use, interventions to reduce side effects, and adverse symptoms to report.

Dietary Considerations: May be taken with food to decrease nausea.

Patient Education: Do not take any new medication during therapy unless approved by prescriber. Take exactly as directed. Avoid alcohol. May cause drowsiness and extreme sedation or somnolence (use caution when driving or engaging in hazardous activities until response to drug is known); postural hypotension (use caution when changing position - rise slowly from sitting or lying position to standing and use caution when climbing stairs); constipation (increased exercise, fluids, fruit, or fiber may help); or urinary frequency. Consult prescriber about persistent adverse effects. **Pregnancy/breast-feeding precautions:** Inform prescriber if you are or intend to become pregnant. Breast-feeding is not recommended.

(Continued)

Pramipexole *(Continued)*

Pregnancy Risk Factor: C

Lactation: Excretion in breast milk unknown/not recommended

Breast-Feeding Considerations: Prolactin secretion may be inhibited.

Administration

Oral: Doses should be titrated gradually in all patients to avoid the onset of intolerable side effects. The dosage should be increased to achieve a maximum therapeutic effect, balanced against the side effects of dyskinesia, hallucinations, somnolence, and dry mouth.

♦ **Pravachol®** *see* Pravastatin *on page 1396*

Pravastatin (PRA va stat in)

U.S. Brand Names Pravachol®

Synonyms Pravastatin Sodium

Pharmacologic Category Antilipemic Agent, HMG-CoA Reductase Inhibitor

Medication Safety Issues

Sound-alike/look-alike issues:

Pravachol® may be confused with Prevacid®, Prinivil®, propranolol

Use Use with dietary therapy for the following:

Primary prevention of coronary events: In hypercholesterolemic patients without established coronary heart disease to reduce cardiovascular morbidity (myocardial infarction, coronary revascularization procedures) and mortality.

Secondary prevention of cardiovascular events in patients with established coronary heart disease: To slow the progression of coronary atherosclerosis; to reduce cardiovascular morbidity (myocardial infarction, coronary vascular procedures) and to reduce mortality; to reduce the risk of stroke and transient ischemic attacks

Hyperlipidemias: Reduce elevations in total cholesterol, LDL-C, apolipoprotein B, and triglycerides (elevations of 1 or more components are present in Fredrickson type IIa, IIb, III, and IV hyperlipidemias)

Heterozygous familial hypercholesterolemia (HeFH): In pediatric patients, 8-18 years of age, with HeFH having LDL-C ≥190 mg/dL **or** LDL ≥160 mg/dL with positive family history of premature cardiovascular disease (CVD) or 2 or more CVD risk factors in the pediatric patient

Mechanism of Action Pravastatin is a competitive inhibitor of 3-hydroxy-3-methylglutaryl coenzyme A (HMG-CoA) reductase, which is the rate-limiting enzyme involved in *de novo* cholesterol synthesis.

Pharmacodynamics/Kinetics

Onset of action: Several days

Peak effect: 4 weeks

Absorption: Rapidly absorbed; average absorption 34%

Protein binding: 50%

Metabolism: Hepatic to at least two metabolites

Bioavailability: 17%

Half-life elimination: ~2-3 hours

Time to peak, serum: 1-1.5 hours

Excretion: Feces (70%); urine (≤20%, 8% as unchanged drug)

Contraindications Hypersensitivity to pravastatin or any component of the formulation; active liver disease; unexplained persistent elevations of serum transaminases; pregnancy; breast-feeding

Warnings/Precautions Secondary causes of hyperlipidemia should be ruled out prior to therapy. Liver function must be monitored by periodic laboratory assessment. Rhabdomyolysis with acute renal failure has occurred. Risk may be increased with concurrent use of other drugs which may cause rhabdomyolysis (including gemfibrozil, fibric acid derivatives, or niacin at doses ≥1 g/day). Temporarily discontinue in any patient experiencing an acute or serious condition predisposing to renal failure secondary to rhabdomyolysis. Use caution in patients with previous liver disease or heavy ethanol use. Treatment in patients <8 years of age is not recommended.

Drug Interactions **Substrate** of CYP3A4 (minor); **Inhibits** CYP2C8/9 (weak), 2D6 (weak), 3A4 (weak)

Cholestyramine: Reduces pravastatin absorption; separate administration times by at least 4 hours.

Clofibrate and fenofibrate: May increase the risk of myopathy and rhabdomyolysis.

Colestipol: Reduces pravastatin absorption; separate administration by 1 hour.

Cyclosporine: Concurrent use may increase the risk of myopathy and rhabdomyolysis.

Gemfibrozil: Increased risk of myopathy and rhabdomyolysis.

Imidazole antifungals (itraconazole, ketoconazole): May modestly increase pravastatin concentrations (AUC).

Niacin: May increase the risk of myopathy and rhabdomyolysis.

P-glycoprotein inhibitors (eg, amiodarone, cyclosporine, ketoconazole): May increase pravastatin concentrations.

Nutritional/Herbal/Ethanol Interactions

Ethanol: Consumption of large amounts of ethanol may increase the risk of liver damage with HMG-CoA reductase inhibitors.

Food: Red yeast rice contains an estimated 2.4 mg lovastatin per 600 mg rice.

Herb/Nutraceutical: St John's wort may decrease pravastatin levels.

Adverse Reactions As reported in short-term trials; safety and tolerability with long-term use were similar to placebo

1% to 10%:

Cardiovascular: Chest pain (4%)

Central nervous system: Headache (2% to 6%), fatigue (4%), dizziness (1% to 3%)

Dermatologic: Rash (4%)

Gastrointestinal: Nausea/vomiting (7%), diarrhea (6%), heartburn (3%)

Hepatic: Transaminases increased (>3x normal on two occasions - 1%)

Neuromuscular & skeletal: Myalgia (2%)

Respiratory: Cough (3%)

Miscellaneous: Influenza (2%)

<1% (Limited to important or life-threatening): Allergy, lens opacity, libido change, memory impairment, muscle weakness, neuropathy, paresthesia, taste disturbance, tremor, vertigo

Postmarketing and/or case reports: Anaphylaxis, angioedema, cholestatic jaundice, cirrhosis, cranial nerve dysfunction, dermatomyositis, erythema multiforme, ESR increase, fulminant hepatic necrosis, gynecomastia, hemolytic anemia, hepatitis, hepatoma, lupus erythematosus-like syndrome, myopathy, pancreatitis, peripheral nerve palsy, polymyalgia rheumatica, positive ANA, purpura, rhabdomyolysis, Stevens-Johnson syndrome, vasculitis

Additional class-related events or case reports (not necessarily reported with pravastatin therapy): Angioedema, cataracts, depression, dyspnea, eosinophilia, erectile dysfunction, facial paresis, hypersensitivity reaction, impaired extraocular muscle movement, impotence, leukopenia, malaise, memory loss, ophthalmoplegia, paresthesia, peripheral neuropathy, photosensitivity, psychic disturbance, skin discoloration, thrombocytopenia, thyroid dysfunction, toxic epidermal necrolysis, transaminases increased, vomiting

Overdosage/Toxicology Treatment is symptomatic.

Dosing

Adults & Elderly:

Hyperlipidemias, primary prevention of coronary events, secondary prevention of cardiovascular events: Oral: Initial: 40 mg once daily; titrate dosage to response (usual range: 10-80 mg) (maximum dose: 80 mg once daily)

Dosage adjustment based on concomitant immunosuppressants (ie, cyclosporine): Oral: Initial: 10 mg/day, titrate with caution (maximum dose: 20 mg/day)

Note: Doses should be individualized according to the baseline LDL-cholesterol levels, the recommended goal of therapy, and patient response; adjustments should be made at intervals of 4 weeks or more; doses may need adjusted based on concomitant medications

Pediatrics:

Heterozygous familial hypercholesterolemia (HeFH): Oral: Children:

8-13 years: 20 mg/day

14-18 years: 40 mg/day

Dosage adjustment based on concomitant immunosuppressants (ie, cyclosporine): Refer to adult dosing.

Note: Doses should be individualized according to the baseline LDL-cholesterol levels, the recommended goal of therapy, and patient response; adjustments should be made at intervals of 4 weeks or more; doses may need adjusted based on concomitant medications

(Continued)

Pravastatin *(Continued)*

Renal Impairment: Initial: 10 mg/day

Hepatic Impairment: Initial: 10 mg/day

Available Dosage Forms Tablet, as sodium: 10 mg, 20 mg, 40 mg, 80 mg

Nursing Guidelines

Assessment: See Contraindications, Warnings/Precautions, and Dosing for use cautions. Assess potential for interactions with other prescriptions, OTC medications, or herbal products patient may be taking (see Drug Interactions). Assess results of laboratory tests (see below) and patient response at beginning of therapy, when increasing dose, and periodically thereafter (see Adverse Reactions and Overdose/Toxicology). Teach patient proper use, possible side effects/appropriate interventions, and adverse symptoms to report (see Patient Education). **Pregnancy risk factor X** - determine that patient is not pregnant before starting therapy. Do not give to females of childbearing age unless capable of complying with barrier contraceptive use. Breast-feeding is contraindicated.

Monitoring Laboratory Tests: Obtain baseline LFTs and total cholesterol profile; creatine phosphokinase due to possibility of myopathy. Repeat LFTs prior to elevation of dose. May be measured when clinically indicated and/or periodically thereafter.

Dietary Considerations: May be taken without regard to meals. Before initiation of therapy, patients should be placed on a standard cholesterol-lowering diet for 6 weeks and the diet should be continued during drug therapy. Red yeast rice contains an estimated 2.4 mg lovastatin per 600 mg rice.

Patient Education: Inform prescriber of all prescriptions, OTC medications, or herbal products you are taking, and any allergies you have. Do not take any new medication during therapy unless approved by prescriber. Take at same time each day. Follow diet and exercise regimen as prescribed. Avoid excess alcohol. You will have periodic blood tests to assess effectiveness. May cause mild nausea or vomiting (small, frequent meals, frequent mouth care, chewing gum, or sucking lozenges may help); diarrhea (buttermilk, boiled milk, or yogurt may help); or headache (see prescriber for analgesic). Report chest pain; CNS changes (memory loss, depression, personality changes); numbness, weakness, tingling, pain, or cramping in extremities or muscles; vision changes; rash; or other persistent adverse reactions. **Pregnancy/breast-feeding precautions:** Inform prescriber if you are pregnant. Consult prescriber for appropriate barrier contraceptive measures to use during and for 1 month following therapy. This drug may cause severe fetal defects. Do not donate blood during or for 1 month following therapy. Do not breast-feed.

Geriatric Considerations: Effective and well tolerated in the elderly. No specific dosage recommendations. Clearance is reduced in older adults, resulting in an increase in AUC between 25% to 50%. However, substantial accumulation is not expected.

The definition of and, therefore, when to treat hyperlipidemia in older adults is a controversial issue. The National Cholesterol Education Program recommends that all adults maintain a plasma cholesterol <160 mg/dL. In elderly patients with one additional risk factor, goal LDL would decrease to <130 mg/dL. Pharmacologic treatment should be reserved for those who are unable to obtain a desirable plasma cholesterol concentration by diet alone and for whom the benefits of treatment are believed to outweigh the potential adverse effects, drug interactions, and cost of treatment.

Pregnancy Risk Factor: X

Pregnancy Issues: Cholesterol biosynthesis may be important in fetal development. Contraindicated in pregnancy. Administer to women of childbearing potential only when conception is highly unlikely and patients have been informed of potential hazards.

Lactation: Enters breast milk/contraindicated

Perioperative/Anesthesia/Other Concerns: Myopathy: Currently-marketed HMG-CoA reductase inhibitors appear to have a similar potential for causing myopathy. Incidence of severe myopathy is about 0.08% to 0.09%. The factors that increase risk include advanced age (especially >80 years), gender (occurs in women more frequently than men), small body frame, frailty, multisystem disease (eg, chronic renal insufficiency especially due to diabetes), multiple medications, **perioperative periods (higher risk when continued during hospitalization for major surgery)**, and drug interactions (use with caution or avoid).

Administration

Oral: May be taken without regard to meals.

Storage: Store at 25°C (77°F); excursions permitted to 15°C to 30°C (59°F to 86°F). Protect from moisture and light.

- **Pravastatin Sodium** *see* Pravastatin *on page 1396*
- **PreCare®** *see* Vitamins (Multiple/Prenatal) *on page 1721*
- **PreCare® Conceive™** *see* Vitamins (Multiple/Prenatal) *on page 1721*
- **PreCare® Prenatal** *see* Vitamins (Multiple/Prenatal) *on page 1721*
- **Precedex™** *see* Dexmedetomidine *on page 501*
- **Pred Forte®** *see* PrednisoLONE *on page 1399*
- **Pred Mild®** *see* PrednisoLONE *on page 1399*

PrednisoLONE (pred NISS oh lone)

U.S. Brand Names AK-Pred®; Bubbli-Pred™; Econopred® Plus; Orapred®; Pediapred®; Pred Forte®; Pred Mild®; Prelone®

Synonyms Deltahydrocortisone; Metacortandralone; Prednisolone Acetate; Prednisolone Acetate, Ophthalmic; Prednisolone Sodium Phosphate; Prednisolone Sodium Phosphate, Ophthalmic

Pharmacologic Category Corticosteroid, Ophthalmic; Corticosteroid, Systemic

Medication Safety Issues

Sound-alike/look-alike issues:

PrednisoLONE may be confused with predniSONE

Pediapred® may be confused with Pediazole®

Use Treatment of palpebral and bulbar conjunctivitis; corneal injury from chemical, radiation, thermal burns, or foreign body penetration; endocrine disorders, rheumatic disorders, collagen diseases, dermatologic diseases, allergic states, ophthalmic diseases, respiratory diseases, hematologic disorders, neoplastic diseases, edematous states, and gastrointestinal diseases; resolution of acute exacerbations of multiple sclerosis

Mechanism of Action Decreases inflammation by suppression of migration of polymorphonuclear leukocytes and reversal of increased capillary permeability; suppresses the immune system by reducing activity and volume of the lymphatic system

Pharmacodynamics/Kinetics

Duration: 18-36 hours

Protein binding (concentration dependent): 65% to 91%; decreased in elderly

Metabolism: Primarily hepatic, but also metabolized in most tissues, to inactive compounds

Half-life elimination: 3.6 hours; End-stage renal disease: 3-5 hours

Excretion: Primarily urine (as glucuronides, sulfates, and unconjugated metabolites)

Contraindications Hypersensitivity to prednisolone or any component of the formulation; acute superficial herpes simplex keratitis; live or attenuated virus vaccines; systemic fungal infections; varicella

Warnings/Precautions Use with caution in patients with hyperthyroidism, cirrhosis, nonspecific ulcerative colitis, hypertension, osteoporosis, thromboembolic tendencies, CHF, convulsive disorders, myasthenia gravis, thrombophlebitis, peptic ulcer, diabetes, or tuberculosis; acute adrenal insufficiency may occur with abrupt withdrawal after long-term therapy or with stress; young pediatric patients may be more susceptible to adrenal axis suppression from topical therapy.

Prolonged use of corticosteroids may result in glaucoma; damage to the optic nerve (not indicated for treatment of optic neuritis), defects in visual acuity and fields of vision, and posterior subcapsular cataract formation may occur. Prolonged use of corticosteroids may also increase the incidence of secondary infection, mask acute infection (including fungal infections) or prolong or exacerbate viral infections. Exposure to chickenpox should be avoided; corticosteroids should not be used to treat ocular herpes simplex. Use following cataract surgery may delay healing or increase the incidence of bleb formation.

Corticosteroids should not be used for cerebral malaria. Because of the risk of adverse effects, systemic corticosteroids should be used cautiously in the elderly, in the smallest possible dose, and for the shortest possible time.

Drug Interactions **Substrate** of CYP3A4 (minor); **Inhibits** CYP3A4 (weak)

Aminoglutethimide: May reduce the serum levels/effects of prednisolone; likely via induction of microsomal isoenzymes.

(Continued)

PrednisoLONE *(Continued)*

Antacids: May increase the absorption of corticosteroids; separate administration by ≥2 hours.

Anticholinesterases: Concurrent use may lead to severe weakness in patients with myasthenia gravis.

Azole antifungals: May increase the serum levels of corticosteroids; monitor.

Barbiturates: May decrease prednisolone levels; monitor.

Calcium channel blockers (nondihydropyridine): May increase the serum levels of corticosteroids; monitor.

CYP3A4 inducers: May decrease the levels/effects of prednisolone. Example inducers include aminoglutethimide, carbamazepine, nafcillin, nevirapine, phenobarbital, and phenytoin.

Cyclosporine: Corticosteroids may increase the serum levels of cyclosporine. In addition, cyclosporine may increase levels of corticosteroids; monitor.

Estrogens: May increase the serum levels of corticosteroids; monitor.

Fluoroquinolones: Concurrent use may increase the risk of tendon rupture, particularly in elderly patients (overall incidence rare).

Isoniazid: Serum concentrations may be decreased by corticosteroids.

Ketoconazole: May decrease metabolism of certain corticosteroids leading to increased levels (up to 60%) and increased risk of adverse effects; monitor.

Neuromuscular-blocking agents: Concurrent use with corticosteroids may increase the risk of myopathy.

Nonsteroidal anti-inflammatory drugs (NSAIDs), aspirin: Concurrent use with corticosteroids may lead to an increased incidence of gastrointestinal adverse effects; use caution.

Phenytoin: May decrease serum levels/effects of prednisolone; monitor

Potassium depleting agents (eg, diuretics, amphotericin B): Concurrent use increases risk of hypokalemia (especially if digitalized); monitor.

Rifampin: May decrease serum levels/effects of prednisolone; monitor.

Salicylates: Salicylates may increase the gastrointestinal adverse effects of corticosteroids.

Skin tests: Corticosteroids may suppress reactions to skin tests.

Vaccines, toxoids: Corticosteroids may suppress the response to vaccinations. The use of live vaccines is contraindicated in immunosuppressed patients. In patients receiving high doses of systemic corticosteroids for ≥14 days, wait at least 1 month between discontinuing steroid therapy and administering immunization.

Warfarin: Corticosteroids may lead to a reduction in warfarin effect; monitor.

Nutritional/Herbal/Ethanol Interactions

Ethanol: Avoid ethanol (may increase gastric mucosal irritation).

Food: Prednisolone interferes with calcium absorption. Limit caffeine.

Herb/Nutraceutical: St John's wort may decrease prednisolone levels. Avoid cat's claw, echinacea (have immunostimulant properties).

Lab Interactions Response to skin tests

Adverse Reactions Frequency not defined.

Ophthalmic formulation:

Endocrine & metabolic: Hypercorticoidism (rare)

Ocular: Conjunctival hyperemia, conjunctivitis, corneal ulcers, delayed wound healing, glaucoma, intraocular pressure increased, keratitis, loss of accommodation, optic nerve damage, mydriasis, posterior subcapsular cataract formation, ptosis, secondary ocular infection

Oral formulation:

Cardiovascular: CHF, edema, hypertension

Central nervous system: Convulsions, headache, insomnia, malaise, nervousness, psychic disorders, vertigo

Dermatologic: Bruising, diaphoresis increased, facial erythema, hirsutism, petechiae, skin test reaction suppression, thin fragile skin, urticaria

Endocrine & metabolic: Carbohydrate tolerance decreased, Cushing's syndrome, diabetes mellitus, growth suppression, hyperglycemia, hypokalemic alkalosis, menstrual irregularities, negative nitrogen balance, pituitary adrenal axis suppression, potassium loss

Gastrointestinal: Abdominal distention, increased appetite, indigestion, nausea, peptic ulcer, ulcerative esophagitis, weight gain

Hepatic: LFTs increased (usually reversible)

Neuromuscular & skeletal: Arthralgia, fractures, intracranial pressure with papilledema (usually after discontinuation), muscle mass decreased, muscle weakness, osteoporosis, steroid myopathy, tendon rupture, weakness

Ocular: Cataracts, exophthalmus, glaucoma, intraocular pressure increased
Respiratory: Epistaxis
Miscellaneous: Impaired wound healing

Overdosage/Toxicology When consumed in high doses for prolonged periods, systemic hypercorticism and adrenal suppression may occur, in those cases discontinuation of the corticosteroid should be done judiciously.

Dosing

Adults: Dose depends upon condition being treated and response of patient. Consider alternate day therapy for long-term therapy. Discontinuation of long-term therapy requires gradual withdrawal by tapering the dose. Patients undergoing unusual stress while receiving corticosteroids, should receive increased doses prior to, during, and after the stressful situation.

Usual dose (range): Oral: 5-60 mg/day

Rheumatoid arthritis: Oral: Initial: 5-7.5 mg/day, adjust dose as necessary

Multiple sclerosis: Oral: 200 mg/day for 1 week followed by 80 mg every other day for 1 month

Conjunctivitis: Ophthalmic (suspension/solution): Instill 1-2 drops into conjunctival sac every hour during day, every 2 hours at night until favorable response is obtained, then use 1 drop every 4 hours.

Dosing adjustment in hyperthyroidism: Prednisolone dose may need to be increased to achieve adequate therapeutic effects.

Elderly: Use lowest effective adult dose. Dose depends upon condition being treated and response of patient; alternate day dosing may be attempted in some disease states.

Pediatrics: Dose depends upon condition being treated and response of patient; dosage for infants and children should be based on severity of the disease and response of the patient rather than on strict adherence to dosage indicated by age, weight, or body surface area. Consider alternate day therapy for long-term therapy. Discontinuation of long-term therapy requires gradual withdrawal by tapering the dose. Patients undergoing unusual stress while receiving corticosteroids, should receive increased doses prior to, during, and after the stressful situation.

Acute asthma: Oral: 1-2 mg/kg/day in divided doses 1-2 times/day for 3-5 days

Anti-inflammatory or immunosuppressive dose: Oral: 0.1-2 mg/kg/day in divided doses 1-4 times/day

Nephrotic syndrome: Oral:

Initial (first 3 episodes): 2 mg/kg/day **or** 60 mg/m^2/day (maximum: 80 mg/day) in divided doses 3-4 times/day until urine is protein free for 3 consecutive days (maximum: 28 days); followed by 1-1.5 mg/kg/dose **or** 40 mg/m^2/dose given every other day for 4 weeks

Maintenance (for frequent relapses): 0.5-1 mg/kg/dose given every other day for 3-6 months

Conjunctivitis: Ophthalmic (suspension/solution): Children: Refer to adult dosing.

Dosing adjustment in hyperthyroidism: Refer to adult dosing.

Renal Impairment: Slightly dialyzable (5% to 20%)

Available Dosage Forms

Solution, ophthalmic, as sodium phosphate: 1% (5 mL, 10 mL, 15 mL) [contains benzalkonium chloride]
AK-Pred®: 1% (5 mL, 15 mL) [contains benzalkonium chloride]

Solution, oral, as sodium phosphate: Prednisolone base 5 mg/5 mL (120 mL)
Bubbli-Pred™: Prednisolone base 5 mg/5 mL (120 mL) [bubble gum flavor]
Orapred®: 20 mg/5 mL (240 mL) [equivalent to prednisolone base 15 mg/5 mL; dye free; contains alcohol 2%, sodium benzoate; grape flavor]
Pediapred®: 6.7 mg/5 mL (120 mL) [equivalent to prednisolone base 5 mg/5 mL; dye free; raspberry flavor]

Suspension, ophthalmic, as acetate: 1% (5 mL, 10 mL, 15 mL) [contains benzalkonium chloride]
Econopred® Plus: 1% (5 mL, 10 mL) [contains benzalkonium chloride]
Pred Forte®: 1% (1 mL, 5 mL, 10 mL, 15 mL) [contains benzalkonium chloride and sodium bisulfite]
Pred Mild®: 0.12% (5 mL, 10 mL) [contains benzalkonium chloride and sodium bisulfite]

Syrup, as base: 5 mg/5 mL (120 mL); 15 mg/5 mL (240 mL, 480 mL)
Prelone®: 15 mg/5 mL (240 mL, 480 mL) [contains alcohol 5%, benzoic acid; cherry flavor]

Tablet, as base: 5 mg

(Continued)

PrednisoLONE *(Continued)*

Nursing Guidelines

Assessment: Assess other medications patient may be taking for effectiveness and interactions. Assess results of laboratory tests, therapeutic effectiveness, and adverse effects according to indications for therapy, dose, route, and duration of therapy. With systemic administration, patients with diabetes should monitor glucose levels closely. Assess knowledge/teach patient appropriate use, interventions to reduce side effects, and adverse symptoms to report. When used for long-term therapy (>10-14 days), do not discontinue abruptly; decrease dosage incrementally.

Monitoring Laboratory Tests: Blood glucose, electrolytes

Dietary Considerations: Should be taken after meals or with food or milk to decrease GI effects; increase dietary intake of pyridoxine, vitamin C, vitamin D, folate, calcium, and phosphorus.

Patient Education: Take exactly as directed; do not increase dose or discontinue abruptly without consulting prescriber. Avoid alcohol. Limit intake of caffeine or stimulants. Prescriber may recommend increased dietary vitamins, minerals, or iron. If you have diabetes, monitor glucose levels closely (antidiabetic medication may need to be adjusted). Inform prescriber if you are experiencing greater-than-normal levels of stress (medication may need adjustment). Some forms of this medication may cause GI upset (oral medication should be taken with meals to reduce GI upset; small frequent meals and frequent mouth care may reduce GI upset). You may be more susceptible to infection (avoid crowds and exposure to infection). Report promptly excessive nervousness or sleep disturbances; any signs of infection (sore throat, unhealed injuries); excessive growth of body hair or loss of skin color; vision changes; excessive or sudden weight gain (>3 lb/week); swelling of face or extremities; respiratory difficulty; muscle weakness; change in color of stools (black or tarry) or persistent abdominal pain; or worsening of condition or failure to improve. **Pregnancy precaution:** Inform prescriber if you are or intend to become pregnant.

Ophthalmic: For ophthalmic use only. Wash hands before using. Tilt head back and look upward. Put drops of suspension inside lower eyelid. Close eye and roll eyeball in all directions. Do not blink for 1/2 minute. Apply gentle pressure to inner corner of eye for 30 seconds. Do not use any other eye preparation for at least 10 minutes. Do not let tip of applicator touch eye; do not contaminate tip of applicator (may cause eye infection, eye damage, or vision loss). Do not share medication with anyone else. Wear sunglasses when in sunlight; you may be more sensitive to bright light. Inform prescriber if condition worsens or fails to improve or if you experience eye pain, disturbances of vision, or other adverse eye response.

Geriatric Considerations: Useful in patients with inability to activate prednisone (liver disease). Because of the risk of adverse effects, systemic corticosteroids should be used cautiously in the elderly, in the smallest possible dose, and for the shortest possible time. For long-term use, monitor bone mineral density and institute fracture prevention strategies. See Pharmacodynamics/kinetics.

Pregnancy Risk Factor: C

Lactation: Enters breast milk/use caution (AAP rates "compatible")

Perioperative/Anesthesia/Other Concerns:

Neuromuscular Effects: ICU-acquired paresis was recently studied in 5 ICUs (3 medical and 2 surgical ICUs) at 4 French hospitals. All ICU patients without pre-existing neuromuscular disease admitted from March 1999 through June 2000 were evaluated (De Jonghe B, 2002). Each patient had to be mechanically ventilated for ≥7 days and was screened daily for awakening. The first day the patient was considered awake was Study Day 1. Patients with severe muscle weakness on Study Day 7 were considered to have ICU-acquired paresis. Among the 95 patients who were evaluable, about 25% developed ICU-acquired paresis. Independent predictors included: female gender, the number of days with ≥2 organ dysfunction, and administration of corticosteroids. Further studies may be required to verify and characterize the association between the development of ICU-acquired paresis and use of corticosteroids. Concurrent use of a corticosteroid and muscle relaxant appear to increase the risk of certain ICU myopathies; avoid or administer the corticosteroid at the lowest dose possible.

Adrenal Insufficiency: Patients will often have steroid-induced adverse effects on glucose tolerance and lipid profiles. When discontinuing steroid therapy in patients on long-term steroid supplementation, it is important that the steroid therapy be discontinued gradually. Abrupt withdrawal may result in adrenal insufficiency with hypotension and hyperkalemia. Patients on long-term steroid supplementation will require higher corticosteroid doses when subject to stress (ie, trauma, surgery, severe infection). Guidelines for glucocorticoid replacement during various surgical procedures has been published (Salem M, 1994, Coursin DB, 2002).

Septic Shock: A recent randomized, double-blind, placebo controlled trial assessed whether low dose corticosteroid administration could improve 28-day survival in patients with septic shock and relative adrenal insufficiency. Relative adrenal insufficiency was defined as an inappropriate response to corticotropin administration (increase of serum cortisol of ≤9 mcg/dL from baseline). Cortisol levels were drawn immediately before corticotropin administration and 30 to 60 minutes afterwards. Three hundred adult septic shock patients requiring mechanical ventilation and vasopressor support were randomized to either hydrocortisone (50 mg IVP every 6 hours) and fludrocortisone (50 mcg tablet daily via nasogastric tube) or matching placebos for 7 days. In patients who did not appropriately respond to corticotropin (nonresponders), there were significantly fewer deaths in the active treatment group. Vasopressor therapy was withdrawn more frequently in this subset of the active treatment group. Adverse events were similar in both groups. Patients who lack adrenal reserve and thus have relative adrenal insufficiency during the stress of septic shock may benefit from physiologic steroid replacement. However, there was a trend for increased mortality in patients who responded to the corticotropin test (increase serum cortisol >9 mcg/dL from baseline). These patients may not benefit from physiologic steroid replacement. Further study is required to better characterize the patient populations who may benefit.

Administration

Oral: Give oral formulation with food or milk to decrease GI effects.

- **Prednisolone Acetate** *see* PrednisoLONE *on page 1399*
- **Prednisolone Acetate, Ophthalmic** *see* PrednisoLONE *on page 1399*
- **Prednisolone and Sulfacetamide** *see* Sulfacetamide and Prednisolone *on page 1581*
- **Prednisolone Sodium Phosphate** *see* PrednisoLONE *on page 1399*
- **Prednisolone Sodium Phosphate, Ophthalmic** *see* PrednisoLONE *on page 1399*

PredniSONE (PRED ni sone)

U.S. Brand Names Prednisone Intensol™; Sterapred®; Sterapred® DS

Synonyms Deltacortisone; Deltadehydrocortisone

Pharmacologic Category Corticosteroid, Systemic

Medication Safety Issues

Sound-alike/look-alike issues:

PredniSONE may be confused with methylPREDNISolone, Pramosone®, prazosin, prednisoLONE, Prilosec®, primidone, promethazine

Use Treatment of a variety of diseases including adrenocortical insufficiency, hypercalcemia, rheumatic, and collagen disorders; dermatologic, ocular, respiratory, gastrointestinal, and neoplastic diseases; organ transplantation and a variety of diseases including those of hematologic, allergic, inflammatory, and autoimmune in origin; not available in injectable form, prednisolone must be used

Unlabeled/Investigational Use Investigational: Prevention of postherpetic neuralgia and relief of acute pain in the early stages

Mechanism of Action Decreases inflammation by suppression of migration of polymorphonuclear leukocytes and reversal of increased capillary permeability; suppresses the immune system by reducing activity and volume of the lymphatic system; suppresses adrenal function at high doses. Antitumor effects may be related to inhibition of glucose transport, phosphorylation, or induction of cell death in immature lymphocytes. Antiemetic effects are thought to occur due to blockade of cerebral innervation of the emetic center via inhibition of prostaglandin synthesis.

Pharmacodynamics/Kinetics

Protein binding (concentration dependent): 65% to 91%

Metabolism: Hepatically converted from prednisone (inactive) to prednisolone (active); may be impaired with hepatic dysfunction

Half-life elimination: Normal renal function: 2.5-3.5 hours

See Prednisolone monograph for complete information.

(Continued)

PredniSONE *(Continued)*

Contraindications Hypersensitivity to prednisone or any component of the formulation; serious infections, except tuberculous meningitis; systemic fungal infections; varicella

Warnings/Precautions Withdraw therapy with gradual tapering of dose, may retard bone growth. Use with caution in patients with hypothyroidism, cirrhosis, CHF, ulcerative colitis, thromboembolic disorders, and patients at increased risk for peptic ulcer disease. Corticosteroids should be used with caution in patients with diabetes, hypertension, osteoporosis, glaucoma, cataracts, or tuberculosis. Use caution in hepatic impairment. Because of the risk of adverse effects, systemic corticosteroids should be used cautiously in the elderly, in the smallest possible dose, and for the shortest possible time.

Drug Interactions Substrate of CYP3A4 (minor); **Induces** CYP2C19 (weak), 3A4 (weak)

Decreased effect:

- Barbiturates, phenytoin, rifampin decrease corticosteroid effectiveness
- Decreases salicylates
- Decreases vaccines
- Decreases toxoids effectiveness

Increased effect/toxicity: NSAIDs: Concurrent use of prednisone may increase the risk of GI ulceration

Nutritional/Herbal/Ethanol Interactions

Ethanol: Avoid ethanol (may increase gastric mucosal irritation)

Food: Prednisone interferes with calcium absorption, Limit caffeine.

Herb/Nutraceutical: St John's wort may decrease prednisone levels. Avoid cat's claw, echinacea (have immunostimulant properties).

Lab Interactions Response to skin tests

Adverse Reactions

>10%:

- Central nervous system: Insomnia, nervousness
- Gastrointestinal: Increased appetite, indigestion

1% to 10%:

- Central nervous system: Dizziness or lightheadedness, headache
- Dermatologic: Hirsutism, hypopigmentation
- Endocrine & metabolic: Diabetes mellitus, glucose intolerance, hyperglycemia
- Neuromuscular & skeletal: Arthralgia
- Ocular: Cataracts, glaucoma
- Respiratory: Epistaxis
- Miscellaneous: Diaphoresis

<1% (Limited to important or life-threatening): Cushing's syndrome, edema, fractures, hallucinations, hypertension, muscle-wasting, osteoporosis, pancreatitis, pituitary-adrenal axis suppression, seizure

Overdosage/Toxicology When consumed in high doses for prolonged periods, systemic hypercorticism and adrenal suppression may occur. In those cases, discontinuation of the corticosteroid should be done judiciously.

Dosing

Adults: Dose depends upon condition being treated and response of patient; consider alternate day therapy for long-term therapy. Discontinuation of long-term therapy requires gradual withdrawal by tapering the dose.

Physiologic replacement: Oral: 4-5 mg/m^2/day

Immunosuppression/chemotherapy adjunct: Oral: Range: 5-60 mg/day in divided doses 1-4 times/day

Allergic reaction (contact dermatitis): Oral:

- Day 1: 30 mg divided as 10 mg before breakfast, 5 mg at lunch, 5 mg at dinner, 10 mg at bedtime
- Day 2: 5 mg at breakfast, 5 mg at lunch, 5 mg at dinner, 10 mg at bedtime
- Day 3: 5 mg 4 times/day (with meals and at bedtime)
- Day 4: 5 mg 3 times/day (breakfast, lunch, bedtime)
- Day 5: 5 mg 2 times/day (breakfast, bedtime)
- Day 6: 5 mg before breakfast

Acute asthma: 1-2 mg/kg/day in divided doses 1-2 times/day for 3-5 days

Asthma maintenance:

Moderate persistent: Inhaled corticosteroid (medium dose) or inhaled corticosteroid (low-medium dose) with a long-acting bronchodilator

Severe persistent: Inhaled corticosteroid (high dose) and corticosteroid tablets or syrup long term: 2 mg/kg/day, generally not to exceed 60 mg/day

Pneumonia due to *Pneumocystis carinii*: Oral:
40 mg twice daily for 5 days **followed by**
40 mg once daily for 5 days **followed by**
20 mg once daily for 11 days or until antimicrobial regimen is completed

Thyrotoxicosis: Oral: 60 mg/day
Note: Dosing adjustment in hyperthyroidism: Prednisone dose may need to be increased to achieve adequate therapeutic effects

Chemotherapy (refer to individual protocols): Oral: Range: 20 mg/day to 100 mg/m²/day

Rheumatoid arthritis: Oral: Use lowest possible daily dose (often ≤7.5 mg/day)

Idiopathic thrombocytopenia purpura (ITP): Oral: 60 mg daily for 4-6 weeks, gradually tapered over several weeks

Systemic lupus erythematosus (SLE): Oral:
Acute: 1-2 mg/kg/day in 2-3 divided doses
Maintenance: Reduce to lowest possible dose, usually <1 mg/kg/day as single dose (morning)

Elderly: Refer to adult dosing; use the lowest effective dose. Oral dose depends upon condition being treated and response of patient. Alternate day dosing may be attempted.

Pediatrics: Note: Dose depends upon condition being treated and response of patient; dosage for infants and children should be based on severity of the disease and response of the patient rather than on strict adherence to dosage indicated by age, weight, or body surface area. Consider alternate day therapy for long-term therapy. Discontinuation of long-term therapy requires gradual withdrawal by tapering the dose.

Physiologic replacement: Oral: Children: 4-5 mg/m²/day

Anti-inflammatory or immunosuppressive dose: Oral: 0.05-2 mg/kg/day divided 1-4 times/day

Acute asthma: Oral: 1-2 mg/kg/day in divided doses 1-2 times/day for 3-5 days
Alternatively (for 3- to 5-day "burst"):
<1 year: 10 mg every 12 hours
1-4 years: 20 mg every 12 hours
5-13 years: 30 mg every 12 hours
>13 years: 40 mg every 12 hours

Asthma long-term therapy (alternative dosing by age): Oral:
<1 year: 10 mg every other day
1-4 years: 20 mg every other day
5-13 years: 30 mg every other day
>13 years: 40 mg every other day

Asthma maintenance: Children ≥5 years: Refer to adult dosing.

Nephrotic syndrome: Oral:
Initial (first 3 episodes): 2 mg/kg/day **or** 60 mg/m²/day (maximum: 80 mg/day) in divided doses 3-4 times/day until urine is protein free for 3 consecutive days (maximum: 28 days); followed by 1-1.5 mg/kg/dose **or** 40 mg/m²/dose given every other day for 4 weeks
Maintenance dose (for frequent relapses): 0.5-1 mg/kg/dose given every other day for 3-6 months

Renal Impairment: Hemodialysis effects: Supplemental dose is not necessary.

Available Dosage Forms

Solution, oral: 1 mg/mL (5 mL, 120 mL, 500 mL) [contains alcohol 5%, sodium benzoate; vanilla flavor]

Solution, oral concentrate (Prednisone Intensol™): 5 mg/mL (30 mL) [contains alcohol 30%]

Tablet: 1 mg, 2.5 mg, 5 mg, 10 mg, 20 mg, 50 mg
Sterapred®: 5 mg [supplied as 21 tablet 6-day unit-dose package or 48 tablet 12-day unit-dose package]
Sterapred® DS: 10 mg [supplied as 21 tablet 6-day unit-dose package or 48 tablet 12-day unit-dose package]

Nursing Guidelines

Assessment: Assess effectiveness and interactions of other medications patient may be taking. Monitor for effectiveness of therapy and adverse reactions according to dose and length of therapy. Assess knowledge/teach patient appropriate use, possible side effects/interventions, and adverse symptoms to report (ie, opportunistic infection, adrenal suppression). Instruct patients with diabetes to monitor serum glucose levels closely; corticosteroids can alter glucose tolerance. Dose may need to be increased if patient is experiencing

(Continued)

PredniSONE *(Continued)*

higher than normal levels of stress. When discontinuing, taper dose and frequency slowly.

Monitoring Laboratory Tests: Blood glucose, electrolytes

Dietary Considerations: Should be taken after meals or with food or milk; increase dietary intake of pyridoxine, vitamin C, vitamin D, folate, calcium, and phosphorus.

Patient Education: Take exactly as directed. Do not take more than prescribed dose and do not discontinue abruptly; consult prescriber. Take with or after meals. Take once-a-day dose with food in the morning. Avoid alcohol. Limit intake of caffeine or stimulants. Maintain adequate nutrition; consult prescriber for possibility of special dietary recommendations. If you have diabetes, monitor serum glucose closely and notify prescriber of changes; this medication can alter hypoglycemic requirements. Notify prescriber if you are experiencing higher than normal levels of stress; medication may need adjustment. Periodic ophthalmic examinations will be necessary with long-term use. You will be susceptible to infection (avoid crowds and exposure to infection). You may experience insomnia or nervousness; use caution when driving or engaging in tasks requiring alertness until response to drug is known. Report weakness, change in menstrual pattern, vision changes, signs of hyperglycemia, signs of infection (eg, fever, chills, mouth sores, perianal itching, vaginal discharge), other persistent side effects, or worsening of condition.

Geriatric Considerations: Because of the risk of adverse effects, systemic corticosteroids should be used cautiously in the elderly, in the smallest possible dose, and for the shortest possible time.

Pregnancy Risk Factor: B

Pregnancy Issues: Crosses the placenta. Immunosuppression reported in 1 infant exposed to high-dose prednisone plus azathioprine throughout gestation. One report of congenital cataracts. Available evidence suggests safe use during pregnancy.

Lactation: Enters breast milk/compatible

Breast-Feeding Considerations: Crosses into breast milk. No data on clinical effects on the infant. AAP considers **compatible** with breast-feeding.

Perioperative/Anesthesia/Other Concerns:

Neuromuscular Effects: ICU-acquired paresis was recently studied in 5 ICUs (3 medical and 2 surgical ICUs) at 4 French hospitals. All ICU patients without pre-existing neuromuscular disease admitted from March 1999 through June 2000 were evaluated (De Jonghe B, 2002). Each patient had to be mechanically ventilated for ≥7 days and was screened daily for awakening. The first day the patient was considered awake was Study Day 1. Patients with severe muscle weakness on Study Day 7 were considered to have ICU-acquired paresis. Among the 95 patients who were evaluable, about 25% developed ICU-acquired paresis. Independent predictors included: female gender, the number of days with ≥2 organ dysfunction, and administration of corticosteroids. Further studies may be required to verify and characterize the association between the development of ICU-acquired paresis and use of corticosteroids. Concurrent use of a corticosteroid and muscle relaxant appear to increase the risk of certain ICU myopathies; avoid or administer the corticosteroid at the lowest dose possible.

Adrenal Insufficiency: Patients will often have steroid-induced adverse effects on glucose tolerance and lipid profiles. When discontinuing steroid therapy in patients on long-term steroid supplementation, it is important that the steroid therapy be discontinued gradually. Abrupt withdrawal may result in adrenal insufficiency with hypotension and hyperkalemia. Patients on long-term steroid supplementation will require higher corticosteroid doses when subject to stress (ie, trauma, surgery, severe infection). Guidelines for glucocorticoid replacement during various surgical procedures has been published (Salem M, 1994, Coursin DB, 2002).

Septic Shock: A recent randomized, double-blind, placebo controlled trial assessed whether low dose corticosteroid administration could improve 28-day survival in patients with septic shock and relative adrenal insufficiency. Relative adrenal insufficiency was defined as an inappropriate response to corticotropin administration (increase of serum cortisol of ≤9 mcg/dL from baseline). Cortisol levels were drawn immediately before corticotropin administration and 30 to 60 minutes afterwards. Three hundred adult septic shock patients requiring mechanical ventilation and vasopressor support were randomized to either hydrocortisone (50 mg IVP every 6 hours) and fludrocortisone (50 mcg tablet daily via nasogastric tube) or matching placebos for 7 days. In patients who did not appropriately respond to corticotropin (nonresponders), there were significantly fewer deaths in the active treatment group. Vasopressor therapy was withdrawn more frequently in this subset of the active treatment group. Adverse events were similar in both groups. Patients who lack adrenal reserve and thus have relative adrenal insufficiency during the stress of septic shock may benefit from physiologic steroid replacement. However, there was a trend for increased mortality in patients who responded to the corticotropin test (increase serum cortisol >9 mcg/dL from baseline). These patients may not benefit from physiologic steroid replacement. Further study is required to better characterize the patient populations who may benefit.

Administration

Oral: Take with food to decrease GI upset.

Related Information

Contrast Media Reactions, Premedication for Prophylaxis *on page 1911*

- Prednisone Intensol™ *see* PredniSONE *on page 1403*
- Pregnyl® *see* Chorionic Gonadotropin (Human) *on page 387*
- Prelone® *see* PrednisoLONE *on page 1399*
- Premarin® *see* Estrogens (Conjugated/Equine) *on page 661*
- Premjact® [OTC] *see* Lidocaine *on page 1033*
- Premphase® *see* Estrogens (Conjugated/Equine) and Medroxyprogesterone *on page 665*
- Prempro™ *see* Estrogens (Conjugated/Equine) and Medroxyprogesterone *on page 665*
- Prenatal 1-A-Day *see* Vitamins (Multiple/Prenatal) *on page 1721*
- Prenatal AD *see* Vitamins (Multiple/Prenatal) *on page 1721*
- Prenatal H *see* Vitamins (Multiple/Prenatal) *on page 1721*
- Prenatal MR 90 Fe™ *see* Vitamins (Multiple/Prenatal) *on page 1721*
- Prenatal MTR with Selenium *see* Vitamins (Multiple/Prenatal) *on page 1721*
- Prenatal Plus *see* Vitamins (Multiple/Prenatal) *on page 1721*
- Prenatal Rx 1 *see* Vitamins (Multiple/Prenatal) *on page 1721*
- Prenatal U *see* Vitamins (Multiple/Prenatal) *on page 1721*
- Prenatal Vitamins *see* Vitamins (Multiple/Prenatal) *on page 1721*
- Prenatal Z *see* Vitamins (Multiple/Prenatal) *on page 1721*
- Prenate Elite™ *see* Vitamins (Multiple/Prenatal) *on page 1721*
- Prenate GT™ *see* Vitamins (Multiple/Prenatal) *on page 1721*
- Preparation H® Hydrocortisone [OTC] *see* Hydrocortisone *on page 873*
- PreserVision® AREDS [OTC] *see* Vitamins (Multiple/Oral) *on page 1720*
- PreserVision® Lutein [OTC] *see* Vitamins (Multiple/Oral) *on page 1720*
- Pretz® [OTC] *see* Sodium Chloride *on page 1545*
- Pretz-D® [OTC] *see* Ephedrine *on page 609*
- Prevacid® *see* Lansoprazole *on page 1006*
- Prevacid® SoluTab™ *see* Lansoprazole *on page 1006*
- Previfem™ *see* Ethinyl Estradiol and Norgestimate *on page 689*
- Prevnar® *see* Pneumococcal Conjugate Vaccine (7-Valent) *on page 1376*
- Prilocaine and Lidocaine *see* Lidocaine and Prilocaine *on page 1042*
- Prilosec® *see* Omeprazole *on page 1264*
- Prilosec OTC™ [OTC] *see* Omeprazole *on page 1264*
- Primacor® *see* Milrinone *on page 1163*
- Primatene® Mist [OTC] *see* Epinephrine *on page 611*
- Primaxin® *see* Imipenem and Cilastatin *on page 894*
- Principen® *see* Ampicillin *on page 160*
- Prinivil® *see* Lisinopril *on page 1047*
- Prinzide® *see* Lisinopril and Hydrochlorothiazide *on page 1051*
- Pristinamycin *see* Quinupristin and Dalfopristin *on page 1455*

Procainamide (proe kane A mide)

U.S. Brand Names Procanbid®

Synonyms PCA (error-prone abbreviation); Procainamide Hydrochloride; Procaine Amide Hydrochloride

(Continued)

Procainamide *(Continued)*

Pharmacologic Category Antiarrhythmic Agent, Class Ia

Medication Safety Issues

Sound-alike/look-alike issues:

Procanbid® may be confused with probenecid

Pronestyl® may be confused with Ponstel®

PCA is an error-prone abbreviation (mistaken as patient controlled analgesia)

Use Treatment of ventricular tachycardia (VT), premature ventricular contractions, paroxysmal atrial tachycardia (PSVT), and atrial fibrillation (AF); prevent recurrence of ventricular tachycardia, paroxysmal supraventricular tachycardia, atrial fibrillation or flutter

Unlabeled/Investigational Use ACLS guidelines:

Intermittent/recurrent VF or pulseless VT not responsive to earlier interventions

Monomorphic VT (EF >40%, no CHF)

Polymorphic VT with normal baseline QT interval

Wide complex tachycardia of unknown type (EF >40%, no CHF, patient stable)

Refractory paroxysmal SVT

Atrial fibrillation or flutter (EF >40%, no CHF) including pre-excitation syndrome

Mechanism of Action Decreases myocardial excitability and conduction velocity and may depress myocardial contractility, by increasing the electrical stimulation threshold of ventricle, His-Purkinje system and through direct cardiac effects

Pharmacodynamics/Kinetics

Onset of action: I.M. 10-30 minutes

Distribution: V_d: Children: 2.2 L/kg; Adults: 2 L/kg; Congestive heart failure or shock: Decreased V_d

Protein binding: 15% to 20%

Metabolism: Hepatic via acetylation to produce N-acetyl procainamide (NAPA) (active metabolite)

Bioavailability: Oral: 75% to 95%

Half-life elimination:

Procainamide (hepatic acetylator, phenotype, cardiac and renal function dependent):

Children: 1.7 hours; Adults: 2.5-4.7 hours; Anephric: 11 hours

NAPA (dependent upon renal function):

Children: 6 hours; Adults: 6-8 hours; Anephric: 42 hours

Time to peak, serum: Capsule: 45 minutes to 2.5 hours; I.M.: 15-60 minutes

Excretion: Urine (25% as NAPA)

Contraindications Hypersensitivity to procaine, other ester-type local anesthetics, or any component of the formulation; complete heart block (except in patients with a functioning artificial pacemaker); second-degree AV block (without a functional pacemaker); various types of hemiblock (without a functional pacemaker); SLE; torsade de pointes; concurrent cisapride use; QT prolongation

Warnings/Precautions Monitor and adjust dose to prevent QT_c prolongation. Watch for proarrhythmic effects. May precipitate or exacerbate CHF. Reduce dosage in renal impairment. May increase ventricular response rate in patients with atrial fibrillation or flutter; control AV conduction before initiating. Correct hypokalemia before initiating therapy. Hypokalemia may worsen toxicity. Use caution in digoxin-induced toxicity (can further depress AV conduction). Reduce dose if first-degree heart block occurs. Use caution with concurrent use of other antiarrhythmics. Avoid use in myasthenia gravis (may worsen condition). Hypersensitivity reactions can occur. Some tablets contain tartrazine; injection may contain bisulfite (allergens).

Potentially fatal blood dyscrasias have occurred with therapeutic doses; close monitoring is recommended during the first 3 months of therapy.

Long-term administration leads to the development of a positive antinuclear antibody (ANA) test in 50% of patients which may result in a drug-induced lupus erythematosus-like syndrome (in 20% to 30% of patients); discontinue procainamide with SLE symptoms and choose an alternative agent

Drug Interactions **Substrate** of CYP2D6 (major)

Amiodarone increases procainamide and NAPA blood levels; consider reducing procainamide dosage by 25% with concurrent use.

Cimetidine increases procainamide and NAPA blood concentrations; monitor blood levels closely or use an alternative H_2 antagonist.

Cisapride and procainamide may increase the risk of malignant arrhythmia; concurrent use is contraindicated.

CYP2D6 inhibitors: May increase the levels/effects of procainamide. Example inhibitors include chlorpromazine, delavirdine, fluoxetine, miconazole, paroxetine, pergolide, quinidine, quinine, ritonavir, and ropinirole.

Neuromuscular blocking agents: Procainamide may potentiate neuromuscular blockade.

Ofloxacin may increase procainamide levels due to an inhibition of renal secretion; monitor levels for procainamide closely.

QT_c-prolonging agents (eg, amiodarone, amitriptyline, bepridil, disopyramide, erythromycin, haloperidol, imipramine, pimozide, quinidine, sotalol, and thioridazine): Effects/toxicity may be increased; use with caution.

Sparfloxacin, gatifloxacin, and moxifloxacin may result in additional prolongation of the QT interval; concurrent use is contraindicated.

Trimethoprim increases procainamide and NAPA blood levels; closely monitor levels.

Nutritional/Herbal/Ethanol Interactions

Ethanol: Avoid ethanol (acute ethanol administration reduces procainamide serum concentrations).

Herb/Nutraceutical: Avoid ephedra (may worsen arrhythmia).

Adverse Reactions

>1%:

Cardiovascular: Hypotension (I.V., up to 5%)

Dermatologic: Rash

Gastrointestinal: Diarrhea (3% to 4%), nausea, vomiting, taste disorder, GI complaints (3% to 4%)

<1% (Limited to important or life-threatening): Agranulocytosis, angioneurotic edema, aplastic anemia, arrhythmia (proarrhythmic effect, new or worsened), bone marrow suppression, cerebellar ataxia, cholestasis, demyelinating polyradiculoneuropathy, depressed myocardial contractility, depression, disorientation, drug fever, granulomatous hepatitis, hallucinations, hemolytic anemia, hepatic failure, hypoplastic anemia, leukopenia, mania, myasthenia gravis (worsened), myocarditis, myopathy, neuromuscular blockade, neutropenia, pancreatitis, pancytopenia, paradoxical increase in ventricular rate in atrial fibrillation/flutter, pericarditis, peripheral neuropathy, pleural effusion, positive ANA, positive Coombs' test, pruritus, pseudo-obstruction, psychosis, pulmonary embolism, QT prolongation (excessive), rash, respiratory failure due to myopathy, second-degree heart block, SLE-like syndrome, thrombocytopenia (0.5%), torsade de pointes, tremor, urticaria, vasculitis, ventricular arrhythmia

Overdosage/Toxicology Procainamide has a low toxic:therapeutic ratio and may easily produce fatal intoxication (acute toxic dose: 5 g in adults). Symptoms of overdose include sinus bradycardia, sinus node arrest or asystole, P-R, QRS, or QT interval prolongation, torsade de pointes (polymorphous ventricular tachycardia), and depressed myocardial contractility, which along with alpha-adrenergic or ganglionic blockade, may result in hypotension and pulmonary edema. Other effects are seizures, coma, and respiratory arrest. Treatment is symptomatic and effects usually respond to conventional therapies. **Note:** Do not use other Type 1A or 1C antiarrhythmic agents to treat ventricular tachycardia. Sodium bicarbonate may treat wide QRS intervals or hypotension. Markedly impaired conduction or high degree AV block, unresponsive to bicarbonate, indicates consideration of a pacemaker.

Dosing

Adults & Elderly: Dose must be titrated to patient's response.

Antiarrhythmic:

Oral: 250-500 mg/dose every 3-6 hours or 500 mg to 1 g every 6 hours extended release; usual dose: 50 mg/kg/24 hours; maximum: 4 g/24 hours

I.M.: 0.5-1 g every 4-8 hours until oral therapy is possible

I.V. (infusion requires use of an infusion pump):

Loading dose: 15-18 mg/kg administered as slow infusion over 25-30 minutes or 100-200 mg/dose repeated every 5 minutes as needed to a total dose of 1 g

Maintenance dose: 1-4 mg/minute by continuous infusion.

Infusion rate: **2 g/250 mL** (I.V. infusion requires use of an infusion pump):

1 mg/minute: 7.5 mL/hour

2 mg/minute: 15 mL/hour

3 mg/minute: 22.5 mL/hour

4 mg/minute: 30 mL/hour

5 mg/minute: 37.5 mL/hour

6 mg/minute: 45 mL/hour

(Continued)

Procainamide *(Continued)*

Intermittent/recurrent VF or pulseless VT:

Initial: 20-30 mg/minute (maximum: 50 mg/minute if necessary), up to a total of 17 mg/kg.

ACLS guidelines: I.V.: Infuse 20 mg/minute until arrhythmia is controlled, hypotension occurs, QRS complex widens by 50% of its original width, or total of 17 mg/kg is given.

Note: Reduce to 12 mg/kg in setting of cardiac or renal dysfunction

I.V. maintenance infusion: 1-4 mg/minute; monitor levels and do not exceed 3 mg/minute for >24 hours in adults with renal failure.

Pediatrics: Must be titrated to patient's response:

Arrhythmias:

Oral: 15-50 mg/kg/24 hours divided every 3-6 hours

I.M.: 50 mg/kg/24 hours divided into doses of $^1/_8$ to $^1/_4$ every 3-6 hours in divided doses until oral therapy is possible

I.V. (infusion requires use of an infusion pump):

Load: 3-6 mg/kg/dose over 5 minutes not to exceed 100 mg/dose; may repeat every 5-10 minutes to maximum of 15 mg/kg/load

Maintenance as continuous I.V. infusion: 20-80 mcg/kg/minute; maximum: 2 g/24 hours

Renal Impairment:

Cl_{cr} 10-50 mL/minute: Administer every 6-12 hours.

Cl_{cr} <10 mL/minute: Administer every 8-24 hours.

Dialysis:

Procainamide: Moderately hemodialyzable (20% to 50%): 200 mg supplemental dose posthemodialysis is recommended.

N-acetylprocainamide: Not dialyzable (0% to 5%)

Procainamide/N-acetylprocainamide: Peritoneal dialysis: Not dialyzable (0% to 5%)

Procainamide/N-acetylprocainamide: Replace by blood level during continuous arteriovenous or venovenous hemofiltration.

Hepatic Impairment: Reduce dose by 50%.

Available Dosage Forms

Capsule, as hydrochloride: 250 mg, 500 mg

Injection, solution, as hydrochloride: 100 mg/mL (10 mL); 500 mg/mL (2 mL) [contains sodium metabisulfite]

Tablet, extended release, as hydrochloride: 500 mg, 750 mg, 1000 mg

Procanbid®: 500 mg, 1000 mg

Nursing Guidelines

Assessment: Assess other medications patient may be taking for effectiveness and interactions. I.V. requires use of infusion pump and continuous cardiac and hemodynamic monitoring. Assess results of laboratory tests, therapeutic effectiveness, and adverse reactions at beginning of therapy, when titrating dosage, and on a regular basis with long-term therapy. **Note:** Procainamide has a low TI and overdose may easily produce severe and life-threatening reactions. Assess knowledge/teach patient appropriate use, interventions to reduce side effects, and adverse symptoms to report.

Monitoring Laboratory Tests: CBC with differential, platelet count

Dietary Considerations: Should be taken with water on an empty stomach.

Patient Education: Oral: Take exactly as directed; do not take additional doses or discontinue without consulting prescriber. Avoid alcohol. You will need regular cardiac checkups and blood tests while taking this medication. You may experience dizziness, lightheadedness, or visual changes (use caution when driving or engaging in tasks requiring alertness until response to drug is known); loss of appetite (small frequent meals, frequent mouth care, chewing gum, or sucking lozenges may help); headaches (prescriber may recommend mild analgesic); or diarrhea (yogurt or boiled milk may help; if persistent consult prescriber). Report chest pain, palpitation, or erratic heartbeat; increased weight or swelling of hands or feet; acute diarrhea; or unusual fatigue and tiredness. **Pregnancy/breast-feeding precautions:** Inform prescriber if you are or intend to become pregnant. Consult prescriber if breast-feeding.

Geriatric Considerations: Monitor closely since clearance is reduced in those >60 years of age. If clinically possible, start doses at lowest recommended dose. Also, elderly frequently have drug therapy which may interfere with the use of procainamide. Adjust dose for renal function in the elderly.

Pregnancy Risk Factor: C

Lactation: Enters breast milk/use caution (AAP rates "compatible")

Breast-Feeding Considerations: Considered compatible by the AAP. However, the AAP stated concern regarding long-term effects and potential for infant toxicity. Use caution and monitor closely if continuing to breast-feed while taking procainamide.

Perioperative/Anesthesia/Other Concerns: In patients with pre-existing cardiovascular disease, the incidence of proarrhythmia and mortality may be increased with Class Ia antiarrhythmic agents.

Procainamide may be used to pharmacologically convert atrial fibrillation to normal sinus rhythm. In this setting, it is important that AV nodal conduction be controlled (eg, digoxin, beta-blocker, calcium channel blocker) prior to cardioversion to inhibit procainamide-induced increases in ventricular response. Patients should be monitored (ECG and BP) in a controlled setting when initiating therapy.

Administration

Oral: Do **not** crush or chew extended release drug products.

I.V.: Must dilute prior to I.V. administration; maximum rate: 50 mg/minute; give around-the-clock to promote less variation in peak and trough serum levels.

Reconstitution: Minimum volume: 1 g/250 mL NS/D_5W

Stability of admixture at room temperature in D_5W or NS is 24 hours. Some information indicates that procainamide may be subject to greater decomposition in D_5W unless the admixture is refrigerated or the pH is adjusted. Procainamide is believed to form an association complex with dextrose - the bioavailability of procainamide in this complex is not known and the complex formation is reversible.

Compatibility: Stable in ½NS, NS, SWFI

Y-site administration: Incompatible with milrinone

Compatibility when admixed: Incompatible with esmolol, ethacrynate, milrinone, phenytoin

Storage: Procainamide may be stored at room temperature up to 27°C; however, refrigeration retards oxidation, which causes color formation. The solution is initially colorless but may turn slightly yellow on standing. Injection of air into the vial causes the solution to darken. Solutions darker than a light amber should be discarded.

Related Information

Management of Postoperative Arrhythmias *on page 1787*

♦ **Procainamide Hydrochloride** *see* Procainamide *on page 1407*

Procaine (PROE kane)

U.S. Brand Names Novocain®

Synonyms Procaine Hydrochloride

Pharmacologic Category Local Anesthetic

Use Produces spinal anesthesia and epidural and peripheral nerve block by injection and infiltration methods

Mechanism of Action Blocks both the initiation and conduction of nerve impulses by decreasing the neuronal membrane's permeability to sodium ions, which results in inhibition of depolarization with resultant blockade of conduction

Pharmacodynamics/Kinetics

Onset of action: 2-5 minutes

Duration (patient, type of block, concentration, and method of anesthesia dependent); 0.5-1.5 hours

Metabolism: Rapidly hydrolyzed by plasma enzymes to para-aminobenzoic acid and diethylaminoethanol (80% conjugated before elimination)

Half-life elimination: 7.7 minutes

Excretion: Urine (as metabolites and some unchanged drug)

Contraindications Hypersensitivity to procaine, PABA, parabens, other ester local anesthetics, or any component of the formulation

Warnings/Precautions Patients with cardiac diseases, hyperthyroidism, or other endocrine diseases may be more susceptible to toxic effects of local anesthetics; some preparations contain metabisulfite

Drug Interactions

Decreased effect of sulfonamides with the PABA metabolite of procaine, chloroprocaine, and tetracaine

Decreased/increased effect of vasopressors, ergot alkaloids, and MAO inhibitors on blood pressure when using anesthetic solutions with a vasoconstrictor

(Continued)

Procaine *(Continued)*

Adverse Reactions

1% to 10%: Local: Burning sensation at site of injection, tissue irritation, pain at injection site

<1% (Limited to important or life-threatening): Aseptic meningitis resulting in paralysis, chills, CNS stimulation followed by CNS depression

Overdosage/Toxicology Treatment is symptomatic and supportive. Termination of anesthesia by pneumatic tourniquet inflation should be attempted when procaine is administered by infiltration or regional injection.

Dosing

Adults & Elderly: Spinal anesthesia, epidural and peripheral nerve block: Injection and infiltration methods: Dose varies with procedure, desired depth, and duration of anesthesia, desired muscle relaxation, vascularity of tissues, physical condition, and age of patient.

Pediatrics: Dose varies with procedure, desired depth, and duration of anesthesia, desired muscle relaxation, vascularity of tissues, physical condition, and age of patient.

Available Dosage Forms Injection, solution, as hydrochloride: 1% [10 mg/mL] (2 mL) [contains sodium bisulfite]; 10% (2 mL) [contains sodium bisulfite]

Nursing Guidelines

Assessment: Monitor response, degree of pain sensation, and injection site. **Epidural:** Monitor CNS status.

Patient Education: The purpose of this medication is to reduce pain sensation. Report local burning or pain at injection site. **Pregnancy/breast-feeding precautions:** Inform prescriber if you are or intend to become pregnant. Consult prescriber if breast-feeding.

Pregnancy Risk Factor: C

Lactation: Excretion in breast milk unknown

Administration

Compatibility: Stable in dextran 6% in dextrose, dextran 6% in NS, D_5LR, $D_5{}^1/_4NS$, $D_5{}^1/_2NS$, D_5NS, D_5W, $D_{10}W$, LR, ½NS, NS

Compatibility when admixed: Incompatible with amobarbital, amphotericin B, chlorothiazide, magnesium sulfate, phenobarbital, phenytoin, sodium bicarbonate

Related Information

Local Anesthetics *on page 1854*

- ♦ **Procaine Amide Hydrochloride** *see* Procainamide *on page 1407*
- ♦ **Procaine Hydrochloride** *see* Procaine *on page 1411*
- ♦ **Procanbid®** *see* Procainamide *on page 1407*
- ♦ **Procardia®** *see* NIFEdipine *on page 1227*
- ♦ **Procardia XL®** *see* NIFEdipine *on page 1227*
- ♦ **Procetofene** *see* Fenofibrate *on page 708*

Prochlorperazine (proe klor PER a zeen)

U.S. Brand Names Compro™

Synonyms Chlormeprazine; Compazine; Prochlorperazine Edisylate; Prochlorperazine Maleate

Pharmacologic Category Antiemetic; Antipsychotic Agent, Typical, Phenothiazine

Medication Safety Issues

Sound-alike/look-alike issues:

Prochlorperazine may be confused with chlorproMAZINE

Compazine® may be confused with Copaxone®, Coumadin®

CPZ (occasional abbreviation for Compazine®) is an error-prone abbreviation (mistaken as chlorpromazine)

Use Management of nausea and vomiting; psychotic disorders including schizophrenia; anxiety

Unlabeled/Investigational Use Behavioral syndromes in dementia

Mechanism of Action Prochlorperazine is a piperazine phenothiazine antipsychotic which blocks postsynaptic mesolimbic dopaminergic D_1 and D_2 receptors in the brain, including the chemoreceptor trigger zone; exhibits a strong alpha-adrenergic and anticholinergic blocking effect and depresses the release of hypothalamic and hypophyseal hormones; believed to depress the reticular activating system, thus affecting basal metabolism, body temperature, wakefulness, vasomotor tone and emesis

Pharmacodynamics/Kinetics

Onset of action: Oral: 30-40 minutes; I.M.: 10-20 minutes; Rectal: ~60 minutes
Peak antiemetic effect: I.V.: 30-60 minutes

Duration: Rectal: 12 hours; Oral: 3-4 hours; I.M., I.V.: Adults: 4-6 hours; I.M.: Children: 12 hours

Distribution: V_d: 1400-1548 L; crosses placenta; enters breast milk

Metabolism: Primarily hepatic; N-desmethyl prochlorperazine (major active metabolite)

Bioavailability: Oral: 12.5%

Half-life elimination: Oral: 3-5 hours; I.V.: ~7 hours

Contraindications Hypersensitivity to prochlorperazine or any component of the formulation (cross-reactivity between phenothiazines may occur); severe CNS depression; coma; pediatric surgery; Reye's syndrome; should not be used in children <2 years of age or <9 kg

Warnings/Precautions May be sedating; use with caution in disorders where CNS depression is a feature. May obscure intestinal obstruction or brain tumor. May impair physical or mental abilities; patients must be cautioned about performing tasks which require mental alertness (eg, operating machinery or driving). Effects with other sedative drugs or ethanol may be potentiated. Use with caution in Parkinson's disease; hemodynamic instability; bone marrow suppression; predisposition to seizures; subcortical brain damage; and in severe cardiac, hepatic, renal or respiratory disease. Caution in breast cancer or other prolactin-dependent tumors (may elevate prolactin levels). May alter temperature regulation or mask toxicity of other drugs. Use caution with exposure to heat. May alter cardiac conduction; life-threatening arrhythmias have occurred with therapeutic doses of phenothiazines. May cause orthostatic hypotension; use with caution in patients at risk of hypotension or where transient hypotensive episodes would be poorly tolerated (cardiovascular disease or cerebrovascular disease). Hypotension may occur following administration, particularly when parenteral form is used or in high dosages.

Phenothiazines may cause anticholinergic effects (eg, constipation, xerostomia, blurred vision, urinary retention); therefore, they should be used with caution in patients with decreased gastrointestinal motility, urinary retention, BPH, xerostomia, or visual problems. Conditions which also may be exacerbated by cholinergic blockade include narrow-angle glaucoma (screening is recommended) and worsening of myasthenia gravis. May cause extrapyramidal symptoms, including pseudoparkinsonism, acute dystonic reactions, akathisia, and tardive dyskinesia (TD). Use caution in the the elderly; incidence of TD may be increased. Children with acute illness or dehydration are more susceptible to neuromuscular reactions (eg, dystonias); use cautiously. May be associated with neuroleptic malignant syndrome (NMS).

Drug Interactions

Acetylcholinesterase inhibitors (central): May increase the risk of antipsychotic-related extrapyramidal symptoms; monitor.

Alpha-/Beta- agonists: May enhance the arrhythmogenic effect of phenothiazines.

Analgesics (narcotic): Phenothiazines may enhance the hypotensive effect of narcotic analgesics.

Antacids: May decrease the absorption of phenothiazines; monitor.

Antidepressants (serotonin reuptake inhibitors/antagonist): Concurrent use may produce increased hypotension.

Anticholinergics: May inhibit the therapeutic response to phenothiazines and excess anticholinergic effects may occur; includes benztropine, trihexyphenidyl, biperiden, and drugs with significant anticholinergic activity (TCAs, antihistamines, disopyramide)

Antihistamines: May enhance the arrhythmogenic effect of phenothiazines.

Antimalarial agents: May increase phenothiazine concentrations.

Antiparkinson's Agents (dopamine agonists such as levodopa): Phenothiazines may inhibit the antiparkinsonian effect of levodopa; avoid this combination.

Attapulgite: May decrease absorption of phenothiazines.

Beta blockers: Serum concentrations of phenothiazines may be increased; phenothiazines may increase hypotensive effects of beta blockers.

CNS depressants: Sedative effects may be additive with phenothiazines; monitor for increased effect; includes barbiturates, benzodiazepines, narcotic analgesics, ethanol and other sedative agents.

Epinephrine: Chlorpromazine (and possibly other low potency antipsychotics) may diminish the pressor effects of epinephrine.

(Continued)

Prochlorperazine *(Continued)*

False Neurotransmitters (guanadrel, methyldopa): Antihypertensive effects may be inhibited by phenothiazines.

Lithium: Phenothiazines may produce neurotoxicity with lithium; this is a rare effect Phenytoin: Concurrent use may increase CNS depression.

Polypeptide antibiotics: Rare cases of respiratory paralysis have been reported with concurrent use of phenothiazines.

Pramlintide: May enhance the anticholinergic effects of phenothiazines.

QT_c-prolonging agents: Effects on QT_c interval may be additive with phenothiazines, increasing the risk of malignant arrhythmias; includes type Ia antiarrhythmics, TCAs, and some quinolone antibiotics (sparfloxacin, moxifloxacin, and gatifloxacin).

Nutritional/Herbal/Ethanol Interactions

Ethanol: Avoid ethanol (may increase CNS depression).

Food: Limit caffeine.

Herb/Nutraceutical: Avoid dong quai, St John's wort (may also cause photosensitization). Avoid kava kava, gotu kola, valerian, St John's wort (may increase CNS depression).

Lab Interactions False-positives for phenylketonuria, pregnancy, urinary amylase, uroporphyrins, urobilinogen

Adverse Reactions Reported with prochlorperazine or other phenothiazines. Frequency not defined

Cardiovascular: Cardiac arrest, hypotension, peripheral edema, Q-wave distortions, T-wave distortions

Central nervous system: Agitation, catatonia, cerebral edema, cough reflex suppressed, dizziness, drowsiness, fever (mild — I.M.), headache, hyperactivity, hyperpyrexia, impairment of temperature regulation. insomnia, neuroleptic malignant syndrome (NMS), paradoxical excitement, restlessness, seizure

Dermatologic: Angioedema, contact dermatitis, discoloration of skin (blue-gray), epithelial keratopathy, erythema, eczema, exfoliative dermatitis (injectable), itching, photosensitivity, rash, skin pigmentation, urticaria

Endocrine & metabolic: Amenorrhea, breast enlargement, galactorrhea, gynecomastia, glucosuria, hyperglycemia, hypoglycemia, lactation, libido (changes in), menstrual irregularity, SIADH

Gastrointestinal: Appetite increased, atonic colon, constipation, ileus, nausea, weight gain, xerostomia

Genitourinary: Ejaculating dysfunction, ejaculatory disturbances, impotence, incontinence, polyuria, priapism, urinary retention, urination difficulty

Hematologic: Agranulocytosis, aplastic anemia, eosinophilia, hemolytic anemia, leukopenia, pancytopenia, thrombocytopenic purpura

Hepatic: Biliary stasis, cholestatic jaundice, hepatotoxicity

Neuromuscular & skeletal: Dystonias (torticollis, opisthotonos, carpopedal spasm, trismus, oculogyric crisis, protusion of tongue); extrapyramidal symptoms (pseudoparkinsonism, akathisia, dystonias, tardive dyskinesia); SLE-like syndrome, tremor

Ocular: blurred vision, cornea and lens changes, lenticular/corneal deposits, miosis, mydriasis, pigmentary retinopathy

Respiratory: Asthma, laryngeal edema, nasal congestion

Miscellaneous: Allergic reactions, diaphoresis

Overdosage/Toxicology Symptoms of overdose include deep sleep, coma, extrapyramidal symptoms, abnormal involuntary muscle movements, seizures, and hypotension. Treatment is symptom-directed and supportive. Do not induce emesis because of risk of aspiration if acute dystonic reaction occurred. Extrapyramidal symptoms may be treated with an anticholinergic such as diphenydramine or benzetropine. Treat hypotension with norephinephrine or phenylephrine. Phenothiazines are not dialyzable.

Dosing

Adults:

Antiemetic:

Oral (tablet): 5-10 mg 3-4 times/day; usual maximum: 40 mg/day; larger doses may rarely be required

I.M. (deep): 5-10 mg every 3-4 hours; usual maximum: 40 mg/day

I.V.: 2.5-10 mg; maximum 10 mg/dose or 40 mg/day; may repeat dose every 3-4 hours as needed

Rectal: 25 mg twice daily

Surgical nausea/vomiting: **Note:** Should not exceed 40 mg/day

I.M.: 5-10 mg 1-2 hours before induction or to control symptoms during or after surgery; may repeat once if necessary

I.V. (administer slow IVP <5 mg/minute): 5-10 mg 15-30 minutes before induction or to control symptoms during or after surgery; may repeat once if necessary

Rectal (unlabeled use): 25 mg

Antipsychotic:

Oral: 5-10 mg 3-4 times/day; titrate dose slowly every 2-3 days; doses up to 150 mg/day may be required in some patients for treatment of severe disturbances

I.M.: Initial: 10-20 mg; if necessary repeat initial dose every 1-4 hours to gain control; more than 3-4 doses are rarely needed. If parenteral administration is still required; give 10-20 mg every 4-6 hours; change to oral as soon as possible.

Nonpsychotic anxiety: *Oral (tablet):* Usual dose: 15-20 mg/day in divided doses; do not give doses >20 mg/day or for longer than 12 weeks

Elderly: Dementia behavior (nonpsychotic, unlabeled use): Initial: 2.5-5 mg 1-2 times/day; increase dose at 4- to 7-day intervals by 2.5-5 mg/day. Increase dosing intervals (twice daily, 3 times/day, etc) as necessary to control response or side effects. Maximum daily dose should probably not exceed 75 mg in the elderly. Gradual increases (titration) may prevent some side effects or decrease their severity. See Geriatric Considerations.

Pediatrics: Not recommended in children <10 kg or <2 years.

Antiemetic:

Oral, rectal: >9 kg: 0.4 mg/kg/24 hours in 3-4 divided doses; **or**

9-13 kg: 2.5 mg every 12-24 hours as needed; maximum: 7.5 mg/day

13.1-17 kg: 2.5 mg every 8-12 hours as needed; maximum: 10 mg/day

17.1-37 kg: 2.5 mg every 8 hours or 5 mg every 12 hours as needed; maximum: 15 mg/day

I.M.: 0.13 mg/kg/dose; change to oral as soon as possible

Antipsychotic: Children 2-12 years (not recommended in children <9 kg or <2 years):

Oral, rectal: 2.5 mg 2-3 times/day; do not give more than 10 mg the first day; increase dosage as needed to maximum daily dose of 20 mg for 2-5 years and 25 mg for 6-12 years

I.M.: 0.13 mg/kg/dose; change to oral as soon as possible

Available Dosage Forms

Injection, solution, as edisylate: 5 mg/mL (2 mL, 10 mL) [contains benzyl alcohol]

Suppository, rectal: 2.5 mg (12s), 5 mg (12s), 25 mg (12s) [may contain coconut and palm oil]

Compro™: 25 mg (12s) [contains coconut and palm oils]

Tablet, as maleate: 5 mg, 10 mg

Nursing Guidelines

Assessment: Assess all other medications patient may be taking. For I.V., continuously monitor blood pressure and heart rate during administration. Monitor blood pressure and heart rate, fluid balance, and dehydration. Monitor for seizures, especially with known seizure disorder. Monitor for excessive sedation, neuromuscular malignant syndrome, autonomic instability (eg, anticholinergic effects), and extrapyramidal symptoms.

Monitoring Laboratory Tests: Baseline liver and kidney function, CBC prior to and periodically during therapy, lipid profile, fasting blood glucose/Hgb A_{1c}; BMI

Dietary Considerations: Increase dietary intake of riboflavin; should be administered with food or water. Rectal suppositories may contain coconut and palm oil.

Patient Education: Take exact amount as prescribed. Do not change brand names. Do not crush or chew tablets. Do not discontinue without consulting prescriber. Avoid alcohol or other sedatives or sleep-inducing drugs. Avoid skin contact with drug; wash immediately with warm soapy water. You may experience appetite changes; small frequent meals may help. Maintain adequate hydration (2-3 L/day of fluids) unless instructed to restrict fluid intake. May cause dizziness, tremors, or visual disturbance (especially during early therapy); use caution when driving or engaging in tasks that require alertness until response to drug is known. Do not change position rapidly (rise slowly). May cause photosensitivity reaction; use sunscreen, wear protective clothing and eyewear, and avoid direct sunlight. Report immediately any changes in gait or muscular tremors. Report unresolved changes in voiding or elimination (constipation or diarrhea), acute dizziness or unresolved sedation, vision changes, palpitations, yellowing of skin or eyes, or changes in color of urine or

(Continued)

Prochlorperazine *(Continued)*

stool (pink or red brown urine is expected). **Pregnancy/breast-feeding precautions:** Inform prescriber if you are or intend to become pregnant. Breast-feeding is not recommended.

Geriatric Considerations: Due to side effect profile (dystonias, EPS) this is not a preferred drug in the elderly for antiemetic therapy.

Pregnancy Issues: Crosses the placenta. Isolated reports of congenital anomalies, however, some included exposures to other drugs. Jaundice, extrapyramidal signs, hyper-/hyporeflexes have been noted in newborns. Available evidence with use of occasional low doses suggests safe use during pregnancy.

Lactation: Excretion in breast milk unknown/use caution

Breast-Feeding Considerations: Other phenothiazines are excreted in human milk; excretion of prochlorperazine is not known.

Perioperative/Anesthesia/Other Concerns: Prochlorperazine is not recommended as an antipsychotic due to inferior efficacy compared to other phenothiazines. Prochlorperazine has a faster onset of action and causes less sedation than promethazine. When compared with ondansetron (4 mg I.V.), prochlorperazine (10 mg I.M.) administered at the end of surgery more effectively reduced postoperative nausea and the need for rescue antiemetics in patients undergoing total hip or knee replacement. In patients undergoing tympanoplasty, prophylactic prochlorperazine (0.02 mg/kg I.M.) administered at the end of surgery was as effective as ondansetron (0.06 mg/kg I.V.) for reducing PONY.

Administration

I.M.:

Inject by deep IM into outer quadrant of buttocks.

I.V.: I.V.: Doses should be given as a short (~30 minute) infusion to avoid orthostatic hypotension; administer at ≤5 mg/minute

Compatibility: Stable in dextran 6% in dextrose, dextran 6% in NS, D_5W, $D_{10}W$, D_5LR, $D_5{}^1/_4NS$, $D_5{}^1/_2NS$, D_5NS, LR, $^1/_2NS$, NS

Y-site administration: Incompatible with aldesleukin, allopurinol, amifostine, amphotericin B cholesteryl sulfate complex, aztreonam, cefepime, etoposide phosphate, fludarabine, foscarnet, filgrastim, gemcitabine, piperacillin/tazobactam

Compatibility in syringe: Incompatible with dimenhydrinate, ketorolac, midazolam, morphine tartrate, pentobarbital, thiopental

Compatibility when admixed: Incompatible with aminophylline, amphotericin B, ampicillin, calcium salts, cephalothin, foscarnet, chloramphenicol, chlorothiazide, floxacillin, furosemide, heparin, hydrocortisone sodium succinate, methohexital, midazolam, penicillin G sodium, phenobarbital, phenytoin, thiopental

Storage:

Injection: Store at <30°C (<86°F). Do not freeze. Protect from light. Clear or slightly yellow solutions may be used.

I.V. infusion: Injection may be diluted in 50-100 mL NS or D_5W.

Suppository, tablet: Store at 15°C to 30°C (59°F to 86°F). Protect from light.

Related Information

Postoperative Nausea and Vomiting *on page 1807*

- **Prochlorperazine Edisylate** *see* Prochlorperazine *on page 1412*
- **Prochlorperazine Maleate** *see* Prochlorperazine *on page 1412*
- **Procrit®** *see* Epoetin Alfa *on page 618*
- **Proctocort®** *see* Hydrocortisone *on page 873*
- **ProctoCream® HC** *see* Hydrocortisone *on page 873*
- **Proctofene** *see* Fenofibrate *on page 708*
- **Procto-Kit™** *see* Hydrocortisone *on page 873*
- **Procto-Pak™** *see* Hydrocortisone *on page 873*
- **Proctosert** *see* Hydrocortisone *on page 873*
- **Proctosol-HC®** *see* Hydrocortisone *on page 873*
- **Proctozone-HC™** *see* Hydrocortisone *on page 873*
- **Prograf®** *see* Tacrolimus *on page 1593*
- **ProHance®** *see* Gadoteridol *on page 793*

Promethazine (proe METH a zeen)

U.S. Brand Names Phenadoz™; Phenergan®; Promethegan™

Synonyms Promethazine Hydrochloride

Pharmacologic Category Antiemetic; Antihistamine; Phenothiazine Derivative; Sedative

Medication Safety Issues

Sound-alike/look-alike issues:

Promethazine may be confused with chlorproMAZINE, predniSONE, promazine

Phenergan® may be confused with Phenaphen®, Phrenilin®, Theragran®

Use Symptomatic treatment of various allergic conditions; antiemetic; motion sickness; sedative; postoperative pain (adjunctive therapy); anesthetic (adjunctive therapy); anaphylactic reactions (adjunctive therapy)

Mechanism of Action Blocks postsynaptic mesolimbic dopaminergic receptors in the brain; exhibits a strong alpha-adrenergic blocking effect and depresses the release of hypothalamic and hypophyseal hormones; competes with histamine for the H_1-receptor; reduces stimuli to the brainstem reticular system

Pharmacodynamics/Kinetics

Onset of action: I.M.: ~20 minutes; I.V.: 3-5 minutes

Peak effect: C_{max}: 9.04 ng/mL (suppository); 19.3 ng/mL (syrup)

Duration: 2-6 hours

Absorption:

I.M.: Bioavailability may be greater than with oral or rectal administration

Oral: Rapid and complete; large first pass effect limits systemic bioavailability

Distribution: V_d: 171 L

Protein binding: 93%

Metabolism: Hepatic; primarily oxidation; forms metabolites

Half-life elimination: 9-16 hours

Time to maximum serum concentration: 4.4 hours (syrup); 6.7-8.6 hours (suppositories)

Excretion: Primarily urine and feces (as inactive metabolites)

Contraindications Hypersensitivity to promethazine or any component of the formulation (cross-reactivity between phenothiazines may occur); coma; treatment of lower respiratory tract symptoms, including asthma; children <2 years of age

Warnings/Precautions Not for SubQ or intra-arterial administration. Injection may contain sodium metabisulfite (may cause allergic reaction). May be sedating; use with caution in disorders where CNS depression is a feature. May impair physical or mental abilities; patients must be cautioned about performing tasks which require mental alertness (eg, operating machinery or driving). Use with caution in Parkinson's disease; hemodynamic instability; bone marrow suppression; subcortical brain damage; and in severe cardiac, hepatic, renal, or respiratory disease. Avoid use in Reye's syndrome. Respiratory fatalities have been reported in children <2 years of age. In children ≥2 years, use the lowest possible dose; other drugs with respiratory depressant effects should be avoided. May lower seizure threshold; use caution in persons with seizure disorders or in persons using narcotics or local anesthetics which may also affect seizure threshold. May alter temperature regulation or mask toxicity of other drugs due to antiemetic effects. May alter cardiac conduction (life-threatening arrhythmias have occurred with therapeutic doses of phenothiazines). May cause orthostatic hypotension; use with caution in patients at risk of hypotension or where transient hypotensive episodes would be poorly tolerated (cardiovascular disease or cerebrovascular disease).

Phenothiazines may cause anticholinergic effects (constipation, xerostomia, blurred vision, urinary retention); therefore, they should be used with caution in patients with decreased gastrointestinal motility, urinary retention, BPH, xerostomia, or visual problems. Conditions which also may be exacerbated by cholinergic blockade include narrow-angle glaucoma (screening is recommended) and worsening of myasthenia gravis. May cause extrapyramidal symptoms, including pseudoparkinsonism, acute dystonic reactions, akathisia, and tardive dyskinesia. May be associated with neuroleptic malignant syndrome (NMS).

Drug Interactions Substrate (major) of CYP2B6, 2D6; **Inhibits** CYP2D6 (weak)

Aluminum salts: May decrease the absorption of phenothiazines; monitor

Amphetamines: Efficacy may be diminished by antipsychotics; in addition, amphetamines may increase psychotic symptoms; avoid concurrent use

Anticholinergics: May inhibit the therapeutic response to phenothiazines and excess anticholinergic effects may occur; includes benztropine, trihexyphenidyl,

(Continued)

Promethazine *(Continued)*

biperiden, and drugs with significant anticholinergic activity (TCAs, antihistamines, disopyramide)

Antihypertensives: Concurrent use of phenothiazines with an antihypertensive may produce additive hypotensive effects (particularly orthostasis)

Bromocriptine: Phenothiazines inhibit the ability of bromocriptine to lower serum prolactin concentrations

CNS depressants: Sedative effects may be additive with phenothiazines; monitor for increased effect; includes barbiturates, benzodiazepines, narcotic analgesics, ethanol, and other sedative agents

CYP2B6 inducers: May decrease the levels/effects of promethazine. Example inducers include carbamazepine, nevirapine, phenobarbital, phenytoin, and rifampin.

CYP2B6 inhibitors: May increase the levels/effects of promethazine. Example inhibitors include desipramine, paroxetine, and sertraline.

CYP2D6 inhibitors: May increase the levels/effects of promethazine. Example inhibitors include chlorpromazine, delavirdine, fluoxetine, miconazole, paroxetine, pergolide, quinidine, quinine, ritonavir, and ropinirole.

Epinephrine: Promethazine may diminish the pressor effects of epinephrine.

Guanethidine and guanadrel: Antihypertensive effects may be inhibited by phenothiazines

Levodopa: Phenothiazines may inhibit the antiparkinsonian effect of levodopa; avoid this combination

Lithium: Phenothiazines may produce neurotoxicity with lithium; this is a rare effect

Propranolol: Serum concentrations of phenothiazines may be increased; propranolol also increases phenothiazine concentrations

Polypeptide antibiotics: Rare cases of respiratory paralysis have been reported with concurrent use of phenothiazines

QT_c-prolonging agents: Effects on QT_c interval may be additive with phenothiazines, increasing the risk of malignant arrhythmias; includes type Ia antiarrhythmics, TCAs, and some quinolone antibiotics (sparfloxacin, moxifloxacin, and gatifloxacin)

Sulfadoxine-pyrimethamine: May increase phenothiazine concentrations

Tricyclic antidepressants: Concurrent use may produce increased toxicity or altered therapeutic response

Trazodone: Phenothiazines and trazodone may produce additive hypotensive effects

Valproic acid: Serum levels may be increased by phenothiazines

Nutritional/Herbal/Ethanol Interactions

Ethanol: Avoid ethanol (may increase CNS depression).

Herb/Nutraceutical: Avoid valerian, St John's wort, kava kava, gotu kola (may increase CNS depression).

Lab Interactions Alters the flare response in intradermal allergen tests

Adverse Reactions

Cardiovascular: Bradycardia, hypertension, nonspecific QT changes, postural hypotension, tachycardia

Central nervous system: Akathisia, catatonic states, confusion, delirium, disorientation, dizziness, drowsiness, dystonias, euphoria, excitation, extrapyramidal symptoms, fatigue, hallucinations, hysteria, insomnia, lassitude, nervousness, neuroleptic malignant syndrome, nightmares, pseudoparkinsonism, sedation, seizure, somnolence, tardive dyskinesia

Dermatologic: Angioneurotic edema, dermatitis, photosensitivity, skin pigmentation (slate gray), urticaria

Endocrine & metabolic: Amenorrhea, breast engorgement, gynecomastia, hyper-/hypoglycemia, lactation

Gastrointestinal: Constipation, nausea, vomiting, xerostomia

Genitourinary: Ejaculatory disorder, impotence, urinary retention

Hematologic: Agranulocytosis, aplastic anemia, eosinophilia, hemolytic anemia, leukopenia, thrombocytopenia, thrombocytopenic purpura

Hepatic: Jaundice

Neuromuscular & skeletal: Incoordination, tremor

Ocular: Blurred vision, corneal and lenticular changes, diplopia, epithelial keratopathy, pigmentary retinopathy

Otic: Tinnitus

Respiratory: Apnea, asthma, nasal congestion, respiratory depression

Overdosage/Toxicology Symptoms of overdose include CNS depression, respiratory depression, possible CNS stimulation, dry mouth, fixed and dilated pupils, and hypotension. Treatment is symptom-directed and supportive. Epinephrine should not be used. Hemodialysis: Not dialyzable (0% to 5%)

Dosing

Adults & Elderly:

Allergic conditions (including allergic reactions to blood or plasma):

Oral, rectal: 25 mg at bedtime **or** 12.5 mg before meals and at bedtime (range: 6.25-12.5 mg 3 times/day)

I.M., I.V.: 25 mg, may repeat in 2 hours when necessary; switch to oral route as soon as feasible

Antiemetic: Oral, I.M., I.V., rectal: 12.5-25 mg every 4-6 hours as needed

Motion sickness: Oral, rectal: 25 mg 30-60 minutes before departure, then every 12 hours as needed

Sedation: Oral, I.M., I.V., rectal: 12.5-50 mg/dose

Pediatrics:

Allergic conditions: Children ≥2 years: Oral, rectal: 0.1 mg/kg/dose (maximum: 12.5 mg) every 6 hours during the day and 0.5 mg/kg/dose (maximum: 25 mg) at bedtime as needed

Antiemetic: Children ≥2 years: Oral, I.M., I.V., rectal: 0.25-1 mg/kg 4-6 times/day as needed (maximum: 25 mg/dose)

Motion sickness: Children ≥2 years: Oral, rectal: 0.5 mg/kg/dose 30 minutes to 1 hour before departure, then every 12 hours as needed (maximum dose: 25 mg twice daily)

Sedation: Children ≥2 years: Oral, I.M., I.V., rectal: 0.5-1 mg/kg/dose every 6 hours as needed (maximum: 50 mg/dose)

Available Dosage Forms [DSC] = Discontinued product

Injection, solution, as hydrochloride: 25 mg/mL (1 mL); 50 mg/mL (1 mL)

Phenergan®: 25 mg/mL (1 mL); 50 mg/mL (1 mL) [contains sodium metabisulfite]

Suppository, rectal, as hydrochloride: 12.5 mg, 25 mg, 50 mg

Phenadoz™: 12.5 mg, 25 mg

Phenergan®: 12.5 mg, 25 mg; 50 mg [DSC]

Promethegan™: 12.5 mg, 25 mg, 50 mg

Syrup, as hydrochloride: 6.25 mg/5 mL (120 mL, 480 mL) [contains alcohol]

Tablet, as hydrochloride: 12.5 mg, 25 mg, 50 mg

Phenergan®: 25 mg [DSC]

Nursing Guidelines

Assessment: See Contraindications, Warnings/Precautions, and Dosing for use cautions. Assess potential for interactions with other prescriptions, OTC medications, or herbal products patient may be taking (see extensive list of Drug Interactions). See Administration for I.V. and I.M. use. Assess for therapeutic effectiveness and adverse response (see Adverse Reactions and Overdose/Toxicology). Use and teach sedation safety measures (side rails up, call light within reach, etc). Teach patient appropriate use (oral), interventions to reduce side effects, and adverse symptoms to report (see Patient Education). Breast-feeding is not recommended.

Dietary Considerations: Increase dietary intake of riboflavin.

Patient Education: Inform prescriber of all prescriptions, OTC medications, or herbal products you are taking, and any allergies you have. Do not take any new medication during therapy unless approved by prescriber (especially anything that may cause CNS depression). Take this drug as prescribed; do not increase dosage. Avoid alcohol. May cause dizziness, drowsiness, or blurred vision (use caution when driving or engaging in tasks requiring alertness until response to drug is known); or nausea, dry mouth, appetite disturbances (small, frequent meals, frequent mouth care, chewing gum, or sucking lozenges may help). Report unusual weight gain, unresolved nausea or diarrhea, chest pain or palpitations, excess sedation or stimulation, or sore throat or respiratory difficulty. **Pregnancy/breast-feeding precautions:** Inform prescriber if you are or intend to become pregnant. Breast-feeding is not recommended.

Geriatric Considerations: Because promethazine is a phenothiazine (and can, therefore, cause side effects such as extrapyramidal symptoms), it is not considered an antihistamine of choice in the elderly.

(Continued)

Promethazine *(Continued)*

Pregnancy Risk Factor: C

Pregnancy Issues: Crosses the placenta. Possible respiratory depression if drug is administered near time of delivery; behavioral changes, EEG alterations, impaired platelet aggregation reported with use during labor. Available evidence with use of occasional low doses suggests safe use during pregnancy.

Lactation: Excretion in breast milk unknown/not recommended

Administration

I.M.: Preferred route of administration; administer into deep muscle

I.V.: I.V. administration is not the preferred route. Solution for injection may be diluted in 25-100 mL NS or D_5W (maximum concentration of 25 mg/mL) and infused over 15-30 minutes at a rate ≤25 mg/minute.

Compatibility: Stable in dextran 6% in dextrose, dextran 6% in NS, D_5W, $D_{10}W$, D_5LR, D_5¼NS, D_5½NS, D_5NS, LR, ½NS, NS

Y-site administration: Incompatible with aldesleukin, allopurinol, amphotericin B cholesteryl sulfate complex, cefazolin, cefepime, cefoperazone, cefotetan, doxorubicin liposome, foscarnet, methotrexate, piperacillin/tazobactam

Compatibility in syringe: Incompatible with cefotetan, chloroquine, diatrizoate sodium 75%, diatrizoate meglumine 52% with diatrizoate sodium 8%, diatrizoate meglumine 34.3% with diatrizoate sodium 35%, dimenhydrinate, heparin, iodipamide meglumine 52%, iothalamate meglumine 60%, iothalamate sodium 80%, ketorolac, pentobarbital, thiopental

Compatibility when admixed: Incompatible with aminophylline, chloramphenicol, chlorothiazide, dimenhydrinate, floxacillin, furosemide, heparin, hydrocortisone sodium succinate, methohexital, penicillin G sodium, pentobarbital, phenobarbital, phenytoin, thiopental

Storage:

Injection: Prior to dilution, store at room temperature; protect from light. Solutions in NS or D_5W are stable for 24 hours at room temperature.

Suppositories: Store refrigerated at 2°C to 8°C (36°F to 46°F).

Tablets: Store at room temperature. Protect from light.

Related Information

Postoperative Nausea and Vomiting *on page 1807*

- **Promethazine Hydrochloride** *see* Promethazine *on page 1417*
- **Promethegan™** *see* Promethazine *on page 1417*
- **Pronap-100®** *see* Propoxyphene and Acetaminophen *on page 1427*

Proparacaine (proe PAR a kane)

U.S. Brand Names Alcaine®; Ophthetic®

Synonyms Proparacaine Hydrochloride; Proxymetacaine

Pharmacologic Category Local Anesthetic, Ophthalmic

Medication Safety Issues

Sound-alike/look-alike issues:

Proparacaine may be confused with propoxyphene

Use Anesthesia for tonometry, gonioscopy; suture removal from cornea; removal of corneal foreign body; cataract extraction, glaucoma surgery; short operative procedure involving the cornea and conjunctiva

Mechanism of Action Prevents initiation and transmission of impulse at the nerve cell membrane by decreasing ion permeability through stabilizing

Pharmacodynamics/Kinetics

Onset of action: ~20 seconds

Duration: 15-20 minutes

Contraindications Hypersensitivity to proparacaine or any component of the formulation

Warnings/Precautions Use with caution in patients with cardiac disease, hyperthyroidism; for topical ophthalmic use only; prolonged use not recommended

Drug Interactions Increased effect of phenylephrine, tropicamide (ophthalmics)

Adverse Reactions

1% to 10%: Local: Burning, stinging, redness

<1% (Limited to important or life-threatening): Allergic contact dermatitis, arrhythmia, blurred vision, CNS depression, conjunctival congestion and hemorrhage, corneal opacification, diaphoresis (increased), epithelium, erosion of the corneal iritis, irritation, keratitis, lacrimation, sensitization

Dosing

Adults & Elderly:

Ophthalmic surgery: Ophthalmic: Instill 1 drop of 0.5% solution in eye every 5-10 minutes for 5-7 doses

Tonometry, gonioscopy, suture removal: Ophthalmic: Instill 1-2 drops of 0.5% solution in eye just prior to procedure

Pediatrics: Children: Refer to adult dosing

Available Dosage Forms Solution, ophthalmic, as hydrochloride: 0.5% (15 mL) [contains benzalkonium chloride]

Nursing Guidelines

Patient Education: May slow wound healing; use sparingly, avoid touching or rubbing the eye until anesthesia has worn off

Pregnancy Risk Factor: C

Administration

Storage: Store under refrigeration at 2°C to 8°C (36°F to 46°F). Protect from light.

♦ Proparacaine Hydrochloride *see* Proparacaine *on page 1420*

♦ Propecia® *see* Finasteride *on page 729*

Propofol (PROE po fole)

U.S. Brand Names Diprivan®

Pharmacologic Category General Anesthetic

Medication Safety Issues

Sound-alike/look-alike issues:

Diprivan® may be confused with Diflucan®, Ditropan®

Use Induction of anesthesia for inpatient or outpatient surgery in patients ≥3 years of age; maintenance of anesthesia for inpatient or outpatient surgery in patients >2 months of age; in adults, for the induction and maintenance of monitored anesthesia care sedation during diagnostic procedures; treatment of agitation in intubated, mechanically-ventilated ICU patients

Unlabeled/Investigational Use Postoperative antiemetic; refractory delirium tremens (case reports); conscious sedation

Mechanism of Action Propofol is a hindered phenolic compound with intravenous general anesthetic properties. The drug is unrelated to any of the currently used barbiturate, opioid, benzodiazepine, arylcyclohexylamine, or imidazole intravenous anesthetic agents.

Pharmacodynamics/Kinetics

Onset of action: Anesthetic: Bolus infusion (dose dependent): 9-51 seconds (average 30 seconds)

Duration (dose and rate dependent): 3-10 minutes

Distribution: V_d: 2-10 L/kg; highly lipophilic

Protein binding: 97% to 99%

Metabolism: Hepatic to water-soluble sulfate and glucuronide conjugates

Half-life elimination: Biphasic: Initial: 40 minutes; Terminal: 4-7 hours (up to 1-3 days)

Excretion: Urine (~88% as metabolites, 40% as glucuronide metabolite); feces (<2%)

Clearance: 20-30 mL/kg/minute; total body clearance exceeds liver blood flow

Contraindications Hypersensitivity to propofol or any component of the formulation; propofol is also contraindicated when general anesthesia or sedation is contraindicated

Warnings/Precautions Use requires careful patient monitoring, should only be used by experienced personnel who are not actively engaged in the procedure or surgery. If used in a nonintubated and/or nonmechanically-ventilated patient, qualified personnel and appropriate equipment for rapid institution of respiratory and/or cardiovascular support must be immediately available.

Use a slower rate of induction and avoid rapid bolus administration in the elderly, debilitated, or ASA III/IV patients. Use with caution in patients who are hypotensive, hypovolemic, hemodynamically unstable, or have abnormally low vascular tone (eg, sepsis). Use caution in patients with severe cardiac disease (ejection fraction <50%) or respiratory disease; may have more profound adverse cardiovascular responses to propofol. Use caution in patients with a history of epilepsy or seizures; risk of seizure during recovery phase. Use caution in patients with increased intracranial pressure or impaired cerebral circulation - substantial decreases in mean arterial pressure and subsequent decreases in cerebral perfusion pressure may occur.

(Continued)

Propofol *(Continued)*

Use caution in patients with hyperlipidemia as evidenced by increased serum triglyceride levels or serum turbidity. Transient local pain may occur during I.V. injection; perioperative myoclonia has occurred. Not recommended for use in obstetrics, including cesarean section deliveries. Safety and efficacy in pediatric intensive care unit patients have not been established. Several deaths associated with severe metabolic acidosis have been reported in pediatric ICU patients on long-term propofol infusion. Concurrent use of fentanyl and propofol in pediatric patients may result in bradycardia.

Abrupt discontinuation prior to weaning or daily wake up assessments should be avoided. Abrupt discontinuation can result in rapid awakening, anxiety, agitation, and resistance to mechanical ventilation; titrate the infusion rate so the patient awakens slowly. Propofol does not have analgesic properties; pain should be treated with analgesic agents, propofol must be titrated separately from the analgesic agent. Propofol emulsion contains soybean oil, egg phosphatide, and glycerol; some formulations also contain sulfites. Some products may contain benzyl alcohol; benzyl alcohol has been associated with the 'gasping syndrome' in neonates and low-birth-weight infants.

Drug Interactions Substrate of CYP1A2 (minor), 2A6 (minor), 2B6 (major), 2C8/9 (major), 2C19 (minor), 2D6 (minor), 2E1 (minor), 3A4 (minor); **Inhibits** CYP1A2 (moderate), 2C8/9 (weak), 2C19 (moderate), 2D6 (weak), 2E1 (weak), 3A4 (strong)

CNS depressants: Additive CNS depression and respiratory depression may necessitate dosage reduction when used with anesthetics, benzodiazepines, opiates, ethanol, phenothiazines.

CYP1A2 substrates: Propofol may increase the levels/effects of CYP1A2 substrates. Example substrates include aminophylline, fluvoxamine, mexiletine, mirtazapine, ropinirole, theophylline, and trifluoperazine.

CYP2B6 inhibitors: May increase the levels/effects of propofol. Example inhibitors include desipramine, paroxetine, and sertraline.

CYP2C8/9 inhibitors: May increase the levels/effects of propofol. Example inhibitors include delavirdine, fluconazole, gemfibrozil, ketoconazole, nicardipine, NSAIDs, pioglitazone, and sulfonamides.

CYP2C19 substrates: Propofol may increase the levels/effects of CYP2C19 substrates. Example substrates include citalopram, diazepam, methsuximide, phenytoin, propranolol, and sertraline.

CYP3A4 substrates: Propofol may increase the levels/effects of CYP3A4 substrates. Example substrates include benzodiazepines, calcium channel blockers, mirtazapine, nateglinide, nefazodone, tacrolimus, and venlafaxine. Selected benzodiazepines (midazolam and triazolam), cisapride, ergot alkaloids, selected HMG-CoA reductase inhibitors (lovastatin and simvastatin), and pimozide are generally contraindicated with strong CYP3A4 inhibitors.

Narcotics: Concomitant use may lead to increased sedative or anesthetic effects of propofol, more pronounced decreases in systolic, diastolic, and mean arterial pressures and cardiac output. Lower doses of propofol may be needed. In addition, fentanyl may cause serious bradycardia when used with propofol in pediatric patients.

Vecuronium: Propofol may potentiate the neuromuscular blockade of vecuronium.

Nutritional/Herbal/Ethanol Interactions Food: EDTA, an ingredient of propofol emulsion, may lead to decreased zinc levels in patients on prolonged therapy (>5 days) or those predisposed to deficiency (burns, diarrhea, and/or major sepsis).

Lab Interactions Increased porphyrin (U); decreased cortisol (S), but does not appear to inhibit adrenal responsiveness to ACTH; decreased cholesterol (S)

Adverse Reactions

>10%:

Cardiovascular: Hypotension (children 17%, adults 3% to 26%)

Central nervous system: Dystonic or choreiform movement (children 17%)

Local: Injection site burning, stinging, or pain (children 10%, adults 18%)

Respiratory: Apnea, lasting 30-60 seconds (children 10%, adults 24%); apnea, lasting >60 seconds (children 5%, adults 12%)

1% to 10%:

Cardiovascular: Hypertension (children 8%), arrhythmia, bradycardia, cardiac output decreased, tachycardia

Central nervous system: Movement (adults)

Dermatologic: Pruritus (children 2%), rash (children 5%)

Endocrine & metabolic: Hyperlipidemia, hypertriglyceridemia

Respiratory: Respiratory acidosis during weaning

<1% (Limited to important or life-threatening): Agitation, amblyopia, anaphylaxis, anaphylactoid reaction, anticholinergic syndrome, asystole, atrial arrhythmia, bigeminy, cardiac arrest, chills, cough, dizziness, delirium; discoloration (green - urine, hair, or nailbeds); dystonia; extremity pain, fever, flushing, hemorrhage, hypersalivation, hypertonia, hypomagnesemia, hypoxia, laryngospasm, leukocytosis, lung function decreased, metabolic acidosis (not associated with "propofol infusion syndrome"), myalgia, nausea, paresthesia, perioperative myoclonia (rarely including convulsions and opisthotonos), phlebitis, postoperative pancreatitis, postoperative unconsciousness with or without increase in muscle tone, premature atrial contractions, premature ventricular contractions, pulmonary edema, rhabdomyolysis, serum triglycerides increased, somnolence, syncope, thrombosis, urine cloudy, vision abnormality, wheezing.

Infusion site reactions include pain, swelling, blisters and/or tissue necrosis following accidental extravasation. **Note:** A "propofol infusion syndrome" has been described in patients receiving high-dose, prolonged infusion; symptoms include severe, sporadic metabolic acidosis and/or lactic acidosis which may be associated with tachycardia, myocardial dysfunction, and/or rhabdomyolysis.

Overdosage/Toxicology

Symptoms of overdose include hypotension, bradycardia, and cardiovascular collapse.

Treatment is symptomatic and supportive. Hypotension usually responds to I.V. fluids and/or Trendelenburg positioning. Parenteral inotropes may be needed. Bradycardia may respond to atropine.

Dosing

Adults: Dosage must be individualized based on total body weight and titrated to the desired clinical effect. Wait at least 3-5 minutes between dosage adjustments to clinically assess drug effects. Smaller doses are required when used with narcotics. The following are general dosing guidelines (see "Symbols and Abbreviations Used in This Handbook" in front section of this book for explanation of ASA classes):

Induction:

General anesthesia:

ASA I or II, <55 years: I.V.: 2-2.5 mg/kg (~40 mg every 10 seconds until onset of induction)

Debilitated, ASA III or IV, hypovolemic: Refer to elderly dosing.

Cardiac anesthesia: I.V.: 0.5-1.5 mg/kg (~20 mg every 10 seconds until onset of induction)

Neurosurgical patients: I.V.: 1-2 mg/kg (~20 mg every 10 seconds until onset of induction)

Maintenance:

ASA I or II, <55 years:

I.V. infusion: Initial: 150-200 mcg/kg/minute for 10-15 minutes; decrease by 30% to 50% during first 30 minutes of maintenance; usual infusion rate: 100-200 mcg/kg/minute (6-12 mg/kg/hour)

I.V. intermittent bolus: 20-50 mg increments as needed

Debilitated, ASA III or IV, hypovolemic: I.V. Infusion: Refer to elderly dosing.

Cardiac anesthesia: I.V. infusion:

Low-dose propofol with primary opioid: 50-100 mcg/kg/minute (see manufacturer's labeling)

Primary propofol with secondary opioid: 100-150 mcg/kg/minute

Neurosurgical patients: I.V. infusion: 100-200 mcg/kg/minute (6-12 mg/kg/hour)

Monitored anesthesia care sedation:

Initiation:

ASA I or II, <55 years: Slow I.V. infusion: 100-150 mcg/kg/minute for 3-5 minutes **or** slow injection: 0.5 mg/kg over 3-5 minutes

Debilitated, neurosurgical, or ASA III or IV patients: Use similar doses to healthy adults; avoid rapid I.V. boluses

Maintenance:

ASA I or II, <55 years: I.V. infusion using variable rates (preferred over intermittent boluses): 25-75 mcg/kg/minute **or** incremental bolus doses: 10 mg or 20 mg

Debilitated, neurosurgical, or ASA III or IV patients: Use 80% of healthy adult dose; **do not** use rapid bolus doses (single or repeated)

ICU sedation in intubated mechanically-ventilated patients: Avoid rapid bolus injection; individualize dose and titrate to response

(Continued)

Propofol *(Continued)*

Continuous infusion: Initial: 0.3 mg/kg/hour (5 mcg/kg/min); increase by 0.3-0.6 mg/kg/hour (5-10 mcg/kg/min) every 5-10 minutes until desired sedation level is achieved; usual maintenance: 0.3-4.8 mg/kg/hour (5-80 mcg/kg/min) or higher. Elderly, debilitated, or ASA III or IV patients: Refer to elderly dosing. Some clinicians recommend daily interruption of infusion to perform clinical evaluation.

Elderly:

General anesthesia:

Induction: Elderly, debilitated, ASA III or IV, hypovolemic: I.V.: 1-1.5 mg/kg (~20 mg every 10 seconds until onset of induction)

Maintenance: Elderly, debilitated, ASA III or IV, hypovolemic: I.V. infusion: 50-100 mcg/kg/minute (3-6 mg/kg/hour)

Monitored anesthesia care sedation:

Initiation: Elderly, debilitated, ASA III or IV, neurosurgical: I.V.: Use doses similar to healthy adults; avoid rapid I.V. boluses

Maintenance: Elderly, debilitated, ASA III or IV, neurosurgical: I.V.: Use 80% of healthy adult dose; **do not** use rapid bolus doses (single or repeated)

ICU sedation in intubated mechanically-ventilated patients: Avoid rapid bolus injection; individualize dose and titrate to response: Continuous infusion: Elderly, debilitated, ASA III or IV: Reduce dose by 80%; reduce dose after adequate sedation established and adjust to response (ie, evaluate frequently to use minimum dose for sedation).

Pediatrics: Dosage must be individualized based on total body weight and titrated to the desired clinical effect; wait at least 3-5 minutes between dosage adjustments to clinically assess drug effects; smaller doses are required when used with narcotics; the following are general dosing guidelines (see "Common Symbols and Abbreviations" in front section of this book for explanation of ASA classes):

General anesthesia:

Induction: I.V.: Children 3-16 years, ASA I or II: 2.5-3.5 mg/kg over 20-30 seconds; use a lower dose for children ASA III or IV

Maintenance: I.V. infusion: Children 2 months to 16 years, ASA I or II: Initial: 200-300 mcg/kg/minute; decrease dose after 30 minutes if clinical signs of light anesthesia are absent; usual infusion rate: 125-150 mcg/kg/minute (range: 125-300 mcg/kg/minute; 7.5-18 mg/kg/hour); children ≤5 years may require larger infusion rates compared to older children.

Available Dosage Forms

Injection, emulsion: 10 mg/mL (20 mL, 50 mL, 100 mL) [contains egg lecithin, and soybean oil; may contain either benzyl alcohol or sodium metabisulfite]

Diprivan®: 10 mg/mL (20 mL, 50 mL, 100 mL) [contains egg lecithin, soybean oil, and disodium edetate]

Nursing Guidelines

Assessment: Dosage and rate of administration should be individualized and titrated to the desired effect, according to relevant clinical factors, premedication, concomitant medications, age, and general condition of patient. Assess other medications for effectiveness and safety. Other drugs that cause CNS depression may increase CNS depression induced by propofol (monitor and adjust dosage as necessary). Continuous monitoring of vital signs, cardiac and respiratory status, and level of sedation is mandatory during infusion and until full consciousness is regained. Safety precautions must be maintained until patient is fully alert. Propofol is an anesthetic; pain must be treated with appropriate analgesic agents. Do not discontinue abruptly (may result in rapid awakening associated with anxiety, agitation, and resistance to mechanical ventilation). Titrate infusion rate so patient awakes slowly. **Note:** After long-term administration, it will take longer for reduction of propofol levels than if propofol is used for short-term anesthesia. For long-term use, monitor fluid levels (intake and output) during and following infusion (urine will be green). Reposition patient and provide appropriate skin care, mouth care, and care of patient's eyes every 2-3 hours while sedated. Provide appropriate emotional and sensory support (auditory and environmental).

Monitoring Laboratory Tests: Serum triglyceride levels should be obtained prior to initiation of therapy (ICU setting) and every 3-7 days thereafter. In patients at risk for renal impairment, urinalysis and urine sediment should be monitored prior to treatment and every other day of sedation.

Diprivan®: Monitor zinc levels in patients predisposed to deficiency (burns, diarrhea, major sepsis) or after 5 days of treatment.

Dietary Considerations: Propofol is formulated in an oil-in-water emulsion. If on parenteral nutrition, may need to adjust the amount of lipid infused. Propofol emulsion contains 1.1 kcal/mL. Soybean fat emulsion is used as a vehicle for propofol. Formulations also contain egg phosphatide and glycerol.

Patient Education: This is an anesthetic. Patient education should be appropriate to individual situation. With long-term use appropriate emotional and sensory support is strongly recommended. Following return of consciousness, do not attempt to change position or rise from bed without assistance. Report immediately any pounding or unusual heartbeat, respiratory difficulty, or acute dizziness. **Breast-feeding precaution:** Do not breast-feed.

Pregnancy Risk Factor: B

Pregnancy Issues: Propofol is not recommended for obstetrics, including cesarean section deliveries. Propofol crosses the placenta and may be associated with neonatal depression.

Lactation: Enters breast milk/not recommended

Perioperative/Anesthesia/Other Concerns: On March 26, 2001, a specific warning was issued concerning the use of propofol in pediatric ICU patients. In the opinion of the FDA, a clinical trial evaluating the use of propofol as a sedative agent in this population was associated with a higher number of deaths as compared to standard sedative agents. The warning reminded healthcare professionals that propofol is not approved in the U.S. for sedation in pediatric ICU patients. There have been several case reports of propofol infusion syndrome in critically-ill adults. Clinical features include circulatory collapse, metabolic acidosis, rhabdomyolysis, hepatomegaly, and hyperkalemia. Preservatives (eg, EDTA or sodium metabisulfite) have been added to some products.

Propofol is a negative inotrope and chronotrope.

Bradycardia may respond to atropine.

Very long-term infusions can result in some tolerance; taper propofol infusions to prevent withdrawal. Caution should be exercised when using high doses (>5 mg/kg/hour) and for long-term (>48 hours).

Administration

I.V.: To reduce pain associated with injection, use larger veins of forearm or antecubital fossa; lidocaine I.V. (1 mL of a 1% solution) may also be used prior to administration. Do not use filter with <5 micron for administration. Tubing and any unused portions of propofol vials should be discarded after 12 hours. Strict aseptic technique must be maintained in handling although a preservative has been added. Do not administer through the same I.V. catheter with blood or plasma. The American College of Critical Care Medicine recommends the use of a central vein for administration in an ICU setting.

Reconstitution: Does not need to be diluted; however, propofol may be further diluted in 5% dextrose in water to a concentration of 2 mg/mL and is stable for 8 hours at room temperature.

Compatibility: Do not mix with other therapeutic agents.

Stable in D_5LR, $D_5{}^1/_4NS$, $D_5{}^1/_2NS$, D_5W, LR

Y-site administration: Incompatible with amikacin, amphotericin B, atracurium, bretylium, calcium chloride, ciprofloxacin, diazepam, digoxin, doxorubicin, gentamicin, methotrexate, methylprednisolone sodium succinate, metoclopramide, minocycline, mitoxantrone, phenytoin, tobramycin, verapamil

Storage: Store at room temperature 4°C to 22°C (40°F to 72°F); refrigeration is not recommended. Protect from light. If transferred to a syringe or other container prior to administration, use within 6 hours. If used directly from vial/prefilled syringe, use within 12 hours. Shake well before use. Do not use if there is evidence of separation of phases of emulsion.

Related Information

Conscious Sedation *on page 1779*
Intravenous Anesthetic Agents *on page 1853*
Postoperative Nausea and Vomiting *on page 1807*

Propoxyphene (proe POKS i feen)

U.S. Brand Names Darvon®; Darvon-N®

Synonyms Dextropropoxyphene; Propoxyphene Hydrochloride; Propoxyphene Napsylate

(Continued)

Propoxyphene *(Continued)*

Pharmacologic Category Analgesic, Narcotic

Medication Safety Issues

Sound-alike/look-alike issues:

Propoxyphene may be confused with proparacaine

Darvon® may be confused with Devrom®, Diovan®

Darvon-N® may be confused with Darvocet-N®

Use Management of mild to moderate pain

Mechanism of Action Propoxyphene is a weak narcotic analgesic which acts through binding to opiate receptors to inhibit ascending pain pathways. Propoxyphene, as with other narcotic (opiate) analgesics, blocks pain perception in the cerebral cortex by binding to specific receptor molecules (opiate receptors) within the neuronal membranes of synapses. This binding results in a decreased synaptic chemical transmission throughout the CNS thus inhibiting the flow of pain sensations into the higher centers. Mu and kappa are the two subtypes of the opiate receptor which propoxyphene binds to cause analgesia.

Pharmacodynamics/Kinetics

Onset of action: 0.5-1 hour

Duration: 4-6 hours

Metabolism: Hepatic to active metabolite (norpropoxyphene) and inactive metabolites; first-pass effect

Half-life elimination: Adults: Parent drug: 6-12 hours; Norpropoxyphene: 30-36 hours

Excretion: Urine (primarily as metabolites)

Contraindications Hypersensitivity to propoxyphene or any component of the formulation

Warnings/Precautions When given in excessive doses, either alone or in combination with other CNS depressants, propoxyphene is a major cause of drug-related deaths; do not exceed recommended dosage; give with caution in patients dependent on opiates, substitution may result in acute opiate withdrawal symptoms. Avoid use in severely depressed or suicidal patients. Tolerance or drug dependence may result from extended use. Propoxyphene should be used with caution in patients with renal or hepatic dysfunction or in the elderly; consider dosing adjustment.

Drug Interactions **Inhibits** CYP2C8/9 (weak), 2D6 (weak), 3A4 (weak)

Decreased effect with charcoal, cigarette smoking

Increased toxicity: CNS depressants may potentiate pharmacologic effects; propoxyphene may inhibit the metabolism and increase the serum concentrations of carbamazepine, phenobarbital, MAO inhibitors, tricyclic antidepressants, and warfarin

Nutritional/Herbal/Ethanol Interactions

Ethanol: Avoid or limit ethanol (may increase CNS depression). Watch for sedation.

Food: May decrease rate of absorption, but may slightly increase bioavailability.

Lab Interactions False-positive methadone test; increased LFTs; decreased glucose (S), 17-OHCS (U)

Adverse Reactions Frequency not defined.

Cardiovascular: Hypotension, bundle branch block

Central nervous system: Dizziness, lightheadedness, sedation, paradoxical excitement and insomnia, fatigue, drowsiness, mental depression, hallucinations, paradoxical CNS stimulation, increased intracranial pressure, nervousness, headache, restlessness, malaise, confusion, dysphoria, vertigo

Dermatologic: Rash, urticaria

Endocrine & metabolic: Hypoglycemia, urinary 17-OHCS decreased

Gastrointestinal: Anorexia, stomach cramps, xerostomia, biliary spasm, nausea, vomiting, constipation, paralytic ileus, abdominal pain

Genitourinary: Urination decreased, ureteral spasms

Hepatic: LFTs increased, jaundice

Neuromuscular & skeletal: Weakness

Ocular: Visual disturbances

Respiratory: Dyspnea

Miscellaneous: Psychologic and physical dependence with prolonged use, histamine release, hypersensitivity reaction

Overdosage/Toxicology Symptoms of overdose include CNS disturbances, respiratory depression, hypotension, pulmonary edema, and seizures. Naloxone, 2 mg I.V. with repeat administration as necessary up to a total of 10 mg, can also be used to reverse toxic effects of the opiate. Charcoal is very effective (>95%) at binding propoxyphene.

Dosing

Adults: Pain management: Oral:

Hydrochloride: 65 mg every 3-4 hours as needed for pain; maximum: 390 mg/day

Napsylate: 100 mg every 4 hours as needed for pain; maximum: 600 mg/day

Elderly: Pain management: Oral:

Hydrochloride: 65 mg every 4-6 hours as needed for pain

Napsylate: 100 mg every 4-6 hours as needed for pain

Pediatrics: Pain management: Oral: Children: Doses for children are not well established; doses of the hydrochloride of 2-3 mg/kg/d divided every 6 hours have been used.

Renal Impairment: Serum concentrations of propoxyphene may be increased or elimination may be delayed. Avoid use in Cl_{cr} <10 mL/minute. Specific dosing recommendations not available for less severe impairment.

Not dialyzable (0% to 5%)

Hepatic Impairment: Serum concentrations of propoxyphene may be increased or elimination may be delayed. Specific dosing recommendations not available.

Available Dosage Forms

Capsule, as hydrochloride (Darvon®): 65 mg

Tablet, as napsylate (Darvon-N®): 100 mg

Nursing Guidelines

Assessment: Assess other medications patient may be taking for effectiveness and interactions. Monitor therapeutic effectiveness, cardio/respiratory and CNS status, adverse reactions and signs of overdose at beginning of therapy and periodically with long-term use. Assess knowledge/teach patient appropriate use, interventions to reduce side effects, and adverse symptoms to report.

Dietary Considerations: May administer with food if gastrointestinal distress occurs.

Patient Education: Take as directed; do not take a larger dose or more often than prescribed. Do not use alcohol, other prescription or OTC sedatives, tranquilizers, antihistamines, or pain medications without consulting prescriber. May cause dizziness, drowsiness, or impaired judgment; avoid driving or engaging in tasks requiring alertness until response to drug is known. If you experience vomiting or loss of appetite, frequent mouth care, small frequent meals, chewing gum, or sucking lozenges may help. Increased fluid intake, exercise, fiber in diet may help with constipation (if unresolved consult prescriber). Report unresolved nausea or vomiting, respiratory difficulty or shortness of breath, or unusual weakness. **Pregnancy/breast-feeding precautions:** Inform prescriber if you are or intend to become pregnant.

Geriatric Considerations: The elderly may be particularly susceptible to the CNS depressant effects of narcotics.

Pregnancy Risk Factor: C/D (prolonged use)

Pregnancy Issues: Withdrawal symptoms have been reported in the neonate following propoxyphene use during pregnancy. Teratogenic effects have also been noted in case reports. Opioid analgesics are considered pregnancy risk factor D if used for prolonged periods or in large doses near term.

Lactation: Enters breast milk/use caution (AAP rates "compatible")

Breast-Feeding Considerations: Propoxyphene and norpropoxyphene are excreted in breast milk.

Perioperative/Anesthesia/Other Concerns: Equivalent dosing: 100 mg of napsylate = 65 mg of hydrochloride

Administration

Oral: Should be administered with glass of water on an empty stomach. Food may decrease rate of absorption, but may slightly increase bioavailability.

Storage: Store at controlled room temperature of 15°C to 30°C (59°F to 86°F).

Propoxyphene and Acetaminophen

(proe POKS i feen & a seet a MIN oh fen)

U.S. Brand Names Balacet 325™; Darvocet A500™; Darvocet-N® 50; Darvocet-N® 100; Pronap-100®

Synonyms Acetaminophen and Propoxyphene; Propoxyphene Hydrochloride and Acetaminophen; Propoxyphene Napsylate and Acetaminophen

(Continued)

Propoxyphene and Acetaminophen *(Continued)*

Pharmacologic Category Analgesic Combination (Narcotic)

Medication Safety Issues

Sound-alike/look-alike issues:

Darvocet-N® may be confused with Darvon-N®

Use Management of mild to moderate pain

Mechanism of Action

Propoxyphene is a weak narcotic analgesic which acts through binding to opiate receptors to inhibit ascending pain pathways

Propoxyphene, as with other narcotic (opiate) analgesics, blocks pain perception in the cerebral cortex by binding to specific receptor molecules (opiate receptors) within the neuronal membranes of synapses. This binding results in a decreased synaptic chemical transmission throughout the CNS thus inhibiting the flow of pain sensations into the higher centers. Mu and kappa are the two subtypes of the opiate receptor to which propoxyphene binds to cause analgesia.

Acetaminophen inhibits the synthesis of prostaglandins in the CNS and peripherally blocks pain impulse generation; produces antipyresis from inhibition of hypothalamic heat-regulating center

Pharmacodynamics/Kinetics See individual agents.

Contraindications Hypersensitivity to propoxyphene, acetaminophen, or any component of the formulation

Warnings/Precautions When given in excessive doses, either alone or in combination with other CNS depressants, propoxyphene is a major cause of drug-related deaths; do not exceed recommended dosage; give with caution in patients dependent on opiates, substitution may result in acute opiate withdrawal symptoms. Avoid use in severely-depressed or suicidal patients. Tolerance or drug dependence may result from extended use.

Propoxyphene should be used with caution in patients with renal or hepatic dysfunction or in the elderly; consider dosing adjustment. Acetaminophen should be used with caution in patients with liver disease; consuming ≥3 alcoholic drinks/day may increase risk of liver damage. Use caution in patients with known G6PD deficiency. Safety and efficacy of this combination have not been established in pediatric patients.

Drug Interactions

Propoxyphene: **Inhibits** CYP2C8/9 (weak), 2D6 (weak), 3A4 (weak)

Acetaminophen: **Substrate** (minor) of CYP1A2, 2A6, 2C8/9, 2D6, 2E1, 3A4; **Inhibits** CYP3A4 (weak)

Also see individual agents.

Nutritional/Herbal/Ethanol Interactions

Based on **propoxyphene** component:

Ethanol: Avoid or limit ethanol (may increase CNS depression). Watch for sedation.

Food: May decrease rate of absorption, but may slightly increase bioavailability.

Based on **acetaminophen** component:

Ethanol: Excessive intake of ethanol may increase the risk of acetaminophen-induced hepatotoxicity. Avoid ethanol or limit to <3 drinks/day.

Food: Rate of absorption may be decreased when given with food.

Herb/Nutraceutical: St John's wort may decrease acetaminophen levels.

Adverse Reactions See individual agents.

Dosing

Adults & Elderly:

Pain management: Oral:

Darvocet A500™, Darvocet-N® 100: 1 tablet every 4 hours as needed; maximum: 600 mg propoxyphene napsylate/day

Darvocet-N® 50: 1-2 tablets every 4 hours as needed; maximum: 600 mg propoxyphene napsylate/day

Note: Formulations contain significant amounts of acetaminophen; intake should be limited to <4 g acetaminophen/day (less in patients with hepatic impairment/ethanol abuse)

Renal Impairment: Serum concentrations of propoxyphene may be increased or elimination may be delayed; specific dosing recommendations not available.

Hepatic Impairment: Serum concentrations of propoxyphene may be increased or elimination may be delayed; specific dosing recommendations not available.

Available Dosage Forms

Tablet: Propoxyphene hydrochloride 65 mg and acetaminophen 650 mg, propoxyphene napsylate 100 mg, and acetaminophen 650 mg

Balacet 325™: Propoxyphene napsylate 100 mg and acetaminophen 325 mg

Darvocet A500™: Propoxyphene napsylate 100 mg and acetaminophen 500 mg [contains lactose]

Darvocet-N® 50: Propoxyphene napsylate 50 mg and acetaminophen 325 mg

Darvocet-N® 100, Pronap-100®: Propoxyphene napsylate 100 mg and acetaminophen 650 mg

Nursing Guidelines

Dietary Considerations: May be taken with food if gastrointestinal distress occurs.

Patient Education: See individual agents. **Pregnancy precaution:** Inform prescriber if you are or intend to become pregnant.

Geriatric Considerations: The elderly may be particularly susceptible to the CNS depressant and constipating effects of narcotics; do not exceed 4 g/day of acetaminophen. See Warnings/Precautions and Dosage. Propoxyphene is not considered the analgesic of choice in the elderly patient when mild-to-moderate pain requires a narcotic analgesic. This is due to the higher incidence of adverse CNS effects seen in this population group. The addiction potential is also a concern; avoid use, if possible.

Pregnancy Risk Factor: C

Pregnancy Issues: Withdrawal symptoms have been reported in the neonate following propoxyphene use during pregnancy. Teratogenic effects have also been noted in case reports. Opioid analgesics are considered pregnancy risk factor D if used for prolonged periods or in large doses near term.

Lactation: Enters breast milk/compatible

Breast-Feeding Considerations: Propoxyphene, norpropoxyphene and acetaminophen are excreted in breast milk. The AAP considers propoxyphene and acetaminophen to be "compatible" with breast-feeding.

Administration

Oral: Should be administered with water on an empty stomach.

Storage: Store at controlled room temperature.

♦ **Propoxyphene Hydrochloride** *see* Propoxyphene *on page 1425*

♦ **Propoxyphene Hydrochloride and Acetaminophen** *see* Propoxyphene and Acetaminophen *on page 1427*

♦ **Propoxyphene Napsylate** *see* Propoxyphene *on page 1425*

♦ **Propoxyphene Napsylate and Acetaminophen** *see* Propoxyphene and Acetaminophen *on page 1427*

Propranolol (proe PRAN oh lole)

U.S. Brand Names Inderal®; Inderal® LA; InnoPran XL™

Synonyms Propranolol Hydrochloride

Pharmacologic Category Antiarrhythmic Agent, Class II; Beta-Adrenergic Blocker, Nonselective

Medication Safety Issues

Sound-alike/look-alike issues:

Propranolol may be confused with Pravachol®, Propulsid®

Inderal® may be confused with Adderall®, Enduron®, Enduronyl®, Imdur®, Imuran®, Inderide®, Isordil®, Toradol®

Inderal® 40 may be confused with Enduronyl® Forte

Use Management of hypertension; angina pectoris; pheochromocytoma; essential tremor; tetralogy of Fallot cyanotic spells; arrhythmias (such as atrial fibrillation and flutter, AV nodal re-entrant tachycardias, and catecholamine-induced arrhythmias); prevention of myocardial infarction; migraine headache; symptomatic treatment of hypertrophic subaortic stenosis

Unlabeled/Investigational Use Tremor due to Parkinson's disease; ethanol withdrawal; aggressive behavior; antipsychotic-induced akathisia; prevention of bleeding esophageal varices; anxiety; schizophrenia; acute panic; gastric bleeding in portal hypertension; thyrotoxicosis

Mechanism of Action Nonselective beta-adrenergic blocker (class II antiarrhythmic); competitively blocks response to $beta_1$- and $beta_2$-adrenergic stimulation which results in decreases in heart rate, myocardial contractility, blood pressure, and myocardial oxygen demand

(Continued)

Propranolol *(Continued)*

Pharmacodynamics/Kinetics

Onset of action: Beta-blockade: Oral: 1-2 hours

Duration: ~6 hours

Distribution: V_d: 3.9 L/kg in adults; crosses placenta; small amounts enter breast milk

Protein binding: Newborns: 68%; Adults: 93%

Metabolism: Hepatic to active and inactive compounds; extensive first-pass effect

Bioavailability: 30% to 40%; may be increased in Down syndrome

Half-life elimination: Neonates and Infants: Possible increased half-life; Children: 3.9-6.4 hours; Adults: 4-6 hours

Excretion: Urine (96% to 99%)

Contraindications Hypersensitivity to propranolol, beta-blockers, or any component of the formulation; uncompensated congestive heart failure (unless the failure is due to tachyarrhythmias being treated with propranolol), cardiogenic shock, bradycardia or heart block (2nd or 3rd degree), pulmonary edema, severe hyperactive airway disease (asthma or COPD), Raynaud's disease; pregnancy (2nd and 3rd trimesters)

Warnings/Precautions Administer cautiously in compensated heart failure and monitor for a worsening of the condition (efficacy of propranolol in CHF has not been demonstrated). Beta-blocker therapy should not be withdrawn abruptly (particularly in patients with CAD), but gradually tapered (over 2 weeks) to avoid acute tachycardia, hypertension, and/or ischemia. Use caution in patient with PVD. Use caution with concurrent use of beta-blockers and either verapamil or diltiazem; bradycardia or heart block can occur. Avoid concurrent I.V. use of both agents. Use cautiously in diabetics because it can mask prominent hypoglycemic symptoms. Can mask signs of thyrotoxicosis. Can cause fetal harm when administered in pregnancy. Use cautiously in hepatic dysfunction (dosage adjustment required). Use care with anesthetic agents which decrease myocardial function. Not indicated for hypertensive emergencies.

Drug Interactions **Substrate** of CYP1A2 (major), 2C19 (minor), 2D6 (major), 3A4 (minor); **Inhibits** CYP1A2 (weak), 2D6 (weak)

Albuterol (and other $beta_2$ agonists): Effects may be blunted by nonspecific beta-blockers.

Alpha-blockers (prazosin, terazosin): Concurrent use of beta-blockers may increase risk of orthostasis.

Aluminum hydroxide: Absorption of propranolol may be decreased.

Cholestyramine, colestipol: Plasma levels of propranolol may be decreased.

Cimetidine increases the plasma concentration of propranolol and its pharmacodynamic effects may be increased.

Clonidine: Hypertensive crisis after or during withdrawal of either agent

CYP1A2 inducers: May decrease the levels/effects of propranolol. Example inducers include aminoglutethimide, carbamazepine, phenobarbital, and rifampin.

CYP1A2 inhibitors: May increase the levels/effects of propranolol. Example inhibitors include amiodarone, ciprofloxacin, fluvoxamine, ketoconazole, norfloxacin, ofloxacin, and rofecoxib.

CYP2D6 inhibitors: May increase the levels/effects of propranolol. Example inhibitors include chlorpromazine, delavirdine, fluoxetine, miconazole, paroxetine, pergolide, quinidine, quinine, ritonavir, and ropinirole.

Diazepam: Metabolism of diazepam may be inhibited; concentrations of diazepam and metabolites may be increased.

Drugs which slow AV conduction (digoxin): Effects may be additive with beta-blockers.

Epinephrine (including local anesthetics with epinephrine): Propranolol may cause hypertension.

Flecainide: Pharmacological activity of both agents may be increased when used concurrently.

Fluoxetine may inhibit the metabolism of propranolol, resulting in cardiac toxicity.

Glucagon: Propranolol may blunt hyperglycemic action.

Haloperidol: Hypotensive effects may be potentiated.

Hydralazine: The bioavailability propranolol (rapid release) and hydralazine may be enhanced with concurrent dosing.

Insulin: Propranolol inhibits recovery and may cause hypertension and bradycardia following insulin-induced hypoglycemia; also masks the tachycardia that usually accompanies insulin-induced hypoglycemia.

Lidocaine: Metabolism of lidocaine may be decreased.

NSAIDs (ibuprofen, indomethacin, naproxen, piroxicam) may reduce the antihypertensive effects of beta-blockers.

Phenothiazines (chlorpromazine, phenothiazine): Plasma levels of propranolol and phenothiazine may both be increased.

Propafenone: May increase the concentrations/effects of propranolol.

Quinidine: May increase plasma levels of propranolol by decreasing metabolism.

Rifampin: May decrease plasma levels of propranolol by increasing metabolism.

Salicylates may reduce the antihypertensive effects of beta-blockers

Serotonin 5-HT_{1D} receptor agonists (such as rizatriptan, zolmitriptan): Propranolol may increase bioavailability of serotonin 5-HT_{1D} receptor agonists.

Sulfonylureas: Beta-blockers may alter response to hypoglycemic agents.

Theophylline: Theophylline clearance may be decreased by propranolol.

Verapamil or diltiazem may have synergistic or additive pharmacological effects when taken concurrently with beta-blockers; avoid concurrent I.V. use of both.

Warfarin: Propranolol may increase bioavailability of warfarin and PT may be increased.

Nutritional/Herbal/Ethanol Interactions

Ethanol: Ethanol may decrease plasma levels of propranolol by increasing metabolism.

Food: Propranolol serum levels may be increased if taken with food. Protein-rich foods may increase bioavailability; a change in diet from high carbohydrate/low protein to low carbohydrate/high protein may result in increased oral clearance.

Cigarette: Smoking may decrease plasma levels of propranolol by increasing metabolism.

Herb/Nutraceutical: Avoid dong quai if using for hypertension (has estrogenic activity). Avoid ephedra, yohimbe, ginseng (may worsen hypertension or arrhythmia). Avoid natural licorice (causes sodium and water retention and increases potassium loss). Avoid garlic (may have increased antihypertensive effect).

Lab Interactions Increased thyroxine (S)

Adverse Reactions Frequency not defined.

Cardiovascular: Bradycardia, CHF, reduced peripheral circulation, chest pain, hypotension, impaired myocardial contractility, worsening of AV conduction disturbance, cardiogenic shock, Raynaud's syndrome, mesenteric thrombosis (rare), syncope

Central nervous system: Mental depression, lightheadedness, amnesia, emotional lability, confusion, hallucinations, dizziness, insomnia, fatigue, vivid dreams, lethargy, cold extremities, vertigo, cognitive dysfunction, psychosis, hypersomnolence

Dermatologic: Alopecia, contact dermatitis, eczematous eruptions, erythema multiforme, exfoliative dermatitis, hyperkeratosis, nail changes, pruritus, psoriasiform eruptions, rash, ulcerative lichenoid, urticaria, Stevens-Johnson syndrome, toxic epidermal necrolysis

Endocrine & metabolic: Hypoglycemia, hyperglycemia, hyperlipidemia, hyperkalemia

Gastrointestinal: Diarrhea, nausea, vomiting, stomach discomfort, constipation, anorexia

Genitourinary: Impotence, proteinuria (rare), oliguria (rare), interstitial nephritis (rare), Peyronie's disease

Hematologic: Agranulocytosis, thrombocytopenia, thrombocytopenic purpura

Neuromuscular & skeletal: Weakness, carpal tunnel syndrome (rare), paresthesia, myotonus, polyarthritis, arthropathy

Ocular: Hyperemia of the conjunctiva, decreased tear production, decreased visual acuity, mydriasis

Respiratory: Wheezing, pharyngitis, bronchospasm, pulmonary edema, respiratory distress, laryngospasm

Miscellaneous: Lupus-like syndrome (rare), anaphylactic/anaphylactoid allergic reaction

Overdosage/Toxicology Symptoms of intoxication include cardiac disturbances, CNS toxicity, bronchospasm, hypoglycemia, and hyperkalemia. The most common cardiac symptoms include hypotension and bradycardia. Atrioventricular block, intraventricular conduction disturbances, cardiogenic shock, and asystole may occur with severe overdose, especially with membrane-depressant drugs (eg, propranolol). CNS effects include convulsions and coma. Respiratory arrest is commonly seen with propranolol and other membrane-depressant and lipid-soluble drugs. Treatment is symptom-directed and supportive.

(Continued)

Propranolol *(Continued)*

Dosing

Adults:

Akathisia: Oral: 30-120 mg/day in 2-3 divided doses

Angina: Oral: 80-320 mg/day in doses divided 2-4 times/day

Long-acting formulation: Initial: 80 mg once daily; maximum dose: 320 mg once daily

Essential tremor: Oral: 20-40 mg twice daily initially; maintenance doses: usually 120-320 mg/day

Hypertension: Initial: 40 mg twice daily; increase dosage every 3-7 days; usual dose: ≤320 mg divided in 2-3 doses/day; maximum daily dose: 640 mg; usual dosage range (JNC 7): 40-160 mg/day in 2 divided doses

Long-acting formulation: Initial: 80 mg once daily; usual maintenance: 120-160 mg once daily; maximum daily dose: 640 mg; usual dosage range (JNC 7): 60-180 mg/day once daily

Hypertrophic subaortic stenosis: Oral: 20-40 mg 3-4 times/day

Long-acting formulation: 80-160 mg once daily

Migraine headache prophylaxis: Oral: Initial: 80 mg/day divided every 6-8 hours; increase by 20-40 mg/dose every 3-4 weeks to a maximum of 160-240 mg/day given in divided doses every 6-8 hours; if satisfactory response not achieved within 6 weeks of starting therapy, drug should be withdrawn gradually over several weeks

Long-acting formulation: Initial: 80 mg once daily; effective dose range: 160-240 mg once daily

Myocardial infarction prophylaxis: Oral: 180-240 mg/day in 3-4 divided doses

Pheochromocytoma: Oral: 30-60 mg/day in divided doses

Tachyarrhythmias:

Oral: 10-30 mg/dose every 6-8 hours

I.V. (in patients having nonfunctional GI tract): 1 mg/dose slow IVP; repeat every 5 minutes up to a total of 5 mg; titrate initial dose to desired response

Thyrotoxicosis:

Oral: 10-40 mg/dose every 6 hours

I.V.: 1-3 mg/dose slow IVP as a single dose

Elderly: Tachyarrhythmias: Initial: 10 mg twice daily; increase dosage every 3-7 days; usual dose range: 10-320 mg given 1-2 times/day. Refer to adult dosing for additional uses.

Pediatrics:

Hypertension:

Oral: Initial: 0.5-1 mg/kg/day in divided doses every 6-12 hours; increase gradually every 5-7 days; maximum: 16 mg/kg/24 hours

I.V.: 0.01-0.05 mg/kg over 1 hour; maximum dose: 10 mg

Migraine headache prophylaxis: Oral: Initial: 2-4 mg/kg/day **or**

≤35 kg: 10-20 mg 3 times/day

>35 kg: 20-40 mg 3 times/day

Tachyarrhythmias:

Oral: Initial: 0.5-1 mg/kg/day in divided doses every 6-8 hours; titrate dosage upward every 3-7 days; usual dose: 2-6 mg/kg/day; higher doses may be needed; do not exceed 16 mg/kg/day or 60 mg/day

I.V.: 0.01-0.1 mg/kg/dose slow IVP over 10 minutes; maximum dose: 1 mg for infants; 3 mg for children

Tetralogy spells:

Oral: Palliation: Initial: 1 mg/kg/day every 6 hours; if ineffective, may increase dose after 1 week by 1 mg/kg/day to a maximum of 5 mg/kg/day, if patient becomes refractory, may increase slowly to a maximum of 10-15 mg/kg/day. Allow 24 hours between dosing changes.

I.V.: 0.01-0.2 mg/kg/dose infused over 10 minutes; maximum initial dose: 1 mg

Thyrotoxicosis: Oral:

2 mg/kg/day, divided every 6-8 hours, titrate to effective dose

Adolescents: Refer to adult dosing.

Renal Impairment:

Not dialyzable (0% to 5%); supplemental dose is not necessary.

Peritoneal dialysis effects: Supplemental dose is not necessary.

Hepatic Impairment: Marked slowing of heart rate may occur in cirrhosis with conventional doses; low initial dose and regular heart rate monitoring.

Available Dosage Forms

Capsule, extended release, as hydrochloride (InnoPran XL™): 80 mg, 120 mg

Capsule, sustained release, as hydrochloride (Inderal® LA): 60 mg, 80 mg, 120 mg, 160 mg

Injection, solution, as hydrochloride (Inderal®): 1 mg/mL (1 mL)

Solution, oral, as hydrochloride: 4 mg/mL (5 mL, 500 mL); 8 mg/mL (500 mL) [strawberry-mint flavor; contains alcohol 0.6%]

Tablet, as hydrochloride (Inderal®): 10 mg, 20 mg, 40 mg, 60 mg, 80 mg

Nursing Guidelines

Assessment: Assess effectiveness and interactions of other medications patient may be taking. Monitor therapeutic effectiveness and adverse reactions when starting or adjusting dosage. I.V. infusion requires hemodynamic monitoring. Monitor serum glucose closely in patients with diabetes. Beta-blockers may alter serum glucose levels. Assess knowledge/teach patient appropriate use, orthostatic precautions, interventions to reduce side effects, and adverse symptoms to report.

Dietary Considerations: Tablets should be taken on an empty stomach; capsules may be taken with or without food, but should always be taken consistently (with food or on an empty stomach)

Patient Education: Take exactly as directed; do not increase, decrease, or discontinue without consulting prescriber. Tablets may be crushed and taken with liquids. Do not chew or crush long-acting forms; take whole. Take at the same time each day. Do not alter dietary intake of protein or carbohydrates without consulting prescriber. You may experience orthostatic hypotension, dizziness, drowsiness, or blurred vision (use caution when driving, climbing stairs, or changing position - rising from sitting or lying to standing; or engaging in tasks requiring alertness until response to drug is known); nausea, vomiting, or stomach discomfort (small frequent meals, frequent mouth care, chewing gum, or sucking lozenges may help); or decreased sexual ability (reversible). If you have diabetes, monitor serum glucose closely. Report unusual swelling of extremities, respiratory difficulty, unresolved cough, unusual weight gain, cold extremities, persistent diarrhea, confusion, hallucinations, headache, nervousness, lack of improvement, or worsening of condition. **Pregnancy/breast-feeding precautions:** Inform prescriber if you are or intend to become pregnant. Consult prescriber if breast-feeding.

Geriatric Considerations: Since bioavailability increased in the elderly, about twofold geriatric patients may require lower maintenance doses, therefore, as serum and tissue concentrations increase $beta_1$ selectivity diminishes; due to alterations in the beta-adrenergic autonomic nervous system, beta-adrenergic blockade may result in less hemodynamic response than seen in younger adults.

Pregnancy Risk Factor: C (manufacturer); D (2nd and 3rd trimesters - expert analysis)

Pregnancy Issues: Propranolol crosses the placenta. Beta-blockers have been associated with bradycardia, hypotension, and IUGR. IUGR is probably related to maternal hypertension. Available evidence suggests beta-blockers are generally safe during pregnancy (JNC 7). Cases of neonatal hypoglycemia have been reported following maternal use of beta-blockers at parturition or during breast-feeding. Monitor breast-fed infant for symptoms of beta-blockade.

Lactation: Enters breast milk/use caution (AAP rates "compatible")

Breast-Feeding Considerations: Propranolol is excreted in breast milk and is considered compatible by the AAP. It is recommended that the infant be monitored for signs or symptoms of beta-blockade (hypotension, bradycardia, etc) with long-term use.

Perioperative/Anesthesia/Other Concerns: Propranolol is not indicated for hypertensive emergencies. It is not significantly removed by hemodialysis.

Myocardial Infarction: Beta-blockers, in general without intrinsic sympathomimetic activity (ISA), have been shown to decrease morbidity and mortality when initiated in the acute treatment of myocardial infarction and continued long-term. In this setting, therapy should be avoided in patients with hypotension, cardiogenic shock, or heart block.

Surgery: Atenolol has also been shown to improve cardiovascular outcomes when used in the perioperative period in patients with underlying cardiovascular disease who are undergoing noncardiac surgery. Bisoprolol in high-risk patients undergoing vascular surgery reduced the perioperative incidence of death from cardiac causes and nonfatal myocardial infarction.

(Continued)

Propranolol *(Continued)*

Atrial Fibrillation: Beta-blocker therapy provides effective rate control in patients with atrial fibrillation.

Withdrawal: Beta-blocker therapy should not be withdrawn abruptly, but gradually tapered over 2 weeks to avoid acute tachycardia and hypertension.

Administration

Oral: Do not crush long-acting forms.

I.V.: I.V. dose is much smaller than oral dose. When administered acutely for cardiac treatment, monitor ECG and blood pressure. May administer by rapid infusion (I.V. push) at a rate of 1 mg/minute or by slow infusion over ~30 minutes. Necessary monitoring for surgical patients who are unable to take oral beta-blockers (prolonged ileus) has not been defined. Some institutions require monitoring of baseline and postinfusion heart rate and blood pressure when a patient's response to beta-blockade has not been characterized (ie, the patient's initial dose or following a change in dose). Consult individual institutional policies and procedures.

Compatibility: Stable in D_5½NS, D_5NS, D_5W, LR, ½NS, NS

Y-site administration: Incompatible with amphotericin B cholesteryl sulfate complex, diazoxide

Compatibility in syringe: Incompatible with HCO_3

Compatibility when admixed: Incompatible with HCO_3

Storage: Protect injection from light. Solutions have maximum stability at pH of 3 and decompose rapidly in alkaline pH. Propranolol is stable for 24 hours at room temperature in D_5W or NS.

- **Propranolol Hydrochloride** *see* Propranolol *on page 1429*
- **Proprinal [OTC]** *see* Ibuprofen *on page 889*
- **Propulsid®** *see* Cisapride *on page 406*
- **Propylene Glycol Diacetate, Acetic Acid, and Hydrocortisone** *see* Acetic Acid, Propylene Glycol Diacetate, and Hydrocortisone *on page 78*
- **Propylene Glycol Diacetate, Hydrocortisone, and Acetic Acid** *see* Acetic Acid, Propylene Glycol Diacetate, and Hydrocortisone *on page 78*
- **2-Propylpentanoic Acid** *see* Valproic Acid and Derivatives *on page 1680*
- **2-Propylvaleric Acid** *see* Valproic Acid and Derivatives *on page 1680*
- **Proquin® XR** *see* Ciprofloxacin *on page 400*
- **Proscar®** *see* Finasteride *on page 729*
- **Prostacyclin** *see* Epoprostenol *on page 622*
- **Prostaglandin E_1** *see* Alprostadil *on page 113*
- **Prostigmin®** *see* Neostigmine *on page 1214*
- **Prostin VR Pediatric®** *see* Alprostadil *on page 113*

Protamine Sulfate (PROE ta meen SUL fate)

Pharmacologic Category Antidote

Medication Safety Issues

Sound-alike/look-alike issues:

Protamine may be confused with ProAmatine®, protamine, Protopam®, Protropin®

Use Treatment of heparin overdosage; neutralize heparin during surgery or dialysis procedures

Unlabeled/Investigational Use Treatment of low molecular weight heparin (LMWH) overdose

Mechanism of Action Combines with strongly acidic heparin to form a stable complex (salt) neutralizing the anticoagulant activity of both drugs

Pharmacodynamics/Kinetics Onset of action: I.V.: Heparin neutralization: ~5 minutes

Contraindications Hypersensitivity to protamine or any component of the formulation

Warnings/Precautions May not be totally effective in some patients following cardiac surgery despite adequate doses; may cause hypersensitivity reaction in patients with a history of allergy to fish (have epinephrine 1:1000 available) and in patients sensitized to protamine (via protamine zinc insulin); too rapid administration can cause severe hypotensive and anaphylactoid-like reactions. Heparin rebound associated with anticoagulation and bleeding has been reported to occur occasionally; symptoms typically occur 8-9 hours after protamine administration, but may occur as long as 18 hours later.

Adverse Reactions Frequency not defined.

Cardiovascular: Sudden fall in blood pressure, bradycardia, flushing, hypotension
Central nervous system: Lassitude
Gastrointestinal: Nausea, vomiting
Hematologic: Hemorrhage
Respiratory: Dyspnea, pulmonary hypertension
Miscellaneous: Hypersensitivity reactions

Overdosage/Toxicology Symptoms of overdose include hypertension. May cause hemorrhage. Doses exceeding 100 mg may cause paradoxical anticoagulation.

Dosing

Adults & Elderly:

Heparin neutralization: I.V.: Protamine dosage is determined by the dosage of heparin; 1 mg of protamine neutralizes 90 USP units of heparin (lung) and 115 USP units of heparin (intestinal); maximum dose: 50 mg

Heparin overdosage, following intravenous administration: I.V.: Since blood heparin concentrations decrease rapidly **after** administration, adjust the protamine dosage depending upon the duration of time since heparin administration as follows: See table.

Time Elapsed	Dose of Protamine (mg) to Neutralize 100 units of Heparin
Immediate	1-1.5
30-60 min	0.5-0.75
>2 h	0.25-0.375

Heparin overdosage, following SubQ injection: I.V.: 1-1.5 mg protamine per 100 units heparin; this may be done by a portion of the dose (eg, 25-50 mg) given slowly I.V. followed by the remaining portion as a continuous infusion over 8-16 hours (the expected absorption time of the SubQ heparin dose)

LMWH overdose (unlabeled use):

Enoxaparin: 1 mg protamine for each mg of enoxaparin; if PTT prolonged 2-4 hours after first dose, consider additional dose of 0.5 mg for each mg of enoxaparin.

Dalteparin or tinzaparin: 1 mg protamine for each 100 anti-Xa int. units of dalteparin or tinzaparin; if PTT prolonged 2-4 hours after first dose, consider additional dose of 0.5 mg for each 100 anti-Xa int. units of dalteparin or tinzaparin.

Note: Antifactor Xa activity never completely neutralized (maximum: ~60% to 75%). Excessive protamine doses may worsen bleeding potential.

Pediatrics: Refer to adult dosing.

Available Dosage Forms Injection, solution, as sulfate [preservative free]: 10 mg/mL (5 mL, 25 mL)

Nursing Guidelines

Assessment: Assess results of laboratory tests and therapeutic effectiveness frequently during therapy. Monitor closely for adverse response. Assess knowledge/teach patient possible side effects and adverse symptoms to report.

Monitoring Laboratory Tests: Coagulation test, aPTT or ACT

Patient Education: Report any respiratory difficulty, rash or flushing, feeling of warmth, tingling or numbness, dizziness, or disorientation. **Pregnancy/breast-feeding precautions:** Inform prescriber if you are pregnant. Consult prescriber if breast-feeding.

Pregnancy Risk Factor: C

Lactation: Excretion in breast milk unknown

Perioperative/Anesthesia/Other Concerns: Monitor vital signs closely during protamine therapy because of possible hypotension during administration.

Anaphylaxis or hypersensitivity responses with acute hypotension to protamine may present with its use, especially in patients with allergies to fish, previous exposure to protamine (through previous use of protamine or protamine-containing insulin), infertile or vasectomized males.

Protamine's reversal of LMWHs is not as complete or predictable as with heparin. Protamine neutralizes the antithrombin activity of LMWHs, but the cationic protein neutralizes the antifactor Xa activity incompletely. A recent case illustrates a failure to reverse enoxaparin (Makris M, 2000). Protamine will not

(Continued)

Protamine Sulfate *(Continued)*

reverse the effects of thrombin inhibitors such as lepirudin, bivalirudin, or argatroban.

Administration

I.V.: For I.V. use only. Administer slow IVP (50 mg over 10 minutes). Rapid I.V. infusion causes hypotension. Reconstitute vial with 5 mL sterile water. Resulting solution equals 10 mg/mL. Inject without further dilution over 1-3 minutes; maximum of 50 mg in any 10-minute period.

Reconstitution: Reconstitute vial with 5 mL sterile water; if using protamine in neonates, reconstitute with preservative-free sterile water for injection; resulting solution equals 10 mg/mL.

Compatibility: Stable in D_5W, NS

Compatibility in syringe: Incompatible with diatrizoate meglumine 52%, diatrizoate sodium 8%, diatrizoate sodium 60%, ioxaglate meglumine 39.3%, ioxaglate sodium 19.6%

Compatibility when admixed: Incompatible with cephalosporins, penicillins

Storage: Refrigerate; avoid freezing. Remains stable for at least 2 weeks at room temperature; preservative-free formulation does not require refrigeration.

- **Protonix®** *see* Pantoprazole *on page 1307*
- **Protopic®** *see* Tacrolimus *on page 1593*
- **Proventil®** *see* Albuterol *on page 96*
- **Proventil® HFA** *see* Albuterol *on page 96*
- **Proventil® Repetabs®** *see* Albuterol *on page 96*
- **Provera®** *see* MedroxyPROGESTERone *on page 1085*
- **Provigil®** *see* Modafinil *on page 1173*
- **Provisc®** *see* Hyaluronate and Derivatives *on page 856*
- **Proxymetacaine** *see* Proparacaine *on page 1420*
- **Prozac®** *see* Fluoxetine *on page 748*
- **Prozac® Weekly™** *see* Fluoxetine *on page 748*
- **PRP-OMP** *see Haemophilus* b Conjugate Vaccine *on page 837*
- **PRP-T** *see Haemophilus* b Conjugate Vaccine *on page 837*
- **23PS** *see* Pneumococcal Polysaccharide Vaccine (Polyvalent) *on page 1378*
- **PS-341** *see* Bortezomib *on page 251*

Pseudoephedrine (soo doe e FED rin)

U.S. Brand Names Biofed [OTC]; Contact® Cold [OTC]; Dimetapp® 12-Hour Non-Drowsy Extentabs® [OTC]; Dimetapp® Decongestant Infant [OTC]; Elix-Sure™ Congestion [OTC]; Genaphed® [OTC]; Kidkare Decongestant [OTC]; Kodet SE [OTC]; Oranyl [OTC]; PediaCare® Decongestant Infants [OTC]; Silfedrine Children's [OTC]; Simply Stuffy™ [OTC]; Sudafed® [OTC]; Sudafed® 12 Hour [OTC]; Sudafed® 24 Hour [OTC]; Sudafed® Children's [OTC]; Sudodrin [OTC]; SudoGest [OTC]; Sudo-Tab® [OTC]

Synonyms *d*-Isoephedrine Hydrochloride; Pseudoephedrine Hydrochloride; Pseudoephedrine Sulfate

Pharmacologic Category Alpha/Beta Agonist

Medication Safety Issues

Sound-alike/look-alike issues:

Dimetapp® may be confused with Dermatop®, Dimetabs®, Dimetane®

Sudafed® may be confused with Sufenta®

Use Temporary symptomatic relief of nasal congestion due to common cold, upper respiratory allergies, and sinusitis; also promotes nasal or sinus drainage

Mechanism of Action Directly stimulates alpha-adrenergic receptors of respiratory mucosa causing vasoconstriction; directly stimulates beta-adrenergic receptors causing bronchial relaxation, increased heart rate and contractility

Pharmacodynamics/Kinetics

Onset of action: Decongestant: Oral: 15-30 minutes

Duration: Immediate release tablet: 4-6 hours; Extended release: ≤12 hours

Absorption: Rapid

Metabolism: Partially hepatic

Half-life elimination: 9-16 hours

Excretion: Urine (70% to 90% as unchanged drug, 1% to 6% as active norpseudoephedrine); dependent on urine pH and flow rate; alkaline urine decreases renal elimination of pseudoephedrine

Contraindications Hypersensitivity to pseudoephedrine or any component of the formulation; with or within 14 days of MAO inhibitor therapy

Warnings/Precautions Use with caution in patients >60 years of age; administer with caution to patients with hypertension, hyperthyroidism, diabetes mellitus, cardiovascular disease, ischemic heart disease, increased intraocular pressure, or prostatic hyperplasia. Elderly patients are more likely to experience adverse reactions to sympathomimetics. Overdosage may cause hallucinations, seizures, CNS depression, and death. When used for self-medication (OTC), notify healthcare provider if symptoms do not improve within 7 days or are accompanied by fever.

Drug Interactions

Decreased effect of methyldopa, reserpine

Increased toxicity: MAO inhibitors may increase blood pressure effects of pseudoephedrine; propranolol, sympathomimetic agents may increase toxicity

Nutritional/Herbal/Ethanol Interactions

Food: Onset of effect may be delayed if pseudoephedrine is taken with food.

Herb/Nutraceutical: Avoid ephedra, yohimbe (may cause hypertension).

Lab Interactions Interferes with urine detection of amphetamine (false-positive)

Adverse Reactions Frequency not defined.

Cardiovascular: Tachycardia, palpitation, arrhythmia

Central nervous system: Nervousness, transient stimulation, insomnia, excitability, dizziness, drowsiness, convulsions, hallucinations, headache

Gastrointestinal: Nausea, vomiting

Genitourinary: Dysuria

Neuromuscular & skeletal: Weakness, tremor

Respiratory: Dyspnea

Miscellaneous: Diaphoresis

Overdosage/Toxicology Symptoms of overdose include seizures, nausea, vomiting, cardiac arrhythmias, hypertension, agitation, hallucinations, and death. There is no specific antidote for pseudoephedrine intoxication. Treatment is primarily supportive.

Dosing

Adults: Nasal congestion: Oral: 30-60 mg every 4-6 hours, sustained release: 120 mg every 12 hours; maximum: 240 mg/24 hours

Elderly: Nasal congestion: 30-60 mg every 6 hours as needed

Pediatrics: Nasal congestion: Oral: General dosing guidelines:

<2 years: 4 mg/kg/day in divided doses every 6 hours

2-5 years: 15 mg every 4-6 hours; maximum: 60 mg/24 hours

6-12 years: 30 mg every 4-6 hours; maximum: 120 mg/24 hours

Renal Impairment: Reduce dose.

Available Dosage Forms

Caplet, extended release, as hydrochloride (Contact® Cold, Sudafed® 12 Hour): 120 mg

Liquid, as hydrochloride: 30 mg/5 mL (120 mL, 480 mL)

Silfedrine Children's: 15 mg/5 mL (120 mL, 480 mL) [alcohol and sugar free; grape flavor]

Simply Stuffy™: 15 mg/5 mL (120 mL) [alcohol free; contains sodium benzoate; cherry berry flavor]

Sudafed® Children's: 15 mg/5 mL (120 mL) [alcohol and sugar free; contains sodium benzoate; grape flavor]

Liquid, oral drops, as hydrochloride:

Dimetapp® Decongestant Infant Drops: 7.5 mg/0.8 mL (15 mL) [alcohol free; contains sodium benzoate; grape flavor]

Kidkare Decongestant: 7.5 mg/0.8 mL (30 mL) [alcohol free; contains benzoic acid and sodium benzoate; cherry flavor]

PediaCare® Decongestant: 7.5 mg/0.8 mL (15 mL) [alcohol free, dye free; contains benzoic acid, sodium benzoate; fruit flavor]

Syrup, as hydrochloride:

Biofed: 30 mg/5 mL (120 mL, 240 mL, 480 mL, 3840 mL) [alcohol free; contains sodium benzoate]

ElixSure™ Congestion: 15 mg/5 mL (120 mL) [grape bubble gum flavor]

Tablet, as hydrochloride: 30 mg, 60 mg

Genaphed®, Kodet SE, Oranyl, Sudafed®, Sudodrin, Sudo-Tab®: 30 mg

SudoGest: 30 mg, 60 mg

Tablet, chewable, as hydrochloride (Sudafed® Children's): 15 mg [sugar free; contains phenylalanine 0.78 mg/tablet; orange flavor]

(Continued)

Pseudoephedrine *(Continued)*

Tablet, extended release, as hydrochloride:
Dimetapp® 12-Hour Non-Drowsy Extentabs®: 120 mg
Sudafed® 24 Hour: 240 mg

Nursing Guidelines

Assessment: Assess effectiveness and interactions of other medications patient may be taking. Monitor effectiveness of therapy and adverse reactions at beginning of therapy and periodically with long-term use. Assess knowledge/ teach patient appropriate use, interventions to reduce side effects, and adverse symptoms to report.

Dietary Considerations: Should be taken with water or milk to decrease GI distress.

Patient Education: Take only as prescribed; do not exceed prescribed dose or frequency. Do not chew or crush timed release forms. Maintain adequate hydration (2-3 L/day of fluids) unless instructed to restrict fluid intake. You may experience nervousness, insomnia, dizziness, or drowsiness (use caution when driving or engaging in tasks requiring alertness until response to drug is known). Report persistent CNS changes (dizziness, tremor, agitation, or convulsions); respiratory difficulty; chest pain, palpitations, or rapid heartbeat; muscle tremor; or lack of improvement or worsening of condition. **Pregnancy/ breast-feeding precautions:** Inform prescriber if you are or intend to become pregnant. Consult prescriber if breast-feeding.

Geriatric Considerations: Elderly patients should be counseled about the proper use of over-the-counter cough and cold preparations. Elderly are more predisposed to adverse effects of sympathomimetics since they frequently have cardiovascular diseases and diabetes mellitus as well as multiple drug therapies. It may be advisable to treat with a short-acting/immediate-release formulation before initiating sustained-release/long-acting formulations.

Pregnancy Risk Factor: C

Lactation: Enters breast milk/use caution (AAP rates "compatible")

Administration

Oral: Do not crush extended release drug product, swallow whole.

♦ Pseudoephedrine, Acetaminophen, and Dextromethorphan *see* Acetaminophen, Dextromethorphan, and Pseudoephedrine *on page 73*

♦ Pseudoephedrine and Loratadine *see* Loratadine and Pseudoephedrine *on page 1060*

♦ Pseudoephedrine and Triprolidine *see* Triprolidine and Pseudoephedrine *on page 1670*

♦ Pseudoephedrine, Dextromethorphan, and Acetaminophen *see* Acetaminophen, Dextromethorphan, and Pseudoephedrine *on page 73*

♦ Pseudoephedrine Hydrochloride *see* Pseudoephedrine *on page 1436*

♦ Pseudoephedrine Sulfate *see* Pseudoephedrine *on page 1436*

♦ Pseudomonic Acid A *see* Mupirocin *on page 1187*

Psyllium (SIL i yum)

U.S. Brand Names Fiberall®; Fibro-Lax [OTC]; Fibro-XL [OTC]; Genfiber® [OTC]; Hydrocil® Instant [OTC]; Konsyl® [OTC]; Konsyl-D® [OTC]; Konsyl® Easy Mix [OTC]; Konsyl® Orange [OTC]; Metamucil® [OTC]; Metamucil® Plus Calcium [OTC]; Metamucil® Smooth Texture [OTC]; Modane® Bulk [OTC]; Natural Fiber Therapy [OTC]; Reguloid® [OTC]; Serutan® [OTC]

Synonyms Plantago Seed; Plantain Seed; Psyllium Hydrophilic Mucilloid

Pharmacologic Category Antidiarrheal; Laxative, Bulk-Producing

Medication Safety Issues

Sound-alike/look-alike issues:
Fiberall® may be confused with Feverall®
Hydrocil® may be confused with Hydrocet®
Modane® may be confused with Matulane®, Moban®
Perdiem® may be confused with Pyridium®

Use Treatment of chronic atonic or spastic constipation and in constipation associated with rectal disorders; management of irritable bowel syndrome; labeled for OTC use as fiber supplement, treatment of constipation

Mechanism of Action Adsorbs water in the intestine to form a viscous liquid which promotes peristalsis and reduces transit time

Pharmacodynamics/Kinetics

Onset of action: 12-24 hours

Peak effect: 2-3 days

Absorption: None; small amounts of grain extracts present in the preparation have been reportedly absorbed following colonic hydrolysis

Contraindications Hypersensitivity to psyllium or any component of the formulation; fecal impaction; GI obstruction

Warnings/Precautions Products must be taken with adequate fluid. Use with caution in patients with esophageal strictures, ulcers, stenosis, or intestinal adhesions; elderly may have insufficient fluid intake which may predispose them to fecal impaction and bowel obstruction.

Drug Interactions Decreased effect of warfarin, digitalis, potassium-sparing diuretics, salicylates, tetracyclines, nitrofurantoin

Adverse Reactions Frequency not defined.

Gastrointestinal: Esophageal or bowel obstruction, diarrhea, constipation, abdominal cramps

Respiratory: Bronchospasm

Miscellaneous: Anaphylaxis upon inhalation in susceptible individuals, rhinoconjunctivitis

Overdosage/Toxicology Symptoms of overdose include abdominal pain, diarrhea, and constipation.

Dosing

Adults & Elderly:

Constipation, IBS: Oral (administer at least 2 hours before or after other drugs): Take 1 dose up to 3 times/day; all doses should be followed with 8 oz of water or liquid

Capsule: 4 capsules/dose (range: 2-6); swallow capsules one at a time

Powder: 1 rounded tablespoonful/dose (1 teaspoonful/dose for many sugar free or select concentrated products) mixed in 8 oz liquid

Tablet: 1 tablet/dose

Wafer: 2 wafers/dose

Pediatrics:

Constipation: Oral (administer at least 2 hours before or after other drugs):

Children 6-11 years: Approximately 1/2 adult dosage

Children ≥12 years: Refer to adult dosing.

Available Dosage Forms

Capsule:

Fibro XL: 675 mg

Metamucil®: 0.52 g [contains potassium 5 mg/capsule; provides 3 g dietary fiber 2.4 g per 6 capsules]

Metamucil® Plus Calcium: 0.42 g [contains potassium 6 mg/capsule; provides dietary fiber 2.1 g and calcium 300 mg per 5 capsules]

Granules (Serutan®): 2.5 g/teaspoon (510 g) [contains sodium benzoate]

Powder: 3.4 g/dose (390 g, 570 g)

Bulk-K: 4.725 g/dose (392 g)

Fiberall®: 3.5 g/dose (454 g) [sugar free; contains phenylalanine; orange flavor]

Fibro-Lax: 4.725 g /dose (140 g, 392g)

Genfiber®: 3.4 g/dose (397 g, 595 g) [regular flavor]

Genfiber®: 3.5 g/dose (283 g) [sugar free; orange flavor]

Hydrocil® Instant: 3.5 g/dose (3.7 g unit-dose packets, 300 g) [sugar free]

Konsyl®: 6 g/dose (6 g unit-dose packets, 300 g, 450 g) [sugar free; contains sodium 4.1 mg/dose; regular flavor]

Konsyl-D®: 3.4 g/dose (6.5 g unit-dose packets, 325 g, 397 g, 500 g) [contains sodium 2.3 mg/dose and dextrose]

Konsyl® Easy Mix: 6 g/dose (6 g unit-dose packets, 250 g) [sugar free; contains sodium 4.4 mg/dose]

Konsyl® Orange: 3.4 g/dose (12 g unit-dose packets, 538 g) [contains sodium 2.3 mg/dose and sucrose; orange flavor]

Konsyl® Orange: 3.4 g/dose (425 g) [sugar free; contains sodium 2.3 mg/dose; orange flavor]

Metamucil®: 3.4 g/dose:

(390 g, 570 g, 870 g) [contains sodium 3 mg and potassium 30 mg per dose; regular flavor]

(570 g, 870 g, 1254 g) [contains sodium 5 mg and potassium 30 mg per dose; orange flavor]

Metamucil® Smooth Texture: 3.4 g/dose:

(unit-dose packets, 609 g, 912 g, 1446 g) [contains sodium 5 mg and potassium 30 mg per dose; orange flavor]

(Continued)

Psyllium *(Continued)*

(300 g, 450 g, 690 g) [contains sodium 4 mg and potassium 30 mg per dose; regular flavor]

(unit-dose packets, 183 g, 300 g, 450 g, 699 g, 1104 g) [sugar free; contains phenylalanine 25 mg, sodium 5 mg, and potassium 30 mg per dose; orange flavor]

Modane® Bulk: 3.4 g/dose (390 g) [contains dextrose; flavor free]

Natural Fiber Therapy: 3.4 g/dose (369 g, 539 g) [natural and orange flavors]

Reguloid®: 3.4 g/dose (300 g, 450 g) [sugar free; regular or orange flavors]; (390 g, 570g) [regular or orange flavors]

Wafers (Metamucil®): 3.4 g/dose (24s) [one dose= 2 wafers; contains sodium 20 mg and potassium 60 mg per dose; apple crisp and cinnamon spice flavors]

Nursing Guidelines

Assessment: See Contraindications, Warnings/Precautions, Drug Interactions, and Dosing for use cautions. Teach patient proper use (according to formulation), possible side effects/appropriate interventions, and adverse symptoms to report (see Patient Education).

Dietary Considerations: Products should be taken with large amount of fluids. Some products contain aspartame, dextrose, or sucrose, as well as additional ingredients. Check individual product information for caloric and nutritional value.

Fiberall® (sugar free formulation) contains phenylalanine.

Metamucil® Smooth Texture (sugar free formulation) contains phenylalanine 25 mg per teaspoonful.

Patient Education: Take as directed. Granules/powder: Mix in large glass of water or juice (8 oz or more) and drink immediately. Maintain adequate hydration (2-3 L/day of fluids), unless instructed to restrict fluid intake. Mix carefully; do not inhale powder. Separate this medication from other medications by at least 1 hour. Results may begin in 12 hours; full results may take 2-3 days. Do not increase dose. Report persistent constipation; watery diarrhea; difficulty, pain, or choking with swallowing; respiratory difficulty; or unusual coughing.

Geriatric Considerations: Elderly may have insufficient fluid intake which may predispose them to fecal impaction and bowel obstruction. Patients should have a 1 month trial, with at least 14 g/day, before effects in bowel function are determined. Bloating and flatulence are mostly a problem in first 4 weeks of therapy.

Pregnancy Risk Factor: B

Lactation: Excretion in breast milk unknown/compatible

Administration

Oral: Inhalation of psyllium dust may cause sensitivity to psyllium (eg, runny nose, watery eyes, wheezing). Drink a full glass of liquid with each dose. Powder must be mixed in a glass of water or juice. Separate dose from other drug therapies.

- **Psyllium Hydrophilic Mucilloid** *see* Psyllium *on page 1438*
- **Pteroylglutamic Acid** *see* Folic Acid *on page 768*
- **Pulmicort Respules®** *see* Budesonide *on page 260*
- **Pulmicort Turbuhaler®** *see* Budesonide *on page 260*
- **Puralube® Tears [OTC]** *see* Artificial Tears *on page 187*
- **PVP-I** *see* Povidone-Iodine *on page 1392*
- **Pyridium®** *see* Phenazopyridine *on page 1342*

Pyridostigmine (peer id oh STIG meen)

U.S. Brand Names Mestinon®; Mestinon® Timespan®; Regonol®

Synonyms Pyridostigmine Bromide

Pharmacologic Category Acetylcholinesterase Inhibitor

Medication Safety Issues

Sound-alike/look-alike issues:

Pyridostigmine may be confused with physostigmine

Mestinon® may be confused with Metatensin®

Regonol® may be confused with Reglan®, Renagel®

Use Symptomatic treatment of myasthenia gravis; antidote for nondepolarizing neuromuscular blockers

Military use: Pretreatment for Soman nerve gas exposure

Mechanism of Action Inhibits destruction of acetylcholine by acetylcholinesterase which facilitates transmission of impulses across myoneural junction

Pharmacodynamics/Kinetics

Onset of action: Oral, I.M.: 15-30 minutes; I.V. injection: 2-5 minutes

Duration: Oral: Up to 6-8 hours (due to slow absorption); I.V.: 2-3 hours

Absorption: Oral: Very poor

Distribution: 19 ± 12 L

Metabolism: Hepatic

Bioavailability: 10% to 20%

Half-life elimination: 1-2 hours; Renal failure: ≤6 hours

Excretion: Urine (80% to 90% as unchanged drug)

Contraindications Hypersensitivity to pyridostigmine, bromides, or any component of the formulation; GI or GU obstruction

Warnings/Precautions Use with caution in patients with epilepsy, asthma, bradycardia, hyperthyroidism, cardiac arrhythmias, or peptic ulcer; adequate facilities should be available for cardiopulmonary resuscitation when testing and adjusting dose for myasthenia gravis; have atropine and epinephrine ready to treat hypersensitivity reactions; overdosage may result in cholinergic crisis, this must be distinguished from myasthenic crisis; anticholinesterase insensitivity can develop for brief or prolonged periods. Safety and efficacy in pediatric patients have not been established.

Regonol® injection contains 1% benzyl alcohol as the preservative (not intended for use in newborns).

Drug Interactions

Aminoglycosides (gentamicin, kanamycin, neomycin, streptomycin): Use of high parenteral doses may intensify/prolong neuromuscular blockade, or lead to resistance of neuromuscular blockade reversal, especially if used with other nondepolarizing neuromuscular-blocking drugs.

Antibiotics (bacitracin, colistin, polymyxin B, sodium colistimethate, tetracycline): Use of high parenteral doses may intensify/prolong neuromuscular blockade, or lead to resistance of neuromuscular blockade reversal, especially if used with other nondepolarizing neuromuscular-blocking drugs.

Beta blockers: Pyridostigmine and beta-blockers may both cause bradycardia and hypotension, effect may be additive; monitor.

Depolarizing neuromuscular-blocking agents (succinylcholine): Increased neuromuscular blocking effect with concomitant use.

Edrophonium: Increased toxicity with concomitant use.

Magnesium: Patients with elevated serum magnesium concentrations may experience enhanced neuromuscular blockage with blocking agents. The reversing effect of pyridostigmine may be compensated.

Quinidine: Recurrent paralysis may occur when quinidine is administered with nondepolarizing neuromuscular-blocking drugs. This may complicate attempts to reverse blockade with pyridostigmine.

Quinolone antibiotics (ciprofloxacin, norfloxacin): Case reports suggest these drugs may exhibit neuromuscular-blocking effects (especially in some patients with myasthenia gravis); monitor.

Lab Interactions Increased aminotransferase [ALT (SGPT)/AST (SGOT)] (S), amylase (S)

Adverse Reactions Frequency not defined.

Cardiovascular: Arrhythmias (especially bradycardia), hypotension, decreased carbon monoxide, tachycardia, AV block, nodal rhythm, nonspecific ECG changes, cardiac arrest, syncope, flushing

Central nervous system: Convulsions, dysarthria, dysphonia, dizziness, loss of consciousness, drowsiness, headache

Dermatologic: Skin rash, thrombophlebitis (I.V.), urticaria

Gastrointestinal: Hyperperistalsis, nausea, vomiting, salivation, diarrhea, stomach cramps, dysphagia, flatulence, abdominal pain

Genitourinary: Urinary urgency

Neuromuscular & skeletal: Weakness, fasciculations, muscle cramps, spasms, arthralgia, myalgia

Ocular: Small pupils, lacrimation, amblyopia

Respiratory: Increased bronchial secretions, laryngospasm, bronchiolar constriction, respiratory muscle paralysis, dyspnea, respiratory depression, respiratory arrest, bronchospasm

Miscellaneous: Diaphoresis (increased), anaphylaxis, allergic reactions

Overdosage/Toxicology Symptoms of overdose include muscle weakness, blurred vision, excessive sweating, tearing and salivation, nausea, vomiting, diarrhea, hypertension, bradycardia, and paralysis. Atropine is the treatment of choice for intoxications manifesting significant muscarinic symptoms. Atropine

(Continued)

Pyridostigmine *(Continued)*

I.V. 2-4 mg every 3-60 minutes should be repeated to control symptoms and then continued as needed for 1-2 days following acute ingestion. Monitor cardiac function and support ventilation.

Dosing

Adults & Elderly:

Myasthenia gravis:

Oral: Highly individualized dosing ranges: 60-1500 mg/day, usually 600 mg/day divided into 5-6 doses, spaced to provide maximum relief

Sustained release formulation: Highly individualized dosing ranges: 180-540 mg once or twice daily (doses separated by at least 6 hours); **Note:** Most clinicians reserve sustained release dosage form for bedtime dose only.

I.M. or slow I.V. Push: To supplement oral dosage pre- and postoperatively during labor and postpartum, during myasthenic crisis, or when oral therapy is impractical): ~1/30th of oral dose; observe patient closely for cholinergic reactions

I.V. infusion: To supplement oral dosage pre- and postoperatively, during labor and postpartum, during myasthenic crisis, or when oral therapy is impractical): Initial: 2 mg/hour with gradual titration in increments of 0.5-1 mg/hour, up to a maximum rate of 4 mg/hour

Pretreatment for Soman nerve gas exposure (military use): Oral: 30 mg every 8 hours beginning several hours prior to exposure; discontinue at first sign of nerve agent exposure, then begin atropine and pralidoxime

Reversal of nondepolarizing muscle relaxants: I.V.: 0.1-0.25 mg/kg/dose; 10-20 mg is usually sufficient (full recovery usually occurs ≤15 minutes, but ≥30 minutes may be required).

Note: Atropine sulfate (0.6-1.2 mg) I.V. immediately prior to pyridostigmine to minimize side effects:

Pediatrics:

Myasthenia gravis:

Oral: Children: 7 mg/kg/24 hours divided into 5-6 doses. Most clinicians reserve sustained release dosage form for bedtime dose only.

I.M., slow I.V. push: Children: 0.05-0.15 mg/kg/dose

Reversal of nondepolarizing muscle relaxants: I.V.: Children: Dosing range: 0.1-0.25 mg/kg/dose (full recovery usually occurs ≤15 minutes, but ≥30 minutes may be required).

Note: Atropine sulfate (0.6-1.2 mg) I.V. immediately prior to pyridostigmine to minimize side effects:

Renal Impairment: Lower dosages may be required due to prolonged elimination; no specific recommendations have been published.

Available Dosage Forms

Injection, solution, as bromide:

Mestinon®: 5 mg/mL (2 mL)

Regonol®: 5 mg/mL (2 mL) [contains benzyl alcohol]

Syrup, as bromide (Mestinon®): 60 mg/5 mL (480 mL) [raspberry flavor; contains alcohol 5%, sodium benzoate]

Tablet, as bromide (Mestinon®): 60 mg

Tablet, sustained release, as bromide (Mestinon® Timespan®): 180 mg

Nursing Guidelines

Assessment: When used to reverse neuromuscular block (anesthesia or excessive acetylcholine), monitor patient safety until full return of neuromuscular functioning. Assess bladder and sphincter adequacy prior to administering medication. Monitor therapeutic effectiveness and adverse reactions (eg, cholinergic crisis). Assess knowledge/teach patient appropriate use (self-injections, oral), interventions to reduce side effects, and adverse symptoms to report.

Patient Education: This drug will not cure myasthenia gravis, but may help reduce symptoms. Use as directed; do not increase dose or discontinue without consulting prescriber. Take extended release tablets at bedtime; do not chew or crush extended release tablets. Maintain adequate hydration (2-3 L/day of fluids) unless instructed to restrict fluid intake. May cause dizziness, drowsiness, or hypotension (rise slowly from sitting or lying position and use caution when driving or climbing stairs); vomiting or loss of appetite (small frequent meals, frequent mouth care, chewing gum, or sucking lozenges may help); or diarrhea (boiled milk, yogurt, or buttermilk may help). Report persistent abdominal discomfort; significantly increased salivation, sweating, tearing, or urination;

flushed skin; chest pain or palpitations; acute headache; unresolved diarrhea; excessive fatigue, insomnia, dizziness, or depression; increased muscle, joint, or body pain; vision changes or blurred vision; or shortness of breath or wheezing.

Geriatric Considerations: See Warnings/Precautions and Adverse Reactions.

Pregnancy Risk Factor: B

Pregnancy Issues: Safety has not been established for use during pregnancy. The potential benefit to the mother should outweigh the potential risk to the fetus. When pyridostigmine is needed in myasthenic mothers, giving dose parenterally 1 hour before completion of the second stage of labor may facilitate delivery and protect the neonate during the immediate postnatal state.

Lactation: Enters breast milk/compatible

Breast-Feeding Considerations: Neonates of myasthenia gravis mothers may have difficulty in sucking and swallowing (as well as breathing). Neonatal pyridostigmine may be indicated by symptoms (confirmed by edrophonium test).

Perioperative/Anesthesia/Other Concerns: Atropine or glycopyrrolate must be administered in combination with pyridostigmine. Large parenteral doses should be accompanied by parenteral atropine. Ephedrine sulfate and potassium chloride have been used orally (in adult patients) to improve response. Extended release products are preferred for use **only** at bedtime for patients who are very weak upon arising.

Administration

Oral: Do **not** crush sustained release tablet.

Storage:

Injection: Protect from light.

Tablet:

30 mg: Store under refrigeration at 2°C to 8°C (36°F to 46°F) and protect from light. Stable at room temperature for up to 3 months.

Mestinon®: Store at 25°C (77°F). Protect from moisture.

♦ Pyridostigmine Bromide *see* Pyridostigmine *on page 1440*

♦ Q-Dryl [OTC] *see* DiphenhydrAMINE *on page 546*

♦ Q-Tussin [OTC] *see* Guaifenesin *on page 834*

♦ Quelicin® *see* Succinylcholine *on page 1573*

♦ Quenalin [OTC] *see* DiphenhydrAMINE *on page 546*

Quetiapine (kwe TYE a peen)

U.S. Brand Names Seroquel®

Synonyms Quetiapine Fumarate

Pharmacologic Category Antipsychotic Agent, Atypical

Medication Safety Issues

Sound-alike/look-alike issues:

Seroquel® may be confused with Serentil®, Serzone®, Sinequan®

Use Treatment of schizophrenia; treatment of acute manic episodes associated with bipolar disorder (as monotherapy or in combination with lithium or valproate)

Unlabeled/Investigational Use Autism, psychosis (children)

Mechanism of Action Mechanism of action of quetiapine (dibenzothiazepine antipsychotic), as with other antipsychotic drugs, is unknown. However, it has been proposed that this drug's antipsychotic activity is mediated through a combination of dopamine type 2 (D_2) and serotonin type 2 (5-HT_2) antagonism. It is an antagonist at multiple neurotransmitter receptors in the brain: serotonin 5-HT_{1A} and 5-HT_2, dopamine D_1 and D_2, histamine H_1, and adrenergic alpha$_1$- and alpha$_2$- receptors; but appears to have no appreciable affinity at cholinergic muscarinic and benzodiazepine receptors.

Antagonism at receptors other than dopamine and 5-HT_2 with similar receptor affinities may explain some of the other effects of quetiapine. The drug's antagonism of histamine H_1-receptors may explain the somnolence observed with it. The drug's antagonism of adrenergic alpha$_1$-receptors may explain the orthostatic hypotension observed with it.

Pharmacodynamics/Kinetics

Absorption: Rapidly absorbed following oral administration

Distribution: V_d: 10 ± 4 L/kg; V_{dss}: ~2 days

Protein binding, plasma: 83%

Metabolism: Primarily hepatic; via CYP3A4; forms two inactive metabolites

Bioavailability: 9% ± 4%; tablet is 100% bioavailable relative to solution

Half-life elimination: Mean: Terminal: ~6 hours

(Continued)

Quetiapine *(Continued)*

Time to peak, plasma: 1.5 hours

Excretion: Urine (73% as metabolites, <1% as unchanged drug); feces (20%)

Contraindications Hypersensitivity to quetiapine or any component of the formulation; severe CNS depression; bone marrow suppression; blood dyscrasias; severe hepatic disease, coma

Warnings/Precautions Patients with dementia-related behavioral disorders treated with atypical antipsychotics are at an increased risk of death compared to placebo. Quetiapine is not approved for this indication.

Has been noted to cause cataracts in animals, lens examination on initiation of therapy and every 6 months is recommended. May be sedating, use with caution in disorders where CNS depression is a feature. Use with caution in Parkinson's disease. Caution in patients with hemodynamic instability; prior myocardial infarction or ischemic heart disease; hypercholesterolemia; thyroid disease; predisposition to seizures; subcortical brain damage; hepatic impairment; severe cardiac, renal, or respiratory disease. May alter temperature regulation or mask toxicity of other drugs due to antiemetic effects. May alter cardiac conduction - life-threatening arrhythmias have occurred with therapeutic doses of antipsychotics. May cause orthostatic hypotension - use with caution in patients at risk of this effect or those who would tolerate transient hypotensive episodes (cerebrovascular disease, cardiovascular disease, or other medications which may predispose). Esophageal dysmotility and aspiration have been associated with antipsychotic use - use with caution in patients at risk of pneumonia (ie, Alzheimer's disease).

May cause anticholinergic effects (confusion, agitation, constipation, xerostomia, blurred vision, urinary retention); therefore, they should be used with caution in patients with decreased gastrointestinal motility, urinary retention, BPH, xerostomia, or visual problems. Conditions which also may be exacerbated by cholinergic blockade include narrow-angle glaucoma (screening is recommended) and worsening of myasthenia gravis. Relative to other antipsychotics, quetiapine has a moderate potency of cholinergic blockade. The risk of extrapyramidal symptoms, tardive dyskinesia, and neuroleptic malignant syndrome (NMS) in association with quetiapine is very low relative to other antipsychotics. May cause hyperglycemia; in some cases may be extreme and associated with ketoacidosis, hyperosmolar coma, or death. Use with caution in patients with diabetes or other disorders of glucose regulation; monitor for worsening of glucose control.

The possibility of a suicide attempt is inherent in psychotic illness or bipolar disorder; use caution in high-risk patients during initiation of therapy. Prescriptions should be written for the smallest quantity consistent with good patient care.

Drug Interactions **Substrate** of CYP2D6 (minor), 3A4 (major)

Acetylcholinesterase inhibitors (central): May increase the risk of antipsychotic-related extrapyramidal symptoms; monitor.

Antihypertensives: Concurrent use with an antihypertensive may produce additive hypotensive effects (particularly orthostasis)

Azole antifungals (fluconazole, itraconazole, ketoconazole): Administration with ketoconazole increases serum concentration of quetiapine by 335%; use with caution.

Cimetidine: May decrease quetiapine's clearance by 20%; increasing serum concentrations.

CNS depressants: Quetiapine may enhance the sedative effects of other CNS depressants; includes antidepressants, benzodiazepines, barbiturates, ethanol, narcotic analgesics, and other sedative agents; monitor for increased effect.

CYP3A4 inducers: CYP3A4 inducers may decrease the levels/effects of quetiapine. Example inducers include aminoglutethimide, carbamazepine, nafcillin, nevirapine, phenobarbital, phenytoin, and rifamycins. Higher maintenance doses of quetiapine may be required.

CYP3A4 inhibitors: May increase the levels/effects of quetiapine. Example inhibitors include azole antifungals, clarithromycin, diclofenac, doxycycline, erythromycin, imatinib, isoniazid, nefazodone, nicardipine, propofol, protease inhibitors, quinidine, telithromycin, and verapamil.

Divalproex: Concomitant use of quetiapine and divalproex increased the mean maximum plasma concentration of quetiapine at by 17% at steady state. The mean oral clearance of valproic acid was increased by 11%.

Levodopa: Quetiapine may inhibit the antiparkinsonian effect of levodopa; monitor.

Lorazepam: Metabolism of lorazepam may be reduced by quetiapine; clearance is reduced 20% in the presence of quetiapine; monitor for increased sedative effect.

Metoclopramide: May increase extrapyramidal symptoms (EPS) or risk.

Phenytoin: Metabolism/clearance of quetiapine may be increased; fivefold changes have been noted. Higher maintenance doses of quetiapine may be required.

Thioridazine: May increase clearance of quetiapine, decreasing serum concentrations; clearance may be increased by 65%.

Nutritional/Herbal/Ethanol Interactions

Ethanol: Avoid ethanol (may cause excessive impairment in cognition/motor function).

Food: In healthy volunteers, administration of quetiapine with food resulted in an increase in the peak serum concentration and AUC (each by ~15%) compared to the fasting state.

Herb/Nutraceutical: St John's wort may decrease quetiapine levels. Avoid valerian, St John's wort, kava kava, gotu kola (may increase CNS depression).

Adverse Reactions

>10%:

Central nervous system: Agitation, dizziness, headache, somnolence

Endocrine & metabolic: Cholesterol increased (11%), triglycerides increased (17%)

Gastrointestinal: Weight gain (≥7% body weight, dose related), xerostomia

1% to 10%:

Cardiovascular: Postural hypotension, tachycardia, palpitation, peripheral edema

Central nervous system: Anxiety, fever, pain

Dermatologic: Rash

Gastrointestinal: Abdominal pain (dose related), constipation, dyspepsia (dose related), anorexia, vomiting, gastroenteritis

Hematologic: Leukopenia

Hepatic: AST increased, ALT increased, GGT increased

Neuromuscular & skeletal: Dysarthria, back pain, weakness, tremor, hypertonia, dysarthria

Ocular: Amblyopia

Respiratory: Rhinitis, pharyngitis, cough, dyspnea

Miscellaneous: Diaphoresis, flu-like syndrome

<1% (Limited to important or life-threatening): Agranulocytosis, anaphylaxis, diabetes mellitus, hyperglycemia, hyperlipidemia, hyponatremia, hypothyroidism, increased appetite, increased salivation, involuntary movements, leukocytosis, neutropenia, photosensitivity, QT prolongation, rash, rhabdomyolysis, SIADH, Stevens-Johnson syndrome, tardive dyskinesia, vertigo

Dosing

Adults:

Schizophrenia/psychosis: Oral: 25-100 mg 2-3 times/day; usual starting dose 25 mg twice daily, increased in increments of 25-50 mg 2-3 times/day on the second or third day. By the fourth day, the dose should be in the range of 300-400 mg/day in 2-3 divided doses. Further adjustments may be made, as needed, at intervals of at least 2 days in adjustments of 25-50 mg twice daily. Usual maintenance range: 150-750 mg/day.

Mania: Oral: Initial: 50 mg twice daily on day 1, increase dose in increments of 100 mg/day to 200 mg twice daily on day 4; may increase to a target dose of 800 mg/day by day 6 at increments of ≤200 mg/day. Usual dosage range: 400-800 mg/day

Note: Dose reductions should be attempted periodically to establish lowest effective dose in patients with psychosis or to establish need to continue treating agitated symptoms in demented older adults. Patients being restarted after 1 week of no drug need to be titrated as above.

Elderly: Lower clearance in elderly patients (40%), resulting in higher concentrations. Dosage adjustment may be required.

Pediatrics: Children and Adolescents:

Autism (unlabeled use): Oral: 100-350 mg/day (1.6-5.2 mg/kg/day)

Psychosis and mania (unlabeled use): Oral: Initial: 25 mg twice daily; titrate as necessary to 450 mg/day

Renal Impairment: No dosage adjustment required: 25% lower mean oral clearance of quetiapine than normal subjects; however, plasma concentrations similar to normal subjects receiving the same dose.

(Continued)

Quetiapine *(Continued)*

Hepatic Impairment: Lower clearance in hepatic impairment (30%), may result in higher concentrations. Dosage adjustment may be required.

Oral: Initial: 25 mg/day, increase dose by 25-50 mg/day to effective dose, based on clinical response and tolerability to patient

Available Dosage Forms Tablet, as fumarate: 25 mg, 100 mg, 200 mg, 300 mg [contains lactose]

Nursing Guidelines

Assessment: Assess other medications patient is taking for effectiveness and interactions (especially drugs affected by P450 enzymes). Assess results of laboratory tests, therapeutic effectiveness, and adverse reactions at beginning of therapy and periodically with long-term use. Evaluate for cataracts before initiating treatment and every 6 months during chronic treatment. Monitor weight prior to initiating therapy and at least monthly. Consider titrating to a different antipsychotic agent for weight gain ≥ 5% of initial weight. Initiate at lower doses and taper dosage slowly when discontinuing. Assess knowledge/teach patient appropriate use, interventions to reduce side effects, and adverse symptoms to report.

Monitoring Laboratory Tests: Fasting lipid profile and fasting blood glucose/Hgb A_{1c} (prior to treatment, at 3 months, then annually)

Dietary Considerations: May be taken with or without food.

Patient Education: Use exactly as directed; do not increase dose or frequency. It may take 2-3 weeks to achieve desired results; do not discontinue without consulting prescriber. Avoid alcohol or caffeine and other prescriptions or OTC medications not approved by prescriber. Maintain adequate hydration (2-3 L/day of fluids) unless instructed to restrict fluid intake. If diabetic, you may experience increased blood sugars. Monitor blood closely. You may experience excess drowsiness, restlessness, dizziness, or blurred vision (use caution driving or when engaging in tasks requiring alertness until response to drug is known); mouth sores or GI upset (small frequent meals, frequent mouth care, chewing gum, or sucking lozenges may help); constipation (increased exercise, fluids, fruit, or fiber may help); or postural hypotension (use caution climbing stairs or when changing position from lying or sitting to standing). Report persistent CNS effects (eg, somnolence, agitation, insomnia); severe dizziness; vision changes; respiratory difficulty; or worsening of condition. **Pregnancy/breast-feeding precautions:** Inform prescriber if you are or intend to become pregnant. Breast-feeding is not recommended.

Geriatric Considerations: (See Warnings/Precautions, Adverse Reactions, and Overdose/Toxicology.) Elderly patients have an increased risk of adverse response to side effects or adverse reactions to antipsychotics.

Pregnancy Risk Factor: C

Lactation: Excretion in breast milk unknown/not recommended

Perioperative/Anesthesia/Other Concerns: Quetiapine has a very low incidence of extrapyramidal symptoms such as restlessness and abnormal movement, and is at least as effective as conventional antipsychotics. For patients who have been off quetiapine for more than 1 week, dose titration is necessary when restarting the medication.

♦ Quetiapine Fumarate *see* Quetiapine *on page 1443*
♦ Quibron®-T *see* Theophylline *on page 1619*
♦ Quibron®-T/SR *see* Theophylline *on page 1619*

Quinapril (KWIN a pril)

U.S. Brand Names Accupril®

Synonyms Quinapril Hydrochloride

Pharmacologic Category Angiotensin-Converting Enzyme (ACE) Inhibitor

Medication Safety Issues

Sound-alike/look-alike issues:

Accupril® may be confused with Accolate®, Accutane®, AcipHex®, Monopril®

Use Management of hypertension; treatment of congestive heart failure

Unlabeled/Investigational Use Treatment of left ventricular dysfunction after myocardial infarction

Mechanism of Action Competitive inhibitor of angiotensin-converting enzyme (ACE); prevents conversion of angiotensin I to angiotensin II, a potent vasoconstrictor; results in lower levels of angiotensin II which causes an increase in plasma renin activity and a reduction in aldosterone secretion; a CNS mechanism may also be involved in hypotensive effect as angiotensin II increases adrenergic outflow from CNS; vasoactive kallikreins may be decreased in conversion to active hormones by ACE inhibitors, thus reducing blood pressure

Pharmacodynamics/Kinetics

Onset of action: 1 hour

Duration: 24 hours

Absorption: Quinapril: ≥60%

Protein binding: Quinapril: 97%; Quinaprilat: 97%

Metabolism: Rapidly hydrolyzed to quinaprilat, the active metabolite

Half-life elimination: Quinapril: 0.8 hours; Quinaprilat: 3 hours; increases as Cl_{cr} decreases

Time to peak, serum: Quinapril: 1 hour; Quinaprilat: ~2 hours

Excretion: Urine (50% to 60% primarily as quinaprilat)

Contraindications Hypersensitivity to quinapril or any component of the formulation; angioedema related to previous treatment with an ACE inhibitor; bilateral renal artery stenosis; patients with idiopathic or hereditary angioedema; pregnancy (2nd and 3rd trimesters)

Warnings/Precautions Anaphylactic reactions can occur. Angioedema can occur at any time during treatment (especially following first dose). Angioedema may involve head and neck (potentially affecting the airway) or the intestine (presenting with abdominal pain). Careful blood pressure monitoring with first dose (hypotension can occur especially in volume-depleted patients). Dosage adjustment needed in renal impairment. Use with caution in hypovolemia; collagen vascular diseases; valvular stenosis (particularly aortic stenosis); hyperkalemia; or before, during, or immediately after anesthesia. Avoid rapid dosage escalation, which may lead to renal insufficiency. Rare toxicities associated with ACE inhibitors include cholestatic jaundice (which may progress to hepatic necrosis) and neutropenia/agranulocytosis with myeloid hyperplasia. If patient has renal impairment, a baseline WBC with differential and serum creatinine should be evaluated and monitored closely during the first 3 months of therapy.

Hypersensitivity reactions may be seen during hemodialysis with high-flux dialysis membranes (eg, AN69). Patients receiving ACE inhibitors have experienced rare life-threatening anaphylactoid reactions during desensitization. Rare hepatic reactions, progressing from cholestatic jaundice to hepatic necrosis, have been reported with ACE inhibitors. Discontinue if marked elevation of hepatic transaminases or jaundice occurs.

Use with caution in unilateral renal artery stenosis and pre-existing renal insufficiency. Deterioration in renal function can occur with initiation.

Drug Interactions

$Alpha_1$ blockers: Hypotensive effect increased.

Aspirin: The effects of ACE inhibitors may be blunted by aspirin administration, particularly at higher dosages (see Cardiovascular Considerations) and/or increase adverse renal effects.

Diuretics: Hypovolemia due to diuretics may precipitate acute hypotensive events or acute renal failure.

Insulin: Risk of hypoglycemia may be increased.

Lithium: Risk of lithium toxicity may be increased; monitor lithium levels, especially the first 4 weeks of therapy.

Mercaptopurine: Risk of neutropenia may be increased.

NSAIDs: May attenuate hypertensive efficacy; effect has been seen with captopril and may occur with other ACE inhibitors; monitor blood pressure. May increase risk of adverse renal effects.

Potassium-sparing diuretics (amiloride, spironolactone, triamterene): Increased risk of hyperkalemia.

Potassium supplements may increase the risk of hyperkalemia.

Quinolones: Absorption may be decreased by quinapril; separate administration by at least 2-4 hours.

Tetracyclines: Absorption may be reduced by quinapril; separate administration by at least 2-4 hours.

Trimethoprim (high dose) may increase the risk of hyperkalemia.

Nutritional/Herbal/Ethanol Interactions Herb/Nutraceutical: Avoid dong quai if using for hypertension (has estrogenic activity). Avoid ephedra, yohimbe, ginseng (may worsen hypertension). Avoid garlic (may have increased antihypertensive effect).

Adverse Reactions Note: Frequency ranges include data from hypertension and heart failure trials. Higher rates of adverse reactions have generally been noted in patients with CHF. However, the frequency of adverse effects associated with placebo is also increased in this population.

(Continued)

Quinapril *(Continued)*

1% to 10%:

Cardiovascular: Hypotension (3%), chest pain (2%), first-dose hypotension (up to 3%)

Central nervous system: Dizziness (4% to 8%), headache (2% to 6%), fatigue (3%)

Dermatologic: Rash (1%)

Endocrine & metabolic: Hyperkalemia (2%)

Gastrointestinal: Vomiting/nausea (1% to 2%), diarrhea (1.7%)

Neuromuscular & skeletal: Myalgias (2% to 5%), back pain (1%)

Renal: Increased BUN/serum creatinine (2%, transient elevations may occur with a higher frequency), worsening of renal function (in patients with bilateral renal artery stenosis or hypovolemia)

Respiratory: Upper respiratory symptoms, cough (2% to 4%; up to 13% in some studies), dyspnea (2%)

<1% (Limited to important or life-threatening): Acute renal failure, agranulocytosis, alopecia, amblyopia, anaphylactoid reaction, angina, angioedema, arrhythmia, arthralgia, depression, dermatopolymyositis, edema, eosinophilic pneumonitis, exfoliative dermatitis, hemolytic anemia, hepatitis, hyperkalemia, hypertensive crisis, impotence, insomnia, MI, orthostatic hypotension, pancreatitis, paresthesia, pemphigus, photosensitivity, pruritus, shock, somnolence, stroke, syncope, thrombocytopenia, vertigo

A syndrome which may include fever, myalgia, arthralgia, interstitial nephritis, vasculitis, rash, eosinophilia and positive ANA, and elevated ESR has been reported with ACE inhibitors. In addition, pancreatitis, hepatic necrosis, neutropenia, and/or agranulocytosis (particularly in patients with collagen-vascular disease or renal impairment) have been associated with many ACE inhibitors.

Overdosage/Toxicology Mild hypotension has been the primary toxic effect seen with acute overdose. Bradycardia may also occur. Hyperkalemia occurs even with therapeutic doses, especially in patients with renal insufficiency and those taking NSAIDs. Treatment is symptom-directed and supportive.

Dosing

Adults:

Hypertension: Oral: Initial: 10-20 mg once daily, adjust according to blood pressure response at peak and trough blood levels; initial dose may be reduced to 5 mg in patients receiving diuretic therapy if the diuretic is continued.

Usual dose range (JNC 7): 10-40 mg once daily

Congestive heart failure or post-MI: Oral: Initial: 5 mg once or twice daily, titrated at weekly intervals to 20-40 mg daily in 2 divided doses; target dose (heart failure): 20 mg twice daily (ACC/AHA 2005 Heart Failure Guidelines)

Elderly: Oral: Initial: 2.5-5 mg/day; increase dosage at increments of 2.5-5 mg at 1- to 2-week intervals; adjust for renal impairment.

Renal Impairment: Lower initial doses should be used; after initial dose (if tolerated), administer initial dose twice daily; may be increased at weekly intervals to optimal response:

Hypertension: Oral: Initial:

Cl_{cr} >60 mL/minute: Administer 10 mg/day

Cl_{cr} 30-60 mL/minute: Administer 5 mg/day

Cl_{cr} 10-30 mL/minute: Administer 2.5 mg/day

Congestive heart failure: Oral: Initial:

Cl_{cr} >30 mL/minute: Administer 5 mg/day

Cl_{cr} 10-30 mL/minute: Administer 2.5 mg/day

Hepatic Impairment: In patients with alcoholic cirrhosis, hydrolysis of quinapril to quinaprilat is impaired; however, the subsequent elimination of quinaprilat is unaltered.

Available Dosage Forms Tablet, as hydrochloride: 5 mg, 10 mg, 20 mg, 40 mg

Nursing Guidelines

Assessment: See Contraindications, Warnings/Precautions, and Dosing for use cautions. Assess potential for interactions with other prescriptions, OTC medications, or herbal products patient may be taking (see Drug Interactions). May be advisable to administer first dose in prescriber's office with careful blood pressure monitoring (hypotension angioedema can occur at any time during treatment, especially following first dose). Assess results of laboratory tests (see below) and patient response at beginning of therapy, when adjusting dose, and periodically with long-term therapy (eg, BP, cardiac status and fluid balance - see Adverse Reactions and Overdose/Toxicology). Teach patient appropriate use, possible side effects/appropriate interventions, and adverse symptoms to report (see Patient Education). **Pregnancy risk factor C/D** - determine that patient is not pregnant prior to beginning therapy. Instruct patient in appropriate use of barrier contraceptives (see Pregnancy Issues). Note breast-feeding caution.

Monitoring Laboratory Tests: CBC, renal function tests, electrolytes If patient has renal impairment, a baseline WBC with differential and serum creatinine should be evaluated and monitored closely during the first 3 months of therapy.

Patient Education: Inform prescriber of all prescriptions, OTC medications, or herbal products you are taking, and any allergies you have. Do not take any new medication during therapy unless approved by prescriber. Take as directed; do not alter dose or discontinue without consulting prescriber. Take first dose at bedtime or when sitting down (hypotension may occur). This drug does not eliminate need for diet or exercise regimen as recommended by prescriber. May cause increased cough (if persistent or bothersome, contact prescriber); postural hypotension (use caution when rising from lying or sitting position or climbing stairs); headache (consult prescriber for approved analgesic); dizziness (use caution when driving or engaging in tasks that require alertness until response to drug is known); nausea or vomiting (small, frequent meals, frequent mouth care, sucking lozenges, or chewing gum may help); or muscle or back pain (consult prescriber for approved analgesic). Immediately report swelling of face, mouth, lips, tongue or throat; chest pain or respiratory difficulty. Report persistent cough; persistent pain in muscles, joints, or back; skin rash; or other persistent adverse reactions. **Pregnancy/breast-feeding precautions:** Inform prescriber if you are or intend to become pregnant. This drug should not be used in the 2nd or 3rd trimester of pregnancy. Consult prescriber for appropriate contraceptive measures if necessary. Consult prescriber if breast-feeding.

Geriatric Considerations: Due to frequent decreases in glomerular filtration (also creatinine clearance) with aging, elderly patients may have exaggerated responses to ACE inhibitors. Differences in clinical response due to hepatic changes are not observed.

Pregnancy Risk Factor: C (1st trimester)/D (2nd and 3rd trimesters)

Pregnancy Issues: ACE inhibitors can cause fetal injury or death if taken during the 2nd or 3rd trimester. Discontinue ACE inhibitors as soon as pregnancy is detected.

Lactation: Enters breast milk/use caution

Perioperative/Anesthesia/Other Concerns: ACE inhibitors decrease morbidity and mortality in patients with asymptomatic and symptomatic left ventricular dysfunction. ACE inhibitors are also indicated in patients postmyocardial infarction in whom left ventricular ejection fraction is <40%.

ACE inhibitor therapy may elicit rapid increases in potassium and creatinine, especially when used in patients with bilateral renal artery stenosis. When ACE inhibition is introduced in patients with pre-existing diuretic therapy who are hypovolemic, the ACE inhibitor may induce acute hypotension. To prevent this, discontinue diuretics 2-3 days prior to initiating quinapril; may restart diuretics if blood pressure is not controlled by quinapril alone. Because of the potent teratogenic effects of ACE inhibitors, these drugs should be avoided, if possible, when treating women of childbearing potential not on effective birth control measures.

Administration

Reconstitution: Unstable in aqueous solutions. To prepare solution for oral administration, mix prior to administration and use within 10 minutes.

Storage: Store at room temperature.

♦ **Quinapril Hydrochloride** *see* Quinapril *on page 1446*

Quinidine (KWIN i deen)

Synonyms Quinidine Gluconate; Quinidine Polygalacturonate; Quinidine Sulfate

Pharmacologic Category Antiarrhythmic Agent, Class Ia

Medication Safety Issues

Sound-alike/look-alike issues:

Quinidine may be confused with clonidine, quinine, Quinora®

Use Prophylaxis after cardioversion of atrial fibrillation and/or flutter to maintain normal sinus rhythm; prevent recurrence of paroxysmal supraventricular tachycardia, paroxysmal AV junctional rhythm, paroxysmal ventricular tachycardia,

(Continued)

Quinidine *(Continued)*

paroxysmal atrial fibrillation, and atrial or ventricular premature contractions; has activity against *Plasmodium falciparum* malaria

Mechanism of Action Class 1a antiarrhythmic agent; depresses phase O of the action potential; decreases myocardial excitability and conduction velocity, and myocardial contractility by decreasing sodium influx during depolarization and potassium efflux in repolarization; also reduces calcium transport across cell membrane

Pharmacodynamics/Kinetics

Distribution: V_d: Adults: 2-3.5 L/kg, decreased with congestive heart failure, malaria; increased with cirrhosis; crosses placenta; enters breast milk

Protein binding:

Newborns: 60% to 70%; decreased protein binding with cyanotic congenital heart disease, cirrhosis, or acute myocardial infarction

Adults: 80% to 90%

Metabolism: Extensively hepatic (50% to 90%) to inactive compounds

Bioavailability: Sulfate: 80%; Gluconate: 70%

Half-life elimination, plasma: Children: 2.5-6.7 hours; Adults: 6-8 hours; prolonged with elderly, cirrhosis, and congestive heart failure

Excretion: Urine (15% to 25% as unchanged drug)

Contraindications Hypersensitivity to quinidine or any component of the formulation; thrombocytopenia; thrombocytopenic purpura; myasthenia gravis; heart block greater than first degree; idioventricular conduction delays (except in patients with a functioning artificial pacemaker); those adversely affected by anticholinergic activity; concurrent use of quinolone antibiotics which prolong QT interval, cisapride, amprenavir, or ritonavir

Warnings/Precautions Monitor and adjust dose to prevent QT_c prolongation. Watch for proarrhythmic effects. May precipitate or exacerbate CHF. Reduce dosage in hepatic impairment. In patients with atrial fibrillation or flutter, block the AV node before initiating. Correct hypokalemia before initiating therapy. Hypokalemia may worsen toxicity. Use may cause digoxin-induced toxicity (adjust digoxin's dose). Use caution with concurrent use of other antiarrhythmics. Hypersensitivity reactions can occur. Can unmask sick sinus syndrome (causes bradycardia). Has been associated with severe hepatotoxic reactions, including granulomatous hepatitis. Hemolysis may occur in patients with G6PD (glucose-6-phosphate dehydrogenase) deficiency. Different salt products are not interchangeable.

Drug Interactions **Substrate** of CYP2C8/9 (minor), 2E1 (minor), 3A4 (major); **Inhibits** CYP2C8/9 (weak), 2D6 (strong), 3A4 (strong)

Amiloride may cause prolonged ventricular conduction leading to arrhythmias.

Amiodarone may increase quinidine blood levels; monitor quinidine levels.

Cimetidine: Increase quinidine blood levels; closely monitor levels or use an alternative H_2 antagonist.

Cisapride and quinidine may increase risk of malignant arrhythmias; concurrent use is contraindicated.

Codeine: Analgesic efficacy may be reduced.

CYP2D6 substrates: Quinidine may increase the levels/effects of CYP2D6 substrates. Example substrates include amphetamines, selected beta-blockers, dextromethorphan, fluoxetine, lidocaine, mirtazapine, nefazodone, paroxetine, risperidone, ritonavir, thioridazine, tricyclic antidepressants, and venlafaxine.

CYP2D6 prodrug substrates: Quinidine may decrease the levels/effects of CYP2D6 prodrug substrates. Example prodrug substrates include codeine, hydrocodone, oxycodone, and tramadol.

CYP3A4 inducers: CYP3A4 inducers may decrease the levels/effects of quinidine. Example inducers include aminoglutethimide, carbamazepine, nafcillin, nevirapine, phenobarbital, phenytoin, and rifamycins.

CYP3A4 inhibitors: May increase the levels/effects of quinidine. Example inhibitors include azole antifungals, clarithromycin, diclofenac, doxycycline, erythromycin, imatinib, isoniazid, nefazodone, nicardipine, propofol, protease inhibitors, telithromycin, and verapamil.

CYP3A4 substrates: Quinidine may increase the levels/effects of CYP3A4 substrates. Example substrates include benzodiazepines, calcium channel blockers, mirtazapine, nateglinide, nefazodone, tacrolimus, and venlafaxine. Selected benzodiazepines (midazolam and triazolam), cisapride, ergot alkaloids, selected HMG-CoA reductase inhibitors (lovastatin and simvastatin), and pimozide are generally contraindicated with strong CYP3A4 inhibitors.

Digoxin blood levels may be increased. Monitor digoxin blood levels.

Metoprolol: Increased metoprolol blood levels.
Mexiletine blood levels may be increased.
Nifedipine blood levels may be increased by quinidine; nifedipine may decrease quinidine blood levels.
Propafenone blood levels may be increased.
Propranolol blood levels may be increased.
QT_c-prolonging agents (eg, amiodarone, amitriptyline, bepridil, disopyramide, erythromycin, haloperidol, imipramine, pimozide, procainamide, sotalol, thioridazine): Effects may be additive; use with caution.
Ritonavir, nelfinavir and amprenavir may increase quinidine levels and toxicity; concurrent use is contraindicated.
Sparfloxacin, gatifloxacin, and moxifloxacin may result in additional prolongation of the QT interval; concurrent use is contraindicated.
Timolol blood levels may be increased.
Urinary alkalinizers (antacids, sodium bicarbonate, acetazolamide) increase quinidine blood levels.
Verapamil and diltiazem increase quinidine blood levels.
Warfarin effects may be increased by quinidine; monitor INR closely during addition or withdrawal of quinidine.

Nutritional/Herbal/Ethanol Interactions

Food: Dietary salt intake may alter the rate and extent of quinidine absorption. A decrease in dietary salt may lead to an increase in quinidine serum concentrations. Avoid changes in dietary salt intake. Quinidine serum levels may be increased if taken with food. Food has a variable effect on absorption of sustained release formulation. The rate of absorption of quinidine may be decreased following the ingestion of grapefruit juice. In addition, CYP3A4 metabolism of quinidine may be reduced by grapefruit juice. Grapefruit juice should be avoided. Excessive intake of fruit juices or vitamin C may decrease urine pH and result in increased clearance of quinidine with decreased serum concentration. Alkaline foods may result in increased quinidine serum concentrations.

Herb/Nutraceutical: St John's wort may decrease quinidine levels. Avoid ephedra (may worsen arrhythmia).

Adverse Reactions

Frequency not defined: Hypotension, syncope

>10%:

Cardiovascular: QT_c prolongation (modest prolongation is common, however, excessive prolongation is rare and indicates toxicity)
Central nervous system: Lightheadedness (15%)
Gastrointestinal: Diarrhea (35%), upper GI distress, bitter taste, diarrhea, anorexia, nausea, vomiting, stomach cramping (22%)

1% to 10%:

Cardiovascular: Angina (6%), palpitation (7%), new or worsened arrhythmia (proarrhythmic effect)
Central nervous system: Syncope (1% to 8%), headache (7%), fatigue (7%), sleep disturbance (3%), tremor (2%), nervousness (2%), incoordination (1%)
Dermatologic: Rash (5%)
Neuromuscular & skeletal: Weakness (5%)
Ocular: Blurred vision
Otic: Tinnitus
Respiratory: Wheezing

<1% (Limited to important or life-threatening): Abnormal pigmentation, acute psychotic reactions, agranulocytosis, angioedema, arthralgia, bronchospasm, cerebral hypoperfusion (possibly resulting in ataxia, apprehension, and seizure), cholestasis, confusion, delirium, depression, drug-induced lupus-like syndrome, eczematous dermatitis, esophagitis, exacerbated bradycardia (in sick sinus syndrome), exfoliative rash, fever, flushing, granulomatous hepatitis, hallucinations, heart block, hemolytic anemia, hepatotoxic reaction (rare), impaired hearing, increased CPK, lichen planus, livedo reticularis, lymphadenopathy, melanin pigmentation of the hard palate, myalgia, mydriasis, nephropathy, optic neuritis, pancytopenia, paradoxical increase in ventricular rate during atrial fibrillation/flutter, photosensitivity, pneumonitis, pruritus, psoriaform rash, QT_c prolongation (excessive), respiratory depression, sicca syndrome, tachycardia, thrombocytopenia, thrombocytopenic purpura, torsade de pointes, urticaria, uveitis, vascular collapse, vasculitis, ventricular fibrillation, ventricular tachycardia, vertigo, visual field loss

Note: Cinchonism, a syndrome which may include tinnitus, high-frequency hearing loss, deafness, vertigo, blurred vision, diplopia, photophobia, headache,
(Continued)

Quinidine *(Continued)*

confusion, and delirium has been associated with quinidine use. Usually associated with chronic toxicity, this syndrome has also been described after brief exposure to a moderate dose in sensitive patients. Vomiting and diarrhea may also occur as isolated reactions to therapeutic quinidine levels.

Overdosage/Toxicology Has a low toxic:therapeutic ratio and may easily produce fatal intoxication (acute toxic dose: 1 g in adults). Symptoms of overdose include sinus bradycardia, sinus node arrest or asystole, P-R, QRS, or QT interval prolongation, torsade de pointes (polymorphous ventricular tachycardia), and depressed myocardial contractility, which along with alpha-adrenergic or ganglionic blockade, may result in hypotension and pulmonary edema. Other effects are anticholinergic (dry mouth, dilated pupils, and delirium) as well as seizures, coma, and respiratory arrest. Treatment is symptomatic and effects usually respond to conventional therapies. **Note:** Do not use other Class 1A or 1C antiarrhythmic agents to treat ventricular tachycardia. Sodium bicarbonate may treat wide QRS intervals or hypotension. Markedly impaired conduction or high degree AV block, unresponsive to bicarbonate, indicates consideration of a pacemaker.

Dosing

Adults & Elderly:

Note: Dosage expressed in terms of the salt: 267 mg of quinidine gluconate = 275 mg of quinidine polygalacturonate = 200 mg of quinidine sulfate.

Test dose for idiosyncratic reaction: Oral, I.M.: 200 mg administered several hours before full dosage (to determine possibility of idiosyncratic reaction)

Antiarrhythmic:

Oral:

Sulfate: 100-600 mg/dose every 4-6 hours; begin at 200 mg/dose and titrate to desired effect (maximum daily dose: 3-4 g)

Gluconate: 324-972 mg every 8-12 hours

I.M.: 400 mg/dose every 4-6 hours

I.V.: 200-400 mg/dose diluted and given at a rate ≤10 mg/minute

Pediatrics:

Note: Dosage expressed in terms of the salt: 267 mg of quinidine gluconate = 200 mg of quinidine sulfate.

Test dose for idiosyncratic reaction (sulfate, oral or gluconate, I.M.): Children: 2 mg/kg or 60 mg/m^2

Antiarrhythmic: Oral (quinidine sulfate): Children: 15-60 mg/kg/day in 4-5 divided doses or 6 mg/kg every 4-6 hours; usual 30 mg/kg/day or 900 mg/m^2/day given in 5 daily doses

I.V. **not** recommended (quinidine gluconate): Children: 2-10 mg/kg/dose given at a rate ≤10 mg/minute every 3-6 hours as needed

Renal Impairment:

Cl_{cr} <10 mL/minute: Administer 75% of normal dose.

Hemodialysis effects: Slightly hemodialyzable (5% to 20%); 200 mg supplemental dose posthemodialysis is recommended; not dialyzable (0% to 5%) by peritoneal dialysis.

Hepatic Impairment: Larger loading dose may be indicated; reduce maintenance doses by 50% and monitor serum levels closely.

Available Dosage Forms

Injection, solution, as gluconate: 80 mg/mL (10 mL) [equivalent to quinidine base 50 mg]

Tablet, as sulfate: 200 mg, 300 mg

Tablet, extended release, as gluconate: 324 mg [equivalent to quinidine base 202 mg]

Tablet, extended release, as sulfate: 300 mg [equivalent to quinidine base 249 mg]

Nursing Guidelines

Assessment: Assess other medications patient may be taking for effectiveness and interactions. I.V. requires use of infusion pump and continuous cardiac and hemodynamic monitoring. Assess results of laboratory tests, therapeutic effectiveness (monitor cardiac functioning closely), and adverse reactions at beginning of therapy, when titrating dosage, and on a regular basis with long-term therapy. **Note:** Quinidine has a low TI and overdose may easily produce severe and life-threatening reactions. Assess knowledge/teach patient appropriate use, interventions to reduce side effects, and adverse symptoms to report.

Monitoring Laboratory Tests: Routine CBC, liver and renal function during long-term administration

Dietary Considerations: Administer with food or milk to decrease gastrointestinal irritation. Avoid changes in dietary salt intake.

Patient Education: Take exactly as directed, around-the-clock; do not take additional doses or discontinue without consulting prescriber. Do not crush, chew, or break sustained release dosage forms. Do not take with grapefruit juice. You will need regular cardiac checkups and blood tests while taking this medication. You may experience dizziness, drowsiness, or visual changes (use caution when driving or engaging in tasks requiring alertness until response to drug is known); abnormal taste, nausea or vomiting, or loss of appetite (small frequent meals, frequent mouth care, chewing gum, or sucking lozenges may help); headaches (prescriber may recommend mild analgesic); or diarrhea (yogurt or boiled milk may help; if persistent consult prescriber). Report chest pain, palpitation, or erratic heartbeat; respiratory difficulty or wheezing; CNS changes (confusion, delirium, fever, consistent dizziness); skin rash; sense of fullness or ringing in ears; or vision changes. **Pregnancy precaution:** Inform prescriber if you are or intend to become pregnant.

Geriatric Considerations: Clearance may be decreased with a resultant increased half-life. Must individualize dose. Bioavailability and half-life are increased in the elderly due to decreases in both renal and hepatic function with age.

Pregnancy Risk Factor: C

Lactation: Enters breast milk/compatible

Administration

Oral: Do not crush, chew, or break sustained release dosage forms. Give around-the-clock to promote less variation in peak and trough serum levels.

I.V.: Give around-the-clock to promote less variation in peak and trough serum levels. Maximum I.V. infusion rate: 10 mg/minute. Minimize use of PVC tubing to enhance bioavailability.

Compatibility: Stable in D_5W, NS

Y-site administration: Incompatible with furosemide

Compatibility when admixed: Incompatible with atracurium

Storage: Do not use discolored parenteral solution.

- ♦ **Quinidine Gluconate** *see* Quinidine *on page 1449*
- ♦ **Quinidine Polygalacturonate** *see* Quinidine *on page 1449*
- ♦ **Quinidine Sulfate** *see* Quinidine *on page 1449*

Quinine (KWYE nine)

Synonyms Quinine Sulfate

Pharmacologic Category Antimalarial Agent

Medication Safety Issues

Sound-alike/look-alike issues:

Quinine may be confused with quinidine

Use In conjunction with other antimalarial agents, suppression or treatment of chloroquine-resistant *P. falciparum* malaria; treatment of *Babesia microti* infection in conjunction with clindamycin

Unlabeled/Investigational Use Prevention and treatment of nocturnal recumbency leg muscle cramps

Mechanism of Action Depresses oxygen uptake and carbohydrate metabolism; intercalates into DNA, disrupting the parasite's replication and transcription; affects calcium distribution within muscle fibers and decreases the excitability of the motor end-plate region; cardiovascular effects similar to quinidine

Pharmacodynamics/Kinetics

Absorption: Readily, mainly from upper small intestine

Protein binding: 70% to 95%

Metabolism: Primarily hepatic

Half-life elimination: Children: 6-12 hours; Adults: 8-14 hours

Time to peak, serum: 1-3 hours

Excretion: Feces and saliva; urine (<5% as unchanged drug)

Contraindications Hypersensitivity to quinine or any component of the formulation; tinnitus, optic neuritis, G6PD deficiency; history of black water fever; thrombocytopenia with quinine or quinidine; pregnancy

Warnings/Precautions Use with caution in patients with cardiac arrhythmias (quinine has quinidine-like activity) and in patients with myasthenia gravis

(Continued)

Quinine *(Continued)*

Drug Interactions Substrate (minor) of CYP1A2, 2C19, 3A4; **Inhibits** CYP2C8/9 (moderate), 2D6 (strong), 3A4 (weak)

CYP2C8/9 substrates: Quinine may increase the levels/effects of CYP2C8/9 substrates. Example substrates include amiodarone, fluoxetine, glimepiride, glipizide, nateglinide, phenytoin, pioglitazone, rosiglitazone, sertraline, and warfarin.

CYP2D6 substrates: Quinine may increase the levels/effects of CYP2D6 substrates. Example substrates include amphetamines, selected beta-blockers, dextromethorphan, fluoxetine, lidocaine, mirtazapine, nefazodone, paroxetine, risperidone, ritonavir, thioridazine, tricyclic antidepressants, and venlafaxine.

CYP2D6 prodrug substrates: Quinine may decrease the levels/effects of CYP2D6 prodrug substrates. Example prodrug substrates include codeine, hydrocodone, oxycodone, and tramadol.

Decreased effect: Phenobarbital, phenytoin, aluminum salt antacids, and rifampin may decrease quinine serum concentrations

Increased toxicity:

- To avoid risk of seizures and cardiac arrest, delay mefloquine dosing at least 12 hours after last dose of quinine
- Beta-blockers + quinine may increase bradycardia
- Quinine may enhance coumarin anticoagulants and potentiate nondepolarizing and depolarizing muscle relaxants
- Quinine may increase plasma concentration of digoxin by as much as twofold; closely monitor digoxin concentrations and decrease digoxin dose with initiation of quinine by ½
- Verapamil, amiodarone, urinary alkalinizing agents, and cimetidine may increase quinine serum concentrations

Nutritional/Herbal/Ethanol Interactions Herb/Nutraceutical: St John's wort may decrease quinine levels.

Lab Interactions Positive Coombs' [direct]

Adverse Reactions

Frequency not defined:

- Central nervous system: Severe headache
- Gastrointestinal: Nausea, vomiting, diarrhea
- Ocular: Blurred vision
- Otic: Tinnitus
- Miscellaneous: Cinchonism (risk of cinchonism is directly related to dose and duration of therapy)

<1% (Limited to important or life-threatening): Anginal symptoms, diplopia, epigastric pain, fever, flushing of the skin, hemolysis in G6PD deficiency, hepatitis, hypersensitivity reactions, hypoglycemia, impaired hearing, nightblindness, optic atrophy, pruritus, rash, thrombocytopenia

Overdosage/Toxicology Symptoms of mild toxicity include nausea, vomiting, and cinchonism. Severe intoxication may cause ataxia, obtundation, convulsions, coma, and respiratory arrest. With massive intoxication quinidine-like cardiotoxicity (hypotension, QRS and QT interval prolongation, AV block, and ventricular arrhythmias) may be fatal. Retinal toxicity occurs 9-10 hours after ingestion (blurred vision, impaired color perception, constriction of visual fields and blindness). Other toxic effects include hypokalemia, hypoglycemia, hemolysis, and congenital malformations when taken during pregnancy. Treatment includes symptomatic therapy with conventional agents. **Note:** Avoid Type 1A and 1C antiarrhythmic drugs. Treat cardiotoxicity with sodium bicarbonate. Dialysis and hemoperfusion procedures are ineffective in enhancing elimination.

Dosing

Adults & Elderly:

Treatment of chloroquine-resistant malaria: Oral: 650 mg every 8 hours for 3-7 days with tetracycline

Suppression of malaria: Oral: 325 mg twice daily and continued for 6 weeks after exposure

Babesiosis: Oral: 650 mg every 6-8 hours for 7 days

Leg cramps: Oral: 200-300 mg at bedtime

Pediatrics:

Treatment of chloroquine-resistant malaria: Oral: Children: 25-30 mg/kg/day in divided doses every 8 hours for 3-7 days with tetracycline (consider risk versus benefit in children <8 years of age)

Babesiosis: Oral: Children: 25 mg/kg/day divided every 8 hours for 7 days

Renal Impairment:

Cl_{cr} 10-50 mL/minute: Administer every 8-12 hours or 75% of normal dose.

Cl_{cr} <10 mL/minute: Administer every 24 hours or 30% to 50% of normal dose.

Not removed by hemo- or peritoneal dialysis; dose for Cl_{cr} <10 mL/minute.

Continuous arteriovenous or venovenous hemofiltration: Dose as for Cl_{cr} 10-50 mL/minute.

Available Dosage Forms

Capsule, as sulfate: 200 mg, 325 mg

Tablet, as sulfate: 260 mg

Nursing Guidelines

Assessment: Assess allergy history prior to beginning therapy. See Contraindications, Warnings/Precautions, and Dosing for use cautions. Assess potential for interactions with other prescriptions, OTC medications, or herbal products patient may be taking (especially digoxin - see Drug Interactions). Assess therapeutic effectiveness (according to purpose for therapy) and adverse reactions (see Adverse Reactions and Overdose/Toxicology). Teach patient appropriate use, possible side effects/interventions, and adverse symptoms to report (see Patient Education). **Pregnancy risk factor X** - determine that patient is not pregnant before starting therapy. Do not give to females of childbearing age unless patient is capable of complying with barrier contraceptive use during and for 2 months following therapy.

Dietary Considerations: May be taken with food.

Patient Education: Inform prescriber of all prescriptions, OTC medications, or herbal products you are taking, and any allergies you have. Do not take any new medication during therapy unless approved by prescriber (avoid use of any aluminum-containing antacids). Take on schedule as directed, with full 8 oz of water. May take with food. Do not crush sustained release preparations. Do not increase dose without consulting prescriber - overdose can cause severe systemic effects. You will need to return for follow-up blood tests. May cause severe headache (consult prescriber for approved analgesic); nausea or vomiting (small, frequent meals, frequent mouth care, chewing gum, or sucking lozenges may help); or diarrhea (buttermilk, boiled milk, or yogurt may help). Report any vision changes (blurring, nightblindness, double vision, etc); ringing in ears; or other persistent side effects. Seek emergency help for chest pain, respiratory difficulty, or seizures. **Pregnancy precautions:** Inform prescriber if you are pregnant. Consult prescriber for appropriate barrier contraceptive measures to use during and for 2 months following therapy. This drug may cause fetal defects. Do not donate blood during or for 1 month following therapy.

Geriatric Considerations: Efficacy in nocturnal leg cramps is not well supported in the medical and pharmacy literature, however, some patients do respond. Nonresponders should be evaluated for other possible etiologies.

Pregnancy Risk Factor: X

Lactation: Enters breast milk/compatible

Administration

Oral: Avoid use of aluminum-containing antacids because of drug absorption problems. Swallow dose whole to avoid bitter taste. May be administered with food.

Storage: Protect from light.

♦ **Quinine Sulfate** *see* Quinine *on page 1453*

♦ **Quintabs [OTC]** *see* Vitamins (Multiple/Oral) *on page 1720*

♦ **Quintabs-M [OTC]** *see* Vitamins (Multiple/Oral) *on page 1720*

Quinupristin and Dalfopristin (kwi NYOO pris tin & dal FOE pris tin)

U.S. Brand Names Synercid®

Synonyms Pristinamycin; RP-59500

Pharmacologic Category Antibiotic, Streptogramin

Use Treatment of serious or life-threatening infections associated with vancomycin-resistant *Enterococcus faecium* bacteremia; treatment of complicated skin and skin structure infections caused by methcillin-susceptible *Staphylococcus aureus* or *Streptococcus pyogenes*

Has been studied in the treatment of a variety of infections caused by *Enterococcus faecium* (not *E. fecalis*) including vancomycin-resistant strains. May also be effective in the treatment of serious infections caused by *Staphylococcus* species including those resistant to methicillin.

(Continued)

Quinupristin and Dalfopristin *(Continued)*

Mechanism of Action Quinupristin/dalfopristin inhibits bacterial protein synthesis by binding to different sites on the 50S bacterial ribosomal subunit thereby inhibiting protein synthesis

Pharmacodynamics/Kinetics

Distribution: Quinupristin: 0.45 L/kg; Dalfopristin: 0.24 L/kg

Protein binding: Moderate

Metabolism: To active metabolites via nonenzymatic reactions

Half-life elimination: Quinupristin: 0.85 hour; Dalfopristin: 0.7 hour (mean elimination half-lives, including metabolites: 3 and 1 hours, respectively)

Excretion: Feces (75% to 77% as unchanged drug and metabolites); urine (15% to 19%)

Contraindications Hypersensitivity to quinupristin, dalfopristin, pristinamycin, or virginiamycin, or any component of the formulation

Warnings/Precautions May cause pain and phlebitis when infused through a peripheral line (not relieved by hydrocortisone or diphenhydramine). Superinfection may occur. As with many antibiotics, antibiotic-associated colitis and pseudomembranous colitis may occur. May cause arthralgias, myalgias, and hyperbilirubinemia. May inhibit the metabolism of many drugs metabolized by CYP3A4. Concurrent therapy with cisapride (which may prolong QT_c interval and lead to arrhythmias) should be avoided.

Drug Interactions Quinupristin: **Inhibits** CYP3A4 (weak)

Cisapride: The manufacturer states that quinupristin/dalfopristin may increase cisapride concentrations and cause QT_c prolongation, and recommends to avoid concurrent use with cisapride.

Cyclosporine: Quinupristin/dalfopristin may increase cyclosporine concentrations; monitor.

Adverse Reactions

>10%:

- Hepatic: Hyperbilirubinemia (3% to 35%)
- Local: Inflammation at infusion site (38% to 42%), local pain (40% to 44%), local edema (17% to 18%), infusion site reaction (12% to 13%)
- Neuromuscular & skeletal: Arthralgia (up to 47%), myalgia (up to 47%)

1% to 10%:

- Central nervous system: Pain (2% to 3%), headache (2%)
- Dermatologic: Pruritus (2%), rash (3%)
- Endocrine & metabolic: Hyperglycemia (1%)
- Gastrointestinal: Nausea (3% to 5%), diarrhea (3%), vomiting (3% to 4%)
- Hematologic: Anemia (3%)
- Hepatic: GGT increased (2%), LDH increased (3%)
- Local: Thrombophlebitis (2%)
- Neuromuscular & skeletal: CPK increased (2%)

<1% (Limited to important or life-threatening): Allergic reaction, anaphylactoid reaction, angina, apnea, arrhythmia, cardiac arrest, coagulation disorder, dysautonomia, dyspnea, encephalopathy, gout, hematuria, hemolytic anemia, hepatitis, hyperkalemia, hypotension, maculopapular rash, mesenteric artery occlusion, myasthenia, neuropathy, pancreatitis, pancytopenia, paraplegia, paresthesia, pericarditis, pleural effusion, pseudomembranous colitis, respiratory distress, seizure, shock, stomatitis, syncope, thrombocytopenia, urticaria

Overdosage/Toxicology Symptoms may include dyspnea, emesis, tremors and ataxia. Treatment is supportive. Not removed by hemodialysis or peritoneal dialysis.

Dosing

Adults & Elderly:

Vancomycin-resistant *Enterococcus faecium*: I.V.: 7.5 mg/kg every 8 hours

Complicated skin and skin structure infection: I.V.: 7.5 mg/kg every 12 hours

Pediatrics: Limited information: Dosages similar to adult dosing have been used in the treatment of complicated skin/soft tissue infections and infections caused by vancomycin-resistant *Enterococcus faecium*

CNS shunt infection due to vancomycin-resistant *Enterococcus faecium*: I.V.: 7.5 mg/kg/dose every 8 hours. Concurrent intrathecal doses of 1-2 mg/day have been administered for up to 68 days.

Renal Impairment: No adjustment is necessary in renal failure, hemodialysis, or peritoneal dialysis.

Hepatic Impairment: Pharmacokinetic data suggest dosage adjustment may be necessary; however, specific recommendations have not been proposed.

Available Dosage Forms Injection, powder for reconstitution:

500 mg: Quinupristin 150 mg and dalfopristin 350 mg

600 mg: Quinupristin 180 mg and dalfopristin 420 mg

Nursing Guidelines

Assessment: Assess effectiveness and interactions of other medications (see Drug Interactions). See Warnings/Precautions and Contraindications for use cautions. See Administration for exact infusion protocols to prevent (or treat) severe venous irritation. Monitor infusion site closely. Monitor therapeutic effectiveness (reduction of infection) and adverse reactions and toxicity (see Adverse Reactions, and Overdose/Toxicology). Assess knowledge/teach patient adverse reactions to report (see Patient Education). Note breast-feeding caution.

Monitoring Laboratory Tests: Culture and sensitivity

Patient Education: This drug can only be administered by intravenous infusion. Report immediately any pain, irritation, redness, burning, swelling at infusion site. You may experience other side effects. Report headache, rash, nausea, vomiting, diarrhea, pain, heat or swelling in muscle areas, especially in lower extremities; respiratory difficulty, tremors, or difficulty speaking. **Breast-feeding precaution:** Consult prescriber if breast-feeding.

Pregnancy Risk Factor: B

Lactation: Excretion in breast milk unknown/use caution

Administration

I.V.: Line should be flushed with 5% dextrose in water prior to and following administration. Incompatible with saline. Infusion should be completed over 60 minutes (toxicity may be increased with shorter infusion). Compatible (Y-site injection) with aztreonam, ciprofloxacin, haloperidol, metoclopramide or potassium chloride when admixed in 5% dextrose in water. Also compatible (Y-site injection) with fluconazole (used as undiluted solution). If severe venous irritation occurs following peripheral administration of quinupristin/dalfopristin diluted in 250 mL 5% dextrose in water, consideration should be given to increasing the infusion volume to 500 mL or 750 mL, changing the infusion site, or infusing by a peripherally inserted central catheter (PICC) or a central venous catheter.

Reconstitution: Reconstitute single dose vial with 5 mL of 5% dextrose in water or sterile water for injection. Swirl gentle to dissolve - do not shake (to limit foam formation). The reconstituted solution should be diluted within 30 minutes. Stability of the diluted solution prior to the infusion is established as 5 hours at room temperature or 54 hours if refrigerated at 2°C to 8°C. Reconstituted solution should be added to at least 250 mL of 5% dextrose in water for peripheral administration (increase to 500 mL or 750 mL if necessary to limit venous irritation). An infusion volume of 100 mL may be used for central line infusions. Do not freeze solution.

Storage: Store unopened vials under refrigeration (2°C to 8°C/36°F to 46°F).

♦ **Quixin™** *see* Levofloxacin *on page 1025*

Rabeprazole (ra BE pray zole)

U.S. Brand Names AcipHex®

Synonyms Pariprazole

Pharmacologic Category Proton Pump Inhibitor; Substituted Benzimidazole

Medication Safety Issues

Sound-alike/look-alike issues:

AcipHex® may be confused with Acephen®, Accupril®, Aricept®

Rabeprazole may be confused with aripiprazole

Use Short-term (4-8 weeks) treatment and maintenance of erosive or ulcerative gastroesophageal reflux disease (GERD); symptomatic GERD; short-term (up to 4 weeks) treatment of duodenal ulcers; long-term treatment of pathological hypersecretory conditions, including Zollinger-Ellison syndrome; *H. pylori* eradication (in combination with amoxicillin and clarithromycin)

Unlabeled/Investigational Use Maintenance of duodenal ulcer

Mechanism of Action Potent proton pump inhibitor; suppresses gastric acid secretion by inhibiting the parietal cell H+/K+ ATP pump

Pharmacodynamics/Kinetics

Onset of action: 1 hour

Duration: 24 hours

Absorption: Oral: Well absorbed within 1 hour

Distribution: 96.3%

Protein binding, serum: 94.8% to 97.5%

Metabolism: Hepatic via CYP3A and 2C19 to inactive metabolites

(Continued)

Rabeprazole *(Continued)*

Bioavailability: Oral: 52%

Half-life elimination (dose dependent): 0.85-2 hours

Time to peak, plasma: 2-5 hours

Excretion: Urine (90% primarily as thioether carboxylic acid); remainder in feces

Contraindications Hypersensitivity to rabeprazole, substituted benzimidazoles (ie, esomeprazole, lansoprazole, omeprazole, pantoprazole), or any component of the formulation

Warnings/Precautions Use caution in severe hepatic impairment; relief of symptoms with rabeprazole does not preclude the presence of a gastric malignancy

Drug Interactions Substrate (major) of CYP2C19, 3A4; **Inhibits** CYP2C19 (moderate), 2DC (weak), 3A4 (weak)

CYP2C19 inducers: May decrease the levels/effects of rabeprazole. Example inducers include aminoglutethimide, carbamazepine, phenytoin, and rifampin.

CYP2C19 substrates: Rabeprazole may increase the levels/effects of CYP2C19 substrates. Example substrates include citalopram, diazepam, methsuximide, phenytoin, propranolol, and sertraline.

CYP3A4 inducers: CYP3A4 inducers may decrease the levels/effects of rabeprazole. Example inducers include aminoglutethimide, carbamazepine, nafcillin, nevirapine, phenobarbital, phenytoin, and rifamycins.

Itraconazole and ketoconazole: Proton pump inhibitors may decrease the absorption of itraconazole and ketoconazole; concurrent use is contraindicated.

Protease inhibitors: Proton pump inhibitors may decrease absorption of some protease inhibitors (atazanavir and indinavir).

Nutritional/Herbal/Ethanol Interactions

Ethanol: Avoid ethanol (may cause gastric mucosal irritation).

Food: High-fat meals may delay absorption, but C_{max} and AUC are not altered.

Adverse Reactions

1% to 10%: Central nervous system: Headache (2.4%)

<1% (Limited to important or life-threatening): Anaphylaxis, agranulocytosis, allergic reactions, alopecia, amnesia, angina, angioedema, apnea, asthma, bradycardia, bundle branch block, cholecystitis, coma, delirium, depression, dysphagia, dyspnea, erythema multiforme, extrapyramidal reaction, gout, hemolytic anemia, interstitial pneumonia, jaundice, leukopenia, MI, neuralgia, neuropathy, pancreatitis, pancytopenia, paresthesia, photosensitivity, pulmonary embolus, QT prolongation, rash, renal calculus, retinal degeneration, rhabdomyolysis, seizure, strabismus, syncope, tachycardia, thrombocytopenia, toxic epidermal necrolysis, Stevens-Johnson syndrome, ventricular tachycardia, vertigo

Overdosage/Toxicology No experience with large overdose; rabeprazole is not dialyzable. Treatment of overdosage should be symptomatic and supportive.

Dosing

Adults & Elderly:

GERD: Oral: 20 mg once daily for 4-8 weeks; maintenance: 20 mg once daily

Duodenal ulcer: Oral: 20 mg/day before breakfast for 4 weeks

Eradication of *H. pylori:* Oral: 20 mg twice daily for 7 days; to be administered with amoxicillin 1000 mg and clarithromycin 500 mg, also given twice daily for 7 days.

Hypersecretory conditions: Oral: 60 mg once daily; dose may need to be adjusted as necessary. Doses as high as 100 mg once daily and 60 mg twice daily have been used.

Renal Impairment: No dosage adjustment required.

Hepatic Impairment:

Mild to moderate: Elimination decreased; no dosage adjustment required.

Severe: Use caution.

Available Dosage Forms Tablet, delayed release, enteric coated, as sodium: 20 mg

Nursing Guidelines

Assessment: Assess other medications, especially those dependent on cytochrome P450 metabolism (eg, digoxin) and those requiring acid environment for absorption (eg, ketoconazole, ampicillin). Monitor therapeutic effectiveness (reduction in symptoms) and adverse reactions and toxicity. Assess knowledge/teach patient appropriate use, interventions to reduce side effects, and adverse reactions to report.

Dietary Considerations: May be taken with or without food; best if taken before breakfast.

Patient Education: Take as directed. Swallow whole, do not crush, split, or chew. Follow recommended diet and activity instructions. Avoid alcohol. You may experience headache (use of mild analgesic may help) or other side effects. Report these to prescriber if they persist. **Breast-feeding precaution:** Breast-feeding is not recommended.

Geriatric Considerations: No difference in efficacy or safety was noted in elderly subjects as compared to younger subjects. No dosage adjustment is necessary in the elderly.

Pregnancy Risk Factor: B

Lactation: Excretion in breast milk unknown/not recommended

Administration

Oral: May be administered with or without food; best if taken before breakfast. Do not crush, split, or chew tablet. May be administered with an antacid.

Storage: Rapidly degraded in acid conditions.

Radiological/Contrast Media (Nonionic)

(ray deo LOG ik al/KON trast MEE dia non eye ON ik)

Synonyms Iohexol; Iopamidol; Ioversol; Metrizamide

Pharmacologic Category Radiopaque Agents

Medication Safety Issues

Sound-alike/look-alike issues:

Optiray® may be confused with Optivar™

Use Enhance visualization of structures during radiologic procedures

Contraindications Known hypersensitivity

Warnings/Precautions Anaphylactic-like reactions and hypotension; acute severe back, leg or groin pain; decision to use contrast enhancement should include consideration of risk of the drug, risk of the procedure, expected benefit of the image and patient's underlying disorder

Drug Interactions

Interleukins: Risk of hypersensitivity reactions may be increased.

Metformin: Risk of metformin-induced acidosis may be increased by iodinated contrast agents. Discontinue metformin prior to contrast exposure and withhold for 48 hours.

Available Dosage Forms [DSC] = Discontinued product

Injection, solution:

Gadoteridol (ProHance®): 279.3 mg/mL (15 mL, 30 mL, 50 mL) [single use vial]; 279.3 mg/mL (20 mL) [prefilled syringe]

Iohexol (Omnipaque®): 140 mg/mL, 180 mg/mL, 210 mg/mL, 240 mg/mL, 300 mg/mL, 350 mg/mL

Iopamidol:

Isovue-128®

Isovue-200®

Isovue-300®

Isovue-370®

Isovue-M 200®

Isovue-M 300®

Ioversol:

Optiray® 160

Optiray® 240

Optiray® 320

Metrizamide: Amipaque® [DSC]

♦ rAHF *see* Antihemophilic Factor (Recombinant) *on page 170*

♦ R-albuterol *see* Levalbuterol *on page 1018*

Ramipril (ra MI pril)

U.S. Brand Names Altace®

Pharmacologic Category Angiotensin-Converting Enzyme (ACE) Inhibitor

Medication Safety Issues

Sound-alike/look-alike issues:

Ramipril may be confused with enalapril, Monopril®

Altace® may be confused with alteplase, Amaryl®, Amerge®, Artane®

Use Treatment of hypertension, alone or in combination with thiazide diuretics; treatment of left ventricular dysfunction after myocardial infarction; to reduce risk of heart attack, stroke, and death in patients at increased risk for these problems

Unlabeled/Investigational Use Treatment of heart failure

(Continued)

Ramipril *(Continued)*

Mechanism of Action Ramipril is an ACE inhibitor which prevents the formation of angiotensin II from angiotensin I and exhibits pharmacologic effects that are similar to captopril. Ramipril must undergo enzymatic saponification by esterases in the liver to its biologically active metabolite, ramiprilat. The pharmacodynamic effects of ramipril result from the high-affinity, competitive, reversible binding of ramiprilat to angiotensin-converting enzyme thus preventing the formation of the potent vasoconstrictor angiotensin II. This isomerized enzyme-inhibitor complex has a slow rate of dissociation, which results in high potency and a long duration of action; a CNS mechanism may also be involved in the hypotensive effect as angiotensin II increases adrenergic outflow from CNS; vasoactive kallikreins may be decreased in conversion to active hormones by ACE inhibitors, thus reducing blood pressure

Pharmacodynamics/Kinetics

Onset of action: 1-2 hours

Duration: 24 hours

Absorption: Well absorbed (50% to 60%)

Distribution: Plasma levels decline in a triphasic fashion; rapid decline is a distribution phase to peripheral compartment, plasma protein and tissue ACE (half-life 2-4 hours); 2nd phase is an apparent elimination phase representing the clearance of free ramiprilat (half-life: 9-18 hours); and final phase is the terminal elimination phase representing the equilibrium phase between tissue binding and dissociation

Metabolism: Hepatic to the active form, ramiprilat

Half-life elimination: Ramiprilat: Effective: 13-17 hours; Terminal: >50 hours

Time to peak, serum: ~1 hour

Excretion: Urine (60%) and feces (40%) as parent drug and metabolites

Contraindications Hypersensitivity to ramipril or any component of the formulation; prior hypersensitivity (including angioedema) to ACE inhibitors; bilateral renal artery stenosis; pregnancy (2nd and 3rd trimesters)

Warnings/Precautions Anaphylactic or anaphylactoid reactions can occur. Angioedema can occur at any time during treatment (especially following first dose). Angioedema may involve head and neck (potentially affecting the airway) or the intestine (presenting with abdominal pain). Careful blood pressure monitoring with first dose (hypotension can occur especially in volume depleted patients). Dosage adjustment needed in renal impairment. Use with caution in hypovolemia; collagen vascular diseases; valvular stenosis (particularly aortic stenosis); hyperkalemia; or before, during, or immediately after anesthesia. Avoid rapid dosage escalation, which may lead to renal insufficiency. Rare toxicities associated with ACE inhibitors include cholestatic jaundice (which may progress to hepatic necrosis) and neutropenia/agranulocytosis with myeloid hyperplasia. If patient has renal impairment then a baseline WBC with differential and serum creatinine should be evaluated and monitored closely during the first 3 months of therapy. Hypersensitivity reactions may be seen during hemodialysis with high-flux dialysis membranes (eg, AN69). Use with caution in unilateral renal artery stenosis and pre-existing renal insufficiency.

Drug Interactions

Alpha$_1$ blockers: Hypotensive effect increased.

Aspirin: The effects of ACE inhibitors may be blunted by aspirin administration, particularly at higher dosages (see Cardiovascular Considerations) and/or increase adverse renal effects.

Diuretics: Hypovolemia due to diuretics may precipitate acute hypotensive events or acute renal failure.

Insulin: Risk of hypoglycemia may be increased.

Lithium: Risk of lithium toxicity may be increased; monitor lithium levels, especially the first 4 weeks of therapy.

Mercaptopurine: Risk of neutropenia may be increased.

NSAIDs: May attenuate hypertensive efficacy; effect has been seen with captopril and may occur with other ACE inhibitors; monitor blood pressure. May increase risk of adverse renal effects or hyperkalemia.

Potassium-sparing diuretics (amiloride, spironolactone, triamterene): Increased risk of hyperkalemia.

Potassium supplements may increase the risk of hyperkalemia.

Trimethoprim (high dose) may increase the risk of hyperkalemia.

Nutritional/Herbal/Ethanol Interactions Herb/Nutraceutical: Avoid dong quai if using for hypertension (has estrogenic activity). Avoid ephedra, yohimbe, ginseng (may worsen hypertension). Avoid garlic (may have increased antihypertensive effect).

Lab Interactions Increases BUN, creatinine, potassium, positive Coombs' [direct]; decreases cholesterol (S); may cause false-positive results in urine acetone determinations using sodium nitroprusside reagent

Adverse Reactions Note: Frequency ranges include data from hypertension and heart failure trials. Higher rates of adverse reactions have generally been noted in patients with CHF. However, the frequency of adverse effects associated with placebo is also increased in this population.

>10%: Respiratory: Cough (increased) (7% to 12%)

1% to 10%:

Cardiovascular: Hypotension (11%), angina (3%), postural hypotension (2%), syncope (2%)

Central nervous system: Headache (1% to 5%), dizziness (2% to 4%), fatigue (2%), vertigo (2%)

Endocrine & metabolic: Hyperkalemia (1% to 10%)

Gastrointestinal: Nausea/vomiting (1% to 2%)

Neuromuscular & skeletal: Chest pain (noncardiac) (1%)

Renal: Renal dysfunction (1%), elevation in serum creatinine (1% to 2%), increased BUN (<1% to 3%); transient elevations of creatinine and/or BUN may occur more frequently

Respiratory: Cough (estimated 1% to 10%)

<1% (Limited to important or life-threatening): Agitation, agranulocytosis, amnesia, anaphylactoid reaction, angina, angioedema, arrhythmia, bone marrow depression, convulsions, depression, dysphagia, dyspnea, edema, eosinophilia, erythema multiforme, hearing loss, hemolytic anemia, hepatitis, hypersensitivity reactions (urticaria, rash, fever), impotence, insomnia, myalgia, MI, neuropathy, onycholysis, pancreatitis, pancytopenia, paresthesia, pemphigoid, pemphigus, photosensitivity, proteinuria, somnolence, Stevens-Johnson syndrome, symptomatic hypotension, syncope, thrombocytopenia, toxic epidermal necrolysis, vertigo

Worsening of renal function may occur in patients with bilateral renal artery stenosis or in hypovolemia. In addition, a syndrome which may include fever, myalgia, arthralgia, interstitial nephritis, vasculitis, rash, eosinophilia and positive ANA, and elevated ESR has been reported with ACE inhibitors. Risk of pancreatitis and/or agranulocytosis may be increased in patients with collagen vascular disease or renal impairment.

Overdosage/Toxicology Mild hypotension has been the primary toxic effect seen with acute overdose. Bradycardia may also occur. Hyperkalemia occurs even with therapeutic doses, especially in patients with renal insufficiency and those taking NSAIDs. Treatment is symptom-directed and supportive.

Dosing

Adults:

Hypertension: Oral: 2.5-5 mg once daily, maximum: 20 mg/day

To reduce the risk of MI, stroke, and death from cardiovascular causes: Oral: Initial: 2.5 mg once daily for 1 week, then 5 mg once daily for the next 3 weeks, then increase as tolerated to 10 mg once daily (may be given as divided dose)

Left ventricular dysfunction postmyocardial infarction: Oral: Initial: 2.5 mg twice daily titrated upward, if possible, to 5 mg twice daily.

Heart failure (unlabeled use): Initial: 1.25-2.5 mg once daily; target dose: 10 mg once daily (ACC/AHA 2005 Heart Failure Guidelines)

Note: The dose of any concomitant diuretic should be reduced. If the diuretic cannot be discontinued, initiate therapy with 1.25 mg. After the initial dose, the patient should be monitored carefully until blood pressure has stabilized.

Elderly: Refer to adult dosing (see Geriatric Considerations). Adjust for renal function for elderly since glomerular filtration rates are decreased; may see exaggerated hypotensive effects if renal clearance is not considered.

Renal Impairment:

Cl_{cr} <40 mL/minute: Administer 25% of normal dose.

Renal failure and hypertension: Administer 1.25 mg once daily, titrated upward as possible.

Renal failure and heart failure: Administer 1.25 mg once daily, increasing to 1.25 mg twice daily up to 2.5 mg twice daily as tolerated.

Available Dosage Forms Capsule: 1.25 mg, 2.5 mg, 5 mg, 10 mg

(Continued)

Ramipril *(Continued)*

Nursing Guidelines

Assessment: See Contraindications, Warnings/Precautions, and Dosing for use cautions. Assess potential for interactions with other prescriptions, OTC medications, or herbal products patient may be taking (see Drug Interactions). May be advisable to administer first dose in prescriber's office with careful blood pressure monitoring (hypotension and angioedema can occur at any time during treatment, especially following first dose). Assess results of laboratory tests (see below) and patient response at beginning of therapy, when adjusting dose, and periodically with long-term therapy (eg, blood pressure, cardiac status and fluid balance - see Adverse Reactions and Overdose/Toxicology). Teach patient appropriate use, possible side effects/appropriate interventions, and adverse symptoms to report (see Patient Education). **Pregnancy risk factor C/D** - see Pregnancy Risk Factor for use cautions; determine that patient is not pregnant prior to beginning therapy. Instruct patient in appropriate use of barrier contraceptives (see Pregnancy Issues). Breast-feeding is not recommended.

Monitoring Laboratory Tests: CBC, renal function tests, electrolytes; if patient has renal impairment, a baseline WBC with differential and serum creatinine should be evaluated and monitored closely during the first 3 months of therapy.

Patient Education: Inform prescriber of all prescriptions, OTC medications, or herbal products you are taking, and any allergies you have. Do not take any new medication during therapy without consulting prescriber. Take as directed; do not alter dose or discontinue without consulting prescriber. Take first dose at bedtime or when sitting down (hypotension may occur). This drug does not eliminate need for diet or exercise regimen as recommended by prescriber. May cause increased cough (if persistent or bothersome, contact prescriber); headache (consult prescriber for approved analgesic); postural hypotension (use caution when rising from lying or sitting position or climbing stairs); dizziness (use caution when driving or engaging in tasks that require alertness until response to drug is known); or nausea or vomiting (small, frequent meals, frequent mouth care, sucking lozenges, or chewing gum may help). Immediately report swelling of face, mouth, lips, tongue or throat; chest pain or irregular heartbeat. Report respiratory difficulty or persistent cough; persistent pain in muscles, joints, or back; or other persistent adverse reactions. **Pregnancy/breast-feeding precautions:** Inform prescriber if you are or intend to become pregnant. This drug should not be used in the 2nd or 3rd trimester of pregnancy. Consult prescriber for appropriate contraceptive measures if necessary. Breast-feeding is not recommended.

Geriatric Considerations: Due to frequent decreases in glomerular filtration (also creatinine clearance) with aging, elderly patients may have exaggerated responses to ACE inhibitors. Differences in clinical response due to hepatic changes are not observed.

Pregnancy Risk Factor: C (1st trimester)/D (2nd and 3rd trimesters)

Pregnancy Issues: ACE inhibitors can cause fetal injury or death if taken during the 2nd or 3rd trimester. Discontinue ACE inhibitors as soon as pregnancy is detected.

Lactation: Excretion in breast milk unknown/not recommended

Breast-Feeding Considerations: The manufacturer states that after single dose studies, ramipril was not excreted in breast milk; however, since the amount excreted with daily dosing is unknown, nursing while taking ramipril is not recommended.

Perioperative/Anesthesia/Other Concerns: A recently completed trial (HOPE), examining the use of ramipril (at a dose of between 2.5-10 mg daily) in patients at high risk for cardiovascular events but who did not have heart failure, documented a significant improvement in cardiovascular outcome in the treated group.

ACE inhibitors decrease morbidity and mortality in patients with asymptomatic and symptomatic left ventricular dysfunction. ACE inhibitors are also indicated in patients postmyocardial infarction in whom left ventricular ejection fraction is <40%.

ACE inhibitor therapy may elicit rapid increases in potassium and creatinine, especially when used in patients with bilateral renal artery stenosis. When ACE inhibition is introduced in patients with pre-existing diuretic therapy who are hypovolemic, the ACE inhibitor may induce acute hypotension. Because of the potent teratogenic effects of ACE inhibitors, these drugs should be avoided, if possible, when treating women of childbearing potential not on effective birth control measures.

Administration

Oral: Capsule is usually swallowed whole, but may be may be mixed in water, apple juice, or applesauce.

Storage: Store at controlled room temperature.

♦ Raniclor™ *see* Cefaclor *on page 326*

Ranitidine (ra NI ti deen)

U.S. Brand Names Zantac®; Zantac 75® [OTC]; Zantac 150™ [OTC]; Zantac® EFFERdose®

Synonyms Ranitidine Hydrochloride

Pharmacologic Category Histamine H_2 Antagonist

Medication Safety Issues

Sound-alike/look-alike issues:

Ranitidine may be confused with amantadine, rimantadine

Zantac® may be confused with Xanax®, Zarontin®, Zofran®, Zyrtec®

Use

Zantac®: Short-term and maintenance therapy of duodenal ulcer, gastric ulcer, gastroesophageal reflux, active benign ulcer, erosive esophagitis, and pathological hypersecretory conditions; as part of a multidrug regimen for *H. pylori* eradication to reduce the risk of duodenal ulcer recurrence

Zantac® 75 [OTC]: Relief of heartburn, acid indigestion, and sour stomach

Unlabeled/Investigational Use Recurrent postoperative ulcer, upper GI bleeding, prevention of acid-aspiration pneumonitis during surgery, and prevention of stress-induced ulcers

Mechanism of Action Competitive inhibition of histamine at H_2-receptors of the gastric parietal cells, which inhibits gastric acid secretion, gastric volume, and hydrogen ion concentration are reduced. Does not affect pepsin secretion, pentagastrin-stimulated intrinsic factor secretion, or serum gastrin.

Pharmacodynamics/Kinetics

Absorption: Oral: 50%

Distribution: Normal renal function: V_d: 1.7 L/kg; Cl_{cr} 25-35 mL/minute: 1.76 L/kg minimally penetrates the blood-brain barrier; enters breast milk

Protein binding: 15%

Metabolism: Hepatic to N-oxide, S-oxide, and N-desmethyl metabolites

Bioavailability: Oral: 48%

Half-life elimination:

Oral: Normal renal function: 2.5-3 hours; Cl_{cr} 25-35 mL/minute: 4.8 hours

I.V.: Normal renal function: 2-2.5 hours

Time to peak, serum: Oral: 2-3 hours; I.M.: ≤15 minutes

Excretion: Urine: Oral: 30%, I.V.: 70% (as unchanged drug); feces (as metabolites)

Contraindications Hypersensitivity to ranitidine or any component of the formulation

Warnings/Precautions Use with caution in patients with hepatic impairment; use with caution in renal impairment, dosage modification required; avoid use in patients with history of acute porphyria (may precipitate attacks); long-term therapy may be associated with vitamin B_{12} deficiency; EFFERdose® formulations contain phenylalanine; safety and efficacy have not been established for pediatric patients <1 month of age

Drug Interactions **Substrate** (minor) of CYP1A2, 2C19, 2D6; **Inhibits** CYP1A2 (weak), 2D6 (weak)

Propantheline: Slight delay and increase in peak ranitidine levels

Triazolam: Ranitidine increases bioavailability of triazolam (10% to 30%), possibly by reducing gastric acidity

Warfarin: May increase or decrease prothrombin time when used concomitantly; monitor

Nutritional/Herbal/Ethanol Interactions

Ethanol: Avoid ethanol (may cause gastric mucosal irritation).

Food: Does not interfere with absorption of ranitidine.

Lab Interactions False-positive urine protein using Multistix®, gastric acid secretion test, skin test allergen extracts, serum creatinine and serum transaminase concentrations, urine protein test

Adverse Reactions Frequency not defined (limited to important or life-threatening):

Cardiovascular: Arrhythmias, vasculitis

(Continued)

Ranitidine *(Continued)*

Central nervous system: Dizziness, hallucinations, headache, mental confusion, somnolence, vertigo

Dermatologic: Erythema multiforme, rash

Gastrointestinal: Pancreatitis

Hematologic: Acquired hemolytic anemia, agranulocytosis, aplastic anemia, granulocytopenia, leukopenia, pancytopenia, thrombocytopenia

Hepatic: Hepatic failure

Miscellaneous: Anaphylaxis, hypersensitivity reactions

Overdosage/Toxicology Symptoms of overdose include abnormal gait, hypotension, and adverse effects seen with normal use. Treatment is primarily symptomatic and supportive.

Dosing

Adults & Elderly:

Duodenal ulcer: Oral: Treatment: 150 mg twice daily, or 300 mg once daily after the evening meal or at bedtime; maintenance: 150 mg once daily at bedtime

Eradication of *Helicobacter pylori*: Oral: 150 mg twice daily; requires combination therapy

Pathological hypersecretory conditions:

Oral: 150 mg twice daily; adjust dose or frequency as clinically indicated; doses of up to 6 g/day have been used

I.V.: Continuous infusion for Zollinger-Ellison: 1 mg/kg/hour; measure gastric acid output at 4 hours, if >10 mEq or if patient is symptomatic, increase dose in increments of 0.5 mg/kg/hour; doses of up to 2.5 mg/kg/hour have been used

Gastric ulcer, benign: *Oral:* 150 mg twice daily; maintenance: 150 mg once daily at bedtime

Erosive esophagitis: *Oral:* Treatment: 150 mg 4 times/day; maintenance: 150 mg twice daily

Prevention of heartburn: *Oral:* Zantac®75 [OTC]: 75 mg 30-60 minutes before eating food or drinking beverages which cause heartburn; maximum: 150 mg in 24 hours; do not use for more than 14 days

Patients not able to take oral medication:

I.M.: 50 mg every 6-8 hours

I.V.: Intermittent bolus or infusion: 50 mg every 6-8 hours

Continuous I.V. infusion: 6.25 mg/hour

Pediatrics:

Duodenal and gastric ulcer:

Oral: Children 1 month to 16 years:

Treatment: 2-4 mg/kg/day divided twice daily; maximum treatment dose: 300 mg/day

Maintenance: 2-4 mg/kg once daily; maximum maintenance dose: 150 mg/day

I.V.: 2-4 mg/kg/day divided every 6-8 hours; maximum: 150 mg/day

GERD and erosive esophagitis: Children 1 month to 16 years:

Oral: 5-10 mg/kg/day divided twice daily; maximum: GERD: 300 mg/day, erosive esophagitis: 600 mg/day

I.V.: 2-4 mg/kg/day divided every 6-8 hours; maximum: 150 mg/day **or as an alternative**

Continuous infusion: Initial: 1 mg/kg/dose for one dose followed by infusion of 0.08-0.17 mg/kg/hour or 2-4 mg/kg/day

Prevention of heartburn: *Oral:* Children ≥12 years: Zantac® 75 [OTC]: 75 mg 30-60 minutes before eating food or drinking beverages which cause heartburn; maximum: 150 mg/24 hours; do not use for more than 14 days

Renal Impairment: Adults: Cl_{cr} <50 mL/minute:

Oral: 150 mg every 24 hours; adjust dose cautiously if needed

I.V.: 50 mg every 18-24 hours; adjust dose cautiously if needed

Hemodialysis: Adjust dosing schedule so that dose coincides with the end of hemodialysis.

Hepatic Impairment: Patients with hepatic impairment may have minor changes in ranitidine half-life, distribution, clearance, and bioavailability; dosing adjustments are not necessary; monitor patient.

Available Dosage Forms

Capsule, as hydrochloride: 150 mg, 300 mg

Infusion, as hydrochloride [premixed in NaCl 0.45%; preservative free] (Zantac®): 50 mg (50 mL)

Injection, solution, as hydrochloride: 25 mg/mL (2 mL, 6 mL)

Zantac®: 25 mg/mL (2 mL, 6 mL, 40 mL) [contains phenol 0.5% as preservative]

Syrup, as hydrochloride: 15 mg/mL (10 mL) [contains alcohol 7.5%; peppermint flavor]

Zantac®: 15 mg/mL (473 mL) [contains alcohol 7.5%; peppermint flavor]

Tablet, as hydrochloride: 75 mg [OTC], 150 mg, 300 mg

Zantac®: 150 mg, 300 mg

Zantac 75® : 75 mg

Zantac 150™: 150 mg

Tablet, effervescent, as hydrochloride (Zantac® EFFERdose®): 25 mg [contains sodium 1.33 mEq/tablet, phenylalanine 2.81 mg/tablet, and sodium benzoate]; 150 mg [contains sodium 7.96 mEq/tablet, phenylalanine 16.84 mg/tablet, and sodium benzoate]

Nursing Guidelines

Assessment: See Contraindications, Warnings/Precautions, and Dosing for use cautions. Assess potential for interactions with other prescriptions, OTC medications, or herbal products patient may be taking (see Drug Interactions). Assess results of laboratory tests (see below) and patient response (see Adverse Reactions and Overdose/Toxicology). Teach patient appropriate use, possible side effects/appropriate interventions, and adverse symptoms to report (see Patient Education). Note breast-feeding caution.

Monitoring Laboratory Tests: AST, ALT, serum creatinine; when used to prevent stress-related GI bleeding, measure the intragastric pH and try to maintain pH >4; occult blood with GI bleeding; monitor renal function and adjust dosage as indicated.

Dietary Considerations: Oral dosage forms may be taken with or without food.

Zantac® EFFERdose®:

Effervescent tablet 25 mg contains sodium 1.33 mEq/tablet and phenylalanine 2.81 mg/tablet

Effervescent tablet 150 mg contains sodium 7.96 mEq/tablet and phenylalanine 16.84 mg/tablet

Patient Education: Inform prescriber of all prescriptions, OTC medications, or herbal products you are taking, and any allergies you have. Do not take any new medication during therapy without consulting prescriber. Take exactly as directed; do not increase dose - may take several days before you notice relief. Allow 1 hour between any other antacids (if approved by prescriber) and ranitidine. Avoid alcohol. Follow diet as prescriber recommends. May cause drowsiness, dizziness, or fatigue (use caution when driving or engaging in tasks requiring alertness until response to drug is known). Report chest pain or irregular heartbeat; skin rash; CNS changes (mental confusion, hallucinations, somnolence); unusual persistent weakness or lethargy; yellowing of skin or eyes; or change in color of urine or stool. **Breast-feeding precaution:** Consult prescriber if breast-feeding.

Geriatric Considerations: H_2 blockers are the preferred drugs for treating PUD in elderly due to cost and ease of administration. These agents are no less or more effective than any other therapy. The preferred agents, due to side effects and drug interaction profile and pharmacokinetics are ranitidine, famotidine, and nizatidine. Treatment for PUD in elderly is recommended for 12 weeks since their lesions are larger; therefore, take longer to heal. Always adjust dose based upon creatinine clearance. Serum half-life is increased to 3-4 hours in elderly patients.

Pregnancy Risk Factor: B

Pregnancy Issues: Ranitidine crosses the placenta, teratogenic effects to the fetus have not been reported. Use with caution during pregnancy.

Lactation: Enters breast milk/use caution

Perioperative/Anesthesia/Other Concerns: Ranitidine causes fewer CNS adverse reactions and drug interactions compared to cimetidine.

Administration

Oral: EFFERdose®: Should not be chewed, swallowed whole, or dissolved on tongue:

25 mg tablet: Dissolve in at least 5 mL (1 teaspoonful) of water; wait until completely dissolved before administering

150 mg tablet: Dissolve each dose in 6-8 ounces of water before drinking

(Continued)

Ranitidine *(Continued)*

I.M.: No dilution is needed

I.V.:

Intermittent bolus: Dilute vials to 2.5 mg/mL; infuse at 4 mL/minute (5 minutes)

Intermittent infusion: Dilute vials to 0.5 mg/mL; infuse at 5-7 mL/minute (15-20 minutes)

Continuous I.V. infusion: Administer at 6.25 mg/hour and titrate dosage based on gastric pH by continuous infusion over 24 hours

Reconstitution: Vials can be mixed with NS or D_5W; solutions are stable for 48 hours at room temperature

Intermittent bolus injection: Dilute to maximum of 2.5 mg/mL

Intermittent infusion: Dilute to maximum of 0.5 mg/mL

Compatibility: Injection: Do not add other medications to premixed bag. Stable in $D_5{}^1\!/_2NS$, D_5W, $D_{10}W$, fat emulsion 10%, LR, NS, sodium bicarbonate 5%

Y-site administration: Incompatible with amphotericin B cholesteryl sulfate complex, hetastarch, insulin (regular)

Compatibility in syringe: Incompatible with hydroxyzine, methotrimeprazine, midazolam, pentobarbital, phenobarbital

Compatibility when admixed: Incompatible with amphotericin B, atracurium, cefamandole, cefazolin, cefoxitin, ceftazidime, cefuroxime, ethacrynate, metaraminol, phytonadione

Storage:

Injection: Vials; Store between 4°C to 30°C (39°F to 86°F); protect from light. Solution is a clear, colorless to yellow solution; slight darkening does not affect potency.

Premixed bag: Store between 2°C to 25°C (36°F to 77°F); protect from light.

EFFERdose® formulations: Store between 2°C to 30°C (36°F to 86°F).

Syrup; Store between 4°C to 25°C (39°F to 77°F); protect from light.

Tablets; Store in dry place, between 15°C to 30°C (59°F to 86°F); protect from light.

- **Ranitidine Hydrochloride** *see* Ranitidine *on page 1463*
- **Rapamune®** *see* Sirolimus *on page 1538*
- **ReAzo [OTC]** *see* Phenazopyridine *on page 1342*
- **Rebetol®** *see* Ribavirin *on page 1475*
- **Rebetron®** *see* Interferon Alfa-2b and Ribavirin *on page 940*
- **Rebif®** *see* Interferon Beta-1a *on page 947*
- **Reclipsen™** *see* Ethinyl Estradiol and Desogestrel *on page 675*
- **Recombinant Hirudin** *see* Lepirudin *on page 1011*
- **Recombinant Plasminogen Activator** *see* Reteplase *on page 1469*
- **Recombinate™** *see* Antihemophilic Factor (Recombinant) *on page 170*
- **Rectacaine [OTC]** *see* Phenylephrine *on page 1350*
- **Red Cross™ Canker Sore [OTC]** *see* Benzocaine *on page 232*
- **Redutemp® [OTC]** *see* Acetaminophen *on page 65*
- **ReFacto®** *see* Antihemophilic Factor (Recombinant) *on page 170*
- **Refludan®** *see* Lepirudin *on page 1011*
- **Refresh® [OTC]** *see* Artificial Tears *on page 187*
- **Refresh Liquigel™ [OTC]** *see* Carboxymethylcellulose *on page 316*
- **Refresh Plus® [OTC]** *see* Carboxymethylcellulose *on page 316*
- **Refresh Tears® [OTC]** *see* Carboxymethylcellulose *on page 316*
- **Regitine [DSC]** *see* Phentolamine *on page 1349*
- **Reglan®** *see* Metoclopramide *on page 1144*
- **Regonol®** *see* Pyridostigmine *on page 1440*
- **Regular Insulin** *see* Insulin Regular *on page 928*
- **Reguloid® [OTC]** *see* Psyllium *on page 1438*
- **Relief® [OTC]** *see* Phenylephrine *on page 1350*
- **Remicade®** *see* Infliximab *on page 910*

Remifentanil (rem i FEN ta nil)

U.S. Brand Names Ultiva®

Synonyms GI87084B

Pharmacologic Category Analgesic, Narcotic

Medication Safety Issues

Sound-alike/look-alike issues:

Remifentanil may be confused with alfentanil

Use Analgesic for use during the induction and maintenance of general anesthesia; for continued analgesia into the immediate postoperative period; analgesic component of monitored anesthesia

Unlabeled/Investigational Use Management of pain in mechanically-ventilated patients

Mechanism of Action Binds with stereospecific mu-opioid receptors at many sites within the CNS, increases pain threshold, alters pain reception, inhibits ascending pain pathways

Pharmacodynamics/Kinetics

Onset of action: I.V.: 1-3 minutes

Distribution: V_d: 100 mL/kg; increased in children

Protein binding: ~70% (primarily $alpha_1$ acid glycoprotein)

Metabolism: Rapid via blood and tissue esterases

Half-life elimination (dose dependent): Terminal: 10-20 minutes; effective: 3-10 minutes

Excretion: Urine

Contraindications Not for intrathecal or epidural administration, due to the presence of glycine in the formulation; hypersensitivity to remifentanil, fentanyl, or fentanyl analogs, or any component of the formulation

Warnings/Precautions Remifentanil is not recommended as the sole agent in general anesthesia, because the loss of consciousness cannot be assured and due to the high incidence of apnea, hypotension, tachycardia and muscle rigidity; it should be administered by individuals specifically trained in the use of anesthetic agents and should not be used in diagnostic or therapeutic procedures outside the monitored anesthesia setting; resuscitative and intubation equipment should be readily available.

Interruption of an infusion will result in offset of effects within 5-10 minutes; the discontinuation of remifentanil infusion should be preceded by the establishment of adequate postoperative analgesia orders, especially for patients in whom postoperative pain is anticipated. Use caution in the morbidly obese.

Drug Interactions

Anesthetics: Synergistic with other anesthetics, may need to decrease thiopental, propofol, isoflurane and midazolam by up to 75%

CNS depressants: Increased effect of CNS depressants

Adverse Reactions

>10%: Gastrointestinal: Nausea, vomiting

1% to 10%:

Cardiovascular: Hypotension (dose dependent), bradycardia (dose dependent), tachycardia, hypertension

Central nervous system: Dizziness, headache, agitation, fever

Dermatologic: Pruritus

Neuromuscular & skeletal: Muscle rigidity (dose dependent)

Ocular: Visual disturbances

Respiratory: Respiratory depression, apnea, hypoxia

Miscellaneous: Shivering, postoperative pain

<1% (Limited to important or life-threatening): Anaphylactic/anaphylactoid reactions, anemia, anxiety, arrhythmia, asystole, bronchospasm, confusion, constipation, CPK-MB increased, diarrhea, dysphagia, electrolyte disorders, hallucinations, heart block, pleural effusion, prolonged emergence from anesthesia, pulmonary edema, syncope, thrombocytopenia, xerostomia

Overdosage/Toxicology

Symptoms of overdose include apnea, chest wall rigidity, seizures, hypoxemia, hypotension and bradycardia

Support of patient's airway, establish an I.V. line, administer intravenous fluids and administer naloxone 2 mg I.V. (0.01 mg/kg for children) with repeat administration as needed up to a total of 10 mg; glycopyrrolate or atropine may be useful for the treatment of bradycardia or hypotension

(Continued)

Remifentanil *(Continued)*

Dosing

Adults: Anesthesia: I.V. continuous infusion: **Note:** Dose should be based on ideal body weight (IBW) in obese patients (>30% over IBW).

Induction of anesthesia: 0.5-1 mcg/kg/minute; if endotracheal intubation is to occur in <8 minutes, an initial dose of 1 mcg/kg may be given over 30-60 seconds

Coronary bypass surgery: 1 mcg/kg/minute

Maintenance of anesthesia: Supplemental bolus dose of 1 mcg/kg may be administered every 2-5 minutes. Consider increasing concomitant anesthetics with infusion rate >1 mcg/kg/minute. Infusion rate can be titrated upward in increments of 25% to 100% or downward in decrements of 25% to 50%. May titrate every 2-5 minutes.

With nitrous oxide (66%): 0.4 mcg/kg/minute (range: 0.1-2 mcg/kg/minute)

With isoflurane: 0.25 mcg/kg/minute (range: 0.05-2 mcg/kg/minute)

With propofol: 0.25 mcg/kg/minute (range: 0.05-2 mcg/kg/minute)

Coronary bypass surgery: 1 mcg/kg/minute (range: 0.125-4 mcg/kg/minute); supplemental dose: 0.5-1 mcg/kg

Continuation as an analgesic in immediate postoperative period: 0.1 mcg/kg/minute (range: 0.025-0.2 mcg/kg/minute). Infusion rate may be adjusted every 5 minutes in increments of 0.025 mcg/kg/minute. Bolus doses are not recommended. Infusion rates >0.2 mcg/kg/minute are associated with respiratory depression.

Coronary bypass surgery, continuation as an analgesic into the ICU: 1 mcg/kg/minute (range: 0.05-1 mcg/kg/minute)

Analgesic component of monitored anesthesia care:

Note: Supplemental oxygen is recommended:

Single I.V. dose given 90 seconds prior to local anesthetic:

Remifentanil alone: 1 mcg/kg over 30-60 seconds

With midazolam: 0.5 mcg/kg over 30-60 seconds

Continuous infusion beginning 5 minutes prior to local anesthetic:

Remifentanil alone: 0.1 mcg/kg minute

With midazolam: 0.05 mcg/kg/minute

Continuous infusion given after local anesthetic:

Remifentanil alone: 0.05 mcg/kg/minute (range: 0.025-0.2 mcg/kg/minute)

With midazolam: 0.025 mcg/kg/minute (range: 0.025-0.2 mcg/kg/minute)

Note: Following local or anesthetic block, infusion rate should be decreased to 0.05 mcg/kg/minute; rate adjustments of 0.025 mcg/kg/minute may be done at 5-minute intervals

Mechanically-ventilated patients: Acute pain (moderate-to-severe) (unlabeled use): 0.6-15 mcg/kg/hour

Elderly: Elderly patients have an increased sensitivity to effect of remifentanil. Doses should be decreased by ½ and titrated.

Pediatrics: Note: Dose should be based on ideal body weight (IBW) in obese patients (>30% over IBW).

Maintenance of anesthesia with nitrous oxide (70%): Children birth to 2 months: Continuous I.V. infusion: 0.4 mcg/kg/minute (range: 0.4-1 mcg/kg/minute); supplemental bolus dose of 1 mcg/kg may be administered, smaller bolus dose may be required with potent inhalation agents, potent neuraxial anesthesia, significant comorbidities, significant fluid shifts, or without atropine pretreatment. Clearance in neonates is highly variable; dose should be carefully titrated.

Maintenance of anesthesia with halothane, sevoflurane or isoflurane: Continuous I.V. infusion: Children 1-12 years: 0.25 mcg/kg/minute (range 0.05-1.3 mcg/kg/minute); supplemental bolus dose of 1 mcg/kg may be administered every 2-5 minutes. Consider increasing concomitant anesthetics with infusion rate >1 mcg/kg/minute. Infusion rate can be titrated upward in increments up to 50% or titrated downward in decrements of 25% to 50%. May titrate every 2-5 minutes.

Available Dosage Forms Injection, powder for reconstitution: 1 mg, 2 mg, 5 mg [contains glycine 15 mg]

Nursing Guidelines

Geriatric Considerations: Elderly patients have an increased sensitivity to effect of remifentanil, therefore, doses should be decreased by ½ and titrated.

Pregnancy Risk Factor: C

Pregnancy Issues: Remifentanil has been shown to cross the placenta. Neonatal respiratory depression and sedation may occur.

Lactation: Excretion in breast milk unknown/use caution

Perioperative/Anesthesia/Other Concerns: Ultra short-acting narcotic that is unique compared to other short-acting narcotics. This agent is not considered suitable as the sole agent for induction; remifentanil should be used in combination with other induction agents; bolus doses are not recommended for sedation cases and in treatment of postoperative pain due to risk of respiratory depression and muscle rigidity; due to remifentanil's short duration of action, when postoperative pain is anticipated, discontinuation of an infusion of remifentanil should be preceded by an adequate postoperative analgesic (ie, fentanyl, morphine).

Elderly patients have an increased sensitivity to effect of remifentanil, doses should be decreased by 1/2 and titrated.

Administration

I.V.: An infusion device should be used to administer continuous infusions. During the maintenance of general anesthesia, I.V. boluses may be administered over 30-60 seconds. Injections should be given into I.V. tubing close to the venous cannula; tubing should be cleared after treatment to prevent residual effects when other fluids are administered through the same I.V. line.

Reconstitution: Prepare solution by adding 1 mL of diluent per 1 mg of remifentanil. Shake well. Further dilute to a final concentration of 20, 25, 50, or 250 mcg/mL.

Compatibility: Stable in D_5LR, D_5NS, D_5W, 1/2NS, NS, SWFI

Incompatible with blood products

Y-site administration: Incompatible with amphotericin B cholesteryl sulfate complex

Storage: Prior to reconstitution, store at 2°C to 25°C (36°F to 77°F). Stable for 24 hours at room temperature after reconstitution and further dilution to concentrations of 20-250 mcg/mL (4 hours if diluted with LR).

Related Information

Narcotic / Opioid Analgesics *on page 1880*

- **Reno-30®** *see* Diatrizoate Meglumine *on page 513*
- **Reno-60®** *see* Diatrizoate Meglumine *on page 513*
- **RenoCal-76®** *see* Diatrizoate Meglumine and Diatrizoate Sodium *on page 514*
- **Reno-Dip®** *see* Diatrizoate Meglumine *on page 513*
- **Renografin®-60** *see* Diatrizoate Meglumine and Diatrizoate Sodium *on page 514*
- **ReoPro®** *see* Abciximab *on page 60*
- **Repan®** *see* Butalbital, Acetaminophen, and Caffeine *on page 280*
- **Replace [OTC]** *see* Vitamins (Multiple/Oral) *on page 1720*
- **Replace with Iron [OTC]** *see* Vitamins (Multiple/Oral) *on page 1720*
- **Requip®** *see* Ropinirole *on page 1495*
- **Resectisol®** *see* Mannitol *on page 1079*
- **Restasis™** *see* CycloSPORINE *on page 465*
- **Restoril®** *see* Temazepam *on page 1601*
- **Restylane®** *see* Hyaluronate and Derivatives *on page 856*
- **Retavase®** *see* Reteplase *on page 1469*

Reteplase (RE ta plase)

U.S. Brand Names Retavase®

Synonyms Recombinant Plasminogen Activator; r-PA

Pharmacologic Category Thrombolytic Agent

Use Management of acute myocardial infarction (AMI); improvement of ventricular function; reduction of the incidence of CHF and the reduction of mortality following AMI

Mechanism of Action Reteplase is a nonglycosylated form of tPA produced by recombinant DNA technology using *E. coli*; it initiates local fibrinolysis by binding to fibrin in a thrombus (clot) and converts entrapped plasminogen to plasmin

Pharmacodynamics/Kinetics

Onset of action: Thrombolysis: 30-90 minutes

Half-life elimination: 13-16 minutes

Excretion: Feces and urine

Clearance: Plasma: 250-450 mL/minute

Contraindications Hypersensitivity to reteplase or any component of the formulation; active internal bleeding; history of cerebrovascular accident; recent intracranial or intraspinal surgery or trauma; intracranial neoplasm, arteriovenous (Continued)

Reteplase *(Continued)*

malformations, or aneurysm; known bleeding diathesis; severe uncontrolled hypertension

Warnings/Precautions Concurrent heparin anticoagulation can contribute to bleeding; careful attention to all potential bleeding sites. I.M. injections and nonessential handling of the patient should be avoided. Venipunctures should be performed carefully and only when necessary. If arterial puncture is necessary, use an upper extremity vessel that can be manually compressed. If serious bleeding occurs then the infusion of anistreplase and heparin should be stopped.

For the following conditions the risk of bleeding is higher with use of reteplase and should be weighed against the benefits of therapy: recent major surgery (eg, CABG, obstetrical delivery, organ biopsy, previous puncture of noncompressible vessels), cerebrovascular disease, recent gastrointestinal or genitourinary bleeding, recent trauma including CPR, hypertension (systolic BP >180 mm Hg and/or diastolic BP >110 mm Hg), high likelihood of left heart thrombus (eg, mitral stenosis with atrial fibrillation), acute pericarditis, subacute bacterial endocarditis, hemostatic defects including ones caused by severe renal or hepatic dysfunction, significant hepatic dysfunction, pregnancy, diabetic hemorrhagic retinopathy or other hemorrhagic ophthalmic conditions, septic thrombophlebitis or occluded AV cannula at seriously infected site, advanced age (eg, >75 years), patients receiving oral anticoagulants, any other condition in which bleeding constitutes a significant hazard or would be particularly difficult to manage because of location.

Coronary thrombolysis may result in reperfusion arrhythmias. Follow standard MI management. Rare anaphylactic reactions can occur. Safety and efficacy in pediatric patients have not been established.

Drug Interactions

Aminocaproic acid (antifibrinolytic agent) may decrease effectiveness.

Drugs which affect platelet function (eg, NSAIDs, dipyridamole, ticlopidine, clopidogrel, IIb/IIIa antagonists) may potentiate the risk of hemorrhage; use with caution.

Heparin and aspirin: Use with aspirin and heparin may increase bleeding. However, aspirin and heparin were used concomitantly with reteplase in the majority of patients in clinical studies.

Warfarin or oral anticoagulants: Risk of bleeding may be increased during concurrent therapy.

Adverse Reactions Bleeding is the most frequent adverse effect associated with reteplase. Heparin and aspirin have been administered concurrently with reteplase in clinical trials. The incidence of adverse events is a reflection of these combined therapies, and are comparable with comparison thrombolytics.

>10%: Local: Injection site bleeding (4.6% to 48.6%)

1% to 10%:

- Gastrointestinal: Bleeding (1.8% to 9.0%)
- Genitourinary: Bleeding (0.9% to 9.5%)
- Hematologic: Anemia (0.9% to 2.6%)

<1% (Limited to important or life-threatening): Allergic/anaphylactoid reactions, cholesterol embolization, intracranial hemorrhage (0.8%)

Other adverse effects noted are frequently associated with MI (and therefore may or may not be attributable to Retavase®) and include arrhythmia, arrest, cardiac reinfarction, cardiogenic shock, embolism, hypotension, pericarditis, pulmonary edema, tamponade, thrombosis

Overdosage/Toxicology Symptoms of overdose include increased incidence of intracranial bleeding. Treatment is supportive.

Dosing

Adults & Elderly:

Acute MI (thrombolysis): I.V.: 10 units I.V. over 2 minutes, followed by a second dose 30 minutes later of 10 units I.V. over 2 minutes; withhold second dose if serious bleeding or anaphylaxis occurs.

Pediatrics: Not recommended

Available Dosage Forms Injection, powder for reconstitution [preservative free]: 10.4 units [equivalent to reteplase 18.1 mg; contains sucrose and polysorbate 80; packaged with sterile water for injection]

Nursing Guidelines

Assessment: See Contraindications, Warnings/Precautions, and Dosing for use cautions. Assess potential for interactions with other prescriptions, OTC medications, or herbal products patient may be taking (especially those medications that may affect coagulation or platelet function - see Drug Interactions). See

Administration specifics for infusion. Neurological status (eg, intracranial hemorrhage), vital signs, and ECG should be monitored prior to, during, and after therapy. Assess infusion site and monitor for hemorrhage during and following therapy (see Adverse Reactions and Overdose/Toxicology). Bedrest and bleeding precautions should be maintained. Avoid I.M. injections and nonessential handling of the patient. Venipunctures should be performed carefully and only when necessary. If arterial puncture is necessary, use an upper extremity vessel that can be manually compressed. Patient instructions determined by patient condition (see Patient Education). Note breast-feeding caution.

Monitoring Laboratory Tests: CBC, PTT, signs and symptoms of bleeding, ECG monitoring

Patient Education: Inform prescriber of all prescriptions, OTC medications, or herbal products you are taking, and any allergies you have. This medication can only be administered by infusion; you will be monitored closely during and after treatment. You will have a tendency to bleed easily; use caution to prevent injury (use electric razor, soft toothbrush, and caution with knives, needles, or anything sharp). Follow instructions for strict bedrest to reduce the risk of injury. If bleeding occurs, report immediately and apply pressure to bleeding spot until bleeding stops completely. Report unusual pain (acute headache, joint pain, chest pain); unusual bruising or bleeding; blood in urine, stool, or vomitus; bleeding gums; vision changes; or respiratory difficulty. **Pregnancy/breast-feeding precautions:** Inform prescriber if you are or intend to become pregnant. Consult prescriber if breast-feeding.

Pregnancy Risk Factor: C

Lactation: Excretion in breast milk unknown/use caution

Administration

I.V.: Infuse over 2 minutes.

Reconstitution: Reteplase should be reconstituted using the diluent, syringe, needle, and dispensing pin provided with each kit.

Storage: Dosage kits should be stored at 2°C to 25°C (36°F to 77°F) and remain sealed until use in order to protect from light.

- Retrovir® *see* Zidovudine *on page 1732*
- Reversol® *see* Edrophonium *on page 596*
- Revex® *see* Nalmefene *on page 1198*
- ReVia® *see* Naltrexone *on page 1202*
- rFVIIa *see* Factor VIIa (Recombinant) *on page 700*
- rGM-CSF *see* Sargramostim *on page 1509*
- r-hCG *see* Chorionic Gonadotropin (Recombinant) *on page 389*
- Rheumatrex® *see* Methotrexate *on page 1127*
- RhIG *see* Rh$_o$(D) Immune Globulin *on page 1471*
- Rhinall [OTC] *see* Phenylephrine *on page 1350*
- Rhinocort® Aqua® *see* Budesonide *on page 260*

Rh$_o$(D) Immune Globulin (ar aych oh (dee) i MYUN GLOB yoo lin)

U.S. Brand Names BayRho-D® Full-Dose; BayRho-D® Mini-Dose; MICRhoGAM®; RhoGAM®; Rhophylac®; WinRho® SDF

Synonyms RhIG; Rho(D) Immune Globulin (Human); RhoIGIV; RhoIVIM

Pharmacologic Category Immune Globulin

Use

Suppression of Rh isoimmunization: Use in the following situations when an Rh$_o$(D)-negative individual is exposed to Rh$_o$(D)-positive blood: During delivery of an Rh$_o$(D)-positive infant; abortion; amniocentesis; chorionic villus sampling; ruptured tubal pregnancy; abdominal trauma; transplacental hemorrhage. Used when the mother is Rh$_o$(D) negative, the father of the child is either Rh$_o$(D) positive or Rh$_o$(D) unknown, the baby is either Rh$_o$(D) positive or Rh$_o$(D) unknown.

Transfusion: Suppression of Rh isoimmunization in Rh$_o$(D)-negative female children and female adults in their childbearing years transfused with Rh$_o$(D) antigen-positive RBCs or blood components containing Rh$_o$(D) antigen-positive RBCs

Treatment of idiopathic thrombocytopenic purpura (ITP): Used in the following nonsplenectomized Rh$_o$(D) positive individuals: Children with acute or chronic ITP, adults with chronic ITP, children and adults with ITP secondary to HIV infection

(Continued)

Rh$_o$(D) Immune Globulin *(Continued)*

Mechanism of Action

Rh suppression: Prevents isoimmunization by suppressing the immune response and antibody formation by Rh$_o$(D) negative individuals to Rh$_o$(D) positive red blood cells.

ITP: Not completely characterized; Rh$_o$(D) immune globulin is thought to form anti-D-coated red blood cell complexes which bind to macrophage Fc receptors within the spleen; blocking or saturating the spleens ability to clear antibody-coated cells, including platelets. In this manner, platelets are spared from destruction.

Pharmacodynamics/Kinetics

Onset of platelet increase: ITP: Platelets should rise within 1-2 days
Peak effect: In 7-14 days

Duration: Suppression of Rh isoimmunization: ~12 weeks; Treatment of ITP: 30 days (variable)

Distribution: V_d: I.M.: 8.59 L

Half-life elimination: 21-30 days

Time to peak, plasma: I.M.: 5-10 days; I.V. (WinRho® SDF): ≤2 hours

Contraindications Hypersensitivity to immune globulins or any component of the formulation; prior sensitization to Rh$_o$(D)

Warnings/Precautions Rare but serious signs and symptoms (eg, back pain, shaking, chills, fever, discolored urine; onset within 4 hours of infusion) of intravascular hemolysis (IVH) have been reported in postmarketing experience in patients treated for ITP. Clinically-compromising anemia, acute renal insufficiency and disseminated intravascular coagulation (DIC) have also been reported. ITP patients should be advised of the signs and symptoms of IVH and instructed to report them immediately.

As a product of human plasma, may potentially transmit disease; screening of donors, as well as testing and/or inactivation of certain viruses reduces this risk. Not for replacement therapy in immune globulin deficiency syndromes. Use caution with IgA deficiency, may contain trace amounts of IgA; patients who are IgA deficient may have the potential for developing IgA antibodies, anaphylactic reactions may occur. Administer I.M. injections with caution in patients with thrombocytopenia or coagulation disorders. Some products may contain maltose, which may result in falsely-elevated blood glucose readings. Use caution with renal dysfunction; may require an infusion rate reduction or discontinuation.

Do not administer I.M. or SubQ for the treatment of ITP; administer dose I.V. only. Safety and efficacy not established in Rh$_o$(D) negative, non-ITP thrombocytopenia, or splenectomized patients. Decrease dose with hemoglobin <10 g/dL; use with extreme caution if hemoglobin <8 g/dL

Rh$_o$(D) suppression: For use in the mother; do not administer to the neonate.

Drug Interactions Live virus vaccines (measles, mumps, polio, rubella): Rh$_o$(D) immune globulin may interfere with the response of live vaccines; vaccines should not be administered within 3 months after Rh$_o$(D).

Lab Interactions Some infants born to women given Rh$_o$(D) antepartum have a weakly positive Coombs' test at birth. Fetal-maternal hemorrhage may cause false blood-typing result in the mother; when there is any doubt to the patients' Rh type, Rh$_o$(D) immune globulin should be administered. WinRho® SDF liquid contains maltose; may result in falsely elevated blood glucose levels with dehydrogenase pyrroloquinolinequinone or glucose-dye-oxidoreductase testing methods. WinRho® SDF contains trace amounts of anti-A, B , C and E; may alter Coombs' tests following administration.

Adverse Reactions Frequency not defined.

Cardiovascular: Hyper-/hypotension, pallor, tachycardia, vasodilation

Central nervous system: Chills, dizziness, fever, headache, malaise, somnolence

Dermatologic: Pruritus, rash

Gastrointestinal: Abdominal pain, diarrhea, nausea, vomiting

Hematologic: Hemoglobin decreased (patients with ITP), intravascular hemolysis (patients with ITP)

Hepatic: LDH increased

Local: Injection site reaction: Discomfort, induration, mild pain, redness, swelling

Neuromuscular & skeletal: Arthralgia, back pain, hyperkinesia, myalgia, weakness

Renal: Acute renal insufficiency

Miscellaneous: Anaphylaxis, diaphoresis, infusion-related reactions

Postmarketing and/or case reports: Signs and symptoms of IVH are associated with treatment for ITP with WinRho® SDF: Anemia (clinically-compromising), DIC

Overdosage/Toxicology No symptoms are likely, however, high doses have been associated with a mild, transient hemolytic anemia. Treatment should be symptom-directed and supportive.

Dosing

Adults:

ITP: WinRho® SDF: I.V.:

Initial: 50 mcg/kg as a single injection, or can be given as a divided dose on separate days. If hemoglobin is <10 g/dL: Dose should be reduced to 25-40 mcg/kg

Subsequent dosing: 25-60 mcg/kg can be used if required to elevate platelet count

Maintenance dosing if patient **did respond** to initial dosing: 25-60 mcg/kg based on platelet and hemoglobin levels:

Maintenance dosing if patient **did not respond** to initial dosing:

Hemoglobin 8-10 g/dL: Redose between 25-40 mcg/kg

Hemoglobin >10 g/dL: Redose between 50-60 mcg/kg

Hemoglobin <8 g/dL: Use with caution

$Rh_o(D)$ suppression: Note: One "full dose" (300 mcg) provides enough antibody to prevent Rh sensitization if the volume of RBC entering the circulation is ≤15 mL. When >15 mL is suspected, a fetal red cell count should be performed to determine the appropriate dose.

Pregnancy:

Antepartum prophylaxis: In general, dose is given at 28 weeks. If given early in pregnancy, administer every 12 weeks to ensure adequate levels of passively acquired anti-Rh

BayRho-D® Full Dose, RhoGAM®: I.M.: 300 mcg

Rhophylac®, WinRho® SDF: I.M., I.V.: 300 mcg

Postpartum prophylaxis: In general, dose is administered as soon as possible after delivery, preferably within 72 hours. Can be given up to 28 days following delivery

BayRho-D® Full Dose, RhoGAM®: I.M.: 300 mcg

Rhophylac®: I.M., I.V.: 300 mcg

WinRho® SDF: I.M., I.V.: 120 mcg

Threatened abortion, any time during pregnancy (with continuation of pregnancy):

BayRho-D® Full Dose, RhoGAM®: I.M.: 300 mcg; administer as soon as possible

Rhophylac®, WinRho® SDF: I.M./I.V.: 300 mcg; administer as soon as possible

Abortion, miscarriage, termination of ectopic pregnancy:

BayRho-D®, RhoGAM®: I.M.: ≥13 weeks gestation: 300 mcg.

BayRho-D® Mini Dose, MICRhoGAM®: <13 weeks gestation: I.M.: 50 mcg

Rhophylac®: I.M., I.V.: 300 mcg

WinRho® SDF: I.M., I.V.: After 34 weeks gestation: 120 mcg; administer immediately or within 72 hours

Amniocentesis, chorionic villus sampling:

BayRho-D®, RhoGAM®: I.M.: At 15-18 weeks gestation or during the 3rd trimester: 300 mcg. If dose is given between 13-18 weeks, repeat at 26-28 weeks and within 72 hours of delivery.

Rhophylac®: I.M., I.V.: 300 mcg

WinRho® SDF: I.M., I.V.:

Before 34 weeks gestation: 300 mcg; administer immediately, repeat dose every 12 weeks during pregnancy

After 34 weeks gestation: 120 mcg, administered immediately or within 72 hours

Abdominal trauma, manipulation:

BayRho-D®, RhoGAM®: I.M.: 2nd or 3rd trimester: 300 mcg. If dose is given between 13-18 weeks, repeat at 26-28 weeks and within 72 hours of delivery.

Rhophylac®: I.M., I.V.: 300 mcg

WinRho® SDF: I.M., I.V.: After 34 weeks gestation: 120 mcg; administer immediately or within 72 hours

Transfusion:

BayRho-D®, RhoGAM®: I.M.: Multiply the volume of Rh positive whole blood administered by the hematocrit of the donor unit to equal the volume of

(Continued)

Rh_o(D) Immune Globulin *(Continued)*

RBCs transfused. The volume of RBCs is then divided by 15 mL, providing the number of 300 mcg doses (vials/syringes) to administer. If the dose calculated results in a fraction, round up to the next higher whole 300 mcg dose (vial/syringe).

WinRho® SDF: Administer within 72 hours after exposure of incompatible blood transfusions or massive fetal hemorrhage.

I.V.: Calculate dose as follows; administer 600 mcg every 8 hours until the total dose is administered:

Exposure to Rh_o(D) positive whole blood: 9 mcg/mL blood

Exposure to Rh_o(D) positive red blood cells: 18 mcg/mL cells

I.M.: Calculate dose as follows; administer 1200 mcg every 12 hours until the total dose is administered:

Exposure to Rh_o(D) positive whole blood: 12 mcg/mL blood

Exposure to Rh_o(D) positive red blood cells: 24 mcg/mL cells

Rhophylac®: I.M., I.V.:20 mcg per 2 mL transfused blood or 1 mL erythrocyte concentrate

Pediatrics: ITP, transfusion: WinRho® SDF: Refer to adult dosing.

Renal Impairment: I.V. infusion: Use caution; may require infusion rate reduction or discontinuation.

Available Dosage Forms

Injection, solution [preservative free]:

BayRho-D® Full-Dose, RhoGAM®: 300 mcg [for I.M. use only]

BayRho-D® Mini-Dose, MICRhoGAM®: 50 mcg [for I.M. use only]

Rhophylac®: 300 mcg/2 mL (2 mL) [1500 int. units; for I.M. or I.V. use]

WinRho® SDF:

120 mcg/~0.5 mL (~0.5 mL) [600 int. units; contains maltose; for I.M. or I.V. use]

300 mcg/~1.3 mL (~1.3 mL) [1500 int. units; contains maltose; for I.M. or I.V. use]

500 mcg/~2.2 mL (~2.2 mL) [2500 int. units; contains maltose; for I.M. or I.V. use]

1000 mcg/~4.4 mL(~4.4 mL) [5000 int. units; contains maltose, for I.M. or I.V. use]

3000 mcg/~13 mL (~13 mL) [15,000 int. units; contains maltose; for I.M. or I.V. use]

Injection, powder for reconstitution [preservative free] (WinRho® SDF):

120 mcg [600 int. units; for I.M. or I.V. use]

300 mcg [1500 int. units; for I.M. or I.V. use]

1000 mcg [5000 int. units; for I.M. or I.V. use]

Nursing Guidelines

Assessment: Assess results of laboratory tests, therapeutic effectiveness, and adverse reactions. Teach patient possible side effects, interventions to reduce side effects, and adverse reactions to report.

Monitoring Laboratory Tests: Patients with suspected IVH should have CBC, haptoglobulin, plasma hemoglobin, urine dipstick, BUN, serum creatinine, liver function tests, DIC-specific tests (D-dimer, fibrin degradation products [FDP] or fibrin split products [FSP]) for differential diagnosis. Clinical response may be determined by monitoring platelets, red blood cell (RBC) counts, hemoglobulin, and reticulocyte levels.

Patient Education: Do not have live virus vaccinations within 3 months of receiving this medication. This medication can only be administered by injection or infusion; report immediately any difficulty breathing, chills, rapid heart beat, back rash, pain, or redness, swelling, or pain at injection site. You may experience headache or mild headache (consult prescriber for appropriate analgesic). Report any acute or persistent adverse effects. **Pregnancy precautions:** Inform prescriber if you are pregnant or plan to become pregnant.

Pregnancy Risk Factor: C

Pregnancy Issues: Animal studies have not been conducted. Available evidence suggests that Rh_o(D) immune globulin administration during pregnancy does not harm the fetus or affect future pregnancies.

Lactation: Does not enter breast milk

Administration

I.M.: Administer into the deltoid muscle of the upper arm or anterolateral aspect of the upper thigh. Avoid gluteal region due to risk of sciatic nerve injury. If large doses (>5 mL) are needed, administration in divided doses at different sites is recommended. **Note:** Do not administer I.M. Rho(D) immune globulin for ITP.

I.V.: WinRho® SDF: Infuse over at least 3-5 minutes; do not administer with other medications

Reconstitution: WinRho® SDF lyophilized powder: Dilute with provided NS only with volumes specified below. Inject diluent slowly into vial and gently swirl until dissolved; do not shake.

I.V. administration:

600 units (120 mcg) vial: 2.5 mL diluent

1500 units (300 mcg) vial: 2.5 mL diluent

5000 units (1000 mcg) vial: 8.5 mL diluent

I.M. administration:

600 units (120 mcg) vial: 1.25 mL diluent

1500 units (300 mcg) vial: 1.25 mL diluent

5000 units (1000 mcg) vial: 8.5 mL diluent (administer into several sites)

Storage: Store at 2°C to 8°C (35°F to 46°F). Do not freeze.

Rhophylac®: Stored at this temperature, Rhophylac® has a shelf life of 36 months. Protect from light.

WinRho® SDF lyophilized powder: Following reconstitution, may store at room temperature for up to 12 hours.

♦ Rho(D) Immune Globulin (Human) *see* Rh_o(D) Immune Globulin *on page 1471*
♦ RhoGAM® *see* Rh_o(D) Immune Globulin *on page 1471*
♦ RhoIGIV *see* Rh_o(D) Immune Globulin *on page 1471*
♦ RhoIVIM *see* Rh_o(D) Immune Globulin *on page 1471*
♦ Rhophylac® *see* Rh_o(D) Immune Globulin *on page 1471*
♦ rHuEPO-α *see* Epoetin Alfa *on page 618*
♦ Ribasphere™ *see* Ribavirin *on page 1475*

Ribavirin (rye ba VYE rin)

U.S. Brand Names Copegus®; Rebetol®; Ribasphere™; Virazole®

Synonyms RTCA; Tribavirin

Pharmacologic Category Antiviral Agent

Medication Safety Issues

Sound-alike/look-alike issues:

Ribavirin may be confused with riboflavin

Use

Inhalation: Treatment of patients with respiratory syncytial virus (RSV) infections; specially indicated for treatment of severe lower respiratory tract RSV infections in patients with an underlying compromising condition (prematurity, bronchopulmonary dysplasia and other chronic lung conditions, congenital heart disease, immunodeficiency, immunosuppression), and recent transplant recipients

Oral capsule:

In combination with interferon alfa-2b (Intron® A) injection for the treatment of chronic hepatitis C in patients with compensated liver disease who have relapsed after alpha interferon therapy or were previously untreated with alpha interferons

In combination with peginterferon alfa-2b (PEG-Intron®) injection for the treatment of chronic hepatitis C in patients with compensated liver disease who were previously untreated with alpha interferons

Oral solution: In combination with interferon alfa 2b (Intron® A) injection for the treatment of chronic hepatitis C in patients ≥3 years of age with compensated liver disease who were previously untreated with alpha interferons or patients ≥18 years of age who have relapsed after alpha interferon therapy

Oral tablet: In combination with peginterferon alfa-2a (Pegasys®) injection for the treatment of chronic hepatitis C in patients with compensated liver disease who were previously untreated with alpha interferons (includes patients with histological evidence of cirrhosis [Child-Pugh class A] and patients with clinically-stable HIV disease)

Unlabeled/Investigational Use Used in other viral infections including influenza A and B and adenovirus

Mechanism of Action Inhibits replication of RNA and DNA viruses; inhibits influenza virus RNA polymerase activity and inhibits the initiation and elongation of RNA fragments resulting in inhibition of viral protein synthesis

Pharmacodynamics/Kinetics

Absorption: Inhalation: Systemic; dependent upon respiratory factors and method of drug delivery; maximal absorption occurs with the use of aerosol generator via endotracheal tube; highest concentrations in respiratory tract and erythrocytes

(Continued)

Ribavirin *(Continued)*

Distribution: Oral capsule: Single dose: V_d 2825 L; distribution significantly prolonged in the erythrocyte (16-40 days), which can be used as a marker for intracellular metabolism

Protein binding: Oral: None

Metabolism: Hepatically and intracellularly (forms active metabolites); may be necessary for drug action

Bioavailability: Oral: 64%

Half-life elimination, plasma:

Children: Inhalation: 6.5-11 hours

Adults: Oral:

Capsule, single dose (Rebetol®, Ribasphere™): 24 hours in healthy adults, 44 hours with chronic hepatitis C infection (increases to ~298 hours at steady state)

Tablet, single dose (Copegus®): 120-170 hours

Time to peak, serum: Inhalation: At end of inhalation period; Oral capsule: Multiple doses: 3 hours; Tablet: 2 hours

Excretion: Inhalation: Urine (40% as unchanged drug and metabolites); Oral capsule: Urine (61%), feces (12%)

Contraindications Hypersensitivity to ribavirin or any component of the formulation; women of childbearing age who will not use contraception reliably; pregnancy

Additional contraindications for oral formulation: Male partners of pregnant women; Cl_{cr}< 50 mL/minute; hemoglobinopathies (eg, thalassemia major, sickle cell anemia); as monotherapy for treatment of chronic hepatitis C; patients with autoimmune hepatitis, anemia, severe heart disease

Refer to individual monographs for Interferon Alfa-2b (Intron® A) and Peginterferon Alfa-2a (Pegasys®) for additional contraindication information.

Warnings/Precautions Negative pregnancy test is required before initiation and monthly thereafter. Avoid pregnancy in female patients and female partners of male patients, during therapy, and for at least 6 months after treatment; two forms of contraception should be used. Elderly patients are more susceptible to adverse effects; use caution. Safety and efficacy have not been established in patients who have failed other alpha interferon therapy, received organ transplants, or been coinfected with hepatitis B or HIV (Copegus® may be used in HIV coinfected patients unless CD4+ cell count is <100 cells/microL). Safety and efficacy have not been established in patients <3 years of age.

Inhalation: Use with caution in patients requiring assisted ventilation because precipitation of the drug in the respiratory equipment may interfere with safe and effective patient ventilation; monitor carefully in patients with COPD and asthma for deterioration of respiratory function. Ribavirin is potentially mutagenic, tumor-promoting, and gonadotoxic. Although anemia has not been reported with inhalation therapy, consider monitoring for anemia 1-2 weeks post-treatment. Pregnant healthcare workers may consider unnecessary occupational exposure; ribavirin has been detected in healthcare workers' urine. Healthcare professionals or family members who are pregnant (or may become pregnant) should be counseled about potential risks of exposure and counseled about risk reduction strategies.

Oral: Severe psychiatric events have occurred including depression and suicidal behavior during combination therapy. Avoid use in patients with a psychiatric history; discontinue if severe psychiatric symptoms occur. Hemolytic anemia is a significant toxicity; usually occurring within 1-2 weeks. Assess cardiac disease before initiation. Anemia may worsen underlying cardiac disease; use caution. If any deterioration in cardiovascular status occurs, discontinue therapy. Use caution in pulmonary disease; pulmonary symptoms have been associated with administration. Discontinue therapy in suspected/confirmed pancreatitis or if hepatic decompensation occurs. Use caution in patients with sarcoidosis (exacerbation reported).

Hemolytic anemia (hemoglobin <10 g/dL) was observed in up to 10% of treated patients in clinical trials when alfa interferons were combined with ribavirin; anemia occurred within 1-2 weeks of initiation of therapy.

Drug Interactions

Antiretroviral (nucleoside): Concomitant use of ribavirin and nucleoside analogues may increase the risk of developing lactic acidosis (includes adefovir, didanosine, lamivudine, stavudine, zalcitabine, zidovudine). Concurrent use with didanosine has been noted to increase the risk of pancreatitis, peripheral neuropathy in addition to lactic acidosis. Suspend therapy if signs/ symptoms of toxicity are present.

Interferons (alfa): Concurrent therapy may increase the risk of hemolytic anemia.

Lamivudine, stavudine: Antagonistic *in vitro*; use with caution (per manufacturer)

Zidovudine: Antagonistic *in vitro*; use with caution (per manufacturer). Concurrent therapy with ribavirin/interferon alfa-2a may cause increased risk of severe anemia and/or severe neutropenia.

Nutritional/Herbal/Ethanol Interactions Food: Oral: High-fat meal increases the AUC and C_{max}.

Adverse Reactions

Inhalation:

1% to 10%:

Central nervous system: Fatigue, headache, insomnia

Gastrointestinal: Nausea, anorexia

Hematologic: Anemia

<1%: Hypotension, cardiac arrest, digitalis toxicity, conjunctivitis, mild bronchospasm, worsening of respiratory function, apnea

Note: Incidence of adverse effects (approximate) in healthcare workers: Headache (51%); conjunctivitis (32%); rhinitis, nausea, rash, dizziness, pharyngitis, and lacrimation (10% to 20%)

Oral (all adverse reactions are documented while receiving combination therapy with interferon alpha-2b or interferon alpha-2a; percentages as reported in adults):

>10%:

Central nervous system: Fatigue (60% to 70%)*, headache (43% to 66%)*, fever (32% to 46%)*, insomnia (26% to 41%), depression (20% to 36%)*, irritability (23% to 32%), dizziness (14% to 26%), impaired concentration (10% to 14%)*, emotional lability (7% to 12%)*

Dermatologic: Alopecia (27% to 36%), pruritus (13% to 29%), dry skin (13% to 24%), rash (5% to 28%), dermatitis (up to 16%)

Gastrointestinal: Nausea (33% to 47%), anorexia (21% to 32%), weight decrease (10% to 29%), diarrhea (10% to 22%), dyspepsia (8% to 16%), vomiting (9% to 14%)*, abdominal pain (8% to 13%), xerostomia (up to 12%), RUQ pain (up to 12%)

Hematologic: Neutropenia (8% to 27%; 40% with HIV coinfection), hemoglobin decreased (25% to 36%), hyperbilirubinemia (24% to 34%), anemia (11% to 17%), lymphopenia (12% to 14%), absolute neutrophil count <0.5 x 10^9/L (5% to 11%), thrombocytopenia (<1% to 14%), hemolytic anemia (10% to 13%), WBC decreased

Neuromuscular & skeletal: Myalgia (40% to 64%)*, rigors (40% to 48%), arthralgia (22% to 34%)*, musculoskeletal pain (19% to 28%)

Respiratory: Dyspnea (13% to 26%), cough (7% to 23%), pharyngitis (up to 13%), sinusitis (up to 12%)*, nasal congestion

Miscellaneous: Flu-like syndrome (13% to 18%)*, viral infection (up to 12%), diaphoresis increased (up to 11%)

*Similar to interferon alone

1% to 10%:

Cardiovascular: Chest pain (5% to 9%)*, flushing (up to 4 %)

Central nervous system: Mood alteration (up to 6%; 9% with HIV coinfection), memory impairment (up to 6%), malaise (up to 6%), nervousness (~5%)*

Dermatologic: Eczema (4% to 5%)

Endocrine & metabolic: Hypothyroidism (up to 5%)

Gastrointestinal: Taste perversion (4% to 9%), constipation (up to 5%)

Genitourinary: Menstrual disorder (up to 7%)

Hepatic: Hepatomegaly (up to 4%)

Neuromuscular & skeletal: Weakness (9% to 10%), back pain (5%)

Ocular: Conjunctivitis (up to 6%), blurred vision (up to 5%)

Respiratory: Rhinitis (up to 8%), exertional dyspnea (up to 7%)

Miscellaneous: Fungal infection (up to 6%)

*Similar to interferon alone

<1% (Limited to important or life-threatening): Aggression, angina, anxiety, aplastic anemia, arrhythmia; autoimmune disorders (systemic lupus erythematosus, rheumatoid arthritis, sarcoidosis); cerebreal hemorrhage, cholangitis, colitis, coma, diabetes mellitus, fatty liver, gastrointestinal bleeding, gout, hepatic dysfunction, hyper-/hypothyroidism, myositis, pancreatitis, peptic ulcer,

(Continued)

Ribavirin *(Continued)*

peripheral neuropathy, psychosis, pulmonary dysfunction, pulmonary embolism, suicidal ideation, suicide, thrombotic thrombocytopenic purpura, thyroid function test abnormalities

Note: Incidence of anorexia, headache, fever, suicidal ideation, and vomiting are higher in children.

Overdosage/Toxicology Treatment is symptom-directed and supportive. Not effectively removed by hemodialysis.

Dosing

Adults & Elderly:

Chronic hepatitis C (in combination with peginterferon alfa-2a): Oral tablet (Copegus®):

Monoinfection, genotype 1,4:

<75 kg: 1000 mg/day, in 2 divided doses for 48 weeks

≥75 kg: 1200 mg/day, in 2 divided doses for 48 weeks

Monoinfection, genotype 2,3: 800 mg/day, in 2 divided doses, for 24 weeks

Coinfection with HIV: 800 mg/day in 2 divided doses for 48 weeks

Note: Also refer to Peginterferon Alfa-2a monograph

Chronic hepatitis C (in combination with interferon alfa-2b): Oral capsule (Rebetol®, Ribasphere™):

Note: Also refer to Interferon Alfa-2b/Ribavirin combination pack monograph

≤75 kg: 400 mg in the morning, then 600 mg in the evening

>75 kg: 600 mg in the morning, then 600 mg in the evening

Note: If HCV-RNA is undetectable at 24 weeks, duration of therapy is 48 weeks. In patients who relapse following interferon therapy, duration of dual therapy is 24 weeks.

Chronic hepatitis C (in combination with peginterferon alfa-2b): Oral capsule (Rebetol®, Ribasphere™): 400 mg twice daily; duration of therapy is 1 year; after 24 weeks of treatment, if serum HCV-RNA is not below the limit of detection of the assay, consider discontinuation.

Pediatrics:

RSV infection: Infants and Children:

Aerosol inhalation: Use with Viratek® small particle aerosol generator (SPAG-2): A concentration of 20 mg/mL (6 g reconstituted with 300 mL of sterile water without preservatives)

Aerosol only: 12-18 hours/day for 3 days, up to 7 days in length

Chronic hepatitis C (in combination with interferon alfa-2b): Oral solution should be used in children 3-5 years of age, children ≤25 kg, or those unable to swallow capsules.

Capsule/oral solution: Children ≥3 years: 15 mg/kg/day in 2 divided doses.

Capsule dosing recommendations:

25-36 kg: 400 mg/day (200 mg morning and evening)

37-49 kg: 600 mg/day (200 mg in the morning and two 200 mg capsules in the evening)

50-61 kg: 800 mg/day (two 200 mg capsules morning and evening)

>61 kg: Refer to adult dosing.

Note: Duration of therapy is 48 weeks in pediatric patients with genotype 1 and 24 weeks in patients with genotype 2,3. Discontinue treatment in any patient if HCV-RNA is not below the limit of detection of the assay after 24 weeks of therapy.

Note: Also refer to Interferon Alfa-2b/Ribavirin combination pack monograph.

Dosage adjustment for toxicity: Oral (capsule, solution, tablet):

Patient without cardiac history:

Hemoglobin <10 g/dL: 7.5 mg/kg/day

Hemoglobin <8.5 g/dL: Refer to adult dosing.

Patient with cardiac history:

Hemoglobin has decreased ≥2 g/dL during any 4-week period of treatment: 7.5 mg/kg/day

Hemoglobin <12 g/dL after 4 weeks of reduced dose: Refer to adult dosing.

Renal Impairment: Cl_{cr} <50 mL/minute: Oral is route contraindicated.

Available Dosage Forms

Capsule (Rebetol®, Ribasphere™): 200 mg

Powder for aerosol (Virazole®): 6 g

Powder for solution, inhalation [for aerosol administration] (Virazole®): 6 g [reconstituted product provides 20 mg/mL]

Tablet (Copegus®): 200 mg

Nursing Guidelines

Assessment: See Contraindications and extensive Warnings/Precautions for use cautions. Handle with care (see Warnings/Precautions and Adverse Effects for healthcare professionals' exposure risks). See Administration - Inhalation and Warnings/Precautions for use with mechanically ventilated patients. Assess results of laboratory tests (see below), respiratory status, and adverse reactions (see Adverse Reactions and Overdose/Toxicology). Teach patient proper use (according to formulation), possible side effects/appropriate interventions, and adverse symptoms to report (see Patient Education). **Pregnancy risk factor X** - determine that patient is not pregnant before beginning treatment. Do not give to women of childbearing age or males who may have intercourse with childbearing women unless both male and female are capable of complying with using two effective forms of contraception during therapy and 6 months following therapy. Breast-feeding is not recommended.

Monitoring Laboratory Tests:

Inhalation: Respiratory function, CBC

Oral: CBC with differential (pretreatment, 2- and 4 weeks after initiation); pretreatment and monthly pregnancy test for women of childbearing age; LFTs, TSH, HCV-RNA after 24 weeks of therapy; ECG in patients with pre-existing cardiac disease

Dietary Considerations: When used in combination with interferon alfa-2b, capsules and solution may be taken with or without food, but always in a consistent manner in regard to food intake (ie, always take with food or always take on an empty stomach). When used in combination with peginterferon alfa 2b, capsules should be taken with food. Tablets should be taken with food.

Patient Education: For oral administration, take as directed. For aerosol use, follow directions for use of aerosol device. Do not allow pregnant women or women of childbearing age to handle medication. Maintain adequate hydration (2-3 L/day of fluids) unless instructed to restrict fluid intake. You will need regular blood tests while taking this drug. You may experience increased susceptibility to infection (avoid crowds and exposure to infection and do not have any vaccinations without consulting prescriber). May cause confusion, impaired concentration, or headache (use cautions when driving or engaging in potentially hazardous tasks until response to drug is known); nausea, vomiting, or anorexia (small, frequent meals, frequent mouth care, chewing gum, or sucking lozenges may help); diarrhea (buttermilk, boiled milk, or yogurt may relieve diarrhea); or loss of hair (reversible). Report rash, infection (fever, chills, unusual bleeding or bruising, infection, or unhealed sores or white plaques in mouth); tingling, weakness, or pain in extremities; or other persistent adverse effects. **Pregnancy/breast-feeding precautions:** Inform prescriber if you are pregnant. Both males and females should use appropriate barrier contraceptive measures during and for 60-90 days following end of therapy. Do not allow family members or friends who are pregnant (or may become pregnant) to handle inhalation powder. This drug may cause serious fetal defects. Consult prescriber for appropriate barrier contraceptive measures. Do not donate blood during or for 6 months following therapy. Breast-feeding is not recommended.

Pregnancy Risk Factor: X

Pregnancy Issues: Produced significant embryocidal and/or teratogenic effects in all animal studies at ~0.01 times the maximum recommended daily human dose. Use is contraindicated in pregnancy. Negative pregnancy test is required before initiation and monthly thereafter. Avoid pregnancy in female patients and female partners of male patients during therapy by using two effective forms of contraception; continue contraceptive measures for at least 6 months after completion of therapy. If patient or female partner becomes pregnant during treatment, she should be counseled about potential risks of exposure. If pregnancy occurs during use or within 6 months after treatment, report to company (800-593-2214).

Lactation: Excretion in breast milk unknown/not recommended

Administration

Oral: Administer concurrently with interferon alfa injection. Capsule should not be opened, crushed, chewed, or broken. Capsules are not for use in children <5 years of age. Use oral solution for children 3-5 years, those ≤25 kg, or those who cannot swallow capsules.

Capsule, in combination with interferon alfa-2b: May be administered with or without food, but always in a consistent manner in regard to food intake.

Capsule, in combination with peginterferon alfa 2b: Administer with food.

Solution, in combination with interferon alfa-2b: May be administered with or without food, but always in a consistent manner in regard to food intake.

(Continued)

Ribavirin *(Continued)*

Tablet: Should be administered with food.

Reconstitution: Inhalation: Do not use any water containing an antimicrobial agent to reconstitute drug. Reconstituted solution is stable for 24 hours at room temperature.

Compatibility: Inhalation: Should not be mixed with other aerosolized medication

Storage:

Inhalation: Store vials in a dry place at 15°C to 25°C (59°F to 78°F).

Oral: Store at 15°C to 30°C (59°F to 86°F). Solution may also be refrigerated at 2°C to 8°C (36°F to 46°F).

- **Ribavirin and Interferon Alfa-2b Combination Pack** *see* Interferon Alfa-2b and Ribavirin *on page 940*
- **Rid-A-Pain Dental Drops [OTC]** *see* Benzocaine *on page 232*
- **rIFN-A** *see* Interferon Alfa-2a *on page 933*
- **rIFN beta-1a** *see* Interferon Beta-1a *on page 947*
- **rIFN beta-1b** *see* Interferon Beta-1b *on page 950*
- **Rimso®-50** *see* Dimethyl Sulfoxide *on page 545*
- **Riomet™** *see* Metformin *on page 1112*
- **Risperdal®** *see* Risperidone *on page 1480*
- **Risperdal® M-Tab®** *see* Risperidone *on page 1480*
- **Risperdal® Consta™** *see* Risperidone *on page 1480*

Risperidone (ris PER i done)

U.S. Brand Names Risperdal®; Risperdal® Consta™; Risperdal® M-Tab®

Synonyms Risperdal M-Tab®

Pharmacologic Category Antipsychotic Agent, Atypical

Medication Safety Issues

Sound-alike/look-alike issues:

Risperidone may be confused with reserpine

Risperdal® may be confused with lisinopril, reserpine

Use Treatment of schizophrenia; treatment of acute mania or mixed episodes associated with bipolar I disorder (as monotherapy or in combination with lithium or valproate)

Unlabeled/Investigational Use Behavioral symptoms associated with dementia in elderly; treatment of Tourette's disorder; treatment of pervasive developmental disorder and autism in children and adolescents

Mechanism of Action Risperidone is a benzisoxazole atypical antipsychotic with mixed serotonin-dopamine antagonist activity that binds to 5-HT_2-receptors in the CNS and in the periphery with a very high affinity; binds to dopamine-D_2 receptors with less affinity. The binding affinity to the dopamine-D_2 receptor is 20 times lower than the 5-HT_2 affinity. The addition of serotonin antagonism to dopamine antagonism (classic neuroleptic mechanism) is thought to improve negative symptoms of psychoses and reduce the incidence of extrapyramidal side effects. $Alpha_1$, $alpha_2$ adrenergic, and histaminergic receptors are also antagonized with high affinity. Risperidone has low to moderate affinity for 5-HT_{1C}, 5-HT_{1D}, and 5-HT_{1A} receptors, weak affinity for D_1 and no affinity for muscarinics or $beta_1$ and $beta_2$ receptors

Pharmacodynamics/Kinetics

Absorption:

Oral: Rapid and well absorbed; food does not affect rate or extent

Injection: <1% absorbed initially; main release occurs at ~3 weeks and is maintained from 4-6 weeks

Distribution: V_d: 1-2 L/kg

Protein binding, plasma: Risperidone 90%; 9-hydroxyrisperidone: 77%

Metabolism: Extensively hepatic via CYP2D6 to 9-hydroxyrisperidone (similar pharmacological activity as risperidone); *N*-dealkylation is a second minor pathway

Bioavailability: Solution: 70%; Tablet: 66%; orally-disintegrating tablets are bioequivalent to tablets

Half-life elimination: Active moiety (risperidone and its active metabolite 9-hydroxyrisperidone)

Oral: 20 hours (mean)

Extensive metabolizers: Risperidone: 3 hours; 9-hydroxyrisperidone: 21 hours

Poor metabolizers: Risperidone: 20 hours; 9-hydroxyrisperidone: 30 hours
Injection: 3-6 days; related to microsphere erosion and subsequent absorption of risperidone

Time to peak, plasma: Oral: Risperidone: Within 1 hour; 9-hydroxyrisperidone: Extensive metabolizers: 3 hours; Poor metabolizers: 17 hours

Excretion: Urine (70%); feces (15%)

Contraindications Hypersensitivity to risperidone or any component of the formulation

Warnings/Precautions Elderly patients with dementia-related behavioral disorders treated with atypical antipsychotics are at an increased risk of cerebrovascular adverse events and death compared to placebo; risk may be increased with dehydration (increased risk of death observed with concurrent furosemide). Risperidone is not approved for the treatment of dementia-related psychosis.

Low to moderately sedating, use with caution in disorders where CNS depression is a feature. Use with caution in Parkinson's disease. Caution in patients with hemodynamic instability; bone marrow suppression; predisposition to seizures; subcortical brain damage; severe cardiac, hepatic, or respiratory disease. Use with caution in renal dysfunction. Esophageal dysmotility and aspiration have been associated with antipsychotic use; use with caution in patients at risk of aspiration pneumonia (ie, Alzheimer's disease). Caution in breast cancer or other prolactin-dependent tumors (elevates prolactin levels). May alter temperature regulation or mask toxicity of other drugs due to antiemetic effects.

May cause orthostasis. Use with caution in patients with cardiovascular diseases (eg, heart failure, history of myocardial infarction or ischemia, cerebrovascular disease, conduction abnormalities). Use caution in patients receiving medications for hypertension (orthostatic effects may be exacerbated) or in patients with hypovolemia or dehydration. May alter cardiac conduction (low risk relative to other neuroleptics); life-threatening arrhythmias have occurred with therapeutic doses of neuroleptics.

May cause anticholinergic effects (confusion, agitation, constipation, xerostomia, blurred vision, urinary retention); therefore, they should be used with caution in patients with decreased gastrointestinal motility, urinary retention, BPH, xerostomia, or visual problems. Conditions which also may be exacerbated by cholinergic blockade include narrow-angle glaucoma (screening is recommended) and worsening of myasthenia gravis. Relative to other neuroleptics, risperidone has a low potency of cholinergic blockade.

May cause extrapyramidal symptoms, including pseudoparkinsonism, acute dystonic reactions, akathisia, and tardive dyskinesia (risk of these reactions is low relative to other neuroleptics, and is dose dependent). Risk of neuroleptic malignant syndrome (NMS) may be increased in patients with Parkinson's disease or Lewy Body Dementia; monitor for symptoms of confusion, obtundation, postural instability and extrapyramidal symptoms. May cause hyperglycemia; in some cases may be extreme and associated with ketoacidosis, hyperosmolar coma, or death. Use with caution in patients with diabetes or other disorders of glucose regulation; monitor for worsening of glucose control.

The possibility of a suicide attempt is inherent in psychotic illness or bipolar disorder; use caution in high-risk patients during initiation of therapy. Prescriptions should be written for the smallest quantity consistent with good patient care.

Drug Interactions **Substrate** of CYP2D6 (major), 3A4 (minor); **Inhibits** CYP2D6 (weak), 3A4 (weak)

Acetylcholinesterase inhibitors (central): May increase the risk of antipsychotic-related extrapyramidal symptoms; monitor.

Antihypertensives: Risperidone may enhance the hypotensive effects of antihypertensive agents

Carbamazepine: Plasma concentrations of risperidone and 9-hydroxyrisperidone were decreased by ~50% with concomitant use. The dose of risperidone may need to be titrated accordingly when carbamazepine is added or discontinued.

Clozapine: Decreases clearance of risperidone, increasing its serum concentrations

CYP2D6 inhibitors: May increase the levels/effects of risperidone. Example inhibitors include chlorpromazine, delavirdine, fluoxetine, miconazole, paroxetine, pergolide, quinidine, quinine, ritonavir, and ropinirole.

Levodopa: At high doses (>6 mg/day), risperidone may inhibit the antiparkinsonian effect of levodopa; avoid this combination when high doses are used

Metoclopramide: May increase extrapyramidal symptoms (EPS) or risk.

Verapamil: May increase the levels and effects of risperidone.

(Continued)

Risperidone *(Continued)*

Valproic acid: Generalized edema has been reported as a consequence of concurrent therapy (case report)

Nutritional/Herbal/Ethanol Interactions

Ethanol: Avoid ethanol (may increase CNS depression).

Herb/Nutraceutical: Avoid kava kava, gotu kola, valerian, St John's wort (may increase CNS depression).

Adverse Reactions

Frequency not defined: Gastrointestinal: Dysphagia, esophageal dysmotility

>10%:

Central nervous system: Insomnia, agitation, anxiety, headache, extrapyramidal symptoms (dose dependent), dizziness (I.M. injection)

Gastrointestinal: Weight gain

Respiratory: Rhinitis (I.M. injection)

1% to 10%:

Cardiovascular: Hypotension (especially orthostatic), tachycardia

Central nervous system: Sedation, dizziness (oral formulation), restlessness, dystonic reactions, pseudoparkinsonism, tardive dyskinesia, neuroleptic malignant syndrome, altered central temperature regulation, nervousness, fatigue, somnolence, hallucination, tremor, hypoesthesia, akathisia

Dermatologic: Photosensitivity (rare), rash, dry skin, seborrhea, acne

Endocrine & metabolic: Amenorrhea, galactorrhea, gynecomastia, sexual dysfunction

Gastrointestinal: Constipation, GI upset, xerostomia, dyspepsia, vomiting, abdominal pain, nausea, anorexia, diarrhea, weight changes

Genitourinary: Polyuria

Neuromuscular & skeletal: Myalgia

Ocular: Abnormal vision

Respiratory: Rhinitis (oral formulation), cough, sinusitis, pharyngitis, dyspnea

<1% (Limited to important or life-threatening): Diabetes mellitus, hyperglycemia, stroke, transient ischemic attack (TIA), anaphylactic reaction, QT_cprolongation

Overdosage/Toxicology Symptoms of overdose include drowsiness, sedation, tachycardia, hypotension, extrapyramidal symptoms (EPS), torsade de pointes, prolonged QT interval, seizures, and cardiopulmonary arrest. Treatment should be symptom-directed and supportive. Gastric decontamination and cardiac monitoring should be initiated. Consider risk of aspiration. Avoid antiarrhythmic therapy known to prolong the QT interval. Avoid vasopressors which may worsen hypotensive effects.

Dosing

Adults:

Bipolar mania: Oral: Recommended starting dose: 2-3 mg once daily; if needed, adjust dose by 1 mg/day in intervals ≥24 hours; dosing range: 1-6 mg/day.

Schizophrenia:

Oral: Initial: 1 mg twice daily; may be increased to 2 mg/day to a target dose of 6 mg/day; usual range: 4-8 mg/day; may be given as a single daily dose once maintenance dose is achieved; daily dosages >6 mg do not appear to confer any additional benefit, and the incidence of extrapyramidal symptoms is higher than with lower doses. Further dose adjustments should be made in increments/decrements of 1-2 mg/day on a weekly basis. Dose range studied in clinical trials: 4-16 mg/day. Maintenance: Target dose: 4 mg once daily (range 2-8 mg/day)

I.M. (Risperdal® Consta™): 25 mg every 2 weeks; some patients may benefit from larger doses; maximum dose not to exceed 50 mg every 2 weeks. Dosage adjustments should not be made more frequently than every 4 weeks.

Note: Oral risperidone (or other antipsychotic) should be administered with the initial injection of Risperdal® Consta™ and continued for 3 weeks (then discontinued) to maintain adequate therapeutic plasma concentrations prior to main release phase of risperidone from injection site.

Tourette's disorder (unlabeled use): Oral: Initial: 0.5 mg; titrate to 2-4 mg/day

Elderly: A starting dose of 0.5 mg twice daily, and titration should progress slowly in increments of no more than 0.5 mg twice daily; increases to dosages >1.5 mg twice daily should occur at intervals of ≥1 week.

Additional monitoring of renal function and orthostatic blood pressure may be warranted. If once-a-day dosing in the elderly or debilitated patient is considered, a twice daily regimen should be used to titrate to the target dose, and this dose should be maintained for 2-3 days prior to attempts to switch to a once-daily regimen.

Pediatrics: Children and Adolescents:

Autism (unlabeled use): Oral: Initial: 0.25 mg at bedtime; titrate to 1 mg/day (0.1 mg/kg/day)

Bipolar disorder (unlabeled use): Oral: Initial: 0.5 mg; titrate to 0.5-3 mg/day

Pervasive developmental disorder (unlabeled use): Oral: Initial: 0.25 mg twice daily; titrate up 0.25 mg/day every 5-7 days; optimal dose range: 0.75-3 mg/day

Schizophrenia (unlabeled use): Oral: Initial: 0.5 mg once or twice daily; titrate as necessary up to 2-6 mg/day

Tourette's disorder (unlabeled use): Refer to adult dosing.

Renal Impairment: Oral: Starting dose of 0.5 mg twice daily; clearance of the active moiety is decreased by 60% in patients with moderate to severe renal disease compared to healthy subjects.

Hepatic Impairment: Oral: Starting dose of 0.5 mg twice daily; the mean free fraction of risperidone in plasma was increased by 35% compared to healthy subjects.

Available Dosage Forms

Injection, microspheres for reconstitution, extended release (Risperdal® Consta™): 25 mg, 37.5 mg, 50 mg [supplied in a dose-pack containing vial with active ingredient in microsphere formulation, prefilled syringe with diluent, needle-free vial access device, and safety needle]

Solution, oral: 1 mg/mL (30 mL) [contains benzoic acid]

Tablet: 0.25 mg, 0.5 mg, 1 mg, 2 mg, 3 mg, 4 mg

Tablet, orally disintegrating (Risperdal® M-Tabs™): 0.5 mg [contains phenylalanine 0.14 mg]; 1 mg [contains phenylalanine 0.28 mg]; 2 mg [contains phenylalanine 0.56 mg]

Nursing Guidelines

Assessment: Assess potential for interactions with other prescriptions, OTC medications, or herbal products patient may be taking. Monitor results of periodic ophthalmic exams. Assess therapeutic effectiveness and adverse reactions at beginning of therapy and periodically with long-term use. Monitor weight prior to initiating therapy and at least monthly. Initiate at lower doses and taper dosage slowly when discontinuing. Teach patient appropriate use, possible side effects, interventions to reduce side effects, and adverse symptoms to report.

Monitoring Laboratory Tests: Fasting lipid profile and fasting blood glucose/ Hgb A_{1c} (prior to treatment, at 3 months, then annually)

Dietary Considerations: May be taken with or without food. Risperdal® M-Tabs™ contain phenylalanine.

Patient Education: Do not take any new medication during therapy unless approved by prescriber. Use exactly as directed; do not increase dose or frequency. It may take several weeks to achieve desired results; do not discontinue without consulting prescriber. Dilute solution with water, milk, or orange juice; do not dilute with beverages containing tannin or pectinate (eg, colas, tea). Avoid alcohol or caffeine unless approved by prescriber. Maintain adequate hydration (2-3 L/day of fluids) unless instructed to restrict fluid intake. If diabetic, you may experience increased blood sugars. Monitor blood sugars closely. You may experience excess sedation, drowsiness, restlessness, dizziness, or blurred vision (use caution driving or when engaging in tasks requiring alertness until response to drug is known); dry mouth, nausea, or GI upset (small frequent meals, frequent mouth care, chewing gum, or sucking lozenges may help); postural hypotension (use caution climbing stairs or when changing position from lying or sitting to standing); or urinary retention (void before taking medication). Report persistent CNS effects (eg, trembling fingers, altered gait or balance, excessive sedation, seizures, unusual muscle or skeletal movements, anxiety, abnormal thoughts, confusion, personality changes); chest pain, palpitations, rapid heartbeat, severe dizziness; swelling or pain in breasts (male and female), altered menstrual pattern, sexual dysfunction; pain or difficulty on urination; vision changes; skin rash or yellowing of skin; respiratory difficulty; or worsening of condition. **Pregnancy/breast-feeding precautions:** Inform prescriber if you are or intend to become pregnant. Do not breast-feed.

Geriatric Considerations: (See Warnings/Precautions, Adverse Reactions, Elderly Dosing, and Overdose/Toxicology.) Elderly patients have an increased risk of adverse response to side effects or adverse reactions to antipsychotics.

(Continued)

Risperidone *(Continued)*

Pregnancy Risk Factor: C

Lactation: Enters breast milk/not recommended

Breast-Feeding Considerations: Risperidone and its metabolite are excreted in breast milk; it is recommended that women not breast feed during therapy or for 12 weeks after the last injection if using Risperdal® Consta™.

Perioperative/Anesthesia/Other Concerns: Risperidone may cause orthostatic hypotension and tachycardia but to a degree which may be less than is seen with other agents (eg, phenothiazines: chlorpromazine, thioridazine). Risperidone may also prolong the QT interval. For these reasons, patient's with cardiovascular disease should be monitored closely while on therapy.

Temazepam (30 mg) can be used to treat risperidone-induced insomnia.

Administration

Oral: Oral solution can be mixed with water, coffee, orange juice, or low-fat milk, but is **not compatible** with cola or tea. May be administered with or without food.

Risperdal® M-Tabs™ should not be removed from blister pack until administered. Using dry hands, place immediately on tongue. Tablet will dissolve within seconds, and may be swallowed with or without liquid. Do not split or chew.

I.M.: Risperdal® Consta™ should be administered I.M. into the upper outer quadrant of the gluteal area. Injection should alternate between the two buttocks. Do not combine two different dosage strengths into one single administration. Do not substitute any components of the dose-pack; administer with needle provided.

Reconstitution: Risperdal® Consta™: Bring to room temperature prior to reconstitution. Reconstitute with provided diluent only. Shake vigorously to mix; will form thick, milky suspension. Following reconstitution, store at room temperature and use within 6 hours. If suspension settles prior to use, shake vigorously to resuspend.

Storage: Risperdal® Consta™: Store in refrigerator at 2°C to 8°C (36°F to 46°F) and protect from light. May be stored at room temperature of 25°C (77°F) for up to 7 days prior to administration.

- ♦ **Ritalin®** *see* Methylphenidate *on page 1137*
- ♦ **Ritalin® LA** *see* Methylphenidate *on page 1137*
- ♦ **Ritalin-SR®** *see* Methylphenidate *on page 1137*
- ♦ **Rituxan®** *see* Rituximab *on page 1484*

Rituximab (ri TUK si mab)

U.S. Brand Names Rituxan®

Synonyms Anti-CD20 Monoclonal Antibody; C2B8; C2B8 Monoclonal Antibody; IDEC-C2B8; Pan-B Antibody

Pharmacologic Category Antineoplastic Agent, Monoclonal Antibody

Medication Safety Issues

Sound-alike/look-alike issues:

Rituxan® may be confused with Remicade®

Use Treatment of relapsed or refractory CD20 positive, B-cell non-Hodgkin's lymphoma (NHL)

Unlabeled/Investigational Use Treatment of autoimmune hemolytic anemia (AIHA) in children; chronic immune thrombocytopenic purpura (ITP); chronic lymphocytic leukemia (CLL) (in combination with chemotherapy); Waldenström's macroglobulinemia (WM); treatment of rheumatoid arthritis

Investigational: Treatment of systemic autoimmune diseases (in addition to rheumatoid arthritis)

Mechanism of Action Rituximab is a monoclonal antibody directed against the CD20 antigen on B-lymphocytes. CD20 regulates cell cycle initiation; and, possibly, functions as a calcium channel. Rituximab binds to the antigen on the cell surface, activating complement-dependent cytotoxicity; and to human Fc receptors, mediating cell killing through an antibody-dependent cellular toxicity.

Pharmacodynamics/Kinetics

Duration: Detectable in serum 3-6 months after completion of treatment; B-cell recovery begins ~6 months following completion of treatment; median B-cell levels return to normal by 12 months following completion of treatment

Absorption: I.V.: Immediate and results in a rapid and sustained depletion of circulating and tissue-based B cells

Half-life elimination: Proportional to dose; wide ranges reflect variable tumor burden and changes in CD20 positive B-cell populations with repeated doses:

>100 mg/m²: 4.4 days (range 1.6-10.5 days)

375 mg/m²:

Following first dose: Mean half-life: 3.2 days (range 1.3-6.4 days)

Following fourth dose: Mean half-life: 8.6 days (range 3.5-17 days)

Excretion: Uncertain; may undergo phagocytosis and catabolism in the reticuloendothelial system (RES)

Contraindications Type I hypersensitivity or anaphylactic reactions to murine proteins or any component of the formulation

Warnings/Precautions Severe and occasionally fatal infusion related reactions (including hypotension, angioedema, bronchospasm, hypoxia and in more severe cases pulmonary infiltrates, acute respiratory distress syndrome, myocardial infarction, ventricular fibrillation, or cardiogenic shock) have been reported during the first 30-120 minutes of the first infusion. Risk factors associated with fatal outcomes include chronic lymphocytic leukemia, female gender, mantle cell lymphoma, or pulmonary infiltrates. Treatment of these reactions is symptomatic. Medications for the treatment of hypersensitivity reactions (eg, epinephrine, antihistamines, corticosteroids) should be available for immediate use. Discontinue infusions in the event of serious or life-threatening cardiac arrhythmias. Mild-to-moderate infusion-related reactions (eg, chills, fever, rigors) occur frequently and are managed through slowing or interrupting the infusion.

Tumor lysis syndrome leading to acute renal failure requiring dialysis may occur 12-24 hours following the first dose. Consider prophylaxis in patients at high risk (high numbers of circulating malignant cells (≥25,000/mm³) or high tumor burden). Severe and sometimes fatal mucocutaneous reactions (lichenoid dermatitis, paraneoplastic pemphigus, Stevens-Johnson syndrome, toxic epidermal necrolysis and vesiculobullous dermatitis) have been reported, occurring from 1-13 weeks following exposure. Patients experiencing severe mucocutaneous skin reactions should not receive further rituximab infusions and should seek prompt medical evaluation. Use caution with cardiac or pulmonary disease and prior cardiopulmonary events. Reactivation of hepatitis B has been reported in association with rituximab (rare); consider screening in high-risk patients. May cause renal toxicity; consider discontinuation with increasing serum creatinine or oliguria. Safety and efficacy in pediatric patients have not been established.

Drug Interactions Monoclonal antibodies: Allergic reactions may be increased in patients who have received diagnostic or therapeutic monoclonal antibodies due to the presence of human antichimeric antibody (HACA).

Adverse Reactions Note: Abdominal pain, anemia, dyspnea, hypotension, and neutropenia are more common in patients with bulky disease.

>10%:

Central nervous system: Fever (53%), chills (33%), headache (19%), pain (12%)

Dermatologic: Rash (15%), pruritus (14%), angioedema (11%)

Gastrointestinal: Nausea (23%), abdominal pain (14%)

Hematologic: Lymphopenia (48%; grade 3/4: 40%; mean duration 14 days), leukopenia (14%; grade 3/4: 4%), neutropenia (14%; grade 3/4: 6%; mean duration 13 days), thrombocytopenia (12%; grade 3/4: 2%)

Neuromuscular & skeletal: Weakness (26%)

Respiratory: Cough (13%), rhinitis (12%)

Miscellaneous: Infection (31%), night sweats (15%)

Mild-to-moderate infusion-related reactions: Chills, fever, rigors, dizziness, hypertension, myalgia, nausea, pruritus, rash and vomiting (first dose 77%; fourth dose 30%; eighth dose 14%)

1% to 10%:

Cardiovascular: Dizziness (10%), hypotension (10%), peripheral edema (8%), hypertension (6%), anxiety (5%), flushing (5%), edema (<5%)

Central nervous system: Agitation (<5%), depression (<5%), insomnia (<5%), malaise (<5%), nervousness (<5%), neuritis (<5%), somnolence (<5%), vertigo (<5%)

Dermatologic: Urticaria (8%)

Endocrine & metabolic: Hyperglycemia (9%), hypoglycemia (<5%)

Gastrointestinal: Diarrhea (10%), vomiting (10%), anorexia (<5%), dyspepsia (<5%), weight loss (<5%)

Hematologic: Anemia (8%; grade 3/4: 3%)

Local: Pain at the injection site (<5%)

(Continued)

Rituximab *(Continued)*

Neuromuscular & skeletal: Arthralgia (10%), back pain (10%), myalgia (10%), arthritis (<5%), hyperkinesia (<5%), hypertonia (<5%), hypoesthesia (<5%), neuropathy (<5%), paresthesia (<5%)

Ocular: Conjunctivitis (<5%), lacrimation disorder (<5%)

Respiratory: Throat irritation (9%), bronchospasm (8%), dyspnea (7%), sinusitis (6%)

Miscellaneous: LDH increased (7%)

Postmarketing and/or case reports: Acute renal failure (associated with tumor lysis syndrome), angina, ARDS, arrhythmia, bronchiolitis obliterans, cardiac failure, cardiogenic shock, fatal infusion-related reactions, hemolytic anemia, hepatic failure, hepatitis, hyperviscosity syndrome (in Waldenström's macroglobulinemia), hypoxia, lichenoid dermatitis, marrow hypoplasia, MI, neutropenia (late onset occurring >40 days after last dose), optic neuritis, pancytopenia, paraneoplastic pemphigus (uncommon), pleuritis, pneumonitis, pure red cell aplasia, renal toxicity, serum sickness, Stevens-Johnson syndrome, toxic epidermal necrolysis, uveitis, vasculitis with rash, ventricular fibrillation, ventricular tachycardia, vesiculobullous dermatitis

Overdosage/Toxicology There has been no experience with overdosage in human clinical trials; single doses higher than 500 mg/m^2 have not been tested

Dosing

Adults & Elderly:

Refer to individual protocols: **Note:** Pretreatment with acetaminophen and diphenhydramine is recommended.

NHL: I.V. infusion: 375 mg/m^2 once weekly for 4-8 weeks

or

100 mg/m^2 I.V. day 1, then 375 mg/m^2 3 times/week for 11 doses has also been reported (cycles may be repeated in patients with refractory or relapsed disease)

Retreatment following disease progression: I.V. infusion: 375 mg/m^2 once weekly for 4 doses

Rheumatoid arthritis (unlabeled use): 1000 mg on days 1 and 15. **Note:** A variety of dosing strategies, including multiple infusions and BSA-adjusted doses have been used in clinical trials, however the relationship between BSA and clearance is not strong. Significant sustained effects noted when used as combination treatment with methotrexate or cyclophosphamide.

Waldenström's macroglobulinemia (unlabeled use): 375 mg/m^2 once weekly for 4 weeks

Combination therapy with ibritumomab: 250 mg/m^2 I.V. day 1; repeat in 7-9 days with ibritumomab

Pediatrics: Note: Pretreatment with acetaminophen and diphenhydramine is recommended.

AIHA, chronic ITP (unlabeled uses): I.V.: 375 mg/m^2 once weekly for 2-4 doses

Available Dosage Forms Injection, solution [preservative free]: 10 mg/mL (10 mL, 50 mL)

Nursing Guidelines

Assessment: Prior to therapy, assess patient history to mouse antibodies (see Monitoring Laboratory Tests). See Contraindications, Warnings/Precautions, and Dosing for use cautions. See Administration for premedication considerations. Assess results of laboratory tests prior to, during, and following therapy (see Monitoring Laboratory Tests). Assess therapeutic effectiveness and adverse reactions (especially infusion-related reactions - see Warnings/Precautions, Adverse Reactions, and Dosing). Teach patient appropriate interventions to reduce side effects and adverse reactions to report. Breast-feeding is contraindicated.

Monitoring Laboratory Tests: CBC with differential and platelets, peripheral CD20+ cells. Patients with elevated HAMA/HACA titers may have an allergic reaction when treated with rituximab or other antibodies from a mouse genetic source.

Patient Education: Inform prescriber of all prescriptions, OTC medications, or herbal products you are taking, and any allergies you have. Do not take any new medication during therapy unless approved by prescriber. This medication can only be administered by infusion. You may experience a reaction during the infusion of this medication including high fever, chills, respiratory difficulty, or congestion. You will be closely monitored and comfort measures provided. Maintain adequate hydration (2-3 L/day of fluids) during entire course of therapy unless instructed to restrict fluid intake. You will be susceptible to infection and people may wear masks and gloves while caring for you to protect you as much as possible (avoid crowds and exposure to infection and do not have any vaccinations without consulting prescriber). May cause dizziness or trembling (use caution until response to medication is known); or nausea or vomiting (small, frequent meals, frequent mouth care may help). Report persistent dizziness, swelling of extremities, unusual weight gain, respiratory difficulty, chest pain or tightness; symptoms of respiratory infection, wheezing or bronchospasms, or respiratory difficulty; unresolved GI effects; skin rash or redness; sore or irritated throat; fatigue, chills, fever, unhealed sores, white plaques in mouth or genital area; unusual bruising or bleeding; or other unusual effects related to this medication. **Pregnancy/breast-feeding precautions:** Inform prescriber if you are or intend to become pregnant. Do not breast-feed.

Pregnancy Risk Factor: C

Lactation: Excretion in breast milk unknown/contraindicated

Breast-Feeding Considerations: The manufacturer recommends discontinuing breast-feeding until circulating levels of rituximab are no longer detectable.

Administration

I.V.: Do **not** administer I.V. push or bolus.

Initial infusion: Start rate of 50 mg/hour; if there is no reaction, increase the rate 50 mg/hour every 30 minutes, to a maximum of 400 mg/hour.

Subsequent infusions: If patient did not tolerate initial infusion follow initial infusion guidelines. If patient tolerated initial infusion, start at 100 mg/hour; if there is no reaction, increase the rate 100 mg/hour every 30 minutes, to a maximum of 400 mg/hour.

Note: If a reaction occurs, slow or stop the infusion. If the reaction abates, restart infusion at 50% of the previous dose.

Reconstitution: Withdraw necessary amount of rituximab and dilute to a final concentration of 1-4 mg/mL with 0.9% sodium chloride or 5% dextrose in water. Gently invert the bag to mix the solution. Do not shake.

Storage: Store vials at refrigeration at 2°C to 8°C (36°F to 46°F); protect vials from direct sunlight. Do not freeze; do not shake. Solutions for infusion are stable at 2°C to 8°C/36°F to 46°F for 24 hours and at room temperature for an additional 24 hours.

Rivastigmine (ri va STIG meen)

U.S. Brand Names Exelon®

Synonyms ENA 713; Rivastigmine Tartrate; SDZ ENA 713

Pharmacologic Category Acetylcholinesterase Inhibitor (Central)

Use Mild to moderate dementia from Alzheimer's disease

Mechanism of Action A deficiency of cortical acetylcholine is thought to account for some of the symptoms of Alzheimer's disease; rivastigmine increases acetylcholine in the central nervous system through reversible inhibition of its hydrolysis by cholinesterase

Pharmacodynamics/Kinetics

Absorption: Fasting: Rapid and complete within 1 hour

Distribution: V_d: 1.8-2.7 L/kg

Protein binding: 40%

Metabolism: Extensively via cholinesterase-mediated hydrolysis in the brain; metabolite undergoes N-demethylation and/or sulfate conjugation hepatically; CYP minimally involved; linear kinetics at 3 mg twice daily, but nonlinear at higher doses

Bioavailability: 40%

Half-life elimination: 1.5 hours

Time to peak: 1 hour

Excretion: Urine (97% as metabolites); feces (0.4%)

Contraindications Hypersensitivity to rivastigmine, other carbamate derivatives, or any component of the formulation

Warnings/Precautions Significant nausea, vomiting, anorexia, and weight loss are associated with use; occurs more frequently in women and during the titration phase. If treatment is interrupted for more than several days, reinstate at the lowest daily dose. Use caution in patients with a history of peptic ulcer disease or concurrent NSAID use. Caution in patients undergoing anesthesia who will receive succinylcholine-type muscle relaxation, patients with sick sinus

(Continued)

Rivastigmine *(Continued)*

syndrome, bradycardia or supraventricular conduction conditions, urinary obstruction, seizure disorders, or pulmonary conditions such as asthma or COPD. There are no trials evaluating the safety and efficacy in children.

Drug Interactions

Anticholinergics: Effects may be reduced with rivastigmine

Antipsychotic agents: Acetylcholinesterase inhibitors (central) may increase the risk of antipsychotic-related extrapyramidal symptoms; monitor.

Beta-blockers without ISA activity: May increase risk of bradycardia

Calcium channel blockers (diltiazem or verapamil): May increase risk of bradycardia

Cholinergic agonists: Effects may be increased with rivastigmine

Cigarette use increases the clearance of rivastigmine by 23%

Digoxin: Increased risk of bradycardia with concurrent use

Neuromuscular blockers: Depolarizing neuromuscular blocking agents effects may be increased with rivastigmine

NSAIDs: Although not seen in clinical studies, patients may be at increased risk for peptic ulcers or gastrointestinal bleeding with concomitant use; monitor

Nutritional/Herbal/Ethanol Interactions

Cigarette use: Increases the clearance of rivastigmine by 23%.

Ethanol: Avoid ethanol (due to risk of sedation; may increase GI irritation).

Food: Food delays absorption by 90 minutes, lowers C_{max} by 30% and increases AUC by 30%.

Adverse Reactions

>10%:

Central nervous system: Dizziness (21%), headache (17%)

Gastrointestinal: Nausea (47%), vomiting (31%), diarrhea (19%), anorexia (17%), abdominal pain (13%)

2% to 10%:

Central nervous system: Fatigue (9%), insomnia (9%), confusion (8%), depression (6%), anxiety (5%), malaise (5%), somnolence (5%), hallucinations (4%), aggressiveness (3%)

Cardiovascular: Syncope (3%), hypertension (3%)

Gastrointestinal: Dyspepsia (9%), constipation (5%), flatulence (4%), weight loss (3%), eructation (2%)

Genitourinary: Urinary tract infection (7%)

Neuromuscular & skeletal: Weakness (6%), tremor (4%)

Respiratory: Rhinitis (4%)

Miscellaneous: Increased diaphoresis (4%), flu-like syndrome (3%)

<2% (Limited to important or life-threatening; reactions may be at a similar frequency to placebo): Acute renal failure, allergic reaction, angina pectoris, aphasia, apnea, apraxia, ataxia, atrial fibrillation, AV block, bradycardia, bronchospasm, bundle branch block, cardiac arrest, cardiac failure, cholecystitis, convulsions, delirium, dysphonia, GI hemorrhage, intestinal obstruction, intracranial hemorrhage, migraine, MI, pancreatitis, peripheral ischemia, peripheral neuropathy, postural hypotension, psychosis, pulmonary embolism, rash, sick sinus syndrome, Stevens-Johnson syndrome, supraventricular tachycardia, thrombocytopenia, thrombophlebitis, thrombosis, urticaria, vomiting (severe) with esophageal rupture (following inappropriate reinitiation of dose)

Overdosage/Toxicology In cases of asymptomatic overdoses, rivastigmine should be held for 24 hours. Cholinergic crisis, caused by significant acetylcholinesterase inhibition, is characterized by severe nausea, vomiting, salivation, sweating, bradycardia, hypotension, respiratory depression, collapse, and convulsions. Treatment is supportive and symptomatic. Dialysis would not be helpful.

Dosing

Adults & Elderly: Alzheimer's dementia: Oral: Initial: 1.5 mg twice daily for 2 weeks; if tolerated, may be increased to 3 mg twice daily; further increases may be attempted no more frequently than every 2 weeks, to 4.5 mg twice daily and then to 6 mg twice daily; maximum dose: 6 mg twice daily. If gastrointestinal adverse events occur, the patient should be instructed to discontinue treatment for several doses then restart at the same or next lower dosage level; antiemetics have been used to control GI symptoms. If treatment is interrupted for longer than several days, restart the treatment at the lowest dose and titrate as previously described.

Renal Impairment: Dosage adjustments are not recommended, however, titrate the dose to the individual's tolerance.

Hepatic Impairment: Clearance is significantly reduced in mild to moderately impaired patients. Although dosage adjustments are not recommended, use lowest possible dose and titrate according to individual's tolerance. May consider waiting >2 weeks between dosage adjustments.

Available Dosage Forms

Capsule: 1.5 mg, 3 mg, 4.5 mg, 6 mg

Solution, oral: 2 mg/mL (120 mL) [contains sodium benzoate]

Nursing Guidelines

Assessment: Assess bladder and sphincter adequacy prior to administering medication. Assess other medications for effectiveness and interactions. Monitor therapeutic effectiveness and adverse reactions at beginning of therapy and regularly with long-term use. Assess cognitive function at periodic intervals. Assess knowledge/teach patient appropriate use, possible side effects/appropriate interventions, and adverse symptoms to report.

Monitoring Laboratory Tests: Cognitive function at periodic intervals

Dietary Considerations: Should be taken with meals.

Patient Education: This drug is not a cure for Alzheimer's disease, but it may reduce the symptoms. Use as directed; do not increase dose or discontinue without consulting prescriber. Swallow capsule whole with meals (do not crush or chew). Liquid can be swallowed directly from syringe or mixed with water, milk, or juice; stir well and drink within 4 hours of mixing. Maintain adequate hydration (2-3 L/day of fluids) unless instructed to restrict fluid intake. Avoid alcohol. May cause dizziness, drowsiness, or postural hypotension (rise slowly from sitting or lying position and use caution when driving or climbing stairs); vomiting or loss of appetite (small frequent meals, frequent mouth care, sucking lozenges, or chewing gum may help); diarrhea (buttermilk, boiled milk, or yogurt may help); or constipation (increased exercise, fluids, fruit, or fiber may help); or urinary frequency. Report persistent abdominal discomfort, diarrhea, or constipation; significantly increased salivation, sweating, tearing, or urination; chest pain, palpitations, acute headache; CNS changes (eg, excessive fatigue, agitation, insomnia, dizziness, confusion, aggressiveness, depression); increased muscle, joint, or body pain; vision changes or blurred vision; shortness of breath, coughing, or wheezing; skin rash; or other persistent adverse reactions. **Breast-feeding precaution:** Consult prescriber if breast-feeding.

Pregnancy Risk Factor: B

Lactation: Excretion in breast milk unknown/use caution

Administration

Oral: Should be administered with meals (breakfast or dinner). Capsule should be swallowed whole. Liquid form is available for patients who cannot swallow capsules (can be swallowed directly from syringe or mixed with water, milk, or juice). Stir well and drink within 4 hours of mixing.

Storage: Store below 77°F (25°C). Store solution in an upright position and protect from freezing.

- **Rivastigmine Tartrate** *see* Rivastigmine *on page 1487*
- **rLFN-α2** *see* Interferon Alfa-2b *on page 936*
- **RMS®** *see* Morphine Sulfate *on page 1177*
- **Robafen® AC** *see* Guaifenesin and Codeine *on page 835*
- **Robaxin®** *see* Methocarbamol *on page 1124*
- **Robinul®** *see* Glycopyrrolate *on page 827*
- **Robinul® Forte** *see* Glycopyrrolate *on page 827*
- **Robitussin® [OTC]** *see* Guaifenesin *on page 834*
- **Rocaltrol®** *see* Calcitriol *on page 289*
- **Rocephin®** *see* Ceftriaxone *on page 353*

Rocuronium (roe kyoor OH nee um)

U.S. Brand Names Zemuron®

Synonyms ORG 946; Rocuronium Bromide

Pharmacologic Category Neuromuscular Blocker Agent, Nondepolarizing

Medication Safety Issues

Sound-alike/look-alike issues:

Zemuron® may be confused with Remeron®

Use Adjunct to general anesthesia to facilitate both rapid sequence and routine endotracheal intubation and to relax skeletal muscles during surgery; to facilitate mechanical ventilation in ICU patients; does not relieve pain or produce sedation

(Continued)

Rocuronium *(Continued)*

Mechanism of Action Blocks acetylcholine from binding to receptors on motor endplate inhibiting depolarization

Pharmacodynamics/Kinetics

Onset of action: Good intubation conditions in 1-2 minutes; maximum neuromuscular blockade within 4 minutes

Duration: ~30 minutes (with standard doses, increases with higher doses)

Metabolism: Minimally hepatic; 17-desacetylrocuronium (5% to 10% activity of parent drug)

Half-life elimination: 60-70 minutes

Excretion: Feces (50%); urine (30%)

Contraindications Hypersensitivity to rocuronium or any component of the formulation

Warnings/Precautions Use with caution in patients with valvular heart disease, pulmonary disease, hepatic impairment; ventilation must be supported during neuromuscular blockade; certain clinical conditions may result in potentiation or antagonism of neuromuscular blockade:

Potentiation: Electrolyte abnormalities, severe hyponatremia, severe hypocalcemia, severe hypokalemia, hypermagnesemia, neuromuscular diseases, acidosis, acute intermittent porphyria, renal failure, hepatic failure

Antagonism: Alkalosis, hypercalcemia, demyelinating lesions, peripheral neuropathies, diabetes mellitus

Increased sensitivity in patients with myasthenia gravis, Eaton-Lambert syndrome; resistance in burn patients (>30% of body) for period of 5-70 days postinjury; resistance in patients with muscle trauma, denervation, immobilization, infection. Cross-sensitivity with other neuromuscular-blocking agents may occur; use extreme caution in patients with previous anaphylactic reactions.

Drug Interactions

Decreased effect: Chronic carbamazepine or phenytoin can shorten the duration of neuromuscular blockade; phenylephrine can severely inhibit neuromuscular blockade

Increased effect: Infusion requirements are reduced 35% to 40% during anesthesia with enflurane or isoflurane

Increased toxicity: Aminoglycosides, vancomycin, tetracyclines, bacitracin

Adverse Reactions

>1%: Cardiovascular: Transient hypotension and hypertension

<1% (Limited to important or life-threatening): Abnormal ECG, acute quadriplegic myopathy syndrome (prolonged use), anaphylaxis, arrhythmia, bronchospasm, edema, hiccups, injection site pruritus, myositis ossificans (prolonged use), nausea, rash, rhonchi, shock, tachycardia, vomiting, wheezing

Overdosage/Toxicology

Symptoms of overdose include prolonged skeletal muscle block, muscle weakness and apnea

Treatment is maintenance of a patent airway and controlled ventilation until recovery of normal neuromuscular block is observed, further recovery may be facilitated by administering an anticholinesterase agent (eg, neostigmine, edrophonium, or pyridostigmine) with atropine, to antagonize the skeletal muscle relaxation; support of the cardiovascular system with fluids and pressors may be necessary

Dosing

Adults & Elderly: Administer I.V.; dose to effect; doses will vary due to interpatient variability; use ideal body weight for obese patients

Tracheal intubation: I.V.:

Initial: 0.6 mg/kg is expected to provide approximately 31 minutes of clinical relaxation under opioid/nitrous oxide/oxygen anesthesia with neuromuscular block sufficient for intubation attained in 1-2 minutes; lower doses (0.45 mg/kg) may be used to provide 22 minutes of clinical relaxation with median time to neuromuscular block of 1-3 minutes; maximum blockade is achieved in <4 minutes

Maximum: 0.9-1.2 mg/kg may be given during surgery under opioid/nitrous oxide/oxygen anesthesia without adverse cardiovascular effects and is expected to provide 58-67 minutes of clinical relaxation; neuromuscular blockade sufficient for intubation is achieved in <2 minutes with maximum blockade in <3 minutes

Maintenance: 0.1, 0.15, and 0.2 mg/kg administered at 25% recovery of control T_1 (defined as 3 twitches of train-of-four) provides a median of 12, 17, and 24 minutes of clinical duration under anesthesia

Rapid sequence intubation: 0.6-1.2 mg/kg in appropriately premedicated and anesthetized patients with excellent or good intubating conditions within 2 minutes

Continuous infusion: Initial: 0.01-0.012 mg/kg/minute only after early evidence of spontaneous recovery of neuromuscular function is evident; infusion rates have ranged from 0.004-0.016 mg/kg/minute.

ICU neuromuscular blockade: 10 mcg/kg/minute; adjust dose to maintain appropriate degree of neuromuscular blockade (eg, 1 or 2 twitches on train-of-four)

Pediatrics: Administer I.V.; dose to effect; doses will vary due to interpatient variability; use ideal body weight for obese patients

Tracheal intubation: I.V.: Children:

Initial: 0.6 mg/kg under halothane anesthesia produce excellent to good intubating conditions within 1 minute and will provide a median time of 41 minutes of clinical relaxation in children 3 months to 1 year of age, and 27 minutes in children 1-12 years

Maintenance: 0.075-0.125 mg/kg administered upon return of T_1 to 25% of control provides clinical relaxation for 7-10 minutes

Available Dosage Forms Injection, solution, as bromide: 10 mg/mL (5 mL, 10 mL)

Nursing Guidelines

Assessment: Only clinicians experienced in the use of neuromuscular blocking agents should administer and/or manage the use of mivacurium. Assess potential for interactions with other prescription or OTC medications or herbal products patient may be taking (eg, other drugs that affect neuromuscular activity may increase/decrease neuromuscular block induced by rocuronium). Dosage and rate of administration should be individualized and titrated to the desired effect, according to relevant clinical factors, premedication, concomitant medication, age, and general condition of the patient. Ventilatory support must be instituted and maintained until adequate respiratory muscle function and/or airway protection are assured. This drug does not cause anesthesia or analgesia; pain must be treated with appropriate agents. Continuous monitoring of vital signs, cardiac and respiratory status, and neuromuscular block (objective assessment with peripheral external nerve stimulator) are mandatory until full muscle tone has returned. Safety precautions must be maintained until full muscle tone has returned. Muscle tone returns in a predictable pattern; starting with diaphragm, abdomen, chest, limbs, and finally muscles of the neck, face, and eyes. **Note:** It may take longer for return of muscle tone in obese or elderly persons or patients with renal or hepatic disease, myasthenia gravis, myopathy, other neuromuscular diseases, dehydration, electrolyte imbalance, or severe acid/base imbalance. Provide appropriate teaching/support prior to, during, and following administration.

Long-term use: Vital signs and fluid levels should be monitored regularly during treatment. Every 2- to 3-hour repositioning, and skin, mouth, and eye care is necessary while patient is sedated. Emotional and sensory support (auditory and environmental) should be provided.

Patient Education: Patient education should be appropriate for patient condition. Reassurance of constant monitoring and emotional support should precede and follow administration. Patients should be reminded as muscle tone returns not to attempt to change position or rise from bed without assistance and to report and skin rash, hives, pounding heartbeat, respiratory difficulty, or muscle tremors. **Pregnancy/breast-feeding precautions:** Inform prescriber if you are pregnant. Consult prescriber if breast-feeding.

Pregnancy Risk Factor: C

Lactation: Excretion in breast milk unknown/use caution

Perioperative/Anesthesia/Other Concerns: Classified as an intermediate duration neuromuscular-blocking agent; do not mix in same syringe with barbiturates.

Critically-Ill Adult Patients: The 2002 ACCM/SCCM/ASHP clinical practice guidelines for sustained neuromuscular blockade in the adult critically-ill patient recommend:

Optimize sedatives and analgesics prior to initiation and monitor and adjust accordingly during course. Neuromuscular blockers do not relieve pain or produce sedation.

(Continued)

Rocuronium *(Continued)*

Protect patient's eyes from development of keratitis and corneal abrasion by administering ophthalmic ointment and taping eyelids closed or using eye patches. Reposition patient routinely to protect pressure points from breakdown. Address DVT prophylaxis.

Concurrent use of a neuromuscular blocker and corticosteroids appear to increase the risk of certain ICU myopathies; avoid or administer the corticosteroid at the lowest dose possible. Reassess need for neuromuscular blocker daily.

Using daily drug holidays (stopping neuromuscular-blocking agent until patient requires it again) may decrease the incidence of acute quadriplegic myopathy syndrome.

Tachyphylaxis can develop; switch to another neuromuscular blocker (taking into consideration the patient's organ function) if paralysis is still necessary.

Atracurium or cisatracurium is recommended for patients with significant hepatic or renal disease, due to organ-independent Hofmann elimination.

Monitor patients clinically and via "Train of Four" (TOF) testing with a goal of adjusting the degree of blockade to 1-2 twitches on based upon the patient's clinical condition.

Administration

I.V.: Administer I.V. only; may be given undiluted as a bolus injection or via a continuous infusion using an infusion pump

Storage: Store under refrigeration (2°C to 8°C), do not freeze; when stored at room temperature, it is stable for 30 days; unlike vecuronium, it is stable in 0.9% sodium chloride and 5% dextrose in water, this mixture should be used within 24 hours of preparation

♦ **Rocuronium Bromide** *see* Rocuronium *on page 1489*

Rofecoxib (roe fe COX ib)

U.S. Brand Names Vioxx® [DSC]

Pharmacologic Category Nonsteroidal Anti-inflammatory Drug (NSAID), COX-2 Selective

Medication Safety Issues

Sound-alike/look-alike issues:

Vioxx® may be confused with Zyvox™

Use Relief of the signs and symptoms of osteoarthritis, rheumatoid arthritis, and juvenile rheumatoid arthritis (JRA); management of acute pain; treatment of primary dysmenorrhea; treatment of migraine attacks

Mechanism of Action Inhibits prostaglandin synthesis by decreasing the activity of the enzyme, cyclooxygenase-2 (COX-2), which results in decreased formation of prostaglandin precursors. Rofecoxib does not inhibit cyclooxygenase-1 (COX-1) at therapeutic concentrations.

Pharmacodynamics/Kinetics

Onset of action: 45 minutes

Duration: Up to >24 hours

Distribution: V_{dss} (apparent): 86-91 L

Protein binding: 87%

Metabolism: Hepatic (99%); minor metabolism via CYP2C8/9 isoenzyme; metabolites inactive

Bioavailability: 93%

Half-life elimination: 17 hours

Time to peak: 2-3 hours

Excretion: Urine (72% as metabolites, <1% as unchanged drug); feces (14% as unchanged drug)

Contraindications Hypersensitivity to rofecoxib or any component of the formulation, aspirin, or other NSAIDs; patients with "aspirin triad" (bronchial asthma, aspirin intolerance, rhinitis); pregnancy (3rd trimester)

Warnings/Precautions Gastrointestinal irritation, ulceration, bleeding, and perforation may occur with NSAIDs (rofecoxib has been associated with rates of these events which are lower than naproxen, a nonselective NSAID); use the lowest effective dose for the shortest duration possible to decrease risk. Use with caution in patients with a history of GI disease (bleeding or ulcers), decreased renal function, hepatic disease, CHF, hypertension, or asthma. Edema, GI irritation, and/or hypertension occur at an increased frequency with chronic use of 50 mg/day. Use with caution in patients with ischemic heart disease; antiplatelet therapies should be considered (rofecoxib is not a substitute for antiplatelet agents).

Anaphylactoid reactions may occur, even with no prior exposure to rofecoxib. Safety and efficacy in pediatric patients <2 years of age and <10 kg, and in cluster headaches have not been established.

Drug Interactions **Substrate** of CYP2C8/9 (minor); **Inhibits** CYP1A2 (weak); **Induces** CYP3A4 (weak)

ACE inhibitors: Antihypertensive effects may be reduced by rofecoxib.

Aspirin: Rofecoxib may be used with low-dose aspirin, however, rates of gastrointestinal bleeding may be increased with coadministration.

Cimetidine increases AUC of rofecoxib by 23%.

Diuretics: Thiazide diuretics, loop diuretics: Effects may be diminished by rofecoxib.

Lithium: Serum concentrations/toxicity may be increased by rofecoxib; monitor.

Methotrexate: Severe bone marrow suppression, aplastic anemia, and GI toxicity have been reported with concomitant NSAID therapy. Selective COX-2 inhibitors appear to have a lower risk of this toxicity, however, caution is warranted.

Rifampin reduces the serum concentration of rofecoxib by ~50%; consider using initial dose of 25 mg/day for osteoarthritis.

Theophylline: Serum concentrations may be increased during therapy with rofecoxib; monitor.

Warfarin: Rofecoxib may increase the INR in patients receiving warfarin and may increase the risk of bleeding complications. However, rofecoxib does not appear to inhibit platelet aggregation.

Nutritional/Herbal/Ethanol Interactions

Ethanol: Avoid ethanol (may increase gastric mucosal irritation)

Food: Time to peak concentrations are delayed when taken with a high-fat meal, however, peak concentration and AUC are unchanged.

Adverse Reactions

2% to 10%:

Cardiovascular: Peripheral edema (4%), hypertension (up to 10%)

Central nervous system: Headache (5%), dizziness (3%)

Gastrointestinal: Diarrhea (7%), nausea (5%), heartburn (4%), epigastric discomfort (4%), dyspepsia (4%), abdominal pain (3%); dry socket (postdental extraction alveolitis 2%)

Genitourinary: Urinary tract infection (3%)

Neuromuscular & skeletal: Back pain (3%), weakness (2%)

Respiratory: Upper respiratory infection (9%), bronchitis (2%), sinusitis (3%)

Miscellaneous: Flu-like syndrome (3%)

0.1% to 2%:

Cardiovascular: Chest pain, upper extremity edema, atrial fibrillation, bradycardia, arrhythmia, palpitation, tachycardia, venous insufficiency, fluid retention

Central nervous system: Anxiety, depression, decreased mental acuity, hypoesthesia, insomnia, neuropathy, migraine, paresthesia, somnolence, vertigo, fever, pain

Dermatologic: Alopecia, atopic dermatitis, basal cell carcinoma, contact dermatitis, pruritus, rash, erythema, urticaria, dry skin

Endocrine & metabolic: Weight gain, hypercholesteremia

Gastrointestinal: Reflux, abdominal distension, abdominal tenderness, constipation, dry mouth, esophagitis, flatulence, gastritis, gastroenteritis, hematochezia, hemorrhoids, oral ulceration, dental caries, aphthous stomatitis

Genitourinary: Breast mass, cystitis, dysuria, menopausal disorder, nocturia, urinary retention, vaginitis, pelvic pain

Hematologic: Hematoma

Hepatic: Transaminases increased >3 times ULN (1%)

Neuromuscular & skeletal: Muscle spasm, sciatica, arthralgia, bursitis, cartilage trauma, joint swelling, muscle cramps, muscle weakness, myalgia, tendonitis, traumatic arthropathy, fracture (wrist)

Ocular: Blurred vision, conjunctivitis

Otic: Otic pain, otitis media, tinnitus

Respiratory: Asthma, cough, dyspnea, pneumonia, respiratory infection, pulmonary congestion, rhinitis, epistaxis, laryngitis, dry throat, pharyngitis, tonsillitis, diaphragmatic hernia

Miscellaneous: Allergy, fungal infection, insect bite reaction, syncope, viral syndrome, herpes simplex, herpes zoster, increased diaphoresis

<2% (Limited to important or life-threatening): Allergy, alopecia, angina, arrhythmia, asthma, atopic dermatitis, atrial fibrillation, blurred vision, decreased mental acuity, depression, dyspnea, esophageal reflux, esophagitis, fluid retention, gastritis, hematochezia, hematoma, hemorrhoids, muscle

(Continued)

Rofecoxib *(Continued)*

cramps, neuropathy, paresthesia, pruritus, rash, somnolence, syncope, tendonitis, tinnitus, transaminases increased (>3 times ULN), urinary retention, urticaria, venous insufficiency, vertigo

<0.1% (Limited to important or life-threatening): Agranulocytosis, aplastic anemia, breast cancer, cholecystitis, colitis, colonic neoplasm, CHF, deep vein thrombosis, duodenal ulcer, gastrointestinal bleeding, hallucinations, intestinal obstruction, lymphoma, MI, pancreatitis, pancytopenia, photosensitivity reaction, prostatic cancer, Stevens-Johnson syndrome, stroke, toxic epidermal necrolysis, transient ischemic attack, unstable angina, urolithiasis

Overdosage/Toxicology Symptoms may include epigastric pain, drowsiness, lethargy, nausea, and vomiting. Gastrointestinal bleeding may occur. Rare manifestations include hypertension, respiratory depression, coma, and acute renal failure. Treatment is symptomatic and supportive. Hemodialysis does not remove rofecoxib.

Dosing

Adults & Elderly:

Osteoarthritis: Oral: 12.5 mg once daily; may be increased to a maximum of 25 mg once daily

Acute pain or dysmenorrhea: Oral: 50 mg once daily as needed (use for longer than 5 days has not been studied)

Migraine attack: Oral: 25 mg once daily, as needed; may be increased to a maximum of 50 mg once daily

Rheumatoid arthritis: Oral: 25 mg once daily

Pediatrics: JRA: Children 2-17 years and ≥10 kg: Oral: 0.6 mg/kg/day (maximum: 25 mg/day)

Renal Impairment: Use in advanced renal disease is not recommended.

Hepatic Impairment: Moderate dysfunction (Child-Pugh score 7-9): Maximum dose: 12.5 mg/day

Available Dosage Forms [DSC] = Discontinued product

Suspension, oral [DSC]: 12.5 mg/5 mL (150 mL); 25 mg/5 mL (150 mL) [strawberry flavor]

Tablet [DSC]: 12.5 mg, 25 mg, 50 mg

Nursing Guidelines

Assessment: Evaluate cardiac risk and potential for GI bleeding prior to prescribing this medication. Assess allergy history (salicylates) prior to beginning therapy. Monitor blood pressure at the beginning of therapy and periodically during use. Assess effectiveness and interactions of other medications patient may be taking (ie, lithium). Assess for signs and symptoms of gastrointestinal bleeding. Monitor effectiveness of therapy and adverse reactions. Assess knowledge/teach patient appropriate use, interventions to reduce side effects, and adverse symptoms to report.

Dietary Considerations: May be taken without regard to meals.

Patient Education: Do not take more than recommended dose. May be taken with food to reduce GI upset. Do not take with antacids. Avoid alcohol, aspirin, and OTC medication unless approved by prescriber. You may experience dizziness, confusion, or blurred vision (avoid driving or engaging in tasks requiring alertness until response to drug is known); or anorexia, nausea, vomiting, taste disturbance, gastric distress (small frequent meals, frequent mouth care, sucking lozenges, or chewing gum may help). GI bleeding, ulceration, or perforation can occur with or without pain; rofecoxib has rates of these events which are lower than nonselective NSAIDs. Stop taking medication and report stomach pain or cramping, unusual bleeding or bruising, or blood in vomitus, stool, or urine immediately. Report persistent insomnia; skin rash; unusual fatigue or easy bruising or bleeding; muscle pain, tremors, or weakness; sudden weight gain; abdominal pain; itching, yellowing of skin; chest pain; changes in hearing (ringing in ears); vision changes; changes in urination pattern; or respiratory difficulty. **Pregnancy/breast-feeding precautions:** Inform prescriber if you are or intend to become pregnant. This drug should not be used in the 3rd trimester of pregnancy. Breast-feeding is not recommended.

Geriatric Considerations: The elderly are at increased risk for adverse effects from NSAIDs. As many as 60% of elderly can develop peptic ulceration and/or hemorrhage asymptomatically. CNS adverse effects such as confusion, agitation, and hallucination are generally seen in overdose or high-dose situations; however, elderly patients may demonstrate these adverse effects at lower doses than younger adults. The elderly are also at increased risk of renal toxicity.

Pregnancy Risk Factor: C/D (3rd trimester)

Pregnancy Issues: In late pregnancy may cause premature closure of the ductus arteriosus.

Lactation: Excretion in breast milk unknown/not recommended

Breast-Feeding Considerations: In animal studies, rofecoxib has been found to be excreted in milk. It is not known whether rofecoxib is excreted in human milk. Because many drugs are excreted in milk, and the potential for serious adverse reactions exists, a decision should be made whether to discontinue nursing or discontinue the drug, taking into account the importance of the drug to the mother.

Perioperative/Anesthesia/Other Concerns: Does not inhibit platelets or prolong bleeding.

- Roferon-A® *see* Interferon Alfa-2a *on page 933*
- Rogaine® Extra Strength for Men [OTC] *see* Minoxidil *on page 1165*
- Rogaine® for Men [OTC] *see* Minoxidil *on page 1165*
- Rogaine® for Women [OTC] *see* Minoxidil *on page 1165*
- Rolaids® [OTC] *see* Calcium Carbonate and Magnesium Hydroxide *on page 294*
- Rolaids® Extra Strength [OTC] *see* Calcium Carbonate and Magnesium Hydroxide *on page 294*
- Romazicon® *see* Flumazenil *on page 739*
- Romilar® AC *see* Guaifenesin and Codeine *on page 835*
- Romycin® *see* Erythromycin *on page 634*

Ropinirole (roe PIN i role)

U.S. Brand Names Requip®

Synonyms Ropinirole Hydrochloride

Pharmacologic Category Anti-Parkinson's Agent, Dopamine Agonist

Medication Safety Issues

Sound-alike/look-alike issues:

Ropinirole may be confused with ropivacaine

Use Treatment of idiopathic Parkinson's disease; in patients with early Parkinson's disease who were not receiving concomitant levodopa therapy as well as in patients with advanced disease on concomitant levodopa; treatment of moderate-to-severe primary Restless Legs Syndrome (RLS)

Mechanism of Action Ropinirole has a high relative *in vitro* specificity and full intrinsic activity at the D_2 and D_3 dopamine receptor subtypes, binding with higher affinity to D_3 than to D_2 or D_4 receptor subtypes; relevance of D_3 receptor binding in Parkinson's disease is unknown. Ropinirole has moderate *in vitro* affinity for opioid receptors. Ropinirole and its metabolites have negligible *in vitro* affinity for dopamine D_1, 5-HT_1, 5-HT_2, benzodiazepine, GABA, muscarinic, alpha$_1$-, alpha$_2$-, and beta-adrenoreceptors. Although precise mechanism of action of ropinirole is unknown, it is believed to be due to stimulation of postsynaptic dopamine D_2-type receptors within the caudate putamen in the brain. Ropinirole caused decreases in systolic and diastolic blood pressure at doses >0.25 mg. The mechanism of ropinirole-induced postural hypotension is believed to be due to D_2-mediated blunting of the noradrenergic response to standing and subsequent decrease in peripheral vascular resistance.

Pharmacodynamics/Kinetics

Absorption: Not affected by food

Distribution: V_d: 525 L

Metabolism: Extensively hepatic via CYP1A2 to inactive metabolites; first-pass effect

Bioavailability: Absolute: 55%

Half-life elimination: ~6 hours

Time to peak: ~1-2 hours; T_{max} increased by 2.5 hours when drug taken with food

Excretion: Clearance: Reduced by 30% in patients >65 years of age

Contraindications Hypersensitivity to ropinirole or any component of the formulation

Warnings/Precautions Syncope, sometimes associated with bradycardia, was observed in association with ropinirole in both early Parkinson's disease (without levodopa) patients and advanced Parkinson's disease (with levodopa) patients. Dopamine agonists appear to impair the systemic regulation of blood pressure resulting in postural hypotension, especially during dose escalation. Parkinson's disease patients appear to have an impaired capacity to respond to a postural challenge; use with caution in patients at risk of hypotension (ie, those receiving antihypertensive drugs) or where transient hypotensive episodes would be poorly

(Continued)

Ropinirole *(Continued)*

tolerated (cardiovascular disease or cerebrovascular disease). Parkinson's patients being treated with dopaminergic agonists ordinarily require careful monitoring for signs and symptoms of postural hypotension, especially during dose escalation, and should be informed of this risk. May cause hallucinations. Use with caution in patients with pre-existing dyskinesia, severe hepatic or renal dysfunction.

Patients treated with ropinirole have reported falling asleep while engaging in activities of daily living; this has been reported to occur without significant warning signs. Monitor for daytime somnolence or pre-existing sleep disorder; caution with concomitant sedating medication; discontinue if significant daytime sleepiness or episodes of falling asleep occur. Patients must be cautioned about performing tasks which require mental alertness (eg, operating machinery or driving). Use with caution in patients receiving other CNS depressants or psychoactive agents. Effects with other sedative drugs or ethanol may be potentiated.

Some patients treated for RLS may experience worsening of symptoms in the early morning hours (rebound) or an increase and/or spread of daytime symptoms (augmentation); clinical management of these phenomena has not been evaluated in controlled clinical trials. Pathologic degenerative changes were observed in the retinas of albino rats during studies with this agent, but were not observed in the retinas of albino mice or in other species. The significance of these data for humans remains uncertain.

Other dopaminergic agents have been associated with a syndrome resembling neuroleptic malignant syndrome on withdrawal or significant dosage reduction after long-term use. Risk of fibrotic complications (eg, pleural effusion/fibrosis, interstitial lung disease) and melanoma has been reported in patients receiving ropinirole; drug causation has not been established.

Drug Interactions Substrate of CYP1A2 (major), 3A4 (minor); **Inhibits** CYP1A2 (weak), 2D6 (strong)

Antipsychotics: May reduce the effect of ropinirole due to dopamine antagonism

Ciprofloxacin: May increase the levels/effects of ropinirole.

CYP1A2 inducers: May decrease the levels/effects of ropinirole. Example inducers include aminoglutethimide, carbamazepine, phenobarbital, and rifampin.

CYP1A2 inhibitors: May increase the levels/effects of ropinirole. Example inhibitors include amiodarone, fluvoxamine, ketoconazole, and rofecoxib.

CYP2D6 substrates: Ropinirole may increase the levels/effects of CYP2D6 substrates. Example substrates include amphetamines, selected beta-blockers, dextromethorphan, fluoxetine, lidocaine, mirtazapine, nefazodone, paroxetine, risperidone, ritonavir, thioridazine, tricyclic antidepressants, and venlafaxine.

CYP2D6 prodrug substrates: Ropinirole may decrease the levels/effects of CYP2D6 prodrug substrates. Example prodrug substrates include codeine, hydrocodone, oxycodone, and tramadol.

Estrogens: May reduce the metabolism of ropinirole; dosage adjustments may be needed; clearance may be reduced by 36%

Metoclopramide: May reduce the effect of ropinirole due to dopamine antagonism

Quinolone antibiotics (specifically ciprofloxacin, norfloxacin, ofloxacin): May inhibit the metabolism of ropinirole.

Nutritional/Herbal/Ethanol Interactions

Ethanol: Avoid ethanol (may increase CNS depression).

Herb/Nutraceutical: Avoid kava kava, gotu kola, valerian, St John's wort (may increase CNS depression).

Adverse Reactions

Data inclusive of trials in both early and late Parkinson's disease (may include levodopa) and restless legs syndrome; frequencies of some adverse effects may be influenced by disease state, particularly in advanced Parkinson's disease:

>10%:

Cardiovascular: Syncope (12%)

Central nervous system: Somnolence (12% to 40%), dizziness (11% to 40%), fatigue (8% to 11%)

Gastrointestinal: Nausea (40% to 60%), vomiting (12%)

Miscellaneous: Viral infection (11%)

1% to 10%:

Cardiovascular: Dependent/leg edema (2% to 7%), orthostasis (1% to 6%), hypertension (2% to 5%), chest pain (4%), flushing (3%), palpitation (3%), peripheral ischemia (3%), hypotension (2%), tachycardia (2%)

Central nervous system: Pain (3% to 8%), confusion (5% to 9%), hallucinations (5% to 10%, dose related), anxiety (6%), pain (5%), hypoesthesia (4%), amnesia (3% to 5%), malaise (3%), paresis (3%), vertigo (2%), yawning (3%), abnormal dreams (3%), insomnia, neuralgia (>1%)

Gastrointestinal: Constipation (5% to 6%), dyspepsia (4% to 10%), abdominal pain (3% to 9%), vomiting (7%), xerostomia (3% to 5%), diarrhea (5%), anorexia (4%), flatulence (2% to 3%), dysphagia (2%), salivation increased (2%), weight loss (2%)

Genitourinary: Urinary tract infection (1% to 5%), impotence (3%)

Hematologic: Anemia (2%)

Hepatic: Alkaline phosphatase increased (3%)

Neuromuscular & skeletal: Falls (10%), arthralgia (4% to 7%), weakness (6%), tremor (6%), hypokinesia (5%), paresthesia (5%), arthritis (3%), muscle cramps (3%)

Ocular: Abnormal vision (6%), xerophthalmia (2%)

Renal: BUN increased (>1%)

Respiratory: Upper respiratory tract infection (9%), pharyngitis (6% to 9%), rhinitis (4%), sinusitis (4%), dyspnea (3%), influenza (3%), cough (3%), nasal congestion (2%)

Miscellaneous: Injury, diaphoresis increased (3% to 7%), viral infection, increased drug level (7%)

<1% (Limited to important or life-threatening): Abnormal coordination, acidosis, agitation, aneurysm, angina, aphasia, asthma, behavioral disorders, bradycardia, bundle branch block, cardiac arrest, cardiac failure, cardiomegaly, cellulitis, cholecystitis, cholelithiasis, choreoathetosis, colitis, coma, conjunctival hemorrhage, dehydration, diabetes mellitus, diverticulitis, Dupuytren's contracture, dysphonia, electrolyte disturbances, eosinophilia, extrapyramidal symptoms, gangrene, gastrointestinal hemorrhage, gastrointestinal ulceration, glaucoma, goiter, gynecomastia, hematuria, hemiparesis, hemiplegia, hepatitis (ischemic), hyperbilirubinemia, hypercholesterolemia, hyperphosphatemia, hyperuricemia, hyper-/hypothyroidism, hyper-/hypotonia, hypoglycemia, hyponatremia; infections (bacterial, viral or fungal); intestinal obstruction, leukocytosis, leukopenia, limb embolism, liver enzymes increased, lymphadenopathy, lymphedema, lymphocytosis, lymphopenia, menstrual abnormalities, mitral insufficiency, MI, neoplasms (various), neuralgia, pancreatitis, paralysis, psychiatric disorders, peripheral neuropathy, photosensitivity, pleural effusion, proteinuria, pulmonary edema, pulmonary embolism, rash, renal calculus, renal failure (acute), seizure, sepsis, SIADH, skin disorders, stomatitis, stupor, subarachnoid hemorrhage, suicide attempt, SVT, tachycardia, thrombocytopenia, thrombosis, tinnitus, tongue edema, torticollis, urticaria, vagina/uterine hemorrhage, ventricular tachycardia, visual disturbances

Overdosage/Toxicology No reports of intentional overdose; symptoms reported with accidental overdosage were agitation, increased dyskinesia, sedation, orthostatic hypotension, chest pain, confusion, nausea, and vomiting. It is anticipated that the symptoms of overdose will be related to its dopaminergic activity. General supportive measures are recommended. Vital signs should be maintained, if necessary. Removal of any unabsorbed material (eg, by gastric lavage) should be considered. Removal by hemodialysis is unlikely.

Dosing

Adults & Elderly:

Parkinson's disease: Oral: The dosage should be increased to achieve a maximum therapeutic effect, balanced against the principal side effects of nausea, dizziness, somnolence and dyskinesia. Recommended starting dose is 0.25 mg 3 times/day; based on individual patient response, the dosage should be titrated with weekly increments as described below:

- Week 1: 0.25 mg 3 times/day; total daily dose: 0.75 mg
- Week 2: 0.5 mg 3 times/day; total daily dose: 1.5 mg
- Week 3: 0.75 mg 3 times/day; total daily dose: 2.25 mg
- Week 4: 1 mg 3 times/day; total daily dose: 3 mg

Note: After week 4, if necessary, daily dosage may be increased by 1.5 mg per day on a weekly basis up to a dose of 9 mg/day, and then by up to 3 mg/day weekly to a total of 24 mg/day

Parkinson's disease discontinuation taper: Ropinirole should be gradually tapered over 7 days as follows: reduce frequency of administration from 3

(Continued)

Ropinirole *(Continued)*

times daily to twice daily for 4 days, then reduce to once daily for remaining 3 days.

Restless Legs Syndrome: Initial: 0.25 mg once daily 1-3 hours before bedtime. Dose may be increased after 2 days to 0.5 mg daily, and after 7 days to 1 mg daily. Dose may be further titrated upward in 0.5 mg increments every week until reaching a daily dose of 3 mg during week 6. If symptoms persist or reappear, the daily dose may be increased to a maximum of 4 mg beginning week 7.

Note: Doses up to 4 mg per day may be discontinued without tapering.

Renal Impairment: Removal by hemodialysis is unlikely.

Available Dosage Forms Tablet: 0.25 mg, 0.5 mg, 1 mg, 2 mg, 3 mg, 4 mg, 5 mg

Nursing Guidelines

Assessment: Assess potential for interactions with other prescriptions, OTC medications, or herbal products patient may be taking. Assess therapeutic effectiveness and adverse responses on a regular basis during therapy. Monitor for CNS depression/somnolence. Teach patient proper use, side effects/appropriate interventions, and adverse reactions to report.

Dietary Considerations: May be taken with or without food.

Patient Education: Take exactly as directed, without regard to food. May cause dizziness, sudden, overwhelming sleepiness (use caution when driving or engaging in tasks that require alertness until response to drug is known); postural hypotension (use caution and avoid quick moves when rising from sitting or lying position, when climbing stairs, or engaging in activities that require quick movements); or nausea, vomiting, lack of appetite, or mouth sores (small frequent meals, frequent mouth care, chewing gum, or sucking lozenges may help). Report unusual and persistent sleepiness; chest pain or palpitations; CNS changes (confusion, hallucinations, amnesia, abnormal dreaming, insomnia); skeletal weakness or increased random tremors or movements, gait changes, or difficulty walking; signs of urinary tract or respiratory infection (pain or burning on urination, pus or blood in urine, or unusual cough and chest tightness); or unusual persistent adverse reactions. **Pregnancy/breast-feeding precautions:** Inform prescriber if you are or intend to become pregnant. Breast-feeding is not recommended.

Pregnancy Risk Factor: C

Lactation: Excretion in breast milk unknown/not recommended

Perioperative/Anesthesia/Other Concerns: If therapy with a drug known to be a potent inhibitor of CYP1A2 is stopped or started during treatment with ropinirole, adjustment of ropinirole dose may be required.

♦ Ropinirole Hydrochloride *see* Ropinirole *on page 1495*

Ropivacaine (roe PIV a kane)

U.S. Brand Names Naropin®

Synonyms Ropivacaine Hydrochloride

Pharmacologic Category Local Anesthetic

Medication Safety Issues

Sound-alike/look-alike issues:

Ropivacaine may be confused with bupivacaine, ropinirole

Use Local anesthetic for use in surgery, postoperative pain management, and obstetrical procedures when local or regional anesthesia is needed

Mechanism of Action Blocks both the initiation and conduction of nerve impulses by decreasing the neuronal membrane's permeability to sodium ions, which results in inhibition of depolarization with resultant blockade of conduction

Pharmacodynamics/Kinetics

Onset of action: Anesthesia (route dependent): 3-15 minutes

Duration (dose and route dependent): 3-15 hours

Metabolism: Hepatic

Half-life elimination: Epidural: 5-7 hours; I.V.: 2.4 hours

Excretion: Urine (86% as metabolites)

Contraindications Hypersensitivity to amide-type local anesthetics (eg, bupivacaine, mepivacaine, lidocaine) or any component of the formulation; septicemia, severe hypotension and for spinal anesthesia, in the presence of complete heart block

Warnings/Precautions Use with caution in patients with liver disease, cardiovascular disease, neurological or psychiatric disorders; it is not recommended for use in emergency situations where rapid administration is necessary

Drug Interactions Substrate of CYP1A2 (major), 2B6 (minor), 2D6 (minor), 3A4 (minor; may be major in cases of 1A2 inhibition/deficiency)

Amiodarone (and other class III antiarrhythmics): Cardiac effects during concomitant therapy may be additive. In addition, amiodarone may decrease th metabolism of ropivacaine. Monitor.

Ciprofloxacin: May increase ropivacaine levels/effects; monitor.

CYP1A2 inhibitors: May increase the levels/effects of ropivacaine. Example inhibitors include ketoconazole, norfloxacin, ofloxacin, and rofecoxib.

Fluvoxamine: May increase ropivacaine levels/effects; monitor.

Adverse Reactions

>5% (dose and route related):

- Cardiovascular: Hypotension, bradycardia
- Central nervous system: Headache
- Dermatologic: Pruritus
- Gastrointestinal: Nausea, vomiting
- Hematologic: Anemia
- Neuromuscular & skeletal: Back pain, paresthesia

1% to 5% (dose related):

- Cardiovascular: Hypertension, tachycardia
- Central nervous system: Dizziness, anxiety, lightheadedness
- Endocrine & metabolic: Hypokalemia
- Genitourinary: Urinary retention
- Neuromuscular & skeletal: Hypoesthesia, rigors, circumoral paresthesia
- Otic: Tinnitus
- Renal: Oliguria
- Respiratory: Dyspnea
- Miscellaneous: Shivering

<1% (Limited to important or life-threatening): Angioedema, apnea (usually associated with epidural block in head/neck region), bronchospasm, cardiac arrest, cardiovascular collapse, dyskinesia, hallucinations, hyperthermia, myocardial depression, MI, rash, seizure, syncope, tinnitus, ventricular arrhythmia

Overdosage/Toxicology Treatment is primarily symptomatic and supportive. Termination of anesthesia by pneumatic tourniquet inflation should be attempted when the agent is administered by infiltration or regional injection. Seizures commonly respond to diazepam, while hypotension responds to I.V. fluids and Trendelenburg positioning. Bradyarrhythmias (when the heart rate is <60) can be treated with I.V. or SubQ atropine 15 mcg/kg. With the development of metabolic acidosis, I.V. sodium bicarbonate 0.5-2 mEq/kg and ventilatory assistance should be instituted. Methemoglobinemia should be treated with methylene blue 1-2 mg/kg in a 1% sterile aqueous solution I.V. push over 4-6 minutes repeated up to a total dose of 7 mg/kg.

Dosing

Adults & Elderly: Dose varies with procedure, onset and depth of anesthesia desired, vascularity of tissues, duration of anesthesia, and condition of patient

Surgical anesthesia:
- Lumbar epidural: 15-30 mL of 0.5% to 1% solution
- Lumbar epidural block for cesarean section:
  - 20-30 mL dose of 0.5% solution
  - 15-20 mL dose of 0.75% solution
- Thoracic epidural block: 5-15 mL dose of 0.5% to 0.75% solution
- Major nerve block:
  - 35-50 mL dose of 0.5% solution (175-250 mg)
  - 10-40 mL dose of 0.75% solution (75-300 mg)
- Field block: 1-40 mL dose of 0.5% solution (5-200 mg)

Labor pain management: Lumbar epidural: Initial: 10-20 mL 0.2% solution; continuous infusion dose: 6-14 mL/hour of 0.2% solution with incremental injections of 10-15 mL/hour of 0.2% solution

Postoperative pain management:
- Lumbar or thoracic epidural: Continuous infusion dose: 6-14 mL/hour of 0.2% solution
- Infiltration/minor nerve block:
  - 1-100 mL dose of 0.2% solution
  - 1-40 mL dose of 0.5% solution

Available Dosage Forms

Infusion, as hydrochloride: 2 mg/mL (100 mL, 200 mL)

Injection, solution, as hydrochloride [preservative free]: 2 mg/mL (10 mL, 20 mL); 5 mg/mL (20 mL, 30 mL); 7.5 mg/mL (20 mL); 10 mg/mL (10 mL, 20 mL)

(Continued)

Ropivacaine *(Continued)*

Nursing Guidelines

Pregnancy Risk Factor: B

Pregnancy Issues: When used for epidural block during labor and delivery, systemically absorbed ropivacaine may cross the placenta, resulting in varying degrees of fetal or neonatal effects (eg, CNS or cardiovascular depression). Maternal hypotension may also result from systemic absorption.

Lactation: Excretion in breast milk unknown/use caution

Perioperative/Anesthesia/Other Concerns: Addition of sodium bicarbonate to local anesthetic solution will increase onset and potency. Only preservative-free solutions should be used for epidural and spinal administration. Although ropivacaine is chemically related to bupivacaine, it is not a racemic mixture (made up of the S-form enantiomer only) and, is less toxic than bupivacaine.

Administration

Storage: Epidural infusions can be used ≤24 hours.

Related Information

Acute Postoperative Pain *on page 1742*

Local Anesthetics *on page 1854*

♦ **Ropivacaine Hydrochloride** *see* Ropivacaine *on page 1498*

Rosiglitazone (roh si GLI ta zone)

U.S. Brand Names Avandia®

Pharmacologic Category Antidiabetic Agent, Thiazolidinedione

Medication Safety Issues

Sound-alike/look-alike issues:

Avandia® may be confused with Avalide®, Coumadin®, Prandin®

Use Type 2 diabetes mellitus (noninsulin dependent, NIDDM):

Monotherapy: Improve glycemic control as an adjunct to diet and exercise

Combination therapy: In combination with a sulfonylurea, metformin, or insulin, or sulfonylurea plus metformin when diet, exercise, and a single agent do not result in adequate glycemic control

Mechanism of Action Thiazolidinedione antidiabetic agent that lowers blood glucose by improving target cell response to insulin, without increasing pancreatic insulin secretion. It has a mechanism of action that is dependent on the presence of insulin for activity.

Pharmacodynamics/Kinetics

Onset of action: Delayed; Maximum effect: Up to 12 weeks

Distribution: V_{dss} (apparent): 17.6 L

Protein binding: 99.8%

Metabolism: Hepatic (99%) via CYP2C8; minor metabolism via CYP2C9

Bioavailability: 99%

Half-life elimination: 3-4 hours

Time to peak, plasma: 1 hour; delayed with food

Excretion: Urine (64%) and feces (23%) as metabolites

Contraindications Hypersensitivity to rosiglitazone or any component of the formulation; active liver disease (transaminases >2.5 times the upper limit of normal at baseline); contraindicated in patients who previously experienced jaundice during troglitazone therapy

Warnings/Precautions Should not be used in diabetic ketoacidosis. Mechanism requires the presence of insulin, therefore use in type 1 diabetes (insulin dependent, IDDM) is not recommended. Use with caution in premenopausal, anovulatory women; may result in resumption of ovulation, increasing the risk of pregnancy. May result in hormonal imbalance; development of menstrual irregularities should prompt reconsideration of therapy. Use with caution in patients with anemia or depressed leukocyte counts (may reduce hemoglobin, hematocrit, and/or WBC). May increase plasma volume and/or increase cardiac hypertrophy. Assess for fluid accumulation in patients with unusually rapid weight gain. Use with caution in patients with edema. Monitor closely for signs and symptoms of heart failure. Not recommended for use in patients with NYHA Class III or IV heart failure, unless serum glucose control outweighs the risk of excessive fluid retention. Discontinue if heart failure develops. Use with caution in patients with elevated transaminases (AST or ALT). Idiosyncratic hepatotoxicity has been reported with another thiazolidinedione agent (troglitazone) and (rarely) with rosiglitazone; discontinue if jaundice occurs. Monitoring should include periodic determinations of liver function. Rosiglitazone has been associated with new onset and/or worsening of macular edema in diabetic patients. Rosiglitazone should be used with caution in patients with a pre-existing macular edema or diabetic retinopathy. Discontinuation of rosiglitazone should be considered in any patient who reports visual deterioration. In addition, ophthalmological consultation should be initiated in these patients. Safety and efficacy in pediatric patients have not been established.

Drug Interactions **Substrate** of CYP2C8/9 (major); **Inhibits** CYP2C8/9 (moderate), 2C19 (weak), 2D6 (weak)

Bile acid sequestrants: May decrease rosiglitazone levels.

CYP2C8/9 inducers: May decrease the levels/effects of rosiglitazone. Example inducers include carbamazepine, phenobarbital, phenytoin, rifampin, rifapentine, and secobarbital.

CYP2C8/9 inhibitors: May increase the levels/effects of rosiglitazone. Example inhibitors include delavirdine, fluconazole, gemfibrozil, ketoconazole, nicardipine, NSAIDs, pioglitazone, and sulfonamides.

CYP2C8/9 substrates: Rosiglitazone may increase the levels/effects of CYP2C8/9 substrates. Example substrates include amiodarone, fluoxetine, glimepiride, glipizide, nateglinide, phenytoin, pioglitazone, sertraline, and warfarin.

Gemfibrozil: Gemfibrozil may increase rosiglitazone levels; a decreased rosiglitazone dose may be warranted

Rifampin: May decrease rosiglitazone levels/effects.

Nutritional/Herbal/Ethanol Interactions

Ethanol: Avoid ethanol (may cause hypoglycemia).

Food: Peak concentrations are lower by 28% and delayed when administered with food, but these effects are not believed to be clinically significant.

Herb/Nutraceutical: Avoid garlic, gymnema (may cause hypoglycemia).

Adverse Reactions

>10%: Endocrine & metabolic: Weight gain, increase in total cholesterol, increased LDL-cholesterol, increased HDL-cholesterol

1% to 10%:

Cardiovascular: Edema (5%)

Central nervous system: Headache (6%), fatigue (4%)

Endocrine & metabolic: Hyperglycemia (4%), hypoglycemia (1%; increased with insulin to 12% to 14%)

Gastrointestinal: Diarrhea (2%)

Hematologic: Anemia (2%)

Neuromuscular & skeletal: Back pain (4%)

Respiratory: Upper respiratory tract infection (10%), sinusitis (3%)

Miscellaneous: Injury (8%)

<1%, postmarketing, and/or case reports: Angioedema, CHF or exacerbation of CHF (increased with insulin to 2% to 3%), transaminases increased, hepatic failure, hepatitis, bilirubin increased, macular edema, pleural effusion, pulmonary edema, urticaria, weight gain (rapid, excessive; usually due to fluid accumulation)

Isolated case reports of hepatotoxic reactions have been reported in patients receiving rosiglitazone; causality not established

Overdosage/Toxicology Experience in overdose is limited. Symptoms may include hypoglycemia. Treatment is supportive.

Dosing

Adults & Elderly: Type 2 diabetes: Oral:

Monotherapy: Initial: 4 mg daily as a single daily dose or in divided doses twice daily. If response is inadequate after 8-12 weeks of treatment, the dosage may be increased to 8 mg daily as a single daily dose or in divided doses twice daily. In clinical trials, the 4 mg twice-daily regimen resulted in the greatest reduction in fasting plasma glucose and Hb A_{1c}.

Combination therapy: When adding rosiglitazone to existing therapy, continue current dose(s) of previous agents:

With sulfonylureas or metformin (or sulfonylurea plus metformin): Initial: 4 mg daily as a single daily dose or in divided doses twice daily. If response is inadequate after 8-12 weeks of treatment, the dosage may be increased to 8 mg daily as a single daily dose or in divided doses twice daily. Reduce dose of sulfonylurea if hypoglycemia occurs. It is unlikely that the dose of metformin will need to be reduced to hypoglycemia.

With insulin: Initial: 4 mg daily as a single daily dose or in divided doses twice daily. Dose of insulin should be reduced by 10% to 25% if the patient reports hypoglycemia or if the plasma glucose falls to <100 mg/dL. Doses of rosiglitazone >4 mg/day are not indicated in combination with insulin.

(Continued)

Rosiglitazone *(Continued)*

Renal Impairment: No adjustment is necessary.

Hepatic Impairment: Clearance is significantly lower in hepatic impairment. Therapy should not be initiated if the patient exhibits active liver disease of increased transaminases (>2.5 times the upper limit of normal) at baseline.

Available Dosage Forms Tablet: 2 mg, 4 mg, 8 mg

Nursing Guidelines

Assessment: Monitor laboratory results closely. Assess other prescriptions, OTC medications, or herbal products patient may be taking. Assess for signs of fluid retention and congestive heart failure. Monitor weight. Monitor response to therapy closely until response is stable. Advise women using oral contraceptives about need for alternative method of contraception. Assess knowledge/teach risks of hyper-/hypoglycemia, its symptoms, treatment, and predisposing conditions. Refer patient to a diabetic educator, if possible. Teach appropriate use of medication, interventions to reduce side effects, and adverse reactions to report.

Monitoring Laboratory Tests: Hemoglobin A_{1c}, serum glucose; liver enzymes (prior to initiation of therapy, then periodically thereafter). Patients with an elevation in ALT >3 times ULN should be rechecked as soon as possible. If the ALT levels remain >3 times ULN, therapy with rosiglitazone should be discontinued.

Dietary Considerations: Management of type 2 diabetes mellitus (noninsulin dependent, NIDDM) should include diet control. May be taken without regard to meals.

Patient Education: May be taken without regard to meals. Follow directions of prescriber. If dose is missed at the usual meal, take it with next meal. Do not double dose if daily dose is missed completely. Monitor urine or serum glucose as recommended by prescriber. More frequent monitoring is required during periods of stress, trauma, surgery, pregnancy, increased activity or exercise. Avoid alcohol. Report chest pain, rapid heartbeat or palpitations, abdominal pain, fever, rash, hypoglycemia reactions, yellowing of skin or eyes, dark urine or light stool, or unusual fatigue or nausea/vomiting. Report unusually rapid weight gain; swelling of ankles, legs, or abdomen; or weakness or shortness of breath. **Pregnancy/breast-feeding precautions:** In anovulatory, premenopausal women, ovulation may occur, increasing the risk of pregnancy. Adequate contraception is recommended. Use alternate means of contraception if using oral contraceptives. Breast-feeding is not recommended.

Pregnancy Risk Factor: C

Pregnancy Issues: Treatment during mid to late gestation was associated with fetal death and growth retardation in animal models. Abnormal blood glucose levels are associated with a higher incidence of congenital abnormalities. Insulin is the drug of choice for the control of diabetes mellitus during pregnancy. In anovulatory, premenopausal women, ovulation may occur, increasing the risk of pregnancy; adequate contraception is recommended.

Lactation: Excretion in breast milk unknown/not recommended

Breast-Feeding Considerations: In animal studies, rosiglitazone has been found to be excreted in milk. It is not known whether rosiglitazone is excreted in human milk. Should not be administered to a nursing woman.

Administration

Storage: Store at 25°C (77°F); excursions permitted to 15°C to 30°C (59°F to 86°F). Protect from light.

Related Information

Perioperative Management of the Diabetic Patient *on page 1794*

Rosiglitazone and Metformin (roh si GLI ta zone & met FOR min)

U.S. Brand Names Avandamet™

Synonyms Metformin and Rosiglitazone; Metformin Hydrochloride and Rosiglitazone Maleate; Rosiglitazone Maleate and Metformin Hydrochloride

Pharmacologic Category Antidiabetic Agent, Biguanide; Antidiabetic Agent, Thiazolidinedione

Use Management of type 2 diabetes mellitus (noninsulin dependent, NIDDM) in patients who are already treated with the combination of rosiglitazone and metformin, or who are not adequately controlled on metformin alone. Used as an adjunct to diet and exercise to lower the blood glucose when hyperglycemia cannot be controlled satisfactorily by diet and exercise alone

Mechanism of Action Rosiglitazone is a thiazolidinedione antidiabetic agent that lowers blood glucose by improving target cell response to insulin, without increasing pancreatic insulin secretion. It has a mechanism of action that is dependent on the presence of insulin for activity. Metformin decreases hepatic glucose production, decreasing intestinal absorption of glucose, and improves insulin sensitivity (increases peripheral glucose uptake and utilization).

Pharmacodynamics/Kinetics See individual agents.

Contraindications Hypersensitivity to rosiglitazone, metformin, or any component of the formulation; renal disease or renal dysfunction (serum creatinine ≥1.5 mg/dL in males or ≥1.4 mg/dL in females, or abnormal creatinine clearance which may also result from conditions such as cardiovascular collapse, acute myocardial infarction, and septicemia); acute or chronic metabolic acidosis with or without coma (including diabetic ketoacidosis); congestive heart failure requiring pharmacologic treatment; active liver disease (including patients with transaminases >2.5 times the upper limit of normal at baseline and/or hepatic dysfunction to a degree which predisposes to lactic acidosis); jaundice during previous troglitazone therapy

Note: Combination product is not appropriate for initial therapy of type 2 diabetes mellitus (noninsulin dependent, NIDDM); temporarily discontinue in patients undergoing radiologic studies in which intravascular iodinated contrast materials are utilized.

Warnings/Precautions Lactic acidosis is a rare, but potentially severe consequence of therapy with metformin. Lactic acidosis should be suspected in any diabetic patient receiving metformin who has evidence of acidosis when evidence of ketoacidosis is lacking. Discontinue metformin in clinical situations predisposing to hypoxemia, including conditions such as cardiovascular collapse, respiratory failure, acute myocardial infarction, acute congestive heart failure, and septicemia.

Metformin is substantially excreted by the kidney. The risk of accumulation and lactic acidosis increases with the degree of impairment of renal function. Patients with renal function below the limit of normal for their age should not receive metformin. In elderly patients, renal function should be monitored regularly; should not be used in any patient ≥80 years of age unless measurement of creatinine clearance verifies normal renal function. Use of concomitant medications that may affect renal function (ie, affect tubular secretion) may also affect metformin disposition. Metformin should be suspended in patients with dehydration and/or prerenal azotemia. Therapy should be suspended for any surgical procedures (resume only after normal intake resumed and normal renal function is verified). Metformin should also be temporarily discontinued for 48 hours in patients undergoing radiologic studies involving the intravascular administration of iodinated contrast materials (potential for acute alteration in renal function).

Avoid use in patients with impaired liver function. Rosiglitazone must be used with caution in patients with elevated transaminases (AST or ALT); avoid use in patients where hepatic dysfunction presents a risk of lactic acidosis. Idiosyncratic hepatotoxicity has been reported with another thiazolidinedione agent (troglitazone) and (rarely) with rosiglitazone; discontinue if jaundice occurs. Monitoring should include periodic determinations of liver function. Patient must be instructed to avoid excessive acute or chronic ethanol use.

Rosiglitazone may cause fluid retention which could exacerbate or lead to heart failure; monitor closely for signs and symptoms of heart failure; not recommended for use in patients with NYHA Class III or IV heart failure. Discontinue if heart failure develops. Use caution in patients with edema. Rosiglitazone requires the presence of endogenous insulin to be active, therefore use in type 1 diabetes (insulin dependent, IDDM) is not recommended. Use rosiglitazone with caution in premenopausal, anovulatory women; may result in resumption of ovulation, increasing the risk of pregnancy. May result in hormonal imbalance; development of menstrual irregularities should prompt reconsideration of therapy. Use rosiglitazone with caution in patients with anemia or depressed leukocyte counts (may reduce hemoglobin, hematocrit, and/or WBC). May increase plasma volume and/or increase cardiac hypertrophy. Rosiglitazone has been associated with new onset and/or worsening of macular edema in diabetic patients. Rosiglitazone should be used with caution in patients with a pre-existing macular edema or diabetic retinopathy. Discontinuation of rosiglitazone should be considered in any patient who reports visual deterioration. In addition, ophthalmological consultation should be initiated in these patients. Safety and efficacy have not been established in pediatric patients.

(Continued)

Rosiglitazone and Metformin *(Continued)*

Drug Interactions Rosiglitazone: **Substrate** of CYP2C8/9 (major); **Inhibits** CYP2C8/9 (moderate), 2C19 (weak), 2D6 (weak)

Also see individual agents.

Nutritional/Herbal/Ethanol Interactions See individual agents.

Adverse Reactions Also see individual agents. Percentages of adverse effects as reported with the combination product.

>10%:

Gastrointestinal: Diarrhea (13%)

Respiratory: Upper respiratory tract infection (16%)

1% to 10%:

Cardiovascular: Edema (4%)

Central nervous system: Headache (7%), fatigue (6%)

Endocrine & metabolic: Hypoglycemia (3%), hyperglycemia (2%)

Hematologic: Anemia (7%)

Neuromuscular & skeletal: Arthralgia (5%), back pain (5%)

Respiratory: Sinusitis (6%)

Miscellaneous: Viral infection (5%)

Overdosage/Toxicology Treatment should be symptom-directed and supportive. Hemodialysis may be effective for the removal of metformin.

Dosing

Adults: Type 2 diabetes mellitus: Oral: Initial dose should be based on current dose of rosiglitazone and/or metformin; daily dose should be divided and given with meals

Patients inadequately controlled on metformin alone: Initial dose: Rosiglitazone 4 mg/day plus current dose of metformin

Patients inadequately controlled on rosiglitazone alone: Initial dose: Metformin 1000 mg/day plus current dose of rosiglitazone

Note: When switching from combination rosiglitazone and metformin as separate tablets: Use current dose

Dose adjustment: Doses may be increased as increments of rosiglitazone 4 mg and/or metformin 500 mg, up to the maximum dose; doses should be titrated gradually.

After a change in the metformin dosage, titration can be done after 1-2 weeks

After a change in the rosiglitazone dosage, titration can be done after 8-12 weeks

Maximum dose: Rosiglitazone 8 mg/metformin 2000 mg daily

Elderly: The initial and maintenance dosing should be conservative, due to the potential for decreased renal function (monitor). Generally, elderly patients should not be titrated to the maximum. Do not use in patients ≥80 years unless normal renal function has been established.

Renal Impairment: Do not use with renal disease or renal dysfunction (serum creatinine ≥1.5 mg/dL in males or ≥1.4 mg/dL in females or abnormal clearance).

Hepatic Impairment: Do not use with active liver disease or ALT >2.5 times the upper limit of normal.

Available Dosage Forms Tablet [film coated]:

1/500: Rosiglitazone 1 mg and metformin hydrochloride 500 mg

2/500: Rosiglitazone 2 mg and metformin hydrochloride 500 mg

4/500: Rosiglitazone 4 mg and metformin hydrochloride 500 mg

2/1000: Rosiglitazone 2 mg and metformin hydrochloride 1000 mg

4/1000: Rosiglitazone 4 mg and metformin hydrochloride 1000 mg

Nursing Guidelines

Assessment: Assess allergy history prior to beginning therapy. See Contraindications, Warnings/Precautions, and Dosing for use cautions. Assess potential for interactions with other prescriptions, OTC medications, or herbal products patient may be taking (eg, anything that may affect glucose levels - see Drug Interactions). Assess results of laboratory tests (see Monitoring Laboratory Tests), therapeutic effectiveness, and adverse response (eg, hypoglycemia, vitamin B_{12} and/or folic acid deficiency - see Adverse Reactions and Overdose/Toxicology) at regular intervals during therapy. Teach patient proper use or refer patient to diabetic educator for instruction, possible side effects/appropriate interventions, and adverse symptoms to report (see Patient Education). Breast-feeding is not recommended.

Monitoring Laboratory Tests: See individual components.

Dietary Considerations: Should be taken with meals. Avoid ethanol. Dietary modification based on ADA recommendations is a part of therapy. Monitor for signs and symptoms of vitamin B_{12} and/or folic acid deficiency; supplementation may be required.

Patient Education: Inform prescriber of all prescriptions, OTC medications, or herbal products you are taking, and any allergies you have. Do not take any new medication during therapy without consulting prescriber. This medication is used to control diabetes; it is not a cure. Take exactly as directed with a meal at the same time(s) each day. Avoid alcohol; may cause severe reaction. Monitor glucose as recommended by prescriber. Maintain regular prescribed dietary intake and exercise routine (consult prescriber or diabetic educator) and always carry a quick source of sugar with you. Contact prescriber immediately if you experience a hypoglycemic reaction. May cause headache, nausea, or diarrhea during first weeks of therapy; consult prescriber if these persist. Report chest pain, rapid heartbeat, or palpitations; hypo- or hyperglycemic reactions; persistent, unusual fatigue; muscle pain or weakness; nausea or vomiting; rapid weight gain; swelling of extremities; or respiratory difficulty. **Pregnancy/breast-feeding precautions:** Inform prescriber if you are or intend to become pregnant. Use alternate means of contraception if using oral contraceptives. Breast-feeding is not recommended.

Pregnancy Risk Factor: C

Pregnancy Issues: Abnormal blood glucose levels are associated with a higher incidence of congenital abnormalities. Insulin is the drug of choice for the control of diabetes mellitus during pregnancy. Safety in pregnant women has not been established. Use during pregnancy only if clearly needed. In anovulatory, premenopausal women, ovulation may occur, increasing the risk of pregnancy; adequate contraception is recommended.

Lactation: Excretion in breast milk unknown/not recommended

Breast-Feeding Considerations: Consider discontinuing rosiglitazone/metformin or discontinue breast-feeding. If Avandamet™ is discontinued and if diet alone is inadequate for controlling blood glucose, consider insulin therapy.

Administration

Oral: Administer with meals. Patients who are NPO may need to have their dose held to avoid hypoglycemia.

Storage: Store at room temperature of 15°C to 30°C (59°F to 86°F). Protect from light.

- ♦ **Rosiglitazone Maleate and Metformin Hydrochloride** *see* Rosiglitazone and Metformin *on page 1502*
- ♦ **Rowasa®** *see* Mesalamine *on page 1105*
- ♦ **Roxanol™** *see* Morphine Sulfate *on page 1177*
- ♦ **Roxanol 100™** *see* Morphine Sulfate *on page 1177*
- ♦ **Roxanol™-T [DSC]** *see* Morphine Sulfate *on page 1177*
- ♦ **Roxicet™** *see* Oxycodone and Acetaminophen *on page 1286*
- ♦ **Roxicet™ 5/500** *see* Oxycodone and Acetaminophen *on page 1286*
- ♦ **Roxicodone™** *see* Oxycodone *on page 1284*
- ♦ **Roxicodone™ Intensol™** *see* Oxycodone *on page 1284*
- ♦ **RP-6976** *see* Docetaxel *on page 557*
- ♦ **RP-59500** *see* Quinupristin and Dalfopristin *on page 1455*
- ♦ **r-PA** *see* Reteplase *on page 1469*
- ♦ **RTCA** *see* Ribavirin *on page 1475*
- ♦ **Rubella, Measles and Mumps Vaccines, Combined** *see* Measles, Mumps, and Rubella Vaccines (Combined) *on page 1082*

Rubella Virus Vaccine (Live) (rue BEL a VYE rus vak SEEN, live)

U.S. Brand Names Meruvax® II

Synonyms German Measles Vaccine

Pharmacologic Category Vaccine

Medication Safety Issues

Sound-alike/look-alike issues:

Meruvax® II may be confused with Attenuvax®

Use Selective active immunization against rubella; vaccination is routinely recommended for persons from 12 months of age to puberty. All adults, both male and female, lacking documentation of live vaccine on or after first birthday, or laboratory evidence of immunity (particularly women of childbearing age and young

(Continued)

Rubella Virus Vaccine (Live) *(Continued)*

adults who work in or congregate in hospitals, colleges, and on military bases) should be vaccinated. Susceptible travelers should be vaccinated.

Note: Trivalent measles - mumps - rubella (MMR) vaccine is the preferred immunizing agent for most children and many adults.

Mechanism of Action Rubella vaccine is a live attenuated vaccine that contains the Wistar Institute RA 27/3 strain, which is adapted to and propagated in human diploid cell culture. Promotes active immunity by inducing rubella hemagglutination-inhibiting antibodies.

Pharmacodynamics/Kinetics Onset of action: Antibodies to vaccine: 2-4 weeks

Contraindications Hypersensitivity to gelatin or any other component of the vaccine; history of anaphylactic reactions to neomycin; individuals with blood dyscrasias, leukemia, lymphomas, or other malignant neoplasms affecting the bone marrow or lymphatic systems; concurrent immunosuppressive therapy; primary and acquired immunodeficiency states; family history of congenital or hereditary immunodeficiency; active/untreated tuberculosis; current febrile illness or active febrile infection; pregnancy

Warnings/Precautions Immediate treatment for anaphylactic/anaphylactoid reaction should be available during vaccine use. Use with caution in patients with thrombocytopenia and those who develop thrombocytopenia after first dose; thrombocytopenia may worsen. Defer vaccine following blood, plasma, or immune globulin (human) administration; children with HIV infection, who are asymptomatic and not immunosuppressed may be vaccinated. Patients with minor illnesses (diarrhea, mild upper respiratory tract infection with or without low-grade fever or other illnesses with low-grade fever) may receive vaccine.

Drug Interactions

Corticosteroids: In patients receiving high doses of systemic corticosteroids for ≥14 days, wait at least 1 month between discontinuing steroid therapy and administering immunization.

Immune globulin, whole blood, plasma: Do not administer together; immune response may be compromised. Defer vaccine administration for ≥3 months.

Immunosuppressant medications: The effect of the vaccine may be decreased, increasing the risk of rubella disease in individuals who are receiving immunosuppressant drugs.

Lab Interactions May depress tuberculin skin test sensitivity

Adverse Reactions All serious adverse reactions must be reported to the U.S. Department of Health and Human Services (DHHS) Vaccine Adverse Event Reporting System (VAERS) 1-800-822-7967.

Frequency not defined.

Cardiovascular: Syncope, vasculitis

Central nervous system: Dizziness, encephalitis, fever, Guillain-Barré syndrome, headache, irritability, malaise, polyneuritis, polyneuropathy

Dermatologic: Angioneurotic edema, erythema multiforme, purpura, rash, Stevens-Johnson syndrome, urticaria

Gastrointestinal: Diarrhea, nausea, sore throat, vomiting

Hematologic: Leukocytosis, thrombocytopenia

Local: Injection site reactions which include burning, induration, pain, redness, stinging, wheal and flare

Neuromuscular & skeletal: Arthralgia/arthritis (variable; highest rates in women, 12% to 26% versus children, up to 3%), myalgia, paresthesia

Ocular: Conjunctivitis, optic neuritis, papillitis, retrobulbar neuritis

Otic: Nerve deafness, otitis media

Respiratory: Bronchial spasm, cough, rhinitis

Miscellaneous: Anaphylactoid reactions, anaphylaxis, regional lymphadenopathy

Dosing

Adults: Immunization: SubQ: Children ≥12 months and Adults: 0.5 mL in outer aspect of upper arm; children vaccinated before 12 months of age should be revaccinated. Recommended age for primary immunization is 12-15 months; revaccination with MMR-II is recommended prior to elementary school.

Pediatrics: Immunization; SubQ: Children ≥12 months: Refer to adult dosing. Children vaccinated before 12 months of age should be revaccinated.

Available Dosage Forms Injection, powder for reconstitution [single dose]: 1000 $TCID_{50}$ (Wistar RA 27/3 Strain) [contains gelatin, human albumin, and neomycin]

Nursing Guidelines

Patient Education: This medication is only given by injection. You may experience burning or stinging at the injection site; joint pain usually occurs 1-10

weeks after vaccination and persists 1-3 days. Notify your prescriber immediately if these effects continue or are severe, or for a high fever, seizures or allergic reaction (respiratory difficulty, hives, weakness, dizziness, fast heartbeat). **Pregnancy/breast-feeding precautions:** Not to be used during pregnancy; do not get pregnant for 28 days after getting the vaccine. Pregnant women should wait until after giving birth to get the vaccine. Consult prescriber if breast-feeding.

Pregnancy Risk Factor: C

Pregnancy Issues: Women who are pregnant when vaccinated or who become pregnant within 28 days of vaccination should be counseled on the theoretical risks to the fetus. The risk of rubella-associated malformations in these women is so small as to be negligible. MMR is the vaccine of choice if recipients are likely to be susceptible to measles or mumps as well as to rubella.

Lactation: Enters breast milk/use caution

Breast-Feeding Considerations: Following vaccination in the mother, rubella virus may be transmitted to the nursing infant via breast milk. Infants may show serologic evidence of infection, however, severe disease is not expected.

Administration

I.V.: Not for I.V. administration.

Storage: Refrigerate, discard reconstituted vaccine after 8 hours; store at 2°C to 8°C (36°F to 46°F); ship vaccine at 10°C; may use dry ice, protect from light.

- ♦ Rubex® *see* DOXOrubicin *on page 576*
- ♦ Rulox *see* Aluminum Hydroxide and Magnesium Hydroxide *on page 122*
- ♦ Rulox No. 1 *see* Aluminum Hydroxide and Magnesium Hydroxide *on page 122*
- ♦ Rum-K® *see* Potassium Chloride *on page 1385*
- ♦ S-2® *see* Epinephrine (Racemic/Dental) *on page 615*
- ♦ Saizen® *see* Somatropin *on page 1555*
- ♦ Salagen® *see* Pilocarpine *on page 1365*
- ♦ Salbutamol *see* Albuterol *on page 96*
- ♦ Salicylazosulfapyridine *see* Sulfasalazine *on page 1586*
- ♦ SalineX® [OTC] *see* Sodium Chloride *on page 1545*

Salmeterol (sal ME te role)

U.S. Brand Names Serevent® Diskus®

Synonyms Salmeterol Xinafoate

Pharmacologic Category Beta$_2$-Adrenergic Agonist

Medication Safety Issues

Sound-alike/look-alike issues:

Salmeterol may be confused with Salbutamol

Serevent® may be confused with Serentil®

Use Maintenance treatment of asthma and in prevention of bronchospasm with reversible obstructive airway disease, including patients with symptoms of nocturnal asthma, who require regular treatment with inhaled, short-acting beta$_2$ agonists; prevention of exercise-induced bronchospasm; maintenance treatment of bronchospasm associated with COPD

Mechanism of Action Relaxes bronchial smooth muscle by selective action on beta$_2$-receptors with little effect on heart rate; because salmeterol acts locally in the lung, therapeutic effect is not predicted by plasma levels

Pharmacodynamics/Kinetics

Onset of action: Asthma: 30-48 minutes, COPD: 2 hours

Peak effect: 2-4 hours, COPD: 3.27-4.75 hours

Duration: 12 hours

Protein binding: 96%

Metabolism: Hepatically hydroxylated

Half-life elimination: 5.5 hours

Excretion: Feces (60%), urine (25%)

Contraindications Hypersensitivity to salmeterol, adrenergic amines, or any component of the formulation; need for acute bronchodilation

Warnings/Precautions Salmeterol is not meant to relieve acute asthmatic symptoms. Acute episodes should be treated with short-acting beta$_2$ agonist. Optimize anti-inflammatory treatment before initiating maintenance treatment with salmeterol. Do not use as a component of chronic therapy without an anti-inflammatory agent. Patient must be instructed to seek medical attention in cases where acute symptoms are not relieved by short-acting beta-agonist (**not** salmeterol) or a previous level of response is diminished. Treatment must not be delayed.

(Continued)

Salmeterol *(Continued)*

Use caution in patients with cardiovascular disease (arrhythmia or hypertension or CHF), convulsive disorders, diabetes, glaucoma, hyperthyroidism, hepatic impairment, or hypokalemia. Beta agonists may cause elevation in blood pressure, heart rate, and result in CNS stimulation/excitation. $Beta_2$ agonists may increase risk of arrhythmia, increase serum glucose, or decrease serum potassium.

In a large, randomized clinical trial (SMART), salmeterol was associated with a small, but statistically significant increase in asthma-related deaths (when added to usual asthma therapy); risk may be greater in African-American patients versus Caucasians.

Do not exceed recommended dose; serious adverse events including fatalities, have been associated with excessive use of inhaled sympathomimetics. Rarely, paradoxical bronchospasm may occur with use of inhaled bronchodilating agents; this should be distinguished from inadequate response. Safety and efficacy have not been established in children <4 years of age.

Drug Interactions Substrate of CYP3A4 (major)

Beta-blockers (nonselective): May antagonize therapeutic effect of salmeterol.

MAO inhibitors: May increase toxicity of salmeterol. Wait 2 weeks after discontinuing MAO inhibitors before initiating salmeterol therapy.

Tricyclic antidepressants (TCAs): May increase toxicity of salmeterol. Wait 2 weeks after discontinuing TCA before initiating salmeterol therapy.

Adverse Reactions

>10%:

Central nervous system: Headache

Endocrine & metabolic: Serum glucose increased, serum potassium decreased

Respiratory: Pharyngitis

1% to 10%:

Cardiovascular: Tachycardia, palpitation, elevation or depression of blood pressure, cardiac arrhythmia

Central nervous system: Nervousness, CNS stimulation, hyperactivity, insomnia, malaise, dizziness

Gastrointestinal: GI upset, diarrhea, nausea

Neuromuscular & skeletal: Tremors (may be more common in the elderly), myalgia, back pain, arthralgia

Respiratory: Upper respiratory infection, cough, bronchitis

<1% (Limited to important or life-threatening): Anaphylactic reaction in patients with severe milk protein allergy (very rare), arrhythmia, atrial fibrillation, hypertension, hypokalemia, immediate hypersensitivity reactions (rash, urticaria, bronchospasm), laryngeal spasm, oropharyngeal irritation, paradoxical bronchospasms

Overdosage/Toxicology Symptoms of overdose include tachycardia, tremor, hypertension, angina, and seizures. Hypokalemia also may occur. Cardiac arrest and death may be associated with abuse of beta-agonist bronchodilators. Treatment includes immediate discontinuation and symptomatic and supportive therapies. Cautious use of beta-adrenergic blocking agents may be considered in severe cases.

Dosing

Adults & Elderly:

Asthma, maintenance and prevention: Inhalation, powder (Serevent® Diskus®): One inhalation (50 mcg) twice daily (~12 hours apart)

Exercise-induced asthma, prevention: One inhalation (50 mcg) at least 30 minutes prior to exercise; additional doses should not be used for 12 hours; should not be used in individuals already receiving salmeterol twice daily

COPD (maintenance treatment of associated bronchospasm): One inhalation (50 mcg) twice daily (~12 hours apart)

Pediatrics: Asthma (maintenance/prevention) and exercise-induced asthma (prevention): Inhalation, powder (Serevent® Diskus®): Children ≥4 years: Refer to adult dosing.

Available Dosage Forms Powder for oral inhalation: 50 mcg (28s, 60s) [delivers 47 mcg/inhalation; contains lactose]

Nursing Guidelines

Assessment: Not for use to relieve acute asthmatic attacks. Assess effectiveness and interactions of other medications patient may be taking. Monitor effectiveness of therapy and adverse reactions at beginning of therapy and periodically with long-term use. Monitor for increased use of short-acting beta$_2$-agonist inhalers; may be marker of a deteriorating asthma condition. For inpatient care, monitor vital signs and lung sounds prior to and periodically during therapy. Assess knowledge/teach patient appropriate use, interventions to reduce side effects, and adverse symptoms to report

Monitoring Laboratory Tests: FEV$_1$, peak flow, and/or other pulmonary function tests

Patient Education: Use exactly as directed (see Administration below). Do not use more often than recommended (excessive use may result in tolerance, overdose may result in serious adverse effects) and do not discontinue without consulting prescriber. Do not use for acute attacks. Maintain adequate hydration (2-3 L/day of fluids) unless instructed to restrict fluid intake. You may experience nervousness, dizziness, or fatigue (use caution when driving or engaging in tasks requiring alertness until response to drug is known); or dry mouth, stomach upset (small frequent meals, frequent mouth care, chewing gum, or sucking hard candy may help). If you have diabetes, check blood sugar; blood glucose level may be increased. Report unresolved GI upset; dizziness or fatigue; vision changes; chest pain, rapid heartbeat, or palpitations; insomnia; nervousness or hyperactivity; muscle cramping, tremors, or pain; unusual cough; or skin rash. **Pregnancy/breast-feeding precautions:** Inform prescriber if you are or intend to become pregnant. Consult prescriber if breast-feeding.

Geriatric Considerations: Geriatric patients were included in four clinical studies of salmeterol; no apparent differences in efficacy and safety were noted in geriatric patients compared to younger adults. Because salmeterol is only to be used for prevention of bronchospasm, patients also need a short-acting beta-agonist to treat acute attacks. Elderly patients should be carefully counseled about which inhaler to use and the proper scheduling of doses; a spacer device may be utilized to maximize effectiveness.

Pregnancy Risk Factor: C

Lactation: Enters breast milk/use caution

Administration

Storage: Inhalation powder (Serevent® Diskus®): Store at controlled room temperature 20°C to 25°C (68°F to 77°F) in a dry place away from direct heat or sunlight. Stable for 6 weeks after removal from foil pouch.

- ♦ **Salmeterol and Fluticasone** *see* Fluticasone and Salmeterol *on page 765*
- ♦ **Salmeterol Xinafoate** *see* Salmeterol *on page 1507*
- ♦ **Salt** *see* Sodium Chloride *on page 1545*
- ♦ **Salt Poor Albumin** *see* Albumin *on page 94*
- ♦ **Sal-Tropine™** *see* Atropine *on page 203*
- ♦ **Sandimmune®** *see* CycloSPORINE *on page 465*
- ♦ **Sandostatin®** *see* Octreotide *on page 1251*
- ♦ **Sandostatin LAR®** *see* Octreotide *on page 1251*
- ♦ **Sani-Supp® [OTC]** *see* Glycerin *on page 826*
- ♦ **Sarafem®** *see* Fluoxetine *on page 748*

Sargramostim (sar GRAM oh stim)

U.S. Brand Names Leukine®

Synonyms GM-CSF; Granulocyte-Macrophage Colony Stimulating Factor; rGM-CSF

Pharmacologic Category Colony Stimulating Factor

Medication Safety Issues

Sound-alike/look-alike issues:

Leukine® may be confused with Leukeran®

Use

Myeloid reconstitution after autologous bone marrow transplantation: Non-Hodgkin's lymphoma (NHL), acute lymphoblastic leukemia (ALL), Hodgkin's lymphoma, metastatic breast cancer

Myeloid reconstitution after allogeneic bone marrow transplantation

Peripheral stem cell transplantation: Metastatic breast cancer, non-Hodgkin's lymphoma, Hodgkin's lymphoma, multiple myeloma

Orphan drug:

Acute myelogenous leukemia (AML) following induction chemotherapy in older adults to shorten time to neutrophil recovery and to reduce the incidence of severe and life-threatening infections and infections resulting in death

(Continued)

Sargramostim *(Continued)*

Bone marrow transplant (allogeneic or autologous) failure or engraftment delay

Safety and efficacy of GM-CSF given simultaneously with cytotoxic chemotherapy have not been established. Concurrent treatment may increase myelosuppression.

Mechanism of Action Stimulates proliferation, differentiation and functional activity of neutrophils, eosinophils, monocytes, and macrophages, as indicated: See table.

Comparative Effects — G-CSF vs GM-CSF

Proliferation/Differentiation	G-CSF (Filgrastim)	GM-CSF (Sargramostim)
Neutrophils	Yes	Yes
Eosinophils	No	Yes
Macrophages	No	Yes
Neutrophil migration	Enhanced	Inhibited

Pharmacodynamics/Kinetics

Onset of action: Increase in WBC: 7-14 days

Duration: WBCs return to baseline within 1 week of discontinuing drug

Half-life elimination: 2 hours

Time to peak, serum: SubQ: 1-2 hours

Contraindications Hypersensitivity to sargramostim, yeast-derived products, or any component of the formulation; concurrent myelosuppressive chemotherapy or radiation therapy. The solution for injection contains benzyl alcohol and should not be used in neonates.

Warnings/Precautions Simultaneous administration, or administration 24 hours preceding/following cytotoxic chemotherapy or radiotherapy is not recommended. Use with caution in patients with pre-existing cardiac problems, hypoxia, fluid retention, pulmonary infiltrates or CHF, renal or hepatic impairment.

Rapid increase in peripheral blood counts: If ANC >20,000/mm^3 or platelets >500,000/mm^3, decrease dose by 50% or discontinue drug (counts will fall to normal within 3-7 days after discontinuing drug)

The manufacturer recommends that precaution be exercised in the usage of sargramostim in any malignancy with myeloid characteristics. Sargramostim can potentially act as a growth factor for any tumor type, particularly myeloid malignancies. Tumors of nonhematopoietic origin may have surface receptors for sargramostim.

There is a "first-dose effect" (refer to Adverse Reactions for details) which is rarely seen with the first dose and does not usually occur with subsequent doses.

Drug Interactions Increased toxicity: Lithium, corticosteroids may potentiate myeloproliferative effects

Adverse Reactions

>10%:

- Cardiovascular: Hypotension, tachycardia, flushing, and syncope may occur with the first dose of a cycle ("first-dose effect"); peripheral edema (11%)
- Central nervous system: Headache (26%)
- Dermatologic: Rash, alopecia
- Endocrine & metabolic: Polydypsia
- Gastrointestinal: Diarrhea (52% to 89%), stomatitis, mucositis
- Local: Local reactions at the injection site (~50%)
- Neuromuscular & skeletal: Myalgia (18%), arthralgia (21%), bone pain
- Renal: Increased serum creatinine (14%)
- Respiratory: Dyspnea (28%)

1% to 10%:

- Cardiovascular: Transient supraventricular arrhythmia; chest pain; capillary leak syndrome; pericardial effusion (4%)
- Central nervous system: Headache
- Gastrointestinal: Nausea, vomiting
- Hematologic: Leukocytosis, thrombocytopenia
- Neuromuscular & skeletal: Weakness
- Respiratory: Cough; pleural effusion (1%)

<1% (Limited to important or life-threatening): Anaphylaxis, anorexia, arrhythmia, constipation, eosinophilia, fever, lethargy, malaise, pericarditis, rigors, sore throat, thrombophlebitis, thrombosis

Overdosage/Toxicology Symptoms of overdose include dyspnea, malaise, nausea, fever, headache, and chills. Discontinue drug and wait for levels to fall. Treatment is supportive. Monitor CBC, respiratory symptoms, and fluid status. Discontinue drug and wait for levels to fall, monitor for pulmonary edema. Toxicity of GM-CSF is dose dependent. Severe reactions such as capillary leak syndrome are seen at higher doses (>15 mcg/kg/day).

Dosing

Adults & Elderly:

I.V. infusion over ≥2 hours or SubQ: **Rounding the dose to the nearest vial size enhances patient convenience and reduces costs without clinical detrement.**

Myeloid reconstitution after peripheral stem cell, allogeneic or autologous bone marrow transplant: I.V.: 250 mcg/m²/day for 21 days to begin 2-4 hours after the marrow infusion or ≥24 hours after chemotherapy or 12 hours after last dose of radiotherapy.

If a severe adverse reaction occurs, reduce or temporarily discontinue the dose until the reaction abates.

If blast cells appear or progression of the underlying disease occurs, disrupt treatment.

Interrupt or reduce the dose by half if ANC is >20,000 cells/mm³

Patients should not receive sargramostim until the postmarrow infusion ANC is <500 cells/mm³.

Neutrophil recovery following chemotherapy in AML: I.V.: 250 mcg/m²/day over a 4-hour period starting approximately day 11 or 4 days following the completion of induction chemotherapy, if day 10 bone marrow is hypoblastic with <5% blasts.

If a second cycle of chemotherapy is necessary, administer ~4 days after the completion of chemotherapy if the bone marrow is hypoblastic with <5% blasts.

Continue sargramostim until ANC is >1500 cells/mm³ for consecutive days or a maximum of 42 days.

Discontinue sargramostim immediately if leukemic regrowth occurs.

If a severe adverse reaction occurs, reduce the dose by 50% or temporarily discontinue the dose until the reaction abates.

Mobilization of peripheral blood progenitor cells: I.V.: 250 mcg/m²/day over 24 hours or SubQ once daily.

Continue the same dose through the period of PBPC collection.

The optimal schedule for PBPC collection has not been established (usually begun by day 5 and performed daily until protocol specified targets are achieved).

If WBC >50,000 cells/mm³, reduce the dose by 50%.

If adequate numbers of progenitor cells are not collected, consider other mobilization therapy.

Postperipheral blood progenitor cell transplantation: I.V.: 250 mcg/m²/day or SubQ once daily beginning immediately following infusion of progenitor cells and continuing until ANC is >1500 for 3 consecutive days is attained.

BMT failure or engraftment delay: I.V.: 250 mcg/m²/day for 14 days

The dose can be repeated after 7 days off therapy if engraftment has not occurred.

If engraftment still has not occurred, a third course of 500 mcg/m²/day for 14 days may be tried after another 7 days off therapy; if there is still no improvement, it is unlikely that further dose escalation will be beneficial.

If a severe adverse reaction occurs, reduce or temporarily discontinue the dose until the reaction abates.

If blast cells appear or disease progression occurs, discontinue treatment.

Pediatrics: Refer to adult dosing.

Available Dosage Forms

Injection, powder for reconstitution: 250 mcg [contains sucrose 10 mg/mL]

Injection, solution: 500 mcg/mL (1 mL) [contains benzyl alcohol and sucrose 10 mg/mL]

Nursing Guidelines

Assessment: See Contraindications, Warnings/Precautions, and Dosing for use cautions. See specific I.V. directions below. Patient must be monitored closely for "first dose effects" (see Adverse Reactions). Assess results of laboratory tests (see below) closely. Assess patient response (eg, fluid balance, CNS

(Continued)

Sargramostim *(Continued)*

response, and GI effects - see Adverse Reactions and Overdose/Toxicology) on a frequent basis. Teach patient use if self-administered (eg, appropriate injection technique and syringe/needle disposal), possible side effects/appropriate interventions, and adverse symptoms to report (see Patient Education). Note breast-feeding caution.

Monitoring Laboratory Tests: To avoid potential complications of excessive leukocytosis (WBC >50,000 cells/mm^3, ANC >20,000 cells/mm^3) a CBC with differential is recommended twice per week during therapy. Sargramostim therapy should be interrupted or the dose reduced by half if the ANC is >20,000 cells/mm^3. Monitoring of renal and hepatic function in patients displaying renal or hepatic dysfunction prior to initiation of treatment is recommended and at least biweekly during sargramostim administration.

Patient Education: I.V.: Immediately report any redness, swelling, pain, or burning at infusion site. You will require frequent blood tests during treatment. May cause bone pain (request analgesic); or nausea and vomiting (small, frequent meals may help); or hair loss (reversible). Report signs or symptoms of edema (eg, swollen extremities, respiratory difficulty, rapid weight gain); onset of severe headache; acute back or chest pain; muscular tremors or seizure activity. **Pregnancy/breast-feeding precautions:** Inform prescriber if you are or intend to become pregnant. Consult prescriber if breast-feeding.

Pregnancy Risk Factor: C

Lactation: Excretion in breast milk unknown

Perioperative/Anesthesia/Other Concerns: Reimbursement Hotline (Leukine®): 1-800-321-4669

Administration

I.V.: Can premedicate with analgesics and antipyretics; control bone pain with non-narcotic analgesics. I.V. infusion should be over at least 2 hours; incompatible with dextrose-containing solutions. An in-line membrane filter should not be used for intravenous injection.

Reconstitution:

Powder for injection: May be reconstituted with preservative free SWFI or bacteriostatic water for injection (with benzyl alcohol 0.9%). Gently swirl to reconstitute; do not shake.

Sargramostim may also be further diluted in 0.9% sodium chloride to a concentration of ≥10 mcg/mL for I.V. infusion administration.

If the final concentration of sargramostim is <10 mcg/mL, 1 mg of human albumin/1 mL of 0.9% sodium chloride (eg, 1 mL of 5% human albumin/50 mL of 0.9% sodium chloride) should be added.

Standard diluent: 25-100 mL NS

Compatibility: Stable in NS, SWFI, bacteriostatic water; **incompatible** with dextrose-containing solutions

Y-site administration: Incompatible with acyclovir, ampicillin, ampicillin/sulbactam, cefoperazone, chlorpromazine, ganciclovir, haloperidol, hydrocortisone sodium phosphate, hydrocortisone sodium succinate, hydromorphone, hydroxyzine, imipenem/cilastatin, lorazepam, methylprednisolone sodium succinate, mitomycin, morphine, nalbuphine, ondansetron, piperacillin, sodium bicarbonate, tobramycin

Storage: Sargramostim should be stored at 2°C to 8°C (36°F to 46°F). Vials should not be frozen or shaken.

Solution for injection: May be stored for up to 20 days at 2°C to 8°C (36°F to 46°F) once the vial has been entered. Discard remaining solution after 20 days.

Powder for injection: Preparations made with SWFI should be administered as soon as possible, and discarded within 6 hours of reconstitution. Preparations made with bacteriostatic water may be stored for up to 20 days at 2°C to 8°C (36°F to 46°F).

I.V. infusion administration: Preparations diluted with NS are stable for 48 hours at room temperature and refrigeration.

Standard diluent: 25-100 mL NS

♦ **Sarnol®-HC [OTC]** *see* Hydrocortisone *on page 873*

♦ **S-Citalopram** *see* Escitalopram *on page 639*

♦ **Scopace™** *see* Scopolamine *on page 1513*

Scopolamine (skoe POL a meen dah RIV ah tives)

U.S. Brand Names Isopto® Hyoscine; Scopace™; Transderm Scōp®

Synonyms Hyoscine Butylbromide; Hyoscine Hydrobromide; Scopolamine Butylbromide; Scopolamine Hydrobromide

Pharmacologic Category Anticholinergic Agent

Medication Safety Issues

Transdermal patch may contain conducting metal (eg, aluminum); remove patch prior to MRI.

Use

Scopolamine hydrobromide:

Injection: Preoperative medication to produce amnesia, sedation, and decrease salivary and respiratory secretions

Ophthalmic: Produce cycloplegia and mydriasis; treatment of iridocyclitis

Oral: Symptomatic treatment of postencephalitic parkinsonism and paralysis agitans; inhibits excessive motility and hypertonus of the genitourinary or gastrointestinal tract in such conditions as the irritable colon syndrome, mild dysentery, diverticulitis, pylorospasm, and cardiospasm

Transdermal: Prevention of nausea/vomiting associated with anesthesia or opiate analgesia; prevention of motion sickness

Scopolamine butylbromide:

Oral/injection: Treatment of smooth muscle spasm of the genitourinary or gastrointestinal tract; injection may also be used to prior to radiological/ diagnostic procedures to prevent spasm

Mechanism of Action Blocks the action of acetylcholine at parasympathetic sites in smooth muscle, secretory glands and the CNS; increases cardiac output, dries secretions, antagonizes histamine and serotonin

Pharmacodynamics/Kinetics

Onset of action: Oral, I.M.: 0.5-1 hour; I.V.: 10 minutes

Peak effect: 20-60 minutes; may take 3-7 days for full recovery; transdermal: 24 hours

Duration: Oral, I.M.: 4-6 hours; I.V.: 2 hours

Absorption: Tertiary salts (hydrobromide) are well absorbed; quaternary salts (butylbromide) are poorly absorbed (local concentrations in the GI tract following oral dosing may be high)

Metabolism: Hepatic

Half-life elimination: 4.8 hours

Excretion: Urine (as metabolites)

Contraindications Hypersensitivity to scopolamine or any component of the formulation; narrow-angle glaucoma; acute hemorrhage; paralytic ileus, GI or GU obstruction; thyrotoxicosis; tachycardia secondary to cardiac insufficiency; myasthenia gravis

Warnings/Precautions Use with caution with hepatic or renal impairment since adverse CNS effects occur more often in these patients; use with caution in infants and children since they may be more susceptible to adverse effects of scopolamine; use with caution in patients with GI obstruction, prostatic hyperplasia (nonobstructive), or urinary retention. Discontinue if patient reports unusual visual disturbances or pain within the eye. Use caution in hiatal hernia, reflux esophagitis, and ulcerative colitis. Scopolamine (hyoscine) hydrobromide should not be interchanged with scopolamine butylbromide formulations; dosages are not equivalent. Transdermal patch may contain conducting metal (eg, aluminum); remove patch prior to MRI.

Drug Interactions

Anticholinergic agents: Adverse anticholinergic effects may be additive with other anticholinergic agents (includes tricyclic antidepressants, antihistamines, and phenothiazines).

CNS depressants: Sedative effects may be additive with scopolamine; use caution.

Nutritional/Herbal/Ethanol Interactions Ethanol: Avoid ethanol (may increase CNS depression).

Adverse Reactions Frequency not defined.

Ophthalmic: Note: Systemic adverse effects have been reported following ophthalmic administration.

Cardiovascular: Vascular congestion, edema

Central nervous system: Drowsiness

Dermatologic: Eczematoid dermatitis

(Continued)

Scopolamine *(Continued)*

Ocular: Blurred vision, photophobia, local irritation, increased intraocular pressure, follicular conjunctivitis, exudate

Respiratory: Congestion

Systemic:

Cardiovascular: Orthostatic hypotension, ventricular fibrillation, tachycardia, palpitation

Central nervous system: Confusion, drowsiness, headache, loss of memory, ataxia, fatigue

Dermatologic: Dry skin, increased sensitivity to light, rash

Endocrine & metabolic: Decreased flow of breast milk

Gastrointestinal: Constipation, xerostomia, dry throat, dysphagia, bloated feeling, nausea, vomiting

Genitourinary: Dysuria

Local: Irritation at injection site

Neuromuscular & skeletal: Weakness

Ocular: Increased intraocular pain, blurred vision

Respiratory: Dry nose

Miscellaneous: Diaphoresis (decreased)

<1% (Limited to important or life-threatening): Anaphylactoid reaction, anaphylaxis, hallucinations, restlessness, retinal pigmentation

Overdosage/Toxicology Symptoms of overdose include dilated pupils, flushed skin, tachycardia, hypertension, and ECG abnormalities. CNS manifestations resemble acute psychosis. CNS depression, circulatory collapse, respiratory failure, and death can occur. For a scopolamine overdose with severe life-threatening symptoms, physostigmine 1-2 mg SubQ or I.V. slowly should be given to reverse toxic effects.

Dosing

Adults & Elderly: Note: Scopolamine (hyoscine) hydrobromide should not be interchanged with scopolamine butylbromide formulations. Dosages are not equivalent.

Scopolamine hydrobromide:

Preoperative:

I.M., I.V., SubQ: 0.3-0.65 mg; may be repeated every 4-6 hours

Transdermal patch: Apply 2.5 cm^2 patch to hairless area behind ear the night before surgery or 1 hour prior to cesarean section (the patch should be applied no sooner than 1 hour before surgery for best results and removed 24 hours after surgery)

Motion sickness: Transdermal: Apply 1 disc behind the ear at least 4 hours prior to exposure and every 3 days as needed; effective if applied as soon as 2-3 hours before anticipated need, best if 12 hours before

Refraction: Ophthalmic: Instill 1-2 drops of 0.25% to eye(s) 1 hour before procedure

Iridocyclitis: Ophthalmic: Instill 1-2 drops of 0.25% to eye(s) up to 4 times/day

Parkinsonism, spasticity, motion sickness: Oral: 0.4-0.8 mg as a range; the dosage may be cautiously increased in parkinsonism and spastic states.

Scopolamine butylbromide:

Gastrointestinal/genitourinary spasm (Buscopan® [CAN]; not available in the U.S.):

Oral: 10-20 mg daily (1-2 tablets); maximum: 6 tablets/day

I.M., I.V., SubQ: 10-20 mg; maximum: 100 mg/day. Intramuscular injections should be administered 10-15 minutes prior to radiological/diagnostic procedures

Pediatrics:

Scopolamine hydrobromide:

Preoperative: I.M., SubQ: 6 mcg/kg/dose (maximum: 0.3 mg/dose) every 6-8 hours

Refraction: Ophthalmic: Instill 1 drop of 0.25% to eye(s) twice daily for 2 days before procedure

Iridocyclitis: Ophthalmic: Instill 1 drop of 0.25% to eye(s) up to 3 times/day

Available Dosage Forms [CAN] = Canadian brand name

Injection, solution, as hydrobromide: 0.4 mg/mL (1 mL)

Injection, solution, as hyoscine-N-butylbromide (Buscopan® [CAN]): 20 mg/mL [not available in U.S.]

Solution, ophthalmic, as hydrobromide (Isopto® Hyoscine): 0.25% (5 mL, 15 mL) [contains benzalkonium chloride]

Tablet, as hyoscine-N-butylbromide (Buscopan® [CAN]): 10 mg [not available in U.S.]

Tablet, soluble, as hydrobromide (Scopace™): 0.4 mg

Transdermal system (Transderm Scōp®): 1.5 mg (4s, 10s, 24s) [releases ~1 mg over 72 hours]

Nursing Guidelines

Assessment: Assess potential for interactions with other prescriptions, OTC medications, or herbal products patient may be taking (eg, ergot-containing drugs). When used preoperatively, safety precautions should be observed and patient should be advised about blurred vision. For all uses, assess therapeutic effectiveness and adverse reactions. Teach patient appropriate use (according to formulation and purpose), interventions to reduce side effects, and adverse symptoms to report. Systemic effects have been reported following ophthalmic administration.

Patient Education: Use as directed. May cause drowsiness, confusion, impaired judgment, or vision changes (use caution when driving or engaging in tasks requiring alertness until response to drug is known); dry mouth, nausea, or vomiting (small frequent meals, frequent mouth care, chewing gum, or sucking lozenges may help); orthostatic hypotension (use caution when climbing stairs and when rising from lying or sitting position); constipation (increased exercise, fluids, fruit, or fiber may help; if not effective consult prescriber); increased sensitivity to heat and decreased perspiration (avoid extremes of heat, reduce exercise in hot weather); or decreased milk if breast-feeding. Report hot, dry, flushed skin; blurred vision or vision changes; difficulty swallowing; chest pain, palpitations, or rapid heartbeat; painful or difficult urination; increased confusion, depression, or loss of memory; rapid or difficult respirations; muscle weakness or tremors; or eye pain. **Pregnancy precaution:** Inform prescriber if you are or intend to become pregnant.

Transdermal: Apply patch behind ear the day before traveling. Wash hands before and after applying, and avoid contact with the eyes. Do not remove for 3 days.

Ophthalmic: Instill as often as recommended. Wash hands before using. Do not let tip of applicator touch eye; do not contaminate tip of applicator (may cause eye infection, eye damage, or vision loss). Sit or lie down, open eye, look at ceiling, and instill prescribed amount of solution. Do not blink for 30 seconds, close eye and roll eye in all directions, and apply gentle pressure to inner corner of eye for 1-2 minutes. Temporary stinging or blurred vision may occur.

Geriatric Considerations: Because of its long duration of action as a mydriatic agent, it should be avoided in elderly patients. Anticholinergic agents are not well tolerated in the elderly and their use should be avoided when possible.

Pregnancy Risk Factor: C

Lactation: Enters breast milk/use caution (AAP rates "compatible")

Perioperative/Anesthesia/Other Concerns: In administering scopolamine, it is important to recognize that lower doses (0.1 mg) may have vagal mimetic effects (ie, increase vagal tone causing paradoxical bradycardia). It is likely that the vagal tonic effects of scopolamine are mediated by blockade of muscarinic receptors at the level of the brain. Disc is programmed to deliver *in vivo* 1 mg over 3 days.

Administration

I.V.:

Hydrobromide: Inject over 2-3 minutes

Butylbromide: Inject at a rate of 1 mL/minute

Storage: Store tablets and/or injection at room temperature of 15°C to 30°C. Protect injection from light.

Hydrobromide injection: Avoid acid solutions, hydrolysis occurs at pH <3

Butylbromide injection: Stable in D_5W, NS, $D_{10}W$, and LR for up to 8 hours

Related Information

Postoperative Nausea and Vomiting *on page 1807*

♦ **Scopolamine Butylbromide** *see* Scopolamine *on page 1513*

♦ **Scopolamine Hydrobromide** *see* Scopolamine *on page 1513*

♦ **Scot-Tussin® Expectorant [OTC]** *see* Guaifenesin *on page 834*

♦ **SDZ ENA 713** *see* Rivastigmine *on page 1487*

♦ **SecreFlo™** *see* Secretin *on page 1516*

Secretin (SEE kre tin)

U.S. Brand Names SecreFlo™

Synonyms Secretin, Human; Secretin, Porcine

Pharmacologic Category Diagnostic Agent

Use Secretin-stimulation testing to aid in diagnosis of pancreatic exocrine dysfunction; diagnosis of gastrinoma (Zollinger-Ellison syndrome); facilitation of ERCP visualization

Mechanism of Action Human and porcine secretin are both synthetically derived products and are equally potent on an osmolar basis. Secretin is a hormone which is normally secreted by duodenal mucosa and upper jejunal mucosa. It increases the volume and bicarbonate content of pancreatic juice; stimulates the flow of hepatic bile with a high bicarbonate concentration; stimulates gastrin release in patients with Zollinger-Ellison syndrome.

Pharmacodynamics/Kinetics

Peak output of pancreatic secretions: ~30 minutes

Duration: At least 2 hours

Distribution: V_d: Human: 2.7 L; Porcine: 2 L

Half-life elimination: Human: 45 minutes; Porcine: 27 minutes

Contraindications Hypersensitivity to secretin or any component of the formulation; acute pancreatitis

Warnings/Precautions Administer test dose to evaluate possible allergy to secretin, particularly in patients with a history of asthma or atopy. Use caution in patients with hepatic disease (including ethanol-induced disease); volume response to secretin may be exaggerated. Response may be blunted in the presence of anticholinergic agents, inflammatory bowel disease, or following vagotomy; blunted response is not indicative of pancreatic disease.

Drug Interactions Anticholinergics: Response to secretin stimulation may be blunted; includes drugs with high anticholinergic activity such as tricyclic antidepressants, phenothiazines, and antihistamines.

Adverse Reactions

1% to 10%:

Cardiovascular: Flushing (1%)

Gastrointestinal: Abdominal discomfort (1%), nausea (1%)

Miscellaneous: Bleeding (sphincterectomy, 1%)

<1% (Limited to important or life-threatening): Abdominal pain, anxiety, bloating, blood pressure decreased, bradycardia (mild), diaphoresis, diarrhea, faintness, fatigue, fever, heart rate increased, leukocytoplastic vasculitis, lightheadedness, numbness/tingling in the extremities, oxygen saturation decreased, pallor, pancreatitis (mild), rash (abdominal), sedation, vomiting, warm sensation (abdomen/face)

Dosing

Adults & Elderly: Note:: A test dose of 0.2 mcg (0.1 mL) is injected to test for possible allergy. Dosing may be completed if no reaction occurs after 1 minute.

Diagnosis of pancreatic dysfunction, facilitation of ERCP: I.V.: 0.2 mcg/kg over 1 minute

Diagnosis of gastrinoma: I.V.: 0.4 mcg/kg over 1 minute

Available Dosage Forms

Injection, powder for reconstitution [human]: 16 mcg

Injection, powder for reconstitution [porcine] (SecreFlo™): 16 mcg

Nursing Guidelines

Monitoring Laboratory Tests: Refer to protocols for collection of pancreatic secretion and/or serum gastrin.

Dietary Considerations: Patients should be in a fasting state (12- to 15-hour fast) prior to testing.

Patient Education: Patients should be in a fasting state (12- to 15-hour fast) prior to testing.

Pregnancy Risk Factor: C

Pregnancy Issues: Reproduction studies have not been conducted.

Lactation: Excretion in breast milk unknown/use caution

Administration

Reconstitution: Add 8 mL NS to yield concentration of 2 mcg/mL; shake vigorously; must be used immediately following reconstitution.

Storage: Prior to reconstitution, store frozen at -20°C. Human product may also be stored under refrigeration for up to 1 year or at room temperature for up to 6 months.

♦ **Secretin, Human** *see* Secretin *on page 1516*

♦ **Secretin, Porcine** *see* Secretin *on page 1516*

♦ **Sectral®** *see* Acebutolol *on page 62*

Selegiline (se LE ji leen)

U.S. Brand Names Eldepryl®

Synonyms Deprenyl; L-Deprenyl; Selegiline Hydrochloride

Pharmacologic Category Anti-Parkinson's Agent, MAO Type B Inhibitor; Antidepressant, Monoamine Oxidase Inhibitor

Medication Safety Issues

Sound-alike/look-alike issues:

Selegiline may be confused with Salagen®, Serentil®, sertraline, Serzone®, Stelazine®

Eldepryl® may be confused with Elavil®, enalapril

Use Adjunct in the management of parkinsonian patients in which levodopa/carbidopa therapy is deteriorating

Unlabeled/Investigational Use Early Parkinson's disease; attention-deficit/hyperactivity disorder (ADHD); negative symptoms of schizophrenia; extrapyramidal symptoms; depression; Alzheimer's disease (studies have shown some improvement in behavioral and cognitive performance)

Mechanism of Action Potent monoamine oxidase (MAO) type-B inhibitor; MAO type B plays a major role in the metabolism of dopamine; selegiline may also increase dopaminergic activity by interfering with dopamine reuptake at the synapse

Pharmacodynamics/Kinetics

Onset of action: Therapeutic: Within 1 hour

Duration: 24-72 hours

Half-life elimination: Steady state: 10 hours

Metabolism: Hepatic to amphetamine and methamphetamine

Contraindications Hypersensitivity to selegiline or any component of the formulation; concomitant use of meperidine

Warnings/Precautions Increased risk of nonselective MAO inhibition occurs with doses >10 mg/day; it is a MAO inhibitor type "B", there should not be a problem with tyramine-containing products as long as the typical doses are employed, however, rare reactions have been reported. Use with tricyclic antidepressants and SSRIs has also been associated with rare reactions and should generally be avoided. Addition to levodopa therapy may result in exacerbation of levodopa adverse effects, requiring a reduction in levodopa dosage. The possibility of a suicide attempt is inherent in major depression and may persist until remission occurs. Use caution in high-risk patients during initiation of therapy. Prescriptions should be written for the smallest quantity consistent with good patient care.

Drug Interactions Substrate of CYP1A2 (minor), 2A6 (minor), 2B6 (major), 2C8/9 (major), 2D6 (minor), 3A4 (minor); **Inhibits** CYP1A2 (weak), 2A6 (weak), 2C8/9 (weak), 2C19 (weak), 2D6 (weak), 2E1 (weak), 3A4 (weak)

Note: Many drug interactions involving selegiline are theoretical, primarily based on interactions with nonspecific MAO inhibitors; at doses <10 mg/day, the risk of these interactions with selegiline may be very low

Amphetamines: MAO inhibitors in combination with amphetamines may result in severe hypertensive reaction or serotonin syndrome; these combinations are best avoided

Anorexiants: Concurrent use of selegiline (high dose) in combination with CNS stimulants or anorexiants may result in serotonin syndrome; these combinations are best avoided; includes dexfenfluramine, fenfluramine, or sibutramine

Barbiturates: MAO inhibitors may inhibit the metabolism of barbiturates and prolong their effect

CNS stimulants: MAO inhibitors in combination with stimulants (methylphenidate) may result in serotonin syndrome; these combinations are best avoided

CYP2B6 inducers: May decrease the levels/effects of selegiline. Example inducers include carbamazepine, nevirapine, phenobarbital, phenytoin, and rifampin.

CYP2B6 inhibitors: May increase the levels/effects of selegiline. Example inhibitors include desipramine, paroxetine, and sertraline.

CYP2C8/9 inducers: May decrease the levels/effects of selegiline. Example inducers include carbamazepine, phenobarbital, phenytoin, rifampin, rifapentine, and secobarbital.

CYP2C8/9 inhibitors: May increase the levels/effects of selegiline. Example inhibitors include delavirdine, fluconazole, gemfibrozil, ketoconazole, nicardipine, NSAIDs, pioglitazone, and sulfonamides.

(Continued)

Selegiline *(Continued)*

Dextromethorphan: Concurrent use of selegiline (high dose) may result in serotonin syndrome; these combinations are best avoided

Disulfiram: MAO inhibitors may produce delirium in patients receiving disulfiram; monitor

Guanadrel and guanethidine: MAO inhibitors inhibit the antihypertensive response to guanadrel or guanethidine; use an alternative antihypertensive agent

Hypoglycemic agents: MAO inhibitors may produce hypoglycemia in patients with diabetes; monitor

Levodopa: MAO inhibitors in combination with levodopa may result in hypertensive reactions; monitor

Lithium: MAO inhibitors in combination with lithium have resulted in malignant hyperpyrexia; this combination is best avoided

Meperidine: Concurrent use of selegiline (high dose) may result in serotonin syndrome; these combinations are best avoided

Nefazodone: Concurrent use of selegiline (high dose) may result in serotonin syndrome; these combinations are best avoided

Norepinephrine: MAO inhibitors may increase the pressor response of norepinephrine (effect is generally small); monitor

Oral contraceptives: Increased selegiline levels have been noted with concurrent administration; monitor

Reserpine: MAO inhibitors in combination with reserpine may result in hypertensive reactions; monitor

SSRIs: Concurrent use of selegiline with an SSRI may result in mania or hypertension; it is generally best to avoid these combinations

Sympathomimetics (indirect-acting): MAO inhibitors in combination with sympathomimetics such as dopamine, metaraminol, phenylephrine, and decongestants (pseudoephedrine) may result in severe hypertensive reaction; these combinations are best avoided

Succinylcholine: MAO inhibitors may prolong the muscle relaxation produced by succinylcholine via decreased plasma pseudocholinesterase

Tramadol: May increase the risk of seizures and serotonin syndrome in patients receiving an MAO inhibitor

Trazodone: Concurrent use of selegiline (high dose) may result in serotonin syndrome; these combinations are best avoided

Tricyclic antidepressants: May cause serotonin syndrome when combined with an MAO inhibitor; avoid this combination

Tyramine: Selegiline (>10 mg/day) in combination with tyramine (cheese, ethanol) may increase the pressor response; avoid high tyramine-containing foods in patients receiving >10 mg/day of selegiline

Venlafaxine: Concurrent use of selegiline (high dose) may result in serotonin syndrome; these combinations are best avoided

Nutritional/Herbal/Ethanol Interactions

Ethanol: Avoid ethanol. Avoid beverages containing tyramine (wine [Chianti and hearty red] and beer).

Food: Selegiline may cause sudden and severe high blood pressure when taken with food high in tyramine (cheeses, sour cream, yogurt, pickled herring, chicken liver, canned figs, raisins, bananas, avocados, soy sauce, broad bean pods, yeast extracts, meats prepared with tenderizers, and many foods aged to improve flavor). Small amounts of caffeine may produce irregular heartbeat or high blood pressure and can interact with this medication for up to 2 weeks after stopping its use.

Herb/Nutraceutical: Avoid valerian, St John's wort, SAMe, kava kava (may increase risk of serotonin syndrome and/or excessive sedation).

Adverse Reactions Frequency not defined.

Cardiovascular: Orthostatic hypotension, hypertension, arrhythmia, palpitation, angina, tachycardia, peripheral edema, bradycardia, syncope

Central nervous system: Hallucinations, dizziness, confusion, anxiety, depression, drowsiness, behavior/mood changes, dreams/nightmares, fatigue, delusions

Dermatologic: Rash, photosensitivity

Gastrointestinal: Xerostomia, nausea, vomiting, constipation, weight loss, anorexia, diarrhea, heartburn

Genitourinary: Nocturia, prostatic hyperplasia, urinary retention, sexual dysfunction

Neuromuscular & skeletal: Tremor, chorea, loss of balance, restlessness, bradykinesia

Ocular: Blepharospasm, blurred vision

Miscellaneous: Diaphoresis (increased)

Overdosage/Toxicology Symptoms of overdose include tachycardia, palpitations, muscle twitching, and seizures. Both hypertension or hypotension can occur with intoxication. While treating hypertension, care is warranted to avoid sudden drops in blood pressure, since this may worsen MAO inhibitor toxicity. Cardiac arrhythmias are best treated with phenytoin or procainamide. Treatment is generally symptom-directed and supportive.

Dosing

Adults: Parkinson's disease: Oral: 5 mg twice daily with breakfast and lunch or 10 mg in the morning

Elderly: Oral: Initial: 5 mg in the morning; may increase to a total of 10 mg/day.

Pediatrics: Children and Adolescents: ADHD (unlabeled use): Oral: 5-15 mg/day

Available Dosage Forms

Capsule, as hydrochloride (Eldepryl®): 5 mg

Tablet, as hydrochloride: 5 mg

Nursing Guidelines

Assessment: Assess effectiveness and interactions of other medications patient may be taking. Monitor therapeutic effectiveness according to rationale for therapy and adverse reactions at beginning of therapy and periodically throughout therapy. Monitor blood pressure. Be alert to thoughts of suicide. Patient should be cautioned against eating foods high in tyramine. Assess knowledge/teach patient appropriate use, interventions to reduce side effects, and adverse symptoms to report.

Patient Education: Take exactly as directed (may be prescribed in conjunction with levodopa/carbidopa); do not change dosage or discontinue without consulting prescriber. Therapeutic effects may take several weeks or months to achieve and you may need frequent monitoring during first weeks of therapy. Take with meals if GI upset occurs, before meals if dry mouth occurs, or after eating if drooling or if nausea occurs. Take at the same time each day. Avoid tyramine-containing foods (low potential for reaction). Maintain adequate hydration (2-3 L/day of fluids) unless instructed to restrict fluid intake; void before taking medication. Do not use alcohol and prescription or OTC sedatives or CNS depressants without consulting prescriber. You may experience drowsiness, dizziness, confusion, or vision changes (use caution when driving, climbing stairs, or engaging in tasks requiring alertness until response to drug is known); orthostatic hypotension (use caution when changing position - rising to standing from sitting or lying); constipation (increased exercise, fluids, fruit, or fiber may help); runny nose or flu-like symptoms (consult prescriber for appropriate relief); or nausea, vomiting, loss of appetite, or stomach discomfort (small frequent meals, frequent mouth care, chewing gum, or sucking lozenges may help). Report unresolved constipation or vomiting; chest pain, palpitations, irregular heartbeat; CNS changes (hallucination, loss of memory, seizures, acute headache, nervousness, thoughts of suicide, etc); painful or difficult urination; increased muscle spasticity, rigidity, or involuntary movements; skin rash; or significant worsening of condition. **Pregnancy/breast-feeding precautions:** Inform prescriber if you are or intend to become pregnant. Consult prescriber if breast-feeding.

Geriatric Considerations: Selegiline is also being studied in Alzheimer's disease, but further studies are needed to assess its usefulness. Do not use at daily doses exceeding 10 mg/day because of the risks associated with nonselective inhibition of MAO.

Pregnancy Risk Factor: C

Lactation: Excretion in breast milk unknown

Perioperative/Anesthesia/Other Concerns: When adding selegiline to levodopa/carbidopa, the dose of the latter can usually be decreased. Studies are investigating the use of selegiline in early Parkinson's disease to slow the progression of the disease. With doses >10 mg/day, selegiline loses MAO type "B" specificity.

♦ **Selegiline Hydrochloride** *see* Selegiline *on page 1517*

♦ **Senexon [OTC]** *see* Senna *on page 1520*

Senna (SEN na)

U.S. Brand Names Black Draught Tablets [OTC]; Evac-U-Gen [OTC]; ex-lax® [OTC]; ex-lax® Maximum Strength [OTC]; Fletcher's® Castoria® [OTC]; Perdiem® Overnight Relief [OTC]; Senexon [OTC]; Senna-Gen® [OTC]; Sennatural™ [OTC]; Senokot® [OTC]; Uni-Senna [OTC]; X-Prep® [OTC] [DSC]

Pharmacologic Category Laxative, Stimulant

Medication Safety Issues

Sound-alike/look-alike issues:

Senexon® may be confused with Cenestin®

Senokot® may be confused with Depakote®

Use Short-term treatment of constipation; evacuate the colon for bowel or rectal examinations

Contraindications Per Commission E: Intestinal obstruction, acute intestinal inflammation (eg, Crohn's disease), colitis ulcerosa, appendicitis, abdominal pain of unknown origin; pregnancy

Warnings/Precautions Not recommended for over-the-counter (OTC) use in patients experiencing stomach pain, nausea, vomiting, or a sudden change in bowel movements which lasts >2 weeks. Not recommended for OTC use in children <2 years of age.

Adverse Reactions Frequency not defined: Gastrointestinal: Nausea, vomiting, diarrhea, abdominal cramps

Dosing

Adults & Elderly:

Bowel evacuation: Oral: OTC labeling: Usual dose: Sennosides 130 mg (X-Prep® 75 mL) between 2-4 PM the afternoon of the day prior to procedure

Constipation: Oral: OTC ranges: Sennosides 15 mg once daily (maximum: 70-100 mg/day, divided twice daily)

Pediatrics:

Bowel evacuation: OTC labeling: Children ≥12 years: Refer to adult dosing.

Constipation: OTC ranges: Children:

2-6 years:

Sennosides: Initial: 3.75 mg once daily (maximum: 15 mg/day, divided twice daily)

Senna concentrate: 33.3 mg/mL: 5-10 mL up to twice daily

6-12 years:

Sennosides: Initial: 8.6 mg once daily (maximum: 50 mg/day, divided twice daily)

Senna concentrate: 33.3 mg/mL: 10-30 mL up to twice daily

≥12 years: Refer to adult dosing.

Available Dosage Forms [DSC] = Discontinued product

Granules (Senokot®): Sennosides 15 mg/teaspoon (60 g, 180 g, 360 g) [cocoa flavor] [DSC]

Liquid:

Senexon: Sennosides 8.8 mg/5 mL (240 mL)

X-Prep®: Sennosides 8.8 mg/5 mL (75 mL) [alcohol free; contains sugar 50 g/75 mL; available individually or in a kit] [DSC]

Liquid concentrate (Fletcher's® Castoria®): Senna concentrate 33.3 mg/mL (75 mL) [alcohol free; contains sodium benzoate; root beer flavor]

Syrup (Uni-Senna): Sennosides 8.8 mg/5 mL (240 mL)[contains alcohol; butterscotch flavor]

Tablet: Sennosides 8.6 mg, 15 mg, 25 mg

ex-lax®: Sennosides USP 15 mg

ex-lax® Maximum Strength: Sennosides USP 25 mg

Perdiem® Overnight Relief: Sennosides USP 15 mg

Sennatural™, Senokot®, Senexon®, Senna-Gen®, Uni-Senna: Sennosides 8.6 mg

Tablet, chewable:

ex-lax®: Sennosides USP 15 mg [chocolate flavor]

Evac-U-Gen: Sennosides 10 mg

Nursing Guidelines

Dietary Considerations: Liquid may be administered with fruit juice or milk to mask taste. X-Prep® liquid contains sugar 50 g/75 mL.

Patient Education: May discolor urine or feces (yellow, brown, pink, red, or violet); may cause dependence with prolonged or excessive use. Bowel movements usually occur within 6-12 hours after a dose. Notify prescriber for failure to have a bowel movement after the first dose or for rectal bleeding. OTC labeling does not recommend for use longer than 1 week, use in children <2 years, or in women who are pregnant or breast-feeding.

Administration

Oral: Once daily doses should be taken at bedtime. Granules may be eaten plain, sprinkled on food, or mixed in liquids

- ♦ Senna and Docusate *see* Docusate and Senna *on page 562*
- ♦ Senna-Gen® [OTC] *see* Senna *on page 1520*
- ♦ Senna-S *see* Docusate and Senna *on page 562*
- ♦ Sennatural™ [OTC] *see* Senna *on page 1520*
- ♦ Senokot® [OTC] *see* Senna *on page 1520*
- ♦ Senokot-S® [OTC] *see* Docusate and Senna *on page 562*
- ♦ Sensorcaine® *see* Bupivacaine *on page 266*
- ♦ Sensorcaine®-MPF *see* Bupivacaine *on page 266*
- ♦ Sensorcaine®-MPF with Epinephrine *see* Bupivacaine and Epinephrine *on page 268*
- ♦ Sensorcaine® with Epinephrine *see* Bupivacaine and Epinephrine *on page 268*
- ♦ Septra® *see* Sulfamethoxazole and Trimethoprim *on page 1582*
- ♦ Septra® DS *see* Sulfamethoxazole and Trimethoprim *on page 1582*
- ♦ Serevent® Diskus® *see* Salmeterol *on page 1507*
- ♦ Seroquel® *see* Quetiapine *on page 1443*
- ♦ Serostim® *see* Somatropin *on page 1555*

Sertraline (SER tra leen)

U.S. Brand Names Zoloft®

Synonyms Sertraline Hydrochloride

Pharmacologic Category Antidepressant, Selective Serotonin Reuptake Inhibitor

Medication Safety Issues

Sound-alike/look-alike issues:

Sertraline may be confused with selegiline, Serentil®

Zoloft® may be confused with Zocor®

Use Treatment of major depression; obsessive-compulsive disorder (OCD); panic disorder; post-traumatic stress disorder (PTSD); premenstrual dysphoric disorder (PMDD); social anxiety disorder

Unlabeled/Investigational Use Eating disorders; generalized anxiety disorder (GAD); impulse control disorders

Mechanism of Action Antidepressant with selective inhibitory effects on presynaptic serotonin (5-HT) reuptake and only very weak effects on norepinephrine and dopamine neuronal uptake. *In vitro* studies demonstrate no significant affinity for adrenergic, cholinergic, GABA, dopaminergic, histaminergic, serotonergic, or benzodiazepine receptors.

Pharmacodynamics/Kinetics

Absorption: Slow

Protein binding: 98%

Metabolism: Hepatic; extensive first-pass metabolism

Bioavailability: 88%

Half-life elimination: Parent drug: 26 hours; Metabolite N-desmethylsertraline: 66 hours (range: 62-104 hours)

Time to peak, plasma: 4.5-8.4 hours

Excretion: Urine and feces

Contraindications Hypersensitivity to sertraline or any component of the formulation; use of MAO inhibitors within 14 days; concurrent use of pimozide; concurrent use of sertraline oral concentrate with disulfiram

Warnings/Precautions

Major psychiatric warnings:

- Antidepressants increase the risk of suicidal thinking and behavior in children and adolescents with major depressive disorder (MDD) and other depressive disorders; consider risk prior to prescribing.
- Closely monitor for clinical worsening, suicidality, or unusual changes in behavior; the child's family or caregiver should be instructed to closely observe the patient and communicate condition with healthcare provider. **Sertraline is not FDA approved for use in children.**
- Adults treated with antidepressants should be observed similarly for clinical worsening and suicidality, especially during the initial few months of a course

(Continued)

Sertraline *(Continued)*

of drug therapy, or at times of dose changes, either increases or decreases. A medication guide should be dispensed with each prescription.

- The possibility of a suicide attempt is inherent in major depression and may persist until remission occurs. Worsening depression and severe abrupt suicidality that are not part of the presenting symptoms may require discontinuation or modification of drug therapy. Use caution in high-risk patients during initiation of therapy.
- Prescriptions should be written for the smallest quantity consistent with good patient care. The patient's family or caregiver should be alerted to monitor patients for the emergence of suicidality and associated behaviors such as anxiety, agitation, panic attacks, insomnia, irritability, hostility, impulsivity, akathisia, hypomania, and mania; patients should be instructed to notify their healthcare provider if any of these symptoms or worsening depression or psychosis occur.
- May worsen psychosis in some patients or precipitate a shift to mania or hypomania in patients with bipolar disorder. Monotherapy in patients with bipolar disorder should be avoided. Patients presenting with depressive symptoms should be screened for bipolar disorder. **Sertraline is not FDA approved for the treatment of bipolar depression.**

Key adverse effects:

- Anticholinergic effects: Relatively devoid of these side effects
- CNS depression: Has a low potential to impair cognitive or motor performance; caution operating hazardous machinery or driving.
- SIADH and hyponatremia: Has been associated with the development of SIADH; hyponatremia has been reported rarely, predominately in the elderly

Concurrent disease:

- Hepatic impairment: Use caution; clearance is decreased and plasma concentrations are increased; a lower dosage may be needed.
- Other concurrent illness: Use caution in patients with certain concomitant systemic illness; due to limited experience.
- Platelet aggregation: May impair platelet aggregation, resulting in bleeding.
- Renal impairment: Use caution; clearance is decreased and plasma concentrations are increased; a lower dosage may be needed.
- Seizure disorders: Use caution with a previous seizure disorder or condition predisposing to seizures such as brain damage or alcoholism.
- Sexual dysfunction: May cause or exacerbate sexual dysfunction.
- Uric acid nephropathy: Use caution in patients at risk of uric acid nephropathy; sertraline acts as a mild uricosuric.
- Weight loss: May cause weight loss. Use caution in patients where weight loss is undesirable.

Concurrent drug therapy:

- Agents which lower seizure threshold: Concurrent therapy with other drugs which lower the seizure threshold.
- Anticoagulants/Antiplatelets: Use caution with concomitant use of NSAIDs, ASA, or other drugs that affect coagulation; the risk of bleeding is potentiated.
- CNS depressants: Use caution with concomitant therapy.
- MAO inhibitors: Potential for severe reaction when used with MAO inhibitors; autonomic instability, coma, death, delirium, diaphoresis, hyperthermia, mental status changes/agitation, muscular rigidity, myoclonus, neuroleptic malignant syndrome features, and seizures may occur.

Special populations:

- Elderly: Use caution in elderly patients.
- Latex sensitivity: Use oral concentrate formulation with caution in patients with latex sensitivity; dropper dispenser contains dry, natural rubber.
- Pediatrics: Monitor growth in pediatric patients.

Special notes:

- Electroconvulsive therapy: May increase the risks associated with electroconvulsive therapy; consider discontinuing, when possible, prior to ECT treatment.
- Withdrawal syndrome: May cause dysphoric mood, irritability, agitation, dizziness, sensory disturbances, anxiety, confusion, headache, lethargy, emotional lability, insomnia, hypomania, tinnitus, and seizures. Upon discontinuation of venlafaxine therapy, gradually taper dose. If intolerable symptoms occur following a decrease in dosage or upon discontinuation of therapy, then resuming the previous dose with a more gradual taper should be considered.

Drug Interactions Substrate of CYP2B6 (minor), 2C8/9 (minor), 2C19 (major), 2D6 (major), 3A4 (minor); **Inhibits** CYP1A2 (weak), 2B6 (moderate), 2C8/9 (weak), 2C19 (moderate), 2D6 (moderate), 3A4 (moderate)

Amphetamines: SSRIs may increase the sensitivity to amphetamines, and amphetamines may increase the risk of serotonin syndrome

Benzodiazepines: Sertraline may inhibit the metabolism of alprazolam and diazepam resulting in elevated serum levels; monitor for increased sedation and psychomotor impairment

Buspirone: Sertraline inhibits the reuptake of serotonin; combined use with a serotonin agonist (buspirone) may cause serotonin syndrome

Carbamazepine: Sertraline may inhibit the metabolism of carbamazepine resulting in increased carbamazepine levels and toxicity; monitor for altered carbamazepine response

Cimetidine: Concurrent use resulted in an increase in sertraline's AUC, C_{max}, and half-life; monitor.

Clozapine: Sertraline may increase serum levels of clozapine; monitor for increased effect/toxicity

Cyclosporine: Sertraline may increase serum levels of cyclosporine (and possibly tacrolimus); monitor

CYP2B6 substrates: Sertraline may increase the levels/effects of CYP2B6 substrates. Example substrates include bupropion, promethazine, propofol, and selegiline.

CYP2C19 inducers: May decrease the levels/effects of sertraline. Example inducers include aminoglutethimide, carbamazepine, phenytoin, and rifampin.

CYP2C19 inhibitors: May increase the levels/effects of sertraline. Example inhibitors include delavirdine, fluconazole, fluvoxamine, gemfibrozil, isoniazid, omeprazole, and ticlopidine.

CYP2C19 substrates: Sertraline may increase the levels/effects of CYP2C19 substrates. Example substrates include citalopram, diazepam, methsuximide, phenytoin, and propranolol.

CYP2D6 inhibitors: May increase the levels/effects of sertraline. Example inhibitors include chlorpromazine, delavirdine, fluoxetine, miconazole, paroxetine, pergolide, quinidine, quinine, ritonavir, and ropinirole.

CYP2D6 substrates: Sertraline may increase the levels/effects of CYP2D6 substrates. Example substrates include amphetamines, selected beta-blockers, dextromethorphan, fluoxetine, lidocaine, mirtazapine, nefazodone, paroxetine, risperidone, ritonavir, thioridazine, tricyclic antidepressants, and venlafaxine.

CYP2D6 prodrug substrates: Sertraline may decrease the levels/effects of CYP2D6 prodrug substrates. Example prodrug substrates include codeine, hydrocodone, oxycodone, and tramadol.

CYP3A4 substrates: Sertraline may increase the levels/effects of CYP3A4 substrates. Example substrates include benzodiazepines, calcium channel blockers, cyclosporine, mirtazapine, nateglinide, nefazodone, sildenafil (and other PDE-5 inhibitors), tacrolimus, and venlafaxine. Selected benzodiazepines (midazolam and triazolam), cisapride, ergot alkaloids, selected HMG-CoA reductase inhibitors (lovastatin and simvastatin), and pimozide are generally contraindicated with strong CYP3A4 inhibitors.

Cyproheptadine: May inhibit the effects of serotonin reuptake inhibitors (fluoxetine); monitor for altered antidepressant response; cyproheptadine acts as a serotonin agonist

Dextromethorphan: Some SSRIs inhibit the metabolism of dextromethorphan; visual hallucinations occurred; monitor for serotonin syndrome

Erythromycin: Serotonin syndrome has been reported when added to sertraline; limited documentation

Haloperidol: Serum concentrations may be increased by sertraline (small increase); monitor

HMG-CoA reductase inhibitors: Sertraline may inhibit the metabolism of lovastatin and simvastatin (metabolized by CYP3A4) resulting in myositis and rhabdomyolysis; although its inhibition is weak, these combinations are best avoided

Lamotrigine: Toxicity has been reported following the addition of sertraline; monitor

Lithium: Patients receiving SSRIs and lithium have developed neurotoxicity; if combination is used, monitor for neurotoxicity

Loop diuretics: Sertraline may cause hyponatremia; additive hyponatremic effects may be seen with combined use of a loop diuretic (bumetanide, furosemide, torsemide); monitor for hyponatremia

(Continued)

Sertraline *(Continued)*

MAO inhibitors: Sertraline should not be used with nonselective MAO inhibitors (isocarboxazid, phenelzine); fatal reactions have been reported; this combination is contraindicated.

Meperidine: Concurrent use may result in serotonin syndrome; these combinations are best avoided

Nefazodone: May increase the risk of serotonin syndrome

NSAIDs: Concomitant use of sertraline and NSAIDs, aspirin, or other drugs affecting coagulation has been associated with an increased risk of bleeding; monitor.

Phenothiazines: Sertraline may inhibit metabolism of thioridazine or mesoridazine, potentially leading to malignant ventricular arrhythmias. Avoid concurrent use. Wait at least 5 weeks after discontinuing sertraline prior to starting thioridazine.

Phenytoin: Sertraline inhibits the metabolism of phenytoin and may result in phenytoin toxicity; monitor for phenytoin toxicity (ataxia, confusion, dizziness, nystagmus, involuntary muscle movement)

Pimozide: Sertraline may increase serum levels of pimozide. Concurrent use is contraindicated.

Ritonavir: Combined use of sertraline with ritonavir may cause serotonin syndrome in HIV-positive patients; monitor

Selegiline: SSRIs have been reported to cause mania or hypertension when combined with selegiline; this combination is best avoided. Concurrent use with SSRIs has been reported to cause serotonin syndrome. As an MAO type B inhibitor, the risk of serotonin syndrome may be less than with nonselective MAO inhibitors.

Sibutramine: May increase the risk of serotonin syndrome with SSRIs; monitor.

SSRIs: Combined use with other drugs which inhibit the reuptake may cause serotonin syndrome

Sumatriptan (and other serotonin agonists): Concurrent use may result in toxicity; weakness, hyper-reflexia, and incoordination have been observed with sumatriptan and SSRIs. In addition, concurrent use may theoretically increase the risk of serotonin syndrome; includes sumatriptan, naratriptan, rizatriptan, and zolmitriptan.

Sympathomimetics: May increase the risk of serotonin syndrome with SSRIs

Tolbutamide: Sertraline may decrease the metabolism of tolbutamide; monitor for changes in glucose control.

Tramadol: Sertraline combined with tramadol (serotonergic effects) may cause serotonin syndrome; monitor

Trazodone: Sertraline may inhibit the metabolism of trazodone resulting in increased toxicity; monitor

Tricyclic antidepressants: Sertraline may inhibit the metabolism of tricyclic antidepressants (amitriptyline, desipramine, imipramine, nortriptyline) resulting is elevated serum levels; if combination is warranted, a low dose of TCA (10-25 mg/day) should be utilized

Tryptophan: Sertraline may inhibit the reuptake of serotonin; combination with tryptophan, a serotonin precursor, may cause agitation and restlessness; this combination is best avoided

Venlafaxine: Sertraline may increase the risk of serotonin syndrome

Warfarin: Sertraline may alter the hypoprothrombinemic response to warfarin; monitor

Zolpidem: Onset of hypnosis may be shortened in patients receiving sertraline; monitor

Nutritional/Herbal/Ethanol Interactions

Ethanol: Avoid ethanol (may increase CNS depression).

Food: Sertraline average peak serum levels may be increased if taken with food.

Herb/Nutraceutical: Avoid valerian, St John's wort, kava kava, gotu kola (may increase CNS depression).

Lab Interactions Increased (minor) triglycerides (S), LFTs; decreased uric acid (S)

Adverse Reactions

>10%:

Central nervous system: Insomnia, somnolence, dizziness, headache, fatigue

Gastrointestinal: Xerostomia, diarrhea, nausea

Genitourinary: Ejaculatory disturbances

1% to 10%:

Cardiovascular: Palpitations

Central nervous system: Agitation, anxiety, nervousness
Dermatologic: Rash
Endocrine & metabolic: Decreased libido
Gastrointestinal: Constipation, anorexia, dyspepsia, flatulence, vomiting, weight gain
Genitourinary: Micturition disorders
Neuromuscular & skeletal: Tremors, paresthesia
Ocular: Visual difficulty, abnormal vision
Otic: Tinnitus
Miscellaneous: Diaphoresis (increased)

<1% (Limited to important or life-threatening): Acute renal failure, agranulocytosis, allergic reaction, angioedema, aplastic anemia, atrial arrhythmia, AV block, blindness, dystonia, extrapyramidal symptoms, gum hyperplasia, gynecomastia, hallucinations, hepatic failure, hypothyroidism, jaundice, lupus-like syndrome, neuroleptic malignant syndrome, oculogyric crisis, optic neuritis, pancreatitis (rare), photosensitivity, priapism, psychosis, pulmonary hypertension, QT_c prolongation, serotonin syndrome, serum sickness, SIADH, Stevens-Johnson syndrome (and other severe dermatologic reactions), thrombocytopenia, vasculitis, ventricular tachycardia (including torsade de pointes)

Additional adverse reactions reported in pediatric patients (frequency >2%): Aggressiveness, epistaxis, hyperkinesia, purpura, sinusitis, urinary incontinence

Overdosage/Toxicology Among 634 patients who overdosed on sertraline alone, 8 resulted in a fatal outcome. Symptoms of overdose include somnolence, vomiting, tachycardia, nausea, dizziness, agitation, and tremor. Treatment is symptomatic and supportive.

Dosing

Adults:

Depression/OCD: Oral: Initial: 50 mg/day

Note: May increase daily dose, at intervals of not less than 1 week, to a maximum of 200 mg/day. If somnolence is noted, give at bedtime.

Panic disorder, PTSD, social anxiety disorder: Oral: Initial: 25 mg once daily; increased after 1 week to 50 mg once daily (see "Note" above)

Premenstrual dysphoric disorder (PMDD): 50 mg/day either daily throughout menstrual cycle **or** limited to the luteal phase of menstrual cycle, depending on physician assessment. Patients not responding to 50 mg/day may benefit from dose increases (50 mg increments per menstrual cycle) up to 150 mg/day when dosing throughout menstrual cycle **or** up to 100 mg day when dosing during luteal phase only. If a 100 mg/day dose has been established with luteal phase dosing, a 50 mg/day titration step for 3 days should be utilized at the beginning of each luteal phase dosing period.

Elderly: Oral: Initial: 25 mg/day in the morning; increase by 25 mg/day increments every 2-3 days if tolerated to 50-100 mg/day; additional increases may be necessary; maximum: 200 mg/day.

Pediatrics:

OCD: Oral: Children:

6-12 years: Initial: 25 mg once daily
13-17 years: Initial: 50 mg once daily
May increase daily dose, at intervals of not less than 1 week, to a maximum: 200 mg/day. If somnolence is noted, give at bedtime.

Renal Impairment: Multiple-dose pharmacokinetics are unaffected by renal impairment.

Hemodialysis effect: Not removed by hemodialysis

Hepatic Impairment: Sertraline is extensively metabolized by the liver. Caution should be used in patients with hepatic impairment. A lower dose or less frequent dosing should be used.

Available Dosage Forms Note: Available as sertraline hydrochloride; mg strength refers to sertraline
Solution, oral concentrate: 20 mg/mL (60 mL) [contains alcohol 12%]
Tablet: 25 mg, 50 mg, 100 mg

Nursing Guidelines

Assessment: Assess other medications patient may be taking for effectiveness and interactions. Assess mental status for worsening of depression, suicidal ideation, anxiety, social functioning, mania, or panic attack (especially during initiation of therapy and when dosage is changed). Taper dosage slowly when discontinuing. Assess knowledge/teach patient appropriate use, interventions to reduce side effects, and adverse symptoms to report. Pediatric patients: Monitor growth pattern.

(Continued)

Sertraline *(Continued)*

Patient Education: Take exactly as directed; do not increase dose or frequency; or discontinue use abruptly. It may take 2-3 weeks to achieve desired results. Take in the morning to reduce the incidence of insomnia. Avoid alcohol, caffeine, and other prescription or OTC medications not approved by prescriber. Maintain adequate hydration (2-3 L/day of fluids) unless instructed to restrict fluid intake. You may experience drowsiness, dizziness, or lightheadedness (use caution when driving or engaging in tasks requiring alertness until response to drug is known); nausea, vomiting, anorexia, or dry mouth (small frequent meals, frequent mouth care, chewing gum, or sucking lozenges may help); postural hypotension (use caution when climbing stairs or changing position from sitting or lying to standing); urinary pattern changes (void before taking medication); or male sexual dysfunction (reversible). Report persistent insomnia or daytime sedation, agitation, nervousness, fatigue; muscle cramping, tremors, weakness, or change in gait; chest pain, palpitations, or swelling of extremities; vision changes or eye pain; hearing changes (ringing in ears); respiratory difficulty or breathlessness; skin rash or irritation; suicidal ideation; or worsening of condition. **Pregnancy/breast-feeding precautions:** Inform prescriber if you are or intend to become pregnant. Breast-feeding is not recommended.

Geriatric Considerations: Sertraline's favorable side effect profile makes it a useful alternative to the traditional tricyclic antidepressants. Its potential stimulation effect and anorexia may be bothersome.

Pregnancy Risk Factor: C

Pregnancy Issues: Nonteratogenic effects including respiratory distress, cyanosis, apnea, seizures, temperature instability, feeding difficulty, vomiting, hypoglycemia, hypo- or hypertonia, hyper-reflexia, jitteriness, irritability, constant crying, and tremor have been reported in the neonate immediately following delivery after exposure of other SSRIs late in the third trimester. Adverse effects may be due to toxic effects of SSRI or drug discontinuation. In some cases, may present clinically as serotonin syndrome. There are no adequate and well-controlled studies in pregnant women. Use during pregnancy only if the potential benefit to the mother outweighs the possible risk to the fetus. If treatment during pregnancy is required, consider tapering therapy during the third trimester.

Lactation: Enters breast milk/not recommended (AAP rates "of concern")

Perioperative/Anesthesia/Other Concerns: Buspirone (15-60 mg/day) may be useful in treatment of sexual dysfunction during treatment with a selective serotonin reuptake inhibitor; may exacerbate tics in Tourette's syndrome.

Administration

Oral: Oral concentrate: Must be diluted before use. Immediately before administration, use the dropper provided to measure the required amount of concentrate; mix with 4 ounces (1/2 cup) of water, ginger ale, lemon/lime soda, lemonade, or orange juice **only**. Do not mix with any other liquids than these. The dose should be taken immediately after mixing; do not mix in advance. A slight haze may appear after mixing; this is normal. **Note:** Use with caution in patients with latex sensitivity; dropper dispenser contains dry natural rubber.

Storage: Tablets and oral solution should be stored at controlled room temperature of 15°C to 30°C (59°F to 86°F).

♦ Sertraline Hydrochloride *see* Sertraline *on page 1521*
♦ Serutan® [OTC] *see* Psyllium *on page 1438*

Sevoflurane (see voe FLOO rane)

U.S. Brand Names Ultane®

Pharmacologic Category General Anesthetic, Inhalation

Medication Safety Issues

Sound-alike/look-alike issues:

Ultane® may be confused with Ultram®

Use Induction and maintenance of general anesthesia

Mechanism of Action Inhaled anesthetics alter activity of neuronal ion channels particularly the fast synaptic neurotransmitter receptors (nicotinic acetylcholine, GABA, and glutamate receptors). Limited effects on sympathetic stimulation including cardiovascular system. Seroflurane does not cause respiratory irritation or circulatory stimulation. May depress myocardial contractility, decrease blood pressure through a decrease in systemic vascular resistance and decrease sympathetic nervous activity.

Pharmacodynamics/Kinetics Sevoflurane has a low blood/gas partition coefficient and therefore is associated with a rapid onset of anesthesia and recovery

Onset of action: Time to induction: Within 2 minutes

Duration: Emergence time: Depends on blood concentration when sevoflurane is discontinued. The rate of change of anesthetic concentration in the lung is rapid with sevoflurane because of its low blood gas solubility (0.63). The 90% decrement time (time required for anesthetic concentration in vessel-rich tissues to decrease by 90%) for sevoflurane is short when the duration of anesthesia is <2 hours but increases dramatically as the duration of administration is lengthened.

Metabolism: 3% to 5% hepatic via CYP2E1

Excretion: Exhaled gases

Contraindications Previous hypersensitivity to sevoflurane, other halogenated anesthetics, or any component of the formulation; known or suspected susceptibility to malignant hyperthermia

Warnings/Precautions Reaction of sevoflurane with CO_2 absorbents that become desiccated within circle breathing equipment can lead to formation of formaldehyde (causing respiratory irritation) and carbon monoxide; maintain fresh absorbent as per manufacturer guidelines regardless of state of colorimetric indicator. Exothermic reaction of sevoflurane with desiccated CO_2 absorbents has been reported to generate extreme heat, smoke and/or fire within breathing circuit. This reaction also leads to formation of a fluorinated byproduct, compound A, which has been reported to cause nephrotoxicity (eg, proteinuria, glycosuria) in animal studies. Compound A-induced renal toxicity is dose- and exposure time-dependent; minimize exposure risk by not exceeding 2 MAC hours and fresh flow rates <2 L/minute (low fresh gas flow rates maximize rebreathing of the anesthetic).

Causes dose-dependent respiratory depression and blunted ventilatory response to hypoxia and hypercapnia. Hypoxic pulmonary vasoconstriction is blunted which may lead to increased pulmonary shunt. May dilate the cerebral vasculature and increase intracranial pressure. Use cautiously in patients with risk of elevation in intracranial pressure. May cause malignant hyperthermia. Use cautiously in patients with renal dysfunction. Use with caution in patients at risk for seizures; seizures have been reported in children and young adults. Monitor for emergence agitation or delirium. Postoperative hepatitis or hepatic dysfunction with or without jaundice has rarely been reported. Safety in patients with severe hepatic dysfunction has not been determined.

Drug Interactions **Substrate** of CYP2A6 (minor), 2B6 (minor), 2E1 (major), 3A4 (minor)

Aminoglycosides: Concomitant use may increase risk of nephrotoxicity.

Antihypertensives: Excessive hypotension may occur with combined use.

Benzodiazepines: Concurrent use may decrease the MAC of sevoflurane.

CYP2E1 inhibitors: May increase the levels/effects of sevoflurane. Example inhibitors include disulfiram, isoniazid, and miconazole.

Neuromuscular-blocking agents (nondepolarizing): Sevoflurane may potentiate the action of nondepolarizing, neuromuscular-blocking agents.

Nitrous oxide: Concurrent use may reduce the anesthetic requirement of sevoflurane.

Opioids: Concurrent use may decrease the MAC of sevoflurane.

Adverse Reactions

>10%:

Cardiovascular: Hypotension (4% to 11% dose dependent)

Central nervous system: Agitation (7% to 15%)

Gastrointestinal: Nausea (25%), vomiting (18%)

Respiratory: Cough increased (5% to 11%)

1% to 10%:

Cardiovascular: Bradycardia (5%), tachycardia (2% to 6%), hypertension (2%)

Central nervous system: Somnolence (8%), dizziness (4%), hypothermia (1%), headache (1%), fever (1%), emergence delirium

Gastrointestinal: Salivation (2% to 4%)

Respiratory: Laryngospasm (2% to 8%), airway obstruction (8%), breath-holding (2% to 5%), apnea (2%)

Miscellaneous: Shivering (6%)

<1% (Limited to important or life-threatening): Acidosis, albuminuria, alkaline phosphatase increased, allergic reactions, ALT/AST increased, amblyopia, anaphylactic/anaphylactoid reaction, arrhythmia, asthenia, atrial arrhythmia, atrial fibrillation, bigeminy, bilirubinemia, bronchospasm, BUN increased,

(Continued)

Sevoflurane *(Continued)*

complete AV block, confusion, conjunctivitis, creatinine increased, crying, dry mouth, dyspnea, fluorosis, glycosuria, hemorrhage, hepatic dysfunction, hepatitis, hiccup, hyperglycemia, hypertonia, hyper-/hypoventilation, hypophosphatemia, hypoxia, insomnia, inverted T wave, jaundice, leukocytosis, LDH increased, liver enzymes increased, malignant hyperthermia, nervousness, oliguria, pain, pharyngitis, pruritus, rash, second degree AV block, seizure, sputum, ST depression, stridor, supraventricular extrasystoles, syncope, taste perversion, thrombocytopenia, urinary retention, ventricular extrasystoles, wheezing

Dosing

Adults: Anesthesia: Inhalation: Minimum alveolar concentration (MAC), the concentration that abolishes movement in response to a noxious stimulus (surgical incision) in 50% of patients, is 2.6% (25 years of age) for sevoflurane. Surgical levels of anesthesia are generally achieved with concentrations from 0.5% to 3%; the concentration at which amnesia and loss of awareness occur is 0.6%.

Minimum alveolar concentrations (MAC) values for surgical levels of anesthesia:

25 years:
- Sevoflurane in oxygen: 2.6%
- Sevoflurane in 65% N_20/35% oxygen: 1.4%

40 years:
- Sevoflurane in oxygen: 2.1%
- Sevoflurane in 65% N_20/35% oxygen: 1.1%

60 years:
- Sevoflurane in oxygen: 1.7%
- Sevoflurane in 65% N_20/35% oxygen: 0.9%

80 years:
- Sevoflurane in oxygen: 1.4%
- Sevoflurane in 65% N_20/35% oxygen: 0.7%

Elderly: Refer to adult dosing. MAC is reduced in the elderly (50% reduction by age 80).

Pediatrics: Anesthesia: Inhalation: Minimum alveolar concentration (MAC), the concentration that abolishes movement in response to a noxious stimulus (surgical incision) in 50% of patients, is 2.6% (25 years of age) for sevoflurane. Surgical levels of anesthesia are generally achieved with concentrations from 0.5% to 3%; the concentration at which amnesia and loss of awareness occur is 0.6%.

Minimum alveolar concentrations (MAC) values for surgical levels of anesthesia:

0 to 1 month old full-term neonates: Sevoflurane in oxygen: 3.3%

1 to <6 months: Sevoflurane in oxygen: 3%

6 months to <3 years:
- Sevoflurane in oxygen: 2.8%
- Sevoflurane in 60% N_20/40% oxygen: 2%

3-12 years: Sevoflurane in oxygen: 2.5%

Renal Impairment: Use with caution in renal insufficiency.

Hepatic Impairment: Use with caution in patients with underlying hepatic conditions.

Available Dosage Forms Liquid for inhalation: 100% (250 mL)

Nursing Guidelines

Pregnancy Risk Factor: B

Breast-Feeding Considerations: Concentrations in breast milk are of no clinical importance 24 hours after anesthesia.

Perioperative/Anesthesia/Other Concerns: When sevoflurane is used in conjunction with desiccated CO_2, isolated reports of fire or extreme heat in the respiratory circuit of anesthesia machines have been reported. Steps that might reduce the risk of these events include: Replace CO_2 absorbent if it has not been used for an extended period of time, shut off anesthesia machine at the end of clinical use or after any case when a subsequent extended period of nonuse is expected, turn off all vaporizers when not in use, verify the integrity of new CO_2 absorbents prior to use, monitor the temperature of the CO_2 absorbent canisters, and monitor the correlation between sevoflurane vaporizer setting and the inspired concentration.

Administration

Storage: Store at 15°C to 30°C (59°F to 86°F).

Related Information

Inhalational Anesthetics *on page 1850*

Sibutramine (si BYOO tra meen)

U.S. Brand Names Meridia®

Synonyms Sibutramine Hydrochloride Monohydrate

Pharmacologic Category Anorexiant

Use Management of obesity, including weight loss and maintenance of weight loss; should be used in conjunction with a reduced-calorie diet

Mechanism of Action Sibutramine and its two primary metabolites block the neuronal uptake of norepinephrine, serotonin, and (to a lesser extent) dopamine. There is no monoamine-releasing (or depleting) activity.

Pharmacodynamics/Kinetics

Absorption: 77%; rapid

Protein binding, plasma: Parent drug and metabolites: >94%

Metabolism: Hepatic; undergoes first-pass metabolism via CYP3A4; forms two primary metabolites (active)

Half-life elimination: Sibutramine: 1 hour; Metabolites: M_1: 14 hours; M_2: 16 hours

Time to peak: Sibutramine: 1.2 hours; Metabolites ($M_1$and M_2): 3-4 hours

Excretion: Primarily urine (77%); feces

Contraindications Hypersensitivity to sibutramine or any component of the formulation; during or within 2 weeks of MAO inhibitors (eg, phenelzine, selegiline) or concomitant centrally-acting appetite suppressants; anorexia nervosa; bulimia nervosa

Warnings/Precautions Use with caution in mild-moderate renal impairment or hepatic dysfunction; not for use in patients with severe renal or hepatic impairment. May cause increase in blood pressure and heart rate; monitor baseline and on-therapy blood pressure and pulse. For patients experiencing a sustained increase in either blood pressure or pulse, dose reduction or discontinuation should be considered. Not recommended for use in patients with uncontrolled or poorly-controlled hypertension, congestive heart failure, coronary heart disease, conduction disorders (arrhythmias), or history of stroke. Use caution with other agents or therapies which stimulate the cardiovascular system.

Mydriasis has been reported; use caution with narrow-angle glaucoma. Seizures have been reported (rarely); use caution with history of seizure disorder. Weight loss may precipitate or exacerbate gallstone formation.

Primary pulmonary hypertension (PPH), a rare and frequently fatal pulmonary disease, has been reported to occur in patients receiving other agents with serotonergic activity which have been used as anorexiants. Although not reported in clinical trials, it is possible that sibutramine may share this potential, and patients should be monitored closely. As sibutramine blocks neuronal serotonin uptake, there is a potential for development of serotonin syndrome if used with other serotonergic agents; concurrent use of serotonergic agents (eg, SSRIs, sumatriptan, dihydroergotamine, dextromethorphan, meperidine, pentazocine, fentanyl, lithium) should be avoided.

Rare cases of bleeding have been reported; use caution in patients with bleeding disorders. Stimulants may unmask tics in individuals with coexisting Tourette's syndrome. Rare reports of depression, suicide and suicidal ideation have been documented in patients on sibutramine. Use caution and monitor closely in patients with history of psychiatric symptoms; it is unknown whether risk of suicidal ideation is increased in adolescent patients. Safety and efficacy have not been established in children <16 years of age.

Drug Interactions Substrate of CYP3A4 (major)

Buspirone: Concurrent use may result in serotonin syndrome; these combinations are best avoided.

CNS stimulants: May increase potential for sibutramine-associated cardiovascular complications or serotonergic effects; includes decongestants, centrally-acting weight loss products, amphetamines, and amphetamine-like compounds.

CYP3A4 inhibitors: May increase the levels/effects of sibutramine. Example inhibitors include azole antifungals, clarithromycin, diclofenac, doxycycline, erythromycin, imatinib, isoniazid, nefazodone, nicardipine, propofol, protease inhibitors, quinidine, telithromycin, and verapamil.

(Continued)

Sibutramine *(Continued)*

Dihydroergotamine: Concurrent use may result in serotonin syndrome; these combinations are best avoided.

Dextromethorphan: Concurrent use may result in serotonin syndrome; these combinations are best avoided.

Lithium: Concurrent use may result in serotonin syndrome; these combinations are best avoided.

MAO inhibitors: Sibutramine should not be used with nonselective MAO inhibitors (isocarboxazid, phenelzine) due to a theoretical risk of serotonin syndrome.

Meperidine: Concurrent use may result in serotonin syndrome; these combinations are best avoided.

Nefazodone: Concurrent use may result in serotonin syndrome; these combinations are best avoided.

Serotonergic agents: Concurrent use may result in serotonin syndrome; includes selective serotonin reuptake inhibitors (eg, sumatriptan, lithium, tryptophan), some opioid/analgesics (eg, meperidine, tramadol), and venlafaxine.

SSRIs: Combined use with other drugs which inhibit the reuptake (sibutramine) may cause serotonin syndrome; avoid these combinations.

Serotonin agonists: Theoretically may increase the risk of serotonin syndrome; includes sumatriptan, naratriptan, rizatriptan, and zolmitriptan.

Tramadol: Sibutramine combined with tramadol (serotonergic effects) may cause serotonin syndrome; monitor.

Trazodone: Sibutramine may inhibit the metabolism of trazodone resulting in increased toxicity; monitor.

Tricyclic antidepressants: Sibutramine may inhibit the metabolism of tricyclic antidepressants (amitriptyline, desipramine, imipramine, nortriptyline) resulting is elevated serum levels; if combination is warranted, a low dose of TCA (10-25 mg/day) should be utilized.

Tryptophan: Sibutramine may inhibit the reuptake of serotonin; combination with tryptophan, a serotonin precursor, may cause agitation and restlessness; this combination is best avoided.

Venlafaxine: Combined use with sibutramine may increase the risk of serotonin syndrome.

Nutritional/Herbal/Ethanol Interactions

Ethanol: Avoid excess ethanol ingestion.

Herb/Nutraceutical: St John's wort may decrease sibutramine levels.

Adverse Reactions

>10%:

- Central nervous system: Headache (30%), insomnia (11%)
- Gastrointestinal: Xerostomia (17%), anorexia (13%), constipation (12%)

1% to 10%:

- Cardiovascular: Tachycardia (3%), vasodilation (2%), hypertension (2%), palpitation (2%), chest pain (2%), edema (1%)
- Central nervous system: Dizziness (7%), nervousness (5%), anxiety (5%), depression (4%), migraine (2%), somnolence (2%), CNS stimulation (2%), emotional lability (1%)
- Dermatologic: Rash (4%), acne (1%), herpes simplex (1%)
- Endocrine & metabolic: Dysmenorrhea (4%), metrorrhagia (1%)
- Gastrointestinal: Appetite increased (9%), nausea (6%), abdominal pain (5%), dyspepsia (5%), gastritis (2%), vomiting (2%), taste perversion (2%), rectal disorder (1%)
- Genitourinary: Urinary tract infection (2%), vaginal *Monilia* (1%)
- Hepatic: Abnormal LFTs (2%)
- Neuromuscular & skeletal: Back pain (8%), weakness (6%), arthralgia (6%), neck pain (2%), myalgia (2%), paresthesia (2%), tenosynovitis (1%), joint disorder (1%)
- Otic: Ear disorder (2%), ear pain (1%)
- Respiratory: Pharyngitis (10%), rhinitis (10%), sinusitis (5%), cough (4%), laryngitis (1%)
- Miscellaneous: Flu-like syndrome (8%), diaphoresis (3%), allergic reactions (2), thirst (2%)

<1% (Limited to important or life-threatening): Bruising, interstitial nephritis, seizure

Frequency not defined:

- Cardiovascular: Peripheral edema
- Central nervous system: Thinking abnormal, agitation, fever
- Dermatologic: Pruritus

Endocrine & metabolic: Menstrual disorders/irregularities
Gastrointestinal: Diarrhea, flatulence, gastroenteritis, tooth disorder
Neuromuscular & skeletal: Arthritis, hypertonia, leg cramps
Ocular: Amblyopia
Respiratory: Bronchitis, dyspnea

Postmarketing and/or case reports (frequency not defined; limited to important or life-threatening): Amnesia, anaphylactic shock, anaphylactoid reaction, anemia, angina, angioedema, arrhythmia, arthrosis, atrial fibrillation, cardiac arrest, cerebrovascular accident, CHF, cholecystitis, cholelithiasis, depression aggravated, GI hemorrhage, goiter, hematuria, hyper-/hypoglycemia, hyper-/hypothyroidism, impotence, intestinal obstruction, intraocular pressure increased, leukopenia, lymphadenopathy, mania, mouth/stomach ulcer, serotonin syndrome, stroke, suicidal ideation, syncope, thrombocytopenia, tongue edema, torsade de pointes, Tourette's syndrome, urinary retention, urticaria, transient ischemic attack, vascular headache, ventricular dysrhythmias

Overdosage/Toxicology Symptoms of overdose include hypertension, tachycardia, headache, and palpitations. Treatment is supportive. Monitor vitals; beta-blockers may be beneficial to control elevated pressure and heart rate; dialysis not likely to be effective.

Dosing

Adults: Obesity: Oral: Initial: 10 mg once daily; after 4 weeks may titrate up to 15 mg once daily as needed and tolerated (may be used for up to 2 years, per manufacturer labeling).

Elderly: Use with caution; adjust dose based on renal or hepatic function.

Renal Impairment: Should not be used in patients with severe renal impairment.

Hepatic Impairment: No adjustment necessary for mild-to-moderate liver failure. Sibutramine should not be used in patients with severe liver failure.

Available Dosage Forms Capsule, as hydrochloride: 5 mg, 10 mg, 15 mg

Nursing Guidelines

Assessment: Assess effectiveness and interactions of other medications patient may be taking. Monitor vital signs, weight, and adverse reactions at start of therapy, when changing dosage, and at regular intervals during therapy. Assess knowledge/teach patient appropriate use, possible side effects, and symptoms to report.

Dietary Considerations: Sibutramine, as an appetite suppressant, is the most effective when combined with a low calorie diet and behavior modification counseling.

Patient Education: Take exactly as directed; do not increase dose or frequency without consulting prescriber. May be taken with meals (do not take at bedtime). Avoid alcohol, caffeine, or OTC medications that act as stimulants. You may experience restlessness, dizziness, sleepiness (use caution when driving or engaging in tasks requiring alertness until response to drug is known); insomnia (taking medication early in morning may help, warm milk, and quiet environment at bedtime may help); increased appetite, nausea or vomiting (small frequent meals, frequent mouth care may help); constipation (increased exercise, fluids, fruit, or fiber may help); diarrhea (buttermilk, boiled milk, or yogurt may help); or altered menstrual periods (reversible when drug is discontinued). Report chest pain, palpitations, or irregular heartbeat; excessive nervousness, excitation, or sleepiness; back pain, muscle weakness, or tremors; CNS changes (acute headache, aggressiveness, restlessness, excitation, sleep disturbances); menstrual pattern changes; rash; blurred vision; runny nose, sinusitis, cough, or respiratory difficulty. **Pregnancy/breast-feeding precautions:** Inform prescriber if you are or intend to become pregnant. Breast-feeding is not recommended.

Pregnancy Risk Factor: C

Lactation: Excretion in breast milk unknown/not recommended

Administration

Oral: May take with or without food.

Storage: Store at room temperature of 15°C to 30°C (59°F to 86°F).

♦ Sibutramine Hydrochloride Monohydrate *see* Sibutramine *on page 1529*
♦ Silace [OTC] *see* Docusate *on page 560*
♦ Siladryl® Allergy [OTC] *see* DiphenhydrAMINE *on page 546*
♦ Siladryl® DAS [OTC] *see* DiphenhydrAMINE *on page 546*
♦ Silafed® [OTC] *see* Triprolidine and Pseudoephedrine *on page 1670*
♦ Silapap® Children's [OTC] *see* Acetaminophen *on page 65*

♦ **Silapap® Infants [OTC]** *see* Acetaminophen *on page 65*
♦ **Silfedrine Children's [OTC]** *see* Pseudoephedrine *on page 1436*
♦ **Silphen® [OTC]** *see* DiphenhydrAMINE *on page 546*
♦ **Siltussin DAS [OTC]** *see* Guaifenesin *on page 834*
♦ **Siltussin SA [OTC]** *see* Guaifenesin *on page 834*
♦ **Silvadene®** *see* Silver Sulfadiazine *on page 1533*

Silver Nitrate (SIL ver NYE trate)

Synonyms $AgNO_3$

Pharmacologic Category Antibiotic, Topical; Cauterizing Agent, Topical; Topical Skin Product, Antibacterial

Use Cauterization of wounds and sluggish ulcers, removal of granulation tissue and warts; aseptic prophylaxis of burns

Mechanism of Action Free silver ions precipitate bacterial proteins by combining with chloride in tissue forming silver chloride; coagulates cellular protein to form an eschar; silver ions or salts or colloidal silver preparations can inhibit the growth of both gram-positive and gram-negative bacteria. This germicidal action is attributed to the precipitation of bacterial proteins by liberated silver ions. Silver nitrate coagulates cellular protein to form an eschar, and this mode of action is the postulated mechanism for control of benign hematuria, rhinitis, and recurrent pneumothorax.

Pharmacodynamics/Kinetics

Absorption: Because silver ions readily combine with protein, there is minimal GI and cutaneous absorption of the 0.5% and 1% preparations

Excretion: Highest amounts of silver noted on autopsy have been in kidneys, excretion in urine is minimal

Contraindications Hypersensitivity to silver nitrate or any component of the formulation; not for use on broken skin, cuts, or wounds

Warnings/Precautions Do not use applicator sticks on the eyes. Prolonged use may result in skin discoloration.

Adverse Reactions Frequency not defined.

Dermatologic: Burning and skin irritation, staining of the skin

Endocrine & metabolic: Hyponatremia

Hematologic: Methemoglobinemia

Overdosage/Toxicology Symptoms of overdose include pain and burning of the mouth, salivation, vomiting, diarrhea, shock, coma, convulsions, and death; blackening of skin and mucous membranes. Absorbed nitrate can cause methemoglobinemia. Fatal dose is as low as 2 g; administer sodium chloride in water (10 g/L) to cause precipitation of silver.

Dosing

Adults & Elderly: Antiseptic: Topical:

Sticks: Apply to mucous membranes and other moist skin surfaces only on area to be treated 2-3 times/week for 2-3 weeks.

Topical solution: Apply a cotton applicator dipped in solution on the affected area 2-3 times/week for 2-3 weeks.

Pediatrics: Antiseptic: Topical: Refer to adult dosing.

Available Dosage Forms

Applicator sticks, topical: Silver nitrate 75% and potassium nitrate 25% (6", 12", 18")

Solution, topical: 10% (30 mL); 25% (30 mL); 50% (30 mL)

Nursing Guidelines

Assessment: Assess knowledge/teach appropriate technique for topical application. Monitor for overuse symptoms.

Monitoring Laboratory Tests: With prolonged use, monitor methemoglobin levels.

Patient Education: Use as directed; do not use more often than instructed. Store container in dry, dark place. Handle with care; silver nitrate stains skin, clothing and utensils. Discontinue and contact prescriber if treated areas worsen or if redness, or irritation develops in surrounding area. **Pregnancy precaution:** Inform prescriber if you are or intend to become pregnant.

Sticks: Apply to mucous membranes and other moist skin surfaces to be treated 2-3 times each week for 2-3 weeks. Not for ophthalmic use.

Solution: Apply to affected area with cotton applicator dipped in solution 2-3 times each week for 2-3 weeks.

Pregnancy Risk Factor: C

Administration

Storage: Must be stored in a dry place. Store in a tight, light-resistant container. Exposure to light causes silver to oxidize and turn brown, dipping in water causes oxidized film to readily dissolve.

Silver Sulfadiazine (SIL ver sul fa DYE a zeen)

U.S. Brand Names Silvadene®; SSD®; SSD® AF; Thermazene®

Pharmacologic Category Antibiotic, Topical

Use Prevention and treatment of infection in second and third degree burns

Mechanism of Action Acts upon the bacterial cell wall and cell membrane. Bactericidal for many gram-negative and gram-positive bacteria and is effective against yeast. Active against *Pseudomonas aeruginosa*, *Pseudomonas maltophilia*, *Enterobacter* species, *Klebsiella* species, *Serratia* species, *Escherichia coli*, *Proteus mirabilis*, *Morganella morganii*, *Providencia rettgeri*, *Proteus vulgaris*, *Providencia* species, *Citrobacter* species, *Acinetobacter calcoaceticus*, *Staphylococcus aureus*, *Staphylococcus epidermidis*, *Enterococcus* species, *Candida albicans*, *Corynebacterium diphtheriae*, and *Clostridium perfringens*

Pharmacodynamics/Kinetics

Absorption: Significant percutaneous absorption of silver sulfadiazine can occur especially when applied to extensive burns

Half-life elimination: 10 hours; prolonged with renal impairment

Time to peak, serum: 3-11 days of continuous therapy

Excretion: Urine (~50% as unchanged drug)

Contraindications Hypersensitivity to silver sulfadiazine or any component of the formulation; premature infants or neonates <2 months of age (sulfonamides may displace bilirubin and cause kernicterus); pregnancy (approaching or at term)

Warnings/Precautions Use with caution in patients with G6PD deficiency, renal impairment, or history of allergy to other sulfonamides; sulfadiazine may accumulate in patients with impaired hepatic or renal function; fungal superinfection may occur; use of analgesic might be needed before application; systemic absorption is significant and adverse reactions may occur

Drug Interactions Decreased effect: Topical proteolytic enzymes are inactivated

Adverse Reactions Frequency not defined.

Dermatologic: Itching, rash, erythema multiforme, discoloration of skin, photosensitivity

Hematologic: Hemolytic anemia, leukopenia, agranulocytosis, aplastic anemia

Hepatic: Hepatitis

Renal: Interstitial nephritis

Miscellaneous: Allergic reactions may be related to sulfa component

Dosing

Adults & Elderly: Antiseptic, burns: Topical: Apply once or twice daily

Pediatrics: Refer to adult dosing.

Available Dosage Forms

Cream, topical: 1% (25 g, 50 mg, 85 g, 400 g)

Silvadene®, Thermazene®: 1% (20 g, 50 g, 85 g, 400 g, 1000 g)

SSD®: 1% (25 g, 50 g, 85 g, 400 g)

SSD® AF: 1% (50 g, 400 g)

Nursing Guidelines

Assessment: Monitor development of granulation. Observe for hypersensitivity reactions in unburned areas. Long-term use over large areas - monitor kidney function, and serum sulfa levels (significant absorption can occur).

Monitoring Laboratory Tests: Serum electrolytes, urinalysis, renal function, CBC in patients with extensive burns on long-term treatment

Patient Education: Usually applied by professional in burn care setting. Patient instruction should be appropriate to extent of burn, patient understanding, etc.

Pregnancy Risk Factor: B

Lactation: For external use

Administration

Storage: Discard if cream is darkened (reacts with heavy metals resulting in release of silver).

Simethicone (sye METH i kone)

U.S. Brand Names Equalizer Gas Relief [OTC]; GasAid [OTC]; Gas-X® [OTC]; Gas-X® Extra Strength [OTC]; Gas-X® Maximum Strength [OTC]; Genasyme® [OTC]; Infantaire Gas Drops [OTC]; Mylanta® Gas [OTC]; Mylanta® Gas (Continued)

Simethicone *(Continued)*

Maximum Strength [OTC]; Mylicon® Infants [OTC]; Phazyme® Quick Dissolve [OTC]; Phazyme® Ultra Strength [OTC]

Synonyms Activated Dimethicone; Activated Methylpolysiloxane

Pharmacologic Category Antiflatulent

Medication Safety Issues

Sound-alike/look-alike issues:

Simethicone may be confused with cimetidine

Mylanta® may be confused with Mynatal®

Mylicon® may be confused with Modicon®, Myleran®

Phazyme® may be confused with Pherazine®

Use Relieves flatulence and functional gastric bloating, and postoperative gas pains

Mechanism of Action Decreases the surface tension of gas bubbles thereby disperses and prevents gas pockets in the GI system

Contraindications Hypersensitivity to simethicone or any component of the formulation

Drug Interactions No data reported

Nutritional/Herbal/Ethanol Interactions Food: Avoid carbonated beverages and gas-forming foods.

Adverse Reactions Frequency not defined: Gastrointestinal: Loose stools

Dosing

Adults & Elderly: Flatulence/bloating: Oral: 40-120 mg after meals and at bedtime as needed, not to exceed 500 mg/day

Pediatrics: Flatulence/bloating: Oral:

Infants: 20 mg 4 times/day

Children <12 years: 40 mg 4 times/day

Children >12 years: Refer to adult dosing.

Available Dosage Forms

Softgels: 125 mg

GasAid, Gas-X® Extra Strength, Mylanta® Gas Maximum Strength: 125 mg

Gas-X® Maximum Strength: 166 mg

Phazyme® Ultra Strength: 180 mg

Suspension, oral drops: 40 mg/0.6 mL (30 mL)

Equalizer Gas Relief, Genasyme®, Infantaire Gas: 40 mg/0.6 mL (30 mL)

Mylicon® Infants: 40 mg/0.6 mL (15 mL, 30 mL) [alcohol free; contains sodium benzoate; available in a nonstaining formula]

Tablet, chewable: 80 mg, 125 mg

Gas-X®: 80 mg [sodium free; peppermint crème or cherry crème flavor]

Gas-X® Extra Strength: 125 mg [peppermint crème or cherry crème flavor]

Genasyme®: 80 mg

Mylanta® Gas: 80 mg [mint flavor]

Mylanta® Gas Maximum Strength: 125 mg [cherry and mint flavors]

Phazyme® Quick Dissolve: 125 mg [contains phenylalanine 0.4 mg per tablet; mint flavor]

Nursing Guidelines

Dietary Considerations: Should be taken after meals.

Patient Education: Some tablets may be chewed thoroughly before swallowing, follow with a glass of water

Pregnancy Risk Factor: C

Administration

Oral: Shake oral suspension (drops) before using; mix with water, infant formula, or other liquids.

- **Simethicone, Aluminum Hydroxide, and Magnesium Hydroxide** *see* Aluminum Hydroxide, Magnesium Hydroxide, and Simethicone *on page 122*
- **Simethicone and Calcium Carbonate** *see* Calcium Carbonate and Simethicone *on page 294*
- **Simply Saline® [OTC]** *see* Sodium Chloride *on page 1545*
- **Simply Saline® Baby [OTC]** *see* Sodium Chloride *on page 1545*
- **Simply Saline® Nasal Moist® [OTC]** *see* Sodium Chloride *on page 1545*
- **Simply Sleep® [OTC]** *see* DiphenhydrAMINE *on page 546*
- **Simply Stuffy™ [OTC]** *see* Pseudoephedrine *on page 1436*
- **Simulect®** *see* Basiliximab *on page 224*

Simvastatin (SIM va stat in)

U.S. Brand Names Zocor®

Pharmacologic Category Antilipemic Agent, HMG-CoA Reductase Inhibitor

Medication Safety Issues

Sound-alike/look-alike issues:

Zocor® may be confused with Cozaar®, Yocon®, Zoloft®

Use Used with dietary therapy for the following:

Secondary prevention of cardiovascular events in hypercholesterolemic patients with established coronary heart disease (CHD) or at high risk for CHD: To reduce cardiovascular morbidity (myocardial infarction, coronary revascularization procedures) and mortality; to reduce the risk of stroke and transient ischemic attacks

Hyperlipidemias: To reduce elevations in total cholesterol, LDL-C, apolipoprotein B, and triglycerides in patients with primary hypercholesterolemia (elevations of 1 or more components are present in Fredrickson type IIa, IIb, III, and IV hyperlipidemias); treatment of homozygous familial hypercholesterolemia

Heterozygous familial hypercholesterolemia (HeFH): In adolescent patients (10-17 years of age, females >1 year postmenarche) with HeFH having LDL-C ≥190 mg/dL **or** LDL ≥160 mg/dL with positive family history of premature cardiovascular disease (CVD), or 2 or more CVD risk factors in the adolescent patient

Mechanism of Action Simvastatin is a methylated derivative of lovastatin that acts by competitively inhibiting 3-hydroxy-3-methylglutaryl-coenzyme A (HMG-CoA) reductase, the enzyme that catalyzes the rate-limiting step in cholesterol biosynthesis

Pharmacodynamics/Kinetics

Onset of action: >3 days

Peak effect: 2 weeks

Absorption: 85%

Protein binding: ~95%

Metabolism: Hepatic via CYP3A4; extensive first-pass effect

Bioavailability: <5%

Half-life elimination: Unknown

Time to peak: 1.3-2.4 hours

Excretion: Feces (60%); urine (13%)

Contraindications Hypersensitivity to simvastatin or any component of the formulation; acute liver disease; unexplained persistent elevations of serum transaminases; pregnancy; breast-feeding

Warnings/Precautions Secondary causes of hyperlipidemia should be ruled out prior to therapy. Liver function must be monitored by laboratory assessment. Rhabdomyolysis with acute renal failure has occurred. Risk is dose-related and is increased with concurrent use of lipid-lowering agents which may cause rhabdomyolysis (gemfibrozil, fibric acid derivatives, or niacin at doses ≥1 g/day), during concurrent use with danazol or strong CYP3A4 inhibitors (including amiodarone, clarithromycin, cyclosporine, erythromycin, telithromycin, itraconazole, ketoconazole, nefazodone, grapefruit juice in large quantities, verapamil, or protease inhibitors such as indinavir, nelfinavir, or ritonavir). Weigh the risk versus benefit when combining any of these drugs with simvastatin. Do not initiate simvastatin-containing treatment in a patient with pre-existing therapy of cyclosporine or danazol, unless the patient has previously demonstrated tolerance to ≥5 mg/day simvastatin. Temporarily discontinue in any patient experiencing an acute or serious major medical or surgical condition which may increase the risk of rhabdomyolysis. Discontinue temporarily for elective surgical procedures. Use caution in patients with renal insufficiency. Use with caution in patients who consume large amounts of ethanol or have a history of liver disease. Safety and efficacy have not been established in patients <10 years or in premenarcheal girls.

Drug Interactions **Substrate** of CYP3A4 (major); **Inhibits** CYP2C8/9 (weak), 2D6 (weak)

Amiodarone may increase the risk of myopathy and rhabdomyolysis; dose of simvastatin should not exceed 20 mg/day.

Antacids: Plasma concentrations may be decreased when given with magnesium-aluminum hydroxide containing antacids (reported with atorvastatin and pravastatin). Clinical efficacy is not altered, no dosage adjustment is necessary

Cholestyramine reduces absorption of several HMG-CoA reductase inhibitors. Separate administration times by at least 4 hours.

Cholestyramine and colestipol (bile acid sequestrants): Cholesterol-lowering effects are additive.

(Continued)

Simvastatin *(Continued)*

Clofibrate and fenofibrate may increase the risk of myopathy and rhabdomyolysis; dose of simvastatin should not exceed 10 mg/day

Cyclosporine: Concurrent use may increase the risk of myopathy and rhabdomyolysis; dose of simvastatin should not exceed 10 mg/day

CYP3A4 inhibitors: May increase the levels/effects of simvastatin. Example inhibitors include azole antifungals, clarithromycin, diclofenac, doxycycline, erythromycin, imatinib, isoniazid, nefazodone, nicardipine, propofol, protease inhibitors, quinidine, telithromycin, and verapamil.

Danazol: May increase risk of myopathy and rhabdomyolysis; dose of simvastatin should not exceed 10 mg/day.

Gemfibrozil: Increased risk of myopathy and rhabdomyolysis; dose of simvastatin should not exceed 10 mg/day.

Grapefruit juice may inhibit metabolism of simvastatin via CYP3A4; avoid high dietary intakes of grapefruit juice.

Niacin (≥1 g/day): Concurrent use may increase the risk of myopathy and rhabdomyolysis; dose of simvastatin should not exceed 10 mg/day.

Verapamil may increase the risk of myopathy and rhabdomyolysis; dose of simvastatin should not exceed 20 mg/day.

Warfarin effects (hypoprothrombinemic response) may be increased; monitor INR closely when simvastatin is initiated or discontinued.

Nutritional/Herbal/Ethanol Interactions

Ethanol: Avoid excessive ethanol consumption (due to potential hepatic effects).

Food: Simvastatin serum concentration may be increased when taken with grapefruit juice; avoid concurrent intake of large quantities (>1 quart/day). Red yeast rice contains an estimated 2.4 mg lovastatin per 600 mg rice.

Herb/Nutraceutical: St John's wort may decrease simvastatin levels.

Adverse Reactions

1% to 10%:

Gastrointestinal: Constipation (2%), dyspepsia (1%), flatulence (2%)

Neuromuscular & skeletal: CPK elevation (>3x normal on one or more occasions - 5%)

Respiratory: Upper respiratory infection (2%)

<1% (Limited to important or life-threatening): Depression, lichen planus, photosensitivity, thrombocytopenia, vertigo

Additional class-related events: Alopecia, anaphylaxis, angioedema, anxiety, cataracts, cholestatic jaundice, depression, dermatomyositis, dyspnea, eosinophilia, erythema multiforme, facial paresis, fulminant hepatic necrosis, gynecomastia, hemolytic anemia, hepatitis, hypersensitivity reaction, impotence, leukopenia, myopathy, ophthalmoplegia, pancreatitis, paresthesia, peripheral nerve palsy, peripheral neuropathy, photosensitivity, polymyalgia rheumatica, psychic disturbance, rash, renal failure (secondary to rhabdomyolysis), rhabdomyolysis, Stevens-Johnson syndrome, systemic lupus erythematosus-like syndrome, thrombocytopenia, thyroid dysfunction, toxic epidermal necrolysis, urticaria, vasculitis, vertigo

Overdosage/Toxicology Very few adverse events. Treatment is symptomatic.

Dosing

Adults: Note: Doses should be individualized according to the baseline LDL-cholesterol levels, the recommended goal of therapy, and the patient's response; adjustments should be made at intervals of 4 weeks or more; doses may need adjusted based on concomitant medications

Homozygous familial hypercholesterolemia: Oral: 40 mg once daily in the evening **or** 80 mg/day (given as 20 mg, 20 mg, and 40 mg evening dose)

Prevention of cardiovascular events, hyperlipidemias: Oral: 20-40 mg once daily in the evening; range: 5-80 mg/day

Patients requiring only moderate reduction of LDL-cholesterol: May be started at 10 mg once daily

Patients requiring reduction of >45% in low-density lipoprotein (LDL) cholesterol: May be started at 40 mg once daily in the evening

Patients with CHD or at high risk for CHD: Dosing should be started at 40 mg once daily in the evening; simvastatin may be started simultaneously with diet

Dosage adjustment for simvastatin with concomitant medications:

Cyclosporine or danazol: Patient must first demonstrate tolerance to simvastatin ≥5 mg once daily: Initial: 5 mg, should **not** exceed 10 mg/day

Fibrates or niacin: Dose should **not** exceed 10 mg/day

Amiodarone or verapamil: Dose should **not** exceed 20 mg/day

Elderly: Oral: Initial: Maximum reductions in LDL-cholesterol may be achieved with daily dose ≤20 mg.

Pediatrics: HeFH: Oral: Children 10-17 years (females >1 year postmenarche): 10 mg once daily in the evening; range: 10-40 mg/day (maximum: 40 mg/day)

Dosage adjustment with concomitant medications: With concomitant cyclosporine, danazol, fibrates, niacin, amiodarone, or verapamil: Refer to adult dosing.

Note: Doses should be individualized according to the baseline LDL-cholesterol levels, the recommended goal of therapy, and the patient's response; adjustments should be made at intervals of 4 weeks or more; doses may need adjusted based on concomitant medications

Renal Impairment: Because simvastatin does not undergo significant renal excretion, modification of dose should not be necessary in patients with mild to moderate renal insufficiency.

Severe renal impairment: Cl_{cr} <10 mL/minute: Initial: 5 mg/day with close monitoring.

Available Dosage Forms Tablet: 5 mg, 10 mg, 20 mg, 40 mg, 80 mg

Nursing Guidelines

Assessment: Use with caution and monitor closely in presence of impaired liver function. Assess potential for interactions with other pharmacological agents or herbal products patient may be taking (eg, gemfibrozil, fibric acid derivatives, niacin may increase risk of myopathy or rhabdomyolysis). Assess LFTs prior to therapy and periodically thereafter. Evaluate therapeutic response (reduction in lipid levels) and adverse reactions on a regular basis (eg, rash, myalgia, blurred vision, abdominal pain, cough) throughout therapy. Teach patient proper use (as adjunct to diet and exercise program), possible side effects/appropriate interventions, and adverse symptoms to report. **Pregnancy risk factor X:** Determine that patient is not pregnant before starting therapy. Do not give to women of childbearing age unless they are capable of complying with effective contraceptive use. Instruct patient in appropriate contraceptive measures.

Monitoring Laboratory Tests: Creatine phosphokinase levels due to possibility of myopathy; serum cholesterol (total and fractionated)

Obtain liver function tests prior to initiation, dose, and thereafter when clinically indicated. Patients titrated to the 80 mg dose should be tested prior to initiation and 3 months after initiating the 80 mg dose. Thereafter, periodic monitoring (ie, semiannually) is recommended for the first year of treatment. Patients with elevated transaminase levels should have a second (confirmatory) test and frequent monitoring until values normalize. Discontinue if increase in ALT/AST is persistently >3 times ULN.

Dietary Considerations: Red yeast rice contains an estimated 2.4 mg lovastatin per 600 mg rice.

Patient Education: Do not take any new medication during therapy without consulting prescriber. Take at same time each day with or without food. Follow cholesterol-lowering diet and exercise regimen as prescribed. Avoid grapefruit juice and excessive alcohol while taking this medication. You will have periodic blood tests to assess effectiveness. May cause mild GI upset (should diminish with use); constipation (increased exercise, fluids, fiber, and fruit may help); headache, dizziness, insomnia (use caution when driving or engaged in potentially hazardous tasks until response to drug in known). Report unusual chest pain, swelling of extremities, weight gain of >5 lb/week, persistent cough; CNS changes (dizziness, memory loss, depression, or vision changes). Contact prescriber immediately with persistent muscle or skeletal pain, joint pain, or numbness, or any sign of allergic reactions (skin rash, difficulty breathing, tightness in throat, choking sensation, swelling of mouth or face). **Pregnancy/breast-feeding precautions:** Inform prescriber if you are pregnant. Do not get pregnant during and for 1 month following therapy. Consult prescriber for appropriate contraceptive measures. This drug may cause severe fetal defects. Do not donate blood during or for 1 month following therapy. Do not breast feed.

Geriatric Considerations: Effective and well tolerated in the elderly. The definition of and, therefore, when to treat hyperlipidemia in the elderly is a controversial issue. The National Cholesterol Education Program recommends that all adults maintain a plasma cholesterol <160 mg/dL. In elderly patients with one additional risk factor, goal LDL would decrease to <130 mg/dL. Pharmacologic treatment should be reserved for those who are unable to obtain a desirable plasma cholesterol concentration by diet alone and for whom the benefits of

(Continued)

Simvastatin *(Continued)*

treatment are believed to outweigh the potential adverse effects, drug interactions, and cost of treatment.

Pregnancy Risk Factor: X

Pregnancy Issues: Cholesterol biosynthesis may be important in fetal development. Contraindicated in pregnancy. Administer to women of childbearing potential only when conception is highly unlikely and patients have been informed of potential hazards.

Lactation: Excretion in breast milk unknown/contraindicated

Breast-Feeding Considerations: Excretion in breast milk is unknown, but would be expected; other medications in this class are excreted in human milk. Breast-feeding is contraindicated.

Perioperative/Anesthesia/Other Concerns: Myopathy: Currently-marketed HMG-CoA reductase inhibitors appear to have a similar potential for causing myopathy. Incidence of severe myopathy is about 0.08% to 0.09%. The factors that increase risk include advanced age (especially >80 years), gender (occurs in women more frequently than men), small body frame, frailty, multisystem disease (eg, chronic renal insufficiency especially due to diabetes), multiple medications, **perioperative periods (higher risk when continued during hospitalization for major surgery)**, and drug interactions (use with caution or avoid).

Administration

Oral: May be taken without regard to meals.

Storage: Tablets should be stored in tightly-closed containers at temperatures between 5°C to 30°C (41°F to 86°F).

♦ **Singulair®** *see* Montelukast *on page 1175*

Sirolimus (sir OH li mus)

U.S. Brand Names Rapamune®

Pharmacologic Category Immunosuppressant Agent

Use Prophylaxis of organ rejection in patients receiving renal transplants, in combination with corticosteroids and cyclosporine (cyclosporine may be withdrawn in low-to-moderate immunological risk patients after 2-4 months, in conjunction with an increase in sirolimus dosage)

Unlabeled/Investigational Use Investigational: Immunosuppression in other forms of solid organ transplantation and peripheral stem cell/bone marrow transplantation

Mechanism of Action Sirolimus inhibits T-lymphocyte activation and proliferation in response to antigenic and cytokine stimulation. Its mechanism differs from other immunosuppressants. It inhibits acute rejection of allografts and prolongs graft survival.

Pharmacodynamics/Kinetics

Absorption: Rapid

Distribution: 12 L/kg (range: 4-20 L/kg)

Protein binding: 92%, primarily to albumin

Metabolism: Extensively hepatic via CYP3A4; P-glycoprotein-mediated efflux into gut lumen

Bioavailability: Oral solution: 14%; Oral tablet: 18%

Half-life elimination: Mean: 62 hours

Time to peak: 1-2hours

Excretion: Feces (91%); urine (2%)

Contraindications Hypersensitivity to sirolimus or any component of the formulation

Warnings/Precautions Immunosuppressive agents, including sirolimus, increase the risk of infection and may be associated with the development of lymphoma. May increase serum lipids (cholesterol and triglycerides). Use with caution in patients with hyperlipidemia. May increase serum creatinine and decrease GFR. Use caution in patients with renal impairment, or when used concurrently with medications which may alter renal function. Monitor renal function closely when combined with cyclosporine; consider dosage adjustment or discontinue in patients with increasing serum creatinine. Has been associated with an increased risk of lymphocele. Cases of interstitial lung disease (eg, pneumonitis, bronchiolitis obliterans organizing pneumonia, pulmonary fibrosis) have been observed; risk may be increased with higher trough levels. Avoid concurrent use of strong CYP3A4 inhibitors or strong inducers of either CYP3A4 or P-glycoprotein. Concurrent use with a calcineurin inhibitor (cyclosporine, tacrolimus) may increase the risk of calcineurin inhibitor-induced hemolytic uremic syndrome/thrombotic thrombocytopenic purpura/thrombotic microangiopathy (HUS/TTP/TMA). Anaphylactic reactions, angioedema and hypersensitivity vasculitis have been reported. May increase sensitivity to UV light; use appropriate sun protection.

Sirolimus is not recommended for use in liver transplant patients; studies indicate an association with an increase risk of hepatic artery thrombosis and graft failure in these patients. Cases of bronchial anastomotic dehiscence have been reported in lung transplant patients when sirolimus was used as part of an immunosuppressive regimen; most of these reactions were fatal. Use in patients with lung transplants is not recommended. Safety and efficacy of cyclosporine withdrawal in high-risk patients is not currently recommended. Safety and efficacy in children <13 years of age, or in adolescent patients <18 years of age considered at high immunological risk, have not been established.

Drug Interactions Substrate of CYP3A4 (major); **Inhibits** CYP3A4 (weak)

Antifungal agents, imidazoles (itraconazole, ketoconazole, voriconazole): May increase the levels/effects of sirolimus. Concurrent use is not recommended.

Calcineurin inhibitors (cyclosporine, tacrolimus): Concurrent therapy may increase the risk of HUS/TTP/TMA.

Clarithromycin: May increase serum concentrations of sirolimus. Concurrent use not recommended.

Cyclosporine capsules (modified) or cyclosporine oral solution (modified) increase C_{max} and AUC of sirolimus during concurrent therapy, and cyclosporine clearance may be reduced during concurrent therapy. Sirolimus should be taken 4 hours after cyclosporine oral solution (modified) and/or cyclosporine capsules (modified).

CYP3A4 inducers: CYP3A4 inducers may decrease the levels/effects of sirolimus. Example inducers include aminoglutethimide, carbamazepine, nafcillin, nevirapine, phenobarbital, phenytoin, and rifamycins. Concurrent use is not recommended.

CYP3A4 inhibitors: May increase the levels/effects of sirolimus. Example inhibitors include azole antifungals, clarithromycin, diclofenac, doxycycline, erythromycin, imatinib, isoniazid, nefazodone, nicardipine, propofol, protease inhibitors, quinidine, telithromycin, and verapamil. Concurrent use is not recommended.

Diltiazem may increase serum concentrations of sirolimus; monitor. Verapamil and nicardipine may share this effect.

Erythromycin: May increase serum concentrations of sirolimus. Concurrent use is not recommended.

P-gp inducers: May decrease serum concentrations of sirolimus.

Rifampin: May decrease serum concentrations of sirolimus. Concurrent use is not recommended.

Vaccines: Vaccination may be less effective and use of live vaccines should be avoided during sirolimus therapy.

Voriconazole: Sirolimus serum concentrations may be increased; concurrent use is contraindicated.

Nutritional/Herbal/Ethanol Interactions

Food: Do not administer with grapefruit juice; may decrease clearance of sirolimus. Ingestion with high-fat meals decreases peak concentrations but increases AUC by 35%. Sirolimus should be taken consistently either with or without food to minimize variability.

Herb/Nutraceutical: St John's wort may decrease sirolimus levels; avoid concurrent use. Avoid cat's claw, echinacea (have immunostimulant properties; consider therapy modifications).

Adverse Reactions Incidence of many adverse effects is dose related

>20%:

Cardiovascular: Hypertension (39% to 49%), peripheral edema (54% to 64%), edema (16% to 24%), chest pain (16% to 24%)

Central nervous system: Fever (23% to 34%), headache (23% to 34%), pain (24% to 33%), insomnia (13% to 22%)

Dermatologic: Acne (20% to 31%)

Endocrine & metabolic: Hypercholesterolemia (38% to 46%), hypophosphatemia (15% to 23%), hyperlipidemia (38% to 57%), hypokalemia (11% to 21%)

Gastrointestinal: Abdominal pain (28% to 36%), nausea (25% to 36%), vomiting (19% to 25%), diarrhea (25% to 42%), constipation (28% to 38%), dyspepsia (17% to 25%), weight gain (8% to 21%)

(Continued)

Sirolimus *(Continued)*

Genitourinary: Urinary tract infection (20% to 33%)
Hematologic: Anemia (23% to 37%), thrombocytopenia (13% to 40%)
Neuromuscular & skeletal: Arthralgia (25% to 31%), weakness (22% to 40%), back pain (16% to 26%), tremor (21% to 31%)
Renal: Increased serum creatinine (35% to 40%)
Respiratory: Dyspnea (22% to 30%), upper respiratory infection (20% to 26%), pharyngitis (16% to 21%)

3% to 20% (Limited to important or life-threatening):
Cardiovascular: Atrial fibrillation, CHF, postural hypotension, syncope, thrombosis, venous thromboembolism
Central nervous system: Anxiety, confusion, depression, emotional lability, neuropathy, somnolence
Dermatologic: Hirsutism, pruritus, skin hypertrophy, rash (10% to 20%)
Endocrine & metabolic: Cushing's syndrome, diabetes mellitus, hypercalcemia, hyperglycemia, hyperphosphatemia, hypocalcemia, hypoglycemia, hypomagnesemia, hyponatremia, hyperkalemia (12% to 17%)
Gastrointestinal: Esophagitis, gastritis, gingival hyperplasia, ileus
Genitourinary: Impotence
Hematologic: TTP, hemolytic-uremic syndrome, hemorrhage, leukopenia (9% to 15%)
Hepatic: Transaminases increased, ascites
Neuromuscular & skeletal: Increased CPK, bone necrosis, tetany, paresthesia
Otic: Deafness
Renal: Acute tubular necrosis, nephropathy (toxic), urinary retention
Respiratory: Asthma, pulmonary edema, pleural effusion
Miscellaneous: Flu-like syndrome, infection, peritonitis, sepsis

Postmarketing and/or case reports: Anaphylactoid reaction, anaphylaxis, anastomotic disruption, angioedema, fascial dehiscence, hepatic necrosis, hypersensitivity vasculitis; interstitial lung disease (pneumonitis, pulmonary fibrosis, and bronchiolitis obliterans organizing pneumonia) with no identified infectious etiology, lymphedema, neutropenia, pancytopenia. In liver transplant patients (not an approved use), an increase in hepatic artery thrombosis and graft failure were noted in clinical trials. In lung transplant patients (not an approved use), bronchial anastomotic dehiscence has been reported. Calcineurin inhibitor-induced hemolytic uremic syndrome/thrombotic thrombocytopenic purpura/thrombotic microangiopathy (HUS/TTP/TMA) have been reported (with concurrent cyclosporine or tacrolimus).

Overdosage/Toxicology Experience with overdosage has been limited. Dose-limiting toxicities include immune suppression. Reported symptoms of overdose include atrial fibrillation. Treatment is supportive, dialysis is not likely to facilitate removal.

Dosing

Adults & Elderly:

Immunosuppression: Oral:

Combination therapy with cyclosporine: For *de novo* transplant recipients, a loading dose of 3 times the daily maintenance dose should be administered on day 1 of dosing. Doses should be taken 4 hours after cyclosporine, and should be taken consistently either with or without food.

Dosing by body weight:

<40 kg: Loading dose: Loading dose: 3 mg/m^2 on day 1, followed by a maintenance dosing of 1 mg/m^2

≥40 kg: Loading dose: 6 mg on day 1; maintenance: 2 mg/day

Maintenance therapy after withdrawal of cyclosporine:

Following 2-4 months of combined therapy, withdrawal of cyclosporine may be considered in low-to-moderate risk patients. Cyclosporine withdrawal in not recommended in high immunological risk patients. Cyclosporine should be discontinued over 4-8 weeks, and a necessary increase in the dosage of sirolimus (up to fourfold) should be anticipated due to removal of metabolic inhibition by cyclosporine and to maintain adequate immunosuppressive effects.

Sirolimus dosages should be adjusted to maintain trough concentrations of 12-24 ng/mL. Dosage should be adjusted at intervals of 7-14 days to account for the long half-life of sirolimus. Considerable increases in dosage may require an additional loading dose, calculated as the difference between the target concentration and the current concentration, multiplied by a factor of 3. Loading doses >40 mg may be administered over two days. Serum concentrations should not be used as the sole basis for dosage adjustment (monitor clinical signs/symptoms, tissue biopsy, and laboratory parameters).

Pediatrics:

Immunosuppression: Children ≥13 years: Oral: Refer to adult dosing.

Renal Impairment: No adjustment is necessary.

Hepatic Impairment: Reduce maintenance dose by approximately 33% in hepatic impairment. Loading dose is unchanged.

Available Dosage Forms

Solution, oral [bottle]: 1 mg/mL (60 mL) [contains ethanol 1.5% to 2.5%; packaged with oral syringes and a carrying case]

Tablet: 1 mg, 2 mg

Nursing Guidelines

Assessment: Assess effectiveness and interactions of other medications. Assess results of laboratory tests at beginning and periodically during therapy, therapeutic effectiveness, and adverse reactions and toxicity. Assess lipid profiles; evaluate the need for medication intervention. Monitor blood pressure and renal function. Assess for signs of fluid retention and infection. Assess knowledge/teach patient appropriate use, interventions to reduce side effects, and adverse reactions to report.

Monitoring Laboratory Tests: Monitor sirolimus levels in pediatric patients, patients ≥13 years of age weighing <40 kg, patients with hepatic impairment, or on concurrent potent inhibitors or inducers of CYP3A4, and/or if cyclosporine dosing is markedly reduced or discontinued. Also monitor serum cholesterol and triglycerides and serum creatinine. Serum drug concentrations should be determined 3-4 days after loading doses; however, these concentrations should not be used as the sole basis for dosage adjustment, especially during withdrawal of cyclosporine (monitor clinical signs/symptoms, tissue biopsy, and laboratory parameters).

Dietary Considerations: Take consistently, with or without food, to minimize variability of absorption.

Patient Education: Do not alter dose or discontinue without consulting prescriber. Do not ever mix sirolimus solution with anything other than water or orange juice (avoid taking with grapefruit juice). May be taken with or without food, but should be taken consistently with regard to food (always on an empty stomach or always with food). Consult prescriber about timing of any other prescribed or OTC medications. Maintain adequate hydration (2-3 L/day of fluids) unless instructed to restrict fluid intake. You will be susceptible to infection (avoid crowds and exposure to infection). If you have diabetes, monitor glucose levels closely (drug may alter glucose levels). Limit exposure to sunlight by wearing protective clothing or sunscreen. You may experience nausea, vomiting, loss of appetite (small frequent meals, good mouth care, chewing gum, or sucking hard candy may help); constipation (increase exercise, fluids, fruit, or fiber may help); or diarrhea (yogurt or buttermilk); or muscle or back pain (mild analgesic). Inform prescriber of any adverse effects including, but not limited to, unresolved GI problems; respiratory difficulty, cough, infection; skin rash or irritation; headache, insomnia, anxiety, confusion, emotional lability; changes in voiding pattern, burning, itching, or pain on urination; persistent bone, joint, or muscle cramping, pain or weakness; chest pain, palpitations, swelling of extremities; weight gain of 3-5 pounds per week; vision changes or hearing; or any other adverse reactions. **Pregnancy/breast-feeding precautions:** Inform prescriber if you are or intend to become pregnant. Breast-feeding is not recommended.

Pregnancy Risk Factor: C

Pregnancy Issues: Effective contraception must be initiated before therapy with sirolimus and continued for 12 weeks after discontinuation.

Lactation: Excretion in breast milk unknown/not recommended

Administration

Oral: The solution should be mixed with at least 2 ounces of water or orange juice. No other liquids should be used for dilution. Patient should drink diluted solution immediately. The cup should then be refilled with an additional 4 ounces of water or orange juice, stirred vigorously, and the patient should drink the contents at once.

Storage:

Oral solution: Protect from light and store under refrigeration, 2°C to 8°C (36°F to 46°F). A slight haze may develop in refrigerated solutions, but the quality of the product is not affected. After opening, solution should be used in 1 month.

(Continued)

Sirolimus *(Continued)*

If necessary, may be stored at temperatures up to 25°C (77°F) for several days after opening (up to 24 hours for pouches and not >15 days for bottles). Product may be stored in amber syringe for a maximum of 24 hours (at room temperature or refrigerated). Solution should be used immediately following dilution.

Tablet: Store at room temperature of 20°C to 25°C (68°F to 77°F). Protect from light.

- SK *see* Streptokinase *on page 1569*
- Skeeter Stik [OTC] *see* Benzocaine *on page 232*
- Sleep-ettes D [OTC] *see* DiphenhydrAMINE *on page 546*
- Sleepinal® [OTC] *see* DiphenhydrAMINE *on page 546*
- Slo-Niacin® [OTC] *see* Niacin *on page 1218*
- Slow FE® [OTC] *see* Ferrous Sulfate *on page 721*
- Slow-Mag® [OTC] *see* Magnesium Chloride *on page 1074*
- Smelling Salts *see* Ammonia Spirit (Aromatic) *on page 143*
- SMZ-TMP *see* Sulfamethoxazole and Trimethoprim *on page 1582*
- Sodium 2-Mercaptoethane Sulfonate *see* Mesna *on page 1108*

Sodium Acetate (SOW dee um AS e tate)

Pharmacologic Category Electrolyte Supplement, Parenteral

Use Sodium source in large volume I.V. fluids to prevent or correct hyponatremia in patients with restricted intake; used to counter acidosis through conversion to bicarbonate

Contraindications Alkalosis, hypocalcemia, low sodium diets, edema, cirrhosis

Warnings/Precautions Avoid extravasation, use with caution in patients with hepatic failure

Adverse Reactions 1% to 10%:

Cardiovascular: Thrombosis, hypervolemia

Dermatologic: Chemical cellulitis at injection site (extravasation)

Endocrine & metabolic: Hypernatremia, dilution of serum electrolytes, overhydration, hypokalemia, metabolic alkalosis, hypocalcemia

Gastrointestinal: Gastric distension, flatulence

Local: Phlebitis

Respiratory: Pulmonary edema

Miscellaneous: Congestive conditions

Dosing

Adults & Elderly:

Note: Sodium acetate is metabolized to bicarbonate on an equimolar basis outside the liver; administer in large volume I.V. fluids as a sodium source. Refer to Sodium Bicarbonate monograph.

Maintenance electrolyte requirements of sodium in parenteral nutrition solutions:

Daily requirements: 3-4 mEq/kg/24 hours or 25-40 mEq/1000 kcal/24 hours

Maximum: 100-150 mEq/24 hours

Available Dosage Forms Injection, solution: 2 mEq/mL (20 mL, 50 mL, 100 mL); 4 mEq/mL (50 mL, 100 mL)

Nursing Guidelines

Dietary Considerations: Sodium and acetate content of 1 g: 7.3 mEq

Pregnancy Risk Factor: C

Administration

I.V.: Must be diluted prior to I.V. administration; infusion hypertonic solutions (>154 mEq/L) via a central line; maximum rate of administration: 1 mEq/kg/hour

Compatibility: Incompatible with acids, acidic salts, alkaloid salts, calcium salts, catecholamines, atropine

Storage: Protect from light, heat, and from freezing.

- Sodium Acid Carbonate *see* Sodium Bicarbonate *on page 1542*
- Sodium Benzoate and Caffeine *see* Caffeine *on page 284*

Sodium Bicarbonate (SOW dee um bye KAR bun ate)

U.S. Brand Names Brioschi® [OTC]; Neut®

Synonyms Baking Soda; $NaHCO_3$; Sodium Acid Carbonate; Sodium Hydrogen Carbonate

Pharmacologic Category Alkalinizing Agent; Antacid; Electrolyte Supplement, Oral; Electrolyte Supplement, Parenteral

Use Management of metabolic acidosis; gastric hyperacidity; as an alkalinization agent for the urine; treatment of hyperkalemia; management of overdose of certain drugs, including tricyclic antidepressants and aspirin

Mechanism of Action Dissociates to provide bicarbonate ion which neutralizes hydrogen ion concentration and raises blood and urinary pH

Pharmacodynamics/Kinetics

Onset of action: Oral: Rapid; I.V.: 15 minutes

Duration: Oral: 8-10 minutes; I.V.: 1-2 hours

Absorption: Oral: Well absorbed

Excretion: Urine (<1%)

Contraindications Alkalosis, hypernatremia, severe pulmonary edema, hypocalcemia, unknown abdominal pain

Warnings/Precautions Rapid administration in neonates and children <2 years of age has led to hypernatremia, decreased CSF pressure and intracranial hemorrhage. **Use of I.V. $NaHCO_3$ should be reserved for documented metabolic acidosis and for hyperkalemia-induced cardiac arrest.** Routine use in cardiac arrest is not recommended. Avoid extravasation, tissue necrosis can occur due to the hypertonicity of $NaHCO_3$. May cause sodium retention especially if renal function is impaired; not to be used in treatment of peptic ulcer; use with caution in patients with CHF, edema, cirrhosis, or renal failure. Not the antacid of choice for the elderly because of sodium content and potential for systemic alkalosis.

Drug Interactions

Decreased effect/levels of lithium, chlorpropamide, methotrexate, tetracyclines, and salicylates due to urinary alkalinization

Increased toxicity/levels of amphetamines, anorexiants, mecamylamine, ephedrine, pseudoephedrine, flecainide, quinidine, quinine due to urinary alkalinization

Nutritional/Herbal/Ethanol Interactions Herb/Nutraceutical: Concurrent doses with iron may decrease iron absorption.

Adverse Reactions Frequency not defined.

Cardiovascular: Cerebral hemorrhage, CHF (aggravated), edema

Central nervous system: Tetany

Gastrointestinal: Belching, flatulence (with oral), gastric distension

Endocrine & metabolic: Hypernatremia, hyperosmolality, hypocalcemia, hypokalemia, increased affinity of hemoglobin for oxygen-reduced pH in myocardial tissue necrosis when extravasated, intracranial acidosis, metabolic alkalosis, milk-alkali syndrome (especially with renal dysfunction)

Respiratory: Pulmonary edema

Overdosage/Toxicology Symptoms of overdose include hypocalcemia, hypokalemia, hypernatremia, and seizures. Treatment is symptom-directed and supportive.

Dosing

Adults & Elderly:

Cardiac arrest: I.V.: Initial: 1 mEq/kg/dose one time; maintenance: 0.5 mEq/kg/dose every 10 minutes or as indicated by arterial blood gases

Note: Routine use of $NaHCO_3$ is not recommended and should be given only after adequate alveolar ventilation has been established and effective cardiac compressions are provided

Metabolic acidosis: I.V.: Dosage should be based on the following formula if blood gases and pH measurements are available:

HCO_3^- (mEq) = 0.2 x weight (kg) x base deficit (mEq/L)

Administer ½ dose initially, then remaining ½ dose over the next 24 hours; monitor pH, serum HCO_3^-, and clinical status

Note: If acid-base status is not available: 2-5 mEq/kg I.V. infusion over 4-8 hours; subsequent doses should be based on patient's acid-base status

Hyperkalemia: I.V.: 1 mEq/kg over 5 minutes

Chronic renal failure: Oral: Initiate when plasma HCO_3^- <15 mEq/L Start with 20-36 mEq/day in divided doses, titrate to bicarbonate level of 18-20 mEq/L

Renal tubular acidosis: Oral:

Distal: 0.5-2 mEq/kg/day in 4-5 divided doses

Proximal: Initial: 5-10 mEq/kg/day; maintenance: Increase as required to maintain serum bicarbonate in the normal range

(Continued)

Sodium Bicarbonate *(Continued)*

Urine alkalinization: Oral: Initial: 48 mEq (4 g), then 12-24 mEq (1-2 g) every 4 hours; dose should be titrated to desired urinary pH; doses up to 16 g/day (200 mEq) in patients <60 years and 8 g (100 mEq) in patients >60 years

Antacid: Oral: 325 mg to 2 g 1-4 times/day

Pediatrics:

Cardiac arrest: I.V.: Infants and Children: 0.5-1 mEq/kg/dose repeated every 10 minutes or as indicated by arterial blood gases; rate of infusion should not exceed 10 mEq/minute; neonates and children <2 years of age should receive 4.2% (0.5 mEq/mL) solution.

Note: Routine use of $NaHCO_3$ is not recommended and should be given only after adequate alveolar ventilation has been established and effective cardiac compressions are provided

Metabolic acidosis: I.V.: Infants and Children: Dosage should be based on the following formula if blood gases and pH measurements are available:

HCO_3^- (mEq) = 0.3 x weight (kg) x base deficit (mEq/L)

Administer ½ dose initially, then remaining ½ dose over the next 24 hours; monitor pH, serum HCO_3^-, and clinical status

Note: If acid-base status is not available: Dose for older Children: 2-5 mEq/kg I.V. infusion over 4-8 hours; subsequent doses should be based on patient's acid-base status.

Chronic renal failure: Oral: Children: Initiate when plasma HCO_3^- <15 mEq/L: 1-3 mEq/kg/day

Renal tubular acidosis, distal: Oral: Children: 2-3 mEq/kg/day

Renal tubular acidosis, proximal: Children: Initial: 5-10 mEq/kg/day; maintenance: Increase as required to maintain serum bicarbonate in the normal range

Urine alkalinization: Oral: Children: 1-10 mEq (84-840 mg)/kg/day in divided doses every 4-6 hours; dose should be titrated to desired urinary pH.

Available Dosage Forms

Granules, effervescent (Brioschi®): 2.69 g/packet (6 g) [unit-dose packets; contains sodium 770 mg/packet; lemon flavor]; 2.69 g/capful (120 g, 240 g) [contains sodium 770 mg/capful; lemon flavor]

Infusion [premixed in sterile water]: 5% (500 mL)

Injection, solution:

4.2% [42 mg/mL = 5 mEq/10 mL] (10 mL)

7.5% [75 mg/mL = 8.92 mEq/10 mL] (50 mL)

8.4% [84 mg/mL = 10 mEq/10 mL] (10 mL, 50 mL)

Neut®: 4% [40 mg/mL = 2.4 mEq/5 mL] (5 mL)

Powder: Sodium bicarbonate USP (120 g, 480 g) [contains sodium 30 mEq per ½ teaspoon]

Tablet: 325 mg [3.8 mEq]; 650 mg [7.6 mEq]

Nursing Guidelines

Assessment: Assess other medications patient may be taking for effectiveness and interactions. **I.V.:** Monitor therapeutic effectiveness, adverse reactions, and infusion site (if extravasation occurs, elevate extravasation site and apply warm compresses). Monitor for signs of fluid retention. Teach patient adverse symptoms to report. **Oral:** Monitor effectiveness of treatment and adverse response. Assess knowledge/teach patient appropriate use, interventions to reduce side effects, and adverse symptoms to report.

Dietary Considerations: Oral product should be administered 1-3 hours after meals.

Sodium content:

Injection: 50 mL, 8.4% = 1150 mg = 50 mEq; each mL of 8.4% $NaHCO_3$ contains 23 mg sodium; 1 mEq $NaHCO_3$ = 84 mg

Granules: 2.69 g packet or capful = 770 mg sodium

Powder: 30 mEq sodium per ½ teaspoon]

Patient Education: Do not use for chronic gastric acidity. Take as directed. Chew tablets thoroughly and follow with a full glass of water, preferably on an empty stomach (2 hours before or after food). Report CNS effects (eg, irritability, confusion); muscle rigidity or tremors; swelling of feet or ankles; respiratory difficulty; chest pain or palpitations; respiratory changes; or tarry stools. **Pregnancy precaution:** Inform prescriber if you are or intend to become pregnant.

Geriatric Considerations: Not the antacid of choice for the elderly because of sodium content and potential for systemic alkalosis (see maximum daily dose under Dosage).

Pregnancy Risk Factor: C

Lactation: Enters breast milk/compatible

Perioperative/Anesthesia/Other Concerns: The use of bicarbonate for the treatment of lactic acidosis has not been proven useful. Increased pCO_2 after bicarbonate administration may result in an acute decrease in intracellular pH. Bicarbonate does not improve any hemodynamic parameters resulting in improved cardiovascular function. Many clinicians do not use bicarbonate in the treatment of lactic acidosis regardless of the patient's pH level.

Administration

Compatibility: Stable in dextran 6% in dextrose, dextran 6% in NS, $D_5{}^1\!/_4$NS, $D_5{}^1\!/_2$NS, D_5NS, D_5W, D_{10}W, ½NS, NS; incompatible with acids, acidic salts, alkaloid salts, calcium salts, catecholamines, and atropine

Y-site administration: Incompatible with allopurinol, amiodarone, amphotericin B cholesteryl sulfate complex, calcium chloride, doxorubicin liposome, idarubicin, imipenem/cilastatin inamrinone, leucovorin, midazolam, nalbuphine, ondansetron, oxacillin, sargramostim, verapamil, vincristine, vindesine, vinorelbine

Compatibility in syringe: Incompatible with etidocaine, glycopyrrolate, mepivacaine, metoclopramide, thiopental

Compatibility when admixed: Incompatible with amiodarone, ascorbic acid injection, carboplatin, carmustine, cefotaxime, ciprofloxacin, cisplatin, dobutamine, dopamine, epinephrine, hydromorphone, imipenem/cilastatin, isoproterenol, labetalol, levorphanol, magnesium sulfate, meropenem, morphine, norepinephrine, pentazocine, procaine, streptomycin, succinylcholine, ticarcillin/clavulanate potassium, vitamin B complex with C

Storage: Store injection at room temperature. Protect from heat and from freezing. Use only clear solutions.

Sodium Chloride (SOW dee um KLOR ide)

U.S. Brand Names Altachlore [OTC]; Altamist [OTC]; Ayr® Baby Saline [OTC]; Ayr® Saline [OTC]; Ayr® Saline No-Drip [OTC]; Breathe Right® Saline [OTC]; Broncho Saline® [OTC]; Deep Sea [OTC]; Entsol® [OTC]; Muro 128® [OTC]; Mycinaire™ [OTC]; NaSal™ [OTC]; Nasal Moist® [OTC]; Na-Zone® [OTC]; Ocean® [OTC]; Oceant® for Kids [OTC]; Pretz® [OTC]; SalineX® [OTC]; Simply Saline® [OTC]; Simply Saline® Baby [OTC]; Simply Saline® Nasal Moist® [OTC]; Syrex; 4-Way® Saline Moisturizing Mist [OTC]; Wound Wash Saline™ [OTC]

Synonyms NaCl; Normal Saline; Salt

Pharmacologic Category Electrolyte Supplement, Oral; Electrolyte Supplement, Parenteral; Lubricant, Ocular; Sodium Salt

Medication Safety Issues

Per JCAHO recommendations, concentrated electrolyte solutions (eg, NaCl >0.9%) should not be available in patient care areas.

High alert medication: The Institute for Safe Medication Practices (ISMP) includes this medication (I.V. formulation) among its list of drugs which have a heightened risk of causing significant patient harm when used in error.

Use

Parenteral: Restores sodium ion in patients with restricted oral intake (especially hyponatremia states or low salt syndrome). In general, parenteral saline uses:

- Bacteriostatic sodium chloride: Dilution or dissolving drugs for I.M., I.V., or SubQ injections
- Concentrated sodium chloride: Additive for parenteral fluid therapy
- Hypertonic sodium chloride: For severe hyponatremia and hypochloremia
- Hypotonic sodium chloride: Hydrating solution
- Normal saline: Restores water/sodium losses
- Pharmaceutical aid/diluent for infusion of compatible drug additives

Ophthalmic: Reduces corneal edema

Oral: Restores sodium losses

Inhalation: Restores moisture to pulmonary system; loosens and thins congestion caused by colds or allergies; diluent for bronchodilator solutions that require dilution before inhalation

Intranasal: Restores moisture to nasal membranes

Irrigation: Wound cleansing, irrigation, and flushing

Unlabeled/Investigational Use Traumatic brain injury (hypertonic sodium chloride)

Mechanism of Action Principal extracellular cation; functions in fluid and electrolyte balance, osmotic pressure control, and water distribution

(Continued)

Sodium Chloride *(Continued)*

Pharmacodynamics/Kinetics

Absorption: Oral, I.V.: Rapid

Distribution: Widely distributed

Excretion: Primarily urine; also sweat, tears, saliva

Contraindications Hypersensitivity to sodium chloride or any component of the formulation; hypertonic uterus, hypernatremia, fluid retention

Warnings/Precautions Use with caution in patients with CHF, renal insufficiency, liver cirrhosis, hypertension, edema; sodium toxicity is almost exclusively related to how fast a sodium deficit is corrected; both rate and magnitude are extremely important; do not use bacteriostatic sodium chloride in newborns since benzyl alcohol preservatives have been associated with toxicity. Wound Wash Saline™ is for single-patient use only.

Drug Interactions Decreased levels of lithium

Adverse Reactions Frequency not defined.

Cardiovascular: Congestive conditions

Endocrine & metabolic: Extravasation, hypervolemia, hypernatremia, dilution of serum electrolytes, overhydration, hypokalemia

Local: Thrombosis, phlebitis, extravasation

Respiratory: Pulmonary edema

Overdosage/Toxicology

Symptoms of overdose include nausea, vomiting, diarrhea, abdominal cramps, hypocalcemia, hypokalemia, hypernatremia

Hypernatremia is resolved through the use of diuretics and free water replacement

Dosing

Adults & Elderly:

GU irrigant: Irrigation: 1-3 L/day by intermittent irrigation

Heat cramps: Oral: 0.5-1 g with full glass of water, up to 4.8 g/day

Replacement: I.V.: Determined by laboratory determinations mEq

Hyponatremia: Sodium deficiency (mEq/kg) = [% dehydration (L/kg)/100 x 70 (mEq/L)] + [0.6 (L/kg) x (140 - serum sodium) (mEq/L)]

To correct acute, serious hyponatremia: mEq sodium = [desired sodium (mEq/L) - actual sodium (mEq/L)] x [0.6 x wt (kg)]; for acute correction use 125 mEq/L as the desired serum sodium; acutely correct serum sodium in 5 mEq/L/dose increments; more gradual correction in increments of 10 mEq/L/day is indicated in the asymptomatic patient

Traumatic brain injury (unlabeled use): I.V.: Hypertonic saline: **Note:** Dosing may vary among institutions. Some protocols include: 7.5%: 250 mL; 23.5%: 30 mL administered over 30 minutes; 2% to 3% as a continuous infusion (some clinicians may mix with sodium acetate to decrease hyperchloremic acidosis). Adjust according to intracranial pressure, serum sodium and chloride, and acid-base status.

Chloride maintenance electrolyte requirement in parenteral nutrition: 2-4 mEq/kg/24 hours or 25-40 mEq/1000 kcals/24 hours; maximum: 100-150 mEq/24 hours

Sodium maintenance electrolyte requirement in parenteral nutrition: 3-4 mEq/kg/24 hours or 25-40 mEq/1000 kcals/24 hours; maximum: 100-150 mEq/24 hours.

Approximate Deficits of Water and Electrolytes in Moderately Severe Dehydration[1]

Condition	Water (mL/kg)	Sodium (mEq/kg)
Fasting and thirsting	100-120	5-7
Diarrhea		
isonatremic	100-120	8-10
hypernatremic	100-120	2-4
hyponatremic	100-120	10-12
Pyloric stenosis	100-120	8-10
Diabetic acidosis	100-120	9-10

[1]A **negative** deficit indicates total body **excess** prior to treatment.

Adapted from Behrman RE, Kleigman RM, Nelson WE, et al, eds, *Nelson Textbook of Pediatrics*, 14th ed, WB Saunders Co, 1992.

Ophthalmic:

Ointment: Apply once daily or more often

Solution: Instill 1-2 drops into affected eye(s) every 3-4 hours

Bronchodilator diluent: Inhalation: 1-3 sprays (1-3 mL) to dilute bronchodilator solution in nebulizer before administration

Nasal congestion: Intranasal: 2-3 sprays in each nostril as needed

Irrigation: Spray affected area

Pediatrics:

Hyponatremia: I.V.: Children: Hypertonic solutions (>0.9%) should only be used for the initial treatment of acute serious symptomatic hyponatremia; maintenance: 3-4 mEq/kg/day; maximum: 100-150 mEq/day; dosage varies widely depending on clinical condition

Replacement: Determined by laboratory determinations mEq

Sodium deficiency (mEq/kg) = [% dehydration (L/kg)/100 x 70 (mEq/L)] + [0.6 (L/kg) x (140 - serum sodium) (mEq/L)]

Children ≥2 years:

Intranasal: Refer to adult dosing.

Irrigation: Refer to adult dosing.

Inhalation: Refer to adult dosing.

Available Dosage Forms

Gel, intranasal:

Ayr® Saline No-Drip: 0.5% (22 mL) [spray gel; contains benzalkonium chloride, benzyl alcohol and soybean oil]

Ayr® Saline: 0.5% (14 g) [contains soybean oil]

Entsol®: 3% (20 g) [contains aloe, benzalkonium chloride, and vitamin E]

Simply Saline® Nasal Moist®: 0.65% (30 g)

Injection, solution [preservative free]: 0.9% (2 mL, 5 mL, 10 mL, 20 mL, 100 mL)

Injection, solution [preservative free, prefilled I.V. flush syringe]: 0.9% (2 mL, 2.5 mL, 3 mL, 5 mL, 10 mL)

Injection, solution: 0.45% (25 mL, 50 mL, 100 mL, 250 mL, 500 mL, 1000 mL); 0.9% (3 mL, 5 mL, 10 mL, 20 mL, 25 mL, 30 mL, 50 mL, 100 mL, 150 mL, 250 mL, 500 mL, 1000 mL); 3% (500 mL); 5% (500 mL)

Syrex: 0.9% (2.5 mL, 5 mL, 10 mL) [prefilled syringe]

Injection, solution [bacteriostatic]: 0.9% (10 mL, 20 mL, 30 mL) [contains benzyl alcohol]

Injection, solution [concentrate]: 14.6% (2.5 mEq/mL) (20 mL, 40 mL); 23.4% (4 mEq/mL) (30 mL, 100 mL, 200 mL, 250 mL)

Ointment, ophthalmic: 5% (3.5 g)

Altachlore, Muro 128®: 5% (3.5 g)

Powder for nasal solution (Entsol®): 3% (10.5 g)

Solution for inhalation: 0.45% (3 mL, 5 mL); 0.9% (3 mL, 5 mL, 15 mL); 3% (15 mL); 10% (15 mL)

Broncho® Saline: 0.9% (90 mL, 240 mL) [for dilution of bronchodilator solutions]

Solution, intranasal: 0.65% (45 mL)

Altamist: 0.65% (60 mL) [spray; contains benzalkonium chloride]

Ayr® Baby Saline: 0.65% (30 mL) [spray/drops; contains benzalkonium chloride]

Ayr® Saline: 0.65% (50 mL) [drops; contains benzalkonium chloride]

Ayr® Saline: 0.65% (50 mL) [mist, contains benzalkonium chloride]

Breathe Right® Saline: 0.65% (44 mL) [spray; contains benzalkonium chloride]

Deep Sea: 0.65% (45 mL) [spray; contains benzalkonium chloride]

Entsol® Mist: 3% (30 mL) [spray; contains benzalkonium chloride]

Entsol® [preservative free]: 3% (100 mL) [spray]

Entsol® [preservative free]: 3% (240 mL) [nasal wash]

Mycinaire™: 0.65% (30 mL) [mist; contains benzalkonium chloride]

Na-Zone®: 0.65% (60 mL) [spray; contains benzalkonium chloride]

NaSal™: 0.65% (15 mL) [drops; contains benzalkonium chloride], (30 mL) [spray; contains benzalkonium chloride]

Nasal Moist®: 0.65% (45 mL) [spray]

Ocean®: 0.65% (45 mL) [mist/spray/drops; contains benzalkonium chloride]; (473 mL) [refill bottle; contains benzalkonium chloride]

Ocean® for Kids: 0.65% (37.5 mL) [drops/spray/stream; contains benzalkonium chloride]

Pretz®: 0.75% (50 mL) [spray; contains benzalkonium chloride and yerba santa]; (240 mL) [irrigation; contains benzalkonium chloride and yerba santa]; (960 mL) [refill bottle; contains benzalkonium chloride and yerba santa]

SalineX®: 0.4% (15 mL) [drops]; (50 mL) [spray]

(Continued)

Sodium Chloride *(Continued)*

Simply Saline®: 0.9% (44 mL, 90 mL) [mist]
Simply Saline® Baby: 0.9% (45 mL) [mist]
4-Way® Saline Moisturizing Mist: 0.74% (30 mL) [alcohol free; contains benzalkonium chloride, eucalyptol, and menthol]
Solution for irrigation: 0.45% (1500 mL, 2000 mL); 0.9% (250 mL, 500 mL, 1000 mL, 1500 mL, 2000 mL, 3000 mL, 4000 mL, 5000 mL)
Wound Wash Saline™: 0.9% (90 mL, 210 mL)
Solution, ophthalmic: 5% (15 mL)
Altachlore: 5% (15 mL, 30 mL)
Muro 128®: 2% (15 mL); 5% (15 mL, 30 mL)

Nursing Guidelines

Patient Education: Blurred vision is common with ophthalmic ointment; may sting eyes when first applied

Pregnancy Risk Factor: C

Administration

Compatibility: Stable in dextran 6% in dextrose, dextran 6% in NS, D_5LR, $D_5{}^1/_4NS$, $D_5{}^1/_2NS$, D_5NS, D_5W, $D_{10}W$, LR, $^1/_2NS$, NS

Sodium Citrate and Citric Acid

(SOW dee um SIT rate & SI trik AS id)

U.S. Brand Names Bicitra®; Cytra-2; Oracit®

Synonyms Modified Shohl's Solution

Pharmacologic Category Alkalinizing Agent, Oral

Use Treatment of metabolic acidosis; alkalinizing agent in conditions where long-term maintenance of an alkaline urine is desirable

Pharmacodynamics/Kinetics

Metabolism: Oxidized to sodium bicarbonate
Excretion: Urine (<5% as sodium citrate)

Contraindications Hypersensitivity to sodium citrate, citric acid, or any component of the formulation; severe renal insufficiency; sodium-restricted diet

Warnings/Precautions Conversion to bicarbonate may be impaired in patients with hepatic failure, in shock, or who are severely ill. Use caution with cardiac failure, hypertension, impaired renal function, and peripheral or pulmonary edema.

Drug Interactions

Decreased effect/levels of lithium, chlorpropamide, salicylates due to urinary alkalinization

Increased toxicity/levels of amphetamines, ephedrine, pseudoephedrine, flecainide, quinidine, quinine due to urinary alkalinization

Adverse Reactions Frequency not defined. Generally well tolerated with normal renal function.

Central nervous system: Tetany
Endocrine & metabolic: Metabolic alkalosis, hyperkalemia
Gastrointestinal: Diarrhea, nausea, vomiting

Overdosage/Toxicology Symptoms of overdose include hypokalemia, hypernatremia, tetany, and seizures. Treatment is symptom-directed and supportive.

Dosing

Adults & Elderly: Systemic alkalization: Oral: 10-30 mL with water after meals and at bedtime

Pediatrics: Systemic alkalization: Oral: Infants and Children: 2-3 mEq/kg/day in divided doses 3-4 times/day **or** 5-15 mL with water after meals and at bedtime

Available Dosage Forms Note: Contains sodium 1 mEq/mL and the equivalent to bicarbonate 1 mEq/mL

Solution, oral: Sodium citrate 500 mg and citric acid 334 mg per 5 mL (480 mL)
Bicitra®: Sodium citrate 500 mg and citric acid 334 mg per 5 mL (480 mL) [sugar free; grape flavor]
Cytra-2: Sodium citrate 500 mg and citric acid 334 mg per 5 mL (480 mL) [alcohol free, dye free, sugar free; grape flavor]
Oracit®: Sodium citrate 490 mg and citric acid 640 mg per 5 mL (15 mL, 30 mL, 500 mL, 3840 mL)

Nursing Guidelines

Assessment: Assess kidney function prior to starting therapy. Monitor cardiac status and serum potassium at beginning of therapy and at regular intervals with long-term therapy. Assess knowledge/teach patient appropriate use, possible side effects, and adverse symptoms to report.

Dietary Considerations: Should be taken after meals to avoid laxative effect.

Patient Education: Take as often as directed, after meals, and at least 2 hours before or after any other medications. Dilute with 1-3 oz of water and follow with additional water; chilling solution prior to taking will help to improve taste. You may experience diarrhea or nausea and vomiting; if severe, contact prescriber. Report CNS changes status (eg, irritability, tremors, confusion); swelling of feet or ankles; respiratory difficulty or palpitations; abdominal pain or tarry stools.

Pregnancy Risk Factor: Not established

Lactation: Excretion in breast milk unknown/compatible

Administration

Oral: Administer after meals. Dilute with 30-90 mL of water to enhance taste. Chilling solution prior to dosing helps to enhance palatability.

Storage: Store at controlled room temperature of 15°C to 30°C (59°F to 86°F). Protect from excessive heat or freezing.

♦ **Sodium Edetate** *see* Edetate Disodium *on page 595*
♦ **Sodium Ferric Gluconate** *see* Ferric Gluconate *on page 718*
♦ **Sodium Hyaluronate** *see* Hyaluronate and Derivatives *on page 856*
♦ **Sodium Hyaluronate-Chrondroitin Sulfate** *see* Chondroitin Sulfate and Sodium Hyaluronate *on page 387*
♦ **Sodium Hydrogen Carbonate** *see* Sodium Bicarbonate *on page 1542*

Sodium Hypochlorite Solution

(SOW dee um hye poe KLOR ite soe LOO shun)

U.S. Brand Names Dakin's Solution; Di-Dak-Sol

Synonyms Modified Dakin's Solution

Pharmacologic Category Disinfectant, Antibacterial (Topical)

Use Treatment of athlete's foot (0.5%); wound irrigation (0.5%); disinfection of utensils and equipment (5%)

Contraindications Hypersensitivity to any component of the formulation

Warnings/Precautions For external use only; avoid eye or mucous membrane contact; do not use on open wounds

Adverse Reactions Frequency not defined.

Dermatologic: Irritating to skin

Hematologic: Dissolves blood clots, delays clotting

Dosing

Adults & Elderly: Disinfectant: Topical: Via irrigation

Pediatrics: Topical irrigation

Available Dosage Forms Solution, topical:

Dakin's: 0.25% (480 mL); 0.5% (480 mL, 3840 mL)

Di-Dak-Sol: 0.0125% (480 mL)

Nursing Guidelines

Assessment: Assess knowledge/teach patient appropriate application and use and adverse symptoms to report.

Patient Education: Use exactly as directed; do not overuse. Avoid contact with eyes. Report worsening of condition or lack of healing. **Pregnancy precaution:** Inform prescriber if you are or intend to become pregnant.

Pregnancy Risk Factor: C

Lactation: For external use

Administration

Storage: Use prepared solution within 7 days.

♦ **Sodium Nafcillin** *see* Nafcillin *on page 1194*
♦ **Sodium Nitroferricyanide** *see* Nitroprusside *on page 1238*
♦ **Sodium Nitroprusside** *see* Nitroprusside *on page 1238*
♦ **Sodium Phosphate and Potassium Phosphate** *see* Potassium Phosphate and Sodium Phosphate *on page 1391*

Sodium Phosphates (SOW dee um FOS fates)

U.S. Brand Names Fleet® Accu-Prep® [OTC]; Fleet® Enema [OTC]; Fleet® Phospho-Soda® [OTC]; Visicol®

Pharmacologic Category Cathartic; Electrolyte Supplement, Oral; Electrolyte Supplement, Parenteral; Laxative, Bowel Evacuant

Use

Oral, rectal: Short-term treatment of constipation and to evacuate the colon for rectal and bowel exams

(Continued)

Sodium Phosphates *(Continued)*

I.V.: Source of phosphate in large volume I.V. fluids and parenteral nutrition; treatment and prevention of hypophosphatemia

Mechanism of Action As a laxative, exerts osmotic effect in the small intestine by drawing water into the lumen of the gut, producing distention and promoting peristalsis and evacuation of the bowel; phosphorous participates in bone deposition, calcium metabolism, utilization of B complex vitamins, and as a buffer in acid-base equilibrium

Pharmacodynamics/Kinetics

Onset of action: Cathartic: 3-6 hours; Rectal: 2-5 minutes

Absorption: Oral: ~1% to 20%

Contraindications Hypersensitivity to sodium phosphate salts or any component of the formulation; congenital megacolon, toxic megacolon, bowel obstruction, bowel perforation, imperforate anus (enema), congestive heart failure, hyperparathyroidism, ascites

Additional product-specific contraindications:

Intravenous phosphate preparation: Should not be used in diseases with high phosphate levels, low calcium levels or hypernatremia.

Oral: Should not be used in patients with kidney disease, unstable angina pectoris, gastric retention, ileus, acute obstruction or pseudo-obstruction, severe chronic constipation, acute colitis, or hypomotility syndrome (ie, hypothyroidism, scleroderma). Should not be used in patients on a sodium-restricted diet.

Warnings/Precautions Use with caution in patients with impaired renal function (oral solution contraindicated), pre-existing electrolyte imbalances (including patients on diuretics which may effect electrolyte levels or dehydration); risk of hypocalcemia, hyperphosphatemia, hypernatremia, and acidosis. Use caution in patients with a history of seizures, concurrent therapy which lowers seizure threshold, or predisposing factors for hyponatremia. If using as a bowel evacuant, correct electrolyte abnormalities before treatment; inadequate fluid intake may lead to excessive fluid loss and hypovolemia. May cause colonic mucosal aphthous ulcerations; use with caution in patients with an acute exacerbation of chronic inflammatory bowel disease, absorption may be enhanced. Use with caution in debilitated patients. Enemas and oral solution are available in pediatric and adult sizes; prescribe by "volume" not "by bottle".

Additional product-specific warnings/precautions:

Enema preparation: Use caution in patients with a colostomy; not for use in children <2 years of age. Enema tips are latex free.

Intravenous preparation: Must be diluted before use; infuse slowly.

Oral solution: Patients receiving >45 mL of oral solution may develop severe electrolyte shifts, even in the absence of medical contraindications. Nephrocalcinosis may occur (rare) during use as a bowel cleanser. Not for use in renally-impaired patients or hyperparathyroidism. Use caution when administered to patients taking angiotensin-receptor blockers or ACE inhibitors. Also use caution in patients receiving diuretics.

Tablet preparation: Prolongation of the QT interval has been reported with use of the tablet formulation; use with caution with other medication known to cause this effect; use caution within 3 months of acute myocardial infarction or cardiac surgery. Do not use with other phosphate-containing products, fatalities have been reported. Not for use in patients <18 years of age.

Drug Interactions

ACE inhibitors or angiotensin-receptor antagonists: May increase the risk of electrolyte disorders or nephrocalcinosis when oral phosphates solution is used as a bowel evacuant. Use caution.

Antacids: Do not give with magnesium- and aluminum-containing antacids which can bind with phosphate.

Bisphosphonates: Increased risk of hypoglycemia with concurrent use.

Diuretics: May increase the risk of electrolyte disorders or nephrocalcinosis when oral phosphates solution is used as a bowel evacuant. Use caution.

Sucralfate: Do not give with sucralfate which can bind with phosphate.

Oral preparations: May affect absorption of other medications due to rapid intestinal peristalsis and watery diarrhea caused by agent

Intravenous preparation: Use caution with thiazide diuretics, may lead to renal damage

Adverse Reactions Frequency not defined.

Cardiovascular: Edema, hypotension

Central nervous system: Dizziness, headache

Endocrine & metabolic: Calcium phosphate precipitation, hypernatremia, hyperphosphatemia, hypocalcemia

Gastrointestinal: Abdominal bloating, abdominal pain, diarrhea, mucosal bleeding, nausea, superficial mucosal ulcerations, vomiting

Renal: Acute renal failure

Postmarketing and/or case reports: Atrial fibrillation following severe vomiting (tablet formulation); nephrocalcinosis (oral solution)

Overdosage/Toxicology Overdose may lead to cardiac arrhythmias, severe electrolyte disturbances, including hyperphosphatemia, hypocalcemia, hypernatremia or hypokalemia. Treat symptomatically.

Dosing

Adults & Elderly:

Normal requirements elemental phosphorus: Oral:

≥19 years: RDA: 700 mg

Hypophosphatemia: It is difficult to provide concrete guidelines for the treatment of severe hypophosphatemia because the extent of total body deficits and response to therapy are difficult to predict. Aggressive doses of phosphate may result in a transient serum elevation followed by redistribution into intracellular compartments or bone tissue. Intermittent I.V. infusion should be reserved for severe depletion situations (<1 mg/dL in adults); large doses of oral phosphate may cause diarrhea and intestinal absorption may be unreliable. I.V. solutions should be infused slowly. Use caution when mixing with calcium and magnesium, precipitate may form. The following dosages are empiric guidelines. **Note:** 1 mmol phosphate = 31 mg phosphorus; 1 mg phosphorus = 0.032 mmol phosphate

Hypophosphatemia treatment: Doses listed as mmol of phosphate:

Intermittent I.V. infusion: Acute repletion or replacement:

Varying dosages: 0.15-0.3 mmol/kg/dose over 12 hours; may repeat as needed to achieve desired serum level **or**

15 mmol/dose over 2 hours; use if serum phosphorus <2 mg/dL **or**

Low dose: 0.16 mmol/kg over 4-6 hours; use if serum phosphorus level 2.3-3 mg/dL

Intermediate dose: 0.32 mmol/kg over 4-6 hours; use if serum phosphorus level 1.6-2.2 mg/dL

High dose: 0.64 mmol/kg over 8-12 hours; use if serum phosphorus <1.5 mg/dL

Oral: 0.5-1 g elemental phosphorus 2-3 times/day may be used when serum phosphorus level is 1-2.5 mg/dL

Maintenance: Doses listed as mmol of phosphate:

Oral: 50-150 mmol/day in divided doses

I.V.: 50-70 mmol/day

Laxative (Fleet®): Rectal: Contents of one 4.5-ounce enema as a single dose, may repeat

Laxative (Fleet® Phospho-Soda®): Oral: Take on an empty stomach; dilute dose with 4 ounces cool water, then follow dose with 8 ounces water; **do not repeat dose within 24 hours**

20-45 mL as a single dose

Bowel cleansing prior to colonoscopy:

Fleet® Phospho-Soda® Accu-Prep™: Oral: Prior to procedure (timing of doses determined by prescriber): One dose is equal to 45 mL (2 doses are recommended): Each dose is diluted as follows:

Mix 45 mL with 120 mL clear liquid; drink, then follow with at least 240 mL of clear liquid; **or**

Mix 15 mL with 240 mL clear liquid; drink, then follow with 240 mL clear liquid; repeat every 10 minutes for a total of 45 mL

Visicol™: Oral: Adults: A total of 40 tablets divided as follows:

Evening before colonoscopy: 3 tablets every 15 minutes for 6 doses, then 2 additional tablets in 15 minutes (total of 20 tablets)

3-5 hours prior to colonoscopy: 3 tablets every 15 minutes for 6 doses, then 2 additional tablets in 15 minutes (total of 20 tablets)

Note: Each dose should be taken with a minimum of 8 ounces of clear liquids. Do not repeat treatment within 7 days. Do not use additional agents, especially sodium phosphate products.

Pediatrics:

Normal requirements elemental phosphorus: Oral:

0-6 months: Adequate intake: 100 mg/day

(Continued)

Sodium Phosphates *(Continued)*

6-12 months: Adequate intake: 275 mg/day
1-3 years: RDA: 460 mg
4-8 years: RDA: 500 mg
9-18 years: RDA: 1250 mg

Note: 1 mmol phosphate = 31 mg phosphorus; 1 mg phosphorus = 0.032 mmol phosphate

Hypophosphatemia treatment: Doses listed as mmol of phosphate:
Acute repletion; Intermittent I.V. infusion:
Children:
Low dose: 0.08 mmol/kg over 6 hours; use if losses are recent and uncomplicated
Intermediate dose: 0.16-0.24 mmol/kg over 4-6 hours; use if serum phosphorus level 0.5-1 mg/dL
High dose: 0.36 mmol/kg over 6 hours; use if serum phosphorus <0.5 mg/dL

Maintenance: Doses listed as mmol of phosphate: Children:
Oral: 2-3 mmol/kg/day in divided doses
I.V.: 0.5-1.5 mmol/kg/day

Laxative (Fleet®): Rectal:
Children 2-<5 years: One-half contents of one 2.25 oz pediatric enema
Children 5-12 years: Contents of one 2.25 oz pediatric enema, may repeat
Children ≥12 years: Refer to adult dosing.

Laxative (Fleet® Phospho-Soda®): Oral: Take on an empty stomach; dilute dose with 4 ounces cool water, then follow dose with 8 ounces water; **do not repeat dose within 24 hours**
Children 5-9 years: 5-10 mL as a single dose
Children 10-12 years: 10-20 mL as a single dose
Children ≥12 years: Refer to adult dosing.

Renal Impairment: Use with caution; ionized inorganic phosphate is excreted by the kidneys. Oral solution is contraindicated in patients with kidney disease.

Available Dosage Forms

Kit (Fleet® Accu-Prep®):
Solution, oral (Fleet® Phosph-Soda®): Monobasic sodium phosphate monohydrate 2.4 g and dibasic sodium phosphate heptahydrate 0.9 g per 5 mL (15 mL) [contains sodium benzoate; kit contains six 15 mL unit-dose containers (equal to two 45 mL doses)]
Pads, anorectal (Fleet® Relief™): Pramoxine hydrochloride 1% and glycerin 12% (4s)

Injection, solution [preservative free]: Phosphorus 3 mmol and sodium 4 mEq per mL (5 mL, 15 mL, 50 mL)

Solution, oral (Fleet® Phospho-Soda®): Monobasic sodium phosphate monohydrate 2.4 g and dibasic sodium phosphate heptahydrate 0.9 g per 5 mL (45 mL, 90 mL) [contains sodium benzoate; unflavored or ginger-lemon flavor]

Solution, rectal [enema]: Monobasic sodium phosphate 19 g and dibasic sodium phosphate 7 g per 118 mL delivered dose (135 mL)
Fleet® Enema: Monobasic sodium phosphate 19 g and dibasic sodium phosphate 7 g per 118 mL delivered dose (135 mL)
Fleet® Enema for Children: Monobasic sodium phosphate 9.5 g and dibasic sodium phosphate 3.5 g per 59 mL delivered dose (68 mL)

Tablet, oral (Visicol®): Sodium phosphate monobasic monohydrate 1.102 g and sodium phosphate dibasic anhydrous 0.398 g [1.5 g total sodium phosphate per tablet]

Nursing Guidelines

Dietary Considerations: Should be taken on an empty stomach with water; a clear liquid diet should be used for 12 hours prior to tablet administration.

Oral solution contains 556 mg (24.17 mEq) sodium/ 5 mL
Whole cow's milk: 0.29 mmol/mL phosphate; 0.025 mEq/mL sodium; 0.035 mEq/mL potassium

Patient Education: May cause diarrhea with the oral preparation; excessive or prolonged use as a laxative may cause dependence. Do not use over-the-counter laxatives when you are nauseated, vomiting, or have abdominal pain, unless directed to by prescriber. Do not use recommended dose more than once in 24 hours. In general, laxative products should not be used for longer than 1 week, unless under guidance of prescriber. Do not use with other laxative products, especially those containing phosphate. **Pregnancy/breast-feeding precautions:** Inform prescriber if you are or intend to become pregnant. Consult prescriber if breast-feeding.

Enemas: Not for oral use. Insert bottle gently into rectum with tip of bottle pointed towards naval; do not force. Squeeze bottle to expel liquid, stop if resistance is felt. Contact prescriber immediately if no liquid is returned following administration, or if rectal bleeding occurs.

Tablets: Undigested or partially-digested tablets of this or other medications may be seen in stool. Take each dose with 8 oz of clear liquids.

Pregnancy Risk Factor: C

Lactation: Use caution in nursing women.

Administration

Compatibility: Y-site administration: Incompatible with ciprofloxacin

Storage: Phosphate salts may precipitate when mixed with calcium salts; solubility is improved in amino acid parenteral nutrition solutions; check with a pharmacist to determine compatibility.

Sodium Polystyrene Sulfonate

(SOW dee um pol ee STYE reen SUL fon ate)

U.S. Brand Names Kayexalate®; Kionex™; SPS®

Pharmacologic Category Antidote

Medication Safety Issues

Sound-alike/look-alike issues:

Kayexalate® may be confused with Kaopectate®

Always prescribe either one-time doses or as a specific number of doses (eg, 15 g q6h x 2 doses). Scheduled doses with no dosage limit could be given for days leading to dangerous hypokalemia.

Use Treatment of hyperkalemia

Mechanism of Action Removes potassium by exchanging sodium ions for potassium ions in the intestine before the resin is passed from the body

Pharmacodynamics/Kinetics

Onset of action: 2-24 hours

Absorption: None

Excretion: Completely feces (primarily as potassium polystyrene sulfonate)

Contraindications Hypersensitivity to sodium polystyrene sulfonate or any component of the formulation; hypernatremia, hypokalemia, obstructive bowel disease

Warnings/Precautions Use with caution in patients with severe CHF, hypertension, edema, or renal failure; avoid using the commercially available liquid product in neonates due to the preservative content; large oral doses may cause fecal impaction (especially in elderly); enema will reduce the serum potassium faster than oral administration, but the oral route will result in a greater reduction over several hours.

Drug Interactions Systemic alkalosis and seizure has occurred after cation-exchange resins were administered with nonabsorbable cation-donating antacids and laxatives (eg, magnesium hydroxide, aluminum carbonate). Digitalis toxicity may occur with hypokalemia.

Adverse Reactions Frequency not defined.

Endocrine & metabolic: Hypernatremia, hypokalemia, hypocalcemia, hypomagnesemia

Gastrointestinal: Anorexia, colonic necrosis (rare), constipation, fecal impaction, intestinal obstruction (due to concretions in association with aluminum hydroxide), nausea, vomiting

Overdosage/Toxicology Symptoms of overdose include hypokalemia including cardiac dysrhythmias, confusion, irritability, ECG changes, muscle weakness, and GI effects. Treatment is supportive, limited to management of fluid and electrolytes.

Dosing

Adults & Elderly: Hyperkalemia:

Oral: 15 g (60 mL) 1-4 times/day

Rectal: 30-50 g every 6 hours

Pediatrics: Hyperkalemia:

Oral: Children: 1 g/kg/dose every 6 hours

Rectal: Children: 1 g/kg/dose every 2-6 hours (in small children and infants, employ lower doses by using the practical exchange ratio of 1 mEq K^+/g of resin as the basis for calculation)

(Continued)

Sodium Polystyrene Sulfonate *(Continued)*

Available Dosage Forms

Powder for suspension, oral/rectal:

Kayexalate®: 15 g/4 level teaspoons (480 g) [contains sodium 100 mg (4.1 mEq)/g]

Kionex™: 15 g/4 level teaspoons (454 g) [contains sodium 100 mg (4.1 mEq)/g]

Suspension, oral/rectal: 15 g/60 mL (60 mL, 120 mL, 200 mL, 500 mL) [contains sodium 1500 mg (65 mEq)/60 mL, sorbitol, and alcohol 0.1%; cherry/caramel flavor]

SPS®: 15 g/60 mL (60 mL, 120 mL, 480 mL) [contains alcohol 0.3%, sodium 1500 mg (65 mEq)/60 mL , and sorbitol; cherry flavor]

Nursing Guidelines

Assessment: Assess results of laboratory tests. Monitor ECG until potassium levels are normal. Monitor for adverse reactions and teach patient interventions and importance of reporting adverse symptoms promptly.

Monitoring Laboratory Tests: Serum electrolytes, calcium, magnesium

Dietary Considerations: Do **not** mix in orange juice. Sodium content of 1 g: 31 mg (1.3 mEq).

Patient Education: Emergency instructions depend on patient's condition. You will be monitored for effects of this medication and frequent blood tests may be necessary. Oral: Take as directed. Mix well with a full glass of liquid (not orange juice). You may experience nausea or vomiting (small frequent meals, frequent mouth care, chewing gum, or sucking lozenges may help); or constipation or fecal impaction (increased dietary fluids and exercise may help). Report persistent constipation or GI distress; chest pain or rapid heartbeat; or mental confusion or muscle weakness. **Pregnancy/breast-feeding precautions:** Inform prescriber if you are pregnant. Consult prescriber if breast-feeding.

Geriatric Considerations: Large doses in the elderly may cause fecal impaction and intestinal obstruction. Best to administer using sorbitol 70% as vehicle.

Pregnancy Risk Factor: C

Lactation: Excretion in breast milk unknown/use caution

Perioperative/Anesthesia/Other Concerns: While sodium polystyrene sulfonate can be used in the treatment of hyperkalemia, if hyperkalemia is associated with ECG changes, more emergent therapy needs to be used (ie, glucose-insulin or calcium). Sodium polystyrene sulfonate should be used with caution in patients with severe heart failure, hypertension, or renal failure. While rectal administration of sodium polystyrene sulfonate achieves a more rapid action, oral administration results in a more sustained potassium reduction.

Administration

Oral: Administer oral (or NG) as ~25% sorbitol solution; never mix in orange juice. Chilling the oral mixture will increase palatability.

Storage: Store prepared suspensions at 15°C to 30°C (59°F to 86°F); store repackaged product in refrigerator and use within 14 days; freshly prepared suspensions should be used within 24 hours; do not heat resin suspension

♦ **Sodium Sulfacetamide** *see* Sulfacetamide *on page 1579*

Sodium Tetradecyl (SOW dee um tetra DEK il)

U.S. Brand Names Sotradecol®

Synonyms Sodium Tetradecyl Sulfate

Pharmacologic Category Sclerosing Agent

Use Treatment of small, uncomplicated varicose veins of the lower extremities

Mechanism of Action Acts by irritation of the vein intimal endothelium and causes thrombosis formation leading to occlusion of the injected vein

Contraindications Hypersensitivity to sodium tetradecyl or any component of the formulation; arterial disease, acute thrombophlebitis; valvular or deep vein incompetence, phlebitis migrans, cellulitis, acute infections; bedridden patients; patients with uncontrolled systemic disease such as diabetes, toxic hyperthyroidism, tuberculosis, asthma, neoplasm, sepsis, blood dyscrasias, and acute respiratory or skin diseases; huge superficial veins with wide open communications to deeper veins; allergic conditions; varicosities caused by abdominal and pelvic tumors (unless tumor has been removed)

Warnings/Precautions Use caution with Buerger's disease or peripheral arteriosclerosis. Avoid extravasation. Observe for hypersensitivity/anaphylactic reaction; emergency resuscitation equipment should be available. Valvular and venous competency should be evaluated prior to use.

Adverse Reactions Frequency not defined.

Central nervous system: Headache
Dermatologic: Discoloration at site of injection, sloughing and tissue necrosis following extravasation
Gastrointestinal: Nausea, vomiting
Local: Pain, itching, or ulceration at injection site
Miscellaneous: Allergic reaction (including hives, asthma, hay fever); anaphylactic shock

Dosing

Adults & Elderly: Sclerosing agent: I.V.: Test dose: 0.5 mL given several hours prior to administration of larger dose; 0.5-2 mL (preferred maximum: 1 mL) in each vein, maximum: 10 mL per treatment session; 3% solution reserved for large varices

Available Dosage Forms Injection, as sulfate: 1% [10 mg/mL] (2 mL) [contains benzyl alcohol]; 3% [30 mg/mL] (2 mL) [contains benzyl alcohol]

Nursing Guidelines

Assessment: Monitor for allergic reaction/anaphylaxis. Have resuscitation equipment available. Monitor injection site for extravasation. Can cause sloughing and necrosis of tissue. Note breast-feeding caution.

Patient Education: A permanent discoloration may remain along the site of the injections. You may experience headache, nausea, and vomiting. Report chest pain or shortness of breath immediately. **Pregnancy/breast-feeding precautions:** Inform prescriber if you are or intend to become pregnant. Consult prescriber before breast-feeding.

Geriatric Considerations: Due to possible contraindications with disease states that may be "out of control," the elderly patient's medical condition must be thoroughly evaluated before use. No specific geriatric data available; see Contraindications.

Pregnancy Risk Factor: C

Lactation: Excretion in breast milk unknown/use caution

Administration

I.V.: Inject slowly.

Compatibility: Incompatible with heparin

Storage: Store at controlled room temperature.

- Sodium Tetradecyl Sulfate *see* Sodium Tetradecyl *on page 1554*
- Solaraze® *see* Diclofenac *on page 521*
- Solarcaine® Aloe Extra Burn Relief [OTC] *see* Lidocaine *on page 1033*
- Solia™ *see* Ethinyl Estradiol and Desogestrel *on page 675*
- Soluble Fluorescein *see* Fluorescein Sodium *on page 742*
- Solu-Cortef® *see* Hydrocortisone *on page 873*
- Solu-Medrol® *see* MethylPREDNISolone *on page 1140*
- Soluvite-F *see* Vitamins (Multiple/Pediatric) *on page 1720*
- Soma® *see* Carisoprodol *on page 316*
- Somatrem *see* Somatropin *on page 1555*

Somatropin (soe ma TROE pin)

U.S. Brand Names Genotropin®; Genotropin Miniquick®; Humatrope®; Norditropin®; Norditropin® NordiFlex®; Nutropin®; Nutropin AQ®; Saizen®; Serostim®; Tev-Tropin™; Zorbtive™

Synonyms Human Growth Hormone; Somatrem

Pharmacologic Category Growth Hormone

Medication Safety Issues

Sound-alike/look-alike issues:
Somatrem may be confused with somatropin
Somatropin may be confused with somatrem, sumatriptan

Use

Children:
Long-term treatment of growth failure due to inadequate endogenous growth hormone secretion (Genotropin®, Humatrope®, Norditropin®, Nutropin®, Nutropin AQ®, Saizen®, Tev-Tropin™)
Long-term treatment of short stature associated with Turner syndrome (Humatrope®, Nutropin®, Nutropin AQ®)
Treatment of Prader-Willi syndrome (Genotropin®)
Treatment of growth failure associated with chronic renal insufficiency (CRI) up until the time of renal transplantation (Nutropin®, Nutropin AQ®)

(Continued)

Somatropin *(Continued)*

Long-term treatment of growth failure in children born small for gestational age who fail to manifest catch-up growth by 2 years of age (Genotropin®)

Long-term treatment of idiopathic short stature (nongrowth hormone-deficient short stature) defined by height standard deviation score (SDS) less than or equal to -2.25 and growth rate not likely to attain normal adult height (Humatrope®, Nutropin®, Nutropin AQ®)

Adults:

AIDS-wasting or cachexia with concomitant antiviral therapy (Serostim®)

Replacement of endogenous growth hormone in patients with adult growth hormone deficiency who meet both of the following criteria (Genotropin®, Humatrope®, Norditropin®, Nutropin®, Nutropin AQ®, Saizen®):

Biochemical diagnosis of adult growth hormone deficiency by means of a subnormal response to a standard growth hormone stimulation test (peak growth hormone ≤5 mcg/L)

and

Adult-onset: Patients who have adult growth hormone deficiency whether alone or with multiple hormone deficiencies (hypopituitarism) as a result of pituitary disease, hypothalamic disease, surgery, radiation therapy, or trauma

or

Childhood-onset: Patients who were growth hormone deficient during childhood, confirmed as an adult before replacement therapy is initiated

Treatment of short-bowel syndrome (Zorbtive™)

Unlabeled/Investigational Use Investigational: Congestive heart failure; AIDS-wasting/cachexia in children (Serostim®)

Mechanism of Action Somatropin is a purified polypeptide hormones of recombinant DNA origin; somatropin contains the identical sequence of amino acids found in human growth hormone; human growth hormone stimulates growth of linear bone, skeletal muscle, and organs; stimulates erythropoietin which increases red blood cell mass; exerts both insulin-like and diabetogenic effects; enhances the transmucosal transport of water, electrolytes, and nutrients across the gut

Pharmacodynamics/Kinetics

Duration: Maintains supraphysiologic levels for 18-20 hours

Absorption: I.M., SubQ: Well absorbed

Metabolism: Hepatic and renal (~90%)

Half-life elimination: Preparation and route of administration dependent

Excretion: Urine

Contraindications Hypersensitivity to growth hormone or any component of the formulation; growth promotion in pediatric patients with closed epiphyses; progression of any underlying intracranial lesion or actively growing intracranial tumor; acute critical illness due to complications following open heart or abdominal surgery; multiple accidental trauma or acute respiratory failure; evidence of active malignancy; use in patients with Prader-Willi syndrome **without** growth hormone deficiency (except Genotropin®) or in patients with Prader-Willi syndrome **with** growth hormone deficiency who are severely obese or have severe respiratory impairment. Saizen® and Norditropin® are contraindicated with proliferative or preproliferative retinopathy.

Warnings/Precautions Use with caution in patients with diabetes or with risk factors for glucose intolerance. Intracranial hypertension has been reported with growth hormone product, funduscopic examinations are recommended; progression of scoliosis may occur in children experiencing rapid growth; patients with growth hormone deficiency may develop slipped capital epiphyses more frequently, evaluate any child with new onset of a limp or with complaints of hip or knee pain; patients with Turner syndrome are at increased risk for otitis media and other ear/hearing disorders, cardiovascular disorders (including stroke, aortic aneurysm, hypertension), and thyroid disease, monitor carefully. Concurrent glucocorticoid therapy may inhibit growth promotion effects; may require dosage adjustment or replacement glucocorticoid therapy in patients with ACTH deficiency. Products may contain benzyl alcohol, m-Cresol or glycerin, some products may be manufactured by recombinant DNA technology using *E. coli* as a host, consult specific product labeling. When administering to newborns, reconstitute with sterile water or saline for injection. Not for I.V. injection.

Fatalities have been reported in pediatric patients with Prader-Willi syndrome following the use of growth hormone. The reported fatalities occurred in patients with one or more risk factors, including severe obesity, sleep apnea, respiratory impairment, or unidentified respiratory infection; male patients with one or more of these factors may be at greater risk. Treatment interruption is recommended in patients who show signs of upper airway obstruction, including the onset of, or increased, snoring. In addition, evaluation of and/or monitoring for sleep apnea and respiratory infections are recommended.

Drug Interactions

Glucocorticoids: May inhibit growth-promoting effects.

Insulin: Growth hormone may induce insulin resistance in patients with diabetes mellitus; monitor glucose and adjust insulin dose as necessary

Adverse Reactions

Growth hormone deficiency: Antigrowth hormone antibodies, carpal tunnel syndrome (rare), fluid balance disturbances, glucosuria, gynecomastia (rare), headache, hematuria, hyperglycemia (mild), hypoglycemia, hypothyroidism, leukemia, lipoatrophy, muscle pain, increased growth of pre-existing nevi (rare), pain/ local reactions at the injection site, pancreatitis (rare), peripheral edema, exacerbation of psoriasis, rash, seizure, weakness

Idiopathic short stature: (From ISS NCGS Cohort; all frequencies <1%): Arthralgia, avascular necrosis, bone growth (abnormal), carpal tunnel syndrome, diabetes mellitus, edema, fracture, gynecomastia, injection site reaction, intracranial hypertension, neoplasm (new onset or recurring), scoliosis (new onset or progression), slipped capital femoral epiphysis, tumor (new onset or recurring). Additional adverse effects noted in product literature (Humatrope®; frequency not established in large cohort): Hip pain, hyperlipidemia, hypertension, hypothyroidism, mylagia, otitis media.

Prader-Willi syndrome: Genotropin®: Aggressiveness, arthralgia, edema, hair loss, headache, benign intracranial hypertension, myalgia; fatalities associated with use in this population have been reported

Turner syndrome: Humatrope®: Surgical procedures (45%), otitis media (43%), ear disorders (18%), hypothyroidism (13%), increased nevi (11%), peripheral edema (7%)

Adult growth hormone replacement: Increased ALT, increased AST, arthralgia, back pain, carpal tunnel syndrome, diabetes mellitus, fatigue, flu-like syndrome, gastritis, gastroenteritis, generalized edema, glucose intolerance, gynecomastia (rare), headache, hypertension, hypoesthesia, hypothyroidism, infection (nonviral), insomnia, joint disorder, laryngitis, myalgia, nausea, increased growth of pre-existing nevi, pain, pancreatitis (rare), paresthesia, peripheral edema, pharyngitis, rhinitis, stiffness in extremities, weakness

AIDS wasting or cachexia (limited): Serostim®: Musculoskeletal discomfort (54%), increased tissue turgor (27%), diarrhea (26%), neuropathy (26%), nausea (26%), fatigue (17%), albuminuria (15%), increased diaphoresis (14%), anorexia (12%), anemia (12%), increased AST (12%), insomnia (11%), tachycardia (11%), hyperglycemia (10%), increased ALT (10%)

Postmarketing and/or case reports: Diabetes, diabetic ketoacidosis, glucose intolerance

Short-bowel syndrome: Zorbtive™: Peripheral edema (69% to 81%), edema (facial: 44% to 50%; peripheral 13%), arthralgia (13% to 44%), injection site reaction (19% to 31%), flatulence (25%), abdominal pain (20% to 25%), vomiting (19%), malaise (13%), nausea (13%), diaphoresis increased (13%), rhinitis (7%), dizziness (6%)

Postmarketing and/or case reports: Carpal tunnel syndrome

Small for gestational age: Genotropin®: Mild, transient hyperglycemia; benign intracranial hypertension (rare); central precocious puberty; jaw prominence (rare); aggravation of pre-existing scoliosis (rare); injection site reactions; progression of pigmented nevi

Overdosage/Toxicology Symptoms of acute overdose may include initial hypoglycemia (with subsequent hyperglycemia), fluid retention, headache, nausea, and vomiting. Long-term overdose may result in signs and symptoms of acromegaly.

Dosing

Adults:

Growth hormone deficiency: To minimize adverse events in older or overweight patients, reduced dosages may be necessary. During therapy, dosage should be decreased if required by the occurrence of side effects or excessive IGF-I levels.

Norditropin®: SubQ: Initial dose ≤0.004 mg/kg/day; after 6 weeks of therapy, may increase dose to 0.016 mg/kg/day

Nutropin®, Nutropin® AQ: SubQ: ≤0.006 mg/kg/day; dose may be increased according to individual requirements, up to a maximum of 0.025 mg/kg/day

(Continued)

Somatropin *(Continued)*

in patients <35 years of age, or up to a maximum of 0.0125 mg/kg/day in patients ≥35 years of age

Humatrope®: SubQ: ≤0.006 mg/kg/day; dose may be increased according to individual requirements, up to a maximum of 0.0125 mg/kg/day

Genotropin®: SubQ: Weekly dosage: ≤0.04 mg/kg divided into 6-7 doses; dose may be increased at 4- to 8-week intervals according to individual requirements, to a maximum of 0.08 mg/kg/week

Saizen®: SubQ: ≤0.005 mg/kg/day; dose may be increased to not more than 0.01 mg/kg/day after 4 weeks, based on individual requirements.

AIDS-wasting or cachexia:

Serostim®: SubQ: Dose should be given once daily at bedtime; patients who continue to lose weight after 2 weeks should be re-evaluated for opportunistic infections or other clinical events; rotate injection sites to avoid lipodystrophy

Daily dose based on body weight:

<35 kg: 0.1 mg/kg
35-45 kg: 4 mg
45-55 kg: 5 mg
>55 kg: 6 mg

Short-bowel syndrome (Zorbtive™): SubQ: 0.1 mg/kg once daily for 4 weeks (maximum: 8 mg/day)

Fluid retention (moderate) or arthralgias: Treat symptomatically or reduce dose by 50%

Severe toxicity: Discontinue therapy for up to 5 days; when symptoms resolve, restart at 50% of dose. If severe toxicity recurs or does not disappear within 5 days after discontinuation, permanently discontinue treatment.

Elderly: Patients ≥65 years of age may be more sensitive to the action of growth hormone and more prone to adverse effects; in general, dosing should be cautious, beginning at low end of dosing range.

Pediatrics:

Growth hormone deficiency:

Genotropin®: SubQ: Weekly dosage: 0.16-0.24 mg/kg divided into 6-7 doses

Humatrope®: I.M., SubQ: Weekly dosage: 0.18 mg/kg; maximum replacement dose: 0.3 mg/kg/week; dosing should be divided into equal doses given 3 times/week on alternating days, 6 times/week, or daily

Norditropin®: SubQ: 0.024-0.034 mg/kg/day, 6-7 times/week

Nutropin®, Nutropin® AQ: SubQ: Weekly dosage: 0.3 mg/kg divided into daily doses; pubertal patients: ≤0.7 mg/kg/week divided daily

Tev-Tropin™: SubQ: Up to 0.1 mg/kg administered 3 times/week

Saizen®: I.M., SubQ: 0.06 mg/kg/dose administered 3 times/week

Note: Therapy should be discontinued when patient has reached satisfactory adult height, when epiphyses have fused, or when the patient ceases to respond. Growth of 5 cm/year or more is expected, if growth rate does not exceed 2.5 cm in a 6-month period, double the dose for the next 6 months; if there is still no satisfactory response, discontinue therapy

Chronic renal insufficiency (CRI): *Nutropin®, Nutropin® AQ:* SubQ: Weekly dosage: 0.35 mg/kg divided into daily injections; continue until the time of renal transplantation

Dosage recommendations in patients treated for CRI who require dialysis:

Hemodialysis: Administer dose at night prior to bedtime or at least 3-4 hours after hemodialysis to prevent hematoma formation from heparin

CCPD: Administer dose in the morning following dialysis

CAPD: Administer dose in the evening at the time of overnight exchange

Turner syndrome: *Humatrope®, Nutropin®, Nutropin® AQ:* SubQ: Weekly dosage: ≤0.375 mg/kg divided into equal doses 3-7 times per week

Prader-Willi syndrome: *Genotropin®:* SubQ: Weekly dosage: 0.24 mg/kg divided into 6-7 doses

Small for gestational age: *Genotropin®:* SubQ: Weekly dosage: 0.48 mg/kg divided into 6-7 doses

Idiopathic short stature:

Humatrope®: SubQ: Weekly dosage: 0.37 mg/kg divided into equal doses 6-7 times per week

Nutropin®, Nutropin AQ®: SubQ: Weekly dosage: Up to 0.3 mg/kg divided into daily doses

AIDS-wasting or cachexia (unlabeled use): *Serostim®:* SubQ: Limited data; doses of 0.04 mg/kg/day were reported in five children, 6-17 years of age; doses of 0.07 mg/kg/day were reported in six children, 8-14 years of age

Renal Impairment: Reports indicate patients with chronic renal failure tend to have decreased clearance; specific dosing suggestions not available

Hepatic Impairment: Clearance may be reduced in patients with severe hepatic dysfunction; specific dosing suggestions are not available.

Available Dosage Forms [DSC] = Discontinued product

Injection, powder for reconstitution [rDNA origin]:

Genotropin® [preservative free]: 1.5 mg [4 int. units/mL] [delivers 1.3 mg/mL] [DSC]

Genotropin® [with preservative]:

5.8 mg [15 int. units/mL] [delivers 5 mg/mL]

13.8 mg [36 int. units/mL] [delivers 12 mg/mL]

Genotropin Miniquick® [preservative free]: 0.2 mg, 0.4 mg, 0.6 mg, 0.8 mg, 1 mg, 1.2 mg, 1.4 mg, 1.6 mg, 1.8 mg, 2 mg [each strength delivers 0.25 mL]

Humatrope®: 5 mg [~15 int. units], 6 mg [18 int. units], 12 mg [36 int. units], 24 mg [72 int. units]

Nutropin® [diluent contains benzyl alcohol]: 5 mg [~15 int. units]; 10 mg [~30 int. units]

Tev-Tropin™: 5 mg [15 int. units/mL] [diluent contains benzyl alcohol]

Saizen® [diluent contains benzyl alcohol]: 5 mg [~15 int. units; contains sucrose 34.2 mg]; 8.8 mg [~26.4 int. units; contains sucrose 60.2 mg]

Serostim®: 4 mg [12 int. units; contains sucrose 27.3 mg]; 5 mg [15 int. units; contains sucrose 34.2 mg]; 6 mg [18 int. units; contains sucrose 41 mg]

Zorbtive™: 8.8 mg [~26.4 int. units; contains sucrose 60.19 mg; packaged with diluent containing benzyl alcohol]

Injection, solution [rDNA origin]:

Norditropin®: 5 mg/1.5 mL (1.5 mL); 15 mg/1.5 mL (1.5 mL) [cartridge]

Norditropin® NordiFlex®: 5 mg/1.5 mL (1.5 mL); 15 mg/1.5 mL (1.5 mL) [prefilled pen]

Nutropin AQ®: 5 mg/mL [~15 int. units/mL] (2 mL) [vial or cartridge]

Nursing Guidelines

Assessment: Assess potential for interactions with other prescriptions, OTC medications, or herbal products patient may be taking. Assess results of laboratory tests, therapeutic effectiveness (according to purpose for use), and adverse reactions Perform funduscopic examinations at initiation of therapy and periodically during treatment; Instruct patients with diabetes to monitor glucose levels closely (may induce insulin intolerance). Instruct patient in proper use if self-administered (storage, reconstitution, injection techniques, and syringe/needle disposal), possible side effects/appropriate interventions, and adverse symptoms to report. Pediatrics: Monitor growth curve: annually determine bone age.

Monitoring Laboratory Tests: Periodic thyroid function tests, periodical urine testing for glucose, somatomedin C (IGF-I) levels; serum phosphorus, alkaline phosphatase and parathyroid hormone. If growth deceleration is observed in children treated for growth hormone deficiency, and not due to other causes, evaluate for presence of antibody formation. Strict blood glucose monitoring in diabetic patients.

Somatrem (Protropin®): Consider changing to somatropin if antibody binding capacity is >2 mg/L

Dietary Considerations:

Prader-Willi syndrome: All patients should have effective weight control (use is contraindicated in severely-obese patients).

Short-bowel syndrome: Intravenous parenteral nutrition requirements may need reassessment as gastrointestinal absorption improves.

Patient Education: This drug can only be administered by injection. If self-administered, you will be instructed by prescriber on proper storage, reconstitution, injection technique, and syringe/needle disposal. Use exactly as prescribed; do not discontinue or alter dose without consulting prescriber. Report immediately any pain, redness, burning, drainage, or swelling at injection site. If you have diabetes, monitor glucose levels closely; this medication may cause an alteration in your insulin levels. May cause side effects which are particular to purpose for use and formulation prescribed; your prescriber will instruct you in particular side effects for your medication. Report immediately unusual or persistent bleeding, excessive fatigue or swelling (edema) of extremities, joint or muscle pain or headache, nausea or vomiting, personality

(Continued)

Somatropin *(Continued)*

changes, or other persistent adverse effects. **Pregnancy/breast-feeding precaution:** Inform prescriber if you are or intend to become pregnant. Breast-feeding is not recommended.

Pregnancy Risk Factor: B/C (depending upon manufacturer)

Lactation: Excretion in breast milk unknown/not recommended

Administration

I.M.: Do not shake; administer SubQ or I.M. (rotate administration sites to avoid tissue atrophy); refer to product labeling. When administering to newborns, reconstitute with sterile water for injection. Cartridge must be administered using the corresponding color-coded NordiPen® injection pen.

Reconstitution:

Genotropin®: Reconstitute with diluent provided.

Genotropin MiniQuick®: Reconstitute with diluent provided. Consult the instructions provided with the reconstitution device.

Humatrope®:

Cartridge: Consult HumatroPen™ User Guide for complete instructions for reconstitution. **Do not use diluent provided with vials.**

Vial: 5 mg: Reconstitute with 1.5-5 mL diluent provided.

Nutropin®: Vial:

5 mg: Reconstitute with 1-5 mL bacteriostatic water for injection.

10 mg: Reconstitute with 1-10 mL bacteriostatic water for injection.

Saizen®: Vial:

5 mg: Reconstitute with 1-3 mL bacteriostatic water for injection or sterile water for injection; gently swirl; do not shake.

8.8 mg: Reconstitute with 2-3 mL bacteriostatic water for injection or sterile water for injection; gently swirl; do not shake.

Serostim®: Vial: Reconstitute with 0.5-1 mL sterile water for injection.

Tev-Tropin™: Reconstitute with 1-5 mL of diluent provided. Gently swirl; do not shake. May use preservative-free NS for use in newborns.

Zorbtive™: 8.8 mg vial: Reconstitute with 1-2 mL bacteriostatic water for injection; use within 14 days

Storage:

Genotropin®: Store at 2°C to 8°C (36°F to 46°F), do not freeze, protect from light

1.5 mg cartridge: Following reconstitution, store under refrigeration and use within 24 hours; discard unused portion

5.8 mg and 13.8 mg cartridge: Following reconstitution, store under refrigeration and use within 21 days

Miniquick®: Store in refrigerator prior to dispensing, but may be stored ≤25°C (77°F) for up to 3 months after dispensing; once reconstituted, solution must be refrigerated and used within 24 hours; discard unused portion

Humatrope®:

Vial: Before and after reconstitution, store at 2°C to 8°C (36°F to 46°F), avoid freezing; when reconstituted with bacteriostatic water for injection, use within 14 days; when reconstituted with sterile water for injection, use within 24 hours and discard unused portion

Cartridge: Before and after reconstitution, store at 2°C to 8°C (36°F to 46°F), avoid freezing; following reconstitution, stable for 14 days under refrigeration. Dilute with solution provided with cartridges **ONLY**; do not use diluent provided with vials

Norditropin®: Store at 2°C to 8°C (36°F to 46°F), do not freeze; avoid direct light

Cartridge: Must be used within 4 weeks once inserted into pen

Prefilled pen: Must be used within 4 weeks after initial injection

Nutropin®: Before and after reconstitution, store at 2°C to 8°C (36°F to 46°F), avoid freezing

Vial: Reconstitute with bacteriostatic water for injection; use reconstituted vials within 14 days; when reconstituted with sterile water for injection, use immediately and discard unused portion

AQ formulation: Use within 28 days following initial use

Saizen®: Prior to reconstitution, store at room temperature 15°C to 30°C (59°F to 86°F); following reconstitution with bacteriostatic water for injection, reconstituted solution should be refrigerated and used within 14 days; when reconstituted with sterile water for injection, use immediately and discard unused portion

Serostim®: Prior to reconstitution, store at room temperature 15°C to 30°C (59°F to 86°F); reconstitute with sterile water for injection; store reconstituted solution under refrigeration and use within 24 hours, avoid freezing. Do not use if cloudy

Tev-Tropin™: Prior to reconstitution, store at 2°C to 8°C (36°F to 46°F). Following reconstitution with bacteriostatic NS, solution should be refrigerated and used within 14 days. Some cloudiness may occur; do not use if cloudiness persists after warming to room temperature.

Zorbtive™: Store unopened vials and diluent at room temperature of 15°C to 30°C (59°F to 86°F). Store reconstituted 8.8 mg vial under refrigeration at 2°C to 8°C (36°F to 46°F); avoid freezing.

- Sominex® [OTC] *see* DiphenhydrAMINE *on page 546*
- Sominex® Maximum Strength [OTC] *see* DiphenhydrAMINE *on page 546*
- Somnote™ *see* Chloral Hydrate *on page 368*

Sorbitol (SOR bi tole)

Pharmacologic Category Genitourinary Irrigant; Laxative, Osmotic

Use Genitourinary irrigant in transurethral prostatic resection or other transurethral resection or other transurethral surgical procedures; diuretic; humectant; sweetening agent; hyperosmotic laxative; facilitate the passage of sodium polystyrene sulfonate through the intestinal tract

Mechanism of Action A polyalcoholic sugar with osmotic cathartic actions

Pharmacodynamics/Kinetics

Onset of action: 0.25-1 hour

Absorption: Oral, rectal: Poor

Metabolism: Primarily hepatic to fructose

Contraindications Anuria

Warnings/Precautions Use with caution in patients with severe cardiopulmonary or renal impairment and in patients unable to metabolize sorbitol; large volumes may result in fluid overload and/or electrolyte changes

Adverse Reactions Frequency not defined.

Cardiovascular: Edema

Endocrine & metabolic: Fluid and electrolyte losses, hyperglycemia, lactic acidosis

Gastrointestinal: Diarrhea, nausea, vomiting, abdominal discomfort, dry mouth

Overdosage/Toxicology Symptoms of overdose include nausea, diarrhea, fluid and electrolyte loss. Treatment is supportive to ensure fluid and electrolyte balance.

Dosing

Adults & Elderly:

Hyperosmotic laxative (as single dose, at infrequent intervals):

Oral: 30-150 mL (as 70% solution)

Rectal enema: 120 mL as 25% to 30% solution

Adjunct to sodium polystyrene sulfonate: 15 mL as 70% solution orally until diarrhea occurs (10-20 mL/2 hours) or 20-100 mL as an oral vehicle for the sodium polystyrene sulfonate resin

When administered with charcoal:

Oral: 4.3 mL/kg of 70% sorbitol with 1 g/kg of activated charcoal every 4 hours until first stool containing charcoal is passed

Transurethral surgical procedures: Irrigation: Topical: 3% to 3.3% as transurethral surgical procedure irrigation

Pediatrics:

Hyperosmotic laxative (as single dose, at infrequent intervals):

Children 2-11 years:

Oral: 2 mL/kg (as 70% solution)

Rectal enema: 30-60 mL as 25% to 30% solution

Children >12 years: Oral, Rectal enema: Refer to adult dosing.

When administered with charcoal: Oral: Children: 4.3 mL/kg of 35% sorbitol with 1 g/kg of activated charcoal

Available Dosage Forms

Solution, genitourinary irrigation: 3% (3000 mL, 5000 mL); 3.3% (2000 mL, 4000 mL)

Solution, oral: 70% (30 mL, 480 mL, 3840 mL)

Nursing Guidelines

Assessment: When used as cathartic, determine cause of constipation before use. Assess knowledge/teach patient about use of nonpharmacological interventions to prevent constipation.

(Continued)

Sorbitol *(Continued)*

Monitoring Laboratory Tests: Electrolytes

Patient Education: Cathartic: Use of cathartics on a regular basis will have adverse effects. Increased exercise, increased fluid intake, or increased dietary fruit and fiber may be effective in preventing and resolving constipation. **Breast-feeding precaution:** Consult prescriber if breast-feeding.

Geriatric Considerations: Causes for constipation must be evaluated prior to initiating treatment. Nonpharmacological dietary treatment should be initiated before laxative use. Sorbitol is as effective as lactulose but is much less expensive.

Pregnancy Risk Factor: C

Lactation: Excretion in breast milk unknown

Administration

Storage: Protect from freezing. Avoid storage in temperatures >150°F.

♦ Soriatane® *see* Acitretin *on page 83*
♦ Sorine® *see* Sotalol *on page 1562*

Sotalol (SOE ta lole)

U.S. Brand Names Betapace®; Betapace AF®; Sorine®

Synonyms Sotalol Hydrochloride

Pharmacologic Category Antiarrhythmic Agent, Class II; Antiarrhythmic Agent, Class III; Beta-Adrenergic Blocker, Nonselective

Medication Safety Issues

Sound-alike/look-alike issues:

Sotalol may be confused with Stadol®
Betapace® may be confused with Betapace AF®
Betapace AF® may be confused with Betapace®

Use Treatment of documented ventricular arrhythmias (ie, sustained ventricular tachycardia), that in the judgment of the physician are life-threatening; maintenance of normal sinus rhythm in patients with symptomatic atrial fibrillation and atrial flutter who are currently in sinus rhythm. Manufacturer states substitutions should not be made for Betapace AF® since Betapace AF® is distributed with a patient package insert specific for atrial fibrillation/flutter.

Mechanism of Action

Beta-blocker which contains both beta-adrenoreceptor-blocking (Vaughan Williams Class II) and cardiac action potential duration prolongation (Vaughan Williams Class III) properties

Class II effects: Increased sinus cycle length, slowed heart rate, decreased AV nodal conduction, and increased AV nodal refractoriness

Class III effects: Prolongation of the atrial and ventricular monophasic action potentials, and effective refractory prolongation of atrial muscle, ventricular muscle, and atrioventricular accessory pathways in both the antegrade and retrograde directions

Sotalol is a racemic mixture of *d*- and *l*-sotalol; both isomers have similar Class III antiarrhythmic effects while the *l*-isomer is responsible for virtually all of the beta-blocking activity

Sotalol has both $beta_1$- and $beta_2$-receptor blocking activity

The beta-blocking effect of sotalol is a noncardioselective [half maximal at about 80 mg/day and maximal at doses of 320-640 mg/day]. Significant beta-blockade occurs at oral doses as low as 25 mg/day.

The Class III effects are seen only at oral doses ≥160 mg/day

Pharmacodynamics/Kinetics

Onset of action: Rapid, 1-2 hours

Peak effect: 2.5-4 hours

Duration: 8-16 hours

Absorption: Decreased 20% to 30% by meals compared to fasting

Distribution: Low lipid solubility; enters milk of laboratory animals and is reported to be present in human milk

Protein binding: None

Metabolism: None

Bioavailability: 90% to 100%

Half-life elimination: 12 hours; Children: 9.5 hours; terminal half-life decreases with age <2 years (may by ≥1 week in neonates)

Excretion: Urine (as unchanged drug)

Contraindications Hypersensitivity to sotalol or any component of the formulation; bronchial asthma; sinus bradycardia; second- and third-degree AV block (unless a functioning pacemaker is present); congenital or acquired long QT syndromes; cardiogenic shock; uncontrolled congestive heart failure. Betapace AF® is contraindicated in patients with significantly reduced renal filtration (Cl_{cr} <40 mL/minute).

Warnings/Precautions Manufacturer recommends initiation (or reinitiation) and doses increased in a hospital setting with continuous monitoring and staff familiar with the recognition and treatment of life-threatening arrhythmias. Dosage of sotalol should be adjusted gradually with 3 days between dosing increments to achieve steady-state concentrations, and to allow time to monitor QT intervals. Some experts will initiate therapy on an outpatient basis in a patient without heart disease or bradycardia, who has a baseline uncorrected QT interval <450 msec, and normal serum potassium and magnesium levels; close EKG monitoring during this time is necessary. ACC/AHA guidelines for management of atrial fibrillation also recommend that for outpatient initiation the patient not have risk factors predisposing to drug-induced ventricular proarrhythmia (Fuster, 2001). Creatinine clearance must be calculated prior to dosing. Use cautiously in the renally-impaired (dosage adjustment required).

Monitor and adjust dose to prevent QT_c prolongation. Concurrent use with other QT_c-prolonging drugs (including Class I and Class III antiarrhythmics) is generally not recommended; withhold for 3 half-lives. Watch for proarrhythmic effects. Correct electrolyte imbalances before initiating (especially hypokalemia and hyperkalemia). Consider pre-existing conditions such as sick sinus syndrome before initiating. Conduction abnormalities can occur particularly sinus bradycardia. Use cautiously within the first 2 weeks post-MI (experience limited). Administer cautiously in compensated heart failure and monitor for a worsening of the condition. Use caution in patients with PVD (can aggravate arterial insufficiency). Beta-blocker therapy should not be withdrawn abruptly (particularly in patients with CAD), but gradually tapered to avoid acute tachycardia, hypertension, and/or ischemia. Use caution with concurrent use of beta-blockers and either verapamil or diltiazem; bradycardia or heart block can occur. Use cautiously in diabetics because it can mask prominent hypoglycemic symptoms. Can mask signs of thyrotoxicosis. Use care with anesthetic agents which decrease myocardial function.

Drug Interactions

Amiodarone: May cause additive effects on QT_c prolongation as well as decreased heart rate, and has been associated with cardiac arrest in patients receiving beta-blockers.

Antacids (aluminum/magnesium) decrease sotalol blood levels; separate administration by 2 hours.

Antiarrhythmics: Concurrent use of Class Ia or Class III antiarrhythmics may result in additive QT_c prolongation; concurrent use is not recommended.

$Beta_2$ agonists: Effects may be diminished by concurrent sotalol; use caution.

Beta-blockers: Due to shared pharmacological effects, heart rate reductions may be additive; concurrent use is not recommended.

Calcium channel blockers: Concurrent use may lead to additive effects on AV conduction, ventricular contractility, and/or hypotension; use caution.

Cisapride: Concurrent use with sotalol increases malignant arrhythmias; contraindicated.

Clonidine: Sotalol may cause rebound hypertension after discontinuation of clonidine.

QT_c-prolonging drugs: Concurrent use may result in additive QT_c prolongation, potentially increasing the risk of malignant arrhythmias. Use of cisapride, mesoridazine, thioridazine, and pimozide with other QT_c-prolonging agents is contraindicated. Concurrent use of sotalol with Class I and Class III antiarrhythmics is not recommended; withhold for 3 half-lives. Use caution with other QT_c-prolonging agents (including bepridil, erythromycin, clarithromycin), fluoroquinolones (including sparfloxacin, gatifloxacin, and moxifloxacin), haloperidol, and TCAs.

Phenothiazines (mesoridazine and thioridazine): Concurrent use may result in additive QT_c prolongation, potentially increasing the risk of malignant arrhythmias; contraindicated.

Pimozide: Concurrent use may result in additive QT_c prolongation, potentially increasing the risk of malignant arrhythmias; contraindicated.

Nutritional/Herbal/Ethanol Interactions

Food: Sotalol peak serum concentrations may be decreased if taken with food.

Herb/Nutraceutical: Avoid ephedra (may worsen arrhythmia).

(Continued)

Sotalol *(Continued)*

Adverse Reactions

>10%:

Cardiovascular: Bradycardia (16%), chest pain (16%), palpitation (14%)

Central nervous system: Fatigue (20%), dizziness (20%), lightheadedness (12%)

Neuromuscular & skeletal: Weakness (13%)

Respiratory: Dyspnea (21%)

1% to 10%:

Cardiovascular: CHF (5%), peripheral vascular disorders (3%), edema (8%), abnormal ECG (7%), hypotension (6%), proarrhythmia (5% in ventricular arrhythmia patients; less than 1% in atrial fibrillation/flutter), syncope (5%)

Central nervous system: Mental confusion (6%), anxiety (4%), headache (8%), sleep problems (8%), depression (4%)

Dermatologic: Itching/rash (5%)

Endocrine & metabolic: Sexual ability decreased (3%)

Gastrointestinal: Diarrhea (7%), nausea/vomiting (10%), stomach discomfort (3% to 6%), flatulence (2%)

Genitourinary: Impotence (2%)

Hematologic: Bleeding (2%)

Neuromuscular & skeletal: Paresthesia (4%), extremity pain (7%), back pain (3%)

Ocular: Visual problems (5%)

Respiratory: Upper respiratory problems (5% to 8%), asthma (2%)

<1% (Limited to important or life-threatening): Alopecia, bronchiolitis obliterans with organized pneumonia (BOOP), cold extremities, diaphoresis, eosinophilia, leukocytoclastic vasculitis, leukopenia, paralysis, phlebitis, photosensitivity reaction, pruritus, pulmonary edema, Raynaud's phenomenon, red crusted skin, retroperitoneal fibrosis, serum transaminases increased, skin necrosis after extravasation, thrombocytopenia, vertigo

Overdosage/Toxicology Symptoms of intoxication include cardiac disturbances, CNS toxicity, bronchospasm, hypoglycemia and hyperkalemia. The most common cardiac symptoms include hypotension and bradycardia; atrioventricular block, intraventricular conduction disturbances, cardiogenic shock, and asystole may occur with severe overdose, especially with membrane-depressant drugs (eg, propranolol); CNS effects include convulsions, coma, and respiratory arrest is commonly seen with propranolol and other membrane-depressant and lipid-soluble drugs.

Treatment includes symptomatic treatment of seizures, hypotension, hyperkalemia and hypoglycemia. Bradycardia and hypotension resistant to atropine, isoproterenol or pacing may respond to glucagon. Wide QRS defects caused by the membrane-depressant poisoning may respond to hypertonic sodium bicarbonate. Repeat-dose charcoal, hemoperfusion, or hemodialysis may be helpful in removal of only those beta-blockers with a small V_d, long half-life, or low intrinsic clearance (acebutolol, atenolol, nadolol, sotalol).

Dosing

Adults & Elderly: Sotalol should be initiated and doses increased in a hospital with facilities for cardiac rhythm monitoring and assessment. Proarrhythmic events can occur after initiation of therapy and with each upward dosage adjustment.

Ventricular arrhythmias (Betapace®, Sorine®): Oral:

Initial: 80 mg twice daily; dose may be increased gradually to 240-320 mg/day; allow 3 days between dosing increments (to attain steady-state plasma concentrations and to allow monitoring of QT intervals).

Usual range: Most patients respond to 160-320 mg/day in 2-3 divided doses.

Maximum: Some patients, with life-threatening refractory ventricular arrhythmias, may require doses as high as 480-640 mg/day; prescribed ONLY when the potential benefit outweighs the increased of adverse events.

Atrial fibrillation or atrial flutter (Betapace AF®): Oral: Initial: 80 mg twice daily

Note: If the initial dose does not reduce the frequency of relapses of atrial fibrillation/flutter and is tolerated without excessive QT prolongation (not >520 msec) after 3 days, the dose may be increased to 120 mg twice daily. This may be further increased to 160 mg twice daily if response is inadequate and QT prolongation is not excessive.

Pediatrics: Sotalol should be initiated and doses increased in a hospital with facilities for cardiac rhythm monitoring and assessment. Proarrhythmic events can occur after initiation of therapy and with each upward dosage adjustment.

Note: The safety and efficacy of sotalol in children have not been established

Supraventricular arrhythmias: Oral: **Note:** Dosing per manufacturer, based on pediatric pharmacokinetic data; wait at least 36 hours between dosage adjustments to allow monitoring of QT intervals

Children ≤2 years: Dosage should be adjusted (decreased) by plotting of the child's age on a logarithmic scale; see graph or refer to manufacturer's package labeling.

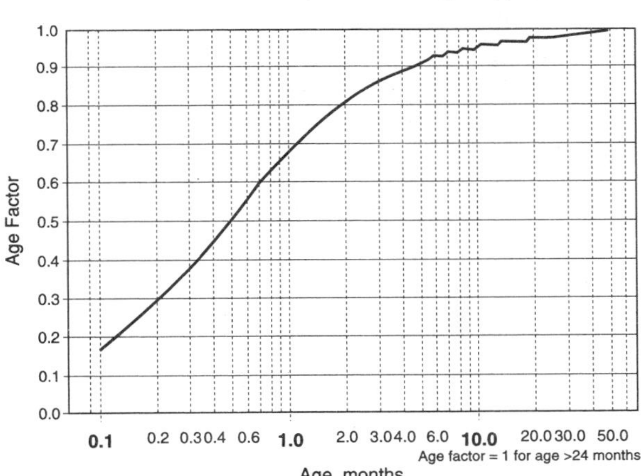

Adapted from U.S. Food and Drug Administration.
http://www.fda.gov/cder/foi/label/2001/2115s3lbl.PDF

Children >2 years: Initial: 90 mg/m^2/day in 3 divided doses; may be incrementally increased to a maximum of 180 mg/m^2/day

Renal Impairment: Adults: Impaired renal function can increase the terminal half-life, resulting in increased drug accumulation. Sotalol (Betapace AF®) is contraindicated per the manufacturer for treatment of atrial fibrillation/flutter in patients with a Cl_{cr} <40 mL/minute.

Ventricular arrhythmias (Betapace®, Sorine®):

Cl_{cr} >60 mL/minute: Administer every 12 hours.

Cl_{cr} 30-60 mL/minute: Administer every 24 hours.

Cl_{cr} 10-30 mL/minute: Administer every 36-48 hours.

Cl_{cr} <10 mL/minute: Individualize dose.

Atrial fibrillation/flutter (Betapace AF®):

Cl_{cr} >60 mL/minute: Administer every 12 hours.

Cl_{cr} 40-60 mL/minute: Administer every 24 hours.

Cl_{cr} <40 mL/minute: Use is contraindicated.

Dialysis: Hemodialysis would be expected to reduce sotalol plasma concentrations because sotalol is not bound to plasma proteins and does not undergo extensive metabolism. Administer dose postdialysis or administer supplemental 80 mg dose. Peritoneal dialysis does not remove sotalol; supplemental dose is not necessary.

Available Dosage Forms

Tablet, as hydrochloride: 80 mg, 80 mg [AF], 120 mg, 120 mg [AF], 160 mg, 160 mg [AF], 240 mg

Betapace® [light blue]: 80 mg, 120 mg, 160 mg, 240 mg

Betapace AF® [white]: 80 mg, 120 mg, 160 mg

(Continued)

Sotalol *(Continued)*

Sorine® [white]: 80 mg, 120 mg, 160 mg, 240 mg

Nursing Guidelines

Assessment: Assess potential for interactions with other prescriptions, OTC medications, or herbal products patient may be taking. Assess blood pressure and heart rate prior to and following first dose and with any change in dosage. Assess results of laboratory tests, therapeutic effectiveness, and adverse effects (eg, cardiac and pulmonary status). Advise patients with diabetes to monitor glucose levels closely (beta-blockers may alter glucose tolerance). Do not discontinue abruptly; dose should be tapered gradually. Teach patient appropriate use, possible side effects/interventions (hypotension precautions), and adverse symptoms to report.

Monitoring Laboratory Tests: Serum magnesium, potassium

Dietary Considerations: Administer on an empty stomach.

Patient Education: Do not take any new medications without consulting prescriber. Take exactly as directed; do not adjust dosage or discontinue without consulting prescriber. Take pulse daily (prior to medication) and follow prescriber's instruction about holding of medication. If you have diabetes, monitor serum sugar closely (drug may alter glucose tolerance or mask signs of hypoglycemia). May cause fatigue, dizziness, lightheadedness, or postural hypotension (use caution when changing position from lying or sitting to standing, when driving, or climbing stairs until response to medication is known); alteration in sexual performance (reversible); nausea or vomiting (small frequent meals, frequent mouth care, sucking lozenges, or chewing gum may help); or diarrhea (boiled milk, buttermilk, or yogurt may help). Report immediately any chest pain, palpitations, irregular heartbeat; swelling of extremities, respiratory difficulty, new cough, or unusual fatigue; persistent nausea, vomiting, or diarrhea; or unusual muscle weakness. **Breast-feeding precaution:** Consult prescriber if breast-feeding.

Geriatric Considerations: Since elderly frequently have Cl_{cr} <60 mL/minute, attention to dose, creatinine clearance, and monitoring is important. Make dosage adjustments at 3-day intervals or after 5-6 doses at any dosage.

Pregnancy Risk Factor: B

Pregnancy Issues: There are no adequate and well-controlled studies in pregnant women. Beta-blockers have been associated with bradycardia, hypotension, and IUGR; IUGR is probably related to maternal hypertension. Sotalol has been shown to cross the placenta, and is found in amniotic fluid; therefore, sotalol should be used during pregnancy only if the potential benefit outweighs the potential risk. Cases of neonatal hypoglycemia have been reported following maternal use of beta-blockers at parturition or during breast-feeding. Monitor breast-fed infant for symptoms of beta-blockade.

Lactation: Enters breast milk/use caution (AAP rates "compatible")

Breast-Feeding Considerations: Sotalol is considered compatible by the AAP. It is recommended that the infant be monitored for signs or symptoms of beta-blockade (hypotension, bradycardia, etc) with long-term use.

Perioperative/Anesthesia/Other Concerns: Withdrawal: Beta-blocker therapy should not be withdrawn abruptly, but gradually tapered to avoid acute tachycardia and hypertension.

Administration

Storage: Store at 25°C (77°F). Excursions permitted to 15°C to 30°C (59°F to 86°F).

- ♦ Sotalol Hydrochloride *see* Sotalol *on page 1562*
- ♦ Sotradecol® *see* Sodium Tetradecyl *on page 1554*
- ♦ Sotret® *see* Isotretinoin *on page 981*
- ♦ SPA *see* Albumin *on page 94*
- ♦ Spacol [DSC] *see* Hyoscyamine *on page 886*
- ♦ Spacol T/S [DSC] *see* Hyoscyamine *on page 886*
- ♦ SPD417 *see* Carbamazepine *on page 306*
- ♦ Spectracef™ *see* Cefditoren *on page 335*

Spironolactone (speer on oh LAK tone)

U.S. Brand Names Aldactone®

Pharmacologic Category Diuretic, Potassium-Sparing; Selective Aldosterone Blocker

Medication Safety Issues

Sound-alike/look-alike issues:

Aldactone® may be confused with Aldactazide®

Use Management of edema associated with excessive aldosterone excretion; hypertension; congestive heart failure; primary hyperaldosteronism; hypokalemia; treatment of hirsutism; cirrhosis of liver accompanied by edema or ascites

Unlabeled/Investigational Use Female acne (adjunctive therapy); hirsutism; hypertension (pediatric); diuretic (pediatric)

Mechanism of Action Competes with aldosterone for receptor sites in the distal renal tubules, increasing sodium chloride and water excretion while conserving potassium and hydrogen ions; may block the effect of aldosterone on arteriolar smooth muscle as well

Pharmacodynamics/Kinetics

Duration of action: 2-3 days

Protein binding: 91% to 98%

Metabolism: Hepatic to multiple metabolites, including canrenone (active)

Half-life elimination: 78-84 minutes

Time to peak, serum: 1-3 hours (primarily as the active metabolite)

Excretion: Urine and feces

Contraindications Hypersensitivity to spironolactone or any component of the formulation; anuria; acute renal insufficiency; significant impairment of renal excretory function; hyperkalemia; pregnancy (pregnancy-induced hypertension - per expert analysis)

Warnings/Precautions Avoid potassium supplements, potassium-containing salt substitutes, a diet rich in potassium, or other drugs that can cause hyperkalemia. Monitor for fluid and electrolyte imbalances. Gynecomastia is related to dose and duration of therapy. Diuretic therapy should be carefully used in severe hepatic dysfunction; electrolyte and fluid shifts can cause or exacerbate encephalopathy. Discontinue use prior to adrenal vein catheterization. When evaluating a heart failure patient for spironolactone treatment, creatinine should be ≤2.5 mg/dL in men or ≤2 mg/dL in women and potassium <5 mEq/L.

Drug Interactions

ACE inhibitors can cause hyperkalemia, especially in patients with renal impairment, potassium-rich diets, or on other drugs causing hyperkalemia; avoid concurrent use or monitor closely.

Cholestyramine can cause hyperchloremic acidosis in cirrhotic patients; avoid concurrent use.

Digoxin's positive inotropic effect may be reduced; serum levels of digoxin may increase.

Mitotane loses its effect; avoid concurrent use.

Potassium supplements may increase potassium retention and cause hyperkalemia; avoid concurrent use.

Salicylates and NSAIDs may interfere with the natriuretic action of spironolactone.

Nutritional/Herbal/Ethanol Interactions

Food: Food increases absorption.

Herb/Nutraceutical: Avoid natural licorice (due to mineralocorticoid activity)

Lab Interactions May cause false elevation in serum digoxin concentrations measured by RIA.

Adverse Reactions Incidence of adverse events is not always reported (mean daily dose 26 mg).

Cardiovascular: Edema (2%, placebo 2%)

Central nervous system: Disorders (23%, placebo 21%) which may include drowsiness, lethargy, headache, mental confusion, drug fever, ataxia, fatigue

Dermatologic: Maculopapular, erythematous cutaneous eruptions, urticaria, hirsutism, eosinophilia

Endocrine & metabolic: Gynecomastia (men 9%; placebo 1%), breast pain (men 2%; placebo 0.1%), serious hyperkalemia (2%, placebo 1%), hyponatremia, dehydration, hyperchloremic metabolic acidosis (in decompensated hepatic cirrhosis), impotence, menstrual irregularities, amenorrhea, postmenopausal bleeding

Gastrointestinal: Disorders (29%, placebo 29%) which may include anorexia, nausea, cramping, diarrhea, gastric bleeding, ulceration, gastritis, vomiting

Hematologic: Agranulocytosis

Hepatic: Cholestatic/hepatocellular toxicity

Renal: Increased BUN concentration

Miscellaneous: Deepening of the voice, anaphylactic reaction, breast cancer

(Continued)

Spironolactone *(Continued)*

Overdosage/Toxicology Symptoms of overdose include drowsiness, confusion, clinical signs of dehydration and electrolyte imbalance, and hyperkalemia. Ingestion of large amounts of potassium-sparing diuretics may result in life-threatening hyperkalemia. This can be treated with I.V. glucose, with concurrent regular insulin. Sodium bicarbonate may also be used as a temporary measure. If needed, Kayexalate® oral or rectal solutions in sorbitol may also be used.

Dosing

Adults: To reduce delay in onset of effect, a loading dose of 2 or 3 times the daily dose may be administered on the first day of therapy. Oral:

Edema, hypokalemia: 25-200 mg/day in 1-2 divided doses
Hypertension (JNC 7): 25-50 mg/day in 1-2 divided doses
Diagnosis of primary aldosteronism: 100-400 mg/day in 1-2 divided doses
Acne in women (unlabeled use): 25-200 mg once daily
Hirsutism in women (unlabeled use): 50-200 mg/day in 1-2 divided doses
CHF, severe (with ACE inhibitor and a loop diuretic ± digoxin): 12.5-25 mg/day; maximum daily dose: 50 mg (higher doses may occasionallly be used). In the RALES trial, 25 mg every other day was the lowest maintenance dose possible.

Note: If potassium >5.4 mEq/L, consider dosage reduction.

Elderly: Oral: Initial: 25-50 mg/day in 1-2 divided doses; increase by 25-50 mg every 5 days as needed. Adjust for renal impairment.

Pediatrics: Administration with food increases absorption. To reduce delay in onset of effect, a loading dose of 2 or 3 times the daily dose may be administered on the first day of therapy.

Edema, hypertension (unlabeled use): Oral: Children 1-17 years: Initial: 1 mg/kg/day divided every 12-24 hours (maximum dose: 3.3 mg/kg/day, up to 100 mg/day)

Diagnosis of primary aldosteronism (unlabeled use): Oral: 125-375 mg/m^2/day in divided doses

Renal Impairment:

Cl_{cr} 10-50 mL/minute: Administer every 12-24 hours.
Cl_{cr} <10 mL/minute: Avoid use.

Available Dosage Forms Tablet: 25 mg, 50 mg, 100 mg

Nursing Guidelines

Assessment: See Contraindications and Warnings/Precautions for use cautions. Diuretic effect may be delayed 2-3 days and antihypertensive effect may be delayed 2-3 weeks (see Dosing to reduce delayed effect). Assess potential for interactions with other prescriptions, OTC medications, or herbal products patient may be taking (see Drug Interactions). Assess results of laboratory tests (see below) and patient response (eg, fluid status and electrolytes - see Adverse Reactions and Overdose/Toxicology). Teach patient appropriate use, possible side effects/appropriate interventions (eg, photosensitivity), and adverse symptoms to report (eg, opportunistic infection - see Patient Education). **Pregnancy risk factor C/D** - see Pregnancy Risk Factor for use cautions; determine that patient is not pregnant before beginning treatment. Instruct patients of childbearing age about necessity for barrier contraceptive measures.

Monitoring Laboratory Tests: Serum electrolytes (potassium, sodium), renal function

Dietary Considerations: Should be taken with food to decrease gastrointestinal irritation and to increase absorption. Excessive potassium intake (eg, salt substitutes, low-salt foods, bananas, nuts) should be avoided.

Patient Education: Inform prescriber of all prescriptions, OTC medications, or herbal products you are taking, and any allergies you have. Do not take any new medication during therapy unless approved by prescriber. Take as directed, with meals. Do not increase dietary potassium. Avoid natural licorice. Weigh yourself weekly at the same time, in the same clothes, and report weight loss >5 lb/week. May cause dizziness, drowsiness, confusion, or headache (use caution when driving or engaging in tasks requiring alertness until response to drug is known); nausea, vomiting, or dry mouth (small, frequent meals, frequent mouth care, sucking lozenges, or chewing gum may help); or decreased sexual ability, gynecomastia, impotence, menstrual irregularities (reversible with discontinuing of medication). Report mental confusion; clumsiness; persistent fatigue, chills, numbness, or muscle weakness in hands, feet, or face; acute persistent diarrhea; breast tenderness or increased body hair in females; breast enlargement or inability to achieve erection in males; chest pain, rapid heartbeat, or palpitations; excessive thirst; or respiratory difficulty. **Pregnancy precaution:** Do not get pregnant while taking this medication. Consult prescriber for appropriate barrier contraceptive measures.

Geriatric Considerations: See Warnings/Precautions. When used in combination with ACE inhibitors, monitor patient for hyperkalemia.

Pregnancy Risk Factor: C/D in pregnancy-induced hypertension (per expert analysis)

Pregnancy Issues: Teratogenic effects were not observed in animal studies; however, doses used were less than or equal to equivalent doses in humans. The antiandrogen effects of spironolactone have been shown to cause feminization of the male fetus in animal studies. Two case reports did not demonstrate this effect in humans however, the authors caution that adequate data is lacking. Diuretics are generally avoided in pregnancy due to the theoretical risk that decreased plasma volume may cause placental insufficiency. Diuretics should not be used during pregnancy in the presence of reduced placental perfusion (eg, pre-eclampsia, intrauterine growth restriction).

Lactation: Enters breast milk/not recommended (AAP rates "compatible")

Breast-Feeding Considerations: The active metabolite of spironolactone has been found in breast milk. Effects to humans are not known; however, this metabolite was found to be carcinogenic in rats. The manufacturer recommends discontinuing spironolactone or using an alternative method of feeding.

Perioperative/Anesthesia/Other Concerns: In severe heart failure, spironolactone (25 mg/day), when combined with maximal standard therapy, resulted in a striking improvement in cardiovascular outcome (*N Engl J Med*, 1999, 341:709-17).

Potassium levels should be monitored in patients on an aldosterone blocker, particularly in those who have underlying renal impairment or concurrent ACE inhibitor therapy.

Administration

Storage: Protect from light.

- Spironolactone and Hydrochlorothiazide *see* Hydrochlorothiazide and Spironolactone *on page 865*
- Sprintec™ *see* Ethinyl Estradiol and Norgestimate *on page 689*
- SPS® *see* Sodium Polystyrene Sulfonate *on page 1553*
- SSD® *see* Silver Sulfadiazine *on page 1533*
- SSD® AF *see* Silver Sulfadiazine *on page 1533*
- Stadol® *see* Butorphanol *on page 282*
- Stadol® NS [DSC] *see* Butorphanol *on page 282*
- Stagesic® *see* Hydrocodone and Acetaminophen *on page 867*
- Staticin® [DSC] *see* Erythromycin *on page 634*
- Sterapred® *see* PredniSONE *on page 1403*
- Sterapred® DS *see* PredniSONE *on page 1403*
- Stimate™ *see* Desmopressin *on page 492*
- Sting-Kill [OTC] *see* Benzocaine *on page 232*
- St. Joseph® Adult Aspirin [OTC] *see* Aspirin *on page 189*
- Streptase® *see* Streptokinase *on page 1569*

Streptokinase (strep toe KYE nase)

U.S. Brand Names Streptase®

Synonyms SK

Pharmacologic Category Thrombolytic Agent

Use Thrombolytic agent used in treatment of recent severe or massive deep vein thrombosis, pulmonary emboli, myocardial infarction, and occluded arteriovenous cannulas

Mechanism of Action Activates the conversion of plasminogen to plasmin by forming a complex, exposing plasminogen-activating site, and cleaving a peptide bond that converts plasminogen to plasmin; plasmin degrades fibrin, fibrinogen and other procoagulant proteins into soluble fragments; effective both outside and within the formed thrombus/embolus

Pharmacodynamics/Kinetics

Onset of action: Activation of plasminogen occurs almost immediately
Duration: Fibrinolytic effect: Several hours; Anticoagulant effect: 12-24 hours
Half-life elimination: 83 minutes
Excretion: By circulating antibodies and the reticuloendothelial system

(Continued)

Streptokinase *(Continued)*

Contraindications Hypersensitivity to anistreplase, streptokinase, or any component of the formulation; active internal bleeding; history of CVA; recent (within 2 months) intracranial or intraspinal surgery or trauma; intracranial neoplasm, arteriovenous malformation, or aneurysm; known bleeding diathesis; severe uncontrolled hypertension

Warnings/Precautions Concurrent heparin anticoagulation can contribute to bleeding; careful attention to all potential bleeding sites. I.M. injections and nonessential handling of the patient should be avoided. Venipunctures should be performed carefully and only when necessary. If arterial puncture is necessary, use an upper extremity vessel that can be manually compressed. If serious bleeding occurs then the infusion of streptokinase and heparin should be stopped.

For the following conditions the risk of bleeding is higher with use of thrombolytics and should be weighed against the benefits of therapy: recent (within 10 days) major surgery (eg, CABG, obstetrical delivery, organ biopsy, previous puncture of noncompressible vessels), cerebrovascular disease, recent (within 10 days) gastrointestinal or genitourinary bleeding, recent trauma (within 10 days) including CPR, hypertension (systolic BP >180 mm Hg and/or diastolic BP >110 mm Hg), high likelihood of left heart thrombus (eg, mitral stenosis with atrial fibrillation), acute pericarditis, subacute bacterial endocarditis, hemostatic defects including ones caused by severe renal or hepatic dysfunction, significant hepatic dysfunction, pregnancy, diabetic hemorrhagic retinopathy or other hemorrhagic ophthalmic conditions, septic thrombophlebitis or occluded AV cannula at seriously infected site, advanced age (eg, >75 years), patients receiving oral anticoagulants, any other condition in which bleeding constitutes a significant hazard or would be particularly difficult to manage because of location.

Coronary thrombolysis may result in reperfusion arrhythmias. Hypotension, occasionally severe, can occur (not from bleeding or anaphylaxis). Follow standard MI management. Rare anaphylactic reactions can occur. Cautious repeat administration in patients who have received anistreplase or streptokinase within 1 year (streptokinase antibody may decrease effectiveness or risk of allergic reactions). Safety and efficacy in pediatric patients have not been established.

Streptokinase is not indicated for restoration of patency of intravenous catheters. Serious adverse events relating to the use of streptokinase in the restoration of patency of occluded intravenous catheters have involved the use of high doses of streptokinase in small volumes (250,000 international units in 2 mL). Uses of lower doses of streptokinase in infusions over several hours, generally into partially occluded catheters, or local instillation into the catheter lumen and subsequent aspiration, have been described in the medical literature. Healthcare providers should consider the risk for potentially life-threatening reactions (hypersensitivity, apnea, bleeding) associated with the use of streptokinase in the management of occluded intravenous catheters.

Drug Interactions

Aminocaproic acid (antifibrinolytic agent) may decrease effectiveness of thrombolytic agents.

Drugs which affect platelet function (eg, NSAIDs, dipyridamole, ticlopidine, clopidogrel, IIb/IIIa antagonists) may potentiate the risk of hemorrhage; use with caution.

Heparin and aspirin: Use with aspirin and heparin may increase bleeding over aspirin and heparin alone. However, aspirin and heparin were used concurrently in the majority of patients in some major clinical studies of streptokinase.

Warfarin or oral anticoagulants: Risk of bleeding may be increased during concurrent therapy.

Nutritional/Herbal/Ethanol Interactions Herb/Nutraceutical: Avoid cat's claw, dong quai, evening primrose, feverfew, red clover, horse chestnut, garlic, green tea, ginseng, ginkgo (all have additional antiplatelet activity).

Adverse Reactions As with all drugs which may affect hemostasis, bleeding is the major adverse effect associated with streptokinase. Hemorrhage may occur at virtually any site. Risk is dependent on multiple variables, including the dosage administered, concurrent use of multiple agents which alter hemostasis, and patient predisposition (including hypertension). Rapid lysis of coronary artery thrombi by thrombolytic agents may be associated with reperfusion-related atrial and/or ventricular arrhythmia.

>10%:

Cardiovascular: Hypotension

Local: Injection site bleeding

1% to 10%:

Central nervous system: Fever (1% to 4%)

Dermatologic: Bruising, rash, pruritus

Gastrointestinal: Gastrointestinal hemorrhage, nausea, vomiting

Genitourinary: Genitourinary hemorrhage

Hematologic: Anemia

Neuromuscular & skeletal: Muscle pain

Ocular: Eye hemorrhage, periorbital edema

Respiratory: Bronchospasm, epistaxis

Miscellaneous: Diaphoresis

<1% (Limited to important or life-threatening): Acute tubular necrosis, allergic reactions, anaphylactic shock, anaphylactoid reactions, anaphylaxis, angioneurotic edema, ARDS, back pain (during infusion), cholesterol embolization, erysipelas-like rash, Guillain-Barré syndrome, hemarthrosis, intracranial hemorrhage, laryngeal edema, morbilliform, Parsonage-Turner syndrome, pericardial hemorrhage, respiratory depression, retroperitoneal hemorrhage, splenic rupture, transaminases increased, urticaria

Additional cardiovascular events associated with use in MI: Asystole, AV block, cardiac arrest, cardiac tamponade, cardiogenic shock, electromechanical dissociation, heart failure, mitral regurgitation, myocardial rupture, pericardial effusion, pericarditis, pulmonary edema, recurrent ischemia/infarction, thromboembolism, ventricular tachycardia

Overdosage/Toxicology Symptoms of overdose include epistaxis, bleeding gums, hematoma, spontaneous ecchymoses, and oozing at the catheter site. If uncontrollable bleeding occurs, discontinue infusion. Whole blood or blood products may be used to reverse bleeding.

Dosing

Adults & Elderly: I.V.:

Note: Antibodies to streptokinase remain for at least 3-6 months after initial dose: See Warnings/Precautions. An intradermal skin test of 100 units has been suggested to predict allergic response to streptokinase. If a positive reaction is not seen after 15-20 minutes, a therapeutic dose may be administered.

Guidelines for acute myocardial infarction (AMI): I.V.: 1.5 million units over 60 minutes

Administration:

Dilute two 750,000 unit vials of streptokinase with 5 mL dextrose 5% in water (D_5W) each, gently swirl to dissolve.

Add this dose of the 1.5 million units to 150 mL D_5W.

This should be infused over 60 minutes; an in-line filter ≥0.45 micron should be used.

Monitor for the first few hours for signs of anaphylaxis or allergic reaction. **Infusion should be slowed if lowering of 25 mm Hg in blood pressure or terminated if asthmatic symptoms appear**.

Note: If heparin is administered, start when aPTT is less than 2 times the upper limit of control; do not use a bolus, but initiate infusion adjusted to a target a PTT of 1.5-2 times the upper limit of control. If heparin is not administered by infusion, initiate 7500-12,500 units SubQ every 12 hours.

Guidelines for acute pulmonary embolism (APE): I.V.: 3 million unit dose over 24 hours

Administration:

Dilute four 750,000 unit vials of streptokinase with 5 mL dextrose 5% in water (D_5W) each, gently swirl to dissolve.

Add this dose of 3 million units to 250 mL D_5W, an in-line filter ≥0.45 micron should be used.

Administer 250,000 units (23 mL) over 30 minutes followed by 100,000 units/hour (9 mL/hour) for 24 hours.

Monitor for the first few hours for signs of anaphylaxis or allergic reaction. **Infusion should be slowed if blood pressure is lowered by 25 mm Hg or if asthmatic symptoms appear**.

Begin heparin 1000 units/hour about 3-4 hours after completion of streptokinase infusion or when PTT is <100 seconds.

Guidelines for thromboses: I.V.: Administer 250,000 units to start, then 100,000 units/hour for 24-72 hours depending on location.

(Continued)

Streptokinase *(Continued)*

Cannula occlusion: 250,000 units into cannula, clamp for 2 hours, then aspirate contents and flush with normal saline; **Not recommended; see Warnings/Precautions**

Pediatrics: Children: Safety and efficacy not established; limited studies have used the following doses.

Thromboses: I.V.: *Chest*, 1998 recommendations: Initial (loading dose): 2000 units/kg followed by 2000 units/kg/hour for 6-12 hours **or** initial (loading dose): 3500-4000 units/kg over 30 minutes followed by I.V. continuous infusion: 1000-1500 units/kg/hour; dose should be individualized based on response.

Clotted catheter: I.V.: **Note:** Not recommended due to possibility of allergic reactions with repeated doses: 10,000-25,000 units diluted in NS to a final volume equivalent to catheter volume; instill into catheter and leave in place for 1 hour, then aspirate contents out of catheter and flush catheter with normal saline.

Available Dosage Forms [DSC] = Discontinued product

Injection, powder for reconstitution: 250,000 int. units; 750,000 int. units; 1,500,000 int. units [DSC]

Nursing Guidelines

Assessment: See Contraindications, Warnings/Precautions, and Dosing for use cautions. **Note:** Streptokinase is not indicated for restoration of patency of intravenous catheters; potentially life-threatening reactions (eg, hypersensitivity, apnea, bleeding) are associated with the use of streptokinase in the management of occluded intravenous catheters. Assess potential for interactions with other prescriptions, OTC medications, or herbal products patient may be taking (especially those medications that may affect coagulation or platelet function - see Drug Interactions). Assess results of laboratory results (see below). See Administration infusion specifics; assess infusion site and monitor for systemic hemorrhage during and following therapy (see Adverse Reactions and Overdose/Toxicology). Neurological status (eg, intracranial hemorrhage), vital signs, and ECG (reperfusion arrhythmias) should be monitored prior to, during, and after therapy. Bedrest and bleeding precautions should be maintained. Avoid I.M. injections and nonessential handling of the patient; venipunctures should be performed carefully and only when necessary. If arterial puncture is necessary, use an upper extremity vessel that can be manually compressed. Patient instructions determined by patient condition (see Patient Education). Note breast-feeding caution.

Monitoring Laboratory Tests: PT, aPTT, platelet count, hematocrit, fibrinogen concentration

Patient Education: Inform prescriber of all prescriptions, OTC medications, or herbal products you are taking, and any allergies you have. This medication can only be administered by infusion; you will be monitored closely during and after treatment: immediately report burning, pain, redness, swelling, or oozing at infusion site, acute headache, joint pain, chest pain, or altered vision, You will have a tendency to bleed easily; use caution to prevent injury (use electric razor, soft toothbrush, and caution with knives, needles, or anything sharp). Follow instructions for strict bedrest to reduce the risk of injury. If bleeding occurs, report immediately and apply pressure to bleeding spot until bleeding stops completely. Report unusual bruising or bleeding; blood in urine, stool, or vomitus; bleeding gums; vision changes; or respiratory difficulty. **Pregnancy/breast-feeding precautions:** Inform prescriber if you are or intend to become pregnant. Consult prescriber if breast-feeding.

Geriatric Considerations: Investigators applied analysis to data for patients ≥75 years of age from two large trials studying the impact of streptokinase on patient outcome after acute myocardial infarction. Their conclusion was that age alone is not a contraindication to the use of streptokinase and that thrombolytic therapy is cost-effective and is beneficial toward the survival of elderly patients. Additional studies are needed to determine if a weight-adjusted dose will maintain efficacy but decrease adverse events such as stroke.

Pregnancy Risk Factor: C

Lactation: Excretion in breast milk unknown

Perioperative/Anesthesia/Other Concerns: Streptokinase can cause hypotension and anaphylaxis or allergic reaction. Heparin should be initiated several hours after completion of streptokinase therapy with close monitoring of the coagulation profile.

Antibodies to streptokinase (even if anistreplase was used) persist for up to 6 months after the initial dose. Therefore, an alternative thrombolytic approach (tissue plasminogen activator) should be used if thrombolytic therapy is needed. Furthermore, patients who have had a recent streptococcal infection (within 6 months) may also manifest hypersensitivity to streptokinase. a hypersensitivity response to urokinase.

Administration

I.M.: Do **not** administer by intramuscular injection.

I.V.: For I.V. or intracoronary use only. Infusion pump is required. Use in-line filter >0.8 micron.

Reconstitution: Reconstituted solutions should be refrigerated and are stable for 24 hours.

Compatibility: Stable in D_5W, NS; **incompatible** with dextrans

Storage: Streptokinase, a white lyophilized powder, may have a slight yellow color in solution due to the presence of albumin. Intact vials should be stored at room temperature. Stability of parenteral admixture at room temperature (25°C) is 8 hours and at refrigeration (4°C) is 24 hours.

♦ Stresstabs® B-Complex [OTC] *see* Vitamin B Complex Combinations *on page 1716*
♦ Stresstabs® B-Complex + Iron [OTC] *see* Vitamin B Complex Combinations *on page 1716*
♦ Stresstabs® B-Complex + Zinc [OTC] *see* Vitamin B Complex Combinations *on page 1716*
♦ Striant® *see* Testosterone *on page 1607*
♦ StrongStart™ *see* Vitamins (Multiple/Prenatal) *on page 1721*
♦ Strovite® Forte *see* Vitamins (Multiple/Oral) *on page 1720*
♦ Stuartnatal® Plus 3™ [OTC] *see* Vitamins (Multiple/Prenatal) *on page 1721*
♦ Stuart Prenatal® [OTC] *see* Vitamins (Multiple/Prenatal) *on page 1721*
♦ Sublimaze® *see* Fentanyl *on page 712*
♦ Subutex® *see* Buprenorphine *on page 270*

Succinylcholine (suks in il KOE leen)

U.S. Brand Names Quelicin®

Synonyms Succinylcholine Chloride; Suxamethonium Chloride

Pharmacologic Category Neuromuscular Blocker Agent, Depolarizing

Use Adjunct to general anesthesia to facilitate both rapid sequence and routine endotracheal intubation and to relax skeletal muscles during surgery; to reduce the intensity of muscle contractions of pharmacologically- or electrically-induced convulsions; does not relieve pain or produce sedation

Mechanism of Action Acts similar to acetylcholine, produces depolarization of the motor endplate at the myoneural junction which causes sustained flaccid skeletal muscle paralysis produced by state of accommodation that developes in adjacent excitable muscle membranes

Pharmacodynamics/Kinetics

Onset of action: I.M.: 2-3 minutes; I.V.: Complete muscular relaxation: 30-60 seconds

Duration: I.M.: 10-30 minutes; I.V.: 4-6 minutes with single administration

Metabolism: Rapidly hydrolyzed by plasma pseudocholinesterase

Contraindications Hypersensitivity to succinylcholine or any component of the formulation; personal or familial history of malignant hyperthermia; myopathies associated with elevated serum creatine phosphokinase (CPK) values; narrow-angle glaucoma, penetrating eye injuries; disorders of plasma pseudocholinesterase

Warnings/Precautions **Use with caution in pediatrics and adolescents** secondary to undiagnosed skeletal muscle myopathy and potential for ventricular dysrhythmias and cardiac arrest resulting from hyperkalemia; use with caution in patients with pre-existing hyperkalemia, paraplegia, extensive or severe burns, extensive denervation of skeletal muscle because of disease or injury to the CNS or with degenerative or dystrophic neuromuscular disease; may increase vagal tone

Drug Interactions

Increased toxicity: Anticholinesterase drugs (neostigmine, physostigmine, or pyridostigmine) in combination with succinylcholine can cause cardiorespiratory

(Continued)

Succinylcholine *(Continued)*

collapse; cyclophosphamide, oral contraceptives, lidocaine, thiotepa, pancuronium, lithium, magnesium salts, aprotinin, chloroquine, metoclopramide, terbutaline, and procaine enhance and prolong the effects of succinylcholine

Prolonged neuromuscular blockade: Inhaled anesthetics; local anesthetics; calcium channel blockers; antiarrhythmics (eg, quinidine or procainamide); antibiotics (eg, aminoglycosides, tetracyclines, vancomycin, clindamycin); immunosuppressants (eg, cyclosporine)

Lab Interactions Increased potassium (S)

Adverse Reactions

>10%:

Ocular: Increased intraocular pressure

Miscellaneous: Postoperative stiffness

1% to 10%:

Cardiovascular: Bradycardia, hypotension, cardiac arrhythmia, tachycardia

Gastrointestinal: Intragastric pressure, salivation

<1% (Limited to important or life-threatening): Acute quadriplegic myopathy syndrome (prolonged use), apnea, bronchospasm, circulatory collapse, erythema, hyperkalemia, hypertension, itching, malignant hyperthermia, myalgia, myoglobinuria, myositis ossificans (prolonged use), rash

Overdosage/Toxicology

Symptoms of overdose include respiratory paralysis and cardiac arrest.

Bradyarrhythmias can often be treated with atropine 0.1 mg (infants). Do not treat with anticholinesterase drugs (eg, neostigmine, physostigmine) since this may worsen its toxicity by interfering with its metabolism.

Dosing

Adults & Elderly: Neuromuscular blockade: Dose to effect; doses will vary due to interpatient variability; use ideal body weight for obese patients

I.M.: 2.5-4 mg/kg, total dose should not exceed 150 mg

I.V.: 1-1.5 mg/kg, up to 150 mg total dose

Maintenance: 0.04-0.07 mg/kg every 5-10 minutes as needed

Continuous infusion: 10-100 mcg/kg/minute (or 0.5-10 mg/minute); dilute to concentration of 1-2 mg/mL in D_5W or NS

Note: Initial dose of succinylcholine must be increased when nondepolarizing agent pretreatment used because of the antagonism between succinylcholine and nondepolarizing neuromuscular blocking agents

Pediatrics: Neuromuscular blockade: I.V.:

Note: Because of the risk of malignant hyperthermia, use of continuous infusions is not recommended in infants and children:

Small Children: Intermittent: Initial: 2 mg/kg/dose one time; maintenance: 0.3-0.6 mg/kg/dose at intervals of 5-10 minutes as necessary

Older Children and Adolescents: Intermittent: Initial: 1 mg/kg/dose one time; maintenance: 0.3-0.6 mg/kg every 5-10 minutes as needed

Hepatic Impairment: Dose should be reduced in patients with severe liver disease.

Available Dosage Forms Injection, solution, as chloride: 20 mg/mL (5 mL, 10 mL); 50 mg/mL (10 mL); 100 mg/mL (10 mL)

Nursing Guidelines

Assessment: Only clinicians experienced in the use of neuromuscular-blocking drugs should administer and/or manage the use of succinylcholine. Dosage and rate of administration should be individualized and titrated to the desired effect, according to relevant clinical factors, premedication, concomitant medications, age, and general condition of patient. Ventilatory support must be instituted and maintained until adequate respiratory muscle function and/or airway protection are assured. Assess other medications for effectiveness and safety. Other drugs that affect neuromuscular activity may increase/decrease neuromuscular block induced by succinylcholine. This drug does not cause anesthesia or analgesia; pain must be treated with appropriate analgesic agents. Continuous monitoring of vital signs, cardiac status, respiratory status, and degree of neuromuscular block (objective assessment with external nerve stimulator) is mandatory during infusion and until full muscle tone has returned. Muscle tone returns in a predictable pattern, starting with limbs, abdomen, chest diaphragm, intercostals, and finally muscles of the neck, face, and eyes. Safety precautions must be maintained until full muscle tone has returned. Provide appropriate patient teaching/support prior to and following administration.

Monitoring Laboratory Tests: Serum potassium and calcium

Patient Education: Patient will usually be unconscious prior to administration. Education should be appropriate to individual situation. Reassurance of constant monitoring and emotional support to reduce fear and anxiety should precede and follow administration. Following return of muscle tone, do not attempt to change position or rise from bed without assistance. Report immediately any skin rash or hives, pounding heartbeat, respiratory difficulty, or muscle tremors. **Pregnancy/breast-feeding precautions:** Inform prescriber if you are pregnant. Consult prescriber if breast-feeding.

Pregnancy Risk Factor: C

Lactation: Excretion in breast milk unknown/use caution

Perioperative/Anesthesia/Other Concerns: Classified as an ultra-short duration neuromuscular-blocking agent; some formulations may contain benzyl alcohol.

Critically-Ill Adult Patients: The 2002 ACCM/SCCM/ASHP clinical practice guidelines for sustained neuromuscular blockade in the adult critically-ill patient recommend:

Optimize sedatives and analgesics prior to initiation and monitor and adjust accordingly during course. Neuromuscular blockers do not relieve pain or produce sedation.

Protect patient's eyes from development of keratitis and corneal abrasion by administering ophthalmic ointment and taping eyelids closed or using eye patches. Reposition patient routinely to protect pressure points from breakdown. Address DVT prophylaxis.

Concurrent use of a neuromuscular blocker and corticosteroids appear to increase the risk of certain ICU myopathies; avoid or administer the corticosteroid at the lowest dose possible. Reassess need for neuromuscular blocker daily.

Using daily drug holidays (stopping neuromuscular-blocking agent until patient requires it again) may decrease the incidence of acute quadriplegic myopathy syndrome.

Tachyphylaxis can develop; switch to another neuromuscular blocker (taking into consideration the patient's organ function) if paralysis is still necessary.

Atracurium or cisatracurium is recommended for patients with significant hepatic or renal disease, due to organ-independent Hofmann elimination.

Monitor patients clinically and via "Train of Four" (TOF) testing with a goal of adjusting the degree of blockade to 1-2 twitches or based upon the patient's clinical condition.

Administration

I.M.: I.M. injections should be made deeply, preferably high into deltoid muscle.

I.V.: May be given by rapid I.V. injection without further dilution.

Compatibility:

Stable in dextran 6% in dextrose, dextran 6% in NS, D_5LR, $D_5{}^1/_4NS$, $D_5{}^1/_2NS$, D_5NS, D_5W, $D_{10}W$, LR, $^1/_2NS$, NS

Y-site administration: Incompatible with thiopental

Compatibility when admixed: Incompatible with methohexital, nafcillin, sodium bicarbonate, thiopental

Storage: Refrigerate at 2°C to 8°C (36°F to 46°F); however, remains stable for ≤3 months unrefrigerated; powder form does not require refrigeration. Stability of parenteral admixture at refrigeration temperature (4°C) is 24 hours in D_5W or NS.

♦ **Succinylcholine Chloride** *see* Succinylcholine *on page 1573*

Sucralfate (soo KRAL fate)

U.S. Brand Names Carafate®

Synonyms Aluminum Sucrose Sulfate, Basic

Pharmacologic Category Gastrointestinal Agent, Miscellaneous

Medication Safety Issues

Sound-alike/look-alike issues:

Sucralfate may be confused with salsalate

Carafate® may be confused with Cafergot®

Use Short-term management of duodenal ulcers; maintenance of duodenal ulcers

Unlabeled/Investigational Use Gastric ulcers; suspension may be used topically for treatment of stomatitis due to cancer chemotherapy and other causes of esophageal and gastric erosions; GERD, esophagitis; treatment of NSAID (Continued)

Sucralfate *(Continued)*

mucosal damage; prevention of stress ulcers; postsclerotherapy for esophageal variceal bleeding

Mechanism of Action Forms a complex by binding with positively charged proteins in exudates, forming a viscous paste-like, adhesive substance. This selectively forms a protective coating that protects the lining against peptic acid, pepsin, and bile salts.

Pharmacodynamics/Kinetics

Onset of action: Paste formation and ulcer adhesion: 1-2 hours

Duration: Up to 6 hours

Absorption: Oral: <5%

Distribution: Acts locally at ulcer sites; unbound in GI tract to aluminum and sucrose octasulfate

Metabolism: None

Excretion: Urine (small amounts as unchanged compounds)

Contraindications Hypersensitivity to sucralfate or any component of the formulation

Warnings/Precautions Successful therapy with sucralfate should not be expected to alter the posthealing frequency of recurrence or the severity of duodenal ulceration; use with caution in patients with chronic renal failure who have an impaired excretion of absorbed aluminum. Because of the potential for sucralfate to alter the absorption of some drugs, separate administration (take other medication 2 hours before sucralfate) should be considered when alterations in bioavailability are believed to be critical

Drug Interactions Decreased effect: Digoxin, phenytoin (hydantoins), warfarin, ketoconazole, quinidine, ciprofloxacin, norfloxacin (quinolones), tetracycline, theophylline; because of the potential for sucralfate to alter the absorption of some drugs, separate administration (take other medications 2 hours before sucralfate) should be considered when alterations in bioavailability are believed to be critical

Note: When given with aluminum-containing antacids, may increase serum/body aluminum concentrations (see Warnings/Precautions)

Nutritional/Herbal/Ethanol Interactions Food: Sucralfate may interfere with absorption of vitamin A, vitamin D, vitamin E, and vitamin K.

Adverse Reactions

1% to 10%: Gastrointestinal: Constipation

<1% (Limited to important or life-threatening): Bezoar formation, hypersensitivity (pruritus, urticaria, angioedema), rash

Overdosage/Toxicology Toxicity is minimal, may cause constipation

Dosing

Adults & Elderly:

Stress ulcer prophylaxis: Oral: 1 g 4 times/day

Stress ulcer treatment: Oral: 1 g every 4 hours

Treatment of duodenal ulcer: Oral:

Initial treatment: 1 g 4 times/day, 1 hour before meals or food and at bedtime for 4-8 weeks, or alternatively 2 g twice daily; treatment is recommended for 4-8 weeks in adults, the elderly will require 12 weeks.

Maintenance/prophylaxis of duodenal ulcer: 1 g twice daily

Stomatitis (unlabeled use): Oral: 1 g/10 mL suspension; swish and spit or swish and swallow 4 times/day.

Pediatrics: Dose not established, doses of 40-80 mg/kg/day divided every 6 hours have been used

Stomatitis (unlabeled use): Oral: Children: 2.5-5 mL (1 g/10 mL suspension), swish and spit or swish and swallow 4 times/day

Renal Impairment: Aluminum salt is minimally absorbed (<5%), however, may accumulate in renal failure.

Available Dosage Forms

Suspension, oral: 1 g/10 mL (10 mL) [DSC]

Carafate®: 1 g/10 mL (420 mL)

Tablet (Carafate®): 1 g

Nursing Guidelines

Assessment: See Contraindications and Warnings/Precautions for use cautions. Assess potential for interactions with other prescriptions, OTC medications, or herbal products patient may be taking (see Drug Interactions). Monitor patient response (see Adverse Reactions and Overdose/Toxicology). Teach patient proper use (eg, timing of other medications), possible side effects (eg, constipation) and interventions, and adverse symptoms to report (see Patient Education) on a regular basis during therapy.

Dietary Considerations: Administer with water on an empty stomach.

Patient Education: Take recommended dose with water on an empty stomach, 1 hour before or 2 hours after meals. Take any other medications at least 2 hours before taking sucralfate. Do not take antacids (if prescribed) within 30 minutes of taking sucralfate. May cause constipation (increased exercise, fluids, fruit, or fiber may help). If constipation persists, consult prescriber for approved stool softener.

Geriatric Considerations: Caution should be used in the elderly due to reduced renal function. Patients with Cl_{cr} <30 mL/minute may be at risk for aluminum intoxication. Due to low side effect profile, this may be an agent of choice in the elderly with PUD.

Pregnancy Risk Factor: B

Lactation: Enters breast milk/compatible

Administration

Oral: Tablet may be broken or dissolved in water before ingestion. Administer with water on an empty stomach.

Storage: Suspension: Shake well. Refrigeration is **not** necessary; do **not** freeze.

♦ Sudafed® [OTC] *see* Pseudoephedrine *on page 1436*

♦ Sudafed® 12 Hour [OTC] *see* Pseudoephedrine *on page 1436*

♦ Sudafed® 24 Hour [OTC] *see* Pseudoephedrine *on page 1436*

♦ Sudafed® Children's [OTC] *see* Pseudoephedrine *on page 1436*

♦ Sudafed PE™ [OTC] *see* Phenylephrine *on page 1350*

♦ Sudafed® Severe Cold [OTC] *see* Acetaminophen, Dextromethorphan, and Pseudoephedrine *on page 73*

♦ Sudafed® Sinus Nighttime [OTC] *see* Triprolidine and Pseudoephedrine *on page 1670*

♦ Sudodrin [OTC] *see* Pseudoephedrine *on page 1436*

♦ SudoGest [OTC] *see* Pseudoephedrine *on page 1436*

♦ Sudo-Tab® [OTC] *see* Pseudoephedrine *on page 1436*

♦ Sufenta® *see* Sufentanil *on page 1577*

Sufentanil (soo FEN ta nil)

U.S. Brand Names Sufenta®

Synonyms Sufentanil Citrate

Pharmacologic Category Analgesic, Narcotic; General Anesthetic

Medication Safety Issues

Sound-alike/look-alike issues:

Sufentanil may be confused with alfentanil, fentanyl

Sufenta® may be confused with Alfenta®, Sudafed®, Survanta®

Use Analgesic supplement in maintenance of balanced general anesthesia

Mechanism of Action Binds to opioid receptors throughout the CNS. Once receptor binding occurs, effects are exerted by opening K+ channels and inhibiting Ca++ channels. These mechanisms increase pain threshold, alter pain perception, inhibit ascending pain pathways; short-acting narcotic

Pharmacodynamics/Kinetics

Onset of action: 1-3 minutes

Duration: Dose dependent

Metabolism: Primarily hepatic

Contraindications Hypersensitivity to sufentanil or any component of the formulation

Warnings/Precautions Sufentanil can cause severely compromised respiratory depression; use with caution in patients with head injuries, hepatic or renal impairment or with pulmonary disease; sufentanil shares the toxic potential of opiate agonists, precaution of opiate agonist therapy should be observed; rapid I.V. infusion may result in skeletal muscle and chest wall rigidity, impaired ventilation, respiratory distress/arrest; nondepolarizing skeletal muscle relaxant may be required

Drug Interactions Substrate of CYP3A4 (major)

CYP3A4 inhibitors: May increase the levels/effects of sufentanil. Example inhibitors include azole antifungals, clarithromycin, diclofenac, doxycycline, erythromycin, imatinib, isoniazid, nefazodone, nicardipine, propofol, protease inhibitors, quinidine, telithromycin, and verapamil.

Increased effect/toxicity with CNS depressants, beta-blockers

(Continued)

Sufentanil *(Continued)*

Adverse Reactions

>10%:

Cardiovascular: Bradycardia, hypotension
Central nervous system: Somnolence
Gastrointestinal: Nausea, vomiting
Respiratory: Respiratory depression

1% to 10%:

Cardiovascular: Cardiac arrhythmia, orthostatic hypotension
Central nervous system: CNS depression, confusion
Gastrointestinal: Biliary spasm
Ocular: Blurred vision

<1% (Limited to important or life-threatening): Bronchospasm, circulatory depression, convulsions, laryngospasm, mental depression, paradoxical CNS excitation or delirium, physical and psychological dependence with prolonged use, rash, urticaria

Overdosage/Toxicology Naloxone 2 mg I.V. (0.01 mg/kg for children) with repeat administration as necessary up to a total of 10 mg; supportive care includes establishment of respiratory change; naloxone may be used to treat respiratory depression; muscular rigidity may also respond to opiate antagonist therapy or to neuromuscular blocking agents

Dosing

Adults & Elderly:

Note: Dose should be based on body weight. In obese patients (ie, >20% above ideal body weight), use lean body weight to determine dosage.

Endotracheal intubation: I.V.: 1-2 mcg/kg with N_2O/O_2; maintenance: 10-25 mcg as needed

Surgical procedures: I.V.: 2-8 mcg/kg with N_2O/O_2; maintenance: 10-50 mcg as needed

Anesthesia: I.V.: 8-30 mcg/kg with 100% O_2 and muscle relaxant produces sleep; at doses ≥8 mcg/kg maintains a deep level of anesthesia; maintenance: 10-50 mcg as needed

Pediatrics:

Anesthesia: I.V.: Children 2-12 years: 10-25 mcg/kg (10-15 mcg/kg most common dose) with 100% O_2, maintenance: up to 1-2 mcg/kg total dose

Available Dosage Forms Injection, solution [preservative free]: 50 mcg/mL (1 mL, 2 mL, 5 mL)

Nursing Guidelines

Patient Education: Do not drive for 24 hours after receiving this medication

Pregnancy Risk Factor: C

Perioperative/Anesthesia/Other Concerns: Sufentanil is a short-acting narcotic, 5-10 times more potent than fentanyl; it is packaged in the same concentration as fentanyl (50 mcg/mL); keep in mind the differences in potency to prevent overdose with sufentanil. Sufentanil may be diluted to decrease concentration; this will decrease the potential for administering excessive doses.

Administration

Compatibility: Stable in D_5W

Y-site administration: Incompatible with lorazepam, phenytoin, thiopental

Compatibility in syringe: Incompatible with diazepam, lorazepam, phenobarbital, phenytoin

Related Information

Acute Postoperative Pain *on page 1742*
Narcotic / Opioid Analgesics *on page 1880*

♦ **Sufentanil Citrate** *see* Sufentanil *on page 1577*
♦ **Sular®** *see* Nisoldipine *on page 1230*
♦ **Sulbactam and Ampicillin** *see* Ampicillin and Sulbactam *on page 163*

Sulfabenzamide, Sulfacetamide, and Sulfathiazole

(sul fa BENZ a mide, sul fa SEE ta mide, & sul fa THYE a zole)

U.S. Brand Names V.V.S.®

Synonyms Triple Sulfa

Pharmacologic Category Antibiotic, Vaginal

Use Treatment of *Haemophilus vaginalis* vaginitis

Mechanism of Action Interferes with microbial folic acid synthesis and growth via inhibition of para-aminobenzoic acid metabolism

Pharmacodynamics/Kinetics
Absorption: Absorption from vagina is variable and unreliable
Metabolism: Primarily via acetylation
Excretion: Urine

Contraindications Hypersensitivity to sulfabenzamide, sulfacetamide, sulfathiazole, or any component of the formulation; renal dysfunction; pregnancy (if near term)

Warnings/Precautions Associated with Stevens-Johnson syndrome; if local irritation or systemic toxicity develops, discontinue therapy

Drug Interactions No data reported

Adverse Reactions Frequency not defined.
Dermatologic: Pruritus, urticaria, Stevens-Johnson syndrome
Local: Local irritation
Miscellaneous: Allergic reactions

Dosing
Adults & Elderly: *Haemophilus vaginalis* vaginitis: Intravaginal: Cream: Insert 1 applicatorful in vagina twice daily for 4-6 days. Dosage may then be decreased to 1/2 to 1/4 of an applicatorful twice daily.

Available Dosage Forms Cream, vaginal: Sulfabenzamide 3.7%, sulfacetamide 2.86%, and sulfathiazole 3.42% (78 g with applicator)

Nursing Guidelines
Assessment: See Contraindications, Warnings/Precautions, and Dosing for use cautions. Assess other medications patient may be taking for effectiveness and interactions (see Warnings/Precautions and Drug Interactions). Teach appropriate administration and adverse symptoms to report (see Patient Education). Note breast-feeding caution.

Patient Education: Inform prescriber of all prescriptions, OTC medications, or herbal products you are taking, and any allergies you have. This medication is only to be inserted into vagina. Use exactly as directed and complete full course of therapy. Follow exact directions for filling applicator with cream. Wash hands before inserting applicator gently into vagina and releasing cream. Wash hands and applicator with soap and water following each application. Discontinue and notify prescriber immediately if burning, irritation, or allergic reaction occurs. **Pregnancy/breast-feeding precautions:** Inform prescriber if you are pregnant before use. Consult prescriber if breast-feeding.

Pregnancy Risk Factor: C (avoid if near term)

Lactation: Excretion in breast milk unknown

Sulfacetamide (sul fa SEE ta mide)

U.S. Brand Names Bleph®-10; Carmol® Scalp; Klaron®; Ovace™

Synonyms Sodium Sulfacetamide; Sulfacetamide Sodium

Pharmacologic Category Antibiotic, Ophthalmic; Antibiotic, Sulfonamide Derivative

Medication Safety Issues
Sound-alike/look-alike issues:
Bleph®-10 may be confused with Blephamide®
Klaron® may be confused with Klor-Con®

Use
Ophthalmic: Treatment and prophylaxis of conjunctivitis due to susceptible organisms; corneal ulcers; adjunctive treatment with systemic sulfonamides for therapy of trachoma
Dermatologic: Scaling dermatosis (seborrheic); bacterial infections of the skin; acne vulgaris

Mechanism of Action Interferes with bacterial growth by inhibiting bacterial folic acid synthesis through competitive antagonism of PABA

Pharmacodynamics/Kinetics
Half-life elimination: 7-13 hours
Excretion: When absorbed, primarily urine (as unchanged drug)

Contraindications Hypersensitivity to sulfacetamide, sulfonamides, or any component of the formulation

Warnings/Precautions Severe reactions to sulfonamides have been reported, regardless of route of administration; reactions may include Stevens-Johnson syndrome, toxic epidermal necrolysis, fulminant hepatic necrosis, or blood dyscrasias. Chemical similarities are present among sulfonamides, sulfonylureas, carbonic anhydrase inhibitors, thiazides, and loop diuretics (except ethacrynic acid). Use in patients with sulfonamide allergy is specifically contraindicated in
(Continued)

Sulfacetamide *(Continued)*

product labeling; however, a risk of cross-reaction exists in patients with allergy to any of these compounds; avoid use when previous reaction has been severe.

Ophthalmic: Inactivated by purulent exudates containing PABA; use with caution in severe dry eye; ointment may retard corneal epithelial healing. For topical application to the eye only; not for injection. Safety and efficacy have not been established in children <2 months of age.

Dermatologic: Use caution if applied to denuded or abraded skin. Some products contain sodium metabisulfite which may cause allergic reactions in certain individuals. For external use only; avoid contact with eyes. Safety and efficacy have not been established in children <12 years of age.

Drug Interactions Decreased effect: Silver, gentamicin (antagonism)

Adverse Reactions Frequency not defined.

Cardiovascular: Edema

Dermatologic: Burning, erythema, irritation, itching, stinging, Stevens-Johnson syndrome

Ocular (following ophthalmic application): Burning, conjunctivitis, conjunctival hyperemia, corneal ulcers, irritation, stinging

Miscellaneous: Allergic reactions, systemic lupus erythematosus

Dosing

Adults & Elderly:

Conjunctivitis: Ophthalmic:

Ointment: Apply to lower conjunctival sac 1-4 times/day and at bedtime

Solution: Instill 1-2 drops several times daily up to every 2-3 hours in lower conjunctival sac during waking hours and less frequently at night; increase dosing interval as condition responds. Usual duration of treatment: 7-10 days

Trachoma: Instill 2 drops into the conjunctival sac every 2 hours; must be used in conjunction with systemic therapy

Acne: Topical: Apply thin film to affected area twice daily

Seborrheic dermatitis: Topical: Apply at bedtime and allow to remain overnight; in severe cases, may apply twice daily. Duration of therapy is usually 8-10 applications; dosing interval may be increased as eruption subsides. Applications once or twice weekly, or every other week may be used to prevent eruptions.

Secondary cutaneous bacterial infections: Topical: Apply 2-4 times/day until infection clears

Pediatrics:

Conjunctivitis: Ophthalmic: Children >2 months: Refer to adult dosing.

Dermatologic: Topical: Children >12 years: Refer to adult dosing.

Available Dosage Forms [DSC] = Discontinued product

Cream, topical, as sodium (Ovace™): 10% (30 g, 60 g)

Foam, topical, as sodium (Ovace™): 10% (50 g, 100 g)

Gel, topical, as sodium (Ovace™): 10% (30 g, 60 g)

Lotion, as sodium:

Carmol® Scalp: 10% (85 g) [contains urea 10%]

Klaron®: 10% (120 mL) [contains sodium metabisulfite]

Ovace™: 10% (180 mL, 360 mL)

Ointment, ophthalmic, as sodium: 10% (3.5 g)

Solution, ophthalmic, as sodium: 10% (15 mL)

Bleph®-10: 10% (5 mL; 15 mL [DSC]) [contains benzalkonium chloride]

Nursing Guidelines

Assessment: Assess for previous sulfonamide allergic reactions (see Warnings/Precautions). Monitor effectiveness of therapy. Assess knowledge/teach patient appropriate use (ophthalmic/topical), interventions to reduce side effects, and adverse symptoms to report (see Patient Education). Note breast-feeding caution.

Patient Education: Use as directed. Complete full course of therapy even if condition appears improved.

Ophthalmic: Store at room temperature. Shake solution before using. Apply prescribed amount as often as directed. Wash hands before using. Do not let tip of applicator touch eye; do not contaminate tip of applicator (may cause eye infection, eye damage, or vision loss). When using solution, tilt head back and look upward. Gently pull down lower lid and put drop(s) in inner corner of eye. When using ointment, place medicine inside the lower lid, close eye, and roll eyeball in all directions. Do not blink for 1/2 minute. Apply gentle pressure to inner corner of eye for 30 seconds. Wipe away excess from skin around eye. Do not use any other eye preparation for at least 10 minutes. Do not share medication with anyone else. May cause sensitivity to bright light (dark glasses may help); temporary stinging or blurred vision may occur. Inform prescriber if you experience eye pain, redness, burning, watering, dryness, double vision, puffiness around eye, vision changes, or other adverse eye response; worsening of condition or lack of improvement within 3-4 days.

Topical: For external use only. Apply a thin film of lotion to affected area as often as directed. Do not cover with occlusive dressing. Report increased skin redness, irritation, or development of open sores; or if condition worsens or does not improve.

Pregnancy/breast-feeding precautions: Inform prescriber if you are pregnant. Consult prescriber if breast-feeding.

Geriatric Considerations: Assess whether patient can adequately instill drops or ointment.

Pregnancy Risk Factor: C

Pregnancy Issues: Use of systemic sulfonamides during pregnancy may cause kernicterus in the newborn; the amount of systemic absorption following topical administration is not known. Use during pregnancy only if clearly needed.

Lactation: Excretion in breast milk unknown/use caution

Breast-Feeding Considerations: The amount of systemic absorption following topical administration is not known. When used orally, small amounts of sulfonamides are excreted in breast milk.

Administration

Compatibility: Incompatible with silver and zinc sulfate. Sulfacetamide is inactivated by blood or purulent exudates.

Storage: Store at controlled room temperature.

Ophthalmic solution: Solution may be used if yellow; do not use if darkened.

Carmol® Scalp treatment: Do not freeze; may be used if slightly discolored.

Sulfacetamide and Prednisolone

(sul fa SEE ta mide & pred NIS oh lone)

U.S. Brand Names Blephamide®

Synonyms Prednisolone and Sulfacetamide

Pharmacologic Category Antibiotic/Corticosteroid, Ophthalmic

Medication Safety Issues

Sound-alike/look-alike issues:

Blephamide® may be confused with Bleph®-10

Vasocidin® may be confused with Vasodilan®

Use Steroid-responsive inflammatory ocular conditions where infection is present or there is a risk of infection; ophthalmic suspension may be used as an otic preparation

Mechanism of Action Interferes with bacterial growth by inhibiting bacterial folic acid synthesis through competitive antagonism of PABA; decreases inflammation by suppression of migration of polymorphonuclear leukocytes and reversal of increased capillary permeability; suppresses the immune system by reducing activity and volume of the lymphatic system

Pharmacodynamics/Kinetics See individual agents.

Drug Interactions Prednisolone: **Substrate** of CYP3A4 (minor); **Inhibits** CYP3A4 (weak)

Decreased effect: Silver, gentamicin, vaccines, toxoids

Adverse Reactions

1% to 10%: Local: Burning, stinging

<1% (Limited to important or life-threatening): Cataracts, Cushing's syndrome, fractures, glaucoma, growth suppression, headache, muscle weakness, nausea, osteoporosis, peptic ulcer, pituitary-adrenal axis suppression, pseudotumor cerebri, psychoses, seizure, skin atrophy, Stevens-Johnson syndrome, vertigo, vomiting

Dosing

Adults & Elderly: Conjunctivitis: Ophthalmic:

Ointment: Apply to lower conjunctival sac 1-4 times/day

Solution, suspension: Instill 1-3 drops every 2-3 hours while awake

Pediatrics: Conjunctivitis: Ophthalmic: Children >2 months: Refer to adult dosing.

(Continued)

Sulfacetamide and Prednisolone *(Continued)*

Available Dosage Forms

Ointment, ophthalmic (Blephamide®): Sulfacetamide sodium 10% and prednisolone acetate 0.2% (3.5 g)

Solution, ophthalmic: Sulfacetamide sodium 10% and prednisolone sodium phosphate 0.25% (5 mL, 10 mL)

Suspension, ophthalmic (Blephamide®): Sulfacetamide sodium 10% and prednisolone acetate 0.2% (5 mL, 10 mL) [contains benzalkonium chloride]

Nursing Guidelines

Assessment: See individual agents.

Patient Education: Eye drops will burn upon instillation. Ointment will cause blurred vision. Do not touch container to eye. Wait at least 10 minutes before using another eye preparation. May cause sensitivity to sunlight. Notify physician if condition does not improve in 3-4 days. **Pregnancy precaution:** Notify prescriber if you are or intend to become pregnant.

Pregnancy Risk Factor: C

♦ **Sulfacetamide Sodium** *see* Sulfacetamide *on page 1579*

Sulfamethoxazole and Trimethoprim

(sul fa meth OKS a zole & trye METH oh prim)

U.S. Brand Names Bactrim™; Bactrim™ DS; Septra®; Septra® DS

Synonyms Co-Trimoxazole; SMZ-TMP; Sulfatrim; TMP-SMZ; Trimethoprim and Sulfamethoxazole

Pharmacologic Category Antibiotic, Miscellaneous; Antibiotic, Sulfonamide Derivative

Medication Safety Issues

Sound-alike/look-alike issues:

Bactrim™ may be confused with bacitracin, Bactine®

Co-trimoxazole may be confused with clotrimazole

Septra® may be confused with Ceptaz®, Sectral®, Septa®

Use

Oral treatment of urinary tract infections due to *E. coli*, *Klebsiella* and *Enterobacter* sp, *M. morganii*, *P. mirabilis* and *P. vulgaris*; acute otitis media in children; acute exacerbations of chronic bronchitis in adults due to susceptible strains of *H. influenzae* or *S. pneumoniae*; treatment and prophylaxis of *Pneumocystis carinii* pneumonitis (PCP); traveler's diarrhea due to enterotoxigenic *E. coli*; treatment of enteritis caused by *Shigella flexneri* or *Shigella sonnei*

I.V. treatment or severe or complicated infections when oral therapy is not feasible, for documented PCP, empiric treatment of PCP in immune compromised patients; treatment of documented or suspected shigellosis, typhoid fever, *Nocardia asteroides* infection, or other infections caused by susceptible bacteria

Unlabeled/Investigational Use Cholera and *Salmonella*-type infections and nocardiosis; chronic prostatitis; as prophylaxis in neutropenic patients with *P. carinii* infections, in leukemics, and in patients following renal transplantation, to decrease incidence of PCP; treatment of *Cyclospora* infection, typhoid fever, *Nocardia asteroides* infection

Mechanism of Action Sulfamethoxazole interferes with bacterial folic acid synthesis and growth via inhibition of dihydrofolic acid formation from para-aminobenzoic acid; trimethoprim inhibits dihydrofolic acid reduction to tetrahydrofolate resulting in sequential inhibition of enzymes of the folic acid pathway

Pharmacodynamics/Kinetics

Absorption: Oral: Almost completely, 90% to 100%

Protein binding: SMX: 68%, TMP: 45%

Metabolism: SMX: N-acetylated and glucuronidated; TMP: Metabolized to oxide and hydroxylated metabolites

Half-life elimination: SMX: 9 hours, TMP: 6-17 hours; both are prolonged in renal failure

Time to peak, serum: Within 1-4 hours

Excretion: Both are excreted in urine as metabolites and unchanged drug

Effects of aging on the pharmacokinetics of both agents has been variable; increase in half-life and decreases in clearance have been associated with reduced creatinine clearance

Contraindications Hypersensitivity to any sulfa drug, trimethoprim, or any component of the formulation; porphyria; megaloblastic anemia due to folate deficiency; infants <2 months of age; marked hepatic damage; severe renal disease; pregnancy (at term)

Warnings/Precautions Use with caution in patients with G6PD deficiency, impaired renal or hepatic function or potential folate deficiency (malnourished, chronic anticonvulsant therapy, or elderly); maintain adequate hydration to prevent crystalluria; adjust dosage in patients with renal impairment. Injection vehicle contains benzyl alcohol and sodium metabisulfite.

Chemical similarities are present among sulfonamides, sulfonylureas, carbonic anhydrase inhibitors, thiazides, and loop diuretics (except ethacrynic acid). Use in patients with sulfonamide allergy is specifically contraindicated in product labeling, however, a risk of cross-reaction exists in patients with allergy to any of these compounds; avoid use when previous reaction has been severe.

Fatalities associated with severe reactions including Stevens-Johnson syndrome, toxic epidermal necrolysis, hepatic necrosis, agranulocytosis, aplastic anemia and other blood dyscrasias; discontinue use at first sign of rash. Elderly patients appear at greater risk for more severe adverse reactions. May cause hypoglycemia, particularly in malnourished, or patients with renal or hepatic impairment. Use with caution in patients with porphyria or thyroid dysfunction. Slow acetylators may be more prone to adverse reactions. Caution in patients with allergies or asthma. May cause hyperkalemia (associated with high doses of trimethoprim). Incidence of adverse effects appears to be increased in patients with AIDS.

Drug Interactions

Sulfamethoxazole: **Substrate** of CYP2C8/9 (major), 3A4 (minor); **Inhibits** CYP2C8/9 (moderate)

Trimethoprim: **Substrate** (major) of CYP2C8/9, 3A4; **Inhibits** CYP2C8/9 (moderate)

ACE Inhibitors and angiotensin receptor antagonists: May increase the risk of hyperkalemia with sulfamethoxazole/trimethoprim.

Amantadine: Concurrent use with sulfamethoxazole/trimethoprim has been associated with toxic delirium (rare).

Cyclosporine: May result in an increased risk of nephrotoxicity when used with sulfamethoxazole/trimethoprim. Sulfonamides may decrease the serum concentrations of cyclosporine.

CYP2C8/9 inducers: May decrease the levels/effects of sulfamethoxazole. Example inducers include carbamazepine, phenobarbital, phenytoin, rifampin, rifapentine, and secobarbital.

CYP2C8/9 substrates: Sulfamethoxazole/trimethoprim may increase the levels/effects of CYP2C8/9 substrates. Example substrates include amiodarone, fluoxetine, glimepiride, glipizide, nateglinide, phenytoin, pioglitazone, rosiglitazone, sertraline, and warfarin.

Dapsone: Trimethoprim may increase the serum concentration of dapsone.

Diuretics, potassium-sparing: May increase the risk of hyperkalemia with sulfamethoxazole/trimethoprim.

Leucovorin: Although occasionally recommended to limit or reverse hematologic toxicity of high-dose sulfamethoxazole/trimethoprim, concurrent use has been associated with a decreased effectiveness in treating *Pneumocystis carinii.*

Methotrexate: Sulfamethoxazole/trimethoprim may increase toxicity of methotrexate (due to displacement from binding sites and/or decreased renal secretion).

Phenytoin: Sulfamethoxazole/trimethoprim may increase phenytoin levels/toxicity. Phenytoin may decrease sulfamethoxazole/trimethoprim levels.

Procainamide: Trimethoprim may decrease the excretion of procainamide.

Pyrimethamine: Concurrent therapy with pyrimethamine (in doses >25 mg/week) may be at increased risk of megaloblastic anemia.

Sulfonylureas: Sulfamethoxazole/trimethoprim may increase the hypoglycemic effect of sulfonylureas; monitor.

Warfarin: Sulfamethoxazole/trimethoprim may increase the hypoprothrombinemic effect of warfarin; monitor INR closely.

Nutritional/Herbal/Ethanol Interactions Herb/Nutraceutical: Avoid dong quai, St John's wort (may also cause photosensitization).

Lab Interactions Increased creatinine (Jaffé alkaline picrate reaction); increased serum methotrexate by dihydrofolate reductase method; does not interfere with RAI method

Adverse Reactions The most common adverse reactions include gastrointestinal upset (nausea, vomiting, anorexia) and dermatologic reactions (rash or urticaria). Rare, life-threatening reactions have been associated with co-trimoxazole,

(Continued)

Sulfamethoxazole and Trimethoprim *(Continued)*

including severe dermatologic reactions and hepatotoxic reactions. Most other reactions listed are rare, however, frequency cannot be accurately estimated.

Cardiovascular: Allergic myocarditis

Central nervous system: Confusion, depression, hallucinations, seizure, aseptic meningitis, peripheral neuritis, fever, ataxia, kernicterus in neonates

Dermatologic: Rashes, pruritus, urticaria, photosensitivity; rare reactions include erythema multiforme, Stevens-Johnson syndrome, toxic epidermal necrolysis, exfoliative dermatitis, and Henoch-Schönlein purpura

Endocrine & metabolic: Hyperkalemia (generally at high dosages), hypoglycemia

Gastrointestinal: Nausea, vomiting, anorexia, stomatitis, diarrhea, pseudomembranous colitis, pancreatitis

Hematologic: Thrombocytopenia, megaloblastic anemia, granulocytopenia, eosinophilia, pancytopenia, aplastic anemia, methemoglobinemia, hemolysis (with G6PD deficiency), agranulocytosis

Hepatic: Hepatotoxicity (including hepatitis, cholestasis, and hepatic necrosis), hyperbilirubinemia, transaminases increased

Neuromuscular & skeletal: Arthralgia, myalgia, rhabdomyolysis

Renal: Interstitial nephritis, crystalluria, renal failure, nephrotoxicity (in association with cyclosporine), diuresis

Respiratory: Cough, dyspnea, pulmonary infiltrates

Miscellaneous: Serum sickness, angioedema, periarteritis nodosa (rare), systemic lupus erythematosus (rare)

Overdosage/Toxicology Symptoms of overdose include nausea, vomiting, GI distress, hematuria, and crystalluria. Bone marrow suppression may occur. Treatment is supportive. Adequate fluid intake is essential. Peritoneal dialysis is not effective and hemodialysis is only moderately effective in removing co-trimoxazole. Leucovorin 5-15 mg/day may accelerate hematologic recovery.

Dosing

Adults & Elderly: Dosage recommendations are based on the trimethoprim component. Double-strength tablets are equivalent to sulfamethoxazole 800 mg and trimethoprim 160 mg.

Urinary tract infection:

Oral: One double-strength tablet every 12 hours for 10-14 days

Duration of therapy: Uncomplicated: 3-5 days; Complicated: 7-10 days

Pyelonephritis: 14 days

Prostatitis: Acute: 2 weeks; Chronic: 2-3 months

I.V.: 8-10 mg TMP/kg/day in divided doses every 6, 8, or 12 hours for up to 14 days with severe infections

Chronic bronchitis: Oral: One double-strength tablet every 12 hours for 10-14 days

Shigellosis:

Oral: One double strength tablet every 12 hours for 5 days

I.V.: 8-10 mg TMP/kg/day in divided doses every 6, 8, or 12 hours for up to 5 days

Travelers' diarrhea: Oral: One double strength tablet every 12 hours for 5 days

Sepsis: I.V.: 20 TMP/kg/day divided every 6 hours

***Pneumocystis carinii*:**

Prophylaxis: Oral: 1 double strength tablet daily or 3 times/week

Treatment: Oral, I.V.: 15-20 mg TMP/kg/day in 3-4 divided doses

Cyclospora (unlabeled use): Oral, I.V.: 160 mg TMP twice daily for 7-10 days

Nocardia (unlabeled use): Oral, I.V.:

Cutaneous infections: 5 mg TMP/kg/day in 2 divided doses

Severe infections (pulmonary/cerebral): 10-15 mg TMP/kg/day in 2-3 divided doses. Treatment duration is controversial; an average of 7 months has been reported.

Note: Therapy for severe infection may be initiated I.V. and converted to oral therapy (frequently converted to approximate dosages of oral solid dosage forms: 2 DS tablets every 8-12 hours). Although not widely available, sulfonamide levels should be considered in patients with questionable absorption, at risk for dose-related toxicity, or those with poor therapeutic response.

Pediatrics: Recommendations are based on the trimethoprim component.

General dosing guidelines: Children >2 months:

Mild-to-moderate infections: Oral: 8-12 mg TMP/kg/day in divided doses every 12 hours

Serious infection:

Oral: 20 mg TMP/kg/day in divided doses every 6 hours

I.V.: 8-12 mg TMP/kg/day in divided doses every 6 hours

Acute otitis media: Oral: 8 mg TMP/kg/day in divided doses every 12 hours for 10 days

Urinary tract infection:

Treatment:

Oral: 6-12 mg TMP/kg/day in divided doses every 12 hours

I.V.: 8-10 mg TMP/kg/day in divided doses every 6, 8, or 12 hours for up to 4 days with serious infections

Prophylaxis: Oral: 2 mg TMP/kg/dose daily or 5 mg TMP/kg/dose twice weekly

***Pneumocystis*:**

Treatment: Oral, I.V.: 15-20 mg TMP/kg/day in divided doses every 6-8 hours

Prophylaxis: Oral, 150 mg TMP/m^2/day in divided doses every 12 hours for 3 days/week; dose should not exceed trimethoprim 320 mg and sulfamethoxazole 1600 mg daily

Alternative prophylaxis dosing schedules include:

150 mg TMP/m^2/day as a single daily dose 3 times/week on consecutive days

or

150 mg TMP/m^2/day in divided doses every 12 hours administered 7 days/week

or

150 mg TMP/m^2/day in divided doses every 12 hours administered 3 times/week on alternate days

Shigellosis:

Oral: 8 mg TMP/kg/day in divided doses every 12 hours for 5 days

I.V.: 8-10 mg TMP/kg/day in divided doses every 6, 8, or 12 hours for up to 5 days

Cyclospora (unlabeled use): Oral, I.V.: 5 mg TMP/kg twice daily for 7-10 days

Renal Impairment:

Cl_{cr} 15-30 mL/minute: Administer 50% of recommended dose.

Cl_{cr} <15 mL/minute: Not recommended

Available Dosage Forms Note: The 5:1 ratio (SMX:TMP) remains constant in all dosage forms.

Injection, solution: Sulfamethoxazole 80 mg and trimethoprim 16 mg per mL (5 mL, 10 mL, 30 mL) [contains propylene glycol ~400 mg/mL, alcohol, benzyl alcohol, and sodium metabisulfite]

Suspension, oral: Sulfamethoxazole 200 mg and trimethoprim 40 mg per 5 mL (480 mL) [contains alcohol]

Septra®: Sulfamethoxazole 200 mg and trimethoprim 40 mg per 5 mL (480 mL) [contains alcohol 0.26% and sodium benzoate; cherry and grape flavors]

Tablet: Sulfamethoxazole 400 mg and trimethoprim 80 mg

Bactrim™: Sulfamethoxazole 400 mg and trimethoprim 80 mg [contains sodium benzoate]

Septra®: Sulfamethoxazole 400 mg and trimethoprim 80 mg

Tablet, double strength: Sulfamethoxazole 800 mg and trimethoprim 160 mg

Bactrim™ DS: Sulfamethoxazole 800 mg and trimethoprim 160 mg [contains sodium benzoate]

Septra® DS: Sulfamethoxazole 800 mg and trimethoprim 160 mg

Nursing Guidelines

Assessment: Assess results of culture and sensitivity tests and patient's allergy history prior to therapy. Assess potential for interactions with other pharmacological agents or herbal products patient may be taking (eg, increased risk of hyperkalemia or nephrotoxicity). Dosage adjustment may be necessary in presence of renal impairment. Assess therapeutic response (according to purpose for use) and adverse effects (reactions are usually rare, however, severe dermatologic and hepatotoxic reactions have been reported). Advise patients with diabetes to monitor glucose levels closely; may cause hypoglycemia. Teach patient possible side effects/appropriate interventions and adverse symptoms to report (eg, rash, persistent gastrointestinal upset).

Monitoring Laboratory Tests: Perform culture and sensitivity testing prior to initiating therapy; serum potassium, creatinine, BUN

Dietary Considerations: Should be taken with 8 oz of water on empty stomach.

(Continued)

Sulfamethoxazole and Trimethoprim *(Continued)*

Patient Education: Do not take any new medication during therapy unless approved by prescriber. Take oral medication with 8 oz of water on an empty stomach, 1 hour before or 2 hours after meals, for best absorption. Finish all medication; do not skip doses. If you have diabetes, you should monitor your glucose levels closely; may cause hypoglycemia. May cause increased sensitivity to sunlight (use sunblock, wear protective clothing and dark glasses, and avoid direct exposure to sunlight); or nausea or vomiting (small frequent meals, frequent mouth care, sucking lozenges, or chewing gum may help). Report immediately rash; palpitations or chest pain; CNS changes (eg, hallucinations, abnormal anxiety, seizures); sore throat, unusual coughing, or shortness of breath; blackened stool; unusual bruising or bleeding; edema; or blood in urine or changes in urinary pattern. **Pregnancy/breast-feeding precautions:** Inform prescriber if you are or intend to become pregnant or breast-feed.

Geriatric Considerations: Elderly patients appear at greater risk for more severe adverse reactions. Adjust dose based on renal function.

Pregnancy Risk Factor: C/D (at term - expert analysis)

Pregnancy Issues: Do not use at term to avoid kernicterus in the newborn and use during pregnancy only if risks outweigh the benefits since folic acid metabolism may be affected.

Lactation: Enters breast milk/contraindicated (AAP rates "compatible with restrictions")

Breast-Feeding Considerations: Sulfonamides are excreted in low concentrations in breast milk. Use during breast feeding in infants <2 months of age is contraindicated according to the manufacturer. The AAP considers use during breast-feeding "compatible" in full term neonates; however, breast-feeding is not recommended if the infant is ill, stressed, or premature **or** if the infant has glucose-6-phosphate dehydrogenase deficiency or hyperbilirubinemia.

Administration

Oral:

May be taken with food and water.

I.V.: Infuse over 60-90 minutes, must dilute well before giving.

Compatibility: Stable in $D_5{}^1/_2$NS, LR, $^1/_2$NS

Y-site administration: Incompatible with fluconazole, midazolam, vinorelbine

Compatibility when admixed: Incompatible with fluconazole, verapamil

Storage:

Injection: Store at room temperature; do not refrigerate. Less soluble in more alkaline pH. Protect from light. Solution must be diluted prior to administration. Following dilution, store at room temperature; do not refrigerate. Manufacturer recommended dilutions and stability of parenteral admixture at room temperature (25°C):

5 mL/125 mL D_5W; stable for 6 hours
5 mL/100 mL D_5W; stable for 4 hours
5 mL/75 mL D_5W; stable for 2 hours

Studies have also confirmed limited stability in NS; detailed references should be consulted.

Suspension, tablet: Store at room temperature; protect from light

Sulfasalazine (sul fa SAL a zeen)

U.S. Brand Names Azulfidine®; Azulfidine® EN-tabs®; Sulfazine; Sulfazine EC

Synonyms Salicylazosulfapyridine

Pharmacologic Category 5-Aminosalicylic Acid Derivative

Medication Safety Issues

Sound-alike/look-alike issues:

Sulfasalazine may be confused with salsalate, sulfaDIAZINE, sulfiSOXAZOLE
Azulfidine® may be confused with Augmentin®, azathioprine

Use Management of ulcerative colitis; enteric coated tablets are also used for rheumatoid arthritis (including juvenile rheumatoid arthritis) in patients who inadequately respond to analgesics and NSAIDs

Unlabeled/Investigational Use Ankylosing spondylitis, collagenous colitis, Crohn's disease, psoriasis, psoriatic arthritis, juvenile chronic arthritis

Mechanism of Action Acts locally in the colon to decrease the inflammatory response and systemically interferes with secretion by inhibiting prostaglandin synthesis

Pharmacodynamics/Kinetics

Absorption: 10% to 15% as unchanged drug from small intestine

Distribution: Small amounts enter feces and breast milk

Metabolism: Via colonic intestinal flora to sulfapyridine and 5-aminosalicylic acid (5-ASA); following absorption, sulfapyridine undergoes N-acetylation and ring hydroxylation while 5-ASA undergoes N-acetylation

Half-life elimination: 5.7-10 hours

Excretion: Primarily urine (as unchanged drug, components, and acetylated metabolites)

Contraindications Hypersensitivity to sulfasalazine, sulfa drugs, salicylates, or any component of the formulation; porphyria; GI or GU obstruction; pregnancy (at term)

Warnings/Precautions Use with caution in patients with renal impairment; impaired hepatic function or urinary obstruction, blood dyscrasias, severe allergies or asthma, or G6PD deficiency; may cause folate deficiency (consider providing 1 mg/day folate supplement). Chemical similarities are present among sulfonamides, sulfonylureas, carbonic anhydrase inhibitors, thiazides, and loop diuretics (except ethacrynic acid). Use in patients with sulfonamide allergy is specifically contraindicated in product labeling, however, a risk of cross-reaction exists in patients with allergy to any of these compounds; avoid use when previous reaction has been severe. Safety and efficacy have not been established in children <2 years of age.

Drug Interactions

Azathioprine, mercaptopurine, sulfasalazine: May increase the risk of myelosuppression (due to TPMT inhibition).

Cyclosporine concentrations may be decreased; monitor levels and renal function

Digoxin's absorption may be decreased

Folic acid's absorption may be decreased

Hydantoin levels may be increased; monitor levels and adjust as necessary

Hypoglycemics: Increased effect of oral hypoglycemics (rare, but severe); monitor blood sugar

Methenamine: Combination may result in crystalluria; avoid use

Methotrexate-induced bone marrow suppression may be increased

NSAIDs and salicylates: May increase sulfonamide concentrations

PABA (para-aminobenzoic acid - may be found in some vitamin supplements): Interferes with the antibacterial activity of sulfonamides; avoid concurrent use

Sulfinpyrazone: May increase sulfonamide concentrations

Thiazide diuretics: May increase the incidence of thrombocytopenia purpura

Thiopental's effect may be enhanced; monitor for possible dosage reduction

Uricosuric agents: Actions of these agents are potentiated

Warfarin and other oral anticoagulants: Anticoagulant effect may be increased; decrease dose and monitor INR closely

Nutritional/Herbal/Ethanol Interactions

Food: May impair folate absorption.

Herb/Nutraceutical: Avoid dong quai, St John's wort (may also cause photosensitization)

Adverse Reactions

>10%:

Central nervous system: Headache (33%)

Dermatologic: Photosensitivity

Gastrointestinal: Anorexia, nausea, vomiting, diarrhea (33%), gastric distress

Genitourinary: Reversible oligospermia (33%)

<3% (Limited to important or life-threatening): Alopecia, anaphylaxis, aplastic anemia, ataxia, crystalluria, depression, epidermal necrolysis, exfoliative dermatitis, granulocytopenia, hallucinations, Heinz body anemia, hemolytic anemia, hepatitis, interstitial nephritis, jaundice, leukopenia, Lyell's syndrome, myelodysplastic syndrome, nephropathy (acute), neutropenic enterocolitis, pancreatitis, peripheral neuropathy, photosensitization, pruritus, rhabdomyolysis, seizure, serum sickness-like reactions, skin discoloration, Stevens-Johnson syndrome, thrombocytopenia, thyroid function disturbance, urine discoloration, urticaria, vasculitis, vertigo

Additional events reported with sulfonamides and/or 5-ASA derivatives: Cholestatic jaundice, eosinophilia pneumonitis, erythema multiforme, fibrosing alveolitis, hepatic necrosis, Kawasaki-like syndrome, SLE-like syndrome, pericarditis, seizure, transverse myelitis

Overdosage/Toxicology Symptoms of overdose include drowsiness, dizziness, anorexia, abdominal pain, nausea, vomiting, hemolytic anemia, acidosis, jaundice, fever, and agranulocytosis. The aniline radical is responsible for hematologic toxicity. High volume diuresis may aid in elimination and prevention of renal

(Continued)

Sulfasalazine *(Continued)*

failure. Leucovorin 5-15 mg/day has been used to speed recovery of bone marrow.

Dosing

Adults & Elderly:

Ulcerative colitis: Oral: Initial: 1 g 3-4 times/day, 2 g/day maintenance in divided doses; may initiate therapy with 0.5-1 g/day

Rheumatoid arthritis: Oral (enteric coated tablet): Initial: 0.5-1 g/day; increase weekly to maintenance dose of 2 g/day in 2 divided doses; maximum: 3 g/day (if response to 2 g/day is inadequate after 12 weeks of treatment)

Pediatrics:

Ulcerative colitis: Oral: Children ≥2 years: Initial: 40-60 mg/kg/day in 3-6 divided doses; maintenance dose: 20-30 mg/kg/day in 4 divided doses

Juvenile rheumatoid arthritis: Oral (enteric coated tablet): Children ≥6 years: 30-50 mg/kg/day in 2 divided doses; Initial: Begin with 1/4 to 1/3 of expected maintenance dose; increase weekly; maximum: 2 g/day typically

Renal Impairment:

Cl_{cr} 10-30 mL/minute: Administer twice daily.

Cl_{cr} <10 mL/minute: Administer once daily.

Hepatic Impairment: Avoid use.

Available Dosage Forms

Tablet (Azulfidine®, Sulfazine): 500 mg

Tablet, delayed release, enteric coated (Azulfidine® EN-tabs®, Sulfazine EC): 500 mg

Nursing Guidelines

Assessment: Assess for allergy history prior to starting therapy. See Contraindications, Warnings/Precautions, and Dosing for use cautions. Assess potential for interactions with other prescriptions, OTC medications, or herbal products patient may be taking (see Drug Interactions). Monitor patient response (see Adverse Reactions and Overdose/Toxicology). Caution patients with diabetes to monitor glucose levels closely (decreased effect of oral hypoglycemic agents). Teach patient proper use, possible side effects/appropriate interventions, and adverse symptoms to report (see Patient Education) on a regular basis during therapy. **Pregnancy risk factor B/D** - see Pregnancy Risk Factor for use cautions. Note breast-feeding caution.

Dietary Considerations: Since sulfasalazine impairs folate absorption, consider providing 1 mg/day folate supplement.

Patient Education: Inform prescriber of all prescriptions, OTC medications, or herbal products you are taking, and any allergies you have. Take as directed, at regular intervals around-the-clock with food. Do not crush, chew, or dissolve coated tablets. Complete full course of therapy even if you are feeling better. Take a missed dose as soon as possible. If almost time for next dose, skip the missed dose and return to your regular schedule. Do not take a double dose. Maintain adequate hydration (2-3 L/day of fluids) to prevent kidney damage unless instructed to restrict fluid intake. If you have diabetes, monitor glucose levels closely (may cause decreased effect of oral hypoglycemic agents). Orange-yellow color of urine is normal. May cause dizziness or headache (use caution when driving or engaging in tasks requiring alertness until response to drug is known); photosensitivity (use sunblock, wear protective clothing and eyewear, and avoid direct sunlight); or nausea, vomiting, or loss of appetite (small, frequent meals, frequent mouth care, sucking lozenges, or chewing gum may help). Report rash; persistent nausea, vomiting, or diarrhea; opportunistic infection (sore throat, fever, vaginal itching or discharge, unusual bruising or bleeding, fatigue); blood in urine or change in urinary pattern; swelling of face, lips, or tongue, tightness in chest, bad cough, blue skin color, or other persistent adverse effects. **Pregnancy/breast-feeding precautions:** Inform prescriber if you are or intend to become pregnant. Consult prescriber if breast-feeding.

Geriatric Considerations: Adjust dose for renal function

Pregnancy Risk Factor: B/D (at term)

Lactation: Enters breast milk/use caution (AAP recommends use "with caution")

Breast-Feeding Considerations: Sulfonamides are excreted in human breast milk and may cause kernicterus in the newborn. Although sulfapyridine has poor bilirubin-displacing ability, use with caution in women who are breast-feeding. The AAP classifies this agent to be used with caution since adverse effects have been reported in nursing infants.

Administration

Oral: GI intolerance is common during the first few days of therapy (give with meals).

Storage: Protect from light.

- Sulfatrim *see* Sulfamethoxazole and Trimethoprim *on page 1582*
- Sulfazine *see* Sulfasalazine *on page 1586*
- Sulfazine EC *see* Sulfasalazine *on page 1586*

Sumatriptan (soo ma TRIP tan SUKS i nate)

U.S. Brand Names Imitrex®

Synonyms Sumatriptan Succinate

Pharmacologic Category Serotonin 5-HT_{1D} Receptor Agonist

Medication Safety Issues

Sound-alike/look-alike issues:

Sumatriptan may be confused with somatropin, zolmitriptan

Use

Oral, SubQ: Acute treatment of migraine with or without aura

SubQ: Acute treatment of cluster headache episodes

Mechanism of Action Selective agonist for serotonin (5-HT_{1D} receptor) in cranial arteries to cause vasoconstriction and reduces sterile inflammation associated with antidromic neuronal transmission correlating with relief of migraine

Pharmacodynamics/Kinetics

Onset of action: ~30 minutes

Distribution: V_d: 2.4 L/kg

Protein binding: 14% to 21%

Metabolism: Hepatic, primarily via MAO-A isoenzyme

Bioavailability: SubQ: 97% ± 16% of that following I.V. injection; Oral: 15%

Half-life elimination: Injection, tablet: 2.5 hours; Nasal spray: 2 hours

Time to peak, serum: 5-20 minutes

Excretion:

Injection: Urine (38% as indole acetic acid metabolite, 22% as unchanged drug)

Nasal spray: Urine (42% as indole acetic acid metabolite, 3% as unchanged drug)

Tablet: Urine (60% as indole acetic acid metabolite, 3% as unchanged drug); feces (40%)

Contraindications Hypersensitivity to sumatriptan or any component of the formulation; patients with ischemic heart disease or signs or symptoms of ischemic heart disease (including Prinzmetal's angina, angina pectoris, myocardial infarction, silent myocardial ischemia); cerebrovascular syndromes (including strokes, transient ischemic attacks); peripheral vascular syndromes (including ischemic bowel disease); uncontrolled hypertension; use within 24 hours of ergotamine derivatives; use within 24 hours of another 5-HT_1 agonist; concurrent administration or within 2 weeks of discontinuing an MAO inhibitor, specifically MAO type A inhibitors; management of hemiplegic or basilar migraine; prophylactic treatment of migraine; severe hepatic impairment; not for I.V. administration

Warnings/Precautions Sumatriptan is indicated only in patients ≥18 years of age with a clear diagnosis of migraine or cluster headache.

Cardiac events (coronary artery vasospasm, transient ischemia, myocardial infarction, ventricular tachycardia/fibrillation, cardiac arrest and death), cerebral/subarachnoid hemorrhage and stroke have been reported with 5-HT_1 agonist administration.

Do not give to patients with risk factors for CAD until a cardiovascular evaluation has been performed; if evaluation is satisfactory, the healthcare provider should administer the first dose and cardiovascular status should be periodically evaluated.

Significant elevation in blood pressure, including hypertensive crisis, has also been reported on rare occasions in patients with and without a history of hypertension. Vasospasm-related reactions have been reported other than coronary artery vasospasm. Peripheral vascular ischemia and colonic ischemia with abdominal pain and bloody diarrhea have occurred.

Use with caution in patients with history of seizure disorder or in patients with a lowered seizure threshold. Safety and efficacy in pediatric patients have not been established.

Drug Interactions Note: Use cautiously in patients receiving concomitant medications that can lower the seizure threshold.

(Continued)

Sumatriptan *(Continued)*

Ergot-containing drugs: Prolong vasospastic reactions; do not use sumatriptan or ergot-containing drugs within 24 hours of each other.

MAO inhibitors (MAO type A inhibitors, nonspecific MAO inhibitors): Reduce sumatriptan clearance; concurrent use is contraindicated; wait at least 2 weeks after discontinuing MAO type A inhibitor to start sumatriptan.

Selegiline: Selegiline is a selective MAO type B inhibitor; while not specifically contraindicated, combination may best be avoided until further study.

SSRIs: Can lead to symptoms of hyper-reflexia, weakness, and incoordination; monitor.

Adverse Reactions

Injection:

>10%:

Central nervous system: Dizziness (12%), warm/hot sensation (11%)

Local: Pain at injection site (59%)

Neuromuscular & skeletal: Tingling (13%)

1% to 10%:

Cardiovascular: Chest pain/tightness/heaviness/pressure (2% to 3%), hyper-/ hypotension (1%)

Central nervous system: Burning (7%), feeling of heaviness (7%), flushing (7%), pressure sensation (7%), feeling of tightness (5%), drowsiness (3%), malaise/fatigue (1%), feeling strange (2%), headache (2%), tight feeling in head (2%), cold sensation (1%), anxiety (1%)

Gastrointestinal: Abdominal discomfort (1%), dysphagia (1%)

Neuromuscular & skeletal: Neck, throat, and jaw pain/tightness/pressure (2% to 5%), mouth/tongue discomfort (5%), weakness (5%), myalgia (2%); muscle cramps (1%), numbness (5%)

Ocular: Vision alterations (1%)

Respiratory: Nasal disorder/discomfort (2%), throat discomfort (3%)

Miscellaneous: Diaphoresis (2%)

Nasal spray:

>10%: Gastrointestinal: Bad taste (13% to 24%), nausea (11% to 13%), vomiting (11% to 13%)

1% to 10%:

Central nervous system: Dizziness (1% to 2%)

Respiratory: Nasal disorder/discomfort (2% to 4%), throat discomfort (1% to 2%)

Tablet:

1% to 10%:

Cardiovascular: Chest pain/tightness/heaviness/pressure (1% to 2%), hyper-/ hypotension (1%), palpitation (1%), syncope (1%)

Central nervous system: Burning (1%), dizziness (>1%), drowsiness (>1%), malaise/fatigue (2% to 3%), headache (>1%), nonspecified pain (1% to 2%, placebo 1%), vertigo (<1% to 2%), migraine (>1%), sleepiness (>1%)

Gastrointestinal: Diarrhea (1%), nausea (>1%), vomiting (>1%), hyposalivation (>1%)

Genitourinary: Hematuria (1%)

Hematologic: Hemolytic anemia (1%)

Neuromuscular & skeletal: Neck, throat, and jaw pain/tightness/pressure (2% to 3%), paresthesia (3% to 5%), myalgia (1%), numbness (1%)

Otic: Ear hemorrhage (1%), hearing loss (1%), sensitivity to noise (1%), tinnitus (1%)

Respiratory: Allergic rhinitis (1%), dyspnea (1%), nasal inflammation (1%), nose/throat hemorrhage (1%), sinusitis (1%), upper respiratory inflammation (1%)

Miscellaneous: Hypersensitivity reactions (1%), nonspecified pressure/tightness/heaviness (1% to 3%, placebo 2%); warm/cold sensation (2% to 3%, placebo 2%)

Route unspecified: <1%: Postmarketing and uncontrolled studies (limited to important or life-threatening): Abdominal aortic aneurysm, abdominal discomfort, abnormal menstrual cycle, abnormal/elevated liver function tests, accommodation disorders, acute renal failure, agitation, anaphylactoid reaction, anaphylaxis, anemia, angioneurotic edema, arrhythmia, atrial fibrillation, bronchospasm, cerebral ischemia, cerebrovascular accident, convulsions, deafness, death, decreased appetite, dental pain, diarrhea, dyspeptic symptoms, dysphagia, dystonic reaction, ECG changes, fluid disturbances (including retention), flushing, gastrointestinal pain, hallucinations, heart block, hematuria, hemolytic anemia, hiccups, hypersensitivity reactions, intestinal obstruction, intracranial pressure increased, ischemic colitis, joint ache, muscle stiffness, nose/throat hemorrhage, numbness of tongue, optic neuropathy (ischemic), pancytopenia, paresthesia, phlebitis, photosensitivity, Prinzmetal's angina, pruritus, psychomotor disorders, pulmonary embolism, rash, Raynaud syndrome, sensation changes, shock, subarachnoid hemorrhage, swallowing disorders, syncope, thrombocytopenia, thrombophlebitis, thrombosis, transient myocardial ischemia, TSH increased, vasculitis, vision loss, xerostomia

Overdosage/Toxicology Single oral doses ≤400 mg, injectable doses ≤16 mg, and nasal doses of 40 mg have been reported without adverse effects. Treatment of overdose should be supportive and symptomatic. Monitor for at least 12 hours or until signs and symptoms subside. It is not known if hemodialysis or peritoneal dialysis is effective.

Dosing

Adults:

Migraine:

Oral: A single dose of 25 mg, 50 mg, or 100 mg (taken with fluids). If a satisfactory response has not been obtained at 2 hours, a second dose may be administered. Results from clinical trials show that initial doses of 50 mg and 100 mg are more effective than doses of 25 mg, and that 100 mg doses do not provide a greater effect than 50 mg and may have increased incidence of side effects. Although doses of up to 300 mg/day have been studied, the total daily dose should not exceed 200 mg. The safety of treating an average of >4 headaches in a 30-day period have not been established.

Intranasal: Single dose of 5, 10, or 20 mg administered in one nostril; a 10 mg dose may be achieved by administration of a single 5 mg dose in each nostril; if headache returns, the dose may be repeated once after 2 hours, not to exceed a total daily dose of 40 mg. The safety of treating an average of >4 headaches in a 30-day period has not been established.

SubQ: 6 mg; a second injection may be administered at least 1 hour after the initial dose, but not more than two injections in a 24-hour period. If side effects are dose-limiting, lower doses may be used.

Cluster headache: Refer to dosing under "Migraine, SubQ"

Renal Impairment: Dosage adjustment is not necessary.

Hepatic Impairment: Bioavailability of oral sumatriptan is increased with liver disease. If treatment is needed, do not exceed single doses of 50 mg. The nasal spray has not been studied in patients with hepatic impairment, however, because the spray does not undergo first-pass metabolism, levels would not be expected to alter. Use of all dosage forms is contraindicated with severe hepatic impairment.

Available Dosage Forms Note: Strength expressed as sumatriptan base

Injection, solution, as succinate: 12 mg/mL (0.5 mL)

Solution, intranasal spray: 5 mg (100 µL unit dose spray device); 20 mg (100 µL unit dose spray device)

Tablet, as succinate: 25 mg, 50 mg, 100 mg

Nursing Guidelines

Assessment: See Contraindications, Warnings/Precautions (clear diagnosis of migraine), and Dosing for use cautions. Assess potential for interactions with other prescriptions, OTC medications, or herbal products patient may be taking (eg, ergot-containing drugs - see Drug Interactions). Assess therapeutic effectiveness and adverse response (see Adverse Reactions and Overdose/Toxicology). Teach patient proper use according to formulation (eg, appropriate injection technique and syringe/needle disposal), possible side effects/appropriate interventions, and adverse symptoms to report (see Patient Education). Note breast-feeding caution.

Patient Education: Inform prescriber of all prescription (including oral contraceptives) and OTC medications or herbal products you are taking, and any allergies you have. Take at first sign of migraine attack. This drug is to be used to reduce your migraine, not to prevent or reduce the number of attacks. Follow exact instructions for use.

Nasal spray: Administer dose into one nostril. If headache returns or is not fully resolved after the first dose, the dose may be repeated after 2 hours. **Do not exceed 40 mg in 24 hours.**

(Continued)

Sumatriptan *(Continued)*

Oral: If headache returns or is not fully resolved after first dose, the dose may be repeated after 2 hours. **Do not exceed 200 mg in 24 hours.** Take whole with fluids.

SubQ: If headache returns or is not fully resolved after first dose, the dose may be repeated after 1 hour. **Do not exceed two injections in 24 hours.**

All forms: Do not take any form of this drug within 24 hours of any other migraine medication without consulting prescriber. May cause dizziness, fatigue, or drowsiness (use caution when driving or engaging in tasks that require alertness until response to drug is known); or nausea or vomiting (small, frequent meals, frequent mouth care, chewing gum, or sucking on lozenges may help). Report chest tightness or pain; excessive drowsiness; acute abdominal pain; skin rash or burning sensation; muscle weakness, soreness, or numbness; respiratory difficulty; or any other persistent adverse reactions. **Pregnancy/breast-feeding precautions:** Inform prescriber if you are or intend to become pregnant. Consult prescriber if breast-feeding.

Geriatric Considerations: Use cautiously in the elderly, particularly since many elderly have cardiovascular disease which would put them at risk for cardiovascular adverse effects. Safety and efficacy in the elderly (>65 years) have not been established. Pharmacokinetic disposition is, however, similar to that in young adults.

Pregnancy Risk Factor: C

Lactation: Enters breast milk/use caution (AAP rates "compatible")

Breast-Feeding Considerations: The amount of sumatriptan an infant would be exposed to following breast-feeding is considered to be small (although the mean milk-to-plasma ratio is ~4.9, weight adjusted doses estimates suggest breast-fed infants receive 3.5% of a maternal dose). Expressing and discarding the milk for 8 hours after a single dose is suggested to reduce the amount present even further. The half-life of sumatriptan in breast milk is 2.22 hours.

Perioperative/Anesthesia/Other Concerns: Sumatriptan should not be used in patients with a history of vasospastic disease, Prinzmetal's angina, or any critical vascular disease.

Administration

Oral: Oral: Should be taken with fluids as soon as symptoms appear.

I.V.: Do **not** administer I.V.; may cause coronary vasospasm.

Storage: Store at 2°C to 20°C (36°F to 86°F). Protect from light.

- **Sumatriptan Succinate** *see* Sumatriptan *on page 1589*
- **Summer's Eve® Medicated Douche [OTC]** *see* Povidone-Iodine *on page 1392*
- **Summer's Eve® SpecialCare™ Medicated Anti-Itch Cream [OTC]** *see* Hydrocortisone *on page 873*
- **Sumycin®** *see* Tetracycline *on page 1613*
- **Supartz™** *see* Hyaluronate and Derivatives *on page 856*
- **Suprane®** *see* Desflurane *on page 491*
- **Surbex-T® [OTC]** *see* Vitamin B Complex Combinations *on page 1716*
- **Sureprin 81™ [OTC]** *see* Aspirin *on page 189*
- **Surfak® [OTC]** *see* Docusate *on page 560*
- **Surgicel®** *see* Cellulose (Oxidized Regenerated) *on page 362*
- **Surgicel® Fibrillar** *see* Cellulose (Oxidized Regenerated) *on page 362*
- **Surgicel® NuKnit** *see* Cellulose (Oxidized Regenerated) *on page 362*
- **Sustiva®** *see* Efavirenz *on page 597*
- **Suxamethonium Chloride** *see* Succinylcholine *on page 1573*
- **Symax SL** *see* Hyoscyamine *on page 886*
- **Symax SR** *see* Hyoscyamine *on page 886*
- **Synercid®** *see* Quinupristin and Dalfopristin *on page 1455*
- **Synthroid®** *see* Levothyroxine *on page 1029*
- **Synvisc®** *see* Hyaluronate and Derivatives *on page 856*
- **Syrex** *see* Sodium Chloride *on page 1545*
- **SyringeAvitene™** *see* Collagen Hemostat *on page 449*
- **T_4** *see* Levothyroxine *on page 1029*

Tacrolimus (ta KROE li mus)

U.S. Brand Names Prograf®; Protopic®

Synonyms FK506

Pharmacologic Category Immunosuppressant Agent; Topical Skin Product

Medication Safety Issues

Sound-alike/look-alike issues:

Prograf® may be confused with Gengraf®

Use

Oral/injection: Potent immunosuppressive drug used in liver or kidney transplant recipients

Topical: Moderate to severe atopic dermatitis in patients not responsive to conventional therapy or when conventional therapy is not appropriate

Unlabeled/Investigational Use Potent immunosuppressive drug used in heart, lung, small bowel transplant recipients; immunosuppressive drug for peripheral stem cell/bone marrow transplantation

Mechanism of Action Suppresses cellular immunity (inhibits T-lymphocyte activation), possibly by binding to an intracellular protein, FKBP-12

Pharmacodynamics/Kinetics

Absorption: Better in resected patients with a closed stoma; unlike cyclosporine, clamping of the T-tube in liver transplant patients does not alter trough concentrations or AUC

Oral: Incomplete and variable; food within 15 minutes of administration decreases absorption (27%)

Topical: Serum concentrations range from undetectable to 20 ng/mL (<5 ng/mL in majority of adult patients studied)

Protein binding: 99%

Metabolism: Extensively hepatic via CYP3A4 to eight possible metabolites (major metabolite, 31-demethyl tacrolimus, shows same activity as tacrolimus *in vitro*)

Bioavailability: Oral: Adults: 7% to 28%, Children: 10% to 52%; Topical: <0.5%; Absolute: Unknown

Half-life elimination: Variable, 21-61 hours in healthy volunteers

Time to peak: 0.5-4 hours

Excretion: Feces (~92%); feces/urine (<1% as unchanged drug)

Contraindications Hypersensitivity to tacrolimus or any component of the formulation

Warnings/Precautions

Oral/injection: Insulin-dependent post-transplant diabetes mellitus (PTDM) has been reported (1% to 20%); risk increases in African-American and Hispanic kidney transplant patients. Increased susceptibility to infection and the possible development of lymphoma may occur after administration of tacrolimus. Nephrotoxicity and neurotoxicity have been reported, especially with higher doses; to avoid excess nephrotoxicity do not administer simultaneously with cyclosporine; monitoring of serum concentrations (trough for oral therapy) is essential to prevent organ rejection and reduce drug-related toxicity; tonic clonic seizures may have been triggered by tacrolimus. A period of 24 hours should elapse between discontinuation of cyclosporine and the initiation of tacrolimus. Use caution in renal or hepatic dysfunction, dosing adjustments may be required. Delay initiation if postoperative oliguria occurs. Use may be associated with the development of hypertension (common). Myocardial hypertrophy has been reported (rare). Each mL of injection contains polyoxyl 60 hydrogenated castor oil (HCO-60) (200 mg) and dehydrated alcohol USP 80% v/v. Anaphylaxis has been reported with the injection, use should be reserved for those patients not able to take oral medications.

Topical: Topical calcineurin agents are considered second-line therapies in the treatment of atopic dermatitis/eczema, and should be limited to use in patients who have failed treatment with other therapies. They should be used for short-term and intermittent treatment using the minimum amount necessary for the control of symptoms should be used.

Infections at the treatment site should be cleared prior to therapy. Patients with atopic dermatitis are predisposed to skin infections, including eczema herpeticum, varicella zoster, and herpes simplex. Discontinue use in patients with unknown cause of lymphadenopathy or acute infectious mononucleosis. Not recommended for use in patients with Netherton's syndrome. Safety not established in patients with generalized erythroderma. The use of Protopic® in children <2 years of age is not recommended, particularly since the effect on immune system development is unknown.

(Continued)

Tacrolimus *(Continued)*

Drug Interactions Substrate of CYP3A4 (major); **Inhibits** CYP3A4 (weak)

Antacids: Separate administration by at least 2 hours

Anticonvulsants: Carbamazepine, phenobarbital, phenytoin: May decrease tacrolimus blood levels.

Azithromycin: May increase tacrolimus serum concentrations (limited documentation); monitor.

Calcium channel blockers (dihydropyridine): May increase tacrolimus serum concentrations; monitor.

Caspofungin: May decrease tacrolimus serum concentrations.

Cisapride (and metoclopramide): May increase serum concentration of tacrolimus

Cyclosporine: Concomitant use is associated with synergistic immunosuppression and increased nephrotoxicity; give first dose of tacrolimus no sooner than 24 hours after last cyclosporine dose. In the presence of elevated tacrolimus or cyclosporine concentration, dosing of the other usually should be delayed longer.

CYP3A4 inducers: CYP3A4 inducers may decrease the levels/effects of tacrolimus. Example inducers include aminoglutethimide, carbamazepine, nafcillin, nevirapine, phenobarbital, phenytoin, and rifamycins.

CYP3A4 inhibitors: May increase the levels/effects of tacrolimus. Example inhibitors include azole antifungals, clarithromycin, diclofenac, doxycycline, erythromycin, imatinib, isoniazid, nefazodone, nicardipine, propofol, protease inhibitors, quinidine, telithromycin, and verapamil.

Ganciclovir: Nephrotoxicity may be additive with tacrolimus; use caution.

Potassium-sparing diuretics: Tacrolimus use may lead to hyperkalemia; avoid concomitant use

Rifabutin, rifampin: May decrease serum levels of tacrolimus.

Sirolimus: May decrease tacrolimus serum concentrations. Concurrent therapy may increase the risk of HUS/TTP/TMA.

St John's wort: May decrease tacrolimus serum concentrations; avoid concurrent use.

Sucralfate: Separate administration by at least 2 hours

Vaccines (live): Vaccine may be less effective; avoid vaccination during treatment if possible

Voriconazole: Tacrolimus serum concentrations may be increased; monitor serum concentrations and renal function. Decrease tacrolimus dosage by 66% when initiating voriconazole.

Nutritional/Herbal/Ethanol Interactions

Ethanol: Localized flushing (redness, warm sensation) may occur at application site of topical tacrolimus following ethanol consumption.

Food: Decreases rate and extent of absorption. High-fat meals have most pronounced effect (35% decrease in AUC, 77% decrease in C_{max}). Grapefruit juice, CYP3A4 inhibitor, may increase serum level and/or toxicity of tacrolimus; avoid concurrent use.

Herb/Nutraceutical: St John's wort: May reduce tacrolimus serum concentrations (avoid concurrent use).

Adverse Reactions

Oral, I.V.:

≥15%:

Cardiovascular: Chest pain, hypertension

Central nervous system: Dizziness, headache, insomnia, tremor (headache and tremor are associated with high whole blood concentrations and may respond to decreased dosage)

Dermatologic: Pruritus, rash

Endocrine & metabolic: Diabetes mellitus, hyperglycemia, hyper-/hypokalemia, hyperlipemia, hypomagnesemia, hypophosphatemia

Gastrointestinal: Abdominal pain, constipation, diarrhea, dyspepsia, nausea, vomiting

Genitourinary: Urinary tract infection

Hematologic: Anemia, leukocytosis, thrombocytopenia

Hepatic: Ascites

Neuromuscular & skeletal: Arthralgia, back pain, weakness, paresthesia

Renal: Abnormal kidney function, increased creatinine, oliguria, urinary tract infection, increased BUN

Respiratory: Atelectasis, dyspnea, increased cough, pleual effusion

<15%:

Cardiovascular: Abnormal ECG (QRS or ST segment abnormal), angina pectoris, cardiopulmonary failure, deep thrombophlebitis, heart rate decreased, hemorrhage, hemorrhagic stroke, hypervolemia, hypotension, generalized edema, peripheral vascular disorder, phlebitis, postural hypotension, tachycardia, thrombosis, vasodilation

Central nervous system: Abnormal dreams, abnormal thinking, agitation, amnesia, anxiety, chills, confusion, depression, dizziness, elevated mood, emotional lability, encephalopathy, hallucinations, nervousness, paralysis, psychosis, quadraparesis, seizure, somnolence

Dermatologic: Acne, alopecia, cellulitis, exfoliative dermatitis, fungal dermatitis, hirsutism, increased diaphoresis, photosensitivity reaction, skin discoloration, skin disorder, skin ulcer

Endocrine & metabolic: Acidosis, alkalosis, Cushing's syndrome, decreased bicarbonate, decreased serum iron, diabetes mellitus, hypercalcemia, hypercholesterolemia, hyperphosphatemia, hypoproteinemia, increased alkaline phosphatase

Gastrointestinal: Anorexia, appetite increased, cramps, duodenitis, dysphagia, enlarged abdomen, esophagitis (including ulcerative), flatulence, gastritis, gastroesophagitis, GI perforation/hemorrhage, ileus, oral moniliasis, pancreatic pseudocyst, rectal disorder, stomatitis, weight gain

Genitourinary: Bladder spasm, cystitis, dysuria, nocturia, oliguria, urge incontinence, urinary frequency, urinary incontinence, urinary retention, vaginitis

Hematologic: Bruising, coagulation disorder, decreased prothrombin, hypochromic anemia, leukopenia, polycythemia

Hepatic: Abnormal liver function tests, ALT/AST increased, bilirubinemia, cholangitis, cholestatic jaundice, GGT increased, hepatitis (including granulomatous), jaundice, liver damage, increase LDH

Neuromuscular & skeletal: Hypertonia, incoordination, joint disorder, leg cramps, myalgia, myasthenia, myoclonus, nerve compression, neuropathy, osteoporosis

Ocular: Abnormal vision, amblyopia

Otic: Ear pain, otitis media, tinnitus

Renal: Albuminuria, renal tubular necrosis, toxic nephropathy

Respiratory: Asthma, bronchitis, lung disorder, pharyngitis, pneumonia, pneumothorax, pulmonary edema, respiratory disorder, rhinitis, sinusitis, voice alteration

Miscellaneous: Abscess, abnormal healing, allergic reaction, crying, flu-like syndrome, generalized spasm, hernia, herpes simplex, peritonitis, sepsis, writing impaired

Limited to important or life-threatening: Acute renal failure, anaphylaxis, ARDS, arrhythmia, atrial fibrillation, atrial flutter, blindness, cardiac arrest, cerebral infarction, coma, deafness, delirium, DIC, hearing loss, hemiparesis, hemolytic-uremic syndrome, hemorrhagic cystitis, hepatic necrosis, hepatotoxicity, leukoencephalopathy, lymphoproliferative disorder (related to EBV), myocardial hypertrophy (associated with ventricular dysfunction; reversible upon discontinuation), MI, neutropenia, pancreatitis (hemorrhagic and necrotizing), pancytopenia, quadriplegia, QT_c prolongation, respiratory failure, seizure, Stevens-Johnson syndrome, syncope, toxic epidermal necrolysis, thrombocytopenic purpura, torsade de pointes, TTP, veno-occlusive hepatic disease, venous thrombosis, ventricular fibrillation. Calcineurin inhibitor-induced hemolytic uremic syndrome/thrombotic thrombocytopenic purpura/thrombotic microangiopathy (HUS/TTP/TMA) have been reported (with concurrent sirolimus).

Topical:

>10%:

Central nervous system: Headache (5% to 20%), fever (1% to 21%)

Dermatologic: Skin burning (43% to 58%), pruritus (41% to 46%), erythema (12% to 28%)

Respiratory: Increased cough (18% children)

Miscellaneous: Flu-like syndrome (23% to 28%), allergic reaction (4% to 12%)

Overdosage/Toxicology Symptoms are extensions of immunosuppressive activity and adverse effects. Symptomatic and supportive treatment is required. Hemodialysis is not effective.

(Continued)

Tacrolimus *(Continued)*

Dosing

Adults & Elderly:

Kidney transplant:

Oral: Initial dose: 0.2 mg/kg/day in 2 divided doses, given every 12 hours; initial dose may be given within 24 hours of transplant, but should be delayed until renal function has recovered; African-American patients may require larger doses to maintain trough concentration

Typical whole blood trough concentrations: Months 1-3: 7-20 ng/mL; months 4-12: 5-15 ng/mL

I.V.: **Note:** I.V. route should only be used in patients not able to take oral medications, anaphylaxis has been reported. Initial dose: 0.03-0.05 mg/kg/day as a continuous infusion; begin no sooner than 6 hours post-transplant, starting at lower end of the dosage range; adjunctive therapy with corticosteroids is recommended; continue only until oral medication can be tolerated

Liver transplant:

Oral: Initial dose: 0.1-0.15 mg/kg/day in 2 divided doses, given every 12 hours; begin oral dose no sooner than 6 hours post-transplant; adjunctive therapy with corticosteroids is recommended; if switching from I.V. to oral, the oral dose should be started 8-12 hours after stopping the infusion

Typical whole blood trough concentrations: Months 1-12: 5-20 ng/mL

I.V.: **Note:** I.V. route should only be used in patients not able to take oral medications, anaphylaxis has been reported. Initial dose: 0.03-0.05 mg/kg/day as a continuous infusion; begin no sooner than 6 hours post-transplant starting at lower end of the dosage range; adjunctive therapy with corticosteroids is recommended; continue only until oral medication can be tolerated

Prevention of graft-vs-host disease: I.V.: 0.03 mg/kg/day as continuous infusion

Atopic dermatitis (moderate to severe): Topical: Apply 0.03% or 0.1% ointment to affected area twice daily; rub in gently and completely; continue applications for 1 week after symptoms have cleared

Pediatrics:

Liver transplant:

Note: Patients without pre-existing renal or hepatic dysfunction have required and tolerated higher doses than adults to achieve similar blood concentrations. It is recommended that therapy be initiated at high end of the recommended adult I.V. and oral dosing ranges; dosage adjustments may be required.

Oral: Initial dose: 0.15-0.20 mg/kg/day in 2 divided doses, given every 12 hours; begin oral dose no sooner than 6 hours post-transplant; adjunctive therapy with corticosteroids is recommended; if switching from I.V. to oral, the oral dose should be started 8-12 hours after stopping the infusion

Typical whole blood trough concentrations: Months 1-12: 5-20 ng/mL

I.V.: **Note:** I.V. route should only be used in patients not able to take oral medications, anaphylaxis has been reported. Initial dose: 0.03-0.05 mg/kg/day as a continuous infusion; begin no sooner than 6 hours post-transplant; adjunctive therapy with corticosteroids is recommended; continue only until oral medication can be tolerated

Moderate-to-severe atopic dermatitis: Topical: Children ≥2 years: Apply 0.03% ointment to affected area twice daily; rub in gently and completely; continue applications for 1 week after symptoms have cleared

Renal Impairment: Evidence suggests that lower doses should be used. Patients should receive doses at the lowest value of the recommended I.V. and oral dosing ranges. Further reductions in dose below these ranges may be required. Tacrolimus therapy should usually be delayed up to 48 hours or longer in patients with postoperative oliguria.

Hemodialysis: Not removed by hemodialysis; supplemental dose is not necessary.

Peritoneal dialysis: Significant drug removal is unlikely based on physiochemical characteristics.

Hepatic Impairment: Use of tacrolimus in liver transplant recipients experiencing post-transplant hepatic impairment may be associated with increased risk of developing renal insufficiency related to high whole blood levels of tacrolimus. The presence of moderate-to-severe hepatic dysfunction (serum bilirubin >2 mg/dL) appears to affect the metabolism of FK506. The half-life of the drug was prolonged and the clearance reduced after I.V. administration. The bioavailability of FK506 was also increased after oral administration. The higher plasma concentrations as determined by ELISA, in patients with severe hepatic dysfunction are probably due to the accumulation of FK506 metabolites of lower activity. These patients should be monitored closely and dosage adjustments should be considered. Some evidence indicates that lower doses could be used in these patients.

Available Dosage Forms

Capsule (Prograf®): 0.5 mg, 1 mg, 5 mg

Injection, solution (Prograf®): 5 mg/mL (1 mL) [contains dehydrated alcohol 80% and polyoxyl 60 hydrogenated castor oil]

Ointment, topical (Protopic®): 0.03% (30 g, 60 g, 100 g); 0.1% (30 g, 60 g, 100 g)

Nursing Guidelines

Assessment: Assess other medications patient may be taking for effectiveness and interactions. Monitor blood pressure frequently. Assess results of laboratory tests prior to, during, and following therapy. Monitor response to therapy and adverse reactions. Patients with diabetes should be advised to monitor glucose levels closely (this medication may alter glucose levels). Monitor/instruct patient on appropriate use, interventions to reduce side effects, to monitor for signs of opportunistic infection, and adverse reactions to report.

Monitoring Laboratory Tests: Renal function, hepatic function, serum electrolytes, glucose. Since pharmacokinetics show great inter- and intrapatient variability over time, monitoring of serum concentrations (trough for oral therapy) has proven helpful to prevent organ rejection and reduce drug-related toxicity. Measure 3 times/week for first few weeks, then gradually decrease frequency as patient stabilizes.

Dietary Considerations: Capsule: Take on an empty stomach; be consistent with timing and composition of meals if GI intolerance occurs (per manufacturer).

Patient Education: Take as directed, on an empty stomach. Be consistent with timing and consistency of meals if GI intolerance occurs (per manufacturer). Do not take within 2 hours before or after antacids. Do not alter dose and do not discontinue without consulting prescriber. Maintain adequate hydration (2-3 L/day of fluids) during entire course of therapy unless instructed to restrict fluid intake. You will be susceptible to infection (avoid crowds and exposure to infection). If you have diabetes, monitor glucose levels closely (drug may alter glucose levels). You may experience nausea, vomiting, loss of appetite (small frequent meals, frequent mouth care may help); diarrhea (boiled milk, yogurt, or buttermilk may help); constipation (increased exercise, fluids, fruit, fluid, or fiber may help; if unresolved, consult prescriber); or muscle or back pain (mild analgesics may be recommended). Report chest pain; acute headache or dizziness; symptoms of respiratory infection, cough, or respiratory difficulty; unresolved GI effects; fatigue, chills, fever, unhealed sores, white plaques in mouth, irritation in genital area; unusual bruising or bleeding; pain or irritation on urination or change in urinary patterns; rash or skin irritation; or other unusual effects.

Topical: Before applying, wash area gently and thoroughly. Apply in thin film to affected area. Do not cover skin with bandages. Wash hands only if not treating skin on the hands. Protect skin from sunlight or exposure to UV light. Consult prescriber if breast-feeding

Pregnancy/breast-feeding precautions: Inform prescriber if you are or intend to become pregnant. Do not breast-feed.

Pregnancy Risk Factor: C

Pregnancy Issues: Tacrolimus crosses the placenta and reaches concentrations four times greater than maternal plasma concentrations. Neonatal hyperkalemia and renal dysfunction have been reported.

Lactation: Enters breast milk/contraindicated

Breast-Feeding Considerations: Concentrations in breast milk are equivalent to plasma concentrations; breast-feeding is not advised.

Perioperative/Anesthesia/Other Concerns:

Additional dosing considerations:

Switch from I.V. to oral therapy: Threefold increase in dose

Pediatric patients: About 2 times higher dose compared to adults

Liver dysfunction: Decrease I.V. dose; decrease oral dose

Renal dysfunction: Does not affect kinetics; decrease dose to decrease levels if renal dysfunction is related to the drug

(Continued)

Tacrolimus *(Continued)*

Tacrolimus is associated with more neurotoxicity, nephrotoxicity, and glucose intolerance but less hypertension, dyslipidemia, gingival hyperplasia, or hirsutism than cyclosporine.

Administration

Oral: If dosed once daily, administer in the morning. If dosed twice daily (not common), doses should be 12 hours apart. If the morning and evening doses differ, the larger dose (differences are never >0.5-1 mg) should be given in the morning. If dosed 3 times/day, separate doses by 8 hours.

I.V.: Administer by I.V. continuous infusion only. Do not use PVC tubing when administering dilute solutions. Tacrolimus is dispensed in a 50 mL glass container with no overfill. It is usually intended to be administered as a continuous infusion over 24 hours.

Reconstitution:

Dilute with 5% dextrose injection or 0.9% sodium chloride injection to a final concentration between 0.004 mg/mL and 0.02 mg/mL.

Storage:

Injection: Prior to dilution, store at 5°C to 25°C (41°F to 77°F). Stable for 24 hours in D_5W or NS in glass or polyolefin containers.

Capsules and ointment: Store at room temperature 25°C (77°F).

- Tagamet® *see* Cimetidine *on page 396*
- Tagamet® HB 200 [OTC] *see* Cimetidine *on page 396*
- Tambocor™ *see* Flecainide *on page 731*

Tamsulosin (tam SOO loe sin)

U.S. Brand Names Flomax®

Synonyms Tamsulosin Hydrochloride

Pharmacologic Category Alpha$_1$ Blocker

Medication Safety Issues

Sound-alike/look-alike issues:

Flomax® may be confused with Fosamax®, Volmax®

Use Treatment of signs and symptoms of benign prostatic hyperplasia (BPH)

Mechanism of Action Tamsulosin is an antagonist of alpha$_{1A}$ adrenoreceptors in the prostate. Smooth muscle tone in the prostate is mediated by alpha$_{1A}$ adrenoreceptors; blocking them leads to relaxation of smooth muscle in the bladder neck and prostate causing an improvement of urine flow and decreased symptoms of BPH. Approximately 75% of the alpha$_1$ receptors in the prostate are of the alpha$_{1A}$ subtype.

Pharmacodynamics/Kinetics

Absorption: >90%

Protein binding: 94% to 99%, primarily to alpha$_1$ acid glycoprotein (AAG)

Metabolism: Hepatic via CYP; metabolites undergo extensive conjugation to glucuronide or sulfate

Bioavailability: Fasting: 30% increase

Distribution: V_d: 16 L

Steady-state: By the fifth day of once-daily dosing

Half-life elimination: Healthy volunteers: 9-13 hours; Target population: 14-15 hours

Time to peak: Fasting: 4-5 hours; With food: 6-7 hours

Excretion: Urine (76%, <10% as unchanged drug); feces (21%)

Contraindications Hypersensitivity to tamsulosin or any component of the formulation; concurrent use with phosphodiesterase-5 (PDE-5) inhibitors including sildenafil (>25 mg), tadalafil (if tamsulosin dose >0.4 mg/day), or vardenafil

Warnings/Precautions Not intended for use as an antihypertensive drug. May cause orthostasis, syncope or dizziness. Patients should avoid situations where injury may occur as a result of syncope. Rule out prostatic carcinoma before beginning therapy with tamsulosin. Intraoperative Floppy Iris Syndrome occurred most often in patients taking their alpha-1 blocker at the time of cataract surgery, but some cases occurred when the alpha-1 blocker blocker was stopped 2-14 days prior to surgery and as long as 5 weeks to 9 months prior to surgery. The benefit of stopping an alpha-1blocker prior to cataract surgery has not been established. Rarely, patients with a sulfa allergy have also developed an allergic reaction to tamsulosin; avoid use when previous reaction has been severe.

Drug Interactions Substrate (major) of CYP2D6, 3A4

Alpha-adrenergic blockers: Risk of hypotension may increase in combination with other alpha-adrenergic blocking agents.

Beta-blockers: Beta-blockers may increase risk of first-dose orthostatic hypotension of tamsulosin

Calcium channel blockers: Risk of hypotension may increase

Cimetidine: Cimetidine may decrease tamsulosin clearance.

CYP2D6 inhibitors: May increase the levels/effects of tamsulosin. Example inhibitors include chlorpromazine, delavirdine, fluoxetine, miconazole, paroxetine, pergolide, quinidine, quinine, ritonavir, and ropinirole.

CYP3A4 inducers: CYP3A4 inducers may decrease the levels/effects of tamsulosin. Example inducers include aminoglutethimide, carbamazepine, nafcillin, nevirapine, phenobarbital, phenytoin, and rifamycins.

CYP3A4 inhibitors: May increase the levels/effects of tamsulosin. Example inhibitors include azole antifungals, clarithromycin, diclofenac, doxycycline, erythromycin, imatinib, isoniazid, nefazodone, nicardipine, propofol, protease inhibitors, quinidine, telithromycin, and verapamil.

Sildenafil, tadalafil, vardenafil: Blood pressure-lowering effects are additive. Use of vardenafil is contraindicated by the manufacturer. Use sildenafil with extreme caution (dose ≤25 mg). Tadalafil may be used when tamsulosin dose is ≤0.4 mg/day.

Nutritional/Herbal/Ethanol Interactions

Food: Fasting increases bioavailability by 30% and peak concentration 40% to 70%.

Herb/Nutraceutical: Avoid saw palmetto (due to limited experience with this combination).

Adverse Reactions

>10%:

Cardiovascular: Studies specific for orthostatic hypotension: Overall, at least one positive test was observed in 16% of patients receiving 0.4 mg and 19% of patients receiving the 0.8 mg dose. "First-dose" orthostatic hypotension following a 0.4 mg dose was reported as 7% at 4 hours postdose and 6% at 8 hours postdose.

Central nervous system: Headache (19% to 21%), dizziness (15% to 17%)

Genitourinary: Abnormal ejaculation (8% to 18%)

Respiratory: Rhinitis (13% to 18%)

1% to 10%:

Cardiovascular: Chest pain (~4%)

Central nervous system: Somnolence (3% to 4%), insomnia (1% to 2%), vertigo (0.6% to 1%)

Endocrine & metabolic: Libido decreased (1% to 2%)

Gastrointestinal: Diarrhea (4% to 6%), nausea (3% to 4%), stomach discomfort (2% to 3%), bitter taste (2% to 3%)

Neuromuscular & skeletal: Weakness (8% to 9%), back pain (7% to 8%)

Ocular: Amblyopia (0.2% to 2%)

Respiratory: Pharyngitis (5% to 6%), cough (3% to 5%), sinusitis (2% to 4%)

Miscellaneous: Infection (9% to 11%), tooth disorder (1% to 2%)

<1% (Limited to important or life-threatening): Allergic reactions (rash, angioedema, pruritus, urticaria) priapism; constipation, intraoperative floppy iris syndrome, orthostasis (symptomatic) (0.2% to 0.4%), palpitation, syncope (0.2% to 0.4%), transaminases increased, vomiting

Overdosage/Toxicology Symptoms of overdose include headache and hypotension. Treatment is supportive.

Dosing

Adults & Elderly: Benign prostatic hyperplasia (BPH): Oral: 0.4 mg once daily ~30 minutes after the same meal each day; dose may be increased after 2-4 weeks to 0.8 mg once daily in patients who fail to respond. If therapy is interrupted for several days, restart with 0.4 mg once daily.

Renal Impairment:

Cl_{cr} ≥10 mL/minute: No adjustment needed.

Cl_{cr} <10 mL/minute: Not studied.

Available Dosage Forms Capsule, as hydrochloride: 0.4 mg

Nursing Guidelines

Assessment: See Contraindications, Warnings/Precautions, and Dosing for use cautions. Assess potential for interactions with other prescriptions, OTC medications, or herbal products patient may be taking (see Drug Interactions). Assess results of laboratory tests, therapeutic effectiveness, and adverse reactions at beginning of therapy and on a regular basis with long-term therapy (see Adverse Reactions and Overdose/Toxicology). When discontinuing, dose should be tapered and blood pressure monitored closely. Teach patient proper

(Continued)

Tamsulosin *(Continued)*

use, possible side effects/appropriate interventions, and adverse symptoms to report (see Patient Education).

Monitoring Laboratory Tests: Periodic lipid panels

Dietary Considerations: Take once daily, 30 minutes after the same meal each day.

Patient Education: Inform prescriber of all prescriptions, OTC medications, or herbal products you are taking, and any allergies you have. Do not take any new medication during therapy unless approved by prescriber. Take as directed; do not skip dose or discontinue without consulting prescriber. Avoid alcohol. Follow recommended diet and exercise program. May cause drowsiness, dizziness, or impaired judgment (use caution when driving or engaging in tasks that require alertness until response to drug is known); postural hypotension (use caution when rising from sitting or lying position or when climbing stairs); nausea (frequent mouth care or sucking lozenges may help); urinary incontinence (void before taking medication); ejaculatory disturbance (reversible, may resolve with continued use); diarrhea (buttermilk, boiled milk, or yogurt may help); palpitations or rapid heartbeat; respiratory difficulty, unusual cough, or sore throat; or other persistent side effects. Report palpitations or rapid heartbeat; respiratory difficulty; muscle weakness, fatigue, or pain; vision changes or hearing; rash; changes in urinary pattern (void before taking medications); or other persistent side effects.

Geriatric Considerations: Metabolism of tamsulosin may be slower, and older patients may be more sensitive to the orthostatic hypotension caused by this medication. A 40% higher exposure (AUC) is anticipated in patients between 55 and 75 years of age as compared to younger subjects (20-32 years).

Pregnancy Risk Factor: B

Lactation: Not indicated for use in women

Perioperative/Anesthesia/Other Concerns: Tamsulosin may induce significant orthostatic hypotension with lightheadedness and possible loss of consciousness.

Administration

Oral: Capsules should be swallowed whole; do not crush, chew, or open.

- ♦ **Tamsulosin Hydrochloride** *see* Tamsulosin *on page 1598*
- ♦ **Tanac® [OTC]** *see* Benzocaine *on page 232*
- ♦ **TAP-144** *see* Leuprolide *on page 1015*
- ♦ **Tapazole®** *see* Methimazole *on page 1122*
- ♦ **Tavist® ND [OTC]** *see* Loratadine *on page 1058*
- ♦ **Taxol®** *see* Paclitaxel *on page 1294*
- ♦ **Taxotere®** *see* Docetaxel *on page 557*
- ♦ **Tazicef®** *see* Ceftazidime *on page 348*
- ♦ **Taztia XT™** *see* Diltiazem *on page 540*
- ♦ **3TC** *see* Lamivudine *on page 999*
- ♦ **3TC, Abacavir, and Zidovudine** *see* Abacavir, Lamivudine, and Zidovudine *on page 58*
- ♦ **TCN** *see* Tetracycline *on page 1613*
- ♦ **Teargen® [OTC]** *see* Artificial Tears *on page 187*
- ♦ **Teargen® II [OTC]** *see* Artificial Tears *on page 187*
- ♦ **Tearisol® [OTC]** *see* Hydroxypropyl Methylcellulose *on page 883*
- ♦ **Tears Again® [OTC]** *see* Artificial Tears *on page 187*
- ♦ **Tears Again® MC [OTC]** *see* Hydroxypropyl Methylcellulose *on page 883*
- ♦ **Tears Again® Gel Drops™ [OTC]** *see* Carboxymethylcellulose *on page 316*
- ♦ **Tears Again® Night and Day™ [OTC]** *see* Carboxymethylcellulose *on page 316*
- ♦ **Tears Naturale® [OTC]** *see* Artificial Tears *on page 187*
- ♦ **Tears Naturale® II [OTC]** *see* Artificial Tears *on page 187*
- ♦ **Tears Naturale® Free [OTC]** *see* Artificial Tears *on page 187*
- ♦ **Tears Plus® [OTC]** *see* Artificial Tears *on page 187*
- ♦ **Tears Renewed® [OTC]** *see* Artificial Tears *on page 187*
- ♦ **Tebamide™** *see* Trimethobenzamide *on page 1668*
- ♦ **Tegretol®** *see* Carbamazepine *on page 306*
- ♦ **Tegretol®-XR** *see* Carbamazepine *on page 306*

Temazepam (te MAZ e pam)

U.S. Brand Names Restoril®

Pharmacologic Category Hypnotic, Benzodiazepine

Medication Safety Issues

Sound-alike/look-alike issues:

Temazepam may be confused with flurazepam, lorazepam

Restoril® may be confused with Vistaril®, Zestril®

Use Short-term treatment of insomnia

Unlabeled/Investigational Use Treatment of anxiety; adjunct in the treatment of depression; management of panic attacks

Mechanism of Action Binds to stereospecific benzodiazepine receptors on the postsynaptic GABA neuron at several sites within the central nervous system, including the limbic system, reticular formation. Enhancement of the inhibitory effect of GABA on neuronal excitability results by increased neuronal membrane permeability to chloride ions. This shift in chloride ions results in hyperpolarization (a less excitable state) and stabilization.

Pharmacodynamics/Kinetics

Distribution: V_d: 1.4 L/kg

Protein binding: 96%

Metabolism: Hepatic

Half-life elimination: 9.5-12.4 hours

Time to peak, serum: 2-3 hours

Excretion: Urine (80% to 90% as inactive metabolites)

Contraindications Hypersensitivity to temazepam or any component of the formulation (cross-sensitivity with other benzodiazepines may exist); narrow-angle glaucoma (not in product labeling, however, benzodiazepines are contraindicated); pregnancy

Warnings/Precautions Should be used only after evaluation of potential causes of sleep disturbance. Failure of sleep disturbance to resolve after 7-10 days may indicate psychiatric or medical illness. A worsening of insomnia or the emergence of new abnormalities of thought or behavior may represent unrecognized psychiatric or medical illness and requires immediate and careful evaluation.

Use with caution in elderly or debilitated patients, patients with hepatic disease (including alcoholics), or renal impairment. Use with caution in patients with respiratory disease, or impaired gag reflex. Avoid use inpatients with sleep apnea.

Causes CNS depression (dose-related) resulting in sedation, dizziness, confusion, or ataxia which may impair physical and mental capabilities. Patients must be cautioned about performing tasks which require mental alertness (eg, operating machinery or driving). Use with caution in patients receiving other CNS depressants or psychoactive agents. Effects with other sedative drugs or ethanol may be potentiated. Benzodiazepines have been associated with falls and traumatic injury and should be used with extreme caution in patients who are at risk of these events (especially the elderly).

Use caution in patients with depression, particularly if suicidal risk may be present. Use with caution in patients with a history of drug dependence. Benzodiazepines have been associated with dependence and acute withdrawal symptoms on discontinuation or reduction in dose (may occur after as little as 10 days). Acute withdrawal, including seizures, may be precipitated after administration of flumazenil to patients receiving long-term benzodiazepine therapy.

Benzodiazepines have been associated with anterograde amnesia. Paradoxical reactions, including hyperactive or aggressive behavior, have been reported with benzodiazepines, particularly in adolescent/pediatric or psychiatric patients. Does not have analgesic, antidepressant, or antipsychotic properties.

Drug Interactions Substrate (minor) of CYP2B6, 2C8/9, 2C19, 3A4

CNS depressants: Sedative effects and/or respiratory depression may be additive with CNS depressants; includes ethanol, barbiturates, narcotic analgesics, and other sedative agents; monitor for increased effect

Theophylline: May partially antagonize some of the effects of benzodiazepines; monitor for decreased response; may require higher doses for sedation

Nutritional/Herbal/Ethanol Interactions

Ethanol: Avoid ethanol (may increase CNS depression).

Food: Serum levels may be increased by grapefruit juice.

Herb/Nutraceutical: St John's wort may decrease temazepam levels. Avoid valerian, St John's wort, kava kava, gotu kola (may increase CNS depression).

(Continued)

Temazepam *(Continued)*

Adverse Reactions

1% to 10%:

Central nervous system: Confusion, dizziness, drowsiness, fatigue, anxiety, headache, lethargy, hangover, euphoria, vertigo
Dermatologic: Rash
Endocrine & metabolic: Decreased libido
Gastrointestinal: Diarrhea
Neuromuscular & skeletal: Dysarthria, weakness
Ocular: Blurred vision
Miscellaneous: Diaphoresis

<1% (Limited to important or life-threatening): Amnesia, ataxia, blood dyscrasias, drug dependence, paradoxical reactions, vomiting

Overdosage/Toxicology Symptoms of overdose include somnolence, confusion, coma, hypoactive reflexes, dyspnea, hypotension, slurred speech, and impaired coordination. Treatment for benzodiazepine overdose is supportive. Flumazenil has been shown to selectively block the binding of benzodiazepines to CNS receptors, resulting in a reversal of benzodiazepine-induced CNS depression but not always respiratory depression due to toxicity.

Dosing

Adults: Insomnia: Oral: 15-30 mg at bedtime

Elderly: 15 mg in elderly or debilitated patients

Available Dosage Forms

Capsule: 15 mg, 30 mg
Restoril®: 7.5 mg, 15 mg, 30 mg

Nursing Guidelines

Assessment: For short-term use. Assess effectiveness and interactions of other medications patient may be taking. Assess for history of addiction (long-term use can result in dependence, abuse, or tolerance) and periodically evaluate need for continued use. After long-term use, taper dosage slowly when discontinuing. For inpatient use, institute safety measures and monitor effectiveness and adverse reactions. For outpatients, monitor therapeutic effectiveness and adverse reactions (eg, CNS depression) at beginning of therapy and periodically with long-term use. Assess knowledge/teach patient appropriate use, interventions to reduce side effects, and adverse symptoms to report. **Pregnancy risk factor X:** Determine that patient is not pregnant before starting therapy. Do not give to sexually-active female patients unless capable of complying with contraceptive use.

Patient Education: Use exactly as directed; do not increase dose or frequency or discontinue without consulting prescriber. Drug may cause physical and/or psychological dependence. May take with food to decrease GI upset. While using this medication, do not use alcohol or other prescription or OTC medications (especially, pain medications, sedatives, antihistamines, or hypnotics) without consulting prescriber. Maintain adequate hydration (2-3 L/day of fluids) unless instructed to restrict fluid intake. You may experience drowsiness, dizziness, lightheadedness, or blurred vision (use caution when driving or engaging in tasks requiring alertness until response to drug is known); or dry mouth or GI discomfort (small frequent meals, frequent mouth care, chewing gum, or sucking lozenges may help). Report CNS changes (confusion, depression, increased sedation, excitation, headache, abnormal thinking, insomnia, or nightmares, memory impairment, impaired coordination); muscle pain or weakness; respiratory difficulty; persistent dizziness, chest pain, or palpitations; alterations in normal gait; vision changes; or ineffectiveness of medication. **Pregnancy/breast-feeding precautions:** Inform prescriber if you are pregnant. Do not get pregnant during or for 1 month following therapy. Consult prescriber for instruction on appropriate contraceptive measures. This drug may cause severe fetal defects. Breast-feeding is not recommended.

Geriatric Considerations: Because of its lack of active metabolites, temazepam is recommended in the elderly when a benzodiazepine hypnotic is indicated. Hypnotic use should be limited to 10-14 days. If insomnia persists, the patient should be evaluated for etiology.

Pregnancy Risk Factor: X

Pregnancy Issues: Benzodiazepines cross the placenta. The association between benzodiazepine exposure and malformations remains controversial. A number of types of malformation have been reported (oral cleft, inguinal hernia, cardiac defects, spina bifida, dysmorphic facial features, skeletal defects); however, confounding factors make a clear association difficult. Overall, the risk to the fetus may be low. Nonteratogenic effects (including neonatal flaccidity, respiratory and feeding problems, and withdrawal symptoms) during the postnatal period have also been reported with benzodiazepine use.

Lactation: Enters breast milk/not recommended (AAP rates "of concern")

Perioperative/Anesthesia/Other Concerns: Chronic use of this agent may increase perioperative benzodiazepine dose needed to achieve desired effect. Abrupt discontinuation after sustained use (generally >10 days) may cause withdrawal symptoms. Benzodiazepines, as a class, may depress respiration; may exacerbate sleep-disordered breathing.

◆ Tenoretic® *see* Atenolol and Chlorthalidone *on page 197*

◆ Tenormin® *see* Atenolol *on page 194*

◆ Tequin® *see* Gatifloxacin *on page 797*

Terazosin (ter AY zoe sin)

U.S. Brand Names Hytrin®

Pharmacologic Category Alpha$_1$ Blocker

Use Management of mild to moderate hypertension; alone or in combination with other agents such as diuretics or beta-blockers; benign prostate hyperplasia (BPH)

Mechanism of Action Alpha$_1$-specific blocking agent with minimal alpha$_2$ effects; this allows peripheral postsynaptic blockade, with the resultant decrease in arterial tone, while preserving the negative feedback loop which is mediated by the peripheral presynaptic alpha$_2$-receptors; terazosin relaxes the smooth muscle of the bladder neck, thus reducing bladder outlet obstruction

Pharmacodynamics/Kinetics

Onset of action: 1-2 hours

Absorption: Rapid

Protein binding: 90% to 95%

Metabolism: Extensively hepatic

Half-life elimination: 9.2-12 hours

Time to peak, serum: ~1 hour

Excretion: Feces (60%); urine (40%)

Contraindications Hypersensitivity to quinazolines (doxazosin, prazosin, terazosin) or any component of the formulation; concurrent use with phosphodiesterase-5 (PDE-5) inhibitors including sildenafil (>25 mg), tadalafil, or vardenafil

Warnings/Precautions Can cause significant orthostatic hypotension and syncope, especially with first dose. Prostate cancer should be ruled out before starting for BPH. Anticipate a similar effect if therapy is interrupted for a few days, if dosage is rapidly increased, or if another antihypertensive drug is introduced.

Drug Interactions

ACE inhibitors: Hypotensive effect may be increased.

Beta-blockers: Hypotensive effect may be increased.

Calcium channel blockers: Hypotensive effect may be increased.

NSAIDs may reduce antihypertensive efficacy.

Sildenafil, tadalafil, vardenafil: Blood pressure-lowering effects are additive. Use of tadalafil or vardenafil is contraindicated by the manufacturer. Use sildenafil with extreme caution (dose ≤25 mg).

Nutritional/Herbal/Ethanol Interactions Herb/Nutraceutical: Avoid dong quai if using for hypertension (has estrogenic activity). Avoid ephedra, yohimbe, ginseng (may worsen hypertension). Avoid saw palmetto. Avoid garlic (may have increased antihypertensive effect).

Adverse Reactions Asthenia, postural hypotension, dizziness, somnolence, nasal congestion/rhinitis, and impotence were the only events noted in clinical trials to occur at a frequency significantly greater than placebo ($p < 0.05$).

>10%:

Central nervous system: Dizziness, headache

Neuromuscular & skeletal: Muscle weakness

1% to 10%:

Cardiovascular: Edema, palpitation, chest pain, peripheral edema (3%), orthostatic hypotension (3% to 4%), tachycardia

Central nervous system: Fatigue, nervousness, drowsiness

Gastrointestinal: Dry mouth

Genitourinary: Urinary incontinence

Ocular: Blurred vision

Respiratory: Dyspnea, nasal congestion

(Continued)

Terazosin *(Continued)*

<1% (Limited to important or life-threatening): Allergic reactions, anaphylaxis, atrial fibrillation, priapism, sexual dysfunction, syncope (0.8%), thrombocytopenia

Overdosage/Toxicology Symptoms of overdose include hypotension, drowsiness, and shock. Treatment is supportive and symptomatic.

Dosing

Adults & Elderly:

Hypertension: Oral: Initial: 1 mg at bedtime; slowly increase dose to achieve desired blood pressure, up to 20 mg/day; usual dose range (JNC 7): 1-20 mg once daily

Benign prostatic hyperplasia: Oral: Initial: 1 mg at bedtime, increasing as needed; most patients require 10 mg day. If no response after 4-6 weeks of 10 mg/day, may increase to 20 mg/day.

Available Dosage Forms Capsule: 1 mg, 2 mg, 5 mg, 10 mg

Nursing Guidelines

Assessment: See Contraindications, Warnings/Precautions, and Dosing for use cautions. Assess potential for interactions with other prescriptions, OTC medications, or herbal products patient may be taking (see Drug Interactions). Assess therapeutic effectiveness (blood pressure) and adverse reactions at beginning of therapy and on a regular basis with long-term therapy (see Adverse Reactions and Overdose/Toxicology). When discontinuing, dose should be tapered and blood pressure monitored closely. Teach patient proper use, possible side effects/appropriate interventions, and adverse symptoms to report (see Patient Education). Note breast-feeding caution.

Dietary Considerations: May be taken without regard to meals at the same time each day.

Patient Education: Inform prescriber of all prescriptions, OTC medications, or herbal products you are taking, and any allergies you have. Do not take any new medication during therapy unless approved by prescriber. Take as directed; at bedtime. Do not skip dose or discontinue without consulting prescriber. Follow recommended diet and exercise program. May cause drowsiness, dizziness, or impaired judgment (use caution when driving or engaging in tasks that require alertness until response to drug is known); postural hypotension (use caution when rising from sitting or lying position or when climbing stairs); dry mouth or nausea (frequent mouth care or sucking lozenges may help); urinary incontinence (void before taking medication); or sexual dysfunction (reversible, may resolve with continued use). Report altered CNS status (eg, fatigue, lethargy, confusion, nervousness); sudden weight gain (weigh yourself in the same clothes at the same time of day once a week); unusual or persistent swelling of ankles, feet, or extremities; palpitations or rapid heartbeat; respiratory difficulty; muscle weakness; or other persistent side effects. **Pregnancy/breast-feeding precautions:** Inform prescriber if you are or intend to become pregnant. Consult prescriber if breast-feeding.

Geriatric Considerations: Adverse reactions such as dry mouth and urinary problems can be particularly bothersome in the elderly.

Pregnancy Risk Factor: C

Lactation: Excretion in breast milk unknown

Terbutaline (ter BYOO ta leen)

U.S. Brand Names Brethine®

Synonyms Brethaire [DSC]; Bricanyl [DSC]

Pharmacologic Category Beta$_2$-Adrenergic Agonist

Medication Safety Issues

Sound-alike/look-alike issues:

Terbutaline may be confused with terbinafine, TOLBUTamide

Use Bronchodilator in reversible airway obstruction and bronchial asthma; tocolytic agent

Unlabeled/Investigational Use Tocolytic agent (management of preterm labor)

Mechanism of Action Relaxes bronchial smooth muscle by action on beta$_2$-receptors with less effect on heart rate

Pharmacodynamics/Kinetics

Onset of action: Oral: 30-45 minutes; SubQ: 6-15 minutes

Protein binding: 25%

Metabolism: Hepatic to inactive sulfate conjugates

Bioavailability: SubQ doses are more bioavailable than oral
Half-life elimination: 11-16 hours
Excretion: Urine

Contraindications Hypersensitivity to terbutaline or any component of the formulation; cardiac arrhythmias associated with tachycardia; tachycardia caused by digitalis intoxication

Warnings/Precautions When used for tocolysis, there is some risk of maternal pulmonary edema, which has been associated with the following risk factors, excessive hydration, multiple gestation, occult sepsis and underlying cardiac disease. To reduce risk, limit fluid intake to 2.5-3 L/day, limit sodium intake, maintain maternal pulse to <130 beats/minute.

Use caution in patients with cardiovascular disease (arrhythmia or hypertension or CHF), convulsive disorders, diabetes, glaucoma, hyperthyroidism, or hypokalemia. Beta agonists may cause elevation in blood pressure, heart rate, and result in CNS stimulation/excitation. $Beta_2$ agonists may increase risk of arrhythmia, increase serum glucose, or decrease serum potassium.

When used as a bronchodilator, optimize anti-inflammatory treatment before initiating maintenance treatment with terbutaline. Do not use as a component of chronic therapy without an anti-inflammatory agent. Only the mildest form of asthma (Step 1 and/or exercise-induced) would not require concurrent use based upon asthma guidelines. Patient must be instructed to seek medical attention in cases where acute symptoms are not relieved or a previous level of response is diminished. The need to increase frequency of use may indicate deterioration of asthma, and treatment must not be delayed.

Do not exceed recommended dose; serious adverse events including fatalities, have been associated with excessive use of inhaled sympathomimetics. Rarely, paradoxical bronchospasm may occur with use of inhaled bronchodilating agents; this should be distinguished from inadequate response.

Drug Interactions

Decreased effect with beta-blockers
Increased toxicity with MAO inhibitors, TCAs

Nutritional/Herbal/Ethanol Interactions Herb/Nutraceutical: Avoid ephedra, yohimbe (may cause CNS stimulation).

Adverse Reactions

>10%:

- Central nervous system: Nervousness, restlessness
- Endocrine & metabolic: Serum glucose increased, serum potassium decreased
- Neuromuscular & skeletal: Trembling

1% to 10%:

- Cardiovascular: Tachycardia, hypertension, pounding heartbeat
- Central nervous system: Dizziness, lightheadedness, drowsiness, headache, insomnia
- Gastrointestinal: Dry mouth, nausea, vomiting, bad taste in mouth
- Neuromuscular & skeletal: Muscle cramps, weakness
- Miscellaneous: Diaphoresis

<1% (Limited to important or life-threatening): Arrhythmia, chest pain, hypokalemia, paradoxical bronchospasm

Overdosage/Toxicology Symptoms of overdose include tachycardia, tremor, hypertension, angina, and seizures. Hypokalemia also may occur. Cardiac arrest and death may be associated with abuse of beta-agonist bronchodilators. Treatment includes immediate discontinuation and symptomatic and supportive therapies. Cautious use of beta-adrenergic blocking agents may be considered in severe cases.

Dosing

Adults & Elderly:

Asthma or bronchoconstriction:

Oral: 5 mg/dose every 6 hours 3 times/day; if side effects occur, reduce dose to 2.5 mg every 6 hours; not to exceed 15 mg in 24 hours.

SubQ: 0.25 mg/dose repeated in 15-30 minutes for one time only; a total dose of 0.5 mg should not be exceeded within a 4-hour period.

Bronchospasm (acute): *Inhalation* (Bricanyl® [CAN] MDI: 500 mcg/puff, *not labeled for use in the U.S.*): One puff as needed; may repeat with 1 inhalation (after 5 minutes); more than 6 inhalations should not be necessary in any 24 hour period. **Note:** If a previously effective dosage regimen fails to provide the usual relief, or the effects of a dose last for >3 hours, medical advice

(Continued)

Terbutaline *(Continued)*

should be sought immediately; this is a sign of seriously worsening asthma that requires reassessment of therapy.

Premature labor (tocolysis):

Acute: I.V. 2.5-10 mcg/minute; increased gradually every 10-20 minutes. Effective maximum dosages from 17.5-30 mcg/minute have been use with caution. Duration of infusion is at least 12 hours.

Maintenance: Oral: 2.5-10 mg every 4-6 hours for as long as necessary to prolong pregnancy depending on patient tolerance

Pediatrics:

Asthma or bronchoconstriction:

Oral: Children:

<12 years: Initial: 0.05 mg/kg/dose 3 times/day, increased gradually as required; maximum: 0.15 mg/kg/dose 3-4 times/day or a total of 5 mg/24 hours

12-15 years: 2.5 mg every 6 hours 3 times/day; not to exceed 7.5 mg in 24 hours

>15 years: 5 mg/dose every 6 hours 3 times/day; if side effects occur, reduce dose to 2.5 mg every 6 hours; not to exceed 15 mg in 24 hours

SubQ: Children:

<12 years: 0.005-0.01 mg/kg/dose to a maximum of 0.3 mg/dose every 15-20 minutes for 3 doses

≥12 years: Refer to adult dosing.

Bronchospasm (acute): *Inhalation:* Bricanyl® [CAN] MDI: 500 mcg/puff, *not labeled for use in the U.S.*): Children ≥6 years: Refer to adult dosing.

Renal Impairment:

Cl_{cr} 10-50 mL/minute: Administer 50% of normal dose.

Cl_{cr} <10 mL/minute: Avoid use.

Available Dosage Forms

Injection, solution, as sulfate: 1 mg/mL (1 mL)

Tablet, as sulfate: 2.5 mg, 5 mg

Additional dosage forms available in Canada: Powder for oral inhalation (Bricanyl® Turbuhaler): 500 mcg/actuation [50 or 200 metered doses]

Nursing Guidelines

Assessment: Respiratory use: Assess effectiveness and interactions of other medications patient may be taking. Monitor therapeutic effectiveness and adverse reactions at beginning of therapy and periodically with long-term use. If diabetic, monitor blood glucose (may cause elevation in serum glucose). For inpatient care, monitor vital signs and lung sounds prior to and periodically during therapy. Assess knowledge/teach patient appropriate use, interventions to reduce side effects, and adverse symptoms to report. **Preterm labor use: Inpatient:** Monitor maternal vital signs; respiratory, fluid status, cardiac, and electrolyte status; frequency, duration, and intensity of contractions; and fetal heart rate. **Outpatient:** Assess knowledge/teach patient appropriate use, interventions to reduce side effects, and adverse symptoms to report.

Monitoring Laboratory Tests: FEV_1, peak flow, and/or other pulmonary function tests; serum potassium, serum glucose (in selected patients)

Tocolysis: If patient receives therapy for more than 1 week, monitor serum glucose.

Patient Education: Use exactly as directed. Do not use more often than recommended (excessive use may result in tolerance, overdose may result in serious adverse effects) and do not discontinue without consulting prescriber. Maintain adequate hydration (2-3 L/day of fluids) unless instructed to restrict fluid intake. If you have diabetes, monitor blood sugar closely. Serum glucose may be elevated. You may experience nervousness, dizziness, or fatigue (use caution when driving or engaging in tasks requiring alertness until response to drug is known); or dry mouth, stomach upset (small frequent meals, frequent mouth care, chewing gum, or sucking hard candy may help). Report unresolved GI upset; dizziness or fatigue; vision changes; sudden weight gain; swelling of extremities; chest pain, rapid heartbeat, or palpitations; insomnia, nervousness, or hyperactivity; muscle cramping, tremors, or pain; unusual cough; or rash (hypersensitivity).

Preterm labor: Notify prescriber immediately if labor resumes or adverse side effects are noted

Pregnancy Risk Factor: B

Lactation: Enters breast milk/compatible

Perioperative/Anesthesia/Other Concerns: $Beta_2$-selective agents lose much of their receptor selectivity when delivered parenterally or orally. Subcutaneous beta-agonist therapy has a deleterious therapeutic to toxicity ratio when compared with inhalation. There is no proven benefit of aerosolized over systemic therapy.

Administration

Oral: Administer around-the-clock to promote less variation in peak and trough serum levels.

I.V.: Use infusion pump.

Compatibility: Stable in D_5W, ½NS, NS

Compatibility when admixed: Incompatible with bleomycin

Storage: Store injection at room temperature. Protect from heat, light, and from freezing. Use only clear solutions. Store powder for inhalation (Bricanyl® Turbuhaler [CAN]) at room temperature between 15°C and 30°C (58°F and 86°F).

♦ **Terramycin® I.M.** *see* Oxytetracycline *on page 1292*

♦ **Tessalon®** *see* Benzonatate *on page 235*

♦ **Testim®** *see* Testosterone *on page 1607*

♦ **Testopel®** *see* Testosterone *on page 1607*

Testosterone (tes TOS ter one)

U.S. Brand Names Androderm®; AndroGel®; Delatestryl®; Depo®-Testosterone; First® Testosterone; First® Testosterone MC; Striant®; Testim®; Testopel®

Synonyms Testosterone Cypionate; Testosterone Enanthate

Pharmacologic Category Androgen

Medication Safety Issues

Sound-alike/look-alike issues:

Testosterone may be confused with testolactone

Testoderm® may be confused with Estraderm®

Transdermal patch may contain conducting metal (eg, aluminum); remove patch prior to MRI.

Use

Injection: Androgen replacement therapy in the treatment of delayed male puberty; male hypogonadism (primary or hypogonadotropic); inoperable female breast cancer (enanthate only)

Pellet: Androgen replacement therapy in the treatment of delayed male puberty; male hypogonadism (primary or hypogonadotropic)

Buccal, topical: Male hypogonadism (primary or hypogonadotropic)

Mechanism of Action Principal endogenous androgen responsible for promoting the growth and development of the male sex organs and maintaining secondary sex characteristics in androgen-deficient males

Pharmacodynamics/Kinetics

Duration (route and ester dependent): I.M.: Cypionate and enanthate esters have longest duration, ≤2-4 weeks

Absorption: Transdermal gel: ~10% of applied dose

Distribution: Crosses placenta; enters breast milk

Protein binding: 98%; bound to sex hormone-binding globulin (40%) and albumin

Metabolism: Hepatic; forms metabolites, including dihydrotestosterone (DHT) and estradiol (both active)

Half-life elimination: 10-100 minutes

Excretion: Urine (90%); feces (6%)

Contraindications Hypersensitivity to testosterone, soy, or any component of the formulation; severe renal or cardiac disease; benign prostatic hyperplasia with obstruction; undiagnosed genital bleeding; males with carcinoma of the breast or prostate; pregnancy

Warnings/Precautions When used to treat delayed male puberty, perform radiographic examination of the hand and wrist every 6 months to determine the rate of bone maturation. May accelerate bone maturation without producing compensating gain in linear growth. Has both androgenic and anabolic activity, the anabolic action may enhance hypoglycemia. Use caution in elderly patients or patients with other demographic factors which may increase the risk of prostatic carcinoma; careful monitoring is required. May cause fluid retention; use caution in patients with cardiovascular disease or other edematous conditions. Prolonged use of orally-active androgens has been associated with serious hepatic effects

(Continued)

Testosterone *(Continued)*

(hepatitis, hepatic neoplasms, cholestatic hepatitis, jaundice). May potentiate sleep apnea in some male patients (obesity or chronic lung disease). Transdermal patch may contain conducting metal (eg, aluminum); remove patch prior to MRI. Gels and buccal system have not been evaluated in males <18 years of age; safety and efficacy of injection have not been established in males <12 years of age.

Drug Interactions Substrate (minor) of CYP2B6, 2C8/9, 2C19, 3A4; **Inhibits** CYP3A4 (weak)

Warfarin: Testosterone may increase the effects warfarin.

Nutritional/Herbal/Ethanol Interactions Herb/Nutraceutical: St John's wort may decrease testosterone levels.

Lab Interactions May cause a decrease in creatinine and creatine excretion and an increase in the excretion of 17-ketosteroids, thyroid function tests.

Adverse Reactions Frequency not defined.

Cardiovascular: Flushing, edema

Central nervous system: Excitation, aggressive behavior, sleeplessness, anxiety, mental depression, headache

Dermatologic: Hirsutism (increase in pubic hair growth), acne

Endocrine & metabolic: Menstrual problems (amenorrhea), virilism, breast soreness, gynecomastia, hypercalcemia, hypoglycemia

Gastrointestinal: Nausea, vomiting, GI irritation

Following buccal administration: Bitter taste, gum edema, gum or mouth irritation, gum tenderness, taste perversion

Genitourinary: Bladder irritability, epididymitis, impotence, priapism, prostatic carcinoma, prostatic hyperplasia, PSA increased (up to 18%), testicular atrophy, urination impaired

Hepatic: Hepatic dysfunction, cholestatic hepatitis, hepatic necrosis

Hematologic: Leukopenia, polycythemia, suppression of clotting factors

Miscellaneous: Hypersensitivity reactions

Dosing

Adults & Elderly:

Inoperable breast cancer (females): I.M.: Testosterone enanthate: 200-400 mg every 2-4 weeks

Male hypogonadism or hypogonadotropic hypogonadism:

Oral (buccal): 30 mg twice daily (every 12 hours) applied to the gum region above the incisor tooth

Pellet (for subcutaneous implantation): Hypogonadism, delayed puberty: 150-450 mg every 3-6 months

Transdermal:

Androderm®: Initial: Apply 5 mg/day once nightly to clean, dry area on the back, abdomen, upper arms, or thighs (do **not** apply to scrotum); dosing range: 2.5-7.5 mg/day; in nonvirilized patients, dose may be initiated at 2.5 mg/day

AndroGel®, Testim®: 5 g (to deliver 50 mg of testosterone with 5 mg systemically absorbed) applied once daily (preferably in the morning) to clean, dry, intact skin of the shoulder and upper arms. AndroGel® may also be applied to the abdomen. Dosage may be increased to a maximum of 10 g (100 mg). **(Do not apply testosterone gel to the genitals.)**

Delayed puberty in males: I.M. (cypionate or enanthate ester) : 50-200 mg every 2-4 weeks for a limited duration

Male hypogonadism: I.M. (cypionate or enanthate ester) 50-400 mg every 2-4 weeks

Pediatrics: Adolescents:

Male hypogonadism:

I.M.:

Initiation of pubertal growth: 40-50 mg/m^2/dose (cypionate or enanthate ester) monthly until the growth rate falls to prepubertal levels

Terminal growth phase: 100 mg/m^2/dose (cypionate or enanthate ester) monthly until growth ceases

Maintenance virilizing dose: 100 mg/m^2/dose (cypionate or enanthate ester) twice monthly

SubQ: Pellet (for subcutaneous implantation): Refer to adult dosing.

Delayed puberty (male):

I.M.: 40-50 mg/m^2/dose monthly (cypionate or enanthate ester) for 6 months

SubQ: Pellet (for subcutaneous implantation): Refer to adult dosing.

Hepatic Impairment: Reduce dose.

Available Dosage Forms

Gel, topical:

AndroGel®:

1.25 g/actuation (75 g) [1% metered-dose pump; delivers 5 g/4 actuations; provides 60 1.25 g actuations; contains ethanol]

2.5 g (30s) [1% unit dose packets; contains ethanol]

5 g (30s) [1% unit dose packets; contains ethanol]

Testim®: 5 g (30s) [1% unit-dose tube; contains ethanol]

Injection, in oil, as cypionate: 200 mg/mL (10 mL)

Depo®-Testosterone: 100 mg/mL (10 mL); 200 mg/mL (1 mL, 10 mL) [contains benzyl alcohol, benzyl benzoate, and cottonseed oil]

Injection, in oil, as enanthate: 200 mg/mL (5 mL)

Delatestryl®: 200 mg/mL (1 mL) [prefilled syringe; contains sesame oil]; (5 mL) [multidose vial; contains sesame oil]

Kit [for prescription compounding testosterone 2%; kits also contain mixing jar and stirrer]:

First® Testosterone:

Injection, in oil: Testosterone propionate 100 mg/mL (12 mL) [contains sesame oil and benzyl alcohol]

Ointment: White petroleum (48 g)

First® Testosterone MC:

Injection, in oil: Testosterone propionate 100 mg/mL (12 mL) [contains sesame oil and benzyl alcohol]

Cream: Moisturizing cream (48 g)

Mucoadhesive, for buccal application [buccal system] (Striant®): 30 mg (10s)

Pellet, for subcutaneous implantation (Testopel®): 75 mg (1 pellet/vial)

Transdermal system (Androderm®): 2.5 mg/day (60s); 5 mg/day (30s) [contains ethanol]

Nursing Guidelines

Assessment: (For use in children see pediatric reference). See Contraindications, Warnings/Precautions, and Dosing for use cautions. Assess potential for interactions with other prescriptions, OTC medications, or herbal products patient may be taking (see Drug Interactions). Assess results of laboratory tests (see below), therapeutic effectiveness (according to purpose for use), and adverse reactions (see Adverse Reactions and Overdose/Toxicology) regularly during therapy. Caution patients with diabetes - may cause hypoglycemic reaction. Teach patient proper use (according to formulation), possible side effects/appropriate interventions, and adverse symptoms to report (see Patient Education). **Pregnancy risk factor X** - determine that patient is not pregnant before beginning treatment. Instruct patients of childbearing age or males who may have intercourse with women of childbearing age on appropriate barrier contraceptive measures. Breast-feeding is contraindicated.

Monitoring Laboratory Tests: Periodic liver function tests, PSA, cholesterol, hemoglobin and hematocrit; radiologic examination of wrist and hand every 6 months (when using in prepubertal children)

Androderm®: Morning serum testosterone levels following application the previous evening

Gel: Morning serum testosterone levels 14 days after start of therapy

Dietary Considerations: Testosterone USP may be synthesized from soy. Food and beverages have not been found to interfere with buccal system; ensure system is in place following eating, drinking, or brushing teeth.

Patient Education: If you have diabetes, monitor serum glucose closely and notify prescriber of changes; this medication may alter hypoglycemic requirements. You may experience acne, growth of body hair, loss of libido, impotence, or menstrual irregularity (usually reversible); nausea or vomiting (small frequent meals, frequent mouth care, sucking lozenges, or chewing gum may help). Report changes in menstrual pattern; enlarged or painful breasts; deepening of voice or unusual growth of body hair; persistent penile erection; fluid retention (swelling of ankles, feet, or hands, respiratory difficulty or sudden weight gain); unresolved changes in CNS (nervousness, chills, insomnia, depression, aggressiveness); altered urinary patterns; change in color of urine or stool; yellowing of eyes or skin; unusual bruising or bleeding; or other persistent adverse reactions.

Transdermal: Androderm®: Apply patch to clean, dry area of skin on the arm, back, or upper buttocks.

Topical gel: AndroGel®, Testim®: Apply gel (preferably in the morning) to clean, dry, intact skin of the shoulder and upper arms (AndroGel® may also be

(Continued)

Testosterone *(Continued)*

applied to the abdomen). Upon opening the packet(s), the entire contents should be squeezed into the palm of the hand and immediately applied to the application site(s). Alternatively, a portion may be squeezed onto palm of hand and applied, repeating the process until entire packet has been applied. Gel is flammable. Application sites should be allowed to dry for a few minutes prior to dressing. Hands should be washed with soap and water after application. **Do not apply testosterone gel to the genitals.**

Pregnancy/breast-feeding precautions: Inform prescriber if you are pregnant. Do not get pregnant during or for 1 month following therapy. Male: Do not cause a female to become pregnant. Male/female: Consult prescriber for instruction on appropriate contraceptive measures. This drug may cause severe fetal defects. Do not breast-feed.

Geriatric Considerations: Geriatric patients may have an increased risk of prostatic hyperplasia or prostatic carcinoma.

Pregnancy Risk Factor: X

Pregnancy Issues: Testosterone may cause adverse effects, including masculinization of the female fetus, if used during pregnancy. Females who are or may become pregnant should also avoid skin-to-skin contact to areas where testosterone has been applied topically on another person.

Lactation: Enters breast milk/contraindicated

Administration

Oral: Striant®: One mucoadhesive for buccal application (buccal system) should be applied to a comfortable area above the incisor tooth. Apply flat side of system to gum. Rotate to alternate sides of mouth with each application. Hold buccal system firmly in place for 30 seconds to ensure adhesion. The buccal system should adhere to gum for 12 hours. If the buccal system falls out, replace with a new system. If the system falls out within 4 hours of next dose, the new buccal system should remain in place until the time of the following scheduled dose. System will soften and mold to shape of gum as it absorbs moisture from mouth. Do not chew or swallow the buccal system. The buccal system will not dissolve; gently remove by sliding downwards from gum; avoid scratching gum.

I.M.: Warm injection to room temperature and shaking vial will help redissolve crystals that have formed after storage. Administer by deep I.M. injection into the upper outer quadrant of the gluteus maximus.

Storage:

Androderm®: Store at room temperature. Do not store outside of pouch. Excessive heat may cause system to burst.

AndroGel®, Delatestryl®, Striant®, Testim®: Store at room temperature.

Depo® Testosterone: Store at room temperature. Protect from light.

Testopel®: Store in a cool location.

◆ Testosterone Cypionate *see* Testosterone *on page 1607*

◆ Testosterone Enanthate *see* Testosterone *on page 1607*

Tetanus Toxoid (Adsorbed) (TET a nus TOKS oyd, ad SORBED)

Pharmacologic Category Toxoid

Medication Safety Issues

Sound-alike/look-alike issues:

Tetanus toxoid products may be confused with influenza virus vaccine and tuberculin products. Medication errors have occurred when tetanus toxoid products have been inadvertently administered instead of tuberculin skin tests (PPD) and influenza virus vaccine. These products are refrigerated and often stored in close proximity to each other.

Use Active immunization against tetanus when combination antigen preparations are not indicated. **Note:** Tetanus and diphtheria toxoids for adult use (Td) is the preferred immunizing agent for most adults and for children after their seventh birthday. Young children should receive trivalent DTaP (diphtheria/tetanus/acellular pertussis), as part of their childhood immunization program, unless pertussis is contraindicated, then TD is warranted.

Mechanism of Action Tetanus toxoid preparations contain the toxin produced by virulent tetanus bacilli (detoxified growth products of *Clostridium tetani*). The toxin has been modified by treatment with formaldehyde so that it has lost toxicity but still retains ability to act as antigen and produce active immunity; the aluminum salt, a mineral adjuvant, delays the rate of absorption and prolongs and enhances its properties; duration ~10 years.

Pharmacodynamics/Kinetics Duration: Primary immunization: ~10 years

Contraindications Hypersensitivity to tetanus toxoid or any component of the formulation

Warnings/Precautions Not equivalent to tetanus toxoid fluid; the tetanus toxoid adsorbed is the preferred toxoid for immunization and Td, TD or DTaP are the preferred adsorbed forms; avoid injection into a blood vessel; allergic reactions may occur; epinephrine 1:1000 must be available; elderly may not mount adequate antibody titers following immunization. Patients who are immunocompromised may have reduced response; may be used in patients with HIV infection. May defer elective immunization during febrile illness or acute infection; defer elective immunization during outbreaks of poliomyelitis. In patients with a history of severe local reaction (Arthus-type) or temperature of >39.4°C (>103°F) following previous dose, do not give further routine or emergency doses of tetanus and diphtheria toxoids for 10 years. Use caution in patients on anticoagulants, with thrombocytopenia, or bleeding disorders (bleeding may occur following intramuscular injection). Contains thimerosal; vial stopper may contain natural latex rubber. This product is not indicated for use in children <7 years of age.

Drug Interactions

Corticosteroids: When used in greater than physiologic doses, corticosteroids lead to decreased effect of vaccine; consider deferring immunization for 1 month after steroid is discontinued.

Immunosuppressive agents: Decreased response to vaccine; consider deferring immunization for 1 month after immunosuppressive agent is discontinued.

Adverse Reactions All serious adverse reactions must be reported to the U.S. Department of Health and Human Services (DHHS) Vaccine Adverse Event Reporting System (VAERS) 1-800-822-7967.

Frequency not defined.

Cardiovascular: Hypotension

Central nervous system: Brachial neuritis, fever, malaise, pain

Gastrointestinal: Nausea

Local: Edema, induration (with or without tenderness), rash, redness, urticaria, warmth

Neuromuscular: Arthralgia, Guillain-Barré syndrome

Miscellaneous: Anaphylactic reaction, Arthus-type hypersensitivity reaction

Dosing

Adults & Elderly:

Primary immunization: I.M.: 0.5 mL; repeat 0.5 mL at 4-8 weeks after first dose and at 6-12 months after second dose

Routine booster dose: Recommended every 10 years

Note: In most patients, Td is the recommended product for primary immunization, booster doses, and tetanus immunization in wound management.

Pediatrics: Children ≥7 years: Refer to adult dosing.

Available Dosage Forms Injection, suspension: Tetanus 5 Lf units per 0.5 mL (0.5 mL) [contains trace amounts of thimerosal]; (5 mL) [contains thimerosal; vial stopper contains latex]

Nursing Guidelines

Patient Education: A nodule may be palpable at the injection site for a few weeks. DT, Td and T vaccines cause few problems; they may cause mild fever or soreness, swelling, and redness where the shot was given. These problems usually last 1-2 days, but this does not happen nearly as often as with DTP vaccine. Sometimes, adults who get these vaccines can have a lot of soreness and swelling where the shot was given.

Pregnancy Risk Factor: C

Administration

I.M.: Inject intramuscularly in the area of the vastus lateralis (midthigh laterally) or deltoid. Do not inject into gluteal area. Shake well prior to withdrawing dose; do not use if product does not form a suspension.

For patients at risk of hemorrhage following intramuscular injection, the ACIP recommends "it should be administered intramuscularly if, in the opinion of the physician familiar with the patients bleeding risk, the vaccine can be administered with reasonable safety by this route. If the patient receives antihemophilia or other similar therapy, intramuscular vaccination can be scheduled shortly after such therapy is administered. A fine needle (23 gauge or smaller) can be used for the vaccination and firm pressure applied to the site (without rubbing) for at least 2 minutes. The patient should be instructed concerning the risk of hematoma from the injection."

Storage: Refrigerate, do not freeze

Tetracaine (TET ra kane)

U.S. Brand Names Pontocaine®; Pontocaine® Niphanoid®

Synonyms Amethocaine Hydrochloride; Tetracaine Hydrochloride

Pharmacologic Category Local Anesthetic

Use Spinal anesthesia; local anesthesia in the eye for various diagnostic and examination purposes; topically applied to nose and throat for various diagnostic procedures

Mechanism of Action Ester local anesthetic blocks both the initiation and conduction of nerve impulses by decreasing the neuronal membrane's permeability to sodium ions, which results in inhibition of depolarization with resultant blockade of conduction

Pharmacodynamics/Kinetics

Onset of action: Anesthetic: Rhinolaryngology: 5-10 minutes

Duration: Rhinolaryngology: ~30 minutes

Metabolism: Hepatic; detoxified by plasma esterases to aminobenzoic acid

Excretion: Urine

Contraindications Hypersensitivity to tetracaine, ester-type anesthetics, aminobenzoic acid, or any component of the formulation; injection should not be used when spinal anesthesia is contraindicated

Warnings/Precautions Use with caution in patients with cardiac disease, hyperthyroidism, abnormal or decreased levels of plasma esterases. Use of the lowest effective dose is recommended. Acutely ill, elderly, debilitated, obstetric patients, or patients with increased intra-abdominal pressure may require decreased doses. Products may contain sodium bisulfite which may cause allergic reactions in some individuals.

Ophthalmic: May delay wound healing. Prolonged use is not recommended. The anesthetized eye should be protected from irritation, foreign bodies, and rubbing to prevent inadvertent damage.

Adverse Reactions Frequency not defined.

Injection: Note: Adverse effects listed are those characteristics of local anesthetics.

Cardiovascular: Cardiac arrest, hypotension

Central nervous system: Chills, convulsions, dizziness, drowsiness, nervousness, unconsciousness

Gastrointestinal: Nausea, vomiting

Neuromuscular & skeletal: Tremors

Ocular: Blurred vision, pupil constriction

Otic: Tinnitus

Respiratory: Respiratory arrest

Miscellaneous: Allergic reaction

Ophthalmic: Ocular: Chemosis, lacrimation, photophobia, transient stinging

With chronic use: Corneal erosions, corneal healing retardation, corneal opacification (permanent), corneal scarring, keratitis (severe)

Overdosage/Toxicology Symptoms of overdose include seizures, respiratory depression, lacrimation, bradycardia, and hypotension. Treatment is supportive.

Dosing

Adults & Elderly:

Short-term anesthesia of the eye: Ophthalmic 0.5% solution: Instill 1-2 drops; prolonged use (especially for at-home self-medication) is not recommended

Spinal anesthesia: Injection: **Note:** Dosage varies with the anesthetic procedure, the degree of anesthesia required, and the individual patient response; it is administered by subarachnoid injection for spinal anesthesia.

Perineal anesthesia: 5 mg

Perineal and lower extremities: 10 mg

Anesthesia extending up to costal margin: 15 mg; doses up to 20 mg may be given, but are reserved for exceptional cases

Low spinal anesthesia (saddle block): 2-5 mg

Topical mucous membranes (rhinolaryngology): Used as a 0.25% or 0.5% solution by direct application or nebulization; total dose should not exceed 20 mg

Available Dosage Forms [DSC] = Discontinued product

Injection, solution, as hydrochloride [preservative free] (Pontocaine®): 1% [10 mg/mL] (2 mL) [contains sodium bisulfite]

Injection, solution, as hydrochloride [premixed in dextrose 6%] (Pontocaine®): 0.3% [3 mg/mL] (5 mL) [DSC]

Injection, powder for reconstitution, as hydrochloride [preservative free] (Pontocaine® Niphanoid®): 20 mg

Solution, ophthalmic, as hydrochloride: 0.5% [5 mg/mL] (15 mL)

Solution, topical, as hydrochloride (Pontocaine®): 2% [20 mg/mL] (30 mL, 118 mL) [for rhinolaryngology]

Nursing Guidelines

Assessment: Note: Tetracaine is 10 times as potent as procaine. Explain use, monitor vital signs, and monitor patient safety before, during, and following use according to formulation used and procedure being done. Caution patient that anesthetic effects of topical or ophthalmic preparation may last for some time after procedure (1-5 hours). Instruct in appropriate safety precautions.

Patient Education: Topical or ophthalmic anesthesia effects may last for some time following use; you will need to observe appropriate safety precautions to prevent injury.

Ophthalmic: Do not rub or touch your eye, scratch your nose, or attempt to apply eye make-up until all sensation returns. May cause temporary rash or stinging when used. Report any ringing in ears, feeling of weakness or faintness, chest pain or palpitation, or increased restlessness. **Pregnancy precaution:** Inform prescriber if you are pregnant.

Topical: Do not eat or drink anything until full sensation returns to lips, mouth, and throat. Use caution with heat or cold; you will not have accurate hot or cold sensation until full effects of anesthesia have worn off.

Pregnancy Risk Factor: C

Lactation: Excretion in breast milk unknown/use caution

Perioperative/Anesthesia/Other Concerns: Tetracaine is ~10 times more potent than procaine.

Administration

Reconstitution:

Solution for injection: Hyperbaric solution: May be made by mixing equal volumes of the 1% solution and $D_{10}W$.

Powder for injection:

Hyperbaric solution: Dissolve 10 mg of Pontocaine® Niphanoid® in 1 mL $D_{10}W$; further dilute with equal volume of spinal fluid. Resulting solution is D_5W with tetracaine 5 mg/mL.

Hypobaric solution: Dissolve 1 mg of Pontocaine® Niphanoid® in 1 mL SWFI.

Storage:

Injection: Store solution under refrigeration. Protect from light.

Ophthalmic and topical solutions: Store under refrigeration at 2°C to 8°C.

Related Information

Local Anesthetics *on page 1854*

♦ **Tetracaine Hydrochloride** *see* Tetracaine *on page 1612*

♦ **Tetracaine Hydrochloride, Benzocaine Butyl Aminobenzoate, and Benzalkonium Chloride** *see* Benzocaine, Butyl Aminobenzoate, Tetracaine, and Benzalkonium Chloride *on page 235*

Tetracycline (tet ra SYE kleen)

U.S. Brand Names Sumycin®

Synonyms Achromycin; TCN; Tetracycline Hydrochloride

Pharmacologic Category Antibiotic, Tetracycline Derivative

Medication Safety Issues

Sound-alike/look-alike issues:

Tetracycline may be confused with tetradecyl sulfate

Achromycin may be confused with actinomycin, Adriamycin PFS®

Use Treatment of susceptible bacterial infections of both gram-positive and gram-negative organisms; also infections due to *Mycoplasma*, *Chlamydia*, and *Rickettsia*; indicated for acne, exacerbations of chronic bronchitis, and treatment of gonorrhea and syphilis in patients that are allergic to penicillin; as part of a multidrug regimen for *H. pylori* eradication to reduce the risk of duodenal ulcer recurrence

Mechanism of Action Inhibits bacterial protein synthesis by binding with the 30S and possibly the 50S ribosomal subunit(s) of susceptible bacteria; may also cause alterations in the cytoplasmic membrane

Pharmacodynamics/Kinetics

Absorption: Oral: 75%

(Continued)

Tetracycline *(Continued)*

Distribution: Small amount appears in bile

Relative diffusion from blood into CSF: Good only with inflammation (exceeds usual MICs)

CSF:blood level ratio: Inflamed meninges: 25%

Protein binding: ~65%

Half-life elimination: Normal renal function: 8-11 hours; End-stage renal disease: 57-108 hours

Time to peak, serum: Oral: 2-4 hours

Excretion: Urine (60% as unchanged drug); feces (as active form)

Contraindications Hypersensitivity to tetracycline or any component of the formulation; do not administer to children ≤8 years of age; pregnancy

Warnings/Precautions Use of tetracyclines during tooth development may cause permanent discoloration of the teeth and enamel, hypoplasia and retardation of skeletal development and bone growth with risk being the greatest for children <4 years and those receiving high doses; use with caution in patients with renal or hepatic impairment (eg, elderly); dosage modification required in patients with renal impairment since it may increase BUN as an antianabolic agent; pseudotumor cerebri has been reported with tetracycline use (usually resolves with discontinuation); outdated drug can cause nephropathy; superinfection possible; use protective measure to avoid photosensitivity

Drug Interactions **Substrate** of CYP3A4 (major); **Inhibits** CYP3A4 (moderate)

Antacids: May decrease tetracycline absorption; separate doses.

Calcium supplements (oral): May decrease tetracycline absorption; separate doses.

CYP3A4 inducers: CYP3A4 inducers may decrease the levels/effects of tetracycline. Example inducers include aminoglutethimide, carbamazepine, nafcillin, nevirapine, phenobarbital, phenytoin, and rifamycins.

CYP3A4 substrates: Tetracycline may increase the levels/effects of CYP3A4 substrates. Example substrates include benzodiazepines, calcium channel blockers, cyclosporine, mirtazapine, nateglinide, nefazodone, sildenafil (and other PDE-5 inhibitors), tacrolimus, and venlafaxine. Selected benzodiazepines (midazolam and triazolam), cisapride, ergot alkaloids, selected HMG-CoA reductase inhibitors (lovastatin and simvastatin), and pimozide are generally contraindicated with strong CYP3A4 inhibitors.

Didanosine: May decrease tetracycline absorption; separate doses.

Digoxin: Tetracyclines may rarely increase digoxin serum levels.

Iron: May decrease tetracycline absorption; separate doses.

Methoxyflurane anesthesia when concurrent with tetracycline may cause fatal nephrotoxicity.

Oral contraceptives: Anecdotal reports suggesting decreased contraceptive efficacy with tetracyclines have been refuted by more rigorous scientific and clinical data.

Quinapril: May decrease tetracycline absorption; separate doses.

Warfarin with tetracyclines may result in increased anticoagulation.

Nutritional/Herbal/Ethanol Interactions

Food: Tetracycline serum concentrations may be decreased if taken with dairy products.

Herb/Nutraceutical: Avoid dong quai, St John's wort (may also cause photosensitization)

Lab Interactions False-negative urine glucose with Clinistix®

Adverse Reactions Frequency not defined.

Cardiovascular: Pericarditis

Central nervous system: Intracranial pressure increased, bulging fontanels in infants, pseudotumor cerebri, paresthesia

Dermatologic: Photosensitivity, pruritus, pigmentation of nails, exfoliative dermatitis

Endocrine & metabolic: Diabetes insipidus syndrome

Gastrointestinal: Discoloration of teeth and enamel hypoplasia (young children), nausea, diarrhea, vomiting, esophagitis, anorexia, abdominal cramps, antibiotic-associated pseudomembranous colitis, staphylococcal enterocolitis, pancreatitis

Hematologic: Thrombophlebitis

Hepatic: Hepatotoxicity

Renal: Acute renal failure, azotemia, renal damage

Miscellaneous: Superinfection, anaphylaxis, hypersensitivity reactions, candidal superinfection

Overdosage/Toxicology Symptoms of overdose include nausea, anorexia, and diarrhea. Treatment is supportive.

Dosing

Adults & Elderly: Antibacterial: Oral:

Systemic infection: Oral: 250-500 mg/dose every 6 hours

Peptic ulcer disease: Eradication of *Helicobacter pylori*: 500 mg 2-4 times/day depending on regimen; requires combination therapy with at least one other antibiotic and an acid-suppressing agent (proton pump inhibitor or H_2 blocker)

Periodontitis: 250 mg every 6 hours until improvement (usually 10 days)

Pediatrics: Antibacterial, systemic: Children >8 years: Oral: 25-50 mg/kg/day in divided doses every 6 hours

Renal Impairment:

Cl_{cr} 50-80 mL/minute: Administer every 8-12 hours.

Cl_{cr} 10-50 mL/minute: Administer every 12-24 hours.

Cl_{cr} <10 mL/minute: Administer every 24 hours.

Slightly dialyzable (5% to 20%) via hemo- and peritoneal dialysis or via continuous arteriovenous or venovenous hemofiltration; supplemental dose is not necessary.

Hepatic Impairment: Avoid use or maximum dose is 1 g/day.

Available Dosage Forms

Capsule, as hydrochloride: 250 mg, 500 mg

Suspension, oral, as hydrochloride (Sumycin®): 125 mg/5 mL (480 mL) [contains sodium benzoate and sodium metabisulfite; fruit flavor]

Tablet, as hydrochloride (Sumycin®): 250 mg, 500 mg

Nursing Guidelines

Assessment: Assess effectiveness and interactions of other medications patient may be taking (see Drug Interactions). Assess results of laboratory tests, therapeutic effectiveness, and adverse reactions (see Adverse Reactions) at beginning of therapy and periodically throughout therapy. Assess knowledge/teach patient appropriate use, interventions to reduce side effects, and adverse symptoms to report (see Patient Education). **Pregnancy risk factor B/D** - see Pregnancy Risk Factor for use cautions - assess knowledge/instruct patient on need to use appropriate barrier contraceptive measures and the need to avoid pregnancy. See Lactation for breast-feeding considerations.

Monitoring Laboratory Tests: Renal, hepatic, and hematologic function; WBC. Perform culture and sensitivity studies prior to initiating therapy to determine the causative organism and its susceptibility to tetracycline.

Patient Education: Take this medication exactly as directed. Take all of the prescription even if you see an improvement in your condition. Do not use more or more often than recommended. Preferable to take on an empty stomach, 1 hour before or 2 hours after meals. Take at regularly scheduled times, around-the-clock. Avoid antacids, iron, or dairy products within 2 hours of taking tetracycline. You may experience photosensitivity (use sunscreen, wear protective clothing and eyewear, and avoid direct sunlight); dizziness or lightheadedness (use caution when driving or engaging in tasks requiring alertness until response to drug is known); or nausea/vomiting (small, frequent meals, frequent mouth care, chewing gum, or sucking lozenges may help). Report rash or intense itching, yellowing of skin or eyes, fever or chills, blackened stool, vaginal itching or discharge, foul-smelling stools, excessive thirst or urination, acute headache, unresolved diarrhea, respiratory difficulty, condition does not improve, or worsening of condition. **Pregnancy/breast-feeding precautions:** Do not get pregnant while taking this medication. Use appropriate barrier contraceptive measures. Breast-feeding is not recommended.

Geriatric Considerations: The role of tetracycline has decreased because of the emergence of resistant organisms. Doxycycline is the tetracycline of choice when one is indicated because of its better GI absorption, less interactions with divalent cations, longer half-life, and the fact that the majority is cleared by nonrenal mechanisms.

Pregnancy Risk Factor: D

Pregnancy Issues: Tetracyclines cross the placenta and enter fetal circulation; may cause permanent discoloration of teeth if used during the last half of pregnancy.

Lactation: Enters breast milk/not recommended (AAP rates "compatible")

Breast-Feeding Considerations: Negligible absorption by infant; potential to stain infants' unerupted teeth

(Continued)

Tetracycline *(Continued)*

Administration

Oral: Oral should be given on an empty stomach (ie, 1 hour prior to, or 2 hours after meals) to increase total absorption. Administer at least 1-2 hours prior to, or 4 hours after antacid because aluminum and magnesium cations may chelate with tetracycline and reduce its total absorption. Administer around-the-clock to promote less variation in peak and trough serum levels.

Storage: Outdated tetracyclines have caused a Fanconi-like syndrome (nausea, vomiting, acidosis, proteinuria, glycosuria, aminoaciduria, polydipsia, polyuria, hypokalemia). Protect oral dosage forms from light.

- Tetracycline Hydrochloride *see* Tetracycline *on page 1613*
- Tetrahydrocannabinol *see* Dronabinol *on page 588*
- Tev-Tropin™ *see* Somatropin *on page 1555*
- Texacort® *see* Hydrocortisone *on page 873*

Thalidomide (tha LI doe mide)

U.S. Brand Names Thalomid®

Pharmacologic Category Angiogenesis Inhibitor; Immunosuppressant Agent; Tumor Necrosis Factor (TNF) Blocking Agent

Medication Safety Issues

Sound-alike/look-alike issues:

Thalidomide may be confused with flutamide

Use Treatment and maintenance of cutaneous manifestations of erythema nodosum leprosum

Unlabeled/Investigational Use Treatment of multiple myeloma; Crohn's disease; graft-versus-host reactions after bone marrow transplantation; AIDS-related aphthous stomatitis; Behçet's syndrome; Waldenström's macroglobulinemia; Langerhans cell histiocytosis; may be effective in rheumatoid arthritis, discoid lupus erythematosus, and erythema multiforme

Mechanism of Action A derivative of glutethimide; mode of action for immunosuppression is unclear; inhibition of neutrophil chemotaxis and decreased monocyte phagocytosis may occur; may cause 50% to 80% reduction of tumor necrosis factor - alpha

Pharmacodynamics/Kinetics

Distribution: V_d: 120 L

Protein binding: 55% to 66%

Metabolism: Nonenzymatic hydrolysis in plasma; forms multiple metabolites

Half-life elimination: 5-7 hours

Time to peak, plasma: 2-6 hours

Excretion: Urine (<1%)

Contraindications Hypersensitivity to thalidomide or any component of the formulation; neuropathy (peripheral); pregnancy or women in childbearing years unless alternative therapies are inappropriate and adequate precautions are taken to avoid pregnancy; patient unable to comply with STEPS™ program.

Warnings/Precautions Effective contraception must be used for at least 4 weeks before initiating therapy, during therapy, and for 4 weeks following discontinuation of thalidomide. May cause sedation; patients must be warned to use caution when performing tasks which require alertness. Use caution in patients with renal or hepatic impairment, neurological disorders, cardiovascular disease, or constipation.

Thalidomide has been associated with the development of peripheral neuropathy, which may be irreversible. Consider immediate discontinuation (if clinically appropriate) in patients who develop neuropathy. Use caution in patients with a history of seizures, concurrent therapy with drugs which alter seizure threshold, or conditions which predispose to seizures. May cause neutropenia; discontinue therapy if absolute neutrophil count decreases to <750/mm^3. Use caution in patients with HIV infection; has been associated with increased viral loads.

May cause orthostasis and/or bradycardia; use with caution in patients with cardiovascular disease or in patients who would not tolerate transient hypotensive episodes. Thrombotic events have been reported (generally in patients with other risk factors for thrombosis [neoplastic disease, inflammatory disease, or concurrent therapy with other drugs which may cause thrombosis]). Safety and efficacy have not been established in children <12 years of age.

Drug Interactions

Anakinra: Thalidomide may be associated with increased risk of serious infection when used in combination with anakinra.

CNS depressants: Thalidomide may enhance the sedative activity of other drugs such as ethanol, barbiturates, reserpine, and chlorpromazine

Drugs which may cause peripheral neuropathy: Use with caution in patients receiving thalidomide.

Drugs which may decrease the efficacy of hormonal contraceptives: Women using any drug which may decrease the serum concentrations and/or efficacy of hormonal contraceptives must use 2 other methods of contraception or abstain from heterosexual contact.

Nutritional/Herbal/Ethanol Interactions

Ethanol: Avoid ethanol (may increase sedation).

Herb/Nutraceutical: Avoid cat's claw (has immunostimulant properties).

Adverse Reactions

Controlled clinical trials: ENL:

>10%:

Central nervous system: Somnolence (37.5%), headache (12.5%)

Dermatologic: Rash (20.8%)

1% to 10% (Limited to important or life-threatening):

Dermatologic: Rash (maculopapular) (4.2%)

Genitourinary: Impotence (8.2%)

HIV-seropositive:

General: An increased viral load has been noted in patients treated with thalidomide. This is of uncertain clinical significance - see Monitoring

>10%:

Central nervous system: Somnolence (36% to 37%), dizziness (18.7% to 19.4%), fever (19.4% to 21.9%), headache (16.7% to 18.7%)

Dermatologic: Rash (25%), maculopapular rash (16.7% to 18.7%), acne (3.1% to 11.1%)

Gastrointestinal: AST increase (2.8% to 12.5%), diarrhea (11.1% to 18.7%), nausea (≤12.5%), oral moniliasis (6.3% to 11.1%)

Hematologic: Leukopenia (16.7% to 25%), anemia (5.6% to 12.5%)

Neuromuscular & skeletal: Paresthesia (may be severe and/or irreversible) (5.6% to 15.6%), weakness (5.6% to 21.9%)

Miscellaneous: Diaphoresis (≤12.5%), lymphadenopathy (5.6% to 12.5%)

1% to 10% (Limited to important or life-threatening): Central nervous system: Agitation (≤9.4%), neuropathy (up to 8% in HIV-seropositive patients)

Postmarketing and/or case reports (limited to important or life-threatening): Acute renal failure, arrhythmia, bradycardia, CML, dyspnea, electrolyte imbalances, erythema multiforme, erythema nodosum, Hodgkin's disease, hypersensitivity, hyperthyroidism, intestinal perforation, lethargy, lymphopenia, mental status changes, myxedema, neutropenia, orthostatic hypotension, pancytopenia, paresthesia, peripheral neuritis, photosensitivity, pleural effusion, psychosis, Raynaud's syndrome, seizure, Stevens-Johnson syndrome, suicide attempt, syncope, thrombosis, toxic epidermal necrolysis, tumor lysis syndrome

Dosing

Adults & Elderly:

Cutaneous ENL: Oral:

Initial dose: 100-300 mg/day taken once daily at bedtime with water (at least 1 hour after evening meal)

Adjustments to initial dose:

Patients weighing <50 kg: Initiate at lower end of the dosing range

Severe cutaneous reaction or previously requiring high dose: May be initiated at 400 mg/day; doses may be divided, but taken 1 hour after meals

Duration and tapering/maintenance:

Dosing should continue until active reaction subsides (usually at least 2 weeks), then tapered in 50 mg decrements every 2-4 weeks

Note: Patients who flare during tapering or with a history or requiring prolonged maintenance should be maintained on the minimum dosage necessary to control the reaction. Efforts to taper should be repeated every 3-6 months, in increments of 50 mg every 2-4 weeks.

Behçet's syndrome (unlabeled use): Oral: 100-400 mg/day

Graft-vs-host reactions (unlabeled use): Oral: 100-1600 mg/day; usual initial dose: 200 mg 4 times/day for use up to 700 days

AIDS-related aphthous stomatitis (unlabeled use): Oral: 200 mg twice daily for 5 days, then 200 mg/day for up to 8 weeks

(Continued)

Thalidomide *(Continued)*

Discoid lupus erythematosus (unlabeled use): Oral: 100-400 mg/day; maintenance dose: 25-50 mg

Pediatrics: Graft-vs-host reactions (unlabeled use): Oral: Children: 3 mg/kg 4 times/day

Available Dosage Forms Capsule: 50 mg, 100 mg, 200 mg

Nursing Guidelines

Assessment: Patient must be capable of complying with STEPS™ program (see Use). Instruct patient on risks of pregnancy, appropriate contraceptive measures (see Patient Education), and necessity for frequent pregnancy testing (schedule pregnancy testing at time of dispensing and give patient schedule in writing). Assess other medications patient may be taking for possible interactions (see Drug Interactions). Monitor closely for signs of neuropathy, neutropenia, and CNS depression. Instruct patient on signs and symptoms to report (see Patient Education), and appropriate interventions for adverse reactions.

Pregnancy risk factor X: Pregnancy test is required within 24 hours prior to beginning therapy, weekly during first month of therapy, and monthly thereafter for all women of childbearing age. Effective contraception with at least two reliable forms of contraception must be used for 1 month prior to beginning therapy, during therapy, and for 1 month following discontinuance of therapy. Women who have undergone a hysterectomy or have been postmenopausal for at least 24 consecutive months are the only exception. Do not prescribe, administer, or dispense to women of childbearing age or males who may have intercourse with women of childbearing age unless both female and male are capable of complying with contraceptive measures. Even males who have undergone vasectomy must acknowledge these risks in writing, and must use a latex condom during any sexual contact with women of childbearing age. Oral and written warnings concerning contraception and the hazards of thalidomide must be conveyed to females and males and they must acknowledge their understanding in writing. Parents or guardians must consent and sign acknowledgment for patients between 12 and 18 years of age following therapy. Breast-feeding is contraindicated.

Monitoring Laboratory Tests: Pregnancy testing is required within 24 hours of initiation of therapy, weekly during the first 4 weeks, then every 4 weeks in women with regular menstrual cycles or every 2 weeks in women with irregular menstrual cycles. In HIV-seropositive patients; monitor viral load after 1 and 3 months, then every 3 months. CBS initially and periodically during therapy. Consider monitoring of sensory nerve application potential amplitudes at baseline and every 6 months to detect asymptomatic neuropathy.

Dietary Considerations: Should be taken at least 1 hour after the evening meal.

Patient Education: You will be given oral and written instructions about the necessity of using two methods of contraception and and the necessity of keeping return visits for pregnancy testing. Do not donate blood while taking this medicine. Male patients should not donate sperm. Avoid extensive handling of capsules; capsules should remain in blister pack until ingestion. If exposed to the powder content from broken capsules or body fluids from patients receiving thalidomide, the exposed area should be washed with soap and water. You may experience postural hypotension (use caution when rising from lying or sitting position); sleepiness; dizziness; headaches; lack of concentration (use caution when driving, climbing stairs, or engaging in tasks requiring alertness until response to drug is known); nausea or vomiting or loss of appetite (small frequent meals, frequent mouth care, chewing gum, or sucking lozenges may help); constipation or diarrhea; oral thrush (frequent mouth care is necessary); or sexual dysfunction (reversible). Report any of the above if persistent or severe. Report chest pain or palpitations or swelling of extremities; back, neck, or muscle pain or stiffness; numbness or pain in extremities; skin rash or eruptions; increased nervousness, anxiety, or insomnia; or any other symptom of adverse reactions. **Pregnancy/breast-feeding precautions:** Do not get pregnant (females) or cause pregnancy (males) during treatment. The use of two forms of contraception are required for 1 month prior to therapy, during therapy, and for 1 month following discontinuation of therapy. Pregnancy tests will be routinely conducted during therapy. Do not breast-feed while taking this medication or for 1 month following discontinuation.

Pregnancy Risk Factor: X

Pregnancy Issues: Embryotoxic with limb defects noted from the 27th to 40th gestational day of exposure; all cases of phocomelia occur from the 27th to 42nd gestational day; fetal cardiac, gastrointestinal, and genitourinary tract abnormalities have also been described. Effective contraception must be used for at least 4 weeks before initiating therapy, during therapy, and for 4 weeks following discontinuation of thalidomide. Males (even those vasectomized) must use a latex condom during any sexual contact with women of childbearing age. Risk to the fetus from semen of male patients is unknown.

Lactation: Excretion in breast milk unknown/not recommended

Breast-Feeding Considerations: Due to the potential for serious adverse reactions in the infant, a decision should be made to discontinue nursing or discontinue treatment with thalidomide.

Administration

Oral: Avoid extensive handling of capsules; capsules should remain in blister pack until ingestion. If exposed to the powder content from broken capsules or body fluids from patients receiving thalidomide, the exposed area should be washed with soap and water.

Storage: Store at 15°C to 30°C (50°F to 86°F). Protect from light. Keep in original package.

- ♦ **Thalitone®** *see* Chlorthalidone *on page 383*
- ♦ **Thalomid®** *see* Thalidomide *on page 1616*
- ♦ **THC** *see* Dronabinol *on page 588*
- ♦ **Theo-24®** *see* Theophylline *on page 1619*
- ♦ **Theochron®** *see* Theophylline *on page 1619*
- ♦ **Theolair™** *see* Theophylline *on page 1619*
- ♦ **Theolair-SR® [DSC]** *see* Theophylline *on page 1619*

Theophylline (thee OFF i lin)

U.S. Brand Names Elixophyllin®; Quibron®-T; Quibron®-T/SR; Theo-24®; Theochron®; Theolair™; Theolair-SR® [DSC]; T-Phyl®; Uniphyl®

Synonyms Theophylline Anhydrous

Pharmacologic Category Theophylline Derivative

Medication Safety Issues

Sound-alike/look-alike issues:

Theolair™ may be confused with Thiola®, Thyrolar®

Use Treatment of symptoms and reversible airway obstruction due to chronic asthma, chronic bronchitis, or COPD

Mechanism of Action Causes bronchodilatation, diuresis, CNS and cardiac stimulation, and gastric acid secretion by blocking phosphodiesterase which increases tissue concentrations of cyclic adenine monophosphate (cAMP) which in turn promotes catecholamine stimulation of lipolysis, glycogenolysis, and gluconeogenesis and induces release of epinephrine from adrenal medulla cells

Pharmacodynamics/Kinetics

Absorption: Oral: Dosage form dependent

Distribution: 0.45 L/kg based on ideal body weight

Metabolism: Children >1 year and Adults: Hepatic; involves CYP1A2, 2E1 and 3A4; forms active metabolites (caffeine and 3-methylxanthine)

Half-life elimination: Highly variable and dependent upon age, liver function, cardiac function, lung disease, and smoking history

Time to peak, serum:

Oral: Liquid: 1 hour; Tablet, enteric-coated: 5 hours; Tablet, uncoated: 2 hours

I.V.: Within 30 minutes

Excretion: Urine

Neonates: 50% unchanged

Children >3 months and Adults: 10% unchanged

Contraindications Hypersensitivity to theophylline or any component of the formulation; premixed injection may contain corn-derived dextrose and its use is contraindicated in patients with allergy to corn-related products

Warnings/Precautions If a patient develops signs and symptoms of theophylline toxicity (eg, persistent, repetitive vomiting), a serum theophylline level should be measured and subsequent doses held. Due to potential saturation of theophylline clearance at serum levels in or (in some patients) less than the therapeutic range, dosage adjustment should be made in small increments (maximum: 25%). Due to wider interpatient variability, theophylline serum level measurements must be used to optimize therapy and prevent serious toxicity. Use with caution in patients

(Continued)

Theophylline *(Continued)*

with peptic ulcer, hyperthyroidism, seizure disorders, hypertension, and patients with cardiac arrhythmias (excluding bradyarrhythmias).

Drug Interactions **Substrate** of CYP1A2 (major), 2C8/9 (minor), 2D6 (minor), 2E1 (major), 3A4 (major); **Inhibits** CYP1A2 (weak)

CYP1A2 inducers: May decrease the levels/effects of theophylline. Example inducers include aminoglutethimide, carbamazepine, phenobarbital, and rifampin.

CYP1A2 inhibitors: May increase the levels/effects of theophylline. Example inhibitors include amiodarone, ciprofloxacin, fluvoxamine, ketoconazole, norfloxacin, ofloxacin, and rofecoxib.

CYP2E1 inhibitors: May increase the levels/effects of theophylline. Example inhibitors include disulfiram, isoniazid, and miconazole.

CYP3A4 inducers: CYP3A4 inducers may decrease the levels/effects of theophylline. Example inducers include aminoglutethimide, carbamazepine, nafcillin, nevirapine, phenobarbital, phenytoin, and rifamycins.

CYP3A4 inhibitors: May increase the levels/effects of theophylline. Example inhibitors include azole antifungals, clarithromycin, diclofenac, doxycycline, erythromycin, imatinib, isoniazid, nefazodone, nicardipine, propofol, protease inhibitors, quinidine, telithromycin, and verapamil.

Nutritional/Herbal/Ethanol Interactions Food: Food does not appreciably affect the absorption of liquid, fast-release products, and most sustained release products; however, food may induce a sudden release (dose-dumping) of once-daily sustained release products resulting in an increase in serum drug levels and potential toxicity. Avoid excessive amounts of caffeine. Avoid extremes of dietary protein and carbohydrate intake. Changes in diet may affect the elimination of theophylline; charbroiled foods may increase elimination, reducing half-life by 50%.

Adverse Reactions

Adverse reactions/theophylline serum level: (Adverse effects do not necessarily occur according to serum levels. Arrhythmia and seizure can occur without seeing the other adverse effects).

15-25 mcg/mL: GI upset, diarrhea, nausea/vomiting, abdominal pain, nervousness, headache, insomnia, agitation, dizziness, muscle cramp, tremor

25-35 mcg/mL: Tachycardia, occasional PVC

>35 mcg/mL: Ventricular tachycardia, frequent PVC, seizure

Uncommon at serum theophylline concentrations ≤20 mcg/mL:

1% to 10%:

Cardiovascular: Tachycardia

Central nervous system: Nervousness, restlessness

Gastrointestinal: Nausea, vomiting

<1% (Limited to important or life-threatening): Insomnia, irritability, seizure, tremor

Overdosage/Toxicology Symptoms of overdose include nausea, vomiting, insomnia, irritability, tachycardia, seizures, tonic-clonic seizures, insomnia, and circulatory failure. If seizures have not occurred, induce vomiting; ipecac syrup is preferred. Do not induce emesis in the presence of impaired consciousness. Repeated doses of charcoal have been shown to be effective in enhancing the total body clearance of theophylline. Do not repeat charcoal doses if an ileus is present. Charcoal hemoperfusion may be considered if serum theophylline levels exceed 40 mcg/mL, the patient is unable to tolerate repeat oral charcoal administrations, or if severe toxic symptoms are present. Clearance with hemoperfusion is better than clearance from hemodialysis. Administer a cathartic, especially if sustained release agents were used. Phenobarbital administered prophylactically may prevent seizures.

Dosing

Adults: Bronchodilation/respiratory stimulant:

Initial dosage recommendation: Loading dose (to achieve a serum concentration of about 10 mcg/mL; loading doses should be given using a rapidly absorbed oral product **not** a sustained release product):

If no theophylline has been administered in the previous 24 hours: 4-6 mg/kg theophylline

If theophylline has been administered in the previous 24 hours: Administer ½ loading dose; 2-3 mg/kg theophylline can be given in emergencies when serum concentrations are not available

On the average, for every 1 mg/kg theophylline given, blood concentrations will rise 2 mcg/mL

Maintenance dose: See table on next page.

Maintenance Dose for Acute Symptoms

Population Group	Oral Theophylline (mg/kg/day)	I.V. Aminophylline
Otherwise healthy nonsmoking adults (including elderly patients)	10 (not to exceed 900 mg/day)	0.5 mg/kg/h
Cardiac decompensation, cor pulmonale, and/or liver dysfunction	5 (not to exceed 400 mg/day)	0.25 mg/kg/h

Note: For continuous I.V. infusion, divide total daily dose by 24 = mg/kg/h.

Bronchodilation: Oral:

Nonsustained release: 16-20 mg/kg/day divided into 4 doses/day

Sustained release: 9-13 mg/kg/day divided into 2-3 doses/day

Note: These recommendations, based on mean clearance rates for age or risk factors, were calculated to achieve a serum concentration of 10 mcg/mL. In healthy adults, a slow-release product can be used (9-13 mg/kg in divided dose). The total daily dose can be divided every 8-12 hours.

Dosage in obese patients: Use ideal body weight for obese patients. Dose should be adjusted further based on serum concentrations. Guidelines for obtaining theophylline serum concentrations are shown in the table under Monitoring Laboratory Tests.

Elderly: Elderly patients should be started with a 25% reduction in the adult dose.

Pediatrics:

Loading dose:

Apnea of prematurity: Neonates: Oral: 4 mg/kg/dose

Treatment of acute bronchospasm: Infants and Children: Oral (to achieve a serum level of about 10 mcg/mL; loading doses should be given using a rapidly absorbed oral product **not** a sustained release product):

If no theophylline has been administered in the previous 24 hours: 5 mg/kg theophylline

If theophylline has been administered in the previous 24 hours: 2.5 mg/kg theophylline may be given in emergencies when serum levels are not available

Note: A modified loading dose (mg/kg) may be calculated (when the serum level is known) by: [Blood level desired - blood level measured] divided by 2 (for every 1 mg/kg theophylline given, the blood level will rise by approximately 2 mcg/mL)

Maintenance dose: See table.

Maintenance Dose for Acute Symptoms

Population Group	Oral Theophylline (mg/kg/day)
Premature infant or newborn to 6 wk (for apnea/bradycardia)[1]	4
6 wk to 6 mo[1]	10
Infants 6 mo to 1 y[1]	12-18
Children 1-9 y	20-24
Children 9-12 y, adolescent daily smokers of cigarettes or marijuana, and otherwise healthy adult smokers <50 y	16
Adolescents 12-16 y (nonsmokers)	13
Otherwise healthy nonsmoking adults (including elderly patients)	10 (not to exceed 900 mg/day)
Cardiac decompensation, cor pulmonale, and/or liver dysfunction	5 (not to exceed 400 mg/day)

[1]**Alternative dosing regimen for full-term infants <1 year of age:**

Total daily dose (mg) = [(0.2 x age in weeks) + 5] x weight (kg)

Postnatal age <26 weeks: Total daily dose divided every 8 hours

Postnatal age >26 weeks: Total daily dose divided every 6 hours

Note: These recommendations, based on mean clearance rates for age or risk factors, were calculated to achieve a serum level of 10 mcg/mL (5 mcg/mL

(Continued)

Theophylline *(Continued)*

for newborns with apnea/bradycardia). In newborns and infants, a fast-release oral product can be used. The total daily dose can be divided every 12 hours in newborns and every 6-8 hours in infants. In children and healthy adults, a slow-release product can be used. The total daily dose can be divided every 8-12 hours.

Note: Use ideal body weight for obese patients

Adjustment of dose: Dose should be further adjusted based on serum levels. Guidelines for drawing theophylline serum levels are shown in the table.

Available Dosage Forms [DSC] = Discontinued product

Capsule, extended release (Theo-24®): 100 mg, 200 mg, 300 mg, 400 mg [24 hours]

Elixir (Elixophyllin®): 80 mg/15 mL (480 mL) [contains alcohol 20%; fruit flavor]

Infusion [premixed in D_5W]: 0.8 mg/mL (500 mL, 1000 mL); 1.6 mg/mL (250 mL, 500 mL); 2 mg/mL (100 mL); 3.2 mg/mL (250 mL); 4 mg/mL (50 mL, 100 mL)

Solution, oral: 80 mg/15 mL (15 mL, 18.75 mL, 500 mL) [dye free, sugar free; contains alcohol 0.4% and benzoic acid; orange flavor]

Tablet, controlled release:

T-Phyl®: 200 mg [12 hours; contains cetostearyl alcohol]

Uniphyl®: 400 mg, 600 mg [24 hours; contains cetostearyl alcohol]

Tablet, extended release: 100 mg, 200 mg, 300 mg, 450 mg

Theochron®: 100 mg, 200 mg, 300 mg [12-24 hours]

Tablet, immediate release:

Quibron®-T: 300 mg

Theolair™: 125 mg, 250 mg

Tablet, sustained release (Quibron®-T/SR): 300 mg [8-12 hours]

Tablet, timed release (Theolair™-SR [DSC]): 300 mg, 500 mg

Nursing Guidelines

Assessment: Assess effectiveness and interactions of other medications patient may be taking. Monitor effectiveness of therapy (respiratory rate, lung sounds, characteristics of cough and sputum) and adverse reactions at beginning of therapy and periodically with long-term use. For inpatient care, monitor vital signs and lung sounds prior to and periodically during therapy. Assess knowledge/teach patient appropriate use, interventions to reduce side effects, and adverse symptoms to report.

Monitoring Laboratory Tests: Therapeutic levels:

Asthma: 10-15 mg/mL (peak level)

Toxic concentration: >20 mg/mL

Dietary Considerations: Should be taken with water 1 hour before or 2 hours after meals. Premixed injection may contain corn-derived dextrose and its use is contraindicated in patients with allergy to corn-related products.

Patient Education: Take exactly as directed; do not exceed recommended dosage. Avoid smoking (smoking may interfere with drug absorption as well as exacerbate condition for which medication is prescribed). If you are smoking when dosage is prescribed; inform prescriber if you stop smoking (dosage may need to be adjusted to prevent toxicity). Preferable to take on empty stomach, 1 hour before or 2 hours after meals, with a full glass of water. Do not chew of crush sustained release forms; capsules may be opened and contents sprinkled on soft food (do not chew beads). Avoid dietary stimulants (eg, caffeine, tea, colas, or chocolate; may increase adverse side effects). Maintain adequate hydration (2-3 L/day of fluids) unless instructed to restrict fluid intake. You may experience nausea, vomiting, or lose of appetite (small frequent meals, frequent mouth care, chewing gum, or sucking lozenges may help). Report acute insomnia or restlessness, chest pain or rapid heartbeat, emotional lability or agitation, muscle tremors or cramping, acute headache, abdominal pain and cramping, blackened stool, or worsening of respiratory condition. **Pregnancy precaution:** Inform prescriber if you are or intend to become pregnant.

Geriatric Considerations: Although there is a great intersubject variability for half-lives of methylxanthines (2-10 hours), elderly as a group have slower hepatic clearance. Therefore, use lower initial doses and monitor closely for response and adverse reactions. Additionally, elderly are at greater risk for toxicity due to concomitant disease (eg, CHF, arrhythmias), and drug use (eg, cimetidine, ciprofloxacin); see Warnings/Precautions and Drug Interactions.

Pregnancy Risk Factor: C

Pregnancy Issues: Theophylline crosses the placenta; adverse effects may be seen in the newborn. Theophylline metabolism may change during pregnancy; monitor serum levels.

Lactation: Enters breast milk/compatible (AAP rates "compatible")

Breast-Feeding Considerations: Irritability may be observed in the nursing infant.

Administration

Oral: Long-acting preparations should be taken with a full glass of water, swallowed whole, or cut in half if scored. Do **not** crush. Extended release capsule forms may be opened and the contents sprinkled on soft foods; do **not** chew beads.

Compatibility: Stable in D_5W

Y-site administration: Incompatible with hetastarch, phenytoin

Compatibility when admixed: Incompatible with ascorbic acid injection, ceftriaxone, cimetidine

- **Theophylline Anhydrous** *see* Theophylline *on page 1619*
- **Theophylline Ethylenediamine** *see* Aminophylline *on page 128*
- **Thera-Flu® Severe Cold Non-Drowsy [OTC] [DSC]** *see* Acetaminophen, Dextromethorphan, and Pseudoephedrine *on page 73*
- **Theragran-M® Advanced Formula [OTC] [DSC]** *see* Vitamins (Multiple/Oral) *on page 1720*
- **Theragran® Heart Right™ [OTC] [DSC]** *see* Vitamins (Multiple/Oral) *on page 1720*
- **Theramycin Z®** *see* Erythromycin *on page 634*
- **Therapeutic Multivitamins** *see* Vitamins (Multiple/Oral) *on page 1720*
- **Theratears®** *see* Carboxymethylcellulose *on page 316*
- **Thermazene®** *see* Silver Sulfadiazine *on page 1533*
- **Thiamazole** *see* Methimazole *on page 1122*

Thiamine (THYE a min)

Synonyms Aneurine Hydrochloride; Thiamine Hydrochloride; Thiaminium Chloride Hydrochloride; Vitamin B_1

Pharmacologic Category Vitamin, Water Soluble

Medication Safety Issues

Sound-alike/look-alike issues:

Thiamine may be confused with Tenormin®, Thorazine®

Use Treatment of thiamine deficiency including beriberi, Wernicke's encephalopathy syndrome, and peripheral neuritis associated with pellagra, alcoholic patients with altered sensorium; various genetic metabolic disorders

Mechanism of Action An essential coenzyme in carbohydrate metabolism by combining with adenosine triphosphate to form thiamine pyrophosphate

Pharmacodynamics/Kinetics

Absorption: Oral: Adequate; I.M.: Rapid and complete

Excretion: Urine (as unchanged drug and as pyrimidine after body storage sites become saturated)

Contraindications Hypersensitivity to thiamine or any component of the formulation

Warnings/Precautions Use with caution with parenteral route (especially I.V.) of administration

Drug Interactions Neuromuscular blocking agents; high carbohydrate diets or I.V. dextrose solutions increase thiamine requirement

Nutritional/Herbal/Ethanol Interactions Food: High carbohydrate diets may increase thiamine requirement.

Lab Interactions False-positive for uric acid using the phosphotungstate method and for urobilinogen using the Ehrlich's reagent; large doses may interfere with the spectrophotometric determination of serum theophylline concentration

Adverse Reactions <1% (Limited to important or life-threatening): Cardiovascular collapse and death, paresthesia

Dosing

Adults & Elderly:

Recommended daily allowance: >14 years: 1-1.5 mg

Thiamine deficiency (beriberi): I.M. or I.V. 5-30 mg/dose 3 times/day (if critically ill); then orally 5-30 mg/day in single or divided doses 3 times/day for 1 month

(Continued)

Thiamine *(Continued)*

Wernicke's encephalopathy: I.V., I.M.: Initial: 100 mg I.V., then 50-100 mg/day I.M. or I.V. until consuming a regular, balanced diet

Dietary supplement (depends on caloric or carbohydrate content of the diet): Oral: 1-2 mg/day

Note: The above doses can be found in multivitamin preparations.

Metabolic disorders: Oral: 10-20 mg/day (dosages up to 4 g/day in divided doses have been used)

Pediatrics:

Recommended daily allowance:

<6 months: 0.3 mg
6 months to 1 year: 0.4 mg
1-3 years: 0.7 mg
4-6 years: 0.9 mg
7-10 years: 1 mg
11-14 years: 1.1-1.3 mg
>14 years: 1-1.5 mg

Thiamine deficiency (beriberi):

Children: I.M., I.V.: 10-25 mg/dose daily (if critically ill), or 10-50 mg/dose orally every day for 2 weeks, then 5-10 mg/dose orally daily for 1 month

Dietary supplement (depends on caloric or carbohydrate content of the diet): Oral:

Infants: 0.3-0.5 mg/day
Children: 0.5-1 mg/day

Note: The above doses can be found in multivitamin preparations

Available Dosage Forms

Injection, solution, as hydrochloride: 100 mg/mL (2 mL)
Tablet, as hydrochloride: 50 mg, 100 mg, 250 mg, 500 mg

Nursing Guidelines

Assessment: Assess knowledge/teach patient appropriate administration (injection technique and needle disposal if I.M. self-administered) and dietary instruction.

Dietary Considerations: Dietary sources include legumes, pork, beef, whole grains, yeast, and fresh vegetables. A deficiency state can occur in as little as 3 weeks following total dietary absence.

Patient Education: Take exactly as directed; do not discontinue without consulting prescriber (deficiency state can occur in as little as 3 weeks). Follow dietary instructions (dietary sources include legumes, pork, beef, whole grains, yeast, fresh vegetables). **Pregnancy precaution:** Inform prescriber if you are or intend to become pregnant.

Pregnancy Risk Factor: A/C (dose exceeding RDA recommendation)

Lactation: Enters breast milk/compatible

Administration

I.M.: Parenteral form may be administered by I.M. or slow I.V. injection.

I.V.: Doses are usually administered over 1-2 minutes.

Compatibility: Stable in dextran 6% in dextrose, dextran 6% in NS, D_5LR, $D_5{}^1/_4NS$, $D_5{}^1/_2NS$, D_5NS, D_5W, $D_{10}W$, fat emulsion 10%, LR, $^1/_2NS$, NS

Storage: Protect oral dosage forms from light.

- **Thiamine Hydrochloride** *see* Thiamine *on page 1623*
- **Thiaminium Chloride Hydrochloride** *see* Thiamine *on page 1623*

Thiopental (thye oh PEN tal)

U.S. Brand Names Pentothal®

Synonyms Thiopental Sodium

Pharmacologic Category Anticonvulsant, Barbiturate; Barbiturate; General Anesthetic

Use Induction of anesthesia; adjunct for intubation in head injury patients; control of convulsive states; treatment of elevated intracranial pressure

Mechanism of Action Short-acting barbiturate with sedative, hypnotic, and anticonvulsant properties. Barbiturates depress the sensory cortex, decrease motor activity, alter cerebellar function, and produce drowsiness, sedation, and hypnosis. In high doses, barbiturates exhibit anticonvulsant activity; barbiturates produce dose-dependent respiratory depression.

Pharmacodynamics/Kinetics

Onset of action: Anesthetic: I.V.: 30-60 seconds
Duration: 5-30 minutes

Distribution: V_d: 1.4 L/kg
Protein binding: 72% to 86%
Metabolism: Hepatic, primarily to inactive metabolites but pentobarbital is also formed
Half-life elimination: 3-11.5 hours; decreased in children

Contraindications Hypersensitivity to thiopental, barbiturates, or any component of the formulation; status asthmaticus; severe cardiovascular disease; porphyria (variegate or acute intermittent); should not be administered by intra-arterial injection

Warnings/Precautions Laryngospasm or bronchospasms may occur; use with extreme caution in patients with reactive airway diseases (asthma or COPD). Use with caution when the hypnotic may be prolonged or potentiated (excessive premedication, Addison's disease, hepatic or renal dysfunction, myxedema, increased blood urea, severe anemia, or myasthenia gravis). Potential for drug dependency exists, abrupt cessation may precipitate withdrawal, including status epilepticus in epileptic patients. Do not administer to patients in acute pain. Use caution in patients with unstable aneurysms, cardiovascular disease, renal impairment, or hepatic disease. Use caution in elderly, debilitated, or pediatric patients. May cause paradoxical responses, including agitation and hyperactivity, particularly in acute pain and pediatric patients. Effects with other sedative drugs or ethanol may be potentiated. May cause respiratory depression or hypotension. Use with caution in hemodynamically unstable patients (hypotension or shock) or patients with respiratory disease. Repeated dosing or continuous infusions may cause cumulative effects. Extravasation or intra-arterial injection causes necrosis due to pH of 10.6, ensure patient has intravenous access.

Drug Interactions

CNS depressants: Sedative effects and/or respiratory depression with barbiturates may be additive with other CNS depressants; monitor for increased effect; includes ethanol, sedatives, antidepressants, narcotic analgesics, and benzodiazepines
Felbamate may inhibit the metabolism of barbiturates and barbiturates may increase the metabolism of felbamate
Methoxyflurane: Barbiturates may enhance the nephrotoxic effects of methoxyflurane

Adverse Reactions Frequency not defined.

Cardiovascular: Bradycardia, hypotension, syncope
Central nervous system: Drowsiness, lethargy, CNS excitation or depression, impaired judgment, "hangover" effect, confusion, somnolence, agitation, hyperkinesia, ataxia, nervousness, headache, insomnia, nightmares, hallucinations, anxiety, dizziness, shivering
Dermatologic: Rash, exfoliative dermatitis, Stevens-Johnson syndrome
Gastrointestinal: Nausea, vomiting, constipation
Hematologic: Agranulocytosis, thrombocytopenia, megaloblastic anemia, immune hemolytic anemia (rare)
Local: Pain at injection site, thrombophlebitis with I.V. use
Renal: Oliguria
Respiratory: Laryngospasm, respiratory depression, apnea (especially with rapid I.V. use), hypoventilation, sneezing, cough, bronchospasm
Miscellaneous: Gangrene with inadvertent intra-arterial injection, anaphylaxis, anaphylactic reactions

Overdosage/Toxicology Symptoms of overdose include respiratory depression, hypotension, shock. Hypotension should respond to I.V. fluids and placement of patient in Trendelenburg position; if necessary, pressors such as norepinephrine may be used; patient may require ventilatory support.

Dosing

Adults & Elderly:

Anesthesia: I.V.:
Induction: 3-5 mg/kg
Maintenance: 25-100 mg as needed

Increased intracranial pressure: I.V.: Children and Adults: 1.5-5 mg/kg/dose; repeat as needed to control intracranial pressure

Seizures: I.V.: 75-250 mg/dose, repeat as needed

Pediatrics:

Anesthesia: I.V.:
Induction:
Infants: 5-8 mg/kg
Children 1-12 years: 5-6 mg/kg
Maintenance: Children: 1 mg/kg as needed

(Continued)

Thiopental *(Continued)*

Increased intracranial pressure: I.V.: Children: 1.5-5 mg/kg/dose; repeat as needed to control intracranial pressure

Seizures: I.V.: Children: 2-3 mg/kg/dose, repeat as needed

Renal Impairment: Cl_{cr} <10 mL/minute: Administer 75% of normal dose.

Note: Accumulation may occur with chronic dosing due to lipid solubility. Prolonged recovery may result from redistribution of thiopental from fat stores.

Available Dosage Forms Injection, powder for reconstitution, as sodium: 250 mg, 400 mg, 500 mg, 1 g

Nursing Guidelines

Dietary Considerations: Sodium content of 1 g (injection): 86.8 mg (3.8 mEq)

Patient Education: Residual sedation following recovery is normal, due to slow release of the drug from lipid depots; patients should not drive or engage in similarly dangerous activities until at least the following day

Pregnancy Risk Factor: C

Perioperative/Anesthesia/Other Concerns: Thiopental switches from linear to nonlinear pharmacokinetics following prolonged continuous infusions.

Administration

I.V.: Avoid extravasation, necrosis may occur

Compatibility: Stable in dextran 6% in dextrose, dextran 6% in NS, D_5¼NS, D_5½NS, D_5W, ½NS, NS; **incompatible** with D_5LR, $D_{10}W$, $D_{10}NS$, LR

Y-site administration: Incompatible with alfentanil, ascorbic acid, atracurium, atropine, diltiazem, dobutamine, dopamine, ephedrine, epinephrine, furosemide, hydromorphone, labetalol, lidocaine, midazolam, nicardipine, norepinephrine, pancuronium, phenylephrine, succinylcholine, sufentanil, vecuronium

Compatibility in syringe: Incompatible with chlorpromazine, dimenhydrinate, diphenhydramine, doxapram, ephedrine, glycopyrrolate, meperidine, morphine, pentazocine, prochlorperazine edisylate, promethazine, sodium bicarbonate

Compatibility when admixed: Incompatible with amikacin, cimetidine, clindamycin, dimenhydrinate, diphenhydramine, droperidol, fentanyl, fibrinolysin (human), hydromorphone, insulin (regular), levorphanol, meperidine, metaraminol, morphine, norepinephrine, penicillin G potassium, prochlorperazine edisylate, promazine, promethazine, succinylcholine

Related Information

Intravenous Anesthetic Agents *on page 1853*

♦ **Thiopental Sodium** *see* Thiopental *on page 1624*

Thioridazine (thye oh RID a zeen)

Synonyms Thioridazine Hydrochloride

Pharmacologic Category Antipsychotic Agent, Typical, Phenothiazine

Medication Safety Issues

Sound-alike/look-alike issues:

Thioridazine may be confused with thiothixene, Thorazine®

Mellaril® may be confused with Elavil®, Mebaral®

Use Management of schizophrenic patients who fail to respond adequately to treatment with other antipsychotic drugs, either because of insufficient effectiveness or the inability to achieve an effective dose due to intolerable adverse effects from those medications

Unlabeled/Investigational Use Psychosis

Mechanism of Action Thioridazine is a piperidine phenothiazine which blocks postsynaptic mesolimbic dopaminergic receptors in the brain; exhibits a strong alpha-adrenergic blocking effect and depresses the release of hypothalamic and hypophyseal hormones

Pharmacodynamics/Kinetics

Duration: 4-5 days

Half-life elimination: 21-25 hours

Time to peak, serum: ~1 hour

Contraindications Hypersensitivity to thioridazine or any component of the formulation (cross-reactivity between phenothiazines may occur); severe CNS depression; circulatory collapse; severe hypotension; bone marrow suppression; blood dyscrasias; coma; in combination with other drugs that are known to prolong the QT_c interval; in patients with congenital long QT syndrome or a history of cardiac arrhythmias; concurrent use with medications that inhibit the metabolism of thioridazine (fluoxetine, paroxetine, fluvoxamine, propranolol, pindolol); patients known to have genetic defect leading to reduced levels of activity of CYP2D6

Warnings/Precautions Thioridazine has dose-related effects on ventricular repolarization leading to QT_c prolongation, a potentially life-threatening effect. Therefore, it should be reserved for patients with schizophrenia who have failed to respond to adequate levels of other antipsychotic drugs. May cause orthostatic hypotension - use with caution in patients at risk of this effect or those who would tolerate transient hypotensive episodes (cerebrovascular disease, cardiovascular disease, or other medications which may predispose).

Highly sedating, use with caution in disorders where CNS depression is a feature. Use with caution in Parkinson's disease. Caution in patients with hemodynamic instability; bone marrow suppression; predisposition to seizures; subcortical brain damage; severe cardiac, hepatic, renal, or respiratory disease. Esophageal dysmotility and aspiration have been associated with antipsychotic use - use with caution in patients at risk of pneumonia (ie, Alzheimer's disease). Caution in breast cancer or other prolactin-dependent tumors (may elevate prolactin levels). May alter temperature regulation or mask toxicity of other drugs due to antiemetic effects.

Phenothiazines may cause anticholinergic effects (confusion, agitation, constipation, xerostomia, blurred vision, urinary retention); therefore, they should be used with caution in patients with decreased gastrointestinal motility, urinary retention, BPH, xerostomia, or visual problems. Conditions which also may be exacerbated by cholinergic blockade include narrow-angle glaucoma (screening is recommended) and worsening of myasthenia gravis. Relative to other neuroleptics, thioridazine has a high potency of cholinergic blockade.

May cause extrapyramidal symptoms, including pseudoparkinsonism, acute dystonic reactions, akathisia, and tardive dyskinesia (risk of these reactions is low relative to other neuroleptics). May be associated with neuroleptic malignant syndrome (NMS). Doses exceeding recommended doses may cause pigmentary retinopathy.

Drug Interactions **Substrate** of CYP2C19 (minor), 2D6 (major); **Inhibits** CYP1A2 (weak), 2C8/9 (weak), 2D6 (moderate), 2E1 (weak)

Acetylcholinesterase inhibitors (central): May increase the risk of antipsychotic-related extrapyramidal symptoms; monitor.

Aluminum salts: May decrease the absorption of phenothiazines; monitor

Amphetamines: Efficacy may be diminished by antipsychotics; in addition, amphetamines may increase psychotic symptoms; avoid concurrent use

Anticholinergics: May inhibit the therapeutic response to phenothiazines and excess anticholinergic effects may occur; includes benztropine, trihexyphenidyl, biperiden, and drugs with significant anticholinergic activity (TCAs, antihistamines, disopyramide)

Antihypertensives: Concurrent use of phenothiazines with an antihypertensive may produce additive hypotensive effects (particularly orthostasis)

Beta-blockers: May increase the risk of arrhythmia; propranolol and pindolol are **contraindicated**

Bromocriptine: Phenothiazines inhibit the ability of bromocriptine to lower serum prolactin concentrations

Carvedilol: Serum concentrations may be increased, leading to hypotension and bradycardia; avoid concurrent use

CNS depressants: Sedative effects may be additive with phenothiazines; monitor for increased effect; includes barbiturates, benzodiazepines, narcotic analgesics, ethanol, and other sedative agents

CYP2D6 inhibitors: May increase the levels/effects of thioridazine. Example inhibitors include chlorpromazine, delavirdine, fluoxetine, miconazole, paroxetine, pergolide, quinidine, quinine, ritonavir, and ropinirole. **Thioridazine is contraindicated with inhibitors of this enzyme.**

CYP2D6 substrates: Thioridazine may increase the levels/effects of CYP2D6 substrates. Example substrates include amphetamines, selected beta-blockers, dextromethorphan, fluoxetine, lidocaine, mirtazapine, nefazodone, paroxetine, risperidone, ritonavir, tricyclic antidepressants, and venlafaxine.

CYP2D6 prodrug substrates: Thioridazine may decrease the levels/effects of CYP2D6 prodrug substrates. Example prodrug substrates include codeine, hydrocodone, oxycodone, and tramadol.

Epinephrine: Chlorpromazine (and possibly other low potency antipsychotics) may diminish the pressor effects of epinephrine

(Continued)

Thioridazine *(Continued)*

Guanethidine and guanadrel: Antihypertensive effects may be inhibited by phenothiazines

Levodopa: Phenothiazines may inhibit the antiparkinsonian effect of levodopa; avoid this combination

Lithium: Phenothiazines may produce neurotoxicity with lithium; this is a rare effect

Metoclopramide: May increase extrapyramidal symptoms (EPS) or risk.

Phenytoin: May reduce serum levels of phenothiazines; phenothiazines may increase phenytoin serum levels

Polypeptide antibiotics: Rare cases of respiratory paralysis have been reported with concurrent use of phenothiazines

Potassium-depleting agents: May increase the risk of serious arrhythmias with thioridazine; includes many diuretics, aminoglycosides, and amphotericin; monitor serum potassium closely

Propranolol: Serum concentrations of phenothiazines may be increased; propranolol also increases phenothiazine concentrations; may also occur with pindolol. **These agents are contraindicated with thioridazine.**

QT_c-prolonging agents: Effects on QT_c interval may be additive with phenothiazines, increasing the risk of malignant arrhythmias; includes type Ia antiarrhythmics, TCAs, and some quinolone antibiotics (sparfloxacin, moxifloxacin and gatifloxacin). **These agents are contraindicated with thioridazine.**

Sulfadoxine-pyrimethamine: May increase phenothiazine concentrations

Trazodone: Phenothiazines and trazodone may produce additive hypotensive effects

Tricyclic antidepressants: Concurrent use may produce increased toxicity or altered therapeutic response

Valproic acid: Serum levels may be increased by phenothiazines

Nutritional/Herbal/Ethanol Interactions

Ethanol: Avoid ethanol (may increase CNS depression).

Herb/Nutraceutical: Avoid kava kava, valerian, St John's wort, gotu kola (may increase CNS depression). Avoid dong quai, St John's wort (may also cause photosensitization).

Lab Interactions False-positives for phenylketonuria, urinary amylase, uroporphyrins, urobilinogen

Adverse Reactions Frequency not defined.

Cardiovascular: Hypotension, orthostatic hypotension, peripheral edema, ECG changes

Central nervous system: EPS (pseudoparkinsonism, akathisia, dystonias, tardive dyskinesia), dizziness, drowsiness, neuroleptic malignant syndrome (NMS), impairment of temperature regulation, lowering of seizure threshold

Dermatologic: Increased sensitivity to sun, rash, discoloration of skin (blue-gray)

Endocrine & metabolic: Changes in menstrual cycle, libido (changes in), breast pain, galactorrhea, amenorrhea

Gastrointestinal: Constipation, weight gain, nausea, vomiting, stomach pain, xerostomia, diarrhea

Genitourinary: Difficulty in urination, ejaculatory disturbances, urinary retention, priapism

Hematologic: Agranulocytosis, leukopenia

Hepatic: Cholestatic jaundice, hepatotoxicity

Neuromuscular & skeletal: Tremor, seizure

Ocular: Pigmentary retinopathy, blurred vision, cornea and lens changes

Respiratory: Nasal congestion

Overdosage/Toxicology Symptoms of overdose include deep sleep, coma, extrapyramidal symptoms, abnormal involuntary muscle movements, hypotension, and arrhythmias.

Immediate cardiac monitoring, including continuous electrocardiographic monitoring, to detect arrhythmias. Avoid use of medications that also prolong the QT_c interval, such as disopyramide, procainamide, and quinidine. Following initiation of essential overdose management, toxic symptom treatment and supportive treatment should be initiated. Hypotension usually responds to I.V. fluids or Trendelenburg positioning. If unresponsive to these measures, the use of a parenteral inotrope may be required (eg, norepinephrine 0.1-0.2 mcg/kg/minute titrated to response); do not use epinephrine or dopamine. Seizures commonly respond to diazepam (I.V. 5-10 mg bolus in adults every 15 minutes if needed up to a total of 30 mg; I.V. 0.25-0.4 mg/kg/dose up to a total of 10 mg in children) or to phenytoin. Avoid barbiturates (may potentiate respiratory depression). Neuroleptics often cause extrapyramidal symptoms (eg, dystonic reactions) requiring management with diphenhydramine 1-2 mg/kg (adults) up to a maximum of 50 mg I.M. or I.V. slow push followed by a maintenance dose for 48-72 hours. When these reactions are unresponsive to diphenhydramine, benztropine mesylate I.V. 1-2 mg (adults) may be effective. These agents are generally effective within 2-5 minutes.

Dosing

Adults:

Schizophrenia/psychosis: Oral: Initial: 50-100 mg 3 times/day with gradual increments as needed and tolerated; maximum: 800 mg/day in 2-4 divided doses

Depressive disorders, dementia: Oral: Initial: 25 mg 3 times/day; maintenance dose: 20-200 mg/day

Elderly: Behavioral symptoms associated with dementia: Oral: Initial: 10-25 mg 1-2 times/day; increase at 4- to 7-day intervals by 10-25 mg/day; increase dose intervals (once daily, twice daily, etc) as necessary to control response or side effects. Maximum daily dose: 400 mg; gradual increases (titration) may prevent some side effects or decrease their severity.

Pediatrics:

Schizophrenia/psychosis: Oral:

Children >2-12 years: Range: 0.5-3 mg/kg/day in 2-3 divided doses; usual: 1 mg/kg/day; maximum: 3 mg/kg/day

Children >12 years: Refer to adult dosing.

Behavior problems: Oral:

Children >2-12 years: Initial: 10 mg 2-3 times/day, increase gradually.

Children >12 years: Refer to adult dosing.

Severe psychoses: Oral:

Children >2-12 years: Initial: 25 mg 2-3 times/day, increase gradually.

Children >12 years: Refer to adult dosing.

Renal Impairment: Not dialyzable (0% to 5%)

Available Dosage Forms Tablet, as hydrochloride: 10 mg, 15 mg, 25 mg, 50 mg, 100 mg, 150 mg, 200 mg

Nursing Guidelines

Assessment: Assess other medications patient is taking for effectiveness and interactions. Review ophthalmic exam and monitor laboratory results, therapeutic effectiveness (mental status, mood, affect, gait), and adverse reactions at beginning of therapy and periodically with long-term use. Monitor for CNS depression/level of sedation. Avoid skin contact with liquid medication; may cause contact dermatitis (wash immediately with warm, soapy water). Initiate at lower doses and taper dosage slowly when discontinuing. Assess knowledge/teach patient appropriate use, interventions to reduce side effects, and adverse symptoms to report.

Monitoring Laboratory Tests: Baseline ECG; serum potassium, lipid profile, fasting blood glucose and Hgb A_{1c}; BMI; do not initiate if QT_c >450 msec

Patient Education: Use exactly as directed; do not increase dose or frequency. Do not discontinue without consulting prescriber. Tablet may be taken with food. Mix oral solution with 2-4 oz of liquid (eg, juice, milk, water, pudding). Do not take within 2 hours of any antacid. Store away from light. Avoid alcohol or caffeine and other prescription or OTC medications not approved by prescriber. Maintain adequate hydration (2-3 L/day of fluids) unless instructed to restrict fluid intake. Avoid skin contact with liquid medication; may cause contact dermatitis (wash immediately with warm, soapy water). May turn urine red-brown (normal). You may experience excess drowsiness, lightheadedness, dizziness, or blurred vision (use caution driving or when engaging in tasks requiring alertness until response to drug is known); nausea, vomiting, or dry mouth (small frequent meals, frequent mouth care, chewing gum, or sucking lozenges may help); constipation (increased exercise, fluids, fruit, or fiber may help); postural hypotension (use caution climbing stairs or when changing position from lying or sitting to standing); urinary retention (void before taking medication); ejaculatory dysfunction (reversible); decreased perspiration (avoid strenuous exercise in hot environments); or photosensitivity (use sunscreen, wear protective clothing and eyewear, and avoid direct sunlight). Report persistent CNS effects (eg, trembling fingers, altered gait or balance, excessive sedation, seizures, unusual movements, anxiety, abnormal thoughts, confusion, personality changes); chest pain, palpitations, rapid heartbeat, severe dizziness; unresolved urinary retention or changes in urinary pattern; altered menstrual pattern, change in libido, swelling or pain in breasts (male or female); vision changes; skin rash, irritation, or changes in color of skin (gray-blue); or

(Continued)

Thioridazine *(Continued)*

worsening of condition. **Pregnancy/breast-feeding precautions:** Inform prescriber if you are or intend to become pregnant. Breast-feeding is not recommended.

Geriatric Considerations: (See Warnings/Precautions, Adverse Reactions, and Overdose/Toxicology.) Elderly patients have an increased risk of adverse response to side effects or adverse reactions to antipsychotics.

Pregnancy Risk Factor: C

Lactation: Excretion in breast milk unknown/not recommended

Administration

Oral: Do not take antacid within 2 hours of taking drug.

Storage: Protect from light.

♦ Thioridazine Hydrochloride *see* Thioridazine *on page 1626*
♦ Thonzonium, Neomycin, Colistin, and Hydrocortisone *see* Neomycin, Colistin, Hydrocortisone, and Thonzonium *on page 1210*
♦ Thorazine® [DSC] *see* ChlorproMAZINE *on page 379*
♦ Thorets [OTC] *see* Benzocaine *on page 232*
♦ Thrombate III® *see* Antithrombin III *on page 173*
♦ Thrombin-JMI® *see* Thrombin (Topical) *on page 1630*

Thrombin (Topical) (THROM bin, TOP i kal)

U.S. Brand Names Thrombin-JMI®

Pharmacologic Category Hemostatic Agent

Use Hemostasis whenever minor bleeding from capillaries and small venules is accessible

Mechanism of Action Catalyzes the conversion of fibrinogen to fibrin

Contraindications Hypersensitivity to thrombin or any component of the formulation

Warnings/Precautions Do not inject, for topical use only

Drug Interactions No data reported

Adverse Reactions 1% to 10%:

Central nervous system: Fever

Miscellaneous: Allergic type reaction

Dosing

Adults & Elderly: Bleeding: Topical: Use 1000-2000 units/mL of solution where bleeding is profuse; apply powder directly to the site of bleeding or on oozing surfaces; use 100 units/mL for bleeding from skin or mucosal surfaces

Available Dosage Forms Powder for reconstitution, topical

Thrombin-JMI®: 5000 units, 20,000 units [packaged with diluent]

Thrombin-JMI® Spray Kit: 20,000 units [packaged with diluent and spray pump]

Thrombin-JMI® Syringe Spray Kit: 20,000 units [packaged with diluent, spray tip, and syringe]

Nursing Guidelines

Patient Education: External use only

Pregnancy Risk Factor: C

Administration

Storage: Refrigerate

♦ Thymoglobulin® *see* Antithymocyte Globulin (Rabbit) *on page 176*
♦ *L*-Thyroxine Sodium *see* Levothyroxine *on page 1029*
♦ Tiazac® *see* Diltiazem *on page 540*

Ticarcillin and Clavulanate Potassium

(tye kar SIL in & klav yoo LAN ate poe TASS ee um)

U.S. Brand Names Timentin®

Synonyms Ticarcillin and Clavulanic Acid

Pharmacologic Category Antibiotic, Penicillin

Use Treatment of infections of lower respiratory tract, urinary tract, skin and skin structures, bone and joint, and septicemia caused by susceptible organisms. Clavulanate expands activity of ticarcillin to include beta-lactamase producing strains of *S. aureus*, *H. influenzae*, *Bacteroides* species, and some other gram-negative bacilli

Mechanism of Action Inhibits bacterial cell wall synthesis by binding to one or more of the penicillin binding proteins (PBPs); which in turn inhibits the final

transpeptidation step of peptidoglycan synthesis in bacterial cell walls, thus inhibiting cell wall biosynthesis. Bacteria eventually lyse due to ongoing activity of cell wall autolytic enzymes (autolysins and murein hydrolases) while cell wall assembly is arrested.

Pharmacodynamics/Kinetics

Ticarcillin: See Ticarcillin monograph.

Clavulanic acid:

Protein binding: 9% to 30%

Metabolism: Hepatic

Half-life elimination: 66-90 minutes

Excretion: Urine (45% as unchanged drug)

Clearance: Does not affect clearance of ticarcillin

Contraindications Hypersensitivity to ticarcillin, clavulanate, any penicillin, or any component of the formulation

Warnings/Precautions Not approved for use in children <12 years of age; use with caution and modify dosage in patients with renal impairment; use with caution in patients with a history of allergy to cephalosporins and in patients with CHF due to high sodium load

Drug Interactions

Aminoglycosides: May be synergistic against selected organisms; physical inactivation of aminoglycosides in the presence of high concentrations of piperacillin and potential toxicity in patients with mild to moderate renal dysfunction

Heparin: Concomitant use with high-dose parenteral penicillins may result in increased risk of bleeding

Methotrexate: Penicillins may increase the exposure to methotrexate during concurrent therapy; monitor.

Neuromuscular blockers: May increase duration of blockade

Oral contraceptives: Anecdotal reports suggesting decreased contraceptive efficacy with penicillins have been refuted by more rigorous scientific and clinical data.

Probenecid: May increase levels of penicillins (ticarcillin)

Tetracyclines: May decrease effectiveness of penicillins (ticarcillin)

Warfarin: Effects of warfarin may be increased

Lab Interactions Positive Coombs' test, false-positive urinary proteins

Some penicillin derivatives may accelerate the degradation of aminoglycosides *in vitro*, leading to a potential underestimation of aminoglycoside serum concentration.

Adverse Reactions Frequency not defined.

Central nervous system: Confusion, convulsions, drowsiness, fever, Jarisch-Herxheimer reaction

Dermatologic: Rash, erythema multiforme, toxic epidermal necrolysis, Stevens-Johnson syndrome

Endocrine & metabolic: Electrolyte imbalance

Gastrointestinal: *Clostridium difficile* colitis

Hematologic: Bleeding, hemolytic anemia, leukopenia, neutropenia, positive Coombs' reaction, thrombocytopenia

Hepatic: Hepatotoxicity, jaundice

Local: Thrombophlebitis

Neuromuscular & skeletal: Myoclonus

Renal: Interstitial nephritis (acute)

Miscellaneous: Anaphylaxis, hypersensitivity reactions

Overdosage/Toxicology Symptoms of overdose include neuromuscular hypersensitivity and seizures. Hemodialysis may be helpful to aid in removal of the drug from blood; otherwise, treatment is supportive or symptom-directed.

Dosing

Adults:

Systemic infections: I.V.: 3.1 g (ticarcillin 3 g plus clavulanic acid 0.1 g) every 4-6 hours; maximum: 18-24 g/day

Urinary tract infections: I.V.: 3.1 g every 6-8 hours

Elderly: I.V.: 3.1 g every 4-6 hours; adjust for renal function.

Pediatrics:

Systemic infections:

Children <60 kg: 200-300 mg of ticarcillin component/kg/day in divided doses every 4-6 hours

Children >60 kg: 3.1 g (ticarcillin 3 g plus clavulanic acid 0.1 g) every 4-6 hours; maximum: 24 g/day

(Continued)

Ticarcillin and Clavulanate Potassium *(Continued)*

Renal Impairment:

Cl_{cr} 30-60 mL/minute: Administer 2 g every 4 hours or 3.1 g every 8 hours.
Cl_{cr} 10-30 mL/minute: Administer 2 g every 8 hours or 3.1 g every 12 hours.
Cl_{cr} <10 mL/minute: Administer 2 g every 12 hours.
Cl_{cr} <10 mL/minute with hepatic dysfunction: 2 g every 24 hours.

Moderately dialyzable (20% to 50%)
Continuous arteriovenous or venovenous hemodiafiltration effects: Dose as for Cl_{cr} 10-50 mL/minute.
Peritoneal dialysis: Administer 3.1 g every 12 hours.
Hemodialysis: Administer 2 g every 12 hours; supplemented with 3.1 g after each dialysis.

Hepatic Impairment: Cl_{cr} <10 mL/minute with hepatic dysfunction: Administer 2 g every 24 hours.

Available Dosage Forms

Infusion [premixed, frozen]: Ticarcillin 3 g and clavulanic acid 0.1 g (100 mL) [contains sodium 4.51 mEq and potassium 0.15 mEq per g]
Injection, powder for reconstitution: Ticarcillin 3 g and clavulanic acid 0.1 g (3.1 g, 31 g) [contains sodium 4.51 mEq and potassium 0.15 mEq per g]

Nursing Guidelines

Assessment: Assess for allergy history prior to starting therapy. See Contraindications and Warnings/Precautions for use cautions. Assess potential for interactions with other prescriptions, OTC medications, or herbal products patient may be taking (see Drug Interactions). Advise patients with diabetes about use of Clinitest®. Assess results of laboratory tests (see below), therapeutic effectiveness, and adverse reactions (eg, hypersensitivity reactions, opportunistic infection - see Adverse Reactions and Overdose/Toxicology). Teach patient possible side effects/appropriate interventions and adverse symptoms to report (see Patient Education).

Monitoring Laboratory Tests: Serum electrolytes, bleeding time, and periodic tests of renal, hepatic, and hematologic function; perform culture and sensitivity before administering first dose.

Dietary Considerations: Sodium content of 1 g: 4.51 mEq; potassium content of 1 g: 0.15 mEq

Patient Education: Inform prescriber of all prescriptions, OTC medications, or herbal products you are taking, and any allergies you have. Do not take any new medication during therapy unless approved by prescriber. This drug can only be given by injection or infusion. Report immediately any redness, swelling, burning, or pain at infusion site or any signs of allergic reaction (eg, respiratory difficulty or swallowing, chest tightness, rash, hives, swelling of lips or mouth). Maintain adequate hydration (2-3 L/day of fluids) unless instructed to restrict fluid intake. If you have diabetes, drug may cause false test results with Clinitest®, consult prescriber for alternative method of glucose monitoring. May cause confusion or drowsiness (use caution when driving or engaging in tasks that require alertness until response to drug is known). Report persistent diarrhea or abdominal pain (do not use antidiarrheal medication without consulting prescriber), fever, chills, unhealed sores, bloody urine or stool, muscle pain, mouth sores, respiratory difficulty, or skin rash; or signs of opportunistic infection (eg, fever, chills, unhealed sores, white plaques in mouth or vagina, purulent vaginal discharge, fatigue).

Geriatric Considerations: When used as empiric therapy or for a documented pseudomonal pneumonia, it is best to combine with an aminoglycoside such as gentamicin or tobramycin. High sodium content may limit use in patients with congestive heart failure. Adjust dose for renal function.

Pregnancy Risk Factor: B

Lactation: Enters breast milk (other penicillins are compatible with breast-feeding)

Administration

I.V.: Infuse over 30 minutes.

Some penicillins (eg, carbenicillin, ticarcillin and piperacillin) have been shown to inactivate aminglycosides *in vitro*. This has been observed to a greater extent with tobramycin and gentamicin, while amikacin has shown greater stability against inactivation. Concurrent use of these agents may pose a risk of reduced antibacterial efficacy *in vivo*, particularly in the setting of profound renal impairment. However, definitive clinical evidence is lacking. If combination penicillin/aminoglycoside therapy is desired in a patient with renal dysfunction, separation of doses (if feasible), and routine monitoring of aminoglycoside levels, CBC, and clinical response should be considered.

Compatibility: Stable in D_5W, LR, NS, SWFI

Y-site administration: Incompatible with alatrofloxacin, amphotericin B cholesteryl sulfate complex

Compatibility when admixed: Incompatible with sodium bicarbonate, aminoglycosides

Storage: Reconstituted solution is stable for 6 hours at room temperature and 72 hours when refrigerated. I.V. infusion in NS is stable for 24 hours at room temperature, 7 days when refrigerated, or 30 days when frozen. Darkening of solution indicates loss of potency of clavulanate potassium.

- Ticarcillin and Clavulanic Acid *see* Ticarcillin and Clavulanate Potassium *on page 1630*
- Tigan® *see* Trimethobenzamide *on page 1668*
- Timentin® *see* Ticarcillin and Clavulanate Potassium *on page 1630*

Timolol (TYE moe lole)

U.S. Brand Names Betimol®; Blocadren®; Istalol™; Timoptic®; Timoptic® OcuDose®; Timoptic-XE®

Synonyms Timolol Hemihydrate; Timolol Maleate

Pharmacologic Category Beta-Adrenergic Blocker, Nonselective; Ophthalmic Agent, Antiglaucoma

Medication Safety Issues

Sound-alike/look-alike issues:

Timolol may be confused with atenolol, Tylenol®

Timoptic® may be confused with Talacen®, Viroptic®

Bottle cap color change:

Timoptic®: Both the 0.25% and 0.5% strengths are now packaged in bottles with yellow caps; previously, the color of the cap on the product corresponded to different strengths.

Use Ophthalmic dosage form used in treatment of elevated intraocular pressure such as glaucoma or ocular hypertension; oral dosage form used for treatment of hypertension and angina, to reduce mortality following myocardial infarction, and for prophylaxis of migraine

Mechanism of Action Blocks both $beta_1$- and $beta_2$-adrenergic receptors, reduces intraocular pressure by reducing aqueous humor production or possibly outflow; reduces blood pressure by blocking adrenergic receptors and decreasing sympathetic outflow, produces a negative chronotropic and inotropic activity through an unknown mechanism

Pharmacodynamics/Kinetics

Onset of action:

Hypotensive: Oral: 15-45 minutes

Peak effect: 0.5-2.5 hours

Intraocular pressure reduction: Ophthalmic: 30 minutes

Peak effect: 1-2 hours

Duration: ~4 hours; Ophthalmic: Intraocular: 24 hours

Protein binding: 60%

Metabolism: Extensively hepatic; extensive first-pass effect

Half-life elimination: 2-2.7 hours; prolonged with renal impairment

Excretion: Urine (15% to 20% as unchanged drug)

Contraindications Hypersensitivity to timolol or any component of the formulation; sinus bradycardia; sinus node dysfunction; heart block greater than first degree (except in patients with a functioning artificial pacemaker); cardiogenic shock; uncompensated cardiac failure; bronchospastic disease; pregnancy (2nd and 3rd trimesters)

Warnings/Precautions Administer cautiously in compensated heart failure and monitor for a worsening of the condition. Beta-blocker therapy should not be withdrawn abruptly (particularly in patients with CAD), but gradually tapered to avoid acute tachycardia, hypertension, and/or ischemia. Use caution with concurrent use of beta-blockers and either verapamil or diltiazem; bradycardia or heart block can occur. Beta-blockers can aggravate symptoms in patients with PVD. Patients with bronchospastic disease should generally not receive beta-blockers; monitor closely if used in patients with potential risk of bronchospasm. Use cautiously in diabetics because it can mask prominent hypoglycemic symptoms. Can mask signs of thyrotoxicosis. Can cause fetal harm when administered in pregnancy. Use cautiously in severe renal impairment: marked hypotension can (Continued)

Timolol *(Continued)*

occur in patients maintained on hemodialysis. Use care with anesthetic agents which decrease myocardial function. Can worsen myasthenia gravis. Similar reactions found with systemic administration may occur with topical administration.

Drug Interactions Substrate of CYP2D6 (major); **Inhibits** CYP2D6 (weak)

Albuterol (and other $beta_2$ agonists): Effects may be blunted by nonspecific beta-blockers.

Alpha-blockers (prazosin, terazosin): Concurrent use of beta-blockers may increase risk of orthostasis.

AV conduction-slowing agents (digoxin): Effects may be additive with beta-blockers.

Clonidine: Hypertensive crisis after or during withdrawal of either agent (not reported with timolol ophthalmic solution)

CYP2D6 inhibitors: May increase the levels/effects of timolol. Example inhibitors include chlorpromazine, delavirdine, fluoxetine, miconazole, paroxetine, pergolide, quinidine, quinine, ritonavir, and ropinirole.

Epinephrine (including local anesthetics with epinephrine): Timolol may cause hypertension.

Glucagon: Timolol may blunt hyperglycemic action.

Insulin and oral hypoglycemics: May mask symptoms of hypoglycemia.

NSAIDs (ibuprofen, indomethacin, naproxen, piroxicam) may reduce the antihypertensive effects of beta-blockers.

Salicylates may reduce the antihypertensive effects of beta-blockers.

Sulfonylureas: Beta-blockers may alter response to hypoglycemic agents.

Verapamil or diltiazem may have synergistic or additive pharmacological effects when taken concurrently with beta-blockers.

Adverse Reactions

Ophthalmic:

>10%: Ocular: Burning, stinging

1% to 10%:

Cardiovascular: Hypertension

Central nervous system: Headache

Ocular: Blurred vision, cataract, conjunctival injection, itching, visual acuity decreased

Miscellaneous: Infection

Systemic:

1% to 10%:

Cardiovascular: Bradycardia

Central nervous system: Fatigue, dizziness

Respiratory: Dyspnea

Frequency not defined (reported with any dosage form):

Cardiovascular: Angina pectoris, arrhythmia, bradycardia, cardiac failure, cardiac arrest, cerebral vascular accident, cerebral ischemia, edema, hypotension, heart block, palpitation, Raynaud's phenomenon

Central nervous system: Anxiety, confusion, depression, disorientation, dizziness, hallucinations, insomnia, memory loss, nervousness, nightmares, somnolence

Dermatologic: Alopecia, angioedema, pseudopemphigoid, psoriasiform rash, psoriasis exacerbation, rash, urticaria

Endocrine & metabolic: Hypoglycemia masked, libido decreased

Gastrointestinal: Anorexia, diarrhea, dyspepsia, nausea, xerostomia

Genitourinary: Impotence, retoperitoneal fibrosis

Hematologic: Claudication

Neuromuscular & skeletal: Myasthenia gravis exacerbation, paresthesia

Ocular: Blepharitis, conjunctivitis, corneal sensitivity decreased, cystoid macular edema, diplopia, dry eyes, foreign body sensation, keratitis, ocular discharge, ocular pain, ptosis, refractive changes, tearing, visual disturbances

Otic: Tinnitus

Respiratory: Bronchospasm, cough, dyspnea, nasal congestion, pulmonary edema, respiratory failure

Miscellaneous: Allergic reactions, cold hands/feet, Peyronie's disease, systemic lupus erythematosus

Overdosage/Toxicology Symptoms of intoxication include cardiac disturbances, CNS toxicity, bronchospasm, hypoglycemia and hyperkalemia. The most common cardiac symptoms include hypotension and bradycardia. Atrioventricular block, intraventricular conduction disturbances, cardiogenic shock, and asystole may occur with severe overdose, especially with membrane-depressant drugs (eg, propranolol). CNS effects including convulsions, coma, and respiratory arrest are commonly seen with propranolol and other membrane-depressant and lipid-soluble drugs. Treatment is symptom-directed and supportive. Timolol is not readily dialyzable.

Dosing

Adults & Elderly:

Glaucoma: Ophthalmic:

Solution: Initial: 0.25% solution, instill 1 drop twice daily; increase to 0.5% solution if response not adequate; decrease to 1 drop/day if controlled; do not exceed 1 drop twice daily of 0.5% solution.

Istalol™: Instill 1 drop (0.5% solution) once daily in the morning.

Gel-forming solution (Timoptic-XE®): Instill 1 drop (either 0.25% or 0.5%) once daily

Hypertension: Oral: Initial: 10 mg twice daily, increase gradually every 7 days, usual dosage: 20-40 mg/day in 2 divided doses; maximum: 60 mg/day.

Prevention of myocardial infarction: Oral: 10 mg twice daily initiated within 1-4 weeks after infarction.

Migraine prophylaxis: Oral: Initial: 10 mg twice daily, increase to maximum of 30 mg/day.

Pediatrics: Children: Ophthalmic: Refer to adult dosing.

Available Dosage Forms Note: Strength expressed as base.

Gel-forming solution, ophthalmic, as maleate: 0.25% (5 mL); 0.5% (2.5 mL, 5 mL)

Timoptic-XE®: 0.25% (5 mL); 0.5% (5 mL)

Solution, ophthalmic, as hemihydrate (Betimol®): 0.25% (5 mL, 10 mL, 15 mL); 0.5% (5 mL, 10 mL, 15 mL) [contains benzalkonium chloride]

Solution, ophthalmic, as maleate: 0.25% (5 mL, 10 mL, 15 mL); 0.5% (5 mL, 10 mL, 15 mL) [contains benzalkonium chloride]

Istalol™: 0.5% (10 mL) [contains benzalkonium chloride and potassium sorbate]

Timoptic®: 0.25% (5 mL, 10 mL); 0.5% (5 mL, 10 mL) [contains benzalkonium chloride]

Solution, ophthalmic, as maleate [preservative free] (Timoptic® OcuDose®): 0.25% (0.2 mL); 0.5% (0.2 mL) [single use]

Tablet, as maleate: 5 mg, 10 mg, 20 mg

Blocadren®: 20 mg

Nursing Guidelines

Assessment: Assess other medications patient may be taking for effectiveness and interactions. Monitor therapeutic effectiveness (according to purpose of therapy) and adverse reactions at beginning of therapy and regularly with long-term therapy. Monitor blood pressure periodically. Assess knowledge/teach patient appropriate use, interventions to reduce side effects, and adverse symptoms to report.

Dietary Considerations: Oral product should be administered with food at the same time each day.

Patient Education: Oral: Take exact dose prescribed; do not increase, decrease, or discontinue dosage without consulting prescriber. Take at the same time each day. If you have diabetes, monitor serum glucose closely. May cause postural hypotension (use caution when rising from sitting or lying position or climbing stairs); dizziness, drowsiness, or blurred vision (use caution when driving or engaging in tasks requiring alertness until response to drug is known); decreased sexual ability (reversible); or nausea or vomiting (small frequent meals or frequent mouth care may help). Report swelling of extremities, respiratory difficulty, or new cough; weight gain (>3 lb/week); unresolved diarrhea or vomiting; or cold blue extremities. **Pregnancy/breast-feeding precautions:** Inform prescriber if you are or intend to become pregnant. Consult prescriber if breast-feeding.

Ophthalmic: For ophthalmic use only. Apply prescribed amount as often as directed. Wash hands before using. Do not let tip of applicator touch eye; do not contaminate tip of applicator (may cause eye infection, eye damage, or vision loss). Tilt head back and look upward. Gently pull down lower lid and put drop(s) inside lower eyelid at inner corner. Close eye and roll eyeball in all directions. Do not blink for ½ minute. Apply gentle pressure to inner corner of eye for 30 seconds. Wipe away excess from skin around eye. Do not use any other eye preparation for at least 10 minutes. Do not share medication with anyone else. Temporary stinging or blurred vision may occur. If using Istalol™, remove contact lenses prior to administration. Lenses may be reinserted 15

(Continued)

Timolol *(Continued)*

minutes following administration. Immediately report any adverse cardiac or CNS effects (usually signifies overdose). Report persistent eye pain, redness, burning, watering, dryness, double vision, puffiness around eye, vision changes, other adverse eye response, worsening of condition or lack of improvement.

Geriatric Considerations: Due to alterations in the beta-adrenergic autonomic nervous system, beta-adrenergic blockade may result in less hemodynamic response than seen in younger adults.

Pregnancy Risk Factor: C (manufacturer); D (2nd and 3rd trimesters - expert analysis)

Pregnancy Issues: Timolol was shown to cross the placenta in an *in vitro* perfusion study. Beta-blockers have been associated with bradycardia, hypotension, hypoglycemia, and intrauterine growth rate (IUGR); IUGR is probably related to maternal hypertension. Available evidence suggests beta-blockers are generally safe during pregnancy (JNC 7). Cases of neonatal hypoglycemia have been reported following maternal use of beta-blockers at parturition or during breast-feeding. Bradycardia and arrhythmia have been reported in an infant following ophthalmic administration of timolol during pregnancy.

Lactation: Enters breast milk/use caution (AAP rates "compatible")

Breast-Feeding Considerations: Timolol is excreted in breast milk following oral and ophthalmic administration, and is considered compatible by the AAP. It is recommended that the infant be monitored for signs or symptoms of beta-blockade (hypotension, bradycardia, etc) with long-term use.

Perioperative/Anesthesia/Other Concerns: It is important to recognize that timolol eye drops may have systemic effects, particularly when patients are also on oral beta-blocker therapy or therapy with other negative chronotropic agents.

Myocardial Infarction: Beta-blockers, in general without intrinsic sympathomimetic activity (ISA), have been shown to decrease morbidity and mortality when initiated in the acute treatment of myocardial infarction and continued long-term. In this setting, therapy should be avoided in patients with hypotension, cardiogenic shock, or heart block.

Surgery: Atenolol has also been shown to improve cardiovascular outcomes when used in the perioperative period in patients with underlying cardiovascular disease who are undergoing noncardiac surgery. Bisoprolol in high-risk patients undergoing vascular surgery reduced the perioperative incidence of death from cardiac causes and nonfatal myocardial infarction.

Withdrawal: Beta-blocker therapy should not be withdrawn abruptly, but gradually tapered to avoid acute tachycardia and hypertension.

Administration

Storage: Ophthalmic drops: Store at room temperature. Protect from light and freezing.

Timoptic Occudose®: Store in the protective foil wrap and use within 1 month after opening foil package.

- ♦ **Timolol and Dorzolamide** *see* Dorzolamide and Timolol *on page 569*
- ♦ **Timolol Hemihydrate** *see* Timolol *on page 1633*
- ♦ **Timolol Maleate** *see* Timolol *on page 1633*
- ♦ **Timoptic®** *see* Timolol *on page 1633*
- ♦ **Timoptic® OcuDose®** *see* Timolol *on page 1633*
- ♦ **Timoptic-XE®** *see* Timolol *on page 1633*
- ♦ **TinBen® [OTC] [DSC]** *see* Benzoin *on page 235*
- ♦ **Tine Test** *see* Tuberculin Tests *on page 1673*

Tinzaparin (tin ZA pa rin)

U.S. Brand Names Innohep®

Synonyms Tinzaparin Sodium

Pharmacologic Category Low Molecular Weight Heparin

Use Treatment of acute symptomatic deep vein thrombosis, with or without pulmonary embolism, in conjunction with warfarin sodium

Mechanism of Action Standard heparin consists of components with molecular weights ranging from 4000-30,000 daltons with a mean of 16,000 daltons. Heparin acts as an anticoagulant by enhancing the inhibition rate of clotting proteases by antithrombin III, impairing normal hemostasis and inhibition of factor Xa. Low molecular weight heparins have a small effect on the activated partial thromboplastin time and strongly inhibit factor Xa. The primary inhibitory activity of tinzaparin is through antithrombin. Tinzaparin is derived from porcine heparin that undergoes controlled enzymatic depolymerization. The average molecular weight of tinzaparin ranges between 5500 and 7500 daltons which is distributed as (<10%) 2000 daltons (60% to 72%) 2000-8000 daltons, and (22% to 36%) >8000 daltons. The antifactor Xa activity is approximately 100 int. units/mg.

Pharmacodynamics/Kinetics

Onset of action: 2-3 hours
Distribution: 3-5 L
Half-life elimination: 3-4 hours
Metabolism: Partially metabolized by desulphation and depolymerization
Bioavailability: 87%
Time to peak: 4-5 hours
Excretion: Urine

Contraindications Hypersensitivity to tinzaparin sodium, heparin, sulfites, benzyl alcohol, pork products, or any component of the formulation; active major bleeding; heparin-induced thrombocytopenia (current or history of)

Warnings/Precautions **Patients with recent or anticipated neuraxial anesthesia (epidural or spinal anesthesia) are at risk of spinal or epidural hematoma and subsequent paralysis.** Consider risk versus benefit prior to neuraxial anesthesia; risk is increased by concomitant agents which may alter hemostasis, as well as traumatic or repeated epidural or spinal puncture, and indwelling epidural catheters. Patient should be observed closely for signs and symptoms of neurological impairment. Not to be used interchangeably (unit for unit) with heparin or any other low molecular weight heparins.

Monitor patient closely for signs or symptoms of bleeding. Certain patients are at increased risk of bleeding. Risk factors include bacterial endocarditis; congenital or acquired bleeding disorders; active ulcerative or angiodysplastic GI diseases; severe uncontrolled hypertension; hemorrhagic stroke; use shortly after brain, spinal, or ophthalmologic surgery; patients treated concomitantly with platelet inhibitors; recent GI bleeding; thrombocytopenia or platelet defects; severe liver disease; hypertensive or diabetic retinopathy; or in patients undergoing invasive procedures. Monitor platelet count closely. Rare cases of thrombocytopenia have occurred. Manufacturer recommends discontinuation of therapy if platelets are <100,000/mm^3.

Safety and efficacy in pediatric patients has not been established. Use with caution in the elderly (delayed elimination may occur). Heparin can cause hyperkalemia by affecting aldosterone; similar reactions could occur with LMWHs. Monitor for hyperkalemia. For subcutaneous injection only, do not mix with other injections or infusions. Clinical experience is limited in patients with BMI >40 kg.

Drug Interactions

Drugs which affect platelet function (eg, aspirin, NSAIDs, dipyridamole, ticlopidine, clopidogrel, sulfinpyrazone, dextran) may potentiate the risk of hemorrhage.

Thrombolytic agents increase the risk of hemorrhage.

Warfarin: Risk of bleeding may be increased during concurrent therapy. Tinzaparin is commonly continued during the initiation of warfarin therapy to assure anticoagulation and to protect against possible transient hypercoagulability

Lab Interactions Asymptomatic increases in AST (SGOT) (8.8%) and ALT (SGPT) (13%) have been reported. Elevations were >3 times the upper limit of normal and were reversible and rarely associated with increases in bilirubin.

Adverse Reactions As with all anticoagulants, bleeding is the major adverse effect of tinzaparin. Hemorrhage may occur at virtually any site. Risk is dependent on multiple variables.

>10%:
- Hepatic: Increased ALT (13%)
- Local: Injection site hematoma (16%)

1% to 10%:
- Cardiovascular: Angina pectoris, chest pain (2%), hyper-/hypotension, tachycardia
- Central nervous system: Confusion, dizziness, fever (2%), headache (2%), insomnia, pain (2%)
- Dermatologic: Bullous eruption, pruritus, rash (1%), skin disorder
- Gastrointestinal: Constipation (1%), dyspepsia, flatulence, nausea (2%), nonspecified gastrointestinal disorder, vomiting (1%)

(Continued)

Tinzaparin *(Continued)*

Genitourinary: Dysuria, urinary retention, urinary tract infection (4%)
Hematologic: Anemia, hematoma, hemorrhage (2%), thrombocytopenia (1%)
Hepatic: Increased AST (9%)
Local: Deep vein thrombosis
Neuromuscular & skeletal: Back pain (2%)
Renal: Hematuria (1%)
Respiratory: Dyspnea (1%), epistaxis (2%), pneumonia, pulmonary embolism (2%), respiratory disorder
Miscellaneous: Impaired healing, infection, unclassified reactions

<1% (Limited to important or life-threatening): Agranulocytosis, allergic purpura, allergic reaction, angioedema, arrhythmia, cholestatic hepatitis, epidermal necrolysis, gastrointestinal hemorrhage, granulocytopenia, hemarthrosis, hematoma, hemoptysis, intracranial hemorrhage, ischemic necrosis, major bleeding, MI, ocular hemorrhage, pancytopenia, priapism, purpura, rash, retroperitoneal/intra-abdominal bleeding, severe thrombocytopenia, skin necrosis, spinal epidural hematoma, Stevens-Johnson syndrome, urticaria, vaginal hemorrhage

Postmarketing and/or case reports: The following adverse effects have been reported in infants of women receiving tinzaparin during pregnancy (relationship has not been established): Cleft palate (one report), optic nerve hypoplasia (one report), trisomy 21 (one report), fetal death/miscarriage, fetal distress, neonatal hypotonia, cutis aplasia of the scalp

Overdosage/Toxicology Overdose may lead to bleeding; bleeding may occur at any site. In case of overdose, discontinue medication, apply pressure to bleeding site if possible, and replace volume and hemostatic blood elements as required. If these measures are ineffective, or if bleeding is severe, protamine sulfate may be administered at 1 mg per every 100 anti-Xa int. units of tinzaparin.

Dosing

Adults & Elderly: Treatment of DVT: SubQ: 175 anti-Xa int. units/kg of body weight once daily. Warfarin sodium should be started when appropriate. Administer tinzaparin for at least 6 days and until patient is adequately anticoagulated with warfarin.

Note: To calculate the volume of solution to administer per dose: Volume to be administered (mL) = patient weight (kg) x 0.00875 mL/kg (may be rounded off to the nearest 0.05 mL)

Renal Impairment: Patients with severe renal impairment had a 24% decrease in clearance, use with caution.

Hepatic Impairment: No adjustment necessary.

Available Dosage Forms Injection, solution, as sodium: 20,000 anti-Xa int. units/mL (2 mL) [contains benzyl alcohol and sodium metabisulfite]

Nursing Guidelines

Assessment: See Contraindications, Warnings/Precautions, and Dosing for use cautions. Assess potential for interactions with other prescriptions, OTC medications, or herbal products patient may be taking (especially anything that will impact coagulation or platelet aggregation - see Drug Interactions). Assess results of laboratory tests (see below), therapeutic effectiveness, and adverse response (eg, thrombolytic reactions - see Adverse Reactions and Overdose/Toxicology). Teach patient use if self-administered (appropriate injection technique and syringe/needle disposal), possible side effects/appropriate interventions (eg, bleeding precautions), and adverse symptoms to report (see Patient Education). **Pregnancy risk factor B:** see Pregnancy Issues. Note breast-feeding caution.

Monitoring Laboratory Tests: CBC including platelet count and hematocrit or hemoglobin, and stool for occult blood; the monitoring of PT and/or PTT is not necessary. Patients receiving both warfarin and tinzaparin should have their INR drawn just prior to the next scheduled dose of tinzaparin.

Patient Education: Inform prescriber of all prescriptions, OTC medications, or herbal products you are taking, and any allergies you have. Do not take any new medication during therapy unless approved by prescriber. This drug can only be administered by injection. Use exactly as directed (if self-administered, follow exact instructions for injection and syringe disposal). Do not alter dosage or discontinue without consulting prescriber. You may have a tendency to bleed easily while taking this drug (brush teeth with soft brush, use waxed dental floss, use electric razor, avoid scissors or sharp knives, and avoid potentially harmful activities). Report immediately any unusual bleeding or bruising (eg, mouth, nose, blood in urine or stool); chest pain or palpitations; confusion, dizziness, or headache; skin rash or itching; GI upset (eg, nausea, vomiting, abdominal pain, acute constipation); warmth, swelling, pain, or redness in calves or other areas; back or muscle pain; respiratory difficulties; or other persistent adverse reactions. **Pregnancy/breast-feeding precautions:** Inform prescriber if you are pregnant or intend to become pregnant. Consult prescriber if breast-feeding.

Pregnancy Risk Factor: B

Pregnancy Issues: There are no adequate and well-controlled studies in pregnant women. Cases of teratogenic effects and/or fetal death have been reported (relationship to tinzaparin not established). Use during pregnancy only if clearly needed. Pregnant women, or those who become pregnant while receiving tinzaparin, should be informed of the potential risks to the fetus.

Lactation: Excretion in breast milk unknown/use caution

Administration

I.V.: Patient should be lying down or sitting. Administer by deep SubQ injection, alternating between the left and right anterolateral and left and right posterolateral abdominal wall. Vary site daily. The entire needle should be introduced into the skin fold formed by the thumb and forefinger. Hold the skin fold until injection is complete. To minimize bruising, do not rub the injection site.

Storage: Store at 25°C (77°F). Excursions permitted to 15°C to 30°C (59°F to 86°F).

- Tinzaparin Sodium *see* Tinzaparin *on page 1636*
- Tisseel® VH *see* Fibrin Sealant Kit *on page 724*
- Titralac™ [OTC] *see* Calcium Carbonate *on page 291*
- Titralac™ Extra Strength [OTC] *see* Calcium Carbonate *on page 291*
- Titralac® Plus [OTC] *see* Calcium Carbonate and Simethicone *on page 294*
- TMP-SMZ *see* Sulfamethoxazole and Trimethoprim *on page 1582*
- TOBI® *see* Tobramycin *on page 1639*
- TobraDex® *see* Tobramycin and Dexamethasone *on page 1643*

Tobramycin (toe bra MYE sin)

U.S. Brand Names AKTob®; TOBI®; Tobrex®

Synonyms Tobramycin Sulfate

Pharmacologic Category Antibiotic, Aminoglycoside; Antibiotic, Ophthalmic

Medication Safety Issues

Sound-alike/look-alike issues:

Tobramycin may be confused with Trobicin®

AKTob® may be confused with AK-Trol®

Nebcin® may be confused with Inapsine®, Naprosyn®, Nubain®

Tobrex® may be confused with TobraDex®

Use Treatment of documented or suspected infections caused by susceptible gram-negative bacilli including *Pseudomonas aeruginosa*; topically used to treat superficial ophthalmic infections caused by susceptible bacteria. Tobramycin solution for inhalation is indicated for the management of cystic fibrosis patients (>6 years of age) with *Pseudomonas aeruginosa*.

Mechanism of Action Interferes with bacterial protein synthesis by binding to 30S and 50S ribosomal subunits resulting in a defective bacterial cell membrane

Pharmacodynamics/Kinetics

Absorption: I.M.: Rapid and complete

Distribution: V_d: 0.2-0.3 L/kg; Pediatrics: 0.2-0.7 L/kg; to extracellular fluid including serum, abscesses, ascitic, pericardial, pleural, synovial, lymphatic, and peritoneal fluids; crosses placenta; poor penetration into CSF, eye, bone, prostate

Protein binding: <30%

Half-life elimination:

Neonates: ≤1200 g: 11 hours; >1200 g: 2-9 hours

Adults: 2-3 hours; directly dependent upon glomerular filtration rate

Adults with impaired renal function: 5-70 hours

Time to peak, serum: I.M.: 30-60 minutes; I.V.: ~30 minutes

Excretion: Normal renal function: Urine (~90% to 95%) within 24 hours

Contraindications Hypersensitivity to tobramycin, other aminoglycosides, or any component of the formulation; pregnancy (injection/inhalation)

Warnings/Precautions Use with caution in patients with renal impairment; pre-existing auditory or vestibular impairment; and in patients with neuromuscular disorders. Dosage modification required in patients with impaired renal function (I.M. & I.V.). Aminoglycosides are associated with significant nephrotoxicity or

(Continued)

Tobramycin *(Continued)*

ototoxicity; the ototoxicity is directly proportional to the amount of drug given and the duration of treatment. Tinnitus or vertigo are indications of vestibular injury. Ototoxicity is often irreversible. Renal damage is usually reversible.

Drug Interactions

Increased effect: Extended spectrum penicillins (synergistic)

Increased toxicity:

Aminoglycosides may potentiate the effects of neuromuscular-blocking agents

Amphotericin B, cephalosporins, loop diuretics, and vancomycin may increase risk of nephrotoxicity

Decreased effect: Tobramycin's efficacy reduced when given concurrently with carbenicillin, ticarcillin, or piperacillin to patients with severe renal impairment (inactivation). Separate administration.

Lab Interactions Some penicillin derivatives may accelerate the degradation of aminoglycosides *in vitro*, leading to a potential underestimation of aminoglycoside serum concentration.

Adverse Reactions

Injection: Frequency not defined:

Central nervous system: Confusion, disorientation, dizziness, fever, headache, lethargy, vertigo

Dermatologic: Exfoliative dermatitis, itching, rash, urticaria

Endocrine & metabolic: Serum calcium, magnesium, potassium, and/or sodium decreased

Gastrointestinal: Diarrhea, nausea, vomiting

Hematologic: Anemia, eosinophilia, granulocytopenia, leukocytosis, leukopenia, thrombocytopenia

Hepatic: ALT, AST, bilirubin, and/or LDH increased

Local: Pain at the injection site

Otic: Hearing loss, tinnitus, ototoxicity (auditory), ototoxicity (vestibular), roaring in the ears

Renal: BUN increased, cylindruria, serum creatinine increased, oliguria, proteinuria

Inhalation:

>10%:

Gastrointestinal: Sputum discoloration (21%)

Respiratory: Voice alteration (13%)

1% to 10%:

Central nervous system: Malaise (6%)

Otic: Tinnitus (3%)

Postmarketing and/or case reports: Hearing loss

Ophthalmic: <1% (Limited to important or life-threatening): Ocular: Conjunctival erythema, lid itching, lid swelling

Overdosage/Toxicology Symptoms of overdose include ototoxicity, nephrotoxicity, and neuromuscular toxicity. Treatment of choice following a single acute overdose appears to be maintenance of urine output of at least 3 mL/kg/hour during the acute treatment phase. Dialysis is of questionable value in enhancing aminoglycoside elimination. If required, hemodialysis is preferred over peritoneal dialysis in patients with normal renal function. Chelation with penicillins is investigational.

Dosing

Adults: Individualization is **critical** because of the low therapeutic index.

Use of ideal body weight (IBW) for determining the mg/kg/dose appears to be more accurate than dosing on the basis of total body weight (TBW). In morbid obesity, dosage requirement may best be estimated using a dosing weight of IBW + 0.4 (TBW - IBW).

Initial and periodic plasma drug levels (eg, peak and trough with conventional dosing) should be determined, particularly in critically-ill patients with serious infections or in disease states known to significantly alter aminoglycoside pharmacokinetics (eg, cystic fibrosis, burns, or major surgery).

I.M., I.V.:

Severe life-threatening infections:

Conventional dosing: 2-2.5 mg/kg/dose every 8-12 hours; to ensure adequate peak concentrations early in therapy, higher initial dosages may be considered in selected patients (eg, edema, septic shock, post-surgery, and/or trauma).

Once-daily dosing: Some clinicians suggest a daily dose of 4-7 mg/kg for all patients with normal renal function; this dose is at least as efficacious with similar, if not less, toxicity than conventional dosing.

Urinary tract infection: 1.5 mg/kg/dose

Synergy (for gram-positive infections): 1 mg/kg/dose

Ocular infections: Ophthalmic:

Ointment: Apply 2-3 times/day; for severe infections, apply every 3-4 hours

Solution: Instill 1-2 drops every 4 hours; for severe infections, instill 2 drops every 30-60 minutes initially, then reduce to less frequent intervals

Pulmonary infections: Inhalation:

Standard aerosolized tobramycin: 60-80 mg 3 times/day

High-dose regimen: 300 mg every 12 hours (do not administer doses <6 hours apart); administer in repeated cycles of 28 days on drug followed by 28 days off drug

Elderly: Dosage should be based on an estimate of ideal body weight.

I.M., I.V.: 1.5-5 mg/kg/day in 1-2 divided doses

I.V.: Once daily or extended interval: 5-7 mg/kg/dose given every 24, 36, or 48 hours based on Cl_{cr} (see Renal Impairment and Geriatric Considerations).

Pediatrics: Individualization is **critical** because of the low therapeutic index

Use of ideal body weight (IBW) for determining the mg/kg/dose appears to be more accurate than dosing on the basis of total body weight (TBW). In morbid obesity, dosage requirement may best be estimated using a dosing weight of IBW + 0.4 (TBW - IBW).

Susceptible systemic infections: I.M., I.V.:

Infants and Children <5 years: 2.5 mg/kg/dose every 8 hours

Children >5 years: 2-2.5 mg/kg/dose every 8 hours

Ocular infection: Ophthalmic: Children ≥2 months: See adult dosing.

Cystic fibrosis:

I.M., I.V.: 2.5-3.3 mg/kg every 6-8 hours

Inhalation:

Standard aerosolized tobramycin: 40-80 mg 2-3 times/day

High-dose regimen (TOBI®): Children ≥6 years: See adult dosing.

Note: Some patients may require larger or more frequent doses if serum levels document the need (eg, cystic fibrosis or febrile granulocytopenic patients). Also see drug level monitoring information in adult dosing,

Renal Impairment: I.M., I.V.:

Conventional dosing:

Cl_{cr} ≥60 mL/minute: Administer every 8 hours.

Cl_{cr} 40-60 mL/minute: Administer every 12 hours.

Cl_{cr} 20-40 mL/minute: Administer every 24 hours.

Cl_{cr} 10-20 mL/minute: Administer every 48 hours.

Cl_{cr} <10 mL/minute: Administer every 72 hours.

High-dose therapy: Interval may be extended (eg, every 48 hours) in patients with moderate renal impairment (Cl_{cr} 30-59 mL/minute) and/or adjusted based on serum level determinations.

Dialyzable; 30% removal of aminoglycosides occurs during 4 hours of HD - administer dose after dialysis and follow levels.

Continuous arteriovenous or venovenous hemofiltration: Dose as for Cl_{cr} of 10-40 mL/minute and follow levels.

Administration via CAPD fluid:

Gram-negative infection: 4-8 mg/L (4-8 mcg/mL) of CAPD fluid

Gram-positive infection (ie, synergy): 3-4 mg/L (3-4 mcg/mL) of CAPD fluid

Administration IVPB/I.M.: Dose as for Cl_{cr} <10 mL/minute and follow levels.

Hepatic Impairment: Monitor plasma concentrations.

Available Dosage Forms

Infusion [premixed in NS]: 60 mg (50 mL); 80 mg (100 mL)

Injection, powder for reconstitution: 1.2 g

Injection, solution: 10 mg/mL (2 mL, 8 mL); 40 mg/mL (2 mL, 30 mL, 50 mL) [may contain sodium metabisulfite]

Ointment, ophthalmic (Tobrex®): 0.3% (3.5 g)

Solution for nebulization [preservative free] (TOBI®): 60 mg/mL (5 mL)

Solution, ophthalmic (AKTob®, Tobrex®): 0.3% (5 mL) [contains benzalkonium chloride]

Nursing Guidelines

Assessment: Assess effectiveness and interactions of other medications patient may be taking. Assess patient's hearing level before, during, and following therapy. Monitor therapeutic effectiveness, laboratory values, and

(Continued)

Tobramycin *(Continued)*

adverse reactions (eg, ototoxicity and nephrotoxicity) at beginning of therapy and periodically throughout therapy. Assess knowledge/teach patient appropriate use, interventions to reduce side effects, and adverse symptoms to report.

Monitoring Laboratory Tests: Urinalysis, BUN, serum creatinine, plasma tobramycin levels (as appropriate to dosing method). Peak levels are drawn 30 minutes after the end of a 30-minute infusion or 1 hour after initiation of infusion or I.M. injection. The trough is drawn just before the next dose. Levels are typically obtained after the third dose in conventional dosing. Perform culture and sensitivity studies prior to initiating therapy to determine the causative organism and its susceptibility to tobramycin. Some penicillin derivatives may accelerate the degradation of aminoglycosides.

Dietary Considerations: May require supplementation of calcium, magnesium, potassium.

Patient Education: Systemic: Maintain adequate hydration (2-3 L/day of fluids) unless instructed to restrict fluid intake. Report decreased urine output, swelling of extremities, respiratory difficulty, vaginal itching or discharge, rash, diarrhea, oral thrush, unhealed wounds, dizziness, change in hearing acuity or ringing in ears, or worsening of condition. **Pregnancy/breast-feeding precautions:** Inform prescriber if you are pregnant. Breast-feeding is not recommended.

Ophthalmic: Use as frequently as recommended; do not overuse. Do not let tip of applicator touch eye; do not contaminate tip of applicator (may cause eye infection, eye damage, or vision loss). Sit down, tilt head back, instill solution or drops inside lower eyelid, and roll eyeball in all directions. Close eye and apply gentle pressure to inner corner of eye for 30 seconds. May experience temporary stinging or blurred vision. Do not use any other eye preparation for 10 minutes. Inform prescriber if condition worsens or does not improve in 3-4 days.

Geriatric Considerations: Aminoglycosides are important therapeutic interventions for susceptible organisms and as empiric therapy in seriously ill patients. Their use is not without risk of toxicity; however, these risks can be minimized if initial dosing is adjusted for estimated renal function and appropriate monitoring is performed. High-dose, once-daily aminoglycosides have been advocated as an alternative to traditional dosing regimens. To date, there is little information on the safety and efficacy of these regimens in persons with a creatinine clearance <60 mL/minute/70 kg. A dosing nomogram based upon creatinine clearance has been proposed. Additional studies comparing high-dose, once-daily aminoglycosides to traditional dosing regimens in the elderly are needed before once-daily aminoglycoside dosing can be routinely adopted to this patient population.

Pregnancy Risk Factor: D (injection, inhalation); B (ophthalmic)

Pregnancy Issues: Aminoglycosides, including tobramycin, cross the placenta. The manufacturers of Nebcin® and TOBI® have a labeled pregnancy category of D based on reports of bilateral congenital deafness in children whose mothers used streptomycin during pregnancy. The risk of teratogenic effects and deafness following *in utero* exposure to tobramycin is considered to be small and some resources consider the pregnancy risk factor to be C. The manufacturer of Tobrex® states that animal studies have not shown harm to the fetus; however, no adequate and well-controlled studies have been conducted in pregnant women.

Lactation: Enters breast milk/not recommended

Breast-Feeding Considerations: Tobramycin is excreted into breast milk. The actual amount following inhalation or topical therapy is not known. The AAP considers a related antibiotic, gentamicin, usually compatible with breast-feeding.

Administration

I.V.: Infuse over 30-60 minutes.

Some penicillins (eg, carbenicillin, ticarcillin and piperacillin) have been shown to inactivate aminglycosides *in vitro*. This has been observed to a greater extent with tobramycin and gentamicin, while amikacin has shown greater stability against inactivation. Concurrent use of these agents may pose a risk of reduced antibacterial efficacy *in vivo*, particularly in the setting of profound renal impairment. However, definitive clinical evidence is lacking. If combination penicillin/aminoglycoside therapy is desired in a patient with renal dysfunction, separation of doses (if feasible), and routine monitoring of aminoglycoside levels, CBC, and clinical response should be considered.

Reconstitution: Dilute in 50-100 mL NS, D_5W for I.V. infusion

Compatibility: Stable in dextran 40 10% in dextrose, D_5NS, D_5W, $D_{10}W$, mannitol 20%, LR, NS

Y-site administration: Incompatible with allopurinol, amphotericin B cholesteryl sulfate complex, cefoperazone, heparin, hetastarch, indomethacin, propofol, sargramostim

Compatibility in syringe: Incompatible with cefamandole, clindamycin, heparin

Compatibility when admixed: Incompatible with cefamandole, cefepime, cefotaxime, cefotetan, floxacillin, heparin, penicillins

Storage:

Injection: Stable at room temperature both as the clear, colorless solution and as the dry powder. Reconstituted solutions remain stable for 24 hours at room temperature and 96 hours when refrigerated.

Ophthalmic solution: Store at 8°C to 27°C (46°F to 80°F).

Solution, for inhalation (TOBI®): Store under refrigeration at 2°C to 8°C (36°F to 46°F); may be stored in foil pouch at room temperature of 25°C (77°F) for up to 28 days. Avoid intense light. Solution may darken over time; however, do not use if cloudy or contains particles.

Related Information

Prevention of Wound Infection and Sepsis in Surgical Patients *on page 1830*

Tobramycin and Dexamethasone

(toe bra MYE sin & deks a METH a sone)

U.S. Brand Names TobraDex®

Synonyms Dexamethasone and Tobramycin

Pharmacologic Category Antibiotic/Corticosteroid, Ophthalmic

Medication Safety Issues

Sound-alike/look-alike issues:

TobraDex® may be confused with Tobrex®

Use Treatment of external ocular infection caused by susceptible gram-negative bacteria and steroid responsive inflammatory conditions of the palpebral and bulbar conjunctiva, lid, cornea, and anterior segment of the globe

Mechanism of Action Refer to individual monographs for Dexamethasone and Tobramycin

Pharmacodynamics/Kinetics

Absorption: Into aqueous humor

Time to peak, serum: 1-2 hours in the cornea and aqueous humor

Contraindications Hypersensitivity to tobramycin, dexamethasone, or any component of the formulation; viral, fungal, or tuberculosis diseases of the eye

Warnings/Precautions Sensitivity to tobramycin may develop; discontinue if sensitivity reaction occurs. Prolonged use of corticosteroids may result in glaucoma; damage to the optic nerve, defects in visual acuity and fields of vision, and posterior subcapsular cataract formation may occur. Prolonged use of corticosteroids may increase the incidence of secondary ocular infection or mask acute infection (including fungal infections); may prolong or exacerbate ocular viral infections; use following cataract surgery may delay healing or increase the incidence of bleb formation. A maximum of 8 g of ointment or 20 mL of suspension should be prescribed initially; patients should be evaluated prior to additional refills. Suspension contains benzalkonium chloride which may be adsorbed by contact lenses; contact lenses should not be worn during treatment of ophthalmic infections. Safety and efficacy have not been established in patients <2 years of age.

Drug Interactions Dexamethasone: **Substrate** of CYP3A4 (minor); **Induces** CYP2A6 (weak), 2B6 (weak), 2C8/9 (weak), 3A4 (weak)

Also see individual agents.

Adverse Reactions Unless otherwise noted, frequency not defined.

Dermatologic: Allergic contact dermatitis, delayed wound healing

Ocular: Cataract formation, conjunctival erythema (<4%), glaucoma, intraocular pressure increased, keratitis, lacrimation, lid itching (<4%), lid swelling (<4%), optic nerve damage, secondary infection

Dosing

Adults & Elderly: Ocular infection/inflammation: Ophthalmic: Instill 1-2 drops of solution every 4 hours; apply ointment 2-3 times/day; for severe infections apply ointment every 3-4 hours, or solution 2 drops every 30-60 minutes initially, then reduce to less frequent intervals

(Continued)

Tobramycin and Dexamethasone *(Continued)*

Pediatrics: Ocular infection/inflammation: Children: Refer to adult dosing.

Available Dosage Forms

Ointment, ophthalmic: Tobramycin 0.3% and dexamethasone 0.1% (3.5 g)

Suspension, ophthalmic: Tobramycin 0.3% and dexamethasone 0.1% (2.5 mL, 5 mL, 10 mL) [contains benzalkonium chloride]

Nursing Guidelines

Assessment: See individual agents.

Patient Education: Shake suspension well before using. Do not touch dropper to eye. Apply light finger pressure on lacrimal sac for one minute following instillation. Notify physician if condition fails to improve or worsens.

Pregnancy Risk Factor: C

Lactation: Excretion in breast milk unknown/use caution

Breast-Feeding Considerations: It is unknown if topical use results in sufficient absorption to produce detectable quantities in breast milk.

♦ **Tobramycin Sulfate** *see* Tobramycin *on page 1639*

♦ **Tobrex®** *see* Tobramycin *on page 1639*

TOLAZamide (tole AZ a mide)

U.S. Brand Names Tolinase® [DSC]

Pharmacologic Category Antidiabetic Agent, Sulfonylurea

Medication Safety Issues

Sound-alike/look-alike issues:

TOLAZamide may be confused with tolazoline, TOLBUTamide

Tolinase® may be confused with Orinase®

Use Adjunct to diet for the management of mild to moderately severe, stable, type 2 diabetes mellitus (noninsulin dependent, NIDDM)

Mechanism of Action Stimulates insulin release from the pancreatic beta cells; reduces glucose output from the liver; insulin sensitivity is increased at peripheral target sites

Pharmacodynamics/Kinetics

Onset of action: 4-6 hours

Duration: 10-24 hours

Protein binding: >98%

Metabolism: Extensively hepatic to one active and three inactive metabolites

Half-life elimination: 7 hours

Excretion: Urine

Contraindications Hypersensitivity to tolazamide, sulfonylureas, or any component of the formulation; type 1 diabetes mellitus (insulin dependent, IDDM) therapy; diabetes complicated by ketoacidosis; pregnancy

Warnings/Precautions False-positive response has been reported in patients with liver disease, idiopathic hypoglycemia of infancy, severe malnutrition, acute pancreatitis, renal dysfunction. Transferring a patient from one sulfonylurea to another does not require a priming dose; doses >1000 mg/day normally do not improve diabetic control. Has not been studied in older patients; however, except for drug interactions, it appears to have a safe profile and decline in renal function does not affect its pharmacokinetics. How "tightly" an elderly patient's blood glucose should be controlled is controversial; however, a fasting blood sugar <150 mg/dL is now an acceptable end point. Such a decision should be based on the patient's functional and cognitive status, how well they recognize hypoglycemic or hyperglycemic symptoms, and how to respond to them and their other disease states.

Chemical similarities are present among sulfonamides, sulfonylureas, carbonic anhydrase inhibitors, thiazides, and loop diuretics (except ethacrynic acid). Use in patients with sulfonylurea allergy is specifically contraindicated in product labeling, however, a risk of cross-reaction exists in patients with allergy to any of these compounds; avoid use when previous reaction has been severe.

Product labeling states oral hypoglycemic drugs may be associated with an increased cardiovascular mortality as compared to treatment with diet alone or diet plus insulin. Data to support this association are limited, and several studies, including a large prospective trial (UKPDS) have not supported an association.

Drug Interactions Increased toxicity: Monitor patient closely; large number of drugs interact with sulfonylureas including salicylates, anticoagulants, H_2 antagonists, TCAs, MAO inhibitors, beta-blockers, thiazides

Nutritional/Herbal/Ethanol Interactions Ethanol: Avoid ethanol (possible disulfiram-like reaction).

Adverse Reactions Frequency not defined.

Central nervous system: Headache, dizziness

Dermatologic: Rash, urticaria, photosensitivity

Endocrine & metabolic: Hypoglycemia, SIADH

Gastrointestinal: Anorexia, nausea, vomiting, diarrhea, constipation, heartburn, epigastric fullness

Hematologic: Aplastic anemia, hemolytic anemia, bone marrow suppression, thrombocytopenia, agranulocytosis

Hepatic: Cholestatic jaundice

Renal: Diuretic effect

Overdosage/Toxicology

Symptoms of overdose include low blood sugar, tingling of lips and tongue, nausea, yawning, confusion, agitation, tachycardia, sweating, convulsions, stupor, and coma

Intoxications with sulfonylureas can cause hypoglycemia and are best managed with glucose administration (oral for milder hypoglycemia or by injection in more severe forms)

Dosing

Adults & Elderly:

Type 2 diabetes: Oral (doses >1000 mg/day normally do not improve diabetic control):

Initial: 100-250 mg/day with breakfast or the first main meal of the day

Fasting blood sugar <200 mg/dL: 100 mg/day

Fasting blood sugar >200 mg/dL: 250 mg/day

Patient is malnourished, underweight, elderly, or not eating properly: 100 mg/day

Adjustment/titration: Increase in increments of 100-250 mg/day at weekly intervals to response. If >500 mg/day is required, give in divided doses twice daily; maximum daily dose: 1 g (doses >1 g/day are not likely to improve control)

Conversion from insulin to tolazamide

10 units day = 100 mg/day

20-40 units/day = 250 mg/day

>40 units/day = 250 mg/day and 50% of insulin dose

Doses >500 mg/day should be given in 2 divided doses

Renal Impairment: Conservative initial and maintenance doses are recommended because tolazamide is metabolized to active metabolites, which are eliminated in the urine.

Hepatic Impairment: Conservative initial and maintenance doses and careful monitoring of blood glucose are recommended.

Available Dosage Forms [DSC] = Discontinued product

Tablet: 100 mg, 250 mg, 500 mg

Tolinase® [DSC]: 100 mg, 250 mg

Nursing Guidelines

Patient Education: This medication is used to control diabetes; it is not a cure. Other components of the treatment plan are important: follow prescribed diet, medication, and exercise regimen. Take exactly as directed; at the same time each day. Do not change dose or discontinue without consulting prescriber. Avoid alcohol while taking this medication; could cause severe reaction. Inform prescriber of all other prescription or OTC medications you are taking; do not introduce new medication without consulting prescriber. Do not take other medication within 2 hours of this medication unless advised by prescriber. If you experience hypoglycemic reaction, contact prescriber immediately; maintain regular dietary intake and exercise routine and always carry quick source of sugar with you. You may be more sensitive to sunlight (use sunscreen, wear protective clothing and eyewear, and avoid direct sunlight). You may experience side effects during first weeks of therapy (headache, nausea, diarrhea, constipation, anorexia); consult prescriber if these persist. Report severe or persistent side effects, extended vomiting or flu-like symptoms, skin rash, easy bruising or bleeding, or change in color of urine or stool. **Pregnancy/breast-feeding precautions:** Do not get pregnant; use appropriate contraceptive measures to prevent possible harm to the fetus. Consult prescriber if breast-feeding.

(Continued)

TOLAZamide *(Continued)*

Pregnancy Risk Factor: D

Pregnancy Issues: Abnormal blood glucose levels are associated with a higher incidence of congenital abnormalities. Insulin is the drug of choice for the control of diabetes mellitus during pregnancy.

Lactation: Excretion in breast milk unknown

Related Information

Perioperative Management of the Diabetic Patient *on page 1794*

♦ Tolinase® [DSC] *see* TOLAZamide *on page 1644*

Tolterodine (tole TER oh deen)

U.S. Brand Names Detrol®; Detrol® LA

Synonyms Tolterodine Tartrate

Pharmacologic Category Anticholinergic Agent

Medication Safety Issues

Sound-alike/look-alike issues:

Detrol® may be confused with Ditropan®

Use Treatment of patients with an overactive bladder with symptoms of urinary frequency, urgency, or urge incontinence

Mechanism of Action Tolterodine is a competitive antagonist of muscarinic receptors. In animal models, tolterodine demonstrates selectivity for urinary bladder receptors over salivary receptors. Urinary bladder contraction is mediated by muscarinic receptors. Tolterodine increases residual urine volume and decreases detrusor muscle pressure.

Pharmacodynamics/Kinetics

Absorption: Immediate release tablet: Rapid; ≥77%

Distribution: I.V.: V_d: 113 ± 27 L

Protein binding: >96% (primarily to alpha$_1$-acid glycoprotein)

Metabolism: Extensively hepatic, primarily via CYP2D6 (some metabolites share activity) and 3A4 usually (minor pathway). In patients with a genetic deficiency of CYP2D6, metabolism via 3A4 predominates. Forms three active metabolites.

Bioavailability: Immediate release tablet: Increased 53% with food

Half-life elimination:

Immediate release tablet: Extensive metabolizers: ~2 hours; Poor metabolizers: ~10 hours

Extended release capsule: Extensive metabolizers: ~7 hours; Poor metabolizers: ~18 hours

Time to peak: Immediate release tablet: 1-2 hours; Extended release tablet: 2-6 hours

Excretion: Urine (77%); feces (17%); excreted primarily as metabolites (<1% unchanged drug) of which the active 5-hydroxymethyl metabolite accounts for 5% to 14% (<1% in poor metabolizers)

Contraindications Hypersensitivity to tolterodine or any component of the formulation; urinary retention; gastric retention; uncontrolled narrow-angle glaucoma; myasthenia gravis

Warnings/Precautions Use with caution in patients with bladder flow obstruction, may increase the risk of urinary retention. Use with caution in patients with gastrointestinal obstructive disorders (ie, pyloric stenosis), may increase the risk of gastric retention. Use with caution in patients with controlled (treated) narrow-angle glaucoma; metabolized in the liver and excreted in the urine and feces, dosage adjustment is required for patients with renal or hepatic impairment. Patients on CYP3A4 inhibitors require lower dose. Safety and efficacy in pediatric patients have not been established.

Drug Interactions **Substrate** of CYP2C8/9 (minor), 2C19 (minor), 2D6 (major), 3A4 (major)

Acetylcholinesterase inhibitors (central): May reduce the therapeutic efficacy of tolterodine.

Anticholinergic agents: Concomitant use with tolterodine may increase the risk of anticholinergic side effects.

Antifungal agents (eg, ketoconazole, fluconazole): May increase the levels/effects of tolterodine; monitor.

CYP2D6 inhibitors: May increase the levels/effects of tolterodine. Example inhibitors include chlorpromazine, delavirdine, fluoxetine, miconazole, paroxetine, pergolide, quinidine, quinine, ritonavir, and ropinirole.

CYP3A4 inducers: CYP3A4 inducers may decrease the levels/effects of tolterodine. Example inducers include aminoglutethimide, carbamazepine, nafcillin, nevirapine, phenobarbital, phenytoin, and rifamycins.

CYP3A4 inhibitors: May increase the levels/effects of tolterodine. Example inhibitors include azole antifungals, clarithromycin, diclofenac, doxycycline, erythromycin, imatinib, isoniazid, nefazodone, nicardipine, propofol, protease inhibitors, quinidine, telithromycin, and verapamil.

Pramlintide: Concomitant use with tolterodine may increase the risk of anticholinergic gastrointestinal adverse effects (eg, reduced gut motility).

Nutritional/Herbal/Ethanol Interactions

Food: Increases bioavailability (~53% increase) of tolterodine tablets, but does not affect the pharmacokinetics of tolterodine extended release capsules; adjustment of dose is not needed. As a CYP3A4 inhibitor, grapefruit juice may increase the serum level and/or toxicity of tolterodine, but unlikely secondary to high oral bioavailability.

Herb/Nutraceutical: St John's wort (*Hypericum*) appears to induce CYP3A enzymes.

Adverse Reactions As reported with immediate release tablet, unless otherwise specified

>10%: Gastrointestinal: Dry mouth (35%; extended release capsules 23%)

1% to 10%:

- Cardiovascular: Chest pain (2%)
- Central nervous system: Headache (7%; extended release capsules 6%), somnolence (3%; extended release capsules 3%), fatigue (4%; extended release capsules 2%), dizziness (5%; extended release capsules 2%), anxiety (extended release capsules 1%)
- Dermatologic: Dry skin (1%)
- Gastrointestinal: Abdominal pain (5%; extended release capsules 4%), constipation (7%; extended release capsules 6%), dyspepsia (4%; extended release capsules 3%), diarrhea (4%), weight gain (1%)
- Genitourinary: Dysuria (2%; extended release capsules 1%)
- Neuromuscular & skeletal: Arthralgia (2%)
- Ocular: Abnormal vision (2%; extended release capsules 1%), dry eyes (3%; extended release capsules 3%)
- Respiratory: Bronchitis (2%), sinusitis (extended release capsules 2%)
- Miscellaneous: Flu-like syndrome (3%), infection (1%)

<1% (Limited to important or life-threatening): Anaphylactoid reactions, angioedema, hallucinations, palpitation, peripheral edema, tachycardia

Overdosage/Toxicology Overdosage with tolterodine can potentially result in severe central anticholinergic effects and should be treated accordingly. ECG monitoring is recommended in the event of overdosage.

Dosing

Adults & Elderly: Treatment of overactive bladder: Oral:

Immediate release tablet: 2 mg twice daily; the dose may be lowered to 1 mg twice daily based on individual response and tolerability

Dosing adjustment in patients concurrently taking CYP3A4 inhibitors: 1 mg twice daily

Extended release capsule: 4 mg once a day; dose may be lowered to 2 mg daily based on individual response and tolerability

Dosing adjustment in patients concurrently taking CYP3A4 inhibitors: 2 mg daily

Renal Impairment: Use with caution (studies conducted in patients with Cl_{cr} 10-30 mL/minute):

Immediate release tablet: 1 mg twice daily

Extended release capsule: 2 mg daily

Hepatic Impairment:

Immediate release tablet: 1 mg twice daily

Extended release capsule: 2 mg daily

Available Dosage Forms

Capsule, extended release, as tartrate (Detrol® LA): 2 mg, 4 mg

Tablet, as tartrate (Detrol®): 1 mg, 2 mg

Nursing Guidelines

Assessment: Assess potential for interactions with other prescriptions, OTC medications, or herbal products patient may be taking (eg, ergot-containing drugs). Assess therapeutic effectiveness and adverse reactions. Teach patient appropriate use (according to formulation and purpose), interventions to reduce side effects, and adverse symptoms to report.

(Continued)

Tolterodine *(Continued)*

Patient Education: Take as directed, preferably with food. Do not break, crush, or chew extended release medication. May cause headache (consult prescriber for a mild analgesic); dizziness, nervousness, or sleepiness (use caution when driving, climbing stairs, or engaging in tasks requiring alertness until response to drug is known); or abdominal discomfort, diarrhea, constipation, nausea, or vomiting (small frequent meals, increased exercise, adequate hydration may help). Report back pain, muscle spasms, alteration in gait, or numbness of extremities; unresolved or persistent constipation, diarrhea, or vomiting; or symptoms of upper respiratory infection or flu. Report immediately any chest pain or palpitations, difficulty urinating, or pain on urination. **Pregnancy/breast-feeding precautions:** Inform prescriber if you are or intend to become pregnant. Breast-feeding is not recommended.

Pregnancy Risk Factor: C

Pregnancy Issues: There are no adequate and well-controlled studies in pregnant women. Use during pregnancy only if the potential benefit to the mother outweighs the possible risk to the fetus.

Lactation: Excretion in breast milk unknown/not recommended

Administration

Storage: Store at 15°C to 30°C (59°F to 86°F). Protect from light.

- ♦ Tolterodine Tartrate *see* Tolterodine *on page 1646*
- ♦ Topicaine® [OTC] *see* Lidocaine *on page 1033*
- ♦ Toposar® *see* Etoposide *on page 695*
- ♦ Toprol-XL® *see* Metoprolol *on page 1150*
- ♦ Toradol® *see* Ketorolac *on page 990*

Torsemide (TORE se mide)

U.S. Brand Names Demadex®

Pharmacologic Category Diuretic, Loop

Medication Safety Issues

Sound-alike/look-alike issues:

Torsemide may be confused with furosemide

Demadex® may be confused with Denorex®

Use Management of edema associated with congestive heart failure and hepatic or renal disease; used alone or in combination with antihypertensives in treatment of hypertension; I.V. form is indicated when rapid onset is desired

Mechanism of Action Inhibits reabsorption of sodium and chloride in the ascending loop of Henle and distal renal tubule, interfering with the chloride-binding cotransport system, thus causing increased excretion of water, sodium, chloride, magnesium, and calcium; does not alter GFR, renal plasma flow, or acid-base balance

Pharmacodynamics/Kinetics

Onset of action: Diuresis: 30-60 minutes

Peak effect: 1-4 hours

Duration: ~6 hours

Absorption: Oral: Rapid

Protein binding, plasma: ~97% to 99%

Metabolism: Hepatic (80%) via CYP

Bioavailability: 80% to 90%

Half-life elimination: 2-4; Cirrhosis: 7-8 hours

Excretion: Urine (20% as unchanged drug)

Contraindications Hypersensitivity to torsemide, any component of the formulation, or any sulfonylureas; anuria

Warnings/Precautions Adjust dose to avoid dehydration. In cirrhosis, avoid electrolyte and acid/base imbalances that might lead to hepatic encephalopathy. Ototoxicity is associated with rapid I.V. administration of other loop diuretics and has been seen with oral torsemide. Do not administer intravenously in less than 2 minutes; single doses should not exceed 200 mg. Hypersensitivity reactions can rarely occur. Monitor fluid status and renal function in an attempt to prevent oliguria, azotemia, and reversible increases in BUN and creatinine. Close medical supervision of aggressive diuresis is required. Monitor closely for electrolyte imbalances particularly hypokalemia and correct when necessary. Coadministration with antihypertensives may increase the risk of hypotension.

Chemical similarities are present among sulfonamides, sulfonylureas, carbonic anhydrase inhibitors, thiazides, and loop diuretics (except ethacrynic acid). Use in patients with sulfonylurea allergy is specifically contraindicated in product labeling, however, a risk of cross-reaction exists in patients with allergy to any of these compounds; avoid use when previous reaction has been severe.

Drug Interactions Substrate of CYP2C8/9 (major); **Inhibits** CYP2C19 (weak)

ACE inhibitors: Hypotensive effects and/or renal effects are potentiated by hypovolemia.

Aminoglycosides: Ototoxicity may be increased.

Anticoagulant activity is enhanced.

Antidiabetic agents: Glucose tolerance may be decreased.

Antihypertensive agents: Effects may be enhanced.

Beta-blockers: Plasma concentrations of beta-blockers may be increased with torsemide.

Chloral hydrate: Transient diaphoresis, hot flashes, hypertension may occur.

Cisplatin: Ototoxicity may be increased.

CYP2C8/9 inducers: May decrease the levels/effects of torsemide. Example inducers include carbamazepine, phenobarbital, phenytoin, rifampin, rifapentine, and secobarbital.

Digitalis: Arrhythmias may occur with diuretic-induced electrolyte disturbances.

Lithium: Plasma concentrations of lithium may be increased; monitor lithium levels.

NSAIDs: Torsemide efficacy may be decreased.

Probenecid: Torsemide action may be reduced.

Salicylates: Diuretic action may be impaired in patients with cirrhosis and ascites.

Thiazides: Synergistic effects may result.

Nutritional/Herbal/Ethanol Interactions Herb/Nutraceutical: Avoid dong quai if using for hypertension (has estrogenic activity). Avoid ephedra, yohimbe, ginseng (may worsen hypertension). Avoid garlic (may have increased antihypertensive effect).

Adverse Reactions

1% to 10%:

Cardiovascular: Edema (1.1%), ECG abnormality (2%), chest pain (1.2%)

Central nervous system: Headache (7.3%), dizziness (3.2%), insomnia (1.2%), nervousness (1%)

Endocrine & metabolic: Hyperglycemia, hyperuricemia, hypokalemia

Gastrointestinal: Diarrhea (2%), constipation (1.8%), nausea (1.8%), dyspepsia (1.6%), sore throat (1.6%)

Genitourinary: Excessive urination (6.7%)

Neuromuscular & skeletal: Weakness (2%), arthralgia (1.8%), myalgia (1.6%)

Respiratory: Rhinitis (2.8%), cough increase (2%)

<1% (Limited to important or life-threatening): Angioedema, atrial fibrillation, GI hemorrhage, hypernatremia hypotension, hypovolemia, rash, rectal bleeding, shunt thrombosis, syncope, ventricular tachycardia

Overdosage/Toxicology Symptoms include electrolyte depletion, volume depletion, hypotension, dehydration, and circulatory collapse. Electrolyte depletion may manifest as weakness, dizziness, mental confusion, anorexia, lethargy, vomiting, and cramps. Treatment is supportive.

Dosing

Adults:

Note: The oral form may be given regardless of meal times. Patients may be switched from the I.V. form to the oral and vice-versa with no change in dose.

Congestive heart failure: Oral, I.V.: 10-20 mg once daily; may increase gradually for chronic treatment by doubling dose until the diuretic response is apparent (for acute treatment. I.V. dose may be repeated every 2 hours with double the dose as needed). **Note:** ACC/AHA 2005 guidelines for chronic heart failure recommend a maximum daily oral dose of 200 mg; maximum single I.V. dose 100-200 mg

Continuous I.V. infusion: 20 mg I.V. load then 5-20 mg/hour

Chronic renal failure: Oral, I.V.: 20 mg once daily; increase as above.

Hepatic cirrhosis: Oral, I.V.: 5-10 mg once daily with an aldosterone antagonist or a potassium-sparing diuretic; increase as above.

Hypertension: Oral, I.V.: 2.5-5 mg once daily; increase to 10 mg after 4-6 weeks if an adequate hypotensive response is not apparent. If still not effective, an additional antihypertensive agent may be added.

Elderly: Usual starting dose should be 5 mg; refer to adult dosing.

Available Dosage Forms

Injection, solution: 10 mg/mL (2 mL, 5 mL)

Tablet: 5 mg, 10 mg, 20 mg, 100 mg

(Continued)

Torsemide *(Continued)*

Nursing Guidelines

Assessment: Assess for allergy to sulfonylurea before beginning therapy. See Contraindications, Warnings/Precautions, and Dosing for use cautions. Assess potential for interactions with other prescriptions, OTC medications, or herbal products patient may be taking (especially anything that may impact fluid balance or increase potential for ototoxicity or hypotension - see Drug Interactions). See Administration for I.V. specifics. Assess results of laboratory tests, therapeutic effectiveness, and adverse response on a regular basis during therapy (eg, dehydration, electrolyte imbalance, postural hypotension - see Adverse Reactions and Overdose/Toxicology). Caution patients with diabetes about closely monitoring glucose levels (glucose tolerance may be decreased). Teach patient appropriate use, possible side effects/appropriate interventions, and adverse symptoms to report (see Patient Education). Note breast-feeding caution.

Monitoring Laboratory Tests: Renal function, electrolytes

Patient Education: Inform prescriber of all prescriptions, OTC medications, or herbal products you are taking, and any allergies you have. Do not take any new medication during therapy unless approved by prescriber. Take as directed, with food or milk (to reduce GI distress), early in the day, or if twice daily, take last dose in late afternoon in order to avoid sleep disturbance and achieve maximum therapeutic effect. Include orange juice or bananas (or other potassium-rich foods) in daily diet. Do not take potassium supplements without consulting prescriber. Weigh yourself each day, at the same time, in the same clothes when beginning therapy, and weekly on long-term therapy; report unusual or unanticipated weight gain or loss. May cause postural hypotension (change position slowly when rising from sitting or lying); transient drowsiness, blurred vision, or dizziness (avoid driving or engaging in tasks that require alertness until response to drug is known); reduced tolerance to heat (avoid strenuous activity in hot weather or excessively hot showers); or constipation (increased exercise and increased dietary fiber, fruit, or fluids may help). Report unusual weight gain or loss (>5 lb/week), swelling of ankles and hands; persistent fatigue; unresolved constipation or diarrhea; weakness, fatigue, or dizziness; vomiting; cramps; change in hearing; or chest pain or palpitations.

Breast-feeding precaution: Consult prescriber if breast-feeding.

Pregnancy Risk Factor: B

Pregnancy Issues: A decrease in fetal weight, an increase in fetal resorption, and delayed fetal ossification has occurred in animal studies.

Lactation: Excretion in breast milk unknown/use caution

Perioperative/Anesthesia/Other Concerns: If given the morning of surgery, it may render the patient volume depleted and blood pressure may be labile during general anesthesia. Torsemide may induce potent diuretic effects and, as with other potent diuretics, electrolytes and volume status needs to be closely monitored.

Equivalent dosing: Torsemide 10-20 mg is approximately equivalent to furosemide 40 mg or bumetanide 1 mg.

Administration

I.V.: I.V. injections should be given over ≥2 minutes.

Compatibility: Stable in D_5W, NS, ½NS

Total Parenteral Nutrition (TOE tal par EN ter al noo TRISH un)

Synonyms Hyperal; Hyperalimentation; Parenteral Nutrition; PN; TPN

Pharmacologic Category Caloric Agent; Intravenous Nutritional Therapy

Use Infusion of nutrient solutions into the bloodstream to support a patient's nutritional need during a time when they are unable to absorb nutrients via the gastrointestinal tract or cannot take adequate nutrition orally or enterally

Contraindications Varies by composition:

Lipid-containing formulations are contraindicated in patients with hypersensitivity to fat emulsion or any component of the formulation; severe egg or legume (soybean) allergies; pathologic hyperlipidemia, lipoid nephrosis, pancreatitis with hyperlipemia

Dextrose is contraindicated in patients with hypersensitivity to corn or corn products; hypertonic solutions in patients with intracranial or intraspinal hemorrhage; glucose-galactose malabsorption syndrome; anuria

Amino acids are contraindicated in patients with hypersensitivity to one or more amino acids; severe liver disease or hepatic coma; anuria

Warnings/Precautions Monitor fluid and electrolyte status carefully. Use with caution in patients at risk for refeeding syndrome. Refeeding syndrome is a medical emergency; it can consist of electrolyte disturbances (eg, potassium, phosphorus), respiratory distress, and cardiac arrhythmias, resulting in cardiopulmonary arrest. It is usually seen in patients with long-standing or severe malnutrition; initiate cautiously; approach goals slowly. Do not overfeed patients; caloric replacement should match as closely as possible to intake. Use caution in patients with diabetes or insulin resistance. Use caution in patients who may be sensitive to volume overload (eg, CHF, renal failure, hepatic failure). Use caution and limit protein in patients with hepatic disease. If TPN is discontinued abruptly, infuse 10% dextrose at same rate and monitor blood glucose for hypoglycemia.

Adverse Reactions Frequency not defined (unless noted).

Endocrine & metabolic: Fluid overload, hyperglycemia, hyper-/hypokalemia, hyper-/hypophosphatemia, metabolic bone disease, nonanion gap metabolic acidosis, refeeding syndrome

Hepatic: Cholestasis, cirrhosis (<1%), gallstones, liver function tests increased, steatosis, triglycerides increased

Renal: Azotemia, BUN increased

Miscellaneous: Bacteremia, catheter-induced infection, exit-site infections

Dosing

Adults: Nutritional supplementation: I.V.:

- Total calories:
  - Normal/mild stress level: 20-25 kcal/kg/day
  - Moderate stress level: 25-30 kcal/kg/day
  - Severe stress level: 30-40 kcal/kg/day
  - Pregnant women in second or third trimester: Add an additional 300 kcal/day
- Fluid: mL/day = 1500 mL for first 20 kg + 20 mL/kg thereafter
- Carbohydrate (dextrose):
  - 5 g/kg/day or 3.5 mg/kg/minute (maximum rate: 4-7 mg/kg/minute)
  - Minimum recommended amount: 400 calories/day or 100 g/day
- Protein (amino acids):
  - Normal/mild stress level: 1-1.2 g/kg/day
  - Moderate stress level: 1.2-1.5 g/kg/day
  - Severe stress level: 1.5-2 g/kg/day
  - Renal failure:
    - With dialysis: 1-1.5 g/kg/day
    - Without dialysis: 0.6-1 g/kg/day
  - Hepatic failure:
    - With encephalopathy: 0.6-1 g/kg/day
    - Without encephalopathy: 1-1.5 g/kg/day
  - Pregnant women in second or third trimester: Add an additional 10-14 g/day
- Fat: Initial: 2.5 g/kg/day (20% to 40% of total calories; do not exceed 60%)

Pediatrics: Nutritional supplementation:

- Neonates: I.V.:
  - Total calories:
    - Term: 90-108 kcal/kg/day
    - Preterm: 100-120 kcal/kg/day
  - Fluid:
    - <1.5 kg: 130-150 mL/kg/day
    - 1.5-2 kg: 110-130 mL/kg/day
    - Term: 100 mL/kg/day
  - Carbohydrate (dextrose):
    - ≥1 kg: Initial: 8 mg/kg/minute; goal: 12-14 mg/kg/minute
    - <1 kg: Initial: 6 mg/kg/min; goal: 12-14 mg/kg/minute
  - Protein (amino acids):
    - Term: Initial: 1.5-2 g/kg/day; goal: 3 g/kg/day
    - ELBW: Initial: 1.5-2 g/kg/day; goal: 3.5-4 g/kg/day
    - Sepsis, hypoxia: Initial: 1 g/kg/day; goal: 3-4g/kg/day
  - Fat:
    - Term: Initial: 1-2 g/kg/day; goal: 3 g/kg/day
    - Preterm: Initial: 0.5-2 g/kg/day; goal: 3 g/kg/day
    - Hyperbilirubinemia, sepsis, severe respiratory distress: Initial: 0.5 g/kg/day; goal: 0.5-1.5 g/kg/day
    - **Note:** Rates can be advanced at 0.5 g/kg/day.
  - Heparin: 1 unit/mL of parenteral nutrition fluids should be added to enhance clearance of lipid emulsions

(Continued)

Total Parenteral Nutrition *(Continued)*

Children: I.V.:
Total calories:
1-7 years: 75-90 kcal/kg/day
7-12 years: 60-75 kcal/kg/day
12-18 years: 30-60 kcal/kg/day
Fluid: 1500 mL/m^2/day
Carbohydrate (dextrose):
1-10 years: Initial: 10% to 12.5%; daily increase: 5% increments (maximum: 15 mg/kg/minute)
>10 years: Initial: 10% to 15%; daily increase: 5% increments (maximum: 8.5 mg/kg/minute)
Protein (amino acids):
1-10 years: Initial: 1-1.5 g/kg/day; daily increase: 1 g/kg/day (maximum: 2-2.5 g/kg/day)
>10 years: Initial: 1-1.5 g/kg/day; daily increase: 1 g/kg/day (maximum: 1.5-2 g/kg/day)
Fat: Initial: 1 g/kg/day; daily increase: 1 g/kg/day (maximum: 3 g/kg/day)

Available Dosage Forms No commercially-available dosage forms; TPN is compounded from optimal combinations of macronutrients (water, protein, dextrose, and lipids) and micronutrients (electrolytes, trace elements, and vitamins) to meet the specific nutritional requirements of a patient.

See Dextrose *on page 511* and Fat Emulsion *on page 705* monographs for additional information.

Administration

I.V.: For I.V. administration only, usually via a central venous catheter; can be administered by continuous infusion over 24 hours or cyclic infusion over 12-14 hours. Cyclic infusion is used with a tapering-up period at the beginning and a tapering-down period at the end to avoid hyper-/hypoglycemia.

Storage: USP Chapter 797 Guidelines consider TPN a medium-risk preparation and state that (in the absence of passing a sterility test) storage period should not exceed 30 hours at room temperature, 7 days at cold temperature, and 45 days in a solid frozen state at -20°C or colder. For patients on home TPN, multiple vitamins should be added prior to TPN administration, due to limited stability of multiple vitamins.

- **tPA** *see* Alteplase *on page 117*
- **T-Phyl®** *see* Theophylline *on page 1619*
- **TPN** *see* Total Parenteral Nutrition *on page 1650*
- **Tracrium®** *see* Atracurium *on page 200*

Tramadol (TRA ma dole)

U.S. Brand Names Ultram®

Synonyms Tramadol Hydrochloride

Pharmacologic Category Analgesic, Non-narcotic

Medication Safety Issues

Sound-alike/look-alike issues:
Tramadol may be confused with Toradol®, Trandate®, Voltaren®
Ultram® may be confused with Ultane®, Voltaren®

Use Relief of moderate to moderately-severe pain

Mechanism of Action Binds to μ-opiate receptors in the CNS causing inhibition of ascending pain pathways, altering the perception of and response to pain; also inhibits the reuptake of norepinephrine and serotonin, which also modifies the ascending pain pathway

Pharmacodynamics/Kinetics

Onset of action: ~1 hour
Duration of action: 9 hours
Absorption: Rapid and complete
Distribution: V_d: 2.5-3 L/kg
Protein binding, plasma: 20%
Metabolism: Extensively hepatic via demethylation, glucuronidation, and sulfation; has pharmacologically active metabolite formed by CYP2D6
Bioavailability: 75%
Half-life elimination: Tramadol: ~6 hours; Active metabolite: 7 hours; prolonged in elderly, hepatic or renal impairment
Time to peak: 2 hours
Excretion: Urine (as metabolites)

Contraindications Hypersensitivity to tramadol, opioids, or any component of the formulation; opioid-dependent patients; acute intoxication with alcohol, hypnotics, centrally-acting analgesics, opioids, or psychotropic drugs

Warnings/Precautions Should be used only with extreme caution in patients receiving MAO inhibitors. May cause CNS depression and/or respiratory depression, particularly when combined with other CNS depressants. Use with caution and reduce dosage when administered to patients receiving other CNS depressants. An increased risk of seizures may occur in patients receiving serotonin reuptake inhibitors (SSRIs or anorectics), tricyclic antidepressants, other cyclic compounds (including cyclobenzaprine, promethazine), neuroleptics, MAO inhibitors, or drugs which may lower seizure threshold. Patients with a history of seizures, or with a risk of seizures (head trauma, metabolic disorders, CNS infection, or malignancy, or during ethanol/drug withdrawal) are also at increased risk.

Elderly patients and patients with chronic respiratory disorders may be at greater risk of adverse events. Use with caution in patients with increased intracranial pressure or head injury. Use tramadol with caution and reduce dosage in patients with liver disease or renal dysfunction. Not recommended during pregnancy or in nursing mothers. Tolerance or drug dependence may result from extended use (withdrawal symptoms have been reported); abrupt discontinuation should be avoided. Tapering of dose at the time of discontinuation limits the risk of withdrawal symptoms. Safety and efficacy in pediatric patients have not been established.

Drug Interactions **Substrate** of CYP2D6 (major), 3A4 (minor)

Amphetamines: May increase the risk of seizures with tramadol.

Carbamazepine: Decreases half-life of tramadol by 33% to 50%.

CYP2D6 inhibitors: May decrease the effects of tramadol. Example inhibitors include chlorpromazine, delavirdine, fluoxetine, miconazole, paroxetine, pergolide, quinidine, quinine, ritonavir, and ropinirole.

Digoxin: Rare reports of digoxin toxicity with concomitant tramadol use.

Linezolid: May be associated with increased risk of seizures (due to MAO inhibition)

MAO inhibitors: May increases the risk of seizures.

Naloxone: May increase the risk of seizures (if administered in tramadol overdose)

Neuroleptic agents: May increase the risk of tramadol-associated seizures and may have additive CNS depressant effects.

Opioids: May increase the risk of seizures, and may have additive CNS depressant effects.

Quinidine: May increase the tramadol serum concentrations.

Selegiline: An increased risk of seizures has been associated with MAO inhibitors. It is not clear if drugs with selective MAO type B inhibition are safer than nonselective agents.

SSRIs: May increase the risk of seizures with tramadol. Includes citalopram, fluoxetine, paroxetine, sertraline.

Tricyclic antidepressants: May increase the risk of seizures.

Warfarin: Concomitant use may lead to an elevation of prothrombin times; monitor.

Nutritional/Herbal/Ethanol Interactions

Ethanol: Avoid ethanol (may increase CNS depression).

Food: Does not affect the rate or extent of absorption.

Herb/Nutraceutical: Avoid valerian, St John's wort, kava kava, gotu kola (may increase CNS depression).

Adverse Reactions Incidence of some adverse effects may increase over time

>10%:

- Central nervous system: Dizziness, headache, somnolence, vertigo
- Gastrointestinal: Constipation, nausea

1% to 10%:

- Cardiovascular: Vasodilation
- Central nervous system: Agitation, anxiety, confusion, coordination impaired, emotional lability, euphoria, hallucinations, malaise, nervousness, sleep disorder, tremor
- Dermatologic: Pruritus, rash
- Endocrine & metabolic: Menopausal symptoms
- Gastrointestinal: Abdominal pain, anorexia, diarrhea, dry mouth, dyspepsia, flatulence, vomiting
- Genitourinary: Urinary frequency, urinary retention

(Continued)

Tramadol *(Continued)*

Neuromuscular & skeletal: Hypertonia, spasticity, weakness
Ocular: Miosis, visual disturbance
Miscellaneous: Diaphoresis

<1% (Limited to important or life-threatening): Allergic reaction, amnesia, anaphylaxis, angioedema, bronchospasm, cognitive dysfunction, creatinine increased, death, depression, dyspnea, gastrointestinal bleeding, liver failure, seizure, serotonin syndrome, Stevens-Johnson syndrome, suicidal tendency, syncope, toxic epidermal necrolysis, vesicles

A withdrawal syndrome may occur with abrupt discontinuation; includes anxiety, diarrhea, hallucinations (rare), nausea, pain, piloerection, rigors, sweating, and tremor. Uncommon discontinuation symptoms may include severe anxiety, panic attacks, or paresthesia.

Overdosage/Toxicology Symptoms of overdose include CNS and respiratory depression, lethargy, coma, seizure, cardiac arrest, and death. Treatment may include naloxone 2 mg I.V. (0.01 mg/kg children) with repeat administration as needed up to 18 mg. Naloxone may increase the risk of seizures in tramadol overdose.

Dosing

Adults:

Moderate to severe chronic pain: Oral: 50-100 mg every 4-6 hours, not to exceed 400 mg/day

Note: For patients not requiring rapid onset of effect, tolerability may be improved by starting dose at 25 mg/day and titrating dose by 25 mg every 3 days, until reaching 25 mg 4 times/day. Dose may then be increased by 50 mg every 3 days as tolerated, to reach dose of 50 mg 4 times/day.

Elderly: Oral: >75 years: 50-100 mg every 4-6 hours not to exceed 300 mg/day; see renal or hepatic dosing.

Renal Impairment: Cl_{cr} <30 mL/minute: Administer 50-100 mg dose every 12 hours; maximum: 200 mg/day.

Hepatic Impairment: Cirrhosis: Recommended dose is 50 mg every 12 hours.

Available Dosage Forms Tablet, as hydrochloride: 50 mg

Nursing Guidelines

Assessment: Assess other medications patient may be taking for additive or adverse interactions. Monitor therapeutic effectiveness and adverse reactions or overdose at beginning of therapy and periodically during therapy. May cause physical and/or psychological dependence. Taper dose when discontinuing to avoid withdrawal symptoms. Assess knowledge/teach patient appropriate use, interventions to reduce side effects, and adverse symptoms to report.

Dietary Considerations: May be taken with or without food.

Patient Education: If self-administered, use exactly as directed; do not increase dose or frequency. Drug may cause physical and/or psychological dependence. While using this medication, do not use alcohol and other prescription or OTC medications (especially pain medications, sedatives, antihistamines, or cough preparations) without consulting prescriber. Maintain adequate hydration (2-3 L/day of fluids) unless instructed to restrict fluid intake. You may experience drowsiness, dizziness, or blurred vision (use caution when driving or engaging in tasks requiring alertness until response to drug is known); nausea, vomiting, or loss of appetite (small frequent meals, frequent mouth care, chewing gum, or sucking lozenges may help); or constipation (increased exercise, fluids, fruit, or fiber may help). Report severe unresolved constipation, respiratory difficulty or shortness of breath, excessive sedation or increased insomnia and restlessness, changes in urinary pattern or menstrual pattern, seizures, muscle weakness or tremors, or chest pain or palpitations. **Pregnancy/breast-feeding precautions:** Inform prescriber if you are or intend to become pregnant. Do not breast-feed.

Geriatric Considerations: One study in the elderly found that tramadol 50 mg was similar in efficacy as acetaminophen 300 mg with codeine 30 mg.

Pregnancy Risk Factor: C

Pregnancy Issues: Tramadol has been shown to cross the placenta. Postmarketing reports following tramadol use during pregnancy include neonatal seizures, withdrawal syndrome, fetal death and stillbirth. Not recommended for use during labor and delivery.

Lactation: Enters breast milk/contraindicated

Breast-Feeding Considerations: Not recommended for postdelivery analgesia in nursing mothers.

Perioperative/Anesthesia/Other Concerns: Tramadol is not any more effective than Tylenol® #3, Darvocet-N® 100, NSAIDs, or Demerol®. It is 5-10 times less potent than morphine and reported to cause less respiratory depression.

Administration

Storage: Store at controlled room temperature of 25°C (77°F).

Related Information

Acute Postoperative Pain *on page 1742*

- Tramadol Hydrochloride *see* Tramadol *on page 1652*
- Tramadol Hydrochloride and Acetaminophen *see* Acetaminophen and Tramadol *on page 70*
- Trandate® *see* Labetalol *on page 996*
- Transderm Scōp® *see* Scopolamine *on page 1513*

Trastuzumab (tras TU zoo mab)

U.S. Brand Names Herceptin®

Pharmacologic Category Monoclonal Antibody

Use

Treatment of metastatic breast cancer whose tumors overexpress the HER-2/*neu* protein

Unlabeled/Investigational Use Treatment of ovarian, gastric, colorectal, endometrial, lung, bladder, prostate, and salivary gland tumors

Mechanism of Action Trastuzumab is a monoclonal antibody which binds to the extracellular domain of the human epidermal growth factor receptor 2 protein (HER-2); it mediates antibody-dependent cellular cytotoxicity against cells which overproduce HER-2

Pharmacodynamics/Kinetics

Distribution: V_d: 44 mL/kg

Half-life elimination: Mean: 5.8 days (range: 1-32 days)

Contraindications Hypersensitivity to trastuzumab, Chinese hamster ovary cell proteins, or any component of the formulation

Warnings/Precautions Hazardous agent - use appropriate precautions for handling and disposal. Congestive heart failure associated with trastuzumab may be severe and has been associated with disabling cardiac failure, death, mural thrombus, and stroke. Left ventricular function should be evaluated in all patients prior to and during treatment with trastuzumab. Discontinuation should be strongly considered in patients who develop a clinically significant decrease in ejection fraction during therapy. Combination therapy which includes anthracyclines and cyclophosphamide increases the incidence and severity of cardiac dysfunction. Extreme caution should be used when treating patients with pre-existing cardiac disease or dysfunction, and in patients with previous exposure to anthracyclines. Advanced age may also predispose to cardiac toxicity.

Serious adverse events, including hypersensitivity reaction (anaphylaxis), infusion reactions (including fatalities), and pulmonary events (including adult respiratory distress syndrome) have been associated with trastuzumab. Most of these events occur within 24 hours of infusion, however, delayed reactions have occurred. Use with caution in pre-existing pulmonary disease. Discontinuation of trastuzumab should be strongly considered in any patient who develops anaphylaxis, angioedema, or acute respiratory distress syndrome. Retreatment of patients who experienced severe hypersensitivity reactions has been attempted (with premedication). Some patients tolerated retreatment, while others experienced a second severe reaction. When used in combination with myelosuppressive chemotherapy, trastuzumab may increase the incidence of neutropenia (moderate-to-severe) and febrile neutropenia.

Drug Interactions

Anthracyclines (ie, doxorubicin): Combined therapy may increase the incidence/severity of cardiac dysfunction.

Cyclophosphamide: Combined therapy may increase the incidence/severity of cardiac dysfunction.

Myelosuppressive agents: Trastuzumab may increase the incidence of neutropenia and/or febrile neutropenia when used in combination with myelosuppressive agents.

Paclitaxel: May result in a decrease in clearance of trastuzumab, increasing serum concentrations.

Adverse Reactions Note: The most common adverse effects are infusion-related, occurring in up to 40% of patients, consisting of fever and chills (mild

(Continued)

Trastuzumab *(Continued)*

to moderate, often with other systemic symptoms). Treatment with acetaminophen, diphenhydramine, and/or meperidine is usually effective.

>10%:

- Central nervous system: Pain (47%), fever (36%), chills (32%), headache (26%)
- Dermatologic: Rash (18%)
- Gastrointestinal: Nausea (33%), diarrhea (25%), vomiting (23%), abdominal pain (22%), anorexia (14%)
- Neuromuscular & skeletal: Weakness (42%), back pain (22%)
- Respiratory: Cough (26%), dyspnea (22%), rhinitis (14%), pharyngitis (12%)
- Miscellaneous: Infection (20%); infusion reaction (40%, chills and fever most common)

1% to 10%:

- Cardiovascular: Peripheral edema (10%), CHF (7%), tachycardia (5%)
- Central nervous system: Insomnia (14%), dizziness (13%), paresthesia (9%), depression (6%), peripheral neuritis (2%), neuropathy (1%)
- Dermatologic: Herpes simplex (2%), acne (2%)
- Genitourinary: Urinary tract infection (5%)
- Hematologic: Anemia (4%), leukopenia (3%)
- Neuromuscular & skeletal: Bone pain (7%), arthralgia (6%)
- Respiratory: Sinusitis (9%)
- Miscellaneous: Flu syndrome (10%), accidental injury (6%), allergic reaction (3%)

<1% (Limited to important or life-threatening): Amblyopia, anaphylactoid reaction, arrhythmia, ascites, cardiac arrest, cellulitis, coagulopathy, deafness, esophageal ulcer, hematemesis, hemorrhage, hepatic failure, hepatitis, hydrocephalus, hypotension, hypothyroidism, ileus, intestinal obstruction, pancreatitis, pancytopenia, pericardial effusion, radiation injury, shock, stomatitis, syncope, vascular thrombosis

Overdosage/Toxicology There is no experience with overdose in human clinical trials. Treatment is supportive.

Dosing

Adults & Elderly:

Metastatic breast carcinoma: I.V.:

Loading dose: 4 mg/kg over 90 minutes; do not administer as an I.V. bolus or I.V. push.

Maintenance dose: 2 mg/kg once weekly (may be infused over 30 minutes if prior infusions are well tolerated).

Renal Impairment: No adjustment is necessary.

Hepatic Impairment: No adjustment necessary.

Available Dosage Forms Injection, powder for reconstitution: 440 mg [packaged with bacteriostatic water for injection; diluent contains benzyl alcohol]

Nursing Guidelines

Assessment: Monitor therapeutic effectiveness and adverse reactions. Monitor vital signs during infusion. Assess knowledge/teach patient interventions to reduce side effects and adverse symptoms to report.

Patient Education: This medication can only be administered by infusion. Report immediately any adverse reactions during infusion (eg, respiratory difficulty, chills, fever, headache, backache, or nausea/vomiting) so appropriate medication can be administered. You will be susceptible to infection (avoid crowds and exposure to infection). You may experience dizziness or weakness (use caution when driving or engaging in tasks requiring alertness until response to drug is known); nausea or vomiting (small frequent meals, frequent mouth care, chewing gum, or sucking lozenges may help); diarrhea (boiled milk, yogurt, or buttermilk may help); or headache, back or joint pain (mild analgesics may offer relief). Report persistent GI effects; sore throat, runny nose, or respiratory difficulty; chest pain, irregular heartbeat, palpitations, swelling of extremities, or unusual weight gain; muscle or joint weakness, numbness, or pain; skin rash or irritation; itching or pain on urination; unhealed sores, white plaques in mouth or genital area, unusual bruising or bleeding; or other unusual adverse effects. **Breast-feeding precaution:** Breast-feeding is not recommended.

Pregnancy Risk Factor: B

Lactation: Excretion in breast milk unknown/not recommended

Breast-Feeding Considerations: It is not known whether trastuzumab is secreted in human milk. Because many immunoglobulins are secreted in milk, and the potential for serious adverse reactions exists, patients should discontinue nursing during treatment and for 6 months after the last dose.

Administration

I.V.: Administered by I.V. infusion; loading doses are infused over 90 minutes; maintenance doses may be infused over 30 minutes if tolerated.

Reconstitution: Reconstitute each vial with 20 mL of bacteriostatic sterile water for injection. Do not shake. If patient has a known hypersensitivity to benzyl alcohol, it may be reconstituted with sterile water for injection. Further dilute in NS prior to administration.

Storage: Store intact vials under refrigeration (2°C to 8°C/36°F to 46°F) prior to reconstitution. Stable for 28 days after reconstitution if refrigerated; do not freeze. If sterile water for injection without preservative is used for reconstitution, it must be used immediately. After dilution in 0.9% sodium chloride for injection in polyethylene bags, solution is stable for 24 hours.

♦ Trasylol® *see* Aprotinin *on page 179*

Trazodone (TRAZ oh done)

U.S. Brand Names Desyrel®

Synonyms Trazodone Hydrochloride

Pharmacologic Category Antidepressant, Serotonin Reuptake Inhibitor/Antagonist

Medication Safety Issues

Sound-alike/look-alike issues:

Desyrel® may be confused with Demerol®, Delsym®, Zestril®

Use Treatment of depression

Unlabeled/Investigational Use Potential augmenting agent for antidepressants, hypnotic

Mechanism of Action Inhibits reuptake of serotonin, causes adrenoreceptor subsensitivity, and induces significant changes in 5-HT presynaptic receptor adrenoreceptors. Trazodone also significantly blocks histamine (H_1) and alpha$_1$-adrenergic receptors.

Pharmacodynamics/Kinetics

Onset of action: Therapeutic (antidepressant): 1-3 weeks; sleep aid: 1-3 hours

Protein binding: 85% to 95%

Metabolism: Hepatic via CYP3A4 to an active metabolite (mCPP)

Half-life elimination: 7-8 hours, two compartment kinetics

Time to peak, serum: 30-100 minutes; delayed with food (up to 2.5 hours)

Excretion: Primarily urine; secondarily feces

Contraindications Hypersensitivity to trazodone or any component of the formulation

Warnings/Precautions Antidepressants increase the risk of suicidal thinking and behavior in children and adolescents with major depressive disorder (MDD) and other depressive disorders; consider risk prior to prescribing. Closely monitor for clinical worsening, suicidality, or unusual changes in behavior; the child's family or caregiver should be instructed to closely observe the patient and communicate condition with healthcare provider. Such observation would generally include at least weekly face-to-face contact with patients or their family members or caregivers during the first 4 weeks of treatment, then every other week visits for the next 4 weeks, then at 12 weeks, and as clinically indicated beyond 12 weeks. Additional contact by telephone may be appropriate between face-to-face visits. Adults treated with antidepressants should be observed similarly for clinical worsening and suicidality, especially during the initial few months of a course of drug therapy, or at times of dose changes, either increases or decreases. A medication guide should be dispensed with each prescription. **Trazodone is not FDA approved for use in children.**

The possibility of a suicide attempt is inherent in major depression and may persist until remission occurs. Monitor for worsening of depression or suicidality, especially during initiation of therapy or with dose increases or decreases. Worsening depression and severe abrupt suicidality that are not part of the presenting symptoms may require discontinuation or modification of drug therapy. Use caution in high-risk patients during initiation of therapy. Prescriptions should be written for the smallest quantity consistent with good patient care. The patient's family or caregiver should be alerted to monitor patients for the emergence of suicidality and associated behaviors such as anxiety, agitation, panic attacks, insomnia, irritability, hostility, impulsivity, akathisia, hypomania, and mania;

(Continued)

Trazodone *(Continued)*

patients should be instructed to notify their healthcare provider if any of these symptoms or worsening depression occur.

May worsen psychosis in some patients or precipitate a shift to mania or hypomania in patients with bipolar disorder. Monotherapy in patients with bipolar disorder should be avoided. Patients presenting with depressive symptoms should be screened for bipolar disorder. **Trazodone is not FDA approved for the treatment of bipolar depression.**

Priapism, including cases resulting in permanent dysfunction, has occurred with the use of trazodone. Not recommended for use in a patient during the acute recovery phase of MI. Trazodone should be initiated with caution in patients who are receiving concurrent or recent therapy with a MAO inhibitor. May cause sedation, resulting in impaired performance of tasks requiring alertness (eg, operating machinery or driving). Sedative effects may be additive with other CNS depressants and ethanol. The degree of sedation is very high relative to other antidepressants. May increase the risks associated with electroconvulsive therapy. Consider discontinuing, when possible, prior to elective surgery. Therapy should not be abruptly discontinued in patients receiving high doses for prolonged periods.

Use with caution in patients at risk of hypotension or in patients where transient hypotensive episodes would be poorly tolerated (cardiovascular disease or cerebrovascular disease). The risk of postural hypotension is high relative to other antidepressants.

Use caution in patients with a previous seizure disorder or condition predisposing to seizures such as brain damage, alcoholism, or concurrent therapy with other drugs which lower the seizure threshold. Use with caution in patients with hepatic or renal dysfunction and in elderly patients. Use with caution in patients with a history of cardiovascular disease (including previous MI, stroke, tachycardia, or conduction abnormalities). However, the risk of conduction abnormalities with this agent is low relative to other antidepressants.

Drug Interactions Substrate of CYP2D6 (minor), 3A4 (major); **Inhibits** CYP2D6 (moderate), 3A4 (weak)

Antipsychotics: Trazodone, in combination with other psychotropics (low potency antipsychotics), may result in additional hypotension (isolated case reports); monitor.

Azole antifungals: Serum concentrations of trazodone may be increased by azole antifungals, via inhibition of CYP3A4. Ketoconazole has been specifically studied. Consider a lower dose of trazodone.

Buspirone: Serotonergic effects may be additive (limited documentation); monitor.

Carbamazepine: Serum concentrations of trazodone may be decreased by carbamazepine, due to induction of CYP3A4. Other CYP inducers are likely to share this effect.

CNS depressants: Sedative effects may be additive with CNS depressants. Includes ethanol, barbiturates, benzodiazepines, narcotic analgesics, and other sedative agents; monitor for increased effect

CYP2D6 substrates: Trazodone may increase the levels/effects of CYP2D6 substrates. Example substrates include amphetamines, selected beta-blockers, dextromethorphan, fluoxetine, lidocaine, mirtazapine, nefazodone, paroxetine, risperidone, ritonavir, thioridazine, tricyclic antidepressants, and venlafaxine.

CYP2D6 prodrug substrates: Trazodone may decrease the levels/effects of CYP2D6 prodrug substrates. Example prodrug substrates include codeine, hydrocodone, oxycodone, and tramadol.

CYP3A4 inducers: CYP3A4 inducers may decrease the levels/effects of trazodone. Example inducers include aminoglutethimide, carbamazepine, nafcillin, nevirapine, phenobarbital, phenytoin, and rifamycins.

CYP3A4 inhibitors: May increase the levels/effects of trazodone. Example inhibitors include azole antifungals, clarithromycin, diclofenac, doxycycline, erythromycin, imatinib, isoniazid, nefazodone, nicardipine, propofol, protease inhibitors, quinidine, telithromycin, and verapamil.

Linezolid: Due to MAO inhibition (see note on MAO inhibitors), this combination should be avoided

MAO inhibitors: Concurrent use may lead to serotonin syndrome; avoid concurrent use or use within 14 days

Meperidine: Combined use, theoretically, may increase the risk of serotonin syndrome

Protease inhibitors: Serum concentrations of trazodone may be increased by protease inhibitors, via inhibition of CYP3A4. Consider a lower dose of trazodone.

Serotonin agonists: Theoretically, may increase the risk of serotonin syndrome; includes sumatriptan, naratriptan, rizatriptan, and zolmitriptan

SSRIs: Combined use of trazodone with an SSRI may, theoretically, increase the risk of serotonin syndrome; in addition, some SSRIs may inhibit the metabolism of trazodone resulting in elevated plasma levels and increased sedation; includes fluoxetine and fluvoxamine (see CYP inhibition); low doses of trazodone appear to represent little risk

Venlafaxine: Combined use with trazodone may increase the risk of serotonin syndrome

Nutritional/Herbal/Ethanol Interactions

Ethanol: Avoid ethanol (may increase CNS depression).

Food: Time to peak serum levels may be increased if trazodone is taken with food.

Herb/Nutraceutical: Avoid valerian, St John's wort, SAMe, kava kava (may increase risk of serotonin syndrome and/or excessive sedation).

Adverse Reactions

>10%:

Central nervous system: Dizziness, headache, sedation

Gastrointestinal: Nausea, xerostomia

Ocular: Blurred vision

1% to 10%:

Cardiovascular: Syncope, hyper-/hypotension, edema

Central nervous system: Confusion, decreased concentration, fatigue, incoordination

Gastrointestinal: Diarrhea, constipation, weight gain/loss

Neuromuscular & skeletal: Tremor, myalgia

Respiratory: Nasal congestion

<1% (Limited to important or life-threatening): Agitation, allergic reactions, alopecia, anxiety, bradycardia, extrapyramidal symptoms, hepatitis, priapism, rash, seizure, speech impairment, tachycardia, urinary retention

Overdosage/Toxicology Symptoms of overdose include drowsiness, vomiting, hypotension, tachycardia, incontinence, coma, and priapism. Treatment is symptom-directed and supportive.

Dosing

Adults:

Depression: Oral: Initial: 150 mg/day in 3 divided doses (may increase by 50 mg/day every 3-7 days); maximum: 600 mg/day

Note: Therapeutic effects may take up to 6 weeks. Therapy is normally maintained for 6-12 months after optimum response is reached to prevent recurrence of depression.

Sedation/hypnotic (unlabeled use): Oral: 25-50 mg at bedtime (often in combination with daytime SSRIs). May increase up to 200 mg at bedtime.

Elderly: Oral: 25-50 mg at bedtime with 25-50 mg/day dose increase every 3 days for inpatients and weekly for outpatients, if tolerated; usual dose: 75-150 mg/day

Pediatrics:

Depression (unlabeled use):

Children 6-12 years: Initial: 1.5-2 mg/kg/day in divided doses; increase gradually every 3-4 days as needed; maximum: 6 mg/kg/day in 3 divided doses

Adolescents: Initial: 25-50 mg/day; increase to 100-150 mg/day in divided doses

Available Dosage Forms Tablet, as hydrochloride: 50 mg, 100 mg, 150 mg, 300 mg

Nursing Guidelines

Assessment: Assess potential and monitor closely for interactions with other prescriptions, OTC medications, or herbal products patient may be taking. Assess results of laboratory tests, therapeutic effectiveness according to rationale for therapy, and adverse reactions at beginning of therapy and periodically with long-term use. Initiate at lower doses and taper dosage slowly when discontinuing (allow 3-4 weeks between discontinuing Desyrel® and starting another antidepressant). Teach patient appropriate use, side effects/appropriate interventions, and adverse symptoms to report.

Monitoring Laboratory Tests: Baseline liver function prior to and periodically during therapy

(Continued)

Trazodone *(Continued)*

Patient Education: Do not take any new medication during therapy unless approved by prescriber. Take exactly as directed; do not increase dose or frequency. It may take 2-4 weeks to achieve desired results. Take after meals. Avoid excessive alcohol and caffeine. Maintain adequate hydration (2-3 L/day of fluids) unless instructed to restrict fluid intake. You may experience drowsiness, lightheadedness, dizziness (use caution when driving or engaging in tasks requiring alertness until response to drug is known); postural hypotension (use caution when climbing stairs or changing position from lying or sitting to standing); nausea, dry mouth (small frequent meals, frequent mouth care, chewing gum, or sucking lozenges may help); constipation (increased exercise, fluids, fruit, or fiber may help); or diarrhea (buttermilk, yogurt, or boiled milk may help). Report persistent dizziness or headache; muscle cramping, tremors, or altered gait; blurred vision or eye pain; chest pain or irregular heartbeat; suicidal ideation; or worsening of condition. Report prolonged or inappropriate erections. **Pregnancy/breast-feeding precautions:** Inform prescriber if you are or intend to become pregnant. Do not breast-feed.

Geriatric Considerations: Very sedating, but little anticholinergic effects.

Pregnancy Risk Factor: C

Lactation: Enters breast milk/use caution (AAP rates "of concern")

Administration

Oral: Dosing after meals may decrease lightheadedness and postural hypotension.

♦ Trazodone Hydrochloride *see* Trazodone *on page 1657*
♦ Trental® *see* Pentoxifylline *on page 1340*
♦ Trexall™ *see* Methotrexate *on page 1127*

Triamcinolone (trye am SIN oh lone)

U.S. Brand Names Aristocort®; Aristocort® A; Aristospan®; Azmacort®; Kenalog®; Kenalog-10®; Kenalog-40®; Nasacort® AQ; Nasacort® HFA; Triderm®; Tri-Nasal®

Synonyms Triamcinolone Acetonide, Aerosol; Triamcinolone Acetonide, Parenteral; Triamcinolone Diacetate, Oral; Triamcinolone Diacetate, Parenteral; Triamcinolone Hexacetonide; Triamcinolone, Oral

Pharmacologic Category Corticosteroid, Adrenal; Corticosteroid, Inhalant (Oral); Corticosteroid, Nasal; Corticosteroid, Systemic; Corticosteroid, Topical

Medication Safety Issues

Sound-alike/look-alike issues:

Kenalog® may be confused with Ketalar®
Nasacort® may be confused with NasalCrom®

TAC (occasional abbreviation for triamcinolone) is an error-prone abbreviation (mistaken as tetracaine-adrenaline-cocaine)

Use

Nasal inhalation: Management of seasonal and perennial allergic rhinitis in patients ≥6 years of age

Oral inhalation: Control of bronchial asthma and related bronchospastic conditions

Oral topical: Adjunctive treatment and temporary relief of symptoms associated with oral inflammatory lesions and ulcerative lesions resulting from trauma

Systemic: Adrenocortical insufficiency, rheumatic disorders, allergic states, respiratory diseases, systemic lupus erythematosus (SLE), and other diseases requiring anti-inflammatory or immunosuppressive effects

Topical: Inflammatory dermatoses responsive to steroids

Mechanism of Action Decreases inflammation by suppression of migration of polymorphonuclear leukocytes and reversal of increased capillary permeability; suppresses the immune system by reducing activity and volume of the lymphatic system; suppresses adrenal function at high doses

Pharmacodynamics/Kinetics

Duration: Oral: 8-12 hours
Absorption: Topical: Systemic
Time to peak: I.M.: 8-10 hours
Half-life elimination: Biologic: 18-36 hours

Contraindications Hypersensitivity to triamcinolone or any component of the formulation; systemic fungal infections; serious infections (except septic shock or tuberculous meningitis); primary treatment of status asthmaticus; fungal, viral, or bacterial infections of the mouth or throat (oral topical formulation)

Warnings/Precautions May cause suppression of hypothalamic-pituitary-adrenal (HPA) axis, particularly in younger children or in patients receiving high doses for prolonged periods. Particular care is required when patients are transferred from systemic corticosteroids to inhaled products due to possible adrenal insufficiency or withdrawal from steroids, including an increase in allergic symptoms. Patients receiving 20 mg per day of prednisone (or equivalent) may be most susceptible. Fatalities have occurred due to adrenal insufficiency in asthmatic patients during and after transfer from systemic corticosteroids to aerosol steroids; aerosol steroids do **not** provide the systemic steroid needed to treat patients having trauma, surgery, or infections. Withdrawal and discontinuation of the corticosteroid should be done slowly and carefully

Use with caution in patients with hypothyroidism, cirrhosis, nonspecific ulcerative colitis and patients at increased risk for peptic ulcer disease. Corticosteroids should be used with caution in patients with diabetes, hypertension, osteoporosis, glaucoma, cataracts, or tuberculosis. Use caution in hepatic impairment. Do not use occlusive dressings on weeping or exudative lesions and general caution with occlusive dressings should be observed; discontinue if skin irritation or contact dermatitis should occur; do not use in patients with decreased skin circulation; avoid the use of high potency steroids on the face.

Because of the risk of adverse effects, systemic corticosteroids should be used cautiously in the elderly, in the smallest possible dose, and for the shortest possible time. Azmacort® (metered dose inhaler) comes with its own spacer device attached and may be easier to use in older patients.

Controlled clinical studies have shown that orally-inhaled and intranasal corticosteroids may cause a reduction in growth velocity in pediatric patients. (In studies of orally-inhaled corticosteroids, the mean reduction in growth velocity was approximately 1 centimeter per year [range 0.3-1.8 cm per year] and appears to be related to dose and duration of exposure.) The growth of pediatric patients receiving inhaled corticosteroids, should be monitored routinely (eg, via stadiometry). To minimize the systemic effects of orally-inhaled and intranasal corticosteroids, each patient should be titrated to the lowest effective dose.

May suppress the immune system, patients may be more susceptible to infection. Use with caution in patients with systemic infections or ocular herpes simplex. Avoid exposure to chickenpox and measles.

Oral topical: Discontinue if local irritation or sensitization should develop. If significant regeneration or repair of oral tissues has not occurred in seven days, re-evaluation of the etiology of the oral lesion is advised.

Drug Interactions

Decreased effect: Barbiturates, phenytoin, rifampin increase metabolism of triamcinolone; vaccine and toxoid effects may be reduced

Increased effect: Salmeterol: The addition of salmeterol has been demonstrated to improve response to inhaled corticosteroids (as compared to increasing steroid dosage).

Increased toxicity: Salicylates may increase risk of GI ulceration

Nutritional/Herbal/Ethanol Interactions

Ethanol: Avoid ethanol (may enhance gastric mucosal irritation).

Food: Triamcinolone interferes with calcium absorption.

Herb/Nutraceutical: Avoid cat's claw, echinacea (have immunostimulant properties).

Adverse Reactions

Systemic: Frequency not defined:

Cardiovascular: CHF, hypertension

Central nervous system: Convulsions, fever, headache, intracranial pressure increased, vertigo

Dermatologic: Bruising, facial erythema, petechiae, photosensitivity, rash, thin/fragile skin, wound healing impaired

Endocrine & metabolic: Adrenocortical/pituitary unresponsiveness (particularly during stress), carbohydrate tolerance decreased, cushingoid state, diabetes mellitus (manifestations of latent disease), fluid retention, growth suppression (children), hypokalemic alkalosis, menstrual irregularities, negative nitrogen balance, potassium loss, sodium retention

Gastrointestinal: Abdominal distention, diarrhea, dyspepsia, nausea, oral *Monilia* (oral inhaler), pancreatitis, peptic ulcer, ulcerative esophagitis, weight gain

Local: Skin atrophy (at the injection site)

(Continued)

Triamcinolone *(Continued)*

Neuromuscular & skeletal: Femoral/humeral head aseptic necrosis, muscle mass decreased, muscle weakness, osteoporosis, pathologic fracture of long bones, steroid myopathy, vertebral compression fractures

Ocular: Cataracts, intraocular pressure increased, exophthalmos, glaucoma

Respiratory: Cough increased (nasal spray), epistaxis (nasal inhaler/spray), pharyngitis (nasal spray/oral inhaler), sinusitis (oral inhaler), voice alteration (oral inhaler)

Miscellaneous: Anaphylaxis, diaphoresis increased, suppression to skin tests

Topical: Frequency not defined:

Dermatologic: Itching, allergic contact dermatitis, dryness, folliculitis, skin infection (secondary), itching, hypertrichosis, acneiform eruptions, hypopigmentation, skin maceration, skin atrophy, striae, miliaria, perioral dermatitis, atrophy of oral mucosa

Local: Burning, irritation

Overdosage/Toxicology When consumed in high doses for prolonged periods, systemic hypercorticism and adrenal suppression may occur. In those cases, discontinuation of the corticosteroid should be done judiciously.

Dosing

Adults & Elderly: The lowest possible dose should be used to control the condition; when dose reduction is possible, the dose should be reduced gradually. Parenteral dose is usually 1/3 to 1/2 the oral dose given every 12 hours. In life-threatening situations, parenteral doses larger than the oral dose may be needed.

Adrenocortical insufficiency: Oral: Range: 4-12 mg/day

Allergic rhinitis (perennial or seasonal):

Nasal spray: 220 mcg/day as 2 sprays in each nostril once daily

Nasal inhaler: Initial: 220 mcg/day as 2 sprays in each nostril once daily; may increase dose to 440 mcg/day (given once daily or divided and given 2 or 4 times/day)

Oral (acute treatment only): Range: 8-12 mg/day

Asthma:

Oral: 8-16 mg/day

Oral inhalation: 200 mcg 3-4 times/day **or** 400 mcg twice daily; maximum dose: 1600 mcg/day

Carditis (acute rheumatic): Oral: Initial: 20-60 mg/day; reduce dose during maintenance therapy

Dermatoses (steroid-responsive, including contact/atopic dermatitis):

Oral: Initial: 8-16 mg/day

Injection:

Acetonide: Intradermal: Initial: 1 mg

Hexacetonide: Intralesional, sublesional: up to 0.5 mg/square inch of affected skin

Topical:

Cream, ointment: Apply thin film to affected areas 2-4 times/day

Spray: Apply to affected area 3-4 times/day

Triamcinolone Dosing

<table>
<tr><th></th><th>Acetonide</th><th>Hexacetonide</th></tr>
<tr><td>Intrasynovial</td><td>5-40 mg</td><td></td></tr>
<tr><td>Intralesional</td><td>1-30 mg (usually 1 mg per injection site); 10 mg/mL suspension usually used</td><td rowspan="2">Up to 0.5 mg/sq inch affected area</td></tr>
<tr><td>Sublesional</td><td>1-30 mg</td></tr>
<tr><td>Systemic I.M.</td><td>2.5-60 mg/dose (usual adult dose: 60 mg; may repeat with 20-100 mg dose when symptoms recur)</td><td></td></tr>
<tr><td>Intra-articular</td><td>2.5-40 mg</td><td>2-20 mg average</td></tr>
<tr><td>large joints</td><td>5-15 mg</td><td>10-20 mg</td></tr>
<tr><td>small joints</td><td>2.5-5 mg</td><td>2-6 mg</td></tr>
<tr><td>Tendon sheaths</td><td>2.5-10 mg</td><td></td></tr>
<tr><td>Intradermal</td><td>1 mg/site</td><td></td></tr>
</table>

Ophthalmic disorders: Oral: 12-40 mg/day

Oral inflammatory lesions/ulcers: Oral topical: Press a small dab (about 1/4 inch) to the lesion until a thin film develops; a larger quantity may be required for coverage of some lesions. For optimal results, use only enough to coat the lesion with a thin film; do not rub in.

Rheumatic or arthritic disorders:

Oral: Range: 8-16 mg/day

Lupus (SLE): Initial: 20-32 mg/day, some patients may need initial doses ≥48 mg; reduce dose during maintenance therapy

Intra-articular (or similar injection as designated):

Acetonide: Intra-articular, intrabursal, tendon sheaths: Initial: Smaller joints: 2.5-5 mg, larger joints: 5-15 mg

Hexacetonide: Intra-articular: Initial range: 2-20 mg/day

I.M.:

Acetonide: Range: 2.5-60 mg/day; Initial: 60 mg

See table on previous page.

Pediatrics:

Allergic rhinitis (perennial or seasonal):

Nasal spray:

Children 6-11 years: 110 mcg/day as 1 spray in each nostril once daily.

Children ≥12 years: Refer to adult dosing.

Nasal inhaler:

Children 6-11 years: Initial: 220 mcg/day as 2 sprays in each nostril once daily

Children ≥12 years: Refer to adult dosing.

Asthma:

Oral: 8-16 mg/day

Oral inhalation:

Children 6-12 years: 100-200 mcg 3-4 times/day **or** 200-400 mcg twice daily; maximum dose: 1200 mg/day

Children >12 years: Refer to adult dosing.

Rheumatic conditions: I.M. (acetonide): Range: 2.5-60 mg/day

Children 6-12 years: Initial: 40 mg

Children ≥12 years: Refer to adult dosing.

Available Dosage Forms

Aerosol for nasal inhalation, as acetonide [CFC free] (Nasacort® [HFA]): 55 mcg/inhalation (9.3 g) [100 doses]

Aerosol for oral inhalation, as acetonide (Azmacort®): 100 mcg per actuation (20 g) [240 actuations]

Aerosol, topical, as acetonide (Kenalog®): 0.2 mg/2-second spray (63 g)

Cream, as acetonide: 0.025% (15 g, 80 g, 454 g); 0.1% (15 g, 80 g, 454 g, 2270 g); 0.5% (15 g)

Aristocort® A: 0.025% (15 g, 60 g); 0.1% (15 g, 60 g); 0.5% (15 g) [contains benzyl alcohol]

Triderm®: 0.1% (30 g, 85 g)

Injection, suspension, as acetonide:

Kenalog-10®: 10 mg/mL (5 mL) [contains benzyl alcohol; not for I.V. or I.M. use]

Kenalog-40®: 40 mg/mL (1 mL, 5 mL, 10 mL) [contains benzyl alcohol; not for I.V. or intradermal use]

Injection, suspension, as hexacetonide (Aristospan®): 5 mg/mL (5 mL); 20 mg/mL (1 mL, 5 mL) [contains benzyl alcohol; not for I.V. use]

Lotion, as acetonide: 0.025% (60 mL); 0.1% (60 mL)

Ointment, topical, as acetonide: 0.025% (15g, 80 g, 454 g); 0.1% (15 g, 80 g, 454 g); 0.5% (15 g)

Aristocort® A: 0.1% (15 g, 60 g)

Paste, oral, topical, as acetonide: 0.1% (5 g)

Solution, spray for nasal inhalation, as acetonide (Tri-Nasal®): 50 mcg/inhalation (15 mL) [120 doses]

Suspension, spray for nasal inhalation, as acetonide (Nasacort® AQ): 55 mcg/inhalation (16.5 g) [120 doses]

Tablet (Aristocort®): 4 mg [contains lactose and sodium benzoate]

Nursing Guidelines

Assessment: Assess other medications patient may be taking for effectiveness and interactions. Assess results of laboratory tests, therapeutic effectiveness, and adverse effects according to indications for therapy, dose, route (systemic or topical), and duration of therapy. With systemic administration, patients with diabetes should monitor glucose levels closely (corticosteroids may alter glucose levels). Assess knowledge/teach patient appropriate use, interventions

(Continued)

Triamcinolone *(Continued)*

to reduce side effects, and adverse symptoms to report. When used for long-term therapy (>10-14 days) do not discontinue abruptly; decrease dosage incrementally.

Dietary Considerations: May be taken with food to decrease GI distress.

Patient Education: Take exactly as directed; do not increase dose or discontinue abruptly without consulting prescriber. Take oral medication with or after meals. Avoid alcohol. Limit intake of caffeine or stimulants. Prescriber may recommend increased dietary vitamins, minerals, or iron. If you have diabetes, monitor glucose levels closely (antidiabetic medication may need to be adjusted). Inform prescriber if you are experiencing greater than normal levels of stress (medication may need adjustment). Some forms of this medication may cause GI upset (oral medication may be taken with meals to reduce GI upset; or small frequent meals and frequent mouth care may reduce GI upset). You may be more susceptible to infection (avoid crowds and exposure to infection). Report promptly excessive nervousness or sleep disturbances; any signs of infection (sore throat, unhealed injuries); excessive growth of body hair or loss of skin color; vision changes; excessive or sudden weight gain (>3 lb/week); swelling of face or extremities; respiratory difficulty; muscle weakness; change in color of stools (black or tarry) or persistent abdominal pain; or worsening of condition or failure to improve. **Pregnancy/breast-feeding precautions:** Inform prescriber if you are or intend to become pregnant. Consult prescriber if breast-feeding.

Aerosol: Shake gently before use. Use at regular intervals, no more frequently than directed. Not for use during acute asthmatic attack. Follow directions that accompany product. Rinse mouth and throat after use to prevent candidiasis. Do not use intranasal product if you have a nasal infection, nasal injury, or recent nasal surgery. If using two products, consult prescriber in which order to use the two products. Report unusual cough or spasm; persistent nasal bleeding, burning, or irritation; or worsening of condition.

Inhalation: Sit when using. Take deep breaths for 3-5 minutes, and clear nasal passages before administration (use decongestant as needed). Hold breath for 5-10 seconds after use, and wait 1-3 minutes between inhalations. Follow package insert instructions for use. Do not exceed maximum dosage. If also using inhaled bronchodilator, use before triamcinolone. Rinse mouth and throat after use to reduce aftertaste and prevent candidiasis.

Topical: For external use only. Not for eyes or mucous membranes or open wounds. Apply in very thin layer to occlusive dressing. Apply dressing to area being treated. Avoid prolonged or excessive use around sensitive tissues, genital, or rectal areas. Inform prescriber if condition worsens (swelling, redness, irritation, pain, open sores) or fails to improve.

Geriatric Considerations: Because of the risk of adverse effects, systemic corticosteroids should be used cautiously in the elderly, in the smallest possible dose, and for the shortest possible time. Azmacort® (metered dose inhaler) comes with its own spacer device attached and may be easier to use in older patients.

Pregnancy Risk Factor: C

Pregnancy Issues: There are no adequate and well-controlled studies in pregnant women, however, triamcinolone is teratogenic in animals; use during pregnancy with caution. Increased incidence of cleft palate, neonatal adrenal suppression, low birth weight, and cataracts in the infant has been reported following corticosteroid use during pregnancy. In general, the use of large amounts, or prolonged use, of topical corticosteroids during pregnancy should be avoided. In the mother, corticosteroids may increase calcium and potassium excretion, elevate blood pressure, and cause salt and water retention.

Lactation: Excretion in breast milk unknown/use caution

Breast-Feeding Considerations: It is not known if triamcinolone is excreted in breast milk, however, other corticosteroids are excreted. Prednisone and prednisolone are excreted in breast milk; the AAP considers them to be "usually compatible" with breast-feeding. Hypertension was reported in a nursing infant when a topical corticosteroid was applied to the nipples of the mother.

Perioperative/Anesthesia/Other Concerns: Triamcinolone is a long-acting corticosteroid with minimal sodium-retaining potential.

Neuromuscular Effects: ICU-acquired paresis was recently studied in 5 ICUs (3 medical and 2 surgical ICUs) at 4 French hospitals. All ICU patients without pre-existing neuromuscular disease admitted from March 1999 through June 2000 were evaluated (De Jonghe B, 2002). Each patient had to be mechanically ventilated for ≥7 days and was screened daily for awakening. The first day the patient was considered awake was Study Day 1. Patients with severe muscle weakness on Study Day 7 were considered to have ICU-acquired paresis. Among the 95 patients who were evaluable, about 25% developed ICU-acquired paresis. Independent predictors included female gender, the number of days with ≥2 organ dysfunction, and administration of corticosteroids. Further studies may be required to verify and characterize the association between the development of ICU-acquired paresis and use of corticosteroids. Concurrent use of a corticosteroid and muscle relaxant appear to increase the risk of certain ICU myopathies; avoid or administer the corticosteroid at the lowest dose possible.

Adrenal Insufficiency: Patients will often have steroid-induced adverse effects on glucose tolerance and lipid profiles. When discontinuing steroid therapy in patients on long-term steroid supplementation, it is important that the steroid therapy be discontinued gradually. Abrupt withdrawal may result in adrenal insufficiency with hypotension and hyperkalemia. Patients on long-term steroid supplementation will require higher corticosteroid doses when subject to stress (ie, trauma, surgery, severe infection). Guidelines for glucocorticoid replacement during various surgical procedures have been published (Salem M, 1994, Coursin DB, 2002).

Septic Shock: A recent randomized, double-blind, placebo controlled trial assessed whether low dose corticosteroid administration could improve 28-day survival in patients with septic shock and relative adrenal insufficiency. Relative adrenal insufficiency was defined as an inappropriate response to corticotropin administration (increase of serum cortisol of ≤9 mcg/dL from baseline). Cortisol levels were drawn immediately before corticotropin administration and 30 to 60 minutes afterwards. Three hundred adult septic shock patients requiring mechanical ventilation and vasopressor support were randomized to either hydrocortisone (50 mg IVP every 6 hours) and fludrocortisone (50 mcg tablet daily via nasogastric tube) or matching placebos for 7 days. In patients who did not appropriately respond to corticotropin (nonresponders), there were significantly fewer deaths in the active treatment group. Vasopressor therapy was withdrawn more frequently in this subset of the active treatment group. Adverse events were similar in both groups. Patients who lack adrenal reserve and thus have relative adrenal insufficiency during the stress of septic shock may benefit from physiologic steroid replacement. However, there was a trend for increased mortality in patients who responded to the corticotropin test (increase serum cortisol >9 mcg/dL from baseline). These patients may not benefit from physiologic steroid replacement. Further study is required to better characterize the patient populations who may benefit.

Administration

Oral: Tablet: Once-daily doses should be given in the morning.

I.M.: Inject I.M. dose deep in large muscle mass, avoid deltoid.

Reconstitution: Injection, suspension: Hexacetonide: Avoid diluents containing parabens or preservatives (may cause flocculation). Diluted suspension stable ~1 week. Suspension for intralesional use, may be diluted with D_5NS, D_{10}NS or SWFI to a 1:1, 1:2, or 1:4 concentration. Solutions for intra-articular use, may be diluted with lidocaine 1% or 2%.

Storage: Store at room temperature. Avoid freezing.
Injection, suspension: Shake well prior to use.
Topical spray: Avoid excessive heat.

- **Triamcinolone Acetonide, Aerosol** *see* Triamcinolone *on page 1660*
- **Triamcinolone Acetonide, Parenteral** *see* Triamcinolone *on page 1660*
- **Triamcinolone Diacetate, Oral** *see* Triamcinolone *on page 1660*
- **Triamcinolone Diacetate, Parenteral** *see* Triamcinolone *on page 1660*
- **Triamcinolone Hexacetonide** *see* Triamcinolone *on page 1660*
- **Triamcinolone, Oral** *see* Triamcinolone *on page 1660*
- **Triaminic® Allerchews™[OTC]** *see* Loratadine *on page 1058*
- **Triaminic® Cough and Sore Throat Formula [OTC]** *see* Acetaminophen, Dextromethorphan, and Pseudoephedrine *on page 73*
- **Triaminic® Thin Strips™ Cough and Runny Nose [OTC]** *see* DiphenhydrAMINE *on page 546*
- **Triamterene and Hydrochlorothiazide** *see* Hydrochlorothiazide and Triamterene *on page 866*

Triazolam (trye AY zoe lam)

U.S. Brand Names Halcion®

Pharmacologic Category Hypnotic, Benzodiazepine

Medication Safety Issues

Sound-alike/look-alike issues:

Triazolam may be confused with alprazolam

Halcion® may be confused with halcinonide, Haldol®

Use Short-term treatment of insomnia

Mechanism of Action Binds to stereospecific benzodiazepine receptors on the postsynaptic GABA neuron at several sites within the central nervous system, including the limbic system, reticular formation. Enhancement of the inhibitory effect of GABA on neuronal excitability results by increased neuronal membrane permeability to chloride ions. This shift in chloride ions results in hyperpolarization (a less excitable state) and stabilization.

Pharmacodynamics/Kinetics

Onset of action: Hypnotic: 15-30 minutes

Duration: 6-7 hours

Distribution: V_d: 0.8-1.8 L/kg

Protein binding: 89%

Metabolism: Extensively hepatic

Half-life elimination: 1.7-5 hours

Excretion: Urine as unchanged drug and metabolites

Contraindications Hypersensitivity to triazolam or any component of the formulation (cross-sensitivity with other benzodiazepines may exist); concurrent therapy with atazanavir, ketoconazole, itraconazole, nefazodone, and ritonavir; pregnancy

Warnings/Precautions Should be used only after evaluation of potential causes of sleep disturbance. Failure of sleep disturbance to resolve after 7-10 days may indicate psychiatric or medical illness. A worsening of insomnia or the emergence of new abnormalities of thought or behavior may represent unrecognized psychiatric or medical illness and requires immediate and careful evaluation. Prescription should be written for a maximum of 7-10 days and should not be prescribed in quantities exceeding a 1-month supply. Abrupt discontinuation after sustained use (generally >10 days) may cause withdrawal symptoms.

An increase in daytime anxiety may occur after as few as 10 days of continuous use, which may be related to withdrawal reaction in some patients. Anterograde amnesia may occur at a higher rate with triazolam than with other benzodiazepines. Use with caution in elderly or debilitated patients, patients with hepatic disease (including alcoholics), or renal impairment. Use with caution in patients with respiratory disease or impaired gag reflex. Avoid use in patients with sleep apnea.

Causes CNS depression (dose-related) resulting in sedation, dizziness, confusion, or ataxia which may impair physical and mental capabilities. Patients must be cautioned about performing tasks which require mental alertness (eg, operating machinery or driving). Use with caution in patients receiving other CNS depressants or psychoactive agents. Effects with other sedative drugs or ethanol may be potentiated. Benzodiazepines have been associated with falls and traumatic injury and should be used with extreme caution in patients who are at risk of these events (especially the elderly).

Use caution with potent CYP3A4 inhibitors, as they may significantly decreased the clearance of triazolam. Use caution in patients with depression, particularly if suicidal risk may be present. Use with caution in patients with a history of drug dependence. Benzodiazepines have been associated with dependence and acute withdrawal symptoms on discontinuation or reduction in dose. Acute withdrawal, including seizures, may be precipitated after administration of flumazenil to patients receiving long-term benzodiazepine therapy.

Paradoxical reactions, including hyperactive or aggressive behavior have been reported with benzodiazepines, particularly in adolescent/pediatric or psychiatric patients. Does not have analgesic, antidepressant, or antipsychotic properties.

Drug Interactions **Substrate** of CYP3A4 (major); **Inhibits** CYP2C8/9 (weak)

CNS depressants: Sedative effects and/or respiratory depression may be additive with CNS depressants; includes ethanol, barbiturates, narcotic analgesics, and other sedative agents; monitor for increased effect

CYP3A4 inducers: CYP3A4 inducers may decrease the levels/effects of triazolam. Example inducers include aminoglutethimide, carbamazepine, nafcillin, nevirapine, phenobarbital, phenytoin, and rifamycins.

CYP3A4 inhibitors: May increase the levels/effects of triazolam. Example inhibitors include azole antifungals, clarithromycin, diclofenac, doxycycline, erythromycin, imatinib, isoniazid, nefazodone, nicardipine, propofol, protease inhibitors, quinidine, telithromycin, and verapamil.

Isoniazid: Isoniazid may increase triazolam levels.

Levodopa: Therapeutic effects may be diminished in some patients following the addition of a benzodiazepine; limited/inconsistent data

Oral contraceptives: May decrease the clearance and increase the half-life of triazolam; monitor for increased triazolam effect

Ranitidine: Ranitidine may increase triazolam levels.

Theophylline: May partially antagonize some of the effects of benzodiazepines; monitor for decreased response; may require higher doses for sedation

Nutritional/Herbal/Ethanol Interactions

Ethanol: Avoid ethanol (may increase CNS depression).

Food: Food may decrease the rate of absorption. Triazolam serum concentration may be increased by grapefruit juice; avoid concurrent use.

Herb/Nutraceutical: St John's wort may decrease levels. Avoid valerian, St John's wort, kava kava, gotu kola (may increase CNS depression).

Adverse Reactions

>10%: Central nervous system: Drowsiness, anteriograde amnesia

1% to 10%:

Central nervous system: Headache, dizziness, nervousness, lightheadedness, ataxia

Gastrointestinal: Nausea, vomiting

<1% (Limited to important or life-threatening): Confusion, depression, euphoria, memory impairment

Overdosage/Toxicology Symptoms of overdose include somnolence, confusion, coma, diminished reflexes, dyspnea, and hypotension. Treatment for benzodiazepine overdose is supportive. Flumazenil has been shown to selectively block the binding of benzodiazepines to CNS receptors, resulting in reversal of benzodiazepine-induced CNS depression but not always respiratory depression.

Dosing

Adults: Note: Onset of action is rapid, patient should be in bed when taking medication.

Insomnia (short-term): Oral: 0.125-0.25 mg at bedtime (maximum dose: 0.5 mg/day)

Dental (preprocedure): Oral: 0.25 mg taken the evening before oral surgery; or 0.25 mg 1 hour before procedure

Elderly: Oral: Insomnia (short-term use): 0.0625-0.125 mg at bedtime; maximum dose: 0.25 mg/day (see Geriatric Considerations)

Hepatic Impairment: Reduce dose or avoid use in cirrhosis.

Available Dosage Forms Tablet: 0.125 mg, 0.25 mg [contains sodium benzoate]

Nursing Guidelines

Assessment: Assess other medications patient may be taking for effectiveness and interactions. Assess for history of addiction; long-term use can result in dependence, abuse, or tolerance; periodically evaluate need for continued use. For inpatient use, institute safety measures and monitor effectiveness and adverse reactions. For outpatients, monitor therapeutic effectiveness and adverse reactions at beginning of therapy and periodically with long-term use. Monitor for CNS depression. Taper dosage slowly when discontinuing. Assess knowledge/teach patient appropriate use, interventions to reduce side effects, and adverse symptoms to report. **Pregnancy risk factor X:** Determine that patient is not pregnant before starting therapy. Do not give to sexually-active female patients unless capable of complying with contraceptive use.

Patient Education: Take exactly as directed; do not increase dose or frequency. Drug may cause physical and/or psychological dependence. Do not use alcohol or other prescription or OTC medications (especially pain medications, sedatives, antihistamines, or hypnotics) without consulting prescriber. Maintain adequate hydration (2-3 L/day of fluids) unless instructed to restrict fluid intake. You may experience drowsiness, lightheadedness, impaired coordination, dizziness, or blurred vision (use caution when driving or engaging in tasks requiring alertness until response to drug is known); nausea, vomiting, or dry mouth (small frequent meals, frequent mouth care, chewing gum, or sucking lozenges may help); constipation (increased exercise, fluids, fruit, or

(Continued)

Triazolam *(Continued)*

fiber may help); altered sexual drive or ability (reversible); or photosensitivity (use sunscreen, wear protective clothing and eyewear, and avoid direct sunlight). Report persistent CNS effects (eg, memory impairment, confusion, depression, increased sedation, excitation, headache, agitation, insomnia or nightmares, dizziness, fatigue, impaired coordination, changes in personality, or changes in cognition); changes in urinary pattern; muscle cramping, weakness, tremors, or rigidity; ringing in ears or visual disturbances; chest pain, palpitations, or rapid heartbeat; excessive perspiration; excessive GI symptoms (cramping, constipation, vomiting, anorexia); or worsening of condition. **Pregnancy/breast-feeding precautions:** Inform prescriber if you are pregnant. Do not get pregnant during or for 1 month following therapy. Consult prescriber for instruction on appropriate contraceptive measures. This drug may cause severe fetal defects. Breast-feeding is not recommended.

Geriatric Considerations: Due to the higher incidence of CNS adverse reactions and its short half-life, this benzodiazepine is not a drug of first choice. For short-term only.

Pregnancy Risk Factor: X

Pregnancy Issues: Benzodiazepines cross the placenta. The association between benzodiazepine exposure and malformations remains controversial. A number of types of malformation have been reported (oral cleft, inguinal hernia, cardiac defects, spina bifida, dysmorphic facial features, skeletal defects); however, confounding factors make a clear association difficult. Overall, the risk to the fetus may be low. Nonteratogenic effects (including neonatal flaccidity, respiratory and feeding problems, and withdrawal symptoms) during the postnatal period have also been reported with benzodiazepine use.

Lactation: Excretion in breast milk unknown/not recommended

Breast-Feeding Considerations: It is not known if triazolam is excreted in breast milk; however, other benzodiazepines are known to be excreted in breast milk. The AAP rates use of related agents as "of concern" and breast-feeding is not recommended.

Perioperative/Anesthesia/Other Concerns: Chronic use of this agent may increase the perioperative benzodiazepine dose needed to achieve desired effect. Abrupt discontinuation after sustained use (generally >10 days) may cause withdrawal symptoms.

Administration

Oral: May take with food. Tablet may be crushed or swallowed whole. Onset of action is rapid, patient should be in bed when taking medication.

- ♦ **Tribavirin** *see* Ribavirin *on page 1475*
- ♦ **Trichloroacetaldehyde Monohydrate** *see* Chloral Hydrate *on page 368*
- ♦ **TriCor®** *see* Fenofibrate *on page 708*
- ♦ **Tricosal** *see* Choline Magnesium Trisalicylate *on page 385*
- ♦ **Triderm®** *see* Triamcinolone *on page 1660*
- ♦ **Triglide™** *see* Fenofibrate *on page 708*
- ♦ **Trileptal®** *see* Oxcarbazepine *on page 1278*
- ♦ **Trilisate® [DSC]** *see* Choline Magnesium Trisalicylate *on page 385*
- ♦ **Trimazide [DSC]** *see* Trimethobenzamide *on page 1668*

Trimethobenzamide (trye meth oh BEN za mide)

U.S. Brand Names Tebamide™; Tigan®; Trimazide [DSC]

Synonyms Trimethobenzamide Hydrochloride

Pharmacologic Category Anticholinergic Agent; Antiemetic

Medication Safety Issues

Sound-alike/look-alike issues:

Tigan® may be confused with Tiazac®, Ticar®

Use Treatment of nausea and vomiting

Mechanism of Action Acts centrally to inhibit the medullary chemoreceptor trigger zone

Pharmacodynamics/Kinetics

Onset of action: Antiemetic: Oral: 10-40 minutes; I.M.: 15-35 minutes
Duration: 3-4 hours
Absorption: Rectal: ~60%
Bioavailability: Oral: 60% to 100%
Half-life elimination: 7-9 hours
Time to peak: Oral: 45 minutes; I.M.: 30 minutes

Excretion: Urine (30% to 50%)

Contraindications Hypersensitivity to trimethobenzamide, benzocaine (or similar local anesthetics), or any component of the formulation; injection contraindicated in children; suppositories contraindicated in premature infants or neonates

Warnings/Precautions May mask emesis due to Reye's syndrome or mimic CNS effects of Reye's syndrome in patients with emesis of other etiologies; use in patients with acute vomiting should be avoided. May cause drowsiness; patient should avoid tasks requiring alertness (eg, driving, operating machinery). May cause extrapyramidal symptoms (EPS) which may be confused with CNS symptoms of primary disease responsible for emesis. Risk of adverse effects (eg, EPS, seizure) may be increased in patients with acute febrile illness, dehydration, or electrolyte imbalance; use caution.

Nutritional/Herbal/Ethanol Interactions Ethanol: Concomitant use should be avoided (sedative effects may be additive).

Adverse Reactions Frequency not defined.

Cardiovascular: Hypotension

Central nervous system: Coma, depression, disorientation, dizziness, drowsiness, EPS, headache, opisthotonos, Parkinson-like syndrome, seizure

Gastrointestinal: Diarrhea

Hematologic: Blood dyscrasias

Hepatic: Jaundice

Neuromuscular & skeletal: Muscle cramps

Ocular: Blurred vision

Miscellaneous: Hypersensitivity reactions

Overdosage/Toxicology Symptoms of overdose include hypotension, seizures, CNS depression, cardiac arrhythmias, disorientation, and confusion. Treatment is symptom-directed and supportive.

Dosing

Adults & Elderly:

Nausea, vomiting:

Oral: 300 mg 3-4 times/day

I.M., rectal: 200 mg 3-4 times/day

Postoperative nausea and vomiting (PONV): I.M.: 200 mg, followed 1 hour later by a second 200 mg dose

Pediatrics: Note: Rectal use is contraindicated in neonates and premature infants.

Nausea, vomiting: Oral, rectal: Children:

<14 kg: 100 mg 3-4 times/day

14-40 kg: 100-200 mg 3-4 times/day

Available Dosage Forms

Capsule, as hydrochloride (Tigan®): 300 mg

Injection, solution, as hydrochloride: 100 mg/mL (2 mL)

Tigan®: 100 mg/mL (2 mL [preservative free], 20 mL)

Suppository, rectal, as hydrochloride: 100 mg, 200 mg

Tebamide™: 100 mg, 200 mg [contains benzocaine]

Tigan®, Trimazide [DSC]: 200 mg [contains benzocaine]

Nursing Guidelines

Assessment: Assess therapeutic effectiveness, and adverse reactions with first dose and on a regular basis during therapy (eg, hypovolemia, angioedema, postural hypotension). Teach patient appropriate use (if self-administered injection, teach injection technique and syringe disposal), possible side effects/ interventions, and adverse symptoms to report.

Patient Education: Do not take any new medication during therapy unless approved by prescriber. Take capsule as directed before meals; do not increase dose and do not discontinue without consulting prescriber. If using injection formulation, follow directions for injection and disposal of syringe. Follow directions for insertion of rectal suppositories. May cause drowsiness or blurred vision (use caution when driving or engaging in tasks that require alertness until response to drug is known) or diarrhea (buttermilk or yogurt may help). Report chest pain or palpitations, persistent dizziness or blurred vision, or CNS changes (disorientation, depression, confusion). **Pregnancy/ breast-feeding precautions:** Inform prescriber if you are or intend to become pregnant. Consult prescriber if breast-feeding.

(Continued)

Trimethobenzamide *(Continued)*

Pregnancy Risk Factor: C

Lactation: Excretion in breast milk unknown

Administration

I.M.: Administer I.M. only. Inject deep into upper outer quadrant of gluteal muscle.

I.V.: Not for I.V. administration.

Storage: Store capsules, injection solution, and suppositories at room temperature.

Related Information

Postoperative Nausea and Vomiting *on page 1807*

- Trimethobenzamide Hydrochloride *see* Trimethobenzamide *on page 1668*

Trimethoprim and Polymyxin B

(trye METH oh prim & pol i MIKS in bee)

U.S. Brand Names Polytrim®

Synonyms Polymyxin B and Trimethoprim

Pharmacologic Category Antibiotic, Ophthalmic

Use Treatment of surface ocular bacterial conjunctivitis and blepharoconjunctivitis

Pharmacodynamics/Kinetics See individual agents.

Contraindications Hypersensitivity to trimethoprim, polymyxin B, or any component of the formulation

Drug Interactions Trimethoprim: **Substrate** (major) of CYP2C8/9, 3A4; **Inhibits** CYP2C8/9 (moderate)

Also see individual agents.

Adverse Reactions 1% to 10%: Local: Burning, stinging, itching, increased redness

Dosing

Adults & Elderly: Conjunctivitis, blepharoconjunctivitis: Ophthalmic: Instill 1-2 drops in eye(s) every 4-6 hours

Available Dosage Forms Solution, ophthalmic: Trimethoprim 1 mg and polymyxin B sulfate 10,000 units per mL (10 mL) [contains benzalkonium chloride]

Nursing Guidelines

Patient Education: Avoid contamination of the applicator tip; contact prescriber if redness, swelling, pain, or irritation persists.

Pregnancy Risk Factor: C

- Trimethoprim and Sulfamethoxazole *see* Sulfamethoxazole and Trimethoprim *on page 1582*
- Trimox® *see* Amoxicillin *on page 144*
- Tri-Nasal® *see* Triamcinolone *on page 1660*
- Trinate *see* Vitamins (Multiple/Prenatal) *on page 1721*
- TriNessa™ *see* Ethinyl Estradiol and Norgestimate *on page 689*
- Trinsicon® *see* Vitamin B Complex Combinations *on page 1716*
- Triple Antibiotic *see* Bacitracin, Neomycin, and Polymyxin B *on page 220*
- Triple Sulfa *see* Sulfabenzamide, Sulfacetamide, and Sulfathiazole *on page 1578*
- Tri-Previfem™ *see* Ethinyl Estradiol and Norgestimate *on page 689*

Triprolidine and Pseudoephedrine

(trye PROE li deen & soo doe e FED rin)

U.S. Brand Names Actifed® Cold and Allergy [OTC]; Allerfrim® [OTC]; Aphedrid™ [OTC]; Aprodine® [OTC]; Genac® [OTC]; Silafed® [OTC]; Sudafed® Sinus Nighttime [OTC]; Tri-Sudo® [OTC]

Synonyms Pseudoephedrine and Triprolidine

Pharmacologic Category Alpha/Beta Agonist; Antihistamine

Medication Safety Issues

Sound-alike/look-alike issues:

Aprodine® may be confused with Aphrodyne®

Use Temporary relief of nasal congestion, decongest sinus openings, running nose, sneezing, itching of nose or throat and itchy, watery eyes due to common cold, hay fever, or other upper respiratory allergies

Mechanism of Action Refer to Pseudoephedrine monograph

Triprolidine is a member of the propylamine (alkylamine) chemical class of H_1-antagonist antihistamines. As such, it is considered to be relatively less sedating than traditional antihistamines of the ethanolamine, phenothiazine, and ethylenediamine classes of antihistamines. Triprolidine has a shorter half-life and duration of action than most of the other alkylamine antihistamines. Like all H_1-antagonist antihistamines, the mechanism of action of triprolidine is believed to involve competitive blockade of H_1-receptor sites resulting in the inability of histamine to combine with its receptor sites and exert its usual effects on target cells. Antihistamines do not interrupt any effects of histamine which have already occurred. Therefore, these agents are used more successfully in the prevention rather than the treatment of histamine-induced reactions.

Pharmacodynamics/Kinetics See Pseudoephedrine monograph.

Contraindications Hypersensitivity to pseudoephedrine or any component of the formulation; MAO therapy, hypertension, coronary artery disease

Warnings/Precautions Not recommended for OTC use for longer than 7 days or if symptoms are accompanied by fever. Consult healthcare provider prior to OTC use with heart disease, hypotension, thyroid disease, diabetes, emphysema, chronic bronchitis, glaucoma, or enlarged prostate. Not for OTC use in children <6 years of age.

Drug Interactions Triprolidine: **Inhibits** CYP2D6 (weak)

Decreased effect of guanethidine, reserpine, methyldopa

Increased toxicity with MAO inhibitors (hypertensive crisis), sympathomimetics, CNS depressants, ethanol (sedation)

Adverse Reactions Frequency not defined.

Cardiovascular: Tachycardia

Central nervous system: Drowsiness, nervousness, insomnia, transient stimulation, headache, fatigue, dizziness

Respiratory: Thickening of bronchial secretions, pharyngitis

Gastrointestinal: Appetite increase, weight gain, nausea, diarrhea, abdominal pain, xerostomia

Genitourinary: Dysuria

Neuromuscular & skeletal: Arthralgia, weakness

Miscellaneous: Diaphoresis

Dosing

Adults & Elderly: Cold, allergy symptoms: Oral:

Syrup: 10 mL every 4-6 hours; do not exceed 4 doses in 24 hours

Tablet: 1 every 4-6 hours; do not exceed 4 doses in 24 hours

Pediatrics: Cold, allergy symptoms: Oral:

Children <12 years:

Syrup:

4 months to 2 years: 1.25 mL 3-4 times/day

2-4 years: 2.5 mL 3-4 times/day

4-6 years: 3.75 mL 3-4 times/day

6-12 years: 5 mL every 4-6 hours; do not exceed 4 doses in 24 hours

Tablet: 1/2 every 4-6 hours; do not exceed 4 doses in 24 hours

Children ≥12 years: Refer to adult dosing.

Available Dosage Forms

Syrup: Triprolidine hydrochloride 1.25 mg and pseudoephedrine hydrochloride 30 mg per 5 mL (120 mL)

Allerfrim®: Triprolidine hydrochloride 1.25 mg and pseudoephedrine hydrochloride 30 mg per 5 mL (120 mL, 480 mL) [contains sodium benzoate]

Aprodine®: Triprolidine hydrochloride 1.25 mg and pseudoephedrine hydrochloride 30 mg per 5 mL (120 mL)

Silafed®: Triprolidine hydrochloride 1.25 mg and pseudoephedrine hydrochloride 30 mg per 5 mL (120 mL, 240 mL)

Tablet (Actifed® Cold and Allergy, Allerfrim®, Aphedrid™, Aprodine®, Genac®, Tri-Sudo®): Triprolidine hydrochloride 2.5 mg and pseudoephedrine hydrochloride 60 mg

Nursing Guidelines

Patient Education: May impair ability to perform hazardous activities requiring mental alertness

Pregnancy Risk Factor: C

- **TripTone® [OTC]** *see* DimenhyDRINATE *on page 544*
- **Trisenox™** *see* Arsenic Trioxide *on page 184*
- **Tri-Sprintec™** *see* Ethinyl Estradiol and Norgestimate *on page 689*
- **Tri-Sudo® [OTC]** *see* Triprolidine and Pseudoephedrine *on page 1670*
- **Trivalent Inactivated Influenza Vaccine (TIV)** *see* Influenza Virus Vaccine *on page 913*
- **Tri-Vi-Flor®** *see* Vitamins (Multiple/Pediatric) *on page 1720*
- **Tri-Vi-Flor® with Iron** *see* Vitamins (Multiple/Pediatric) *on page 1720*

◆ Tri-Vi-Sol® [OTC] *see* Vitamins (Multiple/Pediatric) *on page 1720*
◆ Tri-Vi-Sol® with Iron [OTC] *see* Vitamins (Multiple/Pediatric) *on page 1720*
◆ Trizivir® *see* Abacavir, Lamivudine, and Zidovudine *on page 58*
◆ Trocaine® [OTC] *see* Benzocaine *on page 232*
◆ Tronolane® Suppository [OTC] *see* Phenylephrine *on page 1350*
◆ Tropicacyl® *see* Tropicamide *on page 1672*

Tropicamide (troe PIK a mide)

U.S. Brand Names Mydral™; Mydriacyl®; Tropicacyl®

Synonyms Bistropamide

Pharmacologic Category Ophthalmic Agent, Mydriatic

Use Short-acting mydriatic used in diagnostic procedures; as well as preoperatively and postoperatively; treatment of some cases of acute iritis, iridocyclitis, and keratitis

Mechanism of Action Prevents the sphincter muscle of the iris and the muscle of the ciliary body from responding to cholinergic stimulation

Pharmacodynamics/Kinetics

Onset of action: Mydriasis: ~20-40 minutes; Cycloplegia: ~30 minutes

Duration: Mydriasis: ~6-7 hours; Cycloplegia: <6 hours

Contraindications Hypersensitivity to tropicamide or any component of the formulation; glaucoma

Warnings/Precautions Use with caution in infants and children since tropicamide may cause potentially dangerous CNS disturbances; tropicamide may cause an increase in intraocular pressure

Adverse Reactions Frequency not defined.

Cardiovascular: Edema, tachycardia, vascular congestion

Central nervous system: Headache, parasympathetic stimulations, somnolence

Dermatologic: Eczematoid dermatitis

Gastrointestinal: Dryness of the mouth

Local: Transient stinging

Ocular: Blurred vision, follicular conjunctivitis, increased intraocular pressure, photophobia with or without corneal staining

Overdosage/Toxicology

Symptoms of overdose include blurred vision, urinary retention, tachycardia, cardiorespiratory collapse

Antidote is physostigmine, pilocarpine; anticholinergic toxicity is caused by strong binding of the drug to cholinergic receptors. For anticholinergic overdose with severe life-threatening symptoms, physostigmine 1-2 mg (0.5 mg or 0.02 mg/kg for children) SubQ or I.V., slowly may be given to reverse systemic effects.

Dosing

Adults & Elderly: Note: Individuals with heavily pigmented eyes may require larger doses:

Cycloplegia: Ophthalmic: Instill 1-2 drops (1%); may repeat in 5 minutes

Exam must be performed within 30 minutes after the repeat dose; if the patient is not examined within 20-30 minutes, instill an additional drop

Mydriasis: Ophthalmic: Instill 1-2 drops (0.5%) 15-20 minutes before exam; may repeat every 30 minutes as needed

Pediatrics: Refer to adult dosing.

Available Dosage Forms

Solution, ophthalmic: 0.5% (15 mL); 1% (2 mL, 15 mL) [contains benzalkonium chloride]

Mydriacyl®: 1% (3 mL, 15 mL) [contains benzalkonium chloride]

Mydral™, Tropicacyl®: 0.5% (15 mL); 1% (15 mL) [contains benzalkonium chloride]

Nursing Guidelines

Patient Education: If irritation persists or increases, discontinue use, may cause blurred vision and increased light sensitivity

Pregnancy Risk Factor: C

◆ Trusopt® *see* Dorzolamide *on page 567*
◆ TST *see* Tuberculin Tests *on page 1673*
◆ T-Stat® [DSC] *see* Erythromycin *on page 634*
◆ Tuberculin Purified Protein Derivative *see* Tuberculin Tests *on page 1673*
◆ Tuberculin Skin Test *see* Tuberculin Tests *on page 1673*

Tuberculin Tests (too BER kyoo lin tests)

U.S. Brand Names Aplisol®; Tubersol®

Synonyms Mantoux; PPD; Tine Test; TST; Tuberculin Purified Protein Derivative; Tuberculin Skin Test

Pharmacologic Category Diagnostic Agent

Medication Safety Issues

Sound-alike/look-alike issues:

Aplisol® may be confused with Anusol®, A.P.L.®, Aplitest®, Atropisol®

Tuberculin products may be confused with tetanus toxoid products and influenza virus vaccine. Medication errors have occurred when tuberculin skin tests (PPD) have been inadvertently administered instead of tetanus toxoid products and influenza virus vaccine. These products are refrigerated and often stored in close proximity to each other.

Use Skin test in diagnosis of tuberculosis, cell-mediated immunodeficiencies

Mechanism of Action Tuberculosis results in individuals becoming sensitized to certain antigenic components of the *M. tuberculosis* organism. Culture extracts called tuberculins are contained in tuberculin skin test preparations. Upon intracutaneous injection of these culture extracts, a classic delayed (cellular) hypersensitivity reaction occurs. This reaction is characteristic of a delayed course (peak occurs >24 hours after injection, induration of the skin secondary to cell infiltration, and occasional vesiculation and necrosis). Delayed hypersensitivity reactions to tuberculin may indicate infection with a variety of nontuberculosis mycobacteria, or vaccination with the live attenuated mycobacterial strain of *M. bovis* vaccine, BCG, in addition to previous natural infection with *M. tuberculosis*.

Pharmacodynamics/Kinetics

Onset of action: Delayed hypersensitivity reactions: 5-6 hours

Peak effect: 48-72 hours

Duration: Reactions subside over a few days

Contraindications 250 TU strength should not be used for initial testing

Warnings/Precautions Do not administer I.V. or SubQ; epinephrine (1:1000) should be available to treat possible allergic reactions

Drug Interactions Decreased effect: Reaction may be suppressed in patients receiving systemic corticosteroids, aminocaproic acid, or within 4-6 weeks following immunization with live or inactivated viral vaccines

Adverse Reactions Frequency not defined.

Dermatologic: Ulceration, necrosis, vesiculation

Local: Pain at injection site

Dosing

Adults & Elderly:

Diagnosis of tuberculosis, cell-mediated immunodeficiencies: Intradermal: 0.1 mL about 4" below elbow; use 1/4" to 1/2" or 26- or 27-gauge needle; significant reactions are ≥5 mm in diameter

Interpretation of induration of tuberculin skin test injections: Positive: ≥10 mm; inconclusive: 5-9 mm; negative: <5 mm

Interpretation of induration of Tine test injections: Positive: >2 mm and vesiculation present; inconclusive: <2 mm (give patient Mantoux test of 5 TU/0.1 mL - base decisions on results of Mantoux test); negative: <2 mm or erythema of any size (no need for retesting unless person is a contact of a patient with tuberculosis or there is clinical evidence suggestive of the disease)

Pediatrics: Refer to adult dosing.

Available Dosage Forms Injection, solution: 5 TU/0.1 mL (1 mL, 5 mL)

Nursing Guidelines

Patient Education: Return to physician for reaction interpretation at 48-72 hours

Pregnancy Risk Factor: C

Administration

Storage: Refrigerate; Tubersol® opened vials are stable for up to 24 hours at <75°F

- Tubersol® *see* Tuberculin Tests *on page 1673*
- Tucks® Anti-Itch [OTC] *see* Hydrocortisone *on page 873*
- Tums® [OTC] *see* Calcium Carbonate *on page 291*
- Tums® 500 [OTC] *see* Calcium Carbonate *on page 291*
- Tums® E-X [OTC] *see* Calcium Carbonate *on page 291*

- Tums® Extra Strength Sugar Free [OTC] *see* Calcium Carbonate *on page 291*
- Tums® Smooth Dissolve [OTC] *see* Calcium Carbonate *on page 291*
- Tums® Ultra [OTC] *see* Calcium Carbonate *on page 291*
- Tussin [OTC] *see* Guaifenesin *on page 834*
- Tussi-Organidin® NR *see* Guaifenesin and Codeine *on page 835*
- Tussi-Organidin® S-NR *see* Guaifenesin and Codeine *on page 835*
- T-Vites [OTC] *see* Vitamins (Multiple/Oral) *on page 1720*
- Twelve Resin-K *see* Cyanocobalamin *on page 457*
- Twilite® [OTC] *see* DiphenhydrAMINE *on page 546*
- Twinject™ *see* Epinephrine *on page 611*
- Tylenol® [OTC] *see* Acetaminophen *on page 65*
- Tylenol® 8 Hour [OTC] *see* Acetaminophen *on page 65*
- Tylenol® Arthritis Pain [OTC] *see* Acetaminophen *on page 65*
- Tylenol® Children's [OTC] *see* Acetaminophen *on page 65*
- Tylenol® Cold Day Non-Drowsy [OTC] *see* Acetaminophen, Dextromethorphan, and Pseudoephedrine *on page 73*
- Tylenol® Extra Strength [OTC] *see* Acetaminophen *on page 65*
- Tylenol® Flu Non-Drowsy Maximum Strength [OTC] *see* Acetaminophen, Dextromethorphan, and Pseudoephedrine *on page 73*
- Tylenol® Infants [OTC] *see* Acetaminophen *on page 65*
- Tylenol® Junior [OTC] *see* Acetaminophen *on page 65*
- Tylenol® Sore Throat [OTC] *see* Acetaminophen *on page 65*
- Tylenol® With Codeine *see* Acetaminophen and Codeine *on page 68*
- Tylox® *see* Oxycodone and Acetaminophen *on page 1286*
- UCB-P071 *see* Cetirizine *on page 366*
- UK *see* Urokinase *on page 1674*
- Ulcerease® [OTC] *see* Phenol *on page 1347*
- Ultane® *see* Sevoflurane *on page 1526*
- Ultiva® *see* Remifentanil *on page 1467*
- Ultracet™ *see* Acetaminophen and Tramadol *on page 70*
- Ultra Freeda Iron Free [OTC] *see* Vitamins (Multiple/Oral) *on page 1720*
- Ultra Freeda with Iron [OTC] *see* Vitamins (Multiple/Oral) *on page 1720*
- Ultram® *see* Tramadol *on page 1652*
- Ultra NatalCare® *see* Vitamins (Multiple/Prenatal) *on page 1721*
- Ultraprin [OTC] *see* Ibuprofen *on page 889*
- Ultrase® *see* Pancrelipase *on page 1301*
- Ultrase® MT *see* Pancrelipase *on page 1301*
- Ultra Tears® [OTC] *see* Artificial Tears *on page 187*
- Unasyn® *see* Ampicillin and Sulbactam *on page 163*
- Unicap M® [OTC] *see* Vitamins (Multiple/Oral) *on page 1720*
- Unicap Sr® [OTC] *see* Vitamins (Multiple/Oral) *on page 1720*
- Unicap T™ [OTC] *see* Vitamins (Multiple/Oral) *on page 1720*
- Uniphyl® *see* Theophylline *on page 1619*
- Uni-Senna [OTC] *see* Senna *on page 1520*
- Unisom® Maximum Strength SleepGels® [OTC] *see* DiphenhydrAMINE *on page 546*
- Unithroid® *see* Levothyroxine *on page 1029*
- Urea Peroxide *see* Carbamide Peroxide *on page 311*
- Uristat® [OTC] *see* Phenazopyridine *on page 1342*

Urokinase (yoor oh KIN ase)

U.S. Brand Names Abbokinase® [DSC]

Synonyms UK

Pharmacologic Category Thrombolytic Agent

Use Thrombolytic agent for the lysis of acute massive pulmonary emboli or pulmonary emboli with unstable hemodynamics

Unlabeled/Investigational Use Thrombolytic agent used in treatment of recent severe or massive deep vein thrombosis, myocardial infarction, and occluded I.V. or dialysis cannulas

Mechanism of Action Promotes thrombolysis by directly activating plasminogen to plasmin, which degrades fibrin, fibrinogen, and other procoagulant plasma proteins

Pharmacodynamics/Kinetics

Onset of action: I.V.: Fibrinolysis occurs rapidly

Duration: ≥4 hours

Distribution: 11.5 L

Half-life elimination: 6.4-18.8 minutes

Excretion: Urine and feces (small amounts)

Contraindications Hypersensitivity to urokinase or any component of the formulation; active internal bleeding; history of CVA; recent (within 2 months) intracranial or intraspinal surgery or trauma; intracranial neoplasm, arteriovenous malformation, or aneurysm; known bleeding diathesis; severe uncontrolled hypertension

Warnings/Precautions Concurrent heparin anticoagulation can contribute to bleeding; careful attention to all potential bleeding sites. I.M. injections and nonessential handling of the patient should be avoided. Venipunctures should be performed carefully and only when necessary. If arterial puncture is necessary, use an upper extremity vessel that can be manually compressed. If serious bleeding occurs, then the infusion of urokinase and heparin should be stopped.

For the following conditions the risk of bleeding is higher with use of thrombolytics and should be weighed against the benefits of therapy: recent (within 10 days) major surgery (eg, CABG, obstetrical delivery, organ biopsy, previous puncture of noncompressible vessels), cerebrovascular disease, recent (within 10 days) gastrointestinal or genitourinary bleeding, recent trauma (within 10 days) including CPR, hypertension (systolic BP >180 mm Hg and/or diastolic BP >110 mm Hg), high likelihood of left heart thrombus (eg, mitral stenosis with atrial fibrillation), acute pericarditis, subacute bacterial endocarditis, hemostatic defects including ones caused by severe renal or hepatic dysfunction, significant hepatic dysfunction, pregnancy, diabetic hemorrhagic retinopathy or other hemorrhagic ophthalmic conditions, septic thrombophlebitis or occluded AV cannula at seriously infected site, advanced age (eg, >75 years), patients receiving oral anticoagulants, any other condition in which bleeding constitutes a significant hazard or would be particularly difficult to manage because of location.

Coronary thrombolysis may result in reperfusion arrhythmias. Follow standard MI management. Rare anaphylactoid reactions can occur. Formulated in human albumin; products made from human sources have a theoretical risk of transmitting infectious agents. Safety and efficacy in pediatric patients have not been established.

Drug Interactions

Aminocaproic acid (antifibrinolytic agent) may decrease effectiveness.

Drugs which affect platelet function (eg, aspirin, NSAIDs, dipyridamole, ticlopidine, clopidogrel, IIb/IIIa antagonists) may potentiate the risk of hemorrhage; use with caution.

Heparin: Concurrent use may increase risk of bleeding; use caution.

Warfarin or oral anticoagulants: Risk of bleeding may be increased during concurrent therapy.

Adverse Reactions As with all drugs which may affect hemostasis, bleeding is the major adverse effect associated with urokinase. Hemorrhage may occur at virtually any site. Risk is dependent on multiple variables, including the dosage administered, concurrent use of multiple agents which alter hemostasis, and patient predisposition.

>10%: Local: Injection site: Bleeding (5% decrease in hematocrit reported in 37% patients; most bleeding occurring at external incisions or injection sites, but also reported in other areas)

<1% (Limited to important or life-threatening): Allergic reaction (includes bronchospasm, orolingual edema, urticaria, skin rash, pruritus); cardiac arrest, cerebral vascular accident, chest pain, cholesterol embolism, diaphoresis, hemiplegia, intracranial hemorrhage, retroperitoneal hemorrhage, MI, pulmonary edema, recurrent pulmonary embolism, reperfusion ventricular arrhythmia, stroke, substernal pain, thrombocytopenia, vascular embolization (cerebral and distal); infusion reactions (most occurring within 1 hour) including acidosis, back pain, chills, cyanosis, dyspnea, fever, hyper-/hypotension, hypoxia, nausea, rigors, tachycardia, vomiting

Overdosage/Toxicology Symptoms of overdose include epistaxis, bleeding gums, hematoma, spontaneous ecchymoses, and oozing at the catheter site. In

(Continued)

Urokinase *(Continued)*

the event of overdose, stop the infusion and reverse bleeding with blood products that contain clotting factors.

Dosing

Adults & Elderly:

Acute pulmonary embolism: I.V.: Loading: 4400 int. units/kg over 10 minutes; maintenance: 4400 int. units/kg/hour for 12 hours. Following infusion, anticoagulation treatment is recommended to prevent recurrent thrombosis. Do not start anticoagulation until aPTT has decreased to less than twice the normal control value. If heparin is used, do not administer loading dose. Treatment should be followed with oral anticoagulants.

Deep vein thrombosis (unlabeled use): I.V.: Loading: 4400 units/kg over 10 minutes, then 4400 units/kg/hour for 12 hours

Myocardial infarction (unlabeled use): Intracoronary: 750,000 units over 2 hours (6000 units/minute over up to 2 hours)

Occluded I.V. catheters (unlabeled use):

5000 units in each lumen over 1-2 minutes, leave in lumen for 1-4 hours, then aspirate. May repeat with 10,000 units in each lumen if 5000 units fails to clear the catheter. **Do not infuse into the patient**. Volume to instill into catheter is equal to the volume of the catheter. Will not dissolve drug precipitate or anything other than blood products.

I.V. infusion: 200 units/kg/hour in each lumen for 12-48 hours at a rate of at least 20 mL/hour

Dialysis patient: 5000 units is administered in each lumen over 1-2 minutes; leave urokinase in lumen for 1-2 days, then aspirate.

Pediatrics: Children: Deep vein thrombosis, pulmonary embolus, or occluded catheter: I.V.: Refer to adult dosing.

Available Dosage Forms [DSC] = Discontinued product

Injection, powder for reconstitution: 250,000 int. units [contains human albumin 250 mg and mannitol 25 mg] [DSC]

Nursing Guidelines

Assessment: See Contraindications, Warnings/Precautions, and Dosing for use cautions. Assess potential for interactions with other prescriptions, OTC medications, or herbal products patient may be taking (especially those medications that may affect coagulation or platelet function - see Drug Interactions). Note infusion specifics below; assess infusion site and monitor for systemic hemorrhage during and following therapy (see Adverse Reactions and Overdose/Toxicology). Assess results of laboratory results (see below). Patient should be monitored closely prior to, during, and after therapy (eg, neurological status - intracranial hemorrhage; vital signs; and ECG - reperfusion arrhythmias). Bedrest and bleeding precautions should be maintained. Avoid I.M. injections and nonessential handling of the patient. Venipunctures should be performed carefully and only when necessary. If arterial puncture is necessary, use an upper extremity vessel that can be manually compressed. Patient instructions are determined by patient condition (see Patient Education). Note breast-feeding caution.

Monitoring Laboratory Tests: CBC, platelet count, aPTT, urinalysis

Patient Education: Inform prescriber of all prescriptions, OTC medications, or herbal products you are taking, and any allergies you have. This medication can only be administered by infusion; you will be monitored closely during and after treatment; immediately report burning, pain, redness, swelling, or oozing at infusion site, acute headache, joint pain, chest pain, or altered vision. You will have a tendency to bleed easily; use caution to prevent injury (use electric razor, soft toothbrush, and caution with knives, needles, or anything sharp). Follow instructions for strict bedrest to reduce the risk of injury. If bleeding occurs, report immediately and apply pressure to bleeding spot until bleeding stops completely. Report chest pain, palpitations, irregular heartbeat; unusual bruising or bleeding; blood in urine, stool, or vomiting; bleeding gums; muscle pain; or respiratory difficulty. **Breast-feeding precaution:** Consult prescriber if breast-feeding.

Pregnancy Risk Factor: B

Lactation: Excretion in breast milk unknown/use caution

Perioperative/Anesthesia/Other Concerns: When using thrombolytic therapy in an institution, it is important that the protocol for that institution be followed closely, particularly in terms of dosage, adjunctive heparin therapy, and standard myocardial infarction therapy (eg, aspirin, beta-blocker, ACE inhibitor). Preceding recent thrombolytic therapy must be taken into account when invasive procedures (particularly intravascular procedures) are undertaken. Close clinical monitoring is required to ensure efficacy of therapy. Failure of therapy may require emergent cardiac catheterization and interventional therapy. Reperfusion after successful thrombolysis may be associated with rapid resolution of ECG changes and restoration of cardiac function. However, reperfusion arrhythmias may also manifest.

Administration

I.V.: Solution may be filtered using a 0.22 or 0.45 micron filter during I.V. therapy. Administer using a pump which can deliver a total volume of 195 mL. The loading dose should be administered at 90 mL/hour over 10 minutes. The maintenance dose should be administered at 15 mL/hour over 12 hours. I.V. tubing should be flushed with NS or D_5W to ensure total dose is administered.

Reconstitution: Reconstitute vial with 5 mL sterile water for injection (preservative free) by gently rolling and tilting; do not shake. Contains no preservatives; should not be reconstituted until immediately before using; discard unused portion. Solution will look pale and straw colored. May filter through ≤0.45 micron filter.

Compatibility: Stable in NS

Storage: Prior to reconstitution, store in refrigerator at 2°C to 8°C (36°F to 46°F). Prior to infusion, solution should be further diluted in D_5W or NS.

♦ Uro-KP-Neutral® *see* Potassium Phosphate and Sodium Phosphate *on page 1391*

♦ Urolene Blue® *see* Methylene Blue *on page 1134*

♦ UTI Relief® [OTC] *see* Phenazopyridine *on page 1342*

♦ Vagifem® *see* Estradiol *on page 649*

♦ Vagi-Gard® [OTC] *see* Povidone-Iodine *on page 1392*

Valdecoxib (val de KOKS ib)

U.S. Brand Names Bextra® *[Withdrawn from Market]*

Pharmacologic Category Nonsteroidal Anti-inflammatory Drug (NSAID), COX-2 Selective

Use Relief of signs and symptoms of osteoarthritis and adult rheumatoid arthritis; treatment of primary dysmenorrhea

Mechanism of Action Inhibits prostaglandin synthesis by decreasing the activity of the enzyme, cyclooxygenase-2 (COX-2), which results in decreased formation of prostaglandin precursors. Does not affect platelet function.

Pharmacodynamics/Kinetics

Onset of action: Dysmenorrhea: 60 minutes

Distribution: V_d: 86 L

Protein binding: 98%

Metabolism: Extensively hepatic via CYP3A4 and 2C9; glucuronidation; forms metabolite (active)

Bioavailability: 83%

Half-life elimination: 8-11 hours

Time to peak: 2.25-3 hours

Excretion: Primarily urine (as metabolites)

Contraindications Hypersensitivity to valdecoxib, sulfonamides, or any component of the formulation; patients who have experienced asthma, urticaria, or allergic-type reactions to aspirin or NSAIDs; acute pain following CABG; pregnancy (3rd trimester)

Warnings/Precautions Gastrointestinal irritation, ulceration, bleeding, and perforation may occur with NSAIDs (it is unclear whether valdecoxib is associated with rates of these events which are similar to nonselective NSAIDs). Use with caution in patients with a history of GI disease (bleeding or ulcers) or risk factor for GI bleeding, use lowest dose for shortest time possible. Anaphylactic/anaphylactoid reactions may occur, even with no prior exposure to valdecoxib. Serious dermatologic reactions (including life-threatening Stevens-Johnson syndrome and erythema multiforme) have been reported; discontinue immediately in any patients who develop rash or any signs of hypersensitivity. Risk may be greatest in the first 2 weeks of therapy and in patients with prior sulfonamide allergy. Use with caution in patients with decreased renal function, hepatic disease, CHF, hypertension, fluid retention, dehydration, or asthma. Carefully evaluate individual cardiovascular risk profiles prior to prescribing COX-2 inhibitors. COX-2 inhibitors may not be appropriate in patients with cardiovascular disease or in patients with significant risk factors for cardiovascular disease. Use caution in patients with known or suspected deficiency of cytochrome P450 isoenzyme 2C9. Use in

(Continued)

Valdecoxib *(Continued)*

patients with severe hepatic impairment (Child-Pugh Class C) is not recommended. Use in patients following CABG has been associated with an increase in thromboembolic events, including MI, stroke, DVT, and PE. Safety and efficacy have not been established for patients <18 years of age.

Drug Interactions Substrate (minor) of CYP2C8/9, 3A4; **Inhibits** CYP2C8/9 (weak), 2C19 (weak)

ACE inhibitors: Antihypertensive effects may be decreased by concurrent therapy with NSAIDs; monitor blood pressure.

Angiotensin II antagonists: Antihypertensive effects may be decreased by concurrent therapy with NSAIDs; monitor blood pressure.

Anticoagulants (warfarin, heparin, LMWHs): In combination with NSAIDs, can cause increased risk of bleeding.

Antiplatelet drugs (ticlopidine, clopidogrel, aspirin, abciximab, dipyridamole, eptifibatide, tirofiban): Can cause an increased risk of bleeding.

Azole antifungals: May increase valdecoxib concentrations.

Corticosteroids: May increase the risk of GI ulceration; avoid concurrent use

Cyclosporine: NSAIDs may increase serum creatinine, potassium, blood pressure, and cyclosporine levels; monitor cyclosporine levels and renal function carefully.

Hydralazine: Antihypertensive effect is decreased; avoid concurrent use

Lithium levels can be increased; avoid concurrent use if possible or monitor lithium levels and adjust dose. When NSAID is stopped, lithium will need adjustment again.

Loop diuretics: Diuretic and antihypertensive efficacy is reduced. May be anticipated with any NSAID.

Methotrexate: Severe bone marrow suppression, aplastic anemia, and GI toxicity have been reported with concomitant NSAID therapy. Selective COX-2 inhibitors appear to have a lower risk of this toxicity, however, caution is warranted.

Thiazides: Diuretic efficacy is reduced.

Warfarin: Valdecoxib (40 mg twice daily) may increase plasma warfarin exposure (12% R-warfarin, 15% S-warfarin). May increase the anticoagulant effects of warfarin. Monitor INR closely.

Nutritional/Herbal/Ethanol Interactions

Ethanol: Avoid ethanol (may enhance gastric mucosal irritation).

Food: Time to peak level is delayed by 1-2 hours when taken with high-fat meal, but other parameters are unaffected.

Herb/Nutraceutical: Avoid cat's claw, dong quai, evening primrose, feverfew, garlic, ginger, ginkgo, red clover, horse chestnut, green tea, ginseng (may cause increased risk of bleeding).

Adverse Reactions

2% to 10%:

Cardiovascular: Peripheral edema (2% to 3%), hypertension (2%)

Central nervous system: Headache (5% to 9%), dizziness (3%)

Dermatologic: Rash (1% to 2%)

Gastrointestinal: Dyspepsia (8% to 9%), abdominal pain (7% to 8%), nausea (6% to 7%), diarrhea (5% to 6%), flatulence (3% to 4%), abdominal fullness (2%)

Neuromuscular & skeletal: Back pain (2% to 3%), myalgia (2%)

Otic: Earache, tinnitus

Respiratory: Upper respiratory tract infection (6% to 7%), sinusitis (2% to 3%)

Miscellaneous: Influenza-like symptoms (2%)

<2% (Limited to important or life threatening): Allergy, anaphylaxis, aneurysm, angina, angioedema, aortic stenosis, arrhythmia, atrial fibrillation, bradycardia, breast neoplasm, cardiomyopathy, carotid stenosis, colitis, CHF, convulsion, coronary thrombosis, depression exacerbation, diabetes mellitus, diverticulosis, duodenal ulcer, emphysema, erythema multiforme, esophageal perforation, exfoliative dermatitis, facial edema, gastric ulcer, gastroesophageal reflux, gastrointestinal bleeding, gout, heart block, hepatitis, hiatal hernia, hyperlipemia, hyperparathyroidism, hypertension exacerbation, hypertensive encephalopathy, hypotension, impotence, intermittent claudication, liver function tests increased, lymphadenopathy, lymphangitis, lymphopenia, migraine, mitral insufficiency, MI, myocardial ischemia, neuropathy, osteoporosis, ovarian cyst (malignant), pancreatitis, pericarditis, periorbital swelling, photosensitivity, pneumonia, rash (erythematous, maculopapular, psoriaform), Stevens-Johnson syndrome, syncope, tachycardia, thrombocytopenia, thrombophlebitis, toxic

epidermal necrolysis, unstable angina, urinary tract infection, vaginal hemorrhage, ventricular fibrillation, vertigo

Overdosage/Toxicology Symptoms of overdose may include epigastric pain, drowsiness, lethargy, nausea, and vomiting; gastrointestinal bleeding may occur. Rare manifestations include hypertension, respiratory depression, coma, and acute renal failure. Treatment is symptomatic and supportive. Forced diuresis, hemodialysis, hemoperfusion, and/or urinary alkalinization may not be useful.

Dosing

Adults & Elderly:

Osteoarthritis and rheumatoid arthritis: Oral: 10 mg once daily; **Note:** No additional benefits seen with 20 mg/day

Primary dysmenorrhea: Oral: 20 mg twice daily as needed

Pediatrics: Not indicated for pediatric patients.

Renal Impairment: Not recommended for use in advanced disease.

Hepatic Impairment: Not recommended for use in advanced liver dysfunction (Child-Pugh Class C).

Available Dosage Forms Tablet: 10 mg, 20 mg

Nursing Guidelines

Assessment: Evaluate cardiac risk and potential for GI bleeding prior to prescribing this medication. Assess effectiveness and interactions of other prescription, OTC, or herbal medication patient may be taking. Assess allergy history (salicylates, NSAIDs). Monitor blood pressure at the beginning of therapy and periodically during use. Monitor for effectiveness of therapy and adverse reactions. Assess knowledge/teach patient appropriate use, interventions to reduce possible side effects, and adverse symptoms to report.

Dietary Considerations: May be taken with or without food.

Patient Education: Use exactly as directed. May be taken with food to reduce GI upset. Do not take with antacids. Avoid alcohol, aspirin, or other medication unless approved by prescriber. Maintain adequate hydration (2-3 L/day of fluids) unless instructed to restrict fluid intake. GI bleeding, ulceration, or perforation can occur with or without pain. Stop taking medication and report immediately abdominal tenderness, stomach pain or cramping; unusual bleeding or bruising; or blood in vomitus, stool, or urine. You may experience dizziness, confusion, or blurred vision (avoid driving or engaging in tasks requiring alertness until response to drug is known); or anorexia, nausea, vomiting (small frequent meals, frequent mouth care, chewing gum or sucking lozenges may help). Report any skin rash, muscle aches, unusual fatigue, lethargy, yellowing of skin or eyes, flu-like symptoms, easy bruising or bleeding, sudden weight gain, changes in urinary pattern, respiratory difficulty, shortness of breath, chest pain, or signs of upper respiratory infection. **Pregnancy/breast-feeding precautions:** Inform prescriber if you are or intend to become pregnant. This drug should not be used in the 3rd trimester of pregnancy. Breast-feeding is not recommended.

Geriatric Considerations: The elderly are at increased risk for adverse effects from NSAIDs. As many as 60% of elderly can develop peptic ulceration and/or hemorrhage asymptomatically. CNS adverse effects such as confusion, agitation, and hallucination are generally seen in overdose or high-dose situations; however, elderly patients may demonstrate these adverse effects at lower doses than younger adults. The elderly are also at increased risk of renal toxicity.

Pregnancy Risk Factor: C/D (3rd trimester)

Pregnancy Issues: Use should be avoided in late pregnancy because it may cause premature closure of the ductus arteriosus.

Lactation: Excretion in breast milk unknown/not recommended

Perioperative/Anesthesia/Other Concerns: Valdecoxib does not inhibit platelets or prolong bleeding time.

Administration

Oral: Avoid dehydration. Encourage patient to drink plenty of fluids.

Storage: Store at 15°C to 30°C (59°F to 86°F).

♦ 23-Valent Pneumococcal Polysaccharide Vaccine *see* Pneumococcal Polysaccharide Vaccine (Polyvalent) *on page 1378*

♦ Valium® *see* Diazepam *on page 515*

♦ Valorin [OTC] *see* Acetaminophen *on page 65*

♦ Valorin Extra [OTC] *see* Acetaminophen *on page 65*

♦ Valproate Semisodium *see* Valproic Acid and Derivatives *on page 1680*

♦ Valproate Sodium *see* Valproic Acid and Derivatives *on page 1680*

♦ **Valproic Acid** *see* Valproic Acid and Derivatives *on page 1680*

Valproic Acid and Derivatives

(val PROE ik AS id & dah RIV ah tives)

U.S. Brand Names Depacon®; Depakene®; Depakote® Delayed Release; Depakote® ER; Depakote® Sprinkle®

Synonyms Dipropylacetic Acid; Divalproex Sodium; DPA; 2-Propylpentanoic Acid; 2-Propylvaleric Acid; Valproate Semisodium; Valproate Sodium; Valproic Acid

Pharmacologic Category Anticonvulsant, Miscellaneous

Medication Safety Issues

Sound-alike/look-alike issues:

Depakene® may be confused with Depakote®

Depakote® may be confused with Depakene®, Depakote® ER, Senokot®

Use Monotherapy and adjunctive therapy in the treatment of patients with complex partial seizures; monotherapy and adjunctive therapy of simple and complex absence seizures; adjunctive therapy patients with multiple seizure types that include absence seizures; treatment of acute or mixed manic episodes associated with bipolar disorder; migraine prophylaxis

Mania associated with bipolar disorder (Depakote®)

Migraine prophylaxis (Depakote®, Depakote® ER)

Unlabeled/Investigational Use Behavior disorders (eg, agitation, aggression) in patients with dementia (based on the results of several randomized, controlled trials, there is little evidence to support this use); status epilepticus

Mechanism of Action Causes increased availability of gamma-aminobutyric acid (GABA), an inhibitory neurotransmitter, to brain neurons or may enhance the action of GABA or mimic its action at postsynaptic receptor sites

Pharmacodynamics/Kinetics

Distribution: Total valproate: 11 L/1.73 m^2; free valproate 92 L/1.73 m^2

Protein binding (dose dependent): 80% to 90%

Metabolism: Extensively hepatic via glucuronide conjugation and mitochondrial beta-oxidation. The relationship between dose and total valproate concentration is nonlinear; concentration does not increase proportionally with the dose, but increases to a lesser extent due to saturable plasma protein binding. The kinetics of unbound drug are linear.

Bioavailability: Extended release: 90% of I.V. dose and 81% to 90% of delayed release dose

Half-life elimination: (increased in neonates and with liver disease): Children: 4-14 hours; Adults: 9-16 hours

Time to peak, serum: 1-4 hours; Divalproex (enteric coated): 3-5 hours

Excretion: Urine (30% to 50% as glucuronide conjugate, 3% as unchanged drug)

Contraindications Hypersensitivity to valproic acid, derivatives, or any component of the formulation; hepatic dysfunction; urea cycle disorders

Warnings/Precautions Hepatic failure resulting in fatalities has occurred in patients; children <2 years of age are at considerable risk; other risk factors include organic brain disease, mental retardation with severe seizure disorders, congenital metabolic disorders, and patients on multiple anticonvulsants. Hepatotoxicity has been reported after 3 days to 6 months of therapy. Monitor patients closely for appearance of malaise, weakness, facial edema, anorexia, jaundice, and vomiting; may cause severe thrombocytopenia, inhibition of platelet aggregation and bleeding; tremors may indicate overdosage; use with caution in patients receiving other anticonvulsants.

Cases of life-threatening pancreatitis, occurring at the start of therapy or following years of use, have been reported in adults and children. Some cases have been hemorrhagic with rapid progression of initial symptoms to death.

May cause teratogenic effects such as neural tube defects (eg, spina bifida). Use in women of childbearing potential requires that benefits of use in mother be weighed against the potential risk to fetus, especially when used for conditions not associated with permanent injury or risk of death (eg, migraine).

Hyperammonemic encephalopathy, sometimes fatal, has been reported following the initiation of valproate therapy in patients with known or suspected urea cycle disorders (UCD), particularly those with ornithine transcarbamylase deficiency. Although a rare genetic disorder, UCD evaluation should be considered for the following patients, prior to the start of therapy: History of unexplained encephalopathy or coma; encephalopathy associated with protein load; pregnancy or postpartum encephalopathy; unexplained mental retardation; history of elevated plasma ammonia or glutamine; history of cyclical vomiting and lethargy; episodic extreme irritability, ataxia; low BUN or protein avoidance; family history of UCD or unexplained infant deaths (particularly male); signs or symptoms of UCD (hyperammonemia, encephalopathy, respiratory alkalosis). Patients who develop symptoms of hyperammonemic encephalopathy during therapy with valproate should receive prompt evaluation for UCD and valproate should be discontinued.

Hyperammonemia may occur with therapy and may be present with normal liver function tests. Ammonia levels should be measured in patients who develop unexplained lethargy and vomiting, or changes in mental status. Discontinue therapy if ammonia levels are increased and evaluate for possible UCD.

In vitro studies have suggested valproate stimulates the replication of HIV and CMV viruses under experimental conditions. The clinical consequence of this is unknown, but should be considered when monitoring affected patients.

Anticonvulsants should not be discontinued abruptly because of the possibility of increasing seizure frequency; valproate should be withdrawn gradually to minimize the potential of increased seizure frequency, unless safety concerns require a more rapid withdrawal. Concomitant use with clonazepam may induce absence status.

CNS depression may occur with valproate use. Patients must be cautioned about performing tasks which require mental alertness (operating machinery or driving). Effects with other sedative drugs or ethanol may be potentiated.

Drug Interactions For valproic acid: **Substrate** (minor) of CYP2A6, 2B6, 2C8/9, 2C19, 2E1; **Inhibits** CYP2C8/9 (weak), 2C19 (weak), 2D6 (weak), 3A4 (weak); **Induces** CYP2A6 (weak)

Carbamazepine: Valproic acid may increase, decrease, or have no effect on carbamazepine levels; valproic acid may increase serum concentrations of carbamazepine - epoxide (active metabolite); valproic acid may induce the metabolism of carbamazepine; monitor.

Carbapenem antibiotics (ertapenem, imipenem, meropenem): May decrease valproic acid concentrations to subtherapeutic levels; monitor.

Felbamate: May increase the levels/effects of valproic acid; monitor.

Isoniazid: May decrease valproic acid metabolism (limited documentation).

Lamotrigine: Valproic acid inhibits the metabolism of lamotrigine; combination therapy has been proposed to increase the risk of toxic epidermal necrolysis; monitor.

Macrolide antibiotics: May decrease valproic acid metabolism (limited documentation); includes clarithromycin, erythromycin, troleandomycin; monitor.

Primidone, phenobarbital: Valproic acid appears to inhibit the metabolism of phenobarbital; monitor for increased effect.

Salicylates: May displace valproic acid from plasma proteins, leading to acute toxicity.

Tricyclic antidepressants: Valproate may increase serum concentrations and/or toxicity of tricyclic antidepressants.

Zidovudine: Valproic acid may increase the levels/effects of zidovudine; monitor.

Nutritional/Herbal/Ethanol Interactions

Ethanol: Avoid ethanol (may increase CNS depression).

Food: Food may delay but does not affect the extent of absorption. Valproic acid serum concentrations may be decreased if taken with food. Milk has no effect on absorption.

Herb/Nutraceutical: Avoid evening primrose (seizure threshold decreased)

Lab Interactions Valproic acid may cause abnormalities in liver function tests; false-positive result for urine ketones; accuracy of thyroid function tests

Adverse Reactions

Adverse reactions reported when used as monotherapy for complex partial seizure:

>10%:

Central nervous system: Headache (up to 31%), somnolence (7% to 30%), dizziness (12% to 25%), insomnia (1% to 15%), nervousness (1% to 11%), pain (up to 11%)

Dermatologic: Alopecia (6% to 24%)

Gastrointestinal: Nausea (15% to 48%), vomiting (7% to 27%), diarrhea (7% to 23%), abdominal pain (7% to 23%), dyspepsia (7% to 23%), anorexia (11% to 12%)

Hematologic: Thrombocytopenia (1% to 24%)

Neuromuscular & skeletal: Tremor (1% to 57%), weakness (6% to 27%)

Ocular: Diplopia (up to 16%), amblyopia/blurred vision (8% to 12%)

Miscellaneous: Infection (1% to 20%), flu-like symptoms (1% to 12%)

(Continued)

Valproic Acid and Derivatives *(Continued)*

1% to 10%:

Cardiovascular: Arrhythmia, chest pain, edema, hyper-/hypotension, palpitation, peripheral edema (1% to 8%), postural hypotension, tachycardia, vasodilatation

Central nervous system: Abnormal dreams, agitation, amnesia (5% to 7%), anxiety, catatonic reaction, chills, confusion, depression, emotional lability, hallucinations, hypokinesia, malaise, personality disorder, psychosis, reflexes increased, sleep disorder, speech disorder, tardive dyskinesia, thinking abnormal (up to 6%), vertigo

Dermatologic: Bruising, discoid lupus erythematosus, dry skin, erythema nodosum, furunculosis, macropapular rash, petechia, pruritus, rash, seborrhea, vesiculobullous rash

Endocrine & metabolic: Amenorrhea, dysmenorrhea, hypoproteinemia, metrorrhagia

Gastrointestinal: Dysphagia, eructation, fecal incontinence, flatulence, gastroenteritis, glossitis, gum hemorrhage, hematemesis, appetite increased, mouth ulceration, pancreatitis, periodontal abscess, taste perversion, weight gain (1% to 9%), stomatitis, constipation, dry mouth, tooth disorder, weight loss (up to 6%)

Genitourinary: Cystitis, urinary frequency, urinary incontinence, UTI, vaginitis

Hematologic: Anemia, bleeding time increased, leukopenia

Hepatic: AST/ALT increased

Neuromuscular & skeletal: Abnormal gait, arthralgia, arthrosis, ataxia (up to 8%), back pain (1% to 8%), hypertonia, leg cramps, myalgia, myasthenia, neck rigidity, paresthesia, twitching

Ocular: Abnormal vision, conjunctivitis, dry eye, eye pain, nystagmus (7% to 8%), photophobia

Otic: Deafness, otitis media, tinnitus (1% to 7%)

Respiratory: Bronchitis, epistaxis, hiccup, increased cough, pneumonia, rhinitis, sinusitis

Additional adverse effects: Frequency not defined:

Cardiovascular: Bradycardia

Central nervous system: Aggression, behavioral deterioration, cerebral atrophy (reversible), dementia, encephalopathy (rare), hostility, hyperactivity, hypoesthesia, parkinsonism

Dermatologic: Cutaneous vasculitis, erythema multiforme, photosensitivity, Stevens-Johnson syndrome, toxic epidermal necrolysis (rare)

Endocrine & metabolic: Breast enlargement, galactorrhea, hyperammonemia, hyponatremia, inappropriate ADH secretion, parotid gland swelling, polycystic ovary disease (rare), abnormal thyroid function tests

Genitourinary: Enuresis

Hematologic: Anemia, aplastic anemia, bone marrow suppression, eosinophilia, hematoma formation, hemorrhage, hypofibrinogenemia, intermittent porphyria, lymphocytosis, macrocytosis, pancytopenia

Hepatic: Bilirubin increased, hyperammonemic encephalopathy (in patients with UCD)

Neuromuscular & skeletal: Asterixis, bone pain, dysarthria

Ocular: Seeing 'spots before the eyes'

Renal: Fanconi-like syndrome (rare, in children)

Miscellaneous: Anaphylaxis, carnitine decreased, hyperglycinemia, lupus

Postmarketing and/or case reports: Life-threatening pancreatitis (2 cases out of 2416 patients), occurring at the start of therapy or following years of use, has been reported in adults and children. Some cases have been hemorrhagic with rapid progression of initial symptoms to death. Cases have also been reported upon rechallenge.

Overdosage/Toxicology Symptoms of overdose include coma, deep sleep, motor restlessness, and visual hallucinations. Supportive treatment is necessary. Naloxone has been used to reverse CNS depressant effects, but may block the action of other anticonvulsants.

Dosing

Adults & Elderly:

Seizures:

Oral: Initial: 10-15 mg/kg/day in 1-3 divided doses; increase by 5-10 mg/kg/day at weekly intervals until therapeutic levels are achieved; maintenance: 30-60 mg/kg/day. Adult usual dose: 1000-2500 mg/day. **Note:** Regular release and delayed release formulations are usually given in 2-4 divided doses/day, extended release formulation (Depakote® ER) is usually given once daily. Conversion to Depakote® ER from a stable dose of Depakote® may require an increase in the total daily dose between 8% and 20% to maintain similar serum concentrations.

I.V.: Administer as a 60-minute infusion (≤20 mg/minute) with the same frequency as oral products; switch patient to oral products as soon as possible. Alternatively, rapid infusions have been given: ≤15 mg/kg over 5-10 minutes (1.5-3 mg/kg/minute).

Rectal (unlabeled): Dilute syrup 1:1 with water for use as a retention enema; loading dose: 17-20 mg/kg one time; maintenance: 10-15 mg/kg/dose every 8 hours

Status epilepticus (unlabeled use):

Loading dose: I.V.: 15-25 mg/kg administered at 3 mg/kg/minute

Maintenance dose: I.V. infusion: 1-4 mg/kg/hour; titrate dose as needed based upon patient response and evaluation of drug-drug interactions

Mania:

Oral: 750-1500 mg/day in divided doses; dose should be adjusted as rapidly as possible to desired clinical effect; a loading dose of 20 mg/kg may be used; maximum recommended dosage: 60 mg/kg/day

Extended release tablets: Initial: 25 mg/kg/day given once daily; dose should be adjusted as rapidly as possible to desired clinical effect; maximum recommended dose: 60 mg/kg/day.

Migraine prophylaxis: Oral:

Extended release tablets: 500 mg once daily for 7 days, then increase to 1000 mg once daily; adjust dose based on patient response; usual dosage range 500-1000 mg/day

Delayed release tablets: 250 mg twice daily; adjust dose based on patient response, up to 1000 mg/day

Pediatrics: Seizures: Oral, I.V., Rectal: Children ≥10 years: Refer to adult dosing.

Renal Impairment: A 27% reduction in clearance of unbound valproate is seen in patients with Cl_{cr} <10 mL/minute. Hemodialysis reduces valproate concentrations by 20%, therefore no dose adjustment is needed in patients with renal failure. Protein binding is reduced, monitoring only total valproate concentrations may be misleading.

Hepatic Impairment: Dosage reduction is required. Clearance is decreased with liver impairment. Hepatic disease is also associated with decreased albumin concentrations and 2- to 2.6-fold increase in the unbound fraction. Free concentrations of valproate may be elevated while total concentrations appear normal.

Available Dosage Forms Note: Strength expressed as valproic acid

Capsule, as valproic acid (Depakene®): 250 mg

Capsule, sprinkles, as divalproex sodium (Depakote® Sprinkle®): 125 mg

Injection, solution, as valproate sodium (Depacon®): 100 mg/mL (5 mL) [contains edetate disodium]

Syrup, as valproic acid: 250 mg/5 mL (480 mL)

Depakene®: 250 mg/5 mL (480 mL)

Tablet, delayed release, as divalproex sodium (Depakote®): 125 mg, 250 mg, 500 mg

Tablet, extended release, as divalproex sodium (Depakote® ER): 250 mg, 500 mg

Nursing Guidelines

Assessment: Assess effectiveness and interactions of other medications patient may be taking. **I.V.:** Keep patient under observation, observe safety/seizure precautions, and monitor therapeutic effectiveness (type of seizure activity, force, and duration). Monitor vital signs; neurological, cardiac, and respiratory status. For outpatients, monitor therapeutic effect, laboratory values, and adverse reactions at beginning of therapy and periodically with long-term use. Taper dosage slowly when discontinuing. Assess knowledge/teach patient seizure safety precautions, appropriate use, interventions to reduce side effects, and adverse symptoms to report. **Note:** Valproic acid will alter results of urine ketones (use serum glucose testing) and reduce effectiveness of oral contraceptives (use alternative form of contraception to prevent pregnancy). Some adverse reactions including hepatic failure and thrombocytopenia can occur 3 days to 6 months after beginning therapy.

Monitoring Laboratory Tests: Liver enzymes, CBC with platelets, PT/PTT, serum ammonia (with symptoms of lethargy, mental status change)

(Continued)

Valproic Acid and Derivatives *(Continued)*

Dietary Considerations: Valproic acid may cause GI upset; take with large amount of water or food to decrease GI upset. May need to split doses to avoid GI upset.

Coated particles of divalproex sodium may be mixed with semisolid food (eg, applesauce or pudding) in patients having difficulty swallowing; particles should be swallowed and not chewed

Valproate sodium oral solution will generate valproic acid in carbonated beverages and may cause mouth and throat irritation; do not mix valproate sodium oral solution with carbonated beverages; sodium content of valproate sodium syrup (5 mL): 23 mg (1 mEq)

Patient Education: When used to treat generalized seizures, patient instructions are determined by patient's condition and ability to understand. **Oral:** Take as directed; do not alter dose or timing of medication. Do not increase dose or take more than recommended. Do not crush or chew capsule or enteric-coated pill. While using this medication, do not use alcohol and other prescription or OTC medications (especially pain medications, sedatives, antihistamines, or hypnotics) without consulting prescriber. Maintain adequate hydration (2-3 L/day of fluids) unless instructed to restrict fluid intake. If you have diabetes, monitor serum glucose closely (valproic acid will alter results of urine ketones). Report alterations in menstrual cycle; abdominal cramps, unresolved diarrhea, vomiting, or constipation; skin rash; unusual bruising or bleeding; blood in urine, stool, or vomitus; malaise; weakness; facial swelling; yellowing of skin or eyes; persistent abdominal pain; excessive sedation; or restlessness. **Pregnancy/breast-feeding precautions:** Do not get pregnant while taking this medication; use appropriate contraceptive measures. Consult prescriber if breast-feeding.

Pregnancy Risk Factor: D

Pregnancy Issues: Crosses the placenta. Neural tube, cardiac, facial (characteristic pattern of dysmorphic facial features), skeletal, multiple other defects reported. Epilepsy itself, number of medications, genetic factors, or a combination of these probably influence the teratogenicity of anticonvulsant therapy. Risk of neural tube defects with use during first 30 days of pregnancy warrants discontinuation prior to pregnancy and through this period of possible. Use in women of childbearing potential requires that benefits of use in mother be weighed against the potential risk to fetus, especially when used for conditions not associated with permanent injury or risk of death (eg, migraine).

Lactation: Enters breast milk/use caution (AAP considers "compatible")

Breast-Feeding Considerations: Crosses into breast milk. AAP considers **compatible** with breast-feeding.

Perioperative/Anesthesia/Other Concerns: Extended release tablets have 10% to 20% less fluctuation in serum concentration than delayed release tablets. Extended release tablets are not bioequivalent to delayed release tablets.

Symptoms of overdose include coma, somnolence, motor restlessness, visual hallucinations, and heart block. Naloxone has been used to reverse toxic CNS depressant effects but may block anticonvulsant effects.

Administration

Oral: Do not crush delayed release or extended release drug product or capsules.

I.V.: Depacon®: Following dilution to final concentration, administer over 60 minutes at a rate of ≤20 mg/minute. Alternatively, single doses up to 15 mg/kg have been administered as a rapid infusion over 5-10 minutes (1.5-3 mg/kg/minute).

Reconstitution: Injection should be diluted in 50 mL of a compatible diluent; is physically compatible and chemically stable in D_5W, NS, and LR for at least 24 hours when stored in glass or PVC.

Storage: Store vials at room temperature 15°C to 30°C (59°F to 86°F).

Related Information

Perioperative Management of Patients on Antiseizure Medication *on page 1801*

Valsartan (val SAR tan)

U.S. Brand Names Diovan®

Pharmacologic Category Angiotensin II Receptor Blocker

Medication Safety Issues

Sound-alike/look-alike issues:

Valsartan may be confused with losartan, Valstar™

Diovan® may be confused with Darvon®, Dioval®, Zyban®

Use Alone or in combination with other antihypertensive agents in the treatment of essential hypertension; treatment of heart failure (NYHA Class II-IV); reduction of cardiovascular mortality in patients with left ventricular dysfunction postmyocardial infarction

Mechanism of Action Valsartan produces direct antagonism of the angiotensin II (AT2) receptors, unlike the ACE inhibitors. It displaces angiotensin II from the AT1 receptor and produces its blood pressure lowering effects by antagonizing AT1-induced vasoconstriction, aldosterone release, catecholamine release, arginine vasopressin release, water intake, and hypertrophic responses. This action results in more efficient blockade of the cardiovascular effects of angiotensin II and fewer side effects than the ACE inhibitors.

Pharmacodynamics/Kinetics

Onset of antihypertensive effect: 2 weeks (maximal: 4 weeks)
Distribution: V_d: 17 L (adults)
Protein binding: 95%, primarily albumin
Metabolism: To inactive metabolite
Bioavailability: 25% (range 10% to 35%)
Half-life elimination: 6 hours
Time to peak, serum: 2-4 hours
Excretion: Feces (83%) and urine (13%) as unchanged drug

Contraindications Hypersensitivity to valsartan or any component of the formulation; hypersensitivity to other A-II receptor antagonists; bilateral renal artery stenosis; pregnancy (2nd and 3rd trimesters)

Warnings/Precautions During the initiation of therapy, hypertension may occur, particularly in patients with heart failure or post-MI patients. Avoid use or use a smaller dose in patients who are volume depleted; correct depletion first.

Deterioration in renal function can occur with initiation. Use with caution in unilateral renal artery stenosis and pre-existing renal insufficiency; significant aortic/mitral stenosis. Use caution in patients with severe renal impairment or significant hepatic dysfunction. Monitor renal function closely in patients with severe heart failure; changes in renal function should be anticipated and dosage adjustments of valsartan or concomitant medications may be needed.

Drug Interactions Inhibits CYP2C8/9 (weak)

Lithium: Risk of toxicity may be increased by valsartan; monitor lithium levels.

NSAIDs: May decrease angiotensin II antagonist efficacy; effect has been seen with losartan, but may occur with other medications in this class; monitor blood pressure

Potassium-sparing diuretics (amiloride, potassium, spironolactone, triamterene): Increased risk of hyperkalemia.

Potassium supplements may increase the risk of hyperkalemia.

Trimethoprim (high dose) may increase the risk of hyperkalemia.

Nutritional/Herbal/Ethanol Interactions

Food: Decreases rate and extent of absorption by 50% and 40%, respectively.

Herb/Nutraceutical: Avoid dong quai if using for hypertension (has estrogenic activity). Avoid ephedra, yohimbe, ginseng (may worsen hypertension). Avoid garlic (may have increased antihypertensive effect).

Adverse Reactions

>10%: Central nervous system: Dizziness (2% to 17%)

1% to 10%:

- Cardiovascular: Hypotension (6% to 7%), postural hypotension (2%)
- Central nervous system: Fatigue (2% to 3%)
- Endocrine & metabolic: Serum potassium increased (4% to 10%), hyperkalemia (<1% to 2%)
- Gastrointestinal: Diarrhea (5%), abdominal pain (2%)
- Hematologic: Neutropenia (2%)
- Neuromuscular & skeletal: Arthralgia (3%), back pain (3%)
- Renal: Creatinine increased >50% (4%)
- Respiratory: Cough (3%)
- Miscellaneous: Viral infection (3%)

All indications:

<1% (Limited to important or life-threatening): Allergic reactions, anemia, angioedema, anorexia, anxiety, asthenia, back pain, chest pain, constipation, dyspepsia, dyspnea, flatulence, hematocrit/hemoglobin decreased, hepatitis, impaired renal function, impotence, insomnia, muscle cramps, myalgia, palpitation, paresthesia, pruritus, rhabdomyolysis (rare), rash, renal dysfunction, somnolence, syncope, transaminases increased, vertigo, vomiting, xerostomia

(Continued)

Valsartan *(Continued)*

Overdosage/Toxicology Only mild toxicity (hypotension, bradycardia, hyperkalemia) has been reported with large overdoses (up to 5 g of captopril and 300 mg of enalapril). No fatalities have been reported. Treatment is symptomatic. Not removed by hemodialysis.

Dosing

Adults & Elderly:

Hypertension: Initial: 80 mg or 160 mg once daily (in patients who are not volume depleted); dose may be increased to achieve desired effect; maximum recommended dose: 320 mg/day

Heart failure: Initial: 40 mg twice daily; titrate dose to 80-160 mg twice daily, as tolerated; maximum daily dose: 320 mg

Left ventricular dysfunction after MI: Initial: 20 mg twice daily; titrate dose to target of 160 mg twice daily as tolerated; may initiate ≥12 hours following MI

Renal Impairment:

Cl_{cr} >10 mL/minute: No dosage adjustment necessary.

Dialysis: Not significantly removed.

Hepatic Impairment: Mild to moderate liver disease: ≤80 mg/day

Available Dosage Forms Tablet: 40 mg, 80 mg, 160 mg, 320 mg

Nursing Guidelines

Assessment: Use caution with volume depletion, impaired renal or hepatic function, aortic/mitral stenosis. Assess effectiveness and interactions of other pharmacological agents and herbal products patients may be taking (eg, concurrent use of potassium supplements, ACE inhibitors, potassium-sparing diuretics may increase risk of hyperkalemia). Assess results of laboratory tests at baseline and periodically. Monitor therapeutic effectiveness (reduced hypertension) and adverse response on a regular basis during therapy (eg, dizziness, bradycardia, cough, headache, nausea, hypotension, hyperkalemia). Teach patient appropriate use according to drug form and purpose of therapy, possible side effects/appropriate interventions, and adverse symptoms to report.

Monitoring Laboratory Tests: Baseline and periodic electrolyte panels, renal and liver function, urinalysis

Dietary Considerations: Avoid salt substitutes which contain potassium. May be taken with or without food.

Patient Education: Do not take any new medication during therapy unless approved by prescriber (especially sleep remedies or antisleep, cough or cold remedies, or weight loss products). Take exactly as directed and do not discontinue without consulting prescriber. This drug does not eliminate need for diet or exercise regimen as recommended by prescriber. May cause dizziness, fainting, or lightheadedness (use caution when driving or engaging in tasks that require alertness until response to drug is known); postural hypotension (use caution when rising from lying or sitting position or climbing stairs); diarrhea (boiled milk, buttermilk, or yogurt may help); or decreased libido (will resolve). Report chest pain or palpitations; unrelenting headache; swelling of extremities, face, or tongue; muscle weakness or pain; respiratory difficulty or unusual cough; flu-like symptoms; or other persistent adverse reactions. **Pregnancy/breast-feeding precautions:** Inform prescriber if you are or intend to become pregnant. This drug should not be used in the 2nd or 3rd trimester of pregnancy. Consult prescriber for appropriate contraceptive measures if necessary. Do not breast-feed.

Pregnancy Risk Factor: C/D (2nd and 3rd trimesters)

Pregnancy Issues: Medications which act on the renin-angiotensin system are reported to have the following fetal/neonatal effects: Hypotension, neonatal skull hypoplasia, anuria, renal failure, and death; oligohydramnios is also reported. These effects are reported to occur with exposure during the 2nd and 3rd trimesters. Valsartan should be discontinued as soon as possible after pregnancy is detected.

Lactation: Excretion in breast milk unknown/contraindicated

Perioperative/Anesthesia/Other Concerns: The angiotensin II receptor antagonists appear to have similar indications as the ACE inhibitors. In heart failure, the angiotensin II antagonists are especially useful in providing an alternative therapy in those patients who have intractable cough in response to ACE inhibitor therapy. Candesartan has been studied as an alternative therapy in chronic heart failure patients who cannot tolerate an ACE-I (CHARM-Alternative) and as an added therapy in heart failure patients who are maintained on an ACE-I (CHARM-Added). In both studies the combined endpoint of cardiovascular death or heart failure hospitalizations was significantly improved over the placebo treated group. Similar to ACE inhibitors, pre-existing volume depletion caused by diuretic therapy may potentiate hypotension in response to angiotensin II antagonists. Concomitant NSAID therapy may attenuate blood pressure control; use of NSAIDs should be avoided or limited, with monitoring of blood pressure control. In the setting of heart failure, NSAID use may be associated with an increased risk for fluid accumulation and edema.

Administration

Oral: Administer with or without food.

Storage: Store at controlled room temperature of 15°C to 30°C (59°F to 86°F). Protect from moisture.

Valsartan and Hydrochlorothiazide

(val SAR tan & hye droe klor oh THYE a zide)

U.S. Brand Names Diovan HCT®

Synonyms Hydrochlorothiazide and Valsartan

Pharmacologic Category Angiotensin II Receptor Blocker Combination; Antihypertensive Agent, Combination; Diuretic, Thiazide

Medication Safety Issues

Sound-alike/look-alike issues:

Diovan® may be confused with Darvon®, Dioval®, Zyban®

Use Treatment of hypertension (not indicated for initial therapy)

Pharmacodynamics/Kinetics See individual agents.

Contraindications Hypersensitivity to valsartan, hydrochlorothiazide, thiazides, sulfonamide-derived drugs, or any component of the formulation; anuria; hypersensitivity to other A-II receptor antagonists; bilateral renal artery stenosis; pregnancy (2nd and 3rd trimesters)

Warnings/Precautions Avoid use or use a smaller dose in patients who are volume depleted; correct depletion first. Deterioration in renal function can occur with initiation. Use with caution in unilateral renal artery stenosis and pre-existing renal insufficiency; significant aortic/mitral stenosis. Electrolyte disturbances (hypokalemia, hypochloremic alkalosis, hyponatremia) or increases in cholesterol and triglyceride levels can occur. Use caution with diabetes; may see a change in glucose control. Can cause SLE exacerbation or activation. Use caution with renal or hepatic dysfunction.

Chemical similarities are present among sulfonamides, sulfonylureas, carbonic anhydrase inhibitors, thiazides, and loop diuretics (except ethacrynic acid). Use in patients with sulfonamide allergy is specifically contraindicated in product labeling, however, a risk of cross-reaction exists in patients with allergy to any of these compounds; avoid use when previous reaction has been severe.

Drug Interactions Valsartan: **Inhibits** CYP2C8/9 (weak)

Also see individual agents.

Adverse Reactions Percentages reported with combination product; other reactions have been reported (see individual agents for additional information)

1% to 10%:

Central nervous system: Dizziness (9%; dose related), fatigue (5%)

Gastrointestinal: Diarrhea (3%)

Respiratory: Pharyngitis (3%), cough (3%)

Dosing

Adults & Elderly: Hypertension: Oral: Dose is individualized (combination substituted for individual components); dose may be titrated after 3-4 weeks of therapy.

Usual recommended starting dose of valsartan: 80 mg or 160 mg once daily when used as monotherapy in patients who are not volume depleted

Renal Impairment: Cl_{cr} ≤30 mL/minute: Use of combination not recommended. Contraindicated in patients with anuria.

Hepatic Impairment: Use with caution.

Available Dosage Forms Tablet:

80 mg/12.5 mg: Valsartan 80 mg and hydrochlorothiazide 12.5 mg

160 mg/12.5 mg: Valsartan 160 mg and hydrochlorothiazide 12.5 mg

160 mg/25 mg: Valsartan 160 mg and hydrochlorothiazide 25 mg

Nursing Guidelines

Assessment: See individual agents. **Pregnancy risk factor C/D** - see Pregnancy Risk Factor for use cautions. Assess knowledge/instruct patient on need

(Continued)

Valsartan and Hydrochlorothiazide *(Continued)*

to use appropriate contraceptive measures and the need to avoid pregnancy. Breast-feeding is not recommended.

Patient Education: See individual agents. **Pregnancy/breast-feeding precautions:** Inform prescriber if you are or intend to become pregnant. Breast-feeding is not recommended.

Pregnancy Risk Factor: C/D (2nd and 3rd trimester)

Lactation: Excretion in breast milk unknown/not recommended

Breast-Feeding Considerations: Excretion of valsartan in breast milk is not known and use during nursing is not recommended; hydrochlorothiazide is excreted in breast milk

Related Information

Hydrochlorothiazide *on page 862*
Valsartan *on page 1684*

♦ **Vancocin®** *see* Vancomycin *on page 1688*

Vancomycin (van koe MYE sin)

U.S. Brand Names Vancocin®

Synonyms Vancomycin Hydrochloride

Pharmacologic Category Antibiotic, Miscellaneous

Medication Safety Issues

Sound-alike/look-alike issues:
- I.V. vancomycin may be confused with Invanz®
- Vancomycin may be confused with vecuronium

Use Treatment of patients with infections caused by staphylococcal species and streptococcal species; used orally for staphylococcal enterocolitis or for antibiotic-associated pseudomembranous colitis produced by *C. difficile*

Mechanism of Action Inhibits bacterial cell wall synthesis by blocking glycopeptide polymerization through binding tightly to D-alanyl-D-alanine portion of cell wall precursor

Pharmacodynamics/Kinetics

Absorption: Oral: Poor; I.M.: Erratic; Intraperitoneal: ~38%

Distribution: Widely in body tissues and fluids. except for CSF
- Relative diffusion from blood into CSF: Good only with inflammation (exceeds usual MICs)
- CSF:blood level ratio: Normal meninges: Nil; Inflamed meninges: 20% to 30%

Protein binding: 10% to 50%

Half-life elimination: Biphasic: Terminal:
- Newborns: 6-10 hours
- Infants and Children 3 months to 4 years: 4 hours
- Children >3 years: 2.2-3 hours
- Adults: 5-11 hours; significantly prolonged with renal impairment
- End-stage renal disease: 200-250 hours

Time to peak, serum: I.V.: 45-65 minutes

Excretion: I.V.: Urine (80% to 90% as unchanged drug); Oral: Primarily feces

Contraindications Hypersensitivity to vancomycin or any component of the formulation; avoid in patients with previous severe hearing loss

Warnings/Precautions Use with caution in patients with renal impairment or those receiving other nephrotoxic or ototoxic drugs; dosage modification required in patients with impaired renal function (especially elderly)

Drug Interactions Increased toxicity: Anesthetic agents; other ototoxic or nephrotoxic agents

Adverse Reactions

Oral:

>10%: Gastrointestinal: Bitter taste, nausea, vomiting, stomatitis

1% to 10%:
- Central nervous system: Chills, drug fever
- Hematologic: Eosinophilia

<1% (Limited to important or life-threatening): Interstitial nephritis, ototoxicity, renal failure, skin rash, thrombocytopenia, vasculitis

Parenteral:

>10%:
- Cardiovascular: Hypotension accompanied by flushing
- Dermatologic: Erythematous rash on face and upper body (red neck or red man syndrome)

1% to 10%:
Central nervous system: Chills, drug fever
Hematologic: Eosinophilia
<1% (Limited to important or life-threatening): Ototoxicity, renal failure, thrombocytopenia, vasculitis

Overdosage/Toxicology Symptoms of overdose include ototoxicity and nephrotoxicity. There is no specific therapy for overdose with vancomycin. Care is symptomatic and supportive. Peritoneal filtration and hemofiltration (not dialysis) have been shown to reduce the serum concentration of vancomycin. High flux dialysis may remove up to 25% of the drug.

Dosing

Adults:

Systemic infections: I.V.: Initial dosage recommendation: Normal renal function: 1 g every 12 hours **or** select individualized dosage based on weight (10-15 mg/kg)

Note: Select interval based on estimated Cl_{cr} >60 mL/minute every 12 hours, 40-60 mL/minute every 24 hours, <40 mL/minute every 24 hours; monitor levels.

Prophylaxis for bacterial endocarditis: I.V.:
Dental, oral, or upper respiratory tract surgery: 1 g 1 hour before surgery
GI/GU procedure: 1 g plus 1.5 mg/kg gentamicin 1 hour prior to surgery

CNS infections:
Intrathecal: **Note:** Vancomycin is available as a powder for injection and may be diluted to 1-5 mg/mL concentration in preservative-free 0.9% sodium chloride for administration into the CSF. Dose: Up to 20 mg/day

Antibiotic lock technique (for catheter infections): 2 mg/mL in SWI/NS or D_5W; instill 3-5 mL into catheter port as a flush solution instead of heparin lock. (**Note:** Do not mix with any other solutions.)

Intrathecal: 20 mg/day; vancomycin is available as a powder for injection and may be diluted to 1-5 mg/mL concentration in preservative free 0.9% sodium chloride for administration into the CSF.

Pseudomembranous colitis produced by *C. difficile*: Oral: 125 mg 4 times/day for 10 days. **Note:** Due to the emergence of resistant enterococci, the use of vancomycin is limited in most settings

Elderly: Elderly patients may require greater dosage reduction than expected. Best to individualize therapy; dose (mg/kg/24 hours) = (0.227 x Cl_{cr}) + 5.67. Refer to adult dosing.

Pediatrics:

Systemic infections: Initial dosage recommendation: I.V.:
Neonates:
Postnatal age ≤7 days:
<1200 g: 15 mg/kg/dose every 24 hours
≥1200 g: 10 mg/kg/dose divided every 8 hours
>2000 g: 15 mg/kg/dose every 12 hours
Postnatal age >7 days:
<1200 g: 15 mg/kg/dose every 24 hours
≥1200 g: 10 mg/kg/dose divided every 8 hours
Infants >1 month and Children: 40 mg/kg/day in divided doses every 6 hours

Prophylaxis for bacterial endocarditis: I.V.:
Dental, oral, or upper respiratory tract surgery: 20 mg/kg 1 hour prior to the procedure
GI/GU procedure: 20 mg/kg plus gentamicin 2 mg/kg 1 hour prior to surgery

CNS infections:
Intrathecal: **Note:** Vancomycin is available as a powder for injection and may be diluted to 1-5 mg/mL concentration in preservative-free 0.9% sodium chloride for administration into the CSF
Neonates: 5-10 mg/day
Children: 5-20 mg/day
I.V.: Infants >1 month and Children with staphylococcal central nervous system infection: 60 mg/kg/day in divided doses every 6 hours

Antibiotic lock technique (for catheter infections): 2 mg/mL in SWI/NS or D_5W; instill 3-5 mL into catheter port as a flush solution instead of heparin lock (**Note:** Do not mix with any other solutions)

Pseudomembranous colitis produced by *C. difficile*: Oral:
Neonates: 10 mg/kg/day in divided doses
Children: 40 mg/kg/day in divided doses, added to fluids
Note: Use is restricted in most settings

(Continued)

Vancomycin *(Continued)*

Renal Impairment: Vancomycin levels should be monitored in patients with any renal impairment.

Cl_{cr} >60 mL/minute: Start with 1 g or 10-15 mg/kg/dose every 12 hours.

Cl_{cr} 40-60 mL/minute: Start with 1 g or 10-15 mg/kg/dose every 24 hours.

Cl_{cr} <40 mL/minute: Will need longer intervals; determine by serum concentration monitoring.

Hemodialysis: Not dialyzable (0% to 5%); generally not removed; exception minimal-moderate removal by some of the newer high-flux filters. Dose may need to be administered more frequently. Monitor serum concentrations.

Continuous ambulatory peritoneal dialysis (CAPD): Not significantly removed; administration via CAPD fluid: 15-30 mg/L (15-30 mcg/mL) of CAPD fluid.

Continuous arteriovenous hemofiltration: Dose as for Cl_{cr} 10-40 mL/minute.

Antibiotic lock technique (for catheter infections): 2 mg/mL in SWI/NS or D_5W; instill 3-5 mL into catheter port as a flush solution instead of heparin lock (**Note:** Do not mix with any other solutions).

Hepatic Impairment: Reduce dose by 60%.

Available Dosage Forms

Capsule (Vancocin®): 125 mg, 250 mg

Infusion [premixed in iso-osmotic dextrose] (Vancocin®): 500 mg (100 mL); 1 g (200 mL)

Injection, powder for reconstitution: 500 mg, 1 g, 5 g, 10 g

Nursing Guidelines

Assessment: See Warnings/Precautions and Contraindications for use cautions. Assess effectiveness and interactions of other medications patient may be taking (eg, anything that is ototoxic or nephrotoxic - see Drug Interactions). See specifics below for I.V. administration (eg, premedication and Red Man syndrome). Infusion site must be monitored closely to prevent extravasation. Assess results of laboratory tests (see below), therapeutic effectiveness, and adverse response on a regular basis during therapy (see Adverse Reactions and Overdose/Toxicology). Teach patient appropriate use (oral), possible side effects/appropriate interventions, and adverse symptoms to report (see Patient Education). Note breast-feeding caution.

Monitoring Laboratory Tests: Perform culture and sensitivity studies prior to first dose. Periodic renal function, urinalysis, serum vancomycin concentrations, WBC, audiogram with prolonged use. Obtain drug levels after the third dose unless otherwise directed. Peaks are drawn 1 hour after the completion of a 1- to 2-hour infusion. Troughs are obtained just before the next dose.

Dietary Considerations: May be taken with food.

Patient Education: Inform prescriber of all prescriptions, OTC medications, or herbal products you are taking, and any allergies you have. Do not take any new medication during therapy unless approved by prescriber. With I.V. use, report immediately any chills; pain, swelling, or redness at infusion site; or respiratory difficulty. Take as directed with food, for as long as prescribed. Maintain adequate hydration (2-3 L/day of fluids) unless instructed to restrict fluid intake.

Oral/I.V.: May cause nausea, vomiting, or GI upset (small, frequent meals, frequent mouth care, sucking lozenges, or chewing gum may help). Report rash or hives; chills or fever; persistent GI disturbances; opportunistic infection (sore throat, chills, fever, burning, itching on urination, vaginal discharge, white plaques in mouth); respiratory difficulty; decreased urine output; chest pain or palpitations; changes in hearing or fullness in ears; or worsening of condition.

Pregnancy/breast-feeding precautions: Inform prescriber if you are or intend to become pregnant. Consult prescriber if breast-feeding.

Geriatric Considerations: As a result of age-related changes in renal function and volume of distribution, accumulation and toxicity are a risk in the elderly. Careful monitoring and dosing adjustment is necessary.

Pregnancy Risk Factor: C

Lactation: Enters breast milk/use caution

Breast-Feeding Considerations: Vancomycin is excreted in breast milk but is poorly absorbed from the gastrointestinal tract. Therefore, systemic absorption would not be expected. Theoretically, vancomycin in the GI tract may affect the normal bowel flora in the infant, resulting in diarrhea.

Perioperative/Anesthesia/Other Concerns: The "red man syndrome" (characterized by skin rash and hypotension) is not an allergic reaction, but rather is associated with infusion administered too rapidly. To alleviate or prevent the reaction, infuse vancomycin at a rate of ≥30 minutes for each 500 mg of drug being administered (eg, 1 g over ≥60 minutes; 1.5 g over ≥90 minutes). CVVHD clears vancomycin from the circulation while conventional hemodialysis does not.

Limitations which may contribute to clinical failure include poor lung penetration, slow bactericidal activity against *S. aureus*, limited CNS penetration, high-level resistance to enterococci and *S. aureus*, and limited activity against bacteria that coat prosthetic devices.

Administration

Oral: May be administered with food.

I.M.: Do not administer I.M.

I.V.: Administer vancomycin by I.V. intermittent infusion over at least 60 minutes at a final concentration not to exceed 5 mg/mL.

If a maculopapular rash appears on the face, neck, trunk, and/or upper extremities (Red man syndrome), slow the infusion rate to over 1½ to 2 hours and increase the dilution volume. Hypotension, shock, and cardiac arrest (rare) have also been reported with too rapid of infusion. Reactions are often treated with antihistamines and steroids.

Extravasation treatment: Monitor I.V. site closely; extravasation will cause serious injury with possible necrosis and tissue sloughing. Rotate infusion site frequently.

Reconstitution: Reconstitute vials with 20 mL of SWFI for each 1 g of vancomycin (10 mL/500 mg vial; 20 mL/1 g vial; 100 mL/5 g vial; 200 mL/10 g vial). The reconstituted solution must be further diluted with at least 100 mL of a compatible diluent per 500 mg of vancomycin prior to parenteral administration.

Compatibility: Stable in dextran 6% in NS, D_5LR, D_5NS, D_5W, $D_{10}W$, LR, NS

Y-site administration: Incompatible with albumin, amphotericin B cholesteryl sulfate complex, cefepime, gatifloxacin, heparin, idarubicin, omeprazole

Compatibility in syringe: Incompatible with heparin

Compatibility when admixed: Incompatible with amobarbital, chloramphenicol, chlorothiazide, dexamethasone sodium phosphate, penicillin G potassium, pentobarbital, phenobarbital, phenytoin

Storage: Reconstituted 500 mg and 1 g vials are stable for at either room temperature or under refrigeration for 14 days. **Note:** Vials contain no bacteriostatic agent. Solutions diluted for administration in either D_5W or NS are stable under refrigeration for 14 days or at room temperature for 7 days.

Related Information

Prevention of Wound Infection and Sepsis in Surgical Patients *on page 1830*

♦ **Vancomycin Hydrochloride** *see* Vancomycin *on page 1688*

♦ **Vandazole™** *see* Metronidazole *on page 1154*

♦ **Vanos™** *see* Fluocinonide *on page 741*

♦ **Vaponefrin®** *see* Epinephrine (Racemic/Dental) *on page 615*

♦ **VAQTA®** *see* Hepatitis A Vaccine *on page 850*

Vasopressin (vay soe PRES in)

U.S. Brand Names Pitressin®

Synonyms ADH; Antidiuretic Hormone; 8-Arginine Vasopressin

Pharmacologic Category Antidiuretic Hormone Analog; Hormone, Posterior Pituitary

Medication Safety Issues

Sound-alike/look-alike issues:

Pitressin® may be confused with Pitocin®

Use Treatment of diabetes insipidus; prevention and treatment of postoperative abdominal distention; differential diagnosis of diabetes insipidus

Unlabeled/Investigational Use Adjunct in the treatment of GI hemorrhage and esophageal varices; pulseless ventricular tachycardia (VT)/ventricular fibrillation (VF); vasodilatory shock (septic shock); out-of-hospital asystole

Mechanism of Action Increases cyclic adenosine monophosphate (cAMP) which increases water permeability at the renal tubule resulting in decreased urine volume and increased osmolality; causes peristalsis by directly stimulating the smooth muscle in the GI tract

Pharmacodynamics/Kinetics

Onset of action: Nasal: 1 hour

Duration: Nasal: 3-8 hours; I.M., SubQ: 2-8 hours

(Continued)

Vasopressin *(Continued)*

Metabolism: Nasal/Parenteral: Hepatic, renal

Half-life elimination: Nasal: 15 minutes; Parenteral: 10-20 minutes

Excretion: Nasal: Urine; SubQ: Urine (5% as unchanged drug) after 4 hours

Contraindications Hypersensitivity to vasopressin or any component of the formulation

Warnings/Precautions Use with caution in patients with seizure disorders, migraine, asthma, vascular disease, renal disease, cardiac disease; chronic nephritis with nitrogen retention. Goiter with cardiac complications, arteriosclerosis; I.V. infiltration may lead to severe vasoconstriction and localized tissue necrosis; also, gangrene of extremities, tongue, and ischemic colitis. Elderly patients should be cautioned not to increase their fluid intake beyond that sufficient to satisfy their thirst in order to avoid water intoxication and hyponatremia; under experimental conditions, the elderly have shown to have a decreased responsiveness to vasopressin with respect to its effects on water homeostasis

Drug Interactions

Decreased effect: Lithium, epinephrine, demeclocycline, heparin, and ethanol block antidiuretic activity to varying degrees

Increased effect: Chlorpropamide, phenformin, urea and fludrocortisone potentiate antidiuretic response

Nutritional/Herbal/Ethanol Interactions Ethanol: Avoid ethanol (due to effects on ADH).

Adverse Reactions Frequency not defined.

Cardiovascular: Increased blood pressure, arrhythmia, venous thrombosis, vasoconstriction (with higher doses), chest pain, MI

Central nervous system: Pounding in the head, fever, vertigo

Dermatologic: Urticaria, circumoral pallor

Gastrointestinal: Flatulence, abdominal cramps, nausea, vomiting

Genitourinary: Uterine contraction

Neuromuscular & skeletal: Tremor

Respiratory: Bronchial constriction

Miscellaneous: Diaphoresis

Overdosage/Toxicology Symptoms of overdose include drowsiness, weight gain, confusion, listlessness, and water intoxication. Water intoxication requires withdrawal of the drug. Severe intoxication may require osmotic diuresis and loop diuretics.

Dosing

Adults & Elderly:

Diabetes insipidus:

Note: Dosage is highly variable; titrated based on serum and urine sodium and osmolality in addition to fluid balance and urine output

I.M., SubQ: 5-10 units 2-4 times/day as needed (dosage range 5-60 units/day)

Continuous I.V. infusion: 0.5 milliunit/kg/hour (0.0005 unit/kg/hour); double dosage as needed every 30 minutes to a maximum of 0.01 unit/kg/hour

Intranasal: Administer on cotton pledget, as nasal spray, or by dropper

Abdominal distention: I.M.: 5 units stat, 10 units every 3-4 hours

GI hemorrhage (unlabeled use):

Continuous I.V. infusion: 0.5 milliunits/kg/hour (0.0005 unit/kg/hour); double dosage as needed every 30 minutes to a maximum of 10 milliunits/kg/hour

I.V.: Initial: 0.2-0.4 unit/minute, then titrate dose as needed; if bleeding stops, continue at same dose for 12 hours, taper off over 24-48 hours.

Out-of-hospital asystole (unlabeled use): Adults: I.V.: 40 units; if spontaneous circulation is not restored in 3 minutes, then repeat dose

Pulseless VT/VF (ACLS protocol): I.V.: 40 units (as a single dose only); if no I.V. access, administer 40 units diluted with NS (to a total volume of 10 mL) endotracheally

Vasodilatory shock/septic shock (unlabeled use): I.V.: Vasopressin has been used in doses of 0.01-0.1 units/minute for the treatment of septic shock. Doses >0.05 units/minute may have more cardiovascular side effects. Most case reports have used 0.04 units/minute continuous infusion as a fixed dose.

Pediatrics:

Diabetes insipidus:

Note: Dosage is highly variable; titrated based on serum and urine sodium and osmolality in addition to fluid balance and urine output

I.M., SubQ:

Children: 2.5-10 units 2-4 times/day as needed

Continuous I.V. infusion: Children: 0.5 milliunit/kg/hour (0.0005 unit/kg/hour); double dosage as needed every 30 minutes to a maximum of 0.01 unit/kg/hour

Intranasal: Administer on cotton pledget, as nasal spray, or by dropper

GI hemorrhage (unlabeled use): I.V. infusion: Dilute in NS or D_5W to 0.1-1 unit/mL

Children: Initial: 0.002-0.005 units/kg/minute; titrate dose as needed; maximum: 0.01 unit/kg/minute; continue at same dosage (if bleeding stops) for 12 hours, then taper off over 24-48 hours

Hepatic Impairment: Some patients respond to much lower doses with cirrhosis.

Available Dosage Forms

Injection, solution: 20 units/mL (0.5 mL, 1 mL, 10 mL)

Pitressin®: 20 units/mL (1 mL)

Nursing Guidelines

Assessment: See Warnings/Precautions, Contraindications, and Drug Interactions for use cautions. See specifics below for I.V. or intranasal administration. Infusion site must be monitored closely to prevent extravasation (see Administration). Assess results of laboratory tests (see below), therapeutic effectiveness, and adverse response on a regular basis during therapy (eg, cardiac status, blood pressure, CNS status, fluid balance, signs or symptoms of water intoxication, or intranasal irritation - see Adverse Reactions and Overdose/Toxicology). Teach patient possible side effects/appropriate interventions and adverse symptoms to report (see Patient Education).

Monitoring Laboratory Tests: Serum and urine sodium, urine specific gravity, urine and serum osmolality

Patient Education: Inform prescriber of all prescriptions, OTC medications, or herbal products you are taking, and any allergies you have. Do not take any new medication during therapy unless approved by prescriber. Avoid alcohol. This drug will usually be administered by infusion or injection. Report immediately any redness, swelling, pain, or burning at infusion/injection site. When self-administered follow directions exactly. May cause dizziness, drowsiness (use caution when driving or engaging in potentially hazardous tasks until response to drug is known); nausea, vomiting, cramping (small, frequent meals, frequent mouth care, chewing gum, or sucking lozenges may help), Report persistent nausea, vomiting, abdominal cramps; tremor, acute headache, or dizziness; chest pain or irregular heartbeat; respiratory difficulty or excess perspiration; CNS changes (confusion, drowsiness); or runny nose or painful nasal membranes (intranasal).

Geriatric Considerations: Elderly patients should be cautioned not to increase their fluid intake beyond that sufficient to satisfy their thirst in order to avoid water intoxication and hyponatremia. Under experimental conditions, the elderly have shown to have a decreased responsiveness to vasopressin with respect to its effects on water homeostasis.

Pregnancy Risk Factor: C

Pregnancy Issues: Animal reproduction studies have not been conducted. Vasopressin and desmopressin have been used safely during pregnancy based on case reports.

Lactation: Enters breast milk/use caution

Breast-Feeding Considerations: Based on case reports, vasopressin and desmopressin have been used safely during nursing.

Perioperative/Anesthesia/Other Concerns: Vasopressin (for cardiac resuscitation) may be given by the endotracheal route. Give 40 units; dilute with normal saline to a total volume of 10 mL.

Low-dose vasopressin may be effective for the management of vasodilator shock. Vasopressin binds to different receptors than the catecholamine pressors. Vasoconstrictor effects are through the V_1 vascular receptors. In clinical studies and case reports, vasopressin increased blood pressure, systemic vascular resistance, and urine output. Vasopressin may decrease heart rate and cardiac output, especially at higher doses. Vasopressin has been used in doses of 0.01-0.1 units/minute. Doses >0.05 units/minute may have more cardiovascular effects (decrease cardiac output, asystole, arrhythmias). Vasoconstriction appears to remain effective in severe acidosis. When possible,

(Continued)

Vasopressin *(Continued)*

low-dose vasopressin should be infused via central catheter for the management of vasodilatory shock; peripheral administration has been associated with skin necrosis.

Vasopressin increases factor VIII levels and may be useful in hemophiliacs.

A multicenter, double-blind, randomized, controlled trial evaluated the efficacy of vasopressin or epinephrine when administered to adult patients who suffered an out-of-hospital cardiac arrest (Wenzel V, 2004). For inclusions, patients presented with ventricular fibrillation, pulseless electrical activity, or asystole. They were excluded if they were successfully defibrillated without the administration of a vasopressor, had a terminal illness or had a DNR order, a lack of intravenous access, hemorrhagic shock, pregnancy, cardiac arrest due to trauma or were <18 years of age. Eligible patients were randomized to intravenous vasopressin (40 units) or epinephrine (1 mg). Each patient received an injection of the study drug, if spontaneous circulation was not restored in 3 minutes they received a second dose (same amount) of the same study drug. If there was no response, the managing physician had the option of giving epinephrine. Patients with ventricular fibrillation were randomized if the first three attempts at defibrillation failed; all others were randomized immediately. The primary endpoint was survival to hospital admission; the secondary endpoint was survival to hospital discharge. Five hundred and eighty-nine patients were randomized to vasopressin and five hundred and ninety-seven patients were randomized to epinephrine. There was no significant difference in the rate of hospital admission between the vasopressin group and the epinephrine group if they had ventricular fibrillation (46.2% vs 43% respectively, p: 0.48) or pulseless electrical activity (33.7% vs 30.5% respectively, p: 0.65). Patients with asystole responded significantly better to vasopressin; having higher rates of hospital admission (29% vs 20.3% in the epinephrine group, p: 0.02) and hospital discharge (4.7% vs 1.5% in the epinephrine group, p: 0.04). Patients who failed vasopressin therapy and received additional epinephrine had significant improvement in survival to hospital admission (25.7 % vs 16.4% in the epinephrine group, p: 0.002) and discharge (6.2% vs 1.7%, p: 0.002). Similar patients who were randomized to epinephrine and failed to respond did not improve with additional epinephrine. Cerebral performance among all patients who survived to discharge was similar in both groups. In this trial, vasopressin was superior to epinephrine in patients with asystole. Vasopressin followed by epinephrine may be more effective than epinephrine alone in refractory out-of-hospital cardiac arrest.

A small in-hospital cardiac arrest study evaluated the efficacy of vasopressin or epinephrine in 200 patients. These investigators did not find any differences between the two treatment groups with regard to survival, discharge, or cerebral performance (Stiell IG, 2001).

Administration

I.V.:

GI hemorrhage: Administration requires the use of an infusion pump and should be administered in a peripheral line.

Vasodilatory shock: Administration through a central catheter is recommended.

Infusion rates:

100 units in 500 mL D_5W rate

- 0.1 unit/minute: 30 mL/hour
- 0.2 units/minute: 60 mL/hour
- 0.3 units/minute: 90 mL/hour
- 0.4 units/minute: 120 mL/hour
- 0.5 units/minute: 150 mL/hour
- 0.6 units/minute: 180 mL/hour

Compatibility: Stable in D_5W, NS

Storage: Store injection at room temperature. Protect from heat and from freezing. Use only clear solutions.

♦ Vasotec® *see* Enalapril *on page 601*

♦ VCR *see* VinCRIStine *on page 1710*

Vecuronium (ve KYOO roe ni um)

U.S. Brand Names Norcuron® [DSC]

Synonyms ORG NC 45

Pharmacologic Category Neuromuscular Blocker Agent, Nondepolarizing

Medication Safety Issues

Sound-alike/look-alike issues:

Vecuronium may be confused with vancomycin

Norcuron® may be confused with Narcan®

Use Adjunct to general anesthesia to facilitate endotracheal intubation and to relax skeletal muscles during surgery; to facilitate mechanical ventilation in ICU patients; does not relieve pain or produce sedation

Mechanism of Action Blocks acetylcholine from binding to receptors on motor endplate inhibiting depolarization

Pharmacodynamics/Kinetics

Onset of action:

Good intubation conditions: Within 2.5-3 minutes

Maximum neuromuscular blockade: Within 3-5 minutes

Duration: 20-40 minutes

Metabolism: Active metabolite: 3-desacetyl vecuronium ($1/2$ the activity of parent drug)

Half-life elimination: 51-80 minutes

Excretion: Primarily feces (40% to 75%); urine (30% as unchanged drug and metabolites)

Contraindications Hypersensitivity to vecuronium or any component of the formulation

Warnings/Precautions Ventilation must be supported during neuromuscular blockade; certain clinical conditions may result in potentiation or antagonism of neuromuscular blockade:

Potentiation: Electrolyte abnormalities, severe hyponatremia, severe hypocalcemia, severe hypokalemia, hypermagnesemia, neuromuscular diseases, acidosis, acute intermittent porphyria, renal failure, hepatic failure

Antagonism: Alkalosis, hypercalcemia, demyelinating lesions, peripheral neuropathies, diabetes mellitus

Increased sensitivity in patients with myasthenia gravis, Eaton-Lambert syndrome; resistance in burn patients (>30% of body) for period of 5-70 days postinjury; resistance in patients with muscle trauma, denervation, immobilization, infection; use with caution in patients with hepatic or renal impairment; does not counteract bradycardia produced by anesthetics/vagal stimulation. Cross-sensitivity with other neuromuscular-blocking agents may occur; use extreme caution in patients with previous anaphylactic reactions.

Drug Interactions Increased toxicity/effect with aminoglycosides, ketamine, magnesium sulfate, verapamil, quinidine, clindamycin, furosemide

Adverse Reactions <1% (Limited to important or life-threatening): Bradycardia, circulatory collapse, edema, flushing, hypersensitivity reaction, hypotension, itching, rash, tachycardia, acute quadriplegic myopathy syndrome (prolonged use), myositis ossificans (prolonged use)

Overdosage/Toxicology

Symptoms of overdose include prolonged skeletal muscle weakness and apnea cardiovascular collapse.

Use neostigmine, edrophonium, or pyridostigmine with atropine to antagonize skeletal muscle relaxation; support of ventilation and the cardiovascular system through mechanical means, fluids, and pressors may be necessary.

Dosing

Adults & Elderly:

Neuromuscular blockade: I.V. (do not administer I.M.):

Initial: 0.08-0.1 mg/kg or 0.04-0.06 mg/kg after initial dose of succinylcholine for intubation

Maintenance: 0.01-0.015 mg/kg 25-40 minutes after initial dose, then 0.01-0.015 mg/kg every 12-15 minutes (higher doses will allow less frequent maintenance doses); may be administered as a continuous infusion at 0.8-2 mcg/kg/minute

Pretreatment/priming: Adults: 10% of intubating dose given 3-5 minutes before initial dose

Neuromuscular blockade in ICU patients: Adults: 0.05-0.1 mg/kg bolus followed by 0.8-1.7 mcg/kg/minute once initial recovery from bolus observed or 0.1-0.2 mg/kg/dose every 1 hour

(Continued)

Vecuronium *(Continued)*

Pediatrics:

Neuromuscular blockade: I.V. (do not administer I.M.):

Infants >7 weeks to 1 year: Initial: 0.08-0.1 mg/kg/dose; maintenance: 0.05-0.1 mg/kg/every 60 minutes as needed

Children >1 year: Refer to adult dosing.

Hepatic Impairment: Dose reductions are necessary in patients with liver disease.

Available Dosage Forms Injection, powder for reconstitution, as bromide: 10 mg, 20 mg [may be supplied with diluent containing benzyl alcohol]

Nursing Guidelines

Assessment: Only clinicians experienced in the use of neuromuscular-blocking drugs should administer and/or manage the use of vecuronium. Dosage and rate of administration should be individualized and titrated to the desired effect, according to relevant clinical factors, premedication, concomitant medications, age, and general condition of patient. Ventilatory support must be instituted and maintained until adequate respiratory muscle function and/or airway protection are assured. Assess other medications for effectiveness and safety. Other drugs that affect neuromuscular activity may increase/decrease neuromuscular block induced by vecuronium; monitor and adjust dosage as necessary. This drug does not cause anesthesia or analgesia; pain must be treated with appropriate analgesic agents. Continuous monitoring of vital signs, cardiac status, respiratory status, and degree of neuromuscular block (objective assessment with peripheral external nerve stimulator) is mandatory during infusion and until full muscle tone has returned. Muscle tone returns in a predictable pattern, starting with diaphragm, abdomen, chest, limbs, and finally muscles of the neck, face, and eyes. Safety precautions must be maintained until full muscle tone has returned. **Note:** It may take longer for return of muscle tone in obese or elderly patients or patients with renal or hepatic disease, myasthenia gravis, myopathy, other neuromuscular disease, dehydration, electrolyte imbalance, or severe acid/base imbalance. Provide appropriate patient teaching /support prior to and following administration.

Long-term use: Monitor fluid levels (intake and output) during and following infusion. Reposition patient and provide appropriate skin care, mouth care, and care of patient's eyes every 2-3 hours while sedated. Provide appropriate emotional and sensory support (auditory and environmental).

Patient Education: Patient will usually be unconscious prior to administration. Patient education should be appropriate to individual situation. Reassurance of constant monitoring and emotional support to reduce fear and anxiety should precede and follow administration. Following return of muscle tone, do not attempt to change position or rise from bed without assistance. Report immediately any skin rash or hives, pounding heartbeat, respiratory difficulty, or muscle tremors. **Pregnancy/breast-feeding precautions:** Inform prescriber if you are or intend to become pregnant. Consult prescriber if breast-feeding.

Pregnancy Risk Factor: C

Pregnancy Issues: Use in cesarean section has been reported. Umbilical venous concentrations were 11% of maternal.

Lactation: Excretion in breast milk unknown/use caution

Perioperative/Anesthesia/Other Concerns: Classified as an intermediate duration neuromuscular-blocking agent; produces minimal, if any, histamine release.

Critically-Ill Adult Patients: The 2002 ACCM/SCCM/ASHP clinical practice guidelines for sustained neuromuscular blockade in the adult critically-ill patient recommend:

Optimize sedatives and analgesics prior to initiation and monitor and adjust accordingly during course. Neuromuscular blockers do not relieve pain or produce sedation.

Protect patient's eyes from development of keratitis and corneal abrasion by administering ophthalmic ointment and taping eyelids closed or using eye patches. Reposition patient routinely to protect pressure points from breakdown. Address DVT prophylaxis.

Concurrent use of a neuromuscular blocker and corticosteroids appear to increase the risk of certain ICU myopathies; avoid or administer the corticosteroid at the lowest dose possible. Reassess need for neuromuscular blocker daily.

Using daily drug holidays (stopping neuromuscular-blocking agent until patient requires it again) may decrease the incidence of acute quadriplegic myopathy syndrome.

Tachyphylaxis can develop; switch to another neuromuscular blocker (taking into consideration the patient's organ function) if paralysis is still necessary.

Atracurium or cisatracurium is recommended for patients with significant hepatic or renal disease, due to organ-independent Hofmann elimination.

Monitor patients clinically and via "Train of Four" (TOF) testing with a goal of adjusting the degree of blockade to 1-2 twitches or based upon the patient's clinical condition.

Administration

I.V.: Concentration of 1 mg/mL may be administered by rapid I.V. injection. May further dilute reconstituted vial to 0.1-0.2 mg/mL in a compatible solution for I.V. infusion. Concentration of 1 mg/mL may be used for I.V. infusion in fluid-restricted patients.

Reconstitution: Reconstitute with compatible solution for injection to final concentration of 1 mg/mL.

Compatibility:

Incompatible with alkaline solutions/medications.

Y-Site administration: Incompatible with thiopental

Compatibility in syringe: Incompatible with thiopental

Storage: Store intact vials of powder for injection at room temperature 15°C to 30°C (59°F to 86°F). Vials reconstituted with bacteriostatic water for injection (BWFI) may be stored for 5 days under refrigeration or at room temperature. Vials reconstituted with other compatible diluents (nonbacteriostatic) should be stored under refrigeration and used within 24 hours.

◆ Veetids® *see* Penicillin V Potassium *on page 1328*

◆ Velcade® *see* Bortezomib *on page 251*

◆ Velivet™ *see* Ethinyl Estradiol and Desogestrel *on page 675*

Venlafaxine (VEN la faks een)

U.S. Brand Names Effexor®; Effexor® XR

Pharmacologic Category Antidepressant, Serotonin/Norepinephrine Reuptake Inhibitor

Use Treatment of major depressive disorder; generalized anxiety disorder (GAD), social anxiety disorder (social phobia); panic disorder

Unlabeled/Investigational Use Obsessive-compulsive disorder (OCD); hot flashes; neuropathic pain; attention-deficit/hyperactivity disorder (ADHD)

Mechanism of Action Venlafaxine and its active metabolite o-desmethylvenlafaxine (ODV) are potent inhibitors of neuronal serotonin and norepinephrine reuptake and weak inhibitors of dopamine reuptake. Venlafaxine and ODV have no significant activity for muscarinic cholinergic, H_1-histaminergic, or alpha$_2$-adrenergic receptors. Venlafaxine and ODV do not possess MAO-inhibitory activity.

Pharmacodynamics/Kinetics

Absorption: Oral: 92% to 100%; food has no significant effect on the absorption of venlafaxine or formation of the active metabolite O-desmethylvenlafaxine (ODV)

Distribution: At steady state: Venlafaxine 7.5 ± 3.7 L/kg, ODV 5.7 ± 1.8 L/Kg

Protein binding: Bound to human plasma protein: Venlafaxine 27%, ODV 30%

Metabolism: Hepatic via CYP2D6 to active metabolite, O-desmethylvenlafaxine (ODV); other metabolites include N-desmethylvenlafaxine and N,O-didesmethylvenlafaxine

Bioavailability: Absolute: ~45%

Half-life elimination: Venlafaxine: 3-7 hours; ODV: 9-13 hours; Steady-state, plasma: Venlafaxine/ODV: Within 3 days of multiple-dose therapy; prolonged with cirrhosis (Adults: Venlafaxine: ~30%, ODV: ~60%) and with dialysis (Adults: Venlafaxine: ~180%, ODV: ~142%)

Time to peak:

Immediate release: Venlafaxine: 2 hours, ODV: 3 hours

Extended release: Venlafaxine: 5.5 hours, ODV: 9 hours

Excretion: Urine (~87%, 5% as unchanged drug, 29% as unconjugated ODV, 26% as conjugated ODV, 27% as minor inactive metabolites) within 48 hours

Clearance at steady state: Venlafaxine: 1.3 ± 0.6 L/hour/kg, ODV: 0.4 ± 0.2 L/hour/kg

(Continued)

Venlafaxine *(Continued)*

Clearance decreased with:

Cirrhosis: Adults: Venlafaxine: ~50%, ODV: ~30%

Severe cirrhosis: Adults: Venlafaxine: ~90%

Renal impairment (Cl_{cr} 10-70 mL/minute): Adults: Venlafaxine: ~24%

Dialysis: Adults: Venlafaxine: ~57%, ODV: ~56%; due to large volume of distribution, a significant amount of drug is not likely to be removed.

Contraindications Hypersensitivity to venlafaxine or any component of the formulation; use of MAO inhibitors within 14 days; should not initiate MAO inhibitor within 7 days of discontinuing venlafaxine

Warnings/Precautions

Major psychiatric warnings:

- Antidepressants increase the risk of suicidal thinking and behavior in children and adolescents with major depressive disorder (MDD) and other depressive disorders; consider risk prior to prescribing.
- Closely monitor for clinical worsening, suicidality, or unusual changes in behavior; the child's family or caregiver should be instructed to closely observe the patient and communicate condition with healthcare provider. **Venlafaxine is not FDA approved for use in children.**
- Adults treated with antidepressants should be observed similarly for clinical worsening and suicidality, especially during the initial few months of a course of drug therapy, or at times of dose changes, either increases or decreases. A medication guide should be dispensed with each prescription.
- The possibility of a suicide attempt is inherent in major depression and may persist until remission occurs. Worsening depression and severe abrupt suicidality that are not part of the presenting symptoms may require discontinuation or modification of drug therapy. Use caution in high-risk patients during initiation of therapy.
- Prescriptions should be written for the smallest quantity consistent with good patient care. The patient's family or caregiver should be alerted to monitor patients for the emergence of suicidality and associated behaviors such as anxiety, agitation, panic attacks, insomnia, irritability, hostility, impulsivity, akathisia, hypomania, and mania; patients should be instructed to notify their healthcare provider if any of these symptoms or worsening depression or psychosis occur.
- May worsen psychosis in some patients or precipitate a shift to mania or hypomania in patients with bipolar disorder. Monotherapy in patients with bipolar disorder should be avoided. Patients presenting with depressive symptoms should be screened for bipolar disorder. **Venlafaxine is not FDA approved for the treatment of bipolar depression.**

Key adverse effects:

- CNS depression: Has a low potential to impair cognitive or motor performance; caution operating hazardous machinery or driving.
- SIADH and hyponatremia: Has been associated with the development of SIADH; hyponatremia has been reported rarely, predominately in the elderly
- Weight loss and anorectic effects: Have been observed in both pediatric and adult patients; weight loss was not limited to those experiencing reduced appetite
- Reduced growth rate (pediatric): Small differences in height have been observed in pediatric patients receiving venlafaxine, particularly those <12 years of age, compared to placebo

Concurrent disease:

- Anxiety/Insomnia: May cause increase in anxiety, nervousness, and insomnia.
- Hepatic impairment: Use caution; clearance is decreased and plasma concentrations are increased; a lower dosage may be needed.
- Hypercholesterolemia: May cause increases to serum cholesterol.
- Hypertension/Tachycardia: May cause sustained increase in blood pressure or tachycardia. Use caution in patients with recent history of MI, unstable heart disease, or hyperthyroidism.
- Narrow-angle glaucoma: May cause mydriasis; use caution in patients with increased intraocular pressure or at risk of acute narrow-angle glaucoma.
- Platelet aggregation: May impair platelet aggregation, resulting in bleeding.
- Renal impairment: Use caution; clearance is decreased and plasma concentrations are increased; a lower dosage may be needed.
- Seizure disorders: Use caution with a previous seizure disorder or condition predisposing to seizures such as brain damage or alcoholism.

- Sexual dysfunction: May cause or exacerbate sexual dysfunction.
- Weight loss: May cause weight loss; use caution in patients where weight loss is undesirable.

Concurrent drug therapy:

- Agents which lower seizure threshold: Concurrent therapy with other drugs which lower the seizure threshold.
- Anticoagulants/Antiplatelets: Use caution with concomitant use of NSAIDs, ASA, or other drugs that affect coagulation; the risk of bleeding is potentiated.
- CNS depressants: Use caution with concomitant therapy.
- MAO inhibitors: Potential for severe reaction when used with MAO inhibitors; autonomic instability, coma, death, delirium, diaphoresis, hyperthermia, mental status changes/agitation, muscular rigidity, myoclonus, neuroleptic malignant syndrome features, and seizures may occur.
- Agents causing weight loss or anorectic effects should be avoided.

Special notes:

- Electroconvulsive therapy: May increase the risks associated with electroconvulsive therapy; consider discontinuing, when possible, prior to ECT treatment.
- Withdrawal syndrome: May cause dysphoric mood, irritability, agitation, dizziness, sensory disturbances, anxiety, confusion, headache, lethargy, emotional lability, insomnia, hypomania, tinnitus, and seizures. Upon discontinuation of venlafaxine therapy, gradually taper dose. If intolerable symptoms occur following a decrease in dosage or upon discontinuation of therapy, then resuming the previous dose with a more gradual taper should be considered.

Drug Interactions **Substrate** of CYP2C8/9 (minor), 2C19 (minor), 2D6 (major), 3A4 (major); **Inhibits** CYP2B6 (weak), 2D6 (weak), 3A4 (weak)

Buspirone: Concurrent use may result in serotonin syndrome; these combinations are best avoided

Clozapine: Addition of venlafaxine has been associated with case reports of increased clozapine serum concentrations and seizures.

CYP2D6 inhibitors: May increase the levels/effects of venlafaxine. Example inhibitors include chlorpromazine, delavirdine, fluoxetine, miconazole, paroxetine, pergolide, quinidine, quinine, ritonavir, and ropinirole.

CYP3A4 inducers: CYP3A4 inducers may decrease the levels/effects of venlafaxine. Example inducers include aminoglutethimide, carbamazepine, nafcillin, nevirapine, phenobarbital, phenytoin, and rifamycins.

CYP3A4 inhibitors: May increase the levels/effects of venlafaxine. Example inhibitors include azole antifungals, clarithromycin, diclofenac, doxycycline, erythromycin, imatinib, isoniazid, nefazodone, nicardipine, propofol, protease inhibitors, quinidine, telithromycin, and verapamil.

Haloperidol: Serum levels may be increased during concurrent administration; AUC may be increased by as much as 70%

Indinavir: Serum levels may be reduced by venlafaxine (AUC reduced by 28%); clinical significance unknown

Lithium: Concurrent use may increase risk of serotonin syndrome.

MAO inhibitors: Serotonin syndrome may result when venlafaxine is used in combination or within 2 weeks of an MAO inhibitor; these combinations should be avoided

Meperidine: Concurrent use may increase risk of serotonin syndrome

Mirtazapine: Concurrent use may increase risk of serotonin syndrome

Nefazodone: Concurrent use may increase risk of serotonin syndrome; in addition, nefazodone may inhibit the metabolism of venlafaxine

Selegiline: Concurrent use may predispose to serotonin syndrome; avoid concurrent use.

Serotonin agonists: Theoretically, may increase the risk of serotonin syndrome; includes sumatriptan, naratriptan, rizatriptan, and zolmitriptan

Sibutramine: Concurrent use may increase risk of serotonin syndrome; avoid concomitant use.

SSRIs: Concurrent use may increase risk of serotonin syndrome.

Tramadol: Concurrent use may increase risk of serotonin syndrome.

Trazodone: Concurrent use may increase risk of serotonin syndrome.

Tricyclic antidepressants: Concurrent use may increase risk of serotonin syndrome

Warfarin: Case reports of increased INR when venlafaxine was added to therapy.

Nutritional/Herbal/Ethanol Interactions

Ethanol: Avoid ethanol (may increase CNS effects).

Herb/Nutraceutical: Avoid valerian, St John's wort, SAMe, kava kava, tryptophan (may increase risk of serotonin syndrome and/or excessive sedation).

(Continued)

Venlafaxine *(Continued)*

Lab Interactions Increased thyroid, uric acid, glucose, potassium, AST, cholesterol (S)

Adverse Reactions

>10%:

Central nervous system: Headache (25% to 34%), insomnia (15% to 23%), somnolence (12% to 23%), dizziness (11% to 20%), nervousness (6% to 13%)

Gastrointestinal: Nausea (21% to 37%), xerostomia (12% to 22%), anorexia (8% to 20%), constipation (8% to 15%)

Genitourinary: Abnormal ejaculation/orgasm (2% to 16%)

Neuromuscular & skeletal: Weakness (8% to 17%)

Miscellaneous: Diaphoresis (10% to 14%)

1% to 10%:

Cardiovascular: Vasodilation (3% to 4%); hypertension (dose related; 3% in patients receiving <100 mg/day, up to 13% in patients receiving >300 mg/day); palpitation (3%), tachycardia (2%), chest pain (2%), postural hypotension (1%), edema

Central nervous system: Abnormal dreams (3% to 7%), anxiety (5% to 6%), yawning (3% to 5%), agitation (2% to 4%), chills (3%), confusion (2%), abnormal thinking (2%), depersonalization (1%), depression (1% to 3%), fever, migraine, amnesia, hypoethesia, trismus, vertigo

Dermatologic: Rash (3%), pruritus (1%), bruising

Endocrine & metabolic: Libido decreased (3% to 9%)

Gastrointestinal: Diarrhea (6% to 8%), vomiting (3% to 6%), dyspepsia (5%), abdominal pain (4%), flatulence (3% to 4%), taste perversion (2%), weight loss (1% to 4%), appetite increased, weight gain

Genitourinary: Impotence (4% to 10%), urinary frequency (3%), impaired urination (2%), urinary retention (1%), prostatic disorder

Neuromuscular & skeletal: Tremor (4% to 5%), hypertonia (3%), paresthesia (2% to 3%), twitching (1% to 2%), neck pain, arthralgia

Ocular: Abnormal or blurred vision (4% to 6%), mydriasis (2%)

Otic: Tinnitus (2%)

Respiratory: Pharyngitis (7%), sinusitis (2%), cough increased, dyspnea

Miscellaneous: Infection (6%), flu-like syndrome (6%), trauma (2%)

<1% (Limited to important or life-threatening): Agranulocytosis, anaphylaxis, aplastic anemia, aneurysm, angina pectoris, anuria; arrhythmia (including atrial and ventricular tachycardia, fibrillation and torsade de pointes); arteritis, asthma, ataxia, atelectasis, atrioventricular block, bacteremia, basophilia, bigeminy, biliary pain, bilirubinemia, bleeding time increased, bradycardia, bradykinesia, BUN increased, bundle branch block, carcinoma, cardiovascular disorder (mitral valve and circulatory disturbance), cataract, catatonia, cellulitis, cerebral ischemia, cholelithiasis, congestive heart failure, coronary artery disease, creatinine increased, crystalluria, cyanosis, deafness, DVT, dehydration, delusions, dementia, diabetes mellitus, dystonia, EKG abnormalities (including QT prolongation), electrolyte abnormalities, embolus, eosinophilia, exfoliative dermatitis, erythema multiforme, extrapyramidal symptoms, extrasystoles, facial paralysis, fasciitis, gastrointestinal ulcer, glaucoma, Guillain-Barré syndrome, heart arrest, hematemesis, hematoma; hemorrhage (eye, GI, mucocutaneous, rectal); hepatitis, homicidal ideation, hostility, hyperacusis, hypercalcinuria, hyperchlorhydria, hyper-/hypocholesteremia, hyper-/hypoglycemia, hyperlipemia, hyper-/hypothyroidism, hyperuricemia, hypokalemia, hyponatremia, hypophosphatemia, hypoproteinemia, hypotension, intestinal obstruction, jaundice, kidney function abnormal, larynx edema, leukocytosis, leukoderma, leukopenia, liver enzymes increased, loss of consciousness, lymphadenopathy, lymphocytosis, maculopapular rash, menstrual abnormalities, miliaria, moniliasis, multiple myeloma, myasthenia, myocardial infarct, myoclonus, myopathy, neck rigidity, neuroleptic malignant-like syndrome, neuropathy, neutropenia, osteoporosis, pancytopenia, pleurisy, pneumonia, pyelonephritis, pyuria, rhabdomyolysis, rheumatoid arthritis, seizure, serotonin syndrome, SIADH, skin atrophy, Stevens-Johnson syndrome, suicidal ideation (reported at a frequency up to 2% in children/adolescents with major depressive disorder), suicide attempt, syncope, tendon rupture, thrombocythemia, thrombocytopenia, thrombophlebitis, toxic epidermal necrolysis, withdrawal syndrome

Overdosage/Toxicology Symptoms of overdose include somnolence and occasionally tachycardia. Predominantly occurs in combination with ethanol and/or other drug use. Most overdoses resolve with only supportive treatment, though ECG monitoring would be prudent considering the risk of arrythmia. Use of activated charcoal, inductions of emesis, or gastric lavage should be considered for acute ingestion. Forced diuresis, dialysis, and hemoperfusion not effective due to large volume of distribution.

Dosing

Adults:

Depression:

Immediate-release tablets: 75 mg/day, administered in 2 or 3 divided doses, taken with food; dose may be increased in 75 mg/day increments at intervals of at least 4 days, up to 225-375 mg/day

Extended-release capsules: 75 mg once daily taken with food; for some new patients, it may be desirable to start at 37.5 mg/day for 4-7 days before increasing to 75 mg once daily; dose may be increased by up to 75 mg/day increments every 4 days as tolerated, up to a maximum of 225 mg/day

GAD, social anxiety disorder: *Extended-release capsules:* 75 mg once daily taken with food; for some new patients, it may be desirable to start at 37.5 mg/day for 4-7 days before increasing to 75 mg once daily; dose may be increased by up to 75 mg/day increments every 4 days as tolerated, up to a maximum of 225 mg/day

Panic disorder: *Extended-release capsules:* 37.5 mg once daily for 1 week; may increase to 75 mg daily, with subsequent weekly increases of 75 mg/day up to a maximum of 225 mg/day.

Obsessive-compulsive disorder (unlabeled use): Titrate to usual dosage range of 150-300 mg/day; however, doses up to 375 mg daily have been used; response may be seen in 4 weeks

Neuropathic pain (unlabeled use): Dosages evaluated varied considerably based on etiology of chronic pain, but efficacy has been shown for many conditions in the range of 75-225 mg/day; onset of relief may occur in 1-2 weeks, or take up to 6 weeks for full benefit.

Hot flashes (unlabeled use): Doses of 37.5-75 mg/day have demonstrated significant improvement of vasomotor symptoms after 4-8 weeks of treatment; in one study, doses >75 mg/day offered no additional benefit; however, higher doses (225 mg/day) may be beneficial in patients with perimenopausal depression.

Attention-deficit disorder (unlabeled use): Initial: Doses vary between 18.75 to 75 mg/day; may increase after 4 weeks to 150 mg/day; if tolerated, doses up to 225 mg/day have been used

Note: When discontinuing this medication after more than 1 week of treatment, it is generally recommended that the dose be tapered. If venlafaxine is used for 6 weeks or longer, the dose should be tapered over 2 weeks when discontinuing its use.

Elderly: No specific recommendations for elderly, but may be best to start lower at 25-50 mg twice daily and increase as tolerated by 25 mg/dose. Extended-release formulation: 37.5 mg once daily, increase by 37.5 mg every 4-7 days as tolerated

Pediatrics: ADHD (unlabeled use): Children and Adolescents: Oral: Initial: 12.5 mg/day

Children <40 kg: Increase by 12.5 mg/week to maximum of 50 mg/day in 2 divided doses

Children ≥40 kg: Increase by 25 mg/week to maximum of 75 mg/day in 3 divided doses.

Mean dose: 60 mg or 1.4 mg/kg administered in 2-3 divided doses

Renal Impairment:

Cl_{cr} 10-70 mL/minute: Decrease dose by 25%.

Hemodialysis: Decrease total daily dose by 50% given after completion of dialysis.

Hepatic Impairment: Reduce total dosage by 50%.

Available Dosage Forms

Capsule, extended release (Effexor® XR): 37.5 mg, 75 mg, 150 mg

Tablet (Effexor®): 25 mg, 37.5 mg, 50 mg, 75 mg, 100 mg

Nursing Guidelines

Assessment: Assess other medications patient may be taking for effectiveness and interactions. Monitor for worsening of depression or suicidality, especially during initiation of therapy or with dose increases or decreases. Monitor therapeutic effectiveness according to rationale for therapy and adverse reactions at beginning of therapy and periodically with long-term use. Observe for clinical

(Continued)

Venlafaxine *(Continued)*

worsening, suicidality, or unusual behavior changes; especially during the initial few months of therapy or during dosage changes. Taper dosage slowly when discontinuing. Assess knowledge/teach patient appropriate use, interventions to reduce side effects, and adverse symptoms to report.

Monitoring Laboratory Tests: Cholesterol

Dietary Considerations: Should be taken with food.

Patient Education: Take exactly as directed; do not increase dose or frequency. It may take 2-3 weeks to achieve desired results. Take with food. Extended release capsules should be swallowed whole; do not crush or chew. Alternatively, contents may be emptied onto a spoonful of applesauce and swallowed without chewing. Avoid alcohol, caffeine, and other prescription or OTC medications not approved by prescriber. Maintain adequate hydration (2-3 L/day of fluids) unless instructed to restrict fluid intake. You may experience excess drowsiness or insomnia, lightheadedness, dizziness, or blurred vision (use caution when driving or engaging in tasks requiring alertness until response to drug is known); headache, nausea, vomiting, anorexia, altered taste, dry mouth (small frequent meals, frequent mouth care, chewing gum, or sucking lozenges may help); constipation (increased exercise, fluids, fruit, or fiber may help); diarrhea (buttermilk, yogurt, or boiled milk may help); postural hypotension (use caution when climbing stairs or changing position from lying or sitting to standing); urinary retention (void before taking medication); or sexual dysfunction (reversible). Report persistent CNS effects (eg, insomnia, restlessness, fatigue, anxiety, abnormal thoughts, suicidal ideation, confusion, personality changes, impaired cognitive function); muscle cramping or tremors; chest pain, palpitations, rapid heartbeat, swelling of extremities, or severe dizziness; unresolved urinary retention; vision changes or eye pain; hearing changes or ringing in ears; skin rash or irritation; or worsening of condition. **Pregnancy/breast-feeding precautions:** Inform prescriber if you are or intend to become pregnant. Do not breast-feed.

Geriatric Considerations: Has not been studied exclusively in the elderly, however, its low anticholinergic activity, minimal sedative and hypotensive effects make this a potentially valuable antidepressant in treating elderly with depression. No dose adjustment is necessary for age alone, additional studies are necessary; adjust dose for renal function in the elderly.

Pregnancy Risk Factor: C

Pregnancy Issues: Teratogenic effects were not observed in animal studies. Nonteratogenic effects including respiratory distress, cyanosis, apnea, seizures, temperature instability, feeding difficulty, vomiting, hypoglycemia, hypo- or hypertonia, hyper-reflexia, jitteriness, irritability, constant crying, and tremor have been reported in the neonate immediately following delivery after exposure late in the third trimester. Adverse effects may be due to toxic effects of SNRI or drug discontinuation. There are no adequate and well-controlled studies in pregnant women. Use during pregnancy only if the potential benefit to the mother outweighs the possible risk to the fetus. If treatment during pregnancy is required, consider tapering therapy during the third trimester.

Lactation: Enters breast milk/not recommended

Breast-Feeding Considerations: The manufacturer recommends discontinuing nursing or discontinuing venlafaxine, depending upon the importance of the drug to the mother.

Administration

Oral: Administer with food.

Extended release capsule: Swallow capsule whole; do not crush or chew. Alternatively, contents may be sprinkled on a spoonful of applesauce and swallowed immediately without chewing; followed with a glass of water to ensure complete swallowing of the pellets.

♦ **Venofer®** *see* Iron Sucrose *on page 969*

♦ **Ventolin® HFA** *see* Albuterol *on page 96*

♦ **VePesid®** *see* Etoposide *on page 695*

♦ **Veracolate [OTC]** *see* Bisacodyl *on page 245*

Verapamil (ver AP a mil)

U.S. Brand Names Calan®; Calan® SR; Covera-HS®; Isoptin® SR; Verelan®; Verelan® PM

Synonyms Iproveratril Hydrochloride; Verapamil Hydrochloride

Pharmacologic Category Antiarrhythmic Agent, Class IV; Calcium Channel Blocker

Medication Safety Issues

Sound-alike/look-alike issues:

Verapamil may be confused with Verelan®
Calan® may be confused with Colace®
Covera-HS® may be confused with Provera®
Isoptin® may be confused with Isopto® Tears
Verelan® may be confused with verapamil, Virilon®, Voltaren®

Use Orally for treatment of angina pectoris (vasospastic, chronic stable, unstable) and hypertension; I.V. for supraventricular tachyarrhythmias (PSVT, atrial fibrillation, atrial flutter)

Unlabeled/Investigational Use Migraine; hypertrophic cardiomyopathy; bipolar disorder (manic manifestations)

Mechanism of Action Inhibits calcium ion from entering the "slow channels" or select voltage-sensitive areas of vascular smooth muscle and myocardium during depolarization; produces a relaxation of coronary vascular smooth muscle and coronary vasodilation; increases myocardial oxygen delivery in patients with vasospastic angina; slows automaticity and conduction of AV node.

Pharmacodynamics/Kinetics

Onset of action: Peak effect: Oral: Immediate release: 1-2 hours; I.V.: 1-5 minutes
Duration: Oral: Immediate release tablets: 6-8 hours; I.V.: 10-20 minutes
Protein binding: 90%
Metabolism: Hepatic via multiple CYP isoenzymes; extensive first-pass effect
Bioavailability: Oral: 20% to 35%
Half-life elimination: Infants: 4.4-6.9 hours; Adults: Single dose: 2-8 hours, Multiple doses: 4.5-12 hours; prolonged with hepatic cirrhosis
Excretion: Urine (70%, 3% to 4% as unchanged drug); feces (16%)

Contraindications Hypersensitivity to verapamil or any component of the formulation; severe left ventricular dysfunction; hypotension (systolic pressure <90 mm Hg) or cardiogenic shock; sick sinus syndrome (except in patients with a functioning artificial pacemaker); second- or third-degree AV block (except in patients with a functioning artificial pacemaker); atrial flutter or fibrillation and an accessory bypass tract (WPW, Lown-Ganong-Levine syndrome)

Warnings/Precautions Avoid use in heart failure; can exacerbate condition. Can cause hypotension. Rare increases in liver function tests can be observed. Can cause first-degree AV block or sinus bradycardia. Other conduction abnormalities are rare. Use caution when using verapamil together with a beta-blocker. Avoid use of I.V. verapamil with an I.V. beta-blocker; can result in asystole. Use caution in patients with hypertrophic cardiomyopathy (IHSS). Use with caution in patients with attenuated neuromuscular transmission (Duchenne's muscular dystrophy, myasthenia gravis). Adjust the dose in severe renal dysfunction and hepatic dysfunction. Verapamil significantly increases digoxin serum concentrations (adjust digoxin's dose). May prolong recovery from nondepolarizing neuromuscular-blocking agents.

Drug Interactions **Substrate** of CYP1A2 (minor), 2B6 (minor), 2C8/9 (minor), 2C18 (minor), 2E1 (minor), 3A4 (major); **Inhibits** CYP1A2 (weak), 2C8/9 (weak), 2D6 (weak), 3A4 (moderate)

Alfentanil's plasma concentration is increased. Fentanyl and sufentanil may be affected similarly.

Amiodarone use may lead to bradycardia and decreased cardiac output. Monitor closely if using together.

Aspirin and concurrent verapamil use may increase bleeding times; monitor closely, especially if on other antiplatelet agents or anticoagulants.

Azole antifungals may inhibit the calcium channel blocker's metabolism; avoid this combination. Try an antifungal like terbinafine (if appropriate) or monitor closely for altered effect of the calcium channel blocker.

Barbiturates reduce the plasma concentration of verapamil. May require much higher dose of verapamil.

Beta-blockers may have increased pharmacodynamic interactions with verapamil (see Warnings/Precautions).

Buspirone's serum concentration may increase. May require dosage adjustment.

Calcium may reduce the calcium channel blocker's effects, particularly hypotension.

Carbamazepine's serum concentration is increased and toxicity may result; avoid this combination.

(Continued)

Verapamil *(Continued)*

Cimetidine reduced verapamil's metabolism; consider an alternative H_2 antagonist.

Colchicine: Verapamil may increase colchicine toxicity (especially nephrotoxicity).

Cyclosporine's serum concentrations are increased by verapamil; avoid this combination. Use another calcium channel blocker or monitor cyclosporine trough levels and renal function closely.

CYP3A4 inducers: CYP3A4 inducers may decrease the levels/effects of verapamil. Example inducers include aminoglutethimide, carbamazepine, nafcillin, nevirapine, phenobarbital, phenytoin, and rifamycins.

CYP3A4 inhibitors: May increase the levels/effects of verapamil. Example inhibitors include azole antifungals, clarithromycin, diclofenac, doxycycline, erythromycin, imatinib, isoniazid, nefazodone, nicardipine, propofol, protease inhibitors, telithromycin, and quinidine.

CYP3A4 substrates: Verapamil may increase the levels/effects of CYP3A4 substrates. Example substrates include benzodiazepines, calcium channel blockers, cyclosporine, mirtazapine, nateglinide, nefazodone, sildenafil (and other PDE-5 inhibitors), tacrolimus, and venlafaxine. Selected benzodiazepines (midazolam and triazolam), cisapride, ergot alkaloids, selected HMG-CoA reductase inhibitors (lovastatin and simvastatin), and pimozide are generally contraindicated with strong CYP3A4 inhibitors.

Digoxin's serum concentration is increased; reduce digoxin's dose when adding verapamil.

Doxorubicin's clearance was reduced; monitor for altered doxorubicin's effect.

Erythromycin may increase verapamil's effects; monitor altered verapamil effect.

Ethanol's effects may be increased by verapamil; reduce ethanol consumption.

Flecainide may have additive negative effects on conduction and inotropy.

Grapefruit juice: Verapamil serum concentrations may be increased by grapefruit juice. Avoid concurrent use.

HMG-CoA reductase inhibitors (atorvastatin, cerivastatin, lovastatin, simvastatin): Serum concentration will likely be increased; consider pravastatin/fluvastatin or a dihydropyridine calcium channel blocker. If concurrent use with lovastatin is unavoidable, dose of lovastatin should not exceed 40 mg/day.

Lithium neurotoxicity may result when verapamil is added; monitor lithium levels.

Midazolam's plasma concentration is increased by verapamil; monitor for prolonged CNS depression.

Nafcillin decreases plasma concentration of verapamil; avoid this combination.

Nondepolarizing muscle relaxant: Neuromuscular blockade may be prolonged. Monitor closely.

Prazosin's serum concentration increases; monitor blood pressure.

Quinidine's serum concentration is increased; adjust quinidine's dose as necessary.

Rifampin increases the metabolism of calcium channel blockers; adjust the dose of the calcium channel blocker to maintain efficacy.

Risperidone: Verapamil may increase the levels and effects of risperidone.

Sildenafil, tadalafil, vardenafil: Blood pressure-lowering effects may be additive; use caution.

Tacrolimus's serum concentrations are increased by verapamil; avoid the combination. Use another calcium channel blocker or monitor tacrolimus trough levels and renal function closely.

Theophylline's serum concentration may be increased by verapamil. Those at increased risk include children and cigarette smokers.

Nutritional/Herbal/Ethanol Interactions

Ethanol: Avoid or limit ethanol (may increase ethanol levels).

Food: Grapefruit juice may increase the serum concentration of verapamil; avoid concurrent use.

Herb/Nutraceutical: St John's wort may decrease levels. Avoid dong quai if using for hypertension (has estrogenic activity). Avoid ephedra, yohimbe, ginseng (may worsen arrhythmia or hypertension). Avoid garlic (may have increased antihypertensive effect).

Lab Interactions Increased alkaline phosphatase, CPK, LDH, aminotransferase [AST (SGOT)/ALT (SGPT)] (S)

Adverse Reactions

>10%: Gastrointestinal: Gingival hyperplasia (up to 19%), constipation (12% up to 42% in clinical trials)

1% to 10%:

Cardiovascular: Bradycardia (1.2 to 1.4%), first-, second-, or third-degree AV block (1.2%), CHF (1.8%), hypotension (2.5% to 3%), peripheral edema (1.9%), symptomatic hypotension (1.5% I.V.), severe tachycardia (1%)

Central nervous system: Dizziness (1.2% to 3.3%), fatigue (1.7%), headache (1.2% to 2.2%)

Dermatologic: Rash (1.2%)

Gastrointestinal: Nausea (0.9% to 2.7%)

Respiratory: Dyspnea (1.4%)

<1% (Limited to important or life-threatening): Alopecia, angina, arthralgia, asystole, atrioventricular dissociation, bronchial/laryngeal spasm, cerebrovascular accident, chest pain, claudication, confusion, diarrhea, dry mouth, ecchymosis, electrical mechanical dissociation (EMD), emotional depression, eosinophilia, equilibrium disorders, erythema multiforme, exanthema, exfoliative dermatitis, galactorrhea/hyperprolactinemia, GI obstruction, gingival hyperplasia, gynecomastia, hair color change, impotence, muscle cramps, MI, myoclonus, paresthesia, Parkinsonian syndrome, psychotic symptoms, purpura (vasculitis), rash, respiratory failure, rotary nystagmus, shakiness, shock, somnolence, Stevens-Johnson syndrome, syncope, urticaria, ventricular fibrillation, vertigo

Overdosage/Toxicology Primary cardiac symptoms of calcium blocker overdose include hypotension and bradycardia (second- or third-degree atrioventricular block, or sinus arrest with junctional rhythm). Intraventricular conduction is usually not affected so QRS duration is normal (verapamil does prolong the PR interval).

Noncardiac symptoms include confusion, stupor, nausea, vomiting, metabolic acidosis and hyperglycemia. Following initial gastric decontamination, if possible, repeated calcium administration may promptly reverse depressed cardiac contractility (but not sinus node depression or peripheral vasodilation). Large doses of calcium chloride (up to 1 g/hour for 24 hours) have been used in refractory cases. Glucagon, epinephrine, and amrinone may treat refractory hypotension. Glucagon and epinephrine also increase heart rate (outside the U.S., 4-aminopyridine may be available as an antidote). Dialysis and hemoperfusion are not effective in enhancing elimination although repeat-dose activated charcoal may serve as an adjunct with sustained-release preparations.

Dosing

Adults:

Angina: Oral: Initial: 80-120 mg twice daily (elderly or small stature: 40 mg twice daily); range: 240-480 mg/day in 3-4 divided doses

Hypertension: Oral:

Immediate release: 80 mg 3 times/day; usual dose range (JNC 7): 80-320 mg/day in 2 divided doses

Sustained release: 240 mg/day; usual dose range (JNC 7): 120-360 mg/day in 1-2 divided doses; 120 mg/day in the elderly or small patients (no evidence of additional benefit in doses >360 mg/day).

Extended release:

Covera-HS®: Usual dose range (JNC 7): 120-360 mg once daily (once-daily dosing is recommended at bedtime)

Verelan® PM: Usual dose range: 200-400 mg once daily at bedtime

Arrhythmia (SVT): I.V.: 2.5-5 mg (over 2 minutes); second dose of 5-10 mg (~0.15 mg/kg) may be given 15-30 minutes after the initial dose if patient tolerates, but does not respond to initial dose; maximum total dose: 20 mg

Elderly:

Oral: 120-480 mg/24 hours divided 3-4 times/day

Sustained release: 120 mg/day; adjust dose after 24 hours by increases of 120 mg/day. When switching from immediate release forms, total daily dose may remain the same. Controlled onset: initiate therapy with 180 mg in the evening; titrate upward as needed to obtain desired response and avoiding adverse effects.

Pediatrics: Children: SVT:

I.V.:

<1 year: 0.1-0.2 mg/kg over 2 minutes; repeat every 30 minutes as needed

1-15 years: 0.1-0.3 mg/kg over 2 minutes; maximum: 5 mg/dose, may repeat dose in 15 minutes if adequate response not achieved; maximum for second dose: 10 mg/dose

Oral (dose not well established):

1-5 years: 4-8 mg/kg/day in 3 divided doses **or** 40-80 mg every 8 hours

>5 years: 80 mg every 6-8 hours

(Continued)

Verapamil *(Continued)*

Renal Impairment: Cl_{cr} <10 mL/minute: Administer 50% to 75% of normal dose.

Hepatic Impairment: In cirrhosis, reduce dose to 20% to 50% of normal and monitor ECG.

Available Dosage Forms

Caplet, sustained release (Calan® SR): 120 mg, 180 mg, 240 mg

Capsule, extended release, controlled onset (Verelan® PM): 100 mg, 200 mg, 300 mg

Capsule, sustained release, as hydrochloride (Verelan®): 120 mg, 180 mg, 240 mg, 360 mg

Injection, solution, as hydrochloride: 2.5 mg/mL (2 mL, 4 mL)

Tablet, as hydrochloride: 80 mg, 120 mg

Calan®: 40 mg, 80 mg, 120 mg

Tablet, extended release: 120 mg, 180 mg, 240 mg

Tablet, extended release, controlled onset (Covera-HS®): 180 mg, 240 mg

Tablet, sustained release, as hydrochloride (Isoptin® SR): 120 mg, 180 mg, 240 mg

Nursing Guidelines

Assessment: Assess other medications patient may be taking for effectiveness and interactions. I.V. requires use of infusion pump and continuous cardiac and hemodynamic monitoring. Assess results of laboratory tests, therapeutic effectiveness, and adverse reactions when beginning therapy, when titrating dosage, and periodically during long-term oral therapy. Assess knowledge/teach patient appropriate use (oral), interventions to reduce side effects, and adverse symptoms to report.

Dietary Considerations: Calan® SR and Isoptin® SR products may be taken with food or milk, other formulations may be administered without regard to meals; sprinkling contents of Verelan® or Verelan® PM capsule onto applesauce does not affect oral absorption.

Patient Education: Oral: Take as directed. Do not alter dosage or discontinue therapy without consulting prescriber. Do not crush or chew sustained or extended release forms. Avoid grapefruit juice; avoid (or limit) alcohol and caffeine. You may experience dizziness or lightheadedness (use caution when driving or engaging in tasks requiring alertness until response to drug is known); nausea or vomiting (small frequent meals, frequent mouth care, chewing gum, or sucking lozenges may help); constipation (increased exercise, fluids, fruit, or fiber may help); or diarrhea (buttermilk, boiled milk, or yogurt may help). Report chest pain, palpitations, or irregular heartbeat; unusual cough, respiratory difficulty, or swelling of extremities (feet/ankles); muscle tremors or weakness; confusion or acute lethargy; or skin irritation or rash. **Pregnancy precaution:** Inform prescriber if you are or intend to become pregnant.

Geriatric Considerations: Elderly may experience a greater hypotensive response. Theoretically, constipation may be more of a problem in the elderly. Calcium channel blockers are no more effective in the elderly than other therapies, however, they do not cause significant CNS effects, which is an advantage over some antihypertensive agents. Generic verapamil products which are bioequivalent in young adults may not be bioequivalent in the elderly. Use generics cautiously.

Pregnancy Risk Factor: C

Pregnancy Issues: Crosses the placenta. One report of suspected heart block when used to control fetal supraventricular tachycardia. May exhibit tocolytic effects.

Lactation: Enters breast milk (small amounts)/not recommended

Breast-Feeding Considerations: Crosses into breast milk; manufacturer recommends to discontinue breast-feeding while taking verapamil. AAP considers **compatible** with breast-feeding.

Perioperative/Anesthesia/Other Concerns: I.V. administration, hypertrophic cardiomyopathy, sick sinus syndrome, moderate to severe congestive heart failure, concomitant therapy with beta-blockers or digoxin can all increase incidence of adverse effects. Verapamil should be avoided in patients with left ventricular dysfunction, pulmonary congestion, or heart failure. Verapamil may be administered intravenously in the acute setting to attain ventricular rate control in patients with atrial fibrillation or flutter. Patients that respond, defined in general as at least a 20% decrease in ventricular response rate or attaining a rate <100 beats/minute, can be continued on oral therapy to maintain control. It is important to consider the potential drug interaction with digoxin, as these agents are both used in this setting.

Administration

Oral: Do not crush or chew sustained or extended release products.

Calan® SR, Isoptin® SR: Administer with food.

Verelan®, Verelan® PM: Capsules may be opened and the contents sprinkled on 1 tablespoonful of applesauce, then swallowed without chewing.

I.V.: Rate of infusion: Over 2 minutes

Compatibility: Stable in dextran 40 10% in NS, dextran 75 6% in NS, D_5LR, D_5½NS, D_5NS, D_5W, LR, ½NS, NS

Y-site administration: Incompatible with albumin, amphotericin B cholesteryl sulfate complex, ampicillin, nafcillin, oxacillin, propofol, sodium bicarbonate

Compatibility when admixed: Incompatible with albumin, amphotericin B, floxacillin, hydralazine, trimethoprim/sulfamethoxazole

Storage: Store injection at room temperature. Protect from heat and from freezing. Use only clear solutions. Protect I.V. solution from light.

- **Verapamil Hydrochloride** *see* Verapamil *on page 1702*
- **Verelan®** *see* Verapamil *on page 1702*
- **Verelan® PM** *see* Verapamil *on page 1702*
- **Versed** *see* Midazolam *on page 1158*
- **Viactiv® Multivitamin [OTC]** *see* Vitamins (Multiple/Oral) *on page 1720*
- **Viadur®** *see* Leuprolide *on page 1015*
- **Vibramycin®** *see* Doxycycline *on page 584*
- **Vibra-Tabs®** *see* Doxycycline *on page 584*
- **Vicks® Casero™ [OTC]** *see* Guaifenesin *on page 834*
- **Vicks® DayQuil® Multi-Symptom Cold and Flu [OTC]** *see* Acetaminophen, Dextromethorphan, and Pseudoephedrine *on page 73*
- **Vicks Sinex® 12 Hour [OTC]** *see* Oxymetazoline *on page 1290*
- **Vicks Sinex® 12 Hour Ultrafine Mist [OTC]** *see* Oxymetazoline *on page 1290*
- **Vicks® Sinex® Nasal Spray [OTC]** *see* Phenylephrine *on page 1350*
- **Vicks® Sinex® UltraFine Mist [OTC]** *see* Phenylephrine *on page 1350*
- **Vicodin®** *see* Hydrocodone and Acetaminophen *on page 867*
- **Vicodin® ES** *see* Hydrocodone and Acetaminophen *on page 867*
- **Vicodin® HP** *see* Hydrocodone and Acetaminophen *on page 867*
- **Vicon Forte®** *see* Vitamins (Multiple/Oral) *on page 1720*
- **Vi-Daylin® ADC [OTC] [DSC]** *see* Vitamins (Multiple/Pediatric) *on page 1720*
- **Vi-Daylin® ADC + Iron [OTC] [DSC]** *see* Vitamins (Multiple/Pediatric) *on page 1720*
- **Vi-Daylin® Drops [OTC] [DSC]** *see* Vitamins (Multiple/Pediatric) *on page 1720*
- **Vi-Daylin®/F [DSC]** *see* Vitamins (Multiple/Pediatric) *on page 1720*
- **Vi-Daylin®/F ADC [DSC]** *see* Vitamins (Multiple/Pediatric) *on page 1720*
- **Vi-Daylin®/F ADC + Iron [DSC]** *see* Vitamins (Multiple/Pediatric) *on page 1720*
- **Vi-Daylin®/F + Iron [DSC]** *see* Vitamins (Multiple/Pediatric) *on page 1720*
- **Vi-Daylin® + Iron Drops [OTC] [DSC]** *see* Vitamins (Multiple/Pediatric) *on page 1720*
- **Vi-Daylin® + Iron Liquid [OTC] [DSC]** *see* Vitamins (Multiple/Oral) *on page 1720*
- **Vi-Daylin® Liquid [OTC] [DSC]** *see* Vitamins (Multiple/Oral) *on page 1720*
- **Videx®** *see* Didanosine *on page 528*
- **Videx® EC** *see* Didanosine *on page 528*
- **Vigamox™** *see* Moxifloxacin *on page 1183*

VinBLAStine (vin BLAS teen)

Synonyms NSC-49842; Vinblastine Sulfate; VLB

Pharmacologic Category Antineoplastic Agent, Natural Source (Plant) Derivative; Antineoplastic Agent, Vinca Alkaloid

Medication Safety Issues

Sound-alike/look-alike issues:

VinBLAStine may be confused with vinCRIStine, vinorelbine

Note: Must be dispensed in overwrap which bears the statement "**Do not remove covering until the moment of injection. Fatal if given intrathecally. For I.V. use only.**" Syringes should be labeled: "**Fatal if given intrathecally. For I.V. use only.**"

Use Treatment of Hodgkin's and non-Hodgkin's lymphoma, testicular, lung, head and neck, breast, and renal carcinomas, Mycosis fungoides, Kaposi's sarcoma, histiocytosis, choriocarcinoma, and idiopathic thrombocytopenic purpura

(Continued)

VinBLAStine *(Continued)*

Mechanism of Action Vinblastine binds to tubulin and inhibits microtubule formation, therefore, arresting the cell at metaphase by disrupting the formation of the mitotic spindle; it is specific for the M and S phases. Vinblastine may also interfere with nucleic acid and protein synthesis by blocking glutamic acid utilization.

Pharmacodynamics/Kinetics

Distribution: V_d: 27.3 L/kg; binds extensively to tissues; does not penetrate CNS or other fatty tissues; distributes to liver

Protein binding: 99%

Metabolism: Hepatic to active metabolite

Half-life elimination: Biphasic: Initial: 0.164 hours; Terminal: 25 hours

Excretion: Feces (95%); urine (<1% as unchanged drug)

Contraindications For I.V. use only; **I.T. use may result in death**; hypersensitivity to vinblastine or any component of the formulation; pregnancy

Warnings/Precautions Hazardous agent - use appropriate precautions for handling and disposal. Vinblastine is a moderate vesicant; avoid extravasation. Dosage modification required in patients with impaired liver function and neurotoxicity. Using small amounts of drug daily for long periods may cause neurotoxicity and is therefore not advised. For I.V. use only. **Intrathecal administration may result in death**. Monitor closely for shortness of breath or bronchospasm in patients receiving mitomycin C.

Drug Interactions Substrate of CYP2D6 (minor), 3A4 (major); **Inhibits** CYP2D6 (weak), 3A4 (weak)

CYP3A4 inducers: CYP3A4 inducers may decrease the levels/effects of vinblastine. Example inducers include aminoglutethimide, carbamazepine, nafcillin, nevirapine, phenobarbital, phenytoin, and rifamycins.

CYP3A4 inhibitors: May increase the levels/effects of vinblastine. Example inhibitors include azole antifungals, clarithromycin, diclofenac, doxycycline, erythromycin, imatinib, isoniazid, nefazodone, nicardipine, propofol, protease inhibitors, quinidine, telithromycin, and verapamil.

Mitomycin-C: Previous or simultaneous use with mitomycin-C has resulted in acute shortness of breath and severe bronchospasm within minutes or several hours after vinca alkaloid injection and may occur up to 2 weeks after the dose of mitomycin. Mitomycin-C, in combination with administration of VLB, may cause acute shortness of breath and severe bronchospasm, onset may be within minutes or several hours after VLB injection

Phenytoin may reduce vinblastine serum concentrations.

Nutritional/Herbal/Ethanol Interactions Herb/Nutraceutical: St John's wort may decrease vinblastine levels. Avoid black cohosh, dong quai in estrogen-dependent tumors.

Adverse Reactions

>10%:

Dermatologic: Alopecia

Endocrine & metabolic: SIADH

Gastrointestinal: Diarrhea (less common), stomatitis, anorexia, metallic taste

Hematologic: May cause severe bone marrow suppression and is the dose-limiting toxicity of VLB (unlike vincristine); severe granulocytopenia and thrombocytopenia may occur following the administration of VLB and nadir 5-10 days after treatment

Myelosuppression (primarily leukopenia, may be dose limiting)

Onset: 4-7 days

Nadir: 5-10 days

Recovery: 4-21 days

1% to 10%:

Cardiovascular: Hypertension, Raynaud's phenomenon

Central nervous system: Depression, malaise, headache, seizure

Dermatologic: Rash, photosensitivity, dermatitis

Endocrine & metabolic: Hyperuricemia

Gastrointestinal: Constipation, abdominal pain, nausea (mild), vomiting (mild), paralytic ileus, stomatitis

Genitourinary: Urinary retention

Neuromuscular & skeletal: Jaw pain, myalgia, paresthesia

Respiratory: Bronchospasm

<1% (Limited to important or life-threatening): Hemorrhagic colitis, neurotoxicity (rare; symptoms may include peripheral neuropathy, loss of deep tendon reflexes, headache, weakness, urinary retention, GI symptoms, tachycardia, orthostatic hypotension, convulsions), rectal bleeding

Overdosage/Toxicology Symptoms of overdose include bone marrow suppression, mental depression, paresthesia, loss of deep tendon reflexes, and neurotoxicity. There are no antidotes for vinblastine. Treatment is supportive and symptomatic, including fluid restriction or hypertonic saline (3% sodium chloride) for drug-induced secretion of inappropriate antidiuretic hormone (SIADH).

Dosing

Adults & Elderly: Refer to individual protocols.

Antineoplastic (typical dosages): I.V.: 4-20 mg/m^2 (0.1-0.5 mg/kg) every 7-10 days **or** 5-day continuous infusion of 1.5-2 mg/m^2/day **or** 0.1-0.5 mg/kg/week

Pediatrics: Refer to adult dosing.

Renal Impairment: Not removed by hemodialysis

Hepatic Impairment:

Serum bilirubin 1.5-3.0 mg/dL or AST 60-180 units: Administer 50% of normal dose.

Serum bilirubin 3.0-5.0 mg/dL: Administer 25% of dose.

Serum bilirubin >5.0 mg/dL or AST >180 units: Omit dose.

Available Dosage Forms

Injection, powder for reconstitution, as sulfate: 10 mg

Injection, solution, as sulfate: 1 mg/mL (10 mL) [contains benzyl alcohol]

Nursing Guidelines

Assessment: See Contraindications, Warnings/Precautions, and Dosing for use cautions. Assess potential for interactions with other prescriptions, OTC medications, or herbal products patient may be taking (especially mitomycin - see Drug Interactions). Premedication with antiemetic is advisable. Infusion site must be monitored closely to prevent extravasation (see Administration). Assess results of laboratory tests (see below), therapeutic effectiveness, and adverse reactions prior to each infusion and throughout therapy (see Adverse Reactions and Overdose/Toxicology). Teach patient possible side effects/ appropriate interventions and adverse symptoms to report (see Patient Education). **Pregnancy risk factor D** - determine that patient is not pregnant before beginning treatment. Teach patients of childbearing age, and males who may have intercourse with females of childbearing age, appropriate use of barrier contraceptives. Breast-feeding is not recommended.

Monitoring Laboratory Tests: CBC with differential and platelet count, serum uric acid, hepatic function

Patient Education: Inform prescriber of all prescriptions, OTC medications, or herbal products you are taking, and any allergies you have. Do not take any new medication during therapy unless approved by prescriber. This medication can only be administered by infusion; report immediately any redness, swelling, burning, or pain at infusion site. Maintain adequate hydration (2-3 L/day of fluids) unless instructed to restrict fluid intake, and nutrition (small, frequent meals will help). You will be more susceptible to infection (avoid crowds and exposure to infection and do not have any vaccinations unless approved by prescriber). May cause hair loss (will grow back after therapy); nausea or vomiting (request antiemetic); photosensitivity (use sunscreen, wear protective clothing and eyewear, and avoid direct sunlight); feelings of extreme weakness or lethargy (use caution when driving or engaging in tasks requiring alertness until response to drug is known); or mouth sores (use soft toothbrush, waxed dental floss, and frequent oral care). Report numbness or tingling in fingers or toes (use care to prevent injury); weakness or pain in muscles or jaw; signs of infection (eg, fever, chills, sore throat, burning urination, fatigue); unusual bleeding (eg, tarry stools, easy bruising, blood in stool, urine, or mouth); unresolved mouth sores; skin rash or itching; or respiratory difficulty. **Pregnancy/ breast-feeding precautions:** Do not get pregnant (females) or cause a pregnancy (males) during this therapy. Consult prescriber for appropriate contraceptive measures. Breast-feeding is not recommended.

Pregnancy Risk Factor: D

Lactation: Enters breast milk/not recommended

Administration

I.V.: Vesicant. **Fatal if given intrathecally.** For I.V. administration only, usually as a slow (2-3 minutes) push, or a bolus (5- to 15-minute) infusion. It is occasionally given as a 24-hour continuous infusion.

Reconstitution: Reconstitute to a concentration of 1 mg/mL with bacteriostatic water, bacteriostatic NS, SWFI, NS, or D_5W; for infusion, may be diluted with 50-1000 mL Ns or D_5W.

Compatibility: Stable in D_5W, LR, NS, bacteriostatic water

Y-site administration: Incompatible with cefepime, furosemide

(Continued)

VinBLAStine *(Continued)*

Compatibility in syringe: Incompatible with furosemide

Storage: Store intact vials under refrigeration (2°C to 8°C) and protect from light. Solutions reconstituted in bacteriostatic water or bacteriostatic NS are stable for 21 days at room temperature or under refrigeration.

Note: Must be dispensed in overwrap which bears the statement "Do not remove covering until the moment of injection. Fatal if given intrathecally. For I.V. use only." Syringes should be labeled: **"Fatal if given intrathecally. For I.V. use only."**

♦ **Vinblastine Sulfate** *see* VinBLAStine *on page 1707*

♦ **Vincasar PFS®** *see* VinCRIStine *on page 1710*

VinCRIStine (vin KRIS teen)

U.S. Brand Names Vincasar PFS®

Synonyms LCR; Leurocristine Sulfate; NSC-67574; VCR; Vincristine Sulfate

Pharmacologic Category Antineoplastic Agent, Natural Source (Plant) Derivative; Antineoplastic Agent, Vinca Alkaloid

Medication Safety Issues

Sound-alike/look-alike issues:

VinCRIStine may be confused with vinBLAStine

Oncovin® may be confused with Ancobon®

To prevent fatal inadvertent intrathecal injection, it is recommended that all doses be dispensed in a small minibag. When dispensing vincristine in a syringe, vincristine must be packaged in the manufacturer-provided overwrap which bears the statement **"Do not remove covering until the moment of injection. For intravenous use only. Fatal if given intrathecally."**

Use Treatment of leukemias, Hodgkin's disease, non-Hodgkin's lymphomas, Wilms' tumor, neuroblastoma, rhabdomyosarcoma

Mechanism of Action Binds to tubulin and inhibits microtubule formation; therefore arresting the cell at metaphase by disrupting the formation of the mitotic spindle; it is specific for the M and S phases. Vincristine may also interfere with nucleic acid and protein synthesis by blocking glutamic acid utilization.

Pharmacodynamics/Kinetics

Absorption: Oral: Poor

Distribution: V_d: 163-165 L/m^2; Poor penetration into CSF; rapidly removed from bloodstream and tightly bound to tissues; penetrates blood-brain barrier poorly

Protein binding: 75%

Metabolism: Extensively hepatic

Half-life elimination: Terminal: 24 hours

Excretion: Feces (~80%); urine (<1% as unchanged drug)

Contraindications Hypersensitivity to vincristine or any component of the formulation; **for I.V. use only, fatal if given intrathecally**; patients with demyelinating form of Charcot-Marie-Tooth syndrome; pregnancy

Warnings/Precautions The U.S. Food and Drug Administration (FDA) currently recommends that procedures for proper handling and disposal of antineoplastic agents be considered. Dosage modification required in patients with impaired hepatic function or who have pre-existing neuromuscular disease; avoid extravasation; use with caution in the elderly; avoid eye contamination; observe closely for shortness of breath, bronchospasm, especially in patients treated with mitomycin C. For I.V. use only; **intrathecal administration results in death**; administer allopurinol to prevent uric acid nephropathy; not to be used with radiation.

Drug Interactions Substrate of CYP3A4 (major); **Inhibits** CYP3A4 (weak)

CYP3A4 inducers: CYP3A4 inducers may decrease the levels/effects of vincristine. Example inducers include aminoglutethimide, carbamazepine, nafcillin, nevirapine, phenobarbital, phenytoin, and rifamycins.

CYP3A4 inhibitors: May increase the levels/effects of vincristine. Example inhibitors include azole antifungals, clarithromycin, diclofenac, doxycycline, erythromycin, imatinib, isoniazid, nefazodone, nicardipine, propofol, protease inhibitors, quinidine, telithromycin, and verapamil.

Digoxin plasma levels and renal excretion may decrease with combination chemotherapy including vincristine

Mitomycin-C: Acute pulmonary reactions may occur with mitomycin-C. Previous or simultaneous use with mitomycin-C has resulted in acute shortness of breath and severe bronchospasm within minutes or several hours after vinca alkaloid injection and may occur up to 2 weeks after the dose of mitomycin.

Nifedipine: May increase the levels/effects of vincristine; monitor.

Phenytoin levels may decrease with combination chemotherapy.

Vincristine should be given 12-24 hours before asparaginase to minimize toxicity (may decrease the hepatic clearance of vincristine)

Nutritional/Herbal/Ethanol Interactions Herb/Nutraceutical: St John's wort may decrease vincristine levels.

Adverse Reactions

>10%: Dermatologic: Alopecia (20% to 70%)

1% to 10%:

Cardiovascular: Orthostatic hypotension or hypertension, hyper-/hypotension

Central nervous system: CNS depression, confusion, cranial nerve paralysis, fever, headache, insomnia, motor difficulties, seizure

Intrathecal administration of vincristine has uniformly caused death; vincristine should never be administered by this route. Neurologic effects of vincrisitne may be additive with those of other neurotoxic agents and spinal cord irradiation.

Dermatologic: Rash

Endocrine & metabolic: Hyperuricemia

Gastrointestinal: Abdominal cramps, anorexia, bloating, constipation (and possible paralytic ileus secondary to neurologic toxicity), diarrhea, metallic taste, nausea (mild), oral ulceration, vomiting, weight loss

Genitourinary: Bladder atony (related to neurotoxicity), dysuria, polyuria, urinary retention

Hematologic: Leukopenia (mild), thrombocytopenia

Local: Phlebitis, tissue irritation and necrosis if infiltrated

Neuromuscular & skeletal: Cramping, jaw pain, leg pain, myalgia, numbness, weakness

Peripheral neuropathy: Frequently the dose-limiting toxicity of vincristine. Most frequent in patients >40 years of age; occurs usually after an average of 3 weekly doses, but may occur after just one dose. Manifested as loss of the deep tendon reflexes in the lower extremities, numbness, tingling, pain, paresthesia of the fingers and toes (stocking glove sensation), and "foot drop" or "wrist drop."

Ocular: Optic atrophy, photophobia

<1% (Limited to important or life-threatening): SIADH (rare), stomatitis

Overdosage/Toxicology Symptoms of overdose include bone marrow suppression, mental depression, paresthesia, loss of deep tendon reflexes, alopecia, and nausea. Severe symptoms may occur with 3-4 mg/m^2.

There are no antidotes for vincristine. Treatment is supportive and symptomatic, including fluid restriction or hypertonic saline (3% sodium chloride) for drug-induced secretion of inappropriate antidiuretic hormone (SIADH). Case reports suggest that folinic acid may be helpful in treating vincristine overdose. It is suggested that 100 mg folinic acid be given I.V. every 3 hours for 24 hours, then every 6 hours for 48 hours. This is in addition to supportive care. The use of pyridoxine, leucovorin factor, cyanocobalamin, or thiamine has been used with little success for drug-induced peripheral neuropathy.

Dosing

Adults & Elderly: Note: Doses are often capped at 2 mg; however, this may reduce the efficacy of the therapy and may not be advisable. Refer to individual protocols; orders for single doses >2.5 mg or >5 mg/treatment cycle should be verified with the specific treatment regimen and/or an experienced oncologist prior to dispensing.

Antineoplastic (typical dosages): I.V.: 0.4-1.4 mg/m^2, may repeat every week **or**

0.4-0.5 mg/day continuous infusion for 4 days every 4 weeks **or**

0.25-0.5 mg/m^2/day continuous infusion for 5 days every 4 weeks

Pediatrics: Refer to individual protocols. **Note:** Doses are often capped at 2 mg; however, this may reduce the efficacy of the therapy and may not be advisable. Orders for single doses >2.5 mg or >5 mg/treatment cycle should be verified with the specific treatment regimen and/or an experienced oncologist prior to dispensing.

Antineoplastic (typical dosages): I.V.:

Children ≤10 kg or BSA <1 m^2: Initial therapy: 0.05 mg/kg once weekly then titrate dose

Children >10 kg or BSA ≥1 m^2: 1-2 mg/m^2, may repeat once weekly for 3-6 weeks; maximum single dose: 2 mg

(Continued)

VinCRIStine *(Continued)*

Neuroblastoma: I.V. continuous infusion with doxorubicin: 1 mg/m²/day for 72 hours

Hepatic Impairment:

Serum bilirubin 1.5-3.0 mg/dL or AST 60-180 units: Administer 50% of normal dose.

Serum bilirubin 3.0-5.0 mg/dL: Administer 25% of dose.

Serum bilirubin >5.0 mg/dL or AST >180 units: Omit dose.

Available Dosage Forms Injection, solution, as sulfate: 1 mg/mL (1 mL, 2 mL)

Nursing Guidelines

Assessment: Use caution with impaired liver function (see Warnings/Precautions for specific for use cautions). Assess potential for interactions with other pharmacological agents and herbal products patient may be taking (eg, previous or concurrent use with mitomycin-C can cause severe reaction; see Drug Interactions). Premedication with antiemetic is advisable. Infusion site must be monitored closely to prevent extravasation (vesicant will cause tissue damage and necrosis). May cause severe constipation, paralytic ileus, intestinal obstruction, necrosis, and/or perforation; prophylactic bowel management regimen may be advisable. Assess results of laboratory tests, hepatic function, and adverse reactions prior to each infusion and throughout therapy (eg, CNS [motor difficulties, seizure, depression], neuromuscular [myalgia, cramping], peripheral neuropathy, photophobia; see Adverse Reactions). Teach patient possible side effects/appropriate interventions and adverse symptoms to report (see Patient Education).

Monitoring Laboratory Tests: Serum electrolytes (sodium), hepatic function, CBC, serum uric acid

Patient Education: Do not take any new medication during therapy unless approved by prescriber. This medication can only be administered by infusion; report immediately any redness, swelling, burning, or pain at infusion site. Maintain adequate hydration (2-3 L/day of fluids) unless instructed to restrict fluid intake and nutrition (small frequent meals will help). You will be more susceptible to infection (avoid crowds and exposure to infection and do not have any vaccinations unless approved by prescriber). May cause hair loss (will grow back after therapy); nausea or vomiting (request antiemetic); photosensitivity (use sunscreen, wear protective clothing and eyewear, and avoid direct sunlight); feelings of extreme weakness or lethargy (use caution when driving or engaging in tasks requiring alertness until response to drug is known); or mouth sores (use soft toothbrush, waxed dental floss, and frequent oral care). Report persistent constipation, abdominal pain; numbness or tingling in fingers or toes (use care to prevent injury); weakness, numbness, or pain in muscles or extremities; signs of infection (eg, fever, chills, sore throat, burning urination, fatigue); unusual bleeding (eg, tarry stools, easy bruising, blood in stool, urine, or mouth); unresolved mouth sores; skin rash or itching; or respiratory difficulty. **Pregnancy/breast-feeding precautions:** Do not get pregnant (females) or cause a pregnancy (males) during this therapy. Consult prescriber for appropriate contraceptive measures. Breast-feeding is not recommended.

Pregnancy Risk Factor: D

Lactation: Enters breast milk/not recommended

Administration

I.V.: Vesicant. For I.V. use only. **Fatal if given intrathecally.** Usually administered as slow (1-2 minutes) push or short (10-15 minutes) infusion; 24-hour continuous infusions are occasionally used

Reconstitution: Solutions for I.V. infusion may be mixed in NS or D_5W.

Compatibility: Stable in D_5W, LR, NS

Y-site administration: Incompatible with cefepime, furosemide, idarubicin, sodium bicarbonate

Compatibility in syringe: Incompatible with furosemide

Storage:

Undiluted vials: Store under refrigeration; may be stable for up to 30 days at room temperature

I.V. solution: Diluted in 20-50 mL NS or D_5W, stable for 7 days under refrigeration, or 2 days at room temperature. In ambulatory pumps, solution is stable for 7-10 days at room temperature.

♦ **Vincristine Sulfate** *see* VinCRIStine *on page 1710*

Vinorelbine (vi NOR el been)

U.S. Brand Names Navelbine®

Synonyms Dihydroxydeoxynorvinkaleukoblastine; NVB; Vinorelbine Tartrate

Pharmacologic Category Antineoplastic Agent, Natural Source (Plant) Derivative; Antineoplastic Agent, Vinca Alkaloid

Medication Safety Issues

Sound-alike/look-alike issues:

Vinorelbine may be confused with vinBLAStine

Use Treatment of nonsmall cell lung cancer

Unlabeled/Investigational Use Treatment of breast cancer, ovarian carcinoma, Hodgkin's disease, non-Hodgkin's lymphoma

Mechanism of Action Semisynthetic vinca alkaloid which binds to tubulin and inhibits microtubule formation, therefore, arresting the cell at metaphase by disrupting the formation of the mitotic spindle; it is specific for the M and S phases. Vinorelbine may also interfere with nucleic acid and protein synthesis by blocking glutamic acid utilization.

Pharmacodynamics/Kinetics

Absorption: Unreliable; must be given I.V.

Distribution: V_d: 25.4-40.1 L/kg; binds extensively to human platelets and lymphocytes (79.6% to 91.2%)

Protein binding: 80% to 90%

Metabolism: Extensively hepatic to two metabolites, deacetylvinorelbine (active) and vinorelbine N-oxide

Bioavailability: Oral: 26% to 45%

Half-life elimination: Triphasic: Terminal: 27.7-43.6 hours

Excretion: Feces (46%); urine (18%, 10% to 12% as unchanged drug)

Clearance: Plasma: Mean: 0.97-1.26 L/hour/kg

Contraindications For I.V. use only; **I.T. use may result in death**; hypersensitivity to vinorelbine or any component of the formulation; pregnancy

Warnings/Precautions Hazardous agent - use appropriate precautions for handling and disposal. Avoid extravasation; dosage modification required in patients with impaired liver function and neurotoxicity. Frequently monitor patients for myelosuppression both during and after therapy. Granulocytopenia is dose-limiting. **Intrathecal administration may result in death**. Use with caution in patients with cachexia or ulcerated skin.

Acute shortness of breath and severe bronchospasm have been reported, most commonly when administered with mitomycin. Fatal cases of interstitial pulmonary changes and ARDS have also been reported. May cause severe constipation (grade 3-4), paralytic ileus, intestinal obstruction, necrosis, and/or perforation.

Drug Interactions **Substrate** of CYP2D6 (minor), 3A4 (major); **Inhibits** CYP2D6 (weak), 3A4 (weak)

Cisplatin: Incidence of granulocytopenia is significantly higher than with single-agent vinorelbine.

CYP3A4 inducers: CYP3A4 inducers may decrease the levels/effects of vinorelbine. Example inducers include aminoglutethimide, carbamazepine, nafcillin, nevirapine, phenobarbital, phenytoin, and rifamycins.

CYP3A4 inhibitors: May increase the levels/effects of vinorelbine. Example inhibitors include azole antifungals, clarithromycin, diclofenac, doxycycline, erythromycin, imatinib, isoniazid, nefazodone, nicardipine, propofol, protease inhibitors, quinidine, telithromycin, and verapamil.

Mitomycin-C: Previous or simultaneous use with mitomycin-C has resulted in acute shortness of breath and severe bronchospasm within minutes or several hours after vinca alkaloid injection and may occur up to 2 weeks after the dose of mitomycin.

Nutritional/Herbal/Ethanol Interactions Herb/Nutraceutical: St John's wort may decrease vinorelbine levels.

Adverse Reactions

>10%:

Central nervous system: Fatigue (27%)

Dermatologic: Alopecia (12%)

Gastrointestinal: Nausea (44%, severe <2%), constipation (35%), vomiting (20%), diarrhea (17%)

Emetic potential: Moderate (30% to 60%)

Hematologic: May cause severe bone marrow suppression and is the dose-limiting toxicity of vinorelbine; severe granulocytopenia (90%) may

(Continued)

Vinorelbine *(Continued)*

occur following the administration of vinorelbine; leukopenia (92%), anemia (83%)

Myelosuppressive:

WBC: Moderate - severe

Onset: 4-7d days

Nadir: 7-10 days

Recovery: 14-21 days

Hepatic: Elevated SGOT (67%), elevated total bilirubin (13%)

Local: Injection site reaction (28%), injection site pain (16%)

Neuromuscular & skeletal: Weakness (36%), peripheral neuropathy (20% to 25%)

1% to 10%:

Cardiovascular: Chest pain (5%)

Gastrointestinal: Paralytic ileus (1%)

Hematologic: Thrombocytopenia (5%)

Local: Phlebitis (7%)

Neuromuscular & skeletal: Mild to moderate peripheral neuropathy manifested by paresthesia and hyperesthesia, loss of deep tendon reflexes (<5%); myalgia (<5%), arthralgia (<5%), jaw pain (<5%)

Respiratory: Dyspnea (3% to 7%)

<1% (Limited to important or life-threatening): Anaphylaxis, angioedema, deep vein thrombosis, dysphagia, esophagitis, gait instability, hemorrhagic cystitis, pancreatitis, pulmonary edema, pulmonary embolus, radiation recall (dermatitis, esophagitis), severe peripheral neuropathy (generally reversible), SIADH

Overdosage/Toxicology Symptoms of overdose include bone marrow suppression, mental depression, paresthesia, loss of deep tendon reflexes, and neurotoxicity. There are no antidotes for vinorelbine. Treatment is supportive and symptomatic, including fluid restriction or hypertonic saline (3% sodium chloride) for drug-induced secretion of inappropriate antidiuretic hormone (SIADH).

Dosing

Adults & Elderly: Refer to individual protocols.

Nonsmall cell lung cancer: I.V.:

Single-agent therapy: 30 mg/m^2 every 7 days

Combination therapy with cisplatin: 25 mg/m^2 every 7 days (with cisplatin 100 mg/m^2 every 4 weeks); **Alternatively:** 30 mg/m^2 in combination with cisplatin 120 mg/m^2 on days 1 and 29, then every 6 weeks.

Dosage adjustment in hematological toxicity (based on granulocyte counts):

Granulocytes ≥1500 cells/mm^3 on day of treatment: Administer 100% of starting dose.

Granulocytes 1000-1499 cells/mm^3 on day of treatment: Administer 50% of starting dose.

Granulocytes <1000 cells/mm^3 on day of treatment: Do not administer. Repeat granulocyte count in 1 week. If 3 consecutive doses are held because granulocyte count is <1000 cells/mm^3, discontinue vinorelbine.

Adjustment: For patients who, during treatment, have experienced fever or sepsis while granulocytopenic or had 2 consecutive weekly doses held due to granulocytopenia, subsequent doses of vinorelbine should be:

75% of starting dose for granulocytes ≥1500 cells/mm^3

37.5% of starting dose for granulocytes 1000-1499 cells/mm^3

Renal Impairment: No dose adjustments are required for renal insufficiency.

Hepatic Impairment:

Serum bilirubin ≤2 mg/dL: Administer 100% of starting dose.

Serum bilirubin 2.1-3 mg/dL: Administer 50% of starting dose.

Serum bilirubin >3 mg/dL: Administer 25% of starting dose.

In patients with concurrent hematologic toxicity and hepatic impairment, administer the lower doses determined from the above recommendations under Adult Dosing.

Available Dosage Forms Injection, solution [preservative free]: 10 mg/mL (1 mL, 5 mL)

Nursing Guidelines

Assessment: See Contraindications, Warnings/Precautions, and Dosing for use cautions. Assess potential for interactions with other prescriptions, OTC medications, or herbal products patient may be taking (see Drug Interactions). Premedication with antiemetic is advisable. May cause severe constipation, paralytic ileus, intestinal obstruction, necrosis, and/or perforation; prophylactic bowel management regimen may be advisable. Infusion site must be monitored closely to prevent extravasation (see Administration). Assess results of laboratory tests (see below) and monitor for adverse reactions prior to each infusion and throughout therapy (see Adverse Reactions and Overdose/Toxicology). Teach patient possible side effects/appropriate interventions and adverse symptoms to report (see Patient Education). **Pregnancy risk factor D** - determine that patient is not pregnant before beginning treatment. Teach patients of childbearing age, and males who may have intercourse with females of childbearing age, appropriate use of barrier contraceptives. Breast-feeding is contraindicated.

Monitoring Laboratory Tests: CBC with differential and platelet count, hepatic function

Patient Education: Inform prescriber of all prescriptions, OTC medications, or herbal products you are taking, and any allergies you have. Do not take any new medication during therapy unless approved by prescriber. This medication can only be administered by infusion; report immediately any redness, swelling, burning, or pain at infusion site. Maintain adequate hydration (2-3 L/day of fluids) unless instructed to restrict fluid intake, and nutrition (small, frequent meals will help). You will be more susceptible to infection (avoid crowds and exposure to infection and do not have any vaccinations unless approved by prescriber). May cause hair loss (will grow back after therapy); nausea or vomiting (request antiemetic); photosensitivity (use sunscreen, wear protective clothing and eyewear, and avoid direct sunlight); feelings of weakness or lethargy (use caution when driving or engaging in tasks requiring alertness until response to drug is known); or mouth sores (use soft toothbrush, waxed dental floss and frequent oral care). Report numbness or tingling in fingers or toes (use care to prevent injury); weakness, numbness, or pain in muscles or extremities; signs of infection (eg, fever, chills, sore throat, burning urination, fatigue); unusual bleeding (eg, tarry stools, easy bruising, blood in stool, urine, or mouth); unresolved mouth sores; skin rash or itching; or respiratory difficulty. **Pregnancy/breast-feeding precautions:** Do not get pregnant (females) or cause a pregnancy (males) during this therapy. Consult prescriber for appropriate contraceptive measures. Do not breast-feed.

Pregnancy Risk Factor: D

Lactation: Excretion in breast milk unknown/contraindicated

Administration

I.V.: FATAL IF GIVEN INTRATHECALLY. Administer as a direct intravenous push or rapid bolus, over 6-10 minutes (up to 30 minutes). Longer infusions may increase the risk of pain and phlebitis. Intravenous doses should be followed by 150-250 mL of saline or dextrose to reduce the incidence of phlebitis and inflammation.

Reconstitution: Dilute in 10-50 mL D_5W or NS.

Compatibility: Stable in $D_5{}^1/_2NS$, D_5W, LR, NS, $^1/_2NS$

Y-site administration: Incompatible with acyclovir, allopurinol, aminophylline, amphotericin B, amphotericin B cholesteryl sulfate complex, ampicillin, cefazolin, cefoperazone, cefotetan, ceftriaxone, cefuroxime, co-trimoxazole, fluorouracil, furosemide, ganciclovir, methylprednisolone sodium succinate, mitomycin, piperacillin, sodium bicarbonate, thiotepa

Storage: Store intact vials under refrigeration (2°C to 8°C) and protect from light; vials are stable at room temperature for up to 72 hours. Dilutions in D_5W or NS are stable for 24 hours at room temperature.

♦ **Vinorelbine Tartrate** *see* Vinorelbine *on page 1713*
♦ **Viokase®** *see* Pancrelipase *on page 1301*
♦ **Viosterol** *see* Ergocalciferol *on page 627*
♦ **Vioxx® [DSC]** *see* Rofecoxib *on page 1492*
♦ **Virazole®** *see* Ribavirin *on page 1475*
♦ **Viscoat®** *see* Chondroitin Sulfate and Sodium Hyaluronate *on page 387*
♦ **Visicol®** *see* Sodium Phosphates *on page 1549*
♦ **Visine® L.R. [OTC]** *see* Oxymetazoline *on page 1290*
♦ **Visipaque™** *see* Iodixanol *on page 953*
♦ **Vistaril®** *see* HydrOXYzine *on page 884*
♦ **Vistide®** *see* Cidofovir *on page 391*
♦ **Vita-C® [OTC]** *see* Ascorbic Acid *on page 187*
♦ **Vitaball® [OTC]** *see* Vitamins (Multiple/Pediatric) *on page 1720*
♦ **Vitaball® Wild N Fruity [OTC]** *see* Vitamins (Multiple/Pediatric) *on page 1720*

- ♦ **Vitacon Forte** *see* Vitamins (Multiple/Oral) *on page 1720*
- ♦ **Vitamin C** *see* Ascorbic Acid *on page 187*
- ♦ **Vitamin D_2** *see* Ergocalciferol *on page 627*
- ♦ **Vitamin B_1** *see* Thiamine *on page 1623*
- ♦ **Vitamin B_3** *see* Niacin *on page 1218*
- ♦ **Vitamin B_{12}** *see* Cyanocobalamin *on page 457*

Vitamin B Complex Combinations

(VYE ta min bee KOM pleks kom bi NAY shuns)

U.S. Brand Names Allbee® C-800 [OTC]; Allbee® C-800 + Iron [OTC]; Allbee® with C [OTC]; Apatate® [OTC]; Diatx™; DiatxFe™; Gevrabon® [OTC]; NephPlex® Rx; Nephrocaps®; Nephron FA®; Nephro-Vite®; Nephro-Vite® Rx; Stresstabs® B-Complex [OTC]; Stresstabs® B-Complex + Iron [OTC]; Stresstabs® B-Complex + Zinc [OTC]; Surbex-T® [OTC]; Trinsicon®; Z-Bec® [OTC]

Synonyms B Complex Combinations; B Vitamin Combinations

Pharmacologic Category Vitamin

Medication Safety Issues

Sound-alike/look-alike issues:

Nephrocaps® may be confused with Nephro-Calci®

Surbex® may be confused with Sebex®, Suprax®, Surfak®

Use Supplement for use in the wasting syndrome in chronic renal failure, uremia, impaired metabolic functions of the kidney, dialysis; labeled for OTC use as a dietary supplement

Contraindications Hypersensitivity to any component of the formulation

Warnings/Precautions Adult preparations may contain amounts of iron which should not be used in children.

Nutritional/Herbal/Ethanol Interactions Food: Iron absorption is inhibited by eggs and milk.

Adverse Reactions Frequency not defined.

Central nervous system: Somnolence

Dermatologic: Itching

Gastrointestinal: Bloating, constipation, diarrhea, flatulence, nausea, vomiting

Hematologic: Peripheral vascular thrombosis, polycythemia vera

Neuromuscular & skeletal: Paresthesia

Miscellaneous: Allergic reaction

Dosing

Adults:

Dietary supplement: Oral: One tablet daily

Apatate® liquid: One teaspoonful daily, 1 hour prior to mid-day meal

Gevrabon® liquid: Two tablespoonsful (30 mL) once daily; shake well before use

Renal patients: Oral: One tablet or capsule daily between meals; take after treatment if on dialysis

Nephron FA®: Two tablets once daily, between meals

Available Dosage Forms Content varies depending on product used. For more detailed information on ingredients in these and other multivitamins, please refer to Multivitamin Products.

Nursing Guidelines

Dietary Considerations: May be taken with food to decrease stomach upset.

Pregnancy Risk Factor: A (RDA recommended doses)

Lactation: Enters breast milk/compatible

Related Information

Multivitamin Products *on page 1859*

Vitamin E (VYE ta min ee)

U.S. Brand Names Alph-E [OTC]; Alph-E-Mixed [OTC]; Aquasol E® [OTC]; Aquavit-E [OTC]; d-Alpha-Gems™ [OTC]; E-Gems® [OTC]; E-Gems Elite® [OTC]; E-Gems Plus® [OTC]; Ester-E™ [OTC]; Gamma E-Gems® [OTC]; Gamma-E Plus [OTC]; High Gamma Vitamin E Complete™ [OTC]; Key-E® [OTC]; Key-E® Kaps [OTC]

Synonyms *d*-Alpha Tocopherol; *dl*-Alpha Tocopherol

Pharmacologic Category Vitamin, Fat Soluble

Medication Safety Issues

Sound-alike/look-alike issues:

Aquasol E® may be confused with Anusol®

Use Prevention and treatment of hemolytic anemia secondary to vitamin E deficiency; dietary supplement

Unlabeled/Investigational Use To reduce the risk of bronchopulmonary dysplasia or retrolental fibroplasia in infants exposed to high concentrations of oxygen; prevention and treatment of tardive dyskinesia and Alzheimer's disease

Mechanism of Action Prevents oxidation of vitamin A and C; protects polyunsaturated fatty acids in membranes from attack by free radicals and protects red blood cells against hemolysis

Pharmacodynamics/Kinetics

Absorption: Oral: Depends on presence of bile; reduced in conditions of malabsorption, in low birth weight premature infants, and as dosage increases; water miscible preparations are better absorbed than oil preparations

Distribution: To all body tissues, especially adipose tissue, where it is stored

Metabolism: Hepatic to glucuronides

Excretion: Feces

Contraindications Hypersensitivity to vitamin E or any component of the formulation; I.V. route

Warnings/Precautions May induce vitamin K deficiency; necrotizing enterocolitis has been associated with oral administration of large dosages (eg, >200 units/day) of a hyperosmolar vitamin E preparation in low birth weight infants

Drug Interactions

Cholestyramine (and colestipol): May reduce absorption of vitamin E

Iron: Vitamin E may impair the hematologic response to iron in children with iron-deficiency anemia; monitor

Orlistat: May reduce absorption of vitamin E

Warfarin: Vitamin E may alter the effect of vitamin K actions on clotting factors resulting in an increase hypoprothrombinemic response to warfarin; monitor

Adverse Reactions <1% (Limited to important or life-threatening): Blurred vision, contact dermatitis with topical preparation, gonadal dysfunction

Dosing

Adults & Elderly: One unit of vitamin E = 1 mg *dl*-alpha-tocopherol acetate. Oral:

Recommended daily allowance (RDA): 15 mg (22.5 units); upper limit of intake should not exceed 1000 mg/day

Pregnant female:

≤18 years: 15 mg (22.5 units); upper level of intake should not exceed 800 mg/day

19-50 years: 15 mg (22.5 units); upper level of intake should not exceed 1000 mg/day

Lactating female:

≤18 years: 19 mg (28.5 units); upper level of intake should not exceed 800 mg/day

19-50 years: 19 mg (28.5 units); upper level of intake should not exceed 1000 mg/day

Vitamin E deficiency: 60-75 units/day

Prevention of vitamin E deficiency: Oral: 30 units/day

Cystic fibrosis: Oral: 100-400 units/day

Beta-thalassemia: Oral: 750 units/day

Sickle cell disease: Oral: 450 units/day

Alzheimer's disease: Oral: 1000 units twice daily

Tardive dyskinesia: Oral: 1600 units/day

Superficial dermatologic irritation: Topical: Apply a thin layer over affected area.

Pediatrics: One unit of vitamin E = 1 mg *dl*-alpha-tocopherol acetate. Oral:

Recommended daily allowance (RDA):

Premature infants ≤3 months: 17 mg (25 units)

Infants:

≤6 months: 3 mg (4.5 units)

7-12 months: 4 mg (6 units)

Children:

1-3 years: 6 mg (9 units); upper limit of intake should not exceed 200 mg/day

4-8 years: 7 mg (10.5 units); upper limit of intake should not exceed 300 mg/day

9-13 years: 11 mg (16.5 units); upper limit of intake should not exceed 600 mg/day

(Continued)

Vitamin E *(Continued)*

14-18 years: 15 mg (22.5 units); upper limit of intake should not exceed 800 mg/day

Vitamin E deficiency:

Children (with malabsorption syndrome): 1 unit/kg/day of water miscible vitamin E (to raise plasma tocopherol concentrations to the normal range within 2 months and to maintain normal plasma concentrations)

Prevention of retinopathy of prematurity or BPD secondary to O_2 therapy (AAP considers this use investigational and routine use is not recommended):

Retinopathy prophylaxis: 15-30 units/kg/day to maintain plasma levels between 1.5-2 mcg/mL (may need as high as 100 units/kg/day)

Cystic fibrosis, beta-thalassemia may require higher daily maintenance doses:

Cystic fibrosis: Oral: 100-400 units/day

Beta-thalassemia: Oral: 750 units/day

Available Dosage Forms

Capsule: 400 int. units, 1000 int. units

Key-E® Kaps: 200 int. units, 400 int. units

Capsule, softgel: 200 int. units, 400 int. units, 600 int. units, 1000 int. units

Alph-E: 200 int. units, 400 int. units

Alph-E-Mixed: 200 int. units [contains mixed tocopherols]; 400 int. units [contains mixed tocopherols], 1000 int. units [sugar free; contains mixed tocopherols]

Aqua Gem E®: 200 units, 400 units

d-Alpha-Gems™: 400 int. units [derived from soybean oil]

E-Gems®: 30 int. units, 100 int. units, 200 int. units, 400 int. units, 600 int. units, 800 int. units, 1000 int. units, 1200 int. units [derived from soybean oil]

E-Gems Plus®: 200 int. units, 400 int. units, 800 int. units [contains mixed tocopherols]

E-Gems Elite®: 400 int. units [contains mixed tocopherols]

Ester E™: 400 int. units

Gamma E-Gems®: 90 int. units [also contains mixed tocopherols]

Gamma-E Plus: 200 int. units [contains soybean oil]

High Gamma Vitamin E Complete: 200 int. units [contains soybean oil, mixed tocopherols]

Cream: 50 int. units/g (60 g), 100 int. units/g (60 g), 1000 int. units/120 g (120 g), 30,000 int. units/57g (57g)

Key-E®: 30 int. units/g (60 g, 120 g, 600 g)

Lip balm (E-Gem Lip Care®): 1000 int. units/tube [contains vitamin A and aloe]

Oil, oral/topical: 100 int. units/0.25 mL (60 mL, 75 mL); 1150 units/0.25 mL (30 mL, 60 mL, 120 mL); 28,000 int. units/30 mL (30 mL)

Alph-E: 28,000 int. units/30 mL (30 mL) [topical]

E-Gems®: 100 units/10 drops (15 mL, 60 mL).

Ointment, topical (Key-E®): 30 units/g (60 g, 120 g, 480 g)

Powder (Key-E®): 700 int. units per 1/4 teaspoon (15 g, 75 g, 1000 g) [derived from soybean oil]

Solution, oral drops:15 int. units/0.3 mL (30 mL)

Aquasol E®: 15 int. units/0.3 mL (12 mL, 30 mL) [latex free]

Aquavit-E: 15 int. units/0.3 mL (30 mL) [butterscotch flavor]

Suppository, rectal/vaginal (Key-E®): 30 int. units (12s, 24s) [contains coconut oil]

Tablet: 100 int. units, 200 int. units, 400 int. units, 500 int. units

Key-E®: 200 int. units, 400 int. units

Nursing Guidelines

Assessment: Assess effectiveness and interactions of other medications patient may be taking. Assess knowledge/teach patient appropriate use (according to formulation prescribed) and adverse symptoms to report.

Monitoring Laboratory Tests: Monitor plasma tocopherol concentrations (normal range: 6-14 mcg/mL)

Patient Education: Take exactly as directed; do not take more than the recommended dose. Do not use mineral oil or other vitamin E supplements without consulting prescriber. Report persistent nausea, vomiting, or cramping; or gonadal dysfunction. **Pregnancy precaution:** Inform prescriber if you are pregnant.

Pregnancy Risk Factor: A/C (dose exceeding RDA recommendation)

Lactation: Excretion in breast milk unknown/compatible

Administration

Oral: Swallow capsules whole, do not crush or chew.

Storage: Protect from light.

♦ Vitamin K_1 *see* Phytonadione *on page 1363*

Vitamins (Multiple/Injectable) (VYE ta mins, MUL ti pul/in JEK ti bal)

U.S. Brand Names Infuvite® Adult; Infuvite® Pediatric; M.V.I.®-12 [DSC]; M.V.I. Adult™; M.V.I® Pediatric

Pharmacologic Category Vitamin

Use Nutritional supplement in patients receiving parenteral nutrition or requiring intravenous administration

Contraindications Hypersensitivity to any component of the formulation; pre-existing hypervitaminosis

Warnings/Precautions RDA values are not requirements, but are recommended daily intakes of certain essential nutrients; use with caution in patients with severe renal or hepatic dysfunction or failure. Should not be used prior to testing for megaloblastic anemia. Additional vitamin A may be required in pediatric patients. Some formulations contain aluminum; may reach toxic levels with prolonged administration in renal impairment or immaturity. Some formulations may contain polysorbates which have been associated with the E-Ferol syndrome in low birth weight infants.

Adverse Reactions Frequency not defined.

Cardiovascular: Angioedema, edema

Central nervous system: Agitation, anxiety, dizziness, headache

Dermatologic: Erythema, pruritus, rash, urticaria

Ocular: Diplopia

Respiratory: Dyspnea, wheezing

Miscellaneous: Allergic reactions, anaphylaxis, hypervitaminosis

Overdosage/Toxicology Some formulations contain aluminum; may reach toxic levels with prolonged administration in renal impairment or immaturity. Aluminum doses >4-5 mcg/kg/day are associated with toxicity in patients with renal impairment and in premature neonates.

Dosing

Adults & Elderly: Dietary supplement: I.V. (not for direct infusion): Adult formulation: 10 mL/day added to TPN or ≥500 mL of appropriate solution

Pediatrics: Dietary supplement: I.V. (not for direct infusion):

Children: ≥3 kg to 11 years: Pediatric formulation: 5 mL/day added to TPN or ≥100 mL of appropriate solution

Children >11 years and Adults: Refer to adult dosing.

Available Dosage Forms Content varies depending on product used. For more detailed information on ingredients in these and other multivitamins, please refer to Multivitamin Products.

Nursing Guidelines

Pregnancy Risk Factor: C

Administration

I.V.: Not for direct infusion; solution must be diluted prior to administration.

Reconstitution:

Powder for injection: M.V.I.® Pediatric: Add 5 mL SWFI, D_5W, or NS to vial; swirl gently to dissolve. Must be further diluted prior to administration. Solution is stable for 4 hours prior to final dilution

Solution: Infuvite® Adult, Infuvite® Pediatric, M.V.I.®-12: Solution is provided as 2 separate vials which need combined to provide the usual daily dose following further dilution. Once combined, solution should be immediately added to infusion solution.

Compatibility: Incompatible with alkaline solutions/medications (eg, acetazolamide, chlorothiazide, aminophylline, or bicarbonate), ampicillin, calcium salts, tetracyclines, or fat emulsions

Storage: Store injection at 2°C to 8°C (36°F to 46°F); some components are light sensitive

Related Information

Multivitamin Products *on page 1859*

Vitamins (Multiple/Oral) (VYE ta mins, MUL ti pul/OR al)

U.S. Brand Names Centrum® [OTC]; Centrum® Performance™ [OTC]; Centrum® Silver® [OTC]; Geriation [OTC]; Geritol Complete® [OTC]; Geritol Extend® [OTC]; Geritol® Tonic [OTC]; Glutofac®-MX; Glutofac®-ZX; Gynovite® Plus [OTC]; Hemocyte Plus®; Hi-Kovite [OTC; Iberet® [OTC]; Iberet®-500 [OTC]; Monocaps [OTC]; Multiret Folic 500; Ocuvite® [OTC]; Ocuvite® Extra® [OTC]; Ocuvite® Lutein [OTC]; Olay® Vitamins Complete Women's [OTC]; Olay® Vitamins Complete Women's 50+[OTC]; Olay® Vitamins Even Complexion [OTC]; One-A-Day® 50 Plus Formula [OTC]; One-A-Day® Active Formula [OTC]; One-A-Day® Carb Smart [OTC]; One-A-Day® Cholesterol Plus™ [OTC]; One-A-Day® Essential Formula [OTC]; One-A-Day® Maximum Formula [OTC]; One-A-Day® Men's Formula [OTC]; One-A-Day® Today [OTC]; One-A-Day® Weight Smart [OTC; One-A-Day® Women's Formula [OTC]; Optivite® P.M.T. [OTC]; PreserVision® AREDS [OTC]; PreserVision® Lutein [OTC]; Quintabs [OTC]; Quintabs-M [OTC]; Replace [OTC]; Replace with Iron [OTC]; Strovite® Forte; Theragran® Heart Right™ [OTC] [DSC]; Theragran-M® Advanced Formula [OTC] [DSC]; T-Vites [OTC]; Ultra Freeda Iron Free [OTC]; Ultra Freeda with Iron [OTC]; Unicap M® [OTC]; Unicap Sr® [OTC]; Unicap T™ [OTC]; Viactiv® Multivitamin [OTC]; Vicon Forte®; Vi-Daylin® + Iron Liquid [OTC] [DSC]; Vi-Daylin® Liquid [OTC] [DSC]; Vitacon Forte; Xtramins [OTC]

Synonyms Multiple Vitamins; Therapeutic Multivitamins; Vitamins, Multiple (Oral); Vitamins, Multiple (Therapeutic); Vitamins, Multiple With Iron

Pharmacologic Category Vitamin

Medication Safety Issues

Sound-alike/look-alike issues:

Theragran® may be confused with Phenergan®

Use Prevention/treatment of vitamin and mineral deficiencies; labeled for OTC use as a dietary supplement

Contraindications Hypersensitivity to any component of the formulation; pre-existing hypervitaminosis

Warnings/Precautions RDA values are not requirements, but are recommended daily intakes of certain essential nutrients; use with caution in patients with severe renal or hepatic dysfunction or failure. Adult preparations may contain amounts of ethanol or iron which should not be used in children.

Nutritional/Herbal/Ethanol Interactions Food: Iron absorption is inhibited by eggs and milk.

Lab Interactions Ascorbic acid in the urine can cause false negative urine glucose determinations

Adverse Reactions Refer to individual vitamin monographs.

Dosing

Adults & Elderly: Dietary supplement: Oral: Daily dose of adult preparations varies by product. Generally, 1 tablet or capsule or 5-15 mL of liquid per day. Consult package labeling. Prescription doses may be higher for burn or cystic fibrosis patients.

Available Dosage Forms Content varies depending on product used. For more detailed information on ingredients in these and other multivitamins, please refer to Multivitamin Products.

Nursing Guidelines

Dietary Considerations: May be taken with food to decrease stomach upset.

Patient Education: Do not take more than the recommended dose. May take with food to decrease stomach upset. May cause constipation.

Pregnancy Risk Factor: A (at RDA recommended dose)

Lactation: Enters breast milk/compatible

Administration

Oral: May administer with food to decrease stomach upset.

Related Information

Multivitamin Products *on page 1859*

Vitamins (Multiple/Pediatric) (VYE ta mins, MUL ti pul/pe de AT rik)

U.S. Brand Names ADEKs [OTC]; Centrum® Kids Jimmy Neutron® Complete [OTC]; Centrum® Kids Jimmy Neutron® Extra C [OTC]; Centrum® Kids Rugrats™ Complete [OTC]; Centrum® Kids Rugrats™ Extra C [OTC]; Centrum® Kids Rugrats™ Extra Calcium [OTC]; Flintstones® Complete [OTC]; Flintstones® Plus Calcium [OTC]; Flintstones® Plus Extra C [OTC]; Flintstones® Plus Iron [OTC]; My First Flintstones® [OTC]; One-A-Day® Kids Bugs Bunny and Friends Complete [OTC]; One-A-Day® Kids Bugs Bunny and Friends Plus Extra C [OTC];

One-A-Day® Kids Extreme Sports [OTC]; One-A-Day® Kids Scooby-Doo! Complete [OTC]; One-A-Day® Kids Scooby-Doo! Fizzy Vites [OTC]; One-A-Day® Kids Scooby-Doo! Plus Calcium [OTC]; Poly-Vi-Flor®; Poly-Vi-Flor® With Iron; Poly-Vi-Sol® [OTC]; Poly-Vi-Sol® with Iron [OTC]; Soluvite-F; Tri-Vi-Flor®; Tri-Vi-Flor® with Iron; Tri-Vi-Sol® [OTC]; Tri-Vi-Sol® with Iron [OTC]; Vi-Daylin® ADC [OTC] [DSC]; Vi-Daylin® ADC + Iron [OTC] [DSC]; Vi-Daylin® Drops [OTC] [DSC]; Vi-Daylin®/F [DSC]; Vi-Daylin®/F ADC [DSC]; Vi-Daylin®/F ADC + Iron [DSC]; Vi-Daylin®/F + Iron [DSC]; Vi-Daylin® + Iron Drops [OTC] [DSC]; Vitaball® [OTC]; Vitaball® Wild N Fruity [OTC]

Synonyms Children's Vitamins; Multivitamins/Fluoride

Pharmacologic Category Vitamin

Use Prevention/treatment of vitamin deficiency; products containing fluoride are used to prevent dental caries; labeled for OTC use as a dietary supplement

Contraindications Hypersensitivity to any component of the formulation; pre-existing hypervitaminosis

Warnings/Precautions Not all products can be used in children of all age groups, consult specific product labeling prior to use. Do not exceed recommended doses. Use caution with severe renal or hepatic dysfunction or failure.

Nutritional/Herbal/Ethanol Interactions Food: Iron absorption is inhibited by eggs and milk.

Adverse Reactions Refer to individual vitamin monographs.

Overdosage/Toxicology Chronic overdose of fluoride may result in mottling of tooth enamel and osseous changes.

Dosing

Pediatrics: Daily dose varies by product; refer to package insert for specific product labeling.

Available Dosage Forms Content varies depending on product used. For more detailed information on ingredients in these and other multivitamins, please refer to Multivitamin Products.

Nursing Guidelines

Dietary Considerations: May take with food to decrease stomach upset. Flintstones® Complete contains phenylalanine 4.56 mg/chewable tablet. Flintstones® Plus Calcium contains phenylalanine <4 mg/chewable tablet. One-A-Day® Kids Bugs Bunny and Friends Plus Extra C chewable tablets contain phenylalanine.

Patient Education: May take with food if stomach upset occurs. Constipation may occur.

Administration

Oral: May administer with food to decrease stomach upset. Chewable tablets may be crushed and mixed with food. Oral drops may be mixed with cereal, fruit juice, or food.

Storage: Store at 15°C to 30°C (59°F to 86°F)

Related Information

Multivitamin Products *on page 1859*

Vitamins (Multiple/Prenatal) (VYE ta mins, MUL ti pul/pree NAY tal)

U.S. Brand Names Advanced NatalCare®; A-Free Prenatal; Aminate Fe-90; Anemagen™ OB; Cal-Nate™; CareNate™ 600; Chromagen® OB; Citracal® Prenatal Rx; Duet®; Duet™ DHA; KPN Prenatal; NataChew™; NataFort®; NatalCare® CFe 60 [DSC]; NatalCare® GlossTabs™; NatalCare® PIC; NatalCare® PIC Forte; NatalCare® Plus; NatalCare® Rx; NatalCare® Three; NataTab™ CFe; NataTab™ FA; NataTab™ Rx; Nestabs® CBF; Nestabs® FA; Nestabs® RX; Niferex®-PN; Niferex®-PN Forte; NutriNate®; OB-20; Obegyn®; PreCare®; PreCare® Conceive™; PreCare® Prenatal; Prenatal 1-A-Day; Prenatal AD; Prenatal H; Prenatal MR 90 Fe™; Prenatal MTR with Selenium; Prenatal Plus; Prenatal Rx 1; Prenatal U; Prenatal Z; Prenate Elite™; Prenate GT™; Strong-Start™; Stuartnatal® Plus 3™ [OTC]; Stuart Prenatal® [OTC]; Trinate; Ultra NatalCare®

Synonyms Prenatal Vitamins

Pharmacologic Category Vitamin

Medication Safety Issues

Sound-alike/look-alike issues:

Niferex® may be confused with Nephrox®

PreCare® may be confused with Precose®

Use Nutritional supplement for use prior to conception, during pregnancy, and postnatal (in lactating and nonlactating women)

(Continued)

Vitamins (Multiple/Prenatal) *(Continued)*

Contraindications Hypersensitivity to any component of the formulation; pre-existing hypervitaminosis

Warnings/Precautions Due to calcium content, use caution with kidney stones. Contains iron in amounts which may be toxic to children. Iron supplementation should not be used with hemochromatosis and hemosiderosis. Use caution with severe renal or hepatic dysfunction or failure.

Nutritional/Herbal/Ethanol Interactions Food: Iron absorption is inhibited by eggs and milk.

Adverse Reactions Frequency not defined.

Gastrointestinal: Abdominal pain, constipation, dark stools, diarrhea, nausea, vomiting

Miscellaneous: Allergic reaction

Dosing

Adults & Elderly: Dietary supplement: Oral:

Capsule, tablet: One daily

Powder: 4 teaspoonfuls/day; given once daily or in divided doses; mix 1 teaspoonful in 1 ounce of water

Available Dosage Forms Content varies depending on product used. For more detailed information on ingredients in these and other multivitamins, please refer to Multivitamin Products.

Nursing Guidelines

Dietary Considerations: May be taken with food to decrease stomach upset. Obegyn® powder contains phenylalanine 84 mg/8.25 g. Duet® contains phenylalanine 15 mg/chewable tablet. StrongStart™ contains phenylalanine 6 mg/chewable tablet.

Patient Education: May take with food if stomach upset occurs. Constipation may occur.

Pregnancy Risk Factor: A (in RDA recommended dose)

Lactation: Enters breast milk/compatible

Administration

Oral: May administer with food to decrease stomach upset.

Related Information

Multivitamin Products *on page 1859*

- **Vitamins, Multiple (Therapeutic)** *see* Vitamins (Multiple/Oral) *on page 1720*
- **Vitamins, Multiple With Iron** *see* Vitamins (Multiple/Oral) *on page 1720*
- **Vitrase®** *see* Hyaluronidase *on page 858*
- **Vitrasert®** *see* Ganciclovir *on page 794*
- **Vitrax®** *see* Hyaluronate and Derivatives *on page 856*
- **Viva-Drops® [OTC]** *see* Artificial Tears *on page 187*
- **Vivarin® [OTC]** *see* Caffeine *on page 284*
- **Vivelle®** *see* Estradiol *on page 649*
- **Vivelle-Dot®** *see* Estradiol *on page 649*
- **VLB** *see* VinBLAStine *on page 1707*
- **Volmax® [DSC]** *see* Albuterol *on page 96*
- **Voltaren®** *see* Diclofenac *on page 521*
- **Voltaren Ophthalmic®** *see* Diclofenac *on page 521*
- **Voltaren®-XR** *see* Diclofenac *on page 521*
- **VoSol®** *see* Acetic Acid *on page 78*
- **VoSol® HC** *see* Acetic Acid, Propylene Glycol Diacetate, and Hydrocortisone *on page 78*
- **VoSpire ER™** *see* Albuterol *on page 96*
- **VP-16** *see* Etoposide *on page 695*
- **VP-16-213** *see* Etoposide *on page 695*
- **V.V.S.®** *see* Sulfabenzamide, Sulfacetamide, and Sulfathiazole *on page 1578*

Warfarin (WAR far in)

U.S. Brand Names Coumadin®; Jantoven™

Synonyms Warfarin Sodium

Pharmacologic Category Anticoagulant, Coumarin Derivative

Medication Safety Issues

Sound-alike/look-alike issues:

Coumadin® may be confused with Avandia®, Cardura®, Compazine®, Kemadrin®

High alert medication: The Institute for Safe Medication Practices (ISMP) includes this medication among its list of drugs which have a heightened risk of causing significant patient harm when used in error.

Use Prophylaxis and treatment of venous thrombosis, pulmonary embolism and thromboembolic disorders; atrial fibrillation with risk of embolism and as an adjunct in the prophylaxis of systemic embolism after myocardial infarction

Unlabeled/Investigational Use Prevention of recurrent transient ischemic attacks and to reduce risk of recurrent myocardial infarction

Mechanism of Action Interferes with hepatic synthesis of vitamin K-dependent coagulation factors (II, VII, IX, X)

Pharmacodynamics/Kinetics

Onset of action: Anticoagulation: Oral: 36-72 hours

Peak effect: Full therapeutic effect: 5-7 days; INR may increase in 36-72 hours

Duration: 2-5 days

Absorption: Oral: Rapid

Metabolism: Hepatic

Half-life elimination: 20-60 hours; Mean: 40 hours; highly variable among individuals

Contraindications Hypersensitivity to warfarin or any component of the formulation; hemorrhagic tendencies; hemophilia; thrombocytopenia purpura; leukemia; recent or potential surgery of the eye or CNS; major regional lumbar block anesthesia or surgery resulting in large, open surfaces; patients bleeding from the GI, respiratory, or GU tract; threatened abortion; aneurysm; ascorbic acid deficiency; history of bleeding diathesis; prostatectomy; continuous tube drainage of the small intestine; polyarthritis; diverticulitis; emaciation; malnutrition; cerebrovascular hemorrhage; eclampsia/pre-eclampsia; blood dyscrasias; severe uncontrolled or malignant hypertension; severe hepatic disease; pericarditis or pericardial effusion; subacute bacterial endocarditis; visceral carcinoma; following spinal puncture and other diagnostic or therapeutic procedures with potential for significant bleeding; history of warfarin-induced necrosis; an unreliable, noncompliant patient; alcoholism; patient who has a history of falls or is a significant fall risk; pregnancy

Warnings/Precautions Use care in the selection of patients appropriate for this treatment. Ensure patient cooperation especially from the alcoholic, illicit drug user, demented, or psychotic patient. Use with caution in trauma, acute infection (antibiotics and fever may alter affects), renal insufficiency, prolonged dietary insufficiencies (vitamin K deficiency), moderate-severe hypertension, polycythemia vera, vasculitis, open wound, active TB, history of PUD, anaphylactic disorders, indwelling catheters, severe diabetes, thyroid disease, severe renal disease, and menstruating and postpartum women. Use with caution in protein C deficiency.

Hemorrhage is the most serious risk of therapy. Patient must be instructed to report bleeding, accidents, or falls. Patient must also report any new or discontinued medications, herbal or alternative products used, significant changes in smoking or dietary habits. Necrosis or gangrene of the skin and other tissues can occur (rarely) due to early hypercoagulability. "Purple toes syndrome," due to cholesterol microembolization, may rarely occur (often after several weeks of therapy). Women may be at risk of developing ovarian hemorrhage at the time of ovulation. The elderly may be more sensitive to anticoagulant therapy.

Drug Interactions Substrate of CYP1A2 (minor), 2C8/9 (major), 2C19 (minor), 3A4 (minor); **Inhibits** CYP2C8/9 (moderate), 2C19 (weak)

Acetaminophen: May enhance the anticoagulant effect of warfarin. Most likely to occur with daily acetaminophen doses >1.3 g for >1 week.

Allopurinol: May enhance the anticoagulant effect of warfarin. Reductions in warfarin will likely be required.

Aminoglutethimide: May increase the metabolism, via CYP isoenzymes, of warfarin. Monitor therapy for decreased warfarin effect.

(Continued)

Warfarin *(Continued)*

Amiodarone: May enhance the anticoagulant effect of warfarin. An empiric warfarin dosage reduction of 30% to 50% at the initiation of warfarin may be considered.

Androgens: May enhance the anticoagulant effect of warfarin. Significant reductions in warfarin dosage may be needed during concomitant therapy.

Antifungal agents (imidazole): May decrease the metabolism, via CYP isoenzymes, of warfarin. Monitor for increased therapeutic/toxic effects of warfarin.

Antithyroid agents: May diminish the anticoagulant effects of warfarin. Monitor for decreased therapeutic effects.

Aprepitant: May decrease the serum concentration of warfarin. Monitor closely for 2 weeks following each course of aprecitant.

Azathioprine: May decrease the anticoagulant effect of warfarin. An adjustment in warfarin dose may be needed.

Barbiturates: May increase the metabolism, via CYP isoenzymes, of warfarin. Monitor for decreased therapeutic effect of warfarin. Anticoagulation dosage increase of 30% to 60% may be needed based upon monitored PT.

Bile acid sequestrants: May decrease absorption of warfarin. Separating the administration of doses by >2 hours may reduce the risk of interaction.

Bosentan: May increase metabolism, via CYP isoenzymes, of warfarin. Monitor for decreased effects.

Capecitabine: May decrease metabolism of warfarin. Monitor for evidence of excess anticoagulation.

Carbamazepine: May increase the metabolism, via CYP isoenzymes, of warfarin. Monitor for decreased therapeutic effect of warfarin.

Cephalosporins: May enhance the anticoagulant effect of warfarin. Monitor for increased evidence of bleeding especially in cephalosporins that have NMTT side chain.

Cimetidine: May enhance the anticoagulant effect of warfarin. Monitor for increased therapeutic effects of warfarin.

Contraceptives, hormonal (estrogens and progestins): May diminish the anticoagulant effect of warfarin. Monitor for changes in coagulation status.

COX-2 inhibitor: May enhance the anticoagulant effect of warfarin. Monitor for increased signs and symptoms of bleeding.

CYP2C8/9 inducers (strong): May increase the metabolism of warfarin. Examples of inducers include: Carbamazepine, fosphenytoin, phenobarbital, phenytoin, primidone, rifampin, rifapentine, secobarbital. Monitor for decreased effect of warfarin.

CYP2C8/9 inhibitors (strong): May decrease the metabolism of warfarin. Some examples of inhibitors include: Delavirdine, fluconazole, flurbiprofen, gemfibrozil, ibuprofen, indomethacin, ketoconazole, mefenamic acid, miconazole, nicardipine, pioglitazone, piroxicam, sulfadiazine, sulfisoxazole, tolbutamide. Monitor for increased effect of warfarin.

CYP2C8/9 inhibitors (moderate): May decrease the metabolism of warfarin. Some examples of inhibitors include: Amiodarone, efavirenz, fluvastatin, irbesartan, isoniazid, losartan, omeprazole, pantoprazole, pyrimethamine, quinine, rosiglitazone, sulfamethoxazole, sulfinpyrazone, trimethoprim, warfarin, zafirlukast. Monitor for increased effects of warfarin.

Dicloxacillin: May increase the metabolism, via CYP isoenzymes, of warfarin. Monitor for decreased therapeutic effect of warfarin.

Disulfiram: May increase the serum concentration of warfarin. Monitor for increased therapeutic effects of warfarin.

Drotrecogin Alfa: Warfarin may enhance the adverse/toxic effect of drotrecogin alfa. Monitor for increased risk of bleeding during concomitant therapy. If possible, avoid use of drotrecogin within 7 days of warfarin therapy, or if INR ≥3.

Etoposide: May enhance the anticoagulant effect of warfarin. Monitor for increased effects of warfarin.

Fibric acid derivatives: May enhance the anticoagulant effect of warfarin. Monitor for toxic effects of warfarin; may warrant a 25% to 33% reduction in the warfarin dosage.

Fluconazole: May decrease the metabolism, via CYP isoenzymes, of warfarin. Monitor for increased therapeutic/toxic effects warfarin.

Fluorouracil: May enhance the anticoagulant effect of warfarin. Monitor for increased effects of warfarin.

Glucagon: May enhance the anticoagulant effect of warfarin. Monitor for toxic effects of warfarin, especially if glucagon is administered in high doses.

Glutethimide: May increase the metabolism, via CYP isoenzymes, of warfarin. Consider alternative sedative-hypnotic. Monitor for decreased therapeutic effects of warfarin.

Griseofulvin: May increase the metabolism, via CYP isoenzymes, of warfarin. Monitor for decreased therapeutic effects of warfarin.

HMG-CoA reductase inhibitors: May enhance the anticoagulant effect of warfarin. Monitor for increased effects of warfarin.

Ifosfamide: May enhance the anticoagulant effect of warfarin. Monitor for increased effects of warfarin.

Leflunomide: May enhance the anticoagulant effect of warfarin. Monitor for increased effects of warfarin.

Macrolide antibiotics: May decrease the metabolism, via CYP isoenzymes, of warfarin. Monitor for increased therapeutic effects of warfarin. CYP inhibitors (eg, clarithromycin, erythromycin, and troleandomycin) appear to pose the greatest risk. Azithromycin and telithromycin have also been implicated in a few cases.

Mercaptopurine: May diminish the anticoagulant effect of warfarin. Monitor for decreased therapeutic effects of warfarin.

Metronidazole: May decrease the metabolism, via CYP isoenzymes, of warfarin. If concomitant therapy is necessary, consider an empiric reduction in warfarin dosage of approximately one-third. Monitor for increased therapeutic/toxic effects of warfarin.

Nafcillin: May increase the metabolism of warfarin. Consider choosing an alternative antibiotic if available. Monitor for decreased therapeutic effect of warfarin if nafcillin is initiated. The effects on warfarin dosing may persist long after the nafcillin is discontinued. Close monitoring is required even after nafcillin is discontinued.

NSAID (nonselective): May enhance the anticoagulant effect of warfarin. Monitor for increased signs and symptoms of bleeding.

Orlistat: May enhance the anticoagulant effect of warfarin. Monitor for changes in effects of warfarin.

Phenytoin: May enhance the anticoagulant effect of warfarin. Warfarin may increase the serum concentration of phenytoin. Monitor for increased effects of warfarin and for increased serum concentrations/toxic effects of phenytoin.

Phytonadione: May antagonize the effects of warfarin. Monitor for decreased therapeutic effect of warfarin.

Propafenone: May increase the serum concentration of warfarin. Monitor for increased prothrombin times (PT)/therapeutic effects of warfarin.

Propoxyphene: May decrease the metabolism, via CYP isoenzymes, of warfarin. Monitor for increased prothrombin time/toxic effects of warfarin.

Proton pump inhibitors (omeprazole): May increase the serum concentration of warfarin. Monitor for increased effects of warfarin.

Quinidine: May enhance the anticoagulant effect of warfarin. Monitor for increased prothrombin times (PT)/therapeutic effects of warfarin.

Quinolone antibiotics: May enhance the anticoagulant effect of warfarin. Monitor for increased prothrombin time/toxic effects of warfarin.

Rifamycin derivatives: May increase the metabolism, via CYP isoenzymes, of warfarin. Monitor for decreased prothrombin times (PT)/therapeutic effects of warfarin.

Ropinirole: May enhance the anticoagulant effect of warfarin. Monitor for increased INR/effects of warfarin.

Salicylates: May enhance the anticoagulant effect of warfarin. Monitor for increased signs and symptoms of bleeding if used concomitantly.

Selective serotonin reuptake inhibitors (SSRIs): May enhance the anticoagulant effect of warfarin. Monitor for increased therapeutic/toxic effects of warfarin.

Sulfasalazine: May diminish the anticoagulant effect of warfarin. Monitor for decreased INR/effects of warfarin

Sulfinpyrazone: May decrease the metabolism, via CYP isoenzymes, of warfarin and may decrease the protein binding of warfarin. Monitor for increased prothrombin time (PT)/toxic effects of warfarin.

Sulfonamide derivatives: May enhance the anticoagulant effect of warfarin. Monitor for increased prothrombin time (PT)/toxic effects of warfarin.

Tetracycline derivatives: May enhance the anticoagulant effect of warfarin. Monitor for toxic effects of warfarin.

Thyroid products: May enhance the anticoagulant effect of warfarin. Monitor for increased hypoprothrombinemic effects of warfarin.

Tigecycline: May increase the serum concentration of warfarin. Monitor for increased effects of warfarin.

(Continued)

Warfarin *(Continued)*

Treprostinil: May enhance the adverse/toxic effect of warfarin. Monitor for increased risk of bleeding when used concomitantly.

Tricyclic antidepressants: May enhance the anticoagulant effect of warfarin. Monitor for increased prothrombin times (PT)/toxic effects of warfarin.

Vitamin A: May enhance the anticoagulant effect of warfarin. Monitor for increased prothrombin time (PT)/effects of warfarin.

Vitamin E: May enhance the anticoagulant effect of warfarin. Monitor for increased prothrombin time (PT)/effects of warfarin. Likely only of significant concern with higher doses of vitamin E (eg, 1200 int. units/day).

Voriconazole: May increase the serum concentration of warfarin. Monitor for increased effects (eg, INR, bleeding) of warfarin.

Zafirlukast: May decrease the metabolism, via CYP isoenzymes, of warfarin. Monitor for increased prothrombin time (PT)/effects of warfarin.

Zileuton: May increase the serum concentration of warfarin. Monitor for increased effects of warfarin.

Nutritional/Herbal/Ethanol Interactions

Ethanol: Avoid ethanol. Acute ethanol ingestion (binge drinking) decreases the metabolism of warfarin and increases PT/INR. Chronic daily ethanol use increases the metabolism of warfarin and decreases PT/INR.

Food: The anticoagulant effects of warfarin may be decreased if taken with foods rich in vitamin K. Vitamin E may increase warfarin effect. Cranberry juice may increase warfarin effect.

Herb/Nutraceutical: Cranberry, fenugreek, ginkgo biloba, glucosamine, may enhance bleeding or increase warfarin's effect. Ginseng (American), coenzyme Q_{10}, and St John's wort may decrease warfarin levels and effects. Avoid alfalfa, anise, bilberry, bladderwrack, bromelain, cat's claw, celery, coleus, cordyceps, dong quai, evening primrose oil, fenugreek, feverfew, garlic, ginger, ginkgo biloba, ginseng (American), ginseng (Panax), ginseng (Siberian), grape seed, green tea, guggul, horse chestnut seed, horseradish, licorice, prickly ash, red clover, reishi, same (s-adenosylmethionine), sweet clover, turmeric,and white willow (all have additional antiplatelet activity).

Adverse Reactions As with all anticoagulants, bleeding is the major adverse effect of warfarin. Hemorrhage may occur at virtually any site. Risk is dependent on multiple variables, including the intensity of anticoagulation and patient susceptibility.

Additional adverse effects are often related to idiosyncratic reactions, and the frequency cannot be accurately estimated.

Cardiovascular: Vasculitis, edema, hemorrhagic shock

Central nervous system: Fever, lethargy, malaise, asthenia, pain, headache, dizziness, stroke

Dermatologic: Rash, dermatitis, bullous eruptions, urticaria, pruritus, alopecia

Gastrointestinal: Anorexia, nausea, vomiting, stomach cramps, abdominal pain, diarrhea, flatulence, gastrointestinal bleeding, taste disturbance, mouth ulcers

Genitourinary: Priapism, hematuria

Hematologic: Hemorrhage, leukopenia, unrecognized bleeding sites (eg, colon cancer) may be uncovered by anticoagulation, retroperitoneal hematoma, agranulocytosis

Hepatic: Hepatic injury, jaundice, transaminases increased

Neuromuscular & skeletal: Paresthesia, osteoporosis

Respiratory: Hemoptysis, epistaxis, pulmonary hemorrhage, tracheobronchial calcification

Miscellaneous: Hypersensitivity/allergic reactions

Skin necrosis/gangrene, due to paradoxical local thrombosis, is a known but rare risk of warfarin therapy. Its onset is usually within the first few days of therapy and is frequently localized to the limbs, breast or penis. The risk of this effect is increased in patients with protein C or S deficiency.

"Purple toes syndrome," caused by cholesterol microembolization, also occurs rarely. Typically, this occurs after several weeks of therapy, and may present as a dark, purplish, mottled discoloration of the plantar and lateral surfaces. Other manifestations of cholesterol microembolization may include rash; livedo reticularis; gangrene; abrupt and intense pain in lower extremities; abdominal, flank, or back pain; hematuria, renal insufficiency; hypertension; cerebral ischemia; spinal cord infarction; or other symptom of vascular compromise.

Overdosage/Toxicology Symptoms of overdose include internal or external hemorrhage and hematuria. Avoid emesis and lavage to avoid possible trauma and incidental bleeding. When an overdose occurs, the drug should be immediately discontinued and vitamin K_1 (phytonadione) may be administered, up to 25 mg I.V. for adults. When hemorrhage occurs, fresh frozen plasma transfusions can help control bleeding by replacing clotting factors. In urgent bleeding, prothrombin complex concentrates may be needed.

Management of elevated INR: See table.

Management of Elevated INR

INR	Symptom	Action
Above therapeutic range to <5	No significant bleeding	Lower or hold the next dose and monitor frequently; when INR approaches desired range, may resume dosing with a lower dose if INR was significantly above therapeutic range.
≥5 and <9	No significant bleeding	Omit the next 1or 2 doses; monitor INR and resume with a lower dose when the INR approaches the desired range.
		Alternatively, if there are other risk factors for bleeding, omit the next dose and give vitamin K_1 orally ≤5 mg; resume with a lower dose when the INR approaches the desired range.
		If rapid reversal is required for surgery, then given vitamin K_1 orally 2-4 mg and hold warfarin. Expect a response within 24 hours; another 1-2 mg may be given orally if needed.
≥9	No significant bleeding	Hold warfarin, give vitamin K_1 orally 5-10 mg, expect the INR to be reduced within 24-48 hours; monitor INR and administer additional vitamin K if necessary. Resume warfarin at lower doses when INR is in the desired range.
Any INR elevation	Serious bleeding	Hold warfarin, give vitamin K_1 (10 mg by slow I.V. infusion), and supplement with fresh plasma transfusion or prothrombin complex concentrate (Factor X complex); recombinant factor VIIa is an alternative to prothrombin complex concentrate. Vitamin K_1 injection can be repeated every 12 hours.
Any INR elevation	Life-threatening bleeding	Hold warfarin, give prothrombin complex concentrate, supplemented with vitamin K_1 (10 mg by slow I.V. infusion); repeat if necessary. Recombinant factor VIIa is an alternative to prothrombin complex concentrate.

Note: Use of high doses of vitamin K_1 (10.0-15.0) may cause resistance to warfarin for up to a week. Heparin or low molecular weight heparin can be given until the patient becomes responsive to warfarin. **Reference:** Ansell J, Hirsh J, Poller L et al. "The Pharmacology and Management of the Vitamin K Antagonists," *Chest*, 2004, 126 (3 Suppl):204-33.

Dosing

Adults:

Prevention/treatment of thrombosis/embolism:

I.V. (administer as a slow bolus injection): 2-5 mg/day

Oral: Initial dosing must be individualized. Consider the patient (hepatic function, cardiac function, age, nutritional status, concurrent therapy, risk of bleeding) in addition to prior dose response (if available) and the clinical situation. Start 5-10 mg daily for 2 days. Adjust dose according to INR results; usual maintenance dose ranges from 2-10 mg daily (individual patients may require loading and maintenance doses outside these general guidelines).

Note: Lower starting doses may be required for patients with hepatic impairment, poor nutrition, CHF, elderly, high risk of bleeding, or patients that are debilitated. Higher initial doses may be reasonable in selected

(Continued)

Warfarin *(Continued)*

patients (ie, receiving enzyme-inducing agents and with low risk of bleeding).

Elderly: Oral: Initial dose ≤5 mg. Usual maintenance dose: 2-5 mg/day. The elderly tend to require lower dosages to produce a therapeutic level of anticoagulation (due to changes in the pattern of warfarin metabolism).

Pediatrics:

Prevention/treatment of thrombosis: Oral: Infants and Children: 0.05-0.34 mg/kg/day; infants <12 months of age may require doses at or near the high end of this range; consistent anticoagulation may be difficult to maintain in children <5 years of age.

Hepatic Impairment: Monitor effect at usual doses. The response to oral anticoagulants may be markedly enhanced in obstructive jaundice, hepatitis, and cirrhosis. Prothrombin index should be closely monitored.

Available Dosage Forms

Injection, powder for reconstitution, as sodium (Coumadin®): 5 mg

Tablet, as sodium (Coumadin®, Jantoven™): 1 mg, 2 mg, 2.5 mg, 3 mg, 4 mg, 5 mg, 6 mg, 7.5 mg, 10 mg

Nursing Guidelines

Assessment: Use caution with any condition that increases risk of bleeding (eg, dietary vitamin K or C deficiency, hypertension, open wounds, TB, PUD, diabetes, thyroid or renal disease, recent surgery; see Contraindications and Warnings/Precautions for specific detailed use cautions). Assess potential for interactions with other pharmacological agents and herbal products patient may be taking (especially those medications that may affect coagulation or platelet aggregation; see Drug Interaction). Assess results of laboratory tests closely. Patient should be monitored frequently for adverse reactions (eg, bleeding from any site, rash, urticaria, gastrointestinal upset, abdominal pain, diarrhea, hypersensitivity reaction; see Adverse Reactions). Teach patient possible side effects/appropriate interventions (eg, safety precautions) and adverse symptoms to report (see Patient Education). **Pregnancy risk factor X:** Determine that patient is not pregnant before beginning treatment. Teach patients of childbearing age appropriate use of contraceptives.

Monitoring Laboratory Tests: Prothrombin time (desirable range usually 1.5-2 times the control), hematocrit, INR (desirable range usually 2.0-3.0 with standard therapy, 2.5-3.5 with high-dose therapy)

Dietary Considerations: Foods high in vitamin K (eg, beef liver, pork liver, green tea and leafy green vegetables) inhibit anticoagulant effect. Do not change dietary habits once stabilized on warfarin therapy; a balanced diet with a consistent intake of vitamin K is essential; avoid large amounts of alfalfa, asparagus, broccoli, Brussels sprouts, cabbage, cauliflower, green teas, kale, lettuce, spinach, turnip greens, watercress decrease efficacy of warfarin. It is recommended that the diet contain a CONSISTENT vitamin K content of 70-140 mcg/day. Check with healthcare provider before changing diet.

Patient Education: It is imperative that you inform prescriber of all prescriptions, OTC medications, or herbal products you are taking. Do not take any new medication during therapy unless approved by prescriber. Take exactly as directed; if dose is missed, take as soon as possible. Do not double dose. Follow diet and activity as recommended by prescriber; check with prescriber before changing diet. Avoid alcohol. Do not make major changes in your dietary intake of vitamin K (green vegetables). You will have a tendency to bleed easily while taking this drug (use soft toothbrush, waxed dental floss, electric razor, and avoid scissors or sharp knives and potentially harmful activities). May cause nausea, vomiting, disturbed taste (small frequent meals, frequent mouth care, sucking lozenges, or chewing gum may help). Report any unusual bleeding or bruising (eg, bleeding gums, nosebleed, blood in urine, dark stool, bloody emesis, heavier than usual menses, or menstrual irregularities); skin rash or irritation; unusual fever; persistent nausea or GI upset; pain in joints or back; swelling or pain at injection site, unhealed wounds. **Pregnancy precautions:** Do not get pregnant while taking this medication. Consult prescriber for appropriate contraceptive measures.

Geriatric Considerations: Before committing an elderly patient to long-term anticoagulation therapy, their risk for bleeding complications secondary to falls, drug interactions, living situation, and cognitive status should be considered. A risk of bleeding complications has been associated with increased age.

Pregnancy Risk Factor: X

Pregnancy Issues: Oral anticoagulants cross the placenta and produce fetal abnormalities. Warfarin should not be used during pregnancy because of significant risks. Adjusted-dose heparin can be given safely throughout pregnancy in patients with venous thromboembolism.

Lactation: Does not enter breast milk, only metabolites are excreted (AAP rates "compatible")

Breast-Feeding Considerations: Warfarin does not pass into breast milk and can be given to nursing mothers (AAP rates "compatible"). However, limited data suggests prolonged PT may occur in some infants. Women who are breast-feeding should be carefully monitored to avoid excessive anticoagulation. Evaluation of coagulation tests and vitamin K status of breast-feeding infant is considered prudent.

Perioperative/Anesthesia/Other Concerns: Tube-feeding formulas are often a rich source of vitamin K.

Management of oral anticoagulation prior to surgery: Patients with low risk of thromboembolism: Stop warfarin therapy approximately 4 days before surgery, allow the INR to return to a near normal level, briefly administer postoperative prophylaxis (if the intervention itself creates a higher risk of thrombosis) using low-dose heparin or LMWH, and simultaneously begin warfarin therapy after surgery.

Patients with intermediate risk of thromboembolism: Stop warfarin therapy approximately 4 days before surgery, allow the INR to fall. Initiate low-dose heparin or prophylactic dose of LMWH beginning 2 days before surgery. Then commence full-dose heparin or LMWH, and warfarin therapy after surgery.

Patients with high risk of thromboembolism (eg, a recent [<3 months] history of venous thromboembolism, a mechanical cardiac valve in the mitral position; or an old model of cardiac valve [ball/cage]): Stop warfarin therapy approximately 4 days before surgery, allow the INR to return to a normal level, begin therapy with full-dose heparin or full-dose LMWH as the INR falls (approximately 2 days before surgery). Heparin can be administered as a SubQ injection on an outpatient basis, can then be given as a continuous I.V. infusion after hospital admission in preparation for surgery, and can be discontinued 5 hours before surgery with the expectation that the anticoagulant effect will have worn off at the time of surgery. It is also possible to continue the administration of SubQ heparin or LMWH and to stop therapy 12-24 hours before surgery with the expectation that the anticoagulant effect will be very low or will have worn off by the time of surgery.

Patients with low risk of bleeding: Continue warfarin therapy at a lower dose and operate at an INR of 1.3-1.5, an intensity that has been shown to be safe in randomized trials of gynecologic and orthopedic surgical patients. The dose of warfarin can be lowered 4-5 days before surgery. Warfarin therapy then can be restarted after surgery and supplemented with low-dose heparin or LMWH if necessary.

Heparin-induced Thrombocytopenia (HIT) or Heparin-induced Thrombotic Thrombocytopenia Syndrome (HITTS): When a patient develops HIT/HITTS, do not start warfarin. Rather, a direct thrombin inhibitor should be initiated and continued until platelets return. Warfarin anticoagulation should be postponed in the patient with HIT until substantial recovery of the platelet count has occurred.

Administration

Oral: Do not take with food. Take at the same time each day.

I.V.: Administer as a slow bolus injection over 1-2 minutes. Avoid all I.M. injections.

Reconstitution: Injection is stable for 4 hours at room temperature after reconstitution with 2.7 mL of sterile water (yields 2 mg/mL solution).

Compatibility: Stable in D_5LR, $D_5\frac{1}{2}NS$, D_5NS, D_5W, $D_{10}W$

Y-site administration: Incompatible with aminophylline, bretylium, ceftazidime, cimetidine, ciprofloxacin, dobutamine, esmolol, gentamicin, labetalol, metronidazole, promazine, lactated Ringer's

Compatibility in syringe: Incompatible with heparin

Storage: Protect from light.

♦ Warfarin Sodium *see* Warfarin *on page 1723*
♦ 4-Way® 12 Hour [OTC] *see* Oxymetazoline *on page 1290*
♦ 4-Way® Saline Moisturizing Mist [OTC] *see* Sodium Chloride *on page 1545*

Zafirlukast (za FIR loo kast)

U.S. Brand Names Accolate®

Synonyms ICI-204,219

Pharmacologic Category Leukotriene-Receptor Antagonist

Medication Safety Issues

Sound-alike/look-alike issues:

Accolate® may be confused with Accupril®, Accutane®, Aclovate®

Use Prophylaxis and chronic treatment of asthma in adults and children ≥5 years of age

Mechanism of Action Zafirlukast is a selectively and competitive leukotriene-receptor antagonist (LTRA) of leukotriene D4 and E4 (LTD4 and LTE4), components of slow-reacting substance of anaphylaxis (SRSA). Cysteinyl leukotriene production and receptor occupation have been correlated with the pathophysiology of asthma, including airway edema, smooth muscle constriction and altered cellular activity associated with the inflammatory process, which contribute to the signs and symptoms of asthma.

Pharmacodynamics/Kinetics

Protein binding: >99%, primarily to albumin
Metabolism: Extensively hepatic via CYP2C9
Bioavailability: Reduced 40% with food
Half-life elimination: 10 hours
Time to peak, serum: 3 hours
Excretion: Urine (10%); feces

Contraindications Hypersensitivity to zafirlukast or any component of the formulation

Warnings/Precautions Zafirlukast is not indicated for use in the reversal of bronchospasm in acute asthma attacks, including status asthmaticus. Therapy with zafirlukast can be continued during acute exacerbations of asthma.

Hepatic adverse events (including hepatitis, hyperbilirubinemia, and hepatic failure) have been reported; female patients may be at greater risk. Discontinue immediately if liver dysfunction is suspected. Periodic testing of liver function may be considered (early detection is generally believed to improve the likelihood of recovery). If hepatic dysfunction is suspected (due to clinical signs/symptoms), liver function tests should be measured immediately. Do not resume or restart if hepatic function studies are consistent with dysfunction. Use caution in patients with alcoholic cirrhosis; clearance is reduced.

Rare cases of eosinophilic vasculitis (Churg-Strauss) have been reported in patients receiving zafirlukast (usually, but not always, associated with reduction in concurrent steroid dosage). No causal relationship established. Monitor for eosinophilic vasculitis, rash, pulmonary symptoms, cardiac symptoms, or neuropathy.

An increased proportion of zafirlukast patients >55 years of age reported infections as compared to placebo-treated patients. These infections were mostly mild or moderate in intensity and predominantly affected the respiratory tract. Infections occurred equally in both sexes, were dose-proportional to total milligrams of zafirlukast exposure, and were associated with coadministration of inhaled corticosteroids.

Drug Interactions **Substrate** of CYP2C8/9 (major); **Inhibits** CYP1A2 (weak), 2C8/9 (moderate), 2C19 (weak), 2D6 (weak), 3A4 (weak)

Aspirin: Coadministration of zafirlukast with aspirin results in mean increased plasma levels of zafirlukast by 45%

CYP2C8/9 inducers: May decrease the levels/effects of zafirlukast. Example inducers include carbamazepine, phenobarbital, phenytoin, rifampin, rifapentine, and secobarbital.

CYP2C8/9 substrates: Zafirlukast may increase the levels/effects of CYP2C8/9 substrates. Example substrates include amiodarone, fluoxetine, glimepiride, glipizide, nateglinide, phenytoin, pioglitazone, rosiglitazone, sertraline, and warfarin.

Erythromycin: Coadministration of a single dose of zafirlukast with erythromycin to steady state results in decreased mean plasma levels of zafirlukast by 40% due to a decrease in zafirlukast bioavailability.

Theophylline: Coadministration of zafirlukast at steady state with a single dose of liquid theophylline preparations results in decreased mean plasma levels of zafirlukast by 30%, but no effects on plasma theophylline levels were observed. Cases of increased theophylline serum concentrations have been reported.

Warfarin: Coadministration of zafirlukast with warfarin results in a clinically significant increase in prothrombin time (PT). Closely monitor prothrombin times of patients on oral warfarin anticoagulant therapy and zafirlukast, and adjust anticoagulant dose accordingly.

Nutritional/Herbal/Ethanol Interactions Food: Decreases bioavailability of zafirlukast by 40%.

Adverse Reactions

>10%: Central nervous system: Headache (13%)

1% to 10%:

Central nervous system: Dizziness (2%), pain (2%), fever (2%)

Gastrointestinal: Nausea (3%), diarrhea (3%), abdominal pain (2%), vomiting (2%), dyspepsia (1%)

Hepatic: SGPT increased (2%)

Neuromuscular & skeletal: Back pain (2%), myalgia (2%), weakness (2%)

Miscellaneous: Infection (4%)

<1% (Limited to important or life-threatening): Agranulocytosis, angioedema, arthralgia, bleeding, bruising, edema, eosinophilia (systemic), eosinophilic pneumonia, hepatic failure, hepatitis, hyperbilirubinemia, hypersensitivity reactions, insomnia, malaise, pruritus, rash, urticaria, vasculitis with clinical features of Churg-Strauss syndrome (rare)

Overdosage/Toxicology There is no experience with overdose in humans to date. Treatment is supportive.

Dosing

Adults & Elderly: Asthma: Oral: 20 mg twice daily

Pediatrics: Asthma: Oral:

Children 5-11 years: 10 mg twice daily. Safety and effectiveness have not been established in children <5 years of age.

Children ≥12 years: Refer to adult dosing.

Renal Impairment:

Dosage adjustment not required.

Hepatic Impairment: Clearance of zafirlukast is reduced with a greater C_{max} and AUC of 50% to 60% in patients with alcoholic cirrhosis.

Available Dosage Forms Tablet: 10 mg, 20 mg

Nursing Guidelines

Assessment: Not for use in acute asthma attack. Assess effectiveness and interactions of other medications patient may be taking. Monitor effectiveness of therapy and adverse reactions at beginning of therapy and periodically with long-term use. Monitor for liver dysfunction. Assess knowledge/teach patient appropriate use, interventions to reduce side effects, and adverse symptoms to report.

Monitoring Laboratory Tests: Monitor for improvements in air flow; periodic monitoring of LFTs may be considered (not proved to prevent serious injury, but early detection may enhance recovery)

Dietary Considerations: Should be taken on an empty stomach (1 hour before or 2 hours after meals).

(Continued)

Zafirlukast *(Continued)*

Patient Education: Do not use during acute bronchospasm. Take regularly as prescribed, even during symptom-free periods. This medication should be taken on an empty stomach, 1 hour before or 2 hours after meals. Do not take more than recommended or discontinue use without consulting prescriber. Do not stop taking other antiasthmatic medications unless instructed by prescriber. Avoid aspirin or aspirin-containing medications unless approved by prescriber. You may experience headache, drowsiness, dizziness, or blurred vision (use caution when driving or engaging in tasks requiring alertness until response to drug is known); or gastric upset, nausea, or vomiting (small frequent meals, frequent mouth care, chewing gum, or sucking lozenges may help). Report persistent CNS or GI symptoms; muscle or back pain; weakness, fever, chills; yellowing of skin or eyes; dark urine or pale stool; or skin rash. Contact prescriber immediately if experiencing right upper abdominal pain, nausea, fatigue, itching, flu-like symptoms; swelling of the eyes, face, neck, or throat; anorexia; or worsening of condition. **Breast-feeding precaution:** Do not breast-feed.

Geriatric Considerations: The mean dose (mg/kg) normalized AUC and C_{max} increase and plasma clearance decreases with increasing age. In patients >65 years of age, there is a two- to threefold greater C_{max} and AUC compared to younger adults. Some studies have demonstrated slightly higher adverse effect reports in elderly compared to younger adults: Headache (4.7%), diarrhea and nausea (1.8%), and pharyngitis (1.3%). No changes in dose recommended for elderly.

Pregnancy Risk Factor: B

Lactation: Enters breast milk/contraindicated

Breast-Feeding Considerations: The manufacturer does not recommend breast-feeding due to tumorigenicity observed in animal studies.

Administration

Oral: Administer 1 hour before or 2 hours after meals.

Storage: Store tablets at controlled room temperature (20°C to 25°C; 68°F to 77°F); protect from light and moisture; dispense in original airtight container

- **Zantac®** *see* Ranitidine *on page 1463*
- **Zantac 75® [OTC]** *see* Ranitidine *on page 1463*
- **Zantac 150™ [OTC]** *see* Ranitidine *on page 1463*
- **Zantac® EFFERdose®** *see* Ranitidine *on page 1463*
- **Zaroxolyn®** *see* Metolazone *on page 1147*
- **Z-Bec® [OTC]** *see* Vitamin B Complex Combinations *on page 1716*
- **ZD1033** *see* Anastrozole *on page 168*
- **ZDV** *see* Zidovudine *on page 1732*
- **ZDV, Abacavir, and Lamivudine** *see* Abacavir, Lamivudine, and Zidovudine *on page 58*
- **Zebutal™** *see* Butalbital, Acetaminophen, and Caffeine *on page 280*
- **Zegerid™** *see* Omeprazole *on page 1264*
- **Zemuron®** *see* Rocuronium *on page 1489*
- **Zenapax®** *see* Daclizumab *on page 480*
- **Zephiran® [OTC]** *see* Benzalkonium Chloride *on page 231*
- **Zestoretic®** *see* Lisinopril and Hydrochlorothiazide *on page 1051*
- **Zestril®** *see* Lisinopril *on page 1047*
- **Zetia™** *see* Ezetimibe *on page 699*
- **Ziagen®** *see* Abacavir *on page 56*

Zidovudine (zye DOE vyoo deen)

U.S. Brand Names Retrovir®

Synonyms Azidothymidine; AZT (error-prone abbreviation); Compound S; ZDV

Pharmacologic Category Antiretroviral Agent, Reverse Transcriptase Inhibitor (Nucleoside)

Medication Safety Issues

Sound-alike/look-alike issues:

Azidothymidine may be confused with azathioprine, aztreonam

Retrovir® may be confused with ritonavir

AZT is an error-prone abbreviation (mistaken as azathioprine, aztreonam)

Use Management of patients with HIV infections in combination with at least two other antiretroviral agents; for prevention of maternal/fetal HIV transmission as monotherapy

Unlabeled/Investigational Use Postexposure prophylaxis for HIV exposure as part of a multidrug regimen

Mechanism of Action Zidovudine is a thymidine analog which interferes with the HIV viral RNA dependent DNA polymerase resulting in inhibition of viral replication; nucleoside reverse transcriptase inhibitor

Pharmacodynamics/Kinetics

Absorption: Oral: 66% to 70%

Distribution: Significant penetration into the CSF; crosses placenta

Relative diffusion from blood into CSF: Adequate with or without inflammation (exceeds usual MICs)

CSF:blood level ratio: Normal meninges: ~60%

Protein binding: 25% to 38%

Metabolism: Hepatic via glucuronidation to inactive metabolites; extensive first-pass effect

Half-life elimination: Terminal: 60 minutes

Time to peak, serum: 30-90 minutes

Excretion:

Oral: Urine (72% to 74% as metabolites, 14% to 18% as unchanged drug)

I.V.: Urine (45% to 60% as metabolites, 18% to 29% as unchanged drug)

Contraindications Life-threatening hypersensitivity to zidovudine or any component of the formulation

Warnings/Precautions Often associated with hematologic toxicity including granulocytopenia, severe anemia requiring transfusions, or (rarely) pancytopenia. Use with caution in patients with bone marrow compromise (granulocytes <1000 cells/mm^3 or hemoglobin <9.5 mg/dL); dosage adjustment may be required in patients who develop anemia or neutropenia. Lactic acidosis and severe hepatomegaly with steatosis have been reported, including fatal cases; use with caution in patients with risk factors for liver disease (risk may be increased in obese patients or prolonged exposure) and suspend treatment with zidovudine in any patient who develops clinical or laboratory findings suggestive of lactic acidosis (transaminase elevation may/may not accompany hepatomegaly and steatosis). Prolonged use has been associated with symptomatic myopathy. Reduce dose in patients with renal impairment. Zidovudine has been shown to be carcinogenic in rats and mice.

Drug Interactions Substrate (minor) of CYP2A6, 2C8/9, 2C19, 3A4

Atovaquone: Atovaquone may decrease zidovudine clearance, increasing zidovudine AUC ~35%

Bone marrow suppressants/cytotoxic agents: Concomitant use may increase risk of hematologic toxicity. (May be seen with adriamycin, dapsone, flucytosine, vincristine, vinblastine.)

Doxorubicin: May decrease the antiviral activity of zidovudine (based on *in vitro* data). Avoid concurrent use.

Fluconazole: Fluconazole may decrease clearance and metabolism of zidovudine

Ganciclovir: Concomitant use may increase risk of hematologic toxicities; monitor hemoglobin, hematocrit, and white blood cell count with differential frequently; dose reduction or interruption of either agent may be needed

Interferon-alpha: Concomitant use may increase risk of hematologic toxicities; monitor hemoglobin, hematocrit, and white blood cell count with differential frequently; dose reduction or interruption of either agent may be needed

Phenytoin: Decreased plasma levels of phenytoin may be seen. Phenytoin may decrease clearance of zidovudine.

Probenecid: Probenecid may increase zidovudine levels. Myalgia, malaise, and/or fever and maculopapular rash have been reported with concomitant use.

Ribavirin: Concomitant use of ribavirin and nucleoside analogues may increase the risk of developing lactic acidosis (includes adefovir, didanosine, lamivudine, stavudine, zalcitabine, zidovudine). May decrease the antiviral activity of zidovudine (based on *in vitro* data); avoid concurrent use.

Stavudine: Zidovudine may decrease the antiviral activity of stavudine (based on *in vitro* data). Avoid concurrent use.

Valproic acid: Valproic acid may increase plasma levels of zidovudine; monitor for possible increase in side effects (AUC increased by 80%)

Adverse Reactions

>10%:

Central nervous system: Severe headache (42%), fever (16%)

Dermatologic: Rash (17%)

(Continued)

Zidovudine *(Continued)*

Gastrointestinal: Nausea (46% to 61%), anorexia (11%), diarrhea (17%), pain (20%), vomiting (6% to 25%)
Hematologic: Anemia (23% in children), leukopenia, granulocytopenia (39% in children)
Neuromuscular & skeletal: Weakness (19%)

1% to 10%:
Central nervous system: Malaise (8%), dizziness (6%), insomnia (5%), somnolence (8%)
Dermatologic: Hyperpigmentation of nails (bluish-brown)
Gastrointestinal: Dyspepsia (5%)
Hematologic: Changes in platelet count
Neuromuscular & skeletal: Paresthesia (6%)

<1% (Limited to important or life-threatening): Anaphylaxis, angioedema, aplastic anemia, bone marrow suppression, cardiomyopathy, cholestatic jaundice, confusion, granulocytopenia, gynecomastia, hepatomegaly (with steatosis), hepatotoxicity, lactic acidosis, mania, myopathy, myositis, neurotoxicity, oral pigmentation changes, pancytopenia, rhabdomyolysis, seizure, somnolence, Stevens-Johnson syndrome, tenderness, thrombocytopenia, toxic epidermal necrolysis

Overdosage/Toxicology Symptoms of overdose include nausea, vomiting, ataxia, and granulocytopenia. Erythropoietin, thymidine, and cyanocobalamin have been used experimentally to treat zidovudine-induced hematopoietic toxicity, yet none are presently specified as the agent of choice. Treatment is supportive.

Dosing

Adults & Elderly:

Prevention of maternal-fetal HIV transmission: Maternal (per AIDSinfo guidelines): 100 mg 5 times/day **or** 200 mg 3 times/day **or** 300 mg twice daily. Begin at 14-34 weeks gestation and continue until start of labor.
During labor and delivery, administer zidovudine I.V. at 2 mg/kg over 1 hour followed by a continuous I.V. infusion of 1 mg/kg/hour until the umbilical cord is clamped

HIV infection:
Oral: 300 mg twice daily or 200 mg 3 times/day
I.V.: 1-2 mg/kg/dose (infused over 1 hour) administered every 4 hours around-the-clock (6 doses/day)
Prevention of HIV following needlesticks (unlabeled use): Oral: 200 mg 3 times/day plus lamivudine 150 mg twice daily; a protease inhibitor (eg, indinavir) may be added for high risk exposures; begin therapy within 2 hours of exposure if possible
Note: Patients should receive I.V. therapy only until oral therapy can be administered

Pediatrics:

Prevention of maternal-fetal HIV transmission (in neonates):

Note: Dosing should begin 8-12 hours after birth and continue for the first 6 weeks of life.

Oral:
Full-term infants: 2 mg/kg/dose every 6 hours
Infants ≥30 weeks and <35 weeks gestation at birth: 2 mg/kg/dose every 12 hours; at 2 weeks of age, advance to 2 mg/kg/dose every 8 hours
Infants <30 weeks gestation at birth: 2 mg/kg/dose every 12 hours; at 4 weeks of age, advance to 2 mg/kg/dose every 8 hours

I.V. (infants unable to receive oral dosing):
Full term: 1.5 mg/kg/dose every 6 hours
Infants ≥30 weeks and <35 weeks gestation at birth: 1.5 mg/kg/dose every 12 hours; at 2 weeks of age, advance to 1.5 mg/kg/dose every 8 hours
Infants <30 weeks gestation at birth: 1.5 mg/kg/dose every 12 hours; at 4 weeks of age, advance to 1.5 mg/kg/dose every 8 hours
During labor and delivery, administer zidovudine I.V. at 2 mg/kg over 1 hour followed by a continuous I.V. infusion of 1 mg/kg/hour until the umbilical cord is clamped

Treatment of HIV infection:

Oral: Children 3 months to 12 years:
160 mg/m^2/dose every 8 hours; dosage range: 90 mg/m^2/dose to 180 mg/m^2/dose every 6-8 hours; some Working Group members use a dose of 180

mg/m^2 to 240 mg/m^2 every 12 hours when using in drug combinations with other antiretroviral compounds, but data on this dosing in children is limited

I.V. continuous infusion: 20 mg/m^2/hour

I.V. intermittent infusion: 120 mg/m^2/dose every 6 hours

Renal Impairment: Cl_{cr} <10 mL/minute: May require minor dose adjustment.

Hemodialysis: At least partially removed by hemo- and peritoneal dialysis. Administer dose after hemodialysis or administer 100 mg supplemental dose. During CAPD, dose as for Cl_{cr} <10 mL/minute.

Continuous arteriovenous or venovenous hemodiafiltration effects: Administer 100 mg every 8 hours.

Hepatic Impairment: Reduce dose by 50% or double dosing interval in patients with cirrhosis.

Available Dosage Forms

Capsule (Retrovir®): 100 mg

Injection, solution [preservative free] (Retrovir®): 10 mg/mL (20 mL)

Syrup (Retrovir®): 50 mg/5 mL (240 mL) [contains sodium benzoate; strawberry flavor]

Tablet (Retrovir®): 300 mg

Nursing Guidelines

Assessment: See Warnings/Precautions for specific use cautions (eg, hepatic or renal impairment). Assess potential for interactions with other pharmacological agents and herbal products patient may be taking (eg, increased risk of nephrotoxicity, hepatotoxicity, lactic acidosis; see Drug Interactions). Assess results of laboratory tests and patient response (eg, CNS changes, hematological changes, and gastrointestinal disturbances; see Adverse Reaction) on a regular basis throughout therapy. Teach patient proper use, possible side effects/appropriate interventions, and adverse symptoms to report (see Patient Education).

Monitoring Laboratory Tests: Monitor CBC and platelet count at least every 2 weeks, MCV, serum creatinine kinase, CD4 cell count, viral load

Dietary Considerations: May be taken without regard to food.

Patient Education: Do not take any new medication during therapy unless approved by prescriber. This drug will not cure HIV; use appropriate precautions to prevent spread of HIV to other persons. Take as directed; may be taken without regard to food. Take around-the-clock. Maintain adequate hydration (2-3 L/day of fluids) unless instructed to restrict fluid intake. You may be more susceptible to infection (avoid crowds and exposure to infection and do not have any vaccinations unless approved by prescriber). May cause headache or insomnia; if these persist, notify prescriber. Report unresolved nausea or vomiting; signs of infection (eg, fever, chills, sore throat, burning urination, flu-like symptoms, fatigue); unusual bleeding (eg, tarry stools, easy bruising, or blood in stool, urine, or mouth); pain, tingling, or numbness of toes or fingers; skin rash or irritation; or muscle weakness or tremors. Pregnancy/breast-feeding precautions: Inform prescriber if you are or intend to become pregnant. Breast-feeding is not recommended.

Pregnancy Risk Factor: C

Pregnancy Issues: Zidovudine crosses the placenta. The use of zidovudine reduces the maternal-fetal transmission of HIV by ~70% and should be considered for antenatal and intrapartum therapy whenever possible. The Perinatal HIV Guidelines Working Group considers zidovudine the preferred NRTI for use in combination regimens during pregnancy. In HIV infected mothers not previously on antiretroviral therapy, treatment may be delayed until after 10-12 weeks gestation. Cases of lactic acidosis/hepatic steatosis syndrome have been reported in pregnant women receiving nucleoside analogues. It is not known if pregnancy itself potentiates this known side effect; however, pregnant women may be at increased risk of lactic acidosis and liver damage. Hepatic enzymes and electrolytes should be monitored frequently during the 3rd trimester of pregnancy in women receiving nucleoside analogues. Health professionals are encouraged to contact the antiretroviral pregnancy registry to monitor outcomes of pregnant women exposed to antiretroviral medications (1-800-258-4263 or www.APRegistry.com).

Lactation: Enters breast milk/not recommended

Breast-Feeding Considerations: HIV-infected mothers are discouraged from breast-feeding to decrease potential transmission of HIV.

(Continued)

Zidovudine *(Continued)*

Perioperative/Anesthesia/Other Concerns: Does not reduce risk of transmitting HIV infections. Potential compliance problems, frequency of administration and adverse effects should be discussed with patients before initiating therapy to help prevent the emergence of resistance.

Administration

Oral: Administer around-the-clock to promote less variation in peak and trough serum levels. Oral zidovudine may be administered without regard to food.

I.M.: Do not give I.M.

I.V.: Avoid rapid infusion or bolus injection

Neonates: Infuse over 30 minutes

Adults: Infuse over 1 hour

Reconstitution: Solution for injection should be diluted with D_5W to a concentration of ≤4 mg/mL; the solution is physically and chemically stable for 24 hours at room temperature and 48 hours if refrigerated. Attempt to administer diluted solution within 8 hours, if stored at room temperature or 24 hours if refrigerated to minimize potential for microbially contaminated solutions.

Compatibility: Stable in D_5W, NS; incompatible with blood products and protein solutions

Storage: Store undiluted vials at room temperature and protect from light.

- ♦ **Zidovudine, Abacavir, and Lamivudine** *see* Abacavir, Lamivudine, and Zidovudine *on page 58*
- ♦ **Zilactin-L® [OTC]** *see* Lidocaine *on page 1033*
- ♦ **Zilactin®-B [OTC]** *see* Benzocaine *on page 232*
- ♦ **Zilactin Toothache and Gum Pain® [OTC]** *see* Benzocaine *on page 232*
- ♦ **Zinacef®** *see* Cefuroxime *on page 356*
- ♦ **Zithromax®** *see* Azithromycin *on page 211*
- ♦ **Zithromax® TRI-PAK™** *see* Azithromycin *on page 211*
- ♦ **Zithromax® Z-PAK®** *see* Azithromycin *on page 211*
- ♦ **Zmax™** *see* Azithromycin *on page 211*
- ♦ **Zocor®** *see* Simvastatin *on page 1535*
- ♦ **Zofran®** *see* Ondansetron *on page 1268*
- ♦ **Zofran® ODT** *see* Ondansetron *on page 1268*
- ♦ **Zoladex®** *see* Goserelin *on page 829*
- ♦ **Zoloft®** *see* Sertraline *on page 1521*

Zolpidem (zole PI dem)

U.S. Brand Names Ambien®; Ambien CR™

Synonyms Zolpidem Tartrate

Pharmacologic Category Hypnotic, Nonbenzodiazepine

Medication Safety Issues

Sound-alike/look-alike issues:

Ambien® may be confused with Ambi 10®

Use Short-term treatment of insomnia (sleep onset and/or sleep maintenance)

Mechanism of Action Structurally dissimilar to benzodiazepines. Selective hypnotic effects (with minor anxiolytic, myorelaxant and anticovulsant properties) mediated through selective affinity for the alpha-1 subunit of the omega-1 (benzodiazepine) receptor located on the $GABA_A$ receptor complex. Agonism at this site enhances GABA-ergic chloride conductance hyperpolarizing neuronal membranes thereby reducing the responsiveness to excitatory signals.

Pharmacodynamics/Kinetics

Onset of action: 30 minutes

Duration: 6-8 hours

Absorption: Rapid

Distribution: Very low amounts enter breast milk

Protein binding: 92%

Metabolism: Hepatic, primarily via CYP3A4 (~60%), to inactive metabolites

Half-life elimination: 2.5-2.8 hours (range 1.4-4.5 hours); Cirrhosis: Up to 9.9 hours

Time to peak, plasma: 2 hours; 4 hours with food

Excretion: As metabolites in urine, bile, feces

Contraindications Hypersensitivity to zolpidem or any component of the formulation

Warnings/Precautions Should be used only after evaluation of potential causes of sleep disturbance. Failure of sleep disturbance to resolve after 7-10 days may indicate psychiatric or medical illness. Use with caution in patients with depression. Abnormal thinking and behavioral changes have been associated with sedative-hypnotics. Sedative/hypnotics may produce withdrawal symptoms following abrupt discontinuation. Causes CNS depression, which may impair physical and mental capabilities. Effects with other sedative drugs or ethanol may be potentiated. Use caution in the elderly; dose adjustment recommended. Closely monitor elderly or debilitated patients for impaired cognitive or motor performance. Avoid use in patients with sleep apnea or a history of sedative-hypnotic abuse. Use caution with hepatic impairment; dose adjustment required. Prescriptions should be written for the smallest effective dose (especially in the elderly) and for the smallest quantity consistent with good patient care (especially with depression). Safety and efficacy have not been established in pediatric patients.

Drug Interactions **Substrate** of CYP1A2 (minor), 2C8/9 (minor), 2C19 (minor), 2D6 (minor), 3A4 (major)

Antipsychotics: Sedative effects may be additive with antipsychotics, including phenothiazines; monitor for increased effect

CNS depressants: Sedative effects may be additive with other CNS depressants; monitor for increased effect; includes barbiturates, benzodiazepines, narcotic analgesics, ethanol, and other sedative agents

CYP3A4 inducers: CYP3A4 inducers may decrease the levels/effects of zolpidem. Example inducers include aminoglutethimide, carbamazepine, nafcillin, nevirapine, phenobarbital, phenytoin, and rifamycins.

CYP3A4 inhibitors: May increase the levels/effects of zolpidem. Example inhibitors include azole antifungals, clarithromycin, diclofenac, doxycycline, erythromycin, imatinib, isoniazid, nefazodone, nicardipine, propofol, protease inhibitors, quinidine, telithromycin, troleandomycin, and verapamil.

Rifamycin derivatives: May decrease levels/effects of zolpidem.

Nutritional/Herbal/Ethanol Interactions

Ethanol: Avoid ethanol (may increase CNS depression).

Food: Maximum plasma concentration and bioavailability are decreased with food; time to peak plasma concentration is increased; half-life remains unchanged.

Herb/Nutraceutical: St John's wort may decrease zolpidem levels. Avoid valerian, St John's wort, kava kava, gotu kola (may increase CNS depression).

Lab Interactions Increased aminotransferase [ALT (SGPT)/AST (SGOT)], bilirubin (S); decreased RAI uptake

Adverse Reactions Actual frequency may be dosage form, dose and/or age dependent

>10%: Central nervous system: Dizziness, headache, somnolence

1% to 10%:

Cardiovascular: Blood pressure increased, chest discomfort, palpitation

Central nervous system: Anxiety, apathy, amnesia, ataxia, attention disturbance, body temperature increased, confusion, depersonalization, depression, disinhibition, disorientation, drowsiness, drugged feeling, euphoria, fatigue, fever, hallucinations, hypoesthesia, insomnia, memory disorder, lethargy, lightheadedness, mood swings, stress

Dermatologic: Rash, urticaria, wrinkling

Endocrine & metabolic: Menorrhagia

Gastrointestinal: Abdominal discomfort, abdominal pain, abdominal tenderness, appetite disorder, constipation, diarrhea, dyspepsia, flatulence, gastroenteritis, gastroesophageal reflux, hiccup, nausea, vomiting, xerostomia

Genitourinary: Urinary tract infection

Neuromuscular & skeletal: Arthralgia, back pain, balance disorder, myalgia, neck pain, paresthesia, psychomotor retardation, tremor, weakness

Ocular: Asthenopia, blurred vision, depth perception altered, diplopia, red eye, visual disturbance

Otic: Labyrinthitis, tinnitus, vertigo

Renal: Dysuria

Respiratory: Pharyngitis, sinusitis, throat irritation, upper respiratory tract infection

Miscellaneous: allergy, binge eating, flu-like symptoms

<1% (Limited to important or life-threatening): Abnormal dreams, agitation, anorexia, arthritis, bronchitis, chest pain, cognition decreased, concentrating difficulty, constipation, cough, cystitis, diaphoresis increased, dysarthria, dysphagia, edema, emotional lability, eye irritation, falling, hepatic function abnormalities, hyperglycemia, hypoesthesia, illusion, leg cramps, menstrual

(Continued)

Zolpidem *(Continued)*

disorder, nervousness, pallor, postural hypotension, pruritus, scleritis, speech disorder, stupor, syncope, tachycardia, taste perversion, thirst, urinary incontinence, vaginitis

Overdosage/Toxicology Symptoms of overdose include coma and hypotension. Treatment for overdose is supportive. Rarely is mechanical ventilation required. Flumazenil has been shown to selectively block binding to CNS receptors, resulting in a reversal of CNS depression, but not always respiratory depression. Hemodialysis is not likely to be of benefit.

Dosing

Adults: Insomnia: Oral:

Ambien®: 10 mg immediately before bedtime; maximum dose: 10 mg

Ambien CR™: 12.5 mg immediately before bedtime

Elderly:

Ambien®: 5 mg immediately before bedtime

Ambien CR™: 6.25 mg immediately before bedtime

Renal Impairment: Dose adjustment not required; monitor closely.

Not dialyzable

Hepatic Impairment:

Ambien®: 5 mg

Ambien CR™: 6.25 mg

Available Dosage Forms

Tablet, as tartrate:

Ambien®: 5 mg, 10 mg

Ambien® PAK™ [dose pack]: 5 mg (30s), 10 mg (30s)

Tablet, as tartrate, extended release (Ambien CR™): 6.25 mg, 12.5 mg

Nursing Guidelines

Assessment: For short-term use. Assess effectiveness and interactions of other medications patient may be taking. Assess for history of addiction; long-term use can result in dependence, abuse, or tolerance; periodically evaluate need for continued use. After long-term use, taper dosage slowly when discontinuing. Monitor for CNS depression. For inpatient use, institute safety measures and monitor effectiveness and adverse reactions. For outpatients, monitor for effectiveness of therapy and adverse reactions at beginning of therapy and periodically with long-term use. Assess knowledge/teach patient appropriate use, interventions to reduce side effects, and adverse symptoms to report.

Dietary Considerations: For faster sleep onset, do not administer with (or immediately after) a meal.

Patient Education: Use exactly as directed; do not increase dose or frequency or discontinue without consulting prescriber. Drug may cause physical and/or psychological dependence. While using this medication, do not use alcohol or other prescription or OTC medications (especially, pain medications, sedatives, antihistamines, or hypnotics) without consulting prescriber. Maintain adequate hydration (2-3 L/day of fluids) unless instructed to restrict fluid intake. You may experience drowsiness, dizziness, or blurred vision (use caution when driving or engaging in tasks requiring alertness until response to drug is known); nausea (small frequent meals, frequent mouth care, chewing gum, or sucking lozenges may help); or diarrhea (buttermilk, boiled milk, yogurt may help). Report CNS changes (confusion, depression, increased sedation, excitation, headache, abnormal thinking, insomnia, or nightmares); muscle pain or weakness; respiratory difficulty; chest pain or palpitations; or ineffectiveness of medication. **Breast-feeding precaution:** Consult prescriber if breast-feeding

Geriatric Considerations: In doses >5 mg, there was subjective evidence of impaired sleep on the first post-treatment night. There have been few reports of increased hypotension and/or falls in the elderly with this drug. Can be considered a drug of choice in the elderly when a hypnotic is indicated.

Pregnancy Risk Factor: C

Pregnancy Issues: Children born of mothers taking sedative/hypnotics may be at risk for withdrawal; neonatal flaccidity has been reported in infants following maternal use of sedative/hypnotics during pregnancy.

Lactation: Enters breast milk/not recommended (AAP rates "compatible")

Perioperative/Anesthesia/Other Concerns: Causes less disturbances in sleep stages as compared to benzodiazepines; time spent in sleep stages 3 and 4 are maintained. Zolpidem decreases sleep latency; should not be prescribed in quantities exceeding a 1-month supply.

Administration

Oral: Ingest immediately before bedtime due to rapid onset of action. Ambien CR™ tablets should not be divided, crushed, or chewed.

- ♦ **Zolpidem Tartrate** *see* Zolpidem *on page 1736*
- ♦ **Zorbtive™** *see* Somatropin *on page 1555*
- ♦ **ZORprin®** *see* Aspirin *on page 189*
- ♦ **Zosyn®** *see* Piperacillin and Tazobactam Sodium *on page 1370*
- ♦ **Zovirax®** *see* Acyclovir *on page 86*
- ♦ **Zyban®** *see* BuPROPion *on page 273*
- ♦ **Zydone®** *see* Hydrocodone and Acetaminophen *on page 867*
- ♦ **Zymar™** *see* Gatifloxacin *on page 797*
- ♦ **Zyprexa®** *see* Olanzapine *on page 1259*
- ♦ **Zyprexa® Zydis®** *see* Olanzapine *on page 1259*
- ♦ **Zyrtec®** *see* Cetirizine *on page 366*
- ♦ **Zyvox™** *see* Linezolid *on page 1044*

SPECIAL TOPICS / CONCERNS

TABLE OF CONTENTS

ACUTE POSTOPERATIVE PAIN

Pain in a surgical patient can be due to preexisting disease, the surgical procedure (surgical incision, related drains and tubes, body positioning, immobility, excessive stretching or trauma to a peripheral nerve, postoperative ileus), or a combination of preexisting disease and procedure-related causes. Pain can occur at rest and/or with movement or physical activity. Effective postoperative pain management should provide subjective pain relief, minimize the risk for adverse effects, and allow the patient to return to normal daily activities as soon as possible. In addition, postoperative pain management should minimize the detrimental effects from unrelieved pain which include: thromboembolic and pulmonary complications; impairment of immune function; unnecessary fear, anxiety, and/or suffering; and development of chronic pain.

Preparation should begin before the surgical procedure by performing a pain history and physical exam; treating pre-existing pain and anxiety; and educating the patient about his or her role in reporting pain, reporting analgesic adverse effects, and properly using analgesic modalities (eg, patient controlled analgesia) and nonpharmacological techniques. Then, the pain management plan can be made. The inclusion of pre- and intraoperative analgesics has been shown to provide better pain relief and reduce the need for potent opioid analgesics following surgery.

It is now recommended to utilize a combination of analgesic agents and techniques that work by different mechanisms to provide postoperative analgesia (balanced or multimodal analgesia). Combining analgesics and analgesic techniques provides additive or synergistic analgesia with lower doses compared to monotherapy, potentially minimizing adverse effects. Examples of balanced or multimodal analgesia include a nonsteroidal anti-inflammatory agent (NSAID) or acetaminophen combined with an opioid following outpatient surgery, epidural analgesia with an opioid and a local anesthetic following major abdominal or thoracic surgery, and a peripheral nerve block (using a local anesthetic) with an opioid following shoulder surgery. In some cases, therapy for postoperative pain management actually begins before surgery (eg, preemptive analgesia, peripheral nerve block).

Analgesic drugs can be divided into opioid and nonopioid drugs. Nonopioid analgesics are most commonly used to manage mild and moderate pain. Examples of nonopioid analgesics commonly used to manage postoperative pain include NSAIDs, acetaminophen, and local anesthetics. Ketamine, α_2-receptor agonists (clonidine, dexmedetomidine), tricyclic antidepressants (eg, nortriptyline, amitriptyline), and antiepileptic agents (eg, gabapentin, carbamazepine) are drugs that are often used for other indications but have analgesic properties. Opioids are the mainstay of analgesic therapy for moderate and severe pain. This chapter will review the commonly used drugs in the management of acute postoperative pain.

ACETAMINOPHEN

Acetaminophen, alone or in combination with an opioid or NSAID, is frequently used for treatment of mild to moderate postoperative pain. Acetaminophen most likely provides analgesia by interrupting prostaglandin synthesis in the central nervous system, with no peripheral anti-inflammatory effects. Acetaminophen is generally well tolerated when administered in a daily maximum dose of 4 grams for short-term pain management in adults with normal liver function.

NONSTEROIDAL ANTI-INFLAMMATORY DRUGS (NSAIDs)

NSAIDs are commonly used for postoperative pain management. These agents are frequently the first-line therapy for mild to moderate postoperative pain. The use of NSAIDs for the management of postoperative pain has seen an exponential increase in the past decade, with the entrance of ketorolac (the only parenteral NSAID with an indication for pain) onto the market, and the increase in ambulatory surgical procedures. NSAIDs inhibit the production of prostaglandins by inhibiting cyclooxygenase. These agents have both a peripheral and central effect, with their central effect providing a significant portion of the analgesia and their peripheral effect suppressing postinjury inflammation and subsequent pain. NSAIDs are known to have a morphine-sparing effect and are frequently used in combination with opioids for postoperative pain management.

Adverse Effects

The perioperative limitation of traditional nonselective NSAIDs is most often due to their potential to impair platelet aggregation, which can increase bleeding. Short-term perioperative use of NSAIDs in healthy adults is not expected to become hypovolemic during surgery and should not cause clinically important renal dysfunction. Cases of gastrointestinal bleeding or ulceration have been reported. Careful patient screening is necessary to minimize the risk of these major complications from NSAID therapy. Overall, the risk of adverse effects from NSAID use in postoperative pain management is small and the benefit (good analgesia) is substantial. When considering dosing, analgesia is provided at lower doses (eg, 200 or 400 mg ibuprofen), whereas higher doses (eg, 600 or 800 mg ibuprofen) are necessary to suppress inflammation. If inflammation and swelling are not present, lower doses of NSAIDs should be used to provide analgesia and minimize the occurrence of adverse effects.

TRAMADOL

Tramadol provides analgesia by binding to mu opioid receptors and inhibiting reuptake of norepinephrine and serotonin. Similar to oral opioid-acetaminophen combination products, tramadol is effective for treating moderate pain. Adverse effects that can occur with tramadol include nausea, vomiting, dizziness, and seizures. Tramadol should be used with caution in patients with a history of seizure disorder. Although tramadol is not classified as a controlled substance, physical dependence on tramadol has been reported.

Table 1. Nonopioid Analgesic Agents

Drug	Usual Dose for Adults >50 kg Body Weight	Usual Dose for Adults <50 kg Body Weight
Acetaminophen (Tylenol®)	650 mg q4h or 1000 mg q6h	10-15 mg/kg q4h maximum of 4 g/day
Ibuprofen (Motrin®, others)	400-600 mg q6h	10 mg/kg q6-8h
Ketorolac tromethamine tablets[1] (Toradol®)	10 mg q4-6h to a maximum of 40 mg/d	
Naproxen (Naprosyn®)	250-275 mg q6-8h	5 mg/kg q8h
Naproxen sodium (Anaprox®)	275 mg q6-8h	
Ketorolac tromethamine injection (Toradol®)	60 mg I.M. or 30 mg I.V. initially, then 30 mg q6h, not to exceed 5 days	30 mg I.M. or 15 mg I.V. initially, then 15 mg q6h, not to exceed 5 days

[1]For short-term use only.

Note: Only the above NSAIDs have FDA approval for use as simple analgesics, but clinical experience has been gained with other drugs as well. Doses are for patients with normal renal and hepatic function.

OPIOIDS

Opioids are the mainstay of treatment for moderate to severe postoperative pain management. They are commonly used as the initial analgesic agent in the immediate postoperative period and are continued postoperatively, for days to weeks, for moderate or severe pain. Opioids are administered by the oral, parenteral, or neuraxial route, with the severity of pain and type of surgical procedure dictating the method in which they are administered. Oral opioids, either alone or in combination with acetaminophen, are frequently administered for moderate pain. Parenteral and neuraxial opioids are usually administered for severe pain.

Opioids exert their effects by binding to central opioid receptors. The activity of the specific opioid depends on the actual agent and how well it binds to a given opioid receptor. Unlike NSAIDs and local anesthetics, opioids do not interrupt nociceptive transmission but rather decrease the ability to discern pain.

ACUTE POSTOPERATIVE PAIN *(Continued)*

Opioids are often selected based upon potency, safety, and patient characteristics. Propoxyphene, codeine, and hydrocodone are less potent opioids that are most often used in combination with acetaminophen. These combination products are indicated for mild or moderate pain. Higher doses of these opioids would be required to treat severe pain and would cause significant adverse effects for the patient, including acetaminophen overdose. Morphine, hydromorphone, and fentanyl are potent opioids that can be used alone in a dose that will treat moderate or severe pain. Oxycodone can be used for moderate or severe pain, depending upon the product formulation. When combined with acetaminophen or aspirin, the dose is limited by the amount of acetaminophen or aspirin in the product. Therefore, the dose of oxycodone needed to treat severe pain could not be provided with a combination product. Meperidine undergoes extensive first-pass metabolism, limiting its usefulness as an oral analgesic. High levels of its metabolite, normeperidine, can result in central nervous system excitation ranging from agitation to seizures. Meperidine also inhibits serotonin reuptake, raising concerns about development of the serotonin syndrome particularly if a second serotonergic agent (eg, selective serotonin reuptake inhibitor or SSRI) is concurrently administered. For safety, many hospitals limit the use of meperidine for analgesia. For patients with renal and/or hepatic insufficiency, the doses of most opioids should be reduced. Table 2 represents the most frequently prescribed oral opioids for acute postoperative pain management.

Table 2. Oral Opioids for Acute Postoperative Pain

Drug	Equianalgesic Dose	Effective Adult Dosing[1]	Indication
Hydromorphone	7.5 mg	2-4 mg q4-6h	Severe pain
Codeine[2]	180 mg	15-60 mg q4-6h	Moderate pain
Hydrocodone[2]	30 mg	5-10 mg q4-6h	Moderate pain
Oxycodone[2]	20 mg	5-10 mg q4-6h	Moderate pain
Tramadol	N/A	50-100 mg q4-6h[3]	Moderate pain

[1]For patients with normal renal and hepatic function.

[2]When combined with acetaminophen, aspirin, or ibuprofen.

[3]Not to exceed 400 mg/day in adults or 300 mg/day in patients ≥75 years of age.

Parenteral opioids remain an important component of any analgesic regimen for managing severe postoperative pain in the inpatient and ambulatory setting. Ambulatory surgery patients receive short-acting parenteral analgesics (eg, fentanyl), or limited amounts of morphine, in intermittent bolus doses for treatment of severe pain. The intramuscular route of administration should be avoided if possible due to pain on injection, variability in absorption, and a longer time to peak effect (when compared to intravenous administration). Patient-controlled analgesia (PCA), the self-administered intermittent I.V. administration of an opioid, is the preferred method for administering intravenous (I.V.) opioids for managing postoperative pain. The advantage of PCA over traditional intermittent I.M. or I.V. administration is that the patient reaches his or her ideal level of analgesia more rapidly, has minimal fluctuation within the analgesic range, and has a feeling of control over his or her postoperative pain. The key to using PCA appropriately is adequately educating the patient, assuring that an adequate bolus dose is administered, and making sure the appropriate patient is chosen for PCA administration. PCA is not indicated in a patient who is not able to understand the technique of PCA or press the PCA button, unwilling to assume control of his or her analgesia, or who is obtunded or sedated by his or her illness or medication. Table 3 represents the usual PCA doses of common opioids for the treatment of moderate or severe acute postoperative pain.

Table 3. Usual Adult PCA Opioid Dosing[1]

Drug	Equianalgesic Dose	Loading Dose[2]	PCA Dose	Lockout Interval
Fentanyl	10 mcg	25-100 mcg	10-20 mcg	4-8 min
Hydromorphone (Dilaudid®)	0.2 mg	0.2-1 mg	0.2-0.4 mg	5-10 min
Morphine	1 mg	2-10 mg	1-2 mg	5-10 min

[1]In patients with normal renal and hepatic function.

[2]Titrate in increments to desired level of analgesia or occurrence of excessive adverse effects.

Neuraxial opioid administration is another route that is used for management of moderate or severe acute postoperative pain. Neuraxial administration of opioids works by binding to opioid receptors on the spinal cord. This type of opioid administration can be used to provide analgesia for major abdominal, thoracic, and pelvic procedures, as well as total knee replacements. In these types of surgeries, epidural analgesia often provides better postoperative analgesia than parenteral opioids. Epidural administration of opioids is much more common than intrathecal administration for postoperative pain management. Table 4 represents neuraxial analgesic doses of opioid agonists for the treatment of moderate or severe acute postoperative pain.

Table 4. Usual Neuraxial Opioid Dosing in Adults

Agent	Epidural Bolus Dose	Epidural Continuous Infusion	Intrathecal Bolus Dose
Fentanyl	25-100 mcg	25-100 mcg/h	5-25 mcg
Hydromorphone	1 mg	0.1-0.2 mg/h	–
Morphine	5 mg	0.1-1 mg/h	0.1-0.3 mg
Sufentanil	10-50 mcg	5-30 mcg/h	0.02-0.05 mcg/kg

Adverse Effects

Adverse effects of oral, parenteral, and neuraxial opioid therapy for treatment of acute postoperative pain include sedation, dizziness, nausea, vomiting, pruritus, urinary retention, and respiratory depression. Risk factors for respiratory depression include large doses administered to an opioid-naive patient, pulmonary dysfunction (eg, asthma, obstructive sleep apnea), obesity, low body weight, and concurrent medications that potentiate the respiratory depressant effect of the opioid. The potential for excessive sedation and respiratory depression to occur is greater when parenteral or neuraxial opioids are administered. Monitoring the patient's sedation level is the most effective way to prevent significant opioid-induced respiratory depression.

LOCAL ANESTHETICS

Local anesthetics provide good postoperative analgesia. These agents can be administered by the neuraxial route, as a peripheral nerve block (PNB), or directly into the wound via infiltration. Neuraxial administration is commonly used for acute postoperative pain management for the inpatient, whereas PNB and wound infiltration are more commonly used for the ambulatory surgery patient.

Peripheral nerve blocks of upper and lower extremities (eg, brachial plexus block, femoral nerve block) are often performed to provide intraoperative anesthesia and/or postoperative analgesia. A local anesthetic is injected near or around a nerve or nerve plexus to stop the pain impulses that originate from the surgical site. In addition to sensory fibers, motor and sympathetic fibers are also affected by injection of the local anesthetic solution. Patients undergoing more extensive, and therefore more painful, shoulder, elbow, knee, foot, or ankle surgeries are potential candidates for PNBs. These nerve blocks can be provided by a single injection or a continuous infusion of a local anesthetic to provide postoperative analgesia. Local anesthetic wound infiltration (single injection or a continuous

ACUTE POSTOPERATIVE PAIN *(Continued)*

infusion) before, during, and after surgical procedures has been shown to decrease postoperative pain. Local anesthetics administered epidurally or intrathecally are frequently combined with opioids to provide "balanced analgesia." The most common local anesthetic agents used for intra- and postoperative analgesia are lidocaine, mepivacaine, bupivacaine, and ropivacaine. (Table 5)

Table 5. Common Local Anesthetic Agents and Doses for Intra- and Postoperative Analgesia

Agent	Local Infiltration	Peripheral Nerve Block[1]	Continuous Peripheral Nerve Block	Continuous Epidural Analgesia
Lidocaine	0.5%-1%, 1-50 mL	1.5%-2%, 20 mL	1% at 6-10 mL/h[2]	–
Bupivacaine	0.25%, 1-50 mL	0.25%-0.5%, 30 mL	0.1%-0.2% at 6-10 mL/h[2]	0.05%-0.125% at 4-10 mL/h[3]
Ropivacaine	0.5%, 1-40 mL	0.5%-0.75%, 30 mL	0.15%-0.2% at 6-10 mL/h[2]	0.1%-0.2% at 4-10 mL/h
Mepivacaine	0.5%-1%, 1-50 mL	1.5%-2%, 30 mL	–	–

[1]For a 70 kg patient – doses can vary with the type of block and should not exceed the maximum recommended dose.

[2]For 24-72 hours; some studies have added clonidine 1 mcg/mL.

[3]When administered in combination with fentanyl, sufentanil, hydromorphone, or morphine.

Adverse Effects

The adverse effects most commonly seen with analgesic doses of local anesthetics include hypotension (secondary to sympathetic blockade) and dose-related motor blockade. The potential for CNS and cardiovascular toxicity exists if a large amount of these agents is inadvertently administered systemically.

SUMMARY

The goal of acute postoperative pain management is to provide excellent analgesia with minimal adverse effects. Oftentimes, this is best accomplished with the use of a combination of analgesic agents and techniques that provide analgesia by different mechanisms.

REFERENCES AND RECOMMENDED READING

American Society of Anesthesiologists Task Force on Acute Pain Management, "Practice Guidelines for Acute Pain Management in the Perioperative Setting," *Anesthesiology*, 2004, 100(6):1573-81.

Hartrick CT, "Multimodal Postoperative Pain Management," *Am J Health Syst Pharm*, 2004, 61(Suppl 1):S4-10.

Gilron I, Milne B, and Hong M, "Cyclooxygenase-2 Inhibitors in Postoperative Pain Management: Current Evidence and Future Directions," *Anesthesiology*, 2003, 99(5):1198-208.

Dahl V and Raeder JC, "Non-Opioid Postoperative Analgesia," *Acta Anaesthesiologica Scandinavica*, 2000, 44:1191-203.

Block BM, Liu SS, Rowlingson AJ, et al, "Efficacy of Postoperative Epidural Analgesia: A Meta-Analysis," *JAMA*, 2003, 290(18):2455-63.

Chelly J, Fanelli G, and Casati A, *Continuous Peripheral Nerve Blocks – An Illustrated Guide*, Mosby, 2001 (e-book) **(http://www.harcourt-international.com/e-books/viewbook.cfm?ID=252)**.

Murauski JD and Gonzalez KR, "Peripheral Nerve Blocks for Postoperative Analgesia," *AORN Journal*, 2002, 75:136-47.

ALLERGIC REACTIONS

An allergic drug reaction can be considered an adverse effect involving immunologic mechanisms. True allergic reactions are much less common than nonallergic responses such as side effects and drug-drug interactions. As a result, it is important to carefully evaluate patients who present with allergies to drugs. Patients frequently state an allergy to a drug when the reaction was a predictable side effect (eg, nausea/vomiting with codeine). If a patient presents a history of one or more of the following signs or symptoms after drug administration, an allergic reaction should be assumed until proven otherwise: skin manifestations (pruritus with hives or flushing), facial or oral swelling, shortness of breath, choking, wheezing, and vascular collapse. In these situations, an alternate agent should be selected.

CLASSIFICATION OF ALLERGIC REACTIONS

Allergic reactions can be classified into one of four immunopathologic categories (types I through IV) using the Coombs and Gell Classification System. The following table summarizes the key characteristics of each type of reaction.

Type	Characteristics	Usual Onset	Examples
I - Anaphylactic (IgE mediated)	Requires the presence of IgE specific for drug antigen or other allergen; allergen binds to IgE on basophils and mast cells resulting in release of inflammatory mediators (eg, histamine, serotonin, proteases, bradykinin generating factor, eosinophil chemotactic factors, neutrophil chemotactic factor, leukotrienes, prostaglandins, thromboxanes)	Within 30 minutes	Immediate penicillin reaction Immediate latex reaction Blood products Vaccines Dextran Polypeptide hormones
II - Cytotoxic	Destruction of host cells; cell-associated antigen initiates cytolysis by antigen-specific antibody (IgG or IgM); most often involves blood elements (eg, erythrocytes, leukocytes, platelets)	Usually 5-12 hours	Penicillin, quinidine, phenylbutazone, thiouracils, sulfonamides, methyldopa
III - Immune complex	Antigen-antibody complexes form and deposit on blood vessel walls and activate complement. Result is a serum-sickness-like syndrome.	3-8 hours	Serum sickness; may be caused by penicillins, sulfonamides, I.V. contrast media, hydantoins
IV - Cell mediated (delayed)	Antigens cause activation of lymphocytes (T cells), which release inflammatory mediators	24-48 hours	Graft rejection Latex contact dermatitis Tuberculin reaction

Modified from DiPiro JT and Stafford CT, "Allergic and Pseudoallergic Drug Reactions," *Pharmacotherapy: A Pathophysiologic Approach*, 3rd ed, Stamford CT: Appleton and Lange, 1997, 1675-88.

ANESTHESIA-RELATED AGENTS ASSOCIATED WITH ALLERGY

Certain agents are most often responsible for allergic reactions in surgical patients. These include neuromuscular blocking agents, latex, colloids, hypnotics, antibiotics, benzodiazepines, opioids, local anesthetics, I.V. contrast media, and blood products. The antibiotics most commonly associated with allergic reactions are the sulfonamides, penicillins, and cephalosporins. Propofol contains soybean oil and egg yolk components; in patients with allergies to these items, propofol should be avoided. The ester-type local anesthetics can produce allergic reactions secondary to the metabolite para-aminobenzoic acid. The methylparaben preservative in amide-type local anesthetics may also produce an allergic reaction in

ALLERGIC REACTIONS *(Continued)*

patients sensitive to para-aminobenzoic acid. Sulfites, which are used as preservatives in various drug products, can produce pulmonary complications in patients, occurring more frequently in asthmatics. Cross allergenicity exists between shellfish/seafood and protamine and I.V. contrast media; care should be taken when using these agents in patients with these types of allergies. Special consideration should be given to a patient who presents a personal or family history of allergy to halothane or succinylcholine as this may actually represent an occurrence of malignant hyperthermia.

ANAPHYLAXIS

Anaphylaxis is the most severe form of allergic reaction. It can present as an acute, life-threatening reaction with multiple organ system involvement or it can be more localized in appearance. It has been estimated that 1 in every 2700 hospitalized patients experience drug-induced anaphylaxis. When antibodies are not involved in the process, the reaction is termed anaphylactoid. It is not possible through clinical observation to distinguish between anaphylactic and anaphylactoid reactions. Life-threatening reactions are more likely to occur in patients with a history of allergy, atopy, or asthma. Although these patients are frequently pretreated with corticosteroids, there is no evidence to suggest this practice is effective for preventing true anaphylactic reactions. In a survey examining the incidence of intraoperative anaphylaxis, 70.2% were due to neuromuscular blocking agents, 12.5% due to latex, 4.6% due to colloids, 3.6% due to hypnotics, 2.6% due to antibiotics, 2% due to benzodiazepines, 1.7% due to opioids, 0.7% due to local anesthetics, and 2.8% due to other agents.

Pathophysiology

Anaphylaxis is initiated by an antigen binding to IgE antibodies; however, prior exposure to the antigen or a substance with a similar structure is first required to sensitize the patient to the antigen. The binding of the antigen to the IgE antibodies on the surface of basophils and mast cells causes release of histamine and the chemotactic factors of anaphylaxis. Other chemical mediators (leukotrienes, prostaglandins, kinins) are also released in response to cellular activation. The liberated mediators produce bronchospasm, upper airway edema, vasodilation, increased capillary permeability, and urticaria. The effects of multiple mediators on the heart and peripheral vasculature cause the cardiovascular collapse seen during anaphylaxis. Antigenic challenge in a sensitized individual usually produces immediate clinical manifestations of anaphylaxis; however, the onset may be delayed by up to 30 minutes. The reaction can vary in severity, from minor clinical changes to acute cardiopulmonary collapse.

Signs / Symptoms of Anaphylactic Reaction

The following table lists the signs and symptoms that may indicate an anaphylactic reaction during anesthesia.

Systems	Symptoms	Signs
Cutaneous	Itching, burning	Urticaria (hives), flushing, periorbital edema, perioral edema
Respiratory	Dyspnea, chest tightness	Coughing, wheezing, sneezing, laryngeal edema, decreased pulmonary compliance, pulmonary edema, acute respiratory distress, bronchospasm
Cardiovascular	Dizziness, malaise, retrosternal oppression	Disorientation, diaphoresis, loss of consciousness, hypotension, tachycardia, dysrhythmias, decreased systemic vascular resistance, pulmonary hypertension, cardiovascular collapse

Modified from Levy JH, *Anaphylactic Reactions in Anesthesia and Intensive Care*, Stoneham, Butterworth-Heinemann, 1992.

Treatment of Anaphylactic Reaction

Treatment of a severe, life-threatening anaphylactic reaction must be immediate. Initial therapy should consist of: 1) stop administration of precipitating drug; 2) maintain airway with 100% oxygen; 3) discontinue all anesthetic agents; 4) intravascular volume expansion with crystalloid solution; and 5) epinephrine administration. Secondary therapy consists of administration of antihistamines (eg, diphenhydramine), catecholamine infusions (eg, norepinephrine, epinephrine), inhaled bronchodilators (eg, albuterol) for bronchospasm, corticosteroids (eg, hydrocortisone, methylprednisolone, dexamethasone), and sodium bicarbonate. Patients should be admitted to an ICU for 24 hours following an anaphylactic reaction because of the possibility of recurrent "late-phase" reactions.

REFERENCES AND RECOMMENDED READING

DiPiro JT and Stafford CT, "Allergic and Pseudoallergic Drug Reactions," *Pharmacotherapy: A Pathophysiologic Approach*, 3rd ed, Stamford, CT: Appleton and Lange, 1997, 1675-88.

Levy JH, "Allergy and Anesthesia," Paper presented at the ASA 1996 Annual Refresher Course Lectures, New Orleans, LA, 1996 Oct 20.

ANESTHESIA FOR GERIATRIC PATIENTS

"No skill or art is needed to grow old, but the trick is to endure it." – Goethe

In 1980, people 65 years of age and older made up 12% of the population in the United States but consumed 30% of the healthcare expenditures. By 2040, the elderly will make up about 25% of the population and account for 50% of health-care costs. Because at least half will require surgery, understanding physiologic and pathologic changes in the geriatric population is important to reduce perioperative morbidity and mortality.

In 1961, the perioperative mortality rate in geriatric patients approached 20%. Because of increased understanding of the physiology of aging and improved perianesthetic monitoring, the mortality rate decreased to <5% by 1980, although the mortality associated with emergency surgery is 3-10 times greater than when the same surgery is performed on an elective basis. Improvements in preoperative evaluation, intraoperative management, and postoperative treatment have further reduced morbidity and mortality in geriatric patients.

As a general rule, older people have more pre-existing diseases than younger people do. In addition, geriatric patients have significant alterations in anatomy, physiology, pharmacokinetics, pharmacodynamics, recovery ability, and psychological coping mechanisms. The purpose of this chapter is to identify those major changes which necessitate a modification in perioperative practice. A brief review of major organ systems highlights the natural aging process and the common disease processes that compromise the elderly person.

Figure 1: Changes in physiologic function with age in humans expressed as percentage of mean value at age 30 years.

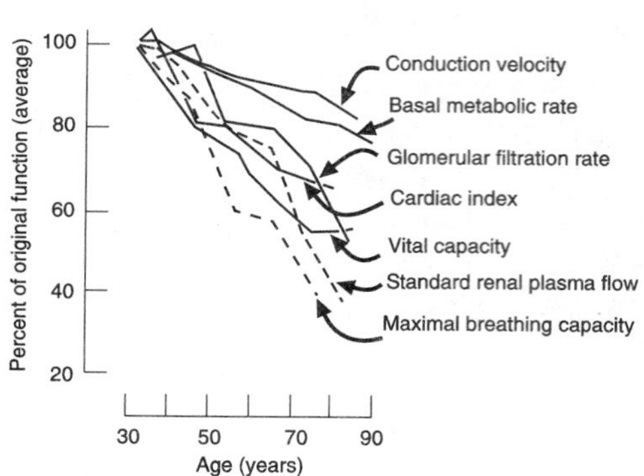

With permission from Miller RD, "Anesthesia for the Elderly," *Anesthesia*, 2nd ed, Miller RD, ed, New York, NY: Churchill Livingstone, 1986, 1802.

CARDIOVASCULAR SYSTEM

Hypertension and atherosclerotic cardiovascular disease occur in more than half of the elderly. Loss of elasticity in arterial walls increases vascular resistance leading to an increase in systolic blood pressure which, in time, produces left ventricular hypertrophy. With aging, the vascular muscular layer is replaced with fibrous tissue and plaque, which cannot stretch, exaggerating the blood pressure rise during systole and fall during diastole. This widened pulse pressure is a marker of compromised compliance in the vessel wall and is associated with increased risk of coronary events.

A decrease in adrenergic activity leads to a slower resting heart rate, a lower maximal heart rate, and a depressed baroreceptor reflex. These physiologic changes associated with aging impair a person's ability to respond to hypovolemia, hypotension, or hypoxemia by attenuating increases in heart rate and cardiac output. A slow circulation time, frequently found in geriatric patients, prolongs onset of action for I.V. drugs (eg, thiopental, propofol, fentanyl), while speeding the induction of anesthesia using inhalational agents (eg, sevoflurane, isoflurane).

Normal Physiologic Changes	Pathophysiologic Changes
Decreased elasticity	Atherosclerosis
Increased afterload	Coronary artery disease
Increased left ventricular hypertrophy	Hypertension
Increased systolic blood pressure	Congestive heart failure
Decreased diastolic blood pressure	Arrhythmias
Decreased adrenergic activity	
Decreased resting heart rate	
Decreased maximum heart rate	
Decreased baroreceptor reflex	
Slowed circulation time	

The development of atherosclerosis is a pathologic process which produces critical coronary stenosis. The development of congestive heart failure and myocardial ischemia compromises cardiac function, which influences other organ systems. Onset of arrhythmias reflects disease of the cardiac conduction system, with atrial fibrillation as the most common arrhythmia. Elderly patients frequently take nitrates, beta-blockers, and calcium channel blockers. Optimization of cardiac function preoperatively, continuing treatment with most chronic cardiac medications, and understanding drug interactions with anesthetics and perioperative medications is important. Knowledge of not only drug action but also physiologic reaction if chronic medications are discontinued is essential. For example, a person receiving beta-blockers following myocardial infarction or for treatment of hypertension may experience rebound hypertension and ventricular arrhythmias with abrupt discontinuation of this medication. The duration of antiplatelet therapy following coronary stenting is not completely understood, with reports of acute thrombosis following discontinuation of the drugs even after one year of administration. The effect this will have on geriatric surgery is not known.

Hypertension is another common cardiovascular disease. Therapy crosses many drug categories. Knowledge about the specific antihypertensive medications and their interactions with anesthetic drugs (eg, clonidine decreases anesthetic drug requirements) is important. Discontinuation of antihypertensive medication can produce preoperative hypertension, with enhanced hemodynamic instability. The decision to continue diuretic therapy preoperatively depends on the patient. Patients prone to congestive heart failure should be maintained on their diuretic therapy, whereas a chronic hypertensive patient receiving a bowel prep for GI surgery does not need additional loss of intravascular volume prior to surgery. Serum potassium may be low in patients taking a thiazide diuretic. This is especially important for people taking digitalis. Although anesthesiologists, cardiologists, and intensivists have over the years expressed concern that maintenance of chronic drug therapy (ie, beta-blockers, calcium channel blockers, ACE inhibitors) may produce complications when combined with anesthetic drugs, current thinking is that maintaining the patient in his optimal state of preoperative hemodynamic control provides the best situation for perianesthetic management. Recently, anesthesiologists echo cardiologists in suggesting that initiation of

ANESTHESIA FOR GERIATRIC PATIENTS *(Continued)*

perioperative beta-blocker therapy for geriatric patients with cardiovascular disease decreases operative morbidity and mortality. Aging also leads to abnormal response to endothelium-dependent vasodilators (ie, acetylcholine) and decreased production of endothelial-derived vasodilator substances (ie, nitric oxide). A poorly controlled hypertensive patient may have a reduced blood volume and will experience tremendous swings in blood pressure during anesthesia and surgery.

RESPIRATORY SYSTEM

A carefully performed history and physical examination can identify patients whose normal pulmonary aging changes have become a pathophysiologic risk. History of recurrent pulmonary infections, smoking, asthma, COPD, and emphysema place patients at high risk for pulmonary complications. Preoperative optimization of pulmonary function (treat infection, stop smoking, bronchodilators) and instruction in the use and importance of incentive spirometry can improve the perioperative pulmonary course. Pulmonary function tests add little to the preoperative evaluation, except for lung resection surgery.

Smoking is a serious problem for the general population. It is more serious in the geriatric population because they have more years of tobacco exposure and more pulmonary damage. Cessation of smoking the day before surgery does two things: a) decreases the level of carbon monoxide in the blood and therefore enhances oxygen carrying capacity, and b) increases bronchial reactivity to stimuli due to the acute withdrawal of nicotine. To improve pulmonary function, the patient must stop smoking at least 6 weeks before surgery. Anatomic and physiologic damage are not reversed, however, the rate of continuing organ dysfunction is reduced to reflect the normal aging process. Supplemental oxygen may be needed in the immediate postoperative period.

Normal Physiologic Changes	Pathophysiologic Changes
Decreased pulmonary elasticity	Emphysema
Decreased alveolar surface, FEV	Chronic bronchitis
Increased V_d, RV, FRC	Pneumonia
Increased closing capacity	Lung cancer
V/Q mismatching	Tuberculosis
Decreased arterial oxygenation	
Increased chest wall rigidity	
Decreased cough	
Blunted response to hypercapnia/ hypoxia	
Progressive kyphosis/scoliosis	
Decreased total lung capacity	

Reduction in elastic recoil of the lung and chest wall, in addition to a decrease in pulmonary blood flow, leads to changes in ventilation:perfusion ratio. Dead space (V_d) increases and small airway collapse occurs during tidal volume ventilation, resulting in decreased gas exchange. This leads to an increase in the alveolar/arterial oxygen gradient and a decrease in arterial oxygen tension. Residual volume (RV) and functional residual capacity (FRC) increase as lung elasticity decreases with a concomitant decrease in forced expiratory volume (FEV). A "rule of thumb" for the normal deterioration of pulmonary function to predict expected change in arterial oxygenation while breathing room air is:

PaO_2 (expected) = 100 - age/4 **or** PaO_2 decreases 0.35 mm Hg per year

CENTRAL NERVOUS SYSTEM

With aging, there is a progressive decrease in cerebral cortical mass and an increase in brain sensitivity to anesthetic agents. The MAC of inhalational anesthetics decreases 40% to 60% by 80 years of age. This occurs not only with inhalational anesthetic gases, but also with intravenous, intrathecal, and epidural drugs. For example, the induction dose of sodium thiopental decreases from 5 mg/kg to 2 mg/kg in the 70 year old patient.

Figure 2: Refers to inhalation, intravenous, and spinal/epidural anesthetic doses

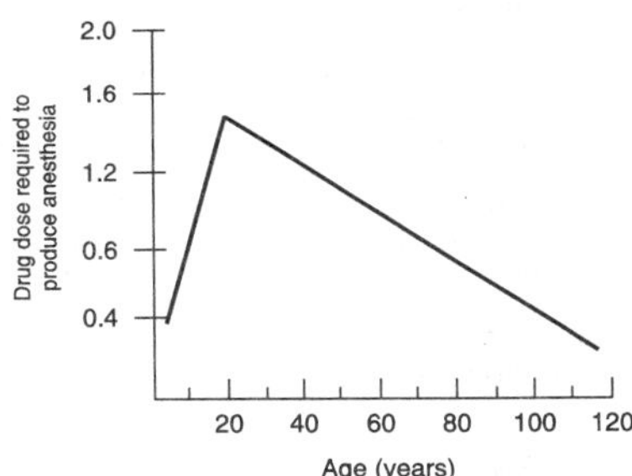

Therefore, it is easy to overdose elderly patients who do not have reserve capacity to overcome the profound side effects of "normal" anesthetic doses. The duration of anesthetics is also prolonged, slowing recovery and increasing postoperative confusion, often for days.

Normal Physiologic Changes	Pathophysiologic Changes
Decreased cerebral cortex	Stroke
Decreased cerebral blood flow (CBF)	Dementia
Decreased cerebral metabolic rate (CMR O_2)	Alzheimer's disease
Prolonged CNS recovery	Memory impairment
Postop confusion	

The blood pressure of patients with cerebrovascular disease should be maintained in the the patient's normal range during and after surgery. Head position should be maintained in the neutral position to prevent occlusion of the carotid or vertebral circulation. Patients with Parkinsonism should continue taking levodopa up to the time of surgery. Drugs with antidopaminergic effects are to be avoided (ie, phenothiazines, butyrophenones). Surgery for patients with recent stroke should be delayed at least 6 weeks to allow for restabilization of the blood-brain barrier and resumption of cerebral autoregulation.

ENDOCRINE SYSTEM

Normal Physiologic Changes	Pathophysiologic Changes
Decreased insulin secretion	Obesity
Increased insulin resistance	Type 2 diabetes mellitus
Decreased thyroid function	Poor wound healing
	Decreased leukocyte function

ANESTHESIA FOR GERIATRIC PATIENTS *(Continued)*

Adult onset diabetes is a common geriatric disease. It affects approximately 35 million people in the United States and is predicted to increase 200% over the next several decades. The severity of the disease and success of glucose management predict end-organ damage. Historically, tight glucose control, the medical management goal for diabetes, could be relaxed in the perioperative period. However, recently there is evidence that tight glucose control in the perioperative and ICU periods improves outcome. These studies show a striking increase in cardiovascular risk with a mild increase in blood glucose concentration. Whether tight glucose control to <110 mg/dL is also important for outpatient surgical patients is not known. It is well known that hyperglycemia decreases wound healing and increases infection; hyperglycemia will also increase the amount of cerebral injury should ischemia occur. However, hypoglycemia can cause cerebral and myocardial ischemia.

For the insulin-controlled diabetic, there is no ideal management protocol. Therapy ranges from withholding all insulin preoperatively vs administering a fraction of the usual dose vs initiation of a continuous dextrose/insulin infusion. Surgery is stressful and blood glucose increases. Without insulin an osmotic glucose diuresis can occur, producing dehydration. Some clinicians feel that the administration of exogenous insulin improves patient outcome by providing the body with a source of energy during this time of stress. The critical aspect of any management regimen is the frequent evaluation of blood glucose levels and appropriate treatment of hyper- or hypoglycemia.

UROLOGIC SYSTEM

Aging decreases renal function as reflected by a reduction in glomerular filtration rate and creatinine clearance. An increase in serum creatinine may not be evident on laboratory tests because total body muscle mass and creatinine production decrease with aging. However, BUN increases on an average of 0.2 mg/dL/year. Decreased ability to concentrate/dilute urine puts the geriatric patient at risk for dehydration/fluid overload. The patient's capacity to metabolize and excrete drugs is also affected.

Normal Physiologic Changes	Pathophysiologic Changes
Decreased renal blood flow	Diabetic nephropathy
Decreased kidney mass	Hypertensive nephropathy
Decreased tubular function	Prostatic enlargement

Elderly males with benign prostatic hypertrophy may experience bladder distention with loss of detrusor muscle tone leading to urinary retention. This can occur with general anesthesia, but is more common with spinal/epidural anesthesia. Neuraxial anesthesia decreases detrusor tone while increasing sphincter tone. Because neuraxial anesthesia produces a sympathectomy and a decrease in blood pressure, fluid administration to maintain normal blood pressure frequently complicates the situation by overdistending the urinary bladder.

Renal blood flow decreases with aging, with a 50% reduction by age 75. This places the geriatric patient at greater risk for perioperative renal damage/failure. Hypotension during anesthesia can further decrease renal perfusion, which can lead to additional renal damage. Maintenance of 0.5 mL/kg/hour urine output is recommended. A decrease in renal blood flow reduces clearance of many drugs, which can prolong drug action and may necessitate a reduction in drug dosage and/or frequency of administration.

GASTROINTESTINAL SYSTEM

Hepatic blood flow decreases with age, as does hepatic protein synthesis and drug metabolism. Gastric emptying also slows, decreasing absorption of orally administered drugs. Many drugs are highly protein bound, therefore a decrease in albumin significantly increases the amount of free drug. Because many drugs are metabolized by the liver, clearance can be decreased. See Pharmacokinetic/ Pharmacodynamic section.

MUSCULOSKELETAL SYSTEM

Normal Physiologic Changes	Pathophysiologic Changes
Decreased muscle mass	Weakness
Decreased joint mobility	Arthritis
Decreased dentition	Airway management problems
Increase osteoporosis	Bone fractures

Changes in the musculoskeletal system pose significant problems in positioning elderly patients. Alterations in skin elasticity and perfusion put patients at risk for ischemic ulcers at pressure points. Restricted joint mobility compounds this problem.

Many geriatric patients are edentulous, which facilitates intubation; however, many others have poor dentition or only a few teeth left, which are critical in supporting their dental bridges. Poor dentition increases the risk of dental trauma. Loss of mandibular bone contour can complicate adequate mask fit, making positive pressure ventilation difficult. Cervical arthritis and temporomandibular problems are not uncommon, as are gastroesophageal reflux and hiatal hernia, which put the patient at risk for inadequate ventilation or aspiration.

Osteoporosis reduces bone density and produces skeletal fragility, especially in postmenopausal women (40% in white females). Hormone replacement therapy in addition to calcium, vitamin D, and exercise, lowers the likelihood of osteoporotic fractures by at least 25%. Estrogen blocks bone resorption by inhibiting cytokine signals necessary for recruitment of bone-resorbing osteoclasts, but has been associated with increased cardiovascular adverse events. Drug therapy (ie, alendronate) also interferes with bone resorption.

The initial dose of muscle relaxant drugs is unchanged, but elderly patients require a decrease in frequency of redosing (due to prolonged elimination). The exceptions to this general rule are drugs that are metabolized in the blood by Hoffman elimination or nonspecific esterases (atracurium, mivacurium, and cisatracurium).

HYPOTHERMIA

Geriatric patients experience more intraoperative hypothermia than younger patients do. The consequences of this include prolonged awakening, slower drug elimination, increased shivering, enhanced coagulation, and increased postoperative metabolic demand associated with increased catabolism. Oxygen demand is increased, and if pulmonary and cardiovascular systems are unable to handle this increased workload, the potential for myocardial ischemia increases. Myocardial oxygen consumption can increase up to 500% with postoperative shivering. Maintenance of intraoperative temperature has been associated with significantly improved wound healing and outcome.

ANESTHESIA FOR GERIATRIC PATIENTS *(Continued)*

PHARMACOKINETICS / PHARMACODYNAMICS

Gastrointestinal absorption of orally administered drugs is affected by aging. There are changes in gastric acidity, intestinal motility, and intestinal perfusion.

Figure 3: Example of increased half-life of diazepam

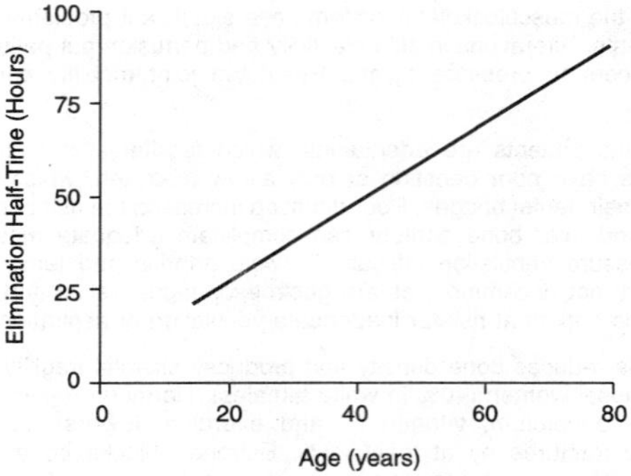

Elimination Half-Time (Hours)
100
75
50
25
0
0 20 40 60 80
Age (years)

Once a drug is absorbed, its pharmacologic action is altered by decreased total body water and increased body fat concentration. Redistribution of drugs from the vessel-rich group is slowed, especially for highly lipid soluble drugs. Decreased hepatic perfusion and drug metabolism by liver microsomal enzymes combined with a reduced renal excretion of drug and/or metabolites can lead to an increased and prolonged drug effect. A decreased number of receptors leads to receptor saturation at substantially lower serum concentration. A decrease in both the amount of plasma protein and the quality of drug-protein binding leads to an increase in free fraction of the drug.

Drug Dosing Adjustments in the Elderly

Drug	Action	Mechanism
Inhalational anesthetics	Decrease dose 40%	↑ sensitivity
I.V. induction drugs[1]	Decrease dose 50%	↑ sensitivity, ↓ clearance/half-life
Antibiotics		
Initial dose	No change	
Repeat doses	Decrease frequency	↓ clearance, ↑ half-life
Muscle relaxants[2]		
Initial bolus	No change	
Repeat bolus	Decrease frequency	↓ clearance, ↑ half-life
Infusion	Decrease dose	↓ clearance, ↑ half-life
Narcotics[3]		
Initial bolus	Decrease dose 50%	↑ sensitivity
Infusion	Decrease dose 30%	↓ clearance, ↑ half-life

[1]Sodium thiopental, propofol, midazolam, etomidate, methohexital.

[2]This does not include muscle relaxants that are metabolized by Hoffman elimination.

[3]This does not include remifentanil.

TYPE OF ANESTH

The debate between regiona
discussion, for no single anest
either the young or the geriatric p
patient, concurrent medical diseases,
the patient's expectations/wishes. The
statement is debated: transurethral rese
extraction, and knee surgery. Traditionally,
regional anesthesia so that mental status
syndrome can be elicited early. Cataract surgery
ophthalmic analgesia providing adequate anesthe
thereby avoiding the physiologic transgressions asso
thesia. Patients with hip and knee surgery performed w
experience an initial 50% reduction in the incidence of deep
pulmonary embolus; however, the 3- to 6-month outcomes we
studies were performed before the intra-/postoperative use of
compression sleeves and low molecular weight heparin. A
comparison has not been made.

Postoperative mental changes attributed to general anesthesia a
uncommon in the elderly; however, the use of heavy sedation during regiona
local anesthesia can also produce a similar prolonged alteration of mental status
The incidence of postoperative cognitive decline (POCD) increases with advanced age. Recent studies suggest that long tern postoperative morbidity and mortality is associated with (1) extent of comorbidieies, (2) duration of intraoperative hypotension, and (3) duration of deep general anesthesia. Drug metabolism and elimination are slowed, producing prolonged sedative effects. It has been proposed that outpatient surgery may disrupt daily habits less and the elderly may actually return to normal faster when in a familiar environment.

EDUCATION FOR GERIATRIC ANESTHESIA

The Anesthesiology Residency Review Committee has mandated that each program provide didactic instruction and clinical experience in managing the geriatric surgical population. The Society for the Advancement of Geriatric Anesthesia (SAGA) was established in 2000 to improve the care of the older person having surgery. There is a joint project between the ASA committee on Geriatric Anesthesia, SAGA, and the American Geriatrics Society (AGS) to develop a curriculum for geriatric anesthesia education. These educational materials can be accessed via the internet.

SUMMARY

The aging process is a progressive alteration of normal physiology over time. This deterioration can significantly alter the patient's response to anesthetics and perioperative medications. Frequently, coexistent with this progressive depression of organ function are superimposed disease processes, which further impair organ function. Geriatric patients present a significant challenge to the physician.

REFERENCES AND RECOMMENDED READING

Apfelbaum JL, Kallar SK, and Wetchler BV, "Adult and Geriatric Patients," *Anesthesia for Ambulatory Surgery*, 2nd ed, Chapter 5, Wetchler BV, ed, JB Lippincott Co, 1995, 272-307.

Bode RH Jr, Lewis KP, Zarich SW, et al, "Cardiac Outcome After Peripheral Vascular Surgery. Comparison of General and Regional Anesthesia," *Anesthesiology*, 1996, 84(1):3-13.

Campbell DN, Lim M, Muir MK, et al, "A Prospective Randomised Study of Local Versus General Anesthesia for Cataract Surgery," *Anaesthesia*, 1993, 48(5):422-8.

Dodds C and Allison J, "Postoperative Cognitive Deficit in the Elderly Surgical Patient," *Br J Anesth*, 1998, 81(3):449-62.

Gottlieb SS, McCarter RJ, and Vogel RA, "Effect of Beta-Blockade on Mortality Among High-Risk and Low-Risk Patients After Myocardial Infarction," *N Engl J Med*, 1998, 339(8):489-97.

Gu W, Pagel PS, Warltier DC, et al, "Modifying Cardiovascular Risk in Diabetes Mellitus,"*Anesthesiology*, 2003, 98(3):774-9.

Kurz A, Sessler DI, and Lenhardt R, "Perioperative Normothermia to Reduce the Incidence of Surgical-Wound Infection and Shorten Hospitalization," *N Engl J Med*, 1996, 334(19):1209-15.

ed)

/ After Noncar-

Role of Epidural

.

sia on Coagula-
6-704.
ardial Ischemia.

ESIA: GENERAL vs REGIONAL

l vs general anesthesia continues to be a topic for
hetic technique has been shown to be better for
atient. The type of anesthesia depends on the
underlying physiology, type of surgery, and
e are several surgeries where the above
tion of the prostate (TURP), cataract
TURP surgery is performed with
changes associated with TURP
s minimally invasive, with local
sia for the procedure and
ciated with general anes-
ith regional anesthesia
vein thrombosis and
re similar. These
lower extremity
modern day

e not
l or

ANESTHESIA CONSIDERATIONS FOR NEUROSURGERY

Various factors must be taken into account for the patient undergoing neurosurgery. These include the surgical procedure being performed; the type of anesthesia to be used; the need for special anesthetic techniques (eg, controlled hypotension); and the effects of the anesthetic agents on brain physiology (cerebral blood flow, cerebral metabolic oxygen requirements, and cerebral vasodilation). This section will review key aspects of the anesthetic management of neurosurgical patients.

PHYSIOLOGY

Cerebral Blood Flow

Cerebral blood flow (CBF) is equal to cerebral perfusion pressure divided by the cerebral vascular resistance. Cerebral perfusion pressure is defined as the difference between mean arterial pressure (MABP) and the greater of intracranial pressure (ICP) or central venous pressure. Autoregulation maintains CBF at a constant level (50 mL/100 g brain/minute) between the MABP of 50 and 150 mm Hg (see Figure A). Various conditions and/or medications can attenuate or abolish autoregulation, making blood flow dependent on MABP; these include the volatile inhalation agents, hypoxia, hypercarbia, and cerebral ischemia. Hypoxia causes cerebral vasodilation and an increase in CBF (see Figure B) while hypocarbia causes a linear decrease in CBF between $PaCO_2$ of 20 and 80 mm Hg (see Figure C).

Cerebral Metabolic Rate

Cerebral metabolic rate ($CMRO_2$) and CBF are directly related; as $CMRO_2$ increases, so does CBF to ensure sufficient substrate is available for metabolic demand (see Figure D). Conditions and/or medications that influence $CMRO_2$ include seizures (↑ $CMRO_2$), temperature (hypothermia ↓ $CMRO_2$), and various anesthetics (eg, volatile inhalation agents ↓ $CMRO_2$).

The Brain's Protective Mechanisms

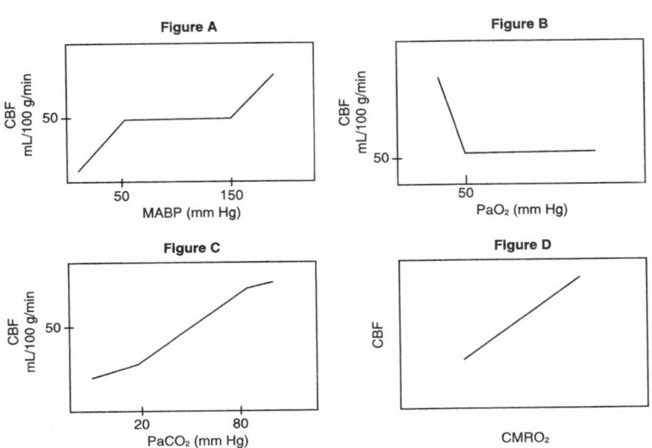

ANESTHESIA CONSIDERATIONS FOR NEUROSURGERY *(Continued)*

Intracranial Pressure

Normal ICP values are between 5 and 15 mm Hg and reflect the relationship between the volume of the cranial vault and intracranial contents. Since the cranial vault is rigid, the capacity of the intracranial contents to adjust to an increasing volume (compliance) will ultimately be exceeded, resulting in a marked increase in ICP with a small increase in volume. Signs and symptoms of increased ICP are found in Table 1. It must be kept in mind that a patient with an increased intracranial volume as a result of a tumor, for example, may be especially sensitive to volume increases secondary to cerebral vasodilation caused by factors such as CO_2 retention or volatile inhalational anesthetic agents. Elevated ICP can be treated by reducing cerebral blood volume, reducing brain tissue volume, or reducing cerebrospinal fluid (CSF) volume (Table 2).

Table 1. Signs and Symptoms of Increased Intracranial Pressure

Headache
Nausea/vomiting
Decreased level of consciousness
Hypertension
Bradycardia
Irregular breathing
Oculomotor (third cranial) nerve palsy
Pupillary dilation
Abducens (sixth cranial) nerve palsy
Hemiparesis or hemiplegia
Coma
Respiratory arrest

Table 2. Treatment of Elevated Intracranial Pressure

Reduction of Cerebral Blood Volume

- Avoid hypoxia and hypercarbia, as they cause cerebral vasodilation
- Hyperventilate to a $PaCO_2$ of 25-30 mm Hg (produces cerebral vasoconstriction)
- Promote venous drainage (eg, elevate head 30 degrees)
- Treat severe hypertension
- Administer medications to produce cerebral vasoconstriction (eg, barbiturates, propofol, etomidate, benzodiazepines)

Reduction of Brain Tissue Volume

- Increase serum osmolality to 305-320 mOsm/L with the administration of mannitol (0.2-1 g/kg I.V.), urea, hypertonic saline
- Administer furosemide (0.5-1 mg/kg I.V.); optimal results seen when combined with mannitol (↓ furosemide dose to 0.15-0.3 mg/kg I.V.)
- Administer steroids (effective for tumors)
- Resection of brain

Reduction of Cerebrospinal Fluid Volume

- Drain CSF through lumbar subarachnoid or ventriculostomy catheter
- Decrease CSF production (furosemide, acetazolamide) and/or increase CSF reabsorption

Cerebrospinal Fluid

The CSF volume in an adult is approximately 150 mL. It is formed in the choroid plexus of the cerebral ventricles (0.35 mL/minute) by the transport of sodium, chloride, and bicarbonate with osmotic movement of water. CSF is absorbed into the venous system of the brain through arachnoid membrane villi. Furosemide and acetazolamide can reduce CSF formation by inhibiting the combined transport of sodium and chloride and by reducing bicarbonate transport, respectively.

EFFECTS OF MEDICATIONS ON BRAIN PHYSIOLOGY

Table 3 lists the effects of select anesthetic agents on cerebral blood flow, cerebral metabolic oxygen requirements, and cerebral vasodilation. In general, inhalational anesthetics decrease cerebral metabolism and increase CBF whereas intravenous agents decrease both cerebral metabolism and blood flow. Of note, ketamine increases oxygen demand and as a result is not commonly used in neuroanesthesia. Isoflurane continues to be an excellent choice for a volatile inhalation agent. Its mild direct vasodilating action is partly offset by its ability to reduce cerebral metabolic rate and subsequently CBF, thereby limiting the net increase in CBF. The newer volatile inhalation agents desflurane and sevoflurane generally appear to act similarly. The nondepolarizing neuromuscular blocking (NMB) agents have no direct effects on CBF and $CMRO_2$ as they do not cross the blood brain barrier; they may have an indirect effect secondary to their effects on heart rate (eg, pancuronium) and blood pressure (eg, tubocurarine) if autoregulation has been abolished. Succinylcholine does increase CBF and $CMRO_2$, but this has minimal clinical impact if administered after a defasciculating dose of a nondepolarizing NMB agent or induction of adequate anesthesia. The vasopressors epinephrine, phenylephrine, and norepinephrine also have no direct cerebral effects but may indirectly increase CBF by increasing cerebral perfusion pressure. The vasodilators nitroglycerin, sodium nitroprusside, and hydralazine can increase CBF and ICP via direct cerebral vasodilation if arterial blood pressure is maintained. Beta-blockers (esmolol, labetalol) do not alter cerebral metabolism or vascular tone.

Table 3. Effects of Anesthetic Agents on Brain Physiology

Medication	Cerebral Blood Flow	Cerebral Metabolic Rate	Direct Cerebral Vasodilation
Inhalation Anesthetic Agents			
Desflurane	↑	↓↓	Yes
Enflurane	↑↑	↓	Yes
Halothane	↑↑↑	↓	Yes
Isoflurane	↑	↓↓	Yes
Nitrous oxide	↑↑/0	↑/0	–
Nitrous oxide with volatile inhalation agent	↑	↑/0	–
Nitrous oxide with intravenous anesthetic agent	0	0	–
Sevoflurane	↑	↓↓	Yes
Intravenous Anesthetic Agents			
Barbiturates	↓↓↓	↓↓↓	No
Etomidate	↓↓↓	↓↓↓	No
Fentanyl	↓/0	↓/0	No
Ketamine	↑↑	↑	Yes
Midazolam	↓↓	↓↓	No
Propofol	↓↓	↓↓	No

ANESTHESIA CONSIDERATIONS FOR NEUROSURGERY *(Continued)*

ELECTROPHYSIOLOGIC MONITORING

Electroencephalogram

The electroencephalogram (EEG) is used to monitor cerebral electrical activity and may allow early detection of ischemia before CBF is not sufficient to maintain tissue viability. It can also be used for localization of epileptic foci. As a general rule, anesthetic effects on the EEG are global in nature in contrast to the focal changes seen with ischemia (see Table 4).

Table 4. EEG Rhythms

Delta	0-0.4 Hz	Deep sleep Deep anesthesia Ischemia
Theta	4-8 Hz	Light sleep Light anesthesia
Alpha	8-13 Hz	Resting and alert
Beta	13-30 Hz	Mental concentration Light sedation

Evoked Potentials

Evoked potentials monitor the functional integrity of ascending sensory pathways and descending motor pathways. Sensory evoked potentials are recorded from the cerebral cortex following peripheral (sensory nerve) stimulation. Motor evoked potentials are recorded from peripheral muscle activity initiated by stimulation of the motor cortex. Evoked potentials are classified by the nerve tract being evaluated (somatosensory, auditory, visual, motor) (see Table 5). The type of evoked potential monitored depends on the area of CNS at risk for intraoperative injury. Evoked potentials are measured in terms of latency (how long it takes the stimulus to reach the recording device) and amplitude (the peak to trough height of the recorded waveform). Because anesthetic agents affect the latency and/or amplitude measurements (Table 6) it is important to obtain a baseline measurement after establishment of anesthesia. Thereafter, the anesthetic regimen should not be altered so that any subsequent decrease in amplitude or increase in latency reflects neuronal ischemia, not a change in depth of anesthesia. Maintaining an adequate depth of anesthesia when monitoring MEPs is difficult, especially since muscle relaxants must be used sparingly to preserve the motor response. Other factors that can alter evoked potentials include hypotension, hypoxia, and hypothermia.

The reader is referred to any major anesthesia text for a further discussion of electrophysiologic monitoring.

Table 5. Evoked Potentials and the Neuronal Tracts They Monitor

Evoked Potential	CNS Tract	Surgical Procedures
SSEP (somatosensory evoked potential)	Sensory neural axis from peripheral nerves to brainstem and cortex	Spinal cord surgery (tumor, scoliosis), carotid endarterectomy, aortic surgery, cerebral aneurysm
BAER (brainstem auditory evoked response)	Brain stem	Acoustic neuroma, posterior fossa lesions, surgery involving cranial nerve VIII or auditory canal
VER (visual evoked response)	Retina, optic chiasm, optic radiation, occipital cortex	Orbit tumors, sphenoid wing meningiomas, supracellular/pituitary tumors, surgery around optic nerve or occipital cortex
MEP (motor evoked potential)	Motor cortex and descending motor tracts	Spinal cord surgery (tumor, scoliosis)

Table 6. Drug Effects on Evoked Potentials

	Amplitude	Latency
I.V. Drugs		
Barbiturates	↓	↑
Benzodiazepines	↓	↑
Droperidol	↓	↑
Etomidate	↑,→	↑,→
Ketamine	↑	→
Narcotics	↓	↑,→
Propofol	↓	↑
Anesthetic Gases		
Inhalational agents (0.5 MAC)	→	→
Inhalational agents (>1 MAC)	↓	↑
Nitrous oxide	↓	→

NEUROSURGICAL PROCEDURES

The following information should be considered when anesthetizing patients undergoing neurosurgical procedures.

Intracranial Tumors

- Assess fluid and electrolyte status. Hypovolemia, which is not uncommon in patients who have been at bedrest and/or treated with mannitol, can predispose the patient to hypotension during induction of anesthesia.
- Care should be taken in premedicating patients as they may be especially sensitive to central nervous system (CNS) depressant drugs; sedatives/analgesics are often not administered until the patient is in the operating room.
- Monitoring should include measurement of arterial blood gases, intra-arterial blood pressure, central venous pressure, and urinary output in addition to the standard monitoring.
- Goals of anesthesia management: Avoid hypertension, hypotension, hypoxia, hypercarbia, and coughing; ICP should not be increased nor CBF compromised.
  - Thiopental, propofol, etomidate, or midazolam are all suitable induction agents.
  - An opioid can be administered to blunt the response to induction.
  - A nondepolarizing NMB agent with minimal cardiovascular effects (eg, vecuronium) should be used if airway management is not considered problematic.
  - A deep level of anesthesia should be established before laryngoscopy/intubation to minimize increases in ICP due to sympathetic stimulation.
  - Hyperventilation to a $PaCO_2$ of 25-30 mm Hg produces cerebral vasoconstriction and decreases intracranial pressure without producing cerebral ischemia.
  - $PaCO_2$ should be normalized near the end of surgery.
  - Long-acting agents should be avoided for the last 1-2 hours of surgery to prevent prolonged wakeup and allow a neurologic examination at the end of surgery.
  - Consider administering lidocaine I.V. 90 seconds before suctioning/extubation to minimize coughing, straining, and hypertension.
  - Before extubation, the patient's ability to protect his/her airway and the adequacy of respiration should be assessed.
  - Hypertension should be treated to minimize bleeding, prevent brain edema, and hematoma; esmolol, sodium nitroprusside, nitroglycerin, nicardipine, and labetalol are suitable options.
  - A neurologic exam should be performed after the patient is extubated.

ANESTHESIA CONSIDERATIONS FOR NEUROSURGERY *(Continued)*

Pituitary Tumors

- ICP may be less of a concern if the tumor is small.
- Endocrine function should be assessed preoperatively.
- Supplemental, short-acting corticosteroid therapy may need to be administered perioperatively.
- With the transcranial approach, ICP may be a concern; measures to control ICP intraoperatively should be instituted.
- Hypertension, tachycardia, arrhythmias, and myocardial ischemia may be seen when phenylephrine and cocaine are used to prepare the nares for the transphenoidal approach.
- At the end of transphenoidal surgery, nasal breathing will not be possible due to nasal packing; make sure the patient is fully conscious before extubation.
- Diabetes insipidus frequently occurs after surgery (within first 12 hours) requiring treatment with I.V. fluids or vasopressin.

Intracranial Aneurysms

- Complications of subarachnoid hemorrhage include increased ICP, aneurysm rebleed, vasospasm, and hydrocephalus.
- Thiopental, propofol, opioids, and volatile inhalation agents (eg, isoflurane) can be used to induce/maintain anesthesia.
- Lidocaine, esmolol, or labetalol can be used during induction to reduce the risk of hypertension and rupture of the aneurysm.
- Following induction, $PaCO_2$ should be maintained between 25 and 35 mm Hg.
- In addition to hyperventilation, osmotic diuresis and CSF drainage may be used to provide a "slack" brain.
- Controlled hypotension may be considered during dissection of the aneurysm.
- Normotension or a slight increase in blood pressure may be employed with temporary "trapping" of the aneurysm.
- EEG or evoked potentials may be used to monitor the safety of temporary occlusion of arteries.
- Mild hypothermia (32°C to 34°C) can improve the brain's ability to tolerate ischemia.
- Treat hyperglycemia because ischemic damage is worse when it occurs with elevated blood glucose levels (>150-180 mg/dL).
- Minimize coughing, straining, hypertension at extubation.
- A neurologic exam should be performed in the operating room.

REFERENCES AND RECOMMENDED READING

Albin MS, ed, *Textbook of Neuroanesthesia With Neurosurgical and Neuroscience Perspectives*, New York, NY: McGraw-Hill, 1997.

Barash PG, Cullen BF, and Stoelting RK, "Neurophysiology and Neuroanesthesia," *Handbook of Clinical Anesthesia*, 2nd ed, Philadelphia, PA: JB Lippincott, 1993, 256-76.

Bendo AA, Kass IS, Hartung J, et al. "Anesthesia for Neurosurgery," Barash PG, Cullen BF, Stoelting RK, eds, *Clinical Anesthesia*, 3rd ed, Philadelphia, PA: Lippincott-Raven, 1997, 699-745.

Cottrell JE and Smith DS, *Anesthesia and Neurosurgery*, 3rd ed, St Louis, MO: Mosby Co, 1994.

Goto T and Kliewer D, "Anesthesia for Neurosurgery," Davison JK, Eckhardt III WF, Perese DA, eds, *Clinical Anesthesia Procedures of the Massachusetts General Hospital*, 4th ed, Boston, MA: Little, Brown and Company, 1993, 368-89.

Shapiro HM and Drummond JC, "Neurosurgical Anesthesia," Miller RD, ed, *Anesthesia*, 4th ed, New York, NY: Churchill Livingstone, 1994, 1897-946.

ANESTHESIA FOR OBSTETRIC PATIENTS IN NONOBSTETRIC SURGERY

Every year 0.75% to 2% of pregnant women undergo a nonobstetric surgical procedure. The major indications for these approximately 75,000 anesthetics are trauma, ovarian cysts, appendicitis, breast tumors, and cervical incompetence. More serious procedures such as cardiopulmonary bypass and cerebral aneurysm clipping are not uncommon. Preoperative, intraoperative, and postoperative care of the pregnant patient is unique because the physician must be concerned about two patients (the mother and the fetus), each with its own special needs.

The physician must take into account the normal physiologic changes of pregnancy, and the possibility of pregnancy-related disease (eg, preeclampsia, HELLP, gestational hypertension, gestational diabetes). Two additional major concerns that must continually be attended to during nonobstetric surgery are the maintenance of uterine perfusion and the prevention of premature labor. In order to understand the importance of these factors, a brief review of the physiologic changes of pregnancy is required.

PHYSIOLOGY OF PREGNANCY

Cardiovascular

Intravascular volume and cardiac output begin to increase during the first trimester and become 30% to 40% above the nonpregnant state by 28 weeks gestational age. Despite this increase in intravascular volume, the mother and fetus are at risk for hypotension which is caused by the gravid uterus compressing the aorta and/or inferior vena cava. This significantly reduces venous return and is called the supine hypotension syndrome. It occurs starting at 20 weeks gestation. The reduction in venous return may or may not be evident as maternal hypotension and puts the fetus at substantial risk of inadequate uteroplacental perfusion even in the asymptomatic mother. The most effective therapy is uterine displacement (ie, lateral position or displace the uterus to the left manually or with a wedge under the right hip). Correct positioning of the pregnant woman is critically important in maintaining adequate uterine blood flow.

Pregnant women are anemic despite a 35% increase in red blood cell mass. This happens because plasma volume, and therefore total blood volume, increases by 50% to 55%, producing a condition called physiologic anemia of pregnancy. Leukocytosis is also present in pregnant women, making the diagnosis of infection more difficult.

Respiratory

During pregnancy, the female experiences a 20% decrease in functional residual capacity concurrent with a 60% increase in oxygen consumption. This places the pregnant female and her infant at risk for hypoxia. Minute ventilation normally increases 50%, with most of this due to an increase in tidal volume. Closing volume (the lung volume at which airways collapse) moves from functional residual capacity into tidal volume ventilation in 30% of parturients, further increasing the risk of hypoxia. Mild hyperventilation reduces $PaCO_2$ by 10 mm Hg with a compensatory decrease in bicarbonate, maintaining a normal pH; therefore, mechanical ventilation with a $PaCO_2$ of 40 mm Hg will produce respiratory acidosis. Positive pressure ventilation can decrease uterine blood flow 25% by reducing venous return. Therefore adequacy of uterine perfusion needs to be evaluated in pregnant women who are mechanically ventilated by monitoring fetal heart tones (eg, looking for loss of beat-to-beat variability, decelerations, fetal bradycardia).

Capillary engorgement increases the possibility of bleeding with the use of oral and nasal airways. The probability of a difficult intubation increases 8-fold during pregnancy; therefore, a smaller size endotracheal tube (6 or 6.5) should be used. Nasal intubations and nasogastric tubes should be avoided if possible.

ANESTHESIA FOR OBSTETRIC PATIENTS IN NONOBSTETRIC SURGERY *(Continued)*

Gastrointestinal

Pregnant women are at risk for aspiration after the first trimester because of increased gastric volume. Gastric emptying is similar in pregnant and nonpregnant patients. It is delayed only during labor, largely because of administration of narcotics. Pregnant patients are at risk for aspiration because of elevation of the stomach and rotation on its axis to the right by the gravid uterus. This leads to incompetence of the lower esophageal sphincter. Up to 80% of pregnant patients experience heartburn.

Use of an oral nonparticulate antacid (ie, sodium citrate, 30 mL) is recommended immediately prior to induction of general anesthesia. Histamine-2 receptor blocker (ie, cimetidine 300 mg I.V., ranitidine 50 mg I.V.) should be given 60-90 minutes prior to induction of general anesthesia to decrease acid production. Metoclopramide (10 mg I.V.) is given to enhance gastric emptying. Intubation should be performed by rapid sequence with cricoid pressure to prevent regurgitation and aspiration.

Renal

Because pregnant females experience an increase in glomerular filtration rate (GFR), their blood urea nitrogen (BUN) and creatinine (Cr) levels are decreased. Therefore, a pregnant woman with high-normal values may have renal insufficiency.

Coagulation

Pregnant women are hypercoagulable with an increase in factors V, VII, VIII, IX, X, XII, and fibrinogen and a decrease in factor XI, XIII, and antithrombin III. Platelet turnover is also increased. They are at risk for deep vein thrombosis (DVT) and pulmonary embolism which accounts for 25% of maternal deaths in the United States annually.

Neurology

Pregnant women have an increased sensitivity to anesthetic agents and other sedative/hypnotic/analgesic drugs because of increased levels of endorphins. Minimum alveolar concentration (MAC) for inhalational anesthetics is decreased 40% and the dose of spinal/epidural drugs also needs to be decreased by a similar amount because of engorgement of epidural veins. It is also thought that the elevated level of circulating progesterone increases neuronal sensitivity (both central and peripheral) to anesthetic/analgesic drugs.

TERATOGENICITY

The incidence of both major and minor anatomic birth defects ranges as high as 7% to 10%. Drug exposure accounts for 2% to 3% and genetic abnormalities for 25% of birth defects, while the etiology for the rest remains unknown. The fetus is most vulnerable to teratogenic drug effects from day 15 to 90 of gestation, when organogenesis is occurring. Unfortunately, many women do not know that they are pregnant during this period.

Drugs are routinely tested in animal teratologic studies; however, there are many examples where extensive animal testing does not correlate with human results. For example, thalidomide was tested in both rats and mice and was not found to be teratogenic; however, the teratogenic effects in the human fetus are profound, especially since no signs of toxicity are present in the mother. Conversely, drugs that are teratogenic in certain animal models, such as steroid therapy, have not exhibited any significant effect on the human fetus. A general statement is that most drugs, at some dose, can be teratogenic in some animal model but few drugs have a proven, clinically significant, teratogenic potential. See FDA Pregnancy Categories *on page 21.*

Possible Teratogens

Alcohol: This teratogen produces fetal alcohol syndrome with an incidence of 2/1000 live births, which is probably an underestimate of the real number. There is a twofold increase in spontaneous abortion, which increases to 5% with heavy alcohol consumption. Gestational alcohol consumption is a leading cause of mental retardation, which exceeds that found with Down syndrome and cerebral palsy. Hyperactivity, speech, language, and hearing difficulties, microcephaly, and abnormal brain development are also common.

Anesthetics: Although there is great concern that anesthetic agents may injure the developing fetus, there is little solid evidence for this. Nitrous oxide inhibits methionine synthetase activity which is involved in thymidine production and subsequent DNA synthesis and cell division. However, recent human studies have shown no effect on fetal outcome. Despite these negative studies, it is still wise to postpone surgery or unnecessary drug therapy until after delivery if possible.

Anticonvulsants: The risk of birth defects increases to 7% in women taking antiepileptic drugs during pregnancy (vs 2% to 3% in controls). The incidence increases in mothers taking higher doses and/or multiple antiseizure drugs. The epoxide metabolites of these drugs appear to produce the fetal abnormalities. Discontinuation of antiseizure drugs may also be dangerous if the fetus is exposed to hypoxia due to maternal seizures.

Benzodiazepines: Retrospective studies from the 1970s showed an increased incidence of cleft lip and palate in infants of mothers who were using benzodiazepines during pregnancy. However, recent epidemiologic studies have been unable to demonstrate this association.

Caffeine: There is no convincing data that caffeine is teratogenic in humans.

Cocaine: Cocaine and heroin exposure of both the mother and the father is associated with fetal microcephaly and other neurologic abnormalities.

Hyperglycemia: Diabetic mothers have a 4% to 12% incidence of major congenital anomalies, which can be significantly reduced to 1.2% when blood glucose levels are tightly controlled during pregnancy.

Marijuana: The placenta acts as a barrier to fetal marijuana exposure. Several studies have demonstrated maternal blood levels of marijuana with nondetectable drug concentration in the cord blood. Cannabinoids are also nonteratogenic in animals.

Retinoids (tretinoin, isotretinoin, etretinate): These drugs are used to treat acne, gram-negative folliculitis, hidradenitis suppurativa, and psoriasis. Teratogenic effects include CNS, cardiac, thymus, craniofacial abnormalities, and spontaneous abortion. Birth control must be practiced when using this class of drugs.

Tobacco: Cigarette smoking during pregnancy is associated with growth retardation. Reports of anencephaly, congenital heart defects, and orofacial clefts have not been confirmed.

Warfarin: Because of its small molecular weight, warfarin easily crosses the placenta. Administration between the 6th and 9th weeks of pregnancy can produce the warfarin embryopathy syndrome which consists of nasal hypoplasia, stippling of uncalcified epiphysis, shortened fingers with nail hypoplasia, low birth weight, and mental retardation in 13% of exposed fetuses.

The two most important factors affecting fetal development are decreased uterine perfusion and hypoxia.

ANESTHESIA FOR OBSTETRIC PATIENTS IN NONOBSTETRIC SURGERY *(Continued)*

GESTATIONAL PHARMACOKINETICS AND PHARMACODYNAMICS

Drugs cross the placenta by simple diffusion. Lipid soluble drugs with low molecular weight (ie, fentanyl, thiopental, isoflurane) cross easily while highly polar water soluble drugs (ie, neuromuscular blocking agents) do not readily cross the placenta. Because fetal pH is lower than maternal pH, the ionized fraction of weak bases (ie, narcotics, local anesthetics) is higher in the fetus than in the mother. This is called "ion trapping." Ion trapping increases total fetal drug level, which will prolong clearance of the drug from the fetus. Ion trapping has been connected with lidocaine (a weak base) and fetal acidosis, leading to "floppy baby syndrome."

PRINCIPLES OF SURGICAL MANAGEMENT

1. **The most important thing is to notify your hospital obstetrician about the case before starting it.**
2. Postpone surgery until the second trimester or delay until after delivery, if possible.
3. Use a nonparticulate antacid preoperatively.
4. Maintain maternal oxygenation and blood pressure.
5. Document fetal heart tones before and after surgery.
6. Monitor for uterine contraction and fetal heart rate intraoperatively whenever possible.
7. Use left uterine displacement during the entire perioperative period.
8. Consider the use of prophylactic tocolytic agents (note that inhalational anesthetic gases are tocolytics)
9. Nonsteroidal anti-inflammatory drugs should not be used after 32 weeks gestational age because of the concern that the ductus may close.
10. Based on gestational age, the obstetrician may give betamethasone prior to surgery to promote fetal lung maturity in case of premature delivery.

The reason to monitor fetal heart tones and uterine contractions is to provide the physician with the opportunity to prevent fetal hypoxia and/or early delivery. Monitoring fetal heart rate will allow the physician to optimize the fetal environment by augmenting oxygen delivery if fetal bradycardia or loss of heart rate variability occurs. Because most anesthetic drugs depress fetal beat-to-beat variability, this monitor of fetal well-being cannot be relied upon until the drug is cleared from the fetus.

Taking care of the pregnant patient for nonobstetric surgery requires recognition of the physiologic changes that accompany pregnancy and the need to treat two patients – the mother and the baby.

Physiologic Changes of Pregnancy

Cardiovascular	Increased cardiac output 50% Increased red blood cell mass 35% Increased plasma volume 55% Physiologic anemia of pregnancy
Pulmonary	Decreased functional reserve capacity (FRC) 20% Increased oxygen consumption ($\dot{V}O_2$) 60% Increased minute ventilation (MV) 50% Increased respiratory rate (RR) 10% Increased tidal volume (V_T) 40% Decreased $PaCO_2$ by 10 mm Hg
Gastrointestinal	Increased gastric volume Decreased gastric pH Incompetent lower esophageal sphincter
Renal	Increased glomerular filtration rate (GFR) Decreased blood urea nitrogen (BUN) Decreased creatinine (Cr)
Coagulation	Increased factors V, VII, VIII, X, XII Increased fibrinogen Decreased factor XI, XIII, and antithrombin III Increased platelet turnover
Neurology	Decreased anesthesia/analgesia drug requirements (35% to 40%) Increased circulating endorphins

REFERENCES AND RECOMMENDED READING

Brodsky JB, Cohen EN, Brown BW Jr, et al, "Surgery During Pregnancy and Fetal Outcome," *Am J Obstet Gynecol*, 1980, 138(8):1165-7.

Chestnut DH, *Obstetric Anesthesia: Principles and Practice*, 2nd ed, Chapter 16, Cohen SE, "Nonobstetric Surgery During Pregnancy," Mosby: Philadelphia, 1999, 279-302.

Cohen EN, Bellville JW, and Brown BS, "Anesthesia, Pregnancy and Miscarriage: A Study of Operating Room Nurses and Anesthetists," *Anesthesiology*, 1971, 35(4):343-7.

Dewan DM and Hoad DD, *Practical Obstetric Anesthesia*, Chapter 20, "Anesthesia for Non-Birth Related Surgery During Pregnancy," WB Saunders Company, Philadelphia: Pennsylvania, 1997, 309-20.

Duncan PG, Pope WD, Cohen MM, et al, "Fetal Risk of Anesthesia and Surgery During Pregnancy," *Anesthesiology*, 1986, 64(6):790-4.

Kaneko M, Saito Y, Kirihara Y, et al, "Pregnancy Enhances the Antinociceptive Effects of Extradural Lignocaine in the Rat," *Br J Anaesth*, 1994, 72(6):657-61.

Liu PL, Warren TM, Ostheimer GW, et al, "Foetal Monitoring in Parturients Undergoing Surgery Unrelated to Pregnancy," *Can Anaesth Soc J*, 1985, 32(5):525-32.

Mazze RI and Kallen B, "Reproductive Outcome After Anesthesia and Operation During Pregnancy: A Register Study of 5405 Cases," *Am J Obstet Gynecol*, 1989, 161(5):1178-85.

Medina VM, Dawson-Basoa ME, and Gintzler AR, "17 Beta-Estradiol and Progesterone Positively Modulate Spinal Cord Dynorphin: Relevance to the Analgesia of Pregnancy," *Neuroendocrinology*, 1993, 58(3):310-5.

Niebyl JR, ed, *Drug Use in Pregnancy*, Philadelphia, PA; Lea & Febiger, 1988.

Palahniuk FJ, Schnider SM, and Eger EI, "Pregnancy Decreases the Requirement for Inhaled Anesthetic Agents," *Anesthesiology*, 1974, 41:82-3.

Pedersen H and Finster M, "Anesthetic Risk in the Pregnant Surgical Patient," *Anesthesiology*, 1979, 51(5):439-51.

Rosenberg L, Mitchell AA, Parsells JL, et al, "Lack of Relation of Oral Clefts to Diazepam Use During Pregnancy," *N Engl J Med*, 1983, 309(21):1282-5.

Schnider SM and Webster GM, "Maternal and Fetal Hazards of Surgery During Pregnancy," *Am J Obstet Gynecol*, 1965, 92:891.

Selye H, "Anesthetic Effect of Steroid Hormones," *Proc Soc Exp Biol Med*, 1941, 46:116-21.

ANESTHESIA FOR PATIENTS WITH LIVER DISEASE

Patients with liver disease pose a significant problem to the perioperative physician. Although the prevalence of clinically significant unsuspected liver disease is 1%, abnormal liver function tests may occur in 33% of screened patients.

The liver is the largest gland in the body, receiving 25% of the cardiac output. While the hepatic artery supplies 25% of the blood flow (and 45% to 50% of the hepatic oxygen supply), the portal vein provides 75% of the blood flow (but only 50% of the oxygen delivery). This unique blood flow circuitry puts the liver at risk for ischemia since half of its oxygen supply is provided by venous blood. Oxygen delivery to this essential organ can be decreased by either an increase in oxygen extraction (reducing portal vein oxygen concentration) or a decrease in arterial blood pressure resulting in a decrease in hepatic artery blood flow.

FUNCTIONS OF THE LIVER

- Glucose homeostasis
  - Glycogen storage
  - Gluconeogenesis
- Fat metabolism (beta oxidation)
- Protein synthesis
  - Albumin, gamma globulin, $alpha_1$-glycoprotein
  - Drug binding
  - Coagulation factors
  - Hydrolysis of ester linkage
- Drug and hormone metabolism
- Bilirubin formation and excretion
- Phagocytize bacteria

PATHOPHYSIOLOGY OF LIVER INJURY

To simplify this presentation, liver disease is divided into two categories: 1) cholestatic disease and 2) parenchymal disease, including acute and chronic hepatitis and cirrhosis.

1. With cholestasis (obstructive jaundice), the liver is unable to secrete bile because of either hepatocellular dysfunction or extrahepatic obstruction. Bilirubin accumulation affects cellular respiration; heme biosynthesis; metabolism of lipids, amino acids, and proteins; and alteration of drug/albumin binding. Coagulation defects occur because of deficient production of vitamin K-dependent factors by the dysfunctional hepatocytes.

   Drugs/conditions that cause cholestasis:

   - Primary biliary cirrhosis
   - Estrogens
   - Methyltestosterone
   - Bile duct gallstones
   - Bile duct stricture
   - Pancreatic cancer obstructing bile duct

2. Hepatic parenchymal disease (ie, hepatitis, cirrhosis) is associated with a hyperdynamic cardiovascular state. Cardiac output increases due to arteriovenous fistulae which decrease systemic vascular resistance and lead to an increased intravascular volume. Blood pressure and heart rate remain normal but portal vein blood flow to the liver is decreased. Hypoxemia occurs because of intrapulmonary shunting (hepatopulmonary syndrome) and ascites can limit diaphragm excursion. The oxygen dissociation curve is shifted to the right and hypoxic pulmonary vasoconstriction is blunted. The patient is anemic due to increased plasma volume, GI bleeding, hemolysis, and malnutrition. Thrombocytopenia occurs from bone marrow depression and hypersplenism. The depressed synthetic function of the liver is manifested by decreased albumin production and prolonged PT and PTT due to

decreased production of factors II, VII, IX, and X. The encephalopathy that appears with acute liver failure is probably due to cerebral edema, while chronic encephalopathy may be caused by decreased elimination of nitrogenous compounds (ie, ammonia). GI bleeding, infection, and excessive use of diuretics increases blood urea nitrogen (BUN). Ascites and peripheral edema are produced by hypoabluminemia and renal reabsorption of urinary sodium. As hepatic dysfunction progresses, hepatorenal syndrome may develop in patients with portal hypertension and ascites. This renal failure is produced by multiple reasons and can be cured by liver transplant.

SOME CAUSES OF HEPATIC INJURY

Viral	Infection
Drugs	NSAIDs
	ACE inhibitors
	Sulfonamides
Other	Reye's syndrome
	Wilson's disease
	Acute fatty liver of pregnancy
	Hemochromatosis
	Cystic fibrosis
	Alpha$_1$-antitrypsin deficiency
	Total parenteral nutrition

LIVER FUNCTION TESTS AND DIFFERENTIAL DIAGNOSIS

Diagnostic Factors	Cholestatic Intrahepatic	Cholestatic Extrahepatic	Parenchymal Hepatocellular
Symptom	Deep jaundice, dark urine, light stools, pruritus	Deep jaundice, dark urine, light stools, pruritus, biliary cholic, cholangitis	Nausea, vomit, fever, anorexia
Physical findings	Tender hepatomegaly	Hepatomegaly, palpable gallbladder	Tender hepatomegaly, ± splenomegaly
Bilirubin, total	>30 mg/dL	<30 mg/dL	↑ conjugated
Transaminases	2-5 fold ↑	>2-3 fold ↑	>5 fold ↑
Alkaline phosphatase	>3-5 fold ↑	<3-5 fold ↑	2-3 fold ↑
Prothrombin time	Prolonged	Prolonged	Prolonged
PT correct with vitamin K	Variable	Yes	No
Causes	Stones, sepsis	Hemolysis, hematoma reabsorption, bili overload from whole blood transfusion	Viral, drugs, sepsis, hypoxemia, cirrhosis

THE EFFECTS OF ANESTHESIA AND SURGERY ON LIVER FUNCTION

Liver injury can occur during surgery either from decreased hepatic oxygen delivery or direct drug toxicity. The most injurious conditions in the perioperative period are hypotension, hypoxemia, and hypovolemia, all which decrease hepatic oxygen delivery. Surgical stress carries a high mortality in patients with severe liver disease, with the greatest insult to the liver occurring with upper abdominal surgery.

Management of the patient with hepatic parenchymal injury requires maintenance of arterial blood pressure and cardiac output to assure adequate hepatic oxygen delivery. When blood flow decreases, the body extracts more oxygen to maintain

ANESTHESIA FOR PATIENTS WITH LIVER DISEASE *(Continued)*

adequate tissue oxygenation. In the normal person, when portal blood flow decreases, hepatic arterial blood flow increases, thereby ensuring adequate oxygen delivery. In the patient with severe hepatic dysfunction, this vascular autoregulation does not occur, leading to reduced hepatic oxygenation.

CLASSIFICATION OF SURGICAL RISK

	Minimal	Mild	Severe
Bilirubin (mg/dL)	<2	2-3	>3
Albumin (g/dL)	>3.5	3-3.5	<3
Prothrombin time (sec prolonged)	1-4	4-6	>6
Encephalopathy	None	Moderate	Severe
Nutrition	Excellent	Good	Poor
Ascites	None	Moderate	Marked

Anesthetic concerns with regional anesthesia include coagulopathy and hypotension. "Halothane hepatitis" is a concern with repeat halothane exposure, with several case reports implicating other inhalational anesthetics. Halothane hepatitis is an immune-mediated response which requires previous exposure and antibody formation against an oxidative trifluoroacetyl halide metabolite of halothane. Genetic susceptibility is probable and it can be fatal.

PHARMACOKINETICS

There are significant changes in the pharmacokinetic profiles of many drugs in the patient with liver disease because the liver is important in metabolism and elimination of drugs. Multiple hepatic enzymes are responsible for drug metabolism, with the cytochrome P450 family of enzymes important in mixed function oxidative reactions.

Albumin is produced solely by the liver, therefore, a decrease in albumin concentration can indicate significant liver disease or malnutrition. Prothrombin time is considered a more sensitive indicator of liver disease than albumin because severe liver disease can affect hepatic synthetic function sufficiently to prolong prothrombin time within 24 hours.

Hepatic drug metabolism and elimination can be classified based on alterations in hepatic blood flow, volume of distribution, and protein binding.

Hepatic blood flow patterns change with hepatic injury. As the liver architecture changes with the development of cirrhosis, portal venous blood is shunted from the liver by collateral channels into the systemic circulation. This blood, along with orally administered drugs absorbed from the GI tract, avoids the hepatic first-pass effect preventing the initial drug metabolism and increasing the amount of drug presented to the central circulation. Blood that passes through the liver has decreased exposure to hepatocyte enzymes because of increased fibrosis and a decrease in number and size of loose endothelial junctions, which limits blood exposure to hepatocytes for drug metabolism. If clearance is high, then changes in hepatic blood flow will significantly alter drug elimination (flow limited drugs). Conversely, clearance is not affected by a decrease in hepatic blood flow for enzyme-limited drugs. The clearance of enzyme-limited drugs may either be protein-binding sensitive (>85% bound) or protein-binding insensitive (<50% bound).

Volume of distribution (V_d) is altered by the development of ascites (which increases the body's total fluid component) and altered hepatic production of plasma proteins. As the volume of distribution increases, drug concentration at steady state decreases. For example, V_d of propranolol and verapamil is doubled in patients with ascites. This condition may lead to an increase in drug half-life and a decrease in drug clearance.

Protein binding is altered with cirrhosis because of a decrease in serum albumin and an accumulation of substances that displace drugs from albumin-binding sites. In this circumstance, the availability of unbound drug increases, leading to greater drug effect. For example, phenytoin is 90% albumin bound. With hypoalbuminemia, the free fraction increases 20% to 30%, which can double or triple unbound active phenytoin, producing drug toxicity; however, this effect may be countered if there is an increase in volume of distribution (V_d) due to ascites. An increase in free unbound drug may also increase clearance, because more drug is available to be metabolized, which can shorten its half-life. The effect of altered protein binding on drug pharmacokinetics is difficult to predict. A simple rule of thumb is that a change in protein binding has a greater effect on drugs that are normally highly protein bound (>60%) compared to poorly bound drugs.

ANESTHESIA FOR PATIENTS WITH LIVER DISEASE
(Continued)

Drug Characteristics in Normal Subjects and Liver Failure Patients

Drug	Protein Binding (%)	Volume of Distribution (V_d) (L/kg)	Half-life (h)	Clearance (Cl) (mL/min)	Effect of Liver Disease on Drug Disposition	Adjustment of Dose
Antibiotics / Antiviral / Antifungal						
Ampicillin	30	0.28	1.0	340	Half-life ↑; V_d ↑; Cl →	None
Cefazolin	84	0.15	1.8	68	Half-life ↓; f_p ↑	None
Cefotetan	83	0.15	3.7	39.5	Negligible unless renal function decreased	None
Cefoxitin	73	0.12	1.0	98	Negligible unless renal function decreased	None
Clindamycin	79	0.58	2.0	160	Half-life slight ↑; V_d →; Cl ↓ 23%; f_p →	Decrease dose in severe cases
Erythromycin	80	0.77	1.6	600	Half-life ↑	Decrease dose in moderate or severe disease
Gentamicin	<5	0.25	2.0	100	Negligible unless renal function decreased	None
Nafcillin	90	0.4	1.0	580	Half-life ↑ but little change; V_d ↓; Cl ↓ 50% to 60%; f_p ?→	Decrease dose in moderate or severe disease
Vancomycin	55	0.4	5.0	80	Half-life ↑; V_d →; Cl ↓	Decrease dose
Analgesic						
Alfentanil	90	0.28	1.5	200	Half-life ↑; V_d →; Cl ↓; f_p ↑ (dose-dependent)	Decrease dose
Fentanyl	80	3.5	4.0	750	Half-life →; V_d →; Cl →	None
Meperidine	65	4.5	4.5	900	Half-life ↑; V_d →; Cl ↓ 50%; f_p →	Decrease oral dose by 50% in cirrhosis or acute viral hepatitis
Methadone	80	4.0	28	150	Half-life ↑ with severe liver disease; Cl →	None or decrease
Morphine	35	3.7	2.0	1200	Half-life →; V_d →; Cl →; f_p →, by some reports f_p ↑	None, but avoid in severe liver disease

Drug Characteristics in Normal Subjects and Liver Failure Patients *(continued)*

Drug	Protein Binding (%)	Volume of Distribution (V_d) (L/kg)	Half-life (h)	Clearance (Cl) (mL/min)	Effect of Liver Disease on Drug Disposition	Adjustment of Dose
Antiepileptic						
Phenytoin	92	0.65	15.0 nonlinear	40	AVH half-life →; Cl →; f_p ↑. Cirrhosis f_p ↑	Decrease dose in moderate to severe liver disease
Phenobarbital	50	0.8	100	8	Half-life ↑; presumed Cl ↓	Decrease with severe liver disease
Antipyretic / Anti-inflammatory						
Dexamethasone	68	0.75	3.25	260	f_p →; V_d →; half-life ↑; Cl ↓	Decrease dose
Ibuprofen	>99	0.15 V area F	2.0	52	Half-life slightly ↑ in severe LD; V_d ?; Cl ?	Decrease in severe liver disease if high doses
Cardiovascular						
Atenolol	<5	0.55	6.5	55-130	Half-life →; V_d →; Cl →	None
Digoxin	30	6.0	35	150	Appears negligible	None
Esmolol	55	1.2	0.15	310/kg	Negligible	None
Labetalol	50	11.5	3.0	1600	Half-life →; V_d ↓; Cl → or ↓; f_p ?, assume ↑	Decrease oral dose; decrease I.V. dose to much smaller extent
Lidocaine	65 nonlinear	1.1	2.0	1000	Half-life ↑; V_d ↑ or →; Cl ↓ ~50%; f_p ? Low therapeutic ratio; decrease in Cl depends on severity of disease	Decrease dose by 50% in severe liver disease
Metoprolol	10	3.2	4.0	800	Half-life ↑; V_d ↑ slightly; Cl ↓ 23%; f_p ?	Decrease dose slightly
Propranolol	95	4.0	4.0	850	Half-life ↑; V_d ↑; Cl ↓ ~60%; f_p ↑. Tremendous decrease in Cl_{int}. Flow/enzyme-limited in cirrhosis	Decrease dose depending on extent of damage
Verapamil	92	6.7	3.5	1570	Half-life ↑; V_d ↑; Cl ↓ 60%; f_p →. Cl_{int} decreases even more than 60%.	Decrease dose by 50% in severe liver disease

ANESTHESIA FOR PATIENTS WITH LIVER DISEASE *(Continued)*

Drug Characteristics in Normal Subjects and Liver Failure Patients *(continued)*

Drug	Protein Binding (%)	Volume of Distribution (V_d) (L/kg)	Half-life (h)	Clearance (Cl) (mL/min)	Effect of Liver Disease on Drug Disposition	Adjustment of Dose
Diuretic						
Furosemide	95	0.15	1.0	170	Half-life ↑ or →; V_d ↑ or →; Cl →; f_p ↑; the change in f_p compensates for decrease in Cl_{int} of liver	None or slight decrease in severe cases
Sedative / Hypnotic						
Diazepam	99	1.2	45	.28	Half-life ↑; V_d ↑; Cl ↓ 50%; f_p ↑. AVH and cirrhosis increase half-life. Large therapeutic index — safe	Single dose, no change; chronic, decrease dose
Flumazenil	40	0.85	0.8	1201	Half-life, Cl, V_d	? Decrease dose
Lorazepam	90	1.3	12.0	53	Half-life ↑; V_d ↑; Cl→; f_p ↑. Neither AVH nor cirrhosis affects drug dosing	None
Methohexital	—	61	2.0	829	No data; assume Cl ↓, half-life↑	Probably decrease dose
Thiopental	85	2.3	9.0	275	Half-life →; V_d →; Cl →; f_p ↑	Uncertain; may need to decrease dose
Midazolam	—	1.3	1.6	624	Half-life ↑; V_d slightly ↑; Cl ↓	Decrease dose

Drug Characteristics in Normal Subjects and Liver Failure Patients *(continued)*

Drug	Protein Binding (%)	Volume of Distribution (V_d) (L/kg)	Half-life (h)	Clearance (Cl) (mL/min)	Effect of Liver Disease on Drug Disposition	Adjustment of Dose
Others						
Atracurium	—	0.16	0.33	385	Half-life →; V_d ↑; Cl →; long half-life of metabolite	Decrease dose if long-term use
Cimetidine	20	1.1	2.3	550	Half-life →; V_d ↑ or ↓ or →; Cl → or ↓; f_p changes assumed unimportant. Drug associated with increased incidence of mental confusion in cirrhotics.	Decrease dose to severe liver disease
Ranitidine	15	1.5	2.3	600	Half-life →; V_d →; Cl →	None
Theophylline	52	0.5	8.0	45	Half-life ↑; V_d → cirrhosis, ↑ hepatitis and cholestasis; Cl ↓ 55%; f_p ↑. Low therapeutic index caution.	Decrease dose by 50%

AVH = acute viral hepatitis; LD = liver disease; fp = fraction of unbound drug; Cl_{int} = intrinsic clearance.

ANESTHESIA FOR PATIENTS WITH LIVER DISEASE *(Continued)*

REFERENCES AND RECOMMENDED READING

Barash PG, Cullen BF, and Stoelting RK, "Anesthesia and the Liver," *Handbook of Clinical Anesthesia*, Philadelphia, PA: JB Lippincott, 1991, 314-24.

Jalan R and Hayes PC, "Hepatic Encephalopathy and Ascites," *Lancet*, 1997, 350(9087):1309-15.

Gelman S, Dillard E, and Bradley EL Jr, "Hepatic Circulation During Surgical Stress and Anesthesia With Halothane, Isoflurane, or Fentanyl," *Anesth Anal*, 1987, 66(10):936-43.

Gelman S and Ernst E, "Role of pH, PCO_2, and O_2 Content of Portal Blood in Hepatic Autoregulation," *Am J Physiol*, 1977, 233(4):E255.

Gelman S, "General Anesthesia and Hepatic Circulation," *Can J Physiol Pharmacol*, 1987, 65(8):1762-79.

Kamath PS, "Clinical Approach to the Patient With Abnormal Liver Test Results," *Mayo Clin Proc*, 1996, 71(11):1089-94.

Krowka MJ, Porayko MK, Plevak DJ, et al, "Hepatopulmonary Syndrome With Progressive Hypoxemia as an Indication for Liver Transplantation: Case Reports and Literature Review," *Mayo Clin Proc*, 1997, 72(1):44-53.

Kubisty CA, Arns RA, Wedlund PJ, et al, "Adjustment of Medication in Liver Failure," *The Pharmacologic Approach to the Critically Ill Patient*, Chernow B, ed, 3rd ed, Baltimore, MD: Williams & Wilkins, 1994, 95-113.

Merritt WT and Gelman S, "Anesthesia for Liver Surgery," *Principles and Practice of Anesthesiology*, Rogers MC, Tinker JH, and Covino BG, eds, Longnecker, DE: Mosby, 1992, 1991-2034.

Neal E, Meffin P, Gregory P, et al, "Enhanced Bioavailability and Decreased Clearance of Analgesics in Patients With Cirrhosis," *Gastroenterology*, 1979, 77(1):96-102.

Powell-Jackson P, Greenway B, and Williams R, "Adverse Effects of Exploratory Laparotomy in Patients With Suspected Liver Disease," *Br J Surg*, 1982, 69(8):449-51.

CONSCIOUS SEDATION

The goal of conscious sedation is to produce a state where: 1) patients are able to tolerate unpleasant procedures; 2) adequate cardiorespiratory function is maintained; and 3) patients are able to respond purposefully to verbal commands and/or tactile stimulation. It is important to remember that sedation occurs over a continuum that can unintentionally progress to deep sedation or even general anesthesia. The American Society of Anesthesiologists (ASA) Task Force on Sedation and Analgesia by Non-Anesthesiologists has recommended that the term "conscious sedation" be replaced with "sedation and analgesia" as this more accurately describes the therapeutic goal desired. When administered appropriately, the ASA Practice Guidelines for Sedation and Analgesia by Non-Anesthesiologists state that sedation/analgesia should "provide benefits of sedation/analgesia while minimizing the associated risks. In children and uncooperative adults, sedation/analgesia may expedite the conduct of procedures that are not particularly uncomfortable but require that the patient not move." Similar to that used by the ASA Task Force, the Joint Commission on Accreditation of Healthcare Organizations' standards and intents for sedation and anesthesia care uses the terminology "moderate sedation/analgesia" instead of conscious sedation. The JCAHO definition of "moderate sedation/analgesia" states that the patient should be able to respond purposefully to verbal commands, either alone or accompanied by light tactile stimulation. It further states that no interventions are required to maintain a patent airway, that spontaneous ventilation is adequate, and that cardiovascular function is usually maintained.

Nonanesthesiologist clinicians who wish to order/administer medications for sedation/analgesia must be trained, demonstrate competency, and receive medical staff privileges to do so.

PATIENT EVALUATION

A presedation assessment, including a relevant patient history and pertinent physical exam, should be performed. The presedation assessment should include:

- Chief complaint/present illness
- Relevant medical/surgical history
- Relevant family history
- Medication history
- Pregnancy status, if appropriate
- Baseline mental status
- Airway assessment
- ASA classification
- Allergies
- Patient's weight and vital signs (HR and rhythm, blood pressure, respiratory rate, temperature, oxygen saturation)
- Previous adverse effects with sedation/analgesia, regional anesthesia, and general anesthesia
- Time/nature of last oral intake (eg, clear liquids >2-3 hours, solids >6-8 hours)
- History of alcohol, tobacco, illicit drug use
- Review of systems (eg, any abnormalities of major organ function)
- Cardiopulmonary examination

A thorough medication history is important to prevent potential drug interactions. For example, meperidine is contraindicated in a patient taking a monoamine oxidase inhibitor (MAOI). It is recommended that the MAOI be discontinued 2 weeks prior to the anticipated administration of meperidine. Opioids and CNS depressants can increase the potential for apnea and oversedation when administered with a benzodiazepine. Other drugs also have the potential to interact with medications used for sedation and analgesia. It is important to check for potential interactions before proceeding with sedation and analgesia. For example, the clearance of diazepam, but not midazolam, is decreased and its half-life increased with cimetidine. Indinavir and saquinavir may inhibit the metabolism of midazolam

CONSCIOUS SEDATION *(Continued)*

and increase the potential for prolonged sedation. Ritonavir can greatly increase the plasma concentrations of midazolam and diazepam; these agents should not be used in patients taking ritonavir.

SEDATION AND ANALGESIA PLAN

A sedation and analgesia plan must be developed and communicated to the patient, family, and other healthcare providers involved with the procedure as well as be documented in the patient's medical record. The plan should be re-evaluated immediately prior to beginning sedation and analgesia.

PATIENT COUNSELING

Patients should be informed of the risks, benefits, and limitations of sedation/analgesia and of potential alternatives. An informed consent form needs to be signed by the patient (or guardian) before proceeding with sedation and analgesia.

MONITORING

The following data should be recorded starting before the procedure and continued during the procedure and recovery period:

- Drugs administered (drug, route, site, time, dose)
- Oxygen saturation (via pulse oximetry)
- Type and amount of I.V. fluid
- Level of consciousness
- Pulmonary ventilation (through observation of spontaneous respiratory activity or auscultation of breath sounds)
- Blood pressure, temperature (pre- and postprocedure), heart rate, and respiratory rate
- ECG for patients with significant cardiovascular disease, ASA class III or IV patients
- Unexpected events
- Status of patient upon completion of the procedure and the start of the recovery period

Minimally, the patient's hemodynamic variables, ventilatory status, and oxygenation status should be documented before the beginning of the procedure, after administration of sedative/analgesic agents, at completion of the procedure, during initial recovery, and at discharge. However, these variables are normally recorded at regular intervals (eg, every 5 minutes) during the procedure. The frequency of vital signs monitoring may need to be individualized on a case-to-case basis. Patients who are chronically or acutely ill or debilitated, or those who deteriorate during the diagnostic or therapeutic procedure may require more frequent measurements of vital signs. The conduct of the procedure may practically preclude monitoring/recording of a given vital sign at a routine interval.

Signs and symptoms of toxicity associated with sedation/analgesia include deep sedation, somnolence, confusion, respiratory depression, apnea, respiratory arrest, hypotension, cardiac arrest, nausea and vomiting, diminished reflexes, impaired coordination, and severe changes in vital signs.

It is critical that an appropriately trained individual other than the person performing the procedure be present to continuously monitor the patient throughout the procedure and recovery.

EQUIPMENT REQUIREMENTS

The following equipment and supplies should be present or readily available (within or adjacent to the procedure room).

- Oxygen source and administration equipment of various types and sizes; supplemental oxygen should be administered when clinically indicated (eg, hypoxemia)
- Suction
- Emergency airway equipment (variety of laryngoscope blades and handles, oral and nasal airways, and various sizes of endotracheal tubes with stylets)
- Means of positive-pressure ventilation (eg, ambu or other resuscitation bag)
- Emergency resuscitation drugs (eg, drugs recommended in the current ACLS guidelines)
- Pharmacologic antagonists (eg, naloxone for opioids, flumazenil for benzodiazepines)
- Intravenous equipment; for patients receiving drugs intravenously, I.V. access should be maintained throughout the whole procedure and until the patient is not at risk for serious adverse events from the drugs administered (eg, cardiorespiratory depression).
- Pulse oximeter
- Noninvasive blood pressure equipment
- ECG
- Telephone

AGENT SELECTION / DOSE TITRATION

Sedatives (eg, midazolam, diazepam, chloral hydrate, droperidol) are routinely used to decrease anxiety and promote somnolence. Analgesics (eg, morphine, meperidine, fentanyl) are routinely used to relieve pain. Combinations of opioids and sedatives may increase the incidence of adverse effects. When used together, each agent should be administered individually in order to allow the desired effect of each agent to be achieved. Propofol should be used with caution for sedation/analgesia. Because of its short half-life, it should be administered by continuous I.V. infusion. Propofol can be used in combination with benzodiazepines and opioids for a synergistic effect.

When given intravenously, sedative/analgesic drugs should be administered in small, incremental doses until the desired effect is achieved (titrate to effect). Please refer to the individual drug monographs for appropriate dosing guidelines. Care must be taken to allow a sufficient time between doses to allow the effect of each dose to be seen. Dosage reductions may be required in the chronically ill or elderly as well as with the concomitant administration of an opioid and sedative agent (eg, benzodiazepine). Additional time should be allowed between doses when drugs are administered by nonintravenous routes (eg, oral, rectal, I.M.) secondary to the time required for drug absorption.

RECOVERY

Patients may continue to be at risk for complications after the procedure and must be monitored (level of consciousness, vital signs, respiratory function) throughout the recovery period until meeting discharge criteria. If a reversal agent has been administered, an appropriate time (up to 2 hours) should have elapsed to ensure that resedation does not occur secondary to the reversal agent's short duration of action when compared to the sedation/analgesia agents used. Patients must be discharged with an accompanying responsible adult. The patient and accompanying adult should be advised (both verbally and in writing) regarding any limitations on the patient's activity (eg, do not operate machinery or drive an automobile for 24 hours), diet, and medication use. In addition, the patient should be given a 24-hour emergency contact telephone number in case problems arise.

CONSCIOUS SEDATION *(Continued)*

QUALITY ASSURANCE

Any unusual occurrences or adverse drug reactions should be reported via the quality assurance program in place for sedation/analgesia. These could include:

- Assisted ventilation required, respiratory rate <8 or periods of apnea at any time during the procedure
- Oxygen saturation decrease ≥10% from preprocedure for ≥5 minutes
- Arrhythmia or hemodynamic instability
- Use of reversal agent
- Procedure stopped or interrupted due to excessive sedation or adverse drug reaction
- Delayed recovery from sedation
- Unanticipated hospital admission or transfer to a higher level of care
- Other clinically significant changes from preprocedure baseline not noted above

REFERENCES AND RECOMMENDED READING

Holland CA, "Conscious Sedation Policy Development and Review," *AANA J*, 1995, 63(3):196-7.

Holzman RS, Cullen DJ, Eichhorn JH, et al, "Guidelines for Sedation by Nonanesthesiologists During Diagnostic and Therapeutic Procedures. The Risk Management Committee of the Department of Anesthesia of Harvard Medical School," *J Clin Anesth*, 1994, 6(4):265-76.

Kaplan RF, "Sedation and Analgesia in Pediatric Patients for Procedures Outside the Operating Room," Paper presented at the ASA 1996 Annual Refresher Course Lectures, New Orleans, LA, October 23, 1996.

Krikorian SA, "Intravenous Conscious Sedation," *US Pharmacist*, 1997, HS26-36.

Malviya S and Voepel-Lewis T, "Sedation of Children Outside the Operating Room," *Progress in Anesthesiology*, 1995, 9:399-411.

"Practice Guidelines for Sedation and Analgesia by Non-Anesthesiologists. A Report by the American Society of Anesthesiologists Task Force on Sedation and Analgesia by Nonanesthesiologists," *Anesthesiology*, 1996, 84(2):459-71.

Revisions to Anesthesia Care Standards, *Comprehensive Accreditation Manual for Hospitals*: Standards and Intents for Sedation and Anesthesia Care, January 1, 2001. Available at: http://www.jcrinc.com/generic.asp?durki=405.

Most Commonly Used Agents for Moderate Sedation in Adults

Medication	Onset of Action	Duration of Action	Adult Dose	Reversal Agent	Comments
Diazepam	P.O.15-30 min I.V.: 3-10 min I.M.: 30-40 min	P.O./I.V.: 6-8 h I.M.: 6-12 h	P.O.: >10 mg I.V.: 2-5 mg (2-5 min) Repeat dosage q10min prn; Max: 0.1-0.2 mg/kg (10 mg)	Flumazenil	
Fentanyl	I.V.: 1-2 min	I.V.: 30-60 min	I.V.: 25-50 mcg (2 min) Repeat dosage q3-5min prn; Max: 500 mcg/4 h	Naloxone	Rapid bolus may cause chest wall rigidity
Flumazenil	I.V.: 1-2 min	I.V.: 1-2 h	I.V.: 0.2 mg (15 sec) Repeat dosage q1min prn; Max: 1 mg		Reversal agent for BZD
Lorazepam	I.V.: 5-10 min I.M.: 30-60 min	I.V.: 4-6 h I.M.: 6-12 h	Slow I.V.: 0.5-2 mg (2 min) Repeat dosage q20min prn; Max: 4 mg	Flumazenil	Hypotension and bradycardia with fast infusion
Meperidine	I.V.: 2-5 min I.M.: 10-15 min	I.V.: 2-3 h I.M.: 3-4 h	I.V.: 25-50 mg (2 min) Repeat dosage q5-10min prn; Max: (1-2 mg/kg) 150 mg	Naloxone	
Methohexital	Immediate	I.V.: 10-20 min	50-120 mg (1% sol 1 mL/5 sec) Repeat 20-40 mg q4-7min prn	None	Use with caution if CV instability, severe liver disease, or asthma
Midazolam	I.V.: 1-5 min I.M.: 5-15 min	I.V.: 30-120 min I.M.: 1-6 h	**<60 y:** Slow I.V.: 1-2.5 mg (2-5 min) Repeat dosage q2min prn; Max: 0.1 mg/kg (10 mg)/h **>60 y or debilitated:** I.V.: 0.5 mg (2-5 min) Repeat dosage q3min prn; Max: 0.05 mg/kg (5 mg)/h	Flumazenil	Hypotension and bradycardia with fast infusion
Morphine	I.V.: 5-10 min I.M.: 15-30 min	I.V.: 2-4 h I.M.: 3-7 h	I.V.: 1-2 mg (5 min) Repeat dosage q3-5min prn; Max: 20 mg	Naloxone	Hypotension due to histamine release
Naloxone	I.V.: 1-2 min	I.V.: 30-60 min	I.V.: 0.4-2 mg (30 sec) Repeat dosage q2-3min prn; Max: 10 mg		Reversal agent for narcotics
Propofol	Immediate	I.V.: 3-10 min	5-10 mcg/kg/min infusion Titrate q5min prn; Max: 50 mcg/kg/min	None	Do not bolus (severe hypotension)

LATEX ALLERGY

The incidence of latex allergy is increasing. This increase has been suggested to be due in part to the implementation of universal precautions by the CDC in 1987 secondary to the AIDS epidemic. **Because of the increased incidence of latex allergy, all patients should be asked about allergic responses to latex products.** For example, patients should be questioned about the presence of swelling or itching of the hands or other areas after contact with rubber gloves, condoms, diaphragms, toys, or other rubber products and about itching or swelling of the lips or mouth after dental exams, blowing up balloons, or after eating bananas, chestnuts, and avocados.

It is important today for healthcare institutions to have a comprehensive plan (including a perioperative component) in place for dealing with the latex allergic patient.

HYPERSENSITIVITY REACTIONS CAUSED BY LATEX

Latex-containing products can produce type I and type IV hypersensitivity reactions.

The type I hypersensitivity reaction is the true "allergic" reaction seen with latex products. Proteins found in the latex promote the production of an antibody of the IgE class which attaches to basophils and mast cells. When the antigen (protein) is encountered again, histamine and other physiologically active mediators are released from mast cells and basophils. The clinical manifestations can include single or multiple system involvement, be mild or severe, range from itching to edema, and from mild hypotension to shock. It has been estimated that 10% of the true anaphylactic reactions during anesthesia are due to latex allergy. These reactions are usually seen 5-30 minutes after induction of anesthesia and start of surgery.

In the type IV reaction, a contact dermatitis is seen. The preservatives, stabilizers, accelerators, and antioxidants used in the latex manufacturing process serve as the antigens for T-cell lymphocytes. The dermatitis produced can be uncomfortable but is not life-threatening.

ROUTES OF EXPOSURE TO LATEX PROTEINS

It is important to consider the route of exposure of the latex protein in allergic patients as this can be a determinant of the type of reaction produced. The following table summarizes major routes of exposure.

Type of Exposure	Reaction
Direct skin contact	Localized or generalized urticaria
Mucous membrane	Rhinitis, conjunctivitis, stomatitis, angioedema; severe anaphylactic reactions and death reported
Inhalation of airborne starch-protein particles	Wheezing, bronchospasm, reduced lung compliance, episodes of desaturation and/or severe hypoxemia
Intravascular absorption of water soluble latex particles from surgical gloves	Sudden tachycardia, severe hypotension, cardiorespiratory collapse

HIGH-RISK PATIENTS

Several groups have been identified as "high-risk" for allergic reactions to latex. Special consideration should be given these individuals.

Healthcare providers. Latex allergy has been reported to be 7.5% for physicians, 5.6% for nurses, and 13.7% for dental personnel. The overall incidence for hospital employees is 1.3% (versus 0.08% for the general population).

Spina bifida patients / patients with congenital urologic abnormalities. An 18% to 40% incidence of latex allergy has been reported for spina bifida patients. These patients are routinely exposed to latex-containing urinary catheters.

Workers in rubber industry. A 10% incidence of latex allergy has been reported.

Patients with a history of atopy. In patients with latex allergy, there is a 35% to 83% incidence of atopy. Patients report allergies to rubber gloves, balloons, and various fruits and foods. Cross-reactivity has been reported with bananas, avocados, kiwis, celery, and chestnuts.

TREATMENT OF ANAPHYLACTIC REACTION

Management of an anaphylactic reaction which is thought to be due to latex allergy is similar to that described earlier. In addition, all latex products should be removed from the surgical field, surgeons must switch to nonlatex gloves, and latex-free tubing should be used for I.V. administration. Further, tests to determine if latex allergy was the cause of the reaction should be performed (eg, RAST, AlaSTAT).

PERIOPERATIVE MANAGEMENT OF A LATEX ALLERGIC PATIENT

No evidence exists to demonstrate that prophylaxis before surgery prevents latex-induced anaphylactic reactions. In spite of this, prophylaxis has been used in patients with a positive history of allergy; one suggested regimen uses diphenhydramine P.O. or I.V. every 6 hours at 13, 7, and 1 hour before surgery, prednisone P.O. every 6 hours at 13, 7, and 1 hour before surgery (hydrocortisone I.V. may be substituted), and ranitidine P.O. or I.V. every 12 hours at 13 and 1 hour before surgery. This regimen is continued for 12 hours after surgery.

The key to perioperative management of the latex allergic patient is to provide a latex-free environment. To accomplish this, the following actions should be taken:

1. Substitute all items with nonlatex alternatives when possible; if there is a question concerning the latex content of a product, the manufacturer should be called.
2. Gloves made of neoprene or other polymers should be used.
3. Latex-based adhesives should be eliminated.
4. Stopcocks should be used for drug administration instead of injection ports on I.V. tubing.
5. Syringes not containing rubber tips on the plunger should be used.
6. Drug products in glass ampuls should be used whenever possible; if a vial must be used, utilize a vial stopper remover so the stopper does not have to be punctured.
7. To reduce exposure to aerosolized glove powder which is a known carrier of latex proteins, schedule the surgery as the first case of the day; some institutions have reserved an O.R. suite for latex allergic patients.

LATEX ALLERGY *(Continued)*

TESTING FOR LATEX ALLERGY

Testing for latex allergy is recommended for high-risk patients. Both *in vitro* and *in vivo* tests are available as seen in the following table.

Test	Type	Description
Skin prick	*in vivo*	Sensitive method to confirm IgE-mediated latex hypersensitivity; correlates well with clinical presence of allergy; high sensitivity (100%), high specificity (99%)
Patch	*in vivo*	Test for type IV hypersensitivity reaction; test performed with 1 inch square of rubber glove; skin observed for contact dermatitis after 48 hours
Radioallergosorbent (RAST)	*in vitro*	Performed on the serum of patients with natural latex as the antigen; used to detect and quantify allergen specific IgE in patient's serum; positive RAST response correlates strongly with *in vivo* allergic response; sensitivity 67% to 82%
AlaSTAT	*in vitro*	Enzyme-linked immunometric assay used to measure latex-specific IgE antibodies; raw natural rubber latex used as source material for AlaSTAT latex allergens; sensitivity 94%, specificity 81%

REFERENCES AND RECOMMENDED READING

Hamid RK, "Latex Allergy: Diagnosis, Management and Safe Equipment," *Refresher Courses in Anesthesiology*, 1996, 24:85-96.

Holzman RS, "Latex Allergy: An Emerging Operating Room Problem," *Anesth Analg*, 1993, 76(3):635-41.

Mostello LA, "The Clinical Significance and Management of Latex Allergy," Paper presented at the ASA 1996 Annual Refresher Course Lectures, New Orleans, LA, 1996 Oct 20.

Senst BL and Johnson RA, "Latex Allergy," *Am J Health Syst Pharm*, 1997, 54(9):1071-5.

Steelman VM, "Latex Allergy Precautions. A Research-Based Protocol," *Nurs Clin North Am*, 1995, 30(3):475-93.

MANAGEMENT OF POSTOPERATIVE ARRHYTHMIAS

Arrhythmias commonly occur in the postoperative setting and can contribute to patient morbidity and mortality. Postoperative supraventricular arrhythmias have been reported to occur in a 3.2% to 13% incidence, depending on the surgical procedure. After cardiac surgery, atrial flutter and fibrillation occur in an even higher incidence (12% to 60%). The presence of serious ventricular arrhythmias (eg, sustained ventricular tachycardia, ventricular fibrillation) after cardiac surgery is becoming uncommon; it is even more so after noncardiac surgery. Patients with structural heart disease are most likely to experience arrhythmias in the postoperative setting. The duration of the arrhythmia, ventricular response rate, and the patient's underlying cardiac function are several of the factors that contribute to the physiologic consequences of an arrhythmia.

CLASSIFICATION OF ARRHYTHMIAS

Arrhythmias can be broadly grouped into tachyarrhythmias and bradyarrhythmias. Tachyarrhythmias are further divided by anatomical origin as either supraventricular or ventricular. Table 1 lists common supraventricular and ventricular arrhythmias. Further classifying tachyarrhythmias into those that do and do not traverse the atrioventricular (AV) node (Table 1) is useful when determining appropriate treatment. For example, pharmacologic agents that slow AV node conduction can be used to control the ventricular response if the arrhythmia traverses the AV node. Bradyarrhythmias include sinus bradycardia, sinoatrial (SA) block, sinus pause, and sinus arrest.

Table 1. Common Supraventricular and Ventricular Arrhythmias

Supraventricular Arrhythmias
Sinus tachycardia
Atrial flutter[1]
Atrial fibrillation[1]
Automatic (ectopic) atrial tachycardia[1]
Multifocal atrial tachycardia[1]
Junctional tachycardia
Atrioventricular nodal re-entrant tachycardias[1]
Atrioventricular reciprocating tachycardias[1]
Ventricular Arrhythmias
Premature ventricular beats
Ventricular tachycardia
Ventricular fibrillation

[1]Traverse the AV node.

PREDISPOSING FACTORS

Factors that predispose patients to postoperative arrhythmias can be found in Table 2. When specifically looking at atrial fibrillation after cardiac surgery, the following conditions may contribute to the development of this arrhythmia: Advanced age, male sex, history of preoperative atrial fibrillation, hypertension, history of congestive heart failure, need for postoperative intra-aortic balloon pump, postoperative pneumonia, ventilation for >24 hours, autonomic imbalance, electrolyte abnormalities, pericardial inflammation, inadequate atrial protection from cardioplegia during bypass, and atrial enlargement from volume overload and impaired hemodynamics encountered in the postoperative period. In the postoperative setting, factors that decrease sympathetic nervous system influence or increase parasympathetic nervous system activity can lead to sinus bradycardia (Table 3). Severe hypoxemia, SA nodal ischemia, and sick sinus syndrome

MANAGEMENT OF POSTOPERATIVE ARRHYTHMIAS *(Continued)*

can also reduce sinus rate. Postoperative ventricular tachycardia or fibrillation usually reflects severe myocardial ischemia, systemic acidemia, or hypoxemia.

An important point to remember is that the genesis of arrhythmias can be multifactorial; caution should be taken not to attribute an arrhythmia to a single factor without fully considering the potential for multiple factors to be at play.

Table 2. Factors Predisposing Patients to Postoperative Arrhythmias

Myocardial ischemia	Acid-base imbalance
Endogenous or exogenous catecholamines	Electrolyte abnormalities
Hypoxemia	Mechanical factors
Hypercarbia	Administration of select medications

Table 3. Factors Predisposing Patients to Sinus Bradycardia

Decrease Sympathetic Activity
- High epidural or spinal anesthesia
- Severe acidemia/hypoxemia
- Withdrawal of stimulus
- Emptying bladder
- Sympatholytic medications (eg, beta-blockers, opioids, local anesthetics)

Increase Parasympathetic Activity
- Increased vagal tone
  - Carotid sinus massage
  - Valsalva maneuver
  - Gagging
  - Increased ocular pressure
  - Bladder distension
  - Pharyngeal stimulation
  - Anxiety/pain (centrally mediated response)
  - Surgery (eg, traction on peritoneum during vascular surgery)
- Parasympathomimetic medications (eg, acetylcholinesterase inhibitors, alpha-adrenergic drugs, opioids, succinylcholine)

PRINCIPLES / GOALS OF TREATMENT

Several principles must be kept in mind when managing patients with postoperative arrhythmias. The most important is to treat the patient and not the electrocardiogram (EKG). Questions one should ask include whether an arrhythmia is truly present (vs an artifact) and whether the rhythm seen on the EKG can account for the patient's condition. The urgency for treatment should then be decided. Items such as the patient's pulse, blood pressure, peripheral perfusion, and the presence of myocardial ischemia and congestive heart failure should be evaluated. For example, prompt electrical cardioversion is indicated in a patient who becomes unconscious or hemodynamically unstable in the presence of a tachyarrhythmia (excluding sinus tachycardia). Treatment should also be instituted if the arrhythmia is a precursor of a more severe arrhythmia. The type of arrhythmia will dictate the goals of therapy. Foremost is the need to establish hemodynamic stability. For tachyarrhythmias, attention is first given to slowing the ventricular response whereas with bradyarrhythmias, the ventricular rate must be increased. Once the patient is hemodynamically stable, restoration of sinus rhythm becomes the goal. If this is not possible, the focus should shift to preventing complications from occurring. In patients without overt cardiac disease, therapy of self-terminating arrhythmias is often not needed.

TREATMENT

Table 4. Common Drugs Used for Postoperative Arrhythmias

Drug	Dose	Indications	Adverse Reactions
Adenosine	6 mg rapid IVP (over 1-2 seconds); if no response within 1-2 minutes then 12 mg IVP; may repeat 12 mg dose if needed	PSVT	Transient heart block, facial flushing, chest pain, hypotension
Amiodarone	150 mg I.V. over 10 minutes, then 1 mg/minute over 6 hours, then 0.5 mg/minute; VF/pulseless VT: 300 mg in 20-30 mL D_5W or NS IVP	VT or VF; rate control and conversion of AF	Hypotension, bradycardia, exacerbation of CHF, QT prolongation, AV nodal arrhythmias
Atropine	0.5-1 mg I.V. every 5 minutes, not to exceed a total of 3 mg or 0.04 mg/kg	Bradycardia or AV block	Excessive tachycardia, myocardial ischemia
Digoxin	10-15 mcg/kg IBW, divide into 2-3 doses over 6 hours (50% of dose initially, 25% of dose 3 hours later, 25% of dose 3 hours later)	Rate control	Arrhythmias, nausea, vomiting
Diltiazem	0.25 mg/kg I.V. over 2 minutes (20 mg average adult dose); if inadequate response after 15 minutes, 0.35 mg/kg I.V. over 2 minutes (25 mg average adult dose); maintenance infusion: 5-15 mg/hour	Rate control	Hypotension, bradycardia, dizziness, exacerbation of CHF, headache
Esmolol	500 mcg/kg I.V. over 1 minute, followed by infusion of 50 mcg/kg/minute; if inadequate response, repeat bolus after 5 minutes and increase infusion by 50 mcg/kg/minute; infusion can be titrated to 300 mcg/kg/minute	Rapid rate control	Hypotension, nausea, dizziness, exacerbation of CHF, bronchospasm (dose >300 mcg/kg/minute)
Ibutilide	1 mg (0.01 mg/kg if <60 kg) I.V. over 10 minutes, may repeat 10 minutes after end of initial infusion	Conversion of AF	QT prolongation, torsade de pointes, headache, hypotension
Lidocaine	1-1.5 mg/kg IVP over 1-1.5 minutes followed by infusion of 1-4 mg/minute (15-50 mcg/kg/minute), repeat bolus of 0.5-1 mg/kg may be required 5-30 minutes after initial bolus	PVBs; VT; VF	CNS (eg, confusion, paresthesias, tremor, ataxia); seizures, sinus arrest
Metoprolol	5 mg IVP over 1 minute, repeat every 2 minutes for 3 doses	Rate control	Bronchospasm, hypotension, exacerbation of CHF
Procainamide	15-18 mg/kg I.V. over 25-30 minutes or 100-200 mg/dose every 5 minutes as needed to a total dose of 1 g; maintenance infusion of 1-6 mg/minute	VT or VF; ventricular premature beats; AF or A flutter	Hypotension, QT prolongation, torsade de pointes, headache

IVP = intravenous push; CHF = congestive heart failure; IBW = ideal body weight; AV = atrioventricular; PSVT = paroxysmal supraventricular tachycardia; AF = atrial fibrillation; A flutter = atrial flutter; VT = ventricular tachycardia; VF = ventricular fibrillation; PVB = premature ventricular beat.

MANAGEMENT OF POSTOPERATIVE ARRHYTHMIAS *(Continued)*

Bradycardia

Treatment of bradycardia centers on the elimination of factors causing autonomic nervous system imbalance. For example, if bradycardia is due to increased vagal tone, the provoking stimulus should be discontinued. No treatment is necessary if the bradycardia is transient and not associated with hemodynamic compromise. If hypotension occurs, atropine or beta-mimetic medications (eg, ephedrine) should be used to restore sinus rhythm. Cardiac pacing may be necessary in some patients.

Heart Block

Treatment for first-degree heart block is not necessary in the absence of hypotension or severe bradycardia. Treatment for Mobitz type I block is necessary only if bundle branch block, bradycardia, or congestive heart failure occurs. Transvenous pacing may be required. The use of a pacemaker is required for a Mobitz type II block as it may progress to complete heart block. Postoperative patients with high grade second- or third-degree atrioventricular block persisting for >7-14 days should be considered for permanent pacemaker implantation.

Sinus Tachycardia

Sinus tachycardia is common postoperatively, is nearly always associated with a physiologic increase in sympathetic nervous system influence, and is usually harmless. Common causes in the postoperative setting include pain, fever, anxiety, hypovolemia, hypoxemia, anemia, and medications. Treatment should be directed at the underlying cause and not the rhythm. For example, I.V. fluids can be administered for hypovolemia, sedatives for anxiety, and analgesics for pain. If the tachycardia constitutes a risk for myocardial ischemia, continuous use of a beta-blocker may be indicated.

Paroxysmal Supraventricular Tachycardia

AV nodal reentry is the most common paroxysmal supraventricular tachycardia. Sinus rhythm may be restored with carotid sinus massage or other vagal maneuvers. Adenosine is the initial drug of choice for this condition secondary to its short half-life (3-10 seconds) which minimizes its side effect potential. In the presence of circulatory insufficiency, cardioversion may be necessary. Beta-blockers or calcium channel blockers can also be used for this arrhythmia.

Atrial Premature Beats

Atrial premature beats occur when ectopic foci in the atria fire before the next expected impulse from the sinus node. The presence of these beats is common, benign (do not cause hemodynamic compromise), and usually requires no treatment.

Atrial Fibrillation

Prophylaxis. A beta-blocker should be administered preoperatively or early in the postoperative period for patients undergoing CABG surgery. Alternatively, amiodarone or sotalol may be considered for prophylaxis. Propafenone can be used as a prophylactic agent but the patient must be free of CAD. Evidence that these agents routinely reduce hospital length of stay and overall cost is currently lacking. Postoperative continuous atrial pacing in post-CABG patients has been demonstrated to reduce the incidence of atrial fibrillation and length of stay.

Treatment. In postsurgical patients who are hemodynamically unstable, direct current cardioversion (DCC) should be performed. In hemodynamically stable patients, the ventricular rate should be controlled with pharmacologic agents; digoxin is appropriate for mildly symptomatic patients. An intravenous beta-blocker or diltiazem should be used when faster ventricular rate control is needed (eg, symptomatic patient). Most patients with postoperative atrial fibrillation will spontaneously convert to sinus rhythm within 48 hours. Digoxin is the least effective and beta-blockers are the most effective for controlling ventricular response during atrial fibrillation. If this is not the case, anticoagulation with heparin should be considered. Ibutilide can be used to pharmacologically convert the patient to normal sinus rhythm. If pharmacologic conversion is not successful, DCC should be performed; it is not necessary to have the post-CABG patient anticoagulated for 3 weeks prior to attempting DCC.

Atrial Flutter

Atrial flutter is rare in postoperative patients. It is managed similar to atrial fibrillation, with some differences. Rapid atrial pacing may be effective in terminating the atrial flutter, especially when combined with a class IA antiarrhythmic agent. Care must be taken when using antiarrhythmic agents because sufficient slowing of the flutter rate may result in 1:1 conduction across the AV node.

Ventricular Premature Beats

Ventricular premature beats (VPBs) commonly occur in patients with or without cardiac disease. VPBs occurring in healthy individuals with no cardiac disease pose little, if any, risk and do not require treatment. The use of antiarrhythmic agents to suppress complex VPBs in patients with cardiac disease is controversial. Historically, lidocaine has been used for VPB suppression, specifically in the setting of acute myocardial infarction, as VPBs were felt to be a warning arrhythmia for ventricular fibrillation. However, warning arrhythmias are no more common in patients who experience ventricular fibrillation than in those who do not. Hence, treatment of the VPBs with an antiarrhythmic agent is not necessary beyond the routine use of beta-blockers. Although beta-blockers may be effective in suppressing VPBs, they are administered in the post-MI population for mortality reduction.

Nonsustained Ventricular Tachycardia

Nonsustained ventricular tachycardia is a common arrhythmia encountered in the ICU and has been extensively studied in cardiac surgery patients. Treatment is usually not necessary in patients with good ventricular function and the arrhythmia is not predictive of adverse outcomes. Monitoring, however, is required as it may be indicative of an underlying problem such as hypoxia, ischemia, or acidosis. In patients with poor postoperative cardiac output or those who have undergone valve replacement and have thick, hypertrophic hearts, there is an increased risk that nonsustained ventricular tachycardia may progress to sustained ventricular tachycardia or to ventricular fibrillation. It is not certain whether antiarrhythmic agents are beneficial in this situation. Antiarrhythmic agents may be useful in patients with nonsustained ventricular tachycardia who are at very high risk due to poor left ventricles or from hemodynamic instability. Amiodarone is most frequently used. Lidocaine and procainamide may be considered.

Sustained Monomorphic Ventricular Tachycardia

This reentrant arrhythmia is commonly seen >48 hours after myocardial infarction. Management depends on its rate, duration, and extent of underlying cardiac disease. In hemodynamically stable patients felt to be at risk for imminent circulatory collapse, amiodarone, lidocaine, or procainamide can be started. Direct current cardioversion is indicated in hemodynamically unstable patients or those with angina.

Sustained Polymorphic Ventricular Tachycardia

This arrhythmia is most commonly seen in patients with myocardial ischemia or infarction. Most episodes of polymorphic ventricular tachycardia terminate spontaneously. They can, however, lead to hemodynamic instability. Treatment is similar to that seen with monomorphic ventricular tachycardia. Direct current cardioversion should be used in unstable patients while antiarrhythmic agents that do not prolong the QT interval should be employed for sustained episodes. In addition to the treatment employed for the arrhythmia, beta-blockers and I.V. nitroglycerin should be used for the coronary disease present.

MANAGEMENT OF POSTOPERATIVE ARRHYTHMIAS *(Continued)*

Torsade de Pointes

This is a rapid form of polymorphic ventricular tachycardia associated with QT prolongation. QT prolongation can be seen with various electrolyte abnormalities (eg, hypomagnesemia, hypokalemia), drugs (eg, type IA or type III antiarrhythmic agents, erythromycin, azole antifungal agents), and conditions such as cerebrovascular accident and hypothyroidism. For an acute episode of torsade de pointes, most patients will require DCC. All patients with suspected torsade de pointes should receive I.V. magnesium (2-6 g I.V. over several minutes followed by continuous infusion of 3-20 mg/minute for 5-48 hours), which suppresses triggered activity, as the benefits of doing so far outweigh the risk associated with it. Patients may also benefit from a short-term isoproterenol infusion until a temporary pacemaker can be inserted to increase ventricular rate.

Ventricular Fibrillation

The presence of postoperative ventricular fibrillation usually indicates severe myocardial ischemia, systemic academia, or hypoxemia. Please refer to the ACLS algorithm for the treatment of ventricular fibrillation.

REFERENCES AND RECOMMENDED READING

Atlee JL, "Perioperative Cardiac Dysrhythmias: Diagnosis and Management," *Anesthesiology*, 1997, 86(6):1397-424.

Bauman JL and Schoen MD, "Arrhythmias", *Pharmacotherapy: A Pathophysiologic Approach*, DiPiro JT, et al, eds, Stamford CT: Appleton & Lange, 1999, 232-64.

Bigatello LM, "The Postanesthesia Care Unit," *Clinical Anesthesia Procedures of the Massachusetts General Hospital*, Hurford WE, et al, eds, Philadelphia PA: Lippincott Williams & Wilkins, 1998, 601-17.

Chow MSS and White CM, "Cardiac Arrhythmias," *Applied Therapeutics: The Clinical Use of Drugs*, Koda-Kimble MA, et al, eds, Philadelphia PA: Lippincott Williams & Wilkins, 2001, 18(1)-18(36).

Daoud EG, Strickberger SA, Man KC, et al, "Preoperative Amiodarone as Prophylaxis Against Atrial Fibrillation After Heart Surgery," *N Engl J Med*, 1997, 337(25):1785-91.

Eagle KA, Berger PB, Calkins H, et al, "ACC/AHA Guideline Update for Perioperative Cardiovascular Evaluation for Noncardiac Surgery - Executive Summary: A Report of the American College of Cardiology/American Heart Association Task Force on Practice Guidelines (Committee to Update the 1996 Guidelines on Perioperative Cardiovascular Evaluation for Noncardiac Surgery)," *J Am Coll Cardiol*, 2002, 39(3):542-53.

Forrest JB, Cahalan MK, Rehder K, et al, "Multicenter Study of General Anesthesia. II. Results," *Anesthesiology*, 1990, 72(2):262-8.

Gomes JA, Ip J, Santoni-Rugiu F, et al, "Oral d,l Sotalol Reduces the Incidence of Postoperative Atrial Fibrillation in Coronary Artery Bypass Surgery Patients: A Randomized, Double-Blind, Placebo-Controlled Study," *J Am Coll Cardiol*, 1999, 34(2):334-9.

Guarnieri T, Nolan S, Gottlieb SO, et al, "Intravenous Amiodarone for the Prevention of Atrial Fibrillation After Open-Heart Surgery: The Amiodarone Reduction in Coronary Heart (ARCH) Trial," *J Am Coll Cardiol*, 1999, 34(2):343-7.

"Guidelines 2000 for Cardiopulmonary Resuscitation and Emergency Cardiovascular Care: An International Consensus on Science," *Circulation*, 2000, 102:Supplement I.

Hillel Z and Thys DM, "Electrocardiography," *Anesthesia*, Miller RD, ed, Philadelphia PA: Churchill Livingstone, 2000, 1231-54.

Hollenberg SM and Dellinger RP, "Noncardiac Surgery: Postoperative Arrhythmias," *Crit Care Med*, 2000, 28(10 Suppl):N145-50.

Mahla E, Rotman B, Rehak P, et al, "Perioperative Ventricular Dysrhythmias in Patients With Structural Heart Disease Undergoing Noncardiac Surgery," *Anesth Analg*, 1998, 86(1):16-21.

Mecca RS, "Postoperative Recovery," *Clinical Anesthesia*, Barash PG, et al, eds, Philadelphia PA: Lippincott Williams & Wilkins, 1997, 1279-303.

Napolitano C, Priori SG, and Schwartz PJ, "Torsade de Pointes. Mechanisms and Management," *Drugs*, 1994, 47(1):51-65.

Ramsay JG, "Cardiac Management in the ICU," *Chest*, 1999, 115(5 Suppl):138S-144S.

Redle JD, Khurana S, Marzan R, et al, "Prophylactic Oral Amiodarone Compared With Placebo for Prevention of Atrial Fibrillation After Coronary Artery Bypass Surgery," *Am Heart J*, 1999, 138(1 Pt 1):144-50.

Rho RW, Bridges CR, and Kocovic D, "Management of Postoperative Arrhythmias," *Semin Thorac Cardiovasc Surg*, 2000, 12(4):349-61.

Tisdale JE, Padhi ID, Goldberg AD, et al, "A Randomized, Double-Blind Comparison of Intravenous Diltiazem and Digoxin for Atrial Fibrillation After Coronary Artery Bypass Surgery," *Am Heart J*, 1998, 135(5 Pt 1):739-47.

VanderLugt JT, Mattioni T, Denker S, et al, "Efficacy and Safety of Ibutilide Fumarate for the Conversion of Atrial Arrhythmias After Cardiac Surgery," *Circulation*, 1999, 100(4):369-75.

White CM, Caron MF, Kalus JS, et al, "Intravenous Plus Oral Amiodarone, Atrial Septal Pacing, or Both Strategies to Prevent Postcardiothoracic Surgery Atrial Fibrillation: The Atrial Fibrillation Suppression Trial II (AFIST II)," *Circulation*, 2003, 108 (Suppl 1):II200-6.

PATIENTS WITH GREATER RISK FOR PULMONARY ASPIRATION

- Pregnant patients
- Diabetic patients
- Obese patients
- Patients with history of gastroesophageal reflux (GER)
- Trauma patients
- Patients with an anticipated difficult airway
- Patients at the extremes of age
- Patients undergoing emergency surgery

Note: Recommended that these patients and any other patients felt to be at risk should be premedicated with a H_2-antagonist, metoclopramide, and/or nonparticulate antacid.

Mallampati Airway Classification[1,2]

Class	Description
1	Faucial pillars, soft palate, and uvula are visible
2	Faucial pillars and soft palate are visible, but uvula is masked by the base of the tongue
3	Only soft palate is visible

[1]Evaluation made with patient sitting upright, the mouth open, and the tongue protruded maximally.

[2]Intubation is predicted to be difficult in patients with class 3 airways.

PERIOPERATIVE MANAGEMENT OF THE DIABETIC PATIENT

Diabetes is a disease that necessitates close consideration in the patient undergoing surgery due to the complexity of the disease and high risk of cardiovascular and/or renal complications. A review of the classification, associated diseases, risks and management of perioperative insulin, oral hypoglycemics, and glucose will be discussed.

CLASSIFICATION

Diabetes mellitus is classified as Type 1 (formerly, insulin-dependent diabetes mellitus) or Type 2 (formerly, noninsulin-dependent diabetes mellitus). The following table describes the general characteristics of the Type 1 and 2 diabetic patient.

	Type 1 (Insulin-Dependent)	**Type 2 (Noninsulin-Dependent)**
Age at onset	Juvenile	Adult
Insulin secretion	Very low	Normal or high
Physical characteristic	Lean	Obese
Response to insulin	Sensitive	Resistant
Ketosis likelihood	High	Low
Hereditary influence	Moderate	Great
Treatment	Insulin	Diet, oral agents, insulin

Characterizations are general; there may be overlap between the two types. Note that Type 2 diabetes may also be treated with insulin.

Modified from Morgan GE and Mikhail MS, "Anesthesia for Patients With Endocrine Disease," *Clinical Anesthesiology*, 2nd ed, Stamford, CT: Appleton and Lange, 1996, 637-49.

ASSOCIATED DISEASES AND PERIOPERATIVE RISKS

In the perioperative setting, mortality and morbidity is higher in both types of diabetes when compared to the nondiabetic patient. Diabetic patients undergoing major surgery will spend approximately 30% to 50% more time in the hospital, compared to a nondiabetic patient.

The perioperative mortality rate of the diabetic patient ranges between 3.7% to 13%. The major causes are secondary to cardiovascular complications and postoperative infections. Increased morbidity in the diabetic patient is secondary to their response to surgical procedures as well as underlying complications caused by the disease state.

ENDOCRINE AND METABOLIC RESPONSE TO SURGERY IN DIABETIC PATIENTS

Endocrine

- Increased secretion of counterregulatory hormones: Catecholamines, glucagon, cortisol (predominantly catabolic hormones), and growth hormone
- Decreased insulin secretion causes a loss of anticatabolic effects of insulin
- Decreased insulin action due to increased insulin resistance secondary to the counterregulatory hormones

Metabolic

- Increased hepatic glucose production leading to hyperglycemia
- Decreased glucose disposal (utilization)
- Increased glucose production secondary to glycogenolysis and gluconeogenesis
- Increased net protein catabolism
- Variable increase in lipolysis with ketone bodies formation
- General increase in metabolic rate and catabolism

Immediate and Long-Term Effects

- Dehydration and hemodynamic instability due to osmotic diuresis and volume loss during surgery
- Loss of lean body mass, negative nitrogen balance, impaired wound healing, decreased resistance to infection
- Loss of adipose tissue and energy reserve from fatty acids
- Deficiency of essential amino acids, vitamins, and minerals

In addition to the above, the diabetic patient is predisposed to disease-state complications. These complications include:

Dermopathy
Macrovascular disease – coronary atherosclerosis, peripheral vascular disease
Microvascular disease – nephropathy, retinopathy
Neuropathy – Distal polyneuropathies, neuromuscular disease, acute mononeuropathy, autonomic neuropathy (gastrointestinal, genitourinary, cardiovascular)

Because many diabetic patients have coronary artery disease, autonomic neuropathies and impaired renal function, their perioperative management must be vigilant in order to prevent significant complications. Furthermore, diabetics may present with asymptomatic cardiac ischemia. If undetected preoperatively, these patients are more likely to have an ischemic event during the perioperative time. If the patient suffers from cardiovascular autonomic neuropathy, he/she will be more likely to experience hypotension during induction of anesthesia, arrhythmias during the surgical procedure, and have an inadequate response to drugs such as atropine when used for treatment of bradycardia. In addition, many diabetic patients are predisposed to dehydration due to osmotic diuresis caused by glycosuria and electrolyte imbalance secondary to renal insufficiency, which can affect intraoperative and postoperative fluid management. It is for these reasons that comprehensive preoperative assessment of the diabetic patient by the physician and/or anesthesiologist is important.

PREOPERATIVE ASSESSMENT

A preoperative evaluation of the diabetic patient undergoing a surgical procedure should include the following:

Identification of Diabetes Type

- Type 1 – absolute need for continual insulin therapy
- Type 2 – associated with increased insulin needs

Determination of Level of Preceding Glycemic Control

- Self-monitoring of blood glucose levels – review blood glucose records
- Review glycosylated hemoglobin levels
- Frequency, timing, and severity of hypoglycemia

Determination of Presence of Diabetic Complications

- Nephropathy – fluid balance, hypotension, drug dosage
- Autonomic aeuropathy – cardiovascular response (arrhythmias, postural hypotension), gastrointestinal (gastroparesis, postoperative nausea or vomiting), bladder dysfunction (urinary retention)
- Retinopathy
- Peripheral vascular disease

Assessment of Operative Risk

- Cardiovascular disease, hypertension, congestive heart failure
- Pulmonary
- Renal
- Hematologic

PERIOPERATIVE MANAGEMENT OF THE DIABETIC PATIENT *(Continued)*

Pharmacological Regimen

- Medication type, dosage, and timing

Anticipated Surgery

- Type of procedure
- Type of anesthesia
- Duration of procedure

Complete blood count, electrolyte panel, renal function, and baseline electrocardiogram should be assessed. If the diabetic patient experiences cardiovascular, autonomic, or renal complications preoperatively, the patient should be optimized before undergoing the surgical procedure. In addition, control of these conditions must be maintained and closely evaluated throughout the surgical procedure to prevent increased morbidity and/or increased mortality.

PERIOPERATIVE INSULIN / GLUCOSE MANAGEMENT

Over the years, the management of perioperative glucose and insulin administration has changed. The one fact that remains consistent, however, is that the perioperative glucose and hypoglycemic agent of choice be diligently managed. The goal is to avoid hypoglycemia and prevent significant hyperglycemia. The usual desire is to maintain blood glucose between 120-180 mg/dL. Perioperative hyperglycemia increases morbidity for the diabetic patient and predisposes the patient to the following: infection, decreased wound healing, worsened neurologic outcome in the face of cerebral ischemia, and loss of metabolic control. Adequate management must start in the preoperative setting and follow through into the postoperative period.

Indications for Insulin Therapy During Major Surgery

Always	All insulin-taking diabetes (Type 1 and Type 2)
	Type 2 treated with diet and/or oral hypoglycemic agents, but with chronic hypoglycemia (fasting blood glucose [FBS] 100 mg/dL and glycosylated hemoglobin [HbA_{1c}] >10%)
Sometimes	Type 2 treated with diet or oral hypoglycemic agents and in acceptable control
	Average fasting blood glucose ≤140 mg/dL GHB >10% Surgery duration - 2 hours Body cavity not invaded Food intake anticipated after operation

INSULIN-TREATED / INSULIN-REQUIRING PATIENTS

Major Surgery

There are two methods for administering insulin in the perioperative setting. The first is administration of 33% to 50% of the patient's normal intermediate-acting insulin dose (ie, NPH) the morning of surgery. This method is sometimes referred to as the "split-dose method." The insulin dose should be administered after arrival at the hospital, after the morning blood glucose level is checked, and after the intravenous line is started for administration of a dextrose infusion. If the patient becomes hypoglycemic (<100 mg/dL) or hyperglycemic (>180 mg/dL) intraoperatively, intravenous dextrose or regular insulin, administered subcutaneously based on a sliding scale, should be given respectively. If insulin is administered as an intravenous bolus, its duration of action is only 20 minutes; therefore requiring frequent glucose evaluations and repeat boluses.

Regular Insulin Dosing Sliding Scale

Blood Glucose (mg/dL)	Regular Insulin (units)
<180	0
180-220	6
221-260	8
261-300	10
>300	12

Because of the potential for either hypoglycemia or hyperglycemia with this method, it is rarely the method of choice for perioperative insulin administration in the patient requiring a lengthy major surgical procedure. This method, however, is still commonly used in the insulin-requiring diabetic undergoing minor surgical procedures.

The second method for perioperative insulin administration is the continuous infusion method. This is a recommended method and is preferred because it allows for a more predictable and accurate way of administering insulin. For the brittle diabetic patient and patients that will have changing insulin requirements, it is advisable to use a separate insulin and dextrose infusion perioperatively.

Guidelines for Perioperative Diabetes Management With a Separate Insulin Infusion

- Insulin: Regular (human) 25 units in 250 mL of normal saline (1 unit/10 mL)
- Intravenous infusion of insulin: Flush 50 mL through line before connecting to patient; piggyback insulin line to perioperative maintenance fluid line
- Perioperative maintenance fluid: Fluids must contain 5% dextrose (rate: 100 mL/hour)
- Blood glucose: Monitor hourly intraoperatively; blood glucose value divided by 150 gives a reasonable estimate of infusion dosage (units/hour):

Blood Glucose	Insulin	
(mg/dL)	(units/h)	(mL/h)
<80	0.0	0.0
81-100	0.5	5.0
101-140	1.0	10
141-180	1.5	15
181-220	2.0	20
221-260	2.5	25
261-300	3.0	30
301-340	4.0	40
>341	5.0	50

- Blood glucose <80 mg/dL: Stop insulin and administer intravenous bolus of 50% dextrose in water (25 mL); once glucose >80 mg/dL, restart insulin infusion. It may be necessary to modify the algorithm.
- Decreased insulin needs: Patients treated with diet or oral agents, or <50 units insulin/day, endocrinologic deficiencies
- Increased insulin needs: Obesity, sepsis, steroid therapy, renal transplant, coronary artery bypass

PERIOPERATIVE MANAGEMENT OF THE DIABETIC PATIENT *(Continued)*

The approximate amount of regular insulin required by the patient can also be determined by the following formula:

units/hour = plasma glucose/150

The combination of insulin and glucose in a single I.V. bag is suitable treatment for those patients whose insulin requirements will remain steady throughout the surgical procedure.

The typical diabetic patient usually requires 0.5-3 units/hour of insulin. However, the following patients have a tendency toward insulin resistance and may require larger doses of insulin:

Obese: 2-3 units/hour of insulin
Sepsis: 3-4 units/hour of insulin
Corticosteroid therapy: 3-4 units/hour of insulin
CABG: 4-6 units/hour of insulin

For all patients receiving an insulin infusion for a major surgical procedure, blood glucose should be monitored every hour during and after the surgical procedure. Potassium levels should also be closely monitored because glucose/insulin will shift potassium intracellularly. For this reason, patients with normal potassium levels should have at least 20 mEq/L of potassium added to their perioperative maintenance fluids and adjust the amount according to the level.

Minor Surgery

For Type 1 diabetic patients undergoing minor surgical procedures or invasive diagnostic procedures, the administration of insulin is similar to that of the major surgical procedures. The "split-dose" insulin administration method is commonly used in this setting. The blood glucose monitoring is, however, less intense. These patients should have their blood glucose monitored every 1-4 hours, which is in contrast to every 1 hour for the patient undergoing a major surgical procedure.

ORAL HYPOGLYCEMIC TREATMENT

The diabetic patient taking an oral hypoglycemic agent for their disease state may be managed similar to the insulin requiring diabetic perioperatively or slightly different, depending on the length and type of surgical procedure. The oral hypoglycemic agent should be stopped before surgery. The following table is a list of the oral hypoglycemic agents currently available, their duration of action, and when they should be discontinued before surgery.

Agent	Duration (h)	Discontinue Prior to Surgery
***Sulfonylureas*, first-generation**		
Chlorpropamide	24-72	24-72 h
Tolazamide	12-24	Day of surgery
Tolbutamide	6-24	Day of surgery
***Sulfonylureas*, second-generation**		
Glimepiride	24	Day of surgery
Glipizide	12-24	Day of surgery
Glyburide	16-24	Day of surgery
Nonsulfonylureas		
Acarbose	?	?
Metformin	12	24-48 h
Pioglitazone	24	24 h
Repaglinide	24	?
Rosiglitazone	12-24	24 h
Troglitazone	24	?

Diabetic patients taking an oral hypoglycemic drug and undergoing a prolonged major surgical procedure should be managed like the insulin-requiring diabetic patient perioperatively. For the diabetic patient taking an oral hypoglycemic agent undergoing minor surgical procedures, the goal is "no glucose - no insulin." These patients should not receive dextrose-containing fluids or insulin, and must have their blood glucose checked before the surgical or invasive diagnostic procedure and again postoperatively. The patient should receive insulin, *if and only if*, the blood glucose is elevated. Regular insulin should be administered subcutaneously based on a sliding scale according to the blood glucose level.

POSTOPERATIVE MANAGEMENT

The immediate postoperative management of the diabetic patient is as critical as the intraoperative management. The following describes the postoperative management of the diabetic patient.

1. Continue perioperative insulin infusion until food is tolerated, then plan new regimen
2. Overlap (30-60 minutes) the initial subcutaneous dose of regular insulin before stopping insulin infusion
3. Type 2 previously treated with diet or oral hypoglycemic agent: Prescribe usual medication if BG is <180 mg/dL; elevated BG may administer regular insulin as per sliding scale; see *Regular Insulin Dosing Sliding Scale* table
4. Insulin-treated diabetics: Prescribe usual regimen or use prior 24- to 48-hour insulin dosage to develop a new basic dose regimen. Dose selected should be 80% to 100% of the previous day's total dose. Insulin requirements may be greater during persistent stress, infection, pain, steroid therapy, or high food intake (total parenteral nutrition); selected basic dose may be given premeal:

    Breakfast (25%) regular insulin

    Lunch (25%) regular insulin

    Dinner (25%) regular insulin

    Bedtime (25%) NPH insulin

   Aim to keep BG in a safe range (120-180 mg/dL)

Premeal Blood Glucose (mg/dL)	Basic Dose (regular insulin)
<80	4 units less
81-120	3 units less
121-180	Basic dose (no adjustment)
181-240	2 units more
241-300	3 units more
>300	4 units more

1. Modify the basic dose regularly (every 1-2 days) according to the sliding scale needs; additional doses of regular insulin may be needed at other times (eg, 10 PM, 2 AM)
2. Establish the most suitable insulin regimen or the patient's previous regimen before patient discharge

PERIOPERATIVE MANAGEMENT OF THE DIABETIC PATIENT *(Continued)*

CONCLUSION

The above recommendations are only guidelines. It is important to realize that the physician must individualize diabetic treatment based on the patient's coexisting diseases, type of diabetes, hypoglycemic agent, and surgical procedure. The health care professional must also remember that the disease-state complications of the diabetic patient (ie, cardiac, renal, fluid/electrolyte abnormalities) are major concerns in the perioperative setting. The associated diseases should always be optimized preoperatively and monitored closely in the intraoperative and postoperative period. Goal should be the prevention of complications as a result of hyperglycemia in the surgical patient.

REFERENCES AND RECOMMENDED READING

Boord JB, Graber AL, Christman JW, et al, "Practical Management of Diabetes in Critically Ill Patients," *Am J Respir Crit Care Med,* 2001, 164(10 Pt 1):1763-7.

Christoperson R, "Anesthesia for Endocrine Surgery," *Principles and Practice in Anesthesiology,* Rogers MC, Tinker JH, Covino BG, et al, St Louis, MO: CV Mosby Co, 1992, 2035-48.

Clement S, Braithwaite SS, Magee MF, et al, "Management of Diabetes and Hyperglycemia in Hospitals," *Diabetes Care,* 2004, 27(2):553-91.

Gavin LA, "Perioperative Management of the Diabetic Patient," *Endocrinol Metab Clin North Am,* 1992, 21(2):457-75.

Jacober SJ and Sowers JR, "An Update on Perioperative Management of Diabetes," *Arch Intern Med,* 1999, 159(20):2405-11.

Marks JB, "Perioperative Management of Diabetes," *Am Fam Physician,* 2003, 67(1):93-100.

Morgan GE and Mikhail MS, "Anesthesia for Patients With Endocrine Disease," *Clinical Anesthesiology,* 2nd ed, Stamford, CT: Appleton and Lange, 1996, 637-49.

Walts LF, Miller J, Davidson MB, et al, "Perioperative Management of Diabetes Mellitus," *Anesthesiology,* 1981, 55(2):104-9.

PERIOPERATIVE MANAGEMENT OF PATIENTS ON ANTISEIZURE MEDICATION

The pathophysiologic conditions that produce seizure activation and the drugs used to treat or prevent it will be discussed in addition to the recommended perioperative management for these situations.

ETIOLOGY OF SEIZURES

Brain injury:	Trauma, surgery, subarachnoid hemorrhage
Hypoxia/ischemia:	Stroke, cardiac arrest, shock, hypotension, hypoxemia, cerebral edema
Infection:	Meningitis, encephalitis, abscess
Metabolic:	Electrolyte abnormalities, hepatic or renal failure, hyperglycemia, hypoglycemia, genetic metabolic abnormalities
Drug toxicity:	Alcohol, cocaine, metrizamide
Pathologic states:	Drug withdrawal, eclampsia, cerebral tumor, AVM, cortical vein thrombosis
Idiopathic epilepsy:	Etiology unknown

TYPES OF SEIZURES

Seizures are recurrent, synchronous, rhythmic firings of cortical neurons. Seizures are classified into five major groups.

Classification of Seizures

1. Generalized seizures
   a. Excitatory (myoclonic, clonic/tonic)
   b. Inhibitors (absence, atonic)
2. Partial seizures
   a. Simple partial
   b. Complex partial
   c. Partial onset with generalization
3. Pseudoseizures
4. Status epilepticus
5. Unclassified seizures

Generalized Seizures

Excitatory seizures occur over the entire brain with no obvious focal onset. They may present with an aura followed by tonic-clonic motor activity. Loss of consciousness occurs along with loss of bladder and bowel sphincter tone. The patient becomes apneic with absence of respiratory effort. During the postictal period, the patient may be somnolent or confused. Seizure treatment is supportive, assuring ventilation/oxygenation and preventing the patient from becoming injured from the motor activity.

Inhibitory seizures include absence seizures (petit mal) and atonic seizures (person loses motor tone and falls down).

PERIOPERATIVE MANAGEMENT OF PATIENTS ON ANTISEIZURE MEDICATION *(Continued)*

Partial Seizures

Partial seizure activity has a focal onset and is frequently asymptomatic (aura or simple seizure). Intracranial EEG recordings are often necessary to identify this type of seizure. Bilateral seizure activity must be sustained for at least 10-30 seconds before a physical manifestation occurs. The clinical response depends on the area of the brain containing the seizure focus (ie, uncontrollable hand moving = precentral gyrus; laughing, crying, fear = limbic; visual light flashes = occipital). These complex seizures are frequently termed psychomotor or temporal lobe seizures. When the seizure activity spreads throughout the entire brain it is called secondary generalization which presents as either tonic or clonic seizures.

Pseudoseizures

Pseudoseizures have no EEG abnormality and are usually attributed to malingering or the psychiatric condition of conversion disorder.

Status Epilepticus

Seizures are usually short-lived; however, when they are prolonged or recur without the patient regaining consciousness, the condition is called status epilepticus. Over 60,000 cases of status epilepticus occur per year in the United States. The longer the episode of untreated or inadequately treated status epilepticus, the more difficult it is to control and the greater the risk of permanent brain damage. Ventilation may need to be controlled since most of the drugs used to treat this condition can produce respiratory insufficiency.

Recommended Acute Intravenous Drug Therapy

1. Diazepam (0.2 mg/kg) or lorazepam (0.1-0.22 mg/kg) in adults. Watch for recurrence of seizures when the benzodiazepine redistributes from the brain, decreasing brain concentration.

   OR

2. Phenytoin (15-20 mg/kg in adults) and the prodrug fosphenytoin (15-20 mg/kg phenytoin equivalents [PE]) effectively treats 41% to 90% of patients. Phenytoin cannot be administered faster than 50 mg/minute without significant hypotension. Fosphenytoin can be administered up to a maximum rate of 150 mg PE/minute. It can be administered at a faster rate than phenytoin because it has fewer cardiovascular side effects.

   OR

3. Phenobarbital (20 mg/kg in adults) is also effective, however, this drug has a prolonged half-life and it is difficult to differentiate between drug-induced sedation vs postictal state vs other CNS concerns.

If these drug therapies are unsuccessful, general anesthesia using an inhalational agent (excluding enflurane, which has the potential to produce EEG seizure activity) can be used. This therapy is a temporizing measure, for upon withdrawal of the anesthetic gas the seizures may recommence.

Unclassified Seizures

Not all seizures are epileptic seizures, for example, alcohol withdrawal or toxic brain injury from liver failure. These seizures usually present with tonic/clonic activity.

SEIZURE CLASSIFICATION AND SUGGESTED DRUG THERAPY

Type	Clinical Features	Drug Therapy
Generalized		
Myoclonic	Isolated clonic jerks	Valproic acid Phenobarbital Clonazepam Topiramate
Absence	Brief loss of consciousness; staring; little or no motor activity	Valproic acid Ethosuximide Clonazepam
Partial		
Simple partial	Focal motor or sensory disturbances	Valproic acid Carbamazepine Gabapentin Phenytoin Fosphenytoin Lamotrigine Topiramate Tiagabine Zonisamide
Complex partial	Aura; bizarre behavior with impaired consciousness	Valproic acid Carbamazepine Gabapentin Phenytoin Fosphenytoin Lamotrigine Topiramate Tiagabine Zonisamide
Status epilepticus	Continual seizure activity	Diazepam Phenytoin Fosphenytoin Phenobarbital

PATHOPHYSIOLOGY OF SEIZURES

As the mechanisms that produce seizure activity become evident, the use of specific antiseizure drugs becomes more logical. It is thought that partial seizures result from a reduction of inhibitory or an increase of excitatory synaptic activity. High frequency neuronal firing also produces seizures. Inactivation of the inner gate of the sodium channel prolongs the time the channels are inactive and inhibits rapid firing. This is probably the mechanism of action for carbamazepine, phenytoin, and valproate.

Another mechanism of seizure modulation involves GABA (gamma amino butyric acid) mediated synaptic inhibition, which reduces neuronal excitability and raises the seizure threshold. Activation of the GABAa receptor inhibits the postsynaptic neuron whereas a decrease in GABA receptor number or activity allows the unopposed excitatory activity to dominate. Benzodiazepines and barbiturates activate GABA receptors. Vigabatrin and valproate reduce the metabolism of GABA, and gabapentin enhances release of GABA from presynaptic cells.

Generalized seizures arise from reciprocal firing between the thalamus and cortex. Thalamic stimulation produces the 3/second spike and wave EEG pattern of absence seizures. These seizures are produced by voltage-regulated calcium currents. Drugs such as ethosuximide, trimethadione, and valproic acid inhibit this low threshold current.

PRINCIPLES OF SEIZURE THERAPY

Determine the cause of the seizure. Initiate therapy with a single drug. If this drug does not provide adequate control, another drug should be substituted. When discontinuing a drug, reduce the dosage gradually to prevent status epilepticus. Monitor for toxicity.

PERIOPERATIVE MANAGEMENT OF PATIENTS ON ANTISEIZURE MEDICATION *(Continued)*

PERIOPERATIVE MANAGEMENT: THE PATIENT WITH EPILEPSY

For patients with epilepsy, it is important to maintain adequate antiseizure drug levels during the perioperative period. Since many seizure medications only exist as oral drugs, this needs to be taken into consideration, especially for long surgical procedures. Patients receiving antiseizure drug therapy are resistant to neuromuscular blocking agents, requiring both higher blood levels and more frequent dosing.

Anesthetic management includes continuation of the anticonvulsant therapy and avoidance of drugs that stimulate seizure activity (enflurane, methohexital). High-dose opioids and etomidate have been implicated in producing seizures; however, these drugs induce muscle hypertonus, producing a myoclonic action which can be mistaken for seizure activity. The only narcotic that has demonstrated seizure activity in humans is meperidine. Its metabolite normeperidine has a long half-life and is a known CNS stimulant. It has produced seizures in patients with renal failure and in cancer patients receiving large doses of meperidine over a prolonged time. It is a central sympathetic stimulant, but it also blocks neuronal NMDA receptor activation. (NMDA receptors are activated by glutamate, the major brain excitatory neurotransmitter.) These drug recommendations are not absolute.

PERIOPERATIVE MANAGEMENT: EXCISION OF SEIZURE FOCUS

When chronic medical therapy is unsuccessful in controlling epileptic seizures, patients may undergo craniotomy for resection of the epileptic foci. For these patients, their antiseizure medications are usually reduced or withdrawn prior to surgery to enhance identification of seizure prone tissue. Craniotomy may be performed under general anesthesia or local anesthesia with I.V. sedation, depending on the surgeon's preference, the patient's ability to cooperate, and the site of the seizure foci. The depth of anesthesia and/or sedation must be light enough not to mask seizure activity (ie, patients should not receive large doses of drugs that depress EEG activity or elevate the seizure threshold). Electrocorticography, or mapping the brain electrical activity using intraoperative cortical surface electrodes, identifies the target areas. Because anticonvulsant medications are discontinued preoperatively, there is a high possibility of stimulating generalized seizure activity, which needs to be treated so the sedated patient does not injure himself. For patients anesthetized with general anesthesia and muscle relaxants, the induced seizure activity may be less obvious. In either case, treatment is needed; however, large doses of long-acting anticonvulsants (eg, phenobarbital) may limit the sensitivity of additional electrocorticography.

PREGNANCY

Stillbirth and infant mortality are higher in epileptic mothers taking antiseizure medication during pregnancy. There is a significant correlation with multidrug therapy and higher blood drug levels. Teratogenicity is greatest for trimethadione. Valproate is associated with spinal bifida and neural tube defects. Carbamazepine is associated with craniofacial defects, fingernail hypoplasia, and developmental delays. The formation of epoxide intermediates from carbamazepine and phenytoin metabolism is associated with fetal malformation. However, this does not mean that every epileptic female should discontinue her antiseizure medications. Pregnant women should continue their antiseizure medication if needed for their safety. The effects of hypoxemia on the fetus from seizure-induced respiratory depression are more dangerous than seizure medication. The recommendations are to keep the dosage as small as possible, administer drugs in divided doses to avoid peak blood levels, and limit therapy to only one drug if at all possible.

ECLAMPSIA

Pregnant women with preeclampsia routinely receive magnesium sulfate seizure prophylaxis treatment even though it is still debatable as to whether magnesium sulfate is an anticonvulsant. Because magnesium blocks calcium entry into myocytes, it causes smooth (vascular, uterine) muscle relaxation with a synergistic interaction with nondepolarizing muscle relaxants (ie, vecuronium, pancuronium). Magnesium is cleared via the kidney and must be given cautiously when renal function is decreased.

SUBARACHNOID HEMORRHAGE / HEAD TRAUMA

Seizures frequently occur with subarachnoid hemorrhage associated with rupture of a cerebral aneurysm or with head trauma. It is routine clinical practice to prophylactically treat these patients with antiseizure medication (primarily phenytoin). The benefit of seizure prophylaxis needs to be weighed against the side effects of the drug therapy.

FEBRILE SEIZURES

Although 2% to 4% of children experience a seizure during a febrile illness, only 2% to 3% of them will develop epilepsy later in life. This is a sixfold higher risk than in the general population. Febrile seizures do **not** have an infectious or metabolic origin within the CNS (eg, not produced by meningitis/encephalitis). Factors associated with this increased risk are pre-existing neurologic disorder, a family history of epilepsy, or a complicated febrile seizure (ie, lasting longer than 15 minutes or followed by another seizure within 24 hours). Fever is usually >102°F. The more rapid the rise in temperature, the greater the likelihood for seizure development. The most common age is between 3 months and 5 years. Adults can also experience febrile seizures. The use of chronic prophylactic antiseizure therapy is questionable because of the drug side effects, especially with regards to cognitive function. Temporary prophylaxis may be useful in subsequent febrile episodes (diazepam 0.33 mg/kg every 8 hours during the fever).

MAJOR ANTISEIZURE DRUGS AND SIDE EFFECTS

Name	Dose-Related Side Effect	Toxic Effect
Carbamazepine	Double vision, lethargy, leukopenia, photosensitivity	Skin rash, blood dyscrasia, hepatic/renal dysfunction, acute intermittent porphyria, Stevens-Johnson syndrome
Diazepam	Depression, lethargy, nystagmus, muscle weakness	Hypotension, respiratory depression
Lamotrigine	Somnolence, diplopia, ataxia	Rash, nausea
Phenobarbital	Irritability, lethargy, hallucinations	Rash, respiratory depression, hypotension
Phenytoin, Fosphenytoin	Ataxia, gingival hyperplasia, hirsutism, nystagmus	Neuropathy, rash, lupus (Stevens-Johnson), blood dyscrasia, hypotension, bradycardia
Tiagabine	Dizziness, CNS depression, tremor, ataxia, myalgia	Hepatic/renal dysfunction
Topiramate	Psychomotor slowing, speech problems, somnolence, weight loss, kidney stones	Metabolic acidosis
Valproic acid	Tremor, somnolence, anorexia, alopecia	Hepatic failure, thrombocytopenia
Zonisamide	Somnolence, dizziness, ataxia	Oligohydrosis, hepatic/renal dysfunction

PERIOPERATIVE MANAGEMENT OF PATIENTS ON ANTISEIZURE MEDICATION *(Continued)*

PHARMACOKINETIC PRINCIPLES

1. Tight capillary endothelial junctions limit the passage of water soluble drugs (eg, phenytoin, carbamazepine) into the brain while permitting the rapid transit of lipid soluble drugs (benzodiazepines, barbiturates).
2. The therapeutic effect obtained from active drug concentration depends on drug absorption and bioavailability (ie, phenytoin binds to enteral feedings, which decrease drug absorption from the gastrointestinal tract).
3. Barbiturates enhance cytochrome P450 enzymes, which increase hepatic metabolism of antiseizure drugs.
4. Most antiseizure drugs are bound to plasma proteins. Therefore, a decrease in protein production in the severely ill patient can acutely increase the concentration of free active drug. Because alcohol and metoclopramide have greater plasma protein binding affinity, the benzodiazepine free fraction will increase with coadministration. It is recommended to assay for free drug rather than for total drug concentration for a better understanding of drug availability/activity.
5. Volume of distribution/redistribution. The first phase of distribution delivers antiseizure drugs directly to the brain for a rapid onset of action. During the second phase of distribution (called redistribution) the drug moves out of the brain and equilibrates with the total body's volume of distribution, thus decreasing brain concentration and diminishing the acute drug effect. During the third phase, the drug moves into adipose tissue and is slowly released into the circulation over time, thus slowly terminating drug concentration following discontinuation of the lipid soluble medication.
6. Metabolism of most antiepileptic drugs follows first order kinetics (ie, a constant rate is metabolized). Phenytoin demonstrates saturation kinetics. When the enzymes responsible for phenytoin become saturated, additional doses are not metabolized at the same rate and higher blood levels occur. This is important because the drug level increases exponentially after enzyme saturation occurs, which is at approximately 10 mcg/mL - the lower therapeutic level for phenytoin.
7. The therapeutic target drug level is the one at which the patient stops seizing. This is the level that provides the best protection from seizures; however, it may not be the best level regarding side effects.

REFERENCES AND RECOMMENDED READING

Litt B and Krauss GL, "Pharmacologic Approach to Acute Seizures and Antiepileptic Drugs P484-506," Chernow B, ed, *The Pharmacologic Approach to the Critically Ill Patient*, 3rd ed, Baltimore, MD: Williams & Wilkins, 1994, 484-506.

McNamara JO, "Drugs Effective in the Therapy of the Epilepsies," Gardman JG, Limbird LE, eds, *Goodman & Gilman's The Pharmacological Basis of Therapeutics*, 9th ed, New York, NY: McGraw Hill, 1996, 461-86.

Miller JW and Anderson HH, "The Effect of N-demethylation on Certain Pharmacologic Actions of Morphine, Codeine, and Meperidine in the Mouse," *J Pharmacol Exp Ther*, 1954, 112(2):191-6.

Rosman NP, Colton T, Labazzo J, et al, "A Controlled Trial of Diazepam Administered During Febrile Illnesses to Prevent Recurrence of Febrile Seizures," *N Engl J Med*, 1993, 329(2):79-84.

Runge JW and Allen FH, "Emergency Treatment of Status Epilepticus," *Neurology*, 1996, 46(6 Suppl 1):S20-3.

Szeto HH, "Accumulation of Normeperidine, An Active Metabolite of Meperidine in Patients With Renal Failure or Cancer," *Ann Int Med*, 1977, 86(6):738-41.

POSTOPERATIVE NAUSEA AND VOMITING

Postoperative nausea and vomiting (PONV) has been called the "biggest little problem" that affects surgical patients. The overall incidence is about 30%, with reports ranging from 0% to over 85%. It is a common postoperative problem and a leading cause of prolonged recovery room stay and unanticipated hospital admission.

The goals of this discussion are:

1. to explain the pathophysiology of PONV
2. to describe the patient risk factors associated with PONV
3. to discuss a rational approach to the prophylaxis and treatment of PONV; and
4. to discuss both commonly used drug treatments and less commonly used therapy

PATHOPHYSIOLOGY OF PONV

Figure 1 presents a simplified scheme of the neural circuits involved in nausea and vomiting. There are four major interconnected centers. Three are located in the medulla: chemoreceptor trigger zone (CTZ), area postrema, and nucleus tractus solitarius. They are jointly identified in this illustration as CTZ. The fourth center, located in the reticular formation, is the vomiting center, whose efferents produce the physical process of vomiting. The vomiting center is reflex activated through the CTZ. The major inputs into the CTZ are metabolic, including hypoglycemia, hypokalemia, and uremia; drugs such as opioid analgesics and chemotherapy agents; and hormones. The CTZ is rich in serotonin type 3 (5-HT_3), histamine type 1 (H_1), muscarinic cholinergic type 1 (M_1), dopamine type 2 (D_2), neurokinin type 1 (NK_1), and mu-opioid receptors. Stimulation of one or more of these receptors can cause nausea and vomiting. Another input to the CTZ is from the vestibular labyrinth via muscarinic (acetylcholine) and histamine receptor activation. If stimulation of the vestibular labyrinth is expected to cause nausea and vomiting following surgery, it makes sense to administer an anticholinergic (eg, transdermal scopolamine) or an antihistamine (eg, diphenhydramine) to prevent it.

Figure 1: Mechanisms of Nausea and Vomiting

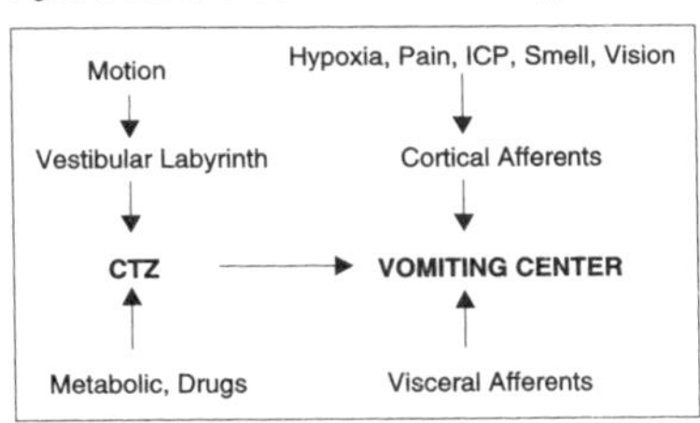

Anxiety, emotions, sights, and smells can activate the vomiting center by stimulating afferents from the cerebral cortex. It is well known that the sights and sounds of nausea and vomiting are quite effective in producing a similar response in a previously comfortable patient.

The last central input to the vomiting center originates in the periphery – the enterochromaffin cells located in the mucosa of the duodenum. They release serotonin, which stimulates vagal afferent nerves to the vomiting center. Therefore, antiserotonin drugs would be appropriate therapy for this vomiting stimulus.

A completely peripheral antinausea action (not presented in figure 1) is mediated via acetylcholine in the GI tract. Drugs such as metoclopramide enhance gastric sensitivity to acetylcholine and increase gastric peristalsis. It is prokinetic drug therapy for nausea and vomiting.

POSTOPERATIVE NAUSEA AND VOMITING *(Continued)*

RISK FACTORS

Risk factors for PONV in adults are listed below. These can be used to identify patients at a higher risk for PONV, which are those who would potentially benefit from prophylactic antiemetic administration.

Table 1. Risk Factors for PONV in Adults

Patient-Specific		
	Gender (female sex)	
	Nonsmoking status	
	Prior PONV	
	History of motion sickness	
Surgical		
	Duration of surgery	ENT surgery
	Breast surgery	Neurosurgery
	Laparoscopic surgery	Strabismus surgery
	Laparotomy	Plastic surgery
Anesthetic		
	Use of volatile anesthetics w/i 0-2 hours	
	Opioid use	
	Nitrous oxide use	
Postoperative		
	Inadequate analgesia	
	Postural hypotension	
	Patient movement	
	Oral fluid consumption	

ASSESSMENT OF RISK

Prophylaxis for PONV is not needed in every patient. Using the risk factors above, several simplified risk factor models have been developed that easily allow the level of risk (eg, low, moderate, high) for PONV to be estimated. Apfel et al used four risk factors in his model (female gender, history of PONV and/or motion sickness, nonsmoking status, and use of postoperative opioids), and was able to demonstrate a 10%, 21%, 39%, 61%, and 79% incidence of PONV with the presence of none, one, two, three, or all four of the risk factors. Koivuranta et al used five predictors in his risk factor model (female gender, history of PONV, history of motion sickness, nonsmoking status, and longer (>60 minutes) surgery) while Sinclair et al used seven predictors (female gender, history of PONV, nonsmoking status, longer duration of surgery, younger age, general anesthesia, and plastic or orthopedic shoulder surgery). These simplified risk models appear to be as good as more complex models but are much easier to use, thereby ensuring better compliance with them.

There does not appear to be a clear consensus on surgery type as an independent risk factor for PONV. Some studies have shown an increased risk of PONV in patients undergoing select surgical procedures while other studies have concluded that surgery type is not an independent risk factor.

REDUCING BASELINE RISK FACTORS

Whenever possible, baseline risk factors should be reduced to decrease the incidence of PONV.

Intraoperatively. Strategies to reduce baseline risk factors include use of propofol for induction and maintenance of anesthesia, use of regional anesthesia, use of hydration, use of supplemental oxygen, avoidance of volatile anesthetics, avoidance of nitrous oxide, minimization of neostigmine use, and minimization of intraoperative and postoperative opioids.

Postoperatively. Although opioids can cause nausea and vomiting, postoperative patients with pain experience nausea and vomiting, and treatment of the pain eliminates this. When these patients are challenged with naloxone, the pain returns and so does the nausea and vomiting. The key is to use the lowest opioid dose that will adequately treat the patient's pain. Inadequate hydration can lead to postural hypotension which can result in PONV. Rapid changes in patient position, or even rapid head movements, will produce PONV, probably via stimulation of the vestibular system. These types of movement in patients should be avoided.

Most recovery room criteria for discharge of ambulatory patients include the requirement for oral fluid consumption. The theory is that if patients can retain oral fluids, they will not become dehydrated due to vomiting when they go home. This practice has been questioned. Schreiner et al divided recovery room patients into two groups (mandatory drinkers and optional drinkers) with PONV significantly less in the latter group (23% vs 14%) and a longer recovery room stay for the mandatory group.

PONV PROPHYLAXIS

The patient's risk level for PONV will dictate whether prophylactic therapy is administered and, if so, how many agents are given to the patient. For example, patients at a low risk (eg, 0-1 risk factors in Apfel's model) for PONV should not receive a prophylactic antiemetic unless vomiting would lead to complications postoperatively. For patients at moderate risk (eg, 2-3 risk factors in Apfel's model) for PONV, a single antiemetic agent should be administered for prophylaxis. For patients at high risk (eg, all 4 risk factors in Apfel's model) for PONV, two or three antiemetic agents should be administered. It is important that these agents be from different classes (have different mechanisms of action).

A PONV Consensus Panel, after reviewing the literature and taking into consideration expert opinion, recommended that droperidol, dexamethasone, and the serotonin receptor antagonists be first-line agents for the prophylaxis of PONV. Droperidol's black box warning has made this agent a less attractive option. Dexamethasone has been shown to be as effective as the serotonin receptor antagonists and droperidol, and may have an advantage in postdischarge nausea and vomiting (PDNV) as its late efficacy seems to be more pronounced. In addition, dexamethasone may offer advantages over traditional antiemetics. When 8 mg of dexamethasone was administered I.V. 90 minutes before laparoscopic cholecystectomy, patients reported less pain, fatigue, nausea, vomiting, and duration of convalescence than patients who received placebo (Bisgaard). A specific serotonin receptor antagonist was not recommended as the panel concluded that there is no evidence of any difference in the safety and efficacy profiles of these agents. The panel stated that these agents can be used alone or in combination depending on PONV risk. It is important to keep in mind that these are general recommendations. One must always consider the specific patient when selecting a prophylactic antiemetic agent. For example, promethazine may be a more appropriate choice for PONV prophylaxis in a patient with motion sickness or who is undergoing surgery affecting the vestibular apparatus.

As a general rule, better efficacy is seen when the prophylactic antiemetic agents are administered at the end of surgery rather than prior to induction. The exception is dexamethasone; it appears to be most effective when administered before induction.

TREATMENT OF PONV

If a patient received no antiemetic prophylaxis and develops nausea and vomiting postoperatively, an appropriate agent (eg, $5\text{-}HT_3$ receptor antagonist) should be administered. Dexamethasone is not recommended for the acute treatment of PONV secondary to its longer onset of action. It has been suggested that treatment doses of the serotonin receptor antagonists can be as low as a quarter of the prophylactic dose. If a patient received one or more prophylactic agents and still develops PONV, a drug from a different class (different mechanism of action) should be used. However, the Consensus Panel's recommendations allow repeat dosing of the serotonin receptor antagonists and droperidol when PONV occurs more than 6 hours after surgery (more than 8 hours for dexamethasone).

POSTOPERATIVE NAUSEA AND VOMITING *(Continued)*

Antiemetic Agents

Antiemetic Drug	Proposed Receptor Site of Action	Usual Dose[1]	Duration of Action	Adverse Effects	Comments and Recommendations for Use
Butyrophenones					
Droperidol (Inapsine®)	D_2	**Adults:** I.V.: 0.625-1.25 mg **Pediatrics:** I.V.: 20-50 mcg/kg	12-24 h	Sedation, hypotension (especially in hypovolemic patients), EPS	Monitor ECG for QT prolongation/ torsade de pointes; duration of action depends on size of dose; antinausea effect greater than antivomiting effect
Phenothiazines					
Prochlorperazine (Compazine®)	D_2	**Adults:** I.V./ I.M.: 5-10 mg P.R.: 25 mg **Pediatrics**[2]**:** P.O.: 0.1 mg/kg I.M.: 0.13 mg/kg P.R.: 2.5 mg	2-6 h (12 h when given P.R.)	Sedation, hypotension (especially in hypovolemic patients), EPS	Effective first-line agent; faster onset and less sedation vs promethazine
Antimuscarinics					
Dimenhydrinate (Dramamine®)	H_1, M_1	**Adults:** I.V./I.M.: 50-100 mg **Pediatrics:** I.V./I.M.: 1.25 mg/kg[4]	6-8 h	Sedation, dry mouth, blurred vision, urinary retention	Good for patients with motion sickness or undergoing surgery affecting the vestibular apparatus
Diphenhydramine (Benadryl®)	H_1, M_1	**Adults:** I.V./I.M.: 12.5-50 mg **Pediatrics:** P.O./I.V.: 1 mg/kg (max: 25 mg for <6 y old)	4-6 h	Sedation, dry mouth, blurred vision, urinary retention	Good for patients with motion sickness or undergoing surgery affecting the vestibular apparatus
Promethazine (Phenergan®)	D_2, H_1, M_1	**Adults:** I.V./I.M./P.R.: 6.25-25 mg **Pediatrics (>2 y):** I.V./I.M./P.R.: 0.25-0.5 mg/kg[3]	4 h	Sedation, hypotension (especially in hypovolemic patients), EPS	Good for patients with motion sickness or undergoing surgery affecting the vestibular apparatus

Antiemetic Agents *(continued)*

Antiemetic Drug	Proposed Receptor Site of Action	Usual Dose[1]	Duration of Action	Adverse Effects	Comments and Recommendations for Use
Scopolamine (Transderm Scōp®)	M_1	**Adults:** 1.5 mg transdermal patch **Pediatrics:** N/A	72 h[5]	Sedation, dry mouth, visual disturbances, dysphoria, confusion, disorientation, hallucinations	Good for patients with motion sickness or undergoing surgery affecting the vestibular apparatus; therapeutic plasma levels are obtained 4 hours after patch is placed; important for patch to be applied/removed correctly
Benzamides					
Metoclopramide (Reglan®)	D_2	**Adults:** I.V.: 20 mg **Pediatrics:** I.V.: 0.25 mg/kg	6-8 h	Sedation, hypotension, EPS	Good if N/V is due to gastric stasis; 10 mg dose not effective for preventing PONV; reduce dose to 5 mg in renal impairment; give slow I.V. push
Serotonin Antagonists					
Dolasetron (Anzemet®)	5-HT_3	**Adults:** I.V.: 12.5 mg **Pediatrics:** I.V.: 0.35 mg/kg	Up to 24 h	Headache, lightheadedness	Much more effective for vomiting than nausea
Granisetron (Kytril®)	5-HT_3	**Adults:** I.V.: 0.35-1 mg **Pediatrics:** Not known	Up to 24 h	Headache, lightheadedness	Much more effective for vomiting than nausea
Ondansetron (Zofran®)	5-HT_3	**Adults:** I.V.: 4 mg **Pediatrics:** I.V.: 0.05-0.1 mg/kg	Up to 24 h	Headache, lightheadedness	Much more effective for vomiting than nausea
Other					
Dexamethasone (Decadron®)	None	**Adults:** I.V.: 4-8 mg **Pediatrics:** I.V.: 0.5-1 mg/kg	Up to 24 h	Watch blood sugar in diabetics; watch for fluid retention in cardiac patients	Well tolerated in healthy patients
Ephedrine	None	**Adults:** I.M.: 0.5 mg/kg **Pediatrics:** N/A	Up to 24 h	Transient elevations in blood pressure	Consider for treatment of PONV when postural hypotension is present; may want to avoid use in patients with hypertension or organic heart disease

POSTOPERATIVE NAUSEA AND VOMITING *(Continued)*

Antiemetic Agents *(continued)*

Antiemetic Drug	Proposed Receptor Site of Action	Usual Dose[1]	Duration of Action	Adverse Effects	Comments and Recommendations for Use
Propofol (Diprivan®)	None	**Adults:** I.V.: 10-20 mg **Pediatrics:** N/A	<10 minutes	Sedation	Very short acting; excessive sedation may be a concern
Trimethobenzamide (Tigan®)	? (probably M_1, D_2)	**Adults:** I.M./P.R.: 200 mg **Pediatrics:** P.R.: 5 mg/kg	6-8 h	Sedation, hypotension, blurred vision	Probably less effective than traditional agents

D_2 = dopamine type 2 receptor; H_1 = histamine type 1 receptor; M_1 = muscarinic cholinergic type 1 receptor; 5-HT_3 = serotonin type 3 receptor; EPS = extrapyramidal symptoms such as motor restlessness or acute dystonia; N/A = not applicable; I.V. = intravenous; I.M. = intramuscular; P.R. = per rectum; P.O. = per os (by mouth); ECG = electrocardiogram; N/V = nausea and/or vomiting.

[1]Pediatric doses should not exceed the adult dose, unless otherwise indicated.

[2]Children >10 kg or 2 years of age only; change from I.M. to oral as soon as possible. When administering P.R., the dosing interval varies from 8-24 hours depending upon the child's weight.

[3]Maximum of 12.5 mg in children <12 years of age.

[4]Children >2 years of age only. Do not exceed 75 mg/dose or 300 mg/day.

[5]Remove after 24 hours. Instruct patients to wash the site where the patch was, as well as their hands, thoroughly.

LESS CONVENTIONAL THERAPY

Stimulation of the P-6 acupuncture point has been shown (Stein; Schlager) to be effective in the prevention of PONV. For both cesarean section and strabismus surgery, this technique decreases PONV when compared to placebo, with no associated drug-induced side effects.

Isopropyl alcohol, when sniffed from a cotton ball or alcohol swab, has been reported to have a significant antiemetic effect (Langevin). The nausea severity score did not change with saline treatment but decreased by 8 points (on a 10-point scale) with alcohol inhalation.

CONCLUSION

It is well known that specific risk factors predispose patients to PONV. These can be classified as patient-specific, surgical, anesthetic, and postoperative. Drug therapy, when tailored to the patient's risk factors, is effective in the prevention or treatment of PONV.

REFERENCES AND RECOMMENDED READING

Aasboe V, Raeder JC, and Groegaard B, "Betamethasone Reduces Postoperative Pain and Nausea After Ambulatory Surgery," *Anesth Analg,* 1998, 87(2):319-23.

Alon E and Himmelseher S, "Ondansetron in the Treatment of Postoperative Vomiting: A Randomized, Double-Blind Comparison With Droperidol and Metoclopramide," *Anesth Analg,* 1992, 75(4):561-5.

Andrews PL, "Physiology of Nausea and Vomiting," *Br J Anaesth,* 1992, 69(Suppl 1):2S-19S.

Aouad MT, Siddik SS, Rizk LB, et al, "The Effect of Dexamethasone on Postoperative Vomiting After Tonsillectomy," *Anesth Analg,* 2001, 92(3):636-40.

Apfel CC, Laara E, Koivuranta M, et al, "A Simplified Risk Score for Predicting Postoperative Nausea and Vomiting: Conclusions From Cross-Validations Between Two Centers," *Anesthesiology,* 1999, 91(3):693-700.

Beattie WS, Lindblad T, Buckley DN, et al, "Menstruation Increases the Risk of Nausea and Vomiting After Laparoscopy. A Prospective Randomized Study," *Anesthesiology,* 1993, 78(2):272-6.

Benedict CR, Arbogast R, Martin L, et al, "Single-Blind Study of the Effects of Intravenous Dolasetron Mesylate Versus Ondansetron on Electrocardiographic Parameters in Normal Volunteers," *J Cardiovasc Pharmacol,* 1996, 28(1):53-9.

Bisgaard T, Klarskov B, Kehlet H, et al, "Preoperative Dexamethasone Improves Surgical Outcome After Laparoscopic Cholecystectomy: A Randomized Double-Blind Placebo-Controlled Trial," *Ann Surg,* 2003, 238(5):651-60.

Borgeat A, Wilder-Smith OH, Saiah M, et al, "Subhypnotic Doses of Propofol Possess Direct Antiemetic Properties," *Anesth Analg,* 1992, 74(4):539-41.

Chen JJ, Frame DG, and White TJ, "Efficacy of Ondansetron and Prochlorperazine for the Prevention of Postoperative Nausea and Vomiting After Total Hip Replacement or Total Knee Replacement Procedures: A Randomized, Double-Blind, Comparative Trial," *Arch Intern Med,* 1998, 158(19):2124-8.

DeSilva PH, Darvish AH, McDonald SM, et al, "The Efficacy of Prophylactic Ondansetron, Droperidol, Perphenazine, and Metoclopramide in the Prevention of Nausea and Vomiting After Major Gynecologic Surgery," *Anesth Analg,* 1995, 81(1):139-43.

Elhakim M, el-Sebiae S, Kaschef N, et al, "Intravenous Fluid and Postoperative Nausea and Vomiting After Day-Case Termination of Pregnancy," *Acta Anaesthesiol Scand,* 1998, 42(2):216-9.

Fan CF, Tanhui E, Joshi S, et al, "Acupressure Treatment for Prevention of Postoperative Nausea and Vomiting," *Anesth Analg,* 1997, 84(4):821-5.

Fujii Y, Toyooka H, and Tanaka H, "Prophylactic Antiemetic Therapy With a Combination of Granisetron and Dexamethasone in Patients Undergoing Middle Ear Surgery," *Br J Anaesth,* 1998, 81(5):754-6.

Gan TJ, Glass PSA, Ginsberg B, et al, "Propofol Patient-Controlled Antiemesis Is a Safe and Effective Method for Treatment of Postoperative Nausea and Vomiting," *Anesthesiology,* 1997, 87:A49.

Gan TJ, Meyer T, Apfel CC, et al, "Consensus Guidelines for Managing Postoperative Nausea and Vomiting," *Anesth Analg,* 2003, 97(1):62-71.

Goll V, Akca O, Greif R, et al, "Ondansetron Is no More Effective Than Supplemental Intraoperative Oxygen for Prevention of Postoperative Nausea and Vomiting," *Anesth Analg,* 2001, 92(1):112-7.

Graczyk SG, McKenzie R, Kallar S, et al, "Intravenous Dolasetron for the Prevention of Postoperative Nausea and Vomiting After Outpatient Laparoscopic Gynecologic Surgery," *Anesth Analg,* 1997, 84(2):325-30.

Harper I, Della-Marta E, Owen H, et al, "Lack of Efficacy of Propofol in the Treatment of Early Postoperative Nausea and Vomiting," *Anaesth Intensive Care,* 1998, 26(4):366-70.

Henzi I, Walder B, and Tramer MR, "Dexamethasone for the Prevention of Postoperative Nausea and Vomiting: A Quantitative Systematic Review," *Anesth Analg,* 2000, 90(1):186-94.

Hovorka J, Korttila K, and Erkola O, "Nitrous Oxide Does Not Increase Nausea and Vomiting Following Gynaecological Laparoscopy," *Can J Anaesth,* 1989, 36(2):145-8.

POSTOPERATIVE NAUSEA AND VOMITING *(Continued)*

Joshi GP, Garg SA, Hailey A, et al, "The Effects of Antagonizing Residual Neuromuscular Blockade by Neostigmine and Glycopyrrolate on Nausea and Vomiting After Ambulatory Surgery," *Anesth Analg,* 1999, 89(3):628-31.

Koivuranta M, Laara E, Snare L, et al, "A Survey of Postoperative Nausea and Vomiting," *Anaesthesia,* 1997, 52(5):443-9.

Kovac AL, O'Connor TA, Pearman MH, et al, "Efficacy of Repeat Intravenous Dosing of Ondansetron in Controlling Postoperative Nausea and Vomiting: A Randomized, Double-Blind, Placebo-Controlled Multicenter Trial," *J Clin Anesth,* 1999, 11(6):453-9.

Langevin A, "Simple, Innocuous, and Inexpensive Treatment for Postoperative Nausea and Vomiting," *Anesth Analg,* 1998, 84:S15.

Lauder GR, McQuillan PJ, and Pickering RM, "Psychological Adjunct to Perioperative Antiemesis," *Br J Anaesth,* 1995, 74(3):266-70.

Liu K, Hsu CC, and Chia YY, "Effect of Dexamethasone on Postoperative Emesis and Pain," *Br J Anaesth,* 1998, 80(1):85-6.

Lonie DS and Harper NJ, "Nitrous Oxide Anaesthesia and Vomiting. The Effect of Nitrous Oxide Anaesthesia on the Incidence of Vomiting Following Gynaecological Laparoscopy," *Anaesthesia,* 1986, 41(7):703-7.

Lopez-Orlando L, Carrascosa F, Pueyo FJ, et al, "Combination of Ondansetron and Dexamethasone in the Prophylaxis of Postoperative Nausea and Vomiting," *Br J of Anaesth,* 1996, 76(6):835-40.

Lussos SA, Bader AM, Thornhill ML, et al, "The Antiemetic Efficacy and Safety of Prophylactic Metoclopramide for Elective Cesarean Delivery During Spinal Anesthesia," *Reg Anesth,* 1992, 17(3):126-30.

Maroof M, Ahmed SM, Khan RM, et al, "Intraoperative Suggestions Reduce Incidence of Posthysterectomy Emesis," *JPMA J Pak Med Assoc,* 1997, 47(8):202-4.

Nelskyla K, Yli-Hankala A, Soikkeli A, et al, "Neostigmine With Glycopyrrolate Does Not Increase the Incidence or Severity of Postoperative Nausea and Vomiting in Outpatients Undergoing Gynaecological Laparoscopy," *Br J Anaesth,* 1998, 81(5):757-60.

Pandit SK, Kothary SP, Pandit UA, et al, "Dose-Response Study of Droperidol and Metoclopramide as Antiemetics for Outpatient Anesthesia," *Anesth Analg,* 1989, 68(6):798-802.

Pueyo FJ, Carrascosa F, Lopez L, et al, "Combination of Ondansetron and Droperidol in the Prophylaxis of Postoperative Nausea and Vomiting," *Anesth Analg,* 1996, 83(1):117-22

Quaynor H and Raeder JC, "Incidence and Severity of Postoperative Nausea and Vomiting Are Similar After Metoclopramide 20 mg and Ondansetron 8 mg Given by the End of Laparoscopic Cholecystectomies," *Acta Anaesthesiol Scand,* 2002, 46(1):109-13.

Rothenberg DM, Parnass SM, Litwack K, et al, "Efficacy of Ephedrine in the Prevention of Postoperative Nausea and Vomiting," *Anesth Analg,* 1991, 72(1):58-61.

Schlager A, Offer T, and Baldissera I, "Laser Stimulation of Acupuncture Point P6 Reduces Postoperative Vomiting in Children Undergoing Strabismus Surgery," *Br J Anaesth,* 1998, 81(4):529-32.

Schreiner MS, Nicolson SC, Martin T, et al, "Should Children Drink Before Discharge From Day Surgery?" *Anesthesiology,* 1992, 76(4):528-33.

Schwartz RH and Beveridge RA, "Marijuana as an Antiemetic Drug: How Useful Is It Today? Opinions From Clinical Oncologists," *J Addict Dis,* 1994, 13(1):54-65.

Scuderi PE, D'Angelo R, Harris L, et al, "Small-Dose Propofol by Continuous Infusion Does Not Prevent Postoperative Vomiting in Females Undergoing Outpatient Laparoscopy," *Anesth Analg,* 1997, 84(1):71-5.

Sinclair DR, Chung F, and Mezei G, "Can Postoperative Nausea and Vomiting Be Predicted?" *Anesthesiology,* 1999, 91(1):109-18.

Stein DJ, Birnbach DJ, Danzer BI, et al, "Acupressure Versus Intravenous Metoclopramide to Prevent Nausea and Vomiting During Spinal Anesthesia for Cesarean Section," *Anesth Analg,* 1997, 84(2):342-5.

Tang J, Wang B, White PF, et al, "The Effect of Timing of Ondansetron Administration on Its Efficacy, Cost-Effectiveness, and Cost-Benefit as a Prophylactic Antiemetic in the Ambulatory Setting," *Anesth Analg,* 1998, 86:274-82.

Tang J, Watcha MF, and White PF, "A Comparison of Costs and Efficacy of Ondansetron and Droperidol as Prophylactic Antiemetic Therapy for Elective Outpatient Gynecologic Procedures," *Anesth Analg,* 1996, 83(2):304-13.

Tramer M, Moore RA, Reynolds DJ, et al, "A Quantitative Systemic Review of Ondansetron in Treatment of Established Postoperative Nausea and Vomiting," *BMJ,* 1997, 314(7087):1088-92.

Wang JJ, Ho ST, Lee SC, et al, "The Prophylactic Effect of Dexamethasone on Postoperative Nausea and Vomiting in Women Undergoing Thyroidectomy: A Comparison of Droperidol With Saline," *Anesth Analg,* 1999, 89(1):200-3.

Yogendran S, Asokumar B, Cheng DC, et al, "A Prospective Randomized Double-Blinded Study of the Effect of Intravenous Fluid Therapy on Adverse Outcomes on Outpatient Surgery," *Anesth Analg,* 1995, 80(4):682-6.

POSTOPERATIVE HYPERTENSION

It has been estimated that the overall incidence of postoperative hypertension (HTN) is approximately 3%. However, a higher incidence is seen with select surgical procedures (Table 1). It has been demonstrated that more than 50% of patients who develop postoperative HTN have pre-existing hypertension. Patients who do not take/receive their antihypertensive medications on the day of surgery are especially prone to present with hypertension postoperatively. Therefore, it is important to counsel patients to take their antihypertensive medications up until their surgical procedures.

Table 1. Incidence of Postoperative Hypertension

Surgery	Incidence
Abdominal aortic surgery	33% to 75%
Coronary artery bypass surgery	30% to 60%
Carotid endarterectomy	9% to 64%
Peripheral vascular surgery	29%
Neurosurgery	7% to 91%
Intraperitoneal or intrathoracic surgery	8%

Postoperative HTN has been defined in various manners (Table 2). A key point to keep in mind is that a diagnosis of postoperative hypertension should be made by considering the patient's preoperative blood pressure. A 20% increase over the baseline often defines treatment threshold; however, as always, each patient must be assessed on an individual basis. Most episodes of postoperative HTN are classified as hypertensive urgency (an increase in systemic arterial pressure without immediate risk of end-organ damage). It can result in various complications, some of them severe (Table 3), but there is no consensus among clinicians about when or how aggressively to treat postsurgical hypertension in the noncardiac surgery patient. Treatment is frequently made at the bedside taking into account the patient's underlying medical conditions. Cardiovascular surgery patients who develop postoperative hypertension are treated aggressively.

Table 2. Definitions of Postoperative Hypertension

- MAP >110 mm Hg
- SBP >160 mm Hg and DBP >90 mm Hg
- BP exceeding preoperative measurements with an increase ≥20% in systolic or diastolic blood pressure

MAP = mean arterial pressure.
SBP = systolic blood pressure.
DBP = diastolic blood pressure.
BP = blood pressure.

Table 3. Complications of Postoperative Hypertension

- Increased myocardial oxygen demand
- Myocardial ischemia
- Ventricular failure
- Rupture of grafts and suture lines
- Postoperative bleeding
- Neurologic defects and intracerebral hemorrhage
- Arrhythmias

POSTOPERATIVE HYPERTENSION *(Continued)*

Patients are most likely to develop blood pressure elevations and tachycardia during the induction of anesthesia. A significant increase in systolic blood pressure (up to 30 mm Hg in normotensive patients; up to 90 mm Hg in uncontrolled hypertensive patients) occurs during the intubation procedure. The recovery period is the next most likely segment where hypertension may occur. Blood pressure increases are usually less dramatic than with induction but occur because of enhanced sympathetic discharge and vascular tone of awakening. Postoperative blood pressure elevations usually begin 30 minutes after the surgery is completed and last for more than 3 hours in 20% of patients.

Other common contributing factors may include pain, anxiety, bladder distension, hypercarbia, hypoxia, fluid overload, hypothermia, antihypertensive withdrawal, and myocardial ischemia. Evaluation and treatment of causes of postoperative hypertension can frequently lower blood pressure. If after treatment, the hypertension has not resolved, antihypertensive drug therapy should be employed. Aggravation of postoperative bleeding, particularly at suture lines is often stated as being an indication for antihypertensive therapy. Systolic pressures ≥180 mm Hg have been associated with increased blood loss from wounds. Short-term injectable therapy in especially likely to be needed for patients who have pre-existing hypertension. Patients whose hypertension was controlled prior to surgery should have their antihypertensive medication reinstated as soon as possible postoperatively.

Patients with postoperative HTN should have their blood pressure frequently monitored. For patients undergoing major surgical procedures, an intra-arterial catheter may still be in place during the early postoperative period and can be used for continuous blood pressure monitoring.

A wide range of parenteral agents is now available for management of postoperative HTN when a patient is not yet tolerating the oral route of administration (Table 4). The drug of choice for a specific patient depends on that patient's circumstances. Table 5 presents some suggested uses for the parenteral agents commonly employed in the treatment of postoperative HTN. The dosages of antihypertensive agents are often titrated to attain a blood pressure value 10% above the patient's normal blood pressure to prevent overshooting the desired value. Unless the situation warrants an immediate reduction in blood pressure (eg, myocardial infarction, dissecting aortic aneurysm, malignant hypertension), the reduction can be achieved over a longer period of time.

Table 4. Select I.V. Agents Used in the Treatment of Postoperative Hypertension

Drug	Dose	Onset	Duration	Mechanism of Action	Potential Adverse Effects
Sodium nitroprusside (Nitropress®)	I.V. infusion: 0.25-0.5 mcg/kg/min initially, titrate every 1-2 min (maximum: 10 mcg/kg/min, limit to <10 min duration)	Immediate	1-2 min	Vasodilator	Nausea, vomiting, muscle twitching, hypotension, sweating, cyanide or thiocyanate toxicity
Nitroglycerin (Tridil®, Nitro-Bid®)	I.V. infusion: 5 mcg/min initially, titrate every 3-5 min by 5-20 mcg/min increments	2-5 min	5-10 min	Vasodilator	Headache, tachycardia, hypotension (especially in volume depleted patients), tolerance
Nicardipine (Cardene®)	I.V. infusion: 5 mg/h initially, titrate every 5-15 min by 2.5 mg/h increments, Nicardipine maintenance: 3 mg/h once blood pressure goals have been met (maximum: 15 mg/h)	5-10 min	15-30 min, up to ≥4 h	Vasodilator	Headache, tachycardia, flushing, phlebitis, hypotension
Enalaprilat (Vasotec®)	Intermittent I.V.: 0.625-1.25 mg every 6 h; use lower dose if hyponatremia, volume depletion, renal failure, or concurrent diuretic therapy in use (maximum: 20 mg/24 h period)	15-30 min	6-12 h	Vasodilator	Hypotension, renal dysfunction, hyperkalemia, angioedema
Hydralazine (Apresoline®)	Intermittent I.V.: 3-20 mg; use lower end of dosing range immediately postoperatively. Can dose every 20-60 min for desired response.	10-20 min	1-4 h	Vasodilator	Headache, flushing, tachycardia, vomiting, aggravation of angina
Fenoldopam (Corlopam®)	I.V. infusion: 0.1-0.3 mcg/kg/min initially, titrate every 15 min by 0.1 mcg/kg/min (maximum: 1.6 mcg/kg/min)	<5 min	30 min	Vasodilator	Headache, flushing, nausea, tachycardia, hypotension

POSTOPERATIVE HYPERTENSION *(Continued)*

Table 4. Select I.V. Agents Used in the Treatment of Postoperative Hypertension *(continued)*

Drug	Dose	Onset	Duration	Mechanism of Action	Potential Adverse Effects
Labetalol (Normodyne®, Trandate®)	Intermittent I.V.: 10-20 mg over 2 min initially; repeat every 10 min (maximum single dose: 80 mg; maximum cumulative dose: 300 mg/day); higher doses may be well tolerated. I.V. infusion: 0.5-4 mg/min initially; titrate every 10 min until desired effect, toxicity, or a cumulative dose of 300 mg in a 24 h period	5-10 min	3-6 h	Alpha and beta blocker	Bronchoconstriction, hypotension, bradycardia, conduction delays, left ventricular dysfunction
Esmolol (Brevibloc®)	I.V. infusion: 250-500 mcg/kg/min for 1 min initially, then 50-100 mcg/kg/min (maximum: 300 mcg/kg/min); can repeat bolus in 5 min and increase infusion by 50 mcg/kg/min	1-2 min	10-30 min	Beta blocker, beta 1 selective	Bronchoconstriction, hypotension, bradycardia, conduction delays, left ventricular dysfunction

Table 5. Suggested Uses for Select I.V. Antihypertensive Agents in Postoperative Hypertension

Drug	Use(s)
Sodium nitroprusside	Most conditions of acute hypertension, especially in patients with CHF. Use caution with high intracranial pressure (in unanesthetized patients ICP can increase), renal dysfunction. Not for patients with acute myocardial ischemia.
Nitroglycerin	Acute hypertension with concurrent CHF, coronary ischemia, postcoronary bypass surgery, or myocardial infarction
Nicardipine	Postoperative HTN in cardiac and noncardiac procedures. Use caution with increased intracranial pressure, acute heart failure.
Enalaprilat	Acute hypertension with concurrent CHF. Use caution with acute myocardial infarction.
Hydralazine	Not recommended for use in postoperative hypertension
Fenoldopam	Postoperative hypertension, where renal blood flow is compromised. Use caution with glaucoma.
Labetalol	Postoperative HTN after aortocoronary bypass surgery, neurosurgical patients with postoperative HTN; acute hypertension associated with MI. Use caution with acute heart failure; asthma; severe sinus bradycardia, heart block, ejection fraction <40% or cardiac index <2.5 L/min/m^2
Esmolol	Hypertension associated with tachycardia, acute aortic dissection. Avoid administration in patients with poor cardiac function or bronchospastic disease

The use of nifedipine capsules sublingually in the treatment of postoperative hypertension is discouraged. Nifedipine capsules have not been approved by the Food and Drug Administration (FDA) for the treatment of any form of hypertension. Further, there is no outcome data demonstrating its effectiveness for this indication. The Sixth Report of the Joint National Committee on Prevention. Detection, Evaluation, and Treatment of High Blood Pressure (JNC VI) states that the routine use of sublingual nifedipine, whenever blood pressure rises beyond a predetermined level in postoperative patients, is unacceptable. In addition, the literature is replete with many reports of serious adverse effects resulting from the sublingual administration of nifedipine (eg, severe hypotension, cerebrovascular ischemia, acute myocardial infarction, conduction disturbances, and death).

REFERENCES AND RECOMMENDED READING

Abdelwahab W, Frishman W, and Landau A, "Management of Hypertensive Urgencies and Emergencies," *J Clin Pharmacol,* 1995, 35(8):747-62.

Chobanian AV, Bakris GI, Black HR, et al, "Seventh Report of the Joint National Committee on Prevention, Detection, Evaluation, and Treatment of High Blood Pressure," *Hypertension,* 2003, 42(6):1206-52.

"Efficacy and Safety of Intravenous Nicardipine in the Control of Postoperative Hypertension," I.V. Nicardipine Study Group, *Chest,* 1991, 99(2):393-8.

Erstad BL and Barletta JF, "Treatment of Hypertension in the Perioperative Patient," *Ann Pharmacother,* 2000, 34(1):66-79.

"Fenoldopam - A New Drug for Parenteral Treatment of Severe Hypertension," *Med Lett Drugs Ther,* 1998, 40(1027):57-8.

Feeley TW and Macario A, "The Postanesthesia Care Unit," *Anesthesia,* 5th ed, Miller RD, ed, Philadelphia, PA: Churchill Livingstone, 2000, 2302-22.

Gal TJ and Cooperman LH, "Hypertension in the Immediate Postoperative Period," *Br J Anaesth,* 1975, 47(1):70-4.

Goldberg ME and Larijani GE, "Perioperative Hypertension," *Pharmacotherapy,* 1998, 18(5):911-4.

POSTOPERATIVE HYPERTENSION *(Continued)*

Graves JW, "Prolonged Continuous Infusion Labetalol: A New Alternative for Parenteral Antihypertensive Therapy," *Crit Care Med,* 1989, 17(8):759-61.

Grossman E, Messerli FH, Grodzicki T, et al, "Should a Moratorium Be Placed on Sublingual Nifedipine Capsules Given for Hypertensive Emergencies and Pseudoemergencies?" *JAMA,* 1996, 276(16):1328-31.

Halpern NA, Goldberg M, Neely C, et al, "Postoperative Hypertension: A Multicenter, Prospective, Randomized Comparison Between Intravenous Nicardipine and Sodium Nitroprusside," *Crit Care Med,* 1992, 20(12):1637-43.

Haas CE and LeBlanc JM, "Acute Postoperative Hypertension: A Review of Therapeutic Options," *Am J Health-Syst Pharm,* 2004, 61:1661-75.

Higgins TL, Yared JP, and Ryan T, "Immediate Postoperative Care of Cardiac Surgical Patients," *J Cardiothorac Vasc Anesth,* 1996, 10(5):643-58.

Laslett L, "Hypertension: Preoperative Assessment and Perioperative Management," *West J Med,* 1995, 162(3):215-9.

Murray MJ, "Perioperative Hypertension: Evaluation and Management," *ASA Refresher Courses in Anesthesiology,* 1998, 26:125-35.

Seltzer JL, Gerson JI, and Grogono AW, "Hypertension in Perioperative Period," *NY J State Med,* 1980, 80(1):29-31.

Shusterman NH, Elliott WJ, and White WB, "Fenoldopam, but not Nitroprusside, Improves Renal Function in Severely Hypertensive Patients With Impaired Renal Function," *Am J Med,* 1993, 95(2):161-8.

"The Sixth Report of the Joint National Committee on Prevention, Detection, Evaluation, and Treatment of High Blood Pressure," *Arch Intern Med,* 1997, 157(21):2413-46.

Udeh EC and Chow MSS, "Acute Hypertension: An Appraisal of New and Old Pharmacologic Agents," *Formulary,* 1996, 31:1178-98.

PREOPERATIVE EVALUATION OF THE CARDIAC PATIENT FOR NONCARDIAC SURGERY

As age increases, so does the prevalence of cardiac disease. Annually, 10% of the United States population has noncardiac surgery, with an overall cardiac morbidity/mortality rate of less than 6% for patients older than 40 years of age undergoing major operations.[1,2] This risk is increased in older patients and those with cardiac disease. The number of patients older than 65 years old presenting for surgery will increase substantially over the next several decades.

The purpose of this chapter is to identify those patients at high risk for postoperative cardiac complications. The preoperative evaluation should stratify patients with preexisting cardiac disease and recommend further workup for those at high risk, while avoiding additional testing for those patients with low potential for postoperative cardiac morbidity or mortality. Preoperative testing should be restricted to those patients in whom the results will affect patient treatment and outcome.

HISTORY OF CARDIAC RISK ASSESSMENTS

Coronary artery disease and congestive heart failure are two clinical conditions closely correlated with postoperative cardiac morbidity (see Table 1). Classic teaching based on the works by Tarhan[3] and Steen[4] in the 1970s reported approximately 30% reinfarction/mortality risk in patients who had surgery within 3 months of their myocardial infarction, decreasing to about 15% if their surgery was within 4-6 months of their MI, and 6% if the surgery was delayed more than 6 months. By 1983, Rao et al reported a reduction in the risk of recurrent MI/cardiac mortality to 6% if operated on within 3 months of a prior MI and 2% if surgery occurred between 4-6 months.[5] Shah confirmed Rao's data of improved cardiac risk in the 1990s.[6] The purposed reasons for this improvement in risk included the intensive postoperative care/monitoring and tight control of hemodynamic variables.

Table 1. Incidence of Perioperative Myocardial Reinfarction

Time Elapsed Since Prior Myocardial Infarction (mo)	Tarhan, et al[1] (%)	Steen, et al[2] (%)	Rao, et al[3] (%)	Shah, et al[4] (%)
0-3	37	27	5.7	4.3
4-6	16	11	2.3	0
>6	5	6		5.7

[1]Tarhan S, Moffitt EA, Taylor WF, et al, "Myocardial Infarction After General Anesthesia," *JAMA*, 1972, 220(11):1451-4.

[2]Steen PA, Tinker JH, and Tarhan S, "Myocardial Infarction After Anesthesia and Surgery," *JAMA*, 1978, 239(24):2566-70.

[3]Rao TL, Jacobs KH, and El-Etr AA, "Reinfarction Following Anesthesia in Patients With Myocardial Infarction," *Anesthesiology*, 1983, 59(6):499-505.

[4]Shah KB, Kleinman BS, Sami H, et al, "Reevaluation of Perioperative Myocardial Infarction in Patients With Prior Myocardial Infarction Undergoing Noncardiac Operations," *Anesth Analg*, 1990, 71(3):231-5.

CARDIAC RISK INDEXES

In the 1970s, Goldman[2] identified nine independent correlates of perioperative cardiac events and assigned them relative value points (see Table 2). The Goldman Cardiac Risk Index). This index stratified patients by cumulative points into four risk classes: Class 1 = 1-5 points (1% to 2% risk of death/major complications. Class II = 6-12 points (5% risk). Class III = 13-25 points (15% risk). Class IV = >25 points (56% risk).

PREOPERATIVE EVALUATION OF THE CARDIAC PATIENT FOR NONCARDIAC SURGERY *(Continued)*

Table 2. Goldman Cardiac Risk Index

Variable	Point Score
History	
Age >70 years	5
Preoperative MI within 6 months	10
Physical examination	
S3 gallop or increased JVP >12	11
Significant valvular aortic stenosis	3
EKG	
Rhythm other than sinus or atrial ectopy	7
PVCs >5/minute at any time	7
General medical status	3
PO_2 <60 or PCO_2 >59	
K^+ <3 or HCO_3 <20	
BUN >50 or creatinine >3	
Chronic liver disease or debilitation	
Operation	
Intraperitoneal, intrathoracic, or aortic	3
Emergency	4
Total possible points	53
Class I	0-5
Class II	6-12
Class III	13-25
Class IV	>25

Adapted from Goldman L, Caldera DL, Nussbaum SR, et al, "Multifactorial Index of Cardiac Risk in Noncardiac Surgical Procedures," *N Engl J Med*, 1977, 297(16):845-50.

In 1999, the Revised Goldman Cardiac Risk Index was developed to simplify risk assessment (using data from approximately 4500 patients) that identified six independent predictors of cardiac complications (see Table 3). Rates of major complications with 0, 1, 2, and 3+ of these factors were 0.4%, 0.9%, 7%, and 11% respectively.[7] Two other indexes focused primarily on high-risk patients. The Detsky risk index[8] added angina and pulmonary edema to Goldman's original criteria, and Eagle Criteria[9] looked at only patients undergoing major vascular surgery. These indexes were more specific to the high-risk population and not very sensitive to patients at the lower risk level.

Table 3. Revised Goldman Cardiac Risk Index

High risk type of surgery
History of ischemic heart disease
History of heart failure
History of cerebrovascular disease
Preoperative treatment with insulin
Preoperative serum creatinine >2 mg/dL

Adapted from Lee TH, Marcantonio ER, Mangione CM, et al, "Derivation and Prospective Validation of a Simple Index for Prediction of Cardiac Risk of Major Noncardiac Surgery," *Circulation*, 1999, 100(10):1043-9.

In 2002, the American College of Cardiology in association with the American Heart Association published practice guidelines to assist anesthesiologists and cardiologists in the preoperative evaluation of the cardiac patient for noncardiac surgery.[10] These guidelines originate from review/evaluation of the literature and provide the physician with a framework for evaluation and management of perioperative cardiac risk.

The perioperative anesthesiologist needs to assess the severity and stability of the patient's cardiac status and determine if additional workup will provide important information prior to the proposed surgery. Following a thorough history and physical examination, the anesthesiologist needs to risk stratify the patient. The predictors of increased perioperative cardiovascular risk, which can lead to myocardial infarction, heart failure, and death, are divided into three categories: **Clinical Predictors**, **Functional Capacity**, and **Risk of Surgical Procedure**. The need for further cardiac workup is based on the patient's classification in these three categories. Preoperative cardiac intervention is rarely indicated to solely decrease surgical risk, unless the intervention is needed regardless of the planned surgical procedure (see Table 4).

Table 4. ACC / AHA Predictors of Perioperative Cardiac Risk (MI, Heart Failure, Death)

Clinical Predictors

Major: Unstable coronary syndromes (including MI within 1 month, unstable or severe angina), decompensated heart failure, high grade AV block, symptomatic ventricular arrhythmias, supraventricular arrhythmias with uncontrolled ventricular rate, and severe valvular disease

Intermediate: Mild angina, previous MI by history or Q waves on ECG, prior heart failure, diabetes – especially insulin dependent, and renal insufficiency (creatinine >2 mg/dL)

Minor: Advanced age, abnormal ECG (LVH, LBBB, ST-T abnormalities), rhythm other than normal sinus, low functional capacity, stroke, uncontrolled HTN

Functional Capacity

1-4 Metabolic equivalents (METs): Able to do activities of daily living, walk 1-2 blocks on level ground, light housework (eg, dusting, washing dishes)

4-10 METs: Able to climb a flight of stairs, walk on level ground at 4 mph, do heavy housework, participate in physical activities like dancing, doubles tennis, golf

>10 METs: Strenuous sports (eg, swimming, football, basketball, skiing, singles tennis)

Risk of Surgical Procedure

High (cardiac risk >5%): Emergent surgery, vascular surgery including aortic and peripheral vascular (due to concurrent coronary artery disease), long procedures with large fluid shifts and/or blood loss

Intermediate (cardiac risk <5%): Carotid endarterectomy, head and neck, intraperitoneal, intrathoracic, orthopedic, and prostate surgery

Low (cardiac risk <1%): Endoscopic, superficial, cataract, and breast procedures

Adapted from Eagle KA, Berger PB, Calkins H, et al, "ACC/AHA Guideline Update for Perioperative Cardiovascular Evaluation for Noncardiac Surgery – Executive Summary: A Report of the American College of Cardiology/American Heart Association Task Force on Practice Guidelines (Committee to Update the 1996 Guidelines on Perioperative Cardiovascular Evaluation for Noncardiac Surgery)," *J Am Coll Cardiol*, 2002, 39(3):542-53.

PREOPERATIVE EVALUATION OF THE CARDIAC PATIENT FOR NONCARDIAC SURGERY *(Continued)*

SUMMARY OF ACA / AHA PREDICTORS OF CARDIAC RISK

A patient is considered at cardiac risk and needs additional cardiac evaluation if he/she has two of the following three conditions:

- Intermediate clinical risk predictor
- Low functional capacity (1-4 METs)
- High-risk surgery

Figure 1 is the complex approach to preoperative cardiac assessment developed by the ACC/AHA task force. It is provided here for completeness. Key points to remember include the following:

Step 1:	If the patient needs emergency surgery, there will be no time for a cardiac evaluation. Careful management of blood pressure, heart rate, and volume status is required intraoperatively. The patient should be risk stratified in the postoperative period and additional cardiac workup performed as indicated.
Step 2:	If the patient has had a coronary artery bypass operation within the past 5 years, or percutaneous coronary intervention between 6 months and 5 years ago, and the clinical status is stable with no ischemia, then additional workup is not needed because the risk of MI is very small.
Step 3:	If the patient has had cardiac evaluation within the last 2 years with good results, and the clinical condition has not changed, the patient does not need additional testing.
Step 4:	If the patient had a previous MI with ongoing evidence of ischemia (unstable angina, CHF, arrhythmias, significant valvular disease), then elective surgery should be postponed until the cardiac condition is treated.
Step 5:	If the patient has intermediate clinical predictors (see Table 1), then the functional capacity and surgery-specific risk are considered. Functional capacity is an excellent predictor of cardiac risk. A MET is equal to the oxygen consumption of a resting 40-year-old, 70 kg male. Perioperative MI and cardiovascular problems are high in patients with poor exercise tolerance (low functional capacity). The surgery specific-risk also contributes to perioperative cardiac morbidity, with very stressful surgical procedures increasing the incidence of cardiac complications. Patients undergoing low risk surgeries do not need additional work-up.
Step 6 and 7:	Patients with intermediate clinical predictors and moderate or excellent functional capacity can undergo intermediate risk surgical procedures without additional concern. Patients with poor functional capacity or with moderate functional capacity but high-risk surgery require additional noninvasive testing.
Step 7:	Patients with minor clinical predictors and moderate or excellent functional capacity can undergo any risk surgery.
Step 8:	Noninvasive testing can lead to invasive testing/therapy or change in medical therapy.

Figure 1. Stepwise Approach to Preoperative Cardiac Assessment

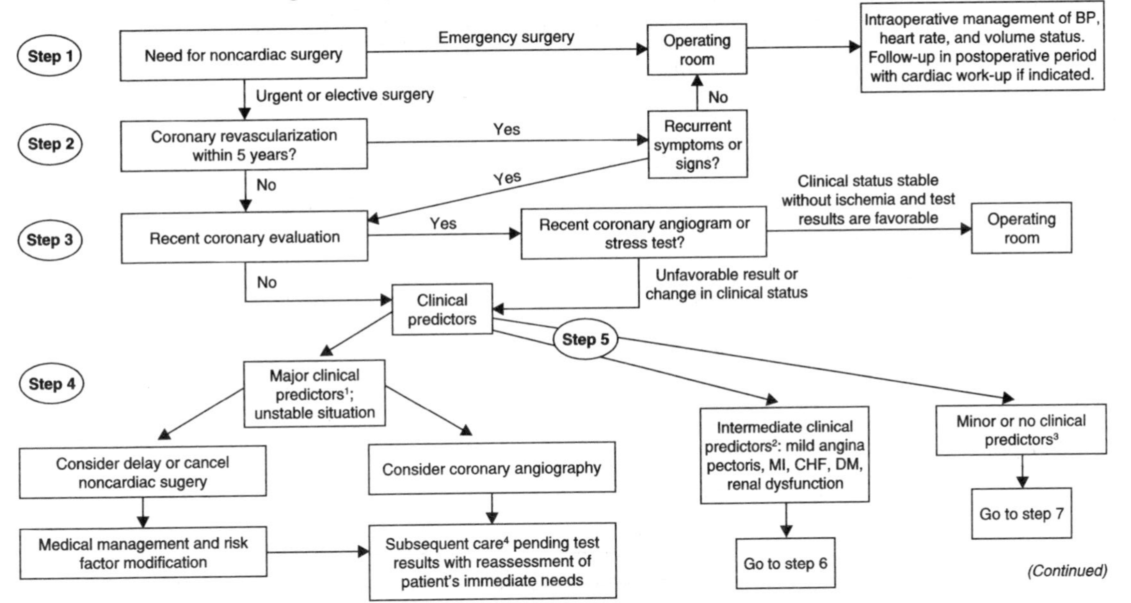

PREOPERATIVE EVALUATION OF THE CARDIAC PATIENT FOR NONCARDIAC SURGERY *(Continued)*

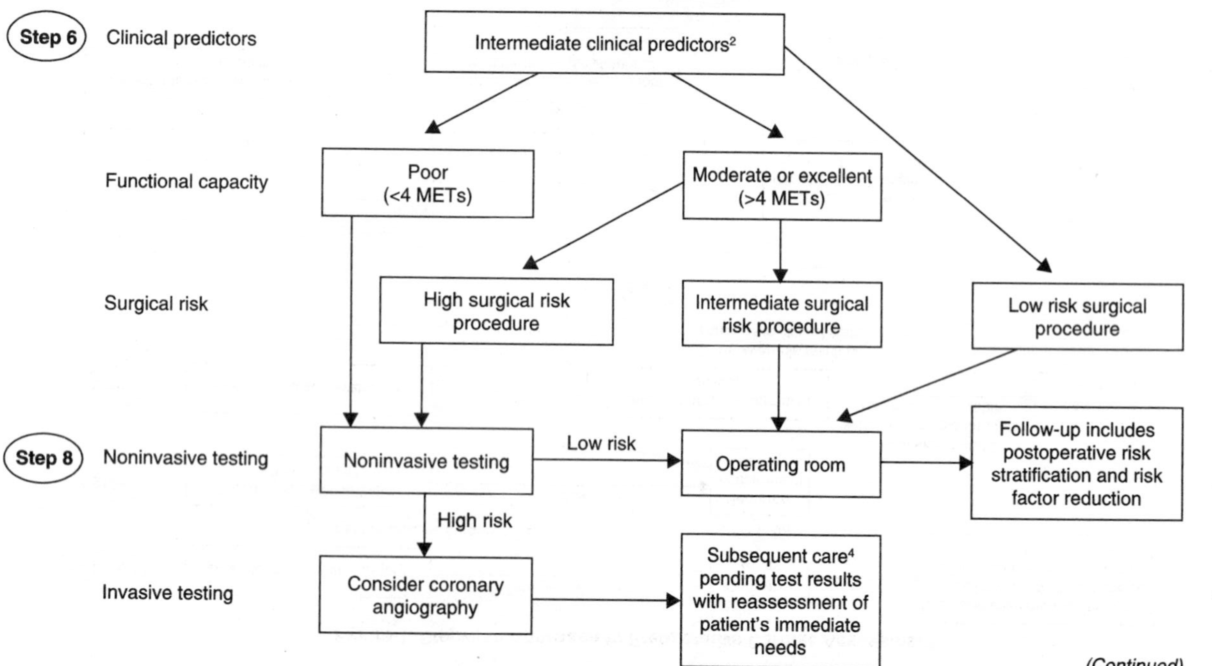

(Continued)

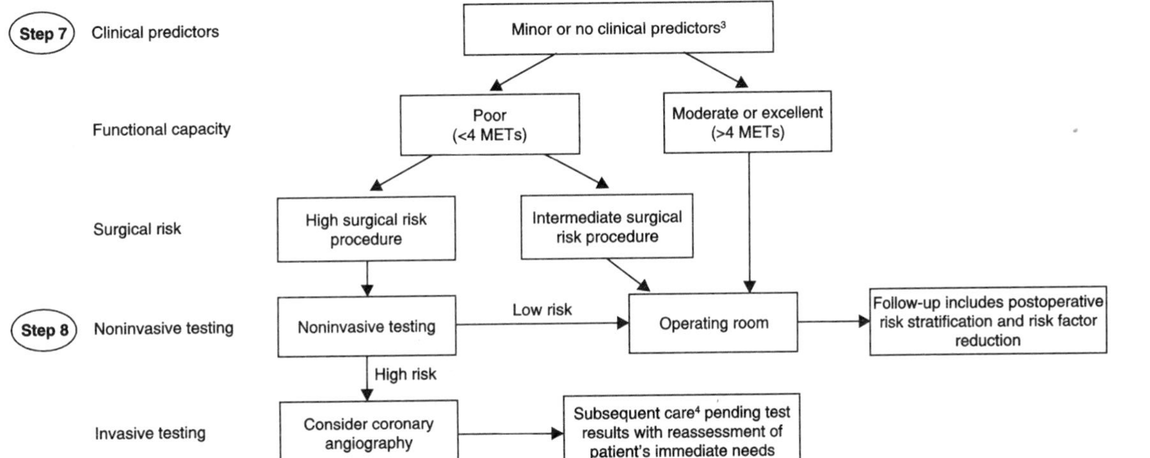

MET = metabolic equivalent.

[1]**Major clinical predictors:** Unstable coronary syndromes; decompensated congestive heart failure; significant arrhythmias; severe valvular disease.

[2]**Intermediate clinical predictors:** Mild angina pectoris; prior myocardial infarction; compensated or prior congestive heart failure; diabetes mellitus; renal insufficiency.

[3]**Minor clinical predictors:** Advanced age; abnormal ECG; rhythm other than sinus; low fuctional capacity; history of stroke; uncontrolled systemic hypertension.

[4]Subsequent care may include cancellation or delay of surgery, coronary revascularization followed by noncardiac surgery, or intensified care.

Adapted from Eagle KA, Berger PB, Calkins H, et al, "ACC/AHA Guideline Update for Perioperative Cardiovascular Evaluation for Noncardiac Surgery - Executive Summary: A Report of the American College of Cardiology/American Heart Association Task Force on Practice Guidelines (Committee to Update the 1996 Guidelines on Perioperative Cardiovascular Evaluation for Noncardiac Surgery)," *J Am Coll Cardiol*, 2002, 39(3):542-53.

PREOPERATIVE EVALUATION OF THE CARDIAC PATIENT FOR NONCARDIAC SURGERY *(Continued)*

REVIEW OF SYSTEMS

Cardiac: With some patients, coronary artery disease is obvious – angina, congestive heart failure, status post CABG, and/or stent placement. However, for many patients the diagnosis is more difficult. Angina may be silent or its functional activity level unclear due to other limiting factors (eg, age, arthritis, muscle wasting). These patients may benefit from further workup (due to low *Functional Capacity*, see Table 4) – unless they are not candidates for myocardial revascularization.

Pulmonary: Obstructive or restrictive disease increases the risk of postoperative respiratory complications. Preoperative symptoms/signs include hypoxemia, hypercapnia, acidosis, increased work of breathing, wheezing, and pneumonia. Preoperative treatment with bronchodilators and steroids may improve pulmonary function and gas exchange. If infection is suspected, antibiotic treatment is essential. Encouragement to stop tobacco use can decrease carboxyhemoglobin and decrease the progression of pulmonary damage.

Diabetes mellitus: Cardiac disease is more common in diabetics, especially those who require insulin. Compounding the risk is the fact that cardiac ischemia symptoms are silent, often not unmasked until a catastrophic event occurs. Chronic tight glucose control (measured by a glycated hemoglobin A_{1c} level <7%) may decrease the severity and rapidity of vascular disease, which has a beneficial effect for critical organs such as brain, heart, lung, and kidney. Aggressive perioperative glucose control, which requires frequent intraoperative evaluation, can improve neurologic outcome. Recent literature has demonstrated a benefit in treating diabetic patients with angiotensin converting enzyme (ACE) inhibitors and/or receptor blockers as demonstrated by a decrease in the incidence of heart failure and proteinuria.

Renal: Azotemia is associated with increased cardiovascular events. Treatment of CHF with fluid restriction and diuretics can produce further worsening of renal function by decrease in glomeruli perfusion. Although treatment with ACE inhibitors and receptor blockers can produce small increases in BUN and creatinine, they should not be discontinued because they have been shown to improve renal function and survival of diabetic patients. Volume status is complicated in dialysis patients, fluctuating from overloaded to dry, depending on frequency of dialysis. A large study has shown that preoperative creatinine >2 mg/dL is an independent predictor of postoperative cardiac complications after noncardiac surgery.[11]

Hematologic: Severe anemia provokes heart failure and myocardial infarction. Although concern for disease transmission via transfusion of blood products exists, a hematocrit <28% is associated with an increased incidence of complications.[12-14] Conditions that increase blood viscosity increase thrombosis. Thrombocytopenia and decreased coagulation factors promote bleeding.

NEW PERIOPERATIVE DRUGS

Beta Blockade: There is substantial evidence that the use of perioperative beta blocker therapy decreases risk of perioperative ischemic cardiac events and long-term mortality.[15] This therapy is especially effective in reducing perioperative mortality in patients with diabetes, left ventricular hypertrophy, coronary artery disease, and renal insufficiency. It has also been shown to decrease the incidence of postoperative atrial fibrillation.[16] Despite solid evidence of their protective effects, they are currently underused in the perioperative period. Part of the reason may be that physicians are concerned about using beta blockers in patients with severe cardiomyopathy, A-V conduction delay, or obstructive pulmonary disease. Additionally, since most anesthesiologists do not direct patient care in the postoperative period, many feel uncomfortable about prescribing this drug category. Another concern is whether all beta blockers possess the same therapeutic profile. This is not currently known. It was initially assumed that beta blockade was beneficial because it reduces heart rate and contractility. It also decreases shear stress and reduces inflammation by decreasing sympathetic tone.[17] The ACC/AHA and the American College of Physicians have recommended that beta blockers be prescribed perioperatively to all patients with a higher risk for perioperative cardiac morbidity.[10] They feel that a cardioselective beta blocker (eg, metoprolol, bisoprolol) should be started days to weeks before surgery with the goal of achieving a resting heart rate of 60 beats/minute. They also support the intraoperative and postoperative use of beta blockade.

Angiotensin converting enzyme (ACE) inhibitors/blockers: The perioperative use of these drugs is still debated. They have been shown to decrease the decline in renal function for patients with diabetes and to improve cardiac function in patients with congestive heart failure. There is some concern about reports of severe intraoperative hypotension with chronic drug administration[18] and several studies have reported increased cardiac and renal complications, although this has not been confirmed by additional studies.

SUMMARY

Preoperative evaluation of the cardiac patient involves careful analysis of the risk factors (clinical predictors, functional capacity, and risk of the surgical procedure). It also involves evaluation of the comorbid disease states that commonly coexist with cardiac dysfunction. The ACC/AHA Guidelines offer the preoperative physician a methodology for the evaluation of these patients.

FOOTNOTES

[1]Goldman L, "Assessment of Perioperative Cardiac Risk," *N Engl J Med*, 1994, 330(10):707-9.

[2]Goldman L, Caldera DL, Nussbaum SR, et al, "Multifactorial Index of Cardiac Risk in Noncardiac Surgical Procedures," *N Engl J Med*, 1977, 297(16):845-50.

[3]Tarhan S, Moffitt EA, Taylor WF, et al, "Myocardial Infarction After General Anesthesia," *JAMA*, 1972, 220(11):1451-4.

[4]Steen PA, Tinker JH, and Tarhan S, "Myocardial Infarction After Anesthesia and Surgery," *JAMA*, 1978, 239(24):2566-70.

[5]Rao TL, Jacobs KH, and El-Etr AA, "Reinfarction Following Anesthesia in Patients With Myocardial Infarction," *Anesthesiology*, 1983, 59(6):499-505.

[6]Shah KB, Kleinman BS, Sami H, et al, "Reevaluation of Perioperative Myocardial Infarction in Patients With Prior Myocardial Infarction Undergoing Noncardiac Operations," *Anesth Analg*, 1990, 71(3):231-5.

[7]Lee TH, Marcantonio ER, Mangione CM, et al, "Derivation and Prospective Validation of a Simple Index for Prediction of Cardiac Risk of Major Noncardiac Surgery," *Circulation*, 1999, 100(10):1043-9.

[8]Detsky AS, Abrams HB, Forbath N, et al, "Cardiac Assessment for Patients Undergoing Noncardiac Surgery. A Multifactorial Clinical Risk Index," *Arch Intern Med*, 1986, 146(11):2131-4.

[9]Eagle KA, Coley CM, Newell JB, et al, "Combining Clinical and Thallium Data Optimizes Preoperative Assessment of Cardiac Risk Before Major Vascular Surgery," *Ann Intern Med*, 1989, 110(11):859-66.

[10]Eagle KA, Berger PB, Calkins H, et al, "ACC/AHA Guideline Update for Perioperative Cardiovascular Evaluation for Noncardiac Surgery – Executive Summary: A Report of the American College of Cardiology/American Heart Association Task Force on Practice Guidelines (Committee to Update the 1996 Guidelines on Perioperative Cardiovascular Evaluation for Noncardiac Surgery)," *J Am Coll Cardiol*, 2002, 39(3):542-53.

[11]Plotkin JS, Benitez RM, Kuo PC, et al, "Dobutamine Stress Echocardiography for Preoperative Cardiac Risk Stratification in Patients Undergoing Orthotopic Liver Transplantation," *Liver Transpl Surg*, 1998, 4(4):253-7.

[12]Hogue CW Jr, Goodnough LT, and Monk TG, "Perioperative Myocardial Ischemic Episodes Are Related to Hematocrit Level in Patients Undergoing Radical Prostatectomy," *Transfusion*, 1998, 38(10):924-31.

[13]Hahn RG, Nilsson A, Farahmand BY, et al, "Blood Haemoglobin and the Long-Term Incidence of Acute Myocardial Infarction After Transurethral Resection of the Prostate," *Eur Urol*, 1997, 31(2):199-203.

[14]Nelson AH, Fleisher LA, and Rosenbaum SH, "Relationship Between Postoperative Anemia and Cardiac Morbidity in High-Risk Vascular Patients in the Intensive Care Unit," *Crit Care Med*, 1993, 21(6):860-6.

[15]Mangano DT, Layug EL, Wallace A, et al, "Effect of Atenolol on Mortality and Cardiovascular Morbidity After Noncardiac Surgery. Multicenter Study of Perioperative Ischemia Research Group," *N Engl J Med*, 1996, 335(23):1713-20.

[16]Jakobsen CJ, Bille S, Ahlburg P, et al, "Perioperative Metoprolol Reduces the Frequency of Atrial Fibrillation After Thoracotomy for Lung Resection," *J Cardiothorac Vasc Anesth*, 1997, 11(6):746-51.

[17]Ohtsuka T, Hamada M, Hiasa G, et al, "Effect of Beta-Blockers on Circulating Levels of Inflammatory and Anti-inflammatory Cytokines in Patients With Dilated Cardiomyopathy," *J Am Coll Cardiol*, 2001, 37(2):412-7.

[18]Brabant SM, Bertrand M, Eyraud D, et al, "The Hemodynamic Effects of Anesthetic Induction in Vascular Surgical Patients Chronically Treated With Angiotensin II Receptor Antagonists," *Anesth Analg*, 1999, 89(6):1388-92.

PREVENTION OF WOUND INFECTION AND SEPSIS IN SURGICAL PATIENTS

Nature of Operation	Likely Pathogens	Recommended Drugs	Adult Dosage Before Surgery[1]
Cardiac	*S. aureus,* *S. epidermidis*	Cefazolin or cefuroxime OR vancomycin[3]	1-2 g I.V.[2] 1.5 g I.V.[2] 1 g I.V.
Gastrointestinal			
Esophageal, gastroduodenal	Enteric gram-negative bacilli, gram-positive cocci	*High risk[4] only:* Cefazolin[5]	1-2 g I.V.
Biliary tract	Enteric gram-negative bacilli, enterococci, clostridia	*High risk[6] only:* Cefazolin[5]	1-2 g I.V.
Colorectal	Enteric gram-negative bacilli, anaerobes, enterococci	*Oral:* Neomycin + erythromycin base[7] OR neomycin + metronidazole[7]	
		Parenteral:	
		Cefotetan or cefoxitin OR cefazolin + metronidazole[5]	1-2 g I.V. 1-2 g I.V. 1-2 g I.V. 0.5-1 g I.V.
Appendectomy, nonperforated	Enteric gram-negative bacilli, anaerobes, enterococci	Cefoxitin or cefotetan OR cefazolin + metronidazole[5]	1-2 g I.V. 1-2 g I.V. 1-2 g I.V. 0.5-1 g I.V.
Ruptured viscus	Enteric gram-negative bacilli, anaerobes, enterococci	Cefoxitin or cefotetan ± gentamicin[5,8]	1-2 g I.V. q6h 1-2 g I.V. q12h 1.5 mg/kg I.V. q8h
Genitourinary	Enteric gram-negative bacilli, enterococci	*High risk[9] only:* Ciprofloxacin	500 mg P.O. or 400 mg I.V.
Gynecologic and Obstetric			
Vaginal, abdominal, or laparoscopic hysterectomy	Enteric gram-negative bacilli, anaerobes, group B streptococci, enterococci	Cefotetan or cefoxitin or cefazolin[5]	1-2 g I.V. 1-2 g I.V 1-2 g I.V
Cesarean section	Same as for hysterectomy	Cefazolin	1-2 g I.V. after cord clamping
Abortion	Same as for hysterectomy	*First trimester, high-risk[10]:*	
		Aqueous penicillin G OR doxycycline	2 mill units I.V. 300 mg P.O.[11]
		Second trimester:	
		Cefazolin	1-2 g I.V.
Head and Neck			
Incisions through oral or pharyngeal mucosa	Anaerobes, enteric gram-negative bacilli, *S. aureus*	Clindamycin + gentamicin OR cefazolin	600-900 mg I.V. 1.5 mg/kg I.V. 1-2 g I.V.
Neurosurgery	*S. aureus,* *S. epidermidis*	Cefazolin OR vancomycin[3]	1-2 g I.V. 1 g I.V.
Ophthalmic	*S. epidermidis,* *S. aureus,* streptococci, enteric gram-negative bacilli, *Pseudomonas*	Gentamicin, tobramycin, ciprofloxacin, gatifloxacin, levofloxacin, moxifloxacin, ofloxacin, or neomycin-gramicidin-polymyxin B	Multiple drops topically over 2-24 hours
		Cefazolin	100 mg subconjunctivally

Nature of Operation	Likely Pathogens	Recommended Drugs	Adult Dosage Before Surgery[1]
Orthopedic			
Total joint replacement, internal fixation of fractures	*S. aureus*, *S. epidermidis*	Cefazolin[12] OR vancomycin[3,12]	1-2 g I.V. 1 g I.V.
Thoracic (Noncardiac)	*S. aureus*, *S. epidermidis*, streptococci, enteric gram-negative bacilli	Cefazolin or cefuroxime OR vancomycin[3]	1-2 g I.V. 1.5 g I.V. 1 g I.V.
Vascular			
Arterial surgery involving a prosthesis, the abdominal aorta, or a groin incision	*S. aureus*, *S. epidermidis*, enteric gram-negative bacilli	Cefazolin OR vancomycin[3]	1-2 g I.V. 1 g I.V.
Lower extremity amputation for ischemia	*S. aureus*, *S. epidermidis*, enteric gram-negative bacilli, clostridia	Cefazolin OR vancomycin[3]	1-2 g I.V. 1 g I.V.

[1]Parenteral prophylactic antimicrobials can be given as a single I.V. dose begun 60 minutes or less before the operation. For prolonged operations, additional intraoperative doses should be given at intervals 1-2 times the half-life of the drug for the duration of the procedure. If vancomycin or a fluoroquinolone is used, the infusion should be started 60-120 minutes before incision in order to minimize the possibility of an infusion reaction close to the time of induction of anesthesia and to have adequate tissue levels at the time of incision.

[2]Some consultants recommend an additional dose when patients are removed from bypass during open-heart surgery.

[3]For hospitals in which methicillin-resistant *S. aureus* and *S. epidermidis* are a frequent cause of postoperative wound infection, for patients previously colonized with MRSA, or for patients allergic to penicillins or cephalosporin. Rapid I.V. administration may cause hypotension, which could be especially dangerous during induction of anesthesia. Even if the drug is given over 60 minutes, hypotension may occur; treatment with diphenhydramine (Benadryl® and others) and further slowing of the infusion rate may be helpful. For procedures in which enteric gram-negative bacilli are likely pathogens, such as vascular surgery involving a groin incision, cefazolin or cefuroxime should be included in the prophylaxis regimen for patients not allergic to cephalosporins; ciprofloxacin, levofloxacin (750 mg), gentamicin, or aztreonam, each one in combination with vancomycin, can be used in patients who cannot tolerate a cephalosporin.

[4]Morbid obesity, esophageal obstruction, decreased gastric acidity, or gastrointestinal motility.

[5]For patients allergic to cephalosporins, clindamycin with either gentamicin, ciprofloxacin, levofloxacin (750 mg), or aztreonam is a reasonable alternative.

[6]Age >70 years, acute cholecystitis, nonfunctioning gallbladder, obstructive jaundice, or common duct stones.

[7]After appropriate diet and catharsis, 1 g of neomycin plus 1 g of erythromycin at 1 PM, 2 PM, and 11 PM or 2 g of neomycin plus 2 g of metronidazole at 7 PM and 11 PM the day before an 8 AM operation.

[8]Therapy is often continued for about 5 days. Ruptured viscus in postoperative setting (dehiscence) requires antibacterials to include coverage of nosocomial pathogens.

[9]Urine culture positive or unavailable, preoperative catheter, transrectal prostatic biopsy, placement of prosthetic material.

[10]Patients with previous pelvic inflammatory disease, previous gonorrhea, or multiple sex partners.

[11]Divided into 100 mg 1 hour before the abortion and 200 mg 30 minutes after.

[12]If a tourniquet is to be used in the procedure, the entire dose of antibiotic must be infused prior to its inflation.

Adapted with permission from "Antimicrobial Prophylaxis for Surgery," *Treatment Guidelines*, 2004, 2(20):28-9.

SUBSTANCE ABUSE AND ANESTHESIA

Substance abuse is a problem that must be considered when evaluating a patient for general surgery under anesthesia. Many agents can potentially interfere with the anesthetics and other agents administered in the perioperative setting. Substances of abuse such as ethanol, central nervous system depressants (opioids, benzodiazepines, barbiturates), and cocaine can all influence the type and the amount of anesthetic administered. Below are brief discussions and tables referring to drugs of abuse and how to perioperatively manage those patients who are abusing the agents.

ETHANOL

Chronic Alcohol Abuse

Chronic ethanol abuse results in induction of the cytochrome P450 system which can affect many of the anesthetic and other medications used perioperatively. Because of this induction, certain agents may need to be dosed more frequently to achieve the desired effect. Larger doses of many of the anesthetic agents are needed in chronic alcohol abusers because of potential cross tolerance. It has been proven that the doses of certain opioids must be significantly increased in the chronic alcoholic to obtain the desired effect. Following is a list of anesthetic drugs that must be altered in the chronic alcoholic.

Agent	Dose
Volatile agents	Increased
Opioids	Increased
Benzodiazepines	Increased
Barbiturates	Increased

Acute Ethanol Abuse

Acute ethanol intoxication causes significant central nervous system (CNS) depression. For those individuals, including chronic alcoholics, undergoing anesthesia while intoxicated, the amount of anesthetic agent used should be decreased.

Agent	Dose
Volatile agents	Decreased
Opioids	Decreased
Benzodiazepines	Decreased
Barbiturates	Decreased

CENTRAL NERVOUS SYSTEM DEPRESSANTS

Patients taking CNS depressants on a chronic basis will frequently need increased doses of certain anesthetic agents. Patients who are taking barbiturates chronically will have enzyme induction and may have an increased requirement for some of the anesthetic agents. Patients on chronic opioids will have an increased requirement for opioids perioperatively. In fact, like chronic alcoholics, patients taking opioids and benzodiazepines chronically, may have a cross tolerance to other agents and the dose of many intravenous anesthetic agents may need to be increased. Following is a list of anesthetic drugs that may need to be altered.

Agent	Dose
Barbiturates	Increased barbiturates
Opioids	Increased - opioids, benzodiazepines (?)
Benzodiazepines	Increased - benzodiazepines, opioids, barbiturates

COCAINE

Cocaine addiction is a common problem in our society. The National Institute of Drug Abuse estimated that there was a fivefold increase in cocaine abuse from the mid 1970s to the mid 1980s. This increased prevalence of cocaine use makes it a significant consideration in the perioperative patient. Acute cocaine use places the surgical candidate in jeopardy of systemic adverse effects and drug interactions. Although the incidence of preoperative patients with a positive urine cocaine screen has not been determined, it is not uncommon for patients to arrive for surgery with a positive screen. It is frequently recommended that preoperative patients with a positive urine toxicology screen wait at least 48-72 hours before undergoing a surgical procedure. Although an increase in morbidity and mortality has occurred in the surgical patient following acute cocaine ingestion, many debates and questions remain as to the time delay for surgery and the potential risks of the surgical procedure in patients with a positive screen. Because a positive urine toxicology screen does not yield precise information on the chronicity or the amount of drug used, more emphasis should be focused on the management of the perioperative effects following acute cocaine administration.

The urine toxicology screen for cocaine detects not only the parent compound but also its metabolites. The metabolites of cocaine include ecgonine methyl ether (EME), benzoylecgonine, and norcocaine. A positive urine toxicology screen occurs up to 48-120 hours after cocaine use. This factor must be kept in mind when evaluating patients with a positive cocaine screen.

Perioperative management of the suspected cocaine intoxicated patient should be aimed at cardiovascular stability. It is very important to have an intravenous antihypertensive available or on board in order to blunt acute hyperdynamic responses. Arrhythmia agents must also be readily available.

For the cocaine intoxicated patient, the dose of many anesthetic agents will need to be increased. Following is a list of anesthetic drugs that must be altered in the cocaine intoxicated patient.

Agent	Dose
Volatile agents	Increased
Opioids	Increased
Benzodiazepines	Increased
Barbiturates	Increased

Management of induction of anesthesia for the cocaine-intoxicated patient should resemble that of the hypertensive patient and the same techniques should be used. The following measures can be taken to prevent the exaggerated increase in blood pressure during intubation from occurring.

Coadminister opioids during induction

- Fentanyl
- Alfentanil
- Remifentanil
- Sufentanil

Administer beta-antagonist during induction

- Esmolol
- Propranolol
- Labetalol
- Metoprolol

Administer topical local anesthetic prior to intubation

For maintenance anesthesia, it is important to avoid halothane in this patient population so as not to increase the risk of arrhythmia secondary to the myocardial sensitivity to catecholamines (epinephrine).

Anesthetic management of the cocaine-intoxicated patient remains an unresolved issue. The anesthesiologist and the surgeon should consider the risk/benefit

SUBSTANCE ABUSE AND ANESTHESIA *(Continued)*

analysis of delaying the procedure. If the surgery is elective, it should be delayed for 48-72 hours or until a negative urine toxicology is achieved. If the procedure is emergent, it need not be postponed and the above precautions and techniques should be considered. It is important to remember, however, that if the procedure occurs, events or medications which exacerbate the adrenergic state should be anticipated or avoided.

APPENDIX TABLE OF CONTENTS

BODY SURFACE AREA OF ADULTS AND CHILDREN

Calculating Body Surface Area in Children

In a child of average size, find weight and corresponding surface area on the boxed scale to the left; or, use the nomogram to the right. Lay a straightedge on the correct height and weight points for the child, then read the intersecting point on the surface area scale. (**Note:** 2.2 lb = 1 kg)

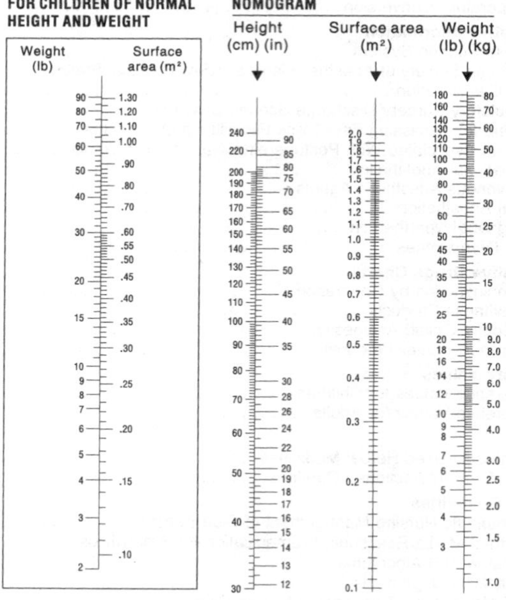

BODY SURFACE AREA FORMULA
(Adult and Pediatric)

$$BSA\ (m^2) = \sqrt{\frac{Ht\ (in) \times Wt\ (lb)}{3131}} \quad \text{or, in metric: } BSA\ (m^2) = \sqrt{\frac{Ht\ (cm) \times Wt\ (kg)}{3600}}$$

References

Lam TK and Leung DT, "More on Simplified Calculation of Body Surface Area," *N Engl J Med*, 1988, 318(17):1130 (Letter).

Mosteller RD, "Simplified Calculation of Body Surface Area", *N Engl J Med*, 1987, 317(17):1098 (Letter).

FORMULAS AND EQUATIONS

CORRECTED SODIUM

Corrected Na^+ = measured Na^+ + [1.5 x (glucose – 150 divided by 100)]

Note: Do not correct for glucose <150.

WATER DEFICIT

Water deficit = 0.6 x body weight [1 – (140 divided by Na^+)]

Note: Body weight is estimated weight in kg when fully hydrated; **Na^+** is serum or plasma sodium. Use corrected Na^+ if necessary. Consult medical references for recommendations for replacement of deficit.

TOTAL SERUM CALCIUM CORRECTED FOR ALBUMIN LEVEL

[(Normal albumin – patient's albumin) x 0.8] + patient's measured total calcium

ACID-BASE ASSESSMENT

Henderson-Hasselbalch Equation

$$pH = 6.1 + \log (HCO_3^- / (0.03)(pCO_2))$$

Alveolar Gas Equation

PIO_2	=	FiO_2 x (total atmospheric pressure – vapor pressure of H_2O at 37°C)
	=	FiO_2 x (760 mm Hg – 47 mm Hg)
PAO_2	=	$PIO_2 - PACO_2 / R$

Alveolar/arterial oxygen gradient = $PAO_2 - PaO_2$

Normal ranges:

Children	15-20 mm Hg
Adults	20-25 mm Hg

where:

PIO_2	=	Oxygen partial pressure of inspired gas (mm Hg) (150 mm Hg in room air at sea level)
FiO_2	=	Fractional pressure of oxygen in inspired gas (0.21 in room air)
PAO_2	=	Alveolar oxygen partial pressure
$PACO_2$	=	Alveolar carbon dioxide partial pressure
PaO_2	=	Arterial oxygen partial pressure
R	=	Respiratory exchange quotient (typically 0.8, increases with high carbohydrate diet, decreases with high fat diet)

Acid-Base Disorders

Acute metabolic acidosis:
$PaCO_2$ expected = 1.5 (HCO_3^-) + 8 ± 2 **or**
Expected decrease in $PaCO_2$ = 1.3 (1-1.5) x decrease in HCO_3^-

Acute metabolic alkalosis:
Expected increase in $PaCO_2$ = 0.6 (0.5-1) x increase in HCO_3^-

Acute respiratory acidosis (<6 h duration):
For every $PaCO_2$ increase of 10 mm Hg, HCO_3 increases by 1 mEq/L

Chronic respiratory acidosis (>6 h duration):
For every $PaCO_2$ increase of 10 mm Hg, HCO_3 increases by 4 mEq/L

Acute respiratory alkalosis (<6 h duration):
For every $PaCO_2$ decrease of 10 mm Hg, HCO_3 decreases by 2 mEq/L

FORMULAS AND EQUATIONS *(Continued)*

Chronic respiratory alkalosis (>6 h duration):

For every $PaCO_2$ decrease of 10 mm Hg, HCO_3 increases by 5 mEq/L

ACID-BASE EQUATION

H^+ (in mEq/L) = (24 x $PaCO_2$) divided by HCO_3^-

Aa GRADIENT

Aa gradient [(713)(FiO_2 – ($PaCO_2$ divided by 0.8))] – PaO_2

Aa gradient	=	alveolar-arterial oxygen gradient
FiO_2	=	inspired oxygen (expressed as a fraction)
$PaCO_2$	=	arterial partial pressure carbon dioxide (mm Hg)
PaO_2	=	arterial partial pressure oxygen (mm Hg)

OSMOLALITY

Definition: The summed concentrations of all osmotically active solute particles.

Predicted serum osmolality =

2 Na^+ + glucose (mg/dL) / 18 + BUN (mg/dL) / 2.8

The normal range of serum osmolality is 285-295 mOsm/L.

Differential diagnosis of increased serum osmolal gap (>10 mOsm/L)

Medications and toxins

Alcohols (ethanol, methanol, isopropanol, glycerol, ethylene glycol)

Mannitol

Calculated Osm

Osmolal gap = measured Osm – calculated Osm

0 to +10: Normal

>10: Abnormal

<0: Probable lab or calculation error

For drugs causing increased osmolar gap, see "Toxicology Information" section in this Appendix.

BICARBONATE DEFICIT

HCO_3^- deficit = (0.4 x wt in kg) x (HCO_3^- desired – HCO_3^- measured)

Note: In clinical practice, the calculated quantity may differ markedly from the actual amount of bicarbonate needed or that which may be safely administered.

ANION GAP

Definition: The difference in concentration between unmeasured cation and anion equivalents in serum.

Anion gap = Na^+ – (Cl^- + HCO_3^-)

(The normal anion gap is 10-14 mEq/L)

Differential Diagnosis of Increased Anion Gap Acidosis

Organic anions

Lactate (sepsis, hypovolemia, seizures, large tumor burden)
Pyruvate
Uremia
Ketoacidosis (β-hydroxybutyrate and acetoacetate)
Amino acids and their metabolites
Other organic acids

Inorganic anions

Hyperphosphatemia
Sulfates
Nitrates

Differential Diagnosis of Decreased Anion Gap

Organic cations

Hypergammaglobulinemia

Inorganic cations

Hyperkalemia
Hypercalcemia
Hypermagnesemia

Medications and toxins

Lithium

Hypoalbuminemia

RETICULOCYTE INDEX

(% retic divided by 2) x (patient's Hct divided by normal Hct) **or**
(% retic divided by 2) x (patient's Hgb divided by normal Hgb)

Normal index: 1.0
Good marrow response: 2.0-6.0

IDEAL BODY WEIGHT CALCULATION

Adults (18 years and older)

IBW (male) = 50 + (2.3 x height in inches over 5 feet)
IBW (female) = 45.5 + (2.3 x height in inches over 5 feet)

IBW is in kg.

Children

a. 1-18 years

$$IBW = \frac{(height^2 \times 1.65)}{1000}$$

IBW is in kg.
Height is in cm.

b. 5 feet and taller

IBW (male) = 39 + (2.27 x height in inches over 5 feet)
IBW (female) = 42.2 + (2.27 x height in inches over 5 feet)

IBW is in kg.

ADJUSTED BODY WEIGHT CALCULATION

Adults (18 years and older)

ABW = IBW + 0.4 (actual body weight – IBW)

Note: This calculation is used in dosing certain medications when patient weighs >20% of his/her IBW. ABW is in kg.

AVERAGE WEIGHTS AND SURFACE AREAS

Average Weight and Surface Area of Preterm Infants, Term Infants, and Children

Age	Average Weight (kg)[1]	Approximate Surface Area (m^2)
Weeks Gestation		
26	0.9-1	0.1
30	1.3-1.5	0.12
32	1.6-2	0.15
38	2.9-3	0.2
40 (term infant at birth)	3.1-4	0.25
Months		
3	5	0.29
6	7	0.38
9	8	0.42
Year		
1	10	0.49
2	12	0.55
3	15	0.64
4	17	0.74
5	18	0.76
6	20	0.82
7	23	0.90
8	25	0.95
9	28	1.06
10	33	1.18
11	35	1.23
12	40	1.34
Adults	70	1.73

[1]Weights from age 3 months and over are rounded off to the nearest kilogram.

MILLIEQUIVALENT AND MILLIMOLE CALCULATIONS

Definitions

mole	=	gram molecular weight of a substance (aka molar weight)
millimole (mM)	=	milligram molecular weight of a substance (a millimole is 1/1000 of a mole)
equivalent weight	=	gram weight of a substance which will combine with or replace one gram (one mole) of hydrogen; an equivalent weight can be determined by dividing the molar weight of a substance by its ionic valence
milliequivalent (mEq)	=	milligram weight of a substance which will combine with or replace one milligram (one millimole) of hydrogen (a milliequivalent is 1/1000 of an equivalent)

Calculations

$$\text{moles} = \frac{\text{weight of a substance (grams)}}{\text{molecular weight of that substance (grams)}}$$

$$\text{millimoles} = \frac{\text{weight of a substance (milligrams)}}{\text{molecular weight of that substance (milligrams)}}$$

$$\text{equivalents} = \text{moles x valence of ion}$$

$$\text{milliequivalents} = \text{millimoles x valence of ion}$$

$$\text{moles} = \frac{\text{equivalents}}{\text{valence of ion}}$$

$$\text{millimoles} = \frac{\text{milliequivalents}}{\text{valence of ion}}$$

$$\text{millimoles} = \text{moles x 1000}$$

$$\text{milliequivalents} = \text{equivalents x 1000}$$

Note: Use of equivalents and milliequivalents is valid only for those substances which have fixed ionic valences (eg, sodium, potassium, calcium, chlorine, magnesium bromine, etc). For substances with variable ionic valences (eg, phosphorous), a reliable equivalent value cannot be determined. In these instances, one should calculate millimoles (which are fixed and reliable) rather than milliequivalents.

MILLIEQUIVALENT CONVERSIONS

To convert mg/100 mL to mEq/L the following formula may be used:

$$\frac{(\text{mg/100 mL}) \times 10 \times \text{valence}}{\text{atomic weight}} = \text{mEq/L}$$

To convert mEq/L to mg/100 mL the following formula may be used:

$$\frac{(\text{mEq/L}) \times \text{atomic weight}}{10 \times \text{valence}} = \text{mg/100 mL}$$

To convert mEq/L to volume of percent of a gas the following formula may be used:

$$\frac{(\text{mEq/L}) \times 22.4}{10} = \text{volume percent}$$

Valences and Atomic Weights of Selected Ions

Substance	Electrolyte	Valence	Molecular Wt
Calcium	Ca^{++}	2	40
Chloride	Cl^{-}	1	35.5
Magnesium	Mg^{++}	2	24
Phosphate	HPO_4^{--} (80%)	1.8	96*
pH = 7.4	$H_2PO_4^{-}$ (20%)	1.8	96*
Potassium	K^{+}	1	39
Sodium	Na^{+}	1	23
Sulfate	SO_4^{--}	2	96*

*The molecular weight of phosphorus only is 31, and sulfur only is 32.

Approximate Milliequivalents — Weights of Selected Ions

Salt	mEq/g Salt	Mg Salt/mEq
Calcium carbonate [$CaCO_3$]	20	50
Calcium chloride [$CaCl_2 \bullet 2H_2O$]	14	74
Calcium gluceptate [$Ca(C_7H_{13}O_8)_2$]	4	245
Calcium gluconate [$Ca(C_6H_{11}O_7)_2 \bullet H_2O$]	5	224
Calcium lactate [$Ca(C_3H_5O_3)_2 \bullet 5H_2O$]	7	154
Magnesium gluconate [$Mg(C_6H_{11}O_7)_2 \bullet H_2O$]	5	216
Magnesium oxide [MgO]	50	20
Magnesium sulfate [$MgSO_4$]	17	60
Magnesium sulfate [$MgSO_4 \bullet 7H_2O$]	8	123
Potassium acetate [$K(C_2H_3O_2)$]	10	98
Potassium chloride [KCl]	13	75
Potassium citrate [$K_3(C_6H_5O_7) \bullet H_2O$]	9	108
Potassium iodide [KI]	6	166
Sodium acetate [$Na(C_2H_3O_2)$]	12	82
Sodium acetate [$Na(C_2H_3O_2) \bullet 3H_2O$]	7	136
Sodium bicarbonate [$NaHCO_3$]	12	84
Sodium chloride [$NaCl$]	17	58
Sodium citrate [$Na_3(C_6H_5O_7) \bullet 2H_2O$]	10	98
Sodium iodine [NaI]	7	150
Sodium lactate [$Na(C_3H_5O_3)$]	9	112
Zinc sulfate [$ZnSO_4 \bullet 7H_2O$]	7	144

POUNDS / KILOGRAMS CONVERSION

1 pound = 0.45359 kilograms
1 kilogram = 2.2 pounds

lb	= kg	lb	= kg	lb	= kg
1	0.45	70	31.75	140	63.50
5	2.27	75	34.02	145	65.77
10	4.54	80	36.29	150	68.04
15	6.80	85	38.56	155	70.31
20	9.07	90	40.82	160	72.58
25	11.34	95	43.09	165	74.84
30	13.61	100	45.36	170	77.11
35	15.88	105	47.63	175	79.38
40	18.14	110	49.90	180	81.65
45	20.41	115	52.16	185	83.92
50	22.68	120	54.43	190	86.18
55	24.95	125	56.70	195	88.45
60	27.22	130	58.91	200	90.72
65	29.48	135	61.24		

TEMPERATURE CONVERSION

Celsius to Fahrenheit = (°C x 9/5) + 32 = °F
Fahrenheit to Celsius = (°F – 32) x 5/9 = °C

°C	= °F	°C	= °F	°C	= °F
100.0	212.0	39.0	102.2	36.8	98.2
50.0	122.0	38.8	101.8	36.6	97.9
41.0	105.8	38.6	101.5	36.4	97.5
40.8	105.4	38.4	101.1	36.2	97.2
40.6	105.1	38.2	100.8	36.0	96.8
40.4	104.7	38.0	100.4	35.8	96.4
40.2	104.4	37.8	100.1	35.6	96.1
40.0	104.0	37.6	99.7	35.4	95.7
39.8	103.6	37.4	99.3	35.2	95.4
39.6	103.3	37.2	99.0	35.0	95.0
39.4	102.9	37.0	98.6	0	32.0
39.2	102.6				

ALDRETE SCORING SYSTEM

Activity	
Able to move 4 extremities voluntarily or on command	2
Able to move 2 extremities voluntarily or on command	1
Not able to move extremities voluntarily or on command	0
Respiration	
Able to deep breathe and cough freely	2
Dyspnea, shallow or limited breathing	1
Apneic	0
Circulation	
Blood pressure ± 20 mm of preanesthesia level	2
Blood pressure ± 20 to 50 mm of preanesthesia level	1
Blood pressure ± 50 mm of preanesthesia level	0
Consciousness	
Fully awake	2
Arousable on calling	1
Not responding	0
Color	
Normal	2
Pale, dusky, blotchy	1
Cyanotic	0

Note: This scoring system is used to determine readiness of patient to be discharged to unit (if inpatient) or to phase II recovery (if outpatient); patients with a score of 9 or above are considered fit for discharge.

Adapted from Aldrete JA and Kroulik D, "A Postanesthetic Recovery Score," *Anes Analg*, 1970, 49:924-34.

AMERICAN SOCIETY OF ANESTHESIOLOGISTS (ASA) PHYSICAL STATUS CLASSIFICATION

Category	Description
ASA 1	Normal, healthy patient
ASA 2	Mild systemic disease — no functional limitation (eg, anemia, chronic bronchitis, controlled hypertension, extremes of age, mild diabetes mellitus, morbid obesity)
ASA 3	Severe systemic disease — definite functional limitation (eg, angina pectoris, diabetes mellitus with vascular complications, history of prior myocardial infarction, obstructive pulmonary disease, poorly controlled hypertension)
ASA 4	Severe systemic disease that is a constant threat to life (eg, advanced pulmonary or hepatic dysfunction, congestive heart failure, heart failure, renal failure)
ASA 5	Moribund patient unlikely to survive 24 hours with or without operation

For procedures performed on an emergency basis, the letter "**E**" should be added to the ASA status.

AMBULATORY SURGERY DISCHARGE SCORING SYSTEMS

Postanesthesia Discharge Scoring System (PADSS) and Modified Postanesthetic Discharge Scoring System (MPADSS)[1]

PADSS	MPADSS	Score
Vital signs	*Vital signs*	
Within 20% of preoperative value	Within 20% of preoperative value	2
Within 20% to 40% of preoperative value	Within 20% to 40% of preoperative value	1
40% of preoperative value	40% of preoperative value	0
Ambulation and mental status	*Ambulation*	
Oriented x 3 **and** has a steady gait	Steady gait/no dizziness	2
Oriented x 3 **or** has a steady gait	With assistance	1
Neither	None/dizziness	0
Pain, or nausea/vomiting	*Nausea/vomiting*	
Minimal	Minimal	2
Moderate	Moderate	1
Severe	Severe	0
Surgical bleeding	*Surgical bleeding*	
Minimal	Minimal	2
Moderate	Moderate	1
Severe	Severe	0
Intake and output	*Pain*	
P.O. fluids **and** voided	Minimal	2
P.O. fluids **or** voided	Moderate	1
Neither	Severe	0

[1]Used to determine readiness of ambulatory surgery patient to be discharged from phase II recovery; patients with a score of 9 or above are considered fit for discharge.

Adapted from Chung F, "Discharge Process," *The Ambulatory Anesthesia Handbook*, Twersky RS, ed, New York, NY: Mosby-Year Book, Inc, 1995, 431-49.

CRITERIA FOR ASSESSING FAST-TRACK ELIGIBILITY IN OUTPATIENTS [ABILITY TO SKIP PHASE I (PACU) RECOVERY]

The patient must meet all the criteria below to be eligible to bypass phase I (PACU) recovery and in the judgment of the anesthesia provider, be capable of transfer to the step-down unit.[1]

- Awake, alert, oriented, responsive (or return to baseline)
- Minimal pain
- Minimal nausea
- No vomiting
- No active bleeding
- Vital signs stable (not likely to require pharmacologic intervention)
- Patient can perform a 5-second head lift if a nondepolarizing neuromuscular blocking agent used
- Oxygen saturation of 94% on room air (3 minutes or longer) **or** return of oxygen saturation to baseline or higher

A minimal score of 12 (with no score <1 in any individual category) is required to bypass phase I (PACU) recovery

	Score
Level of consciousness	
Awake and oriented	2
Arousable with minimal stimulation	1
Responsive only to tactile stimulation	0
Physical activity	
Able to move all extremities on command	2
Some weakness in movement of extremities	1
Unable to voluntarily move extremities	0
Hemodynamic stability	
Blood pressure <15% of baseline mean arterial pressure (MAP)	2
Blood pressure 15% to 30% of baseline MAP	1
Blood pressure >30% below baseline MAP value	0
Respiratory stability	
Able to breathe deeply	2
Tachypnea with good cough	1
Dyspneic with weak cough	0
Oxygen saturation status	
Maintains value >90% on room air	2
Requires supplemental oxygen (nasal prongs)	1
Saturation <90% with supplemental oxygen	0
Postoperative pain assessment	
None or mild discomfort	2
Moderate to severe pain controlled with I.V. analgesics	1
Persistent severe pain	0
Postoperative emetic symptoms	
None or mild nausea with no active vomiting	2
Transient vomiting or retching	1
Persistent moderate to severe nausea and vomiting	0
Total score	**14**

[1]Patients evaluated in the operating room suite using the criteria.

References

Apfelbaum JL, "Current Controversies in Adult Outpatient Anesthesia," ASA Annual Refresher Course Lecture, Dallas, TX, 1999.

White PF and Song D, "New Criteria for Fast-Tracking After Outpatient Anesthesia: A Comparison With the Modified Aldrete's Scoring System," *Anesth Analg*, 1999, 88(5):1069-72.

FACTORS ASSOCIATED WITH POSTOPERATIVE NAUSEA AND VOMITING (PONV)

Patient-Related

Female gender
Obesity
Infants and small children
Surgery during days of menstruation and ovulation
History of previous PONV
History of motion sickness
Gastroparesis
Preoperative anxiety

Surgical Procedure

Children
- Middle ear surgery, eye surgery (especially strabismus surgery), hernia surgery, tonsillectomy/adenoidectomy, otoplasty, orchiopexy

Adults
- Laparoscopic gynecological surgery, extracorporeal shock-wave lithotripsy, abortion, head and neck surgery, gastrointestinal (GI) surgery, ear surgery

Increased incidence with increased duration of surgery

Anesthetic

Premedication with opioids
Inappropriate mask and bag ventilation
Inhalation anesthesia (vs total I.V. anesthesia)
Nitrous oxide-opioid-relaxant technique
Ketamine induction/maintenance
Etomidate induction
Use of anticholinesterase (eg, neostigmine) agents

Postoperative

Pain
Dizziness
Ambulation attempted too early
Changes in position
Hypotension
Oral intake attempted too early
Opioid administration

INHALATIONAL ANESTHETICS

Factors Affecting Minimum Alveolar Concentration (MAC)

Variable	Effect on MAC
Age	
Young	↑
Elderly	↓
Alcohol	
Acute intoxication	↓
Chronic abuse	↑
Anemia	
Hematocrit <10%	↓
Blood pressure	
MAP <40 mm Hg	↓
Drugs	
Anesthetics, local	↓
Barbiturates	↓
Benzodiazepines	↓
Ketamine	↓
Lithium	↓
Opioids	↓
Sympatholytics	
Clonidine	↓
Dexmedetomidine	↓
Sympathomimetics	
Amphetamine	
Acute	↑
Chronic	↓
Cocaine	↑
Ephedrine	↑
MAOI	↑
Verapamil	↓
Electrolytes	
Hypercalcemia	↓
Hypernatremia	↑
Hyponatremia	↓
PaO_2 <40 mm Hg	↓
$PaCO_2$ >95 mm Hg	↓
Pregnancy	↓
Temperature	
Hyperthermia (>42°C)	↑
Hypothermia	↓
Thyroid	
Hyperthyroid	No change
Hypothyroid	No change

Modified from Morgan GE and Mikhail MS, eds, *Clinical Anesthesiology*, East Norwalk, CT: Appleton & Lange, 1992.

Modified from Stoelting RK and Miller RD, eds, *Basics of Anesthesia*, 3rd ed, New York, NY: Churchill Livingstone, 2000.

Effects of Inhalational Anesthetics on Organ Systems

	Desflurane	Enflurane	Halothane	Isoflurane	Nitrous Oxide	Sevoflurane
MAC (%)[1]	6.0	1.68	0.74	1.2	105	2.6
Blood/Gas Partition Coefficient[2]	0.42	1.9	2.4	1.4	0.47	0.63
Cardiovascular						
Blood pressure	↓↓	↓↓	↓↓	↓↓	No change	↓↓
Cardiac output[3]	No change	↓↓	↓	No change	No change	No change
Heart rate	↑	↑	↓	↑	No change	No change
Systemic vascular resistance	↓↓	↓	No change	↓↓	No change	↓
Cerebral						
Blood flow	↑	↑	↑↑	↑	↑↑	↑
Intracranial pressure	↑	↑↑	↑↑	↑	↑	↑
Seizures	↓	↑	↓	↓	↓	↓
Hepatic						
Blood flow	↓	↓↓	↓↓	↓	↓	↓
Metabolism[4]	0.02%	2% to 5%	15% to 50%	0.2%	0.004%	3% to 5%
Neuromuscular						
Nondepolarizing blockade	↑↑↑	↑↑↑	↑↑	↑↑↑	↑	↑↑↑
Renal						
Glomerular filtration rate	?	↓↓	↓↓	↓↓	↓↓	?
Renal blood flow	↓	↓↓	↓↓	↓↓	↓↓	↓
Urinary output	?	↓↓	↓↓	↓↓	↓↓	?

INHALATIONAL ANESTHETICS *(Continued)*

Effects of Inhalational Anesthetics on Organ Systems *(continued)*

	Desflurane	Enflurane	Halothane	Isoflurane	Nitrous Oxide	Sevoflurane
Respiratory						
$PaCO_2$						
Resting	↑	↑↑	↑	↑	No change	↑
Challenge	↑	↑↑	↑	↑	↑	↑
Respiratory rate	↑	↑↑	↑↑	↑	↑	↑
Tidal volume	↓	↓	↓	↓	↓	↓

[1]Minimum alveolar concentration (MAC) = percentage of inspired concentration to prevent 50% of patients from moving to surgical stimulus (ED_{50}).

[2]Solubility of gas in blood at 37°C; less soluble gases have faster onset of action.

[3]Controlled ventilation.

[4]Metabolism = percentage of absorbed anesthetic undergoing metabolism.

Modified from Morgan GE and Mikhail MS, "Clinical Anesthesiology," New York, NY: Lange Medical Books/McGraw-Hill, 1996:138.

INTRAVENOUS ANESTHETIC AGENTS

Agent	Anesthesia Bolus	Anesthesia Maintenance	Sedation Bolus	Sedation Maintenance
Diazepam	0.3-0.6 mg/kg	—	0.04-0.2 mg/kg	—
Etomidate	0.2-0.5 mg/kg	10-20 mcg/kg/min	—	—
Ketamine	1-2 mg/kg	15-75 mcg/kg/min	0.5-1 mg/kg	—
Lorazepam	0.02-0.05 mg/kg	—	0.03-0.05 mg/kg	—
Methohexital	1-2 mg/kg	50-150mcg/kg/min	0.25-1 mcg/kg	10-50 mcg/kg/min
Midazolam	0.2-0.6 mg/kg	0.25-2 mcg/kg/min	0.01-0.1 mg/kg	
Propofol	1.5-2.5 mg/kg	100-200 mcg/kg/min	0.25-1 mcg/kg	25-100 mcg/kg/min
Thiopental	3-5 mg/kg	30-200 mcg/kg/min	0.5-1.5 mg/kg	—

LOCAL ANESTHETICS

Amides – Use / Concentration

Agent	Use	Concentration
Bupivacaine	Infil, PNB, epid, spin	0.25% (infil); 0.25%, 0.5% (PNB); 0.25%, 0.5%, 0.75% (epid); 0.5%, 0.75% (spin)
Etidocaine	Infil, PNB, epid	0.25%, 0.5% (infil); 0.5%, 1% (PNB, epid)
Lidocaine	PNB, epid, infil, spin, topical, bier	1%, 1.5%, 2% (PNB, epid); 5% (spin); 2%, 2.5%, 5% (topical); 0.5%, 1% (infil); 0.5% (bier)
Mepivacaine	Infil, PNB, epid	1% (infil); 1%, 2% (PNB), 1%, 1.5%, 2% (epid)
Prilocaine	Infil, PNB. epid	1%, 2% (infil); 1%, 2%, 3% (PNB, epid)
Ropivacaine	Infil, PNB, epid, spin	0.5% (infil); 0.5% (PNB), 0.5%, 0.75% (epid)

epid = epidural; infil = infiltration; PNB = peripheral nerve block; spin = spinal.

Esters – Use / Concentration

Agent	Use	Concentration
Chloroprocaine	Epid, infil, PNB	1% (infil); 1%, 2% (PNB); 2%, 3% (epid, spin)
Cocaine	Anesthetize and constrict nasal mucosa prior to nasal intubation; nasal surgery; vasoconstriction properties	4% (topical)
Procaine	Infil, PNB, spin	1%, 2% (infil); 5% (spinal)
Tetracaine	Spinal, topical	0.1%, 0.5% (spinal); 2% (topical)

epid = epidural; infil = infiltration; PNB = peripheral nerve block; spin = spinal.

Pharmacodynamics / Kinetics, Maximum Dose, and Toxic Threshold Concentration

Agent	pKa	Protein Binding (%)	Onset	Duration[1] (h)	Maximum Dose (mg/kg)	Toxic Threshold Concentration (mcg/mL)
Bupivacaine	8.1	95	Intermediate	1.5-8.5	2.5	1.6
Chloroprocaine	9.2	<10	Rapid	0.5-1	12	—
Etidocaine	7.7	90-94	Rapid	4-10	4	2.0
Lidocaine	7.8	70-75	Rapid	1-4	5 w/o epi; 7 w/epi	5-6
Mepivacaine	7.6	75	Rapid	2-3	5 w/o epi; 7 w/epi	5-6
Prilocaine	7.8	50	Rapid	2-6	8	5-6
Procaine	8.9	<10	Slow	0.5-1	12	—
Ropivacaine	8.1	95	Intermediate	1.5-9	3	ND
Tetracaine	8.2	75-80	Slow	1-3 (topical)	3	—

[1]Duration of action depends on site of local anesthetic administration.

MALIGNANT HYPERTHERMIA

SIGNS AND SYMPTOMS

Tachycardia (unexplained)	Fever
Increased end-tidal carbon dioxide	Cyanosis
Arrhythmias (ventricular)	Hypoxemia
Acidosis (respiratory, metabolic)	Hyperkalemia
Muscle rigidity	Coagulopathy (eg, DIC)
Tachypnea	Myoglobinuria

THERAPY FOR MALIGNANT HYPERTHERMIA EMERGENCY

CAUTION: This protocol may not apply to every patient and must of necessity be altered according to specific patient needs.

1. Immediately discontinue all inhalation anesthetics and succinylcholine. Hyperventilate with 100% oxygen at high gas flows (≥10 L/minute).
2. In the absence of blood gas analysis, bicarbonate 1-2 mEq/kg should be administered.
3. Dantrolene sodium should be obtained, mixed with 60 mL of sterile water for injection USP (without a bacteriostatic agent), and 2.5 mg/kg administered intravenously. At present, dantrolene is packaged as a lyophilized preparation that contains 20 mg of dantrolene and 3 g mannitol per vial.
4. Simultaneously, cooling should be started by all routes: surface, nasogastric lavage, intravenous cold solutions, wound, and rectally.
5. Arrhythmias will usually respond to treatment of acidosis and hyperkalemia. If they persist or are life-threatening, standard antiarrhythmic agents may be used, with the exception of calcium channel blockers.
6. Administer further doses of dantrolene as necessary titrated to heart rate, muscle rigidity, and temperature. Response to dantrolene should begin to occur in minutes; if not, more drug should be administered. Although the average successful dose of dantrolene is about 2.5 mg/kg, much higher doses may be needed (≥10 mg/kg). Fortunately, dantrolene does not produce significant myocardial depression at these doses.
7. Change anesthetic tubing.
8. Determine and monitor closely urine output, serum potassium, calcium, arterial blood gases, end tidal CO_2, and clotting studies. Hyperkalemia is common in the acute phase of MH and should be treated with intravenous glucose and insulin.
9. Observe the patient in an ICU setting for at least 24 hours since recrudescence of MH may occur, particularly following a case that was difficult to treat.
10. Follow CK, calcium, potassium, and clotting studies until such time as they return.
11. ECG should also be obtained and followed postoperatively.
12. Monitor body temperature closely since overvigorous treatment of MH may lead to hypothermia. Temperature instability may persist for several days after the acute episode. Body temperatures of 41°C to 42°C are compatible with survival and normal brain function if treated promptly.
13. Ensure urine output >1 mL/kg/hour. Consider CVP monitoring because of fluid shifts that may occur.
14. When the patient's condition has stabilized, convert from intravenous to oral dantrolene. Although data are not available regarding optimal doses and duration of treatment with dantrolene after an episode, the patient should probably receive a total dose of 4 mg/kg/day in divided doses for 48 hours postoperatively.
15. Counsel the patient and family regarding MH and further precautions. Refer patient to the Malignant Hyperthermia Association of the United States (MHAUS).

Malignant Hyperthermia Hotline (209) 634-4917

SKIN DERMATOMES

A dermatome is defined as that area of the skin supplied by a single spinal nerve. The body, with the exception of the face, is supplied in sequence by dermatomes C2 through S5. Knowledge of the distribution of spinal nerves is helpful in interpreting the effects of epidural and spinal anesthesia.

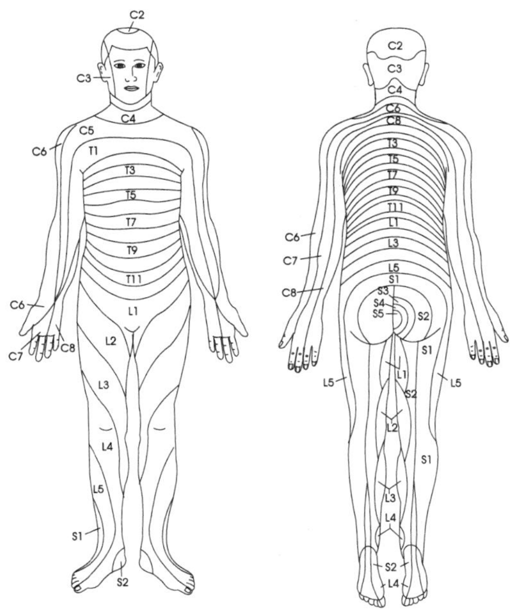

Skin dermatomes corresponding to respective sensory innervation by spinal nerves.

CEPHALOSPORINS BY GENERATION

First Generation	2nd Generation	3rd Generation	4th Generation
Cefadroxil (Duricef®)[1]	Cefaclor (Ceclor®)[1]	Cefdinir (Omnicef®)	Cefepime (Maxipime®)[2]
Cefazolin (Ancef®)	Cefamandole (Mandol®)	Cefixime (Suprax®)[1]	
Cephalexin (Keflex®)[1]	Cefmetazole (Zefazone®)	Cefotaxime (Claforan®)	
Cephalothin (Keflin®)	Ceforanide (Precef®)	Cefpodoxime (Vantin®)[1]	
Cephradine (Anspor®)[1]	Cefotetan (Cefotan®)	Ceftizoxime (Cefizox®)	
	Cefoxitin (Mefoxin®)	Ceftriaxone (Rocephin®)	
	Cefprozil (Cefzil®)[1]	Ceftazidime (Fortaz)[2]	
	Cefuroxime (Zinacef®)[1]		
	Cefuroxime axetil (Ceftin®)		
	Loracarbef (Lorabid®)		

[1]Oral dosage form available.

[2]Antipseudomonal activity notable.

Note: Other brand names or generic products may be available.

MULTIVITAMIN PRODUCTS

Injectable Formulations

Product	A (int. units)	B_1 (mg)	B_2 (mg)	B_6 (mg)	B_{12} (mcg)	C (mg)	D (int. units)	E (int. units)	K (mcg)	Additional Information
Solution										
Infuvite® Adult (per 10 mL)	3300	6	3.6	6	5	200	200	10	150	Supplied as two 5 mL vials. Biotin 60 mcg, folic acid 600 mcg, niacinamide 40 mg, dexpanthenol 15 mg
Infuvite® Pediatric (per 5 mL)	2300	1.6	1.4	1	1	80	400	7	200	Supplied as one 4 mL vial and one 1 mL vial. Biotin 20 mcg, folic acid 140 mcg, niacinamide 17 mg, dexpanthenol 5 mg
M.V.I.®-12 (per 10 mL) [DSC]	3300	3	3.6	4	12.5	100	200	10	–	Supplied as two 5 mL vials or a single 2-chambered 10 mL vial. Biotin 60 mcg, folic acid 400 mcg, niacinamide 40 mg, dexpanthenol 15 mg
M.V.I. Adult™ (per 10 mL)	3300	6	3.6	6	5	200	200	10	150	Supplied as two 5 mL vials or a single 2-chambered 10 mL vial. Also available in a pharmacy bulk package (two 50 mL vials). Biotin 60 mcg, folic acid 600 mcg, niacinamide 40 mg, dexpanthenol 15 mg
Powder for Reconstitution										
M.V.I.® Pediatric	2300	1.2	1.4	1	1	80	400	7	200	Biotin 20 mcg, folic acid 140 mcg, niacinamide 17 mg, dexpanthenol 5 mg, aluminum, polysorbate 80

MULTIVITAMIN PRODUCTS *(Continued)*

Adult Formulations

Product	A (int. units)	B_1 (mg)	B_2 (mg)	B_6 (mg)	B_{12} (mcg)	C (mg)	D (int. units)	E (int. units)	Additional Information
Liquid									
Centrum® [OTC] (per 15 mL)	2500	1.5	1.7	2	6	60	400	30	Biotin 300 mcg, Cr 25 mcg, Fe 9 mg, iodine 150 mcg, Mn 2 mg, Mo 25 mg, niacin 20 mg, pantothenic acid 10 mg, Zn 3 mg; alcohol 5.4%, sodium benzoate (240 mL)
Geriation® [OTC] (per 30 mL)		5	2.5	1	1				Choline 100 mg, Fe 15 mg, iodine 100 mcg, Mg 2 mg, Mn 2 mg, niacinamide 50 mg, pantothenic acid 10 mg, Zn 2 mg; sherry flavor (480 mL)
Geritol® Tonic [OTC] (per 15 mL)		2.5	2.5	0.5					Chlorine bitartrate 50 mg, Fe 18 mg, methionine 25 mg, niacin 50 mg, pantothenic acid 2 mg; sugars 7 g, alcohol 12%, benzoic acid (120 mL, 360 mL)
Strovite® Forte (per 15 mL)	4000	15	17	20	20	300	400	30	Biotin 150 mcg, Cr 50 mcg, Cu 3 mg, Fe 10 mg, folic acid 1 mg, Mg 50 mg, Mn 5 mg, niacinamide 100 mg, pantothenic acid 25 mg, Se 55 mcg, Zn 15 mg; contains aspartame
Vi-Daylin® [OTC] (per 5 mL) [DSC]	2500	1.05	1.2	1.05	4.5	60	400	15	Niacin 13.5 mg; alcohol <0.5%, benzoic acid; lemon/orange flavor (240 mL, 480 mL)
Vi-Daylin® + Iron [OTC] (per 5 mL) [DSC]	2500	1.05	1.2	1.05	4.5	60	400	15	Fe 10 mg, niacin 13.5 mg; alcohol <0.5%, benzoic acid; lemon/orange flavor (240 mL, 480 mL)
Caplet									
Glutofac®-MX (per 1 light purple caplet and 1 dark purple caplet)					10				Ascorbic acid 100 mg, biotin 300 mcg, boron 150 mcg, Ca 425 mg, Cr 200 mcg, dioctyl sodium sulfosuccinate 10 mg, Fe 15 mg, folic acid 800 mcg, iodine 150 mcg, Mg 415 mg, Mn 5 mg, Mo 75 mcg, nickel 5 mcg, pantothenic acid 25 mg, phosphorus 130 mg, potassium 80 mg, Se 100 mcg, tin 10 mcg, vanadium 10 mcg, Zn 35 mg
Glutofac®-ZX	5000	20	20	25	50	500	400	50	Biotin 200 mcg, Ca 66 mg, Cr 200 mcg, Cu 2.5 mg, niacinamide 100 mg, folic acid 1000 mcg, Mg 50 mg, Mn 5 mg, pantothenic acid 25 mg, Se 50 mcg, Zn 20 mg

Adult Formulations *(continued)*

Product	A (int. units)	B_1 (mg)	B_2 (mg)	B_6 (mg)	B_{12} (mcg)	C (mg)	D (int. units)	E (int. units)	Additional Information
Theragran® Heart Right™ [OTC] [DSC]	5000	3	3.4	16	30	120	400	400	Alpha-carotene, beta-carotene, biotin 30 mcg, Ca 55 mg, Cr 50 mcg, cryptoxanthin, Cu 1.5 mg, Fe 4 mg, folic acid as folate 0.6 mg, iodine 150 mcg, lutein, lycopene, Mg 150 mg, Mn 2 mg, Mo 75 mcg, niacin 20 mg, pantothenic acid 10 mg, Se 70 mcg, vitamin K 14 mcg, zeaxanthin, Zn 15 mg
Theragran-M® Advanced Formula [OTC] [DSC]	5000	3	3.4	6	12	90	400	60	Biotin 30 mcg, boron 150 mcg, Ca 40 mg, chloride 7.5 mg, Cr 50 mcg, Cu 2 mg, Fe 9 mg, folic acid 0.4 mg, iodine 150 mcg, Mg 100 mg, Mn 2 mg, Mo 75 mcg, niacin 20 mg, nickel 5 mcg, pantothenic acid 10 mg, phosphorus 31 mg, potassium 7.5 mg, Se 70 mcg, silicon 2 mg, tin 10 mcg, vanadium 10 mcg, vitamin K 28 mcg, Zn 15 mg
Capsule									
Hemocyte Plus®		10	6	5	15	200			Cu 0.8 mg, Fe 106 mg, folic acid 1 mg, Mg 6.9 mg, Mn 1.3 mg, niacinamide 30 mg, pantothenic acid 10 mg, Zn 18.2 mg
Multiret Folic 500		6	6	5	25	500			Calcium pantothenate 10 mg, Fe 525 mg (timed-release), niacinamide 30 mg
Ocuvite® Lutein						60		30	Cu 2 mg, lutein 6 mg, Zn 15 mg
Replace [OTC] (per 2 capsules)	5000	25	25	25	25	60	75	30	Betaine 20 mg, biotin 20 mcg, Ca 180 mg, choline 25 mg, Cr 50 mcg, Cu 0.1 mg, folic acid 400 mcg, inositol 25 mg, iodine 0.225 mg, lemon bioflavonoid complex 50 mg, Mg 90 mg, Mn 2.5 mg, Mo 20 mcg, niacin 40 mg, PABA 12.5 mg, pancreatin 50 mg, pantothenic acid 75 mg, potassium 20 mg, Se 50 mcg, Zn 10 mg
Replace With Iron [OTC] (per 2 capsules)	5000	25	25	25	25	60	75	30	Betaine 20 mg, biotin 20 mcg, Ca 180 mg, choline 25 mg, Cr 50 mcg, Cu 0.1 mg, Fe 10 mg, folic acid 400 mcg, inositol 25 mg, iodine 0.225 mg, lemon bioflavonoid complex 50 mg, Mg 90 mg, Mn 2.5 mg, Mo 20 mcg, niacin 40 mg, PABA 12.5 mg, pancreatin 50 mg, pantothenic acid 75 mg, potassium 20 mg, Se 50 mcg, Zn 10 mg

MULTIVITAMIN PRODUCTS *(Continued)*

Adult Formulations *(continued)*

Product	A (int. units)	B_1 (mg)	B_2 (mg)	B_6 (mg)	B_{12} (mcg)	C (mg)	D (int. units)	E (int. units)	Additional Information
Vicon Forte®	8000	10	5	2	10	150		50	Folic acid 1 mg, Mg 70 mg, Mn 4 mg, niacinamide 25 mg, Zn 80 mg
Vitacon Forte	8000	10	5	2	10	150		50	Folic acid 1 mg, Mg 70 mg, Mn 4 mg, niacinamide 25 mg, Zn 80 mg
Capsule, Softgel									
PreserVision® Lutein [OTC]						226		200	Cu 0.8 mg, lutein 5 mg, Zn 34.8 mg
PreserVision® AREDS [OTC]	14,320					226		200	Cu 0.8 mg, Zn 34.8 mg
Tablet									
Androvite® [OTC] (per 6 tablets)	2500	50	50	100	125	1000	400	400	Betaine 100 mg, boron 3 mg, Cr 200 mcg, Cu 2 mg, Fe 18 mg, folic acid 400 mcg, hesperidin 35 mg, inositol 36 mg, iodine 150 mcg, Mg 500 mg, Mn 10 mg, niacinamide 50 mg, PABA 25 mg, pancreatin 4X 75 mg, pantothenic acid 100 mg, rutin 25 mg, Se 200 mcg, Zn 50 mg
Centrum® [OTC]	3500	1.5	1.7	2	6	60	400	30	Biotin 30 mcg, boron 150 mcg, Ca 162 mg, chloride 72 mg, Cr 120 mcg, Cu 2 mg, Fe 18 mg, folic acid 0.4 mg, iodine 150 mcg, lutein 250 mcg, lycopene 300 mcg, Mg 100 mg, Mn 2 mg, Mo 75 mcg, niacin 20 mg, nickel 5 mcg, pantothenic acid 10 mg, phosphorus 109 mg, potassium 80 mg, Se 20 mcg, silicon 2 mg, tin 10 mcg, vanadium 10 mcg, vitamin K 25 mcg, Zn 15 mg
Centrum® Carb Assist™ [OTC]	3500	4.5	5.1	6	18	120	400	60	Biotin 40 mcg, boron 60 mcg, Ca 100 mg, chloride 72 mg, Cr 120 mcg, Cu 2 mg, Fe 18 mg, folic acid 400 mcg, ginkgo biloba leaf 60 mg, ginseng root 50 mg, iodine 150 mcg, Mg 40 mg, Mo 75 mcg, niacin 40 mg, nickel 5 mcg, pantothenic acid 10 mg, phosphorus 48 mg, potassium 80 mg, Se 70 mcg, silicon 4 mg, tin 10 mcg, vanadium 10 mcg, vitamin K 25 mcg, Zn 15 mg

Adult Formulations *(continued)*

Product	A (int. units)	B_1 (mg)	B_2 (mg)	B_6 (mg)	B_{12} (mcg)	C (mg)	D (int. units)	E (int. units)	Additional Information
Centrum® Performance™ [OTC]	3500	4.5	5.1	6	18	120	400	60	Biotin 40 mcg, boron 60 mcg, chloride 72 mg, folic acid 0.4 mg, Ca 100 mg, Cr 120 mcg, Cu 2 mg, Fe 18 mg, ginkgo biloba leaf 60 mg, ginseng root 50 mg, iodine 150 mcg, Mg 40 mg, Mn 4 mg, Mo 75 mcg, niacin 40 mg, nickel 5 mcg, pantothenic acid 10 mg, phosphorus 48 mg, potassium 80 mg, Se 70 mcg, silicon 4 mg, tin 10 mcg, vanadium 10 mcg, vitamin K 25 mcg, Zn 15 mg
Centrum® Silver® [OTC]	3500	1.5	1.7	3	25	60	400	45	Biotin 30 mcg, boron 150 mcg, Ca 200 mg, chloride 72 mg, Cr 150 mcg, Cu 2 mg, folic acid 0.4 mg, iodine 150 mcg, lutein 250 mcg, lycopene 300 mcg, Mg 100 mg, Mn 2 mg, Mo 75 mcg, niacin 20 mg, nickel 5 mcg, pantothenic acid 10 mg, phosphorus 48 mg, potassium 80 mg, Se 20 mcg, silicon 2 mg, vanadium 10 mcg, vitamin K 10 mcg, Zn 15 mg
Diatx®ZN		1.5	1.5		2	60			Cu 1.5 mg, D-biotin 300 mcg, folic acid 5 mg, niacinamide 20 mg, pantothenic acid 10 mg, Zn 25 mg [gluten free, lactose free, sugar free, yeast free]
Freedavite [OTC]	5000	1.5	1.7	2	6	60	400	30	Biotin 30 mcg, Ca 20 mg, Cu 0.1 mg, Fe 1.8 mg, folic acid 400 mcg, iodine 75 mcg, Mg 8 mg, Mn 0.625 mg, niacinamide 20 mg, pantothenic acid 10 mg, Se 35 mcg, Zn 1.5 mg
Geri-Freeda [OTC]	5000	15	15	15	15	150	400	15	Betaine 10 mg, biotin 15 mcg, Ca 50 mg, choline 10 mg, Cr 60 mcg, Cu 0.5 mg, folic acid 400 mcg, hesperidin 10 mg, inositol 25 mg, iodine 150 mcg, L-lysine 25 mg, Mg 25 mg, Mn 1 mg, niacinamide 50 mg, PABA 10 mg, pantothenic aicd 15 mg, Se 35 mcg, Zn 7.5 mg
Geritol Complete® [OTC]	6100	1.5	1.7	2	6.7	57	400	30	Biotin 44 mcg, Ca 148 mg, chloride 20 mg, Cr 12 mcg, Cu 1.8 mg, Fe 16 mg, folic acid 0.38 mg, iodine 120 mcg, Mg 86 mg, Mn 2.4 mg, Mo 1 mcg, niacin 20 mg, pantothenic acid 13 mg, phosphorous 118 mg, potassium 36 mg, vitamin K 24 mcg, Zn 13.5 mg

MULTIVITAMIN PRODUCTS *(Continued)*

Adult Formulations *(continued)*

Product	A (int. units)	B_1 (mg)	B_2 (mg)	B_6 (mg)	B_{12} (mcg)	C (mg)	D (int. units)	E (int. units)	Additional Information
Geritol Extend® [OTC]	3333	1.2	1.3	2	2.5	55	200	13	Ca 120 mg, Fe 9.5 mg, folic acid 0.2 mg, iodine 130 mcg, Mg 32 mg, niacin 15 mg, phosphorous 98 mg, Se 35 mcg, vitamin K 80 mcg, Zn 14 mg
Gynovite® Plus [OTC] (per 6 tablets)	5000	10	10	20	125	180	400	400	Betaine 100 mg, biotin 125 mcg, boron 3 mg, Ca 500 mg, Cr 200 mcg, Cu 2 mg, Fe 18 mg, folic acid 400 mcg, hesperidin 35 mg, inositol 50 mg, iodine 150 mcg, Mg 600 mg, Mn 10 mg, niacin 20 mg, PABA 25 mg, pancreatin 4X 93 mg, pantothenic acid 10 mg, rutin 25 mg, Se 200 mcg, Zn 15 mg
Hemocyte Plus®		10	6	5	15	200			Cu 0.8 mg, Fe 106 mg, folic acid 1 mg, Mg 6.9 mg, Mn 1.3 mg, niacinamide 30 mg, pantothenic acid 10 mg, Zn 18.2 mg
Hi-Kovite [OTC] (per contents of 1 vitamin tablet plus 1 mineral tablet)	5000	10	10	10	10	200	400	30	Bioflavonoids 10 mg, biotin 30 mcg, Ca 120 mg, Cu 0.5 mg, Fe 9 mg, folic acid 400 mcg, inositol 10 mg, iodine 9 mg, L-lysine 10 mg, Mg 60 mg, Mn 1 mg, niacinamide 100 mg, PABA 10 mg, pantothenic acid 10 mg, potassium 35 mg, Se 17.5 mg, Zn 7.5 mg
Iberet®-500 [OTC]		4.96	5.4	3.7	22.5	500			Fe 95 mg (controlled release), niacin 27.2 mg, pantothenic acid 8.28 mg, sodium 65 mg
Iberet-Folic-500® [OTC]		6	6	5	25	500			Fe 105 mg (controlled release), folic acid 0.8 mg, niacinamde 30 mg, calcium pantothenate 10 mg
Monocaps [OTC]	5000	15	15	15	15	120	400	15	Biotin 15 mcg, Ca 50 mg, Cu 0.1 mg, Fe 14 mg, folic acid 400 mcg, iodine 150 mcg, lecithin 10 mg, L-lysine 10 mg, Mg 30 mg, Mn 1 mg, niacinamide 40 mg, PABA 10 mg, pantothenic acid 15 mg, Se 35 mcg, Zn 3.75 mg
Ocuvite® [OTC]	1000					200		60	Cu 2 mg, lutein 2 mg, Se 55 mcg, Zn 40 mg
Ocuvite® Extra [OTC]	1000		3			300		100	Cu 2 mg, L-glutathione 5 mg, lutein 2 mg, Mn 5 mg, niacinamide 40 mg, Se 55 mcg, Zn 40 mg

Adult Formulations *(continued)*

Product	A (int. units)	B_1 (mg)	B_2 (mg)	B_6 (mg)	B_{12} (mcg)	C (mg)	D (int. units)	E (int. units)	Additional Information
Olay® Vitamins Complete Women's [OTC]	5000	1.5	1.7	2	6	120	400	50	Biotin 30 mcg, boron 150 mcg, Ca 250 mg, chloride 36 mg, coenzyme Q_{10} 2 mg, Cr 120 mcg, Cu 5 mg, Fe 18 mg, folic acid 0.4 mg, iodine 150 mcg, lutein 250 mg, Mg 100 mg, Mn 2 mg, Mo 25 mcg, niacin 20 mg, nickel 5 mcg, pantothenic acid 10 mg, phosphorus 77 mg, potassium 40 mg, Se 25 mcg, silicon 2 mg, vanadium 10 mcg, Zn 15 mg
Olay® Vitamins Complete Women's 50+ [OTC]	5000	3	3.4	4	25	120	400	60	Biotin 30 mcg, boron 150 mcg, Ca 250 mg, chloride 72 mg, coenzyme Q_{10} 2 mg, Cr 120 mcg, Cu 5 mg, folic acid 0.4 mg, iodine 150 mcg, lutein 250 mg, Mg 120 mg, Mn 2 mg, Mo 25 mcg, niacin 20 mg, nickel 5 mcg, pantothenic acid 10 mg, phosphorus 48 mg, potassium 80 mg, Se 50 mcg, silicon 2 mg, vanadium 10 mcg, Zn 22 mg
Olay® Vitamins Even Complexion [OTC]	5000					120	100	60	Cu 2 mg, folic acid 200 mcg, Se 50 mcg, Zn 15 mg
One-A-Day® 50 Plus Formula [OTC]	2500	4.5	3.4	6	25	120	400	33	Biotin 30 mcg, Ca 120 mg, chloride 34 mg, Cr 180 mcg, Cu 2 mg, folic acid 0.4 mg, iodine 150 mcg, Mg 100 mg, Mn 4 mg, Mo 90 mcg, niacin 20 mg, pantothenic acid 15 mg, potassium 37.5 mg, Se 105 mcg, vitamin K 20 mcg, Zn 22.5 mg
One-A-Day® Active Formula [OTC]	5000	4.5	5.1	6	18	120	400	60	American ginseng 55 mg, biotin 40 mcg, boron 150 mcg, Ca 110 mg, chloride 180 mg, Cr 100 mcg, Cu 2 mg, Fe 9 mg, folic acid 0.4 mg, iodine 150 mcg, Mg 40 mg, Mn 2 mg, Mo 25 mcg, niacin 40 mg, nickel 5 mcg, pantothenic acid 10 mg, phosphorus 48 mg, potassium 200 mg, Se 45 mcg, silicon 6 mg, tin 10 mcg, vanadium 10 mcg, vitamin K 25 mcg, Zn 15 mg
One-A-Day® Carb Smart [OTC]	2500	2.2	2.5	3	9	90	400	45	Biotin 450 mcg, Ca 200 mg, Cr 200 mcg, Cu 2 mg, folic acid 400 mcg, Mg 100 mg, Mn 2 mg, Mo 75 mg, niacin 25 mg, pantothenic acid 15 mg, phosphorous 154 mg, potassium 99 mg, Se 105 mcg, vitamin K 25 mcg, Zn 22.5 mg

MULTIVITAMIN PRODUCTS *(Continued)*

Adult Formulations *(continued)*

Product	A (int. units)	B_1 (mg)	B_2 (mg)	B_6 (mg)	B_{12} (mcg)	C (mg)	D (int. units)	E (int. units)	Additional Information
One-A-Day® Cholesterol Plus™ [OTC]	2500	1.5	1.7	2	6	60	400	30	Biotin 50 mcg, Ca 100 mg, Cr 120 mcg, Cu 2 mg, folic acid 400 mcg, iodine 150 mg, Mg 100 mg, Mn 2 mg, Mo 75 mg, niacin 20 mg, pantothenic acid 10 mg, policosanol 10 mg, potassium 99 mg, Se 70 mcg, Zn 15 mg
One-A-Day® Essential Formula [OTC]	5000	1.5	1.7	2	6	60	400	30	Folic acid 0.4 mg, niacin 20 mg, pantothenic acid 10 mg
One-A-Day® Maximum Formula [OTC]	5000	1.5	1.7	2	6	60	400	30	Biotin 30 mcg, boron 150 mcg, Ca 210 mg, chloride 72 mg, Cr 120 mcg, Cu 2 mg, Fe 18 mg, folic acid 0.4 mg, iodine 150 mcg, lycopene 600 mcg, Mg 120 mg, Mn 2 mg, Mo 160 mcg, niacin 20 mg, nickel 5 mcg, pantothenic acid 5 mg, phosphorus 109 mg, potassium 100 mg, Se 105 mcg, silicon 2 mg, tin 10 mcg, vanadium 10 mcg, vitamin K 25 mcg, Zn 15 mg
One-A-Day® Men's Formula [OTC]	3500	1.2	1.7	3	18	90	400	45	Biotin 30 mcg, chloride 34 mg, Cr 150 mcg, Cu 2 mg, folic acid 0.4 mg, iodine 150 mcg, Mg 100 mg, Mn 3.5 mg, Mo 42 mcg, niacin 16 mg, pantothenic acid 10 mg, potassium 37.5 mg, Se 87.5 mcg, vitamin K 20 mcg, Zn 15 mg
One-A-Day® Today [OTC]	3000	1.1	1.7	3	18	75	400	33	Biotin 30 mcg, Ca 240 mg, Cr 120 mcg, Cu 2 mg, folic acid 0.4 mg, Mg 120 mg, Mn 2 mg, niacin 14 mg, pantothenic acid 5 mg, potassium 100 mg, Se 70 mcg, soy extract 10 mg, vitamin K 20 mcg, Zn 15 mg
One-A-Day® Weight Smart [OTC]	2500	1.9	2.125	2.5	7.5	60	400	30	Ca 300 mg, Cr 200 mcg, Cu 2 mg, EGCG 32 mcg, Fe 18 mg, folic acid 400 mcg, Mg 50 mg, Mn 2 mg, niacin 25 mg, pantothenic acid 12.5 mg, Se 70 mcg, vitamin K 80 mcg, Zn 15 mg
One-A-Day® Women's Formula [OTC]	2500	1.5	1.7	2	6	60	400	30	Ca 450 mg, Fe 18 mg, folic acid 0.4 mg, Mg 50 mg, niacin 10 mg, pantothenic acid 5 mg, Zn 15 mg

Adult Formulations *(continued)*

Product	A (int. units)	B_1 (mg)	B_2 (mg)	B_6 (mg)	B_{12} (mcg)	C (mg)	D (int. units)	E (int. units)	Additional Information
Optivite® P.M.T. [OTC] (per 6 tablets)	125,000	25	25	300	60	1500	100	100	Betaine 100 mg, biotin 60 mcg, Ca 125 mg, choline 313 mg, citrus bioflavonioids 250 mg, Cr 100 mcg, Fe 15 mg, folic acid 200 mcg, inositol 24 mg, iodine 75 mcg, Mg 250 mg, Mn 10 mg, niacinamide 25 mg, PABA 25 mg, pancreatin 4X 93 mg, pantothenic acid 25 mg, potassium 48 mg, rutin 25 mg, Se 100 mcg, Zn 25 mg
PreserVision® AREDS [OTC]	14,320					226		200	Cu 0.8 mg, Zn 34.8 mg
Quintabs [OTC]	5000	30	30	30	30	300	400	50	Biotin 30 mcg, folic acid 400 mcg, niacinamide 100 mg, pantothenic acid 30 mg
Quintabs-M [OTC]	5000	30	30	30	30	300	400	50	Biotin 30 mcg, Ca 30 mg, Cu 0.2 mg, Fe 10 mg, folic acid 400 mcg, iodine 150 mcg, Mg 15 mg, Mn 2 mg, niacinamide 100 mg, PABA 10 mg, pantothenic acid 30 mg, Se 35 mcg, Zn 7.5 mg
T-Vites [OTC]		25	25	25	30	100	400		Biotin 30 mcg, folic acid 400 mcg, Mg 100 mg, Mn 0.5 mg, niacinamide 150 mg, pantothenic acid 25 mg, potassium 35 mg, Zn 3.75 mg
Ultra Freeda Iron Free [OTC] (per 3 tablets)	12,500	50	50	50	100	1000	400	200	Bioflavonoids 100 mg, biotin 300 mcg, Ca 250 mg, Cr 200 mcg, folic acid 800 mcg, Mg 100 mg, Mn 10 mg, Mo 12.5 mcg, niacinamide and niacin 100 mg, pantothenic acid 100 mg, potassium 35 mg, Se 100 mcg, Zn 22.5 mg
Ultra Freeda With Iron [OTC] (per 3 tablets)	5000	50	50	50	100	1000	400	200	Bioflavonoids 100 mg, biotin 300 mcg, Ca 250 mg, Cr 200 mcg, Fe 18 mg, folic acid 800 mcg, Mg 100 mg, Mn 10 mg, Mo 12.5 mcg, niacinamide and niacin 100 mg, pantothenic acid 100 mg, potassium 35 mg, Se 100 mcg, Zn 22.5 mg
Unicap Sr.® [OTC]	5000	1.2	1.4	2.2	3	60	200	15	Ca 100 mg, Cu 2 mg, Fe 10 mg, folic acid 400 mcg, iodine 150 mcg, Mg 30 mg, Mn 1 mg, niacin 16 mg, pantothenic acid 10 mg, phosphorus 77 mg, potassium 5 mg, Zn 15 mg

MULTIVITAMIN PRODUCTS *(Continued)*

Adult Formulations *(continued)*

Product	A (int. units)	B_1 (mg)	B_2 (mg)	B_6 (mg)	B_{12} (mcg)	C (mg)	D (int. units)	E (int. units)	Additional Information
Unicap T® [OTC]	5000	10	10	6	18	500	400	30	Cu 2 mg, Fe 18 mg, folic acid 400 mcg, iodine 150 mcg, Mn 1 mg, niacin 100 mg, pantothenic acid 25 mg, potassium 5 mg, Se 10 mg, Zn 15 mg
Xtramins [OTC]	1000	5	2	5	10	50	100	10	Boron 1 mg, Ca 250 mg, Cr 40 mcg, Cu 0.5 mg, d-calcium pantothenate 5 mg, Fe 10 mg, folic acid 400 mcg, iodine 150 mcg, Mg 20 mg, Mn 2 mg, niacinamide 15 mg, PABA 5 mg, potassium 45 mg, Se 30 mcg, Zn 10 mg
Tablet, Chewable									
Centrum® [OTC]	3500	1.5	1.7	2	6	60	400	30	Biotin 45 mcg, Ca 108 mg, Cr 20 mcg, Cu 2 mg, Fe 18 mg, folic acid 0.4 mg, iodine 150 mcg, Mg 40 mg, Mn 1 mg, Mo 20 mcg, niacin 20 mg, pantothenic acid 10 mg, phosphorus 50 mg, vitamin K 10 mcg, Zn 15 mg
Viactiv® Multivitamin [OTC] (softchews)	2500	1.5	1.7	2	6	60	400	33	Biotin 30 mcg, Ca 200 mg, folic acid 400 mcg, niacin 15 mg, pantothenic acid 10 mg; sodium 25 mg; milk chocolate or tropical fruit splash flavors

Ca = calcium, Cr = chromium, Cu = copper, Fe = iron, Mg = magnesium, Mn = manganese, Mo = molybdenum, Se = selenium, Zn = zinc.

Pediatric Formulations

Product	A (int. units)	B_1 (mg)	B_2 (mg)	B_6 (mg)	B_{12} (mcg)	C (mg)	D (int. units)	E (int. units)	Additional Information
Drops									
ADEKs [OTC] (per mL)	3170 (50% as beta carotene)	0.5	0.6	0.6	4	45	400	40	Biotin 15 mcg, niacin 6 mg, pantothenic acid 3 mg, vitamin K 0.1 mg, Zn 5 mg; alcohol free, dye free (60 mL)
Poly-Vi-Flor® 0.25 mg (per mL)	1500	0.5	0.6	0.4	2	35	400	5	**Fluoride 0.25 mg**, niacin 8 mg; fruit flavor (50 mL)
Poly-Vi-Flor® 0.5 mg (per mL)	1500	0.5	0.6	0.4	2	35	400	5	**Fluoride 0.5 mg**, niacin 8 mg; fruit flavor (50 mL)
Poly-Vi-Flor® With Iron 0.25 mg (per mL)	1500	0.5	0.6	0.4		35	400	5	**Fluoride 0.25 mg**, iron 10 mg, niacin 8 mg; fruit flavor (50 mL)
Poly-Vi-Sol® [OTC] (per mL)	1500	0.5	0.6	0.4	2	35	400	5	Niacin 8 mg (50 mL)
Poly-Vi-Sol® With Iron [OTC] (per mL)	1500	0.5	0.6	0.4		35	400	5	Iron 10 mg, niacin 8 mg (50 mL)
Soluvite-F® (per 0.6 mL)	1500					35	400		**Fluoride 0.25 mg**; alcohol free, dye free, orange flavor (57 mL)
Tri-Vi-Flor® 0.25 mg (per mL)	1500					35	400		**Fluoride 0.25 mg**; fruit flavor (50 mL)
Tri-Vi-Flor® With Iron 0.25 mg (per mL)	1500					35	400		**Fluoride 0.25 mg**, iron 10 mg; fruit flavor (50 mL)
Tri-Vi-Sol® [OTC] (per mL)	1500					35	400		Fruit flavor (50 mL)
Tri-Vi-Sol® With Iron [OTC] (per mL)	1500					35	400		Iron 10 mg; fruit flavor (50 mL)
Vi-Daylin® [OTC] (per mL) [DSC]	1500	0.5	0.6	0.4	1.5	35	400	5	Niacin 8 mg; alcohol <0.5%, sugar free, fruit flavor (50 mL)
Vi-Daylin® + Iron [OTC] (per mL) [DSC]	1500	0.5	0.6	0.4		35	400	5	Iron 10 mg, niacin 8 mg; alcohol <0.5%, sugar free, fruit flavor (50 mL)
Vi-Daylin® ADC [OTC] (per mL) [DSC]	1500					35	400		Alcohol <0.5%, sugar free, fruit flavor (50 mL)
Vi-Daylin® ADC + Iron [OTC] (per mL) [DSC]	1500					35	400		Iron 10 mg; benzoic acid, sugar free, fruit flavor (50 mL)
Vi-Daylin®/F (per mL) [DSC]	1500	0.5	0.6	0.4		35	400	5	**Fluoride 0.25 mg**, niacin 8 mg; alcohol <0.1%, benzoic acid, sugar free, fruit flavor (50 mL)
Vi-Daylin®/F + Iron (per mL) [DSC]	1500	0.5	0.6	0.4		35	400	5	**Fluoride 0.25 mg**, iron 10 mg, niacin 8 mg; alcohol <0.1%, benzoic acid, sugar free, fruit flavor (50 mL)
Vi-Daylin®/F ADC (per mL) [DSC]	1500					35	400		**Fluoride 0.25 mg**; sugar free, fruit flavor (50 mL)
Vi-Daylin®/F ADC + Iron (per mL) [DSC]	1500					35	400		**Fluoride 0.25 mg**, iron 10 mg; sugar free, fruit flavor (50 mL)

MULTIVITAMIN PRODUCTS *(Continued)*

Pediatric Formulations *(continued)*

Product	A (int. units)	B_1 (mg)	B_2 (mg)	B_6 (mg)	B_{12} (mcg)	C (mg)	D (int. units)	E (int. units)	Additional Information
Gum									
Vitaball®	5000	1.5	1.7	2	6	60	400	30	Biotin 45 mcg, folic acid 400 mcg, niacinamide 20 mg, pantothenic acid 10 mg; bubble gum, cherry, grape, and watermelon (contains tartrazine) flavors
Vitaball® Wild 'N Fruity [OTC]	5000	1.5	1.7	2	6	240	400	30	Biotin 45 mcg, folic acid 400 mcg, niacinamide 20 mg, pantothenic acid 10 mg; berry, lemon (contains tartrazine), orange, and strawberry flavors
Tablet, Chewable									
ADEKs® [OTC]	9000 (60% as beta carotene)	1.2	1.3	1.5	12	60	400	150	Biotin 50 mcg, folic acid 0.2 mg, niacin 10 mg, pantothenic acid 10 mg, vit K 150 mcg, Zn 7.5 mg; **dye free**
Centrum Kids® Jimmy Neutron™ Complete	5000	1.5	1.7	2	6	60	400	30	Biotin 45 mcg, Ca 108 mg, Cr 20 mcg, Cu 2 mg, Fe 18 mg, folic acid 0.4 mg, iodine 150 mcg, Mg 40 mg, Mn 1 mg, Mo 20 mcg, niacin 20 mg, pantothenic acid 10 mg, phosphorus 50 mg, vitamin K 10 mg, Zn 15 mg; **contains phenylalanine**; cherry, fruit punch, and orange flavors
Centrum Kids® Jimmy Neutron™ Extra C	5000	1.5	1.7	1	5	250	400	15	Ca 108 mg, Cu 0.5 mg, folic aicd 0.3 mg, niacin 13.5 mg, phosphorus 50 mg, sodium 16 mg, Zn 4 mg; **contains phenylalanine**; cherry, fruit punch, and orange flavors
Centrum® Kids Rugrats™ Complete [OTC]	5000	1.5	1.7	2	6	60	400	30	Biotin 45 mcg, Ca 108 mg, Cr 20 mcg, Cu 2 mg, Fe 18 mg, folic acid 0.4 mg, iodine 150 mcg, Mg 40 mg, Mn 1 mg, Mo 20 mcg, niacin 20 mg, pantothenic acid 10 mg, phosphorus 50 mg, vitamin K 10 mg, Zn 15 mg; **contains phenylalanine**; cherry, fruit punch, and orange flavors
Centrum® Kids Rugrats™ Extra C [OTC]	5000	1.5	1.7	1	5	250	400	15	Ca 108 mg, Cu 0.5 mg, folic acid 0.3 mg, niacin 13.5 mg, phosphorus 50 mg, sodium 15 mg, Zn 4 mg; **contains phenylalanine**; cherry, fruit punch, and orange flavors

Pediatric Formulations *(continued)*

Product	A (int. units)	B_1 (mg)	B_2 (mg)	B_6 (mg)	B_{12} (mcg)	C (mg)	D (int. units)	E (int. units)	Additional Information
Centrum® Kids Rugrats™ Extra Calcium [OTC]	5000	1.5	1.7	1	5	60	400	15	Ca 200 mg, Cu 0.5 mg, folic acid 0.3 mg, niacin 13.5 mg, phosphorus 50 mg, Zn 4 mg; **contains phenylalanine**; cherry, fruit punch, and orange flavors
Flintstones® Complete [OTC]	5000	1.5	1.7	2	6	60	400	30	Biotin 40 mcg, Ca 100 mg, Cu 2 mg, Fe 18 mg, folic acid 0.4 mg, iodine 150 mcg, Mg 20 mg, niacin 20 mg, pantothenic acid 10 mg, phosphorus 100 mg, Zn 15 mg; **phenylalanine 4.56 mg**; cherry, grape, and orange flavors
Flintstones® Plus Calcium [OTC]	2500	1.05	1.2	1.05	4.5	60	400	15	Ca 200 mg, folic acid 0.3 mg, niacin 13.5 mg; **phenylalanine <4 mg**; cherry, grape, and orange flavors
Flintstones® Plus Extra C [OTC]	2500	1.05	1.2	1.05	4.5	250	400	15	Folic acid 0.3 mg, niacin 13.5 mg; grape, orange, peach-apricot, raspberry, and strawberry flavors
Flintstones® Plus Iron [OTC]	2500	1.05	1.2	1.05	4.5	60	400	15	Fe 15 mg, folic acid 0.3 mg, niacin 13.5 mg; grape, orange, peach-apricot, raspberry, and strawberry flavors
My First Flintstones® [OTC]	2500	1.05	1.2	1.05	4.5	60	400	15	Folic acid 0.3 mg, niacin 13.5 mg; cherry, grape, and orange flavors
One-A-Day® Kids Bugs Bunny and Friends Complete [OTC]	3000	1.5	1.7	2	6	60	400	30	Biotin 40 mcg, Ca 100 mg, Cu 2 mg, Fe 18 mg, folic acid 0.4 mg, iodine 150 mcg, Mg 20 mg, niacin 15 mg, pantothenic acid 10 mg, phosphorus 100 mg, Zn 12 mg; **contains phenylalanine**; sugar free, fruity flavors
One-A-Day® Kids Bugs Bunny and Friends Plus Extra C [OTC]	2500	1.05	1.2	1.05	4.5	250	400	15	Folic acid 0.3 mg, niacin 13.5 mg, **contains phenylalanine**; sugar free, fruity flavors
One-A-Day® Kids Extreme Sports [OTC]	3000	1.5	1.7	2	6	60	400	30	Biotin 40 mcg, Ca 100 mg, Cu 2 mg, Fe 18 mg, folic acid 0.4 mg, iodine 150 mcg, Mg 20 mg, niacin 15 mg, pantothenic acid 10 mg, phosphorus 100 mg, Zn 12 mg; **contains phenylalanine**
One-A-Day® Kids Scooby-Doo! Complete [OTC]	3000	1.5	1.7	2	6	60	400	30	Biotin 40 mcg, Ca 100 mg, Cu 2 mg, Fe 18 mg, folic acid 0.4 mg, iodine 150 mcg, Mg 20 mg, niacin 15 mg, pantothenic acid 10 mg, phosphorus 100 mg, Zn 12 mg; **contains phenylalanine**; fruity flavors

MULTIVITAMIN PRODUCTS *(Continued)*

Pediatric Formulations *(continued)*

Product	A (int. units)	B_1 (mg)	B_2 (mg)	B_6 (mg)	B_{12} (mcg)	C (mg)	D (int. units)	E (int. units)	Additional Information
One-A-Day® Kids Scooby-Doo! Fizzy Vites [OTC]	1500	0.75	0.85	1	3	170	200	15	Biotin 20 mcg, Ca 50 mg, Cu 1 mg, Fe 9 mg, folic acid 0.2 mg, iodine 75 mcg, Mg 10 mg, niacin 7.5 mg, pantothenic acid 5 mg, phosphorus 50 mg, sodium 20 mg, Zn 6 mg; **contains phenylalanine**; crazy grape, orange pucker, and wild cherry flavors
One-A-Day® Kids Scooby-Doo! Plus Calcium [OTC]	2500	1.05	1.2	1.05	4.5	60	400	15	Ca 200 mg, folic acid 0.3 mg, niacin 13.5 mg; **contains phenylalanine**; fruity flavors
Poly-Vi-Flor® 0.25 mg	2500	1.05	1.2	1.05	4.5	60	400	15	Fluoride 0.25 mg, folic acid 0.3 mg, niacin 13.5 mg; fruity flavor
Poly-Vi-Flor® 0.5 mg	2500	1.05	1.2	1.05	4.5	60	400	15	Fluoride 0.5 mg, folic acid 0.3 mg, niacin 13.5 mg; fruity flavor
Poly-Vi-Flor® 1 mg	2500	1.05	1.2	1.05	4.5	60	400	15	Fluoride 1 mg, folic acid 0.3 mg, niacin 13.5 mg; fruity flavor
Poly-Vi-Flor® 0.25 mg With Iron	2500	1.05	1.2	1.05	4.5	60	400	15	Fluoride 0.25 mg, Cu 1 mg, folic acid 0.3 mg, iron 12 mg, niacin 13.5 mg, Zn 10 mg; fruity flavor
Poly-Vi-Flor® 0.5 mg With Iron	2500	1.05	1.2	1.05	4.5	60	400	15	Fluoride 0.5 mg, Cu 1 mg, folic acid 0.3 mg, iron 12 mg, niacin 13.5 mg, Zn 10 mg; fruity flavor

Ca = calcium, Cr = chromium, Cu = copper, Fe = iron, Mg = magnesium, Mn = manganese, Mo = molybdenum, Zn = zinc.

Prenatal Formulations

Product	A (int. units)	B_1 (mg)	B_2 (mg)	B_6 (mg)	B_{12} (mcg)	C (mg)	D (int. units)	E (int. units)	Additional Information
Caplet									
PreCare® Prenatal		3	3.4	50	12	50	6 mcg	3.5 mg	Ca 250 mg, Cu 2 mg, Fe 40 mg, folic acid 1 mg, Mg 50 mg, Zn 15 mg; dye free
StrongStart™	1000	3	3	20	12	100	400	30	Ca 200 mg, Fe 29 mg, folic acid 1 mg, niacinamide 15 mg, pantothenic acid 7 mg, Zn 20 mg; docusate sodium 25 mg
Capsule									
Anemagen™ OB		1.6	1.8	20	12	60	400	30	Ca 200 mg, Fe 28 mg, folic acid 1 mg; docusate calcium 25 mg
Chromagen OB®		1.6	1.8	20	12	60	400	30	Ca 200 mg, Cu 2 mg, Fe 28 mg, folic acid 1 mg, Mn 2 mg, niacinamide 5 mg, Zn 25 mg; docusate calcium 25 mg
Prenatal H		10	6	5	15	200			Cu 0.8 mg, Fe 106 mg, folic acid 1 mg, Mg 6.9 mg, Mn 1.3 mg, niacinamide 30 mg, pantothenic acid 10 mg, Zn 18.2 mg
Prenatal U		10	6	5	15	200			Cu 0.8 mg, Fe 106.5 mg, folic acid 1 mg, Mn 1.3 mg, niacinamide 30 mg, pantothenic acid 10 mg
Powder									
Obegyn® (per 4 level tsp/8.25 g)	2500 (as palmatate) 2500 (as beta-carotene)	1.7	2	10	12	120	400	60	Biotin 300 mcg, Ca 455 mg, Cu 2 mg, Fe 18 mg, folic acid 1 mg, iodine 150 mcg, Mg 150 mg, niacin 20 mg, pantothenic acid 10 mg, Zn 25 mg; **phenylalanine 84 mg/8.25 g**; orange flavor (495 g/60 doses)
Tablet									
A-Free Prenatal		2	2	1	2	33.3	133.3	10	Calcium 333.3 mg, biotin 10 mcg, Cu 0.1 mg, Fe 9 mg, folic acid 266.6 mcg, Mg 33.3 mg, Mn 0.1 mg, niacinamide 10 mg, pantothenic acid 5 mg, Zn 7.5 mg
Advanced NatalCare®	2700	3	3.4	20	12	120	400	30	Ca 200 mg, Cu 2 mg, Fe 90 mg, folic acid 1 mg, Mg 30 mg, niacinamide 20 mg, Zn 25 mg; docusate sodium 50 mg
Aminate Fe-90	4000	3	3.4	20	12	120	400	30	Ca 250 mg, Cu 2 mg, Fe 90 mg, folic acid 1 mg, iodine 150 mcg, niacinamide 20 mg, Zn 25 mg; docusate sodium 50 mg

MULTIVITAMIN PRODUCTS *(Continued)*

Prenatal Formulations *(continued)*

Product	A (int. units)	B_1 (mg)	B_2 (mg)	B_6 (mg)	B_{12} (mcg)	C (mg)	D (int. units)	E (int. units)	Additional Information
Cal-Nate™	2700	3	3.4	20		120	400	30	Ca 125 mg, Cu 2 mg, Fe 27 mg, folic acid 1 mg, iodine 150 mcg, niacinamide 20 mg, Zn 25 mg; docusate calcium 50 mg
Citracal® Prenatal Rx	2700	3	3.4	20		120	400	30	Ca 125 mg, Cu 2 mg, Fe 27 mg, folic acid 1 mg, iodine 150 mcg, niacinamide 20 mg, Zn 25 mg; docusate sodium 50 mg
Duet®	3000	1.8	4	25	12	120	400	30	Ca 200 mg, Cu 2 mg, Fe 29 mg, folic acid 1 mg, Mg 25 mg, niacinamide 20 mg, Zn 25 mg
KPN Prenatal	2666.6	2	2	1	2	33.3	133.3	10	Ca 333.3 mg, biotin 10 mcg, Cu 0.1 mg, Fe 9 mg, folic acid 266.6 mcg, Mg 33.3 mg, Mn 0.1 mg, niacinamide 10 mg, pantothenic acid 5 mg, Zn 7.5 mg
NatalCare® CFe 60 [DSC]	1000	2	3	10	12	120	400	11	Fe 60 mg, folic acid 1 mg, niacinamide 20 mg
NatalCare® GlossTabs™	2700	3	3.4	20	12	120	400	10	Biotin 30 mcg, Ca 200 mg, Cu 2 mg, Fe 90 mg, folic acid 1 mg, Mg 30 mg, niacinamide 20 mg, pantothenic acid 6 mg, Zn 15 mg; docusate sodium 50 mg
NatalCare® PIC	4000	2.43	3	1.64	3	50	400		Ca 125 mg, folic acid 1 mg, niacinamide 10 mg, polysaccharide-iron complex 60 mg, Zn 18 mg
NatalCare® PIC Forte	5000	3	3.4	4	12	80	400	30	Ca 250 mg, Cu 2 mg, folic acid 1 mg, iodine 200 mcg, Mg 10 mg, niacinamide 20 mg, polysaccharide-iron complex 60 mg, Zn 25 mg
NatalCare® Plus	4000	1.84	3	10	12	120	400	22	Ca 200 mg, Cu 2 mg, Fe 27 mg, folic acid 1 mg, niacinamide 20 mg, Zn 25 mg
NatalCare® Rx	2000	0.75	0.8	2	1.25	40	200	7.5	Biotin 15 mcg, Ca 100 mg, Cu 1.5 mg, folate 0.5 mg, Fe 27 mg, Mg 50 mg, niacin 8.5 mg, pantothenic acid 3.75 mg, Zn 12.5 mg
NatalCare® Three	3000	1.8	4	25	12	120	400	22	Ca 200 mg, Cu 2 mg, Fe 28 mg, folic acid 1 mg, Mg 25 mg, niacinamide 20 mg, Zn 25 mg
NataFort®	1000	2	3	10	12	120	400	11	Fe 60 mg, folic acid 1 mg, niacinamide 20 mg
NataTab™ CFe	4000	3	3	3	8	120	400	30	Ca 200 mg, Fe 50 mg, folic acid 1 mg, iodine 150 mcg, niacin 20 mg, Zn 15 mg

Prenatal Formulations *(continued)*

Product	A (int. units)	B_1 (mg)	B_2 (mg)	B_6 (mg)	B_{12} (mcg)	C (mg)	D (int. units)	E (int. units)	Additional Information
NataTab™ FA	4000	3	3	6	8	120	400	30	Ca 200 mg, Fe 29 mg, folic acid 1 mg, iodine 150 mcg, niacin 20 mg, Zn 15 mg
NataTab™ Rx	4000	3	3	3	8	120	400	30	Biotin 30 mcg, Ca 200 mg, Cu 3 mg, Fe 29 mg, folic acid 1 mg, iodine 150 mcg, Mg 100 mg, niacin 20 mg, pantothenic acid 7 mg, Zn 15 mg
Nestabs® CBF	4000	3	3	3	8	120	400	30	Ca 200 mg, Fe 50 mg, folic acid 1 mg, iodine 150 mcg, niacin 20 mg, Zn 15 mg
Nestabs® FA	4000	3	3	3	8	120	400	30	Ca 200 mg, Fe 29 mg, folic acid 1 mg, iodine 150 mcg, niacin 20 mg, Zn 15 mg
Nestabs® RX	4000	3	3	3	8	120	400	30	Biotin 30 mcg, Ca 200 mg, Cu 3 mg, Fe 29 mg, folic acid 1 mg, iodine 150 mcg, Mg 100 mg, niacin 20 mg, pantothenic acid 7 mg, Zn 15 mg
Niferex®-PN	4000	2.43	3	1.64	3	50	400		Ca 125 mg, folic acid 1 mg, niacinamide 10 mg, polysaccharide-iron complex 60 mg, Zn 18 mg
Niferex®-PN Forte	5000	3	3.4	4	12	80	400	30	Ca 250 mg, Cu 2 mg, folic acid 1 mg, iodine 200 mcg, Mg 10 mg, niacinamide 20 mg, polysaccharide-iron complex 60 mg, Zn 25 mg
OB-20	2000	43	0.5	2.5	2	30	100	15	Biotin 37.5 mcg, Ca 125 mg, Cr 6.25 mcg, Fe 12.5 mg, folic acid 2.5 mg, Mg 37.5 mg, Mn 1.25 mg, niacinamide 5 mg, pantothenic acid 2.5 mg, Se 6.25 mcg, Zn 6.2 mg
PreCare® Conceive™		3	3.4	50	12	60		30	Ca 200 mg, Cu 2 mg, Fe 30 mg, folic acid 1 mg, Mg 100 mg, niacinamide 20 mg, Zn 15 mg
Prenatal 1-A-Day	4000	2	3	3	10	100	400	15	Biotin 100 mcg, Ca 200 mg, Cu 2 mg, Fe 27 mg, folic acid 800 mcg, Mg 60 mg, Mn 2 mg, niacinamide 20 mg, pantothenic acid 10 mg, Zn 15 mg
Prenatal AD	2700	3	3.4	12	120	120	400	30	Ca 200 mg, Cu 2 mg, Fe 90 mg, folic acid 1 mg, Mg 30 mg, niacinamide 20 mg, Zn 25 mg; docusate sodium 50 mg
Prenatal MR 90 Fe™	4000	3	3.4	20	12	120	400	30	Ca 250 mg, Cu 2 mg, Fe 90 mg, folic acid 1 mg, iodine 150 mcg, niacinamide 20 mg, Zn 25 mg; docusate sodium 50 mg

MULTIVITAMIN PRODUCTS *(Continued)*

Prenatal Formulations *(continued)*

Product	A (int. units)	B_1 (mg)	B_2 (mg)	B_6 (mg)	B_{12} (mcg)	C (mg)	D (int. units)	E (int. units)	Additional Information
Prenatal MRT with Selenium	5000	3	3.4	10	12	120	400	30	Biotin 30 mcg, Ca 200 mg, Cr 25 mcg, Cu 2 mg, Fe 27 mg, folic acid 1 mg, iodine 150 mcg, Mg 25 mg, Mn 5 mg, Mo 25 mcg, niacinamide 20 mg, pantothenic acid 10 mg, Se 20 mcg, Zn 25 mg
Prenatal Plus	4000	1.8	3	10	12	120	400	22	Ca 200 mg, Cu 2 mg, Fe 27 mg, folic acid 1 mg, niacinamide 20 mg, Zn 25 mg
Prenatal Rx 1	4000	1.5	1.6	4	2.5	80	400	15	Biotin 30 mcg, Ca 200 mg, Cu 3 mg, Fe 60 mg, folic acid 1 mg, Mg 100 mg, niacinamide 17 mg, pantothenic acid 7 mg, Zn 25 mg
Prenatal Z	3000	1.5	1.6	2.2	2.2	70	400	10	Ca 200 mg, Fe 65 mg, folic acid 1 mg, iodine 175 mcg, Mg 100 mg, niacin 17 mg, Zn 15 mg
Prenate Elite™		3	3.4	20	12	120	400	10	Biotin 300 mcg, Ca 200 mg, Cu 2 mg, Fe 90 mg, folate 1 mg, Mg 30 mg, niacinamide 20 mg, pantothenic acid 6 mg, Zn 15 mg; docusate sodium 50 mg
Prenate GT™	2700	3	3.4	20	12	120	400	10	Biotin 30 mcg, Ca 200 mg, Cu 2 mg, Fe 90 mg, folic acid 1 mg, Mg 30 mg, niacinamide 20 mg, pantothenic acid 6 mg, Zn 15 mg; docusate sodium 50 mg
Stuartnatal® Plus 3™	3000	1.8	4	25	12	120	400	22	Ca 200 mg, Cu 2 mg, Fe 28 mg, folic acid 1 mg, Mg 25 mg, niacinamide 20 mg, Zn 25 mg
Stuart Prenatal®	4000	1.8	1.7	2.6	8	120	400	30	Ca 200 mg, Fe 28 mg, folic acid 0.8 mg, niacin 20 mg, Zn 25 mg
Trinate	3000	1.8	4	25	12	120	400	22	Ca 200 mg, Cu 2 mg, Fe 28 mg, folic acid 1 mg, Mg 25 mg, niacin 20 mg, Zn 25 mg
Ultra NatalCare®	2700	3	3.4	20	12	120	400	30	Ca 200 mg, Cu 2 mg, Fe 90 mg, folic acid 1 mg, iodine 150 mcg, niacinamide 20 mg, Zn 25 mg; docusate sodium 50 mg
Tablet, Chewable									
Duet®	3000	1.8	4	25	12	120	400	30	Ca 100 mg, Cu 2 mg, Fe 29 mg, folic acid 1 mg, Mg 25 mg, niacinamide 20 mg, Zn 25 mg; **phenylalanine 15 mg/tablet**
NataChew™	1000	2	3	10	12	120	400	11	Fe 29 mg, folic acid 1 mg, niacinamide 20 mg; peanut extract, wild berry flavor

Prenatal Formulations *(continued)*

Product	A (int. units)	B_1 (mg)	B_2 (mg)	B_6 (mg)	B_{12} (mcg)	C (mg)	D (int. units)	E (int. units)	Additional Information
NutriNate®	1000	2	3	10	12	120	400	11	Fe 29 mg, folic acid 1 mg, niacinamide 20 mg; wild berry flavor
PreCare®				2		50	6 mcg	3.5 mg	Ca 250 mg, Cu 2 mg, Fe 40 mg, folic acid 1 mg, Mg 50 mg, Zn 15 mg
StrongStart™	1000	1	3	20	15	100	400	30	Ca 200 mg, Fe 29 mg, folic acid 1 mg, niacinamide 15 mg, pantothenic acid 7 mg, Zn 20 mg; **phenylalanine 6 mg/tablet**
Combination Package									
CareNate™ 600 (tablet)	3500	2	3	3	12	60	400	30	Cu 2 mg, Fe 60 mg, folic acid 1 mg, Mg 25 mg, Zn 20 mg; dioctylsulfosuccinate sodium 50 mg Packaged with chewable tablets containing Ca 600 mg; wild berry flavor
Duet™ DHA (tablet)	3000	1.8	4	25	12	120	400	30	Ca 200 mg, Cu 2 mg, Fe 29 mg, folic acid 1 mg, Mg 25 mg, niacinamide 20 mg, Zn 25 mg Packaged with capsules containing Omega-3 fatty acids ≥ DHA 200 mg

Cr = chromium, Cu = copper, Fe = iron, Mg = magnesium, Mn = manganese, Mo = molybdenum, Se = selenium, Zn = zinc.

MULTIVITAMIN PRODUCTS *(Continued)*

Vitamin B Complex Combinations

Product	B_1 (mg)	B_2 (mg)	B_6 (mg)	B_{12} (mcg)	C (mg)	E (int. units)	Additional Information
Caplet							
Allbee® with C [OTC]	15	10.2	5		300		Niacinamide 50 mg, pantothenic acid 10 mg
Allbee® C-800 [OTC]	15	17	25	12	800	45	Niacinamide 100 mg, pantothenic acid 25 mg
Allbee® C-800 + Iron [OTC]	15	17	25	12	800	45	Fe 27 mg, folic acid 0.4 mcg, niacinamide 100 mg, pantothenic acid 25 mg
Capsule							
Trinsicon®				15			C 75 mg, Fe 110 mg, folic acid 0.5 mg, liver-stomach concentrate (containing intrinsic factor and other vitamin B complex factors) 240 mg
Liquid							
Apatate® [OTC] (per 5 mL) [OTC]	15		0.5	25			Cherry flavor (120 mL)
Gevrabon® [OTC] (per 30 mL) [OTC]	5	2.5	1	1			Choline 10 mg, Fe 15 mg, iodine 100 mcg, Mg 2 mg, Mn 2 mg, niacinamide 60 mg, pantothenic acid 10 mg, Zn 2 mg; alcohol, benzoic acid; sherry wine flavor (480 mL)
Softgel							
Nephrocaps®	1.5	1.7	10	6	100		Biotin 150 mcg, folic acid 1 mcg, niacinamide 20 mg, pantothenic acid 5 mg
Tablet							
Diatx™	1.5	1.5	50		60		Biotin 300 mcg, cobalamin 1 mg, folacin 5 mg, niacinamide 20 mg, pantothenic acid 10 mg [dye free, lactose free, sugar free]
DiatxFe™	1.5	1.5	50		60		Biotin 300 mcg, cobalamin 1 mg, ferrous fumarate 304 mg, folacin 5 mg, niacinamide 20 mg, pantothenic acid 10 mg [dye free, lactose free, sugar free]
NephPlex® Rx	1.5	1.7	10	6	60		Biotin 300 mcg, folic acid 1 mg, niacinamide 20 mg, pantothenic acid 10 mg, zinc 12.5 mg
Nephro-Vite®	1.5	1.7	10	6	60		Biotin 300 mcg, folic acid 0.8 mcg, niacinamide 20 mg, pantothenic acid 10 mg
Nephro-Vite® Rx	1.5	1.7	10	6	60		Biotin 300 mcg, folic acid 1 mcg, niacinamide 20 mg, pantothenic acid 10 mg
Nephron FA®	1.5	1.7	10	6	40		Biotin 300 mcg, docusate sodium 75 mg, ferrous fumarate 200 mg, folic acid 1 mg, pantothenic acid 10 mg
Olay® Vitamins Essential Folic Acid w/B_{12} Complex [OTC]		25	25	200		200	Folic acid 600 mcg, Se 50 mcg
Olay® Vitamins Super B-Stress Defense [OTC]	10	10	5	12	500	30	Biotin 100 mcg, folic acid 400 mcg, niacin 100 mg, pantothenic acid 20 mg
Stresstabs® B-Complex [OTC]	10	10	5	12	500	30	Biotin 45 mcg, folic acid 0.4 mcg, niacinamide 100 mg, pantothenic acid 20 mg

Vitamin B Complex Combinations *(continued)*

Product	B_1 (mg)	B_2 (mg)	B_6 (mg)	B_{12} (mcg)	C (mg)	E (int. units)	Additional Information
Stresstabs® B-Complex + Iron [OTC]	10	10	5	12	500	30	Biotin 45 mcg, Fe 18 mg, folic acid 0.4 mcg, niacinamide 100 mg, pantothenic acid 20 mg
Stresstabs® B-Complex + Zinc [OTC]	10	10	5	12	500	30	Biotin 45 mcg, Cu 3 mg, folic acid 0.4 mcg, niacinamide 100 mg, pantothenic acid 20 mg, Zn 23.9 mg
Surbex-T® [OTC]	15	10	5	10	500		Ca 20 mg, niacinamide 100 mg
Z-Bec® [OTC]	15	10.2	10	6	600	45	Niacinamide 100 mg, pantothenic acid 25 mg, Zn 22.5 mg
Tablet, Chewable							
Apatate® [OTC]	15		0.5	25			Cherry flavor

Ca = calcium, Cu = copper, Fe = iron, Mg = magnesium, Mn = manganese, Se = selenium, Zn = zinc.

NARCOTIC / OPIOID ANALGESICS

Dose Equivalents for Opioid Analgesics

Drug	Approximate Equianalgesic Dose	
	Oral	**Parenteral**
Morphine-Like Agonists (mu agonists)		
Morphine	30 mg	10 mg
Oxycodone	20 mg	NA
Hydromorphone (Dilaudid®)	7.5 mg	1.5 mg
Levorphanol (Levo-Dromoran®)	Acute: 4 mg Chronic: 1 mg	Acute: 2 mg Chronic: 1 mg
Meperidine (Demerol®)	300 mg	75 mg
Methadone (Dolophine®, others)	10 mg	5 mg
Oxymorphone (Numorphan®)	NA	1 mg
Mixed Agonist-Antagonists (kappa agonists)		
Butorphanol (Stadol®)	NA	2 mg
Nalbuphine (Nubain®)	NA	10 mg
Pentazocine (Talwin®, others)	50 mg	30 mg
Partial Agonist		
Buprenorphine (Buprenex®)	NA	0.4 mg

Adapted from *Principles of Analgesic Use in the Treatment of Acute Pain and Cancer Pain*, 5th ed, Glenview, IL: American Pain Society, 2003, 16.

AHCPR Usual Starting Dosage for Opioid Analgesics for Moderate to Severe Pain in Opioid-Naive Adults*

Drug	Usual Starting Dose Adults <50 kg		Usual Starting Dose Adults ≥50 kg	
	Oral	Parenteral	Oral	Parenteral
Opioid Agonist				
Morphine[1]	0.3 mg/kg q3-4h	0.1 mg/kg q3-4h	30 mg q3-4h	10 mg q3-4h
Codeine[2] (also in combination with aspirin or acetaminophen)	0.5-1 mg/kg q3-4h	NR	60 mg q3-4h	60 mg q2h (I.M./SubQ)
Hydromorphone[1] (Dilaudid®)	0.06 mg/kg q3-4h	0.015 mg/kg q3-4h	6 mg q3-4h	1.5 mg q3-4h
Levorphanol (Levo-Dromoran®)	0.04 mg/kg q6-8h	0.02 mg/kg q6-8h	4 mg q6-8h	2 mg q6-8h (SubQ)
Meperidine[3] (Demerol®; Meperitab®)	NR	0.74 mg/kg q2-3h	NR	100 mg q3h
Methadone (Dolophine®, others)	0.2 mg/kg q6-8h	0.1 mg/kg q6-8h	20 mg q6-8h	10 mg q6-8h
Oxycodone (Roxicodone®, also in Percocet®, Percodan®, Tylox®, others)	0.2 mg/kg q3-4h	NA	10 mg q3-4h	NA
Oxymorphone[1] (Numorphan®)	NA	NR	NA	1 mg q3-4h
Combination Opioid / NSAID Preparations[4]				
Hydrocodone (in Lorcet®, Lortab®, Vicodin®, others)	0.2 mg/kg q3-4h	NA	10 mg q3-4h	NA
Oxycodone (in Percocet®, Percodan®, Tylox®, others)	0.2 mg/kg q3-4h	NA	10 mg q3-4h	NA
Opioid Agonist-Antagonist and Partial Agonist				
Buprenorphine (Buprenex®)	NA	0.0004 mg/kg q6-8h	NA	0.4 mg q6-8h
Butorphanol (Stadol®)	NA	NR	NA	2 mg q3-4h
Nalbuphine (Nubain®)	NA	0.1 mg/kg q3-4h	NA	10 mg q3-4h
Pentazocine (Talwin®, others)	NR	NR	50 mg q4-6h	NR

Note: Dosage of opiates must be individualized. Lower initial doses may be appropriate in selected patients (consult individual drug monographs).

Caution: Recommended doses do not apply to patients with renal or hepatic insufficiency or other conditions affecting drug metabolism and kinetics.

[1]**Caution:** For morphine, hydromorphone, and oxymorphone, rectal administration is an alternate route for patients unable to take oral medications. Equianalgesic doses may differ from oral and parenteral doses because of pharmacokinetic differences. **Note:** A short-acting opioid should normally be used for initial therapy of moderate to severe pain.

[2]**Caution:** Doses >1.5 mg/kg not recommended. 60 mg oral codeine = 650 mg aspirin or acetaminophen.

[3]For short-term treatment of acute pain only.

[4]**Caution:** Doses of aspirin and acetaminophen in combination opioid/NSAID preparations must also be adjusted to the patient's body weight.

NA = not available; NR = not recommended.

Adapted from Acute Pain Management Guideline Panel, "Acute Pain Management: Operative or Medical Procedures and Trauma," Clinical Practice Guideline, AHCPR Publication No. 92-0032, Rockville, MD: Agency for Health Care Policy and Research, Public Health Service, U.S. Department of Health and Human Services, February 1992.
Available at http://www.ncbi.nlm.nih.gov/books/bv.fcgi?rid=hstat6.chapter.8991, Appendix C.

NARCOTIC / OPIOID ANALGESICS *(Continued)*

Comparative Pharmacokinetics

Drug	Onset (min)	Peak (h)	Duration (h)	Half-Life (h)	Average Dosing Interval (h)		Equianalgesic Doses[1] (mg)	
							I.M.	Oral
Alfentanil	Immediate	ND	ND	1-2	—	—	ND	NA
Buprenorphine	15	1	4-8	2-3			0.4	—
Butorphanol	I.M.: 30-60; I.V.: 4-5	0.5-1	3-5	2.5-3.5	3	(3-6)	2	—
Codeine	P.O.: 30-60; I.M.: 10-30	0.5-1	4-6	3-4	3	(3-6)	120	200
Fentanyl	I.M.: 7-15 I.V.: Immediate	ND	1-2	1.5-6	1	(0.5-2)	0.1	NA
Hydrocodone	ND	ND	4-8	3.3-4.4	6	(4-8)	ND	ND
Hydromorphone	P.O.: 15-30	0.5-1	4-6	2-4	4	(3-6)	1.5	7.5
Levorphanol	P.O.: 10-60	0.5-1	4-8	12-16	6	(6-24)	2 (A) 1 (C)	4 (A) 1 (C)
Meperidine	P.O./I.M./Sub-Q: 10-15 I.V.: ≤5	0.5-1	2-4	3-4	3	(2-4)	75	300
Methadone	P.O.: 30-60; I.V.: 10-20	0.5-1	4-6 (acute); >8 (chronic)	15-30	8	(6-12)	10 (A) 2-4 (C)	20 (A) 2-4 (C)
Morphine	P.O.: 15-60 I.V.: ≤5	P.O./I.M./Sub-Q: 0.5-1; I.V.: 0.3	3-6	2-4	4	(3-6)	10	60[2] (A) 30 (C)
Nalbuphine	I.M.: 30; I.V.: 1-3	1	3-6	5		—	10	—
Oxycodone	P.O.: 10-15	0.5-1	4-6	3-4	4	(3-6)	NA	20
Oxymorphone	5-15	0.5-1	3-6				1	10[3]
Pentazocine	15-20	0.25-1	3-4	2-3	3	(3-6)		
Propoxyphene	P.O.: 30-60	2-2.5	4-6	3.5-15	6	(4-8)	ND	130[4]-200[5]
Remifentanil	1-3	<0.3	0.1-0.2	0.15-0.3	—	—	ND	ND
Sufentanil	1.3-3	ND	ND	2.5-3	—	—	0.02	NA

ND = no data available. NA = not applicable. (A) = acute, (C) = chronic.

[1]Based on acute, short-term use. Chronic administration may alter pharmacokinetics and decrease the oral parenteral dose ratio. The morphine oral-parenteral ratio decreases to ~1.5-2.5:1 upon chronic dosing.

[2]Extensive survey data suggest that the relative potency of I.M.:P.O. morphine of 1:6 changes to 1:2-3 with chronic dosing.

[3]Rectal

[4]HCl salt

[5]Napsylate salt

Adapted from *Principles of Analgesic Use in the Treatment of Acute Pain and Cancer Pain,* 4th ed, Skokie, IL: The American Pain Society, 1999.

Comparative Pharmacology

Drug	Analgesic	Antitussive	Constipation	Respiratory Depression	Sedation	Emesis
Phenanthrenes						
Codeine	+	+++	+	+	+	+
Hydrocodone	+	+++		+		
Hydromorphone	++	+++	+	++	+	+
Levorphanol	++	++	++	++	++	+
Morphine	++	+++	++	++	++	++
Oxycodone	++	+++	++	++	++	++
Oxymorphone	++	+	++	+++		+++
Phenylpiperidines						
Alfentanil	++					
Fentanyl	++			+		+
Meperidine	++	+	+	++	+	
Remifentanil	++			++	+++	++
Sufentanil	+++					
Diphenylheptanes						
Methadone	++	++	++	++	+	+
Propoxyphene	+			+	+	+
Agonist / Antagonist						
Buprenorphine	++	N/A	+++	+++	++	++
Butorphanol	++	N/A	+++	+++	++	+
Nalbuphine	++	N/A	+++	+++	++	++
Pentazocine	++	N/A	+	++	++ or stimulation	++

OVER-THE-COUNTER PRODUCTS

Generic Name	Brand Name	Comments
	Analgesics	
Acetaminophen and aspirin (caffeine in all products)	Excedrin® Extra Strength; Excedrin® Migraine; Fem-Prin®; Genaced™; Pain-Off; Vanquish® Extra Strength Pain Reliever	Relief of mild to moderate pain or fever; avoid alcoholic beverages; take with food or a full glass of water
Acetaminophen and diphenhydramine	Excedrin® P.M.; Legatrin PM®; Tylenol® PM Extra Strength	Relief of mild to moderate pain or sinus headache
Acetaminophen and phenyltolaxamine	Genesec®; Percogesic®; Phenylgesic®	Relief of mild to moderate pain
Capsaicin	Capsagel®; Capzasin-HP®; Zostrix®; Zostrix®-HP	FDA approved for the topical treatment of pain associated with postherpetic neuralgia, rheumatoid arthritis, osteoarthritis, diabetic neuropathy, and postsurgical pain. Unlabeled use: Treatment of pain associated with psoriasis, chronic neuralgias unresponsive to other forms of therapy, and intractable pruritus.
	Antacids, Antiflatulents, or Antiemetics	
Aluminum hydroxide and magnesium carbonate	Gaviscon® Extra Strength; Gaviscon® Liquid	Temporary relief of symptoms associated with gastric acidity
Aluminum hydroxide and magnesium hydroxide	Alamag; Rulox	Antacid; used to treat hyperphosphatemia in renal failure
Aluminum hydroxide and magnesium trisilicate	Gaviscon® Tablet	Temporary relief of hyperacidity
Aluminum hydroxide, magnesium hydroxide, and simethicone	Maalox® Max; Mylanta® Liquid; Mylanta® Maximum Strength Liquid	Temporary relief of hyperacidity associated with gas; may be used for indications associated with other antacids
Calcium carbonate and simethicone	Titralac® Plus	Relief of acid indigestion, heartburn, peptic esophagitis, hiatal hernia, and gas
Dimenhydrinate	Dramamine®; TripTone®	Treatment and prevention of nausea, vertigo, and vomiting associated with motion sickness
Magaldrate and simethicone		Relief of hyperacidity associated with peptic ulcer, gastritis, peptic esophagitis, and hiatal hernia
Simethicone	Alka-Seltzer® Gas Relief; Baby Gasz; Gas-X®; Mylanta Gas®; Mylicon® Infants; Phazyme® Quick Dissolve	Relieves flatulence and functional gastric bloating, and postoperative gas pains
	Antidiarrheals and Laxatives	
Attapulgite	Diasorb®	Symptomatic treatment of diarrhea
Bisacodyl	Bisac-Evac®; Bisacodyl Uniserts®; Dulcolax®; Fleet® Stimulant Laxative	Treatment of constipation; colonic evacuation prior to procedures or examination
Castor oil	Purge®	Preparation for rectal or bowel examination or surgery; rarely used to relieve constipation; also applied to skin as emollient and protectant

Generic Name	Brand Name	Comments
Glycerin	Fleet® Babylax®; Sani-Supp®	Constipation
Lactase enzyme	Lactaid®; Lactrase®	Helps to digest lactose in milk for patients with lactose intolerance; may be administered with meals
Magnesium hydroxide and mineral oil emulsion	Phillip's M-O®	Short-term treatment of occasional constipation
Methylcellulose	Citrucel®; FiberEase™	Adjunct in treatment of constipation
Senna	Senokot®; X-Prep®	Short-term treatment of constipation; evacuate the colon for bowel or rectal examinations; liquid may be administered with fruit juice or milk to mask taste
Sodium phosphate	Fleet® Enema; Fleet® Phospho-Soda®	Short-term treatment of constipation; evacuation of the colon for rectal and bowel exams; source of sodium and phosphorus; treatment and prevention of hypophosphatemia
Cough / Cold or Allergy		
Acetaminophen and pseudoephedrine	Alka-Seltzer Plus® Cold and Sinus Liqui-Gels; Ornex®; Sinus-Relief®; Sinutab® Sinus; Tylenol® Sinus Day Non-Drowsy	Temporary relief of sinus symptoms with no drowsiness
Acetaminophen, chlorpheniramine, and pseudoephedrine	Comtrex®; Sinutab® Tablet; Tylenol® Allergy Sinus; Theraflu® Cold and Sore Throat Night Time	Temporary relief of sinus symptoms
Acetaminophen, dextromethorphan, and pseudoephedrine	Sudafed® Severe Cold; Tylenol® Flu Non-Drowsy Maximum Strength; Vicks® DayQuil® Multi-Symptom Cold and Flu	Relief of cold and flu symptoms with no drowsiness
Brompheniramine and pseudoephedrine	Brofed®; Bromfenex®; Bromfenex® PD	Temporary relief of symptoms of seasonal and perennial allergic rhinitis, and vasomotor rhinitis, including nasal obstruction
Chlorpheniramine	Aller-Chlor®; Chlor-Trimeton®	Relief of perennial and seasonal allergic rhinitis and other allergic symptoms including urticaria
Chlorpheniramine and acetaminophen	Coricidin HBP® Cold & Flu	Symptomatic relief of congestion, headache, aches, and pains of colds and flu
Chlorpheniramine and phenylephrine	Dallergy-JR®; Ed A-Hist®	Temporary relief of nasal congestion and eustachian tube congestion as well as runny nose, sneezing, itching of nose or throat, itchy and watery eyes
Chlorpheniramine and pseudoephedrine	Allerest® Maximum Strength; Deconamine®; Deconamine® SR; PediaCare® Cold and Allergy; Sudafed Sinus & Allergy; Triaminic® Cold and Allergy	Relief of nasal congestion associated with the common cold, hay fever, and other allergies, sinusitis, eustachian tube blockage, and vasomotor and allergic rhinitis
Chlorpheniramine, phenylephrine, and dextromethorphan	Alka-Seltzer Plus® Cold and Cough	Temporary relief of cough due to minor throat and bronchial irritation; relief of nasal congestion, runny nose, and sneezing

OVER-THE-COUNTER PRODUCTS *(Continued)*

Generic Name	Brand Name	Comments
Dexbrompheniramine and pseudoephedrine	Drixoral® Cold & Allergy	Relief of symptoms of upper respiratory mucosal congestion in seasonal and perennial nasal allergies, acute rhinitis, rhinosinusitis, and eustachian tube blockage
Dextromethorphan	Benylin® Adult; Creo-Terpin®; Delsym®; Hold® DM; Robitussin® Maximum Strength Cough; Robitussin® Pediatric; Scot-Tussin DM®; Silphen DM®; Vicks® 44® Cough Relief	Symptomatic relief of coughs caused by minor viral upper respiratory tract infections or inhaled irritants; most effective for a chronic nonproductive cough
Diphenhydramine and pseudoephedrine	Benadryl® Allergy/Sinus	Relief of symptoms of upper respiratory mucosal congestion in seasonal and perennial nasal allergies, acute rhinitis, rhinosinusitis, and eustachian tube blockage
Guaifenesin and pseudoephedrine	Congestac®; Robitussin-PE®; Robitussin® Severe Congestion	Enhances output of respiratory tract fluid and reduces mucosal congestion and edema in nasal passage
Guaifenesin, pseudoephedrine, and dextromethorphan	Maxifed® DM; Robitussin® CF; Touro™ CC; Tri-Vent™ DM	Relief of nasal congestion and cough
Oxymetazoline	Afrin®; Duramist® Plus®; Duration®; Neo-Synephrine® 12-Hour Nasal Solution; Nostrilla®; Visine® L.R.; 4-Way® Long Acting	Symptomatic relief of nasal mucosal congestion and adjunctive therapy of middle ear infections associated with acute or chronic rhinitis, the common cold, sinusitis, hay fever, or other allergies; relief of redness of eye due to minor eye irritations
Phenindamine	Nolahist®	Treatment of perennial and seasonal allergic rhinitis and chronic urticaria
Propylhexedrine	Benzedrex®	Topical nasal decongestant
Pseudoephedrine and dextromethorphan	PediaCare® Decongestant Plus Cough; Robitussin® Maximum Strength Cough & Cold; Vicks® 44D Cough & Head Congestion	Temporary symptomatic relief of nasal congestion due to the common cold, upper respiratory allergies, and sinusitis; promotes nasal or sinus drainage; symptomatic relief of coughs caused by minor viral upper respiratory tract infections or inhaled irritants; most effective for a chronic nonproductive cough
Pseudoephedrine and ibuprofen	Advil® Cold & Sinus; Dristan® Sinus; Motrin® Cold & Sinus; Motrin® Cold, Children's	Temporary symptomatic relief of nasal congestion due to the common cold, upper respiratory allergies, and sinusitis; promotes nasal or sinus drainage; relief of sinus headaches and pains

Generic Name	Brand Name	Comments
Triprolidine and pseudoephedrine	Actifed® Cold and Allergy; Allerfrim®; Allerphed®; Aprodine®; Genac®; Silafed®	Temporary relief of nasal congestion; decongest sinus openings, runny nose, sneezing, itching of nose or throat, and itchy watery eyes due to common cold, hay fever, or other upper respiratory allergies; may cause drowsiness
	Dermatologics	
Aluminum sulfate and calcium acetate	Domeboro®; Pedi-Boro®	Astringent wet dressing for relief of inflammatory conditions of the skin and used to reduce weeping that may occur in dermatitis
Benzoin		Protective application for irritations of the skin; sometimes used in boiling water as steam inhalants for their expectorant and soothing action
Benzoyl peroxide	Del Aqua®; Fostex® 10% BPO; Loroxide®; Neutrogena® Acne Mask; PanOxyl®	Adjunctive treatment of mild to moderate acne vulgaris acne rosacea
Camphor and phenol	Campho-Phenique®	Relief of pain and for minor infections
Chlorophyll	Nullo®	Topically promotes normal healing; relief of pain and inflammation; reduce malodors in wounds, burns, surface ulcers, abrasions, and skin irritations; used orally to control fecal and urinary odors in colostomy, ileostomy, or incontinence
Chloroxine	Capitrol®	Treatment of dandruff or seborrheic dermatitis of the scalp
Coal tar	DHS® Tar; Estar®; Neutrogena® T/Gel; Oxipor® VHC; Pentrax®; Polytar®; PsoriGel®; Zetar®	Topically for controlling dandruff, seborrheic dermatitis, or psoriasis
Coal tar and salicylic acid	Tarsum®; X-Seb™ T	Control seborrheal dermatitis, dandruff
Dibucaine	Nupercainal®	Fast, temporary relief of pain and itching due to hemorrhoids, minor burns, or other minor skin conditions (amide derivative local anesthetic)
Lactic acid	LactiCare®	Lubricate and moisturize the skin counteracting dryness and itching
Lactic acid and ammonium hydroxide	Lac-Hydrin®	Treatment of moderate to severe xerosis and ichthyosis vulgaris
Lanolin, cetyl alcohol, glycerin, petrolatum, and mineral oil	Lubriderm®	Treatment of dry skin
Nonoxynol 9	Delfen®; Emko®; Encare®; Gynol II®; Semicid®; Shur-Seal®	Spermatocide in contraception
Povidone-iodine	Betadine®; Minidyne®	External antiseptic with broad microbicidal spectrum against bacteria, fungi, viruses, protozoa, and yeasts

OVER-THE-COUNTER PRODUCTS *(Continued)*

Generic Name	Brand Name	Comments
Pyrithione zinc	DHS Zinc®; Head & Shoulders® Classic Clean; Zincon®; ZNP® Bar	Relief of itching, irritation, and scalp flaking associated with dandruff and/or seborrheal dermatitis of the scalp
Salicylic acid	Compound W®; DuoFilm®; Freezone®; Gordofilm®; Keralyt®; Mediplast®; Mosco®; Occlusal-HP; Sal-Acid®; Salactic®; Sal-Plant®; Trans-Ver-Sal®; Wart-Off®	Topically used for its keratolytic effect in controlling seborrheic dermatitis or psoriasis of body and scalp, dandruff, and other scaling dermatoses; remove warts, corns, and calluses
Triacetin	Myco-Nail	Fungistat for athlete's foot and other superficial fungal infections
Undecyclenic acid and derivatives	Fungi-Nail®	Treatment of athlete's foot, ringworm, prickly heat, jock itch, diaper rash, and other minor skin irritations
Vitamin A and vitamin D	A and D® Ointment	Temporary relief of discomfort due to chapped skin, diaper rash, minor burns, abrasions, as well as irritations associated with ostomy skin care
Zinc oxide	Balmex®; Desitin®	Protective coating for mild skin irritations and abrasions; soothing and protective ointment to promote healing of chapped skin, diaper rash; if irritation develops, discontinue use and consult a physician; paste is easily removed with mineral oil; for external use only; do not use in eyes
	Dietary Supplements	
Calcium citrate	Citracal®	Adjunct in prevention of postmenopausal osteoporosis; treatment and prevention of calcium depletion
Calcium lactate		Adjunct in prevention of postmenopausal osteoporosis; treatment and prevention of calcium depletion
Calcium phosphate, tribasic	Posture®	Adjunct in prevention of postmenopausal osteoporosis; treatment and prevention of calcium depletion
Ferrous sulfate and ascorbic acid	Fero-Grad 500®	Treatment of iron deficiency in nonpregnant or pregnant adults
Glucose, instant	B-D Glucose®; Glutose®; Insta-Glucose®	Management of hypoglycemia
Glucose polymers	Modical®; Polycose®	Supplies calories for those persons not able to meet the caloric requirement with usual food intake
Magnesium chloride	Slow-Mag®	Correct or prevent hypomagnesemia

Generic Name	Brand Name	Comments
Magnesium gluconate	Magonate®	Dietary supplement for treatment of magnesium deficiencies
Medium chain triglycerides	MCT Oil®	Dietary supplement for those who cannot digest long chain fats; malabsorption associated with disorders such as pancreatic insufficiency, bile salt deficiency, and bacterial overgrowth of the small bowel; induce ketosis as a prevention for seizures (akinetic, clonic, and petit mal)
Polysaccharide-iron complex	Hytinic®; Niferex®; Nu-Iron® 150	Prevention and treatment of iron deficiency anemias
Vitamin B complex	Apatate®	Prevention and treatment of B complex vitamin deficiency
Vitamin B complex with vitamin C	Allbee® With C; Surbex-T®	Supportive nutritional supplementation in conditions in which water-soluble vitamins are required like GI disorders, chronic alcoholism, pregnancy, severe burns, and recovery from surgery
Vitamin B complex with vitamin C and folic acid	Nephrocaps®	Supportive nutritional supplementation in conditions in which water-soluble vitamins are required like GI disorders, chronic alcoholism, pregnancy, severe burns, and recovery from surgery
Zinc sulfate	Orazinc®	Zinc supplement (oral and parenteral); may improve wound healing in those who are deficient
Hemorrhoidal Preparations		
Pramoxine	Proctofoam® NS; Tronolane®	Temporary relief of pain and itching associated with anogenital pruritus or irritation; treatment of dermatosis, minor burns, or hemorrhoids
Witch hazel	Tucks®	After-stool wipe to remove most causes of local irritation; temporary management of vulvitis, pruritus ani, and vulva; help relieve the discomfort of simple hemorrhoids, anorectal surgical wounds, and episiotomies
Ophthalmics		
Artificial tears	Akwa Tears®; AquaSite®; Bion® Tears; HypoTears; Isopto® Tears; Liquifilm® Tears; Moisture® Eyes PM; Murine® Tears; Murocel®; Nature's Tears®; Nu-Tears®; Nu-Tears® II; OcuCoat®; OcuCoat® PF; Puralube® Tears; Refresh®; Refresh® Plus; Teargen®; Tearisol®; Tears Naturale® Free; Tears Naturale® II; Tears Naturale®; Tears Plus®; Tears Renewed®; Ultra Tears®; Viva-Drops®	Ophthalmic lubricant; relief of dry eyes and eye irritation
Balanced salt solution	BSS®	Intraocular irrigating solution; used to soothe and cleanse the eye in conjunction with hard contact lenses

OVER-THE-COUNTER PRODUCTS *(Continued)*

Generic Name	Brand Name	Comments
Benzalkonium chloride	Benza®; Zephiran®	Surface antiseptic and germicidal preservative
Carboxymethyl-cellulose sodium	Refresh Plus®; Theratears®	Preservative-free artificial tear substitute
Glycerin	Osmoglyn®	Reduction of intraocular pressure; reduction of corneal edema; glycerin had been administered orally to reduce intracranial pressure
Naphazoline	AK-Con®; Albalon®; Clear Eyes® ACR; Naphcon®; Privine®	Topical ocular vasoconstrictor; will temporarily relieve congestion, itching, and minor irritation; control hyperemia in patients with superficial corneal vascularity
Naphazoline and antazoline	Vasocon-A®	Topical ocular congestion, irritation, and itching; use with caution in patients with cardiovascular disease
Naphazoline and pheniramine	Naphcon-A®; Opcon A®; Visine® A	Topical ocular vasoconstrictor; use with caution in patients with cardiovascular disease
Phenylephrine and zinc sulfate	Zincfrin®	Soothe, moisturize, and remove redness due to minor eye irritation; discontinue use if ocular pain or visual changes are present after 3 days
Tetrahydrozoline	Eye-Sine™; Geneye®; Murine® Tears Plus; Tyzine®; Visine® Original	Symptomatic relief of nasal congestion and conjunctival congestion
	Oral	
Cetylpyridinium	Cĕpacol® Gold	Temporary relief of sore throat
Cetylpyridinium and benzocaine		Symptomatic relief of sore throat
Gelatin, pectin, and methylcellulose		Temporary relief from minor oral irritations
Phenol	Chloraseptic® Spray; Ulcerease®	Relief of sore throat pain and mouth, gum, and throat irritations
Saliva substitute	Moi-Stir®; Mouthkote®; Salivart®	Relief of dry mouth and throat in xerostomia
	Miscellaneous or Multiple Use	
Sodium chloride	Ayr® Saline; Muro 128®; NaSal™; Nasal Moist®; Ocean®; Pretz®; SalineX®; SeaMist®	Prevention of muscle cramps and heat prostration; restoration of sodium ion in hyponatremia; induce abortion; restore moisture to nasal membranes; GU irrigant; reduction of corneal edema; source of electrolytes and water for expansion of the extracellular fluid compartment

REFERENCE VALUES FOR CHILDREN

		Normal Values
CHEMISTRY		
Albumin	0-1 y	2-4 g/dL
	1 y to adult	3.5-5.5 g/dL
Ammonia	Newborns	90-150 mcg/dL
	Children	40-120 mcg/dL
	Adults	18-54 mcg/dL
Amylase	Newborns	0-60 units/L
	Adults	30-110 units/L
Bilirubin, conjugated, direct	Newborns	<1.5 mg/dL
	1 mo to adult	0-0.5 mg/dL
Bilirubin, total	0-3 d	2-10 mg/dL
	1 mo to adult	0-1.5 mg/dL
Bilirubin, unconjugated, indirect		0.6-10.5 mg/dL
Calcium	Newborns	7-12 mg/dL
	0-2 y	8.8-11.2 mg/dL
	2 y to adult	9-11 mg/dL
Calcium, ionized, whole blood		4.4-5.4 mg/dL
Carbon dioxide, total		23-33 mEq/L
Chloride		95-105 mEq/L
Cholesterol	Newborns	45-170 mg/dL
	0-1 y	65-175 mg/dL
	1-20 y	120-230 mg/dL
Creatinine	0-1 y	≤0.6 mg/dL
	1 y to adult	0.5-1.5 mg/dL
Glucose	Newborns	30-90 mg/dL
	0-2 y	60-105 mg/dL
	Children to adults	70-110 mg/dL
Iron		
	Newborns	110-270 mcg/dL
	Infants	30-70 mcg/dL
	Children	55-120 mcg/dL
	Adults	70-180 mcg/dL
Iron binding	Newborns	59-175 mcg/dL
	Infants	100-400 mcg/dL
	Adults	250-400 mcg/dL
Lactic acid, lactate		2-20 mg/dL
Lead, whole blood		<10 mcg/dL
Lipase		
	Children	20-140 units/L
	Adults	0-190 units/L
Magnesium		1.5-2.5 mEq/L
Osmolality, serum		275-296 mOsm/kg
Osmolality, urine		50-1400 mOsm/kg
Phosphorus	Newborns	4.2-9 mg/dL
	6 wk to 19 mo	3.8-6.7 mg/dL
	19 mo to 3 y	2.9-5.9 mg/dL
	3-15 y	3.6-5.6 mg/dL
	>15 y	2.5-5 mg/dL
Potassium, plasma	Newborns	4.5-7.2 mEq/L
	2 d to 3 mo	4-6.2 mEq/L
	3 mo to 1 y	3.7-5.6 mEq/L
	1-16 y	3.5-5 mEq/L
Protein, total	0-2 y	4.2-7.4 g/dL
	>2 y	6-8 g/dL
Sodium		136-145 mEq/L

REFERENCE VALUES FOR CHILDREN *(Continued)*

		Normal Values
Triglycerides	Infants	0-171 mg/dL
	Children	20-130 mg/dL
	Adults	30-200 mg/dL
Urea nitrogen, blood	0-2 y	4-15 mg/dL
	2 y to adult	5-20 mg/dL
Uric acid	Male	3-7 mg/dL
	Female	2-6 mg/dL
ENZYMES		
Alanine aminotransferase (ALT) (SGPT)	0-2 mo	8-78 units/L
	>2 mo	8-36 units/L
Alkaline phosphatase (ALKP)	Newborns	60-130 units/L
	0-16 y	85-400 units/L
	>16 y	30-115 units/L
Aspartate aminotransferase (AST) (SGOT)	Infants	18-74 units/L
	Children	15-46 units/L
	Adults	5-35 units/L
Creatine kinase (CK)	Infants	20-200 units/L
	Children	10-90 units/L
	Adult male	0-206 units/L
	Adult female	0-175 units/L
Lactate dehydrogenase (LDH)	Newborns	290-501 units/L
	1 mo to 2 y	110-144 units/L
	>16 y	60-170 units/L

Blood Gases

	Arterial	Capillary	Venous
pH	7.35-7.45	7.35-7.45	7.32-7.42
pCO_2 (mm Hg)	35-45	35-45	38-52
pO_2 (mm Hg)	70-100	60-80	24-48
HCO_3 (mEq/L)	19-25	19-25	19-25
TCO_2 (mEq/L)	19-29	19-29	23-33
O_2 saturation (%)	90-95	90-95	40-70
Base excess (mEq/L)	-5 to +5	-5 to +5	-5 to +5

Thyroid Function Tests

Test	Age	Value
T_4 (thyroxine)	1-7 d	10.1-20.9 mcg/dL
	8-14 d	9.8-16.6 mcg/dL
	1 mo to 1 y	5.5-16 mcg/dL
	>1 y	4-12 mcg/dL
FTI	1-3 d	9.3-26.6
	1-4 wk	7.6-20.8
	1-4 mo	7.4-17.9
	4-12 mo	5.1-14.5
	1-6 y	5.7-13.3
	>6 y	4.8-14
T_3 by RIA	Newborns	100-470 ng/dL
	1-5 y	100-260 ng/dL
	5-10 y	90-240 ng/dL
	10 y to adult	70-210 ng/dL
T_3 uptake		35%-45%
TSH	Cord	3-22 μIU/mL
	1-3 d	<40 μIU/mL
	3-7 d	<25 μIU/mL
	>7 d	0-10 μIU/mL

REFERENCE VALUES FOR ADULTS

Automated Chemistry (CHEMISTRY A)

Test	Values	Remarks
SERUM / PLASMA		
Acetone	Negative	
Albumin	3.2-5 g/dL	
Alcohol, ethyl	Negative	
Aldolase	1.2-7.6 IU/L	
Ammonia	20-70 mcg/dL	Specimen to be placed on ice as soon as collected.
Amylase	30-110 units/L	
Bilirubin, direct	0-0.3 mg/dL	
Bilirubin, total	0.1-1.2 mg/dL	
Calcium	8.6-10.3 mg/dL	
Calcium, ionized	2.24-2.46 mEq/L	
Chloride	95-108 mEq/L	
Cholesterol, total	≤200 mg/dL	Fasted blood required – normal value affected by dietary habits. This reference range is for a general adult population.
HDL cholesterol	40-60 mg/dL	Fasted blood required – normal value affected by dietary habits.
LDL cholesterol	<160 mg/dL	If triglyceride is >400 mg/dL, LDL cannot be calculated accurately (Friedewald equation). Target LDL-C depends on patient's risk factors.
CO_2	23-30 mEq/L	
Creatine kinase (CK) isoenzymes		
CK-BB	0%	
CK-MB (cardiac)	0%-3.9%	
CK-MM (muscle)	96%-100%	
CK-MB levels must be both ≥4% and 10 IU/L to meet diagnostic criteria for CK-MB positive result consistent with myocardial injury.		
Creatine phosphokinase (CPK)	8-150 IU/L	
Creatinine	0.5-1.4 mg/dL	
Ferritin	13-300 ng/mL	
Folate	3.6-20 ng/dL	
GGT (gamma-glutamyltranspeptidase)		
male	11-63 IU/L	
female	8-35 IU/L	
GLDH	To be determined	
Glucose (preprandial)	<115 mg/dL	Goals different for diabetics.
Glucose, fasting	60-110 mg/dL	Goals different for diabetics.
Glucose, nonfasting (2-h postprandial)	<120 mg/dL	Goals different for diabetics.
Hemoglobin A_{1c}	<8	
Hemoglobin, plasma free	<2.5 mg/100 mL	
Hemoglobin, total glycosolated (Hb A_1)	4%-8%	
Iron	65-150 mcg/dL	
Iron binding capacity, total (TIBC)	250-420 mcg/dL	
Lactic acid	0.7-2.1 mEq/L	Specimen to be kept on ice and sent to lab as soon as possible.
Lactate dehydrogenase (LDH)	56-194 IU/L	

Automated Chemistry (CHEMISTRY A) *(continued)*

Test	Values	Remarks
Lactate dehydrogenase (LDH) isoenzymes		
LD_1	20%-34%	
LD_2	29%-41%	
LD_3	15%-25%	
LD_4	1%-12%	
LD_5	1%-15%	
Flipped LD_1/LD_2 ratios (>1 may be consistent with myocardial injury) particularly when considered in combination with a recent CK-MB positive result.		
Lipase	23-208 units/L	
Magnesium	1.6-2.5 mg/dL	Increased by slight hemolysis.
Osmolality	289-308 mOsm/kg	
Phosphatase, alkaline		
adults 25-60 y	33-131 IU/L	
adults 61 y or older	51-153 IU/L	
infancy-adolescence	Values range up to 3-5 times higher than adults	
Phosphate, inorganic	2.8-4.2 mg/dL	
Potassium	3.5-5.2 mEq/L	Increased by slight hemolysis.
Prealbumin	>15 mg/dL	
Protein, total	6.5-7.9 g/dL	
SGOT (AST)	<35 IU/L (20-48)	
SGPT (ALT) (10-35)	<35 IU/L	
Sodium	134-149 mEq/L	
Transferrin	>200 mg/dL	
Triglycerides	45-155 mg/dL	Fasted blood required.
Troponin I	<1.5 ng/mL	
Urea nitrogen (BUN)	7-20 mg/dL	
Uric acid		
male	2-8 mg/dL	
female	2-7.5 mg/dL	
CEREBROSPINAL FLUID		
Glucose	50-70 mg/dL	
Protein		
adults and children	15-45 mg/dL	CSF obtained by lumbar puncture.
newborn infants	60-90 mg/dL	
On CSF obtained by cisternal puncture: About 25 mg/dL		
On CSF obtained by ventricular puncture: About 10 mg/dL		
Note: Bloody specimen gives erroneously high value due to contamination with blood proteins		
URINE (24-hour specimen is required for all these tests unless specified)		
Amylase	32-641 units/L	The value is in units/L and **not** calculated for total volume.
Amylase, fluid (random samples)		Interpretation of value left for physician, depends on the nature of fluid.
Calcium	Depends upon dietary intake	
Creatine		
male	150 mg/24 h	Higher value on children and during pregnancy.
female	250 mg/24 h	
Creatinine	1000-2000 mg/24 h	
Creatinine clearance (endogenous)		
male female	85-125 mL/min 75-115 mL/min	A blood sample must accompany urine specimen.
Glucose	1 g/24 h	
5-hydroxyindoleacetic acid	2-8 mg/24 h	

REFERENCE VALUES FOR ADULTS *(Continued)*

Automated Chemistry (CHEMISTRY A) *(continued)*

Test	Values	Remarks
Iron	0.15 mg/24 h	Acid washed container required.
Magnesium	146-209 mg/24 h	
Osmolality	500-800 mOsm/kg	With normal fluid intake.
Oxalate	10-40 mg/24 h	
Phosphate	400-1300 mg/24 h	
Potassium	25-120 mEq/24 h	Varies with diet; the interpretation of urine electrolytes and osmolality should be left for the physician.
Sodium	40-220 mEq/24 h	
Porphobilinogen, qualitative	Negative	
Porphyrins, qualitative	Negative	
Proteins	0.05-0.1 g/24 h	
Salicylate	Negative	
Urea clearance	60-95 mL/min	A blood sample must accompany specimen.
Urea N	10-40 g/24 h	Dependent on protein intake.
Uric acid	250-750 mg/24 h	Dependent on diet and therapy.
Urobilinogen	0.5-3.5 mg/24 h	For qualitative determination on random urine, send sample to urinalysis section in Hematology Lab.
Xylose absorption test		
children	16%-33% of ingested xylose	
FECES		
Fat, 3-day collection	<5 g/d	Value depends on fat intake of 100 g/d for 3 days preceding and during collection.
GASTRIC ACIDITY		
Acidity, total, 12 h	10-60 mEq/L	Titrated at pH 7.

Blood Gases

	Arterial	Capillary	Venous
pH	7.35-7.45	7.35-7.45	7.32-7.42
pCO_2 (mm Hg)	35-45	35-45	38-52
pO_2 (mm Hg)	70-100	60-80	24-48
HCO_3 (mEq/L)	19-25	19-25	19-25
TCO_2 (mEq/L)	19-29	19-29	23-33
O_2 saturation (%)	90-95	90-95	40-70
Base excess (mEq/L)	-5 to +5	-5 to +5	-5 to +5

HEMATOLOGY

Complete Blood Count

Age	Hgb (g/dL)	Hct (%)	RBC (mill/mm^3)	RDW
0-3 d	15.0-20.0	45-61	4.0-5.9	<18
1-2 wk	12.5-18.5	39-57	3.6-5.5	<17
1-6 mo	10.0-13.0	29-42	3.1-4.3	<16.5
7 mo to 2 y	10.5-13.0	33-38	3.7-4.9	<16
2-5 y	11.5-13.0	34-39	3.9-5.0	<15
5-8 y	11.5-14.5	35-42	4.0-4.9	<15
13-18 y	12.0-15.2	36-47	4.5-5.1	<14.5
Adult male	13.5-16.5	41-50	4.5-5.5	<14.5
Adult female	12.0-15.0	36-44	4.0-4.9	<14.5

Age	MCV (fL)	MCH (pg)	MCHC (%)	Plts (x 10^3/mm^3)
0-3 d	95-115	31-37	29-37	250-450
1-2 wk	86-110	28-36	28-38	250-450
1-6 mo	74-96	25-35	30-36	300-700
7 mo to 2 y	70-84	23-30	31-37	250-600
2-5 y	75-87	24-30	31-37	250-550
5-8 y	77-95	25-33	31-37	250-550
13-18 y	78-96	25-35	31-37	150-450
Adult male	80-100	26-34	31-37	150-450
Adult female	80-100	26-34	31-37	150-450

REFERENCE VALUES FOR ADULTS *(Continued)*

WBC and Differential

Age	WBC (x $10^3/mm^3$)	Segs	Bands	Lymphs	Monos
0-3 d	9.0-35.0	32-62	10-18	19-29	5-7
1-2 wk	5.0-20.0	14-34	6-14	36-45	6-10
1-6 mo	6.0-17.5	13-33	4-12	41-71	4-7
7 mo to 2 y	6.0-17.0	15-35	5-11	45-76	3-6
2-5 y	5.5-15.5	23-45	5-11	35-65	3-6
5-8 y	5.0-14.5	32-54	5-11	28-48	3-6
13-18 y	4.5-13.0	34-64	5-11	25-45	3-6
Adults	4.5-11.0	35-66	5-11	24-44	3-6

Age	Eosinophils	Basophils	Atypical Lymphs	No. of NRBCs
0-3 d	0-2	0-1	0-8	0-2
1-2 wk	0-2	0-1	0-8	0
1-6 mo	0-3	0-1	0-8	0
7 mo to 2 y	0-3	0-1	0-8	0
2-5 y	0-3	0-1	0-8	0
5-8 y	0-3	0-1	0-8	0
13-18 y	0-3	0-1	0-8	0
Adults	0-3	0-1	0-8	0

Segs = segmented neutrophils.
Bands = band neutrophils.
Lymphs = lymphocytes.
Monos = monocytes.

Erythrocyte Sedimentation Rates and Reticulocyte Counts

Sedimentation rate, Westergren	Children	0-20 mm/hour
	Adult male	0-15 mm/hour
	Adult female	0-20 mm/hour
Sedimentation rate, Wintrobe	Children	0-13 mm/hour
	Adult male	0-10 mm/hour
	Adult female	0-15 mm/hour
Reticulocyte count	Newborns	2%-6%
	1-6 mo	0%-2.8%
	Adults	0.5%-1.5%

COMMONLY USED HERBAL MEDICINES

The use of herbal medicines by the general population continues to increase. In 1988, retail sales of herbal products was approximately $200 million with this number increasing to $5.1 billion in 1997. If the current trend in herbal medicine use continues, annual sales of $25 billion are expected by the year 2010. A survey of surgical patients performed in 1999 revealed that 17.4% reported taking herbals or nutrachemicals. In this survey, the most common herbs taken were gingko (32.4%), garlic (26.5%), ginger (26.5%), ginseng (14%), and St John's wort (14%). A major problem with herbal medicine use is that patients frequently do not report this use to their healthcare providers. This results in the potential for adverse interactions between the patient's prescription medications and herbal products. Further, the use of herbal medicine may cause problems not anticipated by the healthcare provider (eg, increased bleeding potential) if its use is not communicated. Hence, it is critical that all healthcare providers question patients about herbal use as part of their routine medication history. One may also want to consider having the patient stop taking select herbal medicines up to 2 weeks prior to surgery, if possible, secondary to their potential effects on coagulation (eg, feverfew, garlic, ginger, ginkgo, horse chestnut seed, kava-kava). Although there are hundreds of herbal products available on the market, a relatively small number (10-20) account for the majority of sales. The table that follows lists some of the most commonly used herbal medicines, their traditional uses, and cautions and contraindications with regard to their use. Keep in mind that there are few well-designed studies assessing these products, as they are considered dietary supplements, and as such, are not held to the rigid FDA testing standards for drugs.

Herb	Use(s)	Cautions and Contraindications
Cat's claw *(Unacaria tomentosa)*	– Treatment of allergies, arthritis – Adjunct therapy for AIDS – Adjunct agent for cancer therapy – Immune stimulant – Postradiation therapy – Antiparasitic	– Should not be taken when pregnant, nursing, or by transplant recipients – May see diarrhea or changes in bowel movement – Use with caution in conjunction with anticoagulants (may increase risk of bleeding due to platelet activating factor inhibition) – Use with caution with NSAIDs (may increase risk of GI bleeding)
Cayenne *(Capsicum annuum)*	– **External:** Muscle spasm or soreness, shingles, diabetic neuropathy, cluster headache, osteoarthritis, rheumatoid arthritis – **Internal:** GI tract disorders	– **External:** Potential for skin ulceration and blistering with >2 days' use – **Internal:** Overdose may cause severe hypothermia
Echinacea *(Echinacea purpurea)*	– Prevention and treatment of colds and flu, allergies, infections, tonsillitis, sore throat – Chronic skin complaints	– Should not be administered with immunosuppressants – People with chronic suppressed immunity should not take for extended periods of time (>10-14 days)
Evening primrose oil *(Oenothera biennis)*	– Reduce cholesterol – Allergic/inflammatory conditions – Treatment of PMS	– Reduces platelet aggregation (monitor bleeding times and PT in patients on antiplatelet drugs, warfarin, or other anticoagulant drugs)

COMMONLY USED HERBAL MEDICINES *(Continued)*

Herb	Use(s)	Cautions and Contraindications
Feverfew *(Tanacetum parthenium)*	– Treatment of arthritis – Migraine prophylaxis/ treatment – Antipyretic	– Can inhibit platelet activity and increase bleeding; avoid use in patients on warfarin or other anticoagulants or antiplatelet drugs – Rebound headache with sudden cessation – Avoid in pregnant women (uterine stimulant) – Users may develop aphthous ulcers or GI tract irritation (5% to 15%) – Use with caution when administering with drugs that increase serotonin (eg, fluoxetine, sumatriptan) secondary to increased risk of serotonin syndrome
Garlic *(Allium sativum)*	– Lower cholesterol and blood pressure – Has antiplatelet, antioxidant, and antithrombotic qualities – Prevent infections	– Reduces platelet aggregation and increases fibrinolytic activity; monitor bleeding times and PT in patients on antiplatelet drugs and warfarin – Monitor blood glucose (decreased blood glucose secondary to increased serum insulin levels) – May potentiate antihypertensives – Vasodilator properties
Ginger *(Zingiber officinale)*	– Antinauseant – Antispasmodic	– Potent inhibitor of thromboxane synthetase; may increase bleeding time – May interact with anticoagulant and antiplatelet drugs to increase risk of bleeding – May alter effects of calcium channel blockers (ginger increases calcium uptake by the heart)
Ginkgo *(Ginkgo biloba)*	– Treatment of dementia associated with Alzheimer's disease or other conditions associated with cerebral vascular insufficiency – Treatment of vertigo, headache, tinnitus, depression, peripheral vascular disease, Raynaud's disease	– Ginkgolides inhibit platelet activating factor and antagonize thrombus formation; may enhance bleeding in patients on anticoagulant or antithrombotic therapy
Ginseng *(Panax schinseng)*	– Enhance mental and physical performance – Increase energy, decrease stress – Improve immune function – Adaptogen – Antioxidant	– Use caution in patients on digoxin therapy – Hypoglycemic effect – Ginsenosides inhibit platelet aggregation and enhance fibrinolysis; may interact with warfarin or antiplatelet drugs to increase risk of bleeding – Should not be used in pregnancy or acute infection – May potentiate action of MAOIs

Herb	Use(s)	Cautions and Contraindications
Goldenseal *(Hydrastis canadensis)*	– Diuretic – Hemostatic – Anti-inflammatory – Laxative	– High doses may induce paralysis – Should not be taken during pregnancy or while nursing – Functions as an aquaretic – Functions as an oxytocic
Grape seed extract *(Vitis vinifera)*	– Treatment of allergies, asthma – Improve peripheral circulation – Decrease platelet aggregation, capillary fragility – Improve general circulation – Antioxidant	– Monitor bleeding times and PT in patients on antiplatelet drugs and warfarin
Green tea leaf *(Camellia sinensis)*	– Antioxidant/free radical scavenger – Preventative for cancer and cardiovascular disease – Preventative for atherosclerosis and hypertension – Antibacterial – Lower cholesterol – Platelet inhibition actions	– Use with caution in patients on anticoagulant therapy
Hawthorn *(Crataegus oxyacantha)*	– Treatment for angina, arrhythmias, tachycardia, hypo-/hypertension, irregular heartbeat, peripheral vascular disorders, vascular spasms – Lower cholesterol	– May potentiate digoxin and ACE inhibitors
Horse chestnut seed *(Aesculus hippocastanum)*	– Treatment of varicose veins, hemorrhoids, venous insufficiencies	– Contains coumarin and aescin constituents; use with caution in patients on anticoagulant or antiplatelet therapy (can cause severe bleeding or bruising)
Kava-kava *(Piper methysticum)*	– Anxiolytic – Analgesic – Antidepressant – Insomnia	– Kava lactones (active constituents of kava-kava) potentiate the effects of other CNS depressants such as barbiturates, benzodiazepines, opioids, and anesthetics – Can potentiate ethanol effects – Avoid in endogenous depression – May worsen symptoms of Parkinson's disease (kava-kava antagonizes dopamine)
Licorice root *(Glycyrrhiza glabra)*	– Gastric and duodenal ulcers – Adrenal insufficiency – Expectorant and antitussive	– Contraindicated in many chronic liver conditions, severe kidney insufficiency, hypertension, cardiac disease, hypokalemia – Contraindicated in pregnancy and diabetes – Glycyrrhizic acid in licorice may cause high blood pressure, hypokalemia, and edema

COMMONLY USED HERBAL MEDICINES *(Continued)*

Herb	Use(s)	Cautions and Contraindications
Passionflower vine *(Passiflora incarnata)*	– Sedative and hypnotic – In combination with valerian to produce restful sleep	– May potentiate sedative actions of pharmaceuticals – Use with caution in patients on MAOI therapy – Use with caution with consumption of alcohol
Saw palmetto *(Serenoa repens)*	– Benign prostatic hypertrophy	– Antiestrogen effect (avoid during pregnancy and in patients with breast cancer) – Can cause hypertension and GI disturbances
St John's wort *(Hypericum perforatum)*	– **External:** Herpes simplex 1, minor wounds and burns – **Internal:** Treatment for depression, nervousness, anxiety	– May prolong effects of anesthesia – Photosensitivity in large doses in light-skinned people – Serotonin syndrome that is reversed by decreasing dose – May be prudent to avoid SSRIs, MAOIs, and meperidine – Increases metabolism of many perioperative drugs
Turmeric *(Curcuma longa)*	– Antioxidant – Anti-inflammatory – Antirheumatic – Lower blood lipid levels	– Use with caution if currently taking anticoagulant medications – Use with caution if peptic ulceration is present – Do not use if biliary obstruction is present
Valerian *(Valeriana officinalis)*	– Mild sedative and anxiolytic	– May potentiate the effects of CNS depressants (eg, barbiturates, anesthetics) and anxiolytics – May decrease symptoms of benzodiazepine withdrawal – Many extracts contain alcohol; potential to interact with disulfiram

References

American Society of Anesthesiologists, "Considerations for Anesthesiologists: What You Should Know About Your Patients' Use of Herbal Medicines," 1999 (brochure).

Ang-Lee MK, Moss J, and Yuan CS, "Herbal Medicines and Perioperative Care," *JAMA*, 2001, 286(2):208-16.

Blumenthal M, *The Complete German Commission E Monographs. Therapeutic Guide to Herbal Medicines,* Austin, Texas: American Botanical Council, 1998.

DerMarderosian A, *The Review of Natural Products,* St Louis, MO: Facts and Comparisons, 1999.

Eisenberg DM, Davis RB, Ettner SL, et al, "Trends in Alternative Medicine Use in the United States, 1990-1997: Results of a Follow-up National Survey," *JAMA,* 1998, 280(18):1569-75.

Klepser TB and Klepser ME, "Unsafe and Potentially Safe Herbal Therapies," *Am J Health Syst Pharm,* 1999, 56(2):125-38.

LaValle JB, "Phytotherapy: A Guide to the Safe and Effective Use of Medicinal Herbs," *Pharmacy Practice News,* 1999, 26(11):57-61.

Mahady GB, "Herbal Medicine and Pharmacy Education," *J Amer Pharm Assoc,* 1998, 38:274.

McDermott JH, "Herbal Chart for Healthcare Professionals," *Pharmacy Today,* 1999, 5(8) (centerfold poster).

McLeskey CH, Meyer TA, Baisden CE, et al, "The Incidence of Herbal and Selected Nutrachemical Use in Surgical Patients," *Anesthesiology,* 1999, 91:A1168.

Miller LG, "Herbal Medicinals: Selected Clinical Considerations Focusing on Known or Potential Drug-Herb Interactions," *Arch Intern Med,* 1998, 158(20):2200-11.

Murphy JM, "Preoperative Considerations With Herbal Medicines," *AORN J,* 1999, 69(1):173-5, 177-8, 180-3.

Murray M, *The Healing Power of Herbs: The Enlightened Person's Guide to the Wonders of Medicinal Plants,* Rocklin, CA: Prima Publishing, 1995.

Newall CA, Anderson LA, and Phillipson JD, *Herbal Medicines: A Guide for Health Care Professionals,* London, England: The Pharmaceutical Press, 1996.

Schulz V, Hansel R, and Tyler VE, *Rational Phytotherapy, A Physician's Guide to Herbal Medicine,* New York, NY: Springer, 1998.

Zaglaniczny KL, "An Introduction to Herbal Medicine and Anesthetic Considerations," *Nurse Anesthetist, Forum,* 1999, 2(3):4-5,11.

HERB–DRUG INTERACTIONS / CAUTIONS

Herb	Drug Interaction / Caution
Acidophilus / bifidobacterium	Antibiotics (oral)
Activated charcoal	Vitamins or oral medications may be adsorbed
Alfalfa	Do not use with lupus due to amino acid L-canavanine; causes pancytopenia at high doses; warfarin (alfalfa contains a large amount of vitamin K)
Aloe vera	Caution in pregnancy, may cause uterine contractions; digoxin, diuretics (hypokalemia)
Ashwagandha	May cause sedation and other CNS effects
Asparagus root	Causes diuresis
Barberry	Normal metabolism of vitamin B may be altered with high doses
Birch	If taking a diuretic, drink plenty of fluids
Black cohosh	Estrogen-like component; pregnant and nursing women should probably avoid this herb; also women with estrogen-dependent cancer and women who are taking birth control pills or estrogen supplements after menopause; caution also in people taking sedatives or blood pressure medications
Black haw	Do not give to children <6 years of age (salicin content) with flu or chickenpox due to potential Reye's syndrome; do not take if allergic to aspirin
Black pepper (*Piper nigrum*)	Antiasthmatic drugs (decreases metabolism)
Black tea	May inhibit body's utilization of thiamine
Blessed thistle	Do not use with gastritis, ulcers, or hyperacidity since herb stimulates gastric juices
Blood root	Large doses can cause nausea, vomiting, CNS sedation, low BP, shock, coma, and death
Broom (*Cytisus scoparius*)	MAO inhibitors lead to sudden blood pressure changes
Bugleweed (*Lycopus virginicus*)	May interfere with nuclear imaging studies of the thyroid gland (thyroid uptake scan)
Cat's claw (*Uncaria tomentosa*)	Avoid in organ transplant patients or patients on ulcer medications, antiplatelet drugs, NSAIDs, anticoagulants, immunosuppressive therapy, intravenous immunoglobulin therapy
Chaste tree berry (*Vitex agnus-castus*)	Interferes with actions of oral contraceptives, HRT, and other endocrine therapies; may interfere with metabolism of dopamine-receptor antagonists
Chicory (*Cichorium intybus*)	Avoid with gallstones due to bile-stimulating properties
Chlorella (*Chlorella vulgaris*)	Contains significant amounts of vitamin K
Chromium picolinate	Picolinic acid causes notable changes in brain chemicals (serotonin, dopamine, norepinephrine); do not use if patient has behavioral disorders or diabetes
Cinnabar root (*Salviae miltiorrhizae*)	Warfarin (increases INR)
Deadly nightshade (*Atropa belladonna*)	Contains atropine
Dong quai	Warfarin (increases INR), estrogens, oral contraceptives, photosensitizing drugs, histamine replacement therapy, anticoagulants, antiplatelet drugs, antihypertensives

Herb	Drug Interaction / Caution
Echinacea	Caution with other immunosuppressive therapies; stimulates TNF and interferons
Evening primrose oil	May lower seizure threshold; do not combine with anticonvulsants or phenothiazines
Fennel	Do not use in women who have had breast cancer or who have been told not to take birth control pills
Fenugreek	Practice moderation in patients on diabetes drugs, MAO inhibitors, cardiovascular agents, hormonal medicines, or warfarin due to the many components of fenugreek
Feverfew	Antiplatelets, anticoagulants, NSAIDs
Forskolin, coleonol	This herb lowers blood pressure (vasodilator) and is a bronchodilator and increases the contractility of the heart, inhibits platelet aggregation, and increases gastric acid secretion
Foxglove	Digitalis-containing herb
Garlic	Blood sugar-lowering medications, warfarin, and aspirin at medicinal doses of garlic
Ginger	May inhibit platelet aggregation by inhibiting thromboxane synthetase at large doses; *in vitro* and animal studies indicate that ginger may interfere with diabetics; has anticoagulant effect, so avoid in medicinal amounts in patients on warfarin or heart medicines
Ginkgo biloba	Warfarin (ginkgo decreases blood clotting rate); NSAIDs, MAO inhibitors
Ginseng	Blood sugar-lowering medications (additive effects) and other stimulants
Ginseng (American, Korean)	Furosemide (decreases efficacy)
Ginseng (Siberian)	Digoxin (increases digoxin level)
Glucomannan	Diabetics (herb delays absorption of glucose from intestines, decreasing mean fasting sugar levels)
Goldenrod	Diuretics (additive properties)
Gymnema	Blood sugar-lowering medications (additive effects)
Hawthorn	Digoxin or other heart medications (herb dilates coronary vessels and other blood vessels, also inotropic)
Hibiscus	Chloroquine (reduced effectiveness of chloroquine)
Hops	Those with estrogen-dependent breast cancer should not take hops (contains estrogen-like chemicals); patients with depression (accentuate symptoms); alcohol or sedative (additive effects)
Horehound	May cause arrhythmias at high doses
Horseradish	In medicinal amounts with thyroid medications
Kava	CNS depressants (additive effects, eg, alcohol, barbiturates, etc); benzodiazepines
Kelp	Thyroid medications (additive effects or opposite effects by negative feedback); kelp contains a high amount of sodium
Labrador tea	Plant has narcotic properties, possible additive effects with other CNS depressants
Lemon balm	Do not use with Graves disease since it inhibits certain thyroid hormones

HERB–DRUG INTERACTIONS / CAUTIONS *(Continued)*

Herb	Drug Interaction / Caution
Licorice	Acts as a corticosteroid at high doses (about 1.5 lbs candy in 9 days) which can lead to hypertension, edema, hypernatremia, and hypokalemia (pseudoaldosteronism); do not use in persons with hypertension, glaucoma, diabetes, kidney or liver disease, or those on hormonal therapy; may interact with digitalis (due to hypokalemia)
Lobelia	Contains lobeline which has nicotinic activity; may mask withdrawal symptoms from nicotine; it can act as a polarizing neuromuscular blocker
Lovage	Is a diuretic
Ma huang	MAO inhibitors, digoxin, beta-blockers, methyldopa, caffeine, theophylline, decongestants (increases toxicity)
Marshmallow	May delay absorption of other drugs taken at the same time; may interfere with treatments of lowering blood sugar
Meadowsweet	Contains salicylates
Melatonin	Acts as contraceptive at high doses; antidepressants (decreases efficacy)
Mistletoe	May interfere with medications for blood pressure, depression, and heart disease
L-phenylalanine	MAO inhibitors
Pleurisy root	Digoxin (plant contains cardiac glycosides); also contains estrogen-like compounds; may alter amine concentrations in the brain and interact with antidepressants
Prickly ash (Northern)	Contains coumarin-like compounds
Prickly ash (Southern)	Contains neuromuscular blockers
Psyllium	Digoxin (decreases absorption)
Quassia	High doses may complicate heart or blood-thinning treatments (quassia may be inotropic)
Red clover	May have estrogen-like actions; avoid when taking birth control pills, HRT, people with heart disease or at risk for blood clots, patients who suffer from estrogen-dependent cancer; do not take with warfarin
Red pepper	May increase liver metabolism of other medications and may interfere with high blood pressure medications or MAO inhibitors
Rhubarb, Chinese	Do not use with digoxin (enhanced effects)
St John's wort	Indinavir, cyclosporine, SSRIs or any antidepressants, tetracycline (increases sun sensitivity); digoxin (decreases digoxin concentration); may also interact with diltiazem, nicardipine, verapamil, etoposide, paclitaxel, vinblastine, vincristine, glucocorticoids, cyclosporine, dextromethorphan, ephedrine, lithium, meperidine, pseudoephedrine, selegiline, yohimbine, ACE inhibitors (serotonin syndrome, hypertension, possible exacerbation of allergic reaction)
Saw palmetto	Acts an antiandrogen; do not take with prostate medicines or HRT

Herb	Drug Interaction / Caution
Squill	Digoxin or persons with potassium deficiency; also not with quinidine, calcium, laxatives, saluretics, prednisone (long-term)
Tonka bean	Contains coumarin, interacts with warfarin
Vervain	Avoid large amounts of herb with blood pressure medications or HRT
Wild Oregon grape	High doses may alter metabolism of vitamin B
Wild yam	May interfere with hormone precursors
Wintergreen	Warfarin, increased bleeding
Sweet woodruff	Contains coumarin
Yarrow	Interferes with anticoagulants and blood pressure medications
Yohimbe	Do not consume tyramine-rich foods; do not take with nasal decongestants, PPA-containing diet aids, antidepressants, or mood-altering drugs

THERAPEUTIC NURSING MANAGEMENT OF SIDE EFFECTS

MANAGEMENT OF DRUG-RELATED PROBLEMS

Patients may experience some type of side effect or adverse drug reaction as a result of their drug therapy. The type of effect, the severity, and the frequency of occurrence is dependent on the medication and dose being used, as well as the individual's response to therapy. The following information is presented as helpful tips to assist the patient through these drug-related problems. Pharmacological support may also be required for their management.

Alopecia

- Your hair loss is temporary. Hair usually will begin to grow within 3-6 months of completing drug therapy.
- Your hair may come back with a different texture, color, or thickness.
- Avoid excessive shampooing and hair combing, or harsh hair care products.
- Avoid excessive drying of hair.
- Avoid use of permanents, dyes, or hair sprays.
- Always cover head in cold weather or sunshine.

Anemia

- Observe all bleeding precautions (see Thrombocytopenia).
- Get adequate sleep and rest.
- Be alert for potential for dizziness, fainting, or extreme fatigue.
- Maintain adequate nutrition and hydration.
- Have laboratory tests done as recommended.
- If unusual bleeding occurs, notify prescriber.

Anorexia

- Small frequent meals containing favorite foods may tempt appetite.
- Eat simple foods such as toast, rice, bananas, mashed potatoes, scrambled eggs.
- Eat in a pleasant environment conducive to eating.
- When possible, eat with others.
- Avoid noxious odors when eating.
- Use nutritional supplements high in protein and calories.
- Freezing nutritional supplements sometimes makes them more palatable.
- A small glass of wine (if not contraindicated) may stimulate appetite.
- Mild exercise or short walks may stimulate appetite.
- Request antiemetic medication to reduce nausea or vomiting.

Diarrhea

- Include fiber, high protein foods, and fruits in dietary intake.
- Drink plenty of liquids.
- Buttermilk, yogurt, or boiled milk may be helpful.
- Antidiarrheal agents may be needed. Consult your prescriber.
- Include regular rest periods in your activities.
- Institute skin care regimen to prevent breakdown and promote comfort.

Fluid Retention / Edema

- Elevate legs when sitting.
- Wear support hose.
- Increase physical exercise.
- Maintain adequate hydration; avoiding fluids will not reduce edema.
- Weigh yourself regularly.
- If your prescriber has advised you to limit your salt intake, avoid foods such as ham, bacon, processed meats, and canned foods. Many foods are high in salt content. Read labels carefully.

- Report to prescriber if any of the following occur: sudden weight gain, decrease in urination, swelling of hands or feed, increase in waist size, wet cough, or difficulty breathing.

Headache

- Lie down.
- Use cool cloth on forehead.
- Avoid caffeine.
- Use mild analgesics. Consult prescriber.

Leukopenia / Neutropenia

- Monitor for signs of infections: persistent sore throat, fever, chills, fatigue, headache, flu-like symptoms, vaginal discharge, foul-smelling stools.
- Prevent infection. Maintain strict handwashing at all times. Avoid crowds when possible. Avoid exposure to infected persons.
- Avoid exposure to temperature changes.
- Maintain adequate nutrition and hydration.
- Maintain good personal hygiene.
- Avoid injury or skin breaks.
- Avoid vaccinations (unless recommended by healthcare provider).
- Avoid sunburn.

Nausea and Vomiting

- Eat food served cold or at room temperature. Ice chips are sometimes helpful.
- Drink clear liquids in severe cases of nausea. Avoid carbonated beverages.
- Sip liquids slowly.
- Avoid spicy food. Bland foods are easier to digest.
- Rinse mouth with lemon water. Practice good oral hygiene.
- Avoid sweet, fatty, salty foods and foods with strong odors.
- Eat small frequent meals rather than heavy meals.
- Use relaxation techniques and guided imagery.
- Use distractions such as meals, television, reading, games, etc.
- Sleep during intense periods of nausea.
- Chew gum or suck on hard candy or lozenges.
- Eat in an upright (sitting position), rather than semirecumbent.
- Avoid tight constrictive clothing at meal time.
- Use some mild exercise following light meals rather than lying down.
- Request antiemetic medication to reduce nausea or vomiting.

Postural Hypotension

- Use care and rise slowly from sitting or lying position to standing.
- Use care when climbing stairs.
- Initiate ambulation slowly. Get your bearings before you start walking.
- Do not bend over; always squat slowly if you must pick up something from floor.
- Use caution when showering or bathing (use secure handrails).

Stomatitis

- Perform good oral hygiene frequently, especially before and after meals.
- Avoid use of strong or alcoholic commercial mouthwashes.
- Keep lips well lubricated.
- Avoid tobacco or other products that are irritating to the oral mucosa.
- Avoid hot, spicy, excessively salty foods.
- Eat soft foods and drink adequate fluids.
- Request topical or systemic analgesics for painful ulcerations.
- Be alert for and report signs of oral fungal infections.

THERAPEUTIC NURSING MANAGEMENT OF SIDE EFFECTS *(Continued)*

Thrombocytopenia

- Avoid aspirin and aspirin-containing products.
- Use electric or safety razor and blunt scissors.
- Use soft toothbrush or cotton swabs for oral care. Avoid use of dental floss.
- Avoid use of enemas, cathartics, and suppositories unless approved by prescriber.
- Avoid valsalva maneuvers such as straining at stool.
- Use stool softeners if necessary to prevent constipation. Consult prescriber.
- Avoid blowing nose forcefully.
- Never go barefoot, wear protective foot covering.
- Use care when trimming nails (if necessary).
- Maintain safe environment; arrange furniture to provide safe passageway.
- Maintain adequate lighting in darkened areas to avoid bumping into objects.
- Avoid handling sharp tools or instruments.
- Avoid contact sports or activities that might result in injury.
- Promptly report signs of bleeding; abdominal pain; blood in stool, urine, or vomitus; unusual fatigue; easy bruising; bleeding around gums; or nosebleeds.
- If injection or bloodsticks are necessary, inform healthcare provider that you may have excess bleeding.

Vertigo

- Observe postural hypotension precautions.
- Use caution when driving or using any machinery.
- Avoid sudden position shifts; do not "rush".
- Utilize appropriate supports (eg, cane, walker) to prevent injury.

CONTRAST MEDIA REACTIONS, PREMEDICATION FOR PROPHYLAXIS

American College of Radiology Guidelines for Use of Nonionic Contrast Media

It is estimated that approximately 5% to 10% of patients will experience adverse reactions to administration of contrast dye (less for nonionic contrast). In approximately 1000-2000 administrations, a life-threatening reaction will occur.

A variety of premedication regimens have been proposed, both for pretreatment of "at risk" patients who require contrast media and before the routine administration of the intravenous high osmolar contrast media. Such regimens have been shown in clinical trials to decrease the frequency of all forms of contrast medium reactions. Pretreatment with a 2-dose regimen of methylprednisolone 32 mg, 12 and 2 hours prior to intravenous administration of HOCM (ionic), has been shown to decrease mild, moderate, and severe reactions in patients at increased risk and perhaps in patients without risk factors. Logistical and feasibility problems may preclude adequate premedication with this or any regimen for all patients. It is unclear at this time that steroid pretreatment prior to administration of ionic contrast media reduces the incidence of reactions to the same extent or less than that achieved with the use of nonionic contrast media alone. Information about the efficacy of nonionic contrast media combined with a premedication strategy, including steroids, is preliminary or not yet currently available. For high-risk patients (ie, previous contrast reactors), the combination of a pretreatment regimen with nonionic contrast media has empirical merit and may warrant consideration. Oral administration of steroids appears preferable to intravascular routes, and the drug may be prednisone or methylprednisolone. Supplemental administration of H_1 and H_2 antihistamine therapies, orally or intravenously, may reduce the frequency of urticaria, angioedema, and respiratory symptoms. Additionally, ephedrine administration has been suggested to decrease the frequency of contrast reactions, but caution is advised in patients with cardiac disease, hypertension, or hyperthyroidism. No premedication strategy should be a substitute for the ABC approach to preadministration preparedness listed above. Contrast reactions do occur despite any and all premedication prophylaxis. The incidence can be decreased, however, in some categories of "at risk" patients receiving high osmolar contrast media plus a medication regimen. For patients with previous contrast medium reactions, there is a slight chance that recurrence may be more severe or the same as the prior reaction, however, it is more likely that there will be no recurrence.

General Premedication Regimen

Methylprednisolone	32 mg orally 12 and 2 hours prior to procedure
Diphenhydramine	50 mg orally 1 hour prior to the procedure

Alternative Premedication Regimen

Prednisone	50 mg orally 13, 7, and 1 hour before the procedure
Diphenhydramine	50 mg orally 1 hour before the procedure
Ephedrine	25 mg orally 1 hour before the procedure (except when contraindicated)

CONTRAST MEDIA REACTIONS, PREMEDICATION FOR PROPHYLAXIS *(Continued)*

Unlabeled Use (Nephroprotective)

N-acetylcysteine, P.O.	600 mg orally twice daily on the day before and the day of the scan in addition to hydration with 0.45% saline intravenously

Indications for Nonionic Contrast

- Previous reaction to contrast – premedicate[1]
- Known allergy to iodine or shellfish
- Asthma, especially if on medication
- Myocardial instability or CHF
- Risk for aspiration or severe nausea and vomiting
- Difficulty communicating or inability to give history
- Patients taking beta-blockers
- Small children at risk for electrolyte imbalance or extravasation
- Renal failure with diabetes, sickle cell disease, or myeloma
- At physician or patient request

[1]Life-threatening reactions (throat swelling, laryngeal edema, etc), consider omitting the intravenous contrast.

PEDIATRIC ALS ALGORITHMS

PALS Bradycardia Algorithm

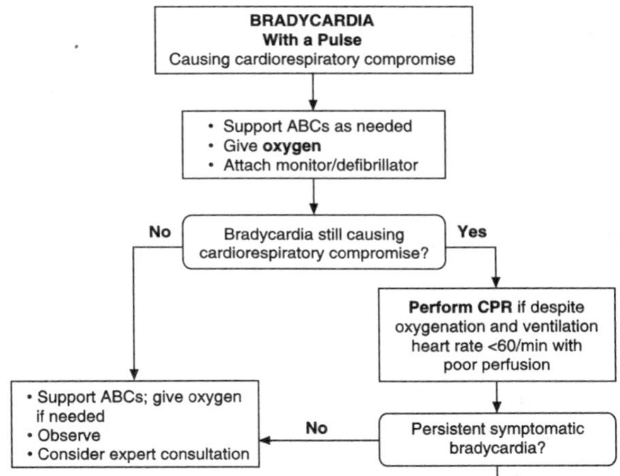

Yes

- **Give epinephrine**
  - I.V./I.O.: 0.01 mg/kg (1:10,000: 0.1 mL/kg)
  - Endotracheal tube: 0.1 mg/kg (1:1000: 0.1 mL/kg)

  Repeat every 3-5 minutes
- **If increased vagal tone or primary AV block:** Give **atropine,** first dose: 0.02 mg/kg, may repeat (Minimum dose: 0.1 mg; maximum total dose for child: 1 mg)
- Consider cardiac pacing

If pulseless arrest develops, go to Pulseless Arrest Algorithm

Reminders

During CPR, push hard and fast (100/min)
Ensure full chest recoil
Minimize interruptions in chest compressions

- Support ABCs
- Secure airway if needed; confirm placement
- Search for and treat possible contributing factors:
  - **H**ypovolemia
  - **H**ypoxia or ventilation problems
  - **H**ydrogen ion (acidosis)
  - **H**ypo-/hyperkalemia
  - **H**ypoglycemia
  - **H**ypothermia
  - **T**oxins
  - **T**amponade, cardiac
  - **T**ension pneumothorax
  - **T**hrombosis (coronary or pulmonary)
  - **T**rauma (hypovolemia, increased ICP)

Adapted from American Heart Association Emergency Cardiovascular Care Committee, "2005 American Heart Association (AHA) Guidelines for Cardiopulmonary Resuscitation (CPR) and Emergency Cardiovascular Care (ECC)," *Circulation*, 2005, 112(24 Suppl):IV-176.

PEDIATRIC ALS ALGORITHMS *(Continued)*

PALS Pulseless Arrest Algorithm

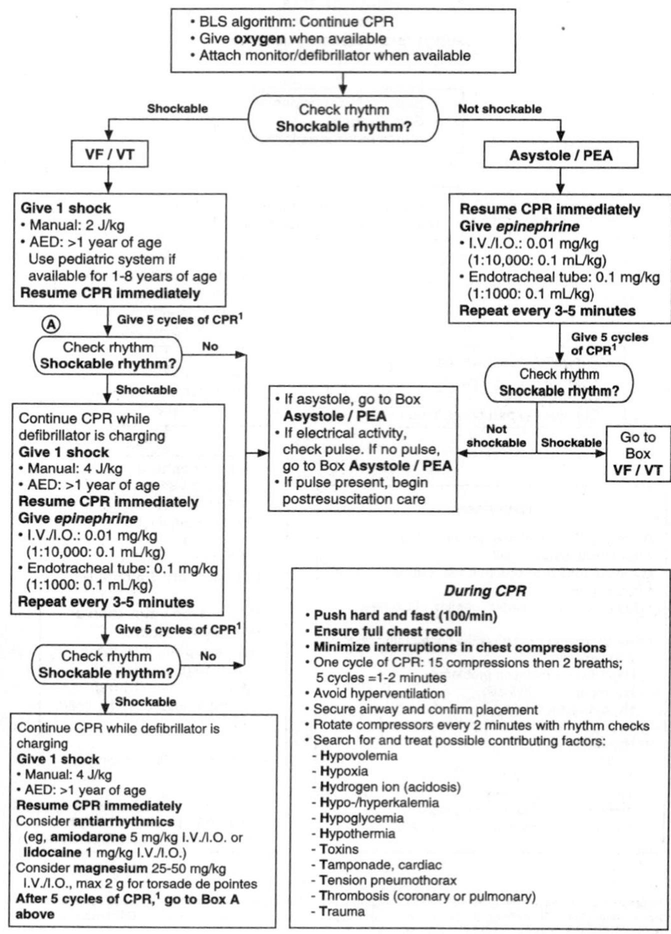

VF = ventricular fibrillation; VT = ventricular tachycardia; PEA = pulseless electrical activity; AED = automated external defibrillator.

[1]After an advanced airway is placed, rescuers no longer deliver "cycles" of CPR. Give continuous chest compressions without pauses for breaths. Give 8-10 breaths/min. Check rhythm every 2 minutes.

Adapted from American Heart Association Emergency Cardiovascular Care Committee, "2005 American Heart Association (AHA) Guidelines for Cardiopulmonary Resuscitation (CPR) and Emergency Cardiovascular Care (ECC)," *Circulation*, 2005, 112(24 Suppl):IV-173.

PALS Tachycardia Algorithm With Pulses and Poor Perfusion

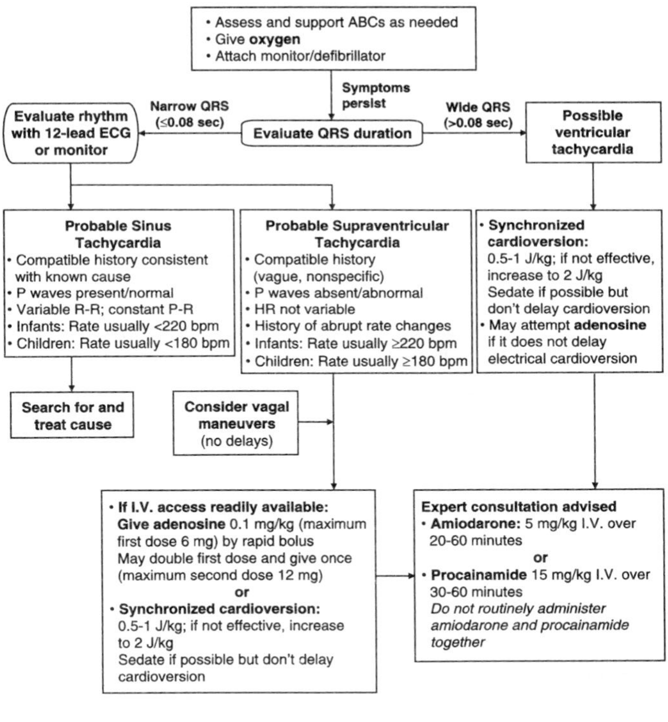

During Evaluation

- Secure, verify airway and vascular access when possible
- Consider expert consultation
- Prepare for cardioversion

Treat possible contributing factors:

- **H**ypovolemia
- **H**ypoxia
- **H**ydrogen ion (acidosis)
- **H**ypo-/hyperkalemia
- **H**ypoglycemia
- **H**ypothermia
- **T**oxins
- **T**amponade, cardiac
- **T**ension pneumothorax
- **T**hrombosis (coronary or pulmonary)
- **T**rauma (hypovolemia)

Adapted from American Heart Association Emergency Cardiovascular Care Committee, "2005 American Heart Association (AHA) Guidelines for Cardiopulmonary Resuscitation (CPR) and Emergency Cardiovascular Care (ECC)," *Circulation*, 2005, 112(24 Suppl):IV-177.

ADULT ACLS ALGORITHMS

Bradycardia Algorithm

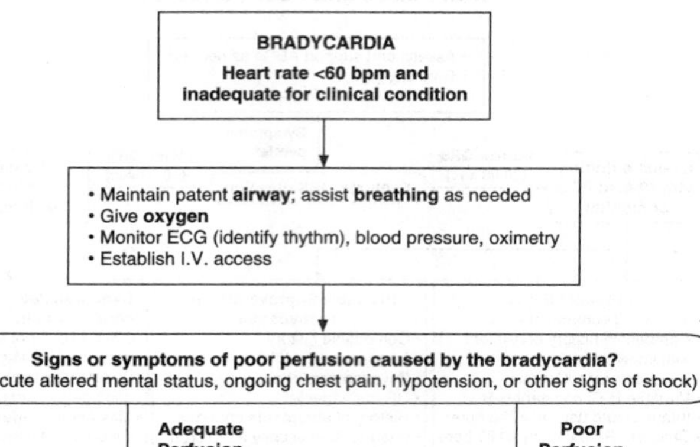

Adequate Perfusion

Observe / Monitor

Poor Perfusion

- **Prepare for transcutaneous pacing;** use without delay for high-degree block (type II second-degree block or third-degree AV block)
- Consider **atropine** 0.5 mg I.V. while awaiting pacer. May repeat to a total dose of 3 mg. If ineffective, begin pacing.
- Consider **epinephrine** (2-10 mcg/min) or **dopamine** (2-10 mcg/kg/min) infusion while awaiting pacer or if pacing ineffective

↓

- Prepare for **transvenous pacing**
- Treat contributing causes
- Consider expert consultation

Reminders

- If pulseless arrest develops, *see* Pulseless Arrest Algorithm
- Search for and treat possible contributing factors:
  - **Hy**povolemia
  - **Hy**poxia
  - **Hy**drogen ion (acidosis)
  - **Hy**po-/hyperkalemia
  - **Hy**poglycemia
  - **Hy**pothermia
  - **T**oxins
  - **T**amponade, cardiac
  - **T**ension pneumothorax
  - **T**hrombosis (coronary or pulmonary)
  - **T**rauma (hypovolemia, increased ICP)

Adapted from American Heart Association Emergency Cardiovascular Care Committee, "2005 American Heart Association (AHA) Guidelines for Cardiopulmonary Resuscitation (CPR) and Emergency Cardiovascular Care (ECC)," *Circulation*, 2005, 112(24 Suppl):IV-68.

ACLS Pulseless Arrest Algorithm

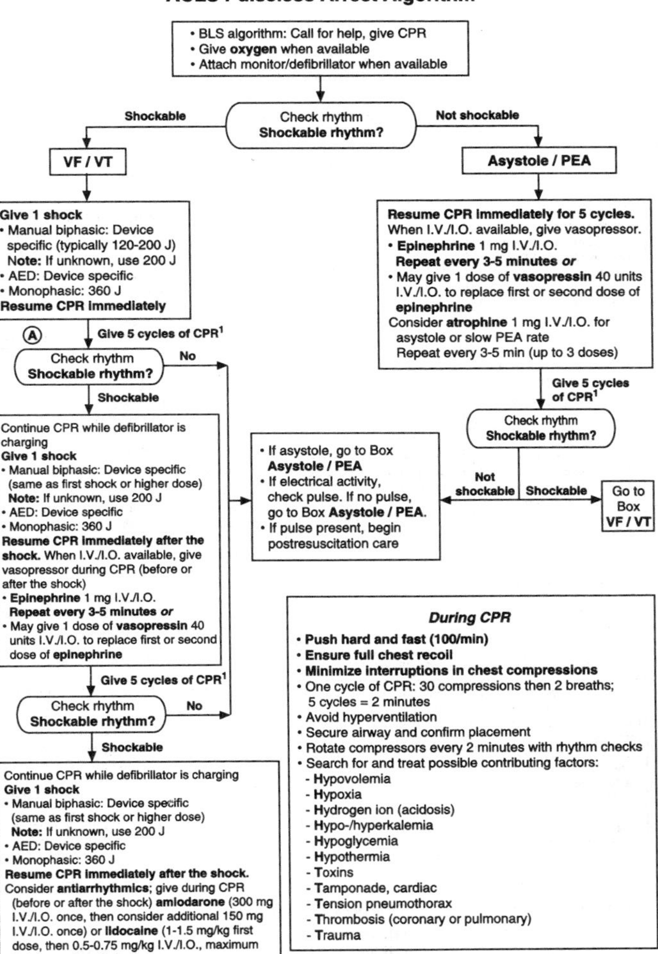

[1]After an advanced airway is placed, rescuers no longer deliver "cycles" of CPR. Give continuous chest compressions without pauses for breaths. Give 8-10 breaths/min. Check rhythm every 2 minutes.

VF = ventricular fibrillation; VT = ventricular tachycardia; PEA = pulseless electrical activity; AED = automated external defibrillator.

Adapted from American Heart Association Emergency Cardiovascular Care Committee, "2005 American Heart Association (AHA) Guidelines for Cardiopulmonary Resuscitation (CPR) and Emergency Cardiovascular Care (ECC)," *Circulation*, 2005, 112(24 Suppl):IV-59.

ADULT ACLS ALGORITHMS *(Continued)*

ACLS Tachycardia Algorithm With Pulses

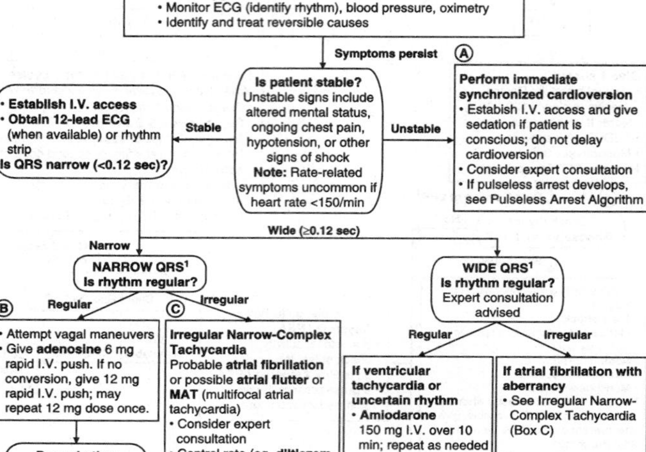

During Evaluation

- Secure, verify airway and vascular access when possible
- Consider expert consultation
- Prepare for cardioversion

Treat possible contributing factors:

- **Hypovolemia**
- **Hypoxia**
- **Hydrogen ion** (acidosis)
- **Hypo-/hyperkalemia**
- **Hypoglycemia**
- **Hypothermia**
- Toxins
- Tamponade, cardiac
- Tension pneumothorax
- Thrombosis (coronary or pulmonary)
- Trauma (hypovolemia)

SVT = supraventricular tachycardia; VT = ventricular tachycardia.

[1]If patient becomes unstable, go to Box A.

Adapted from American Heart Association Emergency Cardiovascular Care Committee, "2005 American Heart Association (AHA) Guidelines for Cardiopulmonary Resuscitation (CPR) and Emergency Cardiovascular Care (ECC)," *Circulation*, 2005, 112(24 Suppl):IV-70.

ORAL MEDICATIONS THAT SHOULD NOT BE CRUSHED

There are a variety of reasons for crushing tablets or capsule contents prior to administering to the patient. Patients may have nasogastric tubes which do not permit the administration of tablets or capsules; an oral solution for a particular medication may not be available from the manufacturer or readily prepared by pharmacy; patients may have difficulty swallowing capsules or tablets; or mixing of powdered medication with food or drink may make the drug more palatable.

Generally, medications which should not be crushed fall into one of the following categories.

- **Extended-Release Products**. The formulation of some tablets is specialized as to allow the medication within it to be slowly released into the body. This is sometimes accomplished by centering the drug within the core of the tablet, with a subsequent shedding of multiple layers around the core. Wax melts in the GI tract. Slow-K® is an example of this. Capsules may contain beads which have multiple layers which are slowly dissolved with time.

  Common Abbreviations for Extended-Release Products

CD	Controlled dose
CR	Controlled release
CRT	Controlled-release tablet
LA	Long-acting
SR	Sustained release
TR	Timed release
TD	Time delay
SA	Sustained action
XL	Extended release
XR	Extended release

- **Medications Which Are Irritating to the Stomach**. Tablets which are irritating to the stomach may be enteric-coated which delays release of the drug until the time when it reaches the small intestine. Enteric-coated aspirin is an example of this.

- **Foul-Tasting Medication**. Some drugs are quite unpleasant to taste so the manufacturer coats the tablet in a sugar coating to increase its palatability. By crushing the tablet, this sugar coating is lost and the patient tastes the unpleasant tasting medication.

- **Sublingual Medication**. Medication intended for use under the tongue should not be crushed. While it appears to be obvious, it is not always easy to determine if a medication is to be used sublingually. Sublingual medications should indicate on the package that they are intended for sublingual use.

- **Effervescent Tablets**. These are tablets which, when dropped into a liquid, quickly dissolve to yield a solution. Many effervescent tablets, when crushed, lose their ability to quickly dissolve.

Recommendations

1. It is not advisable to crush certain medications.
2. Consult individual monographs prior to crushing capsule or tablet.
3. If crushing a tablet or capsule is contraindicated, consult with your pharmacist to determine whether an oral solution exists or can be compounded.

ORAL MEDICATIONS THAT SHOULD NOT BE CRUSHED *(Continued)*

Drug Product	Dosage Form	Dosage Reasons / Comments
Accuhist®	Tablet	Slow release[8]
Accutane®	Capsule	Mucous membrane irritant
Aciphex™	Tablet	Slow release
Adalat® CC	Tablet	Slow release
Adderall XR™	Capsule	Slow release[1]
Advicor®	Tablet	Slow release
Afeditab™ CR	Tablet	Slow release
Aggrenox®	Capsule	Slow release **Note:** Capsule may be opened; contents include an aspirin tablet that may be chewed and dipyridamole pellets that may be sprinkled on applesauce
Alavert™ Allergy Sinus 12 Hour	Tablet	Slow release
Allegra-D®	Tablet	Slow release
Altocor™	Tablet	Slow release
Arthritis Bayer® Time Release	Capsule	Slow release
Arthrotec®	Tablet	Enteric-coated
A.S.A.® Enseals®	Tablet	Enteric-coated
Asacol®	Tablet	Slow release
Ascriptin® A/D	Tablet	Enteric-coated
Ascriptin® Extra Strength	Tablet	Enteric-coated
Augmentin XR™	Tablet	Slow release[2, 8]
Avinza™	Capsule	Slow release[1] (not pudding)
Avodart™	Capsule	Teratogenic potential[9]
Azulfidine® EN-tabs®	Tablet	Enteric-coated
Bayer® Aspirin EC	Caplet	Enteric-coated
Bayer® Aspirin, Low Adult 81 mg	Tablet	Enteric-coated
Bayer® Aspirin, Regular Strength 325 mg	Caplet	Enteric-coated
Biaxin® XL	Tablet	Slow release
Biltricide®	Tablet	Taste[8]
Bisacodyl	Tablet	Enteric-coated[3]
Bontril® Slow-Release	Capsule	Slow release
Calan® SR	Tablet	Slow release[8]
Carbatrol®	Capsule	Slow release[1]
Cardene® SR	Capsule	Slow release
Cardizem®	Tablet	Slow release
Cardizem® CD	Capsule	Slow release[1]
Cardizem® LA	Tablet	Slow release
Cardizem® SR	Capsule	Slow release[1]
Carter's Little Pills®	Tablet	Enteric-coated
Cartia® XT	Capsule	Slow release
Ceclor® CD	Tablet	Slow release
Ceftin®	Tablet	Taste[2] **Note:** Use suspension for children
CellCept®	Capsule, tablet	Teratogenic potential[9]
Charcoal Plus®	Tablet	Enteric-coated
Chloral Hydrate	Capsule	**Note:** Product is in liquid form within a special capsule[2]
Chlor-Trimeton® 12-Hour	Tablet	Slow release[2]
Cipro™	Tablet	Taste[5]
Cipro® XR	Tablet	Slow release
Claritin-D® 12-Hour	Tablet	Slow release
Claritin-D® 24-Hour	Tablet	Slow release

Drug Product	Dosage Form	Dosage Reasons / Comments
Colace®	Capsule	Taste[5]
Colestid®	Tablet	Slow release
Comhist® LA	Capsule	Slow release[1]
Commit™	Lozenge	**Note:** Integrity compromised by chewing or crushing
Compazine® Spansule®	Capsule	Slow release[2]
Concerta®	Tablet	Slow release
Contac® 12-Hour	Tablet	Slow release
Cotazym-S®	Capsule	Enteric-coated[1]
Covera-HS™	Tablet	Slow release
Creon® 5, 10, 20	Capsule	Slow release[1]
Crixivan®	Capsule	Taste **Note:** Capsule may be opened and mixed with fruit puree (eg, banana)
Cytovene®	Capsule	Skin irritant
Cytoxan®	Tablet	**Note:** Drug may be crushed, but maker recommends using injection
Dallergy®	Capsule	Slow release
Dallergy-JR®	Capsule	Slow release
Deconamine® SR	Capsule	Slow release[2]
Defen L.A.®	Tablet	Slow release[8]
Depakene®	Capsule	Slow release mucous membrane irritant[2]
Depakote®	Tablet	Slow release
Depakote® ER	Tablet	Slow release
Desoxyn®	Tablet	Slow release
Desyrel®	Tablet	Taste[5]
Detrol® LA	Capsule	Slow release
Dexedrine® Spansule®	Capsule	Slow release
Diamox® Sequels®	Capsule	Slow release
Dilacor® XR	Capsule	Slow release
Dilatrate-SR®	Capsule	Slow release
Diltia XT®	Capsule	Slow release
Ditropan® XL	Tablet	Slow release
Dolobid®	Tablet	Irritant
Donnatal® Extentab®	Tablet	Slow release[2]
Drisdol®	Capsule	Liquid filled[4]
Drixoral®	Tablet	Slow release[2]
Drixoral® Plus	Tablet	Slow release
Drixoral® Sinus	Tablet	Slow release
Dulcolax®	Capsule	Liquid-filled
Dulcolax®	Tablet	Enteric-coated[3]
Duratuss® G	Tablet	Slow release[9]
Duratuss® GP	Tablet	Slow release[8]
Dynabac®	Tablet	Enteric-coated
DynaCirc® CR	Tablet	Slow release
Easprin®	Tablet	Enteric-coated
EC-Naprosyn®	Tablet	Enteric-coated
Ecotrin® Adult Low Strength	Tablet	Enteric-coated
Ecotrin® Maximum Strength	Tablet	Enteric-coated
Ecotrin® Regular Strength	Tablet	Enteric-coated
E.E.S.® 400	Tablet	Enteric-coated[2]
Effexor® XR	Capsule	Slow release
Efidac/24® Pseudoephedrine	Tablet	Slow release
Efidac® 24	Tablet	Slow release
E-Mycin®	Tablet	Enteric-coated

ORAL MEDICATIONS THAT SHOULD NOT BE CRUSHED
(Continued)

Drug Product	Dosage Form	Dosage Reasons / Comments
Entex® LA	Capsule	Slow release[2]
Entex® PSE	Capsule	Slow release
Entocort™ EC	Capsule	Enteric-coated[1]
Ergomar®	Tablet	Sublingual form[7]
Eryc®	Capsule	Enteric-coated[1]
Ery-Tab®	Tablet	Enteric-coated
Erythrocin Stearate	Tablet	Enteric-coated
Erythromycin Base	Tablet	Enteric-coated
Eskalith CR®	Tablet	Slow release
Evista®	Tablet	Taste; teratogenic potential[9]
Extendryl JR	Capsule	Slow release
Extendryl SR	Capsule	Slow release[2]
Feldene®	Capsule	Mucous membrane irritant
Feosol®	Tablet	Enteric-coated[2]
Feratab®	Tablet	Enteric-coated[2]
Fergon®	Tablet	Enteric-coated
Fero-Grad 500®	Tablet	Slow release
Ferro-Sequels®	Tablet	Slow release
Flagyl ER®	Tablet	Slow release
Flomax®	Capsule	Enteric-coated[1]
Fosamax®	Tablet	Mucous membrane irritant
Fumatinic®	Capsule	Slow release
Geocillin®	Tablet	Taste
Gleevec®	Tablet	Taste[8] **Note:** May be dissolved in mineral oil or apple juice
Glucophage® XR	Tablet	Slow release
Glucotrol® XL	Tablet	Slow release
Gris-PEG®	Tablet	**Note:** Crushing may result in precipitation of larger particles.
Guaifed®	Capsule	Slow release
Guaifed®-PD	Capsule	Slow release
Guaifenex® DM	Tablet	Slow release[8]
Guaifenex® LA	Tablet	Slow release[8]
Guaifenex® PSE	Tablet	Slow release[8]
Guaimax-D®	Tablet	Slow release
Hista-Vent® DA	Tablet	Slow release[8]
Humibid® DM	Tablet	Slow release
Humibid® LA	Tablet	Slow release
Iberet® Filmtab	Tablet	Slow release[2]
Iberet®-500	Tablet	Slow release[2]
Iberet-Folic-500®	Tablet	Slow release
ICAPS® Time Release	Tablet	Slow release
Imdur™	Tablet	Slow release[8]
Inderal® LA	Capsule	Slow release
Inderide® LA	Capsule	Slow release
Indocin® SR	Capsule	Slow release[1,2]
InnoPran XL™	Capsule	Slow release
Ionamin®	Capsule	Slow release
Isoptin® SR	Tablet	Slow release
Isordil® Sublingual	Tablet	Sublingual form[7]
Isosorbide Dinitrate Sublingual	Tablet	Sublingual form[7]
Isosorbide SR	Tablet	Slow release
K+ 8®	Tablet	Slow release[2]

Drug Product	Dosage Form	Dosage Reasons / Comments
K+ 10®	Tablet	Slow release[2]
Kadian®	Capsule	Slow release[1] **Note:** Do not give via N/G tubes
Kaon-Cl®	Tablet	Slow release[2]
K-Dur®	Tablet	Slow release
Klor-Con®	Tablet	Slow release[2]
Klor-Con® M	Tablet	Slow release[2]
Klotrix®	Tablet	Slow release[2]
K-Lyte®	Tablet	Effervescent tablet[6]
K-Lyte/Cl®	Tablet	Effervescent tablet[6]
K-Lyte DS®	Tablet	Effervescent tablet[6]
K-Tab®	Tablet	Slow release[2]
Lescol® XL	Tablet	Slow release
Levbid®	Tablet	Slow release[8]
Levsinex® Timecaps®	Capsule	Slow release
Lexxel®	Tablet	Slow release
Lipram 4500	Capsule	Enteric-coated[1]
Lipram-CR	Capsule	Enteric-coated[1]
Lipram-PN	Capsule	Enteric-coated[1]
Lipram-UL	Capsule	Enteric-coated[1]
Lipram (all products)	Capsule	Slow release[1]
Liquibid-PD	Tablet	Slow release[8]
Lithobid®	Tablet	Slow release
Lodine® XL	Tablet	Slow release
Lodrane® LD	Capsule	Slow release[1]
Mag-Tab® SR	Tablet	Slow release
Maxifed®	Tablet	Slow release
Maxifed® DM	Tablet	Slow release
Maxifed-G®	Tablet	Slow release
Mestinon® Timespan®	Tablet	Slow release[2]
Metadate® CD	Capsule	Slow release[1]
Metadate™ ER	Tablet	Slow release
Methylin™ ER	Tablet	Slow release
Micro-K®	Capsule	Slow release
Motrin®	Tablet	Taste[5]
MS Contin®	Tablet	Slow release[2]
Mucinex®	Tablet	Slow release
Myfortic®	Tablet	Slow release
Naprelan®	Tablet	Slow release
Nasatab® LA	Tablet	Slow release[8]
Nexium®	Capsule	Slow release[1]
Niaspan®	Tablet	Slow release
Nicotinic Acid	Capsule, tablet	Slow release
Nifediac™ CC	Tablet	Slow release
Nitrostat®	Tablet	Sublingual route[7]
Norflex™	Tablet	Slow release
Norpace® CR	Capsule	Slow release form within a special capsule
Oramorph SR®	Tablet	Slow release[2]
Oruvail®	Capsule	Slow release
OxyContin®	Tablet	Slow release
Palgic®-D	Tablet	Slow release[8]
Pancrease®	Capsule	Enteric-coated[1]
Pancrease® MT	Capsule	Enteric-coated[1]
Pancrecarb MS®	Capsule	Enteric-coated[1]
PanMist®-DM	Tablet	Slow release[8]
PanMist®-Jr	Tablet	Slow release[8]

ORAL MEDICATIONS THAT SHOULD NOT BE CRUSHED
(Continued)

Drug Product	Dosage Form	Dosage Reasons / Comments
PanMist®-LA	Tablet	Slow release[8]
Pannaz®	Tablet	Slow release[8]
Papaverine Sustained Action	Capsule	Slow release
Paxil CR™	Tablet	Slow release
Pentasa®	Capsule	Slow release
Perdiem® Fiber Therapy	Granules	Wax coated
PhenaVent™ D	Tablet	Slow release
Plendil®	Tablet	Slow release
Prelu-2®	Capsule	Slow release
Prevacid®	Capsule	Slow release
Prevacid®	Suspension	Slow release **Note:** Contains enteric-coated granules
Prilosec®	Capsule	Slow release
Procainamide HCl SR	Tablet	Slow release
Procanbid®	Tablet	Slow release
Procardia®	Capsule	Delays absorption[2, 5]
Procardia XL®	Tablet	Slow release **Note:** AUC is unaffected.
Profen II®	Tablet	Slow release[8]
Profen II DM®	Tablet	Slow release[8]
Profen Forte™ DM	Tablet	Slow release
Pronestyl®-SR	Tablet	Slow release
Propecia®	Tablet	**Note:** Women who are, or may become, pregnant, should not handle crushed or broken tablets
Proscar®	Tablet	**Note:** Women who are, or may become, pregnant, should not handle crushed or broken tablets
Protonix®	Tablet	Slow release
Quibron-T/SR®	Tablet	Slow release[2]
Rescon-Jr	Tablet	Slow release
Respa-DM®	Tablet	Slow release[8]
Respaire®-120 SR	Capsule	Slow release
Ritalin-SR®	Tablet	Slow release
Rondec-TR®	Tablet	Slow release[2]
Rythmol® SR	Capsule	Slow release
Sinemet® CR	Tablet	Slow release
SINUvent® PE	Tablet	Slow release[8]
Slo-Niacin®	Tablet	Slow release[8]
Slow-Mag®	Tablet	Slow release
Somnote™	Capsule	Liquid filled
Sudafed® 12-Hour	Capsule	Slow release[2]
Sular®	Tablet	Slow release
Symax SR	Tablet	Slow release
Taztia XT™	Capsule	Slow release
Tegretol®-XR	Tablet	Slow release
Temodar®	Capsule	**Note:** If capsules are accidentally opened or damaged, rigorous precautions should be taken to avoid inhalation or contact of contents with the skin or mucous membranes[9]
Tessalon®	Capsule	Slow release
Theo-24®	Tablet	Slow release[2]
Theochron®	Tablet	Slow release
Tiazac®	Capsule	Slow release

Drug Product	Dosage Form	Dosage Reasons / Comments
Topamax®	Capsule	Taste[1]
Topamax®	Tablet	Taste
Touro™ CC	Tablet	Slow release
Touro EX®	Tablet	Slow release
Touro LA®	Tablet	Slow release
Trental®	Tablet	Slow release
TripTone®	Tablet	Slow release
Tylenol® Arthritis Pain	Tablet	Slow release
Tylenol® 8 Hour	Tablet	Slow release
Ultrase®	Capsule	Enteric-coated[1]
Ultrase® MT	Capsule	Enteric-coated[1]
Uniphyl®	Tablet	Slow release
Urocit®-K	Tablet	Wax-coated
Verelan®	Capsule	Slow release[1]
Videx® EC	Capsule	Slow release
Voltaren®-XR	Tablet	Slow release
VoSpire ER™	Tablet	Slow release
Wellbutrin SR®	Tablet	Slow release
Wellbutrin XL™	Tablet	Slow release
Xanax XR®	Tablet	Slow release
Z-Cof LA	Tablet	Slow release[8]
Zephrex LA®	Tablet	Slow release
ZORprin®	Tablet	Slow release
Zyban®	Tablet	Slow release

[1]Capsule may be opened and the contents taken without crushing or chewing; soft food such as applesauce or pudding may facilitate administration; contents may generally be administered via nasogastric tube using an appropriate fluid, provided entire contents are washed down the tube.

[2]Liquid dosage forms of the product are available; however, dose, frequency of administration, and manufacturers may differ from that of the solid dosage form.

[3]Antacids and/or milk may prematurely dissolve the coating of the tablet.

[4]Capsule may be opened and the liquid contents removed for administration.

[5]The taste of this product in a liquid form would likely be unacceptable to the patient; administration via nasogastric tube should be acceptable.

[6]Effervescent tablets must be dissolved in the amount of diluent recommended by the manufacturer.

[7]Tablets are made to disintegrate under the tongue.

[8]Tablet is scored and may be broken in half without affecting release characteristics.

[9]Skin contact may enhance tumor production; avoid direct contact.

Adapted from Mitchell JF, "Oral Dosage Forms That Should Not Be Crushed-2004," available at www.hospitalpharmacyjournal.com.

POTENTIALLY INAPPROPRIATE MEDICATIONS FOR GERIATRICS

Table 1. Critera Independent of Diagnoses or Conditions

Applicable Medication	Summary of Prescribing Concern	Severity
Amiodarone (Cordarone®)	Associated with QT interval problems and risk of provoking torsade de pointes. Lack of efficacy in older adults.	High
Amitriptyline (Elavil®), amitriptyline and chlordiazepoxide (Limbitrol®), and amitriptyline and perphenazine (Triavil®)	Because of its strong anticholinergic and sedation properties, amitriptyline is rarely the antidepressant of choice for elderly patients.	High
Amphetamines (excluding methylphenidate hydrochloride and anorexics)	CNS stimulant adverse effects.	High
Amphetamines and anorexic agents	These drugs have potential for causing dependence, hypertension, angina, and myocardial infarction.	High
Anticholinergics and antihistamines: Chlorpheniramine (Chlor-Trimeton®), diphenhydramine (Benadryl®), hydroxyzine (Vistaril®, Atarax®), cyproheptadine (Periactin), promethazine (Phenergan®), tripelennamine, dexchlorpheniramine (Polaramine®)	All nonprescription and many prescription antihistamines may have potent anticholinergic properties. Nonanticholinergic antihistamines are preferred in elderly patients when treating allergic reactions.	High
Barbiturates (all, except phenobarbital) except when used to control seizures	Are highly addictive and cause more adverse effects than most sedative or hypnotic drugs in elderly patients.	High
Benzodiazepines, long-acting: Chlordiazepoxide (Librium®), amitriptyline and chlordiazepoxide (Limbitrol®), clidinium and chlordiazepoxide (Librax®), diazepam (Valium®), quazepam (Doral®), halazepam (Paxipam®), and chlorazepate (Tranxene®)	These drugs have a long half-life in elderly patients (often several days), producing prolonged sedation and increasing the risk of falls and fractures. Short- and intermediate-acting benzodiazepines are preferred if a benzodiazepine is required.	High
Benzodiazepines, short-acting (doses greater than): Alprazolam (Xanax®) 2 mg; oxazepam (Serax®) 60 mg; lorazepam (Ativan®) 3 mg; temazepam (Restoril®) 15 mg; and triazolam (Halcion®) 0.25 mg	Because of increased sensitivity to benzodiazepines in elderly patients, smaller doses may be effective as well as safer. Total daily doses should rarely exceed the suggested maximums.	High
Chlorpropamide (Diabinese®)	It has prolonged half-life in elderly patients and could cause prolonged hypoglycemia. Additionally, it is the only oral hypoglycemic agent that causes SIADH.	High

Table 1. Critera Independent of Diagnoses or Conditions *(continued)*

Applicable Medication	Summary of Prescribing Concern	Severity
Cimetidine (Tagamet®)	CNS adverse effects including confusion.	Low
Clonidine (Catapres®)	Potential for orthostatic hypotension and CNS adverse effects.	Low
Cyclandelate (Cyclospasmol®)	Lack of efficacy.	Low
Desiccated thyroid	Concerns about cardiac effects. Safer alternatives available.	High
Digoxin (Lanoxin®) (should not exceed >0.125 mg/day except when treating atrial arrhythmias)	Decreased renal clearance may lead to increased risk of toxic effects	Low
Diphenhydramine (Benadryl®)	May cause confusion and sedation. Should not be used as a hypnotic, and when used to treat emergency allergic reactions, it should be used in the smallest possible dose.	High
Dipyridamole, short-acting (Persantine®). Do not consider the long-acting dipyridamole (which has better properties than the short-acting in older adults) except with patients with artificial heart valves	May cause orthostatic hypotension.	Low
Disopyramide (Norpace®, Norpace® CR)	Of all antiarrhythmic drugs, this is the most potent negative inotrope and therefore may induce heart failure in elderly patients. It is also strongly anticholinergic. Other antiarrhythmic drugs should be used.	High
Doxazosin (Cardura®)	Potential for hypotension, dry mouth, and urinary problems.	Low
Doxepin (Sinequan®)	Because of its strong anticholinergic and sedating properties, doxepin is rarely the antidepressant of choice for elderly patients.	High
Ergot mesyloids (Hydergine®) and cyclandelate (Cyclospasmol®)	Have not been shown to be effective in the doses studied.	Low
Estrogens only (oral)	Evidence of the carcinogenic (breast and endometrial cancer) potential of these agents and lack of cardioprotective effect in older women.	Low
Ethacrynic acid (Edecrin®)	Potential for hypertension and fluid imbalances. Safer alternatives available.	Low
Ferrous sulfate >325 mg/day	Doses >325 mg/day do not dramatically increase the amount absorbed but greatly increase the incidence of constipation.	Low
Fluoxetine, daily (Prozac®)	Long half-life of drug and risk of producing excessive CNS stimulation, sleep disturbances, and increasing agitation. Safer alternatives exist.	High

POTENTIALLY INAPPROPRIATE MEDICATIONS FOR GERIATRICS *(Continued)*

Table 1. Critera Independent of Diagnoses or Conditions *(continued)*

Applicable Medication	Summary of Prescribing Concern	Severity
Flurazepam (Dalmane®)	This benzodiazepine hypnotic has an extremely long half-life in elderly patients (often days), producing prolonged sedation and increasing the incidence of falls and fracture. Medium- or short-acting benzodiazepines are preferable.	High
Gastrointestinal antispasmodic drugs: Dicyclomine (Bentyl®), hyoscyamine (Levsin® and Levsinex®), propantheline (Pro-Banthine), belladonna alkaloids (Donnatal® and others), and clidinium and chlordiazepoxide (Librax®)	GI antispasmodic drugs are highly anticholinergic and have uncertain effectiveness. These drugs should be avoided (especially for long-term use).	High
Guanadrel (Hylorel®)	May cause orthostatic hypotension.	High
Guanethidine (Ismelin®)	May cause orthostatic hypotension. Safer alternatives exist.	High
Indomethacin (Indocin® and Indocin® SR)	Of all available NSAIDs, this drug produces the most CNS adverse effects.	High
Isoxsuprine (Vasodilan®)	Lack of efficacy.	Low
Ketorolac (Toradol®)	Immediate and long-term use should be avoided in older persons, since a significant number have asymptomatic GI pathologic conditions.	High
Long-term use of full-dosage, longer half-life, non-COX-selective NSAIDs: Naproxen (Naprosyn®, Avaprox, and Aleve®), oxaprozin (Daypro®), and piroxicam (Feldene®)	Have the potential to produce GI bleeding, renal failure, high blood pressure, and heart failure.	High
Long-term use of stimulant laxatives: Bisacodyl (Dulcolax®), cascara sagrada, and Neoloid except in the presence of opiate analgesic use	May exacerbate bowel dysfunction.	High
Meperidine (Demerol®)	Not an effective oral analgesic in doses commonly used. May cause confusion and has many disadvantages to other narcotic drugs.	High
Meprobamate (Miltown®)	This is a highly addictive and sedating anxiolytic. Those using meprobamate for prolonged periods may become addicted and may need to be withdrawn slowly.	High
Mesoridazine (Serentil®)	CNS and extrapyramidal adverse effects.	High
Methyldopa (Aldomet) and methyldopa and hydrochlorothiazide (Aldoril®)	May cause bradycardia and exacerbate depression in elderly patients.	High

Table 1. Critera Independent of Diagnoses or Conditions *(continued)*

Applicable Medication	Summary of Prescribing Concern	Severity
Methyltestosterone (Android®, Testrad®, Virilon®)	Potential for prostatic hypertrophy and cardiac problems.	High
Mineral oil	Potential for aspiration and adverse effects. Safer alternatives available.	High
Muscle relaxants and antispasmodics: Methocarbamol (Robaxin®), carisoprodol (Soma®), chlorzoxazone (Paraflex®), metaxalone (Skelaxin®), cyclobenzaprine (Flexeril®), and oxybutynin (Ditropan®). Do not consider the extended-release Ditropan® XL.	Most muscle relaxants and antispasmodic drugs are poorly tolerated by elderly patients, since these cause anticholinergic adverse effects, sedation, and weakness. Additionally, their effectiveness at doses tolerated by elderly patients is questionable.	High
Nifedipine, short-acting (Adalat®, Procardia®)	Potential for hypotension and constipation.	High
Nitrofurantoin (Macrodantin®)	Potential for renal impairment. Safer alternatives available.	High
Orphenadrine (Norflex™)	Causes more sedation and anticholinergic adverse effects than safer alternatives.	High
Pentazocine (Talwin®)	Narcotic analgesic that causes more CNS adverse effects, including confusion and hallucinations, more commonly than other narcotic drugs. Additionally, it is a mixed agonist and antagonist.	High
Propoxyphene (Darvon®) and combination products (Darvon® with ASA, Darvon-N®, and Darvocet-N®)	Offers few analgesic advantages over acetaminophen, yet has the adverse effects of other narcotic drugs.	Low
Reserpine at doses >0.25 mg	May induce depression, impotence, sedation, and orthostatic hypotension.	Low
Thioridazine (Mellaril®)	Greater potential for CNS and extrapyramidal adverse effects.	High
Ticlopidine (Ticlid®)	Has been shown to be no better than aspirin in preventing clotting and may be considerably more toxic. Safer, more effective alternatives exist.	High
Trimethobenzamide (Tigan®)	One of the least effective antiemetic drugs, yet it can cause extrapyramidal adverse effects.	High

Adapted from Fick DM, Cooper JW, Wade WE, et al, "Updating the Beers Criteria for Potentially Inappropriate Medication Use in Older Adults: Results of a U.S. Consensus Panel of Experts," *Arch Intern Med,* 2003, 163(22):2716-24.

POTENTIALLY INAPPROPRIATE MEDICATIONS FOR GERIATRICS *(Continued)*

Table 2. Final Criteria Considering Diagnoses or Conditions

Disease or Condition	Drug	Concern	Severity
Anorexia and malnutrition	CNS stimulants: Dextroamphetamine and amphetamine (Adderall®), methylphenidate (Ritalin®), methamphetamine (Desoxyn®), pemolin, and fluoxetine (Prozac®)	Concern due to appetite suppressing effects	High
Arrhythmias	Tricyclic antidepressants (imipramine hydrochloride, doxepin hydrochloride, and amitriptyline hydrochloride)	Concern due to proarrhythmic effects and ability to produce QT interval changes.	High
Bladder outflow obstruction	Anticholinergics and antihistamines, gastrointestinal antispasmodics, muscle relaxants, oxybutynin (Ditropan®), flavoxate (Urispas®), anticholinergics, antidepressants, decongestants, and tolterodine (Detrol®)	May decrease urinary flow, leading to urinary retention.	High
Blood clotting disorders or receiving anticoagulant therapy	Aspirin, NSAIDs, dipyridamole (Persantine®), ticlopidine (Ticlid®), and clopidogrel (Plavix®)	May prolong clotting time and elevate INR values or inhibit platelet aggregation, resulting in an increased potential for bleeding.	High
Chronic constipation	Calcium channel blockers, anticholinergics, and tricyclic antidepressant (imipramine hydrochloride, doxepin hydrochloride, and amitriptyline hydrochloride)	May exacerbate constipation	Low
Cognitive impairment	Barbiturates, anticholinergics, antispasmodics, and muscle relaxants, CNS stimulants: Dextroamphetamine and amphetamine (Adderall®), methylphenidate (Ritalin®), methamphetamine (Desoxyn®), and pemolin	Concern due to CNS-altering effects	High
COPD	Benzodiazepines, long-acting: Chlordiazepoxide (Librium®), amitriptyline and chlordiazepoxide (Limbitrol®), clidinium and chlordiazepoxide (Librax®), diazepam (Valium®), quazepam (Doral®), and chlorazepate (Tranxene®). Beta-blockers: Propranolol	CNS adverse effects. May induce respiratory depression. May exacerbate or cause respiratory depression.	High
Depression	Long-term benzodiazepine use. Sympatholytic agents: Methyldopa (Aldomet), reserpine, and guanethidine (Ismelin)	May produce or exacerbate depression.	High
Gastric or duodenal ulcers	NSAIDs and aspirin (>325 mg) (coxibs excluded)	May exacerbate existing ulcers or produce new/ additional ulcers.	High

Table 2. Final Criteria Considering Diagnoses or Conditions *(continued)*

Disease or Condition	Drug	Concern	Severity
Heart failure	Disopyramide (Norpace®), and high sodium content drugs (sodium and sodium salts [alginate bicarbonate, biphosphate, citrate, phosphate, salicylate, and sulfate])	Negative inotropic effect. Potential to promote fluid retention and exacerbation of heart failure.	High
Hypertension	Phenylpropanolamine hydrochloride (removed from the market in 2001), pseudoephedrine; diet pills, and amphetamines	May produce elevation of blood pressure secondary to sympathomimetic activity.	High
Insomnia	Decongestants, theophylline (Theodur), methylphenidate (Ritalin®), MAOIs, and amphetamines	Concern due to CNS stimulant effects	High
Obesity	Olanzapine (Zyprexa®)	May stimulate appetite and increase weight gain.	Low
Parkinson disease	Metoclopramide (Reglan®), conventional antipsychotics, and tacrine (Cognex®)	Concern due to their antidopaminergic/ cholinergic effects	High
Seizures or epilepsy	Clozapine (Clozaril®), chlorpromazine (Thorazine®), thioridazine (Mellaril®), thiothixene (Navane®)	May lower seizure thresholds.	High
Seizure disorder	Bupropion (Wellbutrin®)	May lower seizure threshold.	High
SIADH/ hyponatremia	SSRIs: Fluoxetine (Prozac®), citalopram (Celexa™), fluvoxamine (Luvox®), paroxetine (Paxil®), and sertraline (Zoloft®)	May exacerbate or cause SIADH.	Low
Stress incontinence	α-Blockers (doxazosin, prazosin, and terazosin), anticholinergic, tricyclic antidepressants (imipramine hydrochloride, doxepin hydrochloride, and amitriptyline hydrochloride), and long-acting benzodiazepines	May produce polyuria and worsening of incontinence	High
Syncope or falls	Short- to intermediate-acting benzodiazepine and tricyclic antidepressants (imipramine hydrochloride, doxepin hydrochloride, and amitriptyline hydrochloride)	May produce ataxia, impaired psychomotor function, syncope, and additional falls.	High

Adapted from Fick DM, Cooper JW, Wade WE, et al, "Updating the Beers Criteria for Potentially Inappropriate Medication Use in Older Adults: Results of a U.S. Consensus Panel of Experts," *Arch Intern Med,* 2003, 163(22):2716-24.

PHARMACOLOGIC CATEGORY INDEX

Antidiuretic Hormone Analog

Antidote

Antidote, Hypoglycemia

Antiemetic

Antiflatulent

Antifungal Agent, Oral

Antifungal Agent, Oral Nonabsorbed

Antifungal Agent, Parenteral

Antifungal Agent, Topical

Antifungal Agent, Vaginal

Antihemophilic Agent

Antihistamine

Urinary Tract Product

Vaccine

Vaccine, Live Virus

Vasoconstrictor

Vasodilator

Vasopressin Analog, Synthetic

Vitamin

Vitamin D Analog

Vitamin, Fat Soluble

Vitamin, Water Soluble

ALPHABETICAL INDEX

NOTES

NOTES